Rosen's Breast Pathology

FOURTH EDITION

Rosen's Breast Pathology

FOURTH EDITION

Syed A. Hoda, MD
Professor
Department of Clinical Pathology and Laboratory Medicine
Weill Cornell Medical College
Attending Pathologist
Department of Pathology and Laboratory Medicine
New York Presbyterian Hospital/Weill Cornell Medical Center
New York, New York

Frederick C. Koerner, MD
Associate Professor
Department of Pathology
Harvard Medical School
Associate Pathologist
Department of Pathology
Massachusetts General Hospital
Boston, Massachusetts

Edi Brogi, MD, PhD
Professor
Department of Clinical Pathology and Laboratory Medicine
Weill Cornell Medical College
E. Lauder Breast and Imaging Center
Director of Breast Pathology
Attending Pathologist
Department of Pathology
Memorial Sloan-Kettering Cancer Center
New York, New York

Paul P. Rosen, MD
Emeritus Professor of Pathology
Department of Pathology and Laboratory Medicine
Weill Cornell Medical College
Cornell University
New York, New York

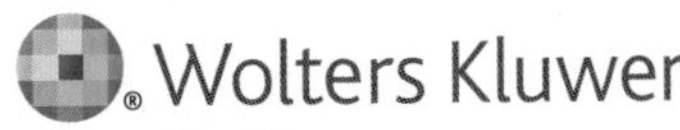

Health

Philadelphia • Baltimore • New York • London
Buenos Aires • Hong Kong • Sydney • Tokyo

Acquisitions Editor: Ryan Shaw
Product Manager: Kate Marshall
Production Product Manager: David Saltzberg
Senior Manufacturing Coordinator: Beth Welsh
Designer: Stephen Druding
Marketing Manager: Dan Dressler
Production Service: S4Carlisle Publishing Services

Two Commerce Square
2001 Market Street
Philadelphia, PA 19103 USA
LWW.com

Printed in China

Library of Congress Cataloging-in-Publication Data

Rosen, Paul Peter, author.
Rosen's breast pathology / Syed A. Hoda, Edi Brogi, Frederick C. Koerner, Paul P. Rosen.—Fourth edition.
p. ; cm.
Breast pathology
Preceded by Rosen's breast pathology / Paul Peter Rosen. 3rd ed. c2009.
Includes bibliographical references and index.
ISBN 978-1-4511-7653-7 (alk. paper)
I. Hoda, Syed A., author. II. Brogi, Edi, author. III. Koerner, Frederick C., author. IV. Title. V. Title: Breast pathology.
[DNLM: 1. Breast Neoplasms—pathology. WP 870]
RC280.B8
616.99'44907—dc23

2013041071

Care has been taken to confirm the accuracy of the information presented and to describe generally accepted practices. However, the authors, editors, and publisher are not responsible for errors or omissions or for any consequences from application of the information in this book and make no warranty, expressed or implied, with respect to the currency, completeness, or accuracy of the contents of the publication. Application of the information in a particular situation remains the professional responsibility of the practitioner.

The authors, editors, and publisher have exerted every effort to ensure that drug selection and dosage set forth in this text are in accordance with current recommendations and practice at the time of publication. However, in view of ongoing research, changes in government regulations, and the constant flow of information relating to drug therapy and drug reactions, the reader is urged to check the package insert for each drug for any change in indications and dosage and for added warnings and precautions. This is particularly important when the recommended agent is a new or infrequently employed drug.

Some drugs and medical devices presented in the publication have Food and Drug Administration (FDA) clearance for limited use in restricted research settings. It is the responsibility of the health care provider to ascertain the FDA status of each drug or device planned for use in their clinical practice.

To purchase additional copies of this book, call our customer service department at (800) 638-3030 or fax orders to (301) 223-2320. International customers should call (301) 223-2300.

Visit Lippincott Williams & Wilkins on the Internet: at LWW.com. Lippincott Williams & Wilkins customer service representatives are available from 8:30 am to 6 pm, EST.

10 9 8 7 6 5 4 3 2 1

CCS1013

Dedication in Prior Editions

To my parents, Beate Caspari-Rosen, MD, and George Rosen, MD, and to the ineffable Mary Sue Rosen.

Dedication for the Fourth Edition

To the esteemed mentors who led us forth, the patients we serve, and the students to whom we entrust the future of breast pathology.

Instruction in medicine is like the culture of the production of the earth. For our natural disposition is, as it were, the soil; the tenets of our teacher are, as it were, the seed; the instruction in youth is like the planting of the seed in the ground at the proper season…and it is time which imparts strength to all things and brings them to maturity.

—FROM *The Law* BY **HIPPOCRATES**

CONTRIBUTORS

Elena Brachtel, MD
Assistant Professor
Department of Pathology
Harvard Medical School
Assistant Pathologist
Department of Pathology
Massachusetts General Hospital
Boston, Massachusetts

Edi Brogi, MD, PhD
Professor
Department of Clinical Pathology and Laboratory Medicine
Weill Cornell Medical College
E. Lauder Breast and Imaging Center
Director of Breast Pathology
Attending Pathologist
Department of Pathology
Memorial Sloan-Kettering Cancer Center
New York, New York

Adriana D. Corben, MD
Assistant Attending Pathologist
Department of Pathology
Memorial Sloan-Kettering Cancer Center
New York, New York

Judith A. Ferry, MD
Associate Professor
Department of Pathology
Harvard Medical School
Director of Hematopathology
Department of Pathology
Massachusetts General Hospital
Boston, Massachusetts

Syed A. Hoda, MD
Professor
Department of Clinical Pathology and Laboratory Medicine
Weill Cornell Medical College
Attending Pathologist
Department of Pathology and Laboratory Medicine
New York Presbyterian Hospital/Weill Cornell Medical Center
New York, New York

Frederick C. Koerner, MD
Associate Professor
Department of Pathology
Harvard Medical School
Associate Pathologist
Department of Pathology
Massachusetts General Hospital
Boston, Massachusetts

Melinda F. Lerwill, MD
Assistant Professor
Department of Pathology
Harvard Medical School
Assistant Pathologist
Department of Pathology
Massachusetts General Hospital
Boston, Massachusetts

Melissa P. Murray, DO
Assistant Attending Pathologist
Department of Pathology
Memorial Sloan-Kettering Cancer Center
New York, New York

Erika Resetkova, MD, PhD
Associate Professor
Breast Pathologist and Cytopathologist
Department of Pathology
M. D. Anderson Cancer Center
Houston, Texas

Paul P. Rosen, MD
Emeritus Professor of Pathology
Department of Pathology and Laboratory Medicine
Weill Cornell Medical College
Cornell University
New York, New York

Aysegul A. Sahin, MD
Professor
Department of Pathology
Chief of Breast Pathology Service
University of Texas M. D. Anderson Cancer Center
Houston, Texas

Yun Wu, MD, PhD
Associate Professor
Department of Pathology
University of Texas
Department of Pathology
M. D. Anderson Cancer Center
Houston, Texas

PREFACE

Not long after I retired from clinical practice in 2010 Jonathan W. Pine, Jr, Senior Executive Editor, contacted me about preparing a fourth edition of *Breast Pathology*. This came as a shock as I had only recently recovered from the effort that produced the third edition and was adjusting to the freedom conferred by retirement. Mr. Pine and I had a very good working relationship in producing the third edition, and being curious to learn what he had in mind, I walked the short distance from my home to the offices of Wolters Kluwer/Lippincott Williams & Wilkins in Philadelphia. As a result of this and subsequent conversations, we arrived at the plan that has given birth to this fourth edition.

After writing the initial edition and revising it twice single-handedly, I am honored that my three colleagues and their associates consented to do the heavy lifting that has been necessary to bring this much-improved Fourth Edition to completion. The book has benefitted greatly from their many decades of experience in the diagnosis of mammary pathology at three of the most prestigious American academic medical centers that are international leaders in the treatment of breast diseases: New York Presbyterian Hospital/Weill Cornell Medical College, Memorial Hospital for Cancer and Allied Diseases/Memorial Sloan-Kettering Cancer Center, and Massachusetts General Hospital/Harvard Medical School.

I have known Syed A. Hoda, MD, for 20 years and worked closely with him for nearly a decade in the Breast Pathology Consultation practice I established at New York Presbyterian Hospital, with the support and encouragement of Daniel M. Knowles, Chairman of Pathology and Laboratory Medicine. I was very pleased that Syed agreed to serve as Editor, taking responsibility for overseeing the project and looking after the innumerable details involved in the creation of a book of this scope. Not the least of these tasks was the final stage of uploading the chapter manuscripts and images as required by the publisher.

Drs. Hoda, Brogi, and Koerner each undertook the revision of approximately one-third of the book, in some instances with the assistance of their associates. While adhering to the basic outline established in prior editions, each chapter has been thoroughly updated to include the most recent information available when the manuscript was completed, as reflected in the substantial number of 2010 to 2013 references cited. In addition to thorough and extensively illustrated descriptions of the surgical pathology and cytology of the breast, the reader will find comprehensive, detailed overviews of the many clinical facets of breast disease, including epidemiology, clinical presentation, diagnostic imaging, molecular/genetic analysis, clinical management, and prognosis. Many new pictures have been added, others have been replaced, and all have been carefully adjusted to enhance image quality. Chapter 40, titled "Lymphoid and Hematopoietic Neoplasms of the Breast," was completely rewritten using contemporary diagnostic terminology by Judith A. Ferry, MD, from Massachusetts General Hospital/Harvard University.

In the Introduction to the third edition to this book, I drew attention to the growing recognition that "altered gene expression is fundamental to neoplastic processes" and noted that "the devil is in the details" of how the exceedingly complex system of gene actions becomes disrupted, resulting in the phenotypic changes in cells and tissues employed by pathologists for diagnosis and estimating prognosis. It has become apparent that the situation is even more complex. Some genotypic alterations are linked to specific neoplasms with similar phenotypic appearances, such as the genetic alterations that underlie the diminished or absent expression of adhesion molecules like E-cadherin in lobular carcinoma or the *ETV6–NTRK3* fusion gene that characterizes secretory carcinoma. On the other hand, an increasing number of genetic alterations of significance for prognosis and treatment, not readily apparent in the histologic phenotype of neoplasms, are being discovered by gene expression profiling, and this is leading to an appreciation of unique characteristics of individual tumors that may render them susceptible to personalized therapies aimed at these targets. Of particular interest is the discovery that some of the genomic alterations found in mammary carcinomas also occur in carcinomas that arise in other organs such as the uterus and ovaries. In view of the rapid advances being made in the study of the molecular biology of breast carcinoma and the growing intersection of the resultant knowledge with diagnostic pathology, it was deemed important to expand this book by adding Chapter 45, titled "Molecular Classification and Testing of Breast Carcinoma," by Drs. Yun Wu and Aysegul A. Sahin from the M. D. Anderson Cancer Center/University of Texas. This chapter provides an introduction to molecular classifications under investigation and predictive molecular tests that are currently used in clinical practice. Data from molecular studies relevant to specific entities can be found in individual chapters. Additional comments about provocative concepts relating to the molecular classification of breast carcinoma that have emerged as a result of gene expression profiling are addressed in a section titled "Molecular versus Morphology for the Classification of Breast Carcinoma: Must It Be Either/Or" in the Introduction.

Histopathologic examination will continue to be the primary basis for the diagnostic classification of mammary lesions in the foreseeable future. Molecular advances used in the past two decades to generate alternative classifications have contributed to defining selected prognostic and therapeutic subgroups within the context of the standard pathologic phenotypic classification presented in this book. It is possible that the pathology report for a mammary carcinoma in the coming decade will include a secondary classification based on molecular markers. Ultimately, it is genotype that serves as the basis for phenotype, and the complex, long-term process of unraveling this relationship will benefit from the work of investigators familiar with both aspects of mammary disease. Surgical pathologists are uniquely qualified to fill this role and to assimilate these advances into routine diagnostic testing for the benefit of patients.

In addition to the extensive revisions and editing of individual chapters by the authors, this book has been subjected to rigorous scrutiny by the publisher's excellent staff throughout the production process. The choice of illustrations, the references listed, the selection of data cited, and the conclusions expressed reflect the experience and opinions of the editors and authors. I had the extraordinary opportunity to read all of the new references as well as to review and edit the manuscripts and pictures of each chapter.

I have also substantially revised and updated the Introduction.

Paul P. Rosen, MD

LIST OF ABBREVIATIONS

A list of the most frequently used abbreviations in this book can be found on page 1351.

LEGENDS FOR COVER IMAGES

Front Cover Image Legends (clockwise from top left): radial sclerosing lesion with ductal hyperplasia, cribriform DCIS (E-cadherin positive) and LCIS (E-cadherin negative) in a duct, secretory carcinoma, and fluorescence *in situ* hybridization (FISH) in secretory carcinoma with separated *red* and *green* signals indicating a disrupted *NTRK3* gene. (Courtesy of Dr. A. John Iafrate and Ms. Clarice Bo-Moon Chang.)

Back Cover Image Legends (clockwise from top left):
partially infarcted adenomyoepithelioma;
metaplastic carcinoma, spindle and squamous type;
reaction to contents of a ruptured breast implant;
solid papillary carcinoma (arrows indicate fibrovascular cores).

PREFACE TO THE FIRST EDITION

1997

He will manage to cure best who has foreseen what is to happen from the present state of matters.

—HIPPOCRATES[1]

The management of diseases of the breast is a multidisciplinary endeavor dependent on the skill and expertise of an array of clinical specialists. In this complex effort, the importance of one or another member of the team for a given patient will vary depending upon the clinical circumstances. At the outset and often at later critical points, an accurate pathologic diagnosis is the crucial element for determining the course of treatment and for estimating prognosis. A thorough knowledge of the pathology of the breast is essential for physicians and other medical personnel who take care of patients with breast diseases. Conversely, the pathologist cloistered in a laboratory, out of touch with patient care, will not be able to provide the clinically meaningful information currently expected of practitioners of this specialty.

The breast appears structurally and functionally to be relatively uncomplicated, but it is the site of a surprisingly broad array of pathologic alterations, many of which are organ-specific. New entities continue to be identified. Our understanding of breast pathology has been substantially amplified by the application of new technology to this effort. Particularly rapid progress has occurred in the past decade as a result of the availability of immunohistochemistry and *in situ* hybridization, which have made it possible to observe the tissue-specific and cell-specific localization of molecular and genetic processes associated with physiologic and pathologic conditions. Yet, it is important not to be blinded by the blizzard of information and to avoid being swept away in the annual flood of "hot topics." All too often, today's hot topic becomes tomorrow's footnote. Ultimately, our understanding of breast pathology is remodeled and enriched by the ongoing process of discovery and thoughtful analysis that contributes to a growing body of knowledge composed of many bits of information from innumerable contributors. This vision embodies the precept of Hippocrates, who wrote:

> *But all these requisites belong of old to Medicine, and an origin and way have been found out, by which many and elegant discoveries have been made, during a length of time, and others will yet be found out, if a person possessed of the proper ability, and knowing those discoveries which have been made, should proceed from them to prosecute his investigations.*[2]

This book provides a comprehensive, extensively illustrated description of breast pathology in a clinical context. Most of the chapters are devoted to specific diseases or disease groupings. The discussion of each topic consists, where relevant, of sections detailing clinical presentation and mammography, epidemiology, gross pathology, microscopic pathology, including electron microscopy and immunohistochemistry, differential diagnosis, treatment, and prognosis. Several chapters deal with broad subjects, such as precancerous breast pathology, staging of carcinoma, biologic markers of prognosis, the pathologic effects of therapy, cytologic and needle core diagnosis, and the pathologic examination of breast specimens.

Illustrations have been selected not only to demonstrate the standard appearance of lesions but also to emphasize the heterogeneity represented by variant forms. Following the manner in which the pathologist encounters them in daily practice, many entities are shown as they appear grossly, in whole-mount histologic sections and, finally, at progressively higher magnification, amplified with immunohistochemistry and other diagnostic procedures.

It is my hope that there is no "pathomythology" in this book. A myth is defined as "an idea that forms part of the beliefs of a group or class but is not founded on fact."[3] *Pathomythology* is a term I use to describe the persistent repetition of hypotheses relating to pathology that are completely contradicted by existing data. Perpetrators of this activity frequently reinforce their myth by quoting themselves or other followers of their belief, eschewing facts that can easily be confirmed by direct observation. One example of pathomythology is the seemingly indestructible idea that the carcinomatous cells of mammary Paget disease arise by transformation of squamous cells in the squamous epithelium that harbors Paget disease. Intraductal carcinoma, which is the source of these carcinoma cells, is detected in virtually every patient with Paget disease, but the pathomythologists rest their case on the very few instances in which duct carcinoma is not discovered. A reasonable explanation for these exceptional cases is offered in this book. Another example of pathomythology is the inaccurate statement that an intraductal component is not found in true medullary carcinoma. Intraductal carcinoma can be found at the periphery of most medullary carcinomas, but the presence or absence of intraductal carcinoma has been shown not to be a criterion for the diagnosis of medullary carcinoma.

Despite diligent attention to detail, it is likely that some errors of omission or commission have occurred in the preparation of this book. The author is responsible for the selection of references and illustrations, for the citation of data from published sources, and for conclusions expressed herein, based on his personal experience and his interpretation of the literature.

Paul P. Rosen, MD

REFERENCES

1. Adams F. The book of prognostics. *The genuine works of Hippocrates.* Baltimore: The Williams & Wilkins Co., 1939:42.
2. Adams F. On ancient medicine. *The genuine works of Hippocrates.* Baltimore: The Williams & Wilkins Co., 1939:1–2.
3. Stein J, ed. *The Random House dictionary of the English language.* New York: Random House, 1973:946.

ACKNOWLEDGMENTS

The majority of the new illustrations in this book were taken from cases seen at the institutions where the Editors and Contributors practice. Thousands of adult women as well as many hundreds of men and children afflicted with breast diseases who cannot be recognized individually are acknowledged for their anonymous contributions to this and prior editions of *Rosen's Breast Pathology*.

The task of turning the manuscript into a finished book has been a cooperative effort. All of the images were digitally enhanced by Ms. Patricia Kuharic in the Medical Art and Photography Department of Weill Cornell Medical College. Her patient and meticulous attention to detail has made an essential contribution to this book. A sincere thank-you is extended to the office staff of each contributor for their vital support, and to residents, fellows, and colleagues who may have provided cases or images that made their way into the book. Dr. Dilip Giri is acknowledged for reviewing portions of the manuscript. Drs. Sonal Varma and Timothy D'Alfonso contributed especially instructive illustrative material.

After Jonathan Pine took on other responsibilities, Ryan Shaw, Acquisitions Editor, became our liason with the publisher, a role he fulfilled efficiently and cheerfully. The production process was ably overseen by Kate Marshall, Product Manager, who guided us and offered many helpful suggestions that have improved the book.

Syed A. Hoda, MD
Paul P. Rosen, MD

CONTENTS

INTRODUCTION

The Pathologist as a Specialist in Breast Carcinoma Care

The development and application of a concept of localized pathology laid the groundwork for modern specialism by providing a number of foci of interest in the field of medicine. Each such focus of interest, that is, a disease or the diseases of an organ or region of the body, provided a nucleus around which could gather the results of clinical and pathological investigation.

—From *The Specialization of Medicine* by **George Rosen, MD**, 1944.

Impressive advances have been made in the past 60 years to detect, treat, and cure breast carcinoma. Major milestones include the development of mammography for early detection, the refinement of image-based needle biopsy of nonpalpable lesions, the introduction of computed tomography (CT) and magnetic resonance imaging (MRI) of the breast, the shift from mastectomy to breast conservation therapy for almost all patients, technologic advances in radiotherapy, improved chemotherapy regimens for primary treatment and as an adjuvant modality, the demonstration that antiestrogenic compounds can inhibit the development and progression of breast carcinoma, the introduction of sentinel lymph node mapping for axillary staging, and technologic advances that make gene expression profiling possible. The growth of medical specialization in the last half of the 20th century has had a profound influence on these accomplishments by fostering multidisciplinary clinical practice and research.

Specialism in all aspects of medical care has revolutionized the role of the surgical pathologist. Rather than fostering professional independence, specialization in medicine has created circumstances in which the specialist, delivering a limited segment of medical care, is increasingly dependent on the assistance of colleagues who have acquired complementary expertise. This situation is epitomized by the multidisciplinary approach that is now standard for treating breast diseases. Inherent in this circumstance is the expectation that each member of the team is capable of delivering optimal specialty care. A corollary effect is the growing pressure for subspecialization in diagnostic pathology in academic centers and in large community hospital centers. This process will be furthered by growing awareness on the part of patients and patient advocacy organizations that accurate and comprehensive pathology diagnosis is fundamental to effective treatment and research in breast diseases.

Even when considered in the context of advances in diagnosis that have been facilitated in recent decades by immunohistochemistry and molecular analysis, microscopic examination of hematoxylin and eosin–stained tissue sections combined with gross inspection remains the most cost-effective diagnostic procedure for breast diseases. Pathologists generate an important part of the information used for therapeutic decisions. The complex multifactorial description of breast pathology now considered to be standard practice has expanded the diagnostic report from a brief one- or two-line statement to a catalog of data that may be several pages in length. Immunohistochemistry makes it possible to determine whether prognostic and therapeutic markers are present by microscopic examination, and these observations are part of the pathologist's report. The expanded role of pathologists in the management of breast diseases requires their active participation as part of the clinical care team. Pathologists who diagnose breast specimens need to be aware of how various components of their reports are relevant to treatment decisions.

Coincidental with these medical developments has been the growing involvement of patients in making decisions about their treatment. This, in turn, has led to greater public awareness of the importance of information contained in pathology reports. For the untrained layperson to read and interpret a pathology report, it is necessary to learn and understand a new vocabulary, a daunting task that is not necessarily made easier by the frequently conflicting and unfiltered information available from the Internet. Surgeons, oncologists, and radiotherapists are experts at interpreting pathology reports for their patients and at explaining the significance of the data. Nonetheless, a substantial number of patients with breast diseases want an explanation from the pathologist who issued the report or they seek out another pathologist, often with specialized expertise, for a second-opinion review. In this way, pathologists increasingly participate in direct patient care and patient education, a vital public service.

SECOND OPINIONS IN BREAST PATHOLOGY

Surgical pathologists in general practice provide accurate diagnoses for the great majority of the breast specimens they encounter without the assistance of intramural or extramural consultation. Nonetheless, pathology departments that do not have a dedicated breast pathology subsection should have a built-in mechanism for obtaining second opinions internally through conferencing or other quality assurance programs. As evidenced by a number of papers published in recent years, there is growing recognition of the importance of having an intradepartmental peer-review quality assurance program in order to minimize diagnostic errors.[1–3] Procedures have been described for internal review shortly after the diagnosis was officially reported[4] and for pre-signout review.[5] For detailed discussions of quality assurance issues in surgical pathology, the reader should consult the aforementioned articles and references cited therein.

In this setting, the individual pathologist or the pathology group in a department may seek an extramural opinion from an expert consultant. This typically occurs when there is a difference of interpretation among pathologists in an institution or the diagnosis is uncertain after internal review. Consultation may also be obtained when the probable diagnosis is one with which there is little or no experience. Another category of consultation results from uncertainty about the diagnosis engendered by a limited or unrepresentative sample, poor histologic preparation, or a pathologic change that appears to be on the borderline between two or more diagnoses. As noted by Leslie et al.,[6] "Second opinions in anatomic pathology are an integral part of quality practice ... frequent consultation between pathologists should be fostered in all practice settings and documented as part of the quality assurance process."

Several studies have demonstrated the important contribution to patient care of second opinion pathology consultations, generally in the context of referrals seen at academic centers. A very encouraging aspect of this practice is the high degree to which the primary diagnosis has been confirmed by the consultant. Epstein et al.[7] reported concordant diagnoses (carcinoma vs. not carcinoma) in 98.7% of 535 prostatic needle biopsies diagnosed as carcinoma. Nonetheless, the six diagnoses not sustained as carcinoma were critically important for the 1.3% of patients. A cost analysis of these results suggested that the saving in medical expenses for the six patients who did not undergo surgery substantially exceeded the cost of reviewing all 535 biopsies. In a subsequent study of 855 core biopsy samples from the prostate gland seen in consultation, Epstein and colleagues[8] reported a 1.2% rate of unconfirmed carcinomas, a result that was virtually identical to their 1996 study. Among 844 cases confirmed to be carcinoma, unreported perineural invasion was detected in 4.3% and unreported periprostatic invasion was found in 0.5%.

A higher rate of discrepancies was found by Abt et al.,[9] who compared the original- and second-opinion diagnoses in a broad range of pathology among 777 patients referred to an academic center. Forty-five diagnostic disagreements (6%) were regarded as clinically significant, and overall the level of agreement was 92.1%. Manion et al.[10] reported a study of 5,629 outside pathology cases examined between 2003 and 2006 as part of the University of Iowa Hospitals and Clinics policy that requires "... second opinion pathology review of pertinent outside material, irrespective of the nature of the specimen or complexity of the case." Major diagnostic disagreements with the potential to change treatment or prognosis were recorded in 132 (2.3%) cases, resulting in changes in clinical management in 68 (1.2%). The most frequent sites of major disagreements were the female reproductive tract, the gastrointestinal tract, and the skin. The largest study to date of discordant pathology was reported by Swapp et al.,[11] who reviewed the records of 71,811 cases seen in consultation at the Mayo Clinic between 2005 and 2010. Major disagreements were recorded in 457 (0.6%) cases. The most frequent sites of discrepant diagnoses were the gastrointestinal tract (17.5%), lymph nodes (16%), and bone/soft tissue (10%). Major disagreements were encountered in 8% of breast cases.

Perkins et al.[12] estimated that diagnoses were inaccurate in 2% to 4% of breast carcinoma cases, including mistaking benign for malignant disease or *vice versa*, over- or underdiagnoses of invasive carcinoma, or misinterpretation of prognostic markers such as human epidermal growth factor/*neu* receptor (HER2/*neu*). In a study restricted to breast carcinomas, Staradub et al.[13] reviewed second-opinion diagnoses on 346 tumors from 340 patients who had been referred to the Sage Comprehensive Breast Program at Northwestern University. Major changes in diagnosis that affected therapy occurred in 30 (7.8%) cases. Among seven discrepant cases with an initial diagnosis of ductal carcinoma *in situ* (DCIS), the second-opinion diagnosis was benign in one and invasive carcinoma in six. Seven other diagnoses were revised from invasive carcinoma to DCIS. Sixteen changes of margin status were documented and in three cases revised margin status coincided with another major change.

Within the United States, several factors have contributed to the growing number of pathology consultations. Much of the increase is generated by patients who seek multiple clinical opinions from different physicians and institutions. Some patients are primarily concerned with confirmation of their diagnosis, and one or more consultations may be obtained directly from pathologists for this reason alone. The involvement of patients is epitomized by a January 17, 2012, *Wall Street Journal* article titled "What If the Doctor Is Wrong?,"[14] which recounts the story of a 47-year-old woman with abdominal tumors. Based on initial tissue samples, it was thought that she had a rare form of ovarian carcinoma. When the patient consulted a major cancer center, further studies led to a diagnosis of lymphoma.

In addition to consultations initiated by pathologists seeking opinions from their colleagues, surgeons, medical oncologists, and other physicians generate some consultations. The review of "outside" pathology slides should be mandatory whenever a patient is referred to a physician for consultation or treatment at an institution other than the one where the primary diagnosis was rendered,[15] a policy referred to by one author as "the pathologist's preventive medicine."[16] The office of the physician seeing a patient in consultation should inform the patient of the necessity of obtaining pathology material for review in a timely manner before the office visit. A policy and procedures should be established for guiding the patient through this process, including instructions as to what material is needed and where it should be sent. The importance of a second review should be explained, and the patient should be informed that there will be a charge for this service.

Slides sent for consultation, regardless of the reason, must be accompanied by documents that confirm the identity of the specimen with the patient and a copy of the pathology/cytology report for each specimen represented, clearly displaying the name of the patient and the accession number corresponding to the slides and paraffin blocks enclosed. It is unacceptable and substandard practice to withhold the pathology report previously obtained from a consultant or second-opinion institution so as not to "bias" the second review. The pathology report provides essential information such as an index of location(s) of the specimen(s) represented by individual slides, a description of the gross appearance of the specimen(s), clinical information provided with the specimen, frozen section interpretations, and details of the originating pathologist's diagnosis. The pathology report must be included even if a final diagnosis had not been reached. When the slides are sent directly from one laboratory to another in relation to a clinical consultation at the recipient institution, the correspondence should include the name of the clinical physician who is being consulted (if known) and detailed billing information. When more than one consultant is involved, it is vital that all consultants examine the same or equivalent material.

MOLECULAR VERSUS MORPHOLOGY FOR THE CLASSIFICATION OF BREAST CARCINOMA: MUST IT BE EITHER/OR?

A host of new classifications of breast carcinoma have emerged from studies using tissue microarray and gene expression profile technology.[17–23] Some of these molecular-based classification schemes have led to the introduction of testing procedures that assign patients to prognostic categories and predict response to therapy, as discussed in Chapter 45. Some of these tests are being used in clinical practice based on analysis of retrospective data. It will take many years before they are fully validated in prospective clinical trials. As the results of additional gene profiling studies are reported, more classifications will no doubt be developed and promoted for various reasons.

The exceptional speed with which the molecular study of breast carcinoma has advanced makes it hazardous to predict circumstances even a few years hence. Nevertheless, the current situation was perhaps best summarized by Rakha and Ellis[22] in their paper titled "Modern Classification of Breast Cancer: Should We Stick with Morphology or Convert to Molecular Profile Characteristics," wherein they observed that the "replacement of conventional classification seems unfounded and incorporation of multigene molecular classifiers to conventional BC [breast carcinoma] classification systems seems more realistic and practical to support more effective tailoring of therapy in the future." In a report titled "Breast Cancer Prognostic Classification in the Molecular Era: The Role of Histological Grade," Rakha et al.[21] concluded that "clinical acceptance of these molecular assays will require them to be more than expensive surrogates for established traditional factors such as histological grade."

A study reported by Sotiriou et al.[24] illustrates how results from gene expression profiling can be complementary to conventional pathologic data. The investigators developed a scoring system or gene expression grade index based on a 97-gene list that correlated patterns of gene expression with histologic grade. A high gene expression grade index was associated with 86% of grade 3 tumors, and a low index was associated with 91% of grade 1 tumors. The contribution of the gene expression index was greatest among grade 2 carcinomas, in which a high index was associated with a significantly greater risk for recurrence than a low index ($p < 0.001$; hazard ratio, 3.61; CI, 2.25 to 5.78).

Finally, there are substantial parts of the world where the technology needed to support a molecular-based description of breast carcinoma is unavailable. This situation is not likely to change soon and will require the continued use of standard morphology-based diagnostic reporting.

It would be wise to observe this rapidly evolving field with a healthy dose of skepticism regarding the likelihood that any of the current molecular-based classification schemes will soon supplant standard pathologic examination as the basis for establishing a diagnosis, estimating prognosis, and for fundamental treatment decisions. At best, molecular data in its current form complement pathologic observations and can "fine tune" therapeutic decisions, especially in intermediate or ambiguous situations.

DCIS BY ANY OTHER NAME IS STILL CARCINOMA

Ever since it was demonstrated in the 1970s and 1980s that mammography screening could detect clinically occult carcinomas of the breast and reduce breast carcinoma mortality, concern has been expressed that screening results in "overdiagnosis" and "overtreatment" because it identifies indolent lesions that are unlikely to have a fatal outcome and could be left untreated. The issue first came to a head in the late 1970s when the early results of the Breast Cancer Diagnosis Demonstration Project (BCDDP) sponsored by the National Cancer Institute (NCI) and the American Cancer Society (ACS) were presented. The BCDDP program, inspired by the breast screening initiative carried out by the Health Insurance Plan of Greater New York (HIP) in the 1960s, consisted of 29 mammography centers in 27 cities across the United States that were created to assess the feasibility of nationwide breast screening by this method. A total of 283,222 women enrolled for five annual screening examinations between 1973 and 1980. The 1977 report revealed that screening on this scale could be accomplished and that clinically occult carcinomas were detected. The program came under fire for leading to "overdiagnosis" and "overtreatment" as evidenced by the large proportion of biopsies from lesions that proved to be benign, the detection of a small number of benign lesions that were misdiagnosed as carcinoma, and treatment for "indolent" carcinomas that might not have become clinically apparent in the patient's lifetime. There was also concern that radiation exposure during screening might induce carcinomas at a later date, but this proved to be of less concern because in subsequent years, advances in mammography technology led to substantially reduced radiation exposure. Many later studies documented the feasibility of mammography screening and also confirmed that it reduced breast carcinoma deaths in the screened populations.[25–30]

Encouraged by the success of breast screening and with the availability of suitable tests, screening for the detection of occult tumors in other organs such as the prostate gland and lungs was introduced, again prompting criticisms of "overdiagnosis" and "overtreatment."[31,32] In this regard, a study that reported a reduction in deaths due to carcinoma of the lung after screening with low-dose CT scans also noted that 96.4% of "positive" screening findings did not prove to be carcinoma, resulting in a large number of diagnostic procedures that did not benefit these individuals.[33]

In March 2012, the NCI sponsored a meeting to once again address concerns that screening results in the "overdiagnosis" of cancer. A report summarizing the conclusions of the participants was published in July, 2013[34] in an article that attracted wide public attention. The authors of the report defined "overdiagnosis" as a diagnosis "...which occurs when tumors are detected that, if left unattended, would not become clinically apparent or cause death. Overdiagnosis, if not recognized, generally leads to overtreatment." It was concluded that "overdiagnosis" most often occurs as a result of screening when clinically asymptomatic, "indolent" cancers are likely to be detected. In this context, the authors defined "cancer" as a disease "...with a *reasonable* (my Italics) likelihood of lethal progression if left untreated." The word "reasonable" was not defined by the authors, but presumably referred to an unspecified risk that a patient would experience a fatal outcome.

The authors also recommended that the word "cancer" should be dropped from what were referred to as "premalignant conditions" such as DCIS that should be renamed "indolent lesions of epithelial origin" under the acronym IDLE conditions. They suggested that this change would remove the frightening connotation associated with "cancer" and reduce "overtreatment" by making it easier to recommend less aggressive therapy for "indolent" lesions. In support of this position, it was argued that not all *in situ* carcinomas in various organs progress to an invasive stage if left untreated, as evidenced by the clinical biology of prostatic (PIN) and cervical (CIN) neoplasia, and that in some instances (e.g., the prostate gland) the invasive neoplasms that ultimately arise are so indolent that they pose little danger in the lifetime of the patient. A corollary of latter argument was that the current tendency to manage all *in situ* carcinomas with equally aggressive treatments results in the overtreatment of some patients who might not have needed the recommended therapy, and may have been harmed by it. Finally, being able to replace costly treatment with observation would reduce healthcare costs. In summary, it was suggested that simply changing the name of a disease would result in important improvements in patient well-being and save money.

Before addressing the foregoing proposal itself, it is necessary to comment on a matter of semantics relating to the words "cancer" and "carcinoma" as they were used by the authors of the aforementioned proposal, as well as many other authors cited among the references in this book. The online Merriam Webster Dictionary defines *cancer* as "a malignant tumor of potentially unlimited growth that expands locally by invasion and systemically by metastasis." *Carcinoma* is defined as "a malignant tumor of epithelial origin." Thus, carcinoma refers to the subset of malignant tumors arising from epithelium, whereas cancer refers to the entire spectrum of malignant tumors, including carcinomas, sarcomas, lymphomas, leukemias, and malignant neoplasms of the central nervous system. Regrettably, Drs. Esserman, Thompson, and Reid confused these terms throughout their paper. Although they were mainly concerned with "overtreatment" relating to screening-detected carcinomas arising at various sites, and pigmented skin lesions, they repeatedly used the words *cancer* and *carcinoma* interchangeably. In the second paragraph of the article, they refer to "breast cancer and prostate cancer" when they appear to mean carcinoma. The authors' misuse of these terms is best appreciated in the following quotation from one of the summary recommendations: "First, premalignant conditions (eg. ductal carcinoma in situ or high-grade prostatic intraepithelial neoplasia) should not be labeled as cancers or neoplasia, nor should the word cancer be in the name." This recommendation is meaningless because the word "cancer" already does not appear in the names of the cited lesions.

It is to be hoped that Drs. Esserman, Thompson, and Reid are not seeking to deny the concept of *in situ* carcinoma generally, and in the breast specifically, by referring to it as a "premalignant" condition. All invasive carcinomas arise from a preinvasive stage of the disease that develops in the epithelium from which the carcinoma originates. The duration of the preinvasive stage is variable, depending on factors that are largely not known. At the histologic level, the cytologic appearance of *in situ* carcinoma cells is often indistinguishable from that of the invasive carcinoma it has given rise to. Molecular studies have shown a high level of concordance in the genetic alterations between these components in a given tumors that consists of DCIS and invasive ductal carcinoma, as discussed in Chapters 11 and 12, as well as Chapters 31 and 32 in the context of lobular carcinoma. Rather than denying the existence of preinvasive carcinoma, what is needed is further study to identify the molecular alterations that endow DCIS (and lobular carcinoma *in situ* [LCIS]) with the ability to invade and metastasize, as well as changes in the patient's "resistance" that might enable these events to occur.

Turning to the flawed proposal, which, if adopted in its current form, would probably be more harmful than beneficial, it is self-evident that changing the name of a disease would not change the disease itself. Despite some general principles that invasive carcinomas appear to have in common, such as epithelial origin and a preinvasive, intraepithelial stage, there are substantial differences between organ sites. Among these differences from a clinical standpoint, accessibility is a critical issue when it comes to treatment. Thus, it is possible to directly observe and follow over time the epithelium of organs with external orifices such as the uterine cervix, the urinary bladder and the gastrointestinal tract. Repeated cytologic samples can be taken from these sites without performing a surgical procedure that removes part of the lesion. These organs, and others such as the prostate gland, can also be monitored with small biopsy samples. As a consequence, it is possible to track preinvasive lesions at these sites in order to distinguish between conditions that can be managed with minimally invasive procedures and those that require more aggressive treatment.

On the other hand, despite repeated efforts to improve mammary ductoscopy, virtually all of the complex glandular structure of the breast where carcinomas arise is not accessible for direct observation, and current imaging technologies only reveal structural alterations without identifying the precise causes of the changes. Sequential imaging that requires repeated radiation exposure only documents the evolution of structural changes. For example, a mass lesion caused by mammary carcinoma usually has an invasive component, but in some circumstances it may consist entirely of noninvasive, intraepithelial carcinoma (DCIS) when excised and thoroughly examined microscopically. If such a tumor were investigated by needle biopsy and the sample proved to be DCIS, there is currently no method (comparable to culposcopy of the uterine cervix) whereby the nature of the remainder of the tumor could be ascertained without removing it entirely. Applying the paradigm of the uterine cervix in the forgoing circumstance would require allowing the mass to remain in the breast and following it with serial imaging studies. If by chance an invasive focus already existed in the mass, this procedure would allow the invasive carcinoma to expand and increase the likelihood of metastatic spread. If left in place, whether indolent or not, the incompletely excised lesion would probably enlarge over time, creating growing anxiety, and yet it might remain entirely noninvasive. This would clearly be an unacceptable way to manage DCIS clinically, and changing the name of the lesion would not solve this conundrum, nor need it change treatment after the diagnosis. Within the limits of our current knowledge, the cornerstone of clinical care for intraepithelial ductal carcinoma of the breast (DCIS) is complete excision and thorough histologic examination of the lesion when it is detected. At present, no procedure short of this can provide the full appreciation of the nature and extent of the lesion that is needed to guide treatment.

In reviewing the proposal to remove the word carcinoma from the intraepithelial, noninvasive stage of ductal carcinoma, one is reminded of the famed manager of the New York Yankees baseball team, Yogi Berra, who is credited with the remark, "It's like déjà vu all over again." In the current context, the effort to delete carcinoma from DCIS repeats the scenario of the 1980s and 1990s when there was a movement to replace LCIS with names such as lobular neoplasia (LN). The very same reasons were put forth for this change as are now offered for removing the word carcinoma from DCIS: changing the name would reduce patient anxiety and lead to less aggressive therapy. One phase of this effort was to promulgate the concept that LCIS was only a marker of breast carcinoma risk and not a precursor to invasive carcinoma. If this were true, mastectomy, then a frequent treatment option after the diagnosis was made by biopsy, would no longer be appropriate.

Research conducted in the past two decades, described in detail in Chapter 31, clearly demonstrated that LCIS is a nonobligate precursor to invasive lobular carcinoma. This means that not every patient with LCIS develops invasive lobular carcinoma in their lifetime, but when it occurs, invasive lobular carcinoma arises from LCIS. It is also well established that patients with LCIS are at increased risk to develop invasive ductal carcinoma that arises independently from the LCIS. In the ensuing years, little progress has been made in distinguishing patients with LCIS who are likely to experience progression to either type of invasive carcinoma from those unlikely to have this outcome. Now, approximately 30 years later, clinical management for LCIS usually consists of medical therapy and clinical observation for a disease that is again widely referred to as LCIS.

Thus, in the case of LCIS, concern with "overtreatment" was expressed in proposals to change the name of the disease, but other factors played a much more important role in creating a new treatment paradigm. Most important of these was a better understanding of the clinical course of the disease that resulted from retrospective long-term follow-up studies of untreated patients published in 1978 and subsequent prospective studies that are described in detail in Chapter 31. Historically, the movement away from mastectomy for the treatment of LCIS coincided with the discovery of hormone receptor proteins, particularly those involved in the response of mammary carcinoma to estrogens and progesterone, and the introduction of selective estrogen receptor modulators (SERMS) such as tamoxifen that have significantly reduced the risk of developing invasive carcinoma in patients with LCIS. While efforts to delete the word "carcinoma" from LCIS may have prompted controversy and drawn attention to the need for changes in therapy, it was better understanding of the clinical and biologic characteristics of the disease, accompanied by new, effective forms of treatment that brought about the desired result.

The foregoing notwithstanding, the concerns expressed by Drs. Esserman, Thompson, and Reid raise an important question about our understanding of the biology of DCIS. Retrospective, long-term follow-up studies described in detail in Chapter 11 demonstrated that if left untreated after a biopsy, about 40% of patients with low-grade DCIS developed invasive carcinoma. Among the remaining majority of patients, the absence of subsequent invasive carcinoma may have been due to complete removal of the DCIS in the diagnostic biopsy sample in some cases. In others, however, it is possible that persistent DCIS remained dormant, either failing to develop the capacity to invade and metastasize or actually regressing, possibly to extinction.

Data from two studies involving a total of 38 women with low-grade micropapillary, papillary, and cribriform DCIS are particularly relevant to this issue.[35,36] Previously overlooked DCIS in these cases was found in the course of reviewing breast biopsies that had been diagnosed originally as benign, a circumstance that attests to the low-grade nature of most of the lesions. With follow-up averaging 21.6 years[35] and 30 years,[36] respectively, invasive carcinoma was found in 16 (48%) of the combined total of 38 patients. In the latter study,[36] the frequency of subsequent carcinoma was 9.1 times expected, with a 95% CI of 4.73 to 17.5. A third, more recent review of biopsies classified as benign found 13 instances of previously unrecognized DCIS (4 low grade, 6 intermediate grade, and 3 high grade).[37] In the course of follow-up, subsequent ipsilateral invasive carcinoma was diagnosed in 6 of the 13 (46%) patients after intervals of 4 to 18 years. In this study, the odds ratio of developing invasive carcinoma in women with DCIS when compared to women with nonproliferative breast disease was 13.5, with a 95% CI of 3.7 to 49.7.

A number of prospective studies of patients with DCIS who had no treatment after a biopsy are also available. The studies differ from the foregoing retrospective studies in two important respects: (1) because the patients were known to have DCIS and were monitored clinically after the initial biopsy, new abnormalities were promptly investigated; and (2) reported clinical follow-up rarely exceeded 5 years.

Two studies described selected patients with clinically occult DCIS that was detected by mammography. In one, 70 patients were followed for a median of 47 months after biopsy-proven DCIS was diagnosed.[38] Among the DCIS lesions, 51% had a comedo (high grade) component and 29% were predominantly comedo-DCIS. During the course of follow-up, invasive carcinomas were detected in 3 (4.3%) patients, and 8 (11.4%) were found to have further evidence of DCIS. Another report describing a selected group of untreated DCIS patients included 59 women.[39] During a median follow-up of 37 months, invasive carcinoma was detected in 4 (6.8%) and additional DCIS in 6 (10.9%).

There are two noteworthy population-based studies of women with DCIS who had no treatment after a diagnostic biopsy. One series consisted of 112 patients with a median follow-up of 53 months during which 5 (4.4%) invasive carcinomas and 19 (17%) instances of DCIS were detected.[40] A smaller study of 21 patients described the finding of invasive carcinoma in 3 (14.3%) patients during a median follow-up of 7 years.[41]

Finally, two prospective studies of women with untreated DCIS detected by mammography screening can be cited. In one report, 38 women with predominantly low-grade cribriform DCIS were followed for a median period of 60 months, during which time 2 (5%) were found to have invasive carcinoma and 3 (8%) had DCIS.[42] The other report described the detection of invasive carcinoma in 1 of 28 (3.8%) women and DCIS in 4 (14.3%) others during a median follow-up of 38 months.[43]

The consequences of short follow-up and clinical monitoring in the foregoing prospective studies are significant. In every instance, subsequent DCIS was detected more frequently than invasive carcinoma. Had the patients not been monitored closely it is highly likely that many of those subsequently found to have DCIS would have developed invasive carcinoma in later years. In fact, it is troubling that the frequency of invasive carcinoma was so high (3.6% to 6.8%) after a median follow-up of only 5 years or less in patients known to have DCIS. This suggests that at least some of these women may have harbored invasive carcinoma when DCIS was first detected, and/or that progression from DCIS to invasion can occur rapidly. In any case, none of the preceding prospective studies can be cited as evidence in favor of the proposal to eliminate the word "carcinoma" from DCIS, or in support of a "treatment" plan based on clinical follow-up alone that underestimates the potential of DCIS to give rise to invasive carcinoma.

In view of the foregoing evidence, and other data presented in Chapter 11, there is an urgent need to better understand the factors involved in the biology of untreated DCIS, especially the low-grade variants of the disease. This will certainly involve intensive molecular studies, including gene expression profiling of DCIS and invasive ductal carcinoma lesions, but it is important not to overlook the role that the "host" environment might play in modulating the evolution of DCIS. As noted above, the same issue pertains to LCIS, and despite more than a decade of investigation, there is still no reliable guide to predicting the likelihood that invasive carcinoma will appear in a particular patient with classical LCIS. *Deleting the word "carcinoma" from DCIS will not solve the fundamental problem. Understating the risk associated with failing to adequately treat low-grade DCIS is likely to create a false sense of security, and might cause significant harm.*

DOES INVASIVE DUCTAL CARCINOMA, NOS, HAVE A FUTURE?

The 2012 World Health Organization (WHO) publication on the classification of mammary carcinoma replaces the term "invasive ductal carcinoma, NOS," with "invasive carcinoma of no special type" because the word "ductal" in this context "...perpetuates the traditional but incorrect concept that these tumors are derived exclusively from mammary ductal epithelium in distinction to lobular carcinomas, which were deemed to have arisen from within lobules, for which there is also no evidence."[44] The muddled thinking of the authors of the WHO book who made these assertions is manifested by the fact that they retained terms such as DCIS, atypical ductal hyperplasia, and invasive lobular carcinoma. We are not convinced that there is merit to the proposed change. As noted in Chapter 12, unless otherwise stated, the term "invasive ductal carcinoma" as used in this book refers to invasive ductal carcinoma, NOS.

This flawed proposal does raise an important issue about the precise microanatomical origin of various lesions included under the broad heading of invasive ductal carcinoma, NOS. The ductal system is a complex series of branching tubules extending from intralobular ductules to the major lactiferous ducts that terminate in the nipple. While the endpoint in the nipple is demarcated histologically by a squamocolumnar junction, the point at which terminal ductular epithelium ends and the secretory glandular epithelium begins is less clearly defined. In fact, this junction appears to be somewhat labile and subject to changes induced by physiologic and/or proliferative factors. Although it is possible that a small percentage of lesions currently categorized as invasive ductal carcinoma, NOS, arise from epithelium that may have attributes associated with secretory lobular epithelium, no reliable basis for distinguishing this subset of carcinomas has been demonstrated.

This issue is confounded by the ability of some *in situ* carcinomas that are classified as DCIS to grow into the glandular compartment of lobules, a process referred to as "lobular cancerization." Conversely, *in situ* carcinomas that arise in the glandular epithelium of lobules, LCIS, may extend into ducts either as the solid proliferation that characterizes florid and pleomorphic LCIS, or as the dispersed cells found in "pagetoid spread." When either of these situations is encountered, classification of the *in situ* carcinoma (and invasive carcinoma if present) is based on the histologic features of the lesion, not on its microanatomic distribution.

The foregoing arguments notwithstanding, the fact that approximately 75% of mammary carcinomas are classified as invasive ductal carcinoma, NOS, is troublesome since within this broad category are subsets of tumors with similar histologic appearances that display diverse clinical attributes. The genetic heterogeneity of these tumors has become the subject of intense investigation, especially in the past decade, leading to the identification of molecular subtypes based of gene expression profiles for estrogen receptor (ER), HER2, epidermal growth factor receptor (EGFR), cytokeratins (CKs), and other markers. At present, the subtypes based on the expression of these markers are referred to as luminal, basal-like, HER2-rich, molecular apocrine, and claudin-low. The complexity of this approach to classification is manifested when a subset of invasive ductal carcinomas, NOS, is classified according to more than one molecular subtype. This is illustrated by the report by Lu et al.,[45] who studied the expression of claudin subtypes in high-grade invasive ductal carcinomas. Claudins are a group of proteins that play an important role in maintaining tight intercellular junctions. The investigators found a significant correlation between the expression of specific claudins and particular molecular subtypes of breast carcinomas (basal-like, luminal, etc.). In addition, low levels of expression for claudins 1, 3, 4, 7, and 8 were detected in 30 of 226 (14%) of tumors (referred to as "claudin low"), 77% of which were basal-like. When compared to patients with "non-claudin low" basal-like carcinomas, those with "claudin-low carcinomas" had a significantly worse recurrence-free survival.

It is noteworthy that the attributes which define some of these molecular subtypes among tumors classified as invasive ductal carcinoma, NOS, are also associated with special types of breast carcinoma that are defined by their distinctive histologic and clinical characteristics.[46] For example, the basal-like subtype characterized as ER(−), PR(−), HER2(−), CK5/6(+), and EGFR(+), which is associated with a relatively unfavorable prognosis among invasive ductal carcinomas, NOS, is also found in prognostically favorable adenoid cystic, medullary, and secretory carcinomas. The relative nonspecific nature of subclassifications of invasive ductal carcinoma, NOS, based on these gene expression profiles is highlighted by the association of the same basal-like attributes with clinically more aggressive metaplastic and pleomorphic lobular special types of breast carcinoma.

Despite these overlapping patterns of gene expression between subsets of invasive ductal carcinoma, NOS, and some special histologic types of mammary carcinoma illustrated by the foregoing examples, gene expression profiling reveals significant and distinctive genomic differences such as the upregulation of genes involved in immune response in medullary carcinomas[47] and the downregulation of genes involved in cell proliferation and migration in adenoid cystic carcinomas.[48]

As Steensma[49] observed, "This is the age of massive genome surveys- at least for a little while longer." Gene expression profiling is really in its infancy and will most likely lead to important, lasting discoveries in the future. The recent finding that carcinomas arising in different organ systems share certain genomic alterations[50] has important therapeutic implications. It is reasonable to predict that genomic studies will eventually lead to stratification of invasive ductal carcinomas NOS, into clinically meaningful subgroups. In the meantime, changing the name of this group of neoplasms without a sound scientific basis will only cause confusion without improving our understanding of the disease. With a little patience, advances in the genomics of breast carcinoma will probably take care of the problem.

Paul P. Rosen, MD

REFERENCES

1. Roy JE, Hunt JL. Detection and classification of diagnostic discrepancies (errors) in surgical pathology. *Adv Anat Pathol* 2010;17:359–365.
2. Smith ML, Raab SS. Directed peer review in surgical pathology. *Adv Anat Pathol* 2012;19:331–337.
3. Raab SS, Swain J, Smith N, et al. Quality and patient safety in the diagnosis of breast cancer. *ClinBiochem2013, http://dx.org/10.1016/j.clinbiochem.2013.04.024.*
4. Renshaw AA, Gould EW. Measuring errors in surgical pathology in real-life practice. Defining what does and does not matter. *Am J Clin Pathol* 2007;127:144–152.

5. Owens SR, Dhir R, Yousem SA, et al. The development and testing of a laboratory information system-driven tool for pre-sign-out quality assurance of random surgical pathology reports. *Am J Clin Pathol* 2010;133:836–841.
6. Leslie KO, Fechner RE, Kempson RL. Second opinions in surgical pathology. *Am J Clin Pathol* 1996;106:S58–S64.
7. Epstein JL, Walsh PC, Sanfilippo F. Clinical and cost impact of second-opinion Pathology. Review of prostate biopsies prior to radical prostatectomy. *Am J Surg Pathol* 1996;20:851–857.
8. Brimo F, Schultz L, Epstein JL. The value of mandatory second opinion review of prostate needle biopsy interpretation before radical prostatectomy. *J Urol* 2010;184:126–130.
9. Abt AB, Abt LG, Oly GJ. The effect of interinstitution anatomic pathology consultation on patient care. *Arch Pathol Lab Med* 1995;119: 514–517.
10. Manion E, Cohen MB, Weydert J. Mandatory second opinion in surgical pathology referral material: clinical consequences of major disagreements. *Am J Surg Pathol* 2008;32:732–737.
11. Swapp RE, Aubry MC, Salomão DR, et al. Outside case review of surgical pathology for referred patients. *Arch Pathol Lab Med* 2013;137:233–240.
12. Perkins C, Balma D, Garcia R, et al. Why current breast pathology practices must be evaluated. A *Susan G. Komen for the Cure* white paper: June 2006. *Breast J* 2007;5:443–447.
13. Staradub VL, Messenger KA, Hao N, et al. Changes in breast cancer therapy because of pathology second opinions. *Ann Surg Oncol* 2002;9:982–987.
14. Landro L. What if the doctor is wrong? *The Wall Street J* Jan 17, 2012.
15. Rosen PP. Review of 'outside' pathology before treatment should be mandatory. *Am J Surg Pathol* 2002;26:1235–1240.
16. Allen TC. Second opinions: pathologists' preventive medicine. *Arch Pathol Lab Med* 2013;137:310–311.
17. Ross JS. Multigene classifiers, prognostic factors, and predictors of breast cancer clinical outcome. *Adv Anat Pathol* 2009;16:204–215.
18. Cianfrocca M, Gradishar W. New molecular classification of breast cancer. *CA Cancer J Clin* 2009;59:303–313.
19. Geyer FC, Reis-Filho JS. Microarray-based gene expression profiling as a clinical tool for breast cancer management: are we there yet? *Int J Surg Pathol* 2009;17:285–302.
20. Schnitt, SJ. Classification and prognosis of invasive breast cancer: from morphology to molecular taxonomy. *Mod Pathol* 2010;23: S60–S64.
21. Rakha, EA, Reis-Filho JS, Baehner F, et al. Breast cancer prognostic classification in the molecular era: the role of histological grade. *Breast Cancer Res* 2010;12:207.
22. Rakha EA, Ellis IO. Modern classification of breast cancer: should we stick with morphology or convert to molecular profile characteristics. *Adv Anat Pathol* 2011;18:255–267.
23. Tamimi RM, Colditz GA, Hazra A, et al. Traditional breast cancer risk factors in relation to molecular subtypes of breast cancer. *Breast Cancer Res Treat* 2011;131:159–167.
24. Sotiriou C, Wirapati P, Loi S, et al. Gene expression profiling in breast cancer: understanding the molecular basis of histologic grade to improve prognosis. *J Natl Cancer Inst* 2006;98:262–272.
25. Berry DA, Cronin KA, Plevritis SK, et al. Effect of screening and adjuvant therapy on mortality from breast cancer. *NEJM* 2005;353: 1784–1792.
26. Ballard-Barbash R, Taplin SH, Yankaskas BC, et al. Breast Cancer Surveillance Consortium: a national mammography screening and outcomes database. *AJR Am J Roengenol* 1997;169:1001–1008.
27. Tabar L, Vitak B, Chen HH, et al. The Swedish Two-County Trial twenty years later: updated mortality results and new insights from long-term follow-up. *Radiol Clin North Am* 2000;38:625–651.
28. Miller AB, To T, Baines CJ, et al. Canadian National Breast Screening Study-2: 13-year results of a randomized trial in women aged 50-59 years. *J Natl Cancer Inst* 2000;92:1490–1499.
29. Nyström L, Andersson I, Bjurstam N, et al. Long-term effects of mammography screening: updated overview of the Swedish randomized trials. *Lancet* 2002;359:909–919.
30. Kalager M, Zelen M, Langmark F, et al. Effect of screening mammography on breast-cancer mortality in Norway. *NEJM* 2010;363:1203–1210.
31. Welch HG, Black WC. Overdiagnosis in cancer. *JNCI* 2010;102: 605–613.
32. Esserman L, Shieh Y, Thompson I. Rethinking screening for breast cancer and prostate cancer. *JAMA* 2009;302:1685–1692.
33. The National Lung Screening Trial Research Team. Reduced lung-cancer mortality with low-dose computed tomographic screening. *NEJM* 2011;365:395–409.
34. Esserman LJ, Thompson IM Jr, Reid, B. Overdiagnosis and overtreatment in cancer. An opportunity for improvement. *JAMA* 2013;310:797–798.
35. Betsill WL Jr, Rosen PP, Lieberman PH, et al. Intraductal carcinoma. Long-term follow-up after treatment by biopsy alone. *JAMA* 1978;239:1863–1869.
36. Page DL, Dupont WD, Rogers LW, et al. Continued local recurrence of carcinoma 15-25 years after a diagnosis of low grade ductal carcinoma in situ of the breast treated by biopsy only. *Cancer* 1982;49:751–758.
37. Collins, LC, Tamimi RM, Baer HJ, et al. Outcome of patients with ductal carcinoma in situ untreated after a diagnostic biopsy: results from the Nurses' Health Study. *Cancer* 2005;103:1778–1784.
38. Schwartz GF, Finkel GC, Garcia JC, et al. Subclinical ductal carcinoma *in situ* of the breast. *Cancer* 1992;70:2468–2474.
39. Hetelekidis S, Collins L, Silver B, et al. Predictors of local recurrence following excision alone for ductal carcinoma *in situ*. *Cancer* 1999;85:427–431.
40. Ottesen GL, Graversen HP, Blichert-Toft M, et al. Ductal carcinoma *in situ* of the female breast. Short-term results of a prospective nationwide study. *Am J Surg Pathol* 1992;16:1183–1196.
41. Ringberg A, Andersson I, Aspegren K, et al. Breast carcinoma *in situ* in 167 women—incidence, mode of presentation, therapy, and follow-up. *Eur J Surg Oncol* 1991;17:466–476.
42. Arnesson L-G, Smeds S, Fagerberg G, et al. Follow-up of two treatment modalities for ductal carcinoma in situ of the female breast. *Br J Surg* 1989;76:672–675.
43. Carpenter R, Boulter PS, Cooke T, et al. Management of screen-detected ductal carcinoma in situ of the female breast. *Br J Surg* 1989;76:564–567.
44. Collins LC, O'Malley F, Visscher D, et al. Encapsulated papillary carcinoma. In: Lakhani SR, Ellis IO, Schnitt SJ, et al., eds. *WHO classification of tumours of the breast* (*IARC WHO Classification of Tumours*, vol. 4). 4th ed. Lyon: World Health Organization-IARC, 2012.
45. Lu, S, Singh K, Mangray S, et al. Claudin expression in high-grade invasive ductal carcinoma of the breast: Correlation with the molecular subtype. *Mod Pathol* 2013;26:485–495.
46. Weigelt B, Geyer FC, Reis-Filho JS. Histological types of breast cancer: how special are they? *Mol Oncol* 2010;4:192–208.
47. Bertucci F, Adelaide J, Debono S, et al. Gene expression profiling shows medullary breast cancer is a subgroup of basal breast cancers. *Cancer Res* 2006;66:4636–4644.
48. Weigelt B, Horlings HM, Kreike B, et al. Refinement of breast cancer classification by molecular characterization of histological special types. *J Pathol* 2008;216:141–150.
49. Steensma DP. The beginning of the end of the beginning in cancer genomics. *NEJM* 2013;368:2138–2140.
50. The Cancer Genome Atlas Research Network. Integrated genomic characterization of endometrial carcinoma. *Nature* 2013;497:67–73.

CHAPTER 1

Anatomy and Physiologic Morphology

SYED A. HODA

EMBRYOLOGY AND DEVELOPMENT OF THE IMMATURE BREAST

Embryology

The breasts develop from the mammary ridges or milk lines, which are thickenings of the epidermis that first appear on the ventral surface of the 5-week fetus. These ridges extend from the axilla to the upper medial region of the thigh. In humans, most of the ridge does not develop further and disappears during fetal development. Persistence of segments of the milk line is the embryologic anlage for ectopic mammary glandular tissue, which occurs most often at the extreme ends of the mammary ridge in the axilla or vulva. Molecular mechanisms guiding embryonic mammary gland development and the potential role of stem cells in normal mammary development and maintenance have been reviewed by Cowin and Wysolmerski[1] and van Keymeuelen et al.,[2] respectively.

Mesenchymal condensation occurs around an epithelial stalk, the breast bud, at the site of mammary development on the chest wall in the 15th week of gestation. Growth of cords of epithelium into the mesenchyme produces a group of solid epithelial columns, each of which gives rise to a lobe in the mammary gland. The papillary layer of the fetal dermis continues to encase these growing epithelial cords, and it ultimately evolves into the vascularized fibrous tissue surrounding individual ducts and their branches of ducts that form lobules. In the fetal breast, epithelial cells that form the breast bud express transforming growth factor α (TGF-α), a mitogen and differentiation factor that may mediate the growth-promoting effect of estrogen on the developing breast.[3] Stromal tissue surrounding the breast bud is rich in TGF-β1, a protein involved in modulating cell–matrix interactions. The basement membrane protein, collagen type IV, is distributed around the basal layer of cells in the breast bud. Early in fetal development, proliferative activity measured by Ki67 immunoreactivity is maximal in the region of the neck of the breast bud, involving epithelial and stromal cells. The development of the fetal breast is characterized by the differential expression of keratins 14, 18, and 19 and of actin in the breast ducts and lobular buds.[4]

Myoepithelial cells appear to arise from basal cells between weeks 23 and 28 of gestation.[5] They play an important role in the branching morphogenesis of the mammary gland through the synthesis of basement membrane constituents such as laminin, type IV collagen, and fibronectin, as well as metalloproteinases and growth factors.[6]

Less cellular, more collagenized stroma that originates in the reticular dermis extends into the breast to encompass lobes and subdivisions of lobes, forming the suspensory ligaments of Cooper that attach the breast parenchyma to the skin.[5] Coincidentally, differentiation of the mesenchyme into fat within the collagenous stroma occurs between weeks 20 and 32. In the last 2 months of gestation, canalization of the epithelial cords occurs, followed by the development of branching lobuloalveolar glandular structures. The mammary pit is a depression in the epidermis where the lactiferous ducts converge. Near birth, the nipple is formed by evagination of the mammary pit. A congenitally inverted nipple is the result of failure of this normal process to occur.

The earliest stages of fetal mammary gland formation appear to be independent of steroid hormones, whereas the actual development of the breast structure after the 15th week is influenced largely by testosterone. In the last weeks of gestation, the fetal breast is responsive to maternal and placental steroid hormones and prolactin, which induce secretory activity. This is manifested after birth by the secretion of colostrum and palpable enlargement of the breast bud. The secretory activity typically subsides and ceases during the first or second month after birth owing to disappearance of maternal hormones from the infant's bloodstream. Thereafter, the gland shrinks and returns to an inactive state in which it is composed of lactiferous ducts that branch somewhat without progressive glandular differentiation, although lobular structures may persist (Fig. 1.1). Endocrine and paracrine factors involved in the "branching morphogenesis" of the mammary gland were reviewed in detail by Sternlicht.[7]

The protein product of the *bcl*-2 gene, which acts to inhibit apoptosis, is maximally expressed in the fetal breast.[8] Immunohistochemical localization of *bcl*-2 has been detected in the basal epithelium of the developing breast bud and in the surrounding stroma of male and female breast tissues. *Bcl*-2 reactivity is lost soon after birth and it is absent from the epithelium of the normal adult breast. These observations suggest that upregulation of *bcl*-2 contributes to morphogenesis of the fetal breast by its inhibitory effect on apoptosis. Further normal breast development does not begin until puberty.

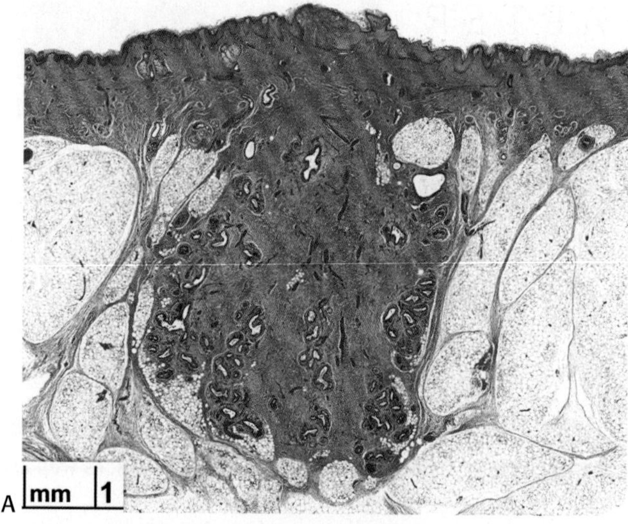

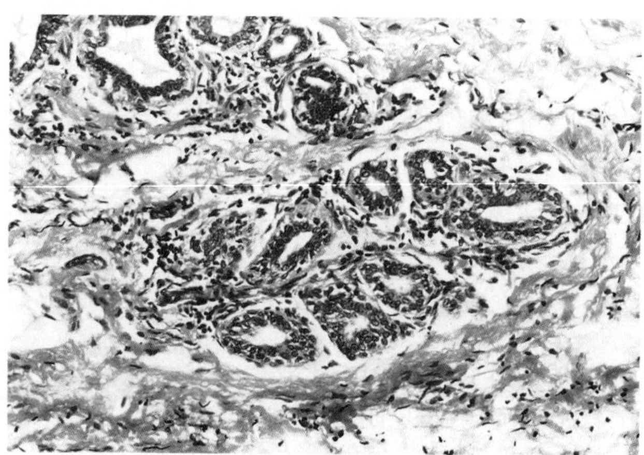

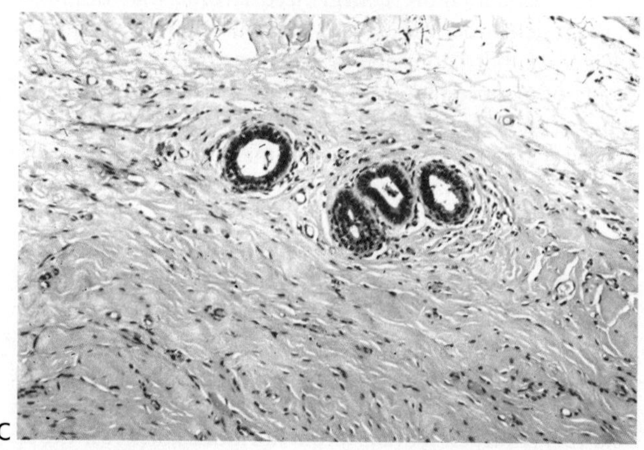

FIG. 1.1. ***Infantile and premenarchal breast.*** **A:** The breast bud in a newborn term female infant. The breast consists of rudimentary lactiferous ducts that branch somewhat without glandular differentiation (Courtesy: Dr D. Beneck). **B:** A lobule in the breast of a 6-month-old girl who had an intraductal papilloma excised. Lobular differentiation at this age reflects the persistent effect of maternal hormones. **C:** Premenarchal breast in an 11-year-old girl. There is no lobular differentiation.

Premature Thelarche

Premature thelarche is the unilateral or bilateral appearance of a discoid subareolar thickening in girls with no other clinical evidence of sexual maturation prior to puberty.[9] The condition may be related to environmental factors, an aberrant response to unusual hormone levels, or due to an activating mutation in the *GNAS* gene that codifies for a subunit of G-stimulating protein.[10] Activation of the *GNAS*-1 gene in premature thelarche may occur in the absence of the other signs such *as café au lait* skin lesions and polyostotic fibrous dysplasia of bone associated with the McCune–Albright syndrome.[10]

The incidence of premature thelarche in white female infants and children up to 7 years old in the United States in 1980 was 20.8 per 100,000,[11] and its prevalence, as reported in 2010 among 318 female children aged 12 to 48 months in a mid-western American hospital, was calculated to be 4.7%.[12] The peak incidence was found between 12 and 17 months of age. The mean basal follicle-stimulating hormone (FSH) level in girls with premature thelarche is higher than that in normal controls and these girls have a greater response to gonadotrophin-releasing hormone.[13] Patients with precocious puberty tend to have normal FSH levels and a normal response to luteinizing hormone–releasing hormone.[14] Klein et al.[15] reported that girls with premature thelarche had significantly higher levels of estradiol than do normal prepubertal girls.

The nodular breast tissue measuring 1.0 to 6.5 cm tends to regress slowly over the subsequent 6 months to 6 years, but in some instances, the hyperplastic breast bud persists until puberty.[11] Curfman et al.[12] reported that breast development persisted in 44% of infants and children with premature thelarche. Volta et al.[16] reported that 60% of girls with premature thelarche that began before age 2 had complete regression prior to the onset of puberty. van Winter et al.[11] reported that follow-up of women who had premature thelarche revealed no predisposition to breast carcinoma and a normal age of menarche. In another series, 14% of girls with premature thelarche developed precocious puberty,[17] a circumstance more likely to occur if the onset of premature thelarche is after 2 years of age.[13] Excision of the tissue that constitutes premature thelarche is contraindicated because this results in amastia.

Histologically, the breast tissue in premature thelarche resembles gynecomastia because it is characterized by epithelial hyperplasia in the duct system with a solid and micropapillary configuration (Fig. 1.2). Growth and branching of the proliferating ducts results in an increased number of duct cross sections surrounded by moderately cellular stroma. Fine-needle aspiration (FNA) cytology reveals a background of myxoid stroma, bipolar stromal cells, and sparse sheets of benign ductal cells.[18]

Premature thelarche should be distinguished from prepubertal breast enlargement, which typically occurs as a

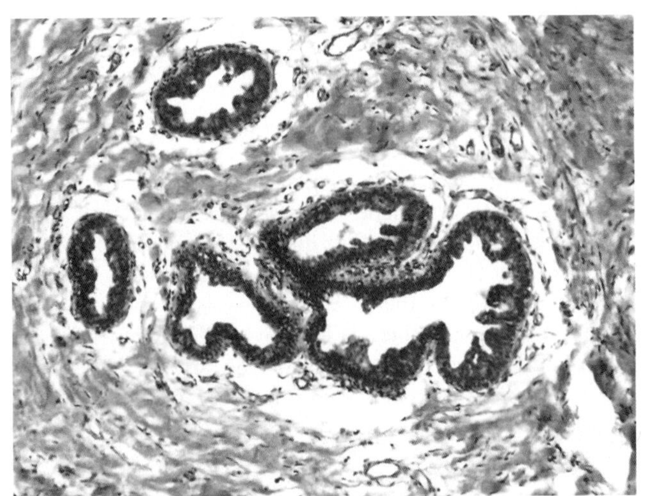

FIG. 1.2. ***Premature thelarche.*** Mild papillary epithelial hyperplasia in a biopsy from 1-year-old girl with unilateral breast enlargement.

result of the accumulation of excess fat and connective tissue in the breast.

ADOLESCENT BREAST DEVELOPMENT

With the onset of cyclical estrogen and progesterone secretion at puberty, adolescent female breast development commences. Growth of ducts that elongate and acquire a thickened epithelium is dependent on estrogens.[19] Differentiation of hormonally responsive, estrogen-dependent periductal stroma also occurs at this time. Growth hormone and glucocorticoids contribute to ductal growth. Terminal duct and lobular differentiation and growth during this period are enhanced primarily by insulin, progesterone, and growth hormone. The lobules are derived from solid masses of cells that form at the ends of terminal ducts. The greatest amount of breast glandular differentiation occurs during puberty, but the process continues for at least a decade and is enhanced by pregnancy[7] (Fig. 1.3). The adolescent male breast consists of fibrofatty tissue and ducts lined by a thin layer of small cuboidal cells (Fig. 1.4).

GROSS ANATOMY OF THE ADULT BREAST

The mature breast has an eccentric configuration, with the long axis diagonally placed on the chest wall largely over the pectoralis major muscle and extending into the axilla as the tail of Spence. The peripheral anatomic boundaries of the breast are not precisely defined, except at the deep surface where the gland overlies the pectoralis fascia. Superficially the breast extends over portions of the serratus anterior muscle laterally, inferiorly over the external oblique muscle and superior rectus sheath, and medially to the sternum. The breast is extremely variable in size, shape, and weight (see Chapter 2).

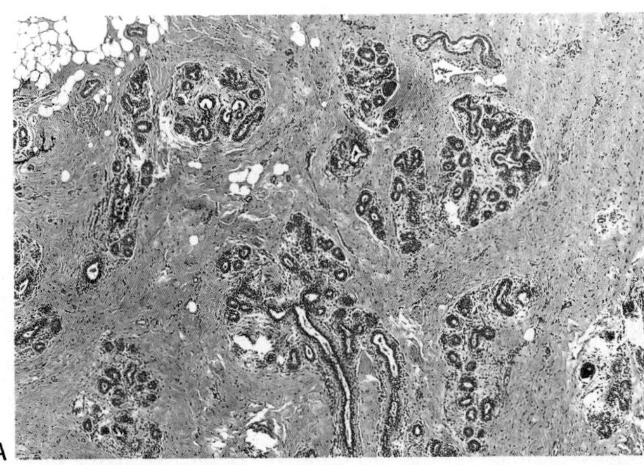

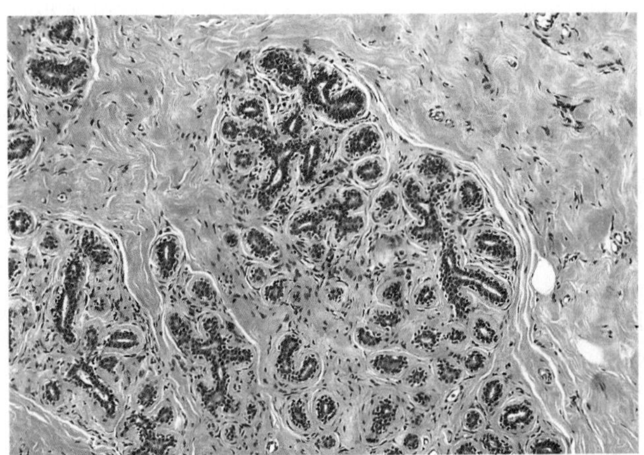

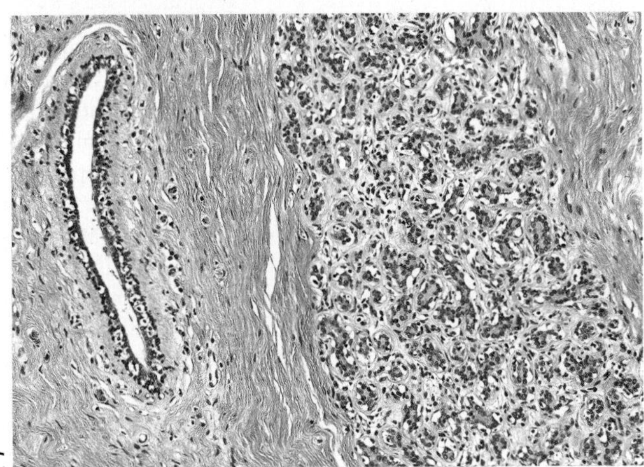

FIG. 1.3. ***Pubertal and adolescent female breast.*** **A:** Biopsy from a 12-year-old girl who had a juvenile fibroadenoma. Menarche was less than 1 year earlier. Lobular architecture is present. **B:** Lobules in a 15-year-old girl consistent with the follicular phase of the menstrual cycle. **C:** Lobule consistent with the luteal phase of the menstrual cycle in a 15-year-old girl.

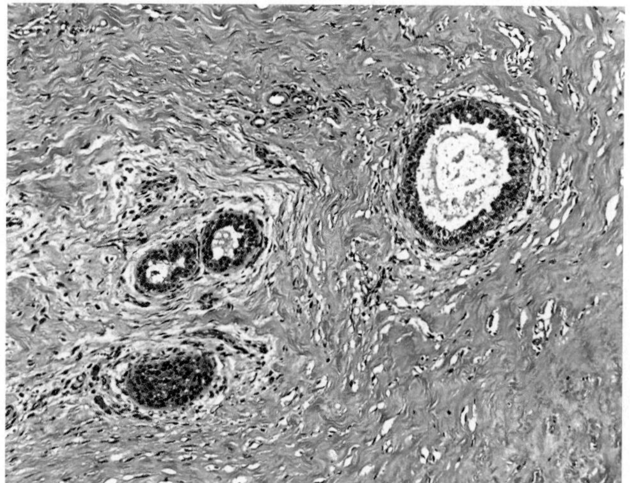

FIG. 1.4. ***Adolescent male breast.*** The thin layer of epithelium shows characteristic cellular crowding, and there is slight dilatation of a duct.

Anatomically, the breast lies in a space within the superficial fascia, although microscopic extensions of glandular parenchyma sometimes traverse these boundaries. Superiorly, this layer is continuous with the cervical fascia, and inferiorly with the superficial abdominal fascia of Cooper. Fibrous strands extend from the dermis into the breast forming the suspensory ligaments of Cooper, which attach the skin and nipple to the breast. Cooper ligaments are more extensive in the upper portions of the breast. Distortion or contraction of the suspensory ligaments by parenchymal lesions may be manifested by skin dimpling or nipple retraction.

The deep membranous layer of the superficial fascia is separated from the fascia of the pectoralis major and serratus anterior muscles by the retromammary or submammary space that contains loose areolar tissue. Extensions of the membranous superficial fascia that traverse the retromammary space act as posterior suspensory ligaments. Microscopic extensions of glandular breast tissue may be found in conjunction with the posterior suspensory ligaments in the retromammary space and, rarely, in the underlying pectoral fascia. Neoplastic or inflammatory infiltration of the retromammary space is clinically associated with fixation of the breast to the chest wall.

The axillary fascia at the dome of the pyramidal axillary space is formed by an extension of the pectoralis major muscle. A fascial layer arising from the lower border of the pectoralis minor muscle joins an extension of the pectoralis major fascia to form the suspensory ligament of the axilla in continuity with the fascia of the latissimus dorsi muscle. An inconstant muscle band in this fascial plane is referred to as the suspensory muscle of the axilla. The fascial boundaries of the axilla provide important landmarks for the *en bloc* dissection of the axillary contents.

ARTERIAL SUPPLY AND VENOUS SYSTEM

The arterial circulation of the breast is derived from the internal thoracic, axillary, and intercostal arteries.[20] There are many individual variations in the relative contributions of these vessels, and patterns of circulation are not necessarily symmetrical in the left and right breasts of an individual.[21] Branches of the internal thoracic artery, which is also commonly referred to as internal mammary artery, provide the major source of arterial circulation in most individuals. These perforating branches traverse the thoracic wall at the sternal border in the first four intercostal spaces. The largest vessel usually lies in the second intercostal space. In about 30% of individuals, the axillary artery is of minor consequence, and in 50% there is little or no dependence on the intercostal arteries.[22] Branches of the arterial circulation within the breast parenchyma do not specifically follow the major duct system.[21]

Venous drainage is more variable than the arterial supply, but it tends to follow the distribution of the arterial circulation.[21] The superficial venous complex consists largely of transverse veins corresponding to branches of the internal thoracic artery. These vessels drain medially into the internal thoracic veins. A minor superficial venous system flows longitudinally toward the suprasternal notch to drain into superficial veins of the neck. Deep venous drainage is largely via perforating branches of the internal thoracic vein. Branches of the axillary vein also contribute to deep venous drainage and are especially prone to variable distribution. Tributaries of the intercostal veins provide a third route for venous drainage, with direct access to the vertebral veins and vertebral plexus.

LYMPHATIC DRAINAGE

A thorough description of the mammary lymphatics was first provided in 1786 by Cruikshank,[23] who referred to lymphatic vessels as "absorbents." He was able to identify the major routes of lymphatic flow from the breast as being along the course of the branches of the external thoracic and internal thoracic veins toward the axilla and internal mammary regions, respectively. Nearly a century later, Sappey[24] employed mercury injection to demonstrate the lymphatic system of the lactating breast and observed drainage that appeared to flow from the parenchyma to the plexus of vessels in the subareolar region now referred to as the subareolar plexus of Sappey. This plexus serves as a pathway for cutaneous lymphatic drainage to the interlobular connective tissue of the breast and subsequently to the parenchymal lymphatic flow.

Various techniques have been used to study the pathways for intramammary lymphatic flow. These include dissection of static injected specimens, x-ray studies of Thorotrast-injected specimens,[25] *in vivo* injection of colloidal gold,[26] *in vivo* injection of a vital dye,[27] and sentinel lymph node mapping with vital dyes and/or radioactive tracers. These investigations have resulted in conflicting observations regarding the pattern and amount of flow from different regions of the breast. In all likelihood, differing observations reflect limitations of the techniques employed and the intrinsic variability in lymphatic drainage between individuals.

Nonetheless, three dominant routes for mammary lymphatic drainage have been identified. The most important of these is to the axilla that receives 75% or more of lymphatic flow into the axillary lymph nodes. Lymph nodes located in the interpectoral fascia constitute Rotter nodes. The most medial group of lymph nodes occurs at the apex of the axilla or level 3. The second pathway via internal lymphatics accounts for less than 25% of lymph flow. These vessels penetrate the pectoralis major and intercostal muscles to the internal thoracic mammary lymph nodes located along the sternal borders of the internal thoracic trunks. A third route for lymph drainage is via the posterior intercostal lymphatics to posterior intercostal lymph nodes in the chest where the ribs and vertebrae articulate. There are additional minor lymphatic channels draining to supraclavicular and infraclavicular lymph nodes as well as to intramammary lymph nodes.[28]

Lymph drainage from any given region in the breast is not limited to one of the foregoing pathways.[26,27] Nonetheless, correlation of patterns of lymph node metastases with the location of primary tumors in the breast suggests that preferential flow exists.[28] For example, in the absence of axillary nodal metastases, the internal mammary lymph nodes are rarely affected, except when the primary tumor arises in the medial or central part of the breast.[29] Conversely, tumors located in the upper outer quadrant are unlikely to metastasize only to internal mammary lymph nodes. Carcinomas that give rise to metastases in Rotter interpectoral lymph nodes are typically located in the upper outer and upper central regions.

Little lymphatic drainage traverses the deep fascia of the breast and the retromammary space. Although minute lymphatic channels have been identified in this fascia, minimal lymph from the mammary gland normally flows in this system. There is also no significant lymphatic flow to the contralateral internal mammary or axillary lymph nodes, but flow via these pathways may be augmented if ipsilateral drainage is obstructed as a result of therapy or by carcinoma.

Studies of sentinel lymph node mapping have provided further information about mammary lymphatic drainage in a physiologic setting and have suggested that a hierarchy exists in the anatomic and functional distribution of lymphatic flow to lymph nodes in the axilla. It is remarkable that this phenomenon can be demonstrated with seemingly equal specificity by injection of a tracer substance in the skin of the breast or in the parenchyma in the vicinity of a carcinoma. A thorough discussion of sentinel lymph node mapping can be found in Chapter 44.

FUNCTIONAL GROSS ANATOMY

The mature adult breast is composed of 15 to 25 grossly defined lobes of varying sizes, corresponding to parenchyma associated with each of the major lactiferous ducts that terminate in the nipple. No obvious landmarks defining the extent of individual lobes are found on inspection at operation or on dissection of the resected breast, and they are not evident in histologic sections. Three-dimensional reconstruction of the ductal system in the breast of a 19-year-old girl revealed that each duct drained an independent territory or "catchment."[30] The total volume drained by a duct and the length of the duct were highly variable. The existence of this functional lobar architecture provides an anatomical framework for treating some benign conditions by major duct excision and certain types of carcinoma by quadrantectomy.

Three-dimensional studies of 72 nipples in mastectomies performed for carcinoma have shown a variable number of nipple duct orifices (range 11 to 48, with a median of 27).[31] In a detailed study of an anatomically normal breast obtained at autopsy, Going and Moffat[31] found that one duct drained 23% of the breast, half of the breast was drained by three ducts, and that 75% was served by the six largest ducts. Three-dimensional reconstruction of a nipple by the same investigators using sequential histologic sections revealed three types of central nipple ducts. Seven of the 27 ducts had a lumen at the skin surface, although some were obstructed by keratin debris. A second group of ducts tapered to a minute lumen that ended in the epidermis in proximity to skin appendage glands. The superficial, narrowed segments of lactiferous ducts resembled the ducts of sweat glands. A third, relatively small group of open ducts appeared to be branches of the seven major patent ducts.

The nipple is covered by stratified squamous epithelium that is not pigmented in the prepubertal breast. Melanin pigmentation develops after menarche and increases during pregnancy, persisting to a variable degree thereafter. Sebaceous glands are present in the skin of the nipple. The areola surrounding the nipple is a ring of skin that undergoes pigmentary changes similar to those of the nipple. This specialized zone of mammary skin contains the glands of Montgomery that are modified sebaceous glands that open via ducts on the surface of the areola through the tubercles of Morgagni. The tubercles of Morgagni are especially visible during pregnancy around the base of the nipple. At this time, the areola appears to be "studded over and rendered unequal by the prominence of glandular follicles, which, varying in number from 12 to 20, project from the surface a sixteenth to an eighth of an inch."[32] The glands of Montgomery enlarge during pregnancy and contribute to a milk-like secretion that moistens the nipple and areola. These glands atrophy after menopause.

The functional glandular and ductal elements of the breast are embedded in fibrofatty tissue, which forms most of the mammary gland. The relative proportion of fat and collagenous stroma varies greatly among individuals and with age and is influenced by physiologic and hormonal factors. The combination of stromal and epithelial components is responsible for the radiographic appearance of breast structure in normal and pathologic states. Premenopausal women benefit from higher sensitivity of mammography performed during the first week of the menstrual cycle when the breast is least dense.[33] The concept that mammographic pattern provides a guide to breast cancer risk, or for recommending preventative therapy, has not been validated; nonetheless, analysis of mammographic images was used to develop a classification scheme based on parenchymal density to predict cancer risk.[34,35]

Magnetic resonance imaging (MRI) provides a more precise method for discriminating between fatty and fibroglandular tissue in the breast without the attendant risk of radiation. By comparing images obtained with mammography and MRI, Lee et al.[36] found a mean fat content of 42.5% (standard deviation [SD] ± 30.3%) in mammograms and 66.5% (SD ± 18%) in MRI images. The ranges of fat content obtained by mammography and MRI were 7.5% to 90% and 17% to 89%, respectively. The correlation coefficient for estimates of fat content obtained by both methods was 0.63, with the strongest correlation ($r = 0.81$) in postmenopausal women. Breast density determined by mammography is increased by exogenous hormone administration,[37] with the greatest effect in postmenopausal women who received continuous combined estrogen–progesterone hormone replacement therapy. (HRT)[38] Estrogen alone causes appreciably less increase in fibroglandular tissue when assessed by mammography[39] or MRI[40] than does combined estrogen–progesterone treatment. When studied by mammography, women receiving "HRT" were found to develop increased breast density that exceeded that of women not using HRT.[41] Breast density remained high with continued HRT use and decreased after therapy was ended. Decreased breast parenchyma has been demonstrated by mammography after tamoxifen therapy.[42] Breast density has been reported to fluctuate by around 7% during the menstrual cycle.[43]

MICROSCOPIC ANATOMY OF THE ADULT BREAST

Lactiferous Ducts

Major lactiferous ducts that exit from the breast terminate in a secretory pore forming the lactiferous duct orifice. The superficial portion of the duct orifice is lined by squamous cells where the duct traverses the epidermis, and squamous epithelium may extend below the epidermis for a short distance into the most terminal portion of the lactiferous duct. The squamocolumnar junction, where the squamous epithelium joins the glandular duct epithelium, is normally distal to a dilated segment of the lactiferous duct, referred to as the lactiferous sinus. Extension of squamous epithelium into or below the lactiferous sinus is a pathologic condition termed *squamous metaplasia* (Fig. 1.5). This may result in obstruction of the affected duct system. The squamocolumnar junction is an important landmark in the pathogenesis of Paget disease.

Lactiferous ducts in the nipple are surrounded by circular and longitudinal arrays of smooth muscle fibers embedded in fibrocollagenous stroma. Some of these muscle fibers attach to the skin of the nipple and areola. Sebaceous glands associated with the overlying skin protrude downward into the superficial stroma of the nipple. The lactiferous ducts extend into the breast through a series of branches diminishing in caliber from the nipple to the terminal ductal–lobular units that are embedded in specialized, hormonally responsive stroma. Extralobular ducts are lined by columnar epithelium that is supported by myoepithelial cells, a basement membrane, and surrounding elastic fibers. In the nonlactating breast, the major ducts cut in cross section have contours marked by folds that create a serrated appearance (Fig. 1.6). The epithelium in the bay-like branches of the duct lumen can give rise to ductules (Fig. 1.7), and fully formed lobules can originate directly from this anatomic arrangement in the nipple or at deeper levels of the mammary duct system[44] (Fig. 1.8).

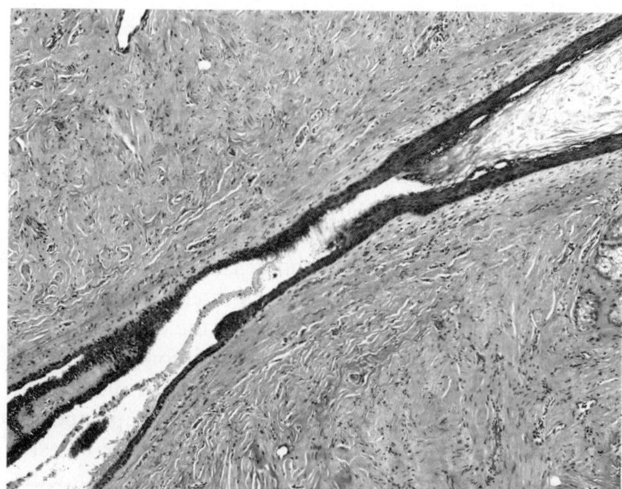

FIG. 1.5. *Major lactiferous duct in nipple with squamous metaplasia. The surface of the nipple is at top right.*

Cells that form the duct epithelium are of two types. The majority are columnar or cuboidal cells lining the lumen. They have cytoplasm endowed with abundant organelles that are involved in secretion. Myoepithelial cells lie between the epithelial layer and the basal lamina, where they form a network of slender processes investing the overlying epithelial cells. The branching network of myoepithelial cell cytoplasmic processes can be seen especially well in scanning electron micrographs[45] (Fig. 1.9). Spindle-shaped ductal myoepithelial cells lie parallel to the long axis of the duct

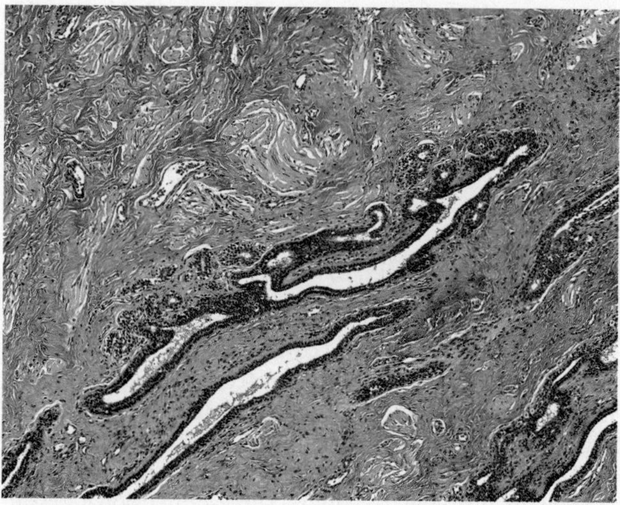

FIG. 1.6. *Major lactiferous duct* with ductular bay-like branches.

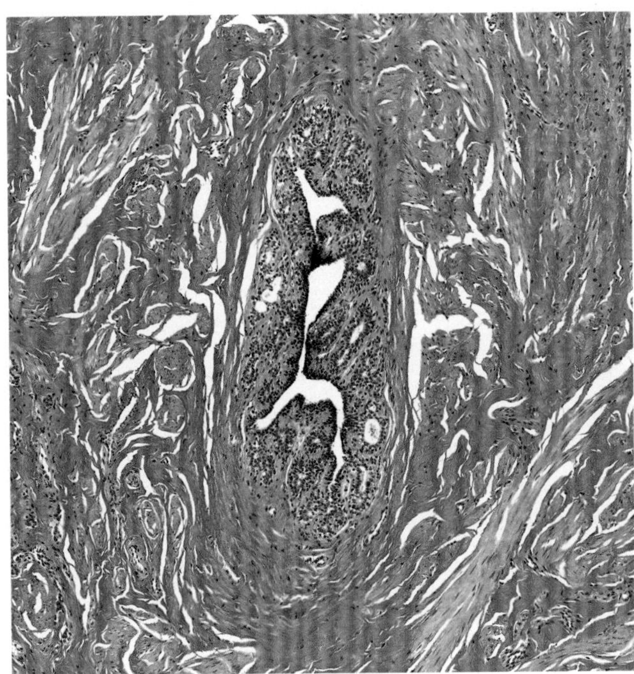

FIG. 1.7. ***Major lactiferous duct*** with ductular branches and early acinar formation.

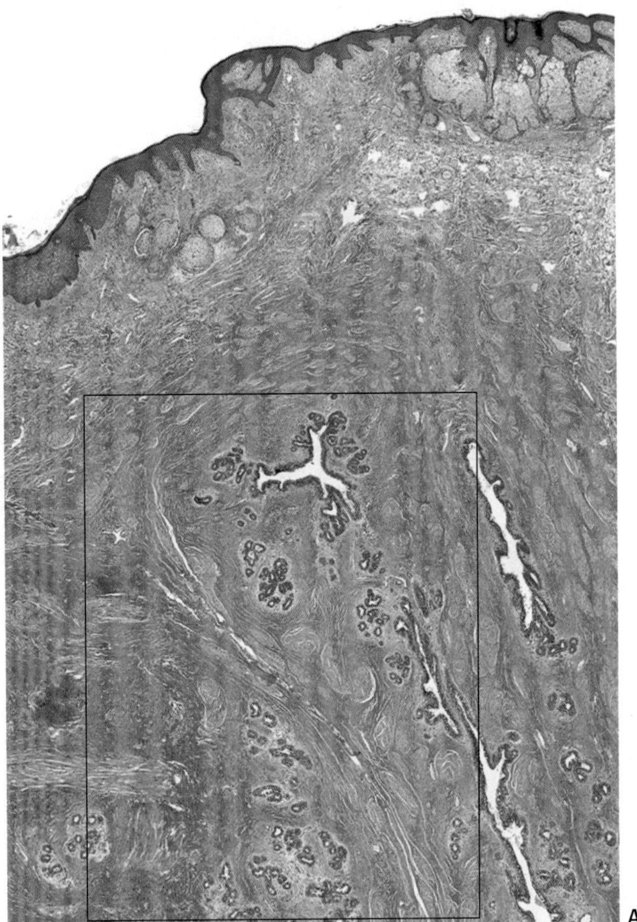

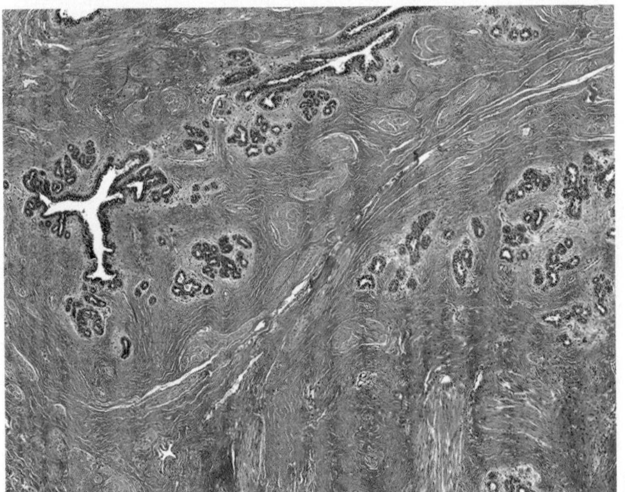

FIG. 1.8. *A*,B: ***Lobules in nipple.*** Major lactiferous duct in nipple with adjacent lobules. Note the specialized intralobular stroma. *Box* in **(A)** indicates area detailed in **(B)**.

and form a continuous layer. Contraction of myoepithelial cells in lobules and around ducts contributes to the flow of milk during lactation.[46]

The histologic appearance and immunoreactivity of myoepithelial cells are variable, especially in pathologic conditions, and depend on the degree to which the myoid or epithelial phenotype is accentuated in a particular situation (Figs. 1.10 and 1.11). Myoepithelial cells usually display nuclear reactivity for p63, which is the most useful marker for detecting these cells in normal and lesional tissues. Epithelioid myoepithelial cells can have reduced p63 reactivity. Other myoepithelial markers discussed elsewhere in this book include actin, calponin, CD10, CK5/6, myosin, and p75.

The apparent absence or near absence of myoepithelial layer, at least as demonstrated by routinely used immunostains, around some mammary cysts that are lined by cytologically benign apocrine epithelium is seemingly inexplicable.[47,48] The need to obtain multiple (at least two) immunostains in the study of myoepithelial cells in benign and malignant lesions of the breast is highlighted by apparently altered patterns of reactivity under various proliferative circumstances.[49,50]

The epithelial–stromal junction consists of the epithelial–myoepithelial layer within the duct, the basal lamina, and a surrounding zone of delimiting fibroblasts and capillaries (Fig. 1.12). Elastic tissue fibers are variably present around normal ducts and these fibers tend to be less pronounced in the premenopausal breast. Farahmand and Cowan[51] were able to detect periductal elastic fibers in 71% of patients younger than 50 years and in 89% of patients older than 50 years. Marked periductal elastic fiber deposition was found in only 3% of normal specimens from women younger than 50 years and in 17% of women older than 50 years. Elastic fibers are largely absent at the lobular level, and, when present, they surround but do not extend into the lobular unit.

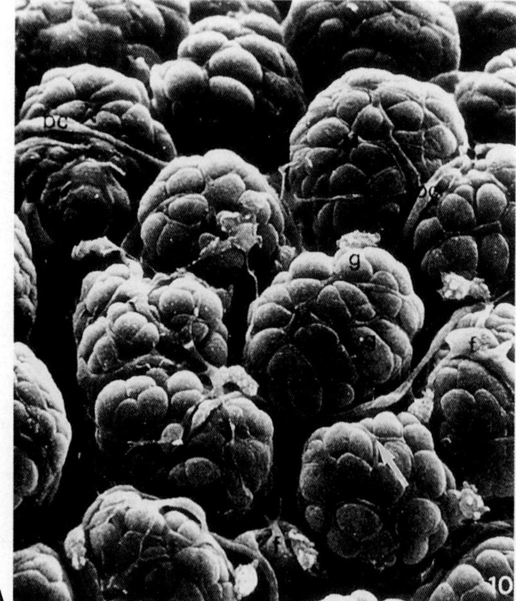

A

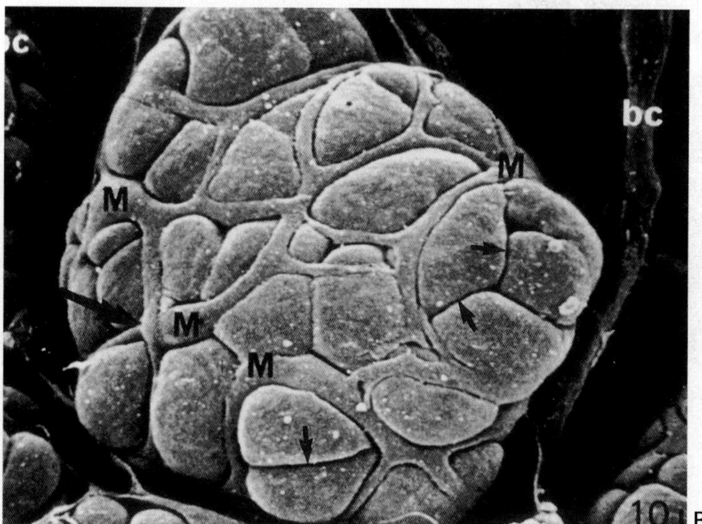

B

FIG. 1.9. ***Scanning electron microscopy of lobules in the rat breast.*** **A:** Connective tissue has been removed by enzyme–HCl digestion to expose rounded glandular cells (*g*) and stellate myoepithelial cells (*large arrow*). Capillaries (*bc*) and fibroblasts (*f*) can be seen. **B:** Magnified view of a lobule with a network of myoepithelial cells (*M*). *Small arrows* indicate boundaries between glandular cells. Blood capillaries (*bc*). (Reprinted with permission from Nagato T, Yoshida H, Yoshida A, et al. A scanning electron microscope study of myoepithelial cells in exocrine glands. *Cell Tissue Res* 1980;209:1–10; copyright Springer-Verlag, 1980.)

In addition to elastic fibers, the normal periductal stroma contains a sparse scattering of lymphocytes, plasma cells, mast cells, and histiocytes. Ochrocytes are periductal histiocytes with cytoplasmic accumulation of lipofuscin pigment (Fig. 1.10). These pigmented cells become more numerous in the postmenopausal breast and in association with inflammatory or proliferative conditions[52] (Fig. 1.13).

Glands of Montgomery

The histologic appearance of the ducts and glands of Montgomery in the subareolar tissues resembles the major lactiferous ducts of the nipple,[53,54] except that the contour tends to be smoother (Fig. 1.14). Serial sections have demonstrated direct connections between lactiferous ducts draining lobular parenchyma and the ducts of Montgomery glands in the tubercle of Morgagni.[55] The epithelium of the ducts connecting

FIG. 1.10. ***Myoid metaplasia in an atrophic lobule.*** Myoepithelial cells with a myoid phenotype around lobular glands.

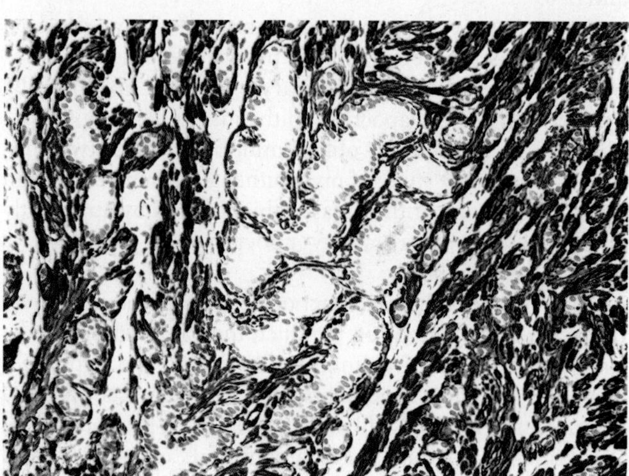

FIG. 1.11. ***Myoid metaplasia in adenosis.*** Myoid myoepithelial cells are immunoreactive for smooth muscle myosin.

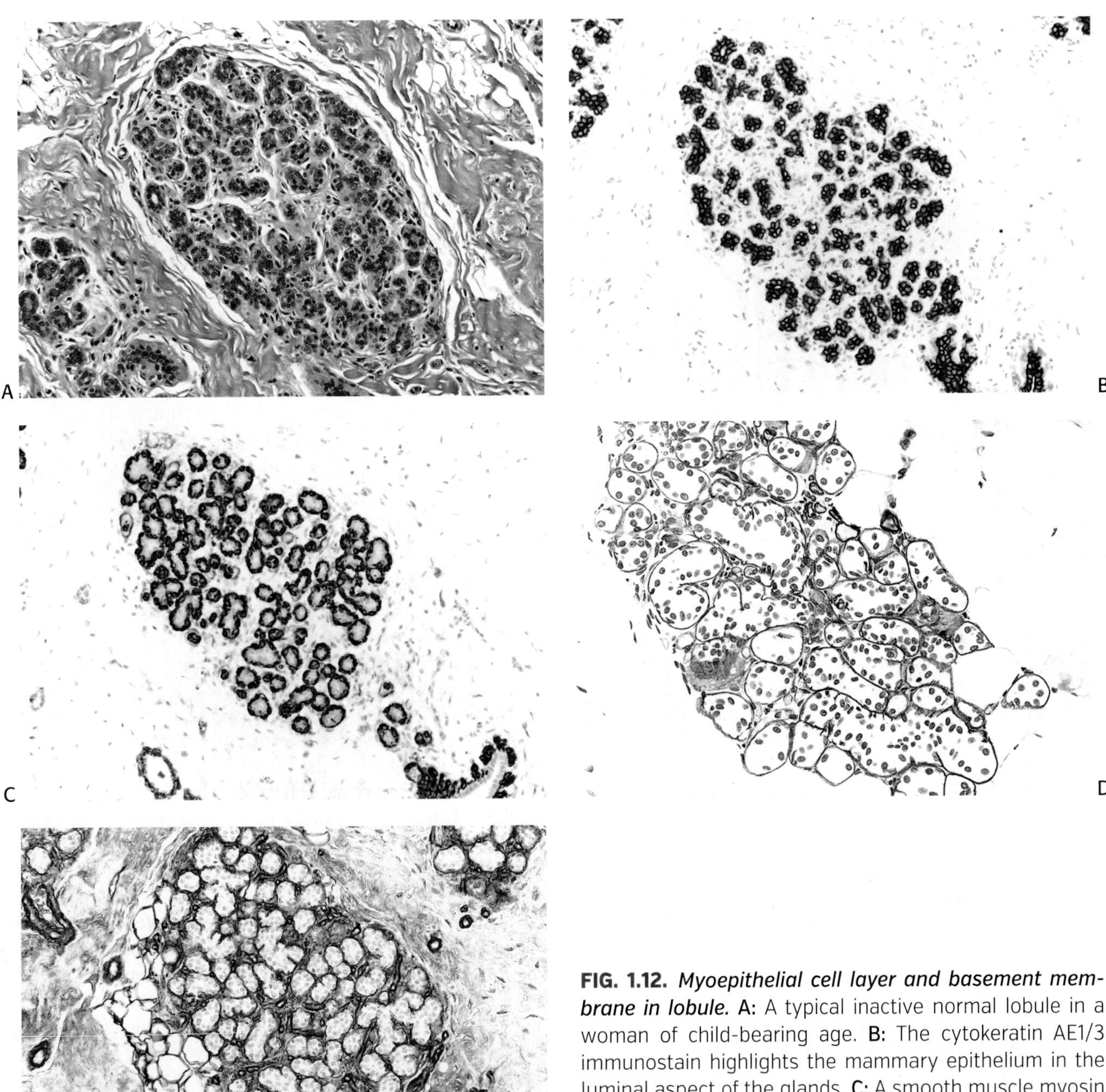

FIG. 1.12. ***Myoepithelial cell layer and basement membrane in lobule.*** **A:** A typical inactive normal lobule in a woman of child-bearing age. **B:** The cytokeratin AE1/3 immunostain highlights the mammary epithelium in the luminal aspect of the glands. **C:** A smooth muscle myosin immunostain shows the myoepithelial cell layer in the abluminal aspect of the gland. **D,E:** A histochemical reticulin stain (D) and a laminin immunostain (E) show the basement membrane surrounding all glands.

breast lobules to the glands of Montgomery is subject to proliferative changes that occur in the lactiferous ducts, including hyperplasia and *in situ* carcinoma.[55] Cystic dilation of a Montgomery gland duct can result in a subareolar mass.

Lobules

Mammary secretion is formed in the lobules that consist of groups of alveolar glands encompassed by specialized vascularized stroma. The alveoli are connected by intralobular ductules that combine to form a single terminal lobular duct that drains into the extralobular duct system. In lobules, alveolar glands are formed along and at the end of intralobular ductules. In whole-mount preparations and in histologic sections, these glandular structures appear as blunt or round saccules protruding from the duct lumen.

The resting lobular gland is lined by a single layer of cuboidal epithelial cells supported by underlying, loosely connected myoepithelial cells. The intralobular stroma contains more capillaries and is less densely collagenized

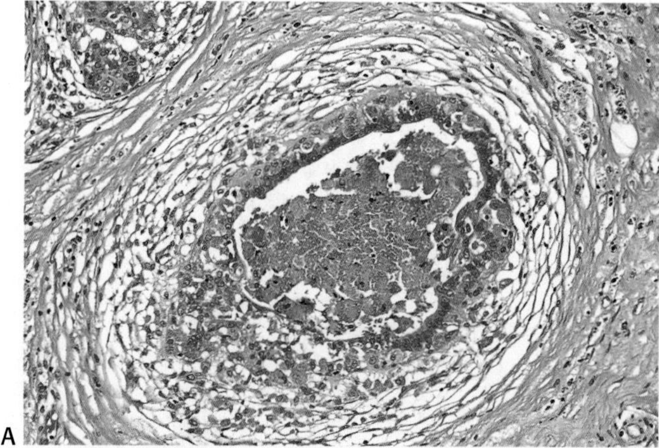

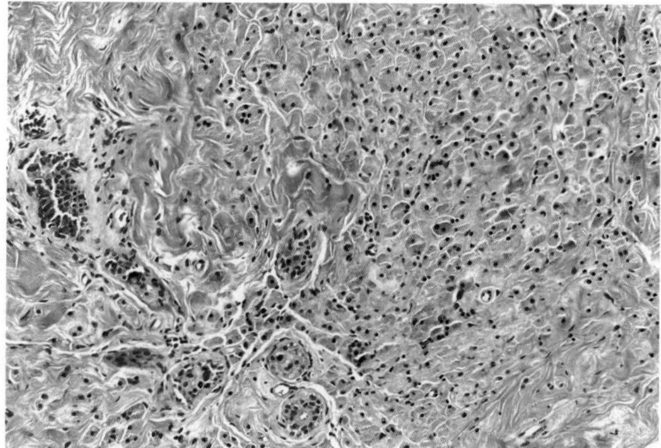

FIG. 1.13. ***Ochrocytes in periductal stroma.*** **A:** Histiocytes with granular, lipofuscin-containing cytoplasm are present in the periductal stroma and in the ductal epithelium in an example of periductal mastitis. **B:** Ochrocytes are seen in the stroma after a complete pathologic response to neoadjuvant chemotherapy for breast carcinoma.

than the interlobular stroma. Ultrastructural studies suggest that, in addition to providing support, the cells in the intralobular stroma also have a paracrine effect on the epithelium. Intralobular stromal fibroblasts are characterized by attenuated cytoplasmic processes that create a network of cell-to-cell connections.[56] These link the delimiting fibroblasts that cover the basement membrane with fibroblasts throughout the lobular stroma. Lymphocytes, plasma cells, macrophages, and mast cells, which normally reside in the lobular stroma, are distributed within the interstices of this fibroblastic network in a manner that results in close apposition of cell surfaces to facilitate cell–cell interaction.[56] Intralobular fibroblasts are reported to be immunoreactive for CD34, an endothelial-associated ligand involved in the cellular attachment of leukocytes in inflammation and immune responses.[57] Morphometric study of the microvascular structure in the preovulatory breast revealed a significant difference between vascularity in lobules and around ducts.[58] Ducts were surrounded by small capillaries, whereas lobules had fewer but larger microvessels.

The normal microscopic anatomy of the lobules is not constant because the structure and histologic appearance of the lobule in the mature breast are subject to changes associated with the menstrual cycle, pregnancy, lactation, exogenous hormone administration, aging, and menopause. Furthermore, there is variation in the functional state of individual lobules regardless of physiologic circumstances, an observation that suggests that individual lobules or groups of lobules in regions of the breast have intrinsic differences in response to hormonal and other stimuli. This is reflected in the substantial variability in labeling indices indicating different proliferative rates among lobules in a given individual.[59] Immunoreactivity for hormone receptors is also variably expressed in lobules.

Genetic alterations manifested by loss of heterozygosity have been detected in histologically normal-appearing lobular epithelium.[60] Genetic changes have been found in epithelial and myoepithelial cells. The frequency of these alterations has not been established, but existing data suggest that they are detected more often in histologically normal lobules from patients with carcinoma than in breasts without carcinoma.

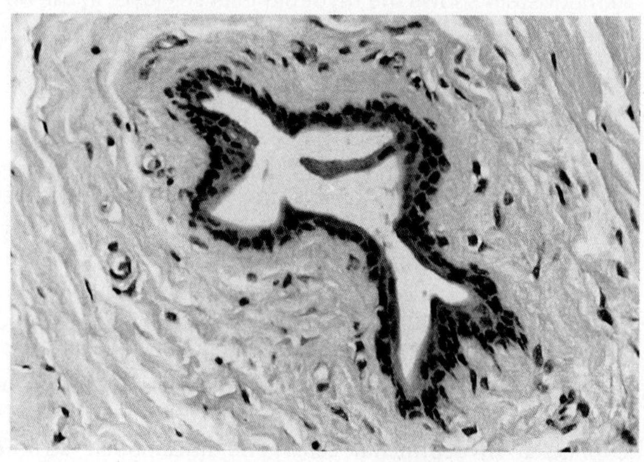

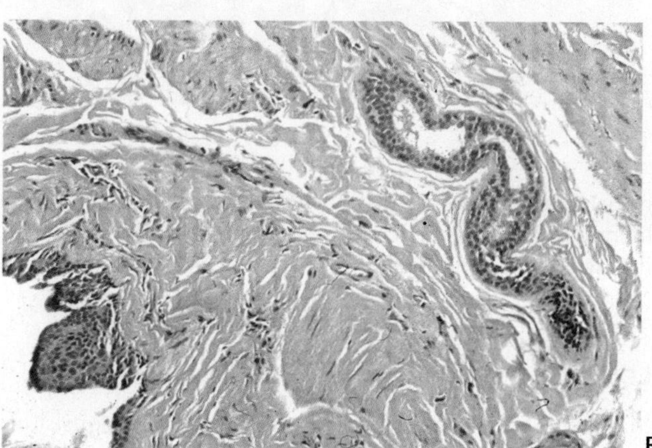

FIG. 1.14. ***Duct of gland of Montgomery.*** **A:** Transverse section. **B:** Longitudinal section.

MENSTRUAL CYCLE

The structural effects of cyclic hormonal changes are manifested clinically by fluctuations in breast size and texture. In general, the breast tends to be the least nodular at mid-cycle in the latter part of the follicular phase (days 8 to 14), making this the optimal time for clinical breast examination. A study of mammograms obtained from women 40 to 49 years of age revealed significantly lower parenchymal density during the follicular phase than during the luteal phase of the menstrual cycle[61] ; however, in a mammographic study of 71 women between the ages of 19 and 49, the mean luteal density exceeded the mean follicular density by 7.1% to 9.2%.[62]

Studies based on water displacement have demonstrated an increase in breast volume during the second half of the normal menstrual cycle of about 100 mL and in the contraceptive-controlled cycle of about 60 mL.[63] Examination by MRI revealed that breast volume was least in the interval from days 6 to 15 of the menstrual cycle, a time characterized by low parenchymal and low water volumes.[64,65] An increase in breast volume between days 16 and 28 was marked by a rise in parenchymal volume and water content that peaked on day 25. A sharp decline in parenchymal and water volume occurred just prior to menses in one study,[64] but others reported elevated water content and fibroglandular content "during menses."[65] These observations indicate that cyclical changes in breast volume involve parenchymal growth as well as fluctuations in water content.[59]

Nodular and diffuse contrast-medium (gadolinium) MRI enhancement has been observed in clinically normal breasts during the course of the menstrual cycle.[66] These foci of enhancement were more frequent in weeks 1 and 4. The rate of enhancement may meet the criteria for a malignant lesion resulting in a false-positive interpretation in a premenopausal woman. This finding is consistent with data obtained by Müller-Schimpfle et al.,[67] who reported that overall parenchymal contrast-medium enhancement was greatest during days 21 to 6 of the cycle, corresponding to the first and fourth weeks, and that enhancement was significantly less during days 7 to 20. This effect was maximal in women 35 to 50 years of age.

The cellular and structural alterations observed histologically in the normal breast during the menstrual cycle were described in detail by Vogel et al.[68] These investigators divided the changes into five phases. However, they noted "that different lobules within the same breast may vary in morphologic appearance. Placing a specimen within a phase required that the most consistent morphology among a population of lobules within several sections be determined."[68]

An *in vitro* study of purified populations of epithelial and myoepithelial cells obtained from reduction mammoplasty specimens revealed notable differences in growth requirements between these cell types.[69] Epidermal growth factor and basic fibroblast growth factor had a mitogenic effect on epithelial cells but not on myoepithelial cells. Insulin was necessary for myoepithelial growth, whereas epithelial cells required fetal calf serum. Reconstitution of lobuloalveolar structures was observed when the two cell types were mixed in a basement membrane matrix. These differences in growth factor requirements probably reflect different physiologic functions, which are also expressed morphologically during the menstrual cycle.

The proliferative phase, days 3 through 7, features the highest rates of epithelial mitoses and of apoptosis.[70,71] This corresponds to a marked decrease in *bcl*-2 expression detected immunohistochemically in lobular gland epithelium at the end of the menstrual cycle in comparison with maximal expression at mid-cycle.[72] The peak time of apoptosis is about 3 days after the peak for mitotic activity.[73] Other investigators who defined this phase as days 0 to 5 reported that "apoptosis and mitosis were by and large absent in this phase."[74]

Lobular glands at this time are lined by crowded, poorly oriented epithelial cells with little or no lumen formation and secretion (Fig. 1.15). Myoepithelial cells are inconspicuous and difficult to distinguish from epithelial cells in hematoxylin and eosin–stained slides. The lobular stroma is relatively dense and hypovascular, with plump fibroblasts ringing lobular glands.

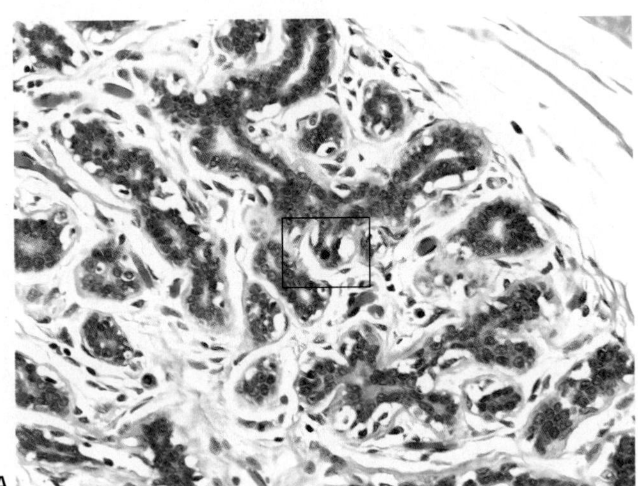

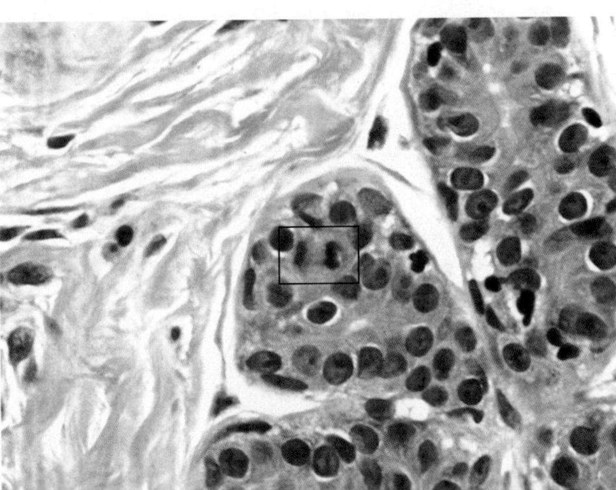

FIG. 1.15. *A,B: **Normal lobule–proliferative phase of menstrual cycle.*** A metaphase mitotic figure is seen in (**A**, *box*), and an anaphase mitosis is seen in (**B**, *box*).

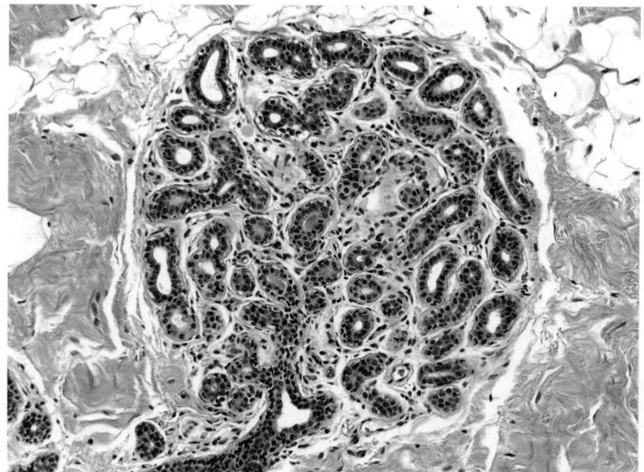

FIG. 1.16. ***Normal lobule–follicular phase of menstrual cycle.*** Lumens are beginning to appear in lobular glands.

Mitotic activity is decreased in the follicular phase (days 8 to 14). At this stage, the myoepithelial cells have a polygonal shape and clear cytoplasm. Epithelial cells become columnar, with increasingly basophilic cytoplasm and basally oriented, darkly stained nuclei (Fig. 1.16). An acinar lumen without secretion is evident. The basal lamina is prominent and there is slight loosening of intralobular stroma.

During the luteal phase, comprising days 15 through 20, myoepithelial cells become more prominent due to increased glycogen accumulation that results in cytoplasmic clearing. Basal cells are more evident at this stage. The glandular lumen is defined by columnar epithelial cells with basophilic cytoplasm. A small amount of secretion is present in a few glands. The basement membrane is attenuated and less prominent, and there is coincidental further loosening of the stroma (Fig. 1.17).

Immunohistochemical study of normal breast tissue during the menstrual cycle revealed peak expression of epidermal growth factor receptor (EGFR) during the luteal phase.[75] EGFR was expressed mainly in the stroma and myoepithelial cells. These observations may reflect a promoting effect of hormones, especially progestins, and suggest that tyrosine kinase receptors play a role in the normal mammary growth and differentiation. Short-term administration of tamoxifen during the luteal phase significantly reduces mitotic activity in normal breast tissue.[76]

The secretory phase corresponding to days 21 through 27 features heightened apocrine secretion with distension of glandular lumens by accumulated secretory material (Fig. 1.18). The epithelium consists of columnar epithelial cells and myoepithelial cells with clear cytoplasm. The basal lamina is thin and the lobular stroma exhibits maximal edema. Venous congestion is evident at the periphery of lobules. Ultrastructural examination of lobular epithelial cells at this phase reveals an increase in endoplasmic reticulum, an enlarged Golgi, and other changes in organelles indicative of active secretion.[77]

In the menstrual phase, comprising days 28 through 3, the stroma once again becomes compact with loss of intralobular edema. Lymphocytes, macrophages, and plasma cells are most conspicuous in the lobular stroma at this stage.[70] Some glandular lumens remain and others appear collapsed. Mitotic activity is absent (Fig. 1.19).

Improved ability to recognize morphologic changes in the breast that are related to the menstrual cycle may become clinically useful in premenopausal women. At present, evidence suggesting that surgery performed during the luteal phase is prognostically advantageous[78,79] remains controversial.[80,81]

Cyclical variation in immunoglobulin (Ig) localization in lobules has been described.[82] Intraluminal IgA and IgM are present in significantly more lobules in the preovulatory, proliferative, and follicular phases (days 4 through 14). No strong intraluminal localization of IgG was found, but weak intraluminal IgG staining was present throughout the menstrual cycle, with no significant difference between pre- and postovulatory phases. There was not a strong correlation between luminal IgA concentration and the number of stromal plasma cells.

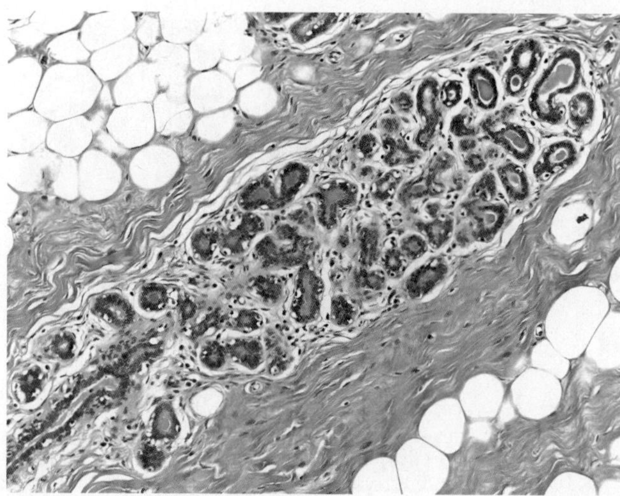

FIG. 1.17. ***Normal lobule–luteal phase of menstrual cycle.*** Myoepithelial cells are conspicuous, and glandular lumens contain scant secretion.

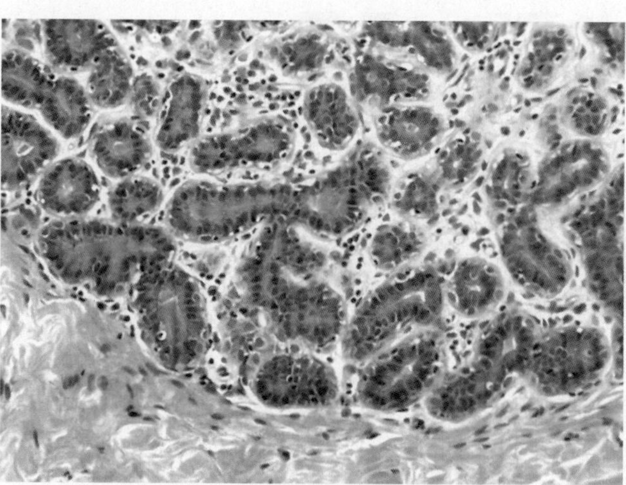

FIG. 1.18. ***Normal lobule–secretory phase of menstrual cycle.*** Stromal edema is evident with a modest mononuclear cell infiltrate. Secretion is present.

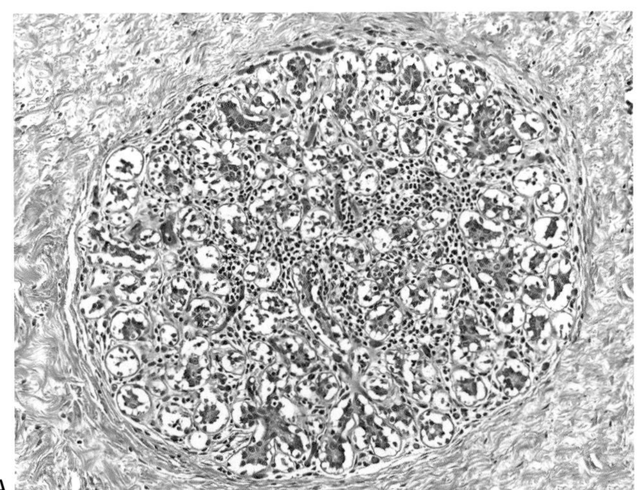
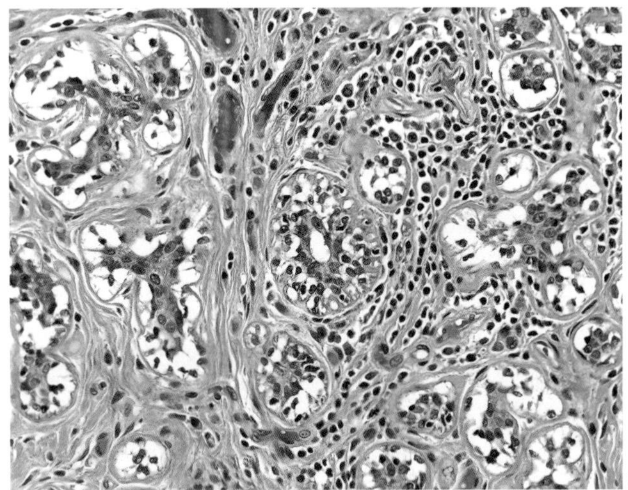

FIG. 1.19. *Normal lobule–menstrual phase of cycle.* A,B: Collapse of lobular glands resulting in a prominent clear cell myoepithelial cell layer. Decreased stromal edema and intralobular round-cell infiltration are present.

Thymidine labeling index (TLI) studies of lobules isolated from normal human breast tissue revealed that the proliferative rate in epithelial cells is higher in the luteal phase than in the follicular phase of the menstrual cycle.[83,84] This effect is seen largely in parous women, and others have reported little difference in TLI during the menstrual cycle in nulliparous women.[85] The difference in TLI between the luteal and follicular phases decreases with age,[86] and there is an overall inverse relationship between TLI and age.[87,88] Analysis of the synthesis phase fraction (SPF) in epithelial cells from normal breast tissue samples by flow cytometry revealed a decreasing SPF with advancing age, such that the SPF in atrophic tissue was approximately 50% less than that in samples from premenopausal women.[89] Similar results have been obtained with 5-bromodeoxyuridine labeling[59] and by using the immunohistochemical proliferation marker Ki67 (MIB-1) on cytologic preparations obtained by FNA from normal volunteers.[90] The mean TLI throughout the menstrual cycle varies from 0% to 11.5%.[83,87] Measurements of paired samples obtained simultaneously from the left and right breasts revealed a highly significant correlation between the SPF determinations in the two breasts.[89] Under normal circumstances, mature myoepithelial cells are not mitotically active.[91]

Estrogen receptors (ERs) and progesterone receptors (PRs) are localized to the nuclei of epithelial cells. Nuclei of approximately 7% of epithelial cells are immunoreactive for ER in normal resting breast tissue, with a higher proportion in lobular than in ductal cells.[92] Considerable heterogeneity exists in nuclear hormone receptor activity among lobules. ER-positive cells are typically distributed singly, surrounded by receptor-negative nuclei in lobules.[93] A significant correlation with increasing age was observed by Shoker et al.,[93] who reported a tendency for positive cells to be "contiguous in patches of variable size." The increase in ER-positive cells remained relatively stable after menopause.

Several groups of investigators have studied the expression of ER and PR in noncarcinomatous breast tissue during different phases of the menstrual cycle in premenopausal women. Employing biochemical analyses of grossly normal-appearing tissue, Silva et al.[94] reported that the greatest frequency of ER positivity and the highest mean concentrations were found during the proliferative phase of the cycle (days 3 to 7), whereas PR was highly expressed in the follicular phase (days 8 to 14). A study of benign epithelial cells obtained by FNA revealed immunohistochemically detectable evidence of nuclear ER in 31% of samples taken during the first half of the menstrual cycle and no ER-positive cells in 33 samples from the second half of the cycle.[95] Others have reported that nuclear ER and PR activity demonstrated by immunohistochemistry in lobular epithelial cells was maximal in the follicular phase.[96] Decreased expression of ER in the luteal phase may be due to downregulation of this protein by the rise in progesterone produced by the corpus luteum.[87] Pujol et al.[97] studied 575 women with breast carcinoma in whom menstrual cycle phases were determined by serum measurements of estradiol, progesterone, FSH, and luteinizing hormone. Expression of ER in a carcinoma was significantly more frequent in the follicular phase (62%) than in the ovulatory phase (52%) or luteal (53%) phase. By contrast, PR expression was more often positive in the ovulatory phase (85%) than in the follicular (78%) and luteal (72%) phases, but these differences were not statistically significant. Other investigators did not find a consistent menstrual cycle–related pattern in the expression of ER and PR in breast carcinomas from premenopausal women.[95,98,99]

Multiple studies have reported variable results regarding the value of timing of surgical procedures for breast carcinoma *vis a vis* phase of menstrual cycle. However, one of the largest studies conducted on the topic by the National Central Cancer Treatment Group (NCCTG) in collaboration with the National Surgical Adjuvant Breast and Bowel Project (NSABP) and the International Breast Cancer Study Group (IBCSG) showed that neither disease-free survival nor overall survival differed between women who underwent surgery during the follicular versus the proliferative phase.[100] Notably, 30% of the patients did not fit either of the two categories in this study.

PREGNANCY

Secretory changes associated with pregnancy occur unevenly throughout the breast. Localized adenomatous lactational hyperplasia, usually encountered in the third trimester, is an extreme manifestation of this phenomenon, which may result in one or more palpable and radiologically detectable masses, called lactational adenomas.[101]

Early in pregnancy, terminal ducts and lobules grow rapidly, resulting in lobular enlargement with variable coincidental depletion of the fibrofatty stroma.[102–106] Stromal vascularity increases, accompanied by infiltration of mononuclear inflammatory cells. More pronounced areolar pigmentation and dilation of superficial cutaneous veins are apparent by the end of the first trimester. At this time, a small amount of secretion may be found in lobular glands (Fig. 1.20).

During the second and third trimesters, lobular growth progresses through the enlargement of cells, as well as by cellular proliferation (Fig. 1.21). Myoepithelial cells remain evident in ducts, but they are largely obscured in lobules by the

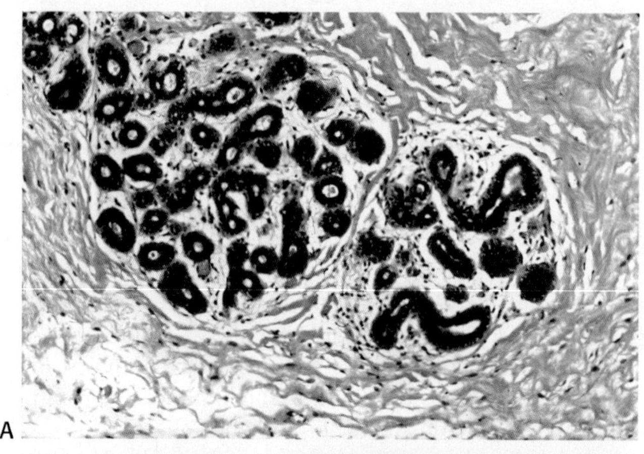
A

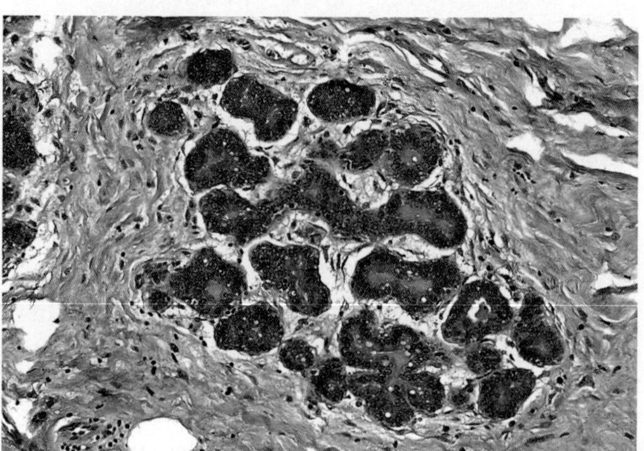
B

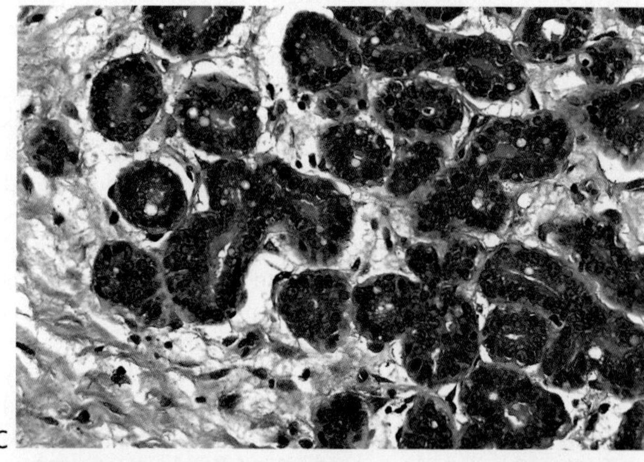
C

FIG. 1.20. ***Lobular hyperplasia in pregnancy–first trimester.*** **A:** An inactive lobule from a woman who was pregnant for 7 weeks. **B,C:** Increased metabolic activity is manifested by cytoplasmic hyperchromasia and nuclear enlargement in this specimen from a 34-year-old woman who was 3 months pregnant.

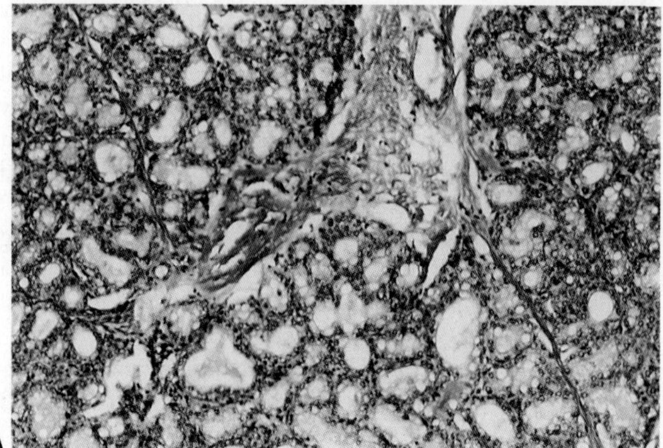
A

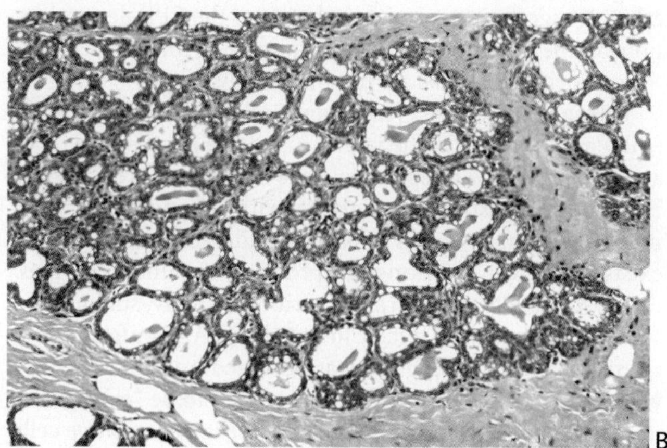
B

FIG. 1.21. ***Lobular hyperplasia in pregnancy–second trimester and early third trimester.*** **A:** Enlarged lobules efface the intervening stroma early in the third trimester. Acinar dilation is evident. **B:** A lobule from early third trimester (7 months) with acinar secretion.

greatly expanded cohort of epithelial cells (Fig. 1.22). The cytoplasm of lobular epithelial cells becomes vacuolated, and secretion is progressively accumulated in distended lobular glands (Figs. 1.23 to 1.25). Glandular expansion through pregnancy and lactation is accompanied by a relative decrease in fibrofatty stroma.

FNA of the lactating breast yields a highly cellular specimen that can contain cohesive glandular clusters as well as dispersed cells (Fig. 1.26). Nuclei are hyperchromatic and often have small nucleoli.

Electron microscopic examination of lactating epithelium reveals organelle-rich cytoplasm with a prominent endoplasmic reticulum, a hypertrophied Golgi apparatus, swollen mitochondria, and abundant secretory material.[105] Myoepithelial cells are flattened and attenuated.

Involution of the breast, after lactation ceases, occurs over a period of about 3 months. Initially, lobular glands are further distended by additional accumulation of milk, which results in attenuation of the epithelial lining (Fig. 1.27). As prolactin levels decrease, secretion of milk ceases, and desquamated, degenerated, lobular epithelial cells are phagocytized. Involution is accompanied by a decrease in the number and size of lobular glands and the apparent reappearance of myoepithelial cells in the lobular epithelium. Fat and collagen are redeposited in the stroma

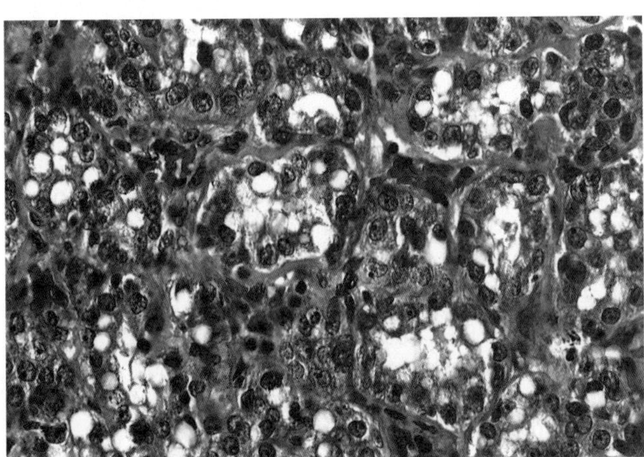

FIG. 1.22. ***Lobular hyperplasia in pregnancy–third trimester.*** Cells forming the lobular glands have abundant vacuolated cytoplasm. There is little secretion and the nuclei have punctate nucleoli.

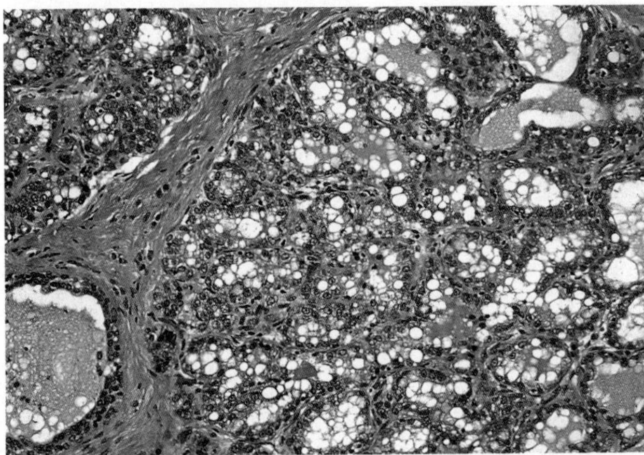

FIG. 1.23. ***Lobular hyperplasia in pregnancy–late third trimester.*** Enlarged nuclei with nucleoli are present. Lactation is evident.

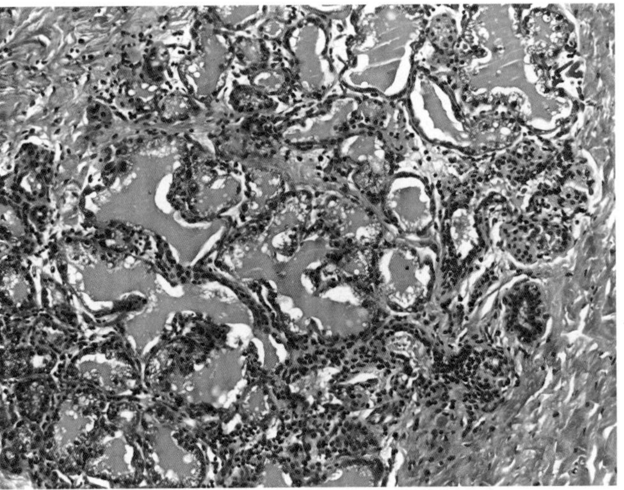

FIG. 1.24. ***Lactating breast.*** Marked distension of lobular glands and accumulation of secretion.

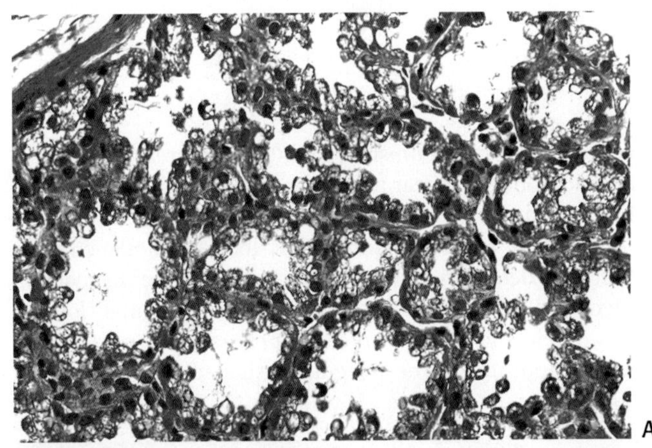

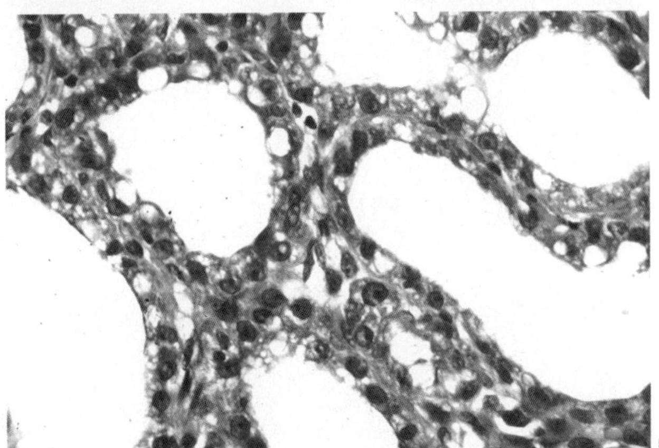

FIG. 1.25. ***Lactating breast.*** **A:** Ectatic lobular glands. **B:** The lactating cells have vacuolated cytoplasm, small nuclei, and nucleoli.

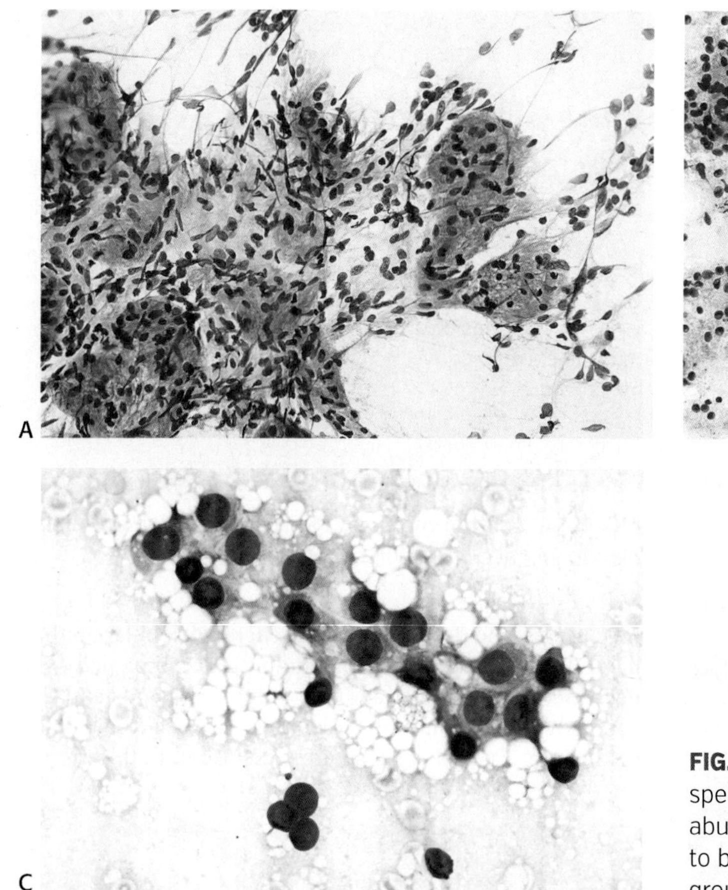

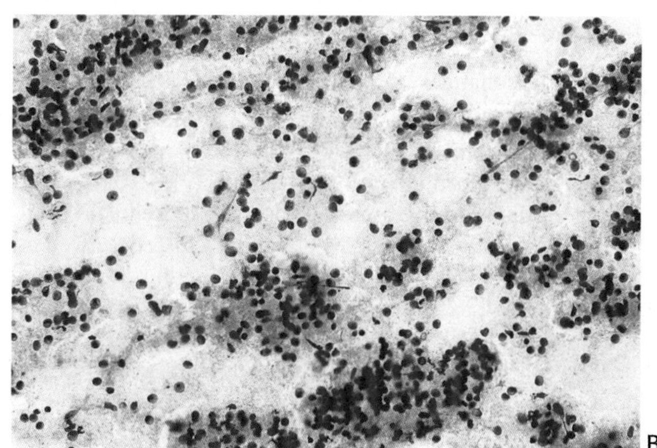

FIG. 1.26. ***Lactating breast–FNA cytology.*** **A–C:** The specimen consists of cohesive glandular elements and abundant dispersed cells. Note that many nuclei appear to be isolated from cytoplasm, and the presence of background secretion.

accompanied by diminished vascularity. Increased numbers of macrophages appear in the stroma during postlactational involution.

Battersby and Anderson[107] described histologic changes that they determined to be characteristic of the postpartum involuted lobule. By comparison with the "normal" lobules of women who were not recently pregnant, the postpartum lobule appeared to be irregularly shaped with a partially angular rather than rounded contour. Intralobular stroma tended to be less distinct in the involuted lobule than in the normal lobule, resulting in a poorly defined border. Intralobular ductules were prominent, and because of concomitant atrophy of lobular epithelium, were the most conspicuous epithelial components in involuted lobules. Lobular changes associated with recent pregnancy were most noticeable within 18 months postpartum.

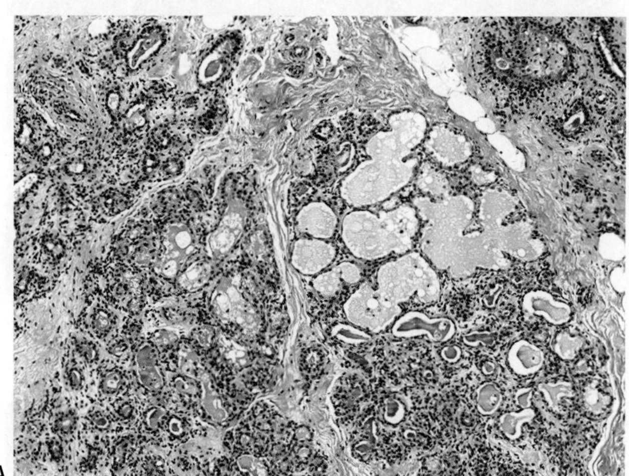

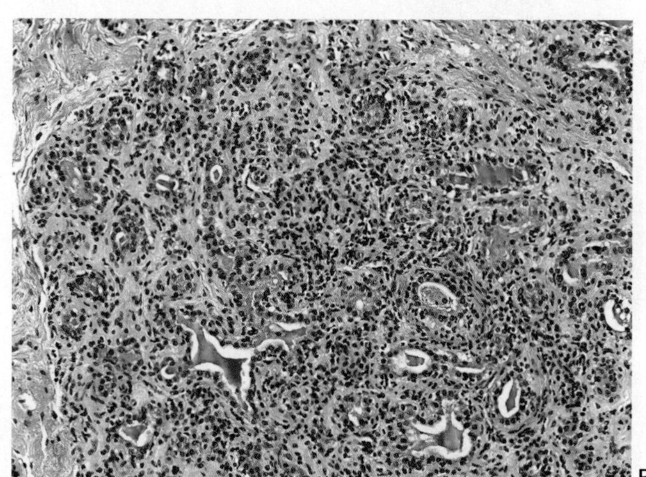

FIG. 1.27. ***Postlactational lobular involution.*** **A:** Some dilated lobular glands with secretion persist. The 32-year-old patient was 9 months postpartum and had stopped nursing 1 month before surgery. **B:** Glandular epithelium is quiescent. Some secretion remains.

MENOPAUSE

Parenchymal changes during and after menopause reflect hormonal alterations that occur at this time. Plasma levels of estrogen and progesterone decline, whereas androgen levels, largely testosterone, are not diminished. The major structural alteration is a decrease in the cellularity and number of lobules, mainly as a result of epithelial atrophy.[108] Coincidental with the loss of glandular epithelium, there is a tendency to thickening of lobular basement membranes and collagenization of intralobular stroma (Fig. 1.28). The process of menopausal atrophy occurs in an uneven fashion, often leaving some lobules relatively unaffected, by comparison with neighboring glands. Atrophy tends to spare myoepithelial cells that frequently persist even in a late stage of the process. Most lobular glands appear to collapse and shrink, but cystic distension may also occur (Fig. 1.29). Minuscule calcifications are sometimes deposited in atrophic lobular glands. In many women older than 65 years of age, lobular integrity is progressively lost, leaving small ducts and glands embedded in fibrocollagenous stroma. The relative proportions of fat and stroma vary greatly in the atrophic breast.

Menopausal mammary atrophy can be attenuated by the administration of HRT after the menopause. Mammographic changes suggestive of physiologic proliferative alterations have been observed in women receiving postmenopausal HRT.[37,109] The effect of HRT on the mammographic appearance of the breast is substantially less in women who have undergone prior breast irradiation.[110] In the nonirradiated breast, the effect of hormone replacement is manifested mainly by increased parenchymal density. This has been observed after treatment with estrogen alone and with estrogen–progesterone combination therapy. Histologic examination does not reveal a consistent pattern. Some patients have lobular differentiation comparable to the premenopausal state (Fig. 1.30), whereas others have prominent cystic or proliferative alterations of ducts and lobules. The findings suggest that the existing epithelial status of the breast is accentuated by exogenous hormone administration. Hargreaves et al.[111] studied the effect of HRT, consisting of estrogens alone or an estrogen–progesterone combination on proliferation and PR expression in the postmenopausal breast. Proliferation was assessed by Ki67 expression. In untreated women, the median Ki67 and PR labeling indices of 0.19 and 4.75, respectively, were unrelated to patient age, duration of menopause, or the presence of either benign or carcinomatous breast disease. HRT caused a significant increase in PR expression but did not significantly alter the Ki67 index.

Arteries in the breast undergo calcifications and atherosclerotic changes comparable to those seen throughout the body with increasing age. The role of these changes as a

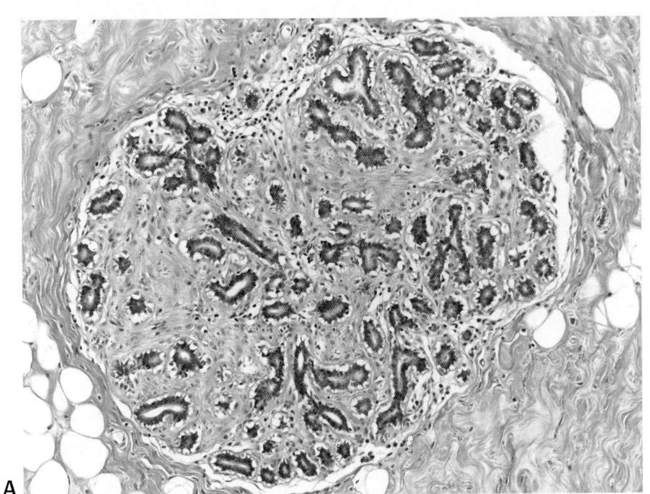

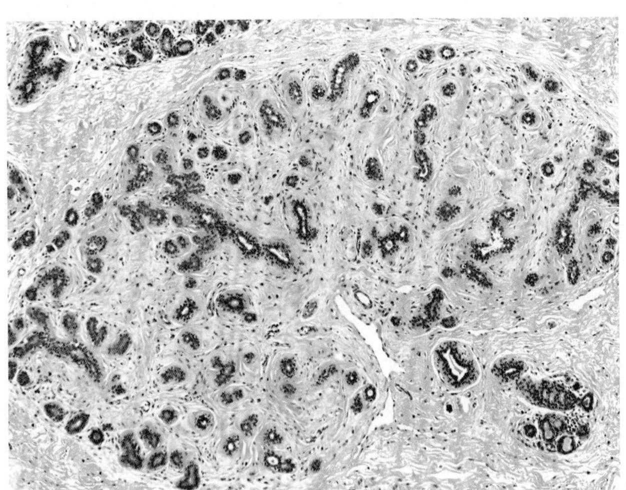

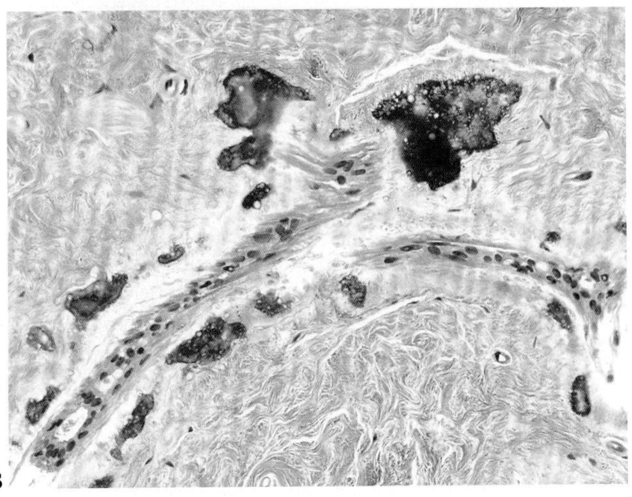

FIG. 1.28. ***Menopausal atrophy of lobule.*** **A–C:** Progressively atrophic lobules with collagenized intralobular stroma and thickened basement membranes around lobular glands. Lobular atrophy at age 58 is seen in **(A)**, age 74 in **(B)**, and age 92 in **(C)**. Note stromal calcification in **(C)** adjacent to lobular ductules.

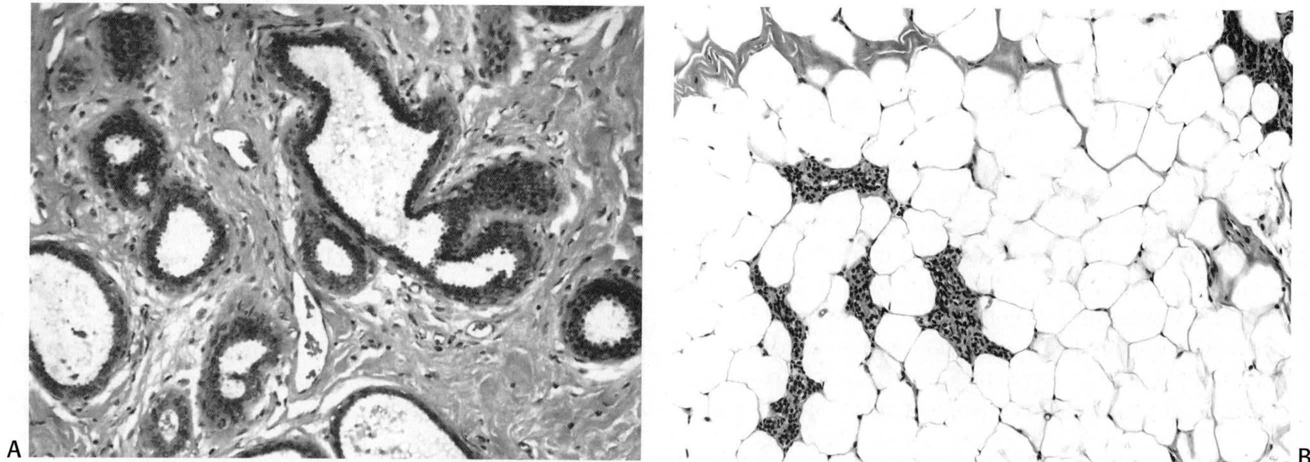

FIG. 1.29. ***Menopausal atrophy of lobule.*** **A:** Microcystic dilation of lobular glands and collagenized intralobular stroma. **B:** Glandular atrophy in fat.

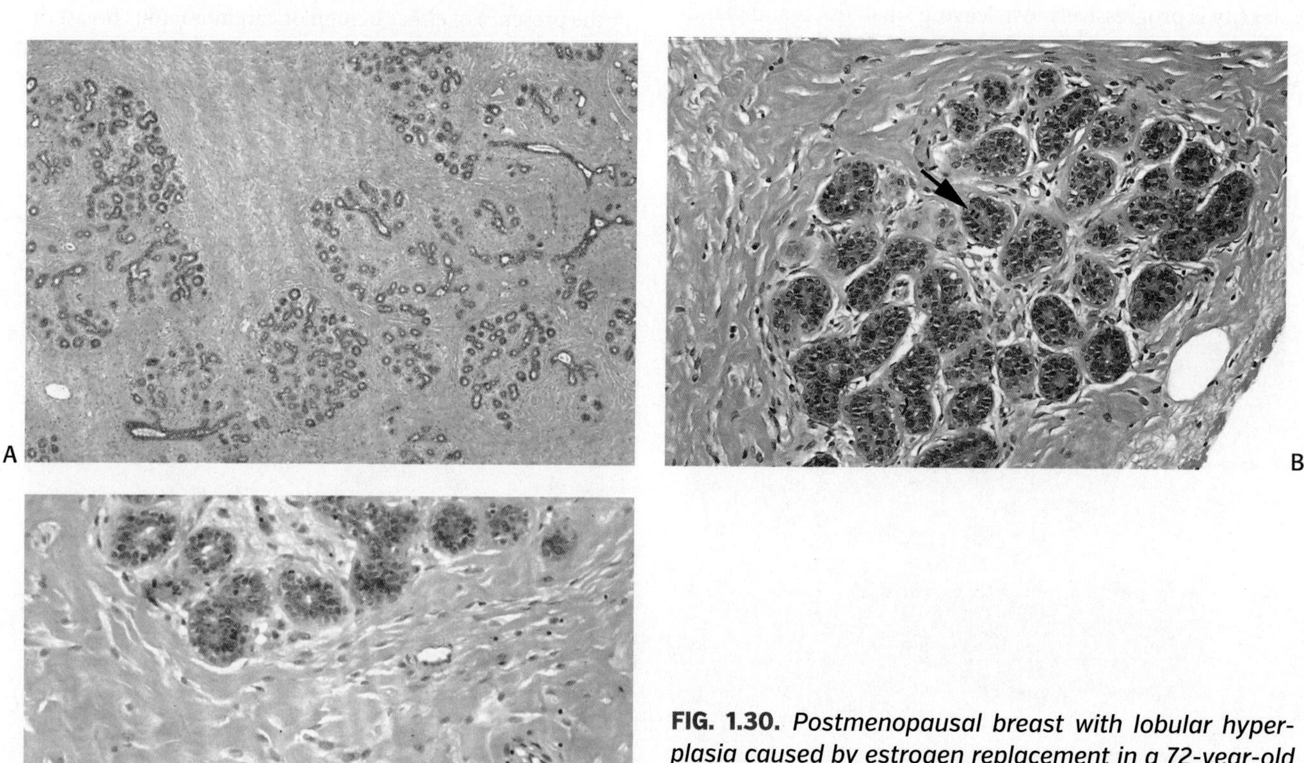

FIG. 1.30. ***Postmenopausal breast with lobular hyperplasia caused by estrogen replacement in a 72-year-old woman.*** **A:** Multiple lobules are evident. **B:** A lobule showing differentiation of intralobular stroma. The glandular epithelium is hyperplastic. A mitotic figure is present (*arrow*). **C:** Pseudoangiomatous hyperplasia is evident in the surrounding stroma.

surrogate marker for coronary and systemic atherosclerosis was reviewed by Shah et al.[112] Their analysis of data from 25 published studies involving 35,542 patients revealed that breast arterial calcification was significantly related to coronary artery disease and cardiovascular disease in the majority of studies. Arterial calcification is most likely to be encountered in the postmenopausal breast.[113,114] Some patients with mammographically detected calcifications have diabetes mellitus, coronary artery disease, and hypertension.[115,116] Arterial calcifications were found in the breasts of 9.1% of 12,239 women 50 to 69 years of age studied in one screening mammography program.[117] This finding was associated with a significantly increased risk of concomitant arteriosclerotic disease, hypertension, and diabetes mellitus. In another screening program, mammary arterial calcification occurred more often in hypertensive than in normotensive women, but the difference was not statistically significant.[113] Calcific arterial sclerosis is usually readily distinguishable from epithelial-associated calcifications in mammograms.

PREGNANCY-LIKE CHANGE

This structural alteration affecting lobules resembles lactational hyperplasia. It occurs in breast tissue from patients who are neither pregnant nor lactating when the specimen is obtained. Most of the patients are pre- or postmenopausal women who had been pregnant, but similar changes have been observed in women who are nulliparous[118,119] and in breast tissue from men treated with estrogens.[120] The reported frequency of finding pregnancy-like change is 1.7% to about 3% in surgical pathology and autopsy series.[118,119,121,122]

The etiology of pregnancy-like change is unknown. Consequently, it is uncertain whether this is a normal physiologic or pathologic alteration. Recent studies have documented cystic hypersecretory hyperplasia and rare instances of carcinoma associated with pregnancy-like hyperplasia (PLH).[123,124] Speculation as to the cause of pregnancy-like change centers on the possibility that the affected lobules remain in a persistent lactating state after pregnancy or that these are lobules that exhibit an idiosyncratic reaction to endogenous hormones, exogenous hormones, medication, or other unidentified substances. Pregnancy-like change can be induced in the rat mammary gland by administering phenothiazine,[125] and similar changes have been found in breast tissue from women receiving this and other medications.[126,127]

Glands and terminal ducts with pregnancy-like change usually contain little secretion, although they are dilated (Fig. 1.31). The glandular cells are swollen with abundant pale-to-clear, finely granular or vacuolated cytoplasm. The nuclei are usually round and stain darkly. Intranuclear vacuoles may be present. The luminal cytoplasmic borders of glandular cells are frayed, and apical cytoplasmic blebs are formed. The nucleus may be contained in a bleb of cytoplasm extruded into the glandular lumen. Diastase-resistant periodic acid–Schiff (PAS) positive granules are present in the cytoplasm, which is also immunoreactive for α-lactalbumin and S-100.[122] The cells express a secretory component and IgA in their cytoplasm, as well as lysozyme and lactoferrin.[128] These features resemble the findings in normal breast lobules in late pregnancy and lactation.

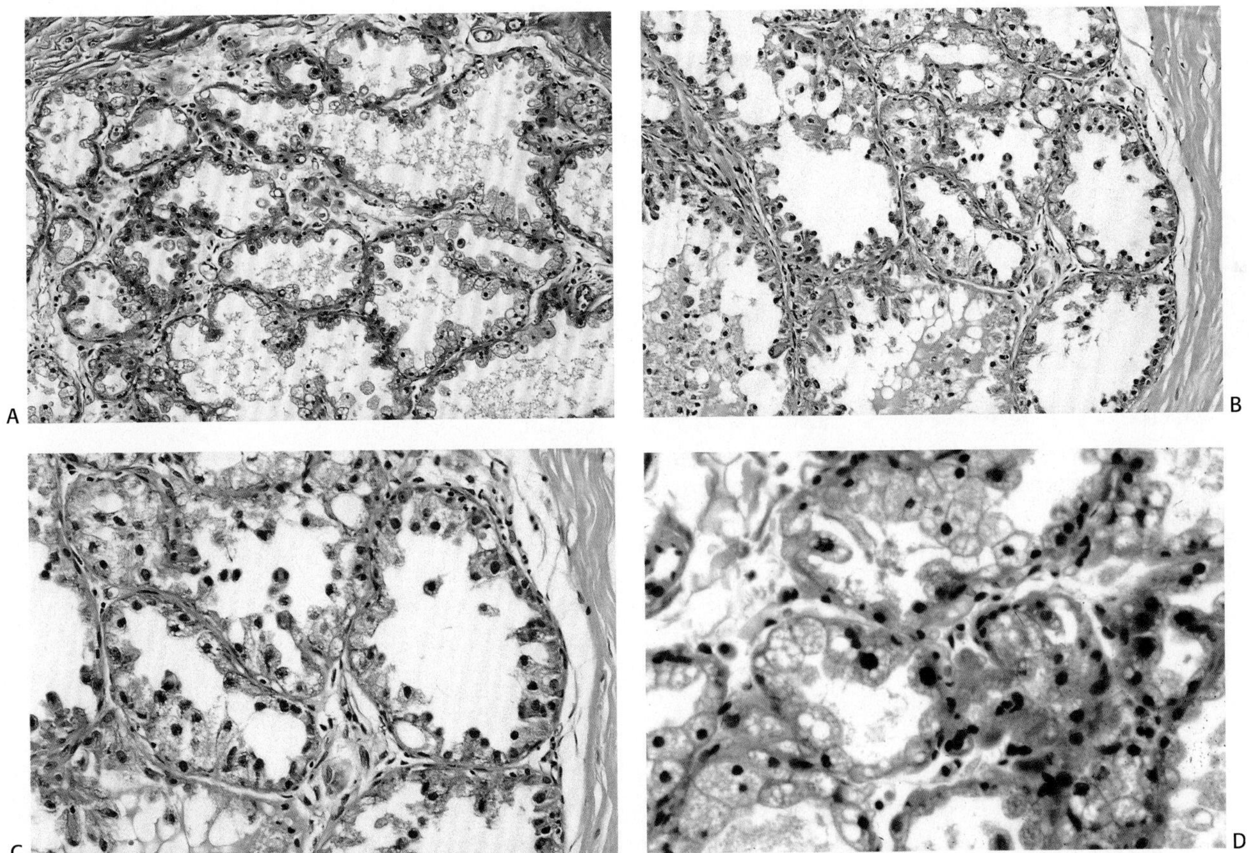

FIG. 1.31. ***Pregnancy-like change.*** **A:** Dilated lobular glands lined by a single layer of cuboidal and columnar cells with dense hyperchromatic nuclei. **B,C:** The glandular cells have finely vacuolated cytoplasm that is frayed at the luminal border. There are extruded nuclei in glandular lumens. **D:** Another example with hyperchromatic nuclei.

In most instances, the epithelium in lobules altered by pregnancy-like change remains one or two cell layers thick, thus simulating the architecture of the truly lactating breast. PLH is the occurrence of pregnancy-like change in hyperplastic epithelium in a non-pregnant woman or a man, (Fig. 1.32). The epithelium is arranged in irregular papillary fronds composed entirely of glandular cells. The glandular lumens in PLH often contain secretion that may accumulate in a laminated fashion and undergo calcification (Figs. 1.33 and 1.34). This lesion may be detected by mammography, leading to sampling by needle core biopsy.[123]

Some examples of PLH feature an atypical epithelial proliferation with substantial nuclear pleomorphism (Fig. 1.35). These instances of *atypical PLH* have been seen most commonly in association with cystic hypersecretory lesions[123] (Figs. 1.36 and 1.37) (see Chapter 24). Rarely carcinoma had been found to arise from atypical PLH, usually in combination with cystic hypersecretory hyperplasia.[124]

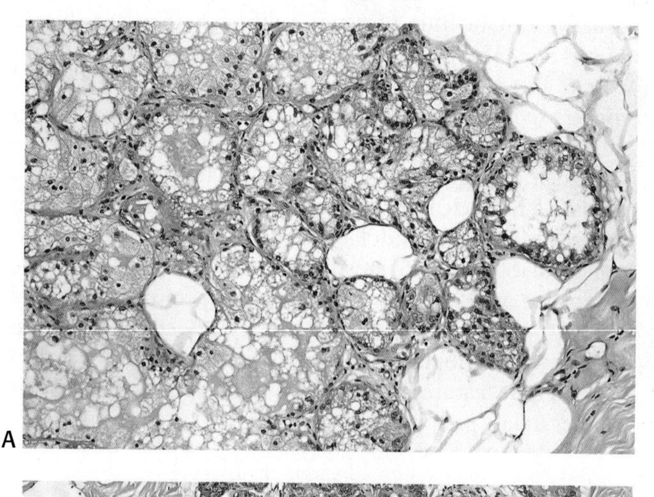

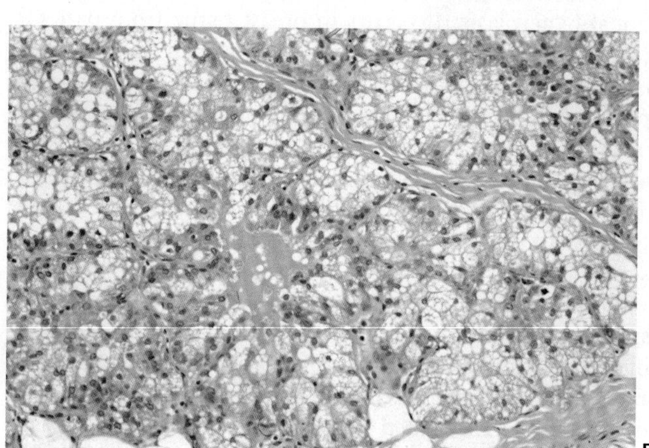

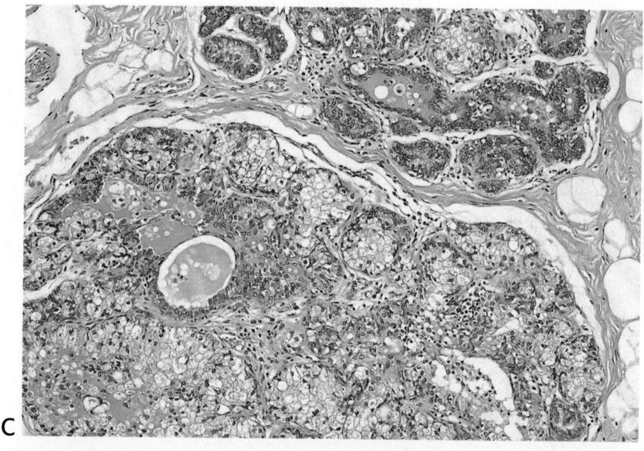

FIG. 1.32. ***Pregnancy-like hyperplasia.*** **A,B:** Hyperplastic cells fill most of the lobular glands, and some secretion is present. **C:** Secretion is present in an intralobular duct. Note the partially involved hyperplastic lobule on the upper right in this specimen from a 60-year-old woman.

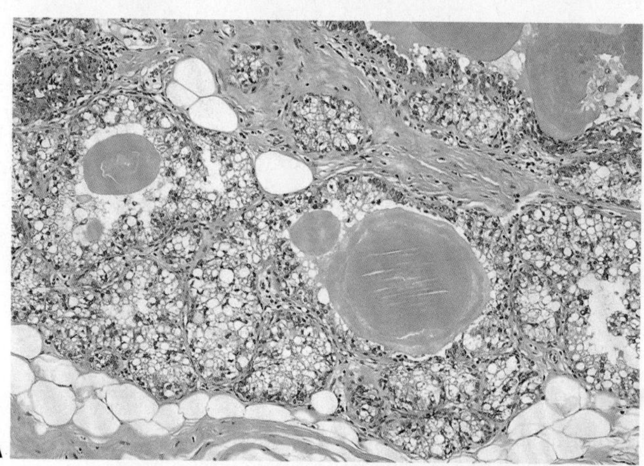

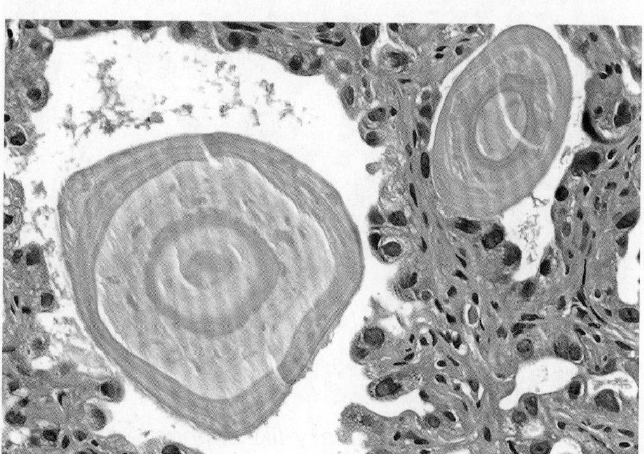

FIG. 1.33. ***Pregnancy-like hyperplasia, laminated secretion.*** **A,B:** Different appearances of laminated deposits of secretion. Cytological atypia is shown in **(B)**.

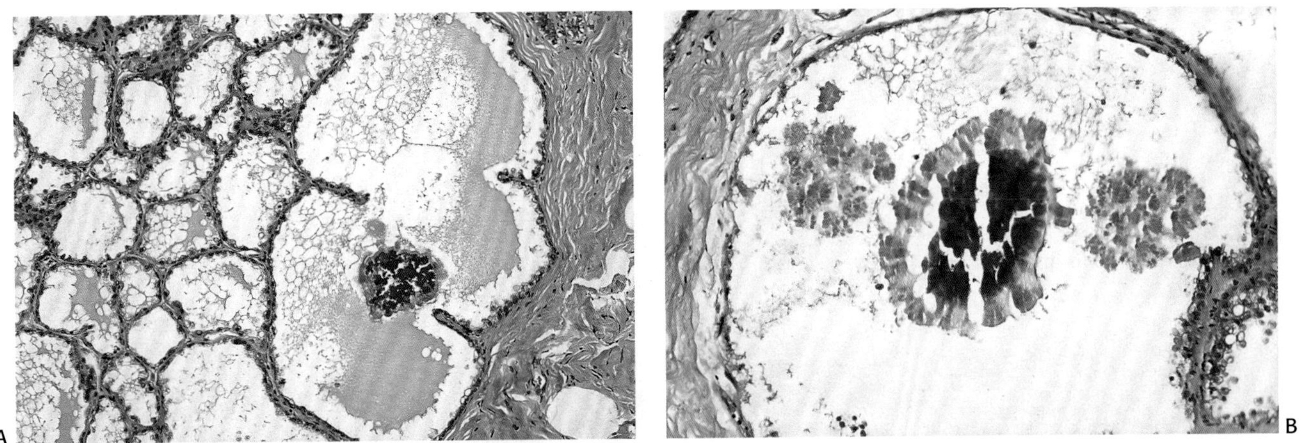

FIG. 1.34. ***Pregnancy-like change, calcifications.*** **A,B:** This distinctive rosette-like calcification is characteristic for pregnancy-like lesions.

Ultrastructural study of PLH revealed features largely similar to the findings in active lactation.[122] However, cells in PLH lack parallel arrays of rough endoplasmic reticulum and abundant swollen mitochondria characteristic of the lactating cell. The mitochondria appear to be shrunken, a feature of postlactational involution.[129] Decapitation secretion, which is responsible for the formation of cytoplasmic blebs in pregnancy-like change, is also an involutional change that differs from the formation of membrane-bound vacuoles in true lactation.

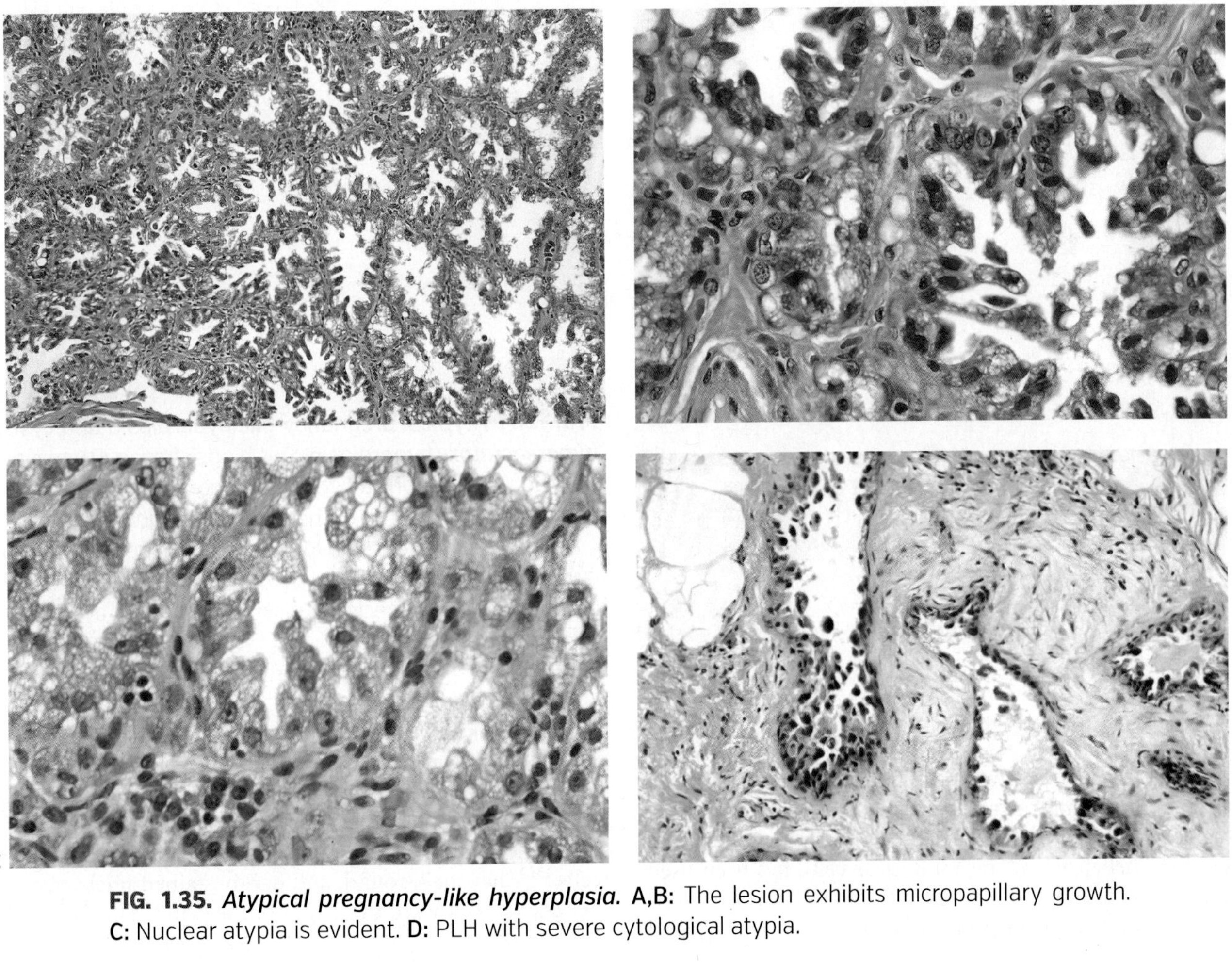

FIG. 1.35. ***Atypical pregnancy-like hyperplasia.*** **A,B:** The lesion exhibits micropapillary growth. **C:** Nuclear atypia is evident. **D:** PLH with severe cytological atypia.

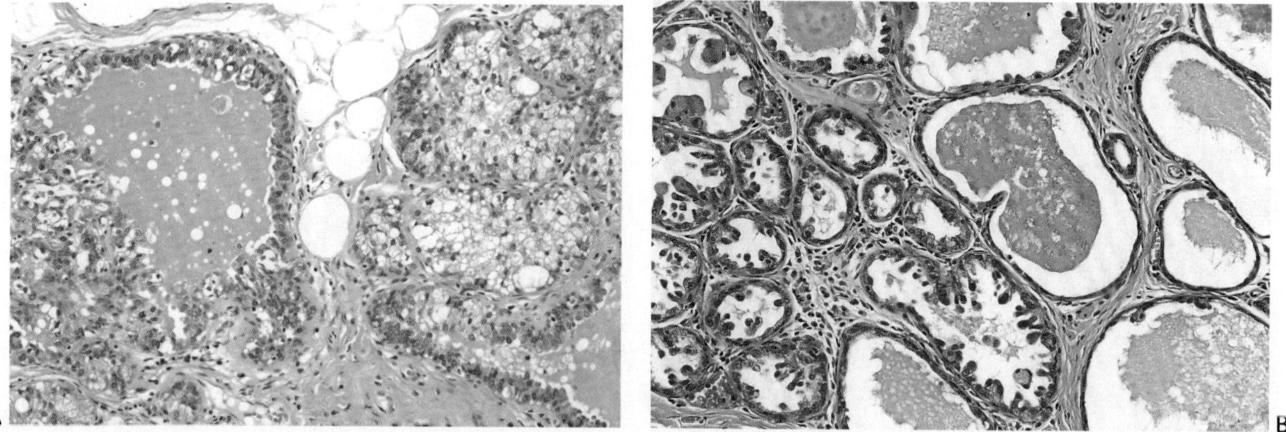

FIG. 1.36. ***Pregnancy-like hyperplasia and cystic hypersecretory hyperplasia.*** **A:** Florid PLH on the *right* and cystic hypersecretory hyperplasia on the *left*. **B:** Atypical cystic hypersecretory hyperplasia (*left*) and cystic hypersecretory hyperplasia (*right*).

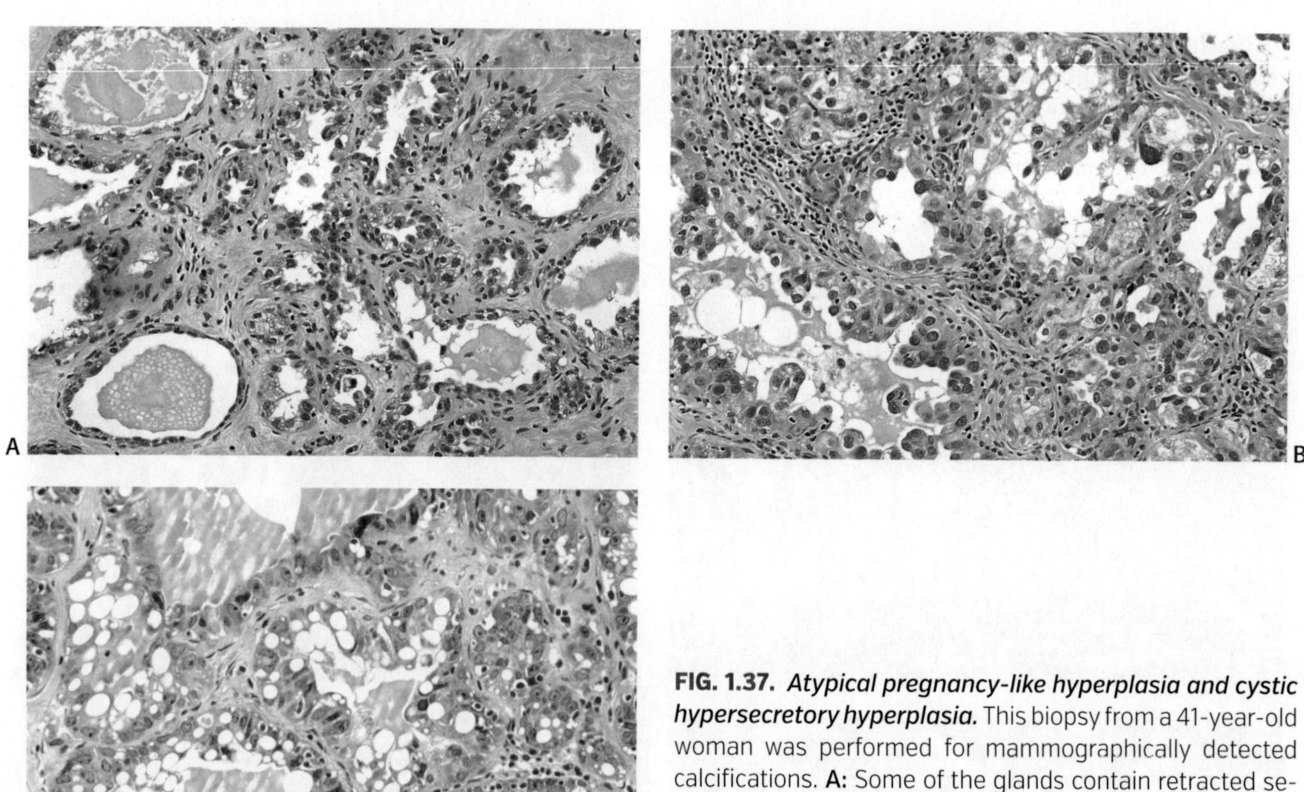

FIG. 1.37. ***Atypical pregnancy-like hyperplasia and cystic hypersecretory hyperplasia.*** This biopsy from a 41-year-old woman was performed for mammographically detected calcifications. **A:** Some of the glands contain retracted secretion typical for cystic hypersecretory hyperplasia. Note nuclear hyperchromasia in the PLH. **B,C:** Other areas in the same biopsy specimen with more severe cytological abnormalities.

CLEAR CELL CHANGE

Clear cell cytologic alteration in lobular and terminal duct epithelium differs microscopically from pregnancy-like change. It has also been referred to as "lamprocytosis," and the term "hellenzellen," meaning clear cells, has been used in the German literature.[130] The affected lobules tend to be larger than adjacent uninvolved lobules. The lobular gland epithelium is composed of swollen cells with abundant clear or pale, finely granular cytoplasm (Fig. 1.38). The cells have well-defined borders. Some glands have dilated lumens with PAS-positive, diastase-resistant secretion, but more often the lobular gland lumens are obliterated by the swollen cells.[131] The small, round, and darkly stained nuclei are often displaced toward the center of the gland. The clear cells

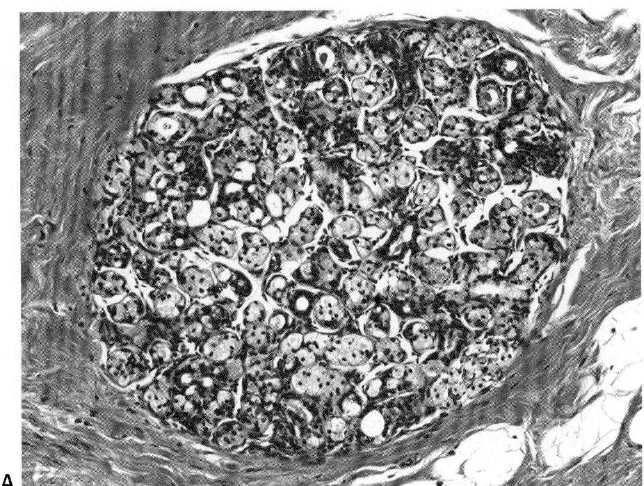

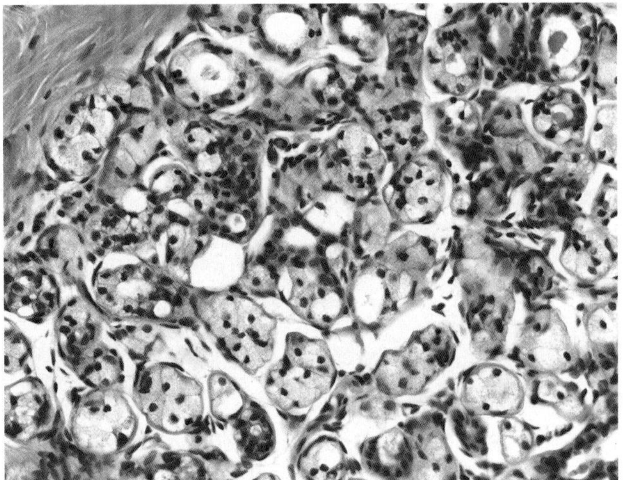

FIG. 1.38. A,B: ***Clear cell change in a lobule.*** The majority of the glands in the lobule are composed of cells with clear cytoplasm. Unaffected portions of the lobule are at its periphery.

are immunoreactive for cytokeratin (Fig. 1.39) but not for actin (Fig. 1.40). The cytoplasm of the clear cells contains diastase-sensitive, PAS-positive glycogen and is usually S-100 positive. The mucicarmine stain is negative, and there is no immunoreactivity for α-lactalbumin.

The etiology and histogenesis of clear cell change are uncertain. The results of special stains and immunohistochemistry suggest that the clear cells are altered epithelial cells. However, clear cell alterations of a less extreme degree affecting myoepithelial cells are not uncommon, leaving open the possibility that fully developed clear cell change is an extreme form of this abnormality (Fig. 1.41). Clear cell change is encountered in pre- and postmenopausal women. There is no association with pregnancy or exogenous hormone use.[127,131] Foci of clear cell change have been identified retrospectively in breast tissue obtained in the 1940s before exogenous hormones were available. Viña and Wells[122] reported finding clear cell change in 15 of 934 (1.6%) biopsies. Specimens that contain clear cell change may harbor carcinoma or benign changes, there being no association with any particular breast lesions.[122] Clear cell change and pregnancy-like change may coexist in the same breast, and, rarely, the two abnormalities seem to overlap in their histologic appearance.

Electron microscopy revealed that the cytoplasm of clear cells contained lipid and protein granules.[131] Dissolution of the former in tissue processing could explain the cytoplasmic clearing, whereas luminal accumulation of protein-associated secretion is the probable source of the PAS-positive material.

The differential diagnosis of clear cell change in breast glands includes pregnancy-like change, cytoplasmic clearing in apocrine metaplasia, cytoplasmic clearing in myoepithelial cells, and lobular involvement by clear cell

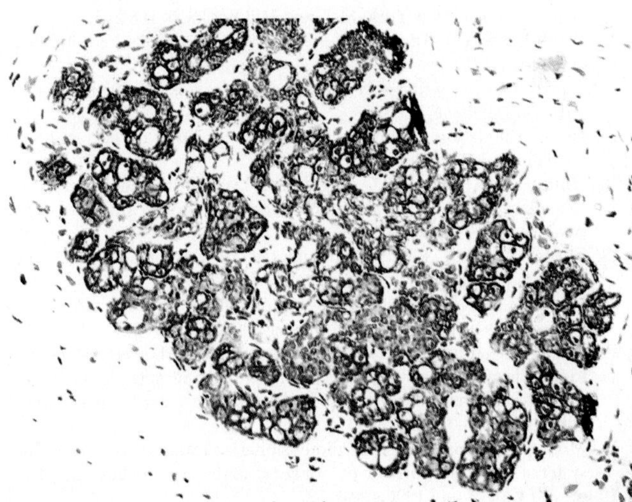

FIG. 1.39. ***Clear cell change in a lobule.*** The clear cells are immunoreactive for cytokeratin.

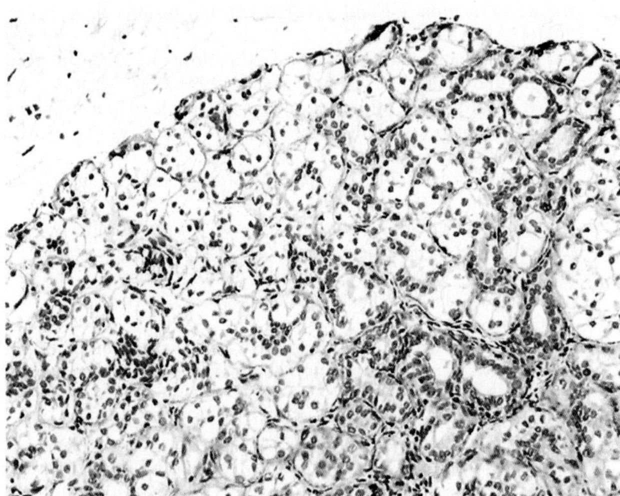

FIG. 1.40. ***Clear cell change in a lobule.*** The clear cells are not immunoreactive for actin.

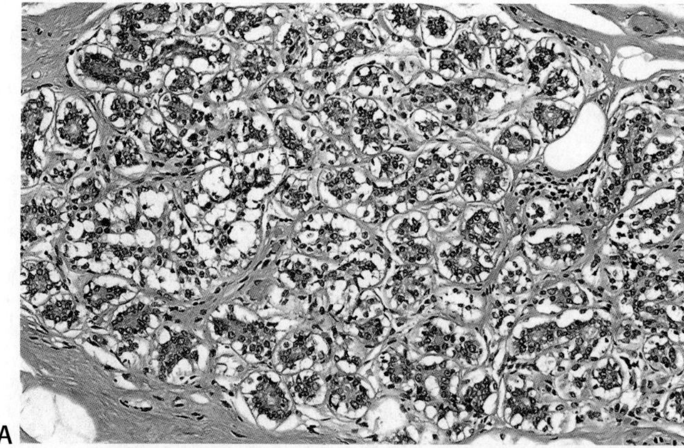

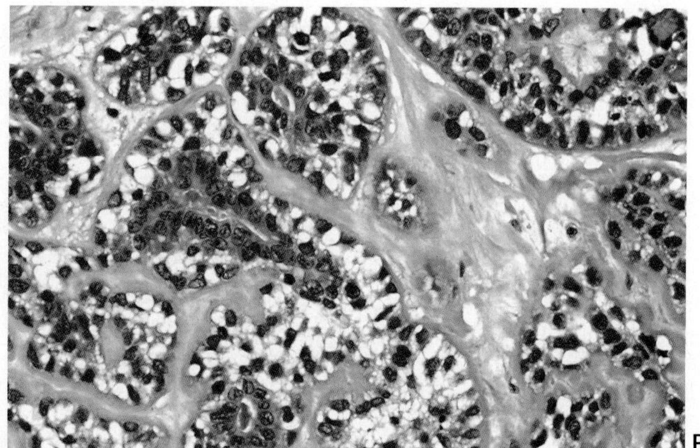

FIG. 1.41. A,B: *Clear cell change in myoepithelial cells.* Clear cell change in adenosis (A) and in an adenomyoepithelioma (B).

carcinoma. These lesions can usually be distinguished in surgical biopsy specimens, but difficulty can be encountered in a needle core biopsy sample. Pregnancy-like change is most readily distinguished from clear cell change because it features "decapitation" secretion at the luminal borders of the cells. Cytoplasmic clearing in apocrine metaplasia is usually a focal change in epithelium that otherwise has the typical features of apocrine metaplasia. Myoepithelial cells with clear cell change retain their position as a layer between the epithelium and the basement membrane. Most instances of clear cell carcinoma have a pronounced intraductal component. Rarely clear cell neoplasms, including renal cell carcinoma and so-called clear cell sarcoma, can metastasize to the breast.[132]

REFERENCES

1. Cowin P, Wysolmerski J. Molecular mechanisms guiding embryonic mammary gland development. *Cold Spring Harb Perspect Biol* 2010;2:a003251.
2. van Keymeulen A, Rocha AS, Ousset M, et al. Distinct stem cells contribute to mammary gland development and maintenance. *Nature* 2011;479:189–193.
3. Osin PP, Anbazhagan R, Bartkova J, et al. Breast development gives insights into breast disease. *Histopathology* 1998;33:275–283.
4. Anbazhagan R, Osin PP, Bartkova J, et al. The development of epithelial phenotypes in the human fetal and infant breast. *J Pathol* 1998;184:197–206.
5. Ham AW, Cormack DH. The breast. *Histology.* 8th ed. Philadelphia: JB Lippincott, 1979:866–874.
6. Adriance MC, Inman JL, Petersen OW, et al. Myoepithelial cells: good fences make good neighbors. *Breast Cancer Res* 2005;7:190–197.
7. Sternlicht MD. Key stages in mammary gland development. The cues that regulate ductal branching morphogenesis. *Breast Cancer Res* 2006;8:201–212.
8. Nathan B, Anbazhagan R, Clarkson P, et al. Expression of BCL-2 in the developing human fetal and infant breast. *Histopathology* 1994;24:73–76.
9. Codner E, Román R. Premature thelarche from phenotype to genotype. *Pediatr Endocrinol Rev* 2008;5:760–765.
10. Román R, Johnson MC, Codner E, et al. Activating GNAS1 gene mutations in patients with premature thelarche. *J Pediatr* 2004;145:218–222.
11. van Winter JT, Noller KL, Zimmerman D, et al. Natural history of premature thelarche in Olmsted County, Minnesota, 1940 to 1984. *J Pediatr* 1990;116:278–280.
12. Curfman AL, Reljanovic SM, McNelis KM, et al. Premature thelarche in infants and toddlers: prevalence, natural history and environmental determinants. *J Pediatr Adolesc Gynecol* 2011;24:338–341.
13. Verrotti A, Ferrari M, Morgese G, Chiarelli F. Premature thelarche: a long-term follow-up. *Gynecol Endocrinol* 1996;10:241–247.
14. Aritaki S, Takagi T, Someya H, et al. A comparison of patients with premature thelarche and idiopathic true precocious puberty in the initial stage of illness. *Acta Paediatrica Japon* 1997;39:21–27.
15. Klein KO, Mericq V, Brown-Dawson JM, et al. Estrogen levels in girls with premature thelarche compared with normal prepubertal girls as determined by an ultrasensitive recombinant cell bioassay. *J Pediatr* 1999;134:190–192.
16. Volta C, Bernasconi S, Cisternino M, et al. Isolated premature thelarche and thelarche variant: clinical and auxological follow-up of 119 girls. *J Endocrinol Invest* 1998;21:180–183.
17. Pasquino AM, Pucarelli I, Passeri F, et al. Progression of premature thelarche to central precocious puberty. *J Pediatr* 1995;126:11–14.
18. Pangarkar MA, Poflee SV, Lele VR. Fine needle aspiration cytology of juvenile hypertrophy of the breast. *Acta Cytol* 1997;41:940–941.
19. Topper YJ, Freeman CS. Multiple hormone interactions in the developmental biology of the mammary gland. *Physiol Rev* 1980;60:1049–1106.
20. Salmon M. Les artères de la glande mammaire. *Ann Anat Pathol* 1939;16:477–500.
21. Cunningham L. The anatomy of the arteries and veins of the breast. *J Surg Oncol* 1977;9:71–85.
22. Skandalakis JE, Grey SW, Rowe JS Jr. *Anatomical complications in general surgery.* New York: McGraw-Hill Book Co, 1983:43.
23. Cruikshank WC. *Anatomy of the absorbing vessels.* 2nd ed. London: G. Nicol, 1790.
24. Sappey MPC. *Description et ichonographie des vaisseaux lymphatiques.* Paris: A. Delahaye, 1885.
25. Gray JH. Relation of lymphatic vessels to spread of cancer. *Br J Surg* 1939;26:462–495.
26. Hultborn KA, Larsson LG, Ragnhult I. Lymph drainage from breast to axillary and parasternal lymph nodes, studied with aid of colloidal. *Acta Radiol* 1955;43:52–64.
27. Turner-Warwick RT. The lymphatics of the breast. *Br J Surg* 1959;46:574–582.
28. Estourgie SH, Nieweg OE, Valdes Olmos RA, et al. Lymphatic drainage patterns from the breast. *Ann Surg* 2004;239:232–237.
29. Shahar KH, Buchholz TA, Delpassand E, et al. Lower and central tumor location correlates with lymphoscintigraphy drainage to the internal mammary lymph nodes in breast carcinoma. *Cancer* 2005;103:1323–3129.
30. Moffat DF, Going JJ. Three dimensional anatomy of complete duct systems in human breast: pathological and developmental implications. *J Clin Pathol* 1996;49:48–52.
31. Going JJ, Moffat DF. Escaping from Flatland: clinical and biological aspects of human mammary duct anatomy in three dimensions. *J Pathol* 2004;203:538–544.

32. Montgomery WF. *An exposition of the signs and symptoms of pregnancy, the period of human gestation, and the signs of delivery.* London: Sherwood, Gilbert and Piper, 1837.
33. Miglioretti DL, Walker R, Weaver DL, et al. Accuracy of screening mammography varies by week of menstrual cycle. *Radiology* 2011;258:372–379.
34. Wolfe JN. Breast patterns as an index of risk for developing breast cancer. *AJR Am J Roentgenol* 1976;126:1130–1139.
35. Saftlas AF, Wolfe JN, Hoover RN, et al. Mammographic parenchymal patterns as indicators of breast cancer risk. *Am J Epidemiol* 1989;129:518–526.
36. Lee NA, Rusinek H, Weinreb J, et al. Fatty and fibroglandular tissue volumes in the breasts of women 20–83 years old: comparison of x-ray mammography and computer-assisted MR imaging. *AJR Am J Roentgenol* 1997;168:501–506.
37. Rand T, Heytmanek G, Seifert M, et al. Mammography in women undergoing hormone replacement therapy. Possible effects revealed at routine examination. *Acta Radiol* 1997;38:228–231.
38. Persson I, Thurfjell E, Holmberg L. Effect of estrogen and estrogen-progestin replacement regimens on mammographic breast parenchymal density. *J Clin Oncol* 1997;15:3201–3207.
39. Marugg RC, van der Mooren MJ, Hendriks JHCL, et al. Mammographic changes in postmenopausal women on hormonal replacement therapy. *Eur Radiol* 1997;7:749–755.
40. Reichenbach JR, Przetak C, Klinger G, et al. Assessment of breast tissue changes on hormonal replacement therapy using MRI: a pilot study. *J Comput Assist Tomogr* 1999;23:407–413.
41. Rutter CM, Mandelson MT, Laya MB, et al. Changes in breast density associated with initiation, discontinuation, and continuing use of hormone replacement therapy. *JAMA* 2001;285:171–176.
42. Son HJ, Oh KK. Significance of follow-up mammography in estimating the effect of tamoxifen in breast cancer patients who have undergone surgery. *AJR Am J Roentgenol* 1999;173:905–909.
43. Chan S, Su MY, Lei FJ, et al. Menstrual cycle-related fluctuations in breast density measured by using three-dimensional MR imaging. *Radiology* 2011;261:744–751.
44. Rosen PP, Tench W. Lobules in the nipple. *Pathol Annu* 1985;20[Pt 1]: 317–322.
45. Nagato T, Yoshida H, Yoshida A, et al. A scanning electron microscope study of myoepithelial cells in exocrine glands. *Cell Tissue Res* 1980;209:1–10.
46. Emerman JT, Vogl AW. Cell size and shape changes in the myoepithelium of the mammary gland during differentiation. *Anat Rec* 1986;216:405–415.
47. Tramm T, Kim JY, Tavassoli FA. Diminished number or complete loss of myoepithelial cells associated with metaplastic and neoplastic apocrine lesions of the breast. *Am J Surg Pathol* 2011;35:202–211.
48. Cserni G. Benign apocrine papillary lesions of the breast lacking or virtually lacking myoepithelial cells—potential pitfalls in diagnosing malignancy. *APMIS* 2012;120:249–252.
49. Hilson JB, Schnitt SJ, Collins LC. Phenotypic alterations in myoepithelial cells associated with benign sclerosing lesions of the breast. *Am J Surg Pathol* 2010;34:896–900.
50. Hilson JB, Schnitt SJ, Collins LC. Phenotypic alterations in ductal carcinoma in situ-associated myoepithelial cells: biologic and diagnostic implications. *Am J Surg Pathol* 2009;33:227–232.
51. Farahmand S, Cowan DF. Elastosis in the normal aging breast. *Arch Pathol Lab Med* 1991;115:1241–1246.
52. Davies JD. Pigmented periductal cells (ochrocytes) in mammary dysplasias: their nature and significance. *J Pathol* 1974;114:205–216.
53. Montagna W, Macpherson EE. Some neglected aspects of the anatomy of human breasts. *J Invest Dermatol* 1974;63:10–16.
54. Schnitt SJ, Goldwyn RM, Slavin SA. Mammary ducts in the areola: implications for patients undergoing reconstructive surgery of the breast. *Plast Reconstr Surg* 1993;92:1290–1293.
55. Smith DM Jr, Peters TG, Donegan WL. Montgomery's areolar tubercle. *Arch Pathol Lab Med* 1982;106:60–63.
56. Eyden BP, Watson RJ, Harris M, et al. Intralobular stromal fibroblasts in the resting human mammary gland: ultrastructural properties and intercellular relationships. *J Submicrosc Cytol Pathol* 1986;18:397–408.
57. Yamazaki K, Eyden BP. Ultrastructural and immunohistochemical observations on intralobular fibroblasts on human breast, with observations on the CD34 antigen. *J Submicrosc Cytol Pathol* 1995;27: 309–323.
58. Naccarato AG, Viacava P, Bocci G, et al. Definition of the microvascular pattern of the normal human adult mammary gland. *J Anat* 2003;203:599–603.
59. Christov K, Chew KL, Ljung B-M, et al. Proliferation of normal breast epithelial cells as shown by *in vivo* labeling with bromodeoxyuridine. *Am J Pathol* 1991;138:1371–1377.
60. Lakhani SR, Chaggar R, Davies S, et al. Genetic alterations in 'normal' luminal and myoepithelial cells of the breast. *J Pathol* 1999;189:496–503.
61. White E, Velentgas P, Mandelson MT, et al. Variation in mammographic breast density by time in menstrual cycle among women aged 40–49 years. *J Natl Cancer Inst* 1998;90:906–910.
62. Morrow M, Chatterton RT Jr, Rademaker AW, et al. A prospective study of variability in mammographic density during the menstrual cycle. *Breast Cancer Res Treat* 2010;121:565–574.
63. Milligan D, Drife JO, Short RV. Changes in breast volume during normal menstrual cycle and after oral contraceptives. *Br Med J* 1975;4:494–496.
64. Fowler PA, Casey CE, Cameron GG, et al. Cyclic changes in composition and volume of the breast during the menstrual cycle, measured by magnetic resonance imaging. *Br J Obstet Gynaecol* 1990;97:595–602.
65. Graham SJ, Stanchev PL, Lloyd-Smith JOA, et al. Changes in fibroglandular volume and water content of breast tissue during the menstrual cycle observed by MR imaging at 1. 5T. *J Magn Reson Imaging* 1995;5:695–701.
66. Kuhl CK, Bieling HB, Gieseke J, et al. Healthy premenopausal breast parenchyma in dynamic contrast-enhanced MR imaging of the breast: normal contrast medium enhancement and cyclical-phase dependency. *Radiology* 1997;203:137–144.
67. Müller-Schimpfle M, Ohmenhäuser K, Stoll P, et al. Menstrual cycle and age: influence on parenchymal contrast medium enhancement in MR imaging of the breast. *Radiology* 1997;203:145–149.
68. Vogel PM, Georgiade NG, Fetter BF, et al. The correlation of histologic changes in the human breast with the menstrual cycle. *Am J Pathol* 1981;104:23–34.
69. Gomm JJ, Coope RC, Browne PJ, et al. Separated human breast epithelial and myoepithelial cells have different growth factor requirements in vitro but can reconstitute normal breast lobuloalveolar structure. *J Cell Physiol* 1997;171:11–19.
70. Longacre TA, Bartow SA. A correlative morphologic study of human breast and endometrium in the menstrual cycle. *Am J Surg Pathol* 1986;10:382–393.
71. Ferguson DJP, Anderson TJ. Morphological evaluation of cell turnover in relation to the menstrual cycle in the "resting" human breast. *Br J Cancer* 1981;4:177–181.
72. Sabourin JC, Martin A, Baruch J, et al. bcl-2 Expression in normal breast tissue during the menstrual cycle. *Int J Cancer* 1994;59:1–6.
73. Anderson TJ, Ferguson JP, Raab GM. Cell turnover in the "resting" human breast: influence of parity, contraceptive pill, age and laterality. *Br J Cancer* 1982;46:376–382.
74. Ramakrishnan R, Khan SA, Badve S. Morphological changes in breast tissue with menstrual cycle. *Mod Pathol* 2002;15:1348–56.
75. Gompel A, Martin A, Simon P, et al. Epidermal growth factor receptor and c-erbB-2 expression in normal breast tissue during the menstrual cycle. *Breast Cancer Res Treat* 1996;38:227–235.
76. Uehara J, Nazário AC, Rodrigues de Lima G, et al. Effects of tamoxifen on the breast in the luteal phase of the menstrual cycle. *Int J Gynaecol Obstet* 1998;62:77–82.
77. Fanger H, Ree HJ. Cyclic changes of human mammary gland epithelium in relation to the menstrual cycle—an ultrastructural study. *Cancer* 1974;34:574–585.
78. Donegan WL, Shah D. Prognosis of patients with breast cancer related to the timing of operation. *Arch Surg* 1993;128:309–313.
79. Badwe RA, Mittra I, Havaldor R. Timing of surgery during the menstrual cycle and prognosis of breast cancer. *J Biosci* 2000;25:113–120.
80. Milella M, Nistico C, Ferraresi V, et al. Breast cancer and timing of surgery during menstrual cycle: a 5-year analysis of 248 premenopausal women. *Breast Cancer Res Treat* 1999;55:259–266.
81. Nomura Y, Kataoka A, Tsuitsui S, et al. Lack of correlation between timing of surgery in relation to the menstrual cycle and prognosis of premenopausal patients with early breast cancer. *Eur J Cancer* 1999;35:1326–1330.
82. McCarty KS Jr, Sasso R, Budwit D, et al. Immunoglobulin localization in the normal human mammary gland: variation with the menstrual cycle. *Am J Pathol* 1982;107:322–326.

83. Potten CS, Watson RJ, Williams GT, et al. The effect of age and menstrual cycle upon proliferative activity of the normal human breast. *Br J Cancer* 1988;58:163–170.
84. Meyer JS. Cell proliferation in normal human breast ducts, fibroadenomas, and other ductal hyperplasias measured by nuclear labeling with tritiated thymidine. Effects of menstrual phase, age, and oral contraceptive hormones. *Hum Pathol* 1977;8:67–81.
85. Masters JRW, Drife JO, Scarisbrick JJ. Cyclic variation of DNA synthesis in human breast epithelium. *J Natl Cancer Inst* 1977;58:1283–1285.
86. Anderson TJ, Battersby S, King RJB, et al. Oral contraceptive use influences resting breast proliferation. *Hum Pathol* 1989;20:1139–1144.
87. Going JJ, Anderson TJ, Battersby S, et al. Proliferative and secretory activity in human breast during natural and artificial menstrual cycles. *Am J Pathol* 1988;130:193–204.
88. Russo J, Calaf G, Roi L, et al. Influence of age and gland topography on cell kinetics of normal human breast tissue. *J Natl Cancer Inst* 1987;72:413–418.
89. Visscher DW, Gingrich DS, Buckley J, et al. Cell cycle analysis of normal, atrophic, and hyperplastic breast epithelium using two-color multiparametric flow cytometry. *Anal Cell Pathol* 1996;12:115–124.
90. Söderqvist G, Isaksson E, von Schoultz B, et al. Proliferation of breast epithelial cells in healthy women during the menstrual cycle. *Am J Obstet Gynecol* 1997;176:123–128.
91. Joshi K, Smith JA, Perusinghe N, et al. Cell proliferation in the human mammary epithelium. Differential contribution by epithelial and myoepithelial cells. *Am J Pathol* 1986;124:199–206.
92. Petersen OW, Hoyer PE, van Deurs B. Frequency and distribution of estrogen receptor-positive cells in normal, nonlactating human breast tissue. *Cancer Res* 1987;47:5748–5751.
93. Shoker BS, Jarvis C, Sibson DR, et al. Oestrogen receptor expression in the normal and pre-cancerous breast. *J Pathol* 1999;188:237–244.
94. Silva JS, Georgiade GS, Dilley WG, et al. Menstrual cycle-dependent variations of breast cyst fluid proteins and sex steroid receptors in the normal human breast. *Cancer* 1983;51:1297–1302.
95. Markopoulos C, Berger U, Wilson P, et al. Oestrogen receptor content of normal breast cells and breast carcinoma throughout the menstrual cycle. *Br Med J* 1988;296:1349–1351.
96. Fabris G, Marchetti E, Marzola A, et al. Pathophysiology of estrogen receptors in mammary tissue by monoclonal antibodies. *J Steroid Biochem Mol Biol* 1987;27:171–176.
97. Pujol P, Daures JP, Thezenas S, et al. Changing estrogen and progesterone receptor patterns in breast carcinoma during the menstrual cycle and menopause. *Cancer* 1998;83:698–705.
98. Weimer DA, Donegan WL. Changes in estrogen and progesterone receptor content of primary breast carcinoma during the menstrual cycle. *Breast Cancer Res Treat* 1987;10:271–278.
99. Smyth CM, Benn DE, Reeve TS. Influence of the menstrual cycle on the concentrations of estrogen and progesterone receptors in primary breast cancer biopsies. *Breast Cancer Res Treat* 1988;11:45–50.
100. Grant CS, Ingle JN, Suman VJ, et al. Menstrual cycle and surgical treatment of breast cancer: findings from the NCCTG N9431 study. *J Clin Oncol*2009;27:3620–3626.
101. Tobin CE, Hendrix TM, Geyer SJ, et al. Breast imaging case of the day. Lobular hyperplasia of pregnancy. *Radiographics* 1996;16:1225–1226.
102. Dawson EK. A histological study of the normal mamma in relation to tumour growth. II. The mature gland in pregnancy and lactation. *Edinburgh Med J* 1935;42:569–598.
103. McCarty KS Jr, Tucker JA. Breast. In: Sternberg SS, ed. *Histology for pathologists*. New York: Raven Press, 1992:893–902.
104. Pitelka DR. The mammary gland. In: *Cell and tissue biology. A textbook of histology*. 6th ed. Baltimore: Urban & Schwarzenberg, 1988:881–898.
105. Salazar H, Tobon H, Josimovich JB. Developmental gestational and postgestational modifications of the human breast. *Clin Obstet Gynecol* 1975;18:113–137.
106. Vorherr H. Human lactation and breast feeding. In: *Lactation*. Vol. IV. New York: Academic Press, 182.
107. Battersby S, Anderson TJ. Histological changes in breast tissue that characterize recent pregnancy. *Histopathology* 1989;15:415–433.
108. Huseby RA, Thomas LB. Histological and histochemical alterations in the normal breast tissues of patients with advanced breast cancer being treated with estrogenic hormones. *Cancer* 1954;7:54–74.
109. Laya MB, Gallagher JC, Schreiman JS, et al. Effect of postmenopausal hormonal replacement therapy on mammographic density and parenchymal pattern. *Radiology* 1995;196:433–437.
110. Margolin FR, Denny SR, Gelfand CA, et al. Mammographic changes after hormone replacement therapy in patients who have undergone breast irradiation. *AJR Am J Roentgenol* 1999;172:147–150.
111. Hargreaves DF, Knox F, Swindell R, et al. Epithelial proliferation and hormone receptor status in the normal post-menopausal breast and the effects of hormone replacement therapy. *Br J Cancer* 1998;78: 945–949.
112. Shah N, Chainani V, Delafontaine P, et al. Mammographically detectable breast arterial calcification and atherosclerosis: a review. *Cardiol Rev* 2013 Apr 11. [Epub ahead of print] PubMed PMID: 23584424.
113. Leinster SJ, Whitehouse GH. Factors which influence the occurrence of vascular calcification in the breast. *Br J Radiol* 1987;60:457–458.
114. Kragel PJ, Aquino MO, Fiorella R, et al. Clinical, radiographic, and pathologic features of medial calcific sclerosis in the breast. *South Med J* 1997;90:518–521.
115. Baum JK, Comstock CH, Joseph L. Intramammary arterial calcifications associated with diabetes. *Radiology* 1980;136:61–62.
116. Moshyedi AC, Puthawala AH, Kurland RJ, et al. Breast arterial calcification: association with coronary artery disease. *Radiology* 1995;194:181–183.
117. van Noord PAH, Beijerinck D, Kemmeren JM, et al. Mammograms may convey more than breast cancer risk: breast arterial calcification and arterio-sclerotic related diseases in women of the DOM cohort. *Eur J Cancer Prev* 1996;5:483–487.
118. Kiaer HW, Andersen JA. Focal pregnancy-like changes in the breast. *Acta Path Microbiol Scand* [A] 1977;85:931–941.
119. Frantz VK, Pickren JW, Melcher GW, et al. Incidence of chronic cystic disease in so-called normal breasts: a study based on 225 postmortem examinations. *Cancer* 1951;4:762–783.
120. Schwartz IS, Wilens SL. The formation of acinar tissue in gynecomastia. *Am J Pathol* 1963;43:797–807.
121. Sandison AT. An autopsy study of the adult human breast. *J Natl Cancer Inst Monogr* 1962;8:58–59.
122. Viña M, Wells CA. Clear cell metaplasia of the breast: a lesion showing eccrine differentiation. *Histopathology* 1989;15:85–92.
123. Shin SJ, Rosen PP. Pregnancy-like (pseudolactational) hyperplasia: a primary diagnosis in mammographically detected lesions of the breast and its relationship to cystic hypersecretory hyperplasia. *Am J Surg Pathol* 2000;24:1670–1674.
124. Shin SJ, Rosen PP. Carcinoma arising from preexisting pregnancy-like and cystic hypersecretory hyperplasia lesions of the breast. A clinicopathologic study of 9 patients. *Am J Surg Pathol* 2004;28:789–793.
125. Pier WJ Jr, Garancis JC, Kuzma JF. Fine structure of tranquilizer-induced changes in rat mammary gland. *Am J Pathol* 1970;60:119–130.
126. Hooper JH, Welch VC, Shackelford RT. Abnormal lactation associated with tranquilizing drug therapy. *JAMA* 1961;178:506–507.
127. Tavassoli FA, Yeh IT. Lactational and clear cell changes of the breast in nonlactating, nonpregnant women. *Am J Clin Pathol* 1987;87:23–29.
128. Al-Sam SZ, Davies JD. Phenotypic expression of immunosecretory function in focal pregnancy-like change in the human breast. *Virchows Arch* [A] 1987;410:515–521.
129. Mills SE, Fraire AE. Pregnancy-like change of the breast. An ultrastructural study. *Diagn Gynecol Obstet* 1981;3:187–191.
130. Skorpil F. Uber das Vorkommen von sog. hellen Zellen (Lamprocyten) in der Milchdruse. *Beitrage Zur Pathol Anat* 1943;108: 378–393.
131. Barwick KW, Kashigarian M, Rosen PP. "Clear-cell" change within duct and lobular epithelium of the human breast. *Pathol Annu* 1982;17[Pt 1]:319–328.
132. Fukada I, Nishimura S, Tanabe M, et al. Clear cell sarcoma of the neck which metastasized to the mammary gland. *Case Rep Oncol* 2013;6:55–61.

CHAPTER 2

Abnormalities of Mammary Development and Growth

SYED A. HODA

Alterations in mammary development and growth can result in a wide variety of morphologic abnormalities. Most such alterations have genetic bases, which remain, as yet, largely unknown.

HYPOPLASIA AND AMASTIA

The most extreme form of mammary hypoplasia (Greek. *hypo*: deficient, *plasis*: molding) is amastia (Gk. *a*: without, *mastos*: breast), that is, the complete failure of one or both breasts, including the nipple, to develop.[1,2] As one of the least common developmental abnormalities, amastia is encountered more often in females than in males. Familial amastia has been documented in instances in which a brother and sister[3] and mother and daughter[4] have been affected. It may be accompanied by developmental defects of the ipsilateral shoulder, chest, and/or arm.[5] Amastia has been reported in the complex genetic defect of *Acrorenal Ectodermal Dysplasia with Lipotrophic Diabetes syndrome*.[6] In addition to amastia, developmental abnormalities in these young women include skeletal and renal defects and hypodontia.

Mammary hypoplasia can occur as a congenital or acquired defect and may be unilateral or bilateral. A diagnosis of unilateral hypoplasia may be made if there is a substantial difference in breast size that far exceeds mild asymmetry and the larger breast is not macromastic. The hypoplastic breast tissue consists of fibrous stroma and ductal structures without acinar differentiation (Fig. 2.1)

Ipsilateral mammary hypoplasia has been reported in conjunction with Becker nevus, a unilateral hairy hyperpigmented lesion,[7,8] although breast abnormalities were not described in the original report by Becker,[9] an American dermatologist. Concurrent hypoplasia of the ipsilateral pectoralis major muscle has also been reported.[10] The pigmented lesions and accompanying mammary hypoplasia occur in males and females.[11] High androgen receptor (AR) levels have been detected in Becker nevi[7,12] but not in the skin from the unaffected contralateral chest.[7]

Hypoplasia or aplasia of the mammary glands and hypoplasia of the nipples occur in the *Ulnar–Mammary syndrome*, a familial genetic abnormality with autosomal dominant inheritance[13–15] caused by mutations in the *TBX3* gene. The latter controls T-box transcription factors,[16] which are important in the morphogenesis of multiple organs.[17] Commonly associated defects include skeletal abnormalities affecting the ulnar rays of the hands, hypoplasia of apocrine glands, and genital anomalies in males. *Poland syndrome*, named after Sir Alfred Poland, a surgeon at Guy's Hospital, London, includes severe congenital defects of the chest and arm combined with mammary hypoplasia, amastia, or athelia.[18] Carcinoma can arise in the hypoplastic breast of women with Poland syndrome.[19,20]

Mammary hypoplasia also occurs in *Turner syndrome*, named after Henry Turner, an American endocrinologist, and in congenital adrenal hyperplasia. Familial hypoplasia of the nipples and athelia (Gk. *a*: without, *thelos*: nipple) associated with mammary hypoplasia has been described in a father and his daughters.[21] Hosokawa et al.[22] described the occurrence of a subcutaneous squamous cyst at the site of unilateral athelia, which suggested that the cystic lesion arose from a maldeveloped nipple.

Acquired mammary hypoplasia has been observed in women who received irradiation of the mammary region in infancy or childhood.[23,24] The most frequent clinical reason for radiation in this age group was the treatment of cutaneous hemangiomas. The degree of hypoplasia was directly related to the radiation dose. Unilateral atrophy of a previously normal breast associated with infectious mononucleosis has been described in a 17-year-old girl.[25] Biopsy revealed "normal" breast tissue. Surgical excision of the prepubertal breast bud, which enlarges in precocious and early breast development, will result in mammary hypoplasia or amastia by removing part or all of the infantile breast anlage. The occurrence of carcinoma arising in an irradiated hypomastic breast has been reported.[26]

MACROMASTIA

Several types of excessive breast growth, as assessed by volume and weight, have been described as forms of macromastia (Gk. *macro*: large, *mastos*: breast). It has been suggested that macromastia, also referred to as gigantomastia (Gk. *gigantikos*: giant), should be defined as excess breast tissue that contributes more than 3% of the patient's total body weight.[27] Breast weight is estimated to be 1 g/cm^3 , but can be rather variable, being mainly density dependent.

Adolescent macromastia occurs as a result of progressive growth over 1 or 2 years during adolescence, resulting

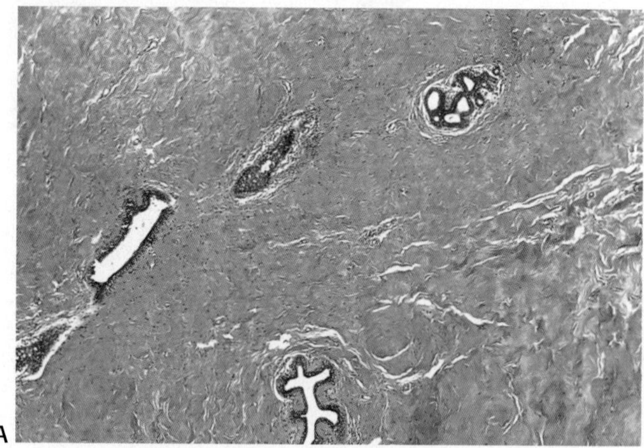

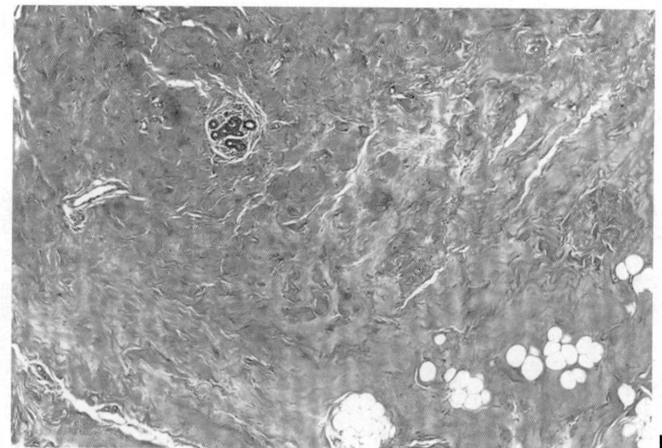

FIG. 2.1. ***Mammary hypoplasia.*** Breast tissue from a 23-year-old woman with unilateral hypoplasia. **A:** Ducts that resemble prepubertal breast in collagenous stroma. **B:** Minimal lobular differentiation.

in breast size that far exceeds normal limits. The breasts do not decrease in size in subsequent years, and breast reduction surgery is invariably required. Although the condition is usually relatively symmetrical, there are instances in which there is substantial disparity in breast size. Histologic examination reveals greatly increased stromal collagen and fat (Fig. 2.2). Epithelial hyperplasia of ducts is present in a minority of cases.[28] Pseudoangiomatous stromal hyperplasia (PASH) is evident in some of these individuals. The stromal cells in one instance of adolescent macromastia, which appears to be PASH in the published illustrations, lacked estrogen receptor (ER) but were positive for progesterone receptor.[29] Biochemical ER assays were negative on tissues from a series of 25 patients (ages 17 to 77 years) who had macromastia not associated with pregnancy.[30]

Gravid (Gk. *gravid*: heavy) *macromastia* develops rapidly, shortly after the onset of pregnancy in the affected individual.[31–33] It occurs in less than 0.01% of pregnancies.[31]

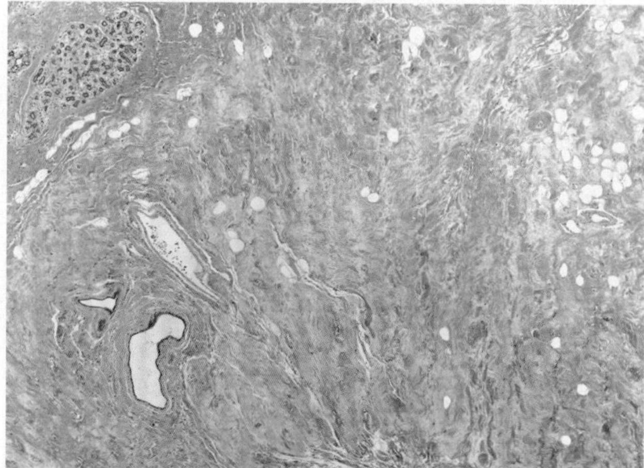

FIG. 2.2. ***Adult macromastia.*** A broad area of moderately edematous interlobular stroma surrounding a normal lobule (upper left) and a duct. The histopathologic findings are less spectacular than the clinical appearance.

The etiology is unknown. Onset very early in pregnancy in some cases has implicated human chorionic gonadotrophin, possibly through a hypersensitivity mechanism. Fetal sex does not appear to be a factor. The majority of women are primiparous, but in some individuals macromastia does not occur until a second or third pregnancy.[31,33,34] Once established, the condition is likely to recur in successive pregnancies, even if the pregnancy terminates in a miscarriage. The chance of recurrence is decreased by reduction mammoplasty, but some patients have required further surgery for regrowth of breast tissue after mastectomy.[33,35] In one case, gravid macromastia involved bilateral axillary breasts and one ectopic thoracic breast, as well as both normally situated glands.[36]

A variety of histopathologic changes have been reported in gravid macromastia. Leis et al.[34] described a case in which the stroma exhibited "marked fibrosis, with bands of dense collagenous tissue and thickening of the intralobular fibrous tissue." Thickening of basement membranes was noted, whereas "ducts and acini demonstrated a two-layered epithelium with apparently inactive cuboidal cells." Fibrosis and collagenization were also noted by Beischer et al.[31] and Kullander.[37] Others have reported fibroadenomas[35,38] and lactational hyperplasia.[39] Several authors have commented on the presence of dilated lymphatics in the breast tissue. PASH is often a prominent feature that is evident in retrospect in published illustrations,[40] although the condition was not described by this term in the reports (see Chapter 38). Pseudohyperparathyroidism has been associated with gravid macromastia.[40] Mastectomy results in prompt remission of the hypercalcemia. Rarely, the clinical presentation of neoplastic conditions such as angiosarcoma or lymphoma in the breast may mimic gravid macromastia.

Mastectomy or breast reduction is usually undertaken after delivery to ameliorate the incapacitating effects of gravid macromastia including pain, depression, and, in some cases, altered pulmonary function. Necrosis of the skin or parenchyma complicated by infection or bleeding may necessitate mastectomy during pregnancy. The concept that hormonal disturbances contribute to the development of gravid macromastia has led to attempts at endocrine treatment, although none has been uniformly effective. There have not been consistent hormonal abnormalities in patients who were studied, and it appears likely that the fundamental problem lies in abnormal responsiveness of the breast tissues.[41] Bromocriptine, a dopamine agonist, has been administered, resulting in reduced prolactin levels in some cases but inconsistent clinical responses.[37,41,42] Treatment with tamoxifen, a selective ER modulator, was not effective in one case.[43]

Penicillamine-induced macromastia has been reported in patients receiving this penicillin-derived chelating agent for the treatment of rheumatoid arthritis,[44] and marked breast enlargement or "hypertrophy" has been observed in women with human immunodeficiency virus infection after treatment with indinavir, a protease inhibitor.[45]

ECTOPIC BREAST TISSUE

The primary milk line develops in the human embryo at 6-week gestation. This line forms a ridge of ectoderm joining the bases of the upper and lower limb buds on either side of the ventral trunk from the mid-axillae through the normal breasts and then inferiorly to the medial groins (Fig. 2.4A).[46] Eventually this ridge atrophies except in the thoracic region from which the orthotopic pair of breast originates. It is likely that any persistence of portions of the mammary ridge results in supernumerary breast tissue. In humans, the presence of multiple breasts, which are present in other mammalian species, may be regarded as atavistic—an evolutionary reversion.

Supernumerary breast tissue may assume multiple forms. Such tissue may be with or without glandular tissue, with or without an areola, or as an areola alone. Polythelia (G. *polys*: many, *thele*: nipple) can be identified at birth; however, supernumerary breast glandular tissue becomes apparent only upon attainment of puberty or with pregnancy.

Ectopic (Gk. *ektopos*: out of place) *breast tissue* occurs along the milk lines, extending bilaterally. In women, the inferior extensions of the milk lines traverse the vulva bilaterally. A study of neonates revealed ectopic or supernumerary nipples in 49 of 2,035 infants (2.4%).[47] Male and female infants were equally affected. Clinically, ectopic breasts are encountered in 1% to 6% of women and considerably less frequently in men.[46,48–50] Approximately 6% of reported cases of ectopic breasts or supernumerary nipples have a familial association, apparently the result of one or more autosomal dominant genes that interfere with regression of the mammary ridges during gestation.[51–54] Male-to-male inheritance has been reported.[55] In one instance, the condition consisted of bilateral axillary breasts limited to females in two generations.[53] Another report described a male child who had accessory breasts on the thorax and abdomen along the milk lines and whose mother also had accessory breast tissue.[51] A study of 156 patients with aberrant mammary tissue diagnosed in a dermatology clinic revealed that 18 patients (11.5%) had a relative with the same condition.[56] Other instances of familial functional ectopic axillary breasts have been reported.[57]

The majority of patients with clinically apparent ectopic breast tissue have unilateral axillary involvement. Bilateral axillary breasts are the second most frequent presentation. Thoracic, abdominal, inguinal, and vulvar ectopic breasts, whether isolated, multiple, or in conjunction with axillary breast tissue, are much less frequent. Polythelia has been associated with a variety of congenital abnormalities, most commonly those of the urogenital system.[58] In a case-control study, 11 of 166 pediatric patients with genitourinary anomalies had polythelia versus 2 of 182 control-group patients (6.6% vs. 1.1%, $p < 0.05$).[59] However, this relationship has not been confirmed by other investigators.[56] Kenny et al.[47] found ultrasound evidence of a renal abnormality in only 1 of 49 neonates with ectopic nipples. Osswald et al.[57] reviewed reported studies of the relationship between accessory mammary tissue and various clinical syndromes.

The clinical presentation of ectopic breasts is highly variable. A complete supernumerary mammary gland with nipple–areola complex is uncommon.[60] Intra-areolar polythelia is a form of accessory breast in which two or more nipples, usually appearing deformed or "dysplastic," occur within the areola.[61] Bilateral intra-areolar polythelia with two nipples in each breast has also been reported.[62] The reported occurrence of intra-areolar polythelia in patients with neurofibromatosis[63] may be the result of mistaking cutaneous neurofibromas of the skin of the areola for accessory nipples.[64]

In some ectopic breasts, the glandular tissue is partly or entirely replaced by fat and may be diagnosed clinically as a lipoma, especially if the nipple and areola are unapparent.[48,65] Physiologic changes may occur during the menstrual cycle, causing swelling of the gland, and occasionally this can be painful. Lactation from ectopic breast tissue has been reported during pregnancy and the postpartum period.[46,66] Spontaneous galactorrhea from an ectopic axillary mammary gland with fully developed nipple was attributed to a pituitary microadenoma in a 28-year-old woman.[67] Her serum prolactin level decreased to normal after treatment with bromocriptine.

The presence of ectopic breast tissue can be confirmed, and lesions arising in these sites can be diagnosed by fine-needle aspiration.[68] The findings in an aspiration smear are variable, depending on the state of development of the tissue. Typically there are clumps and sheets of uniform, cytologically benign duct cells distributed in a monolayered fashion.[69] Proteinaceous secretion and small groups of acinar cells are found in the aspirate of axillary tissue from a lactating patient. Histologic sections of ectopic breast tissue reveal duct and lobular mammary structures, which may display physiologic changes (Fig. 2.3)

Ectopic nipples (Fig. 2.4B) are often located on the anterior chest above or below the normal breast. Most examples of multiple ectopic nipples (polythelia) occur along the milk line without the development of a breast. Ectopic breasts are more common on the left side.[49,60] Examination of 1,691 consecutive neonates in one study revealed ectopic nipples in 24 of 1,000 live births.[70] Others reported frequencies ranging from 1.7%[59] to 3.75%.[49] There are a number of reports of polythelia, with and without familial occurrence, involving men and women, associated with congenital

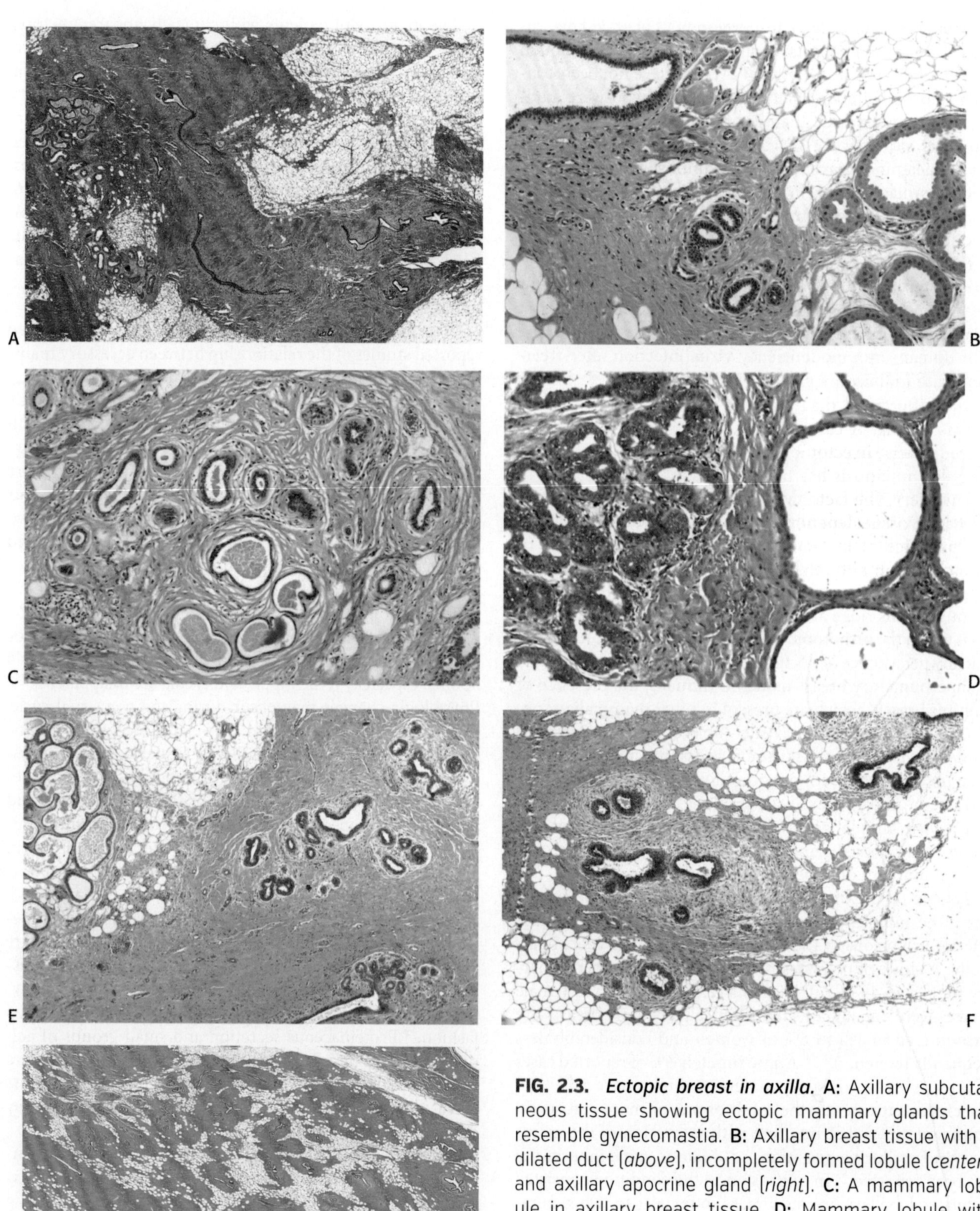

FIG. 2.3. ***Ectopic breast in axilla.*** **A:** Axillary subcutaneous tissue showing ectopic mammary glands that resemble gynecomastia. **B:** Axillary breast tissue with a dilated duct (*above*), incompletely formed lobule (*center*), and axillary apocrine gland (*right*). **C:** A mammary lobule in axillary breast tissue. **D:** Mammary lobule with mild epithelial hyperplasia (*left*) next to a dilated axillary apocrine gland. **E–G:** Gynecomastia-like hyperplasia in axillary ectopic breast tissue. Image **(E)** shows adnexal glands (*left*) and mammary glandular tissue (*right*). **F,G:** Periductal stromal hyperplasia resembling gynecomastia is present.

abnormalities.[71,72] An unusual syndrome is the familial occurrence of intra-areolar polythelia (dysplastic divided nipples) in hypoplastic breasts.[63] Mehregan[73] described the microscopic pathology of 51 examples of ectopic nipple among 360,000 consecutive skin biopsy specimens. The microscopic components included lactiferous ducts and epidermal thickening with pilosebaceous structures sometimes present. Almost all specimens included mammary glandular tissue in the deep dermis (Fig 2.4C).

Benign and malignant disease processes that can occur in the orthotopic breast can also arise in ectopic breast tissue. Syringomatous adenoma occurring in a supernumerary nipple located in the abdominal wall was reported by Page et al.[74] A variety of cutaneous adnexal neoplasms including eccrine syringoma, trichoepithelioma, and microcystic adnexal carcinoma could conceivably be considered in the differential diagnosis of benign glandular tumors in this setting. A carcinoma in the axilla of a male, suspected to arise in ectopic breast tissue, has been reported.[75] Nodular mucinosis has been described in a supernumerary nipple.[76] The fact that the lymphatic drainage of ectopic breast tissue depends on its location probably explains the presence of metastatic carcinoma in a contralateral axillary lymph node that derived from infiltrating lobular carcinoma arising in an accessory mammary gland on the upper anterior chest wall.[77] A full discussion of carcinoma arising in ectopic mammary tissue can be found in Chapter 33.

It has been hypothesized that mammary-like glands located in the anogenital region, specifically in the sulcus between the labia minora and majora, which have been hitherto considered to represent vestiges of the milk ridges, may actually embody a normal constituent of that region; however, such a distinction may be only of academic interest because all lesions that arise in these glands resemble their mammary counterparts.[78]

ABERRANT BREAST TISSUE

Aberrant (Latin. *aberrans*: abnormal) *breast tissue* is defined as mammary glandular parenchyma found in the region of, but beyond, the usual anatomic extent of the milk lines and breasts. Ducts and lobules that make up aberrant breast are structurally normal, but they are not as well organized as in normal or supernumerary breasts. Aberrant breast is, by definition, anatomically separate from the duct system of the breast and it differs in this respect from peripheral extensions

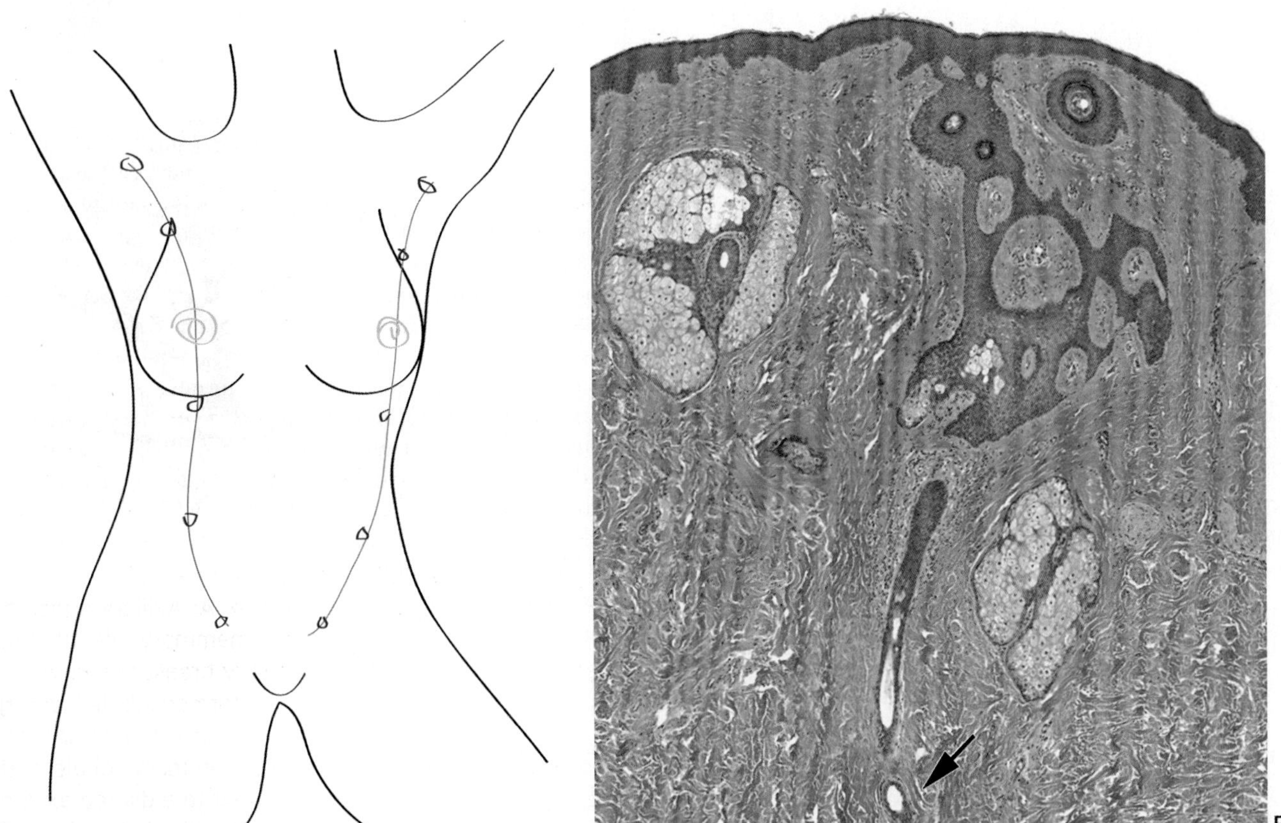

FIG. 2.4. **A:** The "milk line." Usual locations of ectopic nipple and breast along the milk line. **B,C:** Ectopic nipple and breast in axilla. Skin mound of ectopic nipple with underlying lactiferous duct (*arrow*) **(B)**. Deeper portion of dermis with lactiferous ducts and a lobule **(C)**. **D:** Ectopic breast in upper abdomen. Note skin mound with underlying lactiferous ducts and lobules.

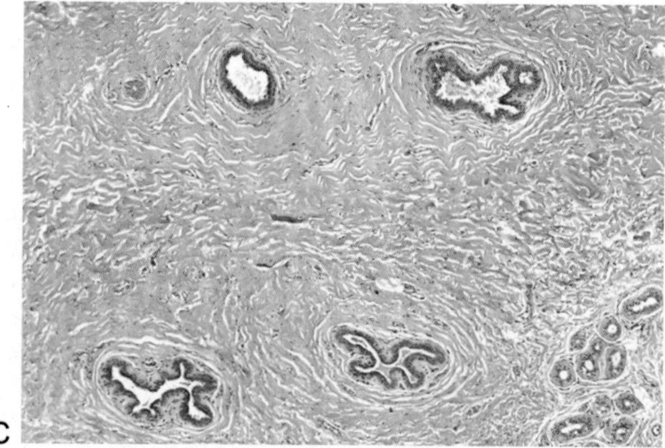

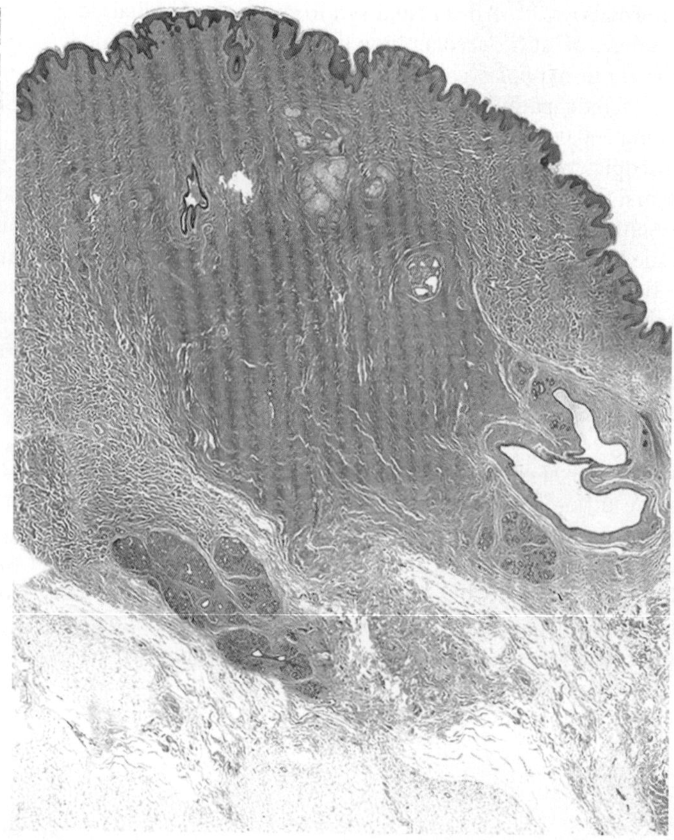

FIG. 2.4. *(Continued)*

of the breast.[79] Aberrant breast tissue does not form a nipple and/or areola and it is usually not clinically apparent unless it becomes the site of a pathologic process or physiologic change such as lactational hyperplasia (see Chapter 33).

The presence of heterotopic (Gk. *heteros*: other, *topos*: place) breast tissue outside the ventrally placed milk ridge, such as on the face, cannot be explained merely by the persistence of the ridge but may be the result of displacement or migration of the milk ridge anlage. The rather well-documented, if embryologically confounding, presence of an ectopic nipple has been reported in the sole of the right foot.[80] The migration theory would explain heterotopic breast-type epithelial inclusion in the atrial tissue of the surgically explanted native heart of a 72-year-old transplant recipient.[81]

THE TRANSSEXUAL BREAST

Female-to-male transsexual conversion involves prolonged androgen administration, which usually begins prior to mastectomy. When compared with normal female breast tissue from reduction mammoplasty operations, the androgen-treated breast had more frequent calcifications.[82] The breast tissue displays stromal collagenization and atrophy of ductal–lobular structures (Fig. 2.5A–C). Cysts and apocrine metaplasia may be present. The expression of estrogen and progesterone receptors and gross cystic disease fluid protein-15 was not significantly different in transsexual breast specimens compared with normal breast specimens.

Male-to-female transsexuals undergo surgical or chemical castration and estrogen therapy. Chemical castration with cyproterone, a progestational agent, is accomplished by blocking ARs. Breast tissue obtained from six patients after 18 months of combined therapy revealed well-developed lobular structures in all cases and pregnancy-like hyperplasia in two patients.[83] Marked reduction of glandular tissue was observed in 93% of breasts examined after long-term testosterone administration in female-to-male transsexuals.[84] Breast carcinoma has been reported in male-to-female transsexuals[85] ; however, proliferative epithelial lesions, including intraductal papilloma, can be encountered in this setting particularly after estrogen therapy (Fig. 2.5D).

The transsexual breast can also be a host to a variety of ailments resulting from cosmetic alterations of the breasts achieved by either surgical or nonsurgical means. Chen et al.[86] described a case of mastitis secondary to self-injection of petroleum jelly in a transsexual.

BREAST ASYMMETRY AND CANCER LATERALITY

Some degree of asymmetry of the normal breasts is nearly universal,[87] and breast carcinoma also has an asymmetrical distribution, being more common in the left than in the right breast. It has been estimated that there is a 5% greater likelihood for breast carcinoma to develop in the left breast and this preferential localization approaches 10% in the lower

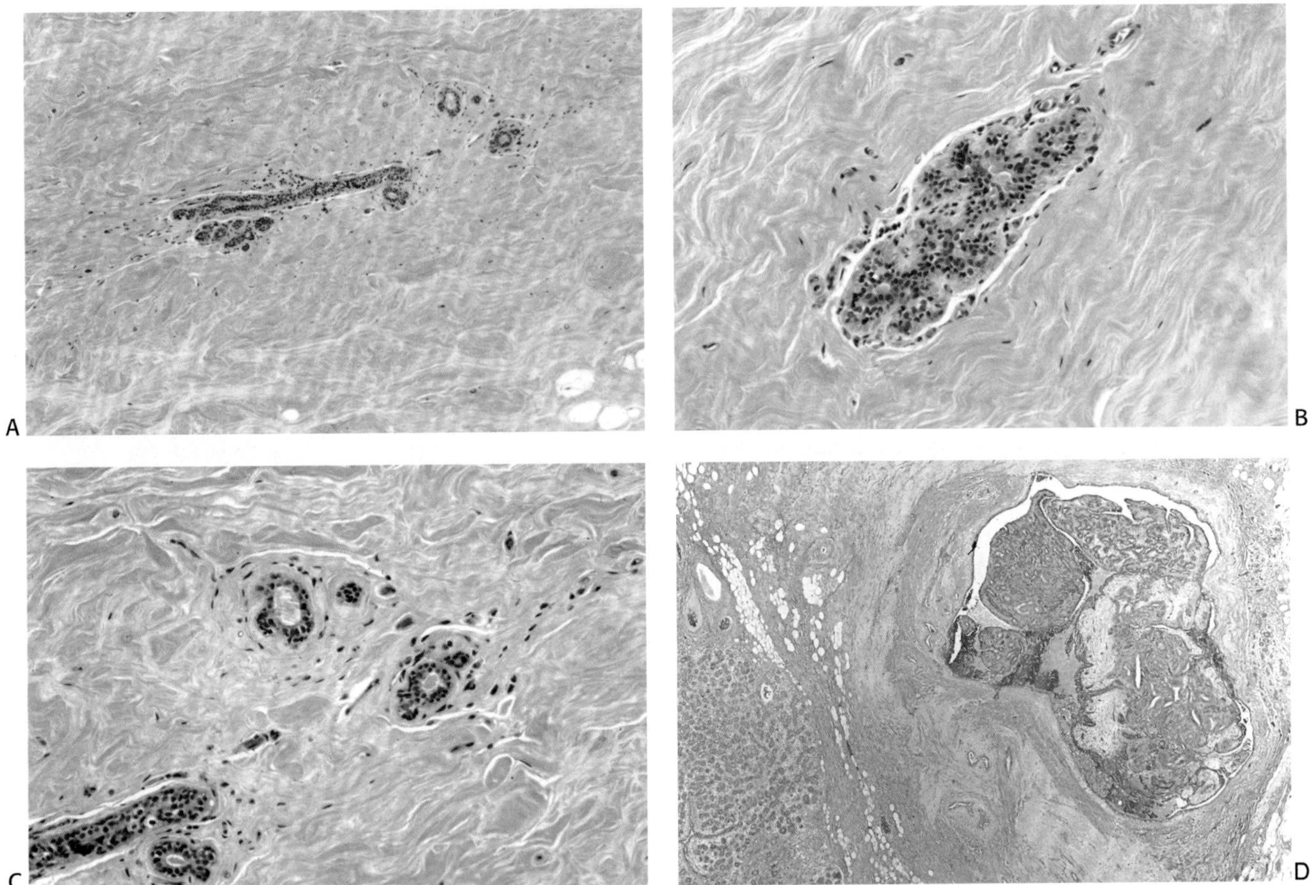

FIG. 2.5. A–C: Male-female transsexual breast. Collagenized stroma with atrophy of ducts and lobules. **D:** Intraductal papilloma in a male-female transsexual breast after estrogen therapy. Note the well-developed mammary lobular unit (lower left).

quadrants.[88,89] Left-sided predominance is even stronger among men.[88,90]

A study by Senie et al.[91] of laterality in 980 consecutive women with unilateral breast carcinoma revealed a left/right ratio of 1.26. Among patients with asynchronous bilateral carcinoma, the left breast was more often the first to be affected and when the carcinomas presented simultaneously, the larger tumor was more often in the left breast. A significant association was found between left-sided presentation and all histologic types except medullary carcinoma. Left breast carcinoma was more frequent among parous than among nulliparous women, especially among those 40 years or older. This report included an analysis of estimated left and right breast volumes in 174 asymptomatic women based on bilateral mammograms that revealed a left/right ratio of 1.23. The left predominance was present in patients older than 35 years who were stratified in 10-year increments. Other studies cited by Senie et al.[91] reported left/right ratios ranging from 0.97 to 1.18.

In an age-matched mammographic study, Scutt et al.[92] showed that more breast volume asymmetry was detected in 250 women with breast cancer than in an equal number of women without breast carcinoma. In a subsequent report, Scutt et al.[93] demonstrated that mammographically calculated breast volume asymmetry was greater in 252 healthy women who later developed breast carcinoma than in 252 women who did not develop breast carcinoma.

Although it seems reasonable to associate left-sided predominance with greater left breast size, it is important to recall that carcinoma develops from the mammary epithelium. Measurements of breast size or volume generally do not provide a quantitative estimate of glandular tissue. To address this issue, Sasano et al.[94] attempted to measure the glandular and total volume of the left breasts of Japanese women in Japan and Hawaii. They reported that the volume of glandular tissue remained unchanged, whereas total breast volume decreased with advancing age in Japanese women and that this effect was not clearly evident among Hawaiian women. Since Sasano et al.[94] could not distinguish between stromal and glandular tissue, these observations raise the possibility that differences in volume might reflect the adipose tissue content of the breasts rather than the stromal–epithelial component.

In addition to differences in breast size, there is evidence to suggest that the breasts of an individual differ in their responses to various stimuli, such as hormones. Differential breast sensitivity is manifested in physiologic and pathologic conditions. Asymmetrical breast hypertrophy has been observed among male and female neonates.[95] This is thought to indicate unequal response of the mammary glands to the hormonal environment *in utero*. Although regression generally occurs within a few weeks of birth, differential sensitivity might be expected to persist. Geschickter[95] also reported that some girls with asymmetric breast growth at puberty had a history of unequal breast size at birth. These observations suggest that differences in sensitivity might be unapparent except during periods of heightened hormonal stimulation such as puberty[96] or pregnancy.

Fluctuations in breast size occur under normal physiologic conditions in adult women. Breast enlargement associated with menses is a widely recognized phenomenon.[97] Although volume alterations during the menstrual cycle are in part due to changes in interstitial fluid, vascular volume, and stroma, epithelial changes also occur (see Chapter 1). More profound glandular growth occurs during pregnancy and lactation, at which time asymmetric breast enlargement is frequently encountered.

A review of somatic asymmetry during embryonic development by Wilting and Hagedorn[98] provides evidence to support the idea that developmental factors could play a significant role in the left-sided predominance of breast carcinoma. Determination of laterality takes place at an early stage in gestation, possibly creating circumstances that make the left breast slightly more susceptible to factors that promote asymmetric development, asymmetric responsiveness of stimuli and to mammary carcinogenesis. As outlined in some detail by Wilting and Hagedorn,[98] progress has been made in unraveling the molecular control of the determination of laterality involving growth and transcription factors some of which are also known to contribute to tumor progression. Future studies may well uncover a link between the asymmetric occurrence of breast carcinoma, the molecular controls of laterality and breast development during embryogenesis, and the responsiveness of breast tissues to oncogenic events.

REFERENCES

Hypoplasia and Amastia

1. Pierre M, Bureau H. A propos de deux case d'absence congenitale d'une glande mammaire. *Ann Chir Plast* 1960;5:137.
2. Trier WC. Complete breast absence. Case report and review of the literature. *Plast Reconstr Surg* 1965;36:430–439.
3. Kowlessar M, Orti E. Complete breast absence in siblings. *Am J Dis Child* 1968;115:91–92.
4. Goldenring H, Crelin ES. Mother and daughter with bilateral congenital amastia. *Yale J Biol Med* 1961;33:466.
5. Zilli L, Stephani G. Unilateral agenesis of the pectoralis muscles associated with mammary hypoplasia. *Friuli Med* 1960;15:1522.
6. Breslau-Siderius EJ, Toonstra J, Baart JA, et al. Ectodermal dysplasia, lipoatrophy, diabetes mellitus, and amastia: a second case of the AREDYLD syndrome. *Am J Med Genet* 1992;44:374–377.
7. Formigón M, Alsina MM, Mascaró JM, et al. Becker's nevus and ipsilateral breast hypoplasia androgen-receptor study in two patients. *Arch Dermatol* 1992;128:992–993.
8. Glinick SE, Alper JC, Bogaars H, et al. Becker's melanosis: associated abnormalities. *J Am Acad Dermatol* 1988;9:509–514.
9. Becker SW. Concurrent melanosis and hypertrichosis in distribution of nevus unis lateris. *Arch Dermatol Syphil* 1949;60:155–160.
10. Moore JA, Schosser RH. Becker's melanosis and hypoplasia of the breast and pectoralis major muscle. *Pediatr Dermatol* 1985;3:34–37.
11. Sharma R, Mishra A. Becker's naevus with ipsilateral areolar hypoplasia in three males. *Br J Dermatol* 1997;136:471–472.
12. Person JR, Longcope C. Becker's nevus: an androgen-mediated hyperplasia with increased androgen receptors. *J Am Acad Dermatol* 1984;10:235–238.
13. Franceschini P, Vardeu MP, Dalforno L, et al. Possible relationship between ulnar-mammary syndrome and split hand with aplasia of the ulna syndrome. *Am J Med Genet* 1992;44:807–812.
14. Gilly E. Absence complête des mammeles chez une femme mere. Atrophie du membre superieur droit. *Courier Med* 1882;32:27–28.
15. Schinzel A. Ulnar-mammary syndrome. *J Med Genet* 1987;24:778–781.
16. Davenport TG, Jerome-Majewski LA, Papaioannou VE. Mammary gland, limb, and yolk sac defects in mice lacking Tbx3, the gene mutated in human ulnar mammary syndrome. *Development* 2003;130:2263–2273.
17. Linden H, Williams R, King J, et al. Ulnar mammary syndrome and TBX3: expanding the phenotype. *Am J Med Genet A* 2009;149A:2809–2812.
18. Shamberger RC, Welch KJ, Upton III J. Surgical treatment of thoracic deformity in Poland's syndrome. *J Pediatr Surg* 1989;24:760–765.
19. Fukushima T, Otake T, Yashima R, et al. Breast cancer in two patients with Poland's Syndrome. *Breast Cancer* 1998;6:127–130.
20. Zhang F, Qi X, Xu Y, et al. Breast cancer and Poland's syndrome: a case report and literature review. *Breast J* 2011;17:196–200.
21. Nelson MM, Cooper CK. Congenital defects of the breast—an autosomal dominant trait. *S Afr Med J* 1982;61:434–436.
22. Hosokawa K, Hata Y, Yano K, et al. Unilateral athelia with a subcutaneous dermoid cyst. *Plast Reconstr Surg* 1987;80:732–733.
23. Fürst CJ, Lundell M, Ahlbäck SO, et al. Breast hypoplasia following irradiation of the female breast in infancy and early childhood. *Acta Oncol* 1989;28:519–523.
24. Kolar J, Bek V, Vrabec R. Hypoplasia of the growing breast after contact x-ray therapy for cutaneous angiomas. *Arch Dermatol* 1967;96:427–430.
25. Haramis HT, Collins RE. Unilateral breast atrophy. *Plast Reconstr Surg* 1995;95:916–919.
26. Funicello A, De Sandre R, Salloum L, et al. Infiltrating ductal carcinoma of the hypomastic breast: a case report. *Am Surg* 1998;64:1037–1039.

Macromastia

27. Dafydd H, Roehl KR, Phillips LG, et al. Redefining gigantomastia. *J Plast Reconstr Aesthet Surg* 2011;64:160–163.
28. Sagot P, Mainguená C, Barrière P, et al. Virginal breast hypertrophy at puberty: a case report. *Eur J Obstet Gynecol Reprod Biol* 1990;34:289–292.
29. Hugh JC, Friedman MH, Danyluk JM, et al. Absence of estrogen receptors in a case of virginal hypertrophy of the breasts related to oral contraceptives. *Breast Dis* 1993;6:143–148.
30. Jabs AD, Frantz AG, Smith-Vaniz A, et al. Mammary hypertrophy is not associated with increased estrogen receptors. *Plast Reconstr Surg* 1990;86:64–66.
31. Beischer NA, Hueston JH, Pepperell RJ. Massive hypertrophy of the breasts in pregnancy: report of 3 cases and review of the literature, "never think you have seen everything." *Obstet Gynecol* 1989;44:234–243.
32. Ship AG, Shulman J. Virginal and gravid mammary gigantism—recurrence after reduction mammoplasty. *Br J Plast Surg* 1971;24:396–401.
33. Williams PC. Massive hypertrophy of the breasts and axillary breasts in successive pregnancies. *Am J Obstet Gynecol* 1957;74:1326–1341.
34. Leis SN, Palmer B, östberg G. Gravid macromastia: case report. *Scand J Plast Reconstr Surg* 1974;8:247.
35. Nolan JJ. Gigantomastia. Report of a case. *Obstet Gynecol* 1962;19:526.
36. Barreto AU. Juvenile mammary hypertrophy. *Plast Reconstr Surg* 1991;87:583–584.
37. Kullander S. Effect of 2 Br-alpha-ergocryptin (CB 154) on serum prolactin and the clinical picture in a case of progressive gigantomastia in pregnancy. *Ann Chir Gynaecol* 1976;65:227.
38. Lewison EF, Jones GS, Trimble FH, et al. Gigantomastia complicating pregnancy. *Surg Gynecol Obstet* 1960;110:215.
39. Wølner-Hanssen P, Palmer B, Sjöberg NO, et al. Case report. Gigantomastia. *Acta Obstet Gynecol Scand* 1981;60:525.
40. Van Heerden JA, Gharib H, Jackson IT. Pseudohyperparathyroidism secondary to gigantic mammary hypertrophy. *Arch Surg* 1988;123:80–82.
41. Taylor PJ, Cumming DC, Corenblum B. Successful treatment of D-penicillamine-induced breast gigantism with danazol. *Br Med J* 1981;282:362.
42. Szczurowicz A, Szymula A. Gravidic macromastia. A problem for the patient and for the doctor. *Clin Exp Obstet Gynecol* 1996;23:177–180.

43. Hedberg K, Karlsson K, Lindstedt G. Gigantomastia during pregnancy: effect of a dopamine agonist. *Am J Obstet Gynecol* 1979;133:928–931.
44. Wolf Y, Pauzner D, Groutz A, et al. Gigantomastia complicating pregnancy. Case report and review of the literature. *Acta Obstet Gynecol Scand* 1995;74:159–163.
45. Lui A, Karter D, Turett G. Another case of breast hypertrophy in a patient treated with indinavir. *Clin Infect Dis* 1998;26:1482.

Ectopic Breast Tissue

46. De Cholnoky T. Supernumerary breast. *Arch Surg* 1939;39:926–941.
47. Kenny RD, Filippo JK, Black EB1. Supernumerary nipples and anomalies in neonates. *Am J Dis Child* 1987;141:987–988.
48. DeCholnoky T. Accessory breast tissue in the axilla. *NY State J Med* 1951;5:2245–2248.
49. Iwai T. A statistical study of the polymastia of the Japanese. *Lancet* 1907;2:753–759.
50. Petrek J, Rosen PP, Robbins GF. Carcinoma of aberrant breast tissue. *Clin Bull* 1980;10:13–15.
51. Cellini A, Offidavi A. Familial supernumerary nipples and breasts. *Dermatology* 1992;185:56–58.
52. Leung AKC. Familial supernumerary nipples. *Am J Med Genet* 1988;31:631–635.
53. Weinberg SK, Motulsky AG. Aberrant axillary breast tissue: a report of a family with six affected women in two generations. *Clin Genet* 1976;10:325–328.
54. Leung AK, Robson WL. Polythelia. *Int J Dermatol* 1989;284:429–433.
55. Tsukahara M, Uchida M, Uchino S, et al. Male to male transmission of supernumerary nipples. *Am J Med Genet* 1997;69:194–195.
56. Urbani CE, Betti R. Familial aberrant mammary tissue: a clinicoepidemiological survey of 18 cases. *Dermatology* 1995;190:207–209.
57. Osswald SS, Osswald MB, Elston M. Ectopic breasts: familial functional axillary breasts and breast cancer arising in an axillary breast. *Cutis* 2011;87:300–304.
58. Meggyessy V, Mehes K. Association of supernumerary nipples with renal anomalies. *J Pediatr* 1987;111:412–413.
59. Ferrara P, Giorgio V, Vitelli O, et al. Polythelia: still a marker of urinary tract anomalies in children? *Scand J Urol Nephrol* 2009;43:47–50.
60. Kajava Y. The proportions of supernumerary nipples in the Finnish population. *Duodecim* 1915;31:143–170.
61. Brightmore T. Bilateral paired nipples. *Br J Surg* 1972;59:55–57.
62. Onesti MG, Anniboletti T, Spinelli G, et al. Bilateral intra-areolar polythelia: report of a rare case. *Aesthetic Plast Surg* 2010;34:381–384.
63. Rintala A, Norio R. Familial intra-areolar polythelia with mammary hypoplasia. *Scand J Plast Reconstr Surg* 1982;16:287–291.
64. Haagensen CD. Anatomy of the mammary gland. *In: Diseases of the breast.* 3rd ed. Philadelphia: WB Saunders, 1986:1–46.
65. Shrotria S, Ghilchik MW. Axillary accessory breasts: a clinicopathological study of 35 patients with axillary masses. *Breast Dis* 1994;7:43–52.
66. O'Hara MF, Page DL. Adenomas of the breast and ectopic breast under lactational influences. *Hum Pathol* 1985;16:707–712.
67. Ünlü;hizaraci K, Bayram F, öztürk M, et al. Unusual presentation of prolactinoma with spontaneous galactorrhoea from ectopic breast tissue. *Clin Endocrinol* 1998;49:136.
68. Das DK, Gupta SK, Mathew SV, et al. Fine needle aspiration cytologic diagnosis of axillary accessory breast tissue, including its physiologic changes and pathologic lesions. *Acta Cytol* 1994;38:130–135.
69. Dey P, Karmakar T. Fine needle aspiration cytology of accessory axillary breasts and their lesions. *Acta Cytol* 1994;38:915–916.
70. Mimouni F, Merlob P, Reisner SH. Occurrence of supernumerary nipples in newborns. *Am J Dis Child* 1983;137:952–953.
71. Hersh JH, Bloom AS, Cromer AO, et al. Does a supernumerary nipple/renal field defect exist? *Am J Dis Child* 1987;141:989–991.
72. Toumbis-Ioannou E, Cohen PR. Familial polythelia. *J Am Acad Dermatol* 1994;30:667–668.
73. Mehregan AH. Supernumerary nipple. A histologic study. *J Cutan Pathol* 1981;8:96–104.
74. Page R, Dittrich L, King R, et al. Syringomatous adenoma of the nipple occurring within a supernumerary breast: a case report. *J Cutan Pathol* 2009;36:1206–1209.
75. Takeyama H, Takahashi H, Tabei I, et al. Malignant neoplasm in the axilla of a male: suspected primary carcinoma of an accessory mammary gland. *Breast Cancer* 2010;17:151–154.
76. Manglik K, Berlingeri-Ramos AC, Boroumand N, et al. Nodular mucinosis of the breast in a supernumerary nipple: case report and review of the literature. *J Cut Pathol* 2010;37:1178–1181.
77. Capobanco G, Spaliviero B, Dessole S, et al. Lymph node axillary metastasis from occult infiltrating lobular carcinoma arising in accessory breast: MRI diagnosis. *Breast J* 2007;13:305–307.
78. Kazakov DV, Spagnolo DV, Stewart CJ, et al. Fibroadenoma and phyllodes tumors of anogenital mammary-like glands: a series of 13 neoplasms including mammary-type juvenile fibroadenoma, fibroadenoma with lactation changes, and neurofibromatosis-associated pseudoangiomatous stromal hyperplasia with multinucleated giant cells. *Am J Surg Pathol* 2010;34:95.

Aberrant Breast Tissue

79. Hicken NF. Mastectomy: clinical and pathological study demonstrating why most mastectomies result in incomplete removal of the mammary gland. *Arch Surg* 1940;40:6–14.
80. Balakrishnan T, Madaree A. Case report: ectopic nipple on the sole of the foot, an unexplained anomaly. *J Plast Reconstr Aesthet Surg* 2010;63:2188–2190.
81. Sasaki K, Parwani AV, Demetris AJ, et al. Heterotopic breast epithelial inclusion of the heart: report of a case. *Am J Surg Pathol* 2010;34:1555–1559.

The Transsexual Breast

82. Burgess HE, Shousha S. An immunohistochemical study of the long-term effects of androgen administration on female-to-male transsexual breast: a comparison with normal female breast and male breast showing gynaecomastia. *J Pathol* 1993;170:37–43.
83. Kanhai RCJ, Hage JJ, van Diest PJ, et al. Short-term and long-term histologic effects of castration and estrogen treatment on breast tissue of 14 male-to-female transsexuals in comparison with two chemically castrated men. *Am J Surg Pathol* 2000;24:74–80.
84. Grynberg M, Fanchin R, Dubost G, et al. Histology of genital tract and breast tissue after long-term testosterone administration in a female-to-male transsexual population. *Reprod Biomed Online* 2010;20:553–558.
85. Ganly I, Taylor EW. Breast cancer in a trans-sexual man receiving hormone replacement therapy. *Br J Surg* 1995;82:341.
86. Chen M, Yalamanchili C, Hamous J, et al. Acute inflammatory response of the male breasts secondary to self-injection of petroleum jelly: a case report. *South Med J.* 2008;101:422–424.

Breast Asymmetry and Cancer Laterality

87. Chan WY, Mathur B, Slade-Sharman D, et al. Developmental breast asymmetry. *Breast J* 2011;17:391–398.
88. Perkins CI, Hotes J, Kohler BA, et al. Association between breast cancer laterality and tumor location, United States 1994–1998. *Cancer Causes Control* 2004;15:637–645.
89. Roychoudhuri R, Putcha V, Moller H. Cancer and laterality: a study of five major paired organs (UK). *Cancer Causes Control* 2006;17:655–662.
90. Goodman MT, Tung KH, Wilkens LR. Comparative epidemiology of breast cancer among men and women in the US, 1996 to 2000. *Cancer Causes Control* 2006;17:127–136.
91. Senie RT, Rosen PP, Lesser ML, et al. Epidemiology of breast carcinoma II: factors related to the predominance of left-sided disease. *Cancer* 1980;46:1705–1713.
92. Scutt D, Manning JT, Whitehouse GH, et al. The relationship between breast asymmetry, breast size and the occurrence of breast cancer. *Br J Radiol* 1997;70:1017–1021.
93. Scutt D, Lancaster GA, Manning JT. Breast asymmetry and predisposition to breast cancer. *Breast Cancer Res* 2006;8:R14.
94. Sasano N, Tatenoh H, Stemmerman G. Volume and hyperplastic lesions of breasts of Japanese women in Hawaii and Japan. *Prev Med* 1978;7:196–204.
95. Geschickter D. *Diseases of the breast Philadelphia: Lippincott,* 1945:111–119.
96. Marshall WA, Tanner JM. Variations in patterns of pubertal changes in girls. *Arch Dis Child* 1969;44:291–303.
97. Mulligan D, Drife JO, Short RV. Changes in breast volume during normal menstrual cycle and after oral contraceptives. *Br Med J* 1975;11:494–496.
98. Wilting J, Hagedorn M. Left-right asymmetry in embryonic development and breast cancer: common molecular determinants? *Curr Med Chem* 2011;18:5519–5527.

CHAPTER 3

Inflammatory and Reactive Tumors

SYED A. HODA

FAT NECROSIS

Fat necrosis in the breast may result from trauma, but it is frequently a consequence of surgery or radiation therapy. Prior to breast-conserving therapy, no specific antecedent exogenous cause was reported in many instances. Trauma was described as the cause of fat necrosis in 32% of patients reported by Haagensen[1] and in 44% of women reported by Adair and Munger.[2] The observation that the clinical features of fat necrosis mimic carcinoma was first emphasized by Lee and Adair[3] in 1920.

Clinical Presentation

Traumatic fat necrosis occurs more frequently in overweight women and in women with pendulous breasts. Haagensen[1] reported a mean age of 52 years with a range from 27 to 80 years. The youngest patient in the Adair and Munger series[2] was 14 years old, with a median age in the 50s.

Patients typically present with a painless mass located superficially in the breast, accompanied by retraction or dimpling of the overlying skin if the lesion is superficially located. The skin may be thickened clinically and radiologically. Fat necrosis most frequently occurs in the subareolar and periareolar regions, but any part of the breast may be affected. Tumors formed by fat necrosis average 2 cm in diameter. They are firm and relatively circumscribed on palpation. The clinical problem of distinguishing between fat necrosis and recurrent or *de novo* carcinoma is especially difficult in patients who have undergone breast-conserving surgery and radiation therapy.[4] Fat necrosis has been reported after various forms of radiation therapy, including external beam, iridium implantation, mammosite, and intraoperative radiation. Massive fat necrosis of the breast has been described as a complication of secondary hyperparathyroidism with mural arterial calcification.[5]

Imaging

Mammographic findings were initially characterized by Leborgne.[6] The manifestations of fat necrosis on mammography, ultrasound, and magnetic resonance imaging (MRI) depend upon its stage of evolution and can thus be highly variable.[7] Mammography usually reveals a spiculated, often poorly defined mass that may contain punctate or large irregular calcifications.[8] Less frequently, the lesion consists of a circumscribed, "oil-filled," partly calcified cyst.[6,9,10] Both patterns may coexist in a single lesion. Attachment to the skin with dimpling and thickening of the skin may be evident on the mammogram. Fat necrosis with calcifications has been detected by mammography in axillary lymph nodes.[11] Sonography demonstrates a discrete mass in almost all cases.[12] The sonographic appearance is variable and is usually accompanied by distortion of the parenchymal architecture. Follow-up examination reveals evolution of the lesion, which decreases in size and becomes solid. On MRI, mammary fat necrosis can exhibit variable appearances and can be mistaken for carcinoma.[13,14] A "black hole" sign on MRI in certain sequences in such scans has been described as a potentially diagnostic finding.[15] Fat necrosis is among the most common causes of false-positive lesions on fludeoxyglucose positron emission tomography (PET) and PET–computerized tomography (CT) scans.[15] In some cases, correlation of clinical findings with mammography, sonography, and MRI is necessary to distinguish between fat necrosis and carcinoma.

Differential Diagnosis

The differential diagnosis of a xanthomatous (lipid-laden) cell infiltrate in the breast includes fat necrosis, granular cell tumor, histiocytoid and lipid-rich carcinomas, and Erdheim–Chester disease. The latter is an infrequent xanthomatous form of non-Langerhans cell histiocytosis that rarely involves the breast (see Chapter 40) and can be mistaken for fat necrosis histologically, especially if the initial clinical manifestation is a breast tumor.[16,17] Nonmammary subcutaneous nodules and osseous lesions are typically present as well. Microscopic examination reveals infiltrates of foamy histiocytes, plasma cells, Touton giant cells, and infrequent epithelioid granulomas. The histiocytes are reactive for CD68 but negative for S-100, CD1a, and cytokeratins.[16]

Gross Pathology

Early in its development, fat necrosis has the appearance of hemorrhage in indurated fat. After several weeks, the affected area becomes demarcated, forming a distinct yellow-gray and focally reddish tumor. Cystic degeneration may develop in the center, resulting in a cavity that contains oily fluid or necrotic fat. Calcification frequently develops in the cyst wall.

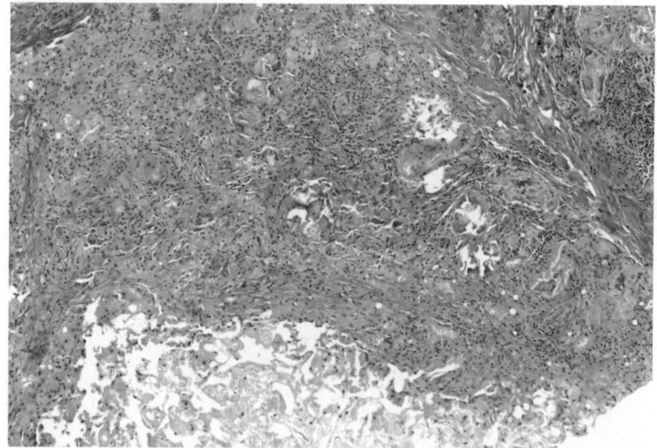

FIG. 3.1. ***"Spontaneous" fat necrosis.*** Histiocytes, giant cells, and hemosiderin deposits in necrotic fat. The patient underwent a needle core biopsy for a palpable mass that had formed a week after sudden onset of localized mastodynia.

Microscopic Pathology

The initial change in fat necrosis is disruption of fat cells accompanied by hemorrhage and an influx of histiocytes. Progression of the lesion is marked by the presence of multinucleated histiocytes and hemosiderin deposition (Fig. 3.1), and later by dystrophic calcification. A variable infiltrate of lymphocytes and plasma cells, sometimes with eosinophils, is present at this stage. Fibrosis develops peripherally as the lesion demarcates, enclosing an area of necrotic fat and cellular debris that may become cystic (Fig. 3.2). In late lesions, reactive inflammatory components replaced by fibrosis contract into a scar, and the tissue may ossify (Fig. 3.2). Loculated degenerated fat or oil (i.e., liquefied lipid) can persist for months or years within a cyst surrounded by such a scar. Squamous metaplasia can develop in the epithelium of ducts and lobules in the area of fat necrosis. Among patients who develop fat necrosis after radiation therapy, cytologic changes attributable to this treatment may be found in contiguous ducts, lobules, and blood vessels. Occasionally, the reactive histiocytic proliferation associated with the process of healing fat necrosis can simulate a spindle cell neoplasm. Such "cellular spindled histiocytic pseudotumors" express histiocyte-associated markers and are typically associated with chronic inflammation and multinucleated giant cells.[4]

Treatment

Excisional biopsy is required when the clinical and radiologic features resemble carcinoma. If there is a distinct history of trauma or prior surgery and characteristic radiologic findings of a demarcated cystic lesion with typical calcifications, excision may not be performed after the diagnosis has been established by fine-needle aspiration (FNA) or needle core biopsy. In such cases, the patient should be monitored by clinical examination and mammography to detect occult carcinoma that might be masked by coexisting fat necrosis.

HEMORRHAGIC NECROSIS AND ANTICOAGULANT THERAPY

Localized hemorrhagic necrosis of the skin and subcutaneous tissue occurs as a complication of some forms of anticoagulant therapy.[18] The first description of this condition in the breast was reported by Flood et al.[19] in 1943. Hemorrhagic necrosis of the breast most often occurs in middle-aged or elderly women treated for thrombophlebitis with warfarin (Coumadin). Within a week after anticoagulation therapy begins, the patient complains of pain and swelling accompanied with blue-black discoloration of the breast. The condition usually progresses despite discontinuation of anticoagulant medication or the administration of vitamin K, eventuating in gangrene of part or all of the breast.[20] After the area of necrosis has become demarcated, surgical treatment consists of local resection or mastectomy.

Hemorrhagic necrosis in the skin and subcutaneous tissue or in the breast has been associated specifically with warfarin anticoagulant therapy. The prothrombin time is usually within the therapeutic range. Heparin does not

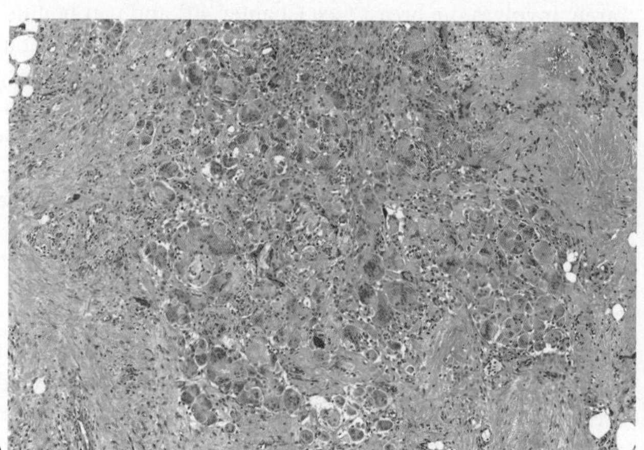

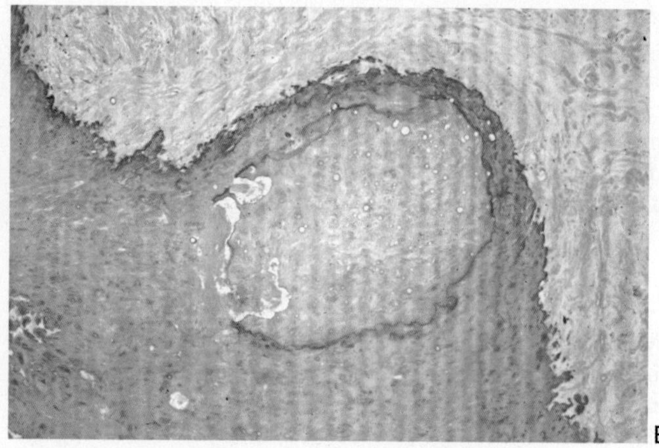

FIG. 3.2. ***Traumatic fat necrosis.*** **A:** Early organizing fat necrosis with numerous multinucleated histiocytes. The lesion is demarcated by fibrosis. **B:** Ossification in scar following fat necrosis.

appear to be a predisposing agent. The clinical features and histopathologic findings suggest a hypersensitivity reaction to the medication, affecting small vessels in the skin and subcutaneous tissue. It has been determined that this syndrome occurs in patients with heterozygous protein C deficiency. In this setting, Coumadin diminishes the formation of vitamin K–dependent coagulation factors, and it also interferes with the synthesis of proteins C and S, and vitamin K–dependent inhibitors of clotting.[21] In some patients, the net effect of these alterations is to promote thrombosis, a situation that leads to hemorrhagic necrosis. Histologic examination of the acutely affected tissue reveals hemorrhagic necrosis and infarction diffusely involving the skin, subcutaneous tissue, and breast parenchyma. Fibrin thrombi are present in small blood vessels, and neutrophils infiltrate the walls of arteries and veins.[22,23] At a later stage, fibrosis and granulomatous inflammation appear as part of the healing process. If due caution is exercised, needle core biopsy of the breast can be safely performed on patients on routine daily anticoagulant therapy, with bruising being the most common complication.[24] The risk of hematoma formation is reduced by using lidocaine with epinephrine for local anesthesia and by applying localized compression to the biopsy site for at least 5 minutes. The successful performance of needle core biopsy in spontaneous intramammary hemorrhage resulting from anticoagulant therapy in which malignancy is also a diagnostic consideration has been described.[25]

BREAST INFARCT

Clinical Presentation

The most frequent form of breast infarct occurs during pregnancy or postpartum. Infarction may develop in lactating glandular parenchyma or in a lactational adenoma. The lesion presents clinically as a discrete mass that is usually asymptomatic, although pain and tenderness are sometimes reported. Because of the association with pregnancy, breast infarcts usually occur in younger women. The firm mass produced by infarcted mammary parenchyma can suggest carcinoma clinically. Axillary lymph node enlargement may coexist with infarcts, presumably resulting from the inflammatory reaction to necrosis. Infarction of accessory breast tissue during pregnancy has been described.[26]

Robitaille et al.[27] found that mammary infarcts could be grouped into broad categories that included lesions that simulated carcinoma and those that did not suggest carcinoma. The former group included infarcts in sclerosing adenosis, papillomas, fibroadenomas, and in pregnancy. Infarcts that did not mimic carcinoma were associated with anticoagulant therapy, infections with abscess formation, and superficial thrombophlebitis.

Gross Pathology

The gross appearance of the excised infarcted tissue is variable. Hemorrhage is seen in lesions of recent onset, whereas older infarcts are typically characterized by one or more areas of relative pallor or yellow discoloration, sometimes bounded by a hyperemic border.

Microscopic Pathology

Microscopic findings are influenced by the duration of the infarct. Hemorrhage and ischemic degeneration with little or no inflammation characterize early lesions. Later stages feature coagulative necrosis with loss of nuclear detail, pallor, and retention of architectural integrity. Liquefactive necrosis is rarely encountered. Infarction is demarcated by a zone of granulation tissue with a variable inflammatory reaction, hemosiderin deposition, and fibrosis. Some authors have described organized or organizing thrombi in areas of infarction or in adjacent tissue,[28,29] but this has not been a constant finding.[30]

The specimen obtained by FNA from a mammary infarct that developed during pregnancy may present a challenging diagnostic problem. The nuclear atypia that reflects the physiologic hyperplasia of lactation may be accentuated in cells that are in early states of ischemic necrosis. Nuclear enlargement and hyperchromasia may be encountered in such cells. At a later stage, these cells will appear poorly preserved and fragmented.

Spontaneous infarction is a rare complication of a fibroadenoma,[31] and such a lesion may mimic carcinoma in imaging studies, especially ultrasonography.[32] "Worrisome" cytologic alterations on FNA from infarcted fibroadenomas can be encountered.[33] Infarction can occur in proliferative lesions other than fibroadenomas such as in florid sclerosing adenosis (Fig. 3.3). This is most likely to occur during pregnancy when the epithelium in sclerosing adenosis may exhibit pronounced hyperplasia, cytologic atypia, and mitotic activity.

Infarcted Papillomas

Papillomas are susceptible to partial or complete infarction, especially lesions in major lactiferous ducts. Infarction occurs in papillomas at any age, but it tends to be more frequent in postmenopausal women, and there is no association with

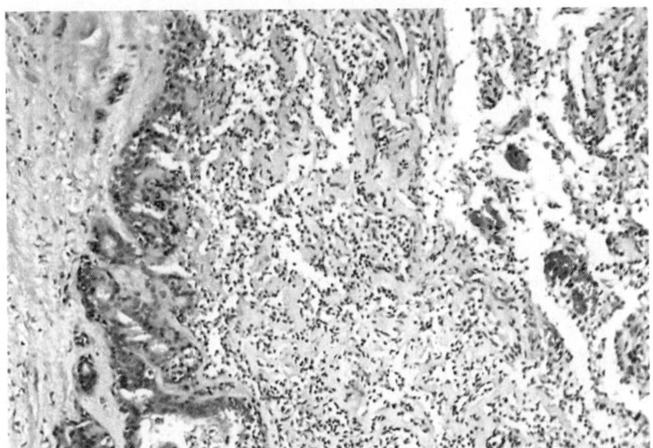

FIG. 3.3. ***Postpartum infarct in sclerosing adenosis.*** A zone of residual epithelium on the left borders on the infarct. Only the nuclei of myoepithelial cells remain in the infarct on the right to outline the spaces formerly occupied by adenosis glands.

pregnancy.[34] Bloody nipple discharge is the most frequent symptom of an infarcted papilloma with or without a mass. Pain is rarely reported. Although infarction of papillomas has been ascribed to ischemia, clinical factors predisposing to this alteration have rarely been documented. A 19-year-old woman with serous nipple discharge and hyperprolactinemia developed bloody nipple discharge after treatment with bromocriptine. Duct excision revealed a partially infarcted papilloma.[35]

Recently infarcted regions in a papilloma exhibit ischemic coagulative necrosis. Structural integrity is usually maintained in such foci, despite progressive loss of cytologic detail. At a late stage, fragmentation of superficial portions of the infarcted tissue occurs. Occasionally, portions of an infarcted papilloma are reduced to intraductal inflammatory polyps consisting of granulation tissue with little or no epithelium. Chronic ischemia and healing of infarcts are marked by fibrosis that may cause considerable distortion of residual entrapped epithelium, producing a pattern that can be mistaken histologically for carcinoma.[34] Squamous metaplasia sometimes develops in the reparative epithelium that proliferates in a papilloma after infarction, and dystrophic calcification may form in the infarcted tissue.[34]

The reliability of immunostaining for evaluating an infarcted papillary lesion is unpredictable and probably depends on the extent of decomposition. In some instances, immunoreactivity for cytokeratin and myoepithelial markers, especially p63, is surprisingly well preserved. When this occurs, it may be possible to "resurrect" the structure of the lesion to a considerable degree.

Infarcted Carcinomas

Infarcted carcinoma is most readily distinguished from infarction of a benign lesion if there is a residual intact component of *in situ* or invasive carcinoma.[36] (Fig. 3.4). The occurrence of rare instances of seemingly totally infarcted carcinoma is more problematic. Many of these lesions have a ghost architecture that is recognizable with a reticulin stain. A sclerotic or thrombosed blood vessel is sometimes identified in the surrounding tissue.[36] Whereas focal necrosis is considered to be an unfavorable prognostic feature of invasive carcinoma, as is encountered in centrally necrotic mammary carcinomas with the basal-like immunophenotype,[37] the prognosis of nearly or totally infarcted carcinoma is not well characterized. Two patients described by Jones et al.[36] had negative lymph nodes and were disease free 12 months after diagnosis.

Treatment and Prognosis

Biopsy, usually excision of the lesion, is often required for the diagnosis of a mammary infarct, although the findings in a needle core biopsy may be suggestive. Infarction occurs more often in benign papillary tumors than in papillary carcinoma. Instances of totally infarcted solid papillary

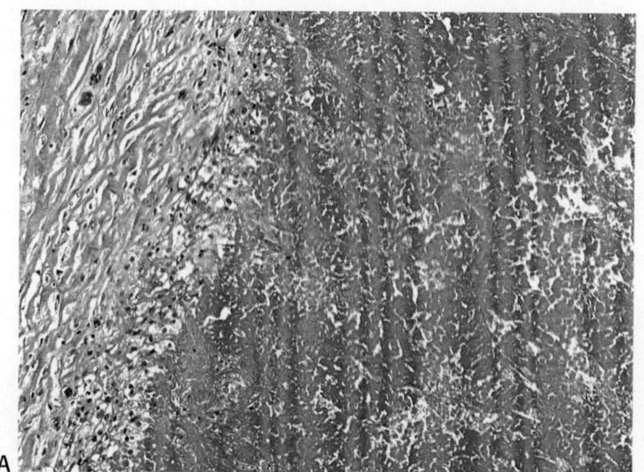

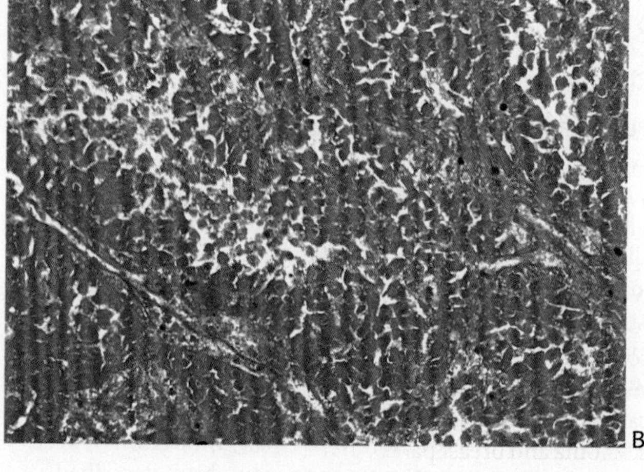

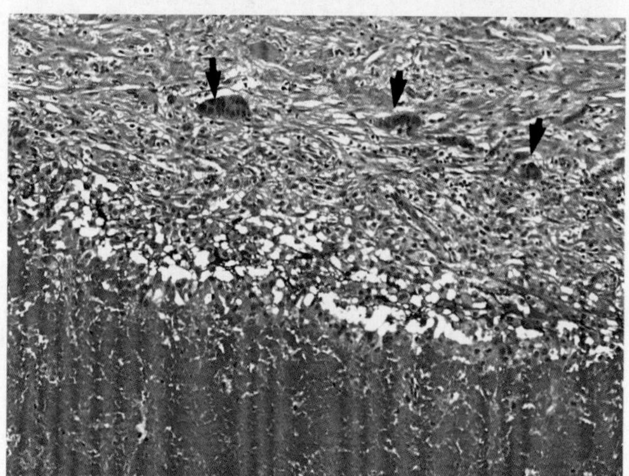

FIG. 3.4. ***Infarcted papillary tumor.*** **A:** The entire lesion is necrotic and surrounded by a granulomatous reaction. **B:** The ghost architecture of the tumor is evident. The abundant epithelial component suggests papillary carcinoma. **C:** Invasive carcinoma persisting in the wall of the tumor (*arrows*).

carcinoma have been encountered. In these cases, the nature of the tumor was determined from the characteristic pattern of fibrovascular stroma. Follow-up data for patients with totally infarcted carcinomas are anecdotal. A favorable prognosis would be expected for a patient with noninvasive, infarcted, solid papillary carcinoma.

Epithelial hyperplasia that is reparative may be found in or near infarcts. Squamous metaplasia also occurs in association with these lesions. There is no documented evidence that proliferative changes related to infarcts are associated with an increased risk for carcinoma.

INFLAMMATORY LESIONS IN PREGNANCY AND LACTATION

Puerperal Mastitis

Puerperal mastitis typically occurs within 2 to 3 weeks of the start of lactation and is usually the result of infection via the mammary duct system. The most common organism is *Staphylococcus aureus* transmitted from the skin or the infant.[38] Accumulation of milk in ducts and lobules creates a microenvironment that fosters bacterial growth. Without prompt antibiotic treatment, the condition may progress to form an abscess, and at a chronic stage, fistulas that require drainage can develop. The histologic appearance of specimens from these lesions depends on the chronicity of the process, varying from acute inflammation, which may be accompanied by focal necrosis, to organized chronic abscesses. Excisional biopsy may be required to control chronic lesions with fistula formation.

Mammary Infarction

Infarction of mammary tissue presents during pregnancy as a discrete, firm tumor that may or may not be tender. The lesion is usually detected in the third trimester or shortly after delivery. The affected area forms a tumor one or more centimeters in diameter that appears distinct from the surrounding hyperplastic parenchyma. Multiple infarcts are uncommon.[39] On cut surface, part or all of the tissue has the yellow color of coagulative necrosis. Grossly and microscopically, the distinction between infarction in a lactational fibroadenoma and breast parenchyma with lactational hyperplasia is not always clear. Infarcts that have been present for several weeks before detection are likely to be surrounded by a granulation tissue reaction in which calcification may occur.[39]

The pathogenesis of pregnancy-related infarcts is uncertain. Although the finding of thrombi in some cases suggests that this may be a factor, no consistent explanation for vascular occlusion has been established, and it is possible that the vascular changes are secondary to infarction initiated by some other mechanism such as localized vasospasm.

Galactoceles

Most galatoceles occur in adult women during pregnancy, but the lesion has been described in male and female infants.[40] A galactocele associated with chronic galactorrhea caused by a pituitary adenoma has been reported.[41] The tumors present as solitary or multiple circumscribed masses that may be unilateral or bilateral. They average about 2 cm in diameter, but galactoceles 5 cm or larger have been described.[41] Mammography reveals a circumscribed density that in many instances has a characteristic appearance consisting of a hypodense upper area and a lower area with density close to that of the surrounding tissue.[42,43] The interface tends to remain horizontal as the patient changes position. The two zones consist of lighter lipid-containing components above the water-based constituents of the fluid. Comparable differences in echogenicity are observed on ultrasound examination.[42]

Necrotic cells and nuclear debris, possibly accompanied by inflammatory cells, are seen in an FNA specimen.[44] Cells with hyperchromatic, atypical-appearing nuclei may suggest carcinoma, but in this inflammatory background, such changes should not be considered definitive. Birefringent crystals were found in the aspirate from one galactocele.[45] Excisional biopsy is diagnostic and provides adequate therapy.

On gross inspection, a galactocele is composed of cysts that contain fluid contents resembling milk and are lined by smooth simple epithelium. Inspissated secretion may be present in the form of soft caseous material. The cysts appear to be formed as a result of duct dilation, and, microscopically, they are lined by cuboidal or flat epithelial cells with cytoplasmic vacuolization owing to lipid accumulation (Fig. 3.5). Apocrine metaplasia may be seen.[40] When intact, the cysts are encompassed by a fibrous wall of varying thickness, with little or no inflammatory reaction. Leakage from a cyst elicits a chronic inflammatory reaction that may be accompanied by fat necrosis.

Most patients are treated by aspiration of the cyst contents. A milk fistula is a rare complication of incomplete surgical excision.[41]

Raynaud Phenomenon

Reynaud phenomenon has been described in the nipple, especially in breast-feeding women.[46] The resultant pain leads to cessation of breast-feeding. Clinical manifestations precipitated by cold and breast-feeding include pain, blanching of the nipple, as well as cracked nipples, ulcers, or blisters of the nipple surface.

PLASMA CELL MASTITIS

Clinical Presentation

The condition known as plasma cell mastitis (PCM) is an extreme form of periductal mastitis that features an intense plasma cell reaction to retained secretion in ducts. Ten patients described by Adair[47] were 29 to 44 years old (average age, 36 years), and all had been pregnant. The average interval between cessation of lactation and the onset of symptoms was 4 years. In the early phase, patients experience the acute onset of mild pain, tenderness, redness, and nipple discharge consisting usually of thick secretion. After the inflammatory symptoms

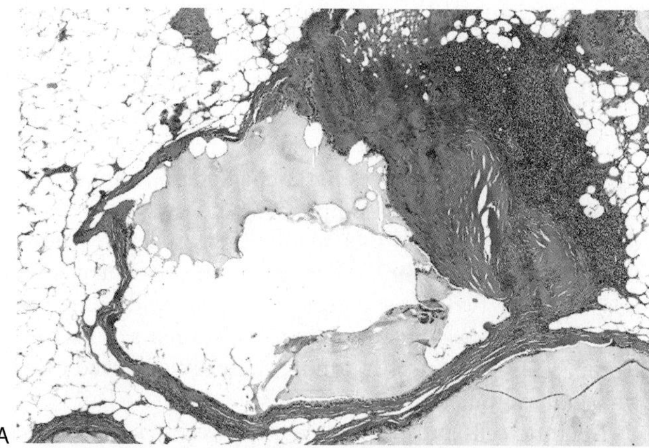

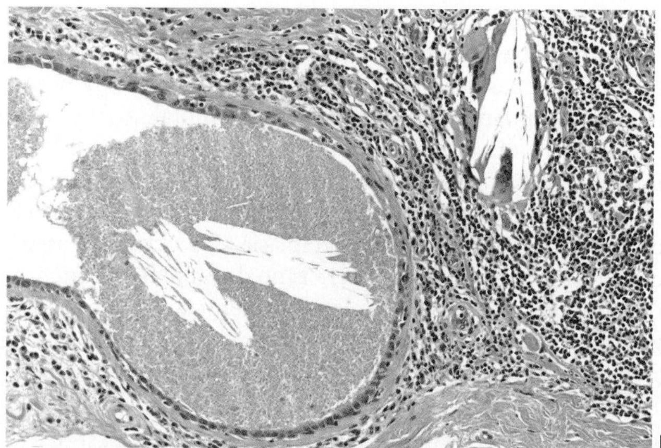

FIG. 3.5. ***Galactocele.*** **A:** Intact cysts. **B:** Cuboidal epithelium with apocrine-type cytoplasmic features lines the cystically dilated duct. Cholesterol crystals are present within and outside the galactocele.

subside, a firm-to-hard mass that can be several centimeters in diameter remains at the site. Nipple discharge usually persists, and nipple retraction is observed in the majority of patients. The mass occurs in the periphery of the breast or in a subareolar location. Axillary lymph nodes are often enlarged.

Gross Pathology

The affected ill-defined area of PCM consists of indurated mammary parenchyma in which there are dilated ducts containing thick, creamy secretion. Some of the affected ducts appear to be cysts. Punctate yellow or golden xanthomatous granulomas may be observed.

Microscopic Pathology

On histologic examination, the feature that distinguishes PCM is a marked, diffuse, plasma cell infiltrate surrounding ducts as well as the lobules. A histiocytic reaction, sometimes with granulomatous features, to desquamated epithelium and lipid material in the ducts is responsible for areas that appear grossly to be xanthomatous and for the comedo-like character of the duct contents[48] (Fig. 3.6). Lymphocytes and neutrophils are variably present, but not in sufficient numbers to obscure the plasma cell reaction. Periductal fibrosis and obliterative proliferation of granulation tissue are not prominent features of PCM.

Treatment and Prognosis

PCM in its acute and mature phases is difficult to distinguish clinically from mammary carcinoma.[49] Redness and edema in the early stage are suggestive of inflammatory carcinoma. The residual nontender mass is easily mistaken for carcinoma on palpation, and the radiologic findings may be interpreted as indicative of carcinoma, especially when calcifications are present. FNA biopsy yields a specimen consisting of inflammatory cells in which plasma cells and histiocytes are especially conspicuous. Hyperplastic epithelial cells that appear atypical can be mistaken for carcinoma in this setting. Similar difficulty is likely to be encountered if the tissue is examined by frozen section. Ultimately, the histologic distinction between PCM and high-grade intraductal carcinoma with central necrosis depends on careful analysis of permanent sections.

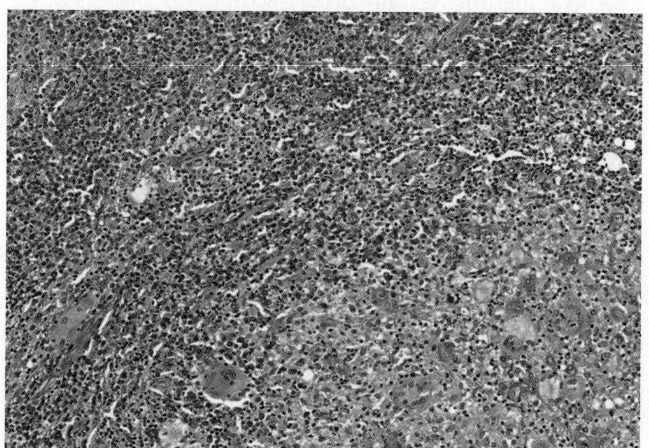

FIG. 3.6. ***So-called plasma cell mastitis.*** An intense infiltrate of lymphocytes and plasma cells surrounding a zone of histiocytic infiltration with xanthomatous features (*lower right*).

Excisional biopsy is recommended as treatment for PCM because cutaneous ulceration and fistulas may develop after the lesion has been incompletely removed. Generally, surgery to remove the mass is performed after the acute phase has subsided. On occasion, the acute phase of PCM may resolve without causing a persistent tumor.

MAMMARY DUCT ECTASIA

The term *mammary duct ectasia* (MDE) was introduced by Haagensen[50] in 1951, but the disease had been recognized at least 30 years earlier. In 1921, Bloodgood[51] included this condition, characterized as “diffuse dilatation of the ducts,” under the heading "chronic cystic mastitis," and he described assisting Halsted in operating on such a patient in 1897. At surgery, a clinically "indefinite palpable tumor beneath the nipple . . . proved to be a dilated duct with a thick wall about the size of a slate pencil (5 mm), tortuous and filled with a brown, granular mass." They did not regard this to be a malignant condition but ". . . concluded that it was safer to perform the complete operation for cancer." Bloodgood[52] later used the term *varicocele of the breast* for cases with prominent subareolar duct dilation. Other names such as mastitis obliterans and comedo mastitis[53] have not been as widely used as MDE, the preferred diagnostic term. The clinical and pathologic features of MDE, granulomatous lobular mastitis (GLM), and PCM are sufficiently different in most cases that these lesions should be distinguishable. In instances where the findings lack specificity, the condition may be diagnosed as mastitis, modified by appropriate descriptive terms. Foci of mild ductal dilatation without associated inflammation occur in elderly women as a normal process of involution of the gland.

The etiology of MDE is not known.[54] Some authors believe that ductal dilation caused by glandular atrophy and involution in postmenopausal women is the primary pathologic process leading to stasis of secretion, which is followed by leakage of lipid material through the walls of the ducts to elicit periductal inflammation.[50,55] Others have concluded that periductal inflammation is the underlying abnormality responsible for duct sclerosis, obliteration, and ectasia.[53,56,57] The latter authors considered stasis caused by ductal obstruction to be the process responsible for inciting the inflammatory reaction that contributed to further obstructive changes as well as to ductal dilation. Parity and breast-feeding are not factors predisposing to the development of MDE.[58] In some cases, squamous metaplasia of the terminal lactiferous duct epithelium results in obstruction that contributes to the development of duct ectasia and eventually to the formation of lactiferous duct fistulas[59,60] (Fig. 3.7).

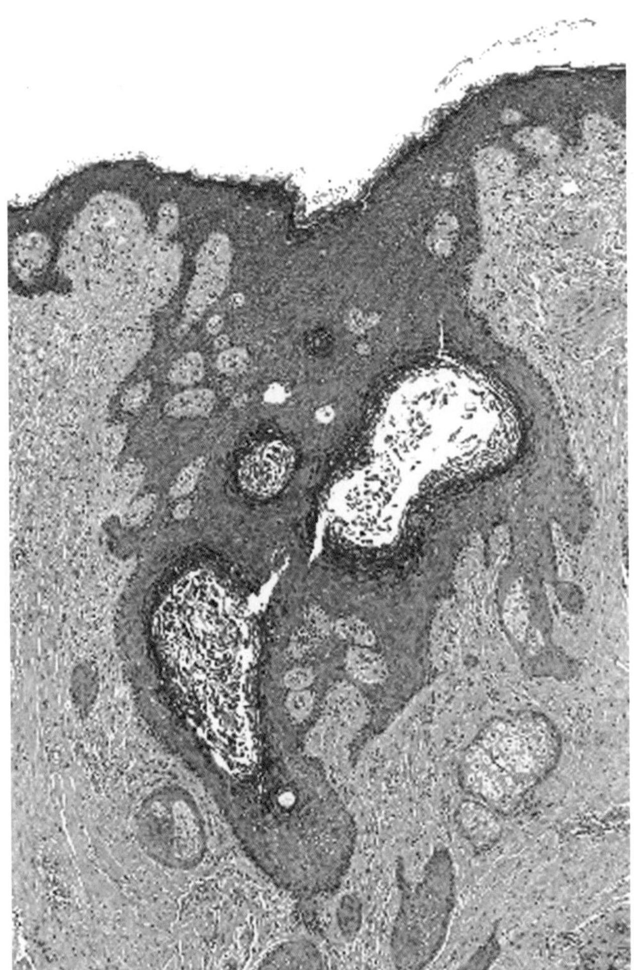

FIG. 3.7. ***Squamous metaplasia of nipple duct.*** Plugs of desquamated keratin fill the terminal portion of a lactiferous duct in the nipple at the site of squamous metaplasia.

Cigarette smoking has been associated with the development of periductal mastitis and MDE, and with an increased risk for fistula formation.[61,62] The mechanism is thought to be mediated through the effects of smoking on the bacterial flora of the mammary ducts.

MDE, galactorrhea, and lipogranulomatous mastitis have been associated with prolonged phenothiazine treatment.[63] MDE was found in three patients who had hyperprolactinemia caused by pituitary adenomas.[64] Slightly elevated serum prolactin was detected in a 3-year-old boy with bilateral MDE.[65] These isolated cases suggest that hyperprolactinemia may play a role in the development of MDE in some patients. Galactorrhea and lactational hyperplasia do not ordinarily precede the development of MDE. The relationship has not been studied sufficiently to determine whether this is more than a sporadic association. MDE has been associated with bilateral extensive ductitis obliterans in diabetic patients.[66]

Clinical Presentation

The earliest symptom is spontaneous, intermittent nipple discharge that is usually clear, yellow, green, or brown. There may be no palpable abnormality. The discharge gives a positive test for blood in about 50% of patients. In more advanced cases, subareolar induration progresses to the formation of a mass. Occasionally, dilated ducts may be palpable as "one or more doughy, wormlike masses beneath the nipple."[52] Pain is usually reported among the early symptoms and tends to be more frequent in young women, whereas nipple inversion or retraction is more often described at a later age.[67] The mean age of patients with pain (39.9 years) or a lump (42.7 years) was younger than that of patients who had painless (47.1 years) and nonpalpable (42.7 years) MDE. Conversely, women with nipple retraction were older (53.4 years) than those without this abnormality (43.4 years). The presence of nipple inversion is generally associated with periductal fibrosis and contracture. Well-established mass lesions may be painful and tender, with the symptoms accentuated in the premenstrual phase of the cycle. When the onset is acute, the clinical findings suggest an abscess. If allowed to persist, the subareolar inflammatory lesion may develop into a fistula.[68]

MDE has been found in women younger than 30[58,69] and older than 80 years of age,[58] but rarely in men.[70]

Approximately two-thirds of the female patients are between 40 and 70 years old. The median age in one series of 34 patients was 44 years.[69] MDE has been reported in children in whom it causes bloody nipple discharge, usually around the age of 3 years with a male-to-male ratio of 3:2.[71]

Mammography reveals a variety of changes associated with MDE. Sweeney and Wylie[72] reported that 12 of 1,437 women who underwent biopsy in a series of screened women had MDE. The mammographic abnormalities included microcalcifications, spiculated masses, and lobulated partially smooth masses. In some instances, the mammographic findings suggested carcinoma. By allowing direct visualization of the ductal system in MDE, ductoscopy can be useful as a guide for excision.[73]

Gross Pathology

At surgery, obviously dilated ducts are identified through a circumareolar incision and removed in a segmental excision with the apex in the nipple. The specimen usually consists of firm breast tissue in which there are prominent ducts that contain pasty or granular secretion. The duct contents vary greatly in color, but most often the secretion is white, cream colored, or brown. Many ducts appear dilated and thick walled as a consequence of periductal fibrosis. Calcification is sometimes apparent grossly in the dilated ducts. Abscess-like yellow necrotic areas can be found in the most severe cases, and these may be the site of cholesterol granulomas and calcification.[48] In addition, the stroma between ducts may be fibrotic and may contain cystically dilated glands.

Microscopic Pathology

The microscopic composition of the duct contents is often varied in a given case. In its most bland form, it consists of eosinophilic, granular, or amorphous, proteinaceous material. Usually, there is an admixture of lipid-containing foam cells (so-called colostrum cells) and desquamated duct epithelial cells (Fig. 3.8).

The origin of foam cells remains controversial. Davies[74,75] concluded that they were macrophages derived from the periductal mononuclear inflammatory infiltrate. Others have suggested that the foam cells are altered epithelial or myoepithelial cells.[76] Derivation of foam cells from altered epithelial or myoepithelial cells may be suggested by the way in which foam cells are sometimes found distributed in the epithelial layer (Fig. 3.9). Myoepithelial and apocrine cells with cytoplasmic clearing bear a superficial resemblance to foam cells. Immunohistochemical study has demonstrated the histiocytic character of foam cells with reactivity for CD68, HAM56, MAC387, lysozyme, and α_1-antitrypsin, and absence of staining for cytokeratins.[77,78] Pagetoid foam cells in the ductal epithelium may display misleading surface cytokeratin staining from the membranes of contiguous epithelial cells or weak reactivity for absorbed antigens such as gross cystic disease fluid protein-15 (GCDFP-15).[78] As a result, they can be mistakenly diagnosed as pagetoid carcinoma cells.

A detailed study of mammary foam cells in the epithelium, in the stroma, and in gland lumens was reported by Damiani et al.[79] Immunohistochemistry revealed that three types of cells were described by the term *foam cell.* Some were epithelial cells, immunoreactive for epithelial membrane antigen and cytokeratin, with apocrine differentiation manifested by the presence of GCDFP-15, demonstrated by immunohistochemistry and *in situ* hybridization. Another group of cells consisted of macrophages with immunoreactivity for MAC387 and CD68. A third cell type with intermediate features was immunoreactive for CD68 and GCDFP-15. These cells also had a peripheral rim of cytokeratin positivity. The latter cells lacked GCDFP-15 mRNA when examined by *in situ* hybridization and probably represent macrophages with adsorbed epithelial antigens.

Histiocytes that contain ceroid pigment were termed *ochrocytes* by Davies[80] (Fig. 3.10). These cells are immunoreactive

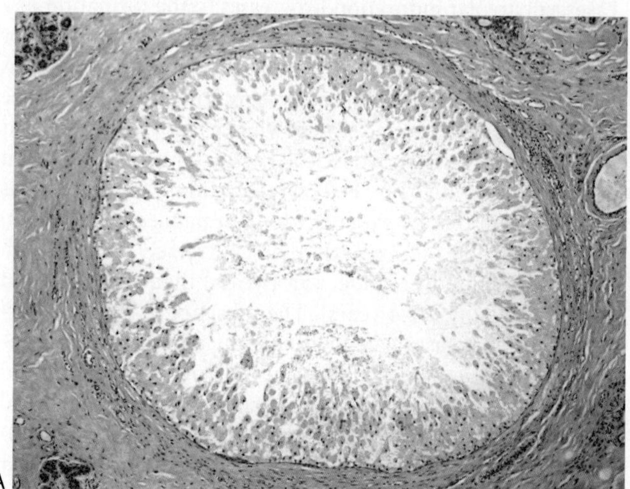

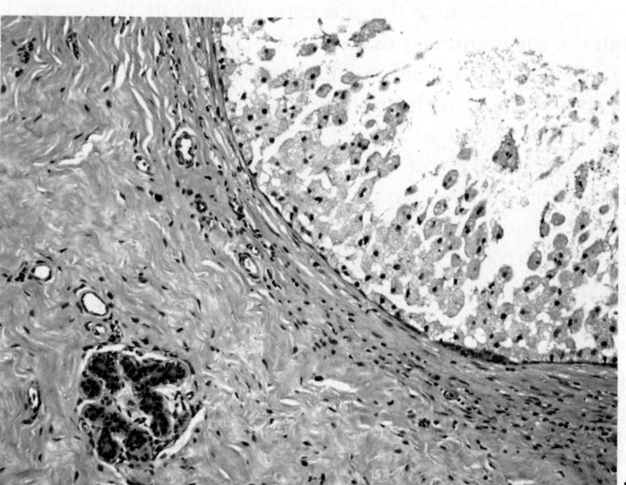

FIG. 3.8. ***Duct stasis.*** **A,B:** The lumen of this cystically dilated duct contains histiocytes. A minimal lymphocytic reaction surrounds the duct.

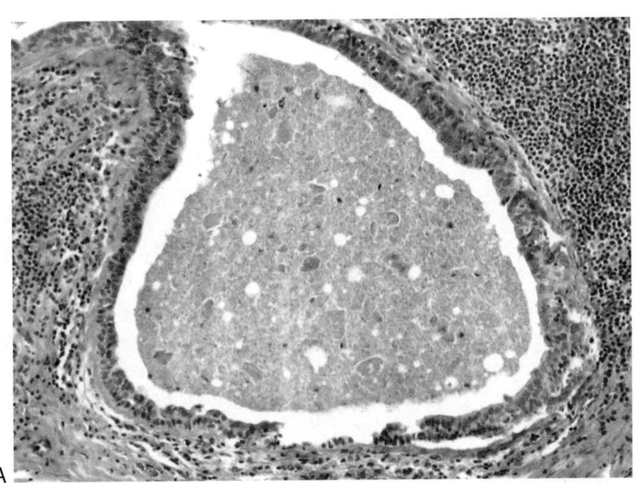

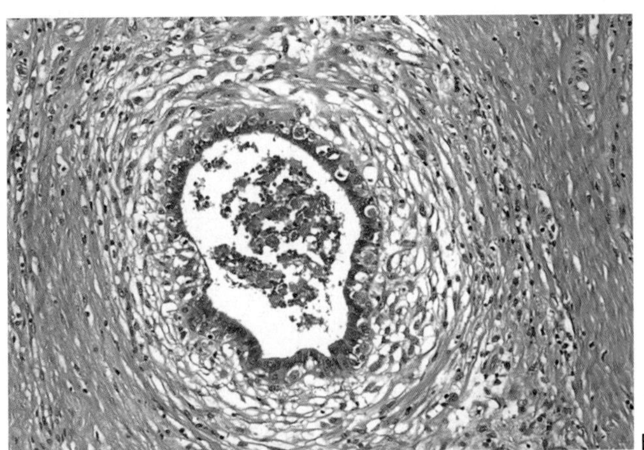

FIG. 3.9. ***Duct stasis.*** **A:** The lumen of this dilated duct contains granular secretion and degenerated epithelial cells. A lymphocytic reaction surrounds the duct. **B:** Histiocytes (ochrocytes) with golden granular cytoplasm are present within the duct epithelium and in the surrounding stroma.

with markers of macrophage differentiation.[81] Hamperl[76] described these foam cells as "fluorocytes" because the pigment is autofluorescent in ultraviolet light. Ochrocytes and foam cells occur within the epithelial–myoepithelial layer of ducts, in periductal tissue and in duct lumens.

Inflammatory changes in the walls of ducts and periductal tissues are a prominent part of the pathologic findings in MDE (Fig. 3.11). Inflammation that features lymphocytes with smaller numbers of plasma cells, neutrophils, and histiocytes is present circumferentially throughout the thickness of the duct and in the periductal stroma. Disruption of ducts is accompanied by discharge of stasis material into the breast, causing a more intense periductal reaction and resulting in abscess formation (Fig. 3.12). There is usually an abundant lipid component that elicits a prominent lipophagic histiocytic reaction bordered by an infiltrate of lymphocytes, plasma cells, neutrophils, and variable numbers of multinucleated histiocytes.

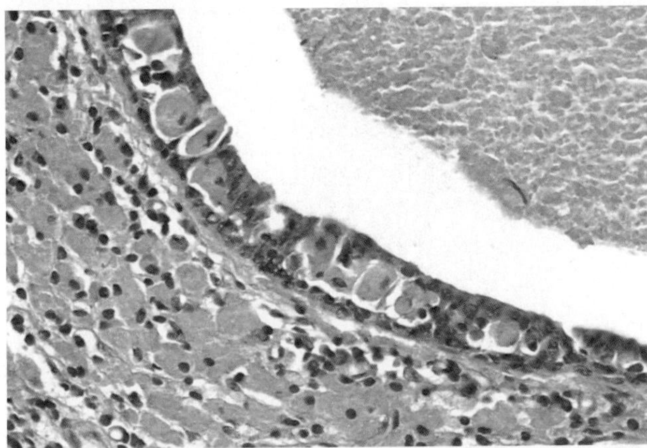

FIG. 3.10. ***Ochrocytes in duct stasis.*** Histiocytes with densely granular cytoplasm (ochrocytes) in the stroma around an ectatic duct and in the epithelium of the duct.

The formation of cholesterol granulomas is an uncommon complication of periductal mastitis.[48,82] Findings on clinical examination and mammography may suggest carcinoma because of the localized nature of the lesion. Histologic examination reveals groups of cholesterol crystals encased by histiocytes and giant cells with surrounding granulomatous zones of histiocytes, lymphocytes, plasma cells, and fibroblastic reaction. The remnants of ectatic ducts can sometimes be identified within cholesterol granulomas as well as in the surrounding tissue.

Periductal fibrosis and hyperelastosis, often with a lamellar distribution, lead to mural thickening in MDE. The inflammatory reaction typically spreads throughout the fibrous periductal collar into the surrounding breast stroma

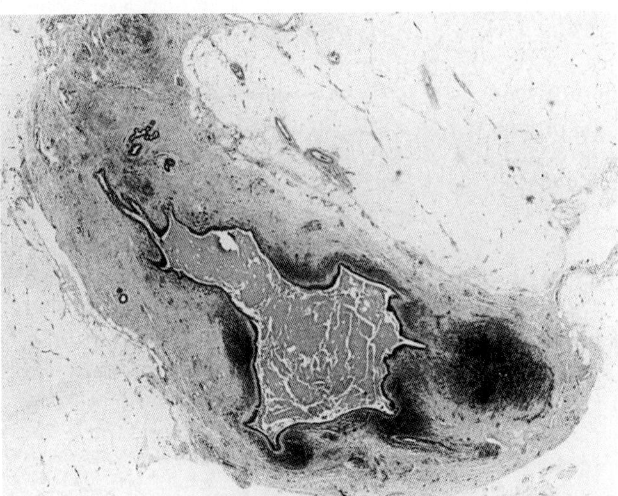

FIG. 3.11. ***Duct ectasia and stasis.*** A dilated duct containing stasis material with nodular periductal lymphocytic infiltrates. (From Rosen PP, Oberman HA. *Tumors of the mammary gland.* [*AFIP Atlas of Tumor Pathology,* 3rd series, vol. 7]. Baltimore: American Registry of Pathology, 1993.)

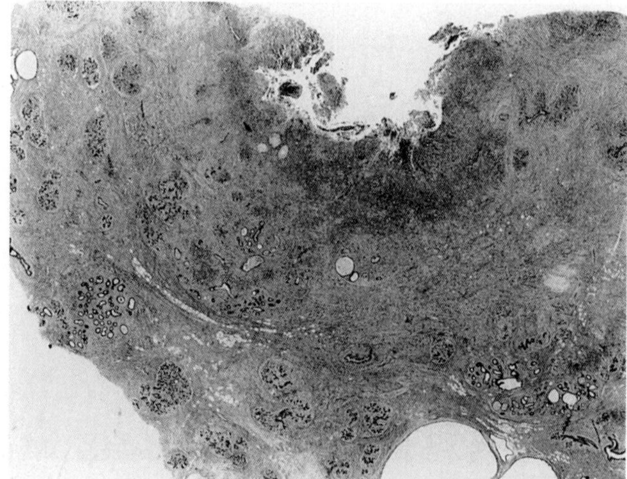

FIG. 3.12. ***Duct ectasia with abscess.*** An abscess associated with duct ectasia is evident in this photograph from the same case as in Fig. 3.11.

(Figs. 3.13 and 3.14). The ductal epithelium is atrophic, flat, and inconspicuous. Epithelial hyperplasia is not a feature of MDE, but it may be found as a component of proliferative breast changes that are coincidentally present.

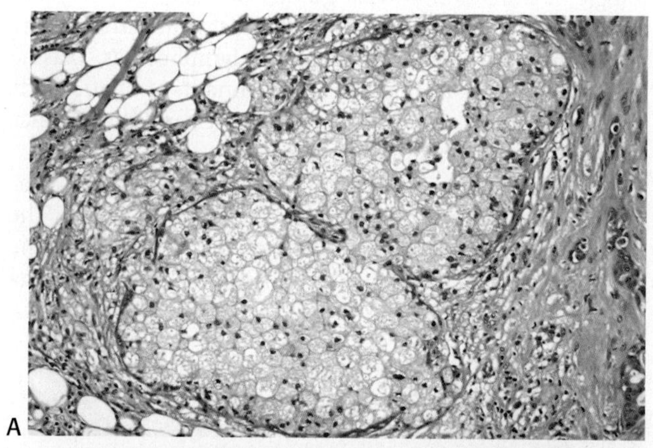

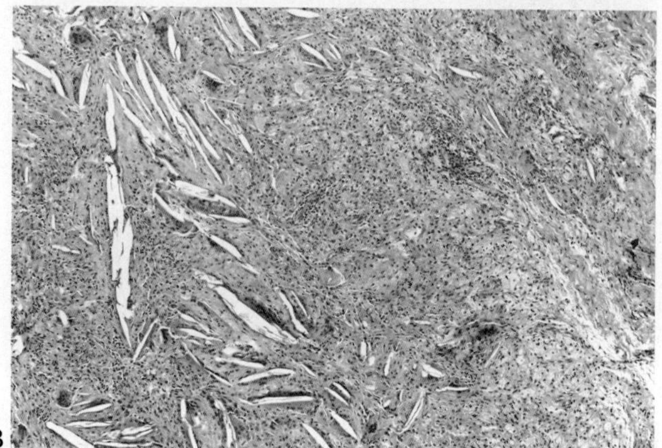

FIG. 3.13. ***Early and late phases of duct ectasia.*** **A:** In the early phase, histiocytes fill the minimally "ectatic" duct. **B:** In the late phase, the duct ruptures with a diffuse histiocytic proliferation. Cholesterol crystals can be prominent (forming the so-called "cholesteroloma").

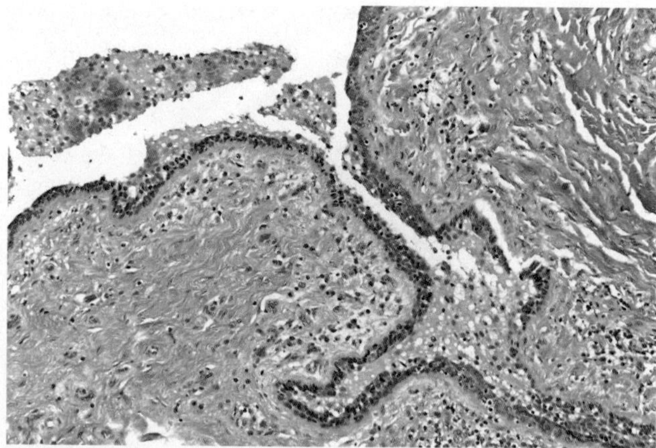

FIG. 3.14. ***Duct ectasia with minimal reactive changes in periductal stroma.*** Mild inflammatory cell infiltrate and capillary proliferation in the region of incipient duct disruption. Histiocytes are present in the duct lumen.

In a late phase, the inflammatory reaction is less conspicuous, but the ducts become encased in a thick laminated layer of hyaline fibrous and elastic tissue.[56] The ductal lumen may be patulous, but in some instances the sclerotic process includes actively proliferating granulation tissue and hyperelastosis that narrows and may totally occlude ducts.[83] The latter configuration has been termed *mastitis obliterans*[47] (Fig. 3.15). Remnants of persisting epithelium may proliferate to form secondary glands within the sclerotic duct, creating a pattern that resembles a recanalized, healed thrombus in a blood vessel. When the epithelium is totally absent, the duct is reduced to a linear fibrous scar. Residual hyperelastotic tissue and histiocytes are sometimes evident, but on occasion the only evidence is a band or ring of eosinophilic collagenous tissue.

The inflammatory reaction is concentrated in and around major lactiferous ducts, but it also extends into peripheral

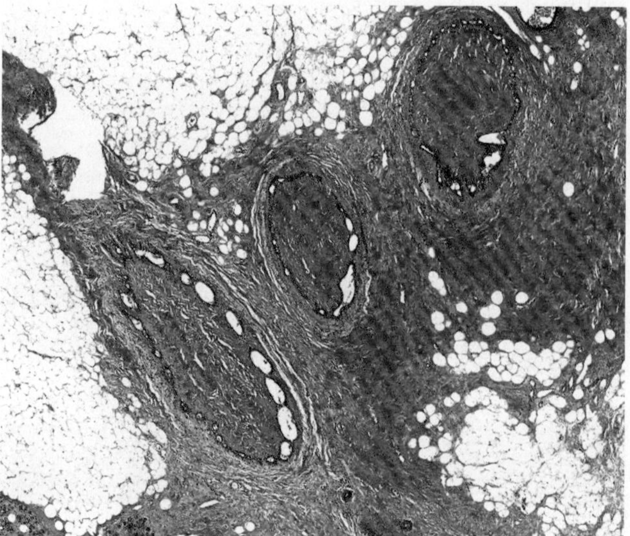

FIG. 3.15. ***Duct ectasia with mastitis obliterans.*** A polyp composed of granulation tissue has obliterated most of the duct lumens.

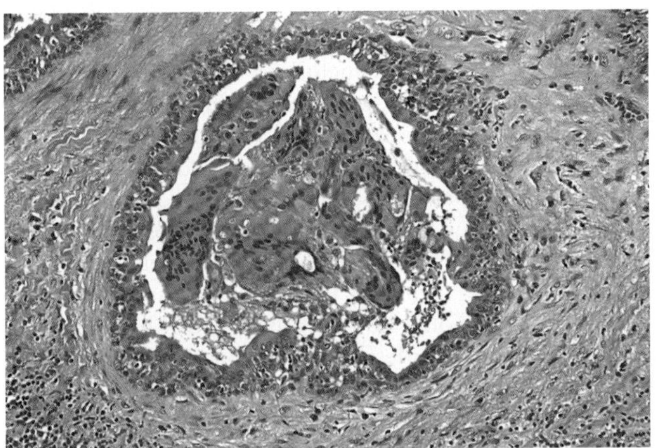

FIG. 3.16. *Duct ectasia with intraluminal multinucleated histiocytes.*

ducts and lobules. This lobulitis typically features a lymphocytic reaction without granulomas. Plasma cells, acinar dilation, and stasis of intralobular secretion are not conspicuous. There is no evidence of lobular hyperplasia or of increased secretory activity in such lobules. Stasis of secretion with mild ectasia may occur in the terminal duct.

An unusual variant of ductal stasis and periductal mastitis features multinucleated histiocytic reaction within the duct lumen, apparently elicited by secretion (Fig. 3.16).

Treatment and Prognosis

The diagnosis of MDE may be suggested by symptoms and clinical findings, but these are not sufficiently specific to exclude carcinoma. Mammography can be helpful, but a radiologic distinction between "comedo" carcinoma and MDE cannot be made with confidence in all cases. The diagnosis is usually established by excising the affected area. A circumareolar incision is used to expose the dilated ducts. These are transected at the base of the nipple and excised with a conical segment of the surrounding tissue. In severe cases, the mass formed by reaction to ruptured ducts is also excised with the affected segmental ducts. Incision and drainage of MDE that has been mistaken clinically for an infection with abscess formation may lead to fistula formation.[69] Asynchronous involvement of the contralateral breast is sometimes encountered. MDE is not associated with an increased risk of subsequent carcinoma of the breast.

GRANULOMATOUS LOBULAR MASTITIS

Numerous pathogenic processes responsible for granulomatous inflammation of the breast can be included under the generic heading of granulomatous mastitis.[84] In the absence of a specific etiologic agent, the term *GLM* has been adopted for these lesions.[85–88] Kessler and Wolloch[89] drew attention to the distinction between granulomatous and PCM. Going et al.[87] recommended the term *GLM* to separate the lesion from granulomatous forms of periductal mastitis. The diagnosis of postlactational granulomatous mastitis[90] is less satisfactory, because the lesion may develop as long as 15 years postpartum.[87]

The etiology of GLM is unknown, although *Corynebacterium* spp. have been implicated (see Chapter 4). No microorganism has been isolated consistently from the tissue, and histochemical stains for pathogens are routinely negative. The perilobular distribution and granulomatous character of the inflammation suggest a cell-mediated reaction to one or more substances concentrated in the secretion of lobular cells, but no specific antigen has been identified. An autoimmune phenomenon seems unlikely in the absence of vasculitis or a prominent plasma cell component in the reactive infiltrate.[90]

Clinical Presentation

The lesion usually appears after, rather than during, pregnancy. Because the mean interval between the last pregnancy and the diagnosis of GLM is 2 years, there does not appear to be an association with breast-feeding. A relationship to oral contraceptive use was suggested in one study in which eight of nine patients had used these medications,[87] and others have reported an increased incidence of GLM in women on oral contraceptives.[91] It is thought that oral contraceptives induce hyperplasia in lobular ductules leading to obstructive desquamation of ductular epithelial cells, distension of ductules, and ultimately a perilobular inflammatory reaction. One patient had hyperprolactinemia associated with phenothiazine treatment, and prolactin levels were reportedly normal in two other patients.[87] Coexistent erythema nodosum was present in one patient.[92]

The age at diagnosis ranged from 17 to 42 years, with a mean of about 33 years in one report.[87] Virtually all patients were parous. Women with GLM typically present with a distinct, firm-to-hard mass that involves any part of the breast but tends to spare the subareolar region. Bilateral involvement is uncommon.[90] Nipple discharge is usually not present. The tumor is sometimes tender. Axillary nodal enlargement and tenderness are rarely encountered. The breast tumors reportedly measure from 1 to 8 cm, averaging nearly 6 cm.

The clinical findings often suggest carcinoma, and mammography may also be described as "suspicious."[90] Focal asymmetric density on mammography and an irregular hypoechoic mass with "tubular extensions" on ultrasound are the most common radiologic presentations.[93] Variable mammographic findings in one study included multiple small masses or asymmetric density without calcification or speculation.[94] The lesions were hypoechoic on sonography, and more of them were detected by the latter method than by mammography. The sonograms were characterized by "multiple clustered, often contiguous tubular hypoechoic lesions."[80]

Gross Pathology

The specimen typically consists of firm-to-hard mammary parenchyma that contains a palpably distinct mass. The margins are less apparent on visual inspection of the cut surface, where the gray-to-tan tissue appears to have a faintly nodular architecture. In some cases, the nodules appear to be small foci of abscess formation. Confluent abscesses are not a characteristic feature of GLM.

Microscopic Pathology

The primary histopathologic change in GLM is a granulomatous inflammatory reaction centered on lobules, a granulomatous lobulitis (Fig. 3.17). Granulomas composed of epithelioid histiocytes, Langhans giant cells accompanied by lymphocytes, plasma cells, and occasional eosinophils are found within and around lobules. The same cellular components are present in FNA smears from these lesions.[95,96] Asteroid bodies are unusual, and Schaumann bodies have not been reported in the giant cells formed in GLM.

With progression of the inflammatory process, confluent granulomas may obscure or obliterate the lobulocentric distribution of the process, particularly toward the central portion of the tumor. Fat necrosis, abscess formation, and fibrosis contribute to effacement of the lobular distribution in confluent lesions[90] (Fig. 3.18). A microcystic space that develops in the center of the abscesses contains no foreign material or demonstrable secretion. It is likely that lipid from degenerating cells contained in these spaces is dissolved during histologic processing of the tissue. A narrow zone of neutrophils usually outlines this space, and neutrophils may accumulate in the lumen. Focal lactational changes can be encountered in lobules in recently parous women. Ducts incorporated in the lesion may become dilated and exhibit periductal or intraductal inflammation, but usually this is relatively inconspicuous. Affected ducts and lobules do not ordinarily contain refractile or birefringent crystalline material or calcifications in GLM. Squamous metaplasia of duct and lobular epithelium is unusual. Vasculitis is not seen in GLM. Stains and cultures for bacteria, acid-fast organisms, and fungi are typically negative. *S. aureus* was isolated from one patient.[87] Corynebacterium-associated GLM is discussed in Chapter 4.

Differential Diagnosis

The differential diagnosis includes a variety of lesions. The distinction between GLM and various other granulomatous inflammatory conditions such as tuberculosis, sarcoidosis, and cat scratch disease can usually be made by correlating the clinical and pathologic findings. Tuberculous mastitis tends to show more eosinophils and necrosis, and idiopathic GLM is commonly associated with relatively more plasma cells.[97] It is critically important that granulomatous reaction in carcinoma also be considered. Although most examples of the latter lesion have areas of easily identified intraductal or invasive carcinoma, the associated carcinoma may be obscured by a pronounced granulomatous reaction.[98] In rare cases, immunohistochemical stains for cytokeratin or other epithelial markers may be necessary to identify carcinoma in this background. Xanthogranulomatous mastitis is characterized mainly by fat necrosis, lipid-laden macrophages (xanthoma cells) admixed with cholesterol crystals, multinucleated giant cells, and it is often related to duct ectasia.[99]

Sarcoidosis should also be considered in the differential diagnosis. Patients presenting with the characteristic clinical and pathologic features of GLM have not had evidence of systemic granulomatous inflammation, and Kveim test in a minority of patients is negative.[87]

Treatment and Prognosis

When the diagnosis of GLM has not been suspected clinically, primary treatment has often been excisional biopsy. Persistence or recurrence of the inflammatory process that may lead to skin ulceration has been described after biopsy,[86,87] but in many patients the disease is self-limiting and controlled by a single operation. Antibiotics may be helpful, especially if secondary infection occurs. Corticosteroids have been effective in resolving the lesions after a specific infectious etiology has been ruled out.[100,101] In some cases,

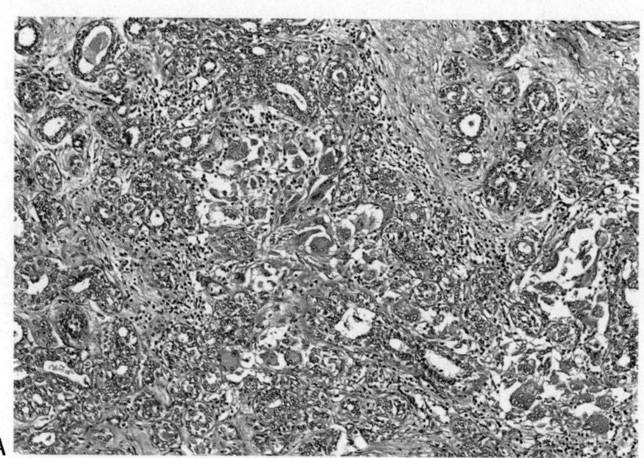

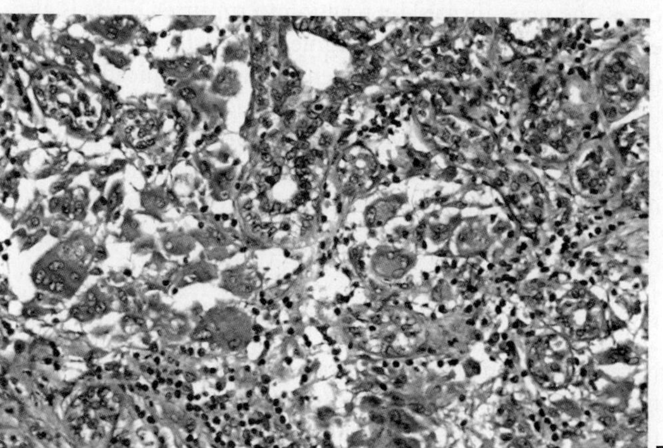

FIG. 3.17. ***Granulomatous lobular mastitis.*** **A,B:** Lobular inflammation with a lymphocytic component involving a lobule. Multinucleated histiocytes are present in the center of the lesion. The lobular architecture is disrupted by this process.

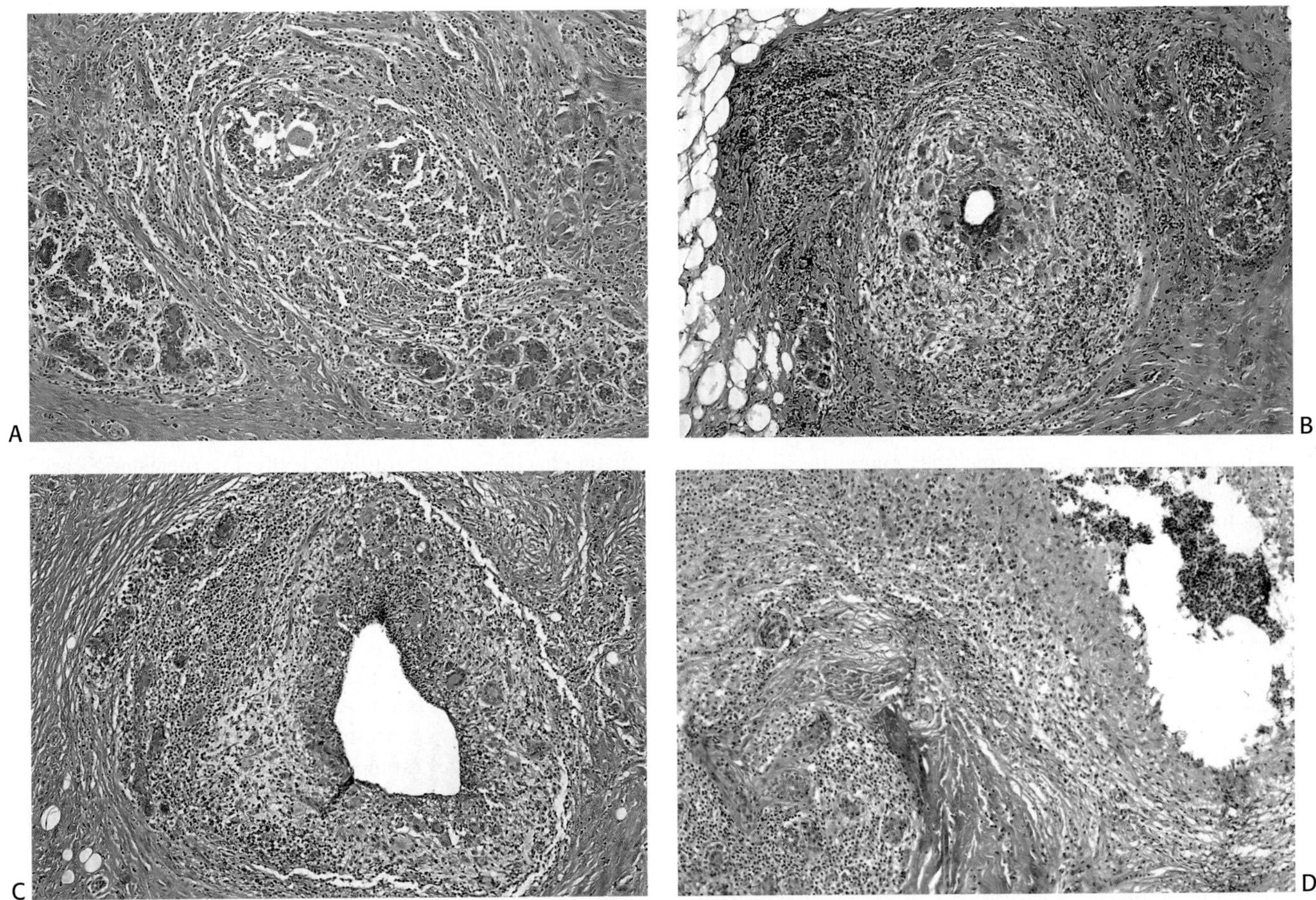

FIG. 3.18. ***Abscesses in granulomatous lobular mastitis.*** These images from a single specimen illustrate progressive destruction of lobules leading to abscess formation. **A:** An early stage in which the inflammatory reaction consists mainly of lymphocytes. **B:** The lobule shown here is entirely engulfed by inflammation with a characteristic lamellar distribution. The lymphoplasmacytic reaction at the periphery surrounds a histiocytic zone with giant cells. A thin layer of neutrophils outlines a central, empty lumen. **C:** Part of the lobule remains on the left in this lesion with a large central vacuole. **D:** Neutrophils are present in the lumen (*right*).

prolonged treatment with steroids is necessary to prevent or control recurrences.[101] Methotrexate has been used successfully in the treatment of "idiopathic granulomatous mastitis" and may be effective in managing GLM that is not responsive to steroids.[102]

SARCOIDOSIS

Clinical Presentation

Systemic sarcoidosis may affect the breast. The women tend to be in their 20s and 30s, reflecting the age distribution of sarcoidosis. One patient with mammary involvement was 65 years old.[103] Mammary lesions are usually detected after the diagnosis has been established on the basis of the typical clinical manifestations of the disease. Only rarely does sarcoidosis present as a primary breast tumor, and then it is usually accompanied by lymph node enlargement.[103,104] The breast lesion caused by mammary sarcoidosis is a firm-to-hard mass that may be mistaken clinically for carcinoma.[105] The mammographic, ultrasound, and MRI characteristics of mammary sarcoidosis are not specific and can be interpreted as suggestive of carcinoma,[106] especially if a spiculated lesion is seen on mammography.[107] Rarely, sarcoidosis produces multiple, bilateral small mammographically detected lesions.[108] In patients with known mammary carcinoma, enlargement of mediastinal lymph nodes and lesions at other sites caused by sarcoidosis that are discovered on a PET scan can be mistaken for metastatic carcinoma.[109,110]

Gross Pathology

The excised specimen consists of firm-to-hard, tan tissue that may have well-defined or indistinct borders. Calcification and necrosis are not features of sarcoidosis involving the breast. Tumors up to 5 cm in diameter have been reported.

Microscopic Pathology

Microscopic examination reveals epithelioid granulomas forming nodules in the mammary parenchyma among lobules and ducts (Fig. 3.19). Multinucleated Langhans giant cells that accompany the granulomas may form asteroid or Schaumann bodies. The lesions do not have caseous necrosis or calcification, and fat necrosis is not found in the surrounding breast. Traces of fibrinoid necrosis may be found in cellular granulomas. A lymphoplasmacytic reaction and fibrosis are present in varying amounts. Isolated granulomas with a sparse lymphocytic reaction can be found in breast tissue that appears grossly to be unaffected. These inconspicuous granulomatous foci tend to be associated with ducts or lobules.

The differential diagnosis includes many specific agents such as tuberculosis, leprosy, brucellosis, other bacterial infections, various fungi and parasitic infestations,[85] and rheumatoid nodules.[111] Lesions caused by miliary tuberculosis may lack caseous necrosis. It is necessary to exclude the presence of acid-fast or other bacteria and fungi with cultures, histochemical stains, and appropriate clinical tests. These studies are indicated even in patients with previously diagnosed sarcoidosis, because they can develop secondary infections, especially when receiving corticosteroid treatment. The diagnosis of mammary sarcoidosis is established by excluding other potential etiologic agents.

Sarcoid-like Lesions and Mammary Carcinoma

Nonnecrotizing sarcoid-like granulomatous inflammation can develop in lymph nodes that are draining organs that harbor carcinoma.[112] This phenomenon has been documented in the lymph nodes of patients with mammary carcinoma who have no clinical evidence of sarcoidosis.[112–114] Bässler and Birke[113] reported sarcoid-like granulomas in axillary lymph nodes from 0.7% of patients with breast carcinoma. Similar granulomatous foci were found in the stroma of 0.3% of mammary carcinomas[113] (Fig. 3.20). Some patients who have sarcoid-like granulomas associated with a carcinoma develop similar lesions in their axillary lymph nodes,[113] but others do not manifest granulomatous lymphadenitis.[115] Systemic manifestations of sarcoidosis may be mistaken clinically or radiologically for metastatic carcinoma in a patient with known mammary carcinoma.[109,110,116]

Histologically, it can be difficult to distinguish carcinoma-associated sarcoid-like reactions from coexistent carcinoma in a patient with sarcoidosis.[117,118] The lymph node lesions of sarcoid and sarcoid-like reactions are histologically similar, especially when the granulomas are composed entirely of epithelioid histiocytes. Both have Langhans giant cells, asteroid and Schaumann bodies, and focal fibrinoid necrosis.[112] Little or no fibrosis is encountered in carcinoma-associated axillary lymph node granulomas, whereas long-standing sarcoidosis is likely to be accompanied by fibrosis.

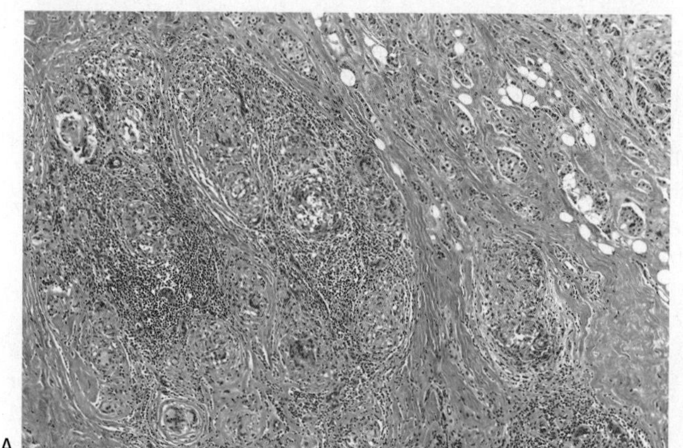

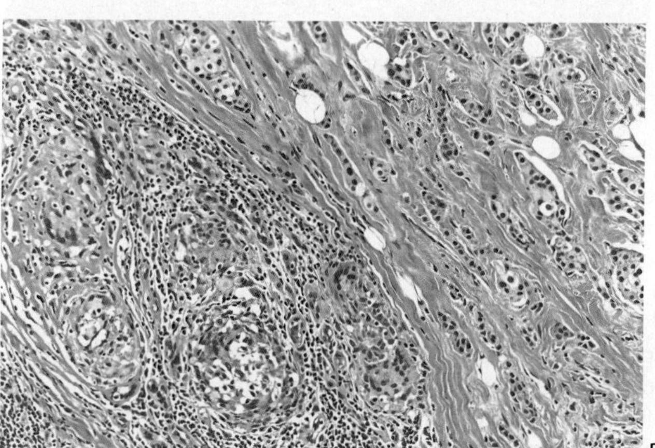

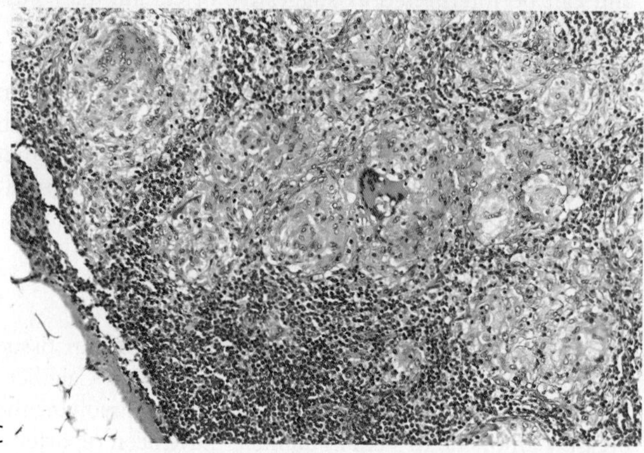

FIG. 3.19. *Sarcoidosis.* **A,B:** Confluent nonnecrotizing granulomas with giant cells lie amidst invasive ductal carcinoma in a patient with sarcoidosis. **C:** The sentinel lymph node shows similar granulomata.

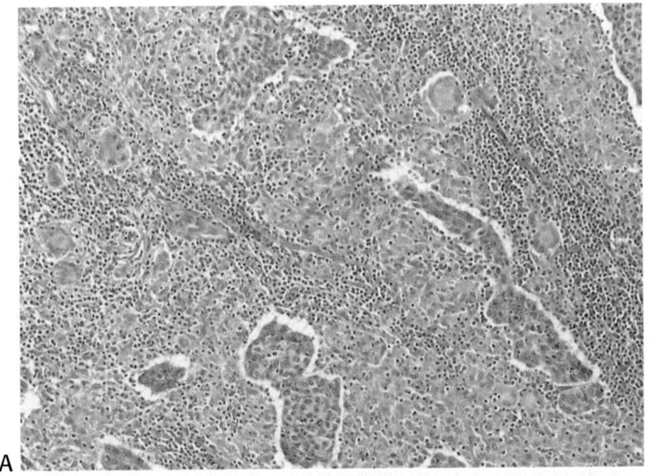

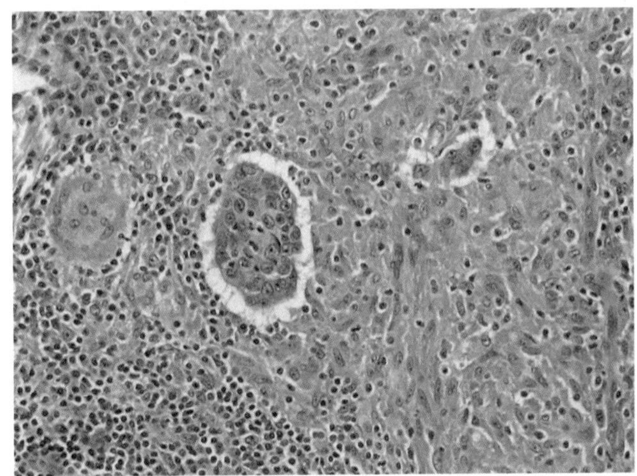

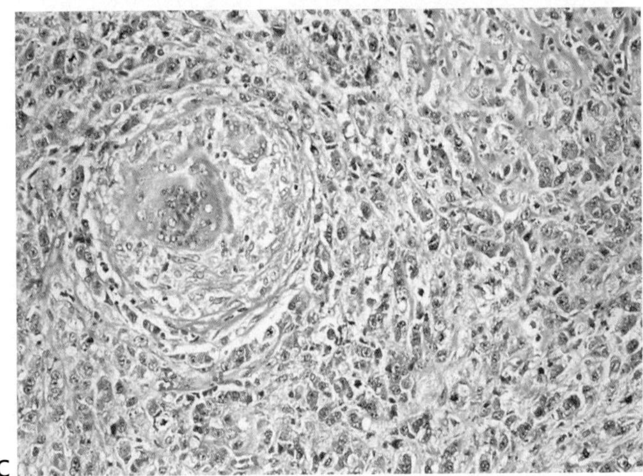

FIG. 3.20. ***Sarcoid-like granulomas in carcinoma.*** **A:** Infiltrating duct carcinoma with granulomatous inflammation. **B:** Histiocytes, lymphocytes, and a giant cell around infiltrating carcinoma. **C:** Granulomatous reaction in metastatic carcinoma in an axillary lymph node.

Within the breast, the carcinoma-associated granulomatous reaction is restricted to the tumor and immediately surrounding mammary parenchyma. Necrosis has been noted in a minority of the carcinomas that had sarcoid-like granulomas. In one case, amyloid deposition accompanied the granulomatous reaction associated with a poorly differentiated carcinoma.[119] Electron microscopy confirmed the presence of tubular amyloid. Collagenization has been described in mammary sarcoid granulomas.[117] Sarcoid-like granulomas were found associated with both tumors in two patients who developed bilateral asynchronous carcinomas within a four-year interval.[94] A granulomatous reaction accompanied the chest wall recurrence in one of these patients.

Treatment and Prognosis

The clinical course of women who have sarcoidosis involving the breast depends on the extent of the underlying disease. The presence of granulomatous inflammation may be suggested in a needle aspirate of the breast, but the cytologic features are not sufficiently specific to distinguish sarcoidosis from other granulomatous lesions.[120] Mammary lesions are adequately managed by excisional biopsy, which is necessary to rule out carcinoma. Patients with advanced sarcoidosis may develop multiple, bilateral lesions. Despite impairment of cellular immunity associated with sarcoidosis and an increased incidence of malignant lymphoma and pulmonary carcinoma, there is no evidence that sarcoidosis influences the risk of developing mammary carcinoma or the prognosis of carcinoma that develops in these women.[121]

SO-CALLED INFLAMMATORY PSEUDOTUMOR

There is no well-characterized lesion of the breast that qualifies for this diagnosis. The diagnosis has been mistakenly applied to a variety of inflammatory lesions as well as benign and malignant neoplasms. Localized nodular lesions in the breast consisting of interlacing bundles of myofibroblastic cells (hence the synonym: inflammatory myofibroblastic tumor) with a prominent infiltrate composed mainly of plasma cells and lymphocytes have been diagnosed as inflammatory pseudotumors (Fig. 3.21).[122–125] Chetty and Govender[124] described three histologic patterns: nodular fasciitis, interlacing fascicles of spindle cells in variably collagenized stroma, and a hypocellular variant composed mainly of hyalinized collagen resembling a scar. The three cases described in their report had varied appearances with differing proportions of these elements.

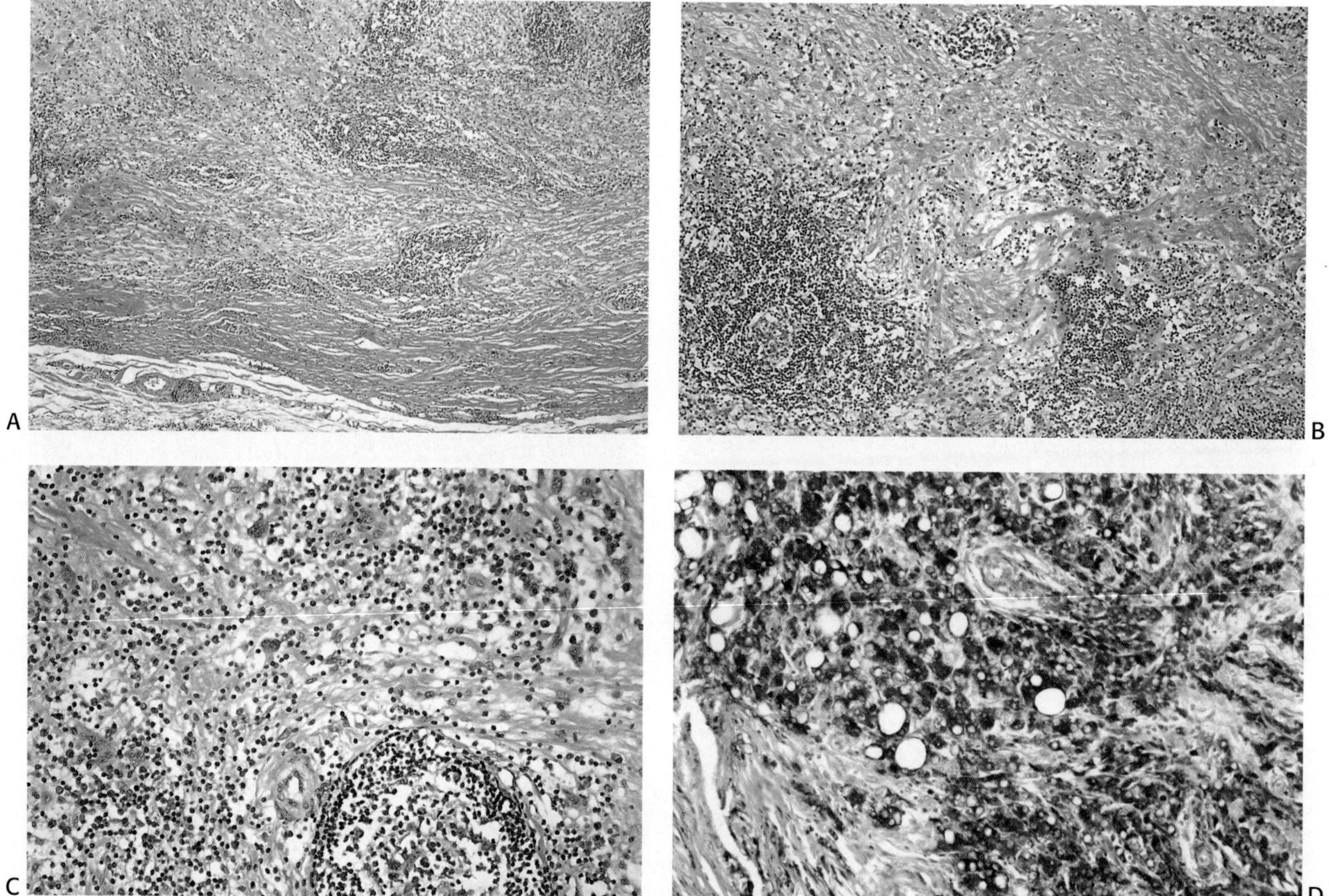

FIG. 3.21. ***Inflammatory pseudotumor.*** **A:** Peripheral fibrosis outlines the lesion. **B:** Lymphocytic infiltrates with germinal center formation in the midst of variably collagenized stroma. **C:** A few multinucleated histiocytes and scattered plasma cells are shown. **D:** Histiocytes are highlighted by the MAC immunostain.

Four reported patients each had a unilateral lesion that did not recur after excision, but follow-up rarely exceeds 1 year.[123,124] Another patient with bilateral tumors developed recurrences in both breasts.[122]

Before the description of the relatively new entity of immunoglobulin G4 (IgG4)-related sclerosing mastitis (*vide infra*), at least one case reported as an "inflammatory pseudotumor" showed elevated serum IgG4.[126] The differential diagnosis includes other lesions rarely encountered in the breast such as Erdheim–Chester disease,[16] previously discussed in the section on Fat Necrosis, and adult-type "juvenile" xanthogranuloma.[127] The latter lesion consists of a prominent spindle cell proliferation associated with multinucleated giant cells, including Touton type, lymphocytes, plasma cells, and xanthomatous histiocytes. The xanthomatous cells are reactive for KP1, MAC387, and PGM1, but negative for S-100 and CD1a.[127]

VASCULITIS

Inflammatory lesions of blood vessels, particularly arteries, are encountered in a variety of systemic disorders that are broadly grouped under the heading of collagen-vascular disease. The breasts may be affected as an example of single-organ vasculitis[128] or as part of multiorgan involvement. The mammary lesions caused by vasculitis often resemble carcinoma clinically. Although there may be some differences in the histopathologic features of the vasculitides associated with various collagen-vascular diseases, the diagnosis of a specific condition is made on the basis of both the clinical and the pathologic findings. Most forms of vasculitis that afflict the breast show fibrinoid vasculitis, in addition to any additional histologic finding. Some of these diseases may be manifested in the breast by mammographically detected dystrophic calcifications.[129] Among all inflammatory vascular conditions, mammary involvement is most frequently associated with granulomatosis with polyangiitis (the erstwhile Wegener granulomatosis).[128]

Giant Cell Arteritis

This condition typically involves the cranial arteries of elderly women who present with temporal headaches, visual impairment, fever, and other symptoms. Anemia and an elevated erythrocyte sedimentation rate (ESR) are usually present. In patients with appropriate symptoms, the diagnosis is confirmed by finding granulomatous arteritis with giant cells and destruction of elastica in a temporal artery biopsy specimen.

Giant cell arteritis limited clinically to the breast was first described by Waugh[130] in 1950, and there have been a number of subsequent case reports.[131–137] The patients have been women 52 to 79 years of age. Almost all presented with one or more palpable breast tumors. An exceptional patient complained of pain and erythema in the upper outer quadrant of one breast.[132] No mass was palpable or evident on a mammogram, and inflammatory carcinoma was suspected clinically. She also had palpable nontender temporal arteries. Biopsy of the breast revealed arteritis. The temporal arteries were not biopsied.

The lesions are bilateral in nearly 50% of cases. The firm-to-hard tender or painful tumors measure from less than 1 to 4 cm. Fixation to the skin was described in several cases, and a few patients had erythema of the skin overlying the lesion that can raise the possibility of inflammatory carcinoma.[138] One patient had nipple retraction, and axillary nodal enlargement has been noted in some cases.[135,139] These features may suggest carcinoma clinically.[135,140] Temporal artery biopsy revealed giant cell arteritis in one patient who had concomitant invasive mammary duct carcinoma and mammary arteritis.[133] A 72-year-old woman with giant cell arteritis of the breast and polymyalgia was found to have necrotizing polyarteritis in a muscle biopsy.[141]

Most patients with giant cell arteritis of the breast have had few systemic symptoms. These may include headache, muscle and joint pain, fever, and night sweats. Mild anemia and an elevated ESR are found in most cases.

The excised specimen consists of ill-defined, rubbery, firm tissue. In one patient with bilateral lesions, each focus of arteritis contained a grossly enlarged, thickened, and thrombosed artery,[130] but in most reports the vascular changes were not grossly evident. Microscopically, granulomatous inflammation involves small- and medium-sized arteries throughout the affected tissue[134,136] (Fig. 3.22). Veins and arterioles are spared. The reactive process consists of a transmural and perivascular infiltrate composed mainly of lymphocytes, histiocytes, and giant cells. Plasma cells, eosinophils, and scattered neutrophils are also seen. Fibrinoid necrosis is not a consistent feature, but fragmentation of the mural elastic fibers is demonstrable with an appropriate stain (Fig. 3.23). Multinucleated giant cells tend to be oriented around these disrupted elastic fibers. In some cases, giant cells are sparse and difficult to detect. The lumen may be narrowed or occluded by a recent blood clot, an organizing thrombus, or by laminated subintimal fibrosis. Calcification commonly develops in vessels that are the site of healed arteritis and these calcified vessels may be seen on a mammogram.[138] The surrounding breast tissue exhibits changes as a consequence of the vascular lesions. These include fibrosis, edema, fat necrosis, and atrophy of glandular elements.

The diagnosis of giant cell arteritis of the breast is made by excisional biopsy. Needle core biopsy may not reveal the diagnostic lesion.[137] The differential diagnosis includes other types of arteritis, phlebitis, infarction related to pregnancy or lactation, and traumatic fat necrosis. Most patients treated with corticosteroids remained free of systemic symptoms with follow-up of 2 years or less. One patient had arteritis in the specimen from a thyroid lobectomy that had been performed for an adenoma shortly after a breast biopsy demonstrated arteritis.[142] Complete resolution of systemic symptoms was reported without steroid therapy in one woman who had bilateral breast involvement.[135]

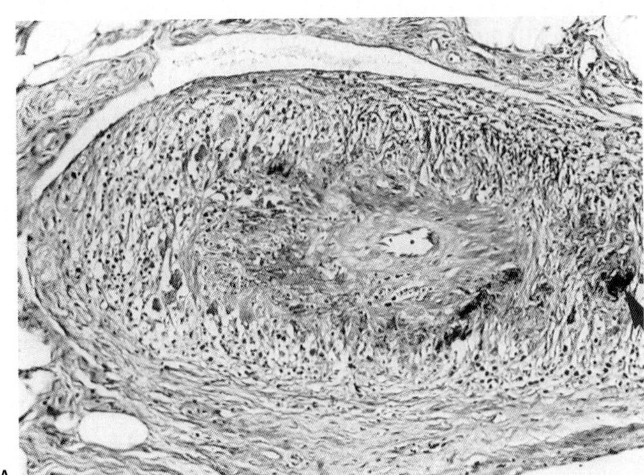

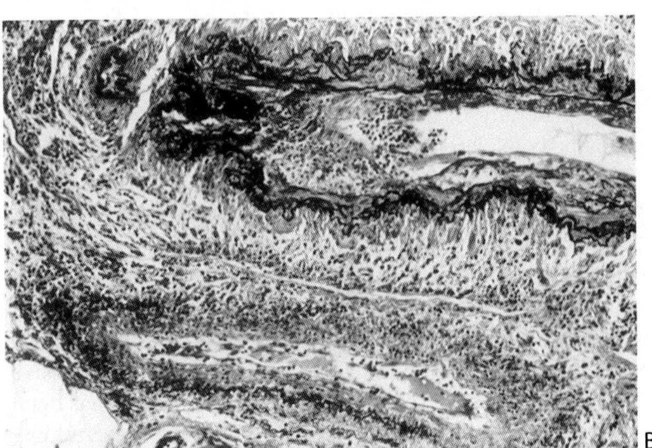

FIG. 3.22. ***Giant cell arteritis.*** **A,B:** Histiocytes, lymphocytes, and giant cells in the wall of an artery **(A)**. The lumen is almost entirely occluded. Irregular calcifications are present (*arrow*). Fragmentation of the internal elastica is evident in the artery. The inflammatory reaction involves a small adjacent vein (elastic van Gieson stain) **(B)**. (From Rosen PP, Oberman HA. *Tumors of the mammary gland.* (*AFIP Atlas of Tumor Pathology,* 3rd series, vol. 7). Baltimore: American Registry of Pathology, 1993.

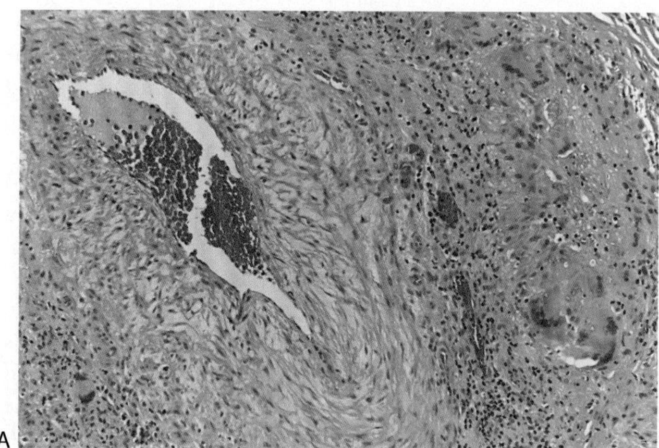

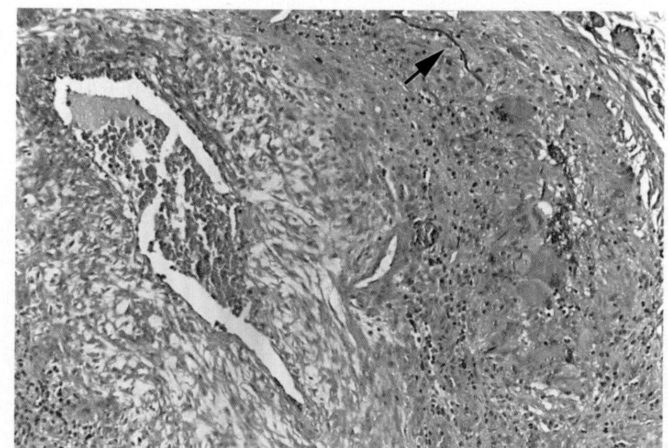

FIG. 3.23. *Giant cell arteritis.* A,B: Fragmentation of the internal elastica is evident in the artery on the elastic van Gieson stain (*arrow*). Note intramural location of the giant cells.

Granulomatosis with Polyangiitis (Wegener Granulomatosis)

The disease known earlier as Wegener granulomatosis is now referred to as granulomatosis with polyangiitis. It is characterized by necrotizing granulomatous vasculitis affecting the upper and lower respiratory tract accompanied by glomerulonephritis.[143] Rarely, the skin, joints, and visceral organs are also involved.[144] The first case of granulomatosis with polyangiitis of the breast was reported by Elsner and Harper[145] in 1969. Additional patients described have been women 40 to 69 years of age[146–151] and a 40-year-old man with bilateral, ulcerated painless breast lesions.[152] The tumor was unilateral in all but one female patient. In two women, the breast tumor was the initial indication of granulomatosis with polyangiitis.[148,150] In four others, systemic manifestations were evident coincidental with[148] or shortly before[145,146,150] detection of a breast mass. Late onset of breast involvement 1 and 6 years after other symptoms has also been described.[149] In a comprehensive review of 27 published cases of breast involvement with granulomatosis with polyangiitis, Allende and Booth[153] noted that the clinical presentation of the lesions, generally in the form of a mass, requires that carcinoma be considered in the differential diagnosis.[128,153,154]

The breast tumor is usually tender. In one case, nipple retraction and *peau d'orange* suggested inflammatory carcinoma.[146] The presence of a breast mass and lung nodules may be misinterpreted clinically as evidence of advanced breast carcinoma. Mammography reveals a distinct dense lesion with an irregular or stellate border.[146] Calcifications are absent. Regression following steroid and immunosuppressive treatment of unresected lesions diagnosed by FNA has been documented with mammography.[146] However, the cytologic findings, consisting of inflammatory cells and evidence of necrosis, are nonspecific. Surgical biopsy is usually necessary to demonstrate necrotizing vasculitis affecting arteries and veins that characterizes this condition. The presence of the underlying vasculitis may not be appreciated when the specimen exhibits prominent fat necrosis.[147] Infarcted portions of the lesion may grossly resemble a carcinoma.[154]

Microscopic examination of the biopsy specimen reveals acute and chronic inflammation of the mammary parenchyma and fat. Arteritis affects small- and medium-sized vessels. Splitting of the elastica is found in larger arteries. Vessels in necrotic areas and in the surrounding breast exhibit inflammatory changes. Granulomatous foci are present in the surrounding breast and at the periphery of infarcted areas with central necrosis (Fig. 3.24). The inflammatory reaction includes multinucleated giant cells, plasma cells, lymphocytes, eosinophils, and neutrophils in varying proportions.

Treatment directed at systemic manifestations of the disease involves steroids, immunosuppressive drugs, and supportive management. Prognosis depends on the severity and extent of systemic involvement. Two of 10 patients described in the literature died of rapidly progressive systemic vasculitis within 6 months.[145,149] The others were reportedly alive with or without evidence of granulomatosis with polyangiitis 2 to 6 years after diagnosis.[146–150]

Polyarteritis

There are several case reports of mammary involvement in polyarteritis.[154–158] In most patients, a unilateral breast lesion was the initial manifestation. One woman with chronic polyarteritis developed a unilateral breast mass 18 years after the onset of her illness.[157] In another case, bilateral involvement caused multiple painful breast nodules.[156] Mammography revealed arterial calcification in a 37-year-old woman who had localized mammary arteritis.[158]

Microscopic examination of the breast biopsy reveals transmural necrotizing vasculitis without a giant cell reaction in the breast parenchyma. Eosinophils may be a prominent component of the mixed inflammatory cell infiltrate. The process involves arterial vessels of varying size, including arterioles, but spares venous channels (Fig. 3.25). Obliteration of vascular lumen during the acute phase is mainly due to the inflammatory process with secondary

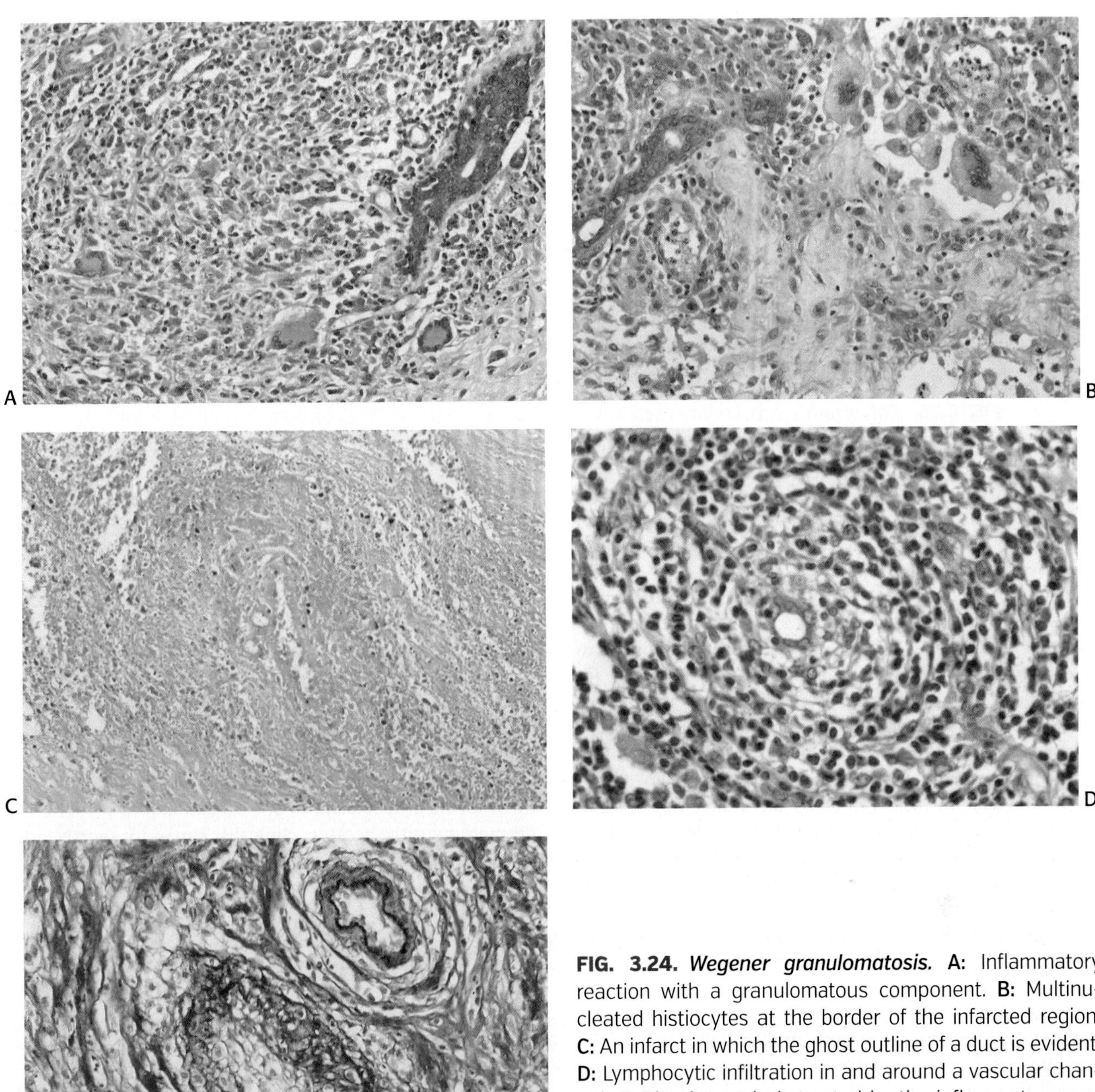

FIG. 3.24. ***Wegener granulomatosis.*** **A:** Inflammatory reaction with a granulomatous component. **B:** Multinucleated histiocytes at the border of the infarcted region. **C:** An infarct in which the ghost outline of a duct is evident. **D:** Lymphocytic infiltration in and around a vascular channel. **E:** Blood vessel obstructed by the inflammatory process (elastic van Gieson stain). (Courtesy of Dr. Wolfgang Schneider [From Göbel U, Kettritz R, Kettritz U, et al. Wegener's granulomatosis masquerading as breast cancer. *Arch Intern Med* 1995;155:205–207, with permission].)

thrombosis. Fibrinoid necrosis may be evident as well. Secondary effects in the surrounding breast resulting from ischemic degeneration include acute and chronic inflammation and fat necrosis.

After a relatively brief follow-up period, all of the patients remained alive, with improvement in systemic symptoms following treatment with corticosteroids. A woman who did not have systemic manifestations of arteritis remained asymptomatic after no treatment other than excision of the breast tumor.[158]

Scleroderma

Scleroderma or systemic sclerosis is one disease in a group of systemic autoimmune rheumatic diseases (SARD), which also includes rheumatoid arthritis, lupus, and dermatomyositis. Scleroderma usually presents with cutaneous and/or visceral symptoms secondary to the effect of the underlying disorder on blood vessels and collagen. Cutaneous involvement of the breast may occur as part of progressive systemic disease. One case report appears to describe an instance of

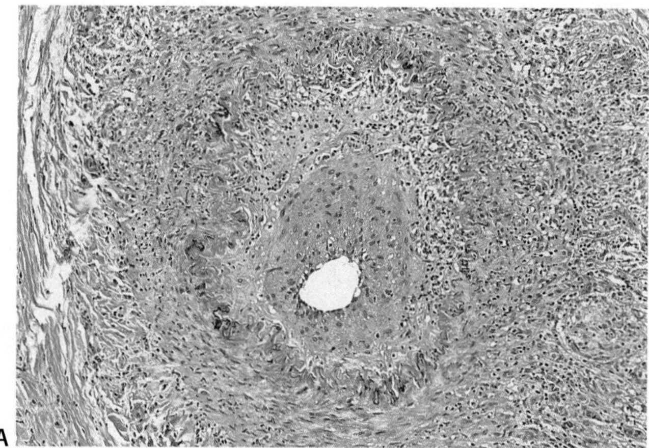

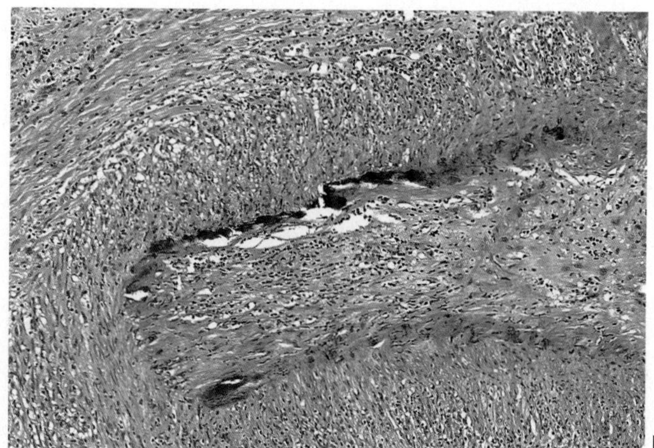

FIG. 3.25. *Polyarteritis.* **A,B:** Fragmentation of the internal elastica and calcification are shown in vessels cut transversely **(A)** and in the long axis **(B)**. Blood vessel lumens are occluded by reactive tissue.

scleroderma diffusely involving the skin and parenchyma of one breast.[159] The patient had no systemic manifestations of scleroderma and no follow-up was given.

There are several case reports of patients with breast carcinoma who developed scleroderma.[160–162] The skin of the breast was involved in at least one of these cases as part of diffuse cutaneous manifestations of the disease.[160] There is evidence for an established relationship between scleroderma and pulmonary carcinoma,[162,163] and breast carcinoma is the second most common malignant neoplasm to arise in this setting.[164] This relationship may be coincidental, but patients with scleroderma and a family history of breast carcinoma may be at increased risk.[165] In about 75% of patients, scleroderma predates mammary carcinoma by an average of about 22 years.[165] Breast carcinoma rarely predates the diagnosis of scleroderma or the two conditions are diagnosed coincidentally. The mean age for the diagnosis of breast carcinoma in patients with scleroderma is about 60 years.[165] The most frequent serologic abnormality is the presence of anticentromere antibodies.

Scleroderma has also been observed in women following breast augmentation with silicone implants after intervals of 2 to 19 years.[166–168] In one case, symptoms of scleroderma regressed after silicone implants were replaced with saline-filled implants.[167] Smooth muscle differentiation has been described in the fibroblastic cells present in cutaneous and visceral sclerodermal lesions.[169] In general, radiation to the breast is avoided in women with breast carcinoma and scleroderma. Interestingly, localized scleroderma (postradiation morphea) is considered to be an "under-recognized" complication of breast irradiation.[170]

Dermatomyositis

Calcification of blood vessels and soft tissues, especially in the extremities, is an important manifestation of dermatomyositis. Cutaneous changes and multiple subcutaneous nodules of both breasts and axillae were described in a 49-year-old woman with long-standing dermatomyositis.[171] Mammography revealed numerous, coarse branching calcifications, similar to those formed in periductal mastitis with duct stasis, and a cluster of punctate calcifications suggestive of carcinoma. With tangential views, it was possible to demonstrate that both types of calcification were situated in the skin and subcutaneous tissue rather than in the breast as it appeared in conventional views. No biopsy was performed.

Several survey studies of patients with dermatomyositis have documented an association with malignant neoplasms.[172–175] Breast carcinoma has been among the more common neoplasms in some series,[172,174] but a study of Japanese patients reported more frequent association with gastric, thyroid, and ovarian carcinomas.[175] Patients often experience remission of their dermatomyositis after treatment for their neoplasm. In one exceptional case, fulminant dermatomyositis became clinically apparent shortly after surgical treatment for a T1N0M0 breast carcinoma.[176]

Other Collagen-Vascular Diseases

Involvement of the breast in patients with *rheumatoid arthritis* is extremely unusual. One case report described a 32-year-old woman with clinically active rheumatoid disease who had a microscopic rheumatoid nodule detected in a breast biopsy performed for symptoms of duct stasis and mastitis.[111]

Weber–Christian disease, also known as "relapsing febrile non-suppurative panniculitis," presents as recurrent subcutaneous nodules accompanied by fever, arthralgias, and malaise. The lesions may or may not be tender. The typical distribution is on the lower extremities and trunk, but mammary involvement has been reported.[177] The excised nodule consists of fat necrosis with a granulomatous reaction. The lesion is usually subcutaneous, but superficial involvement of mammary parenchyma may occur.

Angiopanniculitis presents as a superficial breast mass, fixed to indurated red skin.[178] The age range of the cases reported by Wargotz and Lefkowitz[178] was 36 to 64 years, and all but one patient was female. Two patients had diabetes mellitus. No other systemic conditions were described. The lesions consisted of multiple nonnecrotizing histiocytic granulomas in subcutaneous fat and superficial breast parenchyma (Fig. 3.26). Fat necrosis was present. Small blood vessels and capillaries were infiltrated and rimmed by lymphocytes and histiocytes.

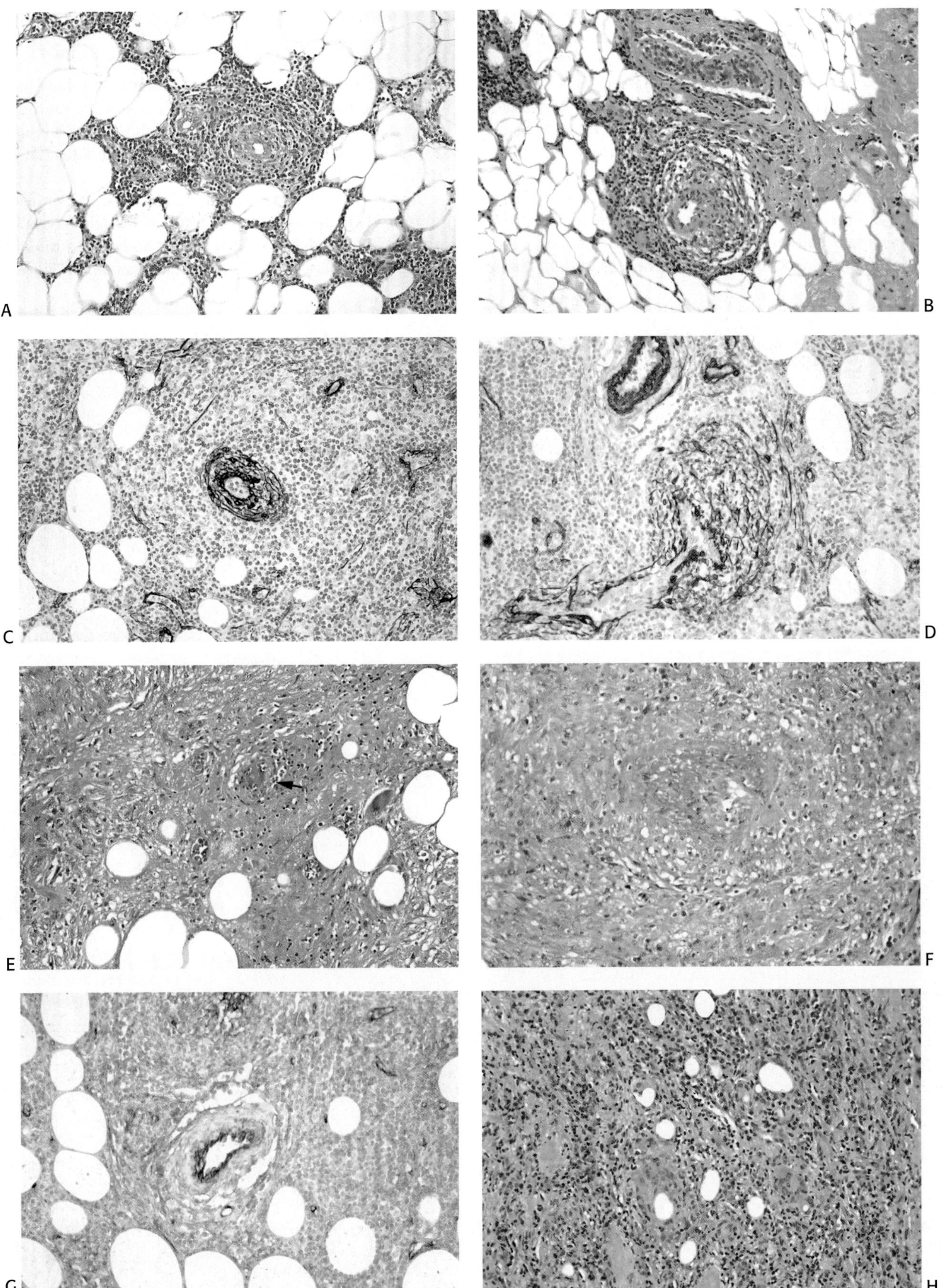

FIG. 3.26. *Angiopanniculitis.* **A,B:** Small arteries surrounded by lymphocytes and histiocytes. Inflammatory cells are present in the vessel walls, but the lumens are patent. **C,D:** Separation of mural smooth muscle layers by inflammatory cells is demonstrated by an antiactin immunostain. **E:** Necrosis of a small artery is shown in the *center* of an area of advanced fat necrosis. **F:** Fibrinoid necrosis in a small blood vessel. **G:** The endothelium of a small blood vessel retains reactivity for factor VIII. **H:** Granulomatous reaction in angiopanniculitis.

Inflammatory changes were not found in larger vessels. Ductal and lobular structures were largely uninvolved by the granulomatous process. Several patients had recurrences in the breast or at other subcutaneous sites. No patient was known to have developed systemic symptoms.

Subcutaneous panniculitis-like T-cell lymphoma can rarely present as a breast lump.[179,180] The clinical presentation consists of single and multiple subcutaneous plaque-like or nodular lesions, most commonly on the legs, but involving other sites including the breasts. Patients may have fever, weight loss, anemia, and coagulation defects that predispose to bleeding. Histologic examination of the lesions reveals infiltrates of T cells and macrophages, with individual fat cells "rimmed" by T cells.

Lupus mastitis is a rare complication of systemic or discoid lupus erythematosus. It can present as a single or multiple subcutaneous or deeply seated masses and often simulates a malignant neoplasm.[181,182] Lymphocytic vasculitis (Fig. 3.27)

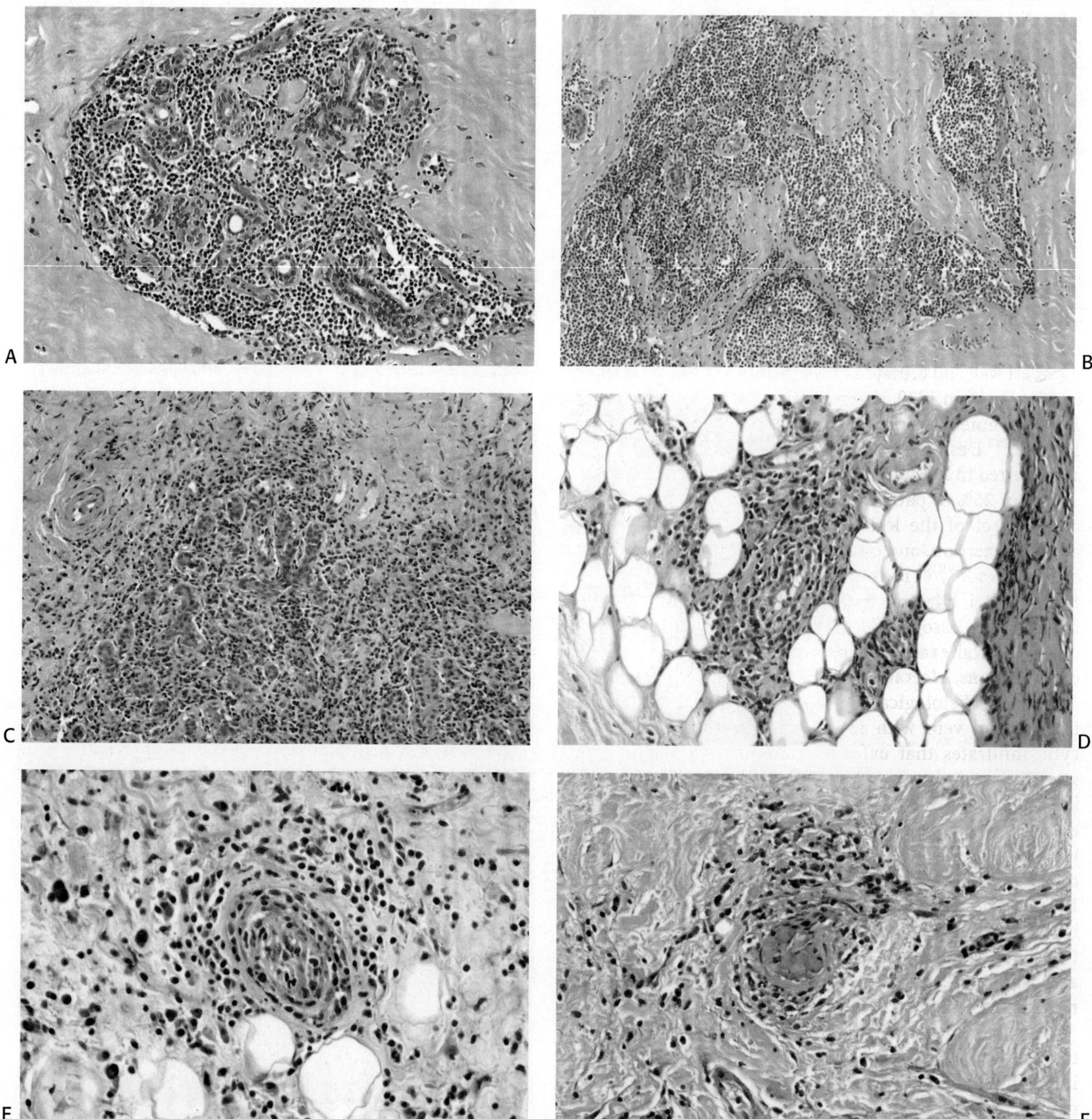

FIG. 3.27. ***Lupus mastitis.*** **A,B:** Lymphocytic lobulitis in a breast biopsy performed for an ill-defined mass in a 39-year-old woman with arthritis and a positive ANA test. Lymphocytic infiltrates involved lobules **(A)** and the stroma **(B)**. **C–F:** Biopsy from a 24-year-old woman with bilateral lupus mastitis showing lymphocytic lobulitis **(C)**, perivascular lymphocytic infiltration **(D,E)**, and vascular necrosis with a fibrin clot **(F)**.

and the formation of germinal centers are frequent features. When studied by immunohistochemistry, the lymphocytic infiltrate is found to consist mainly of CD3+CD4+T cells and CD20 T cells.[182]

Lupus mastitis is a form of lupus panniculitis characterized clinically by nodular lesions and histologically by fat necrosis in various stages of evolution.[183] In some cases, lupus mastitis is manifested by lymphocytic mastopathy distributed mainly in and around lobules. Concentric perivascular fibrosis ("onion-skinning") and hyalinized stromal fibrosis extending around ducts and lobules occur in recurrent lupus.[184,185] Advanced lesions may have considerable calcification. Immunoglobulin deposits can be demonstrated around blood vessels in the lesional tissue. Clinical findings in the skin may mimic inflammatory carcinoma.[185] The radiologic appearance of lupus mastitis is variable and may feature one or more mass lesions and extensive calcifications.[186,187]

Phlebitis

Inflammatory lesions of veins within the breast are rare. The most common form of phlebitis affecting the mammary region is *superficial thrombophlebitis* or *Mondor disease.* The first clinical description of superficial thrombophlebitis of the chest wall and breast has often been attributed to a report by Mondor[188] in 1939. Kaufman[189] reviewed the literature in 1956 and noted descriptions of the syndrome dating back to 1922.[190–192] Despite the earlier reports, the condition is usually referred to as Mondor disease.

About 25% of patients with Mondor disease have been men. Onset of the lesion has been noted after trauma, physical exertion, and operations performed on the breast or chest wall.[193,194] In one case, Mondor disease appeared 8 years after bilateral breast augmentation with silicone implants, an association that may have been coincidental.[195] Clinical examination revealed a 1.5-cm superficial, erythematous, ulcerated nodule that had been present for 3 months. Histologically, the excised tumor contained a thrombosed vein with mural and perivascular lymphocytic infiltrates that extended into the surrounding tissue. A chronic heroin addict who frequently injected her breasts with the drug reportedly developed Mondor disease.[196] Two patients with Mondor disease attributed to a jellyfish sting have been reported.[197] Coexistent mammary carcinoma and Mondor disease have been described.[198–200] In one series, 12.7% of patients with Mondor disease had breast carcinoma.[201] No association with other malignant tumors has been reported, but in one instance Mondor disease was found shortly before diagnosis of small cell carcinoma of the lung that metastasized to the affected breast.[202]

Most patients are between 20 and 40 years of age. Despite the relative youth of female patients with Mondor disease, it has only rarely been reported as a complication of pregnancy.[203] In one series, however, a substantial number of women were multiparous.[194] The left and right breasts are equally affected and, rarely, both breasts may be involved.[204] Physical examination reveals a subcutaneous cord that may be painless or painful and tender. When the area is stretched, as upon elevation of the ipsilateral arm, a groove may be formed along the distribution of the cord. Mondor disease most often involves the upper outer or inframammary portions of the breast and adjacent chest wall. Rarely various other sites of extension have been described, including the cervical region, upper arm, abdomen, and even the groin. These unusual distributions reflect anastomoses in the subcutaneous venous plexus.

The diagnosis of Mondor disease is usually established clinically. The mammographic features of Mondor disease confirm the superficial nature of the process.[205] The typical imaging finding is a linear density, sometimes appearing beaded, that proves to be superficial on tangential films.[206] A biopsy reveals thrombophlebitis of subcutaneous veins characterized by thrombosis with varying stages of organization and recanalization.[204,207] Inflammation of the vein and surrounding tissue tends to be mild in contrast to a relatively brisk fibroblastic proliferation throughout the vessel wall. Abundant stromal mucin, presumably hyaluronic acid, has been observed in the vessel wall during the acute phase of the process.

Subcutaneous thrombophlebitis of the breast and chest wall is a self-limiting condition that resolves over a period of weeks to months after symptomatic treatment. There is no evidence that Mondor disease heralds a malignant visceral neoplasm, and it is only rarely associated with deep venous thrombosis. Antibiotic and anticoagulant therapies are rarely necessary.

PARAFFINOMA

Paraffin injection for cosmetic purposes was first attempted at the turn of the century when testicular prostheses were fashioned by this method in a patient who had undergone orchiectomy for tuberculosis.[208] A variety of other clinical applications were subsequently reported, including breast augmentation.[209] Although paraffin injection was largely abandoned after a relatively short time, it continued as a rare practice mainly in Southeast Asia.[210–213] The use of beeswax and other waxes for breast augmentation has also been described.[214]

Paraffin induces a foreign-body reaction (oleogranuloma or oleogranulomatous mastitis) similar to that caused by other irritating substances injected into the breasts.[212] Within weeks to months, the injected material and consequent reaction form a hard, nodular mass that is likely to distort the breast. Infiltration of the skin has been described, and this may be associated with sinus tract formation accompanied by discharge of paraffin.[215] Drainage of the foreign material to the axilla causes axillary nodal enlargement in most cases.[212] One male patient developed bilateral ulcerations caused by paraffin injected 35 years previously.[216] Another patient developed bilateral carcinoma 30 years after injection of both breasts with paraffin.[211] Mammography reveals a variety of patterns, including a homogeneous mass, a honeycomb appearance, or dense fibrosis with "bizarre" architectural distortion.[210,211,217] Calcifications are flocculent or ring shaped.[217]

SILICONE MASTITIS AND OTHER PATHOLOGY ASSOCIATED WITH BREAST AUGMENTATION

Injection of liquid silicone composed of long-chain polymers of dimethylsiloxane into the breasts for cosmetic augmentation was a fairly widespread practice in the 1960s and 1970s. This procedure was carried out without control in many locations abroad as well as in the United States. The foreign-body inflammatory reaction induced by this material causes either a diffuse process throughout the breast, referred to as silicone mastitis, or nodular lesions, so-called silicone granulomas.[218]

Capsule formation results not only from the foreign-body effect of the implant but also from the seepage of material that it contains. Capsule formation may cause distortion and excess firmness of the breast. Migration of silicone from a silicone gel mammary implant into the soft tissue of the ipsilateral upper arm with secondary neurologic changes has been described.[219] In this case, the distribution of silicone was determined by MRI. Ultrasound is reportedly not effective for detecting leakage of silicone gel within the periprosthetic capsule.[220]

Leakage of silicone gel contained in prostheses causes an inflammatory reaction that is usually less severe than the response to direct silicone injection. The changes tend to be limited to the immediate vicinity of the implant where they contribute to the formation of a capsule.[221] Quantitative measurements of silicone in tissues surrounding such implants have not shown a consistent correlation between silicone concentrations and the overall appearance of the inflammatory reaction.[222,223] The amount of silicone was significantly associated with the intensity of histiocytic reaction but not with calcification or giant cell reaction.[223] Silicone levels are higher in the capsule than in breast tissue surrounding the capsule, regardless of whether the silicone implant is filled with saline or silicone gel.[224] This finding indicates that some of the silicone in tissues derives from the implant itself even if it is filled with saline.

Clinical Presentation

Numerous complications have been observed as a result of liquid silicone injections.[225] These include induration of the skin, draining sinuses, deformity, and the development of firm or hard masses in the breast. The masses may be visible as well as palpable. Migration of injected silicone from a ruptured implant to the chest wall and as far as the groin has been described.[226,227] Addition of oils and other sclerosing agents to the silicone to minimize migration increases the intensity of the reaction in the breast, often causing fixation to the skin and/or pectoral muscle. Expression of silicone from the nipple after rupture of a silicone implant has been reported.[228,229]

Tissue alterations attributable to silicone are detected in the breast and at other sites by many techniques, including mammography, MRI, CT, and gallium-67 scintigraphy.[219,230,231] Screening mammography of 350 women with silicone implants revealed fibrous encapsulation in 257 (73%) patients, periprosthetic calcification in 90 (26%), and silicone leakage in 16 (5%).[231] In one series,[232] mammography and MRI had low sensitivity for detecting implant disruption and silicone leakage, but others have found MRI to be superior to mammography and sonography for detected implant failure.[233,234]

The reaction attributable to silicone mastitis makes it very difficult to detect carcinoma in the breast.[235,236] Clinical examination is complicated by nodularity, skin retraction, hard masses, nipple inversion, and other alterations that may simulate or obscure a carcinoma.[237,238] Axillary lymph node changes have been described as a result of leakage from silicone gel–filled prostheses, as well as after injection of liquid silicone into the mammary parenchyma. Axillary lymph node enlargement secondary to migration of silicone can suggest metastatic carcinoma or disguise metastatic involvement.[239] FNA of silicone lymphadenitis reveals vacuolated histiocytes that contain refractile particles.[240] The pathologic changes of silicone lymphadenitis are discussed in Chapter 43.

The ability to detect carcinoma by mammography is impaired because injected silicone and the associated reaction cause numerous opaque nodules. When an implant is present, special imaging techniques with four or more views may be required to examine the entire breast.[231,241] Calcifications in silicone mastitis are generally irregular and coarse, but fine calcifications resembling those of carcinoma have also been found in silicone mastitis,[242,243] and when present, they should be biopsied.[238] Ultrasonography has not proven to be particularly effective for detecting carcinoma in a breast altered by silicone mastitis.[244] MRI and PET are important procedures for detecting carcinoma in a breast that is distorted by silicone mastitis.[245]

Gross Pathology

A specimen of silicone mastitis consists of firm-to-hard nodular tissue. When bisected, a gritty sensation is noted if there is extensive calcification (Fig. 3.28). Numerous cystic spaces that contain pale yellow or white viscous material are seen on the cut surface after injection of liquid silicone.

Microscopic Pathology

Liquid silicone by itself or with adulterants causes fat necrosis and elicits a foreign-body giant cell reaction (Fig. 3.28). The microscopic features of these processes are not specific for silicone injection. Silicone may also enter the lumens of ducts and lobular glands. During the processing of histologic sections, some of the silicone is lost from the tissue, leaving clear spaces of varying size. The spaces and histiocytes may contain fine particles or crystals of birefringent material, but these are not seen in all cases[222,236] (Fig. 3.29). The presence of silicone can be confirmed by electron microscopy, infrared spectroscopy, atomic absorption spectrophotometry, and other procedures. The accompanying chronic inflammatory reaction and fibrosis vary in intensity.

A B C D

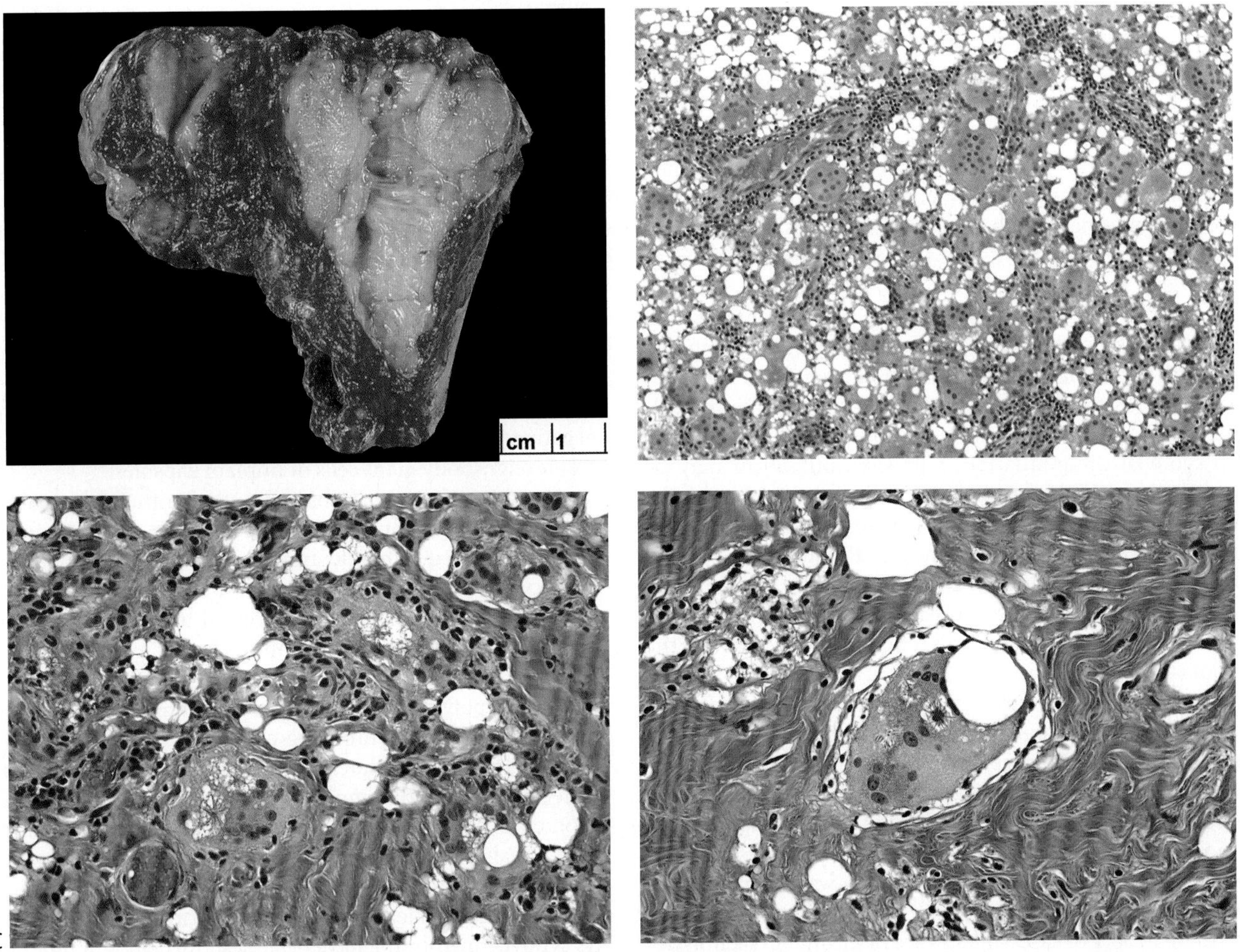

FIG. 3.28. ***Silicone granuloma.*** **A:** Gross specimen containing a nodular silicone granuloma formed after injections of silicone for breast augmentation. **B:** Diffuse granulomatous reaction to silicone. Spaces contained silicone. **C,D:** Asteroid bodies are present in giant cells.

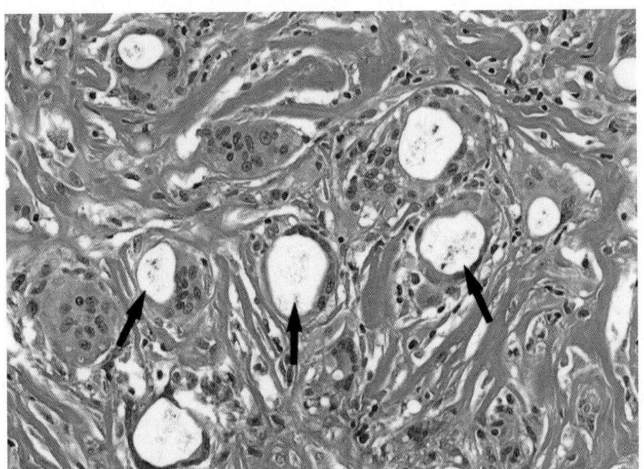

FIG. 3.29. ***Silicone granuloma.*** Birefringent crystalline material (*arrows*) in vacuolated histiocytes in giant cells in a silicone granuloma.

Microscopically, the reactive changes may be mistakenly interpreted as liposarcoma when a history of prior silicone injection is not provided.[243]

The capsule or bursa formed in reaction to silicone-containing implants consists largely of a relatively well-defined band of collagenized fibrous tissue that contains fibroblasts, myofibroblasts, and variable amounts of elastic tissue. The latter components contribute to capsular contracture. Calcification is more likely to occur in the capsule of an implant in place for a decade or longer than in the capsule around a more recent implant.[246] Calcification is found more often in the capsules formed around silicone implants with a thicker wall and Dacron patches typically used in earlier generation implants.[247] Calcification occurs in two forms: "globular aggregates" and true "bone formation." Ultrastructural analysis and other studies confirmed that both types of calcification were composed of hydroxyapatite crystals. The crystals were deposited in an orderly fashion on collagen fibers at sites of bone formation, whereas in globular aggregates they were larger and not related to collagen fibers.

The fine microscopic structure of the capsule is influenced by the surface configuration and composition of the implant.[248] The inflammatory reaction tends to be concentrated on the inner and outer surfaces of the capsule formed around the implant. The outer reaction consists of lymphocytes, plasma cells, histiocytes, and occasional foreign-body giant cells. Fibrohistiocytic cells and multinucleated giant cells are more conspicuous at the interface between the capsule and the prosthesis. A largely fibrous type of capsule consists of layered bands of collagen with a mixed inflammatory cell infiltrate composed mainly of lymphocytes and histiocytes. Fibroblasts are distributed in the collagenous tissue, and calcification is found in some instances. No synovial differentiation is present, but fibrin may be deposited on the inner surface. Other capsules are thicker with a more complex mural structure, and a primitive synovial-like membrane is formed on the surface in contact with the implant. A distinct zone of capillaries develops in a region composed of loosely organized polygonal histiocytic cells incompletely invested by reticulin fibers beneath the synovial-like membrane.

Analysis of tissue removed from capsules formed around silicone breast implants revealed increased amounts of hyaluronic acid when compared with normal breast tissue removed during reconstructive surgery.[249] The inflammatory cells were predominantly T cells and macrophages. Large amounts of interleukin-2 (IL-2) were found in association with the infiltrating lymphocytes. There was no increase in serum levels of hyaluronic acid or of IL-2.[249]

In up to 50% of cases, the surface of the inner reaction develops a more organized structure composed of fibrohistiocytic cells polarized perpendicular to the surface (Figs. 3.30 and 3.31). There is a well-developed reticulin network among these cells. This synovial-like reaction in the bursa has been referred to as synovial metaplasia.[250–252] Synovial metaplasia was most pronounced in capsules examined after the shortest interval between initial placement and removal, an observation suggesting that the occurrence of this change was not dependent on long-term implantation.[253,254] Synovial metaplasia occurs in the capsules formed around smooth and textured implants.[254] The synovial membrane has a flat surface in specimens around smooth implants. An irregular, knob-like surface develops in the capsule around a textured implant[248] (Fig. 3.32).

The lining cells have immunohistochemical properties similar to those of synovial cells including staining for vimentin, α_1-anti-chymotrypsin, lysozyme, and CD68.[250,251,255] Stains for cytokeratins and factor VIII are negative.[252] Reactivity for CD44 was present in macrophages and foreign-body giant cells of implant capsules.[256]

A variety of foreign substances can be found histologically in implant capsules. Liquid silicone droplets form smooth-surfaced refractile, translucent, or clear vacuoles in histiocytes and in the chronic inflammatory cell reaction.[257] Fragments of the implant bag, referred to as *silicone elastomer*, are seen as irregular, nonbirefringent particles, often encompassed by multinucleated foreign-body giant cells. Polyhedral polyurethane crystals will be found in the capsule formed around polyurethane-covered textured implants (Fig. 3.33), and this material may become mixed with silicone from within the implant.[258] These crystals with varied geometric shapes induce a strong granulomatous reaction. Talc has also been detected in tissues associated with breast implant capsules.[259]

Ultrastructural features of the cells forming the metaplastic synovial membrane have been described.[250,252] Studies in experimental animals and in human specimens suggest that the capsular reaction has the functional capacity to transport foreign particulate matter in a manner similar to true synovial membranes.[255] Scanning electron microscopy reveals

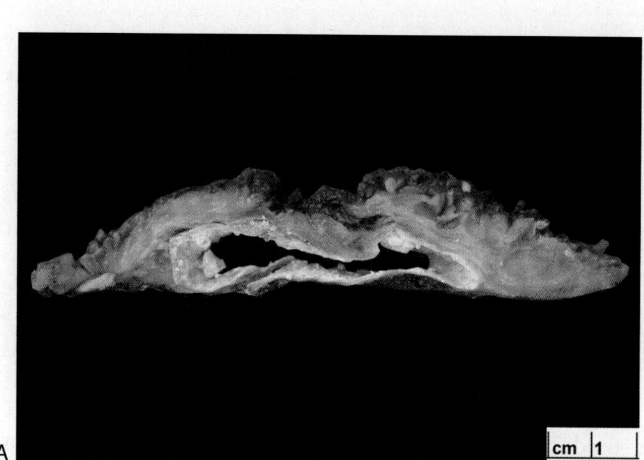

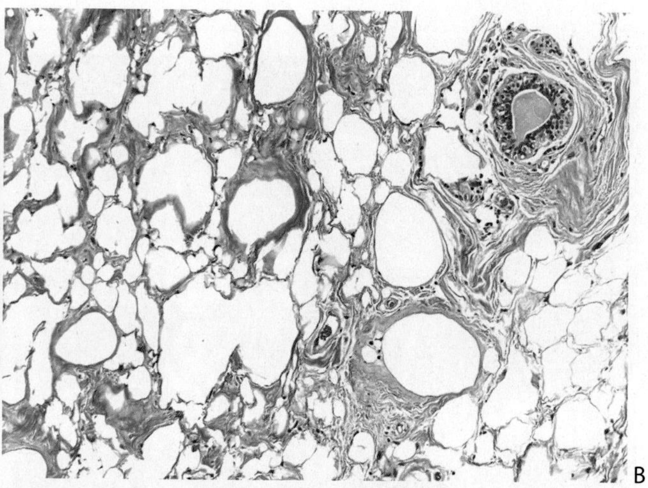

FIG. 3.30. ***Dense fibrosis of capsule around a breast implant.*** **A,B:** Dense reactive fibrosis in the capsule formed around a mammary implant **(A)** resulted from leakage of implant contents. This reaction resulted in capsular "contracture." The implant had been in place for 5 years. The pericapsular mammary tissue showed evidence of implant leakage **(B)**.

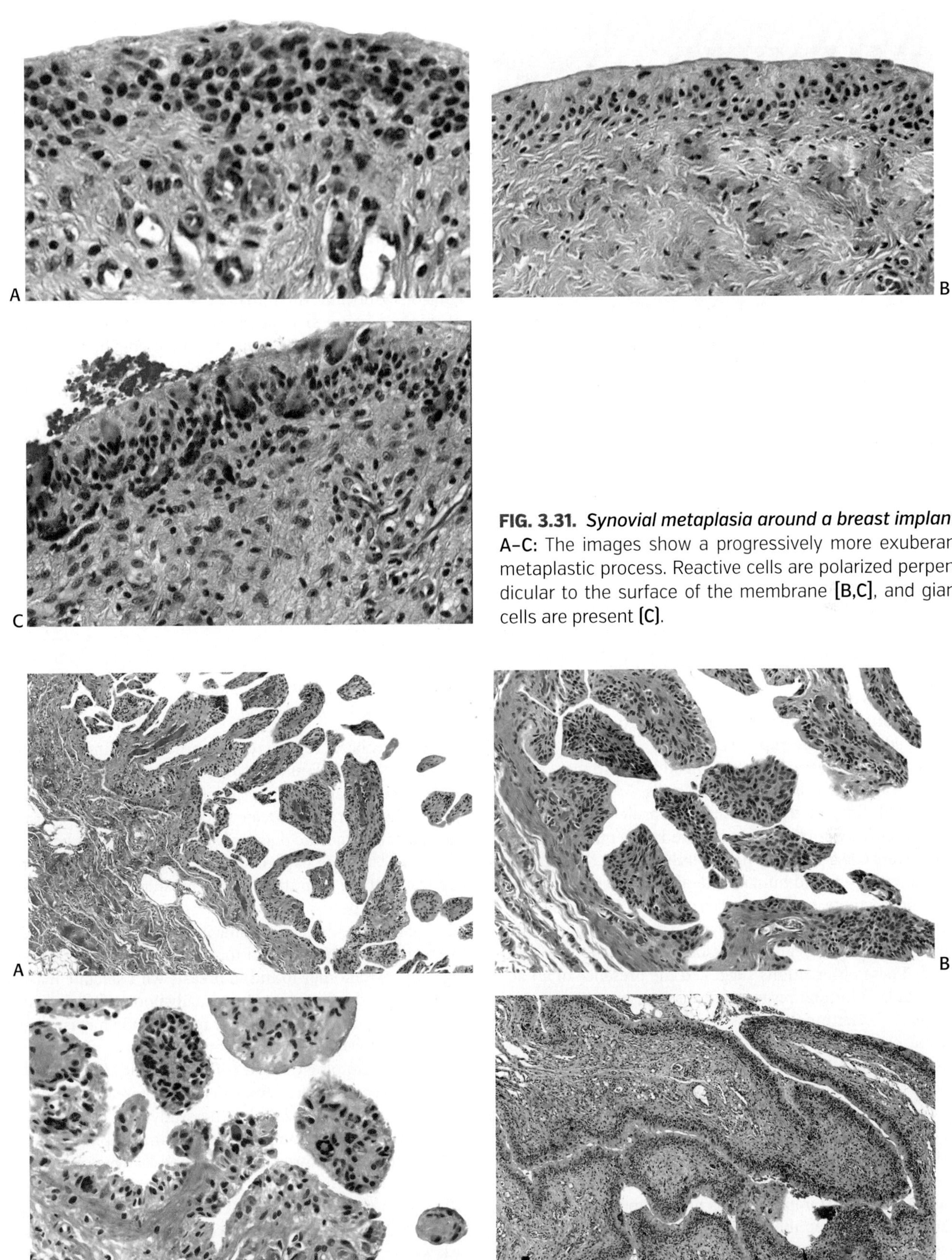

FIG. 3.31. ***Synovial metaplasia around a breast implant.*** **A–C:** The images show a progressively more exuberant metaplastic process. Reactive cells are polarized perpendicular to the surface of the membrane **(B,C)**, and giant cells are present **(C)**.

FIG. 3.32. ***Papillary synovial metaplasia formed around a textured implant*** **(A–D).** Papillary reaction on the inner surface of the capsule **(A–C)**. Multinucleated giant cells **(C)** and chronic inflammation are apparent **(D)**. An exaggerated papillary reaction on the surface of a capsule **(D)**.

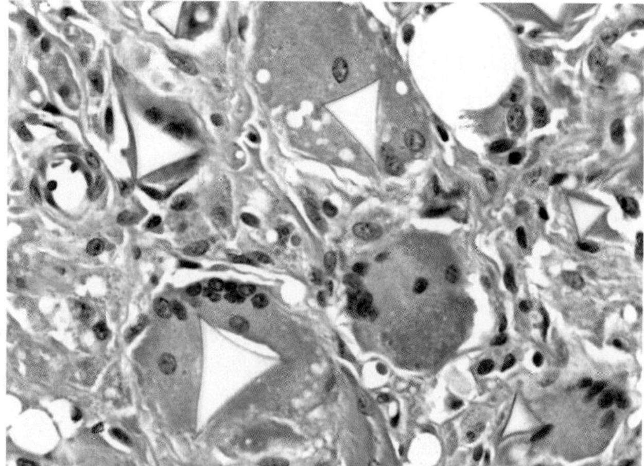

FIG. 3.33. ***Polyurethane-covered implant.*** Triangular polyurethane crystals are present in the granulomatous reaction.

that the layer of synovial metaplasia has a bosselated surface with fine cellular processes directed toward the lumen.[260]

Silicone particles have been identified by light microscopy and other procedures in all layers of the capsule formed around silicone gel implants.[250,261,262] Definitive identification can be made by scanning electron microscopy, backscattered electron imaging with x-ray spectroscopy, or electron probe microanalysis.[262,263] Laser-Raman microspectroscopy has been shown to provide rapid, accurate, and sensitive analysis of silicone and other particulate material associated with breast implants.[264,265]

The mononuclear cell reaction in and around the silicone implant capsule consists largely of T cells,[256,266,267] which are distributed diffusely throughout the capsule[217] and in fluid surrounding the implant.[266] In one study, the majority of the T cells were CD4+, CD29+ helper/inducer cells.[266] These investigators also found human leukocyte antigen (HLA)-DR immunoreactivity in foamy macrophages. HLA-DR+ and CD4+, CD29+ T lymphocytes were present in significantly greater numbers in capsular tissue than in the peripheral blood. These observations suggested the presence of an active cellular immune response in the periprosthetic capsular tissue.[266] Germinal centers were positive for CD20, and plasma cells in the capsule exhibited polyclonal immunoglobulin light chain reactivity.[256]

Most investigators who employed immunohistochemical stains found no evidence of epithelial differentiation in synovial metaplasia. However, rare instances of squamous metaplasia and squamous carcinoma arising from the surface of implant capsules have been reported.[268] Squamous cells lining a breast implant bursa presumably arise from the mammary ductal epithelium damaged during insertion of the implant. Squamous metaplasia is not unusual in breast tissue at a healing surgical site after excisional biopsy, and, rarely, the metaplastic epithelium is observed to grow on the surface of granulation tissue around a biopsy cavity.

Two breast augmentation techniques other than paraffin or silicone injections and placement of silicone implants are polyacrylamide gel injection into the retromammary space and autologous placement of fat obtained by liposuction. The former can elicit an inflammatory response and cause distortion of the breast due to gel migration,[269] and the latter can be associated with fat necrosis that results in the formation of masses composed of liponecrotic pseudocysts with calcification.[270]

Treatment and Prognosis

It may become necessary to perform a total mastectomy to control significant inflammatory or cosmetic complications of injected liquid silicone. Cosmetic results of reconstruction have been unsatisfactory when patients had cutaneous infiltration by silicone. Usually, the effects of leakage from silicone-filled prostheses have been managed by replacing the prosthesis and removing the surrounding contracture. Masses caused by migration of silicone out of the breast are treated by resection when necessary.

Since a carcinoma may be difficult to detect in the presence of silicone mastitis, patients with this condition should have careful clinical follow-up. Women with a strong family history of breast carcinoma or other predisposing factors are candidates for "prophylactic" mastectomy if they have significant silicone mastitis. Slight clinical changes in the breast should be evaluated by mammography, MRI, and biopsy.

Malignant Mammary Neoplasms and Silicone Augmentation

There have been reports of mammary carcinoma arising after injection of liquid silicone into the breast[237,238,240,271] or following leakage from prostheses containing silicone gel.[238] The interval between silicone injection or prosthesis placement and the diagnosis of carcinoma has been 5 to 20 years.[235,238] One patient who developed silicone mastitis as a result of the migration of silicone injected over her sternum to treat pectus excavatum was unexpectedly found to have an invasive duct carcinoma in one breast when bilateral mastectomy was performed for cosmetic reasons.[272] Histologically, carcinomas found in breasts with silicone mastitis have been of the ductal variety, usually poorly differentiated. Most of the patients had axillary lymph node metastases reflecting relatively advanced lesions.

Two epidemiologic studies of women with silicone breast implants have not detected evidence of increased frequency of breast carcinoma.[273,274] In one study, the risk of breast carcinoma among women with silicone implants proved to be significantly lower than expected.[273] This observation suggested that women who underwent augmentation were "drawn from a population already at low risk and that the implants do not substantially increase the risk." The reduced risk was found even in the group with the longest follow-up ranging from 10 to 18 years and at all ages.

Instances of mammary fibromatosis have been described in women with breast prostheses. This observation probably reflects the association between mammary fibromatosis and any type of prior surgical procedure.[275] Fibromatosis accounted for six cases in a series of eight implant-associated mesenchymal tumors.[276] The other neoplasms were a fibrosarcoma and a pleomorphic sarcoma. The latter patient with silicone breast implants had been treated by mastectomy and radiotherapy for breast carcinoma 10 years before the sarcoma was diagnosed. Some of the implants associated with fibromatosis contained saline rather than silicone.

The extraordinary occurrence of angiosarcoma associated with breast augmentation procedures involving silicone and no history of radiation has been reported.[277–279] A long latent period between the augmentation procedures and the clinical manifestations of angiosarcoma was noted in all cases. The association of anaplastic large T-cell lymphoma with silicone breast prostheses[280,281] is discussed in Chapter 40.

Nonneoplastic Diseases and Silicone Augmentation

Isolated case reports have documented the occurrence of systemic scleroderma in women who had silicone-containing breast implants.[282–284] The average interval between implantation and the onset of symptoms was about 8 years.[285] The reported observed frequency of scleroderma associated with silicone breast implants is less than would be by chance alone. A case-control study of a large group of patients failed to detect a significant relationship between silicone breast implants and the risk of developing systemic lupus erythematosus.[286] In 1994, Edelman et al.[287] reviewed all of the then available case reports totaling 40 patients in case series, case-control studies, surveys of plastic surgeons, and cohort studies and found no evidence of an association between silicone breast implants and connective tissue diseases. This conclusion was supported by another review of the subject published in 1997.[288] Weinzweig et al.[224] found no correlation between capsular and breast tissue levels of silicone in patients with and without connective tissue disorders who had either saline or silicone breast implants.

DIABETIC MASTOPATHY

The occurrence of tumor-forming fibrous stromal proliferations in patients with diabetes mellitus was first noted in 1984[289] and subsequently described as mastopathy in insulin-dependent diabetics[290] and diabetic mastopathy.[291] It has been reported that glycosylation and an increase in intermolecular cross-linkages observed in diabetics render collagen resistant to degradation in these patients.[292,293] This process could be responsible for the accumulation of fibrous tissue characteristic of some connective tissue disorders in diabetics, including mastopathy.[289]

The pathologic changes that characterize diabetic mastopathy are not entirely specific for insulin-dependent diabetes mellitus. A review of breast biopsies from patients with diabetes revealed diabetic mastopathy only in those with insulin-dependent disease.[294] However, others have reported the characteristic constellation of pathologic changes in patients who did not have diabetes.[295,296] Nondiabetic autoimmune diseases included hypothyroidism, systemic lupus erythematosus, Sjogren syndrome, and Hashimoto thyroiditis. These reports included men as well as women.

Clinical Presentation

With rare exceptions in men,[291,295,297–299] reported examples of diabetic mastopathy have been in women (Table 3.1). Two male patients described by Weinstein et al.[299] were 42 and 45 years of age at the time of diagnosis. Each had insulin-dependent diabetes mellitus. The palpable retroareolar

TABLE 3.1 Clinical Findings in Diabetic Mastopathy

References	No. Cases	Age Onset Diabetes (yr)	Age Onset Biopsy (yr)	Bilaterality, No. (%) Pts	Retinopathy, No. (%) Pts	Thyroid Disease, No. Pts
Soler and Khardori[289]	12	4–32 (mean, 13)	25–40 (mean, 34)	10 (85)	11 (95)	5 Thyroiditis
Gump and McDermmott[300]	11	8–15 (mean, 12)	27–41 (mean, 35)	5 (46)	–	3 Hypothyroid
Byrd et al.[290]	8	4–19	19–41 (mean, 34)	–	5 (64)	–
Tomaszewski et al.[291]	8	12–33	32–63 (mean, 40)	3 (39)	4 (51)	1 Hypothyroid
Lammie et al.[303]	3	–	31–41 (mean, 36)	1 (34)	–	1 Thyroid microsomal antibodies
Seidman et al.[294]	5	–	34–59 (mean, 47)	0	4	0
Valdez et al.[302]	7	–	30–46 (mean, 38)	–	–	–
TOTAL	**54**	**4–33**	**19–63**	**19 (41)**	**24 (52)**	

masses were clinically and mammographically consistent with gynecomastia. In one case, sonography revealed a hypoechoic tumor. Most female patients were younger than 30, and the majority were 20 years of age or younger when type 1 insulin-dependent diabetes mellitus was diagnosed. A few patients with type 2 diabetes have been described.[291,294] The mean ages at onset of diabetes in two studies were 12 and 13 years.[289,300] Almost all patients were premenopausal when the breast lesions were biopsied. The age when diabetic mastopathy was established by biopsy ranged from 19 to 63 years, with a mean of 34 to 47 years in six studies. The interval between the onset of diabetes and the detection of the breast lesion has averaged about 20 years. Bilateral lesions have been diagnosed in nearly 50% of cases.

The majority of the patients have had complications of juvenile onset diabetes, with severe diabetic retinopathy reported in many cases. In one series, 5 of 12 patients had thyroiditis with elevated serum levels of thyroid microsomal antibodies and enlarged thyroid glands.[289] One woman was thyrotoxic, whereas 11 were euthyroid. None of the patients had antibodies to thyroglobulin. These authors found that 4 patients had neuropathy, and 11 of 12 patients had limited joint mobility indicative of cheiroarthropathy. Hypothyroidism has been reported in some cases.[295,298,300,301] Valdez et al.[302] found no evidence of immunoglobulin heavy chain rearrangement in the lymphocytic infiltrates in seven cases of diabetic mastopathy. The absence of a B-cell clone led these authors to conclude that the patients were not at increased risk for developing lymphoma.

It has been suggested that diabetic mastopathy is one of the manifestations of HLA-associated autoimmune disease. In a series of 13 patients with lymphocytic lobulitis studied by Lammie et al.,[303] only 3 had juvenile onset diabetes. In individual cases, circulating autoantibodies were detected to smooth muscle, parietal cells and thyroid microsomes, and thyroid epithelium. No autoantibodies were detected with the panel used in three cases. HLA typing of DR3, DR4, and DR1 was found in two patients with type 1 diabetes. Others reported that HLA histocompatibility typing did not reveal a distinct subtype.[289]

The initial clinical symptom is a palpable, firm-to-hard tumor detected in one or both breasts. The lesions tend to be ill defined and nontender, and they may suggest carcinoma. The mammogram reveals localized increased density or a heterogeneous parenchymal pattern, but no radiographic changes have been specifically associated with this condition. In some cases, the mammographic appearance of the mass resembles carcinoma or a fibroadenoma.[290,300,304] Breast density associated with diabetic mastopathy could obscure a coexistent lesion such as carcinoma, a setting in which MRI may be useful.[305,306] Spontaneous regression and clinical disappearance of diabetic mastopathy has been reported.[304]

Gross Pathology

The lesions have measured 2.0 to 6.0 cm. Most specimens do not contain a visible tumor, but a distinct firm or hard mass is palpable, and the area of involvement has a firm edge when bisected. The cut surface of the tumor discloses homogeneous white-to-pale gray tissue that may be trabeculated but is often visibly indistinguishable from the surrounding fibrous breast parenchyma (Fig. 3.34). Cysts and other gross alterations of proliferative breast disease are not an integral part of diabetic mastopathy.

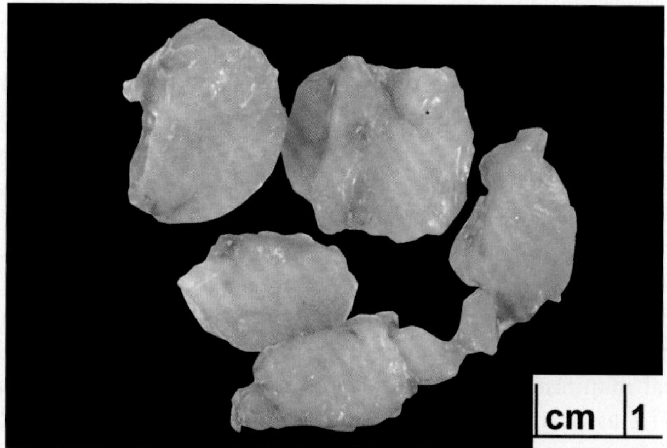

FIG. 3.34. *Diabetic mastopathy.* Gross specimen transected to reveal ill-defined fibrous stroma in diabetic mastopathy.

Microscopic Pathology

The lesional tissue consists of collagenous stroma with keloidal features and an increased concentration of stromal spindle cells when compared with the surrounding breast tissue (Fig. 3.35). Polygonal epithelioid cells are found dispersed in the collagen among spindle cells[294] (Fig. 3.36). The lesional cells, which, in general, show myofibroblastic differentiation, are immunoreactive for CD10, smooth muscle actin (SMA), desmin, CD34, and S-100 protein.[307] Tomaszewski et al.[291] concluded that these cells were specifically associated with diabetic mastopathy and that they

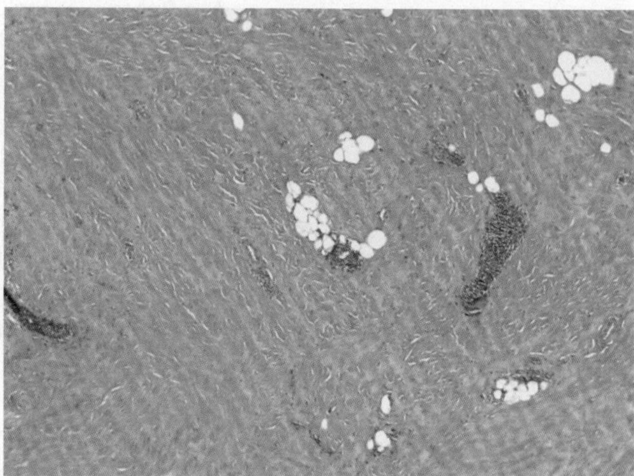

FIG. 3.35. *Diabetic mastopathy.* Histologic section showing typical expansion of the collagenous stroma, which contains prominent myofibroblasts and perivascular lymphocytic infiltrates.

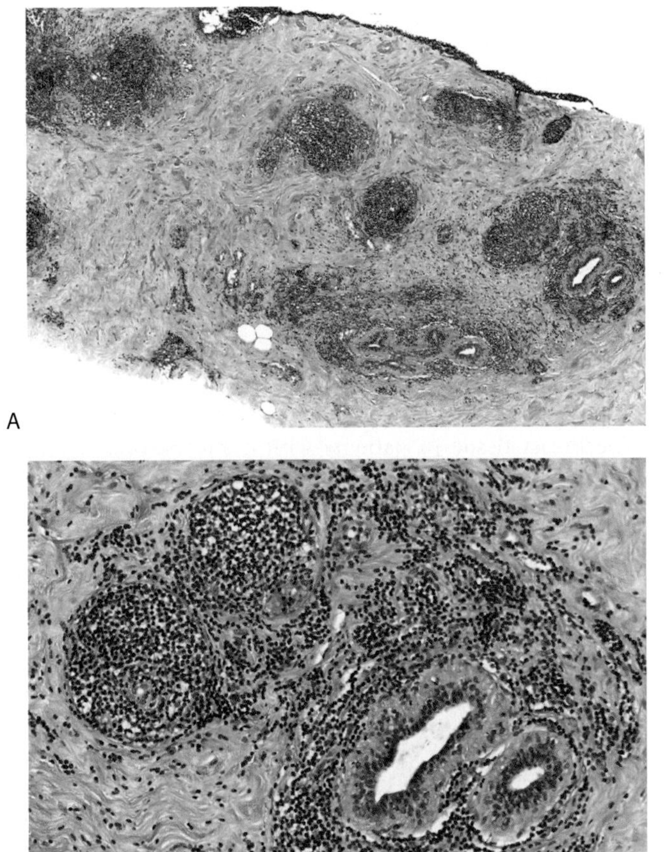

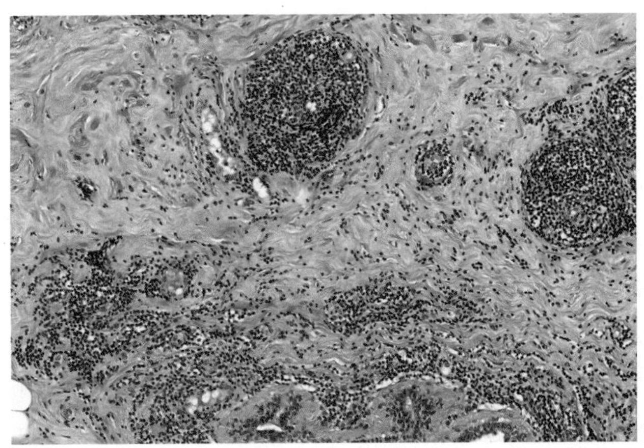

FIG. 3.36. ***Diabetic mastopathy on needle core biopsy.*** **A–C:** Prominent perivascular lymphocytic response in keloid-like stroma.

are absent from nondiabetic lobulitis, but this distinction has not been emphasized by other authors.[303,308] Multinucleated stromal giant cells and mitotic activity are not part of this proliferative process (Fig. 3.37). Mature lymphocytes are clustered circumferentially around small blood vessels throughout the lesion, as well as in and around lobules and ducts (Fig. 3.38). In most instances, diabetic mastopathy has all of the foregoing histologic features, but on occasion, one or more of the typical findings may be absent.[309]

Plasma cells and leukocytes are present in the perivascular infiltrates. Germinal centers are rarely formed. Infarcts, fat necrosis, duct stasis, arteritis, and other inflammatory lesions are not features of diabetic mastopathy. Stromal collagen fibers may appear prominent, but they do not have

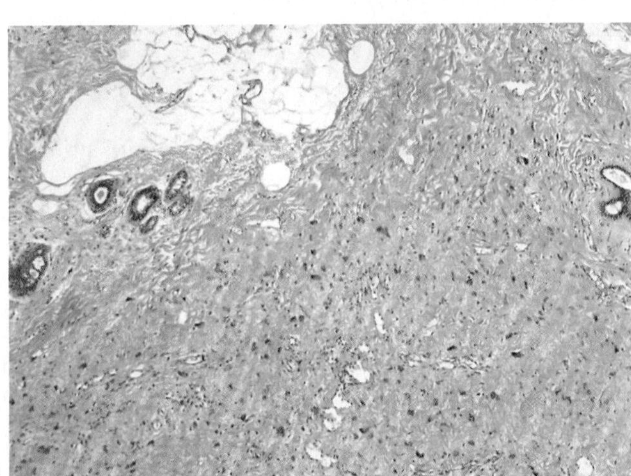

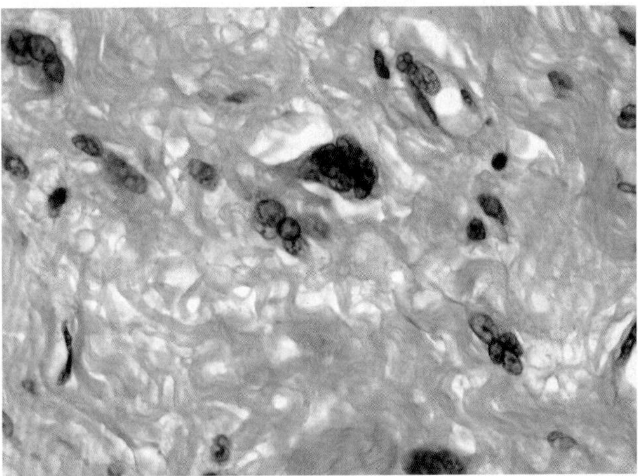

FIG. 3.37. ***Multinucleated stromal giant cells.*** **A:** Localized groups of these cells are an incidental finding unrelated to diabetic mastopathy. **B:** Multinucleated stromal giant cells.

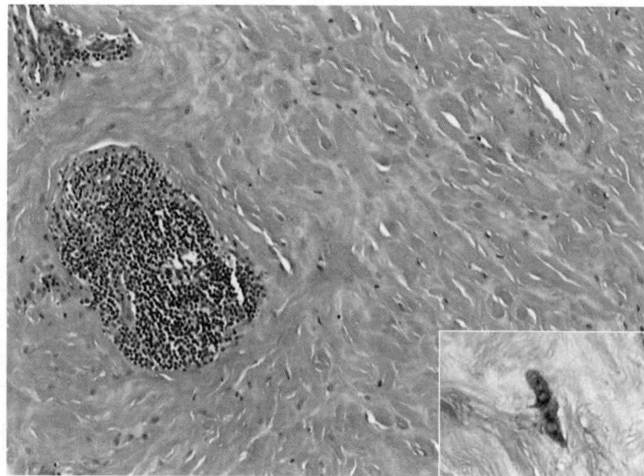

FIG. 3.38. ***Diabetic mastopathy.*** **A,B:** A perivascular infiltrate of mature lymphocytes and myofibroblast [*inset*] proliferation in the surrounding stroma.

a keloidal appearance. Stains for amyloid were negative in two cases, and mast cells have not been present in increased numbers.[290]

The lymphocytic infiltrate is composed predominantly of B cells.[291,303] It has been suggested that the lymphocytic infiltrate composed predominantly of B cells is a feature associated with diabetic mastitis and that nondiabetic mastitis features higher proportions of T cells.[291] However, Schwartz and Strauchen[308] studied eight patients with lesions they characterized as lymphocytic mastopathy, including only one with diabetes mellitus, and reported that the lymphocytic infiltrates in all cases had a B-cell phenotype. Similar results were obtained by Lammie et al.[303] Hunfeld and Bässler[298] compared the stromal and lymphocytic features of diabetic mastopathy and nondiabetic lymphocytic mastitis. Diabetic mastopathy was characterized by greater stromal fibrosis, lobular atrophy, and the presence of epithelioid myofibroblasts in each case. On the other hand, fibrosis tended to be less pronounced, and there were epithelioid myofibroblasts in only one case of lymphocytic mastitis. There was also a more intense B-cell lymphocyte reaction with relatively fewer T cells and macrophages in diabetic mastopathy.

Cytology

FNA cytology may be helpful in monitoring patients with recurrent lesions after a diagnosis of diabetic mastopathy has been established by surgical biopsy.[310] The FNA specimen consists of ductal epithelial cells in clusters, lymphocytes, and epithelioid fibroblasts that are most readily identified if the specimen includes fragments of connective tissues. The diagnosis of diabetic mastopathy by ultrasound-guided needle core biopsy has been reported to be more reliable than FNA.[311]

Treatment and Prognosis

Diabetic mastopathy is generally a self-limited stromal abnormality typically of premenopausal women. Recurrent tumors have occurred in the ipsilateral breast in a minority of cases, and these patients are prone to asynchronous, as well as synchronous, bilateral involvement. Excisional biopsy is adequate treatment. There is no evidence to suggest that diabetic mastopathy predisposes to the development of mammary carcinoma or stromal neoplastic diseases such as fibromatosis. However, patients with diabetic mastopathy can develop mammary carcinoma coincidentally, and therefore any mass that occurs in these women should be subjected to diagnostic assessment.

CYSTIC FIBROSIS

The breast tissue in patients with cystic fibrosis exhibits normal duct and lobular development.[312] Stromal fibrosis with lobular atrophy and ductal sclerosis has been described. There does not appear to be a specific inflammatory lesion. Various epithelial proliferative changes in the breast, including carcinoma, can occur in patients with cystic fibrosis.

Periodic CT scanning has been proposed as a monitoring tool for the assessment of lung disease in patients with cystic fibrosis. However, there has been concern that this would increase the cumulative risk of radiation-induced breast carcinoma, especially in women. Calculations presented by de González et al.[313] estimated the cumulative risk for radiation-induced breast carcinoma after annual lung CT scanning started at 2 years of age to be 26.3 per 100,000 for women with the current median survival of 36 years. For women with a projected median survival by the year 2030 of 50 years, the cumulative risk was estimated to be 275 per 100,000. The total risks for solid malignant neoplasms were 66.2 and 448.8 per 100,000 for women with median survivals of 36 and 50 years, respectively. Although women with a median survival of 50 years had relatively low risks of breast carcinoma of 0.28% and of solid malignant neoplasms of 0.45%, the authors concluded that "routine [CT] monitoring should not be recommended until there is demonstrated benefit that will outweigh these risks."

AMYLOID TUMOR

Amyloid is a group of approximately 25 fibril proteins, which, in certain conditions, deposit in extracellular tissue.[314] Amyloid deposits in the breast have been described in patients with predisposing systemic diseases such as primary amyloidosis,[315,316] rheumatoid arthritis,[317–319] multiple myeloma,[320] and Waldenstrom macroglobulinemia.[321] Some of these patients have had concurrent pulmonary and mammary amyloid tumors.[315,320] The underlying disease is well documented in these cases, and breast involvement, when clinically evident, is invariably a late development. Primary amyloid tumors clinically limited to the breast are uncommon.[322–326] Concurrent pulmonary and mammary amyloid tumors in the absence of an underlying systemic disease are rare.[327] Amyloid has been detected in the stroma of mammary carcinomas, including invasive lobular,[328,329] invasive ductal,[328] and intraductal carcinoma.[330]

Clinical Presentation

Most reported patients with amyloid tumor of the breast have been women.[331] The age at diagnosis ranged from 45 to 86 years. The tumors have usually been solitary, but bilateral involvement has been described.[319,325,332,333] Amyloid tumors may be located in any part of the breast including the axillary tail[317,326] and subareolar region.[318] Involvement of the nipple was described in one case.[331] Most patients report the recent detection of a painless mass.

Clinical examination usually reveals a discrete, firm or hard tumor that is occasionally tender.[327,334] Retraction or dimpling of the overlying skin has been described in patients with lesions located near the skin. Rarely axillary lymphadenopathy may indicate involvement of one or more lymph nodes by amyloidosis.[318] The physical findings may lead to a clinical diagnosis of mammary carcinoma.[318,330] This impression is strengthened if mammographic examination reveals calcifications in the lesion.[316,322,325,332,333,335] This possibility is exemplified by a 51-year-old woman who was found to have ipsilateral breast calcifications 2 years after breast-conserving surgery followed by adjuvant radiation and chemotherapy for a T1N1M0 breast carcinoma.[336] Recurrent carcinoma was suspected clinically, but the sample obtained by needle core biopsy was diagnostic of amyloid tumor. Although the patient had an elevated antinuclear antibody (ANA) titer, she had no systemic evidence of an autoimmune disease. The association of an amyloid tumor with prior irradiation in this case is probably a coincidence.

Gross Pathology

Amyloid tumors of the breast typically measure 2 to 3 cm in diameter. The largest lesion reported was 5 cm.[335] Grossly, the lesion is firm, gray or white, and opalescent. If calcification is present, there may be a gritty sensation when the lesion is incised. Fat and small cysts may be present in breast parenchyma incorporated within the lesion.

Microscopic Pathology

Histologic examination reveals eosinophilic amorphous, homogeneous deposits of amyloid. This material is distributed not only in fat, fibrocollagenous stroma, and blood vessels, but also around ducts and within lobules (Fig. 3.39). Deposits of amyloid around ducts and in lobules are associated with atrophy and obliteration of these glandular components (Fig. 3.40). In adipose tissue, thin ribbons of amyloid may be formed around individual fat cells (Fig. 3.41). These so-called amyloid rings are accentuated when Congo red–stained sections are examined with polarized light.[315,337,338] A variable plasma cell and lymphocytic infiltrate is present in association with the amyloid deposits. Multinucleated giant

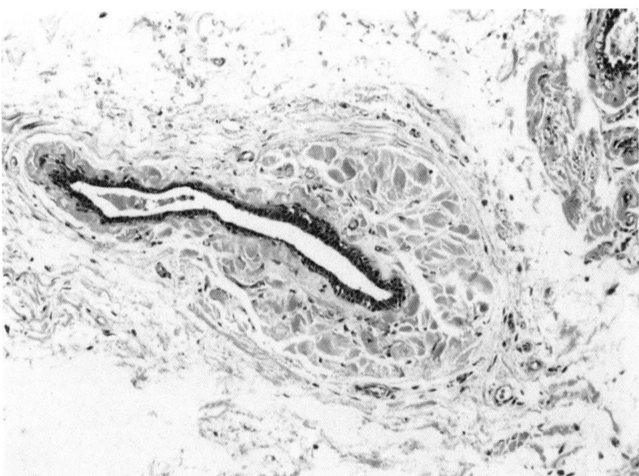

FIG. 3.39. ***Amyloidosis.*** Nodular deposits of amyloid are present in the periductal collagen.

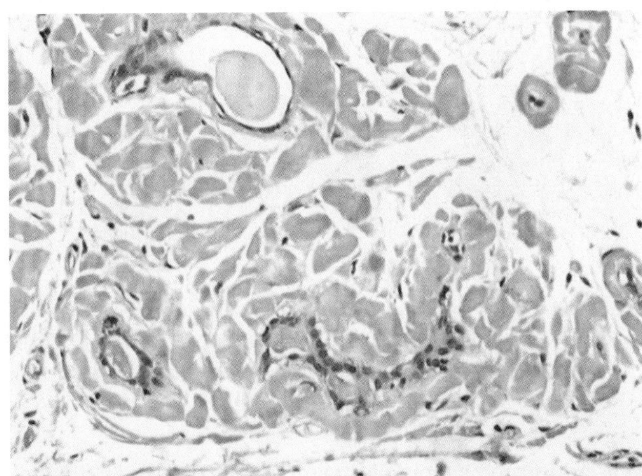

FIG. 3.40. ***Amyloidosis.*** Amyloid is deposited in the basement membranes and collagen surrounding lobular glands and ductules.

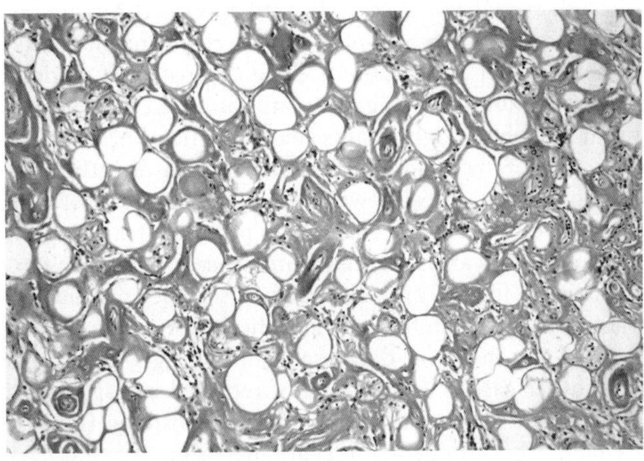

FIG. 3.41. ***Amyloidosis.*** Amyloid rings in fat.

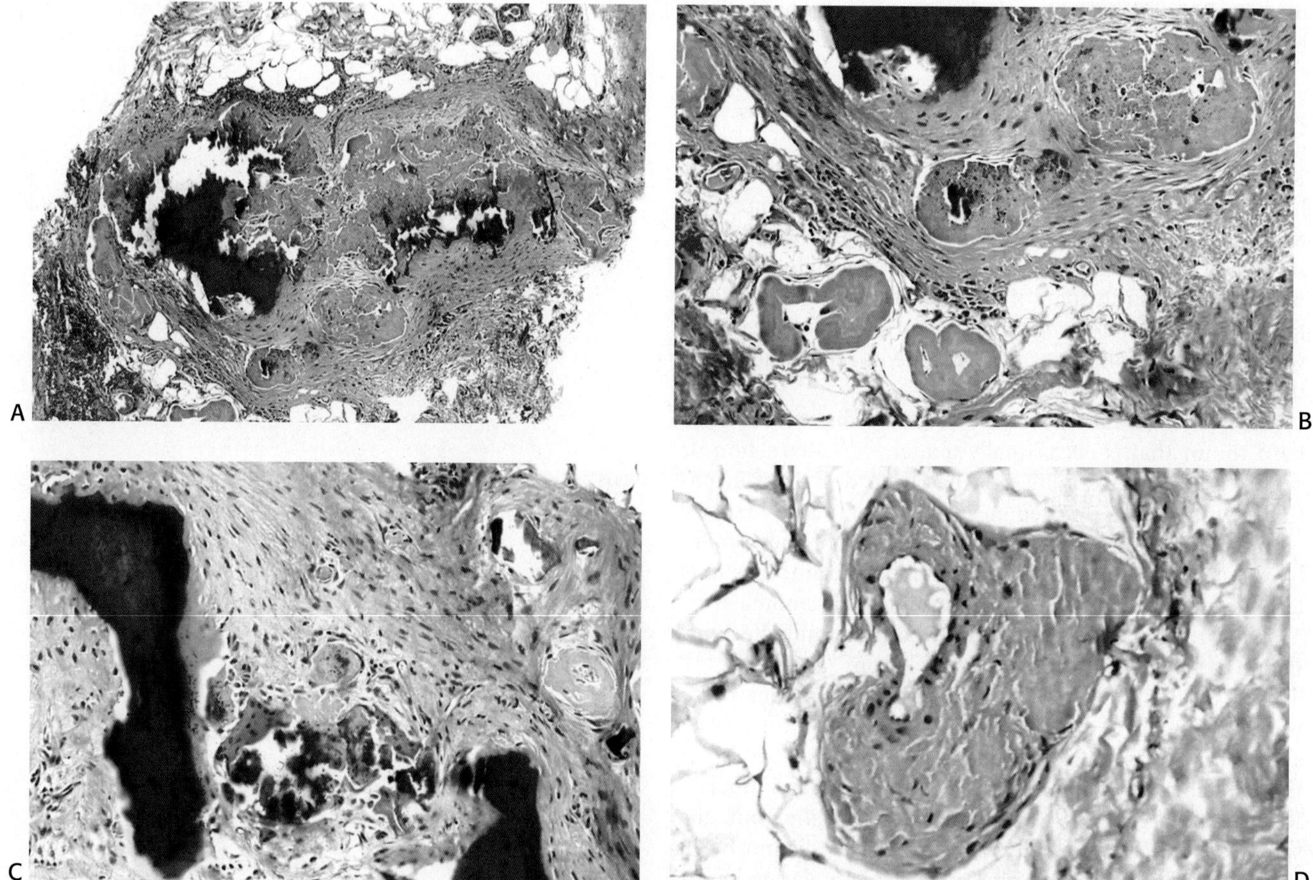

FIG. 3.42. ***Amyloid tumor.*** **A–C:** The lesion is composed of masses of amyloid, fibrosis, multinucleated giant cells, calcifications, and ossification. **D:** Amyloid in the wall of a blood vessel. The amyloid deposits are not associated with epithelial structures in this instance.

cells appear to be a manifestation of a foreign-body–like reaction to the amyloid with prominent granulomatous features (Fig. 3.42). Amyloid deposits in the breast may develop focal calcification, and rarely osseous metaplasia.[339,340]

Amyloid is stained red-orange with alkaline Congo red, and it exhibits apple-green birefringence when the Congo red–stained section is examined with polarized light. Staining with crystal violet results in a strong metachromatic reaction. In most cases, apple-green birefringence has been preserved after incubation of Congo red–stained sections with potassium permanganate, indicating the presence of immunoglobulin light chains characteristic of AL amyloid (Fig. 3.43). Silverman et al.[325] reported that direct immunofluorescence revealed weak staining for IgG, IgM, and kappa and lambda light chains with prominent staining for IgA in bilateral amyloid tumors in one case, and strong focal staining for IgG and lambda chains in the amyloid and plasma cells in another lesion. Others found staining for kappa light chains in one case[324] and for IgG and kappa in another case.[320] In a review of reported cases, Röcken et al.[328] noted that kappa light chain deposits were more frequent than alpha light chain deposits in mammary amyloidosis.

Cytology

Amyloid obtained by FNA appears as refractile or glassy amorphous material in Papanicolaou-stained smears. Metachromasia is evident with a modified Wright stain, and the amyloid appears purple with the May–Grünwald–Giemsa stain.[325] The sparsely cellular smears reveal scattered plasma cells, lymphocytes, spindly stromal cells, epithelial cells, and occasional multinucleated giant cells.

Electron Microscopy

Electron microscopy reveals the presence of straight, nonbranching, haphazardly arranged amyloid fibrils measuring 5 to 12 nm in diameter.[317,322,325,328] The amyloid fibrils are enmeshed to some extent with bands of collagen fibers.

Treatment and Prognosis

Excisional biopsy or needle core biopsy is useful for the diagnosis of amyloid tumor of the breast. The distinction between a primary amyloid tumor and secondary amyloidosis can be made only by careful clinical evaluation to rule

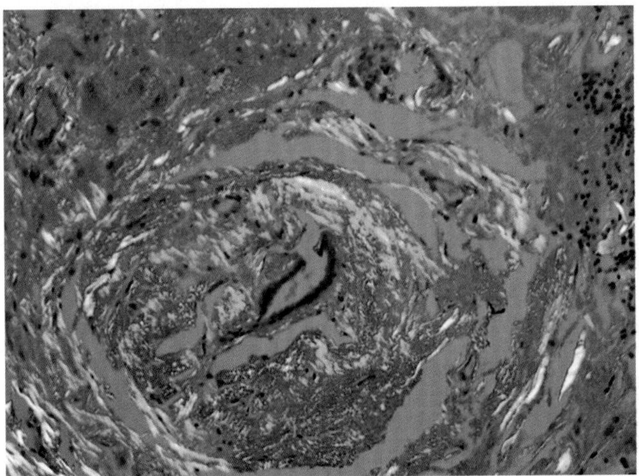

FIG. 3.43. ***Amyloid tumor.*** Apple-green birefringence of amyloid is present in the periductal tissue (Congo red stain with polarized light).

out a systemic condition. This should include a thorough clinical history and physical examination, and appropriate studies of serum proteins and blood, and possibly bone marrow examination. A concurrent hematologic disorder should be excluded in all cases of mammary amyloidosis. In a series of 40 cases of mammary amyloidosis, 22 (55%) were found to have a concomitant hematologic disorder, most commonly mucosal-associated lymphoid tissue lymphoma.[341]

In patients without evidence of concurrent hematologic disorder, most have remained well following an excisional biopsy in the limited follow-up reported to date. However, one woman who presented with bilateral mammary amyloid tumors developed systemic amyloidosis 1 year later,[332] and one woman had bilateral mammary amyloid tumors detected asynchronously over an interval of 10 months.[325] The prognosis of patients with systemic amyloidosis depends on the clinical course of the underlying condition.[341]

NEPHROGENIC SYSTEMIC FIBROSIS

Nephrogenic systemic fibrosis (NSF) is a systemic fibrosing disorder that primarily affects patients with chronic renal insufficiency who are on hemodialysis. NSF is characterized by thickening and hardening of skin of the extremities and trunk, the formation of papules and nodules, and the development of hyperpigmentation and flexion contractures.[342] NSF with swelling and dimpling of both breasts, simulating bilateral inflammatory breast carcinoma, was reported by Solomon and Rosen.[343] In this case, NSF of the breast mimicked inflammatory carcinoma clinically. Microscopic examination revealed thick collagen bundles in the dermis and proliferation of small blood vessels surrounded by a predominant plasma cell infiltrate.

IgG4-RELATED SCLEROSING MASTITIS

Clinical Presentation

IgG4 is the least common of the four subclasses on IgG. Elevated serum titers of IgG4 occur in a variety of IgG4-related diseases that are manifested by the presence of painless tumors. Symptomatology depends on the organ or organs involved. The prototype for this condition is sclerosing pancreatitis (autoimmune pancreatitis). Other common sites of the disease include the salivary glands, orbit, lymph nodes, the thyroid gland, the hepatobiliary tract, and the breast.[344]

Usually measuring 2 cm or more in diameter, the lesions of IgG4-related sclerosing mastitis typically present as one or more painless masses in one or both breasts. Lymphadenopathy in the axilla or other sites may be present. The ages at diagnosis of four female patients described by Cheuk et al.[345] ranged from 37 to 54 years.

Microscopic Pathology

The histologic findings in IgG4-related sclerosing lesions are varied. Those with a pseudolymphomatous pattern feature dense infiltrates of lymphocytes with germinal centers and plasma cells. In this form, sclerosis and inflammation of veins are inconspicuous. Large numbers of IgG4+ plasma cells are detected by immunohistochemistry. Lymphocytes, germinal centers, and plasma cells are less conspicuous in lesions that have prominent sclerotic tissue and phlebitis. A third, mixed pattern has both sclerosis and lymphocytic infiltrates.[344]

As described by Cheuk et al.,[345] the lesions of IgG4-related sclerosing mastitis can have a prominent pseudolymphomatous pattern that does not have a lobulocentric or periductal distribution. The amount and form of sclerosis vary from case to case, consisting of hypocellular stroma with scanty fibroblasts. Granulomas and giant cells are not present. Phlebitis was found in only one of four cases described by Cheuk et al.[345] The lymphoid infiltrate was composed of CD20+ B cells and CD3+ T cells. The density of IgG4+ cells ranged from 272 to 495 per high-power field (HPF), constituting 49% to 85% of all IgG+ cells. Control cases of lymphocytic mastopathy had fewer than five IgG4+ cells per HPF. The concentration of these cells in idiopathic granulomatous mastitis ranged from 5 to 67 per HPF, except in one otherwise indistinguishable case with 398 IgG4+ cells per HPF.

Ogura et al.[346] studied two cases of GLM that had concentrations of 60 and more than 300 IgG4+ cells, respectively. Serum IgG4 was elevated in the latter case. IgG4+ cells were absent from or minimally present in 16 examples of nonspecific lymphocytic and nonlymphocytic mastitis examined by these investigators. A case reported by Zen et al.[126] as an example of "inflammatory pseudotumor" of the breast that featured elevated serum IgG4 and a diffuse infiltrate of IgG4+ plasma cells is probably an example of IgG4-related sclerosing mastitis. It is likely that other cases previously diagnosed as "inflammatory pseudotumor" may be examples of IgG4-related sclerosing mastitis (see Chapter 40).

The diagnosis of IgG4-related sclerosing mastitis requires not only the presence of an increased number of IgG4 plasma cells and elevated serum IgG4, but also the proper histologic findings and the appropriate clinical presentation. Based on limited experience with a small number of fully characterized cases, some lesions may resolve without treatment or after a biopsy has been performed. Recurrence of the breast lesion seems to be uncommon after complete excision, but lymphadenopathy may persist.

REFERENCES

Fat Necrosis

1. Haagensen CD. Traumatic fat necrosis. *Diseases of the breast.* 2nd ed. Philadelphia: W.B. Saunders, 1971:202–211.
2. Adair FE, Munger JT. Fat necrosis of the female breast report of 110 cases. *Am J Surg* 1947;74:117–128.
3. Lee BJ, Adair F. Traumatic fat necrosis of the female breast and its differentiation from carcinoma. *Ann Surg* 1920;72:188–195.
4. Sciallis AP, Chen B, Folpe AL. Cellular spindled histiocytic pseudotumor complicating mammary fat necrosis: a potential diagnostic pitfall. *Am J Surg Pathol* 2012;36:1571–1578.
5. Ilkani R, Gardezi S, Hedayati H, et al. Necrotizing mastopathy caused by calciphylaxis: a case report. *Surgery* 1997;122:967–968.
6. Leborgne R. Esteato necrosis quistica calcificada de la mama. *Torax* 1967;16:172–175.
7. Taboada JL, Stephens TW, Krishnamurthy S, et al. The many faces of fat necrosis in the breast. *AJR Am J Roentgenol* 2009;192:815–825.
8. Hogge JP, Robinson RE, Magnant CM, et al. The mammographic spectrum of fat necrosis of the breast. *Radiographics* 1995;15:1347–1356.
9. Bassett LW, Gold RH, Cove HC. Mammographic spectrum of traumatic fat necrosis: the fallibility of "pathognomonic" signs of carcinoma. *AJR Am J Roentgenol* 1978;130:119–122.
10. Bargum K, Moller Nielsen S. Case report: fat necrosis of the breast appearing as oil cysts with fat-fluid levels. *Br J Radiology* 1993;66:718–720.
11. Hooley R, Lee C, Tocino I, et al. Calcifications in axillary lymph nodes caused by fat necrosis. *AJR Am J Roentgenol* 1996;167:627–628.
12. Soo MS, Kornguth PJ, Hertzberg BS. Fat necrosis in the breast: sonographic features. *Radiology* 1998;206:261–269.
13. Daly CP, Jaeger B, Sill DS. Variable appearances of fat necrosis on breast MRI. *AJR Am J Roentgenol* 2008;191:1374–1380.
14. Trimboli RM, Carbonaro LA, Cartia F, et al. MRI of fat necrosis of the breast: the "black hole" sign at short tau inversion recovery. *Eur J Radiol* 2012;81:e573–e579.
15. Adejolu M, Huo L, Rohren E, et al. False-positive lesions mimicking breast cancer on FDG PET and PET/CT. *AJR Am J Roentgenol* 2012;198:W304–W314.
16. Barnes PJ, Foyle A, Hache KA, et al. Erdheim-Chester disease of the breast: a case report and review of the literature. *Breast J* 2005;11:462–467.
17. Provenzano E, Barter SJ, Wright PA, et al. Erdheim-Chester disease presenting as bilateral clinically malignant breast masses. *Am J Surg Pathol* 2010;34:584–588.

Hemorrhagic Necrosis and Anticoagulant Therapy

18. Verhagen H. Local hemorrhage and necrosis of the skin and underlying tissues, during anticoagulant therapy with dicumarol or dicumacyl. *Acta Medica Scand* 1954;148:453–467.
19. Flood PE, Redish MH, Bocie SJ, et al. Thrombophlebitis migrans disseminata. Report of a case in which gangrene of the breast occurred. *NY J Med* 1943;43:1121–1124.
20. Isenberg JS, Tu Q, Rainey W. Mammary gangrene associated with warfarin ingestion. *Ann Plast Surg* 1996;37:553–555.
21. Rick ME. Protein C and protein S. *JAMA* 1990;263:701–703.
22. Martin BF, Phillips JD. Gangrene of the female breast with anticoagulant therapy: report of two cases. *Am J Clin Pathol* 1970;53: 622–626.
23. Nadelman HL, Kempson RL. Necrosis of the breast: a rare complication of anticoagulant therapy. *Am J Surg* 1966;111:728–737.
24. Somerville P, Seifert PJ, Destounis SV, et al. Anticoagulation and bleeding risk after core needle biopsy. *AJR Am J Roentgenol* 2008;191:1194–1197.
25. Dutta Roy S, Selvachandran SN, Scally J, et al. Appropriateness of breast biopsy in rare cases of spontaneous breast hemorrhage resulting from anticoagulation therapy. *Breast J* 2005;11:363–364.

Breast Infarct

26. Ekeh AP, Marti JR. Spontaneous necrosis of an accessory breast during pregnancy. *Breast Dis* 1996;9:291–293.
27. Robitaille Y, Seemayer TA, Thelmo WL, et al. Infarction of the mammary region mimicking carcinoma of the breast. *Cancer* 1974;33:1183–1189.
28. Lucey JJ. Spontaneous infarction of the breast. *J Clin Pathol* 1975;28:937–943.
29. Newman J, Kahn LB. Infarction of fibroadenoma of the breast. *Brit J Surg* 1973;60:738–740.
30. Hasson J, Pope CH. Mammary infarcts associated with pregnancy presenting as breast tumors. *Surgery* 1961;49:313–316.
31. Toy H, Esen HH, Sonmez FC, et al. Spontaneous Infarction in a fibroadenoma of the breast. *Breast Care (Basel)* 2011;6:54–55.
32. Oh YJ, Choi SH, Chung SY, et al. Spontaneously infarcted fibroadenoma mimicking breast cancer. *J Ultrasound Med* 2009;28:1421–1423.
33. Kavdia R, Kini U. WCAFTI: worrisome cytologic alterations following tissue infarction; a mimicker of malignancy in breast cytology. *Diagn Cytopathol* 2008;36:586–588.
34. Flint A, Oberman HA. Infarction and squamous metaplasia of intraductal papilloma: a benign breast lesion that may simulate carcinoma. *Hum Pathol* 1984;15:764–767.
35. Walker AN, Betsill WL. Infarction of intraductal papilloma associated with hyperprolactinemia. *Arch Pathol Lab Med* 1980;104:280.
36. Jones EL, Codling BW, Oates GD. Necrotic intraduct breast carcinomas simulating inflammatory lesions. *J Pathol* 1973;110:101–103.
37. Yu L, Yang W, Cai X, et al. Centrally necrotizing carcinoma of the breast: clinicopathological analysis of 33 cases indicating its basal-like phenotype and poor prognosis. *Histopathology* 2010;57:193–201.

Inflammatory Lesions in Pregnancy and Lactation

38. Eschenbach DA. Acute postpartum infections. *Emerg Med Clin North Am* 1985;3:87–115.
39. Rickert RR, Rajan S. Localized breast infarcts associated with pregnancy. *Arch Pathol* 1974;97:159–161.
40. Boyle M, Lakhoo K, Ramani P. Galactocele in a male infant: case report and review of literature. *Pediatr Pathol* 1993;13:305–308.
41. Golden GT, Wangensteen SL. Galactocele of the breast. *Am J Surg* 1972;123:271–273.
42. Salvador R, Salvador M, Jimenez JA, et al. Galactocele of the breast: radiologic and ultrasonographic findings. *Br J Radiol* 1990;63:140–142.
43. Gómez A, Mata JM, Donoso L, et al. Galactocele: three distinctive radiographic appearances. *Radiology* 1986;158:43–44.
44. Novotny DB, Maygarden SJ, Shermer RW, et al. Fine needle aspiration of benign and malignant breast masses associated with pregnancy. *Acta Cytol* 1991;35:676–686.
45. Raso DS, Greene WB, Silverman JF. Crystallizing galactocele. A case report. *Acta Cytol* 1997;41:863–870.
46. Lawlor-Smith L, Lawlor-Smith C. Vasospasm of the nipple—a manifestation of Raynaud's phenomenon: case reports. *BMJ* 1997;314:644–645.

So-Called Plasma Cell Mastitis

47. Adair FE. Plasma cell mastitis—a lesion simulating mammary carcinoma. *Arch Surg* 1933;26:735–749.
48. Wilhelmus JL, Schrodt GR, Mahaffey LM. Cholesterol granulomas of the breast. A lesion which clinically mimics carcinoma. *Am J Clin Pathol* 1982;77:592–597.
49. Parsons WH, Henthorne JC, Clark RL Jr. Plasma cell mastitis. Report of five additional cases. *Arch Surg* 1944;49:86–89.

Mammary Duct Ectasia

50. Haagensen CD. Mammary duct ectasia. A disease that may simulate carcinoma. *Cancer* 1951;4:749–761.
51. Bloodgood JC. The pathology of chronic cystic mastitis of the female breast with special consideration of the blue-domed cyst. *Arch Surg* 1921;3:445–542.

52. Bloodgood JC. The clinical picture of dilated ducts beneath the nipple frequently to be palpated as a doughy worm-like mass—the varicocele tumor of the breast. *Surg Gynecol Obstet* 1923;36:486–495.
53. Tice GI, Dockerty MB, Harrington SW. Comedo mastitis: a clinical and pathologic study of data in 172 cases. *Surg Gynecol Obstet* 1948;87:525–540.
54. Rahal RM, de Freitas-Júnior R, Carlos da Cunha L, et al. Mammary duct ectasia: an overview. *Breast J* 2011;17:694–695.
55. Frantz VK, Pickren JW, Melcher GW, et al. Incidence of chronic cystic disease in so-called "normal breasts"; a study based on 225 postmortem examinations. *Cancer* 1951;4:762–783.
56. Davies JD. Inflammatory damage to ducts in mammary dysplasia: a cause of duct dilation. *J Path* 1975;117:47–54.
57. Payne RI, Strauss AF, Glasser RD. Mastitis obliterans. *Surgery* 1943;14:719–727.
58. Dixon JM, Anderson TJ, Lumsden AB, et al. Mammary duct ectasia. *Br J Surg* 1983;70:601–603.
59. Habif DV, Perzin KH, Lipton R, et al. Subareolar abscess associated with squamous metaplasia of lactiferous ducts. *Am J Surg* 1970;119:523–526.
60. Passaro ME, Broughan TA, Sebek BA, et al. Lactiferous fistula. *J Am Coll Surg* 1994;178:29–32.
61. Furlong AJ, Al-Nakib L, Knox WF, et al. Periductal inflammation and cigarette smoke. *J Am Coll Surg* 1994;179:417–420.
62. Bundred NJ, Dover MS, Coley S, et al. Breast abscesses and cigarette smoking. *Br J Surg* 1992;79:58–59.
63. Hunter-Craig ID, Tuddenham EGD, Earle JHO. Lipogranuloma of the breast due to phenothiazine therapy. *Br J Surg* 1970;57:76–79.
64. Shousha S, Backhouse CM, Dawson PM, et al. Mammary duct ectasia and pituitary adenomas. *Am J Surg Pathol* 1988;12:130–133.
65. Stringel G, Perelman A, Jimenez C. Infantile mammary duct ectasia: a cause of blood nipple discharge. *J Pediatr Surg* 1986;21:671–674.
66. Wang Z, Leonard MH Jr, Khamapirad T, et al. Bilateral extensive ductitis obliterans manifested by bloody nipple discharge in a patient with long-term diabetes mellitus. *Breast J* 2007;13:599–602.
67. Rees BI, Gravelle IH, Hughes LE. Nipple retraction in duct ectasia. *Br J Surg* 1977;64:577–580.
68. Khoda J, Lantsberg L, Yegev Y, et al. Management of periareolar abscess and mammillary fistula. *Surg Gynecol Obstet* 1992;175:306–308.
69. Walker JC, Sandison AT. Mammary duct ectasia. *Br J Surg* 1964;51:350–355.
70. Tedeschi LG, McCarthy PE. Involutional mammary duct ectasia and periductal mastitis in a male. *Hum Pathol* 1974;5:232–236.
71. McHoney M, Munro F, Mackinlay G. Mammary duct ectasia in children: report of a short series and review of the literature. *Early Hum Dev* 2011;87:527–530.
72. Sweeney DJ, Wylie EJ. Mammographic appearances of mammary duct ectasia that mimic carcinoma in a screening programme. *Austral Radiol* 1995;39:18–23.
73. Fisher CS, Margenthaler JA. A look into the ductoscope: its role in pathologic nipple discharge. *Ann Surg Oncol* 2011;18:3187–3191.
74. Davies JD. Human colostrum cells: their relation to periductal mononuclear inflammation. *J Pathol* 1974;112:153–160.
75. Davies JD. Periductal foam cells in benign mammary dysplasia. *J Pathol* 1975;117:39–45.
76. Hamperl H. The myothelia (myoepithelial cells). Normal state, regressive changes, hyperplasia, tumors. *Curr Top Pathol* 1970;53:161–220.
77. Dabbs DJ. Mammary ductal foam cells: macrophage immunophenotype. *Hum Pathol* 1993;24:977–981.
78. Tashiro T, Hirokawa M, Sano T. Are mammary pagetoid foam cells histiocytic or epithelial? *Virchows Arch* 2001;439:102–104.
79. Damiani S, Cattani MG, Buonamici L, et al. Mammary foam cells. Characterization by immunohistochemistry and in situ hybridization. *Virchows Arch* 1998;432:433–440.
80. Davies JD. Pigmented periductal cells (ochrocytes) in mammary dysplasias: their nature and significance. *J Pathol* 1974;114:205–216.
81. Dabbs DJ. Mammary ductal foam cells: macrophage immunophenotype for further cells? *Hum Pathol* 1994;25:214–215.
82. Reynolds HE, Cramer HM. Cholesterol granuloma of the breast: a mimic of carcinoma. *Radiology* 1994;191:249–250.
83. Davies JD. Hyperelastosis, obliteration and fibrous plaques in major ducts of the human breast. *J Pathol* 1973;110:13–26.

Granulomatous Lobular Mastitis

84. Fitzgibbons PL. Granulomatous mastitis. *NY State J Med* 1990;90:287.
85. Cohen C. Granulomatous mastitis: a review of 5 cases. *S Afr Med J* 1977;52:15–16.
86. Fletcher A, Magrath IM, Riddell RH, et al. Granulomatous mastitis: a report of seven cases. *J Clin Pathol* 1982;35:941–945.
87. Going JJ, Anderson TJ, Wilkinson S, et al. Granulomatous lobular mastitis. *J Clin Pathol* 1987;40:535–540.
88. Davies JD, Burton PA. Post-partum lobular granulomatous mastitis. *J Clin Pathol* 1983;36:363.
89. Kessler E, Wolloch Y. Granulomatous mastitis: a lesion clinically simulating carcinoma. *Am J Clin Pathol* 1972;58:642–646.
90. Brown KL, Tang PHL. Postlactational tumoral granulomatous mastitis: a localized immune phenomenon. *Am J Surg* 1979;138:326–329.
91. Murthy MSN. Granulomatous mastitis and lipogranuloma of the breast. *Am J Clin Pathol* 1973;60:432–433.
92. Donn W, Rebbeck P, Wilson C, et al. Idiopathic granulomatous mastitis. A report of three cases and review of the literature. *Arch Pathol Lab Med* 1994;118:822–825.
93. Hovanessian Larsen LJ, Peyvandi B, et al. Granulomatous lobular mastitis: imaging, diagnosis, and treatment. *AJR Am J Roentgenol* 2009;193:574–581.
94. Han B-K, Choe YH, Park JM, et al. Granulomatous mastitis: mammographic and sonographic appearances. *AJR Am J Roentgenol* 1999;173:317–320.
95. Kumarasinghe MP. Cytology of granulomatous mastitis. *Acta Cytol* 1997;41:727–730.
96. Kobayashi TK, Sugihara H, Kato M, et al. Cytologic features of granulomatous mastitis. Report of a case with fine needle aspiration cytology and immunocytochemical findings. *Acta Cytol* 1998;42:716–720.
97. Lacambra M, Thai TA, Lam CC, et al. Granulomatous mastitis: the histological differentials. *J Clin Pathol* 2011;64:405–411.
98. Oberman HA. Invasive carcinoma of the breast with granulomatous response. *Am J Clin Pathol* 1987;88:718–721.
99. Koo JS, Jung W. Xanthogranulomatous mastitis: clinicopathology and pathological implications. *Pathol Int* 2009;59:234–240.
100. De Hertogh DA, Rossof AH, Harris AA, et al. Prednisone management of granulomatous mastitis. *N Engl J Med* 1980;308:799–800.
101. Jorgensen MB, Nielsen DM. Diagnosis and treatment of granulomatous mastitis. *Am J Med* 1992;93:97–101.
102. Akbulut S, Yilmaz D, Bakir S. Methotrexate in the management of idiopathic granulomatous mastitis: review of 108 published cases and report of four cases. *Breast J* 2011;17:661–668.

Sarcoidosis

103. Fitzgibbons PL, Smiley DF, Kern WH. Sarcoidosis presenting initially as breast mass: report of two cases. *Hum Pathol* 1985;16:851–852.
104. Banik S, Bishop PW, Ormerod LP, et al. Sarcoidosis of the breast. *J Clin Pathol* 1986;39:446–448.
105. Reitz ME, Seidman I, Roses DF. Sarcoidosis of the breast. *NY State J Med* 1985;85:262–263.
106. Kenzel PP, Hadijuana J, Hosten N, et al. Boeck sarcoidosis of the breast: mammographic, ultrasound, and MR findings. *J Comp Assist Tomogr* 1997;21:439–441.
107. Kirshy D, Gluck B, Brancaccio W. Sarcoidosis of the breast presenting as a spiculated lesion. *AJR Am J Roentgenol* 1999;172:554–555.
108. Nicholson BT, Mills SE. Sarcoidosis of the breast: an unusual presentation of a systemic disease. *Breast J* 2007;13:99–100.
109. Ito T, Okada T, Murayama K, et al. Two cases of sarcoidosis discovered accidentally by positron emission tomography in patients with breast cancer. *Breast J* 2010;16:561–563.
110. Bush E, Lamonica D, O'Connor T. Sarcoidosis mimicking metastatic breast cancer. *Breast J* 2011;17:533–535.
111. Cooper NE. Rheumatoid nodule of the breast. *Histopathology* 1991;19:193–194.
112. Gorton G, Linell F. Malignant tumors and sarcoid reactions in regional lymph nodes. *Acta Radiol* 1957;47:381–392.
113. Bässler R, Birke F. Histopathology of tumour associated sarcoid-like stromal reaction in breast cancer. An analysis of 5 cases with immunohistochemical investigations. *Virchows Arch [A]* 1988;412:231–239.
114. Symmers WS. Localized tuberculoid granulomas associated with carcinoma, their relationship to sarcoidosis. *Am J Pathol* 1951;27:493–521.

115. Oberman HA. Invasive carcinoma of the breast with granulomatous response. *Am J Clin Pathol* 1987;88:718–721.
116. Voravud N, Sneige N, Theriault R, et al. Sarcoidosis and breast cancer. *Breast Dis* 1992;5:191–197.
117. Gansler TS, Wheeler JE. Mammary sarcoidosis. Two cases and literature review. *Arch Pathol Lab Med* 1984;108:673–675.
118. Shah AY, Solomon L, Gumbs MA. Sarcoidosis of the breast coexisting with mammary carcinoma. *NY State J Med* 1990;90:331–333.
119. Santini D, Pasquinelli G, Alberghini M, et al. Invasive breast carcinoma with granulomatous response and deposition of unusual amyloid. *J Clin Pathol* 1992;45:885–888.
120. Bodo M, Döbrössy L, Sugar J. Boeck's sarcoidosis of the breast: cytologic findings with aspiration biopsy cytology. A case clinically mimicking carcinoma *Acta Cytol* 1978;22:1–2.
121. Brincker H, Wilbek E. The incidence of malignant tumours in patients with respiratory sarcoidosis. *Br J Cancer* 1974;29:247–251.

Inflammatory Pseudotumor

122. Yip CH, Wong KT, Samuel D. Bilateral plasma cell granuloma (inflammatory pseudotumour) of the breast. *Aust N Z J Surg* 1997;67:300–303.
123. Pettinato G, Manivel JC, Insabato L, et al. Plasma cell granuloma (inflammatory pseudotumour) of the breast. *Am J Clin Pathol* 1988;90:627–632.
124. Chetty R, Govender D. Inflammatory pseudotumor of the breast. *Pathology* 1997;29:270–271.
125. Haj M, Weiss M, Loberant N, et al. Inflammatory pseudotumor of the breast: case report and literature review. *Breast J* 2003;9:423–425.
126. Zen Y, Kasahara Y, Horita K, et al. Inflammatory pseudotumor of the breast in a patient with a high serum IgG4 level: histologic similarity to sclerosing pancreatitis. *Am J Surg Pathol* 2005;29:275–278.
127. Shin SJ, Scamman W, Gopalan A, et al. Mammary presentation of adult-type "juvenile" xanthogranuloma. *Am J Surg Pathol* 2005;29:827–831.

Vasculitis

128. Hernández-Rodríguez J, Hoffman GS. Updating single-organ vasculitis. *Curr Opin Rheumatol* 2012;24:38–45.
129. Kim SM, Park JM, Moon WK. Dystrophic breast calcifications in patients with collagen diseases. *J Clin Imaging* 2004;28:6–9.
130. Waugh TR. Bilateral mammary arteritis. Report of a case. *Am J Pathol* 1950;26:851–861.
131. Clement PB, Senges H, How AR. Giant cell arteritis of the breast: case report and literature review. *Hum Pathol* 1987;18:1186–1189.
132. Cook DJ, Benson WG, Carroll JJ, et al. Giant cell arteritis of the breast. *CMAJ* 1988;139:513–515.
133. Horne D, Crabtree TS, Lewkonia RM. Breast arteritis in polymyalgia rheumatica. *J Rheumatol* 1987;14:613–615.
134. McKendry RJR, Guindi M, Hill DP. Giant cell arteritis (temporal arteritis) affecting the breast: report of two cases and review of published reports. *Ann Rheum Dis* 1990;49:1001–1004.
135. Polter BT, Housley E, Thomson D. Giant-cell arteritis mimicking carcinoma of the breast. *Br Med J* 1981;282:665–666.
136. Susmano A, Roseman D, Haber MH. Giant cell arteritis of the breast. A unique syndrome. *Arch Intern Med* 1990;150:900–904.
137. Marie I, Audeguy P, François A, et al. Giant cell arteritis presenting as breast lesion: report of a case and review of the literature. *Am J Med Sci* 2008;335:489–491.
138. Kadotani Y, Enoki Y, Itoi N, et al. Giant cell arteritis of the breast: a case report with a review of literatures. *Breast Cancer* 2010;17:225–232.
139. Lau Y, Mak YF, Hui PK, et al. Giant cell arteritis of the breast,. *Aust N Z J Surg* 1996;66:259–261.
140. Pappo I, Beglaibter N, Amir G. Mammary arteritis mimicking cancer. *Eur J Surg* 1992;158:191–193.
141. Dega FJ, Hunder GG. Vasculitis of the breast. An unusual manifestation of polyarteritis. *Arthritis Rheum* 1974;17:973–976.
142. Stephenson TJ, Underwood JCE. Giant cell arteritis: an unusual cause of palpable masses in the breast. *Br J Surg* 1986;73:105.
143. Codman GC, Churg J. Wegener's granulomatosis: pathology and review of the literature. *Arch Path* 1954;58:533–553.
144. Fauci AS, Haynes BF, Katz P, et al. Wegener's granulomatosis: prospective clinical and therapeutic experience with 85 patients in 21 years. *Ann Intern Med* 1983;98:76–85.
145. Elsner B, Harper FB. Disseminated Wegener's granulomatosis with breast involvement. *Arch Pathol* 1969;87:544–547.
146. Deininger HZ. Wegener's granulomatosis of the breast. *Radiology* 1985;154:59–60.
147. Jordan JM, Manning M, Allen, NB. Multiple unusual manifestations of Wegener's granulomatosis: breast mass, microangiopathic hemolytic anemia, consumptive coagulopathy, and low erythrocyte sedimentation rate. *Arthritis Rheum* 1986;29:1527–1531.
148. Jordan JM, Rowe TW, Allen NB. Wegener's granulomatosis involving the breast. Report of three cases and review of the literature. *Am J Med* 1987;83:159–164.
149. Oimoni M, Suehiro I, Mizuno N, et al. Wegener's granulomatosis with intracerebral granuloma and mammary manifestation. *Arch Intern Med* 1980;140:853–854.
150. Pambakian H, Tighe JR. Breast involvement in Wegener's granulomatosis. *J Clin Pathol* 1971;24:343–347.
151. Goulart RA, Mark EJ, Rosen S. Tumefactions as an extravascular manifestation of Wegener's granulomatosis. *Am J Surg Pathol* 1995;19:145–153.
152. Trüeb RM, Pericin M, Kohler E, et al. Necrotizing granulomatosis of the breast. *Br J Dermatol* 1997;137:799–803.
153. Allende DS, Booth CN. Wegener's granulomatosis of the breast: a rare entity with daily clinical relevance. *Ann Diagn Pathol* 2009;13:351–357.
154. Göbel U, Kettritz R, Kettritz U, et al. Wegener's granulomatosis masquerading as breast cancer. *Arch Intern Med* 1995;155:205–207.
155. Matsuoka Y, Yoshino K, Kohno M, et al. Necrotizing angiitis localized to the breasts. *Rynmachi* 1982;22:234–239.
156. McCarty DJ, Imbrigia J, Hung JK. Vasculitis of the breasts. *Arthritis Rheum* 1968;11:796–803.
157. Nishizawa T, Enomoto H, Hino T, et al. Vasculitis of the breast with thrombocytopenia. *J Rheumatol* 1979;5:595–597.
158. Yamashina M, Wilson TK. A mammographic finding in focal polyarteritis nodosa. *Br J Radiol* 1985;58:91–92.
159. Harrison GO, Elliott RL. Scleroderma of the breast: light and electron microscopy study. *Am Surg* 1987;53:526–531.
160. Forbes AM, Woodrow JC, Verbov JL, et al. Carcinoma of the breast and scleroderma: four further cases and a literature review. *Br J Rheumatol* 1989;28:65–69.
161. Papasavvas G, Goodwill CJ. Scleroderma and breast carcinoma. *Br J Rheumatol* 1989;28:366–367.
162. Roumm AD, Medsger TA. Cancer and systemic sclerosis. An epidemiologic study. *Arthritis Rheum* 1985;28:1336–1340.
163. Peters-Golden M, Wise RA, Hochberg M, et al. Incidence of lung cancer in systemic sclerosis. *J Rheumatol* 1985;12:1136–1139.
164. Wooten M. Systemic sclerosis and malignancy: a review of the literature. *Southern Med J* 2008;101:59–62.
165. Lu TY, Hill CL, Pontifex EK, et al. Breast cancer and systemic sclerosis: a clinical description of 21 patients in a population-based cohort study. *Rheumatol Int* 2008;28:895–899.
166. Byron MA, Venning VA, Mowat AG. Postmammoplasty human adjuvant disease. *Br J Rheumatol* 1984;12:227–229.
167. Sahn EE, Garen PD, Silver RM, et al. Scleroderma following augmentation mammoplasty. Report of a case and review of the literature. *Arch Dermatol* 1990;126:1198–1202.
168. Van Nunen SA, Gatenby PA, Basten A. Postmammoplasty connective tissue disease. *Arthritis Rheum* 1982;25:694–697.
169. Sappino A-P, Masouye I, Saurat J-H, et al. Smooth muscle differentiation in scleroderma fibroblastic cells. *Am J Pathol* 1990;137:585–591.
170. Walsh N, Rheaume D, Barnes P, et al. Postirradiation morphea: an underrecognized complication of treatment for breast cancer. *Hum Pathol* 2008;39:1680–1688.
171. Gyves-Ray KM, Adler DD. Dermatomyositis: an unusual cause of breast calcifications. *Breast Dis* 1989;2:195–201.
172. Bonnetblanc JM, Bernard P, Fayol J. Dermatomyositis and malignancy. A multicenter cooperative study. *Dermatologica* 1990;180:212–216.
173. Hidano A, Kaneko A, Arai Y, et al. Survey of the prognosis of DM with special reference to its association with malignancy and pulmonary fibrosis. *J Dermatol* (Tokyo) 1986;13:233–241.
174. Sigurgeirsson B, Lindelöf B, Edhag O, et al. Risk of cancer in patients with dermatomyositis or polymyositis. A population-based study. *N Engl J Med* 1992;326:363–367.
175. Hatada T, Aoki I, Ikeda H, et al. Dermatomyositis and malignancy: case report and review of the Japanese literature. *Tumori* 1996;82:273–275.
176. Abraham Z, Rozenbaum M, Glück Z, et al. Fulminant dermatomyositis after removal of a cancer. *J Dermatol* 1992;19:424–427.
177. Markopoulos CJ, Gogas HJ, Anastassiades OT. Weber-Christian disease with breast involvement. A case report. *Breast Dis* 1994;7:273–276.

178. Wargotz ES, Lefkowitz M. Granulomatous angiopanniculitis of the breast. *Hum Pathol* 1989;20:1084–1088.
179. Sy AN, Lam TP, Khoo US. Subcutaneous panniculitis-like T-cell lymphoma appearing as a breast mass: a difficult and challenging case appearing at an unusual site. *J Ultrasound Med* 2005;24:1453–1460.
180. Schramm N, Pfluger T, Reiser MF, et al. Subcutaneous panniculitis-like T-cell lymphoma with breast involvement: functional and morphological imaging findings. *Br J Radiol* 2010;83:e90–e94.
181. Cernea SS, Kihara SM, Sotto MN, et al. Lupus mastitis. *J Am Acad Dermatol* 1993;29:343–346.
182. Kinonen C, Gattuso P, Reddy VB. Lupus mastitis: an uncommon complication of systemic or discoid lupus. *Am J Surg Pathol* 2010;34: 901–906.
183. Holland NW, McKnight K, Challa VR, et al. Lupus panniculitis (Profundus) involving the breast: report of 2 cases and review of the literature. *J Rheumatol* 1995;22:344–346.
184. Nigar E, Contractor K, Singhal H, et al. Lupus mastitis—a cause of recurrent breast lumps. *Histopathology* 2007;51:847–849.
185. Fernandez-Flores A, Crespo LG, Alonso S, et al. Lupus mastitis in the male breast mimicking inflammatory carcinoma. *Breast J* 2006;12:272–273.
186. Georgian-Smith D, Lawton TJ, Moe RE, et al. Lupus mastitis: radiologic and pathologic features. *AJR Am J Roentgenol* 2002;178:1233–1235.
187. Wani AM, MohdHussain W, Fatani MI, et al. Lupus mastitis-peculiar radiological and pathological features. *Indian J Radiol Imaging* 2009;19:170–172.
188. Mondor H. Tronculite sous-cutanée subaigné de la paroi thoracique antéro-latérale. *Mem Acad Chir* 1939;65:1271–1278.
189. Kaufman PA. Subcutaneous phlebitis of the breast and chest wall. *Ann Surg* 1956;144:847–853.
190. Daniels WB. Superficial thrombophlebitis: new cause of chest pain. *Am J Med Sci* 1932;183:398–401.
191. Fleissinger N, Mathieu P. Thrombophlébitis des veins de la paroi thoraco-abdominale. *Bull Soc Med Hop Paris* 1922;46:352–354.
192. Williams GA. Thoraco-epigastric phlebitis producing dyspnea. *JAMA* 1931;96:2196–2197.
193. Bejanga BI. Mondor's disease: analysis of 30 cases. *J R Coll Surg Edinb* 1992;37:322–324.
194. Green RA, Dowden RV. Mondor's disease in plastic surgery patients. *Ann Plast Surg* 1988;20:231–235.
195. Shousha S, Chun J. Ulcerated Mondor's disease of the breast. *Histopathology* 2008;52:395–396.
196. Cooper RA. Mondor's disease secondary to intravenous drug abuse. *Arch Surg* 1990;125:807–808.
197. Ingram DM, Sheiner HJ, Ginsberg AM. Mondor's disease of the breast resulting from jellyfish sting. *Med J Aust* 1992;157:836–837.
198. Chiedozi LC, Aghahowa JA. Mondor's disease associated with breast cancer. *Surgery* 1988;103:438–439.
199. Miller DR, Cesario TC, Slater LM. Mondor's disease associated with metastatic axillary node. *Cancer* 1985;56:903–904.
200. Vieta JO. Mondor's disease with carcinoma of the breast. *NY State J Med* 1977;77:120–121.
201. Catania S, Zurrida S, Veronesi P, et al. Mondor's disease and breast cancer. *Cancer* 1992;69:2267–2270.
202. Courtney SP, Polacarz S, Raftery AT. Mondor's disease associated with metastatic lung cancer in the breast. *Postgrad Med J* 1989;65:779–780.
203. Terada S, Suzuki N, Uchide K, et al. Imaging study of Mondor's disease in the lactating breast. *Breast Dis* 1996;9:211–216.
204. Skipworth GB, Morris JB, Goldstein N. Bilateral Mondor's disease. *Arch Dermatol* 1967;95:95–97.
205. Tabar L, Dean PB. Mondor's disease: clinical, mammographic and pathologic features. *Breast* 1981;7:18–20.
206. Conant EF, Wilkes AN, Mendelson EB, et al. Superficial thrombophlebitis of the breast (Mondor's disease): mammographic findings. *AJR Am J Roentgenol* 1993;160:1201–1203.
207. Duff P. Mondor disease in pregnancy. *Obstet Gynecol* 1981;58:117–119.

Paraffinoma

208. Gersuny R. Veber eine subcutane prosthese. *Ztschr F Heilkund* 1900;1:199.
209. Boo-Chai K. Paraffinoma. *Plast Reconstruct Surg* 1965;36:101–110.
210. Alagaratnam TT, Ng WF. Paraffinomas of the breast: an oriental curiosity. *Aust N Z J Surg* 1996;66:138–140.
211. Yang WT, Suen M, Ho WS, et al. Paraffinomas of the breast: mammographic, ultrasonographic and radiographic appearances with clinical and histopathological correlation. *Clin Radiol* 1996;51:130–133.
212. Markopoulos C, Mantas D, Kouskos E, et al. Paraffinomas of the breast or oleogranulomatous mastitis—a rare entity. *Breast* 2006;15:540–543.
213. Iyengar R, Saint-Cyr M, Gokaslan T, et al. Breast paraffinoma. *Breast J* 2008;14:504–505.
214. Symmers WStC. Silicone mastitis in "topless" waitresses and some other varieties of foreign-body mastitis. *Br Med J* 1968;3:19–22.
215. Tinckler LF, Stock FE. Paraffinoma of the breast. *Aust N Z J Surg* 1955;25:142–147.
216. Merckx L, Lamote J, Sacre R. Bilateral ulcerating paraffinoma of the breast in a man. *Breast Dis* 1993;6:41–44.
217. Erguvan-Dogan B, Yang WT. Direct injection of paraffin into the breast: mammographic, sonographic and MRI features of early complications. *AJR Am J Roentgenol* 2006;186:888–894.

Silicone Mastitis and Other Pathology Associated with Breast Augmentation

218. Nosanchuk JS. Silicone granuloma in breast. *Arch Surg* 1968;97: 583–585.
219. Persellin ST, Vogler JB III, Brazis PW, et al. Detection of migratory silicone pseudotumor with use of magnetic resonance imaging. *Mayo Clin Proc* 1992;67:891–895.
220. Chilcote WA, Dowden RV, Paushter DM, et al. Ultrasound detection of silicone gel breast implant failure: a prospective analysis. *Breast Dis* 1994;7:307–316.
221. Barker DE, Retsky MI, Shultz S. 'Bleeding' of silicone from bag-gel breast implants, and its clinical relation to fibrous capsule reaction. *Plast Reconstr Surg* 1978;61:836–841.
222. Thomsen JL, Christensen L, Nielsen M, et al. Histologic changes and silicone concentrations in human breast tissue surrounding silicone breast prostheses. *Plast Reconstr Surg* 1990;85:38–41.
223. McConnell JP, Moyer TP, Nixon DE, et al. Determination of silicon in breast and capsular tissue from patients with breast implants performed by inductively coupled plasma emission spectroscopy. Comparison with tissue histology. *Am J Clin Pathol* 1997;107:236–246.
224. Weinzweig J, Schnur PL, McConnell JP, et al. Silicon analysis of breast and capsular tissue from patients with saline or silicone gel breast implants: II. Correlation with connective-tissue disease. *Plast Reconstr Surg* 1998;101:1836–1841.
225. Ellenbogen R, Rubin L. Injectable fluid silicone therapy: human morbidity and mortality. *JAMA* 1975;234:308–309.
226. Capozzi A, DuBou R, Pennisi VR. Distant migration of silicone gel from a ruptured breast implant. *Plast Reconstr Surg* 1978;62:302–303.
227. Travis WE, Balogh K, Abraham JL. Silicone granulomas: report of three cases and review of the literature. *Hum Pathol* 1985;16:19–27.
228. Leibman AJ, Kossoff MB, Kruse BD. Intraductal extension of silicone from a ruptured breast implant. *Plast Reconstr Surg* 1992;89:546–547.
229. Shermis RB, Adler DD, Smith DJ, et al. Intraductal silicone secondary to breast implant rupture. *Breast Dis* 1990;3:17–20.
230. Palestro CJ, Chau P, Goldsmith SJ. Gallium-67 uptake after breast and hip augmentation with silicone. *Clin Nucl Med* 1992;17:897–898.
231. Destouet JM, Monsees BS, Oser RF, et al. Screening mammography in 350 women with breast implants: prevalence and findings of implant complications. *AJR Am J Roentgenol* 1992;159:973–978.
232. Robinson OG Jr, Bradley EL, Wilson DS. Analysis of explanted silicone implants: a report of 300 patients. *Ann Plast Surg* 1995;34:1–7.
233. Gorczyca DP, Sinha S, Ahn CY, et al. Silicone breast implants in vivo: MR imaging. *Radiology* 1992;185:407–410.
234. Morris EA, Dershaw DD. Breast MRI: ready for general use? *Breast J* 1999;5:219–220.
235. Maddox A, Schoenfeld A, Sinnett HD, et al. Breast carcinoma occurring in association with silicone augmentation. *Histopathology* 1993;23:379–382.
236. Winer LH, Sternberg TH, Lehman R, et al. Tissue reactions to injected silicone liquids. *Arch Dermatol* 1964;90:588–593.
237. Lewis CM. Inflammatory carcinoma of the breast following silicone injections. *Plast Reconstr Surg* 1980;66:134–136.
238. Morgenstern L, Gleischman SH, Michel SL, et al. Relation of free silicone to human breast carcinoma. *Arch Surg* 1986;120:573–577.
239. Truong LD, Cartwright J Jr, Goodman MD, et al. Silicone lymphadenopathy associated with augmentation mammoplasty. *Am J Surg Pathol* 1988;12:484–491.
240. Tabatowski K, Elson CE, Johnston WW. Silicone lymphadenopathy in a patient with a mammary prosthesis. Fine needle aspiration cytology,

histology and analytical electron microscopy. *Acta Cytol* 1990;34: 10–14.

241. Eklund GW, Busby RC, Miller SH, et al. Improved imaging of the augmented breast. *AJR Am J Roentgenol* 1988;151:469–473.
242. Koide T, Katayama H. Calcification in augmentation mammoplasty. *Radiology* 1979;130:337–340.
243. Warner E, Lipa H, Pearson D, et al. Silicone mastopathy mimicking malignant disease of the breast in Southeast Asian patients. *Can Med Assoc J* 1991;144:569–571.
244. Rosenbaum JL, Bernardino ME, Thomas JC, et al. Ultrasonic findings in silicone-augmented breasts. *South Med J* 1981;74:455–458.
245. Cheung YC, Su MY, Ng SH, et al. Lumpy silicone-injected breasts: enhanced MRI and microscopic correlation. *Clinical Imaging* 2002;26: 397–404.
246. Peters W, Smith D. Calcification of breast implant capsules: incidence, diagnosis, and contributing factors. *Ann Plast Surg* 1995;34:8–11.
247. Peters W, Pritzker K, Smith D, et al. Capsular calcification associated with silicone breast implants: incidence, determinants, and characterization. *Ann Plast Surg* 1998;41:348–360.
248. Kasper CS. Histologic features of breast capsules reflect surface configuration and composition of silicone bag implants. *Am J Clin Pathol* 1994;102:655–659.
249. Wells AF, Daniels S, Gunasekaran S, et al. Local increase in hyaluronic acid and interleukin-2 in the capsules surrounding silicone breast implants. *Ann Plast Surg* 1994;33:1–5.
250. del Rosario AD, Bui HX, Singh J, et al. True synovial metaplasia of breast implant capsules: a light and electron microscopic study. *Lab Invest* 1994;70:14A.
251. Hameed MR, Erlandson R, Rosen PP. Capsular synovial-like hyperplasia (CSH) around mammary implants similar to detritic synovitis: a morphologic and immunohistochemical study of 15 cases. *Am J Surg Pathol* 1995;19:433–438.
252. Raso DS, Greene WB, Metcalf JS. Synovial metaplasia of a periprosthetic breast capsule. *Arch Pathol Lab Med* 1994;118:249–251.
253. Chase DR, Oberg KC, Chase RL, et al. Pseudoepithelialization of breast implant capsules. *Int J Surg Pathol* 1994;1:151–154.
254. Ko CY, Ahn CY, Ko J, et al. Capsular synovial metaplasia as a common response to both textured and smooth implants. *Plast Reconstr Surg* 1996;97:1427–1435.
255. Emery JA, Hardt NS, Caffee H, et al. Breast implant capsules share synovial transporting capabilities. *Lab Invest* 1994;70:15A.
256. Abbondanzo SL, Young VL, Wei MQ, et al. Silicone gel-filled breast and testicular implant capsules: a histologic and immunophenotypic study. *Mod Pathol* 1999;12:706–713.
257. Emery JA, Spanier SS, Kasnic G Jr, et al. The synovial structure of breast-implant-associated bursae. *Mod Pathol* 1994;7:728–733.
258. Cook PD, Osborne BM, Connor RL, et al. Follicular lymphoma adjacent to foreign body granulomatous inflammation and fibrosis surrounding silicone breast prosthesis. *Am J Surg Pathol* 1995;19:712–717.
259. Kasper CS, Chandler PJ. Talc deposition in skin and tissues surrounding gel-containing prosthetic devices. *Arch Dermatol* 1994; 130:48–53.
260. Raso DS, Crymes LW, Metcalf JS. Histological assessment of fifty breast capsules from smooth and textured augmentation and reconstruction mammoplasty prostheses with emphasis on the role of synovial metaplasia. *Mod Pathol* 1994;7:310–316.
261. Domanskis EJ, Owsley JQ. Histological investigation of the etiology of capsule contracture following augmentation mammoplasty. *Plast Reconstr Surg* 1976;58:689–693.
262. Raso DS, Greene WB. Silicone identification by electron probe microanalysis in periprosthetic breast capsules and distant sites in women with silicone breast implants. *Lab Invest* 1994;70:20A.
263. Hardt NS, Yu LT, La Torre G, et al. Fourier transform infrared microspectroscopy used to identify foreign materials related to breast implants. *Mod Pathol* 1994;7:669–676.
264. Centeno JA, Mullick FG, Panos RG, et al. Laser-Raman microprobe identification of inclusions in capsules associated with silicone gel breast implants. *Mod Pathol* 1999;12:714–721.
265. Pasteris JD, Wopenka B, Freeman JJ, et al. Analysis of breast implant capsular tissue for crystalline silica and other refractile phases. *Plast Reconstr Surg* 1999;103:1273–1276.
266. Katzin WE, Feng LJ. Phenotype of lymphocytes associated with the inflammatory reaction to silicone gel breast implants. *Lab Invest* 1994;70:17A.
267. Raso DS. B and T lymphocytes in periprosthetic breast capsules. *Lab Invest* 1994;70:20A.
268. Kitchen SB, Paletta CE, Shehadi SI, et al. Epithelialization of the lining of a breast implant capsule. *Cancer* 1994;73:1449–1452.
269. Venkataraman S, Hines N, Slanetz PJ. Challenges in mammography: part 2, multimodality review of breast augmentation—imaging findings and complications. *AJR Am J Roentgenol* 2011;197:W 1031–1045.
270. Kim H, Yang EJ, Bang SI. Bilateral liponecrotic pseudocysts after breast augmentation by fat injection: a case report. *Aesthetic Plast Surg* 2012;36:359–362.
271. Timberlake GA, Looney GR. Adenocarcinoma of the breast associated with silicone injections. *J Surg Oncol* 1986;32:79–81.
272. Pennisi, VR. Obscure carcinoma encountered in subcutaneous mastectomy in silicone- and paraffin-injected breasts: two patients. *Plast Reconstr Surg* 1984;74:535–538.
273. Berkel H, Birdsell DC, Jenkins H. Breast augmentation: a risk factor for breast cancer? *N Engl J Med* 1992;326:1649–1653.
274. Deapen DM, Pike MC, Casagrande JT, et al. The relationship between breast cancer and augmentation mammoplasty: an epidemiologic study. *Plast Reconstr Surg* 1986;77:361–368.
275. Rosen PP, Ernsberger D. Mammary fibromatosis. A benign spindle-cell tumor with significant risk for local recurrence. *Cancer* 1989;63:1 363–1369.
276. Balzer BL, Weiss SW. Do biomaterials cause implant-associated mesenchyme tumors of the breast? Analysis of 8 new cases and review of the literature. *Hum Pathol* 2009;40:1564–1570.
277. Kotton DN, Muse VV, Nishino M. Case records of the Massachusetts General Hospital. Case 2-2012. A 63-year-old woman with dyspnea and rapidly progressive respiratory failure. *N Engl J Med* 2012;366:259–269.
278. Saunders ND, Marshall JS, Anderson RC. A case of chest wall angiosarcoma associated with breast implants. *J Thorac Cardiovasc Surg* 2007;134:1076–1077.
279. Takenaka M, Tanaka M, Isobe M, et al. Angiosarcoma of the breast with silicone granuloma: a case report. *Kurume Med J* 2009;56:33–37.
280. Taylor CR, Siddiqi IN, Brody GS. Anaplastic large cell lymphoma occurring in association with breast implants: review of pathologic and immunohistochemical features in 103 cases. *Appl Immunohistochem Mol Morphol* 2013;21:13–20.
281. de Jong D, Vasmel WL, de Boer JP, et al. Anaplastic large-cell lymphoma in women with breast implants. *JAMA* 2008;300:2030–2035.
282. Gutierrez FJ, Espinoza LR. Progressive systemic sclerosis complicated by severe hypertension: reversal after silicone implant removal. *Am J Med* 1990;89:390–392.
283. Spiera H. Scleroderma after silicone augmentation mammoplasty. *JAMA* 1988;260:236–238.
284. Varga J, Schumacher NA, Jimenez SA. Systemic sclerosis after augmentation mammoplasty with silicone implants. *Ann Intern Med* 1989;111:377–383.
285. Englert HJ, Howe GB, Penny R, et al. Scleroderma and silicone breast implants. *Br J Rheumatol* 1994;33:397–399.
286. Strom BL, Reidenberg MM, Freundlich B, et al. Breast silicone and risk of systemic lupus erythematosus. *J Clin Epidemiol* 1994;47:1211–1214.
287. Edelman DA, Grant S, van Os WAA. Autoimmune disease following the use of silicone gel-filled breast implants: a review of the clinical literature. *Semin Arthritis Rheum* 1994;24:183–189.
288. Noone RB. A review of the possible health implications of silicone breast implants. *Cancer* 1997;79:1747–1756.

Diabetic Mastopathy

289. Soler NG, Khardori R. Fibrous disease of the breast, thyroiditis, and cheiroarthropathy in Type I diabetes mellitus. *Lancet* 1984;I:193–195.
290. Byrd BF Jr, Hartmann WH, Graham LS, et al. Mastopathy in insulin-dependent diabetics. *Ann Surg* 1987;205:529–532.
291. Tomaszewski JE, Brooks JSJ, Hicks D, et al. Diabetic mastopathy: a distinctive clinicopathologic entity. *Hum Pathol* 1992;23:780–786.
292. Chang K, Vitto EA, Grant GA, et al. Increased collagen cross-linkages in experimental diabetes. Reversal by beta-amino propionitrile and D-penicillamine. *Diabetes* 1980;29:558–581.
293. Golub LM, Greenwald RA, Zebrowski EJ, et al. The effect of experimental diabetes mellitus on molecular characterization of soluble rat tendon collagen. *Biochem Biophys Acta* 1978;534:73–81.

294. Seidman JD, Schnaper LA, Phillips LE. Mastopathy in insulin-requiring diabetes mellitus. *Hum Pathol* 1994;25:819–824.
295. Ashton MA, Lefkowitz M, Tavassoli FA. Epithelioid stromal cells in lymphocytic mastitis—a source of confusion with invasive carcinoma. *Mod Pathol* 1994;7:49–54.
296. Love JE, Lawton TJ. Diabetic mastopathy in patients with non-diabetic autoimmune disease. *Mod Pathol* 2005;18(Suppl. 1):41A.
297. Lee AHS, Zafrani B, Kafiri G, et al. Sclerosing lymphocytic lobulitis in the male breast. *J Clin Pathol* 1996;49:609–611.
298. Hunfeld KP, Bässler R. Lymphocytic mastitis and fibrosis of the breast in long-standing insulin-dependent diabetics. A histopathologic study on diabetic mastopathy and report of ten cases. *Gen Diagn Pathol* 1997;143:49–58.
299. Weinstein SP, Conant EF, Orel SG, et al. Diabetic mastopathy in men: imaging findings in two patients. *Radiology* 2001;219:797–799.
300. Gump FE, McDermmott J. Fibrous disease of the breast in juvenile diabetes. *NY State J Med* 1990;90:356–357.
301. Pluchinotta AM, Talenti E, Lodovichetti G, et al. Diabetic fibrous breast disease: a clinical entity that mimics cancer. *Eur J Surg Oncol* 1995;21:207–209.
302. Valdez R, Thorson J, Finn WG, et al. Lymphocytic mastitis and diabetic mastopathy: a molecular, immunophenotypic, and clinicopathologic evaluation of 11 cases. *Mod Pathol* 2003;16:223–228.
303. Lammie GA, Bobrow LG, Staunton MDM, et al. Sclerosing lymphocytic lobulitis of the breast—evidence for an autoimmune pathogenesis. *Histopathology* 1991;19:13–20.
304. Bayer U, Horn LC, Schulz HG. Bilateral, tumorlike diabetic mastopathy-progression and regression of the disease during 5-year follow up. Case report. *Eur J Radiol* 1998;26:248–253.
305. Gabriel HA, Feng C, Mendelson EB, et al. Breast MRI for cancer detection in a patient with diabetic mastopathy. *AJR Am J Roentgenol* 2004;182:1081–1083.
306. Tuncbilek N, Karakas HM, Okten O. Diabetic fibrous mastopathy: dynamic contrast-enhanced magnetic resonance imaging findings. *Breast J* 2004;10:359–362.
307. Shousha S. Diabetic mastopathy: strong CD10+ immunoreactivity of the atypical stromal cells. *Histopathology* 2008;52:648–650.
308. Schwartz IS, Strauchen JA. Lymphocytic mastopathy. An autoimmune disease of the breast? *Am J Clin Pathol* 1990;93:725–730.
309. Morgan MC, Weaver MG, Crowe JP, et al. Diabetic mastopathy: a clinicopathologic study of palpable and nonpalpable breast lesions. *Mod Pathol* 1995;8:349–354.
310. Peppoloni L, Buttaro FM, Cristallini EG. Diabetic mastopathy. A report of two cases diagnosed by aspiration cytology. *Acta Cytol* 1997;41:1349–1352.
311. Andrews-Tang D, Diamond AB, Rogers L, et al. Diabetic mastopathy: adjunctive use of ultrasound and utility of core biopsy in diagnosis. *Breast J* 2000;6:183–188.

Cystic Fibrosis

312. Garcia FU, Galindo LM, Holsclaw DSJ. Breast abnormalities in patients with cystic fibrosis: previously unrecognized changes. *Ann Diagn Pathol* 1998;2:281–285.
313. de González AB, Kim KP, Samet JM. Radiation-induced cancer risk from annual computed tomography for patients with cystic fibrosis. *Am J Respir Crit Care Med* 2007;176:970–973.

Amyloid Tumor

314. Westermark P, Benson MD, Buxbaum JN, et al. Amyloid: toward terminology clarification. Report from the Nomenclature Committee of the International Society of Amyloidosis. *Amyloid* 2005;12:1–4.
315. O'Connor CR, Rubinow A, Cohen AS. Primary (AL) amyloidosis as a cause of breast masses. *Am J Med* 1984;77:981–986.
316. Symonds DA, Eichelberger MF, Sager GL. Calcifying amyloidoma of the breast. *South Med J* 1995;88:1169–1172.
317. Cetti R, Reuther K, Hansen JPH, et al. Amyloid tumor of the breast. *Dan Med Bull* 1983;30:34–35.
318. Goonatillake HD, Allsop JR. Amyloid tumour of the breast simulating carcinoma. *Aust N Z J Surg* 1988;58:589–590.
319. Sedeghee SA, Moore SW. Rheumatoid arthritis, bilateral amyloid tumors of the breast and multiple cutaneous nodules. *Am J Clin Pathol* 1974;62:472–476.
320. Hardy TJ, Myerowitz RL, Bender BL. Diffuse parenchymal amyloidosis of lungs and breast. *Arch Pathol Lab Med* 1979;103:583–585.
321. McLellan GL, Steward JH, Balachandran S. Localization of Tc-99m-MDP in amyloidosis of the breast. *Clin Nucl Med* 1981;6:579–580.
322. Fernandez BB, Hernandez FJ. Amyloid tumor of the breast. *Arch Pathol* 1973;95:102–105.
323. Luo J-H, Rotterdam H. Primary amyloid tumor of the breast: a case report and review of the literature. *Mod Pathol* 1997;10:735–738.
324. McMahon RFT, Connolly CE. Amyloid breast tumor. *Am J Surg Pathol* 1987;11:488.
325. Silverman JF, Dabbs DJ, Norris HT, et al. Localized primary (AL) amyloid tumor of the breast. Cytologic, histologic, immunocytochemical and ultrastructural observations. *Am J Surg Pathol* 1986;10:539–545.
326. Walker AN, Fechner RE, Callicott JH Jr. Amyloid tumor of the breast. *Diagn Gynecol Obstet* 1982;4:339–341.
327. Liaw Y-S, Kuo S-H, Yang P-C,et al. Nodular amyloidosis of the lung and the breast mimicking breast carcinoma with pulmonary metastasis. *Eur Respir J* 1995;5:871–873.
328. Röcken C, Kronsbein H, Sletten K, et al. Amyloidosis of the breast. *Virchows Arch* 2002;440:527–535.
329. Sabate JM, Clotet M, Torrubias S, et al. Localized amyloidosis of the breast associated with invasive lobular carcinoma. *Br J Radiol* 2008;81:e252–e254.
330. Munson-Bernardi BD, DePersia LA. Amyloidosis of the breast coexisting with ductal carcinoma in situ. *AJR Am J Roentgenol* 2006;186:54–55.
331. Ganor S, Dollberg L. Amyloidosis of the nipple presenting as pruritus. *Cutis* 1983;31:318.
332. Hecht AH, Tan A, Shen JF. Case report: primary systemic amyloidosis presenting as breast masses, mammographically simulating carcinoma. *Clin Radiol* 1991;44:123–124.
333. Lynch LA, Moriarty AT. Localized primary amyloid tumor associated with osseous metaplasia presenting as bilateral breast masses: cytologic and radiologic features. *Diagn Cytopathol* 1993;9:570–575.
334. Lipper S, Kahn LB. Amyloid tumor. *Am J Surg Pathol* 1978;2:141–145.
335. Tutar E, Onat AM, Aydin A, et al. Amyloid tumor of the breast mimicking breast carcinoma. *South Med J* 2008;101:199–201.
336. Toohey JM, Ismail K, Lonergan D, et al. Amyloidosis of the breast mimicking recurrence in a previously treated early breast cancer. *Australas Radiol* 2007;51:594–596.
337. Pearson B, Rice MM, Dickens KL. Primary systemic amyloidosis. *Arch Pathol* 1941;32:1–10.
338. Libbey CA, Skinner M, Cohen AS. The abdominal fat aspirate for the diagnosis of systemic amyloid. *Arch Intern Med* 1983;143:1549–1552.
339. Yokoo H, Nakazato Y. Primary localized amyloid tumor of the breast with osseous metaplasia. *Pathol Int* 1998;48:545–548.
340. Fernandez-Aguilar S, Sourtzis S, Chaikh A. IgM plasma cell myeloma with amyloidosis presenting as mammary microcalcifications. *APMIS* 2008;116:846–849.
341. Said SM, Reynolds C, Jimenez RE, et al. Amyloidosis of the breast: predominantly AL type and over half have concurrent breast hematologic disorders. *Mod Pathol* 2013;26:232–238.

Nephrogenic Systemic Sclerosis

342. Introcaso CE, Hivnor C, Cowper S, et al. Nephrogenic fibrosing dermopathy-nephrogenic systemic fibrosis: a case series of nine patients and review of the literature . *Int J Dermatol* 2007;46:447–452.
343. Solomon GJ, Rosen PP. Nephrogenic systemic fibrosis mimicking inflammatory breast carcinoma. *Arch Pathol Lab Med* 2007;131:145–148.

IgG4-Related Sclerosing Mastitis

344. Cheuk W, Chan JK. IgG4-related sclerosing disease: a critical appraisal of an evolving clinicopathologic entity. *Adv Anat Pathol* 2010;17: 303–332.
345. Cheuk W, Chan AC, Lam WL, et al. IgG4-related sclerosing mastitis: description of a new member of the IgG4-related sclerosing diseases. *Am J Surg Pathol* 2009;33:1058–1064.
346. Ogura K, Matsumoto T, Aoki Y, et al. IgG4-related tumour-forming mastitis with histological appearances of granulomatous lobular mastitis: comparison with other types of tumour-forming mastitis. *Histopathology* 2010;57:39–45.

CHAPTER 4

Specific Infections

SYED A. HODA

A wide variety of infections caused by fungi, parasites, bacteria, and viruses can afflict the breast. It is distinctly uncommon for the breast to be exclusively involved, and most such diseases involve the breast secondary to systemic involvement.

FUNGAL INFECTIONS

Clinically apparent mycotic infections of the breast are uncommon, even in patients who are immunocompromised as a consequence of an underlying illness or therapy.

Histoplasmosis

Infection with *Histoplasma capsulatum* is endemic in some regions of the United States and in Africa, where many individuals have evidence of healed granulomatous lesions primarily in the lungs, liver, and spleen. Calcified granulomas have been described in the breast, and there have been rare instances of localized mammary *Histoplasma* infection.[1,2] All were in young women. Each patient presented with a single, unilateral mass, which clinically suggested a neoplasm. Two lesions were painful, and inflammatory changes involved the skin in one case.[1] Clinical evaluation in two cases failed to demonstrate evidence of systemic *H. capsulatum* infection, but one patient had an elevated complement fixation test. The excised tumors proved grossly to be multinodular abscesses up to 3 cm in diameter that contained necrotic material. Histologically, as in this reported case, the lesions consist of confluent necrotizing granulomas similar to those of nonspecific granulomatous lobular mastitis in which the 2- to 4-μm yeast forms of *H. capsulatum* can be demonstrated by methenamine silver reaction (Fig. 4.1A–D). Another 55-year-old woman presented with a mass in the lateral mammary region that proved to be enlarged lymph nodes without involvement of breast parenchyma. *H. capsulatum* was isolated in culture and seen in tissue sections.

The diagnosis of histoplasmosis associated with granulomatous mastitis has been reported in a needle core biopsy[3] and in an excisional biopsy in a woman with acquired immunodeficiency syndrome (AIDS).[4]

Blastomycosis

Blastomycosis is endemic in certain regions of the United States and in Africa.[5,6] A 4-cm unilateral breast abscess that contained organisms histologically consistent with the broad-based budding yeasts of *Blastomyces dermatitidis* was excised from the para-areolar region of a 30-year-old woman.[2] She had no other evidence of infection and remained well 8 years later. Mammography reveals well-demarcated lesions. Large nodules may become cavitary with an air–fluid level.[5] The diagnosis is usually made when *Blastomyces* sp. is cultured from skin lesions or from a fine-needle aspiration (FNA) cytology specimen of the breast.[4] One patient also had a tumorous pulmonary lesion and another had a pleural effusion.[5,6] The breast and lung lesions may resolve completely with amphotericin therapy.[5,6]

Cryptococcosis

An extraordinary example of cryptococcal mastitis was described by Symmers.[7] The patient underwent mastectomy for a mistaken diagnosis of mucinous mammary carcinoma. The specimen was preserved in a museum and studied microscopically 61 years after surgery, at which time there was no evidence of carcinoma, but the breast was found to be infected with *Cryptococcus*—an encapsulated yeast with worldwide distribution. The patient died 37 years after mastectomy of an unrelated cause with no evidence of recurrent cryptococcosis. In another case, disseminated cryptococcal infection with involvement of the breasts was detected at autopsy in a patient with systemic lupus erythematosus.[2] Ramos-Barbosa et al.[8] reported mammary cryptococcal infection that presented as a cystic lesion in a 46-year-old woman who was under treatment with corticosteroids for sarcoidosis.

Aspergillosis

Unilateral and bilateral mammary aspergillosis has been reported at the site of prosthetic augmentation implants.[9,10] Involvement of the nipple by *Aspergillus flavus* in a 51-year-old woman apparently followed traumatic rupture of a superficial keratotic cyst.[11]

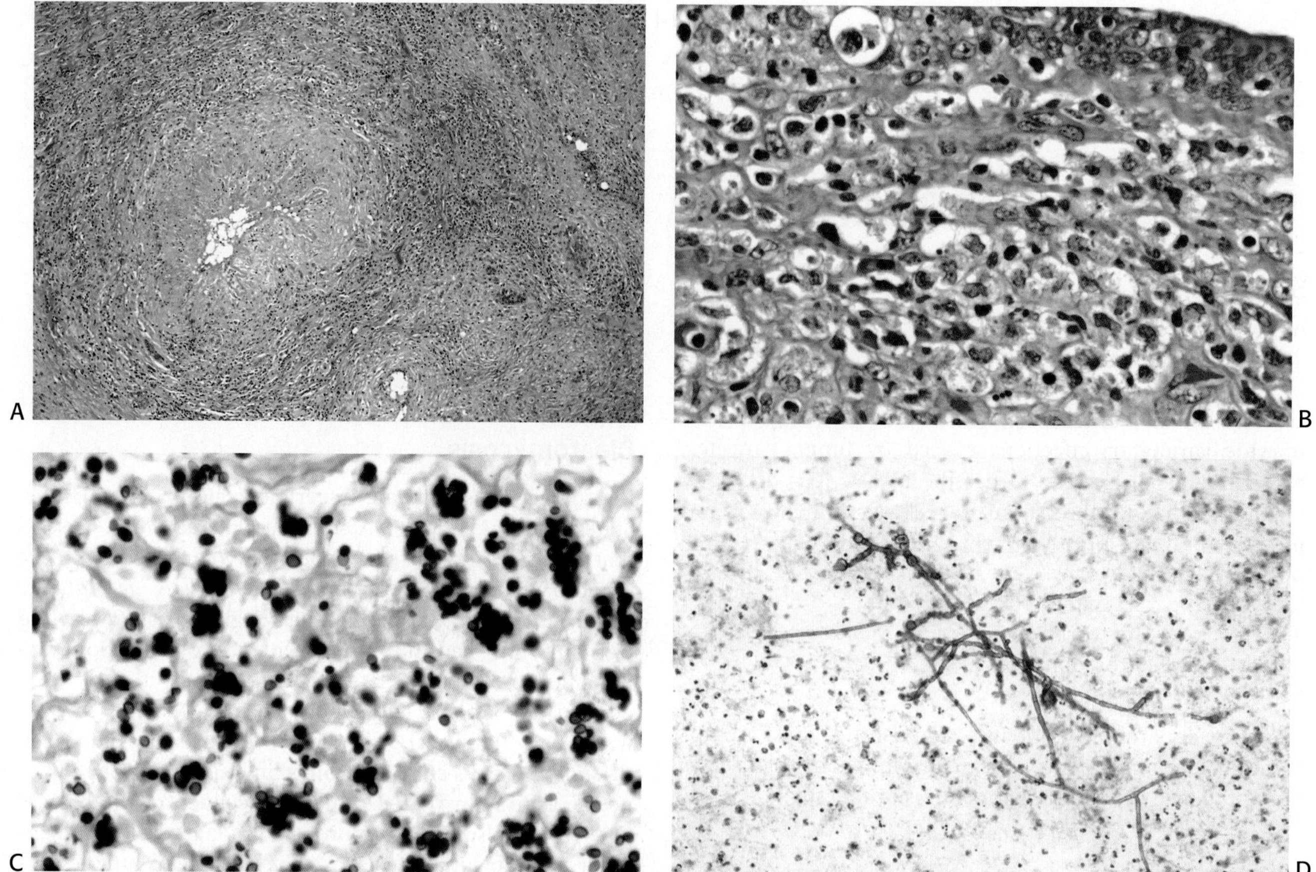

FIG. 4.1. *Mycotic mastitis. Histoplasmosis.* **A,B:** A fibrotic granuloma with mixed inflammatory cell reaction is present amidst breast tissue. **C:** Yeast forms of *H. capsulatum* are evident in the reactive infiltrate around the granuloma on methenamine silver reaction. **D:** *Chromomycosis*. The sample shown was obtained by FNA (Courtesy of Kusum Kapila, MD, and Kusum Verma, MD).

Chromomycosis

Infection of the nipple by *Fonsecaea pedrosoi*, and of mammary skin by *Phialophora verrucosa*, has been described.[12,13] Both fungi cause chromomycosis (also called chromoblastomycosis). On histology, the pigmented yeast forms resemble "copper pennies." The lesion in both cases formed a plaque with crusting. Biopsy revealed epidermal hyperplasia containing characteristic fungal hyphae, which may also be seen in an FNA specimen (Fig. 4.1E).

Coccidioidomycosis

Isolated breast involvement by *Coccidioides immitis* has been reported.[14] The patient was a 60-year-old woman under treatment with prednisone for temporal arteritis. Clinical examination revealed a circumscribed, 1.0-cm breast tumor with sharply defined borders on mammography. The excised mass consisted of a rim of granulation tissue around a necrotic center, which contained spherules characteristic of *C. immitis*. No pulmonary lesions were identified. Pregnancy is a well-recognized factor for the precipitous (and occasionally fatal) dissemination of the disease.[15,16]

PARASITIC INFECTIONS

Filariasis

Mammary filariasis caused most frequently by *Wuchereria bancrofti* has been reported from South America, China, and South Asia, where infection with this organism is endemic.[17,18] Involvement of the breast generally occurs as a late manifestation of low-grade, clinically inapparent infection as evidenced by emigrants and travelers found to have mammary filariasis as late as 3 years[19] and 6 years[20] after last exposure to infection. Microfilariae are sometimes demonstrable in thick blood smear samples taken around midnight, but some investigators have failed to detect microfilaremia in patients with breast lesions.[19,20] Microfilariae have been detected in nipple secretions, suggesting that communication may become established between ducts and dilated, ruptured lymphatics (lymphovarix).[21]

The patient typically presents with a solitary, nontender, painless unilateral breast mass. The upper outer quadrant is the most common site.[17,20] Many of the lesions involve subcutaneous tissue. The resultant hard mass with cutaneous attachment, sometimes accompanied by inflammatory changes, may be clinically indistinguishable from carcinoma.[22] In this setting, axillary nodal enlargement caused by filarial lymphadenitis further complicates the differential diagnosis.[23] In endemic areas, mammary filariasis may be detected coincidentally in patients with breast carcinoma.[18] Viable microfilariae can be detected in the breast by ultrasound examination if they produce a distinctive pattern of movement referred to as the "filaria dance sign."[24] Mammographically detected calcifications attributed to *W. bancrofti* and *Loa loa* infection have been described as having a spiral or serpiginous configuration.[22,25,26]

Microfilariae and gravid adult worms can be detected in fine-needle aspirates from breast lesions (Fig. 4.2).[27] The aspirate usually contains numerous eosinophils as well as other inflammatory cells, and features of a granulomatous reaction may be evident.

The majority of the filaria-associated mammary masses measure between 1 and 3 cm in diameter and are composed of firm, gray or white tissue that tends to merge with the breast parenchyma. Rarely an abscess can develop. Thread-like white worms are sometimes evident grossly in the lesion.[17] Microscopic examination of the excised mass typically reveals adult filarial worms, in varying stages of preservation (Fig. 4.3). Granulomatous reaction is most pronounced in areas of degenerating organisms. Eosinophils are a prominent feature. Degenerative changes may lead to the formation of eosinophilic abscesses (Fig. 4.4).

Female worms are about three times the size of male worms. Eggs in varying stages of maturation are identifiable in the uterus of adult females. Microfilariae may be seen within the uterus and in surrounding inflammatory tissue and appear as nuclei arranged in a linear pattern. Rarely, granulomatous lesions in the breast have contained only microfilariae.[17] Fully degenerated worms are likely to become calcified. Adult worms and microfilariae may also be found in axillary lymph nodes.[17,23]

The diagnosis of mammary involvement by *W. bancrofti* is dependent on the specific microscopic structural features of the worm, eggs, and microfilariae, as well as clinical information. Zoonotic filarial infections of the breast are much less common than those caused by *W. bancrofti*. The microfilariae are transmitted to humans by mosquito vectors, including *Aedes* and *Anopheles* species. Infections of the breast have been reported most often from North America, Europe, and Asia.[28-31] Lesions caused by zoonotic filariasis occur predominantly in the subcutaneous tissue, the conjunctiva, and the lungs.[28]

The organism responsible for most examples of mammary dirofilariasis is *Dirofilaria repens*,[28-31,32] which ordinarily infects cats and dogs, but infestation of humans by *Dirofilaria tenuis*, which primarily infects raccoons, has been reported.[30] The lesions occur in the subcutaneous tissue or superficial mammary parenchyma. Infection of the breast typically presents as a discrete firm to hard nodule that measures approximately 1 cm in diameter. The lesions tend to be

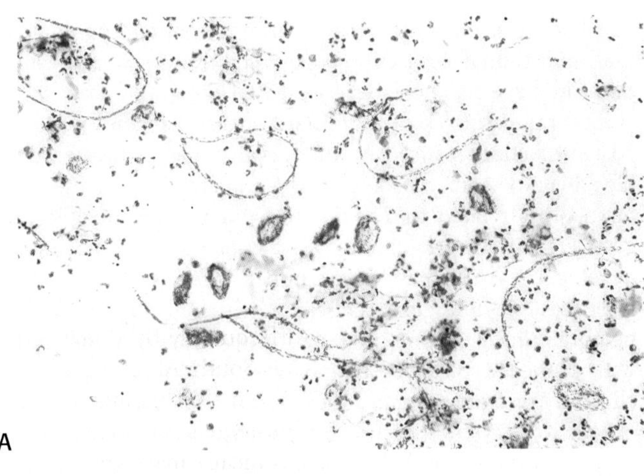

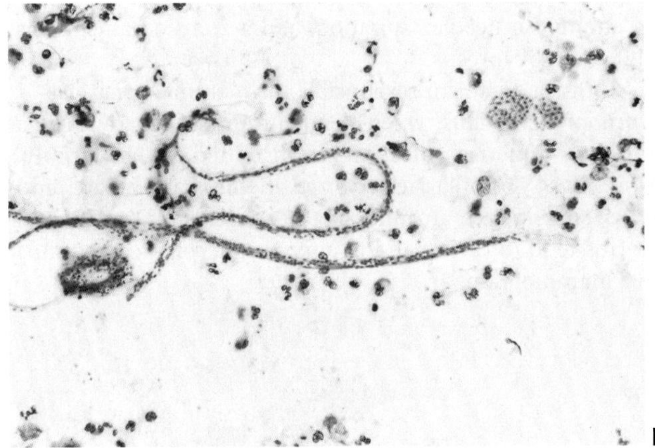

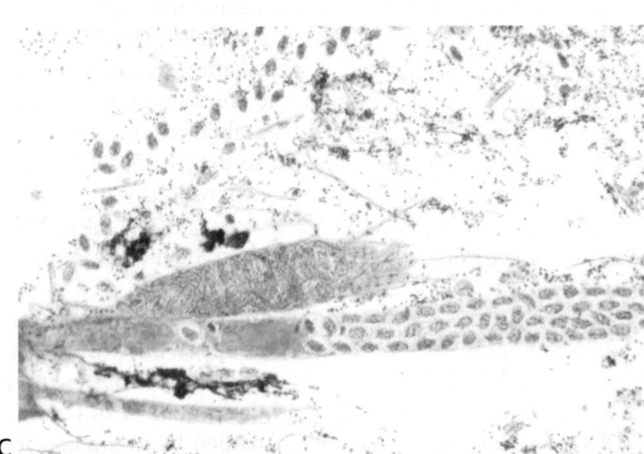

FIG. 4.2. ***Filariasis.*** **A,B:** Microfilariae in the FNA specimen from a breast lesion. **C:** Adult worm (*below*) and microfilariae (*above*) in an FNA sample from a breast tumor caused by *W. bancrofti*. (Courtesy of Kusum Kapila, MD, and Kusum Verma, MD.)

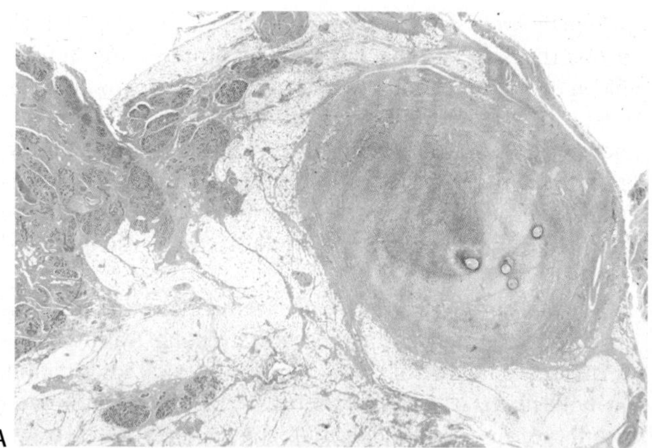

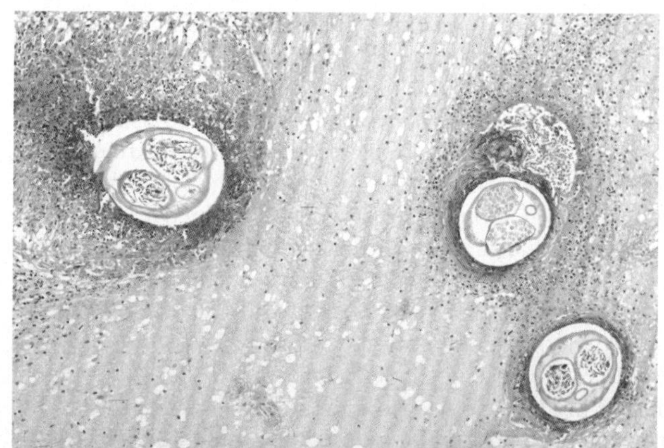

FIG. 4.3. *Filariasis.* **A,B:** An abscess containing cross sections of gravid female *W. bancrofti* in the subcutaneous tissue adjacent to mammary parenchyma.

superficially located. The excised specimen usually consists of a firm fibrous tissue mass with a central cavity (Fig. 4.5) in the subcutaneous or breast tissue. Microscopically, cross sections of the adult worm are found in the central necrotic area accompanied by an intense inflammatory reaction, which includes many eosinophils. A fibrous capsule with lymphocytes, plasma cells, and eosinophils encompasses the necrotic zone. The diagnosis of mammary dirofilariasis is usually not suspected until the excised lesion has been examined microscopically. However, in one case, "a thread-like object was seen projecting from the puncture site" after an attempt at needle aspiration, and a 2-cm organism was pulled out by forceps.[29]

Another organism responsible for mammary filariasis is *Onchocerca volvulus*, which is endemic in sub-Saharan Africa and Latin America. Infection is transmitted by the black fly, *Simulium*. Microfilariae localized in the skin, breast, and other sites induce an inflammatory reaction. Dead filarial worms tend to calcify and to appear as serpiginous strands in a mammogram.[33]

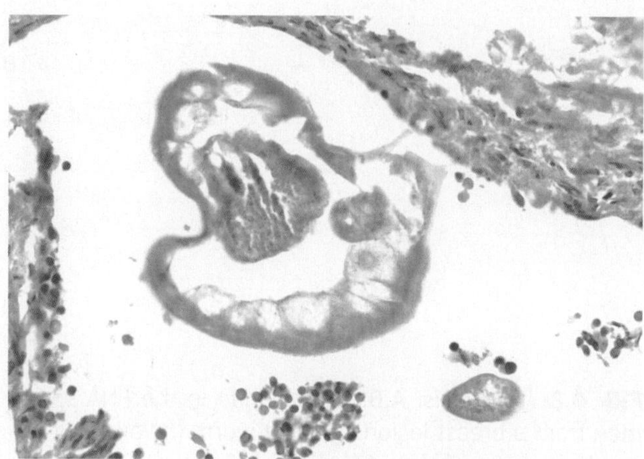

FIG. 4.4. *Filariasis.* A degenerated filarial worm in a breast abscess. (Courtesy of Kusum Kapila, MD, and Kusum Verma, MD.)

Other Parasites

Infection of the breast by *Schistosoma japonicum* has been reported in two women 35 years old[34,35] and in a third who was 50.[36] Calcifications detected by mammography proved to be calcified ova embedded in breast parenchyma in each case. The 50-year-old woman had a painless mass at the site of the mammographic abnormality, which consisted of "branching microcalcifications suggestive of carcinoma *in situ*."[36] The calcified ova found in a biopsy specimen were identified as *S. japonicum*. Similar lesions have also been escribed in the subcutaneous tissue.[37] Mammary parenchymal involvement and cutaneous ulceration by *Schistosoma mansoni* have also been described[38,39] (Fig. 4.6).

Several examples of mammary coenurosis and cysticercosis, infections caused by the larval stages of tapeworms, have been described. Coenurosis results from infestation by tapeworms related to *Taenia* sp., which is responsible for cysticercosis. In one case, a 38-year-old Canadian woman developed a 6-cm mass in the upper inner quadrant of her left breast.[40] At surgery, the lesion, which also involved the pectoral muscle, contained gelatinous material and cysts with scolices typical for tapeworms. An axillary mass that clinically resembled metastatic carcinoma in another patient proved to be cystic coenurus infection caused by *Taenia multiceps*.[41] No source of infection was identified in either case.

Mammary cysticercosis caused by *Taenia solium* has also been reported[42–45] (Fig. 4.7). In a 25-year-old woman, the infestation resulted in the formation of a circumscribed nodule near the areola.[43] Another patient was a 43-year-old woman with a 5-mm nodule in the upper outer quadrant.[42] Both lesions were cystic and contained diagnostic scolices within protruding mural nodules. Clinical examination revealed no other evidence of parasitic infestation in either case.

The breast is a very infrequent site of hydatid cyst formation caused by *Echinococcus granulosus*.[46,47] A review of breast tumors in 915 Saudi Arabian females reported one (0.1%) instance of mammary hydatid cyst.[48] Analysis of 306 surgically resected hydatid cysts in Jordan revealed one (0.35%) female patient with a breast lesion.[49] The lesion typically presents as a firm, discrete mobile mass that may or may

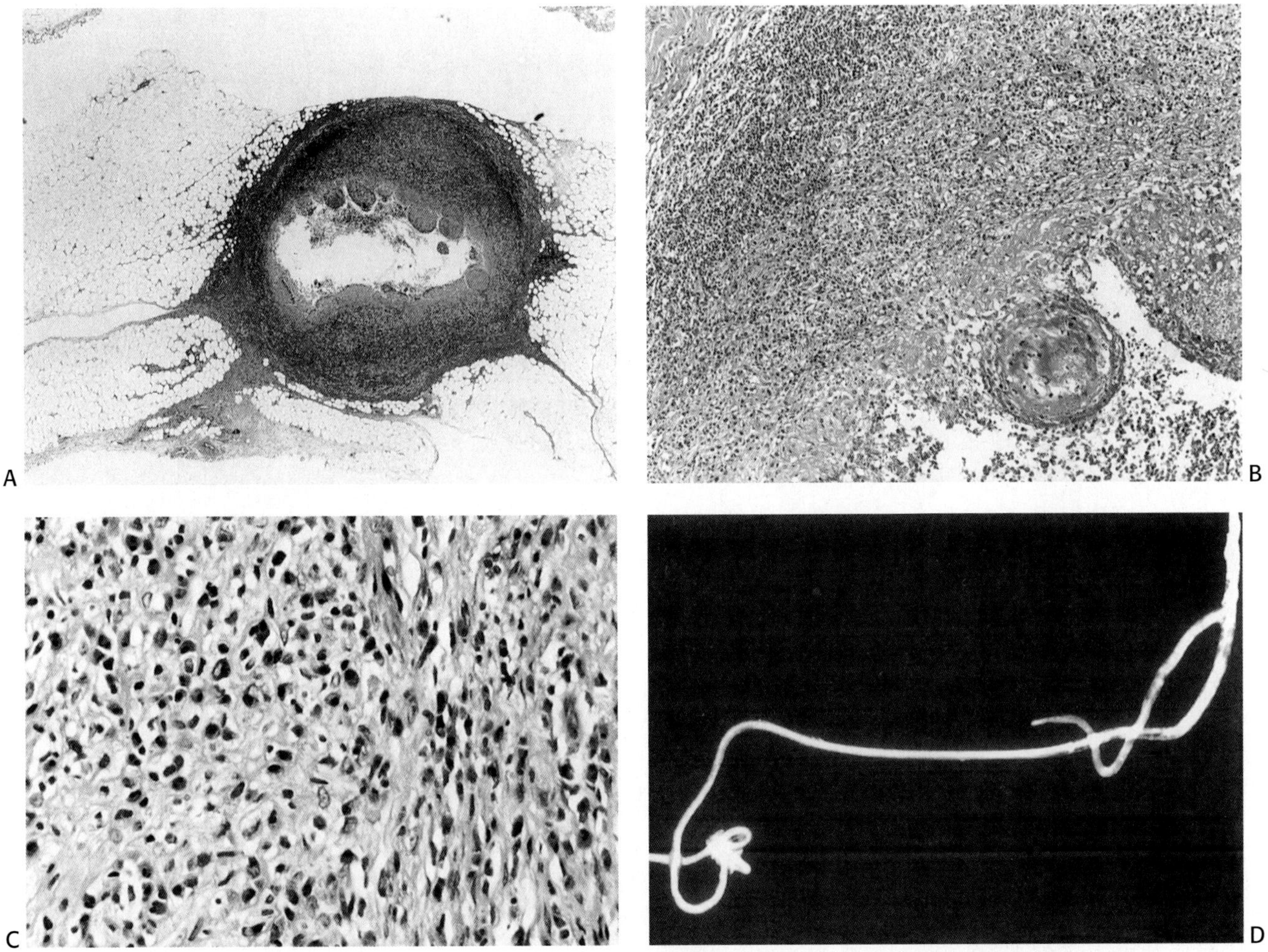

FIG. 4.5. *Filariasis.* **A:** An abscess caused by *Dirofilaria repens* in subcutaneous fat. Mammary lobules are present at the lower edge of the tissue. **B:** The wall of the abscess from the inside out consists of an inner layer of fibrin, the granulomatous reaction, a lymphocytic zone, and peripheral fibrosis. **C:** Granulomatous area in the abscess wall. **D:** Worm removed from the abscess cavity. (Courtesy of Dr. J. Searle.)

not be adherent to the pectoral fascia.[50] Mammography reveals a dense, well-circumscribed tumor within which internal ring structures representing air–fluid levels may be seen. Air–fluid levels and multiple cysts are seen to better advantage by ultrasound.[51] On magnetic resonance (MR) imaging, the hydatid cyst presents as a well-circumscribed cystic lesion

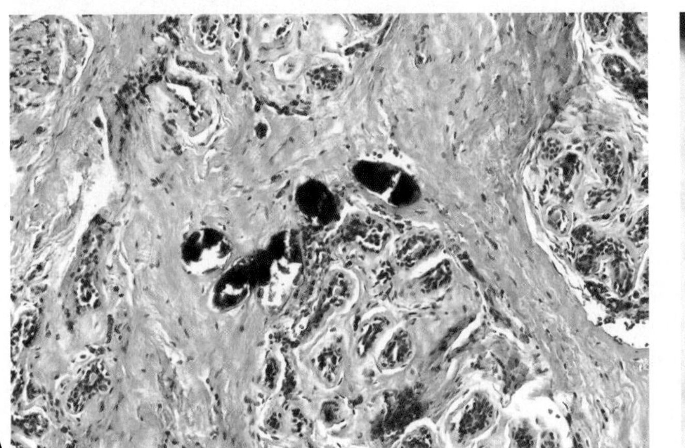

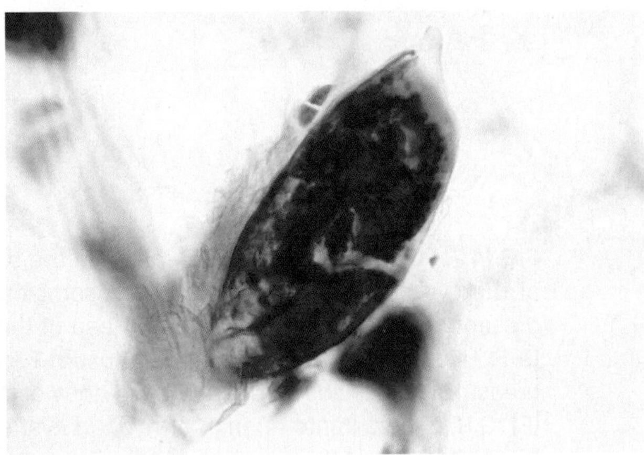

FIG. 4.6. *Schistosomiasis.* **A,B:** Calcified eggs of *Schistosoma mansoni* around breast lobules. (Courtesy of Dr. R. Yantiss.)

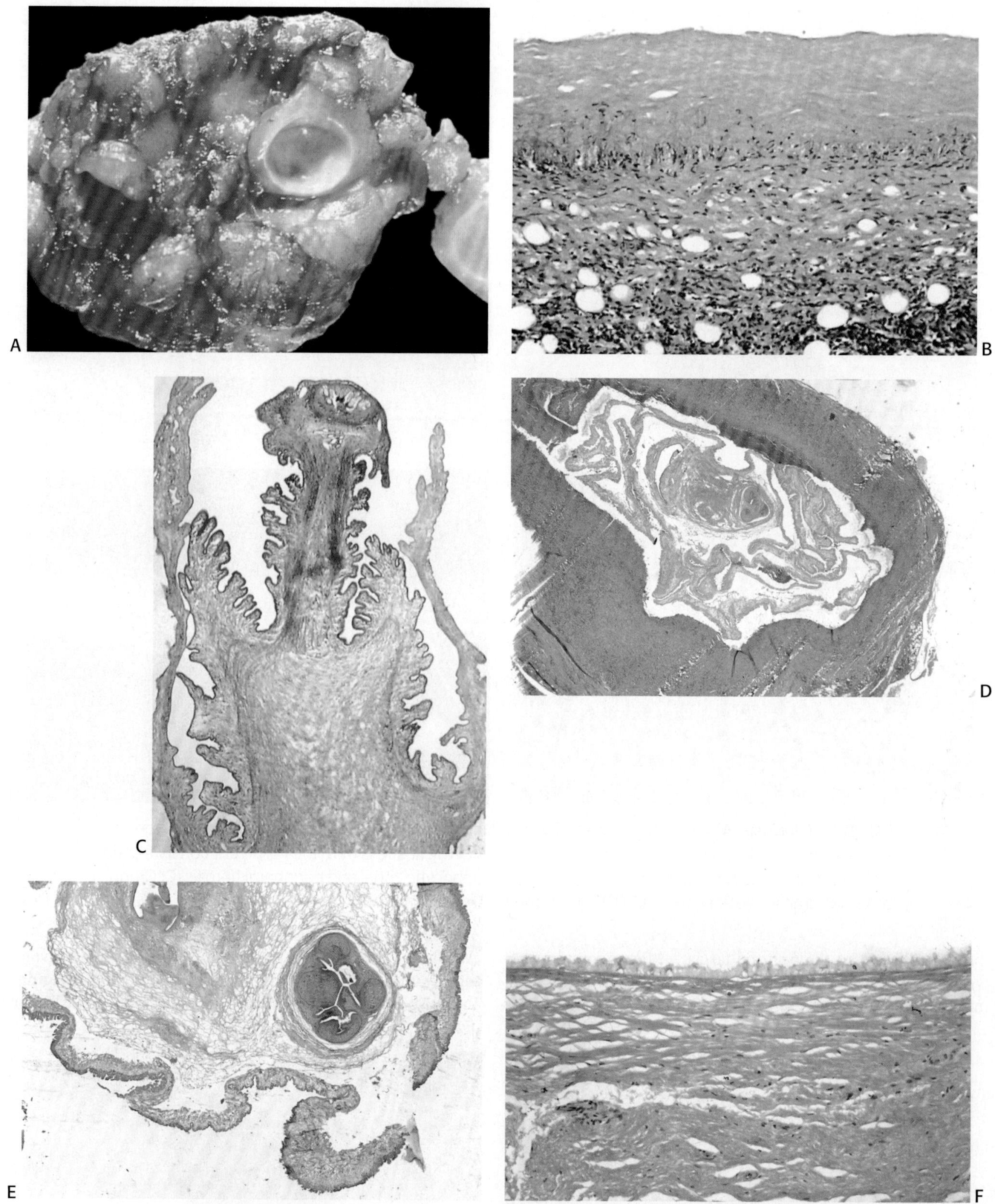

FIG. 4.7. ***Cysticercosis.*** **A–C:** *T. solium* in the breast. (Courtesy of Dr. J. Searle.) Gross appearance of the cyst **(A)**. The wall of the cyst resembles the reaction to a breast implant. Fat necrosis is present outside the cyst wall **(B)**. **C:** Head of the tapeworm with everted scolex found in the cyst. **D–F:** Hydatid cyst. (Courtesy of Dr. Kusum Kapila.) Whole mount section of cyst resected from breast **(D)**, which shows the head and body of the parasite **(E)** and cyst wall with inner membrane **(F)**. **G,H:** The contents of another hydatid cyst showing fragments of breast tissue and the intact head and body of the larval parasite.

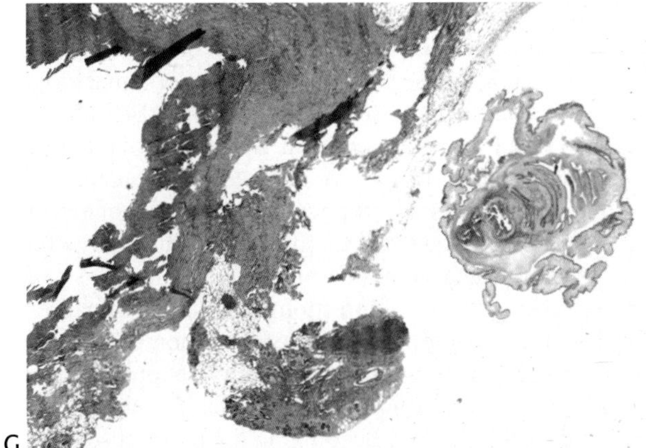

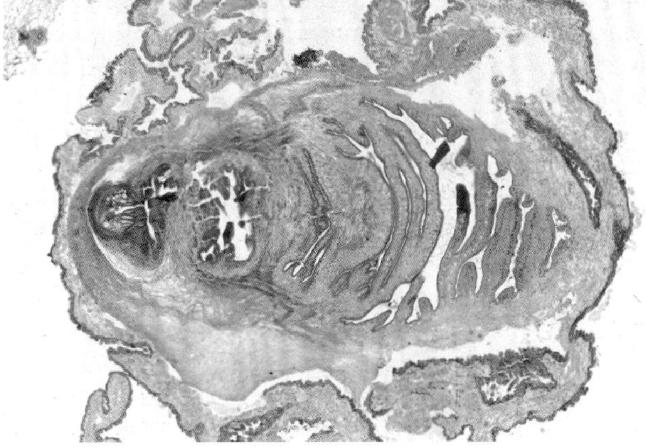

FIG. 4.7. *[Continued]*

with capsular enhancement.[52] The diagnosis of cystic mammary hydatid disease can be made by finding fragments of hydatid membranes and hooklets in the aspirated cyst contents.[51,53,54] Treatment consists of excision of the intact cyst.

Sparganosis, an infection caused by larvae of tapeworms of the genus *Spirometra*, has been reported in the breast.[55,56] The usual hosts for this parasite are dogs and cats. Human infection typically results from ingestion of water or from contaminated raw fish containing *Cyclops*, a microscopic crustacean that harbors the procercoid larval form that migrates to the subcutaneous tissue. The excised mass typically consists of hemorrhagic, necrotic, and sometimes cystic tissue containing larval worms in which there are fine calcifications (Fig. 4.8). In one instance, ultrasonography revealed a "folded band-like hypoechoic structure in an ill-defined heterogeneous hypoechoic mass" in the breast,[57] although in most cases, the parasite is found in the subcutaneous tissue.[58] Mammary sparganosis can present with "migrating" pain.[59]

Dracunculus medinensis, also known as the guinea worm, is the longest nematode that infects humans. The worm forms tumorous granulomatous lesions in the subcutaneous tissue. In one case report, the lesion presented clinically as a breast mass.[60] The excised specimen consisted of a cystic lesion containing four worms 5 to 25 cm in length surrounded by granulomatous inflammation with eosinophils. When calcified, the guinea worm can be detected in a mammogram.[61]

Calcifications in the pectoral muscle that were attributed to *Trichinella* infection have also been found by mammography.[62–64] Although the diagnosis was not confirmed by biopsy, serologic study in one case revealed antibodies for *Trichinella*.[62]

Cutaneous myiasis (maggot infection) caused by larvae of the botfly *Dermatobia hominis* results in a mass lesion accompanied by local inflammation. The mammographic and ultrasound findings in five patients with mammary lesions were reported by de Barros et al.[65] Three tumors were retroareolar, and in two cases, they were more deeply situated in inferior and lateral sites. The mammographically ill-defined tumors measured 0.7 to 2.0 cm. Paired linear microcalcifications were visualized in three lesions. Oval larvae outlined by a hypoechoic zone were demonstrated by ultrasound examination. Although the diagnosis of myiasis will be suggested by a history of origin from or a visit to an endemic area, the clinical findings may mimic inflammatory carcinoma, or the disease can manifest as an ulcerated fungating

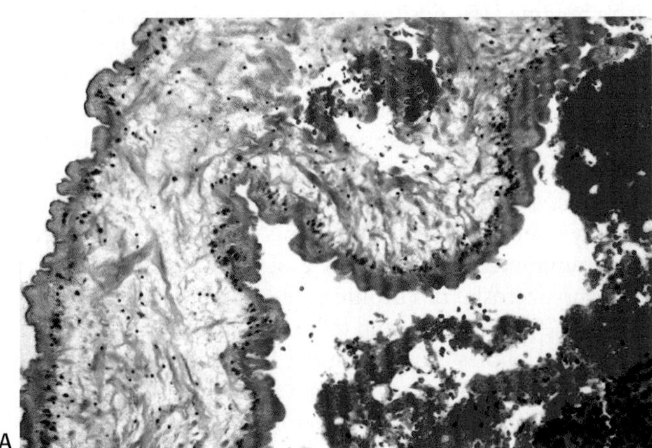

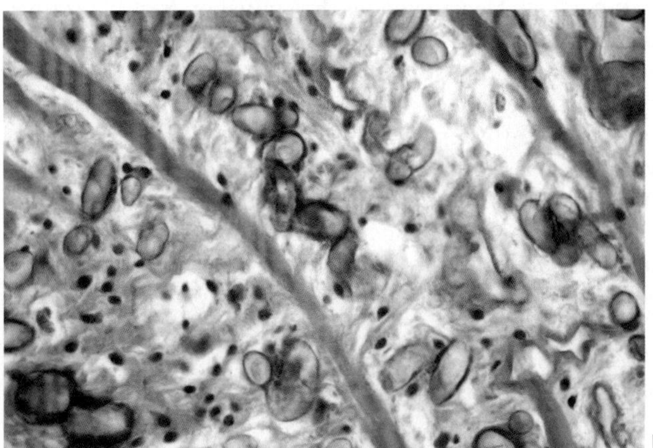

FIG. 4.8. ***Sparganosis.*** **A:** Part of a larval parasite obtained in a needle core biopsy specimen from a partly cystic breast mass. **B:** Magnified view of the interior of the larva showing abundant calcareous bodies.

lesion.[66,67] Another form of cutaneous myiasis that manifests as abscesses with draining sinuses is caused by infestation by larvae of the Tumbu fly (*Cordylobia anthropophaga*) found in sub-Saharan West Africa.[68]

Liesegang rings (*vide infra*) may be mistaken for parasitic ova in an FNA specimen[69] and can appear as calcifications on mammograms.[70]

MYCOBACTERIAL INFECTIONS

The earliest modern clinical report of tuberculosis of the breast is attributed to Sir Astley Cooper in 1829.[71] A review of scrofulous (i.e., tuberculous) mastitis in 1898 provided a detailed description of the lesions.[72] Tuberculosis of the breast remains a serious condition worldwide.[73] Tuberculous mastitis has been encountered with increasing frequency in HIV-positive individuals.[74,75]

Tuberculous mastitis not associated with HIV infection is primarily a disease of premenopausal women that may have a predilection for the lactating breast,[76] but it can affect the female breast at any age and occurs rarely in the male breast.[77] In younger patients, the lesion presents as an abscess, whereas in older women tuberculous infection tends to simulate carcinoma. Unilateral tuberculous mastitis is much more common than involvement of both breasts.[78] Mammary tuberculosis was found in 6 of 1152 (0.52%) consecutive mammographic examinations performed at a university hospital in Saudi Arabia.[79]

Infection of the breast may be the primary manifestation of tuberculosis, but this is uncommon. The breasts are infected secondarily in most patients, even when the presumed primary focus remains clinically inapparent. The majority of patients also have ipsilateral axillary granulomatous lymphadenitis. Retrograde lymphatic flow from the thorax to the axilla could be a mechanism for spread from an inconspicuous primary thoracic focus of mycobacterial infection. Another route of spread from the lungs is via tracheobronchial and paratracheal lymph nodes to internal mammary lymph nodes and then to the subareolar lymphatic plexus. Retrograde spread from infected cervical lymph nodes is also possible. Hematogenous dissemination is also a source of mammary infection. This manner of spread has been observed in patients with AIDS who develop disseminated tuberculosis that includes the breast. Finally, the breast may be involved by extension from primary lung lesions that involve the chest wall or from tuberculous infection originating in bone, cartilage, or the retromammary region of the chest wall.[80–82] Direct inoculation of the nipple via lactiferous ducts, which dilate during lactation, may account for some pregnancy-associated infections.

The diagnosis of tuberculous mastitis is difficult, since the disease has multiple patterns of clinical presentation.[72] The most common form is nodular mastitis, in which the patient develops a slowly growing, solitary mass. The lesion is generally painless but may be tender. The mammographic and clinical appearance of such lesions resembles carcinoma.[76,83] Microcalcifications are usually absent. Ultrasound and MR imaging typically reveal a solid, heterogeneous mass, but cystic encapsulated lesions have been described.[83] Advanced nodular lesions become fixed to the skin and may develop draining sinuses. The combination of a mass in the breast with a sinus tract extending to a superficial bulge and thickened skin was noted as a distinctive feature of mammary tuberculosis in one study.[79] A diffuse type of tuberculous mastitis is characterized by the acute development of multiple painful nodules throughout the breast, producing a pattern that can be mistaken for inflammatory carcinoma.[76,84] The third, sclerosing variety of infection occurs predominantly in elderly women, resulting in diffuse induration of the breast and increased density on mammography.[76] Nipple discharge is most common in the nodular and diffuse forms of the disease. Acid-fast bacilli may be found in the nipple discharge.[85]

The clinical distinction between tuberculous mastitis and mammary carcinoma is further complicated by the occasional coexistence of the lesions in the same breast or in opposite bre asts.[76,86–88] This association is coincidental. Some of these cases may be examples of carcinoma with sarcoid-like granulomas, since tubercle bacilli are not always identified in histological sections or cultured.[86,87] Mammary involvement by tuberculosis and Hodgkin disease has been described in one patient,[89] and another report documents a patient with dermatomyositis treated with corticosteroids, who developed large cell lymphoma and tuberculosis of the breast.[90] Mammary tuberculosis is rarely the presenting manifestation of AIDS.[91] *Mycobacterium tuberculosis* was cultured from FNA material obtained from breast lesions in 7 of 152 patients infected with HIV.[92]

A few examples of atypical mycobacterial infection associated with mammary prosthetic implants have been described. A number of patients with silicone-gel implants have developed infections with various mycobacterial organisms,[93–96] and the infection has also been associated with nipple piercing.[97] Smears of exudate around the implants have usually been positive for acid-fast bacilli. No common source of infection was identified. There have been fewer examples of implant-associated mastitis attributed to *Mycobacterium avium complex* (MAC).[98,99] One HIV-negative patient under treatment with prednisone for systemic lupus developed a breast abscess due to MAC caused by hematogenous spread from a paraspinal abscess.[100] In another instance, a patient who became HIV positive 4 years after bilateral subglandular silicone breast implantation developed MAC infection of one breast.[101] Ten years elapsed between the onset of HIV positivity and clinical evidence of the breast infection.

Grossly, tuberculous mastitis consists of nodular, indurated gray or tan tissue with yellow to white foci of caseous necrosis. Confluent nodular lesions with central cavitation grossly resemble necrotic carcinoma or a suppurative abscess.

Granulomatous lesions in tuberculous mastitis feature caseous necrosis. In chronic cases, fibrosis may be prominent. The granulomas tend to be associated with ducts more than with lobules (Figs. 4.9 and 4.10). Acid-fast bacteria are not detected histologically in most cases.[72]

The diagnosis of granulomatous infection of the breast may be suggested by the findings in a fine-needle aspirate.[83,102–104] In one series from India, 14 of 410 or 3.4% of breast aspiration specimens were consistent with tuberculous mastitis.[103] Tuberculosis was suspected clinically in only

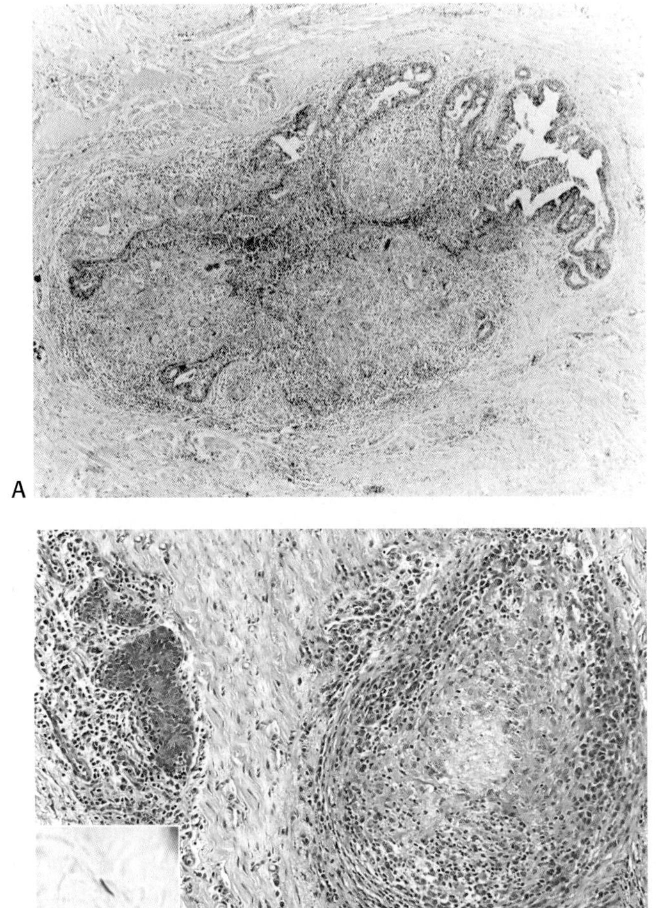

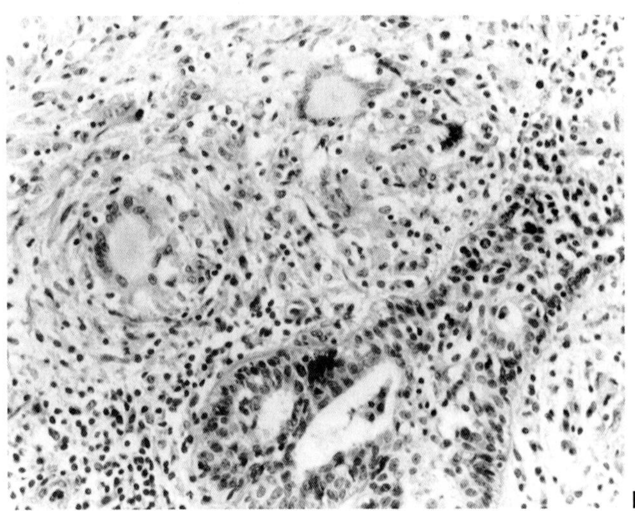

FIG. 4.9. *Tuberculosis.* **A,B:** Granulomas form multiple nodules that distort the wall of a duct, resulting in necrosis of the epithelium **(A)**. Langhans-type giant cells and granulomatous inflammation **(B)**. **C:** A granuloma in the vicinity of inactive mammary glands. Note the absence of giant cells. An acid-fast bacillus found in the granuloma is shown in a Ziehl–Neelsen-stained section seen in the *inset* **(C)**.

two of these cases, and in three cases, the clinical diagnosis was carcinoma. The aspiration cytology specimen consists of epithelioid histiocytes, Langhans giant cells, neutrophils, eosinophils, lymphocytes, and plasma cells. Neutrophils may obscure the granulomatous character of the process in actively inflamed lesions. Calcifications are uncommon.

Cytological examination of nipple discharge shows a nonspecific mixture of foamy histiocytes, neutrophils, and necrotic debris. However, if tuberculous mastitis is suspected, the discharge material should be submitted for culture as well as an acid-fast stain.[103]

Granulomatous mastitis, particularly one associated with cystic degeneration and prominent neutrophilic infiltrate, has been reported with *Corynebacterium*, a Gram-positive bacterium[105–107] (Fig. 4.10). In general, the granulomas of tuberculosis show relatively more prominent eosinophils and necrosis.[108]

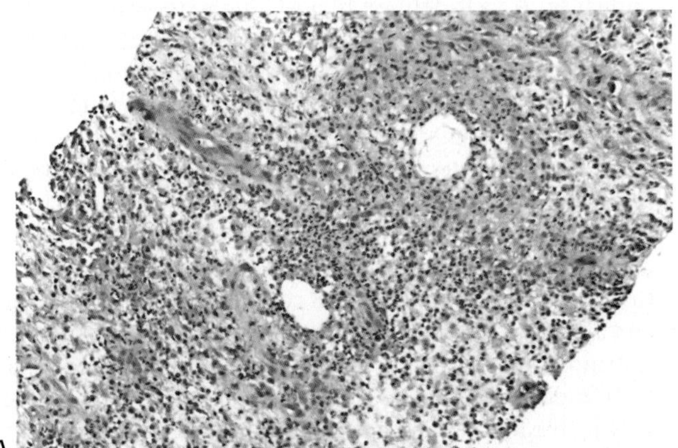

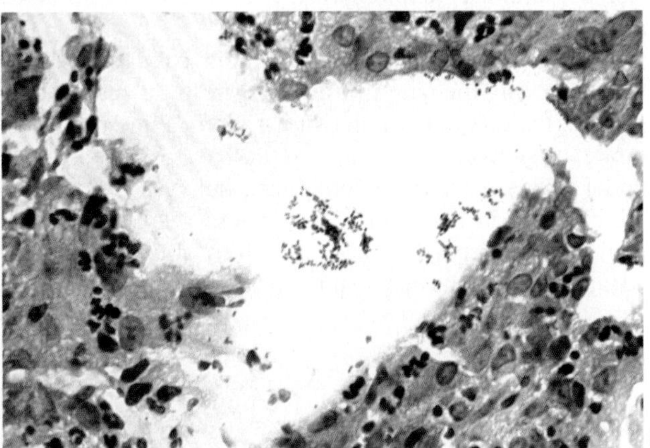

FIG. 4.10. *Necrotizing granulomatous mastitis.* **A:** A lobule has been destroyed by a microabscess with a necrotic center rich in neutrophils. The central microcyst is a characteristic finding in this lesion. **B:** Gram staining showing Gram-positive rods. *Corynebacterium* sp. was cultured.

Surgical biopsy may be necessary to establish a diagnosis of tuberculous mastitis, even if the diagnosis may be suggested by the clinical presentation and the findings in an FNA specimen. Often, the diagnosis is one of exclusion after histochemical studies have been completed, since cultures and the acid-fast staining are negative in most cases. Molecular analysis of material obtained by aspiration or surgical biopsy can be used for the detection of mycobacterial DNA. Mastectomy may be necessary for advanced lesions with extensive sinus formation, but most patients respond to antibiotic regimen after excisional biopsy.[67] Failure to control the lesion has been reported in patients who receive antibiotic therapy without excision of the lesion.

OTHER BACTERIAL INFECTIONS

Actinomycosis

The route of actinomycotic infection is usually via the nipple.[109] One patient was infected by a grain of corn, which was lodged in her nipple during harvesting.[110] Although *Actinomyces israelii* is the most commonly isolated pathogen associated with mammary infection, a variety of strains including *Actinomyces accolens, Actinomyces bovis, Actinomyces neuii, Actinomyces radingae*, and *Actinomyces turicensis* have been implicated.[111,112] A breast abscess attributed to *Actinomyces meyerii* has been associated with chronic periodontal disease.[113] *Paecilomyces variotii* was recovered from the lumen of a saline-filled breast implant removed because of capsular contracture.[114]

Actinomycotic infection of the breast typically presents as an abscess beneath or near the nipple and areola.[115] Sinus tracts develop following incision and drainage when the specific diagnosis is unsuspected clinically, or with progression of the untreated lesion. When a sinus tract does not appear, a chronic abscess may form, creating a hard mass that simulates carcinoma. Axillary nodal enlargement reflects reaction to the inflammatory process more often than spread of actinomycosis to the lymph nodes, but actinomycotic axillary lymphadenitis has been reported.[116] In advanced cases, the infection can spread to the chest wall.[110] Extension of pulmonary actinomycosis to the breast has also been reported.[117]

The diagnosis of mammary actinomycosis is made by demonstrating the Gram-positive organism as filamentous colonies (sulfur granules) in tissue sections, a fine-needle aspirate, or sinus tract drainage. *Actinomyces* can be isolated under anaerobic culture conditions, but positive cultures are obtained in less than 50% of cases.[116] Treatment with penicillin has reportedly been effective,[116] but recurrent or advanced infections may require mastectomy.

Nocardia

Cutaneous and subcutaneous abscesses due to *Nocardia asteroides* occur most frequently as a result of direct percutaneous inoculation from an environmental source. A single case report described a parenchymal mammary abscess due to *N. asteroides* confirmed by culture and surgical excision in a 58-year-old woman with systemic lupus who was receiving immunosuppressive therapy.[118] The source of infection was not determined in this patient. Nocardial infection may develop in lymphopenic patients receiving chemotherapy for breast carcinoma.[119]

Typhoid

Few cases of typhoid (enteric fever) mastitis have been reported. *Salmonella typhi* was isolated from the biopsy specimen obtained from a 32-year-old patient who had a painful breast tumor.[120] She had no gastrointestinal or other symptoms suggestive of typhoid infection. Blood, urine, and stool cultures were negative for *S. typhi*. Radiologic study of the gallbladder was not performed. Histologically, the tissue exhibited nonnecrotizing granulomatous inflammation with no detectable acid-fast bacteria. Gram staining of the tissue was not described, and the patient was lost to follow-up. Another patient was a 43-year-old woman who presented with fever and a 5-cm painful breast mass.[121] Needle biopsy revealed acute inflammation in the breast, and *S. typhi* was isolated from the wound. *S. typhi* was isolated from bilateral breast abscesses in a 35-year-old woman who presented with painful swelling of both breasts in India where the disease is endemic,[122] and unexpectedly from a unilateral breast abscess in a patient from the Bronx in New York.[123] *Salmonella choleraesuis* was isolated from the site of a saline-filled silicone implant removed from a patient 1 month after an episode of diarrhea and vomiting.[124]

Cat Scratch Disease

Granulomatous lesions of cat scratch disease have been described in intramammary lymph nodes and in breast parenchyma.[125,126] All were women 21 to 60 years of age with 1- to 3-cm tumors. Most lesions were in the axillary tail of the breast. One was in the 4-o'clock radius of the left breast. Clinically, these appeared to be intrinsic mammary lesions, and only one of the women also had axillary adenopathy. A well-defined hypoechoic mass was described by ultrasound in one case.[125] Microscopic examination of the excised tumors revealed necrotizing granulomas.

The causative organism is *Bartonella* sp.[127,128] Filamentous and branching Gram-negative Warthin–Starr-positive bacilli may be detected in the necrotic centers of granulomas. The surrounding breast tissue has a lymphoplasmacytic infiltrate without granulomas. Aspiration cytology yields a cellular specimen composed of acute and chronic inflammatory cells with benign epithelial cells.[125] Mammary erythema and axillary adenopathy due to cat scratch disease simulated inflammatory breast carcinoma in a 50-year-old woman with underlying diabetes mellitus.[129] Cat scratch disease involving the breast parenchyma can simulate carcinoma[130,131] or mastitis.[132] Mammary cat scratch disease, confirmed by polymerase chain reaction (PCR) analysis, has been reported after contact with a guinea pig—notwithstanding the name of this disease.[131]

Breast Abscesses

The differential diagnosis of the "red breast" includes various forms of infectious mastitis (including abscess formation and cellulitis), radiation effect, inflammatory dermatoses, inflammatory breast carcinoma, and Paget disease.[133] In this setting, it is imperative to exclude a neoplastic process. Risk factors for the development of breast abscesses include tobacco smoking and nipple piercing.[134,135] However, breast abscesses occur most commonly during lactation.

Lactational mastitis and abscess formation develop as a result of obstruction to the flow in one or more major lactiferous ducts. The initial phases of stasis and mastitis caused by extruded milk are usually sterile. At this stage, the secreted milk has low leukocyte and bacterial counts.[136] Infected lactational mastitis has been characterized by a leukocyte count of more than 10^6 and a bacterial count of more than 10^3 per milliliter. Fever, increased pain, and tenderness herald acceleration of lactational mastitis. Bacteria isolated from nipple discharge are usually skin inhabitants such as *Staphylococcus aureus*, streptococci, and coagulase-negative staphylococci.[136] *S. aureus* is the commonest organism responsible for breast abscesses, and it is isolated in one-half of cases, approximately 10% of which are methicillin-resistant strains.[137] If drainage by needle aspiration and antibiotic therapy are unsuccessful, surgical drainage may be required. Specimens removed in such operations show a mixed acute and chronic inflammatory reaction that may include fat necrosis (Fig. 4.11).

Other strains of bacteria have also been implicated in breast abscesses. A breast abscess caused by *Aeromonas hydrophilia* in an immunocompetent 12-year-old girl with no known predisposing factors was reported by Vine et al.[138] Chagla et al.[139] reported a breast abscess due to *Helcococcus kunzii* in an immunocompetent 57-year-old woman. Breast brucellosis is endemic in the Middle East, and multiple cases from Saudi Arabia have been reported.[140] A 46-year-old Turkish woman with breast and paraspinal abscesses due to brucellosis was successfully treated with systemic antibiotics.[141] Breast abscess due to *Pseudomonas aeruginosa* can culminate in septic shock.[142]

Subareolar abscesses usually occur in nonlactating premenopausal women. The condition is characterized by repeated episodes of abscess formation in the subareolar region. The lesions evolve slowly, eventually rupturing and draining through periareolar sinus tracts. Secondary infection with common skin organisms occurs occasionally, but in some cases, the abscesses are sterile. Subareolar abscesses are the result of duct obstruction caused by squamous metaplasia in the terminal portion of one or more lactiferous ducts.[143] Excision of the affected duct, sinus tract, and abscess is successful in most cases, but recurrences may occur when the process develops in another duct.[144]

Intramammary abscesses have been described as a delayed complication in women treated for breast carcinoma by lumpectomy and radiotherapy.[145] Factors predisposing to infection were the excision of relatively large volumes of tissue and the addition of a radiation boost. Cultures revealed staphylococci and other bacteria of cutaneous origin.

Infection of a polyurethane-coated silicone-gel breast implant site caused by *Clostridium perfringens* has been reported.[146] The cause was probably hematogenous contamination initiated by multiple dental procedures. The origin of *Enterococcus avium* infection of a silicone-gel implant site in another patient was not found.[147]

Breast abscess formation attributable to *Mycobacterium fortuitum*,[148] *Mycobacterium abscessus*,[149] and *Actinomyces turicensis*[150] has been observed following nipple piercing and the insertion of metal rings. *Actinomyces radingae* was identified as the cause of subareolar and axillary abscesses in a 38-year-old man, who presented with bloody nipple discharge.[150]

Necrotizing fasciitis of the breast has been reported as a complication of methylene blue dye injection performed in the course of a sentinel lymph node biopsy procedure.[151] Thus, irradiation, placement of implants, and injections are among the iatrogenic causes (or facilitators) of mammary abscesses.

VIRAL INFECTIONS

Herpes Simplex and Varicella Zoster

Herpes simplex infections of the breast diagnosed cytologically and confirmed by *in situ* hybridization have been reported.[152,153] No patient had a documented underlying

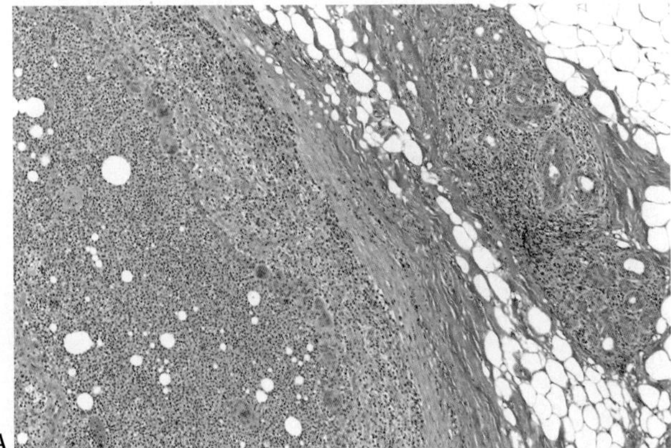

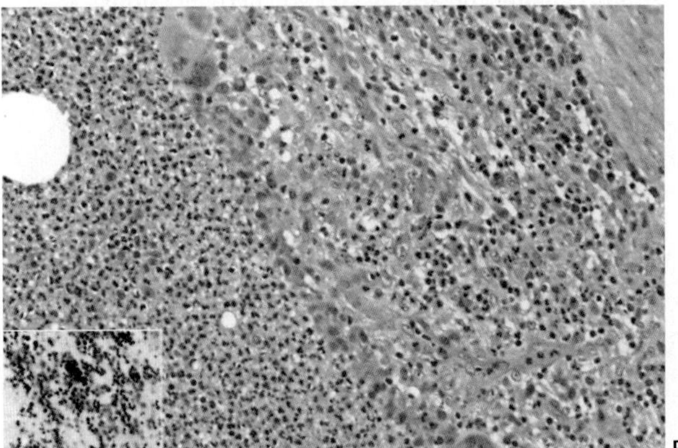

FIG. 4.11. *Staphylococcal abscess.* **A,B:** Purulent mastitis in a 35-year-old woman, who had been breast-feeding until a few weeks prior to the biopsy. The abscess showed Gram-positive cocci [*inset* in **B**]. *S. aureus* was cultured.

immunosuppressive disorder. In one case, herpetic gingivostomatitis was known to be present prior to the onset of bloody nipple discharge and crusting vesicles on the nipple surface. Another patient presented with a nipple lesion.

Mammary infection with varicella (chicken pox) and *Herpes zoster* can assume unusual forms. Cytological changes due to varicella infection were observed in the epithelium of a fibroadenoma in smears from an FNA procedure,[154] and the diagnosis was confirmed by immunostaining and ultrastructural examination.

An unusual case of *Herpes zoster* infection was documented in a 45-year-old patient who had undergone transverse rectus abdominis myocutaneous (TRAM) flap reconstruction following a modified radical mastectomy. The rash showed a "pseudodisseminated" distribution, seemingly crossing multiple dermatomes, following the realignment of intercostal nerves.[155]

HIV Infection

Patients with HIV infection, of which there are approximately 35 million worldwide in 2012, are living longer due to increasingly effective treatment. The breast does not appear to be predisposed to any particular pattern of neoplastic or microbial disease in this setting. Among 46 such individuals (including 34 women) treated in a community hospital setting who presented with breast disease, a malignant tumor was identified in 22% and an infectious process in 17%.[156]

Roca et al.[157] described a 21-year-old woman with HIV infection who developed a breast abscess caused by *P. aeruginosa* that led to fatal septicemia. Massive necrosis of the breast due to *Escherichia coli* puerperal sepsis has been reported in a 26-year-old HIV-positive woman.[158] Another instance of postpartum polymicrobial gangrene of the breast in a HIV-positive patient was treated by mastectomy.[159] A review of mammograms obtained from 67 HIV-infected women compared with age-matched controls revealed significantly larger and denser axillary lymph nodes in the former group.[160] There was no difference in the frequency with which lymph nodes were detected in the axillary region or in the frequency of benign-appearing nodules or calcifications. HIV-associated lymphadenopathy has been reported in an intramammary lymph node.[161] Please see the section on mycobacterial infections in this chapter regarding HIV-related infections.

The issue of whether HIV and AIDS influence the risk of developing breast carcinoma and the grade of carcinomas that occur in this setting remains unresolved.[162–164] Breast carcinoma had been reported in 46 HIV-infected women until 2011, and theories proposing the possible antitumor effect of the infection and antiretroviral treatment have been advanced.[165] Gynecomastia is by far the most common breast disease encountered in HIV-positive males.[156] However, unilateral Bowen disease (squamous cell carcinoma *in situ*) of the nipple in a 41-year-old male with AIDS has been documented.[166]

INCIDENTAL AND ARTIFACTUAL FINDINGS

Cutaneous Infestation by Demodex Mite

Demodex folliculorum is a mite that is typically identified within sebaceous glands in the face, scalp, and eyelids. In a histopathological study of nipples collected at autopsy, *Demodex* mite was identified in 58 (41.4%) of 140 nipples.[167] The mite is only uncommonly encountered in routine surgical pathology practice (Fig. 4.12) and in nipple discharge cytology specimens.[168] *Demodex* infestation of the nipple can occasionally be symptomatic, causing nipple discharge or local discomfort.[168]

Myospherulosis, a Mimic of Parasitic Infestation

Myospherulosis is an artifact formed by an as yet ill-understood interaction of red blood cells and lipid.[169] This reaction results in the formation of a saccular structure (comprising erythrocytes [endo bodies] that lie within cystic spaces [parent bodies]) (Fig. 4.13). Myospherulosis can develop in a variety of organs, including breast,[169,170] wherein it can resemble fungal organisms, especially *Coccidioides immitis*. A history of a prior surgical procedure can usually be elicited.

Liesegang Rings, Another Mimic of Parasitic Infestation

Liesegang rings are spherical deposits similar to corpora amylacea, which occur in breast cysts (Fig. 4.14) and in various

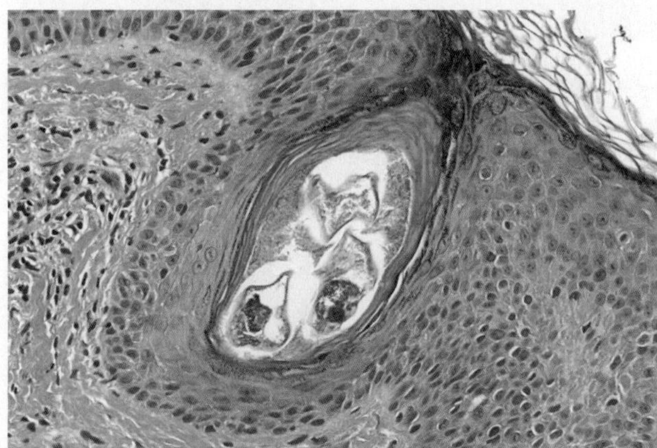

A

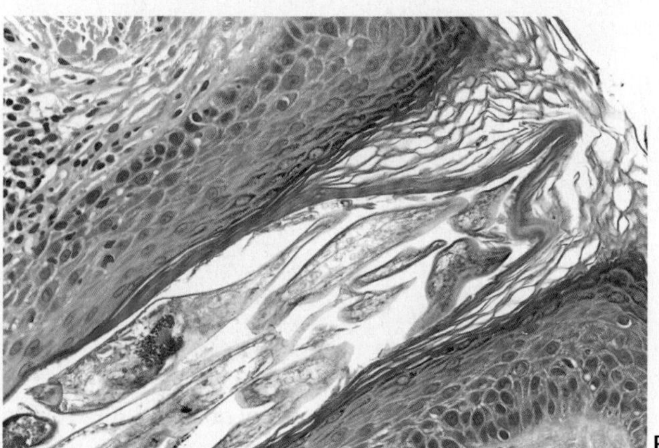

B

FIG. 4.12. ***Demodex infestation.*** **A,B:** Demodex mites are present in the nipple–areolar region. Mites are present in the upper portions of openings of sebaceous units.

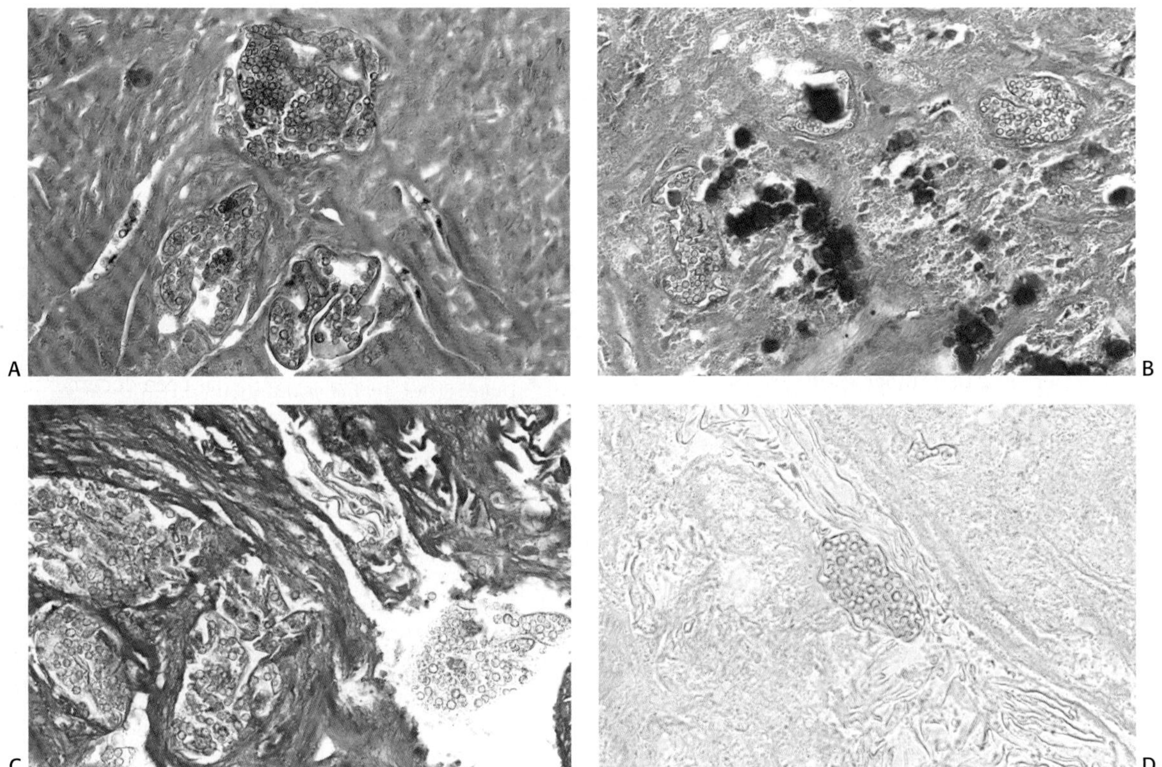

FIG. 4.13. ***Myospherulosis.*** **A,B:** Hematoxylin and eosin–stained sections show myospherulosis, with clustered and tightly packed erythrocytes (endo bodies) in cystic spaces (parent bodies) in necrotic tissue. Myospherulosis is not highlighted by the periodic-acid Schiff (PAS) **(C)** or by the Grocott methenamine silver (GMS) stains **(D)**. The 55-year-old patient who presented with mammographic abnormality had undergone lumpectomy for benign proliferative changes 5 years previously.

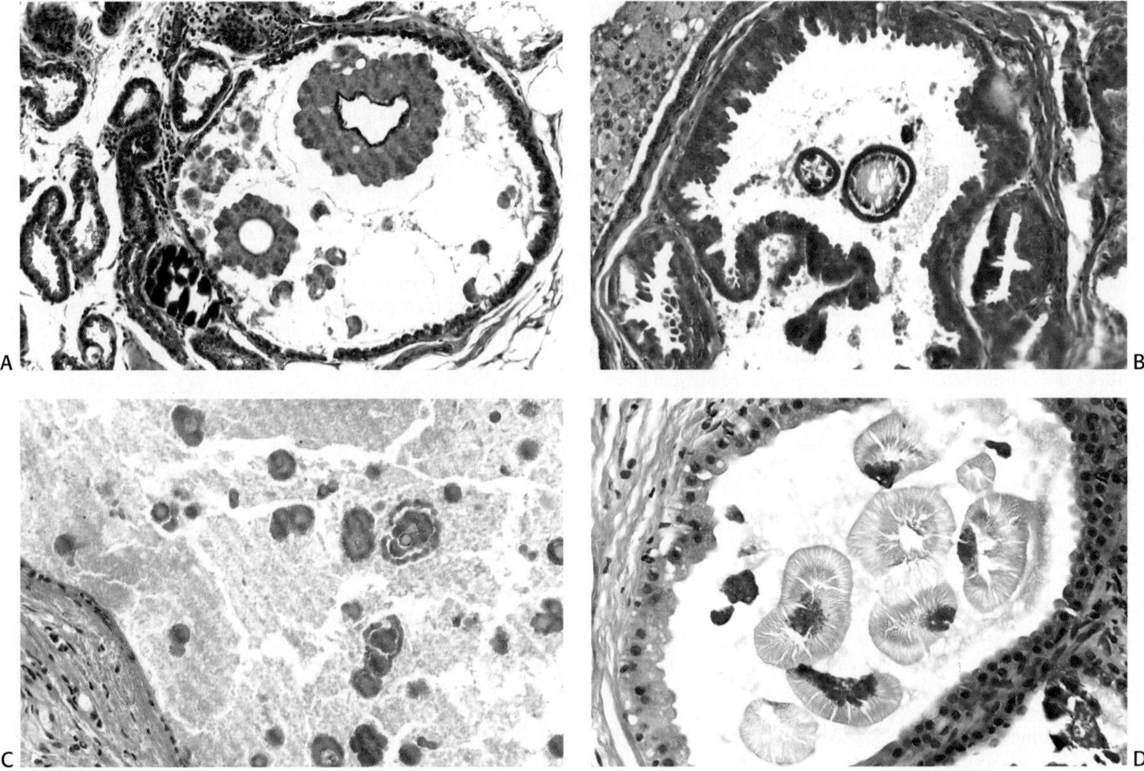

FIG. 4.14. ***Liesegang rings.*** **A–D:** In these four examples, the rings appear rather unlike each other. However, their basic structure is similar, consisting of an amorphous centrally dense, often calcified, nidus surrounded by a striated zone of proteinaceous deposits. Liesegang rings are typically encountered in the breast in benign glands that show either apocrine metaplasia or secretory changes.

other glandular organs. The rings that can be mistaken for parasitic ova are formed by an as yet ill-understood mechanism, whereby various minerals and substances aggregate and segregate. The process can be identified in the *in vitro* and *in vivo* settings. The characteristic structure consists of an amorphous centrally dense nidus with a concentric, seemingly lamellated, corona of proteinaceous material. Liesegang rings in the breast are typically encountered in apocrine cysts or in pregnancy-like hyperplasia.[171] Liesegang rings may calcify and can present as a mammographic abnormality.

REFERENCES

Fungal Infections

1. Osborne BM. Granulomatous mastitis caused by histoplasma and mimicking inflammatory breast carcinoma. *Hum Pathol* 1989;20:47–52.
2. Salfelder K, Schwarz J. Mycotic "pseudotumors" of the breast. *Arch Surg* 1975;110:751–754.
3. Farmer C, Stanley MW, Bardales RH, et al. Mycoses of the breast: diagnosis by fine-needle aspiration. *Diagn Cytopathol* 1995;12:51–55.
4. Payne S, Kim S, Das K, et al. A 36-year-old woman with a unilateral breast mass. Necrotizing granulomatous mastitis secondary to budding yeast forms morphologically consistent with *Histoplasma capsulatum. Arch Pathol Lab Med* 2006;130:e1–e2.
5. Seymour EQ. Blastomycosis of the breast. *AJR Am J Roentgenol* 1982;139:822–823.
6. Propeck PA, Scanlan KA. Blastomycosis of the breast. *AJR Am J Roentgenol* 1996;166:726.
7. Symmers WS. Deep-seated fungal infections currently seen in the histopathologic service of a medical school laboratory in Britain. *Am J Clin Pathol* 1966;46:514–537.
8. Ramos-Barbosa S, Guazzelli LS, Severo LC. Cryptococcal mastitis after corticosteroid therapy. *Rev Soc Bras Med Trop* 2001;37:65–66.
9. Williams K, Walton RL, Bunkis I. Aspergillus colonization associated with bilateral silicone mammary implants. *J Surg Pathol* 1982;71: 260–261.
10. Wright PK, Raine C, Ragbir M, et al. The semi-permeability of silicone: a saline-filled breast implant with intraluminal and pericapsular *Aspergillus flavus. J Plast Reconstr Aesthet Surg* 2006;59:1118–1121.
11. Govindarajan M, Verghese S, Kuruvilla S. Primary *Aspergillus* of the breast. Report of a case with fine needle aspiration cytology diagnosis. *Acta Cytol* 1993;37:234–236.
12. Hiruma M, Ohnishi Y, Ohata H, et al. Chromomycosis of the breast. *Int J Dermatol* 1992;31:184–185.
13. Park SG, Oh SH, Suh SB, et al. A case of chromoblastomycosis with an unusual clinical manifestation caused by *Phialophora verrucosa* on an unexposed area: treatment with a combination of amphotericin B and 5-flucytosine. *Br J Dermatol* 2005;152:560–564.
14. Bocian JJ, Fahmy RN, Michas CA. A rare case of 'coccidioidoma' of the breast. *Arch Pathol Lab Med* 1991;115:1064–1067.
15. Babycos PB, Hoda SA. A fatal case of disseminated coccidioidomycosis in Louisiana. *J La State Med Soc* 1990;142:24–27.
16. Hooper JE, Lu Q, Pepkowitz SH. Disseminated coccidioidomycosis in pregnancy. *Arch Pathol Lab Med* 2007;131:652–625.

Parasitic Infections

17. Chen YH, Qun X. Filarial granuloma of the female breast: a histopathologic study of 131 cases. *Am J Trop Med Hyg* 1981;30:1206–1210.
18. Rangabashyam N, Gnananprakasam D, Krishnaraj B. Spectrum of benign breast lesions in Madras. *J R Coll Surg Edinb* 1983;28:369–373.
19. Lang AP, Luchsinger IS, Rawling EG. Filariasis of the breast. *Arch Pathol Lab Med* 1987;111:757–759.
20. Miller JJ, Moore S. Nodular breast lesion caused by Bancroft's filariasis. *Can Med Assn J* 1965;93:771–774.
21. Lahiri VL. Microfilariae in nipple secretion. *Acta Cytol* 1975;19:154.
22. Choudhury M. Bancroftian microfilaria in the breast clinically mimicking malignancy. *Cytopathology* 1995;6:132–133.
23. Kibbelaar RE, Hol C, Polderman AM, et al. Filaria in an axillary lymph node dissection specimen. *Histopathol* 2000;37:85–86.
24. Dreyer G, Brandão AC, Amaral F, et al. Detection by ultrasound of living adult *Wuchereria bancrofti* in the female breast. *Mem Inst Oswaldo Cruz* 1996;91:95–96.
25. Novak R. Calcifications in the breast in filaria loa infection. *Acta Radiol* 1989;30:507–508.
26. Chow CK, McCarthy JS, Neafie R, et al. Mammography of lymphatic filariasis. *AJR Am J Roentgenol* 1996;167:1425–1426.
27. Kapila K, Verma K. Diagnosis of parasites in fine needle breast aspirates. *Acta Cytol* 1996;40:653–656.
28. Beaver PC, Orihel TC. Human infection with filariae of animals in the United States. *Am J Trop Med Hyg* 1980;29:1018–1019.
29. Bennett IC, Furnival CM, Searle J. Dirofilariasis in Australia: unusual cause of a breast lump. *Aust N Z J Surg* 1989;59:671–673.
30. Gutierrez Y, Paul GM. Breast nodule produced by *Dirofilaria tenuis. Am J Surg Pathol* 1984;8:463–465.
31. Pampiglione S, Franco F, Canestri Trotti G. Human subcutaneous dirofilariasis I: two new cases in Venice: identification of the causal agent as *Dirofilaria repens. Parassitologia* 1982;24:155–165.
32. MacDougall LT, Magoon CC, Fritsche TR. *Dirofilaria repens* manifesting as a breast nodule. *Am J Clin Pathol* 1992;97:625–630.
33. Arribas J, Prieto A, Diaz AC, et al. Calcifications of the breast in *Onchocerca* infection. *Breast J* 2005;11:507.
34. Gorman JD, Champaign JL, Sumida FK, et al. Schistosomiasis involving the breast. *Radiology* 1992;185:423–424.
35. Varin CR, Eisenberg BL, Ladd WA. Mammographic microcalcifications associated with schistosomiasis. *South Med J* 1989;82:1060–1061.
36. Sloan BS, Rickman LS, Blau EM, et al. Schistosomiasis masquerading as carcinoma of the breast. *S Med J* 1996;89:345–347.
37. Fishbon H. A case in which eggs of *Schistosoma japonicum* were demonstrated in multiple skin lesions. *Am J Trop Med* Hyg 1946;26:319–326.
38. Elma CA, Cavalcanti AC, Lima MM, et al. Pseudoneoplastic lesion of the breast caused by *Schistosoma mansoni. Rev Soc Bras Med Trop* 2004;37:63–64.
39. Martin B, Rowland Payne C, Calonje E. An ulcerated plaque on the breast of a young woman. Extragenital bilharziasis cutanea tarda (*Schistosoma mansoni*). *Clin Exp Dermatol* 2010;35:803–804.
40. Benger A, Rennie RP, Roberts JT, et al. A human coenurus infection in Canada. *Am J Trop Med Hyg* 1981;30:638–644.
41. Kurtycz DFI, Alt B, Mack E. Incidental coenurosis: larval cestode presenting as an axillary mass. *Am J Clin Pathol* 1983;80:735–738.
42. Alagaratnam TT, Wing YK, Tuen H. Cysticercosis of the breast. *Am J Trop Med Hyg* 1988;38:601–602.
43. Kunkel JM, Hawksley CZ. Cysticercosis presenting as a solitary dominant breast mass. *Hum Pathol* 1987;18:1190–1191.
44. Conde DM, Kashimoto E, Carvalho LE, et al. Cysticercosis of the breast: an uncommon cause of lumps. *Breast J* 2006;12:179.
45. Bhattacharjee HK, Ramman TR, Agarwal L, et al. Isolated cysticercosis of the breast masquerading as a breast tumour: report of a case and review of literature. *Ann Trop Med Parasitol* 2011;105:455–461.
46. Thurairatnam TP. Echinococcus breast abscess. *Trop Doct* 1992;22:192.
47. Abi F, El Fares I, Khaiz D, et al. Les localisations inhabituelles de kyste hydatique: a propos de 40 cases. *J Chir* (Paris) 1989;126:307–312.
48. Amr SS, Sa'di ARM, Ilahi F, et al. The spectrum of breast diseases in Saudi Arabian females: a 26 year pathological survey at Dhahran Health Center. *Ann Saudi Med* 1995;15:125–132.
49. Amr SS, Amr ZS, Jitawi S, et al. Hydatidosis in Jordan: an epidemiological study of 306 cases. *Ann Trop Med Parasitol* 1994;88:623–627.
50. Geramizadeh B, Makarempour A, Talei A. Primary isolated hydatid cyst of breast. *Breast J* 2011;17:314–316.
51. Vega A, Ortega E, Cavada A, et al. Hydatid cyst of the breast: mammographic findings. *AJR Am J Roentgenol* 1994;162:825–826.
52. Tükel S. Hyatid cyst of the breast: MR imaging findings. *AJR Am J Roentgenol* 1997;168:1386–1387.
53. Epstein NA. Hydatid cyst of the breast: diagnosis by using cytological techniques. *Acta Cytol* 1969;13:420–421.
54. Sagin HB, Kiroglu Y, Aksoy F. Hydatid cyst of the breast diagnosed by fine needle aspiration biopsy. A case report. *Acta Cytol* 1994;38:965–967.
55. Norma SH, Kreutner A Jr. Sparganosis: clinical and pathologic observations in 10 cases. *South Med J* 1980;73:297–300.
56. Chan ABW, Wan SK, Leung S-L, et al. Sparganosis of the breast. *Histopathol* 2004;44:510–511.

57. Chung SY, Park KS, Lee Y, et al. Breast sparganosis: mammographic and ultrasound features. *J Clin Ultrasound* 1995;23:447–451.
58. Koo M, Kim JH, Kim JS, et al. Cases and literature review of breast sparganosis. *World J Surg* 2011;35:573–579.
59. Moon HG, Jung EJ, Park ST. Breast sparganosis presenting as a breast mass with vague migrating pain. *J Am Coll Surg* 2008;207:292.
60. Booth T, Schepps B, Scola FH. *Dracunculus medinensis* infestation of the female breast. A case report. *Breast Dis* 1992;5:45–49.
61. Saleem TB, Ahmed I. "Serpent" in the breast. *J Ayub Med Coll Abbottabad* 2006;18:67–68.
62. Helvie MA, Elson BC, Billi JE, et al. Pectoral muscle microcalcifications shown by mammography in a patient with trichinosis. *Breast Dis* 1995;8:111–113.
63. Valdes PV, Prieto A, Diaz A, et al. Microcalcifications of pectoral muscle in trichinosis. *Breast J* 2005;11:150.
64. Ikeda DM, Sickles EA. Mammographic demonstration of pectoral muscle microcalcifications. *AJR Am J Roentgenol* 1988;151:475–476.
65. de Barros N, D'Avila MS, de Pace Bauab S, et al. Cutaneous myiasis of the breast: mammographic and US features—report of five cases. *Radiology* 2001;218:517–520.
66. Ugwu BT, Nwadiaro PO. *Cordyliobia anthropophagia* mastitis mimicking breast cancer: a case report. *East Afr Med J* 1999;76:115–116.
67. Kwong A, Yiu WK, Chow LW, et al. *Chrysomya bezziana*: a rare infestation of the breast. *Breast J* 2007;13:297–301.
68. Adisa CA, Mbanaso A. Furuncular myiasis of the breast caused by the larvae of the Tumbu fly (*Cordylobia anthropophagia). BMC Surgery* 2004;4:5.
69. Gupta RK. Liesegang rings in fine needle aspirate of breast cysts with predominance of apocrine cells: a study of 14 cases. *Diagn Cytopathol* 2008;36:701–704.
70. Aalaei S, Zarif A, Gattuso P, et al. Liesegang rings. *Breast J* 2005;11:522.

Mycobacterial Infections

71. Cooper AP. *Illustrations of the diseases of the breast.* London: Longman, Rees Co., 1829.
72. Halstead AC, LeCount ER. Tuberculosis of the mammary gland. *Ann Surg* 1898;28:685–707.
73. Hamit HF, Ragsdale TH. Mammary tuberculosis. *J R Soc Med* 1982;75:764–765.
74. Hartstein M, Leaf HL. Tuberculosis of the breast as a presenting manifestation of AIDS. *Clin Infect Dis* 1992;15:692–693.
75. Pantanowitz L, Connolly JL. Pathology of the breast associated with HIV/AIDS. *Breast J* 2002;8:234–243.
76. Tabar L, Kelt K, Nemeth A. Tuberculosis of the breast. *Radiology* 1976;118:587–589.
77. Atiq OT, Reyes CV, Zvetina JR. Male tuberculous mastitis. *Breast Dis* 1992;5:273–275.
78. Ducroz B, Nael LM, Gautier G, et al. Tubreculose mammaire bilatérale: un case. Révue de la literature. *J Gynécol Obstét Biol Réprod (Paris)* 1992;21:484–488.
79. Makanjuola D, Murshid K, Sulaimani A, et al. Mammographic features of breast tuberculosis: the skin bulge and sinus tract sign. *Clin Radiol* 1996;51:354–358.
80. Kappas AM, Bourantas KL, Batsis CP, et al. Chest tuberculosis mimicking breast cancer. *Breast Dis* 1995;8:85–89.
81. Chung SY, Yang I, Bae SH, et al. Tuberculous abscess in retromammary region: CT findings. *J Comp Assist Tomogr* 1996;20:766–769.
82. Greenberg D, Hingston G, Harman J. Chest wall tuberculosis. *Breast J* 1999;5:60–62.
83. Oh KK, Kim JH, Kook SH. Imaging of tuberculous disease involving breast. *Eur Radiol* 1998;8:1475–1480.
84. Sopeña B, Arnillas E, Garcia-Vila LM, et al. Tuberculosis of the breast: unusual clinical presentation of extrapulmonary tuberculosis. *Infection* 1996;24:57–58.
85. Mandal S, Jain S. Purulent nipple discharge: a presenting manifestation of tuberculous mastitis. *Breast J* 2007;13:2005.
86. Grausman RI, Goldman ML. Tuberculosis of the breast: report of nine cases including two cases of co-existing carcinoma and tuberculosis. *Am J Surg* 1945;67:48–56.
87. Miller RE, Salomon PF, West JP. The coexistence of carcinoma and tuberculosis of the breast and axillary lymph nodes. *Am J Surg* 1971;121: 338–340.
88. Rothman GM, Kolkov Z, Meroz A, et al. Breast tuberculosis and carcinoma. *Israel J Med Sci* 1989;25:339–340.
89. Graeme-Cook F, O'Briain S, Daly PA. Unusual breast masses. The sequential development of mammary tuberculosis and Hodgkin's disease of a young woman. *Cancer* 1988;61:1457–1459.
90. Cheng W, Alagaratnam TT, Leung CY, et al. Tuberculosis and lymphoma of the breast in a patient with dermatomyositis. *Aust N Z J Surg* 1993;63:660–661.
91. Hartstein M, Leaf HL. Tuberculosis of the breast as a presenting manifestation of AIDS. *Clin Infect Dis* 1992;15:692–693.
92. Michelow P, Dezube BJ, Pantanowitz L. Fine needle aspiration of breast masses in HIV-infected patients: results from a large series. *Cancer Cytopathol* 2010;118:218–224.
93. Clegg HW, Foster MT, Sanders WE Jr, et al. Infection due to organisms of the *Mycobacterium fortuitum* complex after augmentation mammoplasty: clinical and epidemiologic features. *J Infect Dis* 1983;147:427–433.
94. Toranto IR, Malow JB. Atypical mycobacteria periprosthetic infections—diagnosis and treatment. *Plast Reconstr Surg* 1980;66:226–228.
95. Macadam SA, Mehling BM, Fanning A, et al. Non-tuberculous mycobacterial breast implant infections. *Plast Reconstr Surg* 2007;119:337–344.
96. Wirth GA, Brenner KA, Sundine MJ. Delayed silicone breast implant infection with *Mycobacterium avium-intracellulare. Aesthet Surg J* 2007;27:167–171.
97. Bengualid V, Singh V, Singh H, et al. *Mycobacterium fortuitum* and anaerobic breast abscess following nipple piercing: case presentation and review of the literature. *J Adolesc Health* 2008;42:530–532.
98. Lee D, Goldstein EJC, Zarem HA. Localized *Mycobacterium avium-intracellulare* mastitis in an immunocompetent woman with silicone breast implants. *Plast Reconstr Surg* 1995;95:142–144.
99. Perry RR, Jacques DP, Lesar MSL, et al. *Mycobacterium avium* infection in a silicone-injected breast. *Plast Reconstr Surg* 1985;75:104–106.
100. Brodkin H. Paraspinous abscess with *Mycobacterium avium-intracellulare* in a patient without AIDS. *South Med J* 1991;84:1385–1386.
101. Eliopoulos DA, Lyle G. *Mycobacterium avium* infection in a patient with the acquired immunodeficiency syndrome and silicone breast implants. *South Med J* 1999;92:80–83.
102. Das DK, Sodhani P, Kashyap V, et al. Inflammatory lesions of the breast: diagnosis by fine needle aspiration. *Cytopathology* 1992;3:281–289.
103. Nayar M, Saxena HMK. Tuberculosis of the breast. A cytomorphologic study of needle aspirates and nipple discharges. *Acta Cytol* 1984;28:325–328.
104. Gupta D, Rajwanshi A, Gupta SK, et al. Fine needle aspiration cytology in the diagnosis of tuberculous mastitis. *Acta Cytol* 1999;43:191–194.
105. Ang LM, Brown H. *Corynebacterium accolens* isolated from breast abscess: possible association with granulomatous mastitis. *J Clin Microbiol* 2007;45:1666–1668.
106. Renshaw AA, Derhagopian RP, Gould EW. Cystic neutrophilic granulomatous mastitis: an underappreciated pattern strongly associated with gram-positive bacilli. *Am J Clin Pathol* 2011;136:424–427.
107. Stary CM, Lee YS, Balfour J. Idiopathic granulomatous mastitis associated with Corynebacterium sp. infection. *Hawaii Med J* 2011;70:99–101.
108. Lacambra M, Thai TA, Lam CC, et al. Granulomatous mastitis: the histological differentials. *J Clin Pathol* 2011;64:405–411.
109. Davies JAL. Primary actinomycosis of the breast. *Br J Surg* 1951;38:378–381.
110. Pemberton M. A case of primary actinomycosis of the breast. *Br J Surg* 1942;29:362–363.
111. Attar KH, Waghorn D, Lyons M, et al. Rare species of actinomyces as causative pathogens in breast abscess. *Breast J* 2007;13:501–505.
112. Lacoste C, Escande MC, Jammet P, et al. Breast *Actinomyces neuii* abscess simulating primary malignancy: a case diagnosed by fine-needle aspiration. *Diagn Cytopathol* 2009;37:311–312.
113. Allen JN. *Actinomyces meyerii* breast abscess. *Am J Med* 1987;83:186–187.
114. Young VL, Hertl C, Murray PR, et al. *Paecilomyces variotii* contamination in the lumen of a saline-filled breast implant. *Plast Reconstr Surg* 1995;96:1430–1434.
115. Gogas J, Sechas M, Diamantis S, et al. Actinomycosis of the breast. *Int Surg* 1972;57:664–665.
116. Jain BK, Sehgal VN, Jagdish S, et al. Primary actinomycosis of the breast: a clinical review and a case report. *J Dermatol* 1994;21: 497–500.
117. Pinto MM, Longstreth GB, Khoury GM. Fine needle aspiration of *Actinomyces* infection of the breast. A novel presentation of thoracopleural actinomycosis. *Acta Cytol* 1991;35:409–411.

118. Simpson AJH, Jumaa PA, Das SS. Breast abscess caused by *Nocardia asteroides*. *J Infect* 1995;30:266–267.
119. Apostolakis S, Chalkiadakis I, Ventouri M, et al. Lymphocutaneous nocardiosis in a lymphopenic breast cancer patient under treatment with docetaxel. *Breast J* 2005;11:469.
120. Campbell FC, Eriksson BL, Angorn IB. Localized granulomatous mastitis—an unusual presentation of typhoid. A case report. *S Afr Med J* 1980;57:793–795.
121. Barrett GS, MacDermot J. Breast abscess: a rare presentation of typhoid. *Br Med J* 1972;2:628–629.
122. Singh S, Pandya Y, Rathod J, et al. Bilateral breast abscess: a rare complication of enteric fever. *Indian J Med Microbiol* 2009;27:69–70.
123. Vattipally V, Thatigotla B, Nagpal K, et al. *Salmonella typhi* breast abscess: an uncommon manifestation of an uncommon disease in the United States. *Am Surg* 2011;77:e133–e135.
124. Asaadi M, Suh EDW. Salmonella infection following breast reconstruction. *Plast Reconstr Surg* 1995;96:1749–1750.
125. Chess Q, Santarsieri V Kostroff K, et al. Aspiration cytology of cat scratch disease of the breast. *Acta Cytol* 1990;34:761–762.
126. Lefkowitz M, Wear DJ. Cat-scratch disease masquerading as a solitary tumor of the breast. *Arch Pathol Lab Med* 1989;113:473–475.
127. Regnery RL, Olsom JG, Perkins BA, et al. Serological response to "Rochalimaea henselae" antigen in suspected cat-scratch disease. *Lancet* 1992;339:1443–1445.
128. Batts S, Demers DM. Spectrum and treatment of cat-scratch disease. *Pediatr Infect Dis J* 2004;23:1161–1162.
129. Povoski SP, Spigos DG, Marsh WL. An unusual case of cat-scratch disease from *Bartonella quintana* mimicking inflammatory breast cancer in a 50-year-old woman. *Breast J* 2003;9:497–500.
130. Markaki S, Soiropoulou M, Papaspirou P, et al. Cat-scratch disease presenting as a solitary tumour in the breast: report of three cases. *Eur J Obstet Gynecol Reprod Biol* 2003;106:175–178.
131. Godet C, Roblot F, Le Moal G, et al. Cat-scratch disease presenting as a breast mass. *Scand J Infect Dis* 2004;36:494–495.
132. Gamblin TC, Nobles-James C, Bradley RA, et al. Cat scratch disease presenting as breast mastitis. *Can J Surg* 2005;48:254–255.
133. Froman J, Landercasper J, Ellis R, et al. Red breast as a presenting complaint at a breast center: an institutional review. *Surgery* 2011;149:813–819.
134. Gollapalli V, Liao J, Dudakovic A, et al. Risk factors for development and recurrence of primary breast abscesses. *J Am Coll Surg* 2010;211:41–48.
135. Kapsimalakou S, Grande-Nagel I, Simon M, et al. Breast abscess following nipple piercing: a case report and review of the literature. *Arch Gynecol Obstet* 2010;282:623–626.
136. Thomsen AC, Esperson T, Maigaard S. Course and treatment of milk stasis, non-infectious inflammation of the breast and infectious mastitis in nursing women. *Am J Obstet Gynecol* 1984;149:492–495.
137. Dabbas N, Chand M, Pallet A, et al. Have the organisms that cause breast abscess changed with time? Implications for appropriate antibiotic usage in primary and secondary care. *Breast J* 2010;16:412–415.
138. Vine AJ, Bleiweiss IJ, Mizrachy B. *Aeromonas hydrophila* breast abscess. *Breast Dis* 1994;7:387–391.
139. Chagla AH, Borczyk AA, Facklam RR, et al. Breast abscess associated with *Helcococcus kunzii*. *J Clin Microbiol* 1998;36:2377–2379.
140. Nemenqani D, Yaqoob N, Hafiz M. Fine needle aspiration cytology of granulomatous mastitis with special emphasis on microbiologic correlation. *Acta Cytol* 2009;53:667–671.
141. Gurleyik E. Breast abscess as a complication of human brucellosis. *Breast J* 2006;12:375–376.
142. Harji DP, Rastall S, Catchpole C, et al. Pseudomonal breast infection. *Ann R Coll Surg* 2010;92:W20–W22.
143. Habif DV, Perzin KH, Lipton R, et al. Subareolar abscess associated with squamous metaplasia of lactiferous ducts. *Am J Surg* 1970;119:523–526.
144. Abramson DJ. Mammary duct ectasia, mamillary fistula and subareolar sinuses. *Ann Surg* 1969;169:217–226.
145. Bowers GJ, Prestidge B, Getz JB, et al. Infectious complications in irradiated breasts following conservative breast therapy. *Breast J* 1995;1:295–299.
146. Hunter JG, Padilla M, Cooper-Vastola S. Late *Clostridium perfringens* breast implant infection after dental treatment. *Ann Plast Surg* 1996;36:309–312.
147. Ablaza VJ, La Trenta GS. Late infection of a breast prosthesis with *Enterococcus avium*. *Plast Reconstr Surg* 1998;102:227–230.
148. Lewis CG, Wells MK, Jennings WC. *Mycobacterium fortuitum* breast infection following nipple-piercing, mimicking carcinoma. *Breast J* 2004;10:363–365.
149. Trupiano JK, Sebek BA, Goldfarb J, et al. Mastitis due to *Mycobacterium abscessus* after body piercing. *Clin Infect Dis* 2001;33:131–134.
150. Attar KH, Waghorn D, Lyons M, et al. Rare species of *Actinomyces* as causative pathogens in breast abscess. *Breast J* 2007;13:501–505.
151. Salhab M, Al Sarakbi W, Mokbel K. Skin and fat necrosis of the breast following methylene blue dye injection for sentinel node biopsy in a patient with breast cancer. *Int Semin Surg Oncol* 2005;2:26.

Viral Infections

152. Kobayashi TK, Okamoto H, Yakushiji M. Cytologic detection of herpes simplex virus DNA in nipple discharge by *in situ* hybridization: report of two cases. *Diagn Cytopathol* 1993;9:296–299.
153. Mardi K, Gupta N, Sharma S, et al. Cytodiagnosis of herpes simplex mastitis: report of a rare case. *J Cytol* 2009;26:149–150.
154. Das DK, Rifaat AA, George SS, et al. Morphologic changes in fibroadenoma of breast due to chickenpox: a case report with suspicious cytology in fine needle aspiration smears. *Acta Cytol* 2008;52: 337–343.
155. Tuchman M, Weinberg JM. Monodermatomal *herpes zoster* in a pseudodisseminated distribution following breast reconstruction surgery. *Cutis* 2008;81:71–72.
156. Pantanowitz L, Sen S, Crisi GM, et al. Spectrum of breast disease encountered in HIV-positive patients at a community teaching hospital. *Breast J* 2011;20:303–308.
157. Roca B, C. Vilar, Peréz EV, et al. Breast abscess with lethal septicemia due to *Pseudomonas aeruginosa* in a patient with AIDS. *Presse Med* 1996;25:803–804.
158. Rege SA, Nunes Q, Rajput A, et al. Breast gangrene as a complication of puerperal sepsis. *Arch Surg* 2002;117:1441–1442.
159. Venkatramani V, Pillai S, Marathe S, et al. Breast gangrene in an HIV-positive patient. *Ann R Coll Surg Engl* 2009;91:W13–W14.
160. Solomon SB, Gatewood OMB, Brem RF. HIV infection: analysis of mammographic findings. *Breast J* 1999;5:112–115.
161. Konstantinopoulos PA, Dezube BJ, March D, et al. HIV-associated intramammary lymphadenopathy. *Breast J* 2007;13:192–195.
162. Oluwole SF, Ali AO, Shafaee Z, et al. Breast cancer in women with HIV/AIDS: report of five cases with a review of the literature. *J Surg Oncol* 2005;89:23–27.
163. Voutsadakis IA, Silverman LR. Breast cancer in HIV-positive women: a report of four cases and a review of the literature. *Cancer Invest* 2002;20:590–592.
164. Intra M, Gentilini O, Brenneili F, et al. Breast cancer among HIV-infected patients: the experience of the European Institute of Oncology. *J Surg Oncol* 2005;91:141–142.
165. Palan M, Shousha S, Krell J, Stebbing J. Breast cancer in the setting of HIV. *Pathol Res Int* 2011;2011:925712.
166. Sharma R, Iyer M. Bowen's disease of the nipple in a young man with AIDS: a case report. *Clin Breast Cancer* 2009;9:53–55.

Cutaneous Mite Infestation

167. Val-Bernal JF, Diego C, Rodriguez-Villar D, et al. The nipple-areola complex epidermis: a prospective systematic study in adult autopsies. *Am J Dermatopathol* 2010;32:787–793.
168. Yokoyama T, Yamaguchi R, Itoh T, et al. Detection of *Demodex folliculorum* from nipple discharge. *Diagn Cytopathol* 2013. doi:10.1002/dc.22952.

Artifacts Mimicking Parasitic Infestation

169. Phillip V, Becker K, Bajbouj M, et al. Myospherulosis. *Ann Diagn Pathol* 2013;17(4):383–399.
170. Hata S, Kanomata N, Kozuka Y, et al. Cytologic appearance of myospherulosis of the breast diagnosed by fine-needle aspirates: a clinical, cytological and immunocytochemical study of 23 cases. *Diagn Cytopathol* 2011;39:177–180.
171. Islam MT, Ou JJ, Hansen K, et al. Liesegang-like rings in lactational changes in the breast. *Case Rep Pathol* 2012;2012:268903.

CHAPTER 5

Papilloma and Related Benign Lesions

FREDERICK C. KOERNER

This chapter discusses a heterogeneous group of lesions. Some are fundamentally papillary (intraductal papilloma and subareolar sclerosing papilloma); others are prominently papillary (florid papillomatosis and radial sclerosing lesion [RSL]) or partly papillary (cystic and papillary apocrine metaplasia). Syringomatous adenoma is discussed because it is clinically and histologically part of the differential diagnosis of florid papillomatosis. Collagenous spherulosis, also included here, is a stromal alteration seen in various papillary lesions including papilloma, ductal hyperplasia, and, rarely, adenosis.

PAPILLOMA

Papillomas are discrete benign tumors of the epithelium of mammary ducts. They arise most often from lactiferous ducts in the central part of the breast, but they can occur peripherally in any quadrant. *Intracystic papilloma* is the designation applied to a papilloma in a cystically dilated duct. Large, complex papillomas that have a cystic component have sometimes been referred to as *papillary cystadenomas*, whereas solid, noncystic papillomas have been variously classified as *ductal adenoma*, *solid papilloma*, or *adenomyoepithelioma* (AME). A *solitary papilloma* is a single discrete papillary tumor in one duct. *Multiple papillomas* usually occur in contiguous branches of the ductal system. Solitary papillomas are more common than multiple papillomas. A distinction must be made between intraductal papilloma and papillomatosis (epitheliosis). The latter terms are used to describe usual (conventional) ductal hyperplasia (UDH), the common form of ductal hyperplasia, which may coexist with solitary or multiple papillomas.

Clinical Presentation

In 1951, Haagensen et al.[1] reviewed a series of 367 patients with benign intraductal papillary breast lesions who had been treated at Presbyterian Hospital in New York between 1916 and 1941. After excluding 243 patients with "microscopic papillomas," 14 with incomplete data, and 2 with a papilloma and unrelated nonpapillary carcinoma, the authors concentrated on describing 108 patients treated for gross, benign intraductal papillomas. Microscopic papillomas were characterized as "small multiple papillary projections, with or without fibrous cores, which project into the ducts and cysts of chronic cystic mastitis." By contrast, gross papilloma was defined as a "definite disease entity in which one or more papillomas grow within a relatively localized portion of a duct, or in several adjacent ducts, and attain sufficient size to fill up the duct and become evident grossly."

The study revealed some now well-established features of duct papilloma. The majority (75%) were located in the central part of the breast. Discharge, bloody or nonbloody, was the primary symptom in 72% of cases, but it was less commonly seen with peripheral lesions (29%) than with those in a central duct (86%). Lesions that caused nipple discharge, whether central or peripheral, tended to have a frond-forming papillary configuration, whereas a more solid growth pattern was observed in tumors not associated with a discharge.

Solitary papillomas may occur at any age from infancy to the ninth decade, but they are most frequent in the sixth and seventh decades of life. The tumors usually occur in the subareolar region and come to attention because of a discharge from the nipple. Women with multiple papillomas tend to be younger than women with solitary papillomas and most often present in their 40s and early 50s. Multiple papillomas develop peripherally more often than centrally and typically present as a palpable lesion. Papillomas may occur more frequently in African American women than in women of other ethnic origins.[2]

Papillomas have developed in unusual settings. One report[3] documented the growth of a papilloma in residual breast tissue following a transverse rectus abdominus muscle (TRAM) flap reconstruction. Two publications[4,5] describe the presence of papillomas in ectopic breast tissue in axillary lymph nodes (ALNs) of women with mammary papillomas.

Although papillomas afflict women almost exclusively, the literature contains reports of 26 papillomas in men. Volmer[6] lists the cases described prior to 1985. In 2006, Yamamoto et al.[7] tabulated clinical details of 10 additional cases, and five other examples[8–12] have also been published. The patients range from 7 months[13] to 82 years[14] of age, the range seen in women. Two patients presented during their early teenage years,[8,15] and the author has examined a papilloma from a 15-year-old boy. The presence of several cases in adolescent boys seems a curious coincidence, which might merit further attention. Symptomatic intervals as long as 6 years have been noted.[16] Two patients reported long-term use of phenothiazines.[7,17] One of these patients had an elevated serum prolactin level,[7] and the papillary epithelium in the other case[17] exhibited secretory changes.

Nipple discharge occurs in most patients with a central papilloma. Bloody discharge, more commonly associated with papillary carcinoma, can develop in a papilloma as a result of degenerative changes. A subareolar mass may be palpable in patients with a central solitary papilloma, and a palpable tumor may be the first clinical manifestation of a peripheral papilloma. A papilloma in a 44-year-old man produced a hard, lobulated mass fixed to the chest wall.[10]

Imaging Studies

Cystic, solitary papillary tumors may appear well circumscribed on mammography, but the presence of a cystic component is best appreciated by ultrasonography, which seems to be more sensitive than mammography for the detection of papillomas. Francis et al.[18] reported that 44% of mammograms in their study of 36 women with papillomas were described as normal, whereas only 5% of sonograms appeared normal. These authors also cited similar findings presented in earlier publications. Ductography can also demonstrate the presence of a central papilloma in patients who experience a nipple discharge.[19] Magnetic resonance imaging (MRI) in women with solitary intraductal papillomas and nipple discharge typically reveals duct dilation and the presence of small, oval, smoothly contoured, enhancing intraductal masses,[18,20] but papillomas do not always display these characteristic features. In the study of Kurz et al.,[21] 4 of 20 papillomas had irregular shapes, 3 had irregular or spiculated margins, 8 displayed heterogeneous enhancement, and the characteristics of the time–intensity curves varied. After reviewing images from 15 papillomas, Daniel et al.[22] reported that 7 displayed suspicious morphologic findings such as irregular margins or rim enhancement and that 4 were not evident on the MRI studies.

Cardenosa and Eklund[19] compared the clinical and mammographic findings in patients with solitary and multiple papillomas. The latter group was subdivided into peripheral and central lesions. Most multiple peripheral papillomas were asymptomatic and were detected as a result of mammographic abnormalities, including calcifications, nodules, masses, or various opacities.

After a detailed mammographic and sonographic study of 40 papillary tumors, which were later excised and examined histologically, Lam et al.[23] concluded that "radiologic features are not sufficiently sensitive or specific to differentiate benign from malignant papillary lesions." By using a combination of both imaging modalities, the authors achieved a sensitivity of 61%, a specificity of 33%, a positive predictive value (PPV) of 85%, and a negative predictive value (NPV) of 13%.

Gross Pathology

A part of the mass associated with some solitary papillomas is a cyst formed by the dilated duct in which the papilloma grew (Fig. 5.1). The cyst may contain clear fluid, bloody fluid, or clotted blood. The papilloma usually forms a single mural nodule protruding into the lumen, but occasionally multiple, separate, or aggregated nodules are present (Fig. 5.2). Some papillomas grow as soft, solid friable masses that obliterate the cystic space.

Solitary papillomas are typically bosselated, soft-to-firm tumors that appear gray to reddish brown when examined grossly in the fresh state. The lesions are well circumscribed and appear to be enclosed by a capsule formed by the duct wall and accompanying reactive changes. Multiple associated papillomas can sometimes be appreciated grossly when they form nodules in contiguous dilated ducts (Fig. 5.3).

A

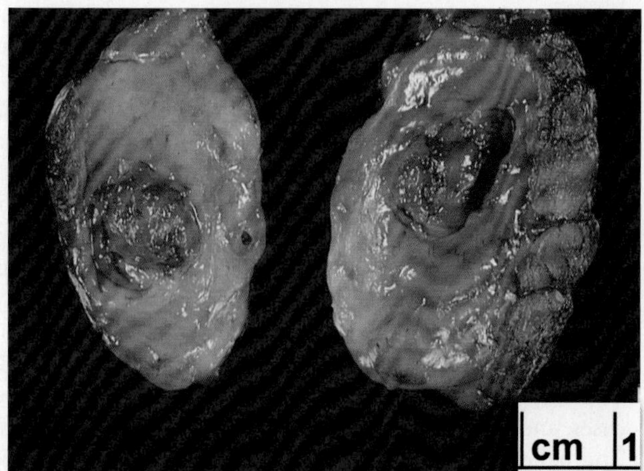

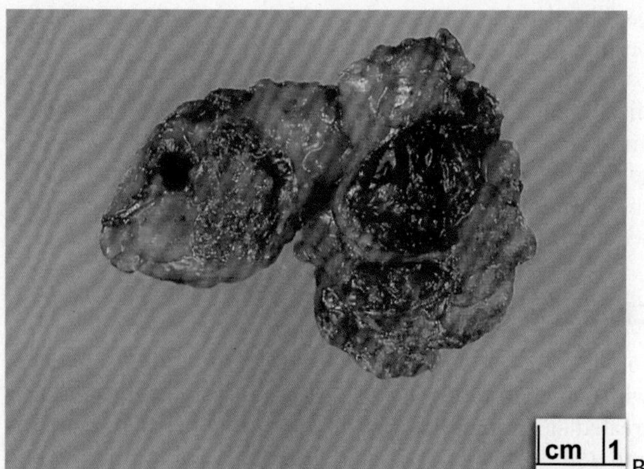

B

FIG. 5.1. ***Papilloma.*** Gross appearance of three lesions. **A:** Intracystic papilloma. **B:** Solid intracystic papilloma virtually filling the cyst lumen. **C:** An everted cystic multinodular papilloma from a 17-year-old girl. **D:** A histologic whole mount of a tumor similar to the one in (**B**).

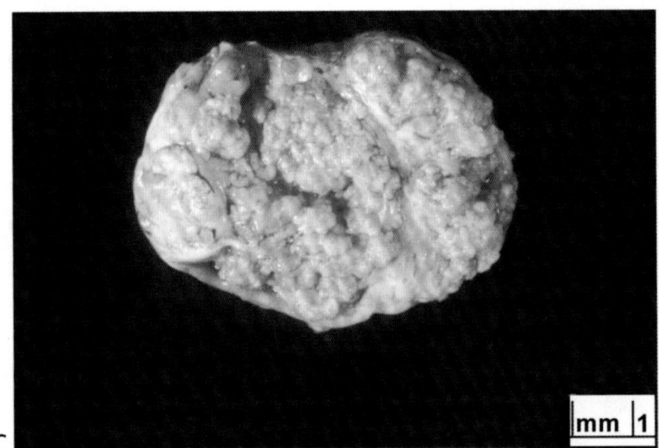

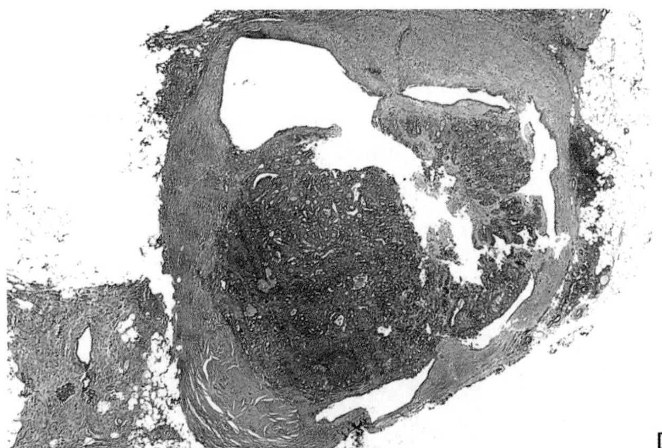

FIG. 5.1. *[Continued]*

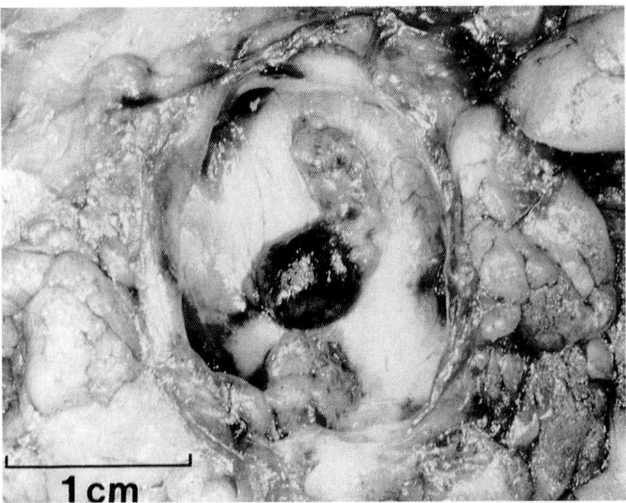

FIG. 5.2. ***Papilloma.*** Gross appearance of an intracystic papilloma consisting of two mural nodules. The cyst wall is a distinct fibrous membrane with a smooth inner surface.

Solitary papillomas may form clinically symptomatic tumors 1 cm or less in diameter in a major lactiferous duct (Fig. 5.4), but the average size is 2 to 3 cm. Benign cystic papillomas may be larger than 10 cm. Tumors formed by multiple papillomas are typically larger than 2 cm.[1,24]

Microscopic Pathology

The basic microscopic structure of a papilloma consists of the proliferation of ductal epithelium supported by frond-forming fibrovascular stroma. The most orderly form of papilloma consists of branching fronds of stroma supporting a layer of epithelium composed of epithelial and myoepithelial cells (Fig. 5.5). The epithelial cells are cuboidal to columnar, and they display little pleomorphism, nuclear hyperchromasia, or mitotic activity. The supporting stroma may arise from a single base or from several foci in the duct wall. Epithelium lining the nonpapillary portion of the duct usually exhibits little or no hyperplasia.

Some papillomas have a more complex structure caused by stromal overgrowth, hyperplasia of the epithelium, or

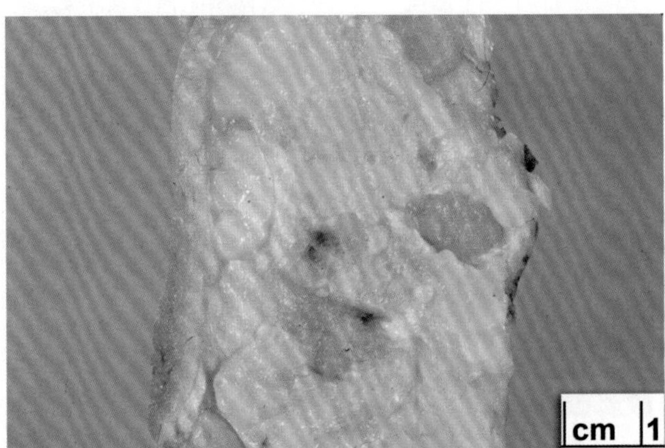

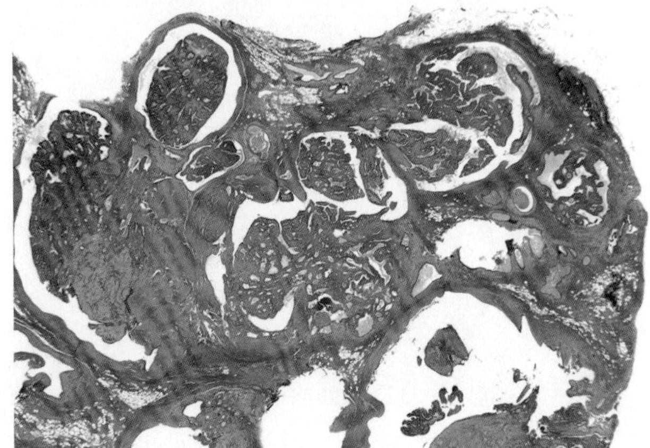

FIG. 5.3. ***Multiple intraductal papillomas.*** **A:** Gross specimen showing multiple papillomas. The two largest lesions are solid, tan tumors. A small cystic papilloma is visible in the center. **B:** A cluster of small intraductal papillomas.

both processes, resulting in fusion of the papillary fronds (Fig. 5.6). The most exaggerated form of this process is the solid intraductal papilloma, in which virtually all the space between fibrovascular stalks is filled by solid sheets of proliferative ductal epithelial cells. More often, secondary lumens are formed within the hyperplastic epithelium, resulting in irregular microlumens, micropapillary fronds, focal solid areas, or heterogeneous combinations of these patterns (Fig. 5.7).

Foci of apocrine metaplasia are not uncommon in papillomas (Fig. 5.8), and rarely most or all of the epithelium is of the apocrine type. When present in the conventional

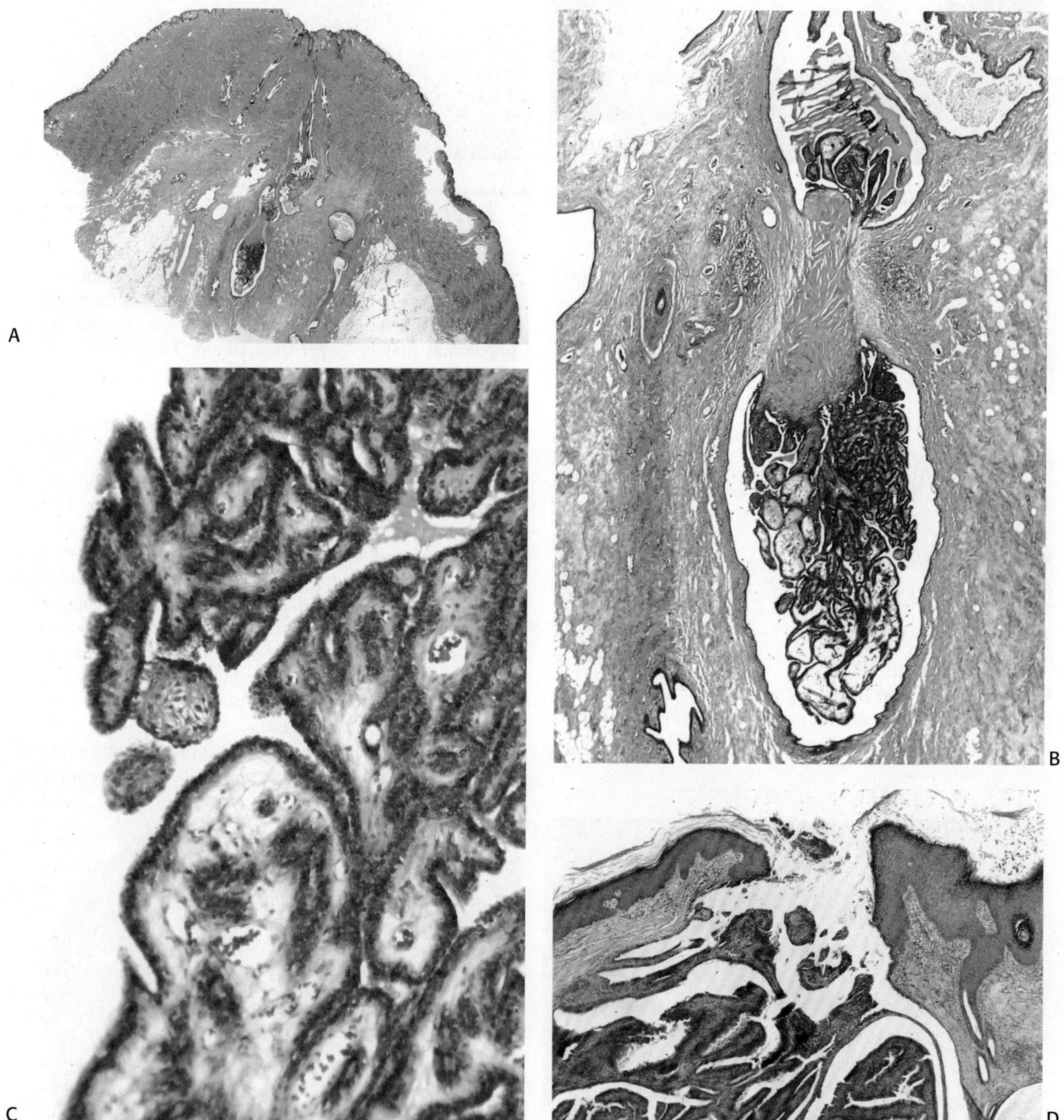

FIG. 5.4. ***Papilloma of lactiferous duct.*** **A,B:** A dumbbell-shaped papilloma with a central zone of fibrosis. **C:** The papillary fronds are composed of somewhat edematous fibrovascular stroma with a thin layer of epithelium on the surface. Similar epithelium lines the lumen of the dilated duct. **D:** A papilloma at the level of a lactiferous duct orifice. **E:** Florid epithelial hyperplasia in a lactiferous duct papilloma.

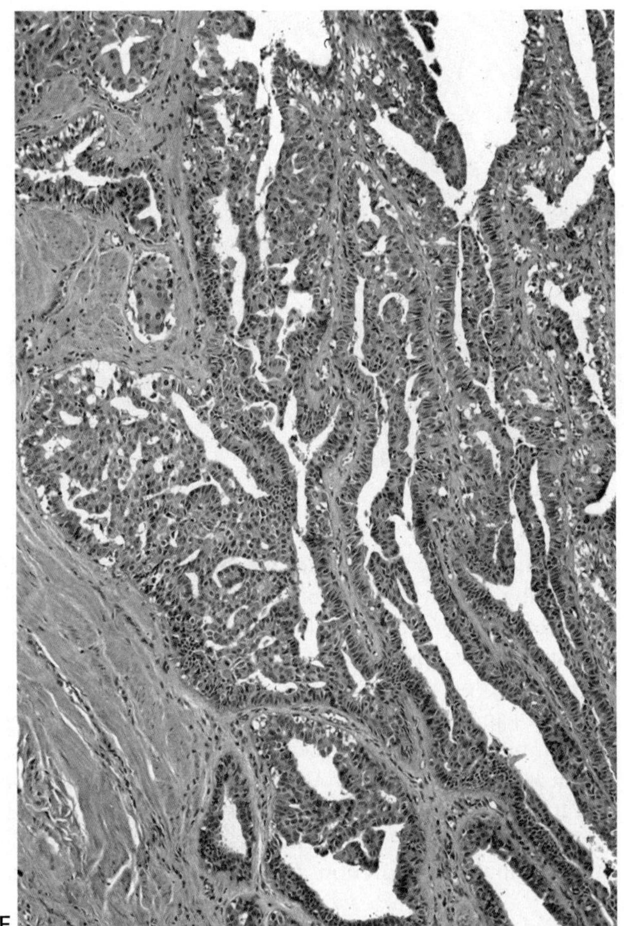

FIG. 5.4. *(Continued)*

papillary configuration, apocrine metaplasia is usually cytologically bland, but apocrine atypia manifested by nuclear pleomorphism and cytoplasmic clearing can be seen in sclerosing papillary tumors. This is especially common when sclerosing adenosis (SA) is incorporated into a papilloma.

The appearance of the fibrovascular stroma varies considerably among papillomas. In some lesions, the stroma is limited to slender inconspicuous strands consisting of thin-walled capillaries and sparse fibroblasts, collagen, and mononuclear cells and forming a network that supports the voluminous epithelium. The distribution of this stroma stands out especially clearly in sections stained for reticulin, vimentin, basement membrane proteins, or vascular markers such as CD34 and CD31. Expansion of the fibrovascular stroma by accumulated histiocytes occurs in papillomas and is an exceedingly rare finding in papillary carcinoma (Fig. 5.9).

Collagenization of the fibrovascular stroma occurs in some papillomas. The papillary architecture is accentuated when this process is limited to the intrinsic papillary structure. If myofibroblastic proliferation accompanies collagenization of the stroma, the papillary arrangement is likely to become distorted. Epithelial elements entrapped in this stroma may simulate invasive carcinoma within or at the periphery of the lesion (Figs. 5.10 and 5.11). In the most extreme situations, fibrous sclerosis is so severe as to virtually obliterate the papilloma, reducing it to a nodular scar containing sparse benign glandular elements (Fig. 5.12). Such a lesion may be difficult to distinguish from a fibroadenoma (FA). This problem is typified by a case report purported to represent an infarcted FA in which the illustrations are highly suggestive of a fibrotic and partially infarcted cystic papilloma.[25]

The epithelium of intraductal papillomas contains a myoepithelial cell layer.[26] Inconspicuous elongated myoepithelial cells with nuclei are flattened along the basement membrane. Hyperplastic myoepithelial cells typically form a prominent layer of cuboidal cells that tend to have relatively clear cytoplasm (Fig. 5.13). Myoepithelial cells in papillomas can be demonstrated with a variety of immunostains.[26,27] When immunostaining is done to detect myoepithelial cells, it is necessary to differentiate stromal and myoepithelial reactivity. Myoepithelial cells are immunoreactive for

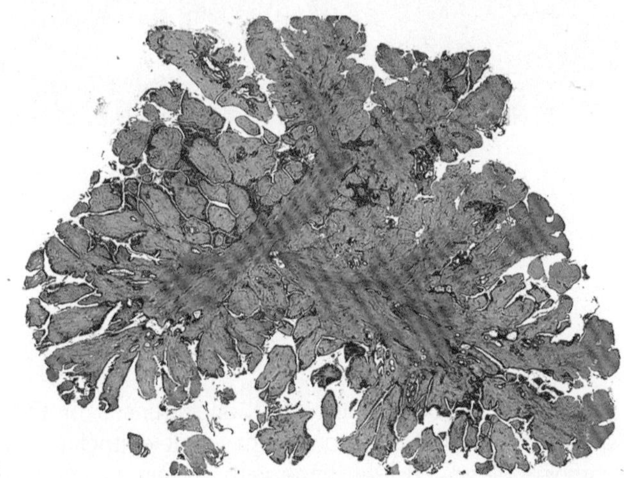

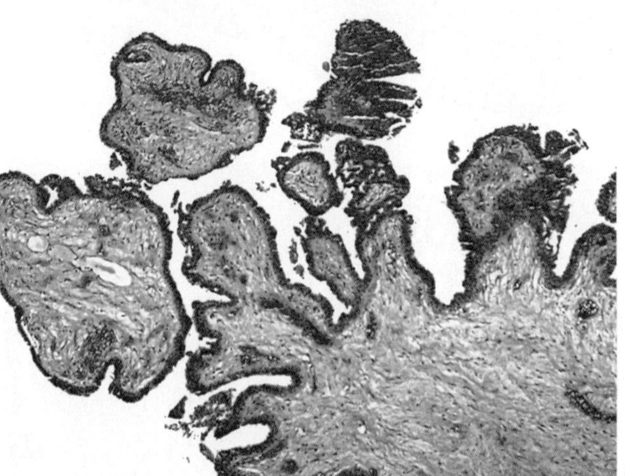

FIG. 5.5. ***Papilloma.*** **A:** This papilloma has dense collagenous stroma. **B:** Epithelium on the surfaces of the fronds is thin. **C:** A thin layer of cuboidal and columnar epithelial cells overlies a continuous layer of myoepithelial cells (*arrows*). **D:** Slight epithelial hyperplasia at the surface of one papillary frond.

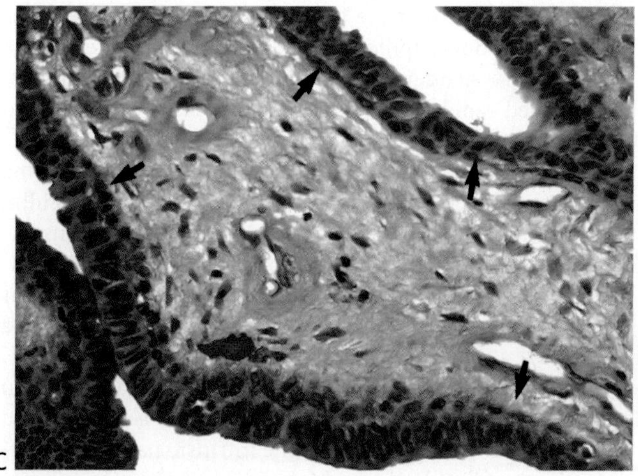

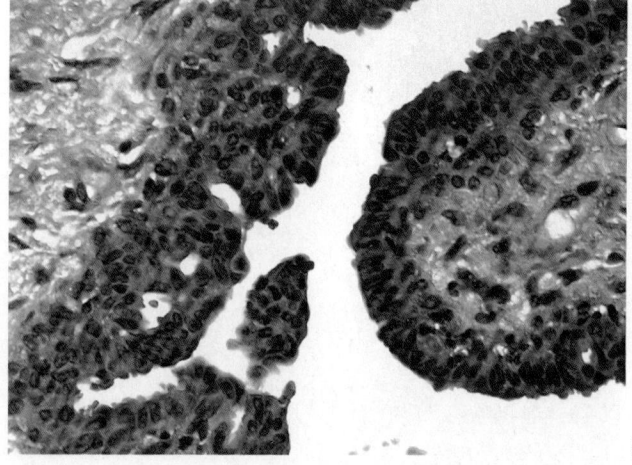

FIG. 5.5. *(Continued)*

actin, calponin, myosin heavy chain, CD10, p63, and CK5/6 (Fig. 5.13). All of these proteins except p63 are cytoplasmic markers, which vary in their proclivity to react with stromal cells. The p63 immunostain localizes in myoepithelial cell nuclei and rarely in the nuclei of epithelial cells in a papillary lesion.[28] Cross-reactivity in stromal cells is not observed. For this reason, it is preferable to include a stain for p63 among those chosen to detect myoepithelial cells. The myoepithelium may become noticeably attenuated and focally undetectable by immunostains in regions of sclerosis in a papilloma. The focal absence of immunoreactive myoepithelium, by itself, is not diagnostic of carcinoma in this setting. When there is marked hyperplasia of myoepithelial cells in a benign papillary tumor, the differential diagnosis includes AME.

Infarction occurs in solitary and in multiple papillomas (Figs. 5.14 and 5.15). No specific cause for the necrosis is evident in most cases. The presence of chronic inflammation and hemosiderin in and around many papillomas suggests that these lesions are prone to transient bleeding secondary to ischemia or incidental trauma. Needling procedures can contribute to infarction and cause fresh hemorrhage,

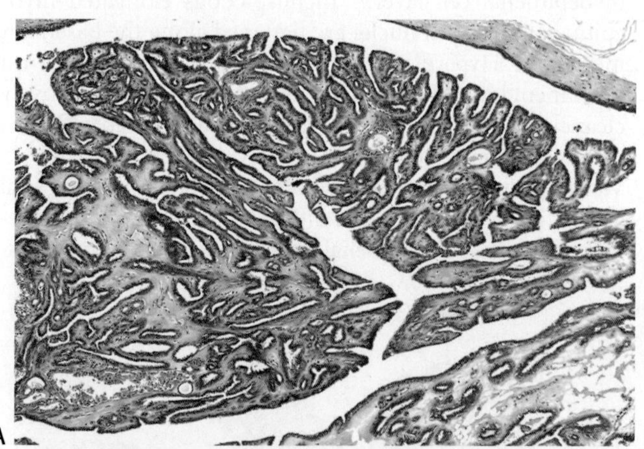

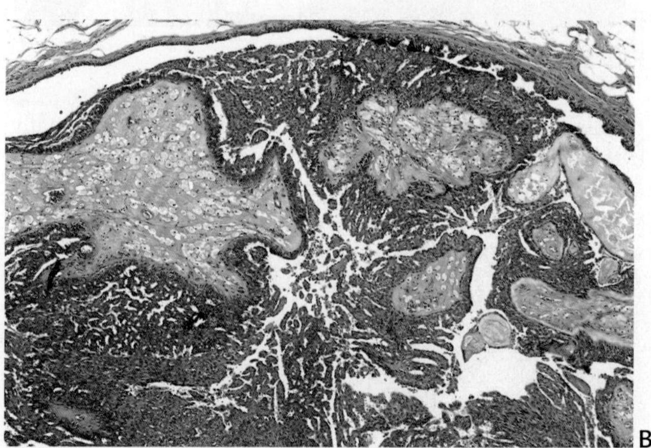

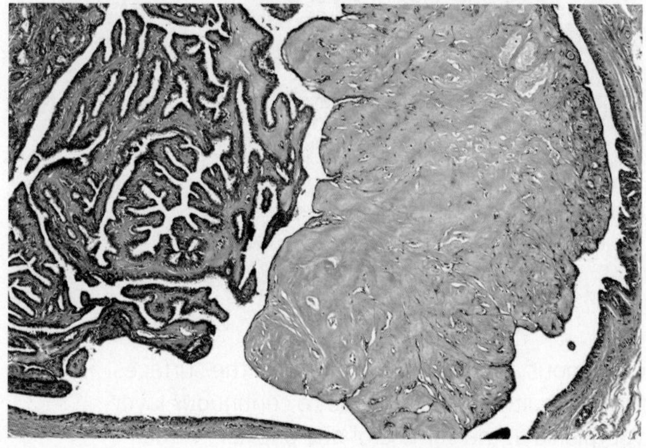

FIG. 5.6. ***Papillomas.*** Histologic appearances of three different tumors. **A:** Papilloma with simple epithelium and complex glands. **B:** Papilloma with prominent epithelial hyperplasia. **C:** Papilloma with complex glands and a discrete nodular area of sclerosis that distorts the underlying papillary architecture.

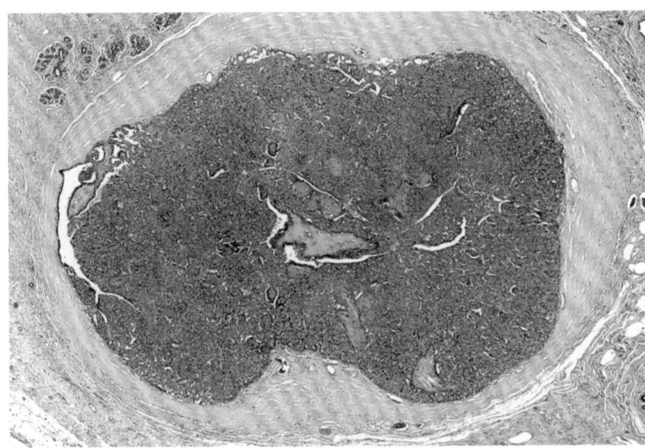

FIG. 5.7. ***Papilloma.*** Florid ductal hyperplasia obscures the papillary architecture of this solid papilloma.

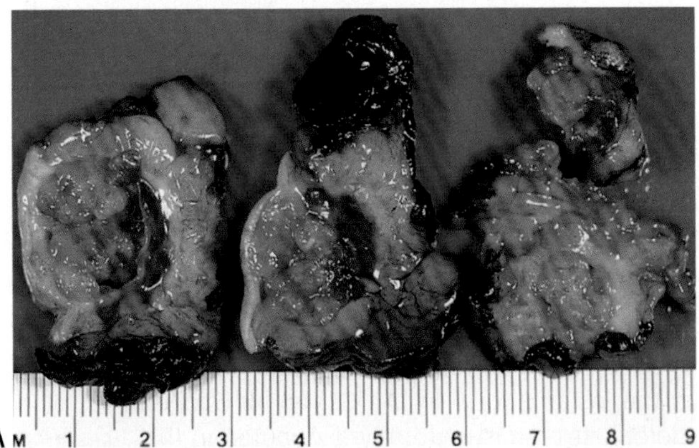

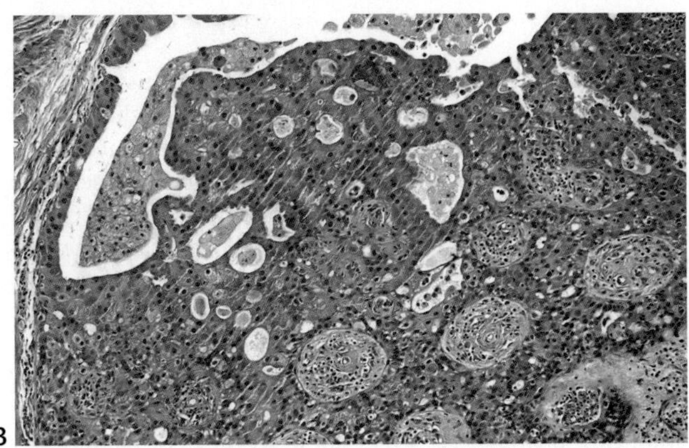

FIG. 5.8. ***Papilloma with apocrine metaplasia.*** **A:** The light brown color of this cystic papillary lesion is typical of tumors with extensive apocrine metaplasia. **B:** Hyperplastic apocrine epithelium on the surface of a papillary frond.

sometimes associated with displaced epithelium. Spontaneous infarction usually involves superficial portions of a papilloma. Rarely, the entire lesion is infarcted either spontaneously or as a consequence of a biopsy. The underlying structure of a fully infarcted papilloma can be demonstrated

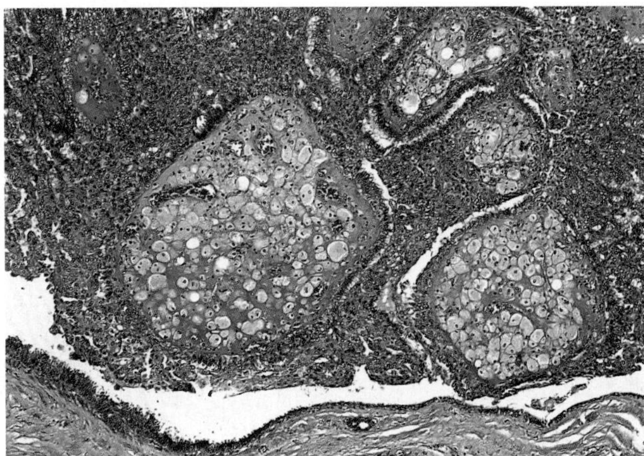

FIG. 5.9. ***Papilloma with stromal histiocytes.*** The fibrovascular stroma is prominent as a result of accumulated histiocytes in a papilloma, which nearly fills a cystically dilated duct. Part of the duct wall is seen at the bottom of the image.

with a reticulin stain. In some infarcted lesions in which degeneration is not advanced, the structure of the epithelium can be displayed more clearly with immunostains such as cytokeratin (CK) and p63.[29] There is no procedure for reliably distinguishing between the completely infarcted epithelium of a papilloma and that of a papillary carcinoma. However, if myoepithelium can be demonstrated in the infarcted tissue, the tumor is more likely to be a papilloma than a papillary carcinoma. Cytologic atypia is commonly found in the partially degenerated epithelium of a papilloma in the vicinity of infarcts. The atypia is usually manifested by nuclear hyperchromasia and pleomorphism. These cytologic abnormalities may lead to an erroneous diagnosis of carcinoma in the fine-needle aspiration (FNA) specimen from an infarcted papilloma[30,31] or in a needle core biopsy specimen.

Squamous metaplasia can occur in the epithelium of a papilloma (Fig. 5.16). It is more likely to be found when there is infarction and probably represents a reactive or reparative process.[32] Rarely, squamous metaplasia constitutes a conspicuous component of the papilloma or of the epithelium lining the cystic portion of the lesion. Extension of squamous metaplasia to the epithelium of adjacent ducts is an uncommon finding.[33] Entrapped metaplastic epithelium in the stromal reaction may simulate metaplastic or squamous carcinoma, and in some instances the distinction between these processes is very difficult.[32] Electron microscopy and immunohistochemistry (IHC) suggest that some examples of squamous metaplasia derive from myoepithelial cells.[34] Sebaceous metaplasia of luminal cells of a papilloma has also been reported.[35]

Intraductal papillomas can be recognized by frozen section (FS), but in most circumstances, it is preferable to rely upon paraffin sections for the diagnosis of papillary tumors. It is sometimes difficult to prepare satisfactory FSs from these fragile lesions or to identify foci of carcinoma that have developed in a papilloma.

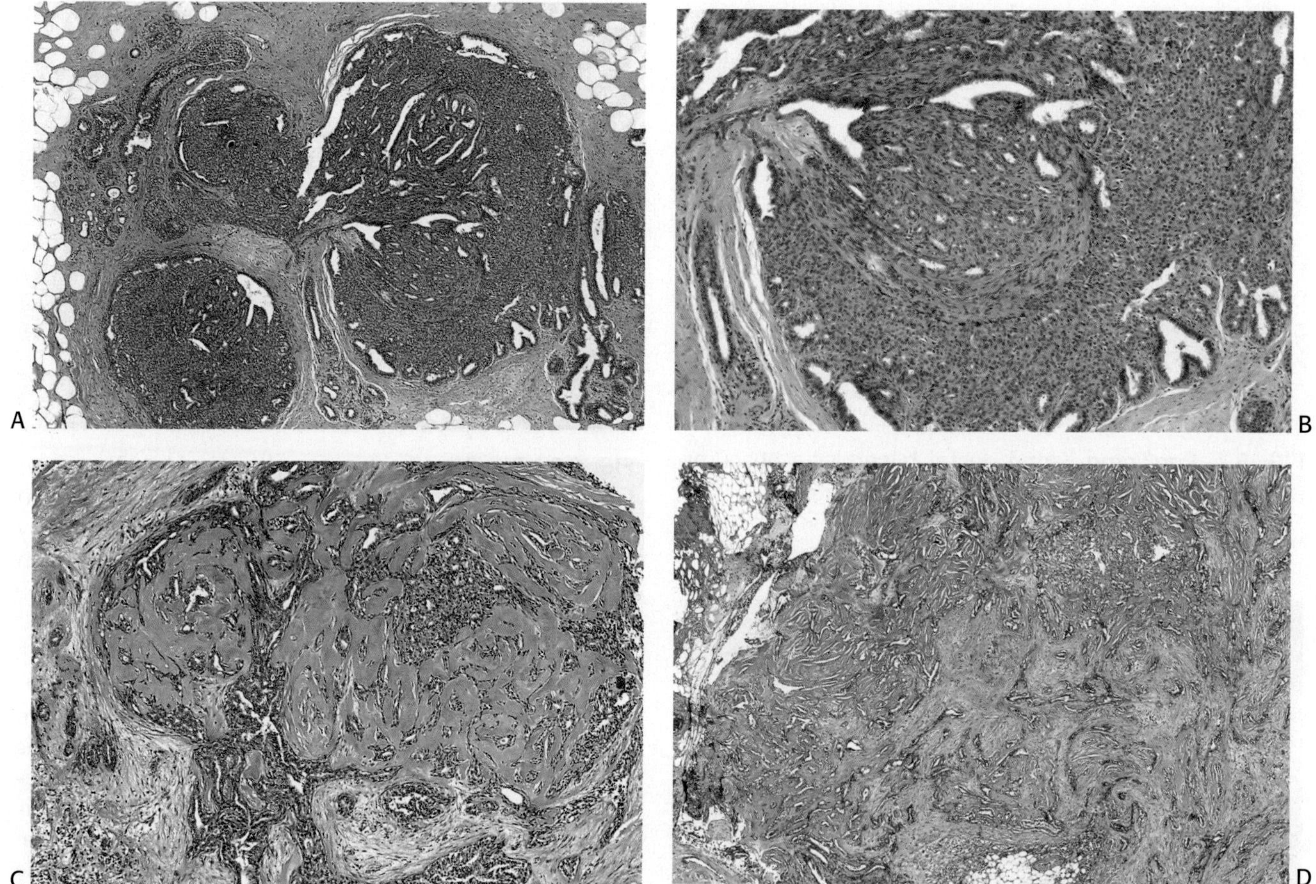

FIG. 5.10. *Papilloma with stromal sclerosis.* **A:** A trilobed solid papilloma showing early central sclerosis. **B:** Florid duct hyperplasia and adenosis in the lesion shown in (A). **C:** Well-developed sclerosis is present throughout this papilloma. **D:** Sclerotic stroma is uniformly distributed in this lesion.

Cytology

The diagnosis of an intraductal papilloma may be suggested by the cytologic findings in an FNA specimen.[36,37] The smear typically has cohesive three-dimensional groups of cytologically benign-appearing cells accompanied by variable amounts of stromal cells, apocrine cells, inflammatory cells, and histiocytes. Two diagnostic problems can arise in this setting.

First, a significant number of lesions classified as papillary on the basis of findings in needle aspiration specimens prove not to exhibit a papillary architecture when excised. Of the 70 cases studied by Simsir et al.[38] in which needle aspiration specimens were classified as papillary, only 31 (44%) showed a papillary architecture when examined histologically. FAs, fibrocystic changes (FCCs), a phyllodes tumor, and carcinomas accounted for the remaining 39 cases. Although usually correctly classified as benign, FAs and FCCs account for the most common discrepancies. Apocrine cells, foamy histiocytes, and bipolar nuclei associated with myoepithelial cells are characteristic of a papilloma. Although one can also observe these cells in aspirates from FAs, the epithelium from the latter lesion tends to be distributed in flat sheets rather than in three-dimensional groups, and it usually has a honeycomb appearance. Furthermore, the epithelial groups from FAs typically lack fibrovascular stroma, and one usually observes fragments of stroma devoid of blood vessels and unassociated with epithelial cells. Most aspirates of FCCs appear less cellular than those from papillomas, and they do not contain branched, three-dimensional cell clusters supported by fibrovascular stroma. These generalizations notwithstanding, many smears do not demonstrate the findings sufficiently clearly that one can make a secure diagnosis of papilloma. Even in retrospect, Simsir et al.[38] could not distinguish the smears of three FAs from those of papillomas. Mak and Field[39] recounted similar observations. The authors studied 56 cases in which smears were interpreted as papillomas. The excision specimens revealed papillomas in 42 (75%) of the cases yielding a PPV of 0.74. FAs, radial scars, and other benign proliferative lesions accounted for 10 discrepancies, atypical ductal hyperplasia (ADH) 2 discrepancies, and tubular carcinomas the remaining two discordant cases.

Second, the cytologic detection of malignancy in a papilloma and the recognition of a papillary carcinoma often prove especially difficult. For example, in the study of FNA

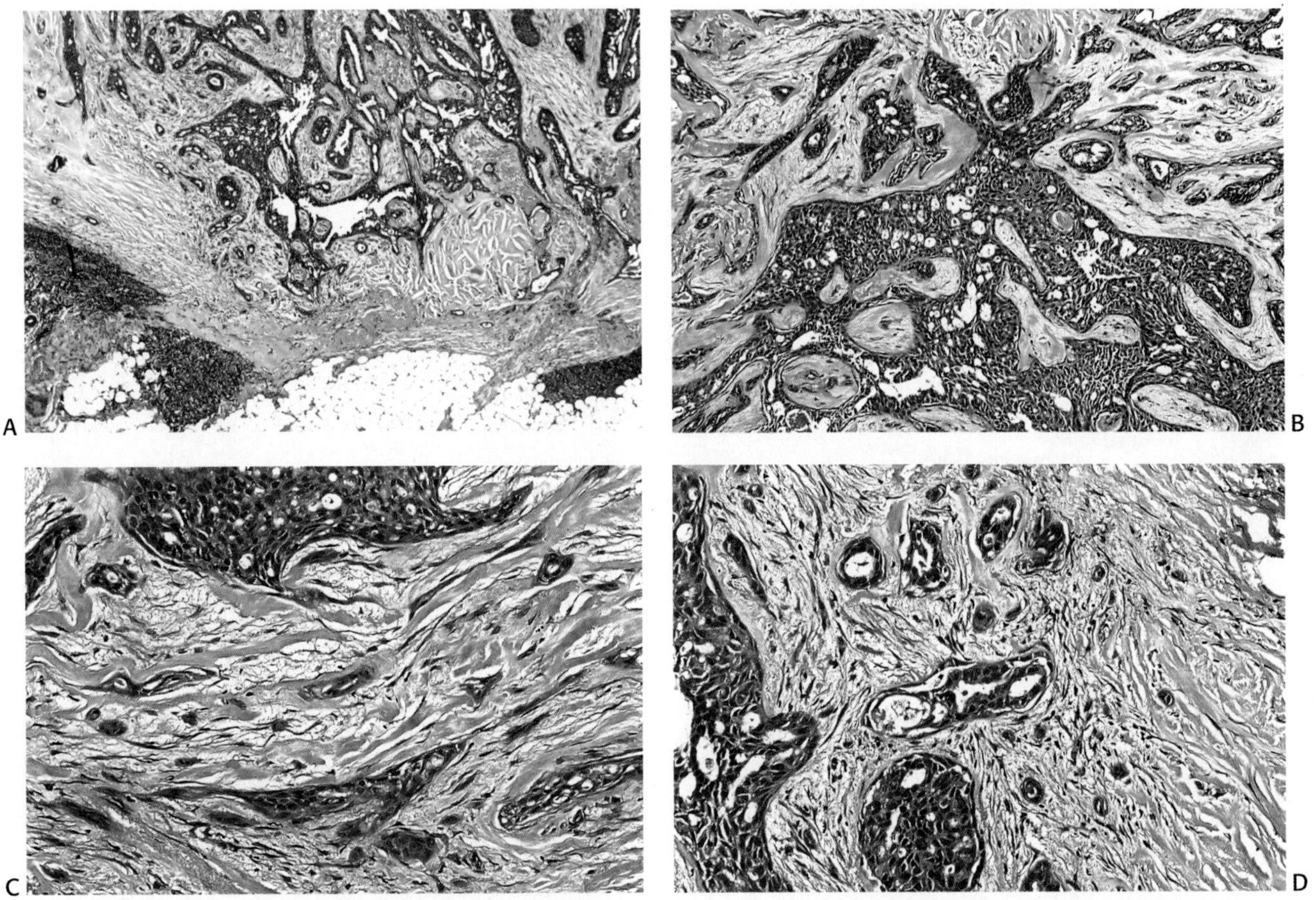

FIG. 5.11. ***Papilloma with stromal sclerosis.*** Images are from one tumor. **A:** The border of the lesion is circumscribed. Note the collections of lymphocytes. **B:** An area near the center of the lesion showing residual papilloma with fenestrated epithelium. **C:** Attenuated epithelium is distributed between layers of myofibroblasts and collagen within the tumor. **D:** This image from the periphery of the lesion shows rounded groups of cells and isolated cells, a characteristic finding at the edges of a papilloma with sclerosis.

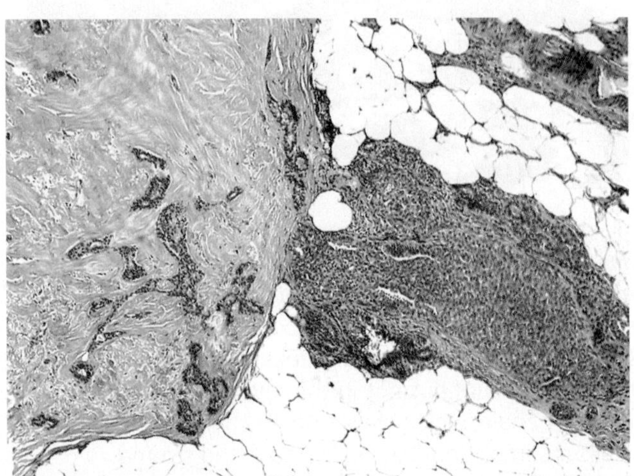

FIG. 5.12. ***Papilloma with extreme stromal sclerosis.*** The main tumor is almost entirely effaced by collagenized stroma. An intraductal papilloma persists in a peripheral duct.

specimens of papillary lesions by Masood et al.,[40] 3 of 21 tumors interpreted as benign papillary lesions proved to be micropapillary ductal carcinoma *in situ* (DCIS) upon study of an excision specimen. Immunostaining may help in the diagnosis of FNA specimens of papillary breast tumors. Chang et al.[41] reported that the percentage of Ki67-positive cells was significantly higher in papillary carcinomas (21.0 ± 19.23%) than in papillomas (6.23 ± 7.25%). These investigators did not find cyclin-D1 reactivity to be a useful differential feature. Staining of cell-block preparations for calponin to reveal myoepithelial cells can provide diagnostic information in certain cases.[42] For further discussion, see Chapter 14.

Core Biopsy

The diagnosis of papillary tumors of the breast by needle core biopsy has been the subject of extensive investigation, and the literature contains more than 40 reports dealing with this topic. Publications by Skandarajah et al.,[43] Bernik et al.,[44] Jung et al.,[45] and Brennan et al.[46] tabulate data from many investigations, and Table 5.1 lists findings from those

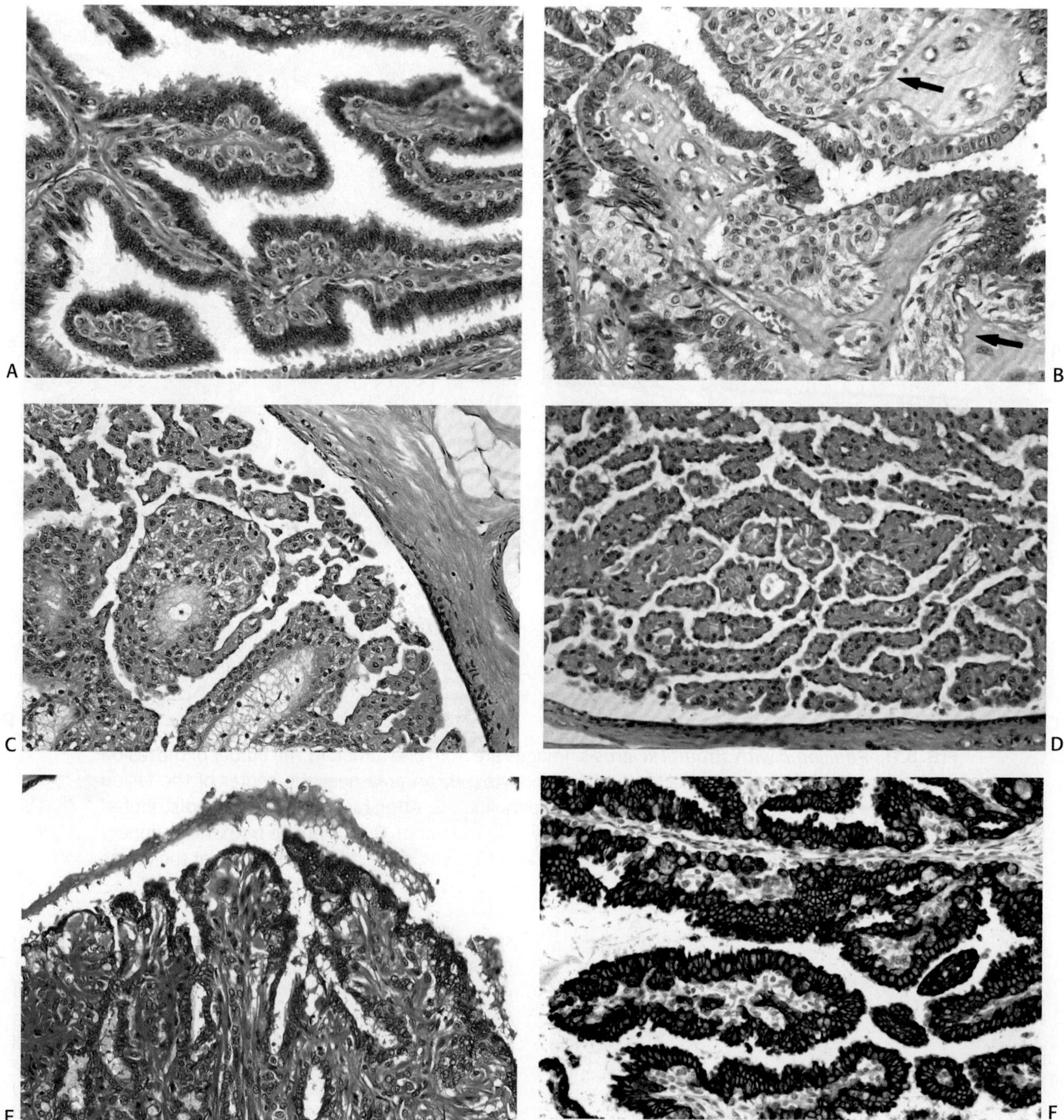

FIG. 5.13. ***Myoepithelial cell hyperplasia.*** **A:** Hyperplastic myoepithelial cells forming an expanded zone beneath the thin epithelium. **B:** The myoepithelial cells have an epithelioid phenotype (*arrows*). **C,D:** Myoepithelial cells with an epithelial phenotype are markedly hyperplastic in these papillomas. The epithelium is reduced to a thin layer of flat cells overlying the multilayered myoepithelium. **E:** A papilloma in which the myoepithelial cells have a striking myoid phenotype and resemble smooth muscle. **F:** The AE1/AE3 immunostain is reactive in the epithelium but not in the myoepithelium. **G:** The myoepithelium is immunoreactive for myosin heavy chain, which shows no reactivity in the epithelium. **H:** Clusters of epithelioid myoepithelial cells resemble lobular carcinoma in the stroma of this papilloma. **I:** Reactivity for E-cadherin in the epithelial and myoepithelial cells is shown. Lobular carcinoma would be E-cadherin negative.

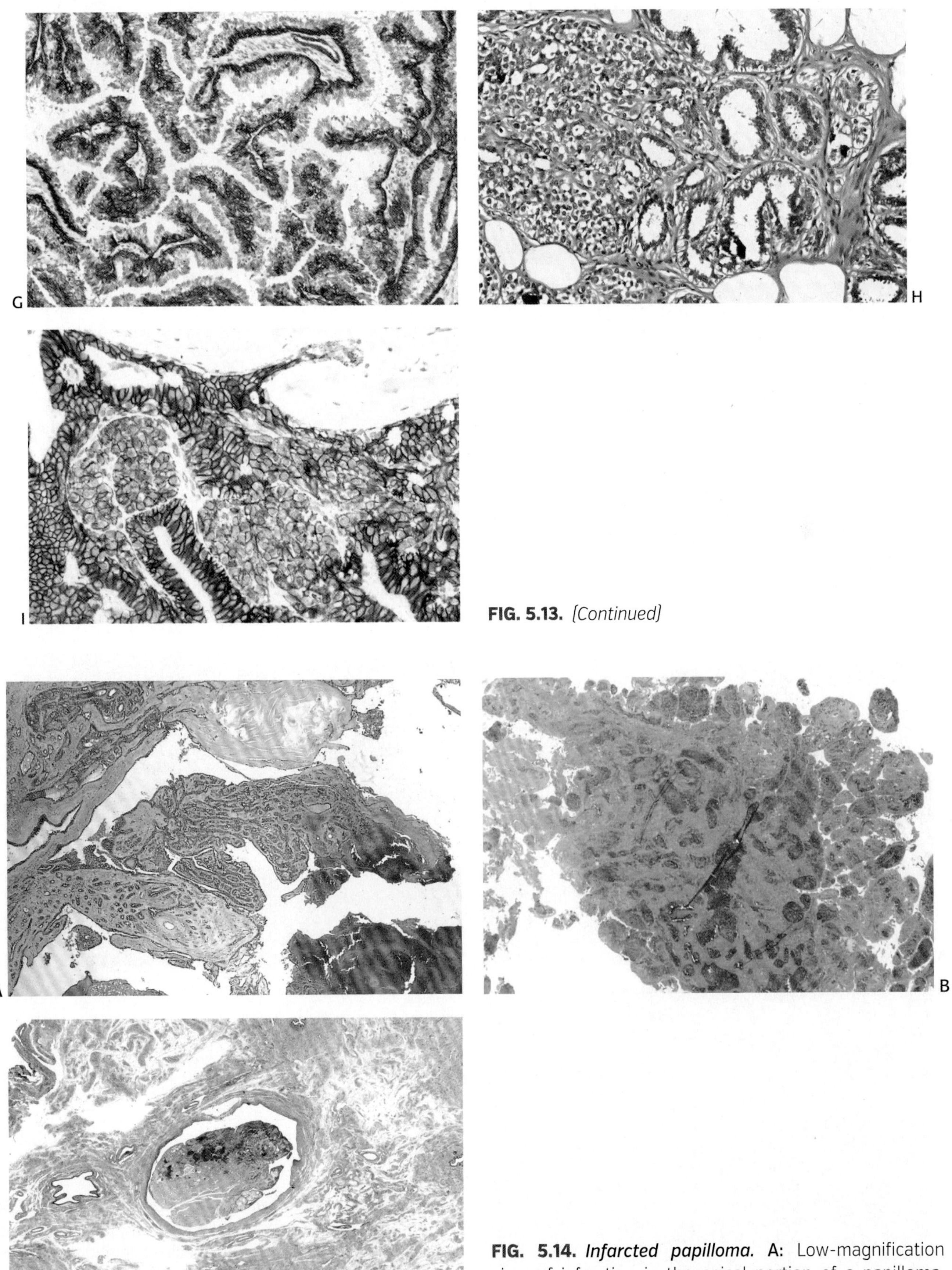

FIG. 5.13. *(Continued)*

FIG. 5.14. ***Infarcted papilloma.*** **A:** Low-magnification view of infarction in the apical portion of a papilloma. **B:** This papillary lesion is entirely infarcted. **C:** A partly infarcted and sclerotic intraductal papilloma.

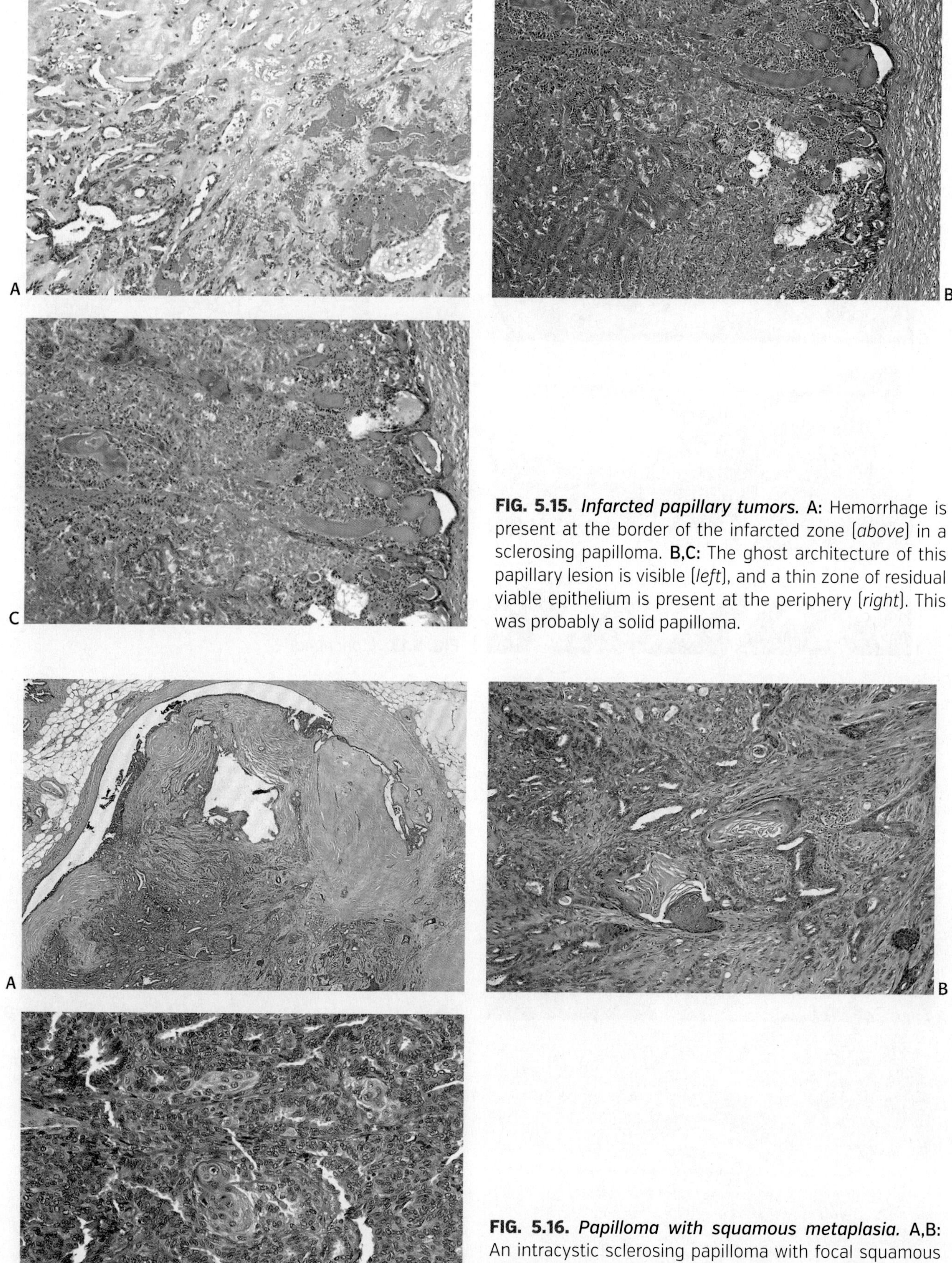

FIG. 5.15. ***Infarcted papillary tumors.*** **A:** Hemorrhage is present at the border of the infarcted zone (*above*) in a sclerosing papilloma. **B,C:** The ghost architecture of this papillary lesion is visible (*left*), and a thin zone of residual viable epithelium is present at the periphery (*right*). This was probably a solid papilloma.

FIG. 5.16. ***Papilloma with squamous metaplasia.*** **A,B:** An intracystic sclerosing papilloma with focal squamous metaplasia. **C:** A small cluster of cells exhibiting squamous differentiation is present in the epithelium of this florid papilloma.

TABLE 5.1 Core Biopsy and Excision of Benign Intraductal Papilloma[a]: A Selected Literature Review

		Excision Findings (%)		
References	**Cases**	**Benign**	**Atypical**	**Malignant**
Rizzo et al.[2]	101	72	19	9
Skandarajah et al.[43]	80	67	14	19
Jung et al.[45]	160	88	6	6
Chang et al.[47]	100	83	13	4
Chang et al.[48]	64	86	11	3
Jaffer et al.[49]	104	84	8	8
Jakate et al.[50]	90	78	13	9
Kil et al.[51]	76	92	0	8
Lu et al.[52]	66	82	12	6
Rizzo et al.[53]	234	73	18	9
Shin[54]	86	79	7	14
Total	**1161**	**80**	**12**	**8**

[a]Benign intraductal papilloma refers to the diagnosis made on the core biopsy sample.

comprising more than 50 cases.[2,43,45,47–54] Interpretation of this body of information is hampered by several factors. First, most studies represent retrospective analyses of cases in which a core biopsy reportedly demonstrated a papilloma. In the early studies, only a few patients underwent excisions, so selection bias may have influenced the results. Second, the designs of the studies have varied widely. Certain ones included retrospective review of histological or radiologic studies, whereas others did not. The histologic classification of the papillary lesions differed, the expertise of the radiologists and pathologists varied, and most studies do not describe in detail the extent of the study of the core biopsy specimens. Statements about the concordance of the radiologic studies and the pathology studies were not included in every report. Finally, during the more than two decades spanned by these studies, the practices of both breast imaging and breast pathology have changed in ways such as the use of vacuum-assisted biopsy methods and immunohistochemical staining, and these advances could have influenced the findings of the studies.

Despite these significant differences in design, a coherent picture has emerged, and two generalizations seem established. First, an excision is usually indicated when a core biopsy specimen of a papillary tumor contains atypical ductal or lobular cells (ADH, atypical lobular hyperplasia [ALH], or lobular carcinoma *in situ* [LCIS]). Between one-third and one-half of such patients will prove to have a carcinoma in an excision specimen. This conclusion mirrors the approach advocated for atypical epithelial proliferations detected in other histologic settings. Second, patients in whom a core biopsy specimen discloses a benign papilloma have a significant likelihood of harboring an atypical epithelial proliferation in an excision specimen. The literature contains data from more than 2,000 core biopsy specimens showing only benign papillomas. Subsequent excision specimens demonstrated benign findings in approximately 80%, atypical ductal or lobular cells (ADH, ALH, or LCIS) in approximately 10%, and DCIS or invasive carcinoma in approximately 10%.

Researchers have attempted to improve the predictive values of the findings present in core biopsy specimens demonstrating benign papillomas by incorporating ancillary clinical, radiologic, or histologic features in their analysis. Scattered reports have identified findings that seem to indicate an increased risk for the presence of atypical cells in an excision specimen; however, other investigations have not borne out the predictive value of these findings in most instances. The literature does suggest that two features may identify patients at elevated risk for atypia: age and size of the lesion. Arora et al.[55] observed an increasing likelihood of an upgrade to malignancy with the increasing age of the patient, and five other studies found that older patients are more likely to have atypical cells discovered on excision.[46,53,56–58] This association notwithstanding, investigators have not discovered an age threshold below which an excision would seem unnecessary.

The size of a papilloma may also influence the likelihood of discovering atypical cells in an excision specimen. In the study of Jung et al.,[45] the presence of a palpable mass indicated an increased likelihood of the detection of carcinoma and so did the presence of a mass on the mammogram. Among studies examining imaging features, two reported that the presence of a mass greater than 1.5 cm detected by sonography[47] or by either sonography or mammography[51] indicated an increased likelihood of carcinoma in a subsequent sample. Another investigation[50] observed that benign papillomas associated with atypia in excision specimens were larger than those that were not. Three other studies did not confirm the predictive nature of the size of the lesion.[49,57,58]

Additional features such as clinical information, radiologic findings, details of the biopsy procedure, and the experience of the radiologists have not improved the predictive values consistently. Many authors stress the need for careful correlation of the radiologic and pathologic findings and point out that lack of correlation accounts for many discrepancies. Nevertheless, in the study by Bernik et al.,[44] 9 of 17 benign papillomas with concordant radiologic studies proved to have ADH in the excision specimen, and 2 of the 17 contained carcinomas. Other authors report the same experience.

Pathologists have searched for way to improve their diagnostic abilities, and both the use of immunohistochemical stains and the expertise of pathologists have come under study. Shah et al.[59] found that the use of immunohistochemical staining for calponin, CK5/6, and p63 allowed pathologists to recognize foci of ADH associated with papillomas. This technique improved the accuracy of all four participating pathologists to the point that they concluded that papillomas lacking atypia "do not require excision in the absence of suspicious clinical/radiological findings." Tse et al.[60] employed staining for estrogen receptor (ER), CK14, and p63 in an attempt to resolve discrepancies encountered in 15 core biopsy specimens. Although the use of these stains reduced the rate of discordance by 69%, the staining results did not eliminate either false-positive or false-negative cases.

The expertise of the pathologist influences the correlation between findings of core biopsy and excision specimens, but even experienced breast pathologists cannot exclude the presence of atypical cells in an excision specimen. In the study of Jakate et al.,[50] diagnoses made by pathologists with fellowship training in breast pathology on core biopsy specimens were less likely to differ from those of the subsequent excision specimen than were diagnoses made by general pathologists; nevertheless, a substantial number of discrepancies remained. An "upgrade" rate of 26.3% was observed for diagnoses made by general pathologists, whereas a rate of 16.3% was observed for breast pathologists. Of the 86 cases in which breast pathologists made a diagnosis of benign papilloma on a core biopsy specimen, 10 excision specimens displayed atypia and 3 showed malignancy.

Several investigations include patients who did not undergo an excision following the diagnosis of benign papilloma on a core biopsy. The authors reported that 7 of the 437 patients (1.6%) included in these studies developed carcinoma. Follow-up periods ranged from 2 to 5 years, and the nature of the follow-up varied. These variations, among many other aspects of the studies, make it impossible to draw secure conclusions about the safety of careful clinical surveillance as an alternative to excision of benign papillomas diagnosed by means of a core biopsy. A conservative approach may prove safe, but investigators have not formulated the criteria to identify either the appropriate patients or the details of the program of surveillance.

Data from the foregoing studies do not provide definitive guidelines for the management of a papilloma without atypia diagnosed by needle core biopsy. A decision as to whether surgical excision should be performed will be influenced by factors such as the size of the lesion, evidence of residual tumor following the biopsy, the ease of mammographic follow-up, family history of breast cancer, and patient concerns. Among women recommended for follow-up without an initial surgical excision, some will require surgical biopsy at a later date. In a series studied by Sexton et al.,[61] 59 of 78 patients (i.e., 75%) with a papilloma diagnosed by needle core biopsy did not undergo surgical biopsy and were followed for 3 to 5 years. Subsequent interval mammographic changes necessitated surgical excision in 10 of the 59 (17%), and 2 (3%) had a subsequent needle core biopsy. All subsequent biopsies were reportedly "benign." This study suggests that up to 20% of patients enrolled in follow-up after a needle core biopsy diagnosis of papilloma will undergo another biopsy within 5 years of the initial procedure. The long-term risk for the development of carcinoma at the site of an incompletely excised papilloma that was sampled by core biopsy has not been determined.

Immunohistochemistry

Immunohistochemical staining of papillomas reveals the results expected for mammary epithelial, myoepithelial, and stromal cells.[26] The epithelial cells in papillomas exhibit nuclear immunoreactivity for ER, which can appear either scattered or diffuse (Fig. 5.17). Most investigations of papillomas using immunohistochemical staining have centered on the differentiation of benign papilloma from papilloma with atypical hyperplasia (atypical papilloma)[59,60] and papillary carcinoma (see Chapter 14).

Electron Microscopy

Electron microscopy reveals the expected ultrastructural features of the cells that compose papillomas.[16,62,63] The epithelial cells have well-developed microvilli on their luminal surfaces and numerous terminal bars and desmosomes between adjacent cells. The nuclear contours appear irregular and invaginated, and the chromatin shows peripheral condensation. The nucleoli sit in the center of the nuclei, they appear round or oval, and they often have irregular borders.

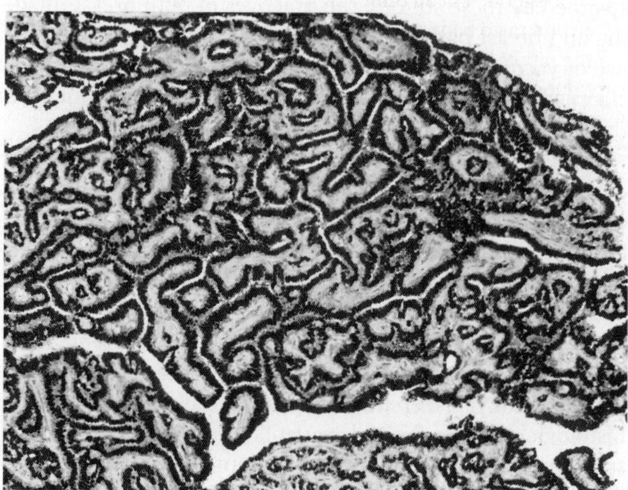

FIG. 5.17. ***Estrogen receptors.*** Immunoreactivity for ER is present in virtually all the epithelial cells.

Cytoplasmic organelles include rough endoplasmic reticulum, free ribosomes, Golgi apparatus, and mitochondria. The cytoplasm contains variable numbers of intermediate filament, lipid droplets, lysosomes, and dense secretory granules. Myoepithelial cells sit between the epithelial cells and the basement membrane. They exhibit polygonal or spindly shapes and possess fusiform nuclei. Myofilaments with dense bodies run parallel to the long axis of the cell, and tonofilaments arranged in thick bundles are arranged in a curvilinear pattern. The basal aspects of the myoepithelial cells often display scalloping. Rare cells display features of both epithelial and myoepithelial cells. A thick basement membrane, which often exhibits splitting and reduplication, separates the epithelium from the stroma.

Other Studies

Clonal analysis based on restriction fragment length polymorphism of the X-linked *phosphoglycerate kinase (PGK)* gene of nine solitary papillomas demonstrated monoclonality in all nine.[64] Furthermore, analysis of widely separated sites of two papillomas showed that the same allele of the *PGK* gene was inactivated at each site. A few studies have contrasted genetic alterations in papillomas with those in papillary carcinoma. Chapter 14 summarizes the findings.

Treatment and Prognosis

The prognosis and treatment of papillomas have been influenced by views about their "precancerous" potential. Because of the widespread belief that the lesion was "precancerous" and that the breast that harbored a papilloma was cancer prone even if the papilloma itself were not malignant, mastectomy was considered appropriate therapy for intraductal papilloma in the first half of the 20th century, as proclaimed in 1922 by Dickinson.[65]

> Every surgeon hesitates to mutilate a woman, and particularly this organ, but every surgeon with a conscience will attack that which is or may become cancer. Benign means "born good," but all tumors of the breast which have this title are apt to go bad and are not to be trusted. . . . Bleeding from the nipple we see associated with them at all times. . . . for tumors only "born good" we have not as yet a definite plan of attack. Some surgeons resect in part; some do a complete plastic subcutaneous resection, and others a radical removal. Can we today say who does wisely?

Bloodgood[66] recommended that papillomas be treated by excision in 1922, but it was not until 1951 that a follow-up study by Haagensen et al.[1] documented the low risk for subsequent carcinoma in women following excision of a papilloma. The latter study reported the follow-up of 72 women, none of whom developed ipsilateral carcinoma after excision of a papilloma. Four women had additional papillomas in the same breast, including three in the area of prior excision. A fifth woman was treated for a contralateral papilloma. Thirty-two patients had been treated initially by mastectomy. In four cases, an erroneous pathologic diagnosis of carcinoma was reported on paraffin sections, and in five cases, an error was made in the interpretation of an FS. From this experience, it was determined that it was not advisable

> to rely upon frozen sections in distinguishing benign from malignant papillary tumors of the breast....Following removal of a satisfactory piece of the lesion the wound is closed and we wait for paraffin sections....We believe that the disadvantage of having to delay and carry out our definitive treatment at a second stage is more than compensated for by the avoidance of the risk of subjecting the patient to the unnecessary radical mastectomy for a benign papilloma.[1]

The "precancerous" significance of papillomas has been the subject of many studies.[67–71] Carter[72] reviewed the subject and concluded that

> ...any of the intraductal papillary tumors may precede invasive carcinoma of the breast. The risk of developing invasive carcinoma increases progressively from those patients with a solitary papilloma with only minor associated changes to those patients with solitary papilloma and associated hyperplastic changes to those patients with multiple papillomas to those patients with intraductal papillary carcinoma.

Sometimes the proximity of mammary carcinoma to a papilloma is such that it is difficult to regard the two lesions as arising separately. In such cases, it is appropriate to conclude that the carcinomatous portion of the lesion arose from the coexisting papilloma. An investigation[73] of 76 solitary papillomas discovered coexisting ductal carcinoma in 12 (16%). Treatment consisted of wide local excision of the papilloma and surrounding tissue, and after a median follow-up of 5.8 years, all patients remained free of disease.

Most follow-up studies of excised papillomas document the low "precancerous" potential of these lesions, but it must be emphasized that there are significant limitations in many of the reports. A substantial number of patients in the earliest studies had their papillomas treated by mastectomy. In some papers, the distinction between papilloma and carcinoma may not have been reliable, and sometimes patients with multiple and solitary papillomas were grouped together. As can be seen in Table 5.2, the reported frequency of carcinoma subsequent to the excision of a papilloma was less than 5%, with nearly half of subsequent carcinomas detected in the opposite breast.[74] MacGrogan and Tavassoli[75] described the follow-up of 119 patients who underwent excision of papillary breast tumors. One of 22 women (4.5%) who had papillomas with "florid hyperplasia" developed invasive carcinoma after an interval of 104 months. Among 40 women who had papillomas with "focal atypia," 2 (5%) developed invasive carcinoma 35 and 162 months later. Atypical papillomas, defined as lesions in which 10% to 32% of the "papilloma's entire surface was involved" by atypical epithelium, were found in 24 women. In the latter group, subsequent carcinomas (two invasive, one intraductal) were diagnosed in three women (12.5%) after intervals of 28 to 145 months. The authors noted that the atypical cells in most cases were confined to the papilloma and that the excision seemed to have removed the entire proliferative population. The study by Cuneo et al.[76] demonstrated similar outcomes: the 5-year risk for the development of noninvasive

TABLE 5.2 Intraductal Papilloma and Carcinoma: A Selected Literature Review

		Carcinomas[a]		
References	**Cases**	**Ipsilateral**	**Contralateral**	**Bilateral**
Haagensen et al.[1]	76	0	0	0
Buhl-Jørgensen et al.[67]	53	3	3	1
Hendrick[68]	207	0	2	0
Kilgore et al.[69]	57	6	2	0
Kraus and Neubecker[70]	19	0	0	0
Lewison and Lyons[71]	23	0	0	0
Carter[72]	64	2	3	1
MacGrogan and Tavassoli[75]	22	0	1	0
Snyder and Chaffin[79]	30	0	0	0
Total	**551**	**11 (2%)**	**11 (2%)**	**2 (0.3%)**

[a]Refers to reported cases of carcinoma diagnosed after excision of a papilloma.

or invasive carcinoma in either breast was 4.6% for patients with a papilloma without atypia and 13% for patients with a papilloma with atypia.

A greater risk for concurrent[77] or subsequent carcinoma has been demonstrated in women with multiple papillomas than in those with solitary papillomas,[78–80] and these women are at risk for developing carcinoma in the contralateral breast.[77] Lewis et al.[81] examined the follow-up of patients with solitary and multiple papillomas treated at the Mayo Clinic. The distribution of patients with respect to the papilloma group was not significantly related to having a family history of breast carcinoma. The risk of developing breast carcinoma after the diagnosis of solitary or multiple papillomas was determined by comparison with an age- and calendar period–matched cohort from Surveillance Epidemiology and End Results (SEER) data. Standardized incidence rates for breast carcinoma were higher for women with solitary (5.11) or multiple (7.01) papillomas accompanied by atypical hyperplasia than for those with solitary (2.04) or multiple (3.01) papillomas without atypia. The mean time to the diagnosis of carcinoma ranged from 4.8 to 6.2 years, being slightly shorted in patients with multiple papillomas.

In general, surgical excision is recommended for palpable papillomas, and it would be prudent for nonpalpable papillomas when part of the lesion is radiographically evident after the needle core biopsy. Ultrasound-guided vacuum-assisted percutaneous removal of six papillomas has been reported.[82]

RADIAL SCLEROSING LESIONS

Terminology

RSLs are proliferative abnormalities that have a stellate configuration radiologically and histologically. Clinical interest in RSLs derives from the realization that these abnormalities may be difficult to distinguish from carcinoma by mammography and the concern that they are precursors of the development of carcinoma.

The existence of these lesions has been recognized throughout most of the 20th century. In 1928, Semb[83] referred to RSLs as rosettes or proliferation centers that might give rise to carcinoma. Bloodgood[84] drew attention to RSLs in a study of "borderline breast tumors," emphasizing diagnostic problems that they present and uncertainty about their precancerous potential.

RSLs have been described by a variety of names introduced since the 1970s. Fenoglio and Lattes[85] described 30 examples, which they termed "sclerosing papillary proliferations" because the lesions had a prominent papillary component. This name has not been met with general acceptance because some of the lesions in this category have little or no papillary element. Fisher et al.[86] suggested the term "nonencapsulated sclerosing lesion," which has the advantage of avoiding issues related to histogenesis. "Infiltrating epitheliosis" has not been widely accepted because it could be misconstrued as indicating an invasive malignant neoplasm.[87] The unpopularity of "indurative mastopathy" is probably attributed to the fact that most of the lesions are too small to be palpable as indurated foci and the vague meaning of the term "mastopathy."[88]

"Radial scar," a widely used name for these lesions, is a translation of "strahlige Narben," the term Hamperl[89] introduced in 1975. This designation refers to the stellate configuration of most of these lesions; it is short, and it avoids terminology that suggests association with particular proliferative ductal lesions. However, use of the word "scar" implies that there is a reparative process in the stroma. Although the stellate configuration has a cicatrix-like appearance, it is possible that the stromal change is an integral part of the proliferative lesion, perhaps enhanced by paracrine growth factors, rather than a reparative process. In this regard, Jacobs et al.[90] compared the "expression of factors involved in vascular stroma formation" in radial scars with invasive carcinomas. When compared with normal breast tissue, the stroma of both radial scars and invasive carcinomas displayed increased vascularity as well as "focally increased expression" of mRNA for collagen type IV, total fibronectin, vascular permeability factor/vascular endothelial growth factor, and other markers. These results provided molecular confirmation of the presence of a vasoproliferative process in both radial scars and invasive carcinomas; however, they did not identify the mechanism by which this process occurs, nor did they necessarily indicate that the same mechanism is involved in both lesions. The term *radial sclerosing lesion*, used here, is preferable because it describes the mammographic and histopathologic appearance of the process without implying histogenesis, and it is sufficiently nonspecific to encompass the many histologic variants included in this category. RSLs are discussed in this chapter devoted to benign papillary tumors because a substantial proportion has a component of papillary ductal proliferation.

Clinical Presentation

Most RSLs are microscopic lesions not detectable by palpation or mammography. They are usually discovered during examination of specimens resected for unrelated indications. Consequently, the distribution of the ages of women with RSLs parallels that of women undergoing breast surgery. RSLs are uncommon before the age of 30 years and most frequent between the ages of 40 and 60 years. The reported frequency of these subclinical lesions varies depending upon the groups of patients studied and the diagnostic criteria. RSLs have been detected in 1.7%,[91] 1.8%,[92] 5.3%,[89] 7.1%,[93] 14%,[94] and 28%[95] of benign breast specimens and in 4%,[86] 16%,[96] and 26%[94] of mastectomy specimens from patients with carcinomas. The broad and overlapping ranges of the frequency of RSLs associated with benign and carcinomatous breasts suggest that RSLs occur with similar frequency in both circumstances. The amount of tissue available for study and the thoroughness with which it is examined are important factors affecting these results. Multiple microscopic RSLs are not uncommon in one breast,[96] and both breasts can be affected.[95] A paper by Anderson and Battersby[97] describes a woman with 80 RSLs in her right breast and 46 in her left breast. RSLs virtually never affect men. One report[98] mentions in passing the presence of a RSL in the breast of a man with breast carcinoma.

Imaging Studies

Most RSLs are smaller than 2 cm when detected radiologically. Typical lesions are characterized by a lucent or dense center, radiating slender strands of tissue, and changes in appearance in different imaging projections[99] (Fig. 5.18A). The ability to visualize a RSL mammographically is enhanced if the lesion is situated in predominantly fatty tissue that provides contrast for the core and radial strands of fibrous stroma containing proliferating epithelium and cysts. In one study of RSLs subjected to stereotactic aspiration biopsy, the average size was 8 mm,[100] and in another report, the size averaged 1.3 cm.[101] Microcalcifications are detected in some but not in all RSLs.[100,102,103] When evident using sonography, RSLs form an irregular hypoechogenic mass with ill-defined borders and diminished posterior acoustic transmission.[104]

Certain radiologic features favor the radiologic diagnosis of a RSL over a stellate carcinoma, but these are not sufficiently distinctive to serve as the basis for a specific diagnosis.[101–103,105,106] MRI may offer valuable diagnostic information. In one study,[107] 18 RSLs did not demonstrate enhancement, whereas 11 of the 12 carcinomas showed irregular areas of focal enhancement with ill-defined borders. These findings led to a specificity of 89%, a sensitivity of 82%, an overall accuracy of 87%, and a K coefficient of 0.97 for the differentiation of RSLs and invasive carcinomas.

Gross Pathology

Most RSLs excised after mammographic localization have gross appearances similar to those of small invasive carcinomas. The nodule is firm and when bisected reveals a pale, retracted center in which there may be white streaks (Fig. 5.18B). Slender bands of pale stroma extend radially into the fat from the core. Small cysts can be appreciated in some lesions. A minority of RSLs lack a distinct stellate gross configuration; instead, they present as ill-defined firm areas or circumscribed nodules.

Microscopic Pathology

Anderson et al.[108] defined the histologic appearance of the RSL or, in their terminology, the "radial scar" as "a distinct histologic structure, characterized by a sclerotic center with a central core containing obliterated duct(s), elastin deposits, and mostly infiltrating tubules and the center is surrounded by a corona of contracted ducts and lobules, which may show different types of proliferative lesions" (Figs. 5.18C–F and 5.19).

The proliferative components that most commonly contribute in differing proportions to RSLs are duct hyperplasia, SA, and cysts (Figs. 5.20 and 5.21). There is a common architectural or structural configuration to RSLs despite the various components. The central nidus is a relatively sclerotic zone composed of fibrosis and elastosis. Abundant elastin in the walls of ducts and throughout the stroma appears as a dense, sometimes granular, eosinophilic or weakly basophilic deposit that can be highlighted by an elastic tissue stain such as Verhoeff or van Gieson. One or more ductal structures within the core appear to be partially or completely obliterated. Sections of a RSL in a relatively early phase of development reveal branching and budding ductal structures in the core. At this stage, the stroma appears relatively cellular with spindle cells distributed around the ductal units and extending along radiating fibrous bands toward the periphery. A light, scattered infiltrate of lymphocytes and plasma cells is found in the stroma. Conspicuous lymphocytic aggregates

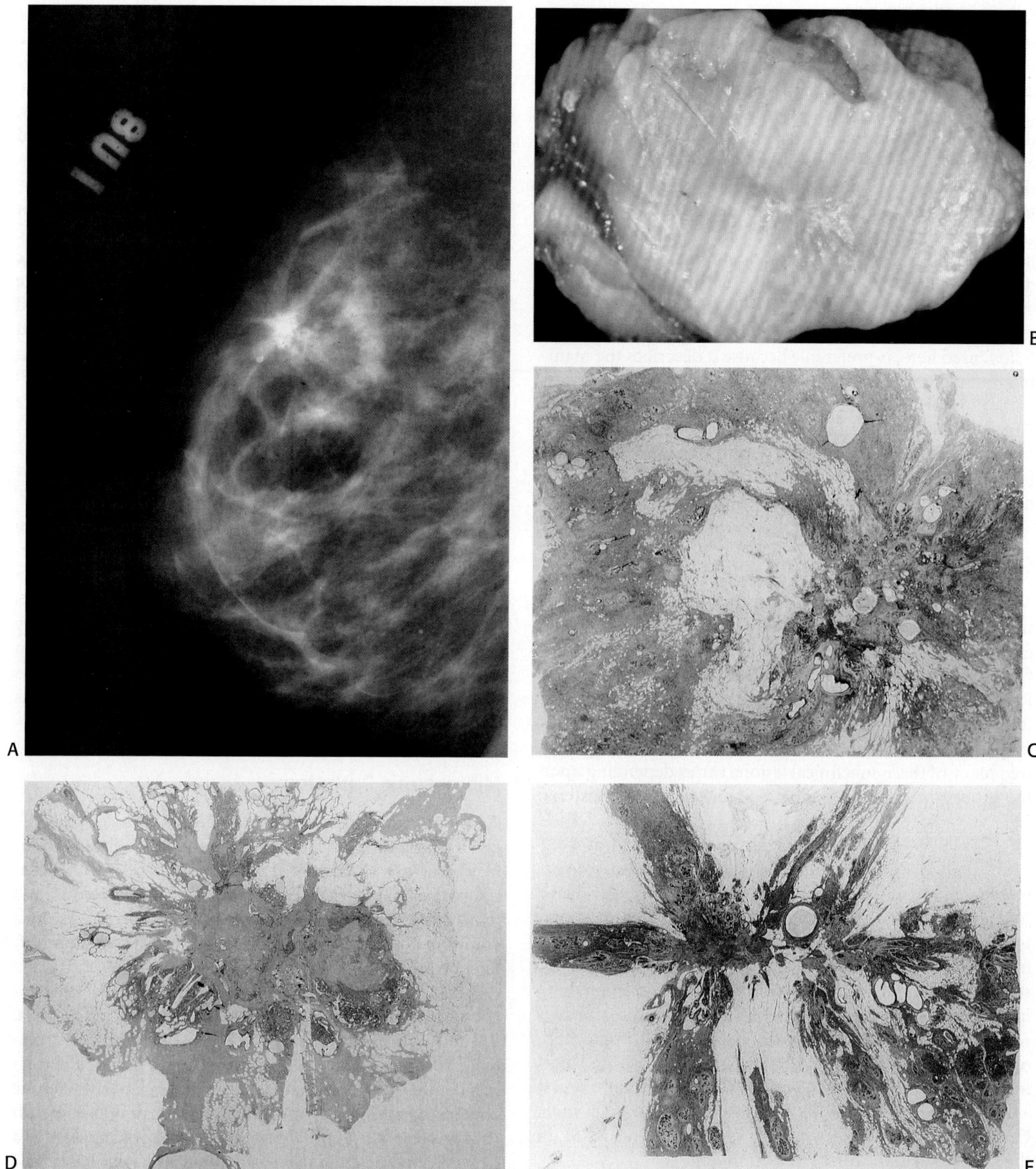

FIG. 5.18. ***Radial sclerosing lesion.*** **A:** Mammogram showing a RSL with a large calcification. **B:** Gross appearance of the lesion seen in (A). The RSL is the stellate whitish lesion near the center of the tissue. **C–F:** Whole-mount histologic sections showing different structural patterns. Relatively ill-defined lesion with multiple cysts (C). Asymmetric, oval lesion with dense central fibrosis. A proliferative component and cysts are present around half of the circumference (D). Lesion with a stellate pattern (E). Ovoid tumor with a contour that is partly smooth and partly stellate (F).

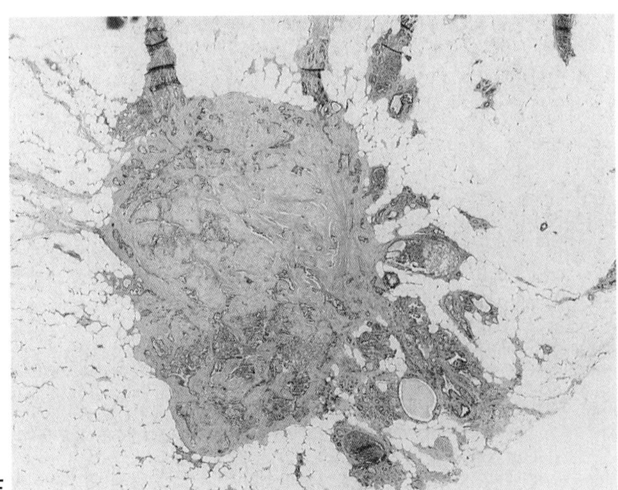

FIG. 5.18. *(Continued)*

are uncommon in the typical RSL, and their presence may indicate a low-grade adenosquamous carcinoma (LGASC) (see Chapter 16). In later stages, the stromal cells are less abundant as the tissue becomes collagenized, and elastosis is more pronounced. Electron microscopy reveals that many of the stromal cells are myofibroblasts,[109] an observation that can be confirmed by IHC.

Small ductules and distorted lobules are distributed between bands of sclerotic tissue radiating from the core into the surrounding stroma. A "corona" of ducts, lobules, and cysts, variably present at the periphery of the lesion, is created by incorporation of these structures from the surrounding tissue (Fig. 5.20). This peripheral zone is not evident around every RSL, and it may appear incomplete or asymmetric owing to intrinsic differences among lesions or as a consequence of asymmetric sectioning. The peripheral zone can also include nonproliferative ducts and lobules, which appear to be drawn toward the core. In some lesions, the "corona" consists mainly or entirely of cysts (Fig. 5.20C). RSLs usually occur as isolated, separate lesions, but on occasion, contiguous foci may be joined to form a larger complex and palpable proliferative lesion in a fashion analogous to the formation of an adenosis tumor.

The fibrous reaction associated with RSLs typically entraps small ductules and, less commonly, nerves. Like nests of epithelium trapped in the stroma at the periphery of a sclerosing papilloma (Fig. 5.11), those in a RSL simulate invasive carcinoma (Figs. 5.21 and 5.22). This is an important consideration when examining needle core biopsy samples (Fig. 5.23). The presence of a myoepithelial cell layer demonstrated with the p63, calponin, or actin immunostains characterizes epithelial entrapment within a RSL and thereby helps to avoid an erroneous diagnosis of invasive carcinoma. Somewhat less than 5% of RSLs demonstrate entrapment of small nerves.[110] They are probably incorporated into RSLs by the same mechanism that is responsible for this phenomenon in other sclerosing lesions[111] (Figs. 5.20C and 5.24).

The epithelium within a RSL can exhibit a range of changes. Apocrine metaplasia frequently occurs in the cystic component of RSLs, and it may occasionally be present more widely in the proliferative component, especially in areas of SA. Clear cell change and nuclear atypia are not uncommon in this apocrine epithelium. Squamous metaplasia is relatively infrequent in RSLs (Fig. 5.25), and those uncommon examples with squamous metaplasia may resemble metaplastic carcinoma, especially the low-grade adenosquamous variant.

Hyperplasia and Carcinoma in RSLs

Ductal proliferations in RSLs can take the form of florid and atypical hyperplasia (Figs. 5.26 and 5.27) as well as DCIS. Duct hyperplasia in a RSL may be solid, cribriform, micropapillary, or any combination of these structural patterns. Focal necrosis occurs in the hyperplastic duct epithelium of about 10% of RSLs (Fig. 5.26). The epithelium with these comedo-like foci is usually indistinguishable from the epithelium in hyperplastic ducts lacking necrosis in the same RSL. The presence of mitoses or necrosis is evidence of atypical hyperplasia in a RSL. Foci of ADH or ALH have been observed in 21%[112] to 51%[113] of RSLs. Often, the significant

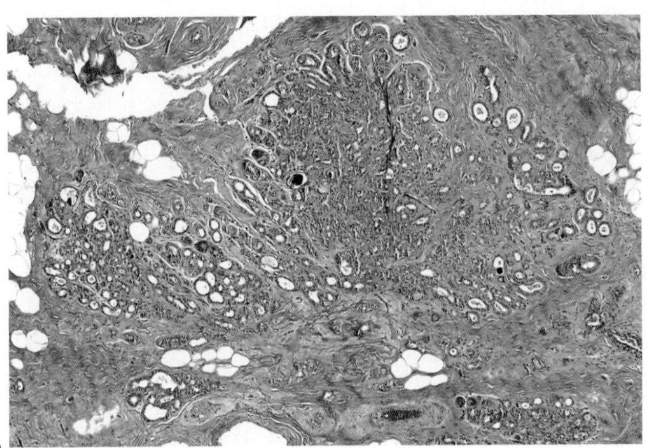

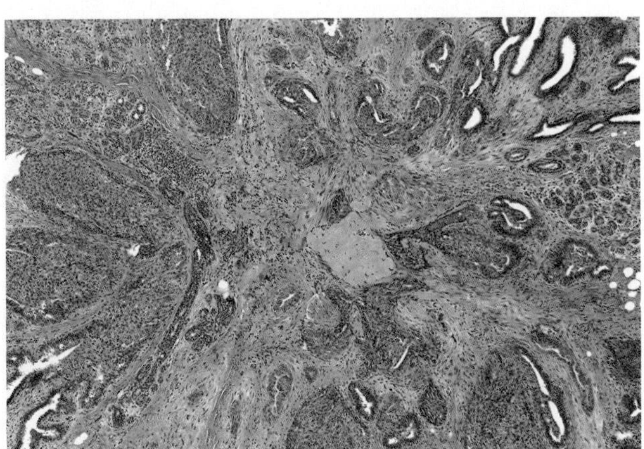

FIG. 5.19. ***Radial sclerosing lesions, elastosis.*** **A:** Foci of SA radiate from the elastotic core. **B:** Florid duct hyperplasia around an elastotic core.

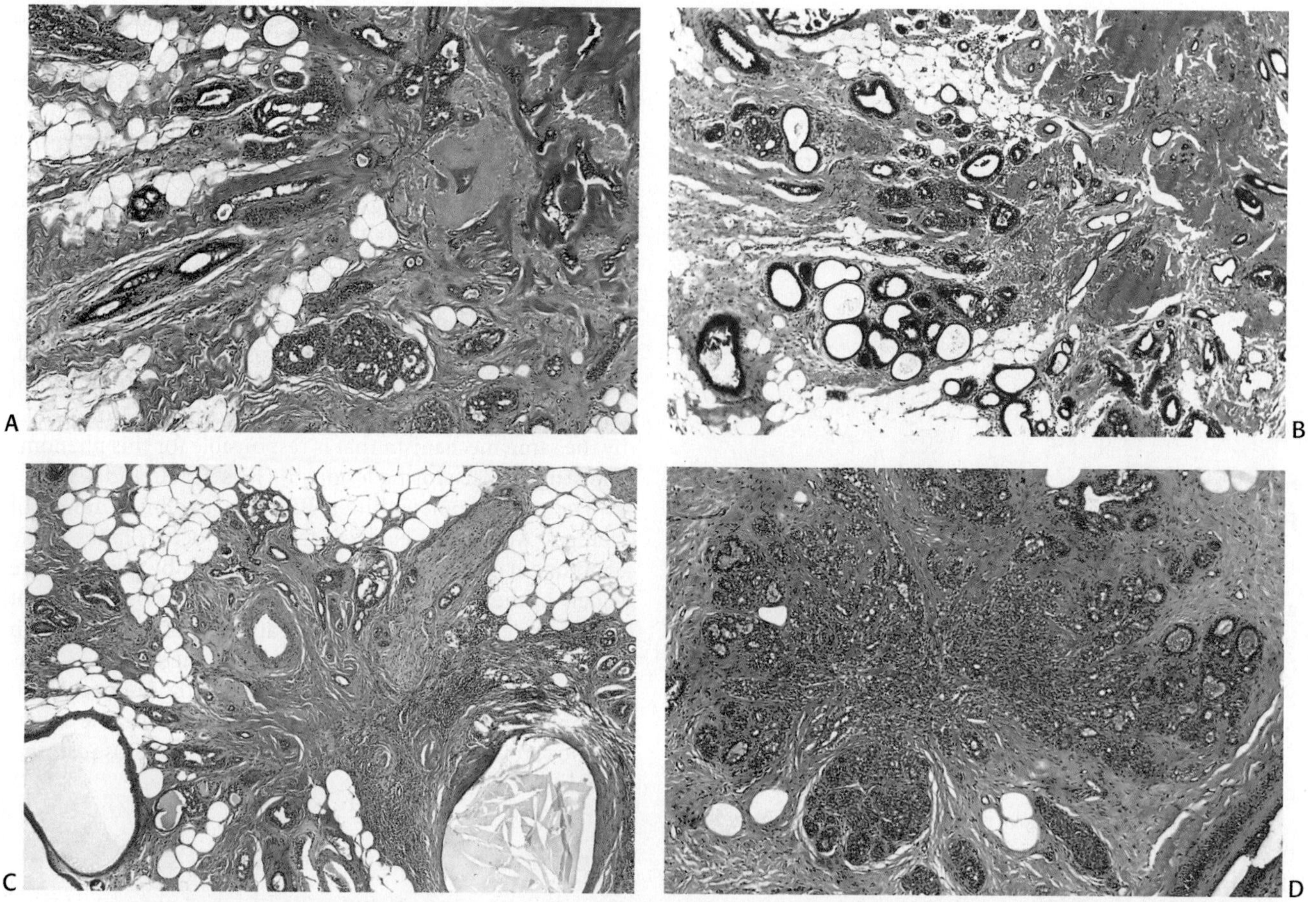

FIG. 5.20. ***Radial sclerosing lesions.*** **A:** The elastotic center is in the *upper right corner*. Mild ductal hyperplasia is present at the periphery. **B:** The elastotic center is in the *upper right corner*. The lesion features adenosis with microcystic dilation of glands. **C:** A RSL with peripheral apocrine cysts and an entrapped nerve (*upper right*). **D:** A RSL composed of SA.

proliferative foci are distributed in multiple tissue fragments in a needle core biopsy specimen. Care should be taken to avoid an erroneous diagnosis of DCIS or invasive carcinoma in this setting. Myoepithelial cells can be demonstrated around the perimeter of most hyperplastic ducts by using immunostains for p63, CD10, smooth muscle myosin-heavy chain (SMM-HC), or actin. However, in the central part of the lesion, myoepithelium may be substantially attenuated and even undetectable around hyperplastic ducts (Fig. 5.23).

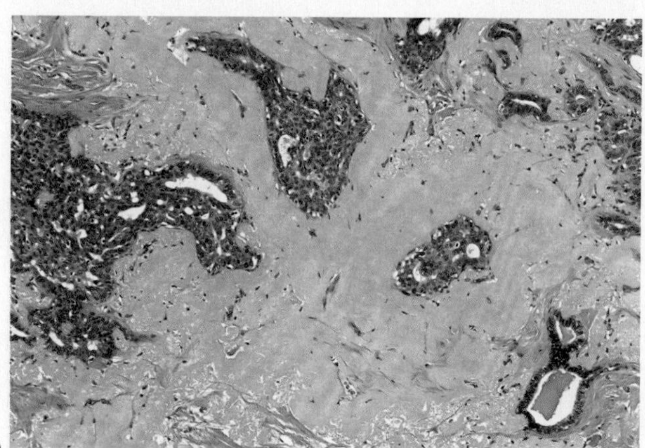

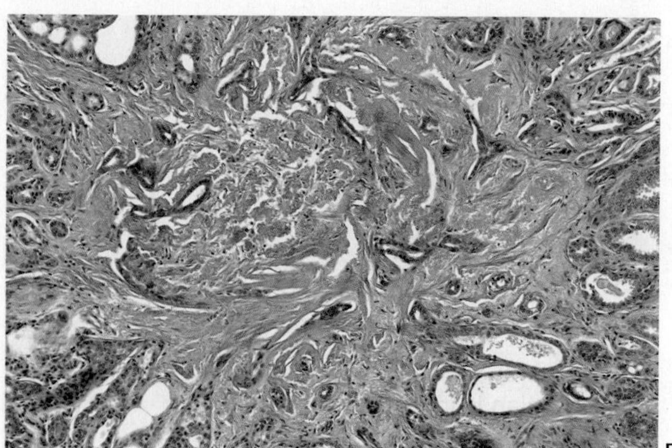

FIG. 5.21. ***Radial sclerosing lesion.*** **A:** Ductal hyperplasia and fibroelastotic stroma. **B:** Adenosis with a pattern that simulates tubular carcinoma.

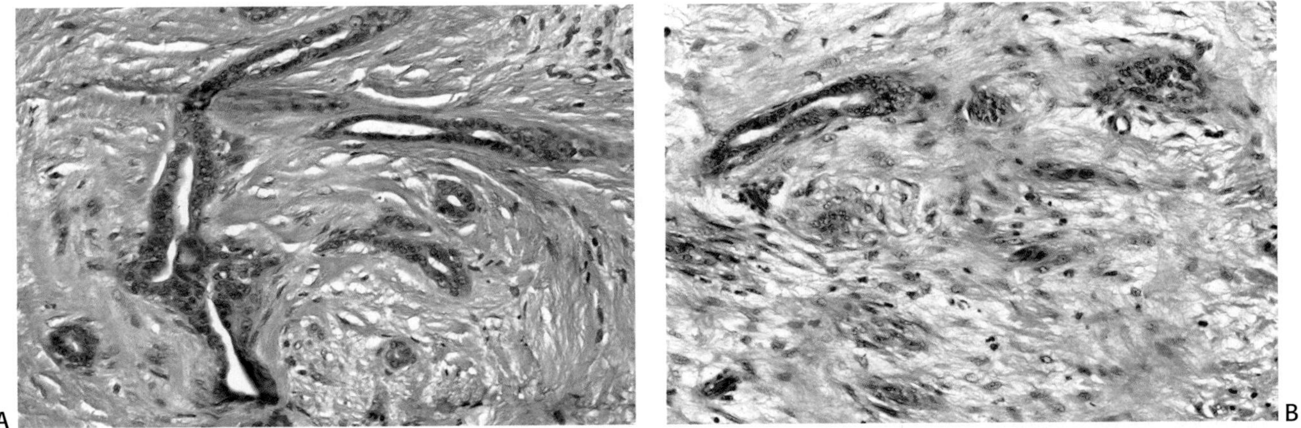

FIG. 5.22. ***Radial sclerosing lesion simulating invasive carcinoma.*** **A:** Irregular ductules in desmoplastic stroma. **B:** The distinction between epithelial and stromal cells is obscured.

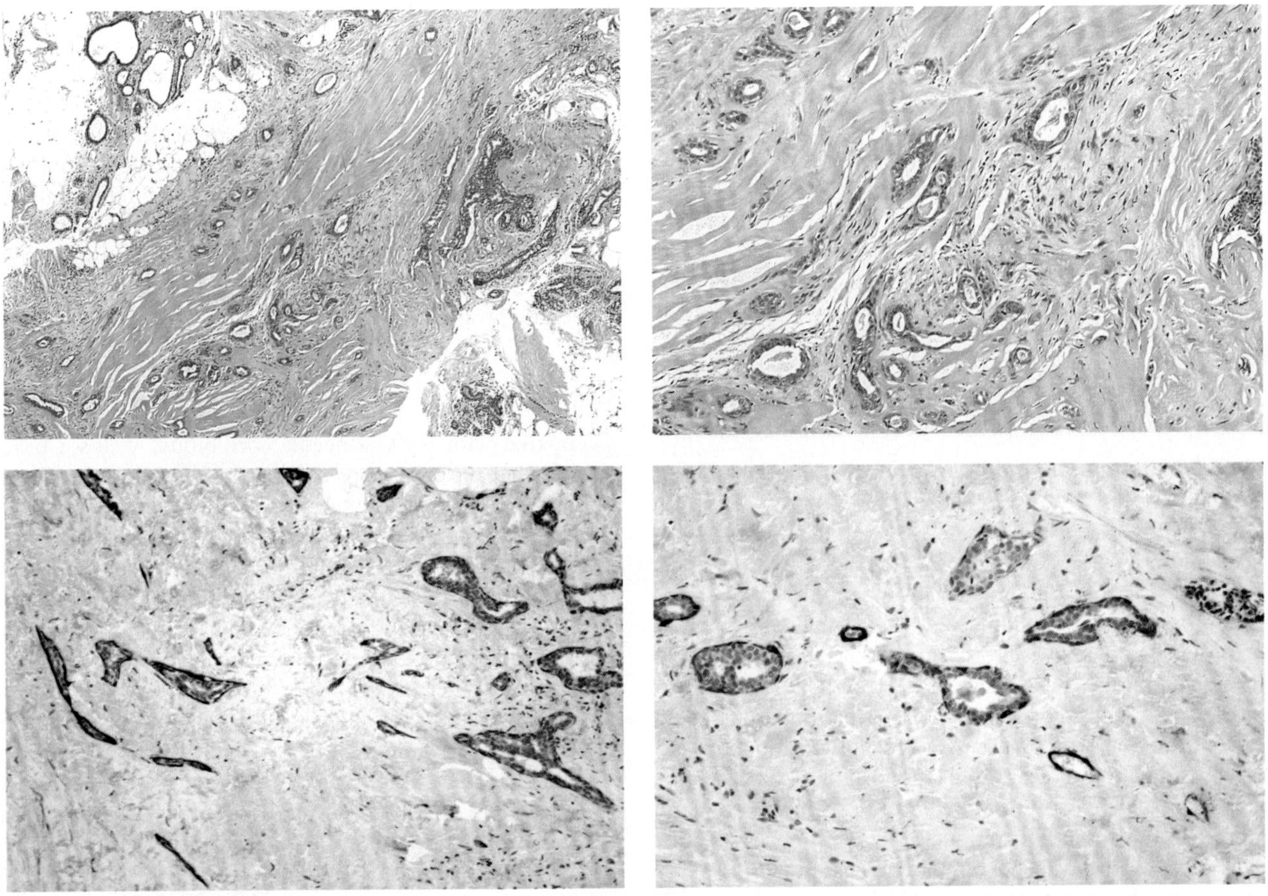

FIG. 5.23. ***Radial sclerosing lesion, needle core biopsy.*** **A:** A low-magnification view of the biopsy sample shows small angular glands in the fibroelastotic stroma. A focus of ductal hyperplasia is present near the *right* border. This specimen was misinterpreted as tubular carcinoma. **B:** Angular glands in the myofibroblastic stromal proliferation. **C:** Actin-positive myoepithelial cells surround these glands in a RSL. **D:** Incomplete and focally absent SMM-HC immunoreactivity in a RSL.

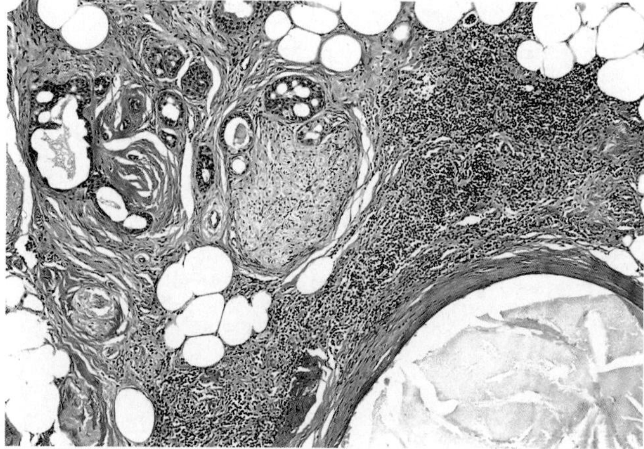

FIG. 5.24. ***Nerve entrapment in a radial sclerosing lesion.*** A nerve is shown in the upper center at the periphery of a RSL. Small glands at the perimeter of the perineurium indent the nerve.

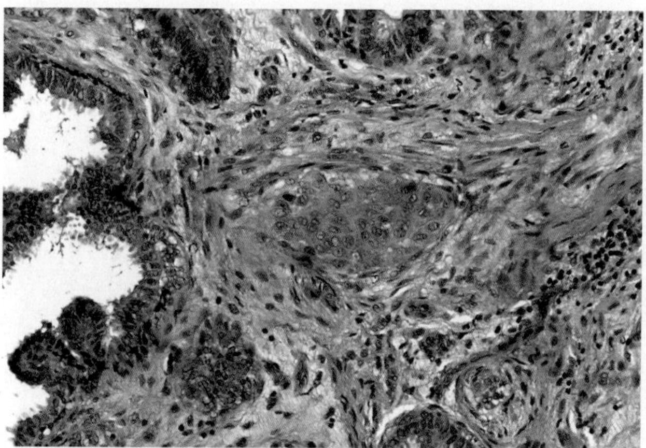

FIG. 5.25. ***Squamous metaplasia in a radial sclerosing lesion.***

The presence of carcinoma, including tubular carcinoma, in RSLs has been well documented,[114] but the literature does not provide a coherent set of estimates of the frequency of this association. Values as high as 31% and 32% have been reported,[112,115] and in one series, 28% of mammographically detected RSLs larger than 1 cm had foci of carcinoma.[116] In this context, it is important to distinguish between carcinomas with a stellate configuration and RSLs with foci of carcinoma. In the absence of residual RSL, it is not possible to prove that an entirely stellate carcinoma arose in a RSL. Carcinoma is most frequently found in RSLs larger than 0.6 cm,[117] and it occurs more often in RSLs from women older than 50 years.[117,118] Both ductal and lobular carcinomas (Fig. 5.28) occur in RSLs, and the frequency of noninvasive carcinomas outweighs that of invasive carcinomas.[110,112,117,118] The carcinomas usually involve only a small region of the RSL, sometimes as little as 5%, and they more frequently occupy the periphery rather than the center.[110,117,118] Commonplace varieties of ductal and lobular carcinomas account for most malignancies seen in RSLs, but LGASCs sometimes develop in the setting of a RSL[119] (see Chapter 16).

The major consideration in the differential diagnosis of RSLs is tubular carcinoma (Fig. 5.23). The glands in tubular carcinoma have round or distinctive angular shapes not ordinarily found in RSLs. The epithelium in tubular carcinomas lacks the myoepithelial layer characteristically present in hyperplastic components in the glands of RSLs. The cystic and apocrine components of RSLs are absent from tubular carcinomas.

FS evaluation is not appropriate for the diagnosis of an excised RSL.[108]

Cytology

FNA cytology provides a sampling of the cellular constituents of a RSL. The finding of benign proliferative epithelium and spindle-shaped stromal cells in conjunction with a characteristic mammographic appearance is presumptive evidence for a diagnosis of RSL.[120] In some instances, it may be difficult to distinguish between the FNA aspirate from a fibroepithelial tumor with epithelial hyperplasia and the aspirate from a RSL. Atypical epithelium and carcinoma can be found in the FNA sample from a RSL. Cells obtained from foci of atypical apocrine metaplasia present a particularly challenging diagnostic problem in an aspiration cytology specimen.[121] Because of the heterogeneous structure of many of these lesions, the FNA sample may not be representative in all cases, and this is not a reliable method for detecting focal carcinoma in RSLs.[116] Orell[122] reported a false-positive rate of 4.3% in RSLs diagnosed by FNA in a mammography-screening program.

Core Biopsy

Compared with FNA, a needle core biopsy yields a tissue sample that offers a more reliable basis for the specific diagnosis of a RSL. Nevertheless, pathologists can still misinterpret nests of hyperplastic epithelium or SA trapped in the stroma of a RSL as invasive carcinoma (Fig. 5.23), and a core biopsy only samples the focus in question, leaving much of the lesion, as well as the tissue around it, histologically unanalyzed. Both limitations can lead to the false exclusion of carcinoma. False-negative rates for RSLs without atypia in the 21 published studies tabulated by Bianchi et al.[123] range from 0% to 40%; the mean rate is 8.3%. DCIS accounts for 60% of the undetected carcinomas, IDC of no special type for 15%, tubular carcinoma for 10%, and other types of invasive and unclassified "carcinomas" for the remainder. These results suggest that incomplete sampling of the lesion rather than misinterpretation of the nature of small glands represents the cause of more than one-half of the discrepancies. The use of the vacuum-assisted technique, the practice of obtaining many samples,[113,124] and close correlation of the radiologic images and the pathologic findings help to minimize the problem of unrepresentative sampling. Four series[106,124–126] contain reports of 133 RSLs diagnosed by means of vacuum-assisted biopsy in which a surgical excision ensued. In only one case did the excision specimen contain a carcinoma

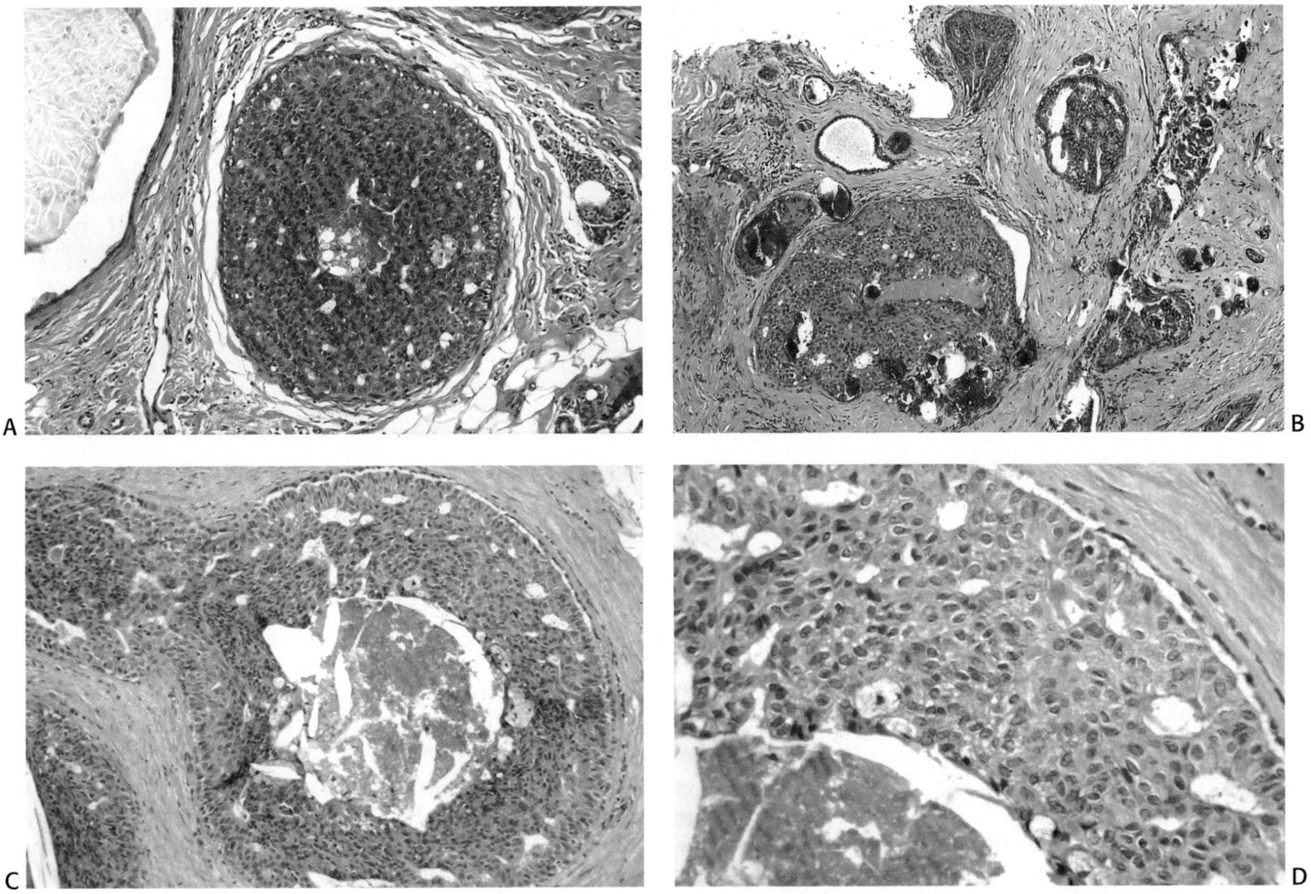

FIG. 5.26. ***Epithelial necrosis in radial sclerosing lesions.*** **A:** A small area of necrosis in the center of a duct with florid hyperplasia at the periphery of a RSL. **B:** A needle core biopsy sample of a RSL with multiple calcifications. ADH is present in the ducts. Necrosis is evident in the center of the largest duct. **C,D:** Central necrosis in florid duct hyperplasia in a RSL. Note irregular microlumens at the periphery of the duct, a characteristic feature of hyperplasia. Myoepithelial cells are evident.

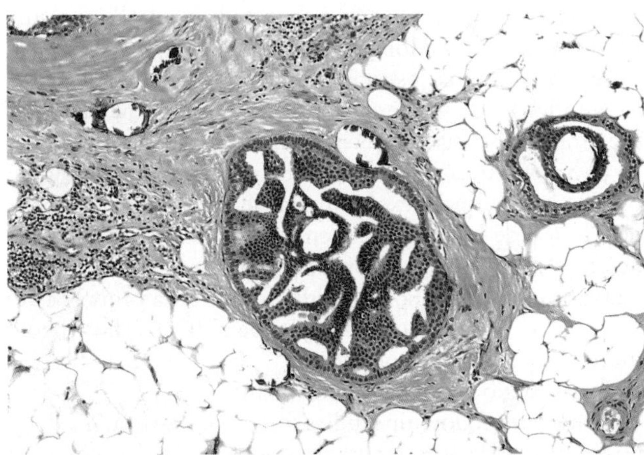

FIG. 5.27. ***Radial sclerosing lesion with atypical duct hyperplasia.*** A duct at the periphery of a RSL shows atypical micropapillary hyperplasia. Note the presence of orderly, cuboidal epithelium at the periphery of the ducts. Calcifications are present in the epithelium and stroma.

(DCIS), and inaccurate sampling of the targeted lesion may explain this solitary discrepancy. It seems that RSLs thoroughly sampled using a vacuum-assisted technique and found lacking in cellular atypia may not require a surgical excision provided that the imaging results comport with the histologic findings.

Published reports have centered on RSLs detected by imaging studies, but the foci sometimes occur as incidental microscopic findings in specimens biopsied for other reasons. In one study[127] of 18 patients with incidental microscopic RSLs without atypia mostly detected using a vacuum-assisted method, surgical excision did not disclose carcinoma in any, but it did reveal the presence of ADH in 6 patients and atypical apocrine adenosis in another.

Finally, radiologists have used the vacuum-assisted technique in an effort to remove RSLs without atypia completely.[128,129] This approach may prove a satisfactory alternative to surgical excision, but extended clinical follow-up and study of a large number of patients are required before reaching that conclusion.

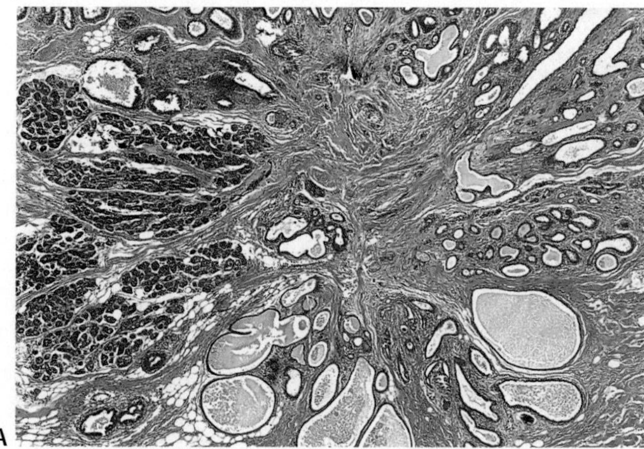

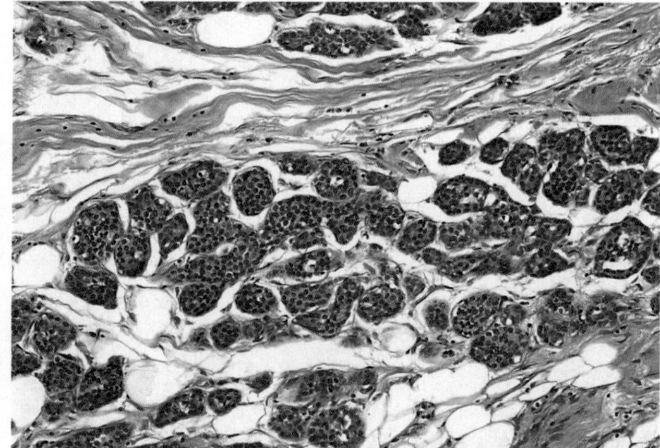

FIG. 5.28. ***Radial sclerosing lesion with LCIS.*** **A:** LCIS occupies glands in the *left* half of this focus. **B:** Magnified view of the LCIS.

Genetic Studies

Iqbal et al.[130] reported that a small percentage of RSLs demonstrate allelic imbalance with respect to chromosome regions 8p and 16q.

Treatment and Prognosis

The presence of carcinoma or atypical hyperplasia in some RSLs has been an important factor in the concern over the precancerous potential of these lesions. Investigators have attempted to determine this potential by studying both morphologic and clinical evidence. On the basis of architectural similarities between RSLs and invasive carcinomas, the belief that RSLs represent a stage in the formation of an invasive carcinoma was most strongly championed by Linell et al.[96] and supported by Fisher et al.[86] Moreover, Wellings and Alpers[94] reported finding RSLs significantly more often in the breasts of women with carcinoma than in the breasts of women without carcinoma. On the other hand, other authors have not found significant differences in the number or frequency of RSLs in the breasts of women with and without carcinoma,[97,131] and the morphologic features of RSLs from the breasts of women with carcinoma do not appear appreciably different from comparable lesions not associated with carcinoma.[97]

Although the results of clinical follow-up studies differ slightly, they have not detected an anatomic link between RSLs and invasive carcinomas. Jacobs et al.[93] conducted a prospective cohort study of 1,396 women with "radial scars" in excision specimens followed for a median of 12 years. The authors calculated a value of 1.8 for the relative risk (RR) for subsequent carcinoma in women with a "radial scar" compared with those not having a "radial scar." The RR was increased by concurrent proliferative changes and was greatest when the "radial scar" coexisted with atypical hyperplasia. Both the size of the "scars" and the number of "scars" influenced the RR for the development of carcinoma. The carcinomas that developed did not preferentially arise in the breasts harboring the "scars"; the carcinomas arose in either breast with equal frequency. The authors concluded that "scars" constitute indicators of an increased risk of the development of breast carcinoma rather than direct precursors of carcinomas in most cases. Several other studies have not observed an increased risk of subsequent carcinomas for women with RSLs. In a retrospective follow-up study of patients after excision of RSLs, Andersen and Gram[91] encountered only one patient with a subsequent carcinoma among 32 women followed for a mean of 19.5 years. Sanders et al.[132] described a retrospective cohort study of 9,556 women among whom 880 (9.2%) were found by review to have one or more "radial scar" lesions. The risk of developing ipsilateral breast carcinoma was directly related to the number of radial scars. When the presence of other proliferative lesions was taken into consideration, the authors observed "that this risk can be largely attributed to the category of coexistent proliferative disease, being greatest when there was atypical hyperplasia". The presence of a "radial scar" "did not significantly increase the risk of carcinoma due to proliferative disease with atypia or atypical hyperplasia existing without a radial scar." Three other studies,[98,133,134] including one[133] involving 439 women followed for a mean interval of 17 years, reached similar conclusions. It seems clear that RSLs frequently coexist with forms of proliferative disease and that the nature of the proliferative disease determines the patients' risk.

It has been suggested that mammographic follow-up rather than surgical excision can be recommended if the RSL in a core biopsy specimen from a mammographically detected nonpalpable lesion does not have atypical hyperplasia or *in situ* carcinoma. Additional criteria proposed are that at least 12 core biopsy samples be obtained showing no more than a RSL without atypia[124] and that the radiologic and pathologic findings be concordant.

Long-term follow-up studies for women with RSLs diagnosed by needle core biopsy and not surgically excised are not available. Based on the current data, excisional biopsy would be prudent when a needle core biopsy sample from a palpable or radiologically detected lesion is diagnostic of RSL with atypia. If the RSL does not have an atypical component and there are no concomitant atypical proliferative lesions, the decision as to whether to recommend excision or follow-up should be made on a case-by-case basis. Factors to consider are prior biopsy findings, other factors predisposing to increased cancer risk such as family history, and ease of clinical or radiologic follow-up.

SUBAREOLAR SCLEROSING DUCT HYPERPLASIA

Subareolar sclerosing duct hyperplasia (SSDH) is a form of sclerosing papilloma that occurs immediately below but not in the nipple.[135] Sclerosing duct hyperplasia can produce a tumor of the central or subareolar breast parenchyma without involving the substance of the nipple. The term *subareolar sclerosing duct hyperplasia* should be reserved for those lesions that constitute a clinicopathologic entity distinct from florid papillomatosis of the nipple.

Clinical Presentation

The age at diagnosis ranges from 26 to 73 years, averaging about 50 years. The left and right breasts are affected with equal frequency; examples of bilateral involvement have not been reported.

The presenting symptom is a mass located beneath the nipple and areola, or both, or in the breast close to the areola. None of the lesions has been within the nipple. Erosion or ulceration of the nipple surface is absent. Nipple retraction may occur, and several patients have experienced bloody discharge. The mammographic findings have not been specific for this lesion and they may suggest carcinoma.

Gross Pathology

The excised lesion is a firm-to-hard, round or oval tumor with indistinct borders measuring as much as 2.0 cm (average 1.2 cm). Yellow streaks may be noted in some examples. Excisions have typically been achieved without incising or removing the nipple, because the lesion is located in the underlying mammary parenchyma. This aspect of the surgical approach is useful in the differential diagnosis of florid papillomatosis and SSDH.

Microscopic Pathology

The histologic structure of SSDH is similar to that of RSLs in other parts of the breast. Sclerosis and elastosis are more marked toward the center of the tumor, whereas duct hyperplasia is most prominent at the periphery. Cartilaginous metaplasia, a rare occurrence in these lesions, typically occurs in the sclerotic core. In some cases, small hyperplastic ducts are seen at the margin, resulting in irregular borders. More often, much of the tumor has a rounded border created by the nodular expansion of confluent large ducts (Figs. 5.29 and 5.30). Scattered mitotic figures may be encountered in the florid hyperplastic epithelium or in hyperplastic myoepithelial cells, which are found throughout much of the lesion. Rarely, focal comedo necrosis is found in the hyperplastic duct epithelium. In contrast to RSLs that occur elsewhere in the breast, SSDH generally lacks cysts, cystic and papillary apocrine change, and squamous metaplasia. Carcinoma rarely arises in SSDH.

Treatment and Prognosis

The tumors should be treated by excisional biopsy, which can usually be performed through a circumareolar incision sparing the nipple. Recurrence may occur after incomplete excision, but in most cases the patients have remained well for up to 4 years after initial treatment. Total mastectomy has been performed when DCIS was present in SSDH or because the lesion was mistakenly diagnosed as carcinoma. At present, there is no evidence that this condition is a risk factor for carcinoma elsewhere in the breast, but longer follow-up will be necessary to evaluate the question fully.

CYSTIC AND PAPILLARY APOCRINE METAPLASIA

Apocrine glands are part of the odoriferous or accessory sex gland system. They are normally present in the skin, particularly in the groin, axilla, and anogenital region. Modified apocrine glands occur in the ears (ceruminous glands) and eyelids (Moll glands). Apocrine glands are morphologically and functionally different from the cutaneous sebaceous and sweat glands. Several observations suggest that cutaneous apocrine glands are responsive to hormonal stimulation in a fashion analogous to the mammary gland. The development of normal apocrine glands is largely delayed until puberty in both sexes. In women, apocrine gland function waxes and wanes somewhat with the phases of the menstrual cycle. Axillary apocrine gland hyperplasia during pregnancy may occasionally produce palpable glandular enlargement, which can be mistaken for a neoplasm or ectopic breast tissue. Increased secretory activity of the axillary apocrine glands has been reported during pregnancy. At present, there is no evidence to indicate that exogenous estrogens contribute to apocrine metaplasia in humans. Comparison of breast tissue of women receiving exogenous estrogen and of untreated women revealed no increase in the frequency of apocrine metaplasia in the treated group.[136]

Cutaneous apocrine gland cells contain abundant pink finely granular cytoplasm, which forms apical tufts or blebs at the luminal surface typical of merocrine secretion. Round, regular nuclei with a punctate nucleolus are located near the base of the cell. At the ultrastructural level, the cytoplasm contains abundant endoplasmic reticulum, mitochondria, intermediate filaments, and secretory vesicles, which are responsible for the granularity observed in hematoxylin and eosin (H&E) sections.[137]

Embryologically, the breasts develop from the anlage that gives rise to apocrine glands, but apocrine glands are not a constituent of the normal microscopic anatomy of the mammary gland. Any benign proliferative lesion may contain cells with apocrine cytologic features. In their most banal form, these metaplastic apocrine cells are indistinguishable from the cells that comprise normal cutaneous apocrine glands.

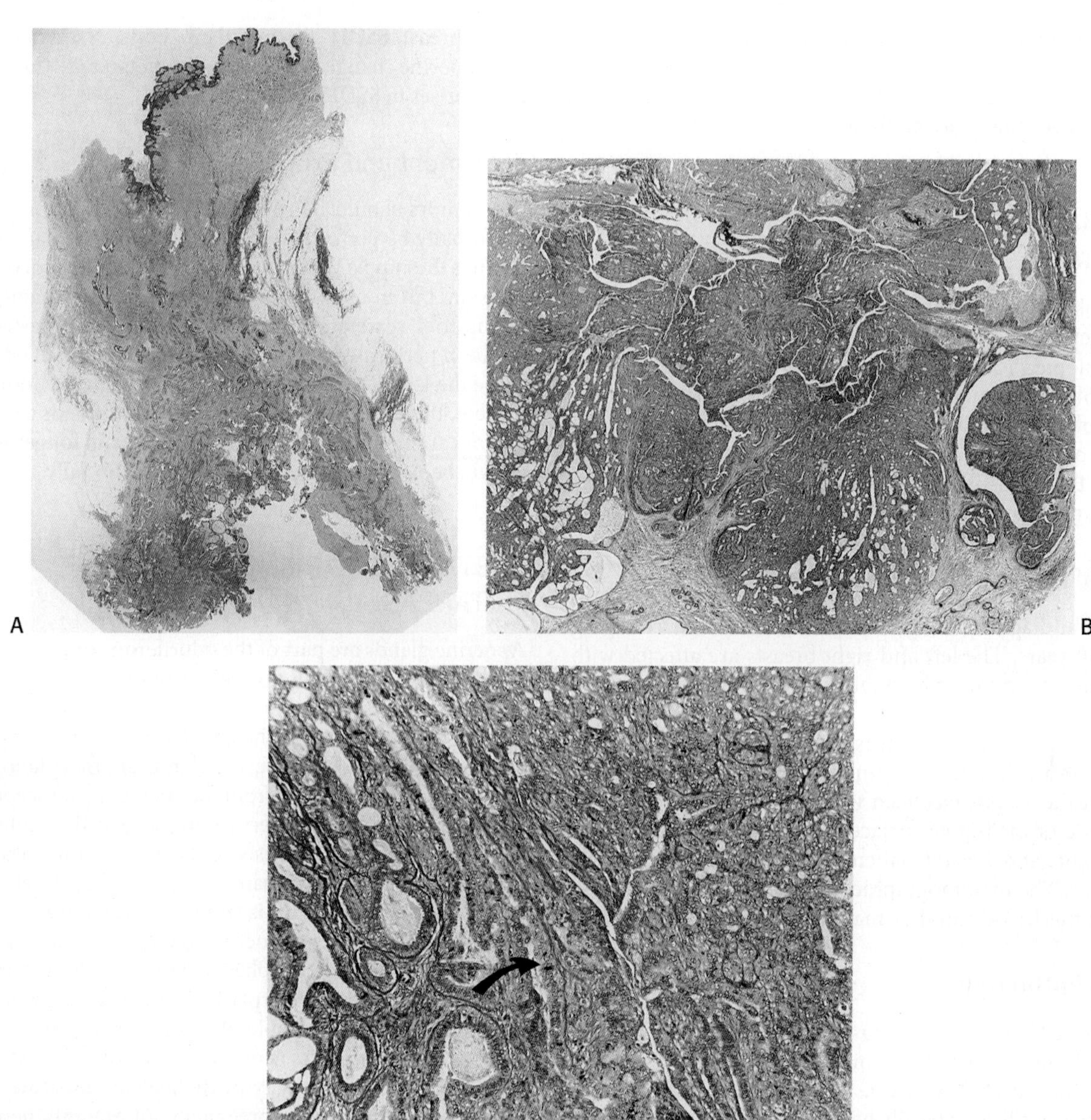

FIG. 5.29. *Subareolar sclerosing duct hyperplasia.* **A:** Whole-mount histologic section of nipple and subareolar tissue with a sclerosing papilloma below rather than in the nipple. **B:** Typical solid growth pattern with focal papillary areas. **C:** The lesion is cellular with occasional mitotic figures (*arrow*). (Reproduced from Rosen PP. Subareolar sclerosing duct hyperplasia of the breast. *Cancer* 1987;59:1927–1930, with permission.)

The proliferative capacity of ordinary apocrine metaplasia is uncertain. The flat apocrine cells lining cysts may be an end stage of cellular differentiation, but studies of the cyst fluid indicate metabolic activity. The fluid in apocrine cysts contains high concentrations of the androgen conjugate dehydroepiandrosterone sulfate,[138] a steroid that is also concentrated in sweat from axillary glands.[139] This finding suggests that the accumulation of the hormone occurs as a result of active transport or synthesis by the cyst epithelium. Mitoses are almost never seen in ordinary apocrine metaplasia, and a low proportion of cells are in S-phase.[140]

Clinical Presentation

Grossly palpable cysts are frequently lined by apocrine epithelium, which can be recognized cytologically in fluid aspirated from the cyst. The fluid tends to have a K^+/Na^+ ratio greater than 1.5, a characteristic of the type I cyst described by Naldoni et al.[141] Type I cysts were significantly associated with low parity and recurrence of cysts but not with a family history of breast carcinoma. There are no clinical features specifically attributable to apocrine cysts. Apocrine metaplasia is frequently present in the epithelial lining of cysts in gross cystic disease.

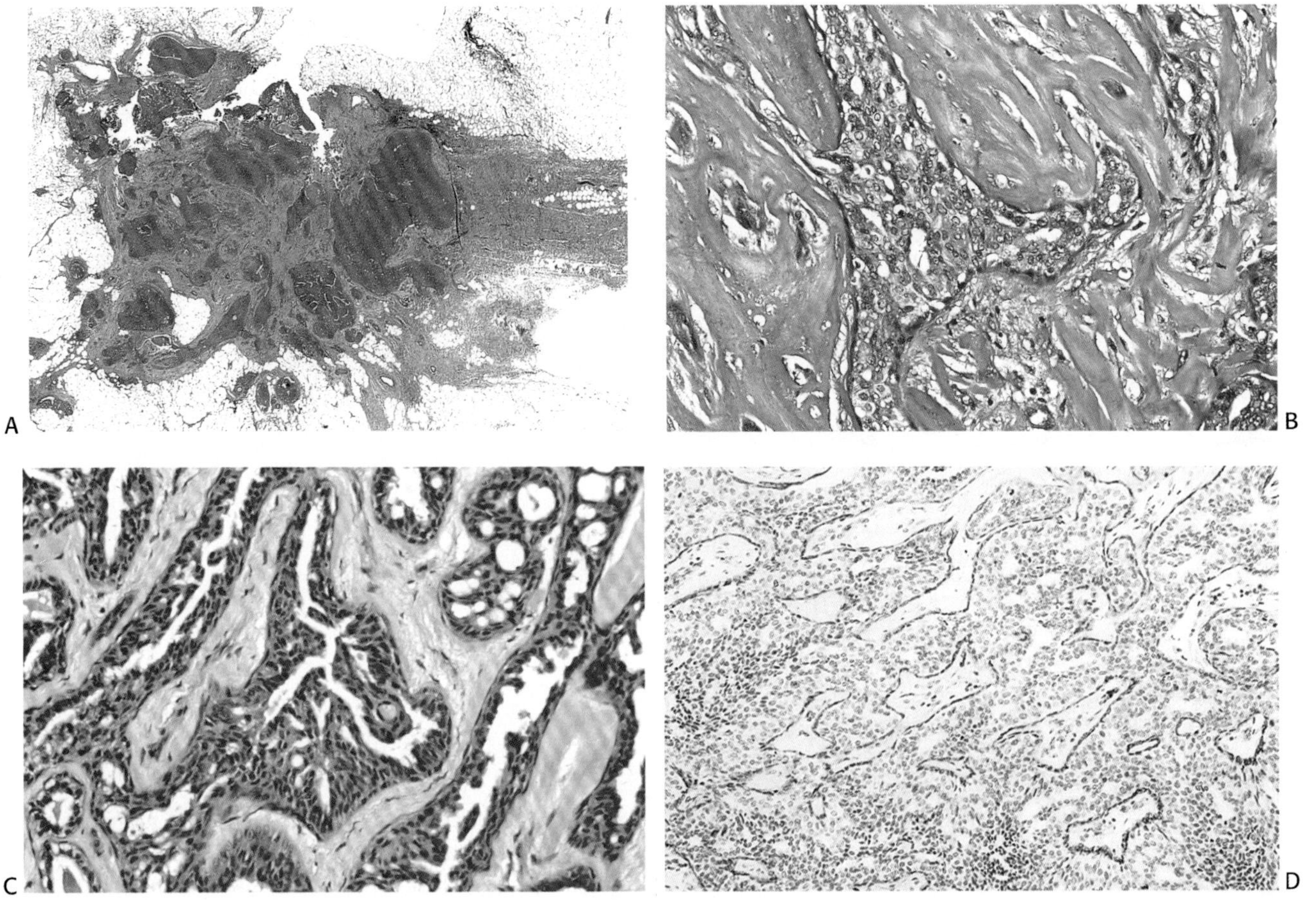

FIG. 5.30. ***Subareolar sclerosing duct hyperplasia.*** **A:** A whole-mount histologic section. The nipple is beyond the *right* border of the image. **B,C:** Foci of ductal hyperplasia with a prominent myoepithelial cell layer and stromal sclerosis. **D:** The intact myoepithelial cell layer, highlighted with the SMM-HC immunostain, outlines the epithelium.

Haagensen[142] reported finding apocrine metaplasia in 78% of 1,169 biopsies performed for gross cystic disease.

Other palpable benign tumors composed of apocrine epithelium are generally divided into two groups: adenomas and papillomas. The distinction between these diagnostic categories is not clear, because illustrations of some lesions reported to be apocrine adenomas have shown a conspicuous papillary component.[143,144] These lesions present as firm, mobile circumscribed tumors that are clinically indistinguishable from their nonapocrine counterparts.

Microscopic foci of apocrine metaplasia are common in the female breast after age 30, and occasionally they may be found in younger women.[145,146] The frequency of microscopic apocrine change is highest in the fifth decade and continues to be greater after age 50 than in younger women, probably reflecting physiologic alterations associated with the menopause. However, there is no consistent increase or decrease in the occurrence of apocrine metaplasia with advancing age beyond 50 years.[145,146] One group of investigators reported that apocrine cysts were significantly more numerous in lower than in upper quadrants of breasts both with and without carcinoma.[145] Apocrine cysts and hyperplasia with apocrine metaplasia were more common in the breasts of American women in New York than in Japanese women in Tokyo.[147]

Gross Pathology

There are no specific gross features associated with apocrine metaplasia. Apocrine foci sometimes exhibit a brown color in the unfixed state (Fig. 5.8).

Microscopic Pathology

Mammary apocrine metaplasia is encountered most frequently in the epithelium of simple cysts. Cystic apocrine metaplasia is composed of flat and cuboidal cells, which may form a single layer or exhibit proliferative change resulting in isolated blunt papillae (Fig. 5.31). The cells are usually evenly spaced, and they contain round nuclei with homogeneous, moderately dense chromatin (Fig. 5.32). There typically is a single central nucleolus. A myoepithelial cell layer is usually readily apparent in cystic and papillary apocrine epithelium. Rarely, the myoepithelium may be inconspicuous

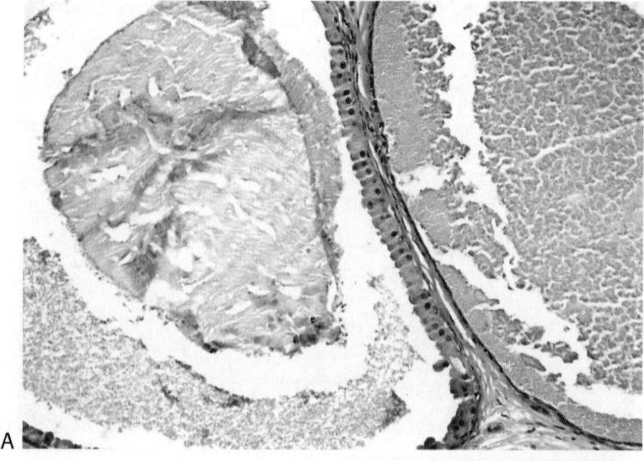

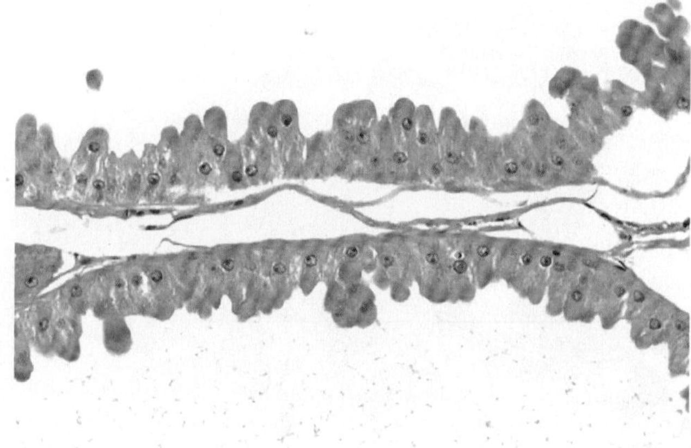

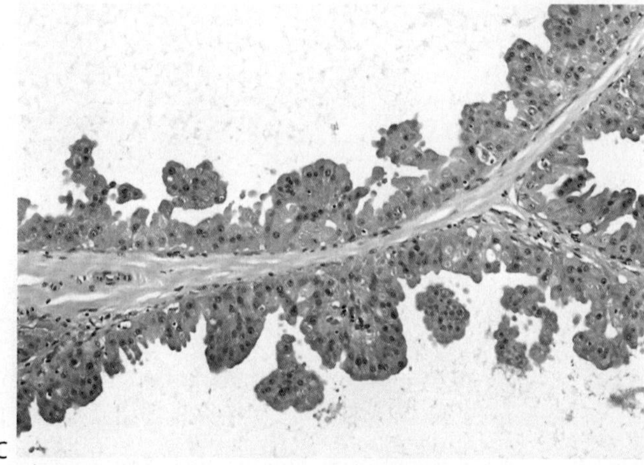

FIG. 5.31. ***Apocrine metaplasia, cystic.*** **A:** Adjacent cysts lined by cuboidal and flat apocrine epithelium. **B:** Minimal papillary hyperplasia of apocrine epithelium. **C:** Micropapillary apocrine hyperplasia in a cyst.

or focally absent in apocrine cysts.[148] Markers that stain the cytoplasm of myoepithelial cells such as calponin or CD10 and the nuclear stain, p63, demonstrate variable patterns of reactivity. This variation may be manifested in a number of ways, which were documented by Tramm et al.[148] These manifestations include increased internuclear distance between myoepithelial cells stained for p63, gaps between calponin immunoreactive myoepithelial cells, and large gaps between myoepithelial cells stained for both p63 and calponin. There were also rare instances in which large gaps were evident between calponin immunoreactive cells but not between cells stained for p63. On the other hand, a substantial number of cases demonstrated large gaps between p63-posistive cells and a continuous layer of cells reactive for calponin. It is clear from these data that any effort to investigate the extent of myoepithelium in apocrine breast lesions must include not only p63 staining but also staining with at least one cytokeratin cytoplasmic marker, an admonition that applies equally to breast tissues generally.

A slight degree of cellular crowding often results in a palisade organization of the epithelium, which may be more than one cell in depth, and florid papillary proliferation can produce more elaborate patterns of hyperplasia with a micropapillary or a branching, true papillary architecture. In extreme cases, this results in the formation of a papilloma composed entirely of apocrine epithelium (Fig. 5.33). Apocrine metaplasia can also be found focally in SA, complex FAs,[149] papillomas,[150] and other benign proliferative abnormalities, including gynecomastia. Nielsen[151] reported finding apocrine metaplasia in 63% of palpable adenosis tumors.

In its proliferative phase, apocrine metaplasia consists of cuboidal to tall columnar cells with eosinophilic cytoplasm. The nuclei are equal in size, round, and basally oriented. "Tufts" or "snouts" of epithelium protrude from the apical surface of the cell into the glandular lumen. The cytoplasm typically is finely granular and uniformly stained, but in rare instances associated with inflammation, coarse granules are conspicuous, possibly as a degenerative change. Metaplastic apocrine epithelium in cysts is prone to regressive changes that may lead to complete disappearance of these cells. This transition is marked by conversion of columnar and cuboidal apocrine epithelium to a flattened layer of cells, which may ultimately be shed into the cyst, leaving only a fibrous shell.

Papillary apocrine change is most often found in cystic apocrine metaplasia associated with other fibrocystic proliferative alterations. The apocrine epithelium is usually arranged in a micropapillary pattern composed of regularly spaced cytologically benign cells (Figs. 5.31 and 5.32). Fibrovascular stroma is absent from or only minimally

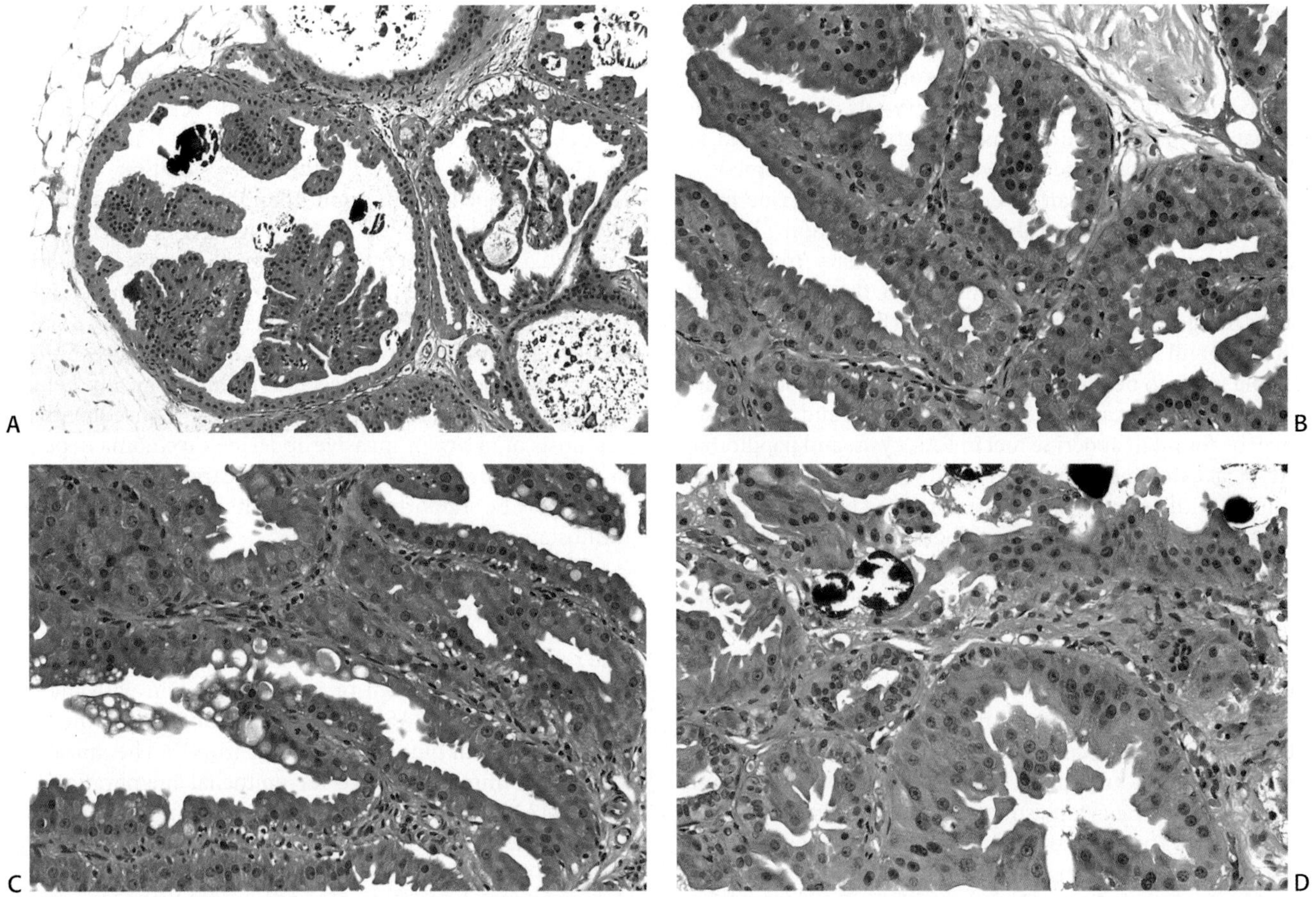

FIG. 5.32. ***Apocrine metaplasia, papillary.*** **A,B:** Complex cystic and papillary apocrine lesions with calcifications. The nuclei are uniform, small, evenly spaced, and generally equidistant from the basement membrane. **C:** Part of the lesion where cytoplasmic vacuoles are present. Nuclei are distributed uniformly and in a single layer. **D:** A focus of apocrine hyperplasia with calcifications. Note slight nuclear heterogeneity, micropapillary growth, multilayered epithelium, and loss of cell polarity with respect to the basement membrane. Images (B–D) are from a single lesion.

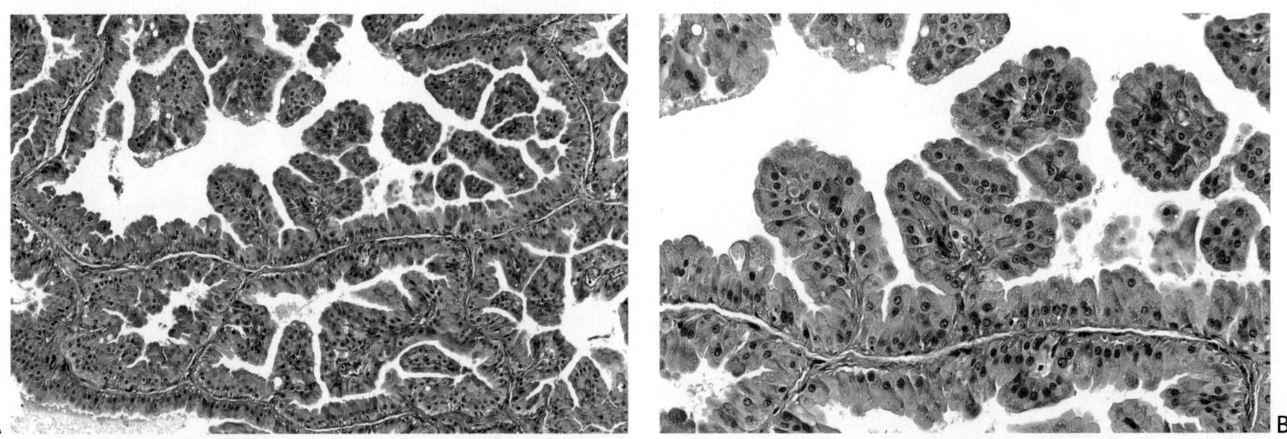

FIG. 5.33. ***Apocrine papilloma.*** **A:** Multiloculated focus of papillary apocrine metaplasia. **B:** Papillary frond with a fibrovascular core and surface epithelium composed of bland apocrine cells. Note the basal position of nuclei in the apocrine cells.

present in these epithelial fronds. Calcifications associated with cystic and papillary apocrine metaplasia may be coarse, basophilic, easily fractured particles of calcium hydroxyapatite or birefringent calcium oxalate crystals (Fig. 5.32). Foci of papillary apocrine metaplasia sometimes coexist with columnar cell lesions, and the two conditions may merge.[152]

Atypical changes can be encountered in apocrine metaplasia in virtually any proliferative configuration.[153] Architectural atypia consists of irregular papillary fronds with little or no stromal support in which the apocrine cells are arranged in a disordered fashion (Fig. 5.34). Epithelial bridges and cribriform areas may be present. Cytologic atypia tends to be more severe in the apocrine epithelium of sclerosing lesions such as SA (see Chapter 7) and RSLs, but it may be found in apocrine foci in FAs, cysts, and papillomas. Atypical cytologic features were present in 71% of adenosis tumors with apocrine metaplasia reported by Nielsen.[151]

Apocrine cells with mild cytologic atypia retain abundant granular eosinophilic cytoplasm and exhibit characteristic "decapitation secretion." Small clear cytoplasmic vacuoles may be found, especially in the nonbasal region of the cell. In comparison with regular apocrine metaplasia, the nuclei in mild apocrine atypia are not spaced at regular intervals, and they may not be basally oriented. Nucleoli are less uniform, they may be eccentric, and an occasional nucleus has more than one nucleolus. With the development of more severe atypia, the cytoplasm of individual cells becomes increasingly vacuolated or clear, and "decapitation" of cytoplasm at the luminal border is lost. Nuclear pleomorphism and hyperchromasia may become striking. Prominent pleomorphic nucleoli characterize the most atypical lesions. The nuclear-to-cytoplasmic ratio increases as apocrine metaplasia becomes more atypical, but the cells generally retain relatively abundant cytoplasm compared with those of nonapocrine epithelium.

When atypical apocrine metaplasia is present, the severity of the change is usually not homogeneous in a given lesion. Cysts and papillary duct hyperplasia, partly or entirely occupied by bland metaplastic apocrine epithelium, are usually found in the vicinity of atypical apocrine metaplasia. The distinction between atypical apocrine metaplasia and apocrine carcinoma is ordinarily not difficult, but this may be a challenging diagnostic problem in the limited sample of a needle core biopsy. In the latter situation, cytologic features may be less important than the growth pattern, especially in sclerosing lesions. A diagnosis of carcinoma is warranted in sclerosing lesions when the atypical apocrine proliferation has the configuration of one of the conventional forms of DCIS.[153] As discussed previously in this section, immunoreactive myoepithelium may be severely attenuated and even undetectable in histologically benign cystic and proliferative apocrine lesions. Consequently, a diagnosis of *in situ* or invasive apocrine carcinoma depends on the structural and cytological appearance of the lesion, which may be supported by the results of myoepithelial immunostains (see Chapter 19).

Immunohistochemistry

The refractile golden brown supranuclear granules that may be seen in the cytoplasm or in vacuoles stain with the periodic acid–Schiff (PAS) reaction, the Sudan black method, and the Prussian blue technique for iron.[140] The apical cytoplasm is immunoreactive for epithelial membrane antigen (EMA), and it stains diffusely with an antibody to gross cystic disease fluid protein-15 (GCDFP-15). The antibody also stains a proportion of normal mammary cells, so a positive reaction for GCDFP-15 does not establish the apocrine nature of a cell. Celis et al.[154] described two other markers, 15-hydroxyprostaglandin dehydrogenase and 3-hydroxymethylglutaryl-CoA reductase, which seem to stain only apocrine cells. Strong cytoplasmic immunohistochemical staining of apocrine cells with an antibody to prolactin has been reported,[155] and immunohistochemical staining reveals that the cytoplasm contains phosphatases, dehydrogenases, and other oxidative enzymes.[156]

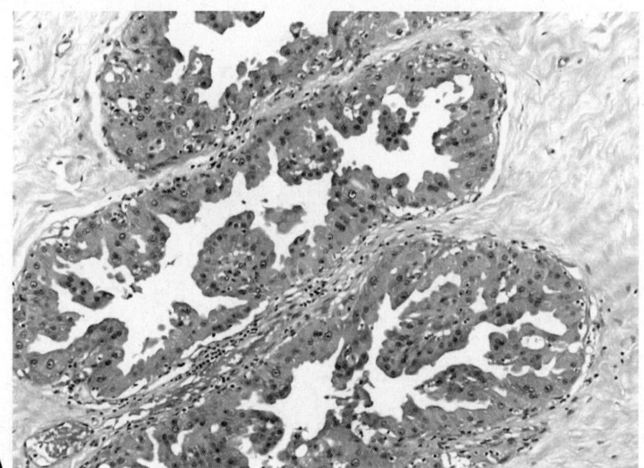
A

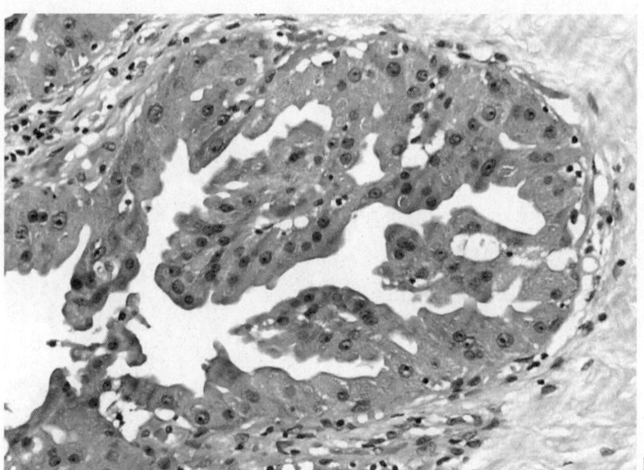
B

FIG. 5.34. ***Papillary apocrine metaplasia with mild atypia.*** **A:** Papillary and micropapillary duct hyperplasia. **B:** Magnified view of **(A)** with atypia manifested by irregular positioning of enlarged nuclei with prominent nucleoli.

Apocrine cells typically do not stain for ER or progesterone receptor (PR), but they consistently stain for androgen receptor (AR).[157–159] Two reports[160,161] described staining for human epidermal growth factor 2 (HER2) along the basal and lateral cell membranes, and one publication described weak staining for epidermal growth factor receptor.[160]

Studies of proliferation of conventional apocrine cells have found Ki67 scores in the range of 0.7%[160,162] to 1.3%,[161] values similar to those of normal mammary cells. Apocrine cells in SA and those growing in papillary configurations have slightly higher proliferative rates (1.5% to 6.6%)[161–163] with higher values associated with atypical apocrine cells. Apocrine cells in all settings show a low apoptotic index.[162] They do not stain for *Bcl-2*,[157,159–161] but they do express other apoptosis-regulating proteins (Bax, Bak, Bcl-x, Bcl-x_L, and Mcl-1).[161,162]

Apocrine cells growing in papillary formations can show alterations in the expression of cell-cycle regulatory proteins such as increased expression of cyclin D1 and p21 and decreased expression of p27.[163] Overexpression of cyclin D1 does not seem to result from gene amplification.[164] Apocrine cells stained for retinoblastoma (Rb) protein and did not stain for p16; the cells in a few cases overexpressed cyclin A.[163]

Apocrine cells tend to stain for c-myc oncoprotein,[161,165,166] but they do not demonstrate amplification of the *c-myc* gene.[166] Significant association between staining for c-myc and Ki67 has been described.[166] In one study, apocrine cells stained for the ras oncoprotein.[165] Only rare apocrine cells demonstrated staining for p53.[157,161]

Genetic Studies

The cytologic changes observed in apocrine metaplasia and apocrine atypia are reflected in the altered DNA content of these cells. Izuo et al.[167] studied apocrine metaplasia by microspectrophotometric measurement of Feulgen-stained paraffin sections. Cutaneous apocrine glands from the vulva used as controls had a diploid DNA content. Although the majority of cells in samples of mammary apocrine metaplasia were diploid, a subset of tetraploid nuclei was found in all specimens. The proportion of tetraploid cells was related to the amount and severity of atypia in the apocrine lesion. One aneuploid lesion reported to exhibit high-grade atypia appears to be an orderly papillary apocrine carcinoma in the authors' illustration. This patient was found to have an invasive mammary carcinoma of unspecified histologic type 2.5 years after the lesion described as apocrine atypia was biopsied. In another investigation,[168] conventional apocrine cells demonstrated DNA indices between 0.9 and 1.1, whereas 2 of 10 cases demonstrating nuclear atypia contained aneuploid stemlines with DNA indices of 1.23 and 1.26. In the study of Elzagheid et al.[169] conventional apocrine cells showed a dominant peak in the diploid region with hyperdiploid and hypodiploid peaks in many cases. The frequency of these other peaks varied with the method of preparation.

Three studies indicate that apocrine cells harbor genetic alterations. In the investigation by Washington et al.,[170] 53% of foci of apocrine metaplasia demonstrated loss of heterozygosity (LOH) at 14 polymorphic loci representing seven chromosomal arms, whereas only approximately 20% of normal lobules and foci showing either adenosis or UDH manifested LOH at the same loci. The authors did not describe the pattern of growth of the apocrine cells. Selim et al.[171] tested examples of both flat and papillary apocrine metaplasia for LOH and allelic imbalance at loci associated with breast carcinomas and discovered that 8 of 41 cases showed LOH or allelic imbalance. Jones et al.[172] used comparative genomic hybridization to search for genetic alterations in papillary apocrine hyperplasia and associated carcinomas. Seven of ten cases of papillary apocrine hyperplasia displayed regions of copy number changes. The most common were losses at 1p, 17q and 22q, and gains at 2q and 13q. Alterations occurred more frequently in coexisting carcinomas, but they often involved the same regions, as well as others. These findings hint at the possibility that proliferative forms of apocrine metaplasia may represent foci of genetic instability that have the potential to evolve into neoplastic proliferations.

Electron Microscopy

Ultrastructural study reveals that the cells in cystic and papillary apocrine metaplasia resemble the cells of normal apocrine glands.[137,140,150,156] Mammary apocrine cells contain numerous mitochondria of variable size and shape, containing sparse, thin, incomplete cristae; abundant endoplasmic reticulum; complex folding of the plasma membrane; short microvilli; and membrane-bound dense lysosomal granules. There is a well-developed Golgi region typically located between the nucleus and the apex of the cell. Junctional complexes are present between adjacent cells.

Treatment and Prognosis

The relationship of apocrine metaplasia to the development of mammary carcinoma is uncertain. In most instances, apocrine metaplasia appears to be part of the fibrocystic complex manifested in cysts with simple or papillary epithelium or as a component of ordinary duct hyperplasia. Cytological and architectural atypia are uncommon in apocrine metaplasia and usually occur in sclerosing proliferative lesions such as adenosis or papilloma, often with a radial scar or adenosis tumor configuration.

Several investigators have reported that they did not find significant differences in the frequency of apocrine metaplasia when breasts with and without carcinoma were compared. In one of the earliest studies, Dawson[173] examined whole sections from 120 carcinomatous breasts and 48 breasts without carcinoma. Apocrine metaplasia was detected in all but 4 of the 168 specimens, leading to the conclusion that apocrine change was not associated with the development of carcinoma. A similar study of "cancerous and noncancerous breasts" was described in 1945 by Foote and Stewart.[174] They observed that apocrine metaplasia was often present in breasts with other "noncancerous proliferative lesions," but found no significant difference in the frequency of apocrine metaplasia between "cancerous and noncancerous breasts."

Although the foregoing anatomic studies of apocrine metaplasia have not shown an association between the frequency of apocrine metaplasia and concurrent carcinoma, some follow-up studies have suggested that apocrine metaplasia may be a predictor for the subsequent development of carcinoma. Haagensen et al.[142] reported a 10-fold greater frequency of carcinoma in women who had apocrine metaplasia in a prior biopsy compared with those in whom apocrine change was absent. The majority of the subsequent carcinomas had "apocrine features," but an origin to apocrine metaplasia was rarely traceable. When compared with Connecticut state incidence figures, patients with apocrine metaplasia had 3.5 times the expected frequency of carcinoma, whereas the risk was only 0.3 times expected when apocrine metaplasia was absent.

A slight overall increase in the number of subsequent carcinomas was observed by Page et al.[175] in women with papillary apocrine change in an antecedent biopsy compared with the expected number of carcinomas based on an age-matched comparison with the Third National Cancer survey. The difference was statistically significant only in women who were older than 45 years when the apocrine lesion was detected. There was also an increased risk in this age group when apocrine metaplasia occurred in duct hyperplasia, but the difference was not statistically significant. A subsequent study by Page et al.[176] confirmed the latter observation, and they concluded that "when characteristic apocrine-type nuclei are present in fairly complex patterns of hyperplasia, they do not represent a worrisome lesion or a reliable risk indicator, particularly if confined to small clusters of cysts or glands."

The precancerous risk of papillary apocrine change depends largely on its association with other proliferative lesions.[177] When compared with a control population, the RR for carcinoma in women who had any type of papillary apocrine change unassociated with atypical hyperplasia was 1.2, and for those with the highly complex type it was 2.4. Neither RR indicated a statistically significant increase in predisposition to develop carcinoma beyond that attributable to concurrent nonapocrine proliferative changes. Tóth et al.[168] reported that atypical duct hyperplasia was present more frequently in breasts with apocrine metaplasia than in those without apocrine change. This effect was seen with simple cysts alone, but it was strongest in association with papillary apocrine cysts.

Histologic evidence of transitions from apocrine metaplasia to apocrine carcinoma has been described. Yates and Ahmed[178] reported a case in which a biopsy showing "florid apocrine metaplasia intermingled with atypical apocrine cells" was followed 19 months later by the finding of a 2.5-cm tumor composed of apocrine carcinoma. Haagensen et al.[142] reported that he had "traced the transformation of benign apocrine metaplasia into apocrine carcinoma in a considerable number of cases." Florid apocrine metaplasia with atypia often coexists with apocrine carcinoma,[179] but very few examples of apocrine carcinoma have been traced to atypical apocrine lesions, and most patients with atypical apocrine hyperplasia have remained well with short-term follow-up.[153]

When carcinoma arises in the opposite breast of a patient with apocrine atypia or apocrine carcinoma, the contralateral carcinoma is not necessarily apocrine.

Specific treatment is not indicated for proliferative lesions with apocrine metaplasia. Most cysts with metaplastic apocrine epithelium collapse and do not re-form after aspiration. The shed epithelium is readily recognized in a cytologic preparation of the fluid. Surgical excision of apocrine cysts is not indicated unless the fluid is bloody, the cysts re-form, or there is atypia in the cytologic specimen. Follow-up of women with breast biopsies that exhibit apocrine metaplasia depends on the overall findings in the specimen and clinical circumstances. Patients with atypical apocrine metaplasia require clinical evaluation comparable to that of women with other atypical proliferative lesions, and the precancerous significance of this abnormality remains uncertain.

FLORID PAPILLOMATOSIS OF THE NIPPLE

Historical Note

Florid papillomatosis of the nipple may have been described as early as 1923 by Miller and Lewis,[180] but the authors provided only a photograph of the gross specimen, which is not diagnostic without histopathologic confirmation. Stowers[181] illustrated an example of florid papillomatosis in 1935. An excellent low-magnification photograph was published in a paper by Haagensen et al.[182] on papillary tumors in 1951. They offered the following commentary:

> In rare cases the papilloma is situated within the portion of a duct traversing the nipple. In this location it may be palpable as a thickening within the nipple, or it may present through the dilated orifice of the duct as a friable granulating lesion... In the intraductal papillary tumor involving the orifice of a nipple duct... the original duct wall has almost disappeared, leaving the epithelial proliferations in a mass of scar tissue suggesting the infiltrative growth of cancer.

It was not until 1955, when Jones[183] published a series of five cases, that the lesion was established as a distinct clinicopathologic entity. Jones reported that "Frank W. Foote has seen three of the most exuberant of these cases and states, 'I think all your cases show a lesion that for many years has been designated in the laboratory as terminal duct papillomatosis.'"

As Jones observed, the growth patterns seen in florid papillomatosis are not specific for this condition. Similar or identical proliferative lesions can be found elsewhere in the breast. However, growth within the nipple produces an unusual clinicopathologic constellation, which may include any or all of the following: erosion of the nipple surface with replacement of the epidermis by glandular epithelium, inflammatory changes, and enlargement of the nipple by a firm tumor mass.

Terminology

The literature is replete with alternative names. Before the lesion was well characterized, Stewart used the terms "adenoma" or "papillomatosis" at various times. Handley and Thackray[184] preferred designating the tumor "adenoma of the nipple." They pointed to the absence of papillary components in some lesions and observed that "the lesion does not in the least resemble either macroscopically or microscopically a typical duct papilloma." They concluded that the lesion resembles an adenoma of sweat gland origin and suggested that it arises as a result of a developmental abnormality of the nipple. Gros and colleagues[185] reached a similar conclusion and recommended the name "l'adénomatose érosive." Perzin and Lattes[186] concluded that the main feature of the lesion is a papillary proliferation when they commented that "in reality, they are essentially composed of an adenomatous proliferation of ductal epithelium with more or less conspicuous papillary foci." They urged that the name "papillary adenoma" be adopted.

None of these other terms is an improvement on the name proposed by Jones, and in some respects the alternatives may be misleading. The term *adenoma* has been applied to a lesion resembling syringoma of the skin.[187–189] Foci of syringomatous differentiation may be associated with florid papillomatosis, but syringomatous adenomas lack the papillary features seen in most examples of florid papillomatosis. Seizing upon the adenomatous feature of a minority of the lesions to justify the term *adenoma* for all cases is no more satisfactory than the original term *florid papillomatosis*, which recognizes duct hyperplasia as the dominant feature in most cases.

Clinical Presentation

Florid papillomatosis occurs only rarely. Perzin and Lattes[186] collected 38 cases from a group of 305,000 surgical specimens, a frequency of 0.0125%, and the lesion was estimated to occur in 1 of 40,000 skin biopsy specimens (0.0025%).[190] Microscopic examination of nipples from mastectomy specimens resected because of breast carcinoma revealed the lesion in 12 of 967 cases (1.24%),[191] which suggests that florid papillomatosis usually exists in a subclinical state.

Approximately one-third of patients were 40 to 50 years old when florid papillomatosis of the nipple was diagnosed,[183–186,192–194] but the reported age at diagnosis ranges from birth[189] to 89 years.[189,190] Approximately 15% of patients were younger than 35, and an equal proportion were older than 65 years. Only a few cases have been reported in adolescents[195–200] and infants.[201] There has not been a predilection for either breast. Bilateral florid papillomatosis is extremely uncommon.[184,202,203] Shioi et al.[204] reported a case of florid papillomatosis arising in breast tissue of the right axilla of an 82-year-old woman. Shinn et al.[205] described a similar case involving the left axilla of a 33-year-old woman and cited four reports of florid papillomatosis involving accessory mammary tissue. In one of the cited cases,[206] the lesion arose in the vicinity of a supernumerary areola but was not connected to it.

Florid papillomatosis of the nipple does not affect men commonly. Three reports appeared in 1965,[197,207,208] and approximately a dozen additional cases were published thereafter. Fernandez-Flores and Suarez-Peñaranda[209] list many of the reports purporting to document florid papillomatosis in men published before 2010. The age at diagnosis ranged from 21[209] to 83 years.[210] The latter man developed florid papillomatosis after receiving diethylstilbestrol over a 10-year period to treat prostatic carcinoma.[210] Since the report of Fernandez-Flores and Suarez-Peñaranda, three additional cases have been described[211–213] ; however, the diagnosis of florid papillomatosis in two of these reports is open to question. One lesion classified as "florid papillomatosis of the male nipple"[213] was a cystic papillary neoplasm, probably a papilloma, in which myoepithelial cells were reportedly demonstrated with stains for "calponin and muscle actin." On the basis of the published photographs in the second case,[212] the lesion appears to have been papillary DCIS involving the nipple rather than DCIS coexisting with florid papillomatosis.

In most cases of florid papillomatosis, the nodules were present for no more than a few months before the patients sought medical attention. However, there are instances on record in which the lesion was reportedly present for 10,[190,192,214] 11,[184] 14,[193] 15,[214] and 20[186] years. The most frequent presenting symptom is discharge, often described as bloody. Pain, itching, or burning sensations are not unusual. Symptoms may worsen late in the menstrual cycle.[184] Small lesions may not cause nipple enlargement, and in these cases palpation usually reveals thickening of the nipple but no discrete mass. In many instances, the nipple appears enlarged, and a mass can be palpated. The surface of the nipple may appear granular, ulcerated, reddened, warty, or crusted. Often these symptoms and clinical findings are mistaken for Paget disease, or the patient is thought to have a papilloma. In most series, florid papillomatosis was rarely considered clinically in the differential diagnosis. There is presently no evidence to indicate that florid papillomatosis is associated with a positive family history or other risk factors for breast carcinoma. However, data on this subject have been incomplete in most studies.

Imaging Studies

Radiologic studies will usually reveal the presence of a mass. The small size and the location within the nipple make it difficult to detect many examples using mammography. Nodules on mammograms typically appear well defined and smoothly contoured,[215,216] but they can also appear ill defined.[217] Sonograms most often reveal a well-defined hypoechoic mass with posterior echo enhancement,[215,216,218] and lateral shadowing may occur. Exceptional cases display irregular contours, lack of sound enhancement, and absence of shadowing. The imaging of such cases can suggest a diagnosis of carcinoma.[217] Increased flow associated with the nodule can be seen with Doppler studies.[218] MRI of three cases[215,216,219] displayed the masses on T1-weighted images, but the findings on T2-weighted images and the dynamic studies varied.

Gross and Microscopic Pathology

Most pathologists who have studied this condition have commented on its heterogeneous histologic features. However, the lesions can be grouped into four categories according to histologic growth pattern. In three subtypes, one structural feature dominates the lesion or is present exclusively, whereas the fourth group consists of tumors with mixed patterns. No prognostic significance can be attached to these subtypes, and there is no evidence that they differ in pathogenesis. Some clinicopathologic correlations have been noted with these categories, and it may be helpful to bear them in mind when faced with a proliferative lesion of the nipple.

1. *Sclerosing papillomatosis pattern.* This lesion typically presents as a discrete tumor. Scaling of the nipple skin may occur, but redness, ulceration, and inflammation are rarely present. About 50% of the patients have nipple discharge that is serous rather than bloody. The preoperative diagnosis is usually papilloma rather than Paget disease or carcinoma.

   Grossly, the nipple contains a firm tumor on palpation, although the margins may not appear well defined. The epidermis may look thickened, white, and scaly. Histologically, the lesion is indistinguishable in many respects from a sclerosing papilloma elsewhere in the breast (Fig. 5.35). Exuberant papillary hyperplasia of ductal epithelium is distorted by an accompanying stromal proliferation within and around the affected ducts. The complex proliferative process is arranged in papillary, solid, tubular, and glandular structures. Foci of myoepithelial cell hyperplasia can usually be identified, but as is generally the case with sclerosing papillary lesions, myoepithelial cells may be inconspicuous or absent in parts of the tumor (Fig. 5.36).

   These lesions exhibit some qualitative and quantitative microscopic differences from the other subtypes of florid papillomatosis. The overlying cutaneous squamous epithelium is usually intact and hyperplastic. Squamous cysts are commonly formed in the terminal portions of lactiferous ducts. Focal comedo-type necrosis may be found in the hyperplastic duct epithelium, sometimes associated with infrequent mitoses in epithelial cells (Fig. 5.36C). Apocrine metaplasia and extension of glandular epithelium to the nipple surface are uncommon and not prominent when present.
2. *Papillomatosis pattern.* Many of these patients complain of bleeding from the nipple. Clinical examination reveals a palpable lesion, which is often described as an induration rather than as a discrete mass (Fig. 5.37). The nipple usually appears ulcerated or inflamed, and the clinical diagnosis of Paget disease or carcinoma is likely.

   A discrete area of induration is evident grossly within the nipple, often extending to the skin surface. Microscopic examination reveals florid papillary hyperplasia of ductal epithelium causing expansion and crowding of the affected ducts (Fig. 5.38). Focal epithelial necrosis and scattered mitotic figures may be found. These tumors lack the stromal proliferation that characterizes the sclerosing papillomatosis type of lesion. Hyperplastic glandular tissue may replace the overlying squamous epithelium over part or all of the apical skin surface of the nipple. Squamous-lined cysts and apocrine metaplasia are not prominent in these lesions.
3. *Adenosis pattern.* These patients may have bloody or serous discharge. One patient had nipple retraction. The lesion produces a discrete nodule within the nipple. The nipple may appear ulcerated, inflamed, and swollen, and the epidermis is usually hyperplastic and intact. The clinical diagnosis is more often papilloma or some other benign lesion rather than Paget disease. Microscopically, the lesion consists of crowded, orderly glandular structures arranged in a pattern that resembles an adenosis tumor in the breast parenchyma (Fig. 5.39). Myoepithelial hyperplasia accompanies the epithelial proliferation. Apocrine metaplasia, hyperplasia of the squamous epithelium, and superficial squamous cysts are rarely present. Mitotic figures and focal necrosis are uncommon.
4. *Mixed proliferative pattern.* Patients with this type of florid papillomatosis may report a variety of symptoms, including scaling, bleeding, pain, burning, and ulceration. Examination usually reveals a mass or nodule in the nipple, and the surface typically appears eroded. The clinical diagnosis is often carcinoma or Paget disease. Microscopic examination reveals varying combinations of the other three patterns (Fig. 5.40). Prominent features present in most cases include superficial squamous metaplasia of ducts with cyst formation, apocrine metaplasia, and acanthosis of the overlying epithelium. Hyperplastic duct epithelium may extend to the nipple surface, accounting for the impression of ulceration. Cystic dilation of ducts is not uncommon near the deep margin of the lesion, where this feature is interspersed with foci of duct hyperplasia. Focal necrosis may be found in duct epithelium. Mitotic activity is minimal. Adenosis occurs in about one-third of these lesions. Rarely, foci with a syringomatous pattern may be found at the edge of the lesion.

Cytology

The diagnosis of florid papillomatosis may be suggested by the cytologic findings in a scraping from the nipple surface.[217,220] FNA yields a cellular specimen containing variable proportions of glandular and myoepithelial cells arranged singly, in clusters, and in sheets or papillary groups.[220–224] In certain respects, the smears resemble those from FAs and papillomas.[224] Apocrine cells, stromal fragments, scant cellular debris, inflammatory cells, and hemosiderin-laden macrophages may be present. The epithelial cells appear uniform, and they contain uniform round or oval nuclei, fine chromatin, and inconspicuous nucleoli. Mitotic figures are not common. Occasional cells can demonstrate slight

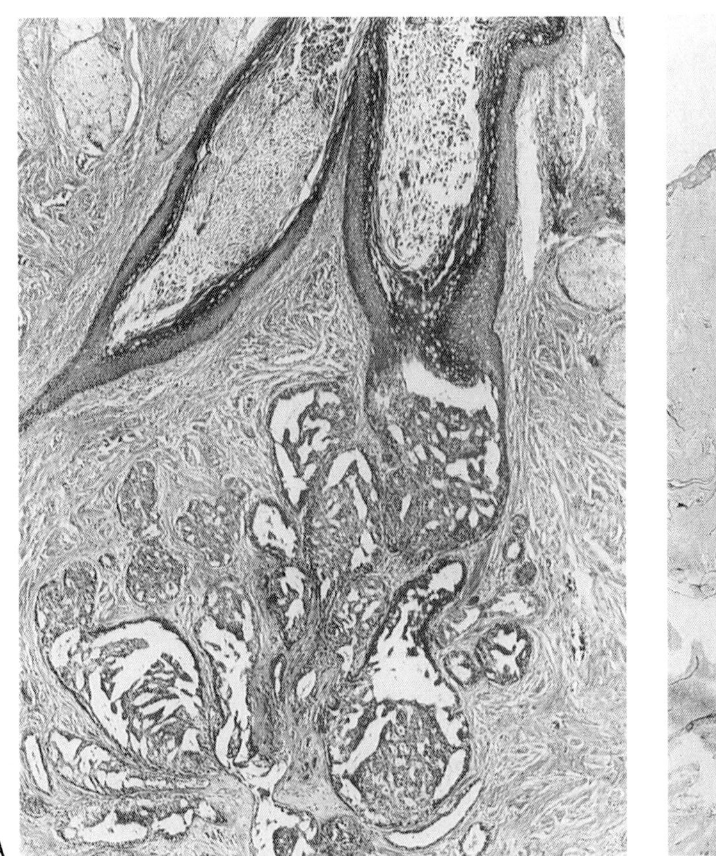

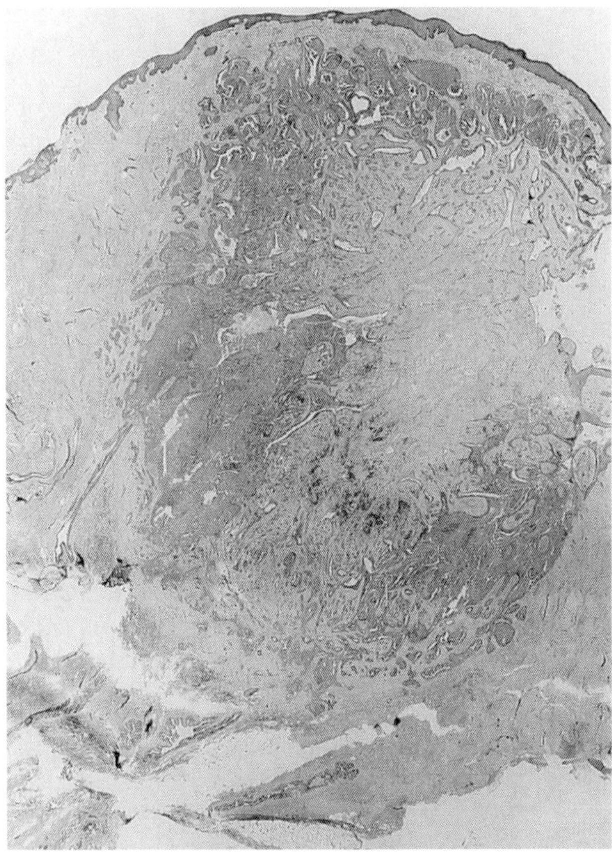

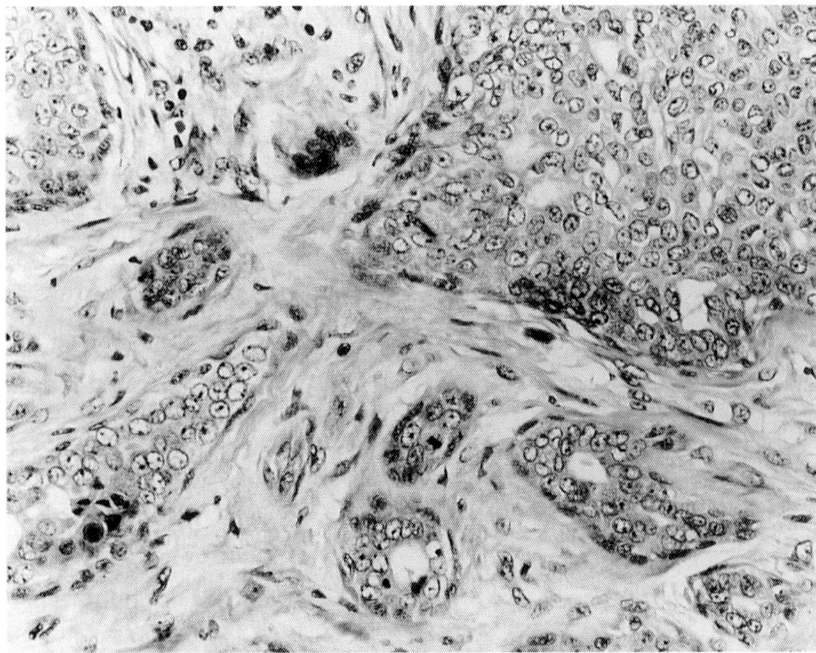

FIG. 5.35. ***Florid papillomatosis, sclerosing papilloma pattern.*** **A:** An early lesion at the squamocolumnar junction of a lactiferous duct and the epidermis. An early phase in the formation of a sclerotic center is evident near the lower border. **B:** Whole-mount histologic section of the nipple lesion with a central area of fibrosis. The irregular border on the *right* is the site of erosion and a prior biopsy. **C:** Ductal hyperplasia and proliferative stroma. (Reproduced from Rosen PP, Caicco JA. Florid papillomatosis of the nipple: a study of 51 patients, including nine having mammary carcinoma. *Am J Surg Pathol* 1986;10:87–101, with permission.)

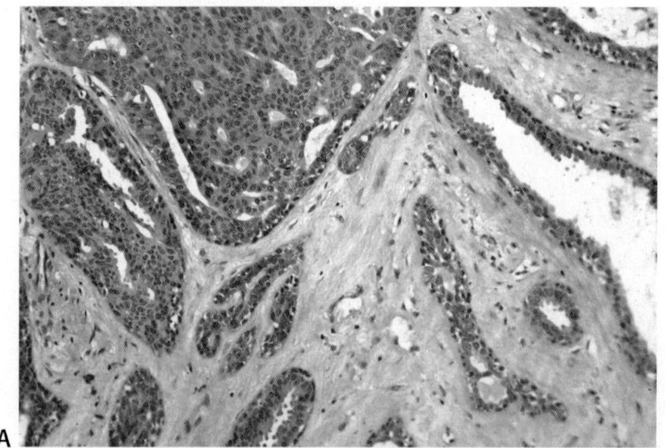

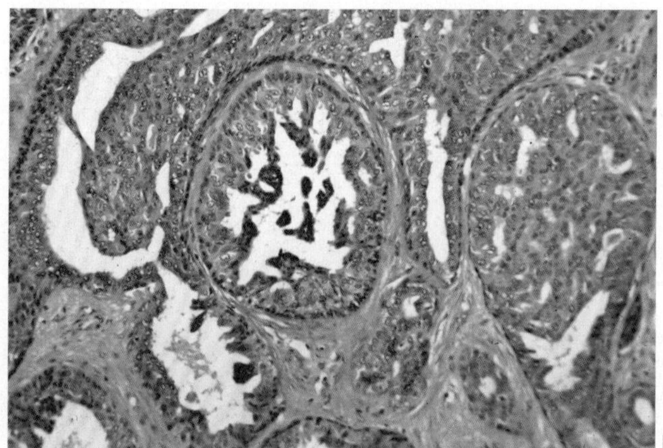

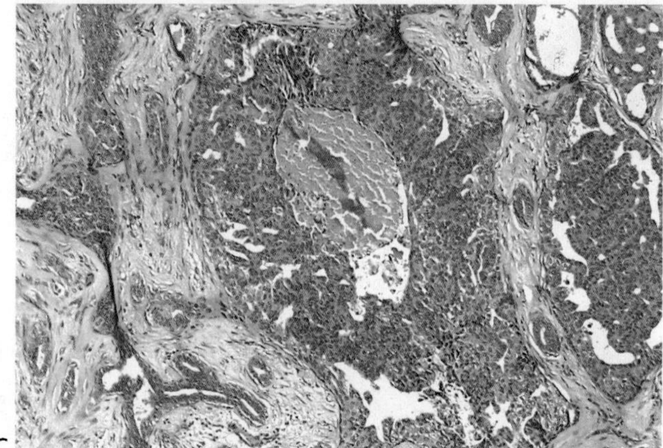

FIG. 5.36. ***Florid papillomatosis, sclerosing papilloma pattern.*** **A,B:** Two foci of florid epithelial hyperplasia with a prominent myoepithelial layer. The sclerotic core is near the *right* border in **(A)**. Micropapillary hyperplasia is shown in **(B)**. **C:** Another lesion with epithelial necrosis.

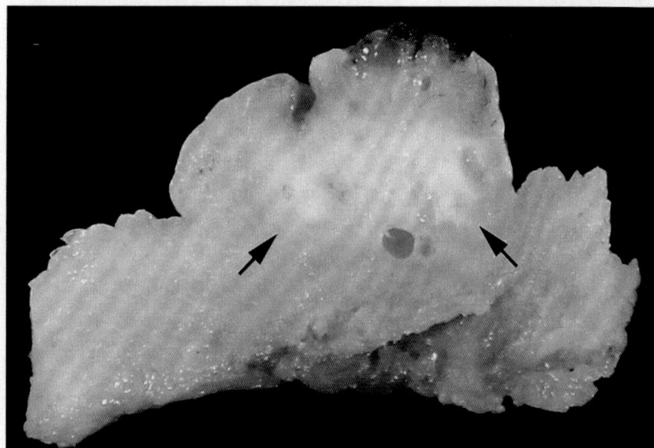

FIG. 5.37. ***Florid papillomatosis of the nipple, papilloma pattern.*** An ill-defined white mass (*arrows*) with small cysts expands the nipple and ulcerates the skin at the tip of the nipple.

pleomorphism or nuclear hyperchromasia.[225] In the setting of a hypercellular smear showing dyshesion and clustering of epithelial cells, the aspiration specimen can be misinterpreted as carcinoma.[217,226]

Immunohistochemistry

Several studies described the results of immunohistochemical staining of cases of florid papillomatosis.[209,213,220,227–229] Although the findings vary somewhat, they present a coherent picture. The cells lining the glands stain for molecules characteristic of luminal cells such as EMA, CK18 (CAM5.2), and MUC1, whereas the cells at the periphery of the glands contain proteins found in myoepithelial cells such as smooth muscle actin (SMA), calponin, and p63. Staining for CK7, keratin AE1/3, S-100, GCDFP-15, and carcinoembryonic antigen (CEA) has yielded variable results. In one case,[209] the epithelial cells stained for keratin 34βE12 but did not stain for CK20. In several examples,[213,220] the cells did not stain for ER, PR, or HER2, and in one case,[209] they failed to stain for AR.

Ki67 stains have yielded values between 2% and 5% in one study[209] and 7.4% in another.[220] The case of Kono et al.[228] demonstrated a geographic variation in the Ki67 index: cells in the deep region had a score of 0.7%, those in the center a score of 6.5%, and those in the superficial region a score of 20.3%.

Two examples of florid papillomatosis studied by flow cytometry[229] proved to be diploid with relatively high SPFs (10.9% and 34.4%), values similar to those found in cases of DCIS (6.4% to 15.8%) included in this investigation.

Electron Microscopy

Electron microscopic study of a single case[229] confirmed the presence of both epithelial and myoepithelial cells. The columnar epithelial cells displayed basal nuclei and apical microvilli. Intercellular connections including junctional complexes joined neighboring cells, and the lucent cytoplasm of the epithelial cells contained scattered organelles. Light and dark myoepithelial cells enclosed the epithelial cells and abutted a continuous basal lamina. The bipolar spindled myoepithelial cells contained abundant endoplasmic reticulum and parallel bundles of intermediate filaments with dense bodies. Scattered junctions were present between myoepithelial cells and epithelial cells, and focal subplasmalemmal densities and widely spaced pinocytotic vesicles were also noted.

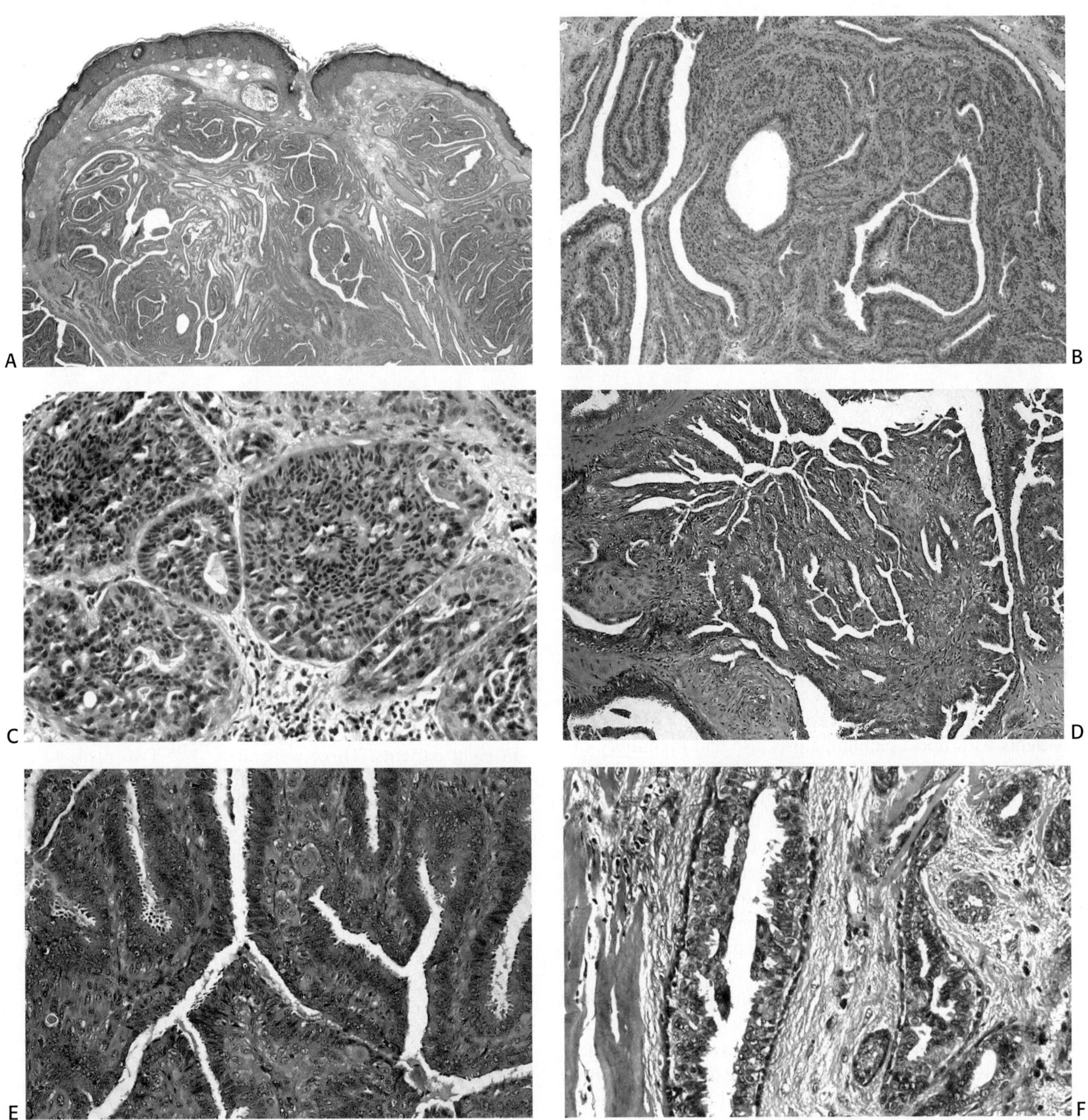

FIG. 5.38. ***Florid papillomatosis, papilloma pattern.*** **A,B:** A papilloma involving lactiferous ducts in the nipple is shown in an excisional biopsy specimen. **C:** Florid ductal hyperplasia with streaming of epithelial cell nuclei in cribriform hyperplasia. **D:** Foci of squamous metaplasia are present in papillary epithelium. **E:** Hyperplasia of epithelial and epithelioid myoepithelial cells. **F:** Micropapillary duct hyperplasia and myoepithelial hyperplasia. **G:** Papillary hyperplasia extends to the lactiferous duct orifice. **H:** Erosion of the epidermis caused by papillary hyperplasia.

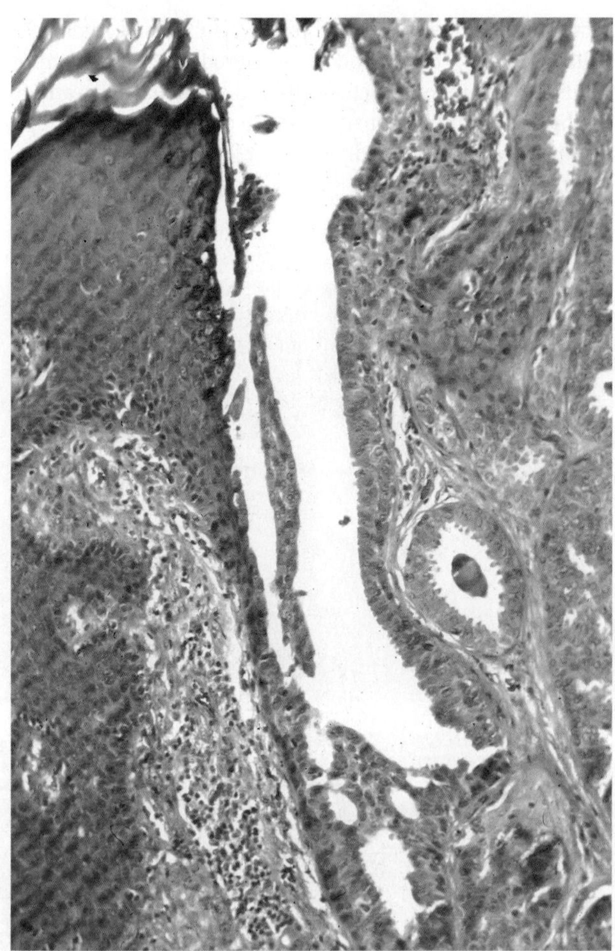

G

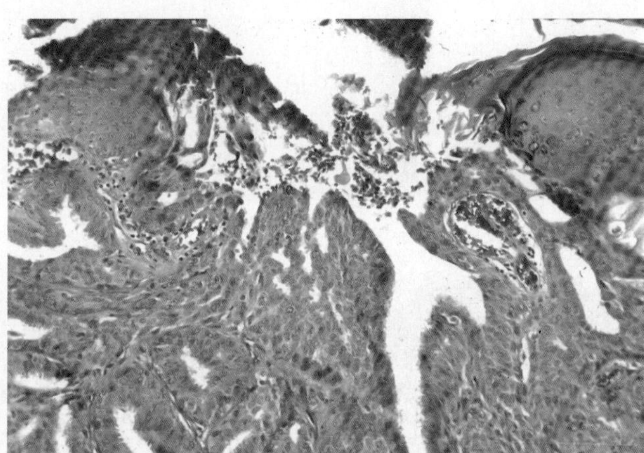

H

FIG. 5.38. *(Continued)*

Relationship to Carcinoma

A review of the literature revealed that 37 of 224 (16.5%) patients with florid papillomatosis also had mammary carcinoma.[214] Nineteen of the 37 patients had carcinoma that arose coincidentally but separately in the same breast. This association is not surprising, since florid papillomatosis of the nipple was reportedly found in 1.2% (12 of 967) of the nipples studied in a review of mastectomy specimens from patients with breast carcinoma.[191] To the extent that they have been described, these coincidental carcinomas have largely been of the ductal variety. One patient had a separate invasive lobular carcinoma.[230]

There were three other reported patients who developed carcinoma in a breast from which florid papillomatosis had been excised previously. One woman was found to have DCIS 10 years later. At mastectomy, she did not have florid papillomatosis of the nipple, and the ALNs were negative. Two years later, she remained well. In another patient, infiltrating ductal carcinoma with metastases in ALNs developed 17 years after resection of a "papillary adenoma."[186] The nipple had no residual papillomatosis. Four years later, she had pulmonary metastases. The third patient was 44 years old when she developed invasive ductal carcinoma with axillary metastases 3 years after excision of florid papillomatosis from the ipsilateral nipple.[214]

Carcinoma arose directly from florid papillomatosis in eight patients. Three were men.[207,214] Two men, 43 and 53 years old, had DCIS arising in florid papillomatosis that was confined to the nipple. Both exhibited nipple enlargement and bloody discharge. Hyperpigmentation of the nipple was evident in one case. Paget disease was seen in the overlying epidermis, and neither patient had evidence of invasive carcinoma (Fig. 5.41). Melanin pigment was present in Paget cells in the patient with hyperpigmentation. Neither mastectomy specimen contained residual carcinoma, nor did the ALNs contain metastatic tumor. One of these men had concurrent contralateral DCIS, which was also treated by mastectomy. The third man, 66 years old, presented with scaling and itching of an enlarged nipple that contained a mass. Examination revealed bilateral gynecomastia. Biopsy yielded a 1.8-cm invasive duct carcinoma arising from florid papillomatosis in the nipple. The overlying nipple epidermis exhibited Paget disease. The remainder of the breast had only gynecomastia, and the ALNs were free of metastases. The patient was well 136 months later. Two other cases purporting to describe carcinoma arising in florid papillomatosis in

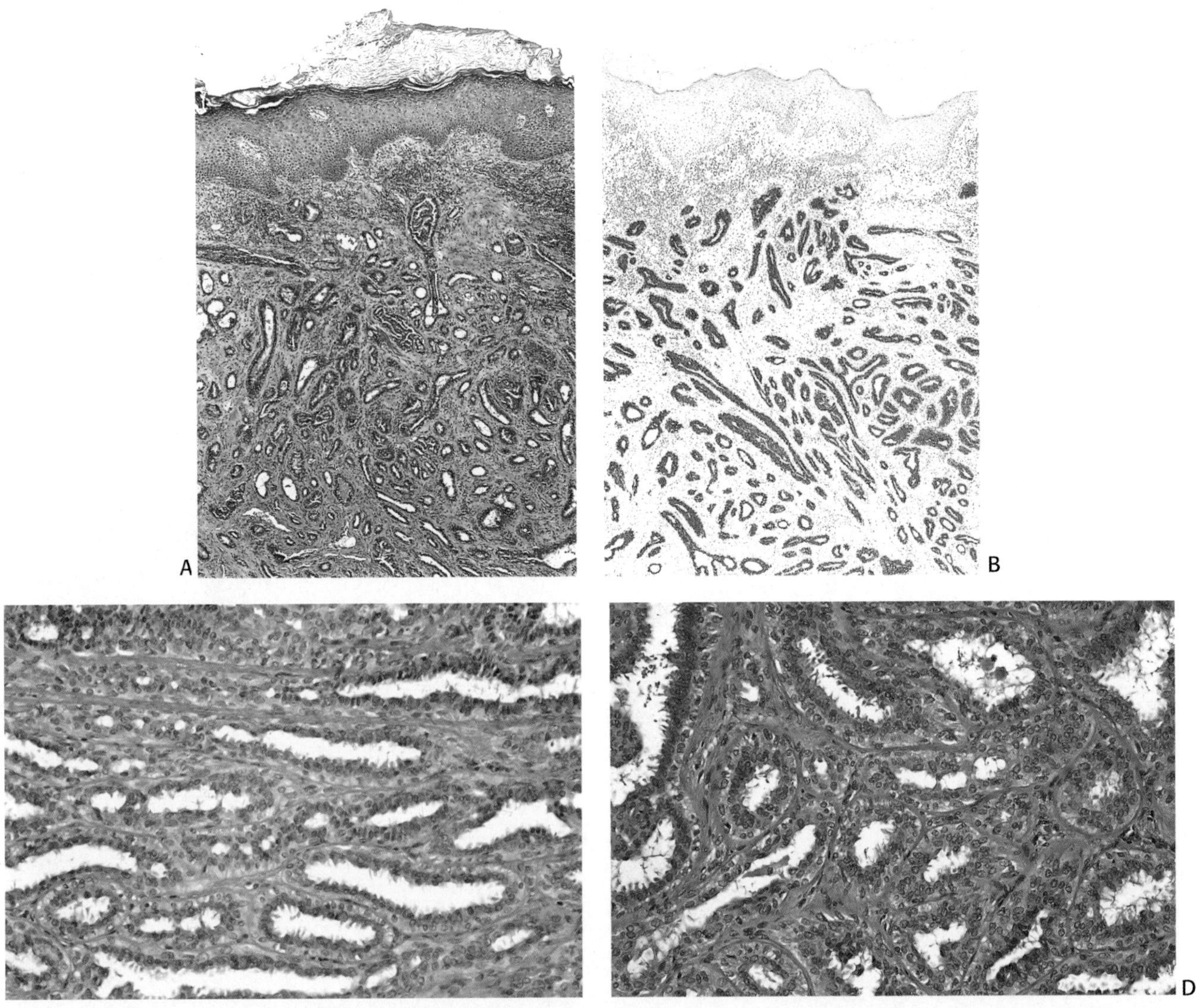

FIG. 5.39. ***Florid papillomatosis, adenosis pattern.*** **A:** The glandular proliferation has an adenosis pattern composed of tubular and oval glands. **B:** The architecture is highlighted by a CAM5.2 CK immunostain. **C,D:** Glandular elements in two lesions with epithelial and myoepithelial hyperplasia.

men[212,231] do not provide convincing evidence of underlying papillomatosis. The lesion illustrated in one report[212] appears to represent papillary DCIS within ducts of the nipple rather than DCIS involving florid papillomatosis. Nine years after an excisional biopsy, the patient presented with invasive ductal carcinoma at the same site. The lesion, described as "an adenoma of the nipple in a male," appears in retrospect to have been entirely a carcinoma.[231] The 74-year-old patient was treated by simple mastectomy. The authors described the specimen: "The nipple was present and adjacent to it was a slightly raised fairly firm nodule approximately 2.5 cm in diameter … on being cut, the nodule was seen to measure 3 cm in diameter. It lay directly beneath the nipple." Hence, there does not seem to have been a lesion in the nipple grossly. The illustrations show areas that appear to be solid carcinoma with an alveolar pattern and foci best interpreted as papillary carcinoma. No follow-up was given.

Five women have reportedly had carcinoma arising directly in florid papillomatosis. Two patients, 43 and 67 years old, had DCIS and IDC, with separate coexistent LCIS in one of these cases.[230] No comment was made about Paget disease in either case. The patients had negative ALNs, and no follow-up was given. Two other women, 52 and 63 years old, had invasive duct carcinoma arising in florid papillomatosis[214] (Fig. 5.42). The younger of these patients did not have Paget disease or other lesions of the breast. She had negative lymph nodes and remained well 2 years later. The older patient had Paget disease of the nipple, a separate focus of intraductal and invasive duct carcinoma in the lower outer quadrant, and metastatic carcinoma in a single ALN. The fifth woman, a 43-year-old patient, developed systemic metastases from invasive duct carcinoma that arose in florid papillomatosis.[232] She had been aware of a tumor in her right nipple for 2 to 3 years prior to seeking medical attention. When examined, there was a 2-cm mass in the nipple, and the ipsilateral ALNs were enlarged. The patient had evidence of systemic metastases, and these were confirmed at autopsy 5 weeks later. The nipple of the right breast contained a lesion that appeared microscopically to be florid papillomatosis. Paget disease was noted in the overlying epidermis, and "in some small areas there was a more florid type of epithelium with a larger nucleoli." Neither breast contained other evidence of carcinoma. Because primary lesions were not found in other organs, it seems likely

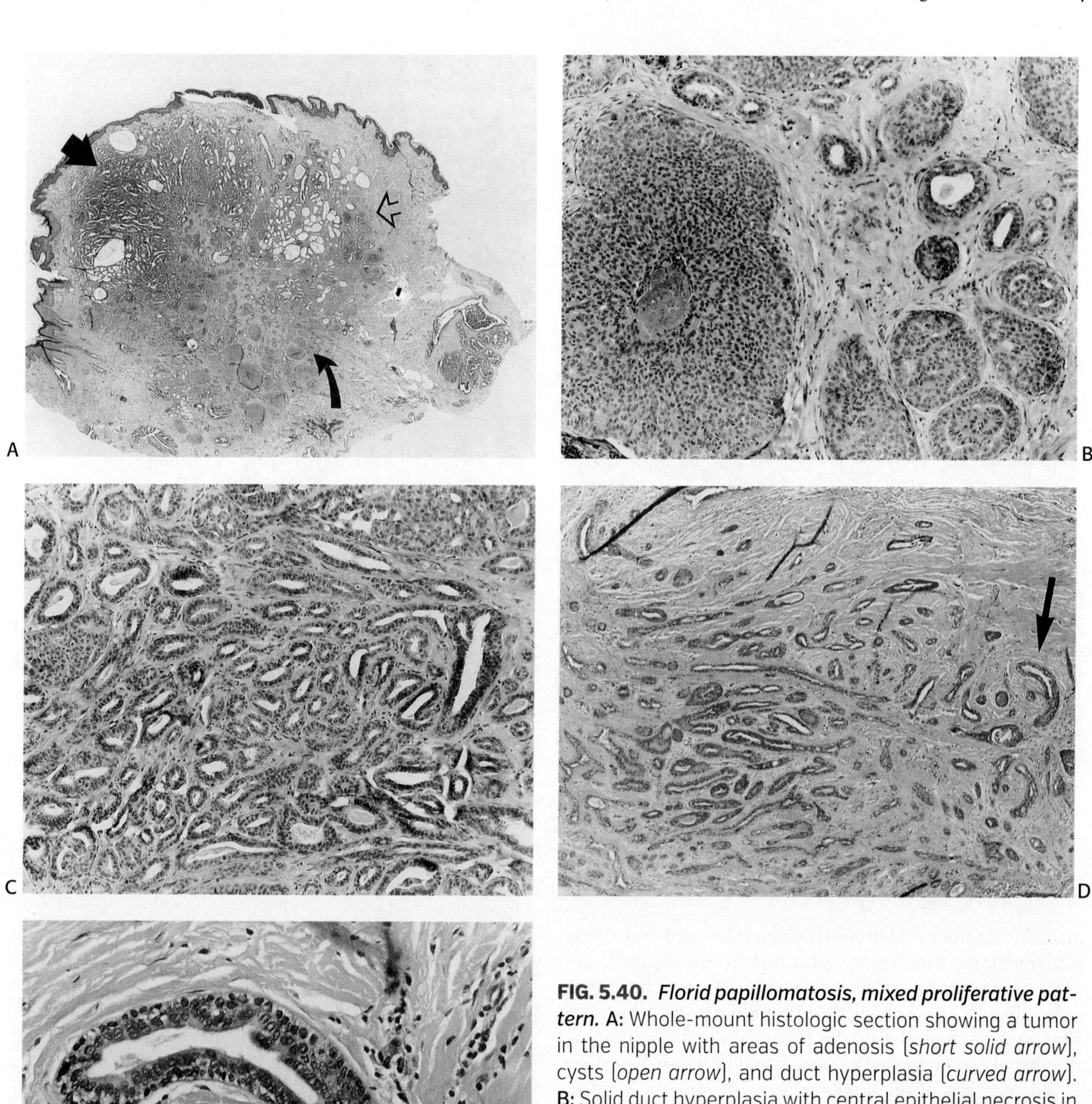

FIG. 5.40. ***Florid papillomatosis, mixed proliferative pattern.*** **A:** Whole-mount histologic section showing a tumor in the nipple with areas of adenosis (*short solid arrow*), cysts (*open arrow*), and duct hyperplasia (*curved arrow*). **B:** Solid duct hyperplasia with central epithelial necrosis in the large duct. **C:** Adenosis. **D,E:** Syringomatous proliferation at the margin of florid papillomatosis. The *arrow* in (**D**) indicates the comma-shaped gland shown enlarged in (**E**). **F,G:** Congenital florid papillomatosis with mixed proliferative pattern in a newborn female infant. Micropapillary duct hyperplasia is shown in (**G**). (**A–E:** Reproduced from Rosen PP, Caicco JA. Florid papillomatosis of the nipple: a study of 51 patients, including nine having mammary carcinoma. *Am J Surg Pathol* 1986;10:87–101, with permission.)

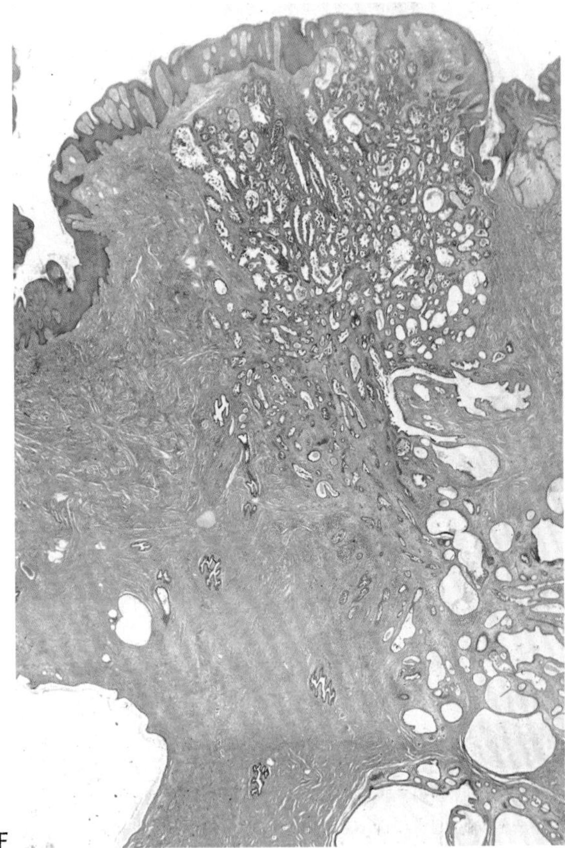

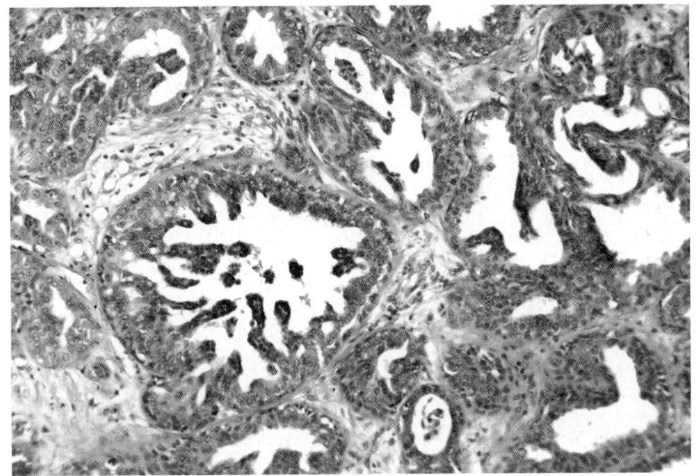

F G

FIG. 5.40. *(Continued)*

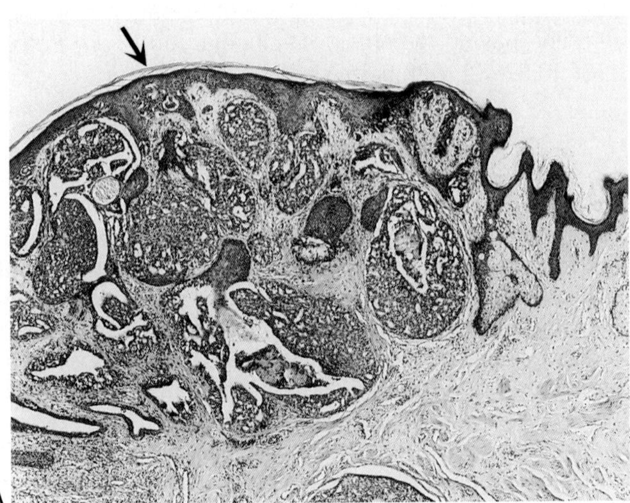

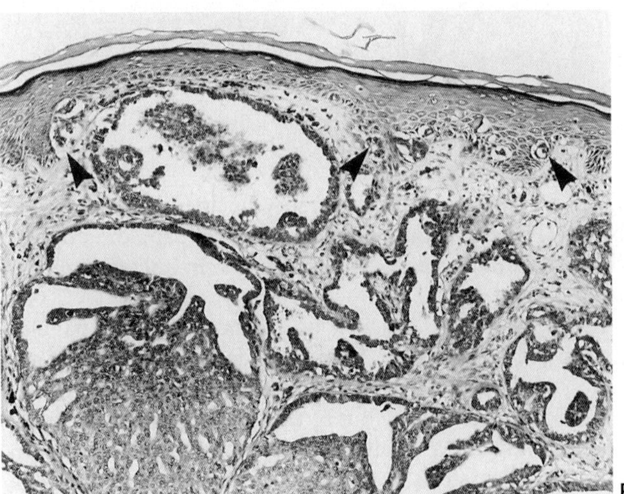

A B

FIG. 5.41. ***DCIS arising in florid papillomatosis.*** **A:** Part of the nipple tumor that contains DCIS as well as duct hyperplasia. Paget disease in the epidermis can be seen (*arrow*). **B:** *Arrowheads* indicate Paget disease in the epidermis overlying duct hyperplasia in another section of the lesion.

that the patient had systemic dissemination of carcinoma, which arose in florid papillomatosis. The experience with this patient is reminiscent of another patient with florid papillomatosis who had ALN metastases, although no definite evidence of carcinoma could be found histologically in the nipple lesion[214] (Fig. 5.43).

Carcinoma of the contralateral breast was described in seven women. Three had bilateral breast carcinoma with

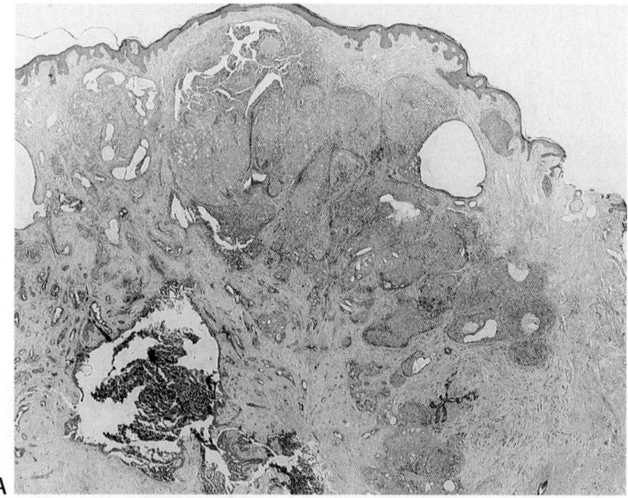

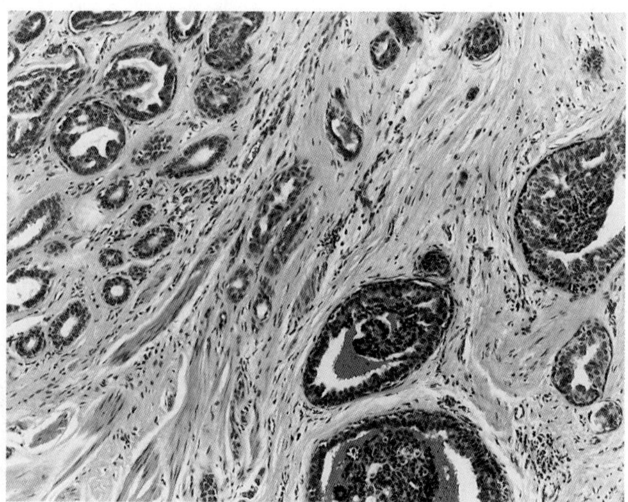

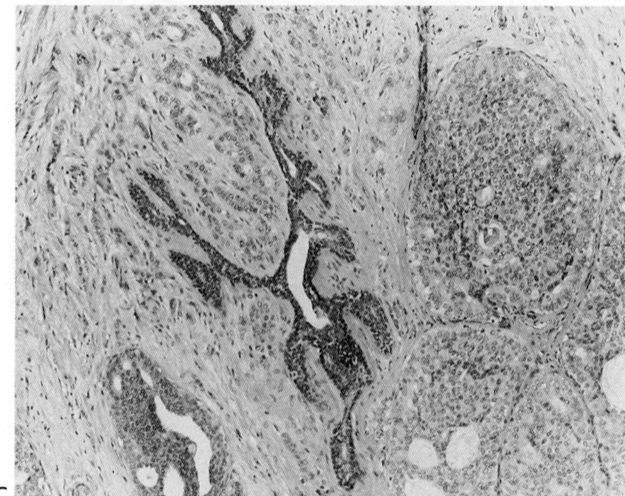

FIG. 5.42. ***Invasive carcinoma in florid papillomatosis.*** **A:** Whole-mount histologic section of a nipple with carcinoma in the *right* half of the lesion. A blood-filled recent biopsy site is evident on the *left*. The area of carcinoma was not sampled in the biopsy, and the lesion was diagnosed as florid papillomatosis. **B:** Papillary epithelial proliferation in the lesion. **C:** Intraductal and infiltrating duct carcinoma around a lactiferous duct in the lesion. [**A,C:** Reproduced from Rosen PP, Caicco JA. Florid papillomatosis of the nipple: a study of 51 patients, including nine having mammary carcinoma. *Am J Surg Pathol* 1986;10:87–101, with permission.]

florid papillomatosis as a separate coincidental lesion in one breast. The other four patients had florid papillomatosis in the nipple of one breast and carcinoma in only the contralateral breast.

Subsequent to the review of 224 cases of florid papillomatosis, which revealed 34 associated carcinomas,[214] 10 additional female patients have been described.[190,233,234] Five had ductal carcinomas, four of which were invasive, present concurrently but clinically and pathologically separate from florid papillomatosis in the same breast. In a sixth case, the patient reportedly had invasive ductal carcinoma in the lower outer quadrant and invasive ductal carcinoma that arose separately in the florid papillomatosis.[234] A seventh patient was reported to have DCIS in florid papillomatosis, but the diagnosis is doubtful because Paget disease was not present.[234] Two patients had invasive ductal carcinoma in the nipple adjacent to and possibly arising from florid papillomatosis.[233] Pathological details were not provided in the final case[190].

These cases raise the question of a pathogenetic relationship between carcinoma and florid papillomatosis of the nipple. In the male breast, both are uncommon lesions. Their coexistence in nearly 50% of men reported to have florid papillomatosis suggests that the latter may be a precancerous tumor in men, especially since the carcinomas seem to have arisen in the nipple lesions. This association may be a reflection of the fact that male breast carcinoma typically arises in the subareolar region. The evidence indicating that florid papillomatosis is precancerous in women is less substantial. Nonetheless, a woman with florid papillomatosis should have both breasts carefully examined clinically and radiologically to exclude an independent concurrent coincidental carcinoma. If the florid papillomatosis lesion is completely excised and found not to harbor carcinoma, the risk of subsequently developing carcinoma in the same breast seems to be relatively low.

As indicated by some of the foregoing case reports, it may be difficult to detect carcinoma arising in florid papillomatosis of the nipple. Hyperplastic areas in the lesions often exhibit atypical features that may include foci with comedonecrosis, as well as cribriform and micropapillary growth patterns, mitoses, and cytologic atypia. In the absence of

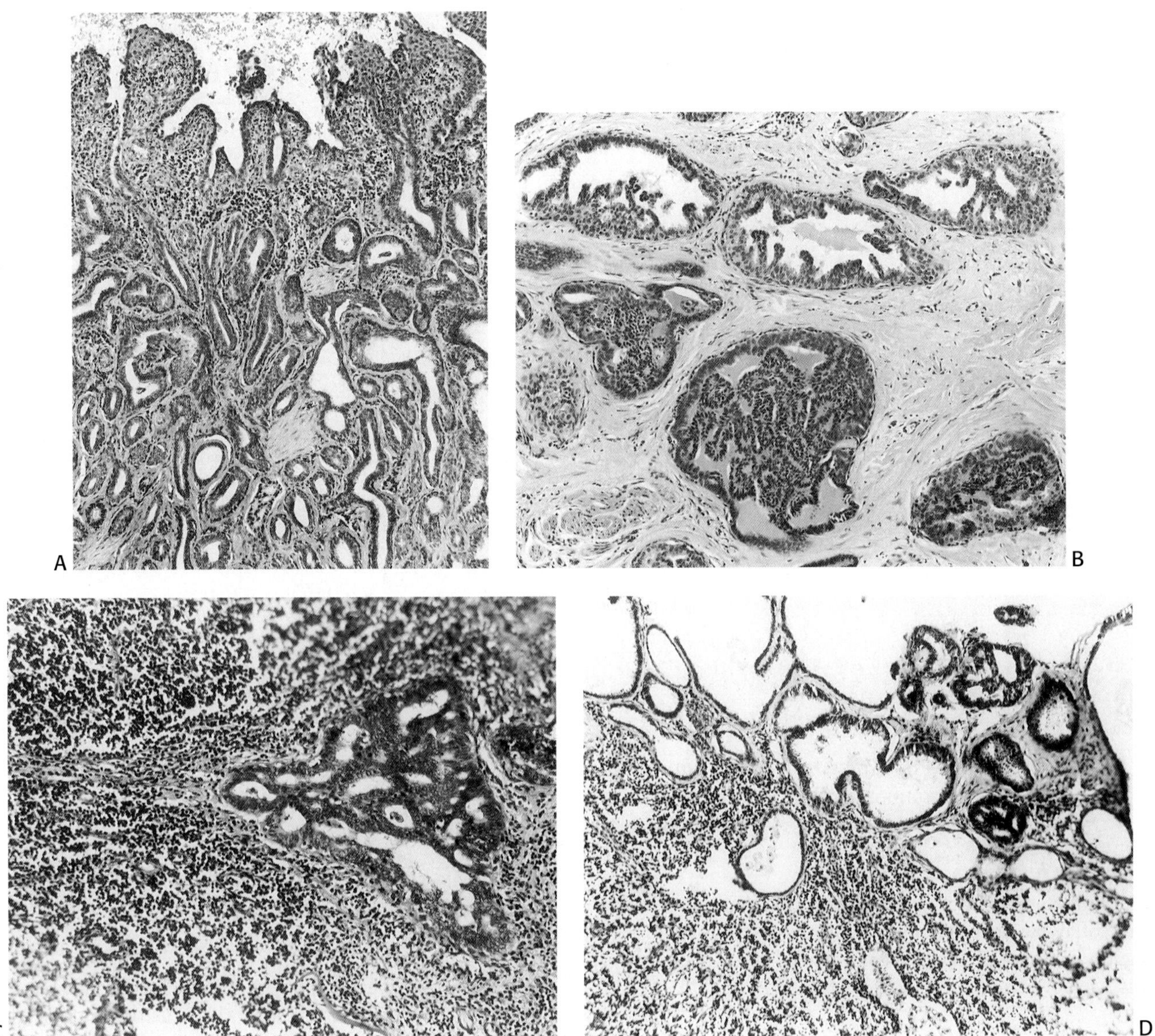

FIG. 5.43. ***Occult carcinoma with lymph node metastases associated with florid papillomatosis.*** **A:** Superficial portion of the lesion with erosion at the surface of the nipple. **B:** The most florid and atypical ductal proliferation found in the tumor. **C,D:** Metastatic carcinoma was found in two lymph nodes, which are illustrated here. [**A–C:** Reproduced from Rosen PP, Caicco JA. Florid papillomatosis of the nipple: a study of 51 patients, including nine having mammary carcinoma. *Am J Surg Pathol* 1986;10:87–101, with permission.]

definitive evidence of invasion, Paget disease of the nipple is the most reliable evidence for a diagnosis of carcinoma arising in florid papillomatosis. The CAM5.2 and CK7 immunostains are helpful for detecting Paget cells, which are selectively immunoreactive for these markers (Fig. 5.44). Paget cells were not detected in any of the larger series of cases of florid papillomatosis regarded as benign, but these studies were published before current immunostains were generally available. When Paget disease is found, underlying areas of DCIS that differ from the rest of the tumor in their growth pattern are usually readily identifiable. Immunostains for myoepithelial markers, especially p63, demonstrate myoepithelium throughout the benign proliferative components of florid papillomatosis. If these immunostains identify ducts that do not have immunoreactive myoepithelium, DCIS may be present, but it must be noted that myoepithelium can be depleted in the central portion of the sclerosing papillary lesion. The differential diagnosis also includes primary invasive ductal carcinoma arising from lactiferous ducts in the nipple without associated florid papillomatosis (Fig. 5.45). In the absence of Paget disease or invasive carcinoma, a diagnosis of DCIS arising in florid papillomatosis is difficult to

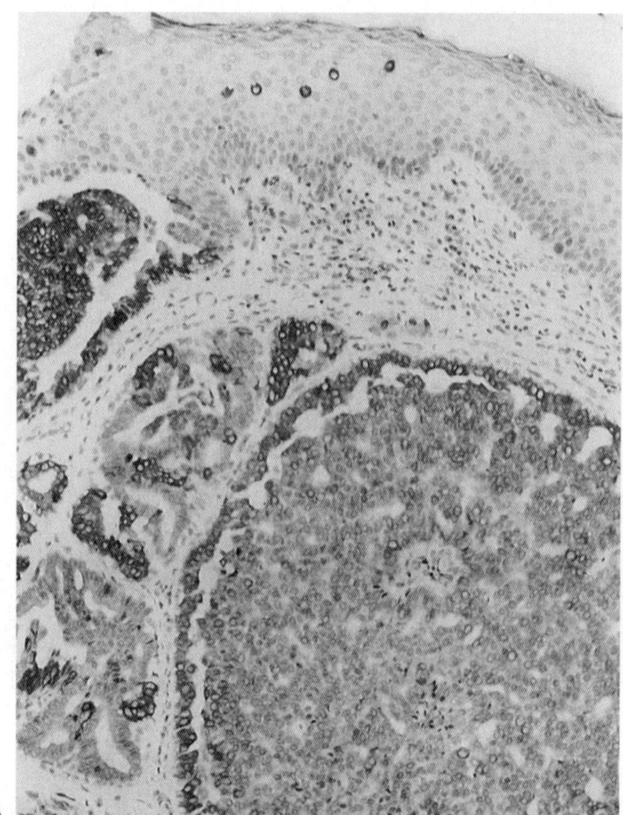

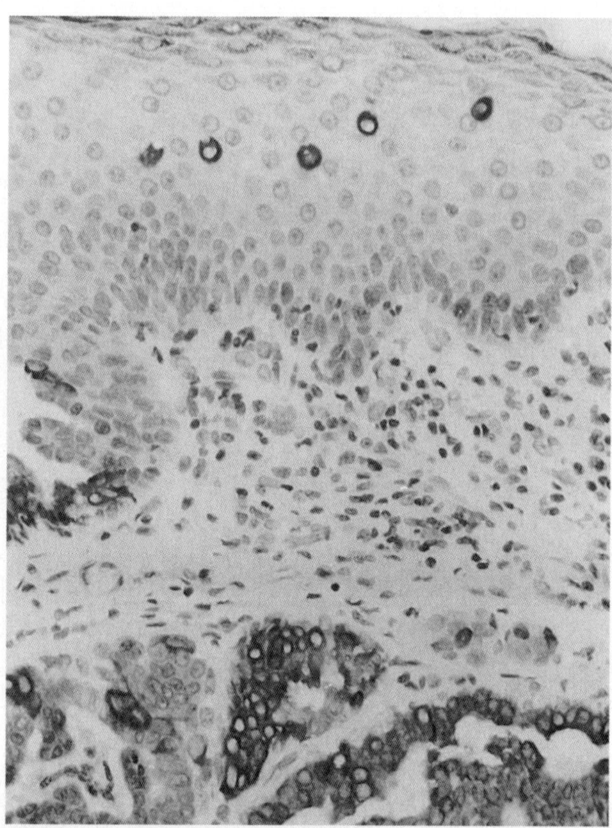

FIG. 5.44. ***Paget disease in florid papillomatosis.*** **A,B:** Five cells are highlighted in the epidermis with the immunostain for CAM5.2. Similar immunoreactive cells representing pagetoid spread of carcinoma are evident focally in the underlying papillary proliferation.

substantiate in routine H&E sections. Regardless of the degree of atypia, a conservative approach to the histologic diagnosis of these lesions is recommended when neither Paget disease nor invasive carcinoma is present.

Treatment and Prognosis

Incisional biopsy and needle biopsy are not satisfactory to exclude the possibility of carcinoma arising in the lesion. In one case seen by the Senior Editor, an incisional biopsy revealed only florid papillomatosis. When excised, the lesion contained an area of invasive ductal carcinoma. Complete excision, which is recommended as definitive treatment, usually requires removal of the nipple. One report[235] described extirpation of the mass following an incision through the nipple. Resection by Mohs microsurgery has been reported,[236,237] and cryosurgery has been used successfully in one case.[238] Treatment of the undeveloped breast poses challenging problems. Excision can damage the breast bud, resulting in abnormal or incomplete breast development, and transection of the large ducts during the surgery can prevent future breast feeding. Local recurrence of florid papillomatosis may occur following subtotal excision,[186,193,201,214] but a substantial number of patients have reportedly remained asymptomatic after incomplete excision. Mastectomy is not indicated as primary treatment of florid papillomatosis unassociated with carcinoma.

SYRINGOMATOUS ADENOMA OF THE NIPPLE

Syringomatous adenoma of the nipple is a benign locally infiltrating neoplasm that has a close histopathologic resemblance to syringomatous tumors commonly found in the skin of the face and other anatomic sites. Related tumors included in this category are locally infiltrating syringomatous tumors of minor salivary glands arising in the lip,[239] microcystic adnexal carcinoma of the skin of the face,[240] and sclerosing sweat gland duct (syringomatous) carcinoma.[241]

The precise anatomic source of the breast lesion is uncertain. The absence of epithelial proliferation in the mammary ducts and the lack of connection with the epidermis in most cases suggest an origin from other structures. Because random sections of nipples taken from breasts removed for mammary carcinoma sometimes reveal sweat gland ducts, it is possible that these structures give rise to syringomatous adenomas.

Early descriptions of this lesion were included in studies of florid papillomatosis of the nipple. Handley and Thackray[242] described an example of syringomatous adenoma in a 39-year-old woman whose biopsy revealed an "adenoma, suggesting a sweat gland origin." Doctor and Sirsat[243] found five syringomatous adenomas in a series of epithelial tumors of the nipple. They concluded that "the lesion designated

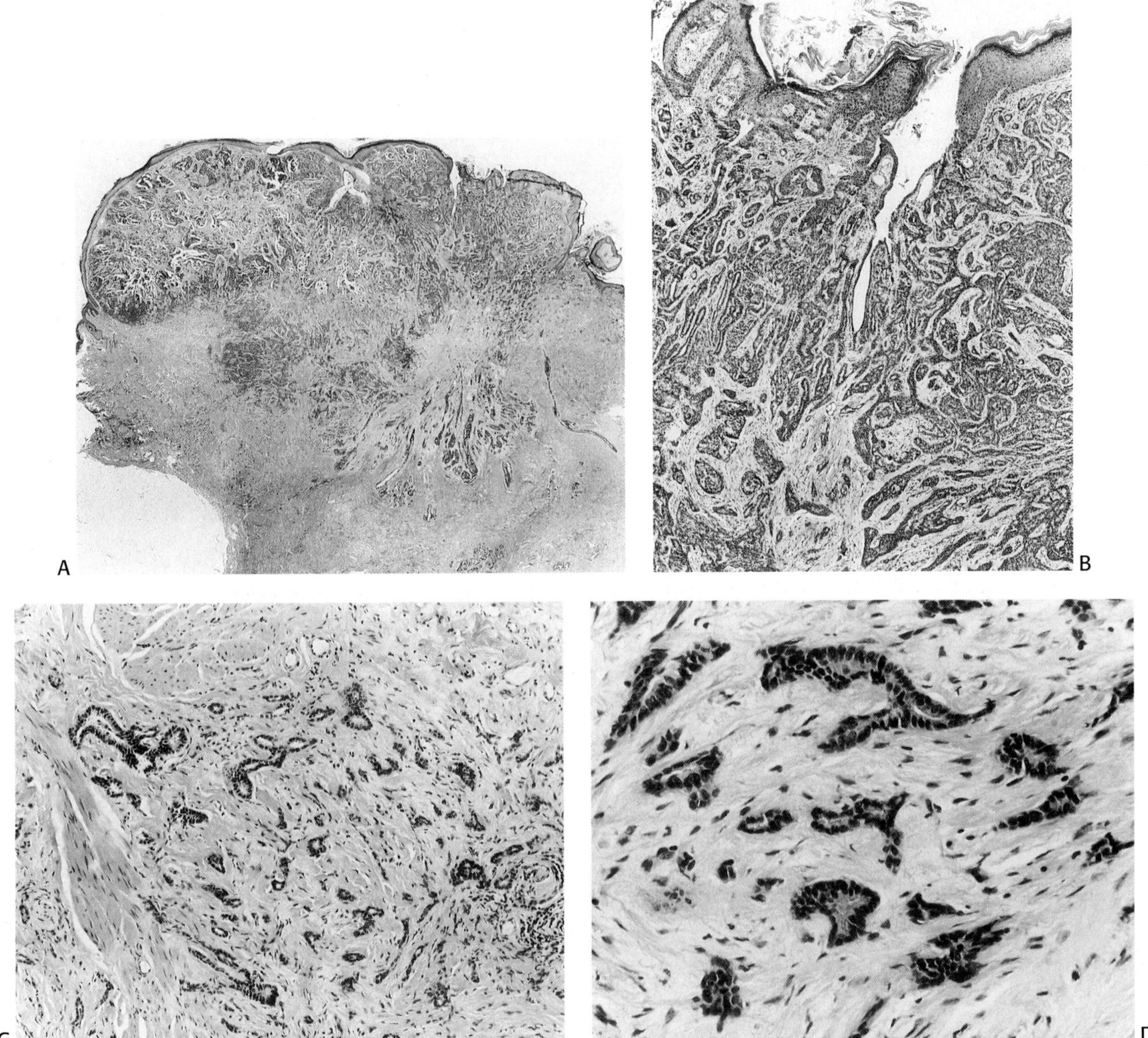

FIG. 5.45. ***Infiltrating carcinoma in the nipple.*** **A:** Whole-mount microscopic section of the nipple containing a tumor composed entirely of carcinoma. **B:** A superficial portion of the carcinoma with papillary features. No Paget disease was present. **C,D:** Invasive duct carcinoma growing as tubular carcinoma and involving smooth muscle of the nipple. (Reproduced from Rosen PP, Caicco JA. Florid papillomatosis of the nipple: a study of 51 patients, including nine having mammary carcinoma. *Am J Surg Pathol* 1986;10:87–101, with permission.)

as florid papillomatosis or adenoma of the nipple does not seem to be one entity, but two distinct lesions…the term florid papillomatosis is applicable to lesions showing a papillomatous pattern and is linked with fibrocystic disease and intracystic papilloma of the breast. The term adenoma of the nipple should be reserved for lesions showing an adenomatous pattern and is related more to the sweat gland tumours."

Rosen[244] described six more cases in 1983 and proposed the term syringomatous adenoma. Additional cases have since been described.[245–254]

Clinical Presentation

The female patients reported since 1983[244,246,249,254,255] ranged from 11 to 76 years of age at diagnosis. The median and mean ages at diagnosis of women were around 40 years. One man was 76 years old.[244] Onset of signs and symptoms within a year prior to diagnosis was usually reported, but a duration of several years has also been described.

Syringomatous adenomas have typically been unilateral lesions affecting either breast with approximately equal frequency. In one case, tumors appeared in both breasts synchronously.[256] Page et al.[257] reported the occurrence of a syringomatous adenoma in a supernumerary nipple. The initial symptom is a mass in the nipple and/or subareolar region. Pain, tenderness, redness, itching, discharge, and/or nipple inversion have been noted in isolated cases. Crusting of the nipple surface owing to hyperkeratosis has been reported, but ulceration and erosion are not features of syringomatous adenoma.

Except for one patient who later died of colon carcinoma,[244] syringomatous adenomas have not been associated with other neoplasms.

Imaging Studies

The results of radiologic imaging studies have varied. Mammography in three cases[248,255,258] demonstrated dense spiculated masses, and in two cases,[248,258] the masses contained calcifications. Another tumor[253] appeared well defined. In three examples, the mammogram showed only calcifications,[256,259] but the relationships between the calcifications and the tumors were not specified. Sonography sometimes shows an irregular mass with heterogeneous internal echoes or posterior acoustical shadowing,[248,250,251,255,258] a well-defined mass,[253] skin thickening,[251] dilated ducts,[247] or calcifications.[256] Ultrasound studies may also fail to demonstrate the lesion.[260]

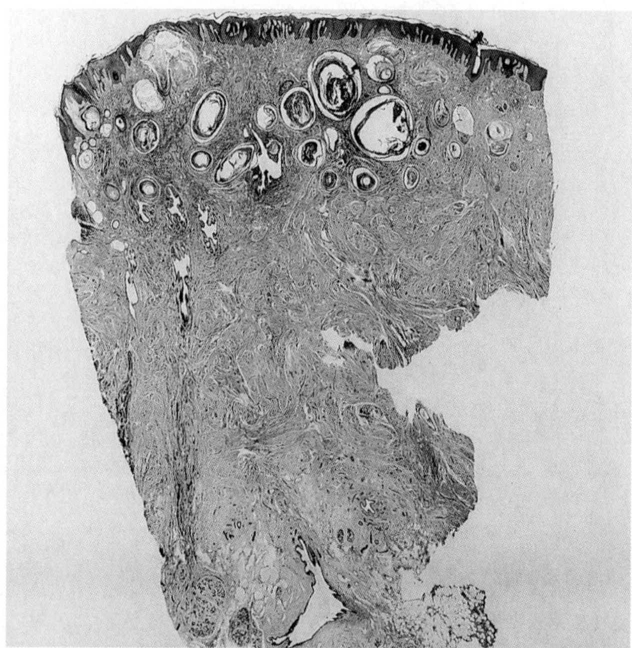

FIG. 5.46. ***Syringomatous adenoma of the nipple.*** A whole-mount microscopic section of the lesion. Keratotic cysts are prominent at this magnification. (Reproduced from Rosen PP. Syringomatous adenoma of the nipple. *Am J Surg Pathol* 1984;7:739–745, with permission.)

Gross Pathology

The excised tumors have measured 1.0 to 3.5 cm, with a mean of 1.7 cm and median of 1.5 cm. Most consist of ill-defined, firm-to-hard, gray, tan, or white tissue. Discrete nodules and microcystic areas have been noted infrequently.

Microscopic Pathology

The lesion consists of tubules, ductules, and strands composed of small, uniform generally basophilic cells infiltrating the dermis and the stroma of the nipple (Fig. 5.46). Hyperplasia of the epidermis is slight in most cases, but occasionally pseudoepitheliomatous hyperplasia may be encountered. Neoplastic glands that proliferate throughout the dermis sometimes appear to be connected to the basal layer of the epidermis.

The ducts, lined by one or more layers of cells, have teardrop, comma-like, and branching shapes with lumens that are either open and round or filled with small uniform cells (Fig. 5.47). Some cells may exhibit cytoplasmic clearing. Mitoses are virtually absent, and the nuclei lack prominent nucleoli and pleomorphism. Flattening of cells around the lumens constitutes evidence of early squamous differentiation, which in a fully developed form, results in keratotic cysts (Fig. 5.48). A foreign-body giant cell reaction may be elicited in the vicinity of ruptured squamous cysts (Fig. 5.48). Calcification is rarely seen in the keratinized epithelium. The lumens of the ducts are empty, or they contain deeply eosinophilic, retracted secretion. The secretion in tubular lumens is PAS positive and sometimes weakly mucicarmine positive[244] (Fig. 5.49).

The adenomatous tubules diffusely infiltrate the periductal stroma of the nipple and may extend into the subareolar breast parenchyma in larger lesions. Invasion into the smooth muscle bundles of the nipple is very common (Fig. 5.47), and occasionally perineural invasion is also observed. The stroma appears to be altered in the vicinity of the infiltrating tubules, because the collagen and fibroblasts tend to be concentrically oriented around the epithelial structures (Fig. 5.47).

Syringomatous glands may be found in proximity to and rarely in direct contact with the epithelium of nipple ducts, ductules and lobules of the breast parenchyma, and the epidermis of the nipple. This appears to be a result of the infiltrative growth pattern of the neoplasm and is not conclusive evidence of origin from any of these structures. Coincidental epithelial hyperplasia of lactiferous ducts or the underlying breast tissue may occasionally be seen, but this is not an intrinsic component of syringomatous adenoma. Paget disease, a manifestation of duct carcinoma, also is not a feature of syringomatous adenoma.

Differential Diagnosis

Several lesions should be considered in the differential diagnosis of syringomatous adenoma of the nipple. Florid papillomatosis is predominantly a hyperplastic epithelial

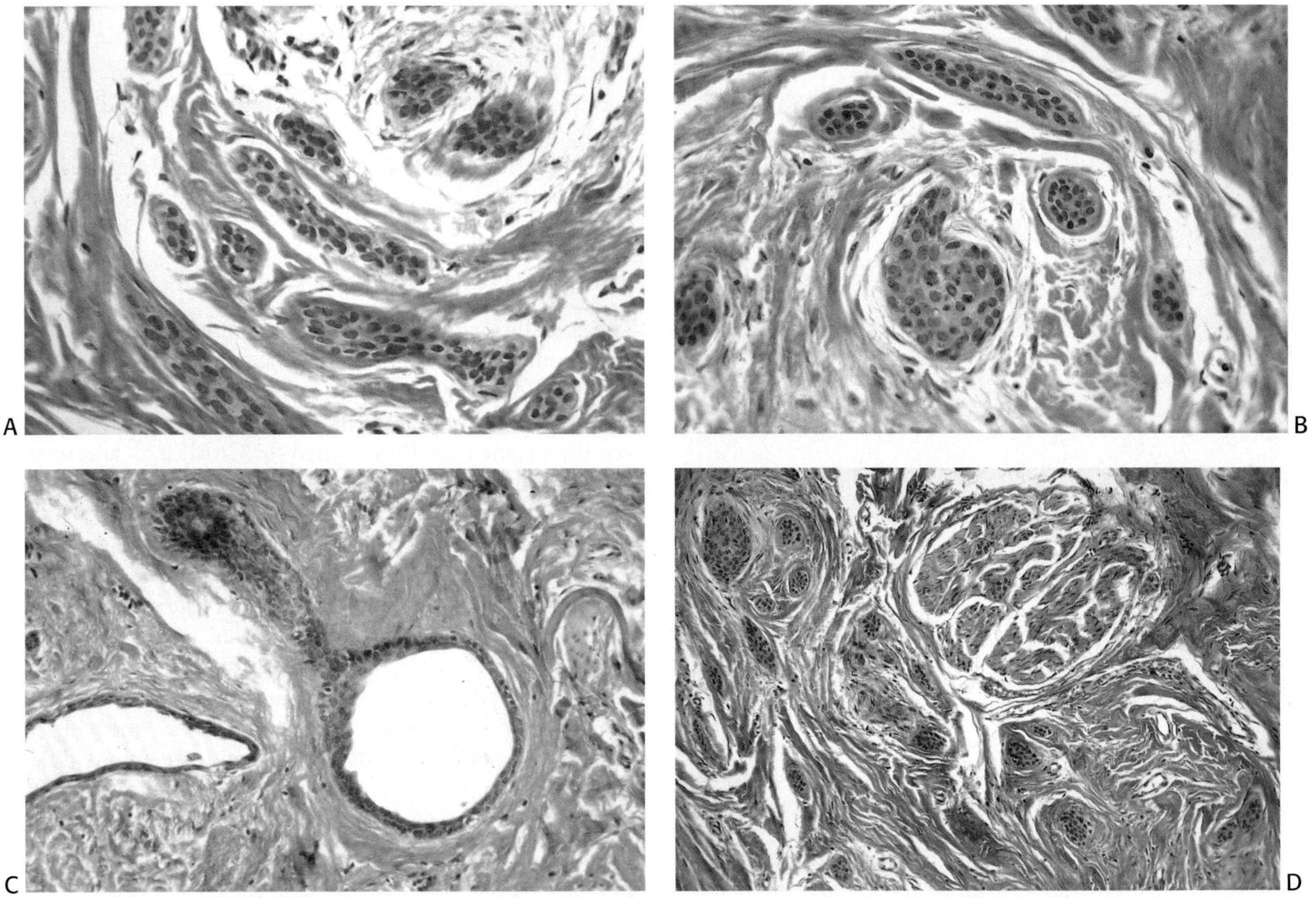

A

B

C

D

FIG. 5.47. ***Syringomatous adenoma.*** **A:** Elongated ductular structures. **B:** Squamous differentiation and a teardrop shape. **C:** Teardrop shape with cystic dilatation. **D:** Infiltration of smooth muscle in the nipple.

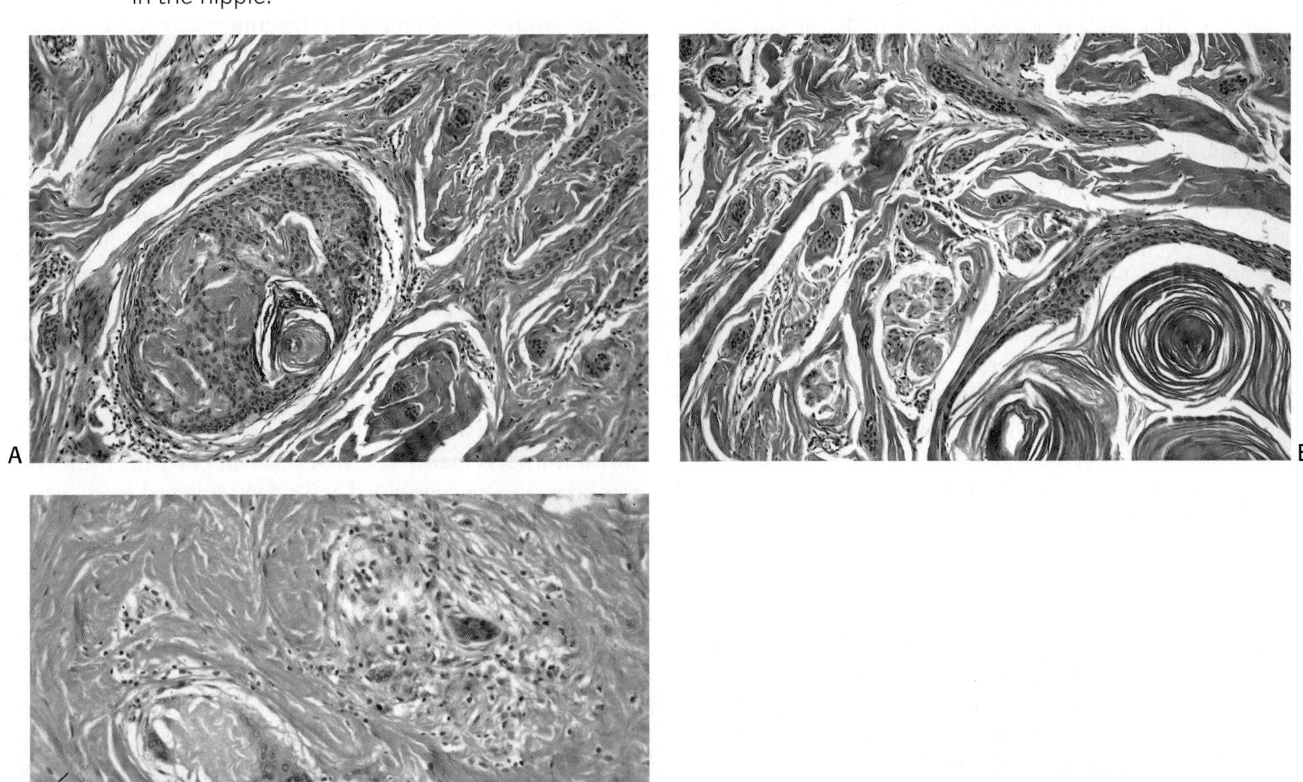

FIG. 5.48. ***Syringomatous adenoma.*** **A,B:** A Solid foci of squamous differentiation. **C:** Granulomatous inflammation elicited by squamous material.

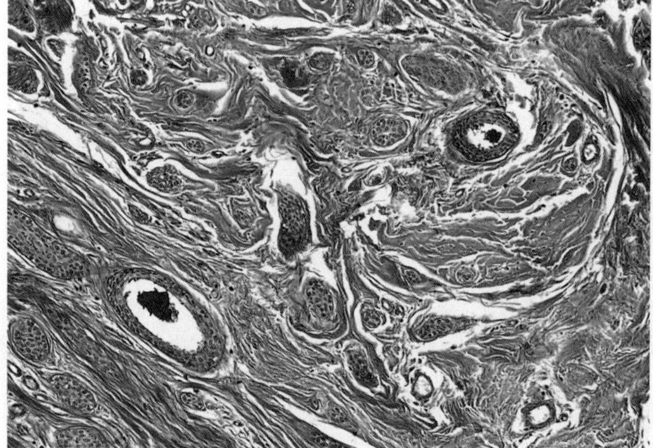

FIG. 5.49. *Syringomatous adenoma.* The secretion in two glands is stained magenta with the PAS reaction.

proliferation of the major lactiferous ducts. Patients with florid papillomatosis tend to be older, they are more likely to have erosion of the nipple with bleeding, and the duration is usually brief compared with syringomatous adenoma. Syringomatous foci are occasionally encountered as a minor component of florid papillomatosis.

Tubular carcinoma sometimes arises in the subareolar region and nipple, where it displays an infiltrative growth pattern that may be difficult to distinguish from syringomatous adenoma. Both invade smooth muscle and around nerves. Features of tubular carcinoma in the nipple that are not seen in syringomatous adenoma include DCIS, Paget disease of the epidermis, and angular glands. Squamous metaplasia and the formation of round glands by ductules that often have a branching pattern, findings seen in syringomatous adenoma, are not features of tubular carcinoma.

Syringomatous adenoma and certain variants of LGASC share certain structural characteristics,[261] and the literature contains two reports[262,263] of tumors classified as syringomatous adenomas in which the findings depict LGASCs. Despite the similarities between syringomatous adenoma and LGASC, the two lesions are not, as has been suggested,[264] part of a single neoplastic process. Syringomatous adenoma arises in the nipple and secondarily involves the breast parenchyma underlying the nipple in almost all cases. LGASC usually develops peripherally, sparing the nipple, although very infrequently it can arise in the subareolar region and involve the nipple.

Cytology

Dahlstrom et al.[258] described the cytologic features of one example of syringomatous adenoma. Moderately cellular smears contained sheets of bland ductal cells and a background of single cells. The ductal cells appeared uniform, and their nuclei contained fine chromatin and inconspicuous nucleoli. The single cells resembled stromal cells, and some had elongated cytoplasmic processes. They possessed plump, oval, moderately pleomorphic nuclei and moderate amounts of basophilic cytoplasm. Fibrillary collagenous tufts occupied a granular background. The smears lacked necrotic material, inflammatory cells, and squamous cells.

Immunohistochemistry

The literature contains only scant, somewhat sketchy, and conflicting results of immunohistochemical staining of this lesion. CEA has been found in the secretion and in the cytoplasm of periluminal cells. The inner cells also express keratin. In one case, they stained for CAM5.2,[258] and in another[250] they reacted with antibodies to clone 34βE12 but did not stain for CK8. Staining for S-100 has yielded either staining of "sparse tumor cells"[249] or a lack of staining.[250,256,258] Jones et al.[254] observed reactivity for actin in the "myoepithelial cells," but other authors did not observe staining for SMA.[250,258] One publication[256] recounts positive reactions for CK5/6, CK7, actin, p63, and E-cadherin, but does not describe the position of the positive cells. The two tumors failed to stain for ER, PR, HER2, CK20, CD117, and p53. The p63 immunostain is reactive in cells with squamous differentiation; therefore, it is not a reliable method for detecting myoepithelium in this lesion.

Electron Microscopy

One publication[254] described a few ultrastructural features of two tumors. They consisted of clusters of cells with irregular nuclei. Some cells contained filaments with focal densities. Well-formed desmosomes and lysosomes were seen.

Treatment and Prognosis

Most patients have been treated by local excision, which required removing the entire nipple in some instances. Reexcision is recommended if the margins appear involved.[264] Total mastectomy is not indicated as primary treatment, although this operation has been performed in a few cases in which the diagnosis was uncertain or because the lesion was incorrectly diagnosed as invasive carcinoma. Local recurrence after incomplete excision has occurred in approximately 30% of cases reported since 1983.[244,245,247,254,255] The time to recurrence has varied from less than 1 year to 8 years. In one case, the lesion was known to have persisted and slowly enlarged for 22 years after initial biopsy, at which time a partial mastectomy was performed for a 3-cm tumor that invaded the breast parenchyma.[244] One patient experienced three recurrences over a 4-year period.[254] None of the patients with lesions correctly diagnosed as syringomatous adenoma has developed metastases in regional lymph nodes or at distant sites. Chang et al.[262] described a case purporting to show a syringomatous adenoma with a few tumor cells in an axillary sentinel lymph node (SLN); however, the published photographs of the mass illustrate LGASC. There is no evidence of an association of syringomatous adenoma and mammary adenocarcinoma.

COLLAGENOUS SPHERULOSIS

Collagenous spherulosis is a structural, histologic alteration of unknown histogenesis that occurs in the epithelium of otherwise well-characterized breast lesions. In this respect, it is analogous to *in situ* carcinoma that might be found in a papilloma, adenosis, or a FA. First described by Clement et al.[265] in 1987, this unusual epithelial proliferation features nodules of eosinophilic or basophilic basement membrane material enclosed in round spaces. Because of a superficial resemblance to adenoid cystic carcinoma (AdCC), adenoid cystic hyperplasia is an alternative name for this condition.[266] Resetkova et al.[267] summarized the clinical and morphologic features of 59 cases identified at a single institution and tabulated data from 61 cases reported prior to 2005.

Clinical Presentation

The clinical presentation of collagenous spherulosis depends upon the nature of the lesion in which it is found. Collagenous spherulosis typically represents an incidental microscopic finding encountered in excision specimens containing other benign proliferations such as papillomas, AMEs, FAs, papillary duct hyperplasia, and SA[267–271] (Figs. 5.50 and 5.51). At times, the collagenous spherulosis may constitute the dominant alteration in the underlying mass.[272,273]

One has difficulty determining the frequency of collagenous spherulosis, because the lesion often goes unrecognized or is misinterpreted as another. During the years between 1987 and 1997, pathologists sought consultative opinions from personnel at the Armed Forces Institute of Pathology regarding 81 cases of collagenous spherulosis.[274] The referring pathologists seemingly overlooked the lesion in approximately one-half the cases and misinterpreted it as a carcinoma or an atypical proliferation in another one-quarter of the cases. Estimates place the frequency of the lesion in the range of less than 1% of excision specimens[275] and 0.2%[276] to 0.5%[277] of cytologic material. Collagenous spherulosis affects women throughout adulthood; the ages of patients in reported cases range from 19[278] to 90 years.[267] The literature does not contain reports of collagenous spherulosis in men.

Imaging Studies

Collagenous spherulosis sometimes comes to clinical attention because of the presence of calcifications or a density on imaging studies or a palpable abnormality. In the series of Resetkova et al.,[267] calcifications led to mammographic detection of the lesion in 17 of 36 cases (47%), a mammographic density or a palpable mass prompted a biopsy in 15 cases (42%), and a mass with calcifications led to the diagnosis in 4 cases (11%). The radiologic imaging does not provide distinctive findings.

Gross Pathology

The small size of most examples of collagenous spherulosis precludes macroscopic recognition of the foci. In one case,[272] the writers described a nodule formed by collagenous spherulosis as an "ovoid, well-circumscribed, unencapsulated, pale tan solid mass measuring 1.0 cm × 0.9 cm." In this instance, the underlying mass was nodular adenosis. Cases of collagenous spherulosis forming a recognizable mass represent spherulosis superimposed on another process such as a papilloma, RSL, or nodular adenosis. It is the underlying process rather than the spherulosis that accounts for the macroscopic abnormality.

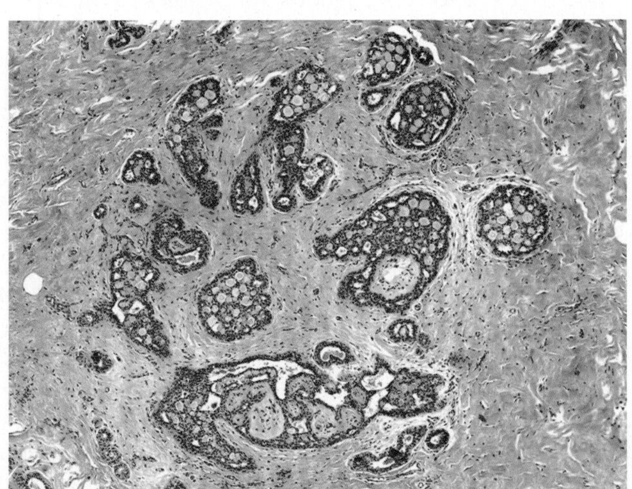

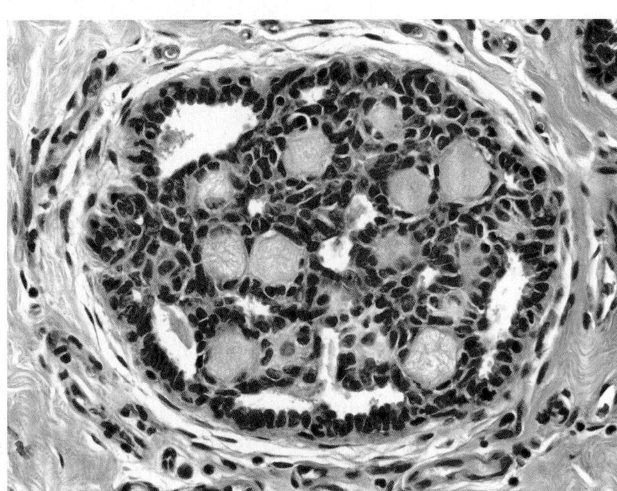

FIG. 5.50. ***Collagenous spherulosis.*** **A:** Hyperplasia in several duct cross sections exhibiting collagenous spherulosis in this small sclerosing papilloma. **B:** The combination of spherules and glandular lumens simulates cribriform growth.

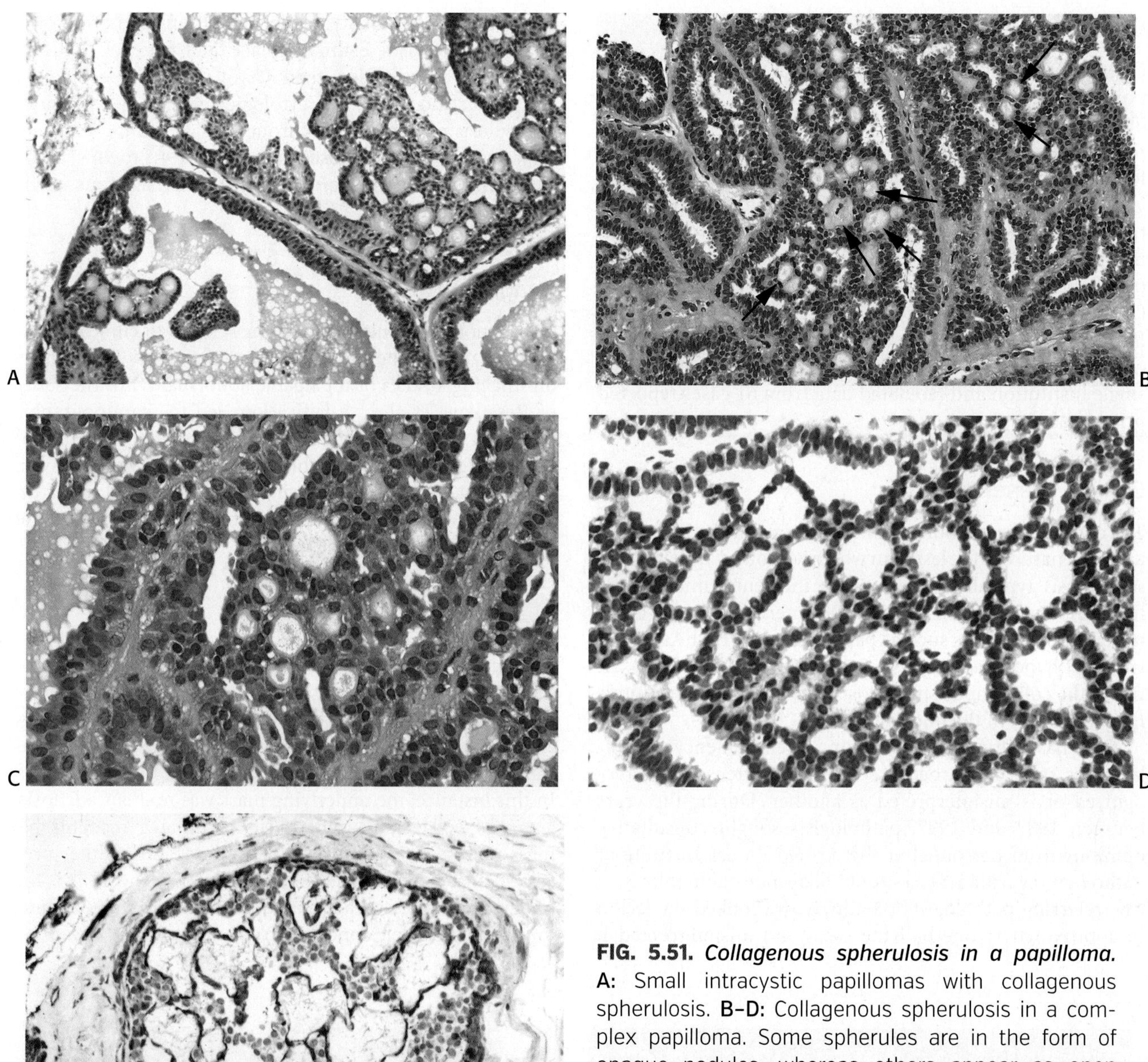

FIG. 5.51. *Collagenous spherulosis in a papilloma.* **A:** Small intracystic papillomas with collagenous spherulosis. **B–D:** Collagenous spherulosis in a complex papilloma. Some spherules are in the form of opaque nodules, whereas others appear as open spaces (*arrows*) surrounded by a border of basement membrane material. **E:** Myoepithelial cells, which are difficult to identify in the H&E section, are highlighted with the SMA stain.

Microscopic Pathology

Spherules composed of acellular material surrounded by epithelial cells constitute the defining features of collagenous spherulosis. The spherules measure 20 to 100 μm in diameter. They have various staining patterns and may be eosinophilic, amphophilic, or nearly transparent. They consist of ground substance and basement membrane material that can calcify (Fig. 5.52). Fibrillar material within spherules rarely has a laminar concentric distribution. More often, stellate fibrils radiate from a central nidus toward the periphery of the spherule. Degenerative changes in the spherule can create a myxoid appearance sometimes accompanied by shrinkage of the outer basement membrane layer, which collapses into the spherule (Figs. 5.52 and 5.53). Immunohistochemical studies and electron microscopy have identified several of the constituents of the spherules including elastin, PAS-positive polysaccharides, and other components of basement membrane, including type IV collagen and laminin[272,275,279,280] (Fig. 5.53).

Two types of cells, myoepithelial cells and luminal cells, contribute to the cellular proliferation in collagenous spherulosis, and the two types of cells give rise to two types of spaces. Myoepithelial cells often constitute the dominant population. They have long spindly shapes, flattened oval hyperchromatic nuclei, and attenuated eosinophilic cytoplasm that is sometimes referred to as a “cuticle.” The

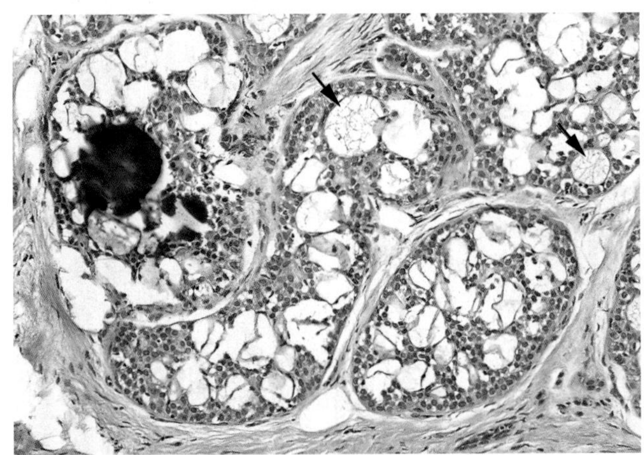

FIG. 5.52. ***Collagenous spherulosis, calcification.*** A large basophilic calcification is shown on the *left*. Fibrillar material is evident in two spherules (*arrows*). Filaments that traverse many empty spaces are strands of basement membrane material with adherent myoepithelial cells, which have collapsed into the spherules. Note myoepithelial cell nuclei associated with the filaments.

myoepithelial cells give rise to the nearly round spaces that enclose the spherules. The attenuated myoepithelial cells may be difficult to identify in H&E sections, but immunostains for actin, p63, CD10, calponin, SMA, or S-100 will highlight them (Fig. 5.54). Small collections of cuboidal luminal cells containing small nuclei, small nucleoli, and dense eosinophilic cytoplasm form glands situated among the myoepithelial cells and the spherules. These glands sometimes contain small amounts of eosinophilic secretory material. This pattern of growth creates an adenoid cystic structural arrangement; however, the lumens of the glandular spaces tend to have more irregular shapes than those of AdCC.

Among the 59 cases studied by Resetkova et al.,[267] collagenous spherulosis was unifocal in 15 (25%) and multifocal in 44 (75%). In the series of Hata et al.,[277] papillomas accounted for 84% of the associated lesions. Atypical epithelial proliferations and carcinomas can supervene in foci of collagenous spherulosis, but coexisting neoplastic proliferations represent independent and unrelated processes.[281] Resetkova et al.[267] observed ADH in 3 of 59 (5%) cases and LCIS in 15 of 59 cases (25%).

With experience, the recognition of collagenous spherulosis does not pose problems, but two neoplastic lesions sometimes enter into consideration. The presence of two types of cells and spherules of basement membrane material bring to mind the diagnosis of AdCC. Immunohistochemical staining using a panel of markers will distinguish the two lesions in most instances. When LCIS colonizes collagenous spherulosis and replaces the luminal cells, an appearance similar to that of low-grade DCIS results (Fig. 5.55).[267,282,283]

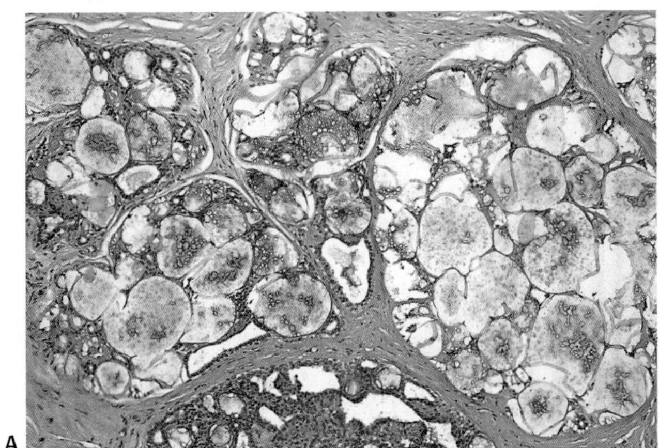

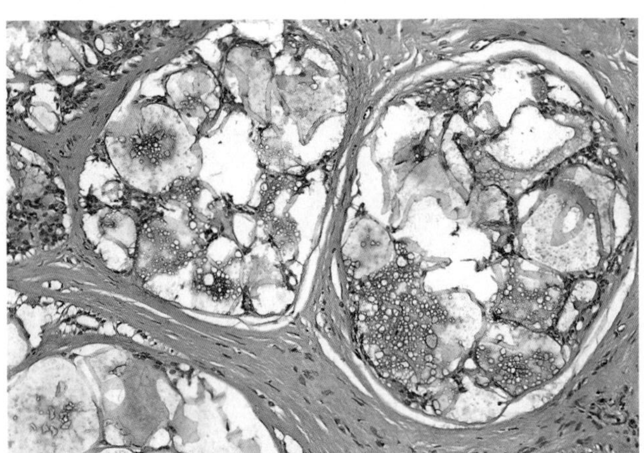

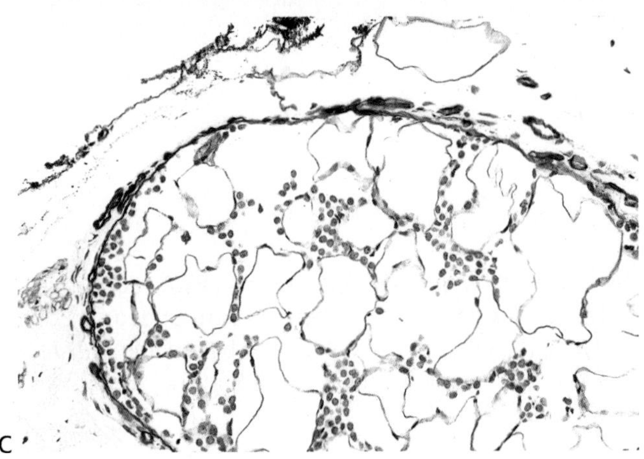

FIG. 5.53. ***Collagenous spherulosis, degenerative.*** **A:** Cystic degeneration has occurred in this example of collagenous spherulosis. Traces of this condition are seen in the papilloma at the lower border. **B:** Epithelial elements are largely absent, the spherule material is basophilic and vesicular, and the basement membranes appear as flaccid filaments. **C:** Basement membranes are highlighted with the immunostain for laminin.

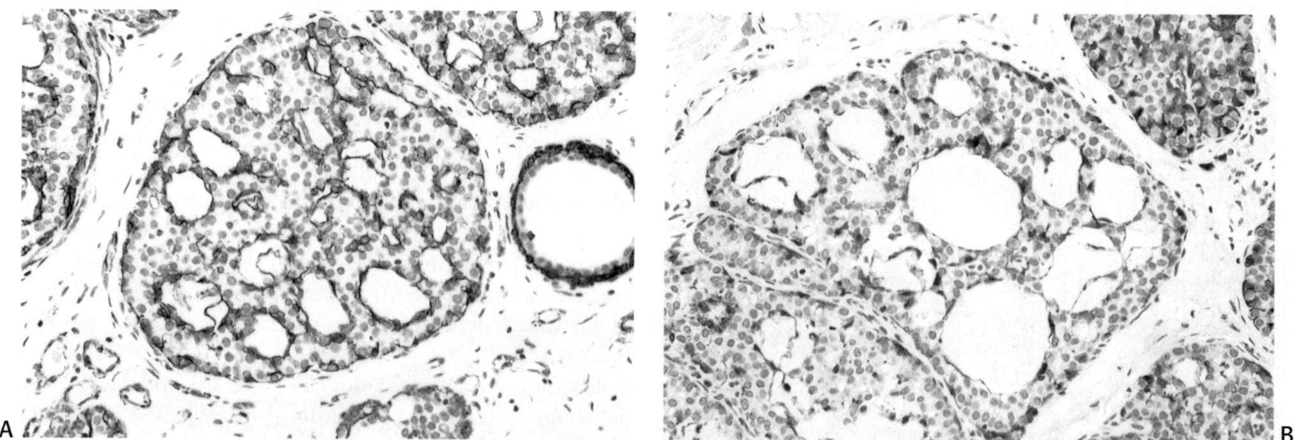

FIG. 5.54. ***Collagenous spherulosis, myoepithelial cells.*** **A:** Spherules are outlined by myoepithelial cells stained for SMA. **B:** Myoepithelial cells are S-100 immunoreactive.

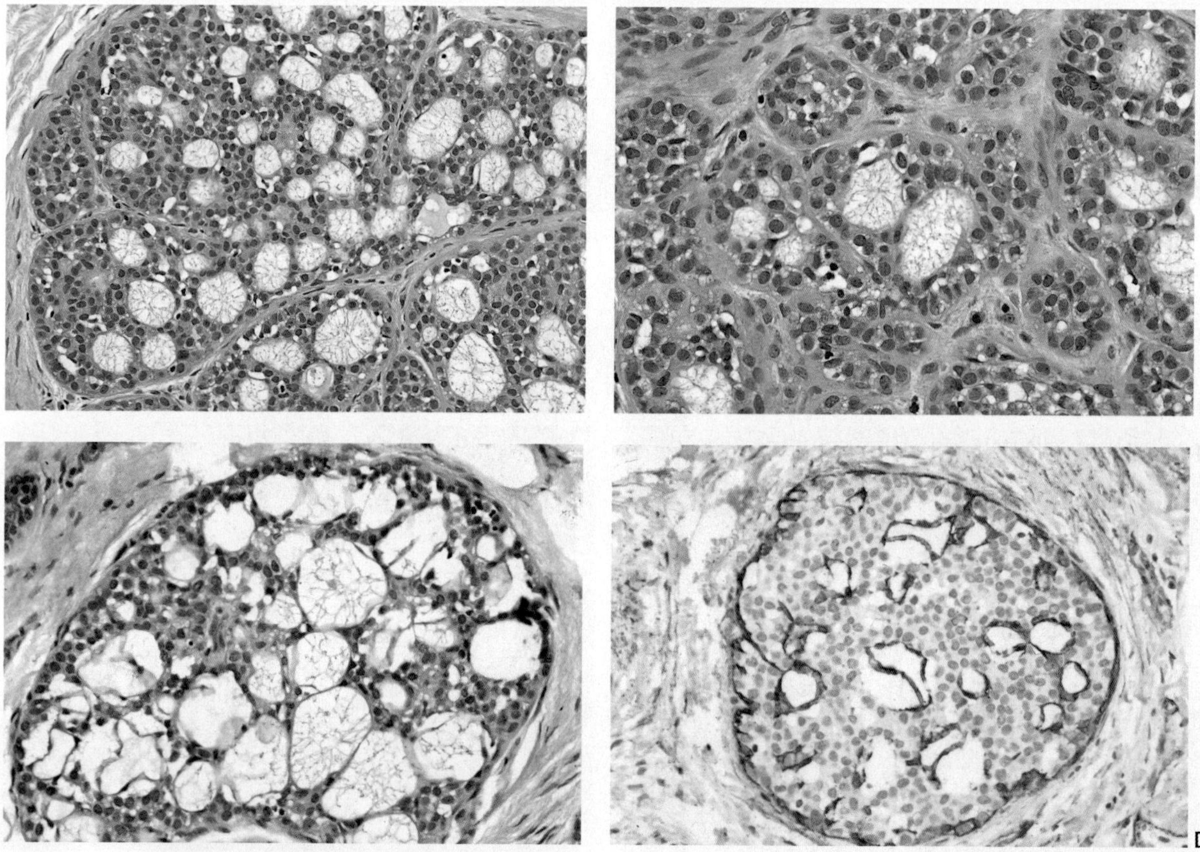

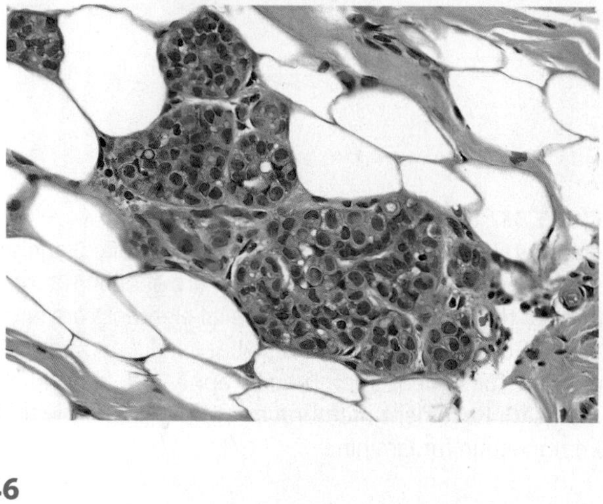

FIG. 5.55. ***Collagenous spherulosis with LCIS.*** **A–C:** Radial fibrillar deposits in spherules surrounded by LCIS. **D:** Myoepithelial cells are highlighted by the immunostain for SMA. **E:** A lobule involved by LCIS in the surrounding tissue.

Cytology

The literature contains only a few reports describing the cytologic findings of collagenous spherulosis. Gangane et al.[269] listed eight studies published prior to 2006 and summarized certain of the clinical and histologic findings. Aspiration of collagenous spherulosis commonly yields moderately cellular smears displaying monolayered cohesive clusters of variable size.[276] The cells display distinct cell borders, uniform round or oval nuclei, finely dispersed chromatin, and inconspicuous nucleoli. The diagnostic feature is the presence of spherules within cell clusters and in isolation. The spherules stain light green with the Papanicolaou stain and pink with a rapid Wright–Giemsa stain. A fibrillary quality can be detected in the spherules when studied with the latter method.[284] Attenuated myoepithelial cells with flattened comma-shaped nuclei surround the spherules frequently (Fig. 5.56). The myoepithelial cells usually form only a single layer. The background contains many bipolar naked nuclei and fibromyxoid stroma. Other elements may be present depending on the nature of the underlying lesion.

The distinction between collagenous spherulosis and AdCC in cytologic material can be problematic. The presence of several layers of cells surrounding spherules and the absence of bipolar naked nuclei in the background, among other findings, would suggest the diagnosis of AdCC rather than collagenous spherulosis.

Immunohistochemistry

The two types of cells stain in the expected ways. The myoepithelial cells stain for proteins such as SMA, p63, and CD10, and the latter antibody sometimes stains the spherules. Luminal cells stain for low-molecular weight CK, ER, and PR. The cells of collagenous spherulosis do not stain for c-kit. By using a panel of these markers, one can distinguish cases of collagenous spherulosis from AdCC. Cabibi et al.[285] found that the cells of collagenous spherulosis stained intensely for CD10, HHF35 actin, ER, and PR, whereas those of AdCC did not. Conversely, the cells of AdCC stained intensely for c-kit, but the cells of collagenous spherulosis did so only weakly. Rabban et al.[286] pointed out that both lesions can express SMA, S-100, and p63 and suggested the use of staining for other myoepithelial proteins. These authors found that the cells of collagenous spherulosis stain intensely for calponin and SMM-HC, and that those of AdCC did not.

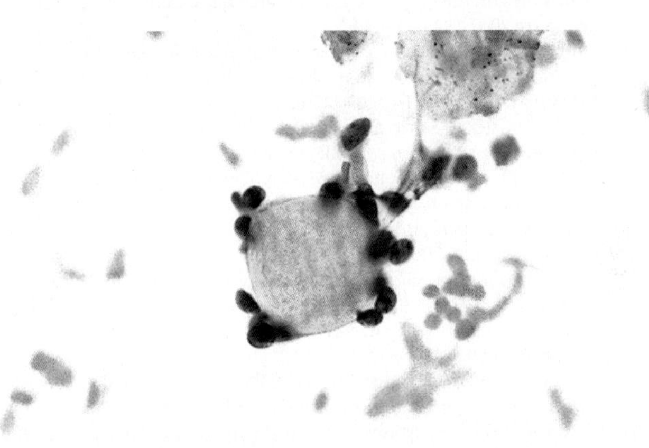

FIG. 5.56. ***Collagenous spherulosis, cytology specimen.*** A spherule in an FNA sample. Myoepithelial cells are adherent to the surface.

Electron Microscopy

Ultrastructural study[272,275,278,280,287] has consistently revealed two types of cells with the expected ultrastructural characteristics. The luminal cells appeared round or oval, and they possessed oval nuclei, prominent nucleoli, sparse organelles, prominent desmosomes, microvilli, and occasional intracytoplasmic lumens. The myoepithelial cells abutted the spherules and contained nuclei, parallel bundles of intracytoplasmic filaments with focal densities, tonofilaments, and hemidesmosomes attaching the cells to basement membrane material. Reduplicated basement membrane material sometimes sat adjacent to the myoepithelial cells. Collagen and basement membrane material comprised the spherules. A few displayed concentric mineralization. One can occasionally observe thin connections between the periductal stroma and the spherules.[287]

Treatment and Prognosis

There is no evidence to indicate that the presence of collagenous spherulosis is associated with precancerous lesions,[265,266] or that it is associated with AdCC. The prognosis and treatment of a patient with collagenous spherulosis depend on the nature of the underlying lesion.

REFERENCES

Papilloma

1. Haagensen CD, Stout AP, Phillips JS. The papillary neoplasms of the breast. I. Benign intraductal papilloma. *Ann Surg* 1951;133:18–36.
2. Rizzo M, Lund MJ, Oprea G, et al. Surgical follow-up and clinical presentation of 142 breast papillary lesions diagnosed by ultrasound-guided core-needle biopsy. *Ann Surg Oncol* 2008;15:1040–1047.
3. Mesurolle B, Kethani K, El-Khoury M, et al. Intraductal papilloma in a reconstructed breast: mammographic and sonographic appearance with pathologic correlation. *Breast* 2006;15:680–682.
4. Dzodic R, Stanojevic B, Saenko V, et al. Intraductal papilloma of ectopic breast tissue in axillary lymph node of a patient with a previous intraductal papilloma of ipsilateral breast: a case report and review of the literature. *Diagn Pathol* 2010;5:17.
5. Ichihara S, Ikeda T, Kimura K, et al. Coincidence of mammary and sentinel lymph node papilloma. *Am J Surg Pathol* 2008;32:784–792.
6. Volmer J. Intraduktales (intrazystisches) Papillom der männlichen Brustdrüse. *Zentralbl Allg Pathol* 1984;129:513–519.
7. Yamamoto H, Okada Y, Taniguchi H, et al. Intracystic papilloma in the breast of a male given long-term phenothiazine therapy: a case report. *Breast Cancer* 2006;13:84–88.
8. Durkin ET, Warner TF, Nichol PF. Enlarging unilateral breast mass in an adolescent male: an unusual presentation of intraductal papilloma. *J Pediatr Surg* 2011;46:e33–e35.
9. Georgountzos V, Ioannidou-Mouzaka L, Tsouroulas M, et al. Benign intracystic papilloma in the male breast. *Breast J* 2005;11:361–362.

10. Shim JH, Son EJ, Kim EK, et al. Benign intracystic papilloma of the male breast. *J Ultrasound Med* 2008;27:1397–1400.
11. Szabó BK, Wilczek B, Saracco A, et al. Solitary intraductal papilloma of the male breast: diagnostic value of galactography. *Breast J* 2003;9:330–331.
12. Radhi JM. Male breast: apocrine ductal papilloma with psammoma bodies. *Breast J* 2004;10:265.
13. Simpson JS, Barson AJ. Breast tumours in infants and children: a 40-year review of cases at a children's hospital. *Can Med Assoc J* 1969;101:100–102.
14. Martorano Navas MD, Rayas Povedano JL, Añorbe Medivil E, et al. Intracystic papilloma in male breast: ultrasonography and pneumocystography diagnosis. *J Clin Ultrasound* 1993;21:38–40.
15. Weshler Z, Sulkes A. Contrast mammography and the diagnosis of male breast cysts. *Clin Radiol* 1980;31:341–343.
16. Hassan MO, Gogate PA, al-Kaisi N. Intraductal papilloma of the male breast: an ultrastructural and immunohistochemical study. *Ultrastruct Pathol* 1994;18:601–609.
17. Sara AS, Gottfried MR. Benign papilloma of the male breast following chronic phenothiazine therapy. *Am J Clin Pathol* 1987;87:649–650.
18. Francis A, England D, Rowlands D, et al. Breast papilloma: mammogram, ultrasound and MRI appearances. *Breast* 2002;11:394–397.
19. Cardenosa G, Eklund GW. Benign papillary neoplasms of the breast: mammographic findings. *Radiology* 1991;181:751–755.
20. Rovno HD, Siegelman ES, Reynolds C, et al. Solitary intraductal papilloma: findings at MR imaging and MR galactography. *AJR Am J Roentgenol* 1999;172:151–155.
21. Kurz KD, Roy S, Saleh A, et al. MRI features of intraductal papilloma of the breast: sheep in wolf's clothing? *Acta Radiol* 2011;52:264–272.
22. Daniel BL, Gardner RW, Birdwell RL, et al. Magnetic resonance imaging of intraductal papilloma of the breast. *Magn Reson Imaging* 2003;21:887–892.
23. Lam WW, Chu WC, Tang AP, et al. Role of radiologic features in the management of papillary lesions of the breast. *AJR Am J Roentgenol* 2006;186:1322–1327.
24. Roy I, Meakins JL, Tremblay G. Giant intraductal papilloma of the breast: a case report. *J Surg Oncol* 1985;28:281–283.
25. Ichihara S, Matsuyama T, Kubo K, et al. Infarction of breast fibroadenoma in a postmenopausal woman. *Pathol Int* 1994;44:398–400.
26. Papotti M, Eusebi V, Gugliotta P, et al. Immunohistochemical analysis of benign and malignant papillary lesions of the breast. *Am J Surg Pathol* 1983;7:451–461.
27. Dabbs DJ, Gown AM. Distribution of calponin and smooth muscle myosin heavy chain in fine-needle aspiration biopsies of the breast. *Diagn Cytopathol* 1999;20:203–207.
28. Stefarefnou D, Batistatou A, Nonni A, et al. p63 Expression in benign and malignant breast lesions. *Histol Histopathol* 2004;19:465–471.
29. Judkins AR, Montone KT, LiVolsi VA, et al. Sensitivity and specificity of antibodies on necrotic tumor tissue. *Am J Clin Pathol* 1998;110:641–646.
30. Kobayashi TK, Ueda M, Nishino T, et al. Spontaneous infarction of an intraductal papilloma of the breast: cytological presentation on fine needle aspiration. *Cytopathology* 1992;3:379–384.
31. Ishihara A, Kobayashi TK. Infarcted intraductal papilloma of the breast: cytologic features with stage of infarction. *Diagn Cytopathol* 2006;34:373–376.
32. Flint A, Oberman HA. Infarction and squamous metaplasia of intraductal papilloma: a benign breast lesion that may simulate carcinoma. *Hum Pathol* 1984;15:764–767.
33. Soderstrom KO, Toikkanen S. Extensive squamous metaplasia simulating squamous cell carcinoma in benign breast papillomatosis. *Hum Pathol* 1983;14:1081–1082.
34. Reddick RL, Jennette JC, Askin FB. Squamous metaplasia of the breast. An ultrastructural and immunologic evaluation. *Am J Clin Pathol* 1985;84:530–533.
35. Jiao YF, Nakamura S, Oikawa T, et al. Sebaceous gland metaplasia in intraductal papilloma of the breast. *Virchows Arch* 2001;438:505–508.
36. Dawson AE, Mulford DK. Benign versus malignant papillary neoplasms of the breast. Diagnostic clues in fine needle aspiration cytology. *Acta Cytol* 1994;38:23–28.
37. Jeffrey PB, Ljung BM. Benign and malignant papillary lesions of the breast. A cytomorphologic study. *Am J Clin Pathol* 1994;101:500–507.
38. Simsir A, Waisman J, Thorner K, et al. Mammary lesions diagnosed as "papillary" by aspiration biopsy: 70 cases with follow-up. *Cancer* 2003;99:156–165.
39. Mak A, Field AS. Positive predictive value of the breast FNAB diagnoses of epithelial hyperplasia with atypia, papilloma, and radial scar. *Diagn Cytopathol* 2006;34:818–823.
40. Masood S, Loya A, Khalbuss W. Is core needle biopsy superior to fine-needle aspiration biopsy in the diagnosis of papillary breast lesions? *Diagn Cytopathol* 2003;28:329–334.
41. Chang JH, Lawson D, Muosunjac MB. Use of proliferation (Ki-67) and G1-cell cycle (cyclin D1) marker in evaluating breast papillary lesions in FNA cell block preparations. *Mod Pathol* 2000;13:31A.
42. Mosunjac MB, Lewis MM, Lawson D, et al. Use of a novel marker, calponin, for myoepithelial cells in fine-needle aspirates of papillary breast lesions. *Diagn Cytopathol* 2000;23:151–155.
43. Skandarajah AR, Field L, Yuen Larn Mou A, et al. Benign papilloma on core biopsy requires surgical excision. *Ann Surg Oncol* 2008;15:2272–2277.
44. Bernik SF, Troob S, Ying BL, et al. Papillary lesions of the breast diagnosed by core needle biopsy: 71 cases with surgical follow-up. *Am J Surg* 2009;197:473–478.
45. Jung SY, Kang HS, Kwon Y, et al. Risk factors for malignancy in benign papillomas of the breast on core needle biopsy. *World J Surg* 2010;34:261–265.
46. Brennan SB, Corben A, Liberman L, et al. Papilloma diagnosed at MRI-guided vacuum-assisted breast biopsy: is surgical excision still warranted? *AJR Am J Roentgenol* 2012;199:W512–W519.
47. Chang JM, Moon WK, Cho N, et al. Risk of carcinoma after subsequent excision of benign papilloma initially diagnosed with an ultrasound (US)-guided 14-gauge core needle biopsy: a prospective observational study. *Eur Radiol* 2010;20:1093–1100.
48. Chang JM, Moon WK, Cho N, et al. Management of ultrasonographically detected benign papillomas of the breast at core needle biopsy. *AJR Am J Roentgenol* 2011;196:723–729.
49. Jaffer S, Nagi C, Bleiweiss IJ. Excision is indicated for intraductal papilloma of the breast diagnosed on core needle biopsy. *Cancer* 2009;115:2837–2843.
50. Jakate K, De Brot M, Goldberg F, et al. Papillary lesions of the breast: impact of breast pathology subspecialization on core biopsy and excision diagnoses. *Am J Surg Pathol* 2012;36:544–551.
51. Kil WH, Cho EY, Kim JH, et al. Is surgical excision necessary in benign papillary lesions initially diagnosed at core biopsy? *Breast* 2008;17:258–262.
52. Lu Q, Tan EY, Ho B, et al. Surgical excision of intraductal breast papilloma diagnosed on core biopsy. *ANZ J Surg* 2012;82:168–172.
53. Rizzo M, Linebarger J, Lowe MC, et al. Management of papillary breast lesions diagnosed on core-needle biopsy: clinical pathologic and radiologic analysis of 276 cases with surgical follow-up. *J Am Coll Surg* 2012;214:280–287.
54. Shin HJ, Kim HH, Kim SM, et al. Papillary lesions of the breast diagnosed at percutaneous sonographically guided biopsy: comparison of sonographic features and biopsy methods. *AJR Am J Roentgenol* 2008;190:630–636.
55. Arora N, Hill C, Hoda SA, et al. Clinicopathologic features of papillary lesions on core needle biopsy of the breast predictive of malignancy. *Am J Surg* 2007;194:444–449.
56. Ahmadiyeh N, Stoleru MA, Raza S, et al. Management of intraductal papillomas of the breast: an analysis of 129 cases and their outcome *Ann Surg Oncol* 2009;16:2264–2269.
57. Sakr R, Rouzier R, Salem C, et al. Risk of breast cancer associated with papilloma. *Eur J Surg Oncol* 2008;34:1304–1308.
58. Ashkenazi I, Ferrer K, Sekosan M, et al. Papillary lesions of the breast discovered on percutaneous large core and vacuum-assisted biopsies: reliability of clinical and pathological parameters in identifying benign lesions. *Am J Surg* 2007;194:183–188.
59. Shah VI, Flowers CI, Douglas-Jones AG, et al. Immunohistochemistry increases the accuracy of diagnosis of benign papillary lesions in breast core needle biopsy specimens. *Histopathology* 2006;48:683–691.
60. Tse GM, Tan PH, Lacambra MD, et al. Papillary lesions of the breast—accuracy of core biopsy. *Histopathology* 2010;56:481–488.
61. Sexton K, Brill YM, Atkins L, et al. Outcome of benign papillary lesions of the breast diagnosed by needle core and mammotome biopsies with 3 to 5 year follow up. *Mod Pathol* 2006;19(Suppl.):42A.
62. Nesland JM, Johannessen JV. Scanning electron microscopy of the human breast and its disorders. *J Submicrosc Cytol* 1984;16:349–357.
63. Tsuchiya S, Takayama S, Higashi Y. Electron microscopy of intraductal papilloma of the breast. Ultrastructural comparison of papillary carcinoma with normal mammary large duct. *Acta Pathol Jpn* 1983;33:97–112.

64. Noguchi S, Motomura K, Inaji H, et al. Clonal analysis of solitary intraductal papilloma of the breast by means of polymerase chain reaction. *Am J Pathol* 1994;144:1320–1325.
65. Dickinson GK. The breast physiologically and pathologically considered with relation to bleeding from the nipple. *Am J Obstet Gynecol* 1922;3:31–34.
66. Bloodgood JC. Benign lesions of the female breast for which operation is not indicated. *JAMA* 1922;78:859–863.
67. Buhl-Jørgesen SE, Fischermann K, Johansen H, et al. Cancer risk in intraductal papilloma and papillomatosis. *Surg Gynecol Obstet* 1968;127:307–313.
68. Hendrick JW. Intraductal papilloma of the breast. *Surg Gynecol Obstet* 1957;105:215–223.
69. Kilgore AR, Fleming R, Ramos MM. The incidence of cancer with nipple discharge and the risk of cancer in the presence of papillary disease of the breast. *Surg Gynecol Obstet* 1953;96:649–660.
70. Kraus FT, Neubecker RD. The differential diagnosis of papillary tumors of the breast. *Cancer* 1962;15:444–455.
71. Lewison EF, Lyons JG Jr. Relationship between benign breast disease and cancer. *AMA Arch Surg* 1953;66:94–114.
72. Carter D. Intraductal papillary tumors of the breast: a study of 78 cases. *Cancer* 1977;39:1689–1692.
73. Greif F, Sharon E, Shechtman I, et al. Carcinoma within solitary ductal papilloma of the breast. *Eur J Surg Oncol* 2010;36:384–386.
74. Rosen PP. Arthur Purdy Stout and papilloma of the breast. Comments on the occasion of his 100th birthday. *Am J Surg Pathol* 1986;10 (Suppl. 1):100–107.
75. MacGrogan G, Tavassoli FA. Central atypical papillomas of the breast: a clinicopathological study of 119 cases. *Virchows Arch* 2003;443:609–617.
76. Cuneo KC, Dash RC, Wilke LG, et al. Risk of invasive breast cancer and ductal carcinoma in situ in women with atypical papillary lesions of the breast. *Breast J* 2012;18:475–478.
77. Ali-Fehmi R, Carolin K, Wallis T, et al. Clinicopathologic analysis of breast lesions associated with multiple papillomas. *Hum Pathol* 2003;34:234–239.
78. Estabrook A. Are patients with solitary or multiple intraductal papillomas at a higher risk of developing breast cancer? *Surg Oncol Clin North Am* 1993;2:45–56.
79. Snyder WH Jr, Chaffin L. Main duct papilloma of the breast. *AMA Arch Surg* 1955;70:680–685.
80. Haagensen CD, Bodian C, Haagensen DE. Multiple intraductal papillomas. In: *Breast carcinoma: risk and detection.* Philadelphia: WB Saunders, 1981:197–237.
81. Lewis JT, Hartmann LC, Vierkant RA, et al. An analysis of breast cancer risk in women with single, multiple, and atypical papilloma. *Am J Surg Pathol* 2006;30:665–672.
82. Wei H, Jiayi F, Qinping Z, et al. Ultrasound-guided vacuum-assisted breast biopsy system for diagnosis and minimally invasive excision of intraductal papilloma without nipple discharge. *World J Surg* 2009;33:2579–2581.

Radial Sclerosing Lesion

83. Semb C. Pathologico-anatomical and clinical investigations of fibroadenomatosis cystica mammae and its relation to other pathological conditions in mamma, especially cancer. *Acta Chir Scand (Suppl)* 1928;64:1–484.
84. Bloodgood JC. Borderline breast tumors: encapsulated and nonencapsulated cystic adenomata, observed from 1890–1931. *Am J Cancer* 1932;16:103–176.
85. Fenoglio C, Lattes R. Sclerosing papillary proliferations in the female breast. A benign lesion often mistaken for carcinoma. *Cancer* 1974;33:691–700.
86. Fisher ER, Palekar AS, Kotwal N, et al. A nonencapsulated sclerosing lesion of the breast. *Am J Clin Pathol* 1979;71:240–246.
87. Azzopardi JG, Ahmed A, Millis RR. *Problems in breast pathology. (Major Problems in Pathology*, vol. 11). Philadelpia: WB Saunders, 1979.
88. Rickert RR, Kalisher L, Hutter RVP. Indurative mastopathy: a benign sclerosing lesion of breast with elastosis which may simulate carcinoma. *Cancer* 1981;47:561–571.
89. Hamperl H. Strahlige Narben und obliterierende Mastopathie Beiträge zur pathologischen Histologie der Mamma. *Virchows Arch A Pathol Anat Histol* 1975;369:55–68.
90. Jacobs TW, Schnitt SJ, Tan X, et al. Radial scars of the breast and breast carcinomas have similar alterations in expression of factors involved in vascular stroma formation. *Hum Pathol* 2002;33:29–38.
91. Andersen JA, Gram JB. Radial scar in the female breast. A long-term follow-up study of 32 cases. *Cancer* 1984;53:2557–2560.
92. Bondeson L, Linell F, Ringberg A. Breast reductions: what to do with all the tissue specimens? *Histopathology* 1985;9:281–285.
93. Jacobs TW, Byrne C, Colditz G, et al. Radial scars in benign breast-biopsy specimens and the risk of breast cancer. *N Engl J Med* 1999;340:430–436.
94. Wellings SR, Alpers CE. Subgross pathologic features and incidence of radial scars in the breast. *Hum Pathol* 1984;15:475–479.
95. Nielsen M, Jensen J, Andersen JA. An autopsy study of radial scar in the female breast. *Histopathology* 1985;9:287–295.
96. Linell F, Ljungberg O, Anderson I. Breast carcinoma: aspects of early stage, progression and related problems. *Acta Pathol Microbiol Scand (Suppl)* 1980;272:1–233.
97. Anderson TJ, Battersby S. Radial scars of benign and malignant breasts: comparative features and significance. *J Pathol* 1985;147:23–32.
98. Patterson JA, Scott M, Anderson N, et al. Radial scar, complex sclerosing lesion and risk of breast cancer. Analysis of 175 cases in Northern Ireland. *Eur J Surg Oncol* 2004;30:1065–1068.
99. Tabar L, Dean PB. Stellate lesions. In: *Teaching atlas of mammography, Second revised edition.* New York: Georg Thieme Verlag, 1985:87–136.
100. Vazquez MF, Mitnick JS, Pressman P, et al. Radial scar: cytologic evaluation by stereotactic aspiration. *Breast Dis* 1994;7:299–306.
101. Adler DD, Helvie MA, Oberman HA, et al. Radial sclerosing lesion of the breast: mammographic features. *Radiology* 1990;176:737–740.
102. Ciatto S, Morrone D, Catarzi S, et al. Radial scars of the breast: review of 38 consecutive mammographic diagnoses. *Radiology* 1993;187:757–760.
103. Orel SG, Evers K, Yeh IT, et al. Radial scar with microcalcifications: radiologic–pathologic correlation. *Radiology* 1992;183:479–482.
104. Cohen MA, Sferlazza SJ. Role of sonography in evaluation of radial scars of the breast. *AJR Am J Roentgenol* 2000;174:1075–1078.
105. Mitnick JS, Vazquez MF, Harris MN, et al. Differentiation of radial scar from scirrhous carcinoma of the breast: mammographic–pathologic correlation. *Radiology* 1989;173:697–700.
106. Linda A, Zuiani C, Furlan A, et al. Radial scars without atypia diagnosed at imaging-guided needle biopsy: how often is associated malignancy found at subsequent surgical excision, and do mammography and sonography predict which lesions are malignant? *AJR Am J Roentgenol* 2010;194:1146–1151.
107. Pediconi F, Occhiato R, Venditti F, et al. Radial scars of the breast: contrast-enhanced magnetic resonance mammography appearance. *Breast J* 2005;11:23–28.
108. Andersen JA, Carter D, Linell F. A symposium on sclerosing duct lesions of the breast. *Pathol Annu* 1986;21(Pt 2):145–179.
109. Battersby S, Anderson TJ. Myofibroblast activity of radial scars. *J Pathol* 1985;147:33–40.
110. Doyle EM, Banville N, Quinn CM, et al. Radial scars/complex sclerosing lesions and malignancy in a screening programme: incidence and histological features revisited. *Histopathology* 2007;50:607–614.
111. Taylor HB, Norris HJ. Epithelial invasion of nerves in benign diseases of the breast. *Cancer* 1967;20:2245–2249.
112. Manfrin E, Remo A, Falsirollo F, et al. Risk of neoplastic transformation in asymptomatic radial scar. Analysis of 117 cases. *Breast Cancer Res Treat* 2008;107:371–377.
113. Cawson JN, Malara F, Kavanagh A, et al. Fourteen-gauge needle core biopsy of mammographically evident radial scars: is excision necessary? *Cancer* 2003;97:345–351.
114. Alvarado-Cabrero I, Tavassoli FA. Neoplastic and malignant lesions involving or arising in a radial scar: a clinicopathologic analysis of 17 cases. *Breast J* 2000;6:96–102.
115. Mokbel K, Price RK, Mostafa A, et al. Radial scar and carcinoma of the breast: microscopic findings in 32 cases. *Breast* 1999;8:339–342.
116. Caneva A, Bonetti F, Manfrin E, et al. Is a radial scar of the breast a premalignant lesion *Mod Pathol* 1997;10(Suppl.):17A.
117. Sloane JP, Mayers MM. Carcinoma and atypical hyperplasia in radial scars and complex sclerosing lesions: importance of lesion size and patient age. *Histopathology* 1993;23:225–231.
118. Farshid G, Rush G. Assessment of 142 stellate lesions with imaging features suggestive of radial scar discovered during population-based screening for breast cancer. *Am J Surg Pathol* 2004;28:1626–1631.
119. Denley H, Pinder SE, Tan PH, et al. Metaplastic carcinoma of the breast arising within complex sclerosing lesion: a report of five cases. *Histopathology* 2000;36:203–209.
120. Mitnick JS, Vazquez MF, Roses DF, et al. Stereotaxic localization for fine-needle aspiration breast biopsy. Initial experience with 300 patients. *Arch Surg* 1991;126:1137–1140.

121. Makunura CN, Curling OM, Yeomans P, et al. Apocrine adenosis within a radial scar: a case of false positive breast cytodiagnosis. *Cytopathology* 1994;5:123–128.
122. Orell SR. Radial scar/complex sclerosing lesion—a problem in the diagnostic work-up of screen-detected breast lesions. *Cytopathology* 1999;10:250–258.
123. Bianchi S, Giannotti E, Vanzi E, et al. Radial scar without associated atypical epithelial proliferation on image-guided 14-gauge needle core biopsy: analysis of 49 cases from a single-centre and review of the literature. *Breast* 2012;21:159–164.
124. Brenner RJ, Jackman RJ, Parker SH, et al. Percutaneous core needle biopsy of radial scars of the breast: when is excision necessary? *AJR Am J Roentgenol* 2002;179:1179–1184.
125. Becker L, Trop I, David J, et al. Management of radial scars found at percutaneous breast biopsy. *Can Assoc Radiol J* 2006;57:72–78.
126. Resetkova E, Edelweiss M, Albarracin CT, et al. Management of radial sclerosing lesions of the breast diagnosed using percutaneous vacuum-assisted core needle biopsy: recommendations for excision based on seven years' of experience at a single institution. *Breast Cancer Res Treat* 2011;127:335–343.
127. Lee KA, Zuley ML, Chivukula M, et al. Risk of malignancy when microscopic radial scars and microscopic papillomas are found at percutaneous biopsy. *AJR Am J Roentgenol* 2012;198:W141–W145.
128. Rajan S, Wason AM, Carder PJ. Conservative management of screen-detected radial scars: role of mammotome excision. *J Clin Pathol* 2011;64:65–68.
129. Tennant SL, Evans A, Hamilton LJ, et al. Vacuum-assisted excision of breast lesions of uncertain malignant potential (B3)—an alternative to surgery in selected cases. *Breast* 2008;17:546–549.
130. Iqbal M, Shoker BS, Foster CS, et al. Molecular and genetic abnormalities in radial scar. *Hum Pathol* 2002;33:715–722.
131. Nielsen M, Christensen L, Andersen J. Radial scars in women with breast cancer. *Cancer* 1987;59:1019–1025.
132. Sanders ME, Page DL, Simpson JF, et al. Interdependence of radial scar and proliferative disease with respect to invasive breast carcinoma risk in patients with benign breast biopsies. *Cancer* 2006;106:1453–1461.
133. Berg JC, Visscher DW, Vierkant RA, et al. Breast cancer risk in women with radial scars in benign breast biopsies. *Breast Cancer Res Treat* 2008;108:167–174.
134. Bunting DM, Steel JR, Holgate CS, et al. Long term follow-up and risk of breast cancer after a radial scar or complex sclerosing lesion has been identified in a benign open breast biopsy. *Eur J Surg Oncol* 2011;37:709–713.

Subareolar Sclerosing Duct Hyperplasia

135. Rosen PP. Subareolar sclerosing duct hyperplasia of the breast. *Cancer* 1987;59:1927–1930.

Cystic and Papillary Apocrine Metaplasia

136. Fechner RE. Benign breast disease in women on estrogen therapy. A pathologic study. *Cancer* 1972;29:273–279.
137. Charles A. An electron microscopic study of the human axillary apocrine gland. *J Anat* 1959;93:226–232.
138. Miller WR, Dixon JM, Forrest AP. Hormonal correlates of apocrine secretion in the breast. *Ann N Y Acad Sci* 1986;464:275–287.
139. Labows JN, Preti G, Hoelzle E, et al. Steroid analysis of human apocrine secretion. *Steroids* 1979;34:249–258.
140. Bussolati G, Cattani MG, Gugliotta P, et al. Morphologic and functional aspects of apocrine metaplasia in dysplastic and neoplastic breast tissue. *Ann N Y Acad Sci* 1986;464:262–274.
141. Naldoni C, Costantini M, Dogliotti L, et al. Association of cyst type with risk factors for breast cancer and relapse rate in women with gross cystic disease of the breast. *Cancer Res* 1992;52:1791–1795.
142. Haagensen CD, Bodian C, Haagensen DE. Apocrine epithelium. In: *Breast carcinoma: risk and detection.* Philadelphia: WB Saunders, 1981:83–105.
143. De Potter CR, Cuvelier CA, Roels HJ. Apocrine adenoma presenting as gynaecomastia in a 14-year-old boy. *Histopathology* 1988;13:697–699.
144. Tesluk H, Amott T, Goodnight JE, Jr. Apocrine adenoma of the breast. *Arch Pathol Lab Med* 1986;110:351–352.
145. Benigni G, Squartini F. Uneven distribution and significant concentration of apocrine metaplasia in lower breast quadrants. *Tumori* 1986;72:179–182.
146. Wellings SR, Alpers CE. Apocrine cystic metaplasia: subgross pathology and prevalence in cancer-associated versus random autopsy breasts. *Hum Pathol* 1987;18:381–386.
147. Schuerch C III, Rosen PP, Hirota T, et al. A pathologic study of benign breast diseases in Tokyo and New York. *Cancer* 1982;50:1899–1903.
148. Tramm T, Kim JY, Tavassoli FA. Diminished number or complete loss of myoepithelial cells associated with metaplastic and neoplastic apocrine lesions of the breast. *Am J Surg Pathol* 2011;35:202–211.
149. Archer F, Omar M. Pink cell (oncocytic) metaplasia in a fibroadenoma of the human breast: electron-microscope observations. *J Pathol* 1969;99:119–124.
150. Pier WJ, Jr, Garancis JC, Kuzma JF. The ultrastructure of apocrine cells in intracystic papilloma and fibrocystic disease of the breast. *Arch Pathol* 1970;89:446–452.
151. Nielsen BB. Adenosis tumour of the breast—a clinicopathological investigation of 27 cases. *Histopathology* 1987;11:1259–1275.
152. Kosemehmetoglu K, Guler G. Papillary apocrine metaplasia and columnar cell lesion with atypia: is there a shared common pathway? *Ann Diagn Pathol* 2010;14:425–431.
153. Carter DJ, Rosen PP. Atypical apocrine metaplasia in sclerosing lesions of the breast: a study of 51 patients. *Mod Pathol* 1991;4:1–5.
154. Celis JE, Gromov P, Moreira JM, et al. Apocrine cysts of the breast: biomarkers, origin, enlargement, and relation with cancer phenotype. *Mol Cell Proteomics* 2006;5:462–483.
155. Kumar S, Mansel RE, Jasani B. Presence and possible significance of immunohistochemically demonstrable prolactin in breast apocrine metaplasia. *Br J Cancer* 1987;55:307–309.
156. Ahmed A. Apocrine metaplasia in cystic hyperplastic mastopathy. Histochemical and ultrastructural observations. *J Pathol* 1975;115: 211–214.
157. Galatica Z. Immunohistochemical analysis of apocrine breast lesions. *Pathol Res Pract* 1997;193:753–758.
158. Selim AG, Wells CA. Immunohistochemical localisation of androgen receptor in apocrine metaplasia and apocrine adenosis of the breast: relation to oestrogen and progesterone receptors. *J Clin Pathol* 1999;52: 838–841.
159. Tavassoli FA, Purcell CA, Bratthauer GL, et al. Androgen receptor expression along with loss of bcl-2, ER, and PR expression in benign and malignant apocrine lesions of the breast: implications for therapy. *Breast J* 1996;2:261–269.
160. Feuerhake F, Unterberger P, Höfter EA. Cell turnover in apocrine metaplasia of the human mammary gland epithelium: apoptosis, proliferation, and immunohistochemical detection of Bcl-2, Bax, EGFR, and c-erbB2 gene products. *Acta Histochem* 2001;103:53–65.
161. Selim AG, El-Ayat G, Wells CA. Expression of c-erbB2, p53, Bcl-2, Bax, c-myc and Ki-67 in apocrine metaplasia and apocrine change within sclerosing adenosis of the breast. *Virchows Arch* 2002;441:449–455.
162. Elayat G, Selim AG, Wells CA. Cell turnover in apocrine metaplasia and apocrine adenosis of the breast. *Ann Diagn Pathol* 2010;14:1–7.
163. Elayat G, Selim AG, Wells CA. Alterations of the cell cycle regulators cyclin D1, cyclin A, p27, p21, p16, and pRb in apocrine metaplasia of the breast. *Breast J* 2009;15:475–482.
164. Elayat G, Selim AG, Gorman P, et al. Cyclin D-1 protein overexpression is not associated with gene amplification in benign and atypical apocrine lesions of the breast. *Pathol Res Pract* 2011;207:75–78.
165. Agnantis NJ, Mahera H, Maounis N, et al. Immunohistochemical study of ras and myc oncoproteins in apocrine breast lesions with and without papillomatosis. *Eur J Gynaecol Oncol* 1992;13:309–315.
166. Selim AG, El-Ayat G, Naase M, et al. C-myc oncoprotein expression and gene amplification in apocrine metaplasia and apocrine change within sclerosing adenosis of the breast. *Breast* 2002;11:466–472.
167. Izuo M, Okagaki T, Richart RM, et al. DNA content in "apocrine metaplasia" of fibrocystic disease of the breast. *Cancer* 1971;27:643–650.
168. Tóth J, Szamel I, Svastics E, et al. Significance of apocrine metaplasia in mammary carcinogenesis. A preliminary morphological and immunohistochemical study. *Ann N Y Acad Sci* 1990;586:238–251.
169. Elzagheid A, Kuopio T, Korhonen AM, et al. Apocrine change in fine-needle aspiration biopsy: nuclear morphometry and DNA image cytometry. *APMIS* 2003;111:898–904.
170. Washington C, Dalbègue F, Abreo F, et al. Loss of heterozygosity in fibrocystic change of the breast: genetic relationship between benign proliferative lesions and associated carcinomas. *Am J Pathol* 2000;157:323–329.
171. Selim AG, Ryan A, El-Ayat G, et al. Loss of heterozygosity and allelic imbalance in apocrine metaplasia of the breast: microdissection microsatellite analysis. *J Pathol* 2002;196:287–291.

172. Jones C, Damiani S, Wells D, et al. Molecular cytogenetic comparison of apocrine hyperplasia and apocrine carcinoma of the breast. *Am J Pathol* 2001;158:207–214.
173. Dawson EK. Sweat carcinoma of the breast. *Edinb Med J* 1932;39: 409–438.
174. Foote FW, Stewart FW. Comparative studies of cancerous versus noncancerous breasts. *Ann Surg* 1945;121:6–53.
175. Page DL, Vander Zwaag R, Rogers LW, et al. Relation between component parts of fibrocystic disease complex and breast cancer. *J Natl Cancer Inst* 1978;61:1055–1063.
176. Page DL, Jensen RA, Dupont WD. Papillary apocrine change of the breast-cancer risk indicator? *Lab Invest* 1994;70(Suppl.):26A.
177. Page DL, Dupont WD, Jensen RA. Papillary apocrine change of the breast: associations with atypical hyperplasia and risk of breast cancer. *Cancer Epidemiol Biomarkers Prev* 1996;5:29–32.
178. Yates AJ, Ahmed A. Apocrine carcinoma and apocrine metaplasia. *Histopathology* 1988;13:228–231.
179. Abati AD, Kimmel M, Rosen PP. Apocrine mammary carcinoma. A clinicopathologic study of 72 cases. *Am J Clin Pathol* 1990;94:371–377.

Florid Papillomatosis of the Nipple

180. Miller EM, Lewis D. The significance of serohemorrhagic or hemorrhagic discharge from the nipple. *JAMA* 1923;81:1651–1657.
181. Stowers JE. The significance of bleeding or discharge from the nipple. *Surg Gynecol Obstet* 1935;61:537–545.
182. Haagensen CD, Stout AP, Phillips JS. The papillary neoplasms of the breast. I. Benign intraductal papilloma. *Ann Surg* 1951;133:18–36.
183. Jones DB. Florid papillomatosis of the nipple ducts. *Cancer* 1955;8:315–319.
184. Handley RS, Thackray AC. Adenoma of nipple. *Br J Cancer* 1962;16: 187–194.
185. Le Gal Y, Gros CM, Bader P. L'adenomatose erosive du mamelon. *Ann Anat Pathol (Paris)* 1959;4:292–304.
186. Perzin KH, Lattes R. Papillary adenoma of the nipple (florid papillomatosis, adenoma, adenomatosis). A clinicopathologic study. *Cancer* 1972;29:996–1009.
187. Doctor VM, Sirsat MV. Florid papillomatosis (adenoma) and other benign tumours of the nipple and areola. *Br J Cancer* 1971;25:1–9.
188. Jones MW, Norris HJ, Snyder RC. Infiltrating syringomatous adenoma of the nipple. A clinical and pathological study of 11 cases. *Am J Surg Pathol* 1989;13:197–201.
189. Rosen PP. Syringomatous adenoma of the nipple. *Am J Surg Pathol* 1983;7:739–745.
190. Brownstein MH, Phelps RG, Magnin PH. Papillary adenoma of the nipple: analysis of fifteen new cases. *J Am Acad Dermatol* 1985;12:707–715.
191. Fisher ER, Gregorio RM, Fisher B, et al. The pathology of invasive breast cancer. A syllabus derived from findings of the National Surgical Adjuvant Breast Project (protocol no. 4). *Cancer* 1975;36:1–85.
192. Nichols FC, Dockerty MB, Judd ES. Florid papillomatosis of nipple. *Surg Gynecol Obstet* 1958;107:474–480.
193. Taylor HB, Robertson AG. Adenomas of the nipple. *Cancer* 1965;18:995–1002.
194. Moulin G, Darbon P, Balme B, et al. Adénomatose érosive du mamelon. A propos de 10 cas avec etude immunohistochimique. *Ann Dermatol Venereol* 1990;117:537–545.
195. Albers SE, Barnard M, Thorner P, et al. Erosive adenomatosis of the nipple in an eight-year-old girl. *J Am Acad Dermatol* 1999;40:834–837.
196. Civatte J, Restout S, Delomenie DC. Adénomatose érosive sur mamelon surnuméraire. *Ann Dermatol Vénéréol* 1977;104:777–779.
197. Miller G, Bernier L. Adenomatose erosive du mamelon. *Can J Surg* 1965;8:261–266.
198. Pettinato G, Manivel JC, Kelly DR, et al. Lesions of the breast in children exclusive of typical fibroadenoma and gynecomastia. A clinicopathologic study of 113 cases. *Pathol Annu* 1989;24(Pt 2):296–328.
199. Tao W, Kai F, Yue Hua L. Nipple adenoma in an adolescent. *Pediatr Dermatol* 2010;27:399–401.
200. Sugai M, Murata K, Kimura N, et al. Adenoma of the nipple in an adolescent. *Breast Cancer* 2002;9:254–256.
201. Clune JE, Kozakewich HP, VanBeek CA, et al. Nipple adenoma in infancy. *J Pediatr Surg* 2009;44:2219–2222.
202. Bergdahl L, Bergman F, Rais O, et al. Bilateral adenoma of nipple. Report of a case. *Acta Chir Scand* 1971;137:583–586.
203. Citoler P, Broer KH, Zippel HH. Doppelseitiges Adenom der Mamille. *Geburtshilfe Frauenheilkd* 1973;33:729–731.
204. Shioi Y, Nakamura SI, Kawamura S, et al. Nipple adenoma arising from axillary accessory breast: a case report. *Diagn Pathol* 2012;7:162.
205. Shinn L, Woodward C, Boddu S, et al. Nipple adenoma arising in a supernumerary mammary gland: a case report. *Tumori* 2011;97:812–814.
206. Palou J, Bordas X, Crego L, et al. Adénome papillaire du mamelon associé a une aréole surnuméraire. *Ann Dermatol Venereol* 1981;108:277–283.
207. Burdick C, Rinehart RM, Matsumoto T, et al. Nipple adenoma and Paget's disease in a man. *Arch Surg* 1965;91:835–839.
208. Shapiro L, Karpas CM. Florid papillomatosis of the nipple. First reported case in a male. *Am J Clin Pathol* 1965;44:155–159.
209. Fernandez-Flores A, Suarez-Peñaranda JM. Immunophenotype of nipple adenoma in a male patient. *Appl Immunohistochem Mol Morphol* 2011;19:190–194.
210. Waldo ED, Sidhu GS, Hu AW. Florid papillomatosis of male nipple after diethylstilbestrol therapy. *Arch Pathol* 1975;99:364–366.
211. Boutayeb S, Benomar S, Sbitti Y, et al. Nipple adenoma in a man: an unusual case report. *Int J Surg Case Rep* 2012;3:190–192.
212. Rao P, Shousha S. Male nipple adenoma with DCIS followed 9 years later by invasive carcinoma. *Breast J* 2010;16:317–318.
213. Tuveri M, Calo PG, Mocci C, et al. Florid papillomatosis of the male nipple. *Am J Surg* 2010;200:e39–e40.
214. Rosen PP, Caicco JA. Florid papillomatosis of the nipple. A study of 51 patients, including nine with mammary carcinoma. *Am J Surg Pathol* 1986;10:87–101.
215. Matsubayashi RN, Adachi A, Yasumori K, et al. Adenoma of the nipple: correlation of magnetic resonance imaging findings with histologic features. *J Comput Assist Tomogr* 2006;30:148–150.
216. Tsushimi T, Enoki T, Takemoto Y, et al. Adenoma of the nipple, focusing on the contrast-enhanced magnetic resonance imaging findings: report of a case. *Surg Today* 2011;41:1138–1141.
217. Fornage BD, Faroux MJ, Pluot M, et al. Nipple adenoma simulating carcinoma. Misleading clinical, mammographic, sonographic, and cytologic findings. *J Ultrasound Med* 1991;10:55–57.
218. Parajuly SS, Peng YL, Zhu M, et al. Nipple adenoma of the breast: sonographic imaging findings. *South Med J* 2010;103:1280–1281.
219. Adusumilli S, Siegelman ES, Schnall MD. MR Findings of nipple adenoma. *AJR Am J Roentgenol* 2002;179:803–804.
220. Kijima Y, Matsukita S, Yoshinaka H, et al. Adenoma of the nipple: report of a case. *Breast Cancer* 2006;13:95–99.
221. Pinto RG, Mandreker S. Fine needle aspiration cytology of adenoma of the nipple. A case report. *Acta Cytol* 1996;40:789–791.
222. Stormby N, Bondeson L. Adenoma of the nipple. An unusual diagnosis in aspiration cytology. *Acta Cytol* 1984;28:729–732.
223. Gupta RK, Dowle CS, Naran S, et al. Fine-needle aspiration cytodiagnosis of nipple adenoma (papillomatosis) in a man and woman. *Diagn Cytopathol* 2004;31:432–433.
224. Sood N, Jayaram G. Cytology of papillary adenoma of the nipple: a case diagnosed on fine-needle aspiration. *Diagn Cytopathol* 1990;6:345–348.
225. Mazzara PF, Flint A, Naylor B. Adenoma of the nipple. Cytopathologic features. *Acta Cytol* 1989;33:188–190.
226. Scott P, Kissin MW, Collins C, et al. Florid papillomatosis of the nipple: a clinico-pathological surgical problem. *Eur J Surg Oncol* 1991;17: 211–213.
227. Diaz NM, Palmer JO, Wick MR. Erosive adenomatosis of the nipple: histology, immunohistology, and differential diagnosis. *Mod Pathol* 1992;5:179–184.
228. Kono S, Kurosumi M, Simooka H, et al. Nipple adenoma found in a mastectomy specimen: report of a case with special regard to the proliferation pattern. *Breast Cancer* 2007;14:234–238.
229. Myers JL, Mazur MT, Urist MM, et al. Florid papillomatosis of the nipple: immunohistochemical and flow cytometric analysis of two cases. *Mod Pathol* 1990;3:288–293.
230. Bhagavan BS, Patchefsky A, Koss LG. Florid subareolar duct papillomatosis (nipple adenoma) and mammary carcinoma: report of three cases. *Hum Pathol* 1973;4:289–295.
231. Richards AT, Jaffe A, Hunt JA. Adenoma of the nipple in a male. *S Afr Med J* 1973;47:581–583.
232. Gudjonsdottir A, Hagerstrand I, Ostberg G. Adenoma of the nipple with carcinomatous development. *Acta Pathol Microbiol Scand A* 1971;79:676–680.
233. Jones MW, Tavassoli FA. Coexistence of nipple duct adenoma and breast carcinoma: a clinicopathologic study of five cases and review of the literature. *Mod Pathol* 1995;8:633–636.
234. Santini D, Taffurelli M, Carolina M, et al. Adenoma of the nipple. A clinico-pathologic study and its relation with carcinoma. *Breast Dis* 1990;3:153–163.

235. Sadanaga N, Kataoka A, Mashino K, et al. An adequate treatment for the nipple adenoma. *J Surg Oncol* 2000;74:171–172.
236. Van Mierlo PL, Geelen GM, Neumann HA. Mohs micrographic surgery for an erosive adenomatosis of the nipple. *Dermatol Surg* 1998;24:681–683.
237. Lee HJ, Chung KY. Erosive adenomatosis of the nipple: conservation of nipple by Mohs micrographic surgery. *J Am Acad Dermatol* 2002;47:578–580.
238. Kuflik EG. Erosive adenomatosis of the nipple treated with cryosurgery. *J Am Acad Dermatol* 1998;38:270–271.

Syringomatous Adenoma of the Nipple

239. Johnston CA, Toker C. Syringomatous tumors of minor salivary gland origin. *Hum Pathol* 1982;13:182–184.
240. Goldstein DJ, Barr RJ, Santa Cruz DJ. Microcystic adnexal carcinoma: a distinct clinicopathologic entity. *Cancer* 1982;50:566–572.
241. Cooper PH, Mills SE, Leonard DD, et al. Sclerosing sweat duct (syringomatous) carcinoma. *Am J Surg Pathol* 1985;9:422–433.
242. Handley RS, Thackray AC. Adenoma of nipple. *Br J Cancer* 1962;16:187–194.
243. Doctor VM, Sirsat MV. Florid papillomatosis (adenoma) and other benign tumours of the nipple and areola. *Br J Cancer* 1971;25:1–9.
244. Rosen PP. Syringomatous adenoma of the nipple. *Am J Surg Pathol* 1983;7:739–745.
245. Carter E, Dyess DL. Infiltrating syringomatous adenoma of the nipple: a case report and 20-year retrospective review. *Breast J* 2004;10: 443–447.
246. Ferrari A, Roncalli M. Adenoma siringomatoso della mammella. *Istocitopatologia* 1984;6:231–234.
247. Kubo M, Tsuji H, Kunitomo T, et al. Syringomatous adenoma of the nipple: a case report. *Breast Cancer* 2004;11:214–216.
248. Toyoshima O, Kanou M, Kintaka N, et al. Syringomatous adenoma of the nipple: report of a case. *Surg Today* 1998;28:1196–1199.
249. Ward BE, Cooper PH, Subramony C. Syringomatous tumor of the nipple. *Am J Clin Pathol* 1989;92:692–696.
250. Odashiro M, Lima MG, Miiji LN, et al. Infiltrating syringomatous adenoma of the nipple. *Breast J* 2009;15:414–416.
251. Oliva VL, Little JV, Carlson GW. Syringomatous adenoma of the nipple—treatment by central mound resection and oncoplastic reconstruction. *Breast J* 2008;14:102–105.
252. Sarma DP, Stevens T. Infiltrating syringomatous eccrine adenoma of the nipple: a case report. *Cases J* 2009;2:9118.
253. Yosepovich A, Perelman M, Ayalon S, et al. Syringomatous adenoma of the nipple: a case report. *Pathol Res Pract* 2005;201:405–407.
254. Jones MW, Norris HJ, Snyder RC. Infiltrating syringomatous adenoma of the nipple. A clinical and pathological study of 11 cases. *Am J Surg Pathol* 1989;13:197–201.
255. Slaughter MS, Pomerantz RA, Murad T, et al. Infiltrating syringomatous adenoma of the nipple. *Surgery* 1992;111:711–713.
256. Mrklić I, Bezić J, Pogorelić Z,et al. Synchronous bilateral infiltrating syringomatous adenoma of the breast. *Scott Med J* 2012;57:121.
257. Page RN, Dittrich L, King R, et al. Syringomatous adenoma of the nipple occurring within a supernumerary breast: a case report. *J Cutan Pathol* 2009;36:1206–1209.
258. Dahlstrom JE, Tait N, Cranney BG, et al. Fine needle aspiration cytology and core biopsy histology in infiltrating syringomatous adenoma of the breast. A case report. *Acta Cytol* 1999;43:303–307.
259. Kim HM, Park BW, Han SH, et al. Infiltrating syringomatous adenoma presenting as microcalcification in the nipple on screening mammogram: case report and review of the literature of radiologic features. *Clin Imaging* 2010;34:462–465.
260. Ku J, Bennett RD, Chong KD, et al. Syringomatous adenoma of the nipple. *Breast* 2004;13:412–415.
261. Rosen PP, Ernsberger D. Low-grade adenosquamous carcinoma. A variant of metaplastic mammary carcinoma. *Am J Surg Pathol* 1987;11:351–358.
262. Chang CK, Jacobs IA, Calilao G, et al. Metastatic infiltrating syringomatous adenoma of the breast. *Arch Pathol Lab Med* 2003;127: e155–e156.
263. Coulthard A, Liston J, Young JR. Case report: infiltrating syringomatous adenoma of the breast—appearances on mammography and ultrasonography. *Clin Radiol* 1993;47:62–64.
264. Jones DB. Florid papillomatosis of the nipple ducts. *Cancer* 1955;8:315–319.

Collagenous Spherulosis

265. Clement PB, Young RH, Azzopardi JG. Collagenous spherulosis of the breast. *Am J Surg Pathol* 1987;11:411–417.
266. Rosen PP. Adenoid cystic carcinoma of the breast. A morphologically heterogeneous neoplasm. *Pathol Annu* 1989;24(Pt 2):237–254.
267. Resetkova E, Albarracin C, Sneige N. Collagenous spherulosis of breast: morphologic study of 59 cases and review of the literature. *Am J Surg Pathol* 2006;30:20–27.
268. Guarino M, Tricomi P, Cristofori E. Collagenous spherulosis of the breast with atypical epithelial hyperplasia. *Pathologica* 1993;85:123–127.
269. Gangane N, Joshi D, Shivkumar VB. Cytological diagnosis of collagenous spherulosis of breast associated with fibroadenoma: report of a case with review of literature. *Diagn Cytopathol* 2007;35:366–369.
270. Ohta M, Mori M, Kawada T, et al. Collagenous spherulosis associated with adenomyoepithelioma of the breast: a case report. *Acta Cytol* 2010;54:314–318.
271. Reis-Filho JS, Fulford LG, Crebassa B, et al. Collagenous spherulosis in an adenomyoepithelioma of the breast. *J Clin Pathol* 2004;57:83–86.
272. Divaris DX, Smith S, Leask D, et al. Complex collagenous spherulosis of the breast presenting as a palpable mass: a case report with immunohistochemical and ultrastructural studies. *Breast J* 2000;6:199–203.
273. Hill P, Cawson J. Collagenous spherulosis presenting as a mass lesion on imaging. *Breast J* 2008;14:301–303.
274. Mooney EE, Kayani N, Tavassoli FA. Spherulosis of the breast. A spectrum of municous and collagenous lesions. *Arch Pathol Lab Med* 1999;123:626–630.
275. Wells CA, Wells CW, Yeomans P, et al. Spherical connective tissue inclusions in epithelial hyperplasia of the breast ("collagenous spherulosis"). *J Clin Pathol* 1990;43:905–908.
276. Sola Pérez J, Pérez-Guillermo M, Bas Bernal A, et al. Diagnosis of collagenous spherulosis of the breast by fine needle aspiration cytology. A report of two cases. *Acta Cytol* 1993;37:725–728.
277. Hata S, Kanomata N, Kozuka Y, et al. Significance of collagenous and mucinous spherulosis in breast cytology specimens. *Cytopathology* 2010;21:157–160.
278. Highland KE, Finley JL, Neill JS, et al. Collagenous spherulosis. Report of a case with diagnosis by fine needle aspiration biopsy with immunocytochemical and ultrastructural observations. *Acta Cytol* 1993;37:3–9.
279. Clement PB. Collagenous spherulosis (Letter to editor). *Am J Surg Pathol* 1987;11:907.
280. Grignon DJ, Ro JY, Mackay BN, et al. Collagenous spherulosis of the breast. Immunohistochemical and ultrastructural studies. *Am J Clin Pathol* 1989;91:386–392.
281. Stephenson TJ, Hird PM, Laing RW, et al. Nodular basement membrane deposits in breast carcinoma and atypical ductal hyperplasia: mimics of collagenous spherulosis. *Pathologica* 1994;86:234–239.
282. Hill P, Cawson J. Collagenous spherulosis with lobular carcinoma in situ: a potential diagnostic pitfall. *Pathology* 2007;39:361–363.
283. Sgroi D, Koerner FC. Involvement of collagenous spherulosis by lobular carcinoma in situ. Potential confusion with cribriform ductal carcinoma in situ. *Am J Surg Pathol* 1995;19:1366–1370.
284. Rey A, Redondo E, Servent R. Collagenous spherulosis of the breast diagnosed by fine needle aspiration biopsy. *Acta Cytol* 1995;39:1071–1073.
285. Cabibi D, Giannone AG, Belmonte B, et al. CD10 and HHF35 actin in the differential diagnosis between collagenous spherulosis and adenoid-cystic carcinoma of the breast. *Pathol Res Pract* 2012;208:405–409.
286. Rabban JT, Swain RS, Zaloudek CJ, et al. Immunophenotypic overlap between adenoid cystic carcinoma and collagenous spherulosis of the breast: potential diagnostic pitfalls using myoepithelial markers. *Mod Pathol* 2006;19:1351–1357.
287. Maluf HM, Koerner FC, Dickersin GR. Collagenous spherulosis: an ultrastructural study. *Ultrastruct Pathol* 1998;22:239–248.

CHAPTER 6

Myoepithelial Neoplasms

EDI BROGI

THE MYOEPITHELIAL CELL

Myoepithelial cells (MECs) comprise part of the normal lining of mammary ducts and lobules.[1] They are interposed between the polarized glandular cells and the underlying basement membrane in the so-called basal cell layer. These cells have contractile properties similar to smooth muscle cells and express smooth muscle–specific proteins such as smooth muscle actin (SMA). Studies of mammary and salivary gland tissue have shown that MECs derive from the ectoderm, whereas smooth muscle cells derive from the mesoderm.[2,3] Differentiation of epithelial cells and MECs has been observed in the terminal end buds of the developing pubertal breast.[4] O'Hare et al.[5] used fluorescence-activated cell sorting to separate epithelial membrane antigen (EMA)-positive luminal cells and CD10-positive MECs from lysates of fresh mammary tissue and studied the cytologic and immunophenotypic characteristics of these two cell types. Additional and more sophisticated methods for purification and study of MECs have also been developed, as reviewed by Clarke et al.[6]

During lactation, mammary MECs contract upon stimulation by oxytocin, resulting in the expression of milk from the nipple ducts. Recent observations[7,8] have demonstrated "tumor-suppressor" properties of MECs that are mediated through physical and paracrine activity. MECs form a barrier between the ductal epithelium composed of luminal cells and the surrounding stroma, thereby preventing direct interaction between the two tissue components. This function is especially important when the glandular epithelium consists of carcinoma *in situ* (CIS). In addition, MECs produce components of the basement membrane, as well as antiangiogenic and antiprotease factors, contributing to maintain a controlled microenvironment that wards off stromal invasion. It has been hypothesized that local chemokines and/or inflammation can result in physical and functional attenuation of the myoepithelial layer, weakening the basement membrane and creating local conditions that are permissive of stromal invasion.[8] On the other end of the spectrum, some investigators hypothesize that MECs, or a population of basal stem cells admixed with MECs, are involved in the development of basal-like mammary carcinomas. However, using a murine model of mammary carcinoma, Molyneux et al.[9] found that deletion of the *BRCA1* gene in the basal cells/MECs led to the development of malignant adenomyoepitheliomas (AMEs). In contrast, deletion of the same gene in the luminal epithelium produced tumors with features of basal-like carcinomas, challenging the hypothesis that basal-like carcinomas derive from basal stem cells presumed to reside in the myoepithelial layer.

This chapter is devoted to a discussion of neoplasms that display the distinctive phenotype of MECs. Carcinomas referred to as "basaloid" or "basal-type" are considered elsewhere in this volume, including in Chapter 12.

MEC Morphology

MECs can have spindle or epithelioid morphology. They are usually inconspicuous, unless they are hyperplastic. In histologic sections, the nucleus of spindle-shaped MECs is located in the center of the cell. It is elongated, with the longest axis parallel to the basement membrane. Although minimally visible in routine hematoxylin and eosin (H&E)–stained sections, the cytoplasm of MECs is readily apparent in sections immunostained for myofilaments such as calponin or SMA. Mammary MECs sometimes acquire polygonal or globoid morphology, with abundant clear cytoplasm and pseudovacuoles. This appearance not only constitutes a physiologic alteration during the luteal phase of the menstrual cycle,[10] but is also commonly found in sclerosing lesions (Fig. 6.1) and in myoepithelial tumors. MECs with clear cytoplasm can mimic atypical lobular hyperplasia (ALH) and classic lobular carcinoma *in situ* (LCIS) with pagetoid growth, but the uniform circumferential distribution at the periphery of the acini is usually sufficient for correct identification. Immunoperoxidase stains for MEC markers can help resolve problematic cases (see also Chapter 31 for a more detailed discussion of this differential diagnosis). Clear cell change and subtle hyperplasia of the MECs are also common in irradiated breast (Fig. 6.1). The pseudovacuoles of MECs lack mucin and do not stain with Alcian blue and periodic acid–Schiff (PAS) stains. Myoepithelial hyperplasia sometimes can nearly obliterate the acinar lumen, resulting in an appearance that mimics classical LCIS or ALH. In these cases, an E-cadherin stain will show expansion by an MEC population with discontinuous and granular membranous reactivity of weaker intensity than in the ductal cells. This pattern of reactivity should not be interpreted as evidence of lobular differentiation, and immunostains for calponin and p63 will complement the diagnosis (Fig. 6.2).

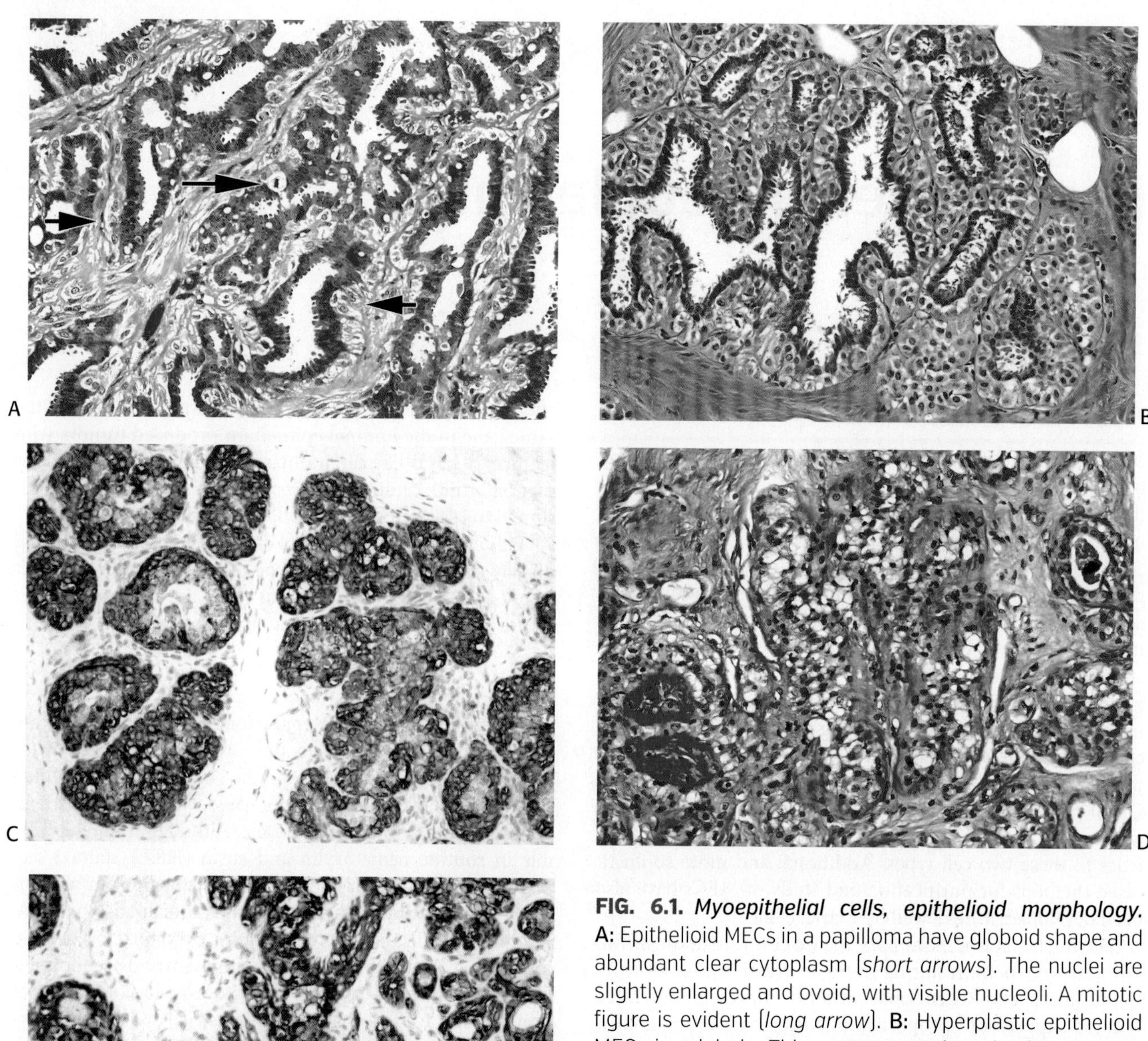

FIG. 6.1. ***Myoepithelial cells, epithelioid morphology.*** **A:** Epithelioid MECs in a papilloma have globoid shape and abundant clear cytoplasm [*short arrows*]. The nuclei are slightly enlarged and ovoid, with visible nucleoli. A mitotic figure is evident [*long arrow*]. **B:** Hyperplastic epithelioid MECs in a lobule. This pattern may be mistaken as pagetoid spread of ALH or classical LCIS. **C:** The MECs in **(B)** are reactive for calponin. **D:** The MECs in this irradiated lobule are slightly hyperplastic and have relatively abundant clear and vacuolated cytoplasm. Almost complete absence of epithelial cells and the thickened basement membranes are consistent with radiation effect. **E:** An immunoperoxidase stain for calponin in the same tissue as in **(D)** highlights the hyperplastic myoepithelium.

Myoid transformation of MECs is commonly observed as an incidental finding in breast tissue from premenopausal and postmenopausal women. When this occurs, the MECs acquire the cytologic and histochemical features of smooth muscle cells, including a more pronounced spindle shape and eosinophilic cytoplasm. Myoid transformation is most frequently encountered around terminal ducts and lobules in the absence of appreciable epithelial proliferation (see Chapter 1) (Fig. 6.3). These changes are not associated with any particular type of tumor and may be found in specimens from patients who had breast tissue sampled for various benign or malignant lesions. Myoid transformation is often present in the foci of sclerosing adenosis, and it may occasionally dominate the process, leading to a leiomyomatous appearance (Fig. 6.4).

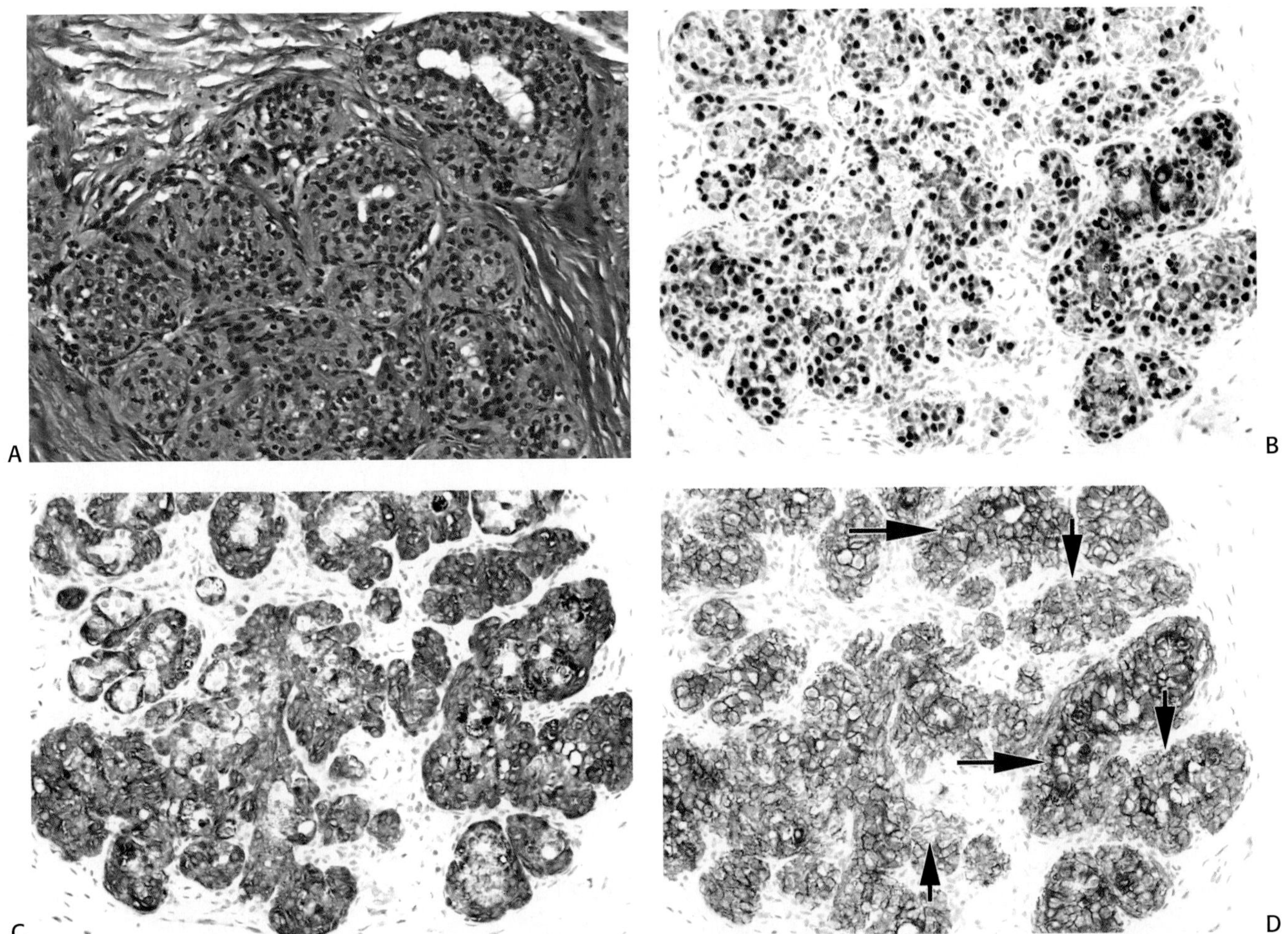

FIG. 6.2. ***Myoepithelial hyperplasia that mimics classical LCIS.*** **A:** In this example of florid myoepithelial hyperplasia, most of the involved acini have no visible lumens, and the overall appearance mimics classic LCIS or ALH. **B:** A p63 immunostain highlights the nuclei of the hyperplastic MECs. **C:** A calponin immunostain decorates the cytoplasm of the hyperplastic MECs. **D:** Membranous immunoreactivity for E-cadherin in the hyperplastic myoepithelium (*short arrows*) is less intense than that in the luminal cells (*long arrows*) lining the acini. Attenuated staining reflects the normal staining pattern of MECs, and it should not be interpreted as suggestive of lobular neoplasia.

Immunohistochemistry

In addition to SMA, the cytoplasm of MECs is also immunoreactive for smooth muscle myosin heavy chain (SMM-HC), calponin, and CD10.[11] S-100 and maspin decorate the cytoplasm and the nucleus of MECs, whereas p75 highlights the cytoplasm and the cell membrane.[11] MECs are characterized by nuclear immunoreactivity for p63, a p53 homolog protein. Glial fibrillary acidic protein (GFAP) and caveolin-1 are myoepithelial antigens less frequently used for the identification of mammary MECs. Epithelial markers such as CK5, 6, 14, and 17, keratin 34βE12, and P-cadherin also stain the mammary MECs. E-cadherin decorates the myoepithelium with a characteristic membranous "dot-like" discontinuous linear pattern. Keratin AE1 does not stain the mammary myoepithelium, whereas AE3 stains the myoepithelium of the mammary ducts but not of the acini.[12] MECs are usually negative for EMA, carcinoembryonic antigen (CEA), and CK8/18.

MECs in Breast Lesions

MECs participate in many benign proliferative processes in the breast, most notably sclerosing adenosis (see Chapter 7) and papillary proliferative lesions of ducts (see Chapter 5). Myoepithelial hyperplasia sometimes accompanies classical LCIS and ALH (see Chapter 31) and is also common in normal and hyperplastic mammary ducts and glands in the irradiated breast. It can also occur focally with no apparent reason (Figs. 6.2 to 6.4). In contrast, MECs are often reduced around ducts involved by ductal carcinoma *in situ* (DCIS) with or without associated invasive carcinoma.

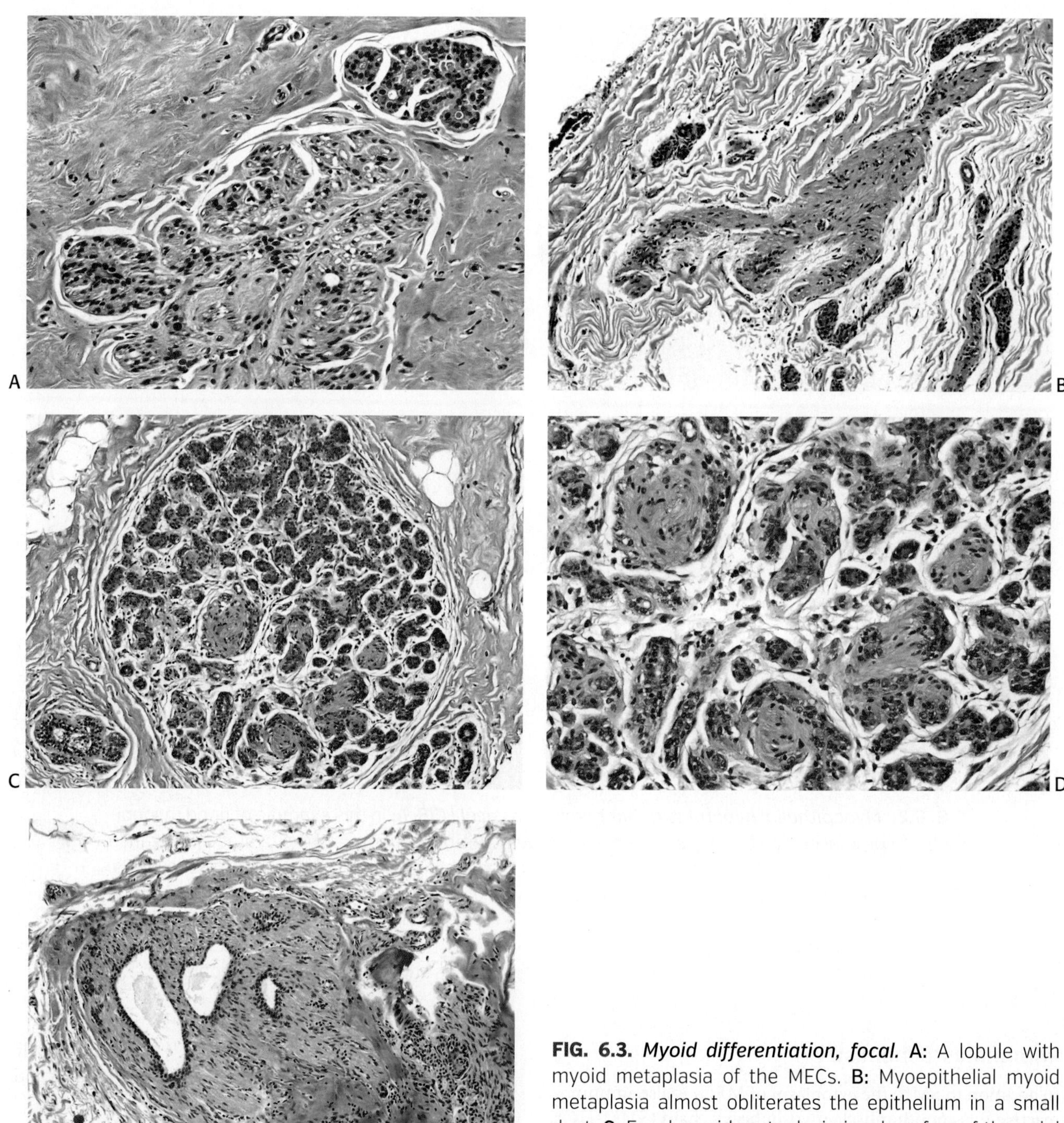

FIG. 6.3. ***Myoid differentiation, focal.*** **A:** A lobule with myoid metaplasia of the MECs. **B:** Myoepithelial myoid metaplasia almost obliterates the epithelium in a small duct. **C:** Focal myoid metaplasia involves few of the acini of a lobule. **D:** Closer view of the myoid foci in image **(C)**. **E:** Another example of myoid metaplasia in a lobule.

Mammary neoplasms composed partly or entirely of MECs are uncommon.[13] The classification of these tumors is complicated by the inherent phenotypic plasticity of MECs. The MECs in the salivary gland epithelium contribute to the histogenesis of pleomorphic adenomas (mixed tumors) and carcinomas that arise in these glands.[14,15] Morphologic similarities between certain tumors of the breast, salivary glands, and skin appendage glands reflect the contribution of MECs to these lesions.

A mammary neoplasm that exhibits epithelial and myoepithelial differentiation is referred to as AME. Most AMEs are benign tumors. When either the epithelial or the myoepithelial component of an adenomyoepitheliomatous tumor is malignant, the appropriate diagnosis is adenocarcinoma arising in an AME or myoepithelial carcinoma, depending on the nature of the malignant component. The term *malignant AME* should be reserved for exceedingly rare neoplasms in which both the epithelial and myoepithelial components

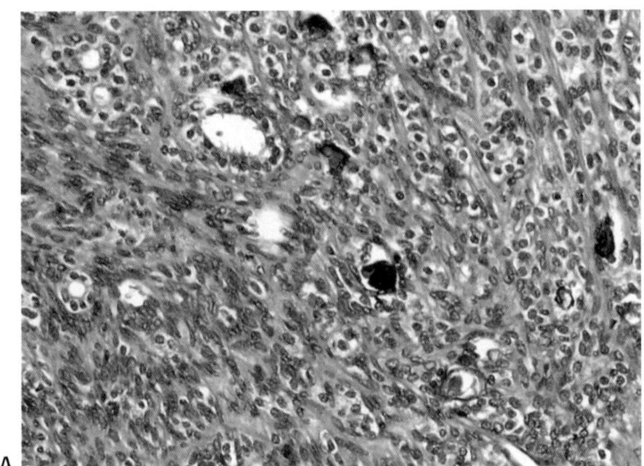

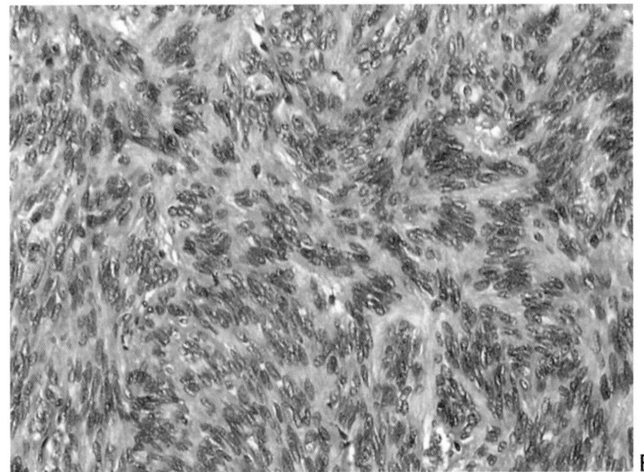

FIG. 6.4. ***Myoid differentiation in sclerosing adenosis.*** **A:** Myoid MECs surround glands with calcifications. **B:** Palisading of spindly MECs in nodular sclerosing adenosis.

are malignant. Unfortunately, these distinctions have not been made in most of the published reports of adenomyoepithelial neoplasms. Classification is further complicated by uncommon tumors that exhibit combined adenomyoepithelial and microglandular adenosis-like (MGA-like) growth patterns.[16,17]

Benign neoplasms composed entirely of MECs are referred to as *myoepitheliomas*. Malignant MEC neoplasms with myoepithelial differentiation have been classified as myoepithelial carcinomas. This term applies to some neoplasms, especially those that qualify as myoepithelial carcinoma arising in an AME. However, the observation that many of the malignant neoplasms classified as metaplastic carcinomas express myoepithelial markers has clouded the distinction between myoepithelial carcinoma and metaplastic carcinoma from a histogenetic standpoint, although these entities are usually histologically distinguishable. Additional discussion of this topic in the context of metaplastic carcinoma can be found in Chapter 16.

ADENOMYOEPITHELIOMA

The first full description of AME of the breast was published in 1970 by Hamperl.[18] With the exception of five studies consisting, respectively, of 6, 13, 18, 27, and 23 cases,[19–23] most reports of AME have been case studies.

Clinical Presentation

Age, Gender, and Genetic Predisposition

Most patients with AME are women of postmenopausal age, but patients as young as 26[20] and 27[21] years have been reported. Two examples of AME have been described in men of age 47[24] and 84 years.[25] No malignant AME has been reported in male patients.

There is no documented evidence of a genetic and/or familial association. A 41-year-old woman with malignant myoepithelioma arising in a mammary AME and multiple gastrointestinal stromal tumors had neurofibromatosis type 1, but no other family member was affected.[26]

Presentation

Most patients present with a solitary, unilateral painless mass. Han and Peng[27] reported one patient with three distinct AMEs, one of which was benign, one atypical, and the third contained DCIS. Most lesions occur in the periphery of the breast, but occasionally they have been found centrally or near the areola,[22,28–34] including AMEs in two male patients.[24,25] Nipple discharge,[32] pain, and tenderness are infrequent. In some cases, the tumor was palpable for nearly a year before excision.[21,22,35] Patients with malignant tumors may describe recent onset or report rapid growth of a long-standing lesion.

Imaging Studies

Mammography typically reveals a single, circumscribed mass that is not easily distinguished from a fibroadenoma. The border of the tumor is usually well circumscribed and sometimes microlobulated. An irregular contour is uncommon.[30,31] In a few instances, the mammographic appearance has been interpreted as suspicious.[30,31,36,37] Radiologically apparent calcifications are exceedingly rare.[27,30,38,39] The presence of pleomorphic calcifications in a benign AME was considered to be a "suspicious" radiologic finding.[40] AMEs examined by mammography usually present as palpable tumors measuring 3 cm or less in diameter,[30] but there have been reports of small nonpalpable AMEs that were detected on mammography alone.[36] Conversely, some palpable AMEs were not apparent in mammograms because they were obscured by superimposed dense breast tissue.[31,38] Since AMEs resemble fibroadenomas mammographically, the lesions may sometimes be left in place and followed with imaging studies.[21]

Sonographically[31,38] AME appears as a solid, round or oval mass (Fig. 6.5) with hypo- or complex echogenic texture. The margin is typically smooth or lobulated, and less often irregular.[31,36] Posterior acoustic enhancement may be present,[36,37] depending on the cellular composition of the tumor (Fig. 6.5). Hypervascularity has been reported in the vicinity of AME,[41] and ectatic ducts may be present. In one case, clustered, small, round calcifications on a screening mammogram proved to be in a nonpalpable 9 × 7 mm well-circumscribed, hypoechoic AME on sonography.[37] Mammographically inapparent AMEs that were detected by sonography were described by Lee et al.[38] and Chang et al.[36] Adjacent duct ectasia is also a common finding. MRI studies are limited and show homogeneous to heterogeneous enhancement with a delayed washout pattern after gadolinium injection.[31,38]

Associated Tumors

Usual types of breast carcinoma can be present separately in a breast that harbors an AME. One of the patients studied by Lee et al.[38] was a 72-year-old woman with two AMEs and a separate focus of DCIS in one breast. Three cases of AME with DCIS have been reported.[27,42,43] Kuroda et al.[44] described a 66-year-old woman with a 3.5-cm invasive duct carcinoma that was adjacent to, but separate from a 0.8-cm AME. A tumor described by Honda and Iyama[45] appears to have been a malignant AME that was invaded by coexisting E-cadherin-negative invasive lobular carcinoma. Metastatic lobular carcinoma was present in axillary lymph nodes. Two years later, a nodule removed from a lung had the histologic appearance of the original AME, and similar lesions were found in both lungs and kidneys 5 years after the initial diagnosis. The biphasic structure of glandular cells surrounded by MECs that was present in the initial AME was also found in the metastatic foci. Da Silva et al.[46] encountered a 0.5-cm AME adjacent to an adenoid cystic carcinoma (AdCC) in an area of tubular adenosis. Another patient reportedly had a breast mass composed of AME and recurrent phyllodes tumor.[47]

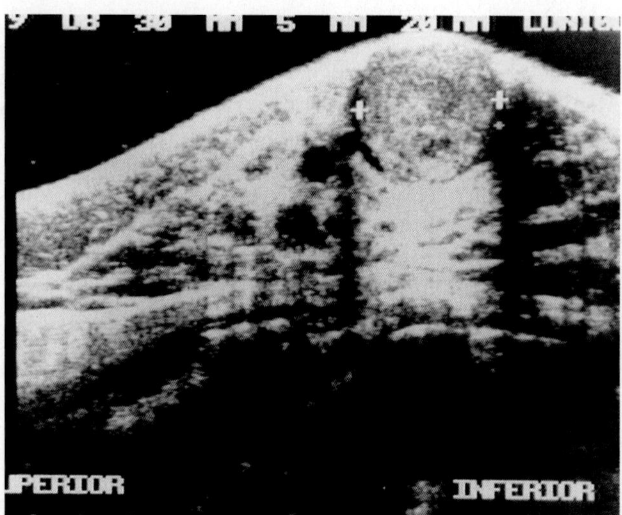

FIG. 6.5. ***Adenomyoepithelioma, imaging.*** This ultrasound image shows a well-circumscribed, slightly inhomogeneous mass in the subareolar region.

Gross Pathology

The gross size of AMEs ranges from 0.5 to 8.0 cm, with an average and median size of about 2.5 cm. With rare exceptions, the tumors have been described as solid, well circumscribed, and firm or hard; lobulation is often noted (Fig. 6.6). Several lesions were described as translucent. The color of the tumor cut surface has been characterized as tan, gray, white, yellow, and pink. Small cysts occur in a minority of cases.[21,22,48] Very large, grossly cystic tumors can occupy a substantial part of the breast (Fig. 6.7). Some tumors have been described as predominantly intracystic.[38,49] There does not appear to be a good correlation between the gross appearance of the tumor and its microscopic composition.

Microscopic Pathology

Benign AME

At low magnification, most AMEs are circumscribed and are composed of aggregated nodules, typically lacking a discrete fibrous capsule. Some AMEs consist of a compact nodular proliferation of epithelial cells and MECs, but most lesions are composed of solid or papillary nodules that often surround a slightly ovoid sclerotic center, in a configuration reminiscent of the petals of a flower (Fig. 6.8). A minority of AMEs consist, for the most part, of intraductal papillary elements, in accordance with the hypothesis that these lesions are variants of intraductal papilloma characterized by myoepithelial expansion (Fig. 6.9). Sometimes the papillary intraductal component extends into ducts outside the main body of the lesion. This characteristic may account for recurrence after a seemingly adequate excision. A minority of AMEs appear to arise from a lobular proliferation or adenosis (Figs. 6.10 and 6.11). Clear

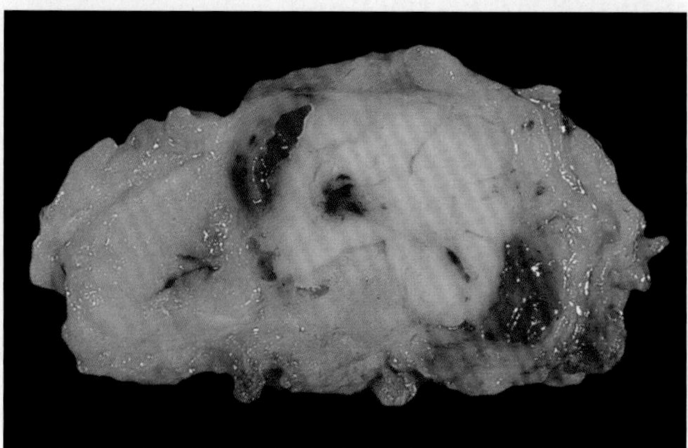

FIG. 6.6. ***Adenomyoepithelioma.*** This bisected tumor is circumscribed and has a nodular architecture. The tumor measures about 2 cm.

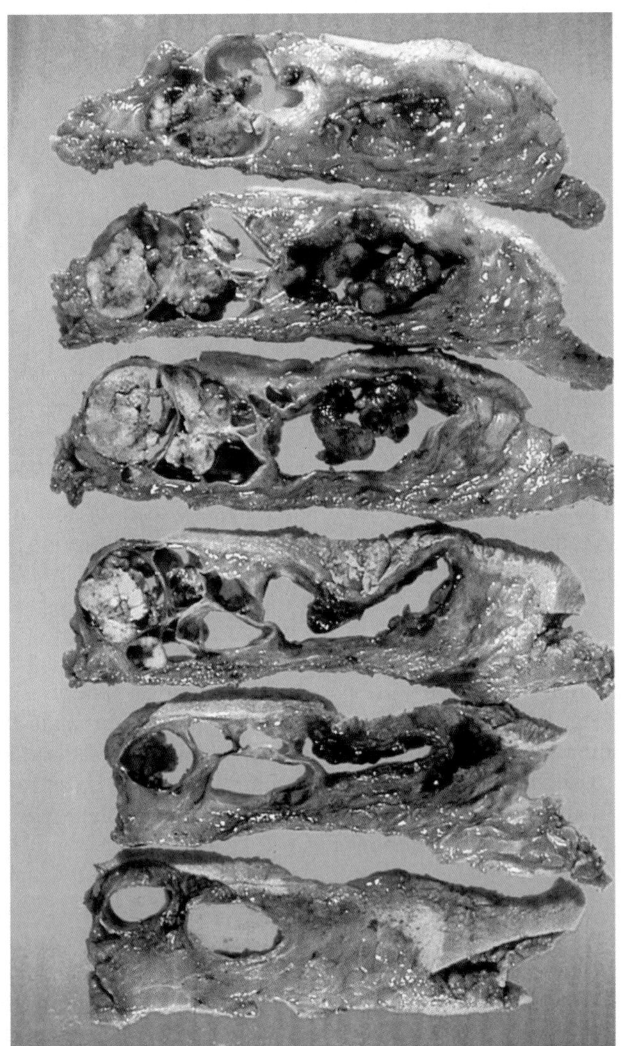
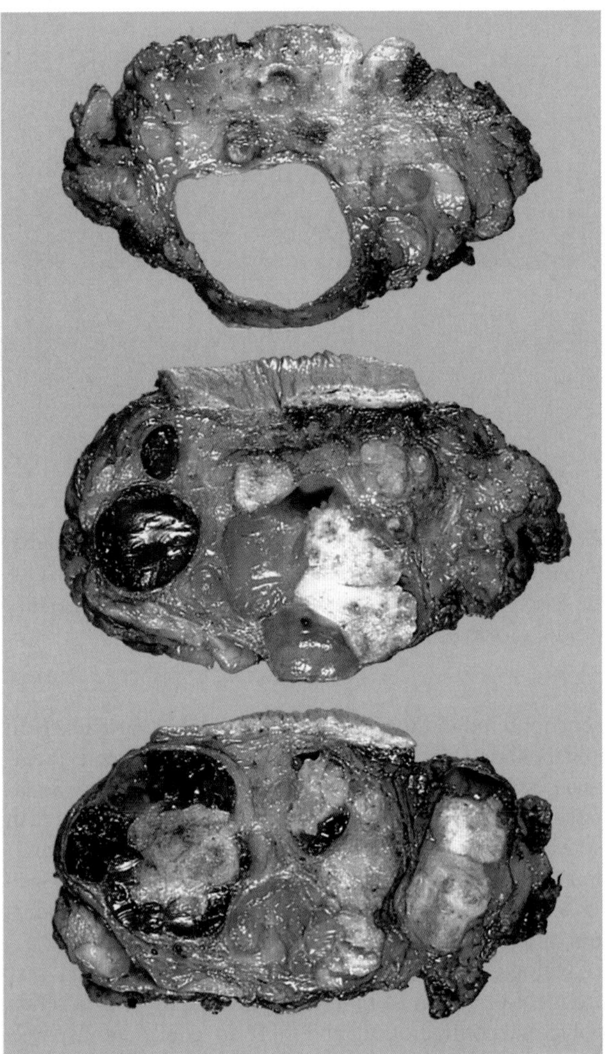

FIG. 6.7. ***Adenomyoepithelioma.*** Two different gross specimens are illustrated. Skin is present on the upper borders of the specimens. **A:** Multiple transverse sections of a mastectomy extensively involved by a multicystic AME with papillary areas. **B:** A solid and cystic multinodular AME that measured about 7 cm in greatest diameter is shown in transverse sections.

cell epithelioid myoepithelial hyperplasia in an AME with the adenosis pattern could be mistaken for invasive carcinoma in a small biopsy sample (Fig. 6.11). The most unusual and exceedingly rare adenosis variant of AME has an infiltrative growth pattern that resembles MGA (Fig. 6.12). However, true MGA is characterized by the absence of myoepithelium (see discussion of MGA in Chapter 7).

The basic structural unit of the typical AME is centered on a small round or oval glandular lumen encompassed by cuboidal epithelial cells. The glands are surrounded by polygonal or spindle-shaped MECs with clear cytoplasm, bounded in turn by basement membrane (Fig. 6.13). The tubular type of AME, the most common microscopic pattern, features a balanced proliferation of round, oval, or tubular glandular elements invested by polygonal MECs with clear cytoplasm. In some tumors, MECs with clear cytoplasm are more numerous than epithelial cells and compress the tubular lumens, resulting in zones virtually devoid of glands (Fig. 6.14). Other lesions feature MECs proliferating in broad bands and trabeculae separated by strands of basement membrane or stroma (Figs. 6.15 and 6.16). The contrast between the dark-staining cytoplasm of the glandular cells and the pale or pink cytoplasm of MECs can be striking and provides a helpful clue to the diagnosis (Fig. 6.17). Small glandular lumens formed within the epithelial areas may have a pattern reminiscent of an endocrine neoplasm. In papillary regions, distinct polygonal MECs accompany the epithelium in its various branches and ramifications.

Metaplasia in AME

The epithelial cells tend to have sparse, darkly stained cytoplasm and hyperchromatic nuclei. In some cases, this produces a plasmacytoid appearance. Apocrine metaplasia may

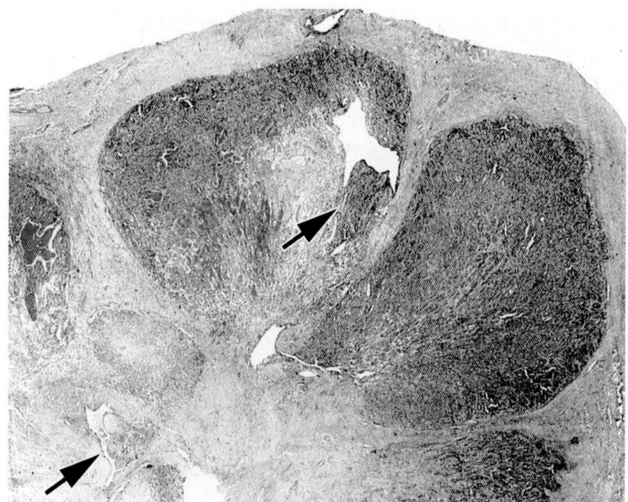

FIG. 6.8. ***Adenomyoepithelioma.*** A whole-mount histologic section in which multiple nodules surround a sclerotic core. There are remnants of ducts with papillary elements (*arrows*).

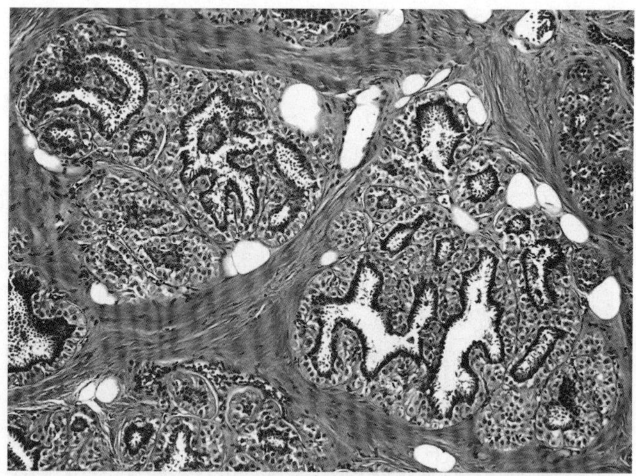

FIG. 6.10. ***Adenomyoepithelial hyperplasia of lobules.*** A group of lobules in which hyperplastic MECs surround the lobular glands, duplicating the pattern found in an AME.

be encountered in the glandular epithelium,[16] particularly in papillary areas (Fig. 6.18). Glands exhibiting sebaceous metaplasia (Fig. 6.19) can occur focally in a minority of cases. Squamous metaplasia (Fig. 6.20) can also occur and sometimes can be florid, raising the differential diagnosis of squamous carcinoma. Cartilaginous metaplasia of the stroma is rarely seen (Fig. 6.21). A previously undescribed AME with mucoepidermoid differentiation has been encountered (Fig. 6.22).

Cytologic atypia and prominent mitotic activity are very infrequent or absent from lesions in which the MECs retain a polygonal configuration, and there are conspicuous papillary areas. Infrequent mitoses can be found in both epithelial and myoepithelial components. Stromal and myoepithelial elements may have an adenoid cystic pattern. This may be manifested by the presence of collagenous spherulosis[29] (Fig. 6.15). Calcifications are rarely present, but some tumors develop central fibrosis or ischemic necrosis leading to calcification (Fig. 6.23). Squamous metaplasia is common in an infarcted AME (Fig. 6.24). The cystic papillary type of AME is very uncommon (Fig. 6.25).

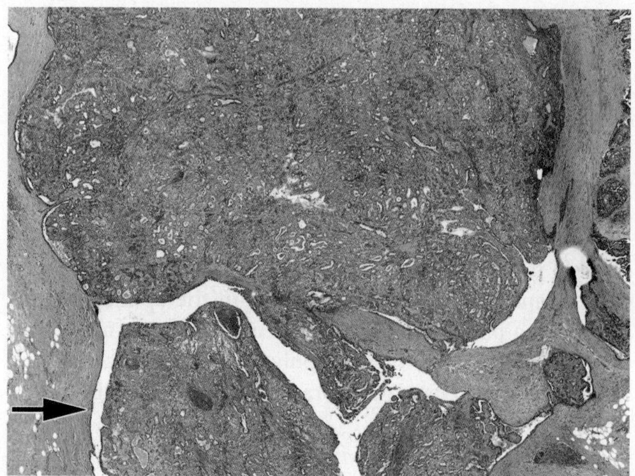

FIG. 6.9. ***Adenomyoepithelioma with papillary area.*** An AME with predominantly solid growth (*top half*) has an area with papillary architecture (*arrow*).

Spindle Cells in AMEs

The extent to which MECs assume a spindly, myoid shape varies greatly. Many AMEs have only limited foci of spindle cell myoid growth (Fig. 6.26). Tumors that are composed entirely of MECs with no identifiable epithelium are classified as myoepitheliomas and discussed separately in this chapter. Usually the myoid areas in an AME consist of a mixture of spindle and polygonal cells. The glandular component may be intermixed with myoid areas, or it may appear to be largely separate (Fig. 6.27). Palisading of spindle cells and alveolar clustering of polygonal MECs are common myoid patterns. The latter configuration has been referred to as the lobulated type *of AME.*[22] An AME of the male breast almost completely composed of spindle cells arranged in a storiform pattern was described by Tamura et al.[24] Despite the spindle cell phenotype, the neoplasm was most strongly reactive for cytokeratin and S-100, with little staining for actin and no vimentin reactivity.

Mammary Lesions Morphologically Related to AME

In addition to papilloma, AME is closely related to ductal adenoma, and some investigators did not to distinguish between the two entities.[48,50,51] Foci of AME can frequently be detected in tubular adenomas. Tumors referred to as *mixed tumors* or *pleomorphic adenomas* of the breast[32,52] are either variants of intraductal papilloma or AME. These lesions occur more frequently in the subareolar region than in the periphery of

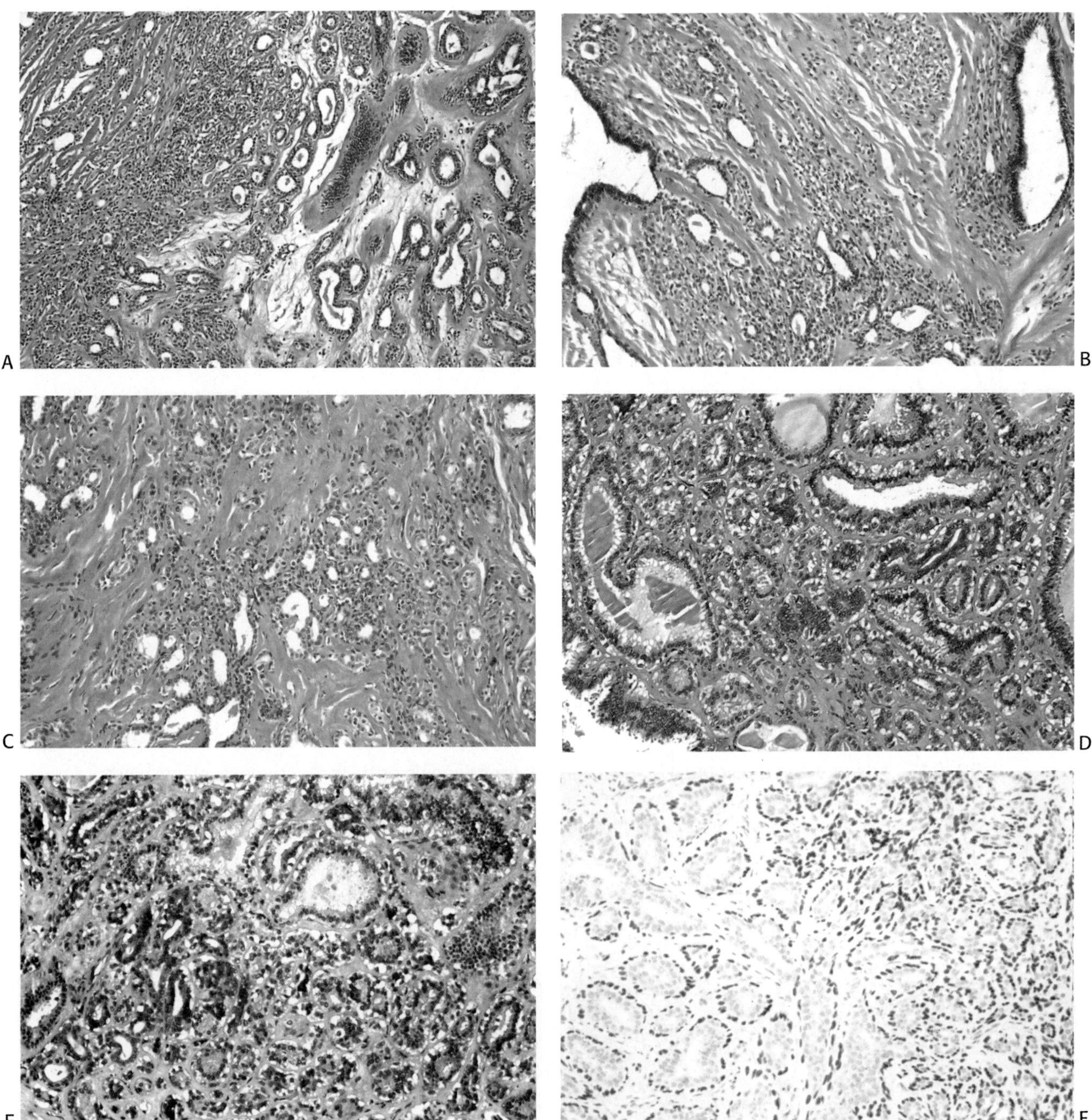

FIG. 6.11. ***Adenomyoepithelioma with adenosis structure.*** **A:** Myoepithelial hyperplasia shown here in sclerosing adenosis is composed of small cells with clear cytoplasm (*left*). Sclerosing adenosis without myoepithelial hyperplasia is shown on the *right*. **B,C:** MECs with clear cytoplasm in sclerosing adenosis. **D,E:** AME with adenosis structure and myoepithelial hyperplasia composed of epithelioid cells with clear cytoplasm around the perimeter of adenosis glands. **F:** MECs are demonstrated in the tumor by the p63 immunostain.

breast and probably arise from large lactiferous ducts.[53,54] Most are solid and circumscribed tumors, but an intracystic mural lesion has been described.[54] Remnants of the underlying epithelial lesion, usually with MEC hyperplasia, can be found in almost all cases.[53,55] A characteristic feature of many so-called mixed tumors in the breast is the formation of collagenized myxoid matrix that is frequently converted into cartilage (Fig. 6.21). Calcification and ossification can occur in some of these tumors as well. Various proliferative patterns are found in these lesions, including foci that resemble cellular mixed tumor of the salivary glands (Fig. 6.28), and areas with distinct papillary component. The epithelium may develop

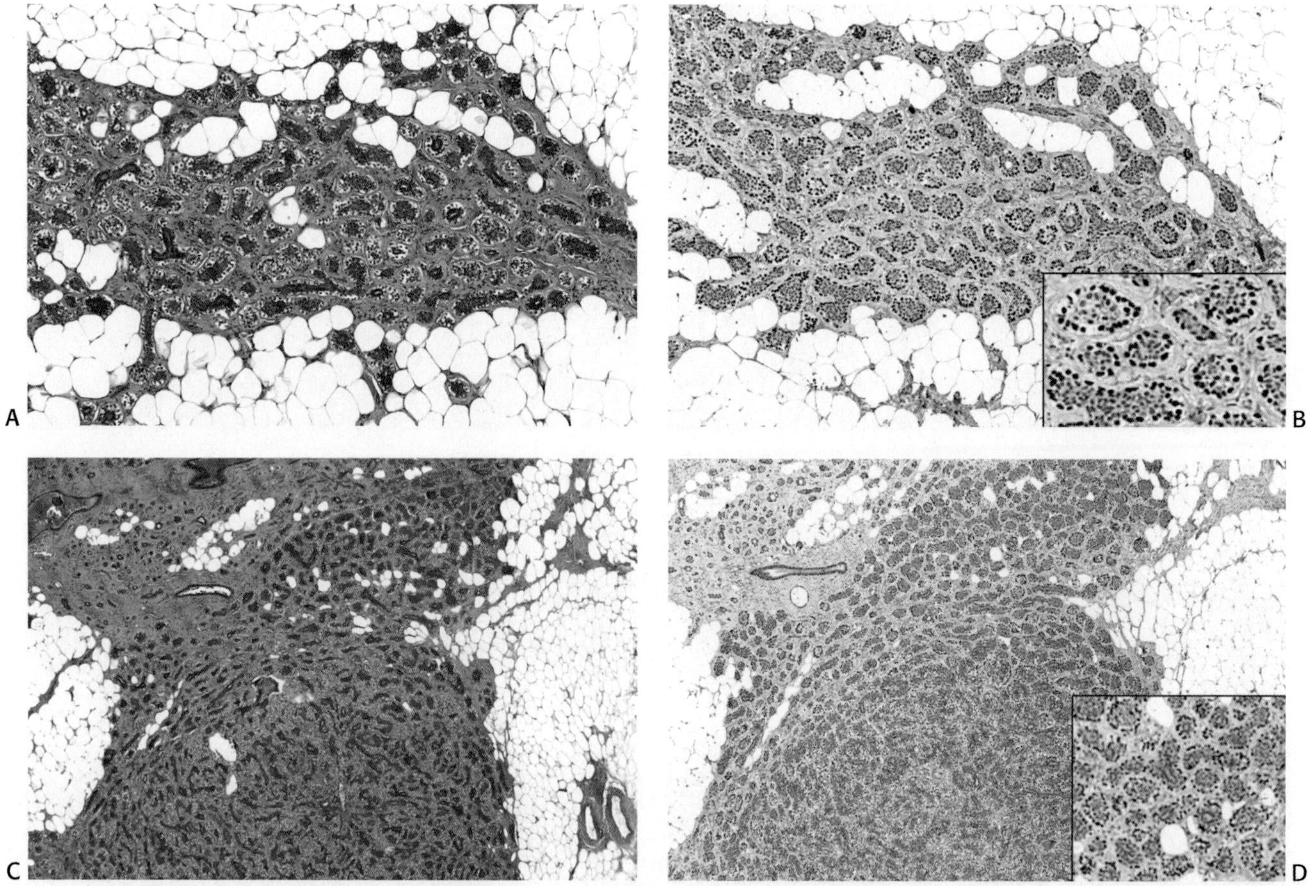

FIG. 6.12. ***Adenomyoepithelioma with microglandular adenosis pattern.*** **A:** Adenosis glands with an infiltrative growth pattern that resembles MGA in fat. Clear cells represent the myoepithelial component. **B:** MEC nuclei in **(A)** are highlighted by the p63 immunostain. **C:** A region with MGA-like infiltrative growth around ducts (*above*) and nodular growth (*below*). **D:** The nuclei of hyperplastic MECs in **(C)** are highlighted by the p63 immunostain.

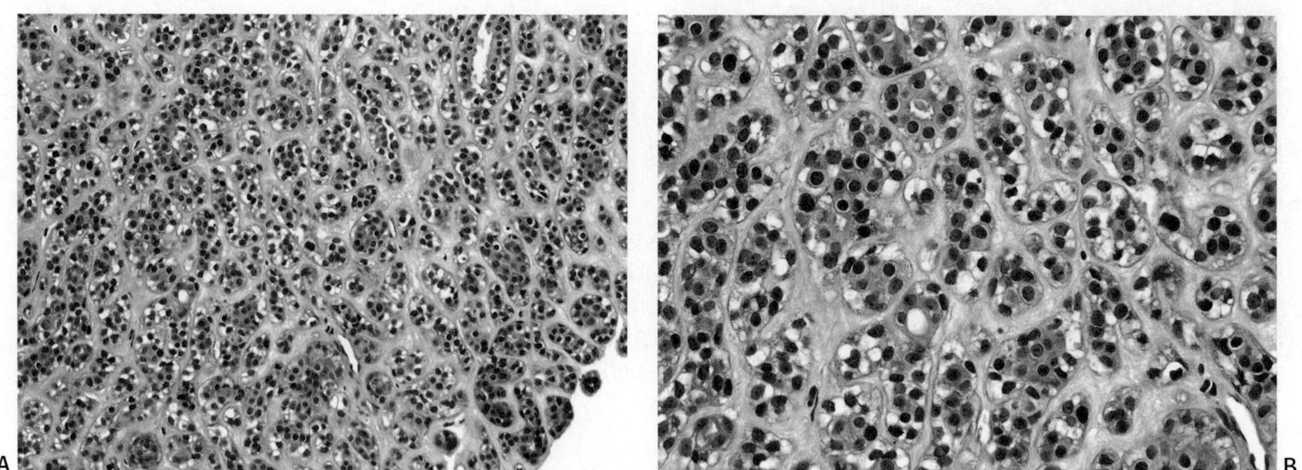

FIG. 6.13. ***Adenomyoepithelioma.*** **A:** This AME shows the characteristic growth pattern in which cords and irregular aggregates of epithelial cells are separated by bands of fibrovascular stroma. **B:** MECs with clear cytoplasm are aligned along the serrated outer edges of epithelial cords. The epithelium has eosinophilic cytoplasm and inconspicuous glandular lumina. The glands are outlined by distinct basement membranes.

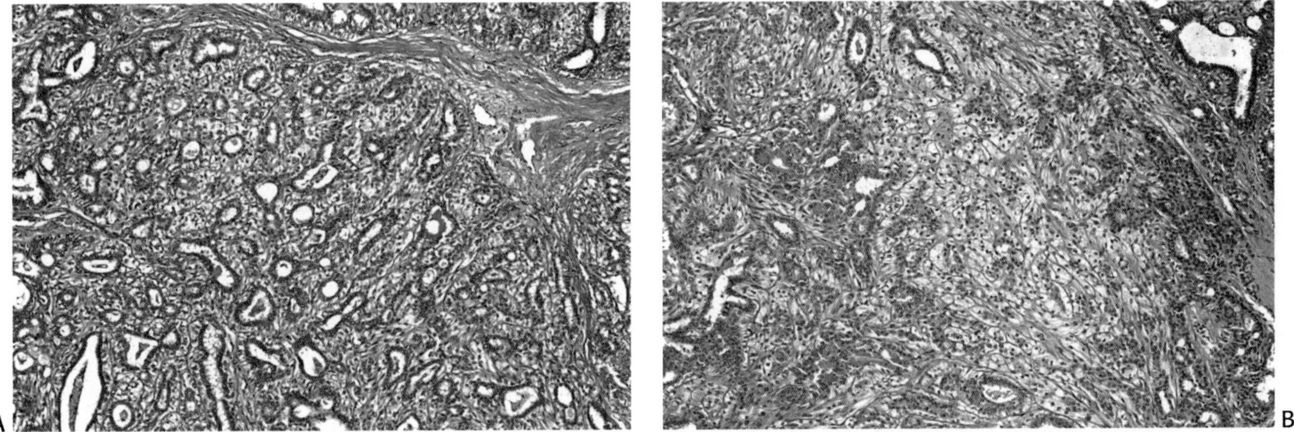

FIG. 6.14. ***Adenomyoepithelioma.*** Two areas in the same tumor are shown. **A:** Balanced glandular and myoepithelial proliferation. **B:** Epithelioid clear cell myoepithelial hyperplasia has displaced glandular structures.

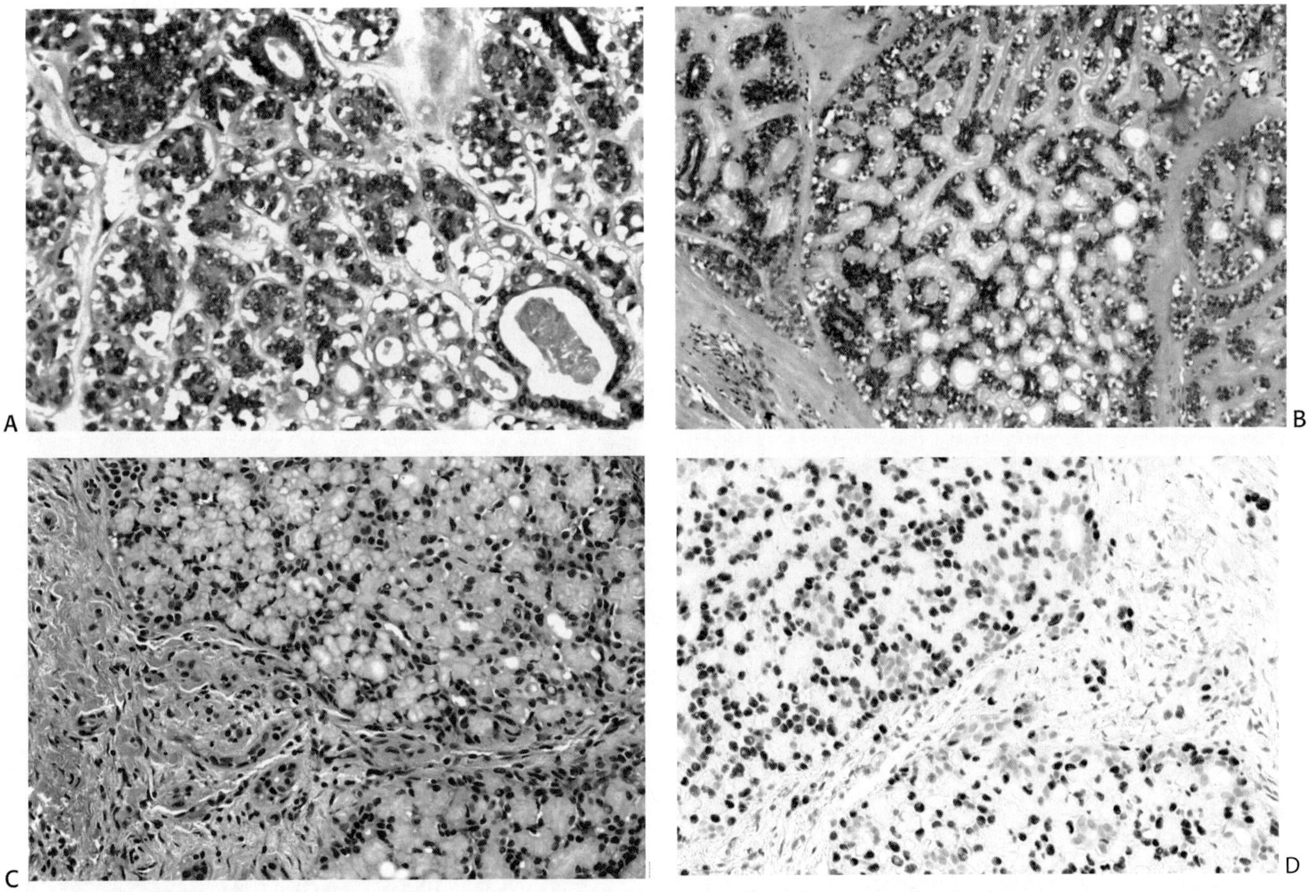

FIG. 6.15. ***Adenomyoepithelioma with sclerotic stroma.*** **A:** Conventional AME structure. **B:** A trabecular growth pattern created by sclerotic stroma in which there are foci of collagenous spherulosis **C:** Another AME with sclerotic collagenous spherulosis. **D:** A p63 immunostain highlights the MECs in the case depicted in **(C)**.

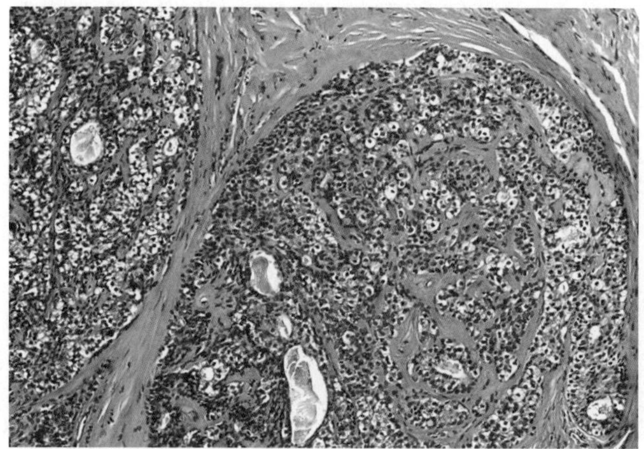

FIG. 6.16. ***Adenomyoepithelioma.*** Epithelioid MECs, many with clear cytoplasm, are arranged in a trabecular pattern.

squamous and sebaceous metaplasia similar to the metaplastic changes that occur in conventional AME (Fig. 6.29). In some of these cases, the differential diagnosis includes metaplastic carcinoma with myxoid/chondroid matrix. The distinction between AME and metaplastic carcinoma rests on the presence of cytologic atypia, increased cellularity, areas of necrosis, evident mitoses, and abnormal expansion of the epithelial or myoepithelial component in metaplastic carcinoma. Cases of pleomorphic adenoma that raised the differential diagnosis of mucinous carcinoma in cytology material[56] and in a surgical specimen[55] have been reported.

Atypical AME

Cytologic atypia of the MECs often occurs in lesions wherein these cells have a predominantly spindle cell morphology and distinctly myoid appearance or abundant clear

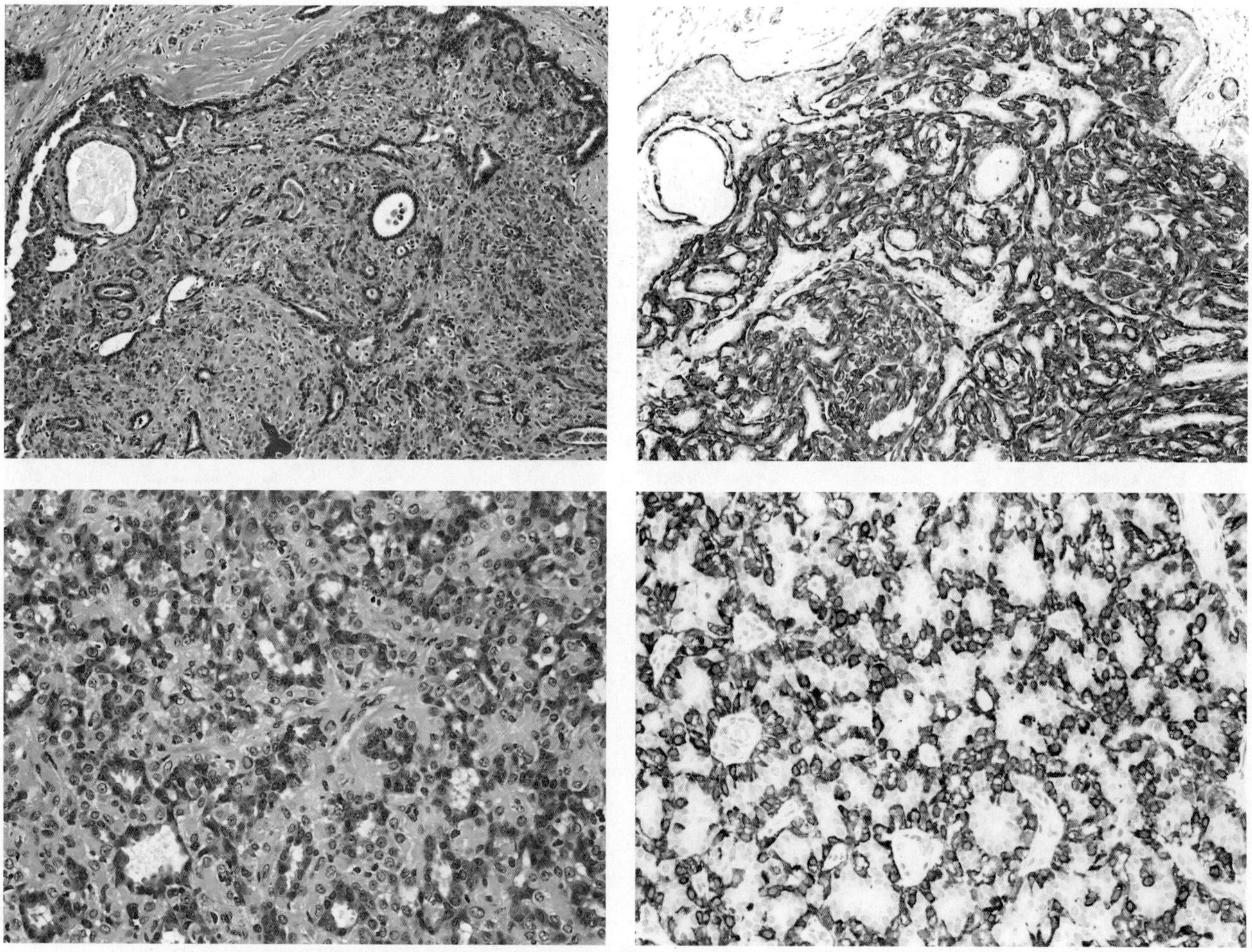

FIG. 6.17. ***Adenomyoepithelioma.*** **A:** Hyperplastic MECs with pale pink cytoplasm surround the intensely blue-stained glandular epithelium of an AME. **B:** A calponin immunostain highlights the hyperplastic myoepithelial component in **(A)**. **C:** MECs with pale pink cytoplasm and plasmacytoid morphology surround the more intensely stained glandular epithelium. This image is representative of a needle core biopsy that had been misdiagnosed as invasive carcinoma. **D:** A calponin stain highlights the MECs in **(C)**. **E:** The myoepithelial nuclei in **(C)** are evident in a p63-immunostained section.

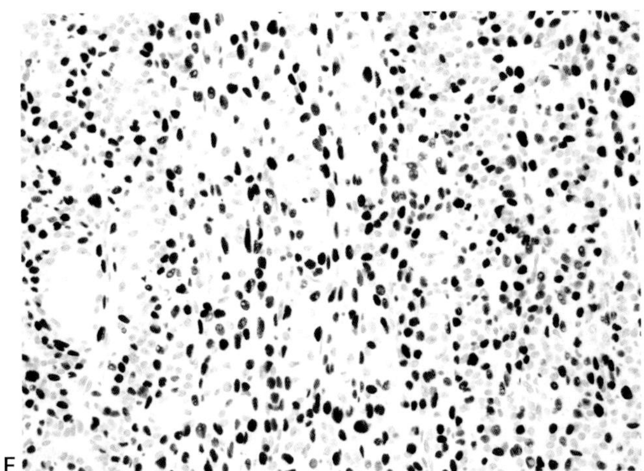

FIG. 6.17. *[Continued]*

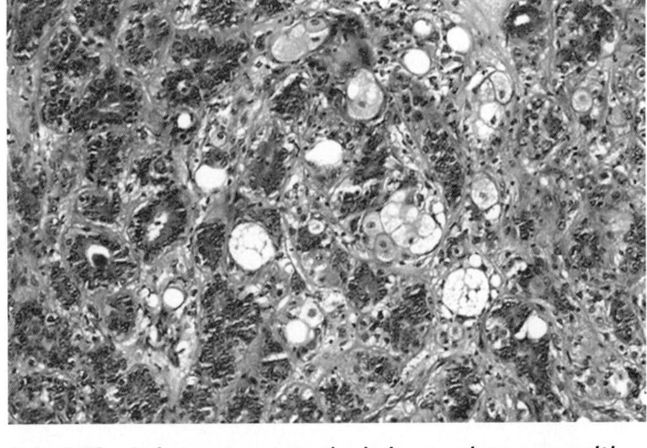

FIG. 6.19. ***Sebaceous metaplasia in an adenomyoepithelioma.*** Sebaceous differentiation manifested by a discrete, round group of cells with clear, vacuolated cytoplasm.

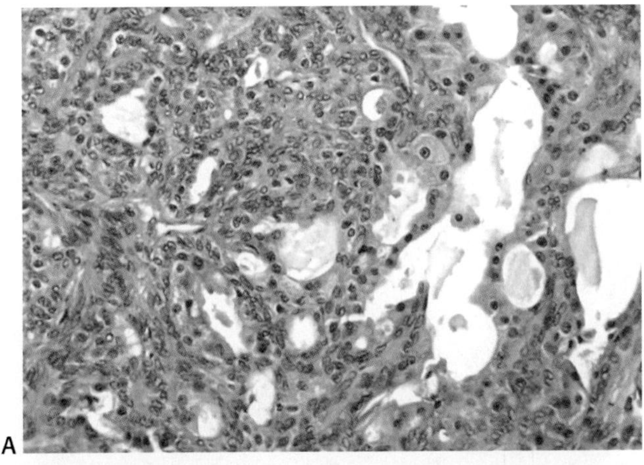

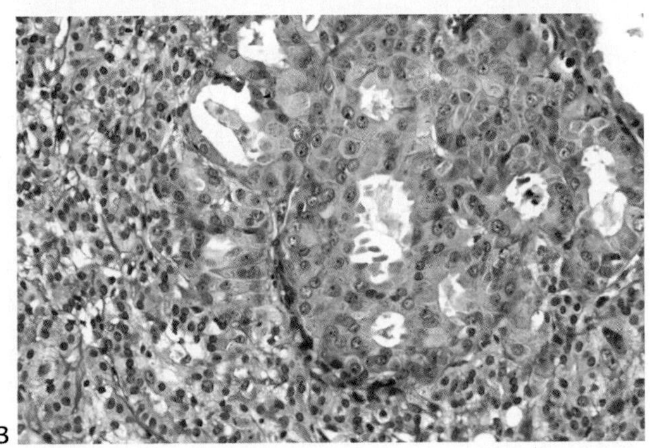

FIG. 6.18. ***Apocrine metaplasia in an adenomyoepithelioma.*** **A:** Apocrine epithelium is evident in the glands. Spindly MECs are present. **B:** Atypical apocrine metaplasia with nuclear atypia surrounded by epithelioid MECs.

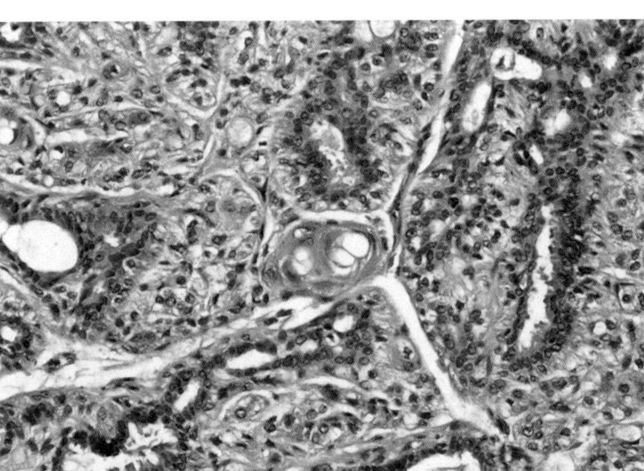

FIG. 6.20. ***Squamous metaplasia in an adenomyoepithelioma.*** Squamous metaplasia in the form of a keratin pearl is seen in the midst of MECs with clear cytoplasm. Squamous and sebaceous metaplasia appears to originate in the MECs.

cytoplasm and nuclear enlargement (Fig. 6.30). In these foci, atypical features include increased mitotic figures, focal nuclear pleomorphism, hyperchromasia, and occasional multinucleated cells. The presence of mitoses in the epithelial and myoepithelial components of an AME at the level of 4 to 5 mitoses per 10 high-power fields (HPFs) is an atypical feature.[23] Myoid hyperplasia may give rise to areas with leiomyomatous features,[2,57] and rarely this process produces leiomyosarcoma.[2] Cytologic atypia and mitotic activity have also been described in the lobulated type of AME.[22] Apocrine atypia is also frequently observed in the epithelial component of an atypical AME (Fig. 6.30).

Malignant Neoplasms Arising in AMEs

Origin of a malignant neoplasm in an AME has been rarely documented. Malignant transformation may be limited to either the epithelial or myoepithelial component, or both

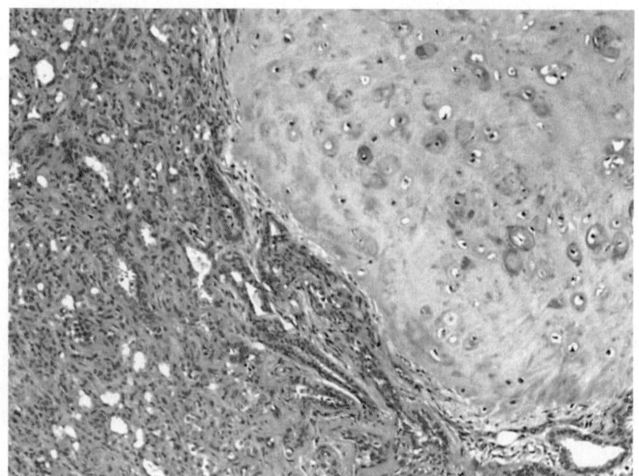

FIG. 6.21. *Cartilaginous metaplasia in an adenomyoepithelioma.*

elements may be involved. The term *malignant AME* should be reserved for biphasic tumors in which both components are malignant, in contrast to cases in which either the myoepithelial or the epithelial component is malignant. Unfortunately, this distinction was not made in most published reports of tumors that were described as malignant AME.

Histologic evidence of malignant growth in an AME includes necrosis, cellular pleomorphism, overgrowth of myoepithelium or epithelium, and invasion at the periphery of the tumor. A high mitotic rate is also a characteristic of a malignant AME (Fig. 6.31). Many of the lesions purported to be malignant AMEs have featured a spindle cell component, and in some instances, the distinction from metaplastic carcinoma is not clear.[58,59] In one case, the malignant component was described as "undifferentiated" and lacked reactivity for cytokeratin and actin,[60] but in other tumors, these cytoskeletal components were immunohistochemically detectable.[61–66] Malignant AMEs with a biphasic growth

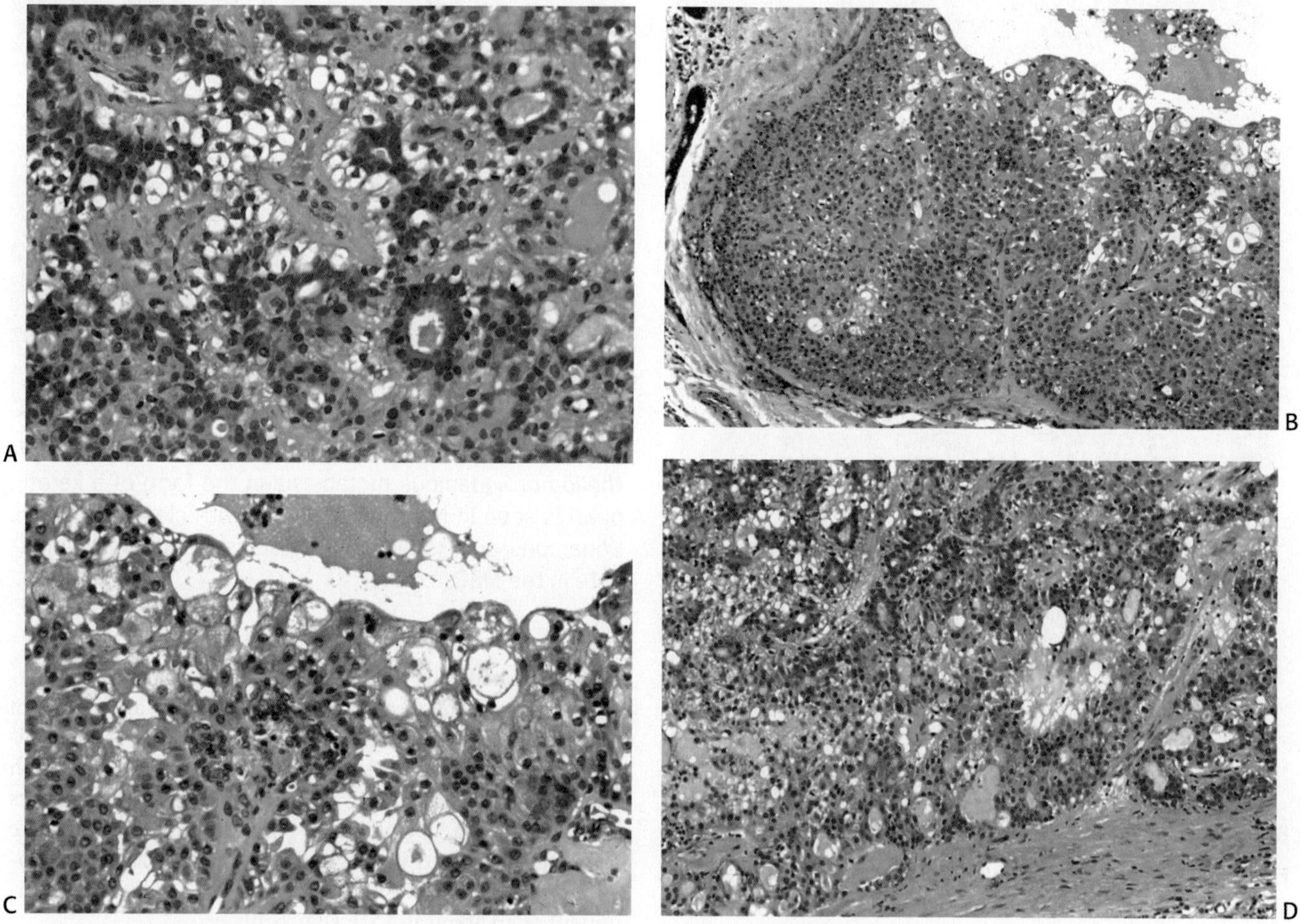

A B C D

FIG. 6.22. ***Adenomyoepithelioma with mucoepidermoid differentiation.*** **A:** A part of the tumor with the typical AME growth pattern. **B,C:** Mucoepidermoid differentiation in a cystic portion of the tumor. **D,E:** Mucinous secretion in glands. **F:** Squamous metaplasia with glandular elements. **G–I:** AME with mucin formed by epithelioid MECs. Vacuolated epithelial cells in the papillary tumor **(G,H)** containing mucin, which is stained magenta by the mucicarmine stain **(I)**. **J:** Collagenous spherulosis in a papillary AME. The basophilic material in spherules surrounded by a distinct basement membrane resembles mucin.

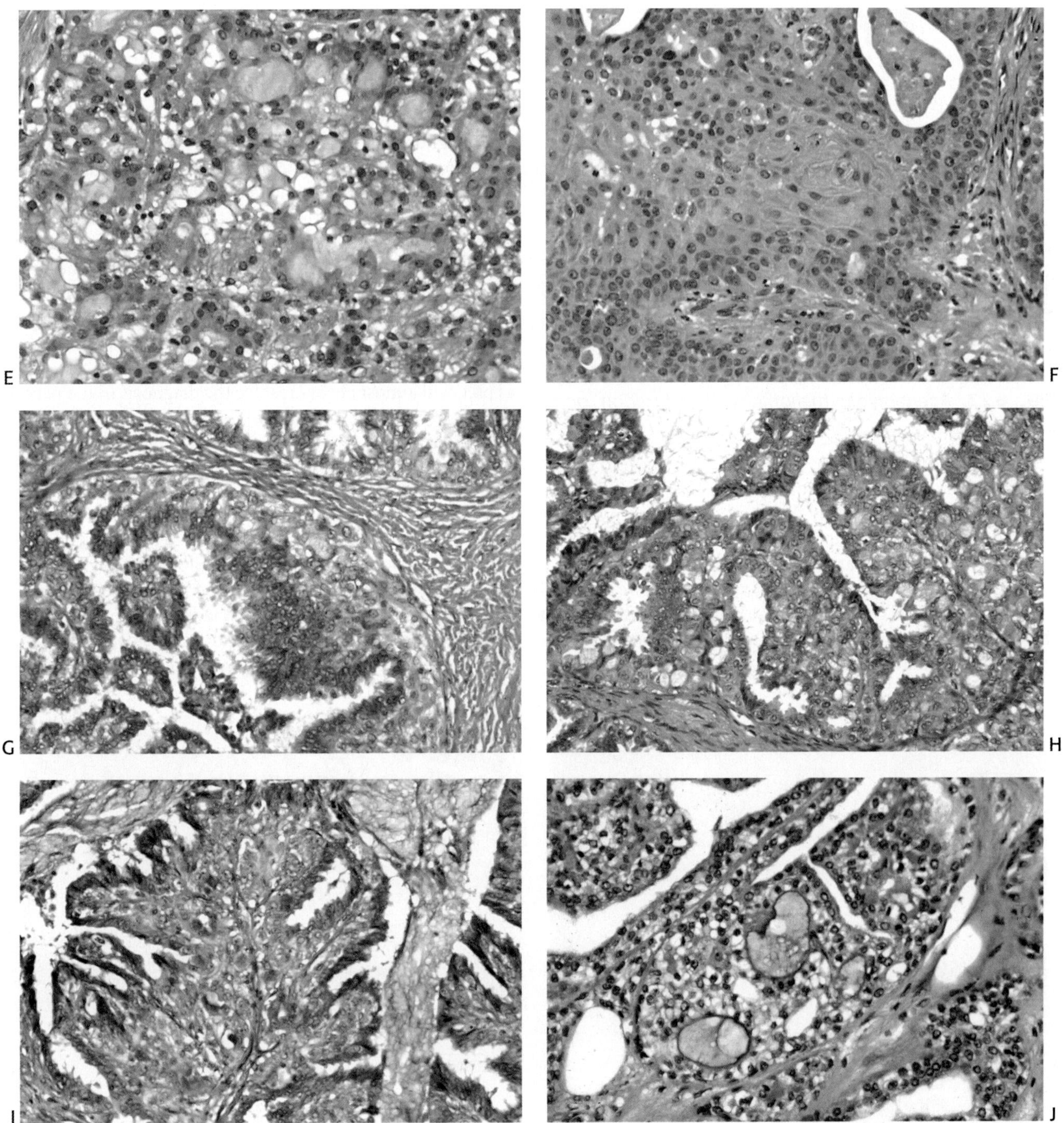

FIG. 6.22. *[Continued]*

pattern in the breast and at metastatic sites have also been reported.[45,64,66–68]

Morphology of Carcinomas Arising in AME Lesions

Various forms of carcinoma have been described in AME, including AdCC,[34] low-grade adenosquamous carcinoma (LGASC),[69,70] acantholytic squamous carcinoma,[70] undifferentiated carcinoma,[60] sarcomatoid carcinoma,[70] invasive ductal carcinoma,[61] undifferentiated carcinoma with heterologous (osteogenic and spindle cell) differentiation,[63] and myoepithelial carcinoma.[62,65,71]

Myoepithelial carcinoma arising in an AME (Figs. 6.32–6.34) is characterized by overgrowth of the myoepithelial component that exhibits mitotic activity and cytologic evidence of carcinoma,[62,65,71,72] often with foci of necrosis.[38] A case report by Jones et al.[65] documented a 3-cm malignant AME that had a substantial malignant spindle cell component with mitoses and necrosis. The tumor gave rise to multiple liver metastases composed entirely of spindle cells.

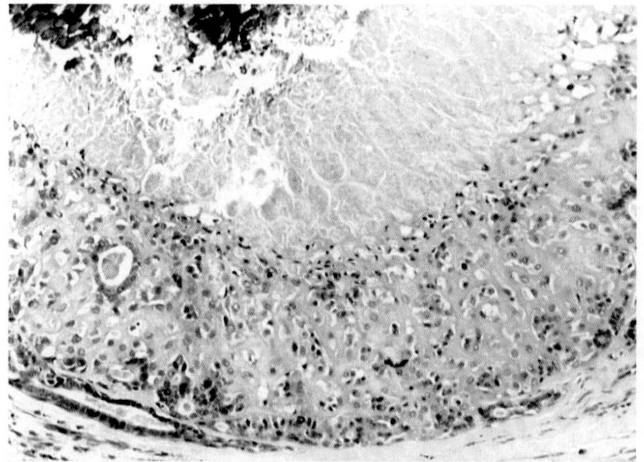

FIG. 6.23. *Adenomyoepithelioma with infarction and calcifications.*

Comparative genomic hybridization (CGH) analysis revealed chromosomal loss of the 11q23–24 and 16q22–23 regions in the epithelial and myoepithelial components of the tumor, a finding that suggests origin from a common precursor; additional losses in 10q25 and 12q24 were limited to the myoepithelial component. The liver metastases shared the same chromosomal alterations as the neoplastic MECs, but showed additional chromosomal losses (2q35–37, 11q23–24, 12q24) and gains (6q12–q16), consistent with genetic progression.

Core Biopsy Diagnosis

The diagnosis of AME may be very challenging in needle core biopsy material.[73] Attention is drawn especially to benign AME in which glandular elements are dispersed amidst spindly MECs, and to tumors that qualify as "pleomorphic adenomas." When seen out of the context of a complete histologic section, a needle core biopsy sample from these benign lesions could be mistaken for invasive carcinoma[73] or phyllodes tumor (Fig. 6.35). If the possibility of a myoepithelial or adenomyoepithelial neoplasm is considered selected appropriate immunostains for myoepithelial markers, such as p63, will almost always resolve the diagnosis in the needle core biopsy sample.

Cytology

Aspiration cytology of an AME yields a cellular specimen composed of relatively large clusters of epithelial cells and MECs, and single cells with epithelioid or spindle morphology.[30,33,74] The clusters are generally cohesive, with a tridimensional configuration and admixed spindle cells[30] (Fig. 6.36). The epithelial cells tend to have deeply staining cytoplasm and prominent round-to-oval nuclei that may be

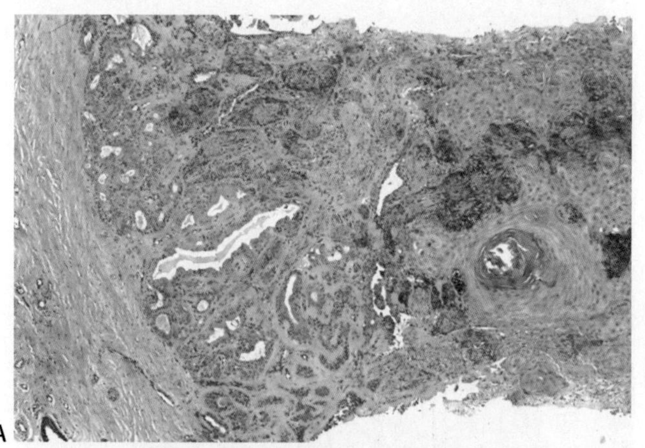

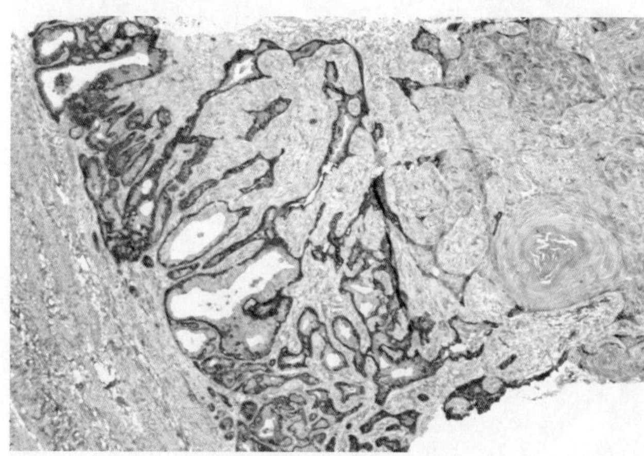

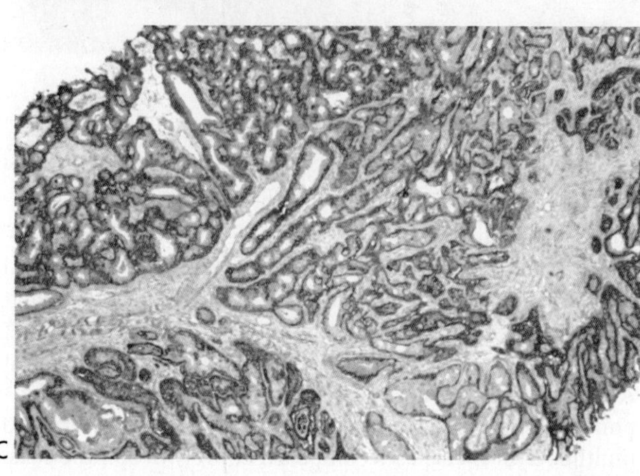

FIG. 6.24. ***Adenomyoepithelioma with infarction.*** **A:** Infarcted AME **B,C:** Myoepithelium is demonstrated in intact regions with the CD10 immunostain.

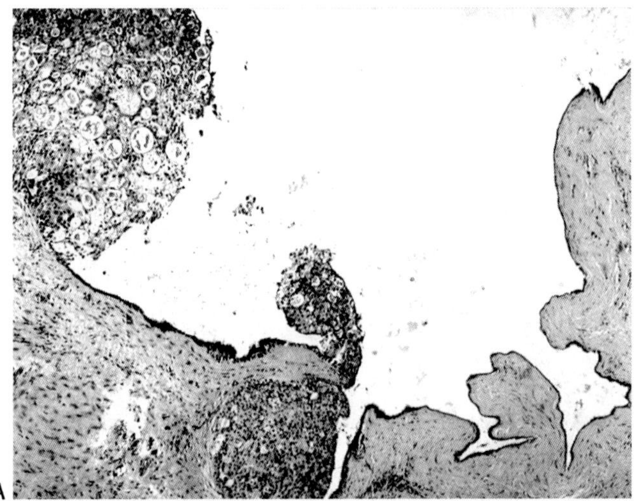

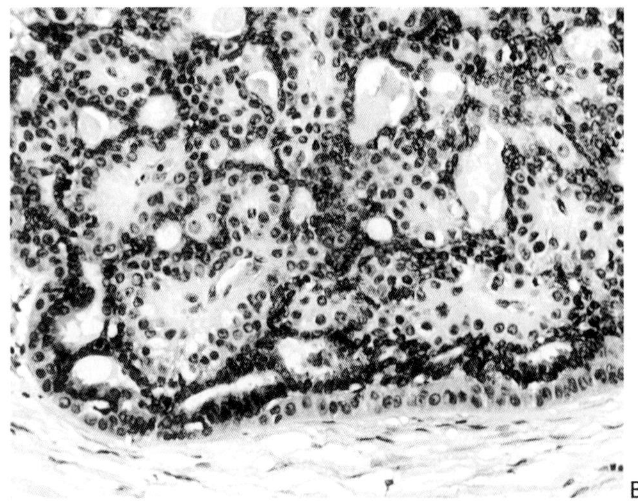

FIG. 6.25. ***Cystic adenomyoepithelioma.*** **A:** At low magnification, nodules of adenomyoepitheliomatous growth protrude from the surface of the cyst, which is otherwise lined by ordinary duct epithelium. **B:** An adenomyoepitheliomatous nodule at the periphery of a duct.

eccentrically placed. Tubule formation was appreciated in only 3/12 (25%) cases in one series.[30] Spindle cells and myxoid fibrillary material are usually present, and the latter is best appreciated on Diff-Quick-stained smears.[30,74] Hyaline globules surrounded by MECs consistent with collagenous spherulosis were found in 4 of 12 cases in one series.[30] In one case, this finding prompted a misdiagnosis as AdCC.

The cytologic features of AME may suggest a diagnosis of carcinoma.[16,30,36,39,49,75,76] Cytologic interpretation as fibroadenoma has also been reported.[30] Iyengar et al.[30] assessed the cytomorphologic findings in fine-needle aspiration (FNA) material from 12 AMEs, including two with features of pleomorphic adenoma. In their study, MECs were either present admixed with epithelium in clusters of different sizes or dispersed as single cells. The MECs showed clear and vacuolated ("soap bubble") cytoplasm in 66% of cases. This feature was best appreciated on Diff-Quick-stained smears and was more difficult to detect in Thin-Prep slides of the same cases. The MECs had intranuclear inclusions in 33% of cases. Other authors have also reported this finding.[77–80] Sparse apocrine cells and foamy macrophages were noted in 25% of cases.

The cytologic findings of pleomorphic adenoma of the breast in an FNA specimen may suggest a phyllodes tumor when numerous bipolar spindle cells are present or metaplastic carcinoma if the aspirate contains abundant metachromatic stroma.[51] Misdiagnosis of pleomorphic adenoma as mucinous carcinoma has also been reported in a case with hypocellular areas composed of abundant translucent and mucoid matrix.[56]

FIG. 6.26. ***Adenomyoepithelioma with myoid cells.*** This lesion has a conspicuous myoid component composed of spindle cells with deeply eosinophilic cytoplasm and a palisading arrangement.

Immunohistochemistry

By and large the diverse cellular components of adenomyoepithelial tumors exhibit the expected histochemical properties. Glands may contain PAS- or mucicarmine-positive secretion, but intracytoplasmic secretion is rarely detectable. In most cases, the secretion is also positive for CEA. The cytoplasm of glandular cells tends to be strongly reactive with antibodies to cytokeratin (Fig. 6.29), and the luminal surfaces of these cells are positive for EMA. Although most of the epithelial cells are S-100 negative, small groups may be strongly reactive for this antigen (Fig. 6.37).

Polygonal and spindle MECs are not reactive for EMA, but focal weak positivity for EMA in the neoplastic MECs of a biphasic malignant AME was reported by Kihara et al.[64] These cells show variable reactivity for cytokeratin. CEA is negative in MECs, although weak CEA positivity was reported in one case.[81] Reactivity for SMM-HC is usually pronounced. The distribution and intensity of staining obtained with anti-actin antibodies is heterogeneous.

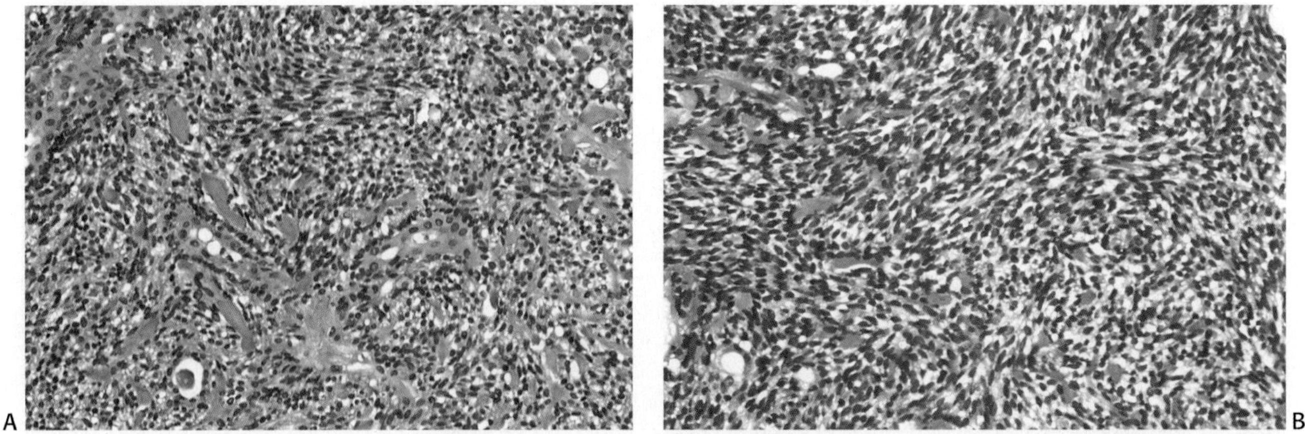

FIG. 6.27. ***Adenomyoepithelioma with spindle cells.*** **A:** Two oval glands in the center and one round gland (*lower left*) are surrounded by a spindly myoepithelial proliferation. **B:** An area with pure spindle cell myoepithelium.

Anti-actin staining tends to be more conspicuous in spindle than in clear polygonal cells. No reactivity for actin is seen in epithelial cells (Fig. 6.37). Some MECs are S-100 positive in virtually all tumors, but the intensity and uniformity of reactivity vary considerably. There does not appear to be a consistent relationship between staining with anti-actin and anti-S-100 antibodies in MECs. Because S-100 reactivity is expressed by glandular and MECs, it is not a specific marker of MECs in AME[82] or in any other breast tumor.

Markers that are relatively specific for MECs include CK5, CD10, myosin, calponin, p75, maspin, and p63. p63 (Figs. 6.15, 6.17, 6.30, and 6.33) is especially helpful because its nuclear localization precludes cytoplasmic cross-reactivity with myofibroblasts that is observed with other markers such as myosin, calponin, SMA, and CD10. The immunophenotype of neoplastic MECs is sometimes different from that of their normal counterpart, and they are not necessarily reactive for all markers. Therefore, a panel of immunostains should be used to maximize the detection of MECs.

The glandular epithelial component of a benign AME displays some nuclear reactivity for estrogen receptor (ER) in most cases, whereas reactivity for progesterone receptor (PR) is often absent. ER and PR are not expressed in the myoepithelial component. Carcinomas arising in AMEs, whether consisting of only epithelial or myoepithelial carcinoma or of the two combined, are usually negative for ER and PR[45,59,64] and for HER2.[45,59]

Electron Microscopy

Several studies have described the ultrastructural features of individual lesions classified as AME.[16,19,33,83–86] In general,

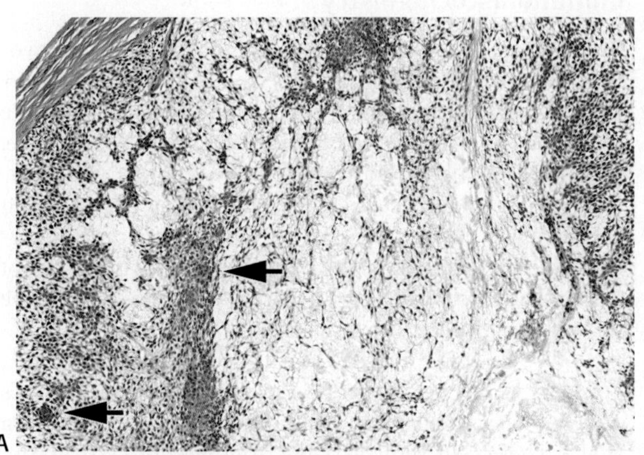

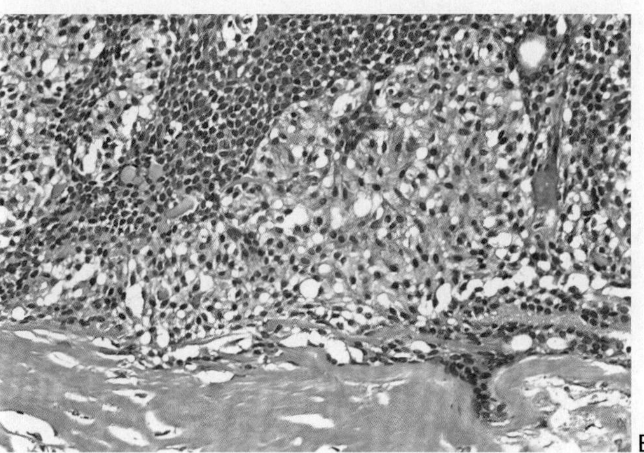

FIG. 6.28. ***Mixed tumor (pleomorphic adenoma).*** **A:** This benign mixed tumor of the breast consists of loose myxoid stroma with admixed spindle cells and scattered glandular elements (*arrows*). **B:** Another example is composed of a myoepithelial proliferation in a myxoid matrix that resembles a cellular mixed tumor.

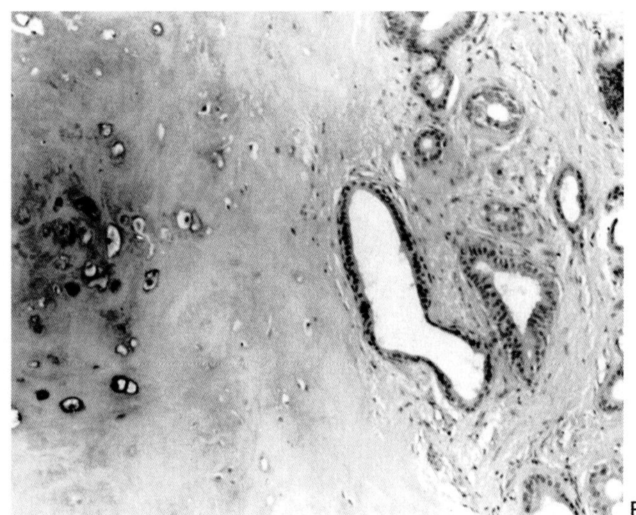

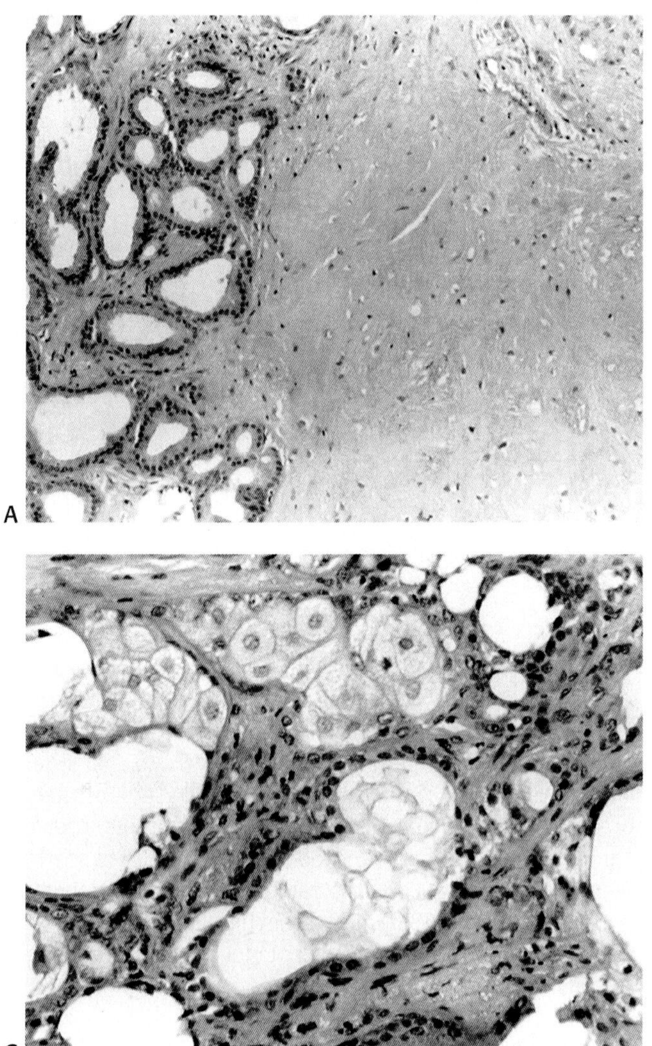

FIG. 6.29. *Mixed tumor (pleomorphic adenoma).* **A:** Collagenized matrix adjacent to glandular elements with an adenosis pattern. **B:** Cartilaginous differentiation in the stroma. **C:** Sebaceous metaplasia of the epithelium.

these reports have documented the presence of epithelial and myoepithelial components in the lesions. Short microvilli are present at the luminal surfaces of the glandular cells that are joined at the luminal edges by tight cell junctions. The cytoplasm of the glandular epithelium contains scattered mitochondria as well as smooth and rough endoplasmic reticulum. Polygonal and spindle-form MECs have desmosomes that may be well or poorly formed, and interdigitating cell processes. Keratin and actin cytofilaments are prominent in the cytoplasm of MECs, sometimes arranged in perinuclear bundles or peripheral arrays. Fusiform densities or condensation zones are commonly found along these arrays of cytofilaments. Distinct basal lamina material is found around and among the MECs.

Genetics and Molecular Studies

Information on the genetic alterations in AME is very limited. Using a diagnostic protocol validated for detection of microsatellite instability in colonic carcinoma, Salto-Tellez et al.[87] detected microsatellite instability for the D17S250 (17q11.2-BRCA1) microsatellite marker and loss of heterozygosity of the *HPC1* gene in one of five AMEs. Gatalica et al.[88] documented a reciprocal translocation t(8:16)(p23;q21) in a 15-cm AME, but could not determine whether this was a constitutional alteration of the patient's genome or specific to the tumor. Using mRNA gene array profiling on the same tumor, the authors detected a greater than twofold change in the mRNA expression of over 800 genes compared with normal tissue. Some of the genes mapping to the translocation point, such as the growth hormone gene, were significantly increased. An increase of some of the corresponding proteins, including growth hormone, was also confirmed immunohistochemically in the tumor compared with normal tissue. Da Silva et al.[46] used high-resolution CGH to study whole genome copy number changes in adjacent lesions consisting of a small AME, an AdCC, and tubular adenosis, and found no common changes. In particular, the small AME yielded no detectable genomic alterations.

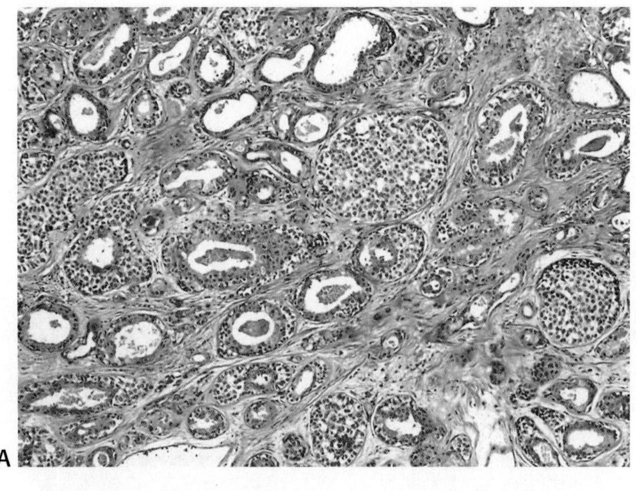

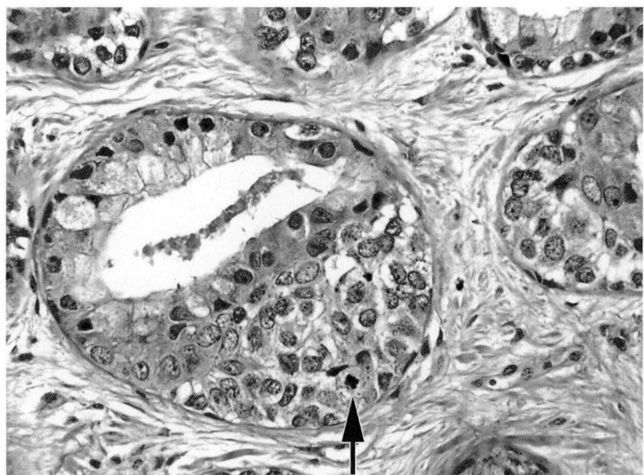

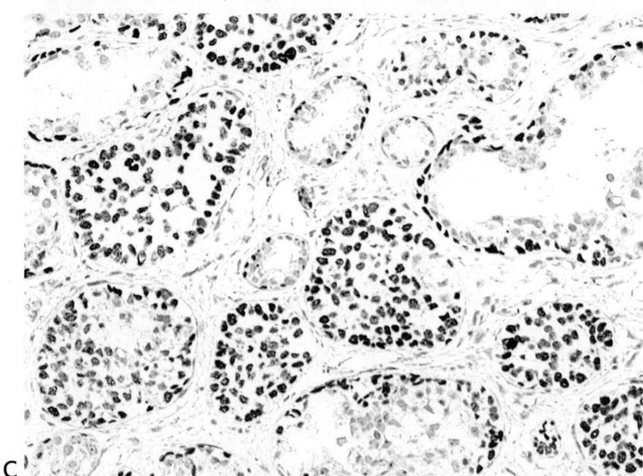

FIG. 6.30. ***Adenomyoepithelioma with atypical myoepithelial cells.*** **A:** The MECs of this AME are expanded, with no evidence of growth beyond the basement membrane of the involved glands. **B:** Nuclear atypia and focal apoptosis (*arrow*) are noted in the MECs. The apocrine glandular cells are also atypical, but show no evidence of hyperplasia. **C:** A p63 immunostain highlights the myoepithelial nuclei. The epithelial cell nuclei are p63 negative.

Treatment and Prognosis

Adenomyoepithelioma

The majority of AMEs are benign tumors that can be treated by local excision.[21] Local recurrence has been reported, usually more than 2 years after the initial excision.[17,20,22] In two cases, two[21] and three[17] episodes of recurrence could be attributed to incomplete excision. The multinodular character of the lesion and peripheral intraductal extension in one of these patients were probably contributory factors.[21] There is no evidence that cytologic atypia or the proportions of spindle and polygonal MECs are related to the risk of local

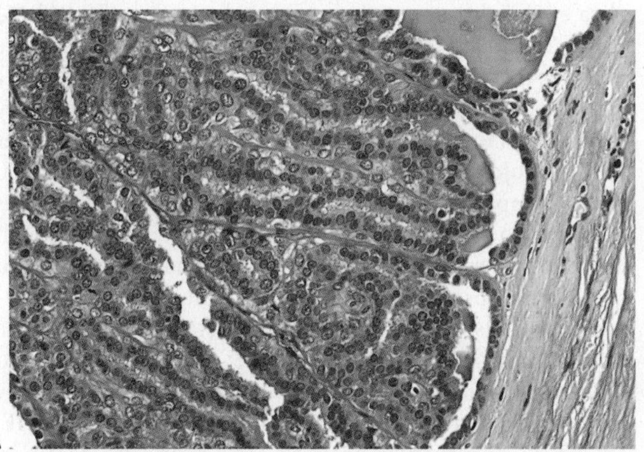

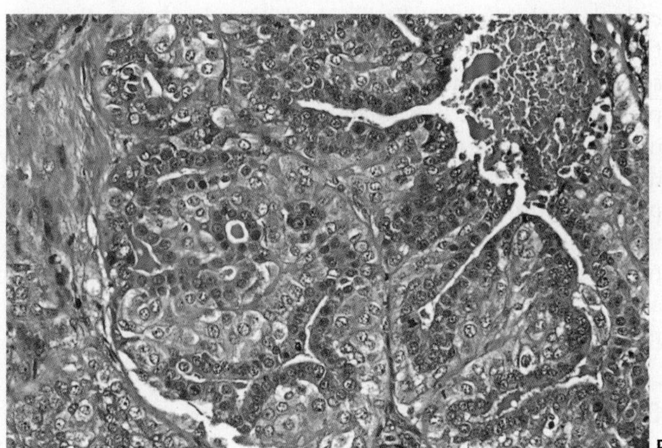

FIG. 6.31. ***Malignant adenomyoepithelioma with epithelial and myoepithelial carcinoma.*** **A:** Neoplastic proliferation of epithelial and MECs with mitotic activity. **B:** Comedonecrosis is present in the epithelial component (*upper right*). Mitotic activity is present.

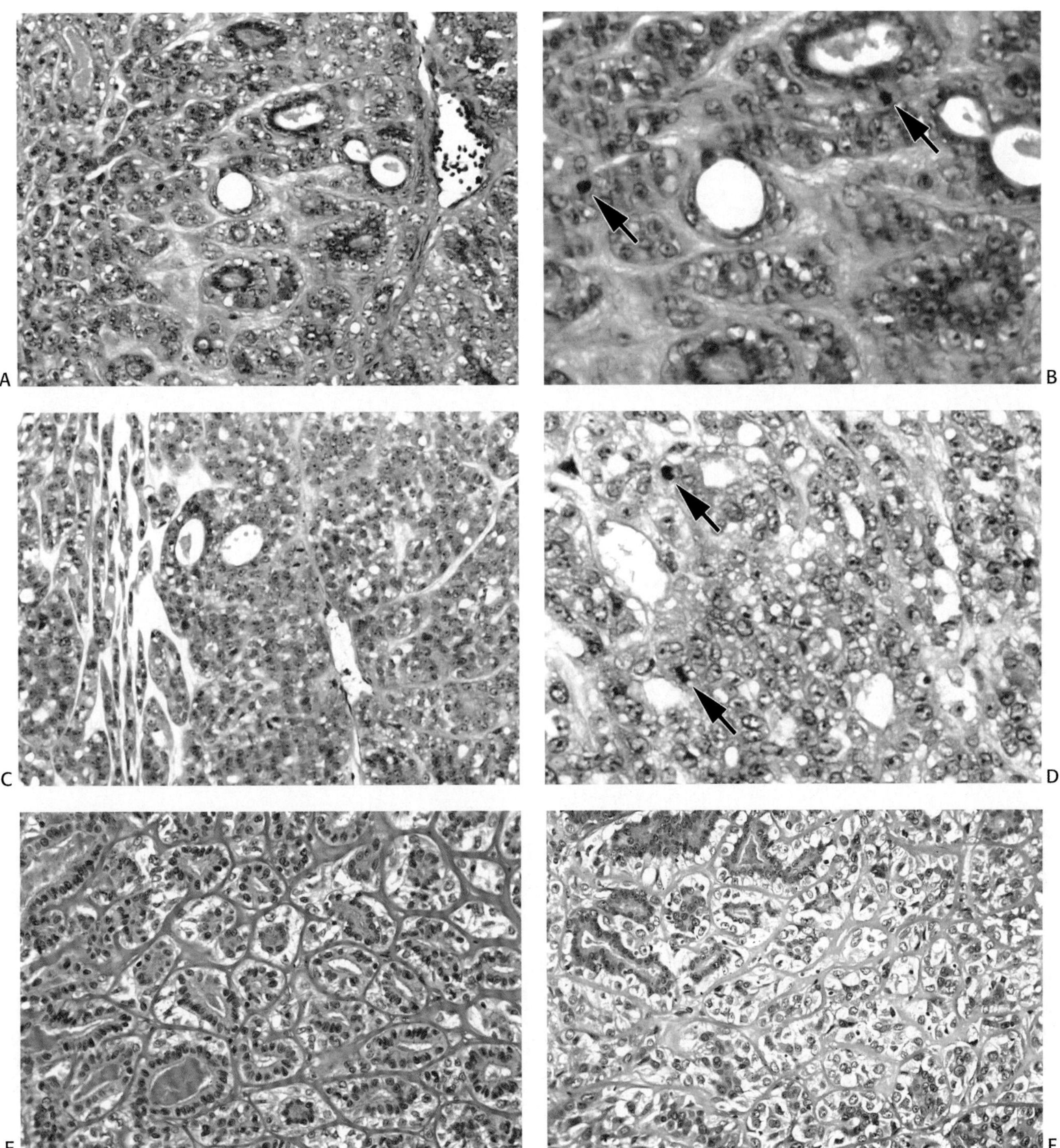

FIG. 6.32. ***Myoepithelial carcinoma arising in adenomyoepithelioma.*** **A:** Overgrowth of MECs in the primary tumor. **B:** An area in **(A)** with mitotic activity (*arrows*) among MECs that have prominent nucleoli. **C:** Part of the primary tumor composed almost entirely of atypical MECs with an epithelial phenotype. **D:** Recurrent tumor growing as myoepithelial carcinoma. The carcinoma cells have prominent nucleoli and frequent mitoses (*arrows*). **E–I:** Images are from a single tumor. AME with myoepithelial hyperplasia **(E)**. Pronounced hyperplasia of atypical MECs is shown displacing glandular epithelial cells **(F)**. A region in which there is nearly complete overgrowth of MECs retaining the fundamental adenomyoepithelial architecture **(G)**. Myoepithelial carcinoma in enlarged alveolar nests **(H)**. Invasive myoepithelial carcinoma **(I,J)**.

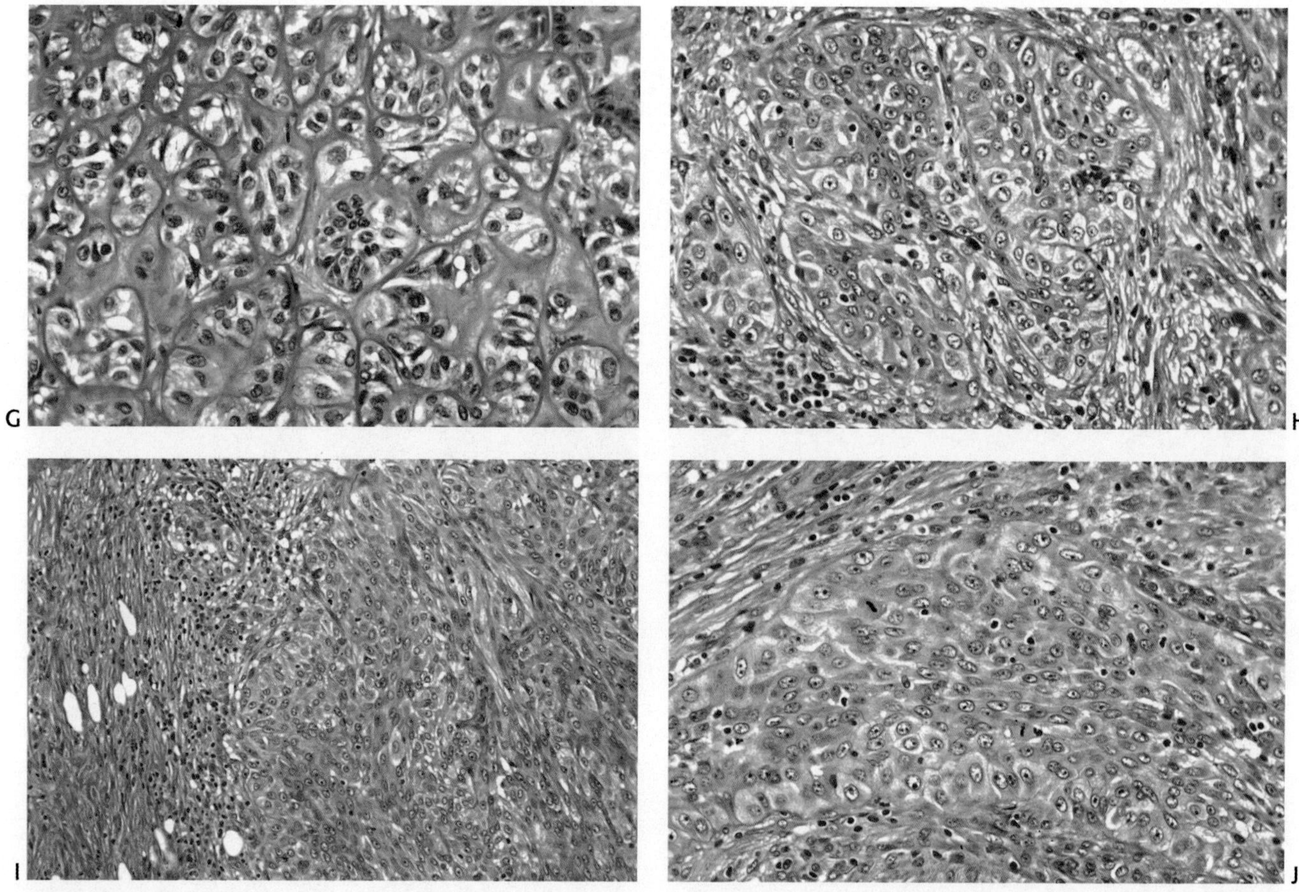

FIG. 6.32. *[Continued]*

recurrence. Carcinoma may be detected as a separate lesion coincidentally or subsequent to excision of an AME.[22] Adenocarcinoma was reportedly found in a recurrent AME.[22]

Surgical reexcision should be performed when the tumor is incompletely excised, especially for multinodular lesions with peripheral intraductal extension. Mastectomy, breast irradiation, and axillary dissection are not appropriate treatment for morphologically benign AME, but may be indicated for those exceptional patients who have malignant tumors arising therein.

Nadelman et al.[89] reported two morphologically "benign" AMEs that developed lung metastases with the same histologic appearance as the primary tumors. In one instance, a 47-year-old woman underwent excision of two breast masses. One was an AME that was resected with a positive margin, and the other was an intraductal papilloma with adenomyoepithelial components that appeared to have been completely excised. Two years later, the patient was found to have multiple AMEs in the ipsilateral breast. After another 2 years, she developed multiple lung nodules. Biopsy of a 1.5-cm pulmonary nodule revealed the same biphasic morphology as the histologically benign-appearing mammary AME, consisting of epithelial cells and MECs. The second patient was a 73-year-old woman who presented with bilateral pulmonary nodules. An excised nodule that was interpreted as metastatic mammary carcinoma led to the discovery of a breast lesion that was diagnosed as a "sclerosing duct papilloma with focal atypical duct hyperplasia." After further study, a diagnosis of AME with spread to the lungs was made.

Malignant AMEs

Carcinomas arising in AMEs should be treated as any other type of breast carcinoma of similar grade and stage. Some morphologically malignant tumors have recurred locally[20,59–61,63,66,90] or resulted in distant metastases and a fatal outcome.[45,60–65,68] Documented sites of metastasis include lung,[63,64] liver,[65] bone,[62] thyroid gland,[68] brain,[61] and kidney.[45] Some patients had distant metastases 1 to 5 months after primary diagnosis,[60,62,64] whereas others developed metastatic disease 12[68] and 15 years[61] after diagnosis of the primary tumor.

MYOEPITHELIOMA AND MYOEPITHELIAL CARCINOMA

Pure myoepithelial neoplasms of the breast are extremely uncommon, and reports are limited to few case studies.

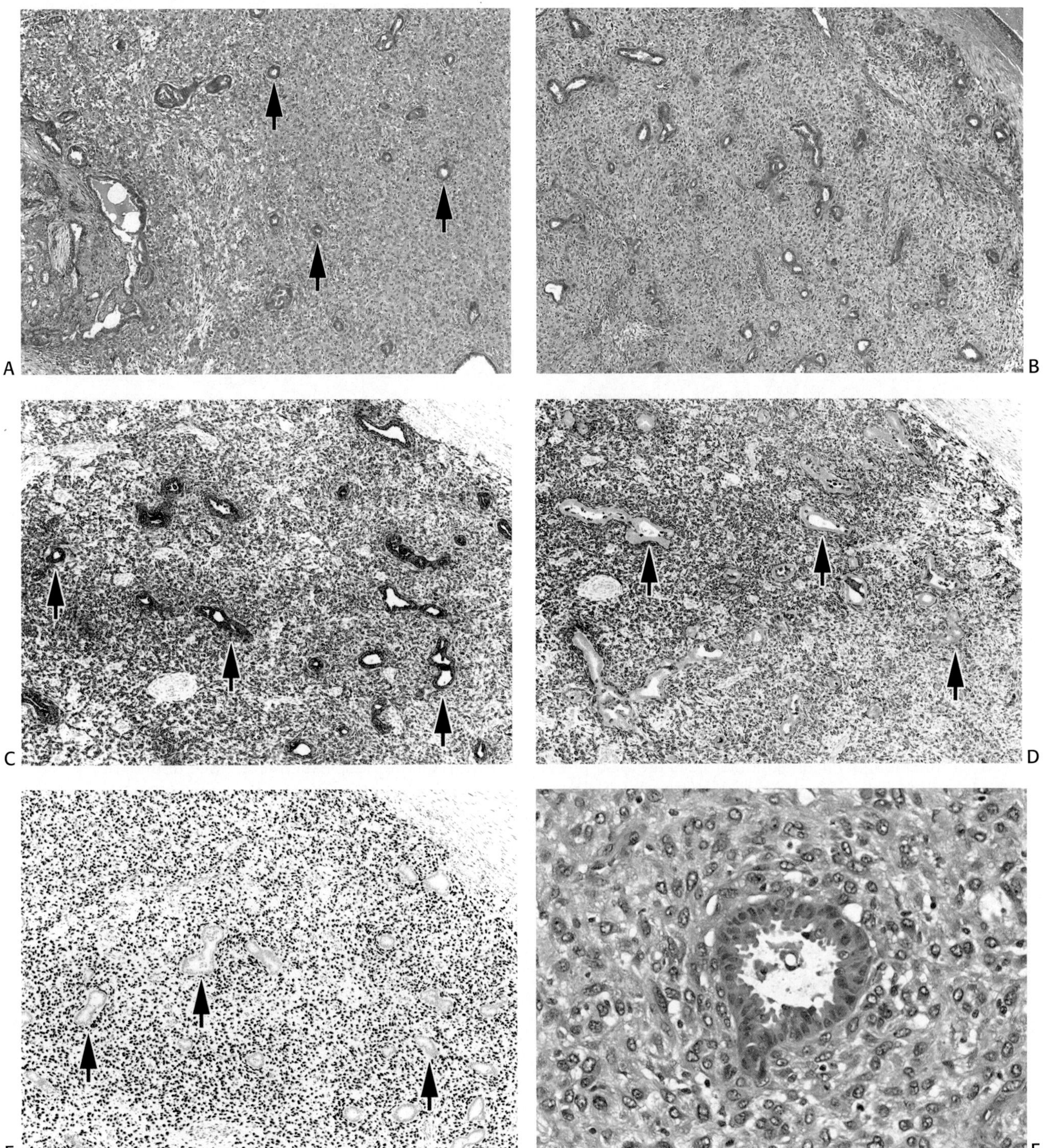

FIG. 6.33. ***Myoepithelial carcinoma arising in adenomyoepithelioma.*** **A:** An infiltrating proliferation of epithelioid myoepithelial carcinoma (*right*) originates from an AME (*left*). Few residual glands are still evident (*arrows*). **B:** The myoepithelial carcinoma appears deceptively circumscribed. Scattered residual glands are evident. **C:** An immunostain for keratin 34βE12 highlights the myoepithelial carcinoma as well as the normal epithelium of few residual adenomyoepithelial glands (*arrows*). **D,E:** The myoepithelial carcinoma is strongly positive for the basal cytokeratin CK5/6 **(D)** and for p63 **(E)**. The residual glands show no reactivity for these two antigens (*arrows*). **F:** A high-power view of the malignant MECs surrounding a residual gland. The pleomorphic neoplastic myoepithelial nuclei are two- or threefold larger than those of the normal epithelium.

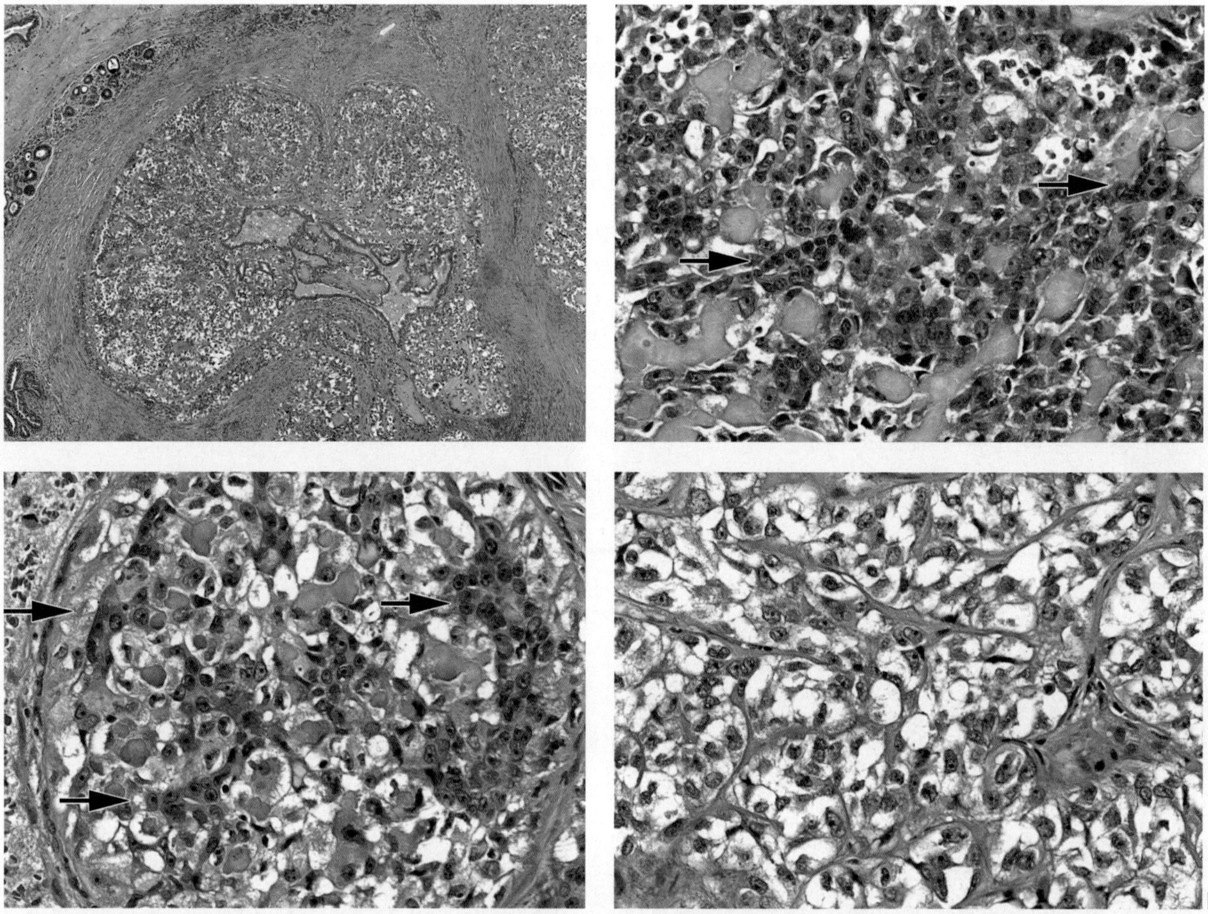

FIG. 6.34. ***Myoepithelial carcinoma arising in adenomyoepithelioma.*** **A:** The carcinoma appears well demarcated from the surrounding normal breast parenchyma. **B:** The myoepithelial carcinoma is focally associated with dense matrix deposits similar to those seen in collagenous spherulosis. Residual atypical glandular cells are also present (*arrows*). **C:** The neoplastic MECs have abundant clear cytoplasm. Residual atypical glandular cells (*arrows*) are not increased in number. **D:** The myoepithelial carcinoma forms solid nests admixed with stroma, with no glandular component. This nesting pattern, typical for a myoepithelial neoplasm, can be misinterpreted as lobular carcinoma.

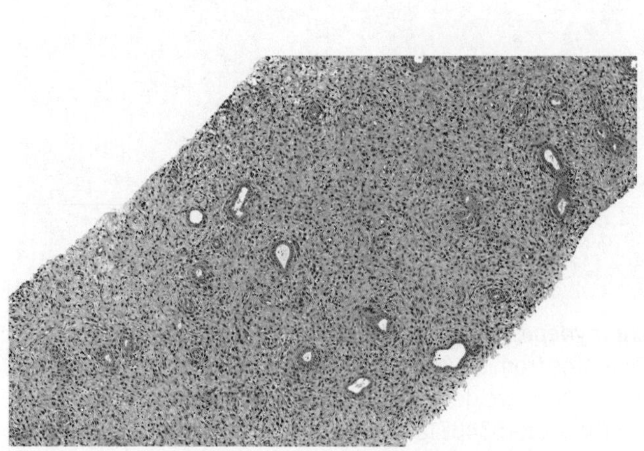

FIG. 6.35. ***Myoepithelial carcinoma arising in adenomyoepithelioma, needle core biopsy.*** The myoepithelial carcinoma in this core biopsy was originally misinterpreted as "cellular stromal proliferation, possibly variant of borderline phyllodes tumor." Images of the myoepithelial carcinoma in the surgical excision specimen are shown in Fig. 6.33.

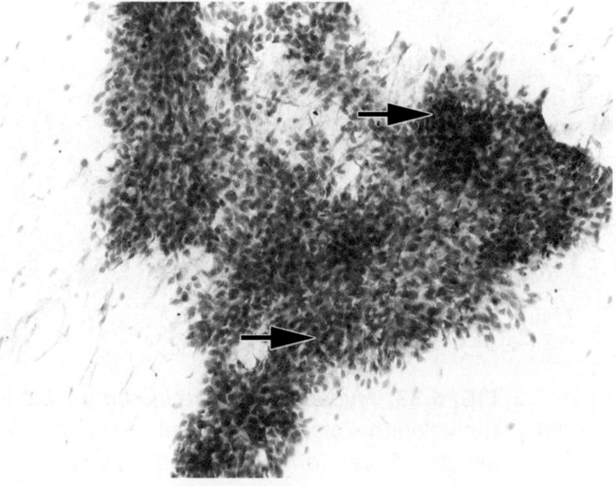

FIG. 6.36. ***Adenomyoepithelioma (pleomorphic adenoma), fine-needle aspiration.*** A tridimensional fragment of spindle cells with rare discernible glandular elements (*arrows*). The differential diagnosis in this case includes a spindle cell lesion, such as a phyllodes tumor. The surgical excision specimen showed a mixed tumor (pleomorphic adenoma) (shown in Fig. 6.28A).

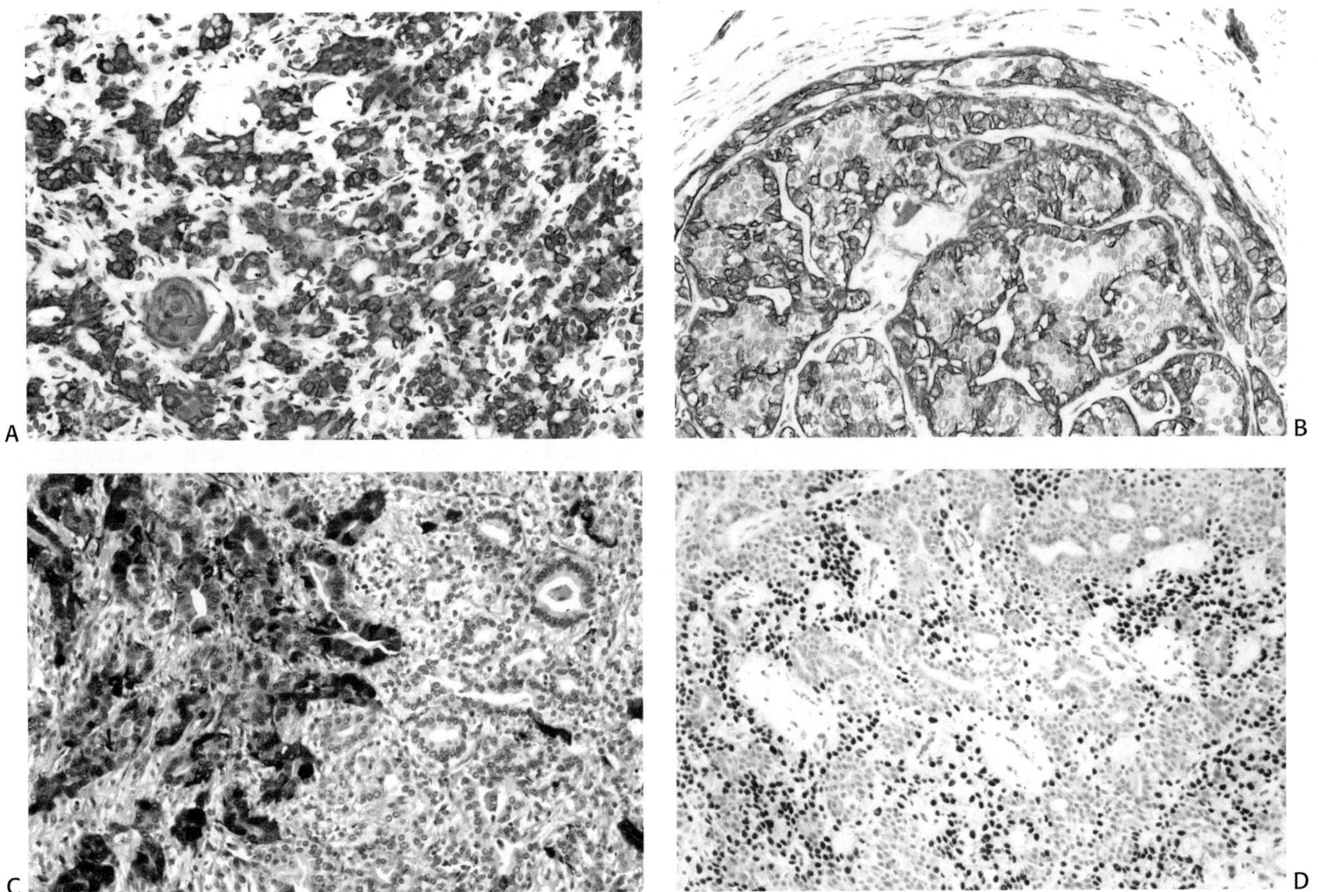

FIG. 6.37. ***Adenomyoepithelioma immunoreactivity.*** **A:** The epithelial cells, including a keratin pearl in the *lower left corner,* are stained with the AE1:AE3 keratin antibody. The MECs are not immunoreactive. **B:** MECs are immunoreactive for actin, which does not stain the epithelial cells. **C:** Focal S-100 immunoreactivity in glandular epithelial cells. **D:** Nuclear reactivity for p63 is localized in MECs.

Myoepithelioma

Myoepithelioma, a tumor comprising almost exclusively benign MECs, is very rare. In 1970, Hamperl[18] described lesions composed of epithelioid and spindly MECs. Leiomyomatous proliferation in these neoplasms may have been coordinated with glandular components, thus retaining adenomyoepitheliomatous features. Toth[91] described a similar lesion that presented as a painful, hard breast tumor. The specimen was grossly nodular and consisted microscopically of dilated ducts "filled with cellular adenomatous intraductal papillomas" in which "the proliferating myoepithelial elements almost filled the ducts… with leiomyoma-like tumors the spindle cells of which formed either bundles or whorl-like patterns." The myoepithelial nature of the spindle cells was confirmed by electron microscopy. After treatment that was evidently limited to the diagnostic excision, the patient was well for approximately 3 years.

Tumors referred to as *muscular*[92] and *myoid hamartomas*[93] (Fig. 6.38) probably arise from myoepithelial hyperplasia. A smooth muscle tumor of the breast that may have arisen secondary to extensive myoid transformation of MECs in sclerosing adenosis was described by Eusebi et al.[94] The patient was a 55-year-old woman who had a 10-cm, nodular, circumscribed tumor present for 8 years. When studied by light and electron microscopy, the lesion was composed largely of smooth muscle cells.

Davies and Riddell[92] noted "the intimate relationship of the smooth muscle to the lobular epithelium" in one of their cases and suggested that "the smooth muscle is of myoepithelial origin." Daroca et al.[93] reported three cases of myoid hamartoma in women 38, 39, and 61 years of age. The tumors were well circumscribed and measured 2.5 to 3.5 cm in greatest dimension. They appeared grossly encapsulated with fat and fibrous stroma. Microscopically, interlacing fascicles of plump spindle cells were distributed in the fibrofatty tissue (Fig. 6.38). The myoid character of these cells was confirmed by strong immunohistochemical reactivity for actin. Electron microscopy in two cases revealed myoid and myoepithelial features. In one tumor, areas of sclerosing adenosis were apparent within the lesion merging with the myoid component. The patients remained well with follow-up of 5 to 13 months after excisional biopsy of these benign tumors.

Spindle cell neoplasms composed entirely of MECs have been described.[86,95–98] The histogenesis of these lesions was

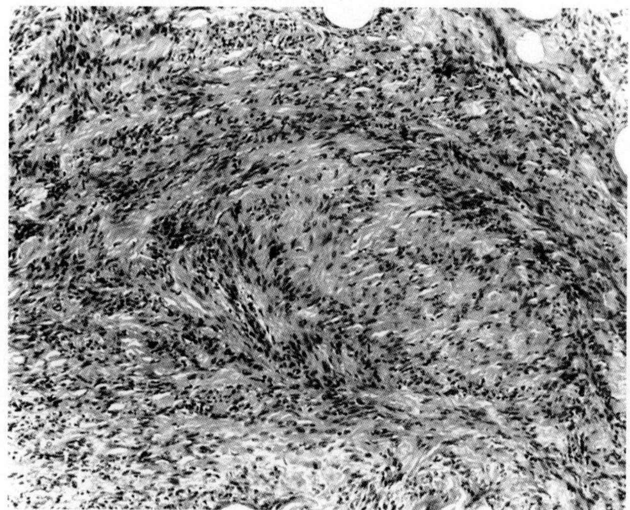

FIG. 6.38. ***Myoid hamartoma.*** Myomatous nodule with palisading of spindle cells. The tumor infiltrates fat at the upper edge of the photograph.

confirmed by electron microscopy and in most instances by immunohistochemistry.[95,96,98] Light microscopy reveals interlacing bundles of spindle cells sometimes arranged in a storiform pattern (Fig. 6.39). The cytoplasm tends to be eosinophilic or sometimes clear. The spindle cells are immunoreactive for actin. In 53-, 54-, and 60-year-old women, three tumors that measured 2.4, 0.9, and 2.8 cm had few or no mitotic figures and a benign clinical course after relatively short follow-up.[86,95,96] Negative axillary nodes were described in one case, and one tumor was ER and PR negative.[86] Cytologic findings in a 4-cm myoepithelioma occurring in a 75-year-old woman have been reported.[99] Some lesions reported in the past as myoepitheliomas with peripheral infiltration into the surrounding fat might have been unrecognized examples of "low-grade" "fibromatosis-like" metaplastic spindle cell carcinoma (see also Chapter 16).

Myoepithelial Carcinoma

A few tumors of the breast composed entirely or almost entirely of malignant spindle cells with myoepithelial/myoid differentiation have been described in the literature as "malignant myoepithelioma[26,97,98,100–102] or "myoepithelial carcinoma."[22,62,71,97,103,104]

Cameron et al.[13] reported a 40-year-old woman with a 5 × 7 cm adenomyoepitheliomatous tumor in which a portion of the lesion was a highly cellular spindle cell neoplasm. One year after treatment by mastectomy, the patient developed a local recurrence involving fat and skeletal muscle consisting entirely of spindle cells with no epithelial structures. The authors stated that "if confronted exclusively with this picture, one would come to the diagnosis 'leiomyosarcoma.'" No follow-up was given.

Numerous mitoses were seen in a 21-cm tumor from an 81-year-old woman[98] and in a 7-cm tumor from a 53-year-old patient.[97] Metastatic carcinoma was found in an axillary lymph node from the former patient, and the latter patient died of pulmonary metastases 6 months after diagnosis. Both malignant myoepithelial neoplasms were negative for ER and PR.

Malignant myoepithelial neoplasms composed of polygonal cells have received less attention than spindle cell myoepithelial tumors. This is remarkable, since MECs frequently have an epithelial configuration within adenomyoepithelial neoplasms of the breast. These lesions typically have an alveolar or nodular growth pattern and they resemble clear cell myoepithelial tumors arising in the salivary glands. These uncommon breast tumors are usually not recognized, and most are probably misclassified as examples of clear cell or AdCC. An invasive clear cell myoepithelial neoplasm that occurred in a 77-year-old woman has been documented by electron microscopy and immunohistochemistry.[105] The 3.5-cm tumor was treated by excisional biopsy only, and no follow-up information was provided. Remarkably high levels of ER (470 fmol/mg protein) were detected in the lesion. Mandal et al.[102] described a fungating 6.0-cm tumor with similar morphology but with triple negative phenotype in a 45-year-old woman. The epithelioid form of invasive myoepithelial carcinoma can sometimes be mistaken for invasive lobular carcinoma[106] (Fig. 6.40).

Buza et al.[71] described 15 myoepithelial carcinomas that were originally classified as a variety of benign and malignant neoplasms. The tumors occurred in women of peri- or postmenopausal age (mean age 69.5 years, range 45 to 86). The mean size was 2.6 cm (range 1.0 to 4.8 cm). Microscopically, the lesions consisted of malignant spindle cells with moderate-to-severe nuclear atypia. In all cases, at least focally, the neoplastic cells appeared to emanate from the myoepithelial layer of few ducts and glands entrapped within the tumor. Focal squamous differentiation was evident in two cases. Mitotic activity ranged from 0 to 9 mitoses per 10 HPFs. An inflammatory infiltrate was present within and at the periphery of the tumors. Associated lesions included three AMEs, one atypical papilloma, ADH, and low-grade DCIS.

Pure spindle cell myoepithelial tumors may be difficult to distinguish by light microscopy from other spindle cell mammary neoplasms. The differential diagnosis includes myofibroblastoma, metaplastic carcinoma, primary spindle cell sarcomas (especially leiomyosarcoma or fibrous histiocytoma), and metastatic spindle and epithelioid tumors such as metastatic malignant melanoma. In most cases, the issue can be resolved by considering the clinical history, as well as careful histologic and immunohistochemical analyses; nowadays electron microscopy is rarely required. The distinction between metaplastic carcinoma and spindle cell myoepithelial neoplasms is not possible on the basis of histochemistry, as the tumors have overlapping immunoprofiles.

Soares et al.[107] described two examples of intralobular myoepithelial carcinoma with spindle cell morphology. In addition, four examples of *in situ* carcinoma with lobular and myoepithelial differentiation have been reported.[108,109] The latter lesions were composed of two distinct cell populations that coexisted in the same expanded acini. One cell

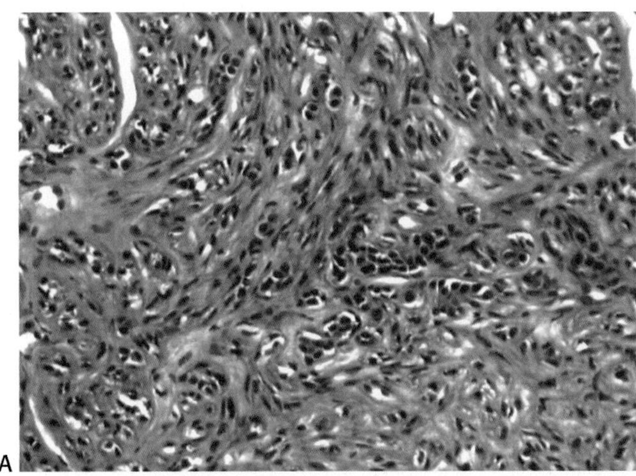
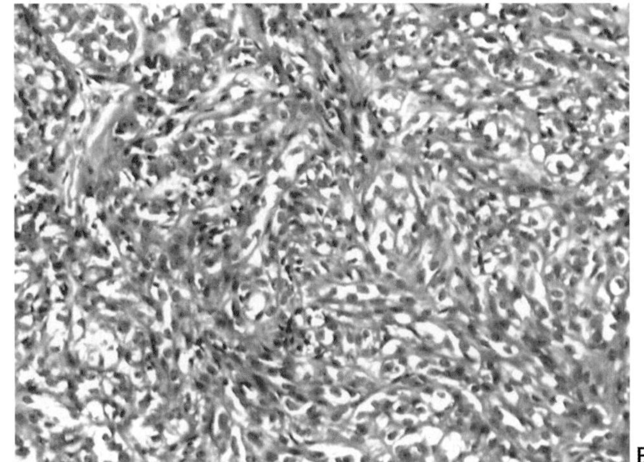

FIG. 6.39. ***Myoepithelioma.*** **A:** Interlacing spindle cells. **B:** Interspersed epithelioid MECs that have clear cytoplasm are present in the tumor arranged in a storiform pattern.

population was positive for E-cadherin and myoepithelial markers, whereas the other population that was located at the periphery of the lesion in one case[109] was negative for the same markers. The biologic significance of these hybrid *in situ* lesions is uncertain. In two of these cases,[108] invasive carcinoma was also present, consisting of a 1.5-cm invasive pleomorphic lobular carcinoma in one case and a minute focus of invasive carcinoma composed of dyshesive cells admixed with desmoplastic stroma in the other.

Immunohistochemistry

Most myoepithelial carcinomas reported by Buza et al.[71] were strongly and diffusely positive for p63, CD10, CK903, and CK5/6. Focal weak to diffuse positivity for calponin, S-100, and SMA was seen in the three cases stained for these markers. All 12 cases tested for ER, PR, and HER2 were triple negative. Epidermal growth factor receptor (EGFR) was strongly positive in 11/12 tumors.

Genetics and Molecular Studies

Jones et al.[104] studied 10 myoepithelial carcinomas of the breast using CGH and found a surprisingly low number of genetic alterations (mean 2.1, range 0 to 4) in these tumors compared with unselected invasive ductal carcinomas (mean 8.6, range 3.6 to 13.8). Most alterations consisted of loss of part of a chromosome, the most common being loss of 16q (3/10 cases), 17p (3/10), 11q (2/10), and 16p (2/10). In one case with coexisting myoepithelial carcinoma and invasive ductal carcinoma, both lesions showed loss of 17p, suggesting origin from a common cell precursor. One case showed gain of 17q and 18p, coupled with loss of 11q and 15q.

MicroRNAs are 21- to 23-nucleotide noncoding RNA molecules that act as post-transcriptional regulators by binding to the complementary sequence in mRNA molecules, favoring their elimination. Bockmeyer et al.[110] reported distinct patterns of microRNA expression in microdissected populations of normal mammary luminal cells and MECs/basal cells. The basal cells/MECs have significantly higher levels of miR-let7C, miR-125b, miR-126, miR-127-3p, miR-143, miR-145, miR-146b-5p, and miR-199a-3p. In contrast, miR-200c and miR-429, which are important in maintaining epithelial cell morphology through positive regulation of the E-cadherin/β-catenin complex, were expressed in the luminal cells. The authors evaluated the microRNA profile of 10 malignant myoepitheliomas of the breast and found it to be consistent with that of MECs and substantially different from that of luminal A, luminal B, and basal carcinomas. The microRNA profile of myoepithelial carcinomas described by Bockmeyer et al.[110] closely mimics that reported by Gregory et al.[111] in metaplastic carcinomas, providing evidence that links myoepithelial carcinomas to metaplastic carcinoma.

Treatment and Prognosis

Two of ten patients with myoepithelial carcinoma studied by Jones et al.[104] had lymph node metastases at initial diagnosis, and one developed an axillary recurrence 6 years after the initial surgery. Four of the seven patients with follow-up information developed metastases in the liver (two patients), lung (one patient), or widespread metastatic involvement, and all four died of disease within a few months to 6 years after the initial diagnosis.

In the study by Buza et al.,[71] the axillary lymph node status was assessed in four patients, and none had lymph node metastases. One of seven patients with follow-up information developed a local recurrence 19 months after the initial diagnosis, and another had lung metastases at 8 months.

The morphologic features, phenotype, and clinical behavior of the myoepithelial carcinomas in these series closely overlap with those of metaplastic spindle cell carcinomas (see Chapter 16).

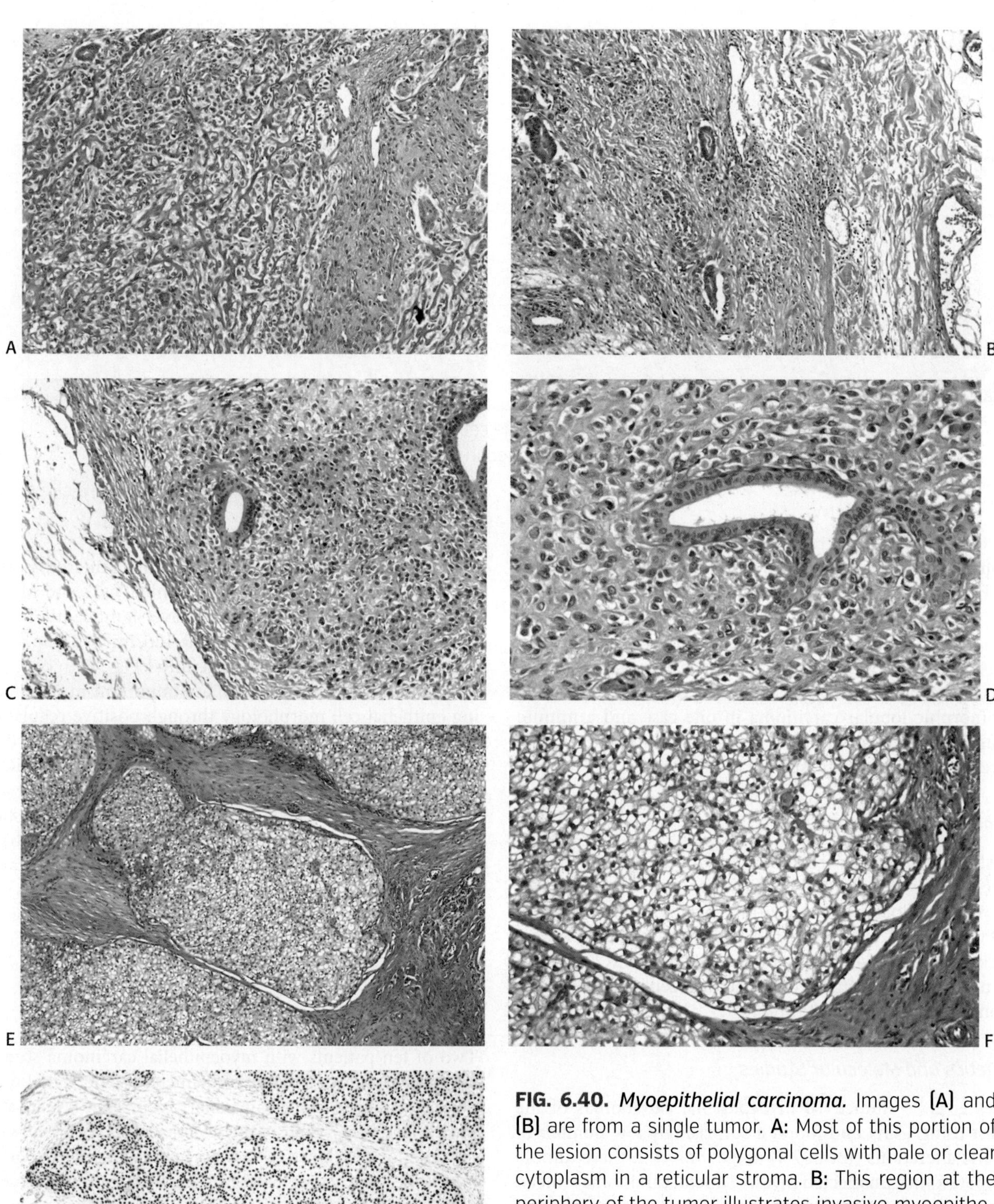

FIG. 6.40. ***Myoepithelial carcinoma.*** Images **(A)** and **(B)** are from a single tumor. **A:** Most of this portion of the lesion consists of polygonal cells with pale or clear cytoplasm in a reticular stroma. **B:** This region at the periphery of the tumor illustrates invasive myoepithelial carcinoma cells. The cells encircling a gland in the *lower center* appear to be *in situ* myoepithelial carcinoma. **C,D:** Invasive myoepithelial carcinoma composed of epithelioid cells with eosinophilic cytoplasm surrounds benign glands. **E,F:** Intraductal myoepithelial carcinoma, clear cell type. **G:** Nuclear p63 immunoreactivity in clear cell myoepithelial intraductal carcinoma.

REFERENCES

1. Gusterson BA, Warburton MJ, Mitchell D, et al. Distribution of myoepithelial cells and basement membrane proteins in the normal breast and in benign and malignant breast diseases. *Cancer Res* 1982;42:4763–4770.
2. Franke WW, Schmid E, Freudenstein C, et al. Intermediate-sized filaments of the prekeratin type in myoepithelial cells. *J Cell Biol* 1980;84:633–654.
3. Joshi K, Smith JA, Perusinghe N, et al. Cell proliferation in the human mammary epithelium. Differential contribution by epithelial and myoepithelial cells. *Am J Pathol* 1986;124:199–206.
4. Rudland PS. Histochemical organization and cellular composition of ductal buds in developing human breast: evidence of cytochemical intermediates between epithelial and myoepithelial cells. *J Histochem Cytochem* 1991;39:1471–1484.
5. O'Hare MJ, Ormerod MG, Monaghan P, et al. Characterization *in vitro* of luminal and myoepithelial cells isolated from the human mammary gland by cell sorting. *Differentiation* 1991;46:209–221.
6. Clarke C, Sandle J, Lakhani SR. Myoepithelial cells: pathology, cell separation and markers of myoepithelial differentiation. *J Mammary Gland Biol Neoplasia* 2005;10:273–280.
7. Barsky SH. Myoepithelial mRNA expression profiling reveals a common tumor-suppressor phenotype. *Exp Mol Pathol* 2003;74:113–122.
8. Pandey PR, Saidou J, Watabe K. Role of myoepithelial cells in breast tumor progression. *Front Biosci* 2010;15:226–236.
9. Molyneux G, Geyer FC, Magnay FA, et al. BRCA1 basal-like breast cancers originate from luminal epithelial progenitors and not from basal stem cells. *Cell Stem Cell* 2010;7:403–417.
10. Longacre TA, Bartow SA. A correlative morphologic study of human breast and endometrium in the menstrual cycle. *Am J Surg Pathol* 1986;10:382–393.
11. Dewar R, Fadare O, Gilmore H, et al. Best practices in diagnostic immunohistochemistry: myoepithelial markers in breast pathology. *Arch Pathol Lab Med* 2011;135:422–429.
12. Sorenson SC, Asch BB, Connolly JL, et al. Structural distinctions among human breast epithelial cells revealed by the monclonal antikeratin antibodies AE1 and AE3. *J Pathol* 1987;153:151–162.
13. Cameron HM, Hamperl H, Warambo W. Leiomyosarcoma of the breast originating from myothelium (myoepithelium). *J Pathol* 1974;114:89–92.
14. Dardick I, van Nostrand AW. Myoepithelial cells in salivary gland tumors—revisited. *Head Neck Surg* 1985;7:395–408.
15. Kahn HJ, Baumal R, Marks A, et al. Myoepithelial cells in salivary gland tumors. An immunohistochemical study. *Arch Pathol Lab Med* 1985;109:190–195.
16. Eusebi V, Casadei GP, Bussolati G, et al. Adenomyoepithelioma of the breast with a distinctive type of apocrine adenosis. *Histopathology* 1987;11:305–315.
17. Young RH, Clement PB. Adenomyoepithelioma of the breast. A report of three cases and review of the literature. *Am J Clin Pathol* 1988;89:308–314.
18. Hamperl H. The myothelia (myoepithelial cells). Normal state; regressive changes; hyperplasia; tumors. *Curr Top Pathol* 1970;53:161–220.
19. Decorsiere J, Thibaut I, Bouissou H. Les proliférations àdenomyoepithéliales du sein. *Ann Pathol* 1988;8:311–316.
20. Loose JH, Patchefsky AS, Hollander IJ, et al. Adenomyoepithelioma of the breast. A spectrum of biologic behavior. *Am J Surg Pathol* 1992;16:868–876.
21. Rosen PP. Adenomyoepithelioma of the breast. *Hum Pathol* 1987;18:1232–1237.
22. Tavassoli FA. Myoepithelial lesions of the breast. Myoepitheliosis, adenomyoepithelioma, and myoepithelial carcinoma. *Am J Surg Pathol* 1991;15:554–568.
23. McLaren BK, Smith J, Schuyler PA, et al. Adenomyoepithelioma: clinical, histologic, and immunohistologic evaluation of a series of related lesions. *Am J Surg Pathol* 2005;29:1294–1299.
24. Tamura G, Monma N, Suzuki Y, et al. Adenomyoepithelioma (myoepithelioma) of the breast in a male. *Hum Pathol* 1993;24:678–681.
25. Berna JD, Arcas I, Ballester A, et al. Adenomyoepithelioma of the breast in a male. *AJR Am J Roentgenol* 1997;169:917–918.
26. Hegyi L, Thway K, Newton R, et al. Malignant myoepithelioma arising in adenomyoepithelioma of the breast and coincident multiple gastrointestinal stromal tumours in a patient with neurofibromatosis type 1. *J Clin Pathol* 2009;62:653–655.
27. Han JS, Peng Y. Multicentric adenomyoepithelioma of the breast with atypia and associated ductal carcinoma in situ. *Breast J* 2010;16:547–549.
28. Jabi M, Dardick I, Cardigos N. Adenomyoepithelioma of the breast. *Arch Pathol Lab Med* 1988;112:73–76.
29. Reis-Filho JS, Fulford LG, Crebassa B, et al. Collagenous spherulosis in an adenomyoepithelioma of the breast. *J Clin Pathol* 2004;57:83–86.
30. Iyengar P, Ali SZ, Brogi E. Fine-needle aspiration cytology of mammary adenomyoepithelioma: a study of 12 patients. *Cancer* 2006;108:250–256.
31. Adejolu M, Wu Y, Santiago L, et al. Adenomyoepithelial tumors of the breast: imaging findings with histopathologic correlation. *AJR Am J Roentgenol* 2011;197:W184–W190.
32. Diaz NM, McDivitt RW, Wick MR. Pleomorphic adenoma of the breast: a clinicopathologic and immunohistochemical study of 10 cases. *Hum Pathol* 1991;22:1206–1214.
33. Vielh P, Thiery JP, Validire P, et al. Adenomyoepithelioma of the breast: fine-needle sampling with histologic, immunohistologic, and electron microscopic analysis. *Diagn Cytopathol* 1993;9:188–193.
34. Van Dorpe J, De Pauw A, Moerman P. Adenoid cystic carcinoma arising in an adenomyoepithelioma of the breast. *Virchows Arch* 1998;432:119–122.
35. Tamura S, Enjoji M, Toyoshima S, et al. Adenomyoepithelioma of the breast. A case report with an immunohistochemical study. *Acta Pathol Jpn* 1988;38:659–665.
36. Chang A, Bassett L, Bose S. Adenomyoepithelioma of the breast: a cytologic dilemma. Report of a case and review of the literature. *Diagn Cytopathol* 2002;26:191–196.
37. Mercado CL, Toth HK, Axelrod D, et al. Fine-needle aspiration biopsy of benign adenomyoepithelioma of the breast: radiologic and pathologic correlation in four cases. *Diagn Cytopathol* 2007;35:690–694.
38. Lee JH, Kim SH, Kang BJ, et al. Ultrasonographic features of benign adenomyoepithelioma of the breast. *Korean J Radiol* 2010;11: 522–527.
39. Howlett DC, Mason CH, Biswas S, et al. Adenomyoepithelioma of the breast: spectrum of disease with associated imaging and pathology. *AJR Am J Roentgenol* 2003;180:799–803.
40. Ruiz-Delgado ML, Lopez-Ruiz JA, Eizaguirre B, et al. Benign adenomyoepithelioma of the breast: imaging findings mimicking malignancy and histopathological features. *Acta Radiol* 2007;48:27–29.
41. Park YM, Park JS, Jung HS, et al. Imaging features of benign adenomyoepithelioma of the breast. *J Clin Ultrasound* 2013;41:218–223.
42. Warrier S, Hwang S, Ghaly M, et al. Adenomyoepithelioma with ductal carcinoma in situ: a case report and review of the literature. *Case Rep Surg* 2013;2013:521417.
43. Ng WK. Adenomyoepithelioma of the breast. A review of three cases with reappraisal of the fine needle aspiration biopsy findings. *Acta Cytol* 2002;46:317–324.
44. Kuroda N, Fujishima N, Ohara M, et al. Coexistent adenomyoepithelioma and invasive ductal carcinoma of the breast: presentation as separate tumors. *Med Mol Morphol* 2008;41:238–242.
45. Honda Y, Iyama K. Malignant adenomyoepithelioma of the breast combined with invasive lobular carcinoma. *Pathol Int* 2009;59:179–184.
46. Da Silva L, Buck L, Simpson PT, et al. Molecular and morphological analysis of adenoid cystic carcinoma of the breast with synchronous tubular adenosis. *Virchows Arch* 2009;454:107–114.
47. Buch A, Rout P, Makhija P. Adenomyoepithelioma with phyllodes tumor—a rare combination in a solitary breast lump. *Indian J Pathol Microbiol* 2006;49:259–261.
48. Gusterson BA, Sloane JP, Middwood C, et al. Ductal adenoma of the breast—a lesion exhibiting a myoepithelial/epithelial phenotype. *Histopathology* 1987;11:103–110.
49. Hikino H, Kodama K, Yasui K, et al. Intracystic adenomyoepithelioma of the breast—case report and review. *Breast Cancer* 2007;14: 429–433.
50. Guarino M, Reale D, Squillaci S, et al. Ductal adenoma of the breast. An immunohistochemical study of five cases. *Pathol Res Pract* 1993;189:515–520.
51. Jensen ML, Johansen P, Noer H, et al. Ductal adenoma of the breast: the cytological features of six cases. *Diagn Cytopathol* 1994;10:143–145.
52. Chen KT. Pleomorphic adenoma of the breast. *Am J Clin Pathol* 1990;93:792–794.
53. Narita T, Matsuda K. Pleomorphic adenoma of the breast: case report and review of the literature. *Pathol Int* 1995;45:441–447.
54. Nevado M, Lopez JI, Dominguez MP, et al. Pleomorphic adenoma of the breast. Case report. *APMIS* 1991;99:866–868.
55. Reid-Nicholson M, Bleiweiss I, Pace B, et al. Pleomorphic adenoma of the breast. A case report and distinction from mucinous carcinoma. *Arch Pathol Lab Med* 2003;127:474–477.
56. Iyengar P, Cody HS III Brogi E. Pleomorphic adenoma of the breast: case report and review of the literature. *Diagn Cytopathol* 2005;33:416–420.
57. Rubin E, Dempsey PJ, Listinsky, CM, et al. Adenomyoepithelioma of the breast: a case report. *Breast Disease* 1995;8:103–109.

58. Van Dorpe J, De Weer F, Bekaert J, et al. Malignant myoepithelioma of the breast. Case report with immunohistochemical study. *Arch Anat Cytol Pathol* 1996;44:193–198.
59. Oka K, Sando N, Moriya T, et al. Malignant adenomyoepithelioma of the breast with matrix production may be compatible with one variant form of matrix-producing carcinoma: a case report. *Pathol Res Pract* 2007;203:599–604.
60. Michal M, Baumruk L, Burger J, et al. Adenomyoepithelioma of the breast with undifferentiated carcinoma component. *Histopathology* 1994;24:274–276.
61. Rasbridge SA, Millis RR. Adenomyoepithelioma of the breast with malignant features. *Virchows Arch* 1998;432:123–130.
62. Chen PC, Chen CK, Nicastri AD, et al. Myoepithelial carcinoma of the breast with distant metastasis and accompanied by adenomyoepitheliomas. *Histopathology* 1994;24:543–548.
63. Simpson RH, Cope N, Skalova A, et al. Malignant adenomyoepithelioma of the breast with mixed osteogenic, spindle cell, and carcinomatous differentiation. *Am J Surg Pathol* 1998;22:631–636.
64. Kihara M, Yokomise H, Irie A, et al. Malignant adenomyoepithelioma of the breast with lung metastases: report of a case. *Surg Today* 2001;31:899–903.
65. Jones C, Tooze R, Lakhani SR. Malignant adenomyoepithelioma of the breast metastasizing to the liver. *Virchows Arch* 2003;442:504–506.
66. Qureshi A, Kayani N, Gulzar R. Malignant adenomyoepithelioma of the breast: a case report with review of literature. *BMJ Case Rep* 2009;2009.
67. Trojani M, Guiu M, Trouette H, et al. Malignant adenomyoepithelioma of the breast. An immunohistochemical, cytophotometric, and ultrastructural study of a case with lung metastases. *Am J Clin Pathol* 1992;98:598–602.
68. Bult P, Verwiel JM, Wobbes T, et al. Malignant adenomyoepithelioma of the breast with metastasis in the thyroid gland 12 years after excision of the primary tumor. Case report and review of the literature. *Virchows Arch* 2000;436:158–166.
69. Van Hoeven KH, Drudis T, Cranor ML, et al. Low-grade adenosquamous carcinoma of the breast. A clinocopathologic study of 32 cases with ultrastructural analysis. *Am J Surg Pathol* 1993;17:248–258.
70. Foschini MP, Pizzicannella G, Peterse JL, et al. Adenomyoepithelioma of the breast associated with low-grade adenosquamous and sarcomatoid carcinomas. *Virchows Arch* 1995;427:243–250.
71. Buza N, Zekry N, Charpin C, et al. Myoepithelial carcinoma of the breast: a clinicopathological and immunohistochemical study of 15 diagnostically challenging cases. *Virchows Arch* 2010;457:337–345.
72. Hungermann D, Buerger H, Oehlschlegel C, et al. Adenomyoepithelial tumours and myoepithelial carcinomas of the breast—a spectrum of monophasic and biphasic tumours dominated by immature myoepithelial cells. *BMC Cancer* 2005;5:92.
73. Zhang C, Quddus MR, Sung CJ. Atypical adenomyoepithelioma of the breast: diagnostic problems and practical approaches in core needle biopsy. *Breast J* 2004;10:154–155.
74. Hock YL, Chan SY. Adenomyoepithelioma of the breast. A case report correlating cytologic and histologic features. *Acta Cytol* 1994;38:953–956.
75. Plaza JA, Lopez JI, Garcia S, et al. Adenomyoepithelioma of the breast. Report of two cases. *Arch Anat Cytol Pathol* 1993;41:99–101.
76. Niemann TH, Benda JA, Cohen MB. Adenomyoepithelioma of the breast: fine-needle aspiration biopsy and histologic findings. *Diagn Cytopathol* 1995;12:245–250.
77. Kurashina M. Fine-needle aspiration cytology of benign and malignant adenomyoepithelioma: report of two cases. *Diagn Cytopathol* 2002;26:29–34.
78. Laforga JB, Aranda FI, Sevilla F. Adenomyoepithelioma of the breast: report of two cases with prominent cystic changes and intranuclear inclusions. *Diagn Cytopathol* 1998;19:55–58.
79. Valente PT, Stuckey JH. Fine-needle aspiration cytology of mammary adenomyoepithelioma: report of a case with intranuclear cytoplasmic inclusions. *Diagn Cytopathol* 1994;10:165–168.
80. Saad RS, Richmond L, Nofech-Mozes S, et al. Fine-needle aspiration biopsy of breast adenomyoepithelioma: a potential false positive pitfall and presence of intranuclear cytoplasmic inclusions. *Diagn Cytopathol* 2012;40:1005–1009.
81. Yahara T, Yamaguchi R, Yokoyama G, et al. Adenomyoepithelioma of the breast diagnosed by a mammotome biopsy: report of a case. *Surg Today* 2008;38:144–146.
82. Gillett CE, Bobrow LG, Millis RR. S100 protein in human mammary tissue—immunoreactivity in breast carcinoma, including Paget's disease of the nipple, and value as a marker of myoepithelial cells. *J Pathol* 1990;160:19–24.
83. Decorsiere J, Bouissou H, Becue J. Problèmes posés par l'adénomyoépithéliome du sein. *Gynecologie* 1985;36:221–227.
84. Weidner N, Levine JD. Spindle-cell adenomyoepithelioma of the breast. A microscopic, ultrastructural, and immunocytochemical study. *Cancer* 1988;62:1561–1567.
85. Zarbo RJ, Oberman HA. Cellular adenomyoepithelioma of the breast. *Am J Surg Pathol* 1983;7:863–870.
86. Erlandson RA, Rosen PP. Infiltrating myoepithelioma of the breast. *Am J Surg Pathol* 1982;6:785–793.
87. Salto-Tellez M, Putti TC, Lee CK, et al. Adenomyoepithelioma of the breast: description of allelic imbalance and microsatellite instability. *Histopathology* 2005;46:230–231.
88. Gatalica Z, Velagaleti G, Kuivaniemi H, et al. Gene expression profile of an adenomyoepithelioma of the breast with a reciprocal translocation involving chromosomes 8 and 16. *Cancer Genet Cytogenet* 2005;156:14–22.
89. Nadelman CM, Leslie KO, Fishbein MC. "Benign," metastasizing adenomyoepithelioma of the breast: a report of 2 cases. *Arch Pathol Lab Med* 2006;130:1349–1353.
90. Pauwels C, De Potter C. Adenomyoepithelioma of the breast with features of malignancy. *Histopathology* 1994;24:94–96.
91. Toth J. Benign human mammary myoepithelioma. *Virchows Arch A Pathol Anat Histol* 1977;374:263–269.
92. Davies JD, Riddell RH. Muscular hamartomas of the breast. *J Pathol* 1973;111:209–211.
93. Daroca PJ Jr, Reed RJ, Love GL, et al. Myoid hamartomas of the breast. *Hum Pathol* 1985;16:212–219.
94. Eusebi V, Cunsolo A, Fedeli F, et al. Benign smooth muscle cell metaplasia in breast. *Tumori* 1980;66:643–653.
95. Bigotti G, Di Giorgio CG. Myoepithelioma of the breast: histologic, immunologic, and electromicroscopic appearance. *J Surg Oncol* 1986;32:58–64.
96. Rode L, Nesland JM, Johannessen JV. A spindle cell breast lesion in a 54-year-old woman. *Ultrastruct Pathol* 1986;10:421–425.
97. Schurch W, Potvin C, Seemayer TA. Malignant myoepithelioma (myoepithelial carcinoma) of the breast: an ultrastructural and immunocytochemical study. *Ultrastruct Pathol* 1985;8:1–11.
98. Thorner PS, Kahn HJ, Baumal R, et al. Malignant myoepithelioma of the breast. An immunohistochemical study by light and electron microscopy. *Cancer* 1986;57:745–750.
99. Nguyen GK, Shnitka TK, Jewell LD. Aspiration biopsy cytology of mammary myoepithelioma. *Diagn Cytopathol* 1987;3:335–338.
100. Fang ZM, Tse RV, Marjoniemi VM, et al. Radioresistant malignant myoepithelioma of the breast with high level of ataxia telangiectasia mutated protein. *J Med Imaging Radiat Oncol* 2009;53:234–239.
101. Noel JC, Simon P, Aguilar SF. Malignant myoepithelioma arising in cystic adenomyoepithelioma. *Breast J* 2006;12:386.
102. Mandal S, Dhingra K, Roy S, et al. Clear cell malignant myoepithelioma—breast presenting as a fungating mass. *Breast J* 2007;13:618–620.
103. Kwon SY, Bae YK, Cho J, et al. Myoepithelial carcinoma with contralateral invasive micropapillary carcinoma of the breast. *J Korean Surg Soc* 2011;81:211–215.
104. Jones C, Foschini MP, Chaggar R, et al. Comparative genomic hybridization analysis of myoepithelial carcinoma of the breast. *Lab Invest* 2000;80:831–836.
105. Cartagena N Jr, Cabello-Inchausti B, Willis I, et al. Clear cell myoepithelial neoplasm of the breast. *Hum Pathol* 1988;19:1239–1243.
106. Fan F, Smith W, Wang X, et al. Myoepithelial carcinoma of the breast arising in an adenomyoepithelioma: mammographic, ultrasound and histologic features. *Breast J* 2007;13:203–204.
107. Soares J, Tomasic G, Bucciarelli E, et al. Intralobular growth of myoepithelial cell carcinoma of the breast. *Virchows Arch* 1994;425:205–210.
108. Del Vecchio M, Foschini MP, Peterse JL, et al. Lobular carcinoma of the breast with hybrid myoepithelial and secretory ("myosecretory") cell differentiation. *Am J Surg Pathol* 2005;29:1530–1536.
109. Shousha S, Knee G. In-situ lobular/myoepithelial neoplasia of the breast. *Histopathology* 2004;45:93–95.
110. Bockmeyer CL, Christgen M, Muller M, et al. MicroRNA profiles of healthy basal and luminal mammary epithelial cells are distinct and reflected in different breast cancer subtypes. *Breast Cancer Res Treat* 2011;130:735–745.
111. Gregory PA, Bert AG, Paterson EL, et al. The miR-200 family and miR-205 regulate epithelial to mesenchymal transition by targeting ZEB1 and SIP1. *Nat Cell Biol* 2008;10:593–601.

CHAPTER 7

Adenosis and Microglandular Adenosis

EDI BROGI

ADENOSIS

Adenosis is a lobulocentric proliferation predominantly derived from the terminal duct lobular unit (TDLU). Larger duct structures are sometimes incorporated into the lesion, but they are less involved than lobules. Epithelial and myoepithelial cells participate in adenosis. Ewing[1] referred to adenosis as "fibrosing adenomatosis." Foote and Stewart[2] subsequently described the lesion as "sclerosing adenomatosis" and "sclerosing adenosis." The earliest clinicopathologic studies of sclerosing adenosis were published in 1949[3] and 1950.[4]

Clinical Presentation

Adenosis occurs most often as part of the spectrum of proliferative alterations commonly referred to as fibrocystic changes. The entire complex may produce a palpable mass, with adenosis accounting for part or most of the lesion. Adenosis limited to isolated lobules that are not part of fibrocystic changes is a microscopic lesion that comes to clinical attention when it harbors mammographically detectable calcifications (Fig. 7.1). Microcalcifications frequently occur in the sclerosing type of adenosis.

Adenosis forms a distinct clinically palpable or radiographically detectable mass when the affected lobules are closely adjacent or merge together to create an adenosis tumor[5] (Figs. 7.2 and 7.3). Patients with adenosis tumor are almost always premenopausal, averaging about 30 years of age at diagnosis. Adenosis tumor is usually smaller than 2 cm. It is rarely attached to the skin, and the lesion is usually a firm, clinically discrete, or ill-defined mass easily mistaken for a fibroadenoma.[3,6,7] A few patients report pain or tenderness.[5,8,9]

Radiology

Non-palpable adenosis tumors that contain calcifications may be detected by mammography (Fig. 7.1). Sonography usually reveals a solid, well-defined tumor.[5] Gill et al.[10] studied the radiologic findings in lesions that contained sclerosing adenosis in needle core biopsy samples. Thirty-three lesions in which sclerosing adenosis represented the major finding were deemed to have concordant radiologic

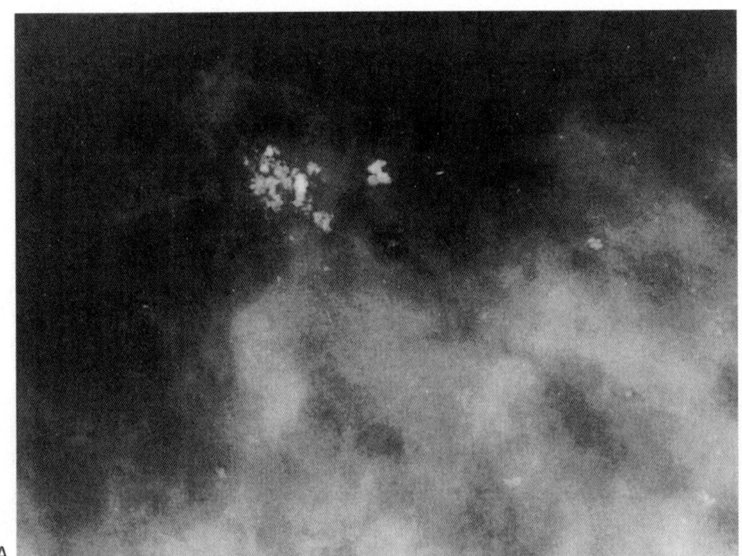

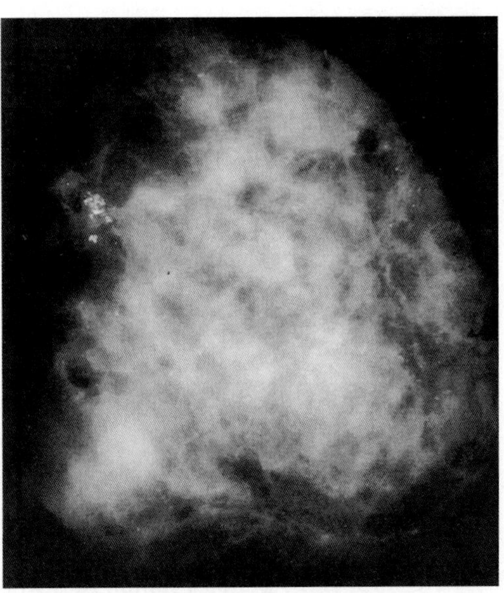

FIG. 7.1. *Adenosis.* **A:** A mammogram showing clustered calcifications that proved to be in sclerosing adenosis. **B:** A specimen radiograph that confirms excision of the calcifications. The safety pin is for orientation.

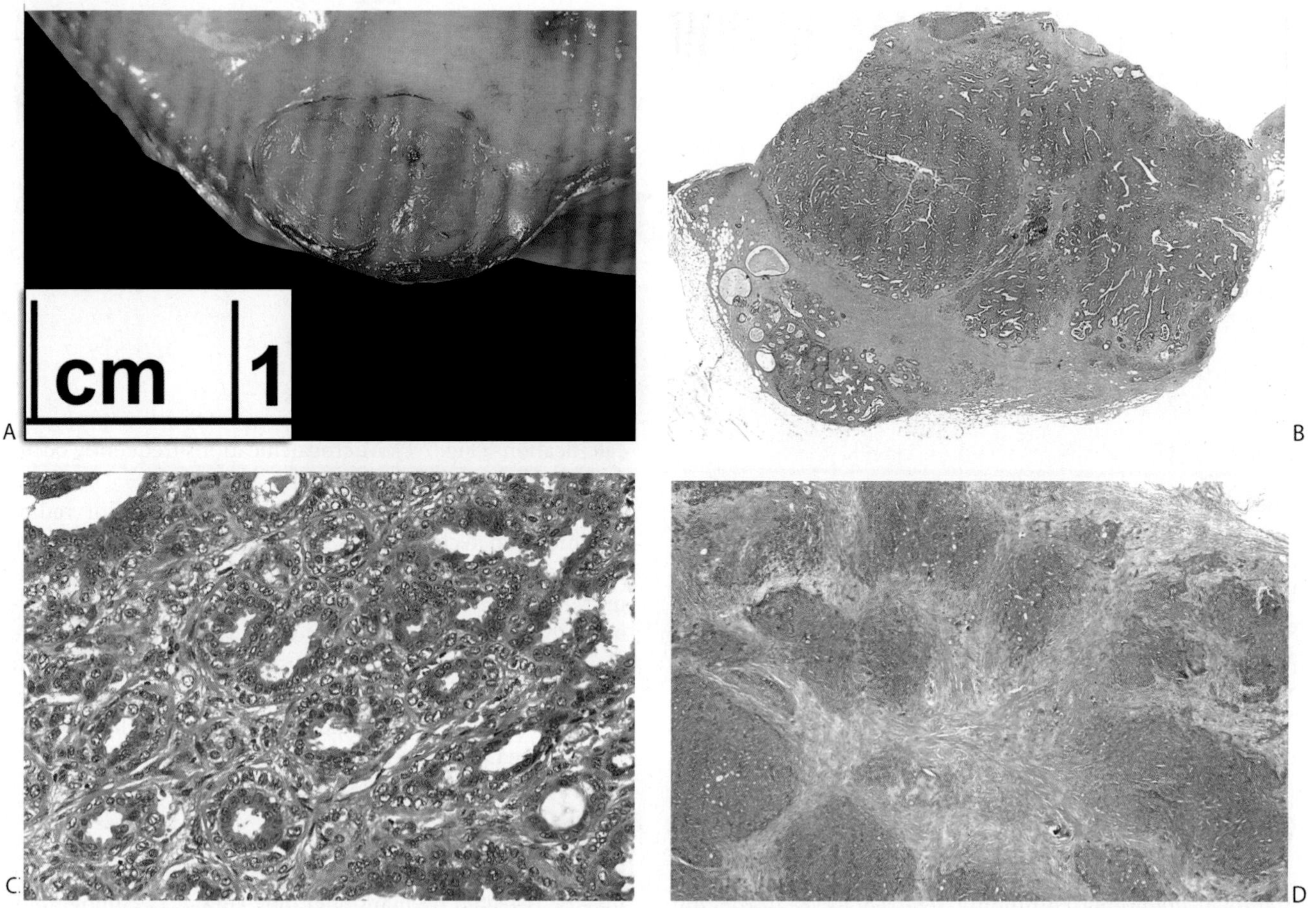

FIG. 7.2. ***Adenosis tumor.*** **A:** A gross specimen with an adenosis tumor composed of beige homogeneous tissue forming an oval, 1-cm nodule. **B:** Whole mount histologic section of the tumor in (A) showing internal nodular architecture. **C:** Florid adenosis with epithelial and myoepithelial hyperplasia in the adenosis tumour is shown in (A) and (B). **D:** Whole-mount histologic section of another tumor formed by confluent nodules.

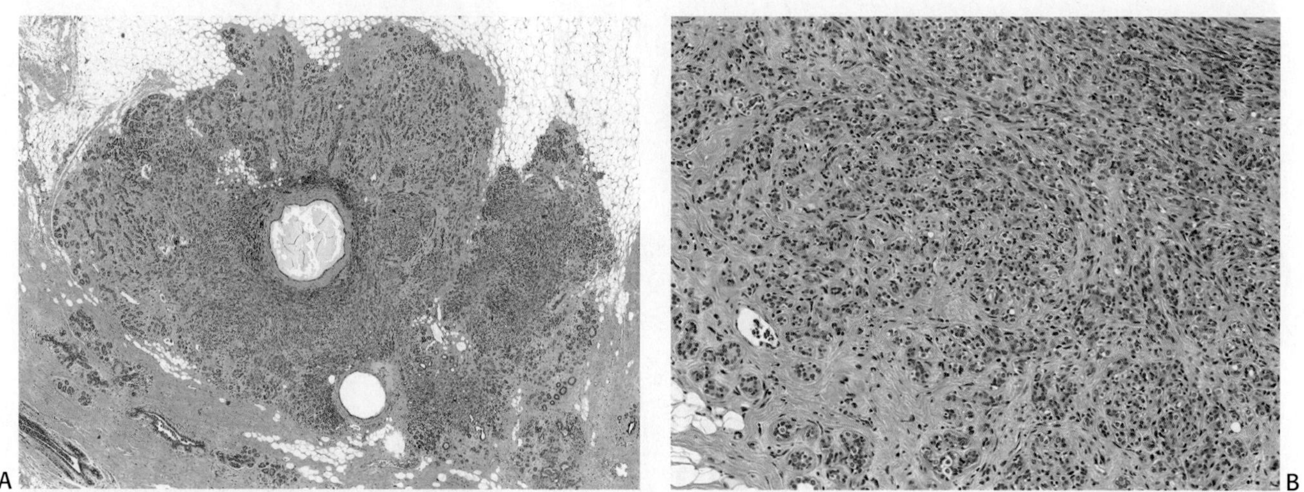

FIG. 7.3. ***Adenosis tumor.*** **A:** A whole-mount histologic section showing a well-circumscribed tumor with microcysts. **B:** Confluent sclerosing adenosis.

and pathologic findings. Seventeen of the 33 lesions were detected radiologically as masses. Ten of 17 (59%) foci were circumscribed on ultrasound and eight by mammography, five had indistinct margins, and two were partially circumscribed. Fifteen of the 33 lesions were detected mammographically as clustered calcifications not associated with a mass. The calcifications were amorphous or indistinct in nine (60%) cases, pleomorphic in four (27%), and punctate in two (13%). In the same study, sclerosing adenosis was a minor component in 44/88 (50%) lesions sampled by core biopsy. Mammographically, ductal carcinoma *in situ* (DCIS) in sclerosing adenosis was associated with pleomorphic calcifications and atypical ductal hyperplasia (ADH) with amorphous calcifications. Taskin et al.[8] evaluated the radiologic findings in 76 breast lesions that yielded a diagnosis of sclerosing adenosis, as either a major or a minor component. The lesions were detected mammographically as masses (25/69, 36%), microcalcifications (25/69, 30%), asymmetrical opacities (15/69, 22%), and architectural distortion (8/69, 12%). The remaining seven lesions were detected by ultrasound. Two lesions appeared as spiculated mammographic and sonographic masses. Sclerosing adenosis was the main finding in 17/37 lesions that underwent needle core biopsy. It constituted a minor component of the lesion in 20/37 (54%) cases in which fibroadenoma (eight cases), fibrocystic changes (seven cases), invasive carcinoma (two cases) and intraductal papilloma, ADH, and DCIS (one case each) were thought to account for the radiologic abnormality. Oztekin et al.[9] described a 37-year-old woman with sclerosing adenosis that presented as bilateral palpable and tender masses with indistinct margins. Multiple oval masses with angulated margins, oriented parallel to the skin, were seen by ultrasound. They had complex posterior acoustic shadowing and mild vascularity on color Doppler ultrasound. Magnetic resonance imaging showed multiple ovoid masses with indistinct borders, intermediate enhancement on T1-weighted and T2-weighted images, and a homogeneous signal.

Gross Pathology

Excised adenosis tumors vary in gross appearance depending upon their microscopic composition (Figs. 7.2 and 7.3). Lesions consisting of florid adenosis with a prominent glandular component are typically well-circumscribed nodules composed of gray or pale tan, firm homogeneous tissue. With increasing sclerosis, adenosis tumors are likely to be grossly less well defined at the borders, multinodular, and more fibrous in appearance. Lesions with abundant calcifications may seem gritty when cut. Gross cyst formation is infrequent. Necrosis and/or infarction are occasionally encountered in an adenosis tumor, usually during pregnancy or lactation.

Nontumorous adenosis in isolated lobules is difficult to detect grossly and it usually mingles with other proliferative lesions. Rarely, minute discrete foci of sclerosing adenosis may be palpated in unfixed breast tissue as fine granules by brushing a finger gently over the cut surface. With tangential light, these foci are sometimes visible as pale tan dots or a granular surface in white breast stroma (Fig. 7.4).

Microscopic Pathology

The structural histologic features described here may be encountered in individual microscopic foci of adenosis and in adenosis tumors. Adenosis tends to have a more prominent glandular pattern in premenopausal women, whereas sclerosis and diminished gland formation are more conspicuous after menopause. In some individual patients, there is very little variability in the spectrum of adenosis, whereas others exhibit diverse patterns.

Florid Adenosis

Florid adenosis is the most cellular type of adenosis. It is characterized by hyperplasia of epithelial and myoepithelial cells. Proliferation of ductules and lobular glands severely distorts and usually effaces the architecture of the underlying lobules. The hyperplastic structures appear to

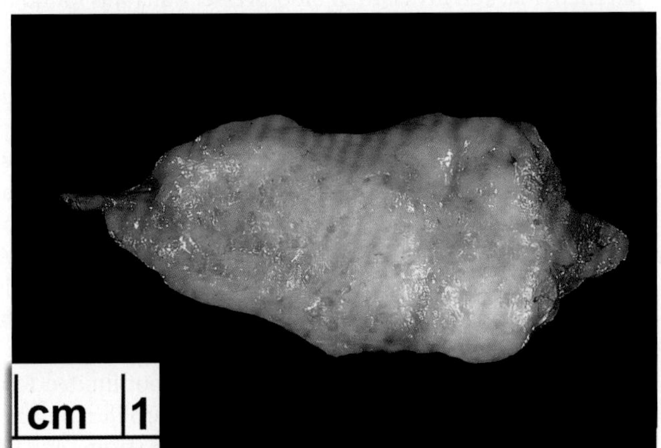

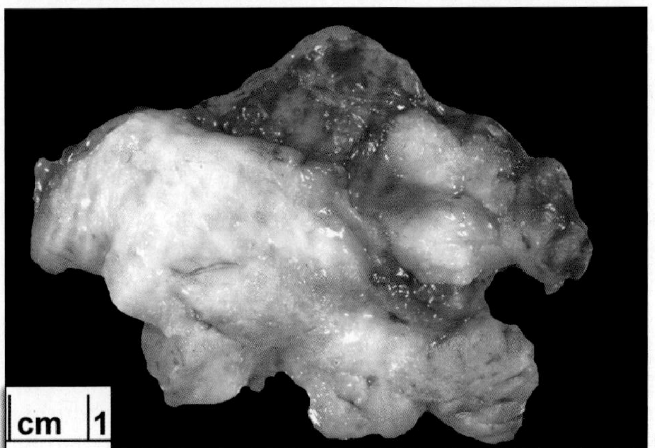

FIG. 7.4. ***Florid adenosis, gross specimen.*** **A:** Multiple tan nodules of florid adenosis on the cut surface of a breast biopsy. **B:** The grainy beige cut surface is an area of florid sclerosing adenosis.

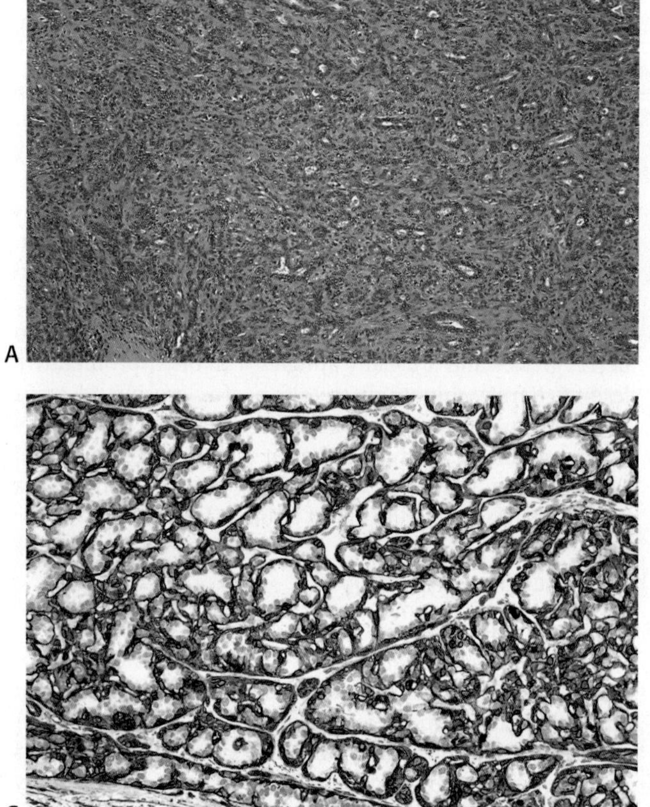

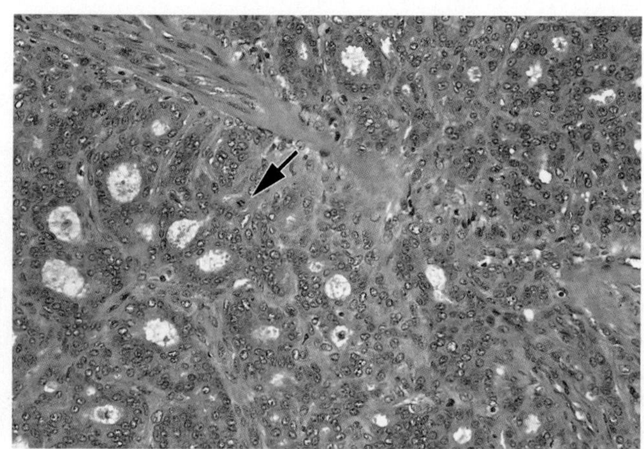

FIG. 7.5. ***Florid adenosis.*** **A:** Confluent growth of adenosis glands not forming distinct lobular structures. **B:** The glandular epithelial cells have vesicular nuclei and distinct nucleoli. Mitosis in a myoepithelial cell is shown (*arrow*). **C:** Myoepithelial cells are highlighted with the myosin immunostain.

be elongated, becoming tortuous and entwined, resulting in many more ductular cross sections than are present in an anatomically normal lobule (Fig. 7.5). In the plane of section, the complex proliferative structure has a swirling pattern, punctuated by glands cut transversely. Some glands may maintain round, open lumens, but the majority of the ductular structures are cut tangentially or longitudinally. They display elongated and often collapsed lumens, usually with smooth, non-angular contours. The caliber of the lumens is relatively constant regardless of the plane of section. Cystic dilation of ductules or glands is not prominent in florid adenosis.

Epithelial cells lining the tubules and glands are flattened, cuboidal, or slightly columnar and are arranged in one or two orderly layers surrounded by myoepithelial cells. Increase in cell size and nuclear pleomorphism can be found in florid adenosis, especially during pregnancy or lactation. Hyperplastic change in the epithelial component of florid adenosis is mirrored by myoepithelial hyperplasia (Figs. 7.2, 7.5, 7.6). Despite an increase of the epithelial elements, mitoses are very infrequent in both epithelial and myoepithelial cells. Mitoses are more numerous during pregnancy. Degeneration of individual cells, manifested by nuclear debris, nuclear pyknosis, and apoptosis, and rarely by geographic areas of necrosis, can be found in pregnancy-associated tumor-forming florid adenosis (Fig. 7.7). Glandular cells with intracytoplasmic mucin vacuoles or signet ring cell morphology are exceedingly rare in florid adenosis and apocrine metaplasia is uncommon. Eosinophilic secretion deposited in the lumens of adenosis glands is typically periodic acid–Schiff (PAS) and mucicarmine-positive. Luminal secretion may undergo calcification, but this phenomenon is less common and less extensive in florid adenosis than in sclerosing adenosis.

Florid adenosis may surround nerves in adjacent breast parenchyma, and invasion of blood vessel walls was found in 10% of the cases in one study.[11]

Sclerosing Adenosis

Sclerosing adenosis is the most common form of adenosis. This glandular proliferation is characterized by preferential preservation of myoepithelial cells and variable atrophy of epithelial cells, accompanied by lobular fibrosis (Fig. 7.8). A swirling lobulocentric pattern is present, but epithelial cells are less conspicuous and the ductular structures are largely attenuated (Figs. 7.8 and 7.9).

In some instances, sclerosing adenosis is not limited to a lobulocentric pattern. When this occurs, the proliferating benign glands display an infiltrative pattern in the stroma and fat that can be mistaken for invasive carcinoma (Fig. 7.10). Sclerosing adenosis with an invasive growth pattern may be particularly difficult to distinguish from infiltrating carcinoma in needle core biopsy samples that often lack the orientation

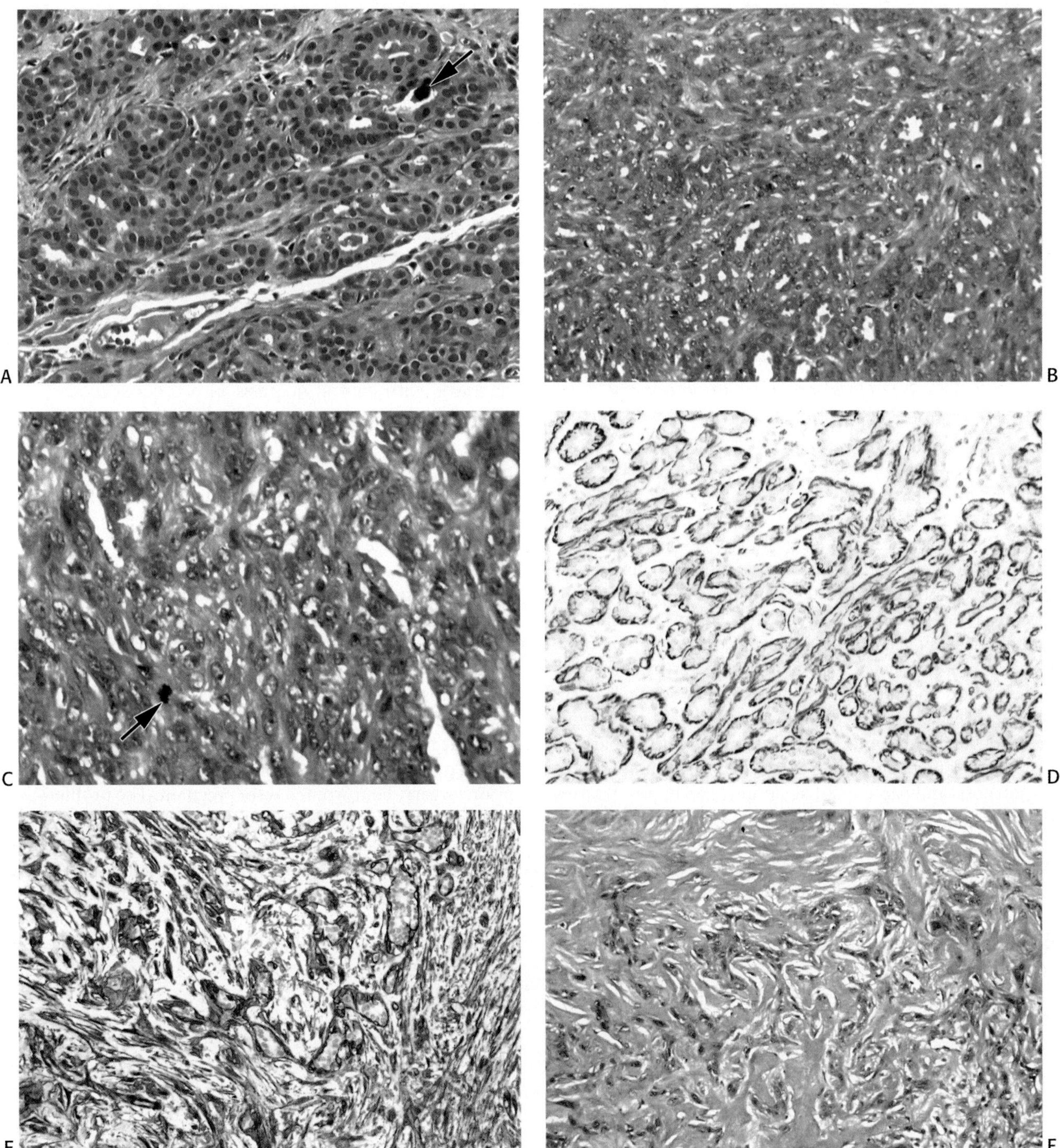

FIG. 7.6. ***Florid adenosis.*** **A:** Adenosis with a prominent glandular pattern and a microcalcification (*arrow*). **B:** Glandular structures are partially effaced by florid epithelial and myoepithelial hyperplasia. **C:** A mitosis in a myoepithelial cell (*arrow*). **D:** Myoepithelial cells are stained for actin (anti-SMA). **E:** Myoepithelial hyperplasia is demonstrated with the SMA immunostain. **F:** A sclerotic area that resembles invasive carcinoma in the tumor shown in **(E)**.

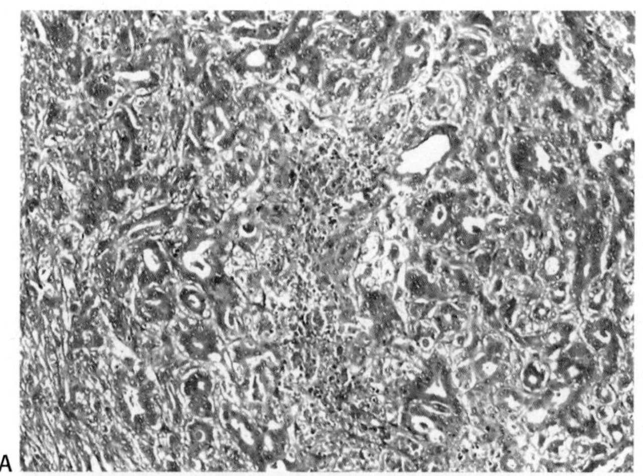

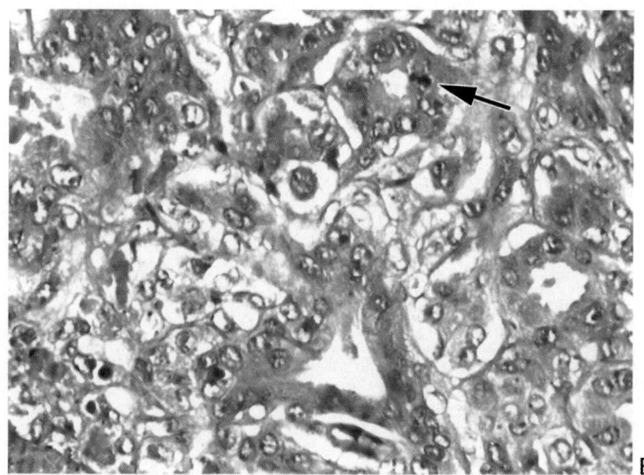

FIG. 7.7. ***Florid adenosis in pregnancy.*** **A:** Florid adenosis with central necrosis in a pregnant woman. **B:** A mitotic figure (*arrow*) and nuclear atypia are present.

provided by adjacent uninvolved breast parenchyma. Epithelial cells may be markedly reduced in number, or even absent, leaving compressed elongated strands of myoepithelial cells (Fig. 7.11). With increasing sclerosis, ductular lumens are progressively obliterated to the point that they may not be recognizable (Fig. 7.12). In contrast, the basement membrane around sclerosing adenosis is usually thickened and often forms a well-delineated eosinophilic layer around the distorted glands and tubules. The persisting myoepithelial cells often display a pronounced spindle shape (myoid phenotype) and are strongly immunoreactive with myoepithelial markers.

Cystically dilated ductules are variably present in sclerosing adenosis and papilloma-like nodular foci of proliferating ductules may protrude into such cystic spaces. This configuration has been referred to as a "glomeruloid structure."[7] Foci of epithelial expansion and/or widely open glands that occur within sclerosing adenosis should be examined closely to rule out epithelial atypia or carcinoma. Calcifications become progressively more numerous with increasing sclerosis, and they are usually small and scattered throughout the lesion. Extremely unusual variants of sclerosing adenosis can show clear cell change (Fig. 7.13) and collagenous spherulosis (Fig. 7.14).

Sclerosing adenosis sometimes infiltrates nerves. The first systematic study of perineural invasion in sclerosing adenosis was reported by Taylor and Norris.[12] Perineural invasion was found in 20 of 1,000 (2%) biopsies with sclerosing adenosis. The median age of the 20 patients with neural involvement was 32 years, and it did not differ significantly from the median age of women with sclerosing adenosis that lacked perineural invasion. Only two of the women had had prior surgery. Four women were pregnant. The proliferative lesions most frequently associated with perineural invasion were sclerosing adenosis and papillomatosis. Histologically benign structures were found around nerves involving the perineurium (Fig. 7.15), and rarely within nerve fibers. After a median follow-up of 7 years, no patient with perineural invasion manifested clinical evidence of carcinoma. The

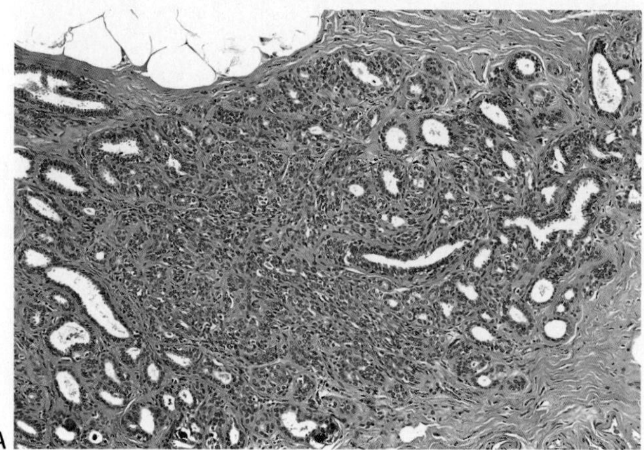

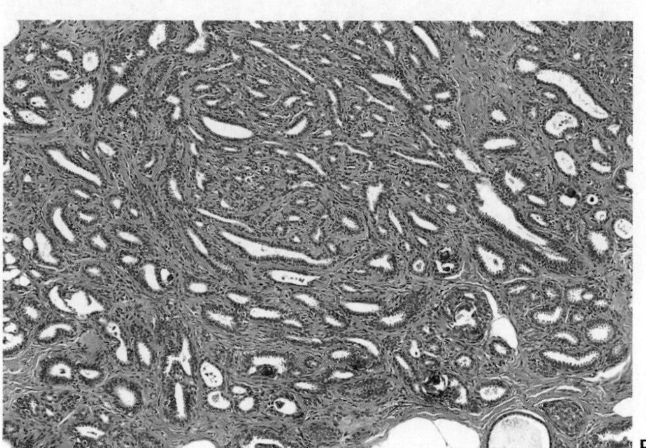

FIG. 7.8. ***Sclerosing adenosis.*** **A:** Swirling pattern with a lobulocentric distribution composed of dilated glands and spindly myoepithelial cells. **B:** Microcalcifications and a tubular growth pattern.

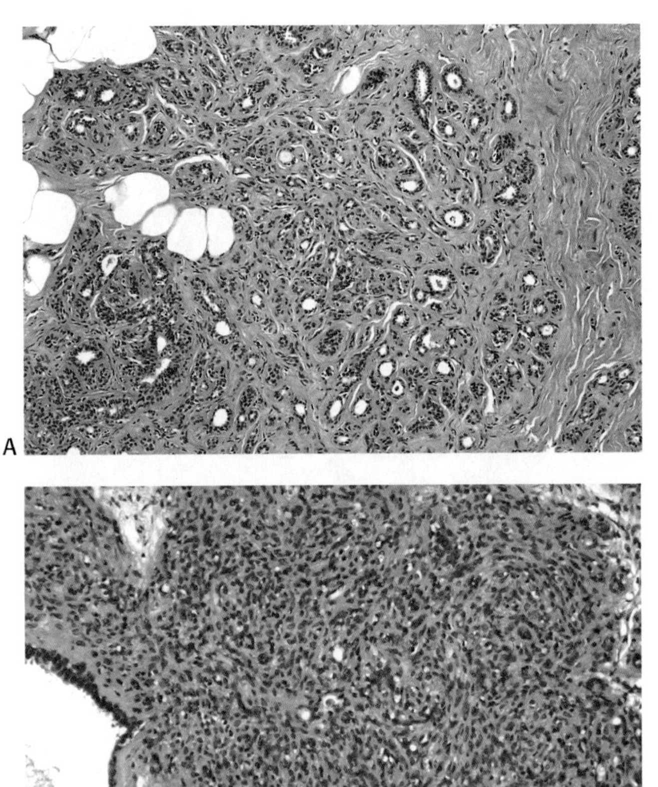

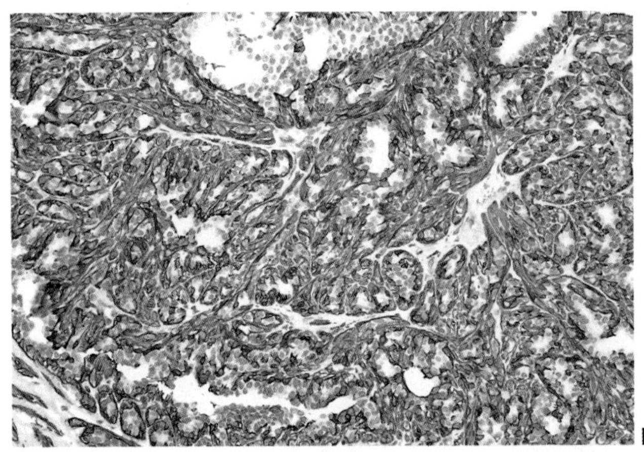

FIG. 7.9. ***Sclerosing adenosis.*** **A:** Well-developed lobular sclerosis, which tends to merge with fat in a postmenopausal woman. **B:** Myoepithelial cell overgrowth is highlighted with the myosin immunostain. **C:** Sclerosing adenosis next to a large duct.

authors found no evidence that the glandular epithelium was in lymphatic or other vascular spaces.

Davies[13] found neural invasion in 4 of 316 (1.3%) cases of mammary "dysplasia." Overall, sclerosing adenosis was present in 25% of the specimens. In three of the four cases, neural invasion had concurrent sclerosing adenosis, and the fourth patient had sclerosing adenosis in a prior biopsy. Nerves were found in 53.5% of biopsies, but not more frequently when there was sclerosing adenosis. Neural invasion was not attributable to prior surgery because only one of the four patients had been operated previously. Sclerosing adenosis penetrated into and focally through the perineurium of affected nerves. Myoepithelial cells were evident in most, but not all, foci of perineural invasion. The glandular elements appeared histologically benign, lacking cytologic atypia or mitotic activity. The patients remained disease free 8 to 38 months after biopsy. Perivascular invasion that simulated the perineural pattern was found in two specimens that did not exhibit perineural invasion.

Apocrine Adenosis

Apocrine metaplasia is relatively common in adenosis, especially in sclerosing adenosis. The resulting configuration, known as apocrine adenosis[7,14] (Fig. 7.16), is often appreciated on low-power examination due to the presence of epithelial cells with more abundant cytoplasm. The cytologic appearance of apocrine adenosis is variable.[15] In some cases, the cells have conventional, pink, finely granular apocrine cytoplasm and regular round nuclei, but often the cytoplasm is gray or slightly amphophilic. When compared with ordinary apocrine metaplasia, atypical features include cytoplasmic clearing or vacuolization, as much as threefold nuclear enlargement, irregular nuclear membrane, and nuclear pleomorphism (Figs. 7.17 and 7.18). Mitotic figures are uncommon in atypical apocrine adenosis, and they are more likely to be present when apocrine carcinoma arises in adenosis. Nuclear hyperchromasia and prominent nucleoli are found in the most extreme examples of apocrine atypia in adenosis.

Florid proliferation of atypical apocrine elements in sclerosing adenosis produces lesions that may be difficult to distinguish from apocrine DCIS.[15,16] Extreme cytologic atypia with readily identifiable mitotic activity and/or a proliferative pattern characteristic of intraductal carcinoma are required to render a diagnosis of apocrine carcinoma *in situ* in this setting. Expression of c-erbB2 (55.6%), p53 (27.8%), Bax (33.3%), and c-myc (100%) has been documented in apocrine adenosis with and without atypia.[17] In the same study, none of the 18 samples tested for bcl-2 showed positive reactivity. Celis et al.[18] assessed immunoreactivity for MRP14/S-100A9, psoriasin/S-100A7, and p53, three

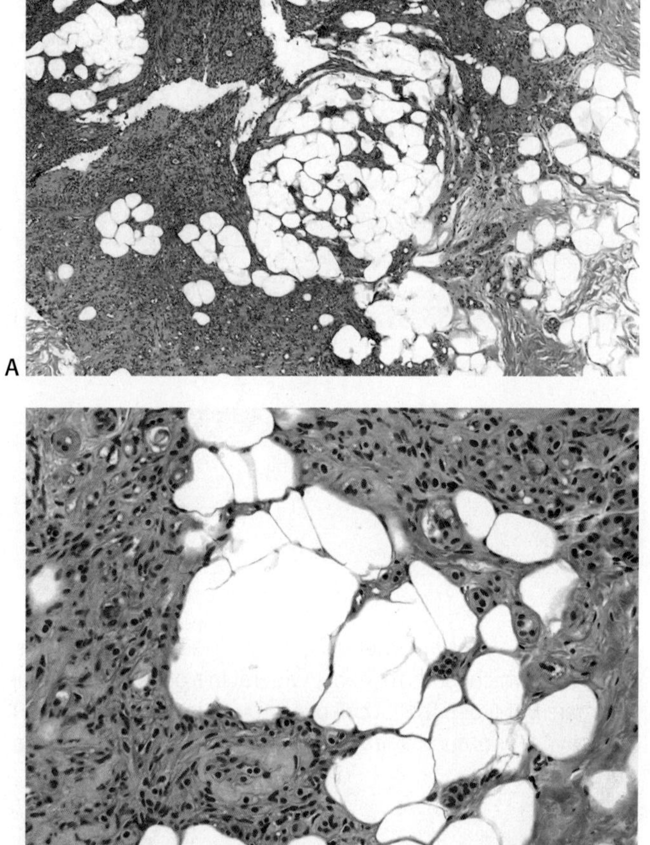

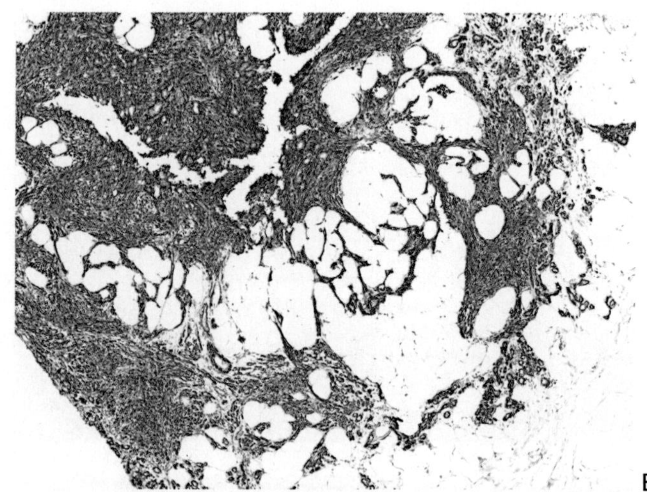

FIG. 7.10. ***Sclerosing adenosis involving fat.*** **A:** Low-power view of sclerosing adenosis extending into fat. Blue dye ink is placed on the surface of the specimen to identify the margin. **B:** A calponin stain highlights the myoepithelial cells in sclerosing adenosis. **C:** Sclerosing adenosis that resembles invasive carcinoma in fat. The cell groups appear to be "packaged" by the stroma. Basement membrane is evident, and myoepithelial cells could be highlighted with an anti-actin stain to rule out stromal invasion.

markers found in invasive apocrine carcinoma, in the apocrine cells present in sclerosing adenosis from 24 patients, 7 of whom also had ipsilateral invasive carcinoma (6 ductal, 1 lobular), and 2 DCIS. In this study, the authors identified apocrine cells based on positivity for 15-prostaglandin dehydrogenase, a protein found in benign and malignant apocrine cells.[19] The apocrine cells with and without atypia present in sclerosing adenosis showed variable positivity for some or all of the markers. Although these results suggest that apocrine adenosis may be a non-obligate precursor of apocrine carcinoma, it has not been determined that oncoprotein expression in apocrine adenosis is associated with a predisposition to develop carcinoma independently of the presence of histologic atypia. Another study[20] found that the median proliferation rate, as assessed by Ki67 staining, was significantly higher in apocrine adenosis compared with normal mammary epithelium (4.5% vs. 1.1%; $p < 0.001$). The same investigators[21] also found apoptosis to be uncommon in apocrine metaplasia and in apocrine adenosis and detected no significant difference between the Ki67 indices of apocrine adenosis with or without atypia (6.6% and 5.2%, respectively).

Tubular Adenosis

Tubular adenosis is characterized by the formation of ductules arranged so that most are cut longitudinally in the plane of the histologic section (Fig. 7.19). The proliferation lacks the lobulocentric distribution of florid or sclerosing adenosis, since the ductules extend in a seemingly haphazard pattern into fibrous mammary stroma and fat, intersecting at different angles. In some instances, there is a dense proliferation of tubular structures that appear to be entwined. Bifurcating tubules and mild cystic dilation of ductules are sometimes observed. Secretion that may calcify is variably present in the ductules. All of the tubular structures have basement membranes and an outer myoepithelial cell layer.[22] These features are important in the distinction between tubular carcinoma and tubular adenosis.

Blunt Duct Adenosis

Blunt duct adenosis (BDA) is a form of terminal duct hyperplasia characterized by abortive lobule formation.[2] The proliferating epithelium forms aggregates of solid or microcystic lobule-like nodules that appear to be the ends of the

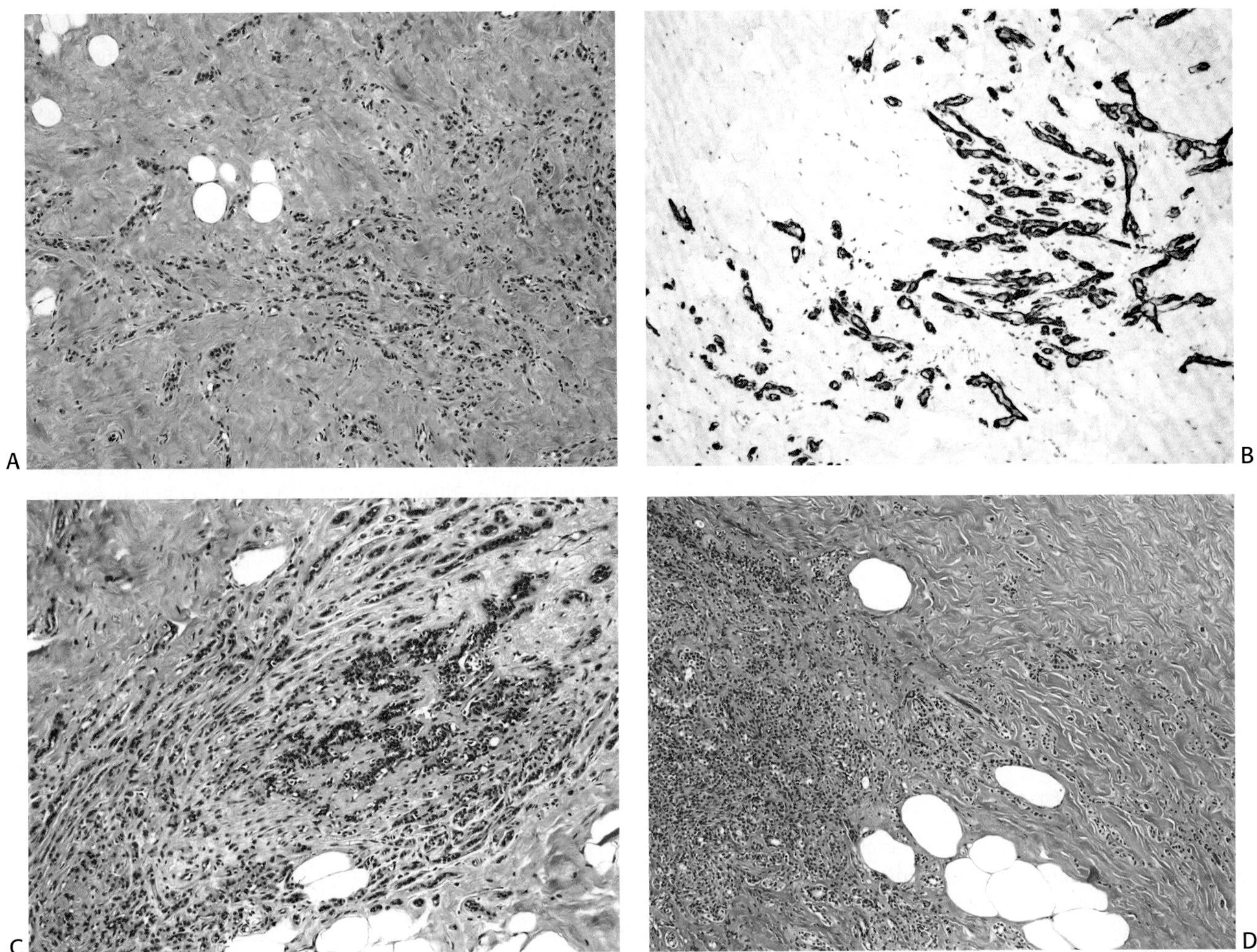

FIG. 7.11. ***Sclerosing adenosis, marked atrophy.*** **A:** Note the linear distribution of myoepithelial cells, which simulates infiltrating lobular carcinoma. **B:** The myoepithelial cells are highlighted with a calponin stain. **C:** Atrophic sclerosing adenosis almost completely surrounds a duct in a pattern that closely mimics invasive lobular carcinoma. Myoepithelial cells were demonstrated by immunohistochemistry. **D:** Atrophic sclerosing adenosis (*left*) adjacent to invasive lobular carcinoma (*right*). The atrophic glands of sclerosing adenosis are arranged in a tight swirling pattern, whereas the invasive lobular carcinoma has more linear distribution. Myoepithelial cells were demonstrated in the sclerosing adenosis but not in the invasive lobular carcinoma.

ductules (Fig. 7.20). The glands are typically round, but they may become irregular when cystic.

Myoepithelial cells in cystic BDA are usually conspicuous and often have abundant clear cytoplasm (Fig. 7.20B, C). Occasionally, the solid type of BDA may be mistakenly diagnosed as atypical lobular hyperplasia (ALH) or lobular carcinoma *in situ* (LCIS). The uniform circumferential distribution around the ductular/acinar structures and the cohesive nature of the proliferation are usually sufficient to identify the cells as predominantly myoepithelial. Immunostains for p63 and E-cadherin will help to resolve any diagnostic uncertainty.

Small lumens are present in some of these lobule-like structures, and they are occasionally cystically dilated (Fig. 7.20B, C). The stroma around the glands of BDA is slightly more expanded, fibrotic, and cellular than usual intralobular stroma and contains few scattered inflammatory cells. BDA sometimes exhibits apocrine metaplasia.

Adenosis in Fibroadenomas

Adenosis in fibroadenomas is usually readily distinguished from carcinoma. Fibroadenomas are likely to develop adenosis, since both lesions arise from the TDLU. Most forms of adenosis occur in fibroadenomas, sometimes accompanied by other proliferative changes such as cystic and papillary apocrine metaplasia. Adenosis may be localized to one part of a fibroadenoma or it may be diffuse, obscuring the underlying fibroepithelial structure. A needle core biopsy of adenosis in a fibroadenoma can simulate the

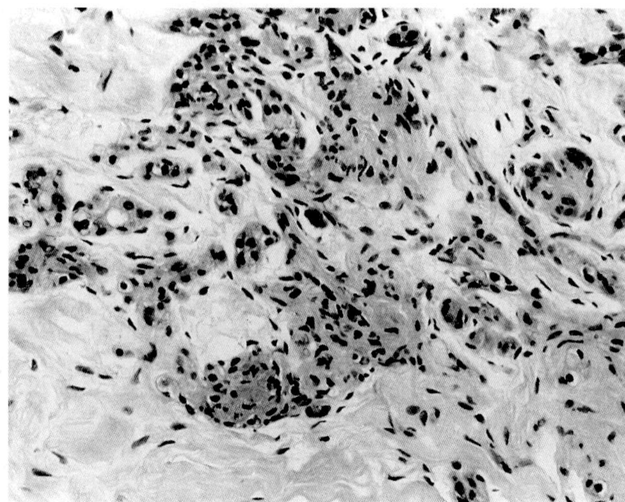

FIG. 7.12. ***Sclerosing adenosis.*** Glandular atrophy with preservation of myoepithelial cells.

appearance of invasive carcinoma (Fig. 7.21). A fibroadenoma with sclerosing adenosis or other components of fibrocystic change is termed a "complex fibroadenoma" (see also Chapter 8).

Differential Diagnosis

The major consideration in the differential diagnosis of adenosis and its variant forms is the distinction between these lesions and invasive carcinoma, especially tubular carcinoma. A discussion of features distinguishing tubular carcinoma from adenosis can be found in Chapter 13, which is devoted to tubular carcinoma. Tubular adenosis infiltrating fat can be especially challenging, as it mimics the infiltrative pattern of a well-differentiated carcinoma. Basement membrane and myoepithelium are usually visible around the pseudoinfiltrating glands in hematoxylin and eosin (H&E)-stained slides. Immunoperoxidase stains for myoepithelial markers can be used in problematic cases.

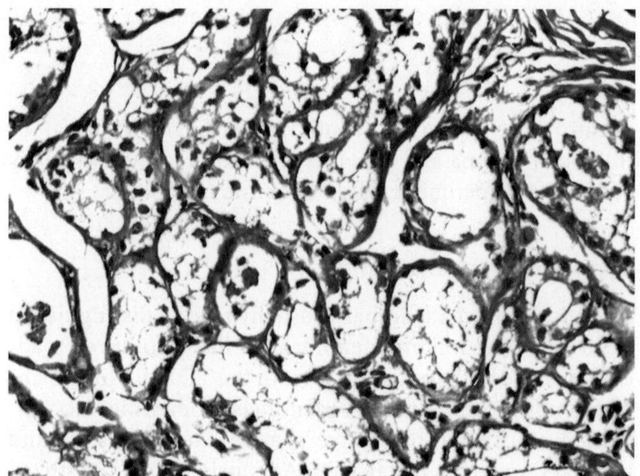

FIG. 7.13. ***Clear cell apocrine metaplasia in sclerosing adenosis.*** The enlarged glands contain voluminous cells with clear cytoplasm. Dark structures in the glands are calcifications.

Carcinoma in Adenosis

Atypical hyperplasia and carcinoma *in situ* can arise in adenosis, or adenosis can be secondarily involved by carcinoma established in the surrounding tissue. Nielsen[7] reported finding CIS in adenosis tumors, as well as in other forms of adenosis. LCIS and DCIS can occur in sclerosing adenosis and in tubular adenosis.

LCIS in Adenosis

The majority of CIS that develops in adenosis is of the lobular type (Figs. 7.19E and 7.22).[23] LCIS usually causes expansion of the epithelial component in adenosis, but in some foci of sclerosing adenosis, the neoplastic process is manifested by pagetoid growth of sparsely distributed discohesive cells.[24] LCIS in adenosis can have signet ring cells that may be highlighted by a mucicarmine stain. The latter stain can be performed to confirm that cytoplasmic mucin is present when cytoplasmic vacuoles are seen in H&E-stained sections. Signet ring cells and stainable intracytoplasmic mucin are not features of benign epithelium in adenosis. Pagetoid LCIS can also be identified in sclerosing adenosis with the E-cadherin stain because the neoplastic cells are not reactive for this marker. In such cases, it is not unusual to also find LCIS in surrounding lobules uninvolved by sclerosing adenosis.

DCIS in Adenosis

DCIS in adenosis is less common than LCIS. In this setting, DCIS can be identified most readily when there is comedo necrosis, if the proliferation has solid, cribriform or papillary architecture, and when there is substantial cytologic atypia in an expanded epithelial component (Figs. 7.23 and 7.24).[7,23] The distinction between atypical apocrine metaplasia and apocrine DCIS in adenosis can be extremely difficult.[15,16,25] Despite considerable cytologic atypia, apocrine metaplasia in adenosis should not be interpreted as carcinoma until there is sufficient epithelial proliferation to form one of the conventional structural patterns of DCIS and/or there is extreme cytologic atypia and/or readily identified mitotic activity. Cytoplasmic clearing or vacuolization occurs in atypical sclerosing apocrine lesions as well as in apocrine carcinoma (see Chapter 19).

Moritani et al.[26] detailed the relationship between sclerosing adenosis and DCIS in 13 cases containing both lesions and observed two distinct patterns. In pattern A, CIS was confined to sclerosing adenosis and did not extend beyond it, whereas in pattern B, CIS involved sclerosing adenosis and the adjacent breast parenchyma. Sclerosing adenosis was significantly larger in pattern A than in pattern B. The authors observed that CIS confined to sclerosing adenosis

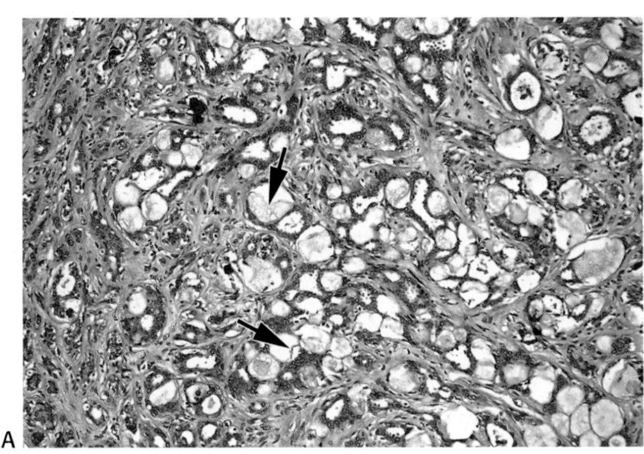

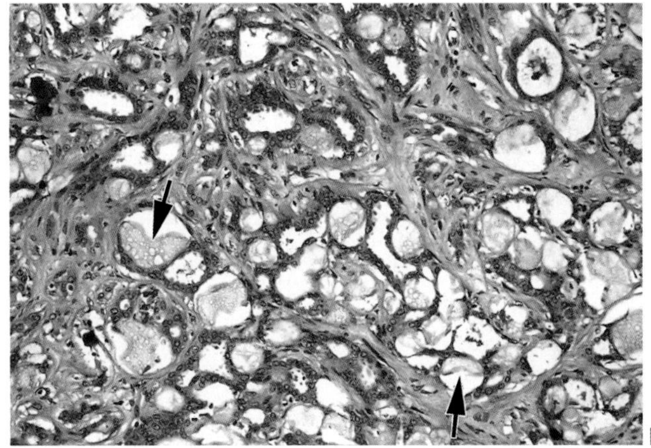

FIG. 7.14. ***Collagenous spherulosis in sclerosing adenosis.*** **A,B:** Degenerative changes are present in the spherules. Detached basement membranes are present in some glandular lumens (*arrows*).

arose within it and was predominantly low grade, whereas CIS in the type B pattern was more heterogeneous, with a tendency to be high grade. In some cases, CIS appeared to arise in adenosis and spread beyond it, but in other instances, the appearance suggested that adenosis was secondarily involved by CIS that originated in the surrounding breast parenchyma.

Adenosis and Stromal Invasion

When LCIS and DCIS involve adenosis, the underlying architecture of adenosis is preserved. The integrity of individual glands in these complex proliferative lesions is sometimes difficult to ascertain based on examination of H&E-stained slides alone, and immunohistochemical studies for basement membranes and myoepithelial cells may be required.[22,27] The p63 immunostain that highlights myoepithelial cell nuclei is preferable in this situation because it avoids cross-reactivity with stromal cells, but this stain should be coupled with staining for a cytoplasmic myoepithelial marker, such as smooth muscle actin (SMA) or calponin (Fig. 7.23). Hilson et al.[28] studied sclerosing lesions with a panel of myoepithelial markers. In cases of sclerosing adenosis, they found no reactivity for calponin in 1/22 (4.5%) lesions, for myosin in 3/21 (14.3%), and for CK5/6 in 4/20 (20%). Reactivity for SMA, CD10, p63, and p75 was documented in all cases tested for these markers. Reticulin or PAS stains can be used to highlight the basement membranes around adenosis glands, but in some cases they can be difficult to interpret. Immunoperoxidase stains for myoepithelial markers are likely to provide more reliable and reproducible results.

Even when the basement membrane and myoepithelial layers appear to be discontinuous, it can be very difficult to confidently diagnose invasion within foci of adenosis. The most convincing evidence for a diagnosis of invasive carcinoma arising in adenosis is the presence of invasive foci extending beyond the adenosis lesion. The invasive carcinoma should have cytologic features duplicating those of the CIS in the adenosis. A focal inflammatory cell infiltrate and reactive stromal changes separating the

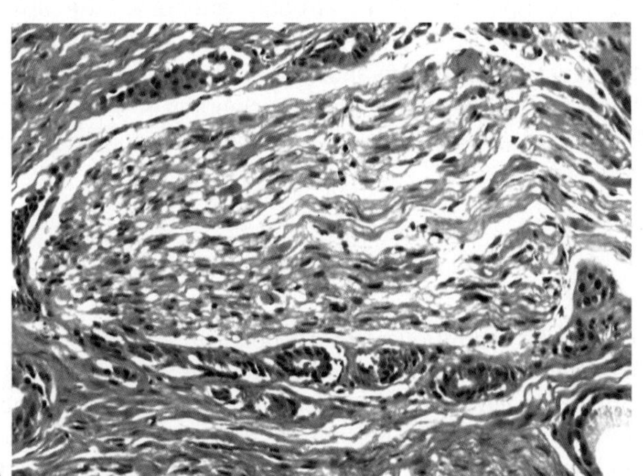

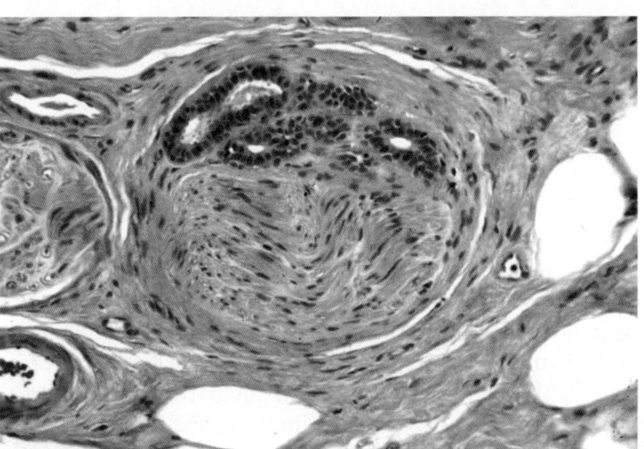

FIG. 7.15. ***Neural invasion.*** **A:** Adenosis glands are wrapped around a nerve. **B:** Adenosis glands are present around this nerve.

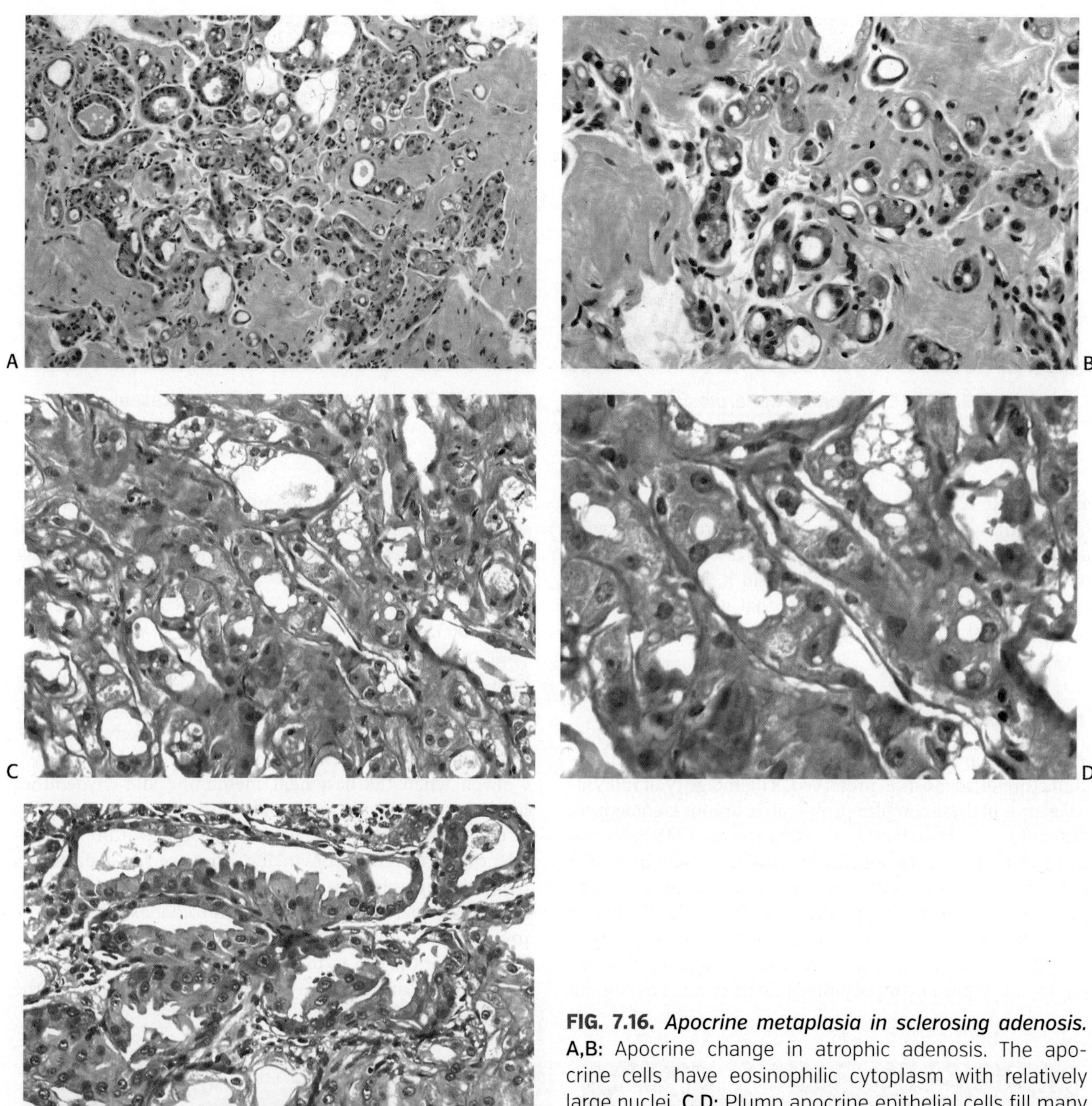

FIG. 7.16. ***Apocrine metaplasia in sclerosing adenosis.*** **A,B:** Apocrine change in atrophic adenosis. The apocrine cells have eosinophilic cytoplasm with relatively large nuclei. **C,D:** Plump apocrine epithelial cells fill many of the glands. Note cytoplasmic clearing in some cells. **E:** Florid apocrine hyperplasia in adenosis (florid apocrine adenosis).

glands often accompany stromal invasion. The glands or cells interpreted as invasive carcinoma should not be accompanied by myoepithelial cells, and basement membrane is largely or completely absent. Finally, the invasive elements should have a distribution and pattern that differ from those of adenosis. Double immunolabeling for cytokeratin and actin can detect isolated invasive carcinoma cells in areas of sclerosing adenosis that are involved by carcinoma.[29]

Cytology

Fine-needle aspiration of an adenosis tumor yields a cellular specimen composed of clusters of epithelial cells; spindly, bipolar, "naked" nuclei of myoepithelial cells; and stromal fragments.[30] The findings resemble the cytologic specimen that may be obtained from a fibroadenoma, but usually lack large, flat sheets of epithelial cells. Immunohistochemical examination of the cytologic specimen reveals

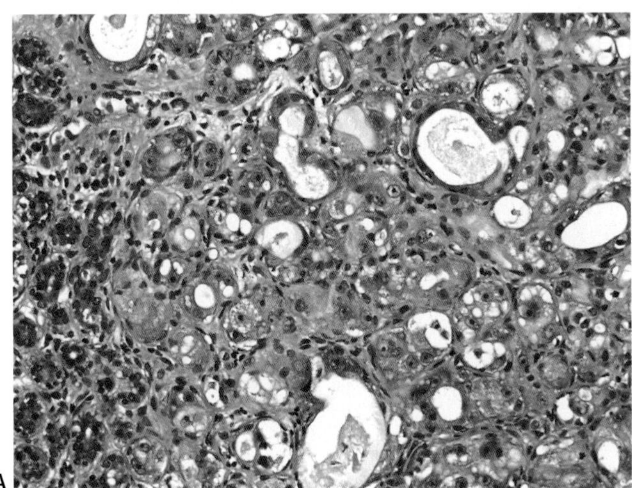

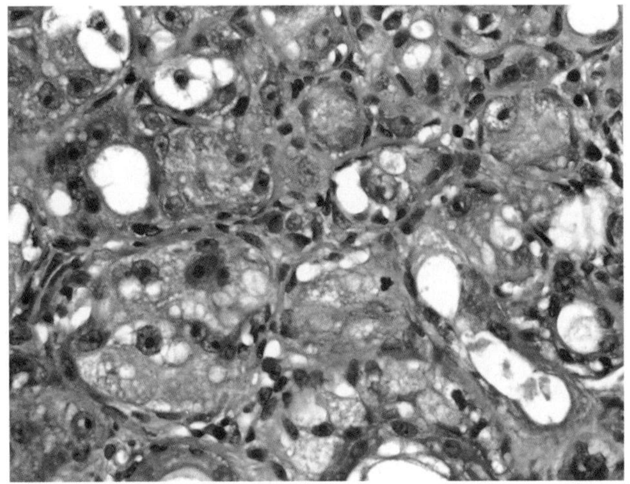

FIG. 7.17. ***Atypical apocrine metaplasia in sclerosing adenosis.*** **A:** The lobular glands are expanded by atypical apocrine cells. Even if the involved acini are enlarged compared with normal [*left*], the number of cells is not increased and no mitosis or necrosis is present. **B:** The atypical apocrine cells show marked nuclear enlargement, prominent nucleoli, and vacuolated cytoplasm.

reactivity for actin, p63, and other myoepithelial markers in bipolar cells.

Electron Microscopy

The ultrastructural features of adenosis tumor are similar to those of sclerosing adenosis.[30,31] Glandular epithelial cells surrounded by myoepithelial cells are supported by a basement membrane that may be thickened by reduplication.[32]

Genetic and Molecular Studies

Information about the genetic features of adenosis is nearly nonexistent. Da Silva et al.[33] studied a case purported to be coexisting tubular adenosis and adenoid cystic carcinoma using comparative genomic hybridization (CGH) and found no evidence of a genomic relationship between the two lesions. However, the so-called tubular adenosis had a complex pattern of genomic alterations that exceeded those of the component described as adenoid cystic carcinoma.

Treatment and Prognosis

Surgical Excision

Excisional biopsy is adequate treatment for adenosis tumor. When adenosis occurs as part of fibrocystic change, microscopic foci may extend beyond the region of palpable clinical involvement. Further excision is not recommended in such cases. If adenosis is diagnosed in a needle core biopsy specimen, surgical excision of the lesional area is recommended

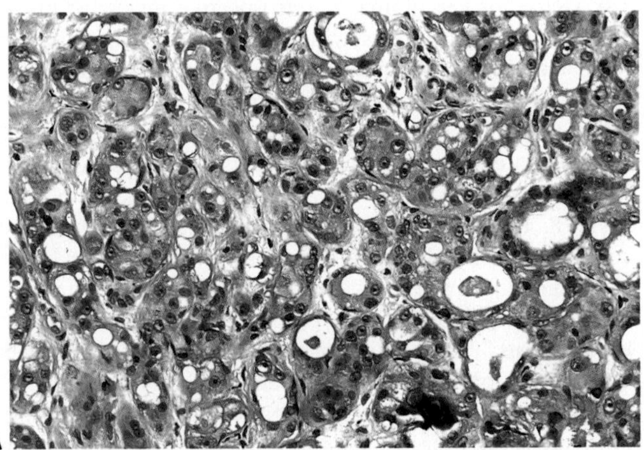

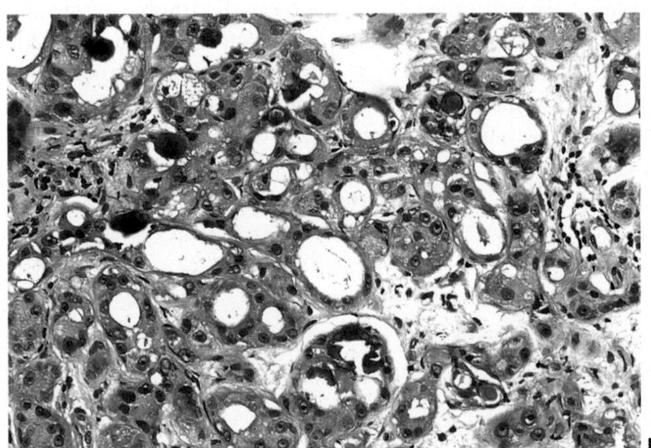

FIG. 7.18. ***Atypical apocrine metaplasia in sclerosing adenosis.*** **A,B:** Numerous calcifications are present. Note the nuclear pleomorphism.

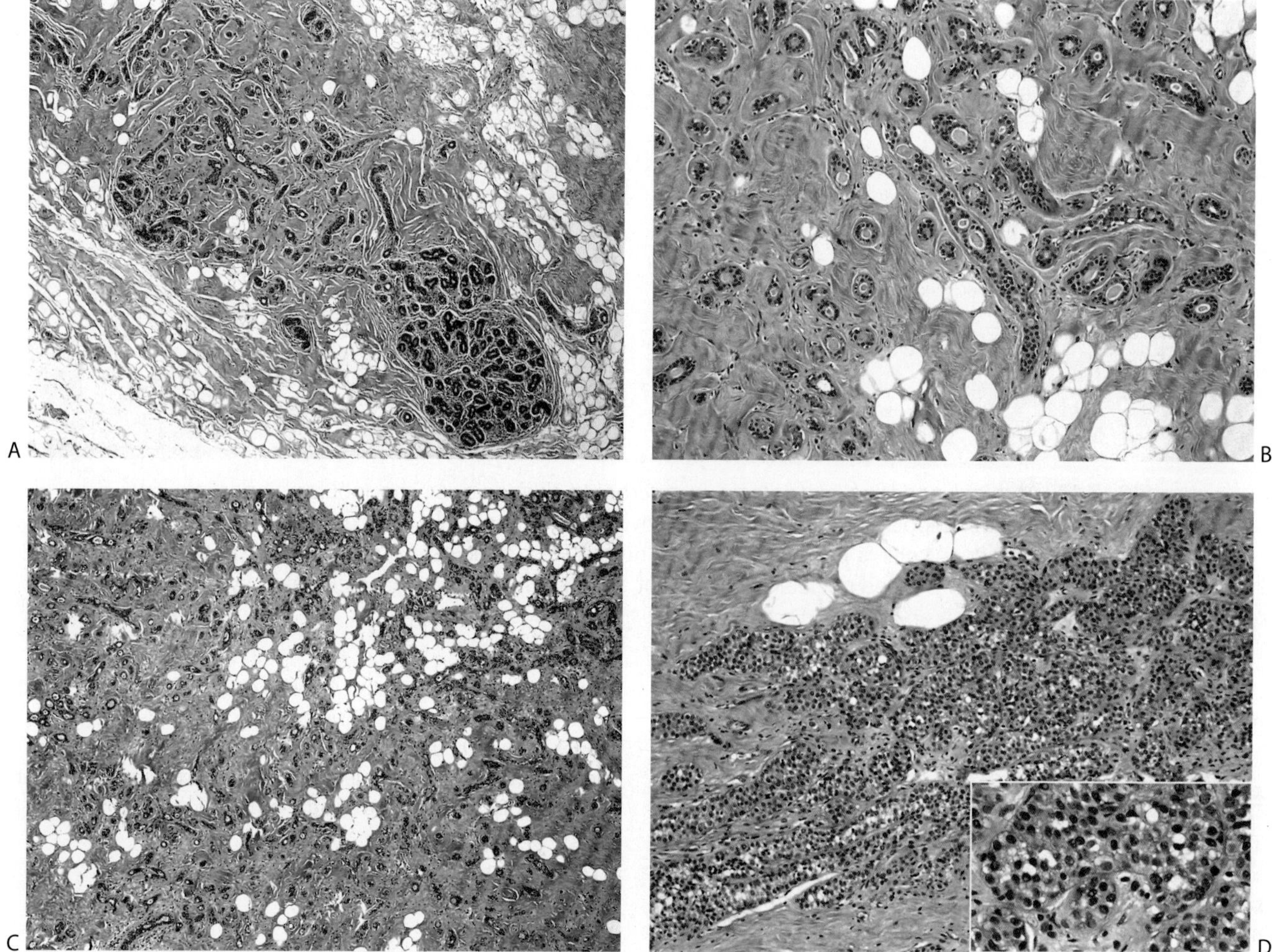

FIG. 7.19. ***Tubular adenosis.*** **A:** A small focus of tubular adenosis (*top*) adjacent to a normal lobule (*bottom*). **B:** A tubular structure cut in the long axis is surrounded by many transversely cut tubules. Note the prominent basement membranes around the tubules. **C:** An example of extensive tubular adenosis with stromal sclerosis. **D:** LCIS in tubular adenosis. LCIS consists of monomorphic cells. A few cells have intracytoplasmic vacuoles indenting the nucleus (*inset*).

to rule out carcinoma if the lesion has radiographically suspicious calcifications, a spiculated contour, and an associated radial sclerosing complex, or if there is florid or atypical epithelial hyperplasia.[10] In the absence of the foregoing features, clinical follow-up may be suggested when the core biopsy of a circumscribed tumor or "non-palpable indistinctly marginated masses" yields sclerosing adenosis.[10] The treatment of carcinoma arising in adenosis depends on the stage and extent of the lesion. In many of these cases, carcinoma is also present in breast tissue outside the area of adenosis.[23,24,26]

Risk of Subsequent Carcinoma

Foote and Stewart[2] studied the frequency of various fibrocystic changes in patients with and without breast carcinoma. They reported that adenosis, especially sclerosing adenosis, was not found more often in breasts with carcinoma, and they concluded that adenosis was not a precursor lesion or risk factor for carcinoma. A retrospective review of breast specimens from patients with and without carcinoma by Kern and Brooks.[34] revealed that sclerosing adenosis was more frequently present in patients who did not have carcinoma. Page et al.[35] did not detect a significantly increased risk associated with sclerosing adenosis in a retrospective follow-up study of women with fibrocystic changes published in 1978. However, subsequent investigations by Page and colleagues[36,37] identified an increased relative risk for breast carcinoma in women with sclerosing adenosis. Jensen et al.[37] found an overall relative risk of 2.1 in women with "sclerosing adenosis." The relative risk decreased to 1.7 in women without concomitant atypical hyperplasia and was not significantly changed by the presence or absence of a family history of breast carcinoma. When sclerosing adenosis was accompanied by atypical hyperplasia, often of the lobular type, the relative risk was 6.7. Others have also reported an increased risk of subsequent carcinoma after a diagnosis of sclerosing

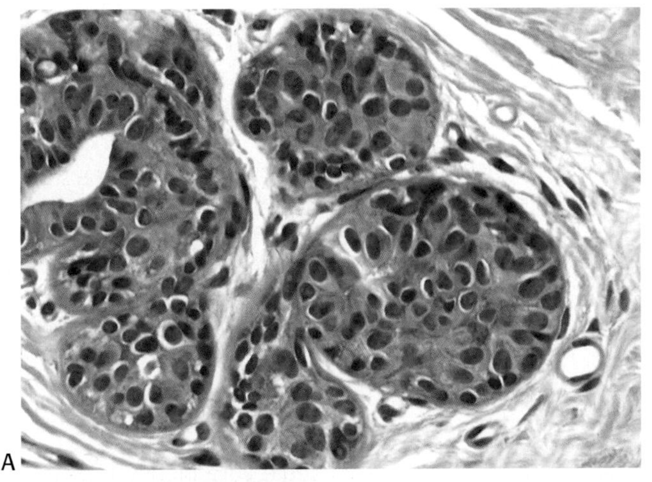

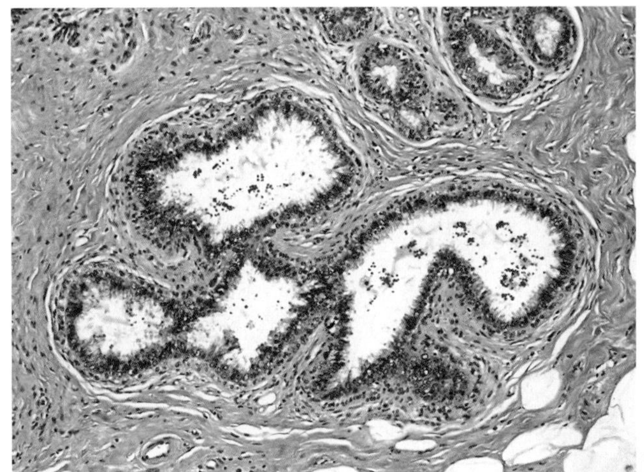

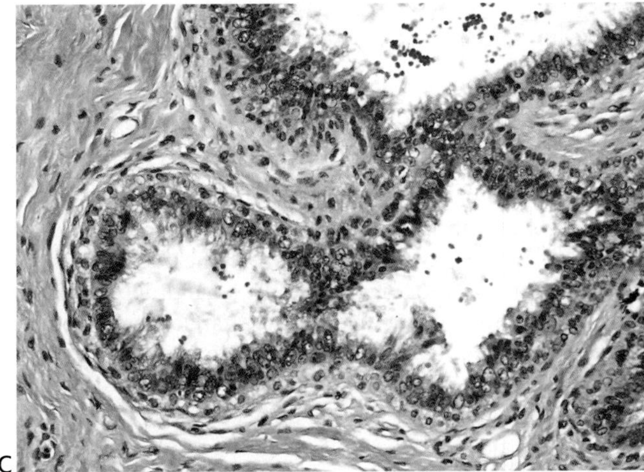

FIG. 7.20. ***Blunt duct adenosis.*** **A:** The glands of solid BDA are filled by a proliferation of cells with variously shaped nuclei. **B,C:** Cystic BDA with columnar epithelial cells and prominent myoepithelial cells.

adenosis.[38–42] Krieger and Hiatt.[42] reported that the overall relative risk compared with control populations for women with adenosis was 2.5. Bodian et al.[38] reported a relative risk of 2.2 for "adenosis" in women without other proliferative changes and no family history of breast carcinoma. Neither of the latter two studies defined "adenosis" or indicated that the data referred to sclerosing adenosis in contrast to florid adenosis. Overall, the risk associated with sclerosing adenosis alone, without atypia, is so small for an individual patient that no intervention is required beyond clinical surveillance.

The precancerous significance of atypical apocrine metaplasia in sclerosing adenosis has been assessed in three studies. Carter and Rosen[15] evaluated 51 patients with sclerosing proliferative lesions that included adenosis with apocrine atypia. After a mean follow-up of 35 months, no subsequent carcinomas were detected. Seidman et al.[16] described 37 patients with a mean follow-up of 8.7 years and reported that 4 (10.8%) patients subsequently developed invasive ductal carcinoma (3 ipsilateral and 1 contralateral). The histologic appearance of the carcinomas (apocrine vs. nonapocrine) was not stated. The relative risk of developing carcinoma was 5.5 (95% confidence interval [CI], 1.9 to 16) compared with age-specific incidence rates. All patients who developed carcinoma were older than 60 years of age when adenosis with apocrine atypia was diagnosed, and the 11 patients in this age group had a relative risk of carcinoma of 14 (95% CI, 4.1 to 48). All carcinomas were diagnosed more than 3 years after the index diagnosis of adenosis, with a mean interval of 5.6 years. In the third study,[43] 37 cases of atypical apocrine adenosis constituted less than 1% of the excisional biopsy specimens obtained from 9,340 women in the Mayo Clinic Benign Breast Disease cohort enrolled between 1967 and 1991. The mean age at diagnosis was 59.3 years for the women with atypical apocrine adenosis versus 51.4 years for all women in the cohort. Three of the 37 women (8%) developed subsequent carcinoma versus 7.8% of women in the entire study cohort. Their age at the time of the index biopsy was 55, 47, and 63 years. Two of the three women developed ipsilateral invasive carcinoma. One invasive ductal carcinoma occurred 4 years after the index biopsy, which also contained ADH. An invasive carcinoma with mixed ductal and lobular morphology developed 18 years after the index biopsy. The third woman developed contralateral DCIS 12 years after the index biopsy. The tumors had no apocrine differentiation, and no atypical apocrine adenosis was present in the background breast parenchyma of all three cases. These results indicate atypical apocrine adenosis to be a rare lesion, at least in the time period studied that preceded the widespread use of needle core biopsy. The authors suggested that atypical apocrine adenosis is probably diagnosed more often nowadays because of the use of needle core biopsy

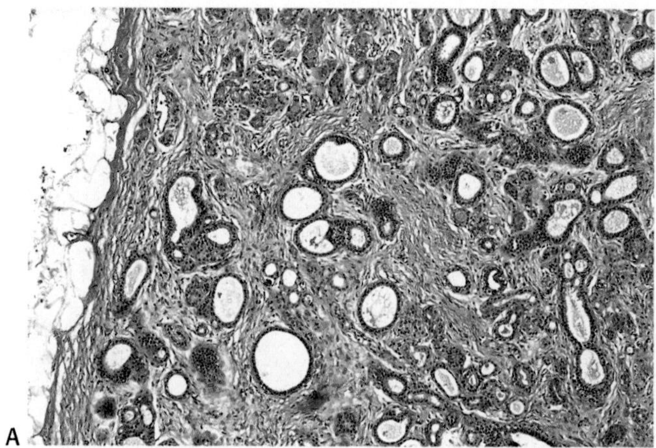

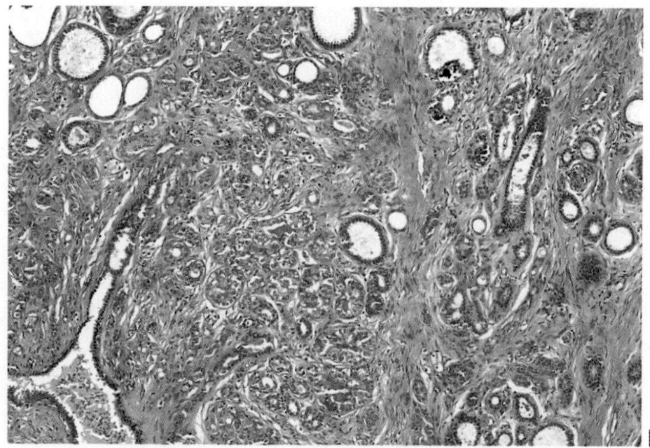

FIG. 7.21. ***Sclerosing adenosis in a fibroadenoma.*** **A:** This picture is from a needle core biopsy sample that was interpreted as invasive ductal carcinoma. **B:** The excised tumor was a fibroadenoma involved extensively by sclerosing adenosis. Cleft-forming fibroadenomatous epithelium is shown at the *lower left*.

technique. In this study, the risk of subsequent carcinoma associated with the diagnosis of atypical apocrine adenosis in breast excision specimens did not appear to differ from that of women with other benign lesions. As noted by Seidman at al.,[16] the Mayo Clinic Benign Breast Disease study also identified an association between older age and the diagnosis of atypical apocrine adenosis, although the results did not specifically suggest a positive relationship between older age and increased incidence of subsequent carcinoma.[43]

MICROGLANDULAR ADENOSIS

Microglandular adenosis (MGA) is a proliferative glandular lesion that mimics carcinoma clinically and pathologically. This entity differs substantially in its structural features from lesions conventionally termed "adenosis." It is included in this chapter because no more suitable placement is readily evident and the word "adenosis" is used to name the lesion.

Although it had been described previously,[44–46] MGA was not well characterized as a clinicopathologic entity until the publication in 1983 of three series totaling 29 patients.[47–49] One patient was probably included in two of these reports.[47,48] More recently, only a handful of examples of MGA without atypia or associated carcinoma were been reported in the English literature in two series[50,51] and one case report.[52]

MGA frequently has areas of atypia (atypical MGA). Carcinoma can also arise in MGA, retaining the MGA structure (CIS arising in MGA), or it can become frankly invasive.

Clinical Presentation

Microglandular Adenosis

All reported patients with MGA have been women, with ages ranging from 28 to 82 years. The majority of the patients were 45 to 55 years old. The presenting symptom in

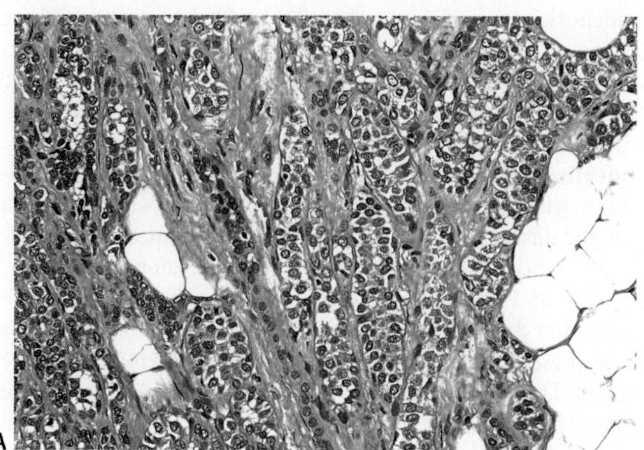

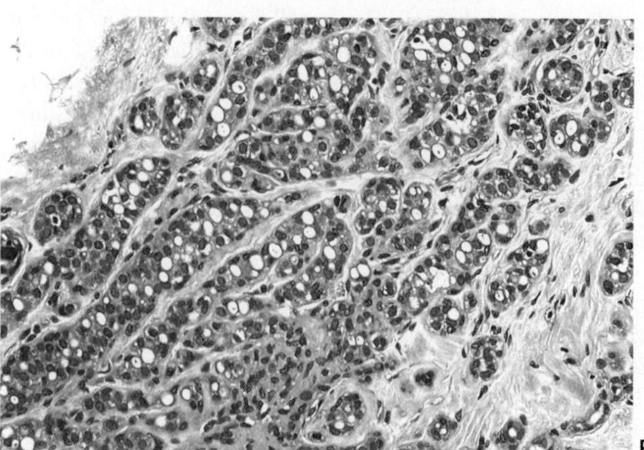

FIG. 7.22. ***Lobular carcinoma in situ in sclerosing adenosis.*** **A:** Trabecular arrangement. **B:** Signet ring cell LCIS in tubular adenosis.

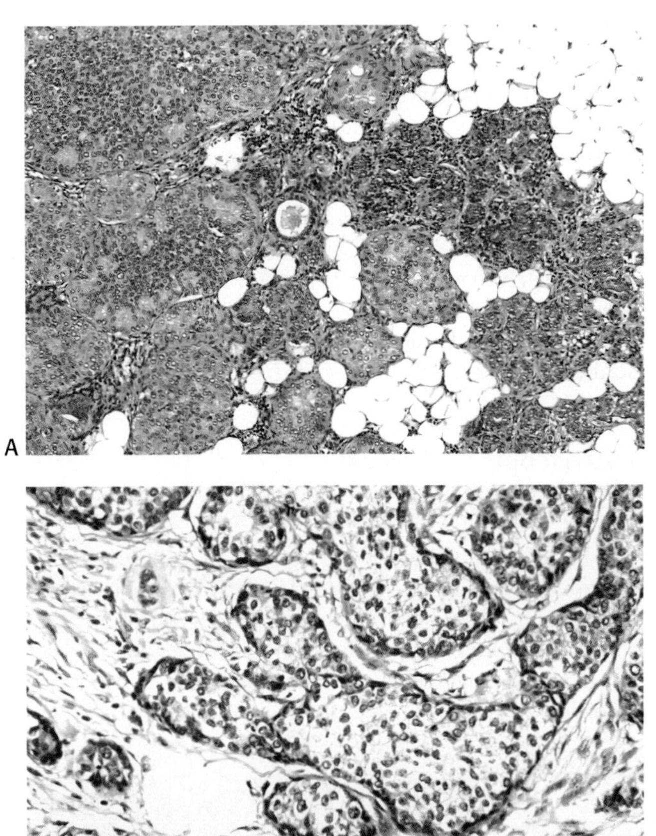

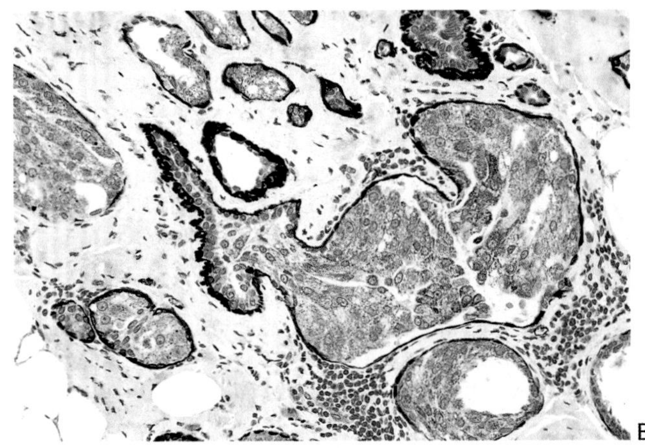

FIG. 7.23. ***Intraductal carcinoma in sclerosing adenosis.*** **A:** Solid intraductal carcinoma with a trace of cribriform growth in adenosis glands. **B:** The myoepithelium is attenuated in the adenosis glands occupied by intraductal carcinoma (anti-SMM-HC). **C:** Adenosis glands distended by intraductal carcinoma.

most instances has been a mass or "thickening" in the breast. Occasionally MGA was one of several lesions responsible for the mass. MGA can be accompanied by cysts and various benign proliferative changes. In one series,[50] MGA was an incidental finding adjacent to fibrocystic changes (one case) or a papilloma (one case) and it formed a 1.9-cm palpable mass in a third case. Kim et al.[52] reported that MGA formed a 2.0-cm palpable mass somewhat fixed to the surrounding tissue and chest wall. The mass can sometimes be painful, and in one case the lesion reportedly changed in size during the menstrual cycles. Duration prior to biopsy has varied from a few weeks to as long as 5 years. A positive family history of breast carcinoma has rarely been mentioned. One patient with MGA had neurofibromatosis.[53] MGA also occurred in a 22-year-old woman with BRCA1 germline mutation (5625G>T mutation in exon 24).[54]

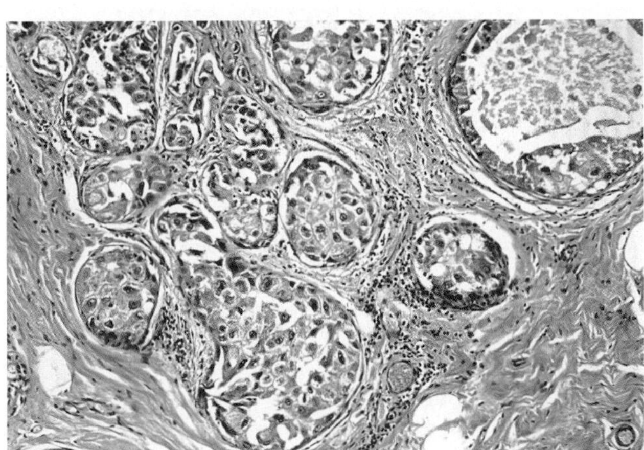

FIG. 7.24. ***Intraductal carcinoma in sclerosing adenosis.*** The enlarged glands contain apocrine intraductal carcinoma. Netrosis is present in one gland (*upper right*).

Atypical MGA and Carcinoma in MGA

The age distribution of atypical MGA and carcinoma arising in MGA are similar to those described for MGA.[50,55–61] These lesions typically present as breast masses. In one study,[61] the median age of patients with MGA and carcinoma was 47 years, ranging from 26 to 68 years, and all patients presented with a mass lesion. Six (43%) had a family history of breast carcinoma.

Radiology

Mammography of MGA may reveal increased density and is sometimes reported to be "suspicious,"[62] but no specific radiologic changes have been described. Rarely, nonpalpable MGA is detected mammographically at the site of an ill-defined density with calcifications, and such a lesion may be sampled by needle core biopsy. None of the three MGA cases reported by Khalifeh et al.[50] was detected mammographically. Ultrasound examination of one case of MGA disclosed an ill-defined hypoechoic mass; the corresponding mammogram showed only dense breasts bilaterally.[52] Another case undetected by mammography was deemed suspicious sonographically.[54] At MRI the lesion consisted of a noncircumscribed mass with moderate early and delayed enhancement and hyperintense T2-weighted images. The radiologic differential diagnosis in this case included FA. On the other hand, atypical MGA and carcinoma arising in MGA appeared mammographically as infiltrative masses.[50] No radiologic abnormality was detected in the breast of a 74-year-old woman who presented with a palpable breast mass consisting of invasive carcinoma arising in MGA.[59]

Gross Pathology

MGA forms an ill-defined infiltrative tumor. As a consequence, the gross size has only rarely been accurately measured, but it has been estimated to range from 3 to 4 cm and can be as large as 20 cm. In some specimens, the process has been described as multifocal or composed of confluent multifocal lesions. Rarely, MGA is an occult lesion 2 cm or less in size that is discovered in a specimen obtained for another abnormality. Cysts and other microscopically detectable proliferative changes often contribute to the grossly evident mass, and in some cases these changes can obscure the true extent of the MGA component. Atypical MGA formed a 6.5-cm mass in one case.[62] Carcinoma arising in MGA forms a moderately hard ill-defined mass with a gray-white cut surface.[57] Some lesions showed chalky yellow streaking or grossly identifiable calcifications.[62] Gelatinous foci were described in two cases.[62]

Microscopic Pathology

Microglandular Adenosis

The basic histologic pattern of MGA is an infiltrative proliferation of small glands in fibrous or fatty mammary stroma (Fig. 7.25). When examined at low magnification, there sometimes appears to be clustering of the glands in nodular, lobule-like aggregates, but most often the distribution is disorderly.

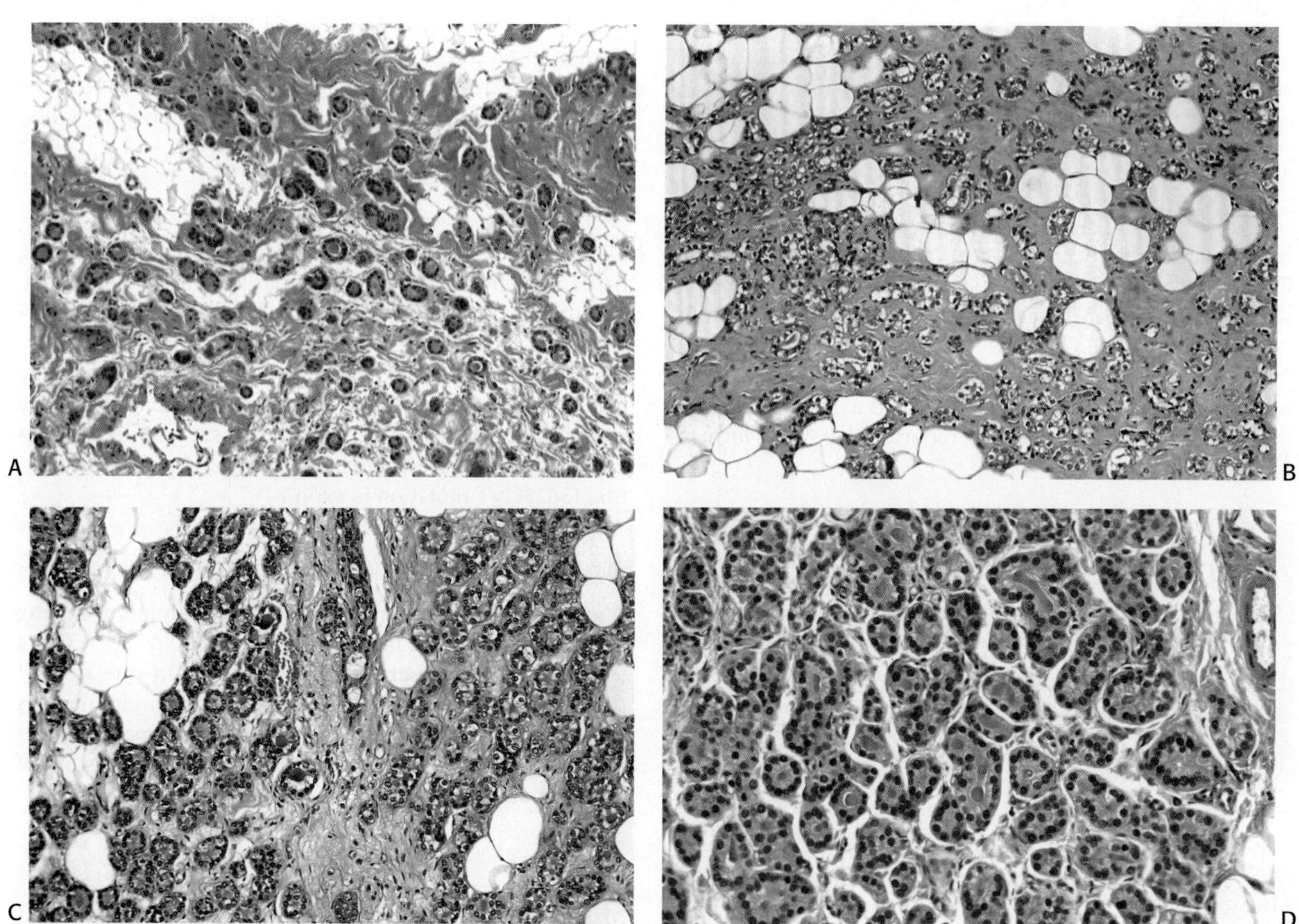

FIG. 7.25. ***Microglandular adenosis.*** **A:** Regular round glands are diffusely distributed in fibrofatty stroma. **B:** The cells in this variant have clear cytoplasm. **C:** The lesion infiltrates fat (*left*) and fibrous stroma (*right*). **D:** A dense glandular proliferation in MGA.

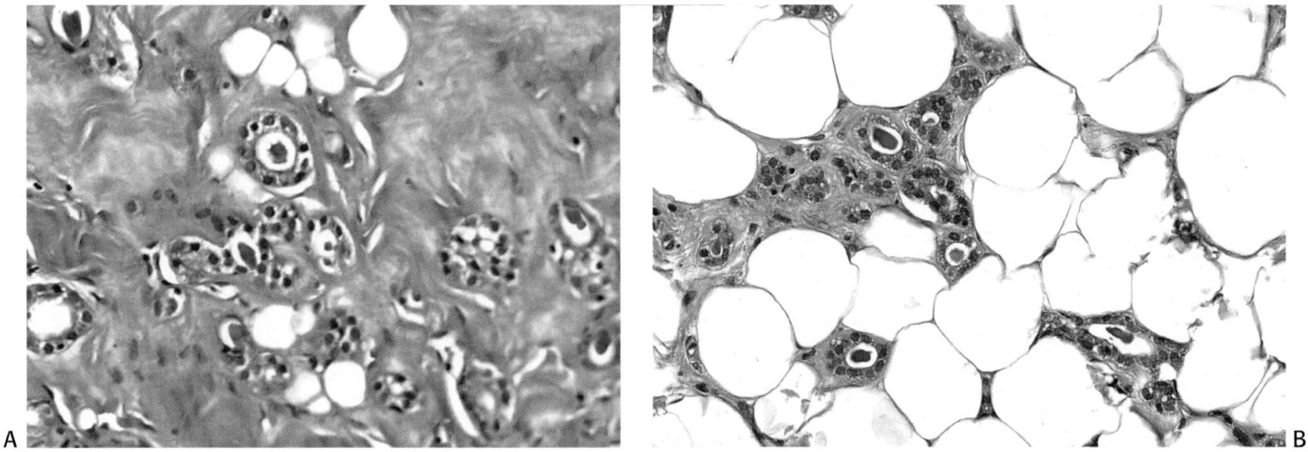

FIG. 7.26. ***Microglandular adenosis.*** **A:** Typical glands composed of uniform cuboidal cells regularly spaced around a lumen containing eosinophilic secretion. Slight cytoplasmic clearing is evident. **B:** MGA in fat is shown.

In its most characteristic form, MGA is composed of small round glands lined by a single layer of flat-to-cuboidal epithelial cells (Figs. 7.25 and 7.26). Each cell has a single round nucleus with an inconspicuous or inapparent nucleolus. The cytoplasm tends to be clear or amphophilic, but pronounced eosinophilia may be encountered, sometimes with cytoplasmic granularity. Inspissated intraluminal secretions often appear as deeply stained and homogeneously eosinophilic globules. This material is usually PAS-positive and diastase-resistant (Fig. 7.27). It is also mucicarmine positive. Occasionally, the intraluminal secretions may calcify, forming small and round calcifications.

Substantial variation in the growth pattern and cytologic appearance of the glands can be encountered in MGA. When elongated, the glands acquire a tubular rather than round configuration. Ordinary MGA may have crowded, "back-to-back" glands, but each acinus remains separate. Areas that resemble MGA can be found in sclerosing adenosis (Fig. 7.28). The glands of MGA lack a myoepithelial layer (Fig. 7.29), but are surrounded by basement membrane that can be highlighted using a reticulin stain or immunoperoxidase stains for laminin and collagen IV (Fig. 7.30).

Atypical MGA

Lesions classified as "atypical" MGA have elements of MGA in its ordinary form as well as foci with a more complex structure and cytologic atypia. Atypical lesions have a heterogeneous mixture of connected microacini and larger, more irregular glands (Fig. 7.31) that tend to be closely packed, and in some cases appear to fuse. Many of the glands of atypical MGA are composed of a single layer of cells, but a few may have stratified epithelium. The epithelial cells tend to be hyperchromatic and pleomorphic with varying amounts of cytoplasm that is clear or eosinophilic. Prominent, coarse, deeply eosinophilic cytoplasmic

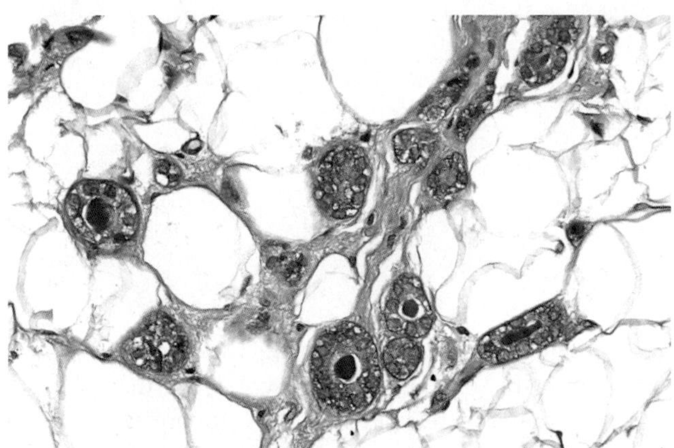

FIG. 7.27. ***Microglandular adenosis.*** Secretion in the lumens reacts positively with the PAS stain, which also highlights the intact basement membranes around glands (PAS reaction).

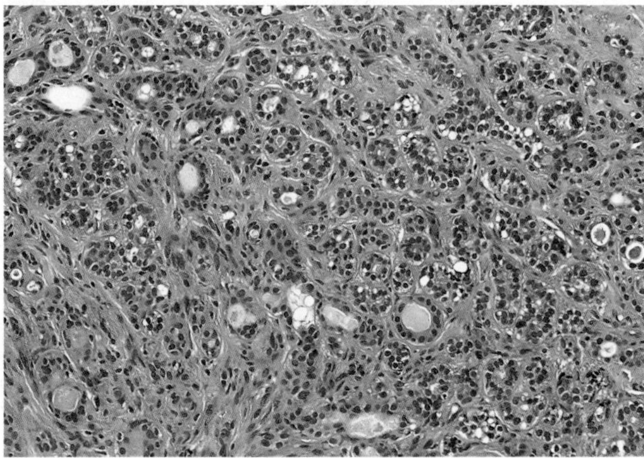

FIG. 7.28. ***Microglandular adenosis and sclerosing adenosis.*** MGA occupying most of this image merges with sclerosing adenosis (*lower left*).

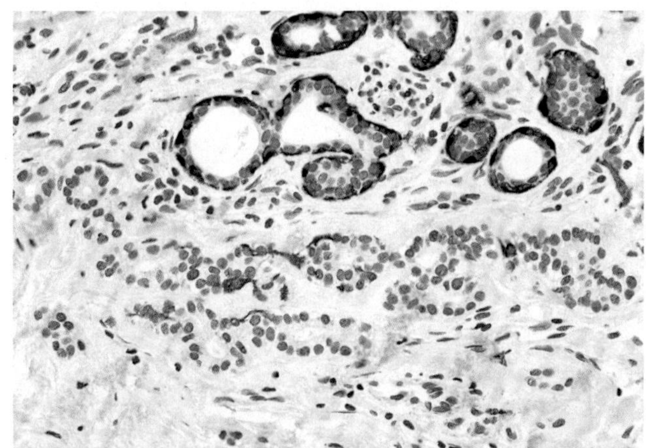

FIG. 7.29. ***Microglandular adenosis.*** Myoepithelial cells are immunoreactive for myosin in adenosis (*above*). No reactivity is seen in MGA (*below*) (anti-SMM-HC).

granules are present in a minority of cases (Fig. 7.32). The latter cytoplasmic appearance is sometimes accompanied by a lymphoplasmacytic reaction that is otherwise not a feature of ordinary MGA. Rare mitoses and focal apoptosis may be present. The more florid epithelial proliferation of atypical MGA produces interconnected budding glandular units with microcribriform nests. When luminal bridging occurs, the monolayered epithelium is replaced by a stratified proliferation that evolves into solid nests of cells. Cartilaginous or chondroid metaplasia sometimes occurs in atypical MGA or when carcinoma arises in MGA (Figs. 7.31 and 7.33).

Carcinoma Arising in MGA

Several studies[49–51,55–58,61–63] and case reports[57,59,60] have described *in situ* and/or invasive carcinoma arising in MGA.

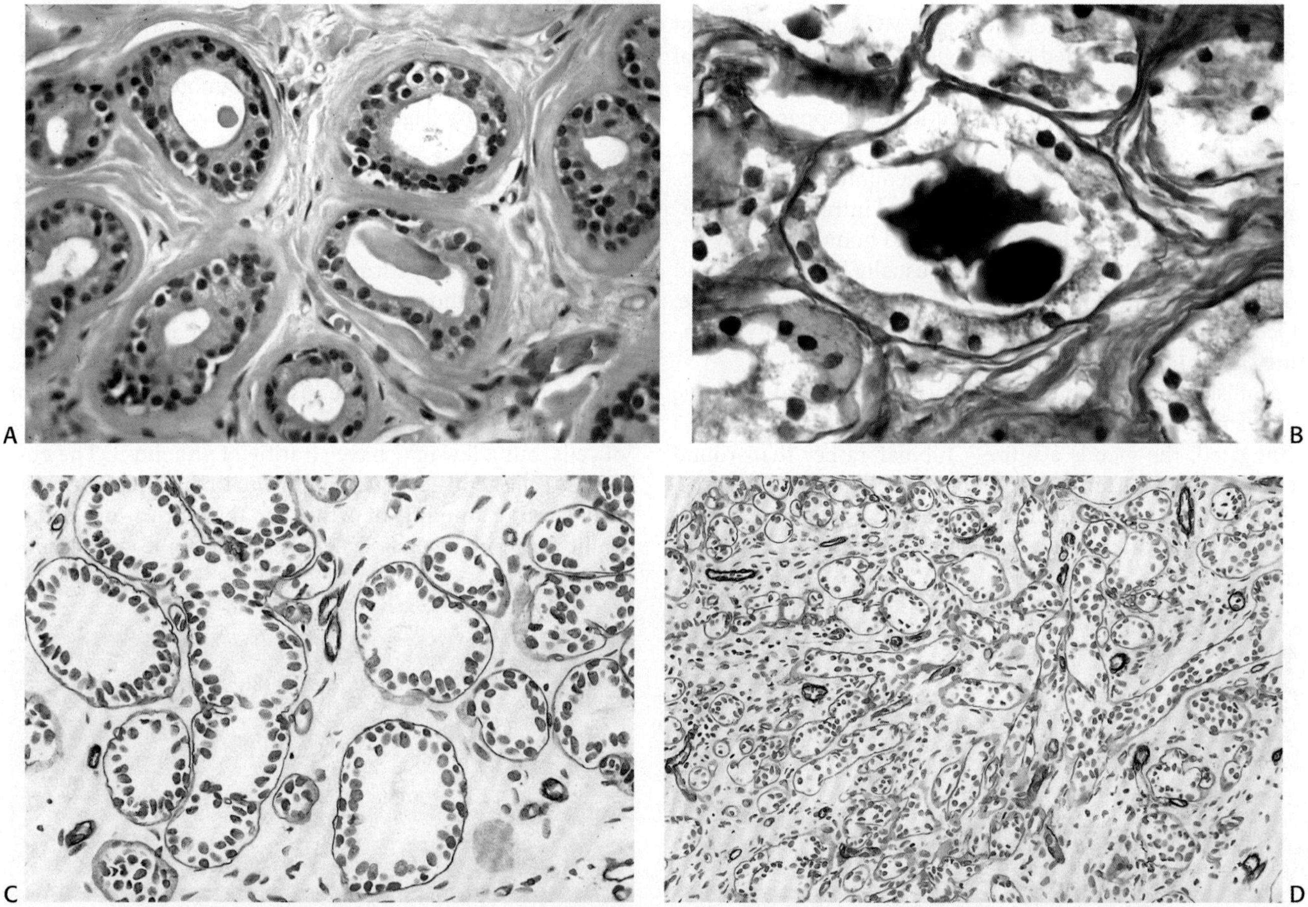

FIG. 7.30. ***Microglandular adenosis.*** **A:** Prominent basement membranes in MGA. **B:** The basement membrane is highlighted by the silver reticulin stain in this example of clear cell MGA. **C:** Laminin reactivity outlines each gland in MGA. **D:** Laminin immunoreactivity in sclerosing adenosis is shown for comparison.

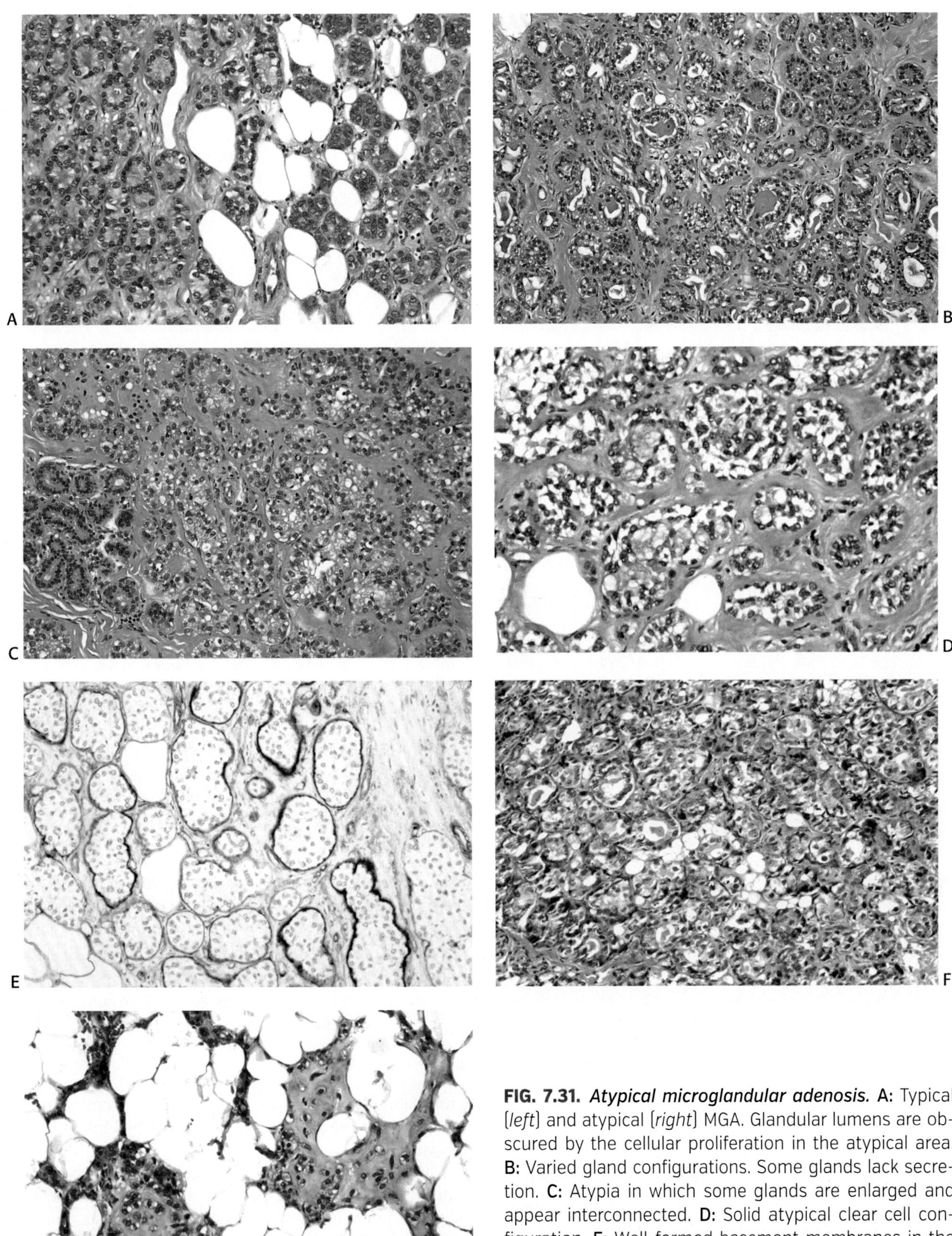

FIG. 7.31. ***Atypical microglandular adenosis.*** **A:** Typical (*left*) and atypical (*right*) MGA. Glandular lumens are obscured by the cellular proliferation in the atypical area. **B:** Varied gland configurations. Some glands lack secretion. **C:** Atypia in which some glands are enlarged and appear interconnected. **D:** Solid atypical clear cell configuration. **E:** Well-formed basement membranes in the lesion shown in (**D**) are demonstrated by the collagen IV immunostain. **F:** Atypical MGA. **G:** Atypical MGA with chondroid metaplasia in fat.

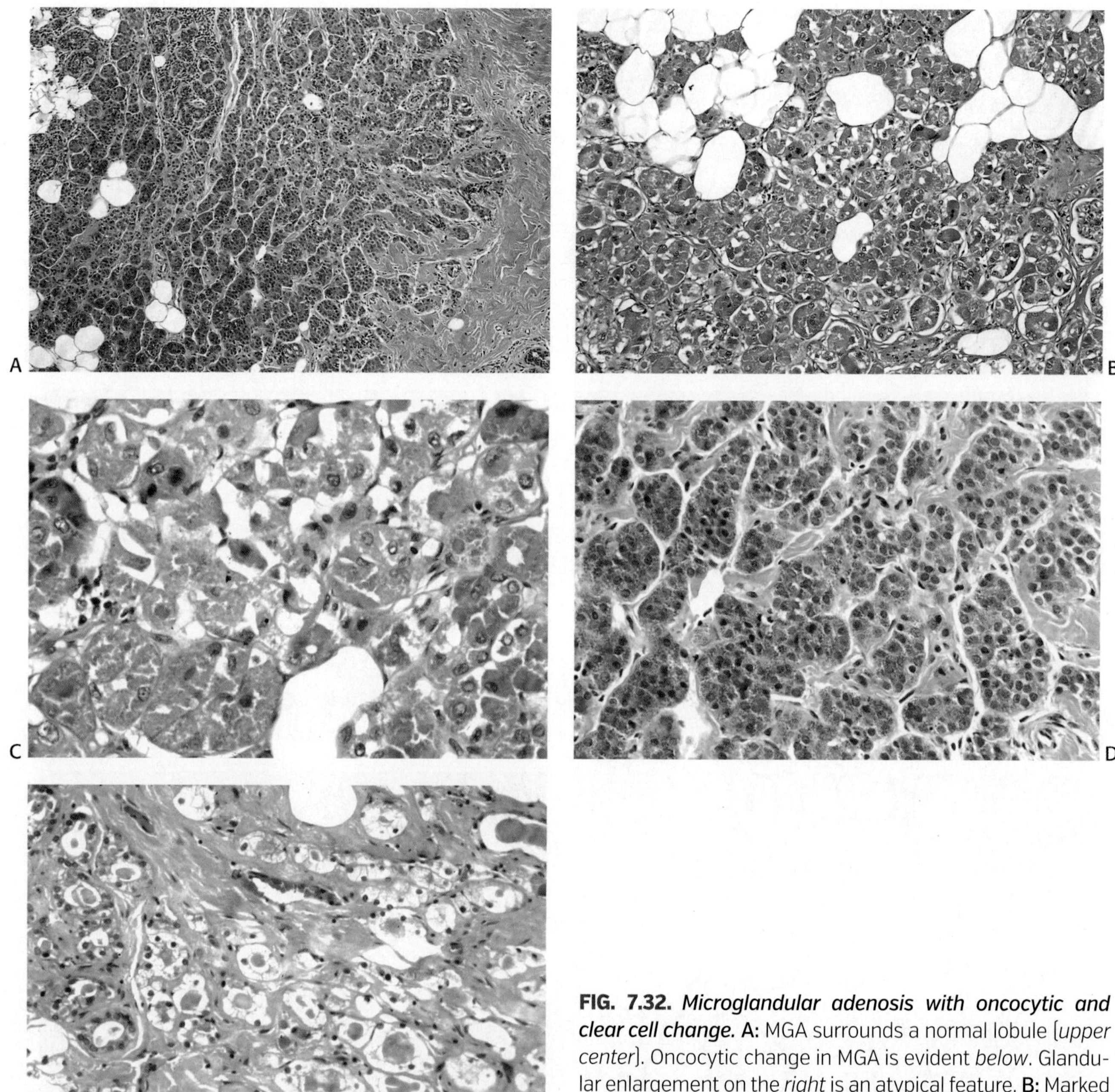

FIG. 7.32. ***Microglandular adenosis with oncocytic and clear cell change.*** **A:** MGA surrounds a normal lobule (*upper center*). Oncocytic change in MGA is evident *below*. Glandular enlargement on the *right* is an atypical feature. **B:** Marked oncocytic change obscures glandular lumens. **C,D:** Cytoplasmic granularity and eosinophilia. **E:** Clear cell change.

Carcinoma in situ in MGA

Structural transitions from MGA to atypical MGA and to intraductal carcinoma are observed in these cases. Extensive sampling can be necessary to find residual foci of MGA without atypia. Duct-forming carcinomatous areas maintain the acinar growth pattern of MGA, but they are enlarged and filled by basaloid cells with a high mitotic rate, substantial cytologic abnormalities, and necrosis. The carcinomatous epithelium may exhibit cytoplasmic features found in MGA, such as secretory activity, cytoplasmic clearing, and prominent granularity (Fig. 7.34). Benign chondromyxoid metaplasia of the stroma has been described in a minority of cases.[62]

CIS arising in MGA can be readily identified because it tends to retain the underlying alveolar growth pattern of the adenosis, but consists of expanded and solid nests. This pattern greatly differs from any of the structural configurations encountered in most ordinary types of DCIS or LCIS, as this *in situ* proliferation has an infiltrative distribution (Figs. 7.35 and 7.36). The nests of CIS arising in MGA are not

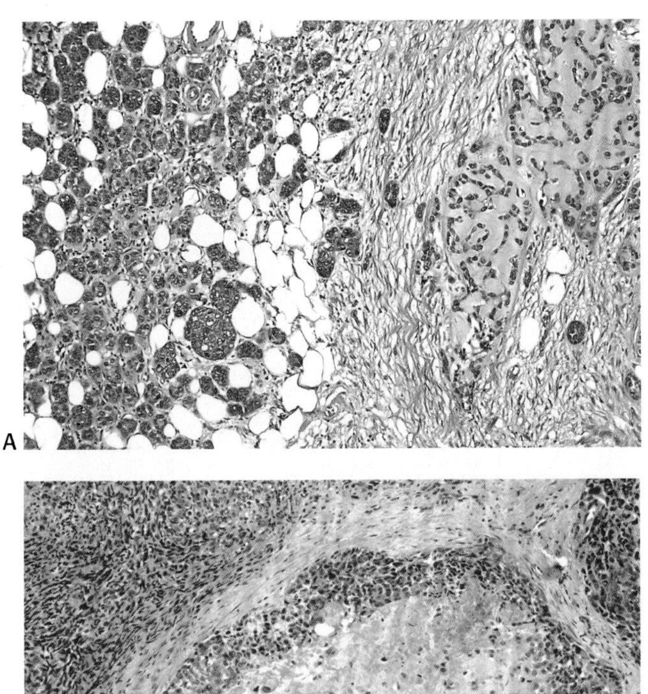

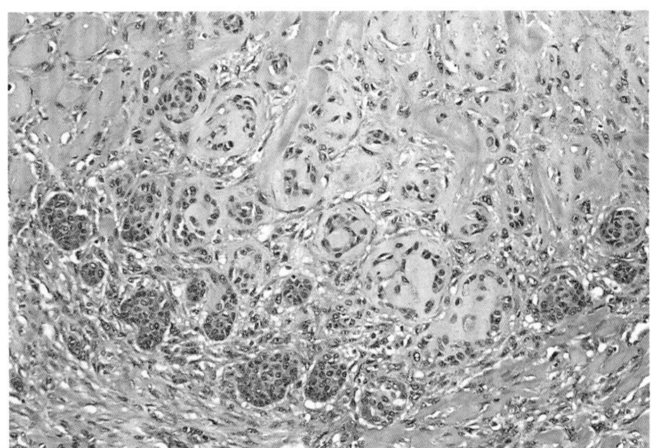

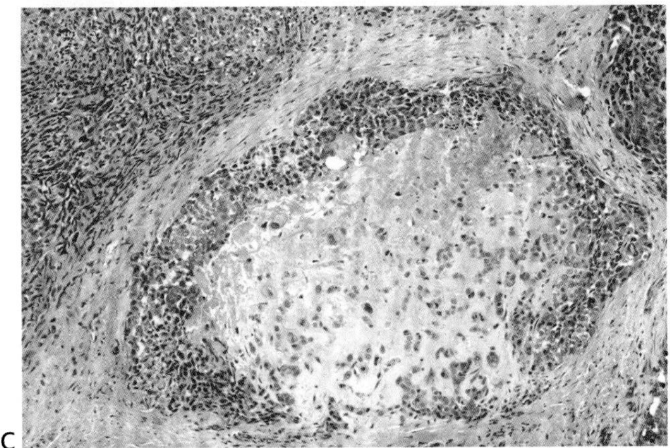

FIG. 7.33. ***Matrix-forming carcinoma arising in microglandular adenosis.*** **A:** MGA on the *left* showing atypia and transition to *in situ* carcinoma. Invasive carcinoma, matrix-forming type, is on the *right*. **B:** Matrix-forming carcinoma is shown arising in carcinoma in MGA. **C:** Chondroid differentiation in high-grade carcinoma that arose in MGA.

regarded as invasive because they are surrounded by basement membrane. The carcinomas frequently have some clear cells, and a few tumors are entirely composed of such cells or of cells with prominent eosinophilic cytoplasmic granularity. These cells are immunoreactive for substances that are found in acinic cell carcinoma, such as amylase, lysozyme, and α_1-antichymotrypsin, as well as S-100 protein.[64] Some tumors classified as acinic cell carcinoma of the breast[64,65] appear to be carcinomas with acinic cell differentiation arising in MGA. A chronic inflammatory infiltrate and a desmoplastic stromal reaction often accompany the development of carcinoma in MGA.

In rare cases, ordinary CIS may coexist with MGA or atypical MGA. Rosen[48] reported two cases of MGA with associated ordinary CIS that consisted of LCIS in one case and DCIS in the other. A case with MGA, invasive carcinoma, and ordinary DCIS (surrounded by basement membrane and myoepithelium) was also part of the series by Geyer et al.[51]

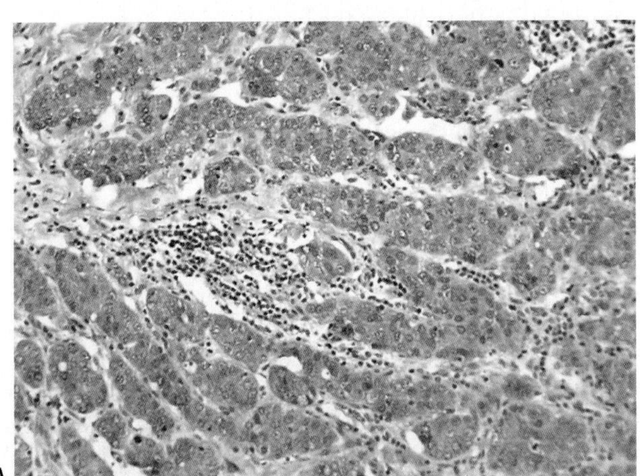

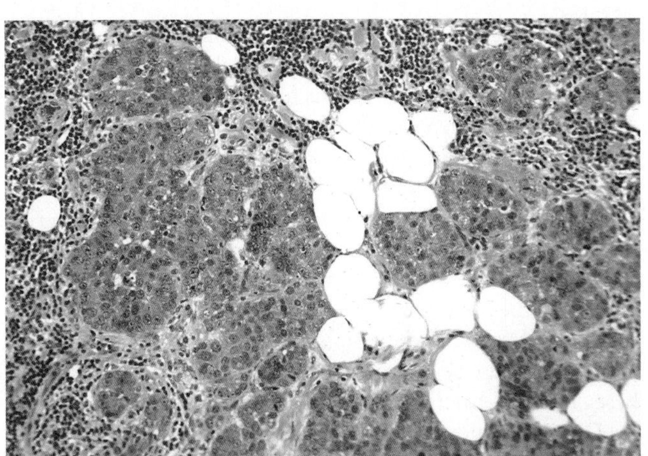

FIG. 7.34. ***Intraductal carcinoma arising in microglandular adenosis.*** **A,B:** Intraductal carcinoma in MGA. Note lymphocytes in the stroma.

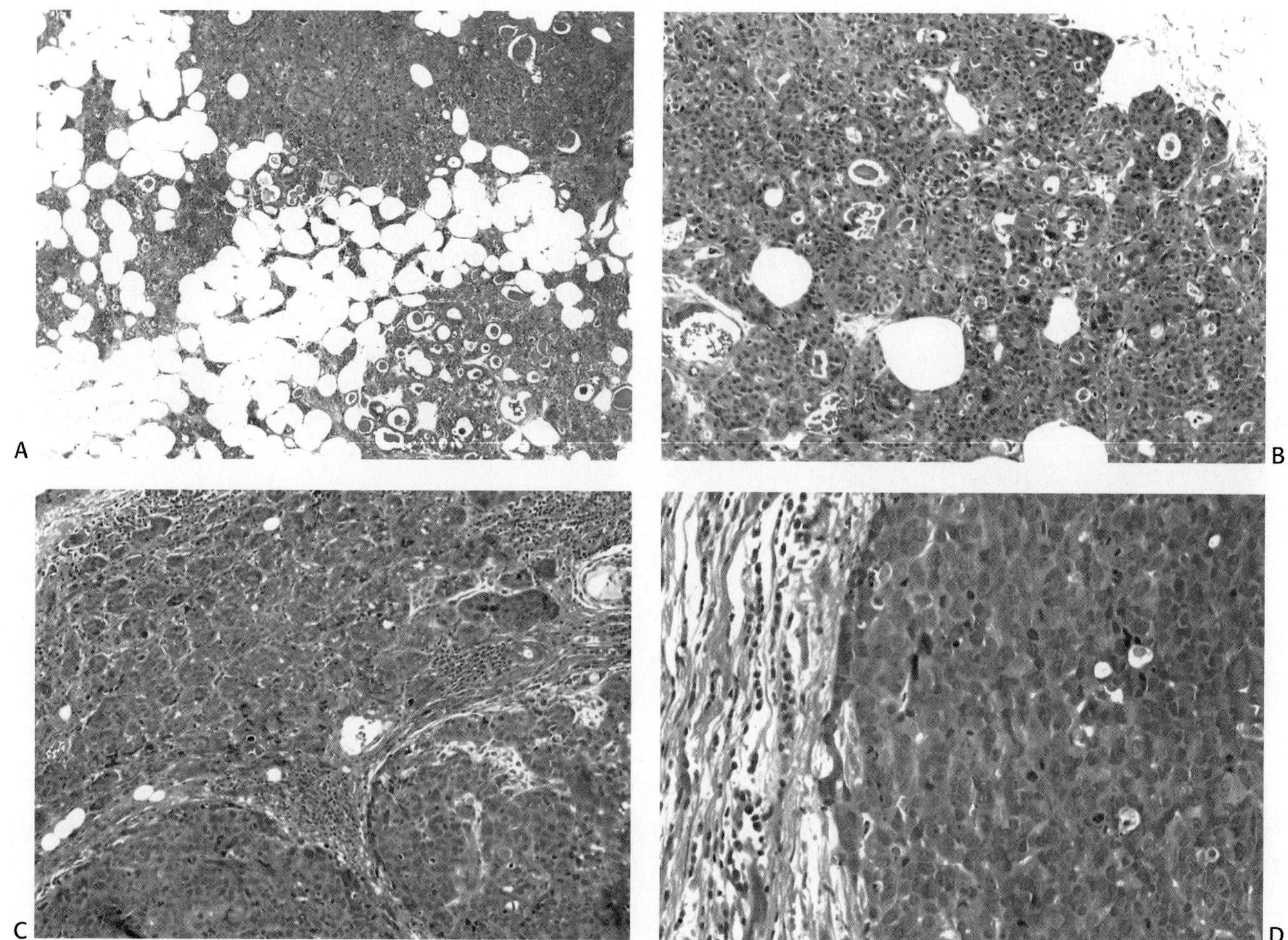

FIG. 7.35. ***Carcinoma arising in microglandular adenosis.*** **A:** Atypical MGA is present in the *lower part* of this picture; the *upper area* depicts carcinoma in MGA. **B:** Atypical MGA. **C:** Carcinoma with adenosis pattern [*upper left*] forming invasive solid nodules [*below*]. The stromal lymphoid infiltrate, seen focally here, is commonly present in this type of carcinoma. **D:** High-grade invasive carcinoma that typifies these lesions.

Invasive Carcinoma Arising in MGA

Invasive carcinoma arising in MGA usually forms microscopic solid tumor masses that are appreciably larger than the surrounding alveolar MGA glands filled by CIS (Fig. 7.35). It often appears that invasive foci are formed by the coalescent growth of expanding alveolar CIS elements. Basement membranes are present in MGA and MGA-associated CIS, but they are disrupted around invasive nests. The invasive foci are typically enveloped by a conspicuous lymphocytic reaction, and necrosis may be present. Mitoses are usually readily apparent in these regions.

Unusual forms of carcinoma, other than the aforementioned high-grade type, are found in association with MGA. These include carcinoma with secretory differentiation (Fig. 7.36), carcinoma with squamous metaplasia, basaloid carcinoma (Fig. 7.37), and adenoid cystic carcinoma. Examples of carcinoma with matrix-forming metaplasia arising in MGA have also been reported[50,51,58] (Fig. 7.33). Paget disease of the nipple has been found associated with carcinoma that involved MGA throughout the breast.

Differential Diagnosis

The histologic differential diagnosis of MGA includes tubular carcinoma and sclerosing adenosis. Tubular carcinoma is usually composed of angular glands of varying size, arranged in a stellate or radial configuration. DCIS is present near some tubular carcinomas and typically has low nuclear grade with micropapillary or cribriform architecture. In some cases, only ADH or columnar cell change with atypia may be present in the surrounding breast, as well as classical LCIS and ALH. Elastosis is not a feature of MGA, but it is often present in tubular carcinoma. Tubular carcinoma glands lack myoepithelial cells and a basement membrane.

Although the foregoing features of tubular carcinoma serve to separate it from MGA in most instances, there are

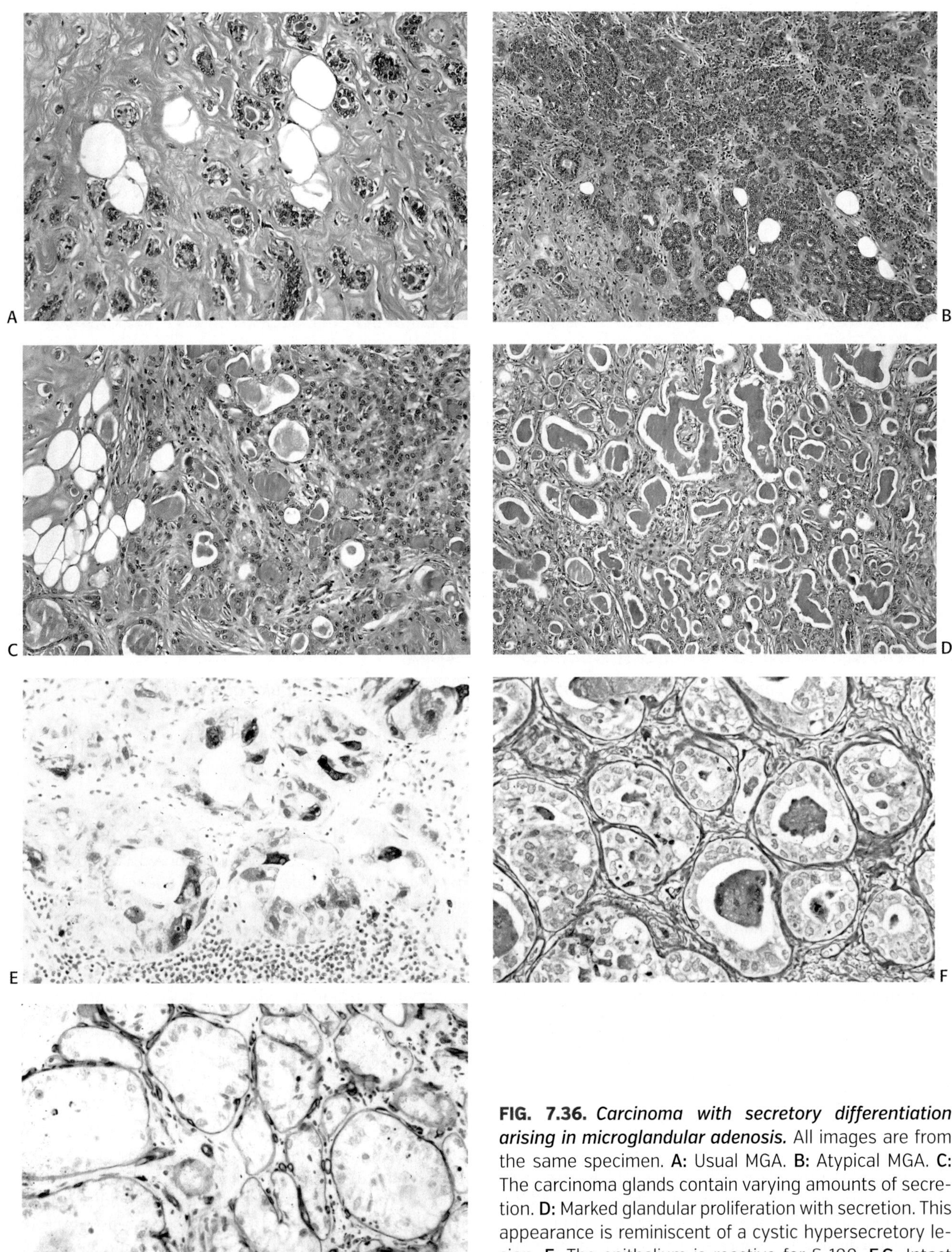

FIG. 7.36. ***Carcinoma with secretory differentiation arising in microglandular adenosis.*** All images are from the same specimen. **A:** Usual MGA. **B:** Atypical MGA. **C:** The carcinoma glands contain varying amounts of secretion. **D:** Marked glandular proliferation with secretion. This appearance is reminiscent of a cystic hypersecretory lesion. **E:** The epithelium is reactive for S-100. **F,G:** Intact basement membranes are demonstrated with the reticulin stain (F) and the laminin immunostain (G).

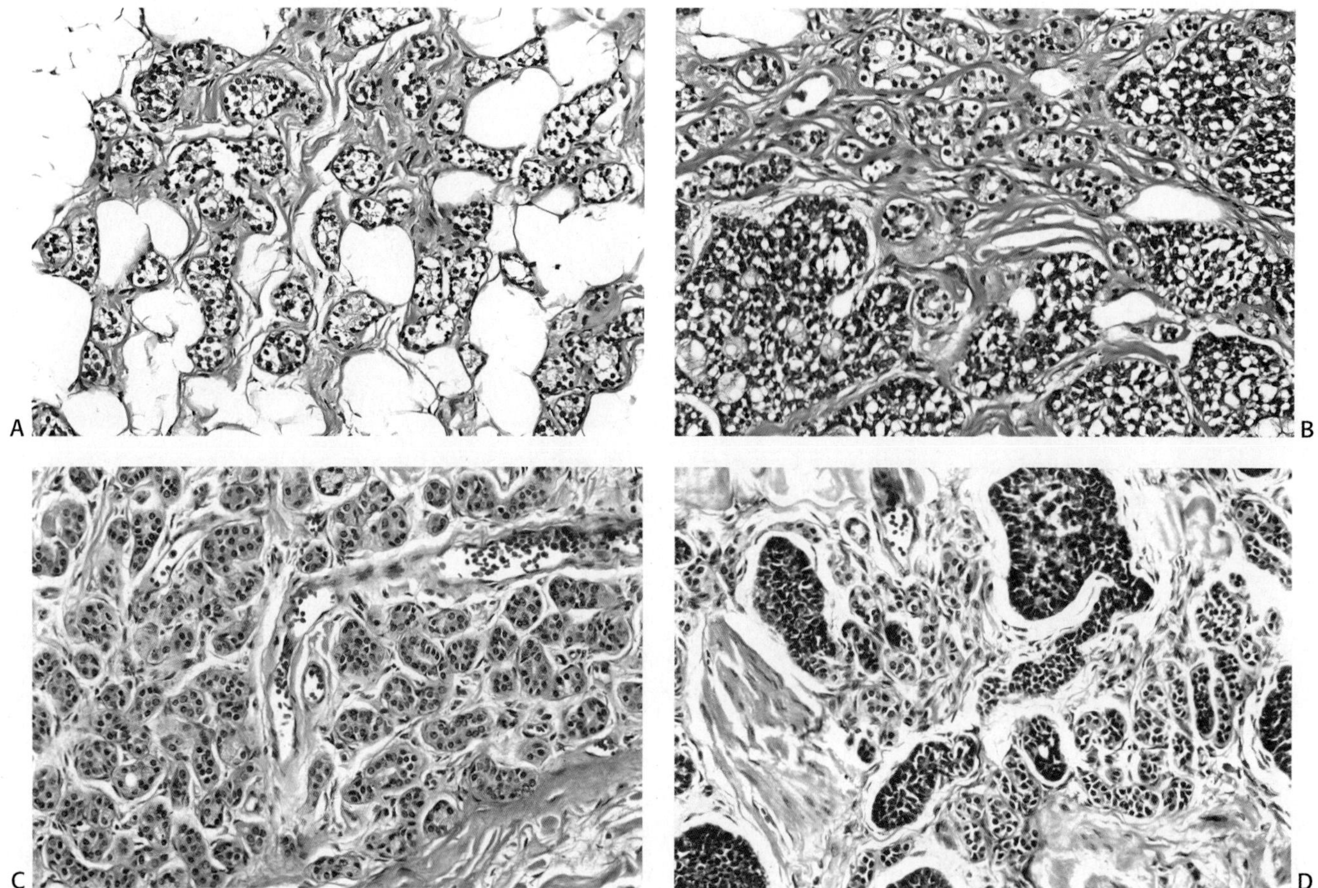

FIG. 7.37. ***Carcinoma with basaloid differentiation arising in microglandular adenosis.*** **A:** Atypical MGA with cytoplasmic clearing. **B:** Carcinoma with basaloid growth in MGA. **C,D:** Compact area of MGA **(C)**, which gave rise to invasive basaloid carcinoma **(D)** in a 48-year-old woman.

situations when the distinction between the two lesions can be difficult. Occasionally, the glands in tubular carcinoma are rounded and the cells have clear or apocrine cytoplasm (see Chapter 13), making it difficult to distinguish them from MGA without the aid of IHC studies (Fig. 7.26). Immunoperoxidase stains for estrogen receptor (ER) and progesterone receptor (PR) that are highly expressed in tubular carcinoma and absent in MGA. S-100 is uniformly positive in MGA (Fig. 7.38) and negative in tubular carcinoma (see the section on Immunohistochemistry in this chapter).

Sclerosing or florid adenosis that may merge with MGA typically features myoepithelial proliferation that often has a spindle cell configuration. The process is usually distinctly lobulocentric, and the compressed glands tend to be arranged in a whorled or laminated fashion within the lobular nodules. Myoepithelial cells in sclerosing or florid adenosis are highlighted with immunostains for p63, calponin, actin, CD10, and other myoepithelial markers. Small areas of round glands growing in a disorderly manner in association with otherwise typical sclerosing adenosis usually have a myoepithelial cell layer, and therefore should be considered part of the sclerosing adenosis process rather than as associated MGA.

Khalifeh et al.[50] reported the histologic findings in 54 cases that had initially been misdiagnosed as MGA. The revised diagnosis included 48 cases of adenosis (21 ordinary adenosis, 17 infiltrating adenosis, 9 adenosis with clear cell changes, and 1 BDA), 2 cases of atypical apocrine metaplasia, and 4 cases with no obvious pathologic abnormality. All glands present in these cases had a complete myoepithelial cell layer, as demonstrated by immunoperoxidase stains for myoepithelial markers.

The differential diagnosis of atypical MGA and of CIS arising in atypical MGA includes invasive carcinoma.

Cytology

The FNA findings in a total of three cases of MGA have been reported by Evans and Hussein[66] and Gherardi et al.[67] The smears were sparsely cellular to hypocellular and contained small, round-to-oval, monotonous cells arranged in tight clusters. The cytoplasm was finely vacuolated or contained small granules. The cells had centrally located nuclei, with round or ovoid shape, uniform size, and finely granular chromatin. No background naked bipolar nuclei were

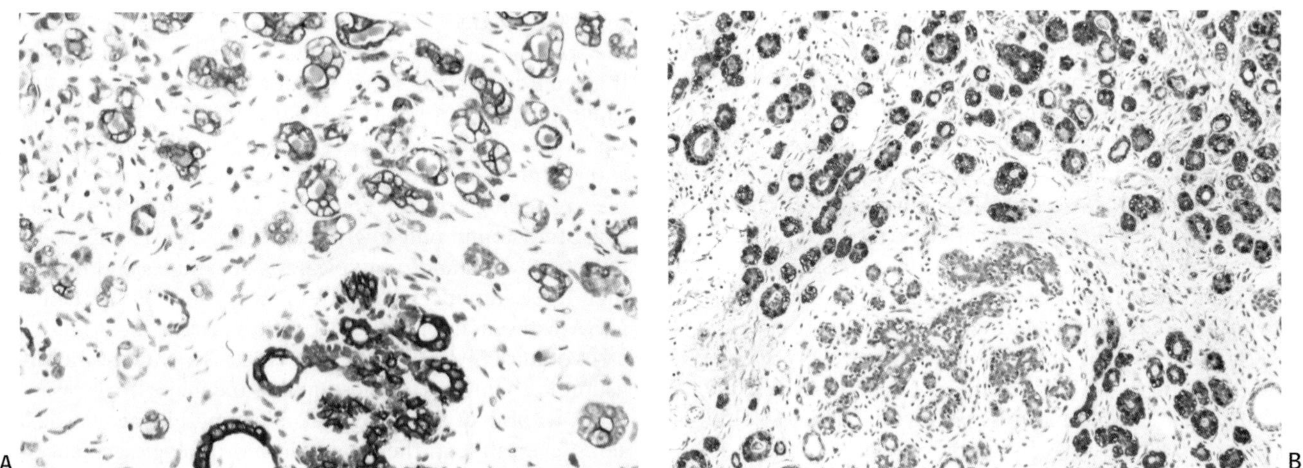

FIG. 7.38. ***Microglandular adenosis.*** **A:** The epithelial cells of a lobule in the lower center display stronger immunoreactivity for cytokeratin than the surrounding MGA glands (anti-AE1). **B:** Strong immunoreactivity for S-100 protein is present in MGA around a nonreactive normal lobule.

identified in the smears. The differential diagnosis in these cases included benign lesions and, in particular, secretory changes.

Immunohistochemistry

The cells forming MGA are strongly immunoreactive for S-100 (Fig. 7.38) and negative for ER, PR, and HER2/*neu*.[61] Immunoperoxidase stains for ER, PR, and S-100 are extremely helpful to solve the differential diagnosis between MGA and tubular carcinoma in morphologically ambiguous cases, as the two lesions show reciprocal patterns of reactivity for these markers. MGA is S-100 positive and ER and PR negative, whereas tubular carcinoma is S-100 negative but ER and PR positive. Eusebi et al.[68] reported that MGA lacks immunoreactivity for gross cystic disease fluid protein-15 (GCDFP-15) and for epithelial membrane antigen (EMA). The absence of EMA was helpful in distinguishing MGA from tubular carcinoma that was consistently EMA positive.

No myoepithelial cells are seen around the glands of MGA in H&E-stained sections and in sections immunohistochemically stained for myoepithelial markers (Fig. 7.29). The glands of MGA, however, are surrounded by basement membrane. The latter is usually visible in H&E-stained sections and is highlighted by immunoreactivity for laminin and type IV collagen. Silver impregnation and PAS stains also reveal a basement membrane ring investing the glands[61,68] (Fig. 7.30). However, immunostains for laminin, collagen IV, and reticulin special stains can all be technically challenging and difficult to interpret, and should be used with extreme caution, because some low-grade carcinomas can also show focal basement membrane. In particular, Cserni[69] detected basement membrane material around the glands of a tubulolobular carcinoma, a morphologic mimic of MGA. This caveat is an important consideration in the diagnosis of the limited sample provided by a needle core biopsy procedure.

MGA is strongly positive for S-100 (Fig. 7.38). Atypical MGA and carcinoma arising in MGA also tend to be S-100 positive, but three separate studies[50,55,56] have reported some reduction in S-100 staining intensity and extent occurring in parallel with increasing severity of the lesion. In MGA, p53 is usually absent in MGA[61] or minimally expressed (less than 3% of cells).[50,56] Khalifeh et al.[50] found positivity for p53 in 5% to 10% of atypical MGA cells and in more than 30% of the cells of carcinoma arising in MGA, but Shin et al.[56] did not observe a substantial difference in the percentage of p53-positive cells in MGA-associated lesions. A few studies[50,55,56] have reported a trend toward increased positivity for the proliferation marker Ki67 together with increasing severity of the lesions. Khalifeh et al.[50] found positivity for Ki67 in fewer than 3% of MGA cells, in 5% to 10% of atypical MGA cells, and in more than 30% of the cells of carcinoma arising in MGA. Shin et al.[56] reported that 5% to 20% of MGA and atypical MGA cells in their series were Ki67 positive (one case with 20% to 90% positivity was the only exception), whereas 5% to 30% of the cells of CIS arising in MGA were Ki67 positive, and even more were positive in invasive carcinoma. In addition, Koenig et al.[55] observed an increasing percentage of Ki67-positive cells in the transition from atypical MGA to CIS arising in MGA and to invasive carcinoma. These data correlate with disease progression going from MGA all the way to invasive carcinoma, and support the hypothesis that MGA is a nonobligate morphologic precursor of invasive breast carcinoma.

MGA, atypical MGA, and carcinoma arising in MGA display a somewhat unique pattern of immunoreactivity for epithelial and basal markers. CK7 was strongly positive in all atypical MGA cases tested by Koenig et al.,[55] whereas CK20 was uniformly negative. Although MGA is negative for EMA in most series, these authors reported that 8/15 cases of atypical MGA, 3/9 of MGA-associated CIS, and 4/6 invasive carcinomas in their series were EMA positive. The basal keratins

CK5/6[50] and 34βE12[55] were also negative in all cases of atypical MGA, CIS, and invasive carcinoma tested for these markers. CK5/6 was negative in 3/3 cases of MGA in another series.[50] In contrast, the luminal keratin CK8/18 was positive in all MGA-related lesions evaluated for this marker in two series.[50,51] Epidermal growth factor receptor (EGFR), another basal marker, decorated 11/11 MGA-related lesions in one series[50] and 13/14 cases in another.[51] Resetkova et al.[60] also reported EGFR positivity in an MGA-related carcinoma. Focal positivity for c-kit was identified in 3/6 cases of carcinoma arising in MGA, two of which were matrix producing and one acinic-like.[50]

Carcinomas derived from MGA do not express ER, PR, and HER2/*neu*,[50,51,55] and only one case has been documented that showed focal ER positivity.[55] The triple negative and EGFR-positive immunoprofile of MGA-associated carcinomas is consistent with the phenotype of basal-like carcinomas as defined by gene array profiling.

Electron Microscopy

Two ultrastructural studies of MGA have been published. The authors of both reports described finding basement membranes surrounded by a loose collagenous layer around the MGA glands.[49,53] The lesion studied by Kay,[53] an example of carcinoma arising in MGA, had glands lined by stratified cells with numerous lysosomal granules.

Genetics and Molecular Studies

More than 30 years after it was fully described, MGA continues to be a fascinating and somewhat puzzling lesion. Its genetic relationship to carcinoma has been the subject of few recent studies. The results suggest that MGA is a nonobligate morphologic precursor of some triple negative invasive carcinomas.

Shin et al.[56] used CGH to evaluate microdissected samples from 17 cases containing one or more MGA-related lesions, including MGA, atypical MGA, and MGA-associated carcinoma. They identified recurrent gains and losses in MGA (2q+, 5q−, 8q+, and 14q−) and atypical MGA (1q+, 5q−, 8q+, 14q−, and 15q−). Few additional alterations were found in MGA-associated carcinomas, including aberrations affecting numerous chromosomal arms. Based on these widespread alterations, together with recurrent loss of 5q and gain of 8q, the authors suggested that MGA-associated carcinomas are related to basal carcinomas. In addition, they identified concordant genetic alterations between MGA, atypical MGA, and MGA-associated carcinoma of the same cases, indicating progression from MGA to the more severe lesions. In particular, MGA, atypical MGA, and MGA-associated carcinoma coexisting in one case were found to be clonally related. The authors also reported c-myc amplification in 3 of 13 cases (32%).

Geyer et al.[51] used high-resolution microarray-based CGH to study 12 MGA-related lesions. One case also contained a basaloid DCIS involving a duct lined by myoepithelium. The authors found genetic alterations in all but three MGA cases, as well as in all samples of atypical MGA and MGA-associated carcinoma. On average, genomic alterations were found in 12% (median 9.2%, range 0.5% to 21.4%) of the genome in MGAs, in 21.4% (median 14.95%, range 9.2% to 46.3%) of the genome of atypical MGAs, and in 28.4% (median 26%, range 9.3% to 61.9%) of the genome of MGA-associated invasive carcinomas. Matched samples from the same patients showed greater concordance of genetic changes than samples from different patients in the same diagnostic category. This study found only low-level gains of the *MYC* locus in 8 out of 13 MGA and/or atypical MGA samples and no focal high-level amplification. Seven cases with a component of MGA without atypia were part of this series, including two cases of pure MGA. Four of the seven cases showed multiple genomic alterations, suggesting that the majority of cases of MGA without atypia are clonal, adenoma-like neoplastic lesions, even though they show no morphologic evidence of atypia.

Treatment and Prognosis

Excisional biopsy is always indicated when a needle core biopsy sample suggests MGA. At present, ordinary MGA is regarded as a morphologically benign proliferative lesion that is properly treated by local excision. Reexcision should be considered if the margins are found to be microscopically involved, since little is known about the long-term course of incompletely excised MGA. In one case, a patient was treated by lumpectomy for intraductal and invasive duct carcinoma arising in MGA.[60] The lumpectomy margins were involved by MGA but not by carcinoma. The patient received no radiation or chemotherapy. A mass detected in the same region of the breast 10 years later proved to be intraductal carcinoma in residual MGA.

The term "atypical" has been introduced to describe some examples of MGA with uncertain biologic potential. Patients with atypical MGA should undergo wide excision with histologically documented negative margins. Reexcision is strongly recommended if the margins of the initial excision are involved, and careful clinical follow-up should be instituted so that treatment can be started promptly should carcinoma develop.

Carcinoma has been found in over 30% of patients with MGA.[50,51,55,56,61,62] In almost all cases, the carcinoma arose within the MGA lesion. The high proportion of cases of MGA associated with carcinoma may be biased by the fact that some instances were identified because of the distinctive growth pattern of the MGA-associated carcinoma. One unusual patient had coincidental but separate foci of MGA and carcinoma in one breast.[49] Another exceptional situation involved a patient with benign MGA in one breast who developed infiltrating duct carcinoma not associated with MGA in the contralateral breast.[61]

In one study,[61] lymph node metastases were found in 3 of 11 axillary dissections (Fig. 7.39). Ten patients treated by mastectomy were recurrence free with median follow-up of 57 months (3 to 108 months). Two of three patients treated by excisional surgery were recurrence free 12 and 105 months later. The third woman had bone metastases at 51 months and was alive at 98 months posttreatment.

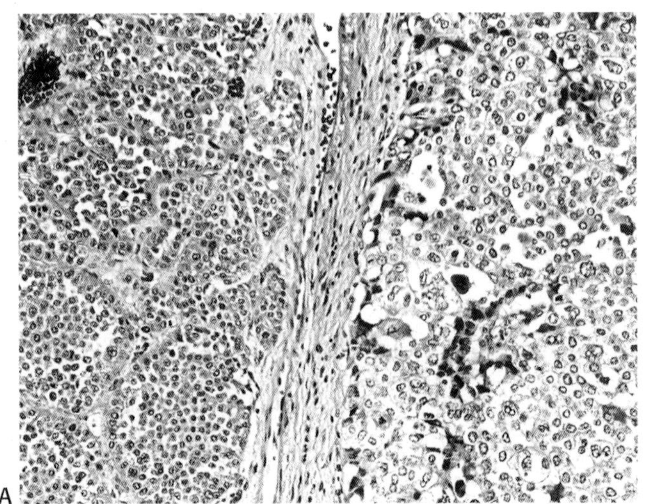
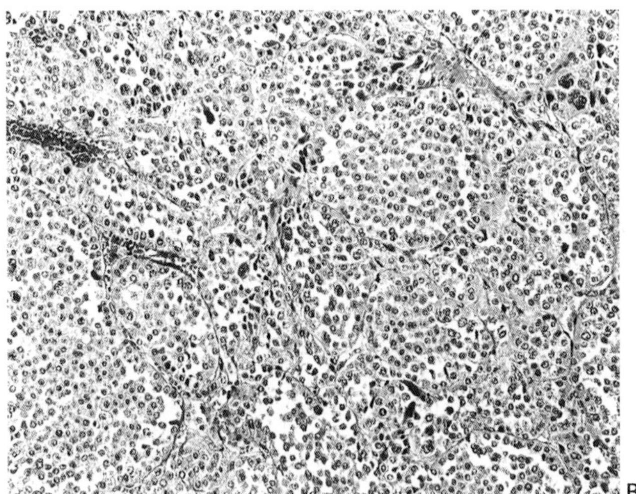

FIG. 7.39. ***Metastatic carcinoma.*** **A:** Invasive carcinoma with two cytologic appearances that arose in MGA. **B:** Carcinoma metastatic from the tumor shown in (**A**) in an axillary lymph node. (Reproduced from Rosen PP. Microglandular adenosis. *Am J Surg Pathol* 1983;7:137–144.)

Khalifeh et al.[50] reported that two of six patients with MGA-associated carcinoma presented with distant metastases. One patient had only bone metastases, whereas the other had widespread systemic involvement, with metastases to axillary lymph nodes, brain, bone, and spinal cord. The metastases were morphologically similar to the primary carcinoma.

On the basis of published reports with limited data and a median follow-up of nearly 5 years, it appears that patients with MGA-associated carcinomas have a relatively favorable outcome despite histopathologic and immunohistochemical features of basal-like carcinoma that is usually associated with a poor prognosis. It is therefore prudent to predicate the treatment of carcinoma arising in MGA on the stage of disease in the individual patient. Because of the insidiously invasive character of MGA, carcinoma arising in this condition is likely to extend microscopically well beyond the grossly apparent tumor. It may, therefore, be difficult to achieve negative margins in some instances. When breast conservation is selected, radiotherapy should be added. Adjuvant chemotherapy is recommended for patients with axillary lymph node metastases or with invasive tumors larger than 1 cm in the absence of nodal metastases.

REFERENCES

Adenosis

1. Ewing J. Epithelial tumors of the breast. *Neoplastic diseases: a textbook on tumors.* Philadelphia: WB Saunders, 1919.
2. Foote FW, Stewart FW. Comparative studies of cancerous versus noncancerous breasts. *Ann Surg* 1945;121:197–222.
3. Urban JA, Adair FE. Sclerosing adenosis. *Cancer* 1949;2:625–634.
4. Heller EL, Fleming JC. Fibrosing adenomatosis of the breast. *Am J Clin Pathol* 1950;20:141–146.
5. Markopoulos C, Kouskos E, Phillipidis T, et al. Adenosis tumor of the breast. *Breast J* 2003;9:255–256.
6. Haagensen C. *Adenosis tumor.* Philadelphia: WB Saunders, 1971.
7. Nielsen BB. Adenosis tumour of the breast—a clinicopathological investigation of 27 cases. *Histopathology* 1987;11:1259–1275.
8. Taskin F, Koseoglu K, Unsal A, et al. Sclerosing adenosis of the breast: radiologic appearance and efficiency of core needle biopsy. *Diagn Interv Radiol* 2011;17:311–316.
9. Oztekin PS, Tuncbilek I, Kosar P, et al. Nodular sclerosing adenosis mimicking malignancy in the breast: magnetic resonance imaging findings. *Breast J* 2011;17:95–97.
10. Gill HK, Ioffe OB, Berg WA. When is a diagnosis of sclerosing adenosis acceptable at core biopsy? *Radiology* 2003;228:50–57.
11. Eusebi V, Azzopardi JG. Vascular infiltration in benign breast disease. *J Pathol* 1976;118:9–16.
12. Taylor HB, Norris HJ. Epithelial invasion of nerves in benign diseases of the breast. *Cancer* 1967;20:2245–2249.
13. Davies JD. Neural invasion in benign mammary dysplasia. *J Pathol* 1973;225–231.
14. Simpson JF, Page DL, Dupont WD. Apocrine adenosis—a mimic of mammary carcinoma. *Surg Pathol* 1990;3:289–299.
15. Carter DJ, Rosen PP. Atypical apocrine metaplasia in sclerosing lesions of the breast: a study of 51 patients. *Mod Pathol* 1991;4:1–5.
16. Seidman JD, Ashton M, Lefkowitz M. Atypical apocrine adenosis of the breast: a clinicopathologic study of 37 patients with 8.7-year follow-up. *Cancer* 1996;77:2529–2537.
17. Selim AG, El-Ayat G, Wells CA. Expression of c-erbB2, p53, Bcl-2, Bax, c-myc and Ki-67 in apocrine metaplasia and apocrine change within sclerosing adenosis of the breast. *Virchows Arch* 2002;441:449–455.
18. Celis JE, Moreira JM, Gromova I, et al. Characterization of breast precancerous lesions and myoepithelial hyperplasia in sclerosing adenosis with apocrine metaplasia. *Mol Oncol* 2007;1:97–119.
19. Celis JE, Gromov P, Moreira JM, et al. Apocrine cysts of the breast: biomarkers, origin, enlargement, and relation with cancer phenotype. *Mol Cell Proteomics* 2006;5:462–483.
20. Elayat G, Selim AG, Wells CA. Cell cycle alterations and their relationship to proliferation in apocrine adenosis of the breast. *Histopathology* 2009;54:348–354.
21. Elayat G, Selim AG, Wells CA. Cell turnover in apocrine metaplasia and apocrine adenosis of the breast. *Ann Diagn Pathol* 2010;14:1–7.
22. Lee KC, Chan JK, Gwi E. Tubular adenosis of the breast. A distinctive benign lesion mimicking invasive carcinoma. *Am J Surg Pathol* 1996;20:46–54.
23. Oberman HA, Markey BA. Noninvasive carcinoma of the breast presenting in adenosis. *Mod Pathol* 1991;4:31–35.
24. Fechner RE. Lobular carcinoma *in situ* in sclerosing adenosis. A potential source of confusion with invasive carcinoma. *Am J Surg Pathol* 1981;5:233–239.

25. Abati AD, Kimmel M, Rosen PP. Apocrine mammary carcinoma. A clinicopathologic study of 72 cases. *Am J Clin Pathol* 1990;94:371–377.
26. Moritani S, Ichihara S, Hasegawa M, et al. Topographical, morphological and immunohistochemical characteristics of carcinoma *in situ* of the breast involving sclerosing adenosis. Two distinct topographical patterns and histological types of carcinoma *in situ*. *Histopathology* 2011;58:835–846.
27. Eusebi V, Collina G, Bussolati G. Carcinoma *in situ* in sclerosing adenosis of the breast: an immunocytochemical study. *Semin Diagn Pathol* 1989;6:146–152.
28. Hilson JB, Schnitt SJ, Collins LC. Phenotypic alterations in myoepithelial cells associated with benign sclerosing lesions of the breast. *Am J Surg Pathol* 2010;34:896–900.
29. Prasad ML, Osborne MP, Hoda SA. Observations on the histopathologic diagnosis of microinvasive carcinoma of the breast. *Anat Pathol* 1998;3:209–232.
30. Silverman JF, Dabbs DJ, Gilbert CF. Fine needle aspiration cytology of adenosis tumor of the breast. With immunocytochemical and ultrastructural observations. *Acta Cytol* 1989;33:181–187.
31. Wellings SR, Roberts P. Electron microscopy of sclerosing adenosis and infiltrating duct carcinoma of the human mammary gland. *J Natl Cancer Inst* 1963;30:269–287.
32. Jao W, Recant W, Swerdlow MA. Comparative ultrastructure of tubular carcinoma and sclerosing adenosis of the breast. *Cancer* 1976;38:180–186.
33. Da Silva L, Buck L, Simpson PT, et al. Molecular and morphological analysis of adenoid cystic carcinoma of the breast with synchronous tubular adenosis. *Virchows Arch* 2009;454:107–114.
34. Kern WH, Brooks RN. Atypical epithelial hyperplasia associated with breast cancer and fibrocystic disease. *Cancer* 1969;24:668–675.
35. Page DL, Vander Zwaag R, Rogers LW, et al. Relation between component parts of fibrocystic disease complex and breast cancer. *J Natl Cancer Inst* 1978;61:1055–1063.
36. Dupont WD, Page DL. Risk factors for breast cancer in women with proliferative breast disease. *N Engl J Med* 1985;312:146–151.
37. Jensen RA, Page DL, Dupont WD, et al. Invasive breast cancer risk in women with sclerosing adenosis. *Cancer* 1989;64:1977–1983.
38. Bodian CA, Perzin KH, Lattes R, et al. Prognostic significance of benign proliferative breast disease. *Cancer* 1993;71:3896–3907.
39. Carter CL, Corle DK, Micozzi MS, et al. A prospective study of the development of breast cancer in 16,692 women with benign breast disease. *Am J Epidemiol* 1988;128:467–477.
40. Hutchinson WB, Thomas DB, Hamlin WB, et al. Risk of breast cancer in women with benign breast disease. *J Natl Cancer Inst* 1980;65:13–20.
41. Kodlin D, Winger EE, Morgenstern NL, et al. Chronic mastopathy and breast cancer. A follow-up study. *Cancer* 1977;39:2603–2607.
42. Krieger N, Hiatt RA. Risk of breast cancer after benign breast diseases. Variation by histologic type, degree of atypia, age at biopsy, and length of follow-up. *Am J Epidemiol* 1992;135:619–631.
43. Fuehrer N, Hartmann L, Degnim A, et al. Atypical apocrine adenosis of the breast: long-term follow-up in 37 patients. *Arch Pathol Lab Med* 2012;136:179–182.

Microglandular Adenosis

44. Linell F, Ljungberg O, Andersson I. Breast carcinoma. Aspects of early stages, progression and related problems. *Acta Pathol Microbiol Scand Suppl* 1980;(272):1–233.
45. McDivitt RW, Stewart FW, Berg JW. *Tumors of the breast. (AFIP Atlas of Tumour Pathology,* 2nd series, vol 2) Bethesda: American Registry of Pathology, 1968.
46. Rosen PP. *Microglandular adenosis.* No AP11-12(1977). Chicago: American Society of Clinical Pathologists, 1978.
47. Clement PB, Azzopardi JG. Microglandular adenosis of the breast—a lesion simulating tubular carcinoma. *Histopathology* 1983;7:169–180.
48. Rosen PP. Microglandular adenosis. A benign lesion simulating invasive mammary carcinoma. *Am J Surg Pathol* 1983;7:137–144.
49. Tavassoli FA, Norris HJ. Microglandular adenosis of the breast. A clinicopathologic study of 11 cases with ultrastructural observations. *Am J Surg Pathol* 1983;7:731–737.
50. Khalifeh IM, Albarracin C, Diaz LK, et al. Clinical, histopathologic, and immunohistochemical features of microglandular adenosis and transition into *in situ* and invasive carcinoma. *Am J Surg Pathol* 2008;32:544–552.
51. Geyer FC, Lacroix-Triki M, Colombo PE, et al. Molecular evidence in support of the neoplastic and precursor nature of microglandular adenosis. *Histopathology* 2012;60:E115–E130.
52. Kim DJ, Sun WY, Ryu DH, et al. Microglandular adenosis. *J Breast Cancer* 2011;14:72–75.
53. Kay S. Microglandular adenosis of the female mammary gland: study of a case with ultrastructural observations. *Hum Pathol* 1985;16:637–641.
54. Sabate JM, Gomez A, Torrubia S, et al. Microglandular adenosis of the breast in a BRCA1 mutation carrier: radiological features. *Eur Radiol* 2002;12:1479–1482.
55. Koenig C, Dadmanesh F, Bratthauer GL, et al. Carcinoma arising in microglandular adenosis: an immunohistochemical analysis of 20 intraepithelial and invasive neoplasms. *Int J Surg Pathol* 2000;8:303–315.
56. Shin SJ, Simpson PT, Da Silva L, et al. Molecular evidence for progression of microglandular adenosis (MGA) to invasive carcinoma. *Am J Surg Pathol* 2009;33:496–504.
57. Shui R, Yang W. Invasive breast carcinoma arising in microglandular adenosis: a case report and review of the literature. *Breast J* 2009;15:653–656.
58. Shui R, Bi R, Cheng Y, et al. Matrix-producing carcinoma of the breast in the Chinese population: a clinicopathological study of 13 cases. *Pathol Int* 2011;61:415–422.
59. Geyer FC, Kushner YB, Lambros MB, et al. Microglandular adenosis or microglandular adenoma? A molecular genetic analysis of a case associated with atypia and invasive carcinoma. *Histopathology* 2009;55:732–743.
60. Resetkova E, Flanders DJ, Rosen PP. Ten-year follow-up of mammary carcinoma arising in microglandular adenosis treated with breast conservation. *Arch Pathol Lab Med* 2003;127:77–80.
61. James BA, Cranor ML, Rosen PP. Carcinoma of the breast arising in microglandular adenosis. *Am J Clin Pathol* 1993;100:507–513.
62. Rosenblum MK, Purrazzella R, Rosen PP. Is microglandular adenosis a precancerous disease? A study of carcinoma arising therein. *Am J Surg Pathol* 1986;10:237–245.
63. Lin L, Pathmanathan N. Microglandular adenosis with transition to breast carcinoma: a series of three cases. *Pathology* 2011;43:498–503.
64. Damiani S, Pasquinelli G, Lamovec J, et al. Acinic cell carcinoma of the breast: an immunohistochemical and ultrastructural study. *Virchows Arch* 2000;437:74–81.
65. Coyne JD, Dervan PA. Primary acinic cell carcinoma of the breast. *J Clin Pathol* 2002;55:545–547.
66. Evans AT, Hussein KA. A microglandular adenosis-like lesion simulating tubular adenocarcinoma of the breast. A case report with cytological and histological appearances. *Cytopathology* 1990;1:311–316.
67. Gherardi G, Bernardi C, Marveggio C. Microglandular adenosis of the breast: fine-needle aspiration biopsy of two cases. *Diagn Cytopathol* 1993;9:72–76.
68. Eusebi V, Foschini MP, Betts CM, et al. Microglandular adenosis, apocrine adenosis, and tubular carcinoma of the breast. An immunohistochemical comparison. *Am J Surg Pathol* 1993;17:99–109.
69. Cserni G. Presence of basement membrane material around the tubules of tubulolobular carcinoma. *Breast Care (Basel)* 2008;3:423–425.

CHAPTER 8

Fibroepithelial Neoplasms

EDI BROGI

SCLEROSING LOBULAR HYPERPLASIA (FIBROADENOMATOID MASTOPATHY)

Clinical Presentation

This benign proliferative lesion presents as a localized tumor spanning up to 8 cm in diameter (mean, approximately 4 cm), usually in the upper outer quadrant of the breast.[1,2] Skin retraction and pain are absent, but the tumor may be tender. The most frequent mammographic finding is a well-defined mass. Microcalcifications may be present.[3] Asymptomatic examples have been detected by mammography.[2] The imaging characteristics are not sufficiently specific to distinguish sclerosing lobular hyperplasia from a fibroadenoma (FA).

Patients range in age from 12[4] to 46[5] years, with a mean age of about 32 years. There is no significant association with oral contraceptive use.

Gross and Microscopic Pathology

The excised specimen is composed of firm, nodular tan tissue with a granular appearance on the cut surface. Microscopic examination reveals enlarged lobules composed of an increased number of intralobular glands. The intralobular stroma is collagenized with loss of stromal mucopolysaccharide, and the interlobular stroma shows variable sclerosis (Fig. 8.1). Individual lobules and groups of lobules have the appearance of miniature FAs with a prominent glandular component. The lobular glands have distinct epithelial and myoepithelial components, each composed of a single layer of cells. Secretory activity may be present, and calcifications are typically not formed.

Sclerosing lobular hyperplasia or fibroadenomatoid mastopathy is found in breast tissue surrounding about 50% of FAs and most phyllodes tumors (PTs).[1] This association suggests that the same or related factors contribute to the pathogenesis of these lesions. The ratio of sclerosing lobular hyperplasia to FA in one series was 9.3:1, a relationship consistent with the hypothesis that some FAs arise as localized foci of accelerated proliferation in a background of sclerosing lobular hyperplasia.[1] Because a FA or PT presents clinically as a dominant mass, its association with sclerosing lobular hyperplasia may be overlooked clinically and pathologically. The occurrence of sclerosing lobular hyperplasia forming a mass by itself is an uncommon event.

Treatment and Prognosis

A diagnosis of sclerosing lobular hyperplasia is usually not made preoperatively, and most of these patients have a clinical diagnosis of FA or fibrocystic change (FCC). Excisional biopsy of the palpable lesion is adequate therapy. There is no systematic follow-up study documenting the frequency of recurrence. Anecdotal experience suggests that recurrence in the form of a FA is very infrequent but that this condition may contribute to the syndrome of multiple recurrent FAs.

FIBROADENOMA

These benign tumors arise from the epithelium and stroma of the terminal duct lobular unit (TDLU). They are the most common breast tumors clinically and pathologically in adolescent and young women.

Risk Factors

Risk factors for developing FAs have not been investigated extensively. Canny et al.[6] carried out a case-control study of 251 women with FAs in Connecticut. Women younger than 45 years with FAs were less likely than controls to have taken contraceptives. This difference was not observed in women older than 45 years when a FA was diagnosed. Conversely, there was a significant positive correlation between FAs and exogenous estrogen replacement therapy regardless of age. The risk of developing a FA among users of oral contraceptives is not related to the extent of epithelial atypia present in the FA.[7] A case-control study of Australian women reported a direct association between contraceptive use before age 20 and the risk of developing a FA.[8] Risk was inversely related to the body mass index and the number of full-term pregnancies. Use of estrogen replacement therapy was not significantly related to the presence of FAs in this series.

Although lesions diagnosed as juvenile FAs have been reported in patients with the Beckwith–Wiedemann syndrome,[9,10] the histologic features of the FA lesions were not described in detail or illustrated, and the clinical appearance was consistent with other entities such as pseudoangiomatous stromal hyperplasia (PASH). In one instance,[9]

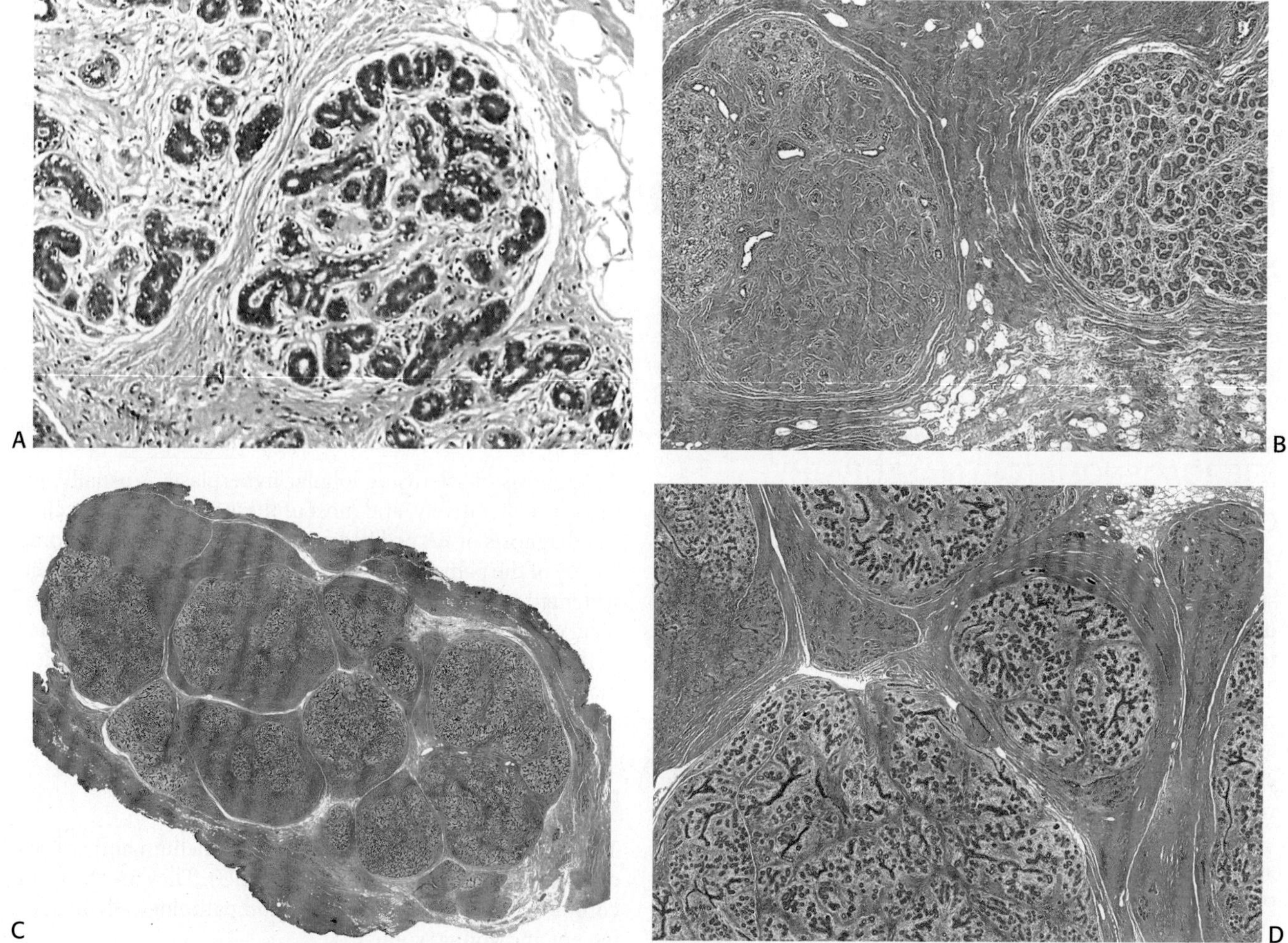

FIG. 8.1. ***Fibroadenomatoid mastopathy (sclerosing lobular hyperplasia).*** **A:** The tumor is composed of enlarged lobules. **B:** In this case, one lobule with sclerotic stroma has the appearance of a small FA. **C,D:** Two views of another example of fibroadenomatoid mastopathy.

a 5-cm unilateral mass excised from the left breast of a 7-month-old girl was diagnosed as "a benign juvenile FA." Ten months later, a recurrent nodule was excised and classified as "a juvenile intracanalicular FA." Another female patient presented with bilateral macromastia at the age of 12.[10] Imaging revealed "multiple, well-defined hyper dense masses in both breasts." Six masses were excised from the right breast, and a left subcutaneous mastectomy yielded a 2185-g specimen. The pathology findings were described as "benign breast parenchyma with epithelial hyperplasia and stromal fibrosis, which was consistent with FAs." It is noteworthy that the authors of the latter case report commented on the similarity of their patient's condition to "juvenile gigantomastia" that is almost always a manifestation of PASH (see Chapter 38).

Multiple bilateral FAs diagnosed simultaneously in two adolescent female identical twins have been described, but the lesions were not subjected to cytogenetic analysis.[11] Women with Carney syndrome may develop myxoid FAs,[12] but it is unknown what percentage of women with myxoid FA also have Carney syndrome.

Rare examples of FAs have been reported in men.[13–18] FAs arising in the male breast usually occur in the context of gynecomastia. Most have been associated with treatment with various medications, such as estrogen or hormone modulators in patients with prostatic carcinoma, hormone treatments in male-to-female transsexuals, and use of spironolactone. It is exceedingly unusual for a FA to arise in the male breast in the absence of gynecomastia and/or the administration of predisposing drugs. Shin and Rosen[19] reported a case of bilateral FAs with digital fibroma-like inclusions in a 66-year-old man treated for prostate carcinoma.

Patients who receive cyclosporin A treatment for immunosuppression after organ transplantation are predisposed to develop FAs.[20–22] The tumors are typically bilateral and multiple. The duration of cyclosporin A treatment prior to the detection of a FA is generally more than a year, with a mean interval of 4.4 ± 1.7 years (range, 1.7 to 7.1 years) in one study.[22] When compared with FAs found in control women who did not undergo transplantation or cyclosporin A treatment, cyclosporin A–related tumors were significantly larger and had a lower longitudinal to anterior–posterior ratio on imaging.[22] Multiple bilateral fibroepithelial lesions developed in a 15-year-old girl maintained for over a year on cyclosporin-based immunosuppressive treatment after liver transplantation for Wilson disease.[23] The largest tumor was 8 cm in size and caused ulceration in the nipple–areolar region. The largest contralateral tumor measured 5 cm. Additional smaller tumor nodules were also present bilaterally. Histologically, the lesions were classified as low-grade (borderline) malignant PTs, but "little" mitotic activity was described, and there was "no apparent heteromorphism of the nuclei," leading the authors to acknowledge difficulty in distinguishing the lesions from FAs. The representative histologic images of this case are highly suggestive of juvenile FA. Iaria et al.[24] reported complete regression of 8/21 FAs in eight renal transplant patients after "cyclosporine" was replaced with "tacrolimus," another immunosuppressive drug. The other FAs remained stable or decreased in size at a mean follow-up of 41.8 months (range 25 to 57). It is unclear whether Epstein–Barr virus is[25] or is not[26] associated with the FAs that develop in immunocompromised patients.

Clinical Presentation

Age and Hormonal Status

The age distribution for FAs ranges from childhood to more than 70 years of age, with a mean age of about 30 years and a median of about 25 years.[27] Less than 5% of women with a FA as their presenting tumor are older than 50 years or are postmenopausal. In a series of 709 consecutive breast biopsies, FA constituted 14% of all lesions, and 44% occurred in postmenopausal women.[28] FAs accounted for 20% of benign masses and 12% of all masses in postmenopausal patients. A study of FAs from premenopausal women found no difference in mitotic index or nuclear volume in FAs obtained in the luteal and secretory menstrual phases.[29] The authors concluded that fibroadenomatous epithelium is independent of the cyclic action of circulating hormones and influenced mainly by paracrine factors. Rego et al.[30] correlated the epithelial changes in FAs with menstrual date reported by the patient and with serum progesterone levels on the day of surgical biopsy. This study found no significant variation in Ki67 indexes in the epithelium of FA in the follicular phase (27.88 ± 27.52 positive nuclei per 1,000 cells) and in the luteal phase (37.88 ± 31.08 positive nuclei per 1,000 cells). The authors concluded that the absence of cyclical proliferative fluctuations in the epithelium of FAs suggests that it represents a neoplasm. Others, however, have observed focal cytologic alterations in the epithelium of FAs compatible with hormonal effect, including secretory changes.[31–33]

Patients with juvenile FAs tend to be younger than the average age for adult FAs, with the majority younger than 20 years of age[34–36] (Fig. 8.2). Juvenile FAs constituted 45% of the tumors in a series of 47 consecutive fibroepithelial lesions in children and adolescent women (age less than 18 years),[36] but tumors with the histologic features of juvenile FA have been found in adult women as old as 72 years.[37] Juvenile FAs can also occur at a very young age. A 3-cm tumor morphologically consistent with juvenile FA has been described in a 16-month-old girl.[38]

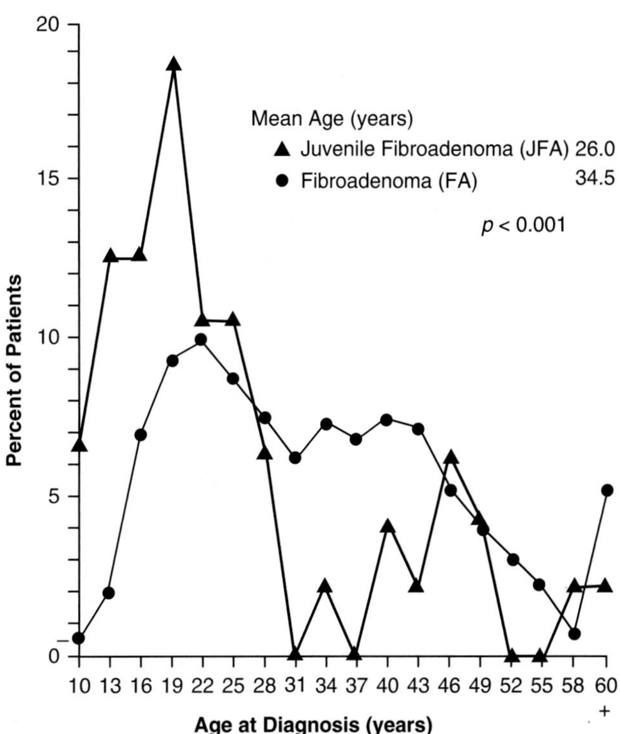

FIG. 8.2. ***Age distribution of typical and juvenile fibroadenomas.*** Juvenile FAs have a lower mean age and biphasic age distribution. [Reprinted from Mies C, Rosen PP. Juvenile fibroadenoma with atypical epithelial hyperplasia. *Am J Surg Pathol* 1987;11:184–190, with permission.]

Patients with complex FA tend to be older than women with noncomplex FAs. Kuijper et al.[39] reported a mean age of 34.5 years. In the series by Sklair-Levy et al.,[40] the median age of patients with complex FA (47 years; range 21 to 69) was significantly higher than the median age of patients with noncomplex FAs (28.5 years; range 12 to 86) ($p < 0.001$).

Clinical Symptoms

In most cases, the presenting symptom is a painless, firm or rubbery, well-circumscribed, solitary mass found by the patient. An increasing percentage of FAs are nonpalpable tumors detected by mammography. The left breast is affected slightly more often than the right, and the single most frequent location is the upper outer quadrant.[27] Multiple FAs occur in about 15% of patients, with equal proportions detected synchronously and metachronously in the same or opposite breast. Foster et al.[27] found that 36% of metachronous FAs developed in the same quadrant as the first FA after a mean interval of about 4 years. FAs can arise in supernumerary breast tissue on the chest wall[33] or in the vulva,[33,41,42] as well as in axillary breast tissue, where they can clinically mimic neoplastic lymphadenopathy.

Most patients with a juvenile FA present with a single, painless, discrete mass that may grow rapidly[36] and sometimes becomes large enough to cause marked asymmetry.

In one study consisting of only African American women ranging in age from 10 to 39 years old, 8 patients had more than one lesion, and 13 had a solitary tumor.[34] The age distribution and median age of individuals with single and multiple tumors were similar at the time of first operation. The frequency of recurrences decreases in early adulthood, and lesions that are not excised may stop growing in adulthood, remaining stable even during pregnancy.[35]

Another uncommon syndrome occurring in adolescence is the metachronous and synchronous development of multiple FAs, usually in both breasts. This condition occurs more often in adolescent African-American girls than in White or Asian girls.[43] Despite repeated excision, new tumors are formed, probably because the breast tissue exhibits diffuse fibroadenomatoid hyperplasia. The familial occurrence of multiple successive FAs has been observed.

Radiology

FAs and cysts may be indistinguishable on palpation and also by mammography (Fig. 8.3). Large and coarse calcifications are not uncommon in FAs after menopause. Most FAs have ultrasound features of a benign tumor. Fleury et al.[44] reported that they could separate usual FAs from complex and hypercellular FAs using sonoelastography. Adamietz et al.[45] reported that sonoelastography could help differentiate FA from PT. All PTs in their study showed an elastic center surrounded by inelastic peripheral tissue (also referred to as "ring sign"), while this pattern was present in only 5% of FAs. These observations need to be validated in larger series. A minority of FAs, including lactating adenomas, have irregular margins, a heterogeneous appearance, and posterior shadowing on ultrasonography, which may suggest a malignant tumor.[46] Yamaguchi et al.[47] reported that FAs with myxoid changes show significantly greater depth-to-width ratio than usual FAs when examined by sonography. In their series, 16/17 lesions sonographically suspicious for mucinous carcinoma due to rapid growth, large size, high depth-to-width ratio, round shape, and internal hyperechogenicity were found to be myxoid FAs at the time of surgical excision.

The magnetic resonance imaging (MRI) appearance of FAs is variable and influenced by the structure and relative proportions of epithelial and stromal components.[48,49] Wurdinger et al.[50] studied 81 FAs using MRI and found that 70.4% had well-defined margins, 90.1% were round or lobulated, 49.4% had heterogeneous internal structure, and 27.2%

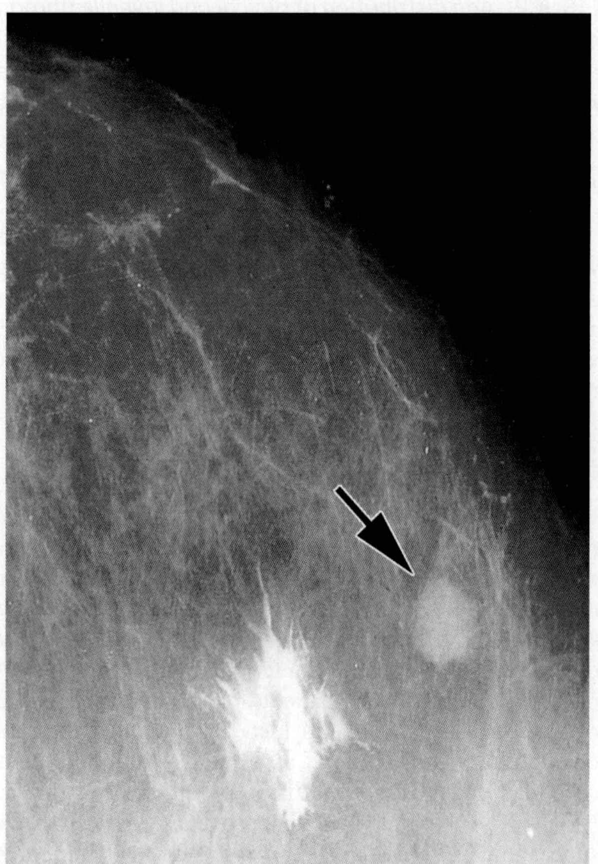

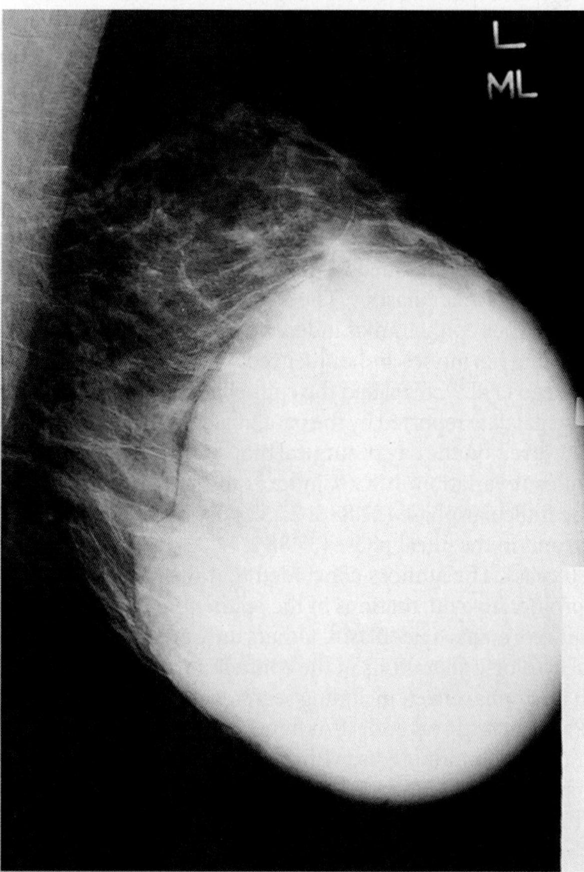

FIG. 8.3. ***Fibroadenoma.*** **A:** The nonpalpable tumor was detected as a homogeneous, oval, circumscribed mass on this mammogram (*arrow*). The stellate white focus is the site of dye injected for localization of the lesion at surgery. **B:** This FA nearly fills the right breast of an 18-year-old girl in a medial-lateral view.

displayed nonenhancing internal septations. After contrast injection, 22.2% of FAs had a suspicious signal intensity–time course. ^{18}F-FDG uptake can occur in a FA undergoing rapid growth and proliferation. A "juvenile FA" positive on ^{111}In-octreotide scan and ^{18}F-FDG-positron emission tomogram/computerized tomogram has been described in a 14-year-old girl with an abdominal neuroendocrine tumor. The histology of the breast tumor was not reported.[51]

Size

Most FAs are not larger than 3 cm (Fig. 8.4). In one series, only 10% of the tumors were larger than 4 cm.[27] FAs larger than 4 cm are significantly more frequent in patients 20 years or younger than in older patients.[27] An occasional tumor may grow to involve most or the entire breast. These tumors, often referred to as adolescent or giant FAs, develop as solitary or multiple masses shortly after puberty[43,52] (Fig. 8.5). One or both breasts can be affected.

In one series, the mean sizes of solitary and multiple juvenile FAs were 2.8 and 2.2 cm, respectively, with the largest tumor measuring 13 cm in a patient with multiple lesions. Others have reported solitary tumors up to 22 cm in diameter.[35]

Sklair-Levy et al.[40] reported that the average size of complex FAs (1.3 ± 0.57 cm; range 0.5 to 2.6) was about half that of usual FAs (2.5 ± 1.44 cm; range 21 to 69) ($p < 0.001$).

Gross Pathology

FAs are often excised by using blunt dissection to peel away the surrounding tissue. The outer surface of a "shelled out" FA has a smooth, bosselated contour. The cut surface of the bisected tumor is composed of bulging, firm, and gray, white, or tan tissue (Fig. 8.4). A minority of FAs have a myxoid or gelatinous appearance. Some tumors appear to be composed of multiple aggregated nodules divided by septa. Extremely rare FAs contain a lipomatous component (fibroadenolipoma) (Fig. 8.4).

On gross examination with a magnifying glass, very fine clefts in the tissue can be identified in the cut surface of some tumors, but these clefts are infrequently pronounced. Discrete round cysts are sometimes present, measuring

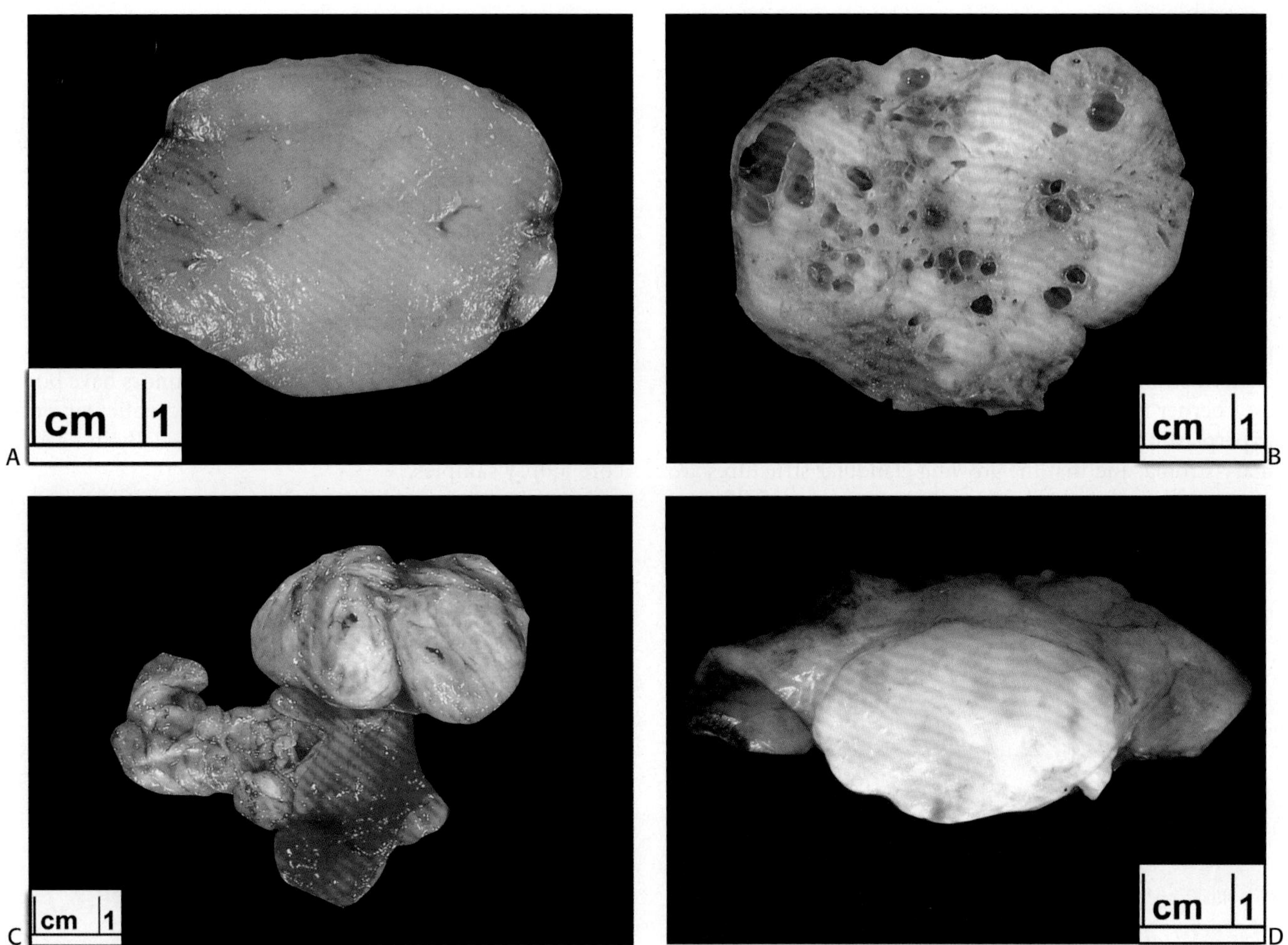

FIG. 8.4. ***Fibroadenomas.*** **A:** Relatively homogenous cut surface. **B:** Multiple cysts are present. **C:** Two adjacent FAs, the larger of which, *above*, is solid in contrast to the smaller, centrally placed, partly cystic tumor. **D:** Gross appearance of FA in which there are patches of adipose tissue.

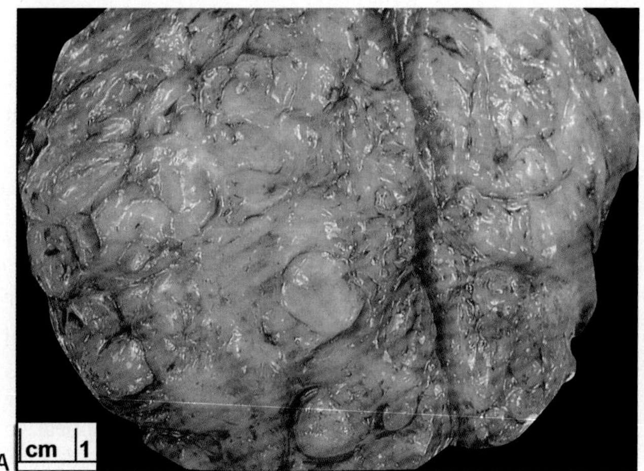

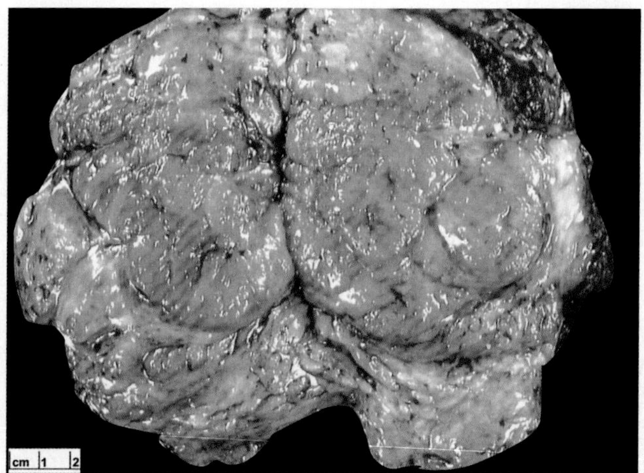

FIG. 8.5. ***Fibroadenomas in young girls.*** **A,B:** The tumors measured more than 10 cm. The cut surface is fleshy and numerous clefts are noted. These FAs could be described as "giant FAs." The patients were 11 and 14 years old.

1 mm to 1 cm or more in diameter, and rarely the tumor is so cystic that it grossly resembles a cystic papilloma (Figs. 8.4 and 8.6).

Juvenile FAs are grossly indistinguishable from the adult variety of the tumor.[34]

Microscopic Pathology

The origin of a FA from the TDLU was elegantly demonstrated by Demetrakopoulos[53] using a serial-section reconstruction technique. The stroma was found to cause numerous invaginations in the walls of branches of the duct within the tumor corresponding to the intracanalicular pattern seen in histologic sections. The significance of specialized stroma in the growth of FAs has been emphasized by Koerner and O'Connell,[54] who suggested that a FA is a hyperplastic lesion of the specialized (intralobular) mammary stroma, and that the growing glandular structures are secondarily distorted by the stromal proliferation. These observations confirm the long-held view that FAs are formed as a result of proliferation of stroma around the terminal duct and within the lobule.[55]

The histologic hallmark of all FAs is concurrent proliferation of glandular and stromal elements. The growth pattern has been referred to as either intracanalicular or pericanalicular. The *intracanalicular pattern* is produced when the stroma is sufficiently abundant to compress ducts into elongated linear branching structures with slit-like lumens (Fig. 8.7A,B). When the ducts are separated by expanded stroma but they retain the original round profile, the architecture has a *pericanalicular pattern* (Fig. 8.7C,D). These structural features have no prognostic or clinical significance, and many tumors have both components. FAs with a prominent intracanalicular pattern may be mistaken for benign PTs, especially in needle core biopsy samples.

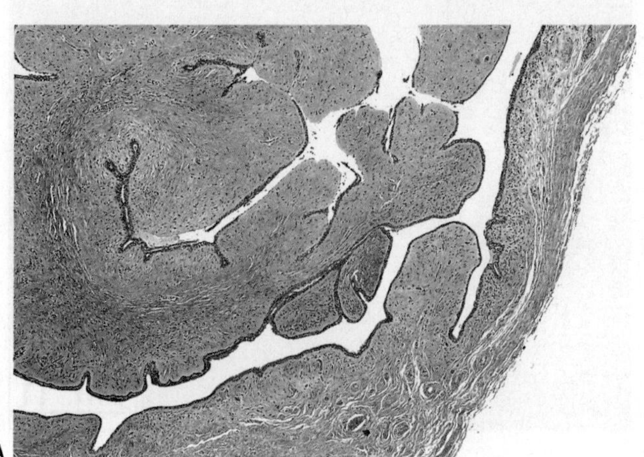

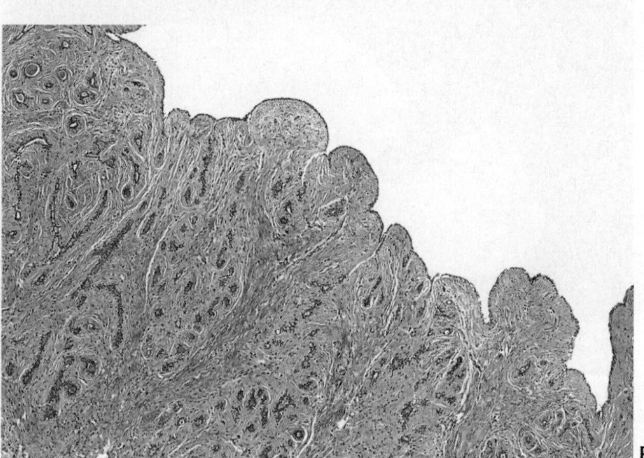

FIG. 8.6. ***Fibroadenomas, cystic.*** **A,B:** Whole-mount sections of cystic FAs. The tumor in **(A)** has fibrotic stroma, and adenosis is shown in **(B)**. These tumors may superficially resemble papillomas, but the fronds are solid, with no discernible fibrovascular cores.

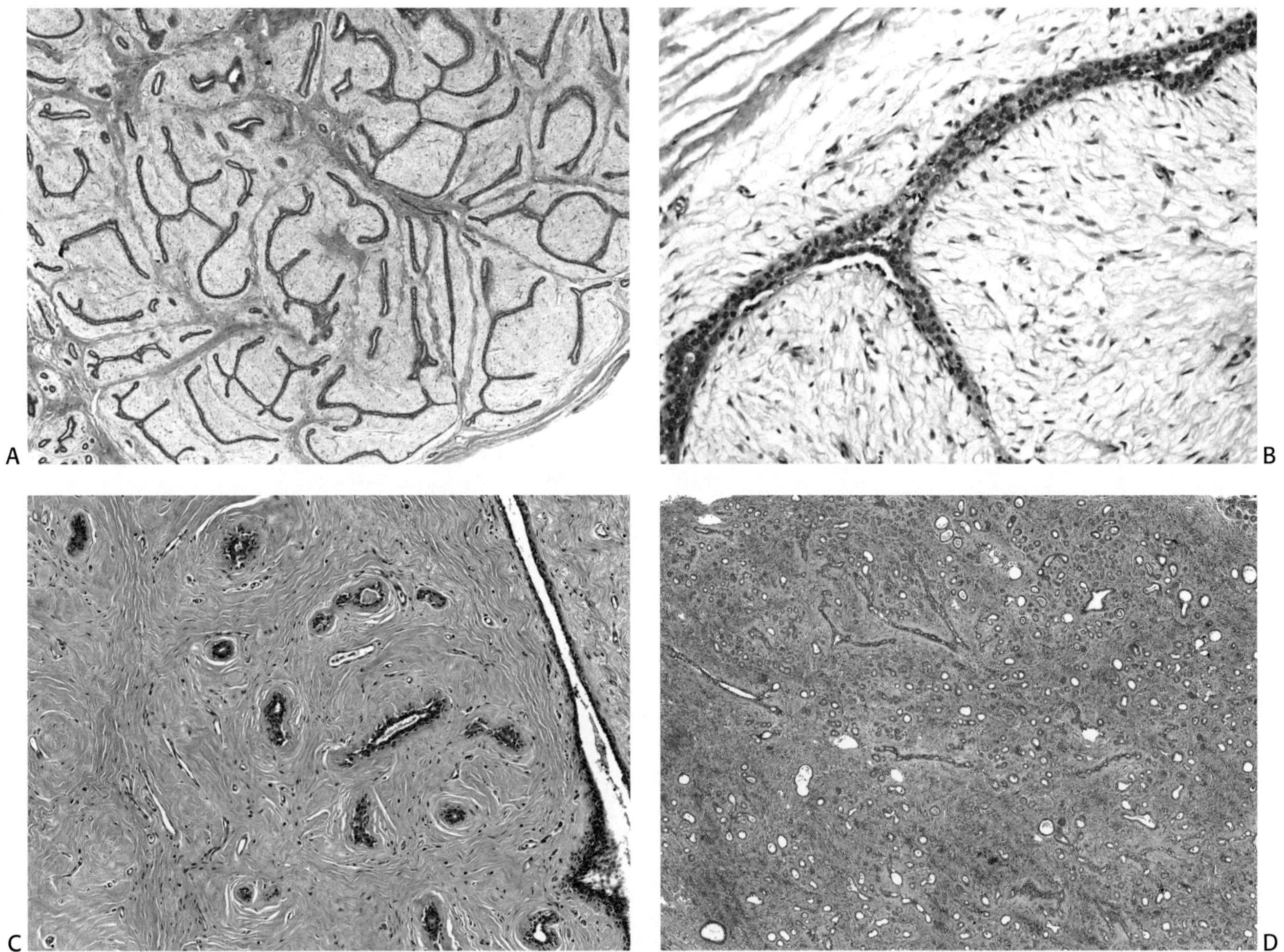

FIG. 8.7. ***Intracanalicular and pericanalicular patterns.*** **A,B:** When the lesional stroma stretches the lobular units and ducts into elongated tubular structures and compresses the glandular lumen, the pattern is referred to as intracanalicular. It commonly occurs in usual (adult-type) FAs, as depicted in this example. **C,D:** When the lesional stroma is expanded but does not bulge into the glandular lumen, and the latter maintains a round outline, the growth pattern is described as pericanalicular. These examples are from an adult-type FA **(C)** and a juvenile FA **(D)**.

Several terms have been used to subclassify FAs. More than 90% of FAs are of the adult/usual type, with the remainder fulfilling criteria for a diagnosis of juvenile FA or other unusual variants of FA. Large or giant FAs are histologically indistinguishable from their counterparts of average size. Tumors described by this term have included benign PT and hamartoma, and the designation of giant FA is best reserved to indicate the clinical presentation rather than a specific pathologic diagnosis.

The appearance of the stroma varies from one FA to another, but it is usually homogeneous in any given lesion. This is an important distinction from PTs that can exhibit considerable stromal heterogeneity, including regions indistinguishable from a FA.

Uncommon forms of stromal differentiation are encountered in a minority of FAs. These include smooth muscle (myoid) metaplasia[56] (Fig. 8.8) and adipose differentiation. Most fibroepithelial tumors with adipose differentiation are PTs.[57] Osteochondroid metaplasia in a FA is very uncommon, and it almost always occurs in postmenopausal women.[58,59]

Giant cells, sometimes with multiple nuclei, are found in the stroma of FAs[60,61] as well as in PTs[61] and other benign breast tumors.[62] The nuclei of multinucleated stromal giant cells may be pleomorphic and hyperchromatic (Fig. 8.9). In some tumors, these cells display a florette-like pattern. In a case studied by the Senior Editor, the giant cells were reactive for CD68, a histiocytic marker, and only a minority of these cells were immunoreactive for actin or CD34. In two FAs with multinucleated stromal cells studied by Ryska et al.,[62] the multinucleated cells were positive for vimentin and CD34; in one case, the cells were also p53 positive. These multinucleated cells have ultrastructural features consistent with fibroblasts. A FA with the multinucleated giant cells has been described in a patient with Li–Fraumeni syndrome.[63] The multinucleated stromal cells in a breast FA from a woman recovering from chicken pox contained ultrastructural evidence of cytoplasmic viral particles.[64] Huo and Gilcrease[65] reported four cases of FA-like lesions with pleomorphic giant cells and focal stromal hypercellularity. One of the four lesions measured 10 cm in

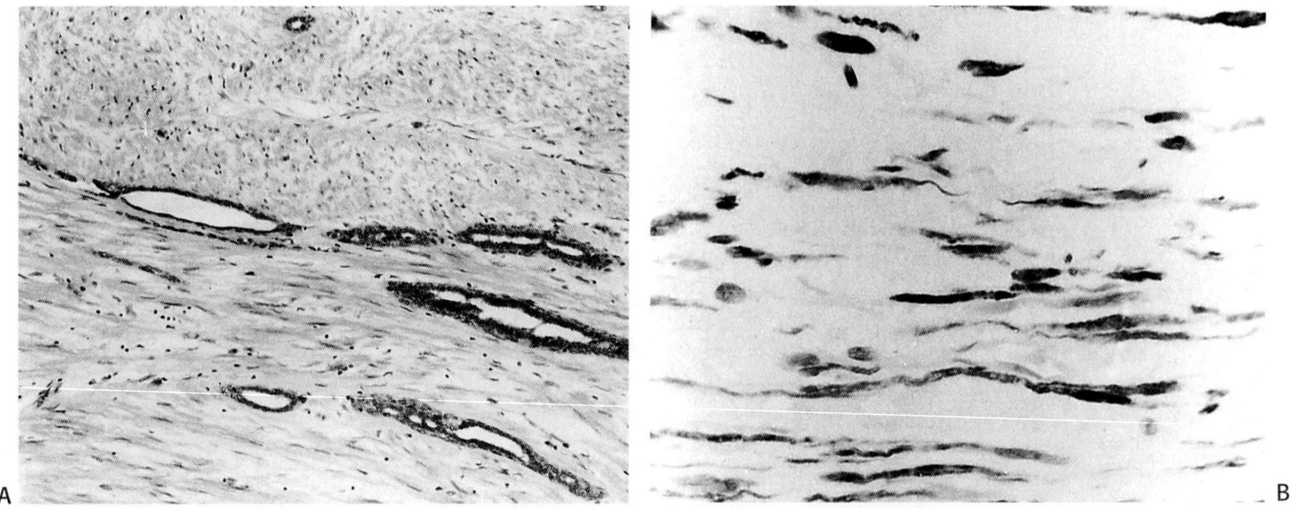

FIG. 8.8. ***Myoid stroma in fibroadenoma.*** **A:** Attenuated ductal structures among bundles of myoid stromal cells. **B:** Immunoreactivity for actin in the stroma detected with the HHF35 antibody.

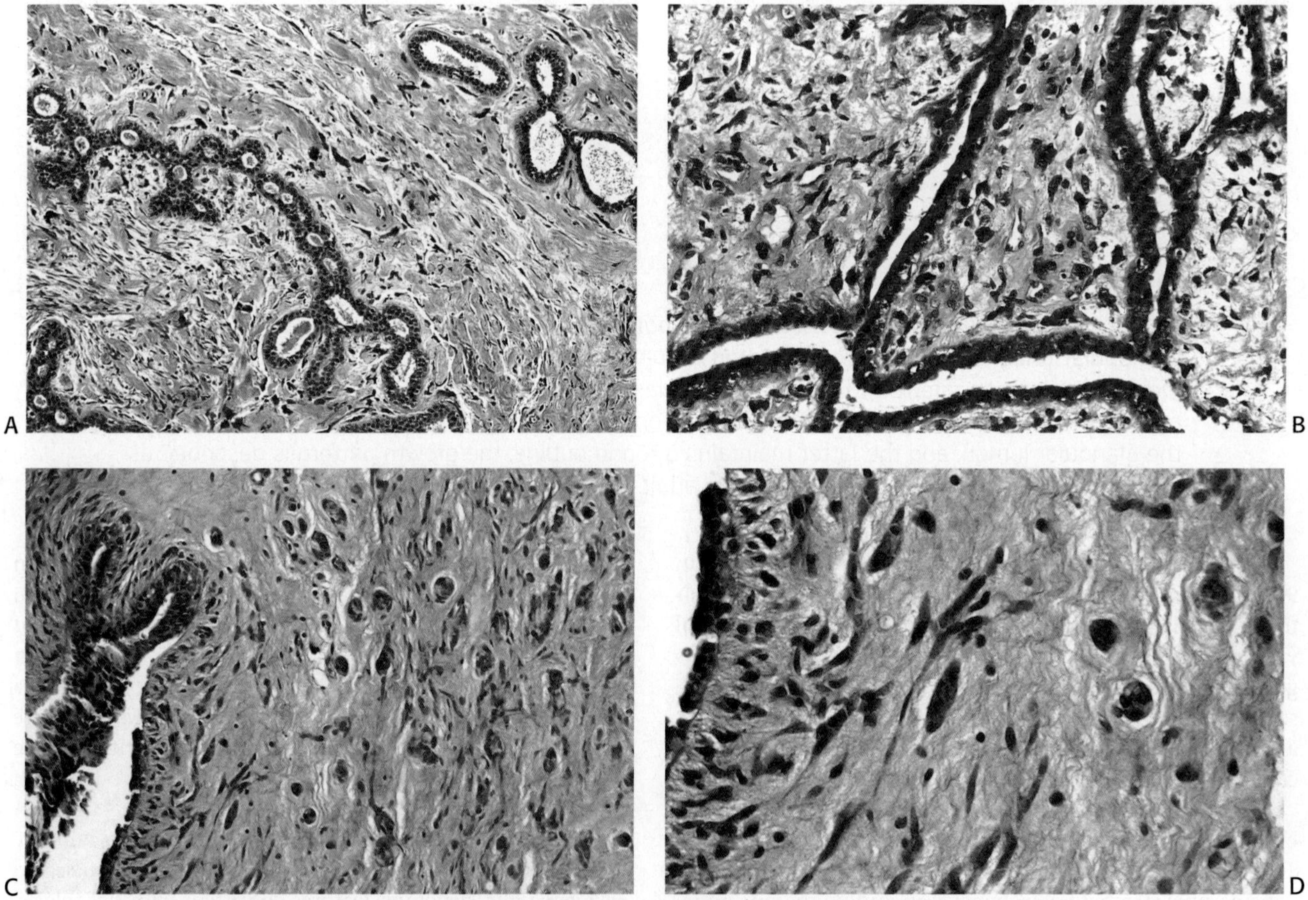

FIG. 8.9. ***Fibroadenoma with stromal giant cells.*** **A:** Cells with hyperchromatic nuclei are present in PASH in a FA. **B:** Multinucleated stromal giant cells in another tumor. **C,D:** Multinucleated stromal cells in a needle core biopsy specimen. The elongated spindle cells in **(D)** simulate invasive carcinoma, but were negative for CK AE1:3 (not shown).

size. It had focally hypercellular stroma, and possibly represented a benign PT. A FA from a patient treated with neoadjuvant chemotherapy for breast carcinoma also showed focal stromal pleomorphism. Clinical follow-up information for three of these patients ranged from 16 to 59 months and was benign in all cases. Despite their atypical cytologic appearance, the presence of multinucleated stromal cells does not appear to influence the clinical course of the lesion. A tumor with the structural features of a FA should not be classified as a PT because the stroma contains multinucleated stromal giant cells.

Two case reports of lesions showing overlapping features of FA and papilloma[66,67] have raised the possibility of a related pathogenesis.

Usual (Adult-Type) FA

The majority of FAs are of adult type. In the average adult FA, the relative proportions of epithelium and stroma are evenly balanced throughout the tumor (Fig. 8.7A), and the density of the stromal cellularity is not related to tumor size. However, FAs from women younger than 20 years of age tend to have more cellular stroma and more proliferative epithelium as a group than do tumors from older women.[36,68] Mitotic figures are extremely unusual in fibroadenomatous stroma. Sparse mitotic activity may be observed in FAs in adolescent girls.[36] Elastic tissue is virtually absent from the stroma of adult FAs. In most instances, the microscopic diagnosis of adult FA is accomplished without difficulty when the tumor has a sharply defined border and the pericanalicular or intracanalicular growth pattern. However, the distinction between FA with cellular stroma and benign PT is sometimes problematic. In these situations, it may be helpful to review the characteristic cytologic features of FAs in formulating the diagnosis. Unfortunately, neoplasms that ultimately recur with the histologic and clinical features of a PT may occasionally present in a form that is histologically indistinguishable from a FA.

The stroma of FA in postmenopausal women tends to be hypocellular and hyalinized, and it often harbors coarse dystrophic calcifications.

Myxoid FA

The stroma of FAs can undergo marked myxoid change (Fig. 8.10). Specimens from such lesions examined by frozen

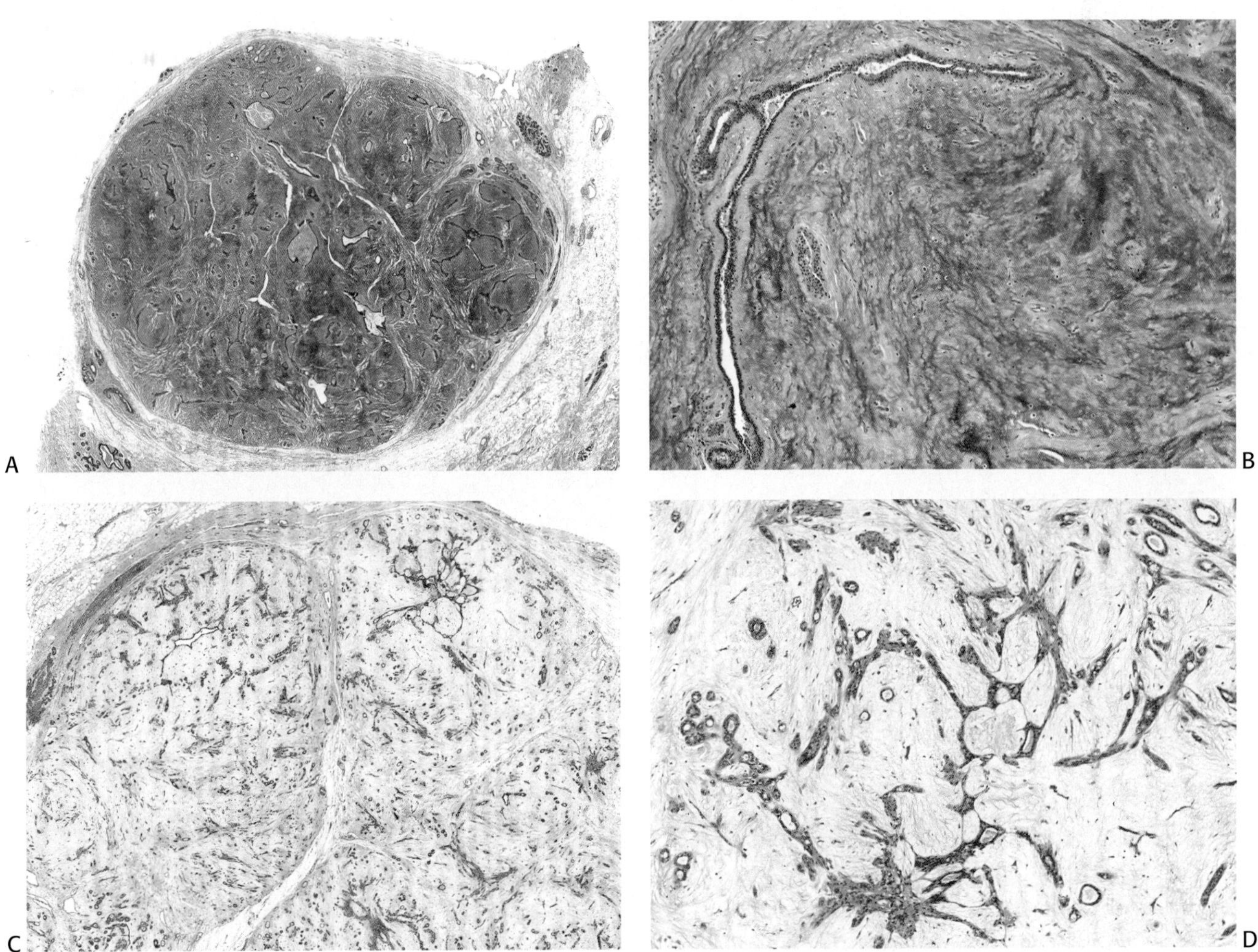

FIG. 8.10. ***Fibroadenoma with myxoid stroma.*** **A:** Myxoid FA has a sharp border with the surrounding breast parenchyma, as shown in this case. This tumor may sometimes raise the differential diagnosis of mucinous carcinoma. **B:** A duct is distended and compressed by the hypocellular myxoid stroma. **C,D:** A myxoid FA with SA.

section, by imprint cytology, by fine-needle aspiration (FNA), or by needle core biopsy may be mistaken for mucinous carcinoma. Myxoid FA and myxomatous stromal masses have been encountered in the familial condition of cutaneous and cardiac myxomas, spotty cutaneous pigmentation, endocrine overactivity, and melanotic schwannomas referred to as Carney syndrome.[12] However, most patients with a myxoid FA do not have a known systemic abnormality.

Complex FA

FAs with sclerosing adenosis (SA), papillary apocrine hyperplasia, cysts, or epithelial calcifications have been designated "complex"[69] (Fig. 8.11). At least one of these histologic features must be present for the lesion to be classified as complex FA. Foci of florid adenosis can also be encountered. Complex FAs constituted 22.7% of 2,458 FAs in one series.[69] A review of 396 FAs from a single institution revealed "complex histologic features" in 40.4% of the tumors.[39] In a series of 63 complex FAs studied by Sklair-Levy et al.,[40] SA was present in 57% of cases, apocrine metaplasia in 8%, and cysts in 1.6%. Calcifications were associated with SA in 9.5% of the cases. Excessive FCCs, especially papillary epithelial hyperplasia and SA, can mask the basic fibroadenomatous nature of a tumor, especially in the limited sample of a needle core biopsy specimen (Fig. 8.11B).

Juvenile FA

Juvenile FAs account for about 4% of all FAs.[34] They are characterized microscopically by stromal cellularity and epithelial hyperplasia (Fig. 8.12). The architecture is more often pericanalicular than intracanalicular, or there is a mixture of these patterns. No appreciable overall differences are found between tumors in patients with solitary and multiple lesions.[35] However, there may be heterogeneity

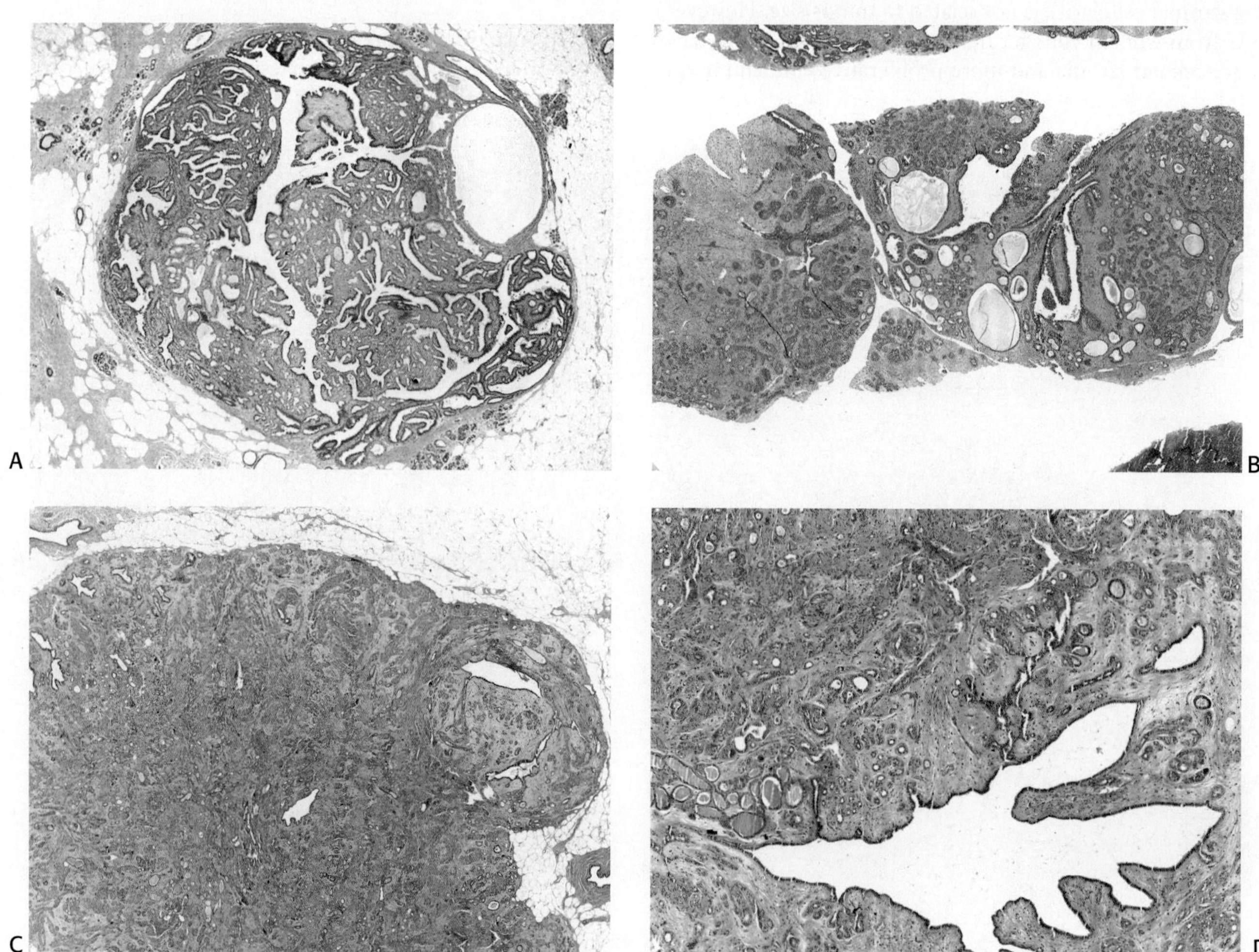

FIG. 8.11. ***Complex fibroadenoma (A,B) and complex fibroadenoma with sclerosing adenosis (C,D).*** **A:** Whole-mount histologic section showing cysts and dark irregular foci of SA. Parts of this complex FA appear papillary. **B:** Excessive FCCs can mask the basic fibroadenomatous nature of the lesion in a limited sample obtained by needle core biopsy. **C:** The fibroadenomatous nature of the lesion is manifested by the elongated ducts. **D:** This example shows extensive sclerotic membrane formation around the glands.

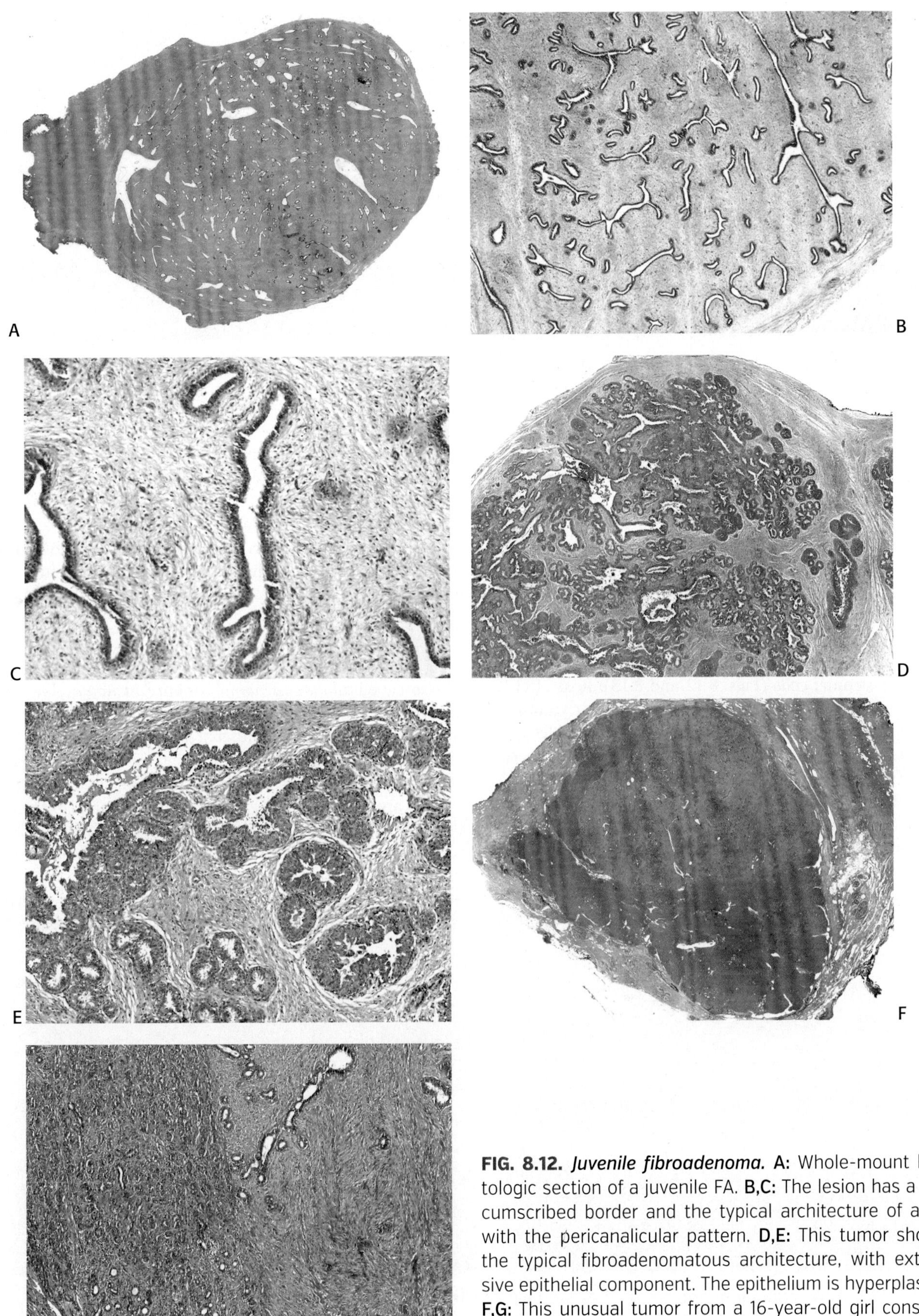

FIG. 8.12. ***Juvenile fibroadenoma.*** **A:** Whole-mount histologic section of a juvenile FA. **B,C:** The lesion has a circumscribed border and the typical architecture of a FA with the pericanalicular pattern. **D,E:** This tumor shows the typical fibroadenomatous architecture, with extensive epithelial component. The epithelium is hyperplastic. **F,G:** This unusual tumor from a 16-year-old girl consists of a fibroadenomatous area coexisting with tubular adenoma. The two components are best appreciated in **(G)**.

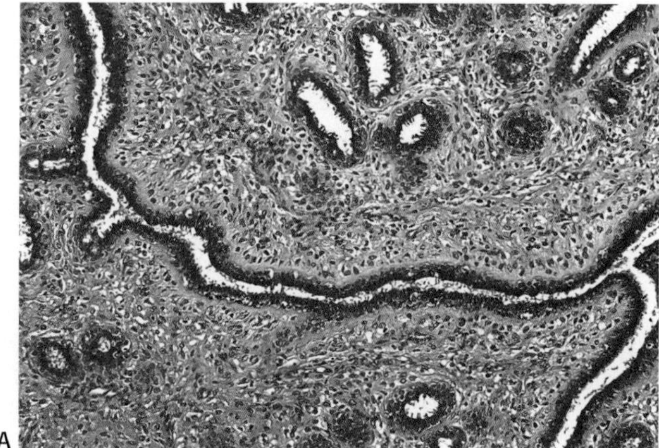

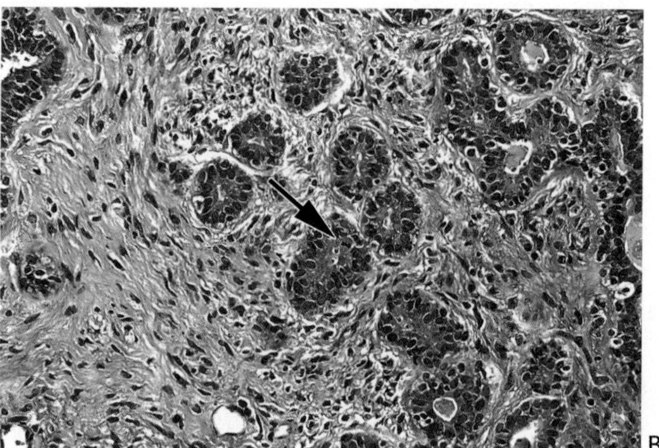

FIG. 8.13. *Juvenile fibroadenoma.* **A:** The stroma is moderately cellular with a slight tendency to condensation around epithelial structures. **B:** Mitotic activity is present in the epithelium (*arrow*).

in the histologic appearance of different tumors from an individual with multiple lesions. The tumor border is usually well defined microscopically, sometimes by a pseudocapsule of compressed parenchyma (Fig. 8.12). Secondary peripheral nodules of fibroadenomatous growth outside the main tumor are encountered in a minority of cases, usually in patients who develop multiple tumors. Mitoses are rarely detected in the stroma of juvenile FAs in adults, but stromal mitoses can be substantial in lesions from adolescents.[36] Little or no atypia and pleomorphism are encountered in the bipolar stromal cells (Figs. 8.12 and 8.13). Ross et al.[36] studied 23 juvenile FAs in women 18 years old or younger. The tumor mean size was 3.1 cm (range, 0.5 to 7). All lesions had circumscribed, noninfiltrative borders and showed pericanalicular growth pattern. The stroma was uniformly cellular, with no separation between intralobular/periglandular stroma and interlobular stroma.

Epithelial elements in a juvenile FA are usually distributed homogeneously. It is exceptional to find a 40× microscopic field occupied entirely by stroma. Ross et al.[36] encountered a few tumors with foci of slight stromal expansion adjacent to gland-rich areas, creating an overall impression of intratumoral heterogeneity that could lead to a diagnosis of PT. In such cases, the uniform quality of the stromal proliferation and lack of nuclear atypia are features critical to reaching the correct diagnosis. Most juvenile FAs feature conspicuous epithelial hyperplasia (see section on epithelium in FA).

Tubular Adenoma

The so-called *tubular adenoma*[70] or *pure adenoma*[71] is a variant of pericanalicular FA with an exceptionally prominent or florid adenosis-like epithelial proliferation (Fig. 8.14). The clinical presentation as a mobile, circumscribed painless mass is indistinguishable from that of an adult FA. These tumors are not associated with pregnancy or oral contraceptive use.[72] They tend to be softer than the average FA, and tan rather than white. Microscopic examination reveals closely approximated round or oval glandular structures composed of a single layer of epithelium supported by a layer of myoepithelial cells. A small amount of secretion is frequently

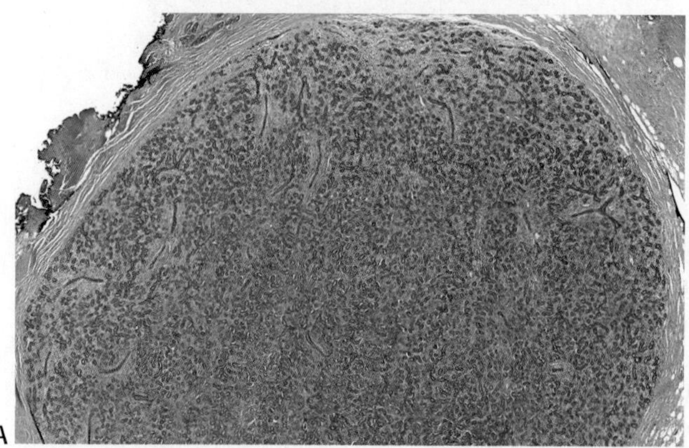

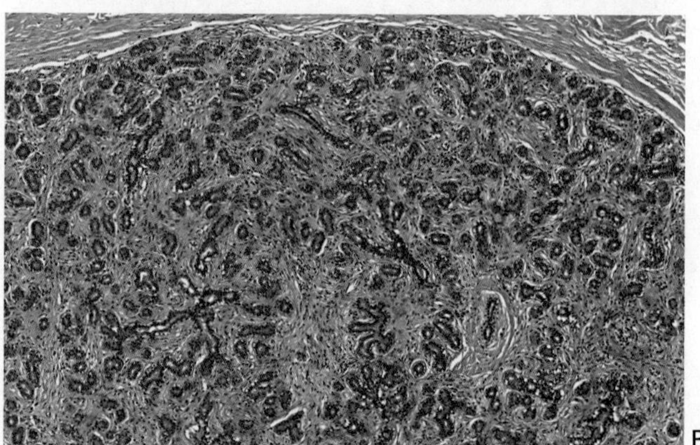

FIG. 8.14. *Tubular adenoma.* **A:** The glandular proliferation has a florid and tight pattern and the lesion resembles a very large lobule. **B:** On closer examination, the glands and tubules are lined by normal epithelium and myoepithelium, in a pattern that resembles tubular adenosis.

present in the glandular lumens, even in tumors from patients who are not pregnant or taking oral contraceptives.[33] This secretion is not immunoreactive for α-lactalbumin.[73]

Other Types of Adenoma

Other so-called adenomas are unrelated to the FA category. *Apocrine adenoma* is a localized nodular focus of prominent papillary and cystic apocrine metaplasia.[74,75] Nodular foci of SA with apocrine metaplasia have been variously termed apocrine adenoma and apocrine adenosis. *Ductal adenoma*[76,77] and *pleomorphic adenoma*[78–80] are variants of intraductal papilloma (discussed in Chapter 5) or adenomyoepithelioma (discussed in Chapter 6).

Infarction in a FA

FAs and lactating adenomas are prone to develop foci of infarction during pregnancy,[81] but infarction has been found in tumors removed from patients who were neither pregnant nor lactating.[82–84] Clinically, the infarcted tumor may be tender or painful. The recent onset of discomfort in a previously painless tumor is suggestive of infarction in a FA.[82,83] The infarcted area can be appreciated grossly as a relatively well-demarcated, pale yellow or white zone of coagulation necrosis. Microscopic examination of the necrotic region reveals the ghostly outline of the underlying structure of the FA in hematoxylin and eosin–stained sections (Fig. 8.15). The architecture of the tissue can be seen to better advantage with a reticulin stain[82] and, if the tissue is not too degenerated, with cytokeratin (CK) stains, AE1:3 in particular. Thrombosed vessels have been detected in some lesions.[83]

Epithelium in FA

The epithelial component of FAs is prone to various alterations. These include foci of minimal epithelial hyperplasia, apocrine metaplasia and squamous metaplasia,[85] cyst formation, and the spectrum of proliferation termed FCC, including apocrine metaplasia, which characterizes complex FA.

Marked epithelial hyperplasia can be encountered in a complex FA or in the absence of a background of FCCs. Generally, these proliferative foci have the same features as hyperplastic lesions outside a FA. Although once attributed to oral contraceptive use,[86] it has been shown that these epithelial changes occur independent of exogenous hormones.[87,88] Secretory hyperplasia sometimes occurs diffusely in FAs during pregnancy,[33] or a preexisting FA may be unaltered.[73] FAs with secretory hyperplasia should be distinguished from the tumor commonly referred to as *lactating adenoma*, which is a compact aggregate of lobules exhibiting secretory hyperplasia (Figs. 8.16 and 8.17). Secretory hyperplasia in the lesional tissue is histologically and ultrastructurally similar to the physiologic changes of pregnancy in the surrounding breast[73,89] (Fig. 8.17). If the tumor is allowed to remain in the breast and excised after delivery, it will be classified as a FA with lactational change. α-Lactalbumin is detectable in the epithelium of lactating adenomas.[73] Involutional change in a lactating adenoma after treatment with bromocriptine has been reported.[89] Tumors with the histologic appearance of lactating adenomas can arise in ectopic breast tissue during pregnancy.[33] One of the most unusual instances of this phenomenon is lactational change in breast tissue present in an ovarian cystic teratoma removed from a 20-year-old woman at the time of cesarean section after a full-term pregnancy.[90] FAs and "tubular adenomas" with focal lactational change are encountered rarely in women who are neither pregnant nor postpartum.[33]

Most juvenile FAs feature conspicuous epithelial hyperplasia that may have a ductal, lobular, or combined ductal–lobular configuration. Several patterns of epithelial proliferation can be found, including laciform, papillary, solid, lobular–terminal ductal, and cribriform[37] (Figs. 8.12 and 8.18). Usually, more than one pattern is present in a given tumor. The laciform pattern features a fenestrated proliferation of ductal epithelial cells that resemble

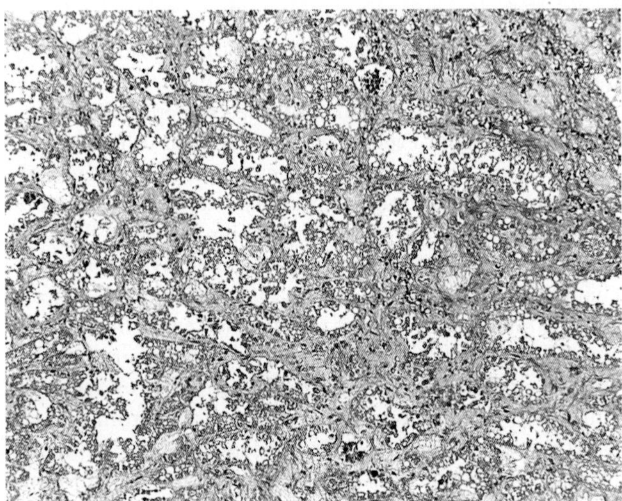

FIG. 8.15. ***Infarcted lactating adenoma.*** Degenerating glands in an infarcted tumor.

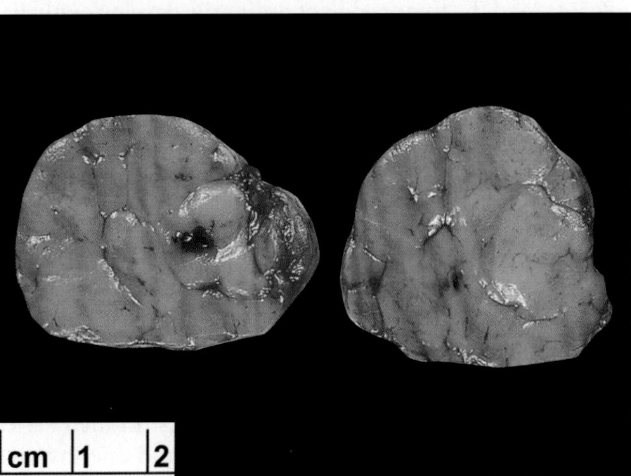

FIG. 8.16. ***Lactating adenoma.*** Gross photograph. The tumor has a compact and fleshy cut surface.

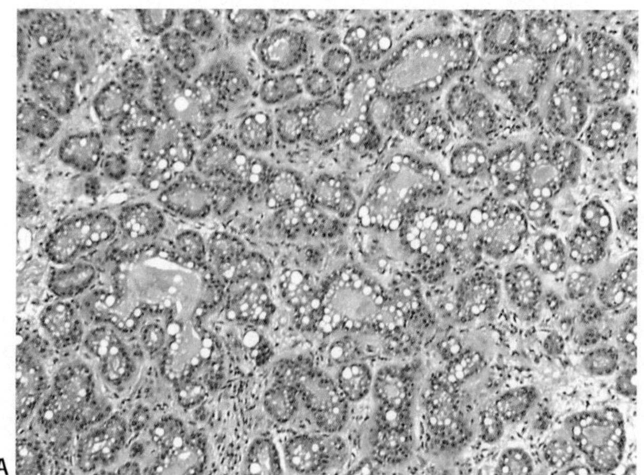
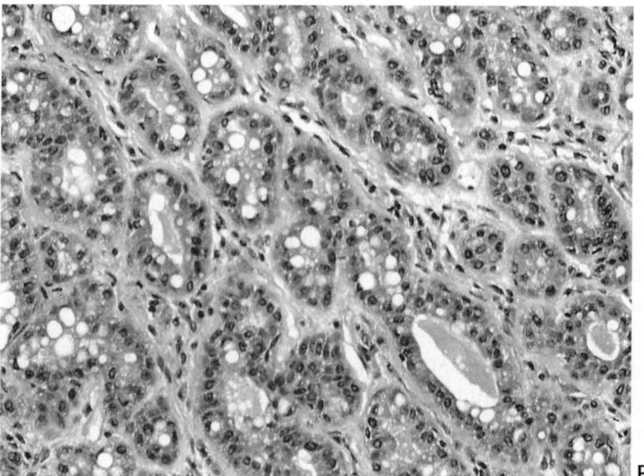

FIG. 8.17. ***Lactating adenoma.*** **A:** The glandular elements are diffusely distributed in sparsely cellular stroma. **B:** The glandular cells have vacuolated cytoplasm.

cribriform ductal carcinoma *in situ* (DCIS). However, in contrast to this form of carcinoma, the epithelium in laciform hyperplasia contains a hyperplastic myoepithelial zone and has the cytologic features of micropapillary hyperplasia, including overlapping, streaming, chromatin condensation, and pyknosis. The papillary type of hyperplasia typically arises in tumors with intracanalicular architecture and may coexist with laciform hyperplasia to create complex branching fronds in dilated duct lumens. A hyperplastic myoepithelial cell layer is typically present. In solid hyperplasia, the epithelium fills expanded duct structures, which have a largely pericanalicular distribution. Instead of the columnar cytology observed in laciform and papillary hyperplasia, solid hyperplasia features round to ovoid cells. The lobular–terminal duct pattern is present when the solid epithelial proliferation branches into lobular radicles.

Mild cellular pleomorphism and cytologic atypia are seen in all histologic patterns of epithelial hyperplasia in juvenile FAs, but tend to be more extreme in solid hyperplasia. Epithelial necrosis is not a feature of the hyperplasia in juvenile FAs, and the tumors do not ordinarily develop epithelial calcifications. Hyperplastic changes are rarely found in the surrounding breast tissue. It is very unusual to find carcinoma in a juvenile FA (Fig. 8.19).

Carcinoma in FA

Lobular and ductal carcinomas can arise in FAs (Figs. 8.20 to 8.22). Ben Hassouna et al.[91] reported two examples of carcinoma involving complex FAs that measured 1.5 and 3 cm in size. The patients were 58 and 28 years old, respectively. Petersson et al.[92] also described an example of low-grade invasive ductal carcinoma arising in a complex FA involved by columnar cell change with atypia and FCCs. In their series of 63 complex FAs, Sklair-Levy et al.[40] found one invasive lobular carcinoma (1.6%) at surgical excision of a lesion in the breast of a 64-year-old woman diagnosed with complex FA and atypical lobular hyperplasia (ALH) at needle core biopsy. We have encountered rare examples of columnar cell change with atypia, atypical ductal hyperplasia (ADH), or low-grade DCIS involving a discrete nodular lesion reminiscent of a complex FA (Fig. 8.23). An example of adenoid cystic carcinoma with squamous metaplasia arising in a FA from a 63-year-old woman has been reported.[93] There are occasional reports of mucinous carcinoma arising in a FA.[91,94] A preexisting FA may delay the detection of an invasive carcinoma arising in the adjacent breast parenchyma (Fig. 8.24). For additional discussion of carcinoma arising in FAs, see Chapter 33.

Cytology

The FNA cytology specimen obtained from a FA typically presents a characteristic combination of epithelial and stromal components.[95–97]

Usual FA

The cytologic findings considered to be diagnostic of a usual (adult-type) FA are abundant bipolar stromal cells (usually seen as bare nuclei), irregular flat sheets of epithelium composed of uniform, evenly spaced polygonal cells, so-called "antler horn" clusters, and fenestrated or "honeycomb" cohesive sheets composed of similar cells. These features are especially useful for distinguishing between the aspirate from a FA and from benign proliferative (fibrocystic) changes. This distinction can be difficult if the FA contains a substantial component of proliferative epithelium. Thirty percent to 50% of aspirates from FA contain foam cells and apocrine cells.[96] Failure to appreciate the cytologic variability that may be found in FNA specimens from FAs can lead to a false suspicion of or misdiagnosis of carcinoma,[98,99] especially when the FNA sample is obtained from a woman of fertile age, as the physiologic alterations characteristic of the luteal phase of the menstrual cycle can occasionally involve the epithelium of a FA. Focal secretory changes can

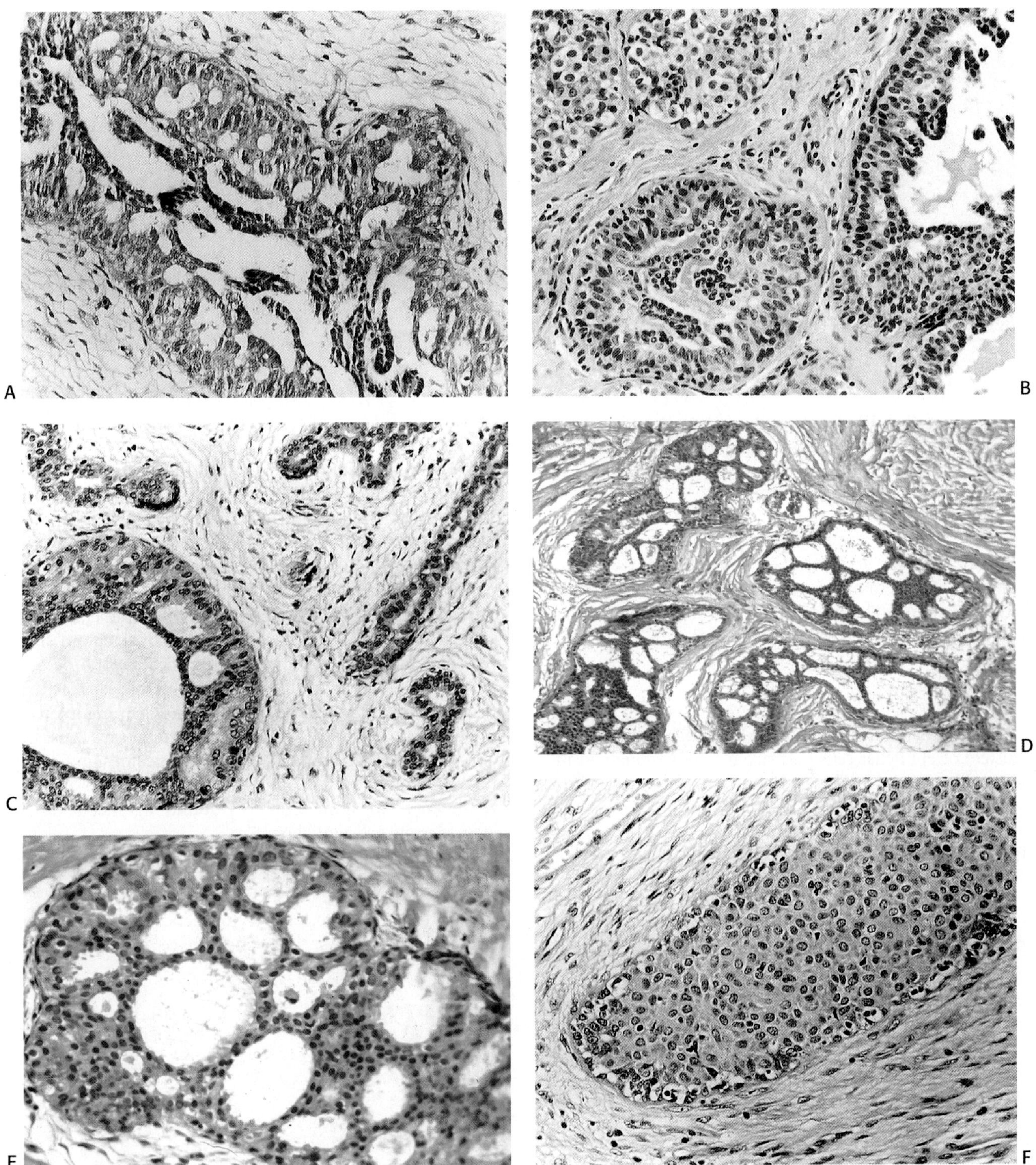

FIG. 8.18. ***Juvenile fibroadenoma, atypical epithelial hyperplasia.*** Patterns of ADH. **A:** Laciform and micropapillary. **B:** Micropapillary and solid. **C–E:** Cribriform. **F:** Solid.

also raise concern in cytology preparations.[31,32] Conversely, careful attention must be paid to atypical cytologic features, since FAs may contain or be adjacent to carcinoma[100] (Fig. 8.24). FNA may induce hemorrhagic infarction in a FA in a nonpregnant patient.[101]

Lactating Adenoma

The aspirate from a lactating adenoma is cellular.[95] It differs from that of a typical FA in lacking "antler horn" and "honeycomb" flat sheets of epithelium. The epithelium is distributed in three-dimensional acinar clusters, and there

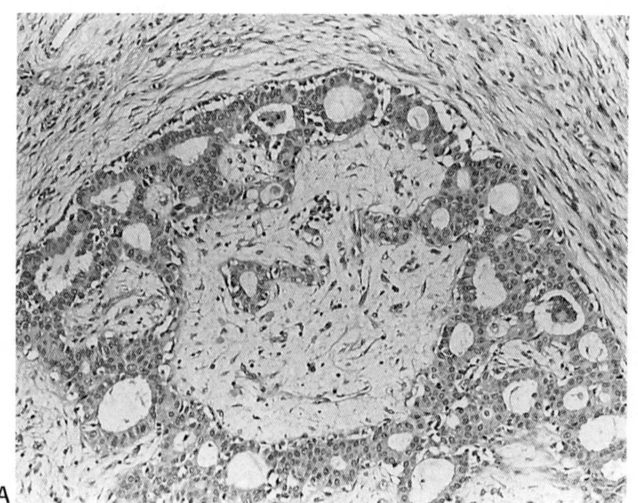

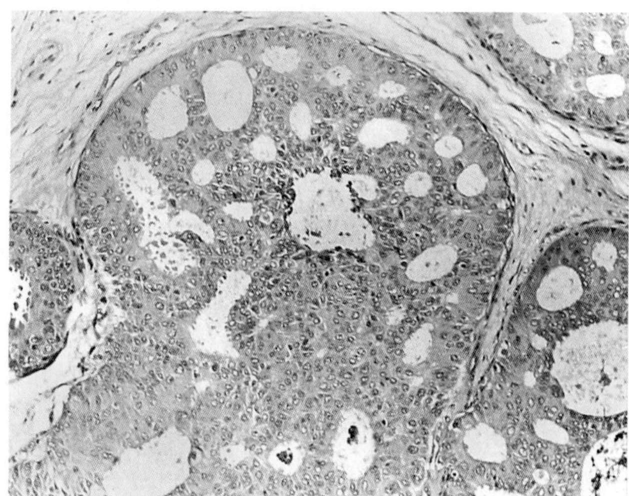

FIG. 8.19. ***Carcinoma in juvenile fibroadenomas.*** **A,B:** The patient was 21 years old with a juvenile FA in which there was cribriform ADH (**A**) and cribriform DCIS (**B**).

is a tendency to cell dyshesion, resulting in many single cells.[102,103] The uniform nuclei have prominent nucleoli, and they often appear to be stripped of cytoplasm. Couplets of naked nuclei are commonly seen in FNA smears from a lactating adenoma. The background may appear foamy, and the cytoplasm of intact cells is vacuolated.

Myxoid FA

The FNA material of a myxoid FA can be cellular, with clusters of epithelial cells and stromal cells embedded in a myxoid background. This appearance can mimic mucinous carcinoma.[32]

Immunohistochemistry

Hormone receptors have been demonstrated in FAs. Estrogen receptor (ER)-α activity is largely confined to the epithelium in most studies.[104–106] Sapino et al.[106] reported finding ER-β in the stroma of FAs, with a significantly lower mean age for ER-β-positive than for ER-β-negative tumors. The extent of ER-α expression correlated with stromal cellularity. Progesterone receptor (PR) is also localized to the stroma[107] but is usually not detected in the epithelium. The stromal cells of FA are variably CD34-positive, and show immunoreactivity for actin in cases with myofibroblastic proliferation. Sawyer et al.[108] documented nuclear reactivity for β-catenin in the stroma of 11/16 FAs; staining intensity ranged from moderate (four cases) to strong (seven cases).

Ki67 indices of FAs and benign PTs were not significantly different in one study,[109] but two separate studies evaluating needle core biopsy material[110,111] found significant differences, despite substantial overlap.

Genetics and Molecular Studies

Investigators have detected cytogenetic abnormalities in 20% to 30% of FAs.[112–116] These have usually involved

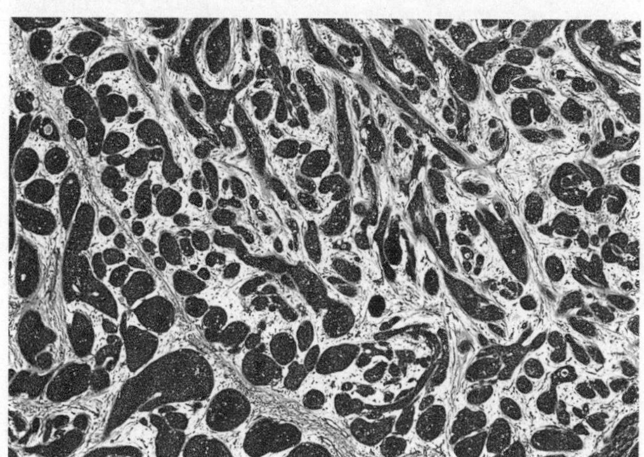

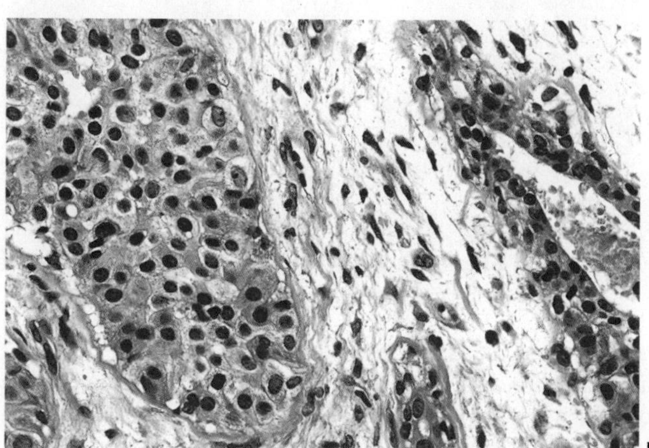

FIG. 8.20. ***Complex fibroadenoma with LCIS.*** **A:** LCIS fills the SA glands of a complex FA. **B:** LCIS fills a duct (*left*) and partially involves another (*right*).

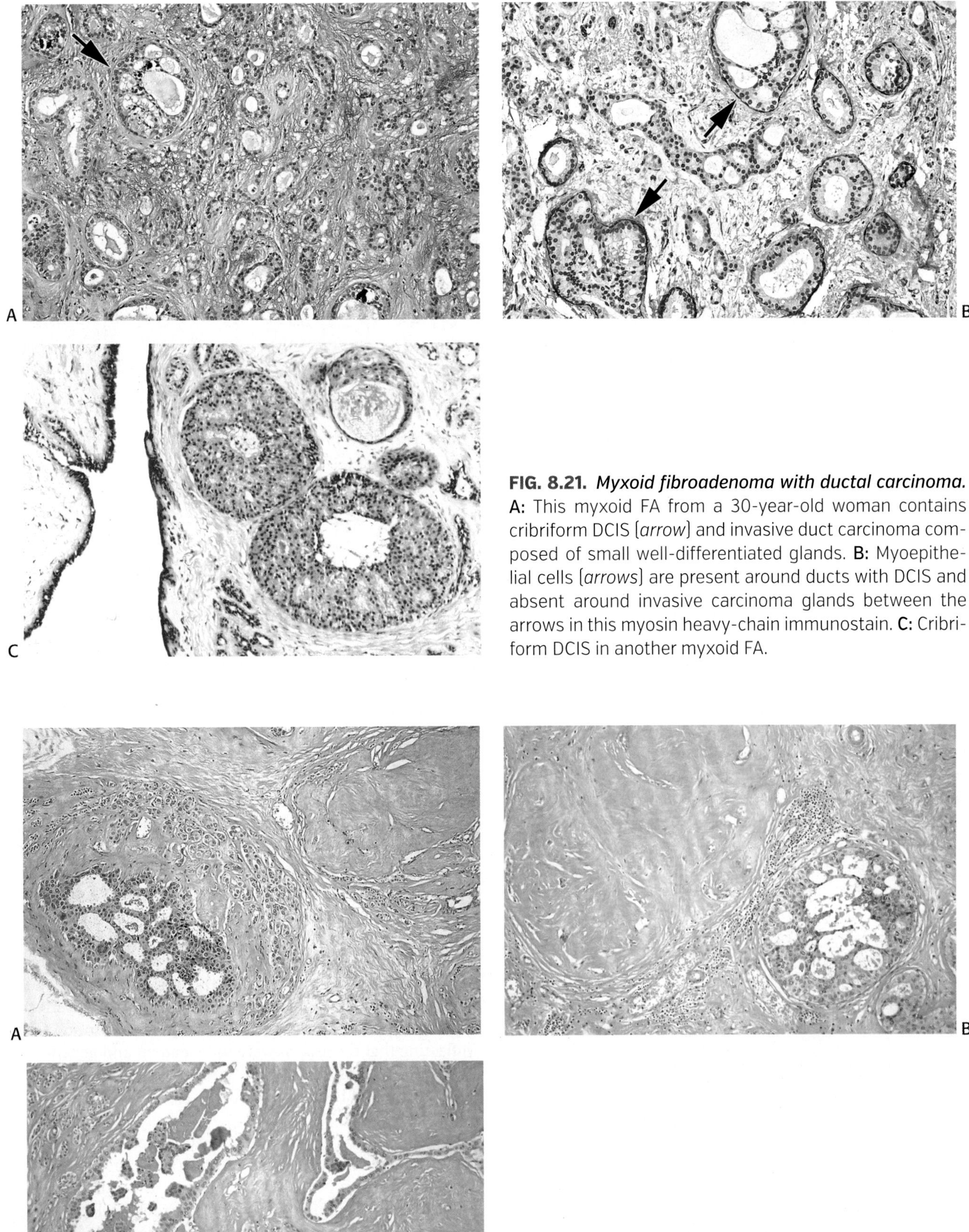

FIG. 8.21. ***Myxoid fibroadenoma with ductal carcinoma.*** **A:** This myxoid FA from a 30-year-old woman contains cribriform DCIS (*arrow*) and invasive duct carcinoma composed of small well-differentiated glands. **B:** Myoepithelial cells (*arrows*) are present around ducts with DCIS and absent around invasive carcinoma glands between the arrows in this myosin heavy-chain immunostain. **C:** Cribriform DCIS in another myxoid FA.

FIG. 8.22. ***Sclerotic fibroadenoma with invasive duct carcinoma.*** **A:** Cribriform DCIS is surrounded by invasive duct carcinoma in a sclerotic FA. **B,C:** Additional foci of DCIS in the sclerotic FA. The patient was a 64-year-old woman.

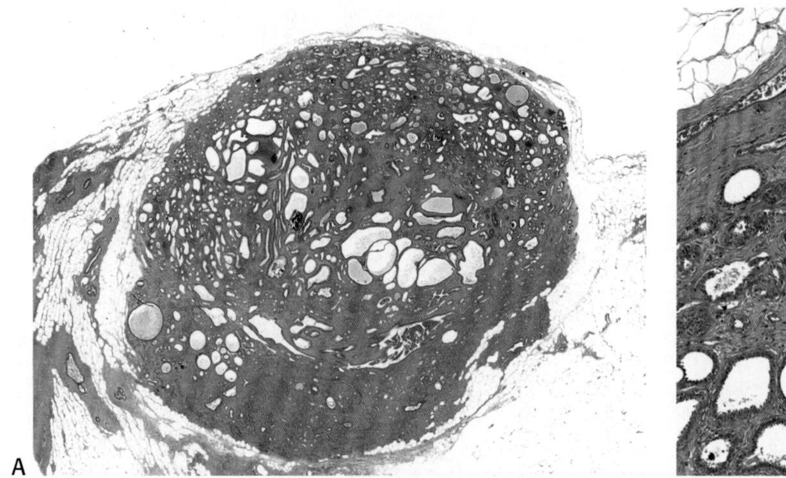

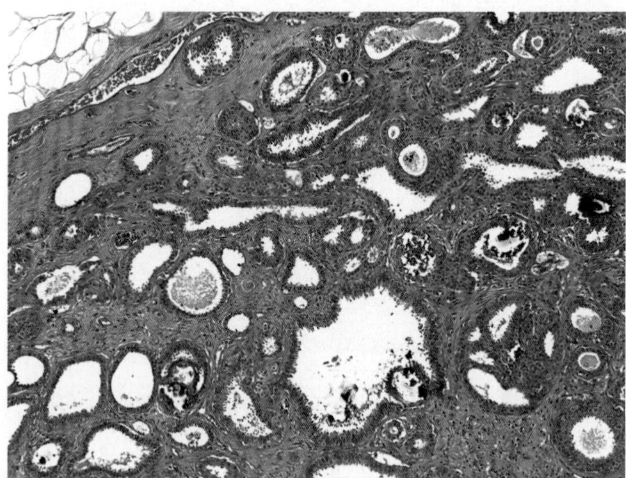

FIG. 8.23. ***Fibroadenomatous nodule with features of complex fibroadenoma, columnar cell change, and atypical ductal hyperplasia.*** **A:** This discrete nodular lesion is a complex FA with numerous cysts. The cysts vary in size but tend to be round and monotonous. **B:** At high magnification, the cysts are lined by columnar cell changes and a few contain small calcifications. A rare gland displays cribriform architecture diagnostic of ADH (*lower right*).

translocations, but no consistent pattern of specific chromosomal alterations has been identified. In one report, cells in three different FAs from a single individual exhibited the same chromosomal change.[112] Conversely, Noguchi et al.[117] assessed X-chromosome polymorphism in 10 FAs and observed that both epithelial and stromal components are polyclonal, a finding that suggests that most FAs are hyperplastic lesions. However, evidence suggesting that a FA may sometimes evolve into a PT was obtained by the same authors[118] from clonal analysis of three tumors initially diagnosed as FAs that recurred as PTs. These tumors were studied for evidence of trinucleotide repeat polymorphism of the X-chromosome-linked androgen receptor (*AR*) gene and random inactivation of the gene by methylation. It was observed that the same allele of the *AR* gene was inactivated in the FA and PT samples

FIG. 8.24. ***Invasive carcinoma adjacent to a sclerotic fibroadenoma.***

from each patient, a result very unlikely to occur in three separate cases by chance alone. Kobayashi et al.[119] used polymerase chain reaction (PCR) for clonal analysis of the stroma in multiple FAs from a single patient and determined that all lesions were polyclonal. Using a similar technique, Kasami et al.[68] detected stromal monoclonality in 1 of 20 (5%) complex FAs and 1 of 25 (4%) simple FAs. The microdissected epithelium was polyclonal in all tumors, including two tumors with monoclonal stroma. The authors commented that "the one monoclonal simple FA was also the only one with mixed features to contain a phyllodes component," an observation that suggests that the sample analyzed as a "simple FA" might have been a FA-like area of a heterogeneous PT.

Wang et al.[120] assessed genome-wide loss of heterozygosity (LOH) in 13 samples of FAs, including metachronous FAs from two patients, and 15 separate PT nodules. They found low levels of LOH (range 0% to 1.5%) in FAs, whereas LOH levels in PTs ranged from 0% to 35.2%. LOH in FAs included the 2q36, 12p13.1–p12.3, and 13q13 regions. Metachronous FAs from the same patient had no common LOH, indicating that the lesions were independent and genetically unrelated. McCulloch et al.[121] also detected LOH in only about 10% of 39 FAs analyzed by PCR and found microsatellite instability in 8% of cases.

Di Vinci et al.[122] demonstrated methylation of the $p16^{INK4a}$ gene promoter in the epithelial and stromal components of 15 FAs, as well as in the adjacent tissue. The authors noted no cytoplasmic staining of p16 in the stromal cells, but p16 nuclear staining appeared substantially decreased in FAs with higher proliferative activity compared with those with a lower proliferation rate. Additional discussion of the genetic alterations found in FAs and of their relationship with PTs has been recently reviewed by Karim et al.[123] Overall, the available data show no evidence of recurrent genetic alterations characteristic of FA. Although most usual FAs are hyperplastic and polyclonal lesions, it appears that a very small percentage consist of neoplasms that, despite having very bland morphology indistinguishable from that of hyperplastic FAs, have the potential to recur and transform into PTs.

Treatment and Prognosis

In the absence of any atypical finding, the management of FA, a benign mass lesion, usually depends on concurrent risk factors and patient's preference.

Surgical Excision

Many solitary FAs are treated by local excision. When the preoperative clinical findings suggest this diagnosis, the tumor can be "shelled out" from the breast, but it is preferable to include at least a thin rim of surrounding normal breast to minimize the need for reexcision in rare instances when the lesion proves to be a PT. There is no evidence that adult-type FAs are prone to local recurrence or that they predispose to the development of PT if incompletely excised. Although complex FAs are usually excised, at present there are no definitive data mandating this practice.

Despite substantial epithelial proliferation, sometimes with considerable atypia, and increased stromal cellularity, follow-up of patients with juvenile FAs has not revealed a predisposition to develop PT or carcinoma subsequently in either breast.[34–36] Excision should be carried out to preserve as much breast tissue as possible, especially in adolescent patients, because near-normal breast development may occur even if removal of very large or multiple tumors leaves a minimal amount of residual uninvolved tissue.[35]

Ultrasound-Guided Vacuum-Assisted Percutaneous Excision

Small FAs measuring 1.5 cm or less may be completely excised in the course of vacuum-assisted ultrasound-guided biopsy.[124] Grady et al.[125] reported the long-term outcome of 52 FAs removed percutaneously under sonographic guidance. The patients were followed with clinical and sonographic evaluation every 6 months. At a median follow-up of 22 months (range 7 to 59), the recurrence rate was 15% (8/52), with an actuarial recurrence rate of 33% at 59 months. None of the recurrent lesions were symptomatic, and only three were palpable. All recurrences pertained to lesions that were greater than 2 cm at initial diagnosis (range 2.1 to 2.8). The authors do not specify whether the recurrent lesions were excised and whether the recurrence consisted only of postsurgical fibrosis or of FA, although they suggest the latter.

Cryoablation

Cryoablation has been investigated as a method for treating FAs instead of surgical excision.[126–128] In a series of 444 FAs treated with cryoablation, the mean pretreatment tumor diameter was 1.8 cm, and 75% of the lesions were palpable.[127] A palpable abnormality was detected in 46% of patients 6 months after treatment and in 35% at 12 months. The finding of a persistent palpable abnormality was related to initial tumor size and occurred more often in women whose index tumors were larger than 2 cm. Kaufman et al.[128] reported the follow-up of 32 FAs from 29 women treated by cryoablation. The average follow-up time was 3.6 years (range 1.3 to 3.8). Three patients complained of local tenderness. The number of palpable lesions decreased from 84% before treatment to 16% after treatment. Four of 15 (27%) FAs larger than 2 cm at presentation were still palpable at follow-up, in contrast to only one of the 17 (6%) tumors smaller than 2 cm. A mammogram showed no evidence of residual mass, architectural distortion, or fibrosis in 15 patients with no residual palpable tumor. In one study,[126] the average sonographic volume of the FAs was 4.2 cm^3 before treatment, and it decreased to 0.7 cm^3 at 12 months follow-up. Two patients underwent removal or biopsy of the residual lesion, which consisted of shrunken hyaline matrix.

Follow-up Without Excision

Because FAs can be quite reliably diagnosed by FNA or needle core biopsy, there has been interest in conservative management consisting of clinical follow-up rather than excision.[129,130] A survey of patient preferences revealed that the majority of women chose excisional biopsy even if they were assured that the lesion was benign by FNA.[129] Semiannual clinical and mammographic follow-up to document stability of the lesion is recommended for women who do not undergo surgical excision after an FNA or needle core biopsy diagnosis of a FA. In one study, the majority of tumors diagnosed clinically as FAs by FNA continued to grow before excision during a predetermined 12-month follow-up period.[130] Gordon et al.[131] concluded that FAs diagnosed by FNA biopsy "may be safely followed up if volume growth rate is less than 16% per month in those younger than 50 years and less than 13% per month in those 50 years or older." Jacklin et al.[132] summarized the features that raise concern for PT in a patient considered clinically to have a FA. These include increasing size of a preexisting tumor, tumor size larger than 3 cm in a patient older than 35 years, lobulated mammographic contour, and ultrasonographic exam showing attenuation or cystic areas in a solid mass.

Risk of Subsequent Carcinoma

Epidemiologic studies suggest that the relative risk (RR) of developing breast carcinoma is increased in women who have had a FA, compared with various control groups. The RR has been reported to be 1.6,[133] 1.7,[134,135] 2.2,[69] and 2.6.[136] Some authors have not excluded patients with synchronous tumors and others have limited their analysis to patients who developed subsequent invasive carcinoma. In two reports,[69,137] the RR was significantly higher for patients with a concurrent FA and benign proliferative changes. Dupont et al.[69] found that increased risk of breast carcinoma was dependent on the presence of proliferative changes in the FA or in the surrounding breast, as well as a family history of breast carcinoma. Proliferative FCCs were reportedly more common near complex than noncomplex FAs. The RR was 3.1 for women who had a FA with cysts, SA, calcifications, or papillary apocrine metaplasia (complex FA). When benign proliferative changes were present in the nonfibroadenomatous breast, the RR was 3.88. For women with a complex FA and a family history of breast carcinoma, the RR was 3.72. The RR associated with complex FA versus noncomplex FA in women without family history of breast carcinoma was not significantly different (2.60 vs. 2.06, respectively).

The risk of upgrade at surgical excision of lesions diagnosed as complex FA at needle core biopsy is low. In a series of 63 complex FAs, 23 were diagnosed at needle core biopsy. A 64-year-old woman with complex FAs and ALH in a needle core biopsy sample that targeted mammographic calcifications had a 0.4-cm invasive lobular carcinoma at surgical excision.[40] The remaining 22 complex FAs were followed clinically and radiologically. One lesion increased in size from 0.8 to 1.4 cm over a period of 2 years (75% increase in maximum diameter) and yielded a benign PT at surgical excision.[40]

PHYLLODES TUMOR

Although PTs may have been described as early as 1774, the lesion was first fully characterized in 1838 by Johannes Müller.[138] The term *cystosarcoma phyllodes* (phyllo = Greek for leaf) was used to emphasize the leaf-like pattern, fleshy and cystic gross appearance of the lesion. Among many other names subsequently applied to the tumor, the only ones currently used are *PT* and *periductal stromal tumor*. The latter term was proposed to emphasize probable origin from specialized periductal stroma, but PT has become the preferred nomenclature. The diagnosis of PT should always include subclassification as *benign, low-grade malignant (borderline), or high-grade malignant PT*. The distinction among these three subgroups is based on the histologic characteristics of the tumors and is predictive of the probable clinical course.

Clinical Presentation

The patient presents with a firm to hard discrete palpable tumor. Large tumors may invade and ulcerate the skin or extend into the chest wall.[139] There are no specific clinical features that reliably distinguish between a FA, a benign PT, and a malignant PT.[140] A diagnosis of PT may be favored clinically if the tumor is larger than 4 cm or if there is a history of rapid growth. Origin in a preexisting FA or malignant transformation of a benign PT is suggested when the patient reports enlargement of a preexisting tumor that was previously stable for a number of years. However, it is exceedingly rare to find convincing morphologic evidence of this process because FA-like areas that appear to be integral parts of the lesion may occur in benign and malignant PTs (see also discussion of genetics and molecular alterations of PTs).

Mass Lesion

PTs usually occur as solitary unilateral masses. Rarely, multifocal PTs have been detected in a single breast,[141,142] or both breasts may be affected.[141,143–147] Unilateral involvement of right and left breasts occurs with similar frequency. Based on Surveillance Epidemiology and End Results (SEER) data, about 28% of malignant PTs involve the upper outer quadrant, 7% the upper inner quadrant, 8% the central area, and 48% overlap two or more quadrants/areas of the breast.[148] Coexistent FAs are found histologically in nearly 40% of cases, but they are not always apparent clinically.[141] Fibroadenomatoid lobular hyperplasia is often present in the surrounding breast tissue.[145] Large tumors may invade and ulcerate the skin or extend into the chest wall.[139]

Age and Pregnancy

PTs have been reported in patients ranging in age from 6 to 86 years.[140,145,149–154] The median age at diagnosis is about 45 years, approximately 20 years older than the median age of patients with FAs. One population-based study reported the highest incidence of PT in women 45 to 49 years old.[155] In a series of 293 PTs treated at Memorial Hospital in New York City,[145] the patient mean age was 41.7 years, and the median age was 42 years (range 11 to 83). The mean age of 124 patients with PT treated at two institutions in Texas and Florida[156] was 44 years (range 15 to 70). In a study based on SEER data from patients with malignant PT,[148] the median age at diagnosis was 50 years (range 12 to 92). PTs are very uncommon in patients younger than 30 years of age. A review of Swedish Cancer Registry data found eight histologically documented PTs in women younger than 25 years old diagnosed from 1960 to 1969.[157] There have been a few reports of PTs in adolescent women.[151,157–167] The majority of PTs in this young age group have been classified as benign, but a few examples of malignant PT have been desc ribed.[158,159,161,163,167] Only rare cases of PT occurring before menarche are reported, including benign,[164] low-grade (borderline),[165,168] and at least two high-grade malignant PTs.[149,163] The youngest reported patient with malignant PT was 6 years old.[149] Bloody nipple discharge was associated with the tumor mass in at least one case.[164]

There are rare reports of malignant PTs occurring during pregnancy,[147,169–172] including at least one case in the first trimester.[173] Successful treatment by surgical excision of a PT diagnosed during pregnancy has been reported.[170] The tumor did not recur during a second pregnancy. A tumor that grew rapidly during hormonal treatment for *in vitro* fertilization was attributed to transformation of a FA to a PT.[174] The diagnosis of a preexisting FA was based on an FNA sample that was consistent with a FA and the presence of areas of FA and malignant PT in the excised tumor. The histologic findings in this case report are similar to those described by Hodges et al.[175]

Ethnicity

A population-based study conducted in Los Angeles County, California, revealed an annual age-adjusted incidence of malignant PT of 2.1 per 1 million women.[155] Analysis by ethnicity documented significantly younger Asian and Latina patients than non-Latina Whites. Foreign-born Latina women from Mexico or the Americas had a three- to fourfold higher risk of PT than did Latina women born in the United States. In a study[148] evaluating SEER data from 821 women diagnosed with malignant PT between 1983 and 2002, most women (77%) were Caucasian, 10% African American, and 13% of other races. The mean age of 124 patients with PT treated at two institutions in Texas and Florida[156] was 44 years (range 15 to 70). Forty-two percent of the patients were Caucasian, 43% Hispanic, 12% Asian, and 3% of other races. There were no racial differences in age at diagnosis. PTs were benign in 49% of the cases, low-grade (borderline) in 35%, and high-grade malignant in 16%. A higher percentage of low-grade and high-grade malignant PTs occurred in Hispanic patients ($p = 0.01$). Tan et al.[146] reported a series of 605 PTs treated at one institution in Singapore between 1992 and 2010. The tumors consisted of 440 (72.7%) benign, 111 (8.4%) low-grade (borderline), and 54 (8.9%) high-grade malignant PTs. The median patient age was 43 years (range 15 to 79). Most patients were of Chinese ethnicity (70.2%). In a study conducted in Australia by Karim et al.,[176] 19/65 (31%) women with PT and 6/9 (67%) women with recurrent PT were of Asian descent. In this study, 32% of the Asian patients developed recurrent disease compared with only 7% of non-Asian patients. These findings led the authors to speculate that women of Asian origin may have a biologic and/or a genetic predisposition to develop PTs.

PTs in Men

Isolated examples of PTs have been described in men.[177–180] Pantoja et al.[180] reported the case of a 70-year-old man with gynecomastia and a large PT that reportedly had been slowly growing for 50 years. The tumor had caused a 12-cm central ulcer. At mastectomy, the breast measured 30 × 30 cm and weighed 8.6 kg. The tumor was described as a focally malignant PT in a giant FA associated with gynecomastia.

Size

The average size of PTs is 4 to 5 cm, ranging from 1 cm to larger than 20 cm.[140,145,146,150,152,153] Although malignant PTs tend to be larger than benign variants, there are many exceptions, with high-grade malignant PTs being smaller than 2 cm and some of the largest lesions being histologically benign. In a study of 293 PTs,[145] tumor size was smaller or equal to 3 cm in 54% of the cases, greater than 3 cm in 43%, and unknown in 3%. Sixty-six percent of benign PTs measured 3 cm or less, whereas 67% of low-grade and high-grade malignant PTs were larger than 3 cm ($p < 0.0001$). In a study of 605 PTs,[146] the mean tumor size was 5.2 cm (range 0.3 to 25). Benign PTs smaller than 5.2 cm represented 56.7% of all tumors in this series, whereas low-grade (borderline) PTs smaller than 5.2 cm were 8.9%, and high-grade malignant PTs only 2.6%. In contrast, benign PTs measuring 5.2 cm or more were only 16.1% of all PTs, whereas low-grade (borderline) malignant PTs of similar size were 9.4%, and high-grade malignant PTs represented 6.3% of all tumors.

Radiology

Mammography reveals a rounded or lobulated, sharply defined opaque mass in most cases[181,182] (Fig. 8.25). Indistinct borders are seen in a minority of cases. Sonographically, the tumor also appears to be well circumscribed, but it is often structurally inhomogeneous due to cysts and epithelium-lined clefts[181] (Fig. 8.25). Calcifications are uncommon and occur with equal frequency in benign and malignant lesions.[182,183] It is not possible to reliably distinguish between benign and malignant PTs by mammography or ultrasonography.[181–183] Using real-time sonoelastography, Adamietz et al.[184] observed an elastic center surrounded by inelastic peripheral tissue ("ring sign") in all eight PTs in their series, but detected the same change only in 5% of FAs. MRI of benign PTs reveals an oval or lobulated shape with internal septations,[185–187] but the features do not allow definitive distinction from FA. Dynamic enhancement is observed after administration of contrast material.[185,187] In a study of 30 tumors, Yabuuchi et al.[188] detected no significant differences in the MRI characteristics of benign and malignant PTs.

Genetic Predisposition

Women with *p53* germline mutation (Li–Fraumeni syndrome) have a significantly increased risk of developing malignant PT ($p = 0.0003$).[189] There is a case report of bilateral PTs in a 28-year-old woman with Poland syndrome, a rare congenital malformation of the chest wall typically associated with breast hypoplasia.[190]

Paraneoplastic Syndromes

Production of insulin-like growth factor II (IGF-II) by a malignant PT was associated with hypoglycemia in at least three cases.[191–193] Two patients had elevated levels of plasma IGF-II that returned to the normal range when the tumors were removed; glycemic values also returned to normal. The third patient died due to hypoglycemic coma.[193] In one case, IGF-II was detected immunohistochemically in the neoplastic stromal cells.[191] A case of malignant PT associated with elevated levels of human chorionic gonadotrophin (HCG) hormone has also been reported.[194] HCG levels dropped from 58 to 2 mIU/ml after mastectomy.

Gross Pathology

The external surface of a PT is well circumscribed but not encapsulated. The tumor may be a single mass or multinodular. PTs with microscopically invasive borders usually appear well circumscribed grossly.

The bisected tumor is composed of firm, bulging, gray to tan tissue (Figs. 8.26 to 8.28). Foci of degeneration, necrosis, and infarction may appear gelatinous or hemorrhagic.

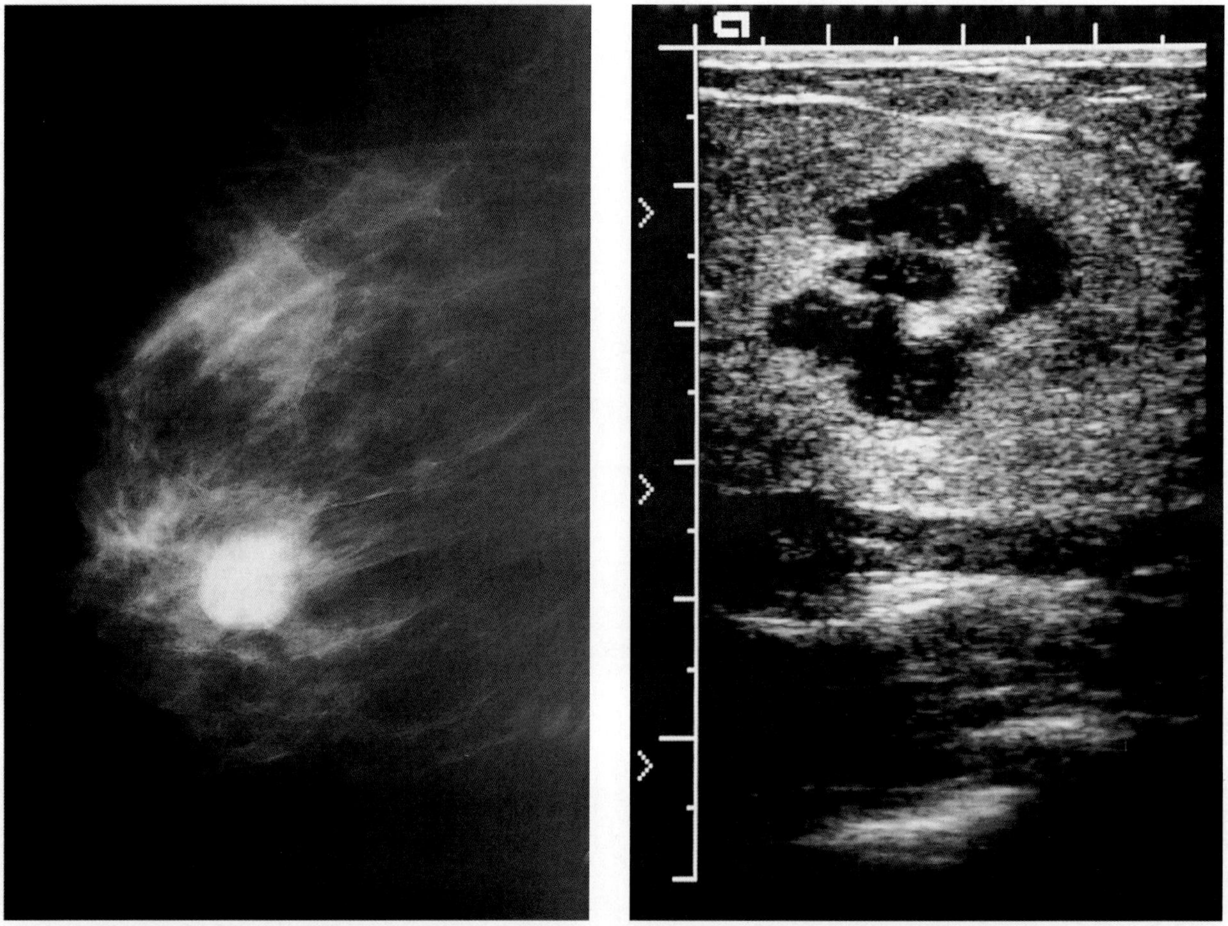

FIG. 8.25. ***Phyllodes tumor, mammography, and ultrasound.*** **A:** This mammogram shows a well-circumscribed tumor, which proved to be a malignant PT with leiomyosarcomatous differentiation. **B:** Inhomogeneous ultrasound transmission in a partly cystic tumor is illustrated.

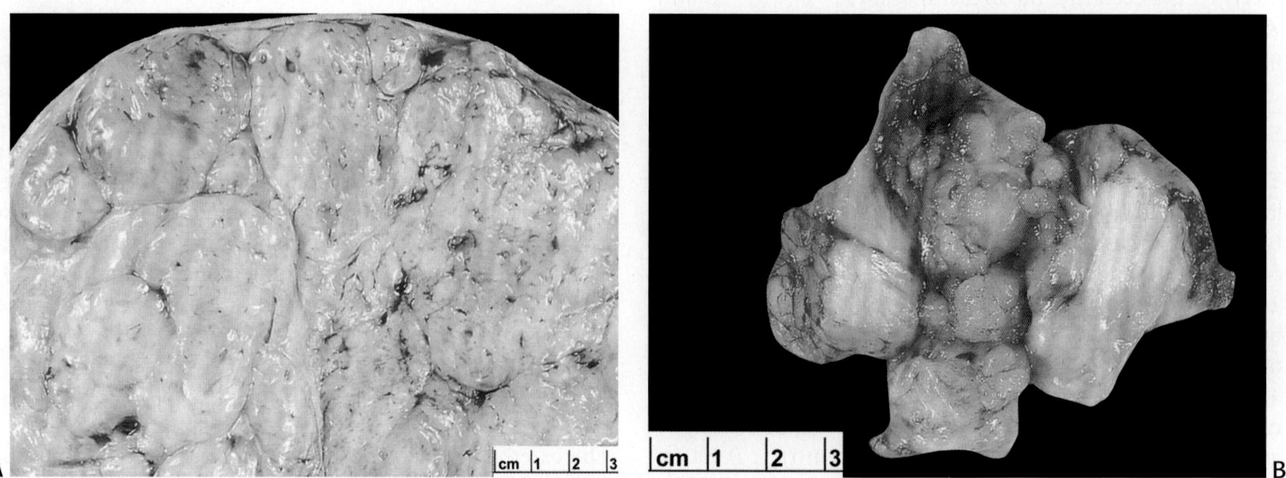

FIG. 8.26. ***Benign phyllodes tumor.*** Gross appearances of transected PT. **A:** Classic phyllodes architecture consisting of dense stroma and interlacing clefts. **B:** A lobulated tumor. **C:** A relatively homogenous tumor with dark foci of infarction. **D:** Whole-mount histologic section of a small benign PT. The tumor margin is slightly ragged in some areas next to fat.

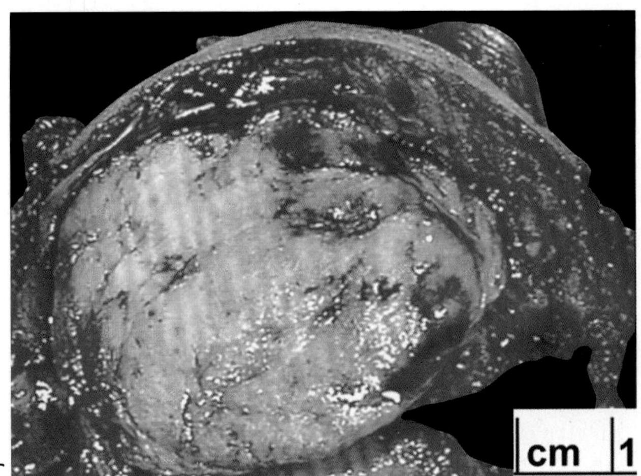

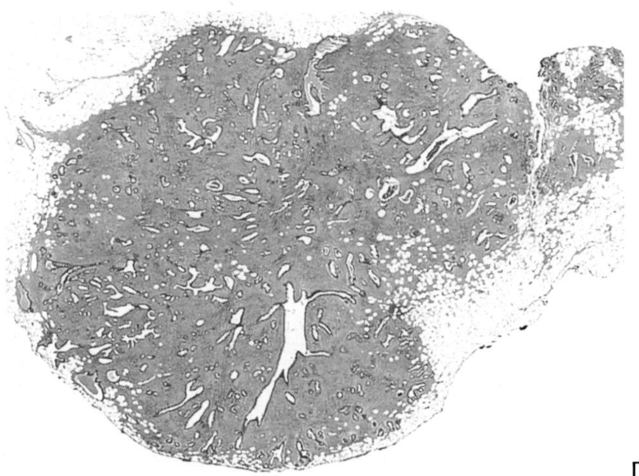

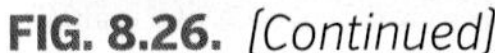

FIG. 8.26. *(Continued)*

These alterations are more common in malignant PTs, but can occur in large benign lesions. Cysts containing keratotic debris may be present. An unusual variant of PT has an exaggerated cystic component resulting in a gross appearance that is difficult to distinguish from a cystic papilloma[195] (Fig. 8.29). PTs with an extensive lipomatous component appear yellow and have fatty consistency grossly (Fig. 8.30).

Microscopic Pathology

The tumors arise from periductal rather than intralobular stroma and usually contain only sparse lobular elements. Most PTs have a heterogeneous histologic appearance. In a number of cases, the intracanalicular pattern of clefts is obscured by hyperplasia of the ductal epithelium, or there may be a conspicuous lobular component.

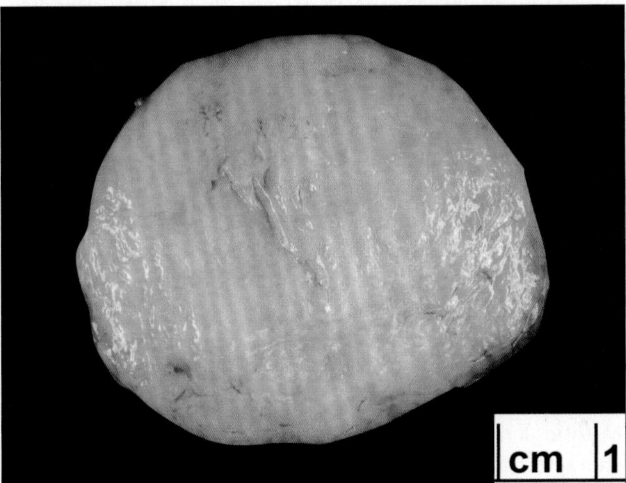

FIG. 8.27. ***Low-grade malignant phyllodes tumor.*** Gross appearance of a transected tumor. The cut surface is fleshy, and a few clefts are visible.

PTs are characterized by expansion and increased cellularity of the stromal component. In some PTs, stromal cellularity is denser in the periductal stroma near the epithelial components. Mitotic activity also tends to be accentuated in this distribution. Stromal mitoses are virtually absent from FAs, and this feature is helpful in the differential diagnosis of benign PTs. A rare subset of PTs with a nodular structure shows prominent periductal stromal proliferation. These have been referred to as "periductal stromal tumors" and subclassified as periductal stromal hyperplasia[196] or periductal stromal sarcoma.[197] However, they are variants of PT that can recur. The recurrent tumors are indistinguishable from conventional PT. Since all PTs are periductal stromal tumors, there is no advantage to referring to a subset of PT by this name. A substantial group of PTs exhibit little or no zonal stromal distribution.

Stromal overgrowth[198] has been defined as absence of an epithelial component in at least one microscopic field at 40× total magnification (10× ocular objective and 4× microscopic lens objective). It is more common in high-grade malignant PTs, but can also occur in low-grade (borderline) PTs. Some authors[145] have also commented on stromal expansion, defined as absence of epithelium in at least one microscopic field at final 100× magnification (10× ocular objective and 10× microscopic lens objective). Stromal expansion is common in low-grade and high-grade malignant PTs. The use of these parameters has intrinsic limitations, as the areas examined can vary slightly depending on the diameter of the objective lenses manufactured by different companies, but it nonetheless provides a useful and practical tool for evaluation of mammary fibroepithelial lesions.

The presence of elongated epithelial-lined clefts is a defining feature associated with PTs (Figs. 8.31 and 8.32). Occasionally, these spaces are dilated, and condensation of the immediately adjacent stroma may be found. The stromal fronds of PT usually project into the dilated clefts with a configuration reminiscent of a geographic peninsula. Each frond is covered by epithelium on three sides and typically has similar or smaller width at the base than at the tip.

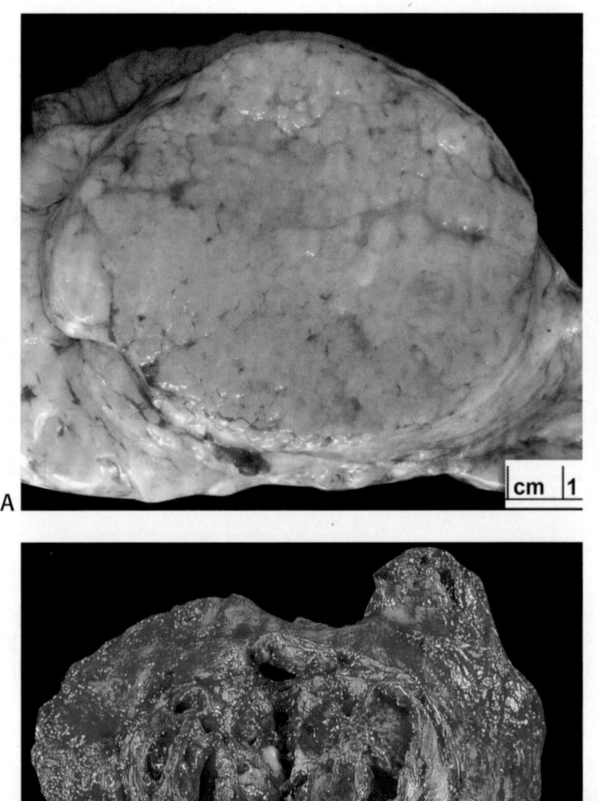

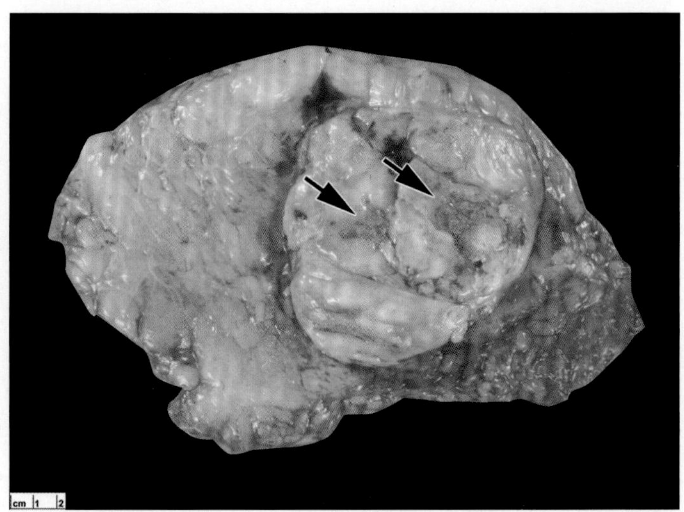

A B C

FIG. 8.28. ***High-grade malignant phyllodes tumor.*** Gross appearances of transected tumors. **A:** The cut surface has a variegated appearance with cysts and clefts. The border appears to be well circumscribed. **B:** Foci of necrosis (*arrows*) stand out from the glistening, fleshy surface. **C:** Extensive necrosis with cysts containing clotted blood.

The fronds of a PT do not fill the dilated clefts and do not appear to mold to one another (Figs. 8.29 and 8.32). The intracanalicular structure of some FAs bears a superficial resemblance to the clefted architecture of benign PTs, and the distinction between the two tumor types may be difficult. This problem is encountered particularly in very large or so-called giant FAs, when tumor size by itself suggests PT, and clefts may be apparent grossly on the cut surface of the tumor. In contrast to PT, the fronds of a FA have a broader base, rarely display the "peninsular" configuration, and completely fill the distended duct lumens, fitting to one another like pieces of a jigsaw puzzle. Histologically, the stroma in intracanalicular FAs tends to be hypocellular and uniform.

Myxoid change in the stroma of PT tends to be patchy and to undergo degenerative changes. PASH occurs in benign and malignant PTs and in some instances is a prominent feature of the lesion (Fig. 8.33). Tan et al.[154] observed PASH in 73.1% and myxoid degeneration in 87.2% of 335 PTs. Rarely, multinucleated stromal giant cells are found in a PT with PASH stroma (Fig. 8.34). These cells were present in 9.3% of 355 PTs studied by Tan et al.,[154] and their number was greater in higher grade lesions. These cells can exhibit lymphophagocytosis. They may express histiocytic immunomarkers such as CD68, as well as p53 and Ki67. Stromal metaplasia can rarely occur in benign PTs and consists of focal lipomatous metaplasia, but it is more common in low-grade (borderline) malignant PTs and most frequent in high-grade malignant PTs. It usually consists of liposarcoma, but rhabdomyosarcoma, angiosarcoma, and osteosarcoma have all been observed. Stromal cellularity is usually heterogeneous in PTs, with foci indistinguishable from FA that abut sharply on more cellular regions (Figs. 8.32 and 8.35). Such areas can lead to the conclusion that the PT arose from a FA, when, in fact, this is an intrinsic feature of some PTs. This variability in structure and stromal cellularity may create substantial difficulty in the accurate classification of some lesions sampled by FNA or needle core biopsy. Some reported instances of malignant clinical behavior or metastases from a "benign" PT are probably a reflection of inaccurate classification of the tumor because of incomplete sampling.

Excisional biopsy is required to grade a PT, a determination based on cytologic atypia, stromal cellularity, mitotic activity, and the microscopic character of the tumor border. Mitotic activity is the most important and often defining characteristic. The subclassification of PT encompasses three groups of lesions, namely benign PT, low-grade (borderline) malignant PT, and high-grade malignant PT. The goal of this classification is to estimate the risk of local recurrence and metastatic spread of a particular tumor.

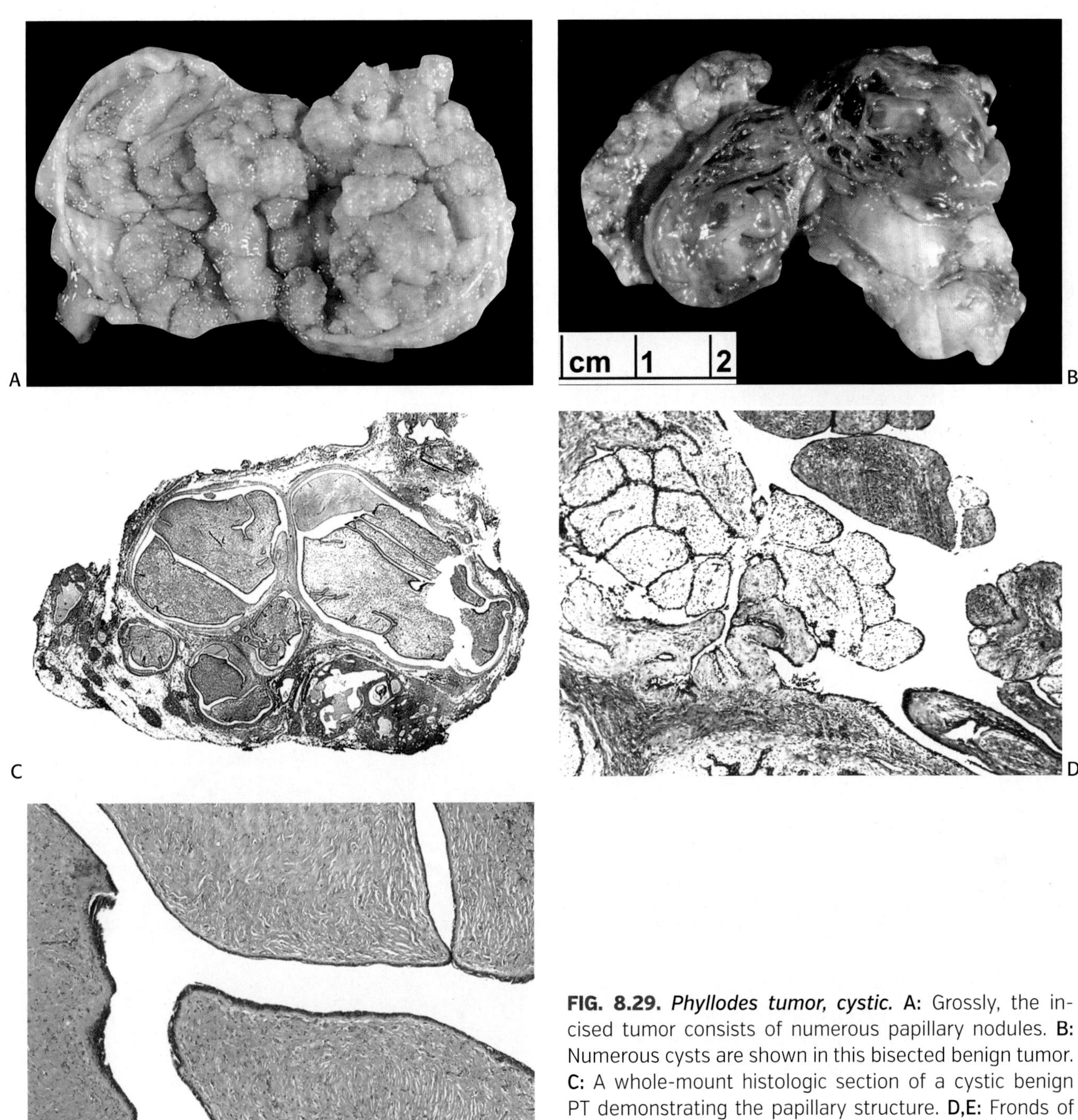

FIG. 8.29. ***Phyllodes tumor, cystic.*** **A:** Grossly, the incised tumor consists of numerous papillary nodules. **B:** Numerous cysts are shown in this bisected benign tumor. **C:** A whole-mount histologic section of a cystic benign PT demonstrating the papillary structure. **D,E:** Fronds of stroma covered by a thin layer of epithelium in benign papillary PTs.

Benign PT

A benign PT is characterized by very few if any stromal mitoses, rarely exceeding 1 to 2 mitoses per 10 high-power fields (HPFs). The 2012 *WHO Classification of Tumours of the Breast*[199] recommends a cutoff of 5 mitoses per 10 HPFs to distinguish between benign and low-grade (borderline) PT. Although it is possible that a PT that has an average of 5 mitoses per 10 HPFs might qualify as benign in the unlikely event that stromal cellularity is low and the tumor border is not infiltrating, the reader is cautioned that the average PT with 5 mitoses per HPF will have a significantly greater risk of local recurrence than a less mitotically active lesion that is classified as benign. For this reason, we would classify a lesion with more than 2 mitoses per 10 HPFs as low-grade malignant (borderline) PT. Modest to marked cellularity with slight to moderate cytologic atypia is present in most benign PTs (Figs. 8.31, 8.32, and 8.36). Stromal expansion and cellularity are typically uniform throughout

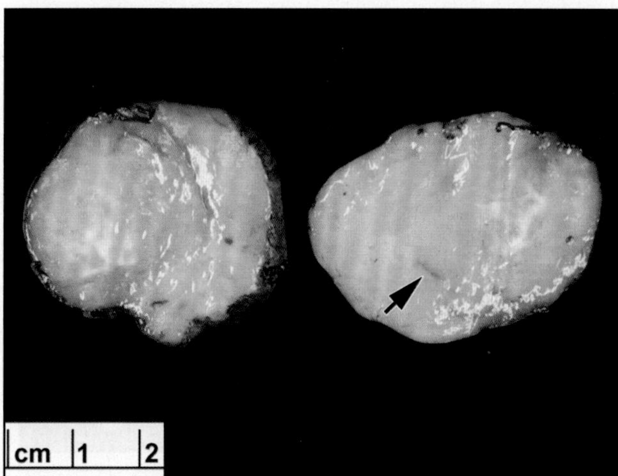

FIG. 8.30. ***Phyllodes tumor with extensive lipomatous component.*** This benign PT showed extensive lipomatous differentiation. The linear tract of a prior core biopsy site is also visible (*arrow*).

the lesion, but as noted previously, these features can be heterogeneous. The degree of epithelial proliferation usually corresponds to the appearance of the stroma. Epithelial hyperplasia is not conspicuous in the average benign PT, but occasionally it can be quite pronounced. The border of the tumor is usually well defined (Figs. 8.31 and 8.32), but invasion may be present in the form of very focal and inconspicuous infiltration at the tumor periphery or of secondary nodules of benign PT around the main tumor (Fig. 8.37). Lipomatous (Figs. 8.38 and 8.39) and osseous metaplasia can occur in the stroma of a benign PT. An extremely unusual example of a benign PT with adipose stromal differentiation that arose in a lipomatous hamartoma has been reported[200] (Fig. 8.40). Multinucleated cells with hyperchromatic nuclei may be present in the stroma (Figs. 8.34 and 8.41). Focal stromal myxoid change is not uncommon in a benign PT, but a tumor composed entirely of this tissue is very unusual. Necrosis is not a feature of benign PT. An unusual benign PT in a 42-year-old woman had stromal cells that contained intracytoplasmic inclusion bodies of the type found in infantile digital fibromatosis[201] (Fig. 8.42). Electron microscopy revealed a mixture of fibroblasts and myofibroblasts. The intracytoplasmic inclusions were closely associated with cytoplasmic microfilaments forming tadpole-like structures. These cells were weakly stained for actin by routine immunohistochemistry (IHC), with no reactivity in the inclusion bodies. After pretreatment with potassium hydroxide in 70% ethanol and 0.1% trypsin, the cells and inclusions were strongly actin positive.

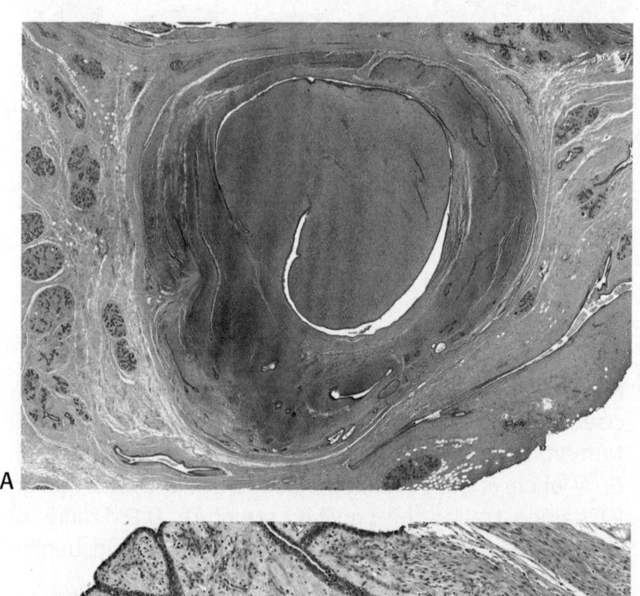

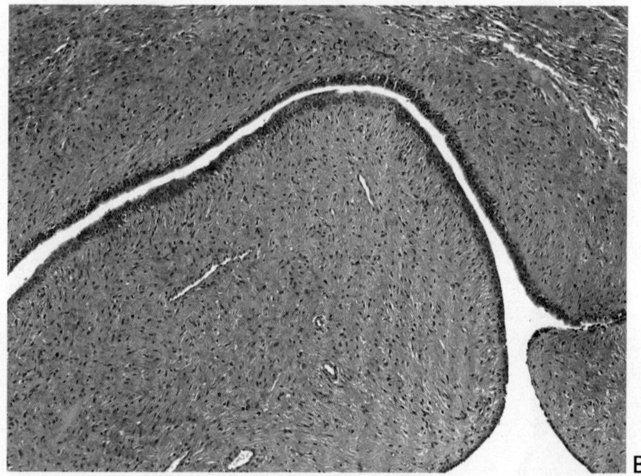

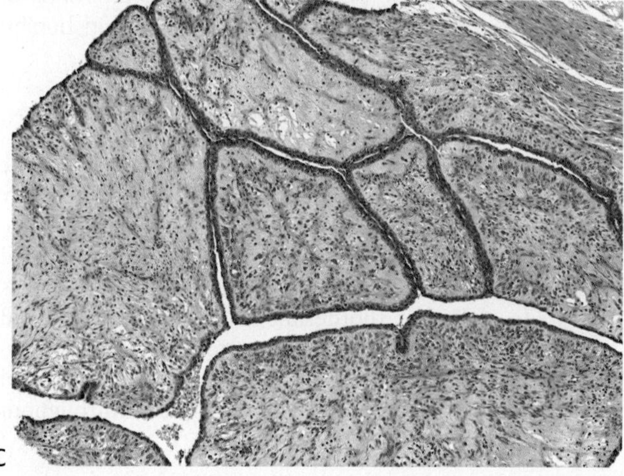

FIG. 8.31. ***Benign phyllodes tumor.*** **A:** A benign PT showing the well-defined interface with the surrounding normal stroma. Note the contrasting stromal cellularity, and an epithelial-lined cleft in the tumor. **B:** Stretched ducts are surrounded by homogeneous stroma in the same case as (A). **C:** Subepithelial stromal condensation and increased vascularity are noted in the fronds of another tumor.

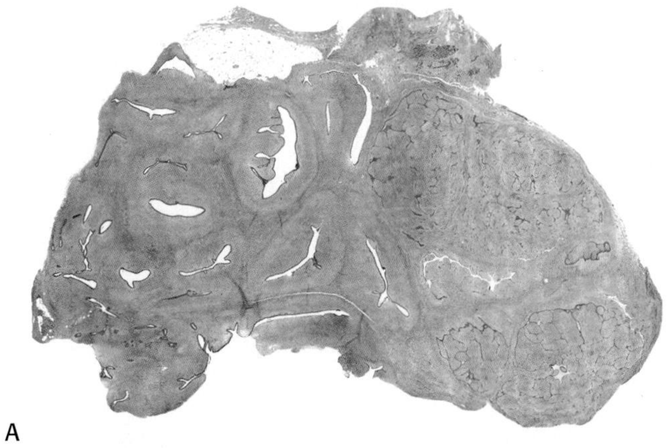

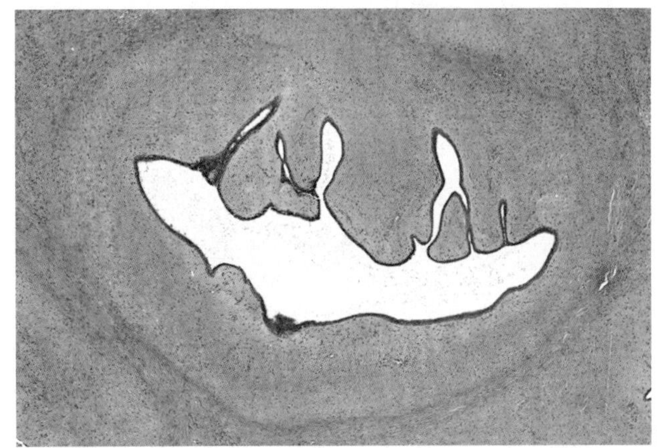

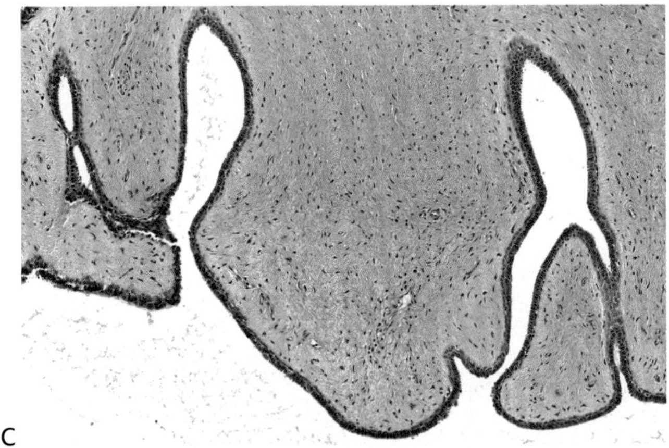

FIG. 8.32. ***Benign phyllodes tumors.*** **A:** Whole-mount section of a benign PT emphasizes the leaf-like architecture and intratumoral heterogeneity. Areas resembling a FA are evident. **B,C:** The stromal proliferation forms a cellular cuff around the duct. The duct lumen is partially filled by the tumor fronds, formed by a relatively bland proliferation of bipolar spindle cells.

Low-Grade Malignant (Borderline) PT

A low-grade malignant (also known as borderline) PT has a microscopically circumscribed or invasive border with satellite nodules, an average of 2 to 5 mitoses per 10 HPFs, and moderate stromal cellularity that is often heterogeneously distributed in the midst of hypocellular areas (Figs. 8.43 to 8.45). The 2012 *WHO Classification of Tumours of the Breast*[199] gives the mitotic activity of a borderline PT as

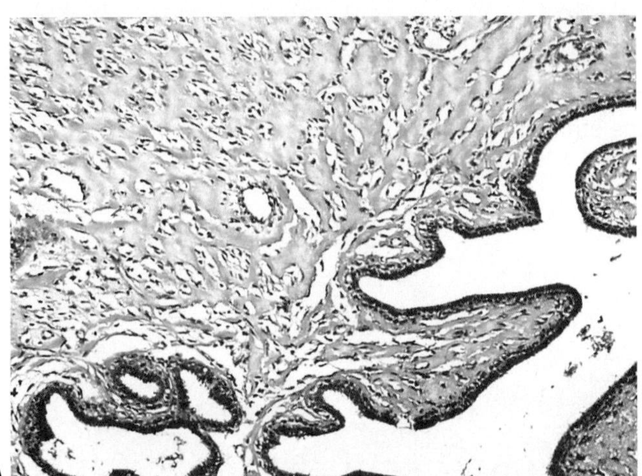

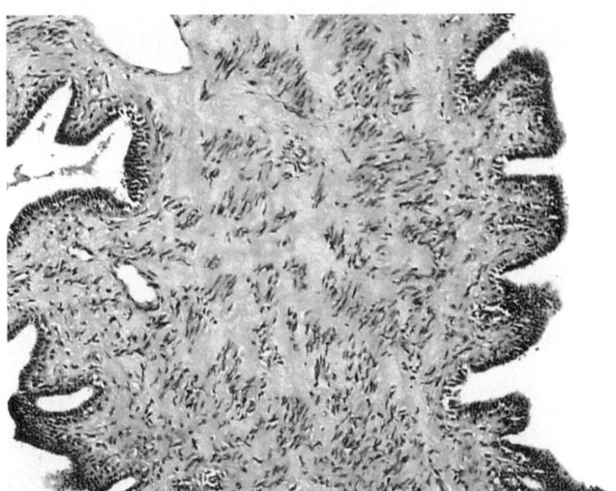

FIG. 8.33. ***Benign phyllodes tumor, variants with myofibroblastic stroma.*** **A:** Stroma in a benign PT with a pseudoangiomatous pattern. **B:** Pseudoangiomatous stroma with myofibroblasts in fascicular arrangement. The fibroepithelial structure has a pseudopapillary configuration. **C:** The pseudoangiomatous structure is highlighted with the SMA immunostain. **D,E:** Myxoid pseudoangiomatous stroma in a benign PT that resembles myxoid myofibroblastoma.

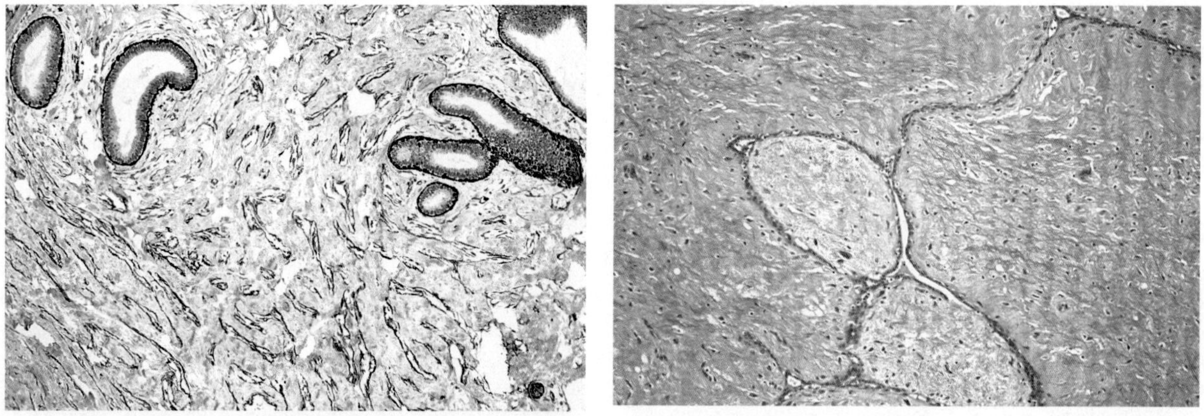

C D 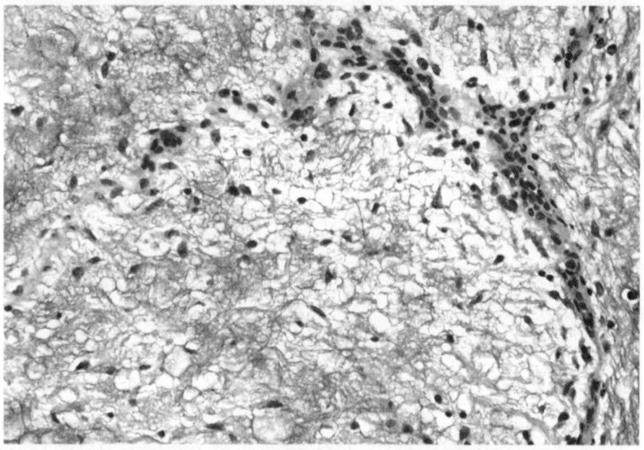 E

FIG. 8.33. *(Continued)*

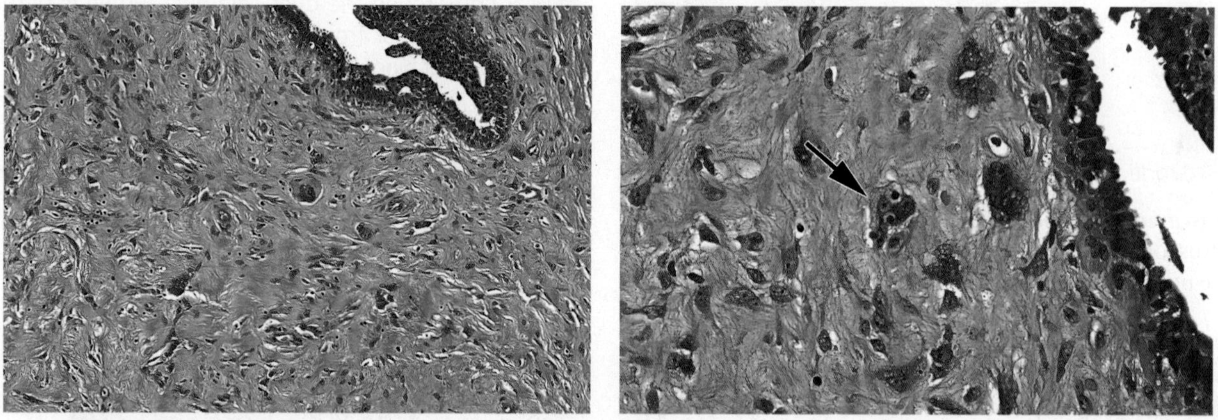

A B

FIG. 8.34. ***Benign phyllodes tumor with pseudoangiomatous stromal hyperplasia and stromal giant cells.*** **A:** Multinucleated cells are present in the stroma. **B:** Lymphophagocytosis is shown in a giant cell (*arrow*).

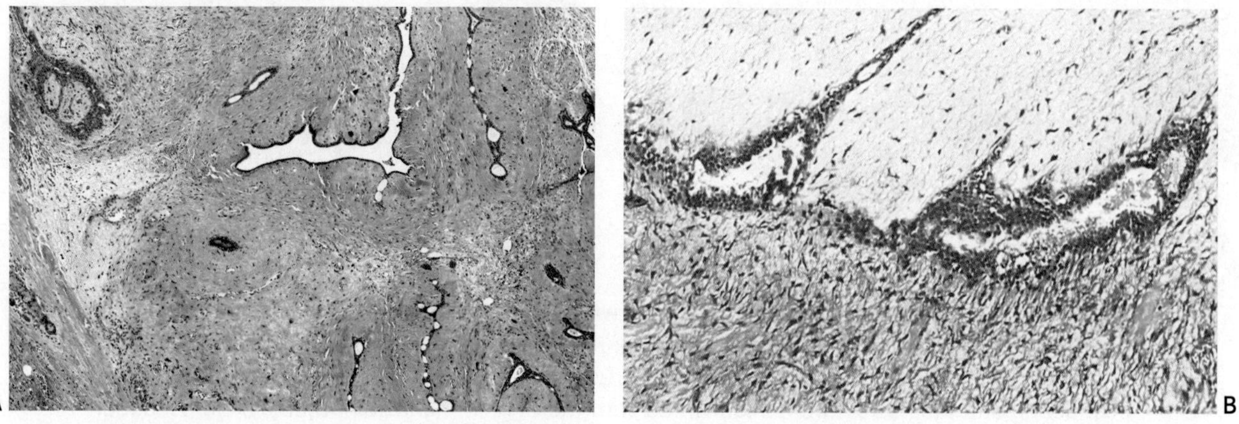

FIG. 8.35. ***Benign phyllodes tumor.*** **A,B:** Examples of stromal heterogeneity in two benign PTs.

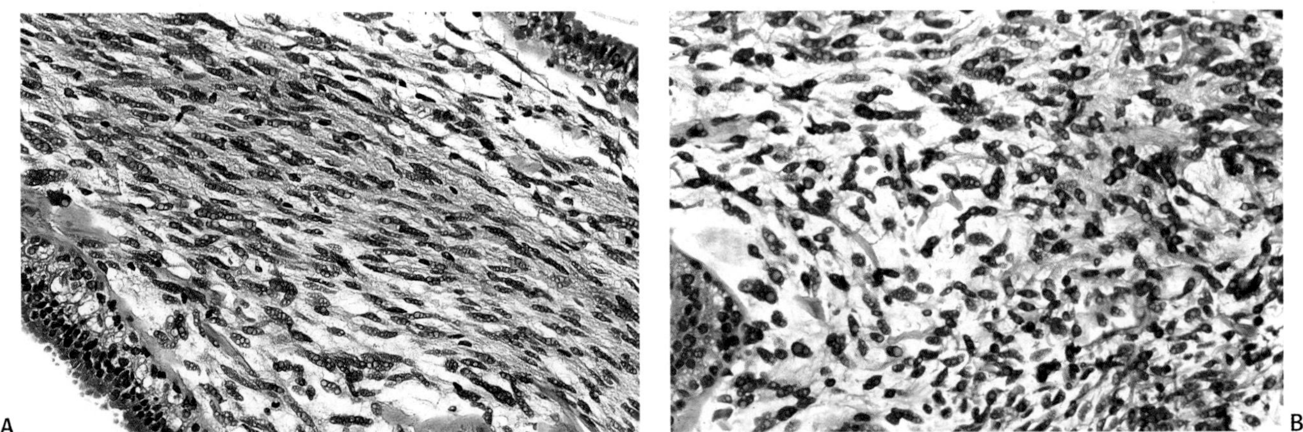

FIG. 8.36. ***Benign phyllodes tumor.*** **A,B:** Characteristic nuclear cytology.

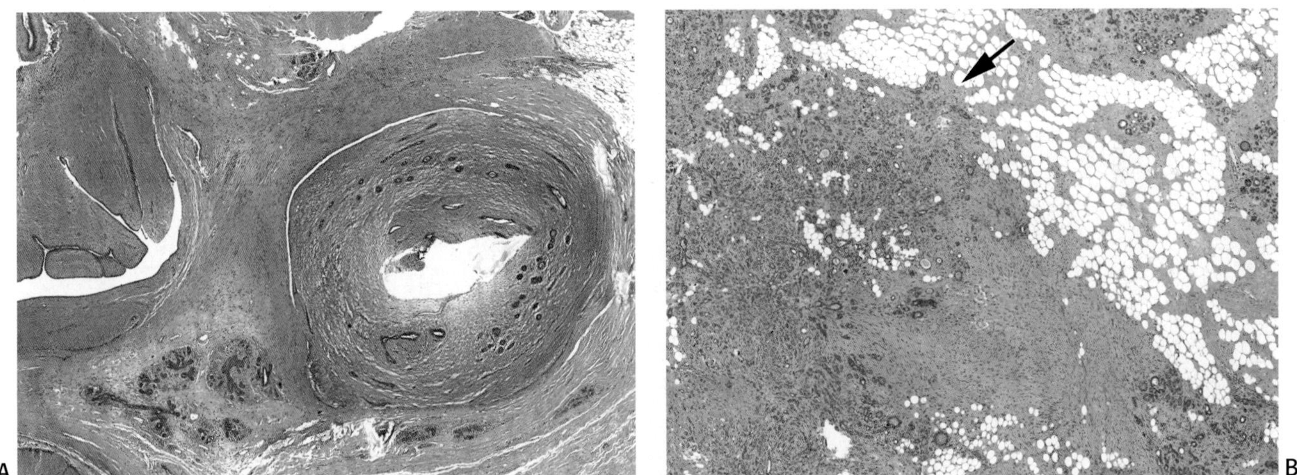

FIG. 8.37. ***Benign phyllodes tumor.*** **A:** This benign PT has a satellite nodule (*right*) separate from the main tumor mass (*left*). **B:** Tumor extending into fat. This unusual variant of PT contains an area of SA (*arrow*).

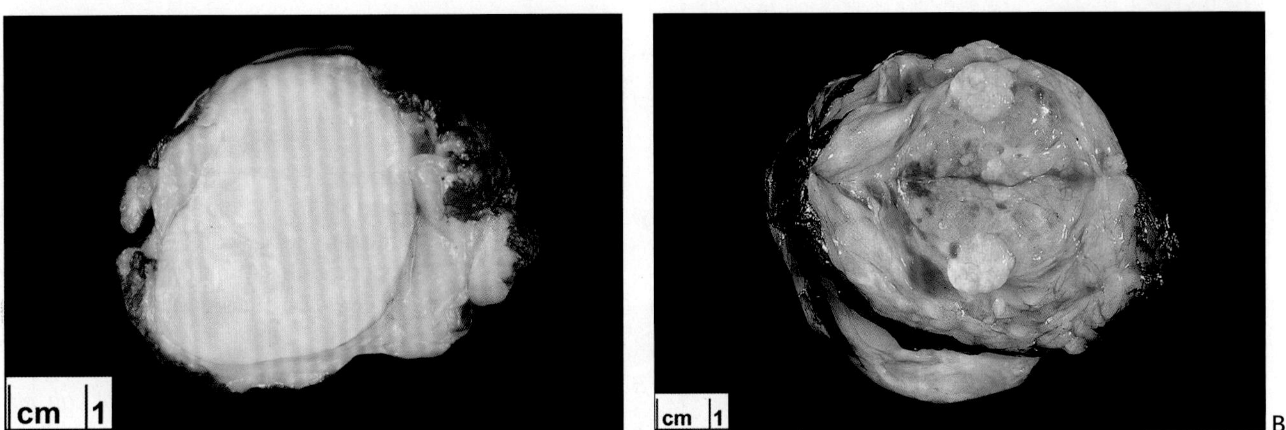

FIG. 8.38. ***Benign phyllodes tumor with lipomatous metaplasia.*** **A:** The entire tumor shows lipomatous differentiation. **B:** The bright yellow nodule in this bisected tumor is an area of lipomatous stromal metaplasia.

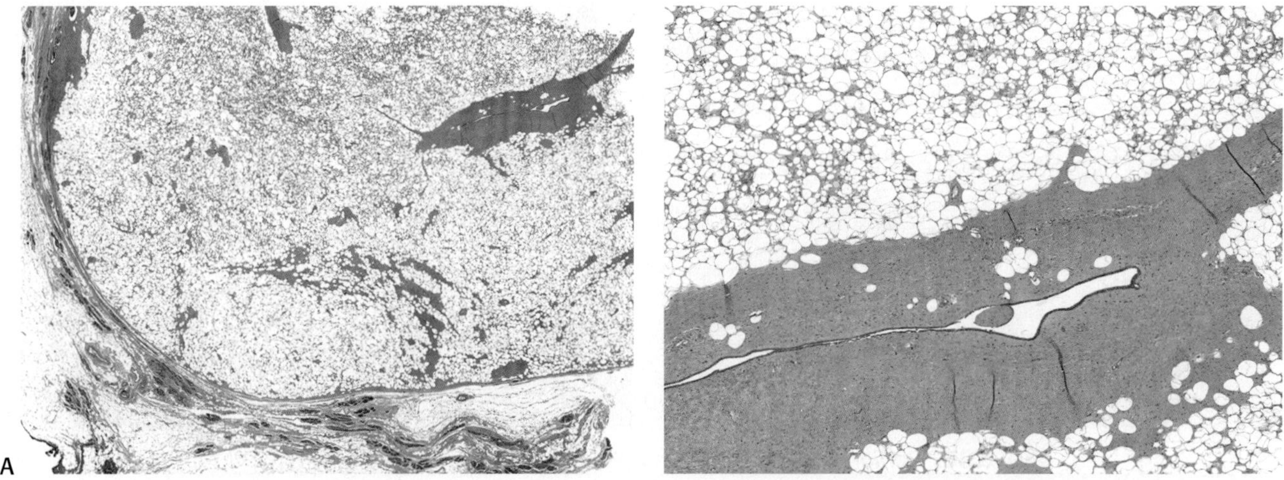

FIG. 8.39. ***Benign phyllodes tumor with lipomatous metaplasia (lipophyllodes tumor).*** **A:** Whole-mount histologic section showing extensive lipomatous transformation of the stroma. **B:** Lipomatous stroma around a stretched out duct.

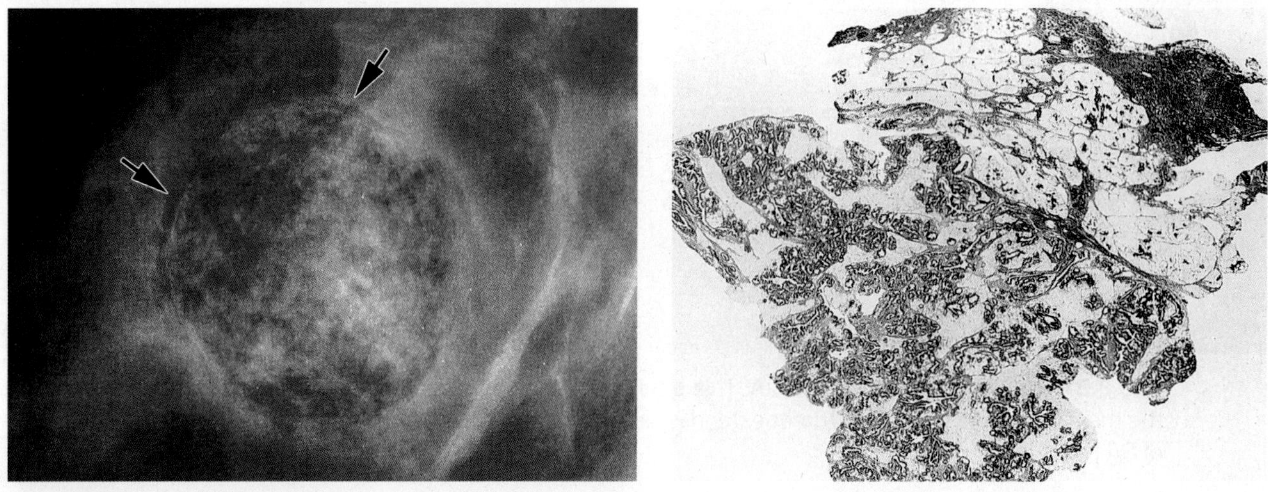

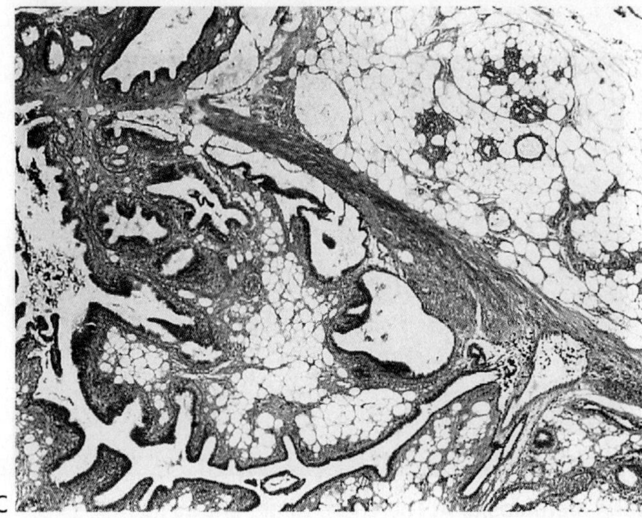

FIG. 8.40. ***Benign phyllodes tumor associated with a lipomatous hamartoma.*** **A:** Magnified view of the mammogram revealing an inhomogeneous tumor with a well-defined border in part demarcated by a zone of decreased density (*arrows*) in the region of the lipomatous hamartoma. **B:** Whole-mount histologic section showing the lipomatous hamartoma *above* and the lipophyllodes tumor *below*. **C:** Lipomatous hamartoma (*above*) and lipophyllodes tumor (*below*). (Reproduced from Rosen PP, Romain K, Liberman L. Mammary cystosarcoma with adipose differentiation (lipophyllodes tumor) arising in a lipomatous hamartoma. *Arch Pathol Lab Med* 1994;118:91–94; Copyright 1994, American Medical Association, with permission.)

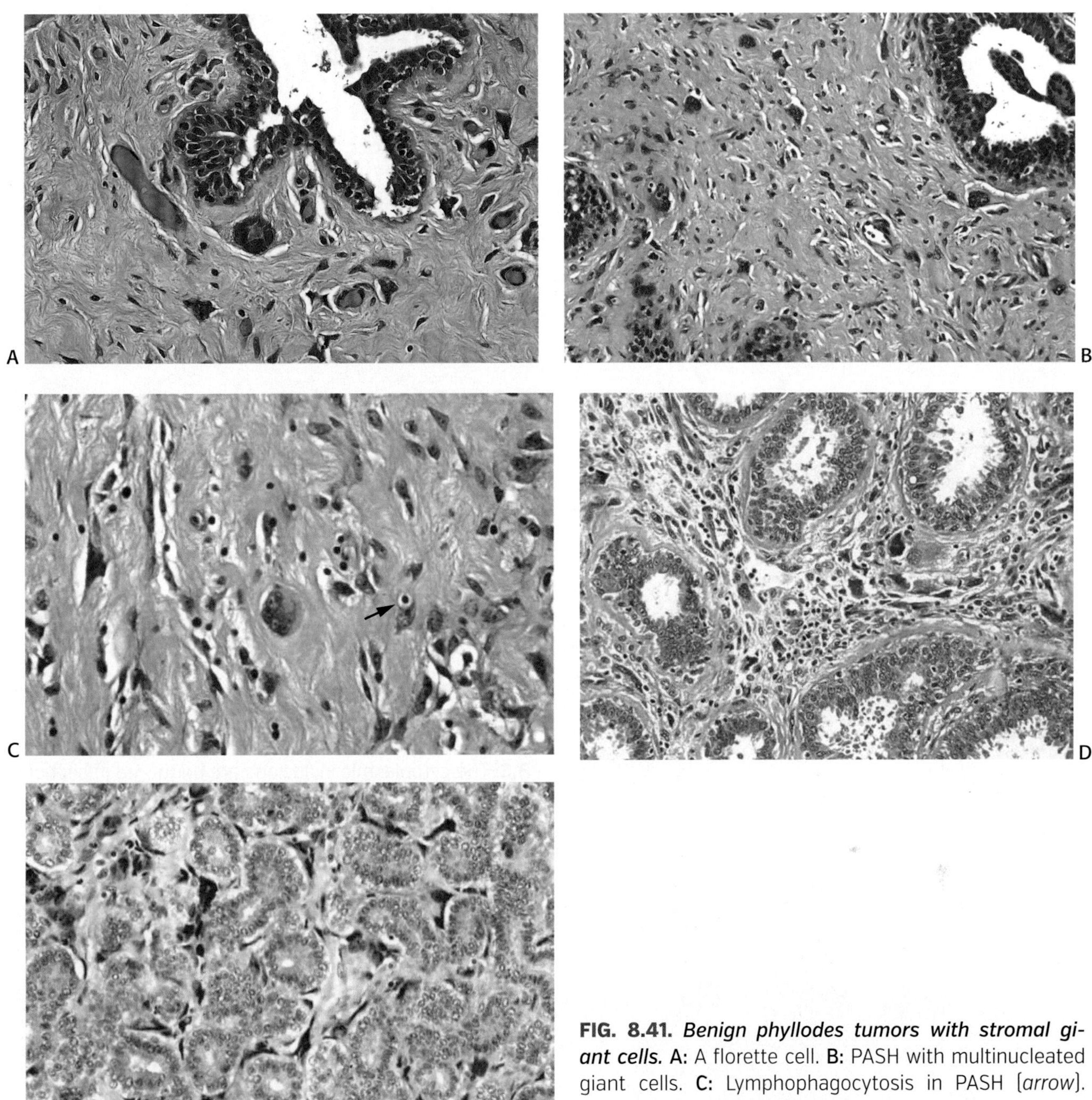

FIG. 8.41. ***Benign phyllodes tumors with stromal giant cells.*** **A:** A florette cell. **B:** PASH with multinucleated giant cells. **C:** Lymphophagocytosis in PASH (*arrow*). **D,E:** Multinucleated stromal cells in a tumor with adenosis proliferation of the epithelium.

5 to 9 mitoses per 10 HPFs. By including lesions with mitotic rates in the 5 to 9 per 10 HPFs in the low-grade malignant (borderline) group, this classification greatly expands the chances of local recurrence in this category, with increased likelihood for a high-grade malignant recurrence and the development of metastases. The spindle cell stroma in many low-grade PTs resembles fibromatosis, low-grade fibrosarcoma, or PASH (Fig. 8.44). Infrequent instances of cartilaginous, osseous, and lipomatous metaplasia have been encountered in low-grade PTs (Fig. 8.45). Focal areas of necrosis may be present.

High-Grade Malignant PT

A fully malignant or high-grade PT typically features hypercellular stroma. Stromal overgrowth is also common. In most cases, this is combined with greater than 5 mitoses per 10 HPFs and an invasive tumor border (Figs. 8.46 and 8.47). The neoplastic stromal cells typically have high-grade and pleomorphic nuclei. In a study by Tan et al.,[154] areas of necrosis were present in 12/31 (39%) malignant PTs. Rarely, the stroma contains specific sarcomatous elements such as angiosarcoma (Fig. 8.48), liposarcoma (Fig. 8.49),

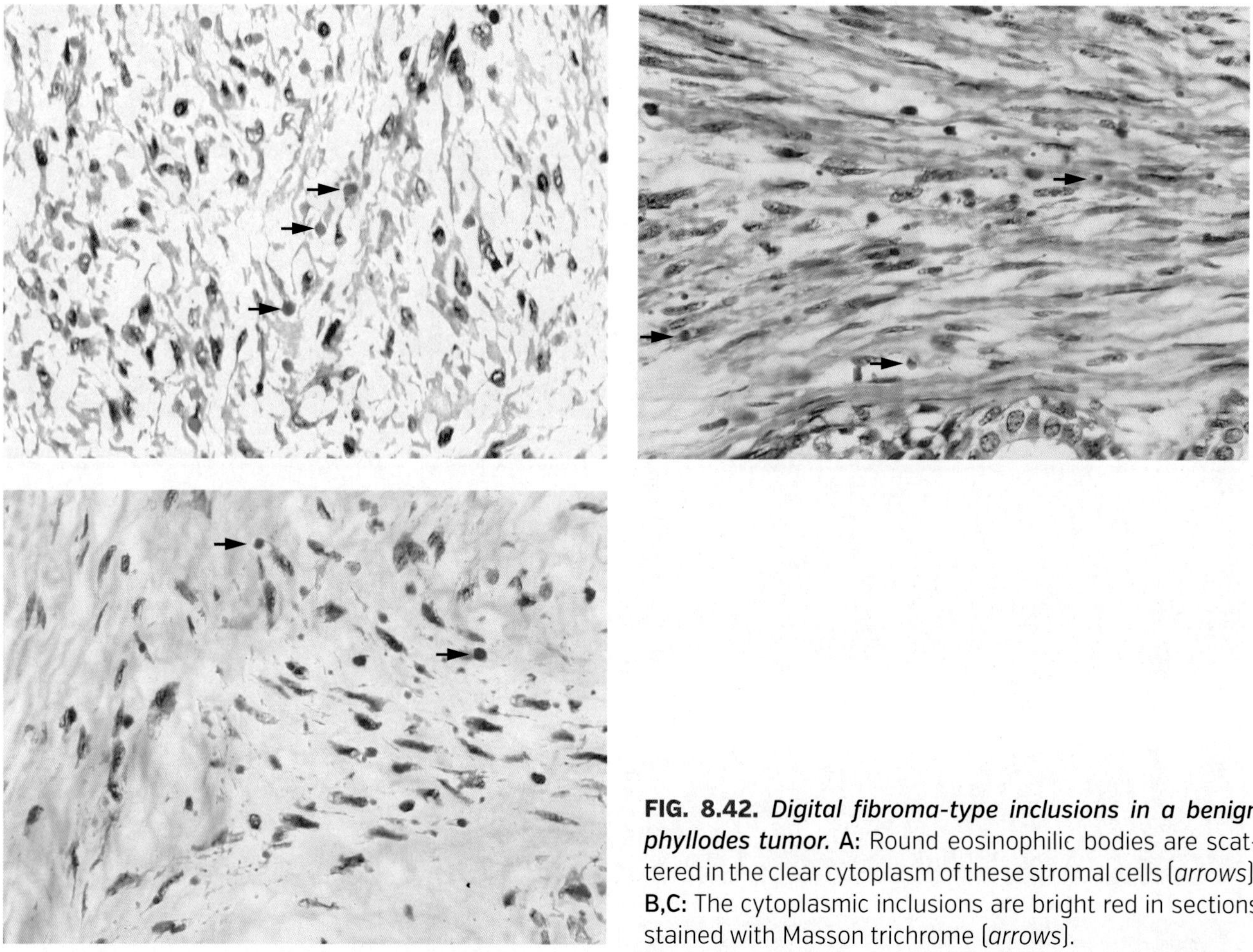

FIG. 8.42. ***Digital fibroma-type inclusions in a benign phyllodes tumor.*** **A:** Round eosinophilic bodies are scattered in the clear cytoplasm of these stromal cells (*arrows*). **B,C:** The cytoplasmic inclusions are bright red in sections stained with Masson trichrome (*arrows*).

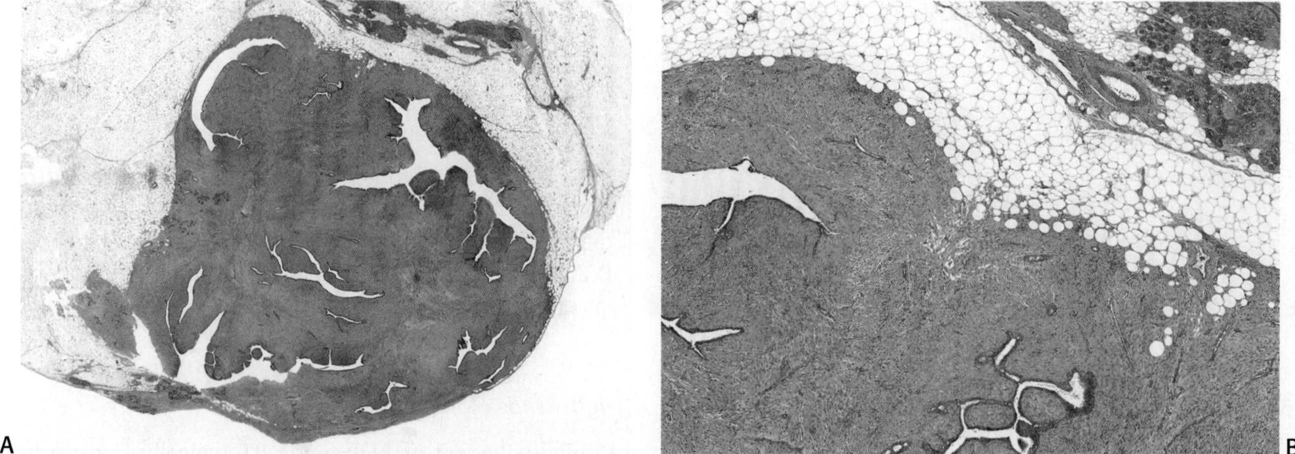

FIG. 8.43. ***Low-grade (borderline) malignant phyllodes tumor.*** **A,B:** The tumor shows stromal expansion and leaf-like architecture. Peripheral infiltration into the adjacent tissue is identified microscopically **(B)**. **C–E:** This tumor shows periductal growth with an exaggerated papillary structure **(C,D)**. The stroma of the neoplastic fronds is hypercellular. Infiltration into the surrounding adipocytes is evident at the tumor periphery **(E)**.

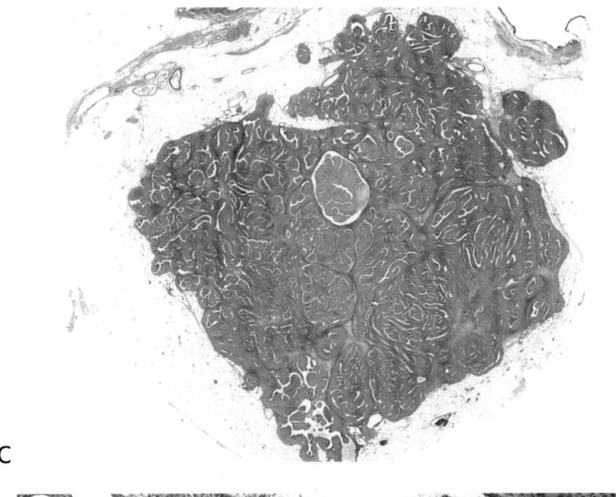

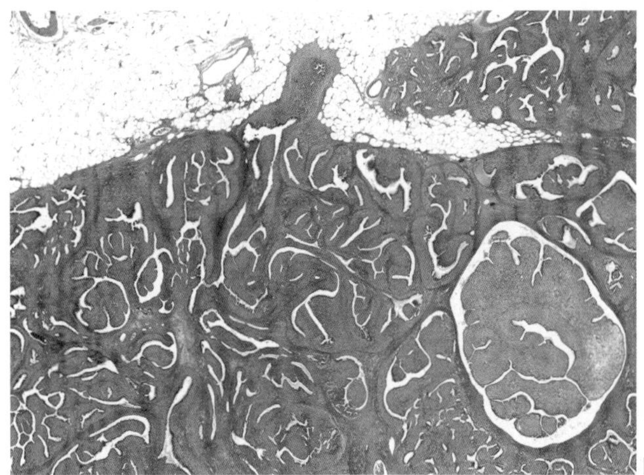

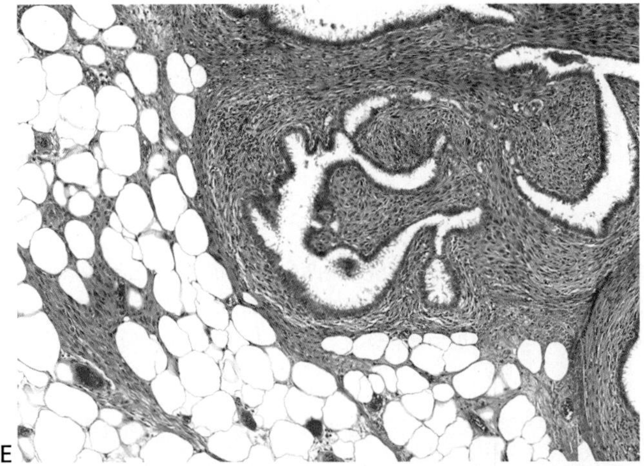

FIG. 8.43. *(Continued)*

chondrosarcoma, myosarcoma, or osteosarcoma[202–205] (Figs. 8.48D and 8.50). Vascular invasion was identified in 3 of 31 high-grade malignant PTs studied by Tan et al.[154]

Epithelium in PTs

Many PTs exhibit epithelial hyperplasia with a variable increase in the thickness of the cuboidal or columnar epithelium lining the slit-like or clefted spaces. Focal or diffuse papillary or cribriform architecture is not uncommon (Fig. 8.51). Myoepithelial hyperplasia can also occur focally. The extent of epithelial hyperplasia tends to parallel the cellularity and mitotic activity of the stroma, but many exceptions to this rule are encountered. Sawyer et al.[206] found epithelial hyperplasia in 60% of 119 PTs, including 8 malignant PTs and 2 with only a sarcomatous component. The hyperplastic changes were marked in 18% of cases and slight in 42%; no epithelial hyperplasia was present in 40% of the cases. Epithelial mitoses were numerous in one case and easy to identify in 20 (18%). Tan et al.[154] found epithelial hyperplasia in 247/335 (74%) PTs. Mild hyperplasia was present in 122/335 (36%) cases, moderate in 94/335 (28%), and severe in 31/335 (9%). Epithelial hyperplasia occurred in 186/250 (74%) of benign PTs and was mild in 98/250 (39%) cases, moderate in 66/250 (26%), and severe in 22/250 (9%). Low-grade (borderline) PTs had the highest rate of epithelial hyperplasia (45/54; 83%), which was mild in 17/54 (31%) cases, moderate in 21/54 (39%), and severe in 7/54 (13%). Epithelial hyperplasia was present in 16/31 (51%) high-grade malignant PTs, and was mild or moderate in 7/31 (22.5%) cases each and severe in 2/31 (6%). Grimes[141] found "marked epithelial hyperplasia" in one-third of benign PTs, including four (13%) with atypia, and in 26% of malignant PTs. The epithelium was described as atypical in 2 of the 13 (15%) cases of malignant PTs with epithelial hyperplasia. In their series of 65 PTs, Karim et al.[176] had 26 cases with usual ductal hyperplasia, another 26 with columnar cell change, 2 with ADH, and 1 with DCIS (Fig. 8.52). Squamous metaplasia of ductal epithelium is found in 3.6%[154] to 10% of PTs[141,150] (Fig. 8.53). Apocrine metaplasia in the epithelium of PTs has been reported (Fig. 8.54).[141,176,207,208] Lobules are occasionally included in or formed in PTs, and they may exhibit proliferative changes, including SA. The presence of lobules can lead to an erroneous diagnosis of FA, especially when lobular hyperplasia is present and stromal cellularity is not greatly increased. In rare instances, the epithelial proliferation in the form of adenosis or papillary hyperplasia can be so extreme that it obscures the underlying

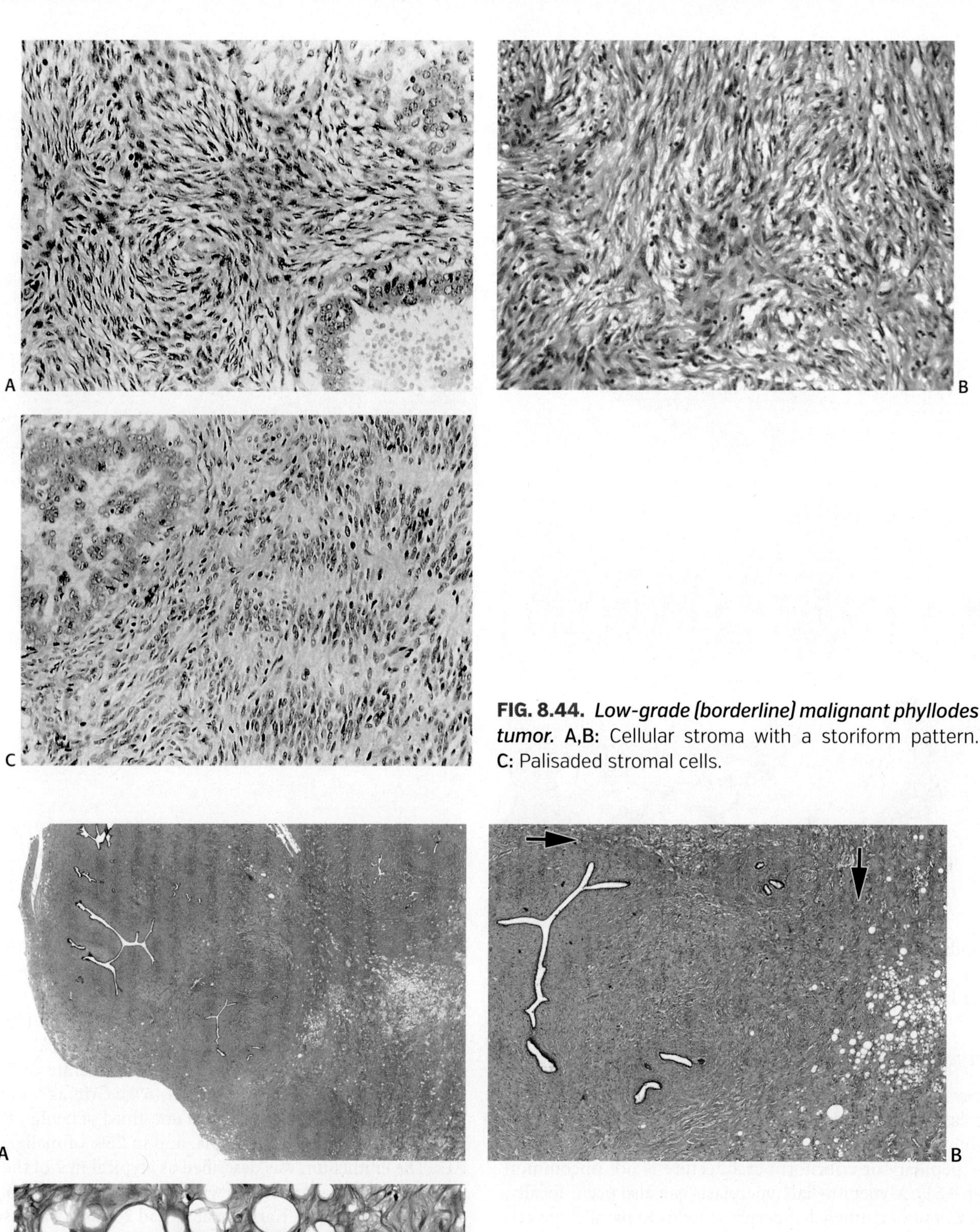

FIG. 8.44. ***Low-grade (borderline) malignant phyllodes tumor.*** **A,B:** Cellular stroma with a storiform pattern. **C:** Palisaded stromal cells.

FIG. 8.45. ***Low-grade (borderline) malignant phyllodes tumor.*** **A,B:** The tumor shows stromal expansion and a liposarcomatous area. Areas of PASH (*arrows*) are present. **C:** A lipoblast is shown.

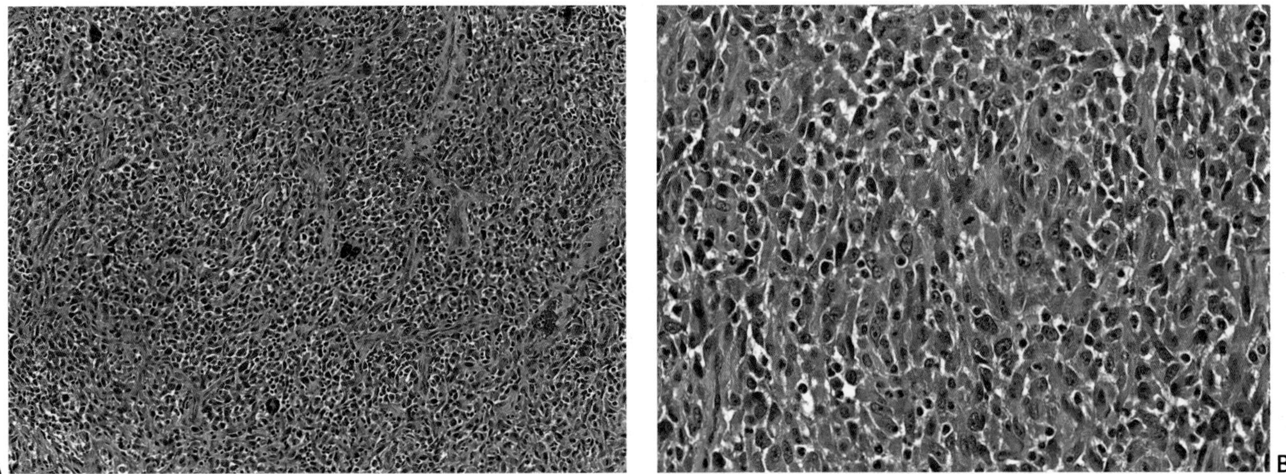

FIG. 8.46. ***High-grade malignant phyllodes tumor.*** **A:** Cellular proliferation of malignant spindle cells. Note high tumor vascularity and scattered anaplastic cells. **B:** The neoplastic cells have high-grade morphology. In a limited needle core biopsy sample, this tumor could be mistaken for a high-grade carcinoma.

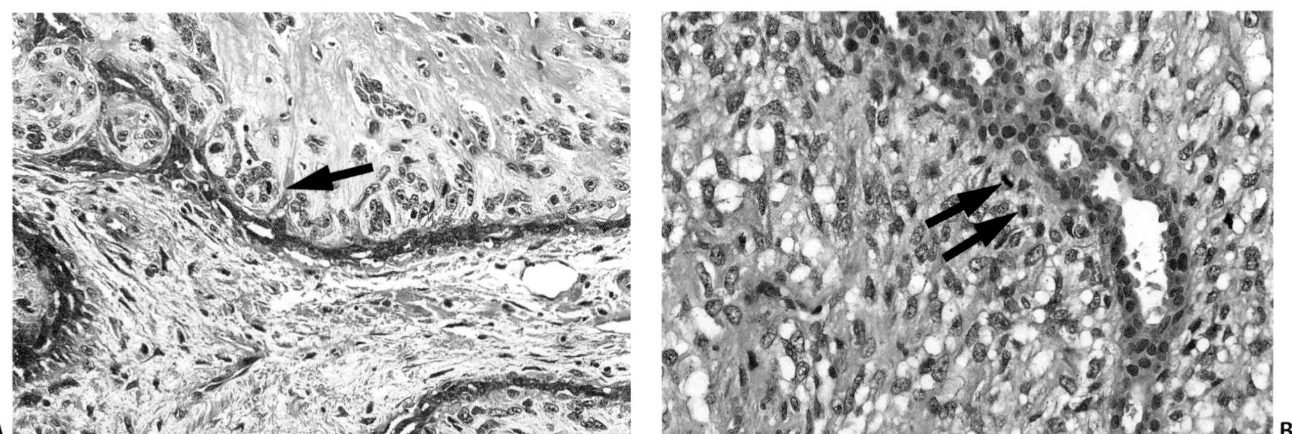

FIG. 8.47. ***High-grade malignant phyllodes tumor.*** **A,B:** Mitotic activity (*arrows*) limited to the subepithelial region in cells with epithelioid **(A)** and spindle cell **(B)** phenotypes.

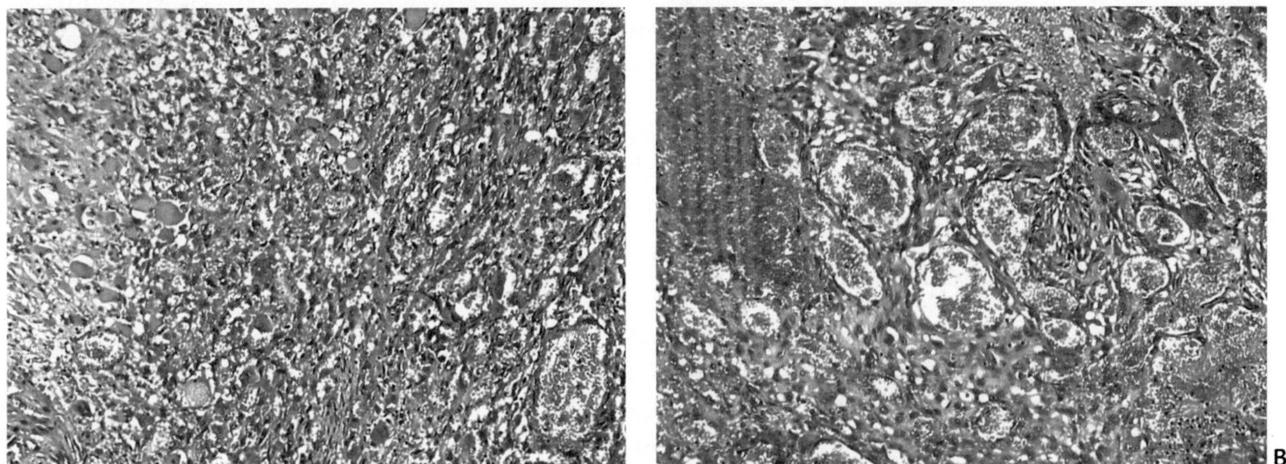

FIG. 8.48. ***Angiosarcoma in high-grade malignant phyllodes tumor.*** **A:** Vasoformative pattern. **B:** Telangiectatic pattern. **C–E:** Another high-grade malignant PT with spindle cell **(C)**, chondrosarcomatous **(D)**, and angiosarcomatous **(E)** components.

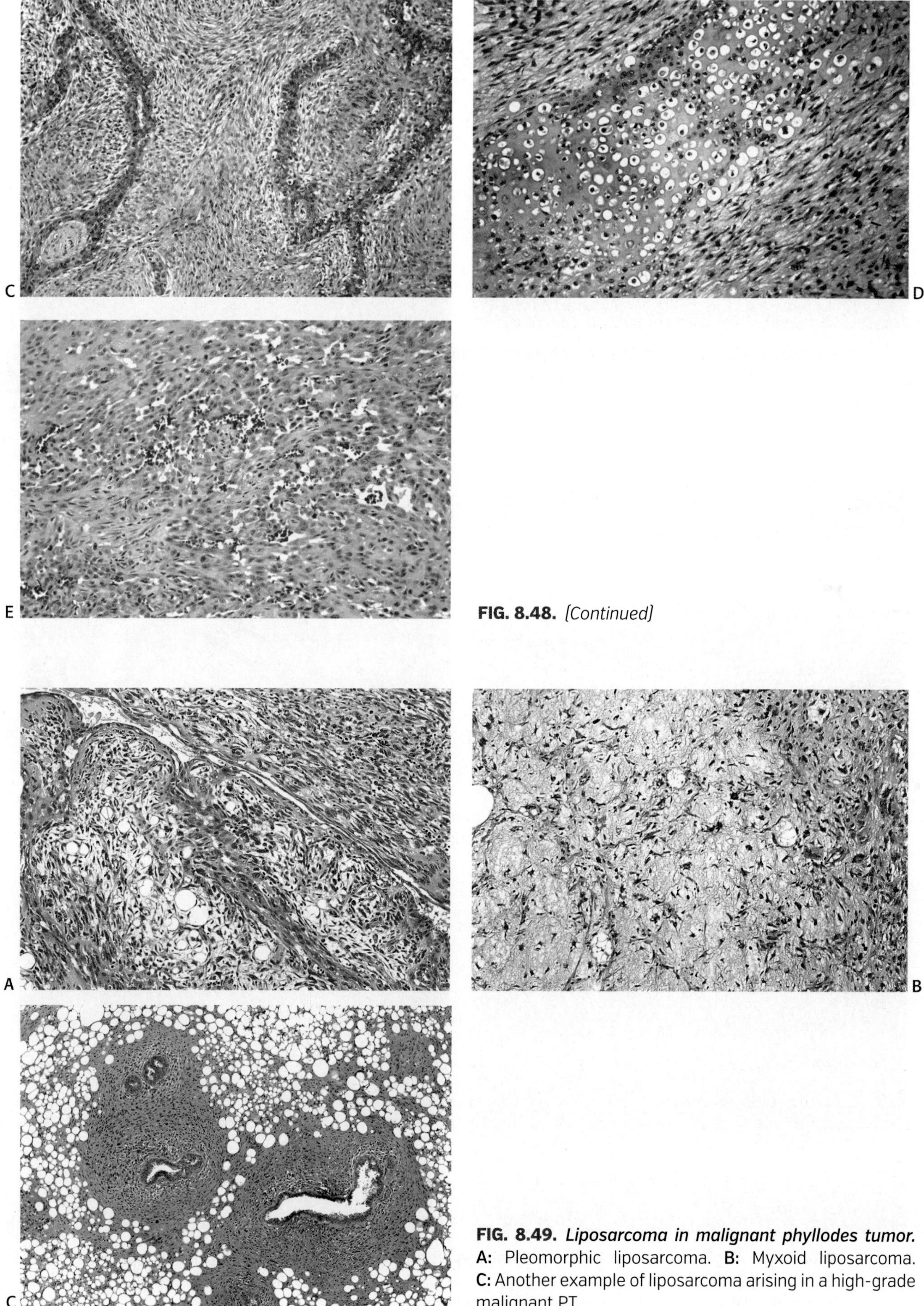

FIG. 8.48. *(Continued)*

FIG. 8.49. ***Liposarcoma in malignant phyllodes tumor.*** **A:** Pleomorphic liposarcoma. **B:** Myxoid liposarcoma. **C:** Another example of liposarcoma arising in a high-grade malignant PT.

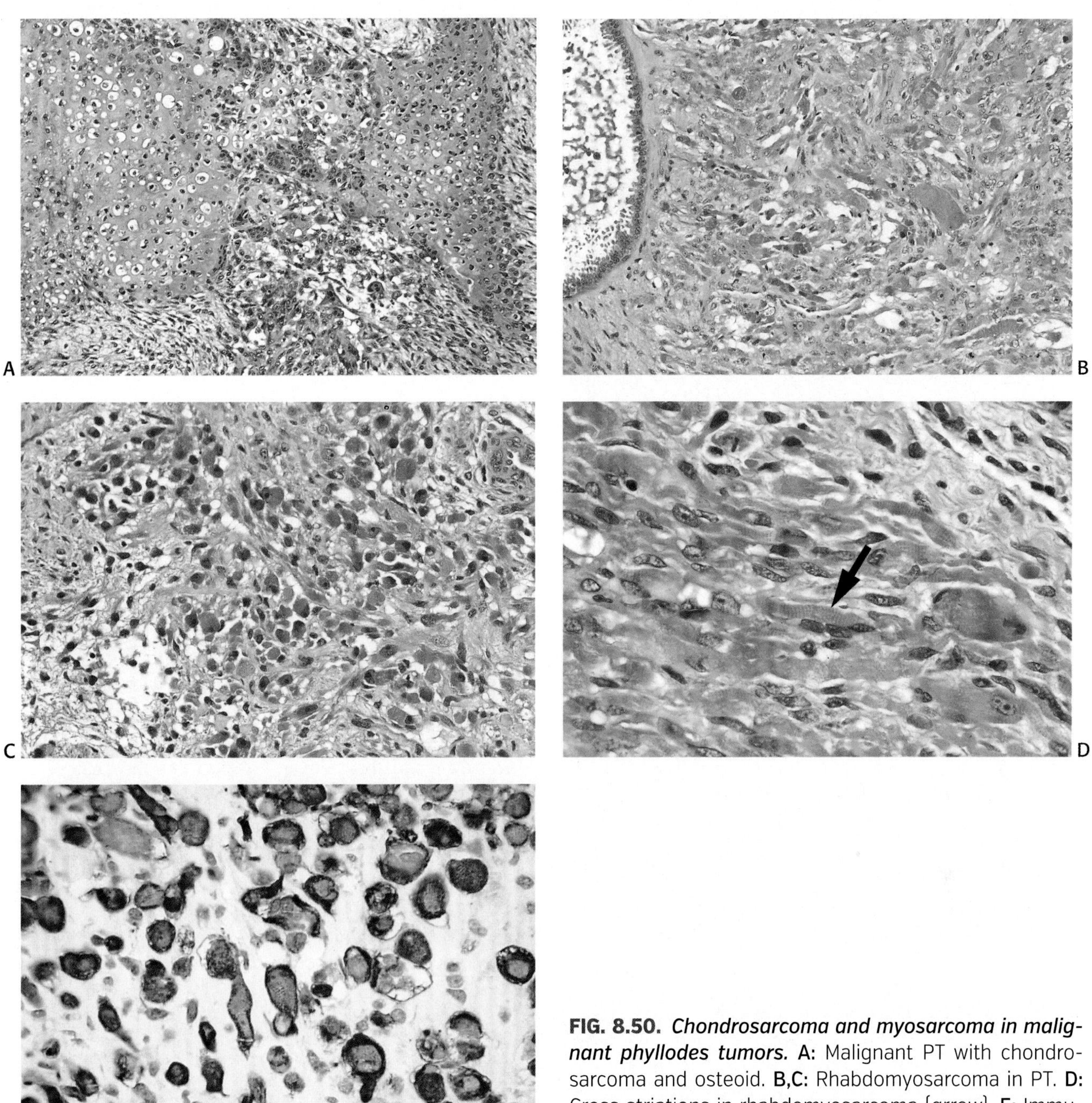

FIG. 8.50. ***Chondrosarcoma and myosarcoma in malignant phyllodes tumors.*** **A:** Malignant PT with chondrosarcoma and osteoid. **B,C:** Rhabdomyosarcoma in PT. **D:** Cross striations in rhabdomyosarcoma (*arrow*). **E:** Immunoreactivity for myoglobin. The rhabdoid tumor cells were also immunoreactivity for desmin (not shown).

PT, and the latter may not be recognized until the tumor recurs (Figs. 8.55 and 8.56). Tumors in which the fundamental phyllodes growth pattern is obscured, typically by an unusual epithelial distribution (PT variants), usually masquerade as papillary neoplasms or as adenosis tumors (Figs. 8.37B, 8.41E, 8.55, and 8.56).

Immunohistochemical and molecular evidence suggests that epithelial alterations may play a role in the pathogenesis of PTs (see sections on immunohistochemistry and genetic and molecular alterations).

Carcinoma in PT

The hyperplastic epithelium in a PT rarely shows cytologic atypia. Atypical epithelial hyperplasia is sometimes extreme, raising the differential diagnosis of intraductal carcinoma (Fig. 8.52). In general, the threshold for the diagnosis of DCIS in a PT should be high. The PT character of the lesion may be overlooked if the stromal component is interpreted as reactive rather than as an intrinsic part of the neoplasm. Epithelial nuclear atypia was marked in 10 (9%) cases reported by Sawyer et al.[206] In the series by Tan et al.,[154] five PTs contained ADH

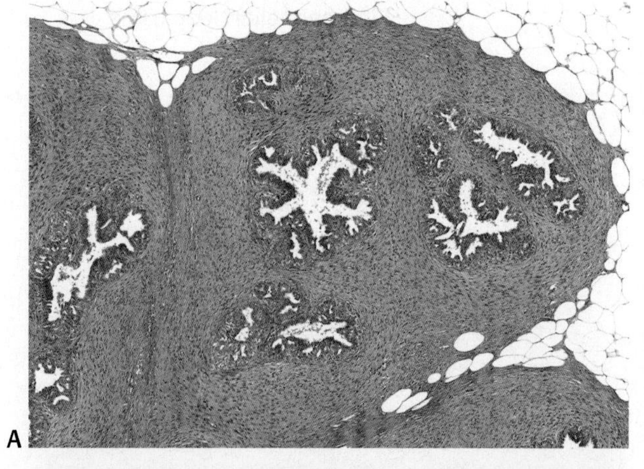

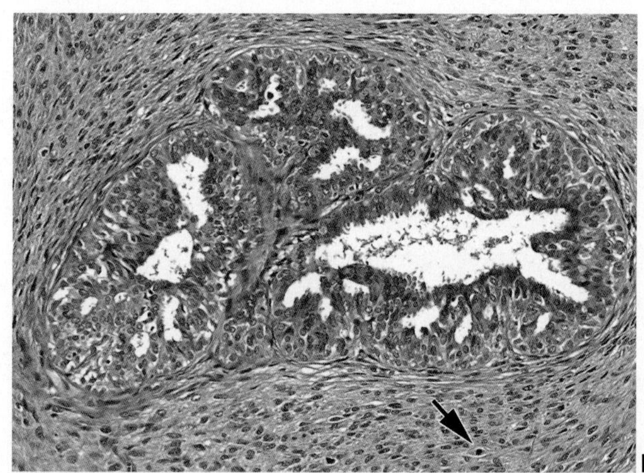

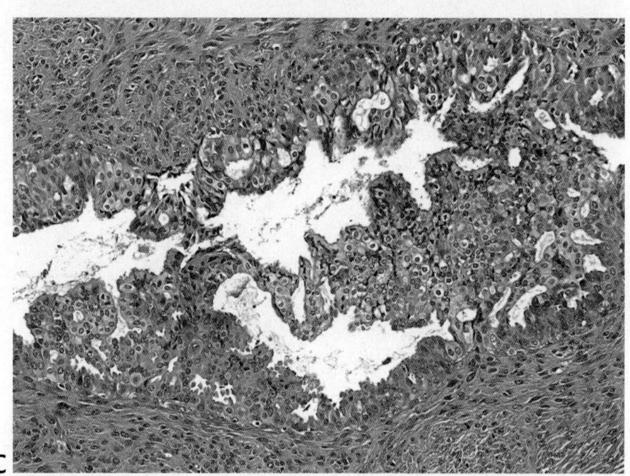

FIG. 8.51. ***Florid and atypical ductal hyperplasia in phyllodes tumor.*** **A:** The epithelium of a low-grade PT shows micropapillary usual ductal hyperplasia. Subtle peripheral invasion of the neoplastic stromal cells into the adjacent fat is also evident. **B:** Usual ductal hyperplasia with pseudocribriform spaces. Note pronounced hyperplasia of myoepithelial cells. A stromal mitosis is evident (*arrow*). **C:** In a different area of the same tumor, the ductal proliferation shows monotonous low-grade cytologic atypia and slightly rigid architecture, consistent with ADH.

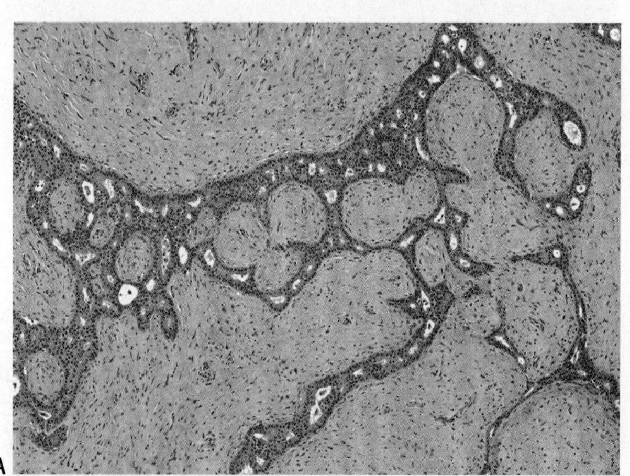

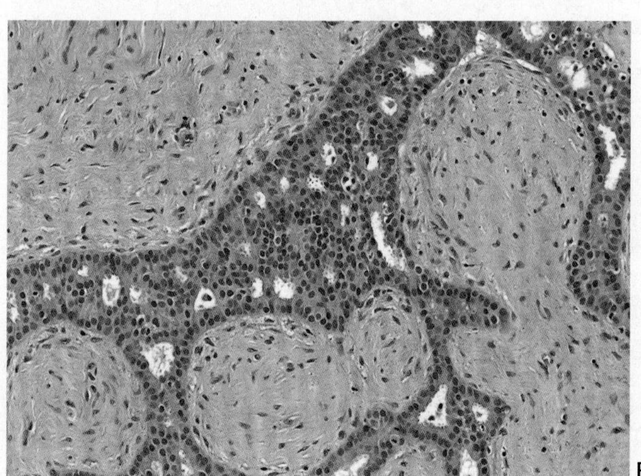

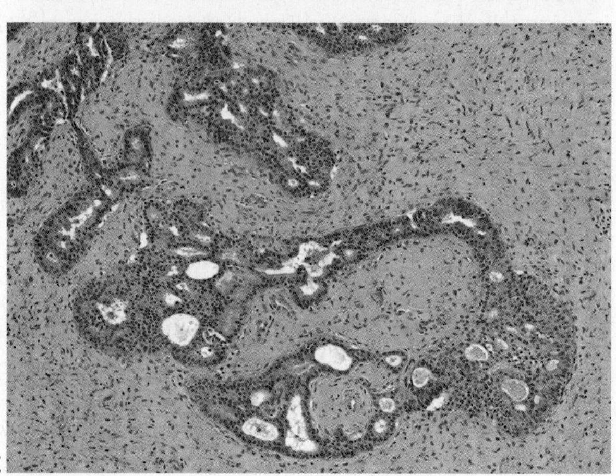

FIG. 8.52. ***Low-grade DCIS in phyllodes tumor.*** **A–C:** Low-grade DCIS with focal cribriform architecture involves multiple ducts. The DCIS was confined to the PT and did not involve the adjacent breast parenchyma. All images are from the same case.

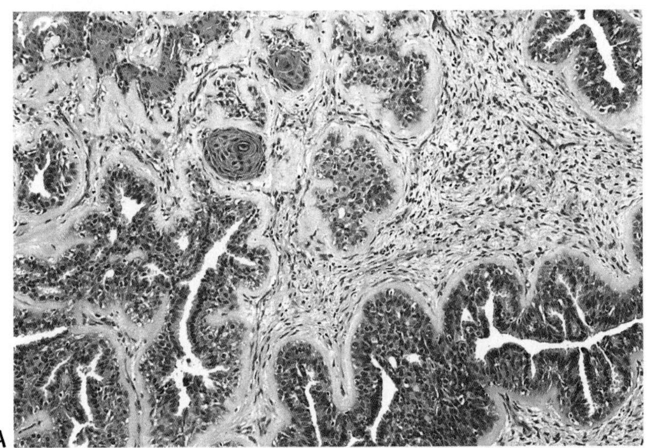

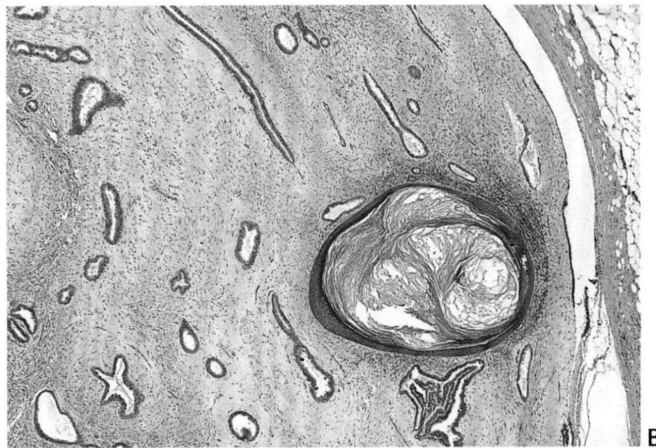

FIG. 8.53. ***Squamous metaplasia in a benign phyllodes tumor.*** **A:** Focal squamous metaplasia associated with florid epithelial hyperplasia. **B:** Cystic squamous metaplasia (both stained with hematoxylin-phloxine-saffranin).

(1.5% of cases); ALH and lobular carcinoma *in situ* (LCIS) were present in one case each (0.03%), and a malignant PT contained DCIS (0.03%). The diagnosis of intraductal or invasive ductal carcinoma in PTs is infrequent.[154,176,209–214] Invasive lobular carcinoma has also been described.[215] Quinlan-Davidson et al.[216] reported a case of tubular carcinoma and LCIS in a low-grade (borderline) PT. Choi et al.[217] described invasive cribriform carcinoma in a malignant PT. Sugie et al.[218] reported a case of invasive carcinoma with squamous differentiation arising in a high-grade malignant PT (Fig. 8.57).

Epithelial alterations have also been documented in the breast parenchyma adjacent to a PT. Tan et al.[154] observed DCIS in the breast parenchyma near a PT in one case, and ADH and ALH in three cases each. The breast parenchyma also showed synchronous FAs, including 5 ipsilateral and 9 contralateral, in 14/355 (3.9%) women.

The subject of carcinoma in FA and PT is discussed further in Chapter 33.

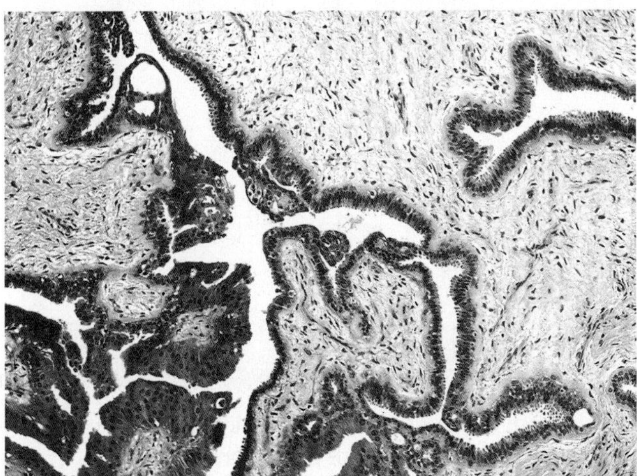

FIG. 8.54. ***Benign phyllodes tumor with apocrine metaplasia (lower left).***

Morphology of Recurrent PT

Ductal elements may be present in locally recurrent PTs in the breast. A postmastectomy chest wall recurrence showing ductal elements probably involves focal residual breast tissue. The morphology of recurrent tumors is usually similar to that of the primary PT,[145,154] but occasionally the recurrent PT differs from the primary and is usually of higher grade. Barrio et al.[145] reported that 6/23 (26%) benign PTs had malignant recurrences. Five of the six original tumors had areas of marked stromal cellularity, three had stromal expansion or marked stromal overgrowth, and two had a high mitotic rate. In the same study,[145] 12 malignant PTs recurred locally, including 9 that recurred with malignant morphology and 2 as benign PT. One recurrence was not classified morphologically. In the series described by Tan et al.,[154] upgrading to the next higher diagnostic category was observed in 14/57 (25%) recurrent cases, but six recurrences had lower grade than the index PT: two high-grade malignant PTs had low-grade (borderline) malignant recurrences, two low-grade malignant (borderline) PTs had benign recurrences, and two high-grade malignant PTs relapsed with benign PT morphology. In a series of 37 recurrent PTs reported by Tan et al.,[219] the recurrent tumor was morphologically similar to the original PT in 24/37 (64.9%) patients. Ten patients (27%) relapsed with a higher grade lesion, including four benign PTs and three low-grade (borderline) PTs that recurred with high-grade malignant PT morphology, and three benign PTs that recurred with low-grade (borderline) malignant PT morphology. Conversely, two low-grade (borderline) malignant PTs relapsed with benign PT morphology. One patient treated by mastectomy for low-grade (borderline) malignant PT developed a contralateral benign PT 4 years later.

Metastatic PTs at distant sites almost always consist entirely of the stromal component. Two case reports claim to demonstrate an epithelial component in lung metastases.[220,221] One of these represents inclusion of pulmonary alveolar tissue in the metastatic lesion.[220] In the other extraordinary case,

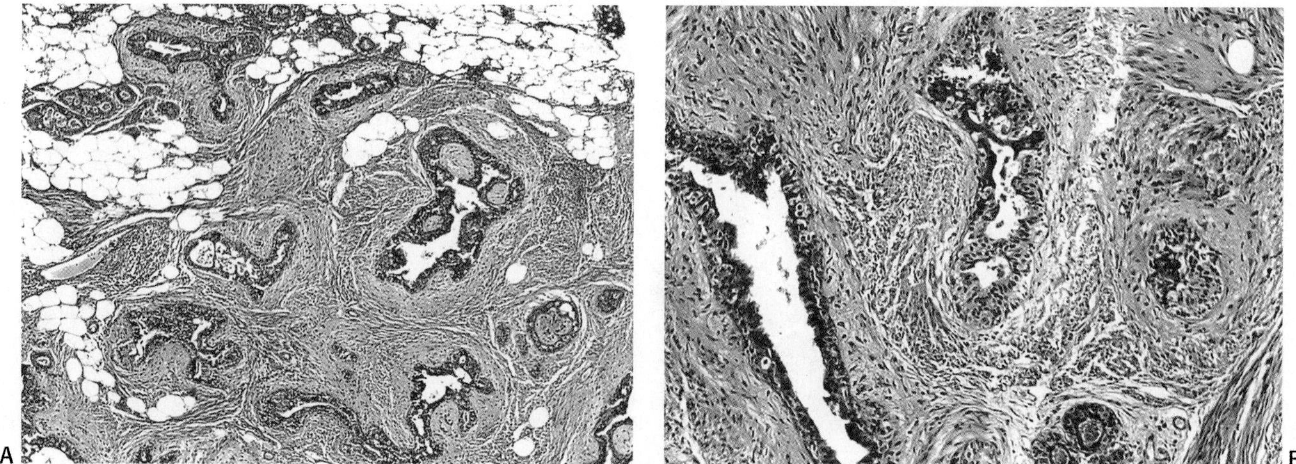

FIG. 8.55. ***Phyllodes tumor variant.*** **A:** The structure of the tumor resembles a radial scar with periductal stromal proliferation, chronic inflammation, and ductal epithelial hyperplasia. These tumors are prone to recur. One patient with this lesion had three recurrences over 10 years with progressive stromal overgrowth. **B:** The stromal proliferation is largely periductal.

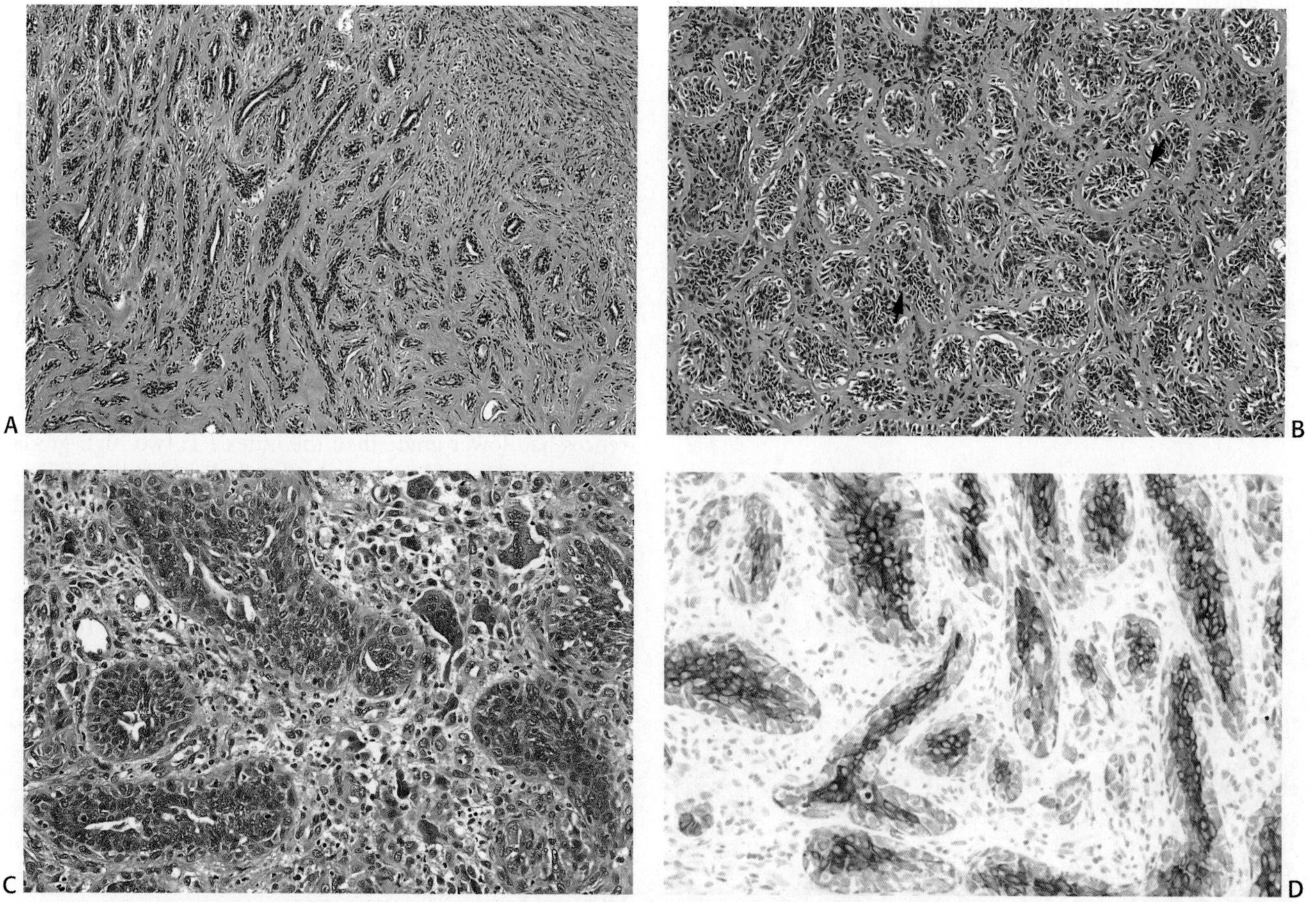

FIG. 8.56. ***Phyllodes tumor variant.*** The three images are from different regions in a single tumor. **A:** Part of the lesion resembles SA. **B:** Glandular hyperplasia accompanied more prominent stroma with osteoclast-like giant cells (*arrows*). **C:** The fully developed lesion has atypical epithelial hyperplasia and malignant stroma with osteoclast-like giant cells. **D:** CK reactivity is much stronger in epithelial than in myoepithelial cells in the glandular elements.

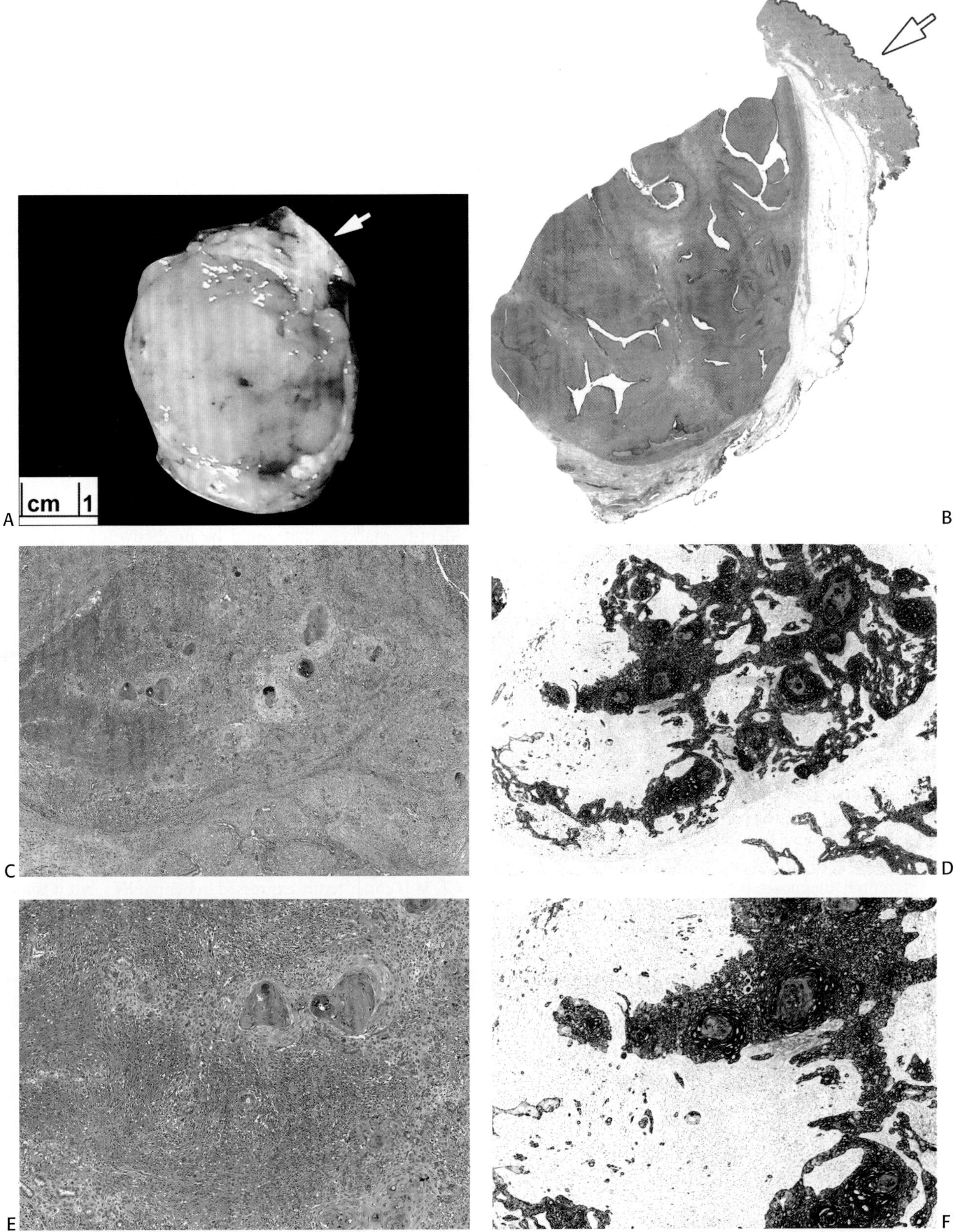

FIG. 8.57. ***High-grade malignant phyllodes tumor with squamous cell carcinoma.*** **A:** Gross photograph of the transected surface of the tumor in the surgical excision specimen. The PT lies just below the skin (*arrow*). **B:** This scan image of the tumor close to the skin (*arrow*) demonstrates the typical leaf-like architecture of a PT. **C:** This area of the PT shows epithelial expansion and squamous metaplasia with keratin cysts. **D:** A CK14 immunostain highlights the irregular outline of the squamous cell carcinoma, as well as few clusters of tumor cells in the stroma. **E:** Closer examination of the squamous proliferation demonstrates marked cytologic atypia, supporting the diagnosis of carcinoma. **F:** CK14 immunostain at the same magnification as **(E)**.

the primary malignant PT exhibited liposarcomatous differentiation with an adenosis-like glandular component.[221] These features were duplicated in lung metastases (Fig. 8.58). The adenosis-like elements in the primary lesion and in the metastases were immunoreactive for gross cystic disease fluid protein 15 (GCDFP-15), and the glandular cells were surrounded by actin-positive myoepithelial cells.

Because most fully malignant PTs are high-grade spindle cell tumors with a fibrosarcomatous pattern, this is the most common appearance encountered in metastatic lesions. Rarely, locally recurrent or metastatic lesions exhibit heterologous differentiation that was not apparent in the primary tumor.[222] Uncommon heterologous sarcomatous elements in the primary tumor such as lipo-,[141,205] chondro-,[141,223] osteo-,[141,224] and leiomyosarcoma[141] can be seen in metastases. In one exceptional case, metastatic malignant PT in the lung exhibited osseous, cartilaginous, and angiosarcomatous elements that had been present in the primary tumor 5 years earlier.[225] Rhabdomyosarcoma was present in the lung metastases from a malignant PT that contained rhabdomyosarcoma.[202] Metastases from a liposarcomatous PT consisted mainly of immature lipoblasts with few adipocytes.[226]

Cytology

The cytologic diagnosis of a PT may be suggested by an aspirate that has an epithelial component typical of a fibroepithelial neoplasm accompanied by excess bipolar stromal cells (Fig. 8.59). Stromal cells with cytoplasm rather than naked bipolar nuclei typify PTs.[227] Cellular stromal fragments are helpful in distinguishing PT from FA.[228–230] Aspiration cytology is an unreliable procedure for the diagnosis of PT in some situations, as pointed out by McDivitt et al.[207] in 1967 and by others.[169,230,231] The reported accuracy rates of FNA for the diagnosis of PT range from 9% to 70%.[169,230,232–234] The differential diagnosis between benign PT and FA is especially difficult. Bipolar nuclei, commonly seen in FNA samples of FA, can also be present in FNA material from a PT.[232] Lesions with marked epithelial hyperplasia may yield an aspirate or needle core biopsy sample in which the stromal element is obscured, and this situation can lead to misdiagnosis of carcinoma[233] or of a FA, if the sample obtained from a heterogeneous tumor has bland epithelium and sparse stromal cells. Scarcity of single epithelial cells, epithelial cohesion, and cell polarity are epithelial features associated with a PT rather than carcinoma in FNA specimens.[233] The aspirate from a malignant PT is likely to contain cellular stromal fragments composed of atypical cells, possibly with mitotic figures. Fragments of stroma with adipose differentiation may be present in the cytologic specimen from a PT with adipose or liposarcomatous differentiation.[235]

Aspiration of a cystic area of squamous metaplasia in a PT may lead to a mistaken diagnosis of a squamous cyst.[236]

Immunohistochemistry

PTs have been a subject of intense investigation by IHC to identify markers that could be predictive of locoregional recurrence, the likelihood that the recurrent lesion will be higher grade, and the propensity to develop distant metastases. The expression of some antigens has been found to correlate with grade and/or recurrence, or with neither, and different studies have sometimes reported different findings. The results pertaining to some broad groups of antigens are discussed below. Karim et al.[237] summarized in table format the results of most immunohistochemical studies on PTs.

Stromal Cell Markers

Actin, CD34, and desmin reactivity are present in the stroma in a variable proportion of cases that exhibit myoid or pseudoangiomatous stromal differentiation of myofibroblasts.[238,239] CD34 is consistently expressed in benign PTs, but it is markedly reduced in high-grade PT.[240–242] In one study,[243] stromal

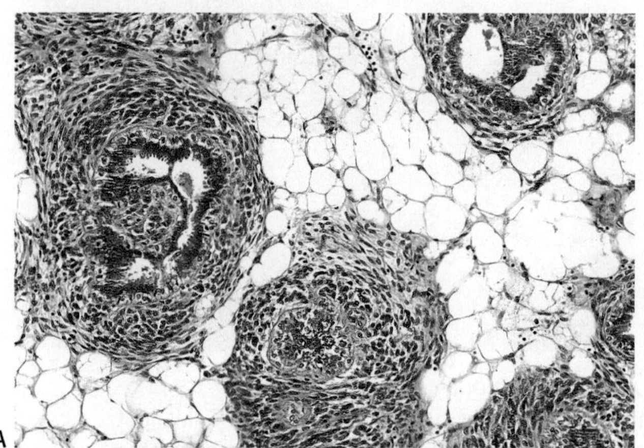
A

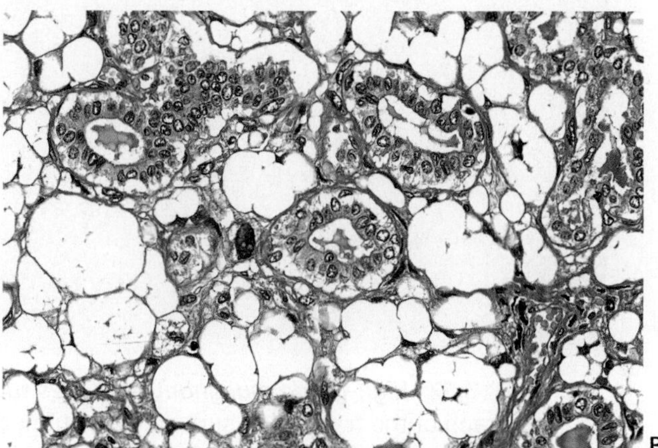
B

FIG. 8.58. ***Malignant phyllodes tumor with metastases of stromal and epithelial components.*** **A:** The primary tumor displayed periglandular malignant spindle cell elements with intervening zones of mature adipose tissue. **B:** Glandular and adipose components were present in the lung metastasis illustrated here. [These images are made from original histologic slides kindly loaned by Drs. Kracht, Sapino, and Bussolati.[221]]

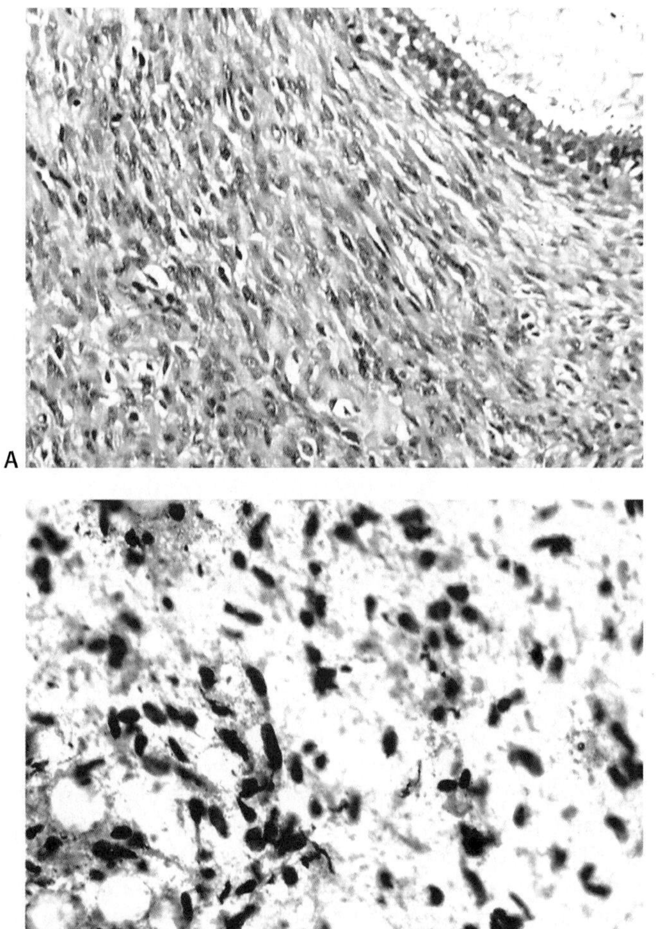

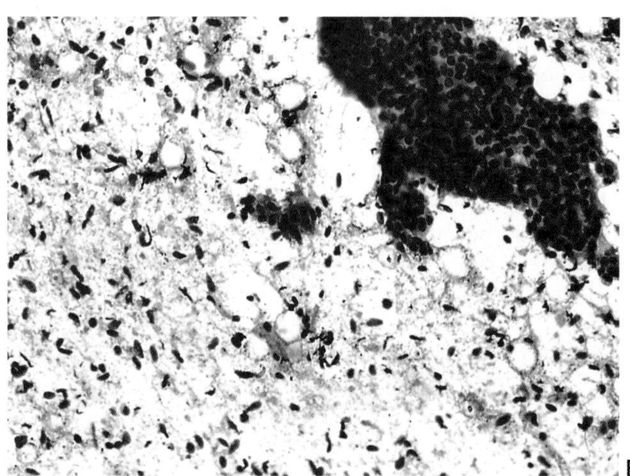

FIG. 8.59. ***Phyllodes tumor, fine-needle aspiration.*** **A:** Histologic section of the low-grade malignant tumor. **B:** Aspiration smear showing numerous bipolar stromal cells and an irregular cluster of epithelial cells. **C:** Stromal cells with hyperchromatic, pleomorphic nuclei.

CD34 was detected in 72.5% of 109 cases, including 78.6% of benign PTs, 66.7% of low-grade, and 44.4% of high-grade malignant PTs. The stromal cells are rarely S-100 positive.

Keratins and p63

Chia et al.[243] evaluated the expression of a panel of CKs (MNF116, 34βE12, CK7, CK14, AE1:3, and CAM5.2) in the stromal component of 109 mammary PTs (70 benign, 30 low grade, and 9 high grade). CK7 showed focal patchy positivity in 1% to 5% of stromal cells in 28.4% of cases, 34βE12 in 22%, MNF116 in 11.9%, AE1:3 in 8.3%, and CAM5.2 and CK14 in 1.8% each. Stromal MNF116 and 34βE12 reactivity decreased significantly with increasing PT grade. The CK-positive cells appeared to be equally distributed in subepithelial and peripheral areas. In the same study, the spindle cell component of 8 metaplastic carcinomas was also CK positive (CK14 100%, MNF116 87.5%, CAM5.2 75%, AE1:3 62.5%, CK7 37.5%, and 34βE12 25%), but none of 8 spindle cell sarcomas and 13 low-grade spindle cell lesions (8 fibromatosis, 4 dermatofibrosarcomas, and 1 myofibroblastoma) showed CK reactivity. Based on these results, the authors recommended cautious interpretation of focal CK positivity in limited material, such as obtained by needle core biopsy, especially in the absence of obvious morphologic findings diagnostic of metaplastic carcinoma or PT. In the same study,[243] no p63 reactivity was identified in the stromal component of PTs.

ER, PR, AR, and HER2

Biochemical analysis detected PR in the stroma of many PTs, whereas only a minority of the tumors showed stromal expression of ER.[244] Tse et al.[245] studied the expression of ER, PR, and AR in 143 PTs by IHC. ER-positive epithelium was present in 83 cases (58%). ER expression correlated with tumor grade (67% in benign PTs, 43% in low-grade PTs, and 47% in high-grade PTs), and was independent of mitotic count. ER reactivity showed a patient age. ER and PR staining demonstrated a strong, inverse correlation with stromal mitoses, and combined ER and PR positivity significantly decreased with increasing severity of the lesion. AR expression was found in less than 5% of the epithelium and stroma of all PTs. Sapino et al.[246] documented ER-β immunoreactivity in the stroma of PTs, including one lesion metastatic to the lung. ER-β expression in PTs was directly correlated with patient age ($p < 0.001$). Shpitz et al.[247] reported epithelial reactivity for HER2, defined as “distinct membrane staining in more than 10% of the cells,” in 61% of PTs, but found no correlation with tumor grade or prognosis. No stromal reactivity for HER2 was observed.

Wingless-Type (Wnt) Pathway, Including β-catenin

Activation of the Wingless-type (Wnt) pathway results in stabilization and nuclear translocation of β-catenin and activates genes involved in embryonic development, cell polarity and adhesion, apoptosis, and tumorigenesis. Nuclear translocation of β-catenin is induced by various factors, including cyclin D1, Wnt5a, and IGF-I and IGF-II. Sawyer et al.[206] documented nuclear β-catenin immunoreactivity in the stroma but not in the epithelium of 72% of 119 PTs. Staining was moderate to strong in 57% of cases, but it was only weak or absent in seven of eight malignant PTs. In the same study,[206] cyclin D1, a marker part of the Wnt activation cascade that is usually not expressed by mammary stromal cells, was present in 47% of PTs and showed a significant correlation with nuclear expression of β-catenin in the stroma ($p < 0.05$). Cyclin D1 decorated the hyperplastic epithelium of PTs in 46% of cases, with moderate to strong reactivity. *In situ* hybridization also documented increased Wnt5a mRNA in the epithelium of PTs. In a subsequent study, Sawyer et al.[248] documented a direct correlation between IGF-I mRNA expression and nuclear β-catenin reactivity in PTs and FAs. In most PTs IGF-I, mRNA was present in the cellular stroma away from the epithelium, but both IGF-I mRNA and nuclear β-catenin were reduced or absent in malignant PTs. IGF-II mRNA was widely expressed in benign and malignant PTs, as well as in FAs. Karim et al.[249] assessed the distribution of a few members of the Wnt pathway, including β-catenin, Wnt1, Wnt5a, E-cadherin, and secreted frizzled related protein 4 (SFRP4) (a Wnt protein receptor) in 34 benign, 23 low-grade, and 8 high-grade PTs. They documented expression of Wnt5a and SFRP4 in the stromal cells, and a significant increase of both proteins with the increased grade of PTs. In this study, membranous reactivity for β-catenin was present in the epithelium of 57% of PTs compared with 75% in the normal epithelium. At the same time, 79% of stromal cells had nuclear staining for β-catenin, and 29% had cytoplasmic staining. The expression of nuclear β-catenin in the stromal cells increased from normal breast to benign PTs to low-grade PTs, but decreased in high-grade PTs. Membranous reactivity for β-catenin in the epithelium of PTs paralleled that of nuclear β-catenin in the stromal cells, suggesting an interaction between the two or a common response to one or more pathogenic stimuli. Taken together, these data suggest a role for epithelial–stromal interactions in the pathogenesis of PTs. Sawyer et al.[206] hypothesized that the morphologically "normal" hyperplastic epithelium of PTs might be genetically altered and could be driving the proliferation of the adjacent stroma. Activation of Wnt5a in the altered epithelium could cause epithelial expression of cyclin D1 and paracrine stromal expression of cyclin D1 and IGF-I, with consequent nuclear translocation of β-catenin in the stromal cells. At the same time, the epithelial proliferation in PTs could be stimulated by the stromal growth. This pathogenetic mechanism would be operating in benign and possibly in low-grade PTs. In high-grade malignant PTs, the neoplastic stromal cells are intrinsically altered and can proliferate independently from the paracrine stimulatory effect of the epithelium. The recurrent observation that in benign and low-grade PTs, mitoses tend to be more frequent in the stroma closer to the epithelium[250] lends support to a possible paracrine function of the epithelium in PTs. Albeit intriguing, this model is based primarily on immunohistochemical data.

CD117/c-kit

The expression of CD117/c-kit, a transmembrane tyrosine kinase receptor and a possible therapeutic target of tyrosine kinase inhibitors, has been extensively evaluated in PTs using IHC. Few studies[240,251–253] have reported c-kit reactivity in PTs, with higher intensity in high-grade malignant PTs than in benign PTs. Tan et al.[254] assessed c-kit immunoreactivity in tissue microarrays of PTs (75% benign PTs, 16% borderline PTs, and 9% malignant PTs) and found positive staining in 17/273 (6%) cases. In this study, c-kit reactivity not only correlated with higher grade morphology ($p = 0.001$) but also with higher recurrence rate (41% vs. 9.3%, respectively) ($p = 0.001$). Bose et al.[255] observed weak c-kit staining in 5% to 30% of the stromal cells in 5/17 (29%) PTs, including 2/5 (40%) recurrent PTs.

However, Djordjevic and Hanna[256] reported that c-kit staining in mammary fibroepithelial lesions (30 benign PTs, 10 borderline PTs, 7 malignant PTs, and 19 FAs) was attributable to infiltrating mast cells, as it had a pattern of reactivity similar to that obtained with toluidine blue stain and tryptase IHC. These authors observed focal c-kit reactivity in the lesional stromal cells only in two PTs (one borderline and one malignant). Neither case had *c-kit* or *PDGFR-α* gene mutations detectable by PCR analysis. Korcheva et al.[257] also found no difference in c-kit staining according to morphologic grade of PTs. Based on these findings and the absence of specific activating mutations, c-kit does not appear to be a suitable target for the treatment of PTs.

p53

Kleer et al.[258] detected focal stromal expression of p53 in 2/7 (29%) benign PTs, in 4/7 (57%) low-grade (borderline) PTs, and in 3/6 (50%) high-grade malignant PTs. p53 staining was almost completely confined to the periductal stroma and did not correlate with tumor size. Few other studies have also used IHC to evaluate the expression of p53 in PTs.[247,254,257,259–268] Differential expression of p53 has been observed in fibroepithelial tumors, with the greatest activity in the periepithelial stroma of high-grade malignant PTs.[262] p53 expression has been correlated with higher grade.[247,254,257,258,261–264,266,269] Gatalica et al.[269] documented a *TP53* gene point mutation in exon 7 in a malignant PT.[269] Korcheva et al.[257] also detected high p53 in malignant PTs, but no *TP53* gene mutations. In the same study, stromal immunoreactivity for murine double minute 2 (MDM2), an E3 ubiquitin ligase involved in p53 degradation, was only weak and sparse, and no *MDM2* gene amplification was detected. p53 reactivity in PTs correlated with reduced survival in at least two studies,[259,266,267] but it was not predictive of tumor recurrence in other series.[247,254,258]

Ki67

Markers of stromal proliferative activity may prove useful not only in the distinction between FAs and PTs, but also in their classification. Ki67 immunoreactivity has been found to correlate with tumor grade in multiple studies.[258,263–265,269–271] In the study by Kocova et al.,[271] the proportion of Ki67-positive tumor cells was significantly higher in malignant than in benign PTs, whereas the difference between the Ki67 indices of benign PTs and FAs was lower. Ki67 expression in greater than 10% of stromal cells was found in 8 of 50 (16%) benign PTs and in 11 of 13 (85%) malignant PTs, a statistically significant difference.[272] Ridgway et al.[273] also reported significantly lower mean Ki67 index in benign PTs (33.31 ± 6.73) than in malignant PTs (76.42 ± 38.55) ($p = 0.007$). Two recent studies have suggested that phospho-histone-3,[257] another marker of mitotic activity, and anaphase-promoting complex 7,[270] a molecule involved in the inactivation of cyclin B, may be more sensitive than Ki67 in distinguishing the spectrum of PTs, but their use has not been validated.

Other Markers

Information about CD10 expression in fibroepithelial lesions is inconsistent. Tse et al.[274] detected positive staining for CD10 in 1 of 3 (33%) FAs, 6 of 102 (6%) benign PTs, 16 of 51 (31%) low-grade (borderline) malignant PTs, and 14 of 28 (50%) high-grade malignant PTs, and demonstrated a statistically significant correlation between stromal CD10 expression and tumor grade. In a study by Al-Masri et al.,[275] the expression of CD10 was higher in malignant PTs and in 6 of 10 PTs that developed distant metastases. Zamenick et al.,[276] however, found no difference in CD10 expression between FAs (60% of cases) and PTs (67% of cases) and concluded that this marker cannot be relied upon to subclassify fibroepithelial lesions.

Kuijper et al.[267] reported that hypoxia-inducible factor 1 (HIF-1), a transcription factor that stimulates angiogenesis in response to hypoxia, is increased in PTs, and its expression correlates significantly with grade, mitotic count, Ki67 index, and p53 accumulation. The expression of vascular epidermal growth factor (VEGF), a powerful angiogenic factor induced by HIF-1, is also an indicator of the grade of a PT. Tse et al.[277] found significantly more intense VEGF reactivity in the stroma of malignant than of benign PTs.

PTs have been found to contain much higher concentrations of endothelin-1 than FAs.[278] This vasoconstrictive peptide stimulates DNA synthesis in vascular smooth muscle cells and in breast stromal cells.[279] Immunohistochemical study revealed that endothelin-1 was localized to the epithelium of PTs and that it was absent from stromal cells in these tumors.[278] This observation suggests that endothelin-1 elaborated by the epithelial component of PTs may have a paracrine function in stimulating proliferation of stromal cells in PTs. Tse et al.[280] found that endothelin-1 expression correlated with atypical histologic features of PTs, including nuclear atypia, stromal cellularity, stromal overgrowth, and pattern of peripheral infiltration.

Electron Microscopy

At the ultrastructural level, the stroma of a PT is composed of cells with features of fibroblasts and myofibroblasts that resemble the normal cellular constituents of the mammary stroma.[239] Electron-dense cytoplasmic bodies, sometimes with a crescentic shape, were described as a distinctive feature by Harris and Khan.[281] These structures appeared to be lysosomal in origin, and they were more numerous in malignant tumors. Various types of cytoplasmic inclusions have been described in other reports.[282,283] Intermediate filaments and dense bodies are observed in myofibroblastic cells.[239] Electron microscopy has not revealed unusual features in the epithelial components of PTs.[239]

Genetics and Molecular Studies

Karim et al.[284] published a detailed review of the molecular mechanisms involved in the pathogenesis of PTs. The limitations of the morphologic classification of PTs for the prognostication of their behavior find explanation in the genetic heterogeneity of these tumors. At present, no chromosomal alterations characteristic of PTs have been identified. Few studies suggest the existence of two main subgroups of PTs with different biologic potential, but there is no consensus on the assignation of low-grade/borderline tumors to the "benign" or "malignant" groups. PTs have proven to be genetically complex, and multiple mechanisms might be involved in the pathogenesis and progression of these lesions. Although some molecular alterations have been correlated with PT recurrence and aggressive behavior, these findings have not been fully validated.

Ploidy and S-Phase Fraction

Layfield et al.[285] reported finding aneuploidy in 75% of benign and in 50% of malignant PTs. Keelan et al.[177] assessed DNA ploidy of 26 primary PTs, including 5 that developed recurrent disease. Sixteen of 21 nonrecurrent PTs were diploid and 5 nondiploid. All five primary PTs that developed recurrence were diploid. Six recurrent PTs and two separate metastases from the same patient were also analyzed: three were diploid and five nondiploid. Jones et al.[286] detected aneuploidy in 3/47 (43%) high-grade malignant PTs, in 3/12 (25%) low-grade (borderline) PTs, and in none of 21 benign PTs, suggesting a positive correlation between aneuploidy and tumor grade.

In the study by Keelan et al.,[177] S-phase fractions (SPFs) of 33 PTs did not differ significantly in relation to recurrence status, even though they tended to be higher in recurrent or metastatic lesions than primary tumors, consistent with the observation that PTs tend to become less differentiated when recurrent. Niezabitowski et al.[287] found that a median SPF higher than 14% was present in 19/39 (48.7%) high-grade malignant PTs compared with 6/70 (8.5%) benign and low-grade malignant PTs combined. Others have observed a trend to a higher recurrence rate in tumors with an S-phase greater than 5%[288,289] and in aneuploid tumors.[288]

Clonality

Few studies have demonstrated clonal origin in PTs.[290,291] Kuijper et al.[292] assessed clonality in the epithelium and stroma of PTs using a PCR assay targeting the human *AR* gene. The stromal component of nine PTs was monoclonal in six cases and polyclonal in three (two benign and one low grade). The morphologically normal or hyperplastic epithelium present in seven PTs was polyclonal in five cases and displayed a nonrandom pattern of inactivation supportive of a monoclonal process in the other two. In the latter cases, both stromal and epithelial components were monoclonal and showed overlapping methylation profiles.

Loss of Heterozygosity

Wang et al.[293] used single-nucleotide polymorphism array analysis to study genome-wide LOH in the stromal component of 11 PTs and 11 FAs. LOH was frequent and often extensive in PTs but rare in FAs. The fractional LOH rate correlated linearly with the mitotic rate. PTs from different patients showed heterogeneous patterns of LOH, and a subset of 22 LOH loci occurred in two or more PTs. LOH at 7p12.3–p13 was significantly more frequent in high-grade PTs than in benign or low-grade tumors ($p = 0.023$), whereas the reverse was true for LOH at 3p24 ($p = 0.038$). In this study, a subset of four PT-specific LOH regions (7p12, 3p24, 10p12, and 9p21) could identify PTs of all grades and distinguish them from FAs. Recurrent PTs shared regions of LOH with the matched primary PT, indicating a clonal origin for recurrent PTs, as well as LOH at additional foci, suggestive of genetic progression in parallel with increasing severity of the histologic changes.

Comparative Genomic Hybridization

Lu et al.[294] analyzed 19 PTs by comparative genomic hybridization (CGH). The most frequent chromosomal gains involved 1q (7/18) and 7q (4/18). Frequent losses involved 3p (6/18), 6q (4/18), and 3q (3/18). Gain of 1q was observed in six cases that developed recurrent disease. A recurrent PT had the same genomic imbalances as the primary tumor. Only one PT without 1q gain developed a recurrence; the latter PT and another recurrent tumor showed loss of the X-chromosome. Five of seven cases with 1q gain had stromal overgrowth, and this association was statistically significant ($p = 0.011$).

Lae et al.[295] studied 30 PTs (9 benign PTs, 12 low-grade, and 9 high-grade malignant PTs) by CGH. They identified recurrent chromosome imbalances in 25/30 (83%) cases, including 55% benign PTs, 91% low-grade, and 100% high-grade malignant PTs ($p = 0.045$). The most frequent chromosomal gains involved 1q (12/30 cases, 40%) and chromosomes 5 (9/30; 30%) and 18 (5/30; 17%). Losses occurred at 13q (7/30; 23%), 6q (9/30; 30%), 10p (8/30; 27%), and 12q (6/30; 17%). Two cases showed high-level gains, one in band 8q24 (site of the *MYC* gene) and the other in bands 7p11 and 12q14 (site of the *MDM2* gene, a negative regulator of p53). Fluorescence *in situ* hybridization (FISH) analysis with a 12q14 probe encompassing *MDM2* found 8 to 10 copies of this gene in the stromal cells, but not in the epithelial component. Amplification of *C-Myc* gene, located in 8q24, was also detected in the stromal component. Each benign PTs had a median of one chromosomal change, whereas low-grade and high-grade malignant PTs had a median of six changes each ($p = 0.003$) and could not be differentiated on the basis of the number of chromosomal alterations. Based on these findings, the authors concluded that chromosomal changes distinguish benign PTs from low-grade and high-grade malignant PTs combined ($p < 0.01$), effectively identifying only two subgroups of PTs.

Lv et al.[296] studied 36 PTs and found that the average number of chromosome copy changes increased with grade (5.58 in benign, 14.08 in low grade, and 12.42 in high grade). Low-grade and high-grade PTs had more chromosomal gains than losses, whereas benign PTs had similar levels. Gains of 4q12 were identified in 12/36 PTs, including 11 low-grade and high-grade malignant tumors, but only in 1 benign PT, suggesting a dichotomous subdivision of PTs. The 4q12 region contains genes for stem cell factor receptor oncogene homolog (*SCFR*), kinase insert domain receptor (*KDR*), and α-fetoprotein (*AFP*). In this study, 1q gain was not associated with a more aggressive clinical course.

Genomic profiling by array CGH[297] showed DNA copy number changes in 10 of 11 PTs, in contrast to none in 3 FAs. The mean of gains and losses were 2.0 and 3.0 per case of PT. Recurrent chromosomal gains most often involved 1q, 2p, 3q, 7p, 8q, and 20, whereas losses involved 1q, 4p, 10, 13, 15q, 16, 17p, 19, and X.

Jones et al.[286] studied frozen samples of 40 PTs and 3 FAs by array CHG. They also analyzed formalin-fixed paraffin-embedded material from 70 additional PTs using a commercial platform for high-throughput genotyping. Low-level gain of 1q was the most frequent alteration. It occurred in two (29%) high-grade and seven (58%) low-grade PTs but not in benign PTs. Other alterations detected in low-grade and high-grade malignant PTs included gain of 5p and chromosome 7 and loss of 9p, 10p, and chromosomes 6 and 13. High-grade malignant PTs had significantly more chromosome 7 and 8 gains than low-grade PTs ($p = 0.009$ and 0.0361, respectively). Low-level gene amplifications were found only in five PTs, and none of the tumors showed high-level gene amplifications. Homozygous deletions were detected in four PTs with low-grade or high-grade morphology, and two involved the 9p21.3 region. Cluster analysis separated the PTs in two groups. One group contained one low-grade and five high-grade PTs and was characterized by gains on chromosome 7. The other group contained two high-grade PTs, all low-grade PTs except one, all benign PTs, and the three FAs. Paired analysis of 19 primary PTs (nine benign, four low-grade, and six high-grade) and their recurrences was performed. Only three recurrences of benign PT showed histologic progression, but six (67%) showed genetic progression, with gain of genetic alterations more common in the low-grade and high-grade malignant group. Additional genetic changes were found in 70% of high-grade or low-grade recurrences. Array CGH of microdissected samples from five PTs with heterogeneous morphology documented intratumoral genetic heterogeneity. Alterations in the 9p21.3 region that contains the cyclin-dependent kinase inhibitor 2A/*p16^{INK4a}* gene (a tumor suppressor gene) were identified in seven high-grade or low-grade PTs and in four recurrent lesions. Loss of *p16^{INK4a}* was documented by IHC in 13/17 PTs with 9p deletion. Methylation of *p16^{INK4a}* was detected in 2/3 high-grade PTs and in 5/5 low-grade PTs. In this study, deletion of 17p (that contains the *TP53* gene) was detected in benign PTs and no *TP53* gene mutations were identified, suggesting that p53 may not be as relevant in the progression of PT as suggested by other studies.

Gene Expression Analysis

Tse et al.[298] used FISH to evaluate amplification of the *epidermal growth factor receptor (EGFR)* gene in 12 PTs (3 benign, 2 low-grade, and 7 high-grade) that showed membranous EGFR immunoreactivity in the neoplastic stromal cells. Low-level amplification (*EGFR/CEP7* ratio of 2.3) was detected only in 1/12 cases (8%). Sawyer et al.[253] found high levels of stromal C-Myc protein in 9/10 malignant PTs compared with 7/20 benign PTs ($p = 0.006$), but only one case showed *MYC* gene amplification. The same authors also reported high levels of c-kit protein in malignant PTs, but sequencing of the *KIT* gene detected no evidence of mutation in five malignant PTs. Two additional studies also found no *KIT*[255,256] or *PDGFR-α*[256] mutations in PTs, including one low-grade and one high-grade PT with stromal reactivity for c-kit.[256]

Using gene array expression profiling to study 23 PTs (12 benign and 11 low-grade or high-grade malignant PTs), Jones et al.[299] identified 162 genes differentially expressed in low-grade and high-grade PTs compared with benign PTs. The mRNA levels of paired box transcription factor 3 (PAX3) and homeobox protein SIX1 (two genes involved in development), transforming growth factor β2 (TGFβ2) (a cytokine and downstream target of PAX3), and high mobility group AT-hook 2 (HMGA2) (a functional DNA transcription factor) were increased in malignant PTs. The corresponding mRNA and/or protein levels were also increased in the neoplastic stroma, as detected by *in situ* hybridization and IHC.

Ang et al.[300] documented overexpression of homeobox protein B13 (HOXB13) mRNA and increased HOXB13 protein in the stroma of high-grade compared with low-grade PTs. In particular, the expression HOXB13 significantly correlated with stromal cellularity ($p = 0.03$) and atypia ($p = 0.039$).

Epigenetic Regulation by Gene Methylation

Huang et al.[301] compared the methylation profiles of 11 genes in 26 FAs and 86 PTs (15 benign, 28 low-grade, and 43 high-grade PTs). They found significantly high methylation of ras-association domain protein-1 gene (*RASSF1A*) (a protein similar to the RAS effector protein) (24.4%) and of twist-related protein 1 (*TWIST1*) (a basic helix–loop–helix transcription factor) (7.1%) in PTs but not in FAs ($p = 0.02$). In particular, *TWIST1* methylation correlated with increasing malignancy in PTs ($p < 0.001$). The authors concluded that determination of the methylation status of *RASSF1* and *TWIST1* may aid in the diagnosis of PTs and that the absence of frequent methylation in FAs supports a nonneoplastic origin. The variable sensitivity of methylation assays limits the use of these tests in clinical practice.

Kim et al.[302] studied promoter methylation of five genes that are frequently methylated in breast cancer, but not in normal breast tissues (glutathione S-transferase pi gene [*GSTP1*]; high in normal 1 [*HIN-1*] [an inhibitor of cell growth]; retinoic acid receptor-β [*RAR-β*]; RASSF1A; and *TWIST1*) in 87 PTs (54 benign, 23 low-grade, and 10 high-grade PTs). The methylation frequency of all genes and the mean number of methylated genes were higher in low-grade and high-grade malignant PTs than in benign PTs. No statistically significant differences in methylation status were detected between low-grade and high-grade malignant PTs. *GSTP1* promoter hypermethylation was associated with loss of GSTP1 protein expression ($p < 0.001$). Based on these results, the authors concluded that methylation profiles segregate PTs into two distinct groups, one consisting of benign PTs and the other of low-grade and high-grade malignant PTs combined.

Origin of PT from FA

The relationship of FA and PT is unclear. PCR analysis of 10 FAs and 5 PTs by Noguchi et al.[291] documented polyclonality in FAs and monoclonality in PTs. In a subsequent study,[303] the same investigators assessed the trinucleotide repeat polymorphism and methylation status of the X-chromosome-linked *AR* gene in three tumors that had been initially diagnosed as FAs and recurred as PTs. The analysis showed that the same allele of the *AR* gene was inactivated in the FA and PT samples from each patient, a result very unlikely to occur in three separate cases by chance alone.

Kuijper et al.[292] assessed clonality in the epithelium and stroma of 19 FAs and 9 PTs using a PCR assay targeting the human *AR* gene. Although the stroma of most FAs was polyclonal, focal areas of stromal expansion in three tumors classified morphologically as FAs were monoclonal, suggesting possible focal progression to PT. However, the picture provided for one of these lesions is consistent with a benign PT. The stromal component of nine PTs was monoclonal in six cases and polyclonal in three (two benign PTs and one low-grade PT).

Hodges et al.[175] studied a tumor that had the histologic features of a malignant PT situated in a FA. Molecular analysis of microdissected samples revealed allelic loss at D75522 in both components and losses at *TP53* and D225264 in the PT part. These data suggest that there was a clonal relationship between the FA and PT, with additional allelic loss consequent to progression from the FA to the PT.

Overall, the data suggesting that PTs may develop from FA remain very limited. Given the intratumoral heterogeneity of PTs, it is possible that examples of FA reported to have evolved into PT consisted of benign PTs with sclerotic stroma and deceptively bland morphology, or that they were inadequately sampled. Nonetheless, the possibility that in rare cases one of the clones in a polyclonal FA may expand and give rise to a PT cannot entirely be ruled out.

Treatment and Prognosis

Because the diagnosis of PT is not anticipated clinically in many cases, surgical excision may be initially incomplete and reexcision is often required.[169] The primary excision and reexcision specimens should be inked and margins thoroughly examined histologically. Mastectomy is indicated as primary therapy if a large high-grade malignant PT cannot be encompassed with a cosmetically acceptable excision. Sentinel lymph node biopsy or axillary lymph node (ALN) dissection is not indicated, unless a concurrent invasive carcinoma is documented in the PT or in the ipsilateral breast.

Surgical Excision

The fundamental principle of therapy for PT is complete excision to prevent local recurrence.[145,146,153,154,169,304–309] According to SEER data[148] from 821 patients with malignant PTs treated between 1983 and 2002, nearly half (48%) of the lesions underwent wide excision and the other half (52%) mastectomy. Women treated with mastectomy were more likely to be 60 years of age or older and have a tumor larger than 5 cm. In one study,[310] the mean size of the tumor was 5.37 ± 2.97 cm for patients who underwent a local excision versus 7.56 ± 4.07 cm for patients initially treated by mastectomy. Guillot et al.[169] reported their experience with 165 patients with PTs (77% benign, 19% low-grade, and 4% high-grade malignant) treated at one European center between 1994 and 2008. In this series, 160 (97%) patients underwent breast-conserving surgery, and only five (3%) had mastectomy as the primary surgical procedure. Six additional patients underwent mastectomy due to incomplete margins in the surgical excision specimen. The patients treated with mastectomy had high-grade (711, 64%) or low-grade malignant (4/11, 36%) PT. In this study, 119 (72%) PTs treated with breast-conserving surgery were excised with a margin of 1 cm or greater. Twenty-four (52%) patients with either a positive or less than a 1-cm margin underwent surgical revision that consisted of reexcision in 74.3% of the cases (combined with oncoplasty in 8.3% of cases) or mastectomy in 25% of the cases. Residual tumor was present in four (16%) cases.

A number of studies recommend surgical excision with at least 1.0-cm margin clearance.[145,308,311–313] A margin of less than 1.0 cm is associated with higher local recurrence in some studies.[154,314] Nonetheless, local recurrences occur in a very small percentage of patients with negative excision margins.

Lymph Node Evaluation

In an SEER data-based series of 1,035 patients with PT,[315] 264 (25.5%) had some type of regional lymphadenectomy, including 9% of patients who had more than 10 lymph nodes removed. In this study, 9/264 (3.4%) patients had lymph node metastases. Twenty of 106 (18.8%) patients studied by Ben Hassouna et al.[308] had axillary clearance, and only 1 had lymph node involvement. In the series by Guillot et al.,[169] none of the 160 patients treated with breast-conserving surgery underwent lymph node evaluation, but 3/5 patients treated with mastectomy also had ALN dissection, and none had metastases. In various other published reports, lymph node metastases were reported in less than 1% of high-grade PTs[141,142,150,316] (Fig. 8.60). A rare case of metastatic PT in a Rotter lymph node has been reported.[317]

Local Recurrence

The classification of PTs as benign, low-grade, or high-grade malignant reflects an estimate of the probable clinical course based on the histologic appearance of the tumor. In 1999, Barth[318] observed that classification of PT as benign, low-grade, and high-grade malignant correlated with local breast recurrence in women who did not undergo mastectomy.

A benign PT will not metastasize and has a low probability for local recurrence after excision, ranging from 11%

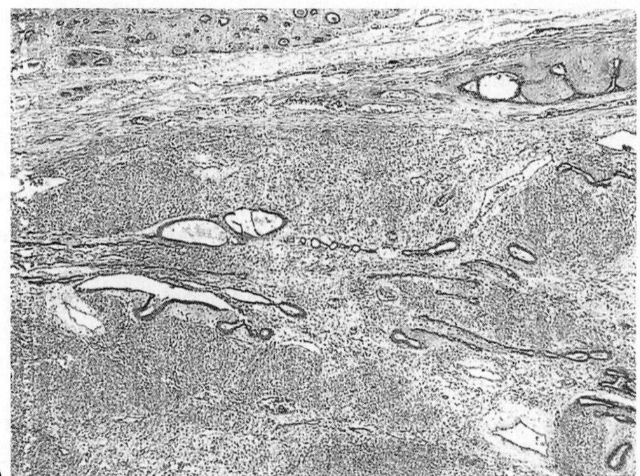

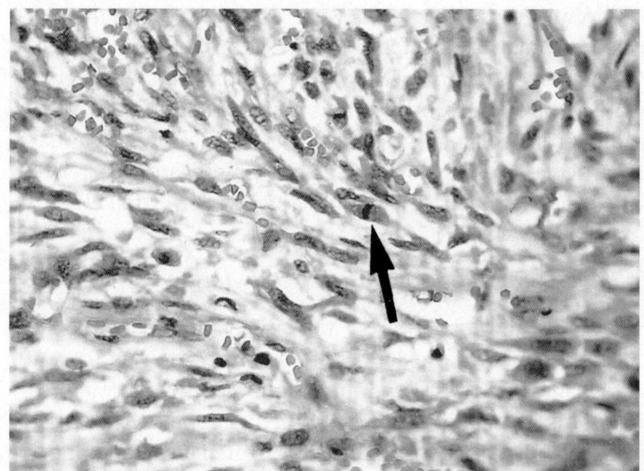

FIG. 8.60. ***Malignant phyllodes tumor with metastases.*** **A:** The primary PT had a circumscribed border and cellular stroma. **B:** Cellular pleomorphism and a mitotic figure (*arrow*) in the primary PT. **C:** Metastatic PT in an ALN at the time of mastectomy. **D:** A subsequent metastasis in the skin of a finger.

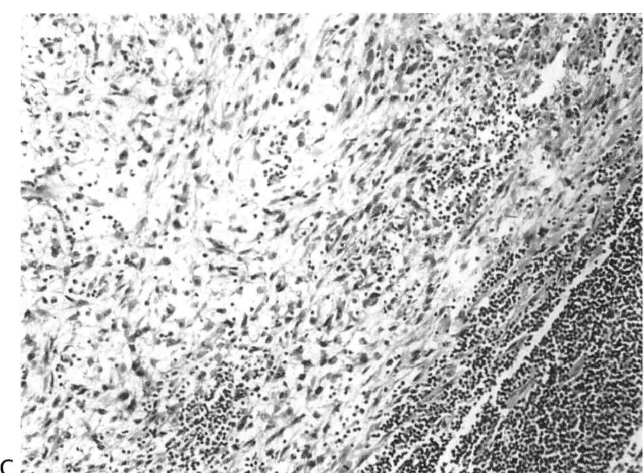

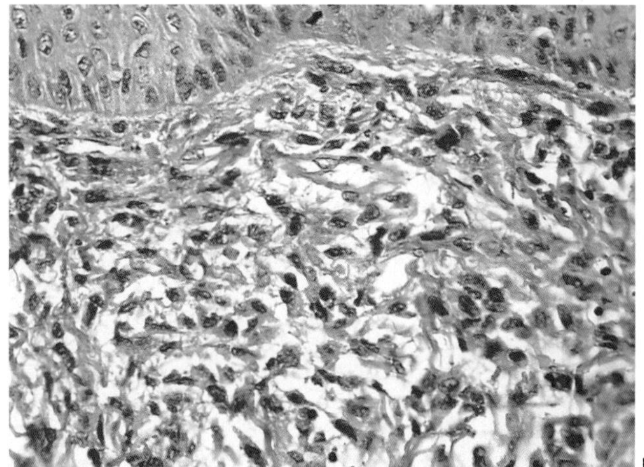

FIG. 8.60. *(Continued)*

to 17%.[145,146,154,311,318] However, some benign PTs may recur with higher grade morphology. Six of 23 (26%) recurrences of benign PTs in the series studied by Barrio et al.[145] had higher grade morphology. In a study by Tan et al.,[146] the recurrence rate of benign PTs was 10.9%; however, 17/48 (35%) tumors recurred with morphology of low-grade PT, and 4/48 (8%) recurred with high-grade malignant morphology. A low-grade malignant PT has a slight probability of metastasis, but the probability of local recurrence ranges from 14% to 25%.[146,154,311] Local recurrence and distant metastases are most common in patients with high-grade malignant PT. Local recurrence occurs in about one-third of cases[146] and tends to present earlier after initial treatment than for benign or low-grade malignant PT.

Primary tumor size may be a factor in the success of local excision because a wider excision may be possible when tumors are small. Zurrida et al.[319] reported that 7/69 (10%) (5/55 benign, 1/11 low-grade, and 1/3 high-grade) PTs treated by enucleation alone recurred locally compared with 9/71 (12.7%) (5/52 benign and 4/12 low-grade) PTs excised with some uninvolved tissue. The local recurrence rate of PTs excised with a broader rim of uninvolved tissue was 8/56 (14.3%) (1/29 benign, 4/18 low grade, and 3/9 high grade). The local recurrence rate was 15% (3/20) for patients treated by mastectomy, and all three patients with recurrence had a high-grade malignant PT. Based on a local recurrence rate of 11/140 (7.9%) for benign PTs, either removed by enucleation or excised with minimal uninvolved tissue, the authors concluded that reexcision may not always be necessary for benign PTs tumors, since most (97/107; 90.65%) patients who had no additional surgery did not develop locally recurrent disease.

Teo et al.[320] retrospectively reviewed the outcome of 44 consecutive Asian women 25 years or younger (median age 20.5 years) who underwent surgical excision of a PT. The mean tumor size was 3.2 ± 1.7 cm. Forty-three tumors were enucleated: two of them had subsequent reexcision for close margins, and one underwent mastectomy for a diagnosis of malignant PT. One patient had wide excision for a low-grade PT. The 44 PTs consisted of 42 (93%) benign PTs (including 15 tumors with positive margins), 2 (4.4%) low-grade, and 1 (2.2%) high-grade malignant PT. At median follow-up of 43 months, none of the patients experienced a recurrence.

Park et al.[321] reported the follow-up of 31 patients with benign PTs who underwent percutaneous excision at the time of ultrasound-guided vacuum-assisted core biopsy. None of the tumors had been sampled before, and they unexpectedly turned out to be benign PTs upon review of the diagnostic and excisional ultrasound-guided core biopsy material. On imaging studies, the tumor size ranged from 0.6 cm to greater than 3 cm. Sonographic and mammographic follow-up evaluation was obtained at 3- to 6-month intervals for a mean follow-up time of 75.9 months (range, 24 to 94 months). A 1.3-cm benign PT recurred at 11 months as a 1.5-cm mass with the same morphology. Although the recurrence rate in this series was relatively low (3.2%), at present percutaneous excision of benign PT does not constitute acceptable practice.

Local recurrence of PT is deleterious, because of the tendency of some PTs to have a higher grade in recurrent lesions than in the primary tumor[145,154,219] and the risk of chest wall invasion (Fig. 8.61). Local recurrences occur in about 10% to 30% of all PT cases, Metastases develop in about 5% to 10% of all PT cases, usually within 3 years of primary treatment,[139,141,145,154,155,169,219,305,306,311,312,322] although occasional instances of late recurrence have been reported.[141,207]

Local recurrence is not a necessary antecedent event to the development of systemic metastases in patients with high-grade malignant PT, and about 40% of patients with a high-grade malignant PT who develop metastases do not experience a local recurrence prior to systemic spread.[150,152,323,324] However, rare instances of benign or low-grade malignant PT that result in distant metastases almost always have had local recurrences with high-grade malignant morphology prior to the appearance of systemic lesions.

Nomogram for Disease Recurrence Prediction

Tan et al.[146] evaluated multiple pathologic parameters in a series of 605 PTs (72.7% benign, 18.4% low grade, and 8.9% high grade) treated at the Singapore General Hospital

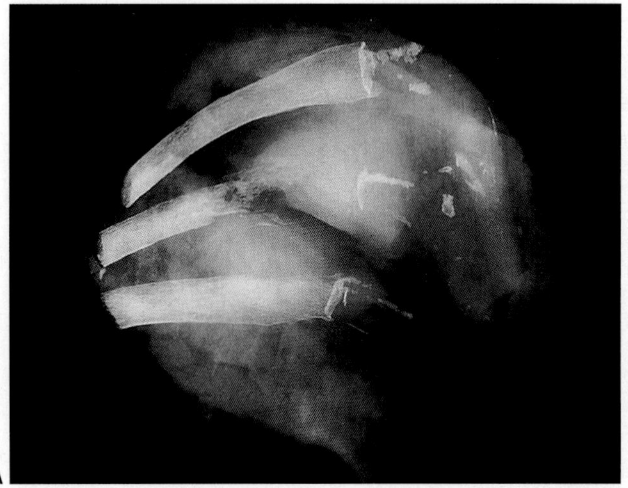
A

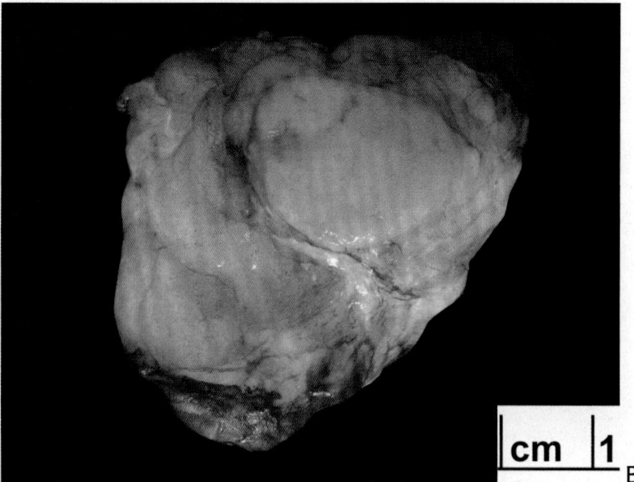

B

FIG. 8.61. ***Locally recurrent phyllodes tumor.*** **A:** Invasion of the chest wall and destruction of ribs by recurrent PT is evident in this x-ray of a surgical specimen. **B:** Recurrent PT in the breast is grossly indistinguishable from a primary tumor.

between 1992 and 2010. In this study, a cutoff of 4 mitoses per 10 HPFs was used to differentiate benign and low-grade PT. Eighty patients developed recurrent disease: 68 had local recurrence, 7 distant metastases, and 5 developed both local and distant recurrence. Twelve women died of disease. Accurate follow-up information was available for 552 patients, with a median follow-up time of 56.9 months. Multivariate analysis showed that nuclear atypia (A), stromal overgrowth (O), and surgical margin status (S) significantly correlated with recurrence-free surgery, whereas mitotic rate (M) approached statistical significance ($p = 0.058$) (the four parameters are summarized by the acronym A.M.O.S.). In this study, the characteristics of tumor borders and stromal hypercellularity were not found to be statistically significant. Based on correlative analysis of histologic parameters, margin status, and clinical events, the authors developed a nomogram for prediction of relapse-free survival (RFS) of patients with PTs. Because local recurrences constituted the most common events, the nomogram is likely to have greater accuracy in predicting locally recurrent disease rather than metastatic spread.

Radiotherapy

A prospective multi-institutional study[325] assessed the recurrence rate in 46 women with PT (35% low-grade and 65% high-grade malignant), including 3 women with a recurrent PT who were treated with adjuvant whole-breast irradiation with boost of the tumor area. The mean tumor size was 3.7 cm, and all tumors were excised with negative margins. After a median follow-up of 56 months, none of the 46 patients developed local recurrence. Two patients (4%) died of metastatic disease at 9 and 14 months from diagnosis. Based on review of the literature showing a local recurrence rate of about 20%, the authors concluded that adjuvant radiotherapy is beneficial, but the validity of this study is limited by small sample size, heterogeneity of cases, and lack of a case-control group. Belkacemi et al.[313] published the experience of the Rare Cancer Network based on the study of 443 women with PT treated between 1971 and 2003. The local recurrence rate was 19%, and the rate of distant metastases 3.4%. In this series, radiotherapy significantly decreased local recurrence ($p = 0.02$) in low-grade and high-grade malignant PTs and was an independent factor in multivariate analysis. In the same type of PTs, mastectomy also achieved better local control than breast-conserving surgery and was the only independent prognostic factor of disease-free survival. At present, post-operative, adjuvant radiotherapy is not part of the standard treatment of PT managed with breast-conserving surgery, especially if the tumor has been excised with negative margins. Radiation may be considered in the management of a primary or recurrent PT that invades beyond the breast into the chest wall.

Chemotherapy

Between 1993 and 2003, Morales-Vasquez et al.[326] used doxorubicin and dacarbazine to treat 17 women with malignant PTs; 23.5% of these patients had undergone breast-conserving surgery, and 24% had positive final resection margin. In a retrospective study, the investigators compared the outcome of patients who received chemotherapy in addition to surgery with that of women with comparable PTs treated with surgery alone during the same period. Thirty-five percent of the patients in the control group underwent breast-conserving surgery, and 36% had final positive margins. Median follow-up was 15 months (range 2 to 81). Seven patients experienced disease recurrence, including one in the control group and six in the treatment group. Recurrence-free survival in the two groups was not significantly different. The five patients who died of disease had received neoadjuvant chemotherapy, and each had developed locally recurrent disease prior to distant metastases. One suspects that the chemotherapy-treated group had features predisposing to a poor clinical outcome that was not ameliorated by the drugs provided to them. Prolonged complete remission (26 and 61 months) was observed in two patients with lung metastases of PT treated with ifosfamide,[327] and palliation was reportedly achieved with combination chemotherapy and radiation in other cases.[328] At present, there is no evidence supporting a beneficial role for adjuvant chemotherapy in the treatment of primary high-grade malignant PT.

Survival

Analysis of 821 patients with malignant PTs recorded in the SEER program with median follow-up of 5.7 years revealed disease-specific survival of 91%, 89%, and 89% at 5, 10, and 15 years, respectively.[148] There was no statistically significant difference in disease-specific survival between patients treated with excisional surgery and those treated with mastectomy.

The overall 5-year survival rate for PT in the series by Grimes[141] was about 90%. A 1999 review by Barth[318] combined survival data from multiple published studies and indicated deaths due to disease in 2 of 600 (0.3%), 7 of 107 (6.6%), and 48 of 240 (20%) patients with benign, low-grade, and high-grade malignant tumors, respectively. In a population-based study of malignant PT with data for the years 1983 to 2002,[148] the estimated cause-specific survival was 91%, 89%, and 89% at 5, 10, and 15 years, and the rates of overall survival for the same periods were 84%, 77%, and 73%, respectively. Deaths due to recurrent or progressive disease occurred in 72 women at a median of 1.8 years (range 1 to 8) after diagnosis. Metastases develop in about 3% to 10% of all PT cases and are usually detected within 3 years of primary treatment.[139,141,145,154,155,169,219,305,306,311,312,322] Most deaths due to metastatic PT are within 5 years of diagnosis.[141,145,154,312,329] Virtually all fatalities occur in patients who have high-grade PTs primarily or who develop recurrences that are high grade. These neoplasms are typically characterized by stromal overgrowth, invasive borders, cellular pleomorphism, and frequent mitoses.[145,154,198,330] Grimes[141] reported that all PTs that resulted in metastases in her series (8 of 100 tumors) had at least 15 mitoses per 50 HPFs in the primary tumors or in a recurrence. Others reported mitotic counts of 11 to 52[329] and 3 to 30[150] per 10 HPFs in tumors that developed metastases. In the study by Tan et al.,[146] margin involvement, atypia and stromal overgrowth were significant predictors of disease recurrence on multivariate analyzis,[146] and mitotic rate was very close to being statistically significant.

Sites of Metastases

The most common sites of distant metastases are the lungs, bone, and heart.[331] One report describes an unusual instance of surgically resected metastatic PT in the lung with intravascular dumbbell extension via the pulmonary vein into the left atrium.[332] Virtually any organ may be found to have metastases, but many of these sites are not apparent ante mortem. Exceptional sites of clinically detected metastases include the mandible,[333] the maxilla,[334] the small bowel,[335] and the central nervous system.[336,337] An unusual case of spontaneous regression of multiple lung metastases clinically presumed to originate from a high-grade malignant PT has been described,[338] but the metastases were not proven by biopsy. Nine months later, the patient developed brain metastases and died of disease.

There appear to be some differences in prognosis also among PTs with different types of stromal differentiation. Several patients with osteogenic or chondrosarcoma have developed systemic metastases,[223,224] but most patients with liposarcomatous PT have remained disease free.[205,226,339,340]

Core Biopsy Diagnosis of Fibroepithelial Lesions

FA rarely poses a challenge on review of core biopsy material. Hyalinized FA with conspicuous epithelial lining may occasionally raise the differential diagnosis of a sclerosed papilloma, but the pseudopapillary fronds lack true fibrovascular cores. Complete excision of the lesion is recommended for definitive evaluation in uncertain cases, as papillomas can harbor atypia or carcinoma.

Excisional biopsy is recommended whenever a needle core biopsy sample has features that raise concern about a possible PT. Findings that favor the diagnosis of PT over that of FA in needle core biopsy material include 2 or more stromal mitoses per 10 HPFs,[341,342] increased stromal cellularity, absence of epithelial elements in at least one microscopic field at 40× final magnification,[342] invasive margins, fragmentation of the tissue cores (a manifestation of the characteristic leaf-like architecture),[343] and presence of adipose tissue admixed with stroma (indicative of peripheral infiltrative growth or a lipophyllodes tumor).[343] Patient age older than 50 to 55 years also favors a diagnosis of PT.[344,345] Epithelial hyperplasia and/or atypia tend to be more common in PT than in FA. If atypical features are noted in the fibroadenomatous epithelium, excision of the tumor with sampling of the surrounding tissue should be performed to assess the epithelial component for evidence of occult carcinoma.

Immunoperoxidase studies have been applied to the diagnosis of fibroepithelial tumors in needle core biopsy samples. Two groups[341,342] performed immunohistochemical stains for Ki67 and topoisomerase I and found that reactivity for these markers had statistically significant correlation with a PT diagnosis. Jacobs et al.[341] reported some overlap between the results in FAs and PTs using both markers (Ki67 index: 1.6, range 0.4 to 4 in FAs vs. 6.0, range 0 to 18 in PTs; topoisomerase II index: 2.8, range 0 to 10 in FAs vs. 7.0, range 1.2 to 29 in PTs), but the results were statistically significant, especially for Ki67 ($p = 0.002$). Jara-Lazaro et al.[342] found that Ki67 and topoisomerase II indexes greater than or equal to 5% and reduced or patchy CD34 staining in the lesional stromal cells present in needle core biopsy material correlated with the diagnosis of PT in the surgical excision specimen. The use of these markers has not been tested prospectively.

The differential diagnosis of PT in a limited needle core biopsy sample often includes other spindle cell lesions such as fibromatosis and metaplastic spindle cell carcinoma. Lacroix-Triki et al.[346] detected nuclear staining for β-catenin in 75% of the epithelial cells and in 94% of the stromal cells of benign PTs, mostly in periductal distribution. β-Catenin nuclear staining was weaker in low-grade and high-grade PTs compared with benign PTs. Nuclear staining for β-catenin was also present in all eight cases of fibromatosis part of the study and was detected focally in 23% of 52 metaplastic carcinomas, including metaplastic spindle cell carcinomas. On the basis of these findings, β-catenin does not appear to be a reliable marker in the evaluation of spindle cell lesions involving the breast.

Chia et al.[243] documented reactivity for multiple CKs (including CK7, MNF116, keratin 34βE12, and AE1:3) in the stromal cells of PTs. CK staining in PTs was usually focal and in a patchy distribution. In the same study, none of the PTs showed reactivity for p63. Awareness of these findings is important for accurate interpretation of the results of IHC on core biopsy material of a mammary spindle cell lesion.

REFERENCES

Fibroadenomatoid Mastopathy (Sclerosing Lobular Hyperplasia)

1. Kovi J, Chu HB, Leffall LD Jr. Sclerosing lobular hyperplasia manifesting as a palpable mass of the breast in young black women. *Hum Pathol* 1984;15:336–340.
2. Poulton TB, de Paredes ES, Baldwin M. Sclerosing lobular hyperplasia of the breast: imaging features in 15 cases. *AJR Am J Roentgenol* 1995;165:291–294.
3. Kamal M, Evans AJ, Denley H, et al. Fibroadenomatoid hyperplasia: a cause of suspicious microcalcification on mammographic screening. *AJR Am J Roentgenol* 1998;171:1331–1334.
4. Kapur P, Rakheja D, Cavuoti DC, et al. Sclerosing lobular hyperplasia of breast: cytomorphologic and histomorphologic features: a case report. *Cytojournal* 2006;3:8.
5. Panikar N, Agarwal S. Sclerosing lobular hyperplasia of the breast: fine-needle aspiration cytology findings—a case report. *Diagn Cytopathol* 2004;31:340–341.
6. Canny PF, Berkowitz GS, Kelsey JL, et al. Fibroadenoma and the use of exogenous hormones. A case-control study. *Am J Epidemiol* 1988;127:454–461.

Fibroadenoma

7. LiVolsi VA, Stadel BV, Kelsey JL, et al. Fibroadenoma in oral contraceptive users: a histopathologic evaluation of epithelial atypia. *Cancer* 1979;44:1778–1781.
8. Yu H, Rohan TE, Cook MG, et al. Risk factors for fibroadenoma: a case-control study in Australia. *Am J Epidemiol* 1992;135:247–258.
9. Raine PA, Noblett HR, Houghton-Allen BW, et al. Breast fibroadenoma and cardiac anomaly associated with EMG (Beckwith-Wiedemann) syndrome. *J Pediatr* 1979;94:633–634.
10. Poh MM, Ballard TN, Wendel JJ. Beckwith–Wiedemann syndrome and juvenile fibroadenoma: a case report. *Ann Plast Surg* 2010;64: 803–806.
11. Morris JA, Kelly JF. Multiple bilateral breast adenomata in identical adolescent Negro twins. *Histopathology* 1982;6:539–547.
12. Carney JA, Toorkey BC. Myxoid fibroadenoma and allied conditions (myxomatosis) of the breast. A heritable disorder with special associations including cardiac and cutaneous myxomas. *Am J Surg Pathol* 1991;15:713–721.
13. Ansah-Boateng Y, Tavassoli FA. Fibroadenoma and cystosarcoma phyllodes of the male breast. *Mod Pathol* 1992;5:114–116.
14. Gupta P, Foshee S, Garcia-Morales F, et al. Fibroadenoma in male breast: case report and literature review. *Breast Dis* 2011;33:45–48.
15. Nielsen BB. Fibroadenomatoid hyperplasia of the male breast. *Am J Surg Pathol* 1990;14:774–777.
16. Uchida T, Ishii M, Motomiya Y. Fibroadenoma associated with gynaecomastia in an adult man. Case report. *Scand J Plast Reconstr Surg Hand Surg* 1993;27:327–329.
17. Kanhai RC, Hage JJ, Bloemena E, et al. Mammary fibroadenoma in a male-to-female transsexual. *Histopathology* 1999;35:183–185.
18. Lemmo G, Garcea N, Corsello S, et al. Breast fibroadenoma in a male-to-female transsexual patient after hormonal treatment. *Eur J Surg Suppl* 2003;588:69–71.
19. Shin SJ, Rosen PP. Bilateral presentation of fibroadenoma with digital fibroma-like inclusions in the male breast. *Arch Pathol Lab Med* 2007;131:1126–1129.
20. Baildam AD, Higgins RM, Hurley E, et al. Cyclosporin A and multiple fibroadenomas of the breast. *Br J Surg* 1996;83:1755–1757.
21. Weinstein SP, Orel SG, Collazzo L, et al. Cyclosporin A-induced fibroadenomas of the breast: report of five cases. *Radiology* 2001;220:465–468.
22. Son EJ, Oh KK, Kim EK, et al. Characteristic imaging features of breast fibroadenomas in women given cyclosporin A after renal transplantation. *J Clin Ultrasound* 2004;32:69–77.
23. Cheng F, Qin JJ, Yu MN, et al. De novo phyllodes tumor in an adolescent female after liver transplantation. *Pediatr Transplant* 2011;15:E12–E14.
24. Iaria G, Pisani F, De Luca L, et al. Prospective study of switch from cyclosporine to tacrolimus for fibroadenomas of the breast in kidney transplantation. *Transplant Proc* 2010;42:1169–1170.
25. Kleer CG, Tseng MD, Gutsch DE, et al. Detection of Epstein-Barr virus in rapidly growing fibroadenomas of the breast in immunosuppressed hosts. *Mod Pathol* 2002;15:759–764.
26. Lau SK, Chen YY, Berry GJ, et al. Epstein-Barr virus infection is not associated with fibroadenomas of the breast in immunosuppressed patients after organ transplantation. *Mod Pathol* 2003;16: 1242–1247.
27. Foster ME, Garrahan N, Williams S. Fibroadenoma of the breast: a clinical and pathological study. *J R Coll Surg Edinb* 1988;33:16–19.
28. Hunter TB, Roberts CC, Hunt KR, et al. Occurrence of fibroadenomas in postmenopausal women referred for breast biopsy. *J Am Geriatr Soc* 1996;44:61–64.
29. Simomoto MM, Nazario AC, Gebrim LH, et al. Morphometric analysis of the epithelium of mammary fibroadenomas during the proliferative and secretory phases of the menstrual cycle. *Breast J* 1999;5:256–261.
30. Rego MF, Navarrete MA, Facina G, et al. Analysis of human mammary fibroadenoma by Ki-67 index in the follicular and luteal phases of menstrual cycle. *Cell Prolif* 2009;42:241–247.
31. Stanley MW, Tani EM, Skoog L. Fine-needle aspiration of fibroadenomas of the breast with atypia: a spectrum including cases that cytologically mimic carcinoma. *Diagn Cytopathol* 1990;6:375–382.
32. Simsir A, Waisman J, Cangiarella J. Fibroadenomas with atypia: causes of under- and overdiagnosis by aspiration biopsy. *Diagn Cytopathol* 2001;25:278–284.
33. O'Hara MF, Page DL. Adenomas of the breast and ectopic breast under lactational influences. *Hum Pathol* 1985;16:707–712.
34. Fekete P, Petrek J, Majmudar B, et al. Fibroadenomas with stromal cellularity. A clinicopathologic study of 21 patients. *Arch Pathol Lab Med* 1987;111:427–432.
35. Pike AM, Oberman HA. Juvenile (cellular) adenofibromas. A clinicopathologic study. *Am J Surg Pathol* 1985;9:730–736.
36. Ross DS, Giri D, Akram M, et al. Fibroepithelial lesions in the breast of adolescent females: a clinicopathological profile of 35 cases. *Mod Pathol* 2012;92(Suppl.):64A.
37. Mies C, Rosen PP. Juvenile fibroadenoma with atypical epithelial hyperplasia. *Am J Surg Pathol* 1987;11:184–190.
38. Shi A, Li S, Xu N, et al. Clinical features and prognosis of a unilateral fibroadenoma of the breast in a 16-month-old female. *Jpn J Clin Oncol* 2011;41:260–264.
39. Kuijper A, Mommers EC, van der Wall E, et al. Histopathology of fibroadenoma of the breast. *Am J Clin Pathol* 2001;115:736–742.
40. Sklair-Levy M, Sella T, Alweiss T, et al. Incidence and management of complex fibroadenomas. *AJR Am J Roentgenol* 2008;190:214–218.
41. Atwal GS, O'Connor SR, Clamp M, et al. Fibroadenoma occurring in supernumerary breast tissue. *Histopathology* 2007;50:513–514.

42. Fisher JH. Fibroadenoma of supernumerary mammary gland tissue in vulva. *Am J Obstet Gynecol* 1947;53:335–337.
43. Oberman HA. Breast lesions in the adolescent female. *Pathol Annu* 1979;14(Pt. 1):175–201.
44. Fleury EF, Rinaldi JF, Piato S, et al. Appearance of breast masses on sonoelastography with special focus on the diagnosis of fibroadenomas. *Eur Radiol* 2009;19:1337–1346.
45. Adamietz BR, Kahmann L, Fasching PA, et al. Differentiation between phyllodes tumor and fibroadenoma using real-time elastography. *Ultraschall Med* 2011;32(Suppl. 2):E75–E79.
46. Sumkin JH, Perrone AM, Harris KM, et al. Lactating adenoma: US features and literature review. *Radiology* 1998;206:271–274.
47. Yamaguchi R, Tanaka M, Mizushima Y, et al. Myxomatous fibroadenoma of the breast: correlation with clinicopathologic and radiologic features. *Hum Pathol* 2011;42:419–423.
48. Stelling CB, Powell DE, Mattingly SS. Fibroadenomas: histopathologic and MR imaging features. *Radiology* 1987;162:399–407.
49. Hochman MG, Orel SG, Powell CM, et al. Fibroadenomas: MR imaging appearances with radiologic–histopathologic correlation. *Radiology* 1997;204:123–129.
50. Wurdinger S, Herzog AB, Fischer DR, et al. Differentiation of phyllodes breast tumors from fibroadenomas on MRI. *AJR Am J Roentgenol* 2005;185:1317–1321.
51. Won KS, Gayed I, Kim EE, et al. Juvenile fibroadenoma of the breast demonstrated on 111in-octreotide SPECT and 18F-FDG PET/CT. *Eur J Nucl Med Mol Imaging* 2007;34:440.
52. Farrow JH, Ashikari H. Breast lesions in young girls. *Surg Clin North Am* 1969;49:261–269.
53. Demetrakopoulos NJ. Three-dimensional reconstruction of a human mammary fibroadenoma. *Q Bull Northwest Univ Med Sch* 1958;32:221–228.
54. Koerner FC, O'Connell JX. Fibroadenoma: morphological observations and a theory of pathogenesis. *Pathol Annu* 1994;29(Pt. 1):1–19.
55. Cheatle GL. Hyperplasia of epithelial and connective tissues in the breast: its relation to fibroadenoma and other pathological conditions. *Br J Surg* 1923:436–455.
56. Goodman ZD, Taxy JB. Fibroadenomas of the breast with prominent smooth muscle. *Am J Surg Pathol* 1981;5:99–101.
57. Powell CM, Rosen PP. Adipose differentiation in cystosarcoma phyllodes. A study of 14 cases. *Am J Surg Pathol* 1994;18:720–727.
58. Spagnolo DV, Shilkin KB. Breast neoplasms containing bone and cartilage. *Virchows Arch A Pathol Anat Histopathol* 1983;400:287–295.
59. Meyer JE, Lester SC, DiPiro PJ, et al. Occult calcified fibroadenomas. *Breast Dis* 1995;8:29–38.
60. Berean K, Tron VA, Churg A, et al. Mammary fibroadenoma with multinucleated stromal giant cells. *Am J Surg Pathol* 1986;10:823–827.
61. Powell CM, Cranor ML, Rosen PP. Multinucleated stromal giant cells in mammary fibroepithelial neoplasms. A study of 11 patients. *Arch Pathol Lab Med* 1994;118:912–916.
62. Ryska A, Reynolds C, Keeney GL. Benign tumors of the breast with multinucleated stromal giant cells. Immunohistochemical analysis of six cases and review of the literature. *Virchows Arch* 2001;439: 768–775.
63. Parham DM, Eccles DM. Fibroadenoma with atypical giant cells occurring in Li Fraumeni Syndrome. *Breast* 2001;10:330–332.
64. Das DK, Rifaat AA, George SS, et al. Morphologic changes in fibroadenoma of breast due to chickenpox: a case report with suspicious cytology in fine needle aspiration smears. *Acta Cytol* 2008;52:337–343.
65. Huo L, Gilcrease MZ. Fibroepithelial lesions of the breast with pleomorphic stromal giant cells: a clinicopathologic study of 4 cases and review of the literature. *Ann Diagn Pathol* 2009;13:226–232.
66. Cummings MC, da Silva L, Papadimos DJ, et al. Fibroadenoma and intraduct papilloma—a common pathogenesis? *Virchows Arch* 2009;455:271–275.
67. Chung A, Scharre K, Wilson M. Intraductal fibroadenomatosis: an unusual variant of fibroadenoma. *Breast J* 2008;14:193–195.
68. Kasami M, Vnencak-Jones CL, Manning S, et al. Monoclonality in fibroadenomas with complex histology and phyllodal features. *Breast Cancer Res Treat* 1998;50:185–191.
69. Dupont WD, Page DL, Parl FF, et al. Long-term risk of breast cancer in women with fibroadenoma. *N Engl J Med* 1994;331:10–15.
70. Moross T, Lang AP, Mahoney L. Tubular adenoma of breast. *Arch Pathol Lab Med* 1983;107:84–86.
71. Persaud V, Talerman A, Jordan R. Pure adenoma of the breast. *Arch Pathol* 1968;86:481–483.
72. Hertel BF, Zaloudek C, Kempson RL. Breast adenomas. *Cancer* 1976;37:2891–2905.
73. James K, Bridger J, Anthony PP. Breast tumour of pregnancy ('lactating' adenoma). *J Pathol* 1988;156:37–44.
74. Baddoura FK, Judd RL. Apocrine adenoma of the breast: report of a case with investigation of lectin binding patterns in apocrine breast lesions. *Mod Pathol* 1990;3:373–376.
75. Tesluk H, Amott T, Goodnight JE Jr. Apocrine adenoma of the breast. *Arch Pathol Lab Med* 1986;110:351–352.
76. Azzopardi JG, Salm R. Ductal adenoma of the breast: a lesion which can mimic carcinoma. *J Pathol* 1984;144:15–23.
77. Gusterson BA, Sloane JP, Middwood C, et al. Ductal adenoma of the breast—a lesion exhibiting a myoepithelial/epithelial phenotype. *Histopathology* 1987;11:103–110.
78. Ballance WA, Ro JY, el-Naggar AK, et al. Pleomorphic adenoma (benign mixed tumor) of the breast. An immunohistochemical, flow cytometric, and ultrastructural study and review of the literature. *Am J Clin Pathol* 1990;93:795–801.
79. Chen KT. Pleomorphic adenoma of the breast. *Am J Clin Pathol* 1990;93:792–794.
80. Soreide JA, Anda O, Eriksen L, et al. Pleomorphic adenoma of the human breast with local recurrence. *Cancer* 1988;61:997–1001.
81. Majmudar B, Rosales-Quintana S. Infarction of breast fibroadenomas during pregnancy. *JAMA* 1975;231:963–964.
82. Delarue JC, Redon H. Les infarctus des fibro-adenomes mammaire. Probleme clinique et pathogenique. *Sem Hop, Paris* 1949;25: 2901–2906.
83. Newman J, Kahn LB. Infarction of fibro-adenoma of the breast. *Br J Surg* 1973;60:738–740.
84. Toy H, Esen HH, Sonmez FC, et al. Spontaneous infarction in a fibroadenoma of the breast. *Breast Care (Basel)* 2011;6:54–55.
85. Salm R. Epidermoid metaplasia in mammary fibro-adenoma with formation of keratin cysts. *J Pathol Bacteriol* 1957;74:221–223.
86. Goldenberg VE, Wiegenstein L, Mottet NK. Florid breast fibroadenomas in patients taking hormonal oral contraceptives. *Am J Clin Pathol* 1968;49:52–59.
87. Fechner RE. Fibroadenomas in patients receiving oral contraceptives: a clinical and pathologic study. *Am J Clin Pathol* 1970;53:857–864.
88. Oberman HA. Hormonal contraceptives and fibroadenomas of breast. *N Engl J Med* 1971;284:984.
89. Terada S, Uchide K, Suzuki N, et al. A lactating adenoma of the breast. *Gynecol Obstet Invest* 1992;34:126–128.
90. Oi RH, Dobbs M. Lactating breast tissue in benign cystic teratoma. *Am J Obstet Gynecol* 1978;130:729–731.
91. Ben Hassouna J, Damak T, Ben Slama A, et al. Breast carcinoma arising within fibroadenomas. Report of four observations. *Tunis Med* 2007;85:891–895.
92. Petersson F, Tan PH, Putti TC. Low-grade ductal carcinoma *in situ* and invasive mammary carcinoma with columnar cell morphology arising in a complex fibroadenoma in continuity with columnar cell change and flat epithelial atypia. *Int J Surg Pathol* 2010;18:352–357.
93. Blanco M, Egozi L, Lubin D, et al. Adenoid cystic carcinoma arising in a fibroadenoma. *Ann Diagn Pathol* 2005;9:157–159.
94. Charfi L, Mrad K, Sellami R, et al. Invasive mucinous carcinoma arising within breast fibroadenoma. *Pathologica* 2008;100:199–201.
95. Bottles K, Taylor RN. Diagnosis of breast masses in pregnant and lactating women by aspiration cytology. *Obstet Gynecol* 1985;66:76S–78S.
96. Bottles K, Chan JS, Holly EA, et al. Cytologic criteria for fibroadenoma. A step-wise logistic regression analysis. *Am J Clin Pathol* 1988;89:707–713.
97. Dejmek A, Lindholm K. Frequency of cytologic features in fine needle aspirates from histologically and cytologically diagnosed fibroadenomas. *Acta Cytol* 1991;35:695–699.
98. Benoit JL, Kara R, McGregor SE, et al. Fibroadenoma of the breast: diagnostic pitfalls of fine-needle aspiration. *Diagn Cytopathol* 1992;8:643–647; discussion 647–648.
99. Troxel DB, Sabella JD. Problem areas in pathology practice. Uncovered by a review of malpractice claims. *Am J Surg Pathol* 1994;18:821–831.
100. Rao S, Latha PS, Ravi A, et al. Ductal carcinoma in a multiple fibroadenoma: diagnostic inaccuracies. *J Cancer Res Ther* 2010;6:385–387.
101. McCutcheon JM, Lipa M. Infarction of a fibroadenoma of breast following fine needle aspiration. *Cytopathology* 1993;4:247–250.
102. Finley JL, Silverman JF, Lannin DR. Fine needle aspiration cytology of breast masses in pregnant and lactating women. *Diagn Cytopathol* 1989;5:255–9.

103. Grenko RT, Lee KP, Lee KR. Fine needle aspiration cytology of lactating adenoma of the breast. A comparative light microscopic and morphometric study. *Acta Cytol* 1990;34:21–26.
104. Giani C, D'Amore E, Delarue JC, et al. Estrogen and progesterone receptors in benign breast tumors and lesions: relationship with histological and cytological features. *Int J Cancer* 1986;37:7–10.
105. Mechtersheimer G, Kruger KH, Born IA, et al. Antigenic profile of mammary fibroadenoma and cystosarcoma phyllodes. A study using antibodies to estrogen- and progesterone receptors and to a panel of cell surface molecules. *Pathol Res Pract* 1990;186:427–438.
106. Sapino A, Bosco M, Cassoni P, et al. Estrogen receptor-beta is expressed in stromal cells of fibroadenoma and phyllodes tumors of the breast. *Mod Pathol* 2006;19:599–606.
107. Rao BR, Meyer JS, Fry CG. Most cystosarcoma phyllodes and fibroadenomas have progesterone receptor but lack estrogen receptor: stromal localization of progesterone receptor. *Cancer* 1981;47:2016–2021.
108. Sawyer EJ, Hanby AM, Poulsom R, et al. Beta-catenin abnormalities and associated insulin-like growth factor overexpression are important in phyllodes tumours and fibroadenomas of the breast. *J Pathol* 2003;200:627–632.
109. Kocova L, Skalova A, Fakan F, et al. Phyllodes tumour of the breast: immunohistochemical study of 37 tumours using MIB1 antibody. *Pathol Res Pract* 1998;194:97–104.
110. Jara-Lazaro AR, Akhilesh M, Thike AA, et al. Predictors of phyllodes tumours on core biopsy specimens of fibroepithelial neoplasms. *Histopathology* 2010;57:220–232.
111. Jacobs TW, Chen YY, Guinee DG Jr, et al. Fibroepithelial lesions with cellular stroma on breast core needle biopsy: are there predictors of outcome on surgical excision? *Am J Clin Pathol* 2005;124:342–354.
112. Calabrese G, Di Virgilio C, Cianchetti E, et al. Chromosome abnormalities in breast fibroadenomas. *Genes Chromosomes Cancer* 1991;3:202–204.
113. Fletcher JA, Pinkus GS, Weidner N, et al. Lineage-restricted clonality in biphasic solid tumors. *Am J Pathol* 1991;138:1199–1207.
114. Stephenson CF, Davis RI, Moore GE, et al. Cytogenetic and fluorescence *in situ* hybridization analysis of breast fibroadenomas. *Cancer Genet Cytogenet* 1992;63:32–36.
115. Rohen C, Staats B, Bonk U, et al. Significance of clonal chromosome aberrations in breast fibroadenomas. *Cancer Genet Cytogenet* 1996;87:152–155.
116. Petersson C, Pandis N, Rizou H, et al. Karyotypic abnormalities in fibroadenomas of the breast. *Int J Cancer* 1997;70:282–286.
117. Noguchi S, Motomura K, Inaji H, et al. Clonal analysis of fibroadenoma and phyllodes tumor of the breast. *Cancer Res* 1993;53:4071–4074.
118. Noguchi S, Yokouchi H, Aihara T, et al. Progression of fibroadenoma to phyllodes tumor demonstrated by clonal analysis. *Cancer* 1995;76:1779–1785.
119. Kobayashi S, Iwase H, Kuzushima T, et al. Consecutively occurring multiple fibroadenomas of the breast distinguished from phyllodes tumors by clonality analysis of stromal tissue. *Breast Cancer* 1999;6:201–206.
120. Wang ZC, Buraimoh A, Iglehart JD, et al. Genome-wide analysis for loss of heterozygosity in primary and recurrent phyllodes tumor and fibroadenoma of breast using single nucleotide polymorphism arrays. *Breast Cancer Res Treat* 2006;97:301–309.
121. McCulloch RK, Sellner LN, Papadimitrou JM, et al. The incidence of microsatellite instability and loss of heterozygosity in fibroadenoma of the breast. *Breast Cancer Res Treat* 1998;49:165–169.
122. Di Vinci A, Perdelli L, Banelli B, et al. p16(^{INK4a}) promoter methylation and protein expression in breast fibroadenoma and carcinoma. *Int J Cancer* 2005;114:414–421.
123. Karim RZ, O'Toole SA, Scolyer RA, et al. Recent insights into the molecular pathogenesis of mammary phyllodes tumours. *J Clin Pathol* 2013;66:496–505.
124. Sperber F, Blank A, Metser U, et al. Diagnosis and treatment of breast fibroadenomas by ultrasound-guided vacuum-assisted biopsy. *Arch Surg* 2003;138:796–800.
125. Grady I, Gorsuch H, Wilburn-Bailey S. Long-term outcome of benign fibroadenomas treated by ultrasound-guided percutaneous excision. *Breast J* 2008;14:275–278.
126. Littrup PJ, Freeman-Gibb L, Andea A, et al. Cryotherapy for breast fibroadenomas. *Radiology* 2005;234:63–72.
127. Nurko J, Mabry CD, Whitworth P, et al. Interim results from the FibroAdenoma Cryoablation Treatment Registry. *Am J Surg* 2005;190:647–651; discussion 651–642.
128. Kaufman CS, Littrup PJ, Freeman-Gibb LA, et al. Office-based cryoablation of breast fibroadenomas with long-term follow-up. *Breast J* 2005;11:344–350.
129. Cant PJ, Madden MV, Close PM, et al. Case for conservative management of selected fibro-adenomas of the breast. *Br J Surg* 1987;74:857–859.
130. Wilkinson S, Anderson TJ, Rifkind E, et al. Fibroadenoma of the breast: a follow-up of conservative management. *Br J Surg* 1989;76:390–391.
131. Gordon PB, Gagnon FA, Lanzkowsky L. Solid breast masses diagnosed as fibroadenoma at fine-needle aspiration biopsy: acceptable rates of growth at long-term follow-up. *Radiology* 2003;229:233–238.
132. Jacklin RK, Ridgway PF, Ziprin P, et al. Optimising preoperative diagnosis in phyllodes tumour of the breast. *J Clin Pathol* 2006;59:454–459.
133. Levi F, Randimbison L, Te VC, et al. Incidence of breast cancer in women with fibroadenoma. *Int J Cancer* 1994;57:681–683.
134. Carter CL, Corle DK, Micozzi MS, et al. A prospective study of the development of breast cancer in 16,692 women with benign breast disease. *Am J Epidemiol* 1988;128:467–477.
135. McDivitt RW, Stevens JA, Lee NC, et al. Histologic types of benign breast disease and the risk for breast cancer. The Cancer and Steroid Hormone Study Group. *Cancer* 1992;69:1408–1414.
136. Krieger N, Hiatt RA. Risk of breast cancer after benign breast diseases. Variation by histologic type, degree of atypia, age at biopsy, and length of follow-up. *Am J Epidemiol* 1992;135:619–631.
137. Hutchinson WB, Thomas DB, Hamlin WB, et al. Risk of breast cancer in women with benign breast disease. *J Natl Cancer Inst* 1980;65:13–20.

Phyllodes Tumor

138. Fiks A. Cystosarcoma phyllodes of the mammary gland—Muller's tumor. For the 180th birthday of Johannes Muller. *Virchows Arch A Pathol Anat Histol* 1981;392:1–6.
139. Browder W, McQuitty JT Jr, McDonald JC. Malignant cystosarcoma phylloides. Treatment and prognosis. *Am J Surg* 1978;136:239–241.
140. Cohn-Cedermark G, Rutqvist LE, Rosendahl I, et al. Prognostic factors in cystosarcoma phyllodes. A clinicopathologic study of 77 patients. *Cancer* 1991;68:2017–2022.
141. Grimes MM. Cystosarcoma phyllodes of the breast: histologic features, flow cytometric analysis, and clinical correlations. *Mod Pathol* 1992;5:232–239.
142. Minkowitz S, Zeichner M, Di Maio V, et al. Cystosarcoma phyllodes: a unique case with multiple unilateral lesions and ipsilateral axillary metastasis. *J Pathol Bacteriol* 1968;96:514–517.
143. Bader E, Isaacson C. Bilateral malignant cystosarcoma phyllodes. *Br J Surg* 1961;48:519–521.
144. Notley RG, Griffiths HJ. Bilateral malignant cystosarcoma phyllodes. *Br J Surg* 1965;52:360–362.
145. Barrio AV, Clark BD, Goldberg JI, et al. Clinicopathologic features and long-term outcomes of 293 phyllodes tumors of the breast. *Ann Surg Oncol* 2007;14:2961–2970.
146. Tan PH, Thike AA, Tan WJ, et al. Predicting clinical behaviour of breast phyllodes tumours: a nomogram based on histological criteria and surgical margins. *J Clin Pathol* 2011;65:69–76.
147. Mrad K, Driss M, Maalej M, et al. Bilateral cystosarcoma phyllodes of the breast: a case report of malignant form with contralateral benign form. *Ann Diagn Pathol* 2000;4:370–372.
148. Macdonald OK, Lee CM, Tward JD, et al. Malignant phyllodes tumor of the female breast: association of primary therapy with cause-specific survival from the Surveillance, Epidemiology, and End Results (SEER) program. *Cancer* 2006;107:2127–2133.
149. Sasa M, Morimoto T, Ii K, et al. A Malignant phyllodes tumor of the breast in a 6-year old girl. *Breast Cancer* 1995;2:71–75.
150. Norris HJ, Taylor HB. Relationship of histologic features to behavior of cystosarcoma phyllodes. Analysis of ninety-four cases. *Cancer* 1967;20:2090–2099.
151. Amerson JR. Cystosarcoma phyllodes in adolescent females. A report of seven patients. *Ann Surg* 1970;171:849–856.
152. Hart WR, Bauer RC, Oberman HA. Cystosarcoma phyllodes. A clinicopathologic study of twenty-six hypercellular periductal stromal tumors of the breast. *Am J Clin Pathol* 1978;70:211–216.
153. Reinfuss M, Mitus J, Smolak K, et al. Malignant phyllodes tumours of the breast. A clinical and pathological analysis of 55 cases. *Eur J Cancer* 1993;29A:1252–1256.

154. Tan PH, Jayabaskar T, Chuah KL, et al. Phyllodes tumors of the breast: the role of pathologic parameters. *Am J Clin Pathol* 2005; 123:529–540.
155. Bernstein L, Deapen D, Ross RK. The descriptive epidemiology of malignant cystosarcoma phyllodes tumors of the breast. *Cancer* 1993;71:3020–3024.
156. Pimiento JM, Gadgil PV, Santillan AA, et al. Phyllodes tumors: race-related differences. *J Am Coll Surg* 2011;213:537–542.
157. Andersson A, Bergdahl L. Cystosarcoma phyllodes in young women. *Arch Surg* 1978;113:742–744.
158. Briggs RM, Walters M, Rosenthal D. Cystosarcoma phylloides in adolescent female patients. *Am J Surg* 1983;146:712–714.
159. Hoover HC, Trestioreanu A, Ketcham AS. Metastatic cystosarcoma phylloides in an adolescent girl: an unusually malignant tumor. *Ann Surg* 1975;181:279–282.
160. Senocak ME, Gogus S, Hicsonmez A, et al. Cystosarcoma phylloides in an adolescent female. *Z Kinderchir* 1989;44:253–254.
161. Rajan PB, Cranor ML, Rosen PP. Cystosarcoma phyllodes in adolescent girls and young women: a study of 45 patients. *Am J Surg Pathol* 1998;22:64–69.
162. Rodriguez Ogando A, Fernandez Lopez T, Rodriguez Castano MJ, et al. Cystosarcoma phyllodes of the breast: a case report in a 12-year-old girl. *Clin Transl Oncol* 2010;12:704–706.
163. Sorelli PG, Thomas D, Moore A, et al. Malignant phyllodes tumor in an 11-year-old premenarchal girl. *J Pediatr Surg* 2010;45:e17–e20.
164. Tagaya N, Kodaira H, Kogure H, et al. A case of phyllodes tumor with bloody nipple discharge in juvenile patient. *Breast Cancer* 1999;6:207–210.
165. Selamzade M, Gidener C, Koyuncuoglu M, et al. Borderline phylloides tumor in an 11-year-old girl. *Pediatr Surg Int* 1999;15:427–428.
166. Blanckaert D, Lecourt O, Loeuille GA, et al. [Phyllodes tumor of the breast in an 11-year-old child]. *Pediatrie* 1988;43:405–408.
167. Ross DS, Giri D, Akram M, et al. Fibroepithelial lesions in the breast of adolescent females: a clinicopathological profile of 35 cases *Mod Pathol* 2012;92(Suppl.):64A.
168. Inder M, Vaishnav K, Mathur DR. Benign breast lesions in prepubertal female children—a study of 20 years. *J Indian Med Assoc* 2001;99:619–620.
169. Guillot E, Couturaud B, Reyal F, et al. Management of phyllodes breast tumors. *Breast J* 2011;17:129–137.
170. Way JC, Culham BA. Phyllodes tumour in pregnancy: a case report. *Can J Surg* 1998;41:407–409.
171. Sharma JB, Wadhwa L, Malhotra M, et al. A case of huge enlargement of cystosarcoma phylloides of breast in pregnancy. *Eur J Obstet Gynecol Reprod Biol* 2004;115:237–239.
172. Aranda C, Sotelo M, Torres A, et al. [Phyllodes tumor and pregnancy. A report of a case]. *Ginecol Obstet Mex* 2005;73:387–392.
173. Blaker KM, Sahoo S, Schweichler MR, et al. Malignant phylloides tumor in pregnancy. *Am Surg* 2010;76:302–305.
174. Pacchiarotti A, Frati P, Caserta D, et al. First case of transformation for breast fibroadenoma to high-grade malignant cystosarcoma in an *in vitro* fertilization patient. *Fertil Steril* 2011;96:1126–1127.
175. Hodges KB, Abdul-Karim FW, Wang M, et al. Evidence for transformation of fibroadenoma of the breast to malignant phyllodes tumor. *Appl Immunohistochem Mol Morphol* 2009;17:345–350.
176. Karim RZ, Gerega SK, Yang YH, et al. Phyllodes tumours of the breast: a clinicopathological analysis of 65 cases from a single institution. *Breast* 2009;18:165–170.
177. Keelan PA, Myers JL, Wold LE, et al. Phyllodes tumor: clinicopathologic review of 60 patients and flow cytometric analysis in 30 patients. *Hum Pathol* 1992;23:1048–1054.
178. Nielsen VT, Andreasen C. Phyllodes tumour of the male breast. *Histopathology* 1987;11:761–762.
179. Reingold IM, Ascher GS. Cystosarcoma phyllodes in a man with gynecomastia. *Am J Clin Pathol* 1970;53:852–856.
180. Pantoja E, Llobet RE, Lopez E. Gigantic cystosarcoma phyllodes in a man with gynecomastia. *Arch Surg* 1976; 111:611.
181. Buchberger W, Strasser K, Heim K, et al. Phylloides tumor: findings on mammography, sonography, and aspiration cytology in 10 cases. *AJR Am J Roentgenol* 1991;157:715–719.
182. Cosmacini P, Zurrida S, Veronesi P, et al. Phyllode tumor of the breast: mammographic experience in 99 cases. *Eur J Radiol* 1992;15:11–14.
183. Liberman L, Bonaccio E, Hamele-Bena D, et al. Benign and malignant phyllodes tumors: mammographic and sonographic findings. *Radiology* 1996;198:121–124.
184. Adamietz BR, Kahmann L, Fasching PA, et al. Differentiation between phyllodes tumor and fibroadenoma using real-time elastography. *Ultraschall Med.* 2011; 32(Suppl. 2):E75–E79.
185. Farria DM, Gorczyca DP, Barsky SH, et al. Benign phyllodes tumor of the breast: MR imaging features. *AJR Am J Roentgenol* 1996;167:187–189.
186. Grebe P, Wilhelm K, Brunier A, et al. [MR tomography of cystosarcoma phylloides. A case report]. *Aktuelle Radiol* 1992;2:376–378.
187. Wurdinger S, Herzog AB, Fischer DR, et al. Differentiation of phyllodes breast tumors from fibroadenomas on MRI. *AJR Am J Roentgenol.* 2005;185:1317–1321.
188. Yabuuchi H, Soeda H, Matsuo Y, et al. Phyllodes tumor of the breast: correlation between MR findings and histologic grade. *Radiology* 2006;241:702–709.
189. Birch JM, Alston RD, McNally RJ, et al. Relative frequency and morphology of cancers in carriers of germline TP53 mutations. *Oncogene* 2001;20:4621–4628.
190. Mojallal A, La Marca S, Shipkov C, et al. Poland syndrome and breast tumor: a case report and review of the literature. *Aesthet Surg J* 2012;32:77–83.
191. Kataoka T, Haruta R, Goto T, et al. Malignant phyllodes tumor of the breast with hypoglycemia: report of a case. *Jpn J Clin Oncol* 1998;28:276–280.
192. Hino N, Nakagawa Y, Ikushima Y, et al. A case of a giant phyllodes tumor of the breast with hypoglycemia caused by high-molecular-weight insulin-like growth factor II. *Breast Cancer* 2010;17:142–145.
193. Aguiar Bujanda D, Rivero Vera JC, Cabrera Suarez MA, et al. Hypoglycemic coma secondary to big insulin-like growth factor II secretion by a giant phyllodes tumor of the breast. *Breast J* 2007;13:189–191.
194. Reisenbichler ES, Krontiras H, Hameed O. Beta-human chorionic gonadotropin production associated with phyllodes tumor of the breast: an unusual paraneoplastic phenomenon. *Breast J* 2009;15:527–530.
195. Horiguchi J, Iino Y, Aiba S, et al. Phyllodes tumor showing intracystic growth: a case report. *Jpn J Clin Oncol* 1998;28:705–708.
196. Coyne JD. Periductal stromal hyperplasia. *Histopathology* 2007;50:814–815.
197. Burga AM, Tavassoli FA. Periductal stromal tumor: a rare lesion with low-grade sarcomatous behavior. *Am J Surg Pathol* 2003;27:343–348.
198. Hawkins RE, Schofield JB, Fisher C, et al. The clinical and histologic criteria that predict metastases from cystosarcoma phyllodes. *Cancer* 1992;69:141–147.
199. Lakhani SR, Ellis IO, Schnitt SJ, et al. *WHO classification of tumours of the breast.* 4th ed. Lyon: World Health Organisation-IARC, 2012.
200. Rosen PP, Romain K, Liberman L. Mammary cystosarcoma with mature adipose stromal differentiation (lipophyllodes tumor) arising in a lipomatous hamartoma. *Arch Pathol Lab Med* 1994;118:91–94.
201. Hiraoka N, Mukai M, Hosoda Y, et al. Phyllodes tumor of the breast containing the intracytoplasmic inclusion bodies identical with infantile digital fibromatosis. *Am J Surg Pathol* 1994;18:506–511.
202. Barnes L, Pietruszka M. Rhabdomyosarcoma arising within a cystosarcoma phyllodes. Case report and review of the literature. *Am J Surg Pathol* 1978;2:423–429.
203. Iihara K, Machinami R, Kubota S, et al. Malignant cystosarcoma phyllodes tumor of the breast mainly composed of chondrosarcoma: a case report. *Gen Diagn Pathol* 1997;142:241–245.
204. Silver SA, Tavassoli FA. Osteosarcomatous differentiation in phyllodes tumors. *Am J Surg Pathol* 1999;23:815–821.
205. Powell CM, Rosen PP, PT. Adipose differentiation in cystosarcoma phyllodes. A study of 14 cases. *Am J Surg Pathol.* 1994;18:720–727.
206. Sawyer EJ, Hanby AM, Rowan AJ, et al. The Wnt pathway, epithelial–stromal interactions, and malignant progression in phyllodes tumours. *J Pathol* 2002;196:437–444.
207. McDivitt RW, Urban JA, Farrow JH. Cystosarcoma phyllodes. *Johns Hopkins Med J* 1967;120:33–45.
208. Salisbury JR, Singh LN. Apocrine metaplasia in phyllodes tumours of the breast. *Histopathology* 1986;10:1211.
209. Grove A, Deibjerg Kristensen L. Intraductal carcinoma within a phyllodes tumor of the breast: a case report. *Tumori* 1986;72:187–190.
210. Knudsen PJ, Ostergaard J. Cystosarcoma phylloides with lobular and ductal carcinoma *in situ*. *Arch Pathol Lab Med* 1987;111: 873–875.
211. Yamaguchi R, Tanaka M, Kishimoto Y, et al. Ductal carcinoma *in situ* arising in a benign phyllodes tumor: report of a case. *Surg Today* 2008;38:42–45.

212. Korula A, Varghese J, Thomas M, et al. Malignant phyllodes tumour with intraductal and invasive carcinoma and lymph node metastasis. *Singapore Med J* 2008;49:e318–e321.
213. Kuo YJ, Ho DM, Tsai YF, et al. Invasive ductal carcinoma arising in phyllodes tumor with isolated tumor cells in sentinel lymph node. *J Chin Med Assoc* 2010;73:602–604.
214. Nomura M, Inoue Y, Fujita S, et al. A case of noninvasive ductal carcinoma arising in malignant phyllodes tumor. *Breast Cancer* 2006;13:89–94.
215. Kodama T, Kameyama K, Mukai M, et al. Invasive lobular carcinoma arising in phyllodes tumor of the breast. *Virchows Arch* 2003;442:614–616.
216. Quinlan-Davidson S, Hodgson N, Elavathil L, et al. Borderline phyllodes tumor with an incidental invasive tubular carcinoma and lobular carcinoma *in situ* component: a case report. *J Breast Cancer* 2011;14:237–240.
217. Choi Y, Lee KY, Jang MH, et al. Invasive cribriform carcinoma arising in malignant phyllodes tumor of breast: a case report. *Korean J Pathol* 2012;46:205–209.
218. Sugie T, Takeuchi E, Kunishima F, et al. A case of ductal carcinoma with squamous differentiation in malignant phyllodes tumor. *Breast Cancer* 2007;14:327–332.
219. Tan EY, Tan PH, Yong WS, et al. Recurrent phyllodes tumours of the breast: pathological features and clinical implications. *ANZ J Surg* 2006;76:476–480.
220. West TL, Weiland LH, Clagett OT. Cystosarcoma phyllodes. *Ann Surg* 1971;173:520–528.
221. Kracht J, Sapino A, Bussolati G. Malignant phyllodes tumor of breast with lung metastases mimicking the primary. *Am J Surg Pathol* 1998;22:1284–1290.
222. Graadt van Roggen JF, Zonderland HM, Welvaart K, et al. Local recurrence of a phyllodes tumour of the breast presenting with widespread differentiation to a telangiectatic osteosarcoma. *J Clin Pathol* 1998;51:706–708.
223. Gisser SD, Toker C. Chondroblastic sarcoma of the breast. *Mt Sinai J Med* 1975;42:232–235.
224. Anani PA, Baumann RP. Osteosarcoma of the breast. *Virchows Arch A Pathol Pathol Anat* 1972;357:213–218.
225. Lubin J, Rywlin AM. Cystosarcoma phyllodes metastasizing as a mixed mesenchymal sarcoma. *South Med J* 1972;65:636–637.
226. Jackson AV. Metastasising liposarcoma of the breast arising in a fibroadenoma. *J Pathol Bacteriol* 1962;83:582–584.
227. Shimizu K, Masawa N, Yamada T, et al. Cytologic evaluation of phyllodes tumors as compared to fibroadenomas of the breast. *Acta Cytol* 1994;38:891–897.
228. Simi U, Moretti D, Iacconi P, et al. Fine needle aspiration cytopathology of phyllodes tumor. Differential diagnosis with fibroadenoma. *Acta Cytol* 1988;32:63–66.
229. Silverman JF, Geisinger KR, Frable WJ. Fine-needle aspiration cytology of mesenchymal tumors of the breast. *Diagn Cytopathol* 1988; 4:50–58.
230. Tse GM, Ma TK, Pang LM, et al. Fine needle aspiration cytologic features of mammary phyllodes tumors. *Acta Cytol* 2002;46:855–863.
231. Ciatto S, Bonardi R, Cataliotti L, et al. Phyllodes tumor of the breast: a multicenter series of 59 cases. Coordinating Center and Writing Committee of FONCAM (National Task Force for Breast Cancer), Italy. *Eur J Surg Oncol* 1992;18:545–549.
232. Shabb NS. Phyllodes tumor. Fine needle aspiration cytology of eight cases. *Acta Cytol* 1997;41:321–326.
233. Dusenbery D, Frable WJ. Fine needle aspiration cytology of phyllodes tumor. Potential diagnostic pitfalls. *Acta Cytol* 1992;36:215–221.
234. Bhattarai S, Kapila K, Verma K. Phyllodes tumor of the breast. A cytohistologic study of 80 cases. *Acta Cytol* 2000;44:790–796.
235. Lee WY, Cheng L, Chang TW. Fine needle aspiration cytology of malignant phyllodes tumor with liposarcomatous stroma of the breast. A case report. *Acta Cytol* 1998;42:391–395.
236. Agarwal J, Kapila K, Verma K. Phyllodes tumor with keratin cysts: a diagnostic problem in fine needle aspiration of the breast. *Acta Cytol* 1991;35:255–256.
237. Karim RZ, O'Toole SA, Scolyer RA, et al. Recent insights into the molecular pathogenesis of mammary phyllodes tumours. *J Clin Pathol.* 2013;66:496–505.
238. Aranda FI, Laforga JB, Lopez JI. Phyllodes tumor of the breast. An immunohistochemical study of 28 cases with special attention to the role of myofibroblasts. *Pathol Res Pract* 1994;190:474–481.
239. Auger M, Hanna W, Kahn HJ. Cystosarcoma phylloides of the breast and its mimics. An immunohistochemical and ultrastructural study. *Arch Pathol Lab Med* 1989;113:1231–1235.
240. Noronha Y, Raza A, Hutchins B, et al. CD34, CD117, and Ki-67 expression in phyllodes tumor of the breast: an immunohistochemical study of 33 cases. *Int J Surg Pathol* 2011;19:152–158.
241. Chen CM, Chen CJ, Chang CL, et al. CD34, CD117, and actin expression in phyllodes tumor of the breast. *J Surg Res* 2000;94:84–91.
242. Moore T, Lee AH. Expression of CD34 and bcl-2 in phyllodes tumours, fibroadenomas and spindle cell lesions of the breast. *Histopathology* 2001;38:62–67.
243. Chia Y, Thike AA, Cheok PY, et al. Stromal keratin expression in phyllodes tumours of the breast: a comparison with other spindle cell breast lesions. *J Clin Pathol* 2012;65:339–347.
244. Rao BR, Meyer JS, Fry CG. Most cystosarcoma phyllodes and fibroadenomas have progesterone receptor but lack estrogen receptor: stromal localization of progesterone receptor. *Cancer* 1981;47:2016–2021.
245. Tse GM, Lee CS, Kung FY, et al. Hormonal receptors expression in epithelial cells of mammary phyllodes tumors correlates with pathologic grade of the tumor: a multicenter study of 143 cases. *Am J Clin Pathol* 2002;118:522–526.
246. Sapino A, Bosco M, Cassoni P, et al. Estrogen receptor-beta is expressed in stromal cells of fibroadenoma and phyllodes tumors of the breast. *Mod Pathol* 2006;19:599–606.
247. Shpitz B, Bomstein Y, Sternberg A, et al. Immunoreactivity of p53, Ki-67, and c-erbB-2 in phyllodes tumors of the breast in correlation with clinical and morphologic features. *J Surg Oncol* 2002;79:86–92.
248. Sawyer EJ, Hanby AM, Poulsom R, et al. Beta-catenin abnormalities and associated insulin-like growth factor overexpression are important in phyllodes tumours and fibroadenomas of the breast. *J Pathol* 2003;200:627–632.
249. Karim RZ, Gerega SK, Yang YH, et al. Proteins from the Wnt pathway are involved in the pathogenesis and progression of mammary phyllodes tumours. *J Clin Pathol* 2009;62:1016–1020.
250. Sawhney N, Garrahan N, Douglas-Jones AG, et al. Epithelial–stromal interactions in tumors. A morphologic study of fibroepithelial tumors of the breast. *Cancer* 1992;70:2115–2120.
251. Tse GM, Putti TC, Lui PC, et al. Increased c-kit (CD117) expression in malignant mammary phyllodes tumors. *Mod Pathol* 2004;17:827–831.
252. Carvalho S, e Silva AO, Milanezi F, et al. c-KIT and PDGFRA in breast phyllodes tumours: overexpression without mutations? *J Clin Pathol* 2004;57:1075–1079.
253. Sawyer EJ, Poulsom R, Hunt FT, et al. Malignant phyllodes tumours show stromal overexpression of c-myc and c-kit. *J Pathol* 2003;200:59–64.
254. Tan PH, Jayabaskar T, Yip G, et al. p53 and c-kit (CD117) protein expression as prognostic indicators in breast phyllodes tumors: a tissue microarray study. *Mod Pathol* 2005;18:1527–1534.
255. Bose P, Dunn ST, Yang J, et al. c-Kit expression and mutations in phyllodes tumors of the breast. *Anticancer Res* 2010;30:4731–4736.
256. Djordjevic B, Hanna WM. Expression of c-kit in fibroepithelial lesions of the breast is a mast cell phenomenon. *Mod Pathol* 2008;21:1238–1245.
257. Korcheva VB, Levine J, Beadling C, et al. Immunohistochemical and molecular markers in breast phyllodes tumors. *Appl Immunohistochem Mol Morphol* 2011;19:119–125.
258. Kleer CG, Giordano TJ, Braun T, et al. Pathologic, immunohistochemical, and molecular features of benign and malignant phyllodes tumors of the breast. *Mod Pathol* 2001;14:185–190.
259. Yonemori K, Hasegawa T, Shimizu C, et al. Correlation of p53 and MIB-1 expression with both the systemic recurrence and survival in cases of phyllodes tumors of the breast. *Pathol Res Pract* 2006;202:705–712.
260. Tse GM, Putti TC, Kung FY, et al. Increased p53 protein expression in malignant mammary phyllodes tumors. *Mod Pathol* 2002;15:734–740.
261. Tse GM, Lui PC, Scolyer RA, et al. Tumour angiogenesis and p53 protein expression in mammary phyllodes tumors. *Mod Pathol* 2003;16:1007–1013.
262. Millar EK, Beretov J, Marr P, et al. Malignant phyllodes tumours of the breast display increased stromal p53 protein expression. *Histopathology* 1999;34:491–496.
263. Erhan Y, Zekioglu O, Ersoy O, et al. p53 and Ki-67 expression as prognostic factors in cystosarcoma phyllodes. *Breast J* 2002;8:38–44.
264. Esposito NN, Mohan D, Brufsky A, et al. Phyllodes tumor: a clinicopathologic and immunohistochemical study of 30 cases. *Arch Pathol Lab Med* 2006;130:1516–1521.

265. Dacic S, Kounelis S, Kouri E, et al. Immunohistochemical profile of cystosarcoma phyllodes of the breast: a study of 23 cases. *Breast J* 2002;8:376–381.
266. Kuijper A, de Vos RA, Lagendijk JH, et al. Progressive deregulation of the cell cycle with higher tumor grade in the stroma of breast phyllodes tumors. *Am J Clin Pathol* 2005;123:690–698.
267. Kuijper A, van der Groep P, van der Wall E, et al. Expression of hypoxia-inducible factor 1 alpha and its downstream targets in fibroepithelial tumors of the breast. *Breast Cancer Res* 2005;7:R808–R818.
268. Koo CY, Bay BH, Lui PC, et al. Immunohistochemical expression of heparan sulfate correlates with stromal cell proliferation in breast phyllodes tumors. *Mod Pathol* 2006;19:1344–1350.
269. Gatalica Z, Finkelstein S, Lucio E, et al. p53 protein expression and gene mutation in phyllodes tumors of the breast. *Pathol Res Pract* 2001;197:183–187.
270. Kang Y, Kim JH, Lee TH, et al. Expression of anaphase-promoting complex7 in fibroadenomas and phyllodes tumors of breast. *Hum Pathol* 2009;40:98–107.
271. Kocova L, Skalova A, Fakan F, et al. Phyllodes tumour of the breast: immunohistochemical study of 37 tumours using MIB1 antibody. *Pathol Res Pract* 1998;194:97–104.
272. Chan YJ, Chen BF, Chang CL, et al. Expression of p53 protein and Ki-67 antigen in phyllodes tumor of the breast. *J Chin Med Assoc* 2004;67:3–8.
273. Ridgway PF, Jacklin RK, Ziprin P, et al. Perioperative diagnosis of cystosarcoma phyllodes of the breast may be enhanced by MIB-1 index. *J Surg Res* 2004;122:83–88.
274. Tse GM, Tsang AK, Putti TC, et al. Stromal CD10 expression in mammary fibroadenomas and phyllodes tumours. *J Clin Pathol* 2005;58:185–189.
275. Al-Masri M, Darwazeh G, Sawalhi S, et al. Phyllodes tumor of the breast: role of CD10 in predicting metastasis. *Ann Surg Oncol* 2012;19:1181–1184.
276. Zamecnik M, Kinkor Z, Chlumska A. CD10+ stromal cells in fibroadenomas and phyllodes tumors of the breast. *Virchows Arch* 2006;448: 871–872.
277. Tse GM, Lui PC, Lee CS, et al. Stromal expression of vascular endothelial growth factor correlates with tumor grade and microvessel density in mammary phyllodes tumors: a multicenter study of 185 cases. *Hum Pathol* 2004;35:1053–1057.
278. Yamashita J, Ogawa M, Egami H, et al. Abundant expression of immunoreactive endothelin 1 in mammary phyllodes tumor: possible paracrine role of endothelin 1 in the growth of stromal cells in phyllodes tumor. *Cancer Res* 1992;52:4046–4049.
279. Schrey MP, Patel KV, Tezapsidis N. Bombesin and glucocorticoids stimulate human breast cancer cells to produce endothelin, a paracrine mitogen for breast stromal cells. *Cancer Res* 1992;52:1786–1790.
280. Tse GM, Chaiwun B, Lau KM, et al. Endothelin-1 expression correlates with atypical histological features in mammary phyllodes tumours. *J Clin Pathol* 2007;60:1051–1056.
281. Harris M, Khan MK. Phyllodes tumour and stromal sarcoma of the breast: an ultrastructural comparison. *Histopathology* 1984;8:315–330.
282. Fernandez BB, Hernanzez FJ, Spindler W. Metastatic cystosarcoma phyllodes: a light and electron microscopic study. *Cancer* 1976;37:1737–1746.
283. Toker C. Cystosarcoma phylloides. An ultrastructural study. *Cancer* 1968;21:1171–1179.
284. Karim RZ, Scolyer RA, Tse GM, et al. Pathogenic mechanisms in the initiation and progression of mammary phyllodes tumours. *Pathology* 2009;41:105–117.
285. Layfield LJ, Hart J, Neuwirth H, et al. Relation between DNA ploidy and the clinical behavior of phyllodes tumors. *Cancer* 1989;64:1486–1489.
286. Jones AM, Mitter R, Springall R, et al. A comprehensive genetic profile of phyllodes tumours of the breast detects important mutations, intratumoral genetic heterogeneity and new genetic changes on recurrence. *J Pathol* 2008;214:533–544.
287. Niezabitowski A, Lackowska B, Rys J, et al. Prognostic evaluation of proliferative activity and DNA content in the phyllodes tumor of the breast: immunohistochemical and flow cytometric study of 118 cases. *Breast Cancer Res Treat* 2001;65:77–85.
288. el-Naggar AK, Ro JY, McLemore D, et al. DNA content and proliferative activity of cystosarcoma phyllodes of the breast. Potential prognostic significance. *Am J Clin Pathol* 1990;93:480–485.
289. Palko MJ, Wang SE, Shackney SE, et al. Flow cytometric S fraction as a predictor of clinical outcome in cystosarcoma phyllodes. *Arch Pathol Lab Med* 1990;114:949–952.
290. Birdsall SH, Summersgill BM, Egan M, et al. Additional copies of 1q in sequential samples from a phyllodes tumor of the breast. *Cancer Genet Cytogenet* 1995;83:111–114.
291. Noguchi S, Motomura K, Inaji H, et al. Clonal analysis of fibroadenoma and phyllodes tumor of the breast. *Cancer Res* 1993;53:4071–4074.
292. Kuijper A, Buerger H, Simon R, et al. Analysis of the progression of fibroepithelial tumours of the breast by PCR-based clonality assay. *J Pathol* 2002;197:575–581.
293. Wang ZC, Buraimoh A, Iglehart JD, et al. Genome-wide analysis for loss of heterozygosity in primary and recurrent phyllodes tumor and fibroadenoma of breast using single nucleotide polymorphism arrays. *Breast Cancer Res Treat* 2006;97:301–309.
294. Lu YJ, Birdsall S, Osin P, et al. Phyllodes tumors of the breast analyzed by comparative genomic hybridization and association of increased 1q copy number with stromal overgrowth and recurrence. *Genes Chromosomes Cancer* 1997;20:275–281.
295. Lae M, Vincent-Salomon A, Savignoni A, et al. Phyllodes tumors of the breast segregate in two groups according to genetic criteria. *Mod Pathol* 2007;20:435–444.
296. Lv S, Niu Y, Wei L, et al. Chromosomal aberrations and genetic relations in benign, borderline and malignant phyllodes tumors of the breast: a comparative genomic hybridization study. *Breast Cancer Res Treat* 2008;112:411–418.
297. Kuijper A, Snijders AM, Berns EM, et al. Genomic profiling by array comparative genomic hybridization reveals novel DNA copy number changes in breast phyllodes tumours. *Cell Oncol* 2009;31:31–39.
298. Tse GM, Lui PC, Vong JS, et al. Increased epidermal growth factor receptor (EGFR) expression in malignant mammary phyllodes tumors. *Breast Cancer Res Treat* 2009;114:441–448.
299. Jones AM, Mitter R, Poulsom R, et al. mRNA expression profiling of phyllodes tumours of the breast: identification of genes important in the development of borderline and malignant phyllodes tumours. *J Pathol* 2008;216:408–417.
300. Ang MK, Ooi AS, Thike AA, et al. Molecular classification of breast phyllodes tumors: validation of the histologic grading scheme and insights into malignant progression. *Breast Cancer Res Treat* 2011;129:319–329.
301. Huang KT, Dobrovic A, Yan M, et al. DNA methylation profiling of phyllodes and fibroadenoma tumours of the breast. *Breast Cancer Res Treat* 2010;124:555–565.
302. Kim JH, Choi YD, Lee JS, et al. Borderline and malignant phyllodes tumors display similar promoter methylation profiles. *Virchows Arch* 2009;455:469–475.
303. Noguchi S, Yokouchi H, Aihara T, et al. Progression of fibroadenoma to phyllodes tumor demonstrated by clonal analysis. *Cancer.* 1995;76:1779–1785.
304. Bartoli C, Zurrida S, Veronesi P, et al. Small sized phyllodes tumor of the breast. *Eur J Surg Oncol* 1990;16:215–219.
305. Hart J, Layfield LJ, Trumbull WE, et al. Practical aspects in the diagnosis and management of cystosarcoma phyllodes. *Arch Surg* 1988;123:1079–1083.
306. McGregor GI, Knowling MA, et al. Sarcoma and cystosarcoma phyllodes tumors of the breast—a retrospective review of 58 cases. *Am J Surg* 1994;167:477–480.
307. Salvadori B, Cusumano F, Del Bo R, et al. Surgical treatment of phyllodes tumors of the breast. *Cancer* 1989;63:2532–2536.
308. Ben Hassouna J, Damak T, Gamoudi A, et al. Phyllodes tumors of the breast: a case series of 106 patients. *Am J Surg* 2006;192:141–147.
309. Asoglu O, Ugurlu MM, Blanchard K, et al. Risk factors for recurrence and death after primary surgical treatment of malignant phyllodes tumors. *Ann Surg Oncol* 2004;11:1011–1017.
310. Fou A, Schnabel FR, Hamele-Bena D, et al. Long-term outcomes of malignant phyllodes tumors patients: an institutional experience. *Am J Surg* 2006;192:492–495.
311. Reinfuss M, Mitus J, Duda K, et al. The treatment and prognosis of patients with phyllodes tumor of the breast: an analysis of 170 cases. *Cancer* 1996;77:910–916.
312. Chaney AW, Pollack A, McNeese MD, et al. Primary treatment of cystosarcoma phyllodes of the breast. *Cancer* 2000;89:1502–1511.
313. Belkacemi Y, Bousquet G, Marsiglia H, et al. Phyllodes tumor of the breast. *Int J Radiat Oncol Biol Phys* 2008;70:492–500.
314. Kapiris I, Nasiri N, A'Hern R, et al. Outcome and predictive factors of local recurrence and distant metastases following primary surgical treatment of high-grade malignant phyllodes tumours of the breast. *Eur J Surg Oncol* 2001;27:723–730.

315. Gullett NP, Rizzo M, Johnstone PA. National surgical patterns of care for primary surgery and axillary staging of phyllodes tumors. *Breast J* 2009;15:41–44.
316. Treves N, Sunderland DA. Cystosarcoma phyllodes of the breast: a malignant and a benign tumor; a clinicopathological study of seventy-seven cases. *Cancer* 1951;4:1286–1332.
317. Harada S, Fujiwara H, Hisatsugu T, et al. Malignant cystosarcoma phyllodes with lymph node metastasis—a case report. *Jpn J Surg* 1987;17:174–177.
318. Barth RJ Jr. Histologic features predict local recurrence after breast conserving therapy of phyllodes tumors. *Breast Cancer Res Treat* 1999;57:291–295.
319. Zurrida S, Bartoli C, Galimberti V, et al. Which therapy for unexpected phyllode tumour of the breast? *Eur J Cancer* 1992;28:654–657.
320. Teo JY, Cheong CS, Wong CY. Low local recurrence rates in young Asian patients with phyllodes tumours: less is more. *ANZ J Surg* 2012;82:325–328.
321. Park HL, Kwon SH, Chang SY, et al. Long-term follow-up result of benign phyllodes tumor of the breast diagnosed and excised by ultrasound-guided vacuum-assisted breast biopsy. *J Breast Cancer* 2012;15:224–229.
322. Hines JR, Murad TM, Beal JM. Prognostic indicators in cystosarcoma phylloides. *Am J Surg* 1987;153:276–280.
323. Blichert-Toft M, Hansen JP, Hansen OH, et al. Clinical course of cystosarcoma phyllodes related to histologic appearance. *Surg Gynecol Obstet* 1975;140:929–932.
324. Oberman HA. Cystosarcoma phyllodes: a clinicopathologic study of hypercellular periductal stromal neoplasms of breast. *Cancer* 1965;18:697–710.
325. Barth RJ Jr, Wells WA, Mitchell SE, et al. A prospective, multi-institutional study of adjuvant radiotherapy after resection of malignant phyllodes tumors. *Ann Surg Oncol* 2009;16:2288–2294.
326. Morales-Vasquez F, Gonzalez-Angulo AM, Broglio K, et al. Adjuvant chemotherapy with doxorubicin and dacarbazine has no effect in recurrence-free survival of malignant phyllodes tumors of the breast. *Breast J* 2007;13:551–556.
327. Hawkins RE, Schofield JB, Wiltshaw E, et al. Ifosfamide is an active drug for chemotherapy of metastatic cystosarcoma phyllodes. *Cancer* 1992;69:2271–2275.
328. Burton GV, Hart LL, Leight GS Jr, et al. Cystosarcoma phyllodes. Effective therapy with cisplatin and etoposide chemotherapy. *Cancer* 1989;63:2088–2092.
329. Pietruszka M, Barnes L. Cystosarcoma phyllodes: a clinicopathologic analysis of 42 cases. *Cancer* 1978;41:1974–1983.
330. Lindquist KD, van Heerden JA, Weiland LH, et al. Recurrent and metastatic cystosarcoma phyllodes. *Am J Surg* 1982;144:341–343.
331. Kessinger A, Foley JF, Lemon HM, et al. Metastatic cystosarcoma phyllodes: a case report and review of the literature. *J Surg Oncol* 1972;4:131–147.
332. Fleisher AG, Tyers FO, Hu D, et al. Dumbbell metastatic cystosarcoma phyllodes of the heart and lung. *Ann Thorac Surg* 1990;49:309–311.
333. Abemayor E, Nast CC, Kessler DJ. Cystosarcoma phyllodes metastatic to the mandible. *J Surg Oncol* 1988;39:235–240.
334. Tenzer JA, Rypins RD, Jakowatz JG. Malignant cystosarcoma phyllodes metastatic to the maxilla. *J Oral Maxillofac Surg* 1988; 46:80–82.
335. Kelly RJ, Barrett C, Swan N, et al. Metastatic phyllodes tumor causing small-bowel obstruction. *Clin Breast Cancer* 2009;9:193–195.
336. Grimes MM, Lattes R, Jaretzki A III. Cystosarcoma phyllodes. Report of an unusual case, with death due to intraneural extension to the central nervous system. *Cancer* 1985;56:1691–1695.
337. Hlavin ML, Kaminski HJ, Cohen M, et al. Central nervous system complications of cystosarcoma phyllodes. *Cancer* 1993;72:126–130.
338. Sadatomo A, Hozumi Y, Shiozawa M, et al. Spontaneous regression of pulmonary metastases from a malignant phyllodes tumor. *Jpn J Clin Oncol* 2011;41:915–917.
339. Oberman HA, Nosanchuk JS, Finger JE. Periductal stromal tumors of breast with adipose metaplasia. *Arch Surg* 1969;98:384–387.
340. Qizilbash AH. Cystosarcoma phyllodes with liposarcomatous stroma. *Am J Clin Pathol* 1976;65:321–327.

Core Biopsy Diagnosis of Fibroepithelial Lesions

341. Jacobs TW, Chen YY, Guinee DG Jr, et al. Fibroepithelial lesions with cellular stroma on breast core needle biopsy: are there predictors of outcome on surgical excision? *Am J Clin Pathol* 2005;124:342–354.
342. Jara-Lazaro AR, Akhilesh M, Thike AA, et al. Predictors of phyllodes tumours on core biopsy specimens of fibroepithelial neoplasms. *Histopathology* 2010;57:220–232.
343. Lee AH, Hodi Z, Ellis IO, et al. Histological features useful in the distinction of phyllodes tumour and fibroadenoma on needle core biopsy of the breast. *Histopathology* 2007;51:336–344.
344. Tsang AK, Chan SK, Lam CC, et al. Phyllodes tumours of the breast-differentiating features in core needle biopsy. *Histopathology* 2011;59:600–608.
345. Morgan JM, Douglas-Jones AG, Gupta SK. Analysis of histological features in needle core biopsy of breast useful in preoperative distinction between fibroadenoma and phyllodes tumour. *Histopathology* 2010;56:489–500.
346. Lacroix-Triki M, Geyer FC, Lambros MB, et al. Beta-catenin/Wnt signalling pathway in fibromatosis, metaplastic carcinomas and phyllodes tumours of the breast. *Mod Pathol* 2010;23:1438–1448.

CHAPTER 9

Ductal Hyperplasia: Usual and Atypical

SYED A. HODA

DEFINING DUCTAL HYPERPLASIA

This chapter is primarily concerned with the histopathology of various degrees and types of ductal hyperplasia. Chapter 10 addresses the concept of hyperplasia as a precancerous condition in greater detail. Chapter 11 is devoted to ductal carcinoma *in situ* (DCIS). Since these topics are intimately related, some subject matter may be covered in more than one chapter. The discussions of ductal hyperplasia and DCIS are presented in separate chapters to emphasize the importance of pathologically distinguishing between these entities in the clinical setting.

Ellis et al.[1] proposed that epithelial hyperplasia of the breast be defined and "identified by a mixture of cell types demonstrated principally by morphology but that could be supported by immunophenotypic diversity and by lack of a dominant epithelial population." It was further suggested that "the distinction of the boundary between hyperplasia and neoplasia in the breast should be recognized . . . [and] . . . is practicable at present . . ." with *in situ* carcinoma "identified by presence of a dominant clonal epithelial cell population that can be identified morphologically by a single cell population having distinctive morphologic, immunophenotypic and molecular genetic characteristics."

For research purposes, it may be useful to view the spectrum of intraductal proliferation as a continuum with no subdivisions. This concept is embodied in the terms mammary intraepithelial neoplasia (MIN)[2] and ductal intraepithelial neoplasia (DIN).[3] Although these alternative classifications replace the word carcinoma with neoplasia, they retain diagnostic groupings intended to distinguish lesions equivalent to hyperplasia, atypical hyperplasia, and DCIS of lower and higher grades. Boundaries are suggested for these groupings with no compelling evidence that they are more biologically or clinically meaningful than the existing classification or that they improve diagnostic reproducibility. The use of the term "neoplasia" for lesions that are generally agreed to be hyperplasia of the usual type (hyperplasia without atypia) is contradictory and confusing.

If ductal carcinoma in the breast evolves in a stepwise fashion comparable to that which has been proposed in other organs such as the colon,[4] then it is likely that some stages in this progression are manifested in the histologic phenotype of intraductal proliferations. Conversely, some significant genotypical alterations may not be manifested in the histologic appearance of lesions. Proliferative foci grouped together under a diagnosis of hyperplasia might consist of genotypically diverse abnormalities with differing risks of carcinoma. The unraveling of this puzzle will be the main focus of research in the realm of "precancerous" breast pathology for years to come. Immunohistochemical and molecular analysis of microdissected samples will be necessary to identify relevant markers, and it is likely that studies based on such tests will eventually be incorporated into diagnostic procedures when the information becomes clinically useful and appropriate technology becomes available.

MOLECULAR CORRELATES OF DUCTAL HYPERPLASIA

Research to date on molecular correlates of usual hyperplasia, atypical hyperplasia, and "precancerous" breast pathology suggests that this is a complex and difficult undertaking. Genetic abnormalities have been detected by chromosomal analysis and by molecular techniques in lesions considered to be benign proliferative breast disease.[5–7] These investigations have employed microdissection to isolate individual ductal lesions for molecular analysis. The results of studies that report loss of heterozygosity (LOH)[6] or monoclonality[8] in atypical ductal hyperplasia (ADH) must be interpreted with caution. Images purported by the investigators to show ADH in these two studies[6,8] could be interpreted by others as DCIS. One may reasonably question whether molecular data should guide interpretation of histologic phenotype or if the reverse interpretation should apply. Nonetheless, it is apparent that molecular analysis is unlikely to resolve the diagnostic issues of interpreting "borderline" lesions in routine histologic sections in the foreseeable future. As long as the primary method for diagnosis is histologic examination, the information gained from molecular studies will become applicable to routine diagnosis only if it results in the identification of one or more specific cancer-associated markers and procedures are developed for studying LOH or other genetic alterations directly *in situ* in tissues.

Ultimately, correlation of molecular alterations in proliferative lesions with clinical outcome will be necessary to determine which phenotypical and genotypical changes are meaningful. Presently, these studies must be retrospective in the sense that the histologic samples to be analyzed have been obtained sometime in the past and patient outcome is determined subsequently without standardized interval follow-up procedures. Prospective studies of the "natural history" of atypical proliferative lesions subjected to molecular analysis are likely to be difficult since the introduction of breast cancer chemoprevention with selective estrogen receptor (ER) modulators and other medications.

The complexity of the task in retrospective analysis is illustrated by several representative investigations. Kasami et al.[9] studied microdissected samples of proliferative breast lesions from eight women. Follow-up ranging from 8 to 25 years was available for four patients. The samples were analyzed for LOH and microsatellite instability (MSI) at 10 loci. In one patient, five loci with MSI and two loci with LOH were found in a lesion described as a papilloma with florid hyperplasia and atypia, whereas 10 other proliferative lesions from this patient showed no genetic alterations or atypia. Three loci of MSI were detected in a proliferative lesion without atypia from another patient. Both patients were well more than 20 years after the biopsies that produced these samples. The authors concluded "that several genetic alterations in proliferative breast disease lesions may not indicate clinically meaningful premalignancy for remaining breast." It is likely that large-scale studies of multiple proliferative lesions from substantial numbers of patients with well-defined follow-up will be needed to detect significant associations between genetic alterations and cancer risk.

One prospective investigation examined the relationship between human epidermal growth factor 2 (HER2) and p53 expression in benign breast lesions, and breast cancer risk in a nested case-control study.[10] The patients were part of the Canadian National Breast Screening Study. Accumulation of p53 protein detected by immunohistochemistry in benign proliferative lesions was associated with an increased risk of developing carcinoma (adjusted odds ratio [OR], 2.5; 95% confidence interval [CI], 1.01 to 6.40). There was not an increased risk associated with HER2 overexpression (adjusted OR, 0.65; 95% CI, 0.27 to 1.53). However, p53 and HER2 are only rarely expressed in hyperplastic lesions, and when present they are usually associated with "borderline" abnormalities that are variously interpreted as atypical hyperplasia or *in situ* carcinoma. Mommers et al.[11] studied the expression of several proliferation and apoptosis-related proteins in foci of usual ductal hyperplasia (UDH). Expression of HER2 and p53 were found in 2% and 8%, respectively, and decreased expression of Bcl-2 was detected in 16%. Other markers with abnormal expression in some examples of usual hyperplasia were cyclin D1, Ki67, p21, and p27. Twenty-three of 91 lesions (25%) expressed more than one abnormal proliferation or apoptosis-related protein.

Studies that report p53 accumulation detected by immunohistochemistry in hyperplastic lesions do not appear well supported by molecular analysis of p53 mutations in these lesions. Done et al.[12] used microdissection to isolate foci of epithelial hyperplasia and DCIS associated with invasive carcinomas with known *p53* mutations. The samples of DCIS had the same *p53* mutations as the corresponding invasive carcinomas, but none of the hyperplasias exhibited any *p53* mutations. The authors did not report immunohistochemical data for these specimens, but the results suggest that *p53* mutations are not a frequent occurrence in hyperplastic lesions, even in a breast that harbors carcinoma with this genetic alteration.

Another complicating factor lies in the reported detection of genetic changes in histologically normal-appearing breast tissues. LOH has been described in cells in microdissected histologically normal lobules obtained from tissue adjacent to breast carcinomas.[13] Gobbi et al.[14] studied the immunohistochemical expression of transforming growth factor-β-receptor II (TGF-β-RII) as a breast cancer risk marker in hyperplastic breast lesions without atypia and in the normal breast. Reduced expression of TGF-β-RII in nonatypical hyperplasia and in adjacent lobules was associated with an increased risk of developing invasive carcinoma in this retrospective study. Expression of HER2 has also been detected in histologically normal breast tissue associated with breast carcinoma. Ratcliffe et al.[15] used a combined *in situ* hybridization and immunohistochemical technique to assess this oncogene and its protein expression. Membrane staining was generally weak when present in normal breast tissue, corresponding to the level of expression in carcinomas lacking HER2 amplification. However, the presence of a signal detected by *in situ* hybridization in scattered nuclei in histologically normal cells may indicate an early stage of amplification preceding histologic evidence of transformation in isolated cells.

These findings raise concern about the specificity of associations between molecular markers and particular types of proliferative lesions. Some alterations may occur in tissues exhibiting little or no proliferative change. Were this to be a widespread phenomenon, then the criteria for selecting samples for analysis that currently concentrate on proliferative abnormalities might need to be revised. Ultimately, a combination of histology, immunohistochemistry, and molecular analysis may lead to a more clinically relevant classification of proliferative ductal lesions than the existing system based entirely on histologic criteria.

The distinction between intraductal hyperplasia and DCIS is obviously important for patient management.[16] In most instances, intraductal proliferations are readily classified by pathologists on the basis of generally accepted histopathologic features as either ductal hyperplasia or *in situ* ductal carcinoma.[17] There exists a subset for which assignment to either of these categories is less certain, and these abnormalities generally qualify as atypical hyperplasia. The existence of these "borderline" lesions, some of which may be diagnosed as hyperplasia or *in situ* carcinoma, depending upon which criteria are employed, is not a compelling reason for abandoning the existing practice of distinguishing pathologically and clinically between UDH, ADH, and DCIS. Studies of interobserver reproducibility in the diagnosis of highly selected examples of these lesions have focused undue attention on the diagnostic problem of "borderline" abnormalities that applies to a small percentage of proliferative breast changes.[2,18,19]

CLINICAL PRESENTATION OF DUCTAL HYPERPLASIA

There are no clinical features specifically associated with ductal hyperplasia. The alterations caused by epithelial proliferation in individual ducts or in multiple branches of a ductal system are typically microscopic in dimension and impalpable and may not harbor calcifications. It follows that specific hyperplastic processes are rarely the targeted lesion in needle core or excisional biopsies of breast. A mass lesion that incorporates elements of ductal hyperplasia may develop if there are coexisting stromal alterations such as pseudoangiomatous stromal hyperplasia (PASH) or if the process is associated with fibrocystic changes that may be detected clinically as a palpable mass or radiographically. In addition to ductal hyperplasia, the lesion complex can include one or more of the following pathologic changes that are discussed individually elsewhere in this book: sclerosing adenosis; cystic and papillary apocrine metaplasia; duct ectasia and associated inflammation; fibrosis, PASH; and lobular hyperplasia.

An important corollary to the lack of clinical indicators specific to ductal hyperplasia is an inability to determine the duration of these lesions. The date on which ductal hyperplasia was biopsied is customarily used as if it were the date of "onset" in follow-up studies. This practice, which is a consequence of inability to determine the preclinical duration of hyperplastic ductal lesions, could be a source of bias in assessing the precancerous significance of proliferative lesions in individual patients.

When clinically evident, ductal hyperplasia most often occurs in an ill-defined palpable area that is described as breast thickening. The nonspecific mammographic manifestations of these changes include altered ductal patterns, parenchymal distortion, nonpalpable mass lesions, calcification, and asymmetry. Calcifications are the most frequent mammographic indication of ADH in the absence of a palpable abnormality.[20–22] Radial sclerosing lesions (RSLs) described on mammography as "radial scars" often have a component of ductal hyperplasia. Some RSLs contain microcalcifications. One of the most distinctive clinicopathologic forms of fibrocystic change with a prominent component of ductal hyperplasia is juvenile papillomatosis, which typically presents as a single, discrete, unilateral mass in women in their teens and early 20s[23] (see Chapter 37).

When the indication for biopsy was a palpable abnormality in the era that preceded the widespread use of mammography, ductal hyperplasia was found in 25% or less of specimens obtained.[24,25] Not more than 5% of these biopsies had ADH. The frequency of atypical abnormalities is somewhat higher among mammographically directed biopsies including surgical excisions and needle core biopsies.[26,27] The yield of ADH in magnetic resonance imaging (MRI)-directed vacuum-assisted core biopsies ranges from 3% to 8% in several studies.[28–30]

Ductal hyperplasia can be found in female patients at virtually any age; however, these proliferative lesions are uncommon before puberty in women and in men at any age. In patients younger than 30 years, most examples of ductal hyperplasia occur either as juvenile papillomatosis[23] or as one of the groups of lesions referred to as papillary duct hyperplasia in children and young women.[31] The majority of women with ductal hyperplasia are between 35 and 60 years of age. A significant subset of these patients have hyperplasia of the columnar cell type, a lesion that is often multifocal and associated with microcalcifications.[32,33] In a study of 10,032 women with benign breast diseases conducted at the Mayo Clinic, the mean age of UDH was 53.9 years and that of ADH was 57.8 years.[34] Ductal hyperplasia becomes less frequent after age 60, and, when present, the growth pattern is usually less florid than in younger women. However, an occasional woman older than 60 years may be found to have extensive proliferative changes with florid ductal hyperplasia. This finding is likely to be accompanied by disproportionately less lobular atrophy than would be expected at this age, or there may be lobular hyperplasia with secretion in lobules. Use of exogenous estrogens can be documented in some of these cases. In general, factors that are associated with the development of breast carcinoma (outlined elsewhere in the book) are also associated with risk of the development of ductal hyperplastic lesions.[35]

GROSS PATHOLOGY OF DUCTAL HYPERPLASIA

There are no grossly apparent pathologic features specifically associated with intraductal hyperplasia. Specimen radiography, and its correlation with clinical mammography, is an important element in the evaluation of needle core and excisional biopsies performed for this group of diseases—primarily to ensure excision of the target lesion (usually calcifications) and to guide sampling for histology in larger specimens.

MICROSCOPIC PATHOLOGY OF UDH

Ductal hyperplasia describes a proliferative condition that is manifested histologically as an increase in the cellularity of ductal epithelium. Since the normal resting epithelium consists of a continuous monolayer of cuboidal to columnar epithelial cells supported by myoepithelial cells, an increase in the cellularity of this two-layer configuration constitutes hyperplasia. Physiologic hyperplasia during pregnancy is manifested by an increase in the number of glandular structures, as well as growth in the thickness of the epithelial layer, especially in lobular glands and ductules that constitute terminal duct lobular units (TDLUs). Concurrent but usually a lesser degree of expansion of the myoepithelium may be present.

Hyperplasia causes an increase in the thickness of the epithelial layer resulting in partial or complete obstruction of the ductal lumen at the site of the proliferative abnormality. If intraductal hyperplasia is traced in serial sections, it is often possible to observe the discontinuous, multifocal nature of the condition along the course of a single duct. Enlargement of the entire affected glandular structure is also frequently observed, in terms of both increased diameter and greater length, resulting in a sinuous structure. Various distortions of the basic ductal architecture occur when hyperplastic ducts become more sinuous or they are incorporated into complex proliferative abnormalities such as papillomas or RSLs. Hyperplasia can extend into branches of a ductal system and frequently involves TDLU structures.

Ductal hyperplasia has been described by names such as epitheliosis[36] and papillomatosis.[37] The former term was applied to "... the solid and quasi-solid benign epithelial proliferation which is found predominantly in small ducts, ductules and lobules."[36] Because it refers to epithelium in general, epitheliosis could be construed to include lobular hyperplasia. Intraductal hyperplasia includes a variable component of proliferative elements that contain some fibrovascular stroma; therefore, the distinction between epitheliosis and papillary hyperplasia is not always clear-cut. Consequently, there is no apparent advantage to replacing the term *ductal hyperplasia* with epitheliosis. Papillomatosis, often used interchangeably with ductal hyperplasia, is a term more appropriately applied to hyperplastic lesions in which a distinct fibrovascular structure supports papillary epithelial hyperplasia. Ductal hyperplasia that is not atypical is referred to as "usual," "regular," or "ordinary" to distinguish it from ADH.

Microanatomic Distribution of UDH

Instances of proliferative lesions originating in major lactiferous ducts or in larger terminal ducts can be readily found to document the capacity of the epithelium of these structures to undergo hyperplastic, atypical hyperplastic, or carcinomatous change. The term *intraductal* as it applies to hyperplasia or *in situ* carcinoma relates to a pattern of epithelial proliferation, as well as its principal site of anatomical distribution.

Studies of breast tissue by subgross dissection suggest that a subset of the proliferative changes commonly described as ductal hyperplasia arise from ductular structures of the lobules.[38] The specific histologic features of hyperplasia arising in a major duct or in the components of an "unfolded" lobule are not readily distinguishable in conventional histologic sections, although the overall structure of the lesion and its microscopic distribution in the breast may suggest the anatomical level of origin.

When subgross dissection is performed, the breast tissue is fixed and processed by a method that makes it possible to study the specimen with a dissecting microscope. The tissue can thus be examined to visualize its three-dimensional structure and abnormalities in the ductal–lobular architecture. Foci of interest can be excised from subgross samples in the form of small tissue blocks and embedded for histologic examination. Microscopic study of these selected specimens has shown that lobular "unfolding" occurs as a result of dilation and stretching of TDLU structures. The dilated structures are typically termed ducts if they are more than three to four times the diameter of a lobular ductule. In some instances, the dilated structures remain clustered together, and there may be remnants of one or more lobules that have participated partially or not at all in the process of unfolding. The ducts formed in some unfolded lobules appear to drift apart so that their origin in a TDLU structure may no longer be apparent in two-dimensional histologic sections.

Whereas many of these dilated structures arising from unfolded TDLU structures maintain continuity with the ductal system, others appear to become isolated and cystic. Some cysts are formed from dilated acinar glands, representing the terminal portions of the intralobular duct system. Others seem to develop in segments of the ductal system, possibly caused by internal ductal obstruction due to hyperplasia or as a result of compression resulting from periductal fibrosis or proliferative changes. It appears that a frequent fate of unfolded TDLU structures is to form cysts or to be the site of hyperplastic changes (Fig. 9.1). This morphogenetic relationship is the probable explanation for the frequent coexistence of the pathologic alterations that constitute fibrocystic changes, including ductal hyperplasia.

Ductal hyperplasia may be limited to one or more isolated foci, or it may involve multiple contiguous foci in a segmental region of the breast. Occasionally, it appears to arise in more than one segmental ductal system. Quantitatively, the amount of hyperplasia in any one duct varies from a minimal increase in the number of cells to complete filling of the duct, with occlusion of the lumen. The size or degree of distension of a duct is not a direct function of the amount of epithelial hyperplasia at that site. Segments of ducts occluded by hyperplastic epithelium may have a relatively small diameter, and ducts that are dilated sometimes exhibit slight hyperplasia.

Cytopathology of UDH

The amount, growth patterns, and anatomical distribution of ductal hyperplasia vary greatly from one patient to another. The structural spectrum of ductal hyperplasia is heterogeneous. Nonetheless, there are certain features that these lesions have in common that are the basis for diagnosis.

The cytologic characteristics of UDH are similar, regardless of the amount of hyperplasia present. The cellular proliferation in ductal hyperplasia often has a syncytial appearance because individual cell borders are inconspicuous (Fig. 9.2). The cytoplasm is amphophilic or weakly eosinophilic and homogeneous. Cytoplasmic vacuolization may occur. True cytoplasmic microlumens that contain secretion that stains positively with the mucicarmine or Alcian blue–periodic acid–Schiff stains are exceedingly unusual in ductal hyperplasia. The presence of intracytoplasmic mucin-containing microlumens is an atypical feature that should occasion careful consideration of a diagnosis of DCIS or pagetoid lobular carcinoma *in situ* (LCIS). In making this determination, it is critical to distinguish between intracytoplasmic vacuoles and small spaces that are remnants of the central duct lumen caught between cells.

The cytoplasmic volume of hyperplastic ductal cells tends to be reduced by comparison with normal ductal cells, causing the nuclear cytoplasmic ratio to be elevated. However, there is little increase, if any, in nuclear size in UDH. Nuclei are round, ovoid to spindly or reniform, depending, in part, on the plane of section. Nuclear spacing is uneven, resulting in areas where the cells appear crowded and nuclei overlap.

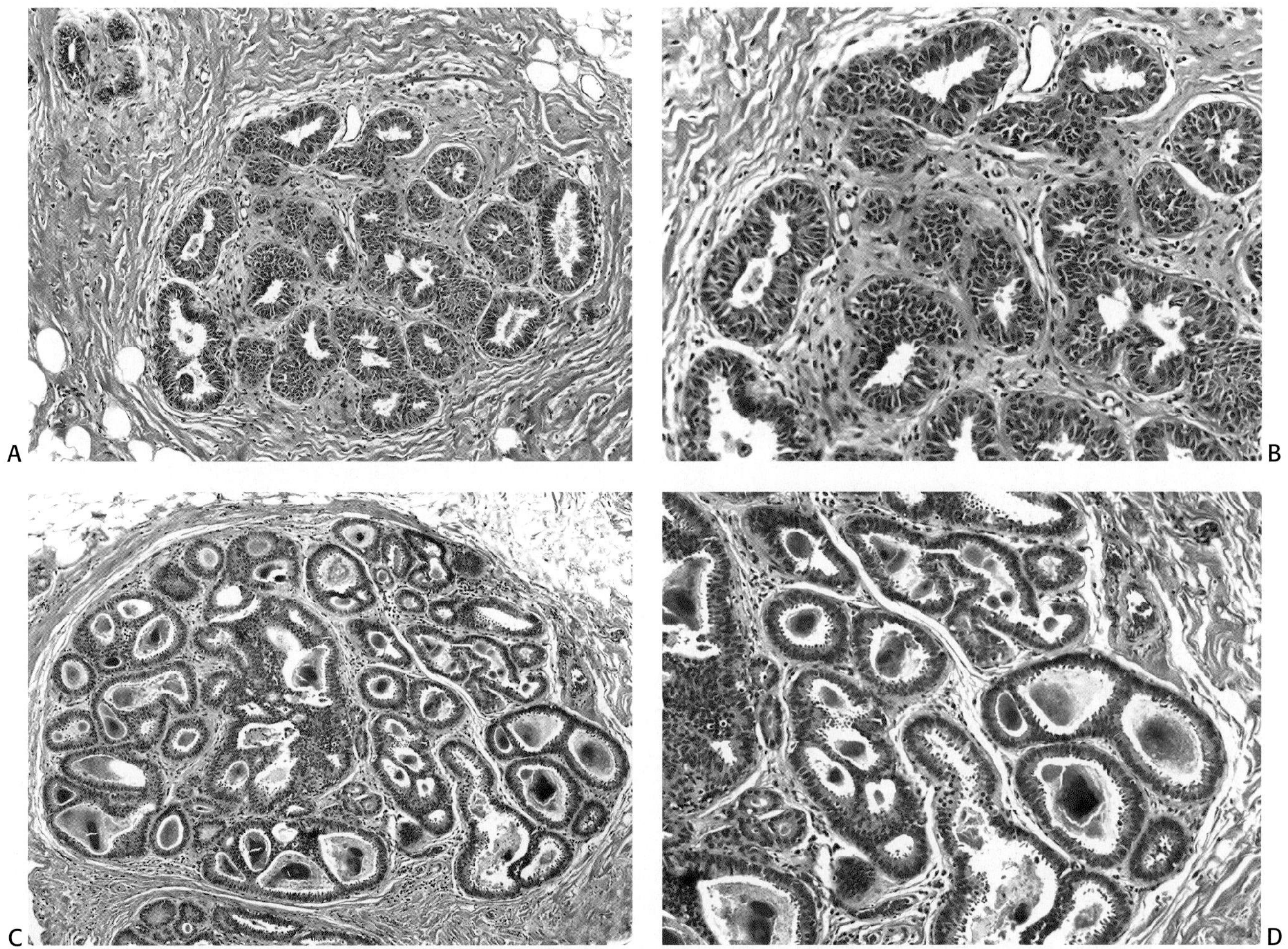

FIG. 9.1. ***Mild ductal hyperplasia in terminal ductal lobular unit.*** **A,B:** Mild ductal hyperplasia with columnar cell features in a terminal ductal lobular structure with minimal cystic dilation of lobules. **C,D:** Mild ductal hyperplasia with columnar cell features in a terminal ductal lobular structure with pronounced cystic dilation of lobules. Note calcific deposits amidst dense secretions.

Nuclear membranes are delicate, and the chromatin pattern is typically uniform. Clear nuclear vesicles that occur in some examples of ductal hyperplasia are intranuclear inclusions of cytoplasm. Some nuclei may display longitudinal grooves. Nucleoli are inapparent or inconspicuous unless there is apocrine metaplasia in the hyperplastic epithelium. Mitotic figures are infrequent, and when present they have a regular configuration.

Qualitative and Quantitative Aspects of UDH

Ductal hyperplasia of the usual type has been subdivided on the basis of qualitative and quantitative criteria into the categories of mild, moderate, and severe or florid. The application of this classification is limited by the fact that disordered epithelial growth with varied structural patterns is a characteristic feature of ductal hyperplasia. As a consequence, hyperplastic epithelium is not uniformly distributed in a stratified fashion that permits easy determination of the number of cell layers. Epithelial thickness is also difficult to judge in tangentially sectioned ducts. Levels of hyperplasia based on epithelial thickness are most reliable when applied to selected nontangential sections of duct structures of sufficient diameter to manifest diagnostic features. Consequently, the classification of ductal hyperplasia based only on epithelial thickness has limitations and may not be applicable in all instances. Nonetheless, some degree of increase in the thickness of ductal epithelium is a characteristic feature of ductal hyperplasia.

In *mild ductal hyperplasia*, the epithelium is three to four cells thick, exclusive of myoepithelium (Figs. 9.1 and 9.3). Mild hyperplasia may affect the entire epithelium circumferentially in a duct cross section, or only a segment of the duct. It usually occurs as a simple flat or slightly papillary increase in epithelial thickness. The diameter of the affected duct is generally not increased.

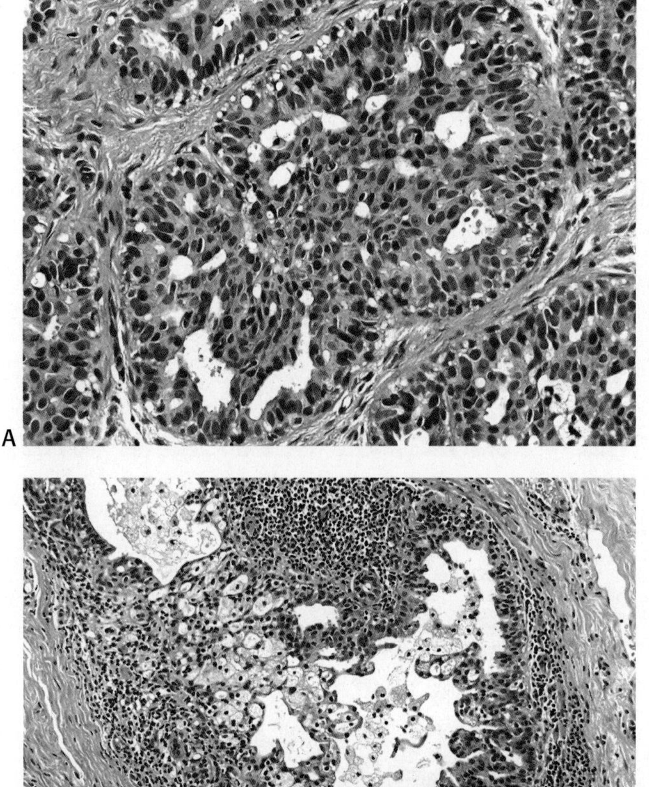

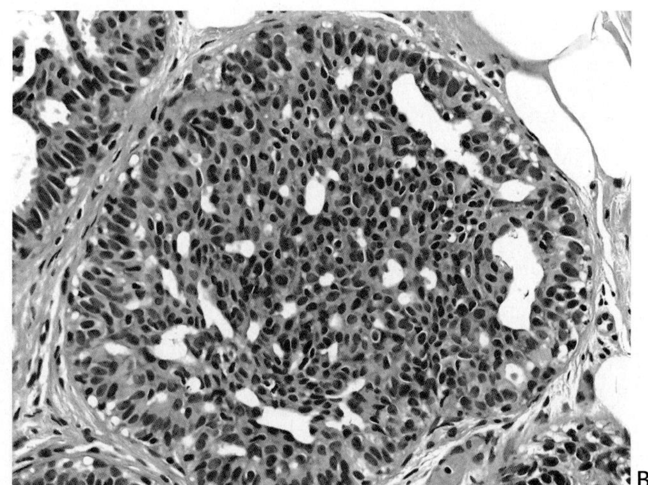

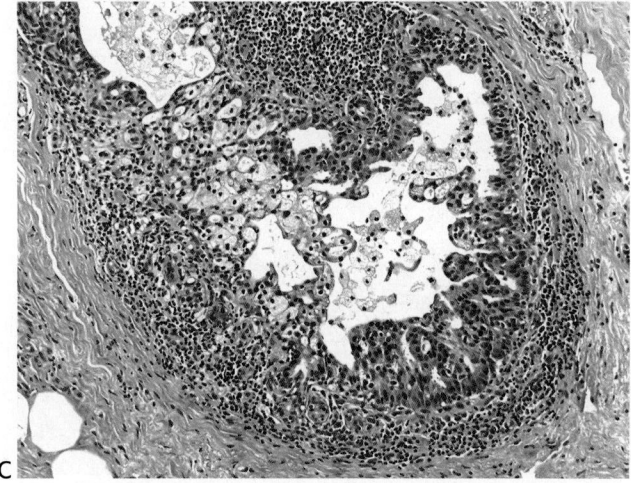

FIG. 9.2. ***Ductal hyperplasia, usual.*** **A:** Streaming of cells is evident in the center of the duct and there are peripheral microlumens. **B:** Note cells with shrunken, hyperchromatic nuclei in the center of the enlarged duct. Peripheral microlumens are shown. **C:** Micropapillary hyperplasia with duct stasis and inflammation.

In *moderate ductal hyperplasia*, the epithelium consistently has a thickness of more than three cell layers. As in mild hyperplasia, the thickened epithelium may be distributed as a flat or papillary layer at the periphery of the duct. In some instances, relatively thin strands of epithelium extend across, or bridge, the lumen, resulting in the formation of secondary glandular lumina in the hyperplastic epithelium (Fig. 9.4). Part of the original ductal lumen usually remains as one or more crescentic spaces at the edge of the duct. The lesional cells around the secondary lumina tend to lie parallel rather than perpendicular to the long axis of the spaces. The diameter of ducts with moderate hyperplasia may be increased compared with unaffected ducts.

Micropapillary ductal hyperplasia is part of the spectrum of moderate ductal hyperplasia (Figs. 9.5 and 9.6). Micropapillary structures typically have a broad base and a narrow apex. The micropapillae are unevenly shaped fronds of hyperplastic epithelium in which the apical cells are smaller and have more condensed nuclei than those in the underlying basal epithelium or in the intervening nonpapillary basal epithelium (Fig. 9.7).

The distinction between moderate and *marked or florid hyperplasia* is not sharp. Lesions are generally placed in the latter category when the affected ducts are appreciably enlarged in comparison with nonhyperplastic counterparts and the lumina are nearly or completely filled by the proliferative epithelium. Squamous metaplasia sometimes develops in moderate and florid hyperplasia (Fig. 9.8). Squamous metaplasia may also be prominent in some cases of gynecomastia that exhibit micropapillary or florid duct hyperplasia. Moderate and severe ductal hyperplasia together constitute the category of ductal hyperplasia without atypia ("ordinary" or "usual" ductal hyperplasia) in the classification of proliferative breast changes used in the assessment of breast cancer risk discussed in Chapter 10.

The nuclei in moderate ductal hyperplasia are often overlapping and may be distributed in a "streaming" fashion. Streaming refers to a growth pattern in which hyperplastic epithelial cells are oriented parallel to their long axes, an appearance most readily appreciated in the distribution of nuclei (Fig. 9.9). Since the cytoplasmic borders of these cells are often indistinct, "streaming" is usually detected as a parallel orientation of oval- or spindle-shaped nuclei. The spectrum of streaming is broad, ranging from subtle foci composed of only a few cells to conspicuous "swirling"

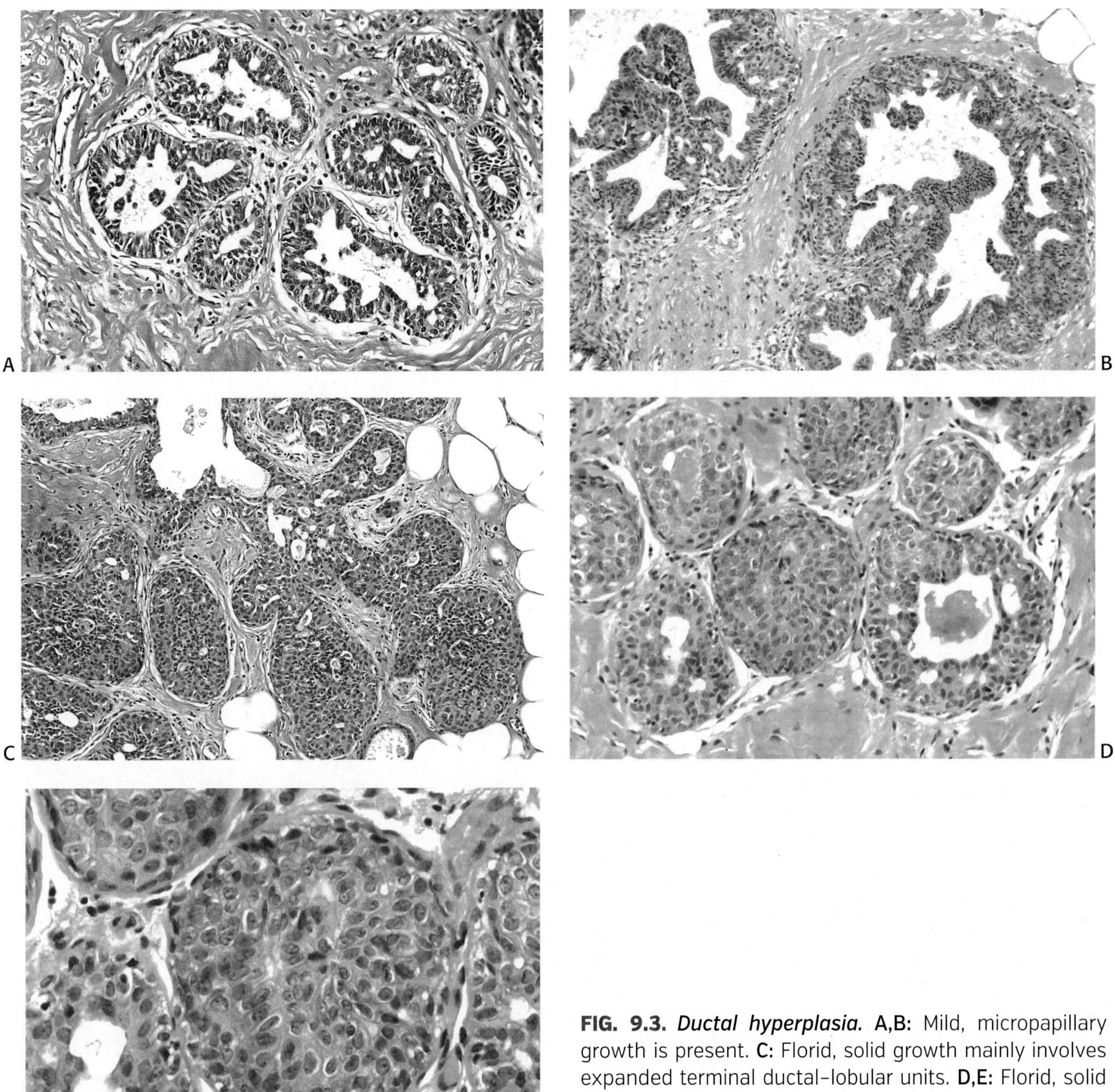

FIG. 9.3. ***Ductal hyperplasia.*** **A,B:** Mild, micropapillary growth is present. **C:** Florid, solid growth mainly involves expanded terminal ductal–lobular units. **D,E:** Florid, solid duct hyperplasia. Note loss of basal orientation of peripheral cells in the ducts.

patterns. Streaming occurs in all types of usual and atypical intraductal hyperplasia. The streaming and swirling of hyperplastic cells is reminiscent of a "school of fish" in appearance and is typically limited to the center of the involved duct space.

The distinction between moderate and florid hyperplasia is not sharp. *Florid ductal hyperplasia* has papillary and bridging growth patterns that are encountered in moderate hyperplasia, but the overall proliferation tends to be more cellular and complex than in moderate hyperplasia. Lesions are generally classified as florid when the affected ducts are appreciably enlarged in comparison with nonhyperplastic counterparts. Foci of florid hyperplasia are more likely to fill the entire duct lumen in a solid or fenestrated (cribriform) fashion. The cells are often distributed in a streaming pattern in solid or in fenestrated areas. The association of the streaming pattern with ductal hyperplasia has been confirmed by computerized morphometric analysis of the orientation of nuclei in proliferative ductal lesions.[39] A part of the original ductal lumen may remain as a crescentic space or spaces at the edge of the duct (Figs. 9.10 to 9.13). The predominantly peripheral distribution of microlumens, also known as "secondary lumens," that characterizes moderate and florid hyperplasia is an important difference from

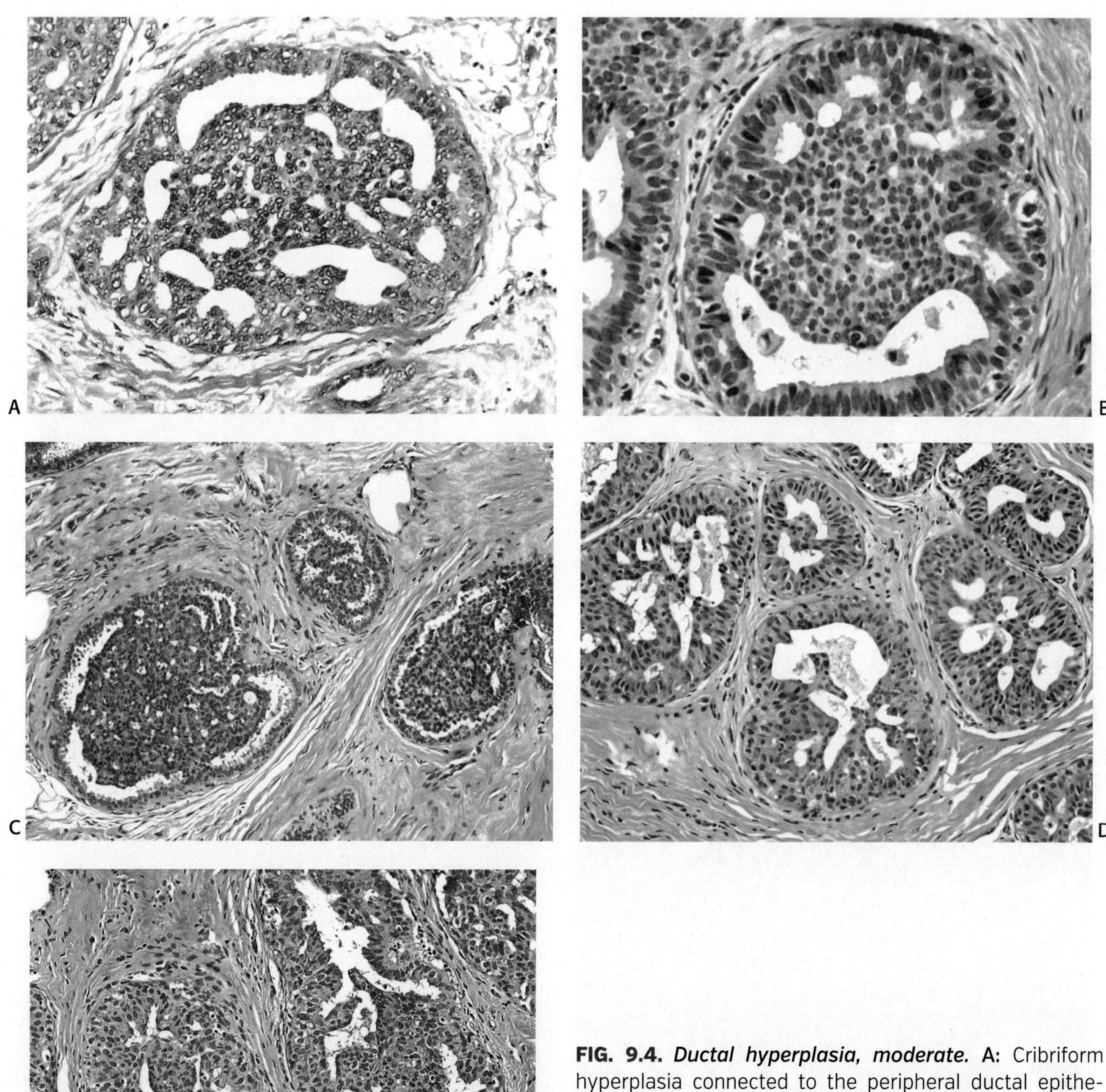

FIG. 9.4. ***Ductal hyperplasia, moderate.*** **A:** Cribriform hyperplasia connected to the peripheral ductal epithelium by strands of cells. **B,C:** A fenestrated growth pattern. Note that cells forming the center of the lesions have relatively sparse cytoplasm and smaller hyperchromatic nuclei. **D,E:** The original duct lumens are subdivided into crescentic and stellate spaces.

cribriform DCIS, wherein microlumens tend to be distributed more evenly across the entire duct cross section.

Necrotic cellular debris is rarely present in hyperplastic ducts, and when found it is usually associated with florid sclerosing papillary hyperplasia. This phenomenon is illustrated in Chapter 5. Hyperplastic ducts with necrosis are cytologically and structurally indistinguishable from adjacent ducts with nonnecrotic hyperplastic epithelium. A distinction should be made between necrosis and the accumulation of dense secretion admixed with minimal cellular detritus and inflammatory cells (Figs. 9.13 and 9.14). Histiocytes or foam cells are found relatively often in hyperplastic duct epithelium that lacks necrosis. The epithelium in florid sclerosing papillary ductal hyperplasia may have isolated mitotic figures as well as focal necrosis, but in this setting this combination is not by itself diagnostic of carcinoma.

The fenestrated (cribriform) growth pattern that occurs in moderate and florid ductal hyperplasia results from the

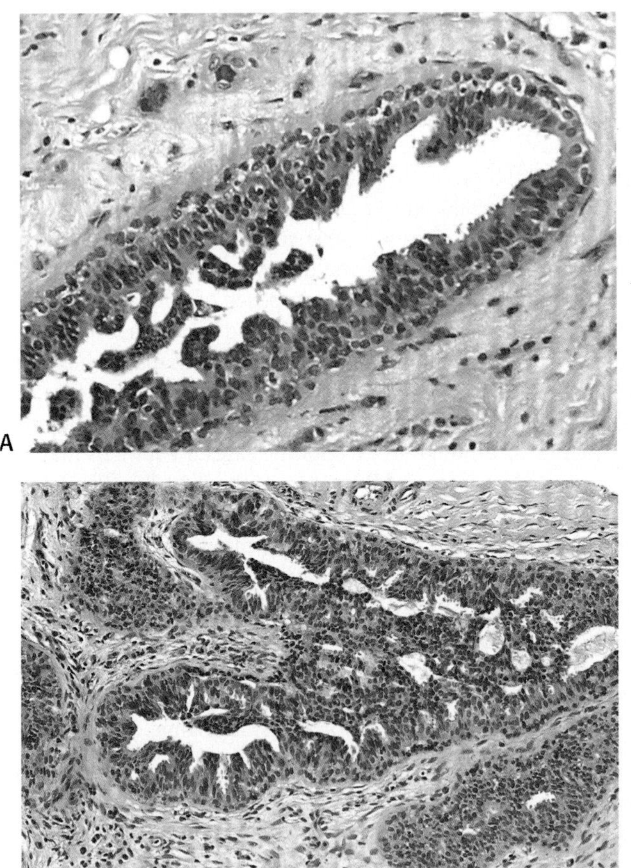

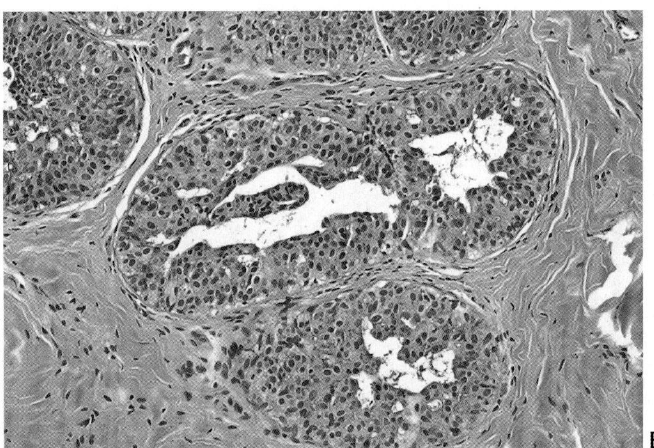

FIG. 9.5. ***Ductal hyperplasia, micropapillary.*** **A:** Ductal epithelium and hyperplastic myoepithelial cells support micropapillary fronds of mildly hyperplastic ductal epithelium. **B:** Micropapillary moderate hyperplasia traverses the duct lumen. **C:** A complex example of micropapillary moderate hyperplasia in which fusion of the epithelial fronds has created a fenestrated structure.

joining of epithelial bridges as they traverse the duct lumen. The fenestrations represent residual portions of the original ductal lumen that have been passively subdivided by the complex arborizing epithelial proliferation. Using a serial-section three-dimensional reconstruction method, Ohuchi et al.[40] demonstrated that the lumens that appear to be separated from each other in a two-dimensional histologic section of intraductal hyperplasia are actually part of a network of channels surrounded by the proliferating epithelium. By contrast, three-dimensional reconstruction of DCIS revealed

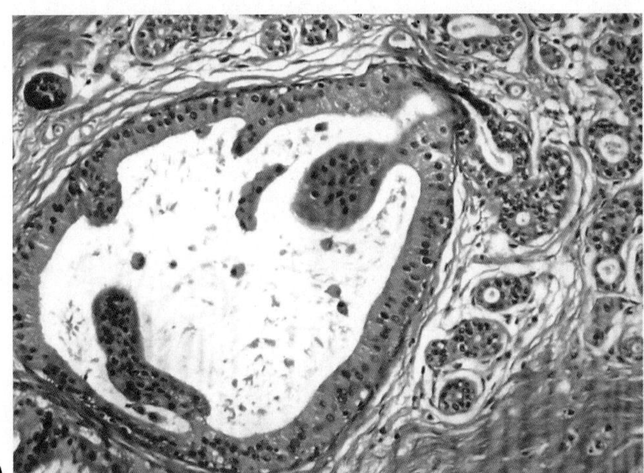

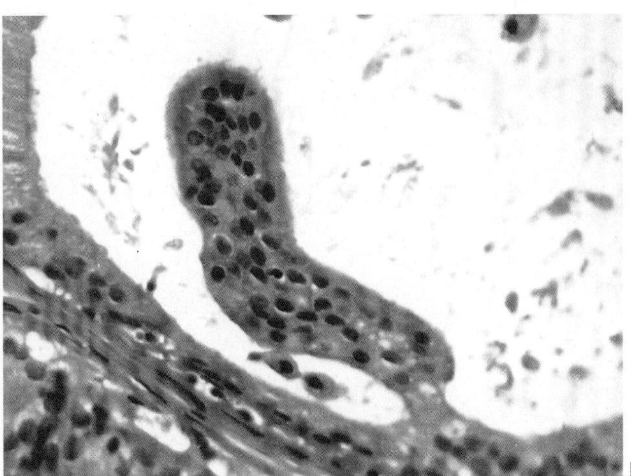

FIG. 9.6. ***Ductal hyperplasia, micropapillary.*** **A:** Micropapillary hyperplasia of apocrine epithelium. Association of the hyperplastic duct with a lobule is evident on the *right*. Note the cuboidal cells with small uniform basally located nuclei at the perimeter of the duct. **B:** Micropapillary apocrine hyperplasia shown in (**A**). Note the small, dark nuclei in the apical region.

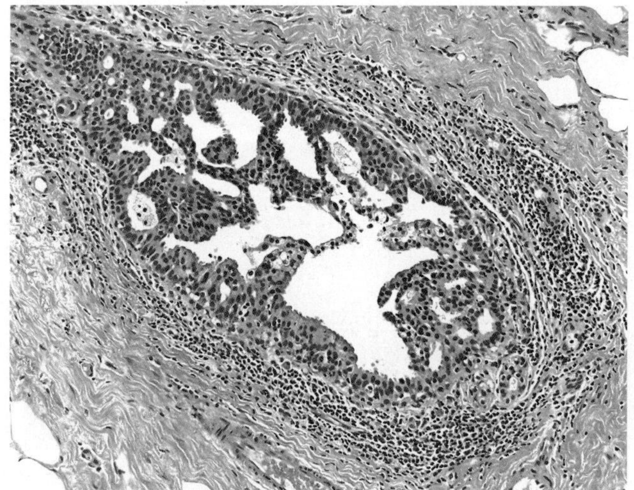

FIG. 9.7. ***Ductal hyperplasia, micropapillary.*** Mild-to-moderate hyperplasia forming interlacing epithelial strands on low columnar ductal epithelium. Cuboidal to low columnar cells with basal nuclei are distributed at the perimeter of the duct.

that the fenestrations in these lesions were newly formed disconnected spaces bordered by polarized neoplastic cells.

The spaces that are found in histologic sections of fenestrated intraductal hyperplasia have distinctive features. The secondary lumens tend to be larger and more numerous at the periphery of the duct than centrally, but variation of this distribution can be encountered (Figs. 9.4, 9.8, 9.11, and 9.12). Cells outlining these spaces are arranged in a haphazard fashion, except at the perimeter of the duct where residual columnar or cuboidal ductal epithelium composed of cells with oriented nuclei sometimes persists (Figs. 9.10 and 9.13). The spaces in a given hyperplastic duct usually have varied shapes rather than being rounded as they tend to be in cribriform carcinoma. In hyperplasia, the spaces may be ovoid, crescentic, irregular, or serpiginous, although in exceptional cases the lumens may be round and larger toward the center of the duct (Fig. 9.15). Cell membranes bordering on the spaces tend to be smooth, or they may present an uneven finely serrated surface that results from cytoplasmic blebs formed by complex folding of the cell membrane and microvilli[41] (Fig. 9.16). Apical blebs that result in a fluffy cytoplasmic border resemble the "snouts" that characterize apocrine cells. In the absence of other apocrine cytologic features, apical cytoplasmic blebs should not be interpreted as a manifestation of apocrine change.

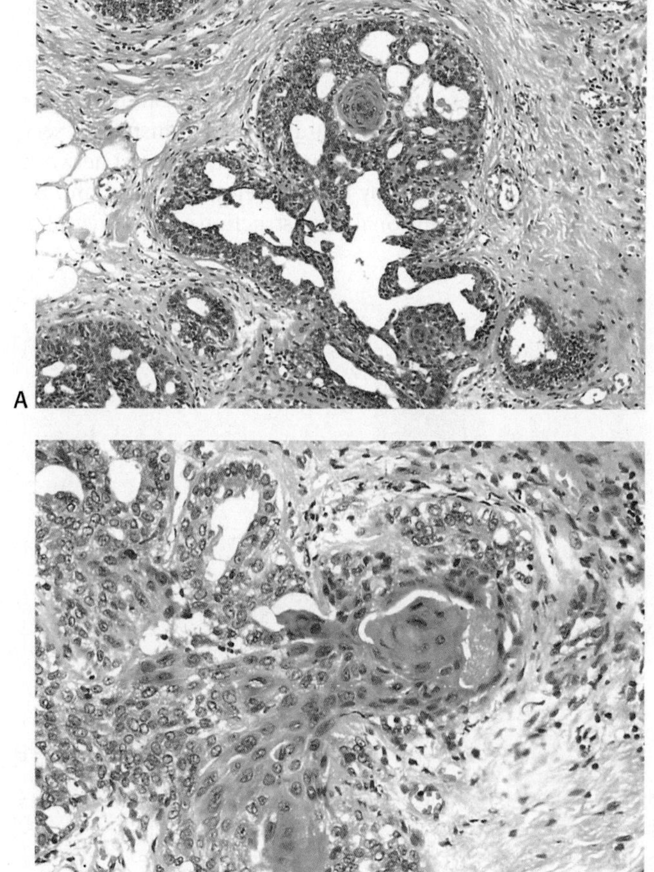

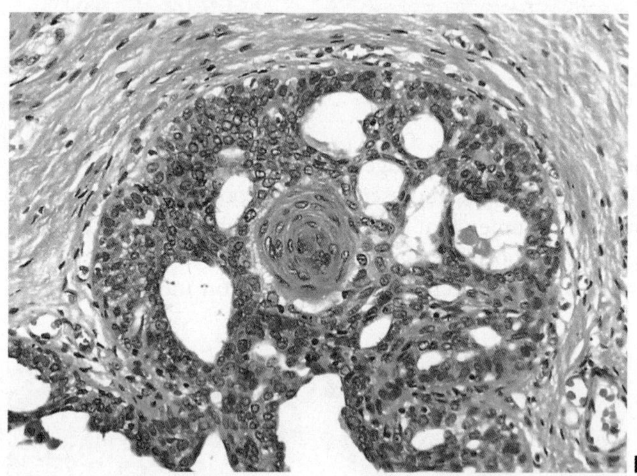

FIG. 9.8. ***Moderate ductal hyperplasia with squamous metaplasia.*** **A,B:** A discrete nodule of metaplastic squamous cells in fenestrated moderate hyperplasia. **C:** Squamous metaplasia blends with the hyperplastic ductal epithelium.

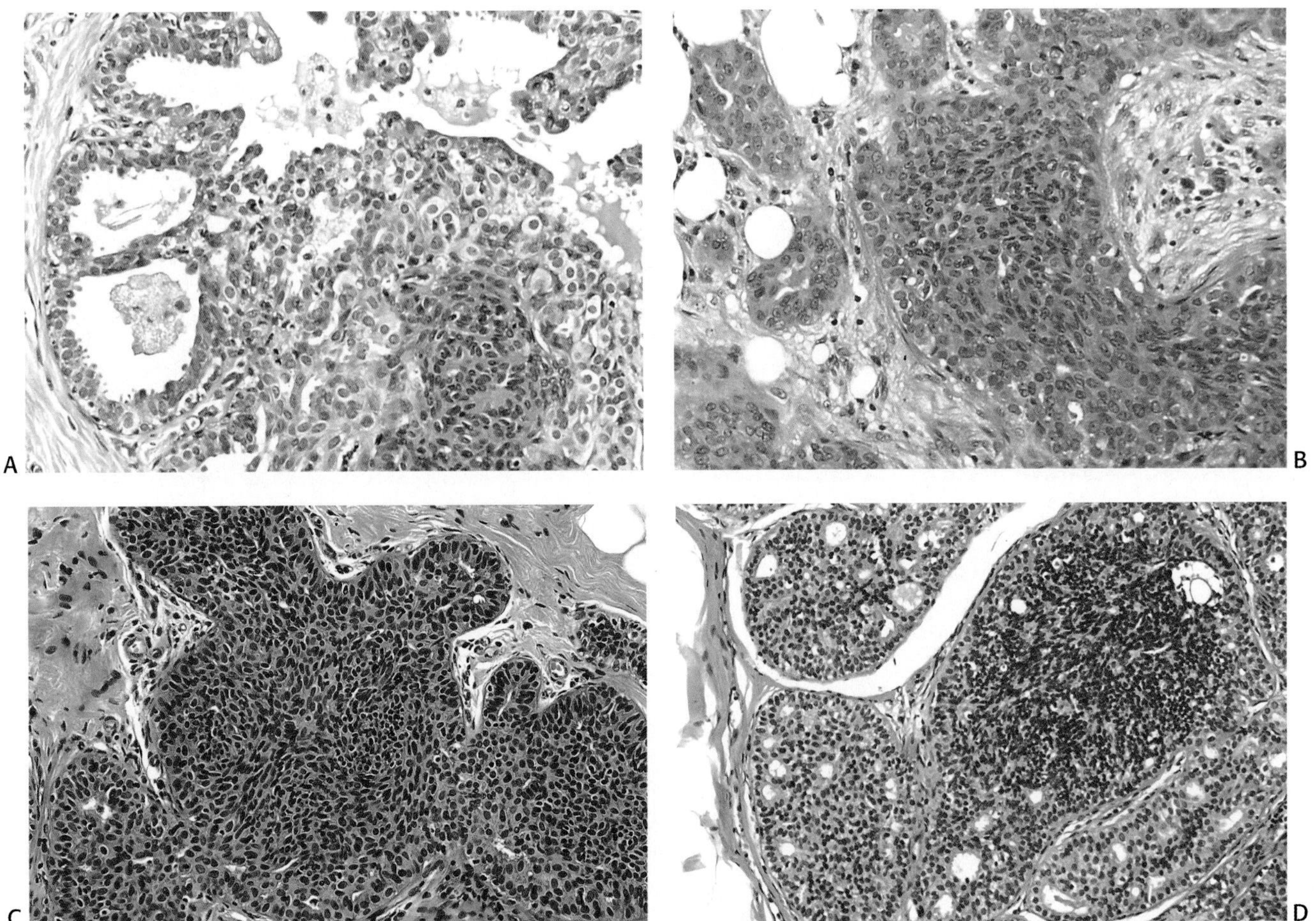

FIG. 9.9. ***Ductal hyperplasia, "streaming."*** **A:** Moderate hyperplasia with a dense area [*lower right*] in which hyperplastic cells have spindle-shaped nuclei in a swirling pattern. **B:** Hyperplastic cells that appear to be "streaming" in the long axis of the duct. **C:** A florid example of streaming with a storiform pattern. **D:** Pronounced streaming in florid hyperplasia. Note overlapping, hyperchromatic nuclei in the central part of the duct.

The spaces formed in intraductal hyperplasia usually appear to be devoid of cells and secretion. Occasionally, there may be histiocytes or lymphocytes present, sometimes with wisps of secretion. Calcification in the form of coarse granular concretions, calcospherites (calcification admixed with proteinaceous secretion), or crystalline deposits are uncommon in UDH unless there is an associated sclerosing component such as adenosis or a radial scar configuration. Columnar cell hyperplastic lesions are an exception to this generalization, since they are prone to form multifocal calcifications with distinctive histologic characteristics as described in subsequent text.

It is usually difficult to detect myoepithelial cells in ductal hyperplasia, except for the layer of these cells that is present at the edge of the duct. Myoepithelial cells may accompany the proliferation into the duct lumen when the fibrovascular stromal framework of solid papillary hyperplasia is present. Immunostains are useful for highlighting the myoepithelium in proliferative ductal lesions. The reactivity of individual myoepithelial markers is unpredictable in a given case, and it is advantageous to employ at least three markers.

p63, a member of the p53 family that is important in the development of epithelial tissues, is the only marker currently available that is localized exclusively in the nuclei of myoepithelial cells. It is not reactive with myofibroblasts or blood vessels.[42] p63 is rarely reactive with scattered epithelial cell nuclei in papillary lesions and ductal hyperplasia. These epithelial cells can be distinguished from myoepithelial cells by their cytologic appearance or their position. Nuclear staining of myoepithelial cells typically produces a string of dots between the epithelium in ducts and lobules and the basement membrane.

Several cytoplasmic markers are available for highlighting the myoepithelium: smooth muscle actin (SMA), smooth muscle myosin-heavy chain (SMM-HC), calponin, CD10, CK5, CK14, and maspin. These markers exhibit variable cross-reactivity with epithelial cells, myofibroblasts, or blood vessels.[43,44] Myofibroblastic reactivity is greatest with SMA or calponin and least with SMM-HC and CD10 (common acute lymphoblastic leukemia antigen [CALLA]).

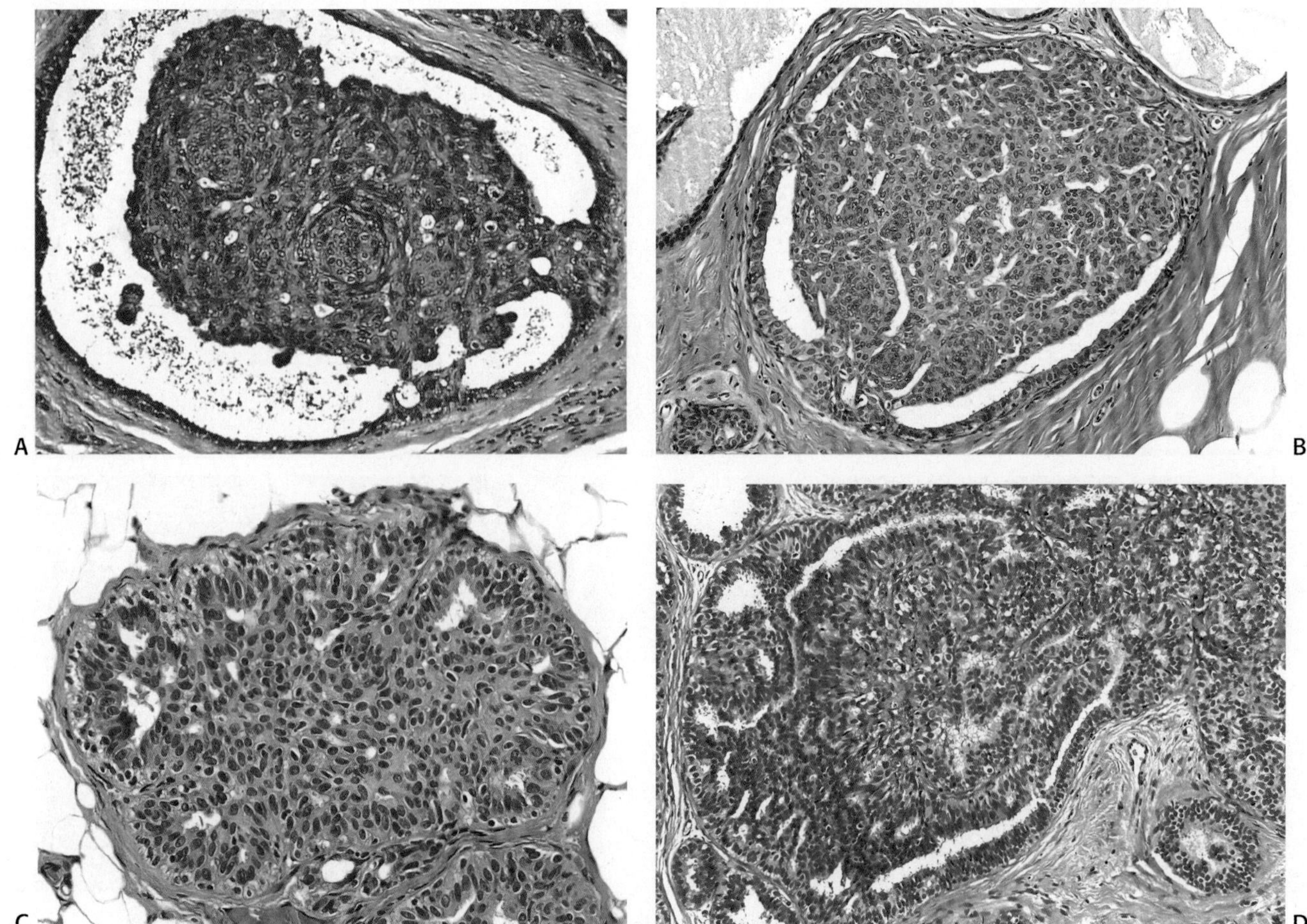

FIG. 9.10. ***Ductal hyperplasia.*** **A:** Polypoid ductal hyperplasia connected to the peripheral duct epithelium at only two points. Note swirling and streaming of the hyperplastic epithelium. **B:** Solid mass of hyperplastic epithelium with several peripheral connections. **C:** Persisting cuboidal ductal cells define the outer borders of slits that remain between points at which the florid hyperplastic epithelium is in contact with the perimeter of the duct. **D:** Peripheral slits remain at only part of the circumference of this duct with papillary hyperplasia.

However, many exceptions can be encountered. For this reason, as well as the variable reactivity of these reagents with myoepithelial cells, it is prudent to employ two or more cytoplasmic markers as well as p63 to evaluate the myoepithelium in a given case.

Myoepithelium is highlighted with immunostains in normal ducts and lobules. When proliferative fibrocystic changes occur in these structures, such as adenosis or ductal hyperplasia, the myoepithelium is usually uniformly present and it may be hyperplastic. Attenuation of myoepithelial cells, which occurs in some hyperplasias, especially sclerosing papillary lesions and ductal hyperplasia with atypia, results in increased space between p63 reactive nuclei compared with the staining pattern in normal structures. In this situation, the presence of the attenuated myoepithelium can usually be demonstrated with one of the cytoplasmic markers for these cells. Because of the stromal proliferation that accompanies many of these lesions, care must be taken not to mistake myofibroblastic reactivity for myoepithelium. Myoepithelium persists, admixed with the neoplastic epithelial proliferation, in some examples of DCIS, where it is usually attenuated. On the other hand, a pronounced degree of intraductal proliferation devoid of myoepithelium that is confirmed with immunostains, in the presence of internal positive controls, is very likely to be *in situ* carcinoma.

Collagenous spherulosis is an unusual finding in ductal hyperplasia and LCIS. In this condition, myoepithelial cells contribute to the formation of spherules of basement membrane material akin to those found in adenoid cystic carcinoma. The center of the spherule can become degenerated, so that it resembles a glandular lumen. Immunostains will demonstrate myoepithelial cells around spherules and distinguish these structures from coexisting true glandular lumina in cribriform hyperplasia and from the lumina

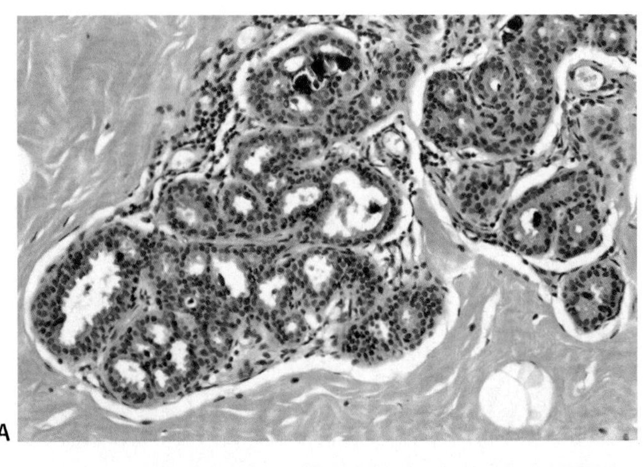
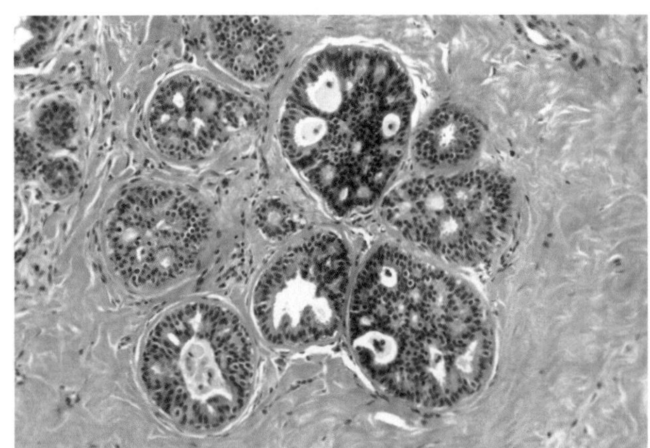
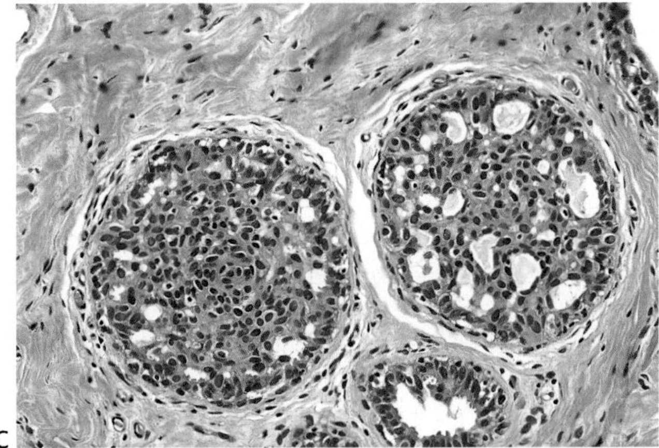

FIG. 9.11. ***Ductal hyperplasia, cribriform.*** **A:** Mild cribriform hyperplasia with calcifications. **B:** Moderate cribriform hyperplasia with peripheral microlumens. Note basal orientation of cells at perimeter of ducts. **C:** Fenestrations are distributed mainly at the periphery of these ducts. Note the swirling pattern in the center of the duct on the *left*.

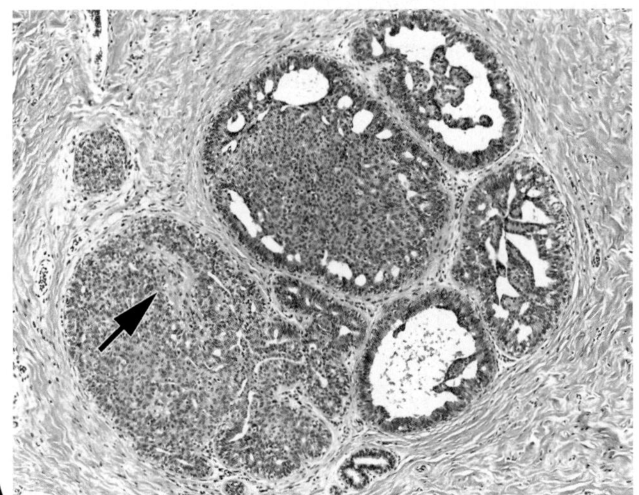
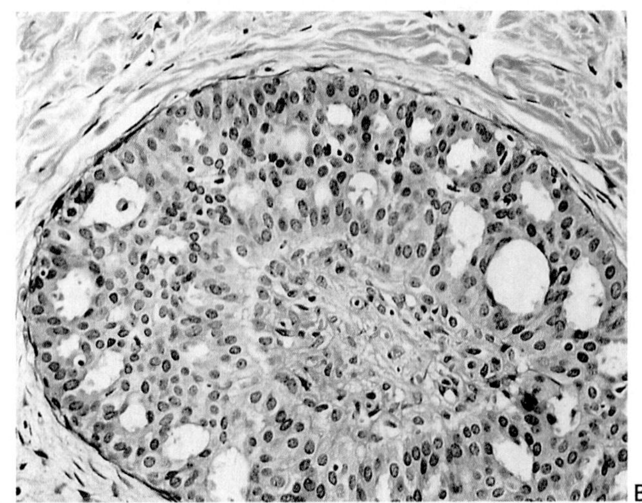

FIG. 9.12. ***Ductal hyperplasia, florid.*** **A:** Columnar ductal epithelium outlines crescentic spaces in glands with florid hyperplasia. A fibrovascular core (*arrow*) is evident in a gland with papillary hyperplasia. **B:** Two rows of fenestrations, one at the periphery and the second centrally, are present around a fibrovascular core.

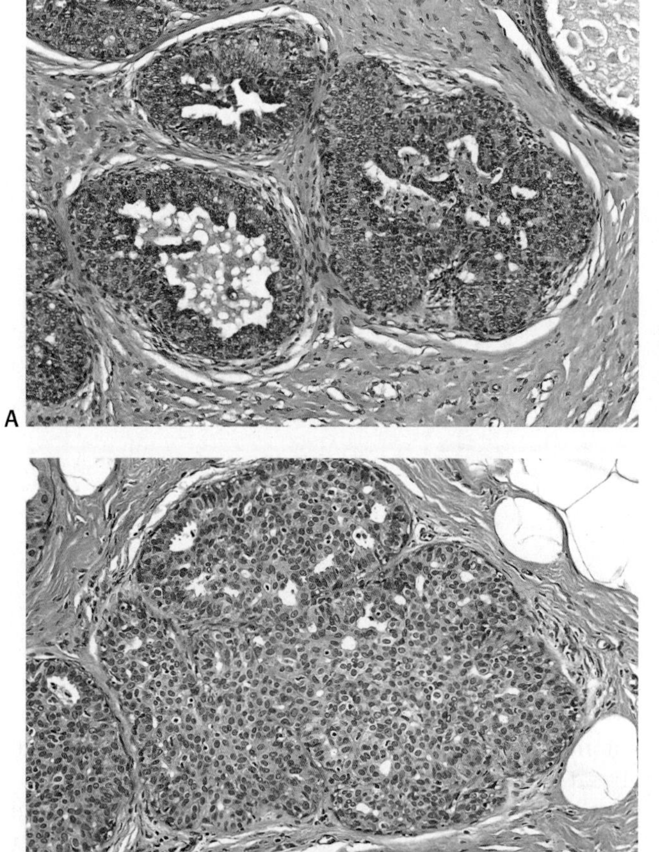

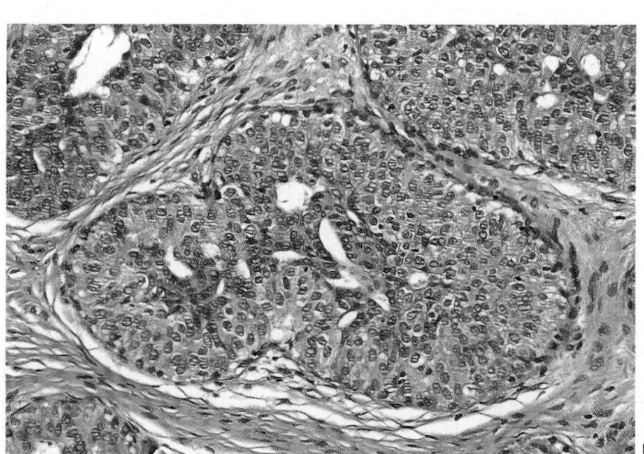

FIG. 9.13. ***Ductal hyperplasia, florid.*** **A:** Moderate hyperplasia. The duct on the *right* borders on florid hyperplasia. It has luminal histiocytes. **B:** Florid hyperplasia in which preexisting ductal epithelium outlines crescentic central spaces. **C:** Florid hyperplasia with a substantial solid component.

in cribriform DCIS. CD117 (c-kit) can be helpful in distinguishing collagenous spherulosis from adenoid cystic carcinoma. The epithelial components of collagenous spherulosis are ER (+), progesterone receptor (PR) (+), and CD117 (−), whereas its myoepithelial component is reactive for p63, CD10, myosin, etc.[45]

MICROSCOPIC PATHOLOGY OF ATYPICAL DUCTAL HYPERPLASIA

There is broad agreement on the general description of ADH as a proliferative lesion that fulfills some but not all criteria for a diagnosis of DCIS. By extension, it can be stated that

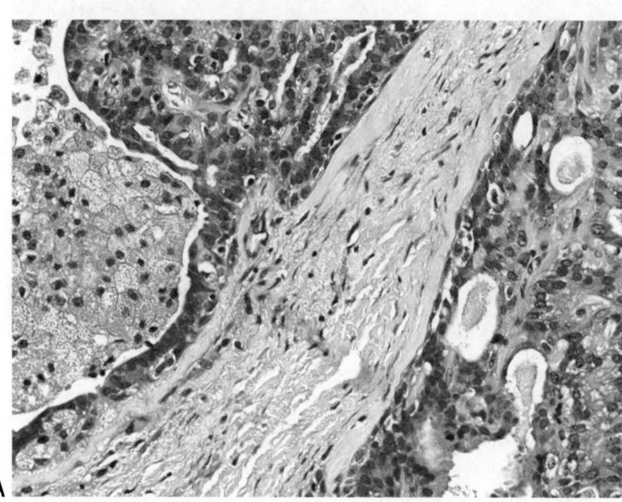

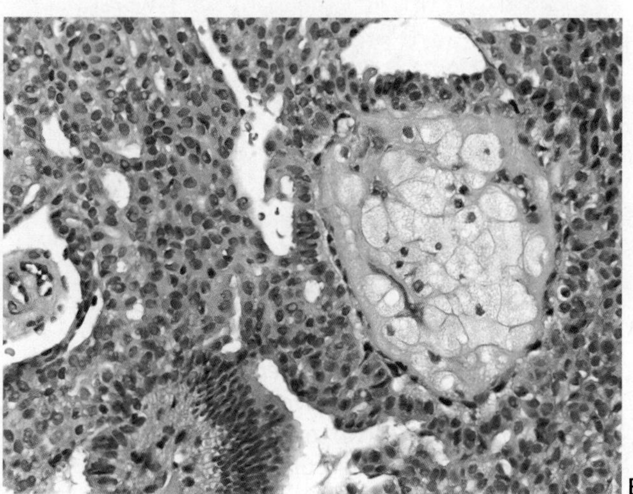

FIG. 9.14. ***Ductal hyperplasia, histiocytes.*** **A:** Aggregates of histiocytes in ductal hyperplasia. **B:** Histiocytes are present within fibrovascular cores in papillary hyperplasia.

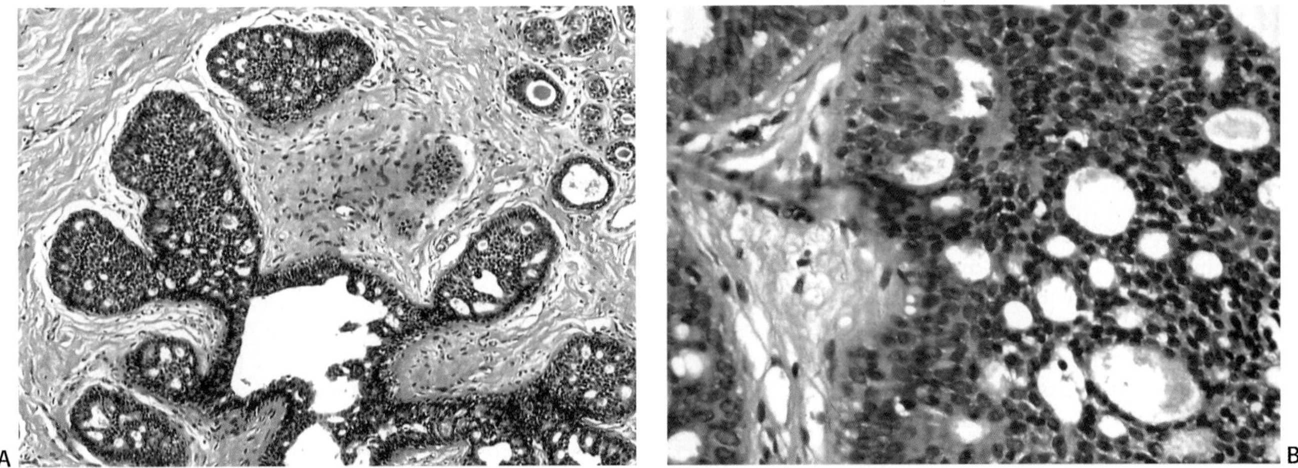

FIG. 9.15. ***Ductal hyperplasia, cribriform.*** **A:** Branches of a large duct showing fenestrated florid hyperplasia. **B:** Microlumens of varying sizes among cells with overlapping nuclei. There is no cellular orientation around the microlumens. Peripheral ductal epithelium has been cut tangentially along the left border of the large duct. Myoepithelial hyperplasia is evident in the *upper left corner*.

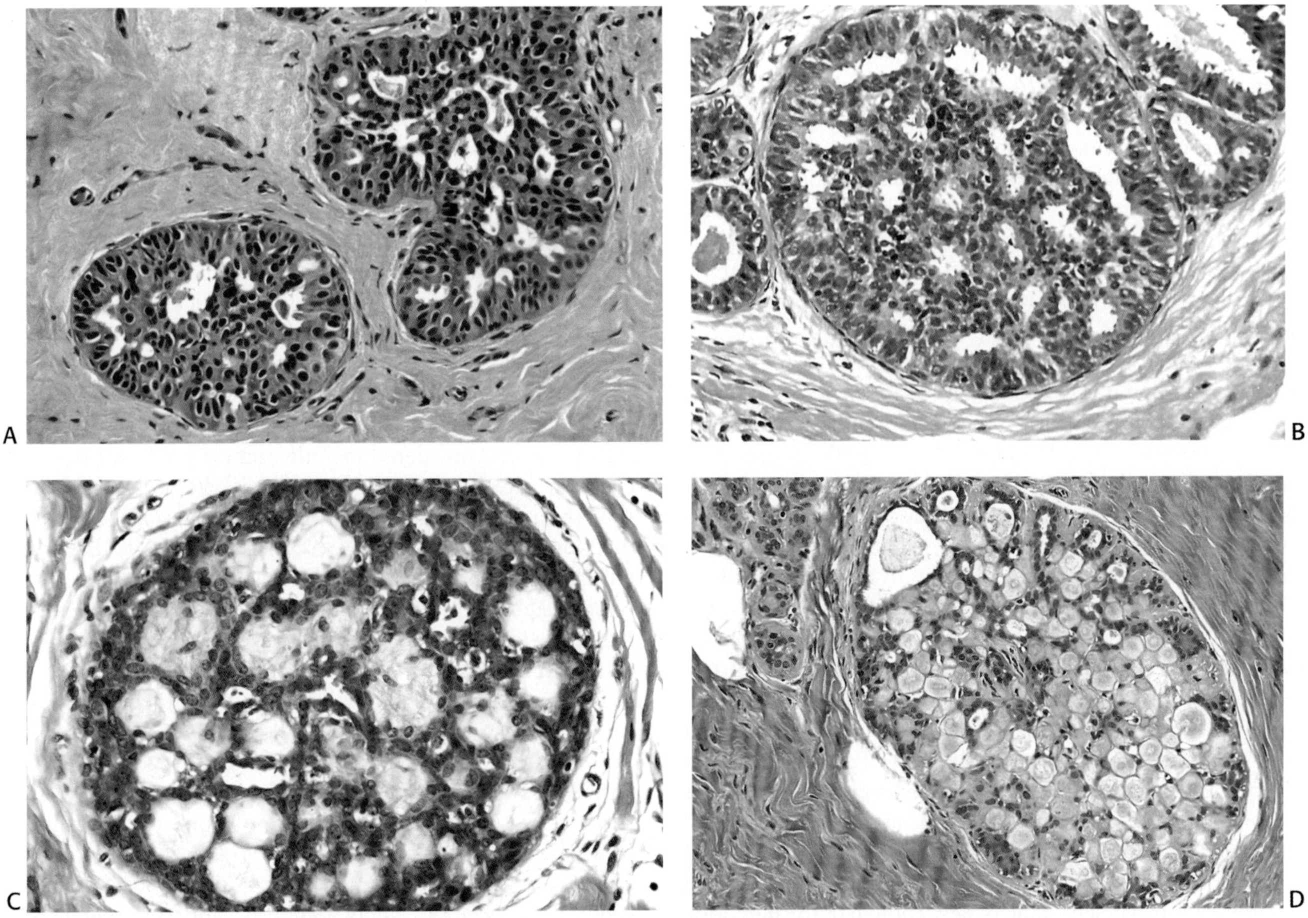

FIG. 9.16. ***Ductal hyperplasia, cribriform.*** **A,B:** Epithelial tufting produces fuzzy edges around microlumens with various shapes at the periphery and in the center of the duct. **C:** Cribriform hyperplasia with collagenous spherulosis such as this may be mistaken for cribriform type of intraductal carcinoma. **D:** Exuberant collagenous spherulosis masks the underlying process of cribriform hyperplasia.

ADH has features of ordinary hyperplasia and of DCIS. The difficulty in arriving at a crisper definition lies in the specifics. In general, these can be considered under two headings: quantitative and qualitative. The former refers to the amount of a proliferative abnormality, whereas the latter is concerned with microscopic structural and cytologic details.

Quantitative Aspects of ADH

Ductal hyperplasia has been distinguished from DCIS on the basis of various quantitative criteria. One of these is the number of duct cross sections that exhibit the abnormality. Others have concentrated on the dimension of the affected area. Some investigators have classified as ADH, proliferative lesions limited to a single duct even if the abnormality is qualitatively consistent with DCIS.[25] This scheme requires at least two fully involved duct cross sections to make a diagnosis of DCIS, and arbitrarily assigns cases with one duct that has the qualitative features of DCIS to the category of atypical hyperplasia.

Tavassoli and Norris[46] emphasized the concept of microscopic dimensions as a fundamental criterion for a diagnosis of ADH. They chose to classify foci measuring less than 2 mm as ADH, regardless of the number of affected duct cross sections, even if the individual ducts qualified as DCIS. The authors stated that they arrived at the 2-mm criterion because "it was at the level of one or more small ducts or ductules measuring around 2 mm in aggregate cross-sectional diameter that most pathologists felt hesitant in diagnosing a lesion as intraductal carcinoma."[47] Elsewhere, Tavassoli and Norris[46] commented that "questions about quantity are raised generally when dispersed lesions add up to from 1.6 to 2.7 mm in aggregate size. Therefore, we arbitrarily chose 2 mm as a cut-off point."

The foregoing quantitative criteria are arbitrary and lack biologic validation. There is no *a priori* reason for choosing two duct cross sections or 2 mm as critical decision points in relation to cancer risk. No published scientific studies have compared the clinical significance of different quantitative criteria. For example, no data exist for the risk to develop subsequent invasive carcinoma in patients whose biopsies contained proliferative lesions qualitatively consistent with DCIS limited to one, two, or three duct cross sections. Regarding the dimensions of the lesion, no analysis comparing foci measuring 1.5, 2.0, 2.5 mm, or larger has been reported.

Technical issues hamper the application of quantitative criteria. What appear to be two contiguous cross sections may prove in serial sections to be part of a single duct, or deeper sections of a single duct lesion may uncover more involved duct cross sections. How close to each other must two duct cross sections be to qualify as contiguous? Quantitative criteria assume that the ducts in question have been sectioned transversely, that is perpendicular to their long axis. Assessing ducts cut longitudinally has not been adequately considered. For example, if the longitudinal dimension of a duct in a section exceeds 2 mm, but the transverse diameter is 1 mm, should this focus be considered DCIS when employing the 2-mm criterion? How is the "aggregate size" of "dispersed lesions" determined to fulfill the 2-mm criterion?

Despite an imaginative effort to address some of these issues through the elaboration of an increasingly complex classification scheme for "DIN," a scientific basis for quantitative criteria remains elusive.[48] In an era of evolving studies that can assess the molecular alterations in the proliferative epithelium of single ducts or even subsets of cells in these structures, the concept of using the size of a proliferative lesion in a histologic section as a fundamental diagnostic criterion is likely to become less meaningful, but lesional size will remain a consideration in therapeutic decision making.

Others have rejected quantitative factors in the diagnosis of ADH. This position was elaborated by Fisher et al.,[49] who stated that "our definition of ADH consists of a ductal epithelial alteration approximating but not unequivocally satisfying the criteria for a diagnosis of DCIS. It does not include arbitrarily established quantities of unequivocal DCIS (less than 2.0 mm or 2 'spaces')." In their study of the prognostic significance of proliferative breast "disease," Bodian et al.[24] reported that ".during the course of many years, DCIS has been diagnosed if the characteristic features are present in only one ductal space."

The role of quantitative factors in the diagnosis of proliferative ductal lesions seems to lie between these extremes. The use of rigid criteria such as two duct cross sections or 2 mm can be justified in a research setting to ensure a homogeneous study group or to assess a particular criterion, but the strict application of these arbitrary rules in a clinical setting is difficult for technical reasons and poorly substantiated by existing data. Nonetheless, given the limitations of current methods for diagnosing intraductal lesions, lesional size is sometimes taken into consideration along with other features in assessing a particular lesion.

Qualitative Aspects of ADH

Other aspects considered include nuclear grade, mitotic activity, architectural structure, the presence of necrosis, and the appearance of associated proliferative lesions. Atypia is diagnosed if a pattern of growth consistent with DCIS is present in part of one duct structure in association with otherwise usual hyperplastic changes. If a carcinoma-like element is more widespread in a duct or partially involves multiple ducts in this or other foci, severe atypia is diagnosed.

A diagnosis of ADH depends upon the presence of structural or cytologic features of DCIS mingling with hyperplasia. Architecturally this may be manifested by a cribriform pattern partially involving a duct (Figs. 9.17 to 9.19). These foci feature sharply defined, round to ovoid spaces outlined by cells with distinct borders and a rigid arrangement. ADH can have a solid growth pattern (Figs. 9.20 to 9.22), and the process can occur in ducts exhibiting apocrine metaplasia (Figs. 9.23 to 9.25).

Cytologic atypia may involve individual cells, focal groups of cells, or the entire population of a proliferative lesion. Atypical features include nuclear enlargement resulting in an increased nuclear-to-cytoplasmic ratio, nuclear hyperchromasia,

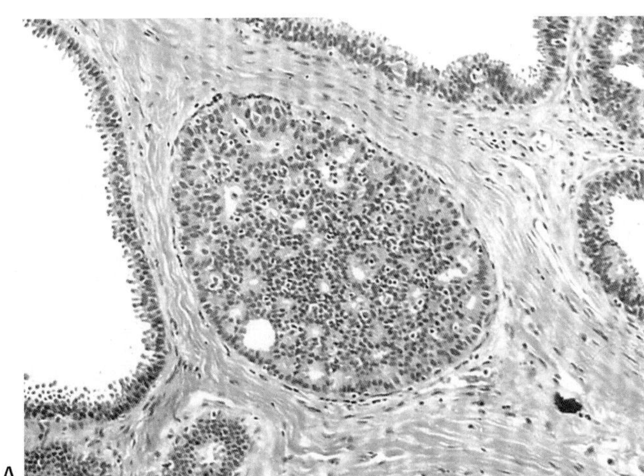

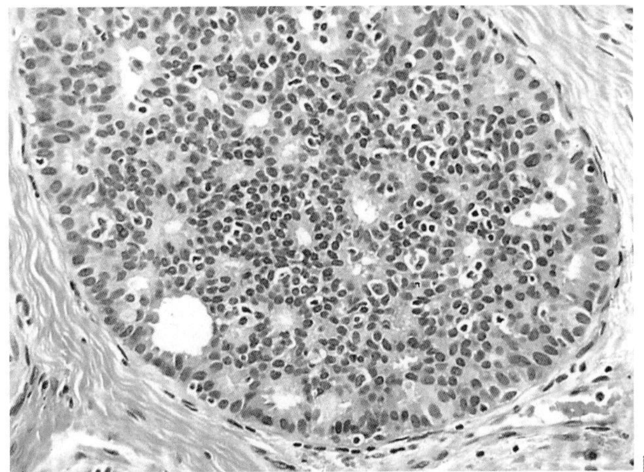

FIG. 9.17. ***Atypical ductal hyperplasia.*** **A:** Cystic CCC and mild CCH are evident in dilated ducts around a focus of atypical cribriform ductal hyperplasia. Stromal calcification is present (*lower right*). **B:** Magnified view of (**A**) showing residual ductal epithelium consisting of low columnar cells with regular basally oriented nuclei around much of the duct circumference. Focally, the epithelium in the duct is composed of cells with relatively abundant cytoplasm that are oriented radially around microlumens most of which are round. The center of the duct contains cells with sparse cytoplasm and small condensed nuclei. Cells tend to be polarized around the microlumens.

an irregular chromatin pattern, or enlarged and pleomorphic nucleoli. Atypical cells may have distinct cell borders, a feature that is especially noticeable when these cells occur singly or in small groups in an otherwise typical hyperplastic focus.

Mitotic activity is exceedingly low in hyperplasia of the usual type. The presence of readily identified mitotic figures is an atypical feature. Prosser et al.[50] reported that the proliferative index of hyperplastic lesions was greater than that in normal breast when measured by MIB-1 immunoreactivity, whereas an apoptotic index determined by the terminal uridine deoxynucleotidyl transferase dUTP nick end labelling (TUNEL) assay tended to be lower in proliferative lesions.

Intracytoplasmic lumina containing mucinous secretion, typically associated with lobular carcinoma in the form of signet ring cells, may also occur in DCIS cells.[51] A minute dot of secretion is often evident in hematoxylin and eosin (H&E)-stained sections in these tiny, sharply defined cytoplasmic lumens. Intracytoplasmic mucin vacuoles can be found in the cells of nonapocrine and apocrine types of DCIS and in papillary and nonpapillary DCIS. The mucinous secretion is highlighted with the Alcian blue and mucicarmine stains. Intracytoplasmic mucin is only rarely present in the cells of ductal hyperplasia. The finding of cells with this feature should be regarded as indicative of an atypical lesion or DCIS depending upon the overall appearance of the proliferation.

COLUMNAR CELL LESIONS AS A FORM OF DUCTAL HYPERPLASIA

Proliferative lesions of the ductal–lobular complex termed "ductal hyperplasia" by Azzopardi[52] have become the subject of closer scrutiny as a result of the widespread use of needle core biopsy to sample mammographically detected lesions with calcifications. These abnormalities are now recognized as being part of a spectrum of lesions described by the terms *columnar cell change* (CCC) and *columnar cell hyperplasia* (CCH).[32,33] Other names that have been offered include atypical cystic lobules,[53] cancerization of lobules and ADH adjacent to DCIS,[54] and columnar alteration with prominent apical snouts and secretion or columnar alteration with prominent apical snouts and secretions (CAPSS).[55] Another group of terms such as flat epithelial atypia and flat DIN has also been used to describe columnar cell lesions.

CCH was described previously as *pretubular hyperplasia*.[56] This name was derived from the observation that patients with tubular carcinoma of the breast often had foci of these lesions distributed in surrounding tissue or sometimes even merging with the carcinomatous lesions. This association suggested that tubular carcinoma might sometimes arise when the hyperplastic lesions transformed to DCIS; hence the term *pretubular hyperplasia*. LCIS is sometimes present.[32]

The adjective pretubular is no longer appropriate for several reasons. Foremost is the growing frequency with which these lesions are being encountered in needle core and surgical biopsy specimens obtained for microcalcifications. In this circumstance, the ductal lesion itself prompts the procedure. Although we should be aware of the possibility of coincidental tubular carcinoma, it is not demonstrated in most of these women, and the risk of subsequent tubular carcinoma is poorly documented.

Unfortunately, none of these names fully describes the microscopic spectrum of the abnormalities. Some foci consist largely of cuboidal or columnar cells, others are

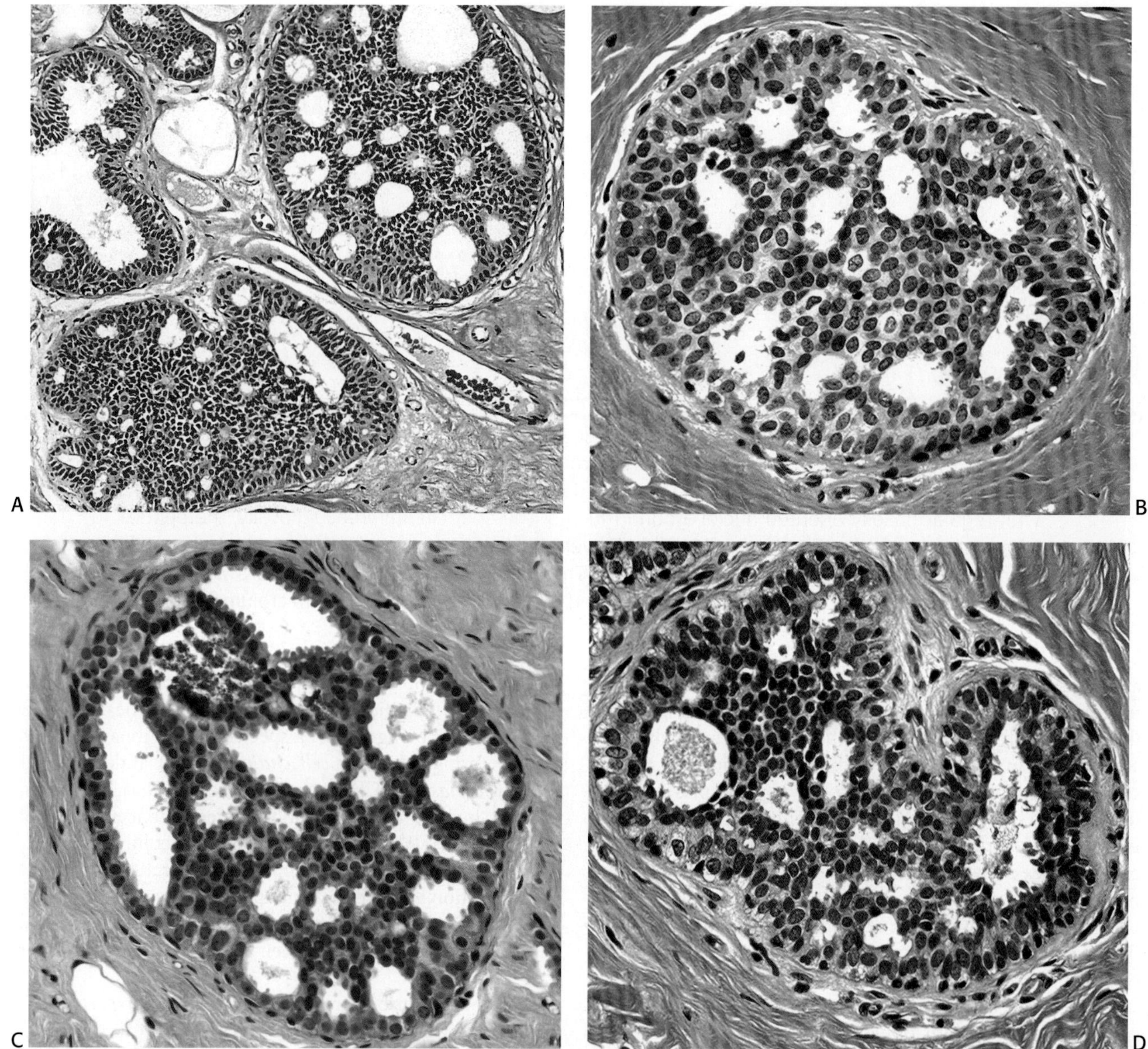

FIG. 9.18. *Atypical ductal hyperplasia.* A–D: The proliferation has a cribriform growth pattern in which microlumens are relatively round. Nuclei are smaller centrally than at the periphery and central nuclei are hyperchromatic. Microlumens are typically nonuniform and are larger at the periphery.

composed of flat cells, and many are comprised of flat, cuboidal, and columnar cells.[57,58] The word "flat" is also used in this context to refer to the flat luminal surface of the epithelium. However, the fact that the epithelium may have mounds and even small papillae renders this an inaccurate term. Finding no advantage in any of the various alternatives, this volume continues to refer to columnar cell lesions as was done in prior editions. In this context, the word "columnar" refers to the usual shape of nonproliferative ductal epithelial cells.

Clinical Presentation of Columnar Cell Hyperplasia

Lubelsky et al.[56] reported that 21% of needle core biopsy specimens obtained for calcifications from mammographically screened women had columnar cell lesions. CCH is a multifocal process that may also be bilateral. It is most often encountered in women 35 to 50 years of age, but CCH can be present after the menopause. CCH rarely produces a palpable abnormality, and it is usually detected mammographically

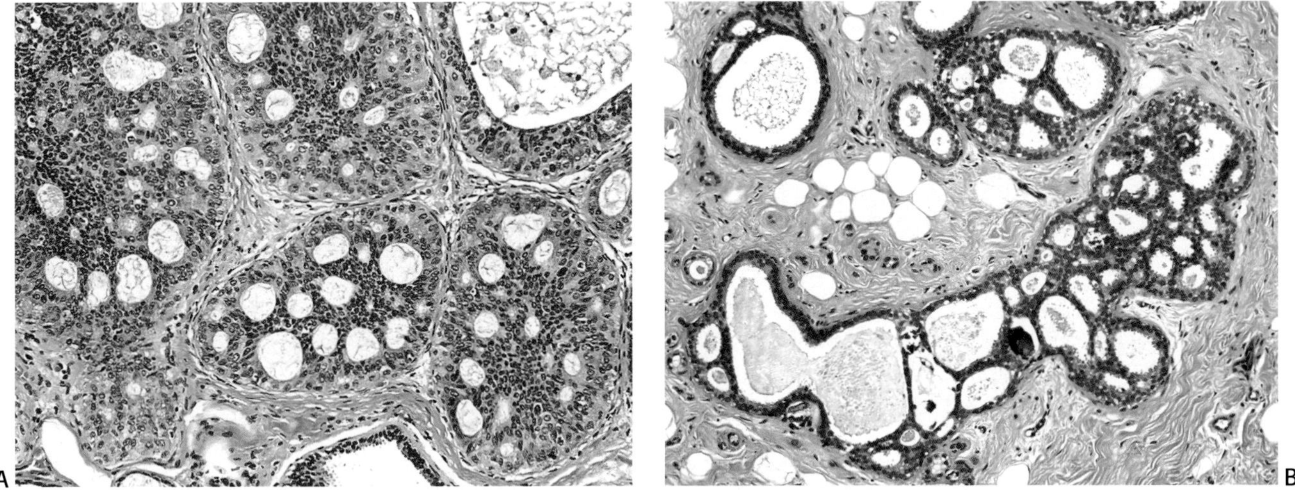

FIG. 9.19. ***Atypical ductal hyperplasia.*** **A:** Cribriform growth in multiple duct cross sections. The centers of the ducts consist of small, crowded cells with overlapping hyperchromatic nuclei. Hyperplastic cells at the periphery of ducts are largely not oriented with respect to the basement membrane. **B:** Polarity of peripheral ductal epithelium is maintained in this lesion, and a calcification is present.

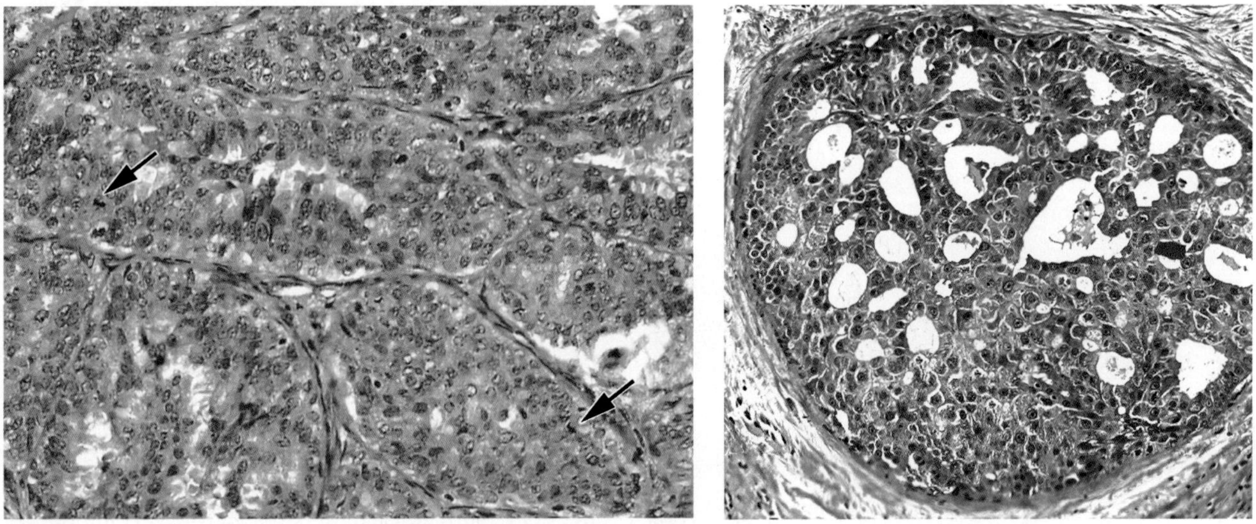

FIG. 9.20. ***Atypical ductal hyperplasia.*** **A:** Mitotic activity (*arrows*) and cellular pleomorphism are depicted. **B:** Irregularly shaped and sized microlumens and minimal cellular pleomorphism are evident. The changes could be considered to be borderline for intraductal carcinoma. **C:** Atypical hyperplasia with a crystalloid in a lobular ductule.

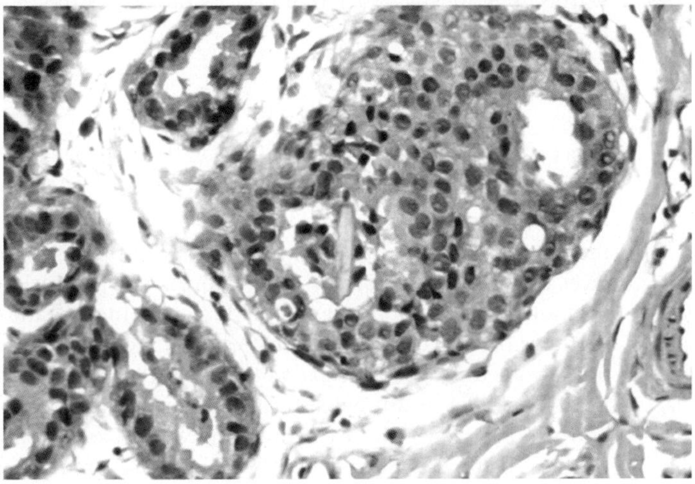

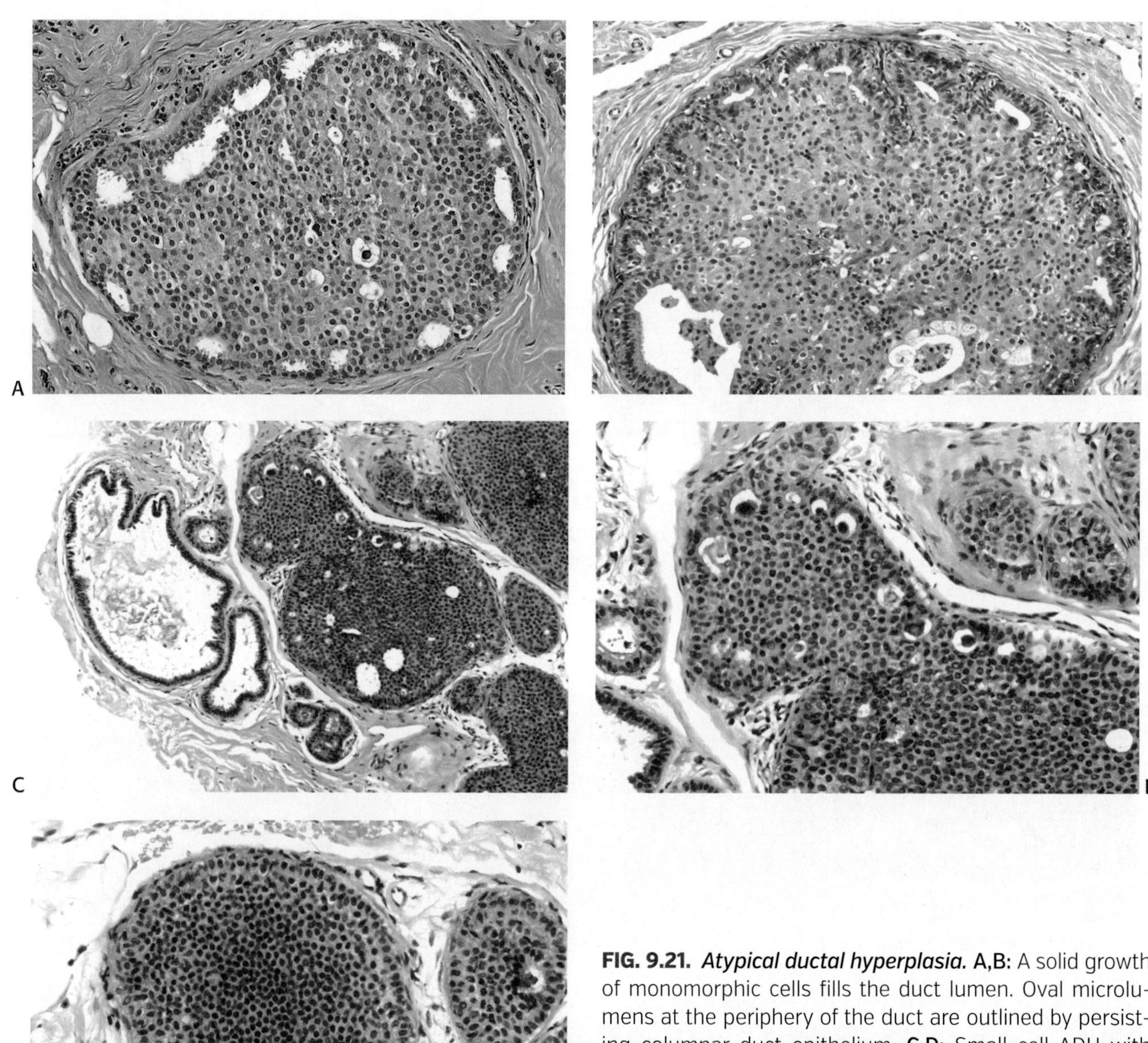

FIG. 9.21. ***Atypical ductal hyperplasia.*** **A,B:** A solid growth of monomorphic cells fills the duct lumen. Oval microlumens at the periphery of the duct are outlined by persisting columnar duct epithelium. **C,D:** Small cell ADH with peripheral, round microlumens that contain calcifications. **E:** Solid small cell ADH without microlumens. Persisting duct epithelium consists of cuboidal to low columnar cells with regular, basally positioned nuclei at the perimeter of the ducts.

because calcifications are frequently formed, becoming the target of needle core biopsy sampling. The fundamental lesion is localized in TDLUs, which become enlarged as a result of epithelial proliferation and cystic dilation.[59]

Microscopic Pathology of Columnar Cell Lesions

The simplest form of this process, *CCC*, features a thin, flat epithelial layer composed of predominantly cuboidal to tall columnar cells distributed in a uniform pattern in variably and irregularly dilated glands. Because the nuclei tend to be relatively large, the cells appear crowded and dark. The nuclei are oriented perpendicular to the underlying basement membrane and myoepithelial cells. The apical cell surfaces usually have apocrine-type cytoplasmic protrusions ("snouts"), and in some cases this is a prominent feature. In the most banal columnar cell lesion, CCC, the epithelium is one to two cells deep and there is little nuclear pleomorphism (Fig. 9.26). Nuclear chromatin is fine. Nucleoli and mitotic figures are exceedingly rare or absent. Calcification is infrequent and usually consists of amorphous

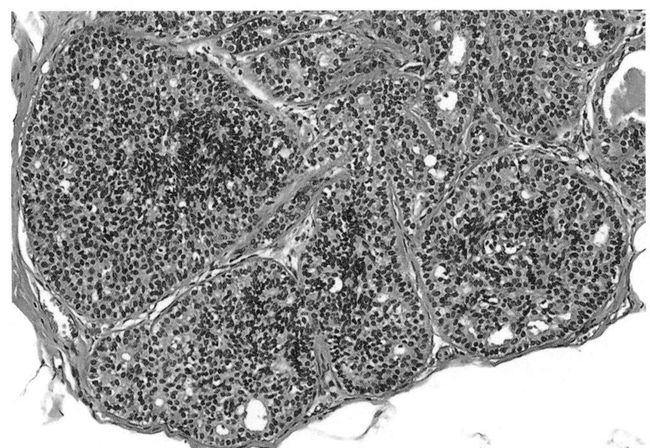

FIG. 9.22. ***Atypical ductal hyperplasia.*** These duct cross sections display variable amounts of growth consisting of nearly solid patches in which there are monomorphic small cells. Areas within the same ducts display streaming and cells with overlapping hyperchromatic nuclei.

granular material (Fig. 9.27). Discrete basophilic calcifications are less common in columnar cell. Myoepithelial cells are inconspicuous.

The cells often express gross cystic disease fluid protein-15 (GCDFP-15), an apocrine marker. They are also immunoreactive for Bcl-2 and ER protein that are typically absent in benign apocrine change.[60] Fine-needle aspiration specimens from columnar cell lesions yield "flat sheets of cells with enlarged nuclei, distinct cell borders, and finely granular cytoplasm."[61] The proliferative activity of columnar cell lesions has been evaluated in the form of Ki67 reactivity.[62] The Ki67 index was significantly lower in CCC (mean, 0.1%) and CCH without atypia (mean, 0.76%) than in normal TDLUs (mean, 2.4%). The Ki67 indices of CCH with flat atypia (mean, 8.2%) and low-grade DCIS (mean, 8.9%) were not significantly different. The highest Ki67 index was found in intermediate- to high-grade DCIS (mean, 25.4%).

Dabbs et al.[61] studied molecular changes in selected microdissected columnar cell lesions and found "a gradient of progressive mutational change" between CCC and invasive carcinoma arising in a background of columnar cell lesions. Mutational changes manifested as LOH at selected loci was absent from CCC and only rarely found in CCH. Increasing LOH was detected across the spectrum of atypical columnar cell hyperplasia (ACH), DCIS, and invasive carcinoma. These results parallel those obtained in noncolumnar cell proliferative duct lesions[63] and appear to support the concept that ADH may, in situations yet to be defined, be a precursor of DCIS and invasive duct carcinoma. The pattern of LOH also parallels the distribution of Ki67 proliferative indices in columnar cell lesions.

CCH is present when the epithelium is more than two cells thick. This is most readily apparent when cellular crowding becomes pronounced and nuclei are not distributed in a single plane relative to the basement membrane. The tendency to "stacking" of nuclei is usually accompanied by nuclear hyperchromasia, and small mounds of cells may be formed in the most cellular regions (Figs. 9.28 and 9.29). Cellular crowding and overlapping is common.

More complex columnar cell proliferative foci comprise lesions described as *ACH*. Mild atypia is usually manifested by the presence of small, and often isolated, foci of micropapillary growth in a background of otherwise usual CCH in dilated glands (Fig. 9.30). The presence of more elaborate growth patterns and cytologic atypia characterize ACH, which, in its most severe form, approaches the appearance of DCIS of the flat micropapillary ("clinging") type[64] (Figs. 9.31 to 9.33). Cytologic atypia is more pronounced than the structural abnormalities (Fig. 9.34), often requiring high-power magnification microscopic evaluation.[65,66] ACH often harbors calcifications.[67]

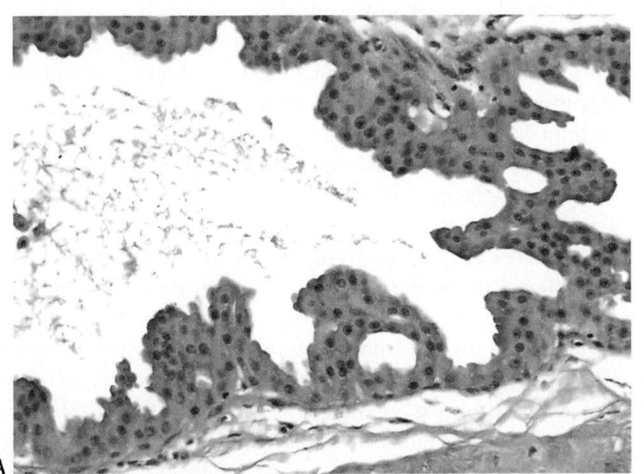

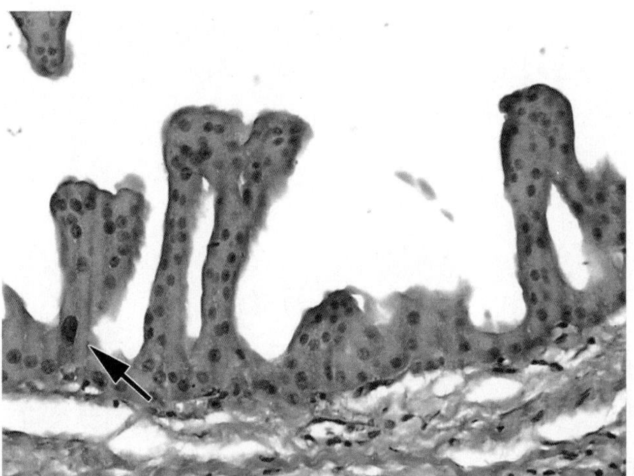

FIG. 9.23. ***Atypical ductal hyperplasia, apocrine.*** **A:** Blunt micropapillary structures composed of cells with small regular nuclei. Atypical features are the pattern and uneven distribution of nuclei. **B:** Elongated micropapillary structures. One large hyperchromatic nucleus is present (*arrow*).

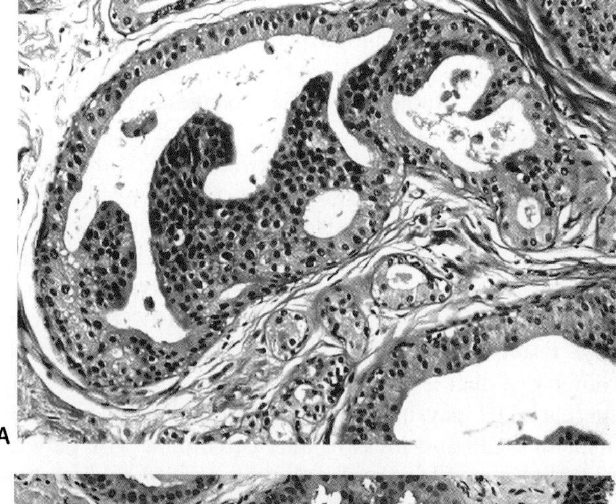

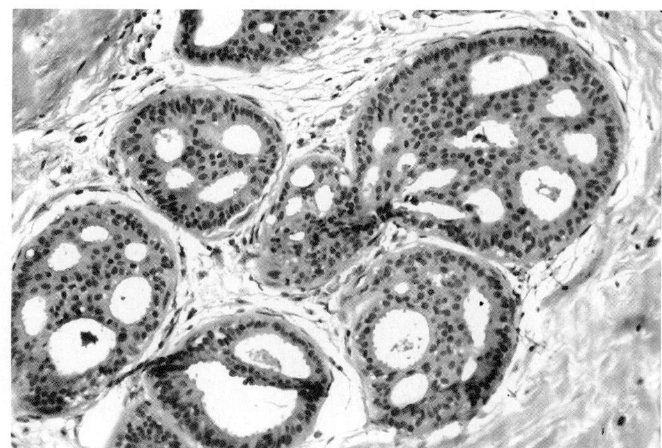

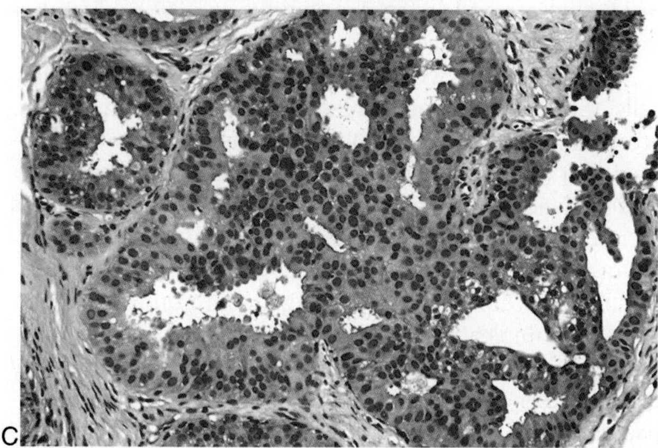

FIG. 9.24. ***Atypical ductal hyperplasia, apocrine.*** **A:** Micropapillary fronds arise from part of the circumference of a duct. The remainder of the duct is lined by regular cuboidal apocrine cells. **B,C:** Atypical cribriform apocrine duct hyperplasia. Note regular cuboidal apocrine cells at the perimeter of ducts.

The lesional cells of ACH are larger than CCC and CCH cells and are much more monotonous. The nuclear-to-cytoplasmic ratio is relatively higher. The nuclear membrane is irregular, chromatin is coarser, minute nucleoli are present, and mitotic figures may be found. ACH may show cellular pseudostratification, mild epithelial tufting with formation of cellular mounds, but neither true micropapillary nor cribriform structures are present.

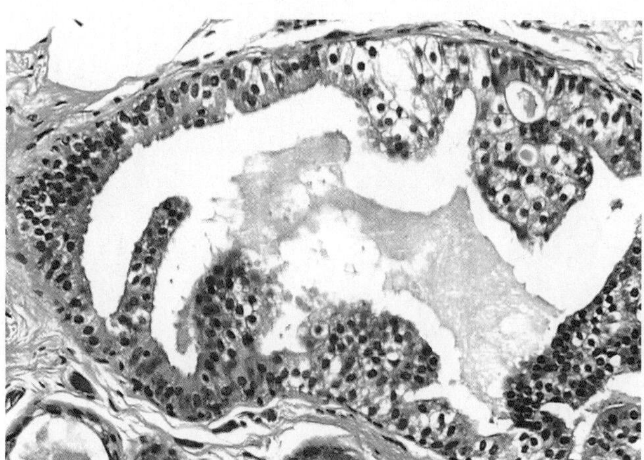

FIG. 9.25. ***Atypical apocrine type of ductal hyperplasia.*** Some cells exhibit cytoplasmic clearing, which is an atypical feature in apocrine epithelium.

When carcinoma arises in CCH, it usually has one of the growth patterns characteristic of DCIS (Figs. 9.35 and 9.36). Rarely, so-called flat micropapillary DCIS with relatively little epithelial complexity is encountered (Fig. 9.37). Atypical lobular hyperplasia (ALH) and LCIS frequently accompany columnar cell abnormalities, and tubular carcinoma may also be present (Fig. 9.38) (see Chapter 13). Hence, columnar cell lesions are part of a triad that includes lobular neoplasia and tubular carcinoma, termed "Rosen Triad."[32,68]

O'Malley et al.[69] reported a high level of interobserver consistency in the diagnosis and classification of columnar cell lesions. The study employed eight pathologists who reviewed a series of images of columnar cell lesions to be classified as atypical or not atypical. Overall agreement on this distinction was 91.8% (95% CI, 84.0% to 96.9%). Tan et al.[70] found a high level of agreement on distinguishing between columnar cell lesions and DCIS, but only moderate agreement on distinguishing between lesions with and without atypia. The lowest level of agreement related to

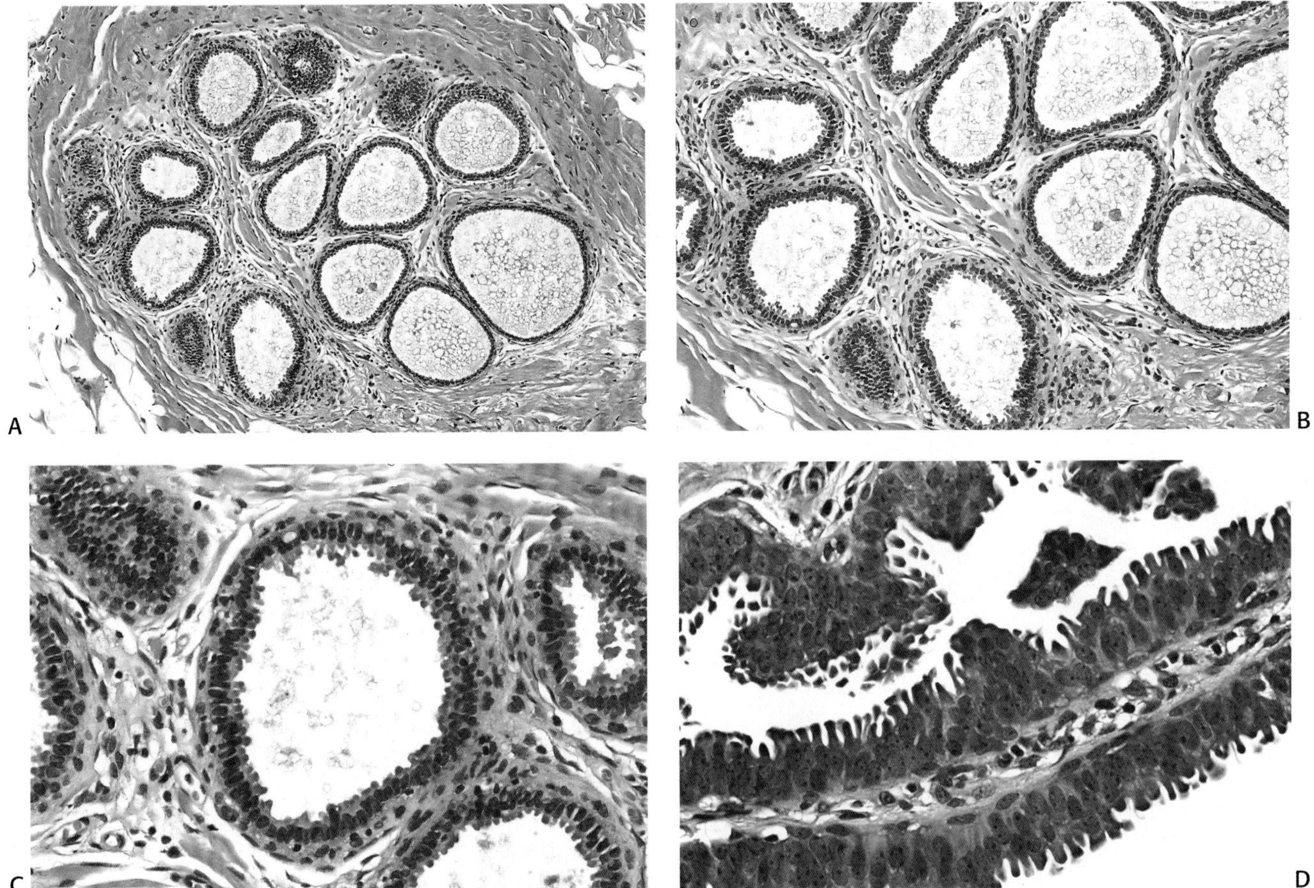

FIG. 9.26. ***Columnar cell change.*** **A,B:** Cystic dilation of lobular ductules that are lined by cuboidal and columnar cells characterized by closely approximated, basally oriented nuclei and luminal cytoplasmic "snouts." The structures are encircled by relatively loose, vascularized stroma. **C,D:** A magnified view of the crowded epithelium, indistinct myoepithelium, and surrounding stroma.

the presence of cytologic atypia in columnar cell lesions. The latter finding underscores the importance of examining columnar cell lesions at intermediate or high magnification because cytologic atypia may be inapparent at low magnification.

Calcifications in Columnar Cell Lesions

Columnar cell lesions develop calcifications in many of the proliferative sites. Two types of calcification are encountered: *crystalline* and *ossifying*. The crystalline type, usually associated with lesions with less atypia, is deeply basophilic, opaque, round, or angular and is prone to fragmentation in the process of histologic sectioning (Figs. 9.27, 9.31 to 9.33, and 9.35). The ossifying type of calcification usually has a rounded, well-defined contour and an internal structure that resembles an ossifying nodule. Within the nodule that has an eosinophilic matrix, basophilic granular calcific deposits are embedded in lacunar-like spaces (Figs. 9.31, 9.35, and 9.39). Ossifying-type calcifications occur throughout the range of CCHs, and they appear to develop in proliferative epithelium, whereas basophilic crystalline deposits are predominantly intraluminal. Both types of calcification can be found in one specimen, and they may occur together in a single proliferative focus. The finding of ossifying-type calcifications is an indication of proliferative activity in CCH, and if they are present in a needle core biopsy specimen, excisional biopsy of the lesional area would be prudent.

Clinical Management of Columnar Cell Lesions

Excisional biopsy is generally recommended when a needle core biopsy specimen contains ACH or if a columnar cell lesion is associated with LCIS or ALH. Guerra-Wallace et al.[71] evaluated patients who underwent surgical excision after a columnar cell lesion was detected in a needle core biopsy specimen. They reported finding carcinoma in 10 of 135 women (7.4%) with CCH without atypia and in 11 of 60 (18.3%) with coexisting atypical hyperplasia. DCIS associated with CCH

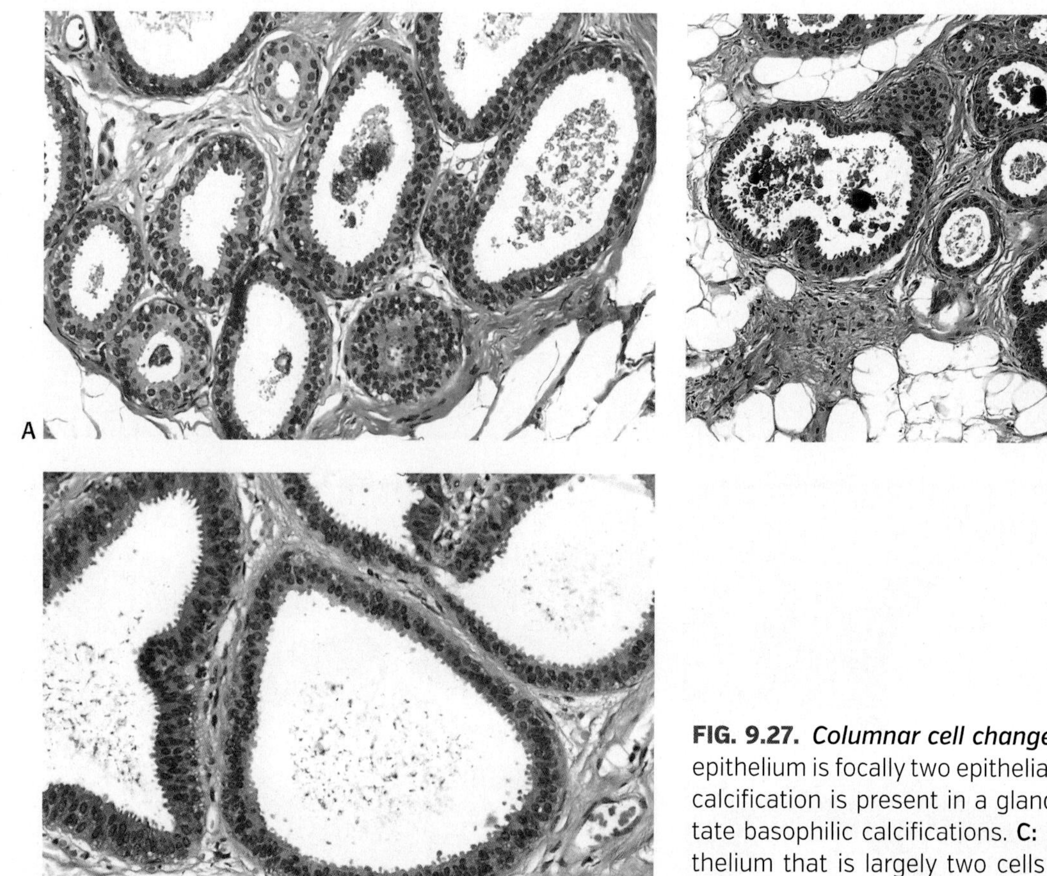

FIG. 9.27. ***Columnar cell change.*** **A:** In this instance, the epithelium is focally two epithelial cells deep, and granular calcification is present in a gland. **B:** Granular and punctate basophilic calcifications. **C:** Nuclear crowding in epithelium that is largely two cells deep. A small epithelial mound is shown in the gland on the *left*.

and ACH tends to have low nuclear grade, micropapillary and cribriform architecture, and lack necrosis.[65] ACH is significantly related to LCIS or ALH,[72] and as stated earlier, it has been associated with invasive lobular carcinoma[73] as well as tubular carcinoma.[32,73–75] There are no studies that have specifically investigated the long-term follow-up of women with ACH.[59] LOH and comparative genomic hybridization assays have demonstrated certain commonality in patterns of genetic alteration in ADH, low-grade DCIS, and invasive carcinoma in the same breast, suggesting that ADH may be a nonobligate precursor lesion. Frequent sites of LOH in ADH include chromosomes 16q, 17p, and 11q13 with losses at 16q

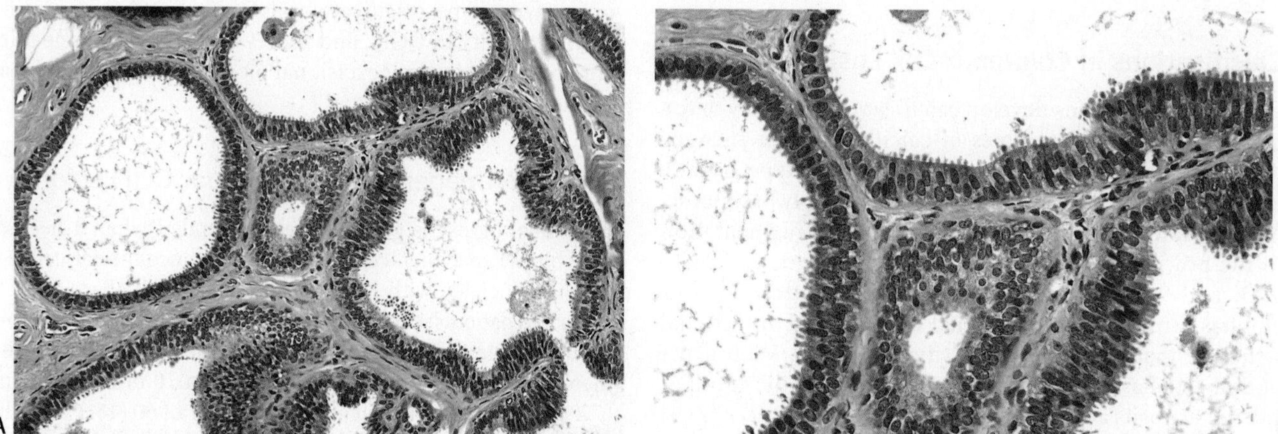

FIG. 9.28. ***Columnar cell hyperplasia.*** **A,B:** Plaque-like areas of epithelium in which overlapping nuclei of columnar cells are multiple cells deep. The myoepithelium is indistinct.

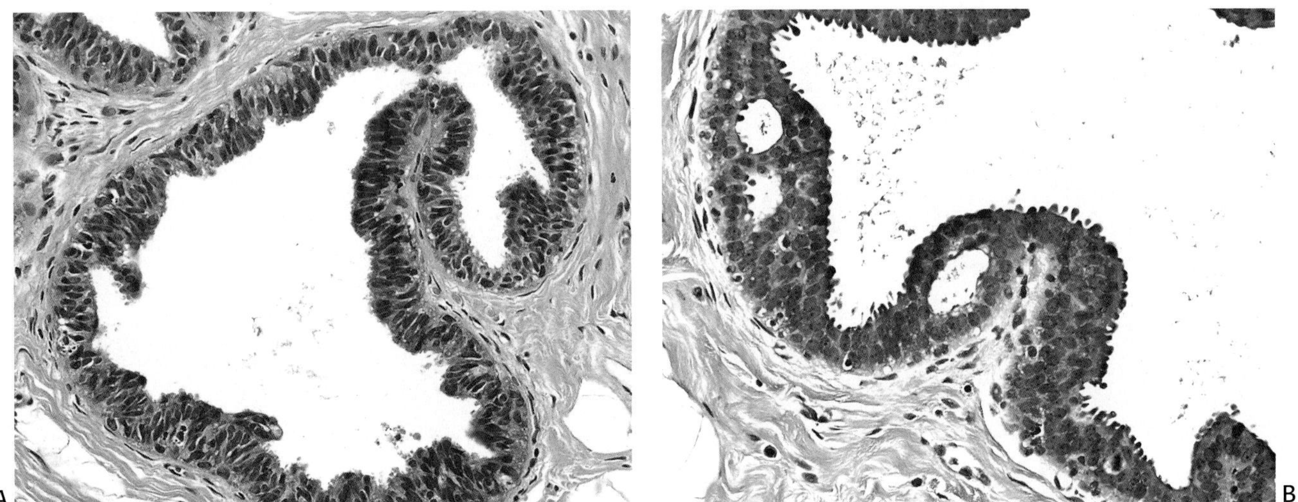

FIG. 9.29. ***Columnar cell hyperplasia.*** **A,B:** The thickened epithelium composed of crowded columnar cells forms small mounds. The myoepithelium is relatively inconspicuous. Note epithelial arches in **(B)**.

being particularly frequent and considered the "hallmark" feature.[76–79]

Immunohistochemistry of Columnar Cell Lesions

The full spectrum of columnar cell lesions is immunoreactive for low-molecular-weight cytokeratins (LMW-CKs) such as CK7 and CK19, and for the broad-spectrum cytokeratin AE1/3. These lesions are typically also strongly and diffusely positive for ER and PR but are negative for high-molecular-weight cytokeratins (HMW-CKs) such as CK5/6 and CK14.[80–82] Columnar cell epithelium is strongly E-cadherin positive and HER2 negative.

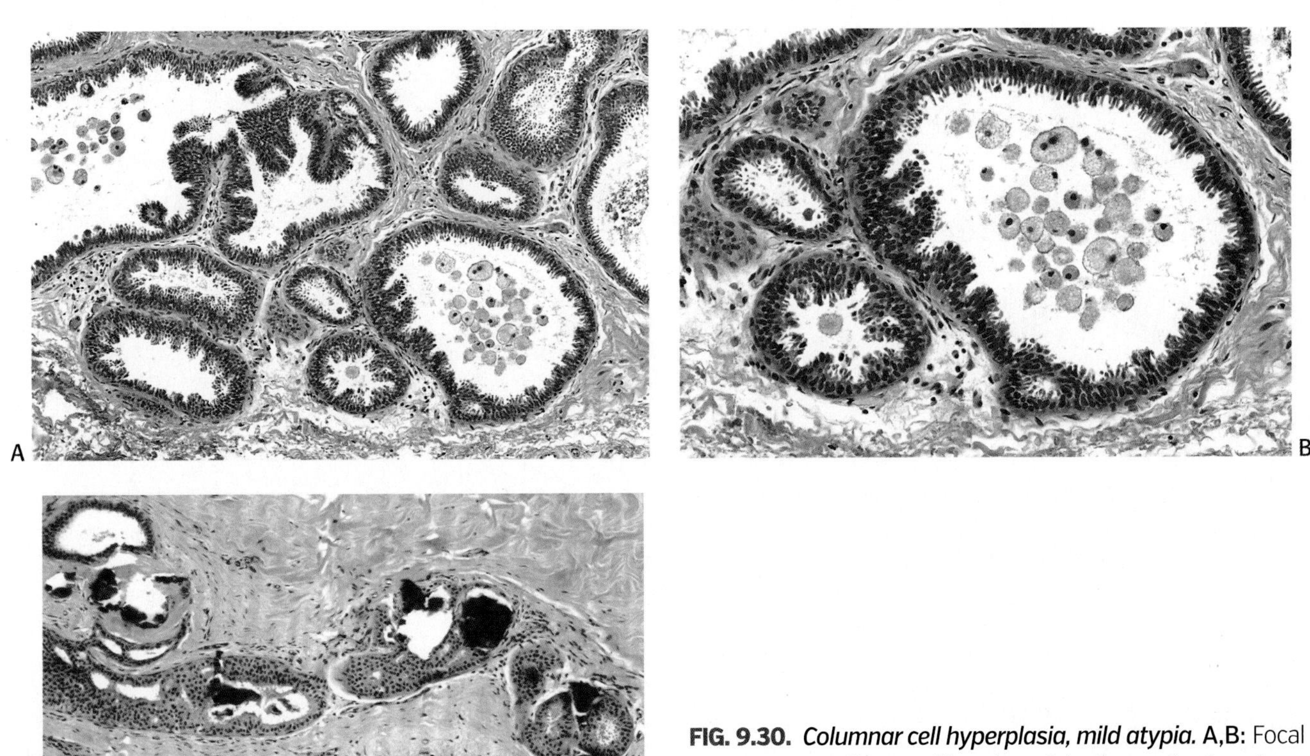

FIG. 9.30. ***Columnar cell hyperplasia, mild atypia.*** **A,B:** Focal blunt micropapillary proliferation of the hyperplastic columnar cell epithelium. Note the marked nuclear hyperchromasia and the high nuclear-to-cytoplasmic ratio. **C:** Mild atypical hyperplasia with large basophilic calcifications and one ossifying calcification (*below*).

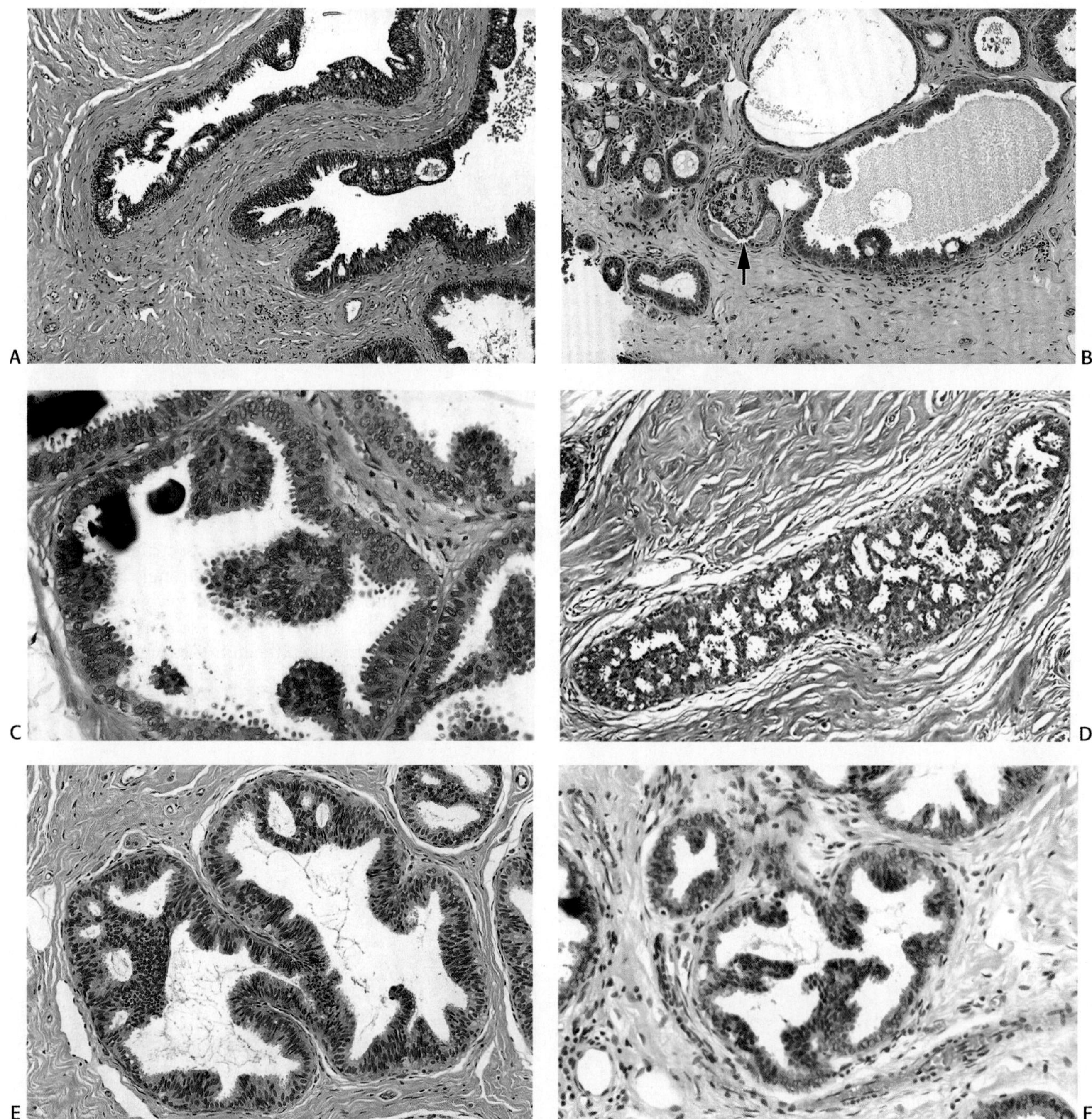

FIG. 9.31. ***Columnar cell hyperplasia, moderate atypia.*** **A–C:** Three examples of atypia with micropapillary architecture with atypia. An "ossifying" calcification (*arrow*) is shown in **(B)**, a section stained with hematoxylin-phloxine-saffranin. Dense basophilic calcifications are shown in **(C)**. **D,E:** Fenestrated atypical micropapillary hyperplasia. **F:** Note hyperchromatic cells at the apices of epithelial fronds in micropapillary hyperplasia.

BORDERLINE LESIONS

The most challenging atypical ductal proliferations, referred to as "borderline" lesions, are subject to varied interpretation because they feature very marked cytologic and architectural atypia (Figs. 9.40 to 9.42). Some of these relatively monomorphic foci retain a minor characteristic of hyperplasia. This would be exemplified by the presence of nuclear overlap, swirling, or streaming in an otherwise typical cribriform DCIS structure formed by rigid epithelial bridges. These slight variations will be disregarded by observers who classify such lesions as DCIS, whereas others may diagnose atypical hyperplasia. Similarly, those who place credence in quantitative criteria will diagnose ADH

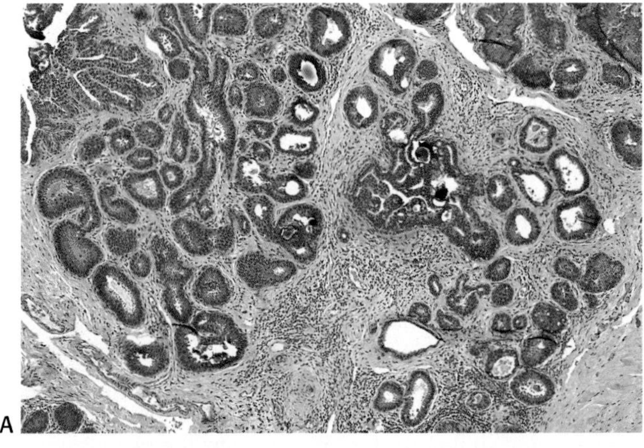

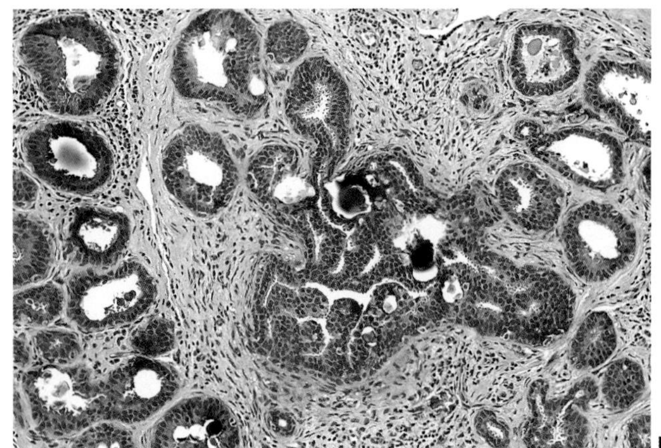

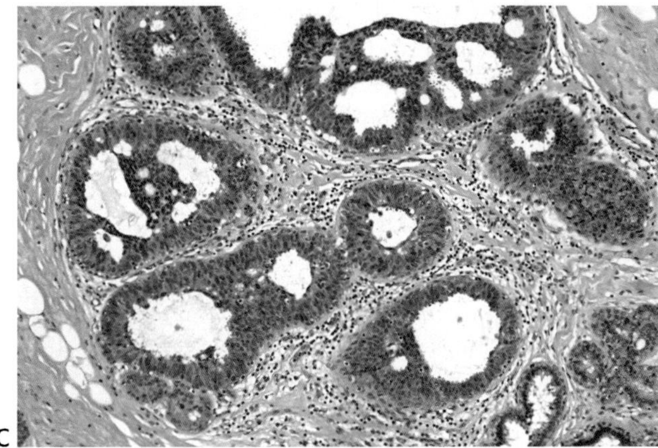

FIG. 9.32. ***Columnar cell hyperplasia, severe atypia.*** **A:** At low magnification, the lesion consists of confluent lobular units with a central focus of papillary proliferation. **B:** The severely atypical epithelium is composed of monomorphic cells uniformly distributed in the micropapillae. CCC is evident in surrounding glandular structures, and calcifications are present. **C:** Thickened epithelium with focal cribriform architecture.

because the extent of a lesion is not sufficient, but others not adhering to these arbitrary rules will diagnose DCIS in the same lesion.

Insufficient emphasis has been placed on diagnosing specific proliferative lesions in the context of the overall spectrum of histologic changes in a biopsy specimen. In a research setting, a pathologist can be required to make a diagnosis that is based only on a focus circled on a single slide or a selected photomicrograph.[2,18,82] This artificial setting, duplicated to some extent in assessing needle core biopsy specimens, is different from the circumstances under which the various diagnostic criteria were originally refined by

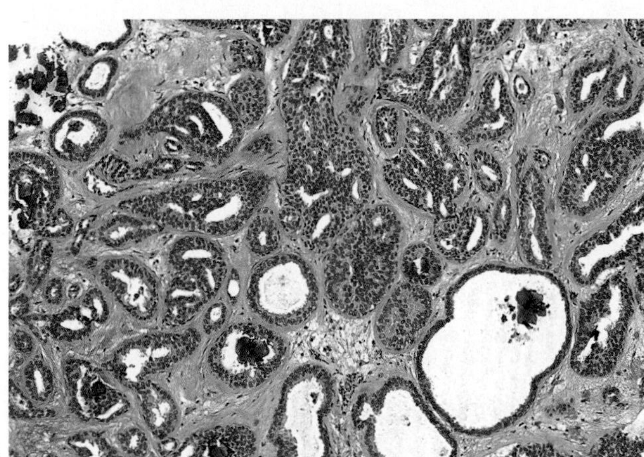

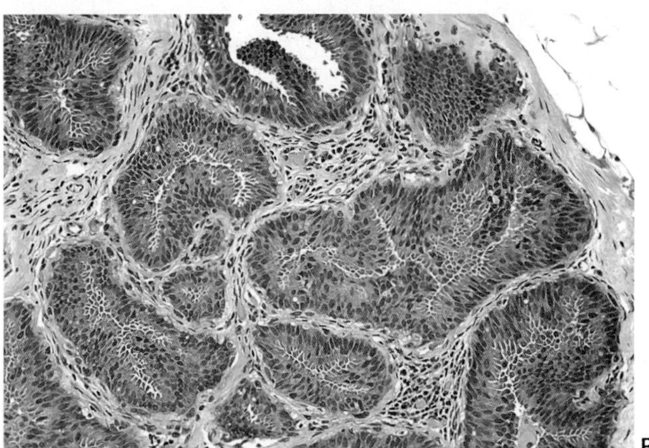

FIG. 9.33. ***Columnar cell hyperplasia, severe atypia.*** **A:** The cribriform growth is composed of monomorphic cells. Microlumens are oval and crescentic rather than round as in cribriform DCIS. CCC and calcifications are also evident. **B:** No mitotic activity is present in this columnar cell proliferation where atypical hyperplastic epithelium fills gland lumens.

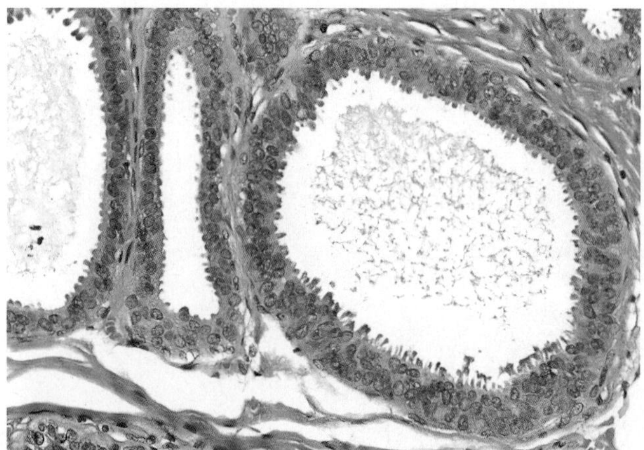

FIG. 9.34. *Columnar cell hyperplasia, mild cytological atypia.*

reviewing multiple histologic sections.[25,27] In clinical practice, the pathologist has an opportunity to examine a case extensively, including recourse to serial sections. Although Elston et al.[82] demonstrated that consistency in diagnosis did not significantly differ when interpretation was confined to specific images compared with assessment of the entire slide, the diagnosis of a "borderline" lesion is usually rendered on the basis of review of multiple slides, even in needle core biopsy material where multiple (at least three) histologic levels should be examined.

As a rule, it is helpful to prepare multiple sections ("recuts") of a tissue sample that contains a borderline focus of ductal proliferation in either needle core or excisional biopsy material. In most instances of DCIS, the lesion will persist, and it may either enlarge or exhibit features considered more readily diagnostic. Conversely, ADH can be diagnosed with greater confidence if the lesion is diminished or it remains unchanged in recut sections. In exceptional cases, features diagnostic of DCIS are present in very few or in only one of a series of sections of a problematic focus.

A review of slides from previous biopsies is often helpful, and should be routinely practiced, if they can be made available. The pathologist should attempt to assemble prior material if faced with a diagnostic problem, although the mobility of patients who are sometimes treated in multiple facilities sometimes makes this a difficult goal to achieve. Whenever possible, the diagnosis of "borderline" intraductal proliferations is best made in the context of the spectrum of pathologic changes present in current and prior specimens. A focus of concern may be found to be substantially more atypical and different qualitatively from the overall proliferative level in a given case, or it may prove to be part of a spectrum of changes lacking distinct histologic boundaries. The former situation would tend to support a diagnosis of DCIS in the lesional area, whereas the latter suggests ADH.

DIAGNOSIS OF ADH IN NEEDLE CORE BIOPSY SPECIMENS

The increasing use of mammography combined with needle core biopsy procedures is presenting pathologists with a growing number of small, limited tissue and cytologic samples from proliferative lesions to interpret. Given the diagnostic difficulties sometimes encountered when such lesions are examined in their entirety in histologic sections, it is not surprising that the fragmentary material obtained by needling procedures often presents a very challenging problem. ADH has been diagnosed in less than 10% of patients subjected to needle core biopsy.[21,22,83–86] In four studies consisting of 323 to 900 patients who underwent a

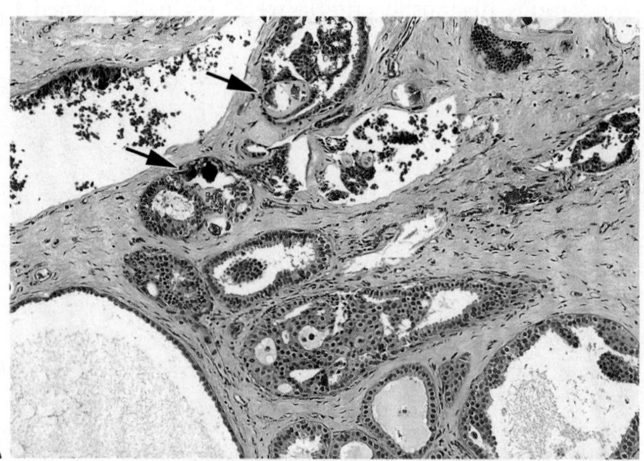

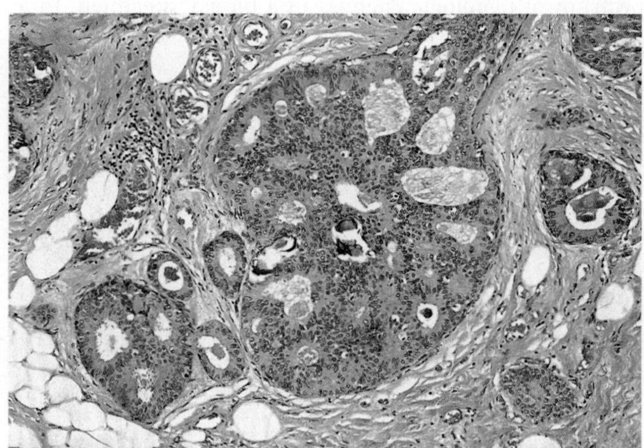

FIG. 9.35. ***Intraductal carcinoma associated with atypical columnar cell hyperplasia.*** **A:** This needle core biopsy specimen was obtained from a focus of nonpalpable mammographically detected calcifications. Basophilic and ossifying-type calcifications are present (*arrows*). Atypical hyperplasia with micropapillary and cribriform structure is apparent (hematoxylin-phloxine-saffranin). **B:** Cribriform intraductal carcinoma that was present in the excisional biopsy specimen obtained after the core biopsy specimen shown in **(A)**.

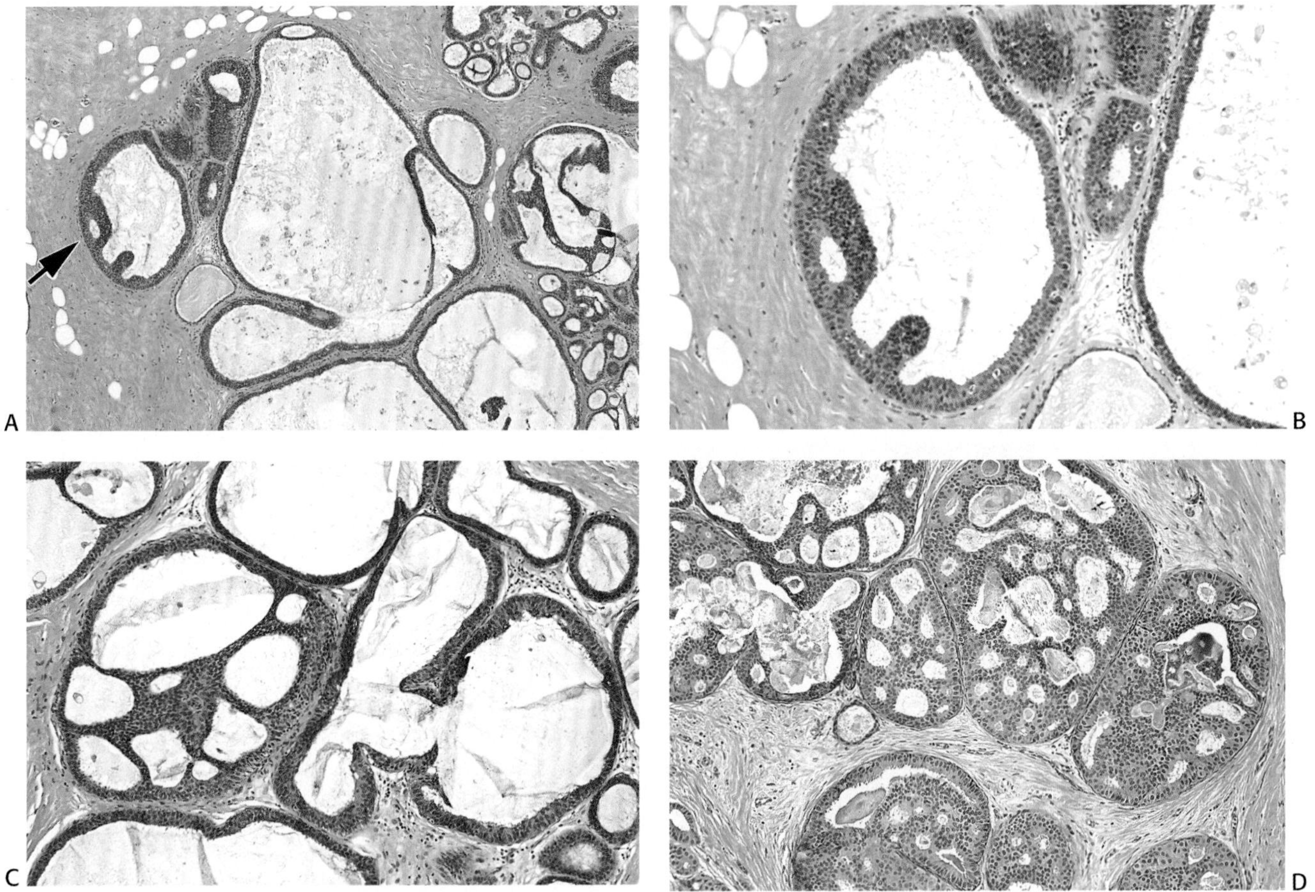

FIG. 9.36. ***Intraductal carcinoma associated with atypical columnar cell hyperplasia.*** **A:** Excisional biopsy revealed multifocal predominantly cystic CCH with focal atypia, shown here with micropapillary architecture (*arrow*). **B:** Magnified view of the atypical focus indicated by an *arrow* in (**A**). **C:** Four years later, repeat biopsy of the same breast performed for calcifications revealed hyperplasia with severe atypia. **D:** Also present in the biopsy shown in (**C**) was cribriform intraductal carcinoma illustrated here.

needle core biopsy of a mammographically detected lesion, the frequencies of ADH were 6.7%, 4.7%, 4.5%, and 4.3%.[87–90] Follow-up surgical biopsy was performed on most of the women with atypical hyperplasia in these reports. Among women who underwent a surgical biopsy, the reported frequencies of DCIS in the specimen were 27%, 12.5%, 33%, and 36%. Invasive carcinoma was found in 14%, 12.5%, 0%, and 11% of patients. In these reports, approximately 25% of surgical biopsies revealed additional foci of ADH. Multiple additional studies, from around the world, consistently display a high "upgrade" rate (18% to 31%).[91–93]

In a series of 74 patients who were diagnosed to have "marked" ADH on needle core biopsy and who underwent subsequent excision, 36 (48.6%) had either invasive or *in situ* carcinoma in the excision.[94] In this series, involvement of an intermediate-sized duct with marked degree of ADH on needle core biopsy and extent of the residual targeted lesion on imaging were significantly associated with finding carcinoma on excision. ADH involving columnar cell lesions and presence of calcification in the needle core biopsy specimen were not predictors of finding carcinoma on excision.

The yield of significant lesions in the excisional biopsy specimen may be somewhat lower after a needle core biopsy diagnosis of ADH if the entire radiologically detected lesion was removed by the core biopsy procedure.[95] The high frequency of carcinoma detected after a diagnosis of ADH in a needle core biopsy sample dictates that surgical excision should be performed promptly in this setting.[21,22]

The reported frequency of ADH in vacuum-assisted MRI-directed core biopsies ranges from 3% to 8%.[28–30] Among patients with ADH detected in vacuum-assisted core biopsy specimens who undergo surgical biopsy, the yield of carcinoma has averaged 34%.[30] The higher yield of subsequent carcinoma, sometimes termed "underestimation of ADH," found in MRI-detected lesions than in mammographically directed biopsies probably reflects the tendency to employ

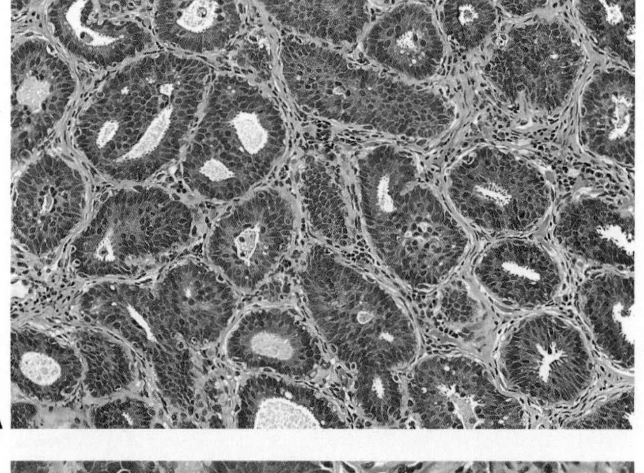
A

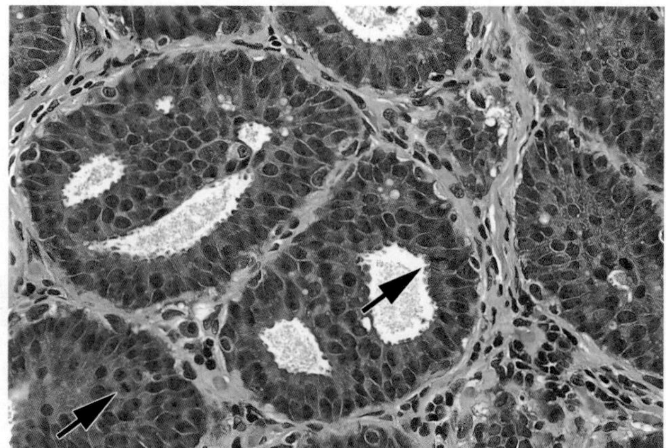
B

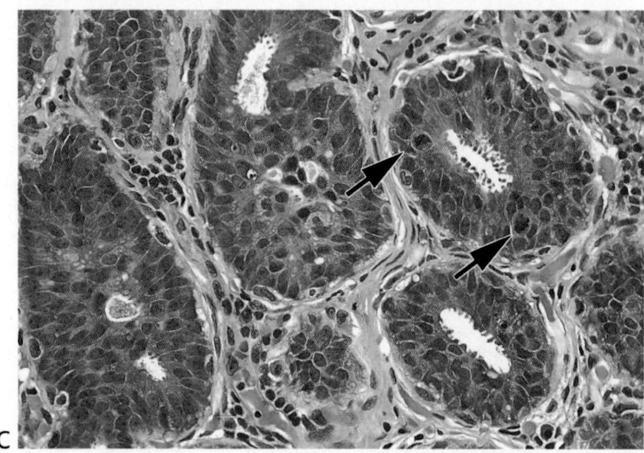
C

FIG. 9.37. ***Intraductal carcinoma associated with atypical columnar cell hyperplasia.*** The sample shown here is from the same biopsy as in Figure. 9.33B, which displayed ACH. **A:** Low-magnification view showing cribriform and flat micropapillary intraductal carcinoma. **B,C:** Intraductal carcinoma with cribriform and flat growth. *Arrows* indicate mitoses.

MRI predominantly in women at higher risk of carcinoma. Almost all of the carcinomas found after ADH was detected by MRI-directed core biopsy have been DCIS.

The management of cases wherein ACH is diagnosed on needle core biopsies remains controversial. Several studies have recommended that excisional biopsies be performed,[96–98] whereas others have suggested that excisional biopsy is not necessary.[99,100] The prudent course of action in this situation is to approach each case in a multidisciplinary manner with clinical, pathologic, and radiologic correlation.[101] It must also be kept in mind that ACH has been linked to low-grade DCIS.[102] Parenthetically, it may be stated that no definite precursor lesion for high-grade DCIS has thus far been identified, although certain types of apocrine lesions are suspected in this regard.[79]

Because of the limited and often fragmented nature of needle core biopsy specimens, some weight may be given to quantitative criteria in assessing these specimens. Pathologists should avoid overinterpreting small biopsy samples. There is temptation to overinterpret small biopsy samples because of the expectation that more lesional tissue remains at the biopsy site. In the diagnosis of needle core biopsy specimens from breast lesions, it must be anticipated that the material seen in the needle core biopsy sample may be the most extreme and potentially the only abnormality present, expressed as "what you see may be all there is." ADH may be diagnosed if detached fragments of abnormal epithelium suggest carcinoma, or if only part of a duct with features of carcinoma is contained in the sample.

The importance of adequate sampling was documented by Jackman et al.[21] who "progressively increased the average number of core samples obtained per lesion and have found a decrease in both the number of ADH lesions and the discordance of ADH lesion." The greater success in diagnosis was attributable to more lesions being diagnosed as DCIS rather than as ADH as a result of more complete sampling.

Molecular markers have been used to study needle core biopsy samples in an effort to predict the likelihood of finding carcinoma in a subsequent excisional biopsy. Tocino et al.[103] evaluated p53 expression in the needle core biopsies from 34 women with ADH. Subsequent surgical biopsy revealed carcinoma in eight (23.5%), including five instances of DCIS and three instances of invasive carcinomas. Mutations in p53 were detected in microdissected samples from seven of the eight (88%) needle core biopsy samples of ADH that were followed by carcinoma at surgery and in 35% of ADH without carcinoma in the subsequent surgical biopsy, a difference that was statistically significant.

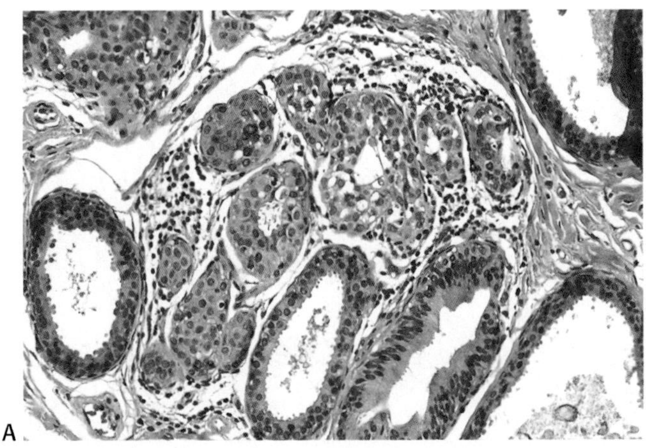

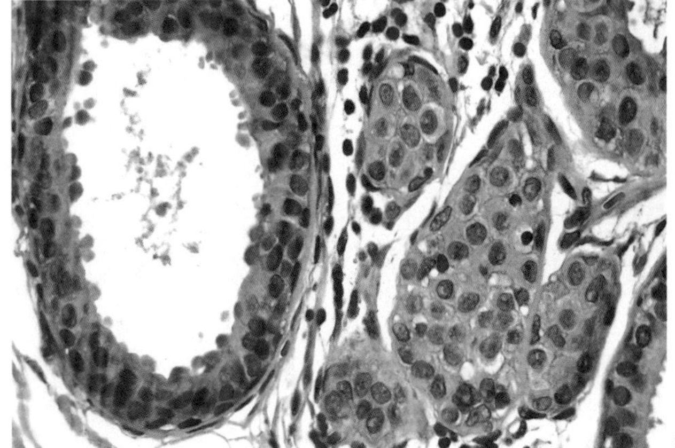

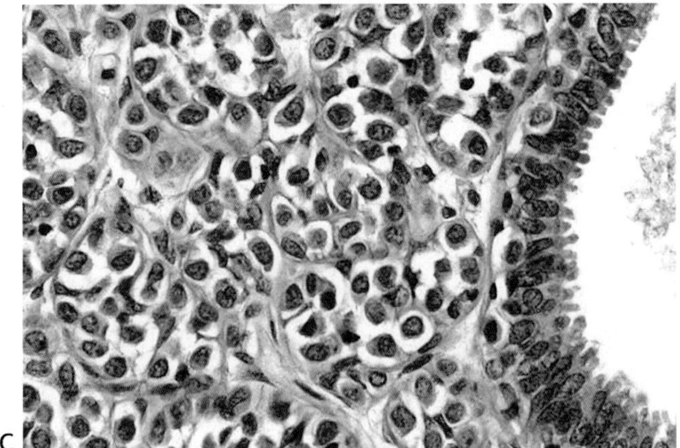

FIG. 9.38. ***LCIS associated with columnar cell change.*** **A:** LCIS is surrounded by cystic ducts with CCC in a 39-year-old woman. **B:** Magnified view of **(A)** showing the mosaic pattern of the monomorphic cells in LCIS. **C:** LCIS next to CCC. Note pagetoid extension of LCIS under the columnar cell epithelium.

USE OF IMMUNOHISTOCHEMISTRY IN THE DIAGNOSIS OF DUCTAL PROLIFERATIVE LESIONS

The use of immunohistochemistry, primarily to assess cytokeratin expression in establishing the diagnosis of ductal proliferative lesions, can only be considered an ancillary technique. In this situation, as in all of surgical pathology, results of immunostaining must be interpreted in the context of all histopathologic findings.

UDH including its florid form is typically immunoreactive for HMW-CKs, generally in a heterogeneous, so-called "mosaic," pattern. The HMW-CKs include CK5, CK6, CK14, CK17, and CK-K903 (34βE12). The cells of ADH, as well as those of most DCIS, are typically negative for HMW-CKs (Fig. 9.43). Staining for ER and PR is heterogeneous in UDH, in contrast to the stronger and more diffuse staining observed in most cases of ADH and low-grade DCIS.[104,105] HER2 immunoreactivity is not encountered in UDH, ADH, and in low-grade DCIS.

ADH-5 is a commercially available antibody cocktail consisting of five antibodies: anti-CK5, anti-CK14 (both HMW-CKs), and two LMW-CKs: anti-CK7, anti-CK18, and anti-p63. This antibody cocktail allows for simultaneous detection of three groups of cells, that is, those epithelial cells that are highlighted by LMW-CKs, others that are decorated by HMW-CK, and myoepithelial cells highlighted by p63. Each of the two groups of CK antibodies uses a different chromogen (DAB: brown; fast red: red) that allows for ready interpretation of cytoplasmic staining. Nuclear p63 positivity identifies myoepithelial cells. UDH shows a mixed pattern of staining with positivity for both groups of CK. Most cases of ADH and DCIS are found to be negative for HMW-CKs and positive for LMW-CKs. The use of this cocktail has been shown to significantly increase diagnostic interobserver agreement among pathologists, compared with H&E alone.[106]

PROGNOSIS AND TREATMENT OF DUCTAL HYPERPLASIA

The prognosis of UDH and ADH is discussed in detail in Chapter 10. The major concern attributable to these lesions is the risk of subsequently developing carcinoma. This risk is greater when there is atypia than if hyperplasia is in the usual category. UDH confers a slight increase in subsequent breast cancer risk in the order of 1.5- to 2-fold. The risk is higher among women with a family history.[107] As stated by the Cancer Committee of CAP, ADH is associated with a moderately increased risk of the subsequent development of invasive carcinoma, with a relative risk (RR) of 3.0 to 5.0.[108] The increased risk of subsequent carcinoma following the finding of UDH, ADH, or ACH applies equally to both breasts.

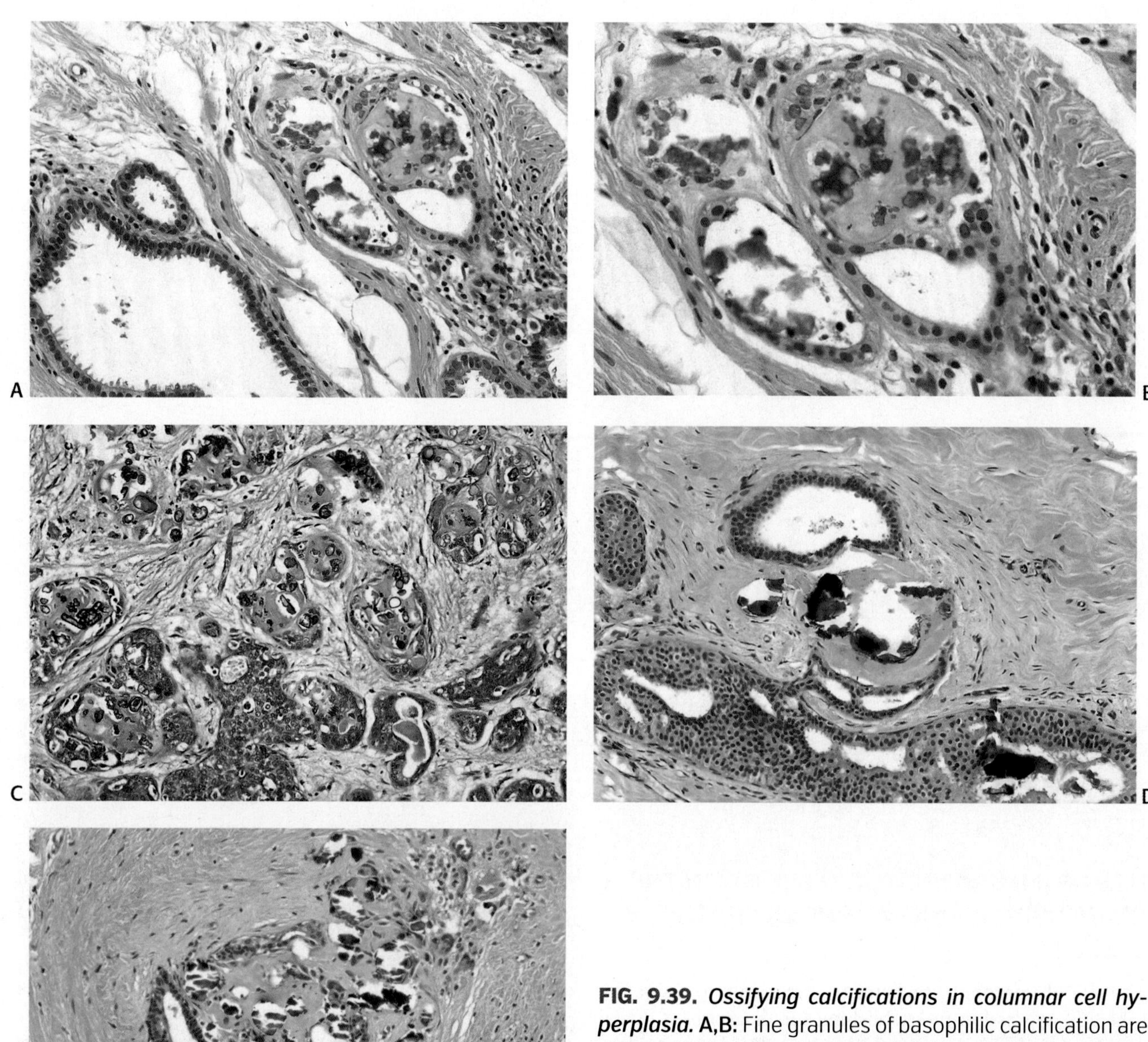

FIG. 9.39. ***Ossifying calcifications in columnar cell hyperplasia.*** **A,B:** Fine granules of basophilic calcification are present in the discrete eosinophilic intraepithelial nodule. **C:** Multiple ossifying calcifications in a single proliferative focus. This is an unusual finding. **D:** A basophilic calcification in ossifying matrix arising in ACH. **E:** Subepithelial ossifying calcification that has spilled into the periductal stroma.

Patients with ductal hyperplasia, especially when there is atypia, are encouraged to participate in a regular follow-up program that employs physician examination, self-examination, and imaging. The goal of this approach is to detect carcinoma at a stage when it would be most amenable to cure. Examinations may be scheduled more frequently for women with atypia, especially if there are associated risk factors such as a family history of breast carcinoma.[109]

Until recently, UDH had been regarded as a precursor lesion of ADH and DCIS. At the molecular level, however, only a few and random chromosomal changes have been encountered in UDH.[7] There are some genomic data to suggest that a minor proportion of UDH lesions may harbor clonal cell populations, indicating that clonal lesions such as ADH may only occasionally arise in this setting. A minority of UDH cases may harbor genomic alterations that may also be observed in ADH,[110] but the majority of these lesions are likely to be "dead-end" proliferations.[111]

Prophylactic bilateral mastectomy may be considered in selected cases, but should be "reserved only for those patients with an extraordinarily high risk, as defined by genetic pedigree analysis demonstrating a hereditary trait or those with severe atypia who find surveillance an unacceptable method of management."[109] If bilateral mastectomy is performed,

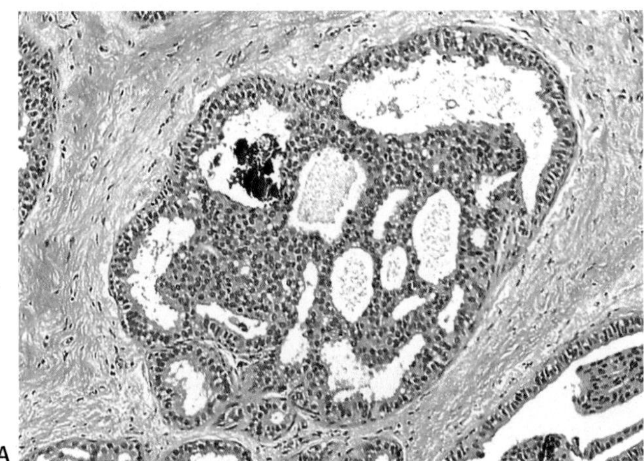

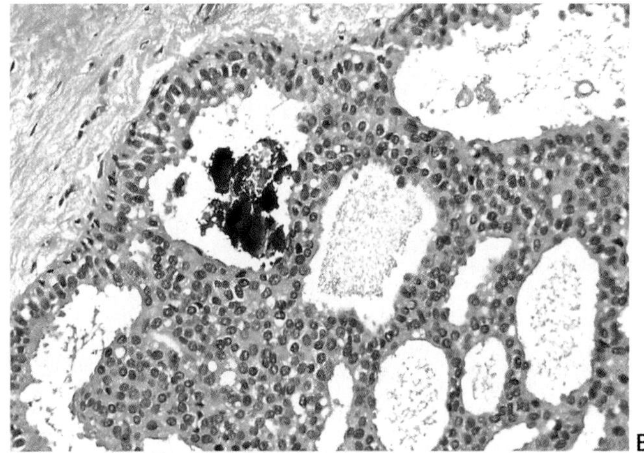

FIG. 9.40. ***Borderline atypical ductal hyperplasia.*** **A,B:** The proliferation in the duct suggests carcinoma. The fragmented calcification is a type found in intraductal carcinoma. **B:** Bands of cells with overlapping nuclei encircling the lumens appear rigid. Ductal epithelium persists focally at the periphery **(B)**.

the operation should be a total mastectomy that includes the axillary tail. It is unlikely that a subcutaneous or nipple-sparing mastectomy will accomplish the goal of entirely removing all breast glandular tissue. Although uncommon, the development of carcinoma in residual breast tissue after a prophylactic mastectomy is a discouraging event.[112] The role of sentinel lymph node biopsy in this situation is discussed in Chapter 44.

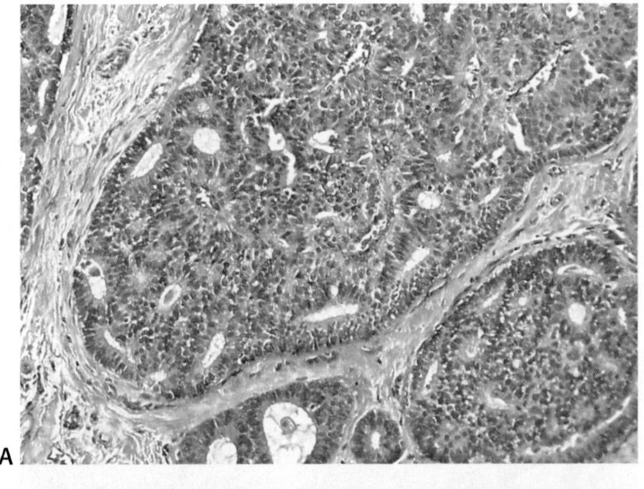

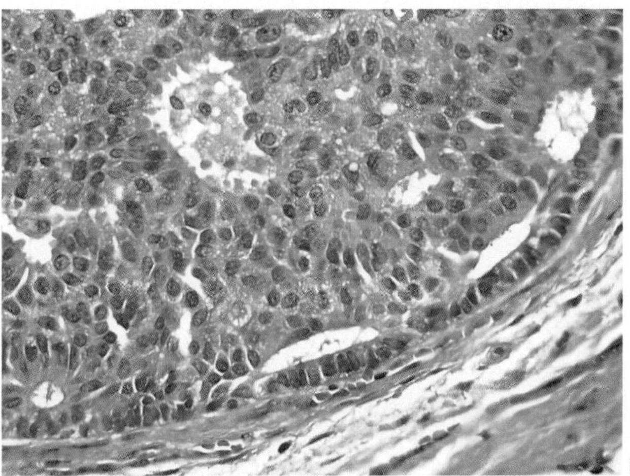

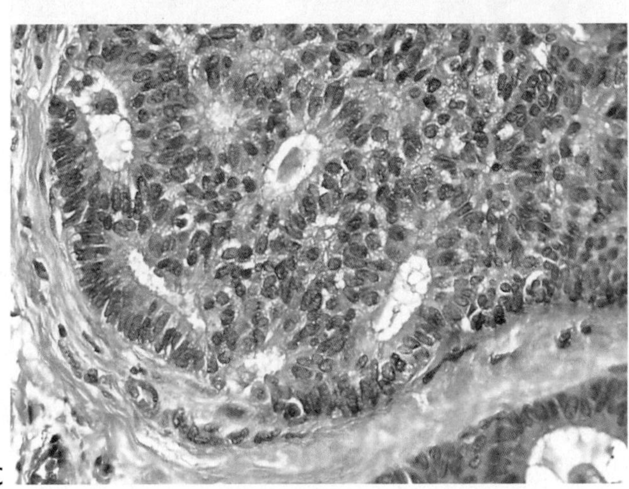

FIG. 9.41. ***Borderline atypical ductal hyperplasia.*** **A:** Hyperplastic epithelium is oriented around microlumens in the duct as well as at the periphery. **B:** Cells are oriented around part of a central microlumen and at the outer borders of peripheral slits. **C:** Microlumens with circumferentially oriented cells.

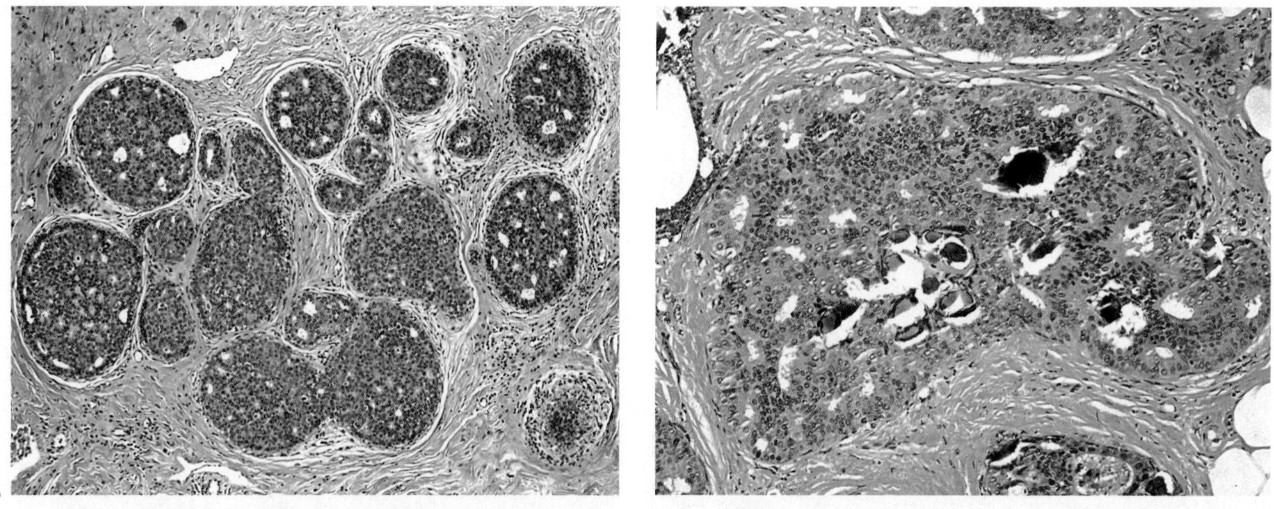

FIG. 9.42. ***Borderline atypical ductal hyperplasia.*** **A:** Atypical cribriform proliferation in an adenosis configuration. Small unaffected glands are evident. **B:** Basophilic and ossifying calcifications are present.

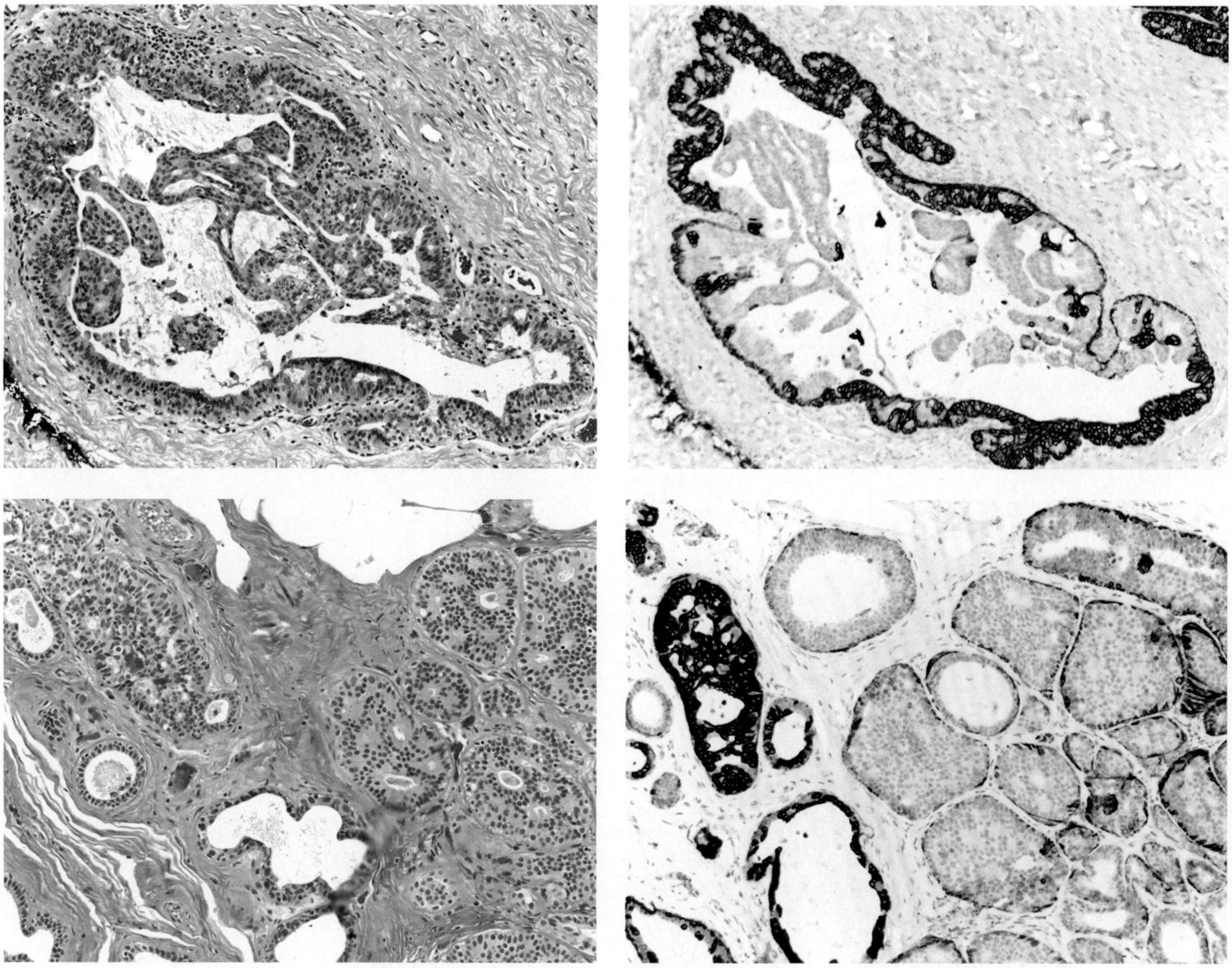

FIG. 9.43. ***Use of HMW-CK in differentiating usual hyperplasia from atypical ductal hyperplasia.*** **A,B:** Usual (nonatypical) hyperplasia is immunoreactive for CK5/6 (an HMW-CK) in a heterogeneous, so-called "mosaic," pattern at the periphery of this duct. ADH of the micropapillary type (at the *center* of the duct) is negative for CK5/6. **C,D:** The cells of ADH, and most but not all forms of DCIS, are typically negative for HMW-CKs. Note positive CK5/6 in the usual hyperplasia (at *left*). HMW-CKs include CK5, CK6, CK14, CK17, and CK-K903 (34βE12).

Tamoxifen, a selective ER modulator, has proven to be effective in the treatment of breast carcinoma and as agent for adjuvant therapy. The use of tamoxifen for primary prevention is supported by the observation that the frequency of contralateral breast carcinoma was reduced by about 35% in women receiving adjuvant tamoxifen therapy for carcinoma in one breast.[113–115] It is believed that the preventive action of tamoxifen is accomplished mainly by interfering with the promoting action of estrogen on proliferative lesions. An effect at the level of initiation is also possible.

A clinical trial of the preventive effects of tamoxifen sponsored by the National Surgical Adjuvant Breast and Bowel Project (NSABP) enrolled more than 13,000 women at high risk of developing breast carcinoma.[116] This randomized study compared women receiving tamoxifen with women given a placebo. There was an 86% reduction in subsequent invasive carcinoma in the treated women with ADH compared with controls.

The estrogen dependence of ductal proliferative lesions is suggested by several observations. Failure to suppress the growth of ER-positive cells may contribute to the progression of hyperplastic foci in some cases. Visscher et al.[117] reported that nuclear ER reactivity was present in significantly more cells in hyperplasias than in normal terminal ductal–lobular units and that nuclear reactivity was even more pronounced in receptor-positive DCIS. Shoker et al.[118] also reported increased ER expression in hyperplastic ductal foci and correlated these findings with increased proliferative activity represented by Ki67 reactivity. A high ratio of ER-α to ER-β detected in hyperplasia of usual type may be a marker of increased breast cancer risk.[119]

It might not be impossible to determine the precise clinical significance, and hence the appropriate management, of various ductal proliferative processes until their molecular pathways are outlined.[110,111] Considerable advances have been made in this regard; for instance, mitochondrial DNA sequencing and phylogenetic tree clustering have revealed direct transitions between some forms of proliferative breast disease and low-grade DCIS.[120] Knowledge of the true incidence and prevalence of proliferative breast diseases in the general population, and the long-term outcome of those who harbor such processes, would also help optimize management. A retrospective study of 2,498 reduction mammoplasties performed from 2006 to 2012 in patients, all without a history of breast carcinoma, showed ADH and "flat epithelial atypia" to be present in 47 (1.9%) patients.[121] This finding provides some data on the prevalence of atypical ductal proliferative disease in this particular setting, if not in the general population. More data are needed in this regard.

REFERENCES

1. Ellis IO, Pinder SE, Lee AH, et al. A critical appraisal of existing classification systems of epithelial hyperplasia and *in situ* neoplasia of the breast with proposals for future methods of categorization: where are we going? *Semin Diagn Pathol* 1999;16:202–208.
2. Rosai J. Borderline epithelial lesions of the breast. *Am J Surg Pathol* 1991;15:209–221.
3. Tavassoli FA. Ductal carcinoma *in situ*: introduction of the concept of ductal intraepithelial neoplasia. *Mod Pathol* 1998;11:140–154.
4. Vogelstein B, Fearon ER, Hamilton SR, et al. Genetic alterations during colorectal-tumor development. *N Engl J Med* 1988;319:525–532.
5. Dietrich CU, Pandis N, Teixeira MR, et al. Chromosome abnormalities in benign hyperproliferative disorders of epithelial and stromal breast tissue. *Int J Cancer* 1995;60:49–53.
6. Lakhani SR, Collins N, Stratton MR, et al. Atypical ductal hyperplasia of the breast: clonal proliferation with loss of heterozygosity on chromosomes 16q and 17p. *J Clin Pathol* 1995;48:611–615.
7. Lakhani SR, Slack DN, Hamoudi RA, et al. Detection of allelic imbalance indicates that a proportion of mammary hyperplasia of usual type are clonal neoplastic proliferations. *Lab Invest* 1996;74:129–135.
8. Rosenberg CL, Larson PS, Romo JD, et al. Microsatellite alterations indicating monoclonality in atypical hyperplasias associated with breast cancer. *Hum Pathol* 1997;28:214–219.
9. Kasami M, Vnencak-Jones CL, Manning S, et al. Loss of heterozygosity and microsatellite instability in breast hyperplasia. No obligate correlation of these genetic alterations with subsequent malignancy. *Am J Pathol* 1997;150:1925–1932.
10. Rohan TE, Hartwick W, Miller AB, et al. Immunohistochemical detection of c-erbB-2 and p53 in benign breast disease and breast cancer risk. *J Natl Cancer Inst* 1998;90:1262–1269.
11. Mommers EC, van Diest PJ, Leonhart AM, et al. Expression of proliferation and apoptosis-related proteins in usual ductal hyperplasia of the breast. *Hum Pathol* 1998;29:1539–1545.
12. Done SJ, Arneson NC, Ozcelik H, et al. p53 Mutations in mammary ductal carcinoma *in situ* but not in epithelial hyperplasias. *Cancer Res* 1998;58:785–789.
13. Deng G, Lu Y, Zlotnikov G, et al. Loss of heterozygosity in normal tissue adjacent to breast carcinomas. *Science* 1996;274:2057–2059.
14. Gobbi H, Dupont WD, Simpson JF, et al. Transforming growth factor-β and breast cancer risk in women with mammary epithelial hyperplasia. *J Natl Cancer Inst* 1999;91:2096–2101.
15. Ratcliffe N, Wells W, Wheeler K, et al. The combination of *in situ* hybridization and immunohistochemical analysis: an evaluation of Her2/*neu* expression in paraffin-embedded breast carcinomas and adjacent normal-appearing breast epithelium. *Mod Pathol* 1997;10:1247–1252.
16. Connolly JL, Schnitt SJ. Benign breast disease. Resolved and unresolved issues. *Cancer* 1993;71:1187–1189.
17. Bodian CA, Perzin KH, Lattes R, et al. Reproducibility and validity of pathologic classifications of benign breast disease and implications for clinical applications. *Cancer* 1993;71:3908–3913.
18. Schnitt SJ, Connolly JL, Tavassoli FA, et al. Interobserver reproducibility in the diagnosis of ductal proliferative breast lesions using standardized criteria. *Am J Surg Pathol* 1992;16:1133–1143.
19. Palli D, Galli M, Bianchi S, et al. Reproducibility of histological diagnosis of breast lesions: results of a panel in Italy. *Eur J Cancer* 1996;32A:603–607.
20. Helvie MA, Hessler C, Frank TS, et al. Atypical hyperplasia of the breast: mammographic appearance and histologic correlation. *Radiology* 1991;179:759–764.
21. Jackman RJ, Nowels KW, Shepard MJ, et al. Stereotaxic large-core needle biopsy of 450 nonpalpable breast lesions with surgical correlation in lesions with cancer or atypical hyperplasia. *Radiology* 1994;193:91–95.
22. Liberman L, Cohen MA, Abramson AF, et al. Atypical ductal hyperplasia diagnosed at stereotaxic core biopsy of breast lesions: an indication for surgical biopsy. *AJR Am J Roentgenol* 1995;164:1111–1113.
23. Rosen PP, Cantrell B, Mullen DL, et al. Juvenile papillomatosis (Swiss cheese disease) of the breast. *Am J Surg Pathol* 1980;4:3–12.
24. Bodian CA, Perzin KH, Lattes R, et al. Prognostic significance of benign proliferative breast disease. *Cancer* 1993;71:3896–3907.
25. Page DL, Rogers LW. Combined histologic and cytologic criteria for the diagnosis of mammary atypical ductal hyperplasia. *Hum Pathol* 1992;23:1095–1097.
26. Rubin E, Visscher DW, Alexander RW, et al. Proliferative disease and atypia in biopsies performed for nonpalpable lesions detected mammographically. *Cancer* 1988;61:2077–2082.
27. Stomper PC, Cholewinski SP, Penetrante RB, et al. Atypical hyperplasia, frequency and mammographic and pathologic relationships in excisional biopsies guided by mammography and clinical examination. *Radiology* 1993;189:667–671.

28. Orel SG, Rosen M, Miles C, et al. MR imaging guided 9-gauge vacuum assisted core needle breast biopsy: initial experience. *Radiology* 2006;238:54–61.
29. Perlet C, Heywang-Kobrunner SH, Heinig A, et al. Magnetic resonance-guided, vacuum-assisted breast biopsy: results from a European multicentre study of 538 lesions. *Cancer* 2006;106:982–990.
30. Liberman L, Holland AE, Marjan D, et al. Underestimation of atypical ductal hyperplasia at MRI-guided 9-gauge vacuum-assisted breast biopsy. *AJR Am J Roentgenol* 2007;188:684–690.
31. Wilson M, Cranor ML, Rosen PP. Papillary duct hyperplasia of the breast in children and young women. *Mod Pathol* 1993;6:570–574.
32. Rosen PP. Columnar cell hyperplasia is associated with lobular carcinoma *in situ* and tubular carcinoma. *Am J Surg Pathol* 1999;23:1561.
33. Rosen PP. Ductal hyperplasia and intraductal hyperplasia. In: *Breast pathology: diagnosis by needle core biopsy*. Philadelphia: Lippincott Williams & Wilkins, 1999:89–92.
34. Hartmann LC, Sellers TA, Frost MH, et al. Benign breast disease and the risk of breast cancer. *N Engl J Med* 2005;353:229–237.
35. Kerlikowske K, Barclay J, Grady D, et al. Comparison of risk factors for ductal carcinoma *in situ* and invasive breast cancer. *J Natl Cancer Inst* 1997;89:76–82.
36. Azzopardi JG, Ahmed A, Millis RR. *Problems in breast pathology*. (*Major problems in pathology*, vol. 11). Philadelphia: WB Saunders, 1979:25.
37. Haagensen CD. *Diseases of the breast*. 3rd ed. Philadelphia: WB Saunders, 1986:118–124.
38. Wellings SR, Jensen HM, Marcum RG. An atlas of subgross pathology of the human breast with special reference to possible precancerous lesions. *J Natl Cancer Inst* 1975;55:231–273.
39. Ozaki D, Kondo Y. Comparative morphometric studies of benign and malignant intraductal proliferative lesions of the breast by computerized image analysis. *Hum Pathol* 1995;26:1109–1113.
40. Ohuchi N, Abe R, Takahashi T, et al. Three-dimensional atypical structure in intraductal carcinoma differentiating from papilloma and papillomatosis of the breast. *Breast Cancer Res Treat* 1985;5:57–65.
41. Ozzello L. Ultrastructure of the human mammary gland. *Pathol Annu* 1971;6:1–59.
42. Barbareschi M, Pecciarini L, Gangi MG, et al. P63, a p53 homologue, is a selective nuclear marker of myoepithelial cells of the human breast. *Am J Surg Pathol* 2001;25:1054–1060.
43. Kalof AN, Tam D, Beatty B, et al. Immunostaining patterns of myoepithelial cells in breast lesions: a comparison of CD10 and smooth muscle myosin heavy chain. *J Clin Pathol* 2004;57:625–629.
44. Lerwill M. Current practical applications of diagnostic immunohistochemistry in breast pathology. *Am J Surg Pathol* 2004;28:1076–1091.
45. Cabibi D, Giannone AG, Belmonte B, et al. CD10 and HHF35 actin in the differential diagnosis between collagenous spherulosis and adenoid-cystic carcinoma of the breast. *Pathol Res Pract* 2012;208:405–409.
46. Tavassoli FA, Norris HJ. A comparison of the results of long-term follow-up for atypical intraductal carcinoma of the breast. *Cancer* 1990;65:518–529.
47. Tavassoli FA. Intraductal hyperplasias, ordinary and atypical. In: *Pathology of the breast*. New York: Elsevier Science, 1992:155–191.
48. Tavassoli FA. *Pathology of the breast*. 2nd ed. Stamford: Appleton & Lange, 1999:205–260.
49. Fisher ER, Costantino J, Fisher B, et al. for the National Surgical Adjuvant Breast and Bowel Project Collaborating Investigators. Pathologic findings from the National Surgical Adjuvant Breast Project (NSABP) Protocol B-17. Intraductal carcinoma (ductal carcinoma *in situ*). *Cancer* 1995;75:1310–1319.
50. Prosser J, Hilsenbeck SG, Fuqua SAW, et al. Cell turnover (proliferation and apoptosis) in normal epithelium and premalignant lesions in the same breast. *Mod Pathol* 1997;10:38.
51. Arapantoni-Dadioti P, Panayiotides J, Georgakila H, et al. Significance of intracytoplasmic lumina in the differential diagnosis between epithelial hyperplasia and carcinoma *in situ* of the breast. *Breast Dis* 1996;9:277–282.
52. Azzopardi JG, Ahmed A, Millis RR. *Problems in breast pathology*. (*Major problems in pathology*, vol. 11). Philadelphia: WB Saunders, 1979:213–214.
53. Oyama T, Maluf H, Koerner F. Atypical cystic lobules: an early stage in the formation of low-grade ductal carcinoma *in situ*. *Virchows Arch* 1999;435:413–421.
54. Goldstein NS, Lacerna M, Vicini F. Cancerization of lobules and atypical ductal hyperplasia adjacent to ductal carcinoma *in situ* of the breast. *Am J Clin Pathol* 1998;110:357–367.
55. Fraser JL, Raza S, Chorny K, et al. Columnar alteration with prominent apical snouts and secretions: a spectrum of changes frequently present in breast biopsies performed for microcalcifications. *Am J Surg Pathol* 1998;22:1521–1527.
56. Lubelsky SM, Bane AL, Shin V, et al. Columnar cell lesions and flat epithelial atypia: incidence and significance in a mammographically screened population. *Mod Pathol* 2005;18(Suppl.):41A.
57. Lakhani SR, Ellis IO, Schnitt SJ, et al. *WHO classification of tumours of the breast*. 4th ed. Lyon: World Health Organization-IARC, 2012.
58. Boulos FI, Dupont WD, Schuyler PA, et al. Clinicopathologic characteristics of carcinomas that develop after a biopsy containing columnar cell lesions: evidence against a precursor role. *Cancer* 2012;118:2372–2377.
59. Schnitt SJ, Vincent-Salomon A. Columnar cell lesions of the breast. *Adv Anat Pathol* 2003;10:113–124.
60. Fraser JL, Pliss N, Connolly JL, et al. Immunophenotype of columnar alteration with prominent apical snouts and secretions (CAPSS). *Mod Pathol* 2000;13:21A.
61. Dabbs DJ, Carter G, Fudge M, et al. Molecular alterations in columnar cell lesions of the breast. *Mod Pathol* 2006;19:344–349.
62. Noel J-C, Fayt I, Fernandes-Aguillar S, et al. Proliferating activity in columnar cell lesions of the breast. *Virchows Arch* 2006;449:617–621.
63. Kaneko M, Arihiro K, Takeshima Y, et al. Loss of heterozygosity and microsatellite instability in epithelial hyperplasia of the breast. *J Exp Ther Oncol* 2002;2:9–18.
64. Jensen KC, Kong CS. Cytologic diagnosis of columnar cell lesions of the breast. *Diagn Cytopathol* 2007;35:73–79.
65. Moinfar F. Flat ductal intraepithelial neoplasia of the breast: a review of diagnostic criteria, differential diagnoses, molecular-genetic findings, and clinical relevance—it is time to appreciate the Azzopardi concept! *Arch Pathol Lab Med* 2009;133:879–992.
66. Lerwill MF. Flat epithelial atypia of the breast. *Arch Pathol Lab Med* 2008;132:615–621.
67. Solorzano S, Mesurolle B, Omeroglu A, et al. Flat epithelial atypia of the breast: pathological–radiological correlation. *AJR Am J Roentgenol* 2011;197:740–746.
68. Brandt SM, Young GQ, Hoda SA. The "Rosen Triad": tubular carcinoma, lobular carcinoma *in situ*, and columnar cell lesions. *Adv Anat Pathol* 2008;15:140–146.
69. O'Malley FP, Mohsin SK, Badve S, et al. Interobserver reproducibility in the diagnosis of flat epithelial atypia of the breast. *Mod Pathol* 2006;19:172–179.
70. Tan PH, Ho BC-S, Selvarajan S, et al. Pathological diagnosis of columnar cell lesions of the breast: are there issues of reproducibility? *J Clin Pathol* 2005;25:705–709.
71. Guerra-Wallace MM, Christensen WN, White RL. A retrospective study of columnar alteration with prominent apical snouts and secretions and the association with cancer. *Am J Surg* 2004;188:395–398.
72. Collins LC, Achacoso NA, Nekhlyudov L, et al. Clinical and pathologic features of ductal carcinoma *in situ* associated with the presence of flat epithelial atypia: an analysis of 543 patients. *Mod Pathol* 2007;20:1149–1155.
73. Abdel-Fatah TM, Powe DG, Hodi Z, et al. High frequency of coexistence of columnar cell lesions, lobular neoplasia, and low-grade ductal carcinoma *in situ* with invasive tubular carcinoma and invasive lobular carcinoma. *Am J Surg Pathol* 2007;31:417–426.
74. Abdel-Fatah TM, Powe DG, Hodi Z, et al. Morphologic and molecular evolutionary pathways of low nuclear grade invasive breast cancers and their putative precursor lesions: further evidence to support the concept of low nuclear grade breast neoplasia family. *Am J Surg Pathol* 2008;32:513–523.
75. Sahoo S, Recant WM. Triad of columnar cell alteration, lobular carcinoma *in situ*, and tubular carcinoma of the breast. *Breast J* 2005;11:140–142.
76. Simpson PT, Gale T, Reis-Filho JS, et al. Columnar cell lesions of the breast: the missing link in breast cancer progression? A morphological and molecular analysis. *Am J Surg Pathol* 2005;29:734–746.
77. O'Connell P, Pekkel V, Fuqua SA, et al. Analysis of loss of heterozygosity in 399 premalignant breast lesions at 15 genetic loci. *J Natl Cancer Inst* 1998;90:697–703.
78. Bombonati A, Sgroi DC. The molecular pathology of breast cancer progression. *J Pathol* 2011;223:307–317.
79. Lopez-Garcia MA, Geyer FC, Lacroix-Triki M, et al. Breast cancer precursors revisited: molecular features and progression pathways. *Histopathology* 2010;57:171–192.

80. Hicks DG, Immunohistochemistry in the diagnostic evaluation of breast lesions. *Appl Immunohistochem Mol Morph* 2011;19:501–505.
81. Yeh IT, Mies C. Application of immunohistochemistry to breast lesions. *Arch Pathol Lab Med* 2008;132:349–358.
82. Elston CW, Sloane JP, Amendoeira I, et al. Causes of inconsistency in diagnosing and classifying intraductal proliferations of the breast. European Commission Working Group on breast screening pathology. *Eur J Cancer* 2000;36:1769–1772.
83. Tocino I, Garcia BM, Carter D. Surgical biopsy findings in patients with atypical hyperplasia diagnosed by stereotaxic core needle biopsy. *Ann Surg Oncol* 1996;3:483–488.
84. Jackman RJ, Birdwell RL, Ikeda DM. Atypical ductal hyperplasia: can some lesions be defined as probably benign after stereotactic 11-gauge vacuum-assisted biopsy, eliminating the recommendation for surgical excision? *Radiology* 2002;224:548–554.
85. Maganini RO, Klem DA, Huston BJ, et al. Upgrade rate of core biopsy-determined atypical ductal hyperplasia by open excisional biopsy. *Am J Surg* 2001;182:355–358.
86. Winchester DJ, Bernstein JR, Jeske JM, et al. Upstaging of atypical ductal hyperplasia after vacuum-assisted 11-guage stereotactic core needle biopsy. *Arch Surg* 2003;138:619–623.
87. Brem RF, Behrndt VS, Sanow L, et al. Atypical ductal hyperplasia: histologic underestimation of carcinoma in tissue harvested from impalpable breast lesions using 11-gauge stereotactically guided directional vacuum-assisted biopsy. *AJR Am J Roentgenol* 1999;172:1405–1407.
88. Moore MM, Hargett CW, Hanks JB, et al. Association of breast cancer with the finding of atypical ductal hyperplasia at core breast biopsy. *Ann Surg* 1997;225:726–731.
89. Gadzala DE, Cederbom GJ, Bolton JS, et al. Appropriate management of atypical ductal hyperplasia diagnosed by stereotactic core needle breast biopsy. *Ann Surg Oncol* 1997;4:283–286.
90. Burbank F. Stereotactic breast biopsy of atypical ductal hyperplasia and ductal carcinoma *in situ* lesions: improved accuracy with directional, vacuum-assisted biopsy. *Radiology* 1997;202:843–847.
91. Flegg KM, Flaherty JJ, Bicknell AM, et al. Surgical outcomes of borderline breast lesions detected by needle biopsy in a breast screening program. *World J Surg Oncol* 2010;8:78.
92. McGhan LJ, Pockaj BA, Wasif N, et al. Atypical ductal hyperplasia on core biopsy: an automatic trigger for excisional biopsy? *Ann Surg Oncol* 2012;19:3264–3269.
93. Chae BJ, Lee A, Song BJ, et al. Predictive factors for breast cancer in patients diagnosed atypical ductal hyperplasia at core needle biopsy. *World J Surg Oncol* 2009;7:77.
94. VandenBussche CJ, Khouri N, Sbaity E, et al. Borderline atypical ductal hyperplasia/low-grade ductal carcinoma *in situ* on breast needle core biopsy should be managed conservatively. *Am J Surg Pathol* 2013;37:913–923.
95. Renshaw AA, Cartagena N, Schenkman RH, et al. Atypical ductal hyperplasia in breast core needle biopsies. *Am J Clin Pathol* 2001;116:92–96.
96. Kunju LP, Kleer CG. Significance of flat epithelial atypia on mammotome core needle biopsy: should it be excised? *Hum Pathol* 2007;38:35–41.
97. Chivukula M, Bhargava R, Tseng G, et al. Clinicopathologic implications of "flat epithelial atypia" in core needle biopsy specimens of the breast. *Am J Clin Pathol* 2009;131:802–808.
98. Rajan S, Sharma N, Dall BJ, et al. What is the significance of flat epithelial atypia and what are the management implications? *J Clin Pathol* 2011;64:1001–1004.
99. Piubello Q, Parisi A, Eccher A, et al. Flat epithelial atypia on core needle biopsy: which is the right management? *Am J Surg Pathol* 2009;33:1078–1084.
100. Senetta R, Campanino PP, Mariscotti G, et al. Columnar cell lesions associated with breast calcifications on vacuum-assisted core biopsies: clinical, radiographic, and histological correlations. *Mod Pathol* 2009;22:762–769.
101. Jara-Lazaro AR, Tse GM, Tan PH. Columnar cell lesions of the breast: an update and significance on core biopsy. *Pathology* 2009;41:18–27.
102. Aulmann S, Elsawaf Z, Penzel R, et al. Invasive tubular carcinoma of the breast frequently is clonally related to flat epithelial atypia and low-grade ductal carcinoma *in situ*. *Am J Surg Pathol* 2009;33:1646–1653.
103. Tocino I, Dillon D, Costa J, et al. Atypical hyperplasia of the breast diagnosed by stereotactic core needle biopsy: correlation of molecular markers with surgical outcome. *Radiology Suppl* 1999;213:289.
104. Otterbach F, Bànkfalvi A, Bergner S, et al. Cytokeratin 5/6 immunohistochemistry assists the differential diagnosis of atypical proliferations of the breast. *Histopathology* 2000;37:232–240.
105. Barr FE, Degnim AC, Hartmann LC, et al. Estrogen receptor expression in atypical hyperplasia: lack of association with breast cancer. *Cancer Prev Res* 2011;4:435–444.
106. Jain RK, Mehta R, Dimitrov R, et al. Atypical ductal hyperplasia: interobserver and intraobserver variability. *Mod Pathol* 2011;24:917–923.
107. Collins LC, Baer HJ, Tamimi RM, et al. The influence of family history on breast cancer risk in women with biopsy-confirmed benign breast disease: results from the Nurses' Health Study. *Cancer* 2006;107:1240–1247.
108. Fitzgibbons PL, Henson DE, Hutter RV. Benign breast changes and the risk for subsequent breast cancer: an update of the 1985 consensus statement. Cancer Committee of the College of American Pathologists. *Arch Pathol Lab Med* 1998;122:1053–1055.
109. Osborne MP, Borgen PI. Atypical ductal and lobular hyperplasia and breast cancer risk. *Surg Oncol Clin N Am* 1993;2:1–11.
110. Gong G, DeVries S, Chew KL, et al. Genetic changes in paired atypical and usual ductal hyperplasia of the breast by comparative genomic hybridization. *Clin Cancer Res* 2001;7:2410–2414.
111. Boecker W, Moll R, Dervan P, et al. Usual ductal hyperplasia of the breast is a committed stem (progenitor) cell lesion distinct from atypical ductal hyperplasia and ductal carcinoma *in situ*. *J Pathol* 2002;198:458–467.
112. Hughes KS, Papa MZ, Whitney T, et al. Prophylactic mastectomy and inherited predisposition to breast carcinoma. *Cancer* 1999;86:1682–1696.
113. Cancer Research Campaign Adjuvant Breast Trial Working Party. Cyclophosphamide and tamoxifen as adjuvant therapies in the management of breast cancer. *Br J Cancer* 1988;57:604–607.
114. Nayfield SG, Karp JE, Ford LG, et al. Potential role of tamoxifen in prevention of breast cancer. *J Natl Cancer Inst* 1991;83:1450–1459.
115. Rutqvist LE, Cedermark B, Glas U, et al. Contralateral primary tumors in breast cancer patients in a randomized trial of adjuvant tamoxifen therapy. *J Natl Cancer Inst* 1991;83:1299–1306.
116. Fisher B, Costantino JP, Wickerham DL, et al. Tamoxifen for prevention of breast cancer: report of the National Surgical Adjuvant Breast and Bowel Project P-1 Study. *J Natl Cancer Inst* 1998;90:1371–1388.
117. Visscher DW, Padiyar N, Long D, et al. Immunohistologic analysis of estrogen receptor expression in breast carcinoma precursor lesions. *Breast J* 1998;4:447–451.
118. Shoker BS, Jarvis C, Clarke RB, et al. Estrogen receptor-positive proliferating cells in the normal and precancerous breast. *Am J Pathol* 1999;155:1811–1815.
119. Shaaban AM, Jarvis C, Moore F, et al. Prognostic significance of estrogen receptor beta in epithelial hyperplasia of usual type with known outcome. *Am J Surg Pathol* 2005;29:1593–1599.
120. Desouki MM, Li Z, Hameed O, et al. Incidental atypical proliferative lesions in reduction mammoplasty specimens: analysis of 2498 cases from 2 tertiary women's health centers. *Hum Pathol* 2013;44:1877–1881.
121. Aulmann S, Braun L, Mietzsch F, et al. Transitions between flat epithelial atypia and low-grade ductal carcinoma *in situ* of the breast. *Am J Surg Pathol* 2012;36:1247–1252.

CHAPTER 10

Precarcinomatous Breast Disease: Epidemiologic, Pathologic, and Clinical Considerations

SYED A. HODA

As advances are made in the diagnosis and treatment of mammary carcinoma, attention has been directed at prevention strategies and to markers of increased risk of developing the disease. The strongest risk factors are genetic predisposition to breast carcinoma (Table 10.1) and antecedent proliferative breast changes documented by biopsy. These factors may be synergistic in their effect on breast carcinoma risk. A wide variety of additional risk factors have been implicated in the pathogenesis of breast carcinoma (Table 10.2).

GENETIC PREDISPOSITION TO BREAST CARCINOMA

Up to 10% of breast carcinomas may be hereditary. The great majority of these carcinomas, approximately 90%, are associated with mutations of breast cancer genes 1 and 2 (*BRCA1* and *BRCA2*), although a significant proportion are caused by *TP53, PTEN, STK11, ATM, BRIP1*, and *PALB2* mutations.[1] Genetic susceptibility is usually manifested clinically by a history of breast carcinoma in one or more female relatives. The risk associated with a positive family history is increased when a maternal first-degree relative is affected, if the relative has premenopausal bilateral breast carcinoma, and if multiple relatives are affected. Other indications of possible hereditary susceptibility include early onset of breast carcinoma, multiple site-specific cancers (e.g., breast and ovarian), and the presence of rare cancers or cancer-associated syndromes.

BRCA1 and *BRCA2* Mutations

Specific chromosomal alterations have been related to breast carcinoma risk as a result of the identification of mutations in the *BRCA1* gene on the long arm of chromosome 17[2–4] and in the *BRCA2* gene located on chromosome 13.[5] *BRCA1* is a pleiotropic DNA damage response protein that functions in both checkpoint activation and DNA repair, whereas *BRCA2* is a mediator of the core mechanism of homologous recombination.[6] The proteins expressed by these genes function together during DNA repair to shield the genome from double-strand DNA damage. Various types of mutations in different segments of these genes have been identified.[5–9] The lifetime risk of developing breast carcinoma as a result of a *BRCA1* mutation has been reported in various studies to be 56% to nearly 90%.[10,11] A slightly lower risk of breast carcinoma associated with *BRCA2* mutations has been reported to be 37% to 84%.[11,12] *BRCA1* may account for up to 45% of cases of hereditary breast carcinoma as well as nearly 90% of patients with combined breast and ovarian carcinoma.[13,14] The lifetime risk of ovarian carcinoma attributed to *BRCA1* mutations is about 45%.[15]

The risks associated with *BRCA1* and *BRCA2* mutations appear to be modified by other genes or genetic alterations, as suggested by a study of genotypes of the androgen receptor (AR).[16] Reproductive factors such as parity and age of first live birth, well-established epidemiologic indicators of breast carcinoma risk, have been shown to interact with familial risk to a slight degree.[17] Parity may influence *BRCA1*-associated breast carcinoma risk.[18] Exogenous factors such as cigarette smoking and oral contraceptive hormones have also been identified as factors that might modify *BRCA1* and/or *BRCA2* penetrance.[19–21] Dietary, environmental, and other as yet undefined factors appear to influence the penetrance of *BRCA1* and *BRCA2* in individual women. This is illustrated by data from a study of 403 *BRCA1* mutation carriers summarized by Rebbeck.[22] Breast carcinoma alone had been diagnosed in 209 (52%) women with a mean age at diagnosis of 42.6 years, but there was a broad range of age (19 to 96 years). Among the other women, 40 (10%) developed ovarian carcinoma, and 22 (5%) had ovarian and breast carcinoma. Nine (7%) of the remaining 132 women who had not developed breast or ovarian carcinoma were older than 70 years. The relationship between particular *BRCA1* and *BRCA2* mutations and susceptibility to breast or ovarian carcinoma or to specific types of carcinoma are under investigation.[23,24]

In the clinical screening situation, 16% of women who had breast carcinoma and reported a family history of breast and/or ovarian carcinoma were found to have detectable

TABLE 10.1 Genetic Predisposition to Breast Carcinoma

Gene	Syndrome	Carcinomas	Other
BRCA1	Breast Ovarian	Breast, ovary	
BRCA2	Breast Ovarian	Breast, ovary, prostate, pancreas	Fanconi anemia in homozygotes
TP53	Li-Fraumeni	Breast, brain, soft tissue, bone, etc.	
PTEN	Cowden	Breast, ovary, thyroid, colon	Adenomas of thyroid, fibroids, gastrointestinal polyps
STKII/LKB1	Peutz-Jegher	Gastrointestinal, breast	Hamartomas of bowel, buccal pigmentation
ATM	Ataxia-Telangiectasia	Breast	Homozygotes: leukemia, lymphoma, cerebellar ataxia, immune deficiency, and telangiectasia
ATM	Site-specific breast	Breast	Low penetrance
MSH2/MLH1	Muir-Torre	Colorectal, breast	

All autosomal dominant.

Adapted from Harris JR, Lippman ME, Morrow M, et al. *Diseases of the breast*. 4th ed. Philadelphia: Wolters Kluwer-Lippincott Williams and Wilkins, 2010:210.

BRCA1 mutations.[25] *BRCA1* mutations were found in 7% women with breast carcinoma and a positive family history. No association was detected between bilateral breast carcinoma in the patient or the number of breast carcinomas in a family and the presence of a *BRCA1* mutation. These data add further support to the notion that *BRCA* mutations have variable penetrance and also suggest that alterations of other *BRCA* gene sites or entirely different genes are responsible for breast carcinoma in some women with a positive family history.

Pathology of *BRCA1* and *BRCA2* Breast Carcinomas

Various reports indicate that *BRCA1*-associated breast carcinomas have distinctive pathologic features, although they are not unique to these patients.[26–29] The intraductal and infiltrating duct carcinomas are typically poorly differentiated (grade 3) and have high-grade nuclei.[30–32] A relatively high frequency of medullary carcinomas and of ductal carcinomas with medullary features has been reported in these patients.[30] The tumors are also characterized by high proliferative rates when studied by flow cytometry or by MIB-1 immunohistochemistry (IHC).[26,28] *BRCA1*-associated breast carcinomas typically do not express estrogen receptor (ER)[26] or human epidermal growth factor 2/*neu* (HER2/*neu*) receptor,[26] but they exhibit p53 nuclear reactivity.[26] Angiogenesis may also be enhanced in *BRCA1*-associated carcinomas.[26]

A study from the Breast Cancer Linkage Consortium examined breast carcinomas from 118 *BRCA1* patients, 78 *BRCA2* patients, 244 non-*BRCA* familial carcinoma patients, and 547 controls.[31] *BRCA1* and *BRCA2* tumors had significantly higher grade than control tumors. Medullary carcinoma was significantly more frequent in the *BRCA1* than in the *BRCA2* and control groups. Lobular carcinoma *in situ* (LCIS) was significantly less frequent in the entire familial carcinoma group than in the controls, but there was not a significant difference between *BRCA1* and *BRCA2* mutation carriers in the frequency of LCIS. *BRCA1* carcinomas had significantly higher mitotic counts and greater pleomorphism than *BRCA2* or control tumors.

In a study of women with carcinomas diagnosed before age 40, Armes et al.[30] found that carcinomas associated with *BRCA1* mutations had significantly higher mitotic rates than carcinomas associated with *BRCA2* mutations and control tumors from women without *BRCA* mutations. *BRCA1*-related carcinomas were also more likely to have necrosis. No differences were observed between the three groups with regard to tumor size, the frequency of or number of nodal metastases, or the presence of lymphatic invasion in the breast.

Using tissue microarrays (TMAs), Palacios et al.[32] compared the immunohistochemical expression of a panel of markers in *BRCA1*-associated (n = 20) and *BRCA2*-associated (n = 18) breast carcinomas to the expression of these markers in breast carcinomas negative for *BRCA1* and *BRCA2* mutations (n = 37). In this study of relatively few cases, there was no statistically significant difference in the distribution of histologic types between the three groups. Non-*BRCA1* and non-*BRCA2* carcinomas were characterized by lower grade, more tubule formation, less nuclear pleomorphism, and fewer mitoses than the combined group of *BRCA1* or *BRCA2* mutation–associated carcinomas. When compared with *BRCA1* mutation tumors alone, the non-*BRCA1* or non-*BRCA2* mutation tumors had significantly less nuclear pleomorphism, fewer mitoses, and more tubule formation. When compared with *BRCA2* mutation tumors, the non-*BRCA1* or non-*BRCA2* tumors

TABLE 10.2 Risk Factors for Breast Carcinoma

	RR
Reproductive factors	
Early menarche	[+]
Age at birth of first child	[++]
Number of births	[+]
Age at menopause	[+]
Breast feeding	[–]
Hormonal factors	
Oral contraceptive (current vs. none)	[+]
Estrogen replacement (10+ yr vs. none)	[+]
Estrogen plus progesterone replacement (>5 yr vs. none)	[++]
High blood estrogen or androgen (postmenopausal)	[+++]
High prolactin	[++]
Nutritional and lifestyle factors	
Obesity (BMI: >30 vs. <25)	
Premenopausal	[–]
Postmenopausal	[+]
Adult weight gain, postmenopausal	[++]
Alcohol (one or more drinks/d vs. none)	[+]
Height (>5 ft 7 in.)	[+]
Physical activity (>3 h/wk)	[–]
Monounsaturated fat vs. saturated fat	[–]
Other factors	
Family history (mother and sister)[a]	[+++]
Family history (first-degree relative)[b]	[++]
Jewish heritage (affirmative vs. negative)	[+]
Ionizing radiation (affirmative vs. negative)	[+]
Benign breast disease (fibrocystic disease vs. none)	[++]

BMI, body mass index; OC, oral contraceptive; RR, relative risk. [+]: 1.1–1.4; [++]: 1.5–2.9; [+++]: 3.0–6.9; [–]: 0.7–0.8.

[a]Two first-degree relatives who have a history of breast cancer before age 65 versus no relative.

[b]First-degree relative who has a history of breast cancer before age 65 versus no relative. [+]: relative risk (RR): 1.1-1.4, [++]: 1.5-2.9, [+++]:3.0-6.9, [-]: 0.7-0.8.

Adapted from Harris JR, Lippman ME, Morrow M, et al. *Diseases of the breast*. 4th ed. Philadelphia: Wolters Kluwer-Lippincott Williams and Wilkins, 2010:279.

were only significantly different in having fewer mitoses. Non-*BRCA1* or non-*BRCA2* mutation tumors had significantly more frequent expression of ER, progesterone receptor (PR), and bcl-2 and less frequent expression of p53 than *BRCA1* mutation–associated carcinomas. They also had a lower proliferation index with the Ki67 immunostain. Non-*BRCA1* or non-*BRCA2* mutation tumors differed from those with *BRCA2* mutations only in having a low Ki67 index. There were no significant differences in the distribution of HER2/*neu* immunoreactivity or amplification of HER2/*neu* by fluorescence *in situ* hybridization (FISH) analysis. There were no instances of HER2/*neu* amplification in the *BRCA1* or *BRCA2* mutation–associated carcinomas. Amplification of C-Myc was significantly more frequent (62.5%) in *BRCA2*-associated carcinomas than in *BRCA1*-associated carcinomas or *BRCA1* or *BRCA2* mutation–negative carcinomas. These results suggested that "*BRCA2* tumors present characteristics intermediate between" *BRCA1* mutation–associated and *BRCA1* or *BRCA2* mutation–negative carcinomas. Bilateral breast carcinomas in *BRCA* mutation carriers tend to have similar patterns of marker expression.[33]

Age at the time of diagnosis influences the histologic features of breast carcinomas in *BRCA1* or *BRCA2* mutation carriers. Using TMA technology, Eerola et al.[34] compared carcinomas from patients younger than 50 years with those from women 50 years or older. Among *BRCA1* carriers, women 50 years and older had significantly fewer grade 3 carcinomas (47.1% vs. 84.4%), fewer ER-negative tumors (25% vs. 83.3%), and fewer p53-positive tumors (7.7% vs. 50%). All medullary carcinomas were in women younger than 50 years. When compared with non-*BRCA1* or non-*BRCA2* mutation carriers, those with *BRCA1* mutations and who were 50 years or older differed significantly only in having more frequent high-grade carcinomas.

The frequency of invasive lobular carcinoma in BRCA-associated patients has been controversial. One review found carcinomas with lobular features and LCIS to be significantly more frequent in women with *BRCA2* mutations than in those with *BRCA1*-associated carcinoma.[27] Armes et al.[30] found that pleomorphic lobular carcinoma was significantly more frequent in women with *BRCA2* than in those with *BRCA1* tumors. When compared with women with sporadic non–BRCA-associated carcinoma, there was not a significantly higher frequency of pleomorphic lobular carcinoma in the *BRCA2* group. Others have reported that there was not a significant difference in the frequency of invasive lobular carcinoma between *BRCA1*, *BRCA2*, and control carcinomas.[31]

BRCA genes might also play a role in the development of breast carcinoma through mechanisms other than gene mutations. These alternative pathways may be the consequence of other genetic alterations, which could have a negative effect on the tumor suppression function of the *BRCA* gene.[35]

Prognosis of *BRCA1*- and *BRCA2*-Associated Breast Carcinomas

The relationship between *BRCA1* and *BRCA2* mutations to breast carcinoma prognosis has been reported by a number of investigators. Some studies found no significant difference between disease-free and overall survival when patients with *BRCA1*-associated and sporadic carcinoma were compared.[29,36,37] Using a different method of analysis, Foulkes et al.[38] reported a statistically significant adverse prognosis among Ashkenazi Jewish women with *BRCA1* mutations compared with women from the same ethnic background, whose tumors did not exhibit *BRCA1* mutations.

Surgery for *BRCA1*- and *BRCA2*-Associated Breast Carcinoma

Because the risk of developing breast carcinoma associated with *BRCA1* and *BRCA2* most likely involves all tissues in both breasts, surgical treatment to substantially reduce or eliminate the risk requires bilateral prophylactic mastectomy.[39] Most of the reports of breast carcinoma occurring at the site of prophylactic mastectomy refer to patients treated by subcutaneous mastectomy. Residual breast tissue is substantially less likely to remain after a complete or total mastectomy with excision of the nipple–areola complex. The age at which the operation is performed influences the benefit derived with the estimated maximal gain in life expectancy from surgery to be in the third decade and little gain at age 60 or later.[40] Among *BRCA1* or *BRCA2* mutation carriers who have not developed breast carcinoma, bilateral prophylactic mastectomy has resulted in a relative risk (RR) reduction of 90% to 100%.[41–44] The efficacy of bilateral mastectomy for carcinoma prevention is influenced by other factors such as the type of surgery performed and whether the patient has also had a bilateral oophorectomy. The breast carcinoma risk reduction attributable to bilateral prophylactic oophorectomy alone ranges from 47% to 68%.[45–47]

Breast conservation therapy is a concern among women with *BRCA1* and *BRCA2* mutations because of the presumed high degree of risk in all breast tissues. Robson et al.[48] compared the outcome of breast-conserving therapy in Ashkenazi Jewish women with and without *BRCA1* or *BRCA2* mutations. Patients with BRCA mutations were younger at the time of diagnosis, they tended to develop ipsilateral breast recurrences more often, and they experienced substantially more frequent contralateral carcinomas. Mutation status was not predictive of distant disease-free survival (DFS) in multivariate analysis.

Haffty et al.[49] reported ipsilateral carcinoma recurrences after breast conservation treatment in 49% of women with BRCA mutation–associated carcinomas and in 21% of women with sporadic carcinomas during a 12-year follow-up. Contralateral carcinoma was diagnosed in 42% of mutation carriers and 9% of sporadic cases. Others have also reported a higher frequency of ipsilateral recurrences in mutation carriers (21.8%) than in sporadic carcinoma cases (12.1%).[50] Metcalfe et al.[51] reported that the risks of contralateral carcinoma with 10 years of follow-up were 43.4% and 34.6%, respectively, in *BRCA1* and *BRCA2* mutation carriers. A prospective follow-up study of 87 *BRCA1* and *BRCA2* mutation carriers who had breast conservation treatment found ipsilateral breast carcinoma recurrence risks of 11.2% and 13.6% after 5 and 10 years of follow-up, respectively.[52] Retrospective analysis of data on 160 *BRCA1* or *BRCA2* mutation carriers reported by Pierce et al.[53] revealed that the incidence of breast recurrence was not significantly increased among mutation carriers who underwent bilateral oophorectomy compared with sporadic controls. The risk of contralateral breast carcinoma in *BRCA1* or *BRCA2* carriers was significantly reduced by tamoxifen therapy, but remained higher than that in the control group.

Nonsurgical Management of *BRCA1*- and *BRCA2*-Associated Breast Carcinoma

One alternative to prophylactic mastectomy is careful clinical follow-up with frequent imaging studies, clinical examination, and breast self-examination. The sensitivity of mammography for detecting carcinoma in BRCA mutation carriers is significantly lower than it is as a general screening modality.[54] Factors that may contribute to lower sensitivity in this setting include the higher density of breast tissue in young women generally and in *BRCA1* or *BRCA2* mutation carriers[55,56] and the high frequency of circumscribed tumors suggestive of benign lesions as opposed to stellate tumors.[56] Tilanus-Linthorst et al.[56] reported finding a statistically significant correlation between false-negative mammography interpretations and "pushing" tumor margins.

The contributions of magnetic resonance imaging (MRI) and positron emission tomography (PET) scanning to early carcinoma detection in high-risk women with documented hereditary breast carcinoma susceptibility have also been investigated. MRI has been demonstrated to have greater sensitivity and specificity for the detection of carcinoma than mammography in *BRCA* mutation carriers or women predicted to be at high risk. In five studies published between 2000 and 2005, the diagnostic sensitivity of MRI ranged from 71.1% to 100%, and the range of specificity was 81% to 95.4%.[57–61] The frequency of axillary lymph node (ALN) metastases in high-risk women with MRI-detected carcinomas ranged from none[57] to 35.3%.[59] The proportion of MRI-detected carcinomas that measured 1 cm or less in these studies ranged from 43.2%[61] to 66.7%.[56] Long-term results of MRI screening in women with *BRCA* mutations are scant; however, the absence of distant recurrences in a series of 24 incident cancers detected on MRI after a median follow-up of 8.4 years since diagnosis is encouraging.[62]

Despite the advantages of MRI for the detection of tumor-forming carcinomas, mammography plays an important role in the surveillance of high-risk women because it is more effective for detecting nontumorous lesions with calcifications such as intraductal carcinoma.[58] Retrospective analysis of a large cohort of women with *BRCA* mutations found that radiation exposure in screening mammography did not result in a greater frequency of carcinoma than in a control population.[63] Nonetheless, the optimal use of mammography and MRI in surveillance of women at high risk may be influenced by patient age, with greater reliance on MRI among younger women and more frequent use of mammography with advancing age. A computer simulation model comparing various annual screening strategies in *BRCA1* and *BRCA2* gene mutation carriers showed annual MRI screening at age 25 and delayed alternating digital mammography starting at age 30 to be the most effective screening strategy.[64]

Chemoprevention in *BRCA1* and *BRCA2* Mutation Carriers

Chemoprevention has been less extensively investigated than mastectomy in *BRCA1* and *BRCA2* mutation carriers. Various strategies are emerging for the prevention of *BRCA* gene mutation–associated breast carcinoma.[65] Chemoprevention of breast carcinoma has been effective in prospective trials of women at high risk of developing breast carcinoma. Tamoxifen has been shown to reduce the risk of developing breast carcinoma in women with several high-risk factors, including a history of one or more first-degree relatives with breast carcinoma.[66,67] The risk reduction was 45% to 49%, depending on the number of affected relatives. The frequency of contralateral carcinoma is also reduced by the use of tamoxifen in adjuvant therapy for ipsilateral carcinoma, and it contributed to lowering the frequency of breast recurrence after conservation therapy.[68] Analysis of competing causes of mortality suggests adjuvant tamoxifen treatment results in a significant decrease in mortality by reducing deaths from contralateral carcinoma and from cardiovascular disease despite predisposing to endometrial carcinoma and thromboembolic events.[66,69]

Narod et al.[70] reported a 50% risk reduction of contralateral carcinoma in *BRCA* mutation carriers who received adjuvant tamoxifen treatment for ipsilateral carcinoma. The risk reduction was greater for *BRCA1* (62%) than for *BRCA2* (37%) mutation carriers. A risk reduction of 84% was observed in women who had prophylactic oophorectomy combined with adjuvant tamoxifen therapy. The fact that this study focused on women who received adjuvant tamoxifen for an index ipsilateral carcinoma suggests that many, if not most of the patients, had an ER-positive ipsilateral carcinoma. Data that specifically examine the role of tamoxifen in the prevention of contralateral breast carcinoma in *BRCA* mutation carriers with an ipsilateral ER-negative carcinoma are presently lacking.

Other Genes Associated with Breast Carcinoma

Several major genes that are less commonly identified than *BRCA1* and *BRCA2* have also been linked to a strong degree of breast carcinoma susceptibility (Table 10.1). These genes are typically involved in cancer syndromes such as *TP53* in the Li-Fraumeni syndrome,[71,72] *PTEN* in Cowden syndrome,[73] and *STK11* in Peutz–Jegher syndrome.[74]

Another group of genes that appears to confer an increased risk of breast carcinoma has been referred to as low-penetrance genes. These genes may account for some instances of nonfamilial or sporadic breast carcinoma. Their influence on breast carcinoma risk is probably mediated through the interaction of other factors such as the metabolism of environmental carcinogens or hormone metabolism. Examples of low-penetrance genes are *GSTM1*, a glutathione-S-transferase, which is involved in carcinogen metabolism,[75,76] and *AIBI*, the Amplified In Breast cancer gene, which is involved in estrogen signal transduction in breast cells.[77]

The Multistep Process of Mammary Carcinogenesis

Genetic changes associated with transitions from normal epithelium to hyperplasia, and ultimately carcinoma, involve a series of events referred to as initiation, transformation, and progression. Few proliferative lesions actually advance through all of these steps to become invasive carcinomas, and it is likely that most never progress beyond early stages of initiation that may be represented in some but not necessarily in all instances by hyperplasia.

The multistep process for the development of breast carcinoma was reviewed by Simpson et al.,[78] who drew attention to the importance of molecular (genotypic) and morphologic (phenotypic) abnormalities. The data suggest that there are two important pathways for carcinogenesis that result in low-grade and high-grade carcinomas, respectively. Low-grade carcinomas are typically ER positive, PR positive, and HER2/*neu* negative and have genetic losses in 16q. On the other hand, high-grade carcinomas are characterized as being positive for HER2/*neu* and negative for ER and PR and as having genetic losses or gains at multiple loci. These authors presented data to support the hypothesis that the majority of low-grade carcinomas are derived from columnar cell hyperplasia and high-grade carcinomas may evolve from apocrine metaplasia. Morphologic support for these ideas can be observed in the frequent coexistence of tubular carcinoma with columnar cell lesions and the frequent presence of apocrine cytologic features in high-grade ductal carcinoma.

One interesting prospect is suggested by studies of markers associated with pulmonary carcinoma. Tockman[79] used IHC to retrospectively examine the distribution of hnRNP and a ceramide related to Lewis-X antigens, two markers associated with carcinoma, in "moderately atypical sputum epithelial cells" preserved in archived cytology specimens. The samples were obtained in a screening program for individuals at high risk of developing pulmonary carcinoma. Expression of the markers was found in atypical cells from 91% of patients who later developed carcinoma and in only 5 of 40 (12.5%) who did not develop carcinoma. A second study employed the same markers to investigate previously treated patients followed for evidence of new primary or recurrent carcinomas.[80] Only 6% of subsequent lung carcinomas were anticipated by finding abnormal cells on routine cytologic examination in this population. Employing quantitative IHC, the authors were able to detect marker overexpression in sputum samples from 92% of patients with second primary carcinomas. The hypothesis underlying the aforementioned investigations of pulmonary carcinoma patients is equally applicable as a model for mammary carcinogenesis. This is based on the concept of field carcinogenesis,[81] which holds that transformation occurs widely in epithelium exposed to a carcinogenic stimulus, but that progression occurs unevenly.

Provocative observations that relate genetic alterations to breast carcinoma risk are reports of loss of heterozygosity (LOH) in morphologically normal lobular glands near breast carcinomas. Deng et al.[82] found that among 10 specimens with LOH at 3p22 to 25 in a breast carcinoma, 6 exhibited the same LOH in histologically normal-appearing lobules taken from tissue surrounding the carcinoma. Corresponding LOH in normal-appearing lobules was found less often for carcinomas that displayed LOH at 17p13.1 and 11p15.5. Larson et al.[83] studied genetic changes represented by LOH in the histologically normal-appearing tissue of women with sporadic breast carcinoma and in women with *BRCA1* gene mutations. LOH was studied in microdissected terminal duct lobular units (TDLUs) from 18 patients with sporadic breast carcinoma, 16 with *BRCA1* mutations and breast carcinoma, and from the breast reduction specimens of 18 women without carcinoma. LOH was detected in TDLU from 5 of 18 (23%) reduction mammoplasty specimens, 15 of 18 (83%) of sporadic carcinoma patients, and 13 of 16 (81%) of *BRCA1* mutation patients ($p = 0.0007$). The adjusted odds ratio (OR) for LOH in TDLU compared with the reduction mammoplasty group was 15.5 for women with sporadic carcinoma and 13.7 for *BRCA1* mutation carriers. The greatest difference was seen in chromosome17q where the ORs for LOH were 12.4 and 4.9 for *BRCA1*-associated and sporadic carcinoma patients, respectively.

Several explanations have been suggested for these findings. One is the possibility that isolated carcinoma cells could be present in seemingly normal lobules as a result of pagetoid spread from the primary tumor. Alternatively, some stages in the process of transformation to carcinoma could occur in cells that retain a "normal" phenotype, prior to the appearance of histologically detectable hyperplasia. The latter scenario includes the possibility that the hyperplastic phenotype can be evanescent or entirely bypassed during carcinogenesis. The absence of hyperplasia at the site of or in the vicinity of some mammary carcinomas is consistent with this hypothesis.

The clonality of histologically normal breast tissue has been investigated by studying the pattern of X-chromosome inactivation in normal contiguous lobules and ducts.[84] The analysis revealed patches of glands with a single X-chromosome inactivated, indicating the existence of discrete clonal regions within the breast. The existence of genetically different but histologically identical-appearing patches of breast glandular parenchyma could provide an explanation for the heterogeneous distribution of proliferative and neoplastic lesions in the breasts. This observation was confirmed by Diallo et al.,[85] who demonstrated the monoclonal origin of TDLU, duct hyperplasia, intraductal papillomas, and intraductal carcinomas and by Larson et al.[86]

Another approach to the study of clonality in the normal breast was described by Lakhani et al.,[87] who performed LOH analysis on colonies of epithelial and myoepithelial cells isolated *in vitro* from fresh breast specimens. LOH present in invasive carcinomas was also identified in adjacent normal-appearing tissue, and under the conditions of the study was not attributable to pagetoid spread of carcinoma cells. LOH was detected in epithelial and myoepithelial cells, providing evidence that the lobule is a clonal structure with both cell types derived from a common stem cell. Analysis of clones derived from normal tissue not in proximity to a carcinoma also revealed LOH. This indicated that genetic alterations that probably occur early in breast development can be heterogeneously distributed in the breast and not limited to a localized region. LOH was also found in epithelial/myoepithelial clones from samples of breast tissue obtained in reduction mammoplasties in the absence of carcinoma.

Clonal analysis has also been applied to the study of bilateral breast carcinomas. Discordant distribution of six immunohistochemical markers in paired samples of bilateral tumors from 51 women reported by Dawson et al.[88] was indicative of independent origin of the carcinomas. Independent clonal origin of bilateral breast carcinomas was also demonstrated by Noguchi et al.[89] Shibata et al.[90] detected different X-chromosome inactivation patterns of the *AR* gene between left and right breast tumors in three patients, indicating independent clonal origin of the neoplasms. Two patients had nonidentical *p53* mutations in both tumors, and in nine instances, *p53* mutations were identified in only one of the two neoplasms. The absence of concordant results with either procedure is further evidence supporting the strong probability that bilateral breast carcinomas are not only clonally independent but that they can arise from genetically distinct epithelial patches, possibly through differing genetic mechanisms.

PROLIFERATIVE (FIBROCYSTIC) BREAST CHANGES

Biopsy-proven benign proliferative or fibrocystic changes, previously referred to as "fibrocystic disease," have been identified as morphologic markers of risk of the development of breast carcinoma. The most extensive studies have been retrospective investigations in which the diagnosis of biopsy specimens was reclassified many years after surgery and correlated with follow-up. Few investigations have been prospective analyses that related the initial diagnostic classification to subsequent outcome. The majority of investigators have analyzed groups consisting of many hundreds or thousands of patients,[91–95] and a few have dealt with highly selected, smaller series.[96–98] A number of observations and conclusions can be drawn from these reports. (See also Chapters 9 and 31 for additional information about atypical ductal hyperplasia [ADH] and atypical lobular hyperplasia [ALH], respectively.)

- **The etiology of proliferative changes in the human breast has received less attention than the precancerous risk associated with these lesions.**

Because of the association of proliferative changes with the development of carcinoma, it is reasonable to speculate that both conditions could have common predisposing factors. This has been borne out by the finding that the risk of biopsy-proven proliferative breast disease is significantly increased by nulliparity, late age of first birth, and late menopause, factors also associated with increased breast carcinoma risk.[99–102] Dietary breast carcinoma risk factors such as high intake of meat fat[102] and caffeine[103] have also been associated with a greater risk of proliferative breast disease. Although most of the foregoing investigations did not specify a relationship with particular proliferative changes, the analysis of meat fat revealed a strong association between frequent consumption and an elevated risk of severe atypia and *in situ* carcinoma.[104] Boyle et al.[103] reported that excess caffeine consumption was associated with ALH and with sclerosing adenosis (SA) accompanied by duct hyperplasia. An inverse relationship between dietary fiber content and the risk of benign proliferative breast disease has been reported.[105,106] A similar relationship was observed between dietary fiber intake and breast density.[107] The mechanism by which dietary fiber influences mammary epithelial proliferation is as yet unknown, but it might involve estrogen metabolism or substances associated with fiber-containing foods such as phytoestrogens.

No consistent association between proliferative changes in the breast and a family history of breast carcinoma has been found,[99,108] although one study reported a slightly higher frequency of atypical hyperplasia in women with a positive family history than among those without.[109] Obesity or excess body mass[100,110] and the use of oral contraceptives[100,101,108] are factors associated with a decreased risk of benign breast disease.

Ionizing radiation is a well-documented cause of breast carcinoma after doses associated with atom bomb exposure, multiple diagnostic x-ray tests, or radiation therapy for benign conditions.[111–113] There was also a significant positive association between radiation exposure from the atomic bomb and the prevalence of proliferative changes, particularly atypical hyperplasia, in the breasts of survivors.[114] The latter association was strongest in women exposed when they were 40 to 49 years old. The increased risk of breast carcinoma after atom bomb radiation exposure occurred largely in women exposed prior to age 40.

- **Surgical and needle core biopsy are currently the most reliable methods for establishing the presence of prognostically significant atypical hyperplasia in individual patients. Fine-needle aspiration (FNA) cytology and mammography are useful adjunctive procedures.**

Needle core biopsy has largely replaced FNA as a method to sample nonpalpable mammographically detected breast lesions, despite emerging opportunities available *via* minimally invasive cytologic sampling.[115] A broad spectrum of pathologic abnormalities is encountered in this biopsy material, including a substantial number of proliferative foci with varying degrees of atypia.[116,117] The mammographic appearance of these lesions is usually not predictive of specific histologic abnormalities, but atypical duct hyperplasia is not infrequently present. Surgical biopsy is indicated if the sampling obtained with a needle core biopsy results in a diagnosis of atypical duct hyperplasia because these abnormalities have been found to be associated with carcinoma in about 25% of cases (see Chapters 9 and 11).

One continuing application of FNA has been in the study of asymptomatic women in families with a known history of breast carcinoma. Employing aspirates from four quadrants, Skolnick et al.[118] compared 77 women from 20 families with two first-degree affected relatives with 31 controls. Proliferative breast disease characterized as the cytologic diagnosis of "moderate to marked ductal hyperplasia or atypical hyperplasia" was found significantly more often (35%) in relatives of breast carcinoma patients than in controls (13%). Genetic analysis suggested that inherited susceptibility was responsible for the proliferative breast changes and for breast carcinoma in the families. Khan et al.[119] did a similar study using FNA to assess the contralateral breasts of 32 women with sporadic breast carcinoma in one breast and 38 control subjects without breast carcinoma. Cytospin preparations prepared from pooled four-quadrant aspirations revealed a significantly higher frequency of proliferative changes and atypical hyperplasia in samples from the contralateral breasts of patients with breast carcinoma. Overall, 40% of the specimens were deemed inadequate because of insufficient cellularity. Low cellularity was significantly more common in control samples and was associated with obesity and age greater than 50 years. An important limitation of these studies is that surgical biopsies were not performed to confirm the cytologic interpretations and to characterize the proliferative lesions histologically.

Mammographic patterns have been studied extensively as possible indicators of breast carcinoma risk. A classification of patterns introduced by Wolfe[120] in the 1970s had four categories, which appeared to be associated with increasing risk. N1 described the predominantly fatty breast with the least risk. Intermediate risk was associated with P1 and P2 mammograms marked by linear densities indicative of a prominent ductal pattern. DY, the highest risk category, described nodular or plaque-like densities referred to in radiologic terms as "mammographic dysplasia." Quantitative classifications based on estimates of the proportion of the breast volume affected by parenchymal patterns such as DY were introduced to improve mammographic risk estimates.[121,122]

Studies of the association between Wolfe mammographic patterns and specific histopathologic findings in the breast did not result in consistent findings. Some investigators reported significant associations between proliferative epithelial changes, epithelial hyperplasia, and radiographic patterns.[123,124] In one study, follow-up of women enrolled in a screening program revealed a 9.7-fold increased risk of subsequent carcinoma *in situ* (CIS) or atypical hyperplasia in women with the greatest mammographic density, compared with women with no mammographic density.[123] They also found a 12.2-fold greater risk of hyperplasia without atypia in the group of women with the greatest density. Urbanski et al.[124] reported a trend to more frequent atypical hyperplasia in women whose concurrent preoperative mammograms showed the greatest mammographic "dysplasia."

Conversely, Moskowitz et al.[125] and Arthur et al.[126] found no association between mammographic pattern and histopathologic changes in concurrent biopsies.

Unfortunately, the foregoing mammography studies and others on this subject are not comparable because of substantial methodologic differences in mammography technology, mammographic classification, and pathology review. It seems likely that a major component of dense mammographic parenchymal patterns is the fibrous stroma, an association noted in some studies.[127,128] Proliferative epithelial lesions are accompanied by increased stromal density to a greater extent in premenopausal than in postmenopausal women. However, premenopausal women with constitutionally dense mammary stroma and abundant glandular tissue lacking proliferative changes may not be distinguishable mammographically.

- **A minority of women with biopsies classified as nonproliferative or proliferative subsequently develop carcinoma in either breast.**

In published reports, the overall proportion of women with an antecedent breast biopsy who later developed breast carcinoma rarely exceeded 10%, even with follow-up of two decades or more. Bodian et al.[129] detected subsequent breast carcinoma in 139 of 1,521 patients (9.1%) with proliferative changes and in 18 of 278 (6.5%) with nonproliferative biopsies within a follow-up period of 21 years. Overall, 8.7% of the patients developed breast carcinoma. In other reports involving at least 1,000 patients, the proportions of women who developed carcinoma after a benign breast biopsy were 2.2%,[130] 2.9%,[91] 4.1%,[131] 4.6%,[132] and 4.9%[96] (Table 10.3). The proportion of patients with subsequent carcinoma tended to increase with length of follow-up, being least in a group followed for fewer than 5 years[133] and highest when follow-up was more than a decade.[91,125,126] This observation is consistent with the rising risk of developing breast carcinoma with advancing age. Against this background, there is evidence that the RR associated with proliferative changes may be attenuated or decrease with time and advancing age.[134]

The frequency of breast carcinoma in previously biopsied women who had proliferative changes exceeds that of unbiopsied normal controls, but only a small proportion of patients with proliferative lesions develop carcinoma. Proliferative breast changes are one of several so-called attributable risk factors, a list that also includes family history of breast carcinoma, parity, age at menarche, age of first birth, and others. An American Cancer Society (ACS) survey published in 1982 found that not more than 30% of women with breast carcinoma had any known attributable risk factor.[135] Data from the first National Health and Nutrition Examination Survey reported in 1995 indicated that approximately 47% (95% confidence interval [CI], 17% to 77%) of breast carcinoma in the study cohort was attributable to known risk factors (first birth after age 20 or nulliparity, family history of breast carcinoma, and high income) and by extrapolation for approximately 41% (95% CI, 2% to 80%) of breast carcinoma in the United States.[136] Consequently, intervention to prevent breast carcinoma limited to women with "precancerous" proliferative changes may have a relatively small impact on the overall frequency of and mortality due to breast carcinoma unless additional therapeutic indications that apply to many more individuals can be identified to select women for chemoprevention therapy.

- **The risk of carcinoma subsequent to unilateral biopsy-proven proliferative changes affects both breasts.**

TABLE 10.3 Frequency of Breast Carcinoma Following Biopsy-Proven Atypical Hyperplasia

References	Length of Follow-Up (Mean or Average, y)	Total No. Patients	Total CA Patients No. (%)	Total No. AH Patients (% AH of Total Patients)	No. of AH Patients with CA	CA in AH patients	
						% AH Patients	% Total CA Patients
Kodlin et al.[130,a]	–	2,931	64 (2.2)	4 (1.7)	3	6.1	4.7
Carter et al.[91]	8.3	16,692	485 (2.9)	1,305 (7.8)	67	5.1	13.8
Dupont and Page[131]	17	3,303	135 (4.1)	232 (7.0)	30	12.9	22.2
Krieger and Hiatt[96,a]	16	2,731	135 (4.9)	52 (1.9)	5	9.6	3.7
Bodian et al.[129]	21	1,799	157 (8.7)	342[b] (19)	33	9.6	21
				272[c]	25	9.1	15.9
			70[d]	8 (5.3)	11.4	5	

AH, atypical hyperplasia; CA, carcinoma.
[a]Atypical hyperplasia defined as Black and Chabon grade 4.[160]
[b]Data below represent subsets of 342.
[c]Hyperplasia with mild atypia.
[d]Hyperplasia with moderate to severe atypia.

The bilaterality of risk was noted by Davis et al.[137] in a review of 297 patients with "cystic disease." These authors also tabulated data from 11 published reports with at least 100 patients who had "cystic disease," showing that 0.7% to 4.9% of patients subsequently developed carcinoma, with 50% of the carcinomas in the contralateral breast.

Krieger and Hiatt[96] found that only 56% of carcinomas that were diagnosed subsequent to a benign biopsy occurred in the previously biopsied breast that had had benign proliferative changes. Laterality of subsequent carcinoma was not significantly influenced by the type of antecedent proliferative change or the age at biopsy. The mean interval to subsequent ipsilateral carcinomas (11.2 years) was less than for contralateral carcinomas (14 years). Page et al.[94] reported that 8 of 18 (44%) carcinomas subsequent to atypical duct hyperplasia and 5 of 16 (31%) carcinomas following ALH occurred in the contralateral breast. Involvement of the contralateral breast in similar proportions of patients was also described by Connolly et al.[138]

An exception to the foregoing reports of bilateral risk was described by Tavassoli and Norris,[98] who found carcinoma in the ipsilateral breast of 10 of 14 (71%) women who had lesions they classified as duct hyperplasia or atypical duct hyperplasia. Although this unusual distribution of laterality could have been a chance event in a relatively small series of cases, it is more likely reflective of the authors' method for defining atypical hyperplasia with a size criterion that can result in classifying some intraductal carcinomas, lesions associated with the greatest increased ipsilateral risk, as atypical hyperplasia.

These data from various sources suggest that the risk of carcinoma is nearly equally divided between the two breasts after proliferative changes are detected in one breast. It appears that epithelial hyperplasia is a marker of a disturbance that may variably affect the entire mammary epithelium. The bilateral risk of subsequent carcinoma associated with proliferative lesions is in striking contrast to the strong tendency for subsequent invasive carcinoma to arise in the ipsilateral breast following intraductal carcinoma. This difference in laterality reflects fundamental biologic changes affecting the mammary epithelium, associated with transitions from marker to precursor, and ultimately to obligate precursor lesions for invasive mammary carcinoma.

- **The chance of developing breast carcinoma is influenced by nonmorphologic factors that may modify the level of risk associated with benign proliferative changes.**

The pathologic findings in a biopsy from an individual patient cannot be viewed out of the clinical context. Age at diagnosis proved to be an additive factor in a study by Carter et al.,[91] who found a sixfold increase in the rate of subsequent breast carcinoma among biopsied patients younger than 46 years with atypical hyperplasia compared with "normal" women. The rate was increased 3.7-fold in women with atypical hyperplasia who were 46 to 55 years of age and 2.3-fold in women older than 55. London et al.[92] also observed an inverse relationship between age and risk in which the RR increased 2.6-fold among premenopausal women who had biopsy-proven atypia compared with postmenopausal subjects. Page et al.[95] reported that the risk associated with ALH was inversely related to age, being greatest in women biopsied before age 45. In the latter study, increased risk attributable to atypical duct hyperplasia was observed only in patients older than 45 years at biopsy.

A history of breast carcinoma among first-degree female relatives is a particularly strong additive factor in women who have atypical hyperplasia. Page et al.[94] and Dupont and Page[139] found that the risk associated with atypical lobular and atypical duct hyperplasia was more than doubled in women with a positive family history compared with the risk without this factor. London et al.[92] found that the increased risk associated with family history was strongest in patients with atypical hyperplasia. RR was not increased by a positive family history in women with nonproliferative biopsies.

Ahmed et al.[140] compared women with breast carcinoma and a prior benign breast biopsy to a cohort of breast carcinoma patients not previously biopsied. Epidemiologic factors that were present significantly more often among women with a prior benign breast biopsy were a positive family history of breast carcinoma and postmenopausal hormone use. Age at the time of breast carcinoma diagnosis was not significantly different between the two groups, and they did not differ significantly with respect to reproductive factors (age at menarche, age of first pregnancy, or the number of pregnancies). Patients with a prior benign breast biopsy were more likely to have lobular carcinoma, smaller tumors, and fewer ALNs with metastatic carcinoma, although the overall frequencies of nodal involvement were not significantly different. The frequency of ER-positive tumors did not differ significantly between the two groups. Patients with prior benign breast disease had a significantly better 10-year DFS than those without a history of benign breast disease. Prior benign biopsies were not reviewed in this study.

- **Among women who have had a benign breast biopsy, the risk of developing subsequent carcinoma is related to the histologic components of the antecedent biopsy.**

In 1978, Page et al.[95] stated that "women with... sclerosing adenosis... were at no greater risk of subsequent carcinoma than women in the general population." Subsequently, the same investigators reported that SA was an additive factor, increasing the risk for women with a family history of breast carcinoma.[141] When assessed independently, SA has been associated with an increased risk in several studies.[98,130,132,139,141,142] Some of these investigators reported a greater increase in risk for relatively small groups of women who had atypical hyperplasia and SA.[97,138,140] Bodian et al.[129] reported a high RR associated with adenosis but no significant difference in risk between patients who had adenosis with or without coexistent atypical hyperplasia.

The RR associated with other proliferative lesions exclusive of atypical hyperplasia is less well documented. Increased risk has been associated with papillary apocrine metaplasia,[94] with "pink cell" metaplasia,[142] and with the presence of microcalcifications detected histologically.[132,139]

A detailed analysis of the relationship of apocrine change to breast carcinoma risk was reported by Page et al.[143] in 1996. Lesions were subdivided on the basis of proliferative pattern into three categories: simple, complex, and highly complex. The RR of developing subsequent carcinoma compared with the expected frequency from the Third National Cancer Survey was slightly increased in women with simple (RR, 1.39) and complex lesions (RR, 1.30), and substantially increased by the presence of highly complex apocrine change (RR, 3.14). Further analysis revealed that atypical hyperplasia in nonapocrine tissue contributed to the risk associated with apocrine change. After exclusion of patients with coexisting atypical hyperplasia, the RRs were 1.29, 0.90, and 2.0 for simple, complex, and highly complex apocrine change, respectively. Although none of these RRs represented a "statistically" significant increase, the RR of highly complex lesions remained substantially higher than the other two categories, and the 95% CIs for patients with complex apocrine change and coexisting atypical hyperplasia (RR, 3.14; 95% CI, 1.3 to 7.6) and for patients without coexisting atypical hyperplasia (RR, 2.0; 95% CI, 0.77 to 7.4) were nearly identical.

The fact that patients in the foregoing study deemed to have highly complex apocrine change exhibited the greatest RR of subsequent carcinoma may have resulted from the inclusion of patients with apocrine intraductal carcinoma in the highly complex apocrine category. The authors acknowledged this with their observation "that patterns within the highly complex category of papillary apocrine change are close to the patterns noted in McDivitt et al.[144] as indicating carcinoma *in situ* of ductal pattern." A further explanation of the distinction between highly complex papillary apocrine change (PAC) and apocrine intraductal carcinoma was offered:

> This is little problem in differential diagnosis, as is usually the case, the alteration of PAC is <2 mm in extent. When the lesion is >4–8 mm in size or has >25% of nuclei with alternate patterns, some form of atypia or low grade DCIS (duct carcinoma *in situ*) may be diagnosed.... We believe that these relatively concise rules foster interobserver agreement in this area, but there is no practical reason to separate simple PAC from complex PAC. Also, the occurrence of highly complex PAC is of practical importance only in avoiding overdiagnosing a borderline lesion, which it is not.

Upon reflection, the report does not provide a crisp distinction between highly complex PAC and apocrine intraductal carcinoma, and the authors themselves suggest that some of the lesions which they included as "highly complex PAC" might be interpreted as intraductal carcinoma. On this basis, highly complex PAC, as described by Page et al.,[143] should be distinguished from a simple and complex PAC, and it is likely that most of the increased RR in highly complex PAC group was attributable to contamination by a subset of women who had apocrine intraductal carcinoma.

A report published in 1998 by the Cancer Committee of the College of American Pathologists defined the RR of breast carcinoma associated with proliferative breast lesions based on published data[145] (Table 10.4).

- **A higher RR is associated with atypical hyperplasia than with other proliferative lesions.**

The proportion of patients who develop carcinoma is highest in the group of women with atypical hyperplasia, intermediate in those with proliferative changes without atypia, and least when there are no proliferative changes (Tables 10.4 and 10.5).

Proliferative changes were identified in 152 (85%) of 1,799 biopsies studied by Bodian et al.[129] Moderate to severe atypia was present in 70 specimens, representing 3.8% of all cases and 4.6% of specimens with proliferative changes. Follow-up revealed that the RR of developing carcinoma compared with the general population represented by data from the Connecticut Tumor Registry was higher in women with any proliferative changes (RR, 2.2) than in those with nonproliferative biopsies (RR, 1.6). Within the group with proliferative changes, the RR ranged from 3.0 for moderate to severe atypia, to 2.3 for mild atypia, and 2.1 for hyperplasia without atypia. These differences in RR were not statistically significant, but the RR of each of the categories of hyperplasia was significantly increased compared with controls. The RRs associated with proliferative changes in ducts and lobules were similar, except for severe atypia where the

TABLE 10.4 Relative Risk of Invasive Carcinoma Associated with Benign Lesions in a Prior Breast Biopsy

• NO INCREASED RISK[a]
Adenosis, other than SA
Duct ectasia
FA lacking complex features
Fibrosis
Mastitis
Hyperplasia without atypia
Cysts, gross or microscopic
Simple apocrine metaplasia without associated or adenosis
Squamous metaplasia
• SLIGHTLY INCREASED RISK (1.5–2.0)
Complex FA
Moderate or florid hyperplasia without atypia
SA
Solitary papilloma without atypical hyperplasia
• MODERATELY INCREASED RISK (4.0–5.0)
ADH
ALH

Based on the study of Fitzgibbons et al.[145]
[a]Relative risk determined by comparison with women who did not have a breast biopsy.

TABLE 10.5 Breast Carcinoma Following Benign Breast Biopsy

References	Length of Follow-up (Average or Mean, y)	No. Patients	No. NP (% Total Patients)	No. CA in NP Patients (% Total Patients)	No. PDWA (% Total Patients)	No. CA in PDWA Patients (% PDWA)	No. AH (% Total Patients)	No. CA in AH Patients (% AH)	No. Total CA (% Total Patients)
Bodian et al.[129]	21	1,799	362 (20)	30 (8.2)	1,095 (60.8)	94 (8.6)	272[a] (15.1)	25 (9.1)	157 (8.7)
							70[b] (3.9)	8 (11.4)	
Dupont and Page[131]	17	3,303	1,378 (41.7)	31 (2.2)	1,693 (51.2)	74 (4.3)	232 (7)	30 (12.9)	135 (4.1)
Carter et al.[91]	8	16,692	6,615 (39.6)	147 (2.2)	8,772 (52.5)	271 (3.1)	1,305 (7.8)	67 (5.1)	485 (2.9)
Moskowitz et al.[133]	~4	1,408	832 (59)	2 (0.02)	503 (35.7)	6 (1.1)	76 (5.3)	5 (6.6)	13 (0.09)

NP, nonproliferative; PDWA, proliferative without atypia; AH, atypical hyperplasia; CA, carcinoma.
[a]All atypical hyperplasias.
[b]Moderate and severe atypical hyperplasias.

risk of ductal lesions (RR, 3.9) was significantly greater than that for severe atypia in lobules (RR, 2.6). Because the combined number of cases with severe atypia in ducts or in lobules was only 70 and five carcinomas occurred in this group, this distinction may not be clinically important because of the few events, even if statistically significant.

Page et al.[94] found the RRs to be 4.7 and 5.8, respectively, for women with atypical duct and ALH compared with women who had nonproliferative biopsies. The RR for women with atypical duct hyperplasia and a family history of breast carcinoma was increased further compared with women with nonproliferative biopsies who had a positive family history.[94] London et al.[92] found the RR of atypical hyperplasia to be 3.7, significantly greater than in women who had proliferative (RR, 1.6) and nonproliferative (RR, 1.0) biopsy samples without atypia. Premenopausal women with atypical hyperplasia had a higher RR (RR, 5.9) than postmenopausal patients (RR, 2.3).

Ma and Boyd[146] undertook a metaanalysis of studies that investigated the association between atypical hyperplasia and breast cancer risk. Fifteen reports between 1960 and 1992 fulfilled the authors' requirements for inclusion in the study, resulting in a total sample size of 182,980 women. The overall OR in comparison with controls for the development of carcinoma in women with atypical hyperplasia was 3.67 (95% CI, 3.16 to 4.26).

- **Regardless of the definition of atypia, the majority of carcinomas subsequent to a benign breast biopsy occur in women who did not have atypical hyperplasia.**

As shown in Table 10.3, the proportion of all subsequent carcinomas that occurred in women with prior biopsy-proven atypical hyperplasia ranged from 3.7% to 22.2%. More than 75% and in some studies more than 90% of subsequent carcinomas developed in women without biopsy-proven antecedent atypical hyperplasia. This conclusion is also supported by several case-control studies.[92,93,147,148] In these reports, subsequent carcinomas were preceded by biopsy-proven atypical hyperplasia in 14.7%[147] to 22.2%[92] of cases, and atypical hyperplasia was present in 2.2%[148] to 10.5%[92] of controls who did not develop carcinoma.

- **Atypical hyperplasia is diagnosed in a small proportion of benign breast biopsies. The frequency of atypia is influenced by the strictness of criteria defining the condition, rarely exceeding 10% of specimens studied.**

In the studies listed in Table 10.3, the frequency of atypical hyperplasia varied from 1.7% to 7.8% of biopsies, except for the report by Bodian et al.,[129] in which 19% of biopsies were classified as atypical hyperplasia. However, most of the latter were classified as mild atypical hyperplasia, and the 70 specimens with moderate to severe atypia constituted only 5.3% of all biopsies in the series.

- **Despite attempts to refine and improve the specificity of definitions of atypical hyperplasia, there are substantial differences in the interpretation of these lesions.**

In 1916, Bloodgood[149] introduced the term *borderline* for lesions about which "both the surgeon and pathologist are in doubt," and he stated that "if women come early we shall find that the borderline group is large." In this prophetic statement, Bloodgood anticipated current circumstances achieved after decades of effort to improve the early detection and diagnosis of breast carcinoma. The emergence of so-called borderline proliferative lesions as a major diagnostic and therapeutic problem is a result of several factors.

These include the widespread use of mammography (which has made it possible to detect many of these abnormalities clinically), epidemiologic studies relating increased risk of developing breast carcinoma to proliferative breast changes, and growing interest in preventing breast carcinoma.

Bloodgood tested the level of agreement among pathologists on the diagnosis of borderline lesions and reported the results of his trial as follows:

> I have submitted over sixty borderline cases to a number of pathologists, and have found that in not a single one has there been uniform agreement as to whether the lesion was benign or malignant. This is no reflection on the diagnostic abilities of the pathologists; it is simply evidence that at the present time there are certain lesions of the breast about which we apparently do not agree from the microscopic appearance only.[149]

Five years later, Bloodgood reported the following conclusion about the diagnosis of proliferative lesions:

> In breast lesions, when good pathologists disagree as to malignancy, the patient lives; when there is agreement, there is always a large percentage of deaths from cancer.[150]

The problem of diagnosing "borderline" lesions persists as illustrated in a report by Bodian et al.[151] To assess diagnostic reproducibility, 63 cases were chosen at random to be interspersed twice in a review of 1,799 biopsies in a manner that was inapparent to the reviewers. There were no disagreements on the diagnosis of intraductal or invasive carcinoma in 5 cases and of lobular neoplasia/LCIS in 10 cases. Disagreements were encountered in 17 of the remaining 48 cases. Interpretations differed in 9 of the 48 cases (19%) with respect to the presence of hyperplasia, resulting in a very low estimated concordance of 0.29. Among 39 cases in which hyperplasia was diagnosed on both reviews, the type of hyperplasia (ductal or lobular) differed in 11 instances. In a separate analysis by the same investigators, 219 of 240 cases (91%) originally diagnosed as hyperplasia without atypia by one pathologist were confirmed by a second pathologist, and 21 were reclassified as having mild or moderate atypia. The authors concluded that there are "sufficient problems with reproducibility of these criteria to suggest caution in making precise risk estimates for specific features of borderline conditions, particularly at the individual patient level."[151]

One of the largest and most complex attempts to assess the reproducibility of the histologic diagnosis of proliferative lesions and carcinomas was conducted in Italy.[152] This project involved 16 pathologists practicing in university or community hospitals in 10 Italian cities. A single set of 82 slides was circulated to the participants "after an initial meeting in which general criteria were discussed." Each case was classified in diagnostic categories employing a slight modification of groupings previously outlined at a consensus meeting in the United States.[153] Diagnostic categories adopted for the study were (1) nonproliferative or proliferative without atypia; (2) atypical ductal and/or lobular hyperplasia; (3) CIS, ductal or lobular; and (4) invasive carcinoma. For analysis, comparisons were made with a standard that was defined as the diagnosis most frequently reported by the panel. The overall kappa value for agreement with the consensus diagnosis was 0.72. High levels of agreement were reached for invasive carcinoma (0.89) and benign lesions without atypia (0.77). Agreement was "relatively good" (0.69) for *in situ* carcinoma and "poor" for atypical hyperplasia (0.33).

A study similar to the one reported by Palli et al.[152] was undertaken in the United States by 10 pathologists from academic and community hospitals.[154] A set of 31 slides representing ductal, lobular, and papillary lesions was reviewed by each participant. Overall agreement on the diagnosis of carcinoma was recorded for 10 (32.3%) cases (kappa, 0.347), on lesion type (ductal, lobular, and papillary) in 17 (54.8%) cases (kappa, 0.789), and for diagnosis in 8 (25.8%) cases (kappa, 0.537).

Pathologists do not differ appreciably from their clinical colleagues in regard to problems of observer reproducibility. The decision-making process that leads a pathologist to classify specific microscopic findings as hyperplasia, atypical hyperplasia, or CIS is similar to that of a radiologist interpreting an x-ray or a clinician presented with a patient's clinical findings and diagnostic tests. The diagnosis or therapeutic decision made in these circumstances is a judgment based on experience applied to data about a specific patient. In the routine diagnostic setting, specific lesions are interpreted in the context of the pathologic changes in all slides from the specimen or specimens. The diagnosis is sometimes influenced by the appearance of associated findings. Consequently, the levels of reproducibility and interobserver disagreement described in various research settings based on selected slides are not directly applicable to routine diagnostic pathology. It is also possible that a variety of factors, including the use of immunohistochemical staining, additional sections, and consideration of corresponding radiologic findings, can influence the level of agreement on the diagnosis of breast biopsies among pathologists.[155]

- **Pathologists can be "trained" to lower the level of their disagreement on the diagnosis of "borderline" lesions, but a degree of uncertainty remains.**

Schnitt et al.[156] demonstrated 58% complete agreement among six pathologists who reviewed a series of proliferative ductal lesions after being trained to employ agreed-upon specified diagnostic criteria. Participants prepared for the review by studying a common set of histologic slides and written definitions of proliferative lesions. After this intensive effort, five of the six pathologists classified 16 of 24 specimens as atypical hyperplasia or CIS. Disagreement between the diagnosis of atypical hyperplasia and CIS occurred in 33% of the cases.

Dupont et al.[147] examined interobserver reproducibility among pathologists who had worked together in one department "for many years." The investigators examined a common set of slides to standardize diagnostic criteria. The two review pathologists agreed on diagnoses in 63% of cases, achieving a kappa statistic of 0.39 described by the authors as "suggesting a fair level of agreement beyond that which would be expected by chance alone."[147] Under these nearly ideal circumstances, the two pathologists did not agree on the interpretation of 37% of the specimens.

The emerging use of digital pathology that allows for instantaneous sharing of "virtual" slides between pathologists is gaining acceptance. This technology has the potential to enhance interobserver agreement.[157,158]

- **There is no consensus presently on criteria that should be adopted and how they should be applied for the distinctions between hyperplasia, atypical hyperplasia, and CIS.**

The lack of consensus is illustrated not only by the previously described problem of observer reproducibility, but also in the definitions employed by various investigators. Pathologists have agreed for decades with the concept that atypical proliferative lesions exhibit some but not all features of CIS, but differences have arisen over specific criteria for the presence and severity of atypia, particularly with respect to qualitative and quantitative aspects of the lesions.[93–95,98,147,159–161] One definition characterizes atypical duct hyperplasia as having "the cytologic and architectural features of the nonnecrotic forms of IDCa [intraductal carcinoma] and the changes may involve two or more ducts or ductules … [but] … the involved ducts/ductules measure less than 2 mm in aggregated diameter."[98] Others require "at least 2 spaces completely involved … " by cells with appropriate cytologic features but do not include a measured dimension in their definition.[94] Differences also exist in regard to definitions of structural growth patterns designated micropapillary and cribriform which are frequently seen in "nonnecrotic" variants of intraductal carcinoma and in hyperplasias.

In view of the foregoing problems in defining proliferative lesions and in diagnostic reproducibility, it has been suggested that the effort to distinguish between atypical hyperplasia and *in situ* carcinoma should be abandoned, and the lesions amalgamated in diagnostic categories might be termed *mammary intraepithelial neoplasia* or *ductal intraepithelial neoplasia*. A precedent for this approach can be found in the uterine cervix, where the term *cervical intraepithelial neoplasia* describes a spectrum of proliferative changes that includes dysplasia and CIS.

There are important clinical differences between the cervix and the mammary glands that limit applying the concept of intraepithelial neoplasia to lesions of the breast. The cervix is accessible to direct observation and nonexcisional methods of sampling that permit correlation of specific cytologic and histologic features of the lesions with clinical progression. In the breast, the absence of equivalent nonexcisional, nondestructive sampling techniques currently makes it impossible to observe and characterize the evolution of individual proliferative epithelial lesions. Furthermore, there appear to be clinical differences in the breast between lesions classified as proliferative and *in situ* carcinoma, especially those arising in the ducts. The risk of subsequent invasive carcinoma is nearly equally distributed for the two breasts after biopsy-proven proliferative changes, whereas carcinoma following intraductal carcinoma tends to occur in the ipsilateral breast. The frequency of subsequent invasive carcinoma is considerably higher after intraductal carcinoma than after lesions usually diagnosed as hyperplasia. Presently it would be prudent to retain the terms *hyperplasia, atypical hyperplasia*, and *in situ carcinoma*, with regard to the breast, since these categories correspond in general terms with the concept that carcinogenesis is a multistage process. Rather than abandoning this concept, we should seek markers that will improve our ability to discriminate among these groups of proliferative change. For additional discussion of this issue, see Chapter 9.

- **The risk of subsequent breast carcinoma attributed to atypical hyperplasia may be exaggerated if this category includes a substantial number of patients with lesions that are regarded as *in situ* carcinoma in some classifications of proliferative lesions.**

In 1978, Page et al.[95] reported finding no significant difference in the risk of subsequent breast carcinoma between biopsies classified as ADH and those described as "ordinary" ductal hyperplasia. To improve the discriminating power of their assessment of proliferative ductal lesions, these investigators redefined the category of ADH by making " … a conscious effort … to exclude the complex and more solid examples of florid hyperplasia and recognize as ADH only those cases with features of DCIS."[134] Application of the revised criteria yielded a significantly increased risk associated with lesions that fulfilled the new definition of atypical hyperplasia. The process of refining morphologic definitions to maximize risk differences was also exemplified by the study of PACs by Page et al.[143] discussed earlier in this chapter. As previously noted, this approach introduces the risk of contaminating the pool of cases classified as atypical hyperplasia with examples of low-grade *in situ* carcinoma.

Bodian et al.[129] noted that the requirement to classify a lesion as atypical hyperplasia if features of intraductal carcinoma were restricted to a single duct could not be met because cases with single duct involvement by intraductal carcinoma had consistently been treated by mastectomy and thus were not available for inclusion in their study. They speculated that the primary difference between their results and those of Dupont and Page[134] related to " … the threshold at which the pathologists recognized various levels of hyperplasia," and that there might be a lower threshold for diagnosing *in situ* carcinoma at their institution.

- **Morphologic criteria for the diagnosis of "atypia" and *in situ* carcinoma, implying increased breast carcinoma risk, may be improved when it is possible to relate proliferative lesions to specific genetic or biochemical markers.**

As stated by London et al.,[92] "the specific characteristics of atypical hyperplasia that confer the highest risk remain unclear." There is currently no laboratory test that serves as a "gold standard" or marker for *in situ* carcinoma of the breast or to distinguish between hyperplasia and CIS.[162] Some interesting observations involving proliferative lesions suggest that significant differences will ultimately be uncovered.

Morphometric analysis of the nuclear cytology of intraductal carcinoma and proliferative ductal lesions has revealed modest differences, and this technique may prove to be a useful quantitative method for assessing the risk associated with various types of hyperplasia.[163,164] The pattern of nuclear distribution in fenestrated duct hyperplasia and in cribriform intraductal carcinoma was studied by Ozaki and Kondo,[165] who calculated the angle of the longest nuclear diameter to a horizon in histologic sections. The nuclear pattern was more often multidirectional in intraductal carcinomas, reflecting "vertical nuclear arrangements toward acinar lumens," whereas hyperplastic lesions featured a more unidirectional nuclear distribution "forming a complex streaming pattern." Morphometric analysis of nuclear cytology could be combined with digital imaging technology for the real-time examination of histologic sections. These results tend to support current histologic criteria for distinguishing between these groups of lesions.

A study of *cell proliferation* in hyperplasias and *in situ* carcinomas using *in vivo* labeling with 5-bromodeoxyuridine (BrdU) found no significant difference between the proliferative fraction of hyperplasia without atypia and atypical hyperplasias.[166] BrdU labeling was significantly increased in *in situ* and invasive carcinomas. When examined by *flow cytometry*, DNA aneuploidy has been found more often in atypical hyperplasia (13%) than in hyperplasia without atypia (7%).[167] Others reported aneuploidy in 30% and 36% of proliferative lesions with atypia and in 30% and 72% of intraductal carcinomas, respectively.[163,168] Similar frequencies of aneuploidy in intraductal and *in situ* lobular carcinoma have been detected in tissues studied by FISH.[169] In the latter study, none of the proliferative lesions exhibited a chromosome gain, and only one example of adenosis had evidence of chromosome 7 monosomy.

Investigations of the role of *oncogenes* in mammary carcinogenesis suggest that activation of *ras* oncogenes occurs at an early stage in the process.[170,171] On the other hand, overexpression of *HER2* oncogene is rarely detected by IHC in hyperplastic lesions.[172–174] Nonetheless, studies using the MTSVI-7 cell line suggest that overexpression of HER2/*neu* can interfere with morphogenesis *in vitro*.[175] Cells transfected with HER2/*neu* failed to form characteristic aggregates to an extent inversely proportional to expression of HER2/*neu*, and this loss of organization was associated with reduced expression of $\alpha_2\beta_1$ integrin.[176]

Weak immunohistochemical membrane staining for HER2/*neu* has been observed in normal breast epithelium, corresponding to the nonamplified level of a single gene copy.[177–179] Two case-control studies have investigated the relevance of HER2/*neu* immunoreactivity in a benign breast biopsy to the risk of subsequent carcinoma. Rohan et al.[180] compared antecedent benign biopsies from 71 women who later developed carcinoma and benign biopsies from 291 women who did not develop carcinoma. Membrane staining for HER2/*neu* was detected in 3 of 71 (4.2%) benign biopsies from study patients and in 14 of 291 (4.7%) control biopsies. The OR for subsequent carcinoma among women with HER2/*neu* detected by IHC in a benign breast biopsy was 0.65 (95% CI, 0.27 to 1.53), indicating no increased risk.

A second case-control study by Stark et al.[181] used IHC and analyzed DNA extracted from archival tissues for HER2/*neu* amplification. None of the benign tissue samples from cases (women who later developed carcinoma) and from controls (no subsequent carcinoma) displayed membrane immunoreactivity for HER2/*neu* in 10% or more of cells. In this study, HER2/*neu* amplification, but not immunohistochemical detection, in a benign breast biopsy was associated with an increased risk of breast carcinoma (OR, 2.2; 95% CI, 0.9 to 5.8). Among women having HER2/*neu* amplification and proliferative benign changes, typical or atypical, the risk was substantially greater (OR, 7.2; 95% CI, 0.9 to 60.8). Immunoreactivity for HER2/*neu* was present in 30% of subsequent carcinomas. These data suggest that HER2/*neu* amplification in benign breast tissue may be a risk factor of subsequent carcinoma, and this effect may interact with the type of benign alteration that is present.

Nuclear *p53 expression* was detected in 12% of 109 *in situ* ductal carcinomas but not in any of 89 samples of benign or hyperplastic tissue studied by Eriksson et al.[167] Mommers et al.[182] found p53 nuclear reactivity in 10 of 124 (8%) examples of ductal hyperplasia with no appreciable difference in the frequency of staining between mild, moderate, and florid lesions. One extensive study of biopsies revealed nuclear p53 staining in 16% of 248 benign specimens.[183] The highest frequency of reactivity was observed in fibroadenomas (FAs) (30%), whereas only 8% of lesions characterized as "fibrocystic disease" were positive. The latter specimens were not subclassified with regard to the types of proliferative changes present. Follow-up revealed subsequent carcinoma in 12% of patients with a p53-positive benign biopsy and in 7% of p53-negative cases, a difference that was not statistically significant.

Data linking *p53* mutations and overexpression with increased breast carcinoma risk have come from several sources. A case-control study conducted by Rohan et al.[180] used IHC to detect p53 overexpression in benign biopsies from 71 study women who later developed breast carcinoma and 288 controls who did not develop carcinoma subsequently. Immunoreactivity for p53 was present in 10 (14%) of the study samples and in 19 (6.6%) of controls. The presence of p53 immunoreactivity in an antecedent breast biopsy was associated with an increased risk of subsequent carcinoma (OR, 2.55; 95% CI, 1.01 to 6.40). The risk was higher when a greater proportion of cells were positive (less than 10% vs. greater than or equal to 10%) and when p53 reactivity coexisted with typical and atypical hyperplasia (OR, 4.62; 95% CI, 1.02 to 20.94). There was no consistent relationship between p53 expression in a benign biopsy and in a subsequent carcinoma. Both were negative in 66.7% of cases and both were positive in 9.8%.

Kamel et al.[184] used FNA to obtain cytologic specimens for p53 immunostaining from women at high risk of developing carcinoma. The cohort included women with a family history of breast carcinoma, prior contralateral carcinoma, or a prior biopsy showing atypical hyperplasia or CIS. Nuclear p53 reactivity was present in 29% of the patients and was highly correlated with the presence of atypical hyperplasia. Five of the seven women who were later found to have intraductal or invasive carcinoma during follow-up had had p53-positive cells in their FNA specimens. Only one of the subsequent carcinomas had a *p53* mutation when microdissected tumor samples were studied by the polymerase chain reaction (PCR).

The foregoing studies indicate that p53 accumulation detected by IHC in benign breast tissue is associated with an increased risk of subsequent carcinoma, and this effect interacts with the presence of hyperplasia to further increase the risk. Mutation of the *p53* gene occurs with greater frequency in breast carcinomas from *BRCA1* carriers than in tumors from noncarriers.[185]

p53 mutations were studied by high-resolution melting (HRM), followed by DNA sequence analysis and by p53 immunostaining in 140 cases of noninvasive breast lesions, including usual hyperplasia, ADH and DCIS, and 240 cases of noninvasive breast lesions.[186] HRM and sequencing analysis detected *p53* mutation positivity in 0%, 12.7%, and 21.6% of cases of usual hyperplasia, ADH, and DCIS, respectively. Immunohistochemical p53 protein expression was detected in none of the usual hyperplasia, 14.6% of ADH, and 31.4% of DCIS cases. *p53* mutation and protein accumulation increased from UDH to ADH to DCIS ($p < 0.05$). The authors concluded that *p53* mutations and p53 accumulation may represent early events in breast carcinogenesis.[186]

The *bcl-2* gene encodes a protein that inhibits apoptosis and participates in the control of cell proliferation. The gene derives its name from B-cell lymphoma. The number 2 refers to its being the second protein described in chromosomal alterations in follicular lymphoma. When studied by IHC, *bcl-2* is found in virtually all normal ductal epithelial cells and ductal hyperplasias.[167,168,171] One study reported no difference in the intensity of reactivity between normal and hyperplastic lesions (typical and atypical), but others reported reduced staining in 16% of hyperplastic foci with differences in intensity not related to the degree of hyperplasia (mild, moderate, and florid). Among intraductal carcinomas, *bcl-2* reactivity was related to the degree of differentiation, being highest in low-grade foci[167] and noncomedo lesions[168] and substantially lower in comedo intraductal carcinoma.[167,168] These observations suggest that loss of *bcl-2* reactivity is not an early event in the evolution of proliferative lesions and the development of intraductal carcinoma. The role of other genes such as *Fas*, involved in promoting apoptosis[187] and *survivin*, an inhibitor of apoptosis,[188] in proliferative breast lesions has received little attention.

Several genes that participate in the regulation of other aspects of the cell cycle have also been investigated in proliferative breast lesions. *Cyclin D1* is involved in controlling progression from G_1 into the S-phase. Cells that overexpress *cyclin D1* show reduced cyclin from G_1 to G_0. Amplification of *cyclin D1* and overexpression of the protein were investigated by differential PCR of microdissected specimens and IHC in benign proliferative lesions and carcinoma by Zhu et al.[189] *Cyclin D1* gene amplification was present in 15% of normal tissues, 19% with epithelial hyperplasia without atypia, 27% with ADH, and 35% with intraductal carcinoma. The corresponding frequencies of overexpression detected by IHC were 13%, 13%, 57%, and 50%. These findings suggest that *cyclin D1* expression can be altered in the absence of a histologically detectable abnormality and that the frequency of altered *cyclin D1* expression as well as amplification tends to increase with the severity of the proliferative abnormality.

In situ hybridization detected increased cyclin D1 mRNA expression in the same proportion (18%) of proliferative lesions without and with atypia. A significantly higher frequency of overexpression was found in intraductal carcinomas: 76% in low-grade lesions and 87% in high-grade lesions.[190] A study of *cyclin D1* overexpression detected by IHC reported an overall frequency of 6%, with no significant difference between mild, moderate, and florid hyperplasia.[182] These data appear to indicate a more abrupt increase in *cyclin D1* overexpression in the transition from hyperplasia to intraductal carcinoma than the foregoing study of Zhu et al.[189] Overall, these investigations demonstrate that *cyclin D1* amplification and overexpression are more strongly associated with intraductal carcinoma than with hyperplasia.

Cyclin D1 expression has been shown to be associated with poorer prognostic features in ER-positive breast cancer.[191]

Growth factors are a group of substances produced locally in tissues that modulate cellular development and may contribute to carcinogenesis. *Epidermal growth factor* (EGF) is a protein involved in the proliferation of normal and neoplastic cells in the breast. The activity of EGF is induced by its interaction with a transmembrane receptor, the *epidermal growth factor receptor* or *EGFR*. Little information is available about expression of EGFR in proliferative breast lesions. EGFR is present in all benign tissues, although when measured biochemically the level of expression appears to be lower than in EGFR-positive breast carcinomas.[192] Specimens classified as benign or fibrocystic have slightly higher EGFR levels than samples of fat and fibrous tissue. Immunohistochemical studies have detected fairly widespread EGFR expression in benign or normal breast tissue samples.[193,194] EGFR positivity is detected in about 45% of breast carcinomas studied by various methods.[195] A noteworthy difference in expression between carcinomas and noncarcinomatous tissues exists in relation to ER. EGFR expression in carcinomas is inversely related to ER expression, being significantly more frequent in ER-negative tumors.[192,193,196,197] On the other hand, EGFR expression is directly related to ER in noncarcinomatous breast samples.[192,195,196] The mechanisms for these differences in expression and their relationship to proliferative breast disease have not been adequately explored.

Nuclear immunoreactivity for *ER* and *PR* can be found in nonneoplastic breast tissue. Specific types of benign lesions do not differ significantly in the frequency of positivity.[198] Khan et al.[199] compared the immunohistochemical expression of ERs and PRs in benign breast tissue from women with and without documented breast carcinoma. There was a significant association between ER positivity in the benign epithelium (not further classified with respect to proliferative activity) and the presence of breast carcinoma. Within various age groups analyzed, the strongest association with concurrent carcinoma was observed in patients with ER (+), PR (−) benign epithelium.

ER plays a critical role in modulating the effect of estrogen on breast epithelial development and growth. This is manifested clinically in part by the observed association between the use of hormone replacement therapy and the risk of benign breast disease, which had a RR of 1.70 (95% CI, 1.06 to 2.72) after 8 years of use in one study.[200] Carcinomas that arise in women using hormone replacement therapy tend to be smaller, better differentiated, and to be less proliferative than tumors that arise in nonusers.[201] These differences are attributable to the association of these prognostic factors with ER-positive but not with ER-negative tumors. Reduced proliferation was observed predominantly in tumors from patients receiving hormone replacement at the time of diagnosis. This finding is consistent with the observation that patients with a breast carcinoma who have used hormone replacement therapy had reduced mortality, with the greatest reduction among those women under treatment at the time of diagnosis.[202]

Changes in *cell polarity* are found histologically in proliferative breast lesions as well as in mammary carcinomas. Hyperplasia is characterized by an increased number of cells that fill part or all of ductal or lobular gland lumens. Common abnormal patterns of cellular distribution in hyperplastic lesions include uneven positioning of cells with respect to the basement membrane, accumulation of cells in a multilayered fashion, polarization of cells around newly formed secondary lumens, and arrays of cells described as "swirling" or "streaming."

Recent studies of proteins associated with *cell adhesion and polarity* have uncovered alterations in these substances that may prove to be markers for classifying proliferative changes and assessing risks for progression to carcinoma.[203] The pattern of expression of genes associated with cell polarity and "apical junction complex" provides confirmation that atypical hyperplasia and ductal CIS are part of tumorigenic multistep process.[204]

Cell surface *receptors for laminin* are important nonintegrin proteins for adhesion to laminin, a component of the basement membrane.[205] They participate in the process whereby epithelial cells are organized around the normal duct lumen. Focal loss of laminin has been observed in the basement membrane region of intraductal carcinomas.[206] Myoepithelial cells appear to exert a tumor suppressor effect by contributing to basement membrane integrity[207] as well as through paracrine factors that inhibit tumor invasion, metastasis, and possibly progression of precancerous epithelial alterations.[208]

The apical and basolateral membrane regions of individual cells have distinctive biochemical and physiologic properties.[209] The presence and distribution of these membrane domains are altered in proliferative lesions. The majority of hyperplastic cells accumulate in and tend to fill glandular lumens, away from the basement membrane. Apical membrane differentiation may be maintained around secondary lumens in hyperplastic epithelium at the surface of the hyperplastic proliferation. However, a substantial number of cells within the solid portions of proliferative foci have no exposure to lumens or to the basement membrane.

Fodrin is a structural protein involved in the maintenance of cell polarity. It has been localized to basolateral cell membranes in normal terminal and intralobular ducts, and in lesions such as SA that are characterized by proliferation of glands with little increase in cell numbers within individual glands. In hyperplastic epithelium that has increased cell numbers, fodrin is found around the entire cell membrane.[210] Circumferential staining of the cell membrane for fodrin has been observed in mammary and colonic carcinomas.[210,211]

Integrins are a family of complex proteins composed of α and β subunits, involved in binding to extracellular matrix and proteins in cell-to-cell adhesion. Their expression in various normal tissues and neoplasms is very complex.[212] Data presently available suggest that an understanding of the distribution of integrins may prove useful in distinguishing between proliferative lesions and carcinoma. Integrin expression in FAs is similar to levels in normal breast tissue, whereas expression is decreased in carcinomas of the breast.[213–215] Zutter et al.[215] observed that the level of integrin mRNA expression detected by *in situ* hybridization was correlated with the degree of differentiation, being lowest in poorly differentiated carcinomas and intermediate in well-to-moderately differentiated tumors. Others have also reported diminished expression of α4 and β6 subunits in carcinomas and in benign breast tissue from patients with carcinoma.[216] The specimens examined did not include examples of "florid epithelial hyperplasia," but the authors suggested that loss of α4β6 expression might be a marker of premalignant change.[216] Downregulation of integrin expression may, in part, be related to loss of contact with basement membranes.

The ability of proliferating epithelial cells to produce *angiogenesis factors* and to induce angiogenesis in surrounding tissue has been demonstrated in hyperplastic mammary lesions, as well as in established carcinomas.[217,218] Bose et al.[219] reported that some types of intraductal carcinoma are characterized by a marked increase in the amount of periductal angiogenesis compared with normal ducts. Heffelfinger et al.[220] reported that periductal vascularity in normal tissue was greater in breasts with invasive carcinoma than in breasts lacking invasive carcinoma. Vascularity was greater around proliferative foci than in normal tissue, and the degree of vascularity increased in proportion to the severity of the lesion (hyperplasia, atypical hyperplasia, or *in situ* carcinoma). These observations suggest that proliferative lesions are capable of inducing angiogenesis and that angiogenesis is not exclusively associated with carcinoma. The extent to which the capacity to produce angiogenesis factors correlates with the morphologic classification of proliferative breast lesions and *in situ* carcinoma remains to be determined.

There is also evidence that alterations in *stromal proteins* may accompany proliferative changes in the breast and carcinomatous transformation. This is illustrated by investigations of tenascin, a matrix glycoprotein. Some forms of tenascin act as antiadhesive molecules. Stromal cells produce predominantly two isoforms of *tenascin* of low (190 kDa) and high (330 kDa) molecular weights.[221] Antiadhesive properties reside largely in the latter isoform, the predominant type found in the activated stroma in some FAs, cystosarcomas, and invasive carcinomas.[221,222] Stroma associated with most benign lesions and atypical hyperplasias expresses mainly the 190-kDa form. Jones et al.[216] reported finding an inverse relationship between integrin and tenascin expression in breast carcinomas. Differences in the distribution of fibronectins have also been observed when stroma from normal and hyperplastic breast tissue was compared with stroma in carcinomas.[223] Specific oncofetal isoforms associated with carcinomas were not found in benign specimens, an observation suggesting that the expression of these markers is associated with carcinomatous transformation.

A number of studies have examined the expression of different *cytokeratins* in proliferative breast lesions and in breast carcinomas. The use of immunohistochemical stains, including CK5/6 and cocktail preparations such as ADH-5 that utilizes CK5, 14, 7, 18, and p63 offers promise for greater interobserver reproducibility if not diagnostic accuracy.[224,225] Normal (luminal) epithelial cells are reactive with antibodies directed against keratins 7, 8, 18, and 19.[226–228] These antibodies reportedly do not stain myoepithelial (basal) cells that are immunoreactive with markers of keratins 5, 6, and14.[226,227] As might be expected, tubular carcinoma is immunoreactive with antibodies to keratins 18 and 19 but not to the 5/14 keratin complex, whereas the latter antibodies are reactive in SA.[226] Hyperplastic proliferative ductal lesions retain a myoepithelial component and are immunoreactive with both types of antibody, but the pattern of staining in intraductal carcinomas is dependent on the degree to which myoepithelium is preserved.[226] Moinfar et al.[229] studied the distribution of reactivity for 34βE12 (K903), an antibody against high-molecular weight cytokeratins CK1, 5, 10, and 14, in normal breast epithelium, proliferative lesions, and in intraductal carcinoma. Reactivity for 34βE12 was stronger and present in a greater proportion of myoepithelial than epithelial cells in normal epithelium. A similar pattern of staining was also observed in hyperplasias, whereas atypical hyperplasia and intraductal carcinoma were characterized by complete or nearly complete absence of epithelial 34βE12 reactivity.

The similarity of cytokeratin staining patterns in lesions classified as atypical duct hyperplasia and as intraductal carcinoma in the study of Moinfar et al.[229] may largely be the result of criteria for defining these groups of lesions rather than a manifestation of intrinsic biologic characteristics. Lesions were classified as atypical intraductal proliferations if "they had the cytologic appearances of low-grade DCIS without recognizable architectural features of DCIS or both cytologic and architectural features suggestive of, but not sufficient for, a diagnosis of DCIS, with partial involvement of one or more ducts... There were cases with atypical intraductal proliferations qualitatively identical to an intraductal carcinoma, quantitatively less than 2 mm in aggregate cross-sectional diameter and therefore insufficient to warrant a diagnosis of carcinoma *in situ*." By definition, the category of ADH differed from intraductal carcinoma not so much because of structural phenotypic differences in the appearance of proliferative foci but largely as a result of quantitative criteria.

- **In view of the clonal nature of carcinoma, quantitative criteria for distinguishing carcinoma from hyperplasia are not biologically meaningful, although lesion size may be relevant clinically to diagnosis and planning treatment.**

Consequently, results from studies such as those of Moinfar et al.[229] and Page et al.[143] regarding apocrine lesions may be misleading by suggesting that there is little difference between atypical hyperplasia and low-grade intraductal carcinoma and proposing that the two groups be merged. By including small intraductal carcinomas among atypical hyperplasias, these investigators, in all likelihood, contaminate the latter group and thereby obscure any biologic differences that might exist. Applying biomarkers in this situation, as for example by Moinfar et al.,[229] inevitably shows little difference in patterns of reactivity between the "atypical hyperplasia" and the intraductal carcinoma groups because the former category includes cases that the authors themselves state have qualitative features of carcinoma. This approach to the study of "precancerous" breast lesions is more likely to fulfill preconceived concepts about the phenotypic characterization of these abnormalities than to contribute to a clinically relevant understanding of their pathobiology.

- **As suggested in the introduction to this chapter, the molecular characterization of mammary epithelium may prove to be as important as, or more significant than, the histologic phenotype. Under these circumstances, much of the current controversy over the classification of proliferative lesions will have less relevance to clinical practice. This will be especially true if important molecular changes associated with transformation are found to be present in cells that do not have an abnormal histologic phenotype, and if progression to carcinoma can occur in such cells with at most a very transient phase corresponding to changes now referred to as "hyperplasia" and "atypia."**

It is clear that there are many elements involved in the conundrum that lies at the heart of the process of neoplastic transformation in the breast. Evidence to date summarized in this chapter suggests that it is unlikely that a single key marker or molecular alteration will emerge as the gold standard for assessing the risk of carcinoma associated with proliferative breast lesions. Instead, the significant information will probably come from a panel of indicators assayed in tissues, blood, or both—most likely molecular biomarkers.[230] The availability of increasingly effective chemoprevention agents as an alternative to surgery combined with data from future studies of cancer risk related to biomarkers may refine histopathologic criteria for risk assessment and identify nonmorphologic markers of risk. Ultimately, such developments are essential, since relatively few women undergo biopsies that yield "benign" tissue that can be used for microscopic risk assessment. The development of reliable biomarkers of risk is likely to be more successful if it is based on the clinical detection of breast carcinoma rather than correlations with intermediate markers of risk such as histologic categories of proliferative lesions. This is because many criteria for stratifying these changes are not strictly limited to histologic morphology and also include factors relevant to making therapeutic decisions such as size of the lesion.

At some point in the future, it is likely that genetic alterations[231,232] and tissue microenvironment may emerge as readily evaluable factors in the genesis of breast carcinoma,[233] and strategies to cause alterations therein may emerge as preventive or therapeutic modalities.

REFERENCES

1. Gage M, Wattendorf D, Henry LR. Translational advances regarding hereditary breast cancer syndromes. *J Surg Oncol* 2012;105:444–451.
2. Friedman LS, Ostermeyer EA, Szabo CI, et al. Confirmation of *BRCA1* by analysis of germline mutations linked to breast and ovarian cancer in ten families. *Nat Genet* 1994;8:399–404.
3. King M-C. Linkage of early-onset familial breast cancer to chromosome 17q21. *Science* 1990;250:1684–1689.
4. Miki Y, Swensen J, Shattuck-Eidens D, et al. A strong candidate for the breast and ovarian cancer susceptibility gene *BRCA1*. *Science* 1994;266:66–71.
5. Wooster R, Bignell G, Lancaster J, et al. Identification of the breast cancer susceptibility gene *BRCA2*. *Nature* 1995;378:789–792.
6. Roy R, Chun J, Powell SN. *BRCA1* and *BRCA2*: different roles in a common pathway of genome protection. *Nat Rev Cancer* 2011;12:68–78.
7. Couch FJ, Weber BL. Mutations and polymorphisms in the familial early-onset breast cancer (*BRCA1*) gene. Breast Cancer Information Core. *Hum Mutat* 1996;8:8–18.
8. Tavtigian SV, Simard J, Rommens J, et al. The complete *BRCA2* gene and mutations in chromosome 13q-linked kindreds. *Nat Genet* 1996;12:333–337.
9. Struewing JP, Brody LC, Erdos MR, et al. Detection of eight *BRCA1* mutations in 10 breast/ovarian cancer families, including 1 family with male breast cancer. *Am J Hum Genet* 1995;57:1–7.
10. Struewing JP, Hartge P, Wacholder S, et al. The risk of cancer associated with specific mutations of *BRCA1* and *BRCA2* among Ashkenazi Jews. *N Engl J Med* 1997;336:1401–1408.
11. Ford D, Easton DF, Stratton M, et al. Genetic heterogeneity and penetrance analysis of the *BRCA1* and *BRCA2* genes in breast cancer families. The Breast Cancer Linkage Consortium. *Am J Hum Genet* 1998;62:676–689.
12. Thorlacius S, Struewing JP, Hartge P, et al. Population-based study of risk of breast cancer in carriers of *BRCA2* mutation. *Lancet* 1998;352:1337–1339.
13. Easton DF, Bishop DT, Ford D, et al. Genetic linkage analysis in familial breast and ovarian cancer: results from 214 families. The Breast Cancer Linkage Consortium. *Am J Hum Genet* 1993;52:678–701.
14. Easton DF, Ford D, Bishop DT. Breast and ovarian cancer incidence in *BRCA1*-mutation carriers. Breast Cancer Linkage Consortium. *Am J Hum Genet* 1995;56:265–271.
15. Ford D, Easton DF, Bishop DT, et al. Risks of cancer in *BRCA1*-mutation carriers. Breast Cancer Linkage Consortium. *Lancet* 1994;343:692–695.
16. Rebbeck TR, Kantoff PW, Krithivas K, et al. Modification of *BRCA1*-associated breast cancer risk by the polymorphic androgen-receptor CAG repeat. *Am J Hum Genet* 1999;64:1371–1377.
17. Andrieu N, Smith T, Duffy S, et al. The effects of interaction between familial and reproductive factors on breast cancer risk: a combined analysis of seven case-control studies. *Br J Cancer* 1998;77:1525–1536.
18. Narod SA, Goldgar D, Cannon-Albright L, et al. Risk modifiers in carriers of *BRCA1* mutations. *Int J Cancer* 1995;64:394–398.
19. Rebbeck TR, Blackwood MA, Walker AH, et al. Association of breast cancer incidence with NAT2 genotype and smoking in *BRCA1* variant carriers. *Am J Hum Genet* 1998;61:A46.
20. Brunet JS, Ghadirian P, Rebbeck TR, et al. Effect of smoking on breast cancer in carriers of mutant *BRCA1* or *BRCA2* genes. *J Natl Cancer Inst* 1998;90:761–766.
21. Ursin G, Henderson BE, Haile RW, et al. Does oral contraceptive use increase the risk of breast cancer in women with *BRCA1/BRCA2* mutations more than in other women? *Cancer Res* 1997;57:3678–3681.
22. Rebbeck TR. Inherited genetic predisposition in breast cancer: a population-based perspective. *Cancer* 1999;86:1673–1681.
23. Grade K, Hoffken K, Kath R, et al. *BRCA1* mutations and phenotype. *J Cancer Res Clin Oncol* 1997;123:69–70.
24. Gayther SA, Mangion J, Russell P, et al. Variation of risks of breast and ovarian cancer associated with different germline mutations of the *BRCA2* gene. *Nat Genet* 1997;15:103–105.
25. Couch FJ, De Shano ML, Blackwood MA, et al. *BRCA1* mutations in women attending clinics that evaluate the risk of breast cancer. *N Engl J Med* 1997;336:1409–1415.
26. Noguchi S, Kasugai T, Miki Y, et al. Clinicopathologic analysis of *BRCA1*- or *BRCA2*-associated hereditary breast carcinoma in Japanese women. *Cancer* 1999;85:2200–2205.
27. Marcus JN, Watson P, Page DL, et al. *BRCA2* hereditary breast cancer pathophenotype. *Breast Cancer Res Treat* 1997;44:275–277.
28. Marcus JN, Watson P, Page DL, et al. Hereditary breast cancer: pathobiology, prognosis, and *BRCA1* and *BRCA2* gene linkage. *Cancer* 1996;77:697–709.
29. Verhoog LC, Brekelmans CT, Seynaeve C, et al. Survival and tumour characteristics of breast-cancer patients with germline mutations of *BRCA1*. *Lancet* 1998;351:316–321.
30. Armes JE, Egan AJM, Southey MC, et al. The histological phenotypes of breast carcinoma occurring before age 40 years in women with and without *BRCA1* or *BRCA2* germline mutations. A population-based study. *Cancer* 1998;83:2335–2345.
31. Lakhani SR, Easton DF, Stratton MR; and the Breast Cancer Linkage Consortium. Pathology of familial breast cancer: differences between breast cancers in carriers of *BRCA1* or *BRCA2* mutations and sporadic cases. *Lancet* 1997;349:1505–1510.
32. Palacios J, Honrado E, Osorio A, et al. Immunohistochemical characteristics defined by tissue microarray of hereditary breast cancer not attributable to *BRCA1* or *BRCA2* mutations: differences from breast carcinomas arising in *BRCA1* and *BRCA2* mutation carriers. *Clin Cancer Res* 2003;9:3606–3614.
33. Weitzel JN, Robson M, Pasini B, et al. A comparison of bilateral breast cancers in BRCA carriers. *Cancer Epidemiol Biomarkers Prev* 2005;14:1534–1538.
34. Eerola H, Heikkila P, Tamminen A, et al. Relationship of patients' age to histopathological features of breast tumors in *BRCA1* and *BRCA2* and mutation-negative breast cancer families. *Breast Cancer Res* 2005;7:R465–R469.
35. Seery LT, Knowlden JM, Gee JM, et al. *BRCA1* expression levels predict distant metastasis of sporadic breast cancers. *Int J Cancer* 1999;84:258–262.
36. Lee JS, Wacholder S, Struewing JP, et al. Survival after breast cancer in Ashkenazi Jewish *BRCA1* and *BRCA2* mutation carriers. *J Natl Cancer Inst* 1999;91:259–263.
37. Verhoog LC, Brekelmans CT, Seynaeve C, et al. Survival in hereditary breast cancer associated with germline mutations of *BRCA2*. *J Clin Oncol* 1999;17:3396–3402.
38. Foulkes WD, Wong N, Brunet JS, et al. Germ-line *BRCA1* mutation is an adverse prognostic factor in Ashkenazi Jewish women with breast cancer. *Clin Cancer Res* 1997;3:2465–2469.
39. Hughes KS, Papa MZ, Whitney T, et al. Prophylactic mastectomy and inherited predisposition to breast carcinoma. *Cancer* 1999;86:1682–1696.
40. Schrag D, Kuntz KM, Garber JE, et al. Decision analysis—effects of prophylactic mastectomy and oophorectomy on life expectancy among women with *BRCA1* or *BRCA2* mutations. *N Engl J Med* 1997;336:1465–1471.
41. Hartmann LC, Sellers TA, Schaid DJ, et al. Efficacy of bilateral prophylactic mastectomy in *BRCA1* and *BRCA2* gene mutation carriers. *J Natl Cancer Inst* 2001;93:1633–1637.

42. Meijers-Heijboer H, van Geel B, van Putten WL, et al. Breast cancer after prophylactic bilateral mastectomy in women with a *BRCA1* or *BRCA2* mutation. *N Engl J Med* 2001;345:159–164.
43. Rebbeck TR, Friebel T, Lynch HT, et al. Bilateral prophylactic mastectomy reduces breast cancer risk in *BRCA1* and *BRCA2* mutation carriers: the PROSE Study Group. *J Clin Oncol* 2004;22:1055–1062.
44. Smith KL, Robson ME. Update on hereditary breast cancer. *Curr Oncol Rep* 2006;8:14–21.
45. Rebbeck TR, Levin AM, Eisen A, et al. Breast cancer risk after bilateral prophylactic oophorectomy in *BRCA1* mutation carriers. *J Natl Cancer Inst* 1999;91:1475–1479.
46. Rebbeck TR, Lynch HT, Neuhausen SL, et al. Prophylactic oophorectomy in carriers of *BRCA1* or *BRCA2* mutations. *N Engl J Med* 2002;346:1616–1622.
47. Kauff ND, Satagopan JM, Robson ME, et al. Risk-reducing salpingo-oophorectomy in women with a *BRCA1* or *BRCA2* mutation. *N Engl J Med* 2002;346:1609–1615.
48. Robson M, Levin D, Federici M, et al. Breast conservation therapy for invasive breast cancer in Ashkenazi women with BRCA gene founder mutations. *J Natl Cancer Inst* 1999;91:2112–2117.
49. Haffty BG, Harold E, Khan AJ, et al. Outcome of conservatively managed early-onset breast cancer by BRCA 1/2 status. *Lancet* 2002;359:1471–1477.
50. Seynaeve C, Verhoog LC, van de Bosch LM, et al. Ipsilateral breast tumour recurrence in hereditary breast cancer following breast-conserving therapy. *Eur J Cancer* 2004;40:1150–1158.
51. Metcalfe K, Lynch HT, Ghadirian P, et al. Contralateral breast cancer in *BRCA1* and *BRCA2* mutation carriers. *J Clin Oncol* 2004;22:2328–2335.
52. Robson M, Svahn T, McCormick B, et al. Appropriateness of breast-conserving treatment of breast carcinoma in women with germline mutations in *BRCA1* or *BRCA2*: a clinic-based series. *Cancer* 2005;103:44–51.
53. Pierce LJ, Levine AM, Rebbeck TR, et al. Ten-year multi-institutional results of breast-conserving surgery and radiotherapy in *BRCA1/2*-associated stage I//II breast cancer. *J Clin Oncol* 2006;24:2437–2443.
54. Brekelmans CT, Seynaeve C, Bartels CC, et al. Effectiveness of breast cancer surveillance in *BRCA1/2* gene mutation carriers and women with high familial risk. *J Clin Oncol* 2001;19:924–930.
55. Carney PA, Miglioretti DL, Yankaskas BC, et al. Individual and combined effects if age, breast density, and hormone replacement therapy use on the accuracy of screening mammography. *Ann Intern Med* 2003;138:168–175.
56. Tilanus-Linthorst M, Verhoog L, Obdeijn IM, et al. A *BRCA1/2* mutation, high breast density and prominent pushing margins of a tumor independently contribute to a frequent false-negative mammography. *Int J Cancer* 2002;102:91–95.
57. Tilanus-Linthorst MM, Obdeijn IM, Bartels KC, et al. First experiences in screening women at high risk for breast cancer with MR imaging. *Breast Cancer Res Treat* 2000;63:53–60.
58. Leach MO, Boggis CR, Dixon AK, et al. Screening with magnetic resonance imaging and mammography of a UK population at high familial risk of breast cancer: a prospective multicentre cohort study (MARIBS). *Lancet* 2005;365:1769–1778.
59. Kuhl CK, Schrading S, Leutner CC, et al. Mammography, breast ultrasound, and magnetic resonance imaging for surveillance of women at high familial risk for breast cancer. *J Clin Oncol* 2005;23:8469–8476.
60. Warner E, Plewes DB, Hill KA, et al. Surveillance of *BRCA1* and *BRCA2* mutation carriers with magnetic resonance imaging, ultrasound, mammography, and clinical breast examination. *JAMA* 2004;292:1317–1325.
61. Kriege M, Brekelmans CT, Boetes C, et al. Efficacy of MRI and mammography for breast-cancer screening in women with familial or genetic predisposition. *N Engl J Med* 2004;351:427–437.
62. Passaperuma K, Warner E, Causer PA, et al. Long-term results of screening with magnetic resonance imaging in women with BRCA mutations. *Br J Cancer* 2012;107:24–30.
63. Narod SA, Lubinski J, Ghadirian P, et al. Screening mammography and risk of breast cancer in *BRCA1* and *BRCA2* mutation carriers: a case-control study. *Lancet Oncol* 2006;7:402–406.
64. Lowry KP, Lee JM, Kong CY, et al. Annual screening strategies in *BRCA1* and *BRCA2* gene mutation carriers: a comparative effectiveness analysis. *Cancer* 2012;118:2021–2030.
65. Euhus DM. New insights into the prevention and treatment of familial breast cancer. *J Surg Oncol* 2011;103:294–298.
66. Fisher B, Costantino JP, Wickerham DL, et al. Tamoxifen for prevention of breast cancer: report of the National Surgical Adjuvant Breast and Bowel Project P-1 Study. *J Natl Cancer Inst* 1998;90:1371–1388.
67. Dalberg K, Johansson H, Johansson U, et al. A randomized trial of long term adjuvant tamoxifen plus postoperative radiation therapy versus radiation therapy alone for patients with early stage breast carcinoma treated with breast-conserving surgery. Stockholm Breast Cancer Study Group. *Cancer* 1998;82:2204–2211.
68. Ragaz J, Coldman A. Survival impact of adjuvant tamoxifen on competing causes of mortality in breast cancer survivors, with analysis of mortality from contralateral breast cancer, cardiovascular events, endometrial cancer, and thromboembolic episodes. *J Clin Oncol* 1998;16:2018–2024.
69. King MC, Wieand S, Hale K, et al. Tamoxifen and breast cancer incidence among women with inherited mutations in *BRCA1* and *BRCA2*: National Surgical Adjuvant Breast and Bowel Project (NSABP-P1) Breast Cancer Prevention Trial. *JAMA* 2001;286:2251–2256.
70. Narod SA, Brunet JS, Ghadirian P, et al. Tamoxifen and risk of contralateral breast cancer in *BRCA1* and *BRCA2* mutation carriers: a case-control study. Hereditary Breast Cancer Clinical Study Group. *Lancet* 2000;356:1876–1881.
71. Li FP, Fraumeni JFJ, Mulvihill JJ, et al. A cancer family syndrome in twenty-four kindreds. *Cancer Res* 1988;48:5358–5362.
72. Birch JM, Hartley AL, Ticker KJ, et al. Prevalence and diversity of constitutional mutations in the p53 gene among 21 Li-Fraumeni families. *Cancer Res* 1994;54:1298–1304.
73. Li J, Yen C, Liaw D, et al. PTEN, a putative protein tyrosine phosphatase gene mutated in human brain, breast, and prostate cancer. *Science* 1997;275:1943–1947.
74. Jenne DE, Reimann H, Nezu J, et al. Peutz-Jeghers syndrome is caused by mutations in a novel serine threonine kinase. *Nat Genet* 1998;18:38–43.
75. Helzlsouer KJ, Selmin O, Huang HY, et al. Association between glutathione S-transferase M1, P1, and T1 genetic polymorphisms and development of breast cancer. *J Natl Cancer Inst* 1998;90:512–518.
76. Maugard CM, Charrier J, Bignon YJ. Allelic deletion at glutathione S-transferase M1 locus and its association with breast cancer susceptibility. *Chem Biol Interact* 1998;111–112:365–375.
77. Rebbeck TR, Kantoff PW, Krithivas K, et al. Modification of breast cancer risk in *BRCA1* mutation carriers by the AIB1 gene. *Proc Am Assoc Cancer Res* 1999;40:1293.
78. Simpson PT, Reis-Filho JS, Gale T, et al. Molecular evolution of breast cancer. *J Pathol* 2005;205:248–254.
79. Tockman MS. Monoclonal antibody detection of premalignant lesions of the lung. In: Fortner JG, Sharp PA, eds. *Accomplishments in cancer research.* Philadelphia: Lippincott-Raven Publishers, 1995:169–177.
80. Tockman MS, Gupta PK, Pressman NJ, et al. Cytometric validation of immunocytochemical observations in developing lung cancer. *Diagn Cytopathol* 1993;9:615–622.
81. Slaughter DP, Southwick HW, Smejkal W. "Field cancerization" in oral stratified squamous epithelium. *Cancer* 1953;6:963–968.
82. Deng G, Lu Y, Zlotnikov G, et al. Loss of heterozygosity in normal tissue adjacent to breast carcinomas. *Science* 1996;274:2057–2059.
83. Larson PS, Schlecter BL, de las Morenas A, et al. Allele imbalance, or loss of heterozygosity, in normal breast epithelium of sporadic breast cancer cases and *BRCA1* gene mutation carriers is increased compared with reduction mammoplasty tissues. *J Clin Oncol* 2005;23:8613–8619.
84. Tsai YC, Lu Y, Nichols PW, et al. Contiguous patches of normal human mammary epithelium derived from a single stem cell: implications for breast carcinogenesis. *Cancer Res* 1996;56:402–404.
85. Diallo R, Schafer K-L, Poremba C, et al. Monoclonality in normal epithelium, hyperplastic and neoplastic lesions of the breast. *Mod Pathol* 2000;13:20A.
86. Larson PS, de Las M, Cupples LA, et al. Genetically abnormal clones in histologically normal breast tissue. *Am J Pathol* 1998;152:1591–1598.
87. Lakhani SR, Chaggar R, Davies S, et al. Genetic alterations in 'normal' luminal and myoepithelial cells of the breast. *J Pathol* 1999;189:496–503.
88. Dawson PJ, Maloney T, Gimotty P, et al. Bilateral breast cancer: one disease or two? *Breast Cancer Res Treat* 1991;19:233–244.
89. Noguchi S, Motomura K, Inaji H, et al. Differentiation of primary and secondary breast cancer with clonal analysis. *Surgery* 1994;115:458–462.

90. Shibata A, Tsai YC, Press MF, et al. Clonal analysis of bilateral breast cancer. *Clin Cancer Res* 1996;2:743–748.
91. Carter CL, Corle DK, Micozzi MS, et al. A prospective study of the development of breast cancer in 16,692 women with benign breast disease. *Am J Epidemiol* 1988;128:467–477.
92. London SJ, Connolly JL, Schnitt SJ, et al. A prospective study of benign breast disease and the risk of breast cancer. *JAMA* 1992;267:941–944.
93. McDivitt RW, Stevens JA, Lee NC, et al. Histologic types of benign breast disease and the risk for breast cancer. *Cancer* 1992;69:1408–1414.
94. Page DL, DuPont WD, Rogers LW, et al. Atypical hyperplastic lesions of the female breast. A long-term follow-up study. *Cancer* 1985;55:2698–2708.
95. Page DL, Van der Zwaag R, Rogers LW, et al. Relation between component parts of fibrocystic disease complex and breast cancer. *J Natl Cancer Inst* 1978;61:1055–1063.
96. Krieger N, Hiatt RA. Risk of breast cancer after benign breast diseases. Variation by histologic type, degree of atypia, age at biopsy, and length of follow-up. *Am J Epidemiol* 1992;135:619–631.
97. Ris H-B, Niederer U, Stirremann H, et al. Long-term follow-up of patients with biopsy-proven benign breast disease. *Ann Surg* 1988;207:404–408.
98. Tavassoli FA, Norris HJ. A comparison of the results of long-term follow-up for atypical intraductal hyperplasia and intraductal hyperplasia of the breast. *Cancer* 1990;65:518–529.
99. Nomura A, Comstock GW, Tonascia JA. Epidemiologic characteristics of benign breast disease. *Am J Epidemiol* 1977;105:505–512.
100. Parazzini F, La Vecchia C, Franceschi S, et al. Risk factors for pathologically confirmed benign breast disease. *Am J Epidemiol* 1984;120:115–122.
101. Sartwell PE, Arthes FG, Tonascia JA. Benign and malignant breast tumours. Epidemiological similarities. *Int J Epidemiol* 1978;7:217–221.
102. La Vecchia C, Parazzini F, Franceschi S, et al. Risk factors for benign breast disease and their relation with breast cancer risk. Pooled information from epidemiologic studies. *Tumori* 1985;71:167–178.
103. Boyle CA, Berkowitz GS, LiVolsi VA, et al. Caffeine consumption and fibrocystic breast disease: a case-control epidemiologic study. *J Natl Cancer Inst* 1984;72:1015–1019.
104. Hislop TG, Band PR, Deschamps M, et al. Diet and histologic types of benign breast disease defined by subsequent risk of breast cancer. *Am J Epidemiol* 1990;131:263–270.
105. Baghurst PA, Rohan TE. Dietary fiber and risk of benign proliferative epithelial disorders of the breast. *Int J Cancer* 1995;63:481–485.
106. Vobecky J, Simard A, Vobecky JS, et al. Nutritional profile of women with fibrocystic breast disease. *Int J Epidemiol* 1993;22:989–999.
107. Brisson J, Verreault R, Morrison AS, et al. Diet, mammographic features of breast tissue, and breast cancer risk. *Am J Epidemiol* 1989;130:14–24.
108. Kelsey JL, Lindfors KK, White C. A case-control study of the epidemiology of benign breast diseases with reference to oral contraceptive use. *Int J Epidemiol* 1974;3:333–340.
109. Page DL, Dupont WD. Proliferative breast disease: diagnosis and implications. *Science* 1991;253:915–916.
110. Cole P, Elwood JM, Kaplan SD. Incidence rates and risk factors of benign breast neoplasms. *Am J Epidemiol* 1978;108:112–120.
111. Mackenzie I. Breast cancer following multiple fluoroscopies. *Br J Cancer* 1965;19:1–8.
112. Mettler FA Jr, Hempelmann LH, Dutton AM, et al. Breast neoplasms in women treated with X rays for acute postpartum mastitis: a pilot study. *J Natl Cancer Inst* 1969;43:803–811.
113. Wanebo CK, Johnson KG, Sato K, et al. Breast cancer after exposure to the atomic bombings of Hiroshima and Nagasaki. *N Engl J Med* 1968;279:667–671.
114. Tokunaga M, Land CE, Aoki Y, et al. Proliferative and nonproliferative breast disease in atomic bomb survivors. Results of a histopathologic review of autopsy breast tissue. *Cancer* 1993;72:1657–1665.
115. Nassar A. Core needle biopsy versus fine needle aspiration biopsy in breast—a historical perspective and opportunities in the modern era. *Diagn Cytopathol* 2011;39:380–388.
116. Parker SH, Burbank F, Jackman RJ, et al. Percutaneous large-core breast biopsy: a multi-institutional study. *Radiology* 1994;193: 359–364.
117. Liberman L, Cohen MA, Abramson AF, et al. Atypical ductal hyperplasia diagnosed at stereotaxic core biopsy of breast lesions: an indication for surgical biopsy. *AJR Am J Roentgenol* 1995;164:1111–1113.
118. Skolnick MH, Cannon-Albright LA, Goldgar DE, et al. Inheritance of proliferative breast disease in breast cancer kindreds. *Science* 1990;250:1715–1720.
119. Khan SA, Masood S, Miller L, et al. Random fine needle aspiration of the breast of women at increased breast cancer risk and standard risk controls. *Breast J* 1998;4:420–425.
120. Wolfe JN. Risk for breast cancer development determined by mammographic parenchymal pattern. *Cancer* 1976;37:2486–2492.
121. Brisson J, Morrison AS, Kopans DB, et al. Height and weight, mammographic features of breast tissue and breast cancer risk. *Am J Epidemiol* 1984;119:371–381.
122. Wolfe JN, Saftlas AF, Salane M. Mammographic parenchymal patterns and quantitative evaluation of mammographic densities: a case-control study. *AJR Am J Roentgenol* 1987;148:1087–1092.
123. Boyd NF, Jensen HM, Cooke G, et al. Relationship between mammographic and histological risk factors for breast cancer. *J Natl Cancer Inst* 1992;84:1170–1179.
124. Urbanski S, Jensen HM, Cooke G, et al. The association of histological and radiological indicators of breast cancer risk. *Br J Cancer* 1988;58:474–479.
125. Moskowitz M, Gartside P, McLauglin C. Mammographic patterns as markers for high-risk benign breast disease and incident cancers. *Radiology* 1980;134:293–295.
126. Arthur JE, Ellis IO, Flowers C, et al. The relationship of "high-risk" mammographic patterns to histological risk factors for development of cancer in the human breast. *Br J Radiol* 1990;63:845–849.
127. Bright RA, Morrison AS, Brisson J, et al. Histologic and mammographic specificity of risk factors for benign breast disease. *Cancer* 1989;64:653–657.
128. Fisher ER, Paleker A, Kim WS, et al. The histopathology of mammographic patterns. *Am J Clin Pathol* 1978;69:421–426.
129. Bodian CA, Perzin KH, Lattes R, et al. Prognostic significance of benign proliferative breast disease. *Cancer* 1993;71:3896–3907.
130. Kodlin D, Winger EE, Morgenstern NL, et al. Chronic mastopathy and breast cancer: a follow-up study. *Cancer* 1977;39:2603–2607.
131. Dupont WD, Page DL. Breast cancer risk associated with proliferative disease, age at first birth, and family history of breast cancer. *Am J Epidemiol* 1987;1225:769–779.
132. Hutchinson WB, Thomas DB, Hamlin WB, et al. Risk of breast cancer in women with benign breast disease. *J Natl Cancer Inst* 1980; 65:13–20.
133. Moskowitz M, Gartside P, Wirman JA, et al. Proliferative disorders of the breast as risk factors for breast cancer in a self-selected screened population: pathologic markers. *Radiology* 1980;134:289–291.
134. Dupont WD, Page DL. Relative risk of breast cancer varies with time since diagnosis of atypical hyperplasia. *Hum Pathol* 1989;20:723–725.
135. Seidman H, Seidman SD, Mushinski MH. A different perspective on breast cancer risk factors: some implications of the nonattributable risk. *Cancer* 1982;32:301–313.
136. Madigan MP, Ziegler RG, Benichou J, et al. Proportion of breast cancer cases in the United States explained by well-established risk factors. *J Natl Cancer Inst* 1995;87:1681–1685.
137. Davis HH, Simons M, Davis JB. Cystic disease of the breast: relationship to carcinoma. *Cancer* 1964;17:957–978.
138. Connolly J, Schnitt S, London S, et al. Both atypical lobular hyperplasia (ALH) and atypical ductal hyperplasia (ADH) predict for bilateral breast cancer risk. *Lab Invest* 1992;66:13A.
139. Dupont WD, Page DL. Risk factors for breast cancer in women with proliferative breast disease. *N Engl J Med* 1985;312:146–151.
140. Ahmed S, Tartter PI, Jothy S, et al. The prognostic significance of previous benign breast disease for women with carcinoma of the breast. *J Am Coll Surg* 1996;183:101–104.
141. Jensen RA, Page DL, Dupont WD, et al. Invasive breast cancer risk in women with sclerosing adenosis. *Cancer* 1989;64:1977–1983.
142. Roberts MM, Jones V, Elton RA, et al. Risk of breast cancer in women with history of benign disease of the breast. *Br Med J* 1984;288: 275–278.
143. Page DL, Dupont WD, Jensen RA. Papillary apocrine change of the breast: associations with atypical hyperplasia and risk of breast cancer. *Cancer Epidemiol Biomarkers Prev* 1996;5:29–32.
144. McDivitt RW, Stewart FW, Berg JW. *Tumors of the breast.* (*AFIP Atlas of Tumour Pathology,* 2nd series, vol 2.). Bethesda: American Registry of Pathology, 1968.

145. Fitzgibbons PL, Henson DE, Hutter RV. Benign breast changes and the risk for subsequent breast cancer: an update of the 1985 consensus statement. Cancer Committee of the College of American Pathologists. *Arch Pathol Lab Med* 1998;122:1053–1055.
146. Ma L, Boyd NF. Atypical hyperplasia and breast cancer risk: a critique. *Cancer Causes Control* 1992;3:517–525.
147. Dupont WD, Parl FF, Hartmann WH, et al. Breast cancer associated with proliferative breast disease and atypical hyperplasia. *Cancer* 1993;71:1258–1265.
148. Palli D, DelTurco MR, Simoncici R, et al. Benign breast disease and breast cancer: a case-control study in a cohort in Italy. *Int J Cancer* 1991;47:703–706.
149. Bloodgood JC. Cancer of the breast. Figures which show that education can increase the number of cures. *JAMA* 1916;66:552–553.
150. Bloodgood JC. The pathology of chronic cystic mastitis of the female breast. *Arch Surg* 1921;111:445–542.
151. Bodian CA, Perzin KH, Lattes R, et al. Reproducibility and validity of pathologic classifications of benign breast disease and implications for clinical applications. *Cancer* 1993;71:3908–3913.
152. Palli D, Galli M, Bianchi S, et al. Reproducibility of histological diagnosis of breast lesions: results of a panel in Italy. *Eur J Cancer* 1996;32A:603–607.
153. Hutter RVP. Consensus meeting on "fibrocytic disease" of the breast precancerous? *Arch Pathol Lab Med* 1986;110:171–173.
154. Palazzo J, Hyslop T. Hyperplastic ductal and lobular lesions and carcinomas *in situ* of the breast: reproducibility of current diagnostic criteria among community- and academic-based pathologists. *Breast J* 1998;4:230–237.
155. Stang A, Trocchi P, Ruschke K, et al. Factors influencing the agreement on histopathological assessments of breast biopsies among pathologists. *Histopathology* 2011;59:939–949.
156. Schnitt SJ, Connolly JL, Tavassoli FA, et al. Interobserver reproducibility in the diagnosis of ductal proliferative lesions using standardized criteria. *Am J Surg Pathol* 1992;16:1133–1143.
157. Al-Janabi S, Huisman A, Van Diest PJ. Digital pathology: current status and future perspectives. *Histopathology* 2012;61:1–9.
158. Shaw EC, Hanby AM, Wheeler K, et al. Observer agreement comparing the use of virtual slides with glass slides in the pathology review component of the POSH breast cancer cohort study. *J Clin Pathol* 2012;65:403–408.
159. Black MM, Barclay THC, Cutler SJ, et al. Association of atypical characteristics of benign breast disease with subsequent risk of breast cancer. *Cancer* 1972;29:338–343.
160. Black MM, Chabon AB. *In situ* carcinoma of the breast. *Pathobiol Annu* 1969;4:185–210.
161. Page DL, Rogers LW. Combined histologic and cytologic criteria for the diagnosis of mammary atypical ductal hyperplasia. *Hum Pathol* 1992;23:1095–1097.
162. Rosen PP. "Borderline" breast lesions. *Am J Surg Pathol* 1991;15: 1100–1102.
163. Crissman JD, Visscher DW, Kubus J. Image cytophotometric DNA analysis of atypical hyperplasias and intraductal carcinomas of the breast. *Arch Pathol Lab Med* 1990;114:1249–1253.
164. King EB, Chew KL, Hom JD, et al. Characterization by image cytometry of duct epithelial proliferative disease of the breast. *Mod Pathol* 1991;4:291–296.
165. Ozaki D, Kondo Y. Comparative morphometric studies of benign and malignant intraductal proliferative lesions of the breast by computerized image analysis. *Hum Pathol* 1995;26:1109–1113.
166. Christov K, Chew KL, Ljung B-M,et al. Cell proliferation in hyperplastic and *in situ* carcinoma lesions of the breast estimated by *in vivo* labeling with bromodeoxyuridine. *J Cell Biochem* 1994;19(Suppl.):165–172.
167. Eriksson ET, Schimmelpenning H, Aspenblad U, et al. Immunohistochemical expression of the mutant p53 protein and nuclear DNA content during the transition from benign to malignant breast disease. *Hum Pathol* 1994;25:1228–1233.
168. Carpenter R, Gibbs N, Matthews J, et al. Importance of cellular DNA content in pre-malignant breast disease and pre-invasive carcinoma of the female breast. *Br J Surg* 1987;74:905–906.
169. Visscher DW, Wallis TL, Crissman JD. Evaluation of chromosome aneuploidy in tissue sections of preinvasive breast carcinomas using interphase cytogenetics. *Cancer* 1996;77:315–320.
170. Kumar R, Sukumar S, Barbacid M. Activation of ras oncogenes preceding the onset of neoplasia. *Science* 1990;248:1101–1104.
171. Ohuchi N, Thor A, Page DL, et al. Expression of the 21,000 molecular weight ras protein in a spectrum of benign and malignant human mammary tissues. *Cancer Res* 1986;46:2511–2519.
172. Allred DC, Clark GM, Molina R, et al. Overexpression of HER-2/neu and its relationship with other prognostic factors change during the progression of *in situ* to invasive breast cancer. *Hum Pathol* 1992;23:974–979.
173. Lodato RF, Maguire HC Jr, Greene MI, et al. Immunohistochemical evaluation of c-erbB-2 oncogene expression in ductal carcinoma *in situ* and atypical ductal hyperplasia of the breast. *Mod Pathol* 1990;3:449–454.
174. De Potter CR, van Daele S, van de Vijver MJ, et al. The expression of the neu oncogene product in breast lesions and in normal fetal and adult human tissues. *Histopathology* 1989;15:351–362.
175. D'Souza B, Berdichevsky F, Kyprianou N, et al. Collagen induced morphogenesis and expression of α_2 integrin subunit is inhibited by c-erbB2 transfected human mammary epithelial cells. *Oncogene* 1993;8:1797–1806.
176. Taylor-Papadimitriou J, D'Souza B, Berdichevsky F, et al. Human models for studying malignant progression in breast cancer. *Eur J Cancer Prev* 1993;2(Suppl.):77–83.
177. Press MF, Cordon-Cardo C, Slamon DJ. Expression of the HER-2/neu proto-oncogene in normal human adult and fetal tissues. *Oncogene* 1990;5:953–962.
178. Natali PG, Nicotra MR, Bigotti A, et al. Expression of the p185 encoded by HER2 oncogene in normal and transformed human tissues. *Int J Cancer* 1990;45:457–461.
179. Ratcliffe N, Wells W, Wheeler K, et al. The combination of *in situ* hybridization and immunohistochemical analysis: an evaluation of Her2/neu expression in paraffin-embedded breast carcinomas and adjacent normal-appearing breast epithelium. *Mod Pathol* 1997;10:1247–1252.
180. Rohan TE, Hartwick W, Miller AB, et al. Immunohistochemical detection of c-erbB-2 and p53 in benign breast disease and breast cancer risk. *J Natl Cancer Inst* 1998;90:1262–1269.
181. Stark A, Hulka BS, Joens S, et al. HER-2/neu amplification in benign breast disease and the risk of subsequent breast cancer. *J Clin Oncol* 2000;18:267–274.
182. Mommers EC, van Diest PJ, Leonhart AM, et al. Expression of proliferation and apoptosis-related proteins in usual ductal hyperplasia of the breast. *Hum Pathol* 1998;29:1539–1545.
183. Younes M, Lebovitz RM, Boomer KE, et al. p53 Accumulation in benign breast biopsy specimens. *Hum Pathol* 1955;26:155–158.
184. Kamel S, Zeiger S, Zalles C, et al. p53 Immunopositivity and gene mutation in a group of women at high risk for breast cancer. *Breast J* 1998;4:396–404.
185. Phillips KA, Nichol K, Ozcelik H, et al. Frequency of p53 mutations in breast carcinomas from Ashkenazi Jewish carriers of *BRCA1* mutations. *J Natl Cancer Inst* 1999;91:469–473.
186. Mao X, Fan C, Wei J, et al. Genetic mutations and expression of p53 in non-invasive breast lesions. *Mol Med Report* 2010;3:929–934.
187. Mullauer L, Mosberger I, Grusch M, et al. Fas ligand is expressed in normal breast epithelial cells and is frequently up-regulated in breast cancer. *J Pathol* 2000;190:20–30.
188. Singh M, Jarboe EA, Shroyer KR. Survivin expression in benign, premalignant and malignant lesions of the breast. *Mod Pathol* 2000;13:47A.
189. Zhu XL, Hartwick W, Rohan T, et al. Cyclin D1 gene amplification and protein expression in benign breast disease and breast carcinoma. *Mod Pathol* 1998;11:1082–1088.
190. Weinstat-Saslow D, Merino MJ, Manrow RE, et al. Overexpression of cyclin D mRNA distinguishes invasive and *in situ* breast carcinomas from non-malignant lesions. *Nat Med* 1995;1:1257–1260.
191. Aaltonen K, Amini RM, Landberg G, et al. Cyclin D1 expression is associated with poor prognostic features in estrogen receptor positive breast cancer. *Breast Cancer Res Treat* 2009;113:75–82.
192. Barker S, Panahy C, Puddefoot JR, et al. Epidermal growth factor receptor and oestrogen receptors in the non-malignant part of the cancerous breast. *Br J Cancer* 1989;60:673–677.
193. van Agthoven T, Timmermans M, Foekens JA, et al. Differential expression of estrogen, progesterone, and epidermal growth factor receptors in normal, benign, and malignant human breast tissues using dual staining immunohistochemistry. *Am J Pathol* 1994;144:1238–1246.
194. Möller P, Mechtersheimer G, Kaufmann M, et al. Expression of epidermal growth factor receptor in benign and malignant primary tumours of the breast. *Virchows Archiv [A]* 1989;414:157–164.

195. Klijn JGM, Berns PMJJ, Schmitz PIM, et al. The clinical significance of epidermal growth factor receptor (EGF-R) in human breast cancer: a review on 5232 patients. *Endocr Rev* 1992;13:3–17.
196. Bolufer P, Miralles F, Rodriguez A, et al. Epidermal growth factor receptor in human breast cancer: correlation with cytosolic and nuclear ER receptors and with biological and histological tumor characteristics. *Eur J Cancer* 1990;26:283–290.
197. Dittadi R, Donisi PM, Brazzale A, et al. Epidermal growth factor receptor in breast cancer. Comparison with nonmalignant breast tissue. *Br J Cancer* 1993;67:7–9.
198. Giri DD, Dundas SAC, Nottingham JF, et al. Oestrogen receptors in benign epithelial lesions and intraduct carcinomas of the breast: an immunohistological study. *Histopathology* 1989;15:575–584.
199. Khan SA, Rogers MAM, Obando JA, et al. Estrogen receptor expression of benign breast epithelium and its association with breast cancer. *Cancer Res* 1994;54:993–997.
200. Rohann TE, Miller AB. Hormone replacement therapy and risk of benign proliferative epithelial disorders of the breast. *Eur J Cancer Prev* 1999;8:123–130.
201. Holli K, Isola J, Cuzick J. Low biologic aggressiveness in breast cancer in women using hormone replacement therapy. *J Clin Oncol* 1998;16:3115–3120.
202. Schairer C, Gail M, Byrne C, et al. Estrogen replacement therapy and breast cancer survival in a large screening study. *J Natl Cancer Inst* 1999;91:264–270.
203. Pignatelli M, Vessey CJ. Adhesion molecules: novel molecular tools in tumor pathology. *Hum Pathol* 1994;25:849–856.
204. Coradini D, Boracchi P, Ambrogi F, et al. Cell polarity, epithelial-mesenchymal transition, and cell-fate decision gene expression in ductal carcinoma *in situ*. *Int J Surg Oncol* 2012;2012:984346.
205. Terranova VP, Rao CN, Kabelic T, et al. Laminin receptor on human breast cancer cells. *Proc Natl Acad Sci USA* 1983;80:444–448.
206. Henning K, Berndt A, Katenkamp D, et al. Loss of laminin-5 in the epithelium-stroma interface: an immunohistochemical marker of malignancy in epithelial lesions of the breast. *Histopathology* 1999;34:305–309.
207. Slade MJ, Coope RC, Gomm JJ, et al. The human mammary gland basement membrane is integral to the polarity of luminal epithelial cells. *Exp Cell Res* 1999;247:267–278.
208. Sternlicht MD, Kedeshian P, Shao ZM, et al. The human myoepithelial cell is a natural tumor suppressor. *Clin Cancer Res* 1997;3:1949–1958.
209. Molitoris BA, Nelson WJ. Alterations in the establishment and maintenance of epithelial cell polarity as a basis for disease processes. *J Clin Invest* 1990;85:3–9.
210. Simpson JF, Page DL. Altered expression of a structural protein (fodrin) within epithelial proliferative disease of the breast. *Am J Pathol* 1992;141:285–298.
211. Younes M, Harris AS, Morrow JS. Fodrin as a differentiation marker: redistributions in colonic neoplasia. *Am J Pathol* 1989;135:1197–1212.
212. Albelda SM. Biology of disease. Role of integrins and other cell adhesion molecules in tumor progression and metastasis. *Lab Invest* 1993;68:4–17.
213. Koukoulis GK, Virtanen I, Korhonen M, et al. Immunohistochemical localization of integrins in the normal, hyperplastic and neoplastic breast. *Am J Pathol* 1991;139:787–799.
214. Zutter MM, Mazoujian G, Santoro SA. Decreased expression of integrin adhesive protein receptors in adenocarcinoma of the breast. *Am J Pathol* 1990;137:863–870.
215. Zutter MM, Krigman HR, Santoro SA. Altered integrin expression in adenocarcinoma of the breast. Analysis by *in situ* hybridization. *Am J Pathol* 1993;142:1439–1448.
216. Jones JL, Critchley DR, Walker RA. Alteration of stromal protein and integrin expression in breast—a marker of premalignant change? *J Pathol* 1992;167:399–406.
217. Brem SS, Jensen HM, Gullino PM. Angiogenesis as a marker of preneoplastic lesions of the human breast. *Cancer* 1978;41:239–244.
218. Folkman J. Tumor angiogenesis factor. *Cancer Res* 1974;34:2109–2113.
219. Bose S, Lesser ML, Rosen PP. Immunophenotype of intraductal carcinoma. *Arch Pathol Lab Med* 1996;120:81–85.
220. Heffelfinger SC, Yassin R, Miller MA, et al. Vascularity of proliferative breast disease and carcinoma *in situ* correlates with histological features. *Clin Cancer Res* 1996;2:1873–1878.
221. Borsi L, Carnemolla B, Nicolò G,et al. Expression of different tenascin isoforms in normal, hyperplastic and neoplastic human breast tissues. *Int J Cancer* 1992;52:688–692.
222. Nicolò G, Salvi S, Oliveri G, et al. Expression of tenascin and of the ED-B containing oncofetal fibronectin isoform in human cancer. *Mech Dev* 1990;32:401–408.
223. Kaczmarek J, Castellani P, Nicolo G, et al. Distribution of oncofetal fibronectin isoforms in normal, hyperplastic and neoplastic human breast tissues. *Int J Cancer* 1994;58:11–16.
224. Nofech-Mozes S, Holloway C, Hanna W. The role of cytokeratin 5/6 as an adjunct diagnostic tool in breast core needle biopsies. *Int J Surg Pathol* 2008;16:399–406.
225. Jain RK, Mehta R, Dimitrov R, et al. Atypical ductal hyperplasia: interobserver and intraobserver variability. *Mod Pathol* 2011;24:917–923.
226. Jarasch E-D, Nagle RB, Kaufmann M, et al. Differential diagnosis of benign epithelial proliferations and carcinomas of the breast using antibodies to cytokeratins. *Hum Pathol* 1988;19:276–289.
227. Gould VE, Koukoulis GK, Jansson DS, et al. Coexpression patterns of vimentin and glial filament protein with cytokeratins in the normal, hyperplastic, and neoplastic breast. *Am J Pathol* 1990;137:1143–1155.
228. Böcker W, Bier B, Ludwig A, et al. Benign proliferative lesions and *in situ* carcinoma of the breast: new immunohistological findings and their biological implications. *Eur J Cancer Prevent* 1993;2(Suppl.): 41–49.
229. Moinfar F, Man YG, Lininger RA, et al. Use of keratin 35BE12 as an adjunct in the diagnosis of mammary intraepithelial neoplasia-ductal type—benign and malignant intraductal proliferations. *Am J Surg Pathol* 1999;23:1048–1058.
230. Allred DC. Molecular biomarkers of risk in premalignancy and breast cancer prevention. *Cancer Prev Res* 2011;4:1947–1952.
231. Wiechmann L, Kuerer HM. The molecular journey from ductal carcinoma *in situ* to invasive breast cancer. *Cancer* 2008;112:2130–2142.
232. Ellis IO. Intraductal proliferative lesions of the breast: morphology, associated risk and molecular biology. *Mod Pathol* 2010;23(Suppl. 2): S1–S7.
233. Bombonati A, Sgroi DC. The molecular pathology of breast cancer progression. *J Pathol* 2011;223:307–317.

CHAPTER 11

Ductal Carcinoma *In Situ*

SYED A. HODA

HISTORICAL BACKGROUND

Ductal carcinoma *in situ* (DCIS), a term that is synonymous with intraductal carcinoma, was defined pathologically early in the 20th century largely by surgeons interested in the microscopic study of tumors they encountered clinically. *In situ*, Latin for "in its place," was first used as a term for noninvasive malignancy by Broders in 1932.[1] Among the first studies of DCIS were those of Warren,[2] a surgeon practicing in Boston. Warren's[2] investigation of "abnormal involution" or cystic disease led him to conclude that carcinoma might develop by transition from hyperplastic duct lesions:

> "It is precisely under these conditions that we most frequently find the combination of abnormal involution and carcinoma. The transition stage is observed when the epithelium no longer confines itself to the cyst cavity, but breaks through the limiting membrane and infiltrates the adjacent structures."

Fundamental pathologic and clinical studies of proliferative ductal lesions of the breast were performed during the early decades of the 20th century by two other surgeons, Sir G. Lenthal Cheatle of King's College Hospital, London, and Joseph Colt Bloodgood (a disciple of Halsted, of the eponymous mastectomy fame) of Johns Hopkins University Hospital, Baltimore, Maryland. The extent to which Bloodgood and Cheatle influenced each other is difficult to ascertain from their published articles that rarely contained references to work other than their own. Contemporaries separated by the Atlantic Ocean, which was figuratively much wider at the time, they seem to have pursued independent routes in their efforts to more clearly distinguish between benign and malignant lesions of the breast.

Cheatle drew heavily upon his own detailed studies of whole-organ sections of the breast to examine the relationships of various lesions to carcinoma as part of a systematic exploration of pathologic processes in the breast. Bloodgood's approach was case oriented, dealing largely with an analysis of patients under his personal care at Johns Hopkins University over several decades. Because of his concern with diagnostic and therapeutic problems prevailing in the operating room at the time, much of Bloodgood's attention was directed to biopsy specimens. He was, therefore, able to relate the morphology of many lesions to clinical follow-up, sometimes of the unresected breast.

Early descriptions of DCIS outlined the major structural patterns of the disease that are recognized today. Micropapillary DCIS was illustrated by Cheatle[3] in 1920 and by Bloodgood[4] in 1921, but this term was not used by either author. Bloodgood[5] also drew attention to the problem of distinguishing between "borderline" hyperplastic lesions and DCIS. Cheatle referred to the micropapillary proliferation as *laciform* and noted the "cartwheel" appearance of carcinoma in a nearby duct. Today, many would describe the "cartwheel" focus as *cribriform*. Muir[6] attributed the term cribriform to Schultz-Brauns'[7] article on breast carcinoma contained in Henke and Lubarsch's 1935 Handbook.

The existence of "comedo" (a term that generally refers to high-grade solid type of DCIS with central necrosis) and cribriform patterns of DCIS is readily apparent in Bloodgood's[8] picture, which illustrated a tumor classified as a comedocarcinoma. The accompanying description provides an interesting historical vignette:

> In 1893, forty-one years ago, I assisted Dr. Halstead in exploring a clinically benign tumor of the breast. The patient was sixty-seven years of age and had observed a small tumor for about eleven months . . . . The moment we cut into and pressed on it, there extruded from its surface many grayish-white, granular cylinders, which I called at that time comedos. From the gross appearance the tumor was diagnosed as malignant, and the radical operation was performed. The nodes were not involved . . . [and] the patient lived nineteen years after operation, dying at age eighty-six.[8]

Bloodgood recognized two types of "comedoadenocarcinoma," which he referred to as "pure comedoadenocarcinoma and comedoadenocarcinoma with areas of fully developed cancer of the breast," the former being entirely intraductal and the latter partly invasive. He observed that large tumors with gross comedo features were more likely to be in the invasive category. Follow-up revealed that 30% of node-negative patients with invasive comedoadenocarcinoma developed metastases and died of the disease.

Bloodgood's[8] 1934 paper described a patient who had a remarkable clinical course. One-year following treatment by excision alone in 1896, the patient developed recurrent carcinoma at the site of prior surgery. A radical mastectomy was then performed. The lymph nodes were negative, and the patient lived more than 15 years without additional recurrence. Because of the apparent curability of the "pure comedo tumor," Bloodgood preferred the term comedo-adenoma. Treatment by local excision was recommended "when the palpable tumor is small and can be completely excised by cutting through normal breast tissue and closing the wound without injury to the symmetry of the breast."[8]

This ranks as one the earliest descriptions of breast conservation surgery for DCIS. Needle aspiration cytologic examination was used by Bloodgood for the diagnosis of breast tumors, especially so that "older women may be spared the complete operation for cancer by an aspiration biopsy, when pure comedo tumor involving a large part of, or the entire breast, is recognized."[8] However, he found that aspiration cytology could not be relied upon for making a distinction between intraductal and invasive carcinoma. In the case of a woman with 1.5-cm lesion,

> The tumor had been aspirated before it was explored and from examination of the stained aspirated cells we could only decide that they suggested a malignant tumor. We did not recognize the comedo tumor.[8]

In 1938, Lewis and Geschickter[9] described 40 patients treated for comedocarcinoma, reporting an 85% 5-year cure rate, with most 5-year survivors having remained well for 10 years. Included were eight women whose initial treatment was only local excision. Six of these eight women developed recurrent carcinoma within 1 to 4 years. Unfortunately, the authors did not distinguish between lesions that were entirely intraductal and those with concomitant invasive carcinoma.

Until about 30 years ago there was little clinical interest in the histologic subtypes of DCIS. This situation most likely derived from the fact that almost all patients were treated by mastectomy and the observation that the lesions rarely consisted of a single growth pattern, for as Cheatle[10] observed, "whole sections reveal that all these varieties may occur in the same mass of disease."

Those interested in the history of DCIS, a disease that has seen an exponential increase in incidence and prevalence in recent decades, will find Fechner's[11] overview to be particularly helpful.

Concepts regarding various aspects of DCIS continue to evolve. Indeed, some observers find it difficult to accept the intraductal neoplastic proliferation of cells as "carcinoma," advocate the use of the acronym DIN, that is, ductal intraepithelial neoplasia, and argue that since N and M categories are not typically applicable for these lesions, there is no reason to retain them within the tumor (size), regional node (involvement), (distant) metastases (TNM) system.[12] Perhaps, as a reflection of the inherent weakness of this argument, the DIN terminology has not gained wide acceptance (and has been eliminated from the latest WHO[13] classification of mammary neoplasms).

CLINICAL PRESENTATION

Frequency

Approximately one-quarter of newly diagnosed breast carcinomas are noninvasive. By American Cancer Society's estimation, there will be 63,300 new cases of DCIS in the United States in 2012; during the same year, there will be 226,870 new cases of invasive breast carcinoma, and about 39,510 women will die of the disease.[14] In 1975, 5.8 American women per 100,000 women were diagnosed with DCIS, and in 2012, the age-adjusted incidence rate of DCIS was 32.5 women per 100,000.[15]

The reported frequency of DCIS in different studies is influenced by clinical circumstances. A review of approximately 1,000 consecutive women treated at a cancer center in the United States in the late 1970s revealed that 5% had DCIS.[16] Data from nine population-based registries included in the National Cancer Institute's Surveillance Epidemiology and End Results (SEER) program for 1975 indicated that 2.9% of patients had DCIS.[17] A review of SEER data published in 1996 demonstrated a striking increase in the incidence of DCIS after 1983.[18] This change was observed in all age groups. Among women 30 to 39 years of age, the average annual increase in the incidence rate changed from 0.3% between 1973 and 1983 to 12.0% between 1983 and 1992. Similar increases were found for women 40 to 49 years of age (0.4% to 17.4%) and for women 50 years and older (5.2% to 18.1%). The estimated total number of cases of DCIS in 1992 was 200% higher than expected based on 1983 rates. In this series, the anatomical distribution of DCIS in the breast was similar to that of invasive carcinomas, with 44% of lesions in the upper-outer quadrant. Further analysis of the SEER data indicated that the estimated number of new cases of DCIS in 1993 was 23,275.[19] Approximately 4,676 were in women 40 to 49 years of age, representing about 15% of breast carcinoma in this age group.

The National Cancer Database reported in 1997 that 3.7% of 31,930 breast carcinomas registered were classified as intraductal.[20] The percentage rose to 7.0% and 9.5%, respectively, in 1990 (65,255 cases) and 1993 (93,915 cases). During the same period, the reported frequency of lobular carcinoma *in situ* (LCIS) was stable, accounting for 1.3% to 1.6% of cases annually.

A population-based study of Danish women in the 1980s revealed that 4% of newly diagnosed carcinomas were intraductal.[21] Review of the records of the Connecticut Tumor Registry revealed a yearly increase in the reported number of patients with DCIS.[22] In 1979, the 33 diagnoses of DCIS represented 1.8% of breast carcinomas, and in 1988 the 200 cases constituted 7.4% of breast carcinomas. Data from the New Mexico Tumor Registry revealed stable incidence values for DCIS in Hispanic White, non–Hispanic White, and Native American women for more than a decade before 1984.[23] Thereafter, the incidence rate increased annually in each ethnic group. In 1994, the incidence rates per 100,000 were 13.8, 9.7, and approximately 7.0, respectively, for non–Hispanic White, Hispanic White, and Native American women. The lower incidence rates in the latter groups may reflect less access to mammography rather than intrinsic ethnic differences in the biology of DCIS. African Americans with DCIS have higher rates of breast carcinoma recurrence, as well as mortality. Analyses of SEER data show that overall mortality is 35% higher in African American versus Caucasian women. The risk of advanced invasive carcinoma was 130% higher in Hispanic and 170% higher in African American versus Caucasian women with DCIS.[24]

The increased age-adjusted incidence of *in situ* breast carcinoma in the United States coincides with a leveling off in the overall age-adjusted incidence of invasive carcinoma and of localized carcinoma, and a decline in the incidence of invasive carcinoma classified as "regional."[25] These changes in incidence by stage have been accompanied by a significant decline in age-adjusted breast carcinoma mortality.[25] The beneficial effects of mammography as a diagnostic or screening modality, and of improved systemic therapy, are reflected in these trends.

Although the incidence of DCIS has steeply escalated over the last few decades, this rise has not been uniform across various histologic types: low-grade DCIS has accounted for the majority of the recent increase in incidence owing to enhanced radiologic detection, whereas the incidence of high-grade DCIS has remained stable.[26]

Risk Factors

Data on epidemiologic risk factors specific to DCIS are limited.[27,28] There appear to be some age-related differences in associations, but overall the risk factors for DCIS and invasive carcinoma appear to be similar.[27] The risk for both lesions increases with age, an association that is stronger for invasive carcinoma. Risk factors for incident DCIS include positive family history.[29] *BRCA* (breast cancer [gene]) mutations were found in 13% of women with DCIS diagnosed before 50 years of age.[30] In the largest analysis of DCIS patients in non–Ashkenazi Jewish women, the prevalence of a *BRCA1/2* mutation was 5.9%.[31] The risk was significantly higher among women younger than 50 years with a personal and family history of breast carcinoma than those 50 years or older.

Mammography and Calcifications

The great majority of currently diagnosed cases of DCIS are nonpalpable and are detected by various radiologic techniques. Mammography is a highly sensitive diagnostic procedure for detecting DCIS.[32] In 2002, it was estimated that about 1 in every 1,300 screening mammograms resulted in a diagnosis of DCIS.[33] Until recently, on initial screening, 8% to 43% of mammographically detected carcinomas were intraductal.[34–40] Twenty-five percent to 30% of nonpalpable carcinomas detected by mammography were intraductal lesions.[37,41–43] In a series of nearly 20,000 patients, 30 of 70 carcinomas (43%) found in biopsies performed only for clustered calcifications detected by mammography were DCIS.[38] Mammographically detected calcifications were found in 72% to 98% of DCIS.[44–47] The proportion of DCIS was not substantially higher in subsequent mammography screening, but some investigators have described a greater frequency of small invasive tumors in later examinations.[34,39]

The interval between screening examinations can influence the clinical characteristics of DCIS detected by mammography.[48] The size of DCIS determined by mammographic measurement was significantly smaller in women examined annually (mean, 1.69 cm; range, 0.3 to 7.7 cm) than in those examined on a biennial (mean, 2.27 cm; range, 0.4 to 10 cm) or triennial (mean, 3.49 cm; range 0.6 to 10 cm) schedule. Comedo-type (high-grade solid) DCIS was significantly more frequent in the biennial (73.7%) than in the annual (46.8%) screening group. Tumor size and nuclear grade were inversely related to the mean sizes for low-, intermediate-, and high-grade lesions determined to be 1.19, 1.85, and 2.82 cm, respectively. The frequency of microinvasion tended to increase with longer intervals between examinations, but the differences were not statistically significant.

Approximately 10% to 15% of DCIS are discovered as incidental lesions in biopsies performed for other indications, usually a palpable abnormality.[32,43,46] Radiologic findings that lead to the detection of a small proportion of "incidental" DCIS are densities and asymmetric soft tissue changes, sometimes with microcalcifications in the noncarcinomatous abnormality. Calcifications alone are more likely to be the mammographic indicator of DCIS in women younger than 50 years, whereas coexistent soft tissue abnormalities are evident more often in women older than 50, a distinction that probably results from variation in overall breast density in these age groups rather than from intrinsic tumor differences.[46]

Relatively specific findings of DCIS on mammograms include microcalcifications of certain types and patterns, that is, the calcifications may be pleomorphic, coarse, and fine and are either clustered or linear in distribution.[47] Calcifications associated with DCIS are generally described as linear "casts" or as granular on mammography (Fig. 11.1). Round or oval, well-circumscribed calcifications are less common in DCIS. Predominantly linear, granular, or mixed types of calcifications occur with approximately equal frequency in DCIS. Calcifications may be clustered, dispersed, or dispersed around clustered foci. Branching calcifications with linear patterns that outline the distribution of one or more ducts may consist of casts or granular particles. The type of calcifications is not related to age at diagnosis or to the size of the area involved mammographically.[46] The level of suspicion for DCIS is a function of the character and the number of calcifications. The majority of DCIS have five or more calcifications.[46]

On mammograms, linear, pleomorphic calcifications are commonly seen in high-grade DCIS, and granular segmental calcifications are typical of lower grade lesions. Ducts afflicted with high-grade DCIS harbor calcifications more often than those with low-grade DCIS. In some cases of low-grade DCIS, the majority of calcifications are in adjacent benign glands. Thus, DCIS may be smaller, larger, or equal to the extent of mammographic calcifications, and calcifications do not always "map-out" DCIS, particularly in lower grade lesions. Despite such nuances, the mammographic distribution of calcifications is commonly used as a guide to the extent of DCIS or the dimensions of the involved area. However, these measurements typically tend to underestimate the size of the lesion compared with careful histologic sampling.[49] When the extents of lesions were measured mammographically and pathologically, discrepancies were found more often between the interpretations for cases that were predominantly cribriform or micropapillary than for high-grade, solid DCIS. A discrepancy of more than 20 mm was found in 44% of pure cribriform–micropapillary lesions,

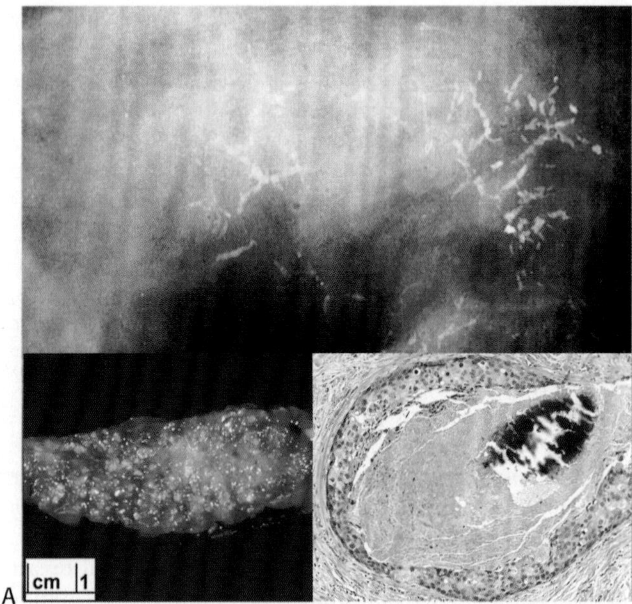

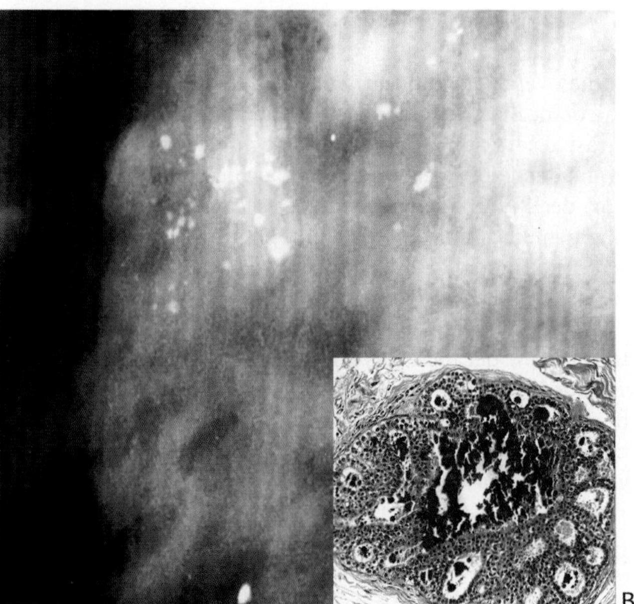

FIG. 11.1. ***DCIS, radiologic–pathologic correlation.*** **A:** Radiograph showing branching linear calcifications found at biopsy to be in high-grade DCIS with necrosis ("comedo" type). *Inset on left*: typical "comedo" appearance on cut section. *Inset on right*: cross section of a duct with high-grade *in situ* carcinoma with central necrosis and calcification. **B:** Clustered, rounded punctate calcifications at the site of cribriform DCIS (*inset*). *Inset* images are from cases other than those shown in the radiographs.

in 12% of pure comedocarcinomas, and in 50% of cases with both patterns.[49] In patients who undergo mastectomy, extension of DCIS to the nipple or subareolar region is more frequent with comedo than with cribriform–micropapillary DCIS.[49] The likelihood of detecting multifocal DCIS radiologically and pathologically is related to the size of the lesion as determined by either procedure.[44,50] Multifocality is appreciably more frequent in lesions larger than 2.0 to 2.5 cm than in smaller foci of DCIS. Carlson et al.[48] reported that the mean size of multifocal DCIS (3.1 cm) was significantly greater than the size of nonmultifocal lesions (1.95 cm).

The mammographic appearance of microcalcifications bears some relationship to the histologic type of the lesion, but, as noted by Stomper and Connolly,[51] "there is considerable overlap, and the predominant histologic subtype cannot be predicted on the basis of the microcalcification type with a high degree of accuracy." Predominantly linear calcifications are found significantly more often in comedocarcinomas than in cribriform, papillary, or solid types, which typically contain granular calcifications.[49,51] Nonetheless, 22% of linear calcifications were associated with noncomedocarcinomas, and 47% of granular calcifications occurred in comedocarcinomas in one series.[51] The presence of extensive casting-type microcalcifications occupying more than one quadrant in a mammogram was associated with high-grade DCIS, multifocal invasive duct carcinoma, and axillary nodal metastases in 33% of 12 patients who had lymph nodes examined.[48]

Image analysis of calcifications has had some success in discriminating between comedo and noncomedo DCIS.[52] Abnormal mammograms without calcifications are more likely to call attention to DCIS of the small cell type than the large cell type, regardless of the growth pattern (solid, cribriform, or mixed) of the lesion.[53] Linear calcifications are a marker of necrosis, and granular calcifications are associated with DCIS without necrosis.[53] DCIS that overexpresses the human epidermal growth factor 2 (*HER2*) oncogene is more likely to have calcifications detected by mammography than is a HER2 negative carcinoma.[54] Extent of mammographic calcifications, presence of either a radiographically or a clinically evident mass, and solid architectural type of DCIS have been demonstrated to be significantly associated with invasion on final excision.[55]

Unusual mammographic presentations of DCIS occur when the lesion has a configuration that suggests a benign tumor or invasive carcinoma. These patterns, reflective of associated soft tissue masses, are found in less than 10% of mammographically detected DCIS.[45,56–59] In one series, 8% of DCIS were represented mammographically by stellate lesions without calcifications,[59] and in another report, 3.6% of DCIS presented as stellate opacities.[56] Three were pure DCIS, and four proved to be DCIS arising in benign radial sclerosing lesions or "radial scars." Microinvasion was found in only one case, despite the radiologic appearance suggesting invasive carcinoma in all instances. At the other end of the spectrum, DCIS may be harbored by radiologically circumscribed lesions and appear to be benign.[57] In addition to carcinoma arising in a fibroadenoma, these are usually examples of solid papillary DCIS or nodular foci of comedocarcinoma. Microinvasion may be present.[57]

Ultrasound Evaluation

Ultrasound is only uncommonly helpful in diagnosing DCIS. In general, "ductal changes" with associated microcalcifications are the most common sonographic findings in about one-third of the cases of high-grade DCIS, and an irregular hypoechoic mass with an indistinct margin is the most frequent finding in about one-third of non–high-grade DCIS cases.[58]

Magnetic Resonance Imaging

Magnetic resonance imaging (MRI) has proven to be an effective method for detecting DCIS, especially lesions that lack calcifications. Menell et al.[60] found that MRI was more sensitive than mammography for detecting DCIS overall and for detecting multifocal DCIS. Lesion detection is based on the finding of contrast enhancement in breast parenchyma after injection of a gadolinium contrast agent compared with the preinjection image.[61–63] Orel et al.[64] described three patterns of enhancement associated with DCIS: ductal, regional, and a peripherally enhancing mass. The mean size of MRI-detected DCIS was 10 mm. Correlation of immunohistochemical studies for vascularity and MRI characteristics of the lesions suggested that tumor angiogenesis contributed to MR enhancement in one series.[61] Contrast-enhanced MRI has proven to be an effective method for the detection of concurrent, unsuspected contralateral carcinoma in women with ipsilateral DCIS.[65]

MRI has higher sensitivity for invasive carcinoma (up to 98%) than for DCIS (sensitivity of 60% to 80%).[66] On MRI, DCIS typically has a non-mass, delayed peak enhancement profile; however, this methodology has a high rate of false negatives. Gadolinium, the contrast media used in MRI, has been shown to accumulate within the intraductal space of DCIS.[67]

Current *indications* for adjunct MRI include the detection of an occult primary tumor, the examination of dense breast tissue, the presence of known *BRCA* mutations, and the detection of chest wall involvement.[68] MRI has two main *roles* in the evaluation of DCIS. The first is assessing the extent of disease, and the other is early detection in breast cancer screening programs.

The sensitivity of MRI for the accurate assessment of DCIS is more than 60%, compared with approximately 55% for mammography and 45% or so for ultrasound[69]; MRI screening may potentially double the probability of carcinoma detection in a high-risk population compared with either mammography or ultrasound alone.[68,70] Owing to the higher detection rate of otherwise occult significant disease on MRI (including so-called "elsewhere carcinoma"), there is a strong association between preoperative MRI performed in women with DCIS and mastectomy.[71]

Palpable DCIS

Prior to the widespread use of mammography, palpable tumors were reportedly present in 50% to 65% of women who had DCIS.[72–74] A study comparing breast carcinomas diagnosed during 1973 to 1974 in Japan and the United States reported a higher frequency of DCIS in Japanese patients and noted that the carcinomas tended to form bulky, palpable tumors in Japanese women.[75] Pandya et al.[74] compared the characteristics of DCIS detected in eras prior to (1969 to 1985) and after the "intensified use of screening" (1986 to 1990) at the Lahey Clinic. The proportion of mammographically detected cases increased from 19% to 80%, whereas palpable lesions decreased from 54% to 12%. The proportion of cases presenting with duct discharge and Paget disease also decreased. Comedo DCIS was found in 7% and 38% of palpable and mammographic lesions, respectively.

Currently, DCIS is not palpable in the majority of patients with this disease.[76] Negative mammograms may be reported in up to 25% of cases, with a sensitivity ranging from 56% in women younger than 40 years to 67% in the 40- to 49-year age group and 76% in those 50 years or older.[32] Nonpalpable lesions are detected because of imaging findings, Paget disease, nipple discharge, or as an incidental finding in a biopsy for a concurrent palpable benign tumor[41,76] (Fig. 11.2). About 25% of biopsy procedures performed for "suspicious" calcifications reveal carcinoma, largely of the intraductal type.[77,78] Duct hyperplasia and sclerosing adenosis (SA) account for the majority of "significant" calcifications that do not prove to be carcinoma. Comedocarcinoma is the type most frequently detected by mammography alone, whereas micropapillary DCIS is more often found as a result of a palpable lesion or other clinical signs.[76]

Frozen Section Evaluation

The diagnosis of DCIS requires histologic sections of excised breast tissue. DCIS can be recognized in frozen sections (FSs), but if any difficulty is encountered, the decision should be immediately deferred to permanent sections because there is a significant risk of trimming away the lesional area if more FSs are made.[79] FS is not appropriate for the diagnosis of mammographically detected, nonpalpable lesions, unless there are exceptional clinical circumstances. In one study of DCIS, 50% of the lesions were diagnosed at the time of FS, 36% were reported to be benign, 8% were deferred, 5% were diagnosed as atypical hyperplasia, and one case was diagnosed as invasive.[80] Approximately 3% of biopsies reported to be benign at FS prove to contain carcinoma when paraffin sections are examined.[79] Because the sampling of a biopsy is limited during surgery, approximately 20% of patients with a FS diagnosis of DCIS prove to have invasion after multiple paraffin sections of the same biopsy specimen were examined.[81]

The use of FS evaluation of margins in breast-conserving surgery has been shown to decrease reoperative rates; however, "technical changes in freezing breast tissue," specifically those with "high adipose content," is a major limitation of such analyses besides the obvious difficulty in interpretation of "atypical ducts."[82] The possibility of "skip lesions" of DCIS must be kept in mind when assessing margins of lumpectomies (and nipple margins in nipple-sparing mastectomies) by FS analyses.[83]

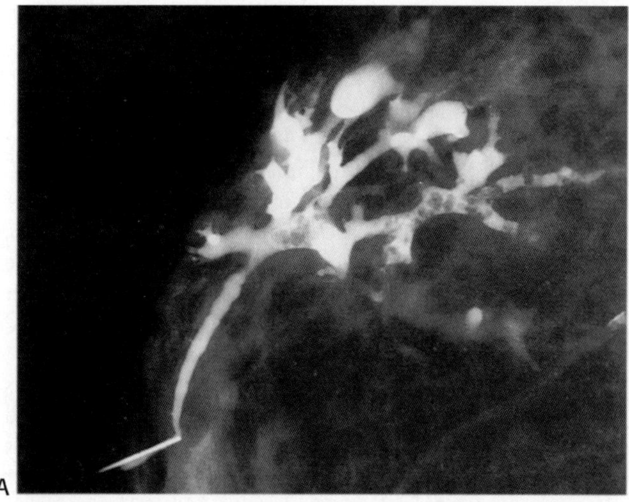

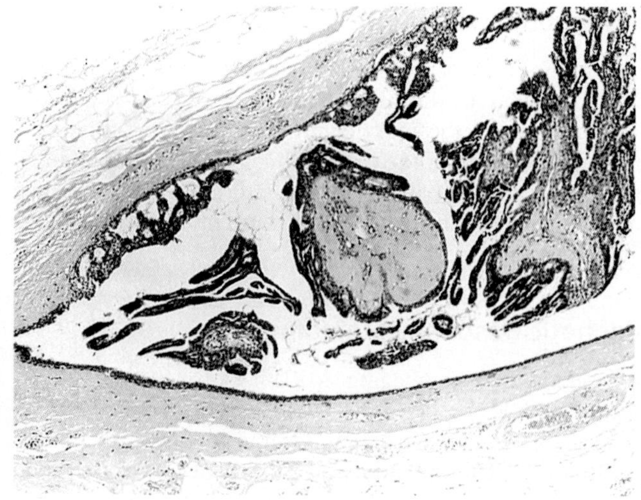

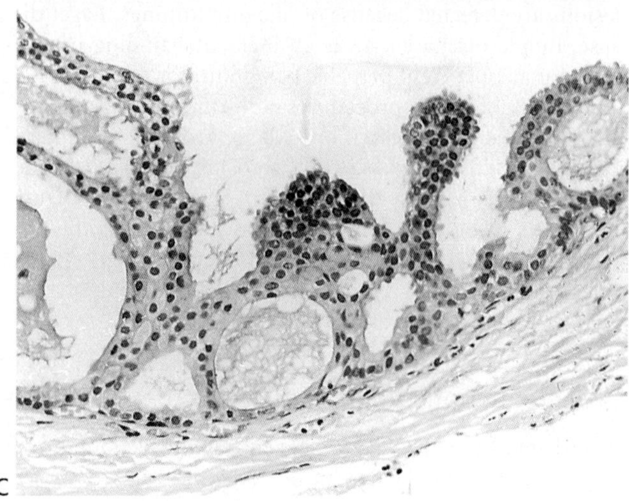

FIG. 11.2. *DCIS.* **A:** Ductogram from an 84-year-old woman with bloody nipple discharge. The cannulated lactiferous duct is seen in the *lower left*. Numerous defects in the white dye in ducts represent intraductal papillary lesions. **B:** Orderly papillary DCIS in the lumen and micropapillary carcinoma at the periphery. **C:** Micropapillary DCIS.

Age at Diagnosis

DCIS occurs throughout the age range of breast carcinoma in women. The mean age at diagnosis of patients in multiple studies was between 50 and 59 years, quite similar to the mean age of women with invasive duct carcinoma.[22,56,62,63] There are no significant differences in the age distributions of structural subtypes of DCIS.[76]

In 2012, in the United States, there is one diagnosis of DCIS for every four diagnoses of invasive breast cancer. For women 50 to 64 years of age, the incidence of DCIS has been estimated to be 88 per 100,000. The risk of DCIS is minimal in women less than 30 years of age and is low in women less than 40 years of age. Thereafter, the risk increases steadily between the ages 40 and 50, increases at a slower rate after age 50, and plateaus after age 60.[15]

A higher recurrence rate is associated with DCIS at a younger age, generally regarded as under 40 years of age; however, breast conservation therapy is possible in smaller, lower grade, and nonnecrotic types of DCIS in which widely negative margins have been achieved.[84] Women with DCIS and a family history of ovarian carcinoma or those who had a BRCAPRO (*BRCA* mutation carrier prediction model) score of more than 10% had a 27% rate of *BRCA1/2* mutation positivity regardless of age at diagnosis.[85] BRCAPRO is a statistically derived score for assessing the probability that an individual carries a germline deleterious mutation of *BRCA1* and *BRCA2* genes, based on family history.

Bilaterality

Limited data are available describing the frequency of bilaterality associated with DCIS in one breast.[86,87] Among 112 patients with DCIS reported by Ashikari et al.,[72] 16 (14%) had concurrent contralateral carcinoma, and 17 (15%) had undergone mastectomy previously for carcinoma. Westbrook and Gallager[73] excluded an unstated number of patients with previous or concurrent contralateral invasive carcinoma from their study of DCIS. Subsequent contralateral biopsies obtained from 14 of the 64 women included in the report revealed DCIS in five and invasion in three others, for an overall frequency of subsequent carcinoma in the opposite breast of 12.5%. The average length of follow-up was not stated. Brown et al.[88] found that 10% of patients with DCIS in one breast had contralateral invasive carcinoma, including three women treated previously for the contralateral lesion and one who subsequently developed contralateral carcinoma. No information about concurrent contralateral biopsies was provided. A population-based study of cases identified in the Connecticut Tumor Registry found that 22% of 217 patients with DCIS in one breast had intraductal or invasive carcinoma in the opposite breast.[22] Overall, 17% of the patients with DCIS also had a nonmammary malignant neoplasm.

A systematic evaluation of the contralateral breast was reported by Urban,[89] who biopsied the opposite breast in 70% of his cases. Among 16 women with DCIS treated between 1966 and 1968, he found that three (19%) had had a prior contralateral mastectomy. There were no patients with simultaneous bilaterality. Ringberg et al.[90] carried out bilateral mastectomy in patients with unilateral carcinoma. The contralateral breast specimens were subjected to a detailed pathologic analysis. Among 23 women with DCIS in one breast, the distribution of contralateral disease was as follows: LCIS, two cases (9%); DCIS, three cases (13%); and invasive carcinoma, two cases (9%). In another study, simultaneous contralateral mastectomy in 25 of 78 patients who had noncomedo DCIS in one breast revealed contralateral DCIS in 3 (12%).[91] The type of DCIS and indications for performing the operation in these cases were not indicated. Schuh et al.[92] reported that 7 of 52 (13%) patients with DCIS had previously undergone a contralateral mastectomy for carcinoma. Simultaneous bilateral carcinoma was found in 3 of the remaining 45 women (7%), including two contralateral invasive lesions and one with LCIS. Schwartz et al.[93] reported that 3 of 47 patients (6%) with nonpalpable DCIS treated by mastectomy had clinically detected DCIS in the opposite breast. Silverstein et al.[87] found bilateral simultaneous or metachronous carcinoma in 22 of 208 patients (11%) with pure or microinvasive DCIS, including 5 (2.4%) with bilateral intraductal lesions. Ciatto et al.[32] reported contralateral carcinoma in 44 of 350 women (13%) with DCIS, including 9 (3%) with synchronous bilateral intraductal, 9 (3%) with synchronous invasive, 2 (6%) with metachronous invasive, and 5 (1.4%) with metachronous DCIS. After excluding synchronous contralateral carcinoma, Ciatto et al.[32] calculated the frequency of metachronous contralateral carcinoma based on breast years at risk to be 8.5%, 5.6 times the expected risk of 1.5% for unilateral breast carcinoma in a normal population.

The occurrence of contralateral carcinoma in women with DCIS was studied in a population-based cancer registry from the state of Washington by Habel et al.[94] The authors identified 1,929 women with DCIS diagnosed in one breast between 1974 and 1993. Contralateral invasive carcinoma developed at a rate twice that of the control population. When contralateral *in situ* carcinoma was found, it was intraductal in 78% of these patients. The detection rate for contralateral DCIS was highest in the first year after diagnosis of the ipsilateral lesion, with a relative risk (RR) compared with controls of 21.4 (95% confidence interval [CI], 11.8 to 38.7). Five years or more after ipsilateral diagnosis, the RR was 3.1 (95% CI, 1.0 to 9.8).

The frequency of subsequent invasive carcinoma in the contralateral breast of women with DCIS was 4.3% in one series, considerably less than that for patients with LCIS.[95] A similar observation was recorded by Habel et al.[94] who found that the RR of contralateral invasive carcinoma was 1.8 (95% CI, 1.4 to 2.4) for women with ipsilateral DCIS and 3.0 (95% CI, 1.7 to 5.1) for women with LCIS compared with a control population. The majority of deaths due to breast carcinoma recorded in patients with DCIS in one breast have been due to invasive carcinoma of the contralateral breast.[32,41,72] Deaths due to contralateral invasive carcinoma were reported in 3.6%,[52] 1.9%,[43] and 1.0%[32] of cases, whereas in two of these studies deaths caused by invasive recurrence in the ipsilateral breast occurred in 2 of 140, or 1.4%,[32] and 2 of 61, or 3.2%,[56] of patients treated with breast conservation.

It is clear from the foregoing review that data regarding bilaterality in women with DCIS in one breast are heavily influenced by methodologic issues relating to how the information was assembled. Clinically apparent synchronous contralateral carcinoma occurs in less than 10% of patients, with at least half also being intraductal. Metachronous subsequent carcinoma occurs more frequently than initial primary DCIS in the general population, with a RR of about 2. Subsequent contralateral invasive carcinoma is responsible for the majority of breast carcinoma deaths in women with ipsilateral DCIS, ranging from 1% to nearly 4%. A small number of deaths are also attributable to ipsilateral invasive recurrences after breast conservation therapy. Contrast-enhanced MRI is an efficient method for detecting occult concurrent contralateral carcinoma in women with ipsilateral DCIS.[65]

GROSS PATHOLOGY

Noncomedo DCIS and nonpapillary DCIS are usually not evident grossly. Comedocarcinoma involving multiple ducts occasionally produces a firm mass (Fig. 11.3). A palpable, high-grade solid type of DCIS with necrosis (i.e., of the

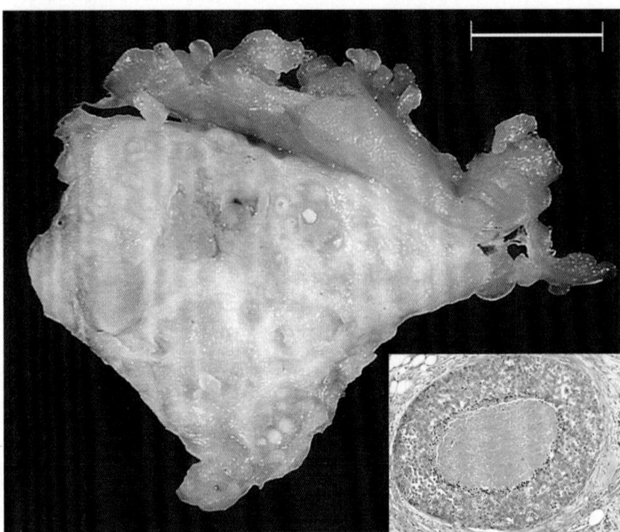

FIG. 11.3. ***DCIS, "comedo."*** Gross biopsy specimen showing numerous round and pale yellow foci of "comedo" type necrosis. *Inset*: cross section of a duct with high-grade *in situ* carcinoma with central necrosis from another case. The latter corresponds to the "comedo" appearance on the cut section of the gross specimen.

comedo type) tends to be a well-defined, tan tumor with white to pale yellow flecks composed of necrotic DCIS (comedos) that extrude from the cut surface when the lesion is compressed. Abundant calcification in the lesion can impart a gritty sensation upon cutting. Although these findings are suggestive of this type of carcinoma, a similar gross appearance is found in some instances of duct ectasia and mastitis.

Most classifications of DCIS have been based on histopathologic features of the lesions, but some investigators have drawn attention to the distinction between grossly apparent and microscopic lesions. Gump et al.[96] studied 70 consecutive patients treated in one institution for lesions classified as DCIS on an initial biopsy. Fifty-four (77%) had carcinomas classified as "gross" because the patient presented with a palpable tumor, nipple discharge, or Paget disease. The majority of these patients (48 of 54 or 89%) had a mass. Microscopic DCIS in 16 (23%) was nonpalpable, and it was detected by mammographic calcifications or it was an incidental finding. Invasive carcinoma was found in six (12%) surgical specimens subsequent to an initial biopsy that revealed gross DCIS, but not in the patients who had microscopic DCIS. Axillary lymph node (ALN) metastases were found in only one patient with a gross lesion, and not in any patient with microscopic DCIS.

A slightly more complex classification based on anatomic distribution was proposed by Andersen et al.[97] They identified three types of growth patterns, which occurred individually or in combinations. "Microfocal" lesions involved "one or a few lobules and/or ducts" measuring up to 5 mm. "Diffuse" DCIS involved a region of 5 to 10 mm or an entire segment of the breast, and the "tumor-forming" type consisted of closely connected glandular structures that occupied an area of 60 to 70 mm, resulting in a palpable mass. Microfocal and diffuse types of DCIS were typically not palpable. A population-based review of cases revealed that 18 of 35 patients (51%) with DCIS had microfocal lesions, 13 (37%) had the diffuse type, and 4 (11%) had tumor-forming DCIS.[21] No ALN metastases were found in any of the patients who had an axillary dissection.

MICROSCOPIC PATHOLOGY

General Histologic Features

The microanatomic site of origin of many DCIS appears to be in the *terminal duct lobular unit* (TDLU). The most convincing evidence for this conclusion comes from the subgross microdissection studies of Wellings et al.[98] Expanded TDLUs sometimes resemble primary or secondary segmental ducts, but their lobular origin is suggested by an excessive number of duct structures within a low-power microscopic field and by the accompanying stroma. Recently characterized columnar cell lesions lend support to this conclusion.

Exceptions can be found to the concept of the TDLU origin of DCIS. For example, it does not readily describe DCIS limited to major central lactiferous ducts, sometimes associated with Paget disease or nipple discharge. Occasionally, random sections disclose foci of DCIS in sections of one or more segmental ducts with no apparent lobular connection even when the lesion is traced with serial sections. The relative frequency of origin from the TDLU or from larger duct structures, and the clinical significance of this distinction remain to be determined.

The microscopic classification of DCIS became the subject of heightened interest after the widespread introduction of breast conservation therapy. Interest in factors associated with the success or failure of this therapy directed attention not only to variants described on the basis of growth pattern, but also to finer cytologic details.

The spectrum of histologic patterns of DCIS in men does not differ appreciably from the appearance of the disease in women. There is a higher proportion of papillary DCIS in men, and comedo DCIS is less frequent than in women.

In standard histologic sections, DCIS is confined within the lumens of ducts and lobules involved in the process. When studied by immunohistochemistry (IHC) for laminin or type IV collagen, basement membranes in DCIS appear intact or focally discontinuous.[99–101] The presence or absence of mitotic figures is not a definitive feature in the diagnosis of DCIS, because mitoses may also be found rarely in normal and hyperplastic epithelium. However, the finding of one or more mitoses per 10 high-power fields (HPFs) suggests DCIS.

Myoepithelium in DCIS

Myoepithelial cells are often retained but attenuated in DCIS, and they are occasionally hyperplastic at the periphery of the duct (Fig. 11.4). Myoepithelial cells do not generally accompany the neoplastic epithelial proliferation within the duct lumen in DCIS except for certain types of carcinoma arising in a papilloma or in solid papillary DCIS.

Experimental evidence suggests that myoepithelial cells may have a paracrine tumor suppressor effect on DCIS, acting to inhibit invasion.[102] Tumor suppression capabilities of myoepithelial cells include inhibition of invasion[103] and of angiogenesis.[104] *In vitro*, myoepithelial cells have been shown to have the capacity to inhibit breast carcinoma cell growth and to induce apoptosis.[105] These tumor-inhibiting properties have been attributed in part to the expression of maspin, a protease inhibitor, by myoepithelial cells.[106] Other tumor suppressor genes expressed by myoepithelial cells include cytokeratin 5 (CK5), smooth muscle actin (SMA), and caveolin-1.[107]

The functional activity of myoepithelial cells in *in situ* carcinoma is significantly changed compared with normal epithelium. These alterations include overexpression of chemokines CXCL12 and CXCL14, which bind to and enhance the invasiveness of carcinoma cells.[108] In particular, CXCL12 and its receptor CXCR4 appear to promote breast carcinoma cell growth and metastases.[109,110]

Cell Types in DCIS

The range of subtle differences in cell type found in DCIS usually engenders little comment, but certain distinct variants have been identified and described by specific names. *Signet*

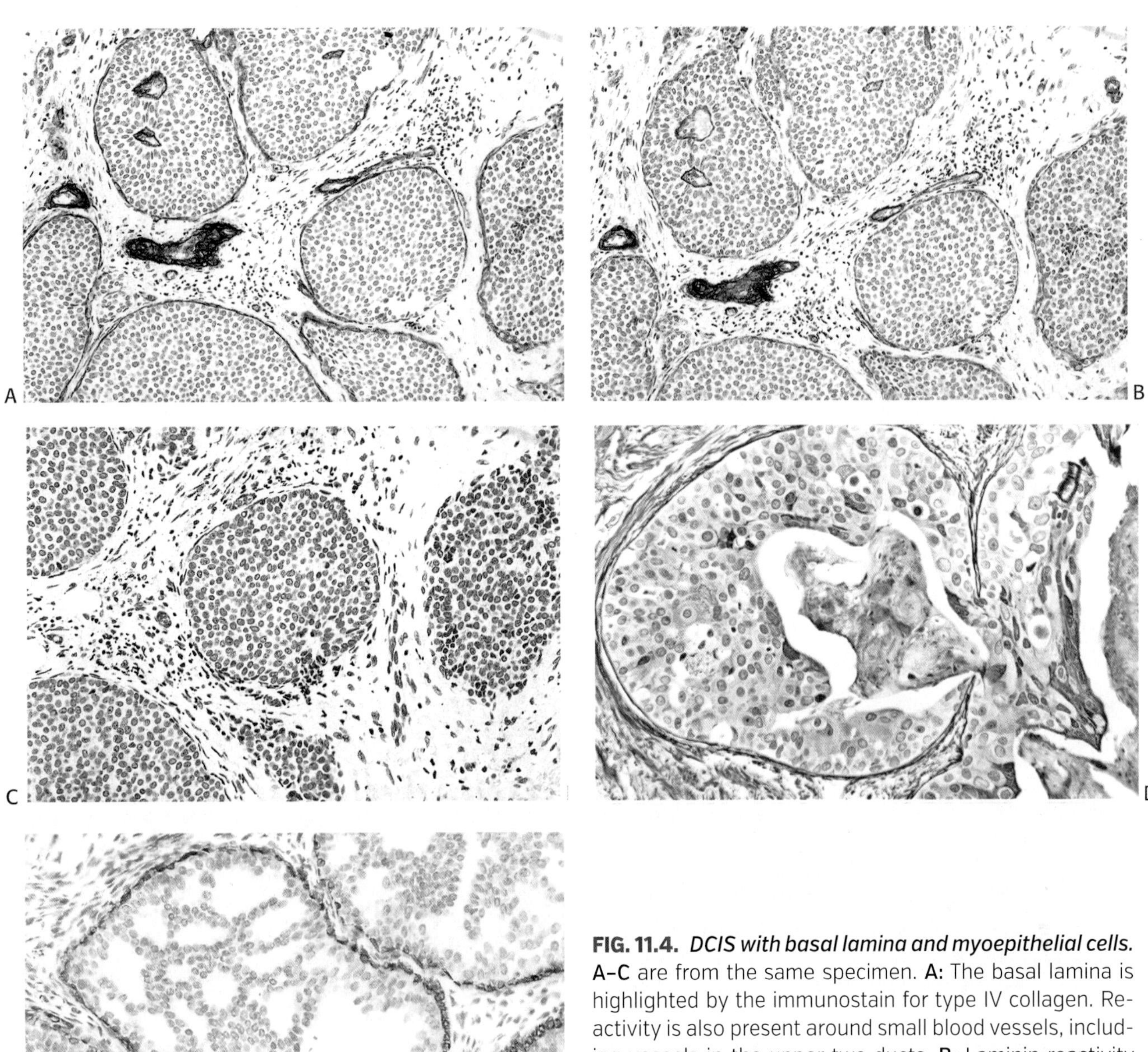

FIG. 11.4. ***DCIS with basal lamina and myoepithelial cells.*** **A–C** are from the same specimen. **A:** The basal lamina is highlighted by the immunostain for type IV collagen. Reactivity is also present around small blood vessels, including vessels in the upper two ducts. **B:** Laminin reactivity shown here has the same distribution as type IV collagen. **C:** There is no reactivity for SMA indicating the absence of myoepithelium in this DCIS. **D:** Basement membrane is highlighted by the reticulin stain. **E:** In this example of cribriform DCIS, myoepithelial cells display reactivity for the SMA.

ring cells, usually associated with lobular carcinoma, also occur in DCIS, most often in the papillary and cribriform types (Fig. 11.5). The presence of signet ring cells with cytoplasmic mucin demonstrated with the mucicarmine, periodic acid–Schiff (PAS), or Alcian blue stains is strong evidence for a diagnosis of DCIS. These cells are present only very rarely in hyperplastic duct lesions. Signet ring cells have eccentric nuclei that are often along the nuclear border, which abuts on the cytoplasmic mucin vacuole. A minute droplet of secretion may be apparent in the vacuole. Intracytoplasmic mucin sometimes imparts a diffuse pale blue color to the cytoplasm of carcinoma cells without forming distinct vacuoles. Nonspecific clear holes in the cytoplasm can be mistaken for signet ring vacuoles. These cytoplasmic defects, sometimes the site of glycogen accumulation, are not reactive with stains for mucin; they usually do not indent the nucleus, and there is ordinarily no secretion evident in the lumen.

Apocrine cytology is encountered in all of the structural types of DCIS (Fig. 11.6). Apocrine DCIS cells have abundant cytoplasm that ranges from granular and eosinophilic

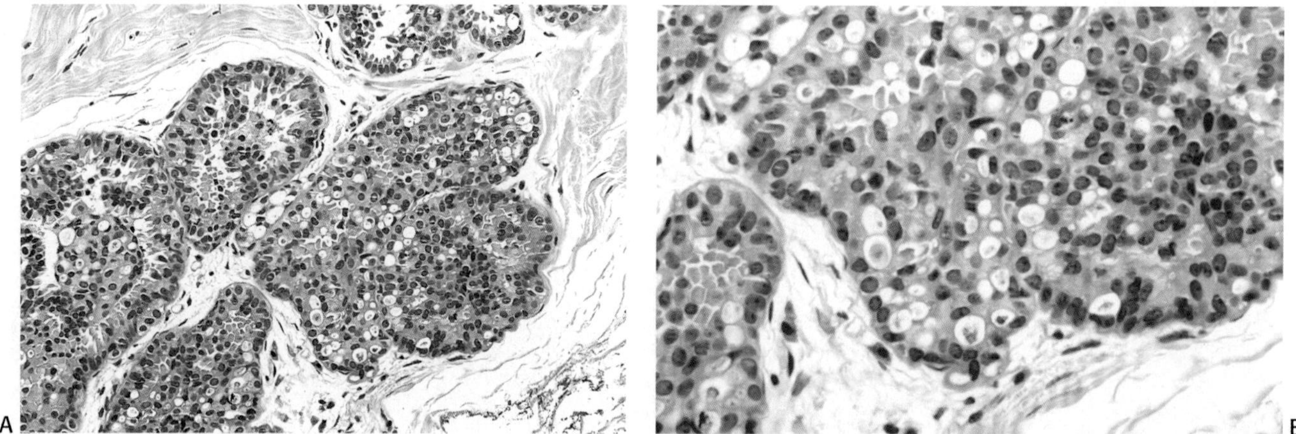

FIG. 11.5. ***DCIS with signet ring cells.*** **A,B:** Many of the tumor cells have cytoplasmic vacuoles that contain condensed secretion.

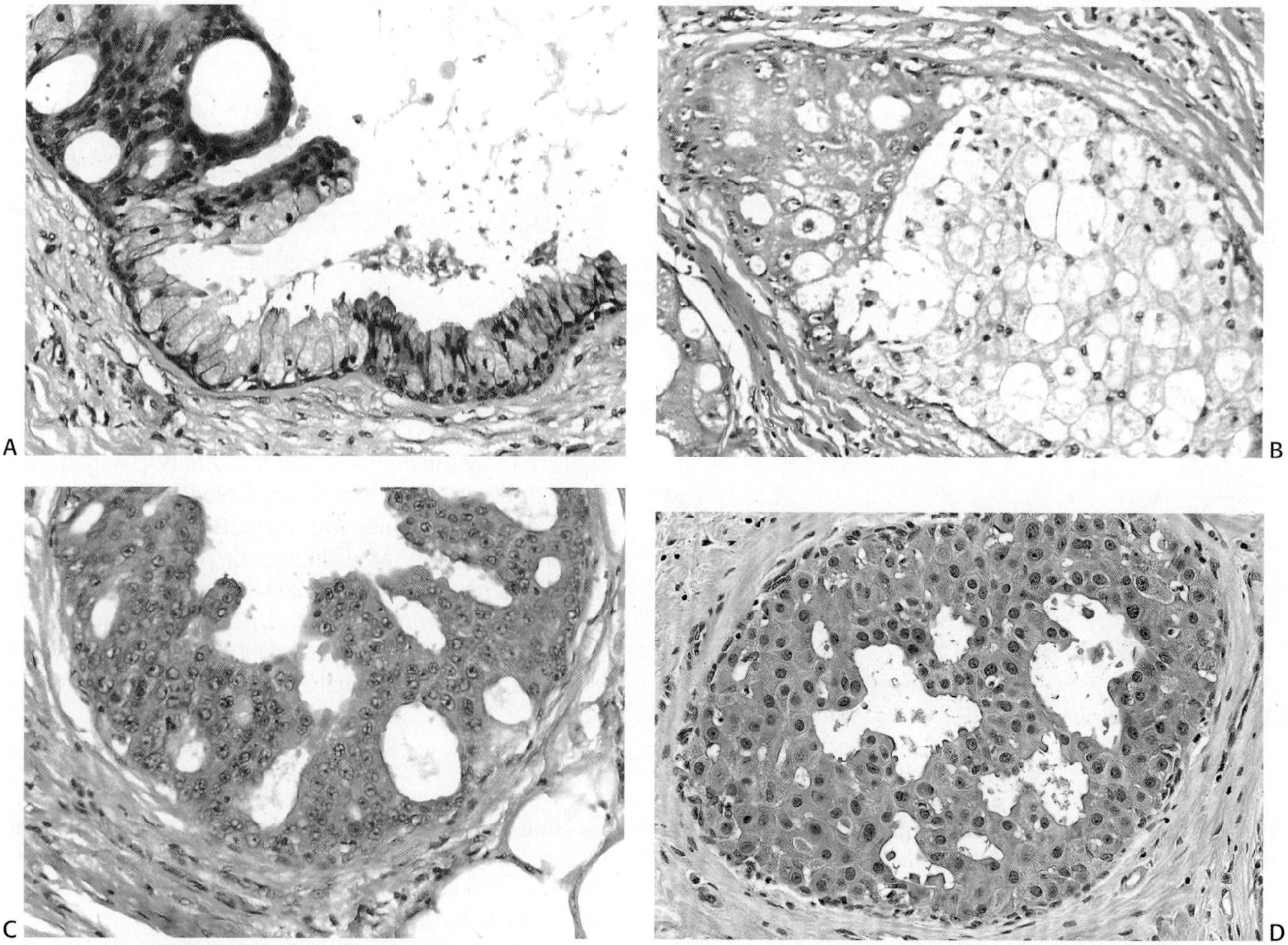

FIG. 11.6. ***DCIS, apocrine.*** **A:** Micropapillary carcinoma, partly clear cell type. **B:** Solid carcinoma, partly clear cell type. **C:** Cribriform carcinoma with high nuclear grade. **D:** Cribriform carcinoma with low and intermediate nuclear grade. **E:** Apocrine carcinoma in enlarged lobular glands with calcification. **F–G:** Apocrine carcinoma of solid type with high nuclear grade and lobular extension **(G)**. Note the periductal **(F)** and intralobular **(G)** lymphocytic infiltrate.

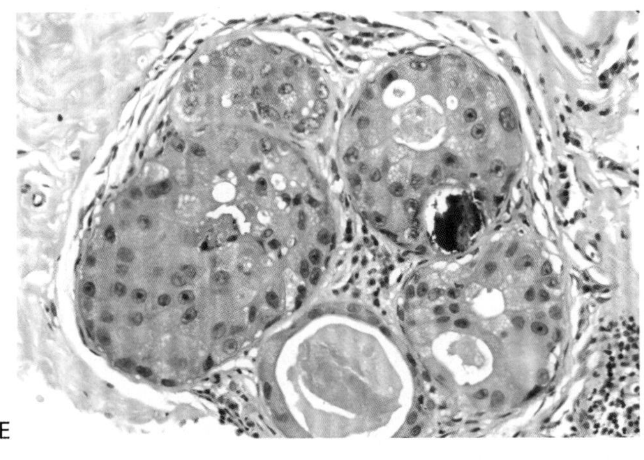
E

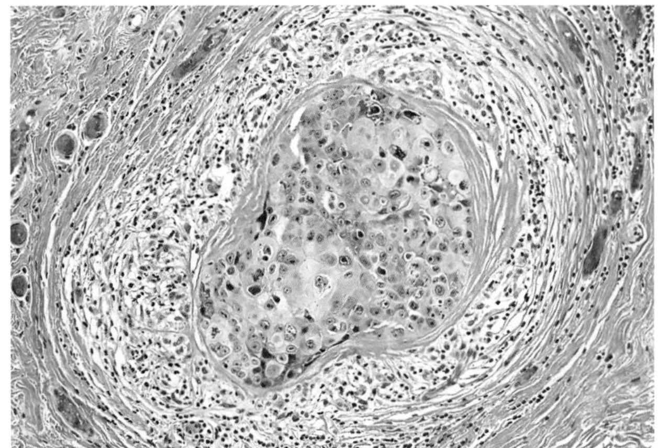
F

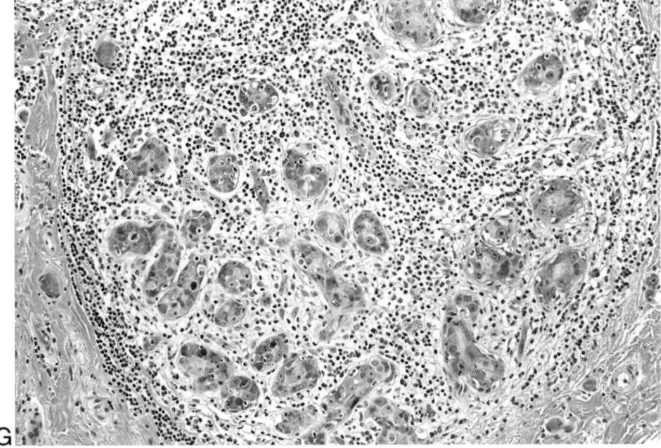
G

FIG. 11.6. *(Continued)*

to vacuolated or clear. There is variable nuclear pleomorphism, sometimes manifested by prominent nucleoli. A more complete discussion of apocrine carcinoma can be found in Chapter 19.

Clear cell DCIS is a poorly defined variant typically encountered with solid and comedo patterns (Fig. 11.7). Some clear cell DCIS are composed of cells with an arrangement described as "mosaic" because of the appearance created by sharply defined cell borders (Fig. 11.7). A subset of lesions classified under this heading includes forms of apocrine carcinoma. The presence of a monomorphic clear cell population is highly suggestive of DCIS. Occasionally, clear cell DCIS are strongly mucicarmine positive. Other clear cell lesions are probably the *in situ* form of lipid-rich or glycogen-rich carcinomas discussed in separate chapters.

Spindle cell DCIS may express neuroendocrine markers such as chromogranin, synaptophysin, and neuron-specific enolase.[111,112] The swirling growth pattern of cells in spindle cell DCIS mimics "streaming," which is characteristically found in usual duct hyperplasia. Spindle cell DCIS often coexists with cribriform DCIS.

Small cell DCIS is extremely uncommon. The growth patterns are typically cribriform and solid or a mixture of these forms. When present by itself, the solid pattern of small cell DCIS can be distinguished from LCIS with the E-cadherin immunostain that demonstrates membrane reactivity in DCIS. E-cadherin staining is absent or fragmented and weak in LCIS. "Neuroendocrine" DCIS is a less aggressive variant of small cell carcinoma (SCC) that is typically characterized by solid growth and spindle cell with fine granular cytoplasm, immunoreactivity for neuroendocrine markers, and a lower proliferation rate than SCC.[112]

The cellular composition of DCIS is typically *monomorphic*. This term has been applied especially to cribriform, solid, and micropapillary carcinomas. In this context, monomorphic means that there is overall homogeneity in the cytologic appearance of the DCIS cells—although there may be minor variation among cells in terms of amount of cytoplasm, nuclear size, etc. Variability in these parameters derives in part from differences in the plane in which they are sectioned. Cell and nuclear shape may be altered by the presence or absence of crowding in one or another part of the duct. The presence of a myoepithelial cell layer is not a consideration in judging whether a ductal proliferation is monomorphic.

Dimorphic variants of DCIS consisting of two distinctly different populations of cells are unusual. The majority of dimorphic DCIS are papillary carcinomas (see Chapter 14). A dimorphic papillary DCIS with a small invasive component of mucinous carcinoma is illustrated in Figure 11.8.

DCIS exhibits considerable tumoral heterogeneity, and in a given patient can have more than a single microscopic structural, cytologic, or immunocytochemical phenotype.[76,113,114] Mixed histologic patterns are found in

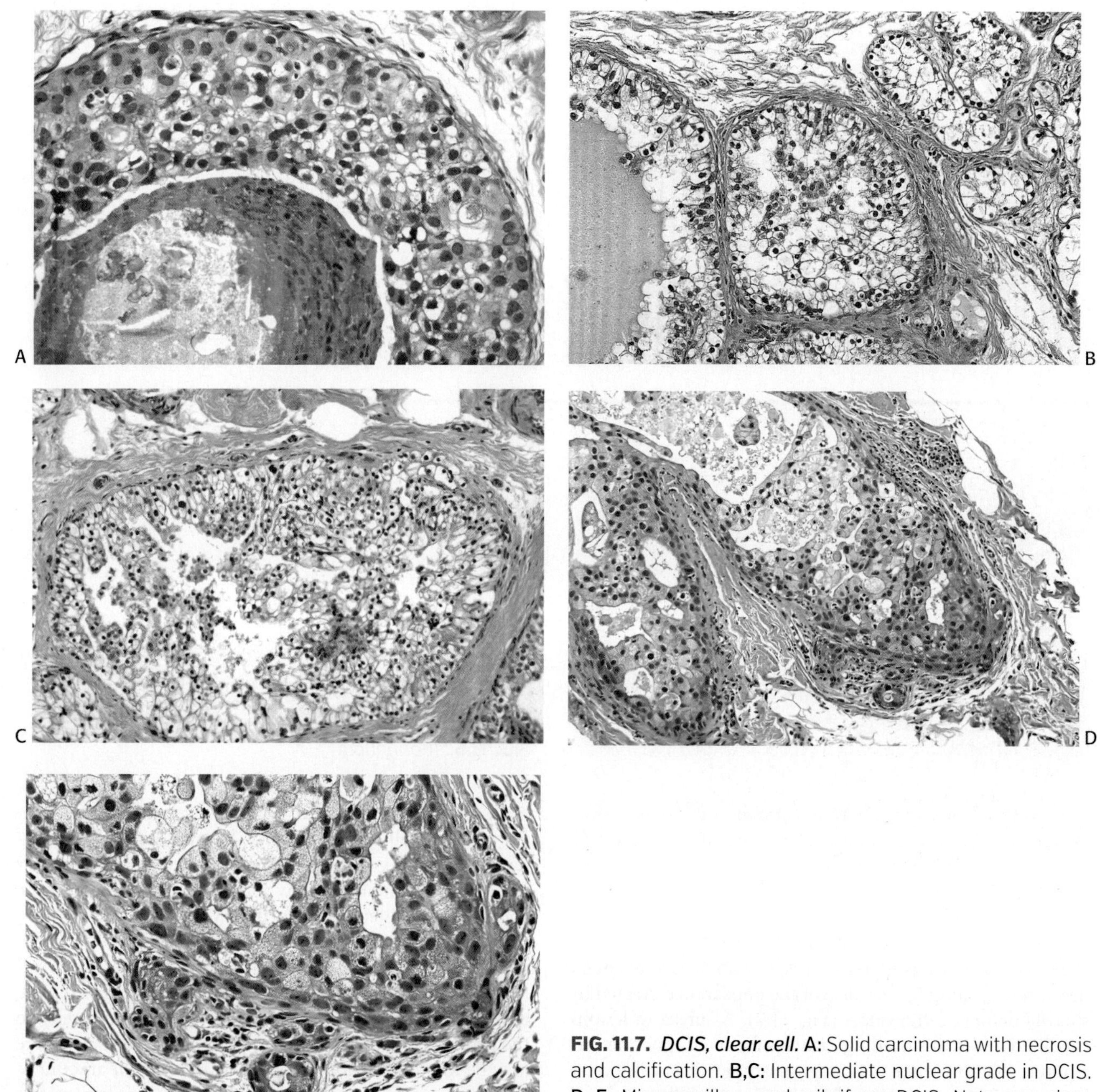

FIG. 11.7. ***DCIS, clear cell.*** **A:** Solid carcinoma with necrosis and calcification. **B,C:** Intermediate nuclear grade in DCIS. **D–E:** Micropapillary and cribriform DCIS. Note apocrine-type cytoplasmic features in some cells.

approximately 50% of cases. Whereas some structural combinations, such as papillary– or micropapillary–cribriform and solid-comedo, occur relatively more often than others, there is considerable heterogeneity with respect to growth patterns.[115] The probability of structural variability increases with the size of the lesion. Needle core biopsy samples may not be representative of the diverse growth patterns in a single case. The histologic diagnosis of DCIS should list the structural types in order of decreasing prominence, placing the dominant pattern first.

Cytologic features, especially at the nuclear level, tend to be more homogeneous than the growth pattern in a given case. Some combinations of growth patterns and cytologic appearances occur more frequently, such as classic comedo DCIS composed of poorly differentiated pleomorphic cells or the low nuclear grade typically present in micropapillary DCIS. Heterogeneity is illustrated by lesions composed of small, cytologically low-grade nuclei growing in a solid pattern or by high-grade nuclei found in some examples of micropapillary DCIS (Fig. 11.9). The presence of two or more structural patterns that have different cytologic features is particularly unusual (Fig. 11.10). Classification schemes developed to take cognizance of the heterogeneous distribution of nuclear grade and necrosis across the spectrum of

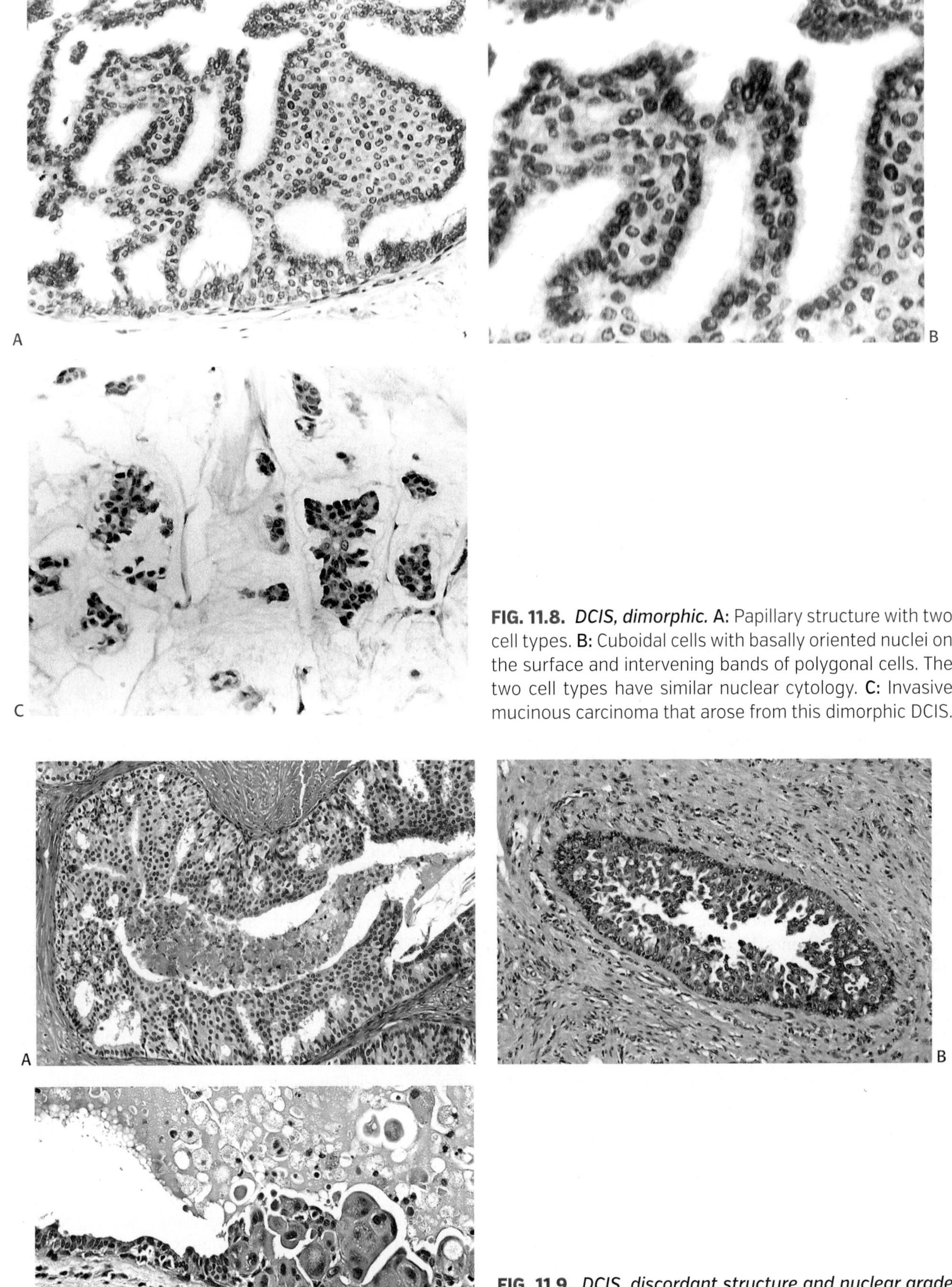

FIG. 11.8. ***DCIS, dimorphic.*** **A:** Papillary structure with two cell types. **B:** Cuboidal cells with basally oriented nuclei on the surface and intervening bands of polygonal cells. The two cell types have similar nuclear cytology. **C:** Invasive mucinous carcinoma that arose from this dimorphic DCIS.

FIG. 11.9. ***DCIS, discordant structure and nuclear grade.*** **A:** Cribriform DCIS with low nuclear grade and necrosis. **B:** Micropapillary DCIS with high nuclear grade. **C:** Flat micropapillary ("clinging") carcinoma with apocrine traits and high nuclear grade.

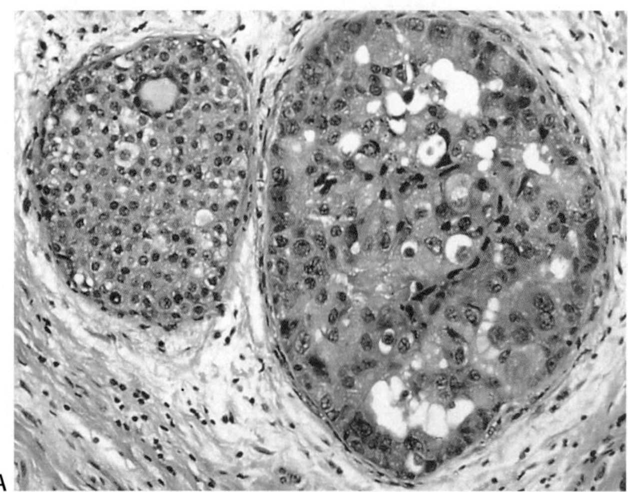

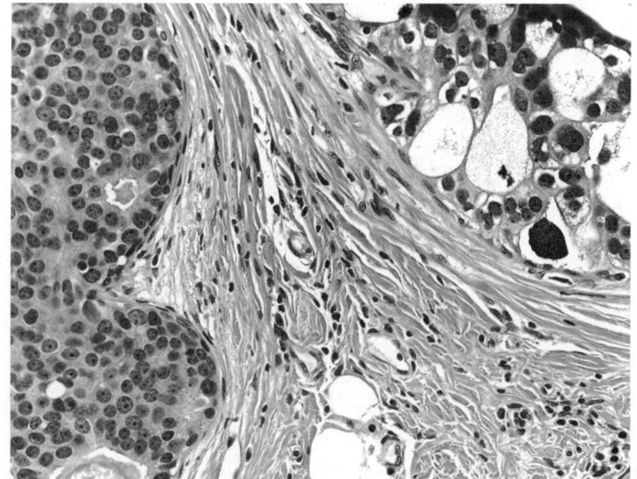

FIG. 11.10. *DCIS.* **A:** The smaller duct contains solid carcinoma with low nuclear grade and the larger duct contains cribriform carcinoma with necrosis and high nuclear grade. **B:** The duct on left contains solid DCIS with intermediate-grade nuclei, and the duct on the *right* shows cribriform DCIS with relatively higher grade nuclei and calcification.

structural patterns are considered subsequent to a discussion of the current conventional structural classification.

Structural Classification of DCIS

Micropapillary DCIS consists of ducts lined by a layer of neoplastic cells giving rise at intervals to papillary fronds or arcuate formations protruding into the duct lumen. When micropapillae are inconspicuous or absent, this type of DCIS has been described as flat or "clinging" because the neoplastic epithelium seems to hug the basement membrane (Fig. 11.11).[116] The papillae are variable in appearance, ranging from short bumps or mounds to long slender processes (Fig. 11.12). The papillae lack a fibrovascular core and are composed of cytologically homogeneous carcinoma cells. Lesions in which the carcinomatous epithelium is supported by fibrovascular stroma should be classified as papillary carcinomas, even if the growth pattern is predominantly micropapillary (Fig. 11.13). Arcuate structures, commonly referred to as Roman bridge (or aqueduct) arches, occur when microlumens are formed under adjacent coalescent fronds or within a mound of neoplastic cells. These fenestrations resemble the lumens formed in cribriform DCIS (Fig. 11.14). In conjunction with micropapillae, these arches are a feature of micropapillary DCIS and do not warrant a diagnosis of cribriform DCIS. In some situations, the micropapillary and cribriform patterns merge (Fig. 11.15). Some samples of micropapillary DCIS develop complex, frond-forming structures without evolving into cribriform growth (Fig. 11.16).

The appearance of the micropapillary fronds varies somewhat with the plane of individual histologic sections. Whereas some micropapillae are cut perpendicular to their long axis, others are seen sectioned tangentially or transversely, resulting in irregular nests of seemingly detached cell clusters in the duct lumen (Fig. 11.16). Ducts with low nuclear grade micropapillary DCIS are usually relatively free of cellular debris or inflammatory cells. Calcifications that are granular, crystalline, or laminated occur particularly when carcinoma arises in a background of columnar cell hyperplasia (CCH) (Fig. 11.11).

In micropapillary DCIS, the normal epithelial layer of the duct is replaced by a single population of neoplastic cells. In any given case, the appearance of the carcinoma cells is relatively homogeneous, but cytologic heterogeneity can occur between individual cases. Most often, micropapillary DCIS is composed of cytologically low-grade homogeneous cells with a high nuclear-to-cytoplasmic ratio and dense, hyperchromatic nuclei (Figs. 11.12, 11.14, and 11.15). The nuclei typically vary little in size, and chromatin density is consistent between cells at the base and tip of micropapillae. Nuclei may be slightly smaller and darker at the surface, but marked disparity in these characteristics is a feature of micropapillary hyperplasia (see Chapter 9). At the margin of the duct, between papillary and arcuate structures, the neoplastic cells are typically arranged in a layer that rarely exceeds three cells in depth. The nuclei of the cells in the epithelium between micropapillae are usually unevenly distributed in relation to the basement membrane (Figs. 11.12, 11.14, and 11.16). Persistent nonneoplastic epithelium between micropapillae is a feature of micropapillary hyperplasia rather than of micropapillary carcinoma. Mitoses are rarely present in low-grade micropapillary DCIS. The carcinoma cells tend to be so crowded and overlapping that their individual borders and cytoplasm cannot be identified. Occasionally, the cells have slightly more abundant cytoplasm, with apocrine-type protrusions at the luminal border. In one variant of this cell type, the nuclei of the tumor cells are contained in cytoplasmic blebs that are extruded into the duct lumen. Low-grade micropapillary DCIS can be found near some tubular carcinomas. These patients often have multifocal CCH with atypia and may also have LCIS

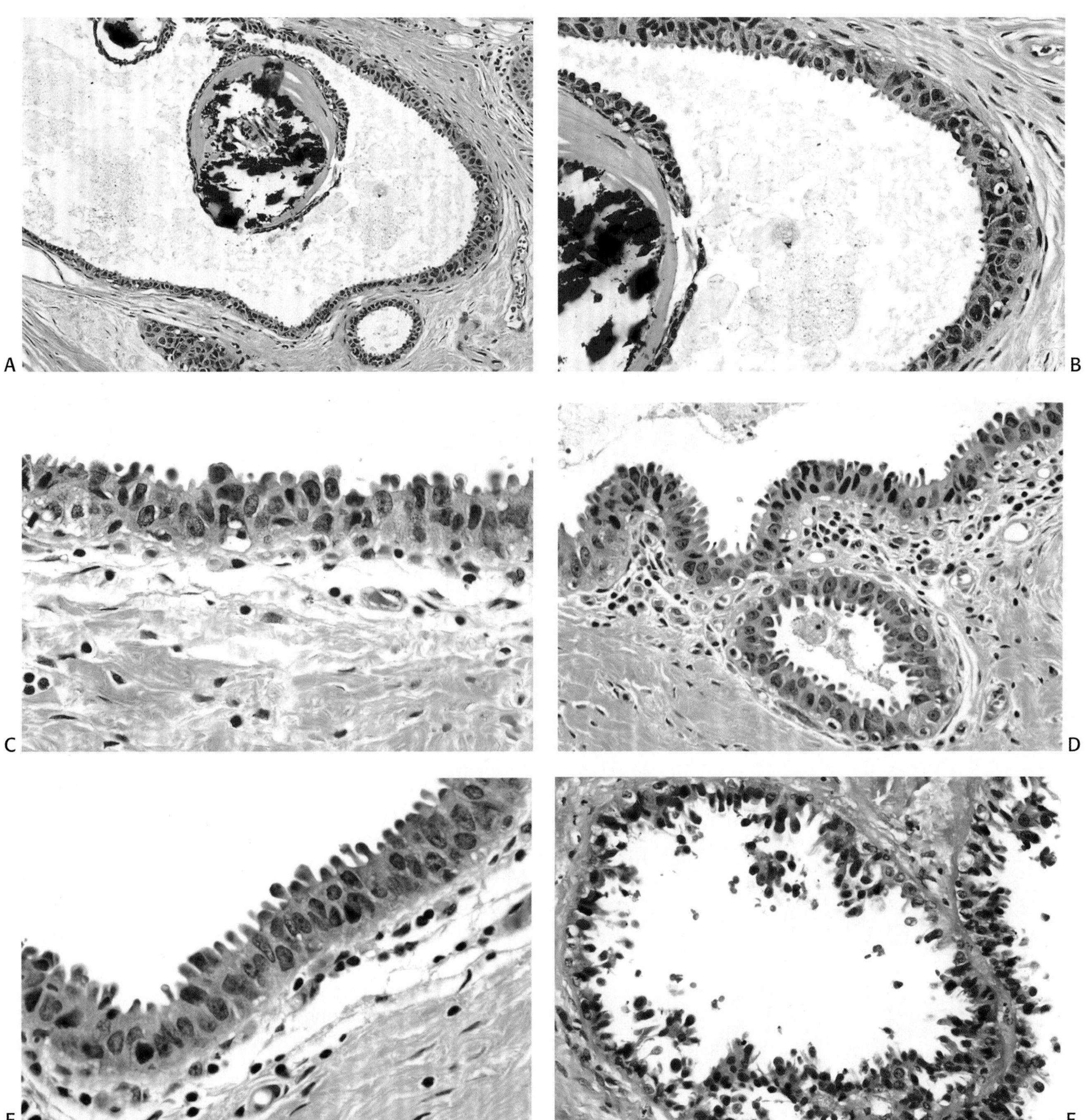

FIG. 11.11. ***DCIS, flat ("clinging") micropapillary type.*** **A:** The papillary structures in this cystically dilated duct contain fractured calcifications of the ossifying type typically associated with columnar cell lesions. **B:** Carcinoma cells with pleomorphic nuclei and a disorderly distribution line the duct and overlie the calcification. **C:** The flat carcinomatous epithelium displays apical apocrine-type cytoplasmic "snouts." **D–F:** Other examples of flat, "clinging" DCIS.

(see Chapter 9). Squamous metaplasia can be encountered in micropapillary DCIS (Fig. 11.17). Clear cell micropapillary DCIS is uncommon (Fig. 11.18).

A minority of micropapillary carcinomas are composed of cells with intermediate- or high- (poorly differentiated) grade cytologic characteristics (Figs. 11.9, 11.16, and 11.19). Cells forming this type of carcinoma differ from those in the conventional micropapillary lesions by being larger, with more abundant cytoplasm. Nuclei are also correspondingly larger, and nucleoli may be apparent. Mitoses can be found in this epithelium, and the cells often have a distinctly apocrine appearance. The cytologically high-grade form of

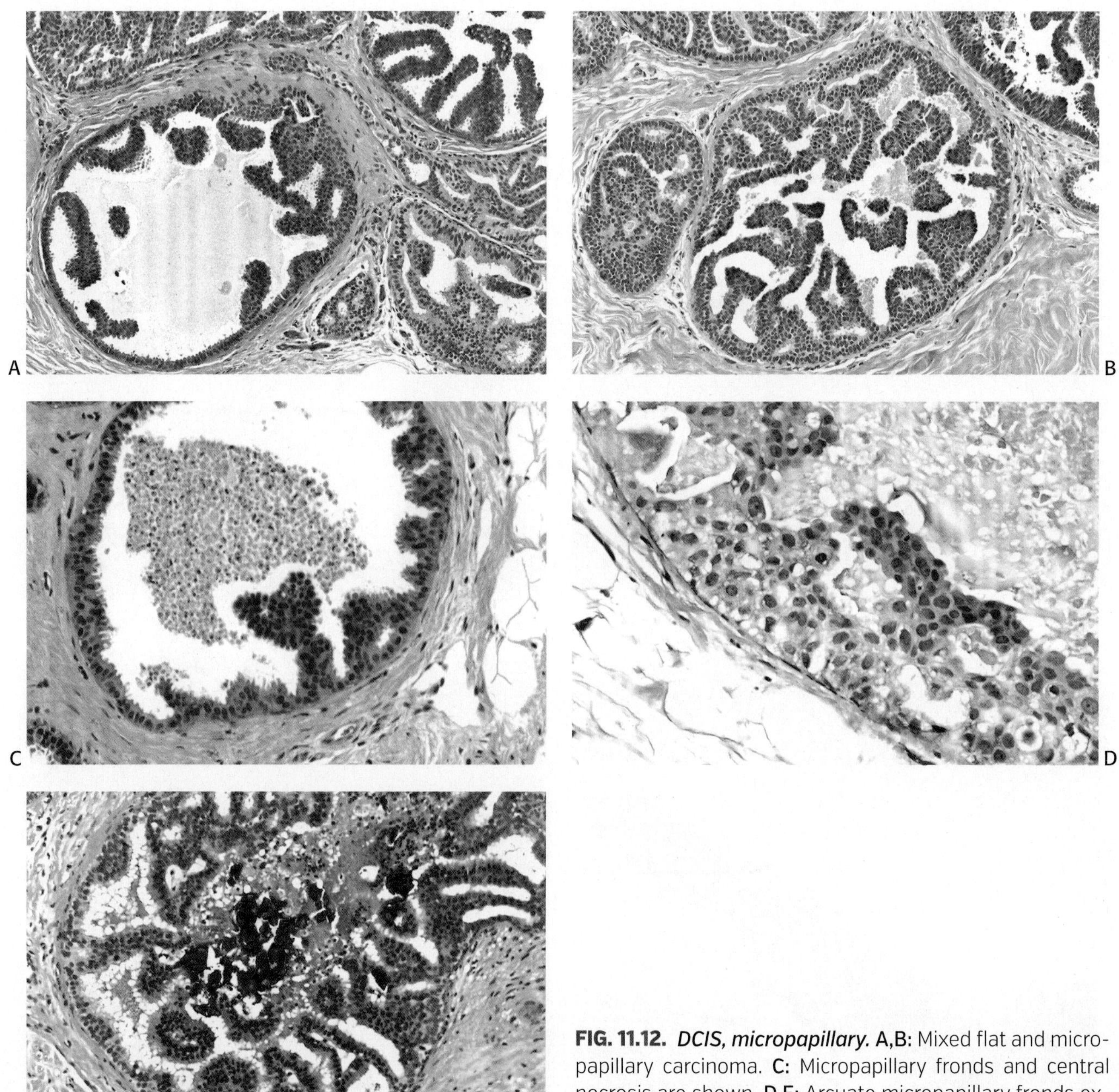

FIG. 11.12. ***DCIS, micropapillary.*** **A,B:** Mixed flat and micropapillary carcinoma. **C:** Micropapillary fronds and central necrosis are shown. **D,E:** Arcuate micropapillary fronds extend into duct lumens. Dense calcific deposits are present in **(E)**.

micropapillary DCIS is more likely to have calcifications than the low-grade variant, and necrotic cellular debris may be found in the duct lumen.

In an interinstitutional study, it was found that high nuclear grade micropapillary DCIS more frequently overexpressed HER2, had a higher proliferation index, displayed necrosis and microinvasion, and was more extensive than those of low- and intermediate-grade nuclei.[117] Furthermore, in the same series, high nuclear grade was found to be the only parameter associated with elevated risk of local recurrence after breast-conserving surgery for micropapillary DCIS.

Two subtypes of micropapillary carcinoma have been given specific designations. *Cystic hypersecretory DCIS* is discussed in Chapter 24. The term *flat micropapillary carcinoma* (so-called "clinging" carcinoma) refers to DCIS with the cytologic appearance of the micropapillary lesion that is lacking in fully developed epithelial fronds (Fig. 11.11). Lesions composed entirely of flat micropapillary DCIS are very uncommon, and more often one or more epithelial fronds or bridges are present. In the absence of calcification or necrosis, flat micropapillary DCIS is easily overlooked microscopically. This type of DCIS is most often found in a background of CCH, which is encountered mainly in

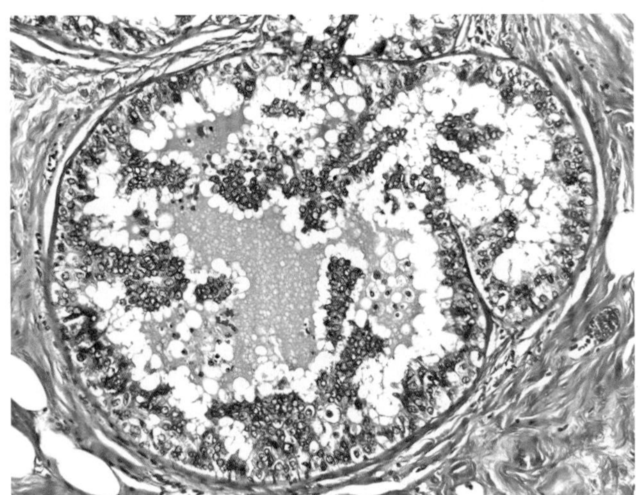

FIG. 11.13. ***DCIS, micropapillary.*** Some epithelial fronds have delicate fibrovascular centers.

women 35 to 55 years of age. The lesions are typically multifocal or multicentric and can be bilateral. Flat micropapillary ("clinging") DCIS should be diagnosed whenever a flat epithelial proliferative process shows relatively small- to medium-sized cells with high-grade round-to-oval nuclei with speckled chromatin. Such neoplastic cells are generally uniform, with centrally placed nuclei within which nucleoli are inconspicuous. So-called "flat epithelial atypia" (in most cases synonymous with atypical CCH) and *low-grade* DCIS of the breast have been shown to share highly homologous molecular and genomic profiles[118]; however, such data can be interpreted as being reflective of the difficulty in distinguishing between the two entities, morphologically as well as by molecular criteria, and the need to be conservative in the diagnosis of low-grade DCIS.

Calcifications with distinctive crystalline, ossifying, and laminated appearances tend to occur in CCH, leading to mammographic detection. Patients with CCH may have tubular carcinoma, LCIS, and invasive lobular carcinoma, as well as micropapillary DCIS.

Cribriform DCIS is a fenestrated epithelial proliferation in which microlumens are formed by neoplastic epithelium that bridges most or all of the duct lumen. Cribriform DCIS can be found at all levels of the main duct system from major ducts to terminal intralobular ductules. Extension into lobular epithelium (so-called "lobular cancerization") or into the main lactiferous ducts of the nipple is uncommon. Markedly dilated ducts with cribriform DCIS can be mistaken for

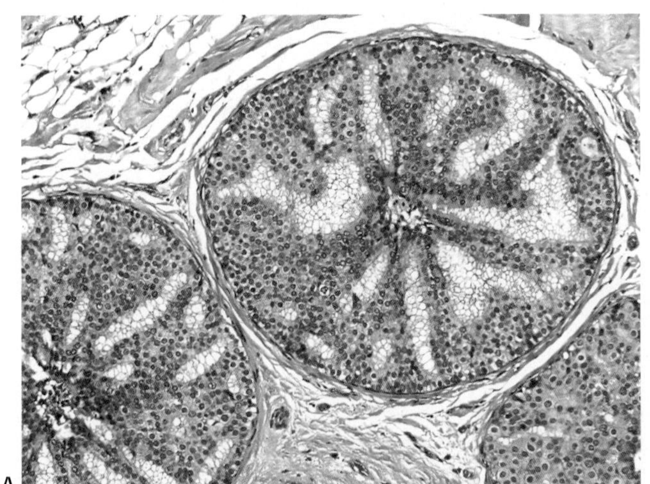

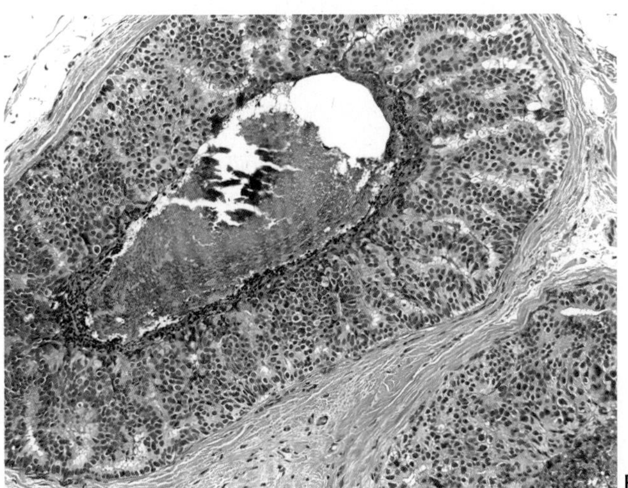

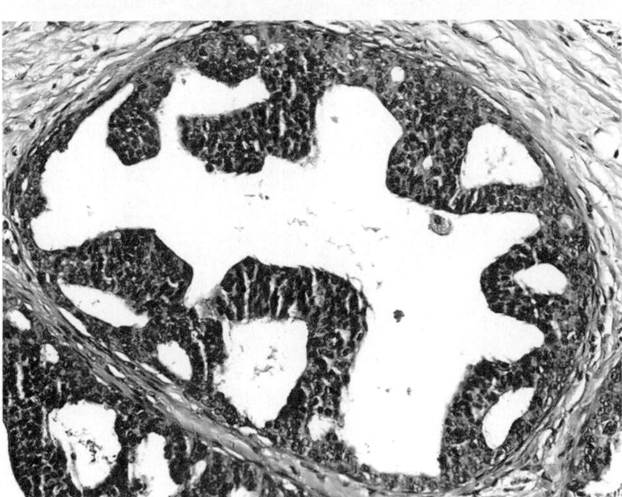

FIG. 11.14. ***DCIS, micropapillary.*** Intraductal micropapillary growth developing cribriform (A,B) and Roman bridge-like (C) structures.

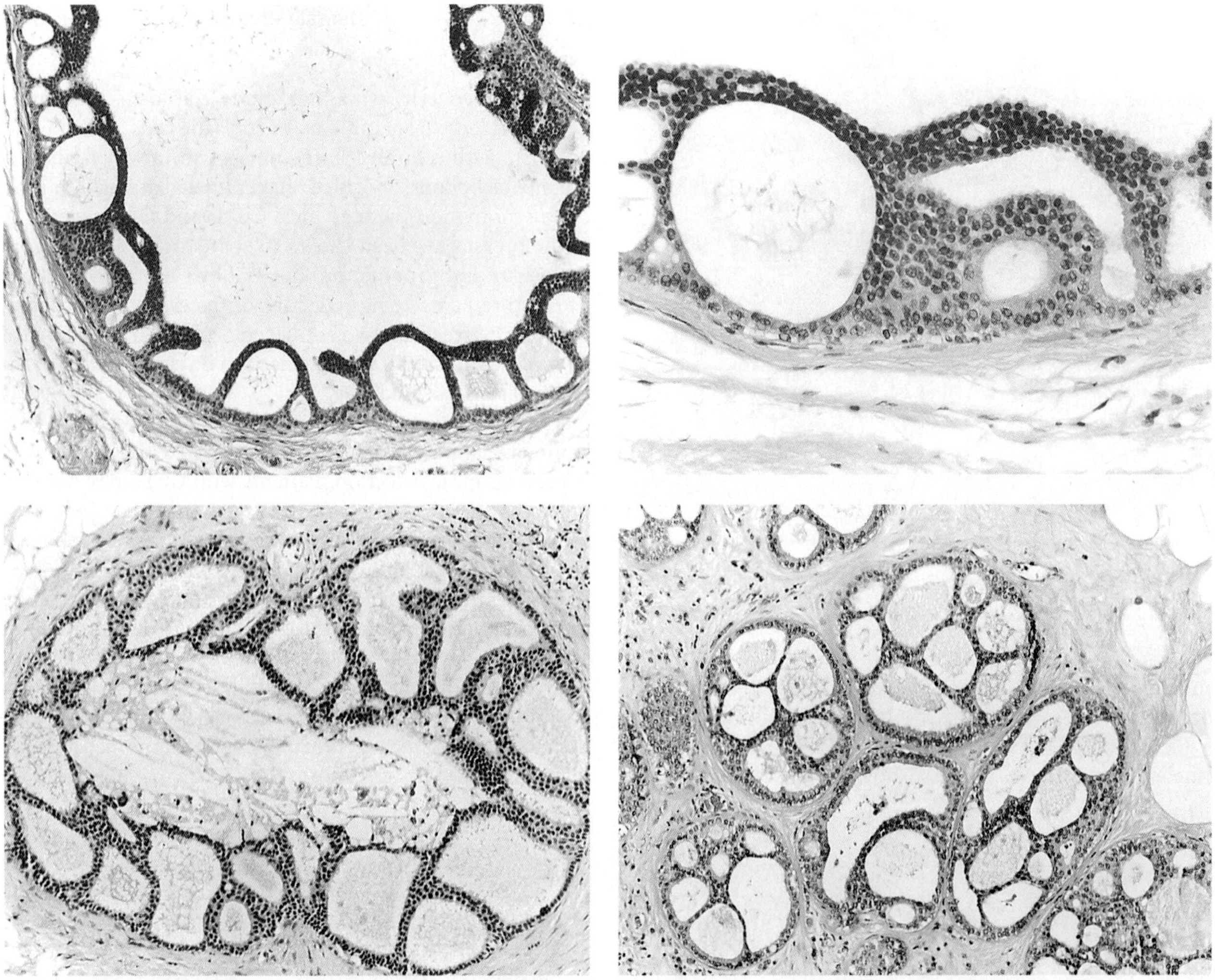

FIG. 11.15. ***DCIS, micropapillary and cribriform.*** **A:** Prominent peripheral micropapillary arches with secondary cribriform microlumina. (From Rosen PP. The pathology of breast carcinoma. In: Harris JR, Hellman S, Henderson IC, Kinne DW, eds. *Breast diseases*. Philadelphia: J.B. Lippincott, 1987:150, with permission.) **B:** Enlarged view of (**A**) showing low-grade nuclei. **C:** Large peripheral arcades which encroach on the lumen that contains histiocytes. (From Rosen PP, Oberman HA. *Tumors of the mammary gland.* (*AFIP Atlas of Tumor Pathology,* 3rd series, vol. 7). Baltimore: American Registry of Pathology, 1993.) **D:** DCIS with a fully developed cribriform structure that can arise in the patient with micropapillary DCIS.

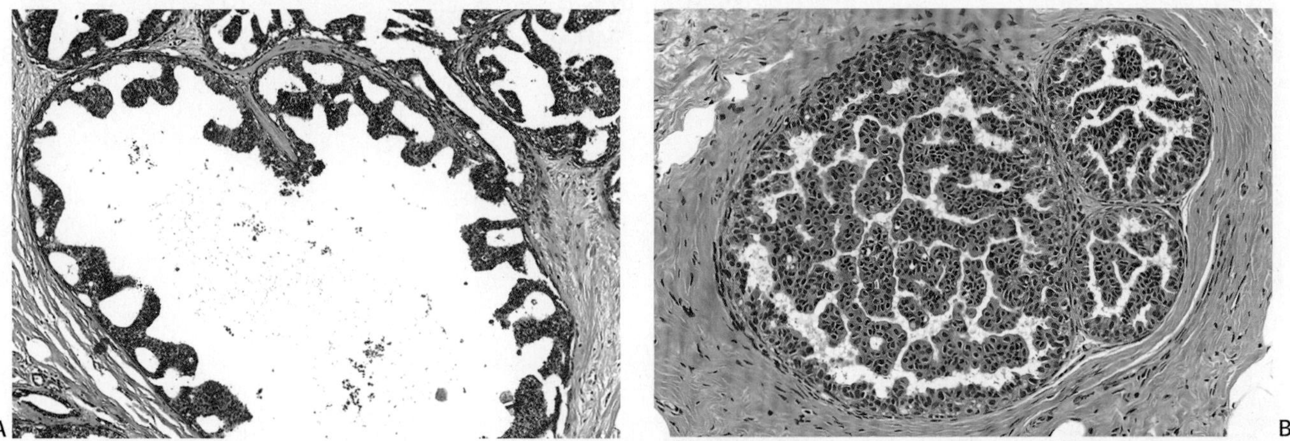

FIG. 11.16. ***DCIS, micropapillary.*** **A:** An example of relatively uncomplicated micropapillary DCIS with apocrine cytology. **B:** Florid micropapillary DCIS with numerous epithelial fronds filling the duct lumen.

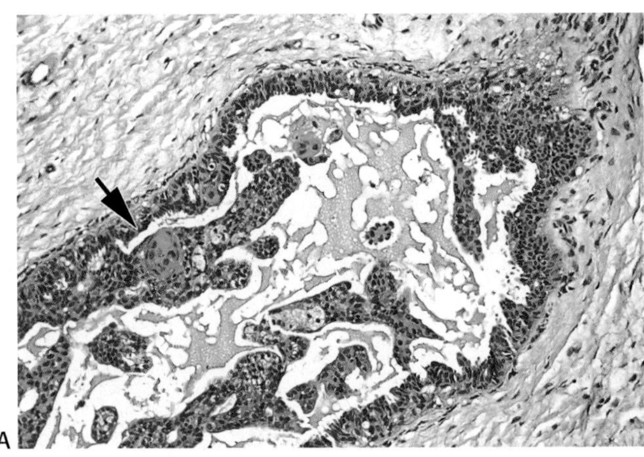

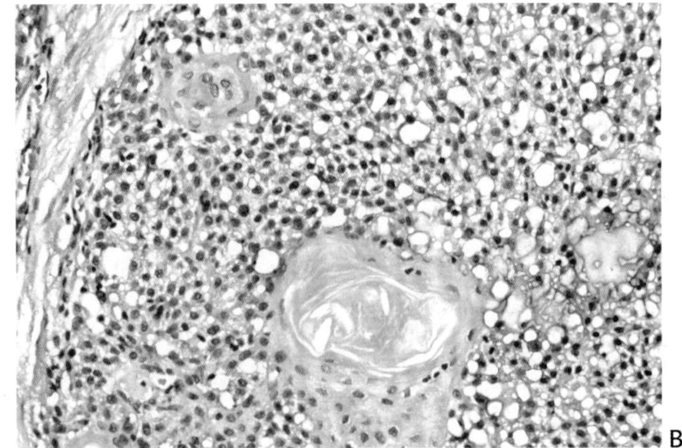

FIG. 11.17. ***DCIS with squamous metaplasia.*** **A:** Isolated foci of squamous metaplasia are present in the micropapillary carcinomatous epithelium (*arrow*). **B:** Squamous metaplasia in solid DCIS.

adenoid cystic carcinoma (AdCC) or a complex papilloma. Collagenous spherulosis that is usually associated with hyperplastic duct lesions can, in rare instances, be involved by DCIS (Fig. 11.20). The resultant structure resembles cribriform DCIS because the spherules simulate microlumens. The presence of collagenous spherulosis can be confirmed with either heavy-chain myosin or SMA immunostain, which will highlight myoepithelial cells at the perimeter of spherules or immunostains for basement membrane components (such as laminin or collagen IV). LCIS can also inhabit collagenous spherulosis. The distinction between intraductal and *in situ* lobular carcinoma in collagenous spherulosis depends on cytologic features of the lesion and can be confirmed with the E-cadherin or p120 immunostains. The appearance of any adjacent coexisting *in situ* carcinoma not in collagenous spherulosis can also be helpful.

The secondary microlumina in cribriform DCIS tend to be round or oval, with smooth luminal edges bordered by cuboidal cells (Fig. 11.21). The distribution of microlumina is variable. In some instances, the spaces are spread across the entire duct or concentrated toward the center. The presence of microlumina entirely at the periphery of the duct is usually an indication of hyperplasia, but this appearance may be mimicked in cribriform DCIS when the center of the duct is destroyed by necrosis (Fig. 11.22). It is a hallmark of cribriform DCIS that the microlumina be surrounded by a homogeneous cell population that is uniformly distributed throughout the duct. The microlumina may contain secretion, small numbers of degenerated or necrotic cells, and punctate calcifications.

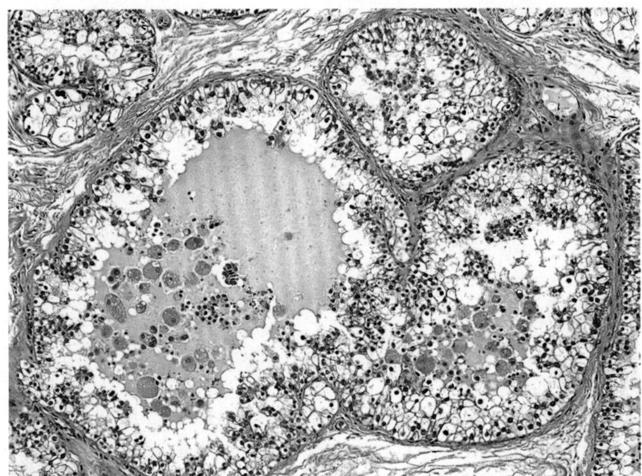

FIG. 11.18. ***DCIS, micropapillary clear cell type.***

Bands of neoplastic cells between and around the microlumina in cribriform DCIS are described as "rigid," a term that refers to the uniform, nonoverlapping, distribution of polygonal cells in contrast to the streaming pattern of overlapping, frequently oval cells in duct hyperplasia (Fig. 11.23). Polarization of the cells in an orderly fashion around the microlumina contributes to the "rigid" appearance. The most orderly type of cribriform DCIS is composed of cuboidal to low columnar monomorphic cells with low nuclear grade. Nucleoli are inconspicuous or absent, and mitoses are rarely encountered. The cells usually have sparse cytoplasm. An apocrine variant is composed of cells with low- to intermediate-grade nuclei and more abundant granular eosinophilic cytoplasm (Fig. 11.24). Secretion is found in some but not all cribriform microlumina, and when present it can form small calcifications. Cribriform DCIS with necrosis, mitotic activity, and poorly differentiated nuclear grade is rare, and these lesions tend to have less well-defined microlumina (Fig. 11.25). The cribriform pattern of carcinoma may either represent DCIS or invasive carcinoma. The latter disease is an uncommon entity that is characterized by an infiltrative pattern of growth (Chapter 26).

In some circumstances, it may be difficult to distinguish between cribriform and other structural subtypes of DCIS, and in these instances the choice is sometimes arbitrary. Fibrovascular stroma and myoepithelial cells are not present in the epithelium of cribriform DCIS, but myoepithelial cells may persist at the periphery of the involved duct (Fig. 11.4). Solid papillary DCIS in which fibrovascular stroma is clearly evident occasionally has a prominent fenestrated pattern that mimics cribriform DCIS. The stromal component of

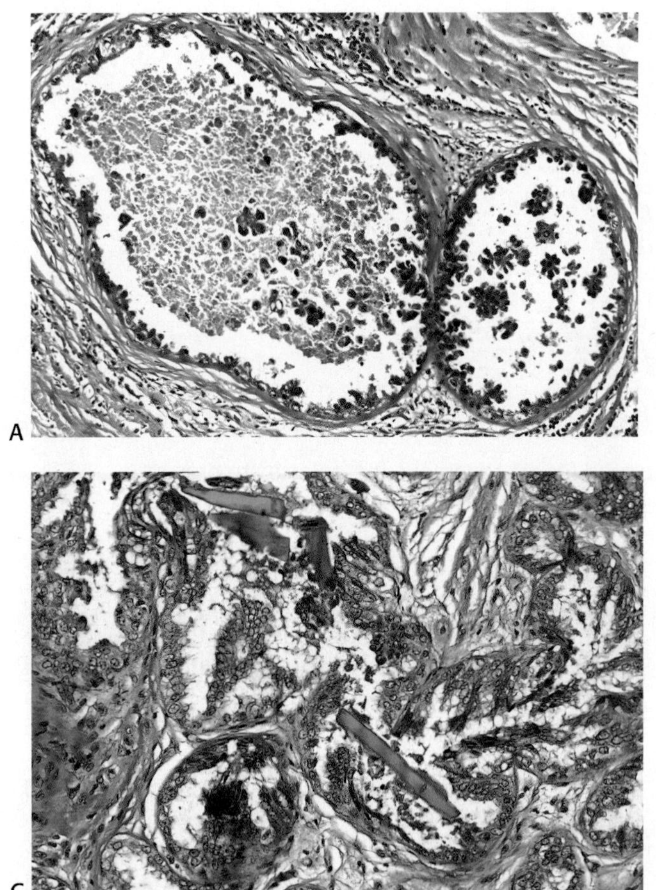

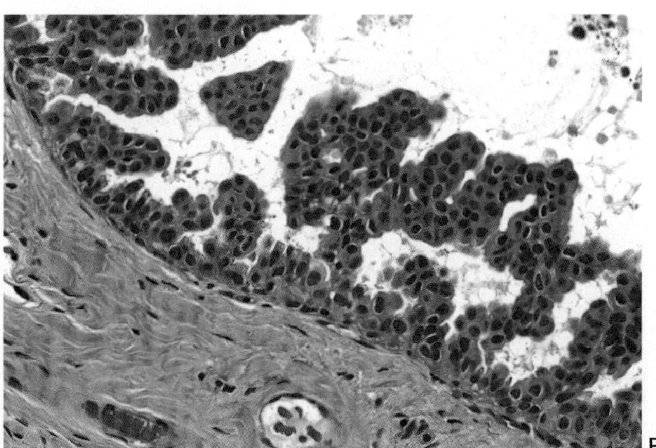

FIG. 11.19. ***DCIS, micropapillary.*** **A:** The cells have high-grade nuclei. There is cellular debris and central necrosis in the ducts. **B:** Apocrine cytology and intermediate nuclear grade. **C:** An unusual micropapillary DCIS with intermediate nuclear grade and crystalloids.

solid papillary DCIS may be quite inconspicuous and easily overlooked. Another ambiguous situation arises when there is prominent secondary lumen formation in micropapillary DCIS (Fig. 11.15). This process can encompass a substantial part of the overall duct lumen. Generally, the growth pattern of micropapillary DCIS is oriented to the circumference of the duct, whereas in cribriform DCIS there is a more even distribution of microlumina across the duct without peripheral orientation. Difficulty in classification also arises when the intraductal proliferation is almost entirely solid with rare microlumina (Fig. 11.26). The differential diagnosis of cribriform DCIS includes other lesions such as AdCC,

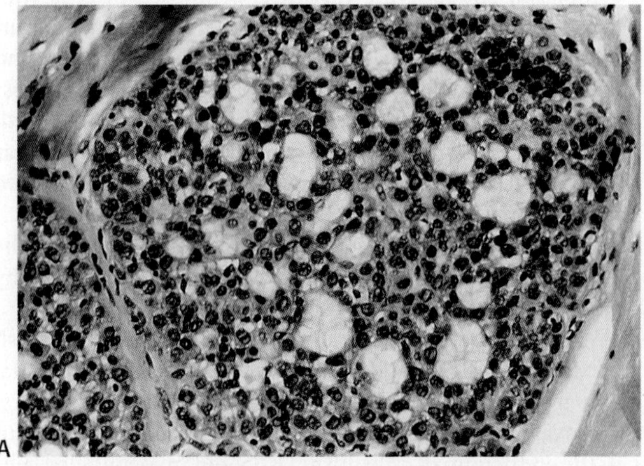

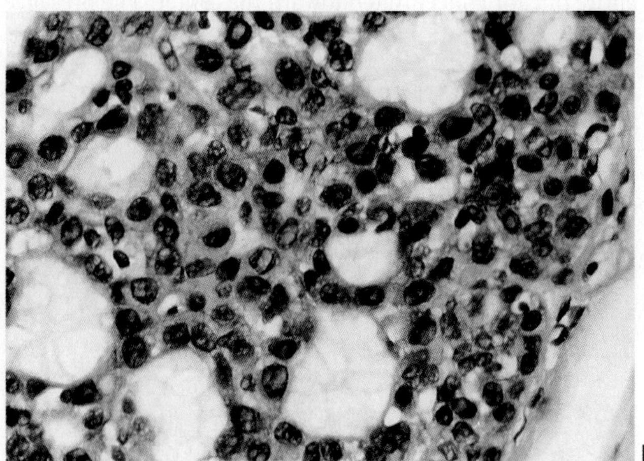

FIG. 11.20. ***DCIS in collagenous spherulosis.*** **A:** The spherules simulate a cribriform pattern. **B:** Stellate fibrils are visible in some spherules. Note the thin bands of basement membrane that define the perimeter of spherules. The carcinoma cells show moderate nuclear pleomorphism and intermediate nuclear grade. The carcinoma cells were immunoreactive for E-cadherin.

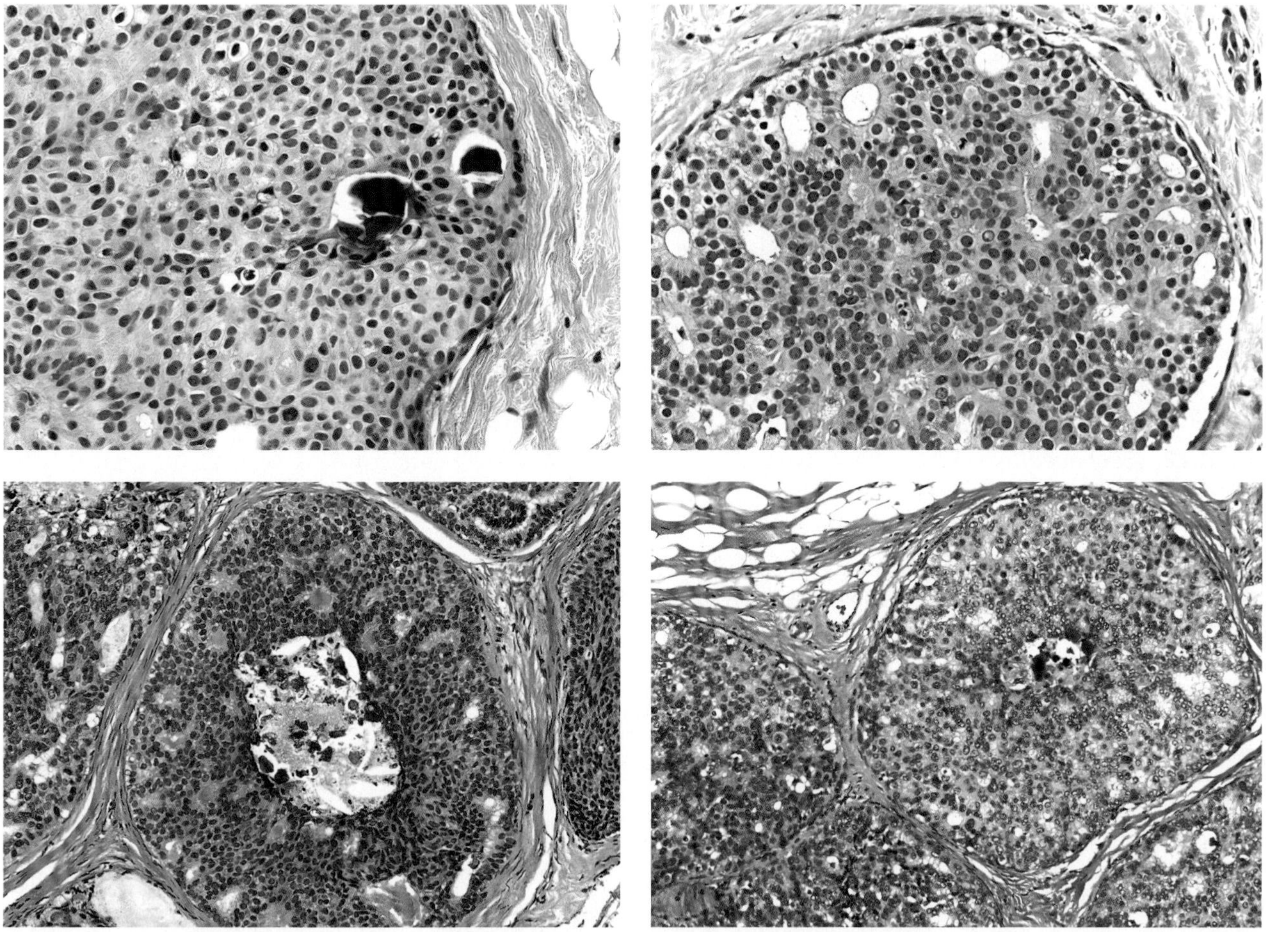

FIG. 11.21. ***DCIS, cribriform.*** **A:** Minimal microlumen formation, some with calcifications. Nuclei are of low grade. **B:** Relatively round microlumina in the distended duct with low-to intermediate-grade nuclei. **C:** Central and peripheral microlumina with central necrosis and calcifications. **D:** Microlumina with irregular contours. There is central necrosis with calcification.

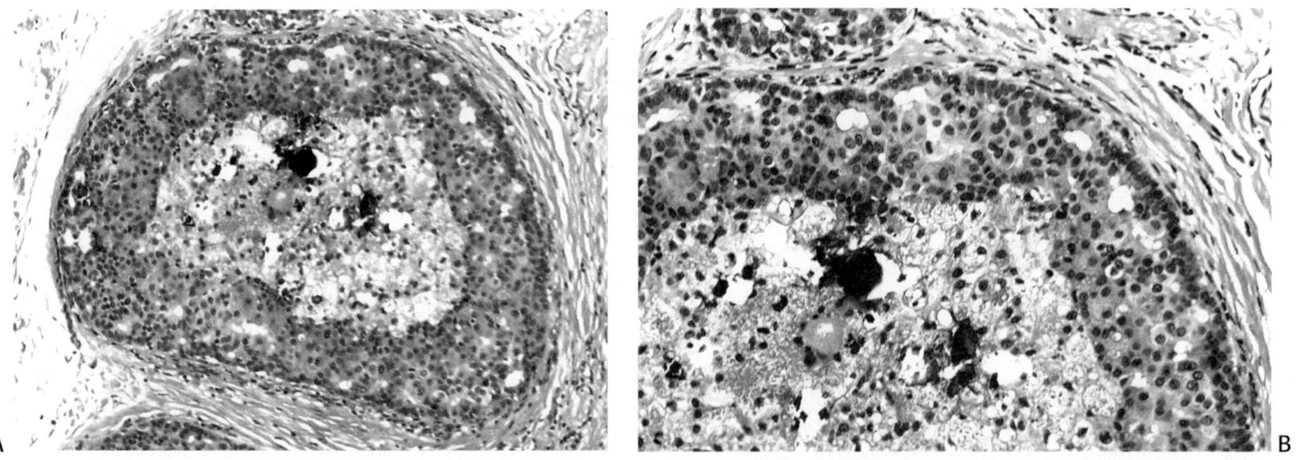

FIG. 11.22. ***DCIS, cribriform.*** **A:** Peripheral microlumina, some of which are slit shaped, and a prominent central lumen with degenerating cells and calcification. **B:** Magnified view showing degenerating tumor cells in the lumen. **C:** Another duct from the same specimen with a conventional cribriform structure. **D:** DCIS with conventional cribriform structure. The duct is filled with histiocytes and calcifications.

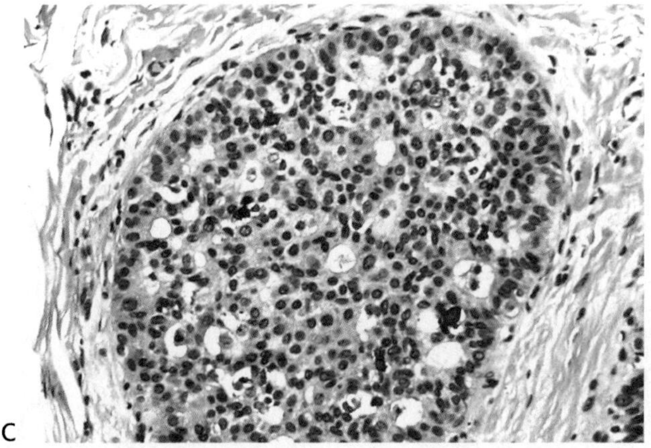

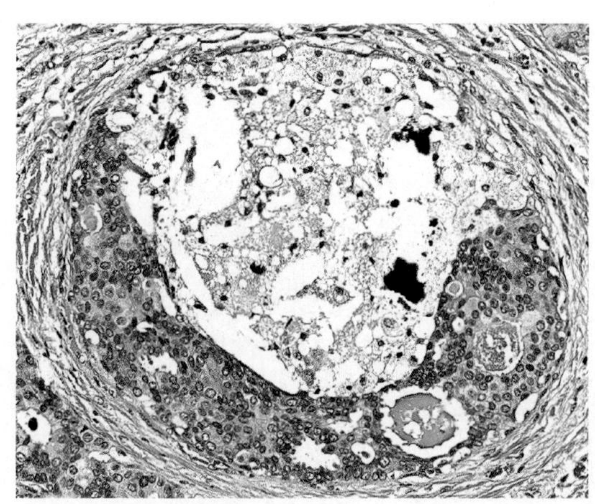

FIG. 11.22. *(Continued)*

invasive cribriform carcinoma, collagenous spherulosis, and atypical ductal hyperplasia (ADH). Applying the "ADH-5" cocktail (a combination of CKs 5/14, 7/18, and p63) in the differential diagnosis of ADH and DCIS has shown promise for improving interobserver and intraobserver agreement; however, the usefulness of this immunostain in a controlled prospective setting remains to be determined.[119]

Comedo DCIS is described classically as a solid growth of large carcinoma cells with poorly differentiated nuclei, central necrosis, calcification, and, in some but not all cases, a high mitotic rate (Fig. 11.27). The myoepithelial cell layer is variably affected and sometimes completely eliminated by the carcinomatous proliferation. In some instances, the myoepithelial cells are hyperplastic with hyperchromatic nuclei,

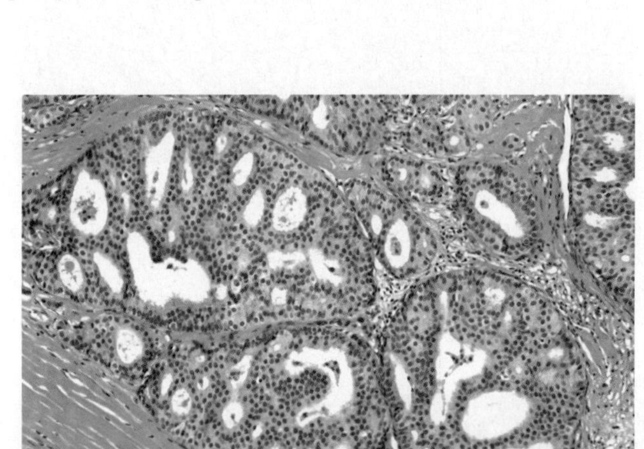

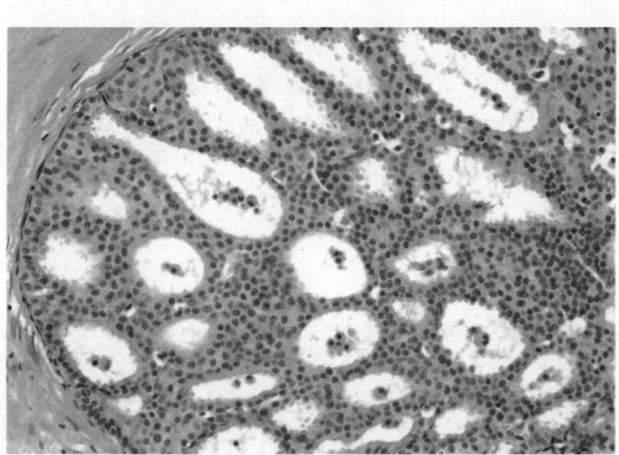

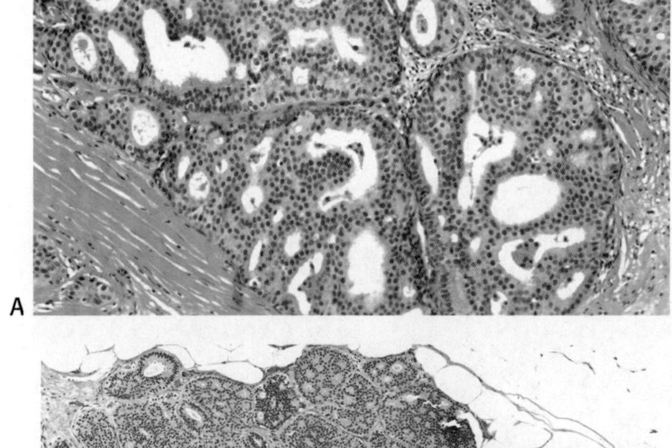

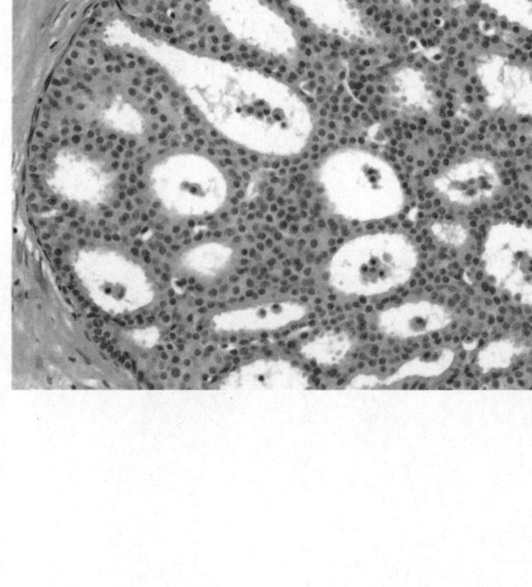

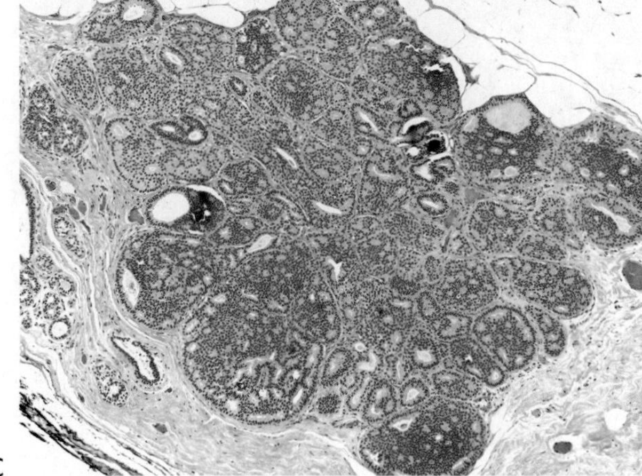

FIG. 11.23. ***DCIS, cribriform.*** **A,B:** Microlumina with various shapes. **C:** A circumscribed lobulated focus of cribriform DCIS with calcifications.

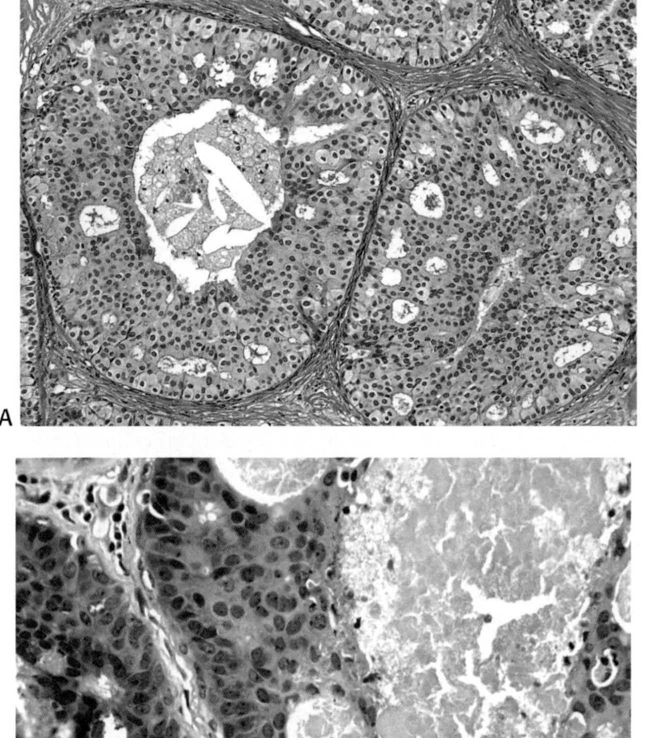

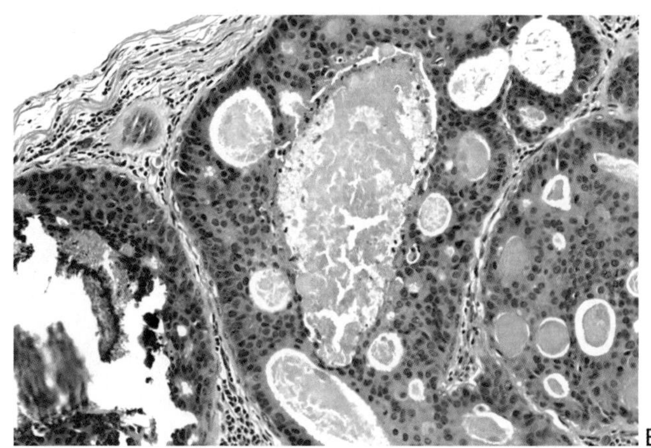

FIG. 11.24. ***DCIS, cribriform.*** **A:** Apocrine features. **B,C:** Low to intermediate nuclear grade with necrosis.

producing a distinct ring between the neoplastic epithelial cells and the basement membrane. This configuration is often accompanied by accentuation of the basement membrane itself, as well as a circumferential periductal collar of desmoplastic stroma. A "cocktail" of antibodies to smooth muscle myosin-heavy chain (SMM-HC) and p63 is especially sensitive for detecting myoepithelium in high-grade DCIS.[120] Elastosis occurs around some ducts with this periductal reaction. Rarely pronounced neovascularity is represented by a partial or complete ring of capillaries external to the basement membrane[101] (Fig. 11.28). A variable inflammatory infiltrate is present in the periductal stroma. In some instances, this consists of lymphocytes and histiocytes in amounts ranging from sparse to very abundant. A more conspicuous granulomatous inflammatory reaction may be elicited in foci where the duct wall is partially disrupted, and it appears that necrotic contents of the duct have been discharged or microinvasion is suspected (Fig. 11.29). Calcification can be

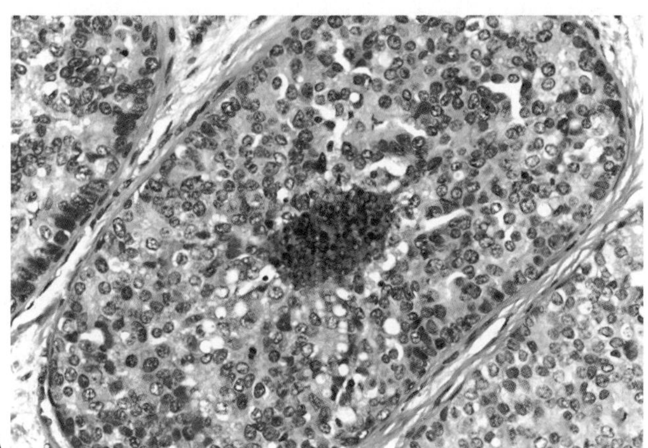

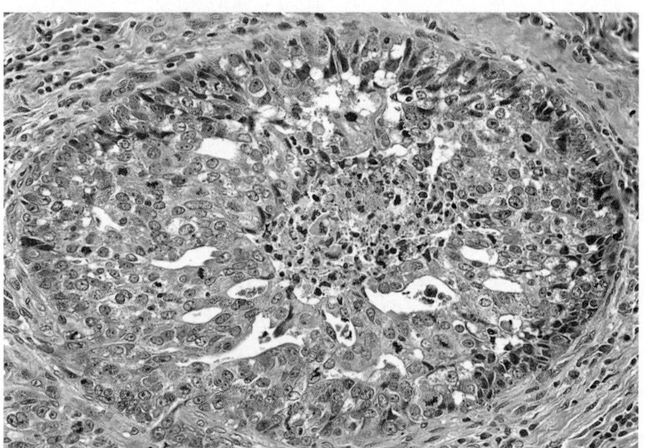

FIG. 11.25. ***DCIS, cribriform.*** **A,B:** The affected ducts show central necrosis, high nuclear grade, and irregularly shaped microlumina.

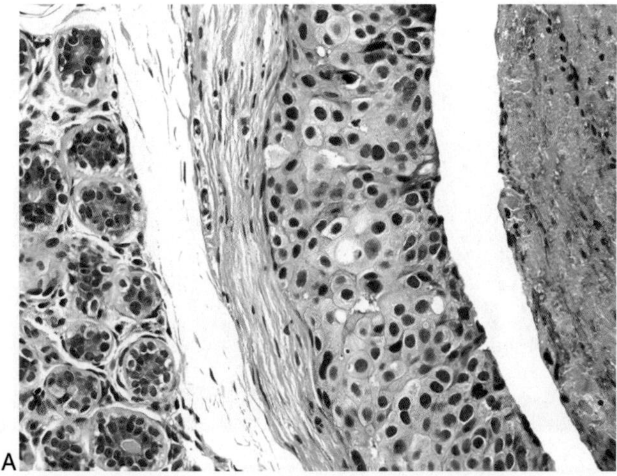

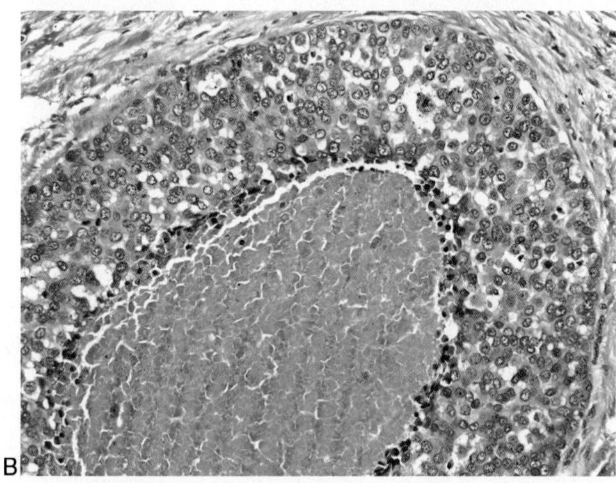

FIG. 11.26. *DCIS, solid.* A,B: Central necrosis is present in these ducts with intermediate nuclear grade. Minute intercellular spaces convey the appearance of microlumina (A).

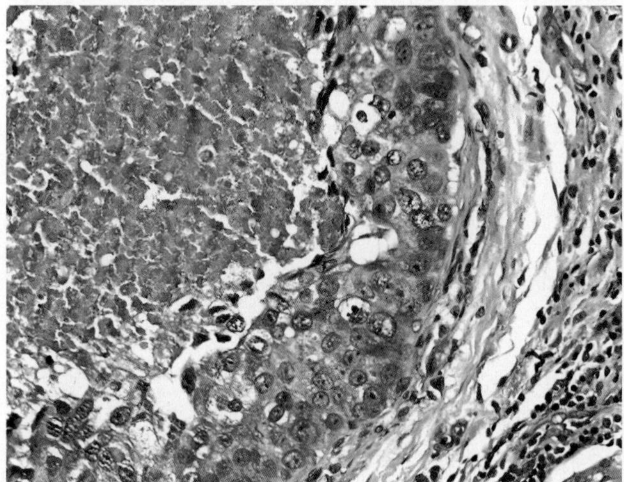

FIG. 11.27. *DCIS, "comedo."* Central necrosis, calcification, and high-grade nuclei are evident.

displaced from the duct into the stroma at such sites. This might be the mechanism responsible for the presence of calcifications in the stroma associated with DCIS when no invasion is evident. Accentuation and duplication of basement membrane components in the form of a thick eosinophilic band may also be evident in such foci (Fig. 11.30).

It is important to distinguish between *comedonecrosis* and the accumulation of secretion accompanied by an inflammatory reaction that occurs in duct stasis. Both conditions are prone to the formation of irregular microcalcifications. Cellular necrosis is rarely seen in duct stasis, and when present the degenerated cells are usually histiocytes. The duct contents in comedocarcinoma consist of necrotic carcinoma cells represented by ghost cells and karyorrhectic nuclear debris, typically with little or no intraductal inflammation. There is a sharp demarcation between viable carcinoma cells at the periphery and the necrotic core (Figs. 11.28 and 11.30). A space may be formed between the surviving cells and the cellular debris, presumably because of shrinkage of the latter during tissue processing. Dying cells at the inner edge of the viable zone have pyknotic nuclei and frayed cytoplasmic borders. The outlines of necrotic carcinoma cells (ghost cells) may be visible in the center of the duct.

Dystrophic calcification develops in the necrotic core. The calcification tends to be finely granular and mixed with cellular debris in some instances, whereas in others, it forms more solid irregular fragments (Fig. 11.27). Calcifications in comedocarcinoma almost always consist of calcium salts, mainly calcium phosphate, rather than crystalline calcium oxalate, which is typically found in benign apocrine lesions. Calcium oxalate calcifications have also been described in apocrine DCIS.[121,122] In routine hematoxylin and eosin (H&E)-stained sections, calcifications are magenta to purple whether in the comedo or other varieties of DCIS. Large calcifications may be fractured in the course of histologic processing, and fragments can be physically pushed by the microtome blade from the duct into the surrounding stroma. Neoplastic epithelium may be coincidentally displaced as well. This artifact is usually readily recognized, because the path of the displaced calcification through the tissue is indicated by one or more linear scratches.

Crystalloids are eosinophilic, noncalcific protein deposits that usually occur in various types of DCIS (Figs. 11.19 and 11.31). They appear to be formed by crystallization of proteins in necrotic debris formed in some DCIS. Rarely, crystalloids are formed in benign breast ducts.[123]

Morphometric analysis has demonstrated a correlation between duct diameter and the presence of necrosis in solid DCIS.[124] In one study, the mean diameter of ducts with necrosis was 470 μm, compared with a mean diameter of 192 μm for solid nonnecrotic duct carcinoma.[124] A diameter of 180 μm proved to be important for distinguishing between ducts with and without necrosis. Necrosis occurred in 94% of ducts greater than 180 μm in diameter and in 34% of smaller ducts. The viable rim of carcinomatous epithelium surrounding the necrotic core averaged 105 μm and exceeded 180 μm in less than 10% of cases. These observations suggest that central necrosis occurs because cells at the center of ducts with

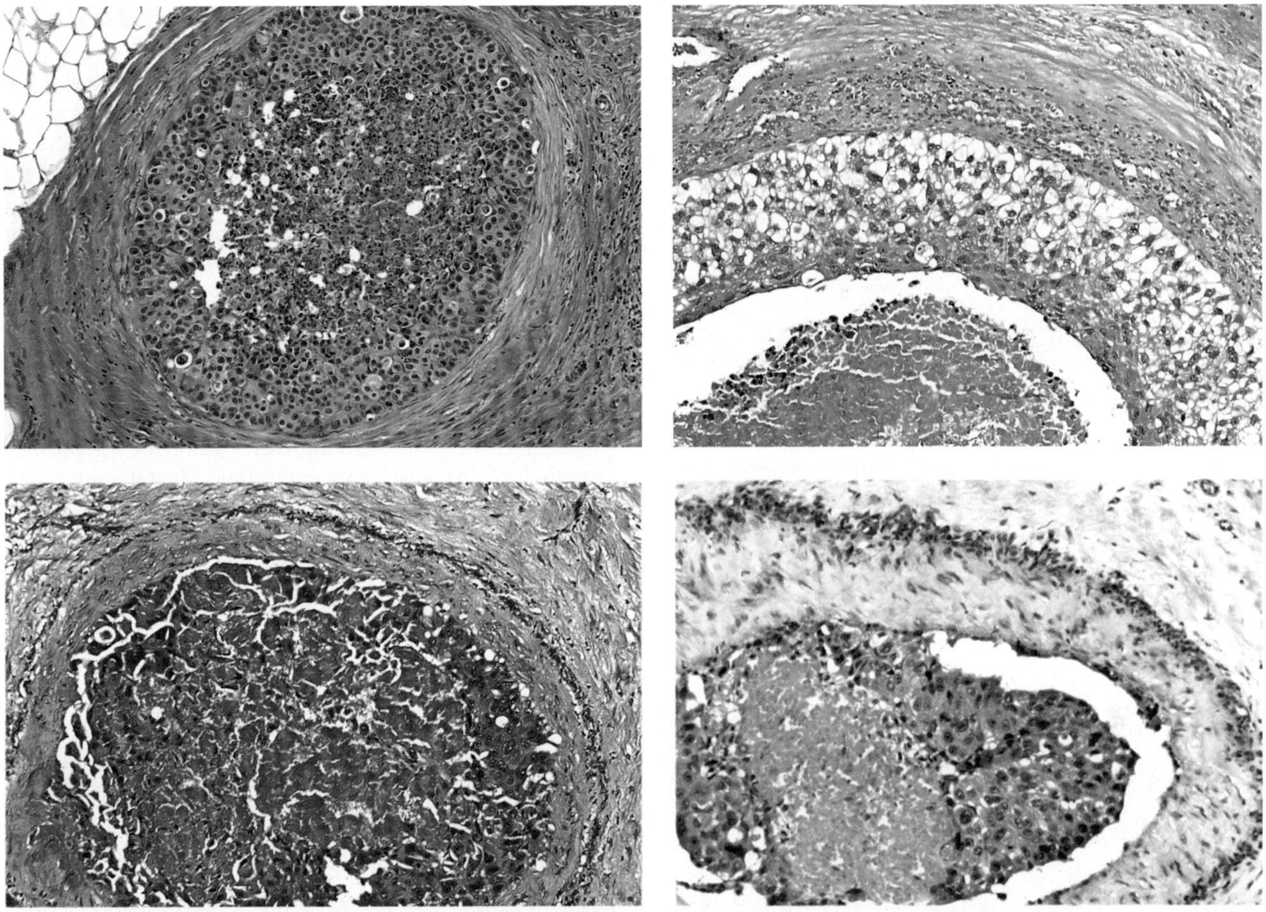

FIG. 11.28. ***DCIS, "comedo," with periductal fibrosis.*** **A:** Solid DCIS with central necrosis and concentric periductal fibrosis. **B:** Prominent periductal neovascularity forms a distinct zone between the comedo DCIS and peripheral concentric fibrosis. **C,D:** A remarkably thick, reduplicated basement membrane forms a broad collar around these ducts between the DCIS and a zone of neovascularization.

an excessive diameter are deprived of one or more essential metabolites, such as oxygen, as a result of limited diffusion in the nonvascularized intraductal neoplastic epithelium. It has been theorized that the presence of a hypoxic compartment in DCIS with comedonecrosis renders this type of DCIS relatively radioresistant and contributes to a high risk of local recurrence after breast conservation and radiotherapy for carcinomas with this feature.[125]

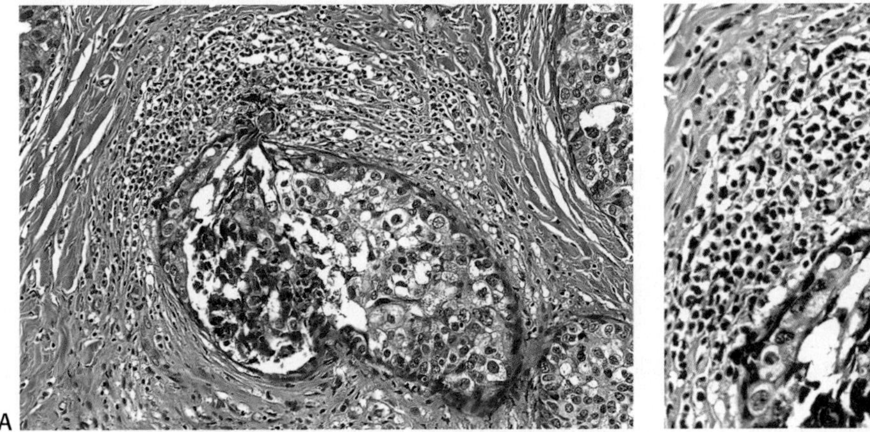

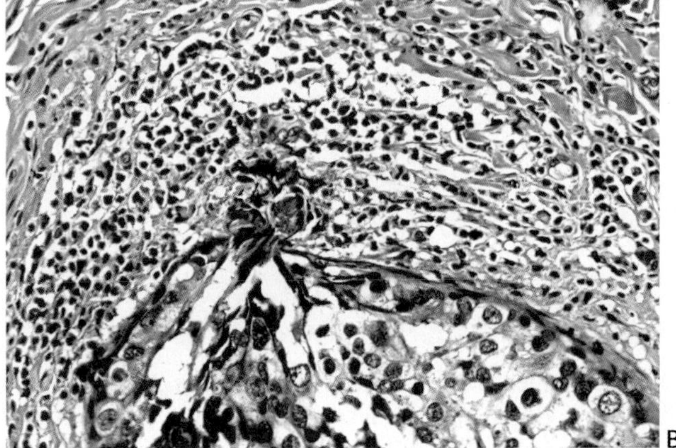

FIG. 11.29. ***DCIS, "comedo" type.*** **A,B:** Periductal lymphocytic reaction is concentrated at a site of possible microinvasion at the upper border of this duct.

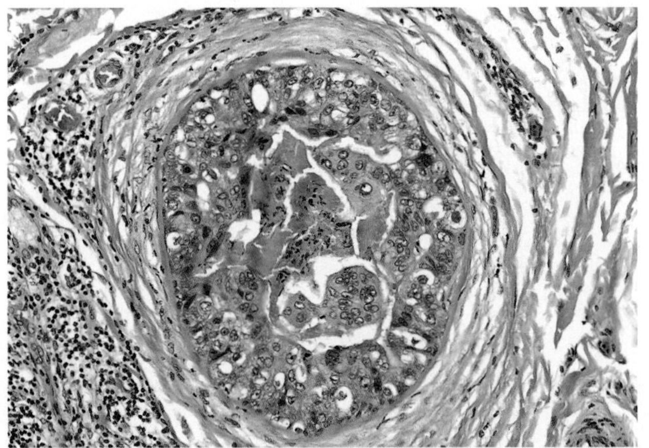

FIG. 11.30. ***DCIS, "comedo" type.*** Note concentric periductal fibrosis, lymphocytic reaction (*left*), and the eosinophilic band at the perimeter of the duct formed by the thickened basement membrane.

Apoptosis, genetically programmed cell death, also appears to contribute to necrosis in comedo and other types of DCIS. Evidence of apoptosis in DCIS is derived from morphologic observations supported by terminal deoxynucleotidyl transferase dUTP nick-end labeling (TUNEL) staining to demonstrate nuclear fragmentation. Morphologic criteria of apoptosis include nuclear shrinkage, condensation of chromatin, nuclear fragmentation, the formation of apoptotic bodies, and the absence of inflammation. Bodis et al.[126] reported that TUNEL-positive staining was present in foci of necrosis with the features of apoptotic cell death in 19 examples of DCIS. No TUNEL staining was found in low-grade DCIS without necrosis. Nuclear immunoreactivity for p53 did not correlate significantly with apoptosis or necrosis.

Harn et al.[127] studied the distribution of apoptosis in intraductal, invasive, and metastatic ductal carcinomas. The apoptosis labeling index determined by the TUNEL method was significantly higher in DCIS than in invasive or metastatic carcinoma. There was also a significant positive

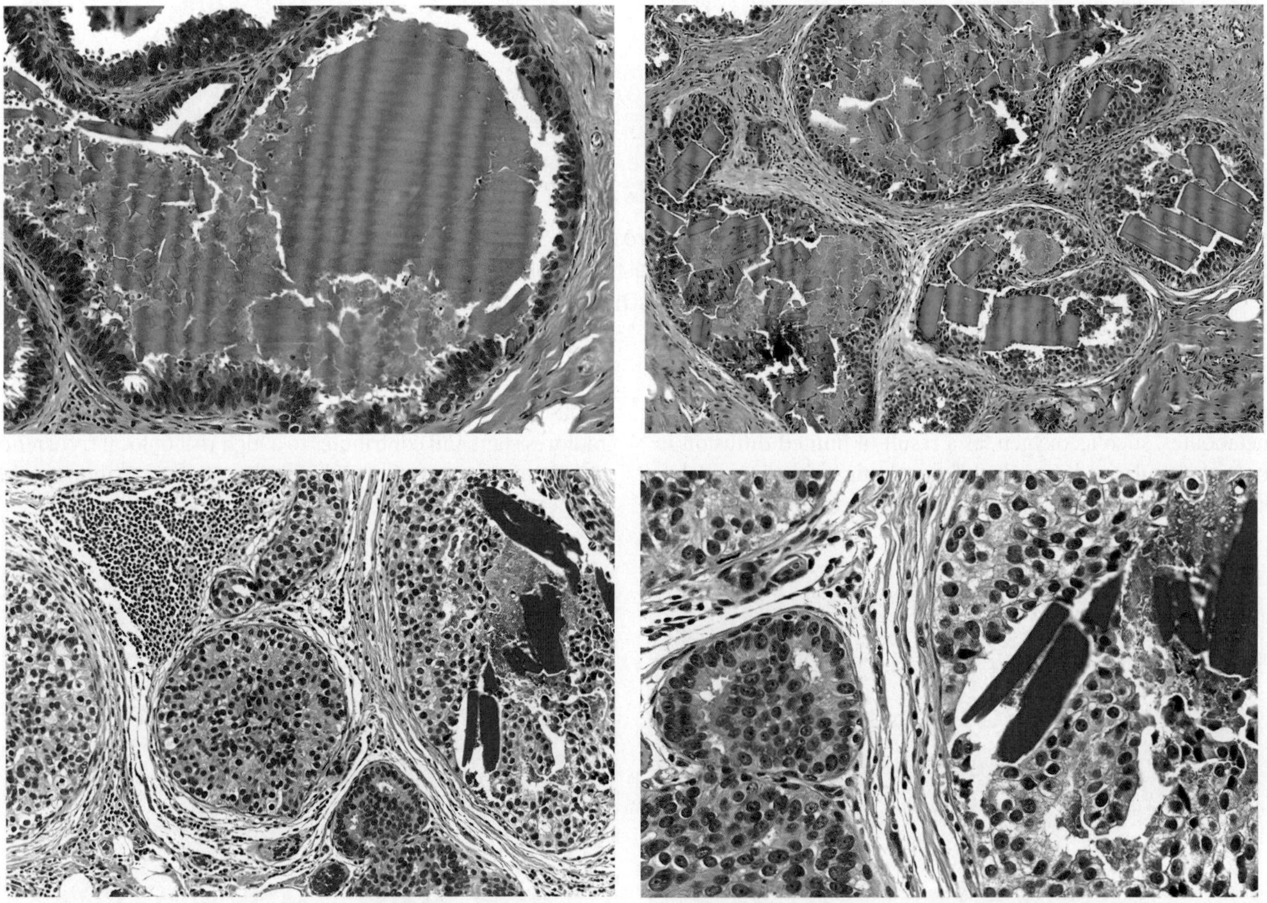

FIG. 11.31. ***DCIS with crystalloids.*** **A:** Small crystalloids are being formed (*upper left*) in the necrotic debris in this duct. **B:** Numerous crystalloids are present in another part of the specimen shown in (A). **C,D:** Cribriform and micropapillary DCIS with crystalloids in another case. **E:** The needle-shaped crystalloids appear transparent in this preparation in which the epithelium and intraductal cellular debris are immunoreactive for epithelial membrane antigen (EMA).

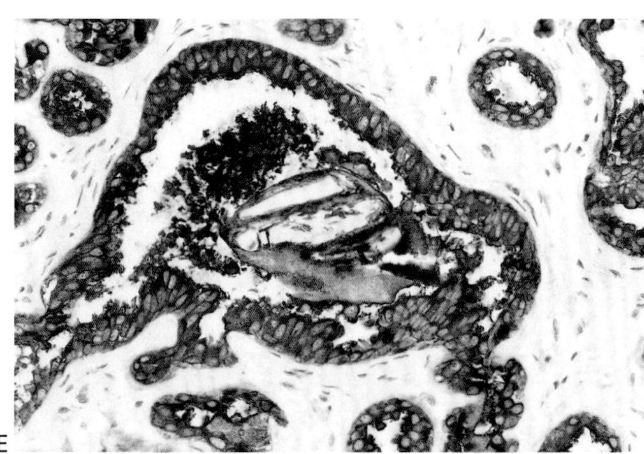

E

FIG. 11.31. *(Continued)*

correlation between the apoptotic index and p53 expression in intraductal and invasive carcinoma, leading the authors to speculate that p53 played a role in the regulation of apoptosis and the development of necrosis in DCIS.

Further evidence that altered control of apoptosis may contribute to necrosis in DCIS comes from studies of *bcl-2 expression.* The *bcl-2* gene located on chromosome 18 plays an important role in regulating growth by inhibiting apoptosis. Bcl-2 expression is inversely related to differentiation as well as to the expression of the estrogen receptor (ER), p53, and HER2 proteins in DCIS.[128] DCIS with biologic features that are most often associated with necrosis are characterized by downregulation of apoptosis inhibiting bcl-2 (Fig. 11.32).

Sneige et al.[129] correlated the frequency of central necrosis in DCIS with nuclear grade. Central necrosis was much more frequent in lesions with poorly differentiated nuclear grade (80%) than in those with intermediate (35%) or low (22%) nuclear grade.

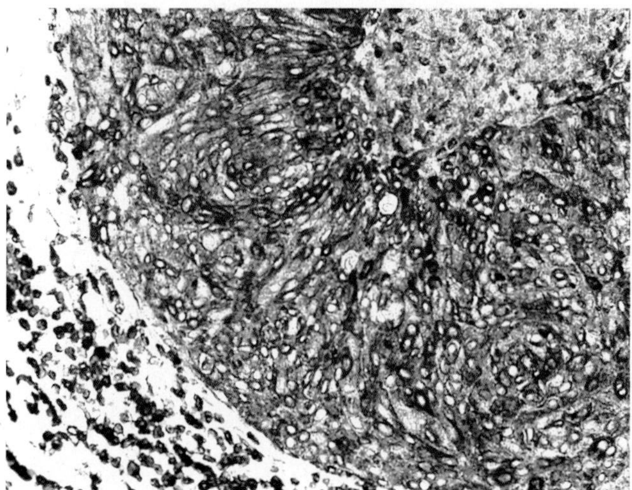

FIG. 11.32. ***DCIS, bcl-2 expression.*** Cytoplasmic and membranous immunoreactivity for bcl-2 is present in DCIS cells. Note cytoplasmic staining in periductal lymphocytes.

Marked periductal fibrosis can, on occasion, be associated with extensive obliteration of DCIS, a process referred to as "healing" by Muir and Aitkenhead[130] (Fig. 11.33). The residual ductal structures typically consist of round-to-oval scars composed of circumferential layers of collagen and elastic tissue. The center of the duct may contain a few residual carcinoma cells, fragments of calcification, or histiocytes. End-stage scars of periductal mastitis may not be distinguishable from those of obliterated comedocarcinoma. After a study of 425 breasts, Davies[131] concluded that ". . . ductal hyperelastosis, obliteration, and fibrous plaques are not limited to breasts that are the seat of carcinoma. Indeed, the prevalence of these three lesions in major ducts that are unaffected by microscopic changes does not differ significantly in 'normal' and carcinomatous breasts." At the other extreme, perhaps also representing the result of host response to the tumor or its products, one can encounter a severe inflammatory reaction that may lead to a mistaken diagnosis of mastitis, because DCIS is masked by the inflammation.

CD10 is a cell-surface metalloproteinase that is expressed in a variety of normal cell types, including mammary myoepithelial cells and lymphoid precursor cells. Stromal CD10 expression has been associated with biologically aggressive carcinomas. In an immunohistochemically analyzed tissue microarray study, no CD10 immunoreactivity was found in the stromal cells of the normal breast; however, CD10 reactivity was detected in the stroma in about 10% of DCIS cases and 50% of invasive carcinoma cases.[132] In this study, CD10 expression correlated significantly with tumor size, stage, grade, nodal involvement, and distant metastases, and was also related to cytoplasmic β-catenin expression in the invasive carcinoma cells.

Secreted protein acid rich in cysteine (SPARC) is a multifunctional glycoprotein that acts through several signaling pathways to regulate extracellular matrix as well as tissue remodeling. It is possible that SPARC and CD10 play an integral role in the development of invasive carcinoma.[133]

Solid DCIS is formed by neoplastic cells that fill most or all of the duct space (Fig. 11.34). Microlumens and papillary structures are absent, but calcifications may be present. Necrosis is not a conspicuous feature of solid DCIS, but small foci may be present in affected ducts (Fig. 11.35). Patients with comedocarcinoma often have coexistent foci of solid DCIS. In contrast to solid intraductal hyperplasia, the polygonal cells are typically of a single type with low to moderate nuclear grade. The cytoplasm has a spectrum of cytologic appearances, including clear, granular, amphophilic and eosinophilic, and apocrine. Myoepithelial cells are variably present at the periphery of ducts involved by solid DCIS.

LCIS, particularly of the florid type, can be mistaken for DCIS; indeed, one description recently proposed for florid LCIS was "solid-type DCIS that lacked E-cadherin expression."[134] Additional immunostains that can be helpful in distinguishing LCIS from DCIS include p120, β-catenin, and high molecular weight cytokeratins.[135]

Papillary DCIS is distinguished by the presence of a fibrovascular stromal architecture supporting one or more of the foregoing structural patterns (see Chapter 14).

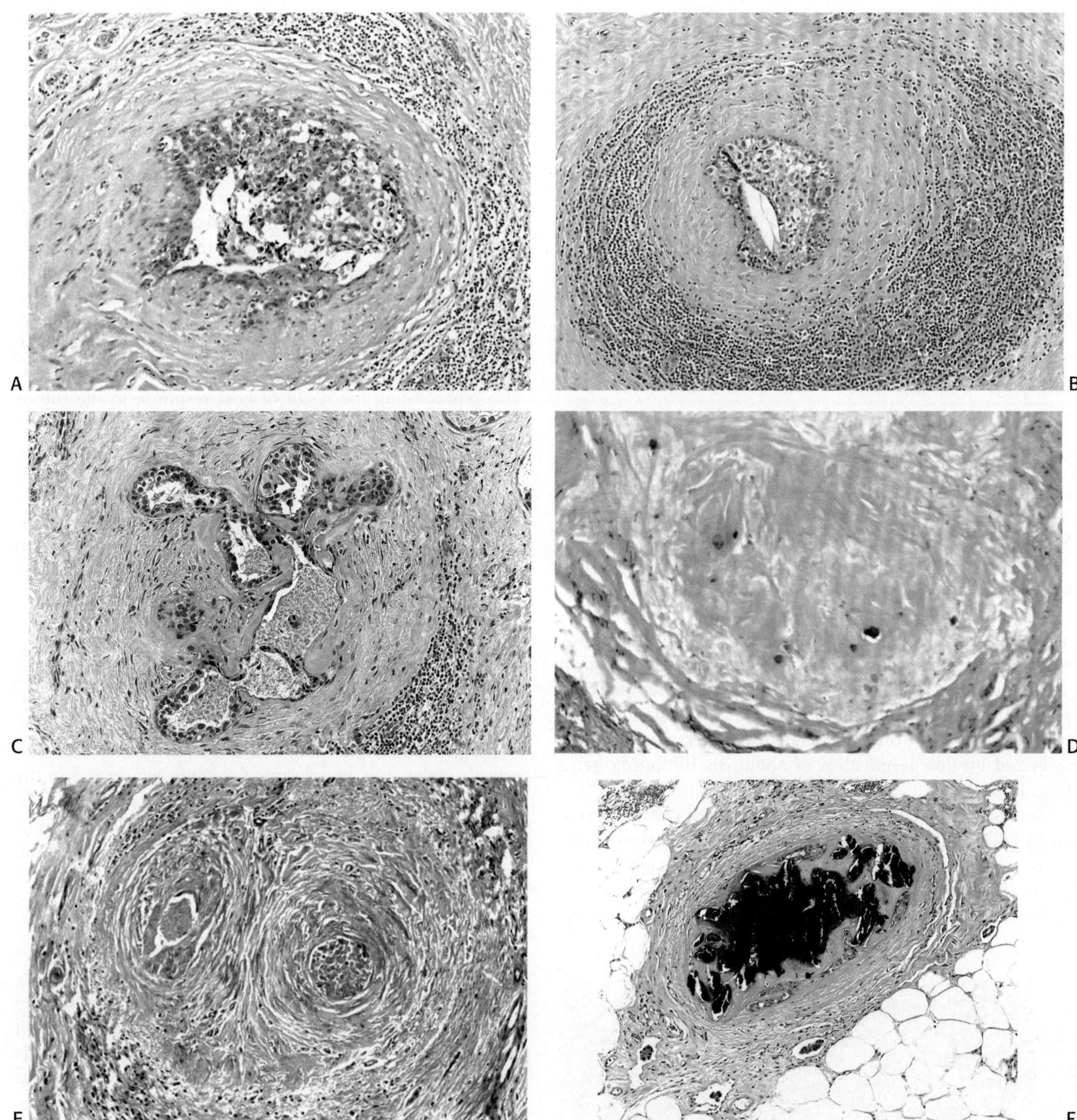

FIG. 11.33. ***DCIS, "healing."*** **A:** Prominent periductal fibrosis and chronic inflammation. **B,C:** Severe periductal fibrosis with lymphocytic reaction. The epithelial element is relatively attenuated (**C**). **D:** Scar composed of collagen and elastin fibers with calcifications at the site of "healed" DCIS. Images (**A–D**) are from a single specimen. **E:** Marked periductal fibrosis with residual necrotic DCIS. **F:** Concentric fibrosis forms a dense calcified scar with sclerosing entrapment of carcinoma cells. Note periductal lymphovascular channel involvement by tumor cells. No invasive carcinoma was identified elsewhere in this case.

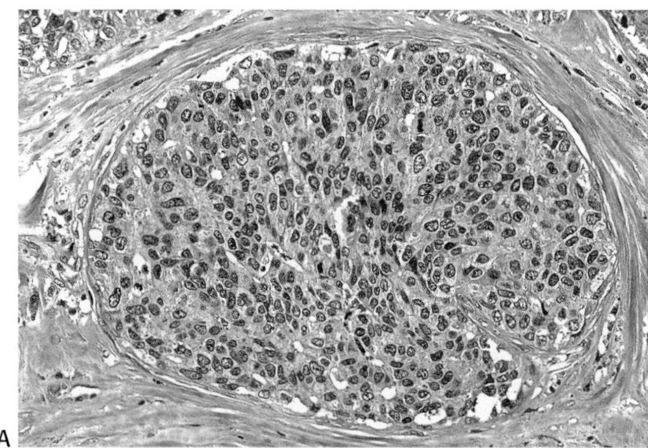

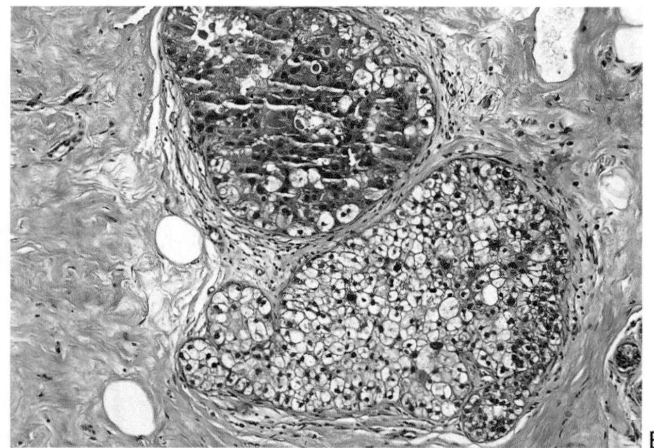

FIG. 11.34. ***DCIS, solid.*** **A:** The duct is filled by a compact growth of carcinoma cells with pleomorphic nuclei of intermediate nuclear grade. **B:** Solid apocrine DCIS with clear cell change.

Some examples of *spindle cell DCIS* are variants of papillary DCIS, but spindle cell growth can be encountered in nonpapillary DCIS (Fig. 11.36). *Small cell DCIS* occurs in association with invasive small cell (oat cell) carcinoma (see Chapter 21) or as an isolated lesion (Fig. 11.37).

DCIS arising in SA assumes the structural configuration of the underlying adenosis and may be mistaken for invasive carcinoma.[136–139] (Fig. 11.38). The majority of these patients are premenopausal. Because SA is fundamentally a lesion formed by altered lobules, this presentation can be viewed as a form of intralobular extension of the ductal lesion. The condition usually occurs focally rather than diffusely and is diagnosed when the proliferative epithelium has the structural and cytologic appearance of DCIS. The growth patterns are usually solid and cribriform (Figs. 11.38 and 11.39). An organoid appearance may result from the alveolar expansion of lobular structures in the adenosis. Microcalcifications may be present in the underlying adenosis or as part of the DCIS. DCIS can be limited to the SA, or there may be foci in the surrounding breast.[137]

The underlying architecture of SA can be appreciated with stains for basement membranes such as PAS, reticulin, or laminin, and immunostains to identify myoepithelial cells such as p63, calponin, CD10, and SMA.[137,139] The antibody for SMM-HC is useful in this circumstance because it is likely to avoid most of the obscuring effect produced by actin reactivity in myofibroblasts encountered with other antiactin antibodies (Fig. 11.39). Rarely, invasive carcinoma can have an adenosis-like pattern that is difficult to distinguish from DCIS in adenosis. In this situation, stains for myoepithelium are useful. Absence of myoepithelium is diagnostic of invasive carcinoma.

Invasive carcinoma arising in SA is difficult to detect unless the invasive component has clearly grown beyond the area of adenosis and has an architectural pattern that differs from that of the adenosis (Figs. 11.40 and 11.41). A double immunostain for cytokeratin and actin can be helpful for identifying

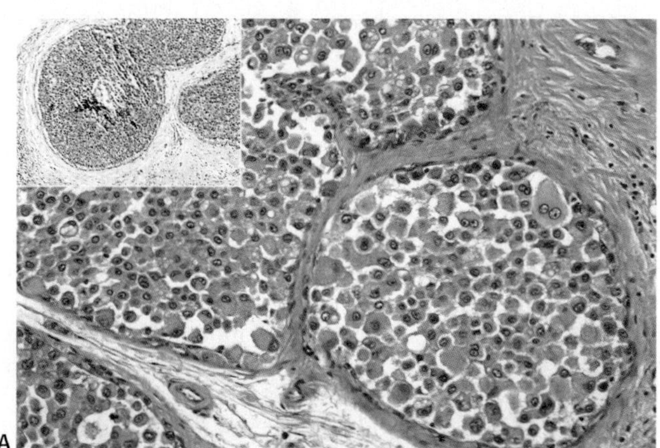

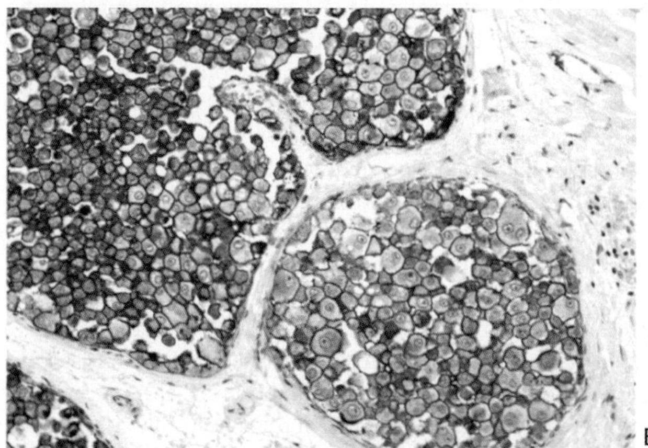

FIG. 11.35. ***DCIS, solid.*** **A:** Apocrine type of solid DCIS with loss of cohesion, with central necrosis (*inset*). The histopathologic appearance simulates pleomorphic LCIS. **B:** DCIS in **(A)** is strongly E-cadherin positive, supporting ductal differentiation.

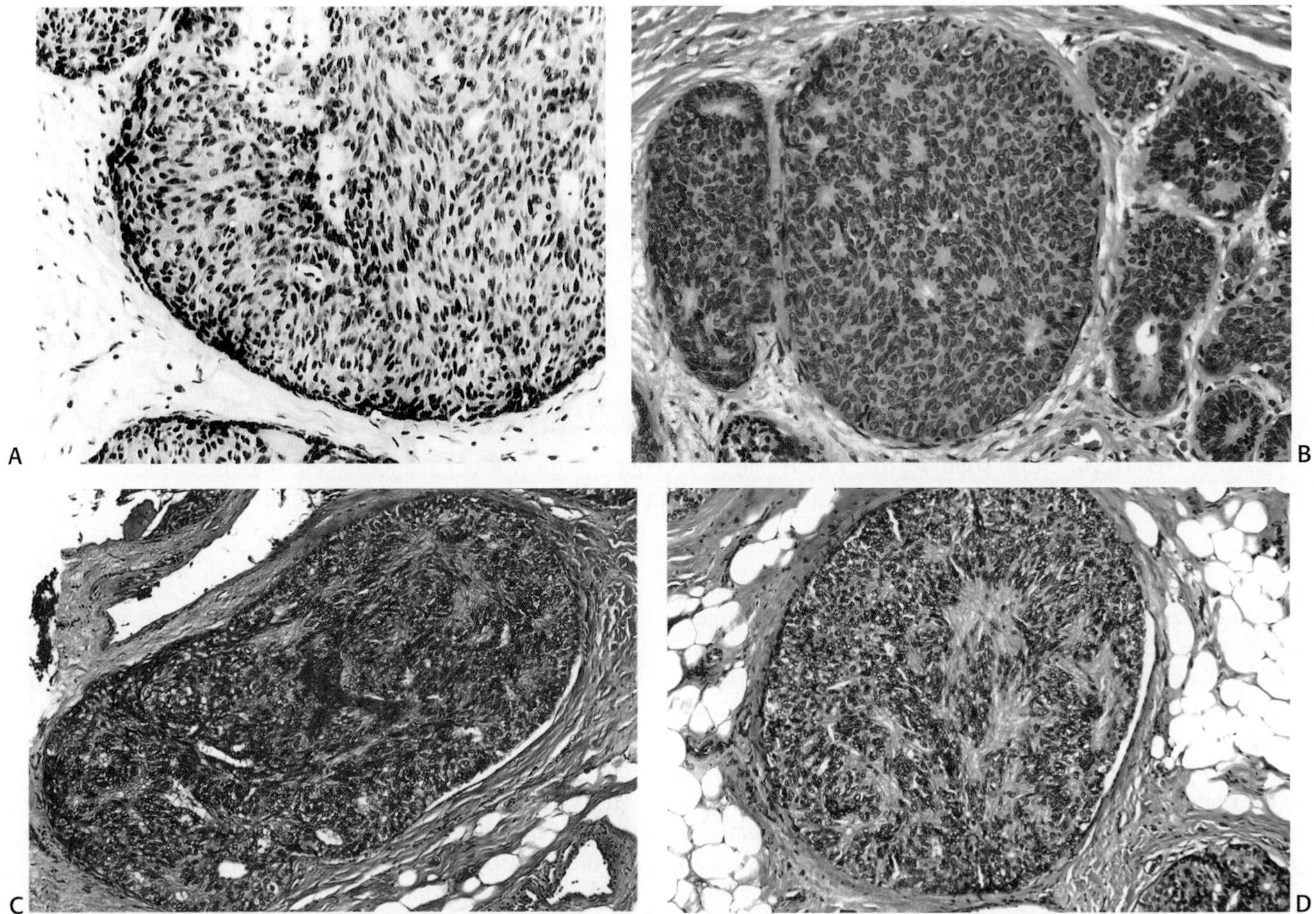

FIG. 11.36. ***DCIS, spindle cell.*** **A:** The carcinoma cells have spindle-shaped nuclei with traces of palisading. **B:** Rosette-like microlumens are present. **C:** Spindle cell carcinoma with a central fibrovascular stromal core. This focus was part of a complex solid papillary carcinoma with an extensive spindle cell component. **D:** Spindle cell DCIS with palisading epithelial cells.

microinvasion when DCIS inhabits SA (Fig. 11.42). In a study of 24 cases of DCIS involving SA, Moritani et al.[140] found that most DCIS that only involved SA were "non-high-grade," whereas DCIS not confined to SA was more often high grade.

Nerves may be incorporated in SA when no carcinoma is present.[141] The presence of this phenomenon when there is DCIS in the adenosis is not indicative of invasion. Neural entrapment has also been observed in areas of sclerosing papillary DCIS not associated with SA.[142]

DCIS has been found to arise near and in *radial sclerosing lesions*, so-called radial scars (Figs. 11.43 and 11.44). The presence of an underlying radial sclerosing lesion (RSL) is indicated by the overall configuration of the lesion and the presence of benign proliferative foci such as duct hyperplasia, cysts, SA, and apocrine metaplasia. DCIS with a stellate growth pattern can present as a RSL(Fig. 11.45). Incomplete samples of radical scar lesions obtained in needle core biopsy specimens are difficult to assess for DCIS or for invasion, and they are likely to be reported as atypical duct hyperplasia.

A diagnosis of radial scar without atypical changes based on a partially sampled lesion on a needle core biopsy does not preclude the finding of carcinoma in the subsequent excision. In a study of 49 cases of radial scar (all without associated atypical epithelial proliferation) that had been diagnosed on needle core biopsy, Bianchi et al.[143] found three cases of DCIS (and one of invasive lobular carcinoma) in the subsequently performed excisional biopsy. However, Resetkova et al.[144] reported no instances of "upgrade" to invasive or *in situ* carcinoma in a study of 19 radial scars diagnosed on needle core biopsy that underwent subsequent excision of the lesion. Another 61 patients with a diagnosis of radial scar on needle core biopsy were followed clinically and radiologically without apparent progression of disease. The authors concluded that ample sampling with larger (11G or 9G) needles and radiologic correlation could obviate the need for excision in radial scars diagnosed on needle core biopsy.[144]

Concurrent intraductal and in situ lobular carcinomas are present when there are separate foci of carcinoma with these histologic features in the breast. This is illustrated by instances in which the lobular lesion with the classical small cell phenotype of lobular carcinoma is limited to TDLUs

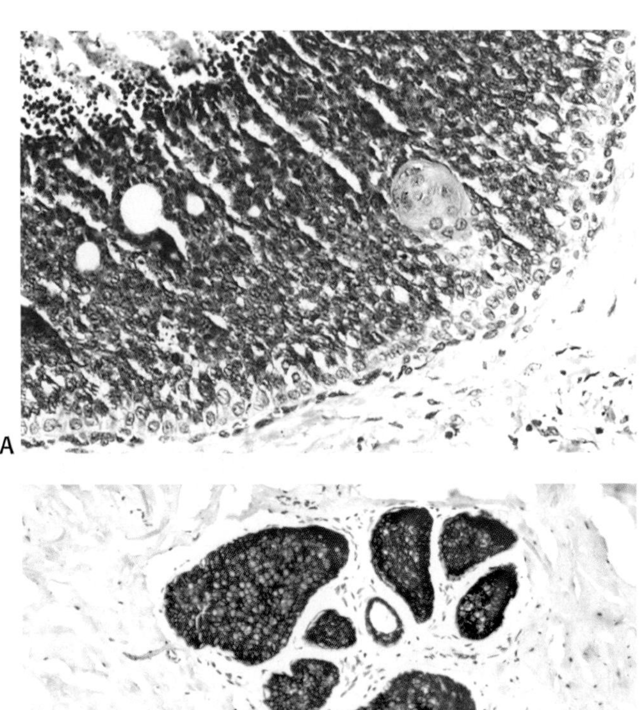

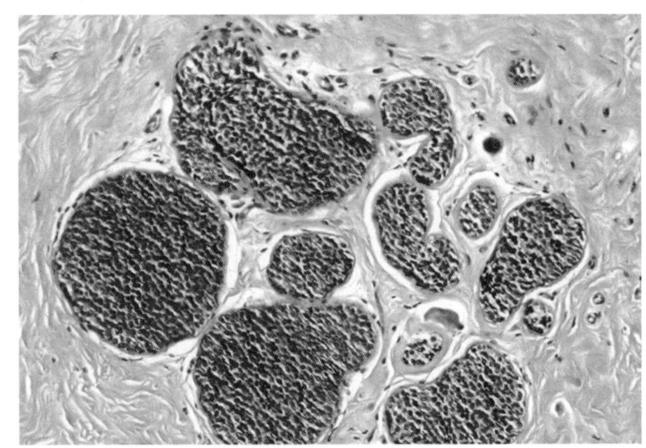

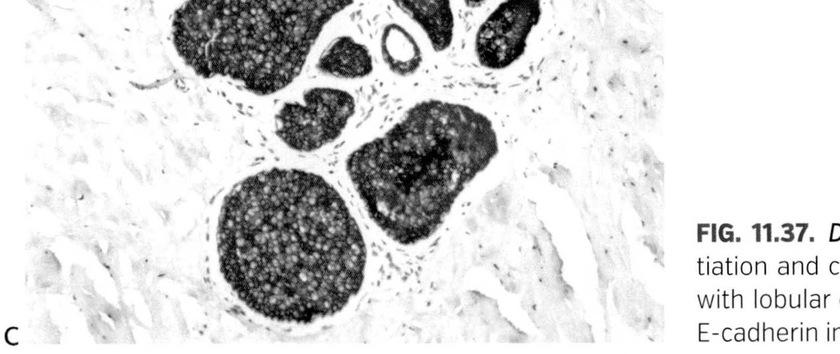

FIG. 11.37. ***DCIS, small cell.*** **A:** Focal squamous differentiation and central necrosis are shown. **B:** Small cell DCIS with lobular extension. **C:** The carcinoma in (**B**) is strongly E-cadherin immunoreactive, indicating ductal type.

that are separate from ducts with the classical features of comedo, papillary, or cribriform DCIS (Fig. 11.46).

In some instances, the distinction is less clear, especially when the proliferation in the ducts and lobules is composed of uniform cells, with cytologically well-differentiated to moderately differentiated nuclei (Fig. 11.47). The difficulty presented by these lesions is whether they should be classified as entirely DCIS with "lobular cancerization" or as LCIS with duct extension. The E-cadherin stain will display strong membrane reactivity if the lesion is DCIS. E-cadherin staining will be reduced and fragmented or absent in LCIS.

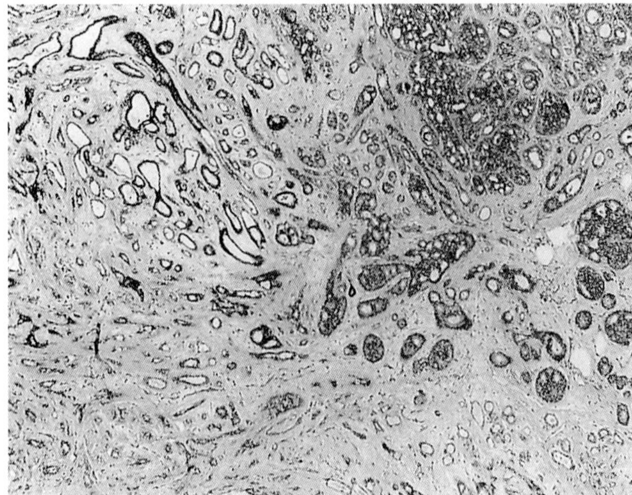

FIG. 11.38. ***DCIS in sclerosing adenosis.*** Cribriform carcinoma is present on the right. SA is present throughout the photograph.

The presence of a cribriform pattern suggests DCIS with lobular extension. Cells with apocrine differentiation are more consistent with ductal carcinoma. Ultimately, some difficult cases defy classification, even after careful consideration of all features and a diagnosis of combined intraductal and *in situ* lobular carcinoma may be made, accompanied by a description of the diagnostic issues presented in the particular instance (Fig. 11.48).

Coexistent intraductal and in situ lobular carcinoma in a single duct-lobular unit constitutes one of the most unusual microscopic patterns of noninvasive breast carcinoma.[145] This diagnosis depends upon finding carcinoma with two distinctly different cytologic and structural patterns in a single duct. In these combined lesions, LCIS with the conventional small cell cytology is typically present within lobular glands as well as in a pagetoid distribution in the duct epithelium (Figs. 11.49 and 11.50). The duct lumen contains a papillary, solid, or cribriform proliferation composed of more pleomorphic cells typically found in

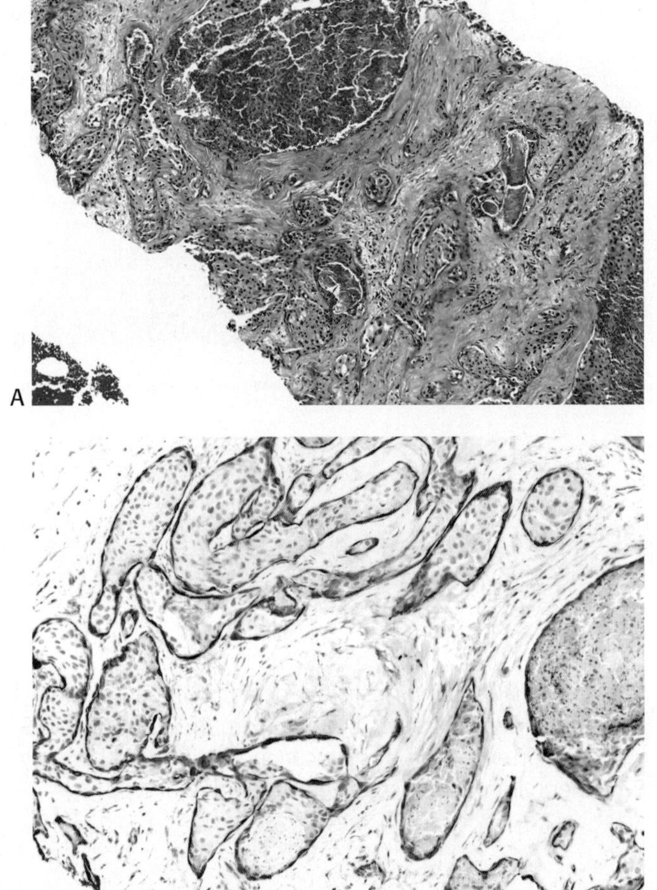

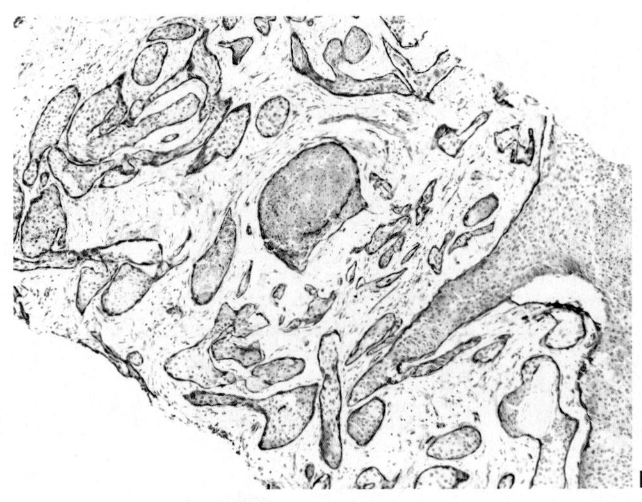

FIG. 11.39. ***DCIS in sclerosing adenosis in a needle core biopsy.*** **A:** DCIS occupies the structure of SA. Groups of carcinoma cells resemble invasive carcinoma cells. Immunostains for SMM-HC **(B)** and SMA **(C)** on sections parallel to **(A)** reveal myoepithelial cells enveloping the groups of carcinoma cells.

DCIS. Coexistent *in situ* lesions have been found in association with invasive duct and invasive lobular carcinoma. This pattern of *in situ* carcinoma should be distinguished from lobular extension of DCIS, so-called lobular cancerization. In the latter condition, the nonneoplastic lobular epithelium is displaced by carcinoma cells with the same cytologic appearance as the DCIS. As outlined earlier, the E-cadherin stain, among others, can be used to identify LCIS in DCIS. Computerized image analysis systems for classifying various noninvasive proliferative and neoplastic lesions on digitized slides are in development, and at this time they have more potential as an educational tool rather than as a stand-alone diagnostic tool.[146]

GRADING OF DCIS

The interval between DCIS and the development of invasive carcinoma is shorter for high-grade DCIS, averaging 5 years, than for low-grade DCIS, which takes a mean period of more than 15 years.[147,148] Grading of DCIS can also be useful for predicting the risk of breast recurrence after conservation therapy. When there is an invasive element associated with DCIS, both components tend to have similar nuclear grades.[149] Grading schemes consisting of two categories (high grade and all others) and three categories (high, intermediate, and low) have been devised for DCIS. The determination of grade is based upon nuclear cytology[150] and the growth pattern. Nuclear grade tends to be relatively constant in a given patient, even when there is substantial variation in architectural pattern.[149] The presence or absence of necrosis may also be considered in grading.

In past decades, DCIS was routinely classified as being of "comedo" or "noncomedo" types. In general, "comedo" carcinoma implied solid type of DCIS with pleomorphic cells bearing high-grade nuclei associated with abundant central necrosis. The term "comedo" referred to necrotic cellular debris that oozed from the cut surfaces of affected ducts when the excised tumor was compressed (i.e., resembling the "comedones" in acne vulgaris). The collective term "noncomedo" DCIS in the premammographic era implied all other types of DCIS. These noncomedo DCIS were rarer,

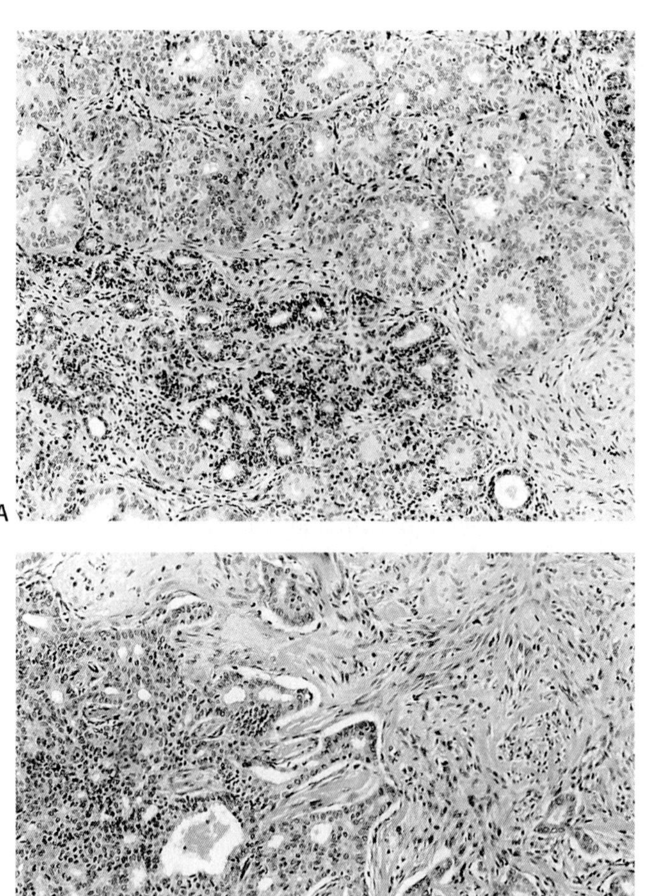

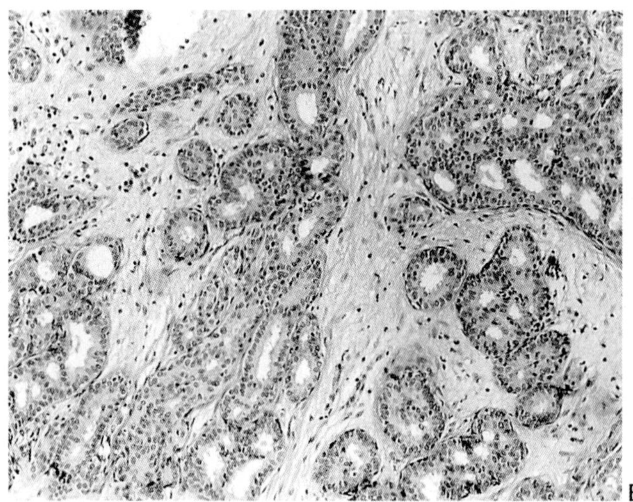

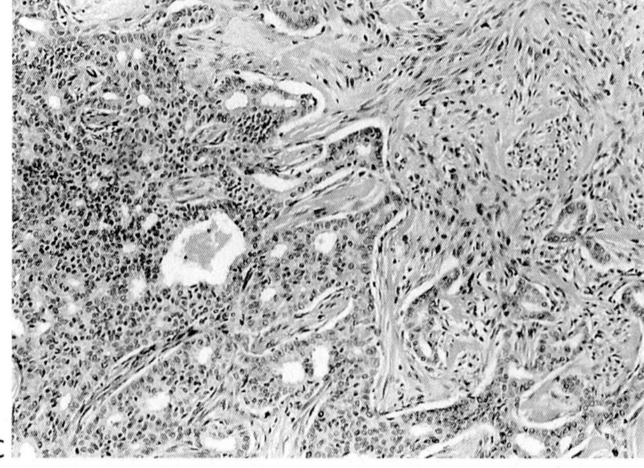

FIG. 11.40. ***DCIS in sclerosing adenosis with invasion.*** **A:** DCIS (*above*) in SA. **B:** Area of sclerosis involved by DCIS. **C:** Invasive cribriform carcinoma originating in SA.

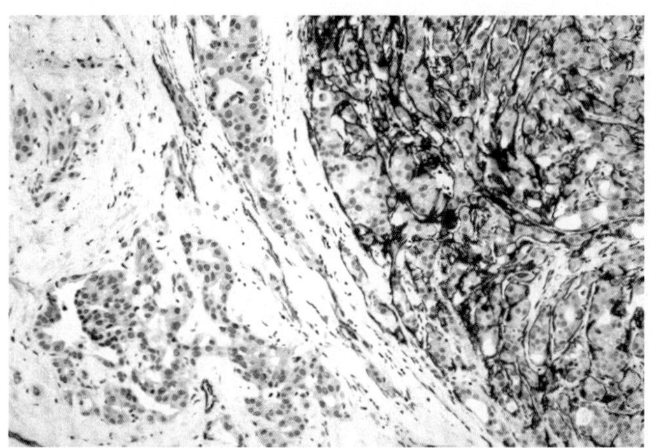

FIG. 11.41. ***Invasive carcinoma arising in sclerosing adenosis.*** DCIS in SA is shown on the *right* in this section prepared with the immunostain for SMM-HC. Invasive carcinoma in the stroma to the *left* of the SA is not encased in actin-positive myoepithelial cells.

were neither palpable nor grossly evident, and were generally of smaller extent with variable histologic type (including cribriform, micropapillary, and papillary) and comprised cells with lower grade nuclei and exhibited no necrosis. Then, as now, a proportion of comedo and noncomedo types of DCIS comprised combinations of growth patterns and nuclear grade.

Comedocarcinoma is "high" grade by definition. Poorly differentiated nuclei, usually accompanied by necrosis, are also infrequently encountered in papillary, micropapillary, and cribriform DCIS[149] (Figs. 11.19, 11.25, and 11.51). DCIS is in the intermediate-grade category when it has a cribriform, solid, or papillary pattern with necrosis but lacks the nuclear anaplasia of comedocarcinoma, or if one of these growth patterns is composed of high-grade carcinoma cells in the absence of necrosis (Figs. 11.9, 11.11, 11.21, and 11.26). Any pattern of DCIS composed of uniform cells without atypia or necrosis is classified as low grade (Figs. 11.2, 11.4, 11.7, 11.15, 11.21, 11.43, and 11.52). A case is usually classified on the basis of the highest grade present.[151] Rarely,

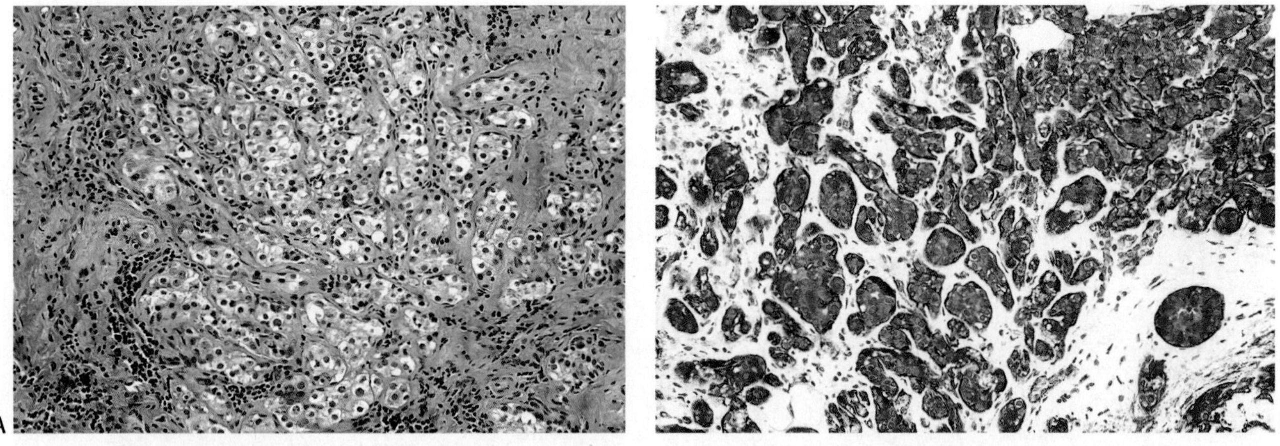

FIG. 11.42. ***DCIS in sclerosing adenosis.*** **A:** This pattern of apocrine DCIS in SA might be mistaken for invasive carcinoma. **B:** The combined cytokeratin (*red*) and actin (*brown*) immunostain demonstrates actin-positive myoepithelial cells around all of the cytokeratin-positive epithelial cells (anti-CK, alkaline phosphatase; anti-SMA).

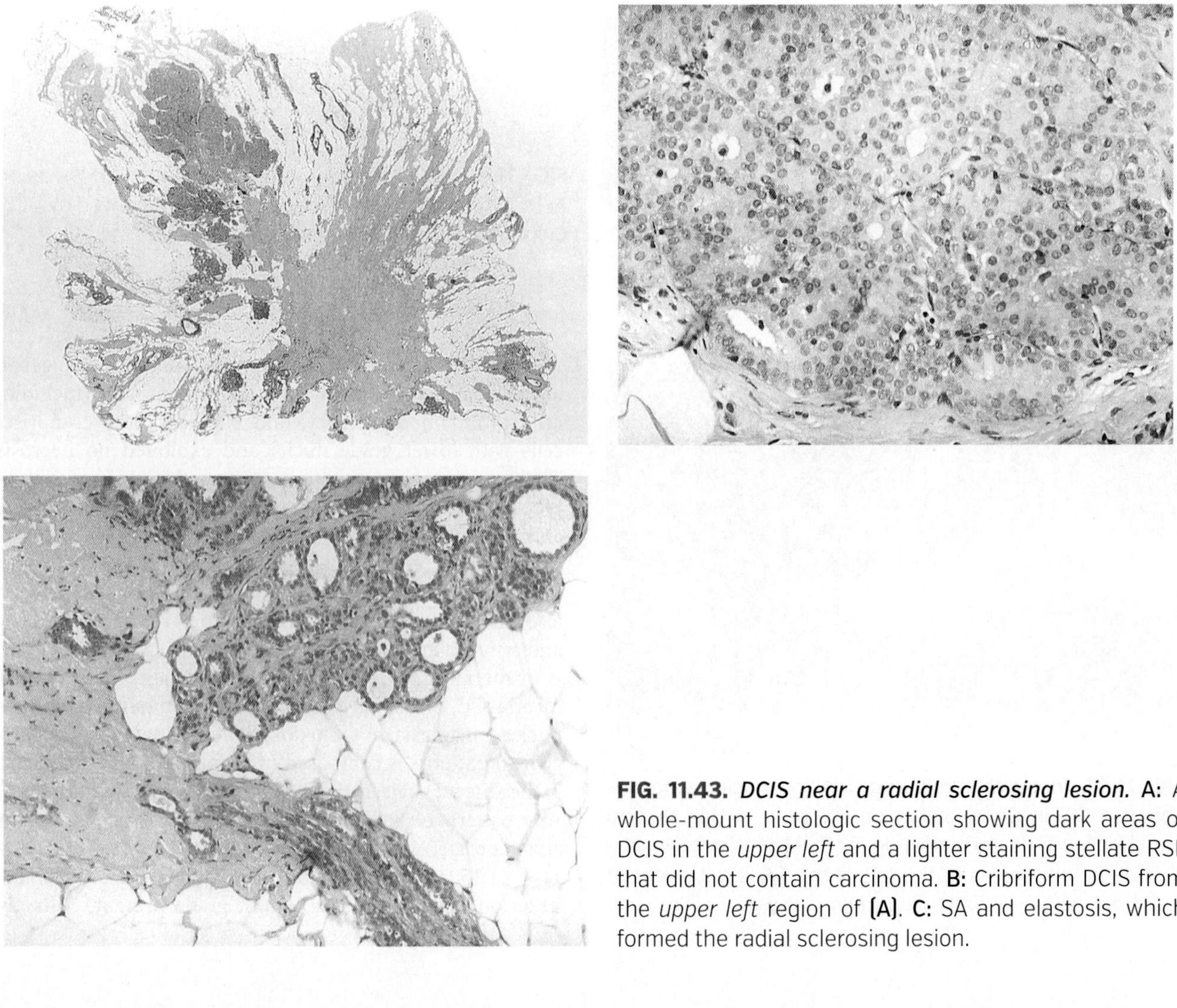

FIG. 11.43. ***DCIS near a radial sclerosing lesion.*** **A:** A whole-mount histologic section showing dark areas of DCIS in the *upper left* and a lighter staining stellate RSL that did not contain carcinoma. **B:** Cribriform DCIS from the *upper left* region of (**A**). **C:** SA and elastosis, which formed the radial sclerosing lesion.

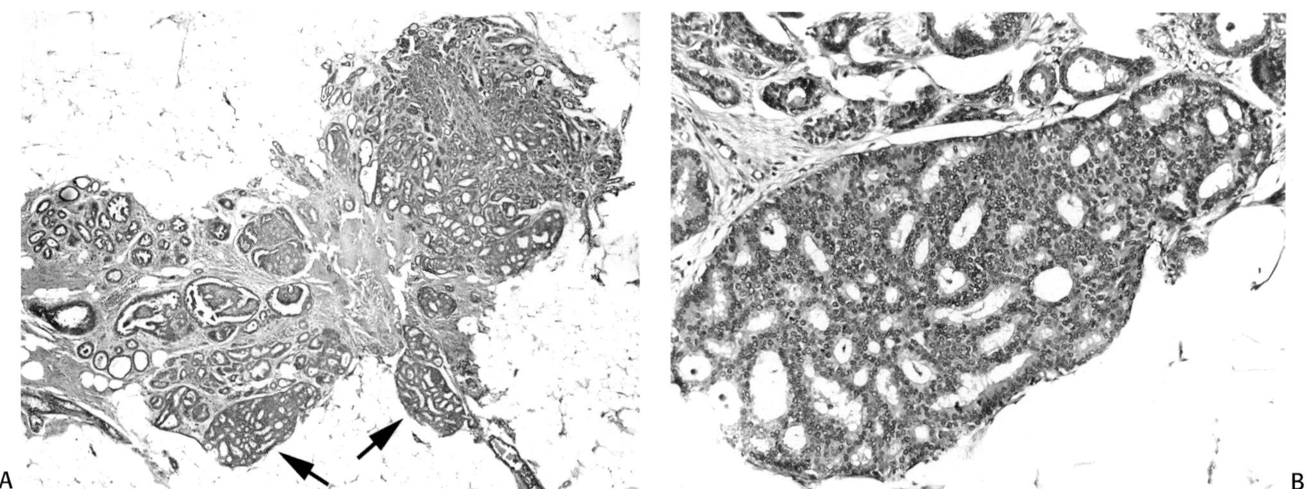

FIG. 11.44. ***DCIS in a radial sclerosing lesion.*** **A:** DCIS of cribriform type (*arrows*) and ductal hyperplasia in a radial sclerosing lesion. **B:** Magnified view of DCIS shown in **(A)**.

high- and low-grade components may coexist in a patient or even in one duct (Figs. 11.10 and 11.53).

Some high-grade DCIS exhibit the basal-like immunophenotype (no reactivity for ER and progesterone receptors [PRs] and for HER2). This form of DCIS is the putative precursor to invasive basal-like ductal carcinoma. Bryan et al.[152] found the basal-like immunophenotype in 4 (6%) of 66 DCIS with high nuclear grade. These DCIS expressed basal cytokeratins and/or epidermal growth factor receptor (EGFR) significantly more often than did high-grade DCIS, which did not have the basal-like immunophenotype.

Silverstein et al.[153] proposed a classification of DCIS based on nuclear grade (high or nonhigh) and the presence or absence of necrosis as part of a prognostic index. Three prognostic categories resulting from consideration of these variables were as follows: Group 1, nonhigh nuclear grade without necrosis; Group 2, nonhigh nuclear grade with necrosis; and Group 3, high nuclear grade with or without necrosis. The Van Nuys Prognostic Index (VNPI, discussed in greater detail below) includes margin status and tumor size as well as these histologic groups.[154] Follow-up revealed a significant correlation between the VNPI and the risk of recurrence in the breast after conservation therapy. VNPI should be used only if margin status and tumor size can be reliably assessed.

Grading has been a component of other classification schemes for assessing the effectiveness of breast conservation therapy in the treatment of DCIS. Including those cited previously, at least six classifications have been proposed.[155] These have been based on some or all of the following features: architecture, nuclear grade, presence or absence of

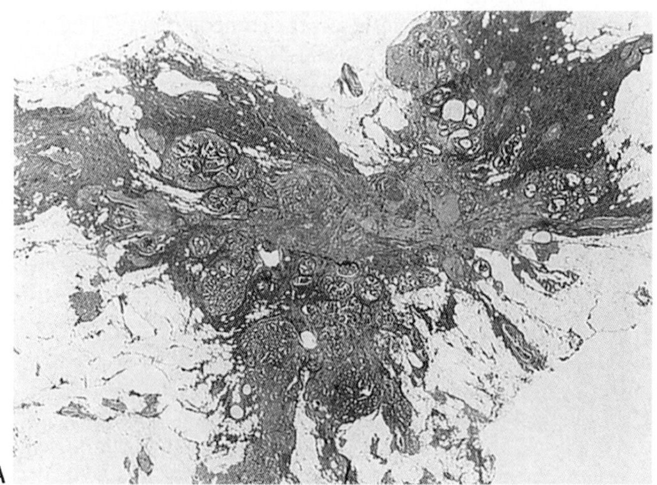

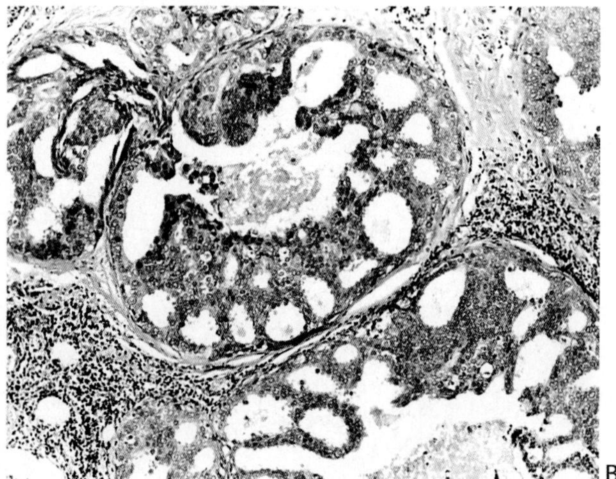

FIG. 11.45. ***DCIS, radial configuration.*** **A:** Stellate lesion with a scleroelastotic center. **B:** Cribriform DCIS shown here is present throughout the tumor.

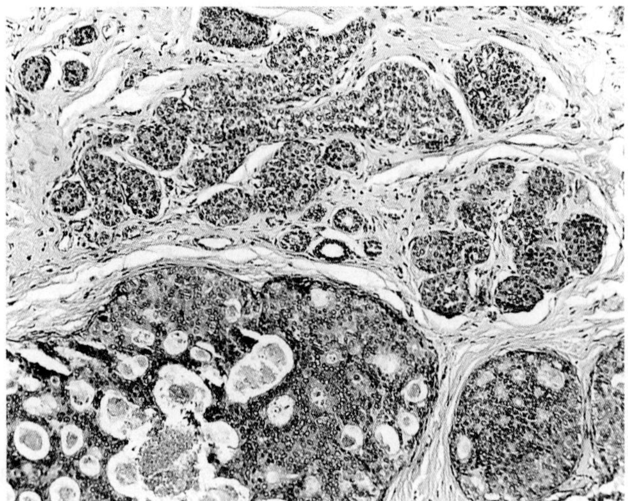

FIG. 11.46. ***Concurrent cribriform intraductal and in situ lobular carcinoma.*** (Reproduced from Rosen PP. Coexistent lobular carcinoma in situ and DCIS in a single lobular-duct unit. *Am J Surg Pathol* 1980;4:241–246, with permission.)

necrosis, lesion size, and cell polarity. Most classifications have emphasized nuclear grade, necrosis, and architecture. Generally, three grades have been proposed: high, intermediate, and low. There is a significant correlation between the grade of DCIS and a corresponding invasive component, if present, regardless of grading system.[155] The grading categories also have significant associations with biologic characteristics of DCIS, especially lesions typically classified as high and low grade. High-grade lesions typically exhibit the following features: absence of ER and PR expressions, aneuploidy, high proliferative rate, periductal angiogenesis, membrane reactivity for HER2, nuclear reactivity for p53, and abnormal bcl-2 expression. Conversely, low-grade DCIS are usually characterized by the following: presence of ERs and PRs, absence of aneuploidy, low proliferative rate, minimal periductal angiogenesis, absence of HER2 and p53 expression, and normal bcl-2 expression. Intermediate-grade DCIS tend to have mixed patterns of biologic marker expression.

No single grading system for DCIS has been demonstrated to be notably superior for anticipating successful breast conservation, and none has gained universal acceptance. A consensus conference convened in 1997 did not endorse any single system of classification, but recommended that a pathology report for DCIS provide information about the descriptive characteristics considered to be necessary in most grading schemes.[156] The three essential elements noted were nuclear grade, necrosis, and architectural pattern(s).

Heterogeneity of nuclear grade is commonly encountered in DCIS; however, it is uncommon for high- and low-grade DCIS to be present in a single lesion. In the 1997 consensus report, nuclear grade was stratified in three categories (Table 11.1). The pathology report should reflect the highest nuclear grade, but may indicate the relative proportions of grade when there is heterogeneity. Necrosis was defined as the "presence of ghost cells and karyorrhectic debris" (Table 11.2). Five architectural patterns were identified: comedo, cribriform, papillary, micropapillary, and solid. It was specified that comedo referred to "solid intraepithelial growth within the basement membrane with central (zonal) necrosis." Such lesions are often but not invariably of high nuclear grade.

Other elements recommended by the 1997 consensus report for inclusion in the diagnosis were lesion "size (extent, distribution)" and margin status. No particular methods for assessing size or margins were suggested.

Interobserver variability is an important consideration in applying a grading system in clinical practice. This issue has been addressed in a limited number of studies, and the results suggest that architectural descriptions (e.g., cribriform, micropapillary, and comedo) are less reproducible than nuclear grade and necrosis.[129,155–157] This probably reflects the heterogeneity of architectural patterns that may be encountered in a single case, whereas nuclear grade tends to be consistent. The description of necrosis can also be a source of disagreement if quantification of necrosis is an element for classifying a lesion as the comedo type.[156] The usual

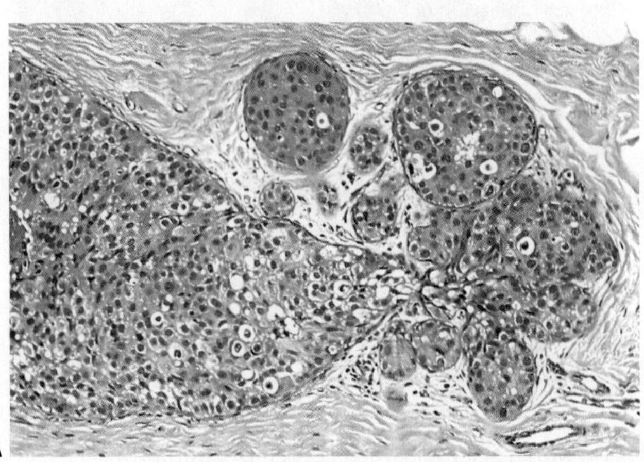

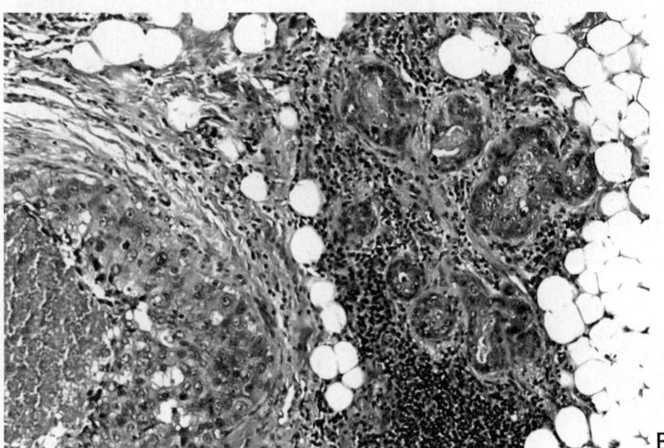

A B

FIG. 11.47. ***Lobular extension of DCIS.*** **A,B:** Solid DCIS extending into lobular glands.

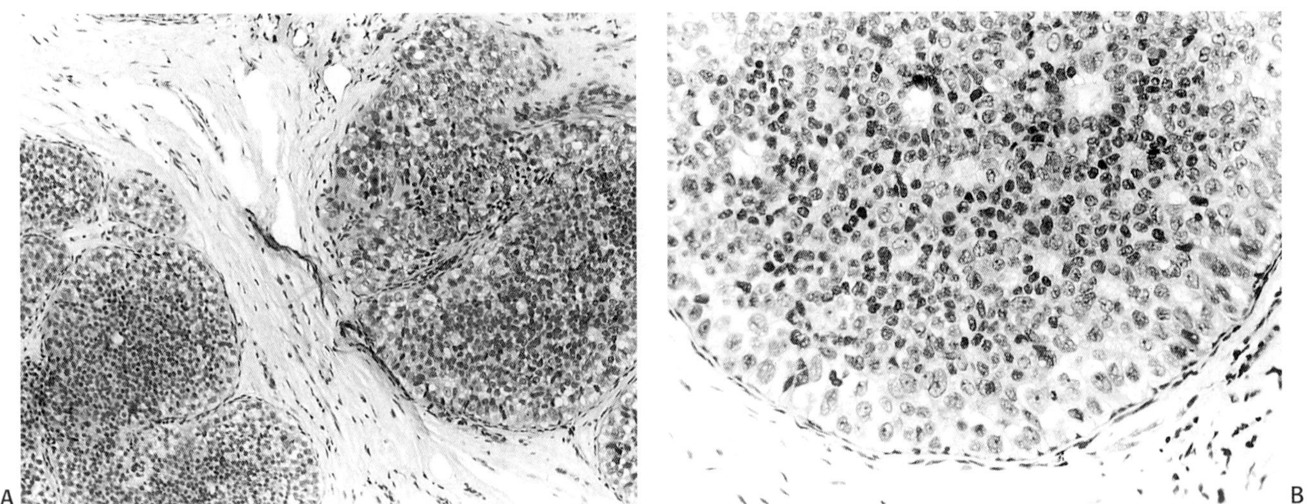

FIG. 11.48. ***In situ carcinoma with ductal and lobular features.*** **A:** Carcinoma in a duct (*right*) and distended lobular glands (*left*). **B:** Small and large cell populations are present. Microlumina have been formed in an area composed of small cells in a duct. The lesion was immunoreactive for E-cadherin.

quantitative descriptors of necrosis are present, focally present, or absent. In the Van Nuys classification system, only the "zonal" type of necrosis classifies DCIS as exhibiting necrosis; however, occasional desquamated or individually necrotic cells do not qualify as DCIS in this scheme.

Sneige et al.[129] studied interobserver reproducibility among six pathologists who assessed nuclear grade, according to Lagios' criteria (Table 11.3), in 125 examples of DCIS. Complete agreement on nuclear grade was reported in 43 cases (35%), and five of six pathologists agreed in 45 (36%). The generalized kappa for distinctions between grades 1 and 2 and between 2 and 3 were 0.29 and 0.48, respectively (standard error = 0.02). These levels of agreement were regarded as fair and moderate by the authors. Pair-wise correlations between individual pathologists and the consensus grade included a range of kappa values from 0.44 to 0.76, with 5 of 6 having values greater than 0.60, representing "substantial" agreement.

Some authors have suggested that apocrine and micropapillary DCIS be listed as separate categories and not included in a three-tiered grading scheme.[157] This proposal appears to derive from perceived difficulty in assigning these lesions to one of the three conventional grades because of inconsistent expression of individual criteria for grading. However, in practice, DCIS with apocrine or micropapillary features express the same range of histologic variation as nonapocrine and nonmicropapillary DCIS, and separate characterization is not recommended. In regard to apocrine lesions, nuclear grade is based on comparison with nuclei in usual benign apocrine metaplasia. The distribution of architectural patterns and necrosis is not different in apocrine and nonapocrine DCIS. Micropapillary DCIS is subject to variations in nuclear grade and to necrosis (illustrated in this chapter), which do not differ from other architectural types of DCIS.

Agreement on DCIS grading has been shown to be achieved more commonly with the Van Nuys classification system, compared with those of Lagios and Holland.[158] Pinder et al.[159] have identified a subdivision of DCIS with "very poor prognosis." This "very high-grade" type of DCIS has high cytonuclear grade, solid (more than 50%) architecture, and extensive comedo-type necrosis (more than 50%). This "novel" classification for DCIS offered better prognostic discrimination for ipsilateral recurrence than "cytonuclear grade" classification alone when applied to cases assembled in a clinical trial.[159]

Preliminary studies show promise in assessing the molecular "grade" of DCIS through the use of array-based comparative genomic hybridization (CGH) and other related techniques. Such molecular profiling has the potential to improve the clinical evaluation of DCIS and is becoming increasingly possible.[160]

ANGIOGENESIS

Studies of the microvascular pattern of capillaries in breast tissue from patients with DCIS have demonstrated increased periductal vascularity associated with some but not all DCIS. The most reliable information has been obtained from histologic sections immunostained with vascular markers such as factor VIII, CD31, or CD34. Increased microvessel size has been observed at sites of DCIS compared with normal breast tissue.[161] Simple hyperplasia has been shown to have a 22-fold greater degree of microvascular density than normal ducts.[162] Neovascularization has been described around DCIS associated with invasive lesions.[163] Periductal neovascularity found around 21 (38%) of 55 examples of pure DCIS studied by Guidi et al.[164] was not related to histologic subtype, the presence of necrosis, proliferative index (PI),

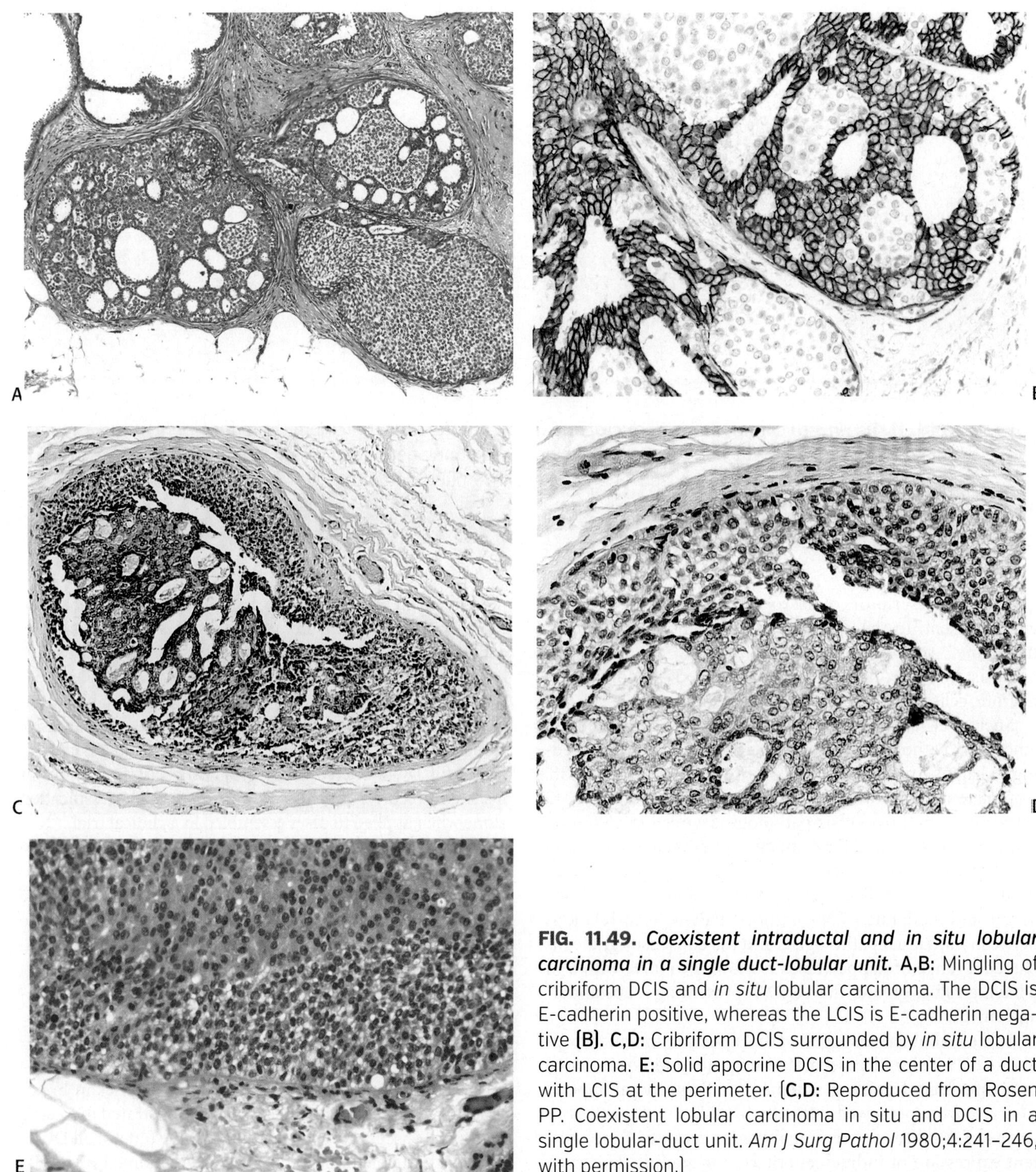

FIG. 11.49. ***Coexistent intraductal and in situ lobular carcinoma in a single duct-lobular unit.*** **A,B:** Mingling of cribriform DCIS and *in situ* lobular carcinoma. The DCIS is E-cadherin positive, whereas the LCIS is E-cadherin negative (**B**). **C,D:** Cribriform DCIS surrounded by *in situ* lobular carcinoma. **E:** Solid apocrine DCIS in the center of a duct with LCIS at the perimeter. (**C,D:** Reproduced from Rosen PP. Coexistent lobular carcinoma in situ and DCIS in a single lobular-duct unit. *Am J Surg Pathol* 1980;4:241–246, with permission.)

or HER2 expression. These authors observed that stromal vascularity was increased in comedo DCIS when there was marked stromal desmoplasia, but the increased vascularity was not specifically periductal in distribution.

Other investigators have also studied the association between the architectural pattern of DCIS and periductal neovascularity. Heffelfinger et al.[165] recorded the distribution of capillaries in contact with the basement membrane of ducts in various conditions, including proliferative changes and DCIS. The mean score for vascularity was increased significantly between normal and proliferative ducts (0.187 vs. 0.836) and between both of these categories and DCIS as a group (1.525). Variations in mean scores were seen in subtypes of DCIS, ranging from 0.962 for micropapillary

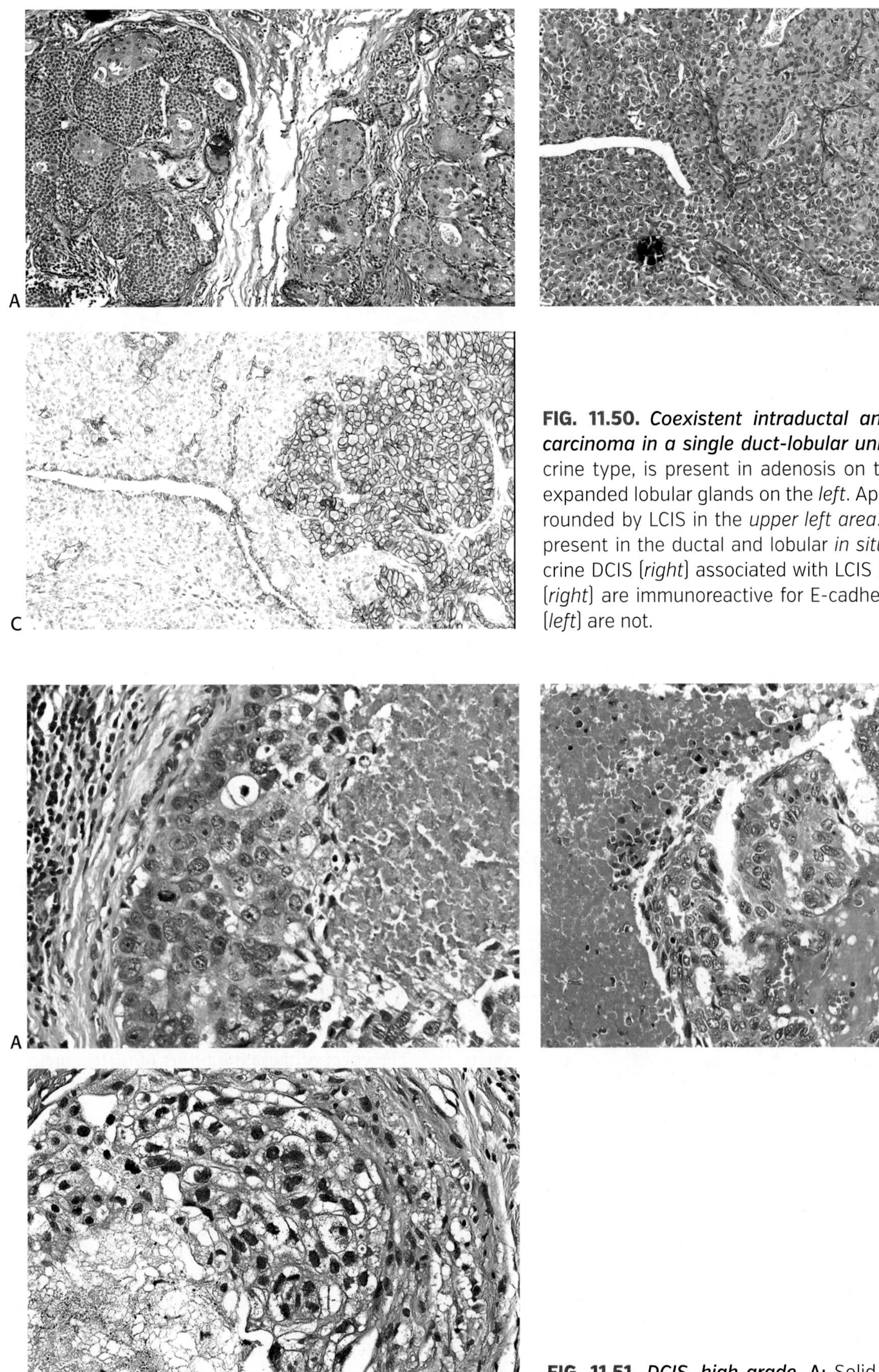

FIG. 11.50. ***Coexistent intraductal and in situ lobular carcinoma in a single duct-lobular unit.*** **A,B:** DCIS, apocrine type, is present in adenosis on the *right*. LCIS fills expanded lobular glands on the *left*. Apocrine DCIS is surrounded by LCIS in the *upper left area*. Calcifications are present in the ductal and lobular *in situ* carcinoma. Apocrine DCIS (*right*) associated with LCIS (*left*). **C:** DCIS cells (*right*) are immunoreactive for E-cadherin, and LCIS cells (*left*) are not.

FIG. 11.51. ***DCIS, high grade.*** **A:** Solid ("comedo") carcinoma. Note mitotic activity. **B:** Papillary carcinoma with necrosis. **C:** Clear cell carcinoma.

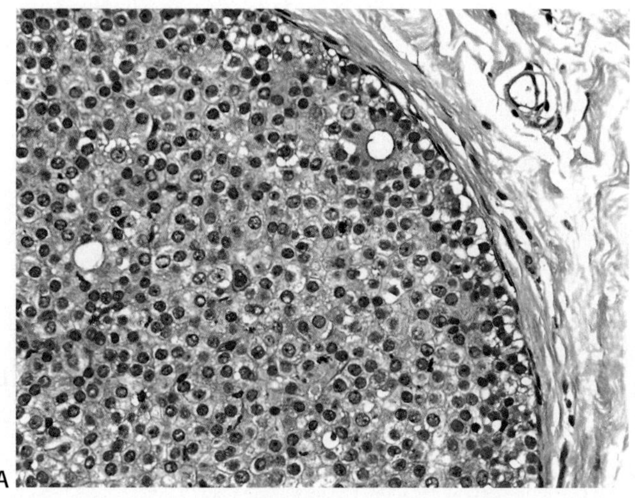
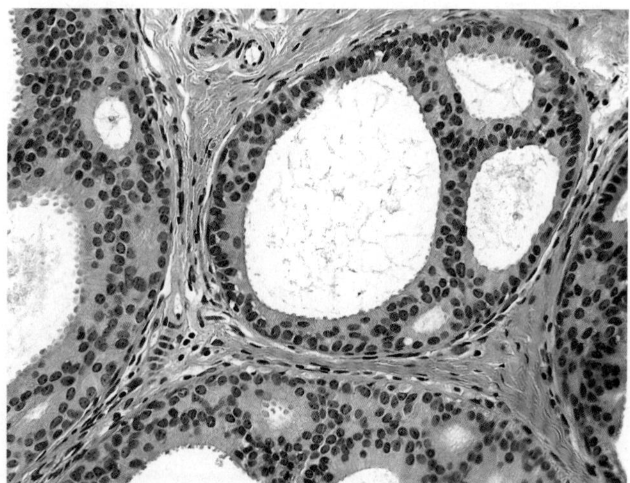

FIG. 11.52. ***DCIS, low grade.*** **A:** Solid DCIS. **B:** Micropapillary architecture.

to 2.216 for comedocarcinoma, but the differences were not statistically significant.

Bose et al.[101] analyzed periductal angiogenesis using factor VIII and CD34 immunostains in comedo and noncomedo types of DCIS. Small capillaries were usually present in the connective tissue, but they were sparse in the region of the basement membrane around normal ducts. New vessel formation associated with DCIS was limited to the region of the basement membrane in ducts with DCIS (Fig. 11.54). Evidence of angiogenesis was found in 80% of DCIS consisting of a ring of neovascularity completely or partially encircling the affected duct. A complete ring was found more often around comedo DCIS, whereas noncomedo lesions tended to have a partial ring or no periductal neovascularity (Figs. 11.28 and 11.54). Using a different method of quantitation, Guidi and Schnitt[166] confirmed that maximal periductal neovascularity was associated

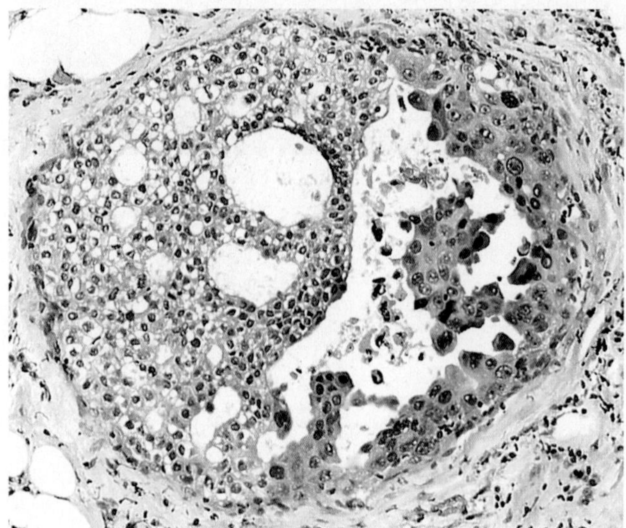

FIG. 11.53. ***DCIS, low and high nuclear grade in a single duct.***

with comedocarcinoma, the expression of HER2, and with a high PI.

Engels et al.[167] compared DCIS with increased stromal vascularity in between affected ducts, which they termed "pattern I" and lesions in which neovascularity formed a dense rim around the basement membrane ("pattern II"). Patterns I and II were present alone in 11% and 16%, respectively, of 75 cases. Increased vascularity with either pattern alone or in combination was associated with high-grade forms of DCIS.

The observed pattern of angiogenesis may be related in part to the fate of myoepithelial cell layer in ducts that develop DCIS. Myoepithelial cells are more likely to persist in low-grade DCIS, and they are usually markedly attenuated or absent in high-grade or comedo DCIS. It has been suggested that myoepithelial cells may exert a tumor suppressor influence on the development or progression of DCIS.[104,168,169] Several lines of evidence appear to support this hypothesis. *In vitro* and *in situ* tissue studies have demonstrated that myoepithelial cells express high amounts of proteinase inhibitors, including maspin, protease nexin II, and α_1-antitrypsin, and that these inhibitory proteins are concentrated in the stroma surrounding ducts.[170,171] The effect of these inhibitors of matrix metalloproteinases is to decrease tumor invasiveness and to reduce angiogenesis.[105,170]

Angiogenesis associated with DCIS may also be modulated by the ability of the neoplastic cells to express angiogenic proteins such as the vascular endothelial growth factor (VEGF). High-grade DCIS and a significantly higher microvessel count have been associated with stronger VEGF mRNA expression detected by *in situ* hybridization.[172]

Vasohibin-1 is a negative feedback regulator of angiogenesis. The status of neovascularization can be determined by the expression of vasohibin-1 mRNA that was more highly expressed in higher grade of DCIS in one study[173]; however, data regarding the degree of angiogenesis in various grades of DCIS are conflicting.[174]

TABLE 11.1 Consensus Committee Recommendation for Nuclear Grading of DCIS

Low Nuclear Grade (NG1)
• Monomorphic (monotonous) appearance
• Size of duct epithelial nuclei or 1.5–2.0 normal red blood cell
• Chromatin diffuse, finely dispersed
• "Occasional nucleoli and mitoses"
• Cells usually polarized
High Nuclear Grade (NG3)
• "Markedly pleomorphic"
• Size usually more than 2.5 duct epithelial nuclei
• Chromatin vesicular with irregular distribution
• "Prominent, often multiple nucleoli"
• "Mitoses may be conspicuous"
Intermediate Nuclear Grade (NG2)
• "Nuclei that are neither NG1 nor NG3"

Based on The Consensus Conference Committee. Consensus Conference on the classification of ductal carcinoma in situ. *Cancer* 1997;80:1798–1802.

BIOMARKERS IN DCIS

A variety of biologic markers have been studied in DCIS. Lari and Kuerer[175] performed a comprehensive review of 622 major studies that had reported on 25 traditional and emerging biologic markers of DCIS and their associated recurrence risk. These studies appeared over a 10-year period beginning late 2000 and included 6,252 patients. The study included hormone receptors, proliferation markers, cell cycle regulation markers, among others. No prospective validation study was identified, and the various studies included in the review suffered from the usual limitations of variations in surgery, radiation, and endocrine therapy. Nonetheless, the review provides considerable information. For the three most common biomarkers, the mean expression rates in DCIS were 68.7 for ER, 59.6% for PR, and 40.1% for HER2.

Estrogen Receptor and Progesterone Receptor

American Society of Clinical Oncology (ASCO) and College of American Pathology (CAP) currently endorse the routine assessment of ER and PR status in all DCIS cases[176]; however, since DCIS is often a lesion of microscopic dimension, little information was available about hormone receptor expression until immunohistochemical methods became available. Biochemical analysis employing homogenized tissue samples contained a substantial proportion of nonneoplastic tissue, and as a consequence, the majority of specimens of DCIS were reportedly receptor negative. In one study, the median level of ER in DCIS was 5 fmol/mg cytosol protein, significantly less than the median of 11 fmol/mg for infiltrating duct carcinoma.[177]

Barnes and Masood[178] described an immunohistochemical study of ER in DCIS in 1990. Nuclear reactivity, usually heterogeneously distributed when present, was found in 75% of pure DCIS, in 73% of DCIS associated with invasive duct carcinoma, and in 100% of 36 examples of atypical duct hyperplasia. Nuclear ER reactivity was less frequent in comedo DCIS than in other variants (Fig. 11.55). The same pattern of ER expression was usually found in the intraductal and in the infiltrating portions of carcinomas with both components. ER positivity was more frequent in tumors

TABLE 11.2 Consensus Committee Recommendation for Reporting Necrosis in DCIS

Comedonecrosis
"Central zone necrosis within a duct, usually exhibiting a linear pattern within ducts if sectioned longitudinally"
Punctate
"Nonzonal type necrosis (foci of necrosis that do not exhibit a linear pattern if longitudinally sectioned)"

Based on The Consensus Conference Committee. Consensus Conference on the classification of ductal carcinoma in situ. *Cancer* 1997;80:1798–1802.

TABLE 11.3 Lagios' Nuclear Grading System

	Low Grade	Intermediate Grade	High Grade
Nuclear Features	**Grade 1**	**Grade 2**	**Grade 3**
Diameter	<2 × rbc	2–2.5 × rbc	>2.5 rbc
Pleomorphism	Absent	More uniform	Prominent
Chromatin	Diffuse	Coarse	Vesicular
Nucleoli	Absent	Inconspicuous	Prominent[a]
Mitoses	Frequent	Infrequent	Rare

[a]Nucleoli not required for grade 3 if pleomorphism and mitoses are prominent.

Modified from Lagios MD. Duct carcinoma in situ: pathology and treatment. *Surg Clin North Am* 1990;70:853–871.

from women older than 55 years than in those from younger patients.

A more detailed analysis of ER IHC was provided by Bur et al.[179] in 1992. They classified 80% of DCIS as ER positive, with a significantly higher frequency of receptor positivity in noncomedo (91%) than in comedo (57%) lesions. The frequencies of ER positivity among variants of noncomedo DCIS did not differ significantly (cribriform, 89%; solid, 94%; micropapillary–papillary, 100%). Cellular features associated with the absence of ER were large cell size, nuclear pleomorphism, and necrosis. These authors also confirmed the observation of Barnes and Masood that ER immunoreactivity was almost always the same in the intraductal and invasive portions of a lesion.

Holland et al.[180] studied the response of DCIS to estrogens in human breast tissue *in vivo* using nude mouse xenografts.

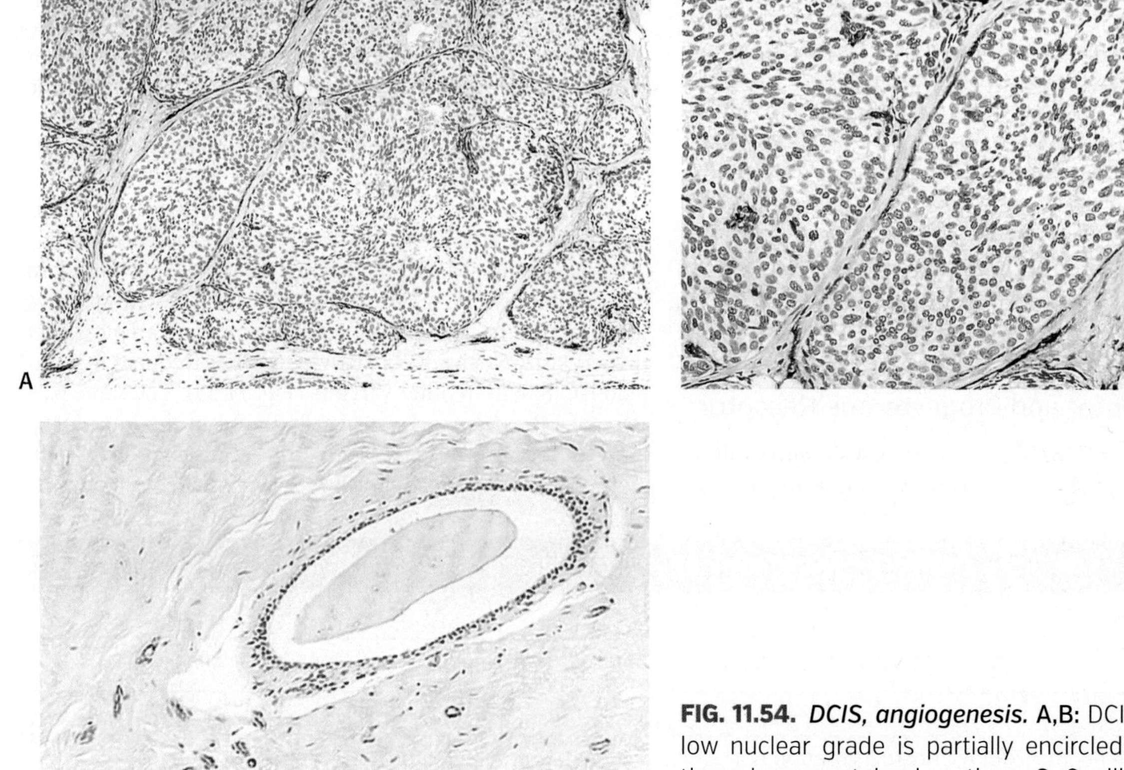

FIG. 11.54. ***DCIS, angiogenesis.*** **A,B:** DCIS, solid type with low nuclear grade is partially encircled by capillaries in these immunostained sections. **C:** Capillaries are present in the stroma, but they are not concentrated around this normal duct (CD34).

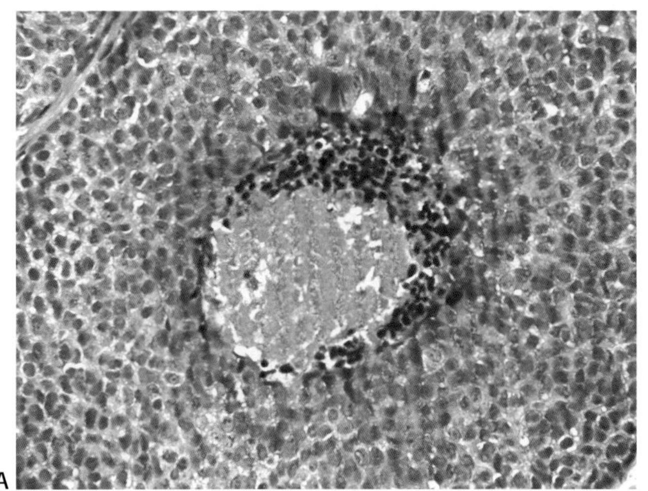

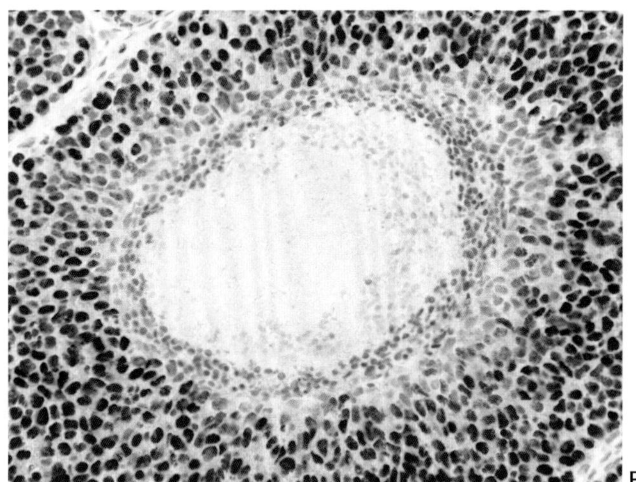

FIG. 11.55. ***DCIS, estrogen receptor.*** **A,B:** Strong and diffuse nuclear immunoreactivity for ER (**B**) in solid DCIS with intermediate-grade nuclei and central necrosis. Nuclear reactivity has been lost in the dying cells around the necrotic center.

Samples of ER-negative comedo DCIS had a high proliferative rate prior to transplantation, and this was maintained but did not increase when xenografts were exposed to estrogen. On the other hand, noncomedo, ER-positive DCIS exhibited increased proliferation after exposure to estrogens, although the proliferative levels did not reach those of the comedo DCIS. These results suggest that ER-negative DCIS is estrogen independent and that antiestrogen therapy may not be beneficial for patients with these lesions.

Hormone receptor expression in DCIS may be a significant factor for local recurrence after breast conservation treatment. Roka et al.[181] reported that DCIS with high nuclear grade and absence of ER had a significantly higher recurrence rate. However, not all high-grade DCIS lack ER expression. Collins and Schnitt[182] found that 14 (12%) of 114 ER-positive DCIS had high nuclear grade and overexpressed HER2 protein. Concurrent ER and HER2 expression was not found in any of the 74 examples of low- and intermediate-grade DCIS, all of which expressed ER and lacked HER2 overexpression.

In general, approximately 75% of DCIS cases show positive nuclear immunoreactivity for ER (ranging from 1% to 100% cells), and a somewhat lower frequency are positive for PR. However, determination of "positivity" of ER and PR in DCIS can be problematic.[183] There are three main scoring methods for ER and PR immunoreactivity. One is the *simple percentage method*, that is, simple proportion of cells staining without regard to intensity. A second is the *histochemical "H" method*, that is, the sum of the percentage of cells with three degrees of staining of cells resulting in a range of 0 to 300. The third, *Allred method*, produces an intensity score between 1 and 3, and a percentage of cells staining compartmentalized in a nonlinear manner using scores between 1 and 5, to yield a final score of between 2 and 8. The Allred and "H" scoring methodologies include assessment of staining intensity, whereas the simple percentage method does not. Optimally, a scoring method utilizing both proportion and intensity of ER staining should be used for DCIS, if only because there is evidence for the value of such assessment in invasive breast cancer. Excellent interobserver agreement has been reported in the use of "H" score for the assessment of ER and PR in invasive breast carcinoma since it provides a "continuous measure of tumor hormone-receptor content" as opposed to the Allred system that has a "limited dynamic range."[184]

The UK breast-screening guidelines recommend the use of less than 5% cells staining for DCIS and the use of the Allred score for invasive cancers.[185] A cutoff point of Allred score 3 for positivity has been used in a study of various phenotypes of DCIS. Baqai and Shousha[186] reviewed 56 cases of pure DCIS. ER positivity was defined as more than 10% of cells showing dark brown nuclear staining (Allred score greater than 4, "H" score of greater than 20). Eighty-eight percent of high-grade DCIS were ER negative. Data from the Sloane Project (named after the late Professor John Sloane of the Royal Liverpool Infirmaray who had a special interest in the pathology of DCIS) show that intermediate and low-grade DCIS are almost invariably ER positive, whereas high-grade DCIS is positive in 69% of cases.[185]

Oncogenes

HER2: Immunohistochemical studies have demonstrated membrane immunoreactivity for the HER2 (HER2) oncogene in 42% to 61% of DCIS.[187–191] (Fig. 11.56). *HER2* gene amplification has been reported in 40% to 48% of DCIS specimens isolated by microdissection and studied by the polymerase chain reaction (PCR).[192,193] Ho et al.[193] found significantly higher frequencies of HER2 amplification in comedo than in noncomedo DCIS (69% vs. 18%) and in lesions with high rather than low nuclear grade (63% vs. 14%). Expression of HER2 occurs in 85% to 100% of comedocarcinomas and is associated with the pleomorphic nuclear cytology in these lesions.[187,191,194]

Most investigators have not detected HER2 in small cell micropapillary and cribriform DCIS.[187,191,195] Using

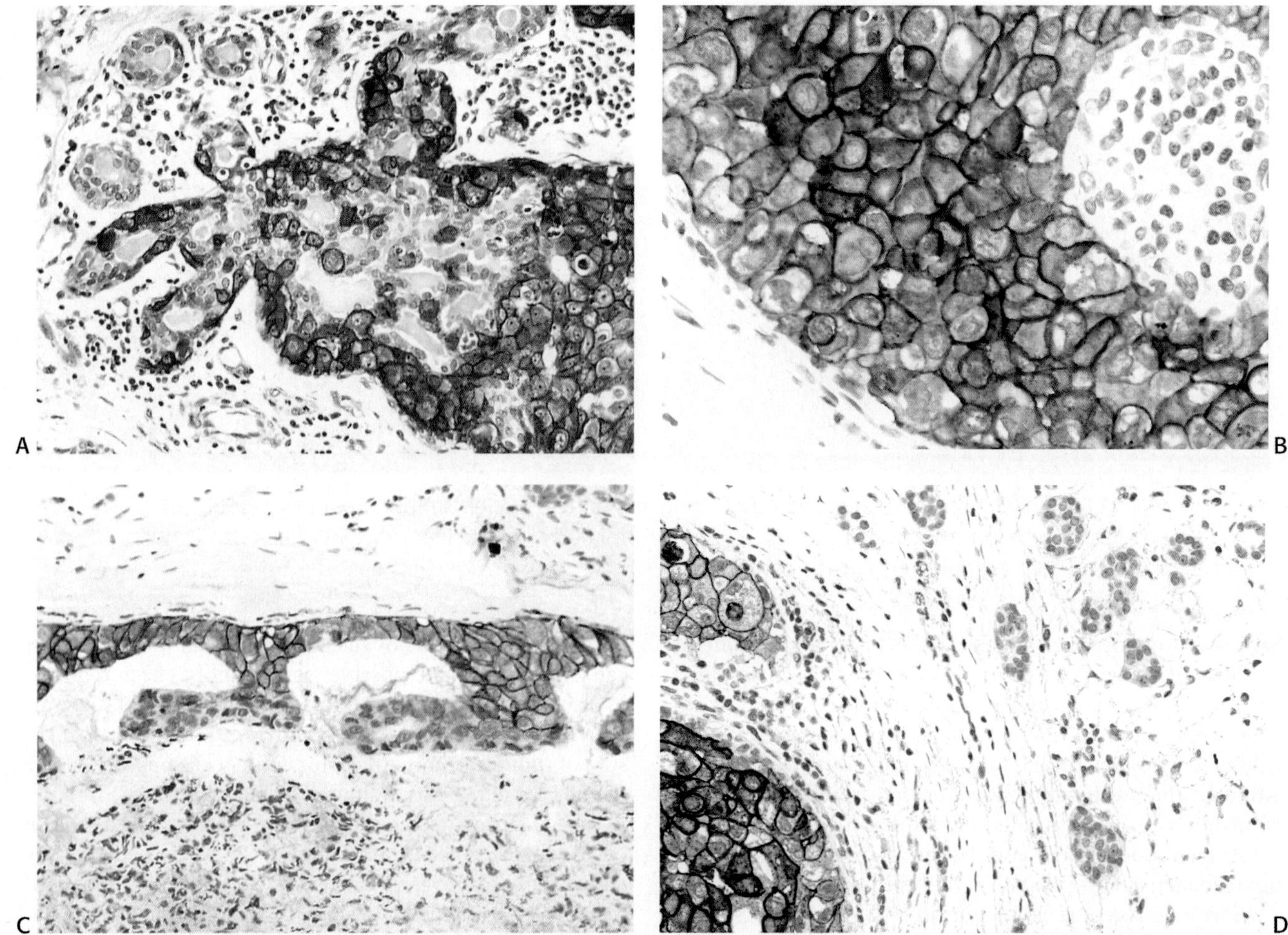

FIG. 11.56. ***DCIS, HER2.*** **A:** HER2 membrane immunoreactivity is present in the DCIS extending into a lobule but not in nonneoplastic epithelial cells. **B:** HER2-positive, solid high-grade DCIS. **C:** HER2-positive micropapillary DCIS with high-grade nuclei and necrosis. **D:** HER2-negative invasive well-differentiated carcinoma (*right*) and HER2-positive solid DCIS (*left*).

actual measurements of nuclear size, Bartkova et al.[187] observed that 94% of DCIS composed of cells with large nuclei (20 μm) were positive for HER2, whereas no membrane reactivity was seen in cells with small nuclei (10 μm). Immunoreactivity was present in 71% of DCIS with intermediate nuclear size (15 μm) and in 91% of lesions composed of cells with mixed nuclear size. In this series, a small number of papillary and clinging DCIS with large nuclei were immunoreactive for HER2. Others have confirmed the finding of HER2 immunoreactivity in 85% of micropapillary or clinging DCIS with large or pleomorphic nuclei.[196] The neoplastic Paget cells in the eponymous disease of the nipple, as well as those of the associated underlying mammary DCIS, are ER negative and HER2 positive in more than 80% of cases.[197]

HER2 immunoreactivity is found more often in DCIS with aneuploid nuclei than in carcinomas with diploid nuclei, an association that correlates well with the reported relationship of HER2 to nuclear size.[190,194] There is also a strong association between positive HER2 reactivity and a high proliferative rate represented by the thymidine and MIB1 labeling indices.[194,198]

The extracellular domain of HER2 can be detected in the serum of patients with invasive breast carcinoma, and this finding has been associated with overexpression in the carcinoma detected by IHC.[199] Serum analysis for HER2 may prove to be a useful method for identifying patients with microinvasive duct carcinoma. Esteva-Lorenzo et al.[200] described a patient with elevated serum extracellular domain of HER2 at the time a breast biopsy demonstrated comedo DCIS that was immunoreactive for HER2. Reexcision performed because carcinoma involved the initial excision margin revealed a microinvasive focus. Thereafter, the serum level of HER2 decreased to normal. No elevation of serum extracellular domain HER2 was detected by these authors in specimens from 8 other patients with DCIS, including 3 with DCIS immunoreactive for HER2, or in 27 patients with benign biopsies. In women with clinically invasive carcinoma, serial HER2 serum levels during the course of chemotherapy did not correlate well with the clinical status of the patients.[201]

Less than 10% of DCIS have been characterized as having the basal-like phenotype on the basis of IHC. These uncommon instances of HER2 (−) high-grade DCIS are not readily distinguished from HER2 (+) high-grade DCIS in routine H&E sections. Livasy et al.[202] studied 245 examples of pure DCIS and found that 19 (7.7%) qualified as basal like: (ER [−], HER2 [−], and EGFR or CK5/6 [+]). This small subset of DCIS displayed a variety of characteristics typically associated with HER2 (+) DCIS, including a high Ki67 index, expression of p53, and comedo histology. Thike et al.[203] examined the DCIS component in 241 triple-negative invasive carcinomas and found that 151 (62.6%) DCIS were of high nuclear grade, and 236 (97.9%) were also triple negative. The basal phenotype, defined by immunoreactivity for CK14, EGFR, and 34βE12, was expressed in 68% in the *in situ* and invasive components of the same case. The authors concluded that triple-negative DCIS is the likely precursor of the corresponding invasive counterpart and that basal-like expression is maintained in the majority of invasive cancers associated with basal-like *in situ* disease.

p53: Investigators employing a monoclonal antibody to wild and mutant forms of the p53 protein have reported nuclear reactivity in 10%,[204] 18.5%,[205] 19.2%,[195] 25.2%,[206] and 37%[207] of DCIS examined (Fig. 11.57). In some studies, expression of p53 was significantly associated with large or pleomorphic cell type, intraductal necrosis, and comedo DCIS,[195,198,204–206] but others did not find a significant correlation between grade or histologic subtype and p53 expression[207] or p53 mutations.[193] Nuclear p53 was found only rarely in small cell DCIS.[206] No p53 reactivity was found in 17 cystic papillary carcinomas studied by O'Malley et al.[204] When present, p53 mutations have been identical in most instances where intraductal and invasive carcinoma samples from a single tumor have been examined.[208] In one study, no p53 mutations were identified in microdissected hyperplastic lesions from patients who had p53 mutations in coexisting intraductal and invasive duct carcinoma.[208]

Carcinomas expressing p53 tend to be ER and PR negative,[198,206] and they show evidence of a higher than median proliferative rate manifested by a relatively high MIB1 labeling index.[198] Molecular analysis using direct sequencing of PCR products revealed mutant p53 protein accumulation in comedo DCIS.[151] There was not a significant trend for coexpression of p53 and HER2 in any subset of carcinoma, despite the independent association of p53 and HER2 with large cell or comedo DCIS in some studies.[189,193,206,209]

Other Markers

The *nm23 gene product* is associated with low metastatic potential in some cell culture systems and in invasive human breast carcinomas.[210] Cytoplasmic immunoreactivity for nm23 is found in normal breast epithelium and in most noninvasive carcinomas.[211] Strong staining was found in LCIS. Comedocarcinomas without associated invasion exhibited more intense nm23 reactivity than comedocarcinomas with invasion, a difference not observed when noncomedo intraductal and invasive carcinoma were compared.[211] These observations suggest that reduced nm23 expression in comedo DCIS may be a marker for the acquisition of invasive characteristics.

The relationship of growth factors and their receptors to the morphology and prognosis of DCIS has not been extensively explored. As noted earlier, *EGFR* expression has been associated with the basal-like phenotype DCIS (Fig. 11.58).

E-cadherin is a cell–cell adhesion molecule expressed by epithelial cells. Loss of expression resulting from mutations in the *E-cadherin* gene has been associated with invasive lobular carcinoma and LCIS. E-cadherin expression may be reduced in DCIS, but it is rarely absent. Vos et al.[212] studied 150 examples of DCIS and detected E-cadherin in all cases with reduced expression in 11%. In one study, there was significantly less expression in high-grade than in low-grade lesions.[213] Bankfalvi et al.[214] also reported reduced E-cadherin reactivity in high-grade DCIS and confirmed the absence of E-cadherin expression in lobular carcinomas. The reduced cell–cell adhesion in high-grade DCIS may contribute to the relatively high frequency of microinvasion observed in these lesions.

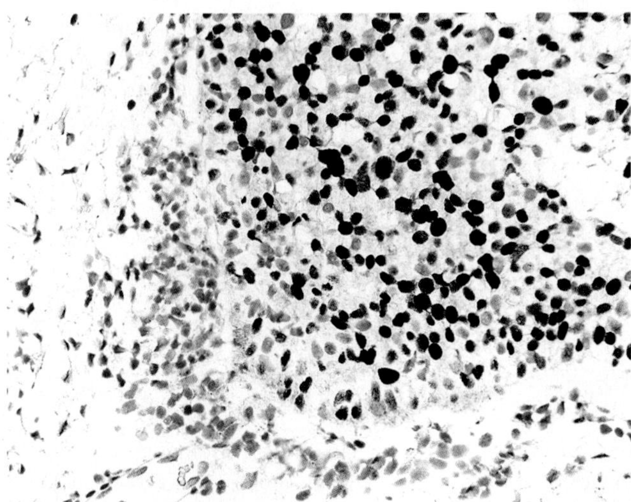

FIG. 11.57. ***DCIS, p53.*** Nuclear immunoreactivity is evident in almost all neoplastic cells in this DCIS with intermediate nuclear grade.

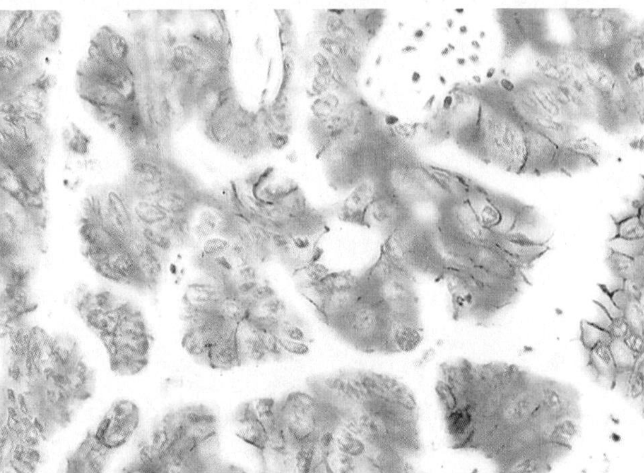

FIG. 11.58. ***DCIS, EGFR.*** Membrane immunoreactivity for EGFR forms slender beaded lines between cells in this DCIS. Background cytoplasmic staining is also evident.

PLOIDY AND PROLIFERATIVE RATE

When studied by flow cytometry, the frequency of aneuploidy in DCIS ranges from 21% to 71%.[215–220] The clinical relevance, and need, for this information has diminished over the years. Aneuploidy has been found in 55% to more than 90% of comedocarcinomas[215,216,218,219] and in 65% of DCIS with high nuclear grade.[217] Image analysis of Feulgen-stained tissue sections revealed aneuploidy in 77.5% of DCIS, predominantly in lesions with high (100%) and intermediate (80%) nuclear grade.[207]

Thymidine labeling and flow cytometry studies demonstrated a significantly higher proliferative rate in comedocarcinoma than in cribriform–micropapillary DCIS.[189,221] All papillary DCIS examined in one series were diploid.[219] Cribriform DCIS tend to be diploid with a low S-phase fraction (SPF).[218,220] Sataloff et al.[220] reported that micropapillary DCIS was typically diploid with a low SPF.

Numerical alterations in individual chromosomes have been studied by fluorescence *in situ* hybridization (FISH) using specific probes. Using this method in paraffin sections of archival tissue samples, Visscher et al.[222] detected chromosomal aneuploidy in 7 to 10 specimens of DCIS. Aneuploidy was more frequent in specimens from patients with concurrent invasive carcinoma. Patterns of aneuploidy consisted of gains only, losses only, or gains and losses involving different chromosomes. Aneuploidy was most frequent for chromosomes 16 and 17. HER2-positive and triple-negative types of DCIS, to a greater degree than the "luminal" types of DCIS, show DNA aneuploidy, as assessed by image analysis.[223]

The proliferative activity in DCIS is now usually analyzed by IHC (Fig. 11.59). Albonico et al.[195] reported the highest PI in lesions of the comedo type. Other types of DCIS had much lower PIs: solid 14.4%, papillary 13.4%, cribriform 4.5%, and micropapillary 0%. DCIS can be graded using

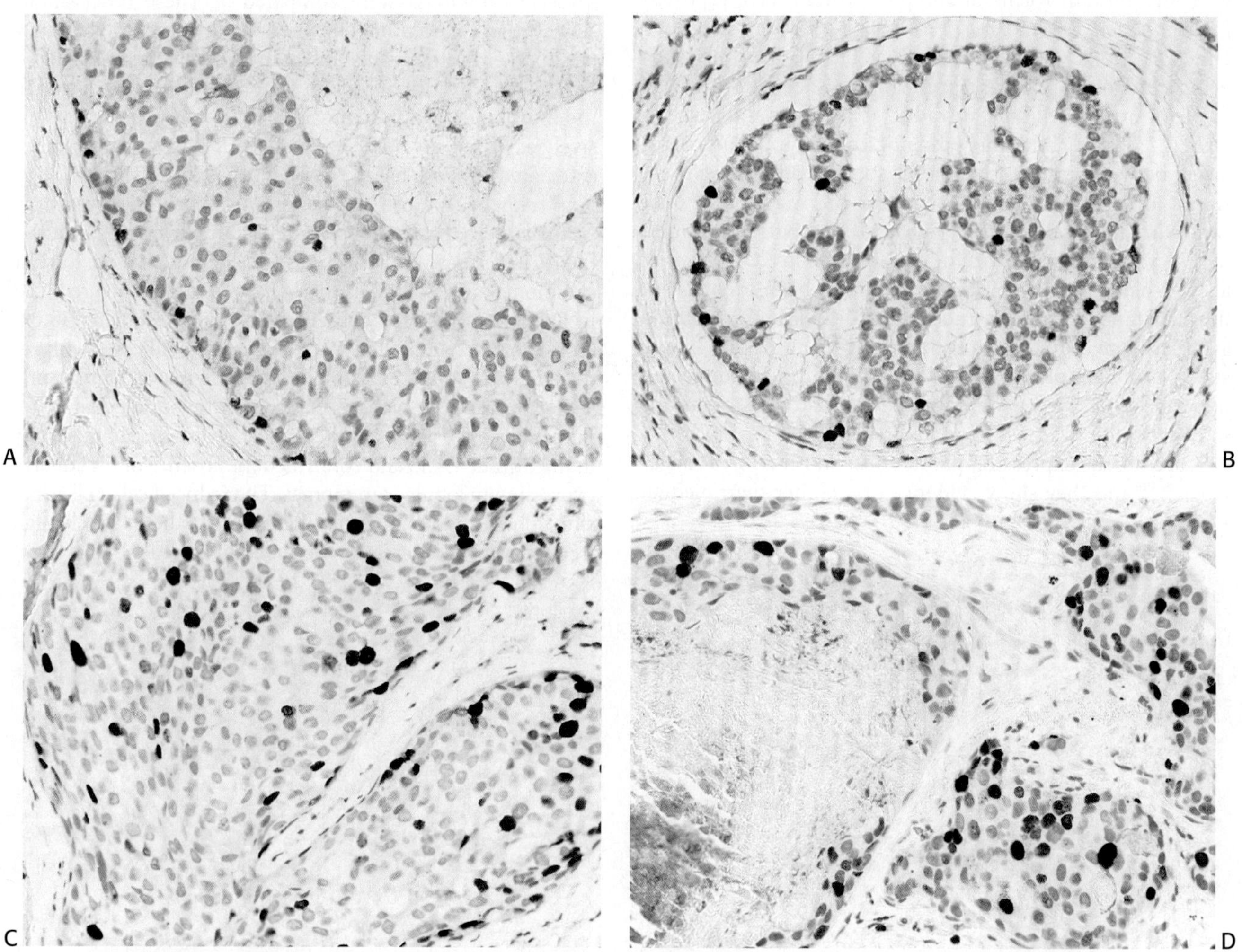

FIG. 11.59. ***DCIS, Ki67 proliferation marker.*** **A:** Nuclear immunoreactivity for Ki67 is present in very few neoplastic cells in the basal region of cribriform DCIS with low-grade nuclei. **B:** Ki67 reactivity observed in less than 10% of cells in this micropapillary DCIS with intermediate-grade nuclei. Nuclear reactivity is mostly localized to the basal region in this example also. **C:** Approximately 10% of the neoplastic cells are Ki67 reactive in this solid DCIS. **D:** Approximately one-third of the neoplastic cells are reactive for Ki67 in this solid high-grade DCIS with necrosis [*left*].

the "nuclear grade + proliferation index" (N + P) system. The N + P methodology utilizes automated assessment of the proliferation index that has been shown to be a reproducible grading system for DCIS as well as for invasive carcinoma.[224] Cases of DCIS that have a high proliferation rate by IHC, and are positive for HER2, confer a higher risk of recurrence, independent of grade and age.[225]

The *bcl-2* gene plays a role in control of cell growth by inhibiting apoptosis (Fig. 11.32). The expression of bcl-2 in DCIS is inversely related to grade. Loss of bcl-2 expression is most pronounced in high-grade DCIS and is directly related to p53 expression.[128] High-grade DCIS exhibit a higher rate of apoptosis (apoptotic index) than low-grade lesions.[226]

CYTOGENETICS AND MOLECULAR GENETICS

Prior to the development of microdissection techniques, few genetic studies of DCIS were reported because of the technical difficulties inherent in isolating the epithelium of these microscopic lesions. DNA extracted from ducts containing DCIS isolated by microdissection has provided the material for the molecular analysis of genetic alterations. Using this method, Radford et al.[227] reported loss of heterozygosity (LOH) on 17p in 29% of DCIS, compared with normal, control DNA. No significant difference in the frequency of LOH was observed among subtypes of DCIS (comedo vs. noncomedo) or in regard to nuclear grade. Another study revealed LOH on chromosome 17p13.1 in 5 of 15 informative cases studied.[228] LOH on 11p15 has been reported in a high proportion of microdissected samples of DCIS.[229] Chuaqui et al.[230] reported finding LOH on 11q13 in 6 (27.3%) of 22 DCIS. All of the lesions with LOH were high grade. LOH was also found in 1 of 11 lesions (9%) classified as atypical duct hyperplasia. The accumulated data suggest that LOH occurs often and early in the development of DCIS and that the sites of LOH are probable loci of one or more tumor suppressor genes.[231,232]

Stratton et al.[233] detected LOH on 16q in 28% and on 17p in 29% of DCIS not associated with invasive lesions. DCIS found in conjunction with invasive carcinomas had a greater frequency of LOH on chromosomes 16q (55%) and 17p (52%). Analysis of intraductal and invasive carcinoma from the same patient has usually but not always shown similar patterns of LOH in both components.[234–237] This is of particular interest because there is also a strong correlation between the distribution of prognostic markers in intraductal and invasive duct carcinoma, usually with identical patterns of expression for hormone receptors, HER2, p53, EGFR, and cyclin D1. Studies by Barsky et al.[238] suggest that DCIS often has many of the biologic characteristics of invasive carcinoma, and they hypothesize that the most significant difference between *in situ* and invasive carcinoma lies in the inhibitory influences of myoepithelial cells. As previously noted, studies performed by these investigators indicated that one or more proteins secreted by myoepithelial cells inhibit invasion and angiogenesis.

A study of alterations in chromosome 1 revealed that the cells in individual ducts from a single specimen of DCIS may have different genetic patterns.[235] Similar observations were reported by Marsh and Varley,[239] who analyzed LOH at 9p in multiple microdissected ducts from individual patients. LOH was found in 12 of 13 cases studied. Loss of at least one marker was detected in all subtypes (comedo, solid, cribriform, and micropapillary), but the most extensive loss was present in comedo and cribriform lesions. The pattern of LOH in DCIS was present in the corresponding invasive carcinoma in some but not all tumors. Aubele et al.[240] applied CGH to microdissected examples of extensive DCIS with small foci of invasive carcinoma. The procedure detected "multiple genetic changes affecting 6 to 19 different chromosomal regions per tumor (mean 13.6 ± 5.4)" in DCIS. "Chromosomal alterations identified in more than one-third of the invasive lesions were mainly identical" to those in the corresponding DCIS, except for gains of DNA on 3p and 12q, which were found more frequently in invasive carcinomas.

A remarkable molecular genetic study of DCIS reported by Waldman et al.[241] employed CGH to detect chromosomal alterations in primary lesions and in subsequent local breast recurrences. Paired samples from 18 patients were studied, with all recurrences being entirely intraductal and detected 16 months to 9.3 years after initial treatment. In 17 cases, the average rate of concordance in chromosomal alterations between paired samples was 81% (range, 65% to 100%), and the pairs of lesions were morphologically similar. One pair of samples had no agreement, having 2 and 20 alterations, respectively. These findings indicate that situations classified as "recurrence" in 17 cases were instances of persistent carcinoma and that the eighteenth patient most likely had two independent foci of DCIS. The mean number of CGH changes was lower in the initial lesions (8.8) than in recurrent DCIS (10.7). The degree of concordance was not significantly related to the time to recurrence.

It is generally accepted that most lower grade invasive breast carcinomas evolve through a series of nonobligatory abnormal stages of preneoplastic and neoplastic growth over an uncertain period of time (most likely several years in duration). These stages are recognized morphologically as hyperplasia, ADH, and DCIS, with the latter two representing the penultimate and ultimate stages of preinvasive neoplastic progression, respectively. Genetic analyses of matched samples of ADH, DCIS, and invasive carcinoma have identified concordant allelic imbalances with similar frequencies, indicating that ADH and DCIS are nonobligate precursors to invasive carcinoma. ADH and low-grade DCIS are characterized by recurrent losses of 16q and 17p, and gain of 1q. The patterns of genetic aberrations in high-grade DCIS are more heterogeneous, with only rare deletions of 16q. The data, thus far, suggest that high-grade DCIS (those that are ER negative and HER positive, express "basal" markers and genomic aberrations) arise either *de novo* or from an as yet unidentified precursor lesion—perhaps related to apocrine lesions or to lesions like microglandular adenosis.[242]

A gene signature of DCIS predictive of potential for either recurrence or invasive carcinoma has, thus far, eluded identification.[243] Livasy et al.[202] identified the "basal-like" profile (i.e., ER negative, HER2 negative, EGFR positive, and

CK5/6 positive) in 8% of DCIS and found it to be associated with unfavorable prognostic variables, including high-grade nuclei, p53 overexpression, and elevated proliferation index.[202] Basal-like DCIS using the immunohistochemical profile of (triple negative, CK5/6 positive and EGFR positive as a surrogate for gene expression profiling) has been shown to have a doubled, yet statistically insignificant, risk of local recurrence and developing invasive cancer compared with other types. In this study of 392 patients, 32 (8.2%) were basal-like.[244]

No significant difference has been detected in the amplification of certain key genes, including *ESR1* that encodes for ER, *CCND1* that encodes for cyclin D1, and *MYC* that encodes for a helix-loop-helix/leucine zipper protein, between DCIS and invasive breast carcinoma.[245] This indicates that these genes are implicated in cancer development but, perhaps, not in the initiation of invasive carcinoma.

NEEDLE CORE BIOPSY

FS examination is not appropriate for a needle core biopsy of a nonpalpable mammographically detected lesion, unless there are exceptional circumstances.[246] Grading of DCIS in paraffin sections of needle core biopsies is generally accurate, but the probability of structural variability increases with the size of the lesion.

Calcifications and necrotic debris may become dislodged in a needle core biopsy specimen, and rarely this material is the only component of DCIS in the sample (Fig. 11.60). In this circumstance, serial sections should be prepared. An excisional biopsy should be considered, even if no epithelial elements of carcinoma are detected in serial sections that show displaced calcification of a type (i.e., amid ghost cells and karyorrhectic debris) that might occur in DCIS. A dislodged fragment of DCIS that becomes embedded in fat or stroma as part of a needle core biopsy sample may be mistaken for invasive carcinoma (Fig. 11.61).

"Healed" DCIS and end-stage periductal mastitis can both result in indistinguishable scarred ductal structures with calcifications (Fig. 11.62). When this type of structure is found in a needle core biopsy specimen, multiple serial sections should be prepared to search for scant foci of carcinoma that may be present. The limited epithelial abnormalities found in some of these cases may result in a diagnosis of ADH. A surgical excision is indicated for the latter diagnosis and in some situations may be appropriate when ductal scars are present without epithelial atypia if the mammographic findings raise concern about carcinoma.

The distinction between invasive carcinoma and SA or radial sclerosing lesions can be challenging in needle core biopsy specimens. This difficulty is compounded when DCIS arises in sclerosing lesions (Fig. 11.63). It is important to consider this potential diagnostic pitfall and to employ immunohistochemical stains to define the distribution of myoepithelial cells in the specimen. Incomplete samples of radial sclerosing lesions obtained in needle core biopsy samples are difficult to assess for intraductal or invasive carcinoma, and they may be reported as atypical hyperplasia.

A needle core biopsy specimen cannot be relied upon to measure the size of a DCIS lesion, even if the procedure is performed for calcifications alone and calcifications are no longer present in a follow-up mammogram. The needle biopsy specimen rarely provides a single intact sample of the lesion, and it is not feasible to reassemble the DCIS foci from multiple samples to obtain a single measurement.

The diagnosis of DCIS in a needle core biopsy specimen does not exclude the possibility of invasive carcinoma in the affected breast. The reported frequency of invasive carcinoma detected in excisional biopsies performed after a needle core biopsy diagnosis of DCIS was 15% to 27%.[247–253] The diagnosis of DCIS without invasion was reported to be more reliable with directional vacuum-assisted biopsy procedure than with the automated needle biopsy system.[249]

The diagnosis of DCIS on needle core biopsies can influence the extent of the subsequent surgery. Dillon et al.[254]

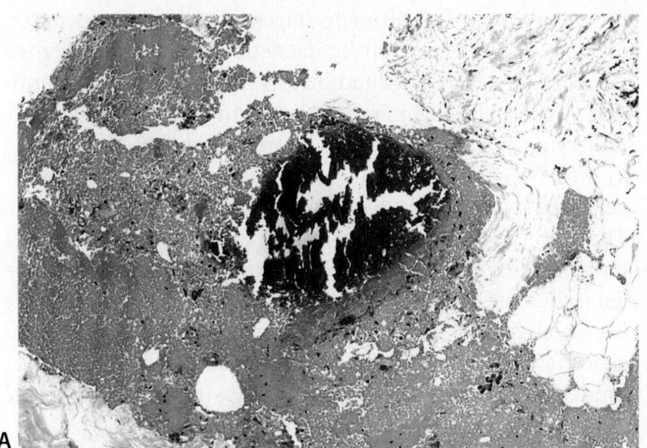

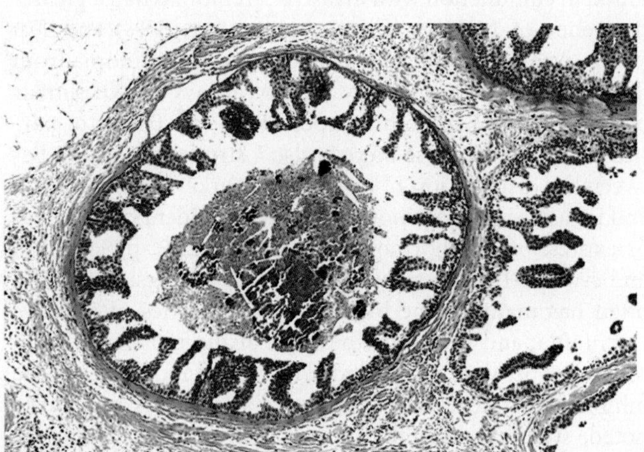

FIG. 11.60. ***DCIS, needle core biopsy.*** **A:** Fragmented calcification surrounded by necrotic debris and sparse isolated atypical cells in blood were the significant findings in a needle core biopsy specimen. **B:** Subsequent surgical excision revealed micropapillary DCIS with calcifications.

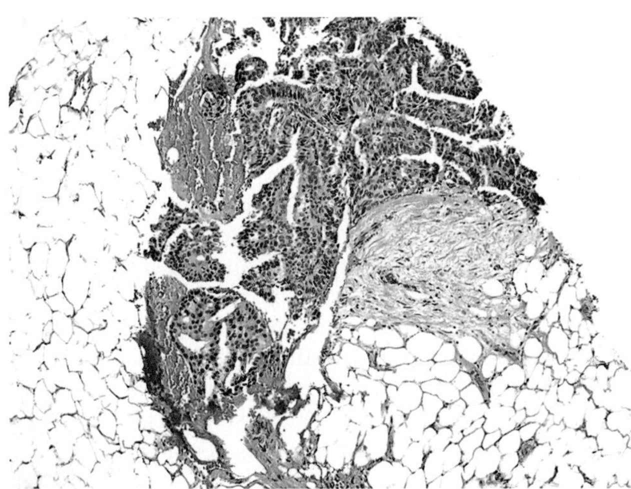

FIG. 11.61. ***DCIS, needle core biopsy with displaced epithelium.*** A fragment of papillary carcinoma is lodged in fat. This is not invasive carcinoma.

reported that patients with a preoperative diagnosis of DCIS rendered on needle core biopsy had a reoperative rate of 36% compared with 65% for those patients who did not ($p = 0.0007$). Furthermore, it has been suggested that findings in needle core biopsies can help in the achievement of negative margins in lumpectomies through the assessment of relative proportion of DCIS in cases of invasive ductal carcinoma. A high proportion of DCIS in the core biopsy specimen have been shown to identify patients at risk of compromised margins in the subsequently performed lumpectomy.[255]

CYTOLOGIC DIAGNOSIS

Fine-needle aspiration (FNA) specimens from DCIS tend to be less cellular than aspirates from invasive carcinomas, and they are more likely to yield insufficient material for diagnosis.[256] These circumstances are especially prone to occur when FNA is performed on a nonpalpable abnormality detected by mammography. Failure to obtain diagnostic material by FNA in this setting is an indication for excisional biopsy. FNA cytologic evaluation is not recommended for assessment of mammographically detected microcalcifications.[257]

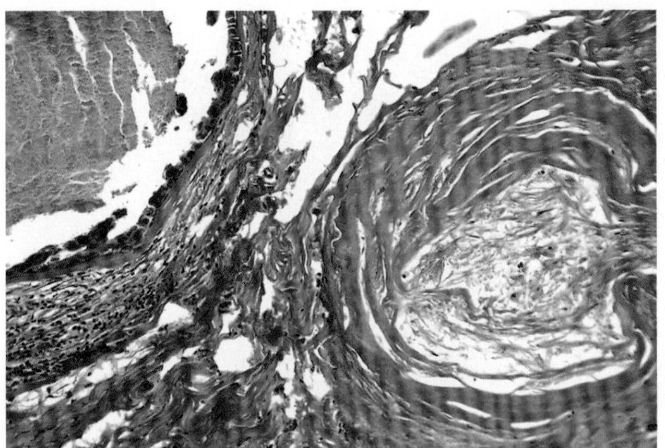

FIG. 11.62. ***DCIS, needle core biopsy with scar.*** Concentric layers of collagen probably represent the scar formed at the site of "healed" DCIS. A dilated duct with a thin layer of DCIS is shown on the *left*.

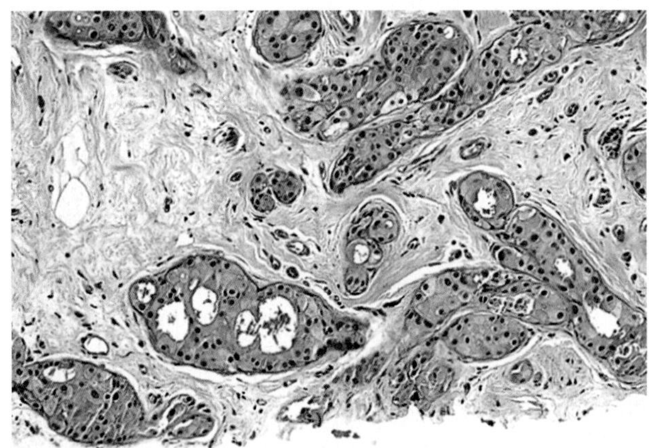

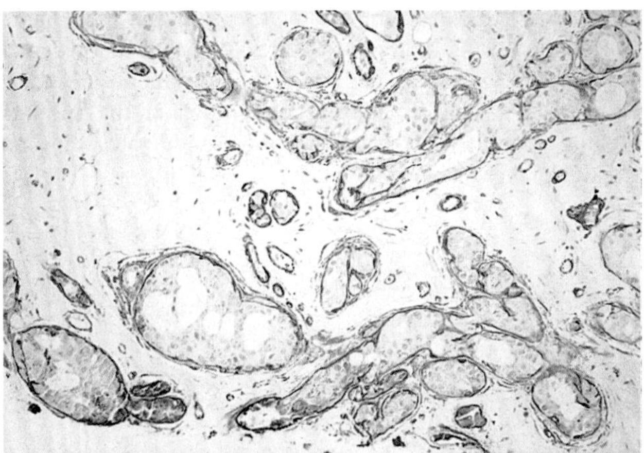

FIG. 11.63. ***DCIS, apocrine type in sclerosing adenosis, needle core biopsy.*** **A:** Apocrine DCIS occupying SA resembles invasive carcinoma. **B:** A section parallel to **(A)** prepared with the immunostain for SMA demonstrating myoepithelial cells around all glandular structures.

When the FNA specimen is diagnostic of carcinoma, the distinction between intraductal and infiltrating ductal carcinoma cannot be made with confidence.[256,258] Correlation with the mammogram is useful, but limitations of sampling make it impossible to exclude the presence of invasive carcinoma in a region outside the site of the FNA procedure or to exclude microinvasion in the region of the FNA. Findings more likely to be associated with intraductal than with invasive carcinoma are admixed cytologically benign epithelial cells and histiocytes. Invasive carcinoma is more likely to be present if carcinoma cells singly or in groups are intimately mingled with adipose tissue, fibrous stroma, or fat cells.

Subclassification of DCIS to distinguish between comedo and noncomedo variants may be suggested by FNA cytology.[258–260] The aspirate from "comedo"-type, that is, solid-type DCIS with high nuclear grade, typically consists of pleomorphic, loosely cohesive cells with poorly differentiated nuclei and prominent nucleoli, sometimes accompanied by mitotic figures. Necrotic debris that may contain calcifications is usually present. Specimens from noncomedo DCIS tend to contain more cohesive three-dimensional cell clusters with a papillary or cribriform configuration, as well as dispersed cells distributed singly or in small groups (Fig. 11.64). Nuclei are intermediate to low grade cytologically, and they usually lack prominent nucleoli. Necrosis and an inflammatory cell background are found much less often in aspirates from noncomedo DCIS.

Although the foregoing cytologic features may be reliable for distinguishing between classic examples of lesions such as solid-type DCIS with high nuclear grade and orderly cribriform DCIS, there are circumstances in which the findings are not clear. This can occur when the intraductal carcinoma has nuclei of variable grade nuclei.

EXTENT OF DCIS

The extent of DCIS ranges from one duct or 0.1 cm to widespread involvement of multiple quadrants of the breast.[261] Although exact determination of the extent of DCIS may be "a wild goose chase,"[262] estimation of its dimension is significant for management purposes. The size of DCIS can be accurately assessed by measuring microscopic extent only when it is present on a single slide.[263] Estimating the size of DCIS from the radiologic extent of calcification or by recording the number blocks can result in either overestimation or underestimation, particularly in cases where the sections are not taken consecutively. It has been suggested that assessment of DCIS using the block method underestimates size with a mean reduction of 33%.

In a study of 33 patients with a histologically proven DCIS by needle biopsy, the mean lesion size was 25.6 histologically, 28.1 mm by MRI, and 27.2 mm on mammography. The correlation coefficient between histopathologic measurement and MRI was 0.831 versus 0.674 between histopathology and mammography. The correlation coefficient

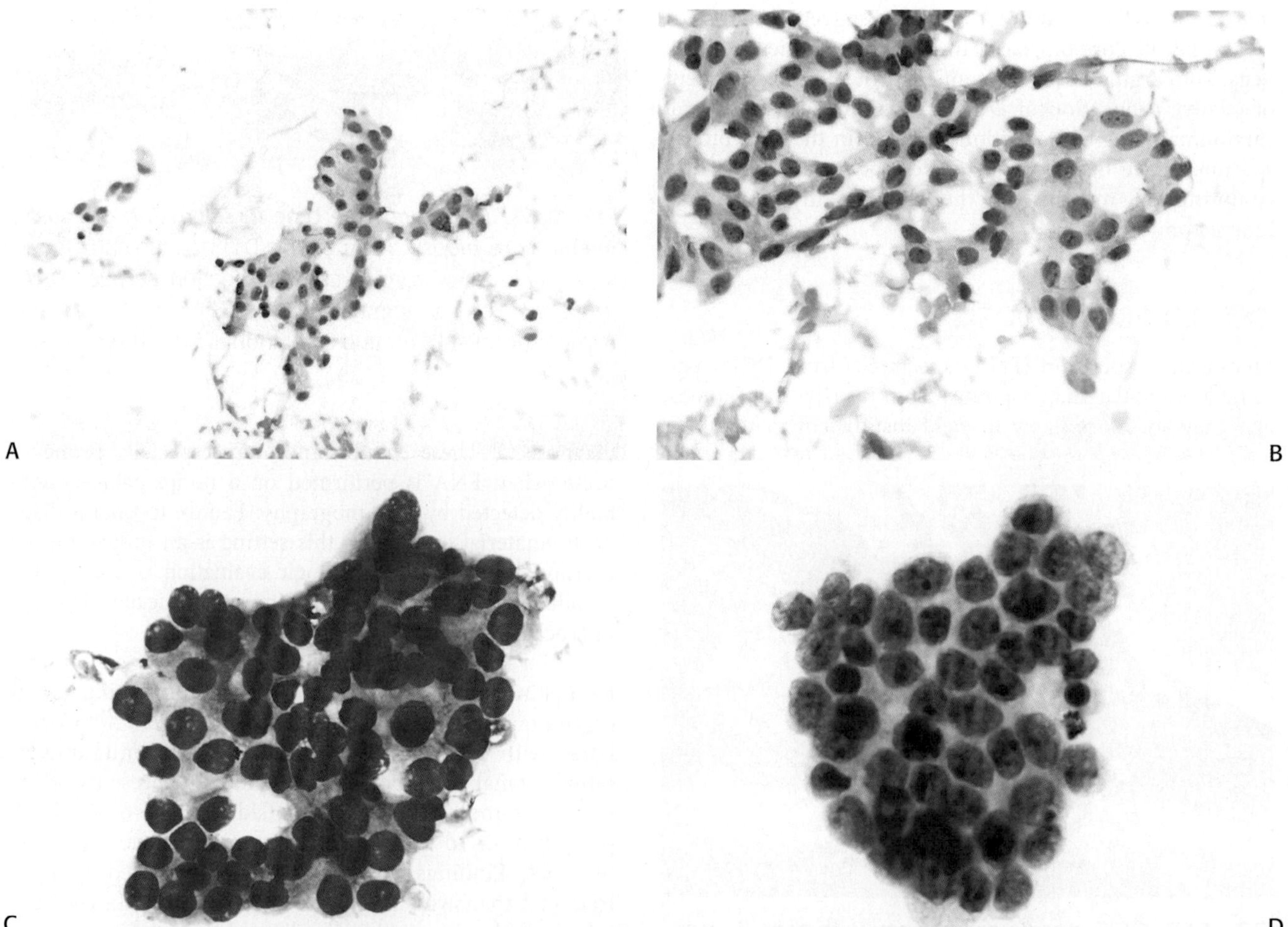

FIG. 11.64. ***DCIS, cribriform, cytology.*** **A:** Irregular flat sheet of cells with a microlumen in an FNA smear. **B:** Three adjacent microlumens are apparent in the epithelium with low-grade nuclear cytology. **C,D:** Epithelial clusters with low-grade nuclei on *ThinPrep* **(C)** and on *Diff-Quik* stain **(D)**.

increased with the nuclear grade of DCIS on mammography, and it increased as the mammographic breast density decreased.[264] Although preoperative imaging has limitations in determining the extent of DCIS, specimen slice radiography can improve these estimates.[265]

It is sometimes possible to determine the size of a lesion microscopically if it is limited to a single group of contiguous ducts (unifocal), especially when the area is confined to the histologic section from a single paraffin block that contains tissue from an excisional biopsy. Reporting the size of the small lesions in this category is confounded by the fact that some authors exclude abnormalities smaller than 2 mm from the diagnosis of DCIS regardless of histologic appearance.[115,266]

A significant proportion of DCIS are multifocal and not confined to a single coherent palpable lesion or to a microscopic focus that will fit in the confines of a single paraffin block. It is noteworthy that the dimensions of a DCIS limited to one standard paraffin block would not ordinarily exceed 2.0 to 2.5 cm or approximately 1 inch. Lagios et al.[267] studied mastectomy specimens from patients with DCIS by a serial subgross method and reported that the frequency of multicentricity and occult invasion was substantially greater for lesions larger than 2.5 cm. It is on the basis of these studies that 2.5 cm came to be viewed as an important size criterion in the selection of patients for breast-conserving therapy. Lagios[268] expressed skepticism about the quantitation of DCIS, observing that "quantitation of DCIS will remain a problem since the association of the extent of DCIS, and the extent of microcalcifications, the only preoperative measure available at present, is quite variable."

Presently, there is no consensus on a method for determining the extent of DCIS on the basis of the proportion of slides showing the lesion. This approach is highly dependent on the completeness of sampling and biopsy size, both of which determine the denominator. This issue would be partially addressed if the denominator were biopsy weight in grams with the numerator representing the number of slides showing DCIS. This calculation would be most useful in situations where all tissue has been processed for histologic examination. Until a standardized method has been validated and widely adopted, the number of sections involved in sequentially taken samples (or at a minimum the proportion of slides with DCIS) will remain a crude measure of the extent of DCIS.

Many patients have more than one diagnostic procedure performed (e.g., needle core biopsy, followed by excision and reexcision of various margins) with DCIS in more than one specimen. It is not practical to reassemble the foci of DCIS from two or more specimens to obtain a single measurement.

For the foregoing reasons, a 1997 consensus report on the classification of DCIS left the issue of size largely unanswered and was unable to address this question.[151] A classification system for DCIS that includes lesion size is currently impractical. Nonetheless, data purportedly describing the "size" of DCIS are reported. The mean size of 227 lesions in one series was 2.1 cm, ranging from 1.5 cm in cribriform to 2.5 cm in comedo DCIS.[269] In a study of cases referred for consultation, Lennington et al.[115] recorded size from the "outside surgical pathology report" for "extensive lesions" but for "smaller, less extensive lesions, size was measured directly from the glass slides." Lesions 2 mm or less in diameter were excluded by definition, because they were classified as atypical hyperplasia. The authors stated that they ". . . recognize the lack of precision, but believe the measurements are usually within 3–5 mm of true extent. There is probably a greater error in larger lesions." This range of error in measuring the size of DCIS is a further impediment to using lesion size as a criterion for distinguishing hyperplasia from DCIS. In the face of these substantial limitations, the authors reported the following distribution of "precise" mean sizes in relation to histologic subtype: all pure DCIS exclusive of micropapillary, 8.5 mm; mixed noncomedo histologic types, 13.1 mm; noncomedo with necrosis, 11.6 mm; comedo, 16.2 mm; and micropapillary, 19.1 mm.[115]

The terms "extensive" intraductal component or "extensive" intraductal carcinoma should not be used as synonyms for widespread DCIS, as these terms have a different clinicopathologic connotation. "Extensive" DCIS ought to be used only when DCIS is associated with invasive carcinoma, and the DCIS therein, constituting more than 25% of the tumor mass, extends beyond the dominant tumor mass into adjacent breast parenchyma.

In sum, sequential sectioning of surgical specimens (optimally conducted with radiologic correlation) is essential for the precise assessment of the extent of DCIS. The consistent practice of sampling in this manner will also optimize observational research on issues relating to size and margins.

MULTICENTRICITY AND MULTIFOCALITY

There is no uniformly accepted definition of *multicentricity* in DCIS. The concept of multicentricity was advanced by Cheatle and Cutler,[10] Cheatle,[270] and Charteris[271] as a result of observations made on whole-organ sections of mastectomy specimens. Carcinoma was considered to be multicentric when there were foci that were separate from the clinically detected tumor. Lagios et al.[272] defined multicentricity as " the presence of separate independent foci of carcinoma within the breast—separate from the lesion which is clinically or mammographically evident, that is, the reference tumor."

Multicentric DCIS is generally defined as that present in multiple quadrants.[273–276] The use of this definition for the term precludes its use in routine lumpectomy specimens, unless the term is used for DCIS separated by 5 cm or some other arbitrary dimension. The rate of multicentricity of DCIS has traditionally been stated to be approximately 25%, with a range from 0% to 75% or so, such a wide range that reflects differences in the definition of the term. For practical purposes, multicentricity refers to foci of carcinoma in distinctly different regions of the breast, usually in two or more quadrants.

Multicentricity should be distinguished from intraepithelial extension within ducts and lobules of a single carcinomatous focus typically limited to one region or quadrant. The latter condition is commonly referred to as *multifocality*. One commonly employed criterion for establishing the presence of multifocality depends on the number of histologic sections that show DCIS. For example, Fisher et al. stated that "ductal carcinoma *in situ* in only one section of two or more obtained from different blocks was considered to be unifocal. Its presence in sections from two or more different blocks was considered multifocal." On the basis of this definition, 329 (60.8%) of 541 evaluable specimens of DCIS were classified as multifocal in data from National Surgical Adjuvant Breast and Bowel Project (NSABP) Protocol B17.[265] Silverstein et al.[269] considered DCIS to be multifocal when "... separate foci of DCIS [duct carcinoma *in situ*] more than 2 cm from primary site . . ." were found in a mastectomy specimen. On the basis of this criterion, multifocality was present in 41 (41%) of 98 breasts examined after mastectomy. Multicentricity, defined as carcinoma outside the index quadrant, was present in 15% of these breasts. Multifocality and multicentricity were not significantly related to the histologic category of DCIS when stratified as comedo and noncomedo type.[269] Hardman et al.[273] found multicentric carcinoma in 27% of mastectomy specimens from patients with carcinoma of the comedo type. Multicentricity was reported in 33%[18] and 37%[274] of mastectomies performed for diverse types of DCIS. A proportion of "multifocal" DCIS, albeit a minor one, may be a product of artifact, because of the inherent problem of two-dimensional viewing of a three-dimensional arborizing disease process.

In an effort to circumvent these technical issues, some investigators have set anatomic limits on the distribution of carcinoma to somewhat arbitrarily distinguish between unicentric and multicentric diseases. For example, carcinoma has been deemed to be multicentric if it is detected in more than one quadrant or if it is 5 cm from the index lesion.[93,274–276] Silverstein et al.[277] classified as multicentric if two foci were separated by more than 2.0 cm.

Schwartz et al.[93,278] studied the frequency of multicentricity in the breasts of patients with DCIS who underwent mastectomy. Multicentricity was defined as "the presence [of] invasive ductal or lobular carcinoma, microinvasive ductal carcinoma, or DCIS in an area or quadrant outside the biopsy site . . . . If the lesion was centrally located, the cancer was considered multicentric only if additional foci of carcinoma were found outside a perimeter of 5 cm from the edge of the nipple and areola."[93] Multicentricity was found in 18 (36%) of 50[93] and 4 (36%) of 11[278] breasts. Multicentricity was more often present in lesions detected because of nipple discharge (71%) or Paget disease (50%) than in those found by mammography (38%).[93] When classified on the basis of the predominant growth pattern, micropapillary DCIS was more often multicentric (86%) than papillary (33%) or comedo (42%) DCIS. No multicentricity was encountered in five cribriform and seven solid DCIS. Bellamy et al.[86] also found multicentricity to be present significantly more often in patients with micropapillary DCIS than in those with other patterns of DCIS.

If the sample provided for histologic diagnosis is an excisional biopsy limited to the region of the index lesion, the material is not suitable for determining whether the patient has multicentric carcinoma. According to some definitions, more than a quadrantectomy is necessary to detect multicentricity. In practice, the distinction between multifocality and multicentricity is difficult to make with certainty in slides prepared by random sampling of breast specimens for diagnostic purposes. Serial sequential sectioning of smaller excisional biopsy specimens facilitates mapping of the extent of disease, and this method should be utilized whenever feasible. Advanced techniques such as stereoscopic dissection and subgross microscopic–radiologic correlative studies are more reliable methods for identifying true multicentricity and multifocality, but they are too costly and time consuming to be practical procedures for routine diagnostic work. Given the limited resources available in most pathology laboratories, it may be unrealistic to expect diagnostic reports on breast biopsies to routinely distinguish multicentricity from multifocality.

It is likely that multifocal and multicentric DCIS will be increasingly detected with growing use of MRI. In a study of 285 patients with newly diagnosed DCIS, MRI examination performed for the evaluation of extent of disease showed separate foci of invasive carcinoma "elsewhere" in the breast, that is, either multicentric or contralateral, in 16 (5.6%) patients.[279] A meta-analysis of 19 studies (n = 2,610) demonstrated that MRI detected additional foci of carcinoma (invasive and/or *in situ*) in 16% of invasive and/or *in situ* carcinoma cases that had not identified by traditional evaluation.[280]

In summary, *multicentric* DCIS refers to its presence in distinctly different regions of the breast, usually in two or more quadrants, whereas *multifocal* DCIS is confined to one quadrant and is generally regarded as that which is spatially closer, with at least some normal breast tissue separating the neoplastic foci. The adjectives, multicentric and multifocal ought not to be used interchangeably owing to the divergent clinical implications of each term.[281]

MICROINVASION

Genomic and phenotypic similarities, among other clinical and pathologic forms of evidence, support the conclusion that DCIS is a nonobligate precursor of invasive ductal carcinoma. Microinvasive carcinoma (abbreviated as T1*mic* in the TNM American Joint Committee on Cancer [AJCC]-Union Internationale Contre le Cancer [UICC] staging system) is the earliest manifestation and stage of invasive mammary ductal carcinoma. The upper limit of the extent of invasion for an invasive carcinoma to qualify for this designation is 0.1 cm (i.e., 1 mm).

Ultrastructural studies have detected foci of discontinuity in the basement membranes of ducts with DCIS,[282,283] and similar observations have been reported in tissues studied by IHC.[284] Breaks in the basement membrane were more common when DCIS was of high nuclear grade with or without necrosis. Carcinoma cells have been observed by electron microscopy protruding through gaps in the basal lamina when invasion was not apparent by light microscopy.[285] In such regions, in H&E sections, the neoplastic epithelium appears to protrude from the duct, coming in contact with the stroma as it remains connected to the intraductal neoplasm. This finding often elicits diagnostic uncertainty. It remains to be determined whether protruding cells detected by electron microscopy or light microscopy still attached to their intraductal counterparts are capable of metastatic spread.

Basement membrane integrity at sites of microinvasion has been investigated by IHC (Fig. 11.65). Barsky et al.[99] detected fragmentation and disruption of basement membranes in areas of microinvasion by employing antibodies to laminin and type IV collagen (Fig. 11.66). Type IV collagen is degraded by type IV collagenase, a metalloproteinase. The active enzyme is absent from normal and proliferative ducts, variably present in comedocarcinoma, and prominent in invasive carcinoma.[286] These and other observations suggest that the ability of carcinoma cells to form latent type IV collagenase and convert it to the active form is an important attribute associated with the invasive phenotype. As noted earlier in this chapter, myoepithelial cells also appear to play a significant role in inhibiting invasion by DCIS.[171] One important function of myoepithelial cells is the elaboration of protease inhibitors that appear to counteract the invasion-promoting effects of metalloproteinases produced by DCIS cells. Another important function of myoepithelial cells in this setting is that they serve as a potential mechanical barrier, along with the basement membrane, between intraductal epithelial cells and periductal stroma.

The type IV collagen molecule consists of a number of distinctive alpha-chain subunits. The cross-linked alpha chains form a macromolecular network, which is a major structural component of the basement membrane. Studies using alpha (IV) chain-specific antibodies and *in situ* hybridization have shown that the expression of selected alpha chains is dependent on the presence of myoepithelial cells.[287] Discontinuous or absent expression of type IV collagen alpha-chain subunits has been observed in invasive carcinomas.[287,288]

The laminin molecule is also composed of cross-linked subunits designated alpha, beta, and gamma chains. Immunohistochemical studies using chain-specific antibodies revealed discontinuous or absent expression of most subunits in invasive carcinomas and no expression of the beta-2 chain.[288]

Microinvasion should be distinguished from minimally invasive carcinoma, a term that refers to invasive lesions less

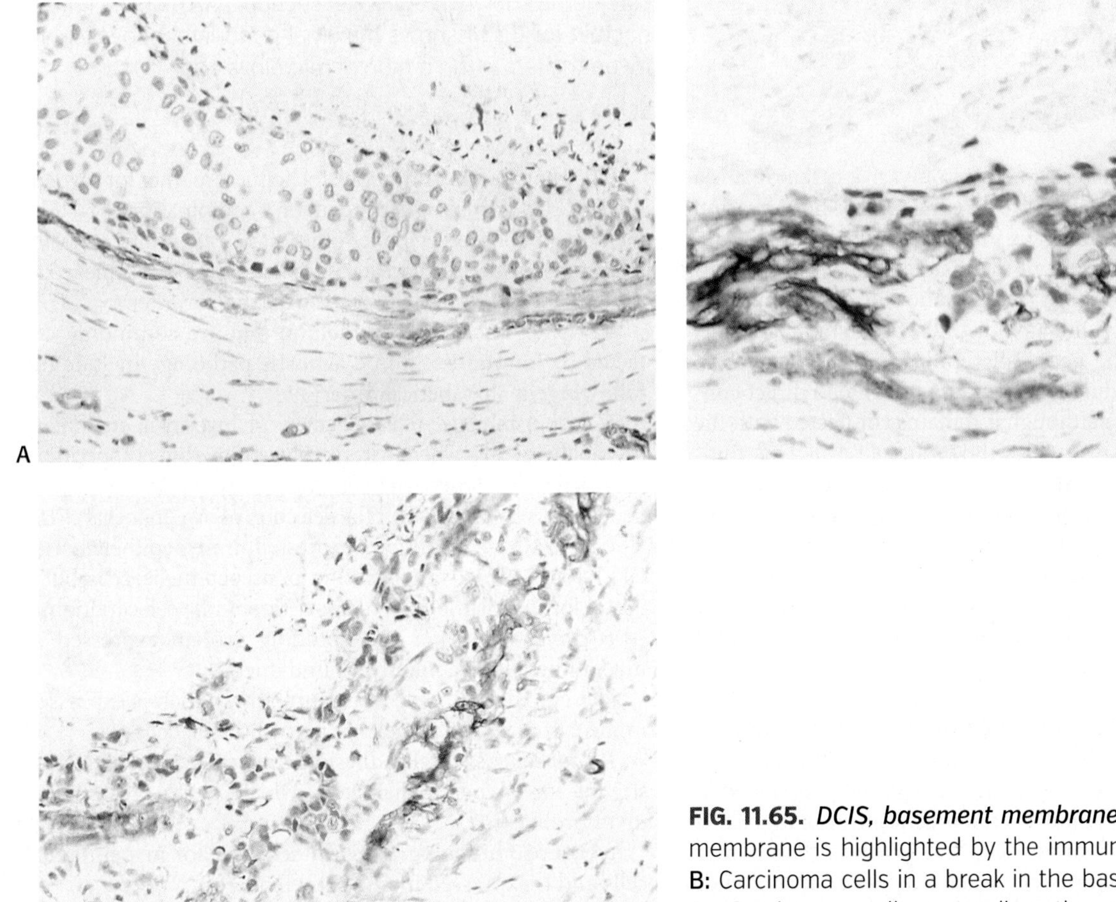

FIG. 11.65. ***DCIS, basement membrane.*** **A:** The basement membrane is highlighted by the immunostain for laminin. **B:** Carcinoma cells in a break in the basement membrane. **C:** Carcinoma cells extending through the basement membrane are in continuity with the intraductal component.

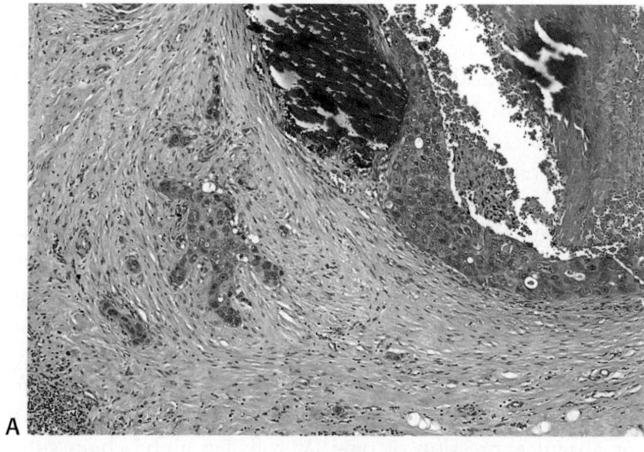

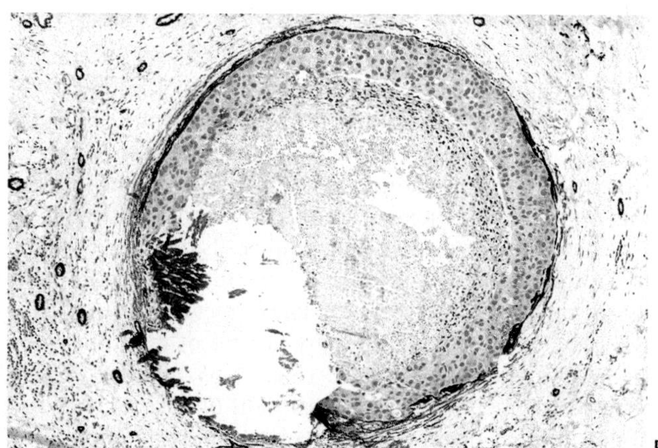

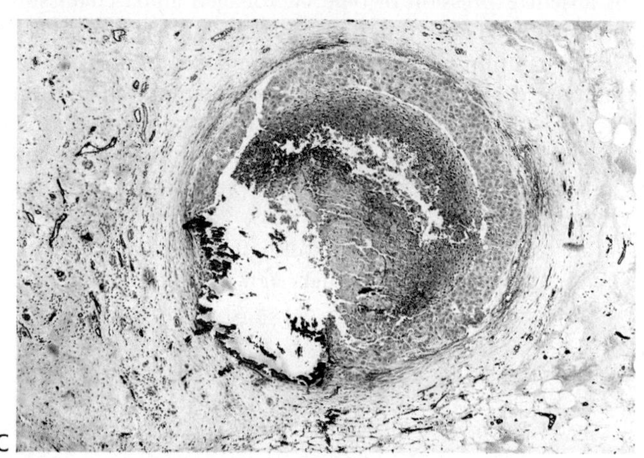

FIG. 11.66. *DCIS, basement membrane and microinvasion.* **A:** DCIS, comedo type with calcification (*right*) and microinvasive carcinoma (*left*). **B:** The immunostain for laminin shows a multilayered basement membrane of variable thickness. The basement membrane is incomplete in the *lower left* region, which is adjacent to the microinvasive carcinoma shown in a parallel section in **(A)**. **C:** The immunostain for CD34 shows maximal periductal neovascularity on the *left* in the region of microinvasion.

than 1.0 cm in diameter.[289–291] Microinvasive carcinoma is a subcategory of minimally invasive carcinoma. Microinvasion is defined as an invasive focus 1 mm or less in greatest extent.

A controversial aspect of the histologic diagnosis of microinvasion relates to the interpretation of ducts that have poorly defined walls with an indistinct basement membrane. In such regions, the neoplastic epithelium may appear to protrude from the duct wall, seeming to come in direct contact with the stroma although it remains connected with the intraductal neoplasm[292] (Figs. 11.29 and 11.67). This finding often elicits diagnostic uncertainty reflected in such caveats as "suspect microinvasion" or "microinvasion cannot be ruled out." Retrospective studies have given no indication that these ambiguous findings are associated with an appreciable risk of systemic metastases, but they may account for some instances in which micrometastases have been detected in sentinel lymph nodes (SLNs) from patients with DCIS.

To qualify for the term *microinvasion*, the cells deemed to be invasive must be distributed in a fashion that does not represent tangential sectioning of a duct or a lobular gland with DCIS (Figs. 11.67 and 11.68). Tangentially sectioned *in situ* carcinoma that simulates microinvasion usually results in compact groups of tumor cells that have a smooth border surrounded by a circumferential layer of cells of stromal and/or myoepithelial origin. These "organoid" foci are distributed in the specialized periductal or intralobular stroma. Immunostains may be helpful in resolving the problem.

The choice of an immunohistochemical marker for myoepithelial cells "should be dependent on a combination of factors, including published evidence of its diagnostic utility, its availability, performance characteristics that have been achieved in a given laboratory, and the specific diagnostic criteria."[293]

The markers or myoepithelium that are commonly detected by immunostain in diagnostic pathology include the following, in alphabetical order:

Calponin inhibits ATPase activity of myosin in mammary myoepithelial cells, wherein it is highly sensitive but not specific as it is reactive in a subset of myofibroblasts. *CD10* is an endopeptide that is relatively sensitive for the detection of myoepithelial cells.

CKs 5, 10, 14, and 17 are expressed in myoepithelial cells. CK-K903 (34βE12) is not specific for myoepithelial cells, but is useful for the diagnosis of metaplastic spindle cell carcinoma.

H-caldesmon is an SMA-binding protein expressed in myoepithelial cells, mainly around ducts.

Maspin is a serine protease inhibitor, which is expressed in the cytoplasm and nuclei of myoepithelial cells.

P-cadherin is a cell adhesion molecule with high sensitivity for myoepithelial cells, which is not reactive in myofibroblasts.

p63, a p53 homolog, is highly sensitive for myoepithelial cells and is expressed in nuclei thereof.

S-100 protein can be identified in a proportion of benign and malignant mammary epithelial cells, as well as myoepithelial cells, and therefore is not useful.

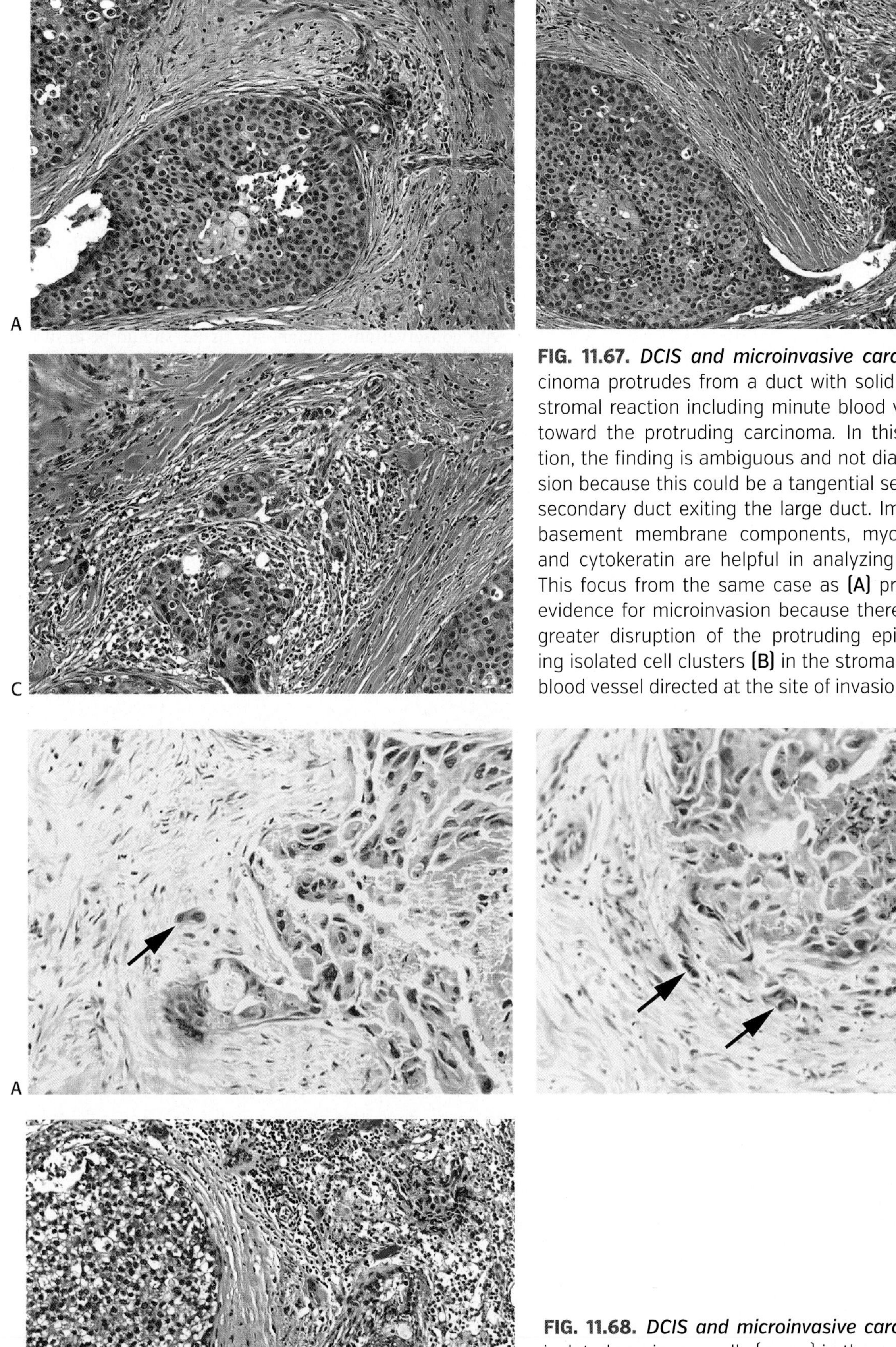

FIG. 11.67. ***DCIS and microinvasive carcinoma.*** **A:** Carcinoma protrudes from a duct with solid DCIS. Note the stromal reaction including minute blood vessels directed toward the protruding carcinoma. In this plane of section, the finding is ambiguous and not diagnostic of invasion because this could be a tangential section of a small secondary duct exiting the large duct. Immunostains for basement membrane components, myoepithelial cells, and cytokeratin are helpful in analyzing such foci. **B,C:** This focus from the same case as **(A)** provides stronger evidence for microinvasion because there appears to be greater disruption of the protruding epithelium including isolated cell clusters **(B)** in the stroma. Note the small blood vessel directed at the site of invasion **(C)**.

FIG. 11.68. ***DCIS and microinvasive carcinoma.*** **A:** Two isolated carcinoma cells (*arrow*) in the periductal stroma adjacent to a tangentially sectioned duct containing DCIS. **B:** Disruption of the basement membrane is evident, and there are carcinoma cells in the periductal stroma (*arrows*). **C:** A larger focus of microinvasion (*upper right*) with a marked lymphocytic reaction.

SMA antibody detects actin filaments in myoepithelial cells, but its specificity is poor since myofibroblasts are also highlighted by SMA. *SMM-HC* detects structural smooth muscle elements in mammary myoepithelial cells but not in myofibroblasts.[185,293]

It is notable that CD10 is expressed uniformly in myoepithelial cells from the terminal duct to acini, and that caldesmon is immunoreactive in myoepithelial cells of large ducts, but is not typically expressed in intralobular ductules and acini.[294] In practical terms, SMM-HC and p63 are the most useful immunostains for the diagnosis of microinvasive carcinoma.

At sites of clear-cut microinvasive ductal carcinoma, tumor cells are distributed singly or as small groups that have irregular shapes reminiscent of conventional invasive carcinoma with no particular orientation (Figs. 11.66 to 11.69). Sometimes the intralobular or periductal stroma appears less dense at sites of microinvasion than in other areas around these structures. Detecting carcinoma cells in the stroma can be difficult when there is a periductal and stromal inflammatory cell reaction. Microinvasion may be suspected at sites where there is a pronounced lymphocytic accumulation near ducts with DCIS (Fig. 11.70). A granulomatous reaction may be elicited at foci of microinvasion.[295] The tumor cells can resemble histiocytes, and it may require immunostains for cytokeratin to confirm the presence of microinvasion. Double immunolabeling for cytokeratin and actin is an elegant method for visualizing foci of microinvasion (Fig. 11.42).[296]

Microinvasion is most often associated with high-grade DCIS, but it may occur in other types of DCIS.[56] Thorough histologic sectioning is recommended for all cases of high-grade DCIS and for other types of DCIS that form a cohesive lesion larger than 2 cm. Serial routine H&E-stained sections, supported by IHC, usually provide the best evidence of microinvasion. Minimal trimming of the block, with conservation of diagnostic tissue, should be ensured in such cases. Care should also be taken to obtain immunostains (including those for cytokeratin, myoepithelial markers, and hormone receptors) early in the evaluation of suspected microinvasion before the sample has been excessively sectioned. At least one H&E slide must always be prepared whenever immunostains are done to study a specimen for microinvasion. Carcinomatous epithelium displaced by needling procedures can usually be distinguished from intrinsic invasive carcinoma (Fig. 11.71). The presence of minute clusters of carcinomatous epithelial cells arranged in a linear manner, typically associated with granulation tissue, fat necrosis, and hemosiderin

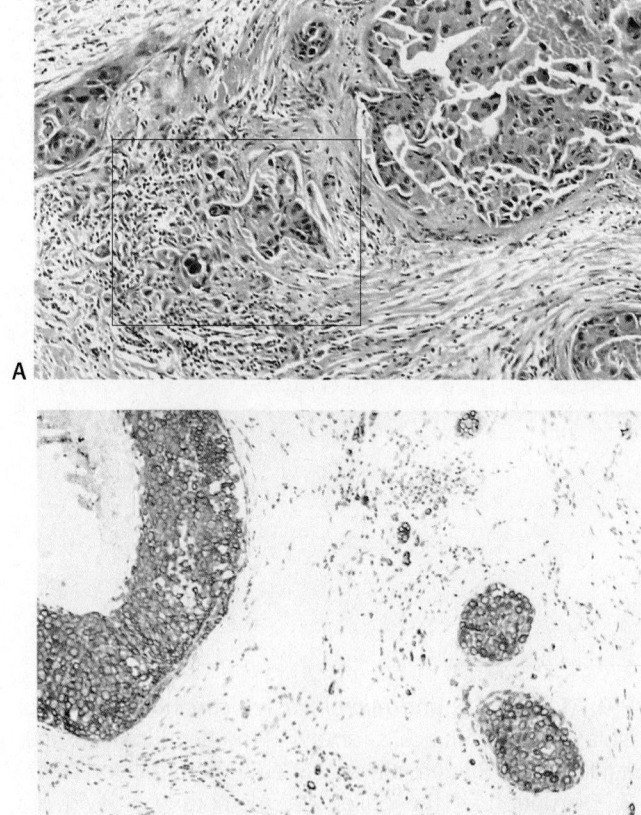

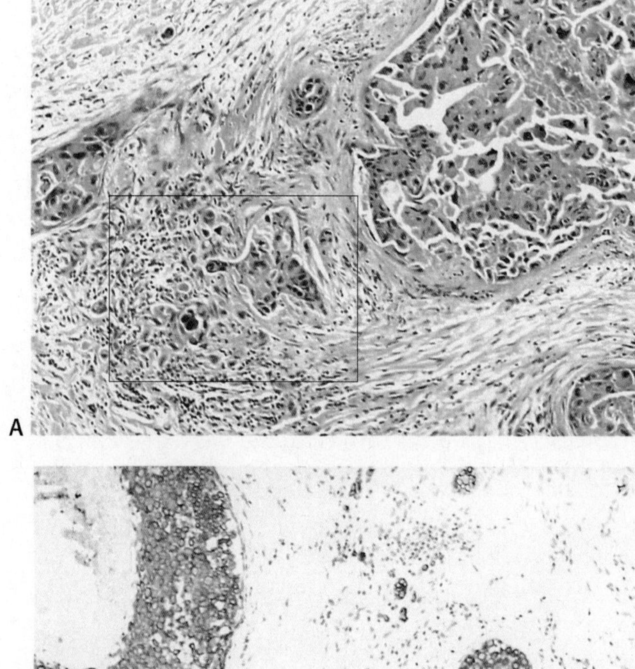

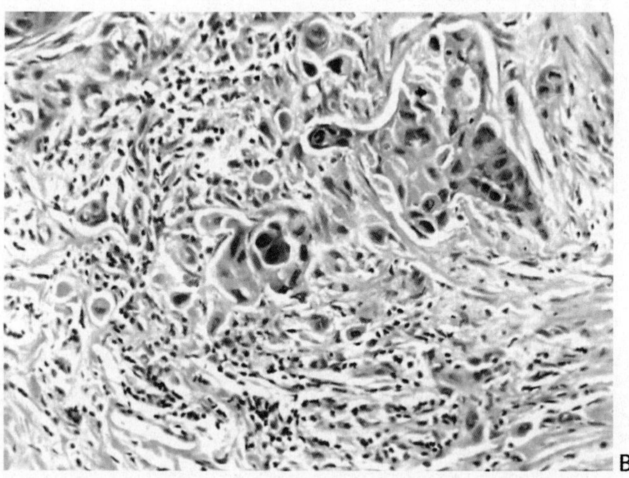

FIG. 11.69. ***DCIS with microinvasive carcinoma.*** **A:** Carcinoma cells in groups and individually in reactive stroma. **B:** Magnified view [of *box* in **[A]**] showing individual carcinoma cells that were partially obscured by the inflammatory reaction. **C:** Invasive carcinoma cells are highlighted by this CAM5.2 immunostain for cytokeratin.

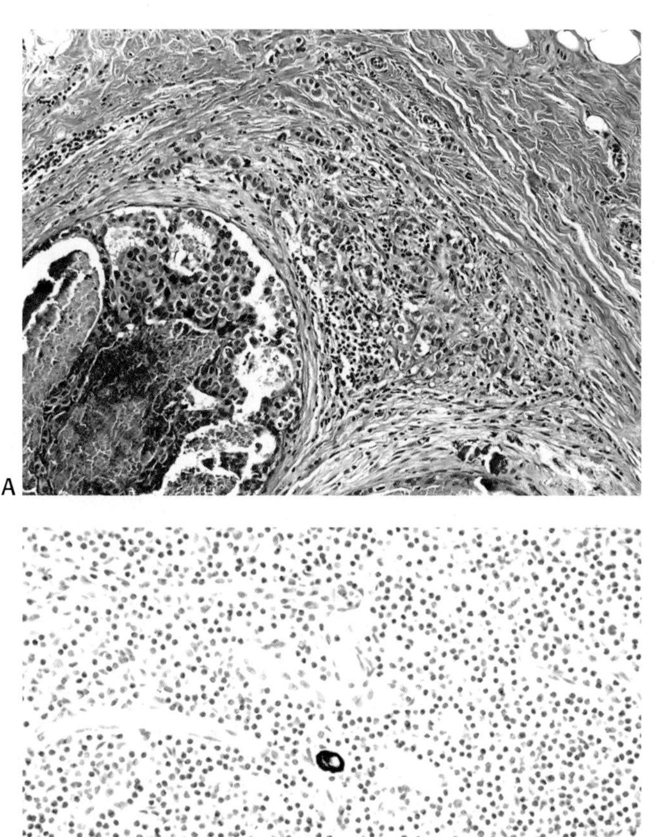

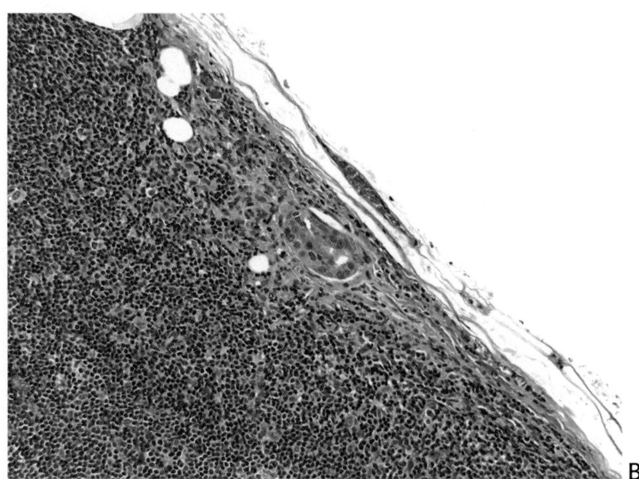

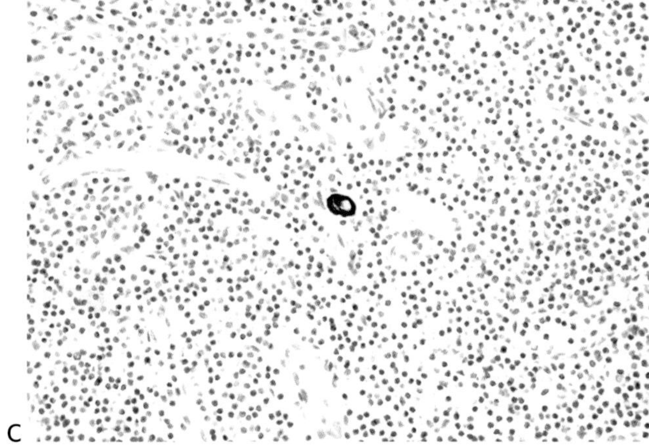

FIG. 11.70. ***DCIS with microinvasive carcinoma and axillary nodal metastasis.*** **A:** DCIS with microinvasion. **B:** A minute subcapsular metastatic deposit (<0.2 cm) was present in one of two sentinel nodes excised in this case. **C:** The cytokeratin AE1/3 immunostain identified one "isolated tumor cell" in the other SLN.

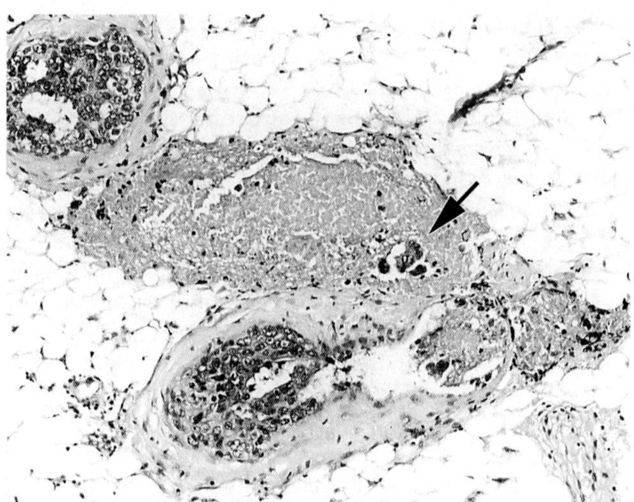

FIG. 11.71. ***DCIS, displaced epithelium.*** Fragment of carcinoma in a fibrin clot (*arrow*) next to DCIS. The site of duct disruption is evident on the *right*. The patient had an FNA biopsy before the surgical excision that yielded this specimen.

deposits, is indicative of traumatic displacement. The presence of carcinoma cells in vascular or lymphatic channels after a needle biopsy of DCIS can be associated with carcinoma cells in ALNs even when intrinsic invasion has not been detected (Fig. 11.72).

If DCIS is found in a needle core biopsy sample, it will require histologic examination of the excised lesional site to rule out coexisting invasive carcinoma. There have been several studies that have identified features of DCIS in core biopsy specimens that were predictive of detecting invasive carcinoma in the subsequent lumpectomy.[254,255] Renshaw[251] reported that invasive carcinoma in the excisional biopsy specimen was significantly associated with cribriform/papillary architecture and necrosis in the DCIS and more than 4 mm of lobular extension. Huo et al.[297] also found lobular extension to be predictive of invasion. Other features of DCIS in a needle core biopsy sample that have been cited as predictive of invasion include the presence of a mass lesion on the imaging study,[254,297–298] high nuclear grade,[299–301] extensive calcifications,[299,300] and a palpable lesion.[300]

The histologic diagnosis of microinvasion is confounded in some instances by the capacity of invasive carcinoma to

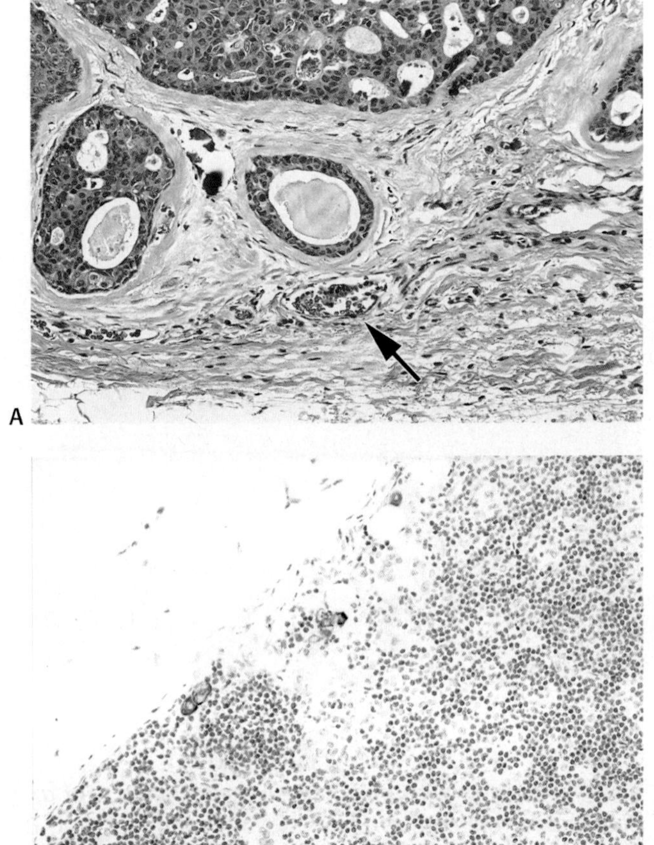

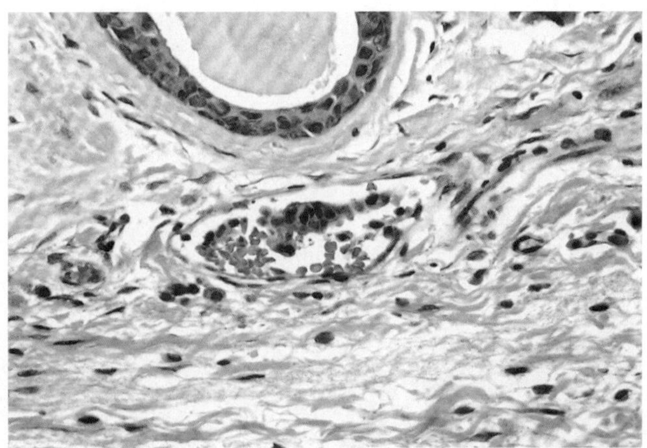

FIG. 11.72. ***DCIS with vascular tumor emboli.*** **A,B:** After a needle core biopsy revealed DCIS, this patient underwent excisional biopsy. The specimen contained cribriform DCIS shown here with carcinoma cells in an adjacent vascular channel (*arrow*). **C:** Isolated cytokeratin (AE1/3) positive cells were present in subcapsular sinuses of the SLNs.

assume a growth pattern that simulates DCIS (Fig. 11.73). This occurrence is most easily appreciated in metastatic deposits at sites outside the breast such as the ALNs and less frequently in visceral metastases. The phenomenon was described by Cowen[302] in 1980 and in a later report, Cowen and Bates[303] reported finding metastatic carcinoma with a DCIS-like appearance in lymph nodes from 35 of 391 patients (9%) with axillary metastases. In two of these cases, no intraductal component was found in the primary tumor, but in the others the "pseudointraductal" carcinoma in metastases resembled DCIS in the primary lesion.

Barsky et al.[304] reported finding DCIS-like metastases in ALNs from 21% of 200 cases. These foci were termed "revertant" DCIS to reflect the hypothesis that this phenomenon is a manifestation of a condition in which metastatic potential is inhibited or reversed by local factors. The authors observed complete concordance between primary and "revertant" DCIS with respect to architectural pattern, nuclear size determined by digital image analysis, and the expression of the prognostic markers p53, HER2, and Ki67. "Revertant" DCIS featured circumferential basement membranes demonstrated by immunoreactivity for laminin and type IV collagen, but lacked myoepithelial cells. The capacity of invasive carcinoma to assume an appearance that resembles its *in situ* counterpart could complicate the diagnosis of microinvasive carcinoma. Cowen and Bates[303] concluded that "since invasive breast carcinoma may mimic intraductal growth, some cases of breast cancer diagnosed histologically as DCIS may, in reality, be invasive." This phenomenon may be responsible for the rare patient found to have axillary nodal metastases, especially as a result of SLN mapping, when the breast appears to be the site of DCIS with no demonstrable invasion.

The difficulties raised by the structural similarities of *in situ* and invasive duct carcinoma are complicated by the results of studies that have demonstrated the presence of basement membrane components around groups of invasive carcinoma cells (Fig. 11.74). Arihiro et al.[305] found immunoreactivity for laminin at sites of invasive carcinoma in 54% of 71 carcinomas. The presence of laminin was associated with a greater degree of tubule formation. These findings correlate with data obtained by Nadji et al.[306] as significantly related to low histologic and nuclear grade.

In light of the foregoing discussion, it is evident that there are instances in which the presence or absence of microinvasion can be difficult to determine with certainty, even with the immunohistochemical reagents currently available. Some guidelines can be suggested based on experience:

1. The presence of myoepithelial cells at the perimeter of neoplastic glands is the most convincing evidence of DCIS, especially if demonstrated with the p63 immunostain.

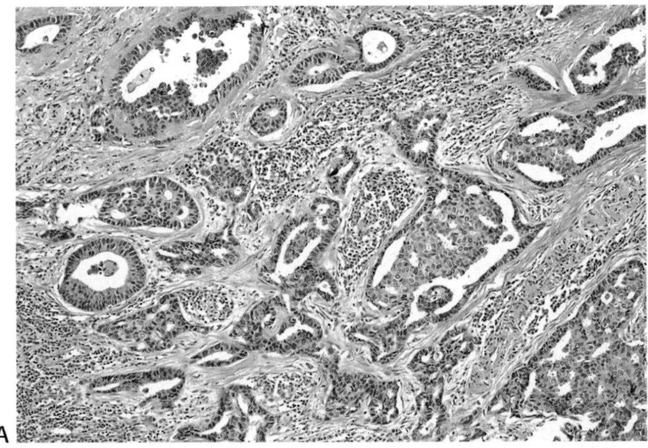

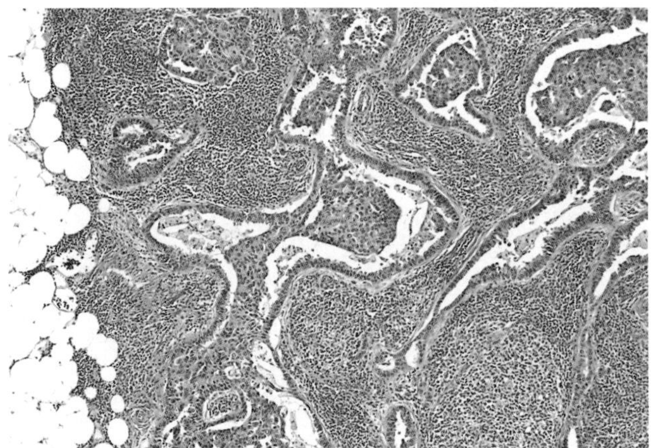

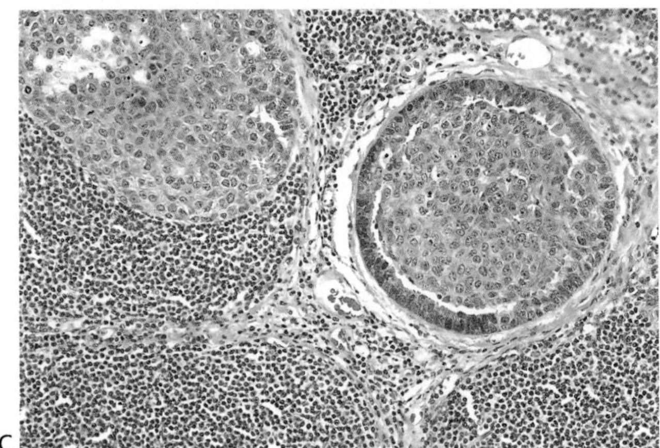

FIG. 11.73. ***Invasive ductal carcinoma with DCIS pattern.*** **A:** Extensive carcinoma with this appearance in the breast was interpreted as DCIS. Immunostains revealed absence of myoepithelial cells and basement membrane around some glandular structures, indicative of an invasive component. **B,C:** Metastatic carcinoma in ALNs duplicated the DCIS-like appearance of the primary invasive tumor.

It is essential to use more than one immunostain, since reactivity is not equally intense with all reagents.

2. The absence of demonstrable immunoreactivity with an appropriate marker usually means that myoepithelial cells are not present, although they can be severely attenuated and difficult to recognize. Loss of the myoepithelial cell layer occurs in some but not all DCIS and in certain types of benign (e.g., cystic apocrine lesions) and noninvasive neoplastic (e.g., some forms of papillary) processes. By itself, absence of myoepithelial cells is not indicative of invasive carcinoma, and the interpretation of this finding depends on the assessment of all histologic appearances of the lesion in the corresponding H&E section.
3. A *new* consecutive H&E section must be prepared whenever immunostains are done for suspected microinvasion. This is necessary because the structure of the lesional tissue changes as additional slides are made.
4. Cytokeratin immunostains are essential for the evaluation of any focus suspected to be the site of microinvasion. It is recommended that at least two different stains be used (e.g., CK7 and AE1/3) because of the variable reactivity of carcinoma cells. Cytokeratin immunostaining highlights the distribution of epithelial cells and distinguishes epithelial cells from histiocytes.
5. Immunostains for basement membrane components, laminin and type IV collagen, are sometimes helpful. Absence of reactivity for both components indicates a strong likelihood of invasive carcinoma, especially if coupled with absence of myoepithelial cells. A reticulin stain may also be helpful in this setting, as well as whenever microglandular adenosis is a diagnostic consideration.
6. Reactivity for one or both basal lamina components in the absence of myoepithelial cells presents the most difficult diagnostic situation that requires assessment of the entire lesion, including multiple H&E levels if possible (see #2). The presence of laminin and type IV collagen favors a diagnosis of *in situ* carcinoma. However, consideration must be given to the possibility that basal lamina may be formed at sites of invasion. With presently available routine diagnostic techniques, the distinction between basal lamina formed at sites of invasion and basement membranes in *in situ* carcinoma cannot be resolved with confidence in all cases.

It is recommended that the term microinvasion be used for invasive lesions 1 mm or less in largest extent. This definition has been adopted by the TNM staging system with the rubric T1*mic* to provide a descriptive identity for these unusually small invasive lesions that are otherwise

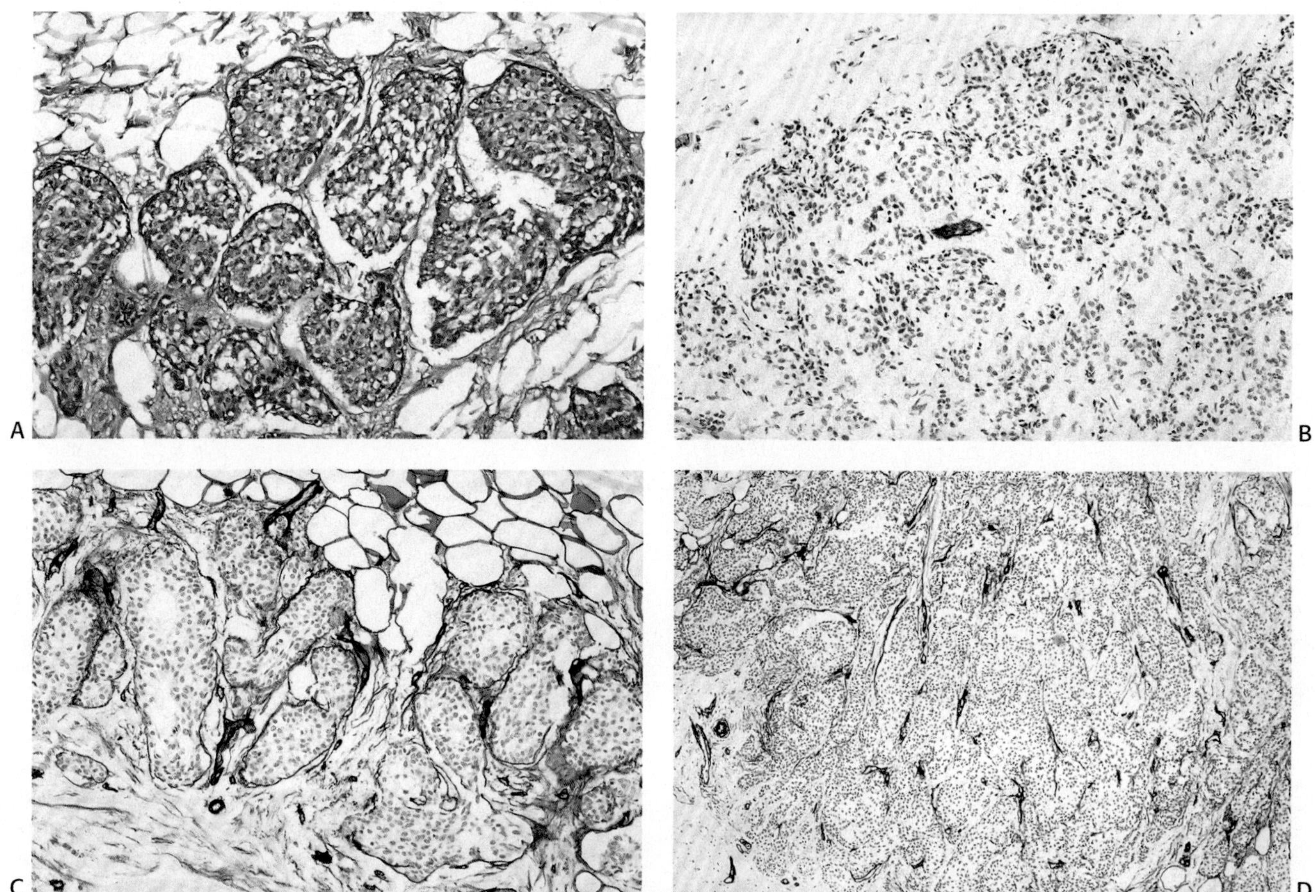

FIG. 11.74. ***Invasive duct carcinoma with formation of basal lamina components. The same tumor is depicted in all images.*** **A:** The carcinoma with an alveolar structure invades fat. There are compressed cells that resemble myoepithelial cells at the perimeter of some of the rounded tumor cell clusters. **B:** The immunostain for actin reveals reactivity in a small central blood vessel but not in the carcinoma, indicating absence of myoepithelial cells. **C:** Alveolar nests of carcinoma cells are encircled here by a thin band of laminin reactivity. **D:** The alveolar groups of carcinoma cells are partially encompassed by reactivity for type IV collagen. Some of the type IV collagen reactivity is associated with small blood vessels in the tumor.

not separately categorized (notably, micrometastasis in a lymph node is designated as N1mi in the TNM system). When multiple foci of microinvasion are present, there is no agreed-upon method for estimating their aggregate extent, and these cases qualify as DCIS with microinvasion; however, the number of microinvasive foci should be reported. Foci of invasion that measure more than 1 mm are diagnosed as invasive ductal carcinoma and reported (and staged) on the basis of the maximal measured extent of invasion.

CLINICAL SIGNIFICANCE OF MICROINVASION

Earlier published reports about microinvasive duct carcinoma had used different definitions of this entity. As a result, comparison of data between these studies must take these differences into consideration.

Solin et al.[307] limited the term microinvasion to a "maximal extent of invasion of less than 2 mm or invasive carcinoma comprising less than 10% of the tumor." ALN metastases were found in 2 (5%) of 39 patients with microinvasion. The majority (67%) had comedocarcinoma, but microinvasion was also found in patients with cribriform, papillary, micropapillary, and solid types of DCIS. After a median follow-up of 55 months, one patient (7%) had developed a distant recurrence, and there were nine instances (24%) of local recurrence in the breast after conservation therapy.

Silverstein et al.[87] employed the term "microinvasion" if "one or two microscopic foci of possible invasion no more than 1 mm in maximum diameter were found or if the pathologists were uncertain as to whether or not a cancerous lobule was tangentially sectioned or infiltrating." Microinvasion as so defined was detected in 28 (13%) of 208 cases. The majority of microinvasive lesions were comedocarcinoma (21 of 28, 75%), representing 20% of intraductal comedocarcinomas. One of the 28 patients (4%) with microinvasive carcinoma had ALN metastases.

Silver and Tavassoli[308] defined microinvasion as "a single focus of invasive carcinoma less than or equal to 2 mm or up to three foci of invasion, each less than or equal to 1 m in greatest dimension" in a study of 38 patients. "Comedo" DCIS was present in 31 (82%), and papillary or other types of DCIS were present in 7 (18%). All patients were treated by mastectomy with axillary dissection, and no lymph node metastases were found. After a mean follow-up of 7.5 years, no patient had developed recurrent breast carcinoma.

de Mascarel et al.[309] subclassified microinvasive duct carcinoma into type 1 (single tumor cells) and type 2 (clusters of tumor cells). Type 1 cases would qualify for classification as *T1mic*, as would some type 2 cases. Among a subset of 20 type 2 cases that were measured, 6 were T1*mic* and 14 had invasive foci of between 2 and 10 mm. None of the 59 type 1 patients who had ALNs removed had nodal metastases. On the other hand, there were nodal metastases in 14 (10%) of the 139 patients with type 2 microinvasion who had ALNs examined. Distant metastases were reported in 2 (3%) of the 72 patients with type 1 microinvasion and in 12 (7%) of 171 with type 2 microinvasion. The survival of patients with type 1 microinvasive carcinoma was similar to that of patients with pure DCIS and significantly better than that of patients with type 2 microinvasion.

Information about patients with microinvasion defined as T1*mic* (less than 1 mm) are becoming increasingly available. Jimenez and Visscher[310] described 75 patients with microinvasion, defined as one focus less than 5 mm or multiple foci with an aggregate diameter of less than 10 mm. Two or more histologically separate foci of invasion were present in 59% of the cases. Microinvasion consisting of isolated cell clusters less than 1 mm was present in 25 cases (33%). ALN dissection performed in 69 cases revealed metastatic carcinoma in five (7%). Two of these patients had invasive foci measuring less than 1 mm (T1*mic*), and in a third case the invasive lesion measured 1.1 mm.

Walker et al.[311] compared the clinical and pathologic features of DCIS detected by mammography to patients who had symptoms, usually a mass or nipple discharge. Microinvasion (T1*mic*) was found in 5 (5%) of 92 mammographically detected and in 10 (13.5%) of 74 symptomatic cases. All but 1 of the 15 DCIS lesions with microinvasion were larger than 2 cm. Most DCIS with microinvasion had a comedo growth pattern or necrosis and high nuclear grade.

By using a double immunostaining procedure for actin and cytokeratin, Prasad et al.[312] were able to confirm microinvasion (T1*mic*) in 21 of 109 cases originally diagnosed as microinvasion or in which microinvasion was suspected. Eighteen lesions were ductal and three were lobular. The carcinoma had high nuclear grade and necrosis in 16 of the 18 (89%) ductal lesions, including 13 (72%) described as comedo type. Axillary dissection performed in 15 patients revealed metastatic carcinoma in two cases, each with one lymph node involved. One of the 18 patients had recurrent carcinoma in the same breast after conservation surgery and radiotherapy, and another developed a chest wall recurrence of invasive duct carcinoma after a mastectomy. There were no systemic metastases after a median follow-up of 28 months.

Microinvasion associated with florid and pleomorphic LCIS may be mistaken for microinvasive *ductal* carcinoma. In the only series of 16 cases reported to date, ALN biopsies (including nine SLN samplings) were performed in 13 cases, with negative results in each, and all patients were alive without evidence of recurrence or of metastases in a mean follow-up of 24 months.[313]

The foregoing data indicate that microinvasion is more likely to be found associated with high-grade, clinically evident DCIS than with low-grade, mammographically detected DCIS. When microinvasion is detected, the frequency of nodal metastases is 10% or less in patients who undergo axillary dissection, and the probability of systemic metastases is 5% or less. Axillary dissection can be avoided in microinvasive duct carcinoma if SLN biopsy is performed. This procedure adds greater precision with less morbidity to the detection of axillary nodal metastases.

SENTINEL LYMPH NODE BIOPSY

SLN biopsy is used to assess axillary nodal status in patients with invasive and *in situ* carcinoma. Routine use of SLN is generally not employed in DCIS, except when there is extensive high-grade DCIS, when invasive carcinoma is suspected, or when mastectomy is performed.[314] The incidence of nodal involvement in patients with DCIS has been reported to range from 0.5% to 1.5%, respectively[253]; however, SLN positivity can be higher in higher grade and more widespread DCIS. In a set of 854 DCIS cases treated at the European Institute of Oncology over more than a decade-long period ending 2006, SLN involvement was detected in 12 (1.4%), consisting of seven cases with micrometastases (less than 0.2 mm) and four patients with isolated tumor cells (ITC).[315] None of the 11 patients who underwent subsequent axillary dissection had additional nodal involvement.[316]

Zavotsky et al.[317] found metastatic carcinoma in the SLN from 2 (14.3%) of 14 patients with DCIS. Completion axillary dissection revealed no other nodal metastases. Dauway et al.[318] cited nine patients with microinvasive carcinoma associated with DCIS (T1*mic*). Three (33%) of these patients had micrometastases detected in an SLN by cytokeratin IHC and no other metastases in a completion axillary dissection. These investigators also reported that 5 (6%) of 86 patients with lesions classified as DCIS had metastases in an SLN. Four of the nodal metastases were detected only by cytokeratin IHC. Four of the five patients had "comedo" DCIS, and the fifth had a 9.5-cm low-grade micropapillary and cribriform lesions. Completion axillary dissection in four cases yielded no additional metastases.

Several additional studies have examined the yield of SLN mapping in intraductal and microinvasive ductal carcinoma. Wilkie et al.[319] found a positive SLN in 27 (5%) of 559 patients with DCIS. Nineteen (70%) of the 27 positive SLNs were detected by IHC. Among 51 women with microinvasive ductal carcinoma, 7 (14%) had a positive SLN, 5 (71%) of which were immunohistochemical findings.

Katz et al.[320] reported finding a positive SLN associated with 8 (7.2%) of 110 breasts with DCIS. In four of these cases, the lymph node was positive only on IHC. No additional nodal metastases were found in two patients who had a subsequent axillary dissection. Two (9.6%) of 21 women with microinvasive ductal carcinoma had a positive SLN, one of which was detected only by IHC. An additional positive lymph node was found in the full axillary dissection in the patient with an H&E-positive SLN.

A positive SLN was found in 4 (10%) of 39 patients with DCIS and in 1 (7%) of 14 patients with microinvasive ductal carcinoma studied by Sakr et al.[321] The SLNs were involved by ITC or micrometastases. Leidenius et al.[322] found that 5 (7%) of 74 patients with DCIS had a positive SLN, including 3 women with ITC. DCIS with a positive SLN were significantly larger (median, 50 mm; range, 45 to 60 mm) than DCIS with negative SLN (median, 18 mm; range, 1 to 110 mm). However, only one of the five patients with a positive SLN had a palpable lesion. The architecture of the DCIS with positive SLN was as follows: cribriform (*n*:2), cribriform and comedo (*n*:1), comedo (*n*:1), and micropapillary (*n*:1).

The results of SLN biopsy in patients who had DCIS diagnosed by needle core biopsy were reported by Huo et al.[323] SLNs were obtained from 103 patients among whom 4 (4%) had one positive lymph node. Three of these patients had invasive carcinoma in their excisional biopsy specimens and metastatic foci in the SLN measuring 0.5 to 6 mm. The fourth patient with DCIS had only ITC in one SLN.

Several conclusions can be drawn from the foregoing studies of SLN mapping in patients with DCIS:

- The frequency of finding a positive SLN in a patient with pure DCIS is 10% or less. Metastatic foci in these cases are likely to be micrometastases or ITC. The risk of having a positive SLN is greater for high-grade, mass-forming, and larger lesions.
- DCIS with microinvasion (T1*mic*) generally has a risk as high as 15% for SLN metastasis, but the frequency in some studies overlaps with the risk in pure DCIS.
- Additional lymph node metastases are rarely found in a completion axillary dissection, with a slightly greater frequency when there is microinvasion.
- If SLN biopsy is being considered as part of the primary surgical management of a patient with DCIS diagnosed in a needle core biopsy specimen, the yield will be higher if the procedure had been performed on patients who were most likely to have invasive carcinoma in the lumpectomy specimen. Risk factors for this "upgraded" diagnosis include the following: high-grade DCIS, necrosis, lobular extension, a palpable or radiographic mass at the site of DCIS, and larger lesion size (median 2.5 vs. 1.5 cm) based on imaging studies.

Disseminated tumor cells have been found in the bone marrow patients with in DCIS. The yield was in 13% (34/266) of patients in one series,[324] and in 21.1% (4/19) in another.[325] The clinical significance of such findings in DCIS, as in invasive carcinoma, is uncertain at this time.

MARGINS OF EXCISION

Microscopic examination of histologic sections is necessary to determine whether DCIS is present at the margin of a surgical biopsy specimen. Macroscopic examination of the gross specimen is unreliable for this purpose, and the use of FSs, while possible, is impractical in most laboratories.[82]

A transected duct containing DCIS that is present at a margin identified by ink applied to the gross specimen or some other standardized marking procedure is reported as a "positive" margin.[326] DCIS involving lobular glands (cancerization of lobules) is considered to be a risk factor of local recurrence and should be reported as a positive margin if present at the margin of the specimen.[327] In cases with a positive margin, the report should indicate the extent of involvement with terms such as *focal* (limited to one or two microscopic fields) or *more than focal*. When the margin is not directly involved, the closest approach of DCIS to the margin should be stated with a measurement in millimeters. The term *close* has been variably defined, but the most frequent usage is for carcinoma within 1 mm of the margin.

Margins of a lumpectomy can be assessed by taking either radial (perpendicular) or shave sections. Shave sections are assessed by obtaining samples of the surface of the post-excision biopsy cavity. Any DCIS found microscopically in this tissue is considered to be indicative of a positive margin.[151] Radial (perpendicular) sections offer the considerable advantage of determination of extent (width) of clearance. A novel combination radial–shave method of margin assessment has been described, but this is a cumbersome and impractical method.[328] The sampling of secondary (biopsy cavity shave) margins has become a popular technique for the assessment of margins.[329] These secondary margins, often all six margins (as of a cube) are taken separately by the surgeon. The technique has been found to decrease the need for reexcision after lumpectomies by one-half.[330]

An aggressive approach to initial resection(s), that is, large resection volume, may avoid positive margins and lower the risk of recurrence or the need for additional surgery. At the present time, the need of radiation therapy is determined by whether or not the margin clearance for DCIS is wide enough. Thus, the apparently opposing goals of negative margins and acceptable cosmetic results have to be balanced. One of the most important determinants of adequate excision may be "excision volume" that may be objectively assessed as the specimen to carcinoma (S:C) ratio.[331,332]

The attainment of negative margins in some cases of DCIS proves to be a Sisyphean task. Significant risk factors for persistently positive margins, encountered in approximately one-quarter to one-third of cases, include multifocality and nodal positivity. In such cases, the use of multiple reexcision biopsies to attain negative margins, often in multiple procedures, is considered to be a "safe" alternative to mastectomy.[333]

Occasionally, it may be difficult to determine whether proliferating ductal epithelial cells at a cauterized surgical margin represents a hyperplastic or neoplastic process. In this setting, immunostaining with high molecular weight cytokeratins (CK5/6 and K903) may be helpful since ADH and

DCIS are negative for high molecular weight cytokeratin, even in epithelia that show marked cautery effect.[334]

In 1999, the DCIS "Consensus Conference" proposed a 10-mm margin as the limit of oncologic safety.[187] Ten years later, there was "consensus" among experts at St. Gallen on avoiding the need to insist on a large (e.g., 1 cm) free margin.[335] In the interim years, various progressively lesser extents of optimal clearance were proposed, that is, 3, 2 to 3, 2, and 1 mm.[336–339] Although the need for negative margins has been assimilated in various guidelines for DCIS management, the absolute need for the attainment of a widely negative margin has been questioned on the basis of the NSABP B1 and B24 trials that only required margins of tumor not touching ink. In this study, only 72 (2.8%) of 2,612 patients treated with breast conservation with and without radiation therapy died of breast carcinoma after 15 years of follow-up.[340] In 2012, Morrow et al.[341] concluded that "bigger is not better" and suggested that a margin with no tumor at the inked surface was satisfactory. This approach places reliance on postsurgical adjuvant radiation and tamoxifen therapy.

Given such fluidity, and divergence, of recommendations in the recent past, it would behoove pathologists to report the pathologic findings in an objective manner, that is, report the presence of tumor at ink as "positive," and the closest distances of tumor to various margins. The use of vague terms (such as "abutting," "near," "approximating," and "free"), without further elaboration, should be avoided.

Innovative approaches such as placement of radioactive "seeds" to enhance tumor localization and thereby ensure adequate margin clearance,[342,343] as well as the intraoperative assessment of surgical margins by the use of radiofrequency spectroscopy during breast-conserving surgery of DCIS,[344] show early promise.

TREATMENT AND PROGNOSIS

Mastectomy

Until the last quarter of the 20th century, the standard treatment for DCIS was mastectomy. Prior to the introduction of modified mastectomy procedures, the operation was a classical radical mastectomy. Even after the widespread adoption of the modified radical mastectomy, an *en bloc* axillary dissection was routinely performed, yielding ALN metastases in only isolated instances.[18,19,73,74] These operations ensured at least a 99% cure rate.[19,73,74,309] Systemic recurrences that occurred in 1% or less of patients after such treatment resulted from contralateral carcinomas or foci of invasion that were undetected.[72,73,345,346] The operation was deemed justified because of the very low local recurrence rate and the presence of unsuspected frankly invasive foci discovered in the mastectomy specimens from about 5% of breasts that had only DCIS in the biopsy specimen.[81,347]

Mastectomy remains a treatment option for patients with DCIS, but it is infrequently indicated under circumstances outlined by a Consensus Conference on the Treatment of *In Situ* Ductal Carcinoma (DCIS).[246] The situations in which mastectomy was recommended were as follows:

1. "Large areas of DCIS of a size that the lesion cannot be removed by an oncologically acceptable excision . . . while still conserving a cosmetically acceptable breast."
2. "Patients with multiple areas of DCIS in the same breast that cannot be encompassed through a single incision."
3. "Patients who cannot undergo radiation therapy because of other medical problems, such as collagen vascular diseases, or prior therapeutic radiation to the chest for another illness, and for whom treatment by excision alone is not appropriate."

Local recurrence on the chest wall is an unusual complication in the treatment of DCIS by total mastectomy. A meta-analysis of published studies reported that the frequency of local recurrence following mastectomy alone was 1.4% (95% CI, 0.7 to 2.1).[348] The recurrent lesion may consist of DCIS,[349] or it may manifest invasion.[350] Some of these recurrences are accompanied by residual breast parenchyma, which may harbor persistent DCIS.[351] Most published descriptions of local recurrence after mastectomy for DCIS do not comment on the presence or absence of breast parenchyma associated with the recurrence. It is essential that persistent breast tissue be looked for and mentioned in the report that describes the specimen from the site of any local recurrence, regardless of whether the primary lesion had been *in situ* or invasive.

Recurrent carcinoma in residual breast tissue constitutes persistence of the original primary tumor or a new primary carcinoma and has a much more favorable prognosis than the more frequent true local recurrence in a mastectomy scar, which is usually a manifestation of systemic metastases. Recurrent carcinoma in persistent breast tissue is adequately treated in most cases by local excision supplemented by radiotherapy and/or systemic chemotherapy, depending upon the size of the lesion and whether invasion is present.[72,352] In one report, the 5- and 10-year survival of patients with an invasive local recurrence after mastectomy for DCIS was 83% and 63%, respectively.[350] This result supports the conclusion that the chest wall recurrences were a manifestation of persistent carcinoma rather than evidence of systemic metastases in a substantial number of these patients.

Recurrence in the preserved nipple is a rare complication of nipple-sparing mastectomy for DCIS. In one instance, recurrence as invasive carcinoma occurred 17 years after a subcutaneous mastectomy that was accompanied by irradiation of the nipple.[353] Additional examples of recurrence in the preserved nipple after subcutaneous mastectomy were described by Price et al.[354] Another unusual type of recurrence consisted of two separate foci of invasive carcinoma at subcutaneous drainage sites 8 years after a patient underwent a modified mastectomy for DCIS.[351] No mammary parenchyma was seen at the sites of recurrence. It was suggested that DCIS cells dislodged at operation persisted at the drain sites and gave rise to recurrent carcinoma.

Recurrent DCIS has been detected as a result of the mammographic appearance of calcifications in residual breast tissue after total mastectomy and saline implant reconstruction.[349] Helvie et al.[355] reported six patients who developed invasive recurrent invasive carcinoma at the mastectomy site after transverse rectus abdominus myocutaneous (TRAM) flap reconstruction. All were described as initially having had extensive DCIS, and four patients had undergone a skin-sparing mastectomy. Five of the recurrent lesions were palpable. Two of four patients who underwent axillary dissection had nodal metastases. The report did not mention whether breast glandular tissue was associated with the recurrent carcinoma lesions.

Introduction to Breast-Conserving Therapy

Despite the widespread reliance on mastectomy, alternative therapies involving excisional surgery and radiotherapy were examined as early as the 1930s. After reviewing the record of his cases of intraductal comedocarcinoma, Bloodgood[8] commented that "the striking feature is that none of the cases of pure comedo adenocarcinoma was associated with metastasis to the axillary nodes, and not a single patient died of cancer." He described four patients with "pure" or noninvasive comedocarcinoma who were "completely excised with postoperative irradiation" and remained well up to 3 years later. These observations led him to conclude that "when the tumor is small and a FS shows a pure comedo neoplasm, it is sufficient to excise only the tumor."[8]

Occasional patients treated by local excision were mentioned in reviews of DCIS published in the 1960s and 1970s. Farrow[356] reported on 25 patients treated by local excision alone. Histologic features of the DCIS were not specified. Further carcinoma developed in the same breast 1 to 8 years after excision in 5 of the 25 women. The subsequent lesions were "within or nearby the previous local excisional site." In 1971, Ashikari et al.[72] mentioned two patients, one of whom refused surgery and a second with a medical contraindication who were treated by local excision and did not develop recurrent carcinoma. Four of 64 patients with DCIS described by Westbrook and Gallager[73] received only radiation therapy after biopsy because of patient preference or comorbid conditions.

The changing trend in the treatment of DCIS in the United States was reported by Winchester et al.[20] in 1997, who analyzed data of more than 39,000 women diagnosed between 1985 and 1993. The use of breast conservation therapy increased from 31% to 54%, and overall 33.4% of patients did not undergo mastectomy during the 8-year interval. Radiotherapy was employed in 38% of patients treated by breast-conserving surgery in 1985 and in 54% in 1993. Axillary dissection was performed in 49% of cases with or without mastectomy, but the frequency of this procedure decreased from 52% in 1985 to 40% in 1993.

Joslyn[357] reviewed SEER data from various regions of the United States from 1973 through 2000 to document trends in the treatment of DCIS. The utilization of breast-conserving surgery increased in all regions surveyed, ranging from 49.5% in Utah to 76.9% in Connecticut for the period from 1997 through 2000. Women younger than 45 years at the time of diagnosis were treated by breast-conserving surgery significantly less often than those 45 years of age and older. Women who received radiotherapy in addition to breast-conserving surgery had significantly lower breast cancer mortality than those treated by breast-conserving surgery alone.

Breast Conservation by Excision Only–Retrospective Data

Long-term follow-up of DCIS treated by local excision alone was documented in several retrospective reports. The patients were identified in reviews of breast biopsies initially deemed to be benign but found to contain foci of DCIS on review. One of the earliest series consisted of eight patients with DCIS detected by Kiaer[358] in a review of patients with "fibroadenomatosis" (proliferative breast changes). "Follow-up revealed that 6 of these 8 patients had died of mammary carcinoma which had become clinically manifest 1-1/2 to 16 years after the first operation."[359] Two of nine patients treated by local excision for DCIS developed breast recurrences in a series described by Millis and Thynne.[359]

Another series consisted of 10 patients, who, in retrospect, had low-grade papillary or micropapillary DCIS identified in 8,609 biopsies from 1940 to 1950.[360] During follow-up averaging 21.6 years, 7 (70%) of the 10 patients were found to have subsequent carcinoma in the same breast after an average interval of 9.7 years. Six of the seven subsequent carcinomas were invasive. Four of these women developed metastatic carcinoma, which was fatal in two instances. In a later report, the series was expanded to 15 patients, 8 (53%) of whom developed subsequent carcinoma.[361] Harvey and Fechner[362] reviewed 879 breast biopsies from 1962 to 1966 reported to be benign. They identified six patients with previously undiagnosed papillary DCIS, all of whom remained well, with four followed for less than 5 years and two for less than 2 years.

Page et al.[363] found 28 women with DCIS treated by excision only in a review of 11,760 biopsies from 1950 to 1968. The DCIS were described as low-grade cribriform and micropapillary types. Invasive carcinoma developed in the ipsilateral breasts of 7 of 25 women who had follow-up of at least 3 years. All subsequent carcinomas were at or near the site of the original intraductal lesion. The observed frequency of subsequent invasive carcinoma was 11 times the expected rate. A second report by these investigators with follow-up averaging nearly 30 years found that 9, or 32%, of 28 women subsequently developed ipsilateral invasive carcinoma.[364] This frequency was 9.1 times expected (95% CI, 4.73 to 17.5). Further investigation of the series with a median follow-up of 31 years revealed invasive carcinoma in 11 (39.3%) of the 28 women. Eight subsequent carcinomas were diagnosed within 15 years of the original biopsy, and three were detected after intervals of 23, 29, and 42 years, respectively.

Eusebi et al.[365] found 28 examples of previously undiagnosed DCIS in a review of 4,397 biopsies performed from 1965 to 1971. Twenty-one of the lesions were forms of micropapillary carcinoma, four were cribriform, one papillary-cribriform, and two had comedocarcinoma. Two patients had ipsilateral recurrences. One of these women who originally had comedocarcinoma developed an invasive recurrence 5 years after biopsy. The other patient was found to have recurrent micropapillary carcinoma 8.8 years after biopsy. In this series, the observed frequency of subsequent carcinoma was 4.3 times (90% CI, 1.1 to 11.1) the expected risk, somewhat higher for nonmicropapillary (5.4) than for micropapillary (3.9) DCIS.

Data from a retrospective review of 1,877 biopsies classified as benign in the Nurses' Health Study were reported in 2007.[147] Previously unrecognized DCIS was identified in 13 specimens (0.7%). Four were classified as low, six as intermediate, and three as high nuclear grade. Architecturally, seven were cribriform, and three were each solid and micropapillary. Carcinoma was clinically diagnosed subsequently in the ipsilateral breast in 10 (77%) of the 13 patients after intervals of 2 to 18 years. DCIS was diagnosed in four cases, 2 to 6 years after the initial biopsy that was interpreted as benign, and six patients were found to have invasive carcinoma after 4 to 18 years. Three patients who did not have clinically diagnosed subsequent carcinoma had follow-up of 21 to 27 years. When compared with women with nonproliferative fibrocystic changes, the odds ratio for the development of subsequent carcinoma was 20.1 (95% CI, 6.1 to 66.5), and for invasive carcinoma it was 13.5 (95% CI, 3.7 to 49.7).

Breast Conservation by Excision Only–Prospective Data

Prior to the emergence of clinical trials, little information was available prospectively about the treatment of DCIS by breast-conserving excision. In 1982, Lagios et al.[267] reported that 3 (15%) of 15 patients treated for DCIS by local excision developed recurrences in the ipsilateral breast during follow-up averaging 44 months. An expanded series consisting of 79 patients with average follow-up of 48 months was reported in 1989.[366] Eight patients had developed recurrent carcinoma, four entirely intraductal, and four invasive. Seven of eight recurrences in the breast were in patients with comedocarcinoma or cribriform carcinoma with comedonecrosis. The eighth recurrence was associated with "intraductal carcinoma with anaplasia." Further information about this series was reported in 1994.[367] At that time, the local failure rate in the conserved breast was 14.7% after a mean follow-up of 106 months. Half of the recurrences were described as "minimally invasive carcinomas," and the others were intraductal. When correlated with histologic features of the initial lesion, the recurrence rate for DCIS of high nuclear grade with comedonecrosis was 30.5%, and for those with intermediate nuclear grade it was 10%. There were no breast recurrences in patients with low-grade DCIS.

After follow-up averaging 39 months, Fisher et al.[368] found a breast recurrence rate of 23% in 22 patients with DCIS treated by excisional biopsy alone. These patients had been entered into a clinical trial for invasive carcinoma in which one of the randomized treatments was excision alone, and the diagnosis was corrected to DCIS during a subsequent pathology review. The same report described recurrences in 2 (7%) of the 29 women with retrospectively diagnosed DCIS who had been randomized to receive radiation therapy. Ciatto et al.[56] reported that infiltrating carcinoma developed in the ipsilateral breast in 7 of 55 women (12.7%) treated only by local excision or quadrantectomy. The DCIS had been detected through routine examinations or mammographic screening in Florence, Italy, from 1968 to 1988. The length of follow-up was not stated.

Several population-based prospective analyses of excisional surgery alone have been reported. The largest series, from Denmark, consisted of 112 women with a median follow-up of 53 months.[369] Recurrent invasive carcinoma occurred in 5 women (4.4%), and 19 (17%) had recurrent DCIS. The initial lesions ranged from 1 to 80 mm, with a median size of 10 mm. Features favoring recurrence were large nuclear size, lesion size greater than 10 mm, and the presence of comedonecrosis regardless of the histologic subtype (solid, micropapillary, or cribriform). Papillary lesions, of which there were few, had a high recurrence rate whether or not comedonecrosis was present. Heterogeneity of growth pattern was found in all but 3 of the 112 lesions. Margin status, evaluable in only about one-third of the cases, did not appear to be a good predictor of recurrence. Recurrences occurred in 33% of cases with negative margins. Review of 132 patients with DCIS diagnosed in Malmo, Sweden, revealed that 3 of 21 women (14%) treated by breast-conserving surgery alone developed ipsilateral invasive carcinoma after a median follow-up of 7 years.[370]

Two additional studies described the follow-up of women with DCIS detected in regional mammography screening programs and treated by excisional surgery alone. Arnesson et al.[371] identified 38 women with lesions detected with a single-view mammography technique, who were treated only by "sector resection" with negative margins. After a median follow-up of 60 months, five (13%) patients had recurrent carcinoma consisting of two invasive and three intraductal lesions. The primary lesions associated with recurrence were 3 to 15 mm in size. Cribriform DCIS preceded the two invasive lesions, whereas comedocarcinoma was followed by recurrent DCIS. Carpenter et al.[372] reported on 28 women with lesions detected through screening mammography and clinical examination. Treatment consisted of quadrantectomy or segmental resection. No data were given about margin status. After a median follow-up of 38 months, five recurrences detected mammographically as microcalcifications in the region of prior excision consisted of one invasive and four intraductal lesions. There was no significant association between the development of recurrent carcinoma and the size of the primary lesions, the size of the excisional biopsy specimen, or the presence of multifocality.

Schwartz et al.[373] selected patients with mammographically detected nonpalpable or incidentally discovered DCIS for treatment by excision alone. Patients were eligible for inclusion if the mammographic diameter of the area of calcifications did not exceed 25 mm. Comedocarcinoma was present to some extent in 51% of the lesions and was the predominant type in 29%. At least two subtypes of DCIS were present in 41% of the cases. The excisions were not consistently studied for margin status. After a median follow-up of 47 months, 11 recurrences were detected in the ipsilateral breasts of 70 women (15.3%), consisting of three invasive and eight intraductal lesions. All recurrent DCIS were detected mammographically because of the appearance of calcifications. Comedocarcinoma was present in 10 of 11 lesions followed by recurrence (one was papillary), and all recurrent DCIS were of the comedo type. There was no correlation between the number of duct cross sections with DCIS in the primary lesion and recurrence.

Another series of clinically selected patients treated by excision alone was reported by Hetelekidis et al.[374] The group consisted of 59 women, almost all of whom had mammographically detected lesions. Local recurrence in the breast was detected in 10 women (17%) 5 to 132 months after excision, with a median interval of 37 months and a 5-year recurrence rate of 10%. Four recurrent lesions were invasive, and six were intraductal. Eight recurrences were at the site of prior excision. Factors associated with local recurrence were high nuclear grade, lesions occupying more than five low-magnification (4×) microscopic fields and tumor 1 mm or less from the margin. Lesion size was the only statistically significant indicator of recurrence. The local recurrence rate was 18% for lesions with poor nuclear grade and less than 10% when nuclear grade was intermediate or well differentiated (p = NS). DCIS involving fewer than five low-power fields had a 3% recurrence rate compared with more extensive lesions with a 17% recurrence rate ($p = 0.02$). The local recurrence rates for negative and close margins were 8% and 25%, respectively.

The foregoing prospective studies suggest that DCIS can be treated successfully by excisional breast-conserving surgery in some cases. Although the majority of these patients will not develop a breast recurrence, about 20% of recurrent lesions are invasive and, therefore, carry the added risk of metastatic spread.

Risk Factors for Breast Recurrences after Conservation Surgery Alone

Data presented in many reports on breast-conserving surgery suggest that pathologic features of DCIS might contribute to the success of treatment by excisional surgery alone. A case-control study by Badve et al.[375] examined the value of five histologic classification schemes for predicting local recurrence in the breast after excisional surgery alone. The exercise involved reviewing slides of excisional biopsies from 43 patients who developed recurrences and from 81 controls matched for age at diagnosis who did not develop a recurrence. The median time to recurrence was 39 months, and for recurrence-free controls median follow-up was 68 months. None of the classifications systems was clearly superior for predicting local recurrence. The characteristics of DCIS most strongly associated with recurrence classification were poorly differentiated histologic grade, the presence of necrosis, and poorly differentiated nuclear grade.

Goonewardene et al.[376] studied the significance of necrosis as a risk factor for local recurrence in 166 women who had been treated for DCIS by excision alone. After an average follow-up of 6.5 years, recurrences were detected in 40 patients (24%) and 12 recurrences were invasive. Substantial necrosis was present in the original DCIS in 70% of the cases with recurrence and in 83% with invasive recurrence. Necrosis was present in only 25% of DCIS not followed by recurrence.

MacDonald et al.[377] retrospectively reviewed 445 patients with DCIS treated by excision alone between 1972 and 2004. In this nonrandomized series of selected patients, 70 (17%) of the women had local breast recurrences, including 26 (6%) that were invasive. Seventy-two of the 79 breast recurrences (91%) were in the same quadrant as the original DCIS. The median follow-up period for all patients was 57 months, and the median time to breast recurrence was 26 months. One patient died of metastatic breast carcinoma, and there were 23 deaths due to other causes. Significant risk factors for local recurrence were margin width of less than 10 mm, age less than 40 years, and high nuclear grade. The hazard ratio (HR) for breast recurrence was 5.39 times greater if the margin widths were less than 10 mm than if they were greater than 10 mm.

Wong et al.[378] described the results of surgery alone with a final margin clearance of at least 10 mm for DCIS in a single-arm prospective trial. The study was limited to patients selected on the basis of the following criteria: predominant grade 1 or 2; mammographic size of less than or equal to 2.5 cm; and final lumpectomy margins clear by 10 mm or more or no DCIS in a reexcision specimen. After a median follow-up of 40 months, 13 of 158 patients (8.2%) enrolled in the study had experienced a breast recurrence. Four recurrences (31%) were invasive, and the remaining recurrences were intraductal. Ten recurrences (77%) were in the same quadrant as the original DCIS. The breast recurrence rate was 2.4% per patient-year with a projected 5-year breast recurrence rate of 12%.

When DCIS has been treated by excision alone, the foregoing data indicate that lesion size greater than 2.5 cm, necrosis, high nuclear grade, and a clear margin of less than 10 mm are factors that predispose to recurrence in the breast. However, as demonstrated by Wong et al.,[378] local breast recurrence may occur after excisional surgery alone, even with a clear margin that exceeds 10 mm.

A commercially available RT-PCR-based multigene assay (Oncotype DX, Genomic Health Inc, Redwood City, CA) is available for DCIS. This test generates a "DCIS score" ranging from 0 to 100. The "score" quantifies the likelihood of 10-year recurrence for *in situ* or invasive carcinoma.[379] The test uses a subset of the 21 genes assessed for the Oncotype DX breast cancer assay for invasive breast carcinoma. It can be performed on formalin-fixed paraffin-embedded tissue using manual microdissection for lesional tissue. The likelihood of local recurrence at 10 years increases continuously with increases in score, and the latter information could potentially help in management decisions.[380]

Breast-Conserving Surgery with Radiotherapy

Radiation therapy has been employed in conjunction with excisional surgery in an effort to improve local control after breast conservation therapy for DCIS. Data are available from a number of prospective investigations of patients treated by excisional surgery with radiation therapy, and from randomized trials comparing the results of excision alone to excision with radiotherapy. Initial reports published in the 1980s described selected patients and noted a recurrence rate in the conserved breast of 10% or less after a median follow-up of approximately 5 years.[381–383] Bornstein et al.[384] reported an actuarial 8-year breast recurrence rate of 27% in a series of 38 selected patients. Five of the eight recurrences were invasive, and one of these women developed metastatic carcinoma. Solin et al.[385] identified 259 women treated in nine institutions in the United States and Europe and found a 10-year actuarial breast failure rate of 16%. Fifty percent of the 28 recurrences were invasive, and four patients developed metastatic carcinoma. A later follow-up report by Solin et al.[386] described an expanded cohort of 1,003 patients from 10 institutions with a median follow-up of 8.5 years (range, 0.2 to 24.6 years). Initial recurrences of carcinoma limited to the breast were documented in 82 patients (8.2%). One additional patient had angiosarcoma (0.1%), and the nature of the breast recurrence was unknown in two cases. The calculated 15-year rates of breast recurrence and systemic metastases were 19% and 3%, respectively. The histology of the 82 initial documented breast carcinoma recurrences was as follows: invasive ductal 46 (57%), intraductal 34 (41%), and other 2 (2%). Five additional patients had invasive breast recurrences concurrently with systemic recurrences. The risk of breast recurrence was significantly lower in women who had a negative surgical margin or were 50 years of age or older at the time of treatment. During the course of follow-up, contralateral breast carcinoma was reported in 71 (7%) patients, and 56 (6%) women had a nonmammary malignant neoplasm.

Two large-scale randomized trials have compared local control in the breast after excision alone and excision plus radiotherapy. The NSABP B17 study revealed a 50% reduction in breast recurrence when radiation was added to lumpectomy.[387] The 12-year risk of breast recurrence was 31.7% with surgery alone and 15.7% for surgery with radiotherapy. A similar randomized trial by the European Organization for Research and Treatment of Cancer (EORTC) yielded a 4-year breast recurrence rate of 16% after surgery alone and 9% when radiation was added to surgery.[388] Updated results from the EORTC study with a median follow-up of 10.5 years revealed a 10-year breast recurrence-free rate of 74% for excision alone and 85% for surgery followed by radiation.[296] The risk reduction attributed to radiotherapy for recurrent DCIS was 48%, and for invasive carcinoma it was 42%.[389] Pathologic features significantly associated with breast recurrence in both treatment groups were intermediate to poorly differentiated grade and cribriform or solid growth.

A low-risk subset of DCIS patients who could be spared radiation treatment was characterized in a prospective Eastern Cooperative Oncology Group and North Central Cancer Treatment Group trial.[339] Patients with either low- or intermediate-grade DCIS spanning less than 2.6 cm or high-grade DCIS measuring less than 1.1 cm who had margin clearance of more than 3 mm and no residual mammographic calcifications were eligible for this 1997 to 2002 trial. In a median follow-up of 6.2 years, the 5-year rate of ipsilateral breast events in 565 patients in the low- or intermediate-grade group was 6.1% (95% CI, 4.1% to 8.2%). With a median follow-up of 6.7 years, the incidence of recurrence for 105 patients in the high-grade stratum was 15.3% (95% CI, 8.2% to 22.5%). Patients with lower grade DCIS and clear margins 3 mm or wider were deemed to have an acceptably low rate of ipsilateral breast events at 5 years without irradiation. Patients with high-grade lesions had a much higher rate of recurrence, suggesting that excision alone would be inadequate.

Although patient outcome is maximized when treatment is tailored to patient and disease characteristics, the number of events prevented per 1,000 radiation-treated women is typically less than 10%.[390] Radiation treatment offers an increase in the chances of successful breast conservation, but this positive feature is somewhat offset by the likelihood that mastectomy will be necessary in the event of recurrence, the detection of a new primary carcinoma, or as a result of various radiation-associated complications.[391]

Accelerated partial breast irradiation, that is, brachytherapy using Mammosite (Hologic, Boxborough, MA), has emerged as a substitute for whole-breast irradiation (including three-dimensional conformal external beam) in the treatment of breast carcinoma.[392,393] Preliminary outcome results indicate similar results regardless of either radiation modality used. A radiotherapy boost to the surgical cavity improves local control in DCIS.[394]

The interpretation of radiation-induced cytologic changes in mammary epithelium may occasionally pose diagnostic difficulty. It should be noted that recurrent disease exhibits a histopathologic appearance that is generally similar to the index lesion.[395] As such, histopathologic review of the previously diagnosed DCIS is critical for the optimal evaluation of all "recurrences."

Risk Factors for Breast Recurrence after Conservation Surgery with Radiotherapy

Factors associated with an increased risk of breast recurrence after surgery alone are also significant for recurrence after surgery and radiotherapy. Necrosis in DCIS or comedo-type DCIS imparts an especially high risk of breast recurrence after breast conservation with radiotherapy. Solin et al.[396] found that the presence of necrosis was a significant risk factor when it occurred in DCIS with poorly differentiated nuclear grade. Kuske et al.[397] reported significantly poorer local control in patients with comedo (75%) than in those with noncomedo (98%) carcinoma, but did not offer a definition of "comedo" DCIS. In the NSABP B17 trial comparing excision alone and excision plus radiotherapy, features associated with increased risk of local recurrence after either form of treatment were the presence of moderate to marked comedonecrosis, regardless of histologic subtype, margins that were positive or indeterminate, multifocality, and a moderate to marked lymphocytic infiltrate.[398] The size of the lesion (less than 10 or greater than or equal to 10 mm) did not prove to be a statistically significant predictor for breast recurrence. Necrosis proved to be the only statistically significant independent risk factor for recurrence in both treatment groups in multivariate analysis.

The VNPI was developed to stratify patients with DCIS, to distinguish between women who are most likely to be treated successfully by breast conservation and those who might be candidates for mastectomy because of a relatively high risk of breast recurrence.[399] The original VNPI was a numerical score of 3 to 9 based on the assessment of three variables: size of DCIS, distance between DCIS and margin, and a pathologic classification based on necrosis and nuclear grade. Each variable was divided into three categories, which were ranked (scored) from most to least favorable as 1 to 3 (Table 11.4). The original VNPI was derived from the sum of scores for individual variables.

Follow-up of patients with DCIS grouped into three VNPI categories (scores 3,4; scores 5,6,7; and scores 8,9) showed significant differences in recurrence-free survival, with the most favorable outcome associated with the lowest scores. Patients were stratified within the VNPI groups according to whether they received radiotherapy in addition to excision. Radiated patients in the VNPI 3,4 group did not differ significantly from those who were not radiated, but radiation appeared to be beneficial in the intermediate VNPI group. Recurrences were "unacceptably" frequent in the VNPI 8,9 group, even when radiotherapy was administered.[399] On the basis of these observations, it was suggested that women with DCIS classified as VNPI 3,4 could be treated by excision alone, that excision with radiotherapy be employed for the VNPI 5 to 7 group, and that mastectomy should be recommended if the VNPI is 8 or 9.

Retrospective studies have not confirmed the VNPI as a prognostic guide for local control of DCIS. For example, de Mascarel et al.[400] found a significant difference in local recurrence between women in the low- and intermediate-risk VNPI groups. In univariate analysis, the local recurrence rate increased with the size of the DCIS, with decrease in distance to the margin, with higher histologic grade, and with the percentage of paraffin blocks involved by DCIS. When these variables were considered in multivariate analysis, the percentage of paraffin blocks with DCIS was the only significant predictor of local recurrence. Boland et al.[401] retrospectively studied 237 patients with DCIS and confirmed that margin width and grade were significant risk factors for breast recurrence. However, when stratified by VNPI, 78% of patients were in the moderate risk group, a result that led the authors to conclude that "the VNPI lacked discriminatory power for guiding further patient management." In this series, margin width was the strongest predictor of successful conservation treatment. When compared with patients who had a clear margin of at least 10 mm, the RR for breast recurrence was 2.5 if the margin was 1 to 9 mm and 22 for a margin of less than 1 mm. Warnberg[402] reported no statistically significant differences in relapse-free survival between patients with DCIS stratified into the three VNPI prognostic groups.

The VNPI should be validated in a prospective randomized trial before acceptance as a basis for clinical practice. This is especially important because of significant concerns about the database from which it was derived. A major issue is the lack of a consistent treatment program illustrated by the following quotation that described the study group[403]:

> Until 1988 all patients with DCIS who elected breast conservation were advised to add breast irradiation to their treatment. Most patients accepted this recommendation; a few refused and were treated with careful clinical follow-up without irradiation. Beginning in 1989, the physicians within The Breast Center were no longer convinced of the overall value of radiation therapy for DCIS, and all breast conservation patients with uninvolved biopsy margins (clear by 1 mm or more) were offered the option of careful clinical follow-up without radiation therapy. Many patients accepted this option; some refused and were treated with breast irradiation. Outside patients with DCIS referred to our radiation oncologists for radiation therapy continued to be treated with radiation therapy in accord with the wishes of their referring physicians.

Other uncontrolled variables included differing radiation schedules and inconsistent boost treatment.[403]

Lesion size was one of the original three variables included in the VNPI. As discussed elsewhere in this chapter, there is no reliable or generally accepted method for measuring the size or extent of DCIS, especially with the precision that is required for the VNPI scoring system. In lesions limited to a single tissue block, it may be possible to distinguish between foci smaller and larger than 15 mm, but the distinction between 15 and 40 mm and larger than 40 mm is likely to be very unreliable. Determining size when DCIS is distributed in more than one tissue block from a single biopsy specimen or if it is in more than one biopsy specimen is very imprecise. The methods for determining lesion extent by counting 4× fields of involvement

TABLE 11.4 The University of Southern California/Van Nuys Prognostic Index (USC/VNPI) Scoring System

Score	1	2	3
Size (mm)	≤15	6–40	≥41
Margins (mm)	≥10	1-9	<1
Pathologic classification	Nonhigh grade	Nonhigh grade	High grade
	(−) necrosis	(−) necrosis	(±) necrosis
Age (yr)	≥61	40–60	≤39

Modified from Silverstein MJ, Lagios MD. Choosing treatment for patients with ductal carcinoma in situ: fine tuning the University of Southern California/Van Nuys Prognostic Index. *J Natl Cancer Inst Monogr* 2010;2010(41):193–196.

or the number of slides with DCIS do not provide measurements suitable for the VNPI.[404,405] There are likely to be many patients for whom a VNPI cannot be determined or for whom the calculated VNPI is of questionable accuracy.

An updated report from the Van Nuys Center published in 1998 did not classify patients according to the VNPI.[406] The series of 707 of nonrandomized patients included 208 women treated by lumpectomy and radiotherapy and 240 treated by excision alone. Breast recurrences were detected in 36 women in each group, representing 17% and 15%, respectively, and approximately half of the recurrences were invasive in each group. Distant metastases were diagnosed in six patients, five of whom had been treated originally by lumpectomy and radiotherapy. Five of the patients (0.7%) in the entire series died of breast carcinoma with four in the radiated group. The median follow-up for the 35 patients who had invasive recurrent carcinoma was 127 months (58 months from initial diagnosis to invasive recurrence and 69 additional months after recurrence). The distant recurrence rate in the subset of 35 patients with invasive recurrence in the breast was 27.1%, and the mortality rate due to breast carcinoma was 14.4% at 8 years.

The VNPI has evolved over the years. In 1995, the Van Nuys classification using a combination of nuclear grade and necrosis was proposed as a tool for the prediction of local recurrence. The 1996 version of VNPI (VNPI-1996) was based upon the *size* of DCIS, its *pathologic grade* and *margins*. The modified University of Southern California (USC)/VNPI-2003 included *age* as the fourth factor to the estimation, although the introduction of age did not appear to cause any significant shift in treatment modalities.

In 2010, the USC-VNPI was fine-tuned further, on the basis of the observations in three times as many patients as were included 15 years previously.[407] The five quantifiable prognostic factors (size, margin width, nuclear grade, comedonecrosis, and age) were retained; however, the recommendations were revised. On the basis of cumulative data that included patients treated as early as 1979, it was concluded that to achieve a local recurrence rate of less than 20% at 12 years, excision alone for patients scoring 4, 5, or 6, and for those with a score of 7 and margin widths of 3 mm or more, would be appropriate. Excision plus radiation therapy would achieve the same goal for patients with a score of 7 with margins less than 3 mm, patients with a score of 8 and margins of 3 mm or more, and patients whose score is 9 with margins of 5 mm or more. Mastectomy was recommended for patients who score 8 and less than 3-mm margins, those with a score 9 and margins less than 5 mm, and for all patients with a score of 10, 11, or 12. As noted above, the VNPI is not evidence based, and its formulation and reformulation have been based on a relatively small retrospective series of cases from a single institution where treatment was not randomized. In fact, it is evident that the treatment program was revised with each reanalysis of the data and lacked consistency throughout the early three decades during which the information was assembled. These factors, changes in the data points used to create the VNPI, and the unreliability of some of the measurements are reasons to be very cautious in accepting the VNPI categories as an absolute basis for making therapeutic decisions.

An attempt to improve the prognostic value of VNPI 2003 through the replacement of nuclear grade by genomic grade index (GGI, a 97-gene measure of histologic tumor grade) to generate the VNPI–GGI index has been described.[408] This unusual (and currently rather impractical) attempt to merge morphologic and molecular information is unlikely to be widely applied. The novel use of USC/VNPI to assess post-mastectomy risk of recurrence has also been proposed.[409]

A nomogram has been established for the risk of relapse after breast-conserving therapy on the basis of 10 predictive factors derived from a Cox multivariate analysis of retrospective data from 1,681 patients who underwent breast-conserving surgery at Memorial Sloan-Kettering Cancer Center in New York.[410] Factors with the greatest influence on the risk of ipsilateral recurrence included age, family history of breast carcinoma, margin status, number of excisions, adjuvant radiation or endocrine therapy, and treatment time period. Notably, neither tumor size nor any of the commonly used biomarkers (ER, PR, and HER2) were included as variables in this nomogram. This is the first nomogram to offer such a decision tool.[410] A recent attempt to validate this nomogram in an independent data set found that it overestimated the risk of recurrence in some subsets of patients.[411]

Breast Conservation for Mammographically Detected DCIS

Few studies have analyzed data based exclusively on mammographically detected DCIS treated by breast conservation with radiotherapy.[404,405] The 10-year breast recurrence rates ranged from 4% to 7% in patients with negative final excision margins to as high as 30% for women with positive or close margins. Time to recurrence appeared to be shorter for patients with positive margins (median 3.6 years) than for those with negative (median 4.3 years) or indeterminate (median 5.2 years) margins.[404] In patients with mammographically detected DCIS, pathologic features such as nuclear grade, necrosis, and architecture (comedo vs. noncomedo) were not significantly related to the risk of local recurrence. The lack of association with pathologic characteristics indicates the importance of stratifying patients by detection modality in the analysis of risk factors for local breast recurrence after conservation therapy.

Age at diagnosis (less than 45 vs. greater than or equal to 45 years) was found to be a significant predictor of local recurrence after breast-conserving surgery with radiation in patients with mammographically detected DCIS.[269] In this study, the 10-year actuarial rate of local failure in the breast was 23.4% for women younger than 45 years when treated and 7.1% among those 45 years or older. The authors were unable to apply the VNPI to their analyses because tumor size could not be determined in 58% of the cases. Pathologic study of the DCIS revealed several factors that might have predisposed the younger women to local recurrence.[412] These included smaller diagnostic biopsy specimens and more frequent lesions with high nuclear grade and necrosis.

Concurrent Proliferative Lesions and Breast Conservation

Adepoju et al.[413] studied the relationship of concurrent atypical duct and lobular hyperplasia and of LCIS to the risk of breast recurrence in women with DCIS treated by breast conservation therapy. Approximately 9.3% of the patients also had microinvasive ductal carcinoma, and about 70% received radiotherapy in addition to surgical excision. Follow-up ranged from 0.3 to 29 years (median, 8.6 years). Eighty patients had concurrent significant proliferative lesions consisting of atypical duct hyperplasia (*n*:54) or atypical lobular hyperplasia (ALH) or LCIS (*n*:10). During the course of follow-up, 43 patients (14%) had breast recurrences, 90% of which were detected by mammography. The risk of local failure was significantly lower in women who had radiotherapy (8.4%) than in those not irradiated (29.5%), and the median time was significantly longer in radiated patients (10 vs. 4.9 years). The presence of concurrent atypical duct or lobular hyperplasia or of LCIS did not have a significant effect on recurrence in the breast with DCIS. However, these lesions were associated with a substantially higher frequency of contralateral carcinoma, which occurred 4.4 times more often in women who had atypical duct hyperplasia associated with DCIS. The 15-year cumulative risk of developing contralateral carcinoma was 19% when atypical duct hyperplasia was present in the ipsilateral breast, and 4.1% when atypical hyperplasia was absent ($p <$ 0.01). An equally large differential was found for ALH and LCIS coexisting with DCIS (15-year cumulative risk, 22.7% vs. 6.5%), but the difference was not statistically significant.

Meta-analysis of Treatment

A meta-analysis of published reports compared recurrence rates for patients with DCIS after treatment with one of three modalities.[348] The summary recurrence rates were 1.4% (95% CI, 0.7 to 2.1), 8.9% (95% CI, 6.8 to 11.0), and 22.5% (95% CI, 16.9 to 28.2), respectively, for mastectomy, lumpectomy with radiotherapy, and lumpectomy alone. The proportions of invasive recurrence in each group were 76%, 50%, and 43%. The nearly threefold higher rate of recurrence after lumpectomy without radiotherapy compared with women who were radiated is especially striking in view of the likelihood that excision alone was most often recommended for patients with low grade, relatively small lesions with negative margins. The authors observed that "patients with risk factors of presence of necrosis, high-grade cytologic features or comedo subtype were found to derive the greatest improvement in local control" from the addition of radiotherapy to conservation surgery.

Selective Estrogen Receptor Modulator in DCIS

The role of Selective Estrogen Receptor Modulators (SERMs), specifically tamoxifen, in managing DCIS has been investigated in the UK/ANZ DCIS trial and also in the NSABP B24 trial. The UK/ANZ Trial comparing radiotherapy and tamoxifen in the treatment of DCIS showed a nonsignificant reduction in all breast events with the addition of tamoxifen and a RR reduction of 22% after 53 months of follow-up.[414]

The NSABP trial on the use of tamoxifen and radiotherapy in DCIS showed benefit, mainly due to reduction in ipsilateral recurrent invasive carcinoma.[415] The 7-year risk of local recurrence in the treated breast after lumpectomy with radiation was reduced from 11.1% without tamoxifen to 7.7% with tamoxifen ($p = 0.02$). The risk of all (ipsilateral and contralateral) breast cancer events was reduced from 16.9% to 10.0% ($p = 0.0003$). DCIS patients received radiotherapy and were then randomized to tamoxifen (20 mg/day) or placebo. After just over 6 years of follow-up, a significant reduction in all new breast cancer events was reported in the tamoxifen group compared with the placebo group. In a recent published follow-up study on the NSABP B24 trial with a median follow-up of 14.5 years,[416] it was reported that adjuvant tamoxifen significantly reduced the ipsilateral, as well as contralateral, risk of DCIS recurrence and/or progression to invasive breast carcinoma by about 50% in patients treated with lumpectomy and radiation, and that the benefit was restricted to patients with ER-positive DCIS (defined as those with an Allred score of 3 or more). Using this cutoff, 76% of DCIS were ER positive. Results for PR were comparatively less predictive of benefit. Thus, patients with ER-positive DCIS treated with tamoxifen (vs. placebo) showed significant decreases in subsequent breast cancer at 10 years (HR, 0.49; $p < 0.001$) and follow-up (HR, 0.60; $p = 0.003$), which remained significant in multivariate analysis (HR, 0.64; $p =$ 0.003). Results were similar, but less significant, when subsequent ipsilateral and contralateral breast carcinomas were considered. Thus, it is likely that SERM therapy will be routinely established in the treatment of appropriately selected ER-positive breast carcinoma patients. Based on data from the NSABP STAR trial, raloxifen offers less protection than tamoxifen for postmenopausal women.[417]

Summary of Treatment Recommendations

Patient survival, the appropriate endpoint for most malignant neoplasms, is the measure by which various therapy regimens are assessed. However, survival is of almost no utility in DCIS since the breast cancer–specific survival in DCIS exceeds 95%, regardless of treatment.[418] The *low mortality* due to DCIS itself is reflected in the 2009 NIH Consensus Statement recommending elimination of the "anxiety-producing term 'carcinoma' from the description of DCIS."[419] Recurrence of disease in either the *in situ* or the invasive form, particularly in the ipsilateral, but also in the contralateral, breast is the most commonly assessed data endpoint. In general, approximately one-half of local recurrences in DCIS cases are invasive carcinoma. Thus, the primary goal of treatment of DCIS is to reduce the risk of local recurrence.

The relatively *high morbidity* of at least some forms of the disease can be assessed by the wide variety of treatment recommendations that are available to any patient with DCIS. In current practice, DCIS is most commonly diagnosed as a result of the detection of a mammographic abnormality on routine screening in asymptomatic women. In such a situation, most patients have relatively limited disease and are eligible for breast conservation (i.e., maximal preservation of disease-free breast). The common breast conservation treatment options include lumpectomy alone, lumpectomy followed by radiation, or mastectomy. An SERM, such as tamoxifen, is the main systemic treatment option. Typically, most patients with DCIS do not require a mastectomy, and the majority of patients in the United States and elsewhere choose breast conservation.[420]

Treatment recommendations for DCIS are made on the basis of clinical and pathologic findings in consultation with the patient. Important considerations include the manner of clinical presentation (e.g., palpable, incidental, or mammographic), extent by mammography, size measured grossly or microscopically when possible, margin status of the lumpectomy, and histologic features of the DCIS such as nuclear grade, growth pattern (e.g., cribriform, comedo, solid, or papillary), and the presence or absence of necrosis. The issue is complicated by the many different combinations of these and other features that can occur in a given case.

Numerous studies cited indicate that margin status and the biologic characteristics of DCIS represented histologically by nuclear grade and the presence or absence of necrosis are the most important predictors of local recurrence in the breast after breast conservation with or without radiotherapy. Tumor size correlates well with the extent of the lesion and thus influences margin status. For example, Cheng et al.[421] reported positive lumpectomy margins in 15%, 28%, and 69% of patients with DCIS lesions measured as less than 1.0 cm, 1.0 to 2.4 cm, and 2.5 cm or larger, respectively. Biologic characteristics, at least partially reflected in the histologic appearance of DCIS, have a complex influence on the success of treatment by affecting the rate of growth (and to some extent the time to detection of clinical recurrences) and radiosensitivity of residual DCIS after lumpectomy. Consequently, it is possible for patients with comparable amounts of incompletely excised residual high-grade (comedo) and low-grade (cribriform) DCIS who receive the same treatment to have similar absolute risks for breast recurrence, but they may differ in time to clinical detection of recurrence, especially of invasive lesions, and in responsiveness to radiotherapy or antiestrogens. Follow-up for more than 10 years of large uniformly treated patient groups with diverse types of DCIS will be needed to reliably assess the interplay of these factors.

Retrospective and prospective randomized studies reviewed in detail in this chapter have demonstrated that radiotherapy after excisional surgery reduces the chance of recurrence in the breast by about 50%. The degree to which a reduced frequency of breast recurrence contributes to overall survival remains to be determined for patients with DCIS. The possibility that there could be a survival advantage conferred by reducing breast recurrences is suggested by a meta-analysis of randomized studies of radiotherapy and breast conservation in women with invasive breast carcinoma that detected this beneficial effect.[422]

The addition of a selective ER modulator such as tamoxifen to breast conservation therapy reduces breast recurrences in women with ER-positive DCIS.[423] In the randomized NSABP B24 trial, the 7-year risk of breast recurrence was 7.7% with lumpectomy and radiation plus tamoxifen and 11.1% after lumpectomy and radiation alone.[387]

From the foregoing review, it is clear that, as a group, patients with DCIS benefit from the addition of radiotherapy to breast-conserving surgery because the breast recurrence rate is reduced by about 50%. Radiotherapy is usually indicated for any of the following circumstances: high-grade DCIS, when margins are close (variously described as 10 mm or less), and for patients younger than 50 years. Tamoxifen may be added for hormone receptor–positive DCIS. Omitting radiotherapy is a consideration for women older than 50 years with a widely clear margin (variously defined as more than 10 mm) and low-grade histology without necrosis. This type of DCIS is very likely to be hormone receptor positive and, therefore, amenable to adjuvant tamoxifen treatment. However, this approach is not without risk as described by Wong et al.,[378] who reported an in-breast recurrence rate of 2.4% per patient-year of follow-up and a projected 5-year breast recurrence rate of 12%.

Mammography is an essential component of the clinical follow-up of women treated by breast-conserving surgery with or without radiotherapy and/or tamoxifen.[248] In one series of 162 women, 33 (20%) developed recurrent ipsilateral carcinoma 6 to 168 months (median, 26) after primary therapy.[424] Review of mammograms from 20 patients with recurrent carcinoma revealed that 17 (85%) of the recurrences were detected solely on the basis of calcifications, which had a pattern similar to that of calcifications seen prior to the initial excision in 82% of cases. DCIS alone was present in 65% of recurrences, whereas 35% also had invasive carcinoma. Particular attention should be paid to the mammographic follow-up of the contralateral breast in women with atypical hyperplasia or LCIS coexisting with DCIS. The role of routine MRI screening in the follow-up of women with DCIS, treated by breast conservation, remains to be determined.

Some patients may choose mastectomy, even if they are candidates for breast conservation. Mastectomy is preferable for the patient with such widespread DCIS that negative margins cannot be achieved with a cosmetically acceptable surgical procedure. Many but not all of these patients have dispersed calcifications on mammography. Lumpectomy with or without radiation will suffice for most women with DCIS limited to a single focus on the basis of pathologic and clinical findings, if the margins of excision are negative, if the lesion is not comedo type with necrosis and high nuclear grade, and if the lesion is small (variously defined as less than 1.0 cm or less than 2.5 cm). Radiation after lumpectomy is recommended regardless of size if the DCIS has high nuclear grade, necrosis, or is distinctively of the comedocarcinoma type, and if the margins are indeterminate or are involved.

The assessment of margins is only a guide to and not a precise measurement of the completeness of excision for DCIS. This was demonstrated by Silverstein et al.,[425] who compared the findings in reexcision specimens from patients who had positive and who had negative margins in their initial excisional biopsy specimens. Although the chance of finding residual DCIS was significantly greater if the original margins were positive, 43% of those with initially negative margins had carcinoma in the reexcision. There was also a higher risk (76%) for residual DCIS if the primary focus was 2.5 cm or larger, but residual carcinoma was present in 57% of reexcisions for lesions smaller than 2.5 cm. Goldstein et al.[426] analyzed the quantitative relationship between the amount of DCIS in a lumpectomy and in the subsequent reexcision. The study was based on 98 patients who had a reexcision performed after a lumpectomy for DCIS. Residual DCIS was present in 52 reexcision specimens (53%). Features that were significantly related to finding DCIS in the reexcision were multifocal involvement of margins by DCIS or by DCIS extending into TDLUs and extensive DCIS represented by the number of slides with the lesion. When DCIS was limited to one or two slides in the initial excision, no DCIS was detected in 62% of reexcisions, whereas DCIS was present in 100% of excisions after initial biopsies with DCIS in more than six slides.

It must be reemphasized that methods for the quantitation of DCIS are imprecise. No method for measuring the size of DCIS has gained wide acceptance. Lagios[267] has observed that "quantitation, or better, estimating the extent of DCIS, should be a collaborative exercise between mammographer and pathologist, but is more a fictional practice than a reliable fact." For this and other reasons summarized by Schnitt et al.,[427] classifications proposed to determine the treatment of DCIS such as the VNPI, which depend on and offer precise size categories, may be viewed, at best, as general guidelines rather than as strict criteria for making therapeutic decisions.

Axillary dissection is not indicated in the majority of patients with DCIS.[428] Some low ALNs may be taken with the axillary tail of the breast in the course of a mastectomy. If the lesion is extensive, DCIS, especially comedo type with marked duct distortion, it would be prudent to perform SLN mapping because of concern for undetected invasion. Micrometastases were detected in axillary SLNs from 4 (4.6%) of 87 patients with DCIS studied by Haigh and Giuliano[429] and in 11 (7.3%) of 150 patients reported by Cox et al.[430] As noted by Haigh and Giuliano,[429] "if metastases are detected, microinvasion can be assumed."

Treatment for the majority of patients with microinvasive duct carcinoma previously described in the literature has been mastectomy, as discussed earlier in this chapter. The outcome overall was relatively favorable after mastectomy, but the studies were not directly comparable because of differing criteria for defining microinvasion. Patients treated by breast conservation therapy were described in several reports with results indicating that this was equally as effective as mastectomy. These and other published reports indicate that the presence of microinvasion, as variously defined in the past or as currently described in the TNM staging system (T1*mic*), probably has little independent impact on the effectiveness of conservation for local control in the breast. The characteristics of the DCIS that are associated with microinvasion, such as high grade, the presence of necrosis, and lesion size, are crucial determinants for treatment. The significance of multiple microinvasive foci is yet to be determined. The finding of microinvasion will lead to ALN staging, often by SLN mapping, in many patients prior to consideration of systemic therapy.[430]

Advances in the understanding of molecular biology of breast carcinoma progression and the development of novel pathway-specific targeted therapy has led to the emergence of molecular-based individually tailored treatment planning for invasive breast carcinoma. Increasing understanding of molecular pathobiology of breast carcinoma progression underlies the potential of molecular-based "tailored" therapy.[431] Thus far, such advances have not affected the practical management of DCIS. However, the routine testing of ER and PR, as well as the emerging adoption of HER2 and gene signature testing, herald the emergence of such a therapeutic approach for DCIS.[432]

Novel approaches for the management of DCIS are under investigation. As hypothesized by Espina and Liotta, "the survival of DCIS cells in the hypoxic, nutrient-dependent intraductal niche could promote genetic instability and the derepression of the invasive phenotype." Thus, "understanding of potential survival mechanisms, such as autophagy, which might be functioning in DCIS lesions, provides strategies for arresting invasion at the premalignant stage."[433] The potential utility of ductoscopy in detecting occult intraductal lesions, and of ductoscopically guided lumpectomy, is under investigation and could potentially lead to more targeted lumpectomy procedures.[434]

The treatment of DCIS continues to evolve[435] and, in at least a proportion of cases, remains a "conundrum."[436] It is likely that various nomograms[415] and molecular marker studies[437] will assume an increasingly significant role in its management. Advances in various forms of radiologic screening, and refinements therein, will likely optimize the detection of DCIS, that is, breast carcinoma in its earliest form.[438,439]

REFERENCES

1. Broders AC. Carcinoma *in situ* contrasted with benign penetrating epithelium. *JAMA* 1932;99:1670–1674.
2. Warren JC. Abnormal involution of the mammary gland with its treatment by operation. *Am J Med Sci* 1907;134:521–535.
3. Cheatle GL. Cysts and primary cancer in cysts of the breast. *Br J Surg* 1920–1921;8:149–166.
4. Bloodgood JC. The pathology of chronic cystic mastitis of the female breast. *Arch Surg* 1921;3:445–542.
5. Bloodgood JC. Border-line breast tumors. *Ann Surg* 1931;93:235–249.
6. Muir R. The evolution of carcinoma of the mamma. *J Pathol Bacteriol* 1941;52:155–172.
7. Schultz-Brauns O. Die geschwulste der Brustbrüse. In: Henke F, Lubarsch O, eds. *Handbuch der speziellen Pathologischen Anatomie und Histologie, VII*. Berlin: Verlag von Julius Springer, 1933.
8. Bloodgood JC. Comedo carcinoma or comedo-adenoma of the female breast. *Am J Cancer* 1934;22:842–853.
9. Lewis D, Geschickter CF. Comedocarcinoma of the breast. *Arch Surg* 1938;36:225–244.
10. Cheatle GL, Cutler M. Tumors of the breast. *Their pathology, symptoms, diagnosis, and treatment.* Philadelphia: JB Lippincott, 1931.
11. Fechner RE. One century of mammary carcinoma *in situ*. What have we learned? *Am J Clin Pathol* 1993;100:654–661.
12. Farante G, Zurrida S, Galimberti V, et al. The management of ductal intraepithelial neoplasia (DIN): open controversies and guidelines of

the Istituto Europeo di Oncologia (IEO), Milan, Italy. *Breast Cancer Res Treat* 2011;128:369–378.
13. Lakhani SR, Ellis IO, Schnitt SJ, et al. *WHO classification of tumours of the breast*. 4th ed. Lyon: World Health Organization-IARC, 2012.
14. www.cancer.org/cancer/breastcancer/detailedguide. Accessed June 30, 2013.
15. Sacchini V, Fortunato L, Cody III HS, et al. Breast ductal carcinoma *in situ*. *Int J Surg Oncol* 2012;2012:753267.
16. Rosen PP. The pathological classification of human mammary carcinoma: past, present and future. *Ann Clin Lab Sci* 1979;9:144–156.
17. Smart CR, Myers MH, Gloecker LA. Implications from SEER data on breast cancer management. *Cancer* 1978;41:787–789.
18. Ernster VL, Barclay J, Kerlikowske K, et al. Incidence of and treatment for ductal carcinoma *in situ* of the breast. *JAMA* 1996;275:913–918.
19. Ernster VL, Barclay J. Increases in ductal carcinoma *in situ* (DCIS) of the breast in relation to mammography: a dilemma. *J Natl Cancer Inst Monogr* 1997;(22):151–156.
20. Winchester DJ, Menck HR, Winchester DP. National treatment trends for ductal carcinoma *in situ* of the breast. *Arch Surg* 1997;132:660–665.
21. Blichert-Toft M, Graversen HP, Andersen J, et al. *In situ* breast carcinomas: a population-based study on frequency, growth pattern, and clinical aspects. *World J Surg* 1988;12:845–851.
22. Ward BA, McKhann CF, Ravikumar TS. Ten-year follow-up of breast carcinoma *in situ* in Connecticut. *Arch Surg* 1992;127:1392–1395.
23. Adams-Cameron M, Gilliland FD, Hunt WC, et al. Trends in incidence and treatment for ductal carcinoma *in situ* in Hispanic, American Indian, and non-Hispanic white women in New Mexico, 1973–1994. *Cancer* 1999;85:1084–1090.
24. Shamliyan T, Wang SY, Virnig BA, et al. Association between patient and tumor characteristics with clinical outcomes in women with ductal carcinoma *in situ*. *J Natl Cancer Inst Monogr* 2010;2010(41):121–129.
25. Chu KC, Tarone RE, Kessler LG, et al. Recent trends in U.S. breast cancer incidence, survival, and mortality rates. *J Natl Cancer Inst* 1996;88:1571–1579.
26. Virnig BA, Tuttle TM, Shamliyan T, et al. Ductal carcinoma *in situ* of the breast: a systematic review of incidence, treatment, and outcomes. *J Natl Cancer Inst* 2010;102:170–178.
27. Kerlikowske K, Barclay J, Grady D, et al. Comparison of risk factors for ductal carcinoma *in situ* and invasive breast cancer. *J Natl Cancer Inst* 1997;89:76–82.
28. Weiss HA, Brinton LA, Brogan D, et al. Epidemiology of *in situ* and invasive breast cancer in women aged under 45. *Br J Cancer* 1996;73:1298–1305.
29. Virnig BA, Wang SY, Shamilyan T, et al. Ductal carcinoma *in situ*: risk factors and impact of screening. *J Natl Cancer Inst Monogr* 2010;2010(41):113–116.
30. Frank TS, Deffenbaugh AM, Reid JE, et al. Clinical characteristics of individuals with germline mutations in BRCA1 and BRCA2: analysis of 10,000 individuals. *J Clin Oncol* 2002;20:1480–1490.
31. Hall MJ, Reid JE, Wenstrup RJ. Prevalence of BRCA1 and BRCA2 mutations in women with breast carcinoma *in situ* and referred for genetic testing. *Cancer Prev Res* (Phila) 2010;3:1579–1585.
32. Ciatto S, Bonardi R, Cataliotti L, et al. Intraductal breast carcinoma. Review of a multicenter series of 350 cases. *Tumori* 1990;76:552–554.
33. Ernster VL, Ballard-Barbash R, Barlow WE, et al. Detection of ductal carcinoma *in situ* in women undergoing screening mammography. *J Natl Cancer Inst* 2002;94:1546–1554.
34. Andersson I. Breast cancer screening in Malmo. *Recent Results in Cancer Res* 1984;90:114–116.
35. Andersson I, Andren L, Hildell J, et al. Breast cancer screening with mammography. A population-based randomized trial with mammography as the only screening mode. *Radiology* 1979;132:273–276.
36. Hendricks JHCL. *Population Screening for Breast Cancer by Means of Mammography in Nijmegen*, 1975–1982. [M.D. Thesis]. Nijmegen University; 1982.
37. Lewis JD, Milbrath JR, Shaffer KA, et al. Implications of suspicious findings in breast cancer screening. *Arch Surg* 1975;110:903–907.
38. Sigfusson BF, Anderson I, Aspergren K, et al. Clustered breast calcifications. *Acta Radiol* 1983;24:273–281.
39. Tabar L, Akerlund E, Gad A. Five-year experience with single-view mammography randomized controlled screening in Sweden. *Recent Results in Cancer Res* 1984;90:105–113.
40. Verbeek ALM, Hendriks JHCL, Holland R, et al. Reduction of breast cancer mortality through mass screening with modern mammography: first results of the Nijmegen Project, 1975–1981. *Lancet* 1984;1:1222–1224.
41. Ciatto S, Cataliotti L, Distante V. Nonpalpable lesions detected with mammography: review of 512 consecutive cases. *Radiology* 1987;165:99–102.
42. Meyer JS. Cell kinetics of histologic variants of *in situ* breast carcinoma. *Breast Cancer Res Treat* 1986;7:171–180.
43. Patchefsky AS, Shaber GS, Schwartz GF, et al. The pathology of breast cancer detected by mass population screening. *Cancer* 1977;40:1659–1670.
44. Dershaw DD, Abramson A, Kinne DW. Ductal carcinoma *in situ*: mammographic findings and clinical implications. *Radiology* 1989;170:411–415.
45. Ikeda DM, Andersson I. Atypical mammographic presentation of ductal carcinoma *in situ*. *Radiology* 1989;172:661–666.
46. Stomper PC, Connolly JL, Meyer JE, et al. Clinically occult ductal carcinoma *in situ* detected with mammography: analysis of 100 cases with radiologic–pathologic correlation. *Radiology* 1989;172:235–241.
47. D'Orsi CJ. Imaging for the diagnosis and management of ductal carcinoma *in situ*. *J Natl Cancer Inst Monogr* 2010;2010(41):214–217.
48. Carlson KL, Helvie MA, Roubidoux MA, et al. Relationship between mammographic screening intervals and size and histology of ductal carcinoma *in situ*. *AJR Am J Roentgenol* 1999;172:313–317.
49. Holland R, Hendriks JHCL, Verbeek ALM, et al. Extent, distribution, and mammographic/histological correlations of breast ductal carcinoma *in situ*. *Lancet* 1990;335:519–522.
50. Lagios MD. Multicentricity of breast carcinoma demonstrated by routine correlated subgross and radiographic examination. *Cancer* 1977;40:1726–1734.
51. Stomper PC, Connolly JL. Ductal carcinoma *in situ* of the breast: correlation between mammographic calcification and tumor subtype. *AJR Am J Roentgenol* 1992;159:483–485.
52. Parker J, Dance DR, Davies DH, et al. Classification of ductal carcinoma *in situ* by image analysis of calcifications from digital mammograms. *Br J Radiol* 1995;68:150–159.
53. Evans A, Pinder S, Wilson R, et al. Ductal carcinoma *in situ* of the breast: correlation between mammographic and pathologic findings. *AJR Am J Roentgenol* 1994;162:1307–1311.
54. Evans AJ, Pinder SE, Ellis IO, et al. Correlations between the mammographic features of ductal carcinoma *in situ* (DCIS) and c-erb-s oncogene expression. *Clin Radiol* 1994;49:559–562.
55. Han JS, Molberg KH, Sarode V. Predictors of invasion and axillary lymph node metastasis in patients with a core biopsy diagnosis of ductal carcinoma *in situ*: an analysis of 255 cases. *Breast J* 2011;17:223–229.
56. Ciatto S, Grazzini G, Iossa A, et al. *In situ* ductal carcinoma of the breast—analysis of clinical presentation and outcome in 156 consecutive cases. *Eur J Surg Oncol* 1990;16:220–224.
57. Mitnick JS, Roses DF, Harris MN, et al. Circumscribed intraductal carcinoma of the breast. *Radiology* 1989;170:423–425.
58. Park JS, Park YM, Kim EK, et al. Sonographic findings of high-grade and non-high-grade ductal carcinoma *in situ* of the breast. *J Ultrasound Med* 2010;29:1687–1697.
59. Reiff DB, Cooke J, Griffin M, et al. Ductal carcinoma *in situ* presenting as a stellate lesion on mammography. *Clin Radiology* 1994;49:396–399.
60. Menell JH, Morris EA, Dershaw DD, et al. Determination of the presence and extent of pure ductal carcinoma *in situ* by mammography and magnetic resonance imaging. *Breast J* 2005;11:382–390.
61. Gilles R, Zafrani B, Guinebretiere J-M,et al. Ductal carcinoma *in situ*: MR imaging-histopathologic correlation. *Radiology* 1995;196:415–419.
62. Orel S, Schnall M, Livolsi V, et al. Suspicious breast lesions: MR imaging with radiologic–pathologic correlation. *Radiology* 1994;190:485–493.
63. Heywang-Köbrunner S. Contrast-enhanced magnetic resonance imaging of the breast. *Invest Radiol* 1994;29:94–104.
64. Orel SG, Mendonca MH, Reynolds C, et al. MR imaging of ductal carcinoma *in situ*. *Radiology* 1997;202:413–420.
65. Pediconi F, Catalano C, Roselli A, et al. Contrast-enhanced MR mammography for evaluation of the contralateral breast in patients with diagnosed unilateral breast cancer or high-risk lesions. *Radiology* 2007;243:670–680.
66. Londero V, Zuiani C, Linda A, et al. High-risk breast lesions at imaging-guided needle biopsy: usefulness of MRI for treatment decision. *AJR Am J Roentgenol* 2012;199:W240–W250.
67. Kuhl CK. Why do purely intraductal cancers enhance on breast MR images? *Radiology* 2009;253:281–283.

68. Howard JH, Bland KI. Current management and treatment strategies for breast cancer. *Curr Opin Obstet Gynecol* 2012;24:44–48.
69. Lehman CD. Magnetic resonance imaging in the evaluation of ductal carcinoma *in situ*. *J Natl Cancer Inst Monogr* 2010;2010(41):150–151.
70. Kuhl C, Weigel S, Schrading S, et al. Prospective multicenter cohort study to refine management recommendations for women at elevated familial risk of breast cancer: the EVA trial. *J Clin Oncol* 2010;28:1450–1457.
71. Itakura K, Lessing J, Sakata T, et al. The impact of preoperative magnetic resonance imaging on surgical treatment and outcomes for ductal carcinoma *in situ*. *Clin Breast Cancer* 2011;11:33–38.
72. Ashikari R, Hajdu SI, Robbins GF. Intraductal carcinoma of the breast (1960–1969). *Cancer* 1971;28:1182–1187.
73. Westbrook KC, Gallager HS. Intraductal carcinoma of the breast. A comparative study. *Am J Surg* 1975;130:667–670.
74. Pandya S, Mackarem G, Lee AKC, et al. Ductal carcinoma *in situ*: the impact of screening on clinical presentation and pathologic features. *Breast J* 1998;4:146–151.
75. Rosen PP, Ashikari R, Thaler H, et al. A comparative study of some pathologic features of mammary carcinoma in Tokyo, Japan and New York, USA. *Cancer* 1977;39:429–434.
76. Patchefsky AS, Schwartz GF, Finkelstein SD, et al. Heterogeneity of intraductal carcinoma of the breast. *Cancer* 1989;63:731–741.
77. Rosen P, Snyder RE, Urban JA, et al. Correlation of suspicious mammograms and X-rays of breast biopsies during surgery. Results in 60 cases. *Cancer* 1973;31:656–660.
78. Snyder R, Rosen P. Radiography of breast specimens. *Cancer* 1971;28:1608–1611.
79. Rosen PP. Frozen section diagnosis of breast lesions. Recent experience with 556 consecutive biopsies. *Ann Surg* 1978;187:17–19.
80. Cheng L, Al-Kaisi NK, Liu AY, et al. The results of intraoperative consultations in 181 ductal carcinomas *in situ* of the breast. *Cancer* 1997;80:75–79.
81. Rosen PP, Senie R, Schottenfeld D, et al. Noninvasive breast carcinoma: frequency of unsuspected invasion and implication for treatment. *Ann Surg* 1979;189:98–103.
82. Jorns JM, Visscher D, Sabel M, et al. Intraoperative frozen section analysis of margins in breast conserving surgery significantly decreases reoperative rates: one-year experience at an ambulatory surgical center. *Am J Clin Pathol* 2012;138:657–669.
83. Tramm T, Zuckerman K, Tavassoli FA. Skip lesion of DIN (DCIS) in the nipple in a case of breast cancer. *Int J Surg Pathol* 2011;19: 817–821.
84. Tunon-de-Lara C, André G, Macgrogan G, et al. Ductal carcinoma *in situ* of the breast: influence of age on diagnostic, therapeutic, and prognostic features. Retrospective study of 812 patients. *Ann Surg Oncol* 2011;18:1372–1379.
85. Bayraktar S, Elsayegh N, Gutierrez Barrera AM, et al. Predictive factors for BRCA1/BRCA2 mutations in women with ductal carcinoma *in situ*. *Cancer* 2012;118:1515–1522.
86. Bellamy COC, McDonald C, Salter DM, et al. Noninvasive ductal carcinoma of the breast: the relevance of histologic categorization. *Hum Pathol* 1993;24:16–23.
87. Silverstein MJ, Waisman JR, Gamagami P, et al. Intraductal carcinoma of the breast (208 cases): clinical factors influencing treatment choice. *Cancer* 1990;66:102–108.
88. Brown PW, Silverman J, Owens E, et al. Intraductal "noninfiltrating" carcinoma of the breast. *Arch Surg* 1976;111:1063–1067.
89. Urban JA. Biopsy of the "normal" breast in treating breast cancer. *Surg Clin North Am* 1969;49:291–301.
90. Ringberg A, Palmer B, Linell F. The contralateral breast at reconstructive surgery after breast cancer operation—a histological study. *Breast Cancer Res Treat* 1982;2:151–161.
91. Griffin A, Frazee RC. Treatment of intraductal breast cancer—noncomedo type. *Am Surg* 1993;59:106–109.
92. Schuh ME, Nemoto T, Penetrante RB, et al. Intraductal carcinoma. Analysis of presentation, pathologic findings, and outcome of disease. *Arch Surg* 1986;121:1303–1307.
93. Schwartz GF, Patchefsky AS, Finklestein SD, et al. Nonpalpable *in situ* ductal carcinoma of the breast. Predictors of multicentricity and microinvasion and implications for treatment. *Arch Surg* 1989;124:29–32.
94. Habel LA, Moe RE, Daling JR, et al. Risk of contralateral breast cancer among women with carcinoma *in situ* of the breast. *Ann Surg* 1997;225:69–75.
95. Webber BL, Heise H, Neifeld JP, et al. Risk of subsequent contralateral breast carcinoma in a population of patients with *in situ* breast carcinoma. *Cancer* 1981;47:2928–2932.
96. Gump FE, Jicha DL, Ozello L. Ductal carcinoma *in situ* (DCIS): a revised concept. *Surgery* 1987;102:790–795.
97. Andersen JA, Nielsen M, Blichert-Toft M. The growth pattern of *in situ* carcinoma in the female breast. *Acta Oncol* 1988;27:739–743.
98. Wellings SR, Jensen HM, Marcum RG. An atlas of subgross pathology of the human breast with special reference to possible precancerous lesions. *J Natl Cancer Inst* 1975;55:231–273.
99. Barsky SH, Siegal GP, Jannotta F, et al. Loss of basement membrane components by invasive tumors but not by their benign counterparts. *Lab Invest* 1983;49:140–147.
100. Henning K, Berndt A, Katenkamp D, et al. Loss of laminin-5 in the epithelium-stroma interface: an immunohistochemical marker of malignancy in epithelial lesions of the breast. *Histopathology* 1999;34:305–309.
101. Bose S, Lesser ML, Norton L, et al. Immunophenotype of intraductal carcinoma. *Arch Pathol Lab Med* 1996;100:81–85.
102. Sternlicht MD, Kedeshian P, Shao ZM, et al. The human myoepithelial cell is a natural tumor suppressor. *Clin Cancer Res* 1997;3:1949–1958.
103. Barsky SH. Myoepithelial mRNA expression profiling reveals a common tumor-suppressor phenotype. *Exp Mol Pathol* 2003;74:113–122.
104. Nguyen M, Lee MC, Wang JL, et al. The human myoepithelial cell displays a multifaceted anti-angiogenic phenotype. *Oncogene* 2000;19:3449–3459.
105. Shao ZM, Nguyen M. Alpaugh ML, et al. The human myoepithelial cell exerts antiproliferative effects on breast carcinoma cells characterized by p21WAF1/CIP1 induction, G2/M arrest, and apoptosis. *Exp Cell Res* 1998;241:394–403.
106. Zou Z, Anisowicz A, Hendrix MJ, et al. Maspin, a serpin with tumor-suppressing activity in human mammary epithelial cells. *Science* 1994;263:526–529.
107. Adriance MC, Inman JL, Peterson OW, et al. Myoepithelial cells: good fences make good neighbors. *Breast Cancer Res* 2005;7:190–197.
108. Allinen M, Beroukhim R, Cai L, et al. Molecular characterization of the tumor microenvironment in breast cancer. *Cancer Cell* 2004;6:17–32.
109. Smith MC, Luker KE, Garbow JR, et al. CXCR4 regulates growth of both primary and metastatic breast cancer. *Cancer Res* 2004;64:8604–8612.
110. Muller A, Homey B, Soto H, et al. Involvement of chemokine receptors in breast cancer metastasis. *Nature* 2001;410:50–56.
111. Kawasaki T, Nakamura S, Sakamoto G, et al. Neuroendocrine ductal carcinoma *in situ* (NE-DCIS) of the breast—comparative clinicopathological study of 20 NE-DCIS cases and 274 non-NE-DCIS cases. *Histopathology* 2008;53:288–298.
112. Farshid G, Moinfar F, Meredith DJ, et al. Spindle cell ductal carcinoma *in situ*. An unusual variant of ductal intra-epithelial neoplasia that simulates ductal hyperplasia or a myoepithelial proliferation. *Virchows Arch* 2001;439:70–77.
113. Allred DC, Wu Y, Mao S, et al. Ductal carcinoma *in situ* and the emergence of diversity during breast cancer evolution. *Clin Cancer Res* 2008;14:370–378.
114. Jansen SA. Ductal carcinoma *in situ*: detection, diagnosis, and characterization with magnetic resonance imaging. *Semin Ultrasound CT MR* 2011;32:306–318.
115. Lennington WJ, Jensen RA, Dalton LW, et al. Ductal carcinoma *in situ* of the breast. Heterogeneity of individual lesions. *Cancer* 1994;73:118–124.
116. Azzopardi JG, Ahmed A, Millis RR. *Problems in breast pathology*. (*Major Problems in Pathology*, vol. 11). Philadelphia: W.B. Saunders, 1979:192–203.
117. Castellano I, Marchiò C, Tomatis M, et al. Micropapillary ductal carcinoma *in situ* of the breast: an inter-institutional study. *Mod Pathol* 2010;23:260–269.
118. Aulmann S, Braun L, Mietzsch F, et al. Transitions between flat epithelial atypia and low-grade ductal carcinoma *in situ* of the breast. *Am J Surg Pathol* 2012;36:1247–1252.
119. Jain RK, Mehta R, Dimitrov R, et al. Atypical ductal hyperplasia: interobserver and intraobserver variability. *Mod Pathol* 2011;24:917–923.
120. Wen P, Marsh WL. SMMHC-p63 cocktail improves detection of myoepithelial layer in high-grade ductal carcinoma *in-situ*. *Mod Pathol* 2005;18(Suppl.):54a–55a.
121. Martin HM, Bateman AC, Theaker JM. Calcium oxalate (Weddellite) crystals within ductal carcinoma *in situ*. *J Clin Pathol* 1999;52:932.

122. Singh N, Theaker JM. Calcium oxalate crystals (Weddellite) within the secretions of ductal carcinoma *in situ*—a rare phenomenon. *J Clin Pathol* 1999;52:145–146.
123. Lomme MM, Steinhoff MM. Intraluminal crystalloids in benign breast ducts. *Breast J* 2005;11:510.
124. Mayr NA, Staples JJ, Robinson RA, et al. Morphometric studies in intraductal breast carcinoma using computerized image analysis. *Cancer* 1991;67:2805–2812.
125. Lindley R, Bulman A, Parsons P, et al. Histologic features predictive of an increased risk of early local recurrence after treatment of breast cancer by local tumor excision and radical radiotherapy. *Surgery* 1989;105:13–20.
126. Bodis S, Siziopikou KP, Schnitt SJ, et al. Extensive apoptosis in ductal carcinoma *in situ* of the breast. *Cancer* 1996;77:1831–1835.
127. Harn HJ, Shen KL, Yueh KC, et al. Apoptosis occurs more frequently in intraductal carcinoma than in infiltrating duct carcinoma of human breast cancer and correlates with altered p53 expression: detected by terminal-deoxynucleotidyl-transferase-mediated dUTP-FITC nick end labelling (TUNEL). *Histopathology* 1997;31:534–539.
128. Quinn CM, Ostrowski JL, Harkins L, et al. Loss of bcl-2 expression in ductal carcinoma *in situ* of the breast relates to poor histological differentiation and to expression of p53 and c-erbB-2 proteins. *Histopathology* 1998;33:531–536.
129. Sneige N, Lagios MD, Schwarting R, et al. Interobserver reproducibility of the Lagios nuclear grading system for ductal carcinoma *in situ*. *Hum Pathol* 1999;30:257–262.
130. Muir R, Aitkenhead AC. The healing of intraduct carcinoma of the mamma. *J Pathol Bacteriol* 1934;38:117–127.
131. Davies JD. Hyperelastosis, obliteration and fibrous plaques in major ducts of the human breast. *J Pathol* 1973;110:13–26.
132. Kim HS, Kim GY, Kim YW, et al. Stromal CD10 expression and relationship to the E-cadherin/beta-catenin complex in breast carcinoma. *Histopathology* 2010;56:708–719.
133. Witkiewicz AK, Freydin B, Chervoneva I, et al. Stromal CD10 and SPARC expression in ductal carcinoma *in situ* (DCIS) patients predicts disease recurrence. *Cancer Biol Ther* 2010;10:391–396.
134. Bagaria SP, Shamonki J, Kinnaird M, et al. The florid subtype of lobular carcinoma *in situ*: marker of precursor for invasive lobular carcinoma. *Ann Surg Oncol* 2011;18:1845–1851.
135. de Deus Moura R, Wludarski SC, Carvalho FM, et al. Immunohistochemistry applied to the differential diagnosis between ductal and lobular carcinoma of the breast. *Appl Immunohistochem Mol Morphol* 2013;21:1–12.
136. Chan JKC, Ng WF. Sclerosing adenosis cancerized by intraductal carcinoma. *Pathology* 1987;19:425–428.
137. Eusebi V, Collina G, Bussolati G. Carcinoma *in situ* in sclerosing adenosis of the breast: an immunocytochemical study. *Semin Diagn Pathol* 1989;6:146–152.
138. Oberman HA, Markey BA. Non-invasive carcinoma of the breast presenting in adenosis. *Mod Pathol* 1991;4:31–35.
139. Ichihara S, Aoyama H. Intraductal carcinoma of the breast arising in sclerosing adenosis. Case report. *Pathol Int* 1994;44:722–726.
140. Moritani S, Ichihara S, Hasegawa M, et al. Topographical, morphological and immunohistochemical characteristics of carcinoma *in situ* of the breast involving sclerosing adenosis. Two distinct topographical patterns and histological types of carcinoma *in situ*. *Histopathology* 2011;58:835–846.
141. Taylor HB, Norris HJ. Epithelial invasion of nerves in benign diseases of the breast. *Cancer* 1967;20:2245–2249.
142. Tsang WYW, Chan JKC. Neural invasion in intraductal carcinoma of the breast. *Hum Pathol* 1992;23:202–204.
143. Bianchi S, Giannotti E, Vanzi E, et al. Radial scar without associated atypical epithelial proliferation on image-guided 14-gauge needle core biopsy: analysis of 49 cases from a single-centre and review of the literature. *Breast* 2012;21:159–164.
144. Resetkova E, Edelweiss M, Albarracin CT, et al. Management of radial sclerosing lesions of the breast diagnosed using percutaneous vacuum-assisted core needle biopsy: recommendations for excision based on seven years of experience at a single institution. *Breast Cancer Res Treat* 2011;127:335–343.
145. Rosen PP. Coexistent lobular carcinoma *in situ* and intraductal carcinoma in a single lobular-duct unit. *Am J Surg Pathol* 1980;4:241–246.
146. Dundar MM, Badve S, Bilgin G, et al. Computerized classification of intraductal breast lesions using histopathological images. *IEEE Trans Biomed Eng* 2011;58:1977–1984.
147. Collins LC, Tamimi RM, Baer HJ, et al. Outcome of patients with ductal carcinoma *in situ* untreated after diagnostic biopsy: results from the Nurses' Health Study. *Cancer* 2005;103:1778–1784.
148. Sanders ME, Schuyler PA, Dupont WD, et al. The natural history of low-grade ductal carcinoma *in situ* of the breast in women treated by biopsy only revealed over 30 years of long-term follow-up. *Cancer* 2005;103:2481–2484.
149. Goldstein NS, Murphy TM. Intraductal carcinoma associated with invasive carcinoma of the breast: a comparison of the two lesions with implications for intraductal carcinoma classification systems. *Am J Clin Pathol* 1996;106:312–318.
150. Shoker BS, Sloane JP. DCIS grading schemes and clinical implications. *Histopathology* 1999;35:393–400.
151. The Consensus Conference Committee. Consensus Conference on the classification of ductal carcinoma *in situ*. *Cancer* 1997;80:1798–1802.
152. Bryan BB, Schnitt SJ, Collins LC. Ductal carcinoma *in situ* with basal-like phenotype: a possible precursor to invasive basal-like breast cancer. *Mod Pathol* 2006;19:617–621.
153. Silverstein MJ, Poller DN, Waisman JR, et al. Prognostic classification of breast ductal carcinoma-*in-situ*. *Lancet* 1995;345:1154–1157.
154. Silverstein MJ, Lagios MD, Craig PH, et al. A prognostic index for ductal carcinoma *in situ* of the breast. *Cancer* 1996;77:2267–2274.
155. Douglas-Jones AG, Gupta SK, Attanoos RL, et al. A critical appraisal of six modern classifications of ductal carcinoma *in situ* of the breast (DCIS): correlation with grade of associated invasive carcinoma. *Histopathology* 1996;29:397–409.
156. Sloane JP, Amendoeira I, Apostolikas N, et al. Consistency achieved by 23 European pathologists in categorizing ductal carcinoma *in situ* of the breast using five classifications. European Commission Working Group on Breast Screening Pathology. *Hum Pathol* 1998;29:1056–1062.
157. Scott MA, Lagios MD, Axelsson K, et al. Ductal carcinoma *in situ* of the breast: reproducibility of histological subtype analysis. *Hum Pathol* 1997;28:967–973.
158. Schuh F, Biazús JV, Resetkova E, et al. Reproducibility of three classification systems of ductal carcinoma *in situ* of the breast using a web-based survey. *Pathol Res Pract* 2010;206:705–711.
159. Pinder SE, Duggan C, Ellis IO, et al. A new pathological system for grading DCIS with improved prediction of local recurrence: results from the UKCCCR/ANZ DCIS trial. *Br J Cancer* 2010;103:94–100.
160. Balleine RL, Webster LR, Davis S, et al. Molecular grading of ductal carcinoma *in situ* of the breast. *Clin Cancer Res* 2008;14: 8244–8252.
161. Ottinetti A, Sapino A. Morphometric evaluation of microvessels surrounding hyperplastic and neoplastic mammary lesions. *Breast Cancer Res Treat* 1988;11:241–248.
162. Tamaki K, Sasano H, Maruo Y, et al. Vasohibin-1 as a potential predictor of aggressive behavior of ductal carcinoma *in situ* of the breast. *Cancer Sci* 2010;101:1051–1058.
163. Weidner N, Semple JP, Welch WR, et al. Tumor angiogenesis and metastasis—correlation in invasive breast cancer. *N Engl J Med* 1991;324:1–8.
164. Guidi AJ, Fischer L, Harris JR, et al. Microvessel density and distribution in ductal carcinoma *in situ* of the breast. *J Natl Cancer Inst* 1994;86:614–619.
165. Heffelfinger SC, Yassin R, Miller MA, et al. Vascularity of proliferative breast disease and carcinoma *in situ* correlates with histological features. *Clin Cancer Res* 1996;2:1873–1878.
166. Guidi AJ, Schnitt SJ. Angiogenesis in preinvasive lesions of the breast. *Breast J* 1996;2:364–369.
167. Engels K, Fox SB, Whitehouse RM, et al. Distinct angiogenic patterns are associated with high-grade *in situ* ductal carcinomas of the breast. *J Pathol* 1997;181:207–212.
168. Sternlicht MD, Barksy SH. The myoepithelial defense: a host defense against cancer. *Med Hypotheses* 1997;48:37–46.
169. Barsky SH, Nguyen M, Grossman DA, et al. Myoepithelial cells limit DCIS metastasis by blocking invasion and angiogenesis. *Mod Pathol* 1997;10:16A.
170. Basset P, Okada A, Chenard MP, et al. Matrix metalloproteinases as stromal effectors of human carcinoma progression: therapeutic implications. *Matrix Biol* 1997;15:535–541.
171. Sternlicht MD, Safarians S, Rivera SP, et al. Characterizations of the extracellular matrix and proteinase inhibitor content of human myoepithelial tumors. *Lab Invest* 1996;74:781–796.

172. Guidi AJ, Schnitt SJ, Fischer L, et al. Vascular permeability factor (vascular endothelial growth factor) expression and angiogenesis in patients with ductal carcinoma *in situ* of the breast. *Cancer* 1997;80:1945–1953.
173. Carpenter PM, Chen WP, Mendez A, et al. Angiogenesis in the progression of breast ductal proliferations. *Int J Surg Pathol* 2011;19:335–341.
174. Adler EH, Sunkara JL, Patchefsky AS, et al. Predictors of disease progression in ductal carcinoma *in situ* of the breast and vascular patterns. *Hum Pathol* 2012;43:550–556.
175. Lari SA, Kuerer HM. Biological markers in DCIS and risk of breast recurrence: a systematic review. *J Cancer* 2011;2:232–261.
176. Hammond ME, Hayes DF, Dowsett M, et al. American Society of Clinical Oncology/College of American Pathologists guideline recommendations for immunohistochemical testing of estrogen and progesterone receptors in breast cancer. *J Clin Oncol* 2010;28:2784–2795.
177. Lesser ML, Rosen PP, Senie RT, et al. Estrogen and progesterone receptors in breast carcinoma: correlations with epidemiology and pathology. *Cancer* 1981;48:299–309.
178. Barnes R, Masood S. Potential value of hormone receptor assay in carcinoma *in situ* of breast. *Am J Clin Pathol* 1990;94:533–537.
179. Bur ME, Zimarowski MJ, Schnitt SJ, et al. Estrogen receptor immunohistochemistry in carcinoma *in situ* of the breast. *Cancer* 1992;69:1174–1181.
180. Holland PA, Knox WF, Potten CS, et al. Assessment of hormone dependence of comedo ductal carcinoma *in situ* of the breast. *J Natl Cancer Inst* 1997;89:1059–1065.
181. Roka S, Rudas M, Taucher S, et al. High nuclear grade and negative estrogen receptor are significant risk factors for recurrence in DCIS. *Eur J Surg Oncol* 2004;30:243–247.
182. Collins LC, Schnitt SJ. HER2 protein overexpression in estrogen receptor-positive ductal carcinoma *in situ* of the breast: frequency and implications for tamoxifen therapy. *Mod Pathol* 2005;18:615–620.
183. Allred DC, Carlson RW, Berry DA, et al. NCCN task force report: estrogen receptor and progesterone receptor testing in breast cancer by immunohistochemistry. *J Natl Compr Cancer Netw* 2009;7(Suppl. 6):S1–S21.
184. Cohen DA, Dabbs DJ, Cooper KL, et al. Interobserver agreement among pathologists for semiquantitative hormone receptor scoring in breast carcinoma. *Am J Clin Pathol* 2012;138:796–802.
185. Walker RA, Hanby A, Pinder SE, et al. Current issues in diagnostic breast pathology. *J Clin Pathol* 2012;65:771–785.
186. Baqai T, Shousha S. Oestrogen receptor negativity as a marker for high-grade ductal carcinoma *in situ* of the breast. *Histopathology* 2003;42:440–447.
187. Bartkova J, Barnes DM, Millis RR, et al. Immunohistochemical demonstration of c-erbB-2 protein in mammary ductal carcinoma *in situ*. *Hum Pathol* 1990;21:1164–1167.
188. Gusterson BA, Machin LG, Gullick WJ, et al. Immunohistochemical distribution of c-erbB-2 in infiltrating and *in situ* breast cancer. *Int J Cancer* 1988;42:842–845.
189. Poller DN, Silverstein MJ, Galea M, et al. Ductal carcinoma *in situ* of the breast: a proposal for a new simplified histological classification association between cellular proliferation and c-erbB-2 protein expression. *Mod Pathol* 1994;7:257–262.
190. Schimmelpenning H, Eriksson ET, Pallis L, et al. Immunohistochemical c-erbB-2 proto-oncogene expression and nuclear DNA content in human mammary carcinoma *in situ*. *Am J Clin Pathol* 1992;97(Suppl. 1):S48–S52.
191. van de Vijver MJ, Peterse JL, Mooi WJ, et al. Neu-protein overexpression in breast cancer. Association with comedo-type ductal carcinoma *in situ* and limited prognostic value in stage II breast cancer. *N Engl J Med* 1988;319:1239–1245.
192. Liu E, Thor A, He M, et al. The HER2 (c-erbB-2) oncogene is frequently amplified in *in situ* carcinomas of the breast. *Oncogene* 1992;7:1027–1032.
193. Ho GH, Calvano JE, Bisogna M, et al. In microdissected ductal carcinoma *in situ*, HER2/neu amplification but not p53 mutation is associated with comedo and high grade ductal carcinoma *in situ*. *Cancer* 2000;89:2153–2160.
194. Barnes DM, Meyer JS, Gonzalez JG, et al. Relationship between c-erbB-2 immunoreactivity and thymidine labelling index in breast carcinoma *in situ*. *Breast Cancer Res Treat* 1991;18:11–17.
195. Albonico G, Querzoli P, Ferretti S, et al. Biological heterogeneity of breast carcinoma *in situ*. *Ann NY Acad Sci* 1996;784:458–461.
196. De Potter CR, Foschini MP, Schelfhout A-M,et al. Immunohistochemical study of neu protein overexpression in clinging *in situ* duct carcinoma of the breast. *Virchows Arch [A]* 1993;422:375–380.
197. Sek P, Zawrocki A, Biernat W, et al. HER2 molecular subtype is a dominant subtype of mammary Paget's cells. An immunohistochemical study. *Histopathology* 2010;57:564–571.
198. Rudas M, Neumayer R, Gnant MFX, et al. p53 protein expression, cell proliferation and steroid hormone receptors in ductal and lobular *in situ* carcinomas of the breast. *Eur J Cancer* 1997;33:39–44.
199. Isola JJ, Holli K, Oksa H, et al. Elevated erbB-2 oncoprotein levels in preoperative and follow-up serum samples define an aggressive disease course in patients with breast cancer. *Cancer* 1994;73:652–658.
200. Esteva-Lorenzo FJ, Paik S, Harris LN. Serum erbB-2 in ductal carcinoma *in situ* of the breast—a marker of microinvasion. *Acta Oncol* 1997;36:651–652.
201. Volas GH, Leitzel K, Teramoto Y, et al. Serial serum c-erbB-2 levels in patients with breast carcinoma. *Cancer* 1996;78:267–272.
202. Livasy CA, Perou CM, Karaca G, et al. Identification of a basal-like subtype of ductal carcinoma *in situ*. *Hum Pathol* 2007;38:197–204.
203. Thike AA, Iqbal J, Cheok PY, et al. Ductal carcinoma *in situ* associated with triple negative invasive breast cancer: evidence for a precursor-product relationship. *J Clin Pathol* 2013;66:665–670.
204. O'Malley FP, Vnencak-Jones CL, Dupont WD, et al. p53 mutations are confined to the comedo type ductal carcinoma *in situ* of the breast. Immunohistochemical and sequencing data. *Lab Invest* 1994;71:67–72.
205. Rajan PB, Scott DJ, Perry RH, et al. p53 protein expression in ductal carcinoma *in situ* (DCIS) of the breast. *Breast Cancer Res Treat* 1997;42:283–290.
206. Poller DN, Bell RJA, Elston CW, et al. p53 protein expression in mammary ductal carcinoma *in situ*: relationship to immunohistochemical expression of estrogen receptor and c-erbB-2 protein. *Hum Pathol* 1993;24:463–468.
207. Leal CB, Schmitt FC, Bento MJ, et al. Ductal carcinoma *in situ* of the breast. Histologic categorization and its relationship to ploidy and immunohistochemical expression of hormone receptors, p53 and c-erbB-2 protein. *Cancer* 1995;75:2123–2131.
208. Done SJ, Arneson NCR, Ozcelik H, et al. p53 mutations in mammary ductal carcinoma *in situ* but not in epithelial hyperplasia. *Cancer Res* 1998;58:785–789.
209. Walker RA, Dearing SJ, Lane DP, et al. Expression of p53 protein in infiltrating and *in-situ* breast carcinomas. *J Pathol* 1991;165:203–211.
210. Barnes R, Masood S, Barker E, et al. Low nm23 protein expression in infiltrating ductal breast carcinomas correlates with reduced patient survival. *Am J Pathol* 1991;139:245–250.
211. Simpson JF, O'Malley F, Dupont WD, et al. Heterogeneous expression of nm23 gene product in noninvasive breast carcinoma. *Cancer* 1994;73:2352–2358.
212. Vos CB, Cleton-Jansen AM, Berx G, et al. E-Cadherin inactivation in lobular carcinoma *in situ* of the breast: an early event in tumorigenesis. *Br J Cancer* 1997;76:1131–1133.
213. Gupta SK, Douglas-Jones AG, Jasani B, et al. E-Cadherin (E-cad) expression in duct carcinoma *in situ* (DCIS) of the breast. *Virchows Arch* 1997;430:23–28.
214. Bankfalvi A, Terpe HJ, Breukelmann D, et al. Immunophenotypic and prognostic analysis of E-cadherin and beta-catenin expression during breast carcinogenesis and tumour progression: a comparative study with CD44. *Histopathology* 1999;34:25–34.
215. Aasmundstad TA, Haugen OA. DNA ploidy in intraductal breast carcinomas. *Eur J Cancer* 1990;26:956–959.
216. Crissman JD, Visscher DW, Kubus J. Image cytophotometric DNA analysis of atypical hyperplasias and intraductal carcinomas of the breast. *Arch Pathol Lab Med* 1990;114:1239–1253.
217. Killeen JL, Namiki H. DNA analysis of ductal carcinoma *in situ* of the breast. A comparison with histologic features. *Cancer* 1991;68:2602–2607.
218. Locker AP, Horrocks C, Gilmour AS, et al. Flow cytometric and histological analysis of ductal carcinoma *in situ* of the breast. *Br J Surg* 1990;77:564–567.
219. Pallis L, Skoog L, Falkmer U, et al. The DNA profile of breast cancer *in situ*. *Eur J Surg Oncol* 1992;18:108–111.
220. Sataloff DM, Russin Vl, Sohn M, et al. DNA flow cytometric analysis in ductal carcinoma *in situ* of the breast. *Breast Dis* 1993;6:195–205.
221. Meyer JE, Kopans DB, Stomper PC, et al. Occult breast abnormalities: percutaneous preoperative needle localization. *Radiology* 1984;150:335–337.

222. Visscher DW, Wallis TL, Crissman JD. Evaluation of chromosome aneuploidy in tissue sections of preinvasive breast carcinomas using interphase cytogenetics. *Cancer* 1996;77:315–320.
223. Sarode VR, Han JS, Morris DH, et al. A comparative analysis of biomarker expression and molecular subtypes of pure ductal carcinoma *in situ* and invasive breast carcinoma by image analysis: relationship of the subtypes with histologic grade, Ki67, p53 overexpression, and DNA ploidy. *Int J Breast Cancer* 2011;2011:217060.
224. Stasik CJ, Davis M, Kimler BF, et al. Grading ductal carcinoma *in situ* of the breast using an automated proliferation index. *Ann Clin Lab Sci* 2011;41:122–130.
225. Rakovitch E, Nofech-Mozes S, Hanna W, et al. HER2/neu and Ki-67 expression predict non-invasive recurrence following breast-conserving therapy for ductal carcinoma *in situ*. *Br J Cancer* 2012;106:1160–1165.
226. Gandhi A, Holland PA, Knox WF, et al. Evidence of significant apoptosis in poorly differentiated ductal carcinoma *in situ* of the breast. *Br J Cancer* 1998;78:788–794.
227. Radford DM, Fair K, Thompson AM, et al. Allelic loss on chromosome 17 in ductal carcinoma *in situ* of the breast. *Cancer Res* 1993;53:2947–2950.
228. Alburquerque A, Kennedy S, Bryant B, et al. LOH on chromosome 17p and 17q in the histologic spectrum of DCIS. *Mod Pathol* 1997;10:15A.
229. Lichy JH, Zavar M, Tsai MM, et al. Loss of heterozygosity on chromosome 11p15 during histological progression in microdissected ductal carcinoma of the breast. *Am J Pathol* 1998;153:271–278.
230. Chuaqui RF, Zhuang Z, Emmert-Buck MR, et al. Analysis of loss of heterozygosity on chromosome 11q13 in atypical ductal hyperplasia and *in situ* carcinoma of the breast. *Am J Pathol* 1997;150:297–303.
231. Chen T, Sahin A, Aldaz CM. Deletion map of chromosome 16q in ductal carcinoma *in situ* of the breast: refining a putative tumor suppressor gene region. *Cancer Res* 1996;56:5605–5609.
232. Fujii H, Szumel R, Marsh C, et al. Genetic progression, histological grade, and allelic loss in ductal carcinoma *in situ* of the breast. *Cancer Res* 1996;56:5260–5265.
233. Stratton MR, Collins N, Lakhani SR, et al. Loss of heterozygosity in ductal carcinoma *in situ* of the breast. *J Pathol* 1995;175:195–201.
234. Radford DM, Phillips NJ, Fair KL, et al. Allelic loss and the progression of breast cancer. *Cancer Res* 1995;55:5180–5183.
235. Munn KE, Walker RA, Varley JM. Frequent alterations of chromosome 1 in ductal carcinoma *in situ* of the breast. *Oncogene* 1995;10:1653–1657.
236. Zhuang Z, Merino MJ, Chuaqui R, et al. Identical allelic loss on chromosome 11q13 in microdissected *in situ* and invasive human breast cancer. *Cancer Res* 1995;55:467–471.
237. James LA, Mitchell ELD, Menasce L, et al. Comparative genomic hybridisation of ductal carcinoma *in situ* of the breast: identification of regions of DNA amplification and deletion in common with invasive breast carcinoma. *Oncogene* 1997;14:1059–1065.
238. Barsky SH, Shao ZM, Bose S. Should DCIS be renamed carcinoma of the ductal system? *Breast J* 1999;5:70–72.
239. Marsh KL, Varley JM. Loss of heterozygosity at chromosome 9p in ductal carcinoma *in situ* and invasive carcinoma of the breast. *Br J Cancer* 1998;77:1439–1447.
240. Aubele M, Mattis A, Zitzelsberger H, et al. Extensive ductal carcinoma *in situ* with small foci of invasive ductal carcinoma: evidence of genetic resemblance by CGH. *Int J Cancer* 2000;85:82–86.
241. Waldman FM, DeVries S, Chew KL, et al. Chromosomal alterations in ductal carcinomas *in situ* and their *in situ* recurrences. *J Natl Cancer Inst* 2000;92:313–320.
242. Lopez-Garcia MA, Geyer FC, Lacroix-Triki M, et al. Breast cancer precursors revisited: molecular features and progression pathways. *Histopathology* 2010;57:171–192.
243. Polyak K. Molecular markers for the diagnosis and management of ductal carcinoma *in situ*. *J Natl Cancer Inst Monogr* 2010;2010(41):210–213.
244. Zhou W, Jirström K, Johansson C, et al. Long-term survival of women with basal-like ductal carcinoma *in situ* of the breast: a population-based cohort study. *BMC Cancer* 2010;10:653.
245. Burkhardt L, Grob TJ, Hermann I, et al. Gene amplification in ductal carcinoma *in situ* of the breast. *Breast Cancer Res Treat* 2010;123:757–765.
246. Schwartz GF, Solin LJ, Olivotto IA, et al. The Consensus Conference on the treatment of *in situ* ductal carcinoma of the breast, April 22–25, 1999. *Hum Pathol* 2000;31:131–139.
247. Jackman RJ, Nowels KW, Shepard MJ, et al. Stereotaxic large-core needle biopsy of 450 nonpalpable breast lesions with surgical correlation in lesions with cancer or atypical hyperplasia. *Radiology* 1994;193:91–95.
248. Liberman L, Dershaw DD, Rosen PP, et al. Stereotaxic core biopsy of breast carcinoma: accuracy at predicting invasion. *Radiology* 1995;194:379–381.
249. Burbank F. Stereotactic breast biopsy of atypical ductal hyperplasia and ductal carcinoma *in situ* lesions: improved accuracy with directional, vacuum-assisted biopsy. *Radiology* 1997;202:843–847.
250. Mendez I, Andreu FJ, Saez E, et al. Ductal carcinoma *in situ* and atypical ductal hyperplasia of the breast diagnosed at stereotactic core biopsy. *Breast J* 2001;7:14–18.
251. Renshaw AA. Predicting invasion in the excision specimen from breast core needle biopsy specimens with only ductal carcinoma *in situ*. *Arch Pathol Lab Med* 2002;126:39–41.
252. Jackman RJ, Burbank F, Parker SH, et al. Stereotactic breast biopsy of nonpalpable lesions: determinants of ductal carcinoma *in situ* underestimation rates. *Radiology* 2001;218:497–502.
253. Tuttle TM, Shamliyan T, Virnig BA, et al. The impact of sentinel lymph node biopsy and magnetic resonance imaging on important outcomes among patients with ductal carcinoma *in situ*. *J Natl Cancer Inst Monogr* 2010;2010(41):117–120.
254. Dillon MF, Quinn CM, McDermott EW, et al. Diagnostic accuracy of core biopsy for ductal carcinoma *in situ* and its implications for surgical practice. *J Clin Pathol* 2006;59:740–743.
255. Dillon MF, Maguire AA, McDermott EW, et al. Needle core biopsy characteristics identify patients at risk of compromised margins in breast conservation surgery. *Mod Pathol* 2008;21:39–45.
256. Wang HH, Ducatman BS, Eick D. Comparative features of ductal carcinoma *in situ* and infiltrating ductal carcinoma of the breast on fine-needle aspiration biopsy. *Am J Clin Pathol* 1989;92:736–740.
257. Willems SM, van Deurzen CH, van Diest PJ. Diagnosis of breast lesions: fine-needle aspiration cytology or core needle biopsy? A review. *J Clin Pathol* 2012;65:287–292.
258. Sneige N, Singletary SE. Fine-needle aspiration of the breast: diagnostic problems and approaches to surgical management. *Pathol Annu* 1994;29(Pt. 1):281–301.
259. Guo HQ, Zhang ZH, Zhao H, et al. Recognizing breast ductal carcinoma *in situ* on fine-needle aspiration: a diagnostic dilemma. *Diagn Cytopathol* 2013;41:710–715.
260. McKee GT, Tildsley G, Hammond S. Cytologic diagnosis and grading of ductal carcinoma *in situ*. *Cancer* 1999;87:203–209.
261. Lester SC, Bose S, Chen YY, et al. Protocol for the examination of specimens from patients with ductal carcinoma *in situ* of the breast. *Arch Pathol Lab Med* 2009;133:15–25.
262. Saqi A, Osborne MP, Rosenblatt R, et al. Quantifying mammary duct carcinoma *in situ*: a wild-goose chase? *Am J Clin Pathol* 2000;113(5 Suppl. 1):S30–S37.
263. Grin A, Horne G, Ennis M, et al. Measuring extent of ductal carcinoma *in situ* in breast excision specimens: a comparison of 4 methods. *Arch Pathol Lab Med* 2009;133:31–37.
264. Marcotte-Bloch C, Balu-Maestro C, Chamorey E, et al. MRI for the size assessment of pure ductal carcinoma *in situ* (DCIS): a prospective study of 33 patients. *Eur J Radiol* 2011;77:462–467.
265. Thomas J, Evans A, Macartney J, et al. Radiological and pathological size estimations of pure ductal carcinoma *in situ* of the breast, specimen handling and the influence on the success of breast conservation surgery: a review of National Surgical Adjuvant Breast Project (NSABP) Protocol B-17. Intraductal carcinoma (ductal carcinoma *in situ*). *Cancer* 1995;75:1310–1319.
266. Tavassoli FA, Norris HJ. A comparison of the results of long-term follow-up for atypical intraductal hyperplasia of the breast. *Cancer* 1990;65:518–529.
267. Lagios MD, Westdahl PR, Margolin FR, et al. Duct carcinoma *in situ*. Relationship of extent of noninvasive disease to the frequency of occult invasion, multicentricity, lymph node metastases, and short-term treatment failures. *Cancer* 1982;50:1309–1314.
268. Lagios MD. Ductal carcinoma *in situ*: biological and therapeutic implications of classification. *Breast J* 1996;2:32–34.
269. Silverstein MJ, Cohlan BF, Gierson ED, et al. Duct carcinoma *in situ*: 227 cases without microinvasion. *Eur J Cancer* 1992;28:630–634.
270. Cheatle GL. Benign and malignant changes in duct epithelium of the breast. *Br J Surg* 1920/1921;8:285–306.

271. Charteris AA. On the changes in the mammary gland preceding carcinoma. *J Pathol* 1930;33:101–117.
272. Lagios MD, Westdahl PR, Rose MR. The concept and implications of multicentricity in breast carcinoma. *Pathol Annu* 1981;16:1123–1130.
273. Hardman PDJ, Worth A, Lee U. The risk of occult invasive breast cancer after excisional biopsy showing in-situ ductal carcinoma of comedo pattern. *Can J Surg* 1989;32:56–60.
274. Ashikari R, Huvos AG, Snyder RE. Prospective study of non-infiltrating carcinoma of the breast. *Cancer* 1977;39:435–439.
275. Gallager HS, Martin JE. Early phases in the development of breast cancer. *Cancer* 1969;24:1170–1178.
276. Morgenstern L, Kaufman PA, Friedman ND. The case against tylectomy for carcinoma of the breast. The factor of multicentricity. *Am J Surg* 1975;130:251–258.
277. Silverstein MJ, Rosser RJ, Gierson ED, et al. Axillary lymph node dissection for intraductal carcinoma: is it indicated? *Cancer* 1987;59:1819–1824.
278. Schwartz GF, Patchefsky AS, Feig SA, et al. Multicentricity of nonpalpable breast cancer. *Cancer* 1980;45:2913–2916.
279. Hollingsworth AB, Stough RG. Multicentric and contralateral invasive tumors identified with pre-op MRI in patients newly diagnosed with ductal carcinoma *in situ* of the breast. *Breast J* 2012;18:420–427.
280. Houssami N, Ciatto S, Macaskill P, et al. Accuracy and surgical impact of magnetic resonance imaging in breast cancer staging: systematic review and meta-analysis in detection of multifocal and multicentric cancer. *J Clin Oncol* 2008;26:3248–3258.
281. Yerushalmi R, Tyldesley S, Woods R, et al. Is breast-conserving therapy a safe option for patients with tumor multicentricity and multifocality? *Ann Oncol* 2012;23:876–881.
282. Ozzello J, Sentipak P. Epithelial-stromal junction of intraductal carcinoma of the breast. *Cancer* 1970;26:1186–1198.
283. Ozzello L. Ultrastructure of intra-epithelial carcinomas of the breast. *Cancer* 1971;28:1508–1515.
284. Rajan PB, Perry RH. A quantitative study of patterns of basement membrane in ductal carcinoma *in situ* (DCIS) of the breast. *Breast J* 1995;1:315–321.
285. Tamimi SO, Ahmed A. Stromal changes in early invasive and non-invasive breast carcinoma: an ultrastructural study. *J Pathol* 1986;150:43–49.
286. Barsky SH, Togo S, Garbisa S, et al. Type IV collagenase immunoreactivity in invasive breast carcinoma. *Lancet* 1983;1:296–297.
287. Nakano S, Iyama K, Ogawa M, et al. Differential tissular expression and localization of type IV collagen alpha-1(IV), alpha-5(IV), and alpha-6(IV) chains and their mRNA in normal breast and in benign and malignant breast tumors. *Lab Invest* 1999;79:281–292.
288. Hewitt RE, Powe DG, Morrell K, et al. Laminin and collagen IV subunit distribution in normal and neoplastic tissues of colorectum and breast. *Br J Cancer* 1997;75:221–229.
289. Frazier TG, Copeland EM, Gallager HS, et al. Prognosis and treatment in minimal breast cancer. *Am J Surg* 1977;133:697–701.
290. Gallager HS, Martin JE. An orientation to the concept of minimal breast cancer. *Cancer* 1971;28:1505–1507.
291. Hutter RVP. The pathologist's role in minimal breast cancer. *Cancer* 1971;28:1527–1536.
292. Ozzello L. The behaviour of basement membranes in intraductal carcinoma of the breast. *Am J Pathol* 1959;35:887–799.
293. Dewar R, Fadare O, Gilmore H, et al. Best practices in diagnostic immunohistochemistry: myoepithelial markers in breast pathology. *Arch Pathol Lab Med* 2011;135:422–429.
294. Pusztaszeri M. *Phenotypic alterations in myoepithelial cells of the breast in normal and pathologic conditions. Am J Surg Pathol* 2010;34:1886.
295. Coyne J, Haboubi NY. Micro-invasive breast carcinoma with granulomatous stromal response. *Histopathology* 1992;20:184–185.
296. Prasad ML, Hyjek E, Giri DD, et al. Double immunolabeling with cytokeratin and smooth-muscle actin in confirming early invasive carcinoma of breast. *Am J Surg Pathol* 1999;23:176–181.
297. Hou L, Sneige N, Hunt KK, et al. Predictors of invasion in patients with core-needle biopsy-diagnosed ductal carcinoma *in situ* and recommendations for a selective approach to sentinel lymph node biopsy in ductal carcinoma *in situ. Cancer* 2006;107:1760–1768.
298. King TA, Farr GH Jr, Cederbom GI, et al. A mass on breast imaging predicts coexisting invasive carcinoma in patients with a core biopsy diagnosis of ductal carcinoma *in situ. Am Surg* 2001;67:907–912.
299. Bagnall MJ, Evans AJ, Wilson AR, et al. Predicting invasion in mammographically detected microcalcification. *Clin Radiol* 2001;56:828–832.
300. Hoorntje LE, Schipper ME, Peeters PH, et al. The finding of invasive cancer after a preoperative diagnosis of ductal carcinoma *in situ*: causes of ductal carcinoma *in situ* underestimates with stereotactic 14-gauge needle biopsy. *Ann Surg Oncol* 2003;10:748–753.
301. Yen TW, Hunt KK, Ross MI, et al. Predictors of invasive breast cancer in patients with an initial diagnosis of ductal carcinoma *in situ*: a guide to selective use of sentinel lymph node biopsy in management of ductal carcinoma *in situ. J Am Coll Surg* 2005;200:516–526.
302. Cowen PN. Recognition of intraduct mammary carcinoma. *J Clin Pathol* 1980;33:797.
303. Cowen PN, Bates C. The significance of intraduct appearances in breast cancer. *Clin Oncol* 1984;10:67–72.
304. Barsky SH, Doberneck SA, Sternlicht MD, et al. 'Revertant' DCIS in human axillary breast carcinoma metastases. *J Pathol* 1997;183:188–194.
305. Arihiro K, Inai K, Kurihara K, et al. Distribution of laminin, type IV collagen and fibronectin in the invasive component of breast carcinoma. *Acta Pathol Japonica* 1993;43:758–764.
306. Nadji M, Nassiri M, Fresno M, et al. Laminin receptor in lymph node negative breast carcinoma. *Cancer* 1999;85:432–436.
307. Solin LJ, Fowble BL, Yeh I-T,et al. Microinvasive ductal carcinoma of the breast treated with breast-conserving surgery and definitive irradiation. *Int J Radiat Oncol Biol Phys* 1992;23:961–968.
308. Silver SA, Tavassoli FA. Mammary ductal carcinoma *in situ* with microinvasion. *Cancer* 1998;82:2382–2390.
309. de Mascarel I, MacGrogan G, Mathoulin-Pelissier S, et al. Breast ductal carcinoma *in situ* with microinvasion. A definition supported by a long-term study of 1248 serially sectioned ductal carcinomas. *Cancer* 2002;94:2134–2142.
310. Jimenez RE, Visscher DW. Clinicopathologic analysis of microscopically invasive breast carcinoma. *Hum Pathol* 1998;29:1412–1419.
311. Walker RA, Dearing SJ, Brown LA. Comparison of pathological and biological features of symptomatic and mammographically detected ductal carcinoma *in situ* of the breast. *Hum Pathol* 1999;30:943–948.
312. Prasad ML, Osborne MP, Giri DD, et al. Microinvasive carcinoma (T1*mic*) of the breast. Clinicopathologic profile of 21 cases. *Am J Surg Pathol* 2000;24:422–428.
313. Ross DS, Hoda SA. Microinvasive (T1*mic*) lobular carcinoma of the breast: clinicopathologic profile of 16 cases. *Am J Surg Pathol* 2011;35:750–756.
314. Shapiro-Wright HM, Julian TB. Sentinel lymph node biopsy and management of the axilla in ductal carcinoma *in situ. J Natl Cancer Inst Monogr* 2010;2010(41):145–149.
315. Moore KH, Sweeney KJ, Wilson ME, et al. Outcomes for women with ductal carcinoma-*in-situ* and a positive sentinel node: a multi-institutional audit. *Ann Surg Oncol* 2007;14:2911–2917.
316. Intra M, Rotmensz N, Veronesi P, et al. Sentinel node biopsy is not a standard procedure in ductal carcinoma *in situ* of the breast: the experience of the European Institute of Oncology on 854 patients in 10 years. *Ann Surg* 2008;247:315–319.
317. Zavotsky J, Hansen N, Brennan MB, et al. Lymph node metastasis from ductal carcinoma *in situ* with microinvasion. *Cancer* 1999;85:2439–2443.
318. Dauway EL, Giuliano R, Pendas S, et al. Lymphatic mapping: a technique providing accurate staging for breast cancer. *Breast Cancer* 1999;6:145–154.
319. Wilkie C, White L, Dupont E, et al. An update of sentinel lymph node mapping in patients with ductal carcinoma *in situ. Am J Surg* 2005;190:563–566.
320. Katz A, Gage I, Evans S, et al. Sentinel lymph node positivity of patients with ductal carcinoma *in situ* or microinvasive breast cancer. *Am J Surg* 2006;191:761–766.
321. Sakr R, Barranger E, Antoine M, et al. Ductal carcinoma *in situ*: value of sentinel lymph node biopsy. *J Surg Oncol* 2006;94:426–430.
322. Leidenius M, Salmenkivi K, von Smitten K, et al. Tumour-positive sentinel node findings in patients with ductal carcinoma *in situ. J Surg Oncol* 2006;94:380–384.
323. Huo l, Resetkova A, Lopez A, et al. Sentinel lymph node (SLN) sampling in patients with core biopsy diagnosis of ductal carcinoma *in situ* (DCIS): UT M.D. Anderson Cancer Center experience and future recommendations. *Mod Pathol* 2006;19(Suppl. 1):30A.
324. Banys M, Gruber I, Krawczyk N, et al. Hematogenous and lymphatic tumor cell dissemination may be detected in patients diagnosed

with ductal carcinoma *in situ* of the breast. *Breast Cancer Res Treat* 2012;131:801–808.

325. Sänger N, Effenberger KE, Riethdorf S, et al. Disseminated tumor cells in the bone marrow of patients with ductal carcinoma *in situ*. *Int J Cancer* 2011;129:2522–2526.
326. Pathology Working Group Breast Cancer Task Force. Standardized management of breast cancer specimens. *Am J Clin Pathol* 1973;60:789–798.
327. Goldstein NS, Lacerna M, Vicini F. Cancerization of lobules and atypical ductal hyperplasia adjacent to ductal carcinoma *in situ* of the breast. *Am J Clin Pathol* 1998;110:357–367.
328. Hodi Z, Ellis IO, Elston CW, et al. Comparison of margin assessment by radial and shave sections in wide local excision specimens for invasive carcinoma of the breast. *Histopathology* 2010;56:573–580.
329. Caughran JL, Vicini FA, Kestin LL, et al. Optimal use of re-excision in patients diagnosed with early-stage breast cancer by excisional biopsy treated with breast-conserving therapy. *Ann Surg Oncol* 2009;16:3020–3027.
330. Guidroz JA, Larrieux G, Liao J, et al. Sampling of secondary margins decreases the need for re-excision after partial mastectomy. *Surgery* 2011;150:802–809.
331. Goldstein SN. Controversies in pathology in early-stage breast cancer. *Semin Radiat Oncol* 2011;21:20–25.
332. Melstrom LG, Melstrom KA, Wang EC, et al. Ductal carcinoma *in situ*: size and resection volume predict margin status. *Am J Clin Oncol* 2010;33:438–442.
333. Coopey S, Smith BL, Hanson S, et al. The safety of multiple re-excisions after lumpectomy for breast cancer. *Ann Surg Oncol* 2011;18:3797–3801.
334. Nayak A, Bhuiya TA. Utility of cytokeratin 5/6 and high-molecular-weight keratin in evaluation of cauterized surgical margins in excised specimens of breast ductal carcinoma *in situ*. *Ann Diagn Pathol* 2011;15:243–249.
335. Goldhirsch A, Ingle JN, Gelber RD, et al. Thresholds for therapies: highlights of the St Gallen International Expert Consensus on the primary therapy of early breast cancer 2009. *Ann Oncol* 2009;20:1319–1329.
336. Hughes LL, Wang M, Page DL, et al. Local excision alone without irradiation for ductal carcinoma *in situ* of the breast: a trial of the Eastern Cooperative Oncology Group. *J Clin Oncol* 2009;27:5319–5324.
337. Vincens E, Alves K, Lauratet B, et al. Margin status in ductal carcinoma *in situ* of the breast (in French). *Bull Cancer* 2008;95:1155–1159.
338. Dunne C, Burke JP, Morrow M, et al. Effect of margin status on local recurrence after breast conservation and radiation therapy for ductal carcinoma *in situ*. *J Clin Oncol* 2009;27:1615–1620.
339. Mansel RE. Ductal carcinoma *in situ*: surgery and radiotherapy. *Breast* 2003;12:447–450.
340. Wapnir IL, Dignam JJ, Fisher B, et al. Long-term outcomes of invasive ipsilateral breast tumor recurrences after lumpectomy in NSABP B-17 and B-24 randomized clinical trials for DCIS. *J Natl Cancer Inst* 2011;103:478–488.
341. Morrow M, Harris JR, Schnitt SJ. Surgical margins in lumpectomy for breast cancer—bigger is not better. *N Engl J Med* 2012;367:79–82.
342. Hughes JH, Mason MC, Gray RJ, et al. A multi-site validation trial of radioactive seed localization as an alternative to wire localization. *Breast J* 2008;14:153–157.
343. Alderliesten T, Loo CE, Pengel KE, et al. Radioactive seed localization of breast lesions: an adequate localization method without seed migration. *Breast J* 2011;17:594–601.
344. Thill M, Röder K, Diedrich K, et al. Intraoperative assessment of surgical margins during breast conserving surgery of ductal carcinoma *in situ* by use of radiofrequency spectroscopy. *Breast* 2011;20:579–580.
345. Kinne DW, Petrek JA, Osborne MP, et al. Breast carcinoma *in situ*. *Arch Surg* 1989;124:33–36.
346. Sunshine JA, Moseley HS, Fletcher WS, et al. Breast carcinoma *in situ*. A retrospective review of 112 cases with minimum 10 year follow-up. *Am J Surg* 1985;150:44–51.
347. Carter D, Smith AL. Carcinoma *in situ* of the breast. *Cancer* 1977;40:1189–1193.
348. Boyages J, Delaney G, Taylor R. Predictors of local recurrence after treatment of ductal carcinoma *in situ*: a meta-analysis. *Cancer* 1999;85:616–628.
349. Clark L, Ritter E, Glazebrook K, et al. Recurrent ductal carcinoma *in situ* after total mastectomy. *J Surg Oncol* 1999;71:182–185.
350. Montgomery RC, Fowble BL, Goldstein LJ, et al. Local recurrence after mastectomy for ductal carcinoma *in situ*. *Breast J* 1998;4:430–436.
351. Finkelstein SD, Sayegh R, Thompson WR. Late recurrence of ductal carcinoma *in situ* at the cutaneous end of surgical drainage following total mastectomy. *Am Surg* 1993;59:410–414.
352. Fisher DE, Schnitt SJ, Christian R, et al. Chest wall recurrence of ductal carcinoma *in situ* of the breast after mastectomy. *Cancer* 1993;71:3025–3028.
353. Srivastava A, Webster DJT. Isolated nipple recurrence seventeen years after subcutaneous mastectomy for breast cancer—a case report. *Eur J Surg Oncol* 1987;13:459–461.
354. Price P, Sinnett HD, Gusterson B, et al. Duct carcinoma *in situ*: predictors of local recurrence and progression in patients treated by surgery alone. *Br J Cancer* 1990;61:869–872.
355. Helvie MA, Wilson TE, Roubidoux MA, et al. Mammographic appearance of recurrent breast carcinoma in six patients with TRAM flap breast reconstructions. *Radiology* 1998;209:711–715.
356. Farrow JH. Current concepts in the detection and treatment of the earliest of the early breast cancers. *Cancer* 1970;25:458–479.
357. Joslyn SA. Ductal carcinoma *in situ*: trends in geographic, temporal, and demographic patterns of care and survival. *The Breast J* 2006;12:20–27.
358. Kiaer W. *Relation of fibroadenomatosis ("Chronic Mastitis") to cancer of the breast.* Copenhagen: Ejnar Munksgaard, 1954:69.
359. Millis RR, Thynne GSJ. *In situ* intraduct carcinoma of the breast: a long term follow-up study. *Br J Surg* 1975;62:957–962.
360. Betsill WL Jr, Rosen PP, Lieberman PH, et al. Intraductal carcinoma. Long-term follow-up after treatment by biopsy alone. *JAMA* 1978;239:1863–1867.
361. Rosen PP, Braun DW Jr, Kinne DW. The clinical significance of pre-invasive breast carcinoma. *Cancer* 1980;46:919–925.
362. Harvey DG, Fechner RE. Atypical lobular and papillary lesions of the breast: a follow-up study of 30 cases. *South Med J* 1978;71:361–364.
363. Page DL, Dupont WD, Rogers LW, et al. Intraductal carcinoma of the breast: follow-up after biopsy only. *Cancer* 1982;49:751–758.
364. Page DL, Dupont WD, Rogers LW, et al. Continued local recurrence of carcinoma 15–25 years after a diagnosis of low grade ductal carcinoma *in situ* of the breast treated only by biopsy. *Cancer* 1995;76:1197–1200.
365. Eusebi V, Foschini MP, Cook MG, et al. Long-term follow-up of *in situ* carcinoma of the breast with special emphasis on clinging carcinoma. *Diagn Pathol* 1989;6:165–173.
366. Lagios MD, Margolin FR, Westdahl PR, et al. Mammographically detected duct carcinoma *in situ*. Frequency of local recurrence following tylectomy and prognostic effect of nuclear grade on local recurrence. *Cancer* 1989;63:618–624.
367. Lagios MD. Evaluation of surrogate endpoint biomarkers for ductal carcinoma *in situ*. *J Cell Biochem* 1994;19(suppl.):186–188.
368. Fisher ER, Sass R, Fisher B, et al. Pathologic findings from the National Surgical Adjuvant Breast Project (Protocol 6). I. Intraductal carcinoma (DCIS). *Cancer* 1986;57:197–208.
369. Ottesen GL, Graversen HP, Blichert-Toft M, et al. Ductal carcinoma *in situ* of the female breast. Short-term results of a prospective nationwide study. *Am J Surg Pathol* 1992;16:1183–1196.
370. Ringberg A, Andersson I, Aspegren K, et al. Breast carcinoma *in situ* in 167 women—incidence, mode of presentation, therapy and follow-up. *Eur J Surg Oncol* 1991;17:466–476.
371. Arnesson L-G, Smeds S, Fagerberg G, et al. Follow-up of two treatment modalities for ductal cancer *in situ* of the breast. *Br J Surg* 1989;76:672–675.
372. Carpenter R, Boulter PS, Cooke T, et al. Management of screen detected ductal carcinoma *in situ* of the female breast. *Br J Surg* 1989;76:564–567.
373. Schwartz GF, Finkel GC, Garcia JC, et al. Subclinical ductal carcinoma *in situ* of the breast. *Cancer* 1992;70:2468–2474.
374. Hetelekidis S, Collins L, Silver B, et al. Predictors of local recurrence following excision alone for ductal carcinoma *in situ*. *Cancer* 1999;85:427–431.
375. Badve S, A'Hern RP, Ward AM, et al. Prediction of local recurrence of ductal carcinoma *in situ* of the breast using five histological classifications: a comparative study with long follow-up. *Hum Pathol* 1998;29:915–923.
376. Goonewardene S, Palazzo J, Cornfield D, et al. Prognostic significance of necrosis in evaluating risk for recurrence of ductal carcinoma *in situ* of the breast and progression to invasive carcinoma: survey of 166 conservatively treated patients. *Am J Clin Pathol* 1999;112:531–532.

377. MacDonald HR, Silverstein MJ, Mabry H, et al. Local control in ductal carcinoma *in situ* treated by excision alone: incremental benefit of larger margins. *Am J Surg* 2005;190:521–525.
378. Wong JS, Kaelin CM, Troyan SL, et al. Prospective study of wide excision alone for ductal carcinoma *in situ* of the breast. *J Clin Oncol* 2006;24:1031–1036.
379. Montague ED. Conservative surgery and radiation therapy in the treatment of operable breast cancer. *Cancer* 1984;53:700–704.
380. Solin LJ, Gray R, Baehner FL. A quantitative multigene RT-PCR assay for predicting recurrence risk after surgical excision alone without irradiation for ductal carcinoma *in situ* (DCIS): a prospective validation study of the DCIS score from ECOG E5194. Presented at: the 2011 CTRC-AACR San Antonio Breast Cancer Symposium; December 6–10, 2011 (Abstract S4–S6).
381. Prat A, Perou CM. Deconstructing the molecular portraits of breast cancer. *Mol Oncol* 2011;5:5–23.
382. Recht A, Danoff BS, Solin LJ, et al. Intraductal carcinoma of the breast: results of treatment with excisional biopsy and irradiation. *J Clin Oncol* 1985;3:1339–1343.
383. Zafrani B, Fourquet A, Vilcoq JR, et al. Conservative management of intraductal breast carcinoma with tumorectomy and radiation therapy. *Cancer* 1986;57:1299–1301.
384. Bornstein BA, Recht A, Connolly JL, et al. Results of treating ductal carcinoma *in situ* of the breast with conservative surgery and radiation therapy. *Cancer* 1991;67:7–13.
385. Solin LJ, Recht A, Fourquet A, et al. Ten-year results of breast-conserving surgery and definitive irradiation for intraductal carcinoma (ductal carcinoma *in situ*) of the breast. *Cancer* 1991;68:2337–2344.
386. Solin LJ, Fourquet A, Vicini FA, et al. Long-term outcome after breast-conservation treatment with radiation for mammographically detected ductal carcinoma *in situ* of the breast. *Cancer* 2005;103:1137–1146.
387. Fisher B, Land S, Mamounas E, et al. Prevention of invasive breast cancer in women with ductal carcinoma *in situ*: an update of the national surgical adjuvant breast and bowel project experience. *Semin Oncol* 2001;28:400–418.
388. Julien JP, Bijker N, Fentiman IS, et al. Radiotherapy in breast-conserving treatment for ductal carcinoma *in situ*: first results of the EORTC randomised phase III trial 10853. EORTC Breast Cancer Cooperative Group and EORTC Radiotherapy Group. *Lancet* 2000;355:528–533.
389. Bijker N, Meijnen P, Peterse JL, et al. Breast-conserving treatment with or without radiotherapy in ductal carcinoma-in-situ: ten-year results of European Organisation for Research and Treatment of Cancer randomized phase III trial 10853—a study by the EORTC Breast Cancer Cooperative Group and EORTC Radiotherapy Group. *J Clin Oncol* 2006;24:3381–3387.
390. Kane RL, Virnig BA, Shamliyan T, et al. The impact of surgery, radiation, and systemic treatment on outcomes in patients with ductal carcinoma *in situ*. *J Natl Cancer Inst Monogr* 2010;2010(41):130–133.
391. Punglia RS, Burstein HJ, Weeks JC. Radiation therapy for ductal carcinoma *in situ*: a decision analysis. *Cancer* 2012;118:603–611.
392. Zauls AJ, Watkins JM, Wahlquist AE, et al. Outcomes in women treated with MammoSite brachytherapy or whole breast irradiation stratified by ASTRO Accelerated Partial Breast Irradiation Consensus Statement Groups. *Int J Radiat Oncol Biol Phys* 2012;82:21–29.
393. Park SS, Grills IS, Chen PY, et al. Accelerated partial breast irradiation for pure ductal carcinoma *in situ*. *Int J Radiat Oncol Biol Phys* 2011;81:403–408.
394. Wong P, Lambert C, Agnihotram RV, et al. Ductal carcinoma *in situ*—the influence of the radiotherapy boost on local control. *Int J Radiat Oncol Biol Phys* 2012;82:e153–e158.
395. Arvold ND, Punglia RS, Hughes ME, et al. Pathologic characteristics of second breast cancers after breast conservation for ductal carcinoma *in situ*. *Cancer* 2012;118:6022–6030.
396. Solin LJ, Yeh I-T, Kurtz J, et al. Ductal carcinoma *in situ* (intraductal carcinoma) of the breast treated with breast-conserving surgery and definitive irradiation. Correlation of pathologic parameters with outcome of treatment. *Cancer* 1993;71:2532–2542.
397. Kuske RR, Bean JM, Garcia DM, et al. Breast conservation therapy for intraductal carcinoma of the breast. *Int J Radiat Oncol Biol Phys* 1993;26:391–396.
398. Fisher ER, Dignam J, Tan-Chiu E, et al. Pathologic findings from the National Surgical Adjuvant Breast Project (NSABP) eight-year update of Protocol B-17: intraductal carcinoma. *Cancer* 1999;86:429–438.
399. Silverstein MJ. Incidence and treatment of ductal carcinoma *in situ* of the breast. *Eur J Cancer* 1997;33:10–11.
400. de Mascarel I, Bonichon F, MacGrogan G, et al. Application of the Van Nuys prognostic index in a retrospective series of 367 ductal carcinomas *in situ* of the breast examined by serial macroscopic sectioning: practical considerations. *Breast Cancer Res Treat* 2000;61:151–159.
401. Boland GP, Chan KC, Knox WF, et al. Value of the Van Nuys Prognostic Index in prediction of recurrence of ductal carcinoma *in situ* after breast-conserving surgery. *Br J Surg* 2003;90:426–432.
402. Warnberg F, Nordgren H, Bergh J, et al. Ductal carcinoma *in situ* of the breast from a population-defined cohort: an evaluation of new histopathological classification systems. *Eur J Cancer* 1999;35:714–720.
403. Silverstein MJ. Ductal carcinoma *in situ* of the breast: the Van Nuys experience by treatment. *Breast J* 1997;3:232–237.
404. Solin LJ, McCormick B, Recht A, et al. Mammographically detected, clinically occult ductal carcinoma *in situ* treated with breast-conserving surgery and definitive breast irradiation. *Cancer J Sci Am* 1996;2:158–165.
405. Fowble B. The results of conservative surgery and radiation for mammographically detected ductal carcinoma *in situ*. *Breast J* 1997;3:238–241.
406. Silverstein MJ, Lagios MD, Martino S, et al. Outcome after invasive local recurrence in patients with ductal carcinoma *in situ* of the breast. *J Clin Oncol* 1998;16:1367–1373.
407. Silverstein MJ, Lagios MD. Choosing treatment for patients with ductal carcinoma *in situ*: fine tuning the University of Southern California/Van NuysPrognostic Index. *J Natl Cancer Inst Monogr* 2010;2010(41):193–196.
408. Altintas S, Toussaint J, Durbecq V, et al. Fine tuning of the Van Nuys prognostic index (VNPI) 2003 by integrating the genomic grade index (GGI): new tools for ductal carcinoma *in situ* (DCIS). *Breast J* 2011;17:343–351.
409. Kelley L, Silverstein M, Guerra L. Analyzing the risk of recurrence after mastectomy for DCIS: a new use for the USC/Van Nuys Prognostic Index. *Ann Surg Oncol* 2011;18:459–462.
410. Rudloff U, Jacks LM, Goldberg JI, et al. Nomogram for predicting the risk of local recurrence after breast-conserving surgery for ductal carcinoma *in situ*. *J Clin Oncol* 2010;28:3762–3769.
411. Yim, Meric-Bernstein F, Kuerer HM, et al. Evaluation of a breast cancer nomogram for predicting risk of ipsilateral breast tumor recurrence in patients with ductal carcinoma *in situ* after local excision. *J Clin Oncol* 2012;30:600–607.
412. Thomas M, Goldstein NS, Vicini FA, et al. The association of age at diagnosis with pathologic features in patients with duct carcinoma *in situ* of the breast. *Mod Pathol* 2000;13:47A.
413. Adepoju LJ, Symmans WF, Babiera GV, et al. Impact of concurrent proliferative high-risk lesions on the risk of ipsilateral breast carcinoma recurrence and contralateral breast carcinoma development in patients with ductal carcinoma *in situ* treated with breast-conserving therapy. *Cancer* 2006;106:42–50.
414. Cuzick J, Sestak I, Pinder SE, et al. Effect of tamoxifen and radiotherapy in women with locally excised ductal carcinoma *in situ*: long-term results from the UK/ANZ DCIS trial. *Lancet Oncol* 2011;12:21–29.
415. Fisher B, Dignam J, Wolmark N, et al. Tamoxifen in treatment of intraductal breast cancer: National Surgical Adjuvant Breast and Bowel Project B-24 randomised controlled trial. *Lancet* 1999;353:1993–2000.
416. Allred DC, Anderson SJ, Paik S, et al. Adjuvant tamoxifen reduces subsequent breast cancer in women with estrogen receptor-positive ductal carcinoma *in situ*: a study based on NSABP protocol B-24. *J Clin Oncol* 2012;30:1268–1273.
417. Vogel VG, Costantino JP, Wickerham DL, et al. Update of the National Surgical Adjuvant Breast and Bowel Project Study of Tamoxifen and Raloxifene (STAR) P-2 Trial: preventing breast cancer. *Cancer Prev Res (Phila)* 2010;3:696–706.
418. Morrow M, O'Sullivan MJ. The dilemma of DCIS. *Breast* 2007;16(Suppl. 2):S59–S62.
419. Allegra CJ, Aberle DR, Ganschow P, et al. National Institutes of Health State-of-the-Science Conference statement: diagnosis and management of ductal carcinoma *in situ*, September 22–24, 2009. *J Natl Cancer Inst* 2010;102:161–169.
420. Cuthli B, Lemanski C, Fourquet A, et al. Breast-conserving surgery with or without radiotherapy vs mastectomy for ductal carcinoma *in situ*: French Survey experience. *Br J Cancer* 2009;100:1048–1054.

421. Cheng L, Al-Kaisi NK, Gordon NH, et al. Relationship between the size and margin status of ductal carcinoma *in situ* of the breast and residual disease. *J Natl Cancer Inst* 1997;89:1356–1360.
422. Early Breast Cancer Trialists Collaborative Group. Effects of radiotherapy and of differences in the extent of surgery for early breast cancer on focal recurrence and on 15-year survival. *Lancet* 2005;366:2087–2106.
423. Allred DC, Bryant J, Land S, et al. Estrogen receptor expression as a predictive marker of the effectiveness of tamoxifen in the treatment of DCIS: findings from NSABP protocol B-24. *Breast Cancer Res Treat* 2002;76:S36.
424. Liberman L, Van Zee KJ, Dershaw DD, et al. Mammographic features of local recurrence in women who have undergone breast-conserving therapy for ductal carcinoma in site. *AJR Am J Roentgenol* 1997;168:489–493.
425. Silverstein MJ, Gierson ED, Colburn WJ, et al. Can intraductal breast carcinoma be excised completely by local excision? *Cancer* 1994;73:2985–2989.
426. Goldstein NS, Kestin L, Vicini F. Pathologic features of initial biopsy specimens associated with residual intraductal carcinoma on reexcision in patients with ductal carcinoma *in situ* of the breast referred for breast-conserving therapy. *Am J Surg Pathol* 1999;23:1340–1348.
427. Schnitt SJ, Harris JR, Smith BL. Developing a prognostic index for ductal carcinoma *in situ* of the breast. Are we there yet? *Cancer* 1996;77:2189–2192.
428. Wood WC. Should axillary dissection be performed in patients with DCIS? *Ann Surg Oncol* 1995;2:193–194.
429. Haigh PI, Giuliano AE. The Coxet al. article reviewed. *Oncology* 1998;12:1293–1294.
430. Cox CE, Haddad F, Bass S, et al. Lymphatic mapping in the treatment of breast cancer. *Oncology* 1998;12:1283–1292.
431. Bombonati A, Sgroi DC. The molecular pathology of breast cancer progression. *J Pathol* 2011;223:307–317.
432. Han K, Nofech-Mozes S, Narod S, et al. Expression of HER2/neu in ductal carcinoma *in situ* is associated with local recurrence. *Clin Oncol (R Coll Radiol)* 2012;24:183–189.
433. Espina V, Liotta LA. What is the malignant nature of human ductal carcinoma *in situ*? *Nature* 2011;11:61–65.
434. Flanagan M, Love S, Hwang ES. Status of intraductal therapy for ductal carcinoma *in situ*. *Curr Breast Cancer Rep* 2010;2:75–82.
435. Bleicher RJ. Ductal carcinoma *in situ*. *Surg Clin North Am* 2013;93:393–410.
436. Berg CD. Resolving the ductal carcinoma *in situ* treatment conundrum. *J Natl Cancer Inst* 2013;105:680–681.
437. Ballehaninna UK, Chamberlain RS. Inclusion of tumor biology molecular markers to improve the ductal carcinoma *in situ* ipsilateral breast tumor recurrence nomogram predictability. *J Clin Oncol* 2011;29:e97–e98.
438. Bleyer A, Welch HG. Effect of three decades of screening mammography on breast-cancer incidence. *N Engl J Med* 2012;367:1998–2005.
439. Baur A, Bahrs SD, Speck S, et al. Breast MRI of pure ductal carcinoma *in situ*: sensitivity of diagnosis and influence of lesion characteristics. *Eur J Radiol* 2013;82:1731–1737.

CHAPTER 12

Invasive Ductal Carcinoma: Assessment of Prognosis with Morphologic and Biologic Markers

SYED A. HODA

INVASIVE DUCTAL CARCINOMA, NOT OTHERWISE SPECIFIED

Invasive ductal carcinoma is the largest group of malignant mammary tumors, comprising approximately 75% of mammary carcinomas.[1,2] Included under this heading are tumors identified previously by such terms as ductal carcinoma with productive fibrosis, scirrhous carcinoma, carcinoma simplex, and a host of other names. A generic term sometimes employed is invasive ductal carcinoma, *not otherwise specified* (NOS), or of no special type (NST). These are useful designations, because they recognize the distinction between the majority of invasive ductal carcinomas and the several infrequent specific "special" forms of ductal carcinoma, such as tubular, medullary, metaplastic, mucinous, and adenoid cystic carcinoma (AdCC). There is accumulating evidence that many of the other 25% of invasive breast carcinomas have not only special phenotypical appearances but also specific genetic attributes; for example, AdCC has the (6;9) MYB-NFIB translocation, secretory carcinoma has the t(12;15) translocation that helps form the *ETV6–NTRK3* fusion gene, and lobular carcinoma exhibits inactivation of the *CDH1* gene[3] that is reflected in the absence of E-cadherin immunoreactivity.

In the latest WHO lexicon,[4] the term invasive *ductal carcinoma* is replaced by *invasive carcinoma of NST*, since in the authors' collective opinion "the use of the term 'ductal' perpetuates the traditional but incorrect concept that these tumors are derived exclusively from mammary ductal epithelium in distinction from lobular carcinomas, which were deemed to have arisen from within lobules, for which there is also no evidence." Nonetheless, the WHO classification retains the term invasive lobular carcinoma, not to mention atypical ductal hyperplasia and ductal carcinoma *in situ* (DCIS). The authors of this volume are not persuaded that this change is warranted at the present time and recommend the continued use of the term "invasive ductal carcinoma" until more compelling evidence is presented. Unless otherwise stated, the term "invasive ductal carcinoma" as used here refers to "invasive ductal carcinoma, NOS." (See *Introduction* for further comments on this issue.)

INVASIVE DUCTAL CARCINOMA WITH MIXED HISTOLOGIC FEATURES

Invasive ductal carcinoma, NOS includes a histologically diverse group of tumors that may express, at least in part, one or more characteristics of the specific types of breast carcinoma but do not constitute pure examples of the individual tumors. Examples of this phenomenon are invasive ductal carcinomas that have limited foci of tubular, medullary, papillary, or mucinous differentiation. When a mixed growth pattern is present in a needle core biopsy, the diagnosis should be descriptive, with final classification reserved for the excisional biopsy. The relatively favorable prognosis associated with some specific histologic types has been found to apply only to those tumors that are composed entirely or in large part of the designated pattern. Where these features are less extensively represented, the tumors are appropriately relegated to the broader group of invasive ductal carcinoma. The prognosis is likely to be that of the dominant invasive ductal carcinoma component. Tumors combining invasive ductal carcinoma with either primary or secondary forms of Paget disease are classified as invasive ductal carcinoma.

Approximately one-third of the lesions characterized as invasive ductal carcinoma in one detailed review of 1,000 carcinomas expressed one or more combined features.[5] Slightly more than one-half of the combined tumors were invasive ductal carcinomas with a tubular carcinoma component. Combinations with invasive lobular carcinoma were detected in 6% of the tumors. Tumors with such combined morphology can either exhibit "hybrid" morphology or show a "mixed" pattern of two (or more) well-defined histologic types. A study by Rakha et al.[6] described the "biologic and clinic characteristics of breast carcinoma with mixed ductal and lobular morphology." The 140 tumors alleged to have "mixed" morphology based on histologic examination alone were 3.6% of all cases studied. However, the identification of a lobular component was evidently not substantiated by the use of the E-cadherin stain in all cases since "absent or reduced E-cadherin" was found only in 70% (47 cases) of the tumors tested. It is clear from this study and many previously cited in the literature that there is a need to reassess carcinomas classified as invasive ductal carcinoma, mixed type with the growing number of markers associated with specific types of carcinoma in an effort to develop a more meaningful subclassification of this heterogeneous entity.

Thus far, no significant prognostic differences have been identified for most of the combined histologic patterns, and, as a consequence, they have frequently been grouped together as invasive ductal carcinoma, NOS. This section considers invasive ductal carcinoma in the context of this broad definition. Reference will be made to specific combined histologic patterns wherever relevant, in this and in other chapters.

DCIS IN INVASIVE DUCTAL CARCINOMA

The growth pattern of a coexisting intraductal component is usually reflected in the structure of the invasive carcinoma. There is a significant association between the grade of DCIS and invasive ductal carcinoma in tumors that have both components.[7] This observation suggests that important prognostic features of the tumor are established in the preinvasive stage and that the clinical course may possibly be predetermined by the component before invasion occurs. Studies of genetic alterations in the intraductal and invasive components of individual tumors have also shown similar patterns of loss of heterozygosity (LOH) in both parts, a finding which further supports this hypothesis.

Tubular carcinoma almost always arises from an orderly micropapillary and/or cribriform DCIS that features cytologically low-grade nuclei and can be associated with classical type of lobular carcinoma *in situ* (LCIS). The intraductal component of medullary carcinoma is typically solid with high-grade nuclei. Invasive poorly differentiated ductal carcinoma tends to develop from solid intraductal carcinoma, with or without necrosis. Comedo-type necrosis may occur in invasive areas of a tumor with high-grade solid DCIS duplicating the intraductal pattern. It can be difficult to distinguish between intraductal and invasive components in such tumors. Foci that resemble DCIS with central necrosis can be encountered in metastatic lesions derived from such tumors.[8]

Moderately differentiated invasive ductal carcinoma most often originates from cribriform or papillary intraductal components. Invasive cribriform carcinoma is a subtype of invasive ductal carcinoma with a prominent cribriform structure. These tumors arise from cribriform DCIS. The presence of invasive components that mimic cribriform intraductal carcinoma can complicate the measurement of the invasive tumor area, and foci with an *in situ* cribriform pattern can occur in metastatic lesions. Invasive carcinomas that are entirely cribriform and those with a mixture of cribriform and tubular components are relatively low grade and have an excellent prognosis. If less-well-differentiated elements are present in the tumor, the prognosis is not as favorable. Invasive cribriform carcinoma is sometimes mistaken for AdCC.[9]

THE COMPLEXITY OF ASSESSING PROGNOSIS

Prognostic and Predictive Factors

Breast carcinoma is a clinically and pathologically heterogeneous disease. As noted by Sistrunk and MacCarty[10] decades ago, "it is impossible to foretell the duration of life of all patients with carcinoma of the breast, because the degree of malignancy varies widely, and persons react differently to the disease."

Innumerable studies have attempted to assess the prognosis of breast carcinoma patients on the basis of clinical and pathologic parameters, and several recommendations for the use of various prognostic and predictive factors from various groups have appeared in recent years.[11,12,13] These and other recommendations regarding prognostic and predictive factors represent the current state of knowledge at the time of publication, based on an analysis of existing data in relation to use in clinical practice, especially for planning therapy and during clinical follow-up. Some factors are recommended and others are not by various organizations and institutions that supported these reviews, but there is not necessarily unanimity in the recommendations set forth in the different documents. And sometimes the conclusion in a report about a particular maker is not clear cut. This latter point is illustrated by the discussion of "flow cytometry-based proliferation markers" in recommendations published by the American Society of Clinical Oncology (ASCO) in 2007.[11] In summary, the document states that "data are insufficient to recommend use of DNA content, S-phase, or other flow cytometry-based markers of proliferation to assign patients to prognostic groupings." Reading further in this section, it becomes apparent that this conclusion was based at least, in part, on concern over "technical variation in flow cytometry determination of S-phase," but "if the flow cytometry–determined S-phase is determined using a validated method, in a laboratory with experience using the technique, it appears that an elevated S-phase fraction (SPF) is associated with a worse outcome." In contrast to the ASCO 2007 recommendations that did not specify the types of specimens analyzed for markers, Rakha and Ellis[12] emphasized the reliability of needle core biopsy samples for the assessment of selected markers, including flow cytometry, for the determination of proliferative activity.

A *prognostic factor* is a characteristic that can be used to estimate the chance of recovery from a disease or its recurrence (e.g., size of tumor), whereas a *predictive factor* is a characteristic that can be used to help predict the response of a particular tumor to a specific treatment (e.g., human epidermal growth factor 2 [HER2]). Because nearly three-fourths of the patients have invasive ductal carcinoma, the characteristics of these tumors have a considerable influence on laboratory, clinical, or pathologic studies of breast carcinoma. The emerging prognostic value of multigene expression assays including Oncotype DX and the 70-gene prognostic signature developed by investigators from Amsterdam will be addressed in Chapter 45.

TABLE 12.1 Percentage Risk of Distant Disease Recurrence Expended at 2, 5, 10, and 15 Years from Diagnosis[a]

Size of Tumor	No. of Lymph Nodes	No. of Patients	No. of Patients Recurred	Total Risk				
					% Risk Expended			
				M	2 yr	5 yr	10 yr	15 yr
All	0	796	177	0.30	20	50	70	85
	1-3	434	232	0.62	45	75	95	99
	>4	360	276	0.86	45	75	90	99
≤2 cm	0	367	56	0.20	15	40	65	80
	1-3	115	36	0.36	20	65	100	100
	≥4	60	43	0.81	30	70	QNS	QNS
>2 cm	0	428	121	0.38	10	50	75	87
	1-3	317	195	0.70	50	75	90	98
	≥4	300	233	0.89	45	75	90	98

QNS, quantity not sufficient (<40 patients).
[a]Calculated from Kaplan-Meier curves.
Reproduced from Heimann R, Hellman S. Clinical progression of breast cancer malignant behavior: what to expect and when to expect it. *J Clin Oncol* 2000;18:591–599, with permission.

Race

Data relating race to prognosis have mainly compared African American and White patients. Overall, African American women have a lower incidence of breast carcinoma than White women; however, the incidence is higher among African American women younger than 40 than among White women in the same age group, and the incidence is reversed in women older than 40.[14,15] African American patients were more likely to have larger tumors and tumors with necrosis. Analysis of a national database composed of more than 115,000 breast carcinoma patients by Edwards et al.[16] revealed that when compared with Whites African American women had a reduced likelihood of cure and had a shorter survival after diagnosis in those who were not cured.

Heterogeneity

The issue of heterogeneity of breast carcinoma was summarized by Heimann and Hellman[17]:

> The varied outcomes of similarly staged patients is most consistent with breast cancer not being a homogeneous disease, but rather a spectrum of disease states that have varying capacities for growth and metastasis . . . .Required of tumors is the development of critical phenotypic attributes: growth, invasion, metastagenicity, and angiogenesis. . . . Recognizing tumor heterogeneity emphasizes the need to determine an individual tumor's place in the evolutionary spectrum. This may be accomplished using clinical features such as size, nuclear grade, and patient age, as well as by examining angiogenesis, metastatic capacity, and proliferation. Identification of the extent of tumor progression with regard to these major tumor phenotypes should allow individual therapy to be fashioned for each patient.

In a subsequent report, Heimann and Hellman[18] analyzed data from approximately 1,500 patients treated by mastectomy without systemic therapy with a median follow-up of 145 months. Analysis revealed that the risk of recurrence ("metastagenicity" or M) and time to recurrence ("virulence" or V) were dependent on tumor size and nodal status. The calculated percentage of risk of recurrence expended in different periods of follow-up revealed an inverse relationship between virulence and the distribution of risk over time (Table 12.1). Among node-positive patients, most of the risk of recurrence was expended in the first 10 years of follow-up, with only 5% to 10% remaining thereafter. In the node-negative group, 30% of the risk of recurrence remained after 10 years. A cured group with a negligible remaining risk of recurrence was identified in each stage group, although the proportion of "cured" patients diminished with greater tumor size and increased nodal involvement.

A similar type of analysis was reported by Blamey et al.,[19] who examined tumor grade as well as size and nodal status. The study included 4,500 patients among whom 1,756 died of breast carcinoma. Presentation of survival curves in logarithmic form revealed two components. The first part of the curve was a relatively rapid decline with a duration determined by tumor grade (grade I, 28 years; grade II, 12 years; grade III, 7 years). Thereafter, an inflection point was reached in each curve to a slow decline that was parallel for all grades. The authors observed that 90% of recurrences occurred within 9, 7, and 5 years for patients with grades I, II, and III tumors, respectively. The rate of death due to breast carcinoma was also influenced by grade, with 90% occurring in 40, 13, and 8 years among patients with grades I, II, and III tumors, respectively. In this study, histologic grade proved to be an additional determinant of "metastagenicity" and "virulence" among patient groups stratified by tumor size and nodal status.

Genetic Factors

A genetic basis for differences in rates of carcinoma progression is suggested by analysis of LOH in primary and locally recurrent lesions. Regitnig et al.[20] studied primary and recurrent tumor specimens from 26 patients and reported that all LOHs identified in the primary tumor were also present in the local recurrence but that there was a significant increase in "total LOH" in recurrent tumors. Early recurrence was associated with LOH at specific loci (TP53 and D5S107). Lymph node metastases were associated with LOH at these sites and also at D35.

The impact on prognosis of mutations in specific genes such as *BRCA1* and *BRCA2* remains under active investigation. BRCA-associated breast carcinomas are significantly more likely than non-BRCA-associated carcinomas to have high histologic grade, lack estrogen receptor (ER) and progesterone receptor (PR) be HER negative, and manifest high a proliferative rate.[20–35] The differences are greatest in BRCA1-associated carcinomas that have higher frequencies of medullary carcinoma, high histologic grade, high mitotic rate, prominent lymphocytic infiltrates, and necrosis than BRCA2-associated carcinomas.[35] Robson et al.[25] found no significant differences in the expression of epidermal growth factor receptor (EGFR), cathepsin-D, bcl-2, p27, p53, or cyclin-D, and there was not a significant difference in relapse-free survival (RFS) or overall survival (OS) between BRCA-associated and non-BRCA-associated tumors, despite the relatively unfavorable tumor characteristics of the former group. Other investigators have found an increased frequency of p53 mutations and lower frequency of HER2/*neu* amplification in BRCA1 carcinomas than in sporadic breast carcinomas.[35] Expression of CK5/6 is increased in BRCA1 but not in BRCA2 carcinomas.[35] Overall BRCA1 carcinomas are characterized by basal-like cell-like histologic and immunohistochemical phenotype that is less often encountered in BRCA2 carcinomas. According to Bane et al.,[36] who compared 157 BRCA2-associated carcinomas with 314 carcinomas not associated with *BRCA1* or *BRCA2* mutations, BRCA2-associated carcinomas are high grade, express luminal cytokeratins significantly more often, and are less likely to overexpress HER2/*neu* protein.

Robson et al.[25] also reported that the presence of a germline *BRCA* mutation did not significantly increase the risk of ipsilateral breast recurrence after breast conservation with lumpectomy and radiotherapy compared with young women not known to have *BRCA* mutations. Patients with *BRCA* germline mutations had a substantial 5-year (11.9%) and 10-year (37.6%) risk of contralateral carcinoma and about 10% developed ovarian carcinoma.

Armes et al.[26] compared the histologic features of BRCA1- and BRCA2-associated breast carcinomas in a population-based study. The cases were drawn from a cohort of Australian women who found to have breast carcinoma before age 40. It is noteworthy that 70% of BRCA1 carriers and 40% of BRCA2 carriers did not have a family history of breast carcinoma in a first- or second-degree relative. When compared with tumors from BRCA2 carriers and age-matched controls, carcinomas in BRCA1 carriers were more often high grade with a higher mitotic rate. They were also more likely to be classified as medullary or atypical medullary carcinomas. Carriers of *BRCA2* mutations had an increased frequency of pleomorphic lobular carcinoma, but in other respects their tumors did not differ significantly from controls in histologic appearance. No follow-up data were provided.

BRCA1-associated invasive carcinomas of the breast are reported to have a significantly lower frequency of associated intraductal carcinoma than sporadic or nonhereditary carcinomas.[24,27] This observation is consistent with the low frequency of pure intraductal carcinoma observed in studies of BRCA1-associated tumors.[28] BRCA2 tumors did not have a significantly different frequency of intraductal carcinoma compared with sporadic control tumors.[24] The detection of BRCA mutations and emerging treatment regimens for patients with this genetic abnormality, such as the use of polyadenosine diphosphate ribose (PARP) polymerase inhibitors, are playing an increasingly significant role in the management of breast carcinoma.[37,38]

Bilaterality

The impact of bilateral breast carcinoma on prognosis has received considerable attention. The increasing use of magnetic resonance imaging (MRI) has enhanced the detection of contralateral breast carcinoma coincidental with a newly diagnosed ipsilateral carcinoma as reported by Berg et al.[39] who found carcinoma in the contralateral breasts of 4.1% (15/367) of women studied with either MRI or positron emission mammography (PEM). MRI detected 14 (93%) and 11 (73%) were visible on PEM. Among women treated by mastectomy, prognosis is similar after unilateral and bilateral diseases, compared on the basis of the higher stage tumor in bilateral cases.[29,30] Several studies that analyzed outcome in women with simultaneous bilateral breast carcinoma treated by breast conservation therapy reported no differences in OS compared with women treated by bilateral mastectomy or in comparison to women treated by unilateral breast conservation.[31–33] When compared with patients with unilateral carcinoma, patients with bilateral carcinoma had a greater frequency of multicentricity in one or both breasts (19% vs. 3%, respectively).[40]

Some reports have noted that patients with simultaneous bilateral breast carcinoma were older than women with unilateral tumors at the time of diagnosis,[34] or that patients with metachronous bilaterality tended to be younger.[41,42] Patients with bilateral carcinoma report a positive family history more often than women with unilateral tumors.[31,43] Lee et al.[33] reported a positive family of breast carcinoma in 28% of women with unilateral tumors and in 40% of patients with bilateral breast carcinoma, a statistically significant difference. The possibility of genetic susceptibility in some cases was suggested by the finding of a 70% incidence of other malignant tumors in women with a first-degree relative affected by breast carcinoma. Testing for *BRCA* mutations was not reported in this series of patients.

Genetic susceptibility to bilateral breast carcinoma is a potential confounding factor in the assessment of long-term prognosis for a patient who presents with unilateral breast carcinoma. Women with germline mutations in the *BRCA1* gene are especially susceptible to contralateral breast carcinoma, with a cumulative risk of nearly 50% by 50 years of age and 64% by 70 years.[44] Among *BRCA2* mutation carriers, the risk of contralateral carcinoma has been calculated to be 37% and 52%, respectively, by ages 50 and 70 years.[45] Age at diagnosis of the ipsilateral carcinoma is a contributing factor, with a risk of contralateral carcinoma of 40% within the subsequent 10 years if the ipsilateral carcinoma was diagnosed before age 50 years.[44] Metcalfe et al.[46] reported that the 10-year risks of subsequent contralateral breast carcinoma in women with ipsilateral carcinoma diagnosed prior to age 49 years, who were not treated with tamoxifen or oophorectomy, were 43.4% and 34.6%, respectively, for *BRCA1* and *BRCA2* mutation carriers.

Increased risk of contralateral breast carcinoma has also been found in women with familial breast carcinoma not attributed to *BRCA1* or *BRCA2* mutation. In a study of 204 women with invasive, familial non-BRCA1/BRCA2 breast carcinoma, Shahedi et al.[47] found a 20-year cumulative risk of contralateral breast carcinoma of 27.3% (95% confidence interval [CI], 15.0 to 37.8) that was significantly greater than the expected risk of 4.9%. The risk of contralateral breast carcinoma was significantly greater if the initial carcinoma was diagnosed prior to age 50 years (41.6%) than after age 50 years or more when ipsilateral carcinoma was diagnosed (10.1%). Adjuvant tamoxifen has been shown to reduce the risk of contralateral carcinoma in *BRCA1/BRCA2* mutation carriers.[48] It is likely that adjuvant anastrozole will also prove to be effective for reducing the occurrence of subsequent contralateral carcinomas in women with a genetic predisposition to develop breast carcinoma.[49]

An increasing proportion of women with unilateral breast cancer are electing to undergo contralateral prophylactic mastectomy. Surveillance Epidemiology and End Results (SEER) data indicate an increase of 150% from 1998 (4.2%) to 2003 (11%) in contralateral prophylactic mastectomies.[50] There was a doubling of such surgeries recorded in New York State Cancer Registry from 1995 to 2005.[51] It is likely that increased perception of the risk of contralateral breast carcinoma contributes to this practice.[52]

Method of Tumor Detection and Screening

The method of tumor detection influences prognosis and disease-free survival (DFS). Among patients diagnosed before widespread mammography screening, tumor detection by clinical examination was associated with a significant reduction in recurrence compared with detection by self-palpation.[53] Screening examinations employing mammography with or without physical examination have been shown to reduce mortality due to breast carcinoma in the screened population. When compared with unscreened controls, a 1985 report of data from a study conducted by the Health Insurance Plan of New York (HIP) revealed a 30% lower death rate due to breast carcinoma among women enrolled in a program of annual breast palpation and mammography.[54] An updated report in 1997 revealed a nearly 25% lower breast cancer mortality among screened women aged 40 to 64 at entry into the study compared with the control group after 18 years.[55] The reduction in mortality, compared with controls, for carcinomas diagnosed when women were in the 40- to 49-year group was 14%, 18 years after entry into the study.

Tabar et al.[56] demonstrated a reduction in mortality of nearly 30% with mammography screening at 2- and 3-year intervals in Sweden. A later analysis of the Swedish, two-county study revealed a 13% difference in breast cancer mortality between women invited and not invited to be screened in the 40- to 49-year age group.[57] In the 50- to 74-year age group, the difference in mortality was 35%, favoring the invited group. The relatively small impact of screening on mortality in the younger age group was attributed to failure to detect high-grade tumors sufficiently early with the screening intervals then being used in the study, and, consequently, more frequent screening was proposed for women younger than 50 years of age.[58,59]

The nationwide Breast Cancer Diagnosis Demonstration Project in the United States resulted in a greater than 50% reduction in "case fatality for all stages. . . . for cases that were screen detected than for cases that were not screen detected."[60] The favorable effect of screening on prognosis has also been documented with 20-year follow-up.[61]

When compared with breast carcinomas presenting clinically, carcinomas detected by screening with mammography tend to be smaller, to be lower grade, and to have fewer nodal metastases.[62–64] This difference is most pronounced in the first or prevalence screening examination.[65] Tumors detected in the first round of mammography screening have been shown to have low S-phase.[66,67] However, the relationship between nodal status and tumor size was similar among patients with carcinomas detected by screening and clinically; the frequency of nodal metastases did not differ significantly according to method of detection within any category of tumor size.[68] Hence, the advantage conferred by screening was dependent on detecting smaller tumors. No differences in the expression of HER2 and EGFR were reported in one study of screen- and clinically detected carcinomas.[63]

"Interval" carcinomas detected between screening examinations have been reported by some to have less favorable prognostic features than screen-detected tumors—such as high S-phase; aneuploidy; larger size; lower ER content[66,69,70]; fewer tubular carcinomas; and more invasive lobular, medullary, and higher grade carcinomas.[71] Although these observations have suggested that interval carcinomas would have a less favorable clinical course than screen-detected tumors,[72] follow-up studies have not consistently revealed a less favorable outcome among women with interval carcinomas.[73,74]

Vitak et al.[70] analyzed patients with prevalent-, incident-, and interval-detected carcinomas using data from the Östergötland county screening program in Sweden. The end points for assessing benefit derived from screening were the time to or frequency of systemic recurrence. The probability of systemic recurrence was significantly greater for women with interval-detected tumors and for women who did not participate in screening than in the screened group. The recurrence rate was significantly higher for interval tumors detected within 1 year of the last screen than for those detected later. These observations support the notion that interval carcinomas as a group tend to be clinically more aggressive than screen-detected tumors. When screen-detected and interval cases with similar characteristics (size, grade, etc.) were compared in multivariate analysis, the method of detection (screening vs. interval) was not significantly related to metastatic potential.

The possibility that a noninvasive diagnostic procedure might also detect prognostically significant biologic features of breast carcinoma has been explored with positron emission tomography (PET) using 2-deoxy-2-fluoro[^{18}F]-d-glucose (FDG) to obtain information about glucose metabolism. Cancer cells exhibit a higher rate of glycolysis than normal cells, and they overexpress the immunohistochemically detected glucose transport molecule, GLUT1, which may be responsible for glucose accumulation.[75] PET has identified breast carcinomas in several studies,[76,77] and it has been effective in distinguishing benign and malignant tumors,[78,79] with a sensitivity of 68% to 94% and a specificity of 84% to 97%.[79] Response of breast carcinoma to preoperative chemotherapy has been evaluated by PET.[80] Oshida et al.[81] studied the differential absorption rate (DAR) of FDG in breast carcinomas by PET and related the calculated DAR to prognosis in 70 patients after a mean follow-up of 41 months. The mean DAR was 2.61 (SD ± 1.61) (range, 0.65 to 9.39). When patients were stratified into two groups with DAR (greater than 3.0 or DAR less than or equal to3.0), patients with high DAR had a significantly worse overall and RFS. DAR proved to be a significant independent indicator of RFS in multivariate analysis. DAR was also significantly related to microvessel density (MVD) in the primary tumors of patients with and without axillary lymph node (ALN) metastases.

Incremental improvements in radiologic techniques have resulted in improved tumor detection rates mainly due to enhanced image quality. The age of onset and frequency of mammographic screening in asymptomatic women without family history of breast carcinoma have been controversial; however, the American Cancer Society recommends annual mammograms beginning at age 40.[82]

Time to Recurrence

The interval to recurrence (DFS or recurrence-free interval) and length of survival are basic measurements of prognosis. In general, these are closely related; hence, factors associated with a high frequency of recurrence correlate with reduced survival. Treatment that delays but does not reduce the overall frequency of recurrence may increase the duration of survival without reducing overall mortality due to the disease. These concepts are supported by a report from Edwards et al.,[83] who analyzed nearly 2,000 patients to assess the relationships between time from treatment to relapse, time from treatment to death, and time from relapse to death. In this series, the time to relapse was not significantly correlated with time from relapse to death. Touboul et al.[84] analyzed 528 patients treated by breast conservation with radiotherapy. In this clinical setting, the risk of distant metastases was related to the incidence of local recurrence. The disease-free interval from the start of treatment to local recurrence influenced survival, so that a shorter interval to local recurrence was associated with shorter OS. Factors predicting local failure and systemic metastases differed. Local recurrence was significantly associated with diagnosis at age 40 years or younger, premenopausal status, two tumor foci rather than one, and extensive intraductal component. The probability of systemic recurrence was significantly related to the number of lymph nodes with metastases, high histologic grade, and presence of local recurrence.

Survival after recurrence is influenced by characteristics of the primary tumor and of the recurrence. The range of reported median survival after recurrence was 11 to 37 months more than a decade ago.[85] Postrecurrence survival has been improved by advances in systemic therapy. Factors associated with shorter postrecurrence survival include short recurrence-free interval, visceral metastases, ER-negative tumor, larger primary tumor size, the presence of axillary nodal metastases at diagnosis, and premenopausal menstrual status at the time of initial treatment.[85–87] Patients with stage I disease at the time of diagnosis are more likely to have an initial recurrence that is locoregional, whereas stage II patients are more likely to have a systemic recurrence initially.[88] If locoregional recurrences are excluded, stage I and stage II patients have similar patterns of recurrence at systemic sites.[88] Systemic adjuvant therapy tends to increase the disease-free interval, and there is evidence that patients given adjuvant therapy relapse in fewer sites.[89]

Local Radiotherapy

Radiotherapy administered to the chest wall after mastectomy or to the breast after lumpectomy reduces the risk of local recurrence at these sites. Whether this beneficial effect on local recurrence is translated into improved OS in patients who receive radiation to the chest wall after mastectomy remains controversial, and the benefit, if any, may not be sufficient to offset potential complications such as cardiovascular disease.[90–92] Data from one study suggest that the survival benefit of reduced local recurrence after mastectomy for node-negative patients at 10 years may be 2%, and 6% for women with axillary nodal metastases.[93] To assess the cardiovascular effects of chest wall radiation, Hojris et al.[94] analyzed data from a trial in which patients were randomized to systemic treatment with or without locoregional radiotherapy after mastectomy. After a median follow-up of 10 years, mortality due to breast carcinoma was lower in the radiated (44.2%) than in the nonradiated group (52.5%). The two groups experienced similar rates of death due to ischemic heart disease. The hazard rate for mortality due to ischemic heart disease in the radiated versus nonradiated group did not increase with time after treatment.

The laterality of carcinoma and subsequent radiotherapy proved to be a significant risk factor of mortality due to myocardial infarction in a study of cancer registry data for U.S. patients treated from 1973 to 1992.[95] The analysis did not distinguish between surgical treatment by lumpectomy or mastectomy. The relative risk (RR) for a fatal myocardial infarction (controlling for age) was 1.17 (95% CI, 1.01 to 13.6) among women with left versus right breast carcinoma. The RR was increased for women treated before age 60 (RR, 1.98; 95% CI, 1.31 to 2.97) but not in women older than 60 years at the time of treatment. The age-related effect was observed in patients with regional disease at diagnosis, but no difference related to age was found for women with local disease. These data suggest that chest wall radiation after left breast carcinoma increases the risk of cardiovascular disease in women younger than 60 years at the time of treatment.

Advances in brachytherapy, exemplified by the development of Accelerated Partial Breast Irradiation (APBI) techniques such as balloon-based MammoSite, offer tumor bed control rate that is at least equal to, and potentially higher than, whole-breast irradiation and have the potential for less radiation to the heart and lungs.[96]

Local Recurrence in Conserved Breast or Chest Wall

In patients treated by breast-conserving surgery and radiation therapy, the time to breast recurrence is significantly related to the risk of systemic metastases and survival at 5 years.[97] Patients with breast recurrences 2 to 4 years after diagnosis have a significantly greater risk of developing systemic metastases and poorer survival than those who manifest breast recurrence more than 4 years after initial treatment.[97,98] The rates of local breast recurrence and distant metastases after breast conservation appear to differ. In one series, the yearly frequency of local breast recurrence was about 1% per year up to 10 years, whereas the probability of systemic metastases was 5% at 2 years and decreased thereafter.[98] Tumor size and ALN metastases were predictors of systemic metastases, but were not related to local recurrence in patients treated by breast conservation.

Whether recurrence in the breast or chest wall is a marker for tumors that are more likely to disseminate or are a source of metastases remains to be determined. The two scenarios are not mutually exclusive, and one or both may apply in individual cases. One study relevant to this issue was described by Schnitt et al.,[99] who reported that breast recurrences were detected in 14 (16%) of 87 patients with node-negative invasive breast carcinoma treated by lumpectomy without radiotherapy. The median follow-up period was 56 months. Tumor size ranged from 2 to 25 mm (median, 9 mm), and 76% of the tumors were detected by mammography alone. All patients underwent reexcision of the initial biopsy site, with residual tumor detected in only two reexcisions, and all had negative final margins of excision. In addition to the 14 patients with local recurrence, 4 other women (11%) had systemic metastases with no prior local recurrences. Breast recurrence was observed in one of these four women after systemic metastases were detected. A comparison group treated with conservation surgery and radiotherapy had no breast recurrences, and the 3-year metastatic rate was 7%. Neither group of patients received systemic adjuvant therapy. These data suggest that local breast recurrence after conservation therapy and systemic metastases are not necessarily linked temporally and may be independent events. Recurrence in the breast after conservation therapy often occurs without clinical evidence of concurrent systemic metastases, and patients may develop systemic metastases when local recurrence is not evident. The "natural history" in these circumstances may be influenced by breast irradiation and adjuvant systemic therapy.

American College of Surgeons Oncology Group's Z0010 was a prospective multicenter trial initiated in 1999 to evaluate occult disease in sentinel lymph nodes (SLNs) and bone marrow of early-stage breast carcinoma patients and to determine factors important in local–regional recurrence (LRR) in patients with negative sentinel nodes by hematoxylin and eosin (H&E) staining. The recently published results of this trial are contributory to the study of local recurrence.[100] Participants included women with biopsy-proven T1–2 breast carcinomas with clinically negative nodes who were treated by lumpectomy and whole-breast radiation. Patients with clinical T1–2N0M0 disease underwent lumpectomy and sentinel node dissection. There was no axillary-specific treatment for H&E-negative sentinel nodes. Of 5,119 patients, 3,904 (76.3%) had H&E-negative sentinel nodes. At median follow-up of 8.4 years, there were 127 local, 20 regional, and 134 distant recurrences. Factors associated with LRR were hormone-receptor–negative disease ($p = 0.0004$) and age at diagnosis of 50 years or less ($p = 0.047$). Hormone-receptor–positive disease and use of chemotherapy were associated with reduced LRR. When local recurrence was included as a time-dependent variable, age at diagnosis of more than 50 years, T2 disease, high tumor grade, and local recurrence were associated with reduced OS.

Early Detection of Recurrence

Most recurrences are documented because patients present with symptoms or they are evident on physical examination.[101,102] The detection of asymptomatic metastases by screening patients with x-ray or laboratory tests during follow-up after primary therapy has resulted in a reduction in the lead time to the diagnosis of recurrence in some[102,103] but not all studies.[104–106] In one study, patients with asymptomatic recurrences detected by screening at scheduled times had a longer postrecurrence survival than patients with symptomatic lesions detected during intervals between scheduled examinations.[107] This may reflect more favorable prognostic features associated with occult recurrences.[102] Routine screening of patients treated by mastectomy using scans, radiography, and laboratory tests to detect asymptomatic, clinically inapparent recurrences has not been shown to improve the OS of patients with breast carcinoma.[102–106] After reviewing the usefulness of routine imaging studies in the follow-up of patients with mammary and colonic carcinoma, Kagan and Steckel[107] concluded that "earlier detection of a local recurrence or metastatic disease through periodic tests in the asymptomatic patient with breast or colon cancer rarely alters the treatment or the outcome." This conclusion must be reconsidered periodically as more effective forms of systemic therapy are developed.

Time Dependency of Prognostic Variables

There is evidence indicating that the prognostic importance of a given pathologic variable does not apply uniformly throughout the course of follow-up, but the time dependency of prognostic variables has not been thoroughly analyzed.[108–110] Some variables are associated with short-term outcome, whereas others appear to exert an effect later. This is illustrated by the observation that the main influence of tumor necrosis on prognosis is manifested early in follow-up.[111] In another study, nuclear grade, nodal status, and peritumoral lymphocytic infiltration were related to prognosis in time-dependent patterns.[112]

Analysis of the long-term follow-up of 462 consecutively treated patients by Nab et al.[113] revealed that the risk of recurrence decreased progressively from 10% in the first 2 years after diagnosis to 1% beyond 10 years. After 10 years, 72% of T1N0 patients were recurrence free, and only 1 of the remaining 79 disease-free women developed a recurrence thereafter. During the first 5 years of follow-up, nodal status and tumor size each had approximately equal significance as prognostic markers. In the 5- to 10-year interval, only tumor size remained prognostically significant.

Arriagada et al.[114] studied a panel of clinicopathologic prognostic factors at 5-year intervals in 2,410 French women with primary operable breast carcinoma and a follow-up of at least 25 years. Tumor size, histologic grade, the number of ALNs with metastases, and age at diagnosis were risk factors for death in the first 5 years of follow-up. The prognostic effect of tumor size, grade, and nodal status declined in the 5- to 10-year follow-up interval, and after 10 to 15 years only age at diagnosis remained significantly related to the risk of death. This analysis did not discriminate death due to breast carcinoma from death due to other causes.

A similar study within a shorter time span reported by Takeuchi et al.[115] involved 1,423 Japanese women analyzed at 2.5-year intervals for 7.5 years. Significant factors for survival in the initial 2.5 years included tumor size, nodal status, age at diagnosis, presence of lymphatic or vascular invasion, and the hormone receptor status of the primary tumor. By 7.5 years, only tumor size and lymphatic or vascular invasion by the primary tumor were prognostically significant in multivariate analysis.

The divergent results with respect to the time dependency of various prognostic factors in the foregoing studies probably reflect differences in treatment, analytical methodology, and other unrecognized factors. Although these reports point to the existence of this phenomenon, considerably more research is needed to more accurately pinpoint how time dependency relates to known prognostic factors.

Combined data from several adjuvant therapy trials under the aegis of the Eastern Cooperative Oncology Group (ECOG) have been analyzed to determine the annual hazard for recurrence in this clinical setting.[116] The peak hazard rate for recurrence occurred 1 to 2 years after diagnosis and the initiation of therapy. A consistent decline in the hazard rate was observed in years 2 to 5, with a more slowly declining rate thereafter through the 12th year. Most patients followed this overall pattern; subsets of patients at greater risk for recurrence, such as women with three or more nodal metastases, had a higher hazard for recurrence at all intervals of follow-up than those at lower risk. For years 5 to 12 after diagnosis, the mean hazard for recurrence was 4.3% per year.

Methods of Analysis: Univariate and Multivariate

Analysis of prognostic variables is typically performed by univariate and multivariate methods. The former approach examines each prognostic factor separately, being influenced by other factors only to the extent that the analysis is restricted by stratification for other variables (e.g., stage, menstrual status). Multivariate analysis compares the relative prognostic importance of the individual variables included in an analysis. A factor that has prognostic significance in univariate analysis may prove not to be significant when assessed in the context of other variables in multivariate analysis.

There have also been attempts to assess combinations of variables as a means for developing a prognostic profile or prognostic index.[117–119] For example, a prognostic model based on SPF, PR status, and tumor size distinguished between node-negative patients with an increased risk of distant relapse and those with an age-adjusted survival similar to a control population.[120] The Nottingham Prognostic Index (NPI) employs tumor size, lymph node status, and histologic grade to stratify patients into significantly different prognostic groups.[121,122] Various methods of grading and ALN staging have been used to determine components of the index.[122] This concept deserves more attention in clinical practice because of the growing interest in a greater variety of clinical, pathologic, and biologic prognostic factors. Because the influence of all prognostic factors in a given case may not be unidirectional (favorable or unfavorable), it is likely that multiple combinations of these variables may be associated with equivalent outcomes.[119]

Impact of Therapy on Prognosis

It is also important to consider the impact of primary treatment on the evaluation of prognostic factors. Radical mastectomy was, until the 1960s, the most widely employed form of primary treatment. A large body of data was accumulated with respect to the importance of stage at diagnosis, type of tumor, and other clinical and morphologic parameters in relation to this form of treatment. Subsequent decades have witnessed major changes in treatment, with a shift from total mastectomy to partial mastectomy, quadrantectomy, or lumpectomy combined with primary radiation therapy and axillary dissection or SLN mapping. The evaluation of prognostic factors has been further complicated by the introduction of neoadjuvant and adjuvant hormonal therapy and chemotherapy for women with nodal metastases and for many patients with uninvolved lymph nodes. At present, reports documenting the follow-up of patients treated with various modalities suggest that pathologic prognostic variables determined to be significant in populations treated by mastectomy are equally relevant to survival and systemic recurrence for patients treated by breast-conserving surgery and radiotherapy.[123,124] The extent to which the prognostic importance of conventional pathologic parameters influences response to neoadjuvant and adjuvant chemotherapy is less certain and should be the subject of investigation. Pinder et al.[125] reported that response to chemotherapy was more favorable in patients with high-grade carcinoma if they had lymph node metastases, but this effect was not evident in node-negative cases.

Changing Incidence and Mortality

Data from the National Cancer Institute (NCI) SEER program have been used to estimate the incidence rate of breast carcinoma and mortality due to the disease in the United States.[126] Between 1973 and 1992, the overall incidence rose from 82.5 per 100,000 women to 110.6, increasing steadily from 1973 to 1987, and stabilizing in the period from 1988 to 1992. From 1973 to 1992, the death rate varied between approximately 26 and 27 per 100,000 women, with a decline to 26.2 in the period from 1989 to 1992. Data from Sweden also documented an increasing incidence of and declining mortality due to breast carcinoma in Malmö compared with the rest of Sweden.[127] The reduction of mortality in Malmö was 43% compared with 12% throughout Sweden.

Data from the NCI summarized in a report titled "Breast Cancer Facts and Figures 2005–2006"[128] indicate that the incidence of female breast carcinoma was constant between 1975 and 1980. The incidence increased by nearly 4% per year from 1980 to 1987 and continued to increase by about 0.3% per year through 2002. Coincidentally, the death rate due to breast cancer rose annually by 0.4% from 1975 to 1990. Between 1990 and 2002, the death rate decreased by 2.3% annually. The annual decline in death due to breast cancer was greater among women younger than 50 years (3.3% per year) than among those 50 years and older (2.0% per year).

The increase in and subsequent stabilization of incidence and the decline in the death rate have been attributed to the combined effects of screening by mammography and clinical examination and improved methods of treatment. A decline in mortality due to breast carcinoma among women born after 1920 has been documented in several countries.[129]

GROSS APPEARANCE

For the most part, there are no clinical features that distinguish invasive ductal carcinoma from other types of invasive carcinoma and some benign tumors. An exception is palpable breast carcinoma associated with Paget disease of the nipple. The underlying invasive carcinoma in these cases is almost always of the ductal type, NOS. However, Paget disease may derive from DCIS limited to the lactiferous ducts without invasion. Coincidentally, there may be a palpable lesion formed by another separate carcinoma, possibly of a different histologic type, such as a tubular carcinoma. Invasive ductal carcinoma occurs throughout the age range of breast carcinoma, being most common in the mid to late 50s.

Invasive ductal carcinoma typically forms a solid tumor. The consistency and appearance of the cut surface vary considerably depending on the composition of the tumor. Cystic change is extremely uncommon in this group of lesions but may be a manifestation of necrosis, sometimes accompanied by hemorrhage in the degenerated area. Noncystic areas of necrosis may be soft and chalky white or hemorrhagic (Fig. 12.1). Carcinomas with a relatively abundant fibrotic stroma can be extremely firm to hard, with a gray to white surface. When there is prominent elastosis of the stroma, yellow tinges may be observed. Chalky white streaks in the tumor are usually indicative of necrosis (Fig. 12.2), calcification, or elastosis. Carcinomas with less abundant stroma that are composed largely of neoplastic cells and inflammatory cells tend to be softer and tan. The cut surfaces of such cellular neoplasms are likely to bulge slightly when incised (Fig. 12.3).

Tumor Size

The measured gross size represented by the largest dimension of a mammary carcinoma is one of the most significant prognostic variables. Numerous studies have shown that survival decreases with increasing tumor size and that there is a coincidental rise in the frequency of axillary nodal metastases.[112,130–132] This phenomenon applies not only to the overall spectrum of primary tumor size, but also within subsets such as those defined by tumor-node-metastasis (TNM) staging. For example, in T1 breast carcinomas (2 cm or less in diameter), there is a significant relationship between size, the frequency of nodal metastases, and prognosis when the tumors are stratified in 5-mm groups.[133,134] Roger et al.[135] reported the following significant ($p < 0.0001$) distribution of the frequency of axillary nodal involvement in relation to tumor size in a series of 534 patients: T1a (0 to 0.5 cm, 3%); T1b (0.6 to 1.0 cm, 10%); (1.1 to 1.5 cm, 21%); and (1.6 to 2.0 cm, 35%). Data from the Breast Cancer Surveillance Consortium for 786,846 women aged 40 to 89 years with breast carcinomas diagnosed by screening mammography revealed negative ALNs in 91.8%, 78.2%, and 57.9% of patients with tumors, which measured 0 to 10 mm, 11 to 20 mm, and 21 to 50 mm, respectively.[136] Prasad et al.[137] investigated the frequency of axillary nodal involvement in patients with T1*mic* carcinoma with invasion measuring 1 mm or less in diameter in 21 patients including 18 with ductal and 3 with lobular carcinomas. Axillary dissection in 15 patients (primary tumor type not specified) revealed a single nodal metastasis in each of two cases.

A detailed analysis of tumor size and nodal status in women with T1 breast carcinoma was reported by Abner

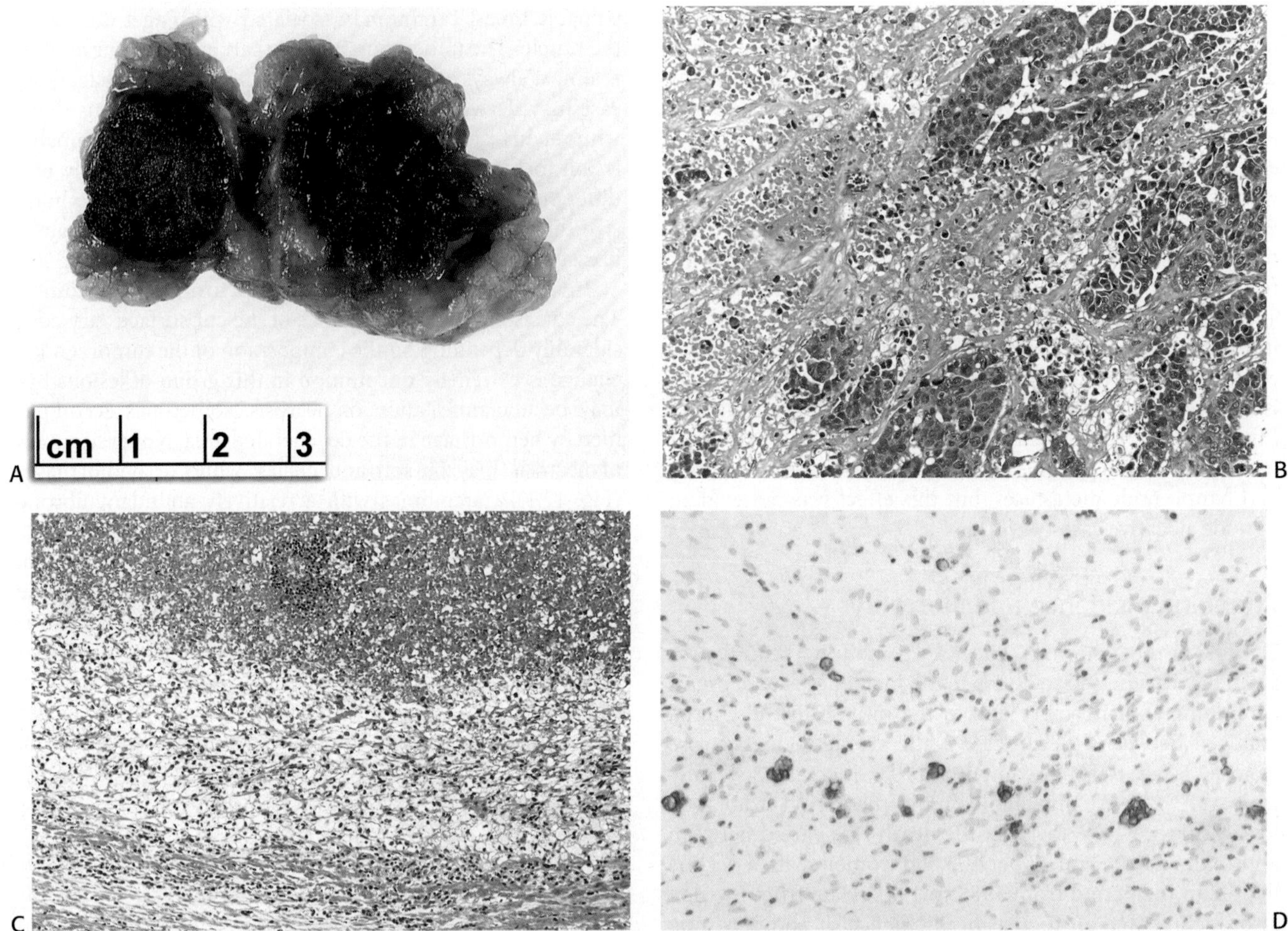

FIG. 12.1. ***Invasive ductal carcinoma.*** **A:** The dark, well-defined area is necrotic invasive carcinoma with hemorrhage. **B:** Pink areas of necrotic tumor contain blue dots of nuclear debris. Remaining islands of residual carcinoma are evident. **C:** Another invasive ductal carcinoma with infarction and peripheral histiocytes. **D:** Isolated carcinoma cells at the border in **[C]** are highlighted by the CK7 cytokeratin immunostain.

et al.,[138] who studied 118 patients treated by breast-onserving surgery and radiation therapy. Macroscopic tumor size and microscopically measured invasive tumor diameter were equal in 22% of cases. The macroscopic size was smaller than microscopic size in 31% and larger in 47% of cases. Overall, 21% of patients had ALN metastases. The 10-year actuarial rate of recurrence-free survival was 91% of N0 patients with tumors measured macroscopically as less than or equal to1.0 cm, compared with 77% for patients with macroscopic tumors measuring 1.1 to 2.0 cm. The rates for tumors measured microscopically were 96% and 72%, respectively. These data indicate somewhat greater prognostic discrimination when T1 tumor size is measured microscopically to define the diameter of the invasive component if the entire invasive tumor fits on one histologic slide.

Analysis of the tumor size of breast carcinomas recorded in SEER registry data revealed a progressive increase in the proportion of smaller tumors between 1975 and 1999.[139] The proportion of carcinomas that measured less than 1 cm rose from less than 10% from 1975 to 1979 to about 25% in 1995 to 1999 among node-negative patients. Among node-positive patients, the proportion with tumors less than 2 cm rose from about 20% to 33% in the same time periods. In both groups, the trends toward smaller tumors were statistically significant. These trends in tumor size distribution were matched by increased relative survival rates in the node-negative and node-positive groups.

Among node-negative patients considered to be at high risk for recurrence (any size tumor, either ER-negative or ER-positive, tumor larger than 2 cm), the addition of systemic chemotherapy resulted in a 34% reduction in the risk of death due to breast carcinoma after 10 years and a 10.1% absolute benefit in OS.[140]

Impact of Tumor Size and Nodal Status on Prognosis

Long-term follow-up is necessary to fully assess the prognosis of patients who had invasive carcinoma with a favorable stage such as T1N0M0 The 20-year OS in a Finish Cancer Registry study was 54% (95% CI, 48% to 60%), and the survival rate corrected for nonbreast carcinoma deaths

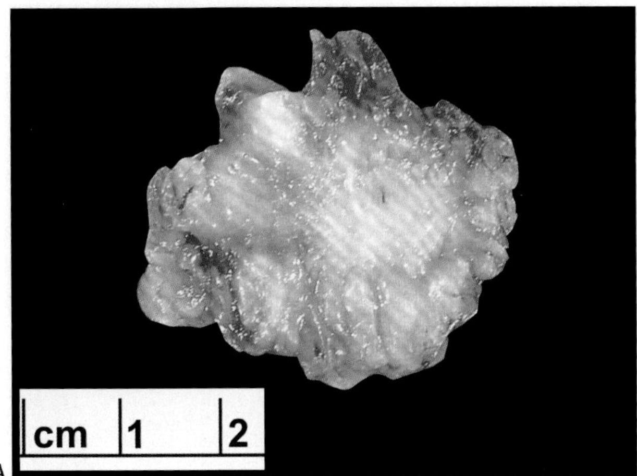

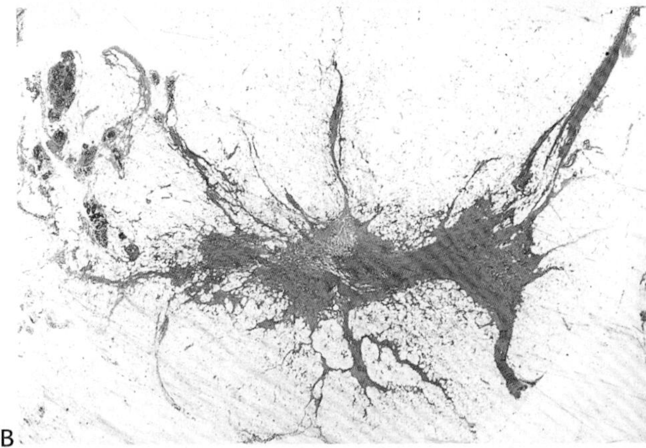

FIG. 12.2. ***Invasive ductal carcinoma.*** **A:** This tumor has a stellate border and chalky white streaks of necrosis. **B:** A whole-mount histologic section of a stellate invasive ductal carcinoma.

was 81% (95% CI, 75% to 87%).[141] In patients with T1a–b tumors, the corrected 20-year survival rate was 92% (95% CI, 86% to 96%), and in the T1c group corrected 20-year survival was 75% (95% CI, 64% to 86%). During the first 15 years of follow-up, the risk of death duc to breast carcinoma was 0.70% per year of follow-up, rising to 0.80%, 1.51%, and 1.19% per year in each of the subsequent 5-year intervals. During the same period, the risk of death due to nonmammary carcinoma was 0.23%, 0.45%, 0.88%, and 0.71% per year in each 5-year period.

The interaction of the number of involved lymph nodes and tumor size is important prognostically in stage II patients. Quiet et al.[142] found that the DFS after mastectomy was 81% in patients with one lymph node metastasis and a tumor 2 cm or smaller, compared with 59% if the tumor was larger than 2 cm.

Measuring the Size of a Unifocal Invasive Ductal Carcinoma

The majority of patients with invasive ductal carcinoma have a single tumor mass clinically and pathologically. Because most carcinomas have asymmetric shapes, the measurement of size is generally reported in terms of the greatest dimension, recorded to the nearest millimeter. It is important that the excised tumor be submitted intact to the pathologist, so that the configuration of the lesion can be assessed by palpation. This makes it possible to bisect the specimen in a plane that exposes the longest dimension. The measurement should be made before samples are taken for frozen section (FS) or any other procedure. When a FS is prepared, the grossly measured diameter may be entered as part of the FS record.

The largest gross diameter of a carcinoma is an approximation of the actual volume of invasive tumor present. Benign tissue with hyperplastic or reactive changes may contribute to the palpable lesion. In some tumors, a considerable part of the mass is composed of invasive carcinoma, whereas in other lesions of comparable gross size, varying proportions of the bulk may be intraductal carcinoma, resulting in a lesser invasive component.[143,144] Measurement of invasive carcinoma exclusive of peripheral extensions of intraductal carcinoma is recommended when it is practical to make this distinction on the basis of histologic sections. In some cases, there is microscopic extension of the invasive component beyond the grossly measurable tumor. These contiguous peripheral invasive elements should be included in the measurement of tumor size, especially in tumors less than 2 cm in greatest dimension when they can be represented by a complete cross section on a histologic slide. If invasive carcinoma is dispersed across the entire tumor dimension in histologic sections, the largest dimension from point to point across the entire invasive diameter is the measured tumor size, even if there are interspersed zones of intraductal carcinoma or benign tissue. A comment can be made to indicate the approximate proportion of the cross-sectional area that is occupied by invasive carcinoma.

It is rarely possible to accurately assess the *in vivo* size of an invasive carcinoma in needle core biopsy samples because it is difficult to ensure that the material represents the largest dimension. When microinvasive ductal carcinoma is found in a needle core biopsy specimen, it is possible that a larger invasive tumor will be found when an excisional biopsy is performed. A small invasive focus may be limited to one of multiple levels prepared from a paraffin block.[145] Correlation of the needle core biopsy sample with the dimensions of a tumor seen on a mammogram can be useful in some circumstances to confirm the gross size of a carcinoma and to assess the contour of the tumor.

One review of tumor sizes determined in mammograms and excised specimens found no evidence that a prior needle core biopsy influenced the final measurement of the tumors.[146] The study evaluated 138 mammographically detected T1 invasive tumors, including 61 sampled by core biopsy prior to excision and 77 excised without a core biopsy. The mean mammographic and pathologic sizes in the two groups were not significantly different (2.3 and 1.96 mm, respectively). However, there are circumstances in which needle core biopsy sampling—particularly with larger vacuum-assisted sampling—removes a substantial portion of a small invasive carcinoma to an extent that the remaining tumor in the excised specimen no longer accurately reflects

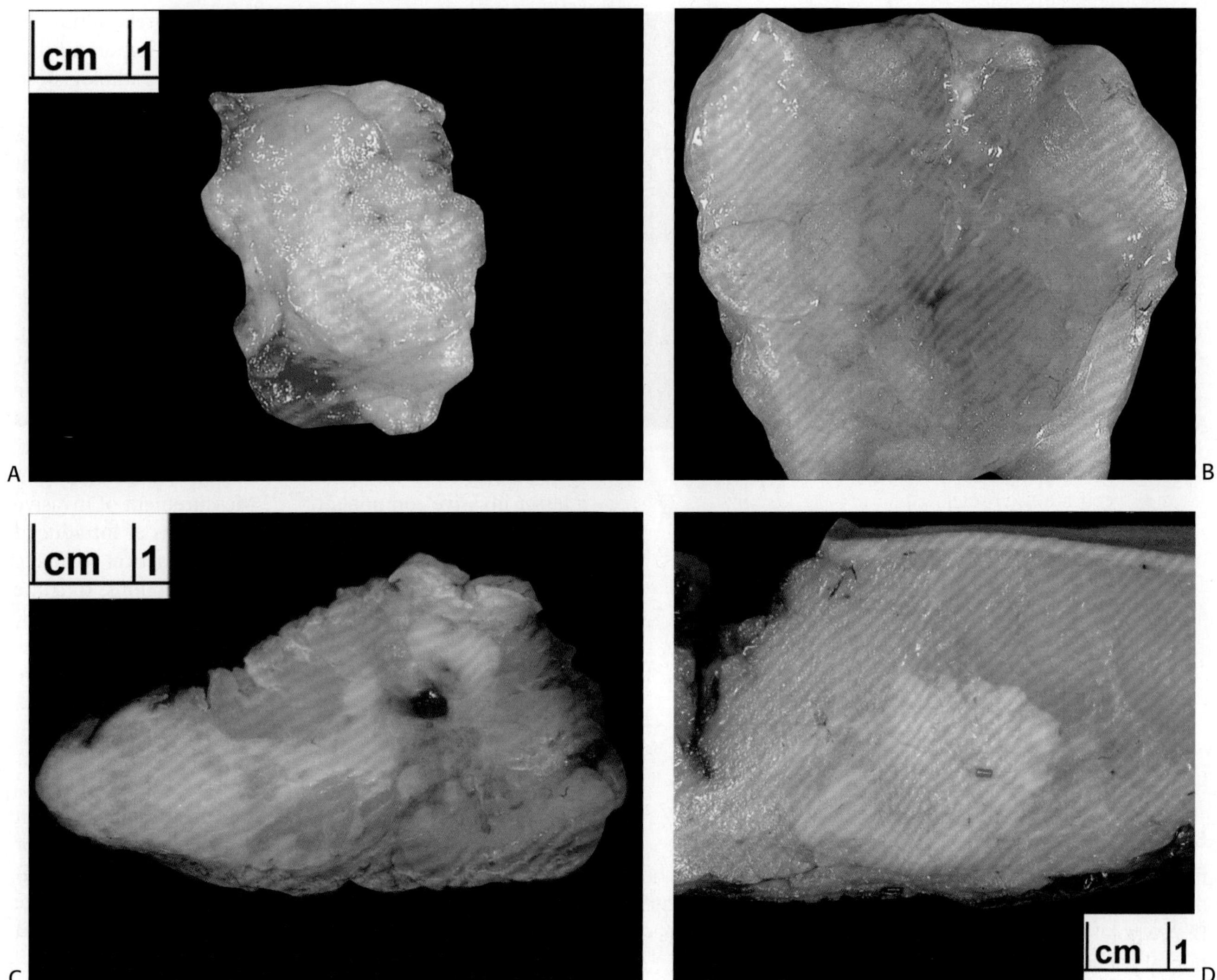

FIG. 12.3. ***Invasive ductal carcinoma.*** **A:** The tumor has a circumscribed border and bulges above the surrounding tissue. **B:** This fleshy invasive ductal carcinoma with central retraction was poorly differentiated and had a lymphocytic infiltrate. **C:** The hemorrhagic cavity in this bisected irregularly shaped invasive ductal carcinoma is the site of a prior needle core biopsy. The various margins are inked in different colors. The deep margin has been marked with orange ink. **D:** This bisected, white, circumscribed invasive ductal carcinoma stands out against the surrounding fat. There is a marker clip in the tumor.

the prebiopsy size. In such situations, size based on imaging studies may be more accurate than pathologic measurements. According to the latest American Joint Committee on Cancer (AJCC) guidelines, in such cases, "either the core biopsy or the excisional biopsy is used for T classification unless imaging dimensions suggest a larger invasive cancer."[147] It is always prudent to review the earlier needle core biopsies with invasive carcinoma whenever "no residual" invasive carcinoma is identified in the subsequently performed excisional biopsy since such cases may rarely represent "false-positive" diagnoses on core biopsy. Furthermore, the greatest extent of invasive carcinoma should be reported in all needle core biopsy specimens since it has been shown that this datum may establish a higher final pathologic T stage—and has been shown by Edwards et al.[148] to do so in 7.5% (15 in a series of 222) cases.

Rakha et al.[149] found no residual carcinoma in 174 of 40,395 (0.43%) patients with a needle core biopsy that was followed by surgery. Eight of the 174 cases were considered false positive because DCIS had been interpreted as invasive carcinoma. In a ninth case, fat necrosis was misdiagnosed as invasive carcinoma. In the remaining 165 cases, review of the core biopsy and excisional biopsy specimens confirmed that the entire lesion had been removed in the initial procedure. The median mammographic size of carcinomas completely removed by the core biopsy procedure was 6 mm (range 3 to 30 mm). In this rare circumstance, the largest dimension of an intact needle core biopsy sample and the mammographic size of the abnormality must be considered in arriving at the T stage.[147]

Measuring the Size of Multifocal or Multicentric Invasive Ductal Carcinoma

A minority of patients have clinically, grossly or microscopically, identifiable multifocal tumor, that is, invasive tumor in the same breast quadrant or multicentric tumor, that is, invasive tumors in more than one quadrant. When clinically apparent, multiple nodules may be sampled by needle core biopsies to confirm this impression.

The 7th edition of the AJCC[147] makes the specific recommendation regarding the pathologic assessment of invasive tumor size, that is pT, that "the microscopic measurement is the most accurate and preferred method to determine pT with a small invasive cancer that can be entirely submitted in one paraffin block" and that "the gross measurement is the most accurate and preferred method to determine pT with larger invasive cancers that must be submitted in multiple paraffin blocks." For smaller tumors, which may be "unapparent to any clinical modalities or gross pathologic examination," pT can be determined "by carefully measuring and recording the relative positions of the tissue samples submitted for microscopic evaluation and determining which contain tumor."

Data obtained by Andea et al.[150] suggest that the aggregate diameter of grossly measurable nodules might be a more accurate guide to prognosis than the current convention of staging on the basis of the largest nodule as recommended in the seventh edition of the AJCC Cancer Staging Manual.[147] In their study, total tumor volumes and surface areas calculated from pathologic measurements were better predictors of nodal status than the diameter of the single largest lesion. When aggregate tumor diameter was calculated, multifocal and unifocal carcinomas of similar size did not differ significantly with respect to nodal status.[151] Coombs and Boyages[152] obtained a similar result in an analysis of 94 patients (11.1%) with multifocal carcinoma in a series of 848 women with breast carcinoma. Axillary nodal metastases were present in 52.1% of patients with multifocal carcinoma and in 37.5% of those with unifocal tumors. When tumor size among those with multifocal carcinoma was based only on the largest lesion, patients with multifocal tumors had more frequent nodal metastases than women with unifocal tumors of equivalent diameter. This difference was substantially diminished when aggregate tumor size was taken into consideration for multifocal tumor cases.

For staging on the basis of the standards set forth by the most recent AJCC Staging Manual, tumor size in patients with multiple simultaneous ipsilateral primary (i.e., multifocal and multicentric) carcinoma should be reported as the largest tumor dimension. The presence and sizes of the smaller tumor(s) should be recorded using the "m" modifier.[147] In clinical practice, it should be appreciated that this rule leads to understaging of tumor size in some cases. Furthermore, the AJCC Tumor Staging Manual[147] does not give clear guidance for determining pT in the presence of multicentric and multifocal invasive carcinomas. One statement referring to "multiple simultaneous ipsilateral primary carcinomas" recommends that "T stage assignment in this setting should be based only on the largest tumor, and the sum of the sizes should not be used." This is followed by the comment that "invasive carcinomas that are in close proximity, but are apparently separate grossly, may represent truly separate tumors or one tumor with a complex shape. Distinguishing these two situations may require judgement and close correlation between pathologic and clinical findings (especially imaging), and preference should be given the modality thought to be the most accurate in a specific case. When macroscopically apparently distinct tumors are very close (e.g., less than 5 mm), especially if they are similar histologically, they are most likely one tumor with a complex shape, and their T category should be based on the largest combined dimension." These guidelines further state that "these criteria apply to multiple macroscopically measurable tumors and do not apply to one macroscopic carcinoma associated with multiple separate microscopic (satellite) foci."

In view of the data provided by Andea et al.[150] and Coombs and Boyages,[152] as well as the imprecise and largely unsubstantiated AJCC recommendations, it would be prudent for the individual pathology report to provide the size (diameter) of the single largest invasive tumor focus and the aggregate size based on the largest diameters of all measurable invasive tumor foci. This information can be provided separately for multiple grossly evident invasive lesions and for foci that are only identified microscopically.

MRI offers a clinical, objective method for determining tumor volume without the necessity for calculations based on pathologic tumor measurements. MRI measurements of tumor diameter correlate more closely with pathologic tumor size than do measurements by mammography, ultrasound, or clinical examination.[153] MRI has also proven to be the most accurate method for measuring tumor size during neoadjuvant chemotherapy.[154] Partridge et al.[155] studied MRI as a method for predicting response to treatment and RFS in 62 patients who received neoadjuvant chemotherapy. Final change in tumor volume determined by MRI was more strongly predictive of RFS ($p = 0.015$) than change in MRI tumor diameter ($p = 0.07$) or change in clinical tumor size ($p = 0.27$). As MRI becomes more universally available, it is possible that primary tumor volume measured by this modality will become an accepted part of the clinical staging of breast carcinoma.

The assessment of invasive size tumor before and after neoadjuvant chemotherapy is discussed in detail in Chapter 41. According to the latest edition of the AJCC Cancer Staging Manual, "pretreatment T is defined as clinical (cT)" since "it is not possible to determine a pretreatment pathologic size." "Post-treatment (ypT) size should be estimated based on the best combination of gross, imaging, and microscopic histologic findings."[147]

Tumor Configuration or Shape

The majority of invasive ductal carcinomas can be described on the basis of gross tumor configuration as stellate (spiculated, infiltrative, radial, serrated), circumscribed (rounded, pushing, encapsulated, smooth), or having a mixed contour (Figs. 12.2 to 12.5). Approximately one-third of the tumors have grossly circumscribed margins. A minority of tumors have indistinct borders and cannot be described in these terms. In general, the gross appearance of the tumor duplicates the configuration visualized by mammography. However, carcinomas that appear to have circumscribed margins grossly or mammographically may exhibit an invasive growth pattern microscopically.

Some investigators have observed a more favorable prognosis associated with circumscribed carcinomas determined by gross inspection or by mammography.[156,157] Infiltrative tumors tend to be larger when detected, and they are more likely to have ALN metastases than those with circumscribed margins.[156–158] Tumors with a stellate configuration with focal necrosis were found to have an especially poor prognosis.[158]

MICROSCOPIC HISTOPATHOLOGIC PROGNOSTIC FACTORS

The histologic appearance of invasive ductal carcinoma is heterogeneous. A number of variables described in this section should be included in the microscopic diagnosis of invasive ductal carcinomas in order to characterize the histologic and prognostic features of a particular tumor. Additional discussion about reporting prognostic features of breast carcinoma can be found in the discussion of specific tumor types.

Grading

Grading of ductal carcinomas is an estimate of differentiation. Unless otherwise indicated, grading is limited to the invasive portion of the tumor. *Nuclear grading* is the cytologic evaluation of tumor nuclei in comparison with the nuclei of normal mammary ductal epithelial cells. Because nuclear grading does not involve an assessment of the growth pattern of the tumor, this procedure is applicable not only to invasive ductal carcinomas but also to other subtypes

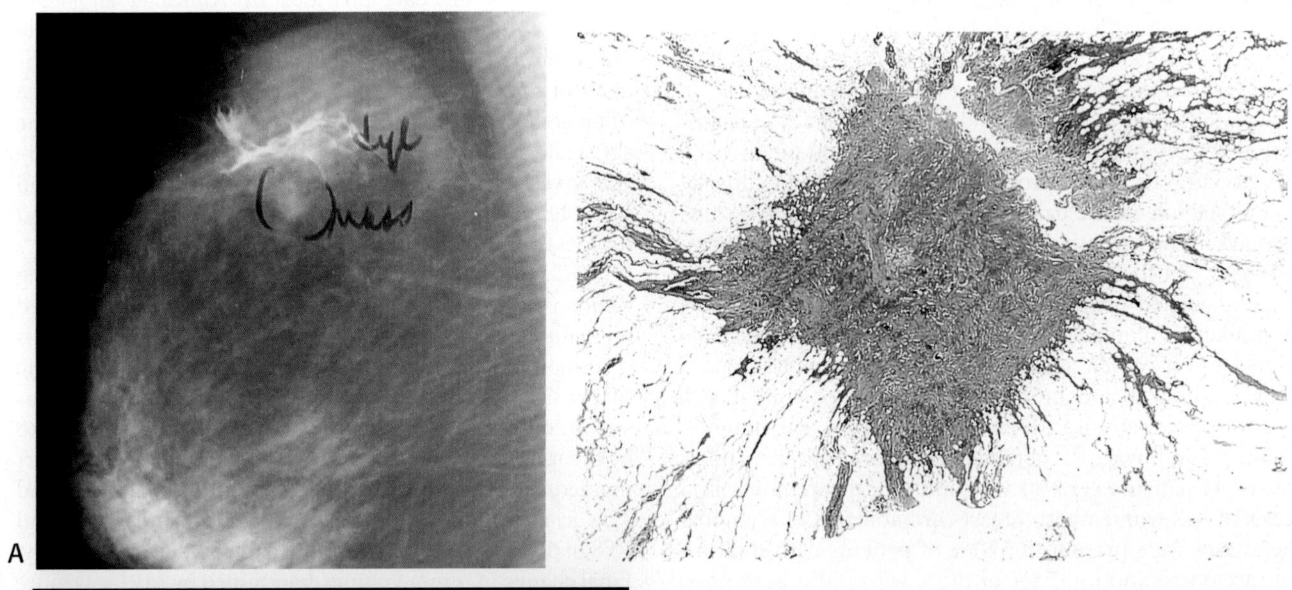

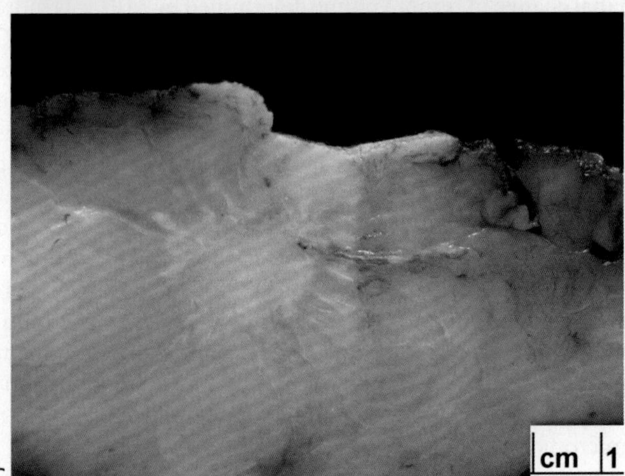

FIG. 12.4. ***Invasive ductal carcinoma.*** **A:** A small, nonpalpable stellate tumor (*circled*) in the upper central area on the mammogram. Dye injected for localization is present above the lesion. **B:** A whole-mount histologic section of the stellate invasive ductal carcinoma in (**A**). **C:** This superficially located stellate invasive ductal carcinoma has involved the nipple, causing it to be retracted.

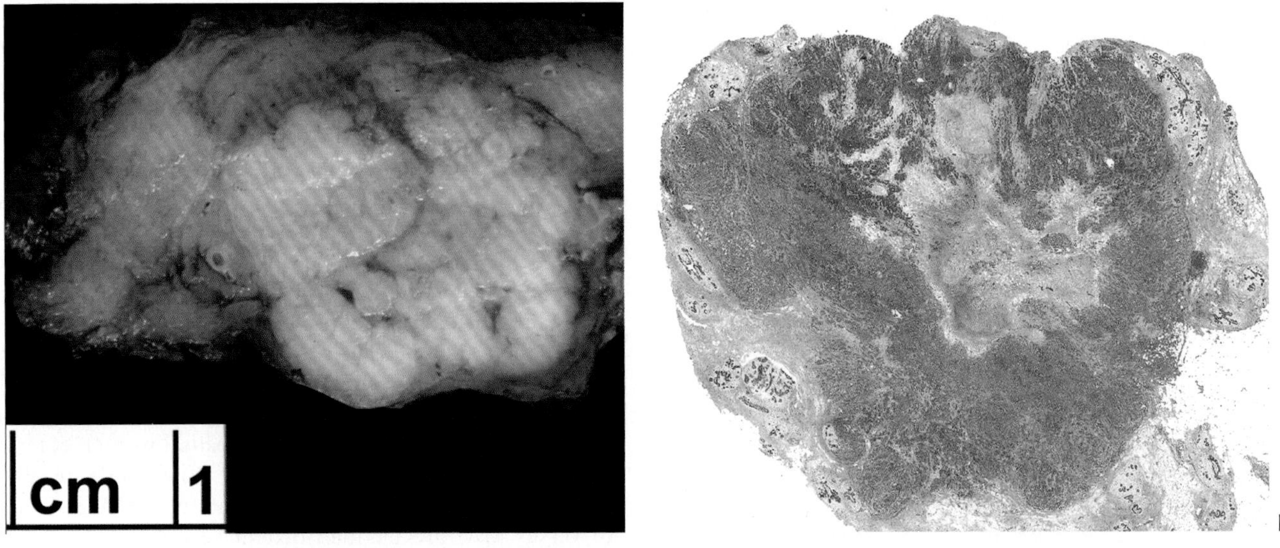

FIG. 12.5. ***Invasive ductal carcinoma.*** **A:** The gross appearance of a bisected circumscribed and lobulated poorly differentiated invasive ductal carcinoma. **B:** A whole-mount histologic section of a multinodular invasive ductal carcinoma with a circumscribed border. The tumor is centrally necrotic and fibrotic.

of mammary carcinoma. The most widely employed system for nuclear grading, introduced by Black and Speer[159] and Cutler et al.,[160] is usually reported in terms of three categories: well differentiated, intermediate, and poorly differentiated (Fig. 12.6). The sequence of numerical designations initially used for nuclear grading was the reverse of the sequence used in histologic grading. Current grading systems employ grades I, II, and III for low, intermediate,

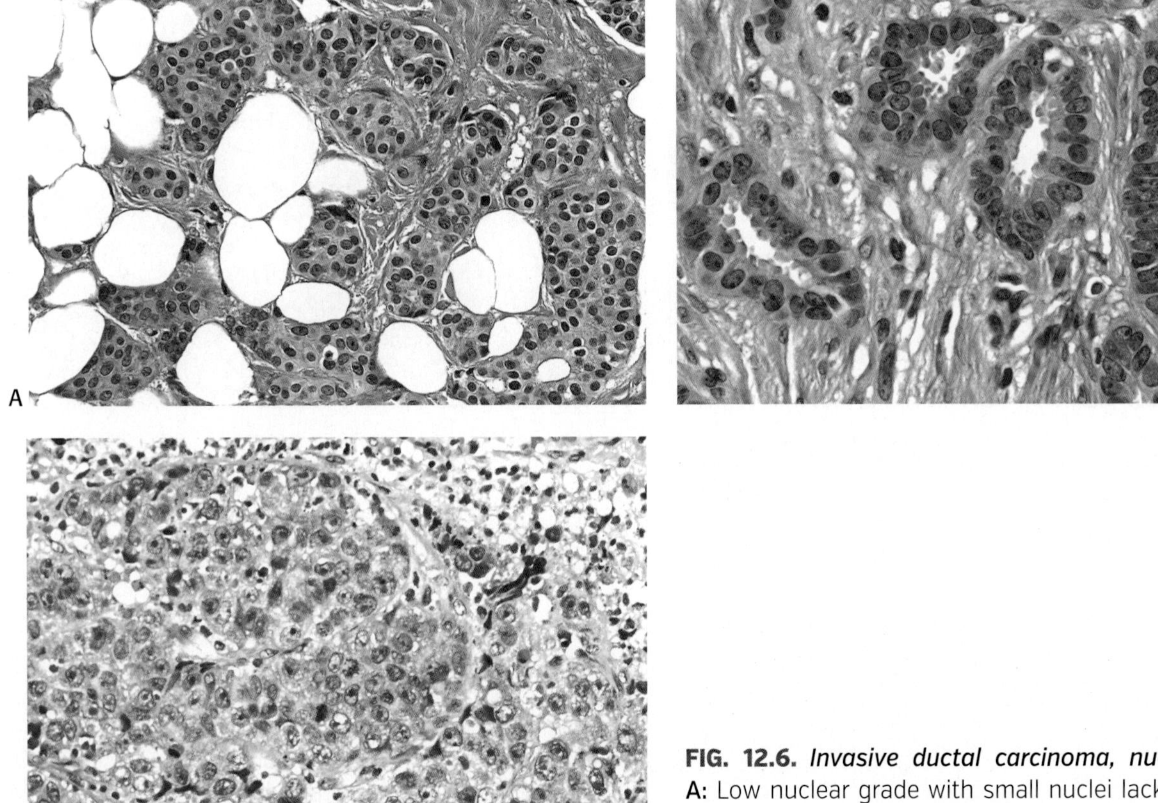

FIG. 12.6. ***Invasive ductal carcinoma, nuclear grade.*** **A:** Low nuclear grade with small nuclei lacking nucleoli. **B:** Intermediate nuclear grade. **C:** High-grade pleomorphic nuclei that have prominent nucleoli.

and high-grade nuclei and for well, intermediate, and poorly differentiated histologic grades, respectively.

Histologic grading describes the microscopic growth pattern of invasive ductal carcinomas, as well as cytologic features of differentiation. The most widely used histologic grading systems are based on criteria established by Bloom,[161] Bloom and Richardson,[162] and Elston and Ellis.[163] The latter system is also known as the Elston–Ellis modification of the Scarff–Bloom–Richardson grading system or the Nottingham combined histologic grade.[164] The parameters measured are (a) the extent of tubule, more accurately duct, formation; (b) nuclear hyperchromasia, pleomorphism, and size; and (c) mitotic rate. Each of the three elements is assigned a score on a scale of 1 to 3, and the final grade is determined from the sums of the scores. Histologic grade is traditionally expressed in three categories: scores 3 to 5, well differentiated (grade I); scores 6 to 7, moderately differentiated (grade II); and scores 8 to 9, poorly differentiated (grade III) (Fig. 12.7). The relative importance of the components in histologic grading is uncertain and, therefore, their values are given equal weight in the foregoing grading schemes.

Mitotic rate was reported to be the most important feature of the Bloom–Richardson grading system by Parham et al.[165] They found that a grading system or prognostic index grade based on mitotic rate and the presence or absence of necrosis was a better predictor of outcome than the Bloom–Richardson grading method. Jannink et al.[166] compared four methods for assessing mitotic activity and concluded that the traditional mitotic activity index (MAI) was preferable because it was "easy to apply and less time consuming." In their report, the MAI was measured in a 0.5 × 0.5-cm area "in the most cellular region at the periphery of the tumor. . . . [selected to] avoid areas of necrosis, inflammation, calcification and large vessels." Counting was done at 400× magnification, and counting was limited to invasive tumor in 10 consecutive fields. When determined by a standardized protocol, MAI proved to be a reliable and reproducible method that added significantly to the prognostic value of lymph node status and tumor size.[167] Baak et al.[168] evaluated the prognostic importance of MAI in a prospective study of Dutch premenopausal women entered into a systemic adjuvant therapy trial. When node-negative patients were compared after stratification by MAI less than 10 versus MAI greater than or equal to 10, MAI was the strongest prognostic factor.

The importance of employing a standardized counting method and, especially, a fixed *field size*, has been emphasized by several observers. Kuopio and Collan[169] demonstrated substantial variation of grading in the Bloom–Richardson system depending on field size and mitotic rate. Variation in field size had the greatest effect on the scoring of mitotic counts (classified as scores 1, 2, or 3 in the Bloom–Richardson system) when the mitotic count per millimeter

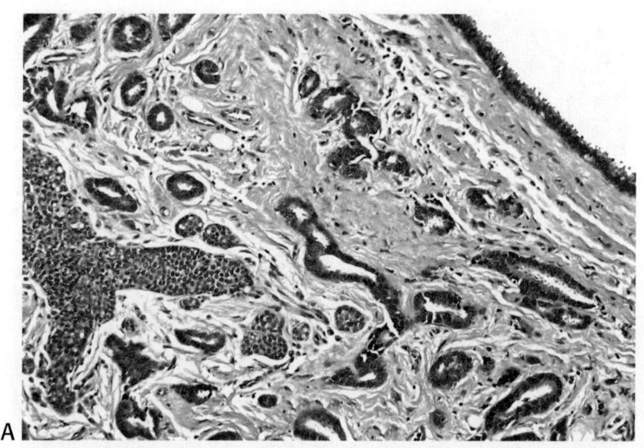

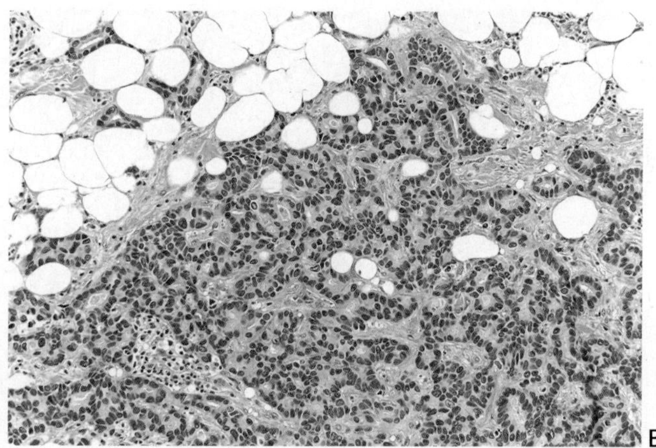

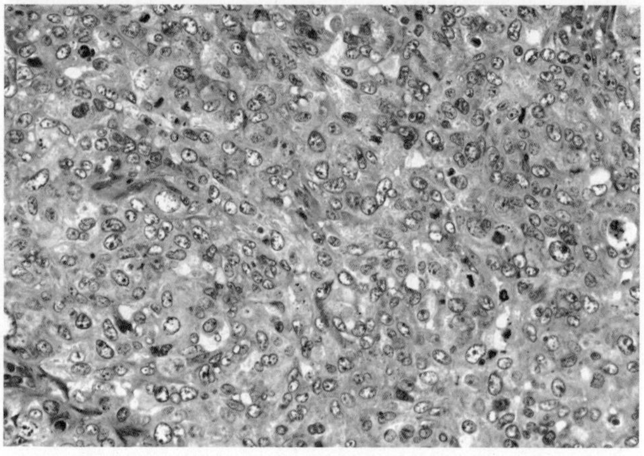

FIG. 12.7. ***Invasive ductal carcinoma, histologic grade.*** **A:** An example of low–histologic grade [tubular] carcinoma with well-formed glands. Note presence of LCIS at *left* and columnar cell change at *right*–forming the Rosen Triad. **B:** An example of moderately differentiated carcinoma with a complex glandular growth pattern. **C:** Poorly differentiated carcinoma with a solid, nonglandular architecture.

squared (mm^2) was between 7 and 20. The larger the field diameter or area measured in mm^2, the greater the probability of obtaining a score of 3 at a given mitotic rate. As a method of overcoming this difficulty, a table has been created listing mitotic rates per 10 high-power fields (HPF) for different microscopes,[163,170] and conversion factors have been developed for converting counts per 10 HPF to counts per mm^2.[171]

The range of *field areas* (mm^2) for 26 combinations of microscope types and eyepieces was tabulated by Ellis and Whitehead.[172] Field areas ranged from 0.071 to 0.385 mm^2 with an objective of 40× in each instance. An important variable in these calculations is the field number, or index, a factor that varies among microscopes and can be obtained from the manufacturer. A table for converting mitotic count and field diameter data to mitotic scores in the modified Bloom–Richardson grading system was devised by Kuopio and Collan.[169]

Another factor influencing mitotic counting is the choice of fields to count. The most widely used approach is to select a cellular invasive region at the periphery of the tumor where mitotic activity is likely to be highest.[141] An alternative method has been used to count mitoses in 10 randomly selected 40× HPF starting from a field previously determined as a "hot spot," that is, found to have "the highest density of mitotic figure."[166]

The definition of *mitotic figure* has also not been standardized. The original Bloom–Richardson grading system considered hyperchromatic nuclei to be mitotic, but subsequent modifications of Bloom–Richardson have introduced more specific criteria for identifying mitoses. The Nottingham histologic grade excludes hyperchromatic nuclei when this is the only mitosis-related feature.[125] van Diest et al.[167] offered detailed specifications for mitotic figures (Table 12.2). It should be noted that the counting of metaphase figures as two separate mitoses, as cited in Table 12.2, in order to achieve comparability with image analysis, is not customarily employed in routine light microscopy where a metaphase figure would be counted as a single mitosis. Mitotic rate is generally underestimated in needle core biopsy specimens—a finding that could be attributed to smaller sample size or technical artifact.[173]

Baehner and Weidner[174] reported improved specificity in mitotic counting by using the mitosis-specific antibody anti-phosphohistone-H3 (PHH3) that tags nuclei in all phases of mitosis. The antibody enhanced recognition of mitotic figures, and the resultant counts were highly correlated with traditional mitotic counts and with Ki67 labeling. Employing immunostains for PHH3 and MIB1 in needle core biopsy samples from invasive carcinomas has been shown to correlate better with mitotic count in the subsequent excised tumors, the gold standard for grading of tumors, than H&E-based mitotic rate.[175]

Several variants of Bloom–Richardson grading have been described. The system of Schauer and Weiss[176] subdivided Bloom–Richardson grade II into two subcategories, resulting in a total of four grades. The modification of Le Doussal et al.[177] created five grades on the basis of nuclear pleomorphism and mitotic index, omitting the degree of structural differentiation. Modification of Bloom–Richardson grading with more rigorous criteria for parameters resulted in the development of the Nottingham histologic grade (Table 12.3).[141,149]

Presently, most methods for grading use the previously cited three-tiered systems for describing tumor structure in

TABLE 12.2 Specifications for Mitotic Figures

Nuclear membrane
"Absent, so cells must have passed the prophase."
Nuclear structure
"Clear, hairy extensions of nuclear material (condensed chromosomes) must be present, either clotted (beginning metaphase), in a plane (metaphase/anaphase), or in separate clots (telophase). Regular extensions with an empty central zone favor a non-mitosis."
Mitotic figure
"Two parallel, clearly separate chromosome clots are to be counted as if they are separate mitoses, however, obvious it is that only one mitotic figure is concerned. This is in view of future automated mitotic figure recognition with image analysis."

From van Diest PJ, Baak JP, Matze-Cok P, et al. Reproducibility of mitosis counting in 2,469 breast cancer specimens: results from the Multicenter Morphometric Mammary Carcinoma Project. *Hum Pathol* 1992;23:603–607, with permission.

TABLE 12.3 Modified Bloom-Richardson Histologic Grading

Tubule formation
Score 1: >75% of tumor has tubules
Score 2: 10%–75% of tumor has tubules
Score 3: <10% tubule formation
Nuclear size
Score 1: Tumor nuclei similar to normal ductal cell nuclei (2–3 × rbc)
Score 2: Intermediate size nuclei
Score 3: Large nuclei, usually vesicular with prominent nucleoli
Mitotic count (per 10 HPF with 40× objective and field area of 0.196 mm^2)
Score 1: 0–7 mitoses
Score 2: 8–14 mitoses
Score 3: 15 or more mitoses

rbc, red blood cells.
From Robbins P, Pinder S, de Klerk N, et al. Histological grading of breast carcinomas: a study of interobserver agreement. *Hum Pathol* 1995;26:873–879, with permission.

terms of tubule formation, nuclear grade, and mitotic count, with the latter usually expressed as the number of mitoses per high-power magnification field (40×). Each element is scored on a scale of 1 to 3, according to criteria of the specific grading system, and the final grade is determined by the sum of the scores. The BloomRichardson and Nottingham histologic grades have similar predictive value and are the most frequently used methods.

The latest AJCC Cancer Staging Manual states that "all invasive carcinomas should be graded"[147] and recommends the Nottingham combined histologic grade, that is, the Elston–Ellis modification to the Scarff–Bloom–Richardson grading system (described above), for this purpose. Approximately one-half of all *symptomatic* invasive breast carcinomas are poorly differentiated, and well-differentiated tumors are least common in this group. Among *screen-detected* invasive breast carcinomas, moderately differentiated tumors are most common (comprising approximately 40%), with well-differentiated and poorly differentiated carcinomas each constituting 30%, respectively (unpublished data from Weill-Cornell Medical Center, New York).

Histologic Grading of Needle Core Biopsy Specimens

Several studies have investigated the accuracy of histologic grading based on needle core biopsy specimens compared with the final grade determined from the excised tumor. The reported concordance rates ranged from 59% to 75%.[177,178] In the same studies, concordance with respect to tumor type ranged from 66.6% to 81.0%. These data suggest that classification and grading of invasive carcinomas based on limited needle core biopsy sample ought to be regarded as provisional. This consideration should be borne in mind when neoadjuvant therapy is administered on the basis of a diagnosis made with a needle core biopsy sample. Tumor heterogeneity, and underestimation of mitotic rate (*vide supra*), are the most common sources of discordant classification and grading between core biopsy and excisional biopsy specimens, but interobserver and intraobserver variations are also factors.

Reproducibility of Grading

The subjective nature of histologic grading has been evaluated in studies of interobserver agreement on the assessment of the components that determine grade and grading its elf.[172,179,180] In one report, the kappa value for tubule formation was 0.64, indicating a substantial level of interobserver agreement on this variable, with lower levels of agreement for mitotic count (kappa = 0.52) and nuclear pleomorphism (kappa = 0.40).[172] Others reported a range of observer agreement for overall modified Bloom–Richardson grading with kappa values of 0.73[181], 0.70[179], and 0.43[180] respectively. Technical factors such as the method of fixation may have a significant influence on the level of observer agreement, which, in one study, was higher for tissues fixed with B5 than with buffered formaldehyde.[181]

It is possible that the architecture of an invasive carcinoma, for example, solid, cribriform, exerts some degree of bias on the assessment of nuclear grade; however, the independent evaluation of tubule formation, nuclear pleomorphism, and mitotic rate in the grading system can circumvent this potential problem.[182]

The clinical importance of histologic grading was aptly summarized by Schumacher et al.,[183] who concluded that "tumor grade is able to separate a small subgroup of patients with very good prognosis and a small subgroup of patients with very poor prognosis. The majority remains in an intermediate group. Here other prognostic factors are necessary to split the patients into groups with different prognoses."

Grading and Prognosis

Pinder et al.[125] analyzed histologic grade as a prognostic factor and as an indicator of response to chemotherapy in an International Breast Cancer Study Group trial involving 465 patients. There was a strong correlation between grading assigned with the Bloom–Richardson and Nottingham systems, although a greater proportion of tumors were classified as grade I with Nottingham grading, and Bloom–Richardson grading identified a greater proportion of tumors as grade III. The authors reported that "no apparent differences in overall and DFS were observed between the two systems."

The histologic and nuclear grades of a given tumor coincide in many but not all invasive ductal carcinomas.[184] There is a significant correlation between nuclear grade and SPF, and it has been suggested that nuclear grade can be used to predict whether a carcinoma has a high SPF.[185] Numerous studies have demonstrated that patients with high-grade or poorly differentiated invasive ductal carcinomas treated by mastectomy had a significantly higher frequency of ALN metastases and of four or more positive lymph nodes, that they developed more systemic recurrences, and that more of them died of metastatic disease than did women with lower grade tumors.[112,133,159–162,186–189] Nuclear and histologic grades have been shown to be useful predictors of prognosis for patients stratified by stage of disease, especially among those without ALN metastases.[133,177,188] The absence of tubule formation is a particularly unfavorable histologic feature when combined with high-grade nuclear cytology.

The impact of grade on prognosis in stage II patients is less clear. Some authors have reported a significant correlation, noting a favorable outcome associated with low-grade lesions.[187,188] However, these analyses have not consistently taken into consideration stratification on the basis of tumor size and the number of affected lymph nodes. In a carefully defined series of stage II, T1N1M0 patients, neither histologic nor nuclear grade was significantly correlated with outcome.[134] On the other hand, a case-control analysis of patients who survived 25 years after radical mastectomy for invasive carcinoma revealed a significantly higher proportion of histologically grade I tumors (43%) among long-term survivors compared with controls matched on the basis of tumor size, number of lymph nodes with metastases, and age at diagnosis.[190]

Histologic grade was reportedly a prognostically significant factor in the response of stage II patients to adjuvant chemotherapy,[191] especially patients who received prolonged rather than perioperative treatment.[122] Higher failure rates were observed in patients with higher grade tumors. This negative effect of grade was independent of nodal status, tumor size, hormone receptors, and several other prognostic factors. Histologic grade was also a significant indicator of response among patients who received endocrine treatment for systemic recurrence.[192,193] Histologic type of tumor (ductal, lobular, or other) was not significantly related to response to treatment.

Histologic grade has been shown to be significantly related not only to the frequency of recurrence and death due to invasive ductal carcinoma, but also to the disease-free interval and overall length of survival after mastectomy regardless of clinical stage.[112] High-grade carcinomas result in early treatment failures, whereas later recurrences are more often observed among low-grade tumors. For this reason, an unequal distribution of patients by grade could significantly influence the results of a randomized trial if this factor is not considered in stratification. The effect would be most marked early in the study.

Increasing tumor grade has been associated with several factors that are related to an increased risk of breast recurrence after conservation therapy including greater tumor size, diagnosis at a relatively young age, and absence of ER expression. Although some investigators found a significant relationship between grade and breast recurrence,[194–196] others concluded that grade was not a significant predictor of breast recurrence.[197–199] In patients with relatively favorable stage I carcinomas treated by lumpectomy without radiotherapy, it has been observed that tumor grade was a significant factor for time to recurrence. Recurrences occurred sooner and with greater frequency after a median follow-up of 58 months in patients with high-grade carcinomas.[99] The prognostic value of the Nottingham grading system is reportedly enhanced by combining lymph node stage and tumor size, assigning equal weight to each to form the NPI.[200] The Kalmar Prognostic Index uses the same factors as the NPI with higher weight, that is, 1.57, given to tumor grade, than to tumor size or to lymph node stage, that is, 0.31 and 0.79, respectively.[201]

Necrosis

The independent prognostic significance of tumor necrosis (Fig. 12.8) has been studied extensively.[108,158,165,202,203] controversy exists about the definition and classification of necrosis, with respect to the amount of necrosis that is considered to be significant as well as the relative distribution of necrosis within intraductal and invasive components of a tumor. There is evidence indicating that the prognostic significance of tumor necrosis is time dependent. For example, Gilchrist et al.[111] found that tumor necrosis, defined as the "presence of confluent necrosis of any dimension in a section of invasive cancer that could be distinguished at intermediate magnification," was a significant predictor of time to recurrence and OS with 10-year follow-up. However, the

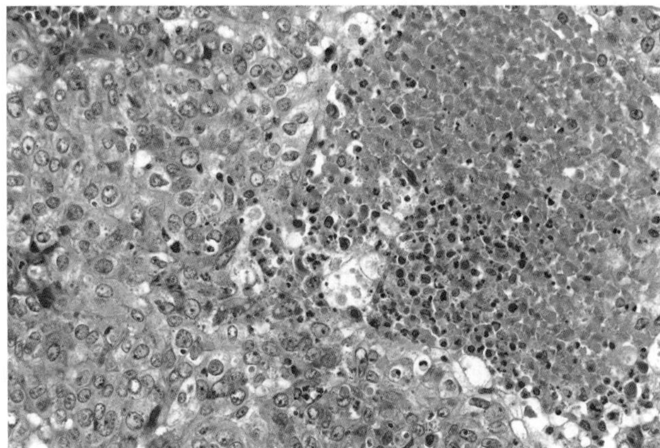

FIG. 12.8. ***Invasive ductal carcinoma.*** Poorly differentiated carcinoma with necrosis on the *right*.

effect was manifested only during the first 2 years of follow-up. For patients who remained disease free beyond 10 years, having had necrosis in the primary tumor no longer was a significant prognostic factor.

Rarely, extensive necrosis destroys most of the tumor, and this process may be so extreme as to leave few or no apparently viable elements (Fig. 12.1). This situation has been encountered in ordinary invasive ductal carcinoma, as well as special tumor types such as papillary carcinoma (see Chapter 14). Jimenez et al.[204] studied 34 "centrally necrotizing carcinomas." The tumors were typically circumscribed, unicentric lesions with a mean size of 2.5 cm. Histologic examination revealed central necrosis surrounded by a narrow rim of viable high-grade carcinoma. Ninety-four percent of tumors were negative for ER and PR. Progression of disease (defined as the development of either a recurrence or fatality) occurred in 24 (71%) patients. Yu et al.[205] studied a group of 33 centrally necrotizing carcinomas, all of which were high grade. Twenty-nine of 33 (87.9%) expressed basal-like markers, and 12 of 26 (46.2%) were positive for myoepithelial markers. Median progression-free survival was 15.5 months. In 12 patients, local recurrence and/or distant metastasis developed. These data add further support to the perception that extensive necrosis is a prognostically unfavorable feature in invasive mammary carcinoma, possibly reflecting a growth rate so rapid that it exceeds tumor sustaining angiogenesis to a substantial degree. Centrally necrotizing carcinomas appear to have a distinctive morphology and basal-like immunophenotype that are associated with a poor prognosis. Such tumors show ring-like enhancement on contrast-enhanced MRI with high intensity in the cystic, necrotic portion on T2-weighted imaging.[206]

Apoptosis, bcl-2, and Telomerase, and Necrosis

Apoptosis is an important mechanism of cell death, and it may be a factor in tumor necrosis. Apoptotic cells are characterized in routine histologic sections by condensation of chromatin and cytoplasm, as well as intra- and extracellular chromatin fragments as small as 2 μm. An apoptotic index (AI) can be determined by counting the number of apoptotic cells using the same method as for a mitotic index.[207] In one study of 288 carcinomas, the AI was significantly related to tumor grade, SPF, mitotic index, and the expression of hormone receptors and p53.[207] High mean AI was associated with poorly differentiated grade, high SPF and high mitotic rate, the absence of hormone receptor expression, and p53 expression.[185] Increased apoptosis has been associated with intraductal carcinoma with high-grade nuclei and necrosis and the concomitant invasive carcinoma.[208] Shen et al.[209] reported that the mean frequency of apoptotic cells determined by the TUNEL method was greater in intraductal than in invasive carcinomas, whereas intraductal carcinoma had a relatively low proliferative rate, a finding suggesting that apoptosis might contribute to maintaining a steady state in intraductal carcinoma. Conversely, the invasive carcinomas featured a higher proliferative rate manifested by Ki67 immunoreactivity and a lower apoptotic rate. When examined in multivariate analysis, apoptosis was not an independent prognostic factor.

Bcl-2, part of the *bcl-2* gene family located at chromosome 18q21, was first identified during studies of the t(14;18) chromosome translocation that occurs in B-cell lymphomas. Individual genes in this family have an inhibiting or promoting effect on cell death. One group of genes, including *bcl-2*, *Bcl-x*, and *MCL1*, suppresses programmed cell death (apoptosis), whereas others, such as *Bax* and *Bak*, promote cell death. These antagonistic functions play an important role in mammary epithelial differentiation and possibly in mammary neoplasia.[210] The mechanism by which *bcl-2* contributes to tumorigenesis is through suppression of apoptosis, thereby conferring a survival advantage on *bcl-2*-expressing cells. The prolonged life span of cells with enhanced *bcl-2* expression may contribute to the greater cellularity of proliferative lesions and increase the risk for these cells to acquire oncogenic genetic changes. p53 induces apoptosis as well as G_1 arrest, downregulates *bcl-2*, and coincidentally upregulates *Bax* to promote apoptosis.[211,212]

Immunohistochemical studies of bcl-2 in tissue reveal cytoplasmic localization. In normal breast tissue, expression is highest in the hormonally regulated lobular epithelium, being maximal at the midpoint in the menstrual cycle.[213] Expression of bcl-2 was reportedly detected in all examples of ADH and LCIS studied by Siziopikou et al.[214] In intraductal carcinoma, bcl-2 expression was found to correlate with the grade of the lesion and to be inversely related to the expression of Bax.[215] Low-grade intraductal carcinomas featured predominate bcl-2 staining relative to Bax, intermediate-grade lesions tended to coexpress both proteins, and high-grade intraductal carcinomas expressed Bax more prominently. Expression of bcl-2 has been detected in 58%,[216] 64%,[217] 68%,[218] 75%,[219] and 79%[220,221] of carcinomas studied (Fig. 12.9). By comparison, Alsabeh at al.[220] found expression in only 5.6% and 8.3% of gastric and pulmonary carcinomas, respectively, and staining of these nonmammary tumors was usually not as intense as in breast carcinomas. bcl-2 expression is significantly associated with the presence of ER and PR.[216,218–224] Some investigators reported an inverse relationship between bcl-2 expression and the immunohistochemical detection of EGFR, HER2, and p53,[217,221–226] whereas others reported no significant association with p53[219,220,227,228] or with transforming growth factor α.[222]

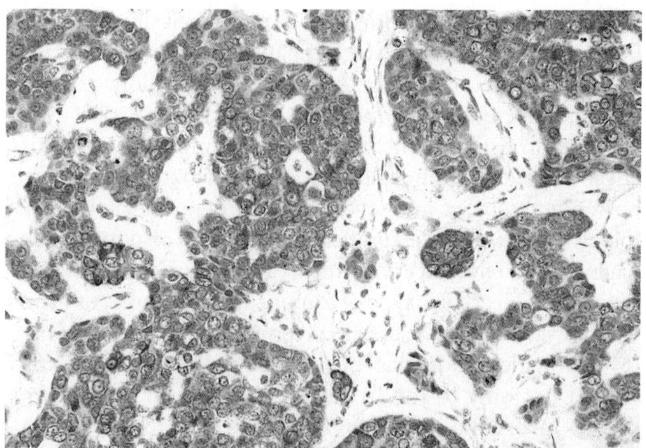

FIG. 12.9. ***Invasive ductal carcinoma, bcl-2.*** Cytoplasmic immunolocalization is shown in a moderately differentiated carcinoma.

The relationship between bcl-2 and proliferative activity in breast carcinoma is not clear. Alsabeh et al.[220] reported that bcl-2 expression was significantly more frequent in breast carcinomas with low MIB1 expression. Joensuu et al.[229] observed bcl-2 expression significantly more often in tumors with a low mitotic count, low S-phase, and a diploid DNA content, and Silvestrini et al.[227] found that bcl-2 staining was inversely related to the thymidine index, another marker of proliferative activity. Gee et al.[222] found no association between bcl-2 and Ki67 proliferative status. Most investigators reported that bcl-2 immunoreactivity was more frequent in low-grade carcinomas.[216,218,220,224,225,229,230] Stage at diagnosis and ALN status were not significantly related to bcl-2 immunoreactivity.[217–219,229,230] An immunohistochemistry (IHC)-based combined Ki67/bcl-2 index has been used to produce a "robust" proliferative index that has been shown to be prognostic in ER-positive tumors.[231]

The relationship of bcl-2 expression to prognosis and response to therapy in breast carcinoma remains uncertain. Because bcl-2 blocks apoptosis, lower levels of apoptosis induced by bcl-2 expression would be expected to result in the accumulation of malignant cells in a carcinoma and thereby have an unfavorable effect on outcome. The subject was reviewed by Zhang et al.,[232] who concluded the following: (a) bcl-2 expression is associated with a better response to hormone therapy and (b) the expression of bcl-2 is a favorable prognostic factor regardless of nodal status. Berardo et al.[233] found that high bcl-2 expression was associated with a significantly improved DFS and OS, and in multivariate analysis bcl-2 expression was associated with a more favorable DFS. Gee et al.[222] found that patients with ER- and bcl-2-positive tumors were particular responsive to endocrine therapies that included an antiestrogen. van Slooten et al.[230] found no association between bcl-2 expression and response to perioperative chemotherapy (5-fluorouracil, doxorubicin, and cyclophosphamide) in node-negative patients. Bonetti et al.[234] reported a higher response rate to chemotherapy among tumors classified as bcl-2 positive with immunostaining in greater than or equal to 40% of tumor cells.

Telomerase is a polymerase that adds telomeric DNA to the ends of chromosomes.[235] This process prevents the shortening of these chromosome ends during replication. In normal cells, the replicating DNA loses terminal segments (telomeres), and with repeated cell divisions shortened telomere length reaches a critical point that signals cessation of division, followed by cell senescence. Increased telomerase activity is associated with telomere repair and may serve as an immortalization marker by inhibiting normal progression to senescence and death.

Telomerase activity has been detected in 79%,[236] 82%,[237,238] and 85%[239] of breast carcinomas studied. In one report, there was no association with lymph node status, tumor size, and hormone receptor status,[236] but others did not confirm these associations.[237] Telomerase has been detected in fibroadenomas[240] and other benign lesions[238] but not in normal tissue samples. High telomerase activity was associated with overexpression of cyclin D1, cyclin E, or both, by Landberg et al.,[239] and with p53 overexpression.[241] Tumors with high telomerase activity had a relatively unfavorable prognosis in node-negative, but not in node-positive patients studied by Roos et al.[241] However, Carey et al.[237] reported that telomerase activity was not predictive of survival regardless of nodal status.

The telomere DNA content of tissues has been measured by a molecular assay. The telomere content of normal tissues decreased with age.[242] The ratio of telomere content in breast carcinomas to the content in nonneoplastic tissues from the same individual ranged from 21% to 93%, averaging 61%.[242] Telomere content in breast carcinomas was inversely related to tumor size, nodal status, and DFS. Hence, high telomere content was associated with smaller tumors, negative ALNs, and improved survival compared with low telomere content. Telomere content did not differ significantly between ductal and lobular carcinomas. Tumors with high telomerase expression, as assessed by quantitative polymerase chain reaction (qPCR) and quantitative reverse transcription–PCR (qRT–PCR), have been found to respond poorly to chemotherapy, but better to endocrine therapy.[243]

In summary, apoptosis, bcl-2, and telomerase play a complex role in controlling the life span of breast carcinoma cells. The interplay of these and other factors such as angiogenesis probably influences the susceptibility of any given carcinoma to develop areas of necrosis. This is a vital area for future investigation since a better understanding of intrinsic biologic factors that promote tumor necrosis could open new avenues for targeted therapy.

Inflammatory Cell Infiltrate

The prognostic significance of inflammatory cells within and around invasive ductal carcinomas has been the subject of considerable interest and some controversy. The reaction consists mainly of mature lymphocytes with a variable admixture of plasma cell, histiocytes, neutrophils, and mast cells (Fig. 12.10). Rarely, plasma cells or eosinophils predominate. Tumors with plasma cell predominance are usually medullary carcinomas or carcinomas with medullary features.[244] The marked lymphoplasmacytic reaction observed in medullary carcinoma also occurs in a minority of nonmedullary invasive ductal carcinomas. A subset of these tumors with some but not all of the features of medullary carcinoma, referred to as infiltrating ductal carcinoma (IFDC) with medullary features, may have a slightly more favorable prognosis than IFDCs generally, but the difference is not statistically significant.[245] Most nonmedullary ductal carcinomas with a prominent lymphocytic reaction tend to be poorly differentiated and have a circumscribed rather than infiltrative

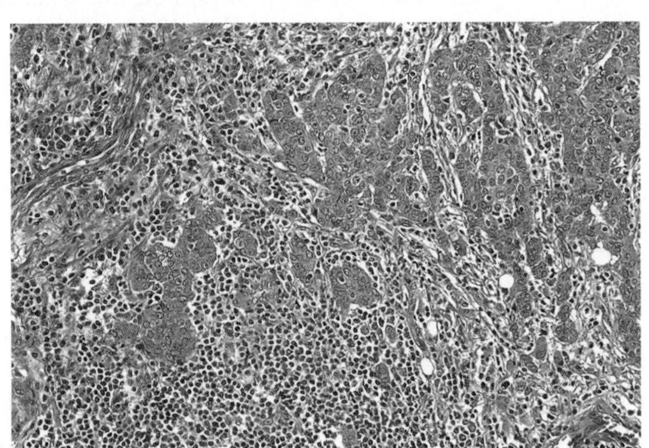

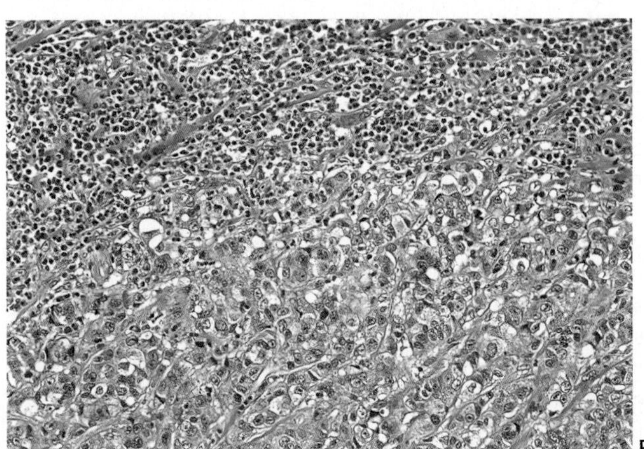

FIG. 12.10. ***Invasive ductal carcinoma.*** **A:** A dense lymphoplasmacytic infiltrate fills the stroma of invasive poorly differentiated ductal carcinoma. **B:** Invasive ductal carcinoma with an unusual stromal infiltrate of eosinophils.

contour. Medullary carcinomas and invasive ductal carcinomas with a marked lymphocytic reaction are almost always ER negative and PR negative. Medullary carcinoma is part of the basal-like group in the gene expression–based molecular taxonomy of breast carcinoma. Marginean et al.[245] reported that the presence of prominent inflammation and poorly differentiated carcinoma cells arranged in anastomosing sheets identified a subset of basal-like carcinomas with a favorable prognosis and that these two features provided "a simplified definition of medullary-like" carcinoma.

Although the favorable prognosis of medullary carcinoma has usually been ascribed to the lymphoplasmacytic reaction that characterizes these tumors, it is thus far less clear that the same conclusion can be drawn about nonmedullary invasive ductal carcinomas. Some investigators have found carcinomas with a "host response" to have a relatively favorable prognosis,[112,160] but others have found no significant difference or have reported a less favorable outcome associated with the presence of a prominent lymphoplasmacytic infiltrate.[13,190,203] The amount or content of inflammatory cells in invasive breast carcinoma does not appear to influence mortality in node-negative breast carcinoma.[246] Subset analysis in one study suggested that the influence of lymphoplasmacytic reaction on prognosis was related to nodal status, tumor grade, and the overexpression of the *HER2* oncogene.[247] In a study of 1,597 patients with invasive carcinomas who received no systemic adjuvant treatment with a median follow-up of 9.5 years, "prominent inflammation" was associated with high histologic grade and with better survival on multivariate analyses.[248]

Studies of the lymphocyte subgroups infiltrating mammary carcinomas indicate that they are largely T lymphocytes[249–251] consisting mainly of T4 (CD4+ helper) and T8 (CD8+ cytotoxic suppressor) cells.[250,251] Employing direct immunofluorescence of FSs, Bilik et al.[249] found that the T4-to-T8 ratio exceeded 1.0 in only 34% of tumors, indicating that T8 cells were more numerous in the majority of carcinomas. Whitford et al.[252] also reported a predominance of T8 cells when lymphocytes were isolated from breast carcinomas and analyzed by flow cytometry. Ordinarily, few B cells are found in benign or in carcinomatous breast tissue, but the proportion of B cells tends to be relatively increased in carcinomas.[253] By applying a variety of procedures including *in situ* hybridization in a small series of cases, Parkes et al.[254] demonstrated that the presence of plasma cells that expressed high levels of immunoglobulin kappa-chain mRNA was associated with a poor prognosis.

The intensity of mast cell infiltration in the substance of or at the periphery of an invasive breast carcinoma was not significantly related to prognosis in a study based on routine histologic sections.[255] Using immunohistochemical staining for c-kit (CD117) as a marker of mast cells in tissue microarrays with 348 invasive breast carcinomas, Dabiri et al.[256] found mast cells in the stroma of 93 (26.7%) of the tumors. The distribution of mast cell–positive cases was not significantly related to axillary nodal status. The presence of stromal mast cells was associated with a significantly more favorable prognosis in patients with negative ALNs, but not in those with axillary nodal metastases. The presence of mast cells was inversely related to the presence of CD68-positive stromal histiocytes. There was no correlation between the presence of mast cells and the status of conventional tumor prognostic markers (ER, PR, and HER2). The influence of tissue mast cells on prognosis may be mediated by substances produced by these cells such as histamine and the cytokine interleukin-4. Inhibition of growth and apoptosis of breast carcinoma cells by interleukin-4 has been reported.[257]

Detection of Lymphatic Tumor Emboli in H&E Sections

Lymphatics are vascular channels lined by endothelium without supporting smooth muscle or elastica (Fig. 12.11).[258,259] Interpretive issues that must be considered in the diagnosis of lymphatic invasion in H&E-stained sections were reviewed by Hoda et al.[260] Most lymphatics do not contain red blood cells, but undoubtedly some blood, that is, vascular, capillaries are included in this definition. The identification of tumor emboli in lymphatic channels in H&E-stained sections without the use of immunostains is more reliable in peritumoral than in intratumoral tissue because shrinkage artifacts that simulate lymphatic channels are more likely to occur in the latter site (Table 12.4). True tumor emboli usually do not conform to the shape of the space in which they are found. When the tumor conforms to the shape of the space it is more likely to represent retraction artifact. It is usually possible to identify endothelial cell nuclei around the perimeter of a true lymphatic channel; absence of this finding may indicate retraction artifact. Some lymphatic channels are adjacent to small blood vessels, but this is an inconstant and unreliable finding. Because immunostains have greatly improved the ability to detect carcinoma in lymphatic and vascular spaces within as well as around an invasive mammary carcinoma, the foregoing guidelines should be supplemented by immunohistochemical examination of the tissue in most cases.

Artifactual spaces can be formed around nests of tumor cells within an invasive carcinoma as a result of tissue shrinkage during incomplete processing, representing the so-called "shrinkage" or "retraction" artifact (Fig. 12.12). Shrinkage artifact, primarily caused by delay to formalin fixation or "cold ischemia" time,[261] is more commonly found in ductal than in lobular carcinomas or in carcinomas with ductal and lobular features.[262] These carcinomas tend to exhibit higher histologic and nuclear grades. Acs et al.[262] found that there was a significant direct correlation between the presence of shrinkage artifact and the presence of lymphatic tumor emboli in node-negative patients. Furthermore, node-negative patients with shrinkage artifact had a significantly higher frequency of distant metastases than patients without shrinkage artifact. These findings led the investigators to suggest that shrinkage artifact may reflect significant aspects of tumor–stromal interaction, possibly related to the formation of lymphatic channels, and not simply a passive phenomenon. The pattern of invasive carcinoma involving pseudoangiomatous stromal hyperplasia (PASH) can stimulate lymphatic invasion. Indeed, the proposal has been made that PASH represents

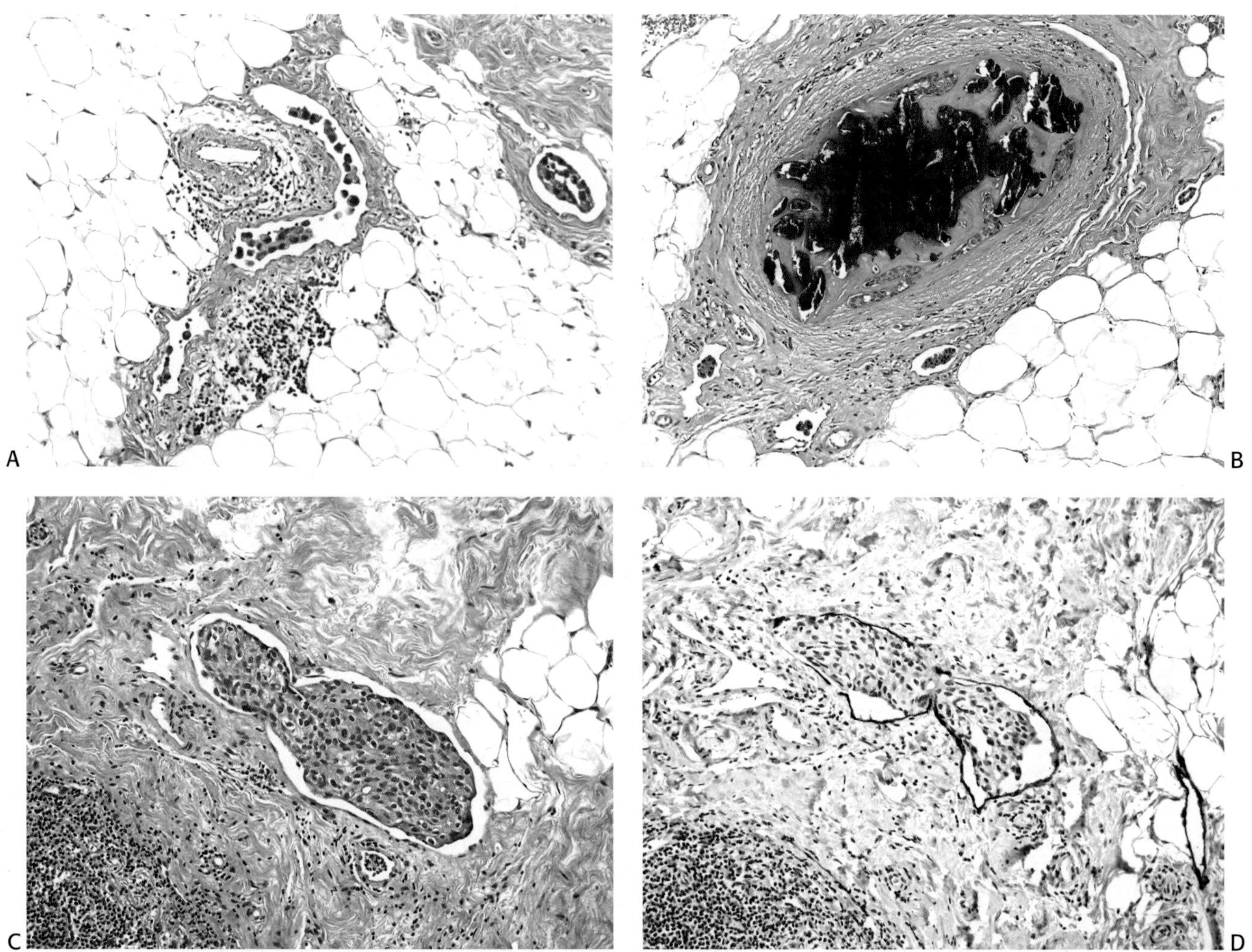

FIG. 12.11. ***Invasive ductal carcinoma, lymphatic channel invasion.*** **A:** Intralymphatic carcinoma is shown next to a small blood vessel. **B:** Carcinoma in lymphatic channels, status-post (s/p) neoadjuvant chemotherapy, around a focus of invasive carcinoma with dense peritumoral sclerosis and calcifications. **C:** A large cluster of carcinoma cells is present in a lymphatic channel. **D:** Cytoplasmic immunoreactivity for CD31 is shown in the endothelial cells lining the lymphatic channel shown in **(C)**.

TABLE 12.4 Diagnostic Criteria for Lymphovascular Involvement

The focus of lymphovascular involvement by tumor should be peritumoral, not intratumoral
Tumor embolus generally does not precisely conform to the shape of the space in which it is found. If it does, then the finding likely represents retraction artifact
Endothelial cell nuclei are present lining the lymphovascular space. If no such nuclei are present, then the finding likely represents retraction artifact
Larger lymphatic channels lie adjacent to blood vessels, that is, artery and vein

From Rosen PP. Tumor emboli in intramammary lymphatics in breast carcinoma: pathologic criteria for diagnosis and clinical significance. *Pathol Annu* 1983;18(Pt 2):215–232.

"pre-lymphatic channels" that communicate with "true" lymphatics[263] and thus form part of intramammary lymphatic labyrinth that facilitates the spread of tumor.[264]

Controversy exists over the presence of intratumoral vascular channels and whether lymphangiogenesis occurs in carcinomas. The availability of antibodies with a purportedly high degree of specificity for lymphatic endothelium has facilitated investigation of these issues. In general, it has been observed that lymphangiogenesis is restricted or absent within breast carcinomas and that lymphatic vessel density is substantially greater in peritumoral than in intratumoral stroma.[265–267]

Detection of Lymphatic Tumor Emboli with Immunostains

Efforts to identify lymphatic spaces by using immunostains associated with blood vessel endothelial cells (factor VIII, CD34, or CD31, and blood group antigens) met with limited

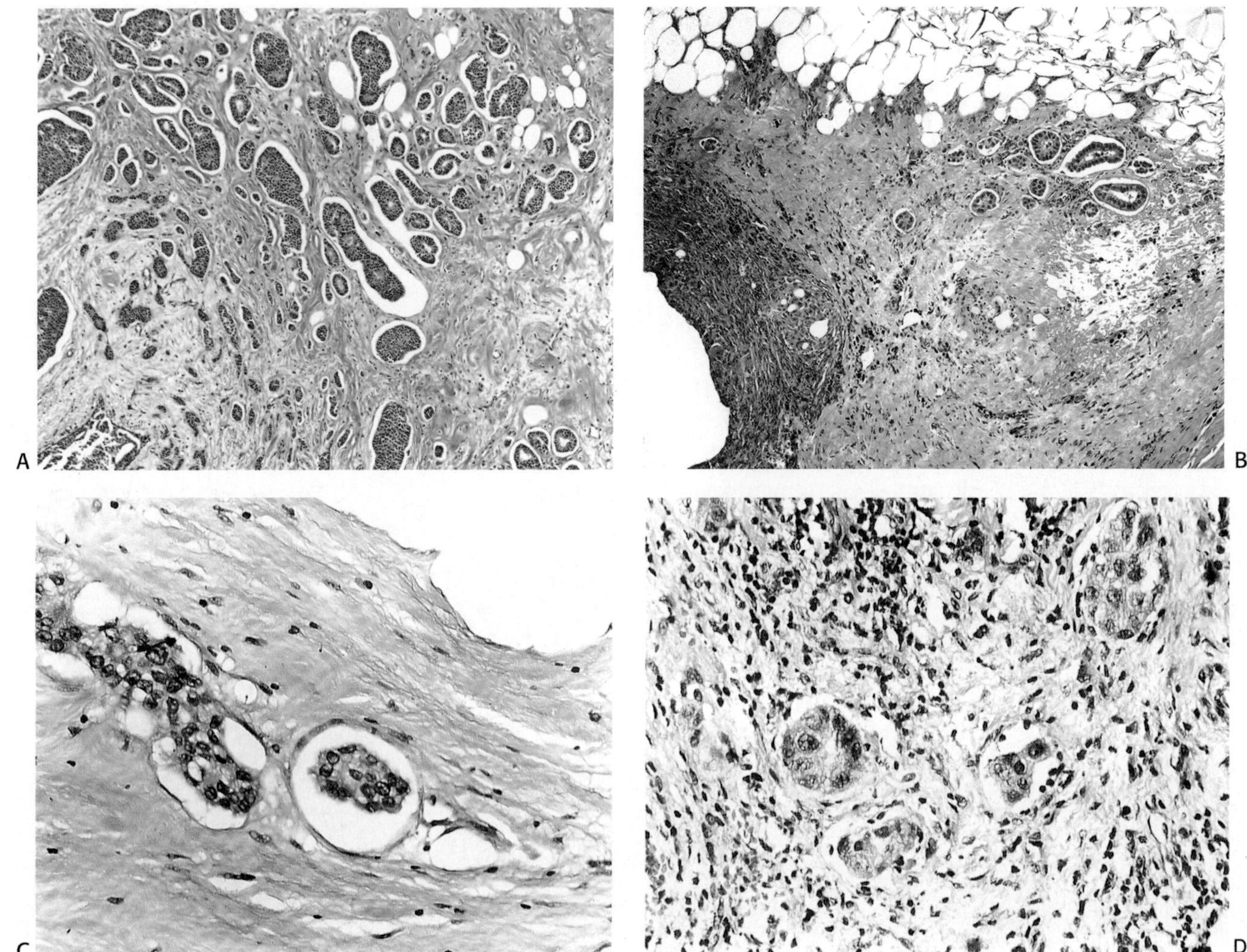

FIG. 12.12. ***Invasive ductal carcinoma, shrinkage artifact.*** **A:** Shrinkage artifact that resembles lymphatic invasion in invasive carcinoma. The groups of carcinoma cells take the shapes of the spaces in which they lie. No endothelial lining of the spaces can be identified. **B:** Groups of displaced carcinoma cells that resemble lymphatic tumor emboli in an invasive carcinoma (s/p needle core biopsy for noninvasive papillary carcinoma). Such foci typically lie along the healing biopsy tract and exhibit shrinkage artifact, and are best interpreted as displaced noninvasive tumor cells. **C:** A shrinkage artifact that resembles lymphatic invasion. The groups of carcinoma cells are attached to the stroma and there is no endothelium. **D:** Groups of carcinoma cells that resemble lymphatic tumor emboli in an invasive carcinoma. Such foci are interpreted as shrinkage artifact.

success,[268–270] because reactivity is strongest in blood vessel endothelium and weaker or absent in lymphatic endothelium. Strong staining of tumor cells for blood group antigens in artifactual spaces can be associated with diffusion of reactivity into the surrounding stroma, and the resultant staining may be most intense at the margin of the space, potentially resulting in a mistaken diagnosis of vascular invasion.[269,271] CD34 and CD31 immunostains are reactive with myofibroblasts and will outline artifactual, nonvascular spaces, and spaces in PASH. Factor VIII antigen has not been consistently demonstrable in all endothelium-lined capillary or lymphatic channels.

D2-40 is a monoclonal antibody directed at podoplanin with a high degree of specificity for the lymphatic endothelium in normal tissues and in the stroma of carcinomas.[271–274] D2-40 is reactive in the endothelium of lymphangiomas,[272,273] angiosarcomas,[272,273] and some hemangiomas.[273] Reactivity for D2-40 is also observed in Kaposi sarcoma[272,273] and the Dabska tumor, that is, endovascular papillary angioendothelioma.[273] A nonneoplastic vascular channel that is D2-40 (+), CD31 (–), and/or CD34 (–) is likely to be a lymphatic space, whereas the reverse immunophenotype (D2-40 [–], CD31 [+], and/or CD34 [+]) is highly associated with a blood vessel channel. In a study using the CD34 and D2-40 antibodies, van den Eynden et al.[275] were able to localize blood vessel (D2-40 [–], CD34 [+]) and lymphatic (D2-40 [+], CD34 [–] or [+]) tumor emboli. Intratumoral and peritumoral sites of lymphovascular invasion were tabulated separately. The presence of axillary nodal metastases was associated with peritumoral but not with intratumoral lymphatic invasion.

Monoclonal and polyclonal antibodies directed at the endothelial hyaluronan receptor 1 (LYVE-1) have also proved to be useful for detecting lymphatic tumor emboli in breast carcinomas.[276,277] In studies with small numbers of cases, the presence of lymphatic tumor emboli detected with the LYVE-1 antibody proved to be associated with the presence of axillary nodal metastases and poorer prognosis.[276,277]

Presently, antibodies to D2-40, LYVE-1, and other endothelial markers such as Fli-1 and ERG can be employed in individual cases where there may be uncertainty about the presence of lymphovascular invasion in diagnostic tissue. A contemporaneous H&E-stained section must always be prepared to ensure correlation of the immunostained sections with the histologic appearance of the tissue. Screening of all breast carcinoma specimens with markers for lymphatic or vascular endothelium can only be regarded as an investigational procedure, the results of which have yet to be correlated with long-term follow-up results. The exclusive use of Wilms tumor 1 (WT-1) as an endothelial marker cannot be advocated since concomitant myoepithelial cell reactivity can be problematic,[278] especially when myoepithelium persists around *in situ* carcinoma in ducts or lobular glands. When this situation is suspected, nuclear reactivity for p63 will distinguish between myoepithelial and endothelial cells that are reactive for WT-1. Indeed, D2-40 immunostaining may also decorate myoepithelial cells; however, such staining is more evident in larger glands and is patchy and less intense than that observed in lymphatic endothelium.[279] Here too, the p63 immunostain can be very helpful.

Prognostic Significance of Lymphatic Tumor Emboli

When studied in H&E sections alone, peritumoral lymphatic tumor emboli are found associated with approximately 15% of invasive ductal carcinomas. The majority of these patients have ALN metastases, but lymphatic tumor emboli are found in the breast surrounding invasive ductal carcinomas in 5% to 10% of patients who have negative lymph nodes in routine H&E slides. The frequency of lymphatic tumor emboli in patients with node-negative invasive carcinoma is higher when immunostains are used to examine the tissues. Mohammed et al.[280] studied 1,005 node-negative tumors with CD34, CD31, and podoplanin/D2-40 to detect blood vessel and lymphatic vessel invasion (LVI). Overall, some form of vascular invasion was found in 218 (22%) of the lesions, consisting of LVI only in 211 (97%) and blood vessel invasion only in 5 (3%). It is remarkable that both types of invasion were found in only two tumors. Among the tumors with LVI, involvement was limited to a peritumoral distribution in 155 and intratumoral channels in 9. LVI was detected in both sites in 49 tumors.

Several studies have shown that peritumoral lymphatic emboli detected in routine H&E sections were prognostically unfavorable in node-negative patients treated by mastectomy[133,203,281–285] and by breast conservation therapy.[286] The deleterious effect was most pronounced in women with T1N0M0 disease. In a 10-year follow-up study of 378 patients treated for T1N0M0 carcinoma, prior to the era of adjuvant chemotherapy, 33% of 30 women with lymphatic emboli identified in routine H&E sections died of disease. Death due to breast carcinoma was observed in only 10% of the 348 women who did not have lymphatic emboli.[133] Another study comparing similar subsets of T1N0M0 patients found recurrences in 32% of those with lymphatic emboli and in 10% of controls.[203] In stage I patients with tumors larger than 2 cm (T2N0M0), those with lymphatic emboli also experienced a higher metastatic rate.[259,269,285] Metastases that developed in node-negative patients who had peritumoral lymphatic emboli tended to occur more than 5 years after diagnosis, and they were almost always systemic. Lymphatic tumor emboli did not predispose to local recurrence in node-negative patients treated by mastectomy, but they were associated with an increased risk of recurrence in the breast after breast conservation therapy.[286] Liljegren et al.[287] reported that the RR for recurrence in the breast after conservation therapy was 1.9 (95% CI, 1.1 to 3.5) in a comparison of women with and without peritumoral lymphatic tumor emboli.

Lymphatic tumor emboli detected with D2-40 immunostain in node-negative patients are also associated with a significant risk of distant but not local recurrence. Arnaout-Alkarain et al.[288] used D2-40 to detect lymphatic tumor emboli in 303 invasive carcinomas from node-negative women with a median follow-up of 7.6 years. Lymphatic invasion was found in 27%, mainly at the perimeter of the carcinomas. Patients with lymphatic tumor emboli detected by this method had a significantly higher frequency of distant recurrence and shorter survival than those without this finding. Mohammed et al.[280] also reported that the presence of LVI detected by immunostains was significantly associated with a shorter disease-free interval, a higher rate of metastases, and reduced survival in univariate and multivariate analyses. There was no significant relationship between the number of foci of LVI and the risk of recurrence or reduced survival.

The effect on prognosis of lymphatic tumor emboli to certain subsets of node-negative patients is controversial.[289,290] Some studies have established that lymphovascular channel involvement has independent prognostic significance in node-negative breast carcinomas, including in the ER-negative and triple-negative groups.[291,292] Lymphatic channel involvement as assessed by D2-40 (+) and p63 (−) in operable T1–2N0M0 invasive carcinomas in women over the age of 55 with a high proliferation rate as defined by phosphohistone H3 of 13 or more has been shown to identify a subgroup with a high risk of distant metastases in one study.[293] Because the nuclei of lymphatic endothelial cells are p63 (−), as opposed to nuclei of myoepithelial cells, which are p63 (+), the lack of nuclear staining confirmed the identity of lymphatic channels in this study.

Data from a study conducted prior to the advent of sentinel mode mapping suggest that the unfavorable effect of lymphatic emboli in lymph node–negative patients is probably not due to occult metastases in their ALNs. Serial sections of lymph nodes detected metastases in 9 of 28 patients originally classified as T1N0M0 with lymphatic tumor emboli in the breast. The recurrence rate was not higher among those with occult nodal metastases than in the subset with truly negative lymph nodes.[290]

The significance of lymphatic tumor emboli for prognosis in patients already proven to have lymph node metastases is uncertain. Among T1N1M0 patients treated by mastectomy prior to the era of adjuvant chemotherapy, lymphatic tumor emboli did not significantly influence DFS at 10 years of follow-up.[134] One group of investigators found that lymphatic invasion did not have an independent effect on DFS at 10 years in patients who received adjuvant chemotherapy.[294] Others have reported significantly lower overall and DFS in stage II patients with "peritumoral vessel invasion" in an adjuvant therapy trial.[295] Analysis of 863 consecutive node-positive patients who received adjuvant therapy at the University of Naples revealed that the presence of lymphatic tumor emboli was a significant, prognostically unfavorable factor in this setting.[285] This effect was independent of the number of lymph nodes with metastases, tumor size, or grade.

The identification of peritumoral lymphatic tumor emboli has also begun to play a role in the management of patients found to have a positive sentinel ALN. Among those who undergo full axillary dissection, the probability of finding metastatic carcinoma in the remaining lymph nodes has proven to be significantly related to primary tumor size, the size of the SLN metastasis, and the presence or absence of peritumoral lymphatic tumor emboli.[296,297] In one study, none of the patients with tumors 1 cm or smaller lacking lymphatic invasion and a sentinel nodal metastasis not larger than 2 mm were found to have nonsentinel nodal metastases.[296] On the other hand, 58% of patients with tumors larger than 1 cm, with lymphatic tumor emboli and a sentinel nodal metastasis larger than 2 mm, had nonsentinel nodal metastases.

Blood Vessel Invasion

Blood vessel invasion, defined as penetration by tumor cells into the lumen of an artery or vein (Fig. 12.13), is almost always coincidental with invasion of lymph vessels.[280,298] These vascular structures can be identified in H&E-stained sections by the presence of a smooth muscle wall supported by elastic fibers. It may be necessary to employ histochemical stains (e.g., orcein or Verhoeff–van Gieson [VVG] stains), which selectively stain elastic tissue to detect this component of the vascular wall. Because elastin fibers are often deposited around ducts that contain intraductal carcinoma within an invasive tumor, the resulting appearance in an elastic tissue stain may be difficult to distinguish from vascular invasion. Immunostains for actin or smooth muscle myosin are useful for defining the smooth muscle structure of blood vessels. Because larger vascular components in the breast usually consist of a paired artery and vein, vascular invasion can be diagnosed with confidence when tumor is detected within one or both of a pair of vessels, as demonstrated by the elastic tissue and appropriate immunostains.

The reported frequency of blood vessel invasion detected in H&E-stained sections varies from about 5% to nearly 50%.[133,134,203,299–301] These widely divergent observations reflect major differences in these studies with respect to the number of patients evaluated, clinical and pathologic characteristics of the study population, and the methods by which blood vessel invasion was identified. Data acquired through the use of immunostains, especially CD31, CD34, D2-40, and podoplanin, indicate that the true frequency of blood vessel invasion is probably around 3%.[280,298] The significance of blood vessel invasion as an independent prognostic factor is difficult to determine because it occurs so infrequently and almost always coexists with lymphatic invasion. In view of these observations, previously published studies based on H&E sections alone that reported more frequent recurrences in patients thought to have blood vessel invasion can no longer be accepted as reliable since the unfavorable outcomes might be attributable to lymphatic invasion and many abnormalities may have been erroneously interpreted as blood vessels.

E-cadherin immunoreactivity provides *de facto* evidence for ductal differentiation of invasive and *in situ* ductal carcinoma, regardless of its phenotype (Fig. 12.14). Blood vessel invasion has been associated with the increased expression of E-cadherin in the intravascular carcinoma in the breast and other sites compared with the extravascular invasive component.[302] This difference between parenchymal and intravascular invasive carcinoma suggests that the biologic properties of the cells may change after entry into the circulatory system. Upregulation of E-cadherin expression in intravascular carcinoma could reflect the absence of inhibitory factors that might be present in the stroma, a stimulatory effect of the intravascular milieu, or the association of E-cadherin expression with other factors involved in vascular invasion.

Quantitation of Lymphovascular Invasion

The quantitation of lymphovascular invasion has not been standardized. Colleoni et al.[303] have defined focal lymphovascular involvement as one focus in one tumor block, moderate involvement as more than focus in one tumor block, and extensive involvement as one or more foci in more than one tumor block. Regardless of the amount of lymphatic invasion, patients whose tumors had this feature were significantly more likely to have positive ALNs than those without lymphatic invasion. Among patients with node-negative carcinoma, the risk of distant metastases was increased regardless of the amount of lymphatic invasion.

Angiogenesis

The angiogenesis associated with breast carcinomas has been of long-standing interest as a prognostic indicator. The capacity of neoplastic[304] and preneoplastic[305,306] tissues

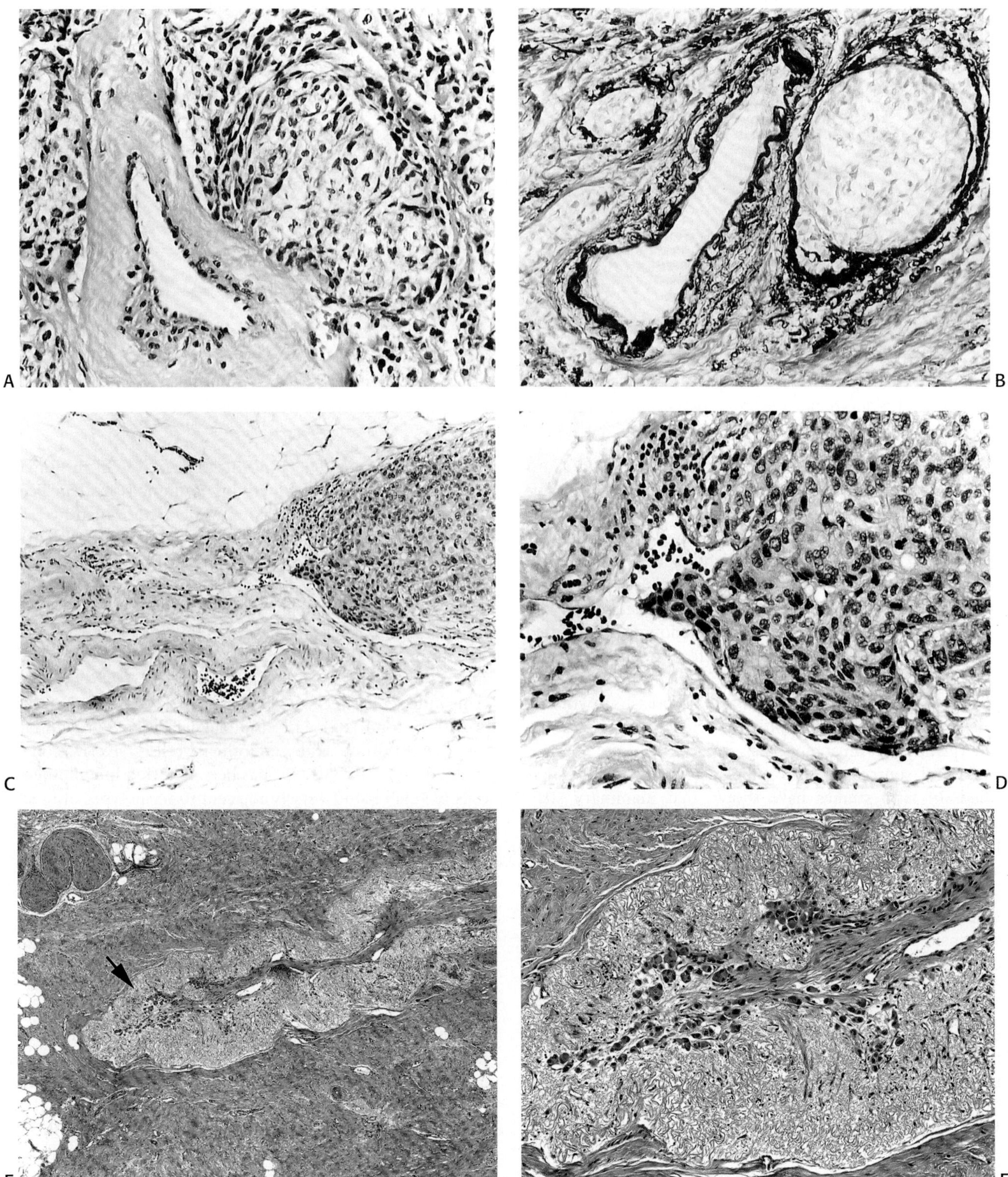

FIG. 12.13. ***Invasive ductal carcinoma, blood vessel invasion.*** **A:** An oval mass of carcinoma in a vein on the *right* is next to a thick-walled artery. **B:** An adjacent section of the focus in **(A)** stained to highlight elastic tissue demonstrating the presence of carcinoma in the vein and an elastic lamina in the artery (van Gieson elastin stain). **C:** On the *right*, carcinoma is present in the lumen of a vein cut longitudinally. **D:** A magnified view of carcinoma in the vein. **E:** Intravascular carcinoma cells (*arrow*), s/p neoadjuvant chemotherapy, in a thrombosed and partially recanalized blood vessel. **F:** A magnified view of carcinoma in the blood vessel.

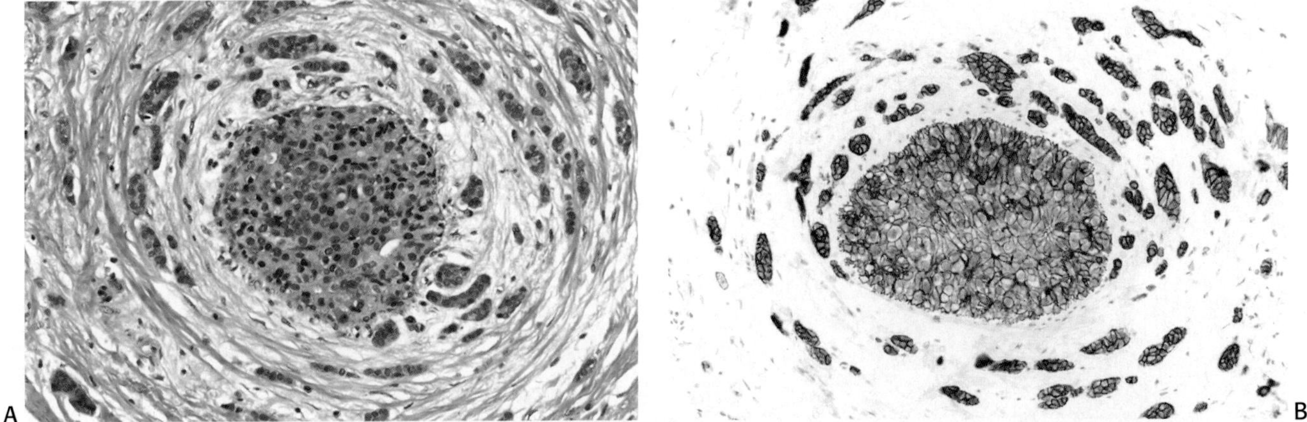

FIG. 12.14. ***Ductal carcinoma simulating lobular carcinoma.*** **A:** An invasive and *in situ* ductal carcinoma mimicking invasive and *in situ* lobular carcinoma. **B:** An E-cadherin immunostain shows characteristic "chicken wire" reactivity in the tumor cells—a result that supports ductal differentiation.

to induce vascular proliferation is well documented. Conversion from *in situ* carcinoma to an enlarging invasive carcinoma is associated with conversion to the angiogenic phenotype. Early expansion of the invasive lesion in the preneovascular stage is guided by a balance between the growth rate and apoptosis, a phenomenon observed in experimental studies at sites of primary tumors and micrometastases.[307]

The acquisition of the angiogenic phenotype is attributed to the overexpression of angiogenic factors such as vascular endothelial growth factor (VEGF), also termed vascular permeability factor (VPF), and basic fibroblast growth factor (bFGF). When studied *in vitro*, VEGF and bFGF have a synergistic effect on angiogenesis.[308]

Several sources of angiogenic factors have been identified. *In vitro* studies have shown that mammary stromal fibroblasts produce VEGF and that expression of this protein is upregulated by exposure of the cells to hypoxic conditions.[309] Angiogenic proteins can be present in the stroma and are produced by inflammatory cells such as macrophages. A significant correlation between stromal cell cathepsin-D reactivity and stromal vascular density has been observed, suggesting that upregulation of matrix proteinases might facilitate invasion and angiogenesis.[310]

VEGF can be detected in the cytoplasm of human breast carcinoma cells by IHC.[311] Anan et al.[312] demonstrated that VEGF mRNA expression determined by the reverse transcription-PCR (RT-PCR) and Southern blotting on samples obtained by fine-needle aspiration (FNA) correlated significantly with neovascularization in invasive ductal carcinomas stained with anti-CD31 antibody.[312] There was a high degree of correlation between VEGF mRNA in the FNA and excision specimens ($r = 0.874$). Expression of VEGF protein and mRNA was higher in invasive ductal than in invasive lobular carcinomas studied by Lee et al.,[313] although MVD in histologic sections did not differ significantly between the tumor types. Expression of VEGF protein and mRNA correlated significantly with MVD in invasive ductal and not in invasive lobular carcinomas, an observation suggesting that other angiogenic factors might play a greater role in invasive lobular carcinoma. The concentration of VEGF in human breast carcinomas measured by immunoassay has been found to correlate with tumoral MVD determined by IHC in the same lesions.[311] The angiogenic phenotype is also promoted by downregulation of inhibitors of angiogenesis such as thrombospondin[314,315] and angiostatin.[316] The tumor suppressor gene *p53* may play a role in controlling the expression of thrombospondin.[315]

Tumor growth is enhanced not only by increased perfusion associated with neovascularization, but also by the paracrine mitogenic effects of growth factors, such as insulin-like growth factor 1 (IGF-1)[315] and platelet-derived growth factor (PDGF) produced by endothelial cells.[317] Expression of receptors for VPF (VEGF) has been detected in endothelial cells in small blood vessels adjacent to some types of breast carcinoma in which tumor cells were found to express VPF mRNA.[318] Inhibition of tumor growth has been achieved experimentally with antibodies to VEGF[319] and to bFGF.[320] The angiogenic phenotype is usually expressed by a subset of cells in a carcinoma. Acquisition of this phenotype may be an important hallmark in the evolution of a carcinoma.

Measurement of Angiogenesis

Pathologic studies of angiogenesis in breast carcinoma have examined the relevance of tumor vascularity to known prognostic markers and to prognosis. To perform such studies, histologic sections of paraffin-embedded tissue are stained with immunohistochemical markers for endothelial cells such as factor VIII (antihuman von Willebrand factor [anti-VWF]), CD34, and CD31 (Fig. 12.15).[321] Comparative studies using these markers of vascular differentiation have not yielded consistent results for determining the optimal method by which angiogenesis should be measured in breast carcinoma. Data from one study indicated that CD31 was the most sensitive reagent and that it gave the highest vessel counts.[321] However, others reported that "anti-CD34 and anti-VWF showed better staining performance than anti-CD31, although the staining results with different antibodies

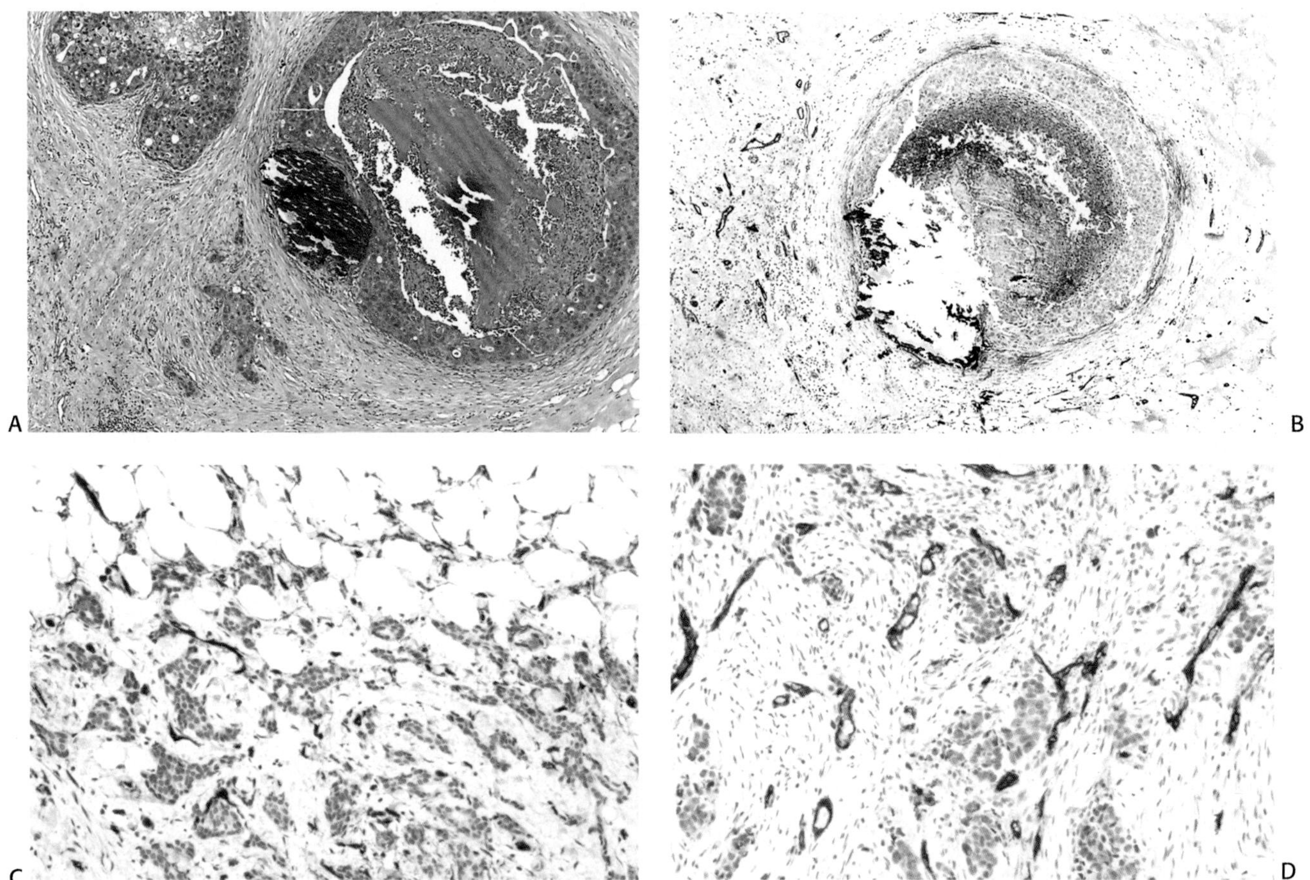

FIG. 12.15. ***Angiogenesis, invasive ductal carcinoma.*** **A:** Microinvasive carcinoma (*lower left*) associated with high-grade intraductal carcinoma, with calcification (*lower left*). **B:** A parallel section of the intraductal carcinoma in **(A)** with the CD34 immunostain shows greater vascularity in the region of the microinvasive carcinoma (*left*) than in the remaining perimeter of the duct. **C:** Angiogenesis is present at the border of this invasive ductal carcinoma. **D:** Intratumoral angiogenesis (all anti-CD34).

were comparable."[322] DualFactor VIII and Ki78 immunostaining highlights actively proliferating vessels.[323]

Employing manual methods, vessel counts are recorded in foci of greatest vascular density, so-called *hotspots*, by counting the number of immunostained structures in a predetermined number of fields at a fixed magnification.[324,325] A significant problem in the method of assessment based on detecting hotspots is the heterogeneity of vascularity within breast carcinomas. Martin et al.[326] studied vascular heterogeneity in breast carcinomas by performing angiograms and comparing the radiographic results with MVD counts in histologic sections of the same tumors. The specimen angiograms revealed two basic patterns of vascularity: an anastomosing pattern exhibiting numerous interconnecting branches and a radiating pattern with relatively few anastomoses. Vascular density in the specimen x-ray images was found to correlate with the histologic assessment of vascularity using CD34 immunostaining. However, vessel counts on three sections from each tumor varied by less than 20% in 70% of cases. An analysis of MVD in three tumor zones (central, intermediate, and peripheral) carried out on 147 invasive ductal carcinomas revealed significantly greater vascularity at the periphery.[327] The average microvessel counts per 200× field were 34.4, 39.4, and 51.5 in the central, intermediate, and peripheral zones, respectively. A study of angiogenesis in multiple blocks from individual carcinomas revealed an average coefficient of variation (CV) of 11.1% for vessel counts in hotspots in different sections from a single paraffin block and a CV of 24.4% when hotspots in sections from different blocks from the same tumor were compared.[328] The authors concluded that "one must carefully scan all the available tumor material in each case for the best spot." Counts based on limited samples such as needle core biopsies or one section of a tumor may be highly misleading.

Numerical microvessel counts have been analyzed by comparing cases above and below the mean number in a given study or by comparing cases with fewer than or more than a mean of microvessels per standardized field (200 or

400×).[323,325,329–333] Recommended methods for reporting vessel counts include Chalkley counting and MVD determined in one hot spot, as the mean of three hot spots, or as the highest count in one of three hot spots. In one study, analysis of microvessel count as a continuous numerical value revealed that more than 80 microvessels provided "the optimal cutoff value for stratifying patients into relatively good and poor prognosis groups." Subjective grading of MVD on a scale of 1 to 4 has also been used.[325] Image analysis has been employed to determine the endothelial area or the surface area that is immunoreactive for a vascular marker.[329,334,335]

Angiogenesis and Prognosis

High MVD has been shown in some studies to be associated with poorer histologic differentiation in invasive ductal carcinomas[310,321,324,335–338] and with a greater probability of axillary nodal metastases.[321,325,336,339,340] Some authors have found high microvessel counts to be associated with greater tumor size,[321,326,338,341] HER2/*neu* expression,[339] ER-negative status,[310,313,322] and age at diagnosis less than 50 years.[332] Others have reported no significant relationship between vessel counts and primary tumor grade,[313,329–332,334,342,343] size,[310,323,324,329–332,334,335,339,343,344] lymph node status,[310,332,334,342,343] the expression of p53[311,330,331,334,337,338] or HER2/*neu*,[321,323,330,334,337,338] or ER status.[330,331,338,339]

Angiogenesis has been reported to be an independent prognostic indicator by some investigators. High microvessel counts have been associated with a poor prognosis in node-negative[324,329,331,332,333,335,344] and in node-positive[329,332,336,344] breast carcinoma. Angiogenesis determined by Chalkley counts proved to be a prognostically significant factor in an adjuvant therapy trial of tamoxifen administered to node-positive patients.[340] However, others have failed to detect a significant relationship with prognosis[322,330,331,335,336,345] or with recurrence in the breast after wide excision and breast conservation.[346]

Substantial methodologic variability may be an important factor in the failure of published studies to detect a consistent relationship between angiogenesis and prognostic factors or prognosis. These technical differences include the use of different markers to highlight vessels (CD31, CD34, and factor VIII), different methods for counting (manual, image analysis), different quantitation methods (average microvessel count per square millimeter vs. highest microvessel count per square millimeter), and variability in microvessel distribution in different parts of a tumor. Hansen et al.[347] examined observer variability using four different methods of vessel counting in tissue sections stained with anti-CD34. The counting methods were Chalkley counting, MVD estimated in one hot spot, the mean MVD in three hot spots, and the highest MVD in one of three hot spots. CVs for intraobserver variability were approximately 20% for each method (14% to 23%). A lower coefficient of interobserver variation was achieved with the Chalkley method (8% to 9%) than with the microvessel methods (30%). Presently, the immunohistochemical assessment of angiogenesis in tissue sections requires further standardization before acceptance as an independent prognostic variable. Emerging automated techniques for the quantification of angiogenesis offer promise in this regard.[348]

Efforts to assess tumor vascularity in patients using MRI with gadolinium enhancement have not yielded consistent results. Buadu et al.[349] reported that the pattern and rate of contrast uptake observed in MRI studies of the breast were directly correlated with the distribution of angiogenesis in the tumors. Two studies reported an association between MRI enhancement and MVD.[350,351] However, there was considerable variability in the measurements, and it was concluded that "MRI cannot be used to predict MVD *in vivo*"[350] and that "gadolinium enhancement of breast lesions is not an accurate predictor of vessel density."[350] A modified dynamic MRI technique with high resolution revealed an association between early signal enhancement with rapid washout of contrast and high tumor vascularity.[352]

Angiogenic Proteins and Prognosis

VEGF and other angiogenesis-related proteins in invasive carcinomas have been evaluated as independent prognostic markers. Linderholm et al.[353] determined cytosolic levels of VEGF in tumors from 525 consecutive, node-negative patients. VEGF level was inversely related to ER and directly correlated with tumor size and grade. Patients with VEGF levels higher than the median had a significantly poorer prognosis after a median follow-up of 46 months. Higher VEGF levels when analyzed as a continuous variable were also prognostically less favorable. Among patients with ER-positive tumors, survival was significantly reduced among those with VEGF expression higher than the median level. A similar association of VEGF and prognosis was reported by Eppenberger et al.,[354] who studied 305 patients with a median follow-up of 37 months. Other angiogenesis factors (angiogenin and bFGF), the plasminogen activator inhibitor 1, and the tumor proteolysis factor urokinase-type plasminogen activator (uPA) were also studied. By multivariate Cox-regression analysis, VEGF and uPA were significantly associated with RFS in node-negative patients. The most favorable RFS was observed in women with tumors classified as VEGF(−)/uPA(−), with intermediate and relatively poor RFS in the groups classified as VEGF(+)/uPA(−) and VEGF(+)/uPA(+), respectively.

Antiangiogenic Therapy

The angiogenic capacity of neoplasms may be a basis for treatment through the use of chemotherapeutic and antiangiogenic agents. Current data indicate that response to conventional forms of chemotherapy is not correlated significantly with tumor angiogenesis. Consequently, tumors with marked angiogenesis do not appear to be more sensitive in the adjuvant setting than tumors with low levels of neovascularization.[338,355] Paulsen et al.[356] reported that MVD was not associated with responsiveness to doxorubicin therapy in patients with locally advanced carcinoma.

Experimental evidence suggests that antiangiogenic therapy may potentiate chemotherapy and inhibit neovascularization of the tumor bed.[357] In an experimental animal model, microtubule inhibitors such as Taxol and 2-methoxyestradiol were able to inhibit neovascularization induced by

VEGF and bFGF.[358] Growth of tumor cells and neovascularity were decreased by the administration of 2-methoxyestradiol in this system. Some antiangiogenic agents such as angiostatin exert their effect by inhibiting endothelial cell proliferation. This is a relatively slow process that requires prolonged administration.[359,360]

Current attempts to interfere with the VEGF pathway have concentrated on the development of monoclonal antibodies to VEGF or VEGF-receptor (VEGFR) and on tyrosine kinase inhibitors.[318] Bevacizumab is a humanized recombinant antibody to VEGF, which is the first of these agents to be approved for clinical trials in combination with chemotherapy. Administration of bevacizumab in conjunction with chemotherapy proved to be more beneficial than chemotherapy alone in a randomized phase III trial involving patients with previously treated metastatic breast carcinoma.[361] Wedam et al.[362] administered bevacizumab in combination with chemotherapy to 21 patients with inflammatory and locally advanced breast carcinoma. Periodic sampling of the tumors revealed significantly increased tumor apoptosis measured by the TUNEL method after bevacizumab alone, which continued after chemotherapy was added. Immunohistochemical examination revealed a median decrease of 66.7% in the expression of phosphorylated VEGFR-2 after bevacizumab and continuation of this decrease in combination with chemotherapy. The addition of bevacizumab to neoadjuvant chemotherapy in patients with triple-negative breast carcinomas significantly increased the rate of pathologic complete response in one study,[363] but others found significant benefit from bevacizumab only in patients with hormone receptor–positive carcinomas.[364] Attempts to identify novel antiangiogenic targets based on gene expression analysis in human breast cancer associated blood vessels are underway.[365]

Perineural Invasion

Carcinomas arising in various organs exhibit a capacity, and in some instances a proclivity, to invade around and into nerves. Perineural invasion (Fig. 12.16) is infrequently observed among invasive mammary carcinomas, perhaps in

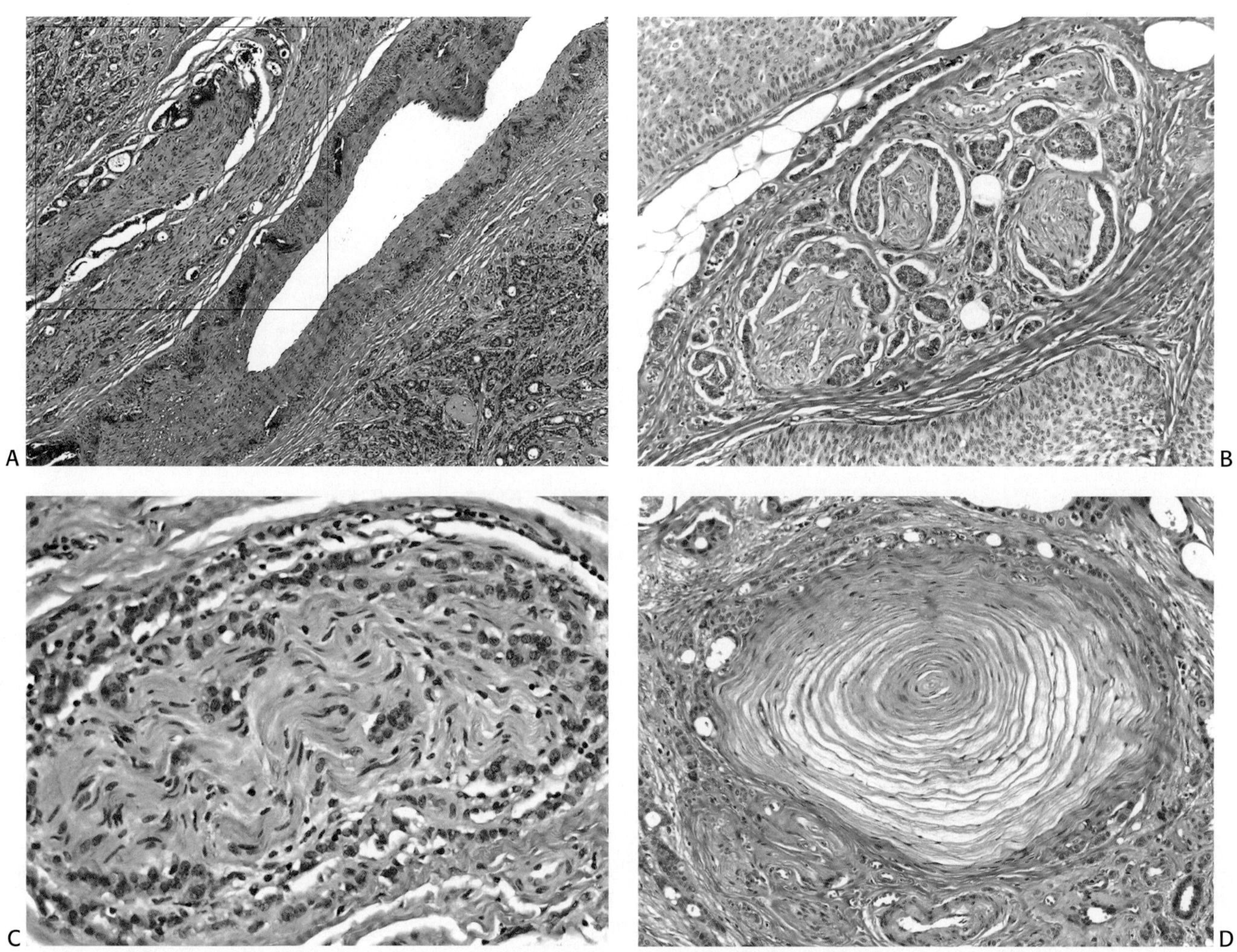

FIG. 12.16. ***Invasive ductal carcinoma, perineural invasion.*** **A:** Carcinoma is present around a large nerve (*box*). **B:** Carcinoma forming thick collars around multiple nerves. **C:** Carcinoma is present around and within a nerve. **D:** Carcinoma is present around a cutaneous Pacinian (lamellar) nerve receptor near the nipple.

part because nerves of notable size are not as numerous in mammary tissues as they are, for example, in prostatic or pancreatic tissues where perineural invasion is more commonly encountered. Perineural invasion can be found in approximately 1% of invasive breast carcinomas.[366] It tends to occur in high-grade tumors, where it is frequently associated with lymphatic tumor emboli, but it has not been proven to have independent prognostic significance.

Stromal Characteristics

Tumors vary considerably with respect to the quantity and qualitative characteristics of their stroma. Extremes are represented by medullary carcinoma, which contains virtually no fibrous stroma, and scirrhous carcinoma characterized by marked collagenization. Despite emerging evidence that suggests that "fibrotic focus" in breast carcinoma confers a worse prognosis,[367] it is not clear that the character of stroma in an invasive ductal carcinoma is an independent prognostic variable. There are strong associations between stromal characteristics and other prognostically significant structural features of breast carcinomas. For example, tumors that contain minimal stromal reaction tend to have the following characteristics: circumscription, high-grade nuclei, poorly differentiated histology, and a prominent lymphoplasmacytic reaction. They also tend to be ER negative. On the other hand, densely fibrotic or scirrhous carcinomas (without necrosis) are more likely to be stellate, to be moderately differentiated, and to have little lymphoplasmacytic reaction. A greater proportion of these lesions are ER positive. The pattern of growth of an invasive carcinoma can be determined by the architecture of the stroma, especially when it grows in PASH (Fig. 12.17).

Attempts to assess the character or composition of stroma in invasive ductal carcinomas have focused on the amount of elastic tissue present. Stromal elastic fibers can be detected using the same stains employed to demonstrate the elastic components in blood vessels (orcein or VVG stains) and by IHC using antibodies to components of elastin.[368] Although elastic tissue is minimally present in normal mammary stroma, increased amounts can be deposited around ducts with benign

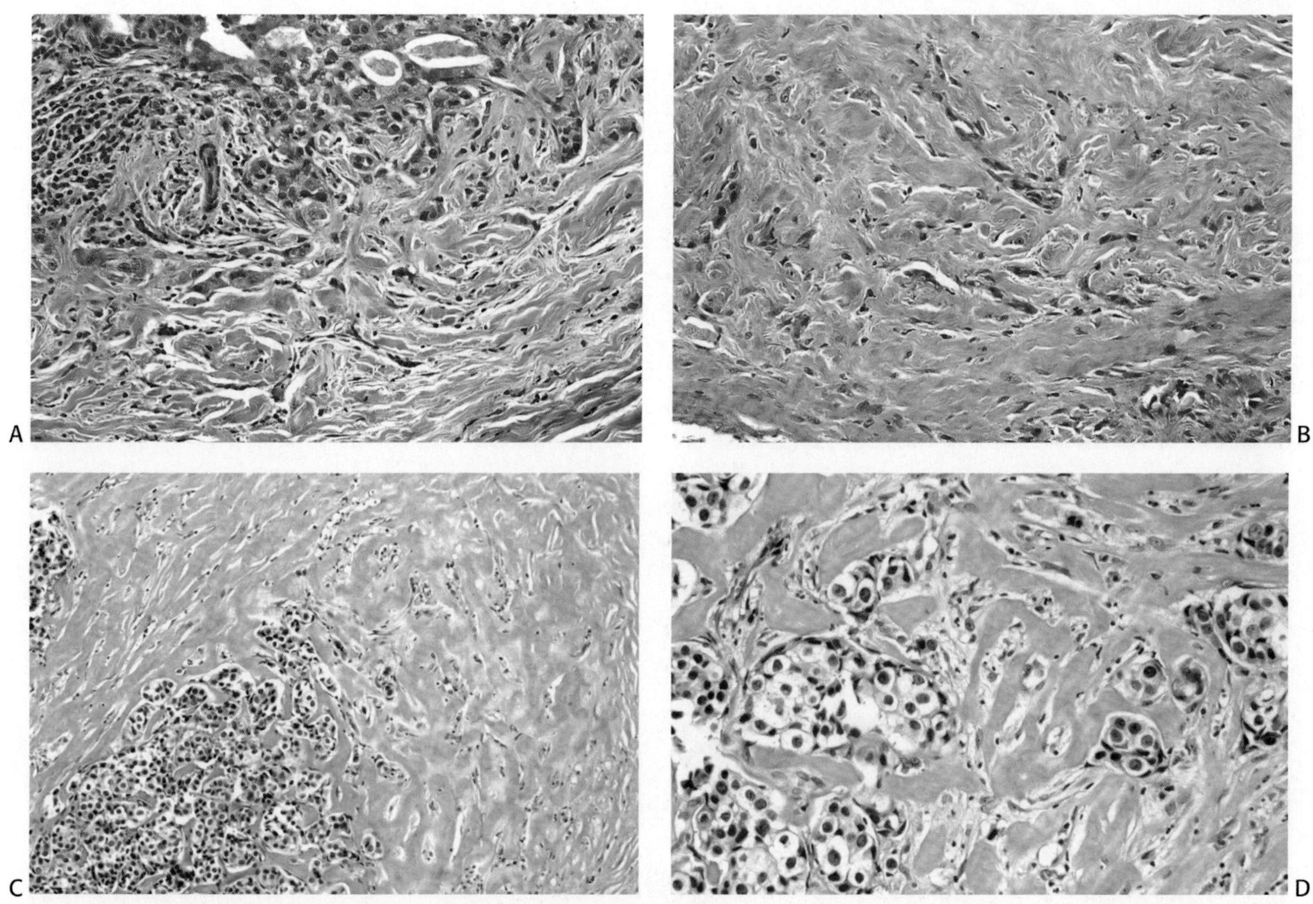

FIG. 12.17. ***Invasive ductal carcinoma in pseudoangiomatous stromal hyperplasia.*** **A:** Moderately differentiated carcinoma on the *left* invades stroma that has pseudoangiomatous features. **B:** Part of the tumor where invasive ductal carcinoma in pseudoangiomatous stroma resembles invasive lobular carcinoma. **C,D:** High-grade invasive ductal carcinoma with linear structure due to growth in pseudoangiomatous stroma.

proliferative breast changes.[369,370] A similar phenomenon occurs around DCIS intraductal carcinoma, particularly when it is present in the invasive portion of the tumor, and to varying degrees in the stroma of invasive carcinoma (Fig. 12.18).

The cellular source of elastin is uncertain. *In vitro* cultured breast carcinoma cells secrete relatively little elastin compared with fibroblasts.[371,372] At the ultrastructural level, elastin fibrils have been found associated with myofibroblasts.[373] Because elastosis can develop in benign proliferative lesions, it is not a specific product of carcinoma cells. It is likely that epithelial cells secrete a factor or factors that induce the production of elastin by stromal cells, thereby contributing to the development of elastosis. The observation that elastotic fibers associated with breast carcinoma bind lectins more strongly than the elastica of blood vessels indicates that they are newly formed and immature.[374] Plasma protease inhibitors including α_1-antitrypsin, α_1-antichymotrypsin, and C1 esterase inhibitor have been detected in elastic tissue associated with carcinoma.[374] These substances contribute to the accumulation of immature elastic fibers by inhibiting elastinolytic enzymes.

In the absence of a widely accepted method for describing elastosis, various grading schemes have been adopted in an effort to convey quantitative estimates of the extent of this process. The frequency of the most extreme or marked degrees of elastosis described in recent reports varied from 17% to 23%, whereas from 12% to 55% of tumors in the same studies were characterized by little or no elastosis.[375,376]

Abundant elastosis is significantly associated with ER positivity.[375–377] The importance of elastosis as an independent prognostic variable remains controversial. Although marked elastosis has been described by some investigators as a favorable prognostic feature,[378,379] others found that elastosis did not correlate with prognosis,[374,375,380] or that abundant elastosis had a negative effect on outcome.[381,382]

Myofibroblastic proliferation occurs to a variable extent in invasive ductal carcinomas. This stromal component is demonstrated with immunostains for actin and CD34. Immunostains for calponin or smooth muscle myosin-heavy chain (SMM-HC) exhibit reactivity in myoepithelial cells, and they are weakly positive or nonreactive in myofibroblasts (Fig. 12.19). Reactivity in myofibroblasts can be a confounding factor when assessing a lesion for possible microinvasion. This is best avoided by using the p63 immunostain that exclusively localizes in the nuclei of myoepithelial cells.

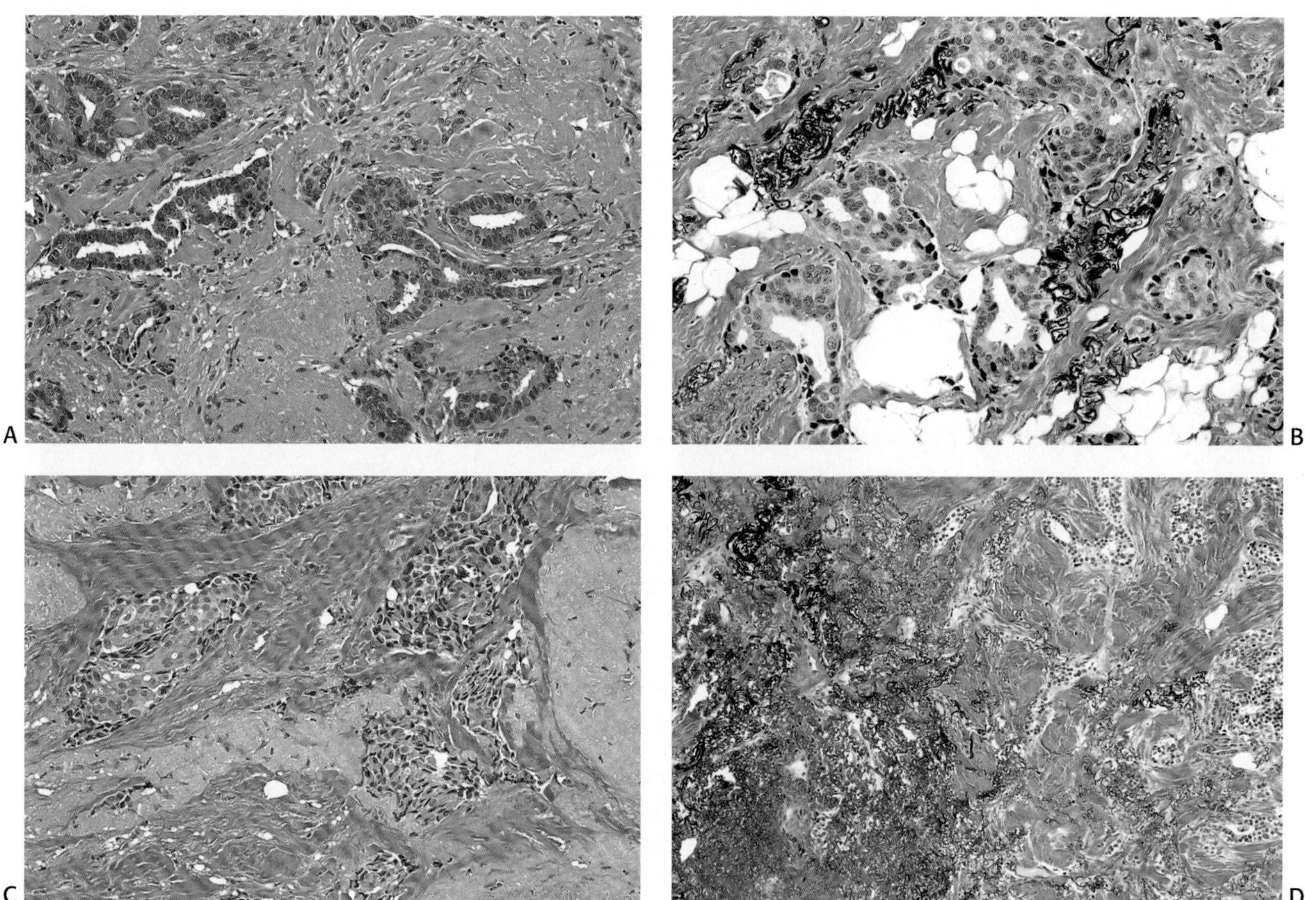

FIG. 12.18. ***Invasive ductal carcinoma, elastosis.*** **A,B:** Fibrillar elastosis blends with collagen fibers in this well-differentiated invasive ductal carcinoma. **C,D:** Coarse elastic fibers stained black are demonstrated in the collagen in the invasive carcinoma in **(B)** and **(D)** (van Gieson elastin stain).

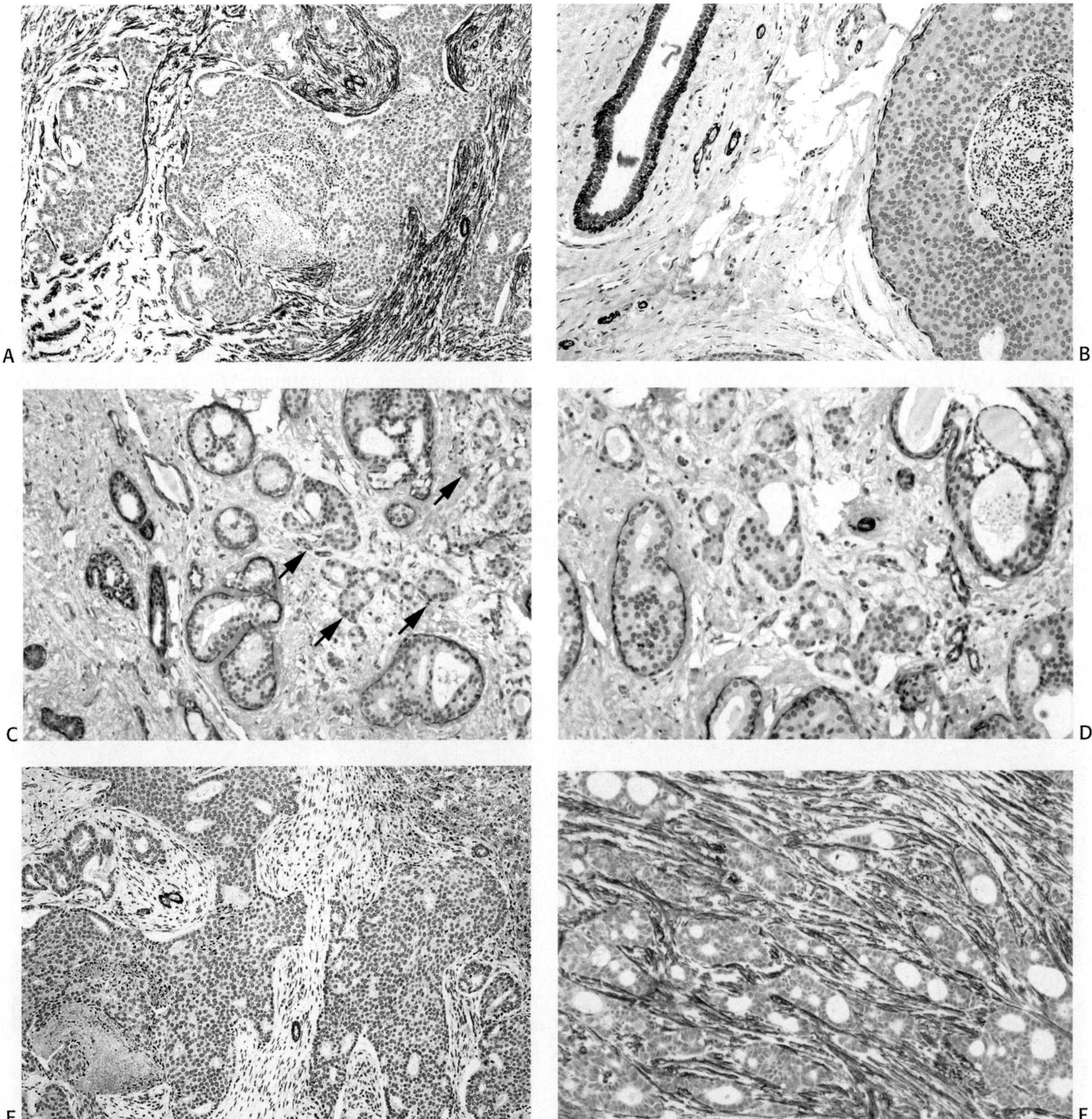

FIG. 12.19. ***Invasive ductal carcinoma, myofibroblastic and myoepithelial reactivity.*** **A:** The immunostain for smooth muscle actin (SMA) reveals myofibroblastic proliferation in the stroma of an invasive ductal carcinoma. In some regions, stromal reactivity simulates myoepithelium. **B:** This immunostain for SMM-HC is reactive in myoepithelial cells in a normal duct (*left*) and intraductal carcinoma (*right*). Stromal reactivity is limited to small blood vessels. **C:** Actin immunoreactivity highlights normal ducts and ducts with intraductal carcinoma. Invasive well-differentiated ductal carcinoma lacks myoepithelial staining (*arrows*). **D:** Actin immunoreactivity is present in myoepithelium around intraductal carcinoma and in vessels. Invasive well-differentiated ductal carcinoma (*center*) lacks myoepithelium. **E:** No myoepithelial cells are present in the invasive ductal carcinoma, and myofibroblasts are not immunoreactive with the SMM-HC antibody. **F:** Marked stromal reactivity for SMA is shown in this moderately differentiated invasive ductal carcinoma. **G:** Invasive, well-differentiated ductal carcinoma with an adenosis pattern. SMA reactivity is limited to small blood vessels and myofibroblasts.

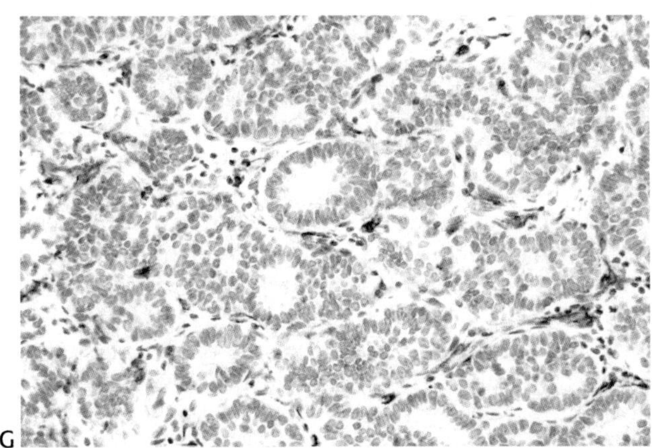

FIG. 12.19. *(Continued)*

Extent of DCIS as a Prognostic Marker

Attention has been directed to the pattern and distribution of DCIS as a prognostic variable in patients with invasive ductal carcinoma. Tumors vary in the relative proportions of intraductal and invasive components, from lesions with only microscopic invasion that is not grossly measurable (Fig. 12.20) to lesions composed entirely of invasive carcinoma.

Although the distribution of DCIS in and around the primary tumor appears to correlate with the risk of recurrence in the breast after lumpectomy and radiation therapy,[383] this feature has no bearing on the risk of systemic recurrence in women treated by breast conservation or mastectomy.[384,385] Recurrence occurs more often in the breast after lumpectomy and radiation therapy in women who have comedo DCIS or when there is extensive DCIS defined as DCIS within and around an invasive tumor that comprises at least 25% of the neoplasm. The increased risk of local recurrence attributable to an extensive DCIS is probably a manifestation of a greater probability of there being carcinoma at or beyond the margin of excision and remaining in the breast. In patients with negative margins, the presence of extensive DCIS does not increase the risk of local recurrence in the breast after breast conservation therapy.[386,387,388]

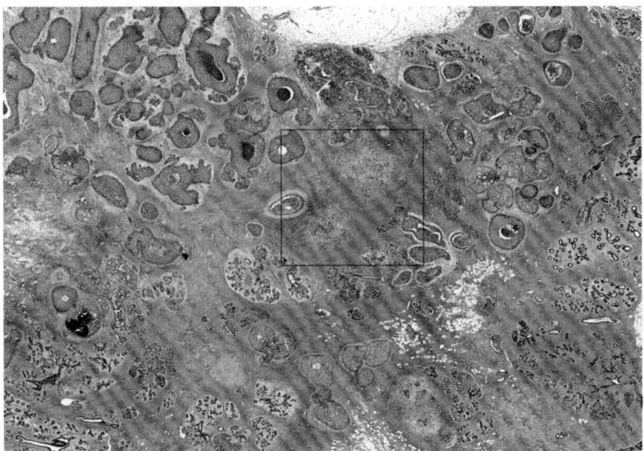

FIG. 12.20. ***Extensive intraductal component of an invasive ductal carcinoma.*** Invasive ductal carcinoma (*box*) lies amidst intraductal carcinoma. The tumor presented as a palpable mass. Invasive carcinoma is present in two minute foci (*upper right* and *lower left* in *box*) that together span approximately 2 mm. The intraductal component of the carcinoma is of the solid type with central necrosis. It constitutes the bulk of the tumor, and widely extends beyond the invasive carcinoma.

Invasive carcinomas with an extensive DCIS component frequently have microcalcifications that help in determining the extent of the lesion on mammography. Lesions with calcifications that extended beyond 3 cm were significantly more likely to have an extensive DCIS component than those with calcifications of lesser extent (90% vs. 54%).[389] In most cases, the mammographic pattern was indicative of a segmental distribution resulting from continuous intraductal spread. This conclusion was supported by a study of the X-chromosome-linked phosphoglycerokinase gene that found a monoclonal pattern of gene expression when multiple areas of DCIS from three cases were analyzed.[390] Molecular analysis of microdissected paired samples of intraductal and invasive components from single tumors found that they had undergone similar chromosomal changes.[391]

The pattern of ductal involvement around invasive ductal carcinomas has been studied by three-dimensional reconstruction using computer graphics.[392] DCIS was usually found extending in a continuous fashion from the invasive tumor into the ductal–lobular system. The direction of involvement was more prominently central than peripheral. Although extension tended to be limited to one ductal system, spread to adjacent ductal segments did occur through anastomosing ductal branches.

Jing et al.[393] studied the biologic characteristics of invasive carcinomas with extensive DCIS. The intraductal component generally had the same pattern of expression as the invasive tumor for c-erbB-2 (HER2) and p53. Overexpression of c-erbB-2 was more frequent in cases with extensive DCIS, and these tumors had significantly more frequent lymphatic tumor emboli or venous invasion.

In one study, there was a significantly greater likelihood that a patient would have extensive DCIS if the preceding needle core biopsy specimen demonstrated DCIS in conjunction with invasive ductal carcinoma.[394] Extensive DCIS was found in 30% of those with intraductal and invasive ductal carcinoma and in none of the patients with invasive ductal carcinoma alone in the core biopsy specimen. Nonetheless, the majority of patients with intraductal and invasive ductal carcinoma in the needle core biopsy specimen did not have extensive DCIS in this report.

The presence of atypical hyperplasia in the breast around an invasive carcinoma does not appear to be associated with an increased risk of tumor recurrence in the breast after conservative surgery with radiation, and it does not correlate significantly with 5- and 10-year survival rates.[395] It is important that minimal involvement of terminal duct-lobular units by *in situ* carcinoma be excluded from the diagnosis of atypical hyperplasia in this setting because the latter circumstance predisposes the patient to an increased risk of breast recurrence after conservation therapy.[388]

Other Histologic Variables

An array of other histologic variables has been assessed as potential prognostic indicators. Among these are the amount and type of mucin produced by the tumor cells, mucopolysaccharide content of tumor stroma, glycogen content of tumor cells, presence of calcifications in the tumor, and the influence of associated benign or atypical proliferative changes in the breast.[395] For the most part, these features have not been correlated strongly with overall prognosis or the risk of recurrence in the breast after breast conservation surgery with radiation.

TUMOR GROWTH RATE

Clinical Assessment of Tumor Growth Rate

Estimates of the growth rate of mammary carcinoma have been made from serial mammography studies. Tabár et al.[57] reported that the mean preclinical state, the "sojourn time," was 2.46 years in women 40 to 49 years of age entered into a breast cancer–screening trial. Mean sojourn time was longer in women 50 to 59 years (3.75 years) and among those 60 to 69 years (7.29) of age at diagnosis. Analysis of data from this study also led the authors to conclude that the rate of tumor progression, manifested by "dedifferentiation" to less well-differentiated grade, larger size, and greater frequency of nodal metastases, was more rapid in women 40 to 49 years of age than in older women. The estimated annual progression rates from size less than 2 cm to size 2 cm or greater were 31%, 22%, and 20% for women 40 to 49, 50 to 59, and 60 to 69 years old, respectively, at entry into the screening program. Annual progression rates from lymph node negative to lymph node positive were 26%, 19%, and 16%, respectively, for the same age groups. Annual progression rates from grades I or II to grade III were 47%, 12%, and 15%, respectively, for these age groups.

Interval carcinomas are defined as tumors diagnosed clinically between screening intervals after a negative screening examination. Vitak et al.[70] reported that in comparison with screen-detected carcinomas, interval carcinomas occurred more often in women 40 to 49 and 50 to 59 years of age on entry into the screening program than in women 60 years or older. Statistically significant unfavorable characteristics of interval carcinomas compared with those of screen-detected tumors were larger size, greater frequency of nodal metastases, fewer stage I tumors, greater frequencies of ER negative or aneuploid carcinomas, and a higher proportion of tumors with high SPF.

Estimates of growth rate have been determined by examining serial mammograms from women who develop carcinoma detected mammographically after a prior "negative" radiographic examination. The radiograph that preceded the diagnostic image is considered to be a "false negative," if on review an abnormality deemed not significant in initial review is found at the site where carcinoma was later detected. Peer et al.[396] used data from serial mammograms to estimate tumor growth rate for incident and interval carcinomas when the prior screening examination was negative. Growth rate expressed as estimated tumor-doubling time was significantly greater in women less than 45 years old on entry into screening (geometric mean in days, 80; 95% CI, 44 to 147) than in those 50 to 70 years (geometric mean, 157; 95% CI, 121 to 204) or in women older than 70 years (geometric mean, 188; 95% CI, 120 to 295). A substantial proportion of carcinomas detected mammographically when no lesion was detectable retrospectively on the antecedent mammogram were *in situ* carcinomas. Other studies have also reported a similar correlation between younger age and shorter doubling time based on screening studies[397,398] or other data.[399] Overall tumor-doubling times reported in these studies, not stratified for age, were 220 days,[397] 174 days,[398] and 115 days.[399] Daly et al.[400] analyzed 25 patients with breast carcinoma detected in a screening program after what proved in retrospect to be a false-negative mammography study. The average mammographic size of false-negative lesions was 6 mm, whereas the average size on mammography of the incident tumors found on subsequent screening examinations was 13.8 mm. The average histologic size of invasive carcinomas detected after false-negative mammography was 16.7 mm (range, 7 to 30 mm).

Determination of SPF and Ploidy by Flow Cytometry

In 1979, Atkin and Kay[401] described the relationship between modal DNA values and prognosis in 1,465 diverse malignant tumors, including some breast carcinomas. Generally, patients whose tumors were in the near-diploid range had a better survival than those with an aneuploid DNA distribution. Subsequently, Auer et al.[402,403] employed FNA biopsies of breast carcinomas to prepare Feulgen-stained smears and reported that the resultant DNA histograms correlated with survival time. In another study also using FNA material, Auer et al.[404] compared the DNA histograms of 18 breast carcinomas and metastases in the same patient. With one exception, little difference in DNA patterns was found between the two specimens from a given patient. When related to ER content, tumors with a near-diploid DNA content tended to be receptor positive, whereas those with aneuploid DNA were likely to be receptor negative.[405]

When measured by flow cytometry, the majority of breast carcinomas in most series have a bimodal distribution of DNA values, with more than 50% of cells in the hyperdiploid range.[406–408] Tumors with a near-diploid DNA distribution tend to be positive for both ER and PR, whereas receptor negativity has been associated with aneuploidy.[406,409,410]

Pathologic studies have shown a close correlation between the cytologic grading of tumor nuclei and DNA ploidy analyzed by flow cytometry.[411,412] Low-grade tumors typically exhibit near-diploid DNA, whereas aneuploidy is most pronounced in tumors with high-grade nuclei. Subtypes of carcinoma that are histologically low grade, such as tubular carcinoma, are usually diploid, whereas medullary carcinoma, which is a cytologically high-grade neoplasm, is generally aneuploid.[413]

The proliferative proportion of cells in DNA synthesis determined by the thymidine labeling index (TLI) has been shown to correlate significantly with prognosis.[414–417] High TLI has been associated with a higher frequency of recurrence, earlier recurrence, and shorter survival after recurrence.[418–421] The unfavorable effect of high TLI was independent of stage at diagnosis,[422–424] but may not be a better guide to prognosis than histologic grade.[417]

Flow cytometry can determine the proliferative fraction (SPF), which is reported to be equivalent to TLI.[425] In 1983, Hedley et al.[426] described a method of preparing paraffin-embedded tissues for flow cytometry DNA analysis. SPF correlated with ploidy to the extent that diploid carcinomas tended to have a lower SPF than aneuploid lesions.[427,428] Tumors with a high SPF tend to be ER negative.[419,428] SPF has been found to correlate with the histologic and cytologic differentiation of ductal carcinomas.[410,428,429] Some investigators reported that ploidy and/or SPF did not correlate with nodal status at the time of initial treatment,[420] but others found a high SPF in node-positive compared with node-negative patients.[421] A reduction in the SPF was found in 25% of nodal metastases from ER-positive tumors. This phenomenon was not apparent when ER-negative tumors were compared with their concurrent nodal metastases.[430]

Owing to the close correlation between tumor grade, SPF, and ploidy, the significance of any one of these features as an independent prognostic factor is difficult to ascertain.[431–434] Although patients with tumors that have a diploid DNA index tend to have a more favorable prognosis,[435–438] "the magnitude of this advantage compared with tumors showing aneuploidy is small."[433] Bergers et al.[439] analyzed DNA ploidy data from breast carcinomas in a prospective study of 1,301 cases, published in 1997, and concluded that "DNA ploidy seems to be of little clinical importance in breast cancer patients compared with other prognostic parameters." A study of DNA ploidy in 393 patients by Pinto et al.,[440] published in 2013, concluded that "along with nodal status and hormone receptor expression, DNA ploidy is an independent predictor of long-term survival. An association between high SPF and increased risk of recurrence has been documented in most studies,[441–445] but others have failed to detect this relationship.[437,446] Hietanen et al.[447] reported that metastatic breast carcinoma with a high SPF was significantly more responsive to chemotherapy than tumors with a low SPF.

Immunohistochemical Assessment of Proliferation

5-Bromodeoxyuridine (BrdU), a thymidine analog, is incorporated into DNA during the S-phase of the cell cycle. Uptake of BrdU after *in vivo* administration to patients[448–450] or *in vitro* incubation of fresh biopsies with BrdU[451,452] can be measured in tissue sections by an immunohistochemical procedure that employs an anti-BrdU antibody,[453–455] or by multiparameter flow cytometry.[449] The results are comparable to those obtained by thymidine labeling.[453,456]

In vivo BrdU administration yielded median labeling indices of 4.2%[449] and 10.3%[399] in two studies based on multiparameter flow cytometry and manual counting of immunohistochemical sections, respectively. Rew et al.[449] found no correlation between the BrdU labeling index, lymph node status, tumor size, and grade. Thor et al.[452] reported that the BrdU labeling index in 460 invasive ductal carcinomas (median, 4%; mean, 6%; range, 0% to 40%) was significantly higher than in 26 invasive lobular carcinomas (median, 3.0%; mean, 3.5%; range, 0% to 12%) when BrdU was considered a continuous variable. BrdU labeling was also significantly associated with tumor grade, tumor size, nodal status, mitotic index, and MIB1 labeling.[452] Weidner et al.[450] also found that *in vivo* BrdU labeling was significantly correlated with histologic grade and with the mitotic count. Although BrdU labeling may be used in a research setting, it is not employed in routine clinical practice at present.

A number of immunocytochemical assays have been developed employing antibodies to cell proliferation–related proteins. These reagents provide a static measure of proliferation at a point in time rather than the proliferative rate. One of these is *Ki67*, a mouse monoclonal antibody to nuclear components of a cell line derived from Hodgkin lymphoma.[457] The antibody reacts with a nuclear antigen expressed in proliferating cells throughout the cell cycle that is absent from quiescent cells.[458] It has been shown that there is a close correlation in breast carcinomas between the Ki67 growth fraction and SPF determined by flow cytometry,[459–462] the TLI,[463] the BrdU index,[464] labeling with MIB1,[465] and mitotic counts.[459,466]

Because Ki67 labeling occurs throughout the non-G_0 portion of the cell cycle, the percentage of positive cells is consistently higher and generally about twice the proportion in S-phase (TLI or BrdU positive). However, Ki67 positivity may not accurately reflect proliferative activity under some circumstances. Ki67 expression may be so low as to be undetectable at the outset of DNA replication, particularly in cells with a long G_1-phase.[467] Cells with proliferation impaired or arrested by suboptimal growth conditions or drug treatment (e.g., tamoxifen) may retain immunohistochemically demonstrable Ki67 antigen. The difference between growth fraction determined by BrdU labeling and Ki67 positivity is accentuated when conditions are altered in a fashion that inhibits proliferation. A statistically significant positive correlation between Ki67 positivity and the number of nucleolar organizer regions in mammary carcinoma nuclei has been reported.[468,469]

The mean value of Ki67-positive cells (3% to 4%) in benign breast lesions is substantially lower than the mean value (16% to 17%) in mammary carcinomas.[463,470] A Ki67 labeling index of 10% or less in a breast carcinoma is generally regarded as "low" and that equal to or more than 10% is considered "high."[471] However, the 2009 Saint Gallen consensus guidelines set "cutoffs" to guide management, that is, proliferation rate, per Ki67, of less than 15% is a "relative indication for endocrine therapy alone," 16% to 30% is "not useful for decision," and greater than 30% constitutes a "relative indication for chemoendocrine therapy."[472] Unfortunately, these "cutoffs" seem rather arbitrary given the lack of standardized assessment, as well as variations in preanalytical specimen handling.

The Ki67 growth fraction is significantly related to grade in most tumors, being highest in poorly differentiated carcinomas, invasive ductal carcinomas with necrosis, and in "triple-negative" carcinomas.[459,462,470,473,474] Trihia et al.[475] concluded that "Ki67 detection represents a valuable tool and is a good objective substitute for mitotic counts when used in a grading system." Invasive lobular and mucinous carcinomas have a low-to-moderate growth fraction, whereas medullary carcinomas have more than 50% Ki67-positive cells. ER-negative and PR-negative tumors tend to have a high Ki67-positive fraction.[470,476] Several studies have reported a significant inverse association between Ki67 staining and disease-free and OS.[466,471,474,477–480] A comparison of screen-detected and interval carcinomas revealed that interval carcinomas had higher Ki67 labeling and higher mitotic rates than tumors detected by screening.[481]

MIB1 is an antibody raised against recombinant parts of the Ki67 antigen that can be employed on microwave-processed paraffin-embedded tissue.[482] A significant correlation between Ki67 expression and MIB1 immunoreactivity was described in three studies,[465,483,484] but Keshgegian and Cnaan[485] reported finding no significant correlation. Pinder et al.[486] reported that high MIB1 labeling was associated with poorly differentiated carcinomas, larger tumor size, earlier recurrence, and poorer survival. Thor et al.[452] found that MIB1 labeling in invasive ductal carcinomas was significantly higher (mean, 32.2%; median, 28.6%; range, 0% to 99%) than in invasive lobular carcinomas (median, 20.8%; mean, 17.8%; range, 2% to 52%). High MIB1 labeling was also associated with diagnosis before age 50, ER negativity, PR negativity, high tumor grade, larger tumor size, and ALN metastases. A strong correlation between MIB1 labeling and DFS was also reported by Arber et al.[487]

Proliferating cell nuclear antigen (PCNA)/cyclin is a nonhistone nuclear protein that serves as a cofactor to DNA polymerase. It is expressed during the late G_1-phase and S-phase of the cell cycle. A number of monoclonal antibodies have been developed to antigenically distinct forms of PCNA, and some of these reagents, applicable to paraffin sections, are commercially available. Staining is localized to nuclei. PCNA positivity is significantly correlated with SPF determined by flow cytometry, and it is higher in aneuploid than in diploid carcinomas.[488]

PCNA staining has been significantly related to tumor size, histologic grade, and mitotic rate.[489] Others confirmed the association with mitotic rate but found no significant association with tumor size or axillary nodal status.[490] In one study, high PCNA scores were associated with a less favorable prognosis than low scores,[490] but another report concluded that the PCNA expression was not a significant indicator of prognosis.[491]

Mitosin is a nuclear phosphoprotein formed during the late G-, S-, G_2-, and M-phases of the cell cycle but not in G_0 phase. Immunohistochemical expression of mitosin was studied by Clark et al.[492] in 386 node-negative tumors. High mitosin expression was associated with an elevated SPF, negative ER and PR, and an unfavorable prognosis.

NUCLEAR MORPHOMETRY

Nuclear morphometry is a method for obtaining quantitative measurements of the size and shape of tumor cell nuclei. Among the parameters commonly recorded in these studies are nuclear diameter, nuclear area, and nuclear perimeter. Careful counts of mitotic activity have also been obtained in some of these studies. Measurements can be made using properly prepared histologic sections[493,494] and on FNA smears.[495–497] Prognostic correlations have been made with the nuclear morphometry of the primary tumor,[493–497] as well as with morphometric features of tumor cell nuclei in axillary nodal metastases.[498] The morphometric feature that most often had a statistically significant association with prognosis was nuclear area.[493,494,496,498,499] Nuclear diameter, a parameter included in the calculation of area, has been significantly related to prognosis,[495,497] as has the frequency of mitoses.[494] Inverse relationships have been observed between mean nuclear area, mean nuclear diameter, mitotic index, and prognosis. Concurrent assessment of nuclear and histologic grading proved prognostically significant in some of these studies.[493,498] Morphometric measurements of tumor cell nuclei do not improve the assessment of prognosis beyond that readily obtained by conventional tumor grading.

THE BASAL-LIKE PHENOTYPE

A subset of mammary carcinomas expresses high-molecular-weight cytokeratins that have been associated mainly but not exclusively with the cells that comprise the myoepithelial or "basal" layer of the mammary gland epithelium.[500] In particular, attention has centered on CK5, CK5/6, CK14, and CK17 that have been referred to as "basal keratins" because of their predominant localization in cells in the basal (myoepithelial) region. Carcinomas of the breast that express one or more of these cytokeratins are described as having a "basal phenotype." Because cells that express basal cytokeratins occur in the glandular as well as the myoepithelial layers of breast glands, it cannot be inferred that a particular carcinoma with the basal immunophenotype arose specifically from the myoepithelium. Hence, terms such as basal or basal-like phenotype refer to the expression of certain cytokeratins and other features rather than histogenesis. It is noteworthy that these carcinomas are not typically immunoreactive with most commonly used noncytokeratin myoepithelial markers such as calponin, CD10, maspin, muscle-specific actin, p63, p75, p-cadherin, smooth muscle actin (SMA), and SMM-HC.[501] In general, carcinomas in this group lack expression of ER, PR, and HER2 (i.e., they are "triple-negative") and they express EGFR. Triple-negative breast carcinomas encompass a varied group of tumors. Expression of basal markers separates a clinically and biologically heterogeneous subgroup that is referred to as basal-like carcinomas[502] within the larger group of triple-negative carcinomas. Presently, there is not universal agreement as to which marker or markers must be present to identify a carcinoma as belonging to the basal-like group. Thus, some investigators have made this assignment on the basis of one cytokeratin, whereas others have required that at least two be expressed. In addition, some studies require that the carcinoma be triple negative and/or express another marker such as EGFR. This lack of a precise definition must be kept in mind when considering published reports that sometimes present conflicting results.

Basal-like carcinomas occur more often in premenopausal women, are more prevalent in women of African descent, and often present as interval carcinomas in mammography screening. Histologically, most such carcinomas are invasive ductal carcinomas with high histologic grade, pushing borders, and prominent inflammatory cell infiltrate (Fig. 12.21).[503] They are prone to develop central necrosis and fibrosis. The *in situ* component of most invasive triple-negative carcinomas, which comprise a substantial fraction of basal-like carcinomas, is also triple negative (97.9% in one series).[504] On FNA cytology material, "triple-negative" carcinomas are mainly characterized by "lymphocytes, ill-defined cell borders and syncytial clusters, tubular/ductal clusters, cytoplasmic vacuoles, and cellular pleomorphism."[505]

El-Rehim et al.[506] studied cytokeratin expression in invasive breast carcinomas, nearly 75% of which were conventional ductal type. The samples were analyzed for cytokeratins associated with luminal epithelium CK7/8, 18, 19 and basal cells (CK5/6, CK14). Four patterns of immunoreactivity were found: luminal phenotype represented by one or more luminal cytokeratins only (71.4%), combined phenotype with luminal and basal markers expressed (27.4%), basal-like phenotype in which only a basal cytokeratin was expressed (0.8%), and a null phenotype that was not reactive for either cytokeratin type (0.4%). These results indicate that breast carcinomas with a pure basal-like immunophenotype as defined in this study are rare. Almost all breast carcinomas express luminal cytokeratins, and among these a minority also expresses basal cytokeratins. These findings are consistent with the observation that only 6% of intraductal carcinomas studied by Bryan et al.[507] had the "triple-negative" basal cell phenotype. An association has been found between the basal phenotype and BRCA1-related carcinomas.[508–510] The basal-like phenotype is infrequently expressed in BRCA2-associated carcinomas.[510]

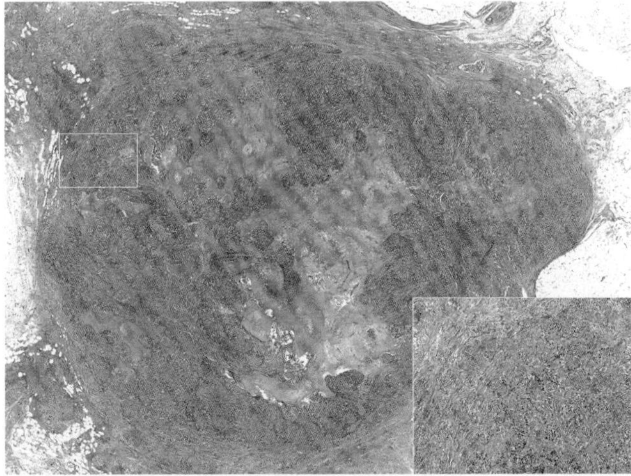

FIG. 12.21. ***Basal-like carcinoma.*** This invasive ductal carcinoma is poorly differentiated, with large central acellular (necrotic) zone. Note the pushing borders. There is a sparse minimal peritumoral chronic inflammatory cell infiltrate (*inset*).

Fulford et al.[511] described histologic features that were associated with the basal-like phenotype among high-grade invasive ductal carcinomas. In this study, the basal-like phenotype was based on the presence of CK14 expression that was found in 88 (19.4%) of 453 tumors examined. The basal-like phenotype was significantly associated with a high mitotic count. Mitotic counts exceeding 40 per 10 HPF occurred in 59% of basal-like phenotype carcinomas and in 30% of nonbasal phenotype carcinomas. The median mitotic counts were basal phenotype, 48, and nonbasal phenotype, 23. Structural features found with significantly greater frequency in carcinomas with the basal phenotype included a partly or completely pushing rather than infiltrative external border, a central scar, necrosis, and a more prominent lymphoid infiltrate. Invasive ductal carcinomas with basal phenotype characteristically do not express ER or PR or HER2. Invasive ductal carcinomas with the basal-like phenotype display increased expression of p53 and EGFR.[512] The combination of ER (−) HER2/*neu* (−) CK5/6 (+) and EGFR (+) has a 76% sensitivity and 100% specificity for the identification of basal-like carcinomas.[513]

Attention has focused on the relationship between the basal-like phenotype and prognosis. In 1987, Dairkee et al.[514] reported that the expression of CK5 and CK17 was associated with early recurrence and reduced survival. More recently, Banerjee et al.[515] compared patients with basal-like carcinomas to a group with non-basal-like carcinomas who were matched for age, nodal status, and tumor grade. The basal-like phenotype was based on the expression of at least one of several cytokeratins (CK5/6, CK14, and CK17). Patients with basal-like carcinomas had significantly higher recurrence rates locally and systemically, as well as significantly shorter disease-free and lower OS rates. The relationship between the basal-like phenotype and chemotherapy response remains to be determined. Banerjee et al.[515] reported that anthracycline-based chemotherapy was less effective in patients with basal-like tumors compared with matched controls. Others have reported greater success with neoadjuvant therapy in women with basal-like carcinomas.[516,517] Haffty et al.[518] reported that the basal-like phenotype was associated with a significantly reduced DFS and poorer OS, but that the basal-like phenotype did not predispose to local breast recurrence after conservative surgery and radiotherapy. In considering these and other studies, it should be noted that diverse criteria used to define the basal-like phenotype in clinical studies include cytokeratin expression, triple-negative status, and other molecular characteristics.[512–514] Standardized criteria for defining the basal-like phenotype as applied in clinical practice have yet to be agreed upon.

A molecular classification of breast carcinoma offers the potential to improve prognostication; however, the traditional histopathology-based tumor classification of breast carcinoma is unlikely to be replaced in the foreseeable future.[519] Despite this avalanche of data, the evaluation of prognosis in patients with mammary carcinoma is still primarily based on fundamental morphologic observations. Biologic variables play an increasingly important role in prognostic evaluation and for tailoring therapy to the characteristics of individual tumors. Indeed, at this time, "molecular profiling currently offers no more than tumor morphology and basic IHC" for assessing prognosis.[520]

ESTROGEN AND PROGESTERONE RECEPTORS

The determination of ER and PR status is a crucial element in the pathologic evaluation of breast carcinomas. The most recent ASCO guidelines on the use of tumor markers recommend that ER and PR should be tested on every primary breast carcinoma, and that metastatic lesions may be tested if the results could influence management.[521]

ER is a nuclear transcription factor that is activated by estrogen. It controls the development and differentiation of normal, hyperplastic, and neoplastic breast epithelial cells. ER is variably expressed in a proportion of ductal cells and in a larger proportion of lobular epithelial cells. There are two forms of ER: ER-alpha (the dominant, and practically, relevant form) encoded by *ESR1* gene and ER-beta encoded by *ESR2* gene. The relative levels of the two forms of ER may have some, as yet indeterminate, impact on the development of breast carcinoma.[522,523]

Approximately 75% of all invasive breast carcinomas are positive for hormone receptors (Fig. 12.22). Slightly more tumors are ER positive than are PR positive. Lower grade invasive carcinomas (including tubular carcinoma, well-differentiated ductal carcinoma, and classical invasive lobular carcinoma) are almost always ER positive and PR positive, as are most moderately differentiated carcinoma. Some rare types of low-grade invasive carcinoma including low-grade adenosquamous carcinoma, AdCC, and secretory carcinoma are typically ER negative.

Two-thirds of invasive cancers in women younger than 50, and approximately three-quarters of those in women

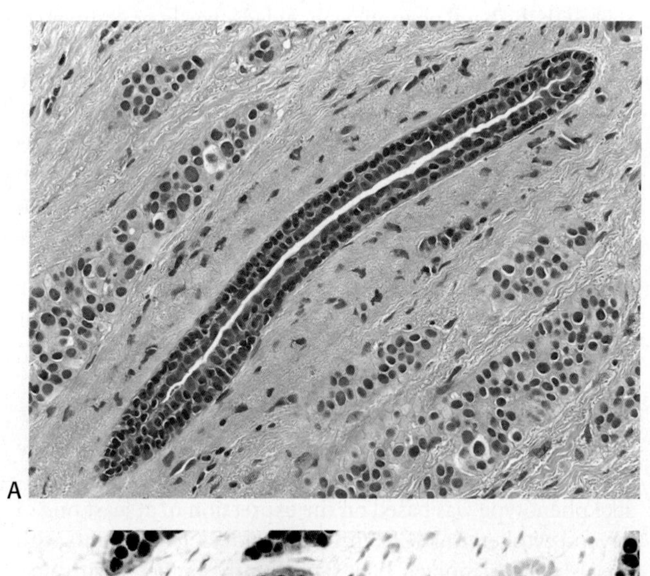

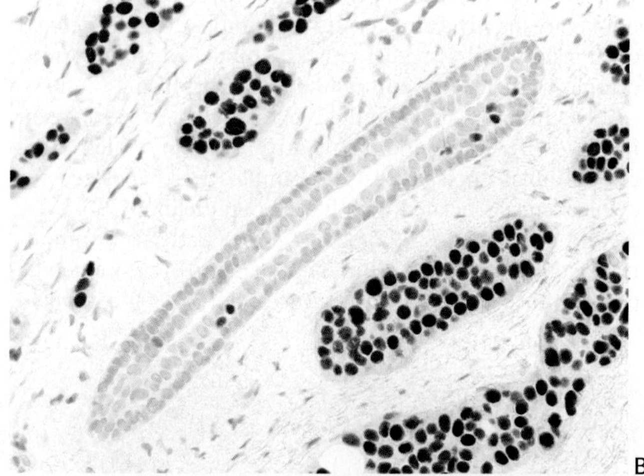

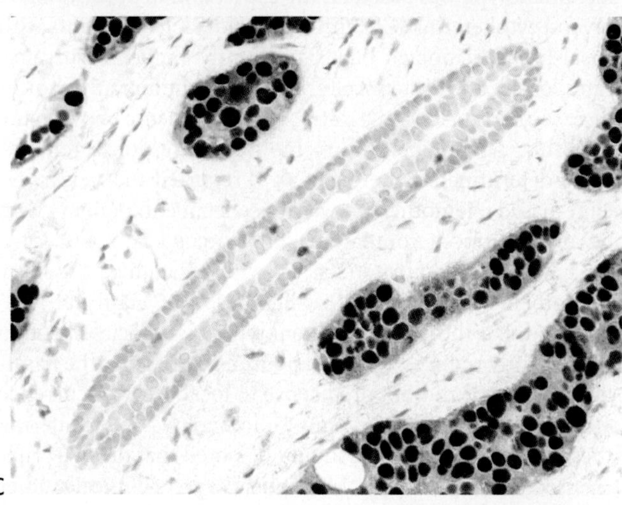

FIG. 12.22. ***Estrogen and progesterone receptor positivity in invasive low-grade ductal carcinoma.*** **A–C:** Invasive tumor cells are strongly and diffusely positive for ERs **(A)**, and PRs **(B)**. Note focal immunoreactivity in the entrapped inactive ductal epithelium.

older than 50, are hormone receptor positive. ER is observed at a consistently higher rate among U.S. Whites and in Asian Americans than in African Americans or Hispanics. Rate of ER positivity in breast carcinoma is higher in screen-detected than in clinically discovered tumors. In general, carcinomas in men are more likely to be ER positive than carcinomas in women. As surgical pathologists know only too well, ER status does not predict metastatic potential of a tumor, but it is generally predictive of a more indolent disease course with a longer time to recurrence. ER-positive tumors tend to metastasize to bone, soft tissues, and in genitourinary organs, whereas ER-negative tumors preferentially migrate to visceral organs and to the brain.[524–528]

Both ER and PR (ER in particular) are relatively weak prognostic factors, but both are strong predictive factors for response to endocrine therapy. Five-year recurrence rates in patients with ER-positive tumors who did not receive systemic therapy after surgery are lower by up to 10% than in patients with ER-negative tumors. Hormone therapies target the ER signaling pathway, either by acting on the receptor itself through selective ER modulators such as tamoxifen, through antagonists that degrade the receptor (e.g., fluvestrant), or by approaches that deprive the receptor of estrogen (e.g., aromatase inhibitor or ovarian ablation). Adjuvant hormonal therapy can diminish the recurrence rate of patients with ER-positive breast carcinomas by as much as 50%. Approximately one-third of patients with ER-positive metastatic disease respond to hormone therapy, and around one-quarter will experience stabilization of disease. Although ER positivity does not always guarantee response to endocrine therapy, ER negativity is almost always associated with lack of response to such treatment.[529–532]

PR is an estrogen-related gene, the expression of which is indicative of a functional ER pathway. The utility of PR as a prognostic factor remains less well established, but there is growing evidence that PR negativity may be a marker of a more aggressive subtype. A subset of patients who have carcinomas that are ER negative and PR positive may respond to hormonal therapy.[533–537]

In current clinical practice, the status of ER and PR is almost always determined by IHC performed on formalin-fixed paraffin-embedded tumor tissue. In principle, IHC testing can be performed on minute samples in needle core biopsy specimens, in archived tissue, and in cells derived from FNA samples. However, multiple preanalytical factors, particularly the duration of tissue fixation and efficiency of antigen retrieval, can affect IHC testing. Guidelines for the testing of hormone receptors and for troubleshooting in the process are available.[538,539]

Harvey et al.[540] showed that the presence of ER immunoreactivity in as few as 1% of tumor cells, even when it is weak, is sufficient to predict benefit from endocrine therapy. A NIH Consensus conference has recommended that any ER staining in a tumor should be sufficient for eligibility to receive endocrine therapy. Mohsin et al.[541] recommended a similar cutoff for PR as well. As stated in the current ASCO/College of American Pathology (CAP) guidelines, ER and PR results can be reported as positive if more than 1% of tumor cells are immunoreactive.[521]

Quantitation of ER/PR Reactivity

Approximately 50% of all invasive carcinomas that are ER positive are also PR positive, 25% or so are ER positive and PR negative, and about 20% are negative for both ER and PR.[542–544] ER negativity and PR positivity are rare, and such a result should be accepted only after the testing is repeated with a similar outcome. Although ER and PR status is generally reported as being positive or negative, it is possible that response rates to endocrine therapies may be related to level of ER and PR concentrations. Therefore, some form of quantitation of ER and PR results is desirable. Ideally, the reporting of ER and PR results should state the approximate percentage of invasive carcinoma cells that show nuclear immunoreactivity, and the average intensity of nuclear staining therein on a scale of 1 to 3. Two formal methods are in use: the Allred score and the "H" score.

The Allred score[540] is calculated by adding two numbers—the first reflects the percentage of positive tumor cells (0 for less than 1%, 2 for 1% to 10%, 3 for 11% to 33%, 4 for 34% to 66%, and 5 for 67% to 100%) and the other reflects the intensity of immunoreactivity (1 for weak, 2 for moderate, and 3 for strong). In the Allred system, the minimum score possible is 2 and the maximum score possible is 8. By definition, there is no Allred score of 1. A total score of between 3 and 8, which represents either 10% weakly staining nuclei, or 1% moderately staining nuclei, is considered ER positive.

The "H" score, and modifications thereof,[545,546] is calculated by multiplying the percentage of positive cells by a factor representing the strength of immunoreactivity (1 for weak, 2 for moderate, and 3 for strong), giving a maximum of 300. A score of less than 50 has generally been considered negative; however, some consider a score of less than 10 to be negative, and a score of 10 to 100 is regarded as weakly positive.[547] Thus, "H" score provides a continuous measure of ER and PR content in a tumor. Cohen et al.[548] have shown a high level of interobserver agreement among pathologists for semiquantitative hormone receptor scoring in breast carcinoma with "H" scoring, and have suggested "universal adoption" of this method.

ER/PR in Recurrent Carcinoma

Hormone receptor status of tumor recurrences or metastases does not always correlate with that of the corresponding primary tumor. This apparent discordance can be attributed to multiple factors, including clonal selection in the metastasis from a heterogeneous cancer, adaptive transformation in the tumor, dedifferentiation of the tumor, or fault in technique. There is an approximately 20% to 30% conversion rate from ER positive to ER negative; however, the reverse, that is, conversion from ER negative to ER positive, is very infrequent.[549–552] As with ER, a significant proportion of PR-positive tumors lose PR expression in their metastases. The hormone receptor status of the metastasis may be more predictive of response than that of the primary tumor. In one study, 74% of patients with ER-positive primary tumors whose recurrent tumors were also ER positive responded to endocrine therapy, whereas only 12% of patients with ER-positive primaries and ER-negative metastases responded.[553]

ER/PR in DCIS

Approximately 75% of DCIS lesions are ER positive, with strong immunoreactivity observed in the majority of tumor cells. Almost all instances of ER-negative DCIS are encountered in lesions with high-grade nuclei. The National Comprehensive Cancer Network practice guidelines include determination of ER in all cases of DCIS,[13] but the latest CAP protocol on DCIS only states that hormone receptor status "may be evaluated" in DCIS.[554] In general, recurrent DCIS has the same immunoprofile as the primary DCIS, but retesting of ER and PR in recurrences could provide potentially significant predictive and prognostic data to clinicians. Each of the two studies that have addressed outcomes of patients with DCIS undergoing hormonal therapy showed that fewer women in the tamoxifen group developed subsequent breast carcinoma: the UK/ANZ study reported 18% versus 14%,[555] and the NSABP B24 study reported a statistically significant difference of 13.4% versus 8.2%.[556] The younger age of the patients in the latter study could have influenced the results, as a smaller benefit was observed in women over the age of 50. After 8.7 years of follow-up, the benefit of tamoxifen, that is, up to 50% reduction in risk seen in a number of categories, was confined to patients whose DCIS was positive for ER, with little reduction in the ER-negative DCIS group.[557] Although PR testing is often "bundled" with ER testing, there are no data showing its relevance in DCIS. The reporting of ER and PR results should ideally state the approximate percentage of DCIS cells that show nuclear staining, and the average intensity of nuclear staining on a scale of 1 to 3. Immunoreactivity in less than 1% of DCIS cells for either ER or PR should be considered negative.

ER/PR RNA Assays

ER and PR results based on RNA assays using qRT–PCR on formalin-fixed paraffin-embedded tissue are offered in the 21-gene Oncotype DX test. ER and PR results obtained with qRT–PCR not only have been shown to correlate with those obtained through IHC but also have been reported to be statistically superior in predicting relapse in tamoxifen-treated ER-positive patients.[558] Nonetheless, it is unlikely that ER and PR testing by IHC will be replaced by molecular techniques as the first-line procedure in the immediate future.[559,560]

HER2

Breast carcinomas result from alterations in molecular genetics that are either inherited or acquired. Carcinoma cells are dependent on such changes for their growth and survival. Thus, these alterations therefore provide targets for therapeutic intervention. Amplification of *HER2* (also known as ERB-B2) gene is the quintessential example of an acquired molecular alteration that promotes the maintenance and growth of carcinoma.

HER2 plays a role in sustaining multiple cancer pathways through improving growth signals, abetting angiogenesis, facilitating mitoses, and enhancing invasive capabilities. Inhibition of HER2 membrane signaling through anti-HER2 antibodies, that is, trastuzamab (Herceptin), or through small molecule inhibitors of HER2 tyrosine kinase activity, that is, lapatinib (Tykerbl), is associated with improved disease outcome in patients with primary and metastatic carcinoma. The major clinical reason to assess HER2 is to select patients who would benefit from treatment with trastuzamab (Herceptin), a monoclonal antibody targeted to HER2. Since these improvements in outcome and the predictive importance of HER2 are so well established, the latest ASCO/CAP guidelines recommend routine testing of HER2 (along with ER and PR) in women diagnosed with primary invasive breast carcinoma.[561] Thus, accurate clinical testing for HER2 is of utmost importance.

Approximately 20% of all invasive breast carcinomas are positive for HER2 (Fig. 12.23). *HER2* gene amplification is a prognostic marker of poor outcome in the absence of adjuvant therapy, independent of nodal status, tumor size, grade, and hormone receptor status.[562–564] It is associated with an increased rate of metastases, decreased time to recurrence, and decreased OS.

As a predictive marker, HER2 has been correlated with response to trastuzamab, lapatinib, anthracycline-based chemotherapy,[565] and paclitaxel-containing regimens.[566] HER2 positivity is indicative of resistance to endocrine modulating therapy. HER2 is a well-documented prognostic factor for outcome in lymph node–negative and -positive tumors.

Since *HER2* gene amplification is directly correlated with HER2 expression levels at the mRNA and protein levels, determination of HER2 status could potentially be made at either of these levels.[561] Techniques available for this purpose that are suitable for use on formalin-fixed paraffin-embedded tissue include fluorescence *in situ* hybridization (FISH), CISH chromogenic *in situ* hybridization, and SISH silver-enhanced *in situ* hybridization to determine gene amplification status. Quantitative real-time RT-PCR (RQ-PCR) and microarray-based RNA expression profile are used to determine HER2 mRNA expression status, and IHC detects HER2 protein overexpression status. The two most common methods in clinical use are detection of HER2/*neu* protein overexpression by using IHC and evaluation of *HER2/neu* gene amplification by FISH.

Two IHC assays for HER2 (Dako Herceptest and Ventana Pathway) and three FISH assays (Abott Pathvysion, Ventana Inform, and Dako PHarmDX) have been approved by the FDA. Both IHC and FISH techniques have advantages and disadvantages. IHC technique is relatively simple, inexpensive, and familiar to most laboratories, and results in a permanent glass slide; but it is only about 90% accurate, dependent on multiple preanalytical factors, and subject to interobserver variation. The FISH technique is relatively insensitive to the vagaries of preanalytical factors and results in a quantitative score. However, it is a relatively advanced and expensive technique that requires specialized equipment and expertise, and results in an impermanent signal.

The 2013 ASCO-CAP HER2 testing guidelines[561] recommend HER2 testing for all newly diagnosed primary or metastatic breast carcinomas and acceptance of the primary assessment of HER2 status using either IHC or ISH (*in situ* hybridization) testing. HER2 results by IHC and ISH testing

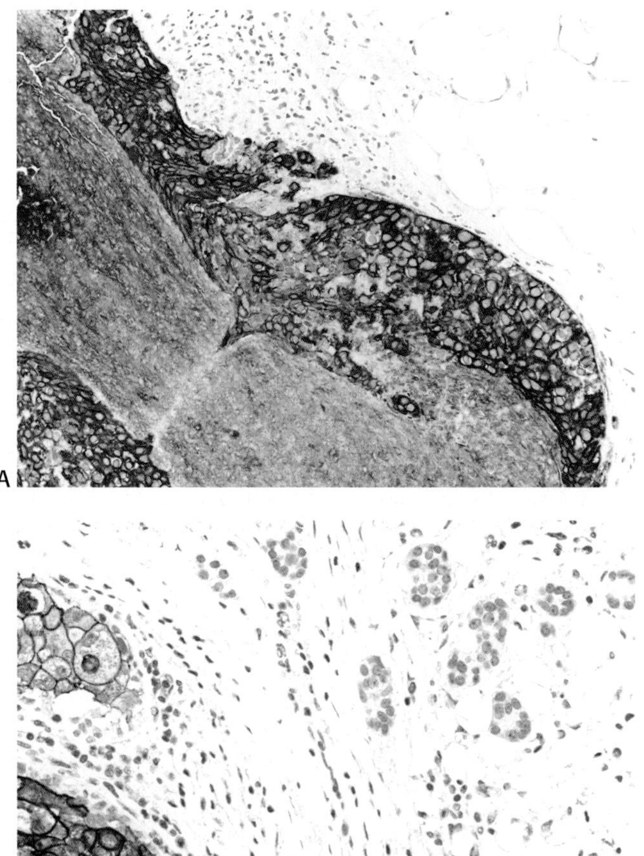

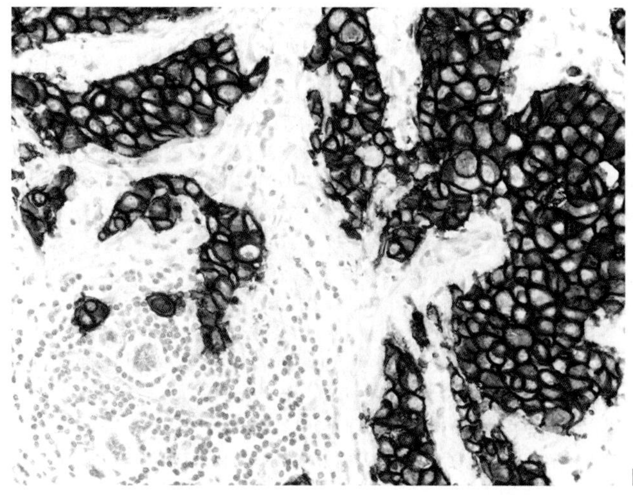

FIG. 12.23. ***HER2 positivity in ductal carcinoma.*** **A:** High-grade intraductal carcinoma cells show 3+ (on a scale of 0 to 3+) immunoreactivity. Tumor cells in a focus suspicious for microinvasion are also equally immunoreactive. **B:** Tumor cells of this poorly differentiated invasive carcinoma show 3+ immunoreactivity. Note lack of immunoreactivity in benign inactive glands and lymphocytes at *bottom left.* **C:** High-grade intraductal carcinoma shows 3+ immunoreactivity, and the associated invasive ductal carcinoma is negative (scored as 0, on a scale of 0 to 3).

are reported as "positive", "equivocal", "negative" or "indeterminate". Per these guidelines, a HER2 test result must be reported as "positive" if there is evidence of protein overexpression, i.e. IHC shows 3+ (on a scale of 0 to 3+) staining, i.e. circumferential membrane staining that is complete and intense "within an area of tumor that amounts to >10% of contiguous and homogeneous tumor cells". Testing criteria further define HER2-positive status when there is evidence of gene amplification (HER2 copy number or HER2/CEP17 ratio by ISH based on counting at least 20 cells within the area). Detailed criteria for interpretation of ISH testing are listed on www.asco.org/guidelines/her2. IHC is considered to be "equivocal", i.e. 2+, based on circumferential membrane staining that is incomplete and/or weak/moderate and within >10% of the invasive tumor cells, or complete and circumferential membrane staining that is intense and within ≤10% of the invasive tumor cells. If the HER2 test result by IHC is reported as equivocal, reflex testing (on same specimen using ISH) or new testing (on new specimen, if available, using IHC or ISH) should be performed. The HER2 test result should be reported as "negative" if IHC is 1+ or 0. 1+ is defined by incomplete membrane staining that is faint/barely perceptible and within >10% of the invasive tumor cells. IHC is reported as 0 when there is no staining observed or incomplete and faint/barely perceptible membrane staining that is in ≤10% of the invasive tumor cells. The HER2 test result is considered "indeterminate" if technical issues prevent one or both tests (IHC and ISH) from being reported as positive, negative, or equivocal. Examples of technical issues include testing performed on inappropriately handled specimens, and those that show crush or edge artifacts. The HER2 test is to be rejected if controls are not as expected, if artifacts involve most of the sample, or if there is strong membrane staining of the internal control, i.e. normal breast ducts. Testing should be repeated if the results are discordant with the corresponding histopathology. The 2013 ASCO-CAP guidelines require that the duration of specimen fixation be between 6 to 72 hours.

HER2 genetic heterogeneity exists if more than 5% but less than 50% of invasive tumor cells have a ratio higher than 2.2 upon FISH testing. A CAP panel has outlined strategies to deal with genetic heterogeneity in HER2 testing in breast carcinoma[567].

The presence of HER2 genetic heterogeneity can result in discordant results by status by FISH and IHC techniques. Breast carcinoma shows protein overexpression in the absence of gene amplification in approximately 3% of cases, suggesting that the former is achieved by means other than through the latter. Polysomy of chromosome 17 can account for some breast carcinoma cases that show 3+ results by IHC but are not HER2 amplified when the HER2/chromosome 17 ratio is evaluated.[568,569]

Given the inevitable, seemingly irreducible, fraction of false-positive and false-negative results with IHC, some authorities recommend FISH testing only for HER2, with IHC used in the less than 5% of breast carcinoma cases wherein FISH results yield equivocal results or otherwise fail. As with ER and PR, the 21-gene Oncotype DX test reports HER2 status of a tumor based on qRT–PCR testing.

HER2 status, as determined in a primary tumor, may or may not change in metastatic tumors.[570,571] As with hormone receptors, such discordance may be due to a variety of factors. Owing to its importance as a predictive factor, HER2 status should be re-evaluated in metastatic tumors that can be readily sampled.

The use of pathologically determined prognostic and predictive factors in breast cancer is an evolving issue, and periodically updated recommendations from organizations such as ASCO should serve as a guide.[11] However, at the present time, no biomarker has been shown to supplant the value of routine histopathologic evaluation of a breast carcinoma.

REFERENCES

1. Rosen PP. The pathological classification of human mammary carcinoma: past, present and future. *Ann Clin Lab Sci* 1979;9:144–156.
2. Tulinius H, Bjarnason O, Sigvaldason H, et al. Tumours in Iceland, 10. Malignant tumours of the female breast. A histological classification, laterality, survival and epidemiological considerations. *APMIS* 1988;96:229–238.
3. Weigelt B, Geyer FC, Reis-Filho JS. Histological types of breast cancer: how special are they? *Mol Oncol* 2010;4:192–208.
4. Lakhani SR, Ellis IO, Schnitt SJ, et al. (Eds). WHO classification of tumours of the breast. (*WHO Classification of Tumours*, vol. 4). 4th ed. Lyon: World Health Organization-IARC, 2012:34.
5. Fisher ER, Gregorio RM, Fisher B, et al. The pathology of invasive breast cancer. A syllabus derived from findings of the National Surgical Adjuvant Breast Project (Protocol No. 4). *Cancer* 1975;36:1–85.
6. Rakha EA, Gill MS, El-Sayed ME, et al. The biological and clinical characteristics of breast carcinoma with mixed ductal and lobular morphology. *Breast Cancer Res Treat* 2009;114:243–250.
7. Gupta SK, Douglas-Jones AG, Fenn N, et al. The clinical behavior of breast carcinoma is probably determined at the preinvasive stage (ductal carcinoma *in situ*). *Cancer* 1997;80:1740–1745.
8. Cowen PN, Bates C. The significance of intraductal appearances in breast cancer. *Clin Oncol* 1984;10:67–72.
9. Wells CA, Ferguson DJP. Ultrastructural and immunocytochemical study of a case of invasive cribriform breast carcinoma. *J Clin Pathol* 1988;41:17–20.
10. Sistrunk WE, MacCarty WC. Life expectancy following radical amputation for carcinoma of the breast: a clinical and pathologic study of 218 cases. *Ann Surg* 1922;75:61–69.
11. Harris L, Fritsche H, Mennel R, et al.; American Society of Clinical Oncology. American Society of Clinical Oncology 2007 update of recommendations for the use of tumor markers in breast cancer. *J Clin Oncol* 2007;25:5287–5312.
12. Rakha EA, Ellis IO. An overview of assessment of prognostic and predictive factors in breast cancer needle core biopsy specimens. *J Clin Pathol* 2007;60:1300–1306.
13. Febbo PG, Ladanyi M, Aldape KD, et al. NCCN Task Force report: evaluating the clinical utility of tumor markers in oncology. *J Natl Compr Canc Netw* 2011;9(Suppl. 5):S1–S32.
14. Anderson WF, Rosenberg PS, Menashe I, et al. Age-related crossover in breast cancer incidence rates between black and white ethnic groups. *J Natl Cancer Inst* 2008;100:1804–1814.
15. Elmore JG, Moceri VM, Carter D, et al. Breast carcinoma tumor characteristics in black and white women. *Cancer* 1998;83:2509–2515.
16. Edwards MJ, Gamel JW, Vaughan WP, et al. Infiltrating ductal carcinoma of the breast: the survival impact of race. *J Clin Oncol* 1998;16:2693–2699.
17. Heimann R, Hellman S. Aging, progression, and phenotype in breast cancer. *J Clin Oncol* 1998;16:2686–2692.
18. Heimann R, Hellman S. Clinical progression of breast cancer malignant behavior: what to expect and when to expect it. *J Clin Oncol* 2000;18:591–599.
19. Blamey RW, Elston CW, Ellis IO. When is a patient cured of breast cancer? *Mod Pathol* 2000;13:18A.
20. Regitnig P, Heckermann H, Moser R, et al. Molecular genetic comparison of primary and recurrent breast carcinoma? Significant increase of loss of heterozygosity (LOH) in the recurrence and specific LOH associated with early recurrence. *Mod Pathol* 2000;13:45A.
21. Robson M, Rajan P, Rosen PP, et al. BRCA-associated breast cancer: absence of a characteristic immunophenotype. *Cancer Res* 1998;58:1839–1842.
22. Karp SE, Tonin PN, Begin LR, et al. Influence of BRCA1 mutations on nuclear grade and estrogen receptor status of breast carcinoma in Ashkenazi Jewish women. *Cancer* 1997;80:435–441.
23. Eisinger F, Stoppa-Lyonnet D, Longy M, et al. Germ line mutation at BRCA1 affects the histoprognostic grade in hereditary breast cancer. *Cancer Res* 1996;56:471–474.
24. Breast Cancer Linkage Consortium. Pathology of familial breast cancer: differences between breast cancers in carriers of BRCA1 and BRCA2 mutations and sporadic cases. *Lancet* 1997;349:1505–1510.
25. Robson M, Savahn T, Mc Cormick B, et al. Appropriateness of breast conserving treatment of breast carcinoma in women with germline mutations in *BRCA1* or *BRCA2*: a clinic-based series. *Cancer* 2005;103:44–51.
26. Armes JE, Egan AJ, Southey MC, et al. The histologic phenotypes of breast carcinoma occurring before age 40 years in women with and without BRCA1 or BRCA2 germline mutations: a population-based study. *Cancer* 1998;83:2335–2345.
27. Jacquemier J, Guinebretiere J-M. Intraductal component and BRCA-1-associated breast cancer. *Lancet* 1996;348:1098.
28. Sun C, Lenoir G, Lynch H, et al. *In-situ* breast cancer and BRCA1. *Lancet* 1996;348:408.
29. Slack NH, Bross ID, Nemoto T, et al. Experiences with bilateral primary carcinoma of the breast. *Surg Gynecol Obstet* 1973;136: 433–440.
30. Schell SR, Montague ED, Spanos WJ, et al. Bilateral breast cancer in patients with initial stage I and II disease. *Cancer* 1982;50:1191–1194.
31. de la Rochefordiere A, Asselain B, Scholl S, et al. Simultaneous bilateral breast carcinomas: a retrospective review of 149 cases. *Int J Radiat Oncol Biol Phys* 1994;30:35–41.
32. Gollamudi SV, Gelman RS, Peiro G, et al. Breast-conserving therapy for stage I–II synchronous bilateral breast carcinoma. *Cancer* 1997;79:1362–1369.
33. Lee MM, Heimann R, Powers P, et al. Efficacy of breast conservation therapy in early stage bilateral breast cancer. *Breast J* 1999;5:36–41.
34. Tulusan AH, Ronay G, Egger H, et al. A contribution to the natural history of breast cancer. V. Bilateral primary breast cancer: incidence, risks and diagnosis of simultaneous primary cancer in the opposite breast. *Arch Gynecol* 1985;237:85–91.
35. Honrado E, Benítez J, Palacios J. The molecular pathology of hereditary breast cancer: genetic testing and therapeutic implications. *Mod Pathol* 2005;18:1305–1320.
36. Bane AL, Beck JC, Bleiweiss I, et al. BRAC2 mutation-associated breast cancers exhibit a distinguishing phenotype based on morphology and molecular profiles from tissue microarraays. *Am J Surg Pathol* 2007;31:121–128.
37. Narod SA. BRCA mutations in the management of breast cancer: the state of the art. *Nat Rev Clin Oncol* 2010;7:702–707.
38. Park SR, Chen A. Poly(adenosine diphosphate-ribose) polymerase inhibitors in cancer treatment. *Hematol Oncol Clin North Am* 2012;26:649–670.
39. Berg WA, Madsen KS, Schilling K, et al. Comparative effectiveness of positron emission mammography and MRI in the contralateral breast of women with newly diagnosed breast cancer. *AJR Am J Roentgenol* 2012;198:219–232.
40. Brown H, Vlastos G, Newman L, et al. Histopathologic features of bilateral and unilateral breast carcinoma: a comparative study. *Mod Pathol* 2000;13:18A.

41. Healey EA, Cook EF, Orav EJ, et al. clinical characteristics and impact on prognosis. *J Clin Oncol* 1993;11:1545–1552.
42. Schwartz AG, Ragheb NE, Swanson GM, et al. Racial and age differences in multiple primary cancers after breast cancer: a population-based analysis. *Breast Cancer Res Treat* 1989;14:245–254.
43. Chaudary MA, Millis RR, Bulbrook RD, et al. Family history and bilateral primary breast cancer. *Breast Cancer Res Treat* 1985;5: 201–205.
44. Verhoog LC, Brekelmans CT, Seynaeve C, et al. Contralateral breast cancer risk is influenced by the age at onset in BRCA1-associated breast cancer. *Br J Cancer* 2000;83:384–386.
45. Easton DF. Cancer risks in BRCA2 mutation carriers. The breast cancer linkage consortium. *J Natl Cancer Inst* 1999; 91:1310–1316.
46. Metcalfe K, Lynch HT, Ghadirian P, et al. Contralateral breast cancer in BRCA1 and BRCA2 mutation carriers. *J Clin Oncol* 2004;22:2328–2335.
47. Shahedi K, Emanuelsson M, Wiklund F, et al. High risk of contralateral breast carcinoma in women with hereditary/familial non-BRCA1/ BRCA2 breast carcinoma. *Cancer* 2006;106:1237–1242.
48. Narod SA, Brunet J-S, Ghadirian P, et al. Tamoxifen and risk of contralateral breast cancer in BRCA1 and BRCA2 mutation carriers: a case control study. *Lancet* 2000;356:1876–1881.
49. Buzdar AIJ, ATAC trialists' group "Arimidex"(anastrozole) versus tamoxifen as adjuvant therapy in postmenopausal women with early breast cancer-efficacy overview. *J Steroid Biochem Mol Biol* 2003;86:399-403.
50. Tuttle TM, Habermann EB, Grund EH, et al. Increasing use of contralateral prophylactic mastectomy for breast cancer patients: a trend toward more aggressive surgical treatment. *J Clin Oncol* 2007;25:5203–5209.
51. McLaughlin CC, Lillquist PP, Edge SB. Surveillance of prophylactic mastectomy: trends in use from 1995 through 2005. *Cancer* 2009;115:5404–5412.
52. Abbott A, Rueth N, Pappas-Varco S, et al. Perceptions of contralateral breast cancer: an overestimation of risk. *Ann Surg Oncol* 2011;18:3129–3136.
53. Senie RT, Lesser M, Kinne DW, et al. Method of tumor detection influences disease-free survival of women with breast carcinoma. *Cancer* 1994;73:1666–1672.
54. Shapiro S, Venet W, Strax P, et al. Selection, follow-up, and analysis in the Health Insurance Plan study: a randomized trial with breast cancer screening. *Natl Cancer Inst Monogr* 1985;67:65–74.
55. Shapiro S. Periodic screening for breast cancer: the HIP Randomized Controlled Trial. Health Insurance Plan. *J Natl Cancer Inst Monogr* 1997;22:27–30.
56. Tabar L, Fagerberg CJ, Gad A, et al. Reduction in mortality from breast cancer after mass screening with mammography. *Lancet* 1985;1:829–832.
57. Tabár L, Chen HH, Fagerberg G, et al. Recent results from the Swedish Two-County Trial: the effects of age, histologic type, and mode of detection on the efficacy of breast cancer screening. *J Natl Cancer Inst Monogr* 1997;22:43–47.
58. Aragon R, Morgan J, Wong JH, et al. Potential impact of USPSTF recommendations on early diagnosis of breast cancer. *Ann Surg Oncol* 2011;18:3137–3142.
59. Tabár L, Duffy SW, Vitak B, et al. The natural history of breast carcinoma: what have we learned from screening? *Cancer* 1999;86:449–462.
60. Morrison AS, Brisson J, Khalid N. Breast cancer incidence and mortality in the breast cancer detection demonstration project. *J Natl Cancer Inst* 1988;80:1540–1547.
61. Lopez MJ, Smart CR. Twenty-year follow-up of minimal breast cancer from the Breast Cancer Detection Demonstration Project. *Surg Oncol Clin N Am* 1997;6:393–401.
62. Anderson TJ, Lamb J, Donnan P, et al. Comparative pathology of breast cancer in a randomised trial of screening. *Br J Cancer* 1991;64:108–113.
63. Cowan WK, Angus B, Henry J, et al. Immunohistochemical and other features of breast carcinomas presenting clinically compared with those detected by cancer screening. *Br J Cancer* 1991;64:780–784.
64. Gibbs NM. Comparative study of the histopathology of breast cancer in a screened and unscreened population investigated by mammography. *Histopathology* 1985;9:1307–1318.
65. Anderson TJ, Alexander F, Chetty U, et al. Comparative pathology of prevalent and incident cancers detected by breast screening. *Lancet* 1986;1:519–523.
66. Arnerlöv C, Emdin SO, Lundgren B, et al. Breast carcinoma growth rate described by mammographic doubling time and S-phase fraction. Correlations to clinical and histopathologic factors in a screened population. *Cancer* 1992;70:1928–1934.
67. Kallioniemi O-P, Kärkkäinen A, Auvinen O, et al. DNA flow cytometric analysis indicates that many breast cancers detected in the first round of mammographic screening have a low malignant potential. *Int J Cancer* 1988;42:697–702.
68. Tabar L, Duffy SW, Krusemo UB. Detection method, tumour size and node metastases in breast cancers diagnosed during a trial of breast cancer screening. *Eur J Cancer Clin Oncol* 1987;23:959–962.
69. von Rosen A, Frisell J, Nilsson R, et al. Histopathologic and cytochemical characteristics of interval breast carcinomas from the Stockholm Mammography Screening Project. *Acta Oncol* 1992;31:399–402.
70. Vitak B, Stal O, Manson JC, et al. Interval cancers and cancers in non-attenders in the Ostergotland Mammographic Screening Programme. Duration between screening and diagnosis, S-phase fraction and distant recurrence. *Eur J Cancer* 1997;33:1453–1460.
71. Ikeda DM, Andersson I, Wattsgård C, et al. Interval carcinomas in the Malmo Mammographic Screening Trial: radiographic appearance and prognostic considerations. *AJR Am J Roentgenol* 1992;159: 287–294.
72. DeGroote R, Rush BF, Milazzo J, et al. Interval breast cancer: a more aggressive subset of breast neoplasias. *Surgery* 1983;94:543–547.
73. Shapiro S, Venet W, Strax P, et al. Ten to fourteen year effect of screening on breast cancer mortality. *J Natl Cancer Inst* 1982;69:349–355.
74. Holmberg LH, Adami HO, Tabar L, et al. Survival in breast cancer diagnosed between mammographic screening examinations. *Lancet* 1986;1:27–30.
75. Brown RS, Wahl RL. Overexpression of glut-1 glucose transporter in human breast cancer. *Cancer* 1993;72:2979–2985.
76. Wahl RL, Cody RL, Hutchins GD, et al. Primary and metastatic breast carcinoma: initial clinical evaluation with PET with the radiolabeled glucose analogue 2-[F-18]-fluoro-2-deoxy-d-glucose. *Radiology* 1991;179:765–770.
77. Bruce DM, Evans NT, Heys SD, et al. Positron emission tomography: 2-deoxy-2-[18F]-fluoro-d-glucose uptake in locally advanced breast cancers. *Eur J Surg Oncol* 1995;21:280–283.
78. Adler LP, Crowe JP, Al-Kaisi NK, et al. Evaluation of breast masses and axillary lymph nodes with [F-18] 2-deoxy-2-fluoro-d-glucose PET. *Radiology* 1993;187:743–750.
79. Avril N, Dose J, Janicke F, et al. Metabolic characterization of breast tumors with positron emission tomography using F-18 fluorodeoxyglucose. *J Clin Oncol* 1996;14:1848–1857.
80. Bassa P, Kim EE, Inoue T, et al. Evaluation of preoperative chemotherapy using PET with fluorine-18-fluorodeoxyglucose in breast cancer. *J Nucl Med* 1996;37:931–938.
81. Oshida M, Uno K, Suzuki M, et al. Predicting the prognoses of breast carcinoma patients with positron emission tomography using 2-deoxy-2-fluoro[18F]- d-glucose. *Cancer* 1998;82:2227–2234.
82. http://www.cancer.org/Healthy/FindCancerEarly/CancerScreening Guidelines/american-cancer-society-guidelines-for-the-early-detection-of-cancer. Accessed August 10, 2012.
83. Edwards MJ, Bonadonna G, Valagussa P, et al. End points in the analysis of breast cancer survival: relapse versus death from tumor. *Surgery* 1998;124:197–202.
84. Touboul E, Buffat L, Belkacémi Y, et al. Local recurrences and distant metastases after breast-conserving surgery and radiation therapy for early breast cancer. *Int J Radiat Oncol Biol Phys* 1999;43:25–38.
85. Vogel CL, Azevedo S, Hilsenbeck S, et al. Survival after first recurrence of breast cancer. The Miami experience. *Cancer* 1992;709:129–135.
86. Aaltomaa S, Lipponen P, Eskelinen M, et al. Prediction of outcome after first recurrence of breast cancer. *Eur J Surg* 1992;158:13–18.
87. Clark GM, Sledge GW Jr, Osborne CK, et al. Survival from first recurrence: relative importance of prognostic factors in 1,015 breast cancer patients. *J Clin Oncol* 1987;5:55–61.
88. Kamby C, Rose C, Ejlertsen B, et al. Stage and pattern of metastases in patients with breast cancer. *Eur J Cancer Clin Oncol* 1987;23:1925–1934.
89. Kamby C, Ejlertsen B, Andersen J, et al. The pattern of metastases in human breast cancer. Influence of systemic adjuvant therapy and impact on survival. *Acta Oncol* 1988;27:715–719.
90. Cuzick J, Stewart H, Rutqvist L, et al. Cause-specific mortality in long-term survivors of breast cancer who participated in trials of radiotherapy. *J Clin Oncol* 1994;12:447–453.

91. Fowble B. Postmastectomy radiation. A modest benefit prevails for high risk patients. *Cancer* 1997;79:1061–1066.
92. Rutqvist LE, Cedermark B, Fornander T, et al. The relationship between hormone receptor content and the effect of adjuvant tamoxifen in operable breast cancer. *J Clin Oncol* 1989;7:1474–1484.
93. Arriagada R, Rutqvist LE, Mattsson A, et al. Adequate locoregional treatment for early breast cancer may prevent secondary dissemination. *J Clin Oncol* 1995;13:2869–2878.
94. Hojris I, Overgaard M, Christensen JJ, et al. Morbidity and mortality of ischaemic heart disease in high-risk breast-cancer patients after adjuvant postmastectomy systemic treatment with or without radiotherapy: analysis of DBCG 82b and 82c randomised trials. Radiotherapy Committee of the Danish Breast Cancer Cooperative Group. *Lancet* 1999;354:1425–1430.
95. Paszat LF, Mackillop WJ, Groome PA, et al. Mortality from myocardial infarction after adjuvant radiotherapy for breast cancer in the surveillance, epidemiology, and end-results cancer registries. *J Clin Oncol* 1998;16:2625–2631.
96. Beitsch PD, Wilkinson JB, Vicini FA, et al. Tumor bed control with balloon-based accelerated partial breast irradiation: incidence of true recurrences versus elsewhere failures in the American Society of Breast Surgery MammoSite(®) Registry Trial. *Ann Surg Oncol* 2012;19:3165–3170.
97. Haffty BG, Reiss M, Beinfield M, et al. Ipsilateral breast tumor recurrence as a predictor of distant disease: implications for systemic therapy at the time of local relapse. *J Clin Oncol* 1996;14:52–57.
98. Veronesi U, Marubini E, Del Vecchio M, et al. Local recurrences and distant metastases after conservative breast cancer treatments: partly independent events. *J Natl Cancer Inst* 1995;87:19–27.
99. Schnitt SJ, Hayman J, Gelman R, et al. A prospective study of conservative surgery alone in the treatment of selected patients with stage I breast cancer. *Cancer* 1996;77:1094–1100.
100. Hunt KK, Ballman KV, McCall LM, et al. Factors associated with local-regional recurrence after a negative sentinel node dissection: results of the ACOSOG Z0010 trial. *Ann Surg* 2012;256:428–436.
101. Mansi JL, Earl HM, Powles TJ, et al. Tests for detecting recurrent disease in the follow-up of patients with breast cancer. *Breast Cancer Res Treat* 1988;11:249–254.
102. Tomin R, Donegan WL. Screening for recurrent breast cancer—its effectiveness and prognostic value. *J Clin Oncol* 1987;5:62–67.
103. Andreoli C, Buranelli F, Campa T, et al. Chest x-ray survey in breast cancer follow-up—a contrary view. *Tumori* 1987;73:463–465.
104. Rutgers EJTh, van Slooten EA, Kluck HM. Follow-up after treatment of primary breast cancer. *Br J Surg* 1989;76:187–190.
105. Stierer M, Rosen HR. Influence of early diagnosis on prognosis of recurrent breast cancer. *Cancer* 1989;64:1128–1131.
106. Wagman LD, Sanders RD, Terz JJ, et al. The value of symptom directed evaluation in the surveillance for recurrence of carcinoma of the breast. *Surg Gynecol Obstet* 1991;172:191–196.
107. Kagan AR, Steckel RJ. Routine imaging studies for the posttreatment surveillance of breast and colorectal carcinoma. *J Clin Oncol* 1991;9:837–842.
108. Freedman LS, Edwards DN, McConnell EM, et al. Histological grade and other prognostic factors in relation to survival of patients with breast cancer. *Br J Cancer* 1979;40:44–45.
109. Lipponen P, Aaltomaa S, Eskelinen M, et al. The changing importance of prognostic factors in breast cancer during long-term follow-up. *Int J Cancer* 1992;51:698–702.
110. Stenkvist B, Bengtsson E, Dahlqvist B, et al. Predicting breast cancer recurrence. *Cancer* 1982;50:2884–2893.
111. Gilchrist KW, Gray R, Fowble B, et al. Tumor necrosis is a prognostic predictor for early recurrence and death in lymph node-positive breast cancer: a 10-year follow-up study of 728 Eastern Cooperative Oncology Group patients. *J Clin Oncol* 1993;11:1929–1935.
112. Yoshimoto M, Sakamoto G, Ohashi Y. Time dependency of the influence of prognostic factors on relapse in breast cancer. *Cancer* 1993;72:2993–3001.
113. Nab HW, Kluck HM, Rutgers EJT, et al. Long-term prognosis of breast cancer: an analysis of 462 patients in a general hospital in south east Netherlands. *Eur J Surg Oncol* 1995;21:42–46.
114. Arriagada R, Le MG, Dunant A, et al. Twenty-five years of follow-up in patients with operable breast carcinoma. Correlation between clinicopathologic factors and the risk of death in each 5-year period. *Cancer* 2006;106:743–750.
115. Takeuchi H, Baba H, Kano T, et al. The time-related changes of the importance of prognostic factors in breast cancer. A sequential multivariate analysis of 1423 Japanese patients. *Breast Cancer Res Treat* 2005;94:273–278.
116. Saphner T, Tormey DC, Gray R. Annual hazard rates of recurrence for breast cancer after primary therapy. *J Clin Oncol* 1996;14:2738–2746.
117. Haybittle JL, Blamey RW, Elston CW, et al. A prognostic index in primary breast cancer. *Br J Cancer* 1982;45:361–366.
118. McGuire WL, Clark GM, Fisher ER, et al. Predicting recurrence and survival in breast cancer. *Breast Cancer Res Treat* 1987;9:27–38.
119. Shek LL, Godolphin W. Model for breast cancer survival: relative prognostic roles of axillary nodal status, TNM stage, estrogen receptor concentration, and tumor necrosis. *Cancer Res* 1988;48:5565–5569.
120. Sigurdsson H, Baldetorp B, Borg Å,et al. Indicators of prognosis in node-negative breast cancer. *N Engl J Med* 1990;322:1045–1053.
121. Galea MH, Blamey RW, Elston CE, et al. The Nottingham Prognostic Index in primary breast cancer. *Breast Cancer Res Treat* 1992;22:207–209.
122. Balslev I, Axelsson CK, Zedeler K, et al. The Nottingham Prognostic Index applied to 9,149 patients from the studies of the Danish Breast Cancer Cooperative Group (DBCG). *Breast Cancer Res Treat* 1994;32:281–290.
123. Tubiana-Hulin M, Le Doussal V, Hacene K, et al. Sequential identification of factors predicting distant relapse in breast cancer patients treated by conservative surgery. *Cancer* 1993;72:1261–1271.
124. Winchester DJ, Menck HR, Winchester DP. The National Cancer Data Base report on the results of a large nonrandomized comparison of breast preservation and modified radical mastectomy. *Cancer* 1997;80:162–167.
125. Pinder SE, Murray S, Ellis IO, et al. The importance of the histologic grade of invasive breast carcinoma and response to chemotherapy. *Cancer* 1998;83:1529–1539.
126. Breast cancer incidence and mortality-United States, 1992. *MMWR Morbid Mortal Wkly Rep* 1996;45:833–851.
127. Garne JP, Aspegren K, Balldin G, et al. Increasing incidence of and declining mortality from breast carcinoma. Trends in Malmö, Sweden, 1961–1992. *Cancer* 1997;79:69–74.
128. American Cancer Society. *Breast cancer facts & figures 2005–2006.* Atlanta: American Cancer Society; 2005:3–7.
129. Hermon C, Beral V. Breast cancer mortality rates are levelling off or beginning to decline in many western countries: analysis of time trends, age-cohort and age-period models of breast cancer mortality in 20 countries. *Br J Cancer* 1996;73:955–960.
130. Adair F, Berg J, Joubert L, et al. Long term follow-up of breast cancer patients. The 30-year report. *Cancer* 1974;33:1145–1150.
131. Say CC, Donegan WL. Invasive carcinoma of the breast: prognostic significance of tumor size and involved axillary lymph nodes. *Cancer* 1974;34:468–471.
132. Smart CR, Myers MH, Gloecker LA. Implications for SEER data on breast cancer management. *Cancer* 1978;41:787–789.
133. Rosen PP, Saigo PE, Braun DW Jr, et al. Predictors of recurrence in stage I ($T_1N_0M_0$) breast carcinoma. *Ann Surg* 1981;193:15–25.
134. Rosen PP, Saigo PE, Braun DW Jr, et al. Prognosis in stage II ($T_1N_1M_0$) breast cancer. *Ann Surg* 1981;194:576–584.
135. Roger V, Beito G, Jolly PC. Factors affecting the incidence of lymph node metastases in small cancers of the breast. *Am J Surg* 1989;157:501–502.
136. Weaver DL, Rosenberg RD, Barlow WE. Pathologic findings from the breast cancer surveillance consortium. Population-based outcomes in women undergoing biopsy after screening mammography. *Cancer* 2006;106:732–742.
137. Prasad ML, Osborne MP, Giri DD, et al. Microinvasive carcinoma (T1mic) of the breast: clinicopathologic profile of 21 cases. *Am J Surg Pathol* 2000;24:422–428.
138. Abner AL, Collins L, Peiro G, et al. Correlation of tumor size and axillary lymph node involvement with prognosis in patients with T1 breast carcinoma. *Cancer* 1998;83:2502–2508.
139. Elkin EB, Hudis C, Begg CB, et al. The effect of changes in tumor size on breast carcinoma survival in the U.S.: 1975–1999. *Cancer* 2005;104:1149–1157.
140. Mansour EG, Gray R, Shatila AH, et al. Survival advantage of adjuvant chemotherapy in high-risk node-negative breast cancer: ten-year analysis—an intergroup study. *J Clin Oncol* 1998;16:3486–3492.

141. Joensuu H, Pylkkanen L, Toikkanen S. Late mortality from pT1N0M0 breast carcinoma. *Cancer* 1999;85:2183–2189.
142. Quiet CA, Ferguson DJ, Weichselbaum RR, et al. Natural history of node-positive breast cancer: the curability of small cancers with a limited number of positive nodes. *J Clin Oncol* 1996;14:3105–3111.
143. Seidman JD, Schnaper LA, Aisner SC. Relationship of the size of the invasive component of the primary breast carcinoma to axillary lymph node metastasis. *Cancer* 1995;75:65–71.
144. Silverberg SG, Chitale AR. Assessment of significance of proportions of intraductal and infiltrating tumor growth in ductal carcinoma of the breast. *Cancer* 1978;32:830–837.
145. Renshaw AA. Minimal (=0.1 cm) invasive carcinoma in breast core needle biopsies. *Arch Pathol Lab Med* 2004;128:996–999.
146. Charles M, Edge SB, Winston JS, et al. Effect of stereotactic core needle biopsy on pathologic measurement of tumor size of T1 invasive breast carcinomas presenting as mammographic masses. *Cancer* 2003;97:2137–2141.
147. American Joint Committee on Cancer. Breast, Chapter 32. In: *AJCC cancer staging manual*, 7th ed. New York: Springer, 2010:347–376.
148. Edwards HD, Oakley F, Koyama T, et al. The impact of tumor size in breast needle biopsy material on final pathologic size and tumor stage: a detailed analysis of 222 consecutive cases. *Am J Surg Pathol* 2013;37:739–744.
149. Rakha EA, El-Sayed ME, Reed J, et al. Screen-detected breast lesions with malignant needle core biopsy diagnoses and no malignancy identified in subsequent surgical excision specimens (potential false-positive diagnosis). *Eur J Cancer* 2009;45:1162–1167.
150. Andea AA, Bouwman D, Wallis T, et al. Correlation of tumor volume and surface area with lymph node status in patients with multifocal/multicentric breast carcinoma. *Cancer* 2004;100:20–27.
151. Andea AA, Wallis T, Newman LA, et al. Pathologic analysis of tumor size and lymph node status in multifocal/multicentric breast carcinoma. *Cancer* 2002;94:1383–1390.
152. Coombs NJ, Boyages J. Multifocal and multicentric breast cancer: does each focus matter? *J Clin Oncol* 2005;23:7497–7502.
153. Berg WA, Gutierrez L, NessAiver MS, et al. Diagnostic accuracy of mammography, clinical examination, US, and MR imaging in preoperative assessment of breast cancer. *Radiology* 2004;233:830–849.
154. Yeh E, Slanetz P, Kopans SB, et al. Prospective comparison of mammography, sonography, and MRI in patients undergoing neoadjuvant chemotherapy for palpable breast cancer. *AJR Am J Roentgenol* 2005;184:868–877.
155. Partridge SC, Gibbs JE, Lu Y, et al. MRI measurements of breast tumor volume predict response to neoadjuvant chemotherapy and recurrence-free survival. *AJR Am J Roentgenol* 2005;184:1774–1781.
156. Gold RH, Main G, Zippin C, et al. Infiltration of mammary carcinoma as an indicator of axillary metastases. A preliminary report. *Cancer* 1972;29:35–40.
157. Lane N, Goksel H, Salerno RA, et al. Clinicopathologic analyses of the surgical curability of breast cancers. A minimum ten year study. *Ann Surg* 1961;153:483–498.
158. Carter D, Pipkin RD, Shepard RH, et al. Relationship of necrosis and tumor border to lymph node metastases and 10 year survival in carcinoma of the breast. *Am J Surg Pathol* 1978;2:39–46.
159. Black MM, Speer FD. Nuclear structure in cancer tissues. *Surg Gynecol Obstet* 1957;105:97–105.
160. Cutler SJ, Black MM, Mork T, et al. Further observations on prognostic factors in cancer of the female breast. *Cancer* 1969;24:653–667.
161. Bloom HJG. Prognosis in carcinoma of the breast. *Br J Cancer* 1950;4:259–288.
162. Bloom HJG, Richardson WW. Histological grading and prognosis in breast cancer. A study of 1049 cases, of which 359 have been followed 15 years. *Br J Cancer* 1957;11:359–377.
163. Elston CW, Ellis IO. Pathological prognostic factors in breast cancer. I. The value of histological grade in breast cancer: experience from a large study with long-term follow-up. *Histopathology* 1991;19:403–410.
164. Rakha EA, El-Sayed ME, Lee AH, et al. Prognostic significance of Nottingham histologic grade in invasive breast carcinoma. *J Clin Oncol* 2008;26:3153–3158.
165. Parham DM, Hagen N, Brown RA. Simplified method of grading primary carcinomas of the breast. *J Clin Pathol* 1992;45:517-520.
166. Jannink I, van Diest PJ, Baak JPA. Comparison of the prognostic value of four methods to assess mitotic activity in 186 invasive breast cancer patients: classical and random mitotic activity assessments with correction for volume percentage of epithelium. *Hum Pathol* 1995;26:1086–1092.
167. van Diest PJ, Baak JPA, Matze-Cok P, et al. Reproducibility of mitosis counting in 2,469 breast cancer specimens: results from the Multicenter Morphometric Mammary Carcinoma Project. *Hum Pathol* 1992;23:603–607.
168. Baak JPA, van Diest PJ, Peterse HL; other MMMCP collaborators. Selection of lymph node negative unfavourable premenopausal breast cancer patients for adjuvant systemic therapy can be done best by the mitotic activity index (MAI). *Mod Pathol* 2000;13:17A.
169. Kuopio T, Collan Y. Still more about counting mitoses. *Hum Pathol* 1996;27:1110–1111.
170. National Co-ordinating Committee for Breast Screening Pathology. *Pathology reporting in breast cancer screening*. 2nd ed. Sheffield: NHSBSP Publications, 1995.
171. Rippey JJ. More about counting mitoses. *Hum Pathol* 1996;27:1109–1110.
172. Ellis PS, Whitehead R. Mitosis counting—a need for reappraisal. *Hum Pathol* 1981;12:3–4.
173. O'Shea AM, Rakha EA, Hodi Z, et al. Histological grade of invasive carcinoma of the breast assessed on needle core biopsy—modifications to mitotic count assessment to improve agreement with surgical specimens. *Histopathology* 2011;59:543–548.
174. Baehner R, Weidner N. Enhanced mitotic figure counting in breast carcinomas using a mitosis-specific antibody: anti-phosphohistone-H3 (PHH3). *Mod Pathol* 2000;13:17A.
175. Kwok TC, Rakha EA, Lee AH, et al. Histological grading of breast cancer on needle core biopsy: the role of immunohistochemical assessment of proliferation. *Histopathology* 2010;57:212–219.
176. Schauer A, Weiss A. Bedeuting des Tumorgrading und der Blutge fäßeinbrche für die Verlaufsbeurteilung des mammacarcinoms bei Stadium-I-Patientinnen. *Verh Dtsch Ges Path* 1981;65:382–394.
177. Le Doussal V, Tubiana-Hulin M, Friedman S, et al. Prognostic value of histologic grade nuclear components of Scarff-Bloom-Richardson (SBR). An improved score modification based on a multivariate analysis of 1262 invasive ductal breast carcinomas. *Cancer* 1989;643:191–1921.
178. de Andra de VP and Gobbi H. Accuracy of typing and grading invasive mammary carcinomas on core needle biopsy compared with the excisional specimen. *Virchows Arch* 2004;445:597–602.
179. Dalton LW, Page DL, Dupont WD. Histologic grading of breast carcinoma. A reproducibility study. *Cancer* 1994;73:2765–2770.
180. Harvey JM, deKlerk NH, Sterrett GF. Histological grading in breast cancer: interobserver agreement, and relation to other prognostic factors including ploidy. *Pathology* 1992;24:63–68.
181. Robbins P, Pinder S, de Klerk N, et al. Histological grading of breast carcinomas: a study of interobserver agreement. *Hum Pathol* 1995;26:873–879.
182. Mora B, Bombari D, Schaefer SC, et al. Tumor architecture exerts no bias on nuclear grading in breast cancer diagnosis. *Virchows Arch* 2012;461:399–403.
183. Schumacher M, Schmoor C, Sauerbrei W, et al. The prognostic effect of histological tumor grade in node-negative breast cancer patients. *Breast Cancer Res Treat* 1993;25:235–245.
184. Goldstein NS, Murphy T. Intraductal carcinoma associated with invasive carcinoma of the breast. A comparison of the two lesions with implications for intraductal carcinoma classification systems. *Am J Clin Pathol* 1996;106:312–318.
185. Dabbs DJ. Ductal carcinoma of breast: nuclear grade as a predictor of S-phase fraction. *Hum Pathol* 1993;24:652–656.
186. Andersen JA, Fischermann K, Hou-Jensen K, et al. Selection of high risk groups among prognostically favorable patients with breast cancer. An analysis of the value of prospective grading of tumor anaplasia in 1048 patients. *Ann Surg* 1981;194:1–3.
187. Henson DE. The histologic grading of neoplasms. *Arch Pathol Lab Med* 1988;112:1091–1096.
188. Hopton DS, Thorogood J, Clayden AD, et al. Histological grading of breast cancer; significance of grade on recurrence and mortality. *Eur J Surg Oncol* 1989;15:25–31.
189. Thoresen S. Histological grading and clinical stage at presentation in breast carcinoma. *Br J Cancer* 1982;46:457–458.
190. Dawson PJ, Ferguson DJ, Karrison T. The pathologic findings of breast cancer in patients surviving 25 years after radical mastectomy. *Cancer* 1982;50:2131–2138.
191. Davis BW, Gelber RD, Goldhirsch A, et al. Prognostic significance of tumor grade in clinical trials of adjuvant therapy for breast cancer with axillary nodal metastases. *Cancer* 1986;58:2662–2670.

192. Masters JRW, Millis RR, Rubens RD. Response to endocrine therapy and breast cancer differentiation. *Breast Cancer Res Treat* 1986;7:31–34.
193. Williams MR, Blamey RW, Todd JH, et al. Histologic grade in predicting response to endocrine treatment. *Breast Cancer Res Treat* 1986;8:165–166.
194. Clarke DH, Le MG, Sarrazin D, et al. Analysis of local-regional relapses in patients with early breast cancer treated by excision and radiotherapy: experience of the Institut Gustave-Roussy. *Int J Radiat Oncol Biol Phys* 1985;11:137–145.
195. Stadler B, Staffen A, Strasser K, et al. Prognostic factors for local recurrence in patients with limited surgery and irradiation of breast cancer. *Strahlenther Onkol* 1990;166:453–456.
196. Locker A, Ellis IO, Morgan DA, et al. Factors influencing local recurrence after excision and radiotherapy for primary breast cancer. *Br J Surg* 1989;76:890–894.
197. Nixon AJ, Schnitt SJ, Gelman R, et al. Relationship of tumor grade to other pathologic features and to treatment outcome of patients with early stage breast carcinoma treated with breast-conserving therapy. *Cancer* 1996;78:426–431.
198. Mate TP, Carter D, Fischer DB, et al. A clinical and histopathologic analysis of the results of conservation surgery and radiation therapy in stage I and II breast carcinoma. *Cancer* 1986;58:1995–2002.
199. Fourquet A, Campana F, Zafrani B, et al. Prognostic factors of breast recurrence in the conservative management of early breast cancer: a 25-year follow-up. *Int J Radiat Oncol Biol Phys* 1989;17:719–725.
200. Lee AH, Ellis IO. The Nottingham prognostic index for invasive carcinoma of the breast. *Pathol Oncol Res* 2008;14:113–115.
201. Sundquist M, Thorstenson S, Brudin L, et al. Applying the Nottingham Prognostic Index to a Swedish breast cancer population. South East Swedish Breast Cancer Study Group. *Breast Cancer Res Treat* 1999;53:1–8.
202. Fisher ER, Palikar AS, Gregorio RM, et al. Pathologic findings from the National Surgical Adjuvant Breast Project (protocol No. 4). IV. Significance of tumor necrosis. *Hum Pathol* 1978;9:523–530.
203. Roses DF, Bell DA, Flotte TJ, et al. Pathologic predictors of recurrence in stage 1 (T1N0M0) breast cancer. *Am J Clin Pathol* 1982;78:817–820.
204. Jimenez RE, Wallis T, Visscher DW. Centrally necrotizing carcinomas of the breast: a distinct histologic subtype with aggressive clinical behavior. *Am J Surg Pathol* 2001;25:331–337.
205. Yu L, Yang W, Cai X, et al. Centrally necrotizing carcinoma of the breast: clinicopathological analysis of 33 cases indicating its basal-like phenotype and poor prognosis. *Histopathology* 2010;57:193–201.
206. Oda K, Satake H, Nishio A, et al. Radiologic–pathologic conferences of the Nagoya University Hospital: centrally necrotizing carcinoma of the breast. *AJR Am J Roentgenol* 2008;190:W237–W239.
207. Lipponen P, Aaltomaa S, Kosma VM, et al. Apoptosis in breast cancer as related to histopathological characteristics and prognosis. *Eur J Cancer* 1994;30A:2068–2073.
208. Nishimura R, Nagao K, Miyayama H, et al. Apoptosis in breast cancer and its relationship to clinicopathological characteristics and prognosis. *J Surg Oncol* 1999;71:226–234.
209. Shen KL, Harn HJ, Ho LI, et al. The extent of proliferative and apoptotic activity in intraductal and invasive ductal breast carcinomas detected by Ki-67 labeling and terminal deoxynucleotidyl transferase-mediated digoxigenin-11-dUTP nick end labeling. *Cancer* 1998;82:2373–2381.
210. Bargou RC, Daniel PT, Mapara MY, et al. Expression of the bcl-2 gene family in normal and malignant breast tissue: low bax-(alpha) expression in tumor cells correlates with resistance towards apoptosis. *Int J Cancer* 1995;60:854–859.
211. Miyashita T, Krajewski S, Krajewska M, et al. Tumor suppressor p53 is a regulator of bcl-2 and bax gene expression *in vitro* and *in vivo*. *Oncogene* 1994;9:1799–1805.
212. Haldar S, Negrini M, Monne M, et al. Down-regulation of bcl-2 by p53 in breast cancer cells. *Cancer Res* 1994;54:2095–2097.
213. Sabourin JC, Martin A, Baruch J, et al. bcl-2 expression in normal breast tissue during the menstrual cycle. *Int J Cancer* 1994;59:1–6.
214. Siziopikou KP, Prioleau JE, Harris JR, et al. bcl-2 Expression in the spectrum of preinvasive breast lesions. *Cancer* 1996;77:499–506.
215. Kapucuoglu N, Losi L, Eusebi V. Immunohistochemical localization of Bcl-2 and Bax proteins in *in situ* and invasive ductal breast carcinomas. *Virchows Arch* 1997;430:17–22.
216. Bhargava V, Kell DL, van de Rijn M, et al. Bcl-2 immunoreactivity in breast carcinoma correlates with hormone receptor positivity. *Am J Pathol* 1994;145:535–540.
217. Silvestrini R, Veneroni S, Daidone MG, et al. The bcl-2 protein: a prognostic indicator strongly related to p53 protein in lymph node-negative breast cancer patients. *J Natl Cancer Inst* 1994;86:499–504.
218. Visscher DW, Sarkar F, Tabaczka P, et al. Clinicopathologic analysis of bcl-2 immunostaining in breast carcinoma. *Mod Pathol* 1996;9:642–646.
219. Hellemans P, van Dam PA, Weyler J, et al. Prognostic value of bcl-2 expression in invasive breast cancer. *Br J Cancer* 1995;72:354–360.
220. Alsabeh R, Wilson CS, Ahn CW, et al. Expression of bcl-2 by breast cancer: a possible diagnostic application. *Mod Pathol* 1995;9:439–444.
221. Leek RD, Kaklamanis L, Pezzella F, et al. bcl-2 in normal human breast and carcinoma, association with oestrogen receptor-positive, epidermal growth factor receptor-negative tumours and *in situ* cancer. *Br J Cancer* 1994;69:135–139.
222. Gee JMW, Robertson JFR, Ellis IO, et al. Immunocytochemical localization of bcl-2 protein in human breast cancers and its relationship to a series of prognostic markers and response to endocrine therapy. *Int J Cancer* 1994;59:619–628.
223. Dueñas-González A, del Mar Abad-Hernández M, Cruz-Hernández J-J, et al. Analysis of bcl-2 in sporadic breast carcinoma. *Cancer* 1997;80:2100–2108.
224. Krajewski S, Thor AD, Edgerton SM, et al. Analysis of bax and bcl-2 expression in p53-immunopositive breast cancers. *Clin Cancer Res* 1997;3:199–208.
225. Barbareschi M, Caffo O, Veronese S, et al. Bcl-2 and p53 expression in node-negative breast carcinoma; a study with long-term follow-up. *Hum Pathol* 1996;27:1149–1155.
226. Geuna M, Palestro G, Malandrone LB, et al. Relationships between proliferative activity and oncogene expression in human breast cancer. *Ann NY Acad Sci* 1996;784:555–563.
227. Silvestrini R, Benini E, Veneroni S, et al. p53 and bcl-2 expression correlates with clinical outcome in a series of node-positive breast cancer patients *J Clin Oncol* 1996;14:1604–1610.
228. Nakopoulou L, Michalopoulou A, Giannopoulou I, et al. bcl-2 Protein expression is associated with a prognostically favourable phenotype in breast cancer irrespective of p53 immunostaining. *Histopathology* 1999;34:310–319.
229. Joensuu H, Pylkkänen L, Toikkanen S. Bcl-2 immunoreactivity and long-term survival in breast cancer. *Am J Pathol* 1994;145: 1191–1198.
230. van Slooten H-J, Clahsen PC, van Dierendonck JH, et al. Expression of BCL-2 in node-negative breast cancer is associated with various prognostic factors, but does not predict response to one course of perioperative chemotherapy. *Br J Cancer* 1996;74:78–85.
231. Ali HR, Dawson SJ, Blows FM, et al. A Ki67/BCL2 index based on immunohistochemistry is highly prognostic in ER-positive breast cancer. *J Pathol* 2012;226:97–107.
232. Zhang GJ, Kimijima I, Tsuchiya A, et al. The role of bcl-2 expression in breast carcinomas (Review). *Oncol Rep* 1998;5:1211–1216.
233. Berardo MD, Elledge RM, de Moor C, et al. bcl-2 and apoptosis in lymph node positive breast carcinoma. *Cancer* 1998;82:1296–1302.
234. Bonetti A, Zaninelli M, Leone R, et al. bcl-2 But not p53 expression is associated with resistance to chemotherapy in advanced breast cancer. *Clin Cancer Res* 1998;4:2331–2336.
235. Greider CW, Blackburn EH. Telomeres, telomerase and cancer. *Sci Am* 1996;274:92–97.
236. Nawaz S, Hashizumi TL, Markham NE, et al. Telomerase expression in human breast cancer with and without lymph node metastases. *Am J Clin Pathol* 1997;107:542–547.
237. Carey LA, Kim NW, Goodman S, et al. Telomerase activity and prognosis in primary breast cancers. *J Clin Oncol* 1999;17:3075–3081.
238. Winnikow EP, Medeiros LR, Edelweiss MI, et al. Accuracy of telomerase in estimating breast cancer risk: a systematic review and meta-analysis. *Breast* 2012;21:1–7.
239. Landberg G, Nielsen NH, Nilsson P, et al. Telomerase activity is associated with cell cycle deregulation in human breast cancer. *Cancer Res* 1997;57:549–554.
240. Poremba C, Shroyer KR, Frost M, et al. Telomerase is a highly sensitive and specific molecular marker in fine-needle aspirates of breast lesions. *J Clin Oncol* 1999;17:2020–2026.

241. Roos G, Nilsson P, Cajander S, et al. Telomerase activity in relation to p53 status and clinico-pathological parameters in breast cancer. *Int J Cancer* 1998;79:343–348.
242. Fordyce CA, Heaphy CM, Bisoffi M, et al. Telomere content correlates with stage and prognosis in breast cancer. *Breast Cancer Res Treat* 2006;99:193–202.
243. Lu L, Zhang C, Zhu G, et al. Telomerase expression and telomere length in breast cancer and their associations with adjuvant treatment and disease outcome. *Breast Cancer Res.* 2011;13:R56.
244. Alderson MR, Hamlin I, Staunton MD. The relative significance of prognostic factors in breast carcinoma. *Br J Cancer* 1971;25:646–656.
245. Marginean F, Rakha EA, Ho BC, et al. Histological features of medullary carcinoma and prognosis in triple-negative basal-like carcinomas of the breast. *Mod Pathol* 2010;23:1357–1363.
246. Löfdahl B, Ahlin C, Holmqvist M, et al. Inflammatory cells in node-negative breast cancer. *Acta Oncol* 2012;51:680–686.
247. Pupa SM, Bufalino R, Invernizzi AM, et al. Macrophage infiltrate and prognosis in c-erbB-2-overexpressing breast carcinomas. *J Clin Oncol* 1996;14:85–94.
248. Rakha EA, Aleskandarany M, El-Sayed ME, et al. The prognostic significance of inflammation and medullary histological type in invasive carcinoma of the breast. *Eur J Cancer* 2009;45:1780–1787.
249. Bilik R, Mor C, Haraz B, et al. Characterization of T-lymphocyte subpopulations infiltrating breast cancer. *Cancer Immunol Immunother* 1989;28:143–147.
250. Horny H-P, Horst H-A. Lymphoreticular infiltrates in invasive ductal breast cancer. A histological and immunohistological study. *Virchows Arch [A]* 1986;409:275–286.
251. Whiteside TL, Miescher S, Hurlimann J, et al. Clonal analysis and *in situ* characterization of lymphocytes infiltrating human breast carcinomas. *Cancer Immunol Immunother* 1986;23:169–173.
252. Whitford P, Mallon EA, George WD, et al. Flow cytometric analysis of tumour infiltrating lymphocytes in breast cancer. *Br J Cancer* 1990;62:971–975.
253. Zuk JA, Walker RA. Immunohistochemical analysis of HLA antigens and mononuclear infiltrates of benign and malignant breast. *J Pathol* 1987;152:275–285.
254. Parkes H, Collis T, Baildam A, et al. *In situ* hybridization and S_1 mapping show that the presence of infiltrating plasma cells is associated with poor prognosis in breast cancer. *Br J Cancer* 1988;58:715–722.
255. Fisher ER, Sass R, Watkins G, et al. Tissue mast cells in breast cancer. *Breast Cancer Res Treat* 1985;5:285–291.
256. Dabiri S, Huntsman D, Makretsov N, et al. The presence of stromal mast cells identifies a subset of invasive breast cancers with a favorable prognosis. *Mod Pathol* 2004;17:690–695.
257. Gooch JL, Lee AV, Yee D. Interleukin 4 inhibits growth and induces apoptosis in human breast cancer cells. *Cancer Res* 1998;58:4199–4205.
258. Gilchrist KW, Gould VE, Hirschl S, et al. Interobserver variation in the identification of breast carcinoma in intramammary lymphatics. *Hum Pathol* 1982;13:170–172.
259. Rosen PP. Tumor emboli in intramammary lymphatics in breast carcinoma: pathologic criteria for diagnosis and clinical significance. *Pathol Annu* 1983;18(Part 2):215–232.
260. Hoda SA, Hoda RS, Merlin S, et al. Issues relating to lymphovascular invasion in breast carcinoma. *Adv Anat Pathol* 2006;13:308–315.
261. Khoury T. Delay to formalin fixation alters morphology and immunohistochemistry for breast carcinoma. *Appl Immunohistochem Mol Morphol* 2012;20:531–542.
262. Acs G, Dumoff KL, Solin LJ, et al. Extensive retraction artifact correlates with lymphatic invasion and nodal metastasis and predicts poor outcome in early stage breast carcinoma. *Am J Surg Pathol* 2007;31:129–140.
263. Asioli S, Eusebi V, Gaetano L, et al. The pre-lymphatic pathway, the roots of the lymphatic system in breast tissue: a 3D study. *Virchows Arch* 2008;453:401–406.
264. Damiani S, Eusebi V, Peterse JL. Malignant neoplasms infiltrating pseudoangiomatous' stromal hyperplasia of the breast: an unrecognized pathway of tumour spread. *Histopathology* 2002;41:208–215.
265. Agarwal B, Saxena R, Morimiya A, et al. Lymphangiogenesis does not occur in breast cancer. *Am J Surg Pathol* 2005;29:1449–1455.
266. Williams CS, Leek RD, Robson AM, et al. Absence of lymphangiogenesis and intratumoral lymph vessels in human metastatic breast cancer. *J Pathol* 2003;200:195–206.
267. Vlengel MM, Bos R, van der Groep P, et al. Lack of lymphangiogenesis during breast carcinogenesis. *J Clin Pathol* 2004;57:746–751.
268. Hanau CA, Machera H, Miettinen M. Immunohistochemical evaluation of vascular invasion in carcinomas with five different markers. *Appl Immunohistochem* 1993;1:46–50.
269. Lee AKC, DeLellis RA, Wolfe HJ. Intramammary lymphatic invasion in breast carcinomas. Evaluation using ABH isoantigens as endothelial markers. *Am J Surg Pathol* 1986;10:589–594.
270. Saigo PE, Rosen PP. The application of immunohistochemical stains to identify endothelial-lined channels in mammary carcinoma. *Cancer* 1987;59:51–54.
271. Ordonez NG, Brooks T, Thompson S, et al. Use of *Ulex Europaeus* agglutinin I in the identification of lymphatic and blood vessel invasion in previously stained microscopic slides. *Am J Surg Pathol* 1987;11:543–550.
272. Kahn HJ, Bailey D, Marks A. Monoclonal antibody D2-40, a new marker of lymphatic endothelium, reacts with Kaposi's sarcoma and a subset of angiosarcomas. *Mod Pathol* 2002;15:434–440.
273. Fukunaga M. Expression of D2-40 in lymphatic endothelium of normal tissues and in vascular tumors. *Histopathology* 2005;46:396–402.
274. Schacht V, Dadras SS, Johnson LA, et al. Up-regulation of the lymphatic marker podoplanin, a mucin-type transmembrane glycoprotein, in human squamous cell carcinomas and germ cell tumors. *Am J Pathol* 2005;166:913–921.
275. van den Eynden GG, van der Auwera I, van Laere SJ, et al. Distinguishing blood and lymph vessel invasion in breast cancer: a prospective immunohistochemical study. *Br J Cancer* 2006;94:1643–1649.
276. Kato T, Prevo R, Steers G, et al. A quantitative analysis of lymphatic vessels in human breast cancer, based on LYVE-I immunoreactivity. *Br J Cancer* 2005;93:1168–1174.
277. Bono P, Wasenius V-M, Lundin J, et al. High LYVE-I positive lymphatic vessel numbers are associated with poor outcome in breast cancer. *Clin Cancer Res* 2004;10:7144–7149.
278. Li JH, Man YG. Dual usages of single Wilms' tumor 1 immunohistochemistry in evaluation of breast tumors: a preliminary study of 30 cases. *Cancer Biomark.* 2009;5:109–116.
279. Rabban JT, Chen YY. D2-40 expression by breast myoepithelium: potential pitfalls in distinguishing intralymphatic carcinoma from *in situ* carcinoma. *Hum Pathol* 2008;39:175–183.
280. Mohammed RA, Martin SG, Mahmmod AM, et al. Objective assessment of lymphatic and blood vascular invasion in lymph node-negative breast carcinoma: findings from a large case series with long-term follow-up. *J Pathol* 2011;223:358–365.
281. Bettelheim R, Penman HG, Thornton-Jones H, et al. Prognostic significance of peritumoral vascular invasion in breast cancer. *Br J Cancer* 1984;50:771–777.
282. Fracchia AA, Rosen PP, Ashikari R. Primary carcinoma of the breast without axillary lymph node metastases. *Surg Gynecol Obstet* 1980;151:375–378.
283. Merlin C, Gloor F, Hardmeier T, et al. Hat die intrammarare lymphangiosis carcinomatosa bein nodel-negativen mammakarziom eine prognostische bedeutung? *Schweiz Med Wochenschr* 1980;110:605–606.
284. Nime F, Rosen PP, Thaler H, et al. Prognostic significance of tumor emboli in intramammary lymphatics in patients with mammary carcinoma. *Am J Surg Pathol* 1977;1:25–30.
285. Lauria R, Perrone F, Carlomagno C, et al. The prognostic value of lymphatic and blood vessel invasion in operable breast cancer. *Cancer* 1995;76:1772–1778.
286. Clemente CG, Boracchi P, Andreola S, et al. Peritumoral lymphatic invasion in patients with node-negative mammary ductal carcinoma. *Cancer* 1992;69:1396–1403.
287. Liljegren G, Holmberg L, Bergh J, et al. 10-Year results after sector resection with or without postoperative radiotherapy for stage I breast cancer: a randomized trial. *J Clin Oncol* 1999;17:2326–2333.
288. Arnaout-Alkarain A, Kahn HJ, Narod SA, et al. Significance of lymph vessel invasion identified by the endothelial lymphatic marker D2-40 in node negative breast cancer. *Mod Pathol* 2007;20:183–191.
289. Freedman GM, Li T, Polli LV, et al. Lymphatic space invasion is not an independent predictor of outcomes in early stage breast cancer treated by breast-conserving surgery and radiation. *Breast J* 2012;18:415–419.
290. Rakha EA, Martin S, Lee AH, et al. The prognostic significance of lymphovascular invasion in invasive breast carcinoma. *Cancer* 2011;118:3670–3680.

291. Mohammed RA, Ellis IO, Mahmmod AM, et al. Lymphatic and blood vessels in basal and triple-negative breast cancers: characteristics and prognostic significance. *Mod Pathol* 2011;24:774–785.
292. Gudlaugsson E, Skaland I, Undersrud E, et al. D2-40/p63 defined lymph vessel invasion has additional prognostic value in highly proliferating operable node negative breast cancer patients. *Mod Pathol* 2011;24:502–511.
293. Rosen PP, Saigo PE, Braun DW Jr, et al. Occult axillary lymph node metastases from breast cancers with intramammary lymphatic tumor emboli. *Am J Surg Pathol* 1982;6:639–641.
294. Fisher ER, Sass R, Fisher B. Pathologic findings from the National Surgical Adjuvant Project for breast cancers (Protocol No. 4). X. Discriminants of tenth year treatment failure. *Cancer* 1984;53:712–723.
295. Davis BW, Gelber R, Goldhirsch A, et al. Prognostic significance of peri-tumoral vessel invasion in clinical trials of adjuvant therapy for breast cancer with axillary lymph node metastases. *Hum Pathol* 1985;16:1212–1218.
296. Weiser MR, Montgomery LL, Tan LK, et al. Lymphovascular invasion enhances the prediction of non-sentinel node metastases in breast cancer patients with positive sentinel nodes. *Ann Surg Oncol* 2001;8:145–149.
297. Turner RR, Chu U, Qi K, et al. Pathologic features associated with nonsentinel lymph node metastases in patients with metastatic breast carcinoma in a sentinel lymph node. *Cancer* 2000;89:574–581.
298. Mohammed RA, Martin SG, Gill MS, et al. Improved methods of detection of lymphovascular invasion demonstrate that it is the predominant method of vascular invasion in breast cancer and has important clinical consequences. *Am J Surg Pathol* 2007;31:1825–1833.
299. Bell JR, Friedell GH, Goldenberg IS. Prognostic significance of pathologic findings in human breast carcinoma. *Surg Gynecol Obstet* 1969;129:258–262.
300. Sampat MB, Sirsat MV, Gangadharan P. Prognostic significance of blood vessel invasion in carcinoma of the breast in women. *J Surg Oncol* 1977;9:623–632.
301. Weigand RA, Isenberg WM, Russo J, et al. Blood vessel invasion and axillary lymph node involvement as prognostic indicators for human breast cancer. *Cancer* 1982;50:962–696.
302. Cowley GP, Smith MEF. Modulation of E-cadherin expression and morphological phenotype in the intravascular component of adenocarcinomas. *Int J Cancer* 1995;60:325–329.
303. Colleoni M, Rotmensz N, Maisonneuve P, et al. Prognostic role of the extent of peritumoral vascular invasion in operable breast cancer. *Ann Oncol* 2007;18:1632–1640.
304. Folkman J. What is the evidence that tumors are angiogenesis dependent? *J Natl Cancer Inst* 1990;82:4–6.
305. Folkman J, Watson K, Ingber D, et al. Induction of angiogenesis during the transition from hyperplasia to neoplasia. *Nature* 1989;339:58–61.
306. Jensen HM, Chen I, DeVault MR, et al. Angiogenesis induced by "normal" human breast tissue: a probable marker for precancer. *Science* 1982;218:293–295.
307. Holmgren L, O'Reilly MS, Folkman J. Dormancy of micrometastases: balanced proliferation and apoptosis in the presence of angiogenesis suppression. *Nature Med* 1995;1:149–153.
308. Pepper MS, Ferrara N, Orci L, et al. Potent synergism between vascular endothelial growth factor and basic fibroblast growth factor in the induction of angiogenesis *in vitro*. *Biochem Biophys Res Commun* 1992;189:824–831.
309. Hlatky L, Tsionou C, Hahnfeldt P, et al. Mammary fibroblasts may influence breast tumor angiogenesis via hypoxia-induced vascular endothelial growth factor up-regulation and protein expression. *Cancer Res* 1994;54:6083–6086.
310. Gonzalez-Vela MC, Garijo MF, Fernandez F, et al. Cathepsin D in host stromal cells is associated with more highly vascular and aggressive invasive breast carcinoma. *Histopathology* 1999;34:35–42.
311. Toi M, Kondo S, Suzuki H, et al. Quantitative analysis of vascular endothelial growth factor in primary breast cancer. *Cancer* 1996;77:1101–1106.
312. Anan K, Morisaki T, Katano M, et al. Preoperative assessment of tumor angiogenesis by vascular endothelial growth factor mRNA expression in homogenate samples of breast carcinoma: fine-needle aspirates vs. resection samples. *J Surg Oncol* 1997;66:257–263.
313. Lee AH, Dublin EA, Bobrow LG, et al. Invasive lobular and invasive ductal carcinoma of the breast show distinct patterns of vascular endothelial growth factor expression and angiogenesis. *J Pathol* 1998;185:394–401.
314. Rastinejad F, Polverini P, Bouck NP. Regulation of the activity of a new inhibitor of angiogenesis by a cancer suppressor gene. *Cell* 1989;56:345–355.
315. Dameron KM, Volpert OV, Tainsky MA, et al. Control of angiogenesis in fibroblasts by p53 regulation of thrombospondin-1. *Science* 1994;265:1582–1584.
316. O'Reilly MS, Holmgren L, Shing Y, et al. Angiostatin: a novel angiogenesis inhibitor that mediates the suppression of metastases by a Lewis lung carcinoma. *Cell* 1994;79:315–328.
317. Rak JW, St Croix BD, Kerbel RS. Consequences of angiogenesis for tumor progression, metastasis and cancer therapy. *Anti-Cancer Drugs* 1995;6:3–18.
318. Brown LF, Berse B, Jackman RW, et al. Expression of vascular permeability factor (vascular endothelial growth factor) and its receptors in breast cancer. *Hum Pathol* 1995;26:86–91.
319. Kim KJ, Li B, Winer J, et al. Inhibition of vascular endothelial growth factor-induced angiogenesis suppresses tumour growth *in vivo*. *Nature* 1993;362:841–844.
320. Hori A, Sasada R, Matsutani E, et al. Suppression of solid tumor growth by immunoneutralizing monoclonal antibody against human basic fibroblast growth factor. *Cancer Res* 1991;51:6180–6184.
321. Horak ER, Leek R, Klenk N, et al. Angiogenesis, assessed by platelet/endothelial cell adhesion molecule antibodies, as indicator of node metastases and survival in breast cancer. *Lancet* 1992;340: 1120–1124.
322. Siitonen SM, Haapasalo HK, Rantala IS, et al. Comparison of different immunohistochemical methods in the assessment of angiogenesis: lack of prognostic value in a group of 77 selected node-negative breast carcinomas. *Mod Pathol* 1995;8:745–752.
323. Arnes JB, Stefansson IM, Straume O, et al. Vascular proliferation is a prognostic factor in breast cancer. *Breast Cancer Res Treat* 2012;133:501–510.
324. Gasparini G, Gullick WJ, Bevilacqua P, et al. Human breast cancer: prognostic significance of the c-erbB-2 oncoprotein compared with epidermal growth factor receptor, DNA ploidy, and conventional pathologic features. *J Clin Oncol* 1992;10:686–695.
325. Weidner N, Gasparini G. Determination of epidermal growth factor receptor provides additional prognostic information to measuring tumor angiogenesis in breast carcinoma patients. *Breast Cancer Res Treat* 1994;29:97–107.
326. Martin L, Holcombe C, Green B, et al. Is a histological section representative of whole tumour vascularity in breast cancer? *Br J Cancer* 1997;76:40–43.
327. Jitsuiki Y, Hasebe T, Tsuda H, et al. Optimizing microvessel counts according to tumor zone in invasive ductal carcinoma of the breast. *Mod Pathol* 1999;12:492–498.
328. de Jong JS, van Diest PJ, Baak JPA. Methods in laboratory investigation. Heterogeneity and reproducibility of microvessel counts in breast cancer. *Lab Invest* 1995;73:922–926.
329. Simpson JF, Ahn C, Battifora H, et al. Endothelial area as a prognostic indicator for invasive breast carcinoma. *Cancer* 1996;77:2077–2085.
330. Costello P, McCann A, Carney DN, et al. Prognostic significance of microvessel density in lymph node negative breast carcinoma. *Hum Pathol* 1995;26:1181–1184.
331. Axelsson K, Ljung B-ME, Moore II, DH,et al. Tumor angiogenesis as a prognostic assay for invasive ductal breast carcinoma. *J Natl Cancer Inst* 1995;87:997–1008.
332. Ogawa Y, Chung Y-S, Nakata B, et al. Microvessel quantitation in invasive breast cancer by staining for factor VIII-related antigen. *Br J Cancer* 1995;71:1297–1301.
333. Obermair A, Kurz C, Czelwenka K, et al. Microvessel density and vessel invasion in lymph-node negative breast cancer: effect on recurrence-free survival. *Int J Cancer* 1995;62:126–131.
334. Charpin C, Devictor B, Bergeret D, et al. CD31 quantitative immunocytochemical assays in breast carcinomas. Correlation with current prognostic factors. *Am J Clin Pathol* 1995;103:443–448.
335. Goulding H, Nik Abdul Rashid NF, Robertson JF, et al. Assessment of angiogenesis in breast carcinoma: an important factor in prognosis? *Hum Pathol* 1995;26:1196–1200.
336. Harris AL, Horak E. Growth factors and angiogenesis in breast cancer. Recent results. *Cancer Res* 1993;127:35–41.
337. Bevilacqua P, Barbareschi M, Verderio P, et al. Prognostic value of intratumoral microvessel density, a measure of tumor angiogenesis, in

node-negative breast carcinoma—results of a multiparametric study. *Breast Cancer Res Treat* 1995;36:205–217.
338. Gasparini G. Clinical significance of the determination of angiogenesis in human breast cancer: update of the biological background and overview of the Vicenza studies. *Eur J Cancer* 1996;32A:2485–2493.
339. Toi M, Inada K, Suzuki H, et al. Tumor angiogenesis in breast cancer: its importance as a prognostic indicator and the association with vascular endothelial growth factor expression. *Breast Cancer Res Treat* 1995;36:193–204.
340. Gasparini G, Fox SB, Verderio P, et al. Determination of angiogenesis adds information to estrogen receptor status in predicting the efficacy of adjuvant tamoxifen in node-positive breast cancer patients. *Clin Cancer Res* 1996;2:1191–1198.
341. Heimann R, Ferguson D, Powers C, et al. Angiogenesis as a predictor of long-term survival for patients with node-negative breast cancer. *J Natl Cancer Inst* 1996;88:1764–1769.
342. Miliaras D, Kamas A, Kalekou H. Angiogenesis in invasive breast carcinoma: is it associated with parameters of prognostic significance? *Histopathology* 1995;26:165–169.
343. Kato T, Kimura T, Miyakawa R, et al. Clinicopathologic study of angiogenesis in Japanese patients with breast cancer. *World J Surg* 1997;21:49–56.
344. Toi M, Kashitani J, Tominaga T. Tumor angiogenesis is an independent prognostic indicator in primary breast carcinoma. *Int J Cancer* 1993;55:371–374.
345. Sightler HE, Borowsky AD, Dupont WD, et al. Evaluation of tumor angiogenesis as a prognostic marker in breast cancer. *Lab Invest* 1994;70:22A.
346. Cohen P, Guidi A, Harris J, et al. Microvessel density and local recurrence in patients with early stage breast cancer treated by wide excision above (WEA). *Lab Invest* 1994;70:14A.
347. Hansen S, Grabau DA, Rose C, et al. Angiogenesis in breast cancer: a comparative study of the observer variability of methods for determining microvessel density. *Lab Invest* 1998;78:1563–1573.
348. Mikalsen LT, Dhakal HP, Bruland OS, et al. Quantification of angiogenesis in breast cancer by automated vessel identification in CD34 immunohistochemical sections. *Anticancer Res* 2011;31:4053–4060.
349. Buadu LD, Murakami J, Murayama S, et al. Breast lesions: correlation of contrast medium enhancement patterns on MR images with histopathologic findings and tumor angiogenesis. *Radiology* 1996;200:639–649.
350. Stomper PC, Winston JS, Herman S, et al. Angiogenesis and dynamic MR imaging gadolinium enhancement of malignant and benign breast lesions. *Breast Cancer Res Treat* 1997;45:39–46.
351. Buckley DL, Drew PJ, Mussurakis S, et al. Microvessel density of invasive breast cancer assessed by dynamic Gd-DTPA enhanced MRI. *J Magn Reson Imaging* 1997;7:461–464.
352. Esserman L, Hylton N, George T, et al. Contrast-enhanced magnetic resonance imaging to assess tumor histopathology and angiogenesis in breast carcinoma. *Breast J* 1999;5:13–21.
353. Linderholm B, Tavelin B, Grankvist K, et al. Vascular endothelial growth factor is of high prognostic value in node-negative breast carcinoma. *J Clin Oncol* 1998;16:3121–3128.
354. Eppenberger U, Kueng W, Schlaeppi JM, et al. Markers of tumor angiogenesis and proteolysis independently define high- and low-risk subsets of node-negative breast cancer patients. *J Clin Oncol* 1998;16:3129–3136.
355. Penault-Llorca F, Sun ZZ, Viens P, et al. Tumor angiogenesis is not a predictive marker of responsiveness to conventional adjuvant chemotherapy. *Mod Pathol* 1997;10:23A.
356. Paulsen T, Aas T, Borressen A-L. Angiogenesis does not predict clinical response to doxorubicin monotherapy in patients with locally advanced breast cancer (Letter to Editor). *Int J Cancer (Pred Oncol)* 1997;74:138–140.
357. Teicher BA, Holden SA, Ara G, et al. Potentiation of cytotoxic cancer therapies by TNP-470 alone and with other anti-angiogenic agents. *Int J Cancer* 1994;57:920–925.
358. Klauber N, Parangi S, Flynn E, et al. Inhibition of angiogenesis and breast cancer in mice by the microtubule inhibitors 2-methoxyestradiol and taxol. *Cancer Res* 1997;57:81–86.
359. Brem H, Goto F, Budson A, et al. Minimal drug resistance after prolonged antiangiogenic therapy with AGM-1470. *Surg Forum* 1994;45:674–677.
360. Hicklin DL, Ellis LM. Role of the vascular endothelial growth factor pathway in tumor growth and angiogenesis. *J Clin Oncol* 2005;23:1011–1027.
361. Miller KD, Chap LI, Holmes FA, et al. Randomized phase III trial of capecitabine compared with bevacizumab plus capecitabine in patients with previously treated metastatic breast cancer. *J Clin Oncol* 2005;23:792–799.
362. Wedam SB, Low JA, Yang SX, et al. Antiangiogenic and antitumor effects of bevacizumab in patients with inflammatory and locally advanced breast cancer. *J Clin Oncol* 2006;24:769–777.
363. von Minckwitz G, Eidtmann H, Rezai M, et al. Neoadjuvant chemotherapy and bevacizumab for HER2-negative breast cancer. *N Engl J Med* 2012;366:299–309.
364. Bear HD, Tang G, Rastogi P, et al. Bevacizumab added to neoadjuvant chemotherapy for breast cancer. *N Engl J Med* 2012;366:310–320.
365. Jones DT, Lechertier T, Mitter R, et al. Gene expression analysis in human breast cancer associated blood vessels. *PLoS One* 2012;7(10):e44294.
366. Karak SG, Quatrano N, Buckley J, et al. Prevalence and significance of perineural invasion in invasive breast carcinoma. *Conn Med* 2010;74:17–21.
367. Mujtaba SS, Ni YB, Tsang JY, et al. Fibrotic focus in breast carcinomas: relationship with prognostic parameters and biomarkers. *Ann Surg Oncol* 2013;20:2842–2849.
368. Uchiyama S, Fukuda Y. Abnormal elastic fibers in elastosis of breast carcinoma. Ultrastructural and immunohistochemical studies. *Acta Pathol Jpn* 1989;39:245–253.
369. Davies JD. Hyperelastosis, obliteration and fibrous plaques in major ducts of the human breast. *J Pathol* 1973;110:13–26.
370. Reyes MG, Bazile DB, Tosch T, et al. Periductal elastic tissue of breast cancer. *Arch Pathol Lab Med* 1982;106:610–614.
371. Douglas JG, Shivas AA. The origins of elastosis in breast carcinoma. *J R Coll Surg Edinb* 1974;19:89–93.
372. Kao RT, Hall J, Stern R. Collagen and elastin synthesis in human stroma and breast carcinoma cell lines; modulation by extracellular matrix. *Connect Tissue Res* 1986;14:245–255.
373. Mera SL, Davies JD. Elastosis in breast carcinoma: I. Immunohistochemical characterization of elastic fibres. *J Pathol* 1987;151:103–110.
374. Davies JD, Mera SL. Elastosis in breast carcinoma: II. Association of protease inhibitors with immature elastic fibres. *J Pathol* 1987;151:317–324.
375. Humeniuk V, Forrest APM, Hawkins RA, et al. Elastosis and primary breast cancer. *Cancer* 1983;52:1448–1452.
376. Rasmussen BB, Pedersen BV, Thorpe SM, et al. Elastosis in relation to prognosis in primary breast carcinoma. *Cancer Res* 1985;45:1428–1430.
377. Masters JRW, Sangster K, Hawkins RA, et al. Elastosis and estrogen receptors in human breast cancer. *Br J Cancer* 1976;33:342–343.
378. Shivas AA, Douglas JG. The prognostic significance of elastosis in breast carcinoma. *J R Coll Surg Edinb* 1972;17:315–320.
379. Tamura S, Enjoji M. Elastosis in neoplastic and non-neoplastic tissues from patients with mammary carcinoma. *Acta Pathol Jpn* 1988;38:1537–1546.
380. Robertson AJ, Brown RA, Cree IA, et al. Prognostic value of measurement of elastosis in breast carcinoma. *J Clin Pathol* 1981;34:738–743.
381. Anastassiades OT, Bouropoulou V, Kontogeorgos G, et al. Ductal elastosis in infiltrating carcinoma of the breast. *Pathol Res Pract* 1979;165:411–421.
382. Glaubitz LC, Bowen JH, Cox ED, et al. Elastosis in human breast cancer. Correlation with sex steroid receptors and comparison with clinical outcome. *Arch Pathol Lab Med* 1984;108:27–30.
383. Schnitt SJ, Connolly JL, Harris JR, et al. Pathologic predictors of early local recurrences in Stage I and II breast cancer treated by primary radiation therapy. *Cancer* 1984;53:1049–1057.
384. Rosen PP, Kinne DW, Lesser ML, et al. Are prognostic factors for local control of breast cancer treated by primary radiotherapy significant for patients treated by mastectomy? *Cancer* 1986;57:1415–1420.
385. Joura EA, Lösch A, Kainz CH, et al. Infiltrating ductal carcinoma of the breast: extensive intraductal component has no impact on lymph node involvement and survival. *Anticancer Res* 1995;15:2285–2286.
386. Hurd TC, Sneige N, Allen PK, et al. Impact of extensive intraductal component on recurrence and survival in patients with stage I and II breast cancer treated with breast conservation therapy. *Ann Surg Oncol* 1997;4:119–124.

387. Schnitt SJ, Abner A, Gelman R, et al. The relationship between microscopic margins of resection and the risk of local recurrence in patients with breast cancer treated with breast-conserving surgery and radiation therapy. *Cancer* 1994;74:1746–1751.
388. Goldstein SN. Controversies in pathology in early-stage breast cancer. *Semin Radiat Oncol* 2011;21:20–25.
389. Stomper PC, Connolly JL. Mammographic features predicting an extensive intraductal component in early-stage infiltrating ductal carcinoma. *AJR Am J Roentgenol* 1992;158:269–272.
390. Noguchi S, Aihara T, Koyama H, et al. Discrimination between multicentric and multifocal carcinomas of the breast through clonal analysis. *Cancer* 1994;74:872–877.
391. Aubele M, Mattis A, Zitzelsberger H, et al. Extensive ductal carcinomas *in situ* with small foci of invasive ductal carcinoma: evidence of genetic resemblance by CGH. *Int J Cancer* 2000;85:82–86.
392. Ohtake T, Abe R, Kimijima I, et al. Intraductal extension of primary invasive breast carcinoma treated by breast-conservation surgery. Computer graphic three-dimensional reconstruction of the mammary ductal-lobular systems. *Cancer* 1995;76:32–45.
393. Jing X, Kakudo K, Murakami M, et al. Intraductal spread of invasive breast carcinoma has a positive correlation with c-erb B-2 overexpression and vascular invasion. *Cancer* 1999;86:439–448.
394. Dzierzanowski M, Melville KA, Barnes PJ, et al. Ductal carcinoma *in situ* in core biopsies containing invasive breast cancer: correlation with extensive intraductal component and lumpectomy margins. *J Surg Oncol* 2005;90:71–76.
395. Fowble B, Hanlon AL, Patchefsky A, et al. The presence of proliferative breast disease with atypia does not significantly influence outcome in early-stage invasive breast cancer treated with conservative surgery and radiation. *Int J Radiat Oncol Biol Phys* 1998;42: 105–115.
396. Peer PG, van Dijck JA, Hendriks JH, et al. Age-dependent growth rate of primary breast cancer. *Cancer* 1993;71:3547–3551.
397. von Fournier D, Weber E, Hoeffken W, et al. Growth rate of 147 mammary carcinomas. *Cancer* 1980;45:2198–2207.
398. Kuroishi T, Tominaga S, Morimoto T, et al. Tumor growth rate and prognosis of breast cancer mainly detected by mass screening. *Jpn J Cancer Res* 1990;81:454–462.
399. Tabbane F, Bahi J, Rahal K, et al. Inflammatory symptoms in breast cancer. Correlations with growth rate, clinicopathologic variables, and evolution. *Cancer* 1989;64:2081–2089.
400. Daly CA, Apthorp L, Field S. Second round cancers: how many were visible on the first round of the UK National Breast Screening Programme, three years earlier? *Clin Radiol* 1998;53:25–28.
401. Atkin NB, Kay R. Prognostic significance of modal DNA value and other factors in malignant tumors based on 1465 cases. *Br J Cancer* 1979;40:210–221.
402. Auer GU, Caspersson TO, Wallgren AS. DNA content and survival in mammary carcinomas. *Anal Quant Cytol Histol* 1980;2:162–165.
403. Auer GU, Eriksson E, Azavedo E, et al. Prognostic significance of nuclear DNA content in mammary adenocarcinomas in humans. *Cancer Res* 1984;44:394–396.
404. Auer GU, Falenius AG, Erhardt KY, et al. Progression of mammary adenocarcinomas as reflected by nuclear DNA content. *Cytometry* 1984;5:420–425.
405. Auer GU, Caspersson TO, Gustaffson SA, et al. Relationship between nuclear DNA distribution and estrogen receptors in human mammary carcinomas. *Anal Quant Cytol Histol* 1980;2:280–284.
406. Bichel P, Paulsen HS, Andersen J. Estrogen receptor content and ploidy of human mammary carcinomas. *Cancer* 1982;50:1771–1774.
407. Chessevent A, Daver A, Bertrand G, et al. Comparative flow DNA analysis of different cell suspensions in the breast carcinomas. *Cytometry* 1984;5:263–267.
408. Sven-Borje E, Langstrom E, Baldetorp B, et al. Flow cytometric DNA analysis in primary breast carcinomas and clinicopathologic correlations. *Cytometry* 1984;5:408–419.
409. Cornelisse CJ, de Koning HR, Moolenaar AJ, et al. Image and flow cytometric analysis of DNA content in breast cancer. Relation to estrogen receptor content and lymph node involvement. *Anal Quant Cytol Histol* 1984;6:9–18.
410. Raber MN, Barlogie B, Latreille J, et al. Ploidy, proliferative activity and estrogen receptor content in human breast cancer. *Cytometry* 1982;3:36–41.
411. Fisher B, Gunduz N, Constantino J, et al. DNA flow cytometric analysis of primary operable breast cancer. Relation of ploidy and S-phase fraction to outcome of patients in NSABP B-04. *Cancer* 1991;68:1465–1475.
412. Frierson HF Jr. Grade and flow cytometric analysis of ploidy for infiltrating ductal carcinomas. *Hum Pathol* 1993;24:24–29.
413. Cook DL, Weaver DL. Comparison of DNA content, S-phase fraction, and survival between medullary and ductal carcinoma of the breast. *Am J Clin Pathol* 1995;104:17–22.
414. Meyer JS, Friedman E, McCrate M, et al. Prediction of early course of breast carcinomas by thymidine labeling. *Cancer* 1983;51:1879–1886.
415. Meyer JS, McDivitt RW, Stone KR, et al. Practical breast carcinoma cell kinetics; review and update. *Breast Cancer Res Treat* 1984;4:79–88.
416. Tubiana M, Pejovic MH, Chavaudra N, et al. The long-term prognostic significance of the thymidine labeling index in breast cancer. *Int J Cancer* 1984;33:441–445.
417. Tubiana M, Pejovic MH, Koscielny S, et al. Growth rate, kinetics of tumor cell proliferation and long-term outcome in human breast cancer. *Int J Cancer* 1989;44:17–22.
418. Meyer JS, Prey MV, Babcock DS, et al. Breast carcinoma cell kinetics, morphology, stage and host characteristics. A thymidine labelling study. *Lab Invest* 1986;54:41–51.
419. Paradiso A, Mangia A, Barletta A, et al. Heterogeneity of intratumour proliferative activity in primary breast cancer: biological and clinical aspects. *Eur J Cancer* 1995;31A:911–916.
420. Klintenberg C, Stal O, Nordenskjold B, et al. Proliferative index, cytosol estrogen receptor and axillary nodal status as prognostic predictors in human mammary carcinoma. *Breast Cancer Res Treat* 1986;7(suppl.):99–106.
421. Silvestrini R, Daidone MG, Valagussa P, et al. ^{3}H-Thymidine-labeling index as a prognostic indicator in node-positive breast cancer. *J Clin Oncol* 1990;8:1321–1326.
422. Fossa SD, Thorud E, Vaage S, et al. DNA cytometry of primary breast cancer. A comparison of microspectrophotometry and flow cytometry and different preparation methods for flow cytometric measurements. *Acta Pathol Microbiol Immunol Scand (A)* 1983;91:235–243.
423. Hedley DW, Friedlander ML, Taylor IW, et al. Method for analysis of cellular DNA content of paraffin-embedded pathological material using flow cytometry. *J Histochem Cytochem* 1983;31:1333–1335.
424. Meyer JS, Hixon B. Advanced stage and early relapse of breast carcinomas associated with high thymidine labeling indices. *Cancer Res* 1979;39:4042–4047.
425. Moran RE, Black M, Alpert L, et al. Correlation of cell-cycle kinetics, hormone receptors, histopathology and nodal status in human breast cancer. *Cancer* 1984;54:1586–1590.
426. Olszewski W, Darzynkiewicz A, Rosen PP, et al. Flow cytometry of breast carcinoma: I. Relation of DNA ploidy level to histology and estrogen receptor. *Cancer* 1981;48:980–984.
427. Olszewski W, Darzynkiewicz Z, Rosen PP, et al. Flow cytometry of breast carcinoma. II. Relation of tumor cell cycle distribution to histology and estrogen receptor. *Cancer* 1981;48:985–988.
428. McDivitt RW, Stone KR, Craig B, et al. A proposed classification of breast cancer based on kinetic information derived from a comparison of risk factors in 168 primary operable breast cancers. *Cancer* 1986;57:269–276.
429. Dressler LG, Seamer LC, Owens MA, et al. DNA flow cytometry and prognostic factors in 1331 frozen breast cancer specimens. *Cancer* 1988;61:420–427.
430. Olszewski W, Darzynkiewicz Z, Rosen PP, et al. Flow cytometry of breast carcinoma. III. Possible altered kinetics in axillary node metastases. *Anal Quant Cytol Histol* 1982;4:275–278.
431. Frierson HF Jr. Ploidy analysis and S-phase fraction determination by flow cytometry of invasive adenocarcinomas of the breast. *Am J Surg Pathol* 1991;15:358–367.
432. Batsakis JG, Sneige N, El-Naggar AK. Flow cytometric (DNA content and S-phase fraction) analysis of breast cancer. *Cancer* 1993;71:2151–2153.
433. Hedley DW, Clark GM, Cornelisse CJ, et al. Consensus review of the clinical utility of DNA cytometry in carcinoma of the breast. *Cytometry* 1993;14:482–485.
434. O'Reilly SM, Richards MA. Is DNA flow cytometry a useful investigation in breast cancer? *Eur J Cancer* 1992;28:504–507.
435. Ellis CN, Frey ES, Burnette JJ, et al. The content of tumor DNA as an indicator of prognosis in patients with T1N0M0 and T2N0M0 carcinoma of the breast. *Surgery* 1989;106:133–138.

436. Keyhani-Rofagha S, O'Toole RV, Farrar WB, et al. Is DNA ploidy an independent prognostic indicator in infiltrative node-negative breast adenocarcinoma? *Cancer* 1990;65:1577–1582.
437. Witzig TE, Ingle JN, Cha SS, et al. DNA ploidy and the percentage of cells in S-phase as a prognostic factors for women with lymph node negative breast cancer. *Cancer* 1994;74:1752–1761.
438. Toikkanen S, Joensuu J, Klemi P. Nuclear DNA content as a prognostic factor in T1-2N0 breast cancer. *Am J Clin Pathol* 1990;93:471–479.
439. Bergers E, Baak JPA, van Diest PJ, et al. Prognostic value of DNA ploidy using flow cytometry in 1301 breast cancer patients: results of the prospective multicenter morphometric mammary carcinoma project. *Mod Pathol* 1997;10:762–768.
440. Pinto AE, Pereira T, Santos M, et al. DNA ploidy is an independent predictor of survival in breast invasive ductal carcinoma: a long-term multivariate analysis of 393 patients. *Ann Surg Oncol* 2012;20:1530–1537.
441. Bosari S, Lee AKC, Tahan SR, et al. DNA flow cytometric analysis and prognosis of axillary lymph nodes-negative breast carcinoma. *Cancer* 1992;70:1943–1950.
442. Camplejohn RS, Ash CM, Gillett CE, et al. The prognostic significance of DNA flow cytometry in breast cancer: results from 881 patients treated in a single centre. *Br J Cancer* 1995;71:140–145.
443. Clark GM, Mathieu M-C, Owens MA, et al. Prognostic significance of S-phase fraction in good-risk, node-negative breast cancer patients. *J Clin Oncol* 1992;10:428–432.
444. Haffty BG, Toth M, Flynn S, et al. Prognostic value of DNA flow cytometry in the locally recurrent, conservatively treated breast cancer patient. *J Clin Oncol* 1992;10:1839–1847.
445. Stål O, Dufmats M, Hatschek T, et al. S-Phase fraction is a prognostic factor in stage I breast carcinoma. *J Clin Oncol* 1993;11:1717–1722.
446. Stanton PD, Cooke TG, Oakes SJ, et al. Lack of prognostic significance of DNA ploidy and S phase fraction in breast cancer. *Br J Cancer* 1992;66:925–929.
447. Hietanen P, Blomqvist C, Wasenius V-M,et al. Do DNA ploidy and S-phase fraction in primary tumour predict the response to chemotherapy in metastatic breast cancer? *Br J Cancer* 1995;71:1029–1032.
448. Goodson III WH, Ljung B-M, Moore II DH, et al. Tumor labeling indices of primary breast cancers and their regional lymph node metastases. *Cancer* 1993;71:3914–3919.
449. Rew DA, Campbell ID, Taylor I, et al. Proliferation indices of invasive breast carcinomas after *in vivo* 5-bromo-2'-deoxyuridine labelling: a flow cytometric study of 75 tumours. *Br J Surg* 1992;79:335–339.
450. Weidner N, Moore II DH, Ljung B-M,et al. Correlation of bromodeoxyuridine (BRDU) labeling of breast carcinoma cells with mitotic figure content and tumor grade. *Am J Surg Pathol* 1993;17:987–994.
451. Meyer JS, Nauert J, Koehm S, et al. Cell kinetics of human tumors by *in vitro* bromodeoxyuridine labeling. *J Histochem Cytochem* 1989;37:1449–1454.
452. Thor AD, Liu S, Moore DH, et al. Comparison of mitotic index, *in vitro* bromodeoxyuridine labeling, and MIB-1 assays to quantitate proliferation in breast cancer. *J Clin Oncol* 1999;17:470–477.
453. Gratzner HG. Monoclonal antibody to 5-bromo- and 5-iododeoxyuridine: a new reagent for detection of DNA replication. *Science* 1982;218:474–475.
454. Lloveras B, Edgerton S, Thor AD. Evaluation of *in vitro* bromodeoxyuridine labeling of breast carcinomas with the use of a commercial kit. *Am J Clin Pathol* 1991;95:41–47.
455. Sasaki K, Ogino T, Takahashi M. Immunological determination of labelling index on human tumor tissue sections using monoclonal anti-BrdU antibody. *Stain Technol* 1986;61:155–161.
456. Meyer JS, Koehm SL, Hughes JM, et al. Bromodeoxyuridine labeling for S-phase measurement in breast carcinoma. *Cancer* 1993;71:3531–3540.
457. Gerdes J, Schwab U, Lemke H, et al. Production of a mouse monoclonal antibody reactive with a human nuclear antigen associated with cell proliferation. *Int J Cancer* 1983;31:13–20.
458. Gerdes J, Lemke H, Baisch H, et al. Cell cycle analysis of cell proliferation-associated human nuclear antigen defined by the monoclonal antibody Ki-67. *J Immunol* 1984;133:1710–1715.
459. Isola JJ, Helin HJ, Helle MJ, et al. Evaluation of cell proliferation in breast carcinoma. Comparison of Ki-67 immunohistochemical study, DNA flow cytometric analysis, and mitotic count. *Cancer* 1990;65:1180–1184.
460. Sahin AA, Ro JY, El-Naggar AK, et al. Tumor proliferative fraction in solid malignant neoplasms. A comparative study of Ki-67 immunostaining and flow cytometric determinations. *Am J Clin Pathol* 1991;96:512–519.
461. Vielh P, Chevillard S, Mosseri V, et al. Ki67 index and S-phase fraction in human breast carcinomas. Comparison and correlations with prognostic factors. *Am J Clin Pathol* 1990;94:681–686.
462. Urruticoechea A, Smith IE, Dowsett M. Proliferation marker Ki-67 in early breast cancer. *J Clin Oncol* 2005;23:7212–7220.
463. Kamel OW, Franklin WA, Ringus JC, et al. Thymidine labeling index and Ki-67 growth fraction in lesions of the breast. *Am J Pathol* 1989;134:107–113.
464. Sasaki K, Matsumura K, Tsuji T, et al. Relationship between labeling indices of Ki-67 and BrdU in human malignant tumors. *Cancer* 1988;62:989–993.
465. Barbareschi M, Girlando S, Mauri FM, et al. Quantitative growth fraction evaluation with MIB1 and Ki67 antibodies in breast carcinomas. *Am J Clin Pathol* 1994;102:171–175.
466. Sahin AA, Ro J, Ro JY, et al. Ki-67 immunostaining in node-negative stage I/II breast carcinoma. Significant correlation with prognosis. *Cancer* 1991;68:549–557.
467. van Dierendonck JH, Keijzer R, van de Velde CJH, et al. Nuclear distribution of the Ki-67 antigen during the cell cycle: comparison with growth fraction in human breast cancer cells. *Cancer Res* 1989;49:2999–3006.
468. Dervan PA, Magee HM, Buckley C, et al. Proliferating cell nuclear antigen counts in formalin-fixed paraffin-embedded tissue correlate with Ki-67 in fresh tissue. *Am J Clin Pathol* 1992;97(Suppl.1): S21–S28.
469. Raymond WA, Leong AS-Y. Nuclear organizer regions relate to growth fractions in human breast carcinoma. *Hum Pathol* 1989;20:741–746.
470. Gerdes J, Lelle RJ, Pickartz H, et al. Growth fractions in breast cancers determined in situ with monoclonal antibody Ki-67. *J Clin Path* 1986;39:977–980.
471. Aleskandarany MA, Rakha EA, Macmillan RD, et al. MIB1/Ki-67 labelling index can classify grade 2 breast cancer into two clinically distinct subgroups. *Breast Cancer Res Treat* 2011;127:591–599.
472. Goldhirsch A, Ingle JN, Gelber RD, et al. Thresholds for therapies: highlights of the St Gallen International Expert Consensus on the primary therapy of early breast cancer 2009. *Ann Oncol* 2009;20:1319–1329.
473. Kuenen-Boumeester V, Van Der Kwast ThH, van Laarhoven HAJ, et al. Ki-67 staining in histologic subtypes of breast carcinoma and fine needle aspiration smears. *J Clin Pathol* 1991;44:208–210.
474. Munzone E, Botteri E, Sciandivasci A, et al. Prognostic value of Ki-67 labeling index in patients with node-negative, triple-negative breast cancer. *Breast Cancer Res Treat* 2012;134:277–282.
475. Trihia H, Murray S, Price K. Ki-67 expression in breast carcinoma. Its association with grading systems, clinical parameters, and other prognostic factors—a surrogate marker? *Cancer* 2003;97:1321–1331.
476. Veronese SM, Gambacorta M. Detection of Ki-67 proliferation rate in breast cancer. Correlation with clinical and pathologic features. *Am J Clin Pathol* 1991;95:30–34.
477. Bouzubar N, Walker KJ, Griffiths K, et al. Ki67 immunostaining in primary breast cancer: pathological and clinical associations. *Br J Cancer* 1989;59:943–947.
478. Lelle RJ, Heidenreich W, Stauch G, et al. The correlation of growth fractions with histologic grading and lymph node status in human mammary carcinoma. *Cancer* 1987;59:83–88.
479. Weikel W, Beck T, Mitze M, et al. Immunohistochemical evaluation of growth fractions in human breast cancers using monoclonal antibody Ki-67. *Breast Cancer Res Treat* 1991;18:149–154.
480. Pierga J-Y, Leroyer A, Viehl P, et al. Long term prognostic value of growth fraction determination by Ki-67 immunostaining in primary operable breast cancer. *Breast Cancer Res Treat* 1996;37:57–64.
481. Porter PL, El-Bastawissi AY, Mandelson MT, et al. Breast tumor characteristics as predictors of mammographic detection: comparison of interval- and screen-detected cancers. *J Natl Cancer Inst* 1999;91: 2020–2028.
482. Cattoretti G, Becker MH, Key G, et al. Monoclonal antibodies against recombinant parts of the Ki-67 antigen (MIB 1 and MIB 3) detect proliferating cells in microwave-processed formalin-fixed paraffin sections. *J Pathol* 1992;168:357–363.
483. McCormick D, Chong H, Hobbs C, et al. Detection of the Ki-67 antigen in fixed and wax-embedded sections with the monoclonal antibody MIB1. *Histopathology* 1993;22:355–360.

484. Remmele W, Mühlfait V, Keul HG. Estimation of the proliferative activity of human breast cancer tissue by means of the Ki-67 and MIB-1 antibodies—comparative studies on frozen and paraffin sections. *Virchows Arch* 1995;426:435–439.
485. Keshgegian AA, Cnaan A. Proliferation markers in breast carcinoma. Mitotic figure count, S-phase fraction, proliferating cell nuclear antigen, Ki-67 and MIB1. *Am J Clin Pathol* 1995;104:42–49.
486. Pinder SE, Wencyk P, Sibbering DM, et al. Assessment of the new proliferation marker MIB1 in breast carcinoma using image analysis: associations with other prognostic factors and survival. *Br J Cancer* 1995;71:146–149.
487. Arber JM, Riggs MW, Arber DA. Correlation among MIB-1, paraffin section proliferation index, and recurrence in low stage breast carcinoma. *Appl Immunohistochem* 1997;5:117–124.
488. Visscher DW, Wykes S, Kubus J, et al. Comparison of PCNA/cyclin immunohistochemistry with flow cytometric S-phase fraction in breast cancer. *Breast Cancer Res Treat* 1992;22:111–118.
489. Frierson HF Jr. Immunohistochemical analysis of proliferating cell nuclear antigen (PCNA) in infiltrating ductal carcinomas: comparison with clinical and pathologic variable. *Mod Pathol* 1993;6:290–294.
490. Tahan SR, Neuberg DS, Dieffenbach A, et al. Prediction of early relapse and shortened survival in patients with breast cancer by proliferating cell nuclear antigen score. *Cancer* 1993;71:3552–3559.
491. Haerslev T, Jacobsen GK, Zedeler K. Correlation of growth fraction by Ki-67 and proliferating cell nuclear antigen (PCNA) immunohistochemistry with histopathological parameters and prognosis in primary breast carcinomas. *Breast Cancer Res Treat* 1996;37:101–113.
492. Clark GM, Allred DC, Hilsenbeck SG, et al. Mitosin (a new proliferation marker) correlates with clinical outcome in node-negative breast cancer. *Cancer Res* 1997;57:5505–5508.
493. Baak JPA, VanDop H, Kurver PHJ, et al. The value of morphometry to classic prognosticators in breast cancer. *Cancer* 1985;56:374–382.
494. Abdalla F, Boder J, Markus R, et al. Correlation of nuclear morphometry of breast cancer in histological sections with clinicopathological features and prognosis. *Anticancer Res* 2009;29:1771–1776.
495. Kuenen-Boumeester V, Hop WCJ, Blonk DE, et al. Prognostic scoring using cytomorphometry and lymph node status of patients with breast carcinoma. *Eur J Cancer Clin Oncol* 1984;20:337–345.
496. Stenkvist B, Bengtsson E, Eriksson O, et al. Correlation between cytometric features and mitotic frequency in human breast carcinoma. *Cytometry* 1981;1:287–291.
497. Zajdela A, DeLaRiva LS, Ghossein NA. The relation of prognosis to the nuclear diameter of breast cancer cells obtained by cytologic aspiration. *Acta Cytol* 1979;23:75–80.
498. Maehle B, Thoresen S, Skjaerve R, et al. Mean nuclear area and histological grade of axillary node tumor in breast cancer. Relation to prognosis. *Br J Cancer* 1982;46:95–100.
499. van der Linden HC, Baak JPA, Lindeman J, et al. Morphometry and breast cancer. II. Characterization of breast cancer cells with high malignant potential in patients with spread to lymph nodes: preliminary results. *J Clin Pathol* 1986;39:603–609.
500. Gusterson BA, Ross DT, Heath VJ, et al. Basal cytokeratins and their relationship to the cellular origin and functional classification of breast cancer. *Breast Cancer Res* 2005;7:143–148.
501. Dewar R, Fadare O, Gilmore H, et al. Best practices in diagnostic immunohistochemistry: myoepithelial markers in breast pathology. *Arch Pathol Lab Med* 2011;135:422–429.
502. Rakha EA, Elsheikh SE, Aleskandarany MA, et al. Triple-negative breast cancer: distinguishing between basal and nonbasal subtypes. *Clin Cancer Res* 2009;15:2302–2310.
503. Badve S, Dabbs DJ, Schnitt SJ, et al. Basal-like and triple-negative breast cancers: a critical review with an emphasis on the implications for pathologists and oncologists. *Mod Pathol* 2011;24:157–167.
504. Thike AA, Iqbal J, Cheok PY, et al. Ductal carcinoma *in situ* associated with triple negative invasive breast cancer: evidence for a precursor-product relationship. *J Clin Pathol* 2013;66:665–670.
505. Bonzanini M, Morelli L, Bonandini EM, et al. Cytologic features of triple-negative breast carcinoma. *Cancer Cytopathol* 2012;120:401–409.
506. El-Rehim DMA, Pinder SE, Paish CE, et al. Expression of luminal and basal cytokeratins in human breast carcinoma. *J Pathol* 2004;203:661–671.
507. Bryan BB, Schnitt SJ, Collins LC. Ductal carcinomas *in situ* with basal-like phenotype: a possible precursor to invasive basal-like cancer. *Mod Pathol* 2006;19:617–621.
508. Sorlie T, Perou CM, Tibshirani R, et al. Gene expression pattern of breast carcinoma distinguishing tumor subclasses with clinical implications. *Proc Natl Acad Sci USA* 2001;98:10869–10874.
509. Foulkes WD, Stefansson IM, Chappnis PO, et al. Germline BRCA1 mutations and a basal phenotype in breast cancer. *J Natl Cancer Inst* 2003;95:1482–1485.
510. Laakso M, Loman N, Borg A, et al. Cytokeratin 5/14-positive breast cancer: true basal phenotype confined to BRCA1 tumors. *Mod Pathol* 2005;18:1321–1328.
511. Fulford LG, Easton DF, Reis-Filho JS, et al. Specific morphological features predictive for the basal phenotype in grade 3 invasive ductal carcinoma of breast. *Histopathology* 2006;49:22–34.
512. Korsching E, Packeisen J, Agelopoulos K, et al. Cytogenetic alterations and cytokeratin expression patterns in breast cancer: integrating a new model of breast differentiation into cytogenetic pathways of breast carcinogenesis. *Lab Invest* 2002;82:1525–1533.
513. Nielsen TO, Hsu FD, Jensen K, et al. Immunohistochemical and clinical characterization of the basal-like subtype of invasive breast carcinoma. *Clin Cancer Res* 2004;10:5367–5374.
514. Dairkee SH, Mayall BH, Smith HS, et al. Monoclonal marker that predicts early recurrence of breast cancer. *Lancet* 1987;1:514.
515. Banerjee S, Reis-Filho JS, Ashley S, et al. Basal-like breast carcinomas: clinical outcome and response to chemotherapy. *J Clin Pathol* 2006;59:729–735.
516. Carey LA, Dees EC, Sawyer LR, et al. The triple negative paradox: primary tumor chemosensitivity of the basal-like breast cancer phenotype. *Breast Cancer Res Treat* 2004;80:1023.
517. Rouzier R, Perou CM, Symmons WF, et al. Breast cancer molecular subtypes respond differently to perioperative chemotherapy. *Clin Cancer Res* 2005;11:5678–5685.
518. Haffty BG, Yang Q, Reiss M, et al. Local-regional relapse and distant metastasis in conservatively managed triple negative early stage breast cancer. *J Clin Oncol* 2006;24:265.
519. Rakha EA, Ellis IO. Modern classification of breast cancer: should we stick with morphology or convert to molecular profile characteristics. *Adv Anat Pathol* 2011;18:255–267.
520. Weigelt B, Reis-Filho JS. Molecular profiling currently offers no more than tumour morphology and basic immunohistochemistry. *Breast Cancer Res* 2010;12(Suppl. 4):S5.
521. Hammond ME, Hayes DF, Dowsett M, et al. American Society of Clinical Oncology/College Of American Pathologists guideline recommendations for immunohistochemical testing of estrogen and progesterone receptors in breastcancer. *J Clin Oncol* 2010;28:2784–2795.
522. Dressman MA, Walz TM, Lavedan C, et al. Genes that co-cluster with estrogen receptor alpha in microarray analysis of breast biopsies. *Pharmacogenomics J* 2001;1:135–141.
523. Shaaban AM, O'Neill PA, Davies MP, et al. Declining estrogen receptor-beta expression defines malignant progression of human breast neoplasia. *Am J Surg Pathol* 2003;27:1502–1512.
524. Anderson WF, Chatterjee N, Ershler WB, et al. Estrogen receptor breast cancer phenotypes in the surveillance, epidemiology, and end results database. *Breast Cancer Res Treat* 2002;76:27–36.
525. Clark GM, Osborne CK, McGuire WL. Correlations between estrogen receptor, progesterone receptor, and patient characteristics in human breast cancer. *J Clin Oncol* 1984;2:1102–1109.
526. Chu KC, Anderson WF. Rates for breast cancer characteristics by estrogen and progesterone receptor status in the major racial/ethnic groups. *Breast Cancer Res Treat* 2002;74:199–211.
527. Joslyn SA. Hormone receptors in breast cancer: racial differences in distribution and survival. *Breast Cancer Res Treat* 2002;73:45–59.
528. Ernst MF, Roukema JA, Coebergh JW, et al. Breast cancers found by screening: earlier detection, lower malignant potential or both? *Breast Cancer Res Treat* 2002;76:19–25.
529. Muir D, Kanthan R, Kanthan SC. Male versus female breast cancers. A population-based comparative immunohistochemical analysis. *Arch Pathol Lab Med* 2003;127:36–41.
530. Sui M, Huang Y, Park BH, et al. Estrogen receptor alpha mediates breast cancer cell resistance to paclitaxel through inhibition of apoptotic cell death. *Cancer Res* 2007;67:5337–5344.
531. Crowe JP, Hubay CA, Pearson OH, et al. Estrogen receptor status as a prognostic indicator for stage I breast cancer patients. *Breast Cancer Res Treat* 1982;2:171–176.
532. Fisher B, Redmond C, Fisher ER, et al. Relative worth of estrogen or progesterone receptor and pathologic characteristics of differentiation

as indicators of prognosis in node negative breast cancer patients: findings from National Surgical Adjuvant Breast and Bowel Project Protocol B-06. *J Clin Oncol* 1988;6:1076–1087.
533. Bardou VJ, Arpino G, Elledge RM, et al. Progesterone receptor status significantly improves outcome prediction over estrogen receptor status alone for adjuvant endocrine therapy in two large breast cancer databases. *J Clin Oncol* 2003;21:1973–1979.
534. Creighton CJ, Kent Osborne C, van de Vijver MJ, et al. Molecular profiles of progesterone receptor loss in human breast tumors. *Breast Cancer Res Treat* 2009;114:287–299.
535. Dowsett M, Houghton J, Iden C, et al. Benefit from adjuvant tamoxifen therapy in primary breast cancer patients according oestrogen receptor, progesterone receptor, EGF receptor and HER2 status. *Ann Oncol* 2006;17:818–826.
536. Schmidt M, Bremer E, Hasenclever D, et al. Role of the progesterone receptor for paclitaxel resistance in primary breast cancer. *Br J Cancer* 2007;96:241–247.
537. Arpino G, Weiss H, Lee AV, et al. Estrogen receptor-positive, progesterone receptor-negative breast cancer: association with growth factor receptor expression and tamoxifen resistance. *J Natl Cancer Inst* 2005;97:1254–1261.
538. Gown AM. Current issues in ER and HER2 testing by IHC in breast cancer. *Mod Pathol* 2008;21(Suppl. 2):S8–S15.
539. Yaziji H, Taylor CR, Goldstein NS, et al. Consensus recommendations on estrogen receptor testing in breast cancer by immunohistochemistry. *Appl Immunohistochem Mol Morphol* 2008;16:513–520.
540. Harvey JM, Clark GM, Osborne CK, et al. Estrogen receptor status by immunohistochemistry is superior to the ligand-binding assay for predicting response to adjuvant endocrine therapy in breast cancer. *J Clin Oncol* 1999;17:1474–1481.
541. Mohsin SK, Weiss H, Havighurst T, et al. Progesterone receptor by immunohistochemistry and clinical outcome in breast cancer: a validation study. *Mod Pathol* 2004;17:1545–1554.
542. Rimm DL, Giltnane JM, Moeder C, et al. Bimodal population or pathologist artifact? *J Clin Oncol* 2007;25:2487–2488.
543. Collins LC, Botero ML, Schnitt SJ. Bimodal frequency distribution of estrogen receptor immunohistochemical staining results in breast cancer: an analysis of 825 cases. *Am J Clin Pathol* 2005;123:16–20.
544. Nadji M, Gomez-Fernandez C, Ganjei-Azar P, et al. Immunohistochemistry of estrogen and progesterone receptors reconsidered: experience with 5,993 breast cancers. *Am J Clin Pathol* 2005;123:21–27.
545. Leake R, Barnes D, Pinder S, et al. Immunohistochemical detection of steroid receptors in breast cancer: a working protocol. UK Receptor Group, UK NEQAS, The Scottish Breast Cancer Pathology Group, and The Receptor and Biomarker Study Group of the EORTC. *J Clin Pathol* 2000;53:634–735.
546. McCarty KS Jr, Miller LS, Cox EB, et al. Estrogen receptor analyses. Correlation of biochemical and immunohistochemical methods using monoclonal antireceptor antibodies. *Arch Pathol Lab Med* 1985;109:716–721.
547. Shousha S. Oestrogen receptor status of breast carcinoma: Allred/H score conversion table. *Histopathology* 2008;53:346–347.
548. Cohen DA, Dabbs DJ, Cooper KL, et al. Interobserver agreement among pathologists for semiquantitative hormone receptor scoring in breast carcinoma. *Am J Clin Pathol* 2012;138:796–802.
549. Spataro V, Price K, Goldhirsch A, et al. Sequential estrogen receptor determinations from primary breast cancer and at relapse: prognostic and therapeutic relevance. The International Breast Cancer Study Group (formerly Ludwig Group). *Ann Oncol* 1992;3:733–740.
550. Branković-Magić M, Janković R, Nesković-Konstantinović Z, et al. Progesterone receptor status of breast cancer metastases. *J Cancer Res Clin Oncol* 2002;128:55–60.
551. Hull DF III, Clark GM, Osborne CK, et al. Multiple estrogen receptor assays in human breast cancer. *Cancer Res* 198;43:413–416.
552. Munzone E, Curigliano G, Rocca A, et al. Reverting estrogen-receptor-negative phenotype in HER-2-overexpressing advanced breast cancer patients exposed to trastuzumab plus chemotherapy. *Breast Cancer Res* 2006;8:R4.
553. Kuukasjärvi T, Kononen J, Helin H, et al. Loss of estrogen receptor in recurrent breast cancer is associated with poor response to endocrine therapy. *J Clin Oncol* 1996;14:2584–2589.
554. http://www.cap.org/apps/docs/committees/cancer/cancer_protocols/2012/BreastDCIS_12protocol_3100.pdf. Accessed April 9, 2013.
555. Houghton J, George WD, Cuzick J, et al. Radiotherapy and tamoxifen in women with completely excised ductal carcinoma *in situ* of the breast in the UK, Australia, and New Zealand: randomised controlled trial. *Lancet* 2003;362:95–102.
556. Fisher B, Land S, Mamounas E, et al. Prevention of invasive breast cancer in women with ductal carcinoma *in situ*: an update of the National Surgical Adjuvant Breast and Bowel Project experience. *Semin Oncol* 2001;28:400–418.
557. Fisher B, Dignam J, Wolmark N, et al. Tamoxifen in treatment of intraductal breast cancer: National Surgical Adjuvant Breast and Bowel Project B-24 randomised controlled trial. *Lancet* 1999;353:1993–2000.
558. Oh DS, Troester MA, Usary J, et al. Estrogen-regulated genes predict survival in hormone receptor-positive breast cancers. *J Clin Oncol* 2006;24:1656–1664.
559. Abba MC, Hu Y, Sun H, et al. Gene expression signature of estrogen receptor alpha status in breast cancer. *BMC Genomics* 2005;6:37.
560. Badve SS, Baehner FL, Gray RP, et al. Estrogen- and progesterone-receptor status in ECOG 2197: comparison of immunohistochemistry by local and central laboratories and quantitative reverse transcription polymerase chain reaction by central laboratory. *J Clin Oncol* 2008;26:2473–2481.
561. Wolff AC, Hammond ME, Hicks DG, et al. Recommendations for human epidermal growth factor receptor 2 testing in breast cancer: ASCO/CAP clinical practice guideline update [published online ahead of print October 7, 2013]. *J Clin Oncol*. PubMed PMID: 24101045.
562. Slamon DJ, Clark GM, Wong SG, et al. Human breast cancer: correlation of relapse and survival with amplification of the HER-2/neu oncogene. *Science* 1987;235:177–182.
563. Slamon DJ, Godolphin W, Jones LA, et al. Studies of the HER-2/neu proto-oncogene in human breast and ovarian cancer. *Science* 1989;244:707–712.
564. Kallioniemi OP, Holli K, Visakorpi T, et al. Association of c-erbB-2 protein over-expression with high rate of cell proliferation, increased risk of visceral metastasis and poor long-term survival in breast cancer. *Int J Cancer* 1991;49:650–655.
565. Muss HB, Thor AD, Berry DA, et al. c-erbB-2 Expression and response to adjuvant therapy in women with node-positive early breast cancer. *N Engl J Med* 1994;330:1260–1266.
566. Hayes DF, Thor AD, Dressler LG, et al. HER2 and response to paclitaxel in node-positive breast cancer. *N Engl J Med* 2007;357:1496–1506.
567. Vance GH, Barry TS, Bloom KJ, et al. Genetic heterogeneity in HER2 testing in breast cancer: panel summary and guidelines. *Arch Pathol Lab Med* 2009;133:611–612.
568. Lal P, Salazar PA, Ladanyi M, et al. Impact of polysomy 17 on HER-2/neu immunohistochemistry in breast carcinomas without HER-2/neu gene amplification. *J Mol Diagn* 2003;5:155–159.
569. Ma Y, Lespagnard L, Durbecq V, et al. Polysomy 17 in HER-2/neu status elaboration in breast cancer: effect on daily practice. *Clin Cancer Res* 2005;11:4393–4399.
570. Tapia C, Savic S, Wagner U, et al. HER2 gene status in primary breast cancers and matched distant metastases. *Breast Cancer Res* 2007;9:R31.
571. Lower EE, Glass E, Blau R, Harman S. HER-2/neu expression in primary and metastatic breast cancer. *Breast Cancer Res Treat* 2009;113:301–306.

CHAPTER 13

Tubular Carcinoma

EDI BROGI

Tubular carcinoma is a distinct type of mammary carcinoma, first recognized nearly 150 years ago.[1] The term "tubular" refers to the unique morphology of this tumor, which consists of simple neoplastic tubules lined by a single layer of cells with a structure that closely resembles normal mammary ductules.[2,3]

Pure tubular carcinoma constitutes less than 2% of all breast carcinomas.[4–11] It tends to have small size and is relatively more frequent among T1 tumors. In one series, 5% of 382 T1N0M0 breast carcinomas were tubular.[12] When further stratified by size, tubular carcinomas represented 9% of lesions 1.0 cm or smaller versus only 2% of carcinomas spanning 1.1 to 2.0 cm.[12] Liu et al.[13] reported that 97% of 71 tubular carcinomas were smaller than 2 cm (pT1). In a series by Rakha et al.,[14] 59% of 102 tubular carcinomas were smaller than 1 cm, 37% measured 1 to 2 cm, and only 4% were larger than 2 cm.

CLINICAL PRESENTATION

Imaging

Tubular carcinomas are often nonpalpable and are usually detected mammographically as irregular mass lesions. The conclusion that screening mammography has resulted in an increase in the frequency of this type of carcinoma being diagnosed is supported by many studies. Tubular carcinomas constituted 8% of invasive carcinomas spanning 1.0 cm or less detected in the Breast Cancer Detection Demonstration Projects.[15] In one U.S. screening program, tubular carcinomas were 7% of 138 breast cancers; all tubular carcinomas were detected by mammography, but only 30% of them were evident clinically.[16] A study correlating breast carcinoma histology and method of detection found that 83% of 41 tubular carcinomas had been detected mammographically, 12% were self-detected by the patient, and only 5% were found at clinical examination.[17] Louwman et al.[10] reviewed data for Dutch women aged 50 to 64 years with breast carcinoma diagnosed between 1988 and 2004. They found that tubular carcinoma constituted 8% of 9,259 screen-detected carcinomas, 2% of 5,413 interval carcinomas, and 2.1% of 6,710 carcinomas in women who did not undergo screening mammography. Similar results were obtained in Great Britain, where Nagtegaal et al.[18] found that tubular carcinomas were 8.4% of screen-detected carcinomas, 2% of interval carcinomas, and 2.1% of carcinomas in women not participating in a mammographic screening program, respectively.

Mammographic findings can be suggestive of tubular carcinoma, but are not specific. The radiologic differential diagnosis of tubular carcinoma includes benign sclerosing lesions such as radial scar or sclerosing adenosis (SA), as well as well-differentiated invasive duct carcinoma. In one study, the average radiographic size of nonpalpable tubular carcinomas was 0.8 cm and that of palpable lesions 1.2 cm.[19] Most tubular carcinomas are spiculated (Fig. 13.1), and they often harbor calcifications.[20] Rounded lesions, densities with indistinct borders or calcifications in the absence of a mass rarely prove to be tubular carcinoma. Radiologically, tubular carcinoma and radial scar are nearly indistinguishable, as both lesions have similar growth patterns and tubular carcinoma can arise in a radial scar.[21,22] Ultrasonography is also helpful in detecting tubular carcinoma, especially small lesions that are inapparent mammographically.[23] No features specific for tubular carcinoma have been reported in magnetic resonance imaging studies.

Age

Among women, the age at diagnosis of tubular carcinoma ranges from 24 to 92 years.[7,8,10,13,14,24–28] In one series,[27] 75% of tumors were diagnosed in women between ages 50 and 79 years. A study based on Surveillance Epidemiology and End Results (SEER) data for breast carcinomas reported that 73.6% of 4,477 tubular carcinomas diagnosed in the United States from 1992 and 2007 occurred in women 50 to 79 years old, 17.5% in women 40 to 49 years old, 6.9% in women older than 80 years, and only 2% in women 30 to 39 years old.[11] Tubular carcinoma of the male breast has been reported,[24,25,29] but this tumor constitutes less than 1% of male breast carcinomas.[30,31]

Family History

Tubular carcinoma was associated with a 40% frequency of positive family history of breast carcinoma among first-degree relatives in one study.[32] This association may reflect selective factors related to the specific population studied, which included many women who had mammography performed because they had a positive family history. Others have not found a disproportionately high frequency of positive family history among relatives of women treated for tubular carcinoma.

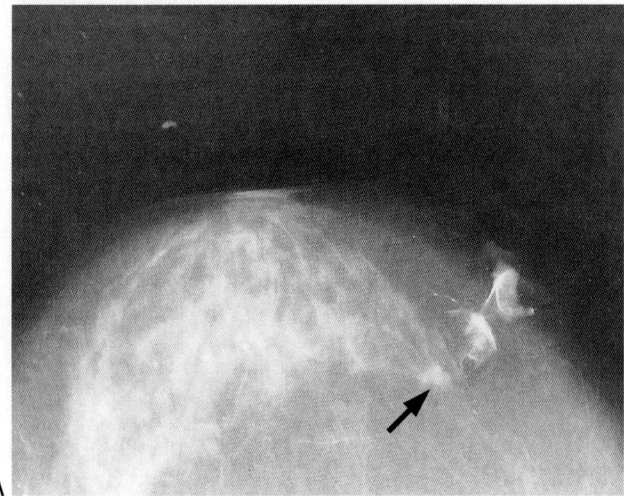

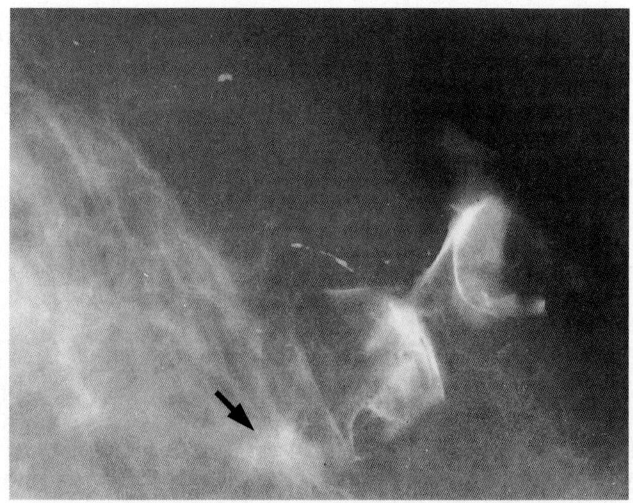

FIG. 13.1. ***Tubular carcinoma, radiology.*** **A:** A mammogram showing a nonpalpable tumor near the right border (*arrow*) of the breast parenchyma. **B:** Magnified view of the stellate carcinoma near the lower border (*arrow*) of the image and two wisps of dye injected for surgical localization.

Ethnicity and Menstrual Status

In a multicenter population-based case-control study conducted in five metropolitan areas of the United States, 80.5% of tubular carcinomas occurred in Caucasian/White women,[33] and an epidemiologic study based on SEER data reported that 90% of patients with tubular carcinomas were non–Hispanic White women.[11] The remaining patients were almost equally distributed, respectively, among women of African American (3.6%), Asian/Pacific Islander (3.5%), Hispanic White (2.3%), and American Indian/Alaska Native (0.5%) race or ethnicity.[11]

A family history of breast carcinoma in a first-degree relative tripled the risk of tubular carcinoma in premenopausal women, but was not significantly related to the occurrence of tubular carcinoma in postmenopausal patients.[33] At least two studies have reported a two- to threefold increase in the risk of having tubular carcinoma in postmenopausal women who used hormone replacement therapy.[33,34]

Clinical Duration and Position in the Breast

Occasionally, a palpable lesion has reportedly been present for a substantial period before biopsy, or a relatively long duration can be established by retrospective review of mammograms, but the median duration prior to histologic diagnosis is about 2 months.[24–26]

Rarely, superficial tumors may be fixed to the skin, producing retraction signs. Tubular carcinoma usually occurs in peripheral portions of the breast, and nipple discharge is an infrequent presenting symptom.[7] However, tubular carcinoma can arise near the major lactiferous ducts in the nipple or slightly lower in the subareolar region and raise the differential diagnosis of florid papillomatosis of the nipple. In this setting, the finding of Paget disease supports the diagnosis of tubular carcinoma (Fig. 13.2). Paget disease is very rarely found in association with tubular carcinoma not involving the nipple, except when coexistent DCIS separately involves the latter.

Stage and Lymph Node Metastases

A compilation of Netherlands registry data found that 70% of 3,456 patients with tubular carcinoma presented at stage I, 26% as stage II, 2% as stage III, and 1% as stage IV.[10] According to SEER data, 90.5% of women diagnosed with tubular carcinoma presented at stage I, 8.9% at stage II, 0.4% at stage III, and 0.2% at stage IV.[11]

The average frequency of axillary lymph node (ALN) metastases resulting from tubular carcinoma is about 10%,[4,7,12,24–26,35–40] ranging from none[7,35] to 29%.[21] A meta-analysis of 680 patients in published reports found axillary nodal metastases in 6.6% of those with pure tubular carcinoma and in 25% with "mixed" tubular carcinoma.[41] Tubular carcinomas were only 1.5% of all carcinomas in a series of 142 patients with T1N1M0 disease.[15]

Affected lymph nodes are usually in the low axilla (level I), and only exceptionally are more than three lymph nodes involved.[24] Fedko et al.[42] found lymph node metastases in 5 (5.4%) of 93 patients with pure tubular carcinoma and known lymph node status: 2 patients had macrometastases, and the other 3 had micrometastases. Two additional patients had lymph nodes occupied by isolated tumor cells (N0(i+)).[42] The size of the primary tumor ranged from 0.9 to 1.5 cm. Bradford et al.[40] reported that 13.3% of patients with tubular carcinoma 1 cm or larger had axillary nodal metastases. On the other hand, Green et al.[37] reported that three tubular carcinomas with nodal metastases were smaller than 1 cm, including one 0.4-mm lesion. In a retrospective analysis of sentinel lymph node (SLN) biopsy in 234 patients with tubular carcinoma treated at nine different French institutions,[43] the procedure successfully identified one or more lymph nodes in 229/234 (98%) cases. Pathologic evaluation

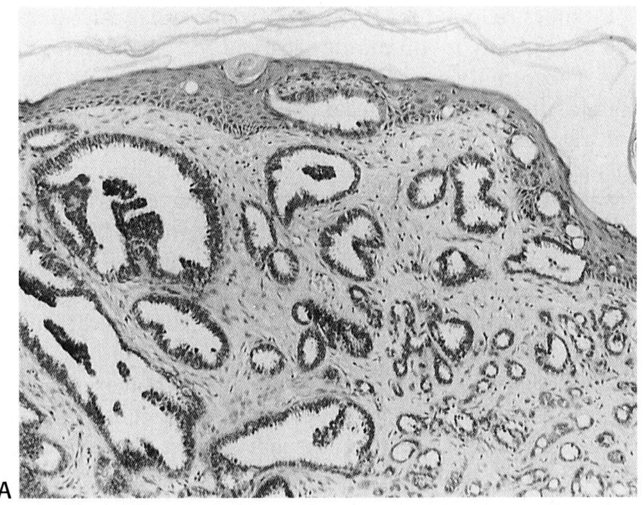

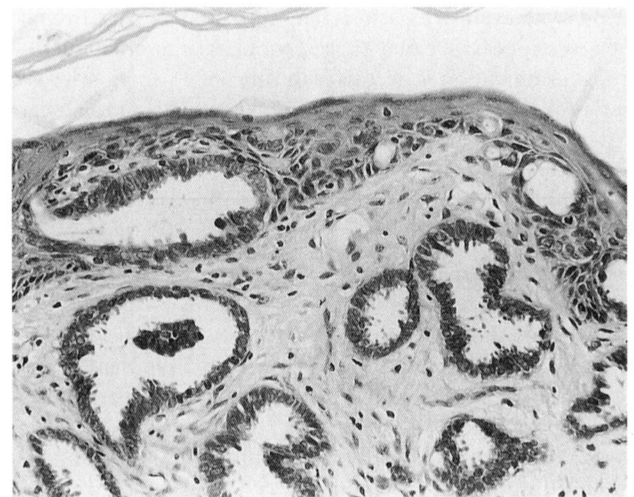

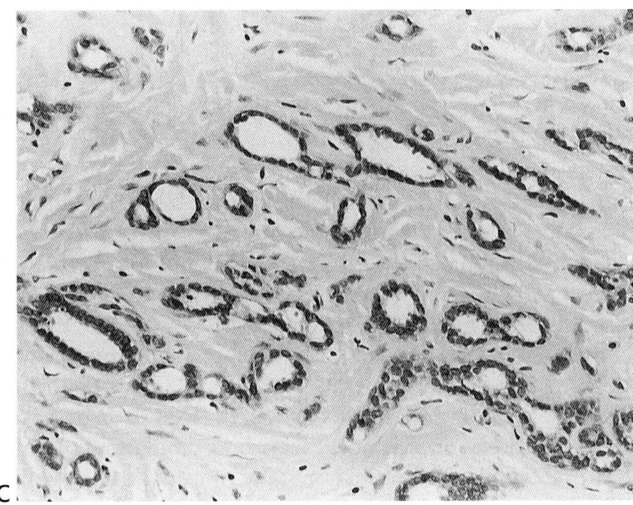

FIG. 13.2. ***Tubular carcinoma in the nipple.*** **A:** Invasive glands of tubular carcinoma in the nipple extending to the epidermis. **B:** Paget disease composed of tubular carcinoma glands. **C:** Typical carcinomatous glandular units of the type seen in the *lower right-hand corner* of **(A)**.

of SLNs included routine stained sections and cytokeratin stains at three levels. Six of 234 (2.5%) patients had macrometastases, 15/234 (6.4%) had micrometastases, and 2/234 (0.8%) had isolated tumor cells (N0(i+)). The median size of the tubular carcinomas was 9.59 mm (range, 1 to 22). The median size of tumors with SLN metastases (either macro- or micrometastases) was 12.17 versus 9.39 mm for tumors without lymph node metastases ($p = 0.005$). On multivariate analysis, pathologic tumor size greater than 10 mm was the only parameter significantly associated with lymph node metastases ($p = 0.007$). In this study, all patients with macrometastatic carcinoma had a tumor greater than 1 cm.

GROSS PATHOLOGY

Grossly, tubular carcinoma forms an ill-defined firm to hard mass. When bisected, the lesion is often stellate and infiltrating, and the cut surface is likely to retract, becoming depressed in relation to the surrounding nonneoplastic tissue (Fig. 13.3). Most tumors are described as gray to white, but

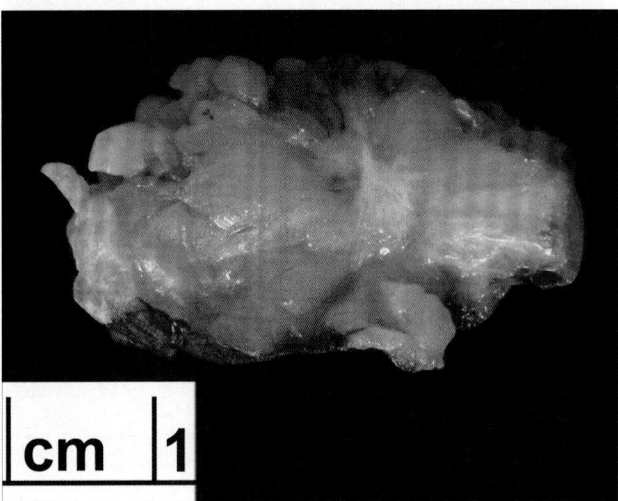

FIG. 13.3. ***Tubular carcinoma, gross pathology.*** The cut surface of a small tubular carcinoma has stellate appearance. It is slightly retracted and depressed in relation to the surrounding nonneoplastic tissue.

lesions with extensive elastosis may appear tan or pale. Even if the gross appearance may suggest tubular carcinoma, microscopic examination is necessary to rule out a benign sclerosing lesion such as sclerosing papillomatosis with a radial scar pattern or an invasive ductal carcinoma of no special type.

Size

Most tubular carcinomas are 2 cm or less in diameter, but tumors as large as 4 cm have been described,[4,6,7,24–26,44] and in one study the largest tumor spanned 12 cm.[45] In some instances, tumors reported to be larger than 5 cm may be examples of coalescent multifocal lesions. Some investigators have reported that 67%[27] to 87%[24] of tubular carcinomas were 1 cm or smaller. In the latter study,[24] the median size of 90 "pure" tubular carcinomas was 0.8 cm. Fifty-two percent of ductal carcinomas with tubular features were 1 cm or less. The median size of mixed duct and tubular lesions was 1.1 cm.[24]

MICROSCOPIC PATHOLOGY

Microscopically, tubular carcinoma consists of a haphazard proliferation of small glands and tubules. The overall configuration tends to be stellate with ill-defined borders. Most of the glands and tubules are simple and lined by a single layer of neoplastic epithelium. "Tubularity" of a carcinoma can be expressed as the percentage of all tumor cells that directly line the lumens of the neoplastic glands.[46] The diagnosis of tubular carcinoma is made when either the entire tumor or nearly all of it exhibits tubular growth pattern. Although there is no agreement on the lowest percentage of tubules required for the diagnosis of tubular carcinoma, 90% tubularity is commonly regarded as a "practical" cutoff. Focal multilayering of the epithelium or a more complex architecture are features compatible with the diagnosis of tubular carcinoma only if limited to a minority of the glands. When a tubular component involves less than 90% of a carcinoma, the lesion is often referred to as a "mixed" tubular carcinoma or ductal carcinoma with tubular features. These tumors form a very heterogeneous group with respect to the proportion of the tubular component and also in regard to the degree of differentiation of the nontubular element.

The glands of tubular carcinoma may have virtually any shape, but irregular shapes and angular contours predominate (Fig. 13.4). They usually have a widely patent lumen that is best appreciated at low-power examination. The neoplastic epithelium is cuboidal or columnar and has round to oval nuclei that tend to be basally oriented and show low-grade atypia. The neoplastic cells are usually homogeneous within a given lesion, but scattered glands show some variation in the height of the lining epithelium, with nearly flat epithelium adjacent to elongated columnar cells (Fig. 13.5). The cytoplasm is usually amphophilic or infrequently clear. It is commonly quite abundant, but can be scant. Cytoplasmic tufts or "snouts" are often present at the luminal cell border (Fig. 13.5). Eosinophilic cytoplasm and apical intracytoplasmic granules characteristic of apocrine differentiation are infrequent in a pure tubular carcinoma. Nucleoli are inconspicuous or inapparent, often somewhat peripheral in the nucleus and adjacent to the nuclear membrane. Mitoses are rarely seen, and necrosis is absent. Very uncommon variants of tubular carcinoma feature mucin secretion or apocrine differentiation[47] (Fig.13.6).

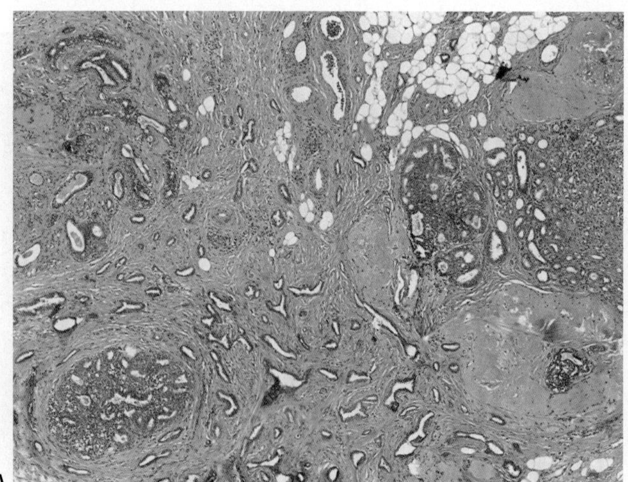

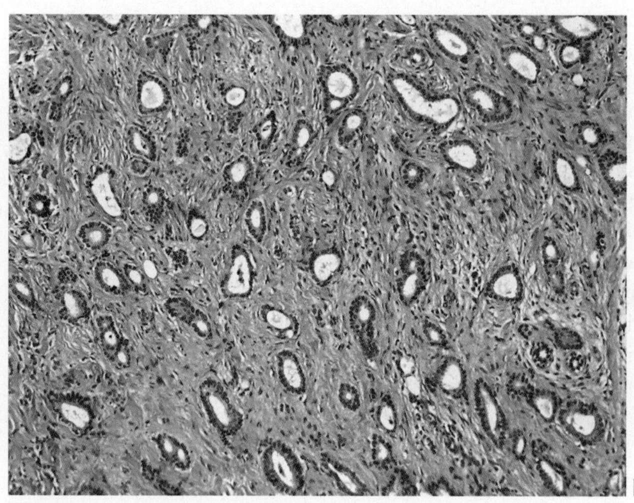

FIG. 13.4. ***Tubular carcinoma, various glandular patterns.*** **A:** Medium-power view of tubular carcinoma infiltrating between lobules involved by SA. The neoplastic glands have open lumens, in contrast to the compressed lumens of the tubules of SA. **B:** Oval and angular glands in moderately cellular stroma. **C:** Predominantly angular glands in core biopsy material. **D:** Round glands. This pattern resembles MGA.

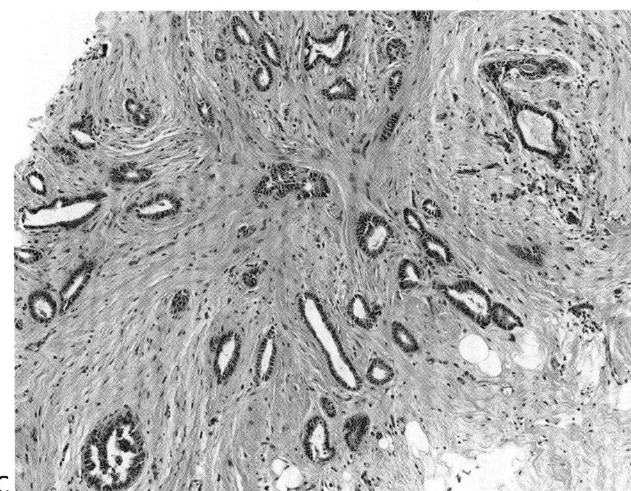

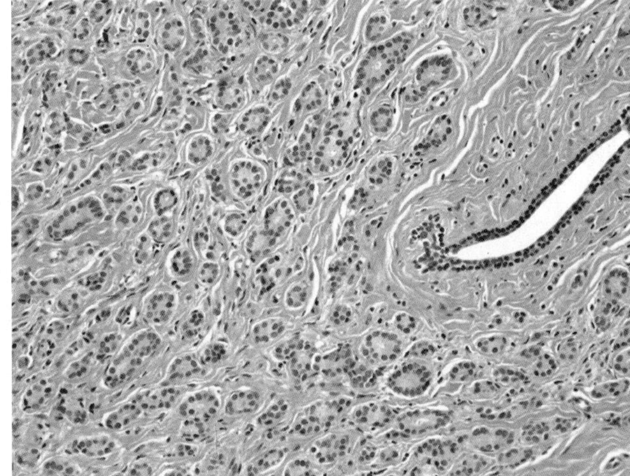

FIG. 13.4. *(Continued)*

The stroma between the glands of tubular carcinoma often differs from the stroma in the surrounding nonneoplastic breast tissue, providing a subtle but useful clue to the presence of tubular carcinoma at low-power examination. The stroma admixed with tubular carcinoma is usually rich in myofibroblasts, abundant elastic tissue, and myxoid matrix[48,49] (Figs. 13.4 and 13.5); it tends to be abundant and separates the neoplastic glands more widely than in nontubular well-differentiated ductal carcinomas. Elastosis has been regarded as a hallmark of tubular carcinoma (Fig. 13.5),[48,49] but it is not present in all cases and can also be a prominent feature of nontubular carcinomas and of some benign lesions, particularly those with the "radial scar" pattern.

Calcifications are detected microscopically in at least 50% of tubular carcinomas. They may be present in the lumen of the neoplastic glands (Fig. 13.5) and in the stroma admixed with the tumor, as well as in the associated intraductal carcinoma component and in adjacent glands with low-grade atypia.

Tubular carcinoma does not elicit a notable lymphocytic reaction. Perineural invasion is uncommon (Fig. 13.7). Blood vessel invasion and lymphatic tumor emboli are virtually never seen except after needling procedures (Fig. 13.8).

Precursor Lesions Associated with Tubular Carcinoma

Ductal carcinoma *in situ* (DCIS) has been described in 21% to 84% of tubular carcinomas.[6,24,25,38,50] The DCIS typically has papillary, micropapillary, or cribriform patterns or shows a mixed pattern[24] (Figs. 13.9 and 13.10). In a significant number of cases, the intraductal proliferation associated with tubular carcinoma, and from which carcinoma appears to have arisen, is histologically indistinguishable from atypical ductal hyperplasia (ADH). Tubular carcinoma may arise from or in association with a benign proliferative lesion with a radial scar configuration.[51,52]

Tubular carcinoma frequently develops in breast tissue involved by a multifocal alteration of the terminal ductal–lobular units usually referred to as "columnar cell change (CCC)" (Figs. 13.9 and 13.10). This lesion was previously designated informally as "pretubular" hyperplasia.[53] The spectrum of columnar cell lesions ranges from CCC and columnar cell hyperplasia (CCH) without atypia through CCC and/or hyperplasia with atypia to DCIS. Atypical CCH is also referred to as "flat epithelial atypia" (FEA). Cystic dilatation of the involved acini is a characteristic feature of these lesions, and Goldstein and O'Malley[44] referred to carcinoma in this setting as "cancerization of small ectatic ducts of the breast by DCIS cells with apocrine snouts." Cytomorphologic features common to all phases of CCC with atypia are nuclear hyperchromasia and a high nuclear-to-cytoplasmic ratio. Apical snouts are also frequently present at the luminal borders of ducts and ductules. The most subtle expression of this condition consists of a monostratified layer of cuboidal or low columnar cells, with the foregoing cytologic features. CCH is characterized by crowding of cells that become increasingly compressed and columnar, and display haphazard arrangement of the nuclei with respect to the basement membrane. Atypical CCH shows low-grade atypia with round to oval nuclei with smooth nuclear contour and finely dispersed homogeneous chromatin. Rare inconspicuous nucleoli are often seen abutting the nuclear membrane. The presence of blunt micropapillae or cribriform growth composed of the same proliferative cells with "streaming" or condensation of cells toward the lumen is often associated with atypical CCH, transitioning into ADH. The acini affected by CCCs may contain dense intraluminal flocculent secretions that often undergo calcification, forming small basophilic deposits. These laminated concretions are often detected mammographically as fine punctate clustered calcifications of indeterminate significance. DCIS with low nuclear grade and cribriform or micropapillary architecture often arises in the background of CCCs, whereas high-grade DCIS is extremely rare in this setting.[54,55]

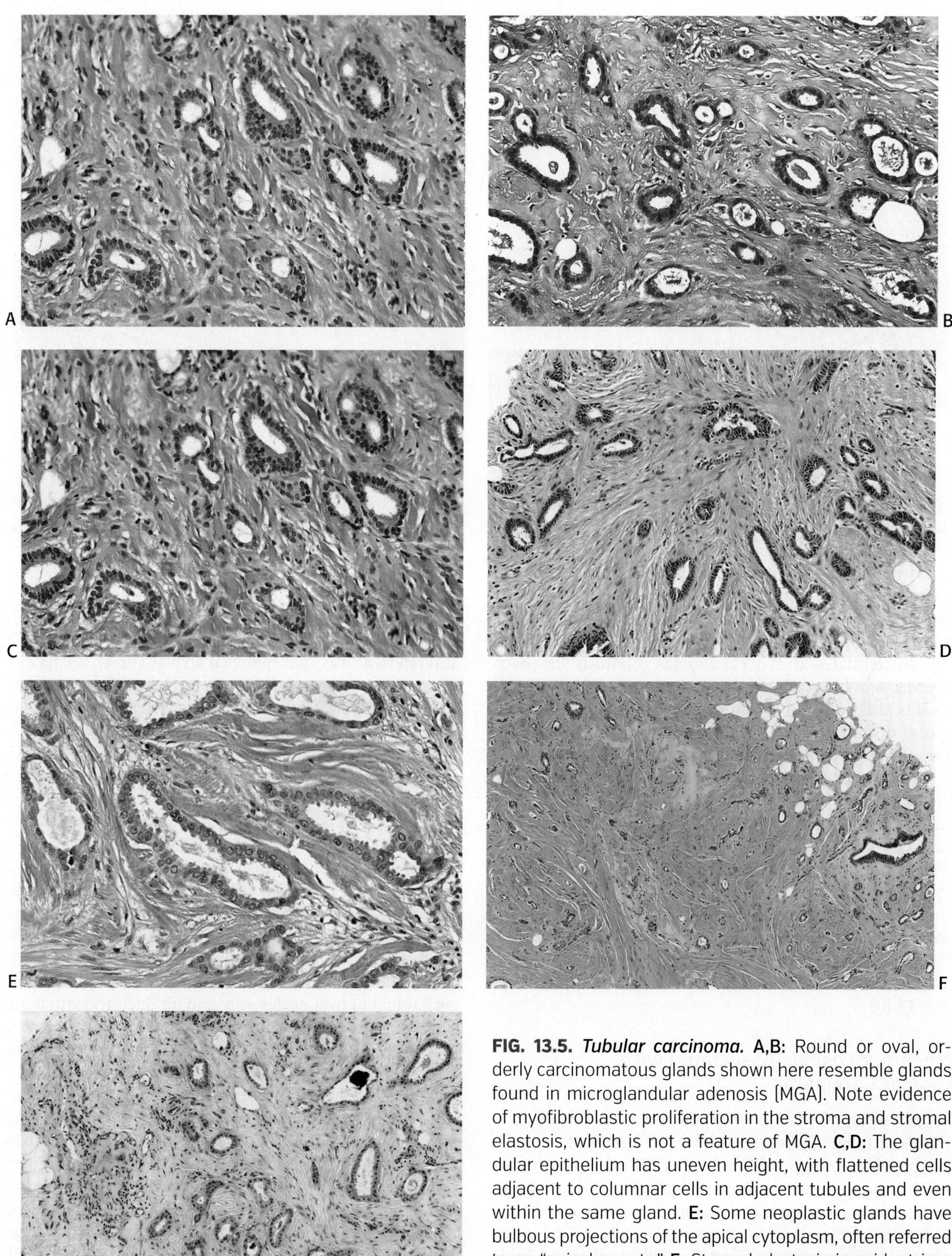

FIG. 13.5. ***Tubular carcinoma.*** **A,B:** Round or oval, orderly carcinomatous glands shown here resemble glands found in microglandular adenosis (MGA). Note evidence of myofibroblastic proliferation in the stroma and stromal elastosis, which is not a feature of MGA. **C,D:** The glandular epithelium has uneven height, with flattened cells adjacent to columnar cells in adjacent tubules and even within the same gland. **E:** Some neoplastic glands have bulbous projections of the apical cytoplasm, often referred to as "apical snouts." **F:** Stromal elastosis is evident in a tubular carcinoma with MGA-like glands. **G:** Minute calcifications are present in the lumens of neoplastic glands.

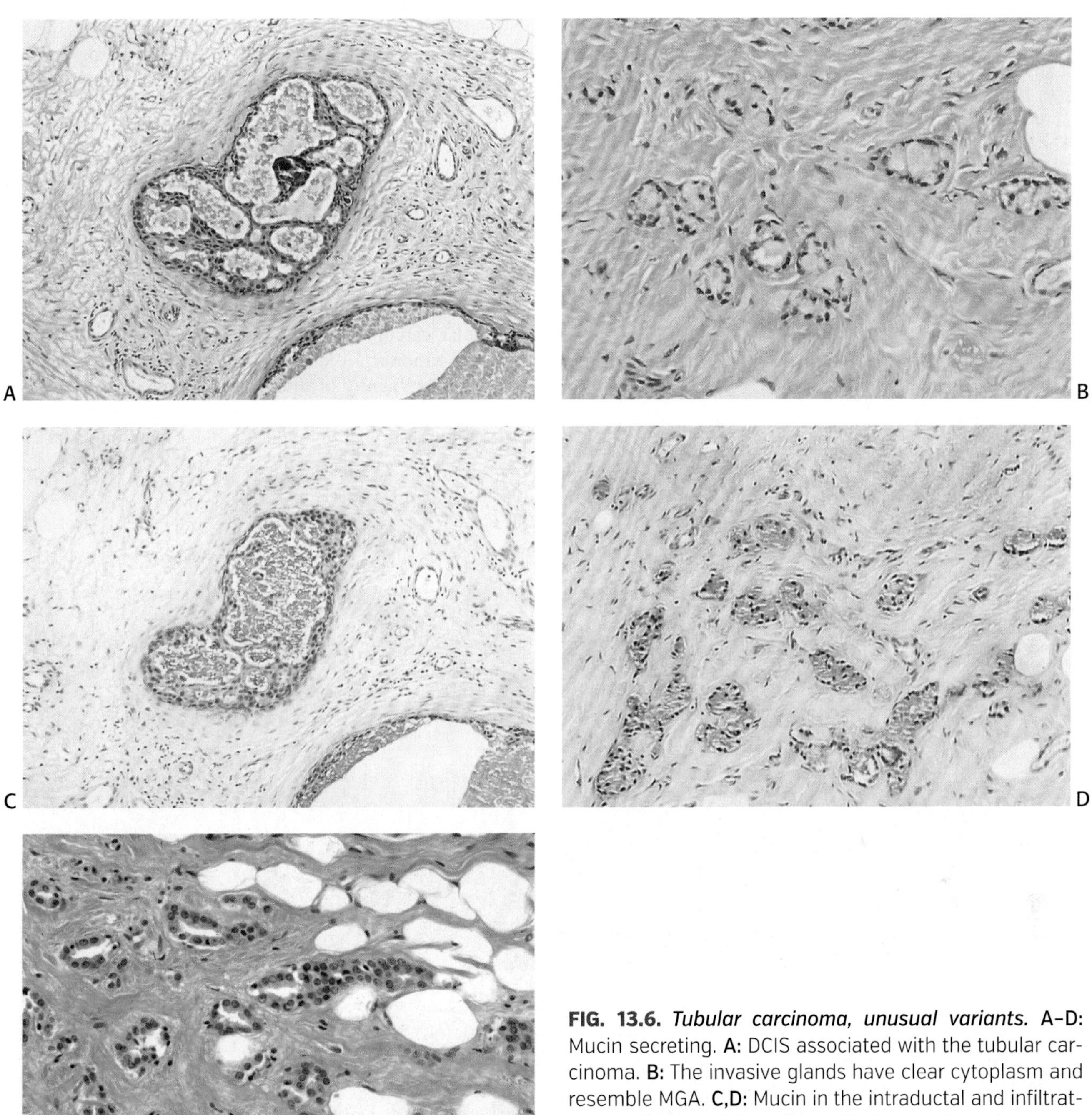

FIG. 13.6. ***Tubular carcinoma, unusual variants.*** **A–D:** Mucin secreting. **A:** DCIS associated with the tubular carcinoma. **B:** The invasive glands have clear cytoplasm and resemble MGA. **C,D:** Mucin in the intraductal and infiltrating carcinoma stains pink with the mucicarmine stain. **E:** Apocrine type. Tubular carcinoma glands with apocrine cytology.

Columnar cell lesions are associated with classical lobular carcinoma *in situ* (LCIS) (Figs. 13.9 and 13.10), as well as with tubular carcinoma and tubulolobular carcinoma (described later).[53,56,57] This complex has been referred to as the "Rosen triad."[58] In one study,[50] 8/14 (57%) tubular carcinomas had associated CCCs with atypia (FEA), 7/14 (50%) had micropapillary ADH, 3/14 (21%) had low nuclear grade DCIS, and 4/14 (29%) had lobular neoplasia. Only 2 of 18 (11%) size-matched, well-differentiated nontubular ductal carcinomas had associated CCC with atypia (FEA). Rakha et al.[14] observed that tubular carcinoma was associated more frequently with columnar cell lesions (93%) than with usual ductal hyperplasia (18%) or high-grade DCIS (1%). Columnar cell alterations were associated with 24 (89%) of 27 tubular carcinoma studies by Aulmann et al.[55] and showed atypia in 22 cases. Low-grade DCIS was present in 37% of cases, and foci of lobular neoplasia in 11%.[55]

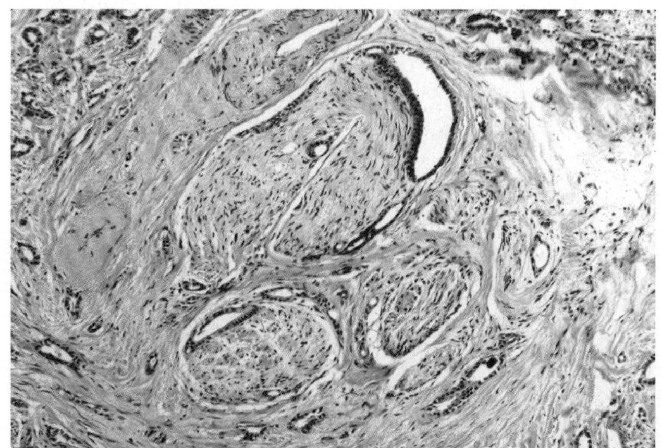

FIG. 13.7. ***Tubular carcinoma.*** Perineural invasion is evident around the perimeter of nerves, and one carcinomatous gland is present in the nerve.

Because CCH is prone to develop calcifications, often at multiple sites, it is a relatively common finding in needle core biopsy samples from women with mammographically detected calcifications. Excisional biopsy should be performed after a needle core biopsy diagnosis of CCH with atypia, or if the follow-up mammogram shows residual calcifications. (Additional discussion and illustrations of CCH with and without atypia can be found in Chapter 9.)

Coexistent classical LCIS has been described in 0.7% to 40% of patients with tubular carcinoma.[6,24–26,50] In retrospect, a subset of the invasive lesions previously classified as tubular carcinoma would be classified now as tubulolobular carcinoma.[37] When present, classical LCIS is usually found in the vicinity of tubular carcinoma, but it has also been identified separately in the same breast or in the contralateral breast. Foci of atypical lobular hyperplasia (ALH)

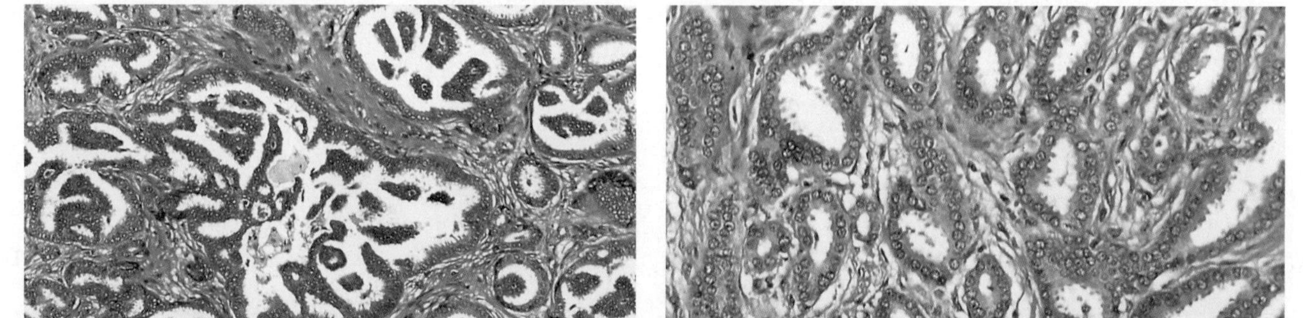

FIG. 13.8. ***Tubular carcinoma, needling effect.*** **A:** The intraductal component is micropapillary. **B:** Tubular carcinoma. **C:** Displaced epithelium in the needle track with hemorrhage. **D:** Clusters of carcinoma cells in dilated vascular channels, probably derived from the papillary intraductal component.

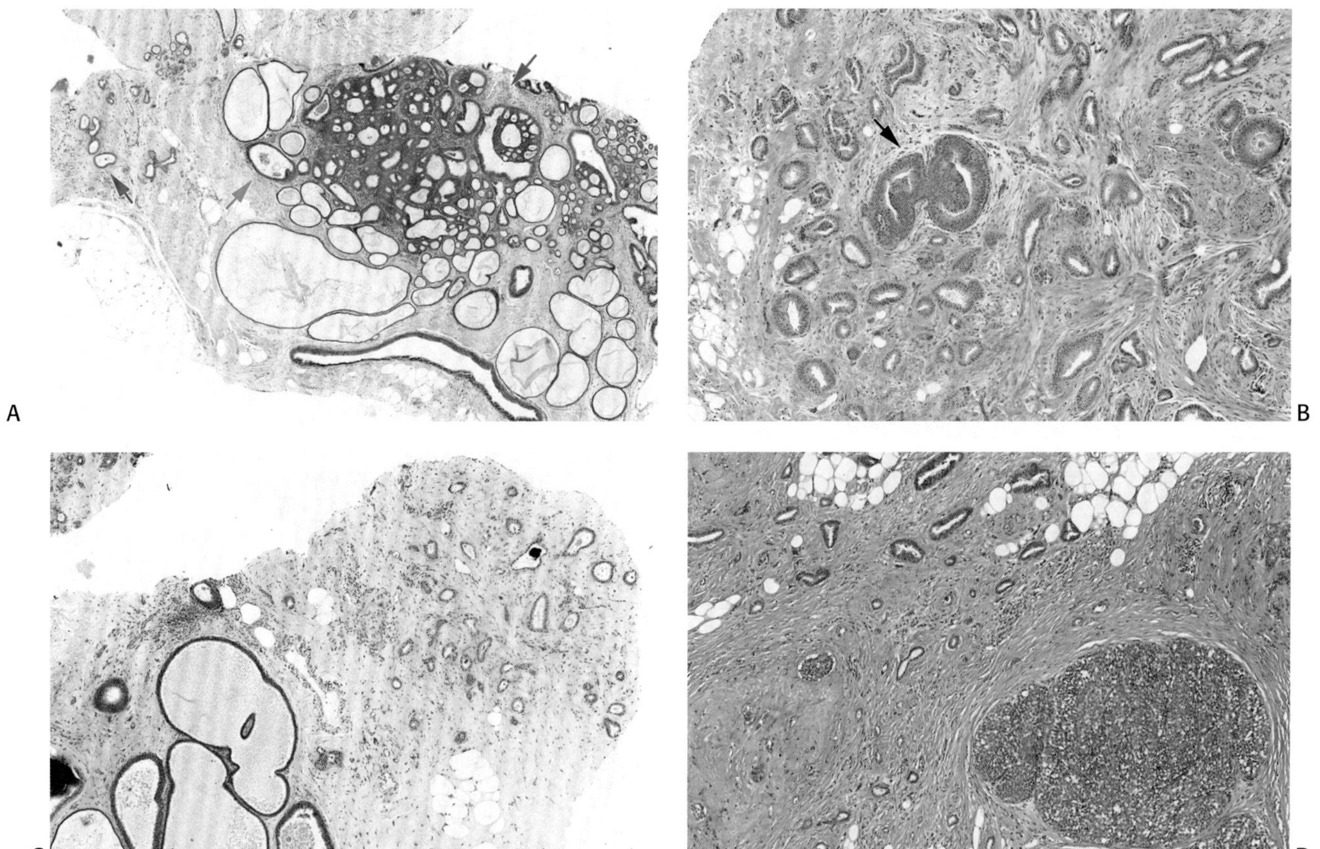

FIG. 13.9. ***Tubular carcinoma and precursor lesions.*** **A:** Rare and inconspicuous glands of tubular carcinoma (*red arrow*) are adjacent to a focus of intraductal low-grade neoplasia, ranging from columnar cells to columnar cells with atypia (*green arrow*), ADH and low-nuclear grade DCIS (*blue arrow*). **B:** A focus of CCC with atypia (*arrow*) is admixed with tubular carcinoma. **C:** A small focus of tubular carcinoma is adjacent to CCC (*lower left*) in a needle core biopsy. A calcification is present in the lumen of a tubular carcinoma gland. **D:** A lobule involved by LCIS is adjacent to tubular carcinoma. Note that the neoplastic glands range from large and angular, with hyperchromatic nuclei, to small and round.

(Fig. 13.10) are often present, whether in association with or without fully developed classical LCIS. Lobular proliferative lesions are so commonly encountered in association with tubular carcinoma that their presence may be regarded as secondary evidence supporting a diagnosis of tubular carcinoma (Figs. 13.9 and 13.10).

Multifocal Tubular Carcinoma and Contralateral Carcinoma

Most patients with tubular carcinoma present clinically with a single mass detected by mammography. When studied pathologically, however, 10% to 20% of patients have multifocal tubular carcinomas growing as separate foci in one or more quadrants.[23,37] These are not intramammary metastases, since one does not find associated lymphatic tumor emboli and DCIS is often present in the individual carcinomatous areas.

The frequency and prognostic significance of multifocal tubular carcinoma have not been carefully evaluated. Although several studies have described multifocal tubular carcinoma, the data are difficult to interpret because some authors have tabulated the intraductal portion of the tubular carcinoma as if it were a separate carcinoma.[32] Between 10% and 56% of patients with tubular carcinoma had independent foci of carcinoma elsewhere in the same breast[6,24,26,32,38] consisting of various types of *in situ* and/or invasive carcinoma. Twenty (16.7%) of 120 patients treated by mastectomy had tubular carcinoma remaining at the biopsy site, 6 (5%) had a second separate infiltrating carcinoma, 4 (3.3%) had multifocal DCIS, and 3 (2.5%) had LCIS.[24] Mitnick et al.[23] found invasive lobular carcinoma (ILC) in 7% of patients with tubular carcinoma.

The reported frequency of contralateral carcinoma varies from 0% to 38%.[7,13,24–26,32,36] Despite the relatively common coexistence of tubular and LCIS, infiltrating duct carcinomas

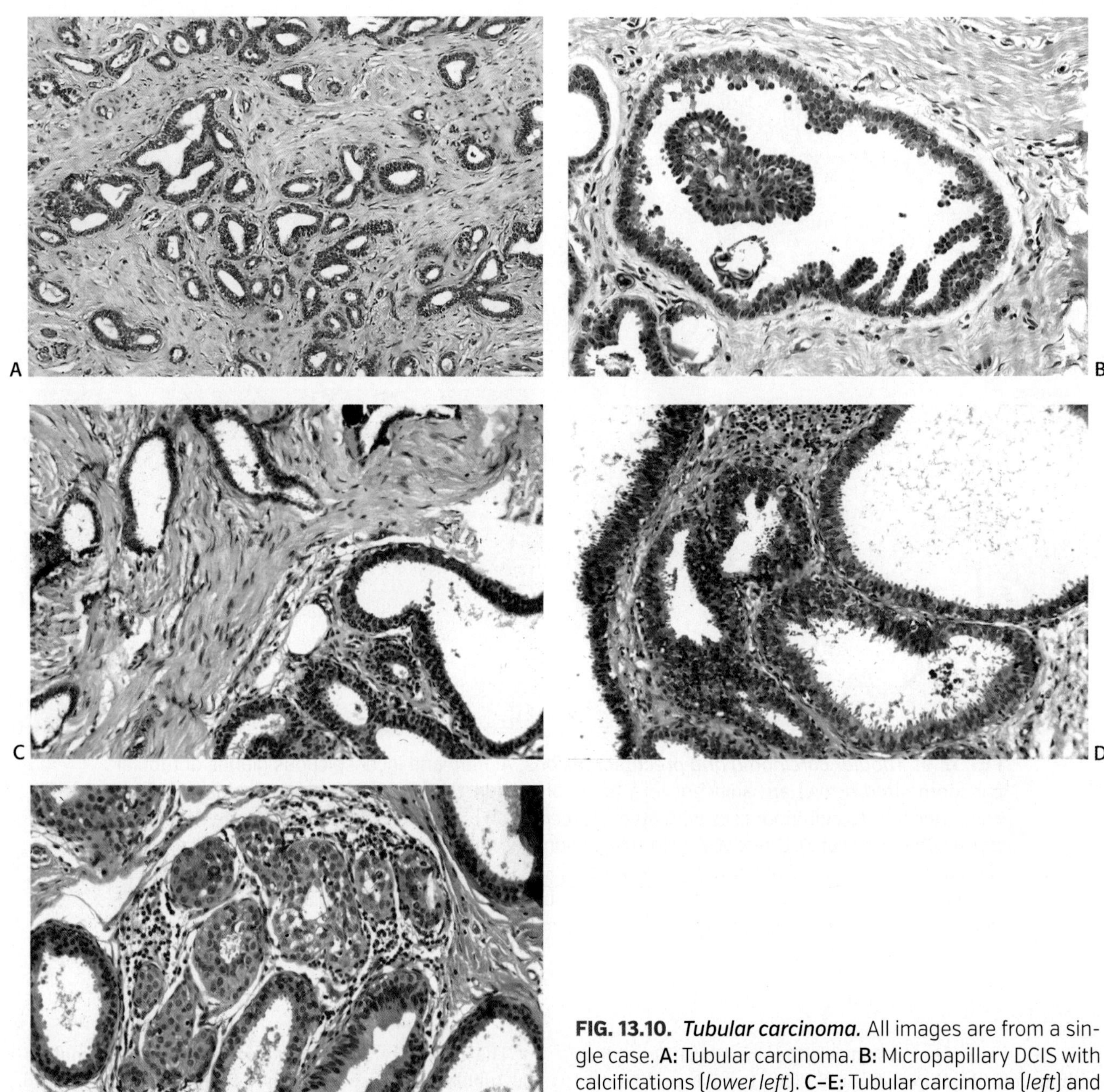

FIG. 13.10. ***Tubular carcinoma.*** All images are from a single case. **A:** Tubular carcinoma. **B:** Micropapillary DCIS with calcifications (*lower left*). **C–E:** Tubular carcinoma (*left*) and CCH (*right*) in (**C**) are associated with flat micropapillary DCIS in (**D**) and LCIS in (**E**).

are the most common contralateral tumors. Bilateral tubular carcinoma is uncommon.[7,26,38]

DIFFERENTIAL DIAGNOSIS

Microglandular Adenosis

Small tubular carcinomas (less than 1 cm) composed of round or oval glands of relatively uniform caliber may resemble microglandular adenosis (MGA)[59,60] (Fig. 13.4). However, MGA typically has a diffuse infiltrative growth pattern rather than the localized growth found in tubular carcinoma, and the glands tend to be small and round or oval throughout, with no angular contours. The epithelium of MGA is typically cuboidal, with uniform height and pale to clear cytoplasm, whereas the epithelium of tubular carcinoma has columnar morphology with apical snouts, but it can also consist of more cuboidal to flat cells. Columnar and flat cells sometimes coexist in the same gland of tubular carcinoma (Fig. 13.5). The lumen of the glands of MGA is open, but not overtly distended, and often contains dense homogeneous eosinophilic secretion that may

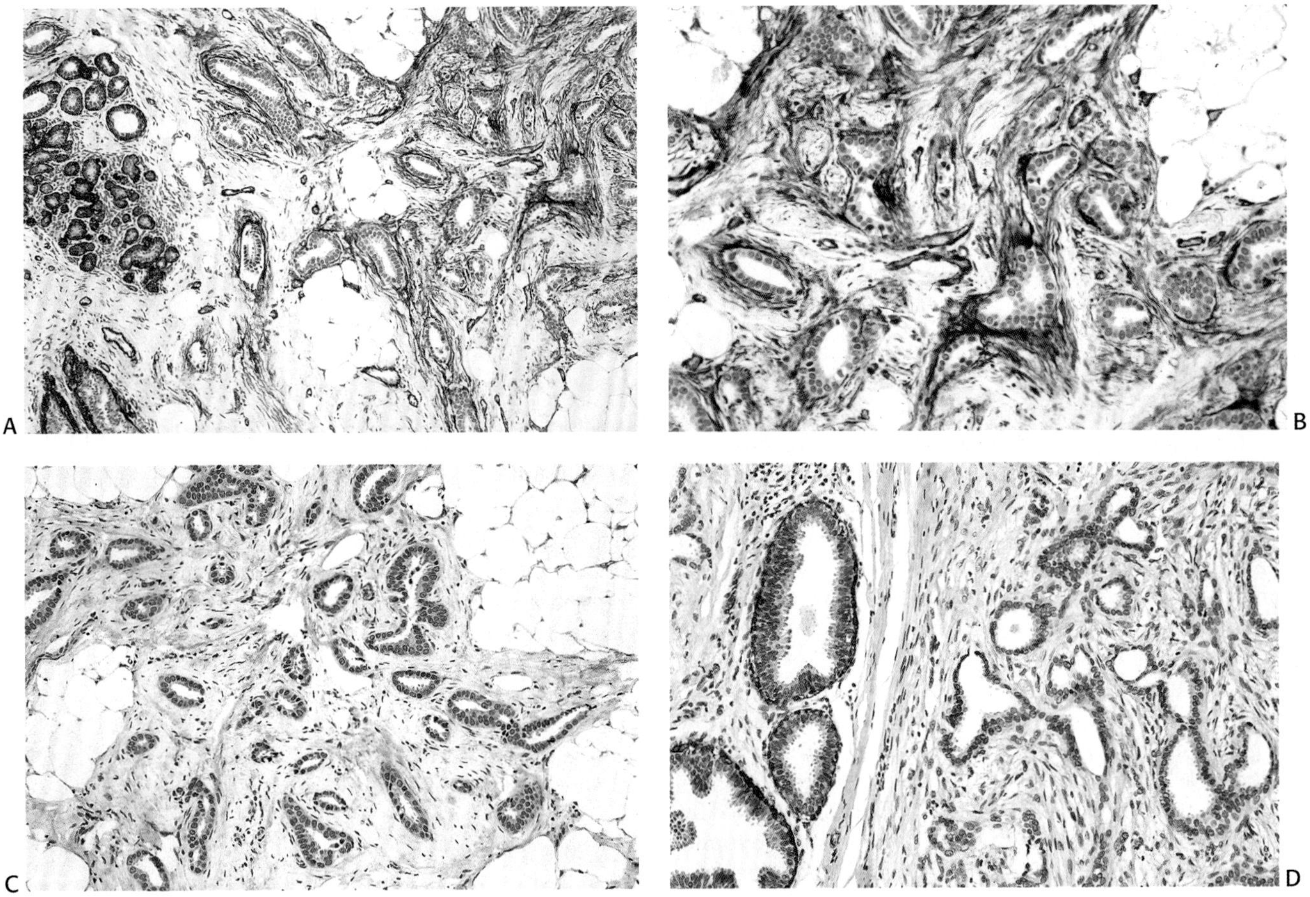

FIG. 13.11. ***Tubular carcinoma.*** **A:** The immunostain for smooth muscle actin (SMA) shows reactivity in myoepithelial cells around lobular glands in adenosis (*left*) and in myofibroblasts in the carcinoma (*right*). **B:** Magnified view of **(A)** showing tubular carcinoma with stromal myofibroblastic reactivity. **C:** No reactivity was seen when the same tumor is stained here for smooth muscle myosin-heavy chain (SMM-HC). **D:** Another specimen in which myoepithelial cells around ducts are stained for SMM-HC (*left*), and reactivity is absent from the carcinoma (*right*).

undergo calcification. Tubular carcinoma and MGA are devoid of myoepithelium, as demonstrated by immunostains for myoepithelial markers such as p63, CD10, and calponin (Fig. 13.11). Basement membrane completely surrounds the glands of MGA and can be easily detected in hematoxylin and eosin (H&E)-stained slides. Reticulin and periodic acid–Schiff (PAS) histochemical stains or immunoperoxidase stains for collagen IV or laminin highlight the basement membrane around the glands of MGA. Laminin, type IV collagen, and basement membrane proteoglycan were not detected around the neoplastic glands of tubular carcinoma in one series of nine cases,[61] and other investigators also reported lack of laminin[62] and type IV collagen[63] around the neoplastic glands of tubular carcinoma. It should be noted, however, that some investigators have found basement membrane, though attenuated, incomplete and/or focally disrupted, in association with many invasive carcinomas, and particularly those that are well differentiated[64,65] (Fig. 13.12). It is therefore prudent not to rest the distinction between tubular carcinoma and MGA uniquely

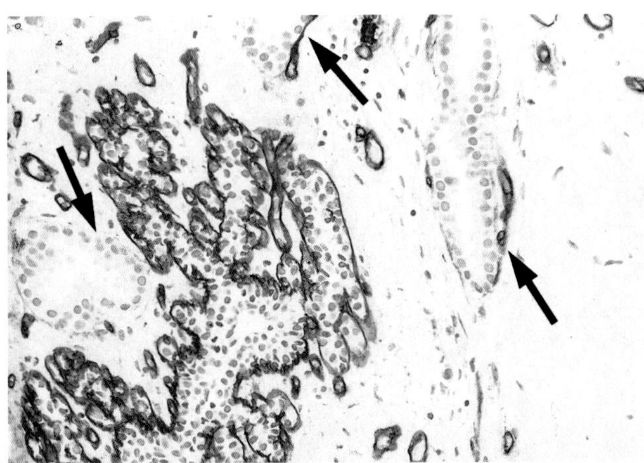

FIG. 13.12. ***Tubular carcinoma.*** This section stained with an anti-type IV collagen antibody reveals immunoreactivity in the basement membranes of lobular glands on the *left* and immunoreactivity associated with vascular channels around two carcinomatous glands (*arrows*).

on the presence of basement membrane. In difficult cases, the differential diagnosis between these two lesions can be solved using immunoperoxidase stains for S-100 protein, which decorates MGA but not tubular carcinoma, and for estrogen receptor (ER) and progesterone receptor (PR), both of which are usually strongly positive in tubular carcinoma and always negative in MGA.[66]

Sclerosing Adenosis and Radial Sclerosing Lesions

The microscopic architecture of tubular carcinoma must be distinguished from that of SA. SA has a lobulocentric proliferative pattern, and at low magnification it is almost always possible to identify individual altered lobules composed of whorled glands and tubules. Tubular carcinoma does not have a lobulocentric configuration, but it can be multicentric, as discussed later in this chapter.

At higher magnification, SA consists of compact whorled, elongated, and mostly compressed glands. Few round, oval, or angular glands with open lumens of varying size are usually dispersed in these foci, but the glands are not as widely open as in tubular carcinoma. All glands and tubules of SA are surrounded by spindly myoepithelium that is absent in the glands of tubular carcinoma.

Radial sclerosing lesions (RSLs) are composed of adenosis and duct hyperplasia or papilloma, often accompanied by cysts. Varying proportions of these components are found in individual lesions, and some consist entirely of adenosis or of papilloma. Stromal elastosis is a feature of many RSLs, especially those in which adenosis is not a prominent component. Although myoepithelial cells are usually evident in routine H&E-stained sections, sometimes they can be markedly attenuated or focally inapparent in the areas of dense sclerosis. In difficult cases, myoepithelium can be visualized with the aid of immunostains.[63] Nuclear p63 protein is the most specific myoepithelial antigen, as it (almost exclusively) decorates normal myoepithelial nuclei and does not cross-react with stromal myofibroblasts. Most other myoepithelial markers are cytoplasmic and include calponin, SMA, CD10, CK5, CK5/6, and SMM-HC. The cytoplasmic myoepithelial antigens display variable cross-reactivity with myofibroblasts (Fig. 13.11) and can be substantially attenuated in the myoepithelium of a sclerosing lesion.[67] For optimal assessment, it is therefore advised to use a panel of myoepithelial antigens inclusive of p63 and calponin and/or SMA, as these markers are least attenuated in sclerosing lesions.[67] This is especially important when dealing with a needle core biopsy sample where contextual information from the surrounding tissue can be limited or not available. A contemporaneous H&E recut should also always be prepared.[68]

Well-Differentiated Invasive Ductal Carcinoma

In well-differentiated nontubular ductal carcinoma, the pattern of glandular growth is largely tubular, but areas composed of glands lined by two or more cell layers represent more than 10% of the lesion. Some glands show micropapillary tufts, transluminal bridges, or abortive cribriform arrangements (Figs. 13.13 and 13.14). An occasional mitotic figure may be encountered, and there is a tendency to greater cytologic pleomorphism, with the neoplastic epithelium showing intermediate nuclear grade nearly throughout. The intraductal component associated with well-differentiated nontubular duct carcinoma is more likely to be cribriform than micropapillary.

TUBULOLOBULAR CARCINOMA

A carcinoma with areas of invasive lobular and tubular carcinoma is referred to as *tubulolobular carcinoma* (Fig. 13.15). Tubulolobular carcinomas range from 0.3 to 2.5 cm in greatest dimension (mean, about 1.3 cm).[37,69,70] These tumors display varying proportions of tubular and ILC. In one study evaluating 11 cases, tubular and lobular carcinoma were nearly equally present in 3 (27%), lobular carcinoma was predominant in 5 (46%), and the tubular pattern was more pronounced in 3 (27%).[70]

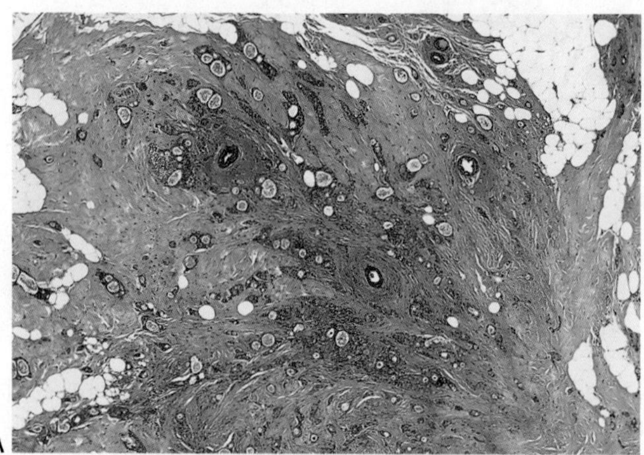

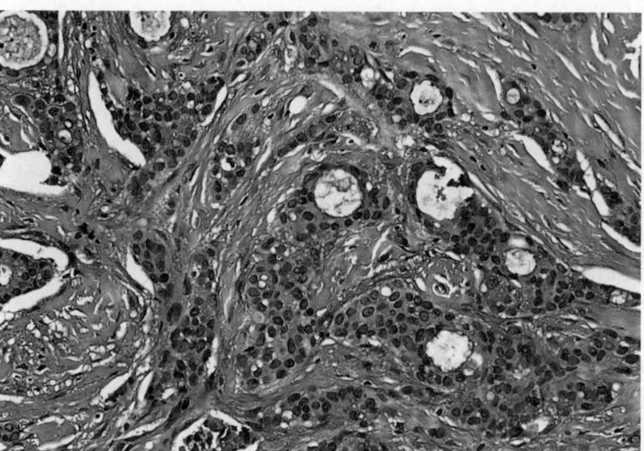

FIG. 13.13. ***Well-differentiated invasive duct carcinoma.*** **A,B:** This carcinoma has a radial sclerosing configuration. Stromal elastosis is evident.

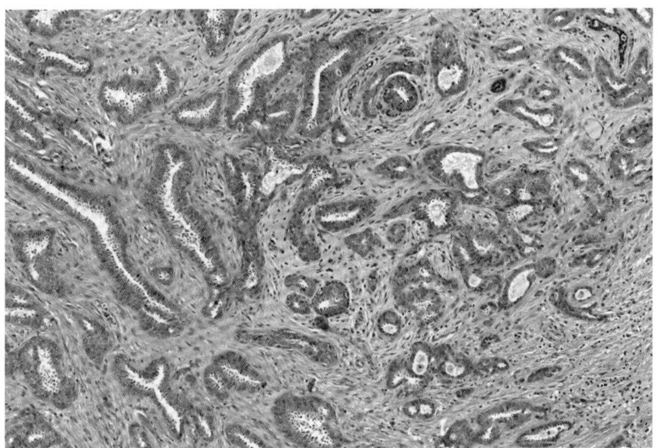

FIG. 13.14. ***Well-differentiated invasive duct carcinoma.*** This carcinoma shows merging of the glands in a complex configuration.

Multifocality, more frequent in tubulolobular carcinoma than in pure tubular carcinoma, was found in 19%[69] and 29%[37] of tubulolobular carcinomas in two studies. By comparison, the frequency of multifocality in pure tubular carcinomas was 10%[69] and 20%.[37]

Tubulolobular carcinoma has been regarded as a variant of tubular carcinoma by some authors, and as a form of ILC by others. The unifying concept of low-grade epithelial mammary neoplasia identifies tubulolobular carcinoma as a morphologic variant of invasive carcinoma in this spectrum of lesions.[56,57]

The observation that almost all tubulolobular carcinomas in three studies were E-cadherin positive supports ductal histogenesis, since loss of E-cadherin reactivity is associated with ILC.[69–71] E-cadherin immunoreactivity was found in invasive tubular and invasive lobular components, even in tumors wherein the lobular pattern was more prominent. In one study, α-catenin and β-catenin were expressed in 50% and 62.5% of tubulolobular carcinomas, respectively.[71] Esposito et al.[70] detected membranous reactivity for α-, β-, and χ-catenin in all tubulolobular and tubular carcinomas they studied. Infiltrating lobular carcinomas displayed cytoplasmic staining for β- and χ-catenin but no reactivity for α-catenin. In this study, all tubular and tubulolobular carcinomas had membranous reactivity for E-cadherin, whereas membranous E-cadherin reactivity is usually absent in lobular carcinomas. Wheeler et al.[69] found that 25 of 27 tubulolobular carcinomas were immunoreactive for the high–molecular weight cytokeratin K903, a marker that has been associated with lobular differentiation,[72,73] but the specificity of this reaction is not uniformly accepted. Overall the mixed immunophenotype of tubulolobular carcinoma reflects the ductal and lobular histologic components of this tumor, with the preponderance of evidence favoring ductal histogenesis.

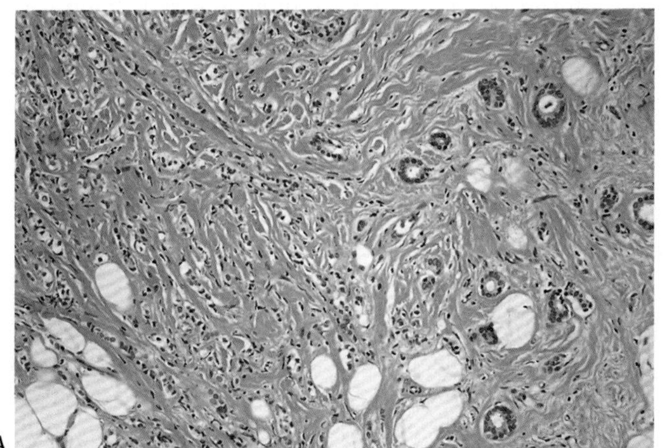

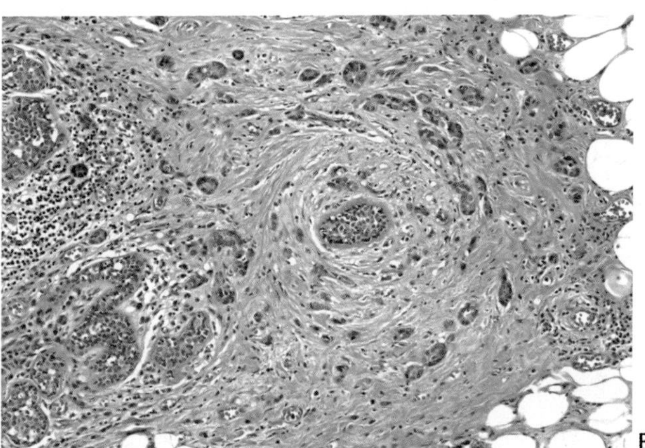

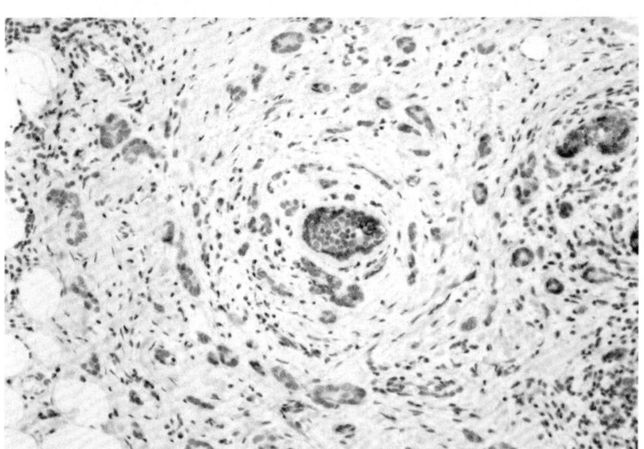

FIG. 13.15. ***Tubulolobular carcinoma.*** **A:** Invasive carcinoma with the linear growth pattern and signet ring cells of lobular carcinoma (*left*) and the round glands of tubular carcinoma (*right*). **B,C:** Tubulolobular carcinoma growing circumferentially around a duct (*center*). Tubular carcinoma and ILC elements are not reactive in the E-cadherin immunostain (**C**). Focal E-cadherin reactivity is seen at the perimeter of the central duct and in a lobular gland (*right*). E-cadherin–negative cells in the duct lumen represent LCIS.

Three-dimensional modeling of tubular and tubulolobular carcinomas has revealed cavitary glandular structures connected by a network of slender, solid cords of single cells.[74] The connecting network of single cells in tubulolobular carcinomas consists of longer strands, which might account for the histologic pattern suggestive of ILC in a ductal lesion.

In situ carcinoma associated with tubulolobular carcinoma consists of classical LCIS, DCIS, or classical LCIS and DCIS.[37,69,70] DCIS alone is found more often in association with pure tubular carcinoma than with tubulolobular carcinoma, whereas tubulolobular carcinoma is more likely to be accompanied by classical LCIS only.[37,69]

The rate of ALN metastases in patients with tubulolobular carcinomas is higher than for tubular carcinoma,[37,69,70] amounting to about 30% of patients who undergo an axillary dissection[37] (Fig. 13.16). The presence of multifocal carcinoma at the primary site appears to predispose patients with tubular and tubulolobular carcinoma to developing ALN metastases, perhaps because of the greater tumor volume associated with multifocality. ALN metastases were found in 21%[4] and 29%[26] of patients with duct carcinomas with tubular features (mixed tubular carcinomas). In the latter study, 21% of patients with a stage II mixed tubular tumor had metastatic carcinoma in more than three lymph nodes.

Presently, patients with tubulolobular carcinoma should be viewed as having a good prognosis that is closer to that of pure tubular carcinoma[37,69,70] than to that of ILC.[37,69,70]

DIAGNOSIS OF TUBULAR CARCINOMA IN NEEDLE CORE BIOPSY MATERIAL

Because of the limited sampling provided by a needle core biopsy, the diagnosis of pure tubular carcinoma is often uncertain in this material, especially when only a small portion of the lesion is present in the tissue cores. The differential diagnosis with the benign lesions described above can be particularly difficult on needle core biopsy material, as contextual information from the surrounding breast parenchyma is not available or very limited. Pure tubular morphology in core biopsy samples provides no guarantee of the same morphology in the rest of the lesion. Greater confidence in a diagnosis of "pure" tubular carcinoma by needle core biopsy can be obtained by correlating the pathologic and radiologic findings, especially if it is determined that the radiologic target lesion has been completely or nearly completely removed by the biopsy procedure. Nonetheless, it is prudent practice to indicate in the needle core biopsy report that the final classification of the carcinoma will depend on the findings in the core and excisional biopsies.

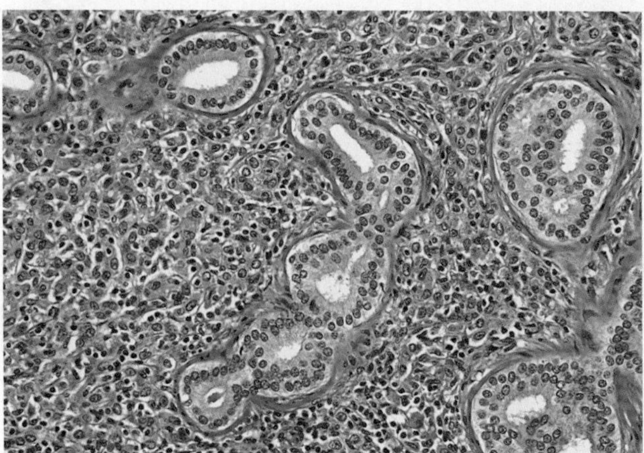

FIG. 13.16. ***Metastatic tubulolobular carcinoma in a lymph node.*** Tubular carcinoma glands are separate from lobular carcinoma in this lymph node metastasis.

IMMUNOHISTOCHEMISTRY

More than 90% of tubular carcinomas express ER.[13,14,35,36,75,76] Nuclear reactivity for PR has been detected in 69% to 75% of tubular carcinomas.[13,14,76–78] Oakley et al.[79] reported that none of 55 tubular carcinomas studied by fluorescence *in situ* hybridization exhibited *HER2/neu* gene amplification. All tubular carcinomas studied by Rakha et al.[14] were negative for HER2/neu or p53, but 3/27 (11.11%) tubular carcinomas in another series[13] were classified as HER2/neu positive, although the criteria for assessing HER2/neu positivity were not specified. Considering the bland histomorphology and very indolent behavior of tubular carcinoma, it is very unlikely that this tumor carries *HER2/neu* gene amplification or overexpresses the HER2/neu protein. It is therefore recommended to carefully reassess the morphologic diagnosis for any carcinoma classified as tubular type that is reported found to be HER2/neu positive.

Almost all tubulolobular carcinomas are immunoreactive for ER and PR,[37,70] and they are only rarely HER2/neu positive.[70]

ELECTRON MICROSCOPY

Electron microscopy of tubular carcinoma typically demonstrates a monolayer of uniform cells, although slight stratification within the neoplastic gland can occur. Myoepithelial cells are scarce or absent.[80,81] Observations regarding the basement membrane have been inconsistent, but it is usually described as absent, incompletely formed, or discontinuous.[80,81] Microvilli are seen at the luminal cell surface in the neoplastic glands. The tumor cells are joined by numerous desmosomes and well-formed terminal bars. The cytoplasm contains mitochondria, rough endoplasmic reticulum, tonofilaments that may have a perinuclear distribution, and occasional cytoplasmic secretory lumina. Collagen and elastic fibers are present in the stroma.

CYTOLOGY

Cytologic samples of tubular carcinomas contain glandular cells with mild to moderate nuclear atypia, usually arranged in relatively tight clusters with angular outline, small groups of 4 to 10 cells, and scattered single cells.[82,83]

In some of the clusters, the polarized arrangement of the neoplastic cells may outline a glandular lumen, and tubular clusters and focal cribriform structures may occur. The tubular structures are often described as angulated or have a shape resembling that of an extended finger, a sleeve, or a test tube. The neoplastic cells have slightly enlarged nuclei, about 1.5 to 2 times the size of a red blood cell, with smooth nuclear membrane and uniform chromatin. Minute nucleoli are sometimes encountered. Small laminated calcifications may occur. Background bipolar stromal nuclei can be present, but no myoepithelial nuclei are admixed with the neoplastic tubules. Scattered actin-positive bipolar cells in the aspirate from tubular carcinoma are likely to be myofibroblasts from the stroma; small fragments of desmoplastic stroma may also be present. Cytologically, the differential diagnosis of tubular carcinoma includes fibroadenoma and proliferative changes with or without atypia. In contrast to tubular carcinoma, a fine-needle aspiration (FNA) sample of a fibroadenoma contains dispersed bipolar myofibroblasts and myoepithelial cells present as either dispersed cells or are admixed with benign epithelial cell clusters. The aspirate of benign proliferative changes shows a wider range of cells, including ductal, myoepithelial, and apocrine cells.

Cangiarella et al.[84] assessed the diagnostic features in FNA material from 21 tubular carcinomas. Features suggestive of tubular carcinoma included smears of moderate to high cellularity, angular cellular clusters with sharp borders and peripheral oval epithelial cells, scattered single cells with minimal cytologic atypia, and absence or paucity of bipolar nuclei. Lamb and McGoogan[85] compared the findings in cytology specimens of 31 tubular carcinomas and 22 RSLs with overlapping clinical features and comparable size. This study revealed substantial difficulty in distinguishing between the two lesions based on evaluation of cytologic material alone. Twenty-five of the tubular carcinomas (81%) were interpreted as malignant or suspicious, two (6%) as benign, and four (13%) as acellular. Cytologic material from nine (41%) of the RSLs had initially been misdiagnosed as suspicious or diagnostic of carcinoma, whereas 46% had been diagnosed as benign, and three (13%) as acellular. Mitnick et al.[23] reported greater accuracy in diagnosing tubular carcinoma by needle core biopsy than by FNA.

Tubulolobular carcinoma is suggested by an aspirate that demonstrates signet ring cells and the features of tubular carcinoma.[86]

GENETICS AND MOLECULAR STUDIES

The relationship between tubular carcinoma and less well-differentiated forms of IDC is an unresolved issue. Because some ductal carcinomas have tubular and nontubular elements, it has been speculated that some tubular carcinomas "dedifferentiate" over time. One approach to this question has been to compare the molecular features of tubular and nontubular carcinomas. In a study of 18 pure tubular carcinomas sampled by laser microdissection and investigated by comparative genomic hybridization, Waldman etal.[87] detected an average of 3.6 chromosomal alterations per tumor. Tubular carcinomas had significantly fewer chromosomal alterations overall and significantly fewer 16q gains compared with a group of nontubular invasive duct carcinomas. The authors concluded that pure tubular carcinomas are a "genetically distinct group of invasive breast cancers that probably do not progress to a more aggressive subtype of ductal cancer."[87] However, the data cited by Waldman et al.[87] do not exclude the possibility that "dedifferentiation" might occur over time in some tubular carcinomas.

Recent studies have evaluated the genetic alterations of tubular carcinoma. Loss of 16q, the most frequent chromosomal abnormality, is also found in other low-grade mammary epithelial neoplastic lesions, including CCC with atypia, ADH, low-grade DCIS, ALH, classical LCIS, well-differentiated IDC, tubulolobular carcinoma, and invasive cribriform carcinoma.[57] Aulmann et al.[55] documented loss of heterozygosity in tubular carcinoma, involving the long arm of chromosome 16 as well as chromosomes 8p21, 3p14, 1p36, and 11q14, and a high degree of homologous allelic losses with CCCs with atypia and low-grade DCIS. Using comparative genomic hybridization, Riener et al.[88] found loss of the *CDH13* locus on chromosome 16q in 86% of 23 tubular carcinomas. The *CDH13* gene encodes a cell surface glycoprotein, member of the cadherin family.[88] Although tubular carcinoma and well-differentiated IDC share a number of genetic alterations, comparative transcriptomic analysis of these two tumors has revealed some differences; in particular, tubular carcinoma shows upregulation of *ESR1*, *CREBBP1*, and *NCOR1* signals, all of which are part of ER-driven signaling pathways, and high expression of *INPP4B*, an enzyme involved in phosphatidylinositol signaling.[89]

PATHOLOGY OF LYMPH NODE METASTASES

The lymph node metastases of tubular carcinoma tend to reproduce the tubular growth pattern of the primary tumor. Metastatic deposits may involve the lymph node capsule or parenchyma (Fig. 13.17). Cserni[90] has reported a rare pattern of axillary involvement consisting of micrometastases with perinodal extracapsular extension in eight patients with well-differentiated carcinoma, including three with tubular carcinoma (Fig. 13.18). In this setting, extracapsular extension was not associated with worse prognosis.[90] The lymph node metastases of tubular carcinoma can simulate benign glandular inclusions, but the absence of p63- and/or calponin-positive myoepithelium around the neoplastic glands supports the diagnosis of metastatic carcinoma. Endosalpingiosis involving an ALN may also closely resemble metastatic tubular carcinoma.[91] The use of myoepithelial stains can be misleading in this setting, as endosalpingiosis has no myoepithelial layer. Ciliated cells and intercalated "peg" cells are essential features of endosalpingiosis (Fig. 13.19). Nuclear reactivity for Wilms tumor 1 (WT-1) and PAX8 may be used to confirm the morphologic impression.[91] Rarely, metastases

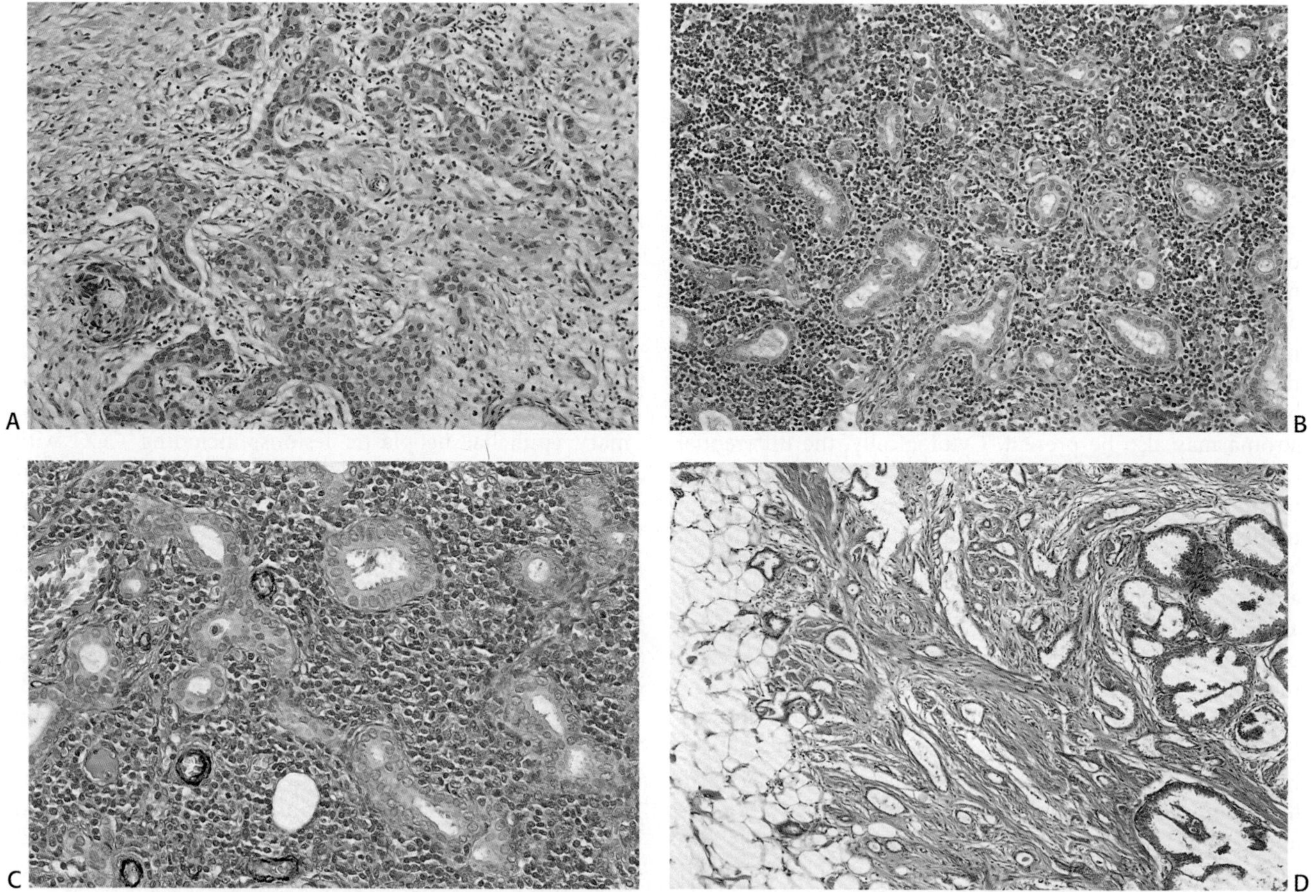

FIG. 13.17. ***Metastatic tubular carcinoma in lymph node.*** All images are from the same case. **A:** Lumpectomy was performed for the moderately differentiated invasive duct carcinoma shown here. **B:** SLN mapping revealed metastatic carcinoma of the tubular type in the SLN. All other lymph nodes were free of metastases. **C:** The immunostain for SMA shows reactivity in small blood vessels in the lymph node but not around the metastatic glands. **D:** Extensive further sampling of the lumpectomy disclosed a separate, previously inapparent tubular carcinoma, which was responsible for the lymph node metastasis.

of tubular carcinoma are less well differentiated or resemble infiltrating lobular carcinoma.

TREATMENT AND PROGNOSIS

For decades, patients with pure and mixed tubular carcinomas were treated by modified or radical mastectomy. Less than 10% of patients in larger series were treated by excisional surgery with or without adjuvant radiotherapy. In a series of patients with T1N0 breast carcinoma treated by modified or radical mastectomy and followed for a median of 18 years, there were no recurrences among patients with tubular carcinoma.[92]

Presently, patients with unifocal pure tubular carcinoma are most often treated with breast conservation therapy. According to SEER data, most (82.4%) patients with tubular carcinoma diagnosed between 1992 and 2007 underwent breast-conserving surgery, and only 17% had a mastectomy; no information was available about the remaining 0.5% of patients.[11] About two-thirds (64.3%) of patients received adjuvant radiation treatment.[11] In this epidemiologic study, the hazard ratio of breast cancer–specific mortality in patients 50 years or older with ER- or PR-positive tumors was 0.58 for tubular carcinoma compared with IDC, not otherwise specified. Liu et al.[13] also reported that patients with tubular carcinoma treated with breast conservation therapy had a lower rate of distant metastases (1% vs. 13%) and a lower rate of breast cancer–specific death (1% vs. 10%) than patients with IDC.[13] Neither of these studies, however, included careful histopathologic review of the original diagnosis that may have resulted in the erroneous attribution of a few deaths to tubular carcinoma.

When the histologic diagnosis of tubular carcinoma is restricted to tumors that consist entirely or almost entirely of tubular elements, tubular carcinoma has a very good prognosis.[4–7,13,14,24–26,28,42,76,77,92] A review of several follow-up studies[6,7,21,22,38,78,88] describing more than 400 women with pure tubular carcinoma revealed that 3.0% had recurrences

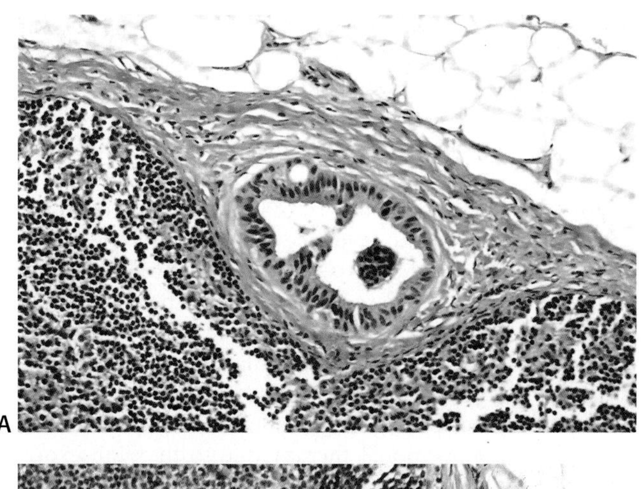

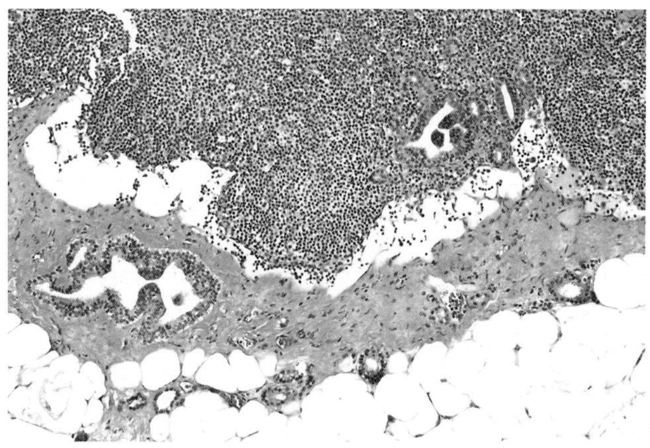

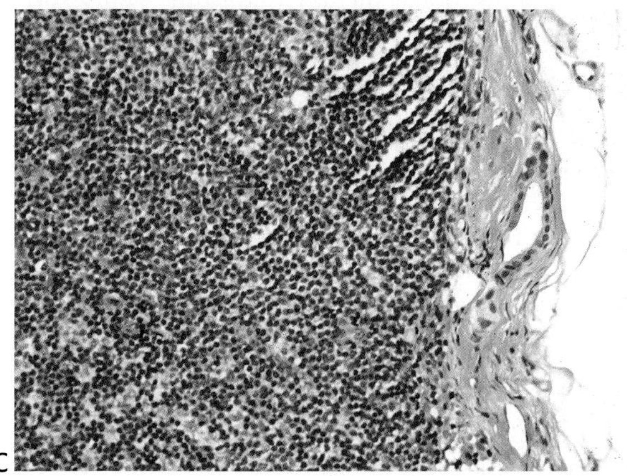

FIG. 13.18. ***Metastatic tubular carcinoma.*** Patterns of metastases in ALNs that are sometimes mistaken for benign glandular inclusion. **A:** Metastatic carcinoma in the lymph node capsule. **B:** Metastatic carcinoma in cortical lymphoid tissue. Focal extracapsular extension is present. In patients with metastatic tubular carcinoma, this finding does not seem to be associated with worse prognosis. **C:** Metastatic tubular carcinoma consisting of a single gland in the lymph node capsule.

due to the tubular carcinoma. Six of the women had recurrent carcinoma in the same breast following simple excision after an interval of 2 to 22 years. One of these six women also had axillary nodal metastases when the breast recurrence was detected, but none were reported to have developed systemic metastases after a mastectomy was performed to treat the mammary recurrence.

Livi et al.[28] reported on a series of 307 patients with a histologically verified diagnosis of tubular carcinoma. All patients were treated at an Italian university hospital from 1976 and 2001; the median follow-up time was 8.4 years. Most (80%) patients treated with breast-conserving surgery also received adjuvant radiotherapy, and 35% had tamoxifen treatment. Only 21 women (7%) received chemotherapy,

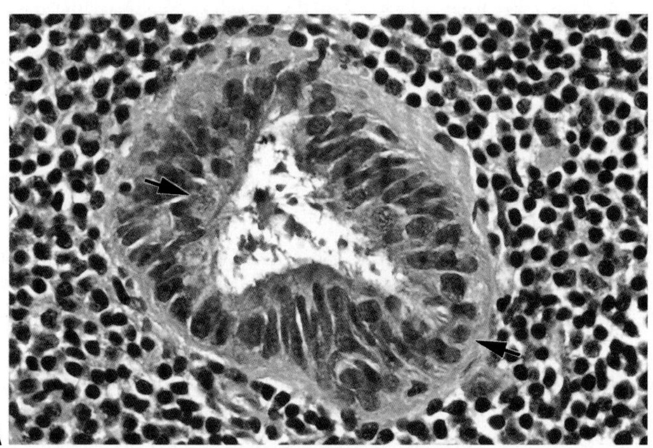

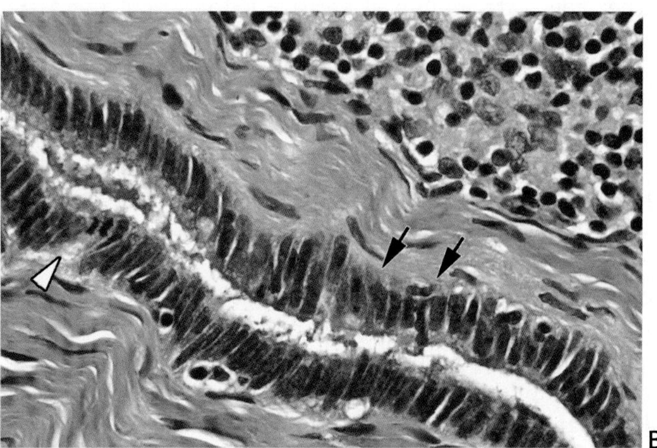

FIG. 13.19. ***Endosalpingiosis in axillary lymph nodes mimics metastatic tubular carcinoma.*** **A:** A few cells have cilia and a terminal bar (*arrows*). **B:** The finding of mitotic activity (*arrowhead*) may raise the suspicion of metastatic carcinoma, but the cells show terminal bars and cilia (*arrows*) that characterize endosalpingiosis.

including 15 with lymph node metastases. Twelve patients experienced local recurrence of carcinoma after a median time of 4.1 years, including two patients with chest wall recurrences, nine with in-breast recurrences (three in the same quadrant as the index cancer, five in another quadrant, and one multicentric), and one patient with a recurrence in the supraclavicular fossa.[28]

Rakha et al.[14] compared the outcomes and local recurrences of 102 histologically confirmed tubular carcinomas and 212 grade 1 IDCs. The median follow-up time was 127 months. Local recurrences developed in seven (6.9%) patients with tubular carcinoma, all of whom had been initially treated by wide local excision. Two of the seven patients had also received adjuvant radiotherapy, but none was treated with adjuvant systemic treatment. In contrast, 53 (25.1%) patients with grade 1 IDC developed a local recurrence and 9% died of disease. In this study, tubular carcinoma patients had a longer disease-free survival (DFS) and breast carcinoma–specific survival than those with grade 1 IDC, even when analysis was limited to tumors 1 cm or smaller. Histologic tumor type and tumor size, but not lymphovascular invasion, lymph node metastasis, and ER status, were independent predictors of DFS in multivariate analysis.[14]

These studies confirm the good prognosis of tubular carcinoma diagnosed based on strict histomorphologic criteria. In particular, no deaths attributable to tubular carcinoma have been reported in series with careful histologic review of the tumor.[5,14,26,28,37,39,76,92] Death due to metastatic mammary carcinoma in several patients with bilateral carcinoma has been attributable to a less well-differentiated contralateral carcinoma when one breast had a tubular carcinoma.[21,88] Recurrences have been reported in up to 32% of patients with mixed tubular carcinoma, and 6% to 28% of these patients reportedly died of metastatic mammary carcinoma.[6,7,88]

SLN mapping is usually performed in patients with tubular carcinoma, even though the chances of lymph node involvement are low. SLN biopsy should always be performed if the tumor is larger than 1 cm,[43] tubulolobular carcinoma, when there are multifocal invasive lesions, or if there are other indications that suggest axillary nodal metastases.

Adjuvant radiotherapy is currently administered to most patients with tubular carcinoma treated with breast-conserving surgery.[93] In one series,[94] there were no breast recurrences among 21 patients with tubular carcinoma treated by lumpectomy and radiotherapy with median follow-up of 9.4 years. Bradford et al.[40] reported no breast or systemic recurrences in 38 women treated by excision, including 17 who did not have breast irradiation. Only 20% of patients treated with breast-conserving surgery in the largest series of tubular carcinoma published to date[28] did not receive adjuvant radiotherapy. In a prospective study,[95] six patients with stage I tubular carcinoma and no histologic evidence of extensive DCIS or lymphovascular invasion were treated by wide excision to a microscopic margin of at least 1cm and received no adjuvant radiation or systemic therapy. No specific information on the size of the tubular carcinomas was provided. Three of the six patients (50%) developed a local recurrence within 5 years. These results support the use of adjuvant radiotherapy in patients with tubular carcinoma treated by breast-conserving surgery. Patients with multifocal tubular carcinoma, coexistent extensive DCIS, or evidence of other invasive lesions in the breast should always have radiotherapy after excision, or they may require mastectomy.

In view of the extremely favorable prognosis of tubular carcinoma, there is no evidence that adjuvant chemotherapy is beneficial, except possibly for women with multifocal carcinoma or tumors larger than 3 cm, if there are axillary metastases, or if there is also a less well-differentiated carcinoma in the ipsilateral or contralateral breast. Information regarding the benefit of adjuvant hormonal therapy is very limited, but patients with tubular carcinoma could be candidates for hormonal therapy due to the high expression of ER. In one retrospective series, only a third (35%) of patients with tubular carcinoma received tamoxifen.[28] Adjuvant hormonal treatment in the form of tamoxifen, or aromatase inhibitors for postmenopausal women, is now often recommended.

Patients with mixed tubular carcinomas should receive treatment appropriate for an infiltrating ductal carcinoma of the grade of the nontubular component as determined by tumor size and stage. This is likely to include postoperative radiotherapy and systemic adjuvant therapy if the tumor is larger than 1 cm.

REFERENCES

1. Cornil V, Ranvier L. *Manuel d'histologie pathologique.* Paris: Germer-Baillière, 1869:1167–1170.
2. Foote FW Jr. Surgical pathology of cancer of the breast. In: Parsons W, ed. *Cancer of the breast.* Springfield: Charles C. Thomas, 1959:37–38.
3. McDivitt R, Stewart F, Berg J. *Tumors of the breast.* (*AFIP Atlas of Tumor Pathology,* 2nd series, vol. 2.) Bethesda: American Registry of Pathology, 1968:89–90.
4. Carstens PH. Tubular carcinoma of the breast. A study of frequency. *Am J Clin Pathol* 1978;70:204–210.
5. Carstens PH, Greenberg RA, Francis D, et al. Tubular carcinoma of the breast. A long term follow-up. *Histopathology* 1985;9:271–280.
6. Cooper HS, Patchefsky AS, Krall RA. Tubular carcinoma of the breast. *Cancer* 1978;42:2334–2342.
7. Peters GN, Wolff M, Haagensen CD. Tubular carcinoma of the breast. Clinical pathologic correlations based on 100 cases. *Ann Surg* 1981;193:138–149.
8. Rosen PP. The pathological classification of human mammary carcinoma: past, present and future. *Ann Clin Lab Sci* 1979;9:144–156.
9. Northridge ME, Rhoads GG, Wartenberg D, et al. The importance of histologic type on breast cancer survival. *J Clin Epidemiol* 1997;50:283–290.
10. Louwman MW, Vriezen M, van Beek MW, et al. Uncommon breast tumors in perspective: incidence, treatment and survival in the Netherlands. *Int J Cancer* 2007;121:127–135.
11. Li CI. Risk of mortality by histologic type of breast cancer in the United States. *Horm Cancer* 2010;1:156–165.
12. Rosen PP, Saigo PE, Braun DW Jr, et al. Predictors of recurrence in stage I (T1N0M0) breast carcinoma. *Ann Surg* 1981;193:15–25.
13. Liu GF, Yang Q, Haffty BG, et al. Clinical-pathologic features and long-term outcomes of tubular carcinoma of the breast compared with invasive ductal carcinoma treated with breast conservation therapy. *Int J Radiat Oncol Biol Phys* 2009;75:1304–1308.
14. Rakha EA, Lee AH, Evans AJ, et al. Tubular carcinoma of the breast: further evidence to support its excellent prognosis. *J Clin Oncol* 2010;28:99–104.

15. Beahrs O, Shapiro S, Smart C. Report of the working group to review the National Cancer Institute—American Cancer Society Breast Cancer Detection Demonstration Projects. *J Natl Cancer Inst* 1979;62:640–709.
16. Feig SA, Shaber GS, Patchefsky A, et al. Analysis of clinically occult and mammographically occult breast tumors. *AJR Am J Roentgenol* 1977;128:403–408.
17. Newcomer LM, Newcomb PA, Trentham-Dietz A, et al. Detection method and breast carcinoma histology. *Cancer* 2002;95:470–477.
18. Nagtegaal ID, Allgood PC, Duffy SW, et al. Prognosis and pathology of screen-detected carcinomas: how different are they? *Cancer* 2011;117:1360–1368.
19. Leibman AJ, Lewis M, Kruse B. Tubular carcinoma of the breast: mammographic appearance. *AJR Am J Roentgenol* 1993;160:263–265.
20. Elson BC, Helvie MA, Frank TS, et al. Tubular carcinoma of the breast: mode of presentation, mammographic appearance, and frequency of nodal metastases. *AJR Am J Roentgenol* 1993;161:1173–1176.
21. Vega A, Garijo F. Radial scar and tubular carcinoma. Mammographic and sonographic findings. *Acta Radiol* 1993;34:43–47.
22. Frouge C, Tristant H, Guinebretiere JM, et al. Mammographic lesions suggestive of radial scars: microscopic findings in 40 cases. *Radiology* 1995;195:623–625.
23. Mitnick JS, Gianutsos R, Pollack AH, et al. Tubular carcinoma of the breast: sensitivity of diagnostic techniques and correlation with histopathology. *AJR Am J Roentgenol* 1999;172:319–323.
24. McDivitt RW, Boyce W, Gersell D. Tubular carcinoma of the breast. Clinical and pathological observations concerning 135 cases. *Am J Surg Pathol* 1982;6:401–411.
25. Oberman HA, Fidler WJ Jr. Tubular carcinoma of the breast. *Am J Surg Pathol* 1979;3:387–395.
26. Deos PH, Norris HJ. Well-differentiated (tubular) carcinoma of the breast. A clinicopathologic study of 145 pure and mixed cases. *Am J Clin Pathol* 1982;78:1–7.
27. Vo T, Xing Y, Meric-Bernstam F, et al. Long-term outcomes in patients with mucinous, medullary, tubular, and invasive ductal carcinomas after lumpectomy. *Am J Surg* 2007;194:527–531.
28. Livi L, Paiar F, Meldolesi E, et al. Tubular carcinoma of the breast: outcome and loco-regional recurrence in 307 patients. *Eur J Surg Oncol* 2005;31:9–12.
29. Taxy JB. Tubular carcinoma of the male breast: report of a case. *Cancer* 1975;36:462–465.
30. Heller KS, Rosen PP, Schottenfeld D, et al. Male breast cancer: a clinicopathologic study of 97 cases. *Ann Surg* 1978;188:60–65.
31. Norris HJ, Taylor HB. Carcinoma of the male breast. *Cancer* 1969;23:1428–1435.
32. Lagios MD, Rose MR, Margolin FR. Tubular carcinoma of the breast: association with multicentricity, bilaterality, and family history of mammary carcinoma. *Am J Clin Pathol* 1980;73:25–30.
33. Li CI, Daling JR, Malone KE, et al. Relationship between established breast cancer risk factors and risk of seven different histologic types of invasive breast cancer. *Cancer Epidemiol Biomarkers Prev* 2006;15:946–954.
34. Flesch-Janys D, Slanger T, Mutschelknauss E, et al. Risk of different histological types of postmenopausal breast cancer by type and regimen of menopausal hormone therapy. *Int J Cancer* 2008;123:933–941.
35. Berger A, Miller S, Harris M. Axillary dissection for tubular carcinoma of the breast. *Breast J* 1996;2:204–208.
36. Winchester DJ, Sahin AA, Tucker SL, et al. Tubular carcinoma of the breast. Predicting axillary nodal metastases and recurrence. *Ann Surg* 1996;223:342–347.
37. Green I, McCormick B, Cranor M, et al. A comparative study of pure tubular and tubulolobular carcinoma of the breast. *Am J Surg Pathol* 1997;21:653–657.
38. Carstens PH, Huvos AG, Foote FW Jr, et al. Tubular carcinoma of the breast: a clinicopathologic study of 35 cases. *Am J Clin Pathol* 1972;58:231–238.
39. Rosen PP, Saigo PE, Braun DW, et al. Prognosis in stage II (T1N1M0) breast cancer. *Ann Surg* 1981;194:576–584.
40. Bradford W, Christensen W, Fraser H. Treatment of pure tubular carcinoma of the breast. *Breast J* 1998;4:437–440.
41. Papadatos G, Rangan AM, Psarianos T, et al. Probability of axillary node involvement in patients with tubular carcinoma of the breast. *Br J Surg* 2001;88:860–864.
42. Fedko MG, Scow JS, Shah SS, et al. Pure tubular carcinoma and axillary nodal metastases. *Ann Surg Oncol* 2010;17(Suppl. 3):338–342.
43. Dejode M, Sagan C, Campion L, et al. Pure tubular carcinoma of the breast and sentinel lymph node biopsy: a retrospective multi-institutional study of 234 cases. *Eur J Surg Oncol* 2013;39:248–254.
44. Goldstein NS, O'Malley BA. Cancerization of small ectatic ducts of the breast by ductal carcinoma *in situ* cells with apocrine snouts: a lesion associated with tubular carcinoma. *Am J Clin Pathol* 1997;107:561–566.
45. Andersen JA, Carter D, Linell F. A symposium on sclerosing duct lesions of the breast. *Pathol Annu* 1986;21(Pt. 2):145–179.
46. Stalsberg H, Hartmann WH. The delimitation of tubular carcinoma of the breast. *Hum Pathol* 2000;31:601–607.
47. Eusebi V, Betts CM, Bussolati G. Tubular carcinoma: a variant of secretory breast carcinoma. *Histopathology* 1979;3:407–419.
48. Egger H, Dressler W. A contribution to the natural history of breast cancer. I. Duct obliteration with periductal elastosis in the centre of breast cancers. *Arch Gynecol* 1982;231:191–198.
49. Tremblay G. Elastosis in tubular carcinoma of the breast. *Arch Pathol* 1974;98:302–307.
50. Kunju LP, Ding Y, Kleer CG. Tubular carcinoma and grade 1 (well-differentiated) invasive ductal carcinoma: comparison of flat epithelial atypia and other intra-epithelial lesions. *Pathol Int* 2008;58:620–625.
51. Linell F, Ljungberg O. Breast carcinoma. Progression of tubular carcinoma and a new classification. *Acta Pathol Microbiol Scand A* 1980;88:59–60.
52. Linell F, Ljungberg O, Andersson I. Breast carcinoma. Aspects of early stages, progression and related problems. *Acta Pathol Microbiol Scand Suppl* 1980;1–233.
53. Rosen PP. Columnar cell hyperplasia is associated with lobular carcinoma *in situ* and tubular carcinoma. *Am J Surg Pathol* 1999;23:1561.
54. Collins LC, Achacoso NA, Nekhlyudov L, et al. Clinical and pathologic features of ductal carcinoma *in situ* associated with the presence of flat epithelial atypia: an analysis of 543 patients. *Mod Pathol* 2007;20:1149–1155.
55. Aulmann S, Elsawaf Z, Penzel R, et al. Invasive tubular carcinoma of the breast frequently is clonally related to flat epithelial atypia and low-grade ductal carcinoma *in situ*. *Am J Surg Pathol* 2009;33:1646–1653.
56. Abdel-Fatah TM, Powe DG, Hodi Z, et al. High frequency of coexistence of columnar cell lesions, lobular neoplasia, and low grade ductal carcinoma *in situ* with invasive tubular carcinoma and invasive lobular carcinoma. *Am J Surg Pathol* 2007;31:417–426.
57. Abdel-Fatah TM, Powe DG, Hodi Z, et al. Morphologic and molecular evolutionary pathways of low nuclear grade invasive breast cancers and their putative precursor lesions: further evidence to support the concept of low nuclear grade breast neoplasia family. *Am J Surg Pathol* 2008;32:513–523.
58. Brandt SM, Young GQ, Hoda SA. The "Rosen Triad": tubular carcinoma, lobular carcinoma *in situ*, and columnar cell lesions. *Adv Anat Pathol* 2008;15:140–146.
59. Rosen PP. Microglandular adenosis. A benign lesion simulating invasive mammary carcinoma. *Am J Surg Pathol* 1983;7:137–144.
60. Shen SS, Sahin AA. Invasive ductal carcinoma of the breast with a microglandular adenosis pattern. *Ann Diagn Pathol* 2004;8:39–42.
61. Ekblom P, Miettinen M, Forsman L, et al. Basement membrane and apocrine epithelial antigens in differential diagnosis between tubular carcinoma and sclerosing adenosis of the breast. *J Clin Pathol* 1984;37:357–363.
62. Flotte TJ, Bell DA, Greco MA. Tubular carcinoma and sclerosing adenosis: the use of basal lamina as a differential feature. *Am J Surg Pathol* 1980;4:75–77.
63. Joshi MG, Lee AK, Pedersen CA, et al. The role of immunocytochemical markers in the differential diagnosis of proliferative and neoplastic lesions of the breast. *Mod Pathol* 1996;9:57–62.
64. Visscher DW, Sarkar FH, Sakr W, et al. Immunohistologic analysis of invasive phenotype in breast carcinoma. A clinicopathologic study. *Pathol Res Pract* 1993;189:867–872.
65. Kitayama J, West R, Jensen K. Comparison of immunohistochemical stains for myoepithelial cells versus collagen type IV in invasive ductal carcinomas and ductal carcinoma *in situ* of the breast. *Abstract 181, USCAP meeting 2012 March 19–23, Vancouver, Canada*. 2012.
66. Khalifeh IM, Albarracin C, Diaz LK, et al. Clinical, histopathologic, and immunohistochemical features of microglandular adenosis and transition into *in situ* and invasive carcinoma. *Am J Surg Pathol* 2008;32:544–552.
67. Hilson JB, Schnitt SJ, Collins LC. Phenotypic alterations in myoepithelial cells associated with benign sclerosing lesions of the breast. *Am J Surg Pathol* 2010;34:896–900.
68. Hoda SA, Rosen PP. Contemporaneous H&E sections should be standard practice in diagnostic immunopathology. *Am J Surg Pathol* 2007;31:1627.

69. Wheeler DT, Tai LH, Bratthauer GL, et al. Tubulolobular carcinoma of the breast: an analysis of 27 cases of a tumor with a hybrid morphology and immunoprofile. *Am J Surg Pathol* 2004;28:1587–1593.
70. Esposito NN, Chivukula M, Dabbs DJ. The ductal phenotypic expression of the E-cadherin/catenin complex in tubulolobular carcinoma of the breast: an immunohistochemical and clinicopathologic study. *Mod Pathol* 2007;20:130–138.
71. Kuroda H, Tamaru J, Takeuchi I, et al. Expression of E-cadherin, alpha-catenin, and beta-catenin in tubulolobular carcinoma of the breast. *Virchows Arch* 2006;448:500–505.
72. Bratthauer GL, Miettinen M, Tavassoli FA. Cytokeratin immunoreactivity in lobular intraepithelial neoplasia. *J Histochem Cytochem* 2003;51:1527–1531.
73. Bratthauer GL, Moinfar F, Stamatakos MD, et al. Combined E-cadherin and high molecular weight cytokeratin immunoprofile differentiates lobular, ductal, and hybrid mammary intraepithelial neoplasias. *Hum Pathol* 2002;33:620–627.
74. Marchio C, Sapino A, Arisio R, et al. A new vision of tubular and tubulo-lobular carcinomas of the breast, as revealed by 3-D modelling. *Histopathology* 2006;48:556–562.
75. Masood F, Barwick KW. Estrogen receptor expression of the less common breast carcinomas. *Am J Clin Pathol* 1990;93:437.
76. Diab SG, Clark GM, Osborne CK, et al. Tumor characteristics and clinical outcome of tubular and mucinous breast carcinomas. *J Clin Oncol* 1999;17:1442–1448.
77. Colleoni M, Rotmensz N, Maisonneuve P, et al. Outcome of special types of luminal breast cancer. *Ann Oncol* 2012;23:1428–1436.
78. Fasano M, Vamvakas E, Delgado Y, et al. Tubular carcinoma of the breast: immunohistochemical and DNA flow cytometric profile. *Breast J* 1999;5:252–255.
79. Oakley GJ III, Tubbs RR, Crowe J, et al. HER-2 amplification in tubular carcinoma of the breast. *Am J Clin Pathol* 2006;126:55–58.
80. Erlandson RA, Carstens PH. Ultrastructure of tubular carcinoma of the breast. *Cancer* 1972;29:987–995.
81. Harris M, Ahmed A. The ultrastructure of tubular carcinoma of the breast. *J Pathol* 1977;123:79–83.
82. Dawson AE, Logan-Young W, Mulford DK. Aspiration cytology of tubular carcinoma. Diagnostic features with mammographic correlation. *Am J Clin Pathol* 1994;101:488–492.
83. Fischler DF, Sneige N, Ordonez NG, et al. Tubular carcinoma of the breast: cytologic features in fine-needle aspirations and application of monoclonal anti-alpha-smooth muscle actin in diagnosis. *Diagn Cytopathol* 1994;10:120–125.
84. Cangiarella J, Waisman J, Shapiro RL, et al. Cytologic features of tubular adenocarcinoma of the breast by aspiration biopsy. *Diagn Cytopathol* 2001;25:311–315.
85. Lamb J, McGoogan E. Fine needle aspiration cytology of breast in invasive carcinoma of tubular type and in radial scar/complex sclerosing lesions. *Cytopathology* 1994;5:17–26.
86. Boppana S, Erroll M, Reiches E, et al. Cytologic characteristics of tubulolobular carcinoma of the breast. *Acta Cytol* 1996;40:465–471.
87. Waldman FM, Hwang ES, Etzell J, et al. Genomic alterations in tubular breast carcinomas. *Hum Pathol* 2001;32:222–226.
88. Riener MO, Nikolopoulos E, Herr A, et al. Microarray comparative genomic hybridization analysis of tubular breast carcinoma shows recurrent loss of the CDH13 locus on 16q. *Hum Pathol* 2008;39:1621–1629.
89. Lopez-Garcia MA, Geyer FC, Natrajan R, et al. Transcriptomic analysis of tubular carcinomas of the breast reveals similarities and differences with molecular subtype-matched ductal and lobular carcinomas. *J Pathol* 2010;222:64–75.
90. Cserni G. Axillary sentinel lymph node micrometastases with extracapsular extension: a distinct pattern of breast cancer metastasis? *J Clin Pathol* 2008;61:115–118.
91. Corben AD, Nehhozina T, Garg K, et al. Endosalpingiosis in axillary lymph nodes: a possible pitfall in the staging of patients with breast carcinoma. *Am J Surg Pathol* 2010;34:1211–1216.
92. Rosen PR, Groshen S, Saigo PE, et al. A long-term follow-up study of survival in stage I (T1N0M0) and stage II (T1N1M0) breast carcinoma. *J Clin Oncol* 1989;7:355–366.
93. Sullivan T, Raad RA, Goldberg S, et al. Tubular carcinoma of the breast: a retrospective analysis and review of the literature. *Breast Cancer Res Treat* 2005;93:199–205.
94. Haffty B, Perrotta P, Ward B. Conservatively treated breast cancer: outcome by histologic subtype. *Breast J* 1997;3:7–14.
95. Lim M, Bellon JR, Gelman R, et al. A prospective study of conservative surgery without radiation therapy in select patients with Stage I breast cancer. *Int J Radiat Oncol Biol Phys* 2006;65:1149–1154.

CHAPTER 14

Papillary Carcinoma

FREDERICK C. KOERNER

FREQUENCY

Papillary carcinoma is an uncommon form of ductal carcinoma in which the neoplastic cells grow on an arborizing fibrovascular skeleton. Early writers did not use the term *papillary*, in a consistent way, nor did they maintain a clear distinction between the noninvasive and invasive forms of this type of carcinoma. The many and varied definitions of papillary carcinoma have included ductal carcinoma *in situ* (DCIS) with papillary features in multiple ducts, solitary papillary tumors, cystic papillary carcinomas, and invasive carcinomas with a papillary growth pattern.[1,2] Consequently, the literature contains only scant secure data concerning the frequency of this lesion. In a group of carcinomas from 383,146 women in the 1973 to 1998 Surveillance Epidemiology and End Results (SEER) registry, papillary carcinoma accounts for only 0.6%.[3] McDivitt et al.[4] wrote that invasive papillary carcinoma constituted approximately 1.5% of the cases of operable invasive carcinoma seen at Memorial Sloan-Kettering Cancer Center, and Fisher et al.[1] classified 2.1% of the carcinomas studied in National Surgical Adjuvant Breast and Bowel Project (NSABP) protocol #4 as invasive papillary carcinoma. Among radiologically detected carcinomas, invasive papillary carcinoma accounted for 0.04% in one series[5] and 2.8% in another.[6] Papillary carcinoma was found in 2 of 169 women (1.2%) who were at least 75 years old when breast carcinoma was diagnosed.[7] A greater percentage of male breast carcinomas are papillary, accounting for 2.6% of 2,537 carcinomas in the 1973 to 1998 SEER registry,[3] 2.7% of a series of 187 cases in Denmark,[8] and 8% of a group of 113 tumors seen at the Armed Forces Institute of Pathology.[9]

RELATIONSHIP BETWEEN PAPILLOMA AND PAPILLARY CARCINOMA

The relationship between benign and malignant papillary tumors of the breast has long been a controversial subject. As early as 1922, Bloodgood[10] classified papilloma as a benign condition best managed by local excision. However, other authors, who concluded that papillomas frequently give rise to carcinoma, advocated simple mastectomy to treat breast papilloma.[11–13] In 1946, Foote and Stewart[14] commented that surrounding some lesions "... in which the presence of noninfiltrating papillary carcinoma is quite obvious, there will be additional outlying or adjacent foci in which the degree of structural change is distinctly less advanced and this leads one to believe that preexisting papillomatosis had been present and had undergone malignant transformation."

A differing point of view was expressed by Stout[15] in 1952, when he made the following comment at the Second National Cancer Conference:

> Intraductal papillomas are altogether benign and the papillary carcinomas altogether malignant. I have never been able to detect cancer cells intermingled with the cells of a benign papilloma. Therefore in the breast I cannot say I have ever observed what may be interpreted as a carcinoma arising in a benign papilloma. Are benign papillomas precancerous lesions? It is almost impossible to get convincing evidence pro and con on this question for once a papilloma has been removed there is no further chance for that particular one to become malignant.

However, Stout and coworkers[16] acknowledged that *in situ* carcinoma could reside in a papilloma when he stated:

> Recognizable nodules of papillary carcinoma almost never show traces of benign intraductal proliferations, so that in doubtful cases if there are microscopic cells which one might be tempted to consider cancerous within an otherwise benign papillary tumor ... either these are not cancer cells, or if one chooses to regard them as such, the condition is comparable to cancer *in situ*. Because we have no proof that this condition has ever led to the development of true *clinical cancer*, we have classified tumors showing epithelial proliferations of this sort with the rest of the benign intraductal papillary tumors.

One must presume that Stout used the term "clinical cancer" to mean invasive carcinoma. Because papillary lesions with *in situ* carcinoma did not produce metastases, he evidently chose to classify them as papillomas, but it is clear from the foregoing quotation that he did appreciate the fact that areas with carcinomatous features could be found within benign appearing papillary tumors.[17] He recognized the difficulties inherent in proving that carcinoma may have arisen from a previously excised papillary lesion[18]:

> Most attempts to determine the incidence of cancer development from intraductal papillomas by follow-up studies are fruitless because when discovered the papilloma is

> removed. All that can then be demonstrated is that . . . the rate of breast cancer development in either breast following it is no higher than the expected breast cancer development rate for a comparable age group and time period.

Stout and Stewart took part in a study of lesions that had been diagnosed as benign intraductal papillomas from 125 patients treated at the New York Hospital.[19] Carcinoma was subsequently detected in the ipsilateral breast of seven patients, typically in proximity to the lesion previously described as a papilloma. The investigators agreed that five lesions originally diagnosed as papillomas had actually been carcinomas. A sixth tumor was confirmed to be a papilloma, and the seventh prior lesion was not reviewed.

A solitary papilloma that has been excised and not found to contain carcinoma or severely atypical hyperplasia is not a precancerous lesion. The risk of detecting carcinoma subsequently in the same breast is low. Overall, fewer than 5% of patients reportedly have developed breast carcinoma after excision of a papilloma, and nearly one-half of the subsequent carcinomas were detected in the opposite breast. In some cases, the proximity of mammary carcinoma and a papilloma is such that they must be regarded as parts of a single lesion. Mingling of the two processes is evidence of carcinoma arising in a papilloma. Usually, the carcinomatous component in these lesions is DCIS. Papillary tumors that have progressed to invasion rarely contain areas of papilloma. A greater risk for the development of carcinoma has been associated with the presence of multiple papillomas and with papillomas that contain *in situ* carcinoma (see Chapter 5).

CLINICAL PRESENTATION

Age

The literature does not contain well-established reliable information concerning the epidemiologic features of patients with papillary carcinoma. The tumor usually occurs in adults beyond the age of 50 years, and, on average, women with papillary carcinoma are older than women with other types of breast carcinoma. In a review of 35 cases, Fisher et al.[1] stated that "The lesion occurs with a significantly high frequency among . . . postmenopausal women." Other publications echo this observation.[6,20] Small series and case reports document the occurrence of papillary carcinomas in women as young as 29 years[21] and as old as 91 years.[22] Grabowski et al.[23] calculated a mean age of approximately 70 years using cases in the California Cancer Registry classified as intracystic papillary carcinoma. Men with papillary carcinoma span the same range of ages. According to Fisher et al.,[1] papillary carcinoma occurs more commonly in "non-Caucasians."

Location

Nearly 50% of papillary carcinomas arise in the central part of the breast, and as a consequence, nipple discharge has been described in 22% to 34% of patients.[24,25] Bleeding from the nipple occurs in a higher percentage of patients with papillary carcinoma than in women with a papilloma. Paget disease is rarely found in association with papillary carcinoma, but may be present if the lesion arises from major lactiferous ducts within the nipple or if there are additional foci of DCIS in the nipple. Most papillary carcinomas have a slow growth rate. Patients have reported the presence of a discharge or a mass for prolonged periods, and a duration of symptoms for a year or more before presentation is not unusual.[24–27]

Imaging Studies

Invasive papillary carcinomas present varied radiologic findings. Mammograms often display a multinodular pattern of increased density in a segmental distribution,[5,6] and the nodules sometimes occupy only a single quadrant.[5,6] Solitary masses also occur frequently.[20] The masses typically appear round, oval, or lobulated,[5,20,28] and their borders may be either well defined[5,22] or ill defined.[20,29] The differential diagnosis for a well-defined mass includes fibroadenoma (FA), benign cystic lesions, medullary carcinoma, and mucinous carcinoma. Coarse, irregular calcifications may develop in areas of sclerosis or resolved hemorrhage in papillomas or in papillary carcinomas. Calcifications are not abundant in most papillary carcinomas, and when present, they tend to be punctate and associated with the intraductal component.[22] In one case,[30] the calcifications appeared "rod like." The sonographic features of papillomas and papillary carcinomas overlap.[31,32] Sonography of invasive papillary carcinomas typically demonstrates masses that appear well defined, solid or mixed solid and cystic, inhomogeneous, and hypoechogenic with posterior enhancement.[5,20,30] The presence of a nonparallel orientation, echogenic halo, posterior acoustic enhancement, and calcifications suggests the diagnosis of papillary carcinoma rather than papilloma.[32] Magnetic resonance imaging (MRI) of one case[33] yielded T1-weighted images showing an irregular mass with moderately decreased signal intensity; on T2-weighted images, the carcinoma appeared hypointense. After gadolinium injection, mild and inhomogeneous enhancement was noted. Other cases of invasive and noninvasive papillary carcinoma did not demonstrate specific findings.[34] In fact, MRI failed to detect 2 of 13 papillary carcinomas and classified 6 of the remaining 11 as benign or probably benign. Extension of papillary carcinoma into adjacent ducts cannot be reliably assessed by mammography. Galactography may be used to examine patients who have nipple discharge to determine whether papillary lesions are multicentric.[35] Filling defects in ducts outlined in a galactogram may be due to papillomas or papillary carcinoma.

Clinically detectable enlargement of axillary lymph nodes (ALNs) is unusual except in patients with massive tumors, which tend to develop areas of hemorrhagic necrosis.

GROSS PATHOLOGY

The gross appearance of papillary carcinomas varies considerably depending on the relative proportions of cystic and solid components (Fig. 14.1). The average clinically

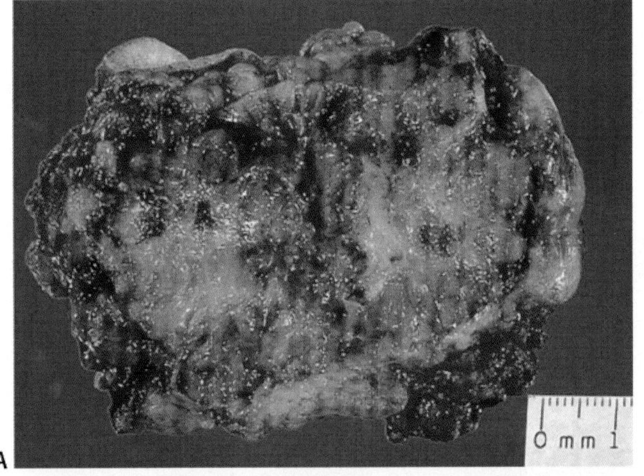

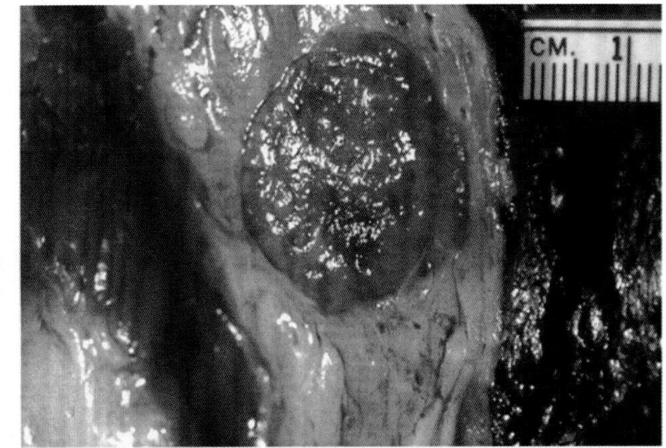

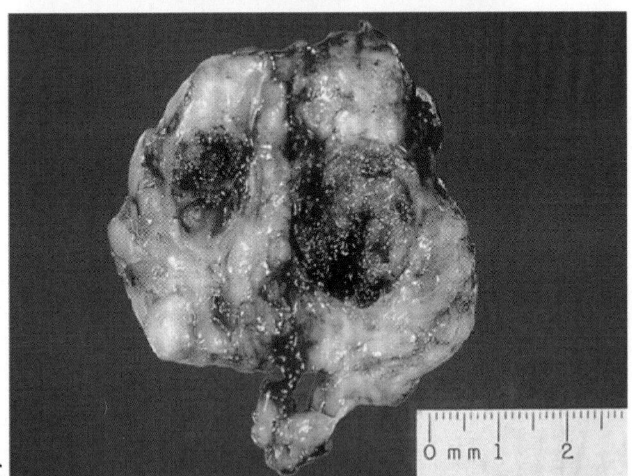

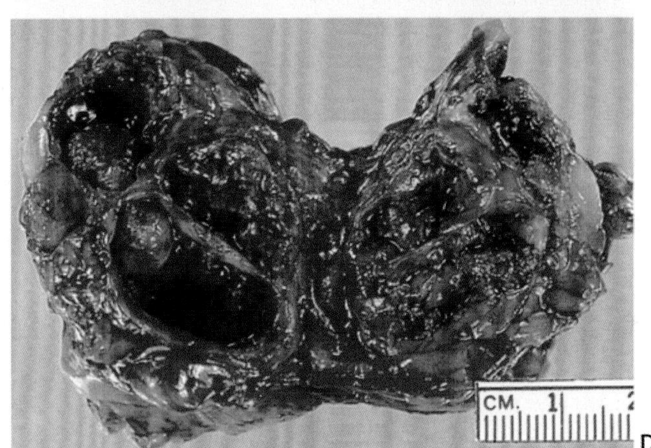

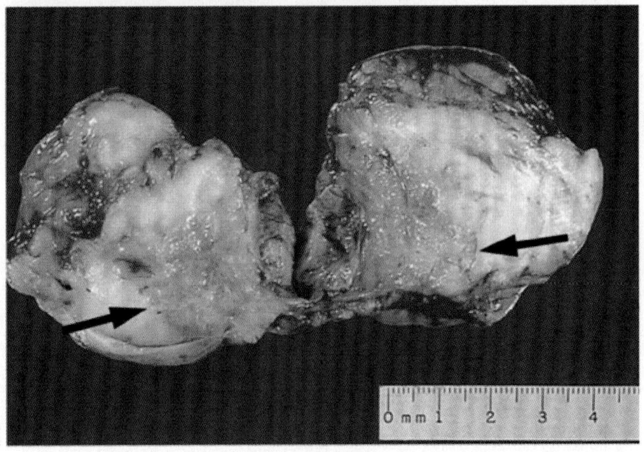

FIG. 14.1. ***Papillary carcinoma.*** Various gross appearances. **A:** Solid tumor with a lobulated contour and central fibrosis. **B:** A brown, bulging solid papillary carcinoma with no cystic component. **C:** Solid intracystic tumor. **D:** Multiloculated cystic tumor with intracystic papillary nodules. **E:** Cystic papillary carcinoma with a large invasive component represented by the tan areas (*arrows*).

determined size of tumors is 2 to 3 cm. Papillary carcinomas are usually well circumscribed grossly, and they may even appear encapsulated (Fig. 14.2). The tumor is soft to moderately firm, depending upon the extent of fibrosis. Bleeding into the tumor can impart a dark brown or hemorrhagic appearance, but the carcinomas are usually described as tan or gray. Needle aspiration or needle core biopsy can produce more hemorrhage than occurs in a nonpapillary mammary carcinoma because of the friable character of many papillary lesions, especially those without fibrosis or healed prior hemorrhage.

MICROSCOPIC PATHOLOGY

The term "papillary" describes carcinomas in which the underlying microscopic pattern is predominantly frond forming (Fig. 14.3). Although most of these tumors are large enough to form a palpable mass, the diagnosis is also applicable to microscopic lesions that have a papillary structure (Fig. 14.4). Many papillary carcinomas have cystic areas, but cyst formation is not necessary for the diagnosis of papillary carcinoma. Foote and Stewart[14] observed that "in some areas the cell

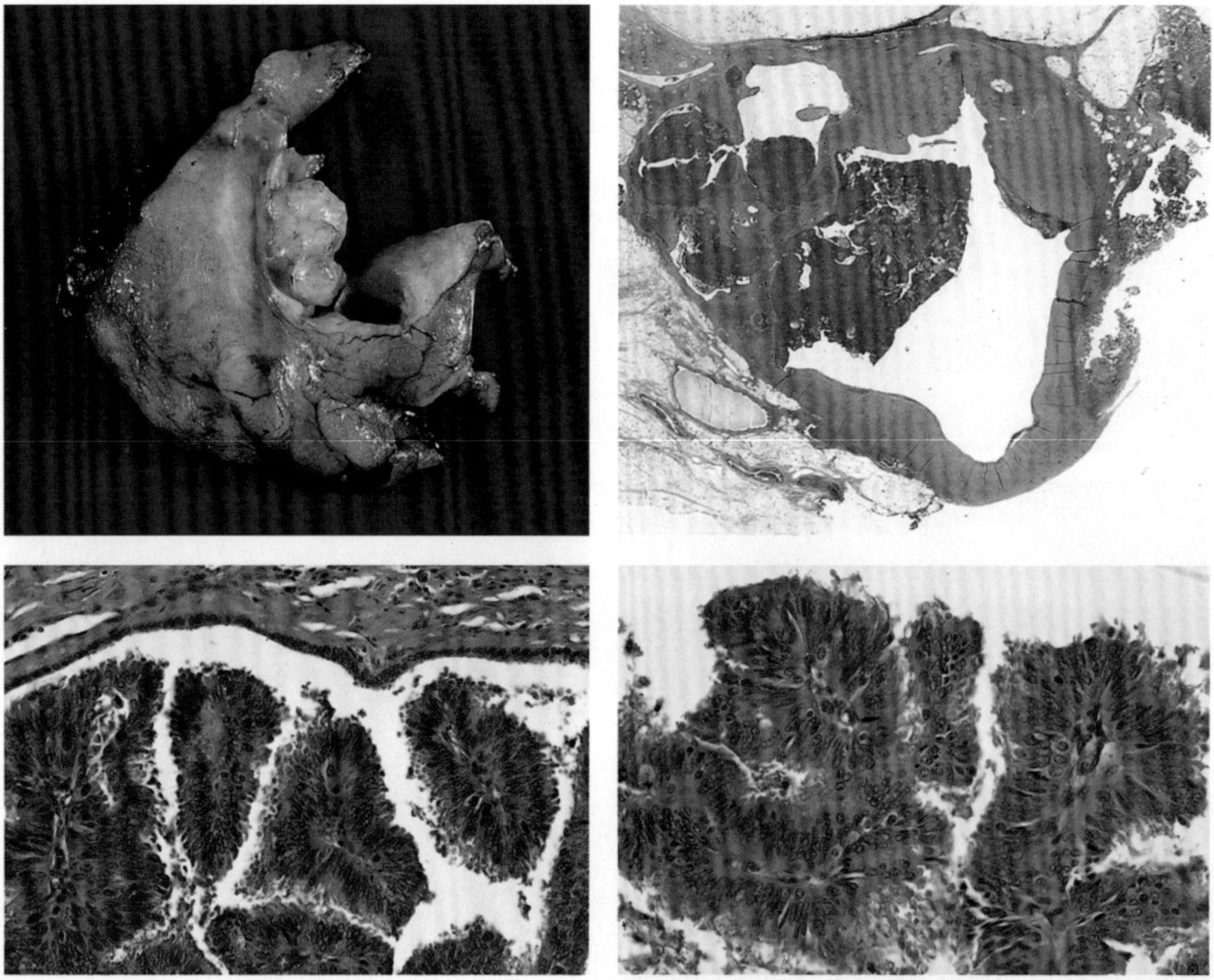

FIG. 14.2. ***Papillary carcinoma, cystic.*** **A:** The tumor forms a tan nodule, which protrudes into the cyst. **B:** A whole-mount histologic section of a similar specimen showing a nodular papillary tumor protruding into the cyst lumen and the thick fibrous cyst wall. **C,D:** Histologic appearance of an orderly papillary carcinoma.

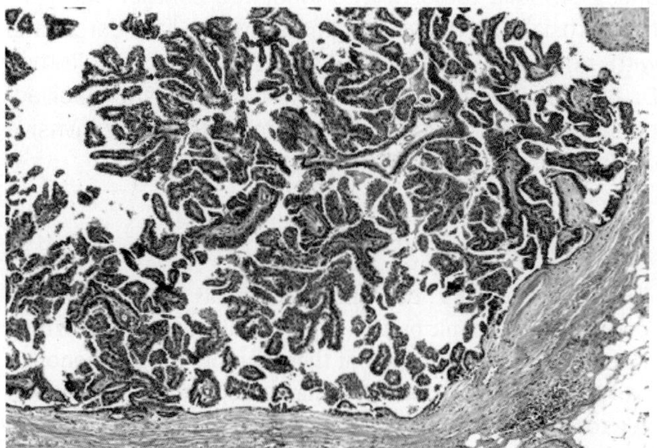

FIG. 14.3. ***Papillary carcinoma.*** Low magnification reveals the characteristic formation of fronds.

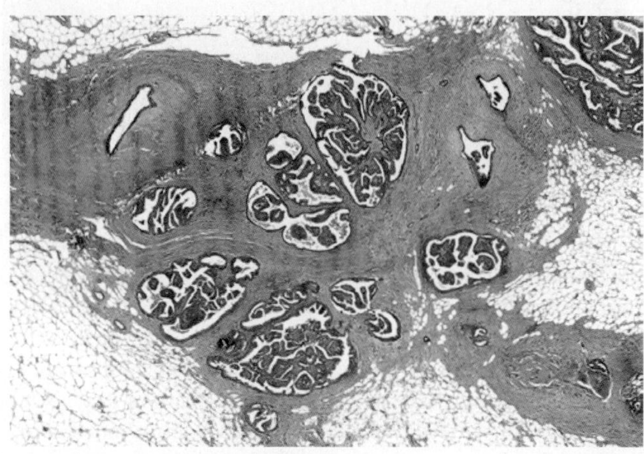

FIG. 14.4. ***Papillary carcinoma.*** A nonpalpable focus that has a radial scar configuration.

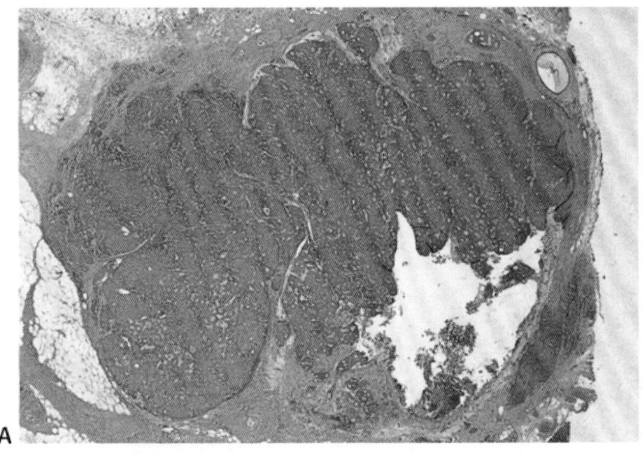

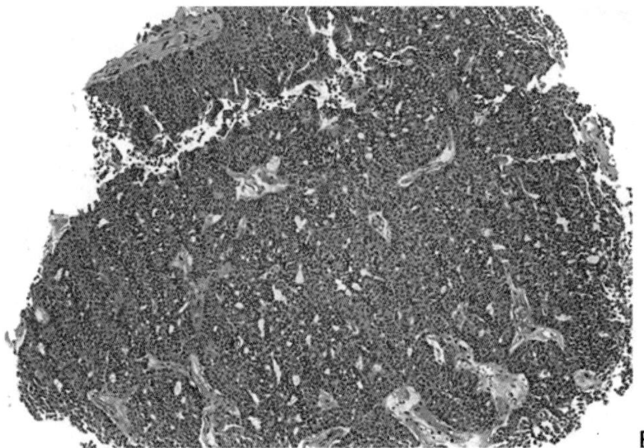

FIG. 14.5. ***Solid papillary carcinoma.*** **A:** A whole mount showing the multinodular circumscribed tumor. A defect in the tumor is the site of a needle core biopsy. **B:** The needle core biopsy specimen, which contains branching fibrovascular stroma.

proliferation becomes so dense that basic papillary properties are overgrown." Such a tumor is classified as *solid papillary carcinoma* (Fig. 14.5). The underlying papillary nature of these lesions is defined by a branching network of fibrovascular stroma, but there are no spaces between individual papillary fronds.

NONINVASIVE PAPILLARY CARCINOMA

The histologic features of *in situ* papillary carcinomas contrast with those of their benign counterparts, papillomas. The distinction between the two lesions is determined by their cytologic and microscopic attributes. In 1962, Kraus and Neubecker[36] set forth often quoted criteria for distinguishing benign from malignant papillary tumors. The histologic characteristics enumerated by Kraus and Neubecker are summarized in Table 14.1; however, numerous exceptions and structural variations complicate the application of these criteria.

The fundamental principle in evaluating papillary tumors is to determine whether the epithelium between adjacent fibrovascular cores has features diagnostic of DCIS. The space between the fibrovascular cores can be likened to a duct lumen bounded by these stromal elements and the epithelium covering the cores to the epithelium lining a duct. The cytologic and architectural attributes of the epithelial cells growing on the stromal cores determine that the nature of the papillary tumor and other, ancillary, findings will often help to substantiate the diagnosis.

Cell Types

Benign luminal and myoepithelial cells make up the epithelium of a papilloma, whereas malignant ductal cells comprise the entire epithelial population of most papillary carcinomas. As a result of uneven stratification and loss of polarity with respect to stromal elements within the lesion (Fig. 14.6), the carcinoma cells of papillary carcinoma grow in a less orderly fashion than do the benign cells of papillomas. They usually do not form two consistently arranged layers composed of distinct cell types. Instead, the carcinoma cells demonstrate

TABLE 14.1 Criteria of Kraus and Neubecker[36] for the Diagnosis of Papillary Breast Lesions[a]

Histologic Feature	Papilloma	Papillary Carcinoma
1. Cell types	Epithelial/myoepithelial	Epithelial
2. Nuclei	Normochromatic	Hyperchromatic
3. Apocrine metaplasia	Present	Absent
4. Glandular pattern	Complex	Cribriform
5. Stroma	Prominent Fibrosis with epithelial entrapment	Delicate or absent Stroma invaded in invasive lesions
6. Adjacent ducts	Hyperplasia	Intraductal carcinoma
7. Associated SA	Sometimes present	Usually absent

[a]See text for detailed discussion and interpretation of these criteria.

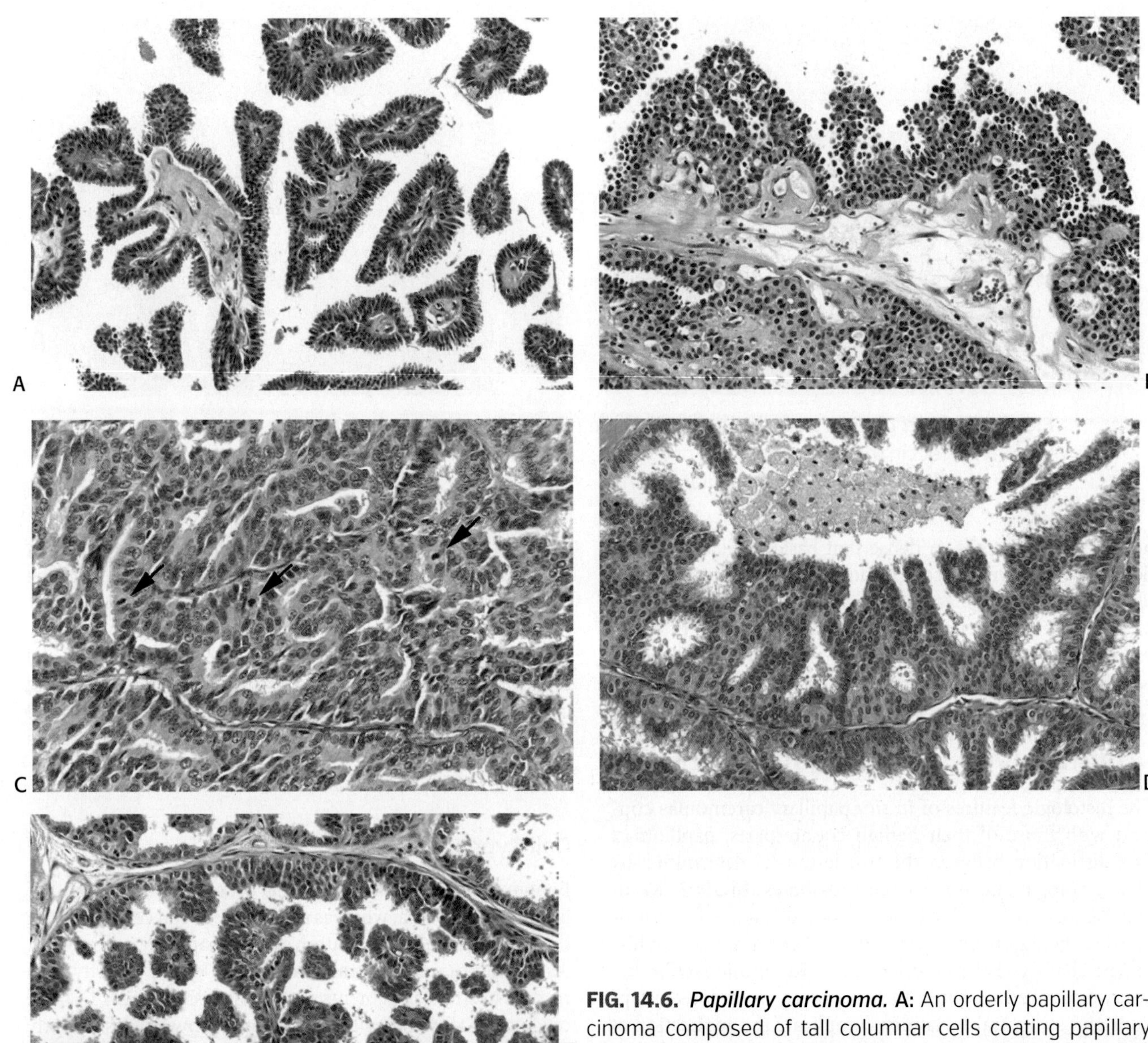

FIG. 14.6. ***Papillary carcinoma.*** **A:** An orderly papillary carcinoma composed of tall columnar cells coating papillary fronds. **B:** Disorderly arrangement of neoplastic epithelial cells with hyperchromatic nuclei on a papillary frond. **C:** Cells with large nuclei and frequent mitotic figures (*arrows*) on a delicate frond. **D:** Cribriform carcinoma on the fibrovascular stroma of a papillary tumor. **E:** Micropapillary carcinoma.

papillary, micropapillary or filiform, cribriform, reticular, or solid growth patterns (Fig. 14.7).

Myoepithelial cells that are distributed relatively uniformly and proportionately with the epithelium in benign papillary lesions are usually overgrown in papillary carcinomas. However, the finding of myoepithelial cells in some parts of a papillary lesion is not inconsistent with a diagnosis of carcinoma.[37–39] Myoepithelial cells are prominent mainly in residual areas of a papilloma that has given rise to a papillary carcinoma, and they tend to be less conspicuous or absent in the carcinomatous areas (Fig. 14.8).

Nuclei

The malignant cells of papillary carcinomas demonstrate the same cytologic features as those of commonplace DCIS. Although the cellular attributes vary according to the grade of the carcinoma, common alterations include an increase in the size of the cell and enlargement of its nucleus. In common, low-grade papillary carcinomas, the cells appear uniform, but those of the uncommon high-grade papillary carcinomas demonstrate conspicuous cellular pleomorphism. The nuclei are characteristically hyperchromatic regardless of cytologic grade, and there is usually a high

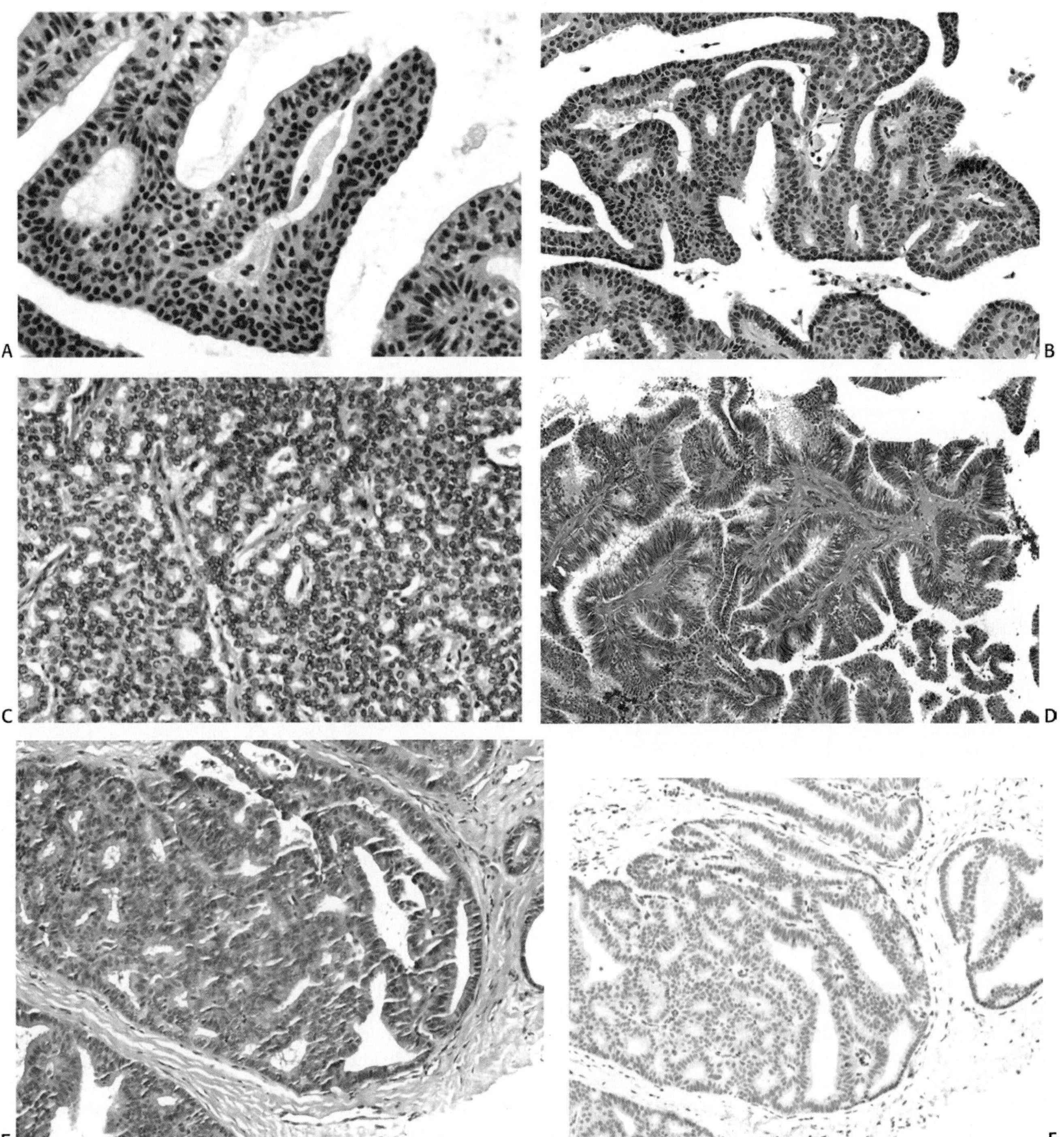

FIG. 14.7. ***Papillary carcinoma.*** Architectural growth patterns. **A:** Micropapillary. **B:** Trabecular. **C:** Solid papillary with cribriform glands. **D:** Papillary. **E,F:** Papillary carcinoma with cribriform structure. Absence of myoepithelium is evident in the p63 immunostain **(F)**.

nuclear-to-cytoplasmic ratio. The mitotic figures vary in number , and they are more numerous in carcinomas that exhibit the most severe cytologic atypia. Mitotic activity is uncommon in papillomas. The presence of more than one mitosis in 10 high-magnification (40×) fields suggests the diagnosis of papillary carcinoma.

Apocrine Metaplasia

The tumor cells sometimes have secretory "snouts" at the luminal surface. The cytoplasm is typically amphophilic, but eosinophilic cells are found in a number of lesions. Papotti et al.[37] found apocrine cells that were immunoreactive

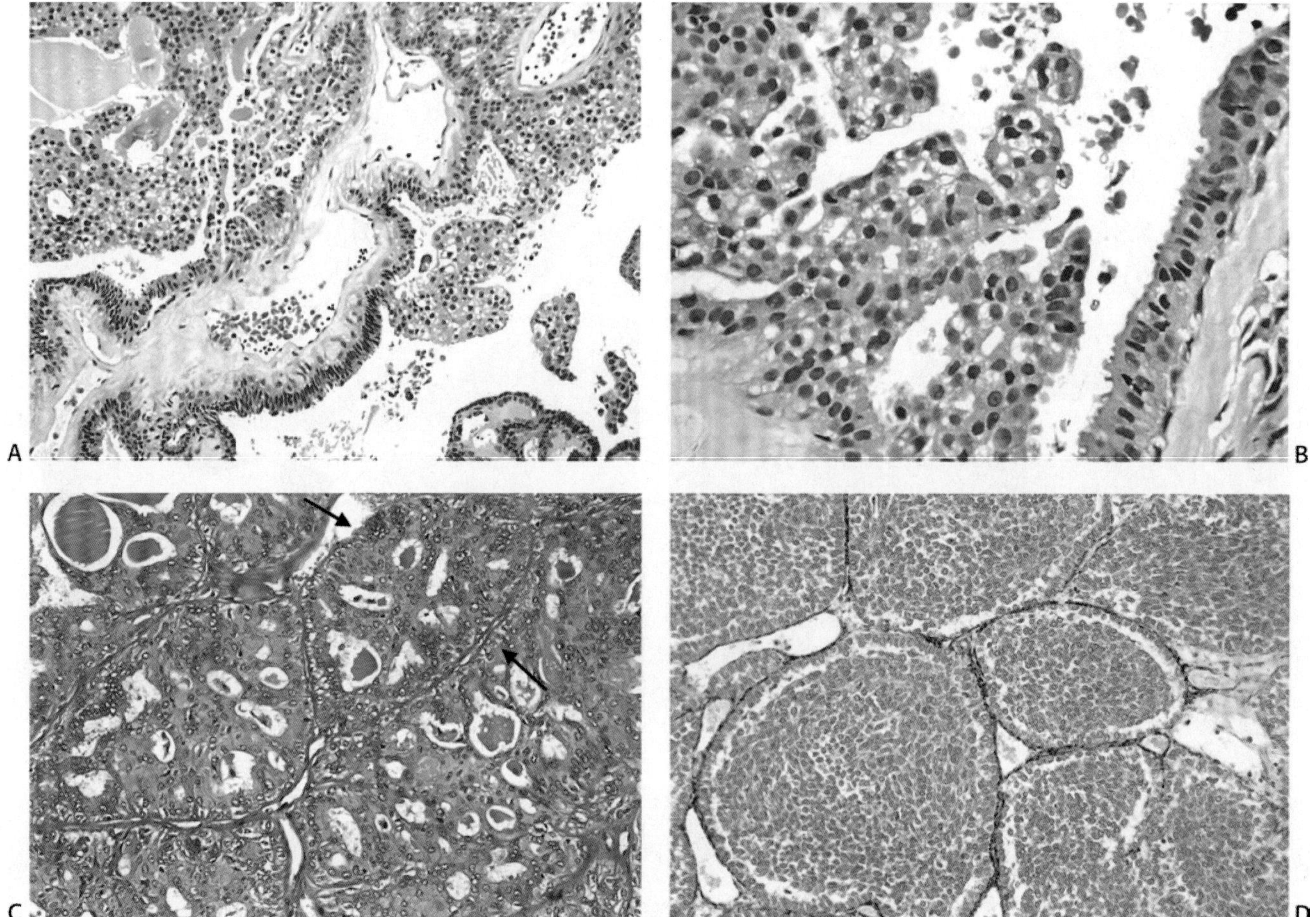

FIG. 14.8. ***Papillary carcinoma.*** **A:** Solid areas of carcinoma are distributed on the surfaces of the fronds of an underlying papilloma. **B:** Myoepithelial cells are seen in epithelium of the papilloma on the *right*, and they are absent in the papillary carcinoma on the *left*. **C:** Papillary carcinoma with cribriform structure and myoepithelial cells (*arrows*). **D:** Solid papillary carcinoma with spindle cell growth in which attenuated myoepithelial cells are highlighted by an immunostain for SMA.

for gross cystic disease fluid protein-15 (GCDFP-15) in 75% of papillomas and in 50% of papillary carcinomas. Apocrine areas in a papillary carcinoma exhibit cytologic atypia consistent with the rest of the tumor and, in that way, differ from the bland foci of apocrine metaplasia commonly encountered in papillomas (Fig. 14.9). The presence of cytologically benign apocrine elements is invariably associated with a papilloma rather than a papillary carcinoma.

Glandular Pattern

Describing the epithelium of papillomas, Kraus and Neubecker[36] introduced the term *complex glandular pattern* to refer to the compact, back-to-back arrangement of proliferative glands within the stalk of a papilloma. The authors noted that this close crowding of glands ". . . was often a source of confusion in that it superficially resembled the cribriform pattern of carcinoma."[36] The cribriform pattern characteristic of low-grade DCIS does occur in papillary carcinomas frequently. To distinguish the "complex glandular pattern" seen in papillomas from the cribriform spaces of papillary carcinoma, one should examine the tissue separating the individual acinar structures. Thin strands of collagen and slender capillaries surround each of the glands that compose the "complex glandular pattern," whereas the spaces formed in cribriform carcinomas lack these connective stromal elements.

Stroma

Supporting fibrovascular stroma is present in virtually all papillary carcinomas, but it tends to be less conspicuous in carcinomas than in benign papillary lesions because of the dominance of the epithelial component in carcinomas. A minority of papillary carcinomas have areas in which there are relatively broad fibrous stalks of extensive sclerosis, and consequently the character of the stroma within the lesion is not by itself a reliable diagnostic feature (Fig. 14.10).

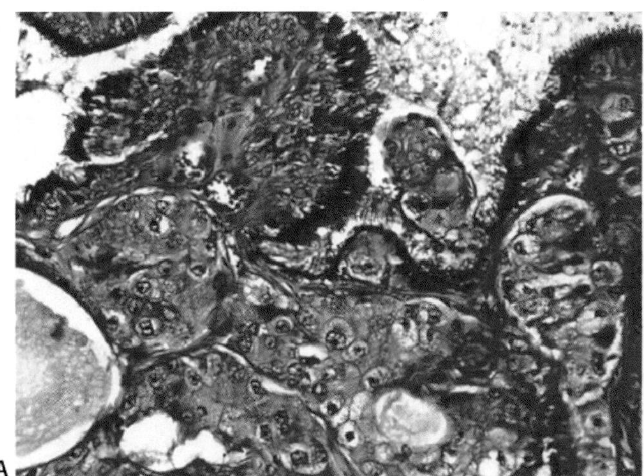

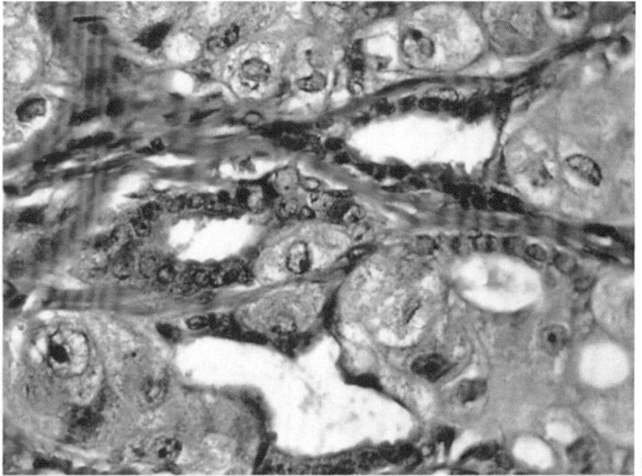

FIG. 14.9. ***Papillary carcinoma.*** **A:** Residual epithelium of a papilloma is present on the surface of these fronds, which are occupied by apocrine carcinoma (*below*). **B:** Apocrine carcinoma has almost completely replaced the benign epithelium of this papillary tumor leaving a few glands composed of benign epithelium.

Scaring frequently occurs in the periphery of papillary tumors. This process can entrap both benign glands and those harboring *in situ* carcinoma. The resulting appearance simulates the look of invasive carcinoma and makes the recognition of minimal invasion difficult.

Adjacent Ducts

Carcinoma usually extends into ducts at the periphery of a papillary carcinoma. When the interpretation of an orderly papillary tumor is difficult, careful examination of the surrounding ducts can be extremely helpful. The presence of foci of papillary, cribriform, or comedocarcinoma is usually evidence that *in situ* carcinoma is also present in the papillary tumor. In the same way, study of an epithelial proliferation situated on the wall of the duct harboring a papillary tumor can shed light on the nature of the epithelial cells within the papillary portion.

Sclerosing Adenosis

In almost one-half of the papillomas studied by Kraus and Neubecker,[36] the surrounding tissue displayed sclerosing adenosis (SA), and it protruded into ducts and simulated papillomas in a few instances. SA does not coexist with papillary carcinomas commonly.

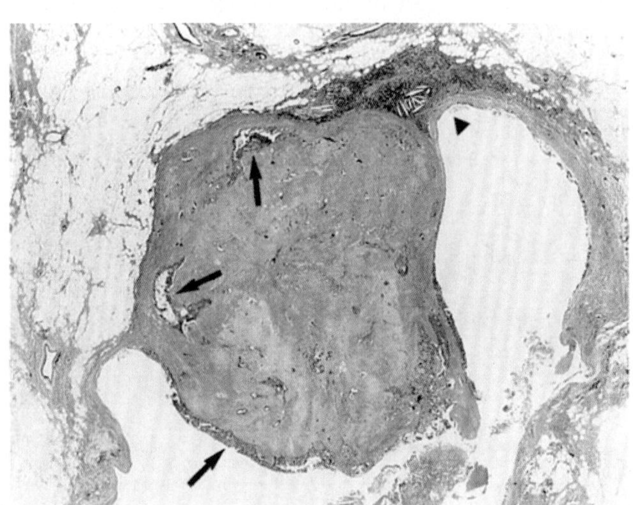

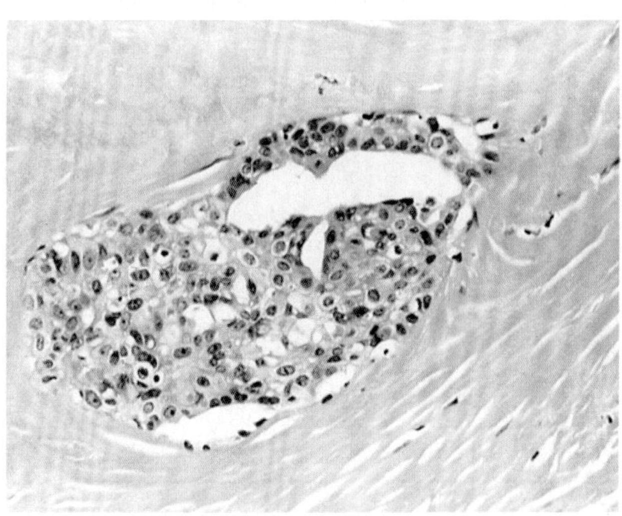

FIG. 14.10. ***Papillary carcinoma with sclerosis.*** **A:** A whole-mount histologic section of a cystic papillary carcinoma that has been reduced to a fibrotic nodule with a few neoplastic glands and a thin layer of residual carcinoma on the surface (*arrows*). Chronic inflammation and fat necrosis are evident at the *upper* border of the tumor. **B:** A carcinomatous gland within the fibrotic tumor.

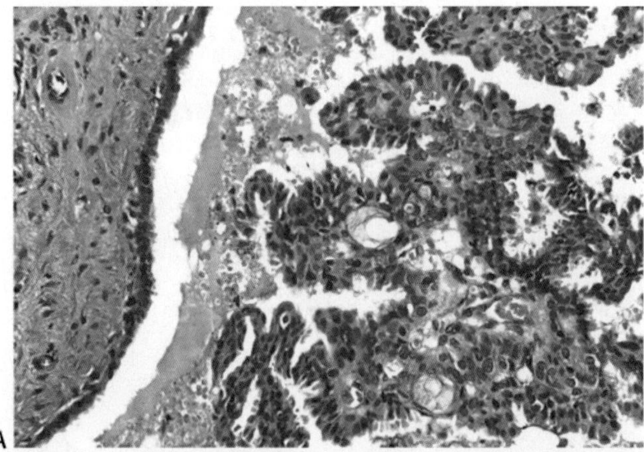

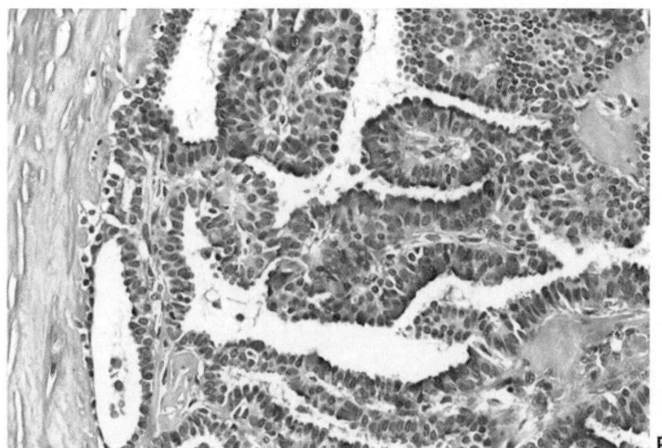

FIG. 14.11. ***Papillary carcinoma with mucin secretion.*** **A:** *Blue* mucin vacuoles are present in the epithelium. **B:** The mucin is stained blue with the Alcian blue/PAS reaction.

Mucin Secretion

There is a broad range of mucin secretion demonstrable in papillary carcinomas with the mucicarmine, Alcian blue, and periodic acid–Schiff (PAS) stains (Fig. 14.11). Some papillary carcinomas have no detectable intracellular mucin. In the majority, mucin secretion is not prominent, but a small number of papillary carcinomas have signet ring cells (Fig. 14.12) or abundant and diffuse intracellular mucin secretion (Fig. 14.13). The accumulation of abundant extracellular mucin creates a pattern that resembles invasive mucinous carcinoma, but does not represent invasion when confined within the tumor (Fig. 14.14).

Microcalcifications

Microcalcifications found in many papillary carcinomas are usually distributed in the glandular portions of the lesion, but they may also be found in the papillary stroma. Calcifications also form in the stroma of papillomas, so neither the presence nor the pattern of calcification provides reliable diagnostic information.

Residual Papilloma

Papillary carcinoma that has arisen in a papilloma sometimes retains areas of papilloma that appear benign or atypical, as well as having foci of more cellular proliferation diagnostic of carcinoma (Figs. 14.8, 14.9, and 14.15). Small areas of papilloma in such lesions are of little consequence, and they should not impede the recognition of the carcinomatous element. In some instances, the diagnosis of papillary carcinoma can be "a 'shadow land' even for the most experienced pathologist,"[40] a situation that Foote and Stewart[14] referred to as "a zone of altered cell growth where the diagnosis of carcinoma versus atypical papillomatosis

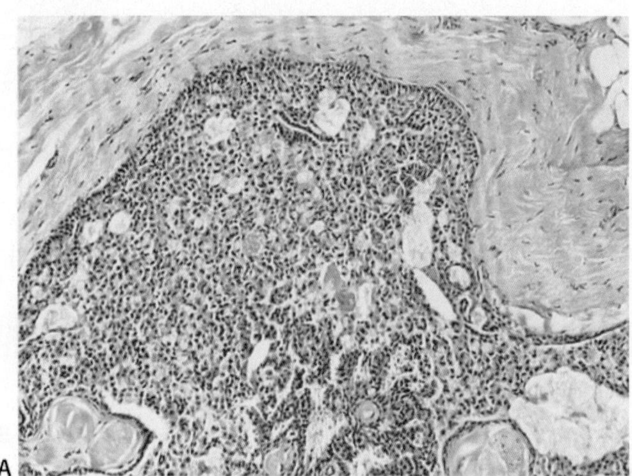

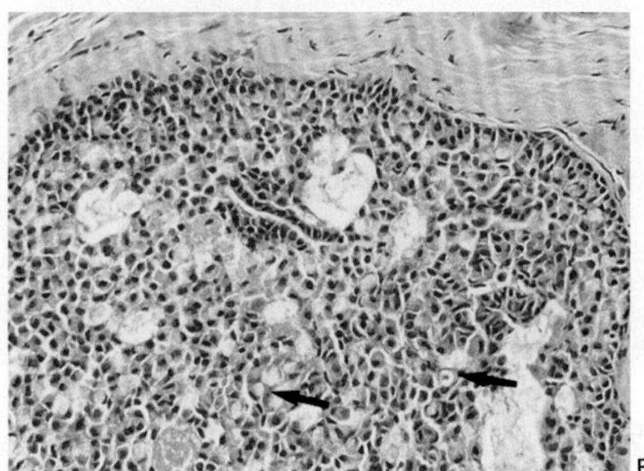

FIG. 14.12. ***Papillary carcinoma with signet ring cells.*** **A:** The cells with clear cytoplasm were strongly reactive with the mucicarmine stain and focally positive with the Grimelius stain. **B:** Signet ring cells (*arrows*).

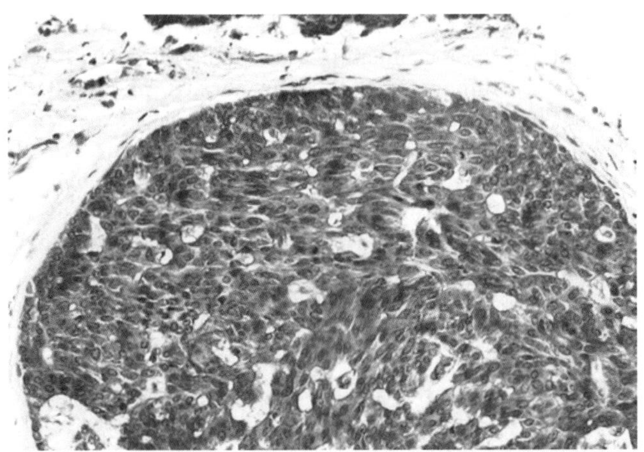

FIG. 14.13. ***Solid papillary carcinoma with mucin.*** The spindle cells show diffuse magenta staining with the mucicarmine stain.

is a question of occult distinction and must be accepted or rejected on grounds of faith in the pathologist or lack of it." "Borderline" papillary lesions that fit this description often have modest or substantial areas of benign papillary proliferation as well as more cellular and atypical components. To make a diagnosis of carcinoma in the latter setting, it is necessary to find one or more low-power microscopic fields where the growth pattern and cytologic appearance constitute one of the established patterns of DCIS. Some authors have illustrated focal DCIS in papillomas, but classified these lesions as "papillomas with atypical ductal hyperplasia."[41,42] In one of these studies, the relative risk for "subsequent carcinoma" in women with such papillomas was more than four times the risk of women with papillomas that lacked atypical ductal hyperplasia/DCIS.[42] Underdiagnosis of such lesions is likely to result in inadequate treatment that is reflected in the outcomes of patients in these reports.

Three-Dimensional Structure

Three-dimensional reconstruction of the microscopic structure of papillary lesions has revealed some interesting differences between papillomas and papillary carcinomas.[43,44] In papillomas and usual ductal hyperplasia (UDH), the luminal spaces between the proliferating epithelial cells form a complex but diffusely anastomosing continuous network of channels. On the other hand, in DCIS, the luminal spaces tend to be separate, and they do not form a continuous network. These elegant and painstaking studies have resulted in a more complete appreciation of the structural differences between hyperplastic and carcinomatous papillary lesions.

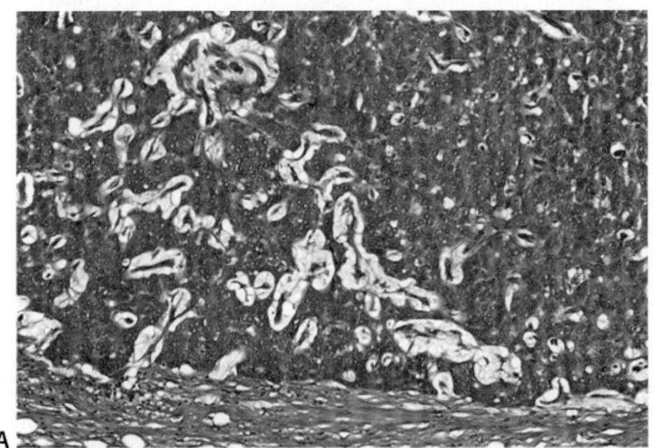

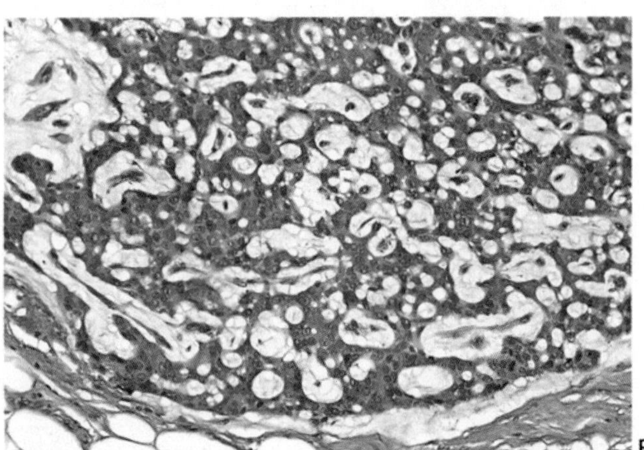

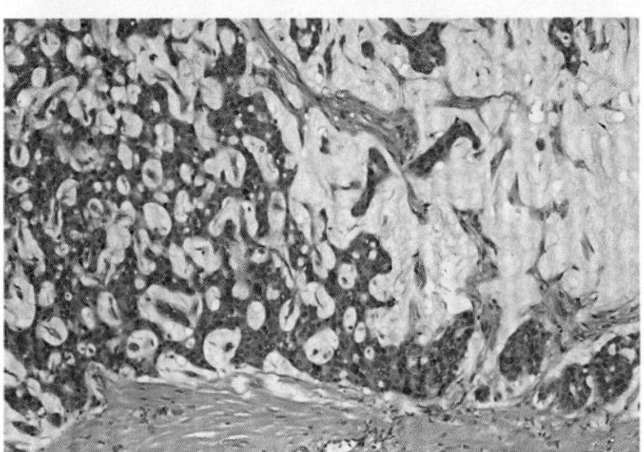

FIG. 14.14. ***Solid papillary carcinoma with extracellular mucin.*** These images from a single tumor illustrate progressive accumulation of extracellular mucin. **A:** Extracellular mucin is concentrated around fibrovascular structures rather than in gland lumens. **B:** Further expansion of the mucin is evident including at the interface of the tumor and stroma [*below*]. Vascular structures remain in virtually every mucin collection. **C:** Coalescent areas of mucin on the *right* contain the basic papillary vascular pattern. Note the retained sharply defined border *below*.

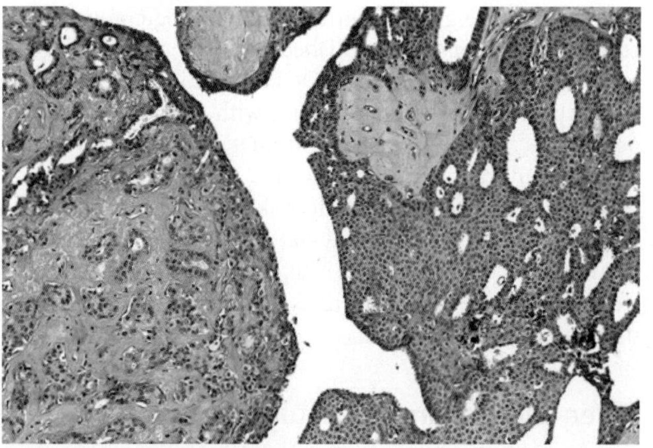

FIG. 14.15. ***Papillary carcinoma arising in a papilloma.*** A portion of the underlying papilloma is evident in the *left* of the field. Carcinoma *in situ* covers fronds in the *right* of the field.

Cystic Papillary Fluid

In additional to histologic study, biochemical analysis of the fluid from cystic papillary lesions may be helpful in the differential diagnosis between cystic papilloma and papillary carcinoma. Matsuo et al.[45] found an elevated carcinoembryonic antigen (CEA) content in aspirated fluid from a 10-cm cystic breast tumor. CEA was demonstrated immunohistochemically in the carcinoma cells in the resected specimen. Another study compared CEA and human epidermal growth factor 2 (HER2) protein levels in fluid from 6 cystic papillomas, 6 papillary carcinomas, and 42 gross cysts.[46] Five of the six carcinomas (83%) had elevated levels of both proteins compared with two (33%) of the papillomas and two (5%) of gross cysts.

INVASIVE PAPILLARY CARCINOMA

Evidence of Invasion

The growth patterns found in areas of frankly invasive papillary carcinoma usually constitute variations on the architecture of the carcinoma in the underlying *in situ* papillary tumor (Fig. 14.16). The cytologic characteristics of the invasive component also resemble those of the *in situ* portion of the lesion, in some cases including apocrine features. Cribriform, comedo, tubular, and mucinous foci may also be present. The invasive element may grow partly or entirely as mucinous

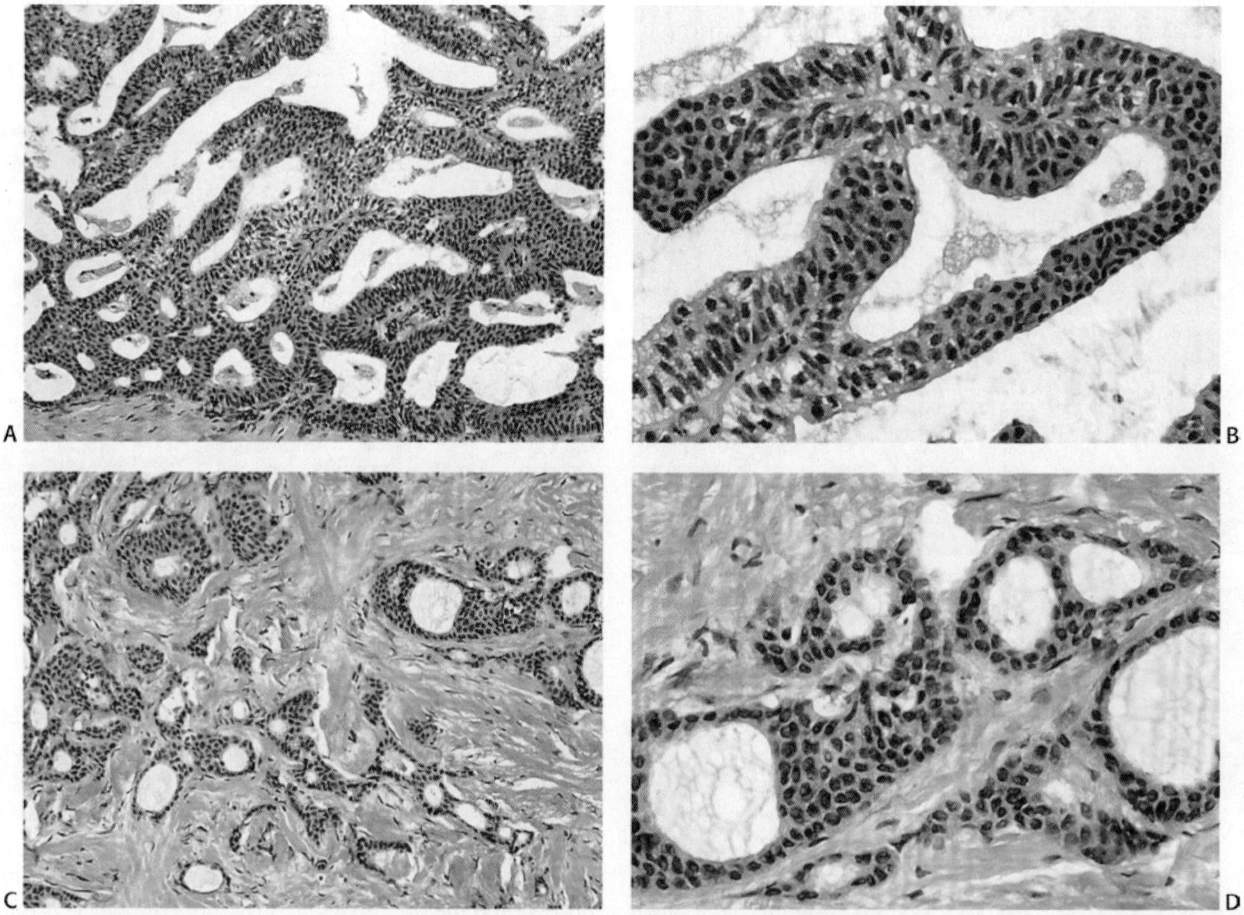

FIG. 14.16. ***Invasive papillary carcinoma.*** **A:** *In situ* papillary carcinoma. **B:** The carcinoma cells in (A) have dark cytologically low-grade nuclei and eosinophilic cytoplasm. **C:** Invasive cribriform carcinoma that arose in the papillary carcinoma. **D:** The cytologic features of the invasive component resemble the papillary *in situ* carcinoma.

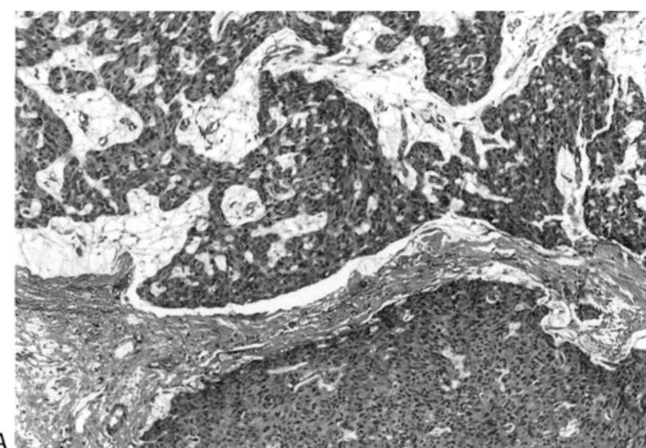
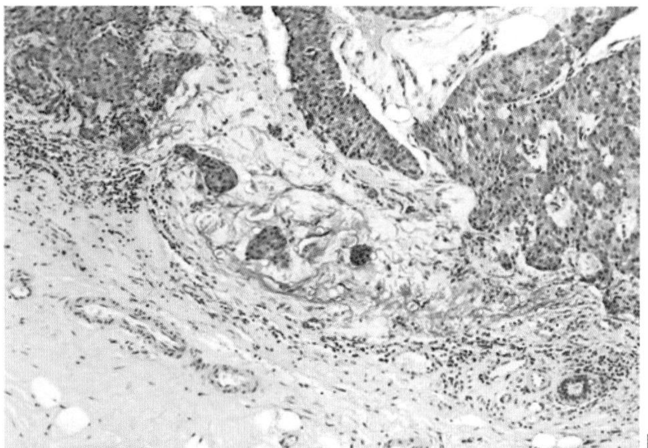

FIG. 14.17. ***Papillary carcinoma, invasive mucinous.*** **A:** Extracellular mucin in a solid papillary carcinoma confined to the tumor (*above*) does not constitute invasive carcinoma (see Fig. 14.14). **B:** Small clusters of carcinoma cells and mucin in the peritumoral stroma represent invasive mucinous carcinoma (mucicarmine stain).

carcinoma, an occurrence usually associated with solid papillary carcinoma. Mucinous differentiation in solid papillary carcinoma is manifest not only by the presence of intracellular and intraluminal mucin but also by the accumulation of extracellular mucin in limited amounts between the neoplastic epithelium and adjacent stroma (Fig. 14.14). This phenomenon can occur within the tumor, adjacent to fibrovascular stalks, and at the border of the tumor. The resultant small pools of mucin are not interpreted as invasive mucinous carcinoma unless they contain detached neoplastic cells. Larger accumulations may surround or disrupt portions of the epithelium, and the resultant appearance is interpreted as invasive mucinous carcinoma when carcinoma cells surrounded by mucin extend into the adjacent stroma (Fig. 14.17).

Clusters of invasive papillary carcinoma cells are particularly prone to shrinkage artifact, and they often appear to lie in spaces, creating the appearance of lymphatic tumor emboli. When one applies strict criteria for the diagnosis of lymphatic invasion, most such foci prove to be artifactual.[47]

The invasive nature of many papillary carcinomas appears obvious, but the recognition of minimally invasive papillary carcinoma can be difficult. Many papillary carcinomas are bounded by zones of fibrosis, recent or resolved hemorrhage, and chronic inflammation, and similar alterations may occur within the lesion. Papillary or glandular clusters of epithelial cells routinely found within these areas present a challenging problem (Fig. 14.18). If one recalls that similar patterns of epithelial dispersal can occur in sclerotic portions of benign papillary lesions, it is possible to determine that these do not constitute foci of invasion in most cases. Groups of neoplastic cells distributed parallel to layers of reactive stroma at the border of a papillary carcinoma usually represent entrapped *in situ* epithelium rather than invasive carcinoma. An actin immunostain is sometimes helpful in this situation, although staining of reactive myofibroblasts can complicate the interpretation. Myofibroblastic staining is avoided if the p63 immunostain is used, but this procedure is useful only if the p63 stain reveals myoepithelium throughout the papillary tumor. Isolated invasive carcinoma cells can be identified with a cytokeratin immunostain. In general, the most reliable histologic evidence of frank invasion is extension of tumor beyond the zone of reactive changes into the mammary parenchyma and fat (Figs. 14.17, 14.19, and 14.20).

Effects of Needling Procedures

Papillary lesions that have been subjected to fine-needle aspiration (FNA) or needle core biopsy prior to excision can exhibit iatrogenic alterations that complicate the determination of invasion. Hemorrhage is commonly found in and around the tumor grossly. The best microscopic clues to such manipulation of the tumor are the presence of fresh

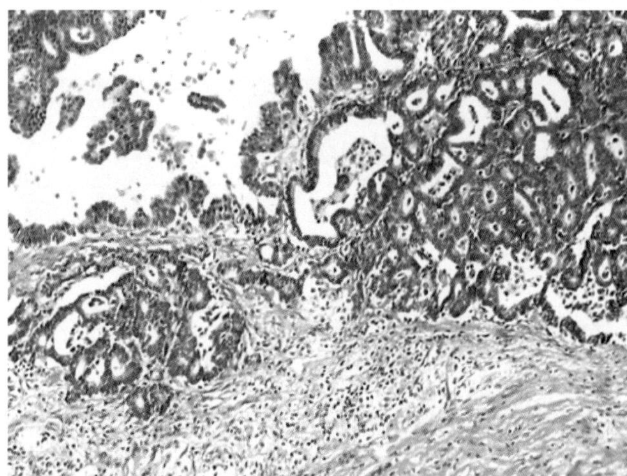

FIG. 14.18. ***Papillary carcinoma, possibly microinvasive.*** Epithelial nest in the fibrous wall around a papillary carcinoma. Irregular epithelial islands with this cribriform pattern are suggestive of invasion but could be part of the intracystic lesion trapped in the cyst wall.

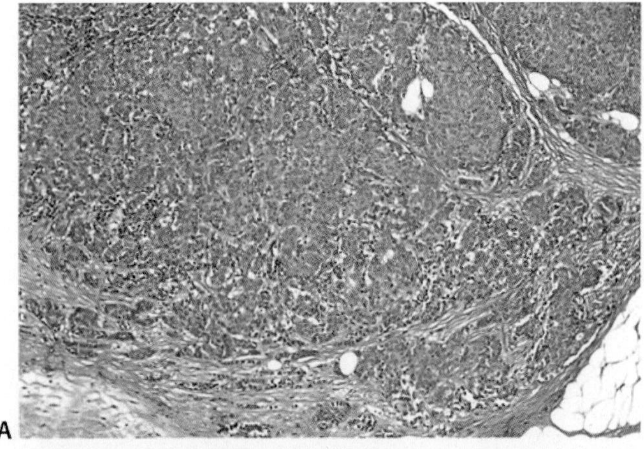

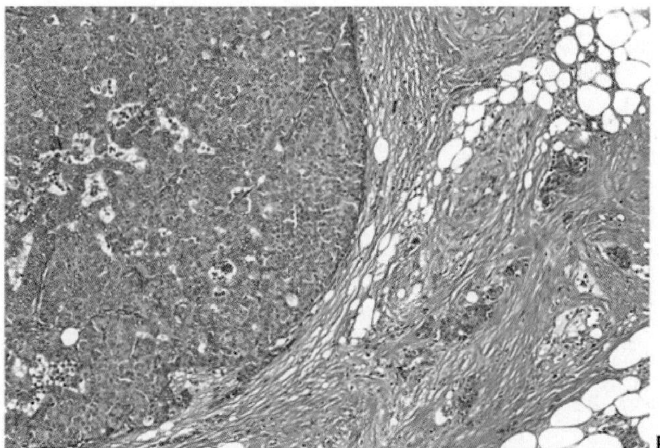

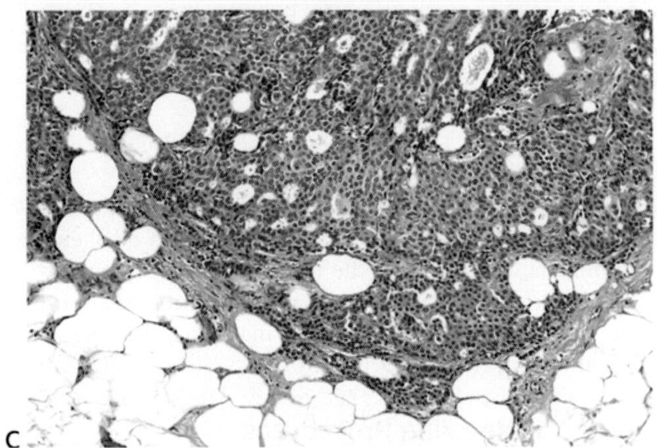

FIG. 14.19. ***Papillary carcinoma, invasive.*** **A:** The solid papillary growth pattern is disrupted at the periphery of this tumor (*below*), where glands are arranged parallel to the reactive stromal tissue (*lower left* and *center*) and form irregular masses (*lower right*). These foci are very suggestive of invasion, especially on the *lower right*. Immunostains to assess the vascular pattern, basement membranes, and the presence of myoepithelial cells are helpful in the questionable region. **B:** Nests of invasive carcinoma cells are present in fibrofatty tissue (*right*) outside a solid papillary carcinoma. **C:** Carcinoma with a microcribriform pattern invades fat.

hemorrhage and acute inflammation associated with "unnatural" fragmentation of the lesion. Tumor cells can be found singly or in clusters deposited in areas of hemorrhage and along the course of the needle tracks (Fig. 14.21). As long as it is known that the lesion was recently biopsied, these detached cells are best regarded as the result of trauma rather than as evidence of invasion. Sometimes epithelial cells are also seen in capillary or lymphatic channels after needle aspiration (Fig. 14.22). This uncommon finding should be described in the pathology report and may be regarded as a manifestation of invasive carcinoma in some instances.[48] Epithelial displacement associated with needling procedures is discussed more extensively in Chapter 44.

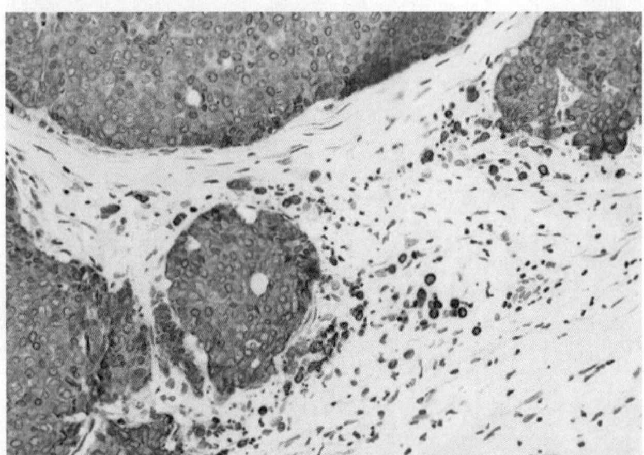

FIG. 14.20. ***Papillary carcinoma, microinvasive.*** Isolated microinvasive carcinoma cells are highlighted in the peritumoral stroma by a cytokeratin immunostain (CAM5.2).

One unusual pattern of true invasion found in solid papillary carcinomas simulates epithelial displacement resulting from needling procedures. This type of invasion is characterized by the presence of one or more irregular cohesive sheets of carcinoma cells in fat or stroma surrounding the tumor without the reactive stromal changes that ordinarily accompany invasive carcinoma (Fig. 14.23). These invasive carcinomatous foci abut sharply on normal fat cells or less often on collagenous stroma in a fashion that superficially suggests that they were "pushed" or artifactually displaced to this location. In this situation, the features that favor true invasion are the absence at this site of evidence of a prior procedure such as hemorrhage, fat necrosis, a needle track, or tissue disruption. Perhaps the most telling observation is the intimate mingling of carcinoma cells and normal tissue, especially in fat, where individual adipose cells may be found in the sheet of carcinoma cells. Carcinoma cells may be "molded" around fat cells within or at the border of such foci (Fig. 14.24).

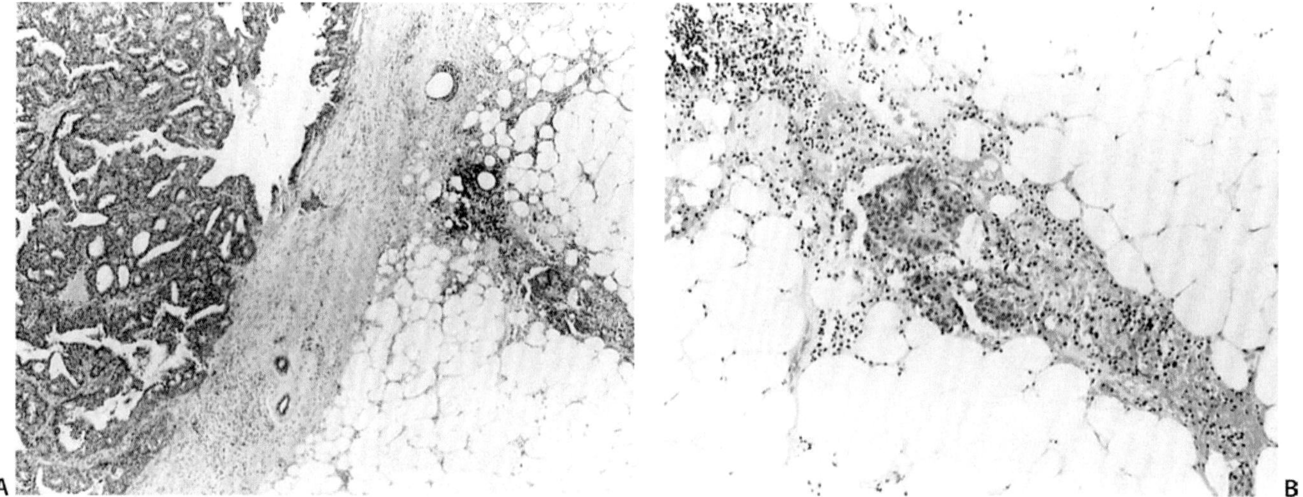

FIG. 14.21. ***Papillary carcinoma, needle biopsy.*** **A:** *In situ* papillary carcinoma surrounded by a thick capsule. The track of a needle aspiration biopsy is evident on the *right*. At this plane of section the site of penetration into the tumor is not seen. **B:** Carcinomatous papillary epithelium displaced in the needle track.

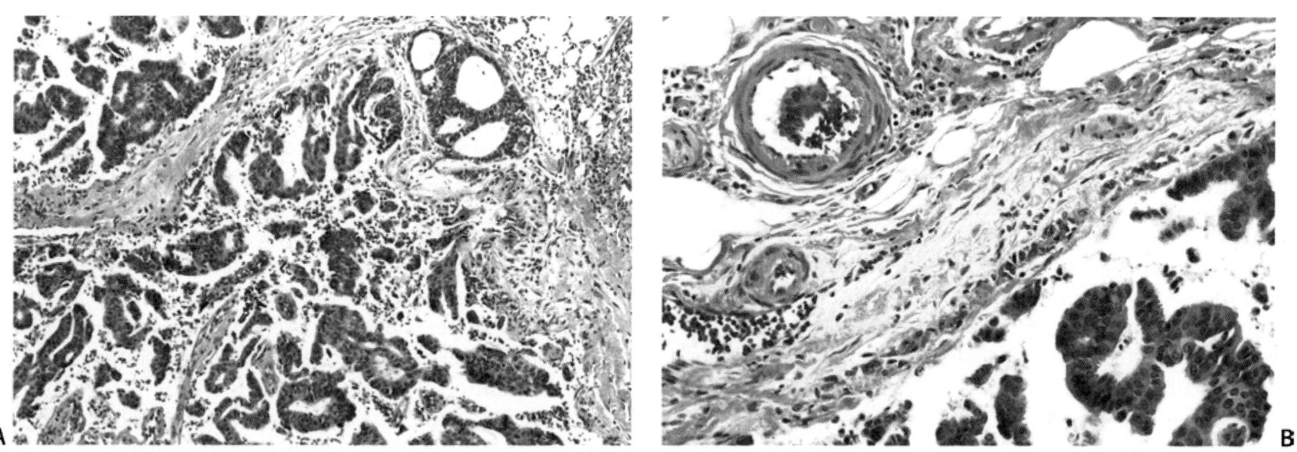

FIG. 14.22. ***Papillary carcinoma, needle biopsy.*** **A:** Tumor disruption and hemorrhage. **B:** Disrupted papillary neoplasm (*below*) and a fragment of papillary epithelium in a blood vessel (*above*).

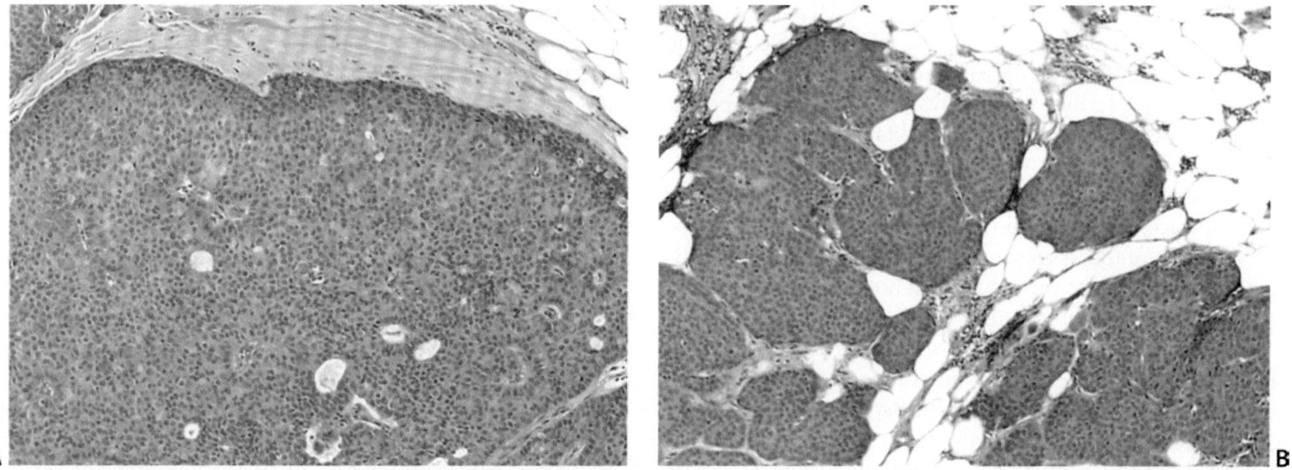

FIG. 14.23. ***Solid papillary carcinoma with invasion.*** **A:** Solid papillary carcinoma. This portion of the tumor is intraductal. **B:** Invasive carcinoma in fat without reactive stroma. Note the absence of tissue disruption, hemorrhage, and fat necrosis, which characterize a needle track.

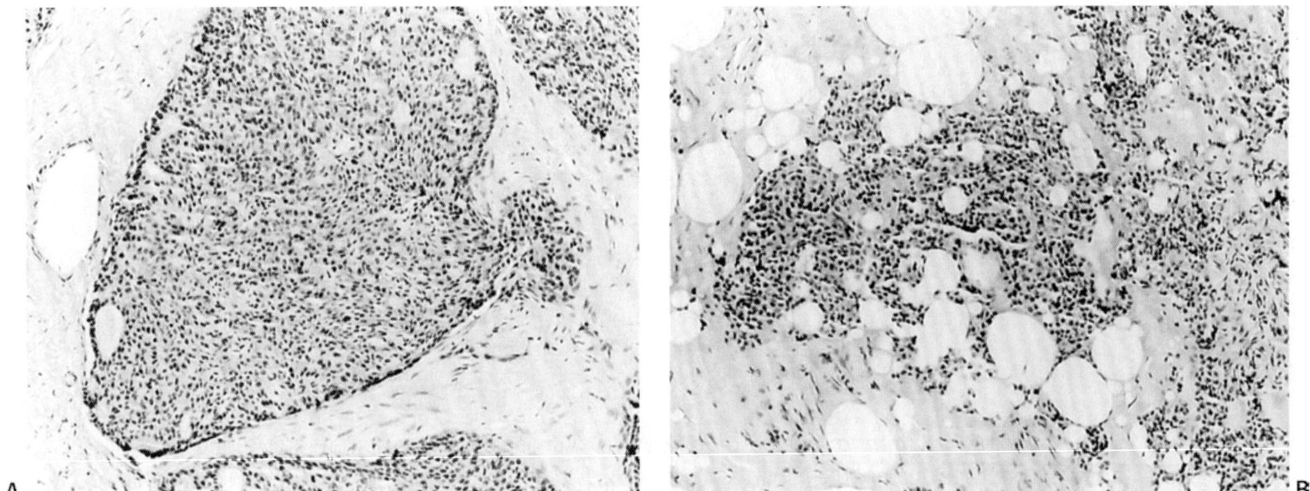

FIG. 14.24. ***Solid papillary carcinoma with invasion.*** **A:** The solid portion of the tumor with a knob of epithelium protruding into the stroma. By itself, this phenomenon does not constitute definitive evidence of invasion. **B:** Irregular groups of invasive carcinoma cells mingle with fat and fibrous stroma at the periphery of the tumor. No preoperative or intraoperative needling procedure was performed in this case.

VARIANT PATTERNS OF PAPILLARY CARCINOMA

Classical invasive papillary carcinomas consist of a population of malignant ductal cells forming a more or less compact mass and dissecting into the surrounding tissue in an arborizing manner. Differences in the manner of growth or the characteristics of the neoplastic cells give rise to several variant patterns of *in situ* and invasive papillary carcinoma.

(Intra)cystic Papillary Carcinoma

Physicians have known of the existence of predominantly cystic papillary carcinomas since the middle of the 19th century, but the lesion did not become well defined until 100 years later, when Gatchell et al.[49] and Czernobilsky[50] published studies of cases from the Mayo Clinic and the Hospital of the University of Pennsylvania, respectively. Czernobilsky described the features of this form of papillary carcinoma as "... a large, usually solitary hemorrhagic cyst surrounded by a fibrous wall into which projects a predominantly papillary adenocarcinoma which often also lines the inner surface of the cyst and the absence of extensive tumor involvement of the tissues surrounding the cyst favor the diagnosis of intracystic carcinoma." In both reports, this form of carcinoma constituted 0.5% of mammary carcinomas; however, a subsequent study by McKittrick et al.[51] reported a frequency of 2.0%, and among a large group of Swedish and Hungarian women,[52] intracystic papillary carcinoma accounted for 1.3% of breast carcinomas.

The age of patients with cystic papillary carcinoma ranges from 21[49] to 94 years,[51] and the lesion affects both women and men. Cases in men have attracted special interest,[53–65] and one notes the large proportion of reports in the Japanese literature.[56] In one series,[66] intracystic papillary carcinoma accounted for 5% of breast carcinoma in men. The ages of men with cystic papillary carcinoma cluster in the seventh and eighth decades with just a few cases beyond the age of 80 years.[55] Patients usually report especially long symptomatic intervals. In one case,[67] the patient noted the appearance of the mass 10 years prior to presentation, and in another, complaints persisted for 59 years before the patient sought medical attention.[49]

Most cystic papillary carcinomas appear well defined on a mammogram,[55,58,60,68] but two cases displayed slightly ill-defined margins,[62] and two others appeared lobulated.[30,59] Calcifications occur in only a minority of cases.[62] The calcifications appear linear, amorphous, or stippled. Ultrasonography reveals a complex, predominantly cystic mass with posterior enhancement and one or more mural nodules. Serial studies of one case demonstrated growth of the nodule.[55] Intracystic carcinomas usually consist of just one cyst, but multilocular examples have been described.[29,53,58,64,68] Computerized tomography scans reveal the cyst[69] and may show an inner mass.[64] MRI has the ability to demonstrate both the cystic and the solid components,[29,58,63] and it can highlight regions of invasion.[29] Dynamic MRI studies may yield findings that suggest a malignant neoplasm.[63,70] Pneumocystography highlights the intracystic tumor and thickening of the cyst wall.[52,53]

Classical cystic carcinomas present a characteristic macroscopic appearance. They usually measure several centimeters; however, dimensions as large as 18 cm have been recorded,[67] and McKittrick et al.[51] noted that the masses involved the entire breasts in five women. Cystic papillary carcinomas in men have spanned from 1.5[62] to 10 cm,[61] and they have usually involved the subareolar region. Czernobilsky[50] described the typical macroscopic appearance of intracystic carcinoma thus: "The cyst was surrounded by a thick fibrous wall in most instances. A striking feature in almost all of the cysts was the presence of dark brown blood clots within the lumen and on the cyst wall often presenting the appearance of a typical chocolate cyst. More or less papillary, often friable tumors projected into the cyst lumen . . . . The inner surface of these cysts was usually ragged and covered by a mixture of tumor, old blood, and what appeared grossly as granulation tissue."

The carcinomas can become fixed to the skin, invade it, and even ulcerate.[51] Two men experienced nipple retraction.[58,61] Large cystic papillary carcinomas should be examined carefully to separate the tumor tissue for microscopic study. The membrane that constitutes the cyst wall is formed of fibrous tissue, reactive inflammatory infiltrates, and varying amounts of proliferating epithelium. Residual papillary tumor can usually be found on the luminal surface or in the cyst wall. It is important that such areas be sampled extensively, since they may contain foci of invasion (Fig. 14.25).

Aspiration of the cystic component of a cystic papillary carcinoma usually yields "murky brown"[71] or frankly bloody fluid, but one can also encounter straw-colored fluid.[52] With the passage of time, the fluid usually reaccumulates, sometimes rapidly. The fluid can contain cells with features diagnostic of malignancy,[58,62] but more often, cytologic examination does not permit a definitive diagnosis.[52,56]

Despite the distinctive macroscopic appearance of intracystic carcinoma, it does not exhibit distinguishing microscopical features. The cytologic[57] and histologic features do not differ from those of conventional invasive papillary carcinoma. Thus, the diagnosis of intracystic carcinoma reflects a specific manner of growth of a carcinoma rather than a consistent constellation of histologic features. Foote and Stewart[14] made this point in 1946, when they wrote that intracystic carcinoma is a variant of papillary carcinoma, ". . . more distinctly a gross than a microscopic entity." One must also keep in mind that the formation of a large cyst harboring a papillary tumor does not itself establish the diagnosis of intracystic papillary carcinoma, for papillomas can produce an identical macroscopic appearance.[69,72–77]

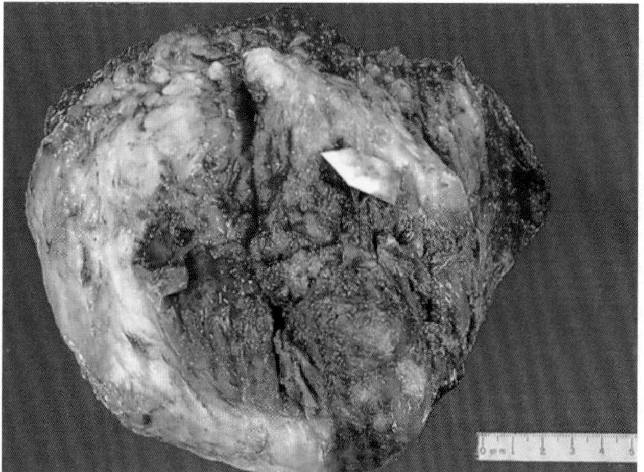

FIG. 14.25. ***Cystic papillary carcinoma.*** An opened cystic tumor that contains blood clot, tan mural nodules of papillary carcinoma below the arrow, and a focus of invasive carcinoma indicated by the arrow.

The interpretation of the findings of recent studies of carcinomas classified as intracystic papillary carcinomas has become nearly impossible for two reasons. First, many investigators have not required the presence of the macroscopic appearance recorded in the seminal publications to render a diagnosis of intracystic papillary carcinoma. Thus, the entity no longer has a precise pathologic definition. Second, writers have proposed several new terms to replace the designation, *intracystic papillary carcinoma*. For example, Lefkowitz et al.[26] suggested the diagnosis of *intraductal papillary carcinoma* to emphasize the presumed noninvasive aspect of the lesion, Leal et al.[78] offered the alternative term, *encysted papillary carcinoma*, Hill and Yeh[79] proposed the designation of *encapsulated papillary carcinoma*, and Grabowski et al.[23] used several of these terms synonymously. The authors of the *WHO Classification of Tumors of the Breast*[80] have eliminated the term *intracystic carcinoma* from their classification scheme, preferring the category of *encapsulated papillary carcinoma*. As a result of the laxity in the application of the classical diagnostic criteria and the variable and changing diagnostic terminology, most recently reported examples of intracystic papillary carcinomas do not meet the classical definition of that entity; in fact, most probably represent conventional papillary carcinomas with a cystic component.

The original studies of intracystic papillary carcinoma and the few subsequent ones that adhere to the classical diagnostic features reveal a few consistent attributes. First, the histologic characteristics of the carcinomas vary. Czernobilsky[50] described three patterns: well-differentiated papillary adenocarcinoma, moderately differentiated partly papillary and partly solid adenocarcinoma, and poorly differentiated mostly solid adenocarcinoma. Gatchell et al.[49] also observed several patterns of growth and all grades of malignancy. Seal et al.[81] described five intracystic carcinomas with purely apocrine features, and Laforga et al.[82] detailed another purely apocrine cystic papillary tumor that the authors classified as malignant on the basis of the absence of myoepithelial cells using immunohistochemical staining. Second, besides growing within the distended space and on its wall, the carcinoma cells frequently extend into neighboring ducts and may invade the parenchyma surrounding the cyst.[50,51,78,83] The frequency of these events varies from 35%[50] to 50%.[83] The associated *in situ* or invasive carcinomas tend to display low or intermediate grade, but they usually do not exhibit a papillary architecture. Finally, one does not usually find myoepithelial cells at the periphery of the carcinomas.[83] This finding, among others, led Calderaro et al.[83] to reconsider the presumed noninvasive nature of this lesion and to favor ". . . its classification as a low grade invasive carcinoma."

Encapsulated Papillary Carcinoma

The term *encapsulated papillary carcinoma* is an alternative designation that encompasses both of the now well-established categories of intracystic and solid papillary carcinoma. The designation arose from immunohistochemical studies of myoepithelial markers by Hill and Yeh.[79] After studying a series of papillary carcinomas, the investigators found five with "no or only focal staining of the basal" myoepithelial cell layer for calponin, smooth muscle myosin-heavy chain (SMM-HC), and p63. The absence of myoepithelial reactivity led these authors to suggest that such carcinomas are "part of a spectrum of progression intermediate between *in situ* and invasive disease," and the writers proposed the term "encapsulated papillary carcinoma." In a similar study, Collins et al.[84] used staining for five myoepithelial markers (calponin, p63, CD10, CK5/6, and SMM-HC) to investigate the distribution of myoepithelial cells in 22 tumors that had been classified as "intracystic papillary carcinomas." On the basis of the illustrations provided and the gross descriptions that referred to "circumscribed," "soft," and "focally hemorrhagic nodules," with no mention of a cystic component, these carcinomas seem to have been *solid* rather than "intracystic" papillary carcinomas. All of the 22 tumors were devoid of myoepithelial reactivity with the five immunostain markers. The authors argued that the carcinomas did not represent a form of DCIS and concurred with the suggestion of Hill and Yeh[79] that the tumors be called encapsulated papillary carcinomas. Subsequent investigators and the contributors to the fourth edition of the *WHO Classification of Tumors of the Breast* have taken up this usage.[80,85]

The infiltrative nature of encapsulated papillary carcinoma remains open to much discussion and spirited controversy. Because the rounded contours of the nests of carcinoma cells resemble distended ducts and acini, traditional thinking regards such foci as noninvasive carcinoma. However, the results of immunohistochemical staining for myoepithelial cells by Hill and Yeh[79] and Collins et al.[84] have called that notion into question. Although Hill and Yeh[79] worded their opinions cautiously, they seem to suggest that these carcinomas represent a peculiar form of invasive carcinoma. Apparently in agreement, Collins et al.[84] pointed out that "... these lesions have striking histologic similarities to encapsulated papillary thyroid carcinomas, tumors about which the invasive nature is undisputed." On the other hand, the writers caution, "... we believe it is most prudent ... to avoid categorization of such lesions as frankly invasive papillary carcinomas."

Other groups have addressed this question by evaluating the presence of myoepithelial cells, type IV collagen, histologic features, or matrix metalloproteinases (MMPs). Esposito et al.[86] used immunohistochemical staining for both myoepithelial cells and type IV collagen to define the presence of basement membrane. The workers failed to detect myoepithelial cells at the periphery of most encapsulated papillary carcinomas, but 65% of the carcinomas showed strong staining for type IV collagen and 35% displayed moderate staining for the protein. The authors concluded that "... [encapsulated papillary carcinomas] are confined within an intact basement membrane and are thus *in situ* carcinomas." Wynveen et al.[87] carried out staining for both myoepithelial cells and type IV collagen in 40 cases. The authors did not observe myoepithelial cells in 33 of the 40 (82.5%) carcinomas and observed only focal staining with one or more of the five myoepithelial markers in the remaining seven cases. The investigators observed discontinuous staining for type IV collagen in 97% of the cases, and one lymph node containing metastatic carcinoma showed "strong and continuous 3+ positivity around most nests of metastatic carcinoma." As a consequence, Wynveen et al.[87] concluded that "... this tumor most likely represents a spectrum of *in situ* and [invasive carcinoma] with predominance of the latter." Rakha et al.[85] collected morphologic data from 207 encapsulated papillary carcinomas and immunohistochemical findings from a subset of them. The immunohistochemical stains did not reveal more than an "occasional" myoepithelial cell at the periphery of the 45 papillary carcinomas studied. Eight of the study cases demonstrated invasion of stroma, fat, or skeletal muscle, and the authors noted that "... all these invasive foci maintained their cystic papillary morphology with absence of surrounding myoepithelial cells, and some of the intramuscular foci were surrounded by fibrous capsule with basement membrane–like (type IV collagen and laminin positive) material similar to that seen around localized [encapsulated papillary carcinomas]." Rakha et al.[85] concluded that "... most [encapsulated papillary carcinomas] are indolent invasive carcinoma, with a small proportion that may be *in situ*." Finally, in a subsequent publication, Rakha et al.[88] studied 17 encapsulated papillary carcinomas for the presence of invasion-associated proteinases. The workers found that the encapsulated papillary carcinomas expressed MMP-1 and MMP-9 at levels higher than those seen in cases of DCIS and at levels comparable to those of invasive carcinomas. On the other hand, the levels of expression of MMP-2 and MMP-7 in encapsulated papillary carcinoma resembled those seen in cases of DCIS rather than the levels characteristic of invasive carcinomas. Although the results of these several studies seem generally consistent, pathologists have not reached a consensus on their interpretation, and the question about the invasive nature of encapsulated papillary carcinoma remains open to further study and discussion.

The state "intermediate between *in situ* and invasive disease" posited by Hill and Yeh[79] and the notion that these tumors represent invasive but not "frankly invasive" carcinomas suggested by Collins et al.[84] seem puzzling. Pathologists traditionally regard the attributes, *in situ* and invasive, as nonoverlapping and mutually exclusive conditions similar to other pairs of qualities such as *finite* and *infinite*, *complete* and *incomplete*, and *in motion* and *at rest*. It is difficult to imagine a state intermediate between *in situ* and invasive, and to suggest that an intermediate form exists would seem to blur the distinction between the two. It is true that there are examples of cystic and solid types of papillary carcinoma that elicit uncertainty as to the presence of an invasive component. However, it has not yet been demonstrated that among these uncertain tumors there is an identifiable subset with a propensity to cause metastases in the absence of an evident invasive component.

The fundamental flaw in the argument that the absence of myoepithelial cells in encapsulated papillary carcinoma is indicative of an invasive neoplasm lies in the failure of proponents of this position to fully acknowledge that the majority of papillary carcinomas, whether *in situ* or invasive, are characterized by the absence of these cells. Therefore, failure to detect myoepithelial cells in a papillary breast tumor does not by itself define any part of the lesion as invasive. In this circumstance, investigators have not clearly indicated whether the diagnosis, "encapsulated papillary carcinoma," should apply to all papillary carcinomas that are entirely devoid of myoepithelial cells or only to those where invasion is suspected. No mention has been made of the classification of lesions that partially lack myoepithelium or of papillary carcinomas endowed with myoepithelium that have foci suspicious for invasion. In addition, the adjective "encapsulated" suggests encasement, just the reverse of suspected invasion. As discussed above, advocates of the term "encapsulated papillary carcinoma" have failed to provide a compelling argument for why this name is preferable to solid papillary carcinoma, a well-defined existing diagnostic term that adequately describes lesions that are referred to as "encapsulated papillary carcinoma."

Our inability to detect the presence of invasion in some papillary carcinomas with confidence reflects the limitations of existing knowledge and technology. This conundrum will probably not be resolved until future research discovers one or more markers that specifically distinguish between *in situ* and invasion carcinoma cells, an advance that would focus attention on the tumor cells themselves rather than on their pattern of growth by which invasion is presently determined. At present, it is preferable to simply describe a papillary carcinoma as cystic, solid, or a combination of cystic and solid and to state that invasion is present, absent, or indeterminate (e.g., "suspected"; "cannot be ruled out").

Dimorphic Papillary Carcinoma

Lefkowitz et al.[26] drew attention to the presence of cuboidal cells with abundant clear or faintly eosinophilic cytoplasm in papillary carcinomas (Fig. 14.26). These cells were located mainly near the basement membrane singly, in small clusters, or in broad sheets, a distribution that suggested myoepithelial origin. Occasionally, the polygonal cells with pale cytoplasm were numerous, creating solid and cribriform regions beneath the superficial columnar epithelium. The appearance of the polygonal cells contrasted strikingly with that of the conventional columnar epithelial cells and brought to mind the appearance of the pagetoid spread of carcinoma. Despite the difference in cytoplasmic features between the clear cells and the columnar carcinomatous cells, the nuclei of the two cell types were similar. Both cell types are immunoreactive for cytokeratin, and there is no reactivity for smooth muscle actin (SMA) or p63 in the polygonal cells. Both cell types are of epithelial origin, and this pattern is referred to as "dimorphic" papillary carcinoma. Polygonal dimorphic carcinoma cells should not be mistaken in hematoxylin and eosin (H&E)-stained sections for residual myoepithelial cells in a papillary lesion.

Solid Papillary Carcinoma with Endocrine Differentiation

Neoplasms with a characteristic papillary and cystic structure are readily recognized as papillary carcinoma, but the existence of a solid variant of papillary carcinoma is less widely appreciated.[89] These tumors are found in ducts completely filled by a solid neoplastic proliferation. They are usually well circumscribed and often multinodular. The presence of a delicate network of fibrovascular stroma distributed in an arborizing pattern throughout the compact epithelium is the hallmark of solid papillary carcinoma (Figs. 14.5 and 14.27). Collagenization and sclerosis of stroma around and among the ducts are present to a variable degree, in some cases producing a pattern with features of a radial sclerosing lesion (Fig. 14.4). Most, if not all lesions described in the foregoing discussion of tumors referred to in the literature as "encapsulated papillary carcinomas" are in reality examples of the previously well-characterized solid papillary carcinoma repackaged with a different name.

Many solid papillary carcinomas display histologic features suggesting the presence of endocrine characteristics (see Chapter 20). First brought to attention by Cross et al.[90] and Azzopardi et al.,[91] solid papillary carcinoma with endocrine

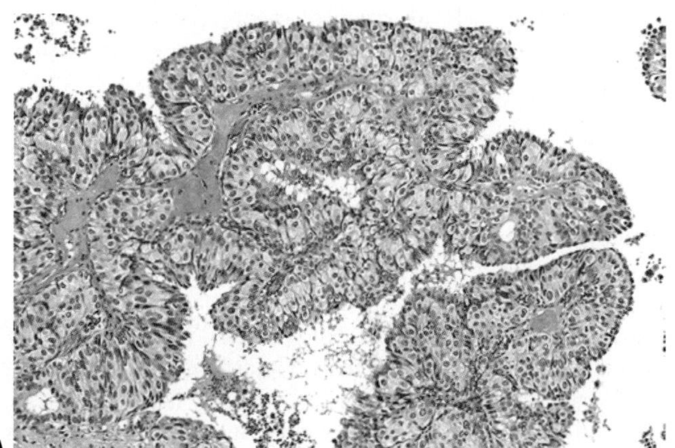

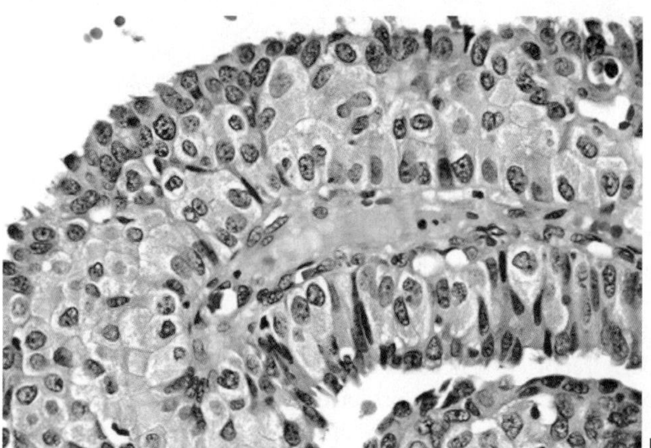

FIG. 14.26. ***Dimorphic papillary carcinoma.*** **A:** The cells covering this papillary frond consist of a thin layer of small epithelial cells overlying a collection of larger cells with pale cytoplasm. **B:** Cuboidal epithelial cells overlie columnar or polygonal cells on the papillary fronds.

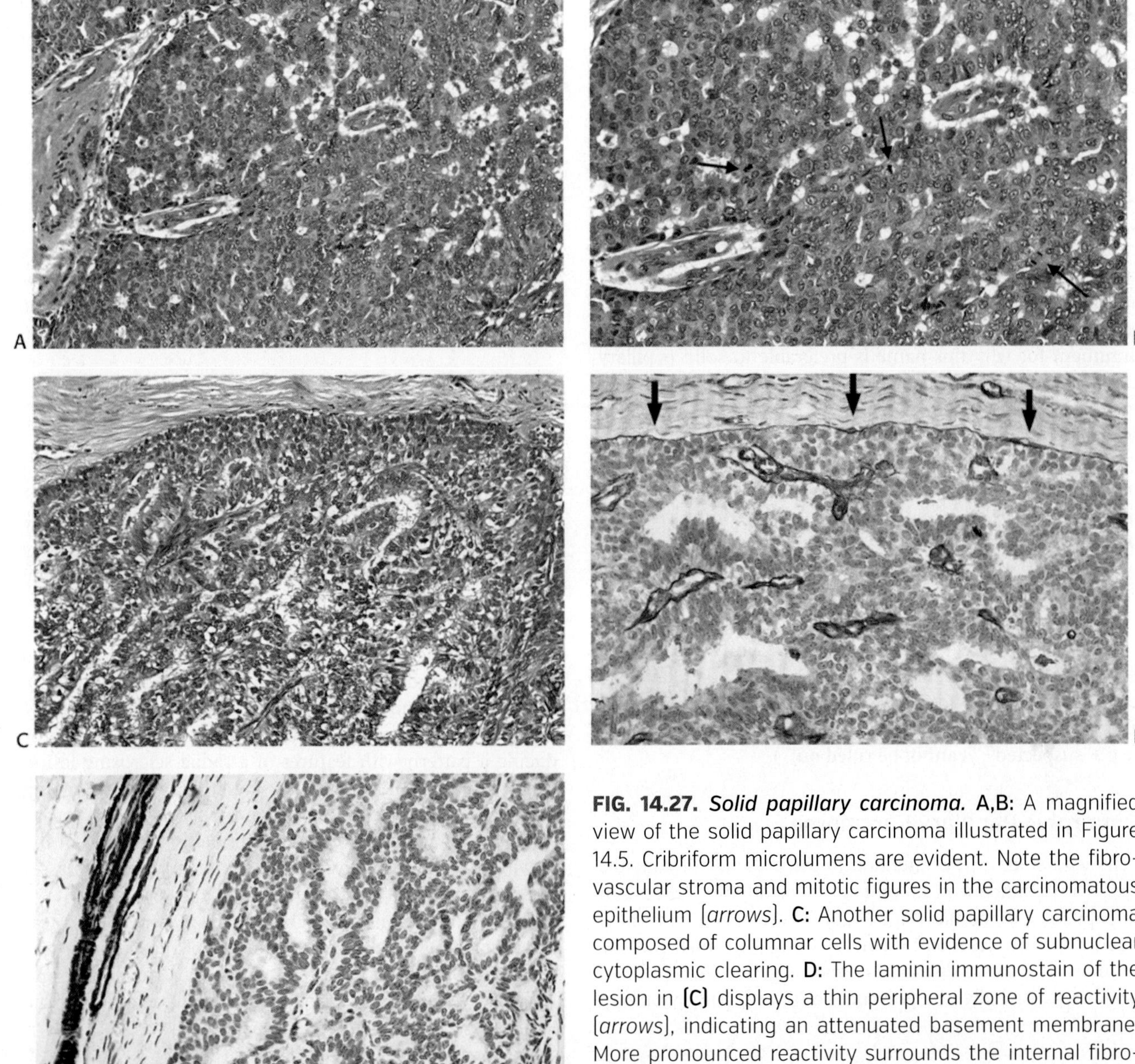

FIG. 14.27. ***Solid papillary carcinoma.*** **A,B:** A magnified view of the solid papillary carcinoma illustrated in Figure 14.5. Cribriform microlumens are evident. Note the fibrovascular stroma and mitotic figures in the carcinomatous epithelium (*arrows*). **C:** Another solid papillary carcinoma composed of columnar cells with evidence of subnuclear cytoplasmic clearing. **D:** The laminin immunostain of the lesion in **(C)** displays a thin peripheral zone of reactivity (*arrows*), indicating an attenuated basement membrane. More pronounced reactivity surrounds the internal fibrovascular stroma. **E:** Absence of myoepithelial cells in the carcinoma is evident in this immunostain for SMA. A small blood vessel on the *left* is immunoreactive.

differentiation accounts for approximately 1% to 2% of breast carcinomas.[92] With one exception,[93] all patients have been women. Although the ages of patients ranged from 30 to 105 years,[93] most presented during their seventh or eighth decade of life, and mean ages from 61.0[94] to 72.3 years[95] have been reported. The carcinoma typically involved just one breast, but bilateral tumors have been observed.[93,95,96]

The carcinomas usually appear well circumscribed and often multinodular. They often do not suggest a malignant neoplasm to the unaided eye. Pathologists usually described them as well defined and fleshy or firm but not hard. Shades of yellow, pink, and tan were recorded often. Episodes of hemorrhage can impart a red or deep brown color. Examples have spanned from 0.2[95] to 15.0 cm.[93] The mean sizes calculated from data in two series are 2.04[92] and 2.08 cm.[96]

On histologic study, the noninvasive and invasive components display identical cytologic and architectural characteristics. In most cases, the neoplastic cells demonstrate low-grade atypia and appear only slightly larger than their normal counterparts. They display oval to spindle shapes; occasionally, the spindle morphology predominates.[97] In many cases, the nuclei resemble hyperplastic nuclei: they have slightly irregular shapes, folds and grooves, granular chromatin, and uniform small nucleoli. The nuclei in other tumors look like those of commonplace low-grade ductal carcinoma. The cytoplasm usually appears eosinophilic or amphophilic and granular (Fig. 14.28). Intermediate- and high-grade cytologic features occur in a minority of cases.[93] The stroma within the cellular masses varies from delicate strands of collagen surrounding dilated capillaries to broad, blunt fronds composed of acellular, hyalinized collagen.

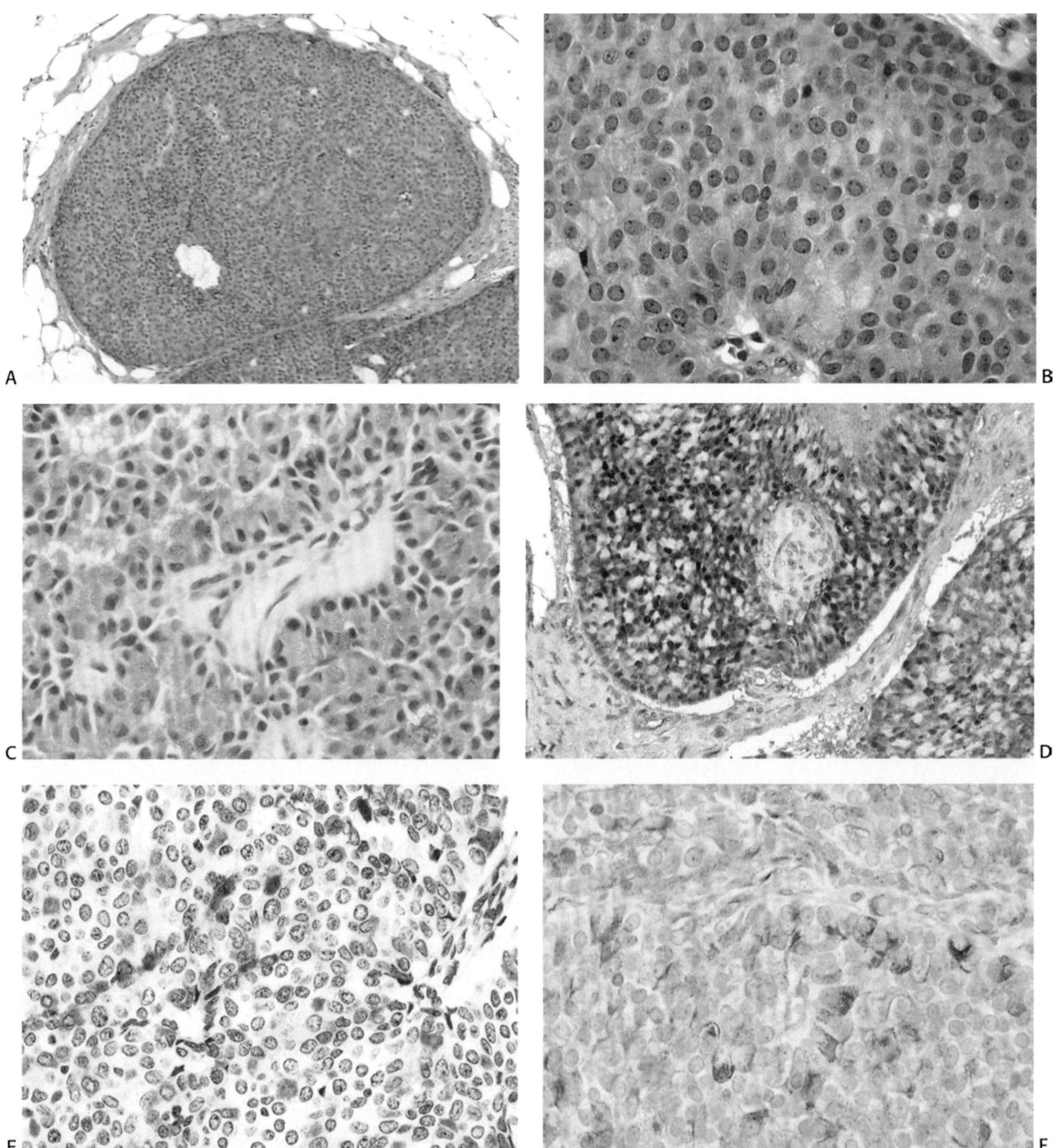

FIG. 14.28. ***Solid papillary carcinoma with endocrine differentiation.*** **A:** Fibrovascular cores containing capillaries are scattered through this solid papillary carcinoma. **B:** The tumor cells have amphophilic finely granular cytoplasm and focal intracytoplasmic mucin. **C:** A positive reaction for mucin is present in the cytoplasm of most carcinoma cells (mucicarmine stain). **D:** Immunoreactivity for NSE. **E:** Immunoreactivity for synaptophysin. **F:** Grimelius-positive black granules are present in many tumor cells (Grimelius stain).

Many solid papillary carcinomas have areas with an organoid growth pattern in which solid masses of cells are outlined by a peripheral zone of palisaded cells. Occasionally, solid areas are broken up into ribbons or trabeculae of neoplastic cells by prominent fibrovascular stroma. One often detects both intracellular mucin in minuscule droplets within the cytoplasm and extracellular mucin in pools between the stroma and the neoplastic cells. Massive accumulation of intracellular mucin creates signet ring cells.[97] Frequent mitotic figures are characteristic, but calcifications, cribriform spaces, and comedonecrosis are not. Uncommon variants of solid papillary carcinoma include glycogen-rich clear cell tumors (Fig. 14.29), spindle cell tumors (Fig. 14.30), and carcinomas with mucoepidermoid features (Fig. 14.31).

Cytologic preparations obtained by needle aspiration, smearing of a nipple discharge, or direct scraping typically yield cellular preparations showing loose cellular aggregates and intact single cells.[98–100] Yamada et al.[101] tabulated the findings in 20 cases. The neoplastic cells appear polygonal or cuboidal, and they contain round or oval nuclei that vary slightly in size and bland chromatin. The cytoplasm appears variably eosinophilic. An eccentric position of the nucleus creates a plasmacytoid appearance. Thin capillaries corresponding to the delicate fibrovascular stroma can be seen.

Ultrastructural study of 12 cases[90,96,97,102,103] revealed cells with abundant cytoplasm and numerous granules of several types: small (180 to 390 nm) electron-dense granules, large (790 to 880 nm) electron-dense granules, and flocculent granules measuring 330 to 550 nm. The granules were thought to represent neurosecretory granules, lysosomes, and mucin granules, respectively. Other cellular organelles observed include tonofilaments, desmosomes, rough endoplasmic reticulum, and microvilli on the luminal borders of a few cells.[96]

Cellular evidence of endocrine differentiation can take the form of a positive reaction with the Grimelius stain,[92] immunoreactivity for chromogranin, synaptophysin, or neuron-specific enolase (NSE),[92,95,96,104] or the detection of dense core granules.[96] Solid papillary carcinomas demonstrate consistent receptor, oncogene, and proliferative profiles. They virtually always stain for estrogen receptor (ER) (Fig. 14.32) and most stain for progesterone

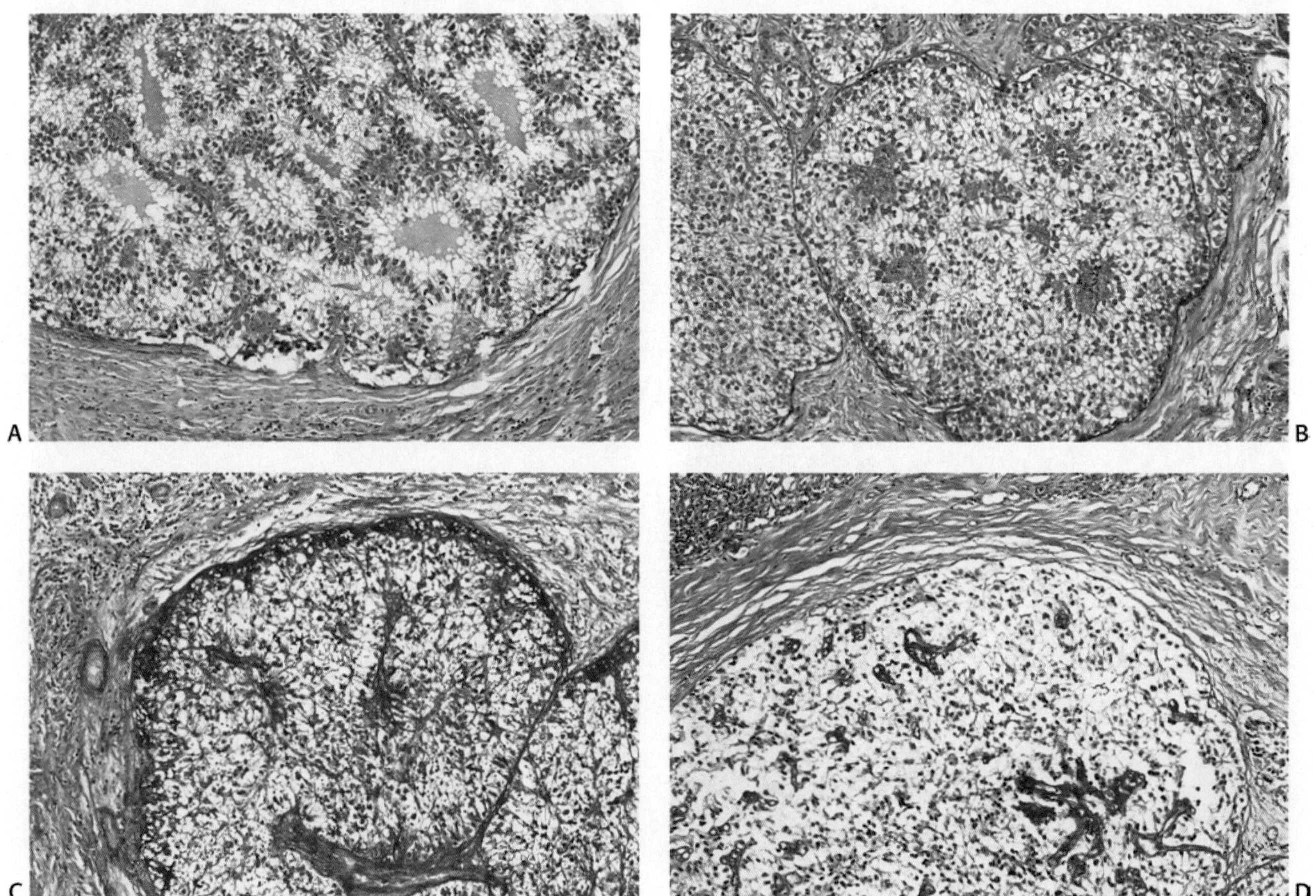

FIG. 14.29. ***Solid papillary carcinoma, glycogen-rich clear cell type.*** All images are from a single tumor in a 29-year-old woman. **A:** Columnar cells with clear cytoplasm are arranged on fibrovascular stroma outlining glands that contain secretion. **B:** Another region in the tumor with solid, non–gland-forming growth. **C:** The tumor cells contain PAS-positive material. **D:** PAS staining has been abolished by diastase.

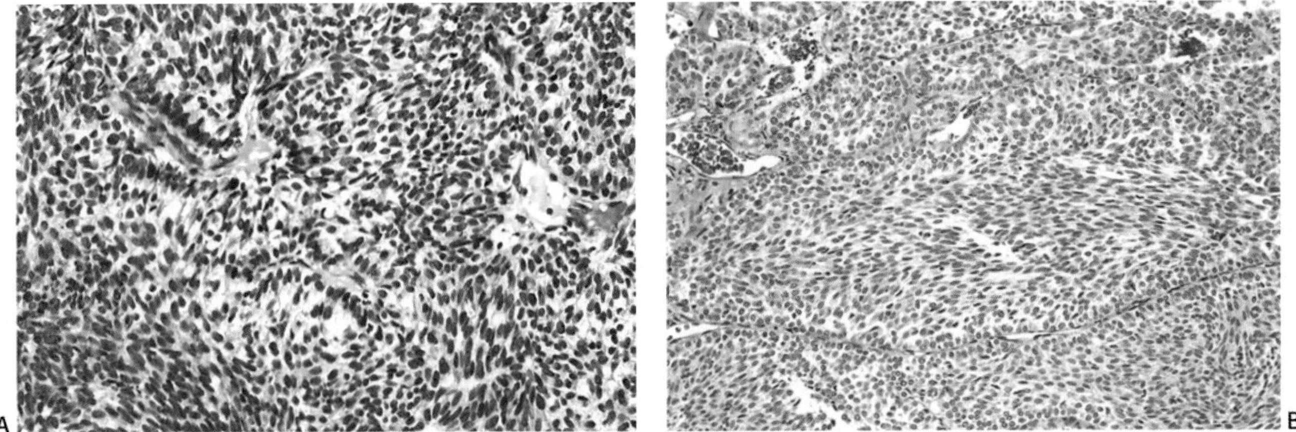

FIG. 14.30. ***Solid papillary carcinoma, spindle cell type.*** **A:** Palisading of spindle cells is evident around fibrovascular cores. **B:** Pronounced spindle cell growth is shown.

receptor (PR).[92,93,95,96] They do not show HER2 overexpression.[92,93,96,99] The cases described by Tsang and Chan[96] did not stain for p53, nor did the cases described by Hardisson et al.,[99] but 10 of 20 cases studied by Otsuki et al.[92] showed staining for the protein in 2% to 29% of the tumor cells. Ki67 scores less than 5% have been recorded.[96,99]

Because the recognition of invasion by solid papillary carcinoma with endocrine differentiation often poses problems, pathologists have sought help from the results of immunohistochemical staining for proteins found in myoepithelial cells. Loss of myoepithelium can be used to distinguish some papillary carcinomas from papillomas,[105] but by itself this phenomenon is not a basis for separating *in situ* from invasive papillary carcinomas. In the case of solid papillary carcinoma, the presence of myoepithelium around the entire circumference of the lesion supports the diagnosis of solid papillary DCIS. Focal or even complete absence of peripheral myoepithelium in a solid papillary carcinoma

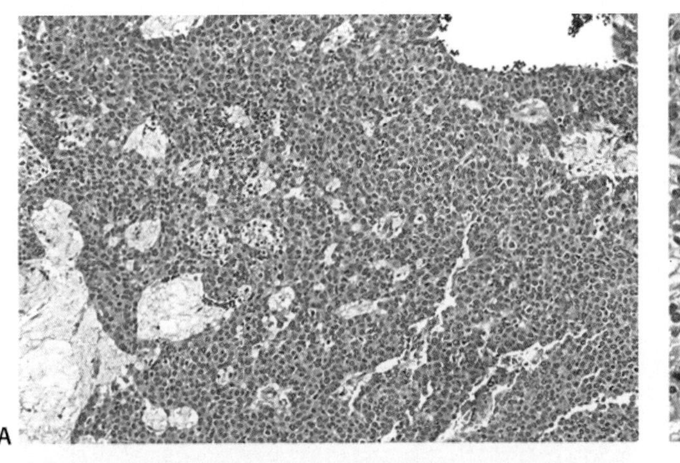

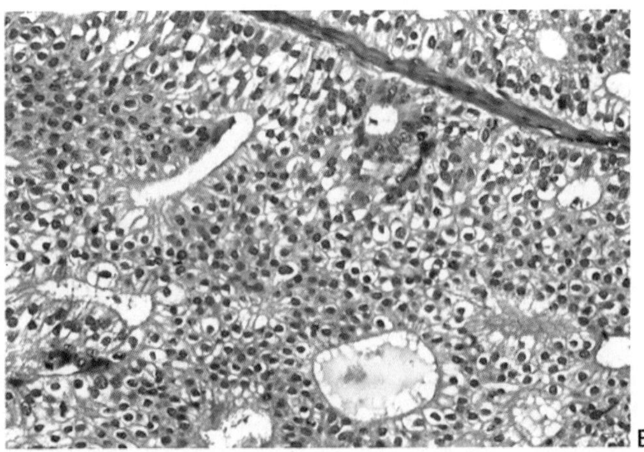

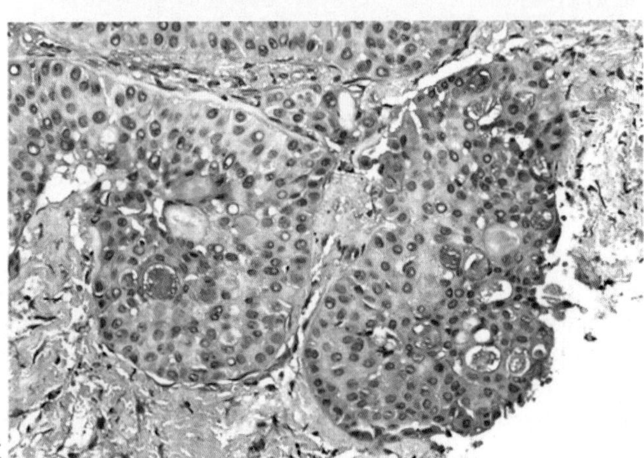

FIG. 14.31. ***Solid papillary carcinoma, mucoepidermoid type.*** **A:** The tumor consists of solid masses of polygonal tumor cells with inconspicuous fibrovascular structures. Extracellular mucin is shown in the *lower left corner*. **B:** The tumor cells form glands and exhibit distinct cell borders. Nuclei are small and low grade. Cytoplasmic vacuolization is variably present. **C:** The mucicarmine stain demonstrates mucin in gland lumens and in the cytoplasm of tumor cells in mucoepidermoid epithelium.

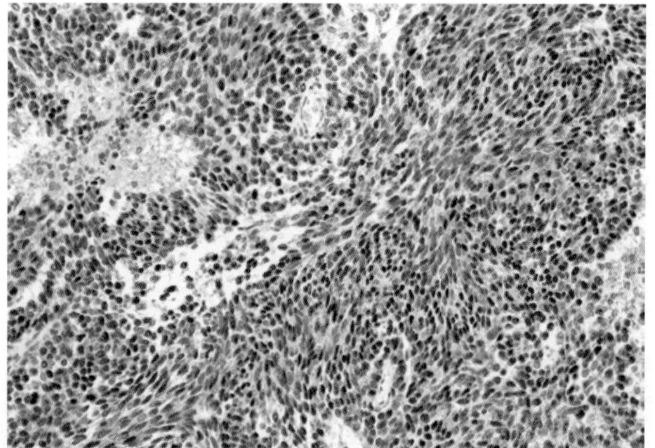

FIG. 14.32. ***Solid papillary carcinoma with ER.*** Nuclear immunoreactivity is demonstrated in a spindle cell lesion.

renders the tumor "indeterminate for invasion."[94] However, the actual structure of the tumor must also be considered, with the best evidence for invasion being a localized change in the growth pattern, such as focal *cribriform, tubular,* or *mucinous carcinoma,* which extends beyond the perimeter of the tumor. Absence of myoepithelium around a solid papillary carcinoma that retains a smooth peripheral contour is not definitive evidence of invasion. It is sometimes helpful to use one or more cytokeratin immunostains to detect individual invasive carcinoma cells that may have extended beyond the perimeter of an apparently circumscribed solid papillary carcinoma.

Solid papillary carcinoma with endocrine differentiation frequently coexists with conventional types of invasive carcinoma. Among the 34 invasive carcinomas in the series of Nassar et al.,[93] 50% consisted of pure or mixed colloid carcinomas, and 30% were neuroendocrine-like carcinomas. Invasive ductal carcinoma, not otherwise specified, invasive lobular carcinoma, and tubular carcinoma accounted for the remaining tumors. Nineteen of the 20 carcinomas studied by Tsang and Chan[96] were colloid or neuroendocrine-like carcinomas or composites of these two types; the single remaining tumor was a small cell carcinoma.

Breast Tumor Resembling the Tall Cell Variant of Papillary Thyroid Carcinoma

In 2003, Eusebi et al.[106] described five examples of a variety of breast carcinoma composed of cells resembling those of the tall cell variant of papillary thyroid carcinoma, and subsequent publications added details of another seven cases.[107–110] The ages of the patients ranged from 45 to 80 years.[109]

The tumor does not present distinctive clinical or macroscopic features, but histologic study reveals carcinoma cells arranged in solid, papillary, and cribriform aggregates (Fig. 14.33). The glands typically contain densely eosinophilic, homogeneous material with scalloped borders, which

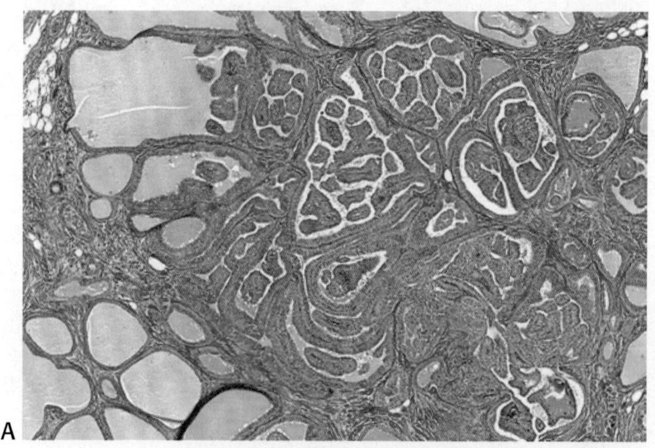

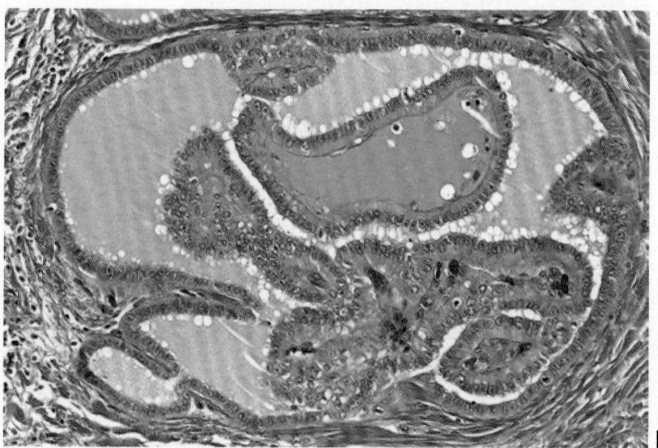

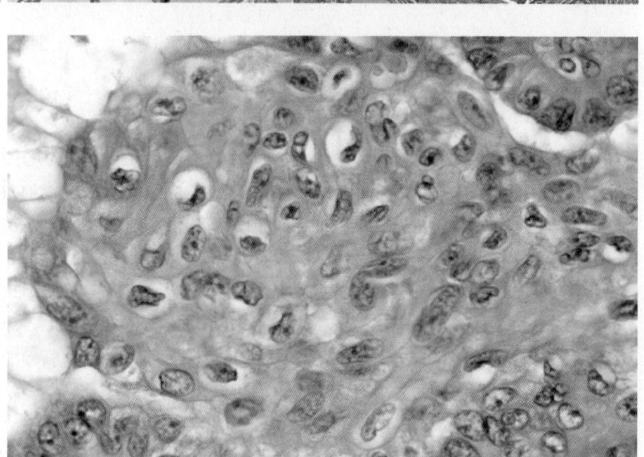

FIG. 14.33. ***Papillary carcinoma thyroid like.*** **A:** This papillary carcinoma forms fronds and spaces containing eosinophilic material. **B:** A single layer of columnar cells covers the stromal core. The eosinophilic material displays scalloping that is analogous to thyroid colloid. **C:** The carcinoma cells possess irregular notched and folded nuclei, pale and granular chromatin, and small nucleoli.

resembles thyroid colloid. In this respect, the appearance bears a resemblance to hypersecretory carcinoma growing in a papillary configuration. The neoplastic cells have columnar to cuboidal shapes, slightly pleomorphic oval nuclei, and eosinophilic granular cytoplasm. The nuclei usually occupy the basal aspect of the cells, but they can also sit next to the luminal membranes. The nuclei exhibit angular contours, grooves, and eosinophilic pseudoinclusions, and some nuclei exhibit clearing. Several, but not all, cases have contained psammoma bodies. Using immunohistochemical techniques, most examples have stained for mitochondria and CK7. Staining for epithelial membrane antigen (EMA), GCDFP-15, and CK19 has disclosed variable results, and so has staining for ER and PR. The carcinoma cells do not stain for TTF-1 or thyroglobulin, nor do they display mutations of the *RET* protooncogene[111] or the *BRAF* gene.[108]

The nuclear characteristics and pattern of growth so closely resemble those of certain papillary thyroid carcinomas that the original authors stated, ". . . without the help of immunohistochemistry for thyroid transcription factor 1 and thyroglobulin, the differential diagnosis would have been virtually impossible."[106] Complicating the differential diagnosis even more is the report of a case of metastatic tall cell papillary thyroid carcinoma involving the breast.[112] Two patients with mammary tumors developed metastatic disease, one in the skull[108] and one in an intramammary lymph node,[110] but no patient has reportedly died of the carcinoma. Despite the morphologic resemblances between this type of papillary breast carcinoma and the tall cell variant of papillary thyroid carcinoma, evidence does not suggest an association between the two types of carcinoma. Masood et al.[109] suggested renaming the breast lesion *tall cell variant of papillary breast carcinoma*.

CYTOLOGY

In view of the difficulty sometimes encountered distinguishing papillomas from papillary carcinomas in histologic sections, it is not surprising that diagnostic problems arise in aspiration cytology and needle core biopsy specimens from these lesions.[113] Needle aspiration specimens present two difficulties. First, a significant number of lesions classified as papillary on the basis of findings in aspiration specimens prove not to exhibit a papillary architecture when excised. Of the 70 cases studied by Simsir et al.[114] in which masses were classified as papillary on the basis of needle aspiration specimens, only 31 (44%) showed a papillary architecture when examined histologically. FAs, fibrocystic changes, a phyllodes tumor, and carcinomas accounted for the remaining 39 cases. Chapter 5 presents a more detailed discussion of the problem of establishing the papillary nature of a mass by cytologic study.

Cytopathologists also find it difficult to differentiate benign papillary tumors from malignant ones, and opinions vary concerning the utility of this endeavor. For example, Gomez-Aracil et al.[115] stated: "We suggest that papillary carcinoma of the breast can be diagnosed by cytology and differentiated from papilloma," and Kumar et al.[116] and Michael and Buschmann[117] agree. On the other hand, Prathiba et al.[118] concluded that "cytomorphological features alone are inadequate for the precise diagnosis of papillary lesions of the breast," a point echoed by Tse et al.[119] and Jeffrey and Ljung.[120]

Despite this difference in opinion, all of the foregoing authors agreed that certain cytologic features suggest the diagnosis of papillary carcinoma in aspirated specimens. These features fall into four categories: overall cellularity, quantity and cellular characteristics of cell clusters, quantity and cellular characteristics of single cells, and features of the papillary fragments.[119] Papillary carcinomas usually yield hypercellular specimens[57,72,78,121–124] containing single cells, cell clusters, and three-dimensional papillary fragments in greater numbers than usually seen in smears from papillomas. The delicate, thin fragments consist of slender fibrovascular cores containing capillaries,[122] which are covered by a monomorphous population of disorderly epithelial cells. The papillary fragments exhibit a complex architecture, in which numerous thin fronds project in different directions.[117]

Unlike the cells in smears from papillomas, which consist of both epithelial and myoepithelial cells, the epithelial cells in aspirates from papillary carcinomas constitute a monomorphous population.[72,125] They typically have low to tall columnar shapes. Dei Tos et al.[122] stressed the uniformity of the epithelial cell population and the columnar shape of the cells thus: ". . . when facing a papillary breast lesion, such monotonous appearance should strongly suggest a malignant process. Low to tall columnar cells are invariably present in all our cases. This finding, evaluated together with the other parameters, could be regarded as a useful marker of papillary neoplasia." The observations of Naran et al.[124] support this conclusion.

The detection of cytologic atypia in individual cells and those composing the clusters can be difficult. The cells within the clusters may contain hyperchromatic nuclei and show disorderly stratification.[121] Naran et al.[124] appreciated moderate anisokaryosis and vesicular, rounded, naked nuclei in each of the 11 cases that they studied, and Gomez-Aracil et al.[115] noted nuclear atypia in all of their 15 cases. The rounded or oval nuclei appeared enlarged, and they demonstrated mild anisokaryosis, occasional hyperchromatism, mild thickening of their membranes, and small nucleoli. Nayar et al.[76] observed hyperchromatic elongated nuclei in two papillary carcinomas. Jeffrey and Ljung[120] appreciated mild atypia in three of five cases and more advanced atypia in the remaining two. On the other hand, Kline and Kannan[123] detected nuclear irregularities only after diligent searches. Kumar et al.[116] noted the frequent presence of strips of palisading tall and low cuboidal epithelial cells "resembling clusters of bananas." Many of the columnar cells contained prominent eosinophilic cytoplasmic granules located at both poles of the cells. Other investigators did not observe these granules.[115,118,126] Smears of papillary carcinomas usually do not contain the bipolar naked nuclei or apocrine cells commonly seen in aspirations from papillomas. Signet ring cells and extracellular mucin can be present if the papillary carcinoma has mucinous differentiation. These features may be a clue to the diagnosis of spindle cell, argyrophilic, mucin-producing papillary carcinoma.[127]

Infarction of a papilloma can lead to cytological changes mimicking those seen in papillary carcinomas. Dawson and Mulford[121] studied two infarcted papillomas and observed marked nuclear atypia in the setting of an inflammatory and necrotic background.

These observations notwithstanding, the accuracy of the cytologic diagnosis of papillary lesions does not seem acceptable. Tse et al.[119] report an accuracy of 65% for the diagnosis of papilloma with a false-positive rate of 23% and an accuracy of 45% for the diagnosis of papillary carcinoma with a false-negative rate of 27%.

CORE BIOPSY SPECIMENS

The distinction between a papilloma and a papillary carcinoma is often difficult when examining the tissue fragments obtained by needle core biopsy.[128] On occasion, a core biopsy will provide diagnostic tissue[59]; however, because carcinoma may only focally involve a papillary tumor, the absence of this element in a core biopsy specimen might simply be due to incomplete sampling of the lesion. It should also be noted that fragments of florid hyperplasia may suggest *in situ* carcinoma when seen out of context such as in a core biopsy sample and that epithelial clusters entrapped in the stromal fragments of a benign sclerosing papillary lesion can mimic invasive carcinoma.[129]

Excision is recommended when a papillary tumor is suspected on the basis of an FNA specimen and when a needle core biopsy sample reveals a papillary tumor.

IMMUNOHISTOCHEMISTRY AND MOLECULAR STUDIES

Many immunohistochemical studies of papillary lesions center on the distinction between papillary carcinomas and papillomas.[130] Several investigations have examined the expression of cytokeratin molecules, mostly of the high molecular weight or basal type. These cytokeratins are identified with immunostains for CK5/6, CK14, and 34βE12, which are reactive with hyperplastic ductal cells and myoepithelial cells but show decreased or absent reactivity in conventional DCIS. When using this approach to analyze papillary tumors, one must keep in mind that most normal mammary luminal cells, including those within papillomas, do not stain for high molecular weight cytokeratins using conventional immunohistochemical methods. Staining for these proteins finds its most reliable use in distinguishing UDH occurring in a papilloma from atypical or malignant ductal proliferations with a papillary growth pattern. Rabban et al.[131] reported that there was no reactivity for CK5/6 in the epithelium of 14 solid papillary carcinomas. CK5/6 antibodies did stain residual nonneoplastic epithelial cells and myoepithelial cells in the carcinomas, and they stained hyperplastic ductal cells strongly. The antibodies were strongly reactive in the epithelium of duct hyperplasia. Tan et al.[132] reported that immunostaining for CK5/6 had higher sensitivity and specificity for distinguishing papillomas from papillary carcinomas than staining for CK14 and 34βE12. The authors developed an immunoscore calculated by multiplying the percentage of cells stained and their staining intensity. The mean immunoscores for CK5/6, CK14, and 34βE12 in papillomas (107.6, 186.6, and 113.1, respectively) and papillary carcinomas (12.0, 29.6, and 34.5, respectively) were significantly different. When Tse et al.[133] used a threshold of moderate to strong staining of 50% or more of the epithelial cells, they observed that the presence of reactivity for CK14 "becomes 100% specific in identifying benign epithelial proliferation within a papilloma." It is evident from these results that the expression of these proteins, especially CK5/6, is greatly diminished or absent in most papillary carcinomas, but that their focal, weak presence does not exclude the diagnosis of papillary carcinoma. If a diagnosis of papillary carcinoma is being contemplated for a papillary tumor in which there is strong epithelial expression of CK5/6, CK14, or 34βE12, the diagnosis should be reconsidered.

Investigators have also studied the presence and distribution of myoepithelial cells in an effort to distinguish papillary carcinomas from papillomas. When present, myoepithelial cells can usually be recognized in H&E-stained sections of papillary lesions, but immunohistochemical staining offers the most reliable method for detecting myoepithelial cells. Cytoplasmic markers associated with myoepithelium include S-100, CK14, 34βE12, CD10, SMA, calponin, CK5/6, and SMM-HC. The cytoplasmic markers sometimes cross-react with stromal myofibroblasts and vascular structures. The degree to which this cross-reactivity will occur is unpredictable and quite variable with respect to individual markers. Thus, there may be considerable stromal reactivity for SMA in a given case and greater myoepithelial specificity for CD10 in the same tissue. The nuclear marker p63 is relatively specific for myoepithelial cells. It exhibits no cross-reactivity for stromal cells, but it can be expressed in the nuclei of epithelial cells in a papillary lesion.[134,135] These p63-positive epithelial cells can be readily distinguished from myoepithelium by their position in the epithelium. Whenever possible, it is prudent to employ a panel of several markers when evaluating myoepithelium in a papillary tumor to compensate for issues of variable staining and cross-reactivity with stromal elements. Such a panel should always include p63 and representative cytoplasmic markers such as CD10, calponin, SMM-HC, and SMA. A contemporary H&E-stained recut should be prepared at the same time as the immunostains to appreciate any new structural characteristics of the tumor, which may appear in the immunostained sections.

Raju et al.[105] examined the expression of SMA, 34βE12, and S-100 and found that the absence of staining for SMA distinguished all 18 papillary carcinomas from all 25 papillomas. Staining for the other two proteins did not provide clear-cut differentiation of the two lesions. Papotti et al.[37] used an antiactin antiserum and observed similar results. Hill and Yeh[79] found that four invasive papillary carcinomas did not stain for calponin, SMM-HC, or p63, whereas all 23 papillomas did so. Tse et al.[133] used staining for SMA, p63, CD10, and CK14 to highlight myoepithelial cells in 100 papillomas and 68 papillary carcinomas. Expression of the p63 protein proved the most sensitive method to detect myoepithelial cells. The investigators found them in 99 of 100 papillomas but only 2 of 9 invasive papillary carcinomas. Although most invasive papillary carcinomas lack myoepithelial cells, the latter result makes clear that the presence of myoepithelial cells does not exclude the diagnosis of papillary carcinoma. Ichihara et al.[136] detected myoepithelial cells in most "atypical papillomas" and about one-half of papillary carcinomas, and Tse et al.[133] noted myoepithelial cells in approximately one-third of *in situ* papillary carcinomas and two-thirds of papillomas overrun by DCIS. Moritani et al.[104] found that 6 of 21 (29%) of solid papillary carcinomas contained a layer of myoepithelial cells similar to that seen in papillomas.

Staining to reveal the distribution of both epithelial and myoepithelial cells or to define the properties of an epithelial proliferation may help pathologists reach the proper diagnosis in problematic cases. For example, using sequential staining for 34βE12 and p63, Ichihara et al.[136] demonstrated the neoplastic population in 8 "atypical papillomas" and 15 papillary carcinomas and differentiated these tumors from 9 of 10 papillomas with UDH. Douglas-Jones et al.[137] stained 129 core biopsy specimens of papillary tumors for CK5/6, calponin, and p63. The staining results allowed a panel of four pathologists to improve their rate of agreement regarding the diagnosis from 44% to 91%. The overall weighted kappa values rose from 0.696 to 0.954. Grin et al.[138] combined staining for CK5 and ER in an attempt to identify the presence of atypical cells in core biopsy specimens of papillary tumors. The investigators defined high expression of CK5 as staining of more than 20% of the cells and high expression of ER as staining of more than 90% of the cells. The workers observed that papillomas exhibited high expression of CK5 and low expression of ER, whereas atypical proliferations demonstrate the opposite findings. The use of this observation allowed the authors to classify 15 of 15 papillomas and 14 of 15 atypical papillary tumors correctly compared with the findings of excision specimens.

Carcinomas described in small series or case reports have stained for CEA and EMA.[54,61] It was reported that areas of papilloma were negative for CEA, but that cytoplasmic CEA was present in carcinomatous portions of the same papillary tumors.[37,39] The latter authors concluded that "CEA-positive myoepithelial cell-free carcinomatous areas can be anatomically associated with and even present inside the benign-looking papillary lesions." The observations were seen "as evidence of a malignant transformation of intraductal papillomas, or less likely, of their 'cancerization' by ductal carcinoma." As noted previously, fluid aspirated from cystic papillary carcinomas is more likely to contain increased amounts of CEA than fluid from cystic papillomas.[46]

Two investigations[139,140] suggested that the majority of the epithelial cells in papillomas express CD44, whereas only a small number of those in papillary carcinomas contain the protein. Tse et al.[140] report a sensitivity of 45%, a specificity of 92%, and an accuracy of 62% for the results of immunohistochemical for CD44. Troxell et al.[135] did not observe a difference in the CD44 staining of papillomas and papillary carcinoma. Most papillary carcinomas do not stain for epidermal growth factor receptor (EGFR), caveolin 1, caveolin 2, or nestin.[141]

Papillary carcinomas typically express ER (Fig. 14.34A)[78,83,85,87,141] and the estrogen-regulated proteins, PR,[83,87,141] bcl-2, cathepsin-D (Fig. 14.34B), and cyclin D1. The carcinomas typically do not stain for HER2.[55,59,63,64,70,78,83,85,87,141,142] Tumors composed of apocrine cells have not stained for ER, PR, or HER2.[81–83] Saddik et al.[143] found that a significantly ($p < 0.0001$) greater proportion of cells expressed cyclin D1 in papillary carcinomas than in papillomas. The percentage of cyclin D1–positive cells was 89% ± 18% (range, 53% to 98%) in papillary carcinomas and 8% ± 7% (range, 0% to 19%) in papillomas. A statistically significant difference ($p = 0.01$) was also observed for Ki67 immunoreactivity, but the values for papillary carcinoma (13% ± 6%; range, 9% to 23%) and for papillomas (8% ± 2%; range,

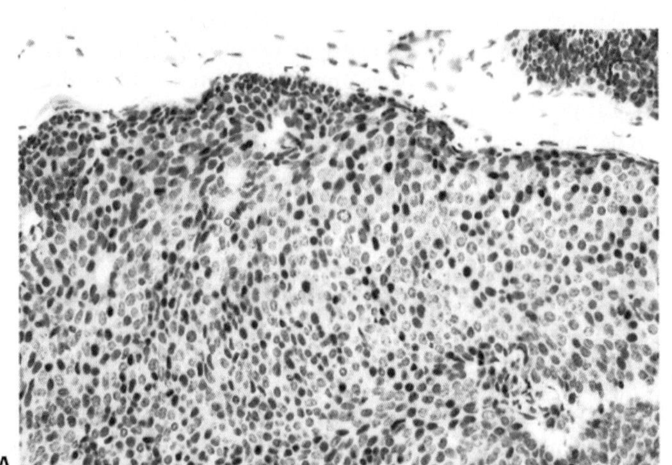

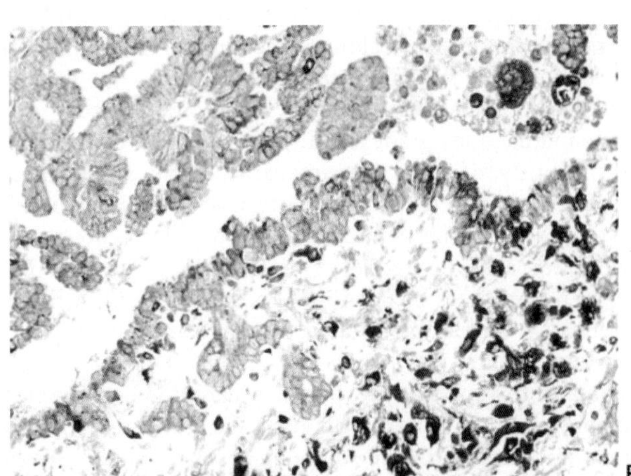

FIG. 14.34. ***Papillary carcinoma.*** **A:** Nuclear immunoreactivity for ER in solid papillary carcinoma. **B:** Cytoplasmic immunoreactivity for cathepsin-D in papillary carcinoma cells and in stromal histiocytes *lower right.*

6% to 12%) showed some overlap, making this a less reliable diagnostic criterion. In other investigations, most carcinomas have shown a low growth fraction measured by thymidine labeling index,[144,145] proliferating cell nuclear antigen (PCNA) index (less than 10% positive cells),[142] or Ki67 scores.[63,78,82,141,143] However, uncommon, high-grade carcinomas can display a high PCNA index,[142] and they may express p53.[141,142]

Flow cytometry has not been helpful in distinguishing between benign and malignant papillary tumors. All benign lesions were diploid in one study,[146] and only 1 of 15 borderline lesions and 5 of 19 papillary carcinomas were aneuploid. Six of eight papillary carcinomas in one investigation demonstrated low-degree aneuploid stemlines, a tetraploid stemline, and a diploid stemline.[125]

GENETIC STUDIES

Molecular analysis of DNA isolated from papillomas and papillary carcinomas has demonstrated both similarities and significant differences. Di Cristofano et al.[147] detected loss of heterozygosity (LOH) at loci 16p13 and 16q21 in both papillomas and papillary carcinomas, whereas only the carcinomas demonstrated LOH at locus 16q23. Other investigators, who studied several loci of 16p13, reported finding LOH in 6 of 10 (60%) papillomas with florid hyperplasia, in 8 of 10 (80%) carcinomas arising in papillomas, and in 2 of 6 (33%) papillary carcinomas.[148] LOH on chromosome 16q was found in 8 of 12 (67%) cystic papillary carcinomas and in 7 of 11 (64%) of low-grade invasive duct carcinomas, but not in any of 11 papillomas studied.[149] A single intracystic papillary carcinoma from a man aged 64 years did not demonstrate LOH on chromosome 16q.[64] Oikawa et al.[150] found greater genomic alterations (including copy number change and LOH) in papillary carcinomas than in papillomas. Chromosomal regions at 3p21.31, 3p14.2, and 20q13.13 were altered most frequently.

Microarray-based comparative genomic hybridization of 63 papillary carcinomas[141] revealed several findings. First, the carcinomas belong to the luminal group of breast carcinomas. Second, they display fewer gene copy number alterations than invasive ductal carcinomas of no special type matched for grade and ER content (12.1% vs. 16.9%, respectively, of BACs showing gains, losses, or amplifications). Although the general pattern of alterations did not differ between the two groups, the papillary carcinomas exhibited a lower frequency of 1q whole-arm gains and whole-arm losses of 6q, 17p, 19p, and 22q and a higher frequency of 19p gains than did the carcinomas in the control group. Third, like low-grade ER-positive carcinomas of no special type, papillary carcinomas frequently displayed mutations in the *PIK3CA* gene. Finally, the genomic profiles of the solid, encapsulated, and conventional types of papillary carcinoma appeared to be similar, leading the authors to suggest that the three varieties of papillary carcinoma "may constitute histologic variants of the same entity."[141]

Papillary carcinomas do not show evidence of the *RET* rearrangements found in papillary thyroid carcinomas despite the frequent presence of shared morphologic features such as nuclear overlap and nuclear grooves.[151]

ELECTRON MICROSCOPY

Electron microscopy generally confirms the light microscopic characteristics of papillary carcinoma and is not regarded as particularly helpful in evaluating difficult cases.[152,153] The carcinoma cells have columnar to cuboidal shapes, and they contain large, dense, and frequently nuclei and cytoplasm with abundant organelles. Myoepithelial cells in papillary carcinomas number considerably fewer than those in benign papillary lesions. Papillomas tend to have abundant, well-formed microvilli at the luminal surfaces of epithelial cells, whereas in some papillary carcinomas, microvilli are less abundant, stunted, and poorly formed.[152] Intracytoplasmic lumens have been described in the cells of papillary carcinoma.[153] The cystic carcinomas reported by Ramos et al.[61] and De Rosa et al.[54] exhibited membrane-bound, dense core secretory granules. One tumor containing electron-dense membrane-bound granules failed to stain for NSE, S-100, vasoactive intestinal peptide, corticotropin, calcitonin, lactalbumin, and bombesin.[61]

TREATMENT AND PROGNOSIS

Changing terminology, disagreement about the invasive properties of the lesions, lack of pathologic details in many reports, and great variation in the evaluation and treatment of patients make it impossible to draw secure and detailed conclusions about the clinical behavior of papillary carcinomas. Nevertheless, several generalizations emerge. First, seemingly noninvasive cystic papillary carcinomas that lack conventional forms of both DCIS and invasive carcinoma metastasize only rarely. When metastases develop, they tend to form small deposits in just one or two ALNs, and the growth pattern of the primary tumor is often duplicated in metastatic foci. For example, the seminal publication by Carter et al.[2] described 18 patients with noninvasive cystic papillary carcinoma who had simple mastectomies and 11 others who were treated by mastectomy and axillary dissection. None of the latter group had axillary metastases. Several other groups[78,81,87,129,154,155] report the lack of metastases in patients with "pure intracystic papillary carcinoma." On the other hand, Lefkowitz et al.[26] described the case of a 71-year-old woman with intraductal papillary carcinoma lacking both DCIS and invasive carcinoma, who had two positive lymph nodes at the time of mastectomy. Mulligan and O'Malley[156] reported two patients with encapsulated papillary carcinoma without conventional invasive carcinoma who had metastatic carcinoma in ALNs. In one patient, one of three sentinel lymph nodes (SLNs) contained three micrometastases; micrometastases involved 2 of 11 lymph nodes from the second patient. A micrometastasis occupied one SLN from 1 of 11 similar patients studied by Esposito et al.[86] Distant spread from a pure intracystic papillary carcinoma represents an extraordinary event. Wynveen et al.[87] report the only case in the literature. This patient experienced a recurrence of pure intracystic papillary carcinoma 8 years after primary excision and radiation therapy. Following the recurrence, she did not receive further therapy, and bone metastases appeared 9 years later (17 years after the original diagnosis).

Second, even when treated only by excision, seemingly noninvasive cystic papillary carcinomas lacking conventional *in situ* and invasive carcinoma do not recur often. Recurrence in the breast after a mistaken diagnosis of cystic papillary carcinoma as a papilloma or after breast conservation therapy for a correctly diagnosed tumor typically occurs more than 3 years after initial treatment. The group of patients studied by Carter et al.[2] included seven with intracystic papillary carcinoma alone treated only with diagnostic excision, and none of these patients developed recurrences. Hill and Yeh[79] reported the same experience. In contrast, several investigators[78,83,87,154,155] have noted local recurrences following limited surgery. Wynveen et al.[87] described three such occurrences; two recurrent carcinomas grew as intracystic papillary carcinomas, and the third as a conventional invasive ductal carcinoma. One of 14 similar patients studied by Solorzano et al.[155] experienced a recurrence 42 months following excision; it took the form of a 0.7-cm pure intracystic papillary carcinoma. The recurrence described by Leal et al.,[78] which came to attention 5 years after excision, appeared to be identical to the original tumor. A conventional invasive ductal carcinoma of no special type recurred in one patient in the study of Calderaro et al.[83] Fayanju et al.[154] did not describe the morphologic features of the carcinoma that recurred 34 months following excision in one patient. Lefkowitz et al.[26] reported chest wall recurrences following mastectomies in four women with intracystic papillary carcinomas. Three recurrences were invasive papillary carcinomas, and the fourth was a conventional invasive ductal carcinoma. The evidence in certain studies notwithstanding, it seems clear that pure intracystic papillary carcinoma has the potential for local recurrence following excision or mastectomy.

Third, the presence of either conventional DCIS or invasive carcinoma associated with intracystic papillary carcinoma may indicate a heightened risk for local recurrence or systemic dissemination, but opinions about this point differ. Carter et al.[2] concluded that the presence of conventional DCIS or invasive ductal carcinoma indicates an increased likelihood for local recurrence. Their study group included four patients with intracystic papillary carcinoma and conventional DCIS. One of the four developed a recurrence of the intracystic papillary carcinoma, and two developed ipsilateral invasive carcinoma. Fifteen patients had intracystic papillary carcinomas and invasive duct carcinoma, and 2 of the 15 presented with ALN metastases. Solorzano et al.[155] report similar findings. Two of three patients with locally recurrent disease had either invasive carcinoma or DCIS associated with intracystic papillary carcinoma, and one patient with an axillary recurrence and another with bone metastases had concomitant DCIS. Lefkowitz et al.[26] reached the opposite conclusion: "data in this study suggest that patients with [intracystic papillary carcinoma] have an increased probability of chest wall recurrence or distant metastases compared with patients with other noncomedo intraductal carcinomas, but the presence of DCIS does not increase this risk of recurrence or distant metastases." Wynveen et al.[87] echo this point of view: "we did not observe an association between the presence of DCIS near [intracystic papillary carcinoma] and higher recurrence rate." The findings of Fayanju et al.[154] do not seem to support the conclusion of Carter et al., either. The investigators studied 21 patients with pure intracystic papillary carcinoma, 18 patients with intracystic papillary carcinoma and DCIS, and 6 patients with intracystic papillary carcinoma with microinvasion. One patient in the first group experienced a local recurrence, and one patient in the second group developed pulmonary metastases, but none of the patients in the third group suffered from recurrent carcinoma. Rakha et al.[85] did not detect an association between the presence of concurrent DCIS and recurrence or metastasis.

Fourth, the prognosis of patients with invasive cystic papillary carcinoma is very favorable, even in women who have axillary nodal metastases.[1,155] When they occur, local and metastatic recurrences of invasive cystic papillary carcinoma often become clinically apparent more than 5 years after diagnosis. These patients are subject to the same tendency to "late" recurrence as are women with mucinous carcinoma. The literature contains only three instances of death from this tumor. Czernobilsky[50] described two women with pure intracystic papillary carcinoma who died of metastatic breast carcinoma, and Fayanju et al.[154] documented the death of a woman with intracystic papillary carcinoma and accompanying DCIS, who developed pulmonary metastases. Another patient with intracystic papillary carcinoma and DCIS died of metastatic breast carcinoma, but histologic study of the metastatic foci was not available,[85] and one patient with intracystic papillary carcinoma and invasive carcinoma died with a clinical diagnosis of cerebral and pulmonary metastases.[78] Six patients in three other series[26,86,155] developed visceral metastases but remained alive at the time of the publication of these reports. Using data from the California Cancer Registry, Grabowski et al. studied the outcome of 917 cases of intracystic papillary carcinoma. The investigators did not review the histologic material; however, using reports, the workers classified 47% of the cases as noninvasive and 53% as invasive and 90% of the invasive carcinomas as localized. The authors found that the relative cumulative survival rates of patients with noninvasive papillary carcinoma and invasive papillary carcinoma did not differ significantly. After 5 years, the values were 101.3% and 93.9%, respectively, and after 10 years, 96.8% and 94.4%, respectively.

Finally, the prognosis for patients with solid papillary carcinomas is relatively favorable, but not to the degree observed for patients with cystic papillary carcinomas. In most cases described in the literature, the patients remained free of metastatic carcinoma, but ALN and systemic metastases developed at a noticeable rate. In about one-half the reported cases, the axillary metastases resembled the primary solid papillary carcinoma; in the others, coexisting invasive carcinomas gave rise to the metastatic foci. For example, 1 of the 4 patients reported by Tse and Ma[157] also had an invasive endocrine carcinoma that spread to 5 of 15 ALNs. Among the seven patients with solid papillary carcinoma described by Nicolas et al.,[94] two patients developed axillary metastases from associated invasive ductal carcinomas. One patient had macrometastases in two of five lymph nodes, and the other had isolated tumor cells in several of six SLNs. Nassar et al.[93] provide the largest experience. Among a group of 30 women with solid papillary carcinoma and invasive carcinoma who underwent ALN examination, 6 had evidence of metastatic disease, and the number of positive nodes ranged from 1 to 10. Three of the six invasive carcinomas displayed neuroendocrine characteristics, one was a colloid carcinoma, one a mixed neuroendocrine and colloid carcinoma, and the last a conventional carcinoma of no special type. The cytologic characteristics of the cells in the lymph nodes mirrored those of the invasive carcinomas.

Local recurrences have developed in seven patients. Five of 28 patients developed chest wall recurrences at intervals between 4 and 10 years following diagnosis,[93] 1 patient in the series of Tsang and Chan[96] suffered a chest wall recurrence, and so did 1 patient described by Maluf et al.[97] Systemic metastases have been documented in eight patients. Nassar et al.[93] cited six patients who experienced visceral and osseous metastasis, Nicolas et al.,[94] one patient with sternal and pulmonary metastases, and Maluf and Koerner[95] another patient with pulmonary spread. Six deaths have been attributed to solid papillary carcinomas.[93] The deaths took place between 1 and 10 years from the time of diagnosis. One patient had had axillary nodal metastases, but five did not. The invasive components of the primary tumors measured less than 0.5 cm in three cases and 1 to 2 cm in two cases. In one case, the size was not specified. Including both the invasive and noninvasive components, the tumor sizes ranged from 1 to 8 cm with a mean of 3 cm.

The definitive treatment of patients with papillary carcinomas has ranged from diagnostic excision to modified radical mastectomy, and a minority of patients have received irradiation and systemic therapy. This variation in treatment coupled with uncertainties regarding the interpretation of certain histologic findings makes it impossible to formulate well-founded treatment recommendations. Complete excision of the carcinoma would seem prudent in all cases. For patients with invasive cystic papillary carcinoma, features such as the patient's age and the size and grade of the invasive component could help to determine the need for sampling or removal of ALNs and for the use of irradiation and systemic therapy. On the basis of the results presented by Nassar et al.,[93] it may be advisable to offer systemic adjuvant hormonal and/or chemotherapy to patients with invasive solid papillary carcinoma regardless of nodal status.

REFERENCES

1. Fisher ER, Palekar AS, Redmond C, et al. Pathologic findings from the National Surgical Adjuvant Breast Project (protocol no. 4). VI. Invasive papillary cancer. *Am J Clin Pathol* 1980;73:313–322.
2. Carter D, Orr SL, Merino MJ. Intracystic papillary carcinoma of the breast. After mastectomy, radiotherapy or excisional biopsy alone. *Cancer* 1983;52:14–19.
3. Giordano SH, Cohen DS, Buzdar AU, et al. Breast carcinoma in men: a population-based study. *Cancer* 2004;101:51–57.
4. McDivitt RW, Stewart FW, Berg JW. *Tumors of the breast. (AFIP Atlas of Tumor Pathology*, 2nd series, vol. 2). Bethesda: American Registry of Pathology, 1968.
5. Schneider JA. Invasive papillary breast carcinoma: mammographic and sonographic appearance. *Radiology* 1989;171:377–379.
6. Mitnick JS, Vazquez MF, Harris MN, et al. Invasive papillary carcinoma of the breast: mammographic appearance. *Radiology* 1990;177:803–806.
7. Schaefer G, Rosen PP, Lesser ML, et al. Breast carcinoma in elderly women: pathology, prognosis, and survival. *Pathol Annu* 1984;19(Pt 1):195–219.
8. Visfeldt J, Scheike O. Male breast cancer. I. Histologic typing and grading of 187 Danish cases. *Cancer* 1973;32:985–990.
9. Norris HJ, Taylor HB. Carcinoma of the male breast. *Cancer* 1969;23:1428–1435.
10. Bloodgood J. Benign lesions of female breast for which operation is not indicated *JAMA* 1922;78:859–863.
11. Estes AC, Phillips C. Papilloma of lacteal duct. *Surg Gynecol Obstet* 1949;89:345–348.
12. Gray HK, Wood GA. Significance of mammary discharge of cases of papilloma of the breast: a clinical and pathologic study. *Arch Surg* 1941;42:203–208.
13. Kilgore AR, Fleming R, Ramos MM. The incidence of cancer with nipple discharge and the risk of cancer in the presence of papillary disease of the breast. *Surg Gynecol Obstet* 1953;96:649–660.
14. Foote FW Jr, Stewart FW. A histologic classification of carcinoma of the breast. *Surgery* 1946;19:74–99.
15. Stout AP. Diagnosis of benign, borderline and malignant lesions of the breast. *Proceedings of the Second National Cancer Conference 1952.* Cincinnati: American Cancer Society, 1954:179–183.
16. Haagensen CD, Stout AP, Phillips JS. The papillary neoplasms of the breast. I. Benign intraductal papilloma. *Ann Surg* 1951;133:18–36.
17. Rosen PP. Arthur Purdy Stout and papilloma of the breast. Comments on the occasion of his 100th birthday. *Am J Surg Pathol* 1986;10(suppl. 1):100–107.
18. Stout AP. The relationships of benign lesions of the breast to cancer. *J Natl Med Assoc* 1954;46:375–381.
19. Moore SW, Pearce J, Ring E. Intraductal papilloma of the breast. *Surg Gynecol Obstet* 1961;112:153–158.
20. McCulloch GL, Evans AJ, Yeoman L, et al. Radiological features of papillary carcinoma of the breast. *Clin Radiol* 1997;52:865–868.
21. Baykara M, Coskun U, Demirci U, et al. Intracystic papillary carcinoma of the breast: one of the youngest patient in the literature. *Med Oncol* 2010;27:1427–1428.
22. Soo MS, Williford ME, Walsh R, et al. Papillary carcinoma of the breast: imaging findings. *AJR Am J Roentgenol* 1995;164:321–326.
23. Grabowski J, Salzstein SL, Sadler GR, et al. Intracystic papillary carcinoma: a review of 917 cases. *Cancer* 2008;113:916–920.
24. Carter D. Intraductal papillary tumors of the breast: a study of 78 cases. *Cancer* 1977;39:1689–1692.
25. Haagensen CD. *Diseases of the breast.* Philadelphia: W.B. Saunders, 1971:528–544.
26. Lefkowitz M, Lefkowitz W, Wargotz ES. Intraductal (intracystic) papillary carcinoma of the breast and its variants: a clinicopathological study of 77 cases. *Hum Pathol* 1994;25:802–809.
27. Hunter CE Jr, Sawyers JL. Intracystic papillary carcinoma of the breast. *South Med J* 1980;73:1484–1486.
28. Estabrook A, Asch T, Gump F, et al. Mammographic features of intracystic papillary lesions. *Surg Gynecol Obstet* 1990;170:113–116.
29. Knelson MH, el Yousef SJ, Goldberg RE, et al. Intracystic papillary carcinoma of the breast: mammographic, sonographic, and MR appearance with pathologic correlation. *J Comput Assist Tomogr* 1987;11:1074–1076.
30. Silva R, Ferrozzi F, Paties C. Invasive papillary carcinoma in elderly women: sonographic and mammographic features. *AJR Am J Roentgenol* 1992;159:898–899.

31. Ganesan S, Karthik G, Joshi M, et al. Ultrasound spectrum in intraductal papillary neoplasms of breast. *Br J Radiol* 2006;79:843–849.
32. Kim TH, Kang DK, Kim SY, et al. Sonographic differentiation of benign and malignant papillary lesions of the breast. *J Ultrasound Med* 2008;27:75–82.
33. Blaumeiser B, Tjalma WA, Verslegers I, et al. Invasive papillary carcinoma of the male breast. *Eur Radiol* 2002;12:2207–2210.
34. Linda A, Londero V, Mazzarella F, et al. Rare breast neoplasms: is there any peculiar feature on magnetic resonance mammography? *Radiol Med* 2007;112:850–862.
35. Tobin CE, Hendrix TM, Resnikoff LB, et al. Breast imaging case of the day. Multicentric intraductal papillary carcinoma. *Radiographics* 1996;16:720–722.
36. Kraus FT, Neubecker RD. The differential diagnosis of papillary tumors of the breast. *Cancer* 1962;15:444–455.
37. Papotti M, Eusebi V, Gugliotta P, et al. Immunohistochemical analysis of benign and malignant papillary lesions of the breast. *Am J Surg Pathol* 1983;7:451–461.
38. Murad TM, Swaid S, Pritchett P. Malignant and benign papillary lesions of the breast. *Hum Pathol* 1977;8:379–390.
39. Papotti M, Gugliotta P, Ghiringhello B, et al. Association of breast carcinoma and multiple intraductal papillomas: an histological and immunohistochemical investigation. *Histopathology* 1984;8:963–975.
40. Snyder WH Jr, Chaffin L. Main duct papilloma of the breast. *AMA Arch Surg* 1955;70:680–685.
41. Raju U, Vertes D. Breast papillomas with atypical ductal hyperplasia: a clinicopathologic study. *Hum Pathol* 1996;27:1231–1238.
42. Page DL, Salhany KE, Jensen RA, et al. Subsequent breast carcinoma risk after biopsy with atypia in a breast papilloma. *Cancer* 1996;78:258–266.
43. Ohuchi N, Abe R, Kasai M. Possible cancerous change of intraductal papillomas of the breast. A 3-D reconstruction study of 25 cases. *Cancer* 1984;54:605–611.
44. Ohuchi N, Abe R, Takahashi T, et al. Three-dimensional atypical structure in intraductal carcinoma differentiating from papilloma and papillomatosis of the breast. *Breast Cancer Res Treat* 1985;5:57–65.
45. Matsuo S, Eto T, Soejima H, et al. A case of intracystic carcinoma of the breast: the importance of measuring carcinoembryonic antigen in aspirated cystic fluid. *Breast Cancer Res Treat* 1993;28:41–44.
46. Inaji H, Koyama H, Motomura K, et al. Simultaneous assay of ErbB-2 protein and carcinoembryonic antigen in cyst fluid as an aid in diagnosing cystic lesions of the breast. *Breast Cancer* 1994;1:25–30.
47. Rosen PP. Tumor emboli in intramammary lymphatics in breast carcinoma: pathologic criteria for diagnosis and clinical significance. *Pathol Annu* 1983;18(Pt 2):215–232.
48. Youngson BJ, Cranor M, Rosen PP. Epithelial displacement in surgical breast specimens following needling procedures. *Am J Surg Pathol* 1994;18:896–903.
49. Gatchell FG, Dockerty MB, Clagett OT. Intracystic carcinoma of the breast. *Surg Gynecol Obstet* 1958;106:347–352.
50. Czernobilsky B. Intracystic carcinoma of the female breast. *Surg Gynecol Obstet* 1967;124:93–98.
51. McKittrick JE, Doane WA, Failing RM. Intracystic papillary carcinoma of the breast. *Am Surg* 1969;35:195–202.
52. Tabár L, Péntek Z, Dean PB. The diagnostic and therapeutic value of breast cyst puncture and pneumocystography. *Radiology* 1981;141:659–663.
53. Andrés B, Aguilar J, Torroba A, et al. Intracystic papillary carcinoma in the male breast. *Breast J* 2003;9:249–250.
54. De Rosa G, Giordano G, Boscaino A, et al. Intracystic papillary carcinoma of the male breast. A case report (histochemical, immunohistochemical and ultrastructural study). *Tumori* 1992;78:37–42.
55. Gupta D, Torosian MH. Intracystic breast carcinoma in a male: unusual case presentation and literature review. *Oncol Rep* 2002;9:405–407.
56. Imoto S, Hasebe T. Intracystic papillary carcinoma of the breast in male: case report and review of the Japanese literature. *Jpn J Clin Oncol* 1998;28:517–520.
57. Joshi N, Pande C. Papillary carcinoma of the male breast diagnosed by fine needle aspiration cytology. *Indian J Pathol Microbiol* 1998;41:103–106.
58. Kihara M, Mori N, Yamauchi A, et al. A case of intracystic papillary carcinoma with a multilocular cyst of the breast in male. *Breast Cancer* 2004;11:409–412.
59. Kinoshita T, Fukutomi T, Iwamoto E, et al. Intracystic papillary carcinoma of the breast in a male patient diagnosed by core needle biopsy: a case report. *Breast* 2005;14:322–324.
60. Pacelli A, Bock BJ, Jensen EA, et al. Intracystic papillary carcinoma of the breast in a male patient diagnosed by ultrasound-guided core biopsy: a case report. *Breast J* 2002;8:387–390.
61. Ramos CV, Boeshart C, Restrepo GL. Intracystic papillary carcinoma of the male breast. Immunohistochemical and ultrastructural study. *Arch Pathol Lab Med* 1985;109:858–861.
62. Sonksen CJ, Michell M, Sundaresan M. Case report: intracystic papillary carcinoma of the breast in a male patient. *Clin Radiol* 1996;51:438–439.
63. Tochika N, Takano A, Yoshimoto T, et al. Intracystic carcinoma of the male breast: report of a case. *Surg Today* 2001;31:806–809.
64. Yoshida M, Mouri Y, Yamamoto S, et al. Intracystic invasive papillary carcinoma of the male breast with analyses of loss of heterozygosity on chromosome 16q. *Breast Cancer* 2010;17:146–150.
65. Sinha S, Hughes RG, Ryley NG. Papillary carcinoma in a male breast cyst: a diagnostic challenge >*Ann R Coll Surg Engl* 2006;88:W3–W5.
66. Heller KS, Rosen PP, Schottenfeld D, et al. Male breast cancer: a clinicopathologic study of 97 cases. *Ann Surg* 1978;188:60–65.
67. Appu S, Valentine R, Swann J. Intracystic papillary carcinoma of the breast. *ANZ J Surg* 2001;71:440–441.
68. Fallentin E, Rothman L. Intracystic carcinoma of the male breast. *J Clin Ultrasound* 1994;22:118–120.
69. Kihara M, Miyauchi A. Intracystic papilloma of the breast forming a giant cyst. *Breast Cancer* 2010;17:68–70.
70. Amemiya T, Oda K, Satake H, et al. A case of intracystic papillary carcinoma accompanying widespread ductal carcinoma *in situ*. *Breast Cancer* 2007;14:312–316.
71. Squires JE, Betsill WL Jr. Intracystic carcinoma of the breast: a correlation of cytomorphology, gross pathology, microscopic pathology and clinical data. *Acta Cytol* 1981;25:267–271.
72. Bardales RH, Suhrland MJ, Stanley MW. Papillary neoplasms of the breast: fine-needle aspiration findings in cystic and solid cases. *Diagn Cytopathol* 1994;10:336–341.
73. Weshler Z, Sulkes A. Contrast mammography and the diagnosis of male breast cysts. *Clin Radiol* 1980;31:341–343.
74. Georgountzos V, Ioannidou-Mouzaka L, Tsouroulas M, et al. Benign intracystic papilloma in the male breast. *Breast J* 2005;11:361–362.
75. Martorano Navas MD, Rayas Povedano JL, Añorbe Medivil E, et al. Intracystic papilloma in male breast: ultrasonography and pneumocystography diagnosis. *J Clin Ultrasound* 1993;21:28–40.
76. Nayar R, De Frias DV, Bourtsos EP, et al. Cytologic differential diagnosis of papillary pattern in breast aspirates: correlation with histology. *Ann Diagn Pathol* 2001;5:34–42.
77. Shim JH, Son EJ, Kim EK, et al. Benign intracystic papilloma of the male breast. *J Ultrasound Med* 2008;27:1397–1400.
78. Leal C, Costa I, Fonseca D, et al. Intracystic (encysted) papillary carcinoma of the breast: a clinical, pathological, and immunohistochemical study. *Hum Pathol* 1998;29:1097–1104.
79. Hill CB, Yeh IT. Myoepithelial cell staining patterns of papillary breast lesions: from intraductal papillomas to invasive papillary carcinomas. *Am J Clin Pathol* 2005;123:36–44.
80. Collins LC, O'Malley F, Visscher D, et al. Encapsulated papillary carcinoma. In: Lakhani SR, Ellis IO, Schnitt SJ, et al., eds. *WHO classification of tumours of the breast.* (*WHO Classification of Tumours*, vol. 4). 4th ed. Lyon: World Health Organization-IARC, 2012.
81. Seal M, Wilson C, Naus GJ, et al. Encapsulated apocrine papillary carcinoma of the breast—a tumour of uncertain malignant potential: report of five cases. *Virchows Arch* 2009;455:477–483.
82. Laforga JB, Gasent JM, Sanchez I. Encapsulated apocrine papillary carcinoma of the breast: case report with clinicopathologic and immunohistochemical study. *Diagn Cytopathol* 2011;39:288–293.
83. Calderaro J, Espie M, Duclos J, et al. Breast intracystic papillary carcinoma: an update. *Breast J* 2009;15:639–644.
84. Collins LC, Carlo VP, Hwang H, et al. Intracystic papillary carcinomas of the breast: a reevaluation using a panel of myoepithelial cell markers. *Am J Surg Pathol* 2006;30:1002–1007.
85. Rakha EA, Gandhi N, Climent F, et al. Encapsulated papillary carcinoma of the breast: an invasive tumor with excellent prognosis. *Am J Surg Pathol* 2011;35:1093–1103.
86. Esposito NN, Dabbs DJ, Bhargava R. Are encapsulated papillary carcinomas of the breast *in situ* or invasive? A basement membrane study of 27 cases. *Am J Clin Pathol* 2009;131:228–242.

87. Wynveen CA, Nehhozina T, Akram M, et al. Intracystic papillary carcinoma of the breast: an *in situ* or invasive tumor? Results of immunohistochemical analysis and clinical follow-up. *Am J Surg Pathol* 2011;35:1–14.
88. Rakha EA, Tun M, Junainah E, et al. Encapsulated papillary carcinoma of the breast: a study of invasion associated markers. *J Clin Pathol* 2012;65:710–714.
89. Rosen PP, Oberman HA. Papillary carcinoma. In: *Tumors of the mammary gland.* (*AFIP Atlas of Tumor Pathology*, 3rd series, vol. 7.) Baltimore: American Registry of Pathology, 1993.
90. Cross AS, Azzopardi JG, Krausz T, et al. A morphological and immunocytochemical study of a distinctive variant of ductal carcinoma *in-situ* of the breast. *Histopathology* 1985;9:21–37.
91. Azzopardi JG, Muretto P, Goddeeris P, et al. 'Carcinoid' tumours of the breast: the morphological spectrum of argyrophil carcinomas. *Histopathology* 1982;6:549–569.
92. Otsuki Y, Yamada M, Shimizu S, et al. Solid-papillary carcinoma of the breast: clinicopathological study of 20 cases. *Pathol Int* 2007;57:421–429.
93. Nassar H, Qureshi H, Adsay NV, et al. Clinicopathologic analysis of solid papillary carcinoma of the breast and associated invasive carcinomas. *Am J Surg Pathol* 2006;30:501–507.
94. Nicolas MM, Wu Y, Middleton LP, et al. Loss of myoepithelium is variable in solid papillary carcinoma of the breast. *Histopathology* 2007;51:657–665.
95. Maluf HM, Koerner FC. Solid papillary carcinoma of the breast. A form of intraductal carcinoma with endocrine differentiation frequently associated with mucinous carcinoma. *Am J Surg Pathol* 1995;19:1237–1244.
96. Tsang WY, Chan JK. Endocrine ductal carcinoma *in situ* (E-DCIS) of the breast: a form of low-grade DCIS with distinctive clinicopathologic and biologic characteristics. *Am J Surg Pathol* 1996;20:921–943.
97. Maluf HM, Zukerberg LR, Dickersin GR, et al. Spindle-cell argyrophilic mucin-producing carcinoma of the breast. Histological, ultrastructural, and immunohistochemical studies of two cases. *Am J Surg Pathol* 1991;15:677–686.
98. Boran MD, de Saint Hilaire PJ, Leveugle-Pin J, et al. Fine needle aspiration cytology of a solid papillary carcinoma of the breast. A case report with immunohistochemical studies. *Acta Cytol* 1998;42:725–728.
99. Hardisson D, Gonzalez-Peramato P, Perna C, et al. Fine needle aspiration cytology of solid papillary carcinoma of the breast. A report of four cases. *Acta Cytol* 2003;47:259–264.
100. Yin H, Schinella R. Cytologic characteristics of endocrine ductal carcinoma *in situ* of the breast. A case report. *Acta Cytol* 2002;46: 873–876.
101. Yamada M, Otsuki Y, Shimizu S, et al. Cytological study of 20 cases of solid-papillary carcinoma of the breast. *Diagn Cytopathol* 2007;35:417–422.
102. Kanbayashi C, Oka K, Hakozaki H, et al. Solid papillary carcinoma of the breast: report of two cases. *Ultrastruct Pathol* 2001;25:147–152.
103. Dickersin GR, Maluf HM, Koerner FC. Solid papillary carcinoma of breast: an ultrastructural study. *Ultrastruct Pathol* 1997;21:153–161.
104. Moritani S, Ichihara S, Kushima R, et al. Myoepithelial cells in solid variant of intraductal papillary carcinoma of the breast: a potential diagnostic pitfall and a proposal of an immunohistochemical panel in the differential diagnosis with intraductal papilloma with usual ductal hyperplasia. *Virchows Arch* 2007;450:539–547.
105. Raju UB, Lee MW, Zarbo RJ, et al. Papillary neoplasia of the breast: immunohistochemically defined myoepithelial cells in the diagnosis of benign and malignant papillary breast neoplasms. *Mod Pathol* 1989;2:569–576.
106. Eusebi V, Damiani S, Ellis IO, et al. Breast tumor resembling the tall cell variant of papillary thyroid carcinoma: report of 5 cases. *Am J Surg Pathol* 2003;27:1114–1118.
107. Chang SY, Fleiszer DM, Mesurolle B, et al. Breast tumor resembling the tall cell variant of papillary thyroid carcinoma. *Breast J* 2009;15:531–535.
108. Cameselle-Teijeiro J, Abdulkader I, Barreiro-Morandeira F, et al. Breast tumor resembling the tall cell variant of papillary thyroid carcinoma: a case report. *Int J Surg Pathol* 2006;14:79–84.
109. Masood S, Davis C, Kubik MJ. Changing the term "breast tumor resembling the tall cell variant of papillary thyroid carcinoma" to "tall cell variant of papillary breast carcinoma". *Adv Anat Pathol* 2012;19:108–110.
110. Tosi AL, Ragazzi M, Asioli S, et al. Breast tumor resembling the tall cell variant of papillary thyroid carcinoma: report of 4 cases with evidence of malignant potential. *Int J Surg Pathol* 2007;15:14–19.
111. Eusebi V, Tallini G, Rosai J. Nuclear alterations and RET/PTC activation. *Am J Surg Pathol* 2004;28:974–975.
112. Fiche M, Cassagnau E, Aillet G, et al. Métastase mammaire d'un carcinome papillaire á cellules hautes de la thyroïde. *Ann Pathol* 1998;18:130–132.
113. Saad RS, Kanbour-Shakir A, Syed A, et al. Sclerosing papillary lesion of the breast: a diagnostic pitfall for malignancy in fine needle aspiration biopsy. *Diagn Cytopathol* 2006;34:114–118.
114. Simsir A, Waisman J, Thorner K, et al. Mammary lesions diagnosed as "papillary" by aspiration biopsy: 70 cases with follow-up. *Cancer* 2003;99:156–165.
115. Gomez-Aracil V, Mayayo E, Azua J, et al. Papillary neoplasms of the breast: clues in fine needle aspiration cytology. *Cytopathology* 2002;13:22–30.
116. Kumar PV, Talei AR, Malekhusseini SA, et al. Papillary carcinoma of the breast. Cytologic study of nine cases. *Acta Cytol* 1999;43: 767–770.
117. Michael CW, Buschmann B. Can true papillary neoplasms of breast and their mimickers be accurately classified by cytology? *Cancer* 2002;96:92–100.
118. Prathiba D, Rao S, Kshitija K, et al. Papillary lesions of breast—an introspect of cytomorphological features. *J Cytol* 2010;27:12–15.
119. Tse GM, Ma TK, Lui PC, et al. Fine needle aspiration cytology of papillary lesions of the breast: how accurate is the diagnosis? *J Clin Pathol* 2008;61:945–949.
120. Jeffrey PB, Ljung BM. Benign and malignant papillary lesions of the breast. A cytomorphologic study. *Am J Clin Pathol* 1994;101:500–507.
121. Dawson AE, Mulford DK. Benign versus malignant papillary neoplasms of the breast. Diagnostic clues in fine needle aspiration cytology. *Acta Cytol* 1994;38:23–28.
122. Dei Tos AP, Della Giustina D, Bittesini L. Aspiration biopsy cytology of malignant papillary breast neoplasms *Diagn Cytopathol* 1992;8:580–584.
123. Kline TS, Kannan V. Papillary carcinoma of the breast. A cytomorphologic analysis. *Arch Pathol Lab Med* 1986;110:189–191.
124. Naran S, Simpson J, Gupta RK. Cytologic diagnosis of papillary carcinoma of the breast in needle aspirates. *Diagn Cytopathol* 1988;4:33–37.
125. Corkill ME, Sneige N, Fanning T, et al. Fine-needle aspiration cytology and flow cytometry of intracystic papillary carcinoma of breast. *Am J Clin Pathol* 1990;94:673–680.
126. Jayaram G, Elsayed EM, Yaccob RB. Papillary breast lesions diagnosed on cytology. Profile of 65 cases. *Acta Cytol* 2007;51:3–8.
127. Burgan AR, Frierson HF Jr, Fechner RE. Fine-needle aspiration cytology of spindle-cell argyrophilic mucin-producing carcinoma of the breast. *Diagn Cytopathol* 1996;14:238–242.
128. Rosen PP. *Breast pathology: diagnosis by needle core biopsy*. Philadelphia: Lippincott William & Wilkins, 1999:21–42, 135–146.
129. Harris KP, Faliakou EC, Exon DJ, et al. Treatment and outcome of intracystic papillary carcinoma of the breast. *Br J Surg* 1999;86:1274.
130. Tse GM, Tan PH, Moriya T. The role of immunohistochemistry in the differential diagnosis of papillary lesions of the breast. *J Clin Pathol* 2009;62:407–413.
131. Rabban JT, Koerner FC, Lerwill MF. Solid papillary ductal carcinoma *in situ* versus usual ductal hyperplasia in the breast: a potentially difficult distinction resolved by cytokeratin 5/6. *Hum Pathol* 2006;37:787–793.
132. Tan PH, Aw MY, Yip G, et al. Cytokeratins in papillary lesions of the breast: is there a role in distinguishing intraductal papilloma from papillary ductal carcinoma *in situ*? *Am J Surg Pathol* 2005;29: 625–632.
133. Tse GM, Tan PH, Lui PC, et al. The role of immunohistochemistry for smooth-muscle actin, p63, CD10 and cytokeratin 14 in the differential diagnosis of papillary lesions of the breast. *J Clin Pathol* 2007;60:315–320.
134. Stefanou D, Batistatou A, Nonni A, et al. p63 Expression in benign and malignant breast lesions. *Histol Histopathol* 2004;19:465–471.
135. Troxell ML, Masek M, Sibley RK. Immunohistochemical staining of papillary breast lesions. *Appl Immunohistochem Mol Morphol* 2007;15:145–153.

136. Ichihara S, Fujimoto T, Hashimoto K, et al. Double immunostaining with p63 and high-molecular-weight cytokeratins distinguishes borderline papillary lesions of the breast. *Pathol Int* 2007;57:126–132.
137. Douglas-Jones A, Shah V, Morgan J, et al. Observer variability in the histopathological reporting of core biopsies of papillary breast lesions is reduced by the use of immunohistochemistry for CK5/6, calponin and p63. *Histopathology* 2005;47:202–208.
138. Grin A, O'Malley FP, Mulligan AM. Cytokeratin 5 and estrogen receptor immunohistochemistry as a useful adjunct in identifying atypical papillary lesions on breast needle core biopsy. *Am J Surg Pathol* 2009;33:1615–1623.
139. Saddik M, Lai R. CD44s as a surrogate marker for distinguishing intraductal papilloma from papillary carcinoma of the breast. *J Clin Pathol* 1999;52:862–864.
140. Tse GM, Tan PH, Ma TK, et al. CD44s is useful in the differentiation of benign and malignant papillary lesions of the breast. *J Clin Pathol* 2005;58:1185–1188.
141. Duprez R, Wilkerson PM, Lacroix-Triki M, et al. Immunophenotypic and genomic characterization of papillary carcinomas of the breast. *J Pathol* 2012;226:427–441.
142. Lanzafame S, Emmanuele C, Torrisi A, et al. Correlated expression of BCL-2 protein, estrogen receptor, cathepsin D and low growth fraction (PCNA) in intracystic papillary breast carcinoma. *Pathol Res Pract* 1998;194:541–547.
143. Saddik M, Lai R, Medeiros LJ, et al. Differential expression of cyclin D1 in breast papillary carcinomas and benign papillomas: an immunohistochemical study. *Arch Pathol Lab Med* 1999;123:152–156.
144. Meyer JS, Bauer WC, Rao BR. Subpopulations of breast carcinoma defined by S-phase fraction, morphology, and estrogen receptor content. *Lab Invest* 1978;39:225–235.
145. Masood S, Barwick K. Estrogen receptor expression of the less common breast carcinomas. *Am J Clin Pathol* 1990;93:437.
146. Tiltman AJ. DNA ploidy in papillary tumours of the breast. *S Afr Med J* 1989;75:379–380.
147. Di Cristofano C, Mrad K, Zavaglia K, et al. Papillary lesions of the breast: a molecular progression? *Breast Cancer Res Treat* 2005;90:71–76.
148. Lininger RA, Zhuang Z, Man Y-G, et al. LOH at 16p13 detected in microdissected papillary neoplasms of the breast and their precursors. *Mod Pathol* 1997;10:22A.
149. Tsuda H, Uei Y, Fukutomi T, et al. Different incidence of loss of heterozygosity on chromosome 16q between intraductal papilloma and intracystic papillary carcinoma of the breast. *Jpn J Cancer Res* 1994;85:992–996.
150. Oikawa M, Nagayasu T, Yano H, et al. Intracystic papillary carcinoma of breast harbors significant genomic alteration compared with intracystic papilloma: genome-wide copy number and LOH analysis using high-density single-nucleotide polymorphism microarrays. *Breast J* 2011;17:427–430.
151. Hameed O, Perry A, Banerjee R, et al. Papillary carcinoma of the breast lacks evidence of RET rearrangements despite morphological similarities to papillary thyroid carcinoma. *Mod Pathol* 2009;22:1236–1242.
152. Ahmed A. Ultrastructural aspects of human breast lesions. *Pathol Annu* 1980;15:411–443.
153. Tsuchiya S, Takayama S, Higashi Y. Electron microscopy of intraductal papilloma of the breast. Ultrastructural comparison of papillary carcinoma with normal mammary large duct. *Acta Pathol Jpn* 1983;33:97–112.
154. Fayanju OM, Ritter J, Gillanders WE, et al. Therapeutic management of intracystic papillary carcinoma of the breast: the roles of radiation and endocrine therapy. *Am J Surg* 2007;194:497–500.
155. Solorzano CC, Middleton LP, Hunt KK, et al. Treatment and outcome of patients with intracystic papillary carcinoma of the breast. *Am J Surg* 2002;184:364–368.
156. Mulligan AM, O'Malley FP. Metastatic potential of encapsulated (intracystic) papillary carcinoma of the breast: a report of 2 cases with axillary lymph node micrometastases. *Int J Surg Pathol* 2007;15:143–147.
157. Tse GM, Ma TK. Fine-needle aspiration cytology of breast carcinoma with endocrine differentiation. *Cancer* 2000;90:286–291.

CHAPTER 15

Medullary Carcinoma

FREDERICK C. KOERNER

Mammary carcinomas have been described as "medullary" for nearly a century. Initially, the term was employed clinically and pathologically for large, solid carcinomas with a papillary or fleshy macroscopic appearance. Included in this group were tumors characterized by a marked lymphoid reaction and a favorable prognosis referred to as cystic neomammary carcinoma by Geschickter.[1] At Memorial Hospital in New York City, these tumors were termed "bulky adenocarcinomas" until the name "medullary carcinoma" was proposed in the 1940s.[2,3] As classically envisioned, medullary carcinoma is a well-circumscribed carcinoma composed of poorly differentiated cells with scant stroma and prominent lymphoid infiltration. The term *atypical medullary carcinoma* was introduced in 1975[4] to describe carcinomas that have features generally suggestive of medullary carcinoma but lack one or more of the defining histologic characteristics. These tumors are now classified as *invasive ductal carcinomas with medullary features.*

The diagnosis of medullary carcinoma seems to have lost favor during the past decade or two. Many pathologists, including those at large referral centers, feel uncertain about the recognition and the application of the classical diagnostic criteria. A poor level of diagnostic reducibility and uncertainty about the clinical ramifications of this diagnosis add to pathologists' reluctance to classify carcinomas as medullary. The editors and contributors to the 4th edition of the *WHO Classification of Tumours of the Breast* recommend that "classic [medullary carcinoma], atypical [medullary carcinoma], and invasive carcinoma NST with medullary features be grouped within the category of carcinomas with medullary features."[5] The short discussion that follows this recommendation does not offer criteria to distinguish among the members of this group. This movement away from classifying certain carcinomas as medullary seems regrettable and premature. Well-conducted clinical follow-up studies continue to demonstrate the favorable prognosis afforded by this type of breast carcinoma. It would be a shame to abandon the diagnosis of medullary carcinoma at the moment when contemporary genomic studies offer the hope of a greater understanding of this tumor. Such studies might discover a molecular signature that identifies those members of the group of "carcinomas with medullary features" that have a relatively more favorable prognosis; they might reveal consistent genetic alterations that underlie the formation of medullary carcinomas, and they might elucidate the molecular mechanisms responsible for the favorable clinical behavior of medullary carcinomas. With such information in hand, pathologists could then study the histologic characteristics of these tumors and, possibly, describe a set of robust criteria that define medullary carcinoma. Until investigators have explored this group of tumors at the genetic level, it seems preferable to continue to classify certain carefully characterized carcinomas as medullary.

CLINICAL PRESENTATION

Frequency

Medullary carcinomas constitute fewer than 5% of most series of breast carcinomas,[6–11] but frequencies as high as 7% have been reported.[12–15] A review of 524 consecutive patients with T1N0 and T1N1 breast carcinomas treated from 1964 to 1970 found that medullary carcinoma comprised 2% of both groups.[16,17]

Epidemiology

In epidemiologic studies, medullary carcinoma was detected relatively more frequently in Japanese women in Japan than in Caucasian women in the United States[18–20] and more commonly in African American women than in Caucasian women in the United States.[21–24] An analysis of data from a large number of women beyond the age of 50 years with breast carcinoma demonstrated an elevated risk of medullary carcinoma among African American and certain groups of Asian and Hispanic women compared with the risk faced by non–Hispanic Caucasian women. Puerto Rican women had the greatest risk, 7.7 times that of non–Hispanic Caucasian women, and Native American women followed with a risk of 4.7 times that of non–Hispanic Caucasian women.[25] Maier et al.[6] also noted more medullary carcinomas in "non-Caucasians."

Family History

Maternal breast carcinoma was reportedly more frequent among women with medullary carcinoma than among women with other types of carcinoma, whereas very few of their sisters had breast carcinoma.[26] A detailed analysis of the family pedigrees of patients with medullary carcinoma did not reveal an increased risk of neoplastic disease, including breast carcinoma compared with the families of patients with tubular or invasive ductal carcinoma.[27]

Medullary carcinoma afflicts adults of all ages. Patients as young as 21 years[28] and as old as 95 years[6] have developed medullary carcinoma. This broad range of ages notwithstanding, patients with medullary carcinoma tend to be relatively young. Moore and Foote[3] found that 59% of their patients were younger than 50 years, and in other series, 40%[13] and 60%[29] of patients were younger than 50 years. The mean age in several series ranged from 45 to 54 years.[6,7,9,11,28–33] A study of 159 women aged 35 years or less with breast carcinoma found that 11% had medullary carcinomas.[34] Medullary carcinoma is relatively uncommon in elderly patients,[35] and it occurs in the male breast only very rarely.

Clinical Location of Tumor

The anatomic distribution of medullary carcinoma in the breast does not differ significantly from that of breast carcinomas in general. Multicentricity, defined as microscopic foci of carcinoma outside the primary quadrant, is uncommon in patients with medullary carcinoma. It was found in 10% of 58 cases in one series.[36] Medullary carcinoma arising in the axillary tail is difficult to distinguish from metastatic carcinoma in a lymph node.[37] Medullary carcinoma is not especially common among patients with bilateral mammary carcinoma. On the other hand, bilateral carcinoma has been found in 3% to 12% of patients with medullary carcinoma.[6,8,35,36] Synchronous or metachronous medullary carcinoma involving both breasts is very uncommon.[28,36]

Clinical Presentation of Axillary Lymph Nodes

Ipsilateral axillary lymph nodes (ALNs) tend to be enlarged on clinical examination in patients with medullary carcinoma even when there are no nodal metastases. This phenomenon, which may complicate clinical staging,[38] can also be encountered in patients with invasive ductal carcinomas with medullary features.[39] Microscopically, the lymph nodes have a lymphoplasmacytic infiltrate, germinal center hyperplasia, and sinus histiocytosis. On average, the number of lymph nodes evident in axillary dissection specimens from patients with medullary or atypical medullary carcinoma is greater than for other types of carcinoma.[39] This difference probably results from the greater ease of finding enlarged hyperplastic lymph nodes.

Imaging Studies

Mammograms of medullary carcinomas typically demonstrate a uniformly dense, round or oval mass with indistinct or lobulated borders and lacking calcifications.[40] Because they have circumscribed margins, medullary carcinomas can be mistaken radiologically for fibroadenomas.[7,41] The findings apparent on ultrasound studies vary from one case to the next. Medullary carcinoma most commonly displays a hypoechogenic mass with an inhomogeneous echotexture, a microlobulated or indistinct border, and posterior enhancement.[40] Medullary carcinomas that have undergone cystic degeneration can exhibit a complex pattern of echoes.[41,42] Invasive ductal carcinomas with medullary features tend to have an irregular margin on ultrasonography.[42] By magnetic resonance imaging, the carcinomas are iso- or hypointense on T1-weighted images and iso- or hyperintense on T2-weighted images. The masses usually have oval or lobular shapes and smooth borders, and they often exhibit rim enhancement. Time–intensity curves display a rapid initial rise in enhancement and a plateau or washout pattern.[40,43] Kopans and Rubens[44] and Tominaga et al.[43] emphasized that radiologic findings cannot differentiate medullary carcinoma from circumscribed non-medullary carcinoma (Figs. 15.1 and 15.2).

GROSS PATHOLOGY

Early descriptions[1,3] of medullary carcinoma emphasized its large size, a characteristic exemplified by the term "bulky carcinoma" once used for this tumor. The passage of time has not improved upon the description written by Drs. Foote and Stewart[2]: "They are commonly quite bulky, measuring 4, 5 and 6 cm in diameter, and now and then these dimensions are doubled. They are rounded or globoid, cut with little resistance, and although not encapsulated these tumors are distinctly circumscribed and present a smooth periphery. On cut section the exposed surface bulges above the level of the surrounding tissue, the tumor is soft, and chalky streaks are unexpected. Where the *carcinoma* is fully viable it is grayish white, but as a group these tumors are quite prone to spontaneous hemorrhage and necrosis, and for this reason may present variegated coloring."

In contemporary times, the size distribution of grossly measured medullary carcinomas is not appreciably different from that of conventional invasive ductal carcinomas (IDC); several series report a median size of 2.0 to 3.2 cm.[8,12,28] These smaller examples of medullary carcinoma do not display signs of advanced disease such as ulceration of the skin and fixation to the chest wall as did large, bulky tumors described in the earliest descriptions of medullary carcinoma.

The typical intact medullary carcinoma is a moderately firm discrete tumor that one can easily mistake for a fibroadenoma (Fig. 15.3). A distinct margin outlines the tumor when bisected and distinguishes it from the surrounding breast tissue (Fig. 15.4). In larger lesions, particularly those with prominent cystic areas, peripheral fibrosis may suggest encapsulation (Fig. 15.5). Some small medullary carcinomas have poorly circumscribed borders.[30] The peripheral areas of ill-defined medullary carcinomas have an intense lymphoplasmacytic reaction that extends well beyond the perimeter of the carcinoma; consequently, gross circumscription is supportive of but necessary for a diagnosis of medullary carcinoma. Some non-medullary infiltrating

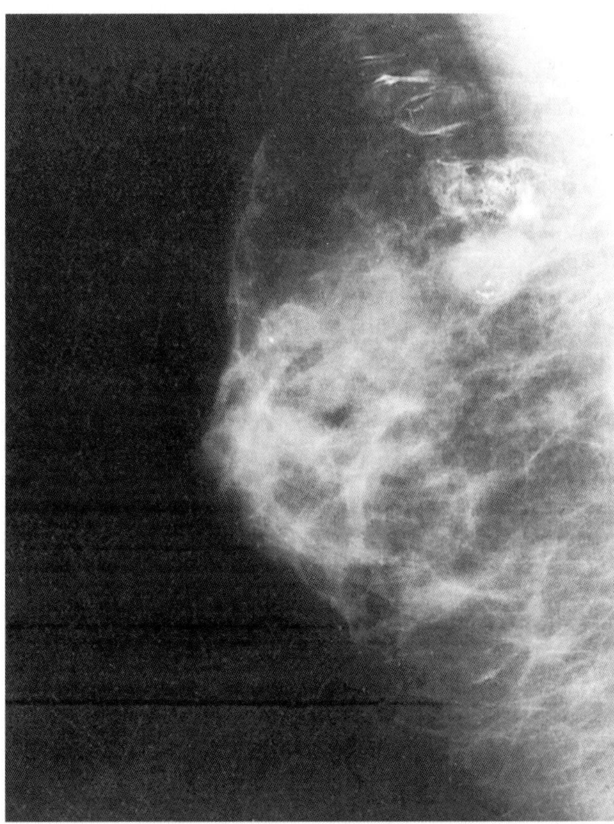

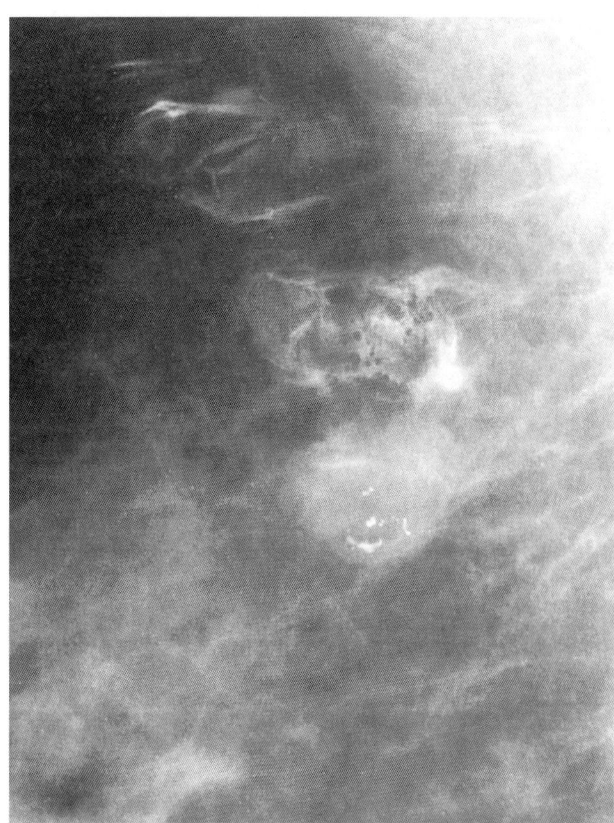

FIG. 15.1. ***Medullary carcinoma, mammography.*** **A:** The tumor is an oval circumscribed mass. **B:** Dye injected into the breast for localization is present *above* the tumor, which contains coarse calcifications.

carcinomas are as well circumscribed as typical medullary carcinomas (Fig. 15.6).

The cut surface of the fresh specimen and whole-mount histologic sections reveal that a medullary carcinoma has a lobulated or nodular internal structure (Figs. 15.5 and 15.7). One can occasionally find secondary nodules at the periphery of the main tumor or appreciate that the mass is composed of coalescent nodules (Fig. 15.8). The pale brown to gray tumor is softer than the average breast carcinoma, and it tends to bulge above the surrounding parenchyma rather than to display the retracted appearance of the commonplace invasive ductal carcinoma. In 1956, Richardson[13] noted that "The tumour tissue looks moister and more succulent than that of

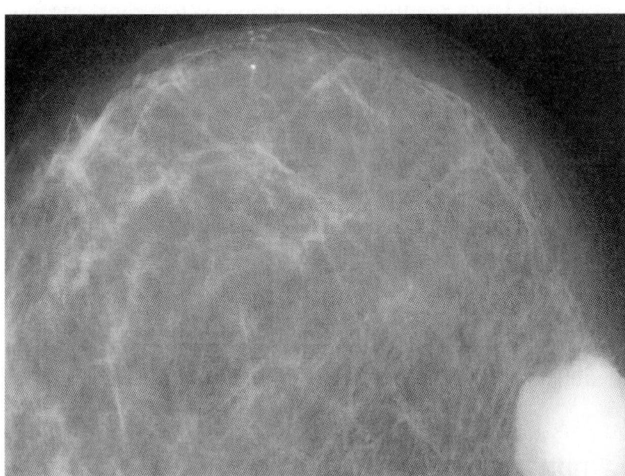

FIG. 15.2. ***Circumscribed non-medullary carcinoma, mammography.*** Histologic examination of the circumscribed tumor revealed an infiltrating duct carcinoma with medullary features.

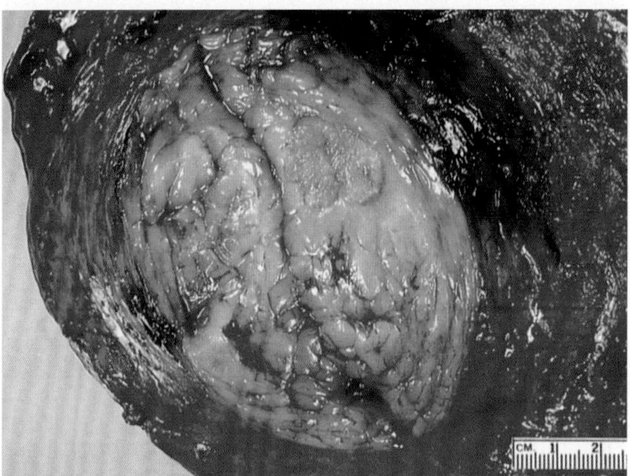

FIG. 15.3. ***Medullary carcinoma, gross specimen.*** The nodular tumor has a circumscribed border and lobulated cut surface.

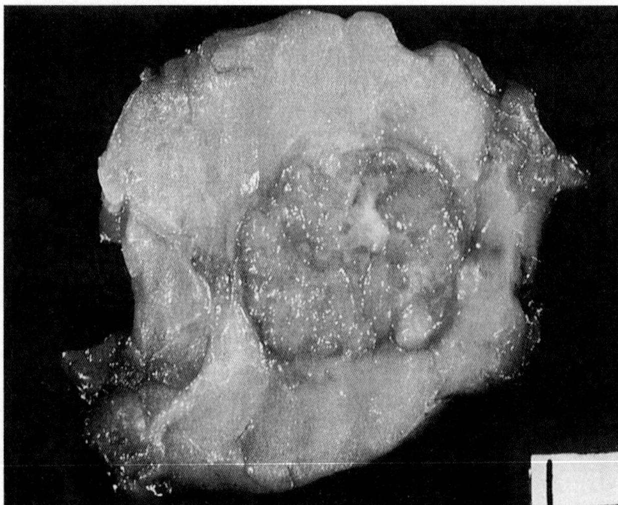

FIG. 15.4. ***Medullary carcinoma, gross specimen.*** The tumor protrudes above the surrounding tissue. The borders are circumscribed, and the cut surface reveals internal nodularity. (Reproduced from Rosen PP, Oberman HA. *Tumors of the mammary gland.* (*AFIP Atlas of Tumor Pathology*, 3rd series, vol. 7). Baltimore: American Registry of Pathology, 1993, with permission.)

other types of breast carcinoma." Hemorrhage and necrosis occur at times, even in medullary carcinomas smaller than 2 cm; however, the extent of necrosis is directly related to tumor size: as the extent of necrosis increases, so, too, does the likelihood that the tumor will develop cystic foci (Fig. 15.9). Prominent cystic degeneration is seen only in tumors larger than 5 cm (Fig. 15.10). The necrotic tissue sometimes has a caseous, granular appearance. Fragmented tumor in the cavity of a cystic medullary carcinoma may be grossly indistinguishable from a cystic papillary carcinoma.

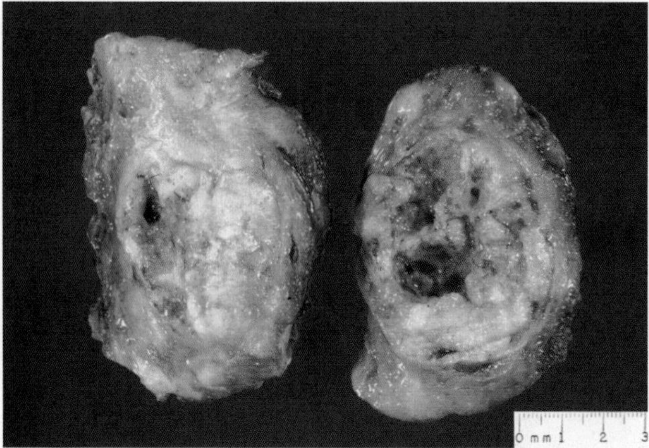

FIG. 15.5. ***Medullary carcinoma, gross specimen.*** Cystic degeneration is apparent. A pseudocapsule is evident at the lower border of the tumor. The tumor protrudes above the surrounding tissue, and the internal structure is nodular.

MICROSCOPIC PATHOLOGY

It is necessary to adhere strictly to defined morphologic criteria if the diagnosis of medullary carcinoma is to be predictive of a relatively favorable prognosis.[6,30] The gross appearance of a tumor may lead one to suspect medullary carcinoma, and occasionally this may be taken into consideration in deciding how to classify a lesion with borderline features; however, the diagnosis ultimately depends upon the microscopic characteristics of the tumor. Overdiagnosis of medullary carcinoma has been reported in several reviews. This phenomenon usually results from a failure to limit the diagnosis to lesions that fulfill all diagnostic criteria.[8,28,30,45,46]

Investigators have reported substantial interobserver and intraobserver variability in the diagnosis of medullary carcinoma.[45,47,48] This variation has led to the suggestion that histologic criteria for the diagnosis be modified; however, the favorable prognosis attributed to true medullary carcinoma is not observed in cases classified according to modified criteria.[49] Jensen et al.[50] compared three systems for defining medullary carcinoma and invasive ductal carcinoma with medullary features. The criteria set forth by Ridolfi et al.[30] proved more reliable for detecting survival differences between true medullary, atypical medullary, and non-medullary carcinomas than the modified definitions set forth by Tavassoli[51] and by Pedersen.[49] Marginean et al.[52] also proposed a simplified set of criteria for the diagnosis of medullary carcinoma. The specific diagnosis of medullary carcinoma will be improved by increased familiarity with and strict adherence to the diagnostic criteria already established. In doubtful situations, a tumor should not be classified as a medullary carcinoma.

Medullary carcinoma is defined by a constellation of histopathologic features initially enumerated by Foote and Stewart[2] and Moore and Foote.[3] These features include prominent lymphoplasmacytic reaction, noninvasive microscopic circumscription, growth in sheets (syncytial pattern), poorly differentiated nuclear grade, and a high mitotic rate. A tumor must display all of these definitive characteristics to be classified as a medullary carcinoma. When most but not all of the needed components are present, the tumor may be termed an *IDC with medullary features.* Tumors in this category have a syncytial growth pattern and certain other histologic features of medullary carcinoma, but deviate from the definitive appearance by demonstrating one or more of the following structural variations: invasive growth at the periphery; sparse or diminished lymphoplasmacytic reaction; well-differentiated nuclear cytology; low mitotic rate; and conspicuous glandular, trabecular, or papillary growth with fibrosis. Invasive ductal carcinomas with medullary features can display immunohistochemical findings seen in typical medullary carcinomas, but they do so less frequently.

Lymphoplasmacytic Infiltrate

The lymphoplasmacytic reaction must involve the periphery and be present diffusely in the substance of the tumor. In most medullary carcinomas, the internal lymphoplasmacytic infiltrate tends to be limited to fibrovascular stroma

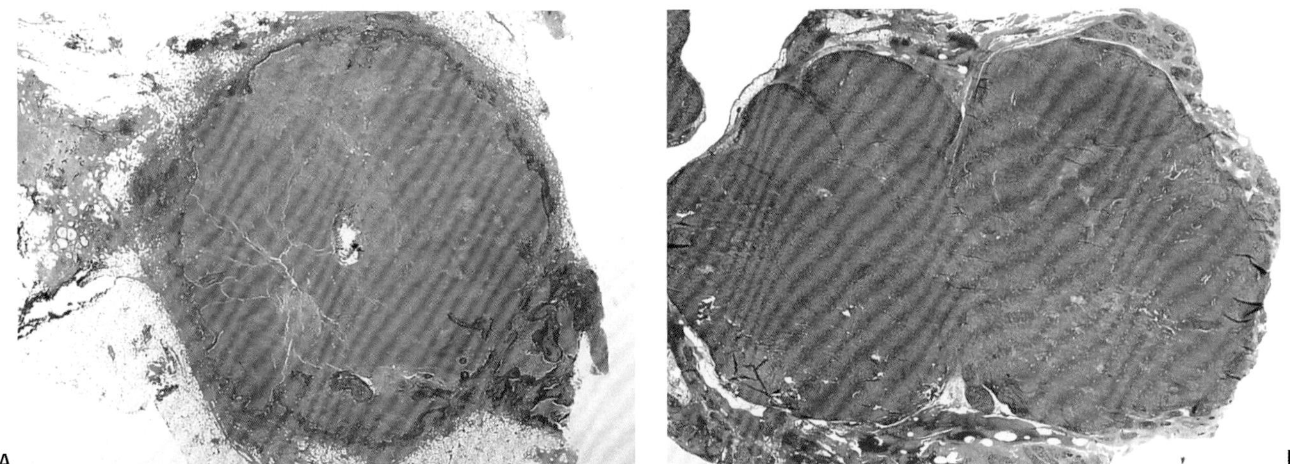

FIG. 15.6. ***Circumscribed non-medullary carcinomas.*** Whole-mount histologic sections. **A:** Carcinoma with extensive central infarction and peripheral lymphocytic reaction. **B:** A bilobed diffuse infiltrating duct carcinoma with focal peripheral lymphocytic infiltration represented by the discontinuous, thin blue line at the border.

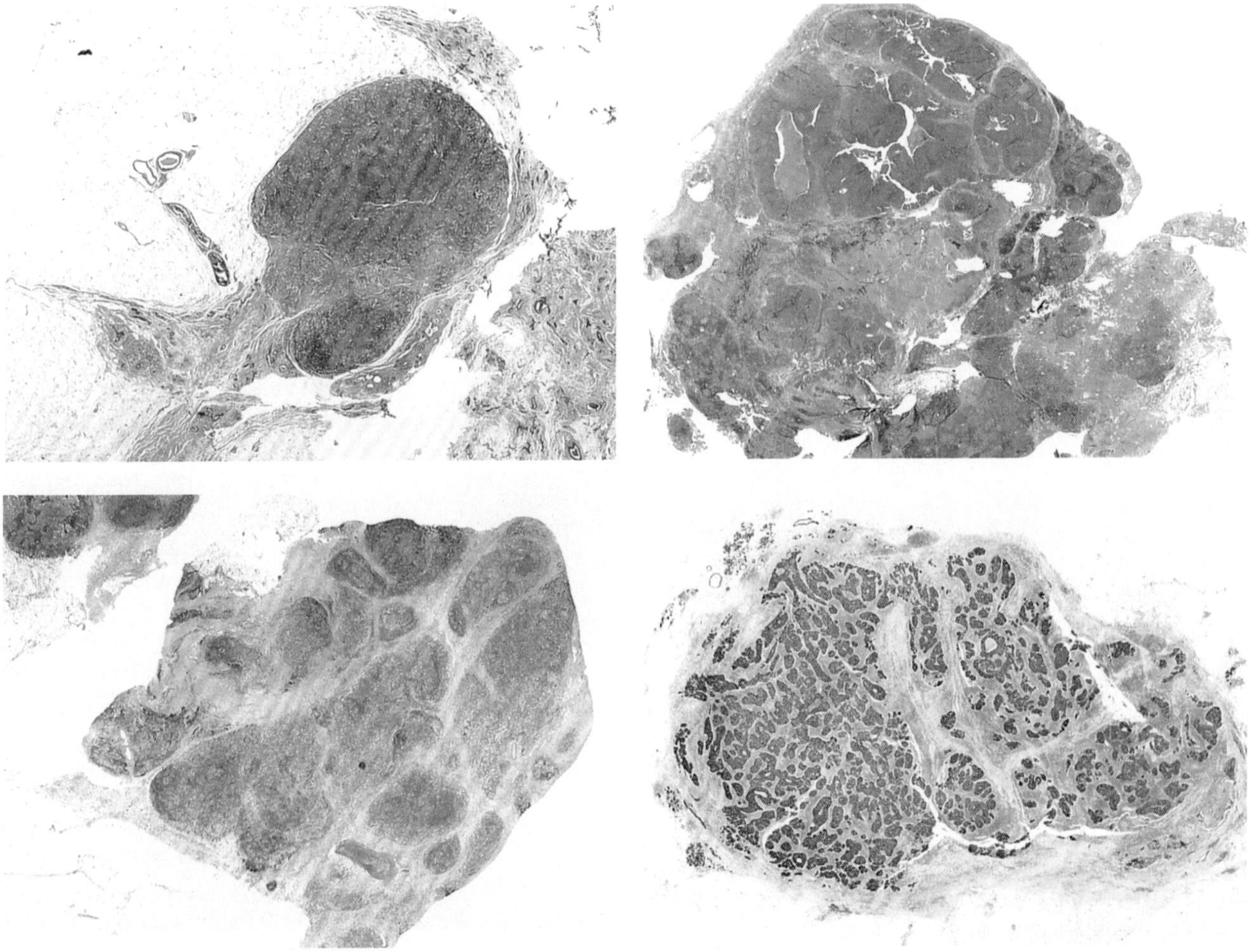

FIG. 15.7. ***Medullary carcinoma, nodular structure.*** Whole-mount histologic sections. **A–C:** Illustrations of varying complexity in the nodular structure of three different tumors. **D:** Epithelial areas within the nodules are stained brown by the immunoreaction for cytokeratin AE1/AE3.

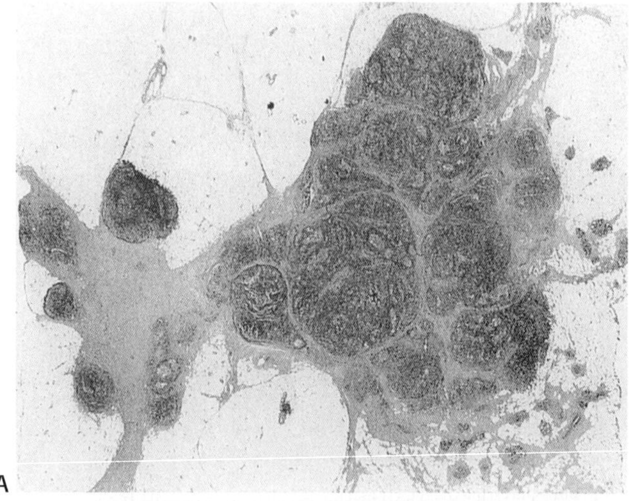

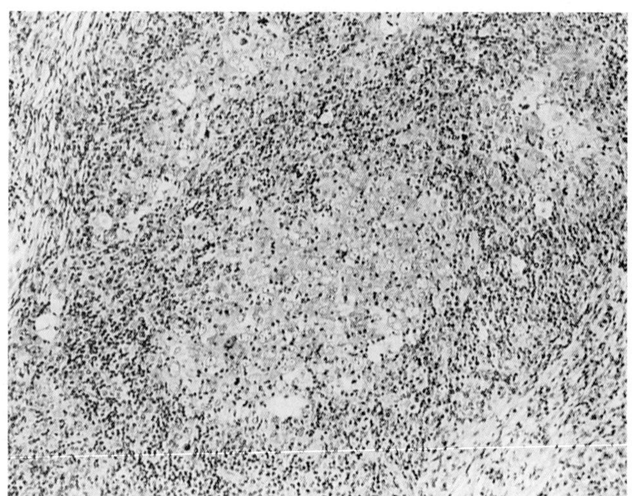

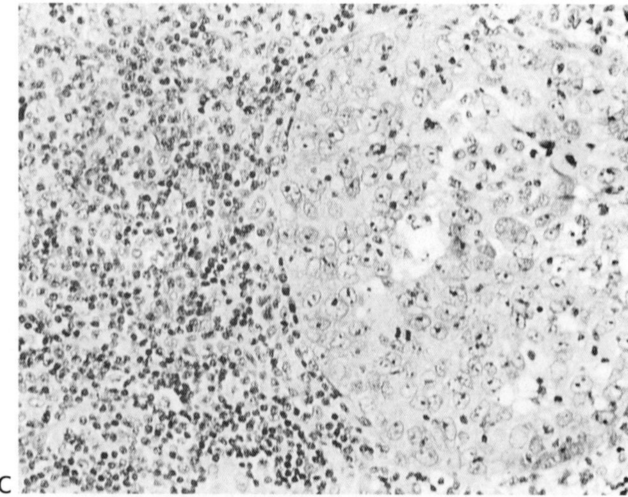

FIG. 15.8. ***Medullary carcinoma, peripheral nodules.*** **A:** In addition to multiple coalescent nodules forming the main tumor, smaller circumscribed nodules of tumor are evident on the left. **B,C:** The histologic appearance of carcinoma in one of the secondary tumor nodules on the *left* in (**A**) showing poorly differentiated carcinoma with a syncytial pattern and a lymphocytic reaction. Carcinoma merges with the lymphocytes in (**B**), whereas in (**C**) the carcinoma is sharply circumscribed.

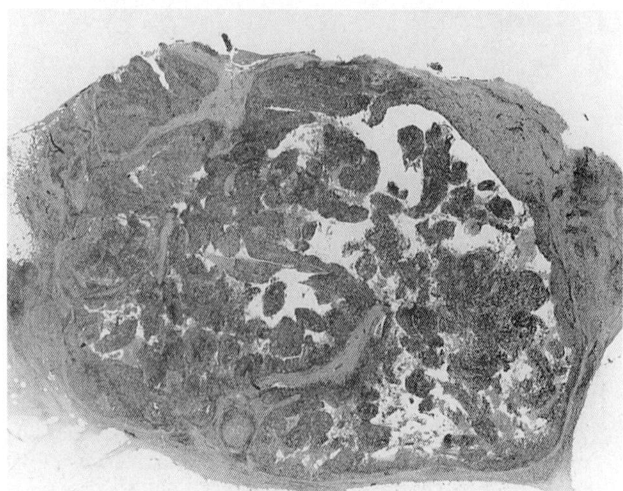

FIG. 15.9. ***Medullary carcinoma, cystic degeneration.*** The internal nodular structure is evident in areas of cystic degeneration in this whole-mount histologic section. The tumor has a papillary appearance.

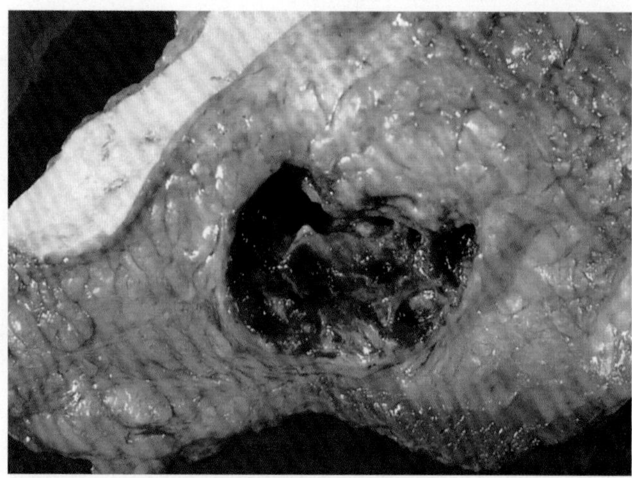

FIG. 15.10. ***Medullary carcinoma, cystic.*** The gross appearance of the tumor in a mastectomy specimen.

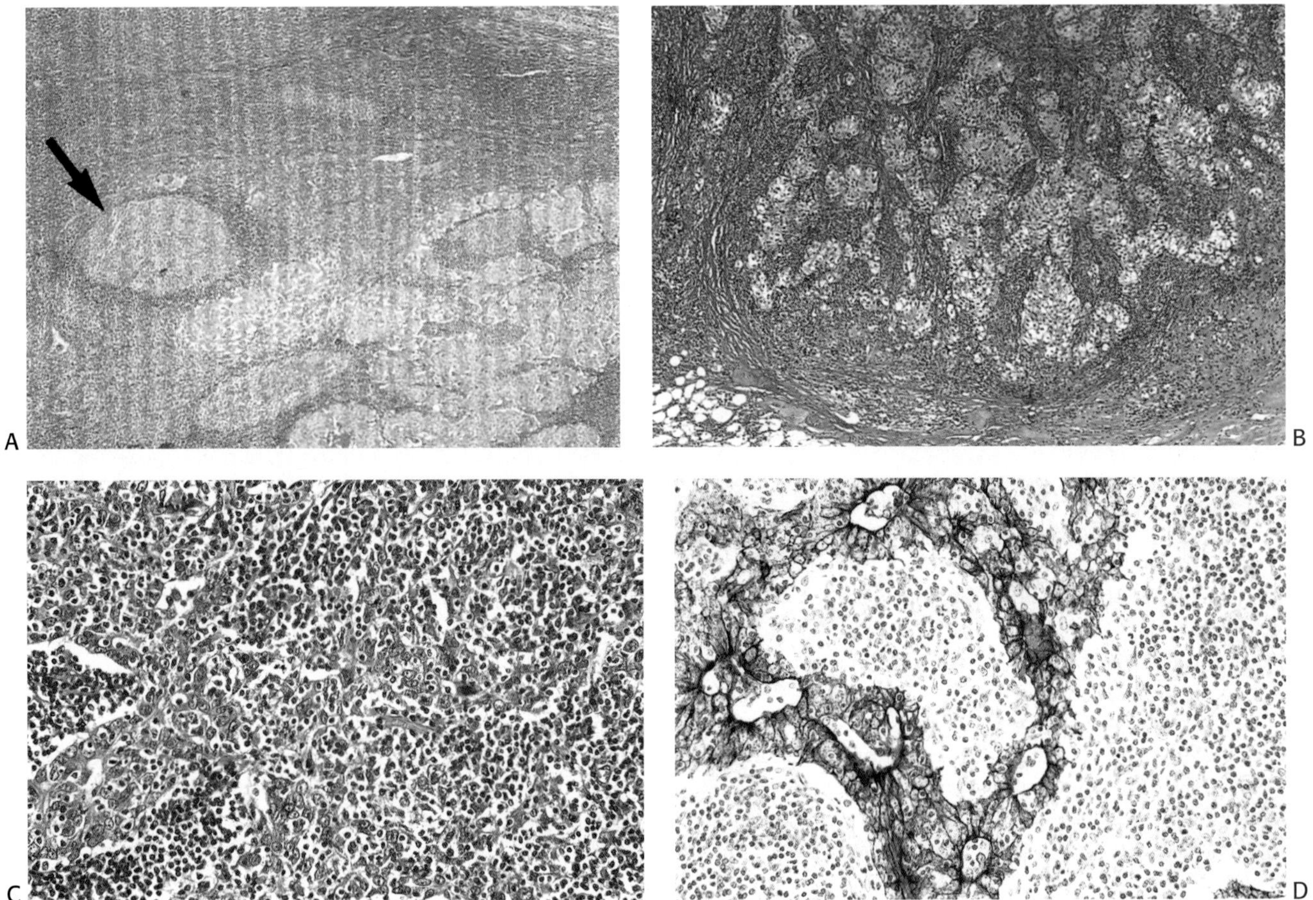

FIG. 15.11. ***Medullary carcinoma, lymphoplasmacytic reaction.*** **A:** Syncytial sheets of carcinoma cells surrounded by a diffuse lymphocytic reaction. The germinal center is an unusual occurrence (*arrow*). **B:** Lymphocytic reaction around groups of carcinoma cells in nodular aggregates. **C:** Lymphocytic reaction mingles with and obscures the carcinoma cells, creating an appearance that resembles lymphoepithelioma. **D:** The carcinoma cells are highlighted with the CK immunostain.

between syncytial zones of tumor cells. A minority of medullary carcinomas seem to be largely devoid of stroma, and the lymphoplasmacytic infiltrate mingles intimately with carcinoma cells[12] (Fig. 15.11). Pathologists sometime refer to such lesions as lymphoepithelioma-like carcinomas. One can find it difficult to differentiate such a tumor from metastatic carcinoma in a lymph node.

At the periphery of the tumor, there may be some variation in the amount of lymphocytic reaction, but it should be at least moderately intense at the interface of the carcinoma with mammary parenchyma and in the adjacent tissue. In the usual case, the lymphoplasmacytic reaction encompasses surrounding ducts and lobules occupied by *in situ* carcinoma (Fig. 15.12). The reactive process also tends to involve more distant ducts and lobules, which do not contain identifiable tumor cells (Fig. 15.13). These secondary peripheral alterations are so common in medullary carcinoma that the diagnosis may be questioned when they are absent.

The lymphoplasmacytic infiltrate may be composed almost entirely of either lymphocytes or plasma cells, but most often there is a mixture of these cells[12] (Fig. 15.14). Bässler et al.[12] reported that lymphocytes predominated at the periphery of medullary carcinomas, whereas plasma cells represented the preponderant inflammatory cell in the center of the carcinoma. Intense lymphoplasmacytic infiltrates can occur in non-medullary infiltrating duct carcinomas; however, when plasma cells predominate, the tumor is more likely to be a medullary carcinoma. A few neutrophils, eosinophils, and monocytes can be found, especially when there is necrosis or cystic degeneration, but never do they dominate in a medullary carcinoma. Rarely, the lymphocytic infiltrate gives rise to germinal centers within the tumor or the surrounding tissue (Figs. 15.11, 15.14 and 15.15). Hence, the presence of germinal centers cannot be relied upon as evidence that one is dealing with metastatic carcinoma in a lymph node in the breast or in the axilla.

Microscopic Circumscription

Noninvasive microscopic circumscription refers to the appearance of the border of the infiltrating carcinoma rather than the periphery of the surrounding lymphoplasmacytic reaction. In medullary carcinoma, the edge of the tumor should have a smooth, rounded contour that appears

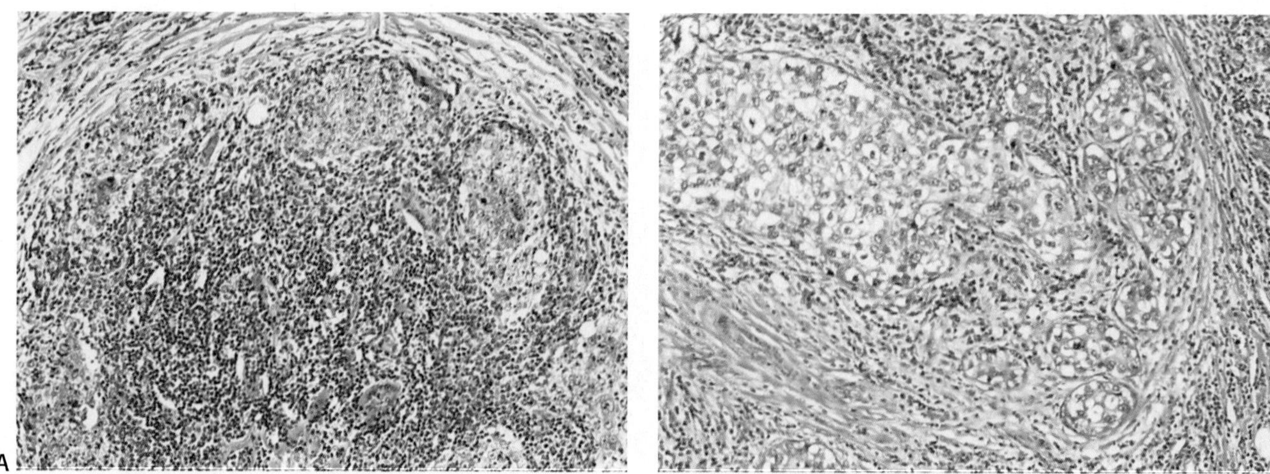

FIG. 15.12. ***Medullary carcinoma, lobular extension.*** **A:** Carcinoma cells have replaced most of the normal epithelium in this lobule at the periphery of a medullary carcinoma. A few clusters of dark nonneoplastic cells remain. A lymphocytic reaction is apparent in and around the lobule. **B:** Intraepithelial carcinoma in an intralobular ductule and in lobular glands with a lymphocytic reaction.

to push aside the breast parenchyma and fat rather than to infiltrate it (Figs. 15.16 and 15.17). Consequently, nonneoplastic glandular or fatty breast tissue should not be found within the main body of the invasive portion of the tumor. In assessing this feature, it is important to distinguish between ducts, lobules, or islands of fat cells trapped in the surrounding lymphoplasmacytic reaction of medullary carcinoma and the same structures invaded by non-medullary invasive carcinoma (Fig. 15.18). In the latter instance, the tumor typically lacks the cohesive syncytial structure of medullary carcinoma, and the tumor cells tend to invade in trabecular, dendritic, or dispersed patterns.

Syncytial Structure

Syncytial structure requires that most of the tumor growth (variously defined as 75% or more of the histologically sampled areas) be arranged in broad irregular sheets or islands in which the borders of individual cells are indistinct (Fig. 15.19). The histology sometimes resembles a poorly differentiated epidermoid carcinoma (Fig. 15.20). This comparison is particularly apt because traces of epidermoid differentiation are not unusual in medullary carcinomas, and some of these tumors have well-formed foci of squamous metaplasia. A tumor that is otherwise characteristic may be accepted as a medullary carcinoma if it has minor components of trabecular, glandular, alveolar, or papillary growth (Fig. 15.21). Such regions may have a diminished lymphoplasmacytic infiltrate and fibrosis and thus appear distinct from the medullary growth pattern. It has been reported that overall survival (OS) and relapse-free survival (RFS) are directly related to the extent of the syncytial component.[53] Although there was not a significant difference in outcome between patients with 75% and 90% syncytial growth, survival was diminished when less than 75% of a tumor was syncytial, and the difference was most marked at or below the 50% level. These data justify the currently employed requirement for at least a 75% syncytial component.

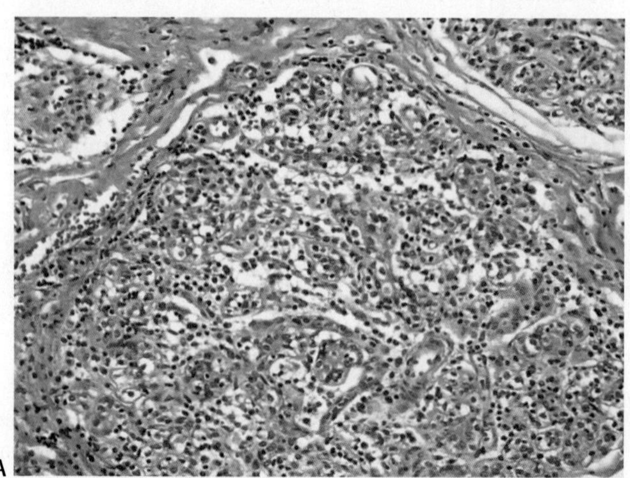

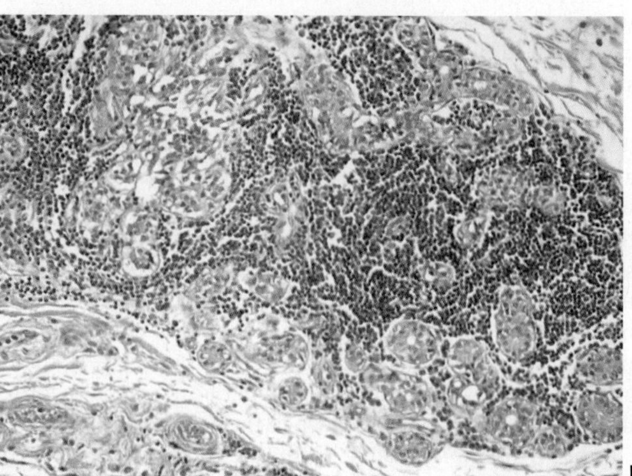

FIG. 15.13. ***Medullary carcinoma, lobular lymphocytic reaction.*** **A,B:** Lymphocytic reaction in lobules at the periphery of a medullary carcinoma. No carcinoma is evident.

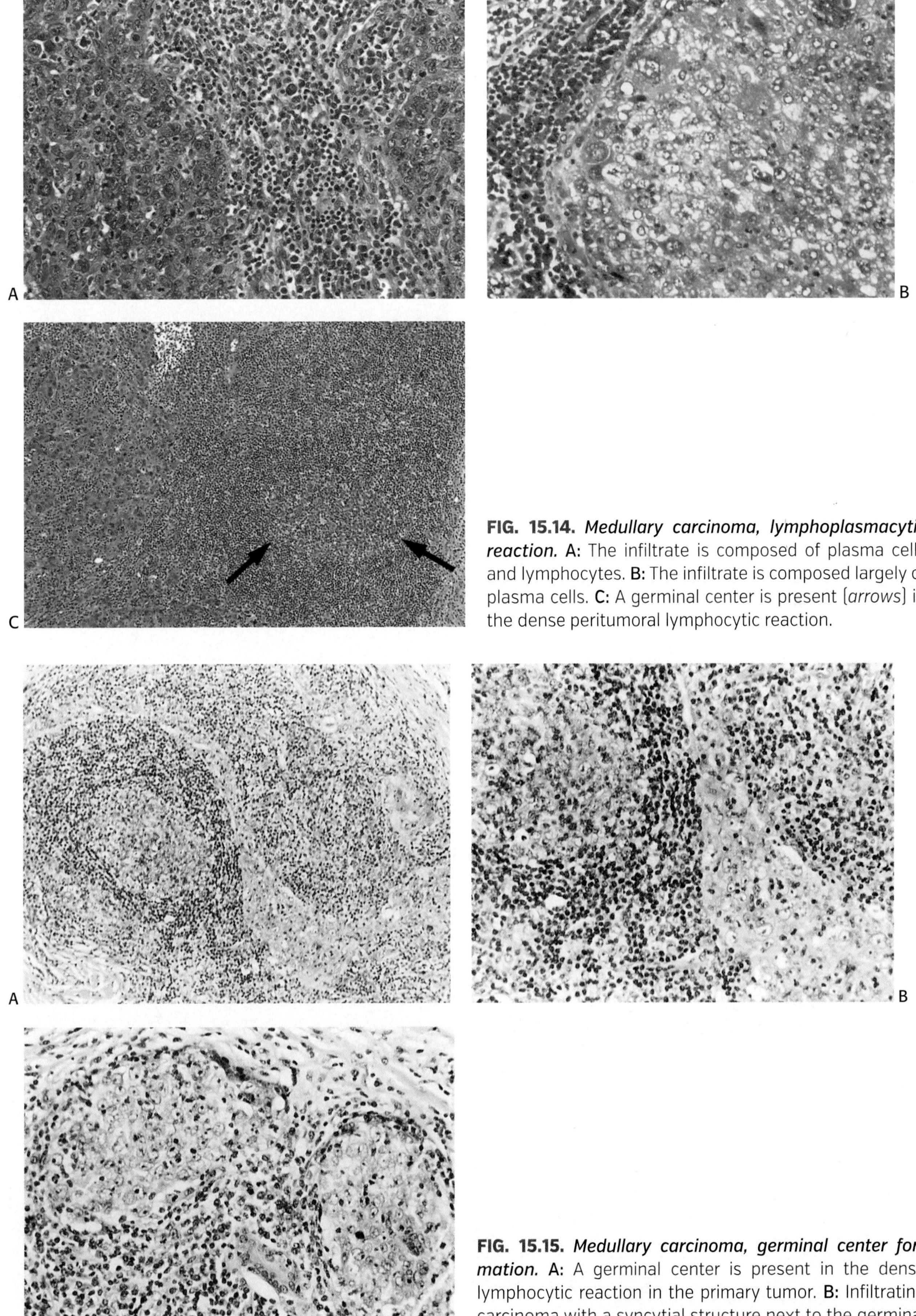

FIG. 15.14. ***Medullary carcinoma, lymphoplasmacytic reaction.*** **A:** The infiltrate is composed of plasma cells and lymphocytes. **B:** The infiltrate is composed largely of plasma cells. **C:** A germinal center is present (*arrows*) in the dense peritumoral lymphocytic reaction.

FIG. 15.15. ***Medullary carcinoma, germinal center formation.*** **A:** A germinal center is present in the dense lymphocytic reaction in the primary tumor. **B:** Infiltrating carcinoma with a syncytial structure next to the germinal center. **C:** *In situ* carcinoma in the epithelium of a lobule next to the tumor.

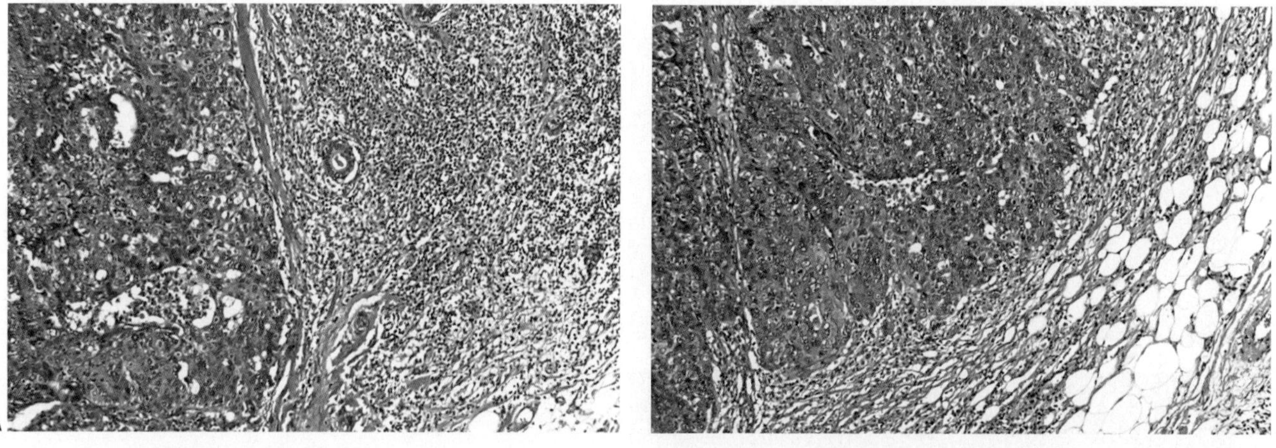

FIG. 15.16. ***Medullary carcinoma, tumor border.*** **A:** Carcinoma is confined to syncytial masses with a lymphocytic reaction at the tumor border. **B:** Carcinoma is confined to syncytial growth within the lymphocytic reaction. The lymphocytic reaction, not the carcinoma, merges with the fat.

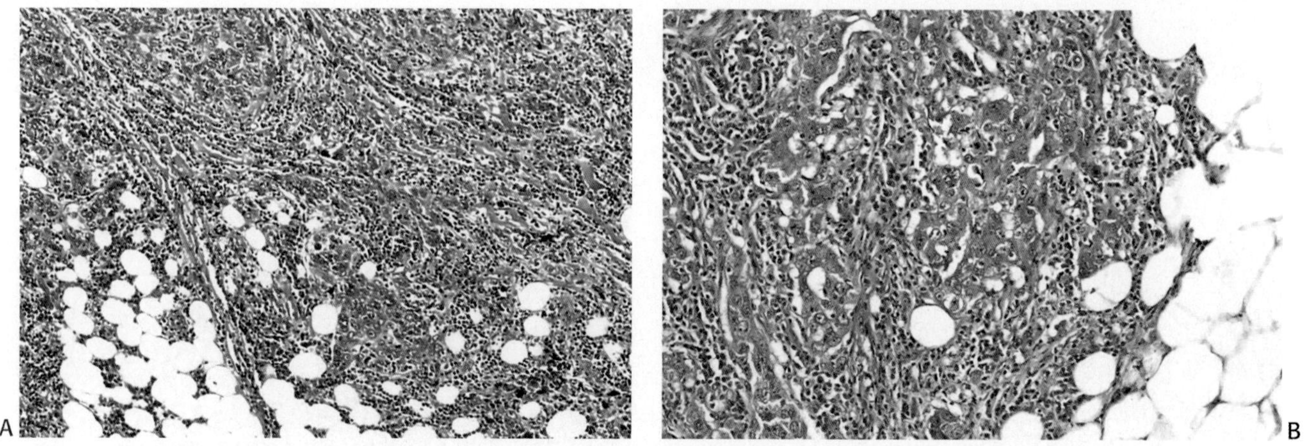

FIG. 15.17. ***Non-medullary invasive duct carcinoma, tumor border.*** **A:** Fat cells surrounded by carcinoma represent a manifestation of invasive growth. **B:** This pattern of carcinoma and lymphocytes invading fat is not compatible with a diagnosis of medullary carcinoma.

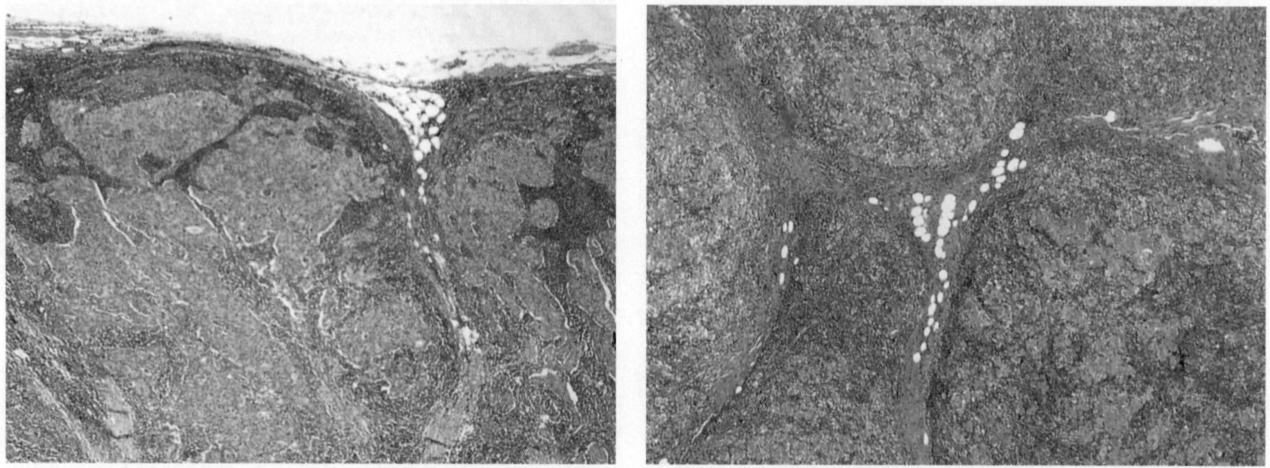

FIG. 15.18. ***Medullary carcinoma, tumor border.*** **A,B:** Fibrofatty stroma is trapped between the tumor nodules, but each nodule has a sharply circumscribed border.

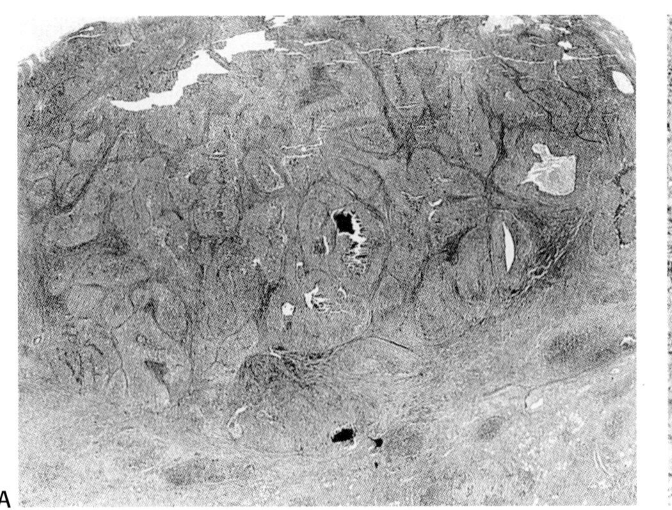
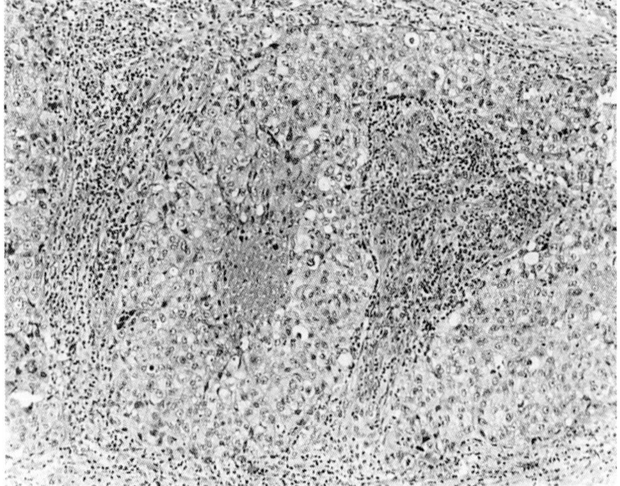

FIG. 15.19. ***Medullary carcinoma, syncytial growth.*** **A:** The syncytial growth in this medullary carcinoma has created a serpentine architecture. Dark calcifications have been formed in two foci of necrosis. **B:** Interlacing bands of carcinoma cells in a lymphoplasmacytic reaction. Focal necrosis is evident in the center of the carcinomatous epithelium.

Nuclear Grade and Mitoses

Poorly differentiated nuclear grade and high mitotic rate are interrelated characteristics of medullary carcinoma. Typically, the tumor cells have pleomorphic nuclei with coarse chromatin and prominent nucleoli (Fig. 15.22). Pyknotic nuclei of degenerating cells are easily found, as are mitotic figures (Fig. 15.23). Regarding the latter, Richardson[13] observed that ". . . seldom are there less than four per high power field, and abnormal forms are common."

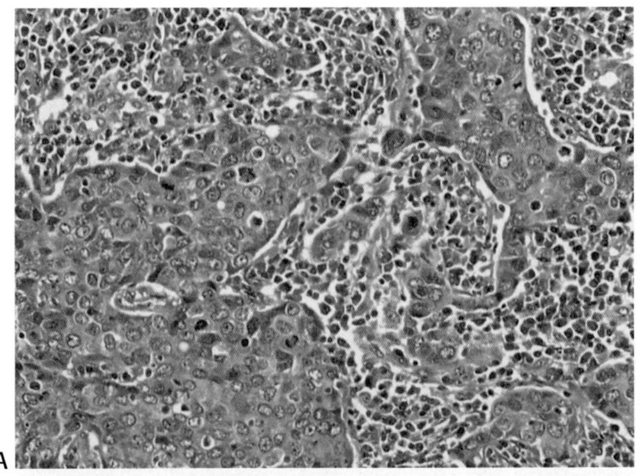
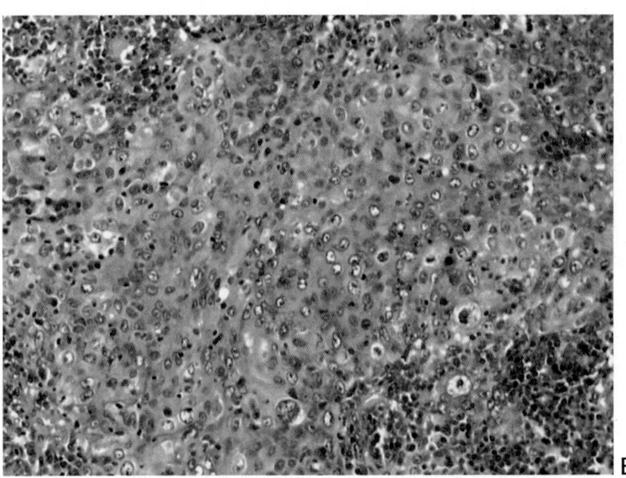
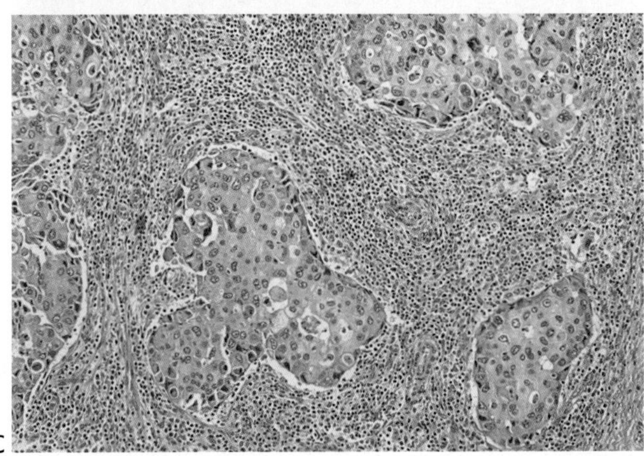

FIG. 15.20. ***Medullary carcinoma, syncytial growth.*** **A:** The carcinoma is distributed in sharply defined bands separated by stroma permeated predominantly by plasma cells. The cytoplasmic borders of individual carcinoma cells are not seen. **B:** Diffuse cytoplasmic eosinophilia that hints at squamous differentiation (see Fig. 15.26A). **C:** Islands of syncytial carcinoma cells surrounded by lymphocytes.

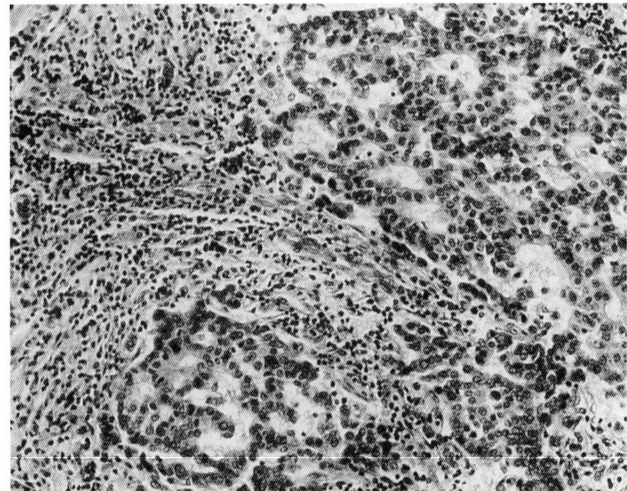

FIG. 15.21. ***Medullary carcinoma, glandular differentiation.*** Isolated foci of glandular differentiation such as this may be found in medullary carcinoma.

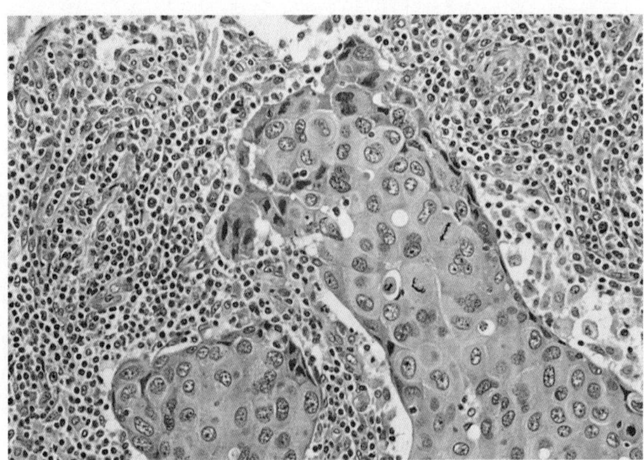

FIG. 15.22. ***Medullary carcinoma, poorly differentiated nuclear grade.*** This carcinoma has mitotic figures and pleomorphic nuclei with nucleoli.

A number of other microscopic features may be found in some medullary carcinomas. The presence of one or more of these secondary histopathologic characteristics is helpful to confirm a diagnosis of medullary carcinoma, but the diagnosis does not depend on the presence of any of them. These ancillary microscopic features include *in situ* carcinoma, squamous metaplasia, pseudosarcomatous metaplasia, and necrosis.

Ductal Carcinoma *In Situ*

Ductal carcinoma *in situ* (DCIS) is found at the periphery of a substantial number of medullary carcinomas (Fig. 15.24). The DCIS often has a comedo or solid growth pattern, and it only rarely contains calcifications. It is also not unusual for the carcinoma cells to involve the epithelium of lobules (lobular extension of ductal carcinoma), thereby creating foci of *in situ* carcinoma in lobules. Foci of intraductal and intralobular carcinoma tend to be seen more frequently with increasing tumor size, and they are accompanied by the same prominent mononuclear cell infiltrate that occurs in the main tumor. This mononuclear infiltrate can be so intense that it obscures the presence of subtle extension of ductal carcinoma into the lobular epithelium. However, close inspection reveals that these lobules contain cells with the same poorly differentiated nuclei as the invasive portion of the medullary carcinoma.

The frequent occurrence of *in situ* carcinoma associated with medullary carcinomas conflicts with the widespread and oft-repeated belief that the *absence* of DCIS represents one of the defining characteristics of medullary carcinoma.[4] This mistaken belief probably took its origin from the second series of the *Atlas of Tumor Pathology*, in which McDivitt et al.[54] wrote: "The cytologic pattern of medullary carcinomas has rarely been seen when the tumor is still intraductal." The writers seem to state that medullary carcinoma does not commonly exist purely as an intraductal proliferation. Misinterpretation of this sentence led to the assertion that the presence of DCIS does not comport with the diagnosis of medullary carcinoma. Ridolfi

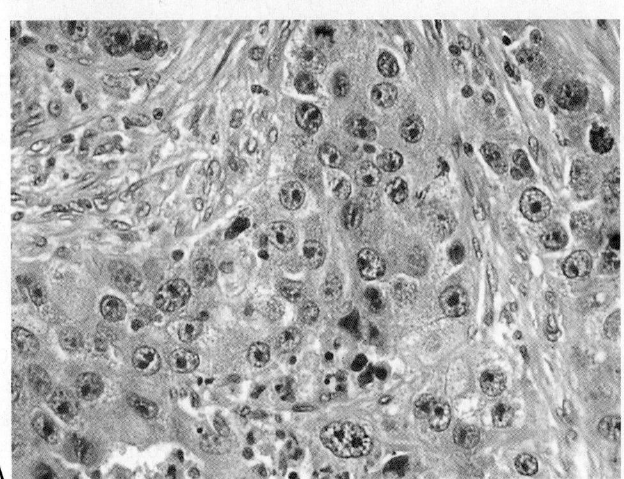

A

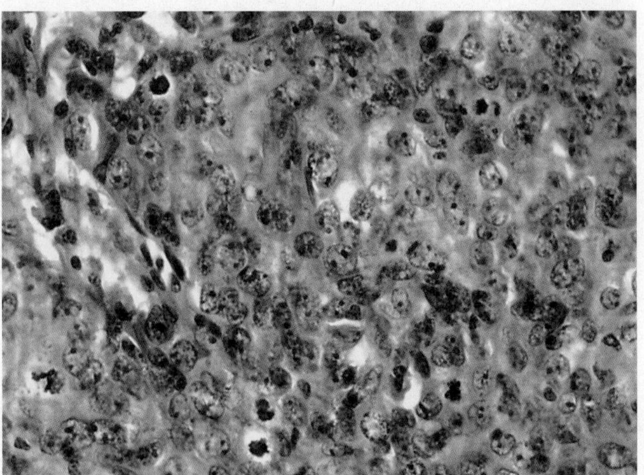

B

FIG. 15.23. ***Medullary carcinoma, poorly differentiated nuclear grade.*** **A:** Prominent nucleoli. **B:** Multiple nucleoli and numerous mitoses.

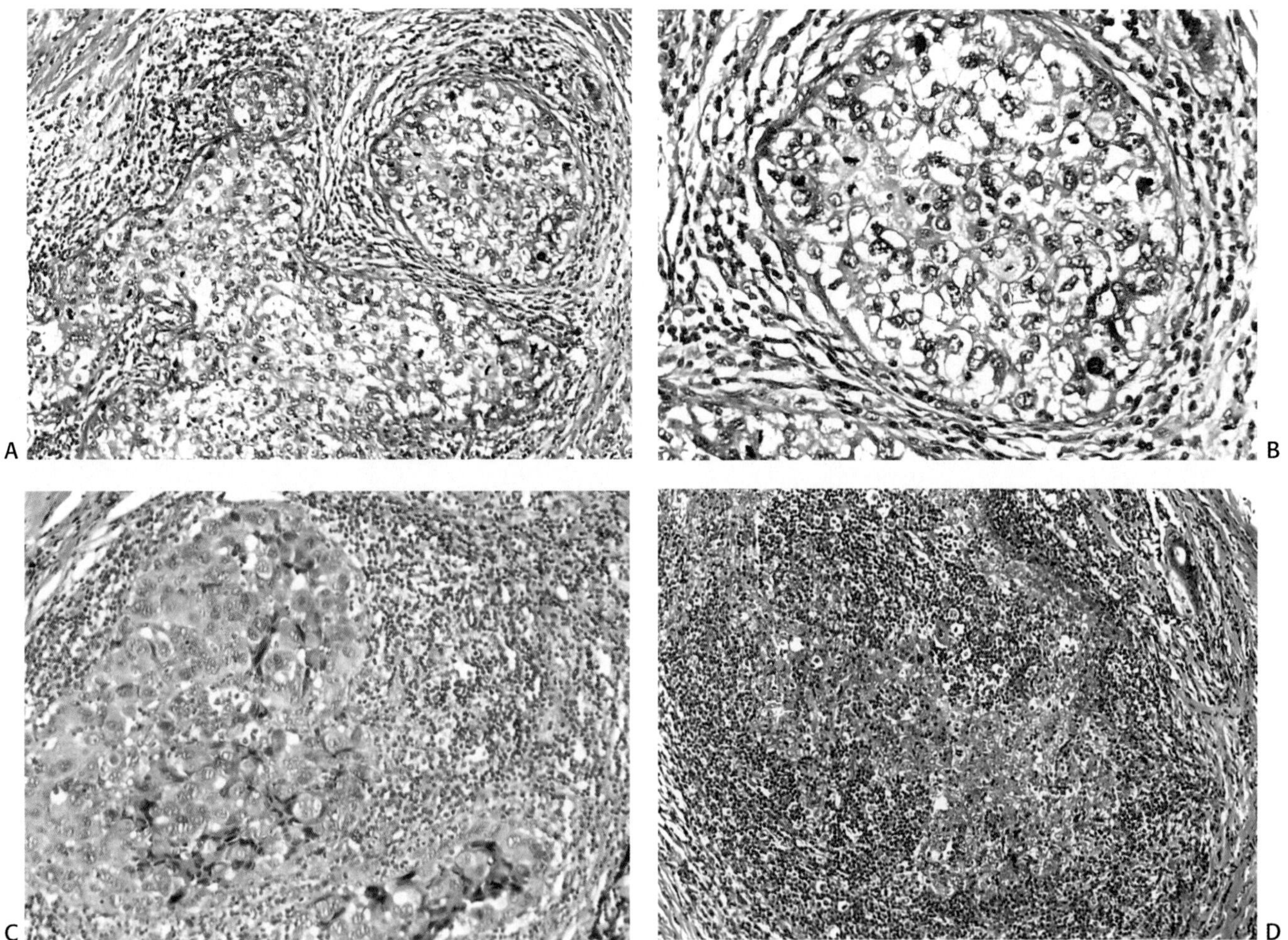

FIG. 15.24. ***Medullary carcinoma, intraductal.*** **A:** Intraductal carcinoma at the periphery of a medullary carcinoma. **B:** Enlarged view of **(A)** showing intraductal carcinoma that has the cytologic features of medullary carcinoma. **C:** This sharply outlined focus of carcinoma surrounded by a lymphocytic reaction may have been the site of intraductal carcinoma, but the basement membrane is no longer evident. **D:** At this stage, it is difficult to distinguish between intraductal and invasive carcinoma. Basement membrane components are not usually demonstrable with immunostains in such foci.

et al.[30] made specific study of this contention and concluded that "Survival of patients with medullary lesions that were characterized as atypical *only* because of intraductal areas was excellent. Consequently, the presence of intraductal and/or intralobular carcinoma with the cytologic features of medullary carcinoma should probably be considered a characteristic of medullary carcinoma." Wargotz et al.[28] and Marginean et al.[52] reached the same conclusion. On the basis of these studies, one must conclude that the presence of DCIS does not exclude the diagnosis of typical medullary carcinoma.

Around the main tumor mass, expansile growth of *in situ* carcinoma in ducts and lobules leads to the formation of secondary peripheral tumor nodules that have the appearance of small "satellite" medullary carcinomas (Fig. 15.25). Fat and mammary stroma may persist between nodules at the margin of the tumor. One should not interpret the presence of these marginal nodular foci and intervening stroma as evidence of invasive growth. Coalescence of these enlarging nodules and their incorporation into the expanding main mass is responsible for the grossly nodular appearance of medullary carcinomas. With the high rate of division of the carcinoma cells, this phenomenon probably contributes to the rapid growth of medullary carcinomas.

Rarely one may encounter a lesion consisting only of DCIS with the histologic features of DCIS found at the periphery of a medullary carcinoma. Typically, such foci have the poorly differentiated cytology that characterizes medullary carcinoma, a comedo growth pattern, and an intense lymphocytic reaction that can obscure the duct margin, thereby creating difficulty in evaluating the lesion for invasion. There is no definite proof that these lesions constitute an *in situ* form of medullary carcinoma, but this possibility can be inferred from uncommon examples of medullary carcinoma composed largely of DCIS with only a minor invasive component.

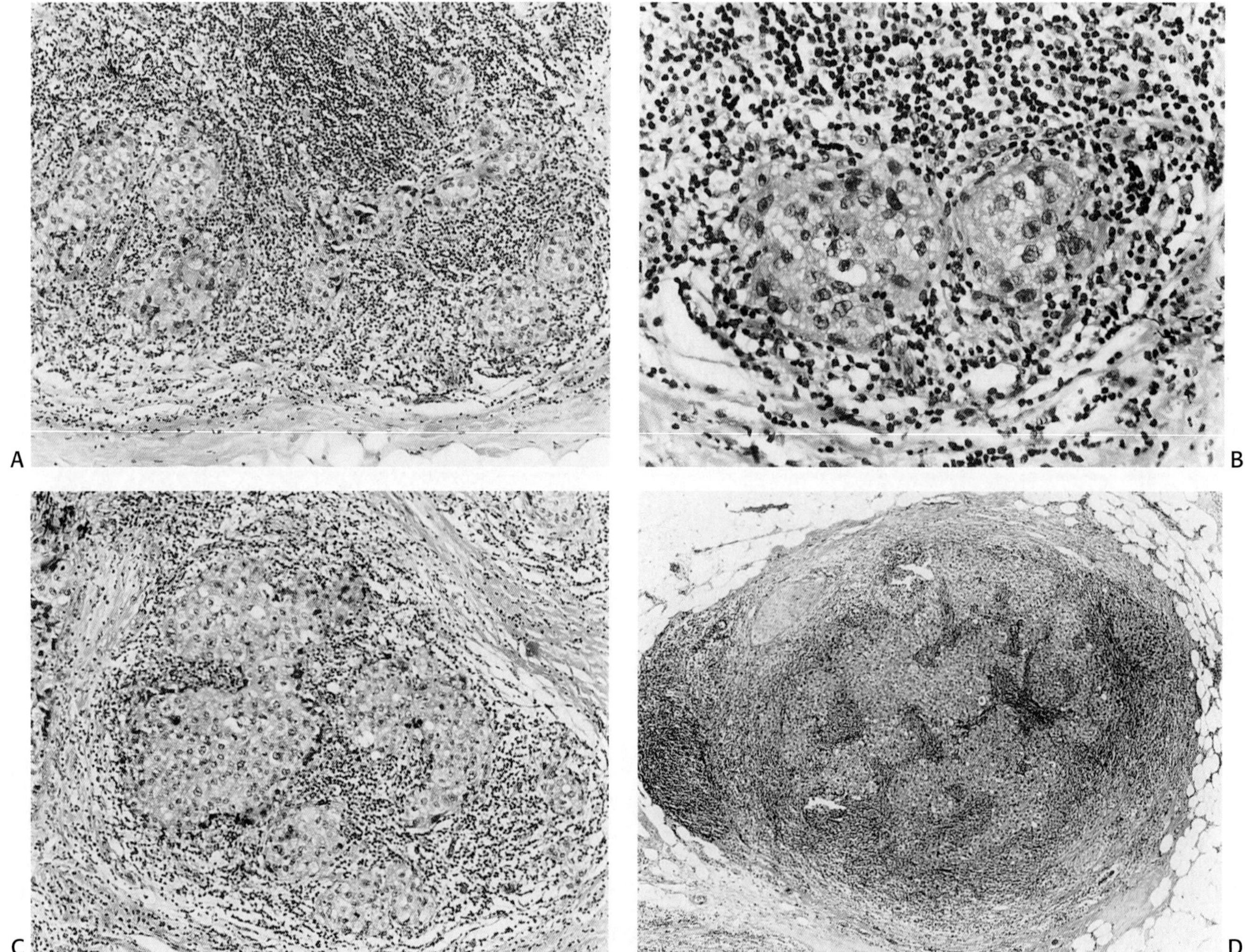

FIG. 15.25. ***Medullary carcinoma, evolution of lobular extension to form a secondary nodule.*** **A:** Intraepithelial carcinoma in a lobule adjacent to a medullary carcinoma. **B:** Magnified view of lobular glands depicted in the lower right corner of **(A)**. **C:** Expanded intralobular glands and ductules forming serpiginous nests of carcinoma cells with a syncytial arrangement. **D:** A fully developed secondary nodule formed by one or more expanded lobules like the one shown in **(C)**.

Metaplasia

Metaplastic changes occur in a minority of medullary carcinomas, and they usually involve only a part of the lesion. Squamous metaplasia has been found in 16% of medullary carcinomas,[30] whereas osseous, cartilaginous, and spindle cell metaplasia are much less common (Figs. 15.26 and 15.27). It is not clear whether bizarre epithelial giant cell areas found in an otherwise typical medullary carcinoma represent a metaplastic variant or a degenerative change (Fig. 15.28).

Necrosis

Necrosis develops in medullary carcinomas initially within zones of syncytial epithelial growth (Fig. 15.29). Expansion of these microscopic foci leads to the formation of small clefts and eventually to gross cystic areas. The pattern resembles the process of cystic degeneration sometimes seen in squamous carcinomas. Necrosis is often found in conjunction with squamous metaplasia in medullary carcinomas.

NEEDLE CORE BIOPSY

A diagnosis of medullary carcinoma cannot be made with certainty on the basis of a needle core biopsy specimen because of the limited sampling that this method provides. It is appropriate to report that the sample raises the possibility of medullary carcinoma and to indicate that final classification will depend upon evaluation of the excised specimen.

CYTOLOGY

Specimens obtained by needle aspiration are usually very cellular (Fig. 15.30), and they typically display three features in varying degrees: large pleomorphic cells, bizarre naked

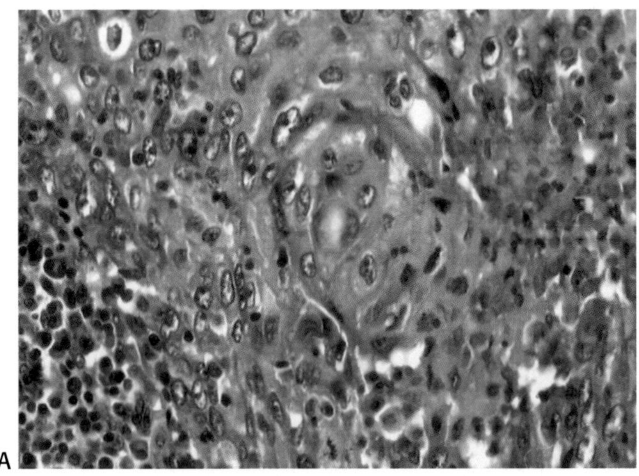

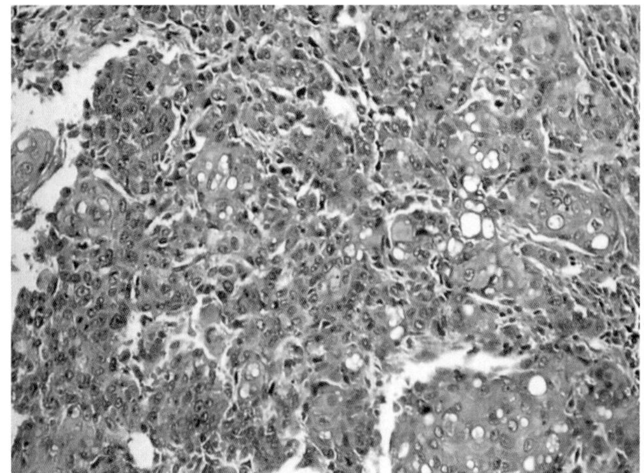

FIG. 15.26. ***Medullary carcinoma, squamous metaplasia.*** **A:** A poorly formed squamous pearl in the tumor depicted in Fig. 15.20B. **B:** A larger focus of squamous metaplasia.

nuclei, and lymphocytes.[55] One observes large, poorly differentiated carcinoma cells that are distributed individually and in syncytial sheets. The cells typically measure 15 to 25 μm, and they feature large pleomorphic nuclei with prominent nucleoli and modest or large amounts of cytoplasm. Large and bizarre naked nuclei occur, also. Numerous lymphocytes, plasma cells, and neutrophils occupy much of the background. Blood and necrotic debris may be evident when the tumor is cystic.[56] Inflammatory debris from a cystic medullary carcinoma may obscure the degenerated tumor cells and lead to the mistaken diagnosis of an abscess or an infected cyst. The diagnosis of medullary carcinoma may be suggested by the findings in a fine-needle aspiration (FNA) smear, but it is impossible to distinguish classic medullary carcinoma from IDC with medullary features by this method.

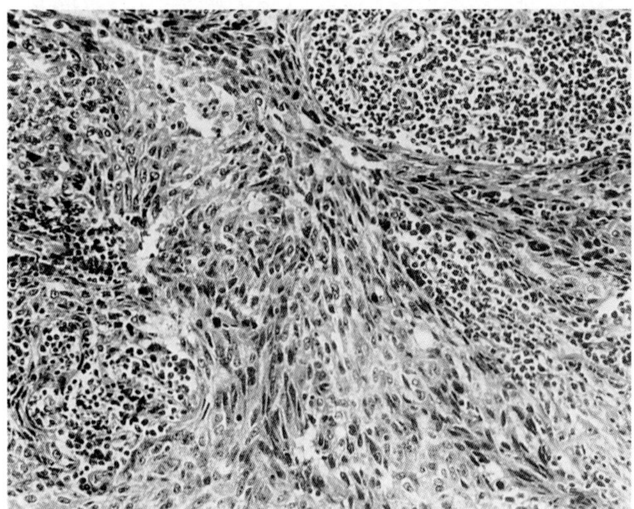

FIG. 15.27. ***Medullary carcinoma, spindle cell change.*** [Reproduced from Ridolfi R, Rosen P, Port A, et al. Medullary carcinoma of the breast. A clinicopathologic study with 10-year follow-up. *Cancer* 1977;40:1365–1385, with permission.]

IMMUNOHISTOCHEMISTRY

Cytokeratin

Most medullary carcinomas express keratin and stain with the AE1/AE3 cocktail. Investigators have tested examples of medullary carcinoma for the presence of specific keratin molecules such as cytokeratin 4 (CK4), CK5/6, CK7, CK14, CK8/18, CK19, and CK20,[31,57–59] but the results have varied strikingly. For example, Tot[58] reported that 25% of typical medullary carcinomas stain for CK5/6, but Vincent-Salomon et al.[59] detected the molecule in 94% of the cases in their study group.

The variability of results makes it difficult to detect consistent patterns; nevertheless, two conclusions seem secure. First, CK8/18 is the most commonly expressed cytokeratin molecule in medullary carcinoma, and one can detect it in 84%[57] to 100%[58] of cases. One can detect CK14 in 12%[58] to 55%[59] of medullary carcinomas, but medullary carcinomas only rarely express CK20.[58] Second, one cannot rely on the expression of any of the types of cytokeratin to distinguish medullary carcinomas from non-medullary carcinomas. For instance, Larsimont et al.[60] studied the expression of CK19 in medullary and non-medullary carcinomas. None of the 12 medullary carcinomas expressed the protein, whereas 23 of 29 high-grade non-medullary carcinomas and all of 12 low-grade carcinomas were reactive. Other workers, in contrast, did not observe a significant difference in the expression of CK19 between medullary and poorly differentiated non-medullary carcinomas.[58,61,62] The investigators used different antibodies, and this difference may explain the variation in their results.[61] Differences in results may also arise because of variation within the neoplastic population. Tot et al.,[58] for example, discovered differences between the cytokeratin staining of primary medullary carcinomas and their metastases in 4 of the 10 cases tested.

Vimentin

Vimentin expression has been observed in 18%[63] to 78%[64] of medullary carcinomas. Holck et al.[63] observed the protein

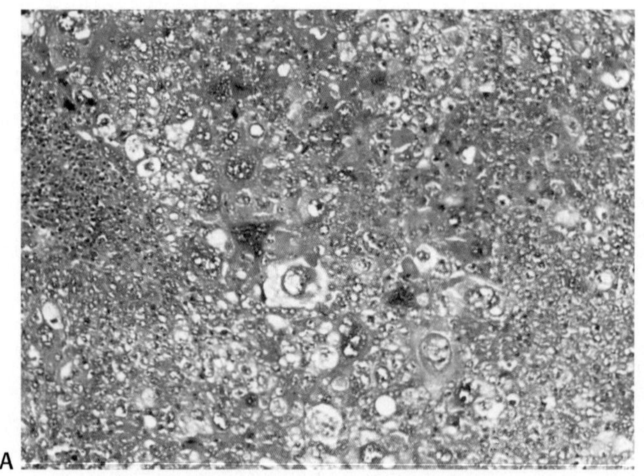

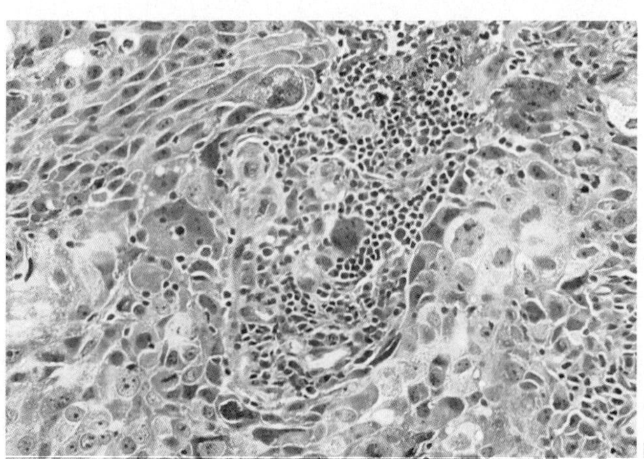

FIG. 15.28. ***Medullary carcinoma, giant cells.*** **A:** Many enlarged carcinoma cells have single or multiple cytologically atypical nuclei. **B:** Syncytial giant cells with bizarre hyperchromatic nuclei.

more frequently in medullary carcinomas and ductal carcinomas with medullary features than in ordinary invasive ductal carcinomas; however, the difference did not prove statistically significant. Flucke et al.[31] report similar findings. The presence or absence of vimentin did not prove to be prognostically significant in the study of Holck et al.[63]

Other Cellular Markers

Immunoreactivity for epithelial membrane antigen and E-cadherin are frequently demonstrable in medullary carcinoma cells, but the cells do not stain for mammaglobin.[65] Investigators have tested small numbers of medullary

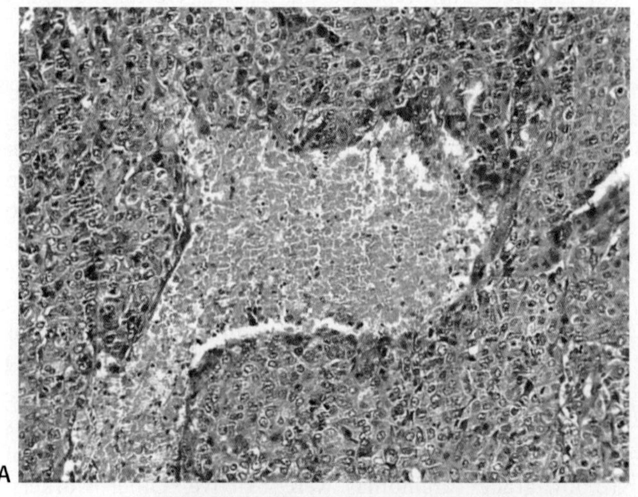

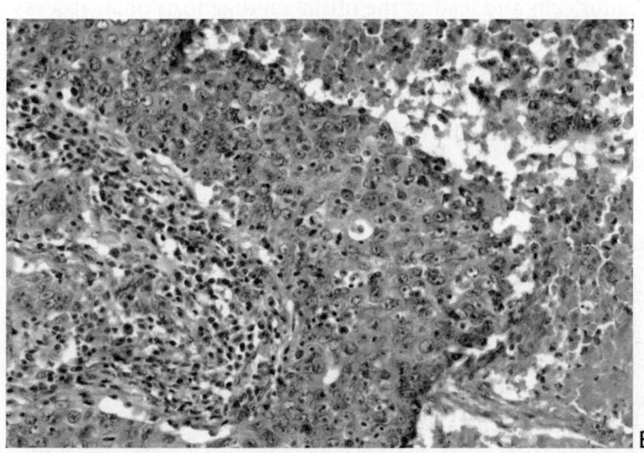

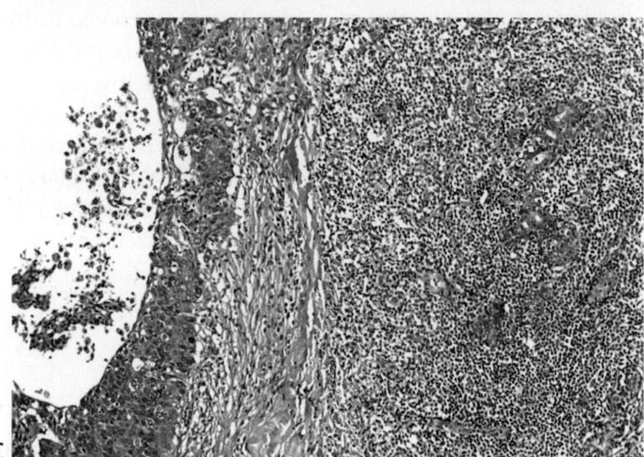

FIG. 15.29. ***Medullary carcinoma, necrosis.*** **A,B:** Comedo necrosis in the carcinoma. **C:** Cystic degeneration resulting from extensive necrosis.

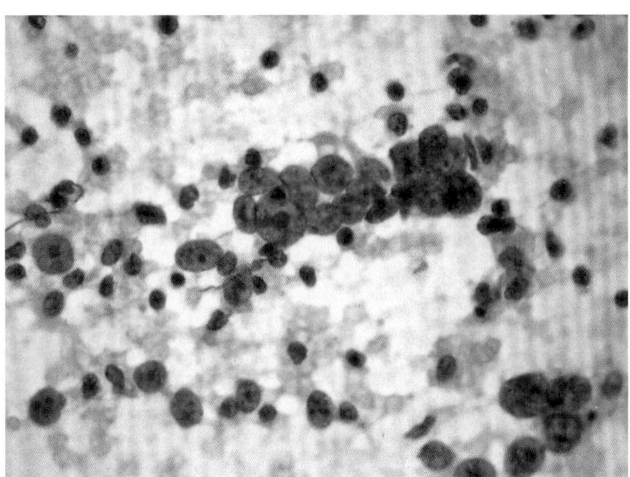

FIG. 15.30. ***Medullary carcinoma, fine-needle aspiration cytology.*** Poorly differentiated carcinoma cells singly and in small groups with lymphocytes scattered in the background.

carcinomas for the presence of many other proteins: p63, AP-2α, AP-2γ, CD56, CD138,[31] aurora B, bcl-2, cyclin D1, muc 1,[57] and c-kit.[59] These individual studies have not demonstrated sufficiently distinctive patterns in the expressions of these proteins that one could use them to distinguish medullary carcinomas from and non-medullary carcinomas.

Hormone Receptors

Fewer than 10% of medullary carcinomas are estrogen receptor (ER)- or progesterone receptor (PR) positive when analyzed biochemically,[66] an observation confirmed by immunohistochemical studies.[57,67,68] This feature is consistent with clinical experience that metastatic medullary carcinoma is relatively unresponsive to endocrine therapy.[69] Only a small percentage of medullary carcinoma express the human epidermal growth factor 2 (HER2).[31,57,70,71]

Basal-Like Immunophenotype

The presence of vimentin, CK5/6, and CK14[58,59] in medullary carcinomas led several investigators to examine the possibility that the tumors express other proteins associated with basal/myoepithelial cells such as P-cadherin, epidermal growth factor receptor (EGFR), smooth muscle actin, and S-100 protein.[31,57] Jacquemier et al.[57] found P-cadherin in 97% of medullary carcinoma and only 64% of non-medullary grade 3 invasive ductal carcinomas. Flucke et al.[31] also observed P-cadherin in 87% of medullary carcinomas, but the workers did not observe a difference in the expression of the molecule between medullary and non-medullary carcinomas. Epidermal growth factor occurs in 42%[31] to 71%[57] of medullary carcinomas. Jacquemier et al.[57] observed that 71% of medullary carcinomas expressed EGFR, whereas only 37% of invasive ductal carcinoma did so, and Vincent-Salomon et al.[59] reported similar results. Smooth muscle actin has been detected in 25%[31] to 34%[57] of medullary carcinomas. Jacquemier et al.[57] found that 44% of medullary carcinomas expressed the S-100 protein (Fig. 15.31), but only 24% of non-medullary high-grade ductal carcinomas did so. Rodríguez-Pinilla et al.[72] observed that carcinomas classified as invasive ductal carcinoma with medullary features displayed immunohistochemical features characteristic of basal-like carcinomas more often than did high-grade conventional invasive ductal carcinoma (62.9% vs. 18.9% of cases).

p53

Several investigations devoted to medullary carcinomas[57,59,64,71,73–75] and several others that included just a few medullary carcinomas without specifying the criteria used to make this diagnosis[76,77] demonstrated that the majority of medullary carcinomas exhibited nuclear accumulation of p53 (Fig. 15.32A). The frequency ranged from 46%[78] to 87%,[73] and two groups[64,73] noted that most of the malignant cells stained for the protein. In two studies,[57,75] expression of p53 occurred at a significantly greater frequency in medullary carcinomas than in conventional high-grade invasive ductal carcinomas, and another study[64] documented a difference between the two groups but did not report the results of a statistical test for the significance of this difference. One group failed to detect a difference in the expression of p53.[78] The investigators observed the protein in 46% of medullary carcinomas and 44% of non-medullary carcinomas. Invasive ductal carcinomas with medullary features might accumulate p53 less frequently than *bona fide* medullary carcinomas,[57,73–75] but the observed lower rates probably do not reach statistical significance. Two investigations[74,75] failed to demonstrate prognostic significance of the presence of nuclear p53 as measured by either disease-free survival (DFS) or OS.

Accumulation of the p53 protein usually indicates the presence of a mutation in the *p53* gene. Study of a small number of tumors classified as medullary and conventional carcinomas without reexamination of the diagnostic material discovered mutations of the *p53* gene in 39% of the

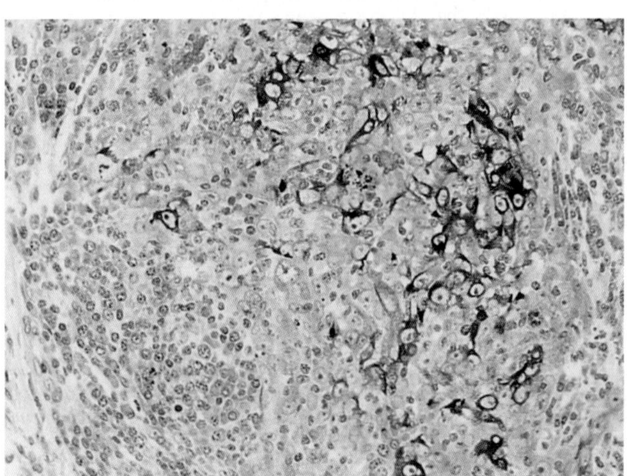

FIG. 15.31. ***Medullary carcinoma, S-100 protein.*** Many of the carcinoma cells are S-100 positive.

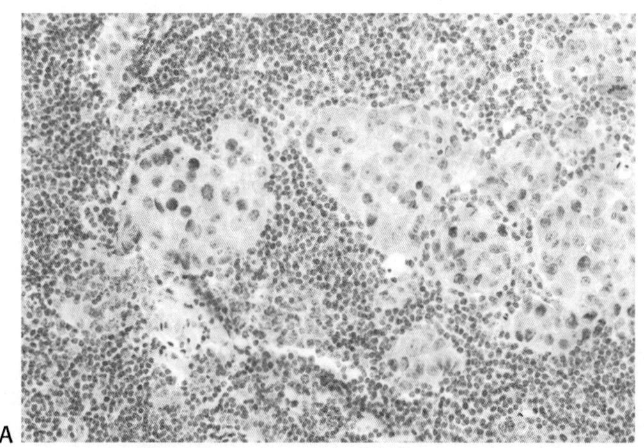

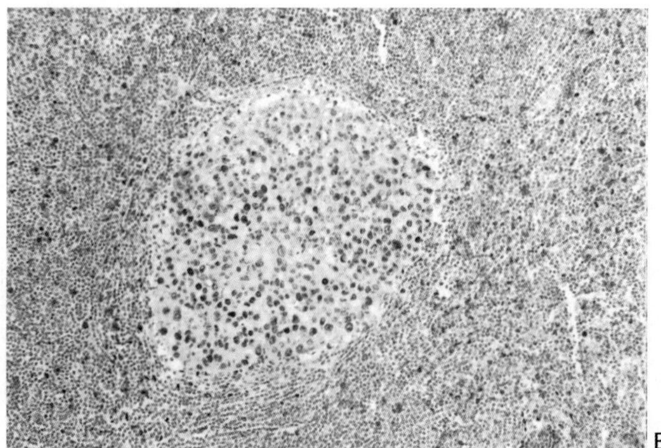

FIG. 15.32. ***Medullary carcinoma, proliferative and oncogene markers.*** **A:** Some tumor cell nuclei are immunoreactive for p53. This tumor had no reactivity for HER2 or hormone receptors. **B:** A high proliferative index indicated by nuclear reactivity for Ki67.

medullary carcinomas and 26% of the conventional ductal carcinomas.[77] Analysis of the *p53* gene in a group of carefully selected medullary carcinomas and invasive ductal carcinomas with medullary features disclosed mutations in the *p53* gene in 100% of the medullary carcinomas, but only 25% of invasive ductal carcinoma with medullary features.[73] The latter frequency matches that of *p53* mutations in conventional invasive ductal carcinomas. A subsequent investigation discovered mutations of the *p53* gene in 77% of medullary carcinomas.[59] These studies indicate that mutation of the *p53* gene and subsequent accumulation of the defective protein occurs in most medullary carcinomas.

Taken together, these observations indicate that medullary carcinomas belong to the family of basal-like breast carcinomas and that these markers cannot distinguish medullary carcinomas from non-medullary basal-like carcinomas on a case-by-case basis.

Growth Rate

As measured by thymidine incorporation,[79] flow cytometry,[80,81] and MIB1 staining[57,71,77] (Fig. 15.32B), medullary carcinoma has one of the highest growth rates among breast carcinomas. This observation supports the clinical observations of rapid growth of medullary carcinomas in certain cases. Medullary carcinomas have significantly higher apoptotic indices determined by the terminal deoxynucleotidyl transferase dUTP nick-end labeling method.[78]

Medullary carcinomas typically overexpress cyclin E. Berglund et al.[82] found high levels of the protein in 87% of medullary carcinomas. Overexpression of cyclin E in a breast carcinoma cell line led to upregulation of genes associated with cell proliferation, and functional assays demonstrated increased cell adhesion, diminished motility, decreased invasion, and alteration of the cytoskeletal proteins of the cyclin E overexpressing cells. The authors suggest that these molecular alterations might explain the "pushing" margin of medullary carcinomas.

Lymphoplasmacytic Infiltrate

Because the inflammatory cell infiltrate might contribute to the favorable prognosis of medullary carcinoma,[83] the immunohistochemical characteristics of the lymphoplasmacytic reaction have been the subject of several studies.[84–87] IgG cells predominate in medullary carcinomas and in IDC.[57,85] Substantial numbers of IgA cells may also be found in non-medullary IDC and less often in medullary carcinomas.[85] Immunoglobulin-containing cells in the lymphoplasmacytic infiltrate associated with normal breast tissue, benign tumors, and hyperplastic lesions tend to be of the IgA type.[85,88] Kuroda et al.[86] reported that medullary carcinomas have few natural killer cells as evidenced by low CD56 antibody reactivity. CD8-positive lymphocytes exceeded CD4-positive T lymphocytes. The tumors contained relatively high proportions of cytotoxic TIA-1 and granzyme B–positive cells, a feature that could be relevant to the favorable prognosis of the tumor. Lymphocytes infiltrating medullary and non-medullary carcinomas are predominantly peripheral T lymphocytes.[84,89] There do not appear to be significant differences between medullary and IDCs in the distribution of antigenic phenotypes of lymphocytes.[84,89] However, medullary and atypical medullary carcinomas are characterized by significantly increased numbers of activated cytotoxic lymphocytes that may play a role in prognosis.[90]

Yazawa et al.[91] reported a high frequency of HLA-DR-positive lymphocytes in medullary carcinomas. There was correspondingly strong HLA-DR reactivity in the carcinoma cells. The authors speculated that HLA-DR expression was linked to the favorable prognosis of medullary carcinoma. These authors also found that non-medullary carcinomas that expressed HLA-DR had a relatively better prognosis compared with HLA-DR-negative tumors. Lazzaro et al.[92] noted strong expression of HLA-DR, and Reyes et al.[65] used expression of this molecule to confirm the diagnosis of medullary carcinoma based on conventional histologic criteria.

Epstein–Barr Virus

The microscopic features of medullary carcinoma with an exceptionally abundant lymphoplasmacytic reaction resemble those of lymphoepithelial carcinomas that arise at other sites.[93] These and other characteristics have suggested that the Epstein–Barr virus (EBV) might play a role in pathogenesis of medullary carcinoma; however, a study of 10 tumors using immunohistochemistry, *in situ* hybridization, and the polymerase chain reaction failed to detect evidence of EBV.[94] A lymphoepithelioma-like tumor studied by Naidoo and Chetty[93] was also negative for EBV. This lesion was accompanied by sclerosing lymphocytic lobulitis in the surrounding breast tissue.

ELECTRON MICROSCOPY

Electron microscopy has not yielded consistent findings in medullary carcinoma.[95–98] This inconsistency may reflect either a failure to adhere to rigorous diagnostic criteria in some cases or an intrinsic variability in the tumors. The ultrastructural findings are not sufficiently specific to be regarded as diagnostic, but one can draw certain conclusions. Light and dark cells, differing in cytoplasmic density, have been described by most authors. Both types of cells contain the usual cellular organelles. The dark cells tend to have more organelles, especially rough endoplasmic reticulum, whereas free polyribosomes are more numerous in the light cells.[96] The cells also contain lipid droplets and granules of glycogen, and the occasional presence of tonofilaments may be evidence of squamous differentiation.[96] Intracytoplasmic lumens lined by microvilli may be found, but they are present much less often than in other types of breast carcinoma. Desmosomes are found with varying frequency, and cellular interdigitations occur in small numbers.[98] Myoepithelial cells are scant or absent, and there is little basal lamina.[95] Migrating lymphocytes have been observed in the endothelium of vascular channels in tumor stroma. Two studies have failed to find distinctive ultrastructural differences between the tumor cells of medullary and atypical medullary carcinomas.[96,99]

GENETIC AND MOLECULAR STUDIES

Medullary carcinomas are typically aneuploid or polyploid.[80,100] Cytogenetic studies have revealed the presence of trisomy 18 in a few medullary carcinomas,[101,102] but this mutation has also been found in other types of breast carcinoma.[103] Medullary carcinomas frequently display losses and gains of genetic material,[104] but they do not seem to display microsatellite instability when classified by either classical[104,105] or alternative criteria.[106]

Medullary carcinomas have a number of features in common with breast-cancer-1-(BRCA1)-associated breast carcinomas, including relatively young age at diagnosis, poorly differentiated histology, lymphocytic infiltration, absence of hormone receptors, and frequent p53 alterations. A study of BRCA1-associated breast carcinomas revealed that 6 of 32 tumors (19%) were true medullary carcinomas, a significantly higher frequency than observed among non–BRCA1-associated control tumors.[107] Marcus et al.[108] reported that medullary carcinomas represented 13% of carcinomas in families with BRCA1 mutations and that IDC with medullary features accounted for an additional 13% of tumors in their study. In the investigation of Lakhani et al.,[109] medullary carcinomas accounted for 11% of the carcinomas in patients with BRCA1 mutations, and the Breast Cancer Linkage Consortium[110] observed medullary carcinoma in 13% of patients with BRCA1 mutations. Two studies[111,112] detected lower frequencies, which did not differ significantly from those observed for sporadic breast carcinomas.

One can find BRCA1 mutations in patients with medullary carcinoma more frequently than in patients with other varieties of breast carcinoma. Malone et al.[113] found BRCA1 mutations in 5 of 21 (23.8%) women with medullary carcinoma and in 17 of 285 (6%) women with non-medullary tumors. All patients included in the latter study underwent BRCA1 testing because of a family history of breast carcinoma or early onset of breast carcinoma. Osin et al.[114] found BRCA1 mutations in 6 of 25 (25%) medullary carcinomas. Immunohistochemical staining failed to detect the BRCA1 protein in 24 of 35 medullary carcinomas (67%), whereas only 2 of 30 control cases (6%) demonstrate complete absence of staining. Iau et al.[115] found BRCA1 mutations in 14% of typical medullary carcinomas. Eisinger et al.,[107] tested 18 medullary carcinomas selected from a hospital-based registry without knowledge of the family history and discovered BRCA1 nonsense mutations in two tumors (11%), seven times the frequency of these alterations in the general population. In neither case did the patient report a family history suggestive of heritable breast carcinoma. The 11% detection rate is higher than that encountered when using early onset as a criterion for genetic testing. These findings make clear that medullary carcinomas occur more frequently in women with BRCA1 mutations and that the presence of a medullary carcinoma sometimes heralds the presence of a BRCA1 mutation. The latter observation suggests that the diagnosis of medullary carcinoma could represent an indication for *BRCA* testing.[116]

One study[117] of the methylation status of the BRCA1 promoter detected hypermethylation in 8 of 12 medullary carcinomas. This finding indicates that epigenetic mechanisms may account for the absence of the BRCA1 protein in certain medullary carcinomas.

Two genetic studies provide evidence that medullary carcinomas constitute a specific subtype of basal-like carcinoma. Vincent-Salomon et al.[59] compared medullary carcinomas and non-medullary basal-type invasive ductal carcinomas using high-density array comparative genomic hybridization profiles. The investigators found that the two types of carcinoma shared genomic alterations such as 1q and 8q gains and X losses, but that they differed in other genetic alterations. The medullary carcinomas displayed a greater rate of gains and losses compared with the basal-like carcinomas, and the former exhibited more frequent 10p, 9p, and 16q gains; 4p losses; and 1q, 8p, 10p, and 12p amplicons than the latter.

Bertucci et al.[71] used whole-genome oligonucleotide microarrays to compare the gene expression profiles of medullary carcinomas and conventional invasive ductal carcinomas. The investigators discovered that 95% of medullary carcinomas displayed a profile similar to that of basal-like carcinomas. However, medullary carcinomas and basal-like carcinomas did not demonstrate identical expression profiles. When compared with basal-like invasive ductal carcinomas, medullary carcinomas demonstrated overexpression of 269 genes and underexpression of 265 genes. The overexpressed genes cluster in groups related to the immune response, extrinsic apoptosis pathway, and antigen processing and presentation. Many genes in the immune response group regulate T cells, and the data suggested that a T_H1-based immunoprofile characterizes medullary carcinoma. Underexpressed genes include those involved in the architecture and remodeling of the cytoskeleton, those coding for smooth muscle–specific proteins, and those involved in cell invasiveness. Finally, the workers observed a significant overexpression of genes located in the 12p13 and the 6p21.3 regions among the genes overexpressed in medullary carcinomas. These findings allowed the investigators to identify a gene expression signature that could distinguish medullary carcinomas from other basal-like breast carcinomas. With a median follow-up of 41 months, the patients with medullary carcinomas identified by this gene expression signature experienced a higher DFS rate than those with conventional basal-like carcinomas. A subsequent study[118] confirmed the sensitivity of the gene expression signature and demonstrated that the expression profile could separate non-medullary basal-like carcinomas into two groups. Patients with basal-like carcinomas expressing the profile seen in medullary carcinomas experienced a greater rate of DFS than those with carcinomas that did not demonstrate the gene expression signature. By identifying those high-grade carcinomas with a favorable prognosis, the use of this profile might allow pathologists to identify morphologic findings associated with this improved outcome and thereby to refine the histologic criteria for the diagnosis of medullary carcinoma.

PROGNOSIS

Overall, a high proportion of patients treated for medullary carcinoma survive without recurrence after treatment by modified or radical mastectomy. In an early description of the tumor, Moore and Foote[3] stated that only 11.5% of their patients with medullary carcinoma died of the tumor within 5 years. This favorable outcome was especially striking because 42% of the patients had ALN metastases. The series includes nine women, each of whom had a single lymph node metastasis and survived disease-free for 5 years. The results described by Richardson[13] several years later confirmed the observations of Moore and Foote. The 5-year DFS of their 99 patients treated with mastectomy, some with radiation, was 78%, with death due to disease in only 10%. Ten-year follow-up was available for 47 patients. OS in this subset was 64% with only eight deaths (17%) due to breast carcinoma and nine deaths (19%) due to other causes. Axillary metastases occurred in 45% of the entire series, but these patients were found to have a much more favorable prognosis than stage II patients with ordinary types of breast carcinoma. In the study conducted by Bloom et al.,[15] the 20-year DFS rate for stage I patients treated with mastectomy was 95%. For women with stage II medullary carcinoma treated with mastectomy and radiation, it was 61% in contrast to the 13% observed for "other types of breast cancer."[15]

Several later studies refined the diagnostic criteria for medullary carcinoma and confirmed the favorable prognosis of this type of tumor.[8–10,28,30,32,119,120] Five of these series include a pathologic review of all cases recorded as medullary carcinoma or as invasive ductal carcinoma with medullary features.[8,28,30,32,120] As a consequence of these reviews, fewer than 50% of the lesions were accepted as true medullary carcinomas, and the remaining cases were diagnosed as invasive ductal carcinomas with medullary features or invasive ductal carcinomas. Patients with medullary carcinoma proved to have a statistically significant more favorable prognosis than those in either of the other two groups (Fig. 15.33). Although the outcome of patients with invasive ductal carcinoma with medullary features was slightly better than the prognosis of women with usual invasive ductal carcinoma, the difference did not prove to be statistically significant in five of the series.[8,9,28,30,120]

An examination of data from the Surveillance Epidemiology and End Results (SEER) program was undertaken to determine tumor-related survival and the likelihood of cure for patients with different histologic types of breast carcinoma.[119] Analysis of 163,808 patients revealed 2,908 (3%) with stage I and 1,654 (2.4%) with stage II medullary carcinoma. Patients with medullary carcinoma had relatively high "cured fractions" of 82% and 64% for stages I and II, respectively. The median survival times for uncured patients dying of their carcinomas were 4 and 3 years for stages I and II, respectively. These times were relatively short compared with those for other histologic types of carcinoma.

Patients with medullary carcinoma tend to have a lower overall frequency of ALN metastases than patients with invasive ductal carcinoma with medullary features or usual invasive ductal carcinoma.[8,9,11,28,30,32] The prognosis of patients with small, node-negative medullary carcinoma is particularly favorable, with a DFS of 90% or better.[28,30] When nodal metastases are present, they typically involve no more than three lymph nodes.[8,28,32,74,120] The survival results for stage II, T1N1M0 medullary carcinoma have also been exceptionally good at 10 and 20 years of follow-up. Although stage II medullary carcinoma patients have a more favorable prognosis than equivalent patients with non-medullary carcinoma, tumor size and nodal status are still significant determinants of DFS.[32] Patients whose medullary carcinomas are larger than 3 cm or who have four or more involved lymph nodes have high recurrence rates that are not appreciably different from the recurrence rates of patients with usual invasive ductal carcinoma.[30]

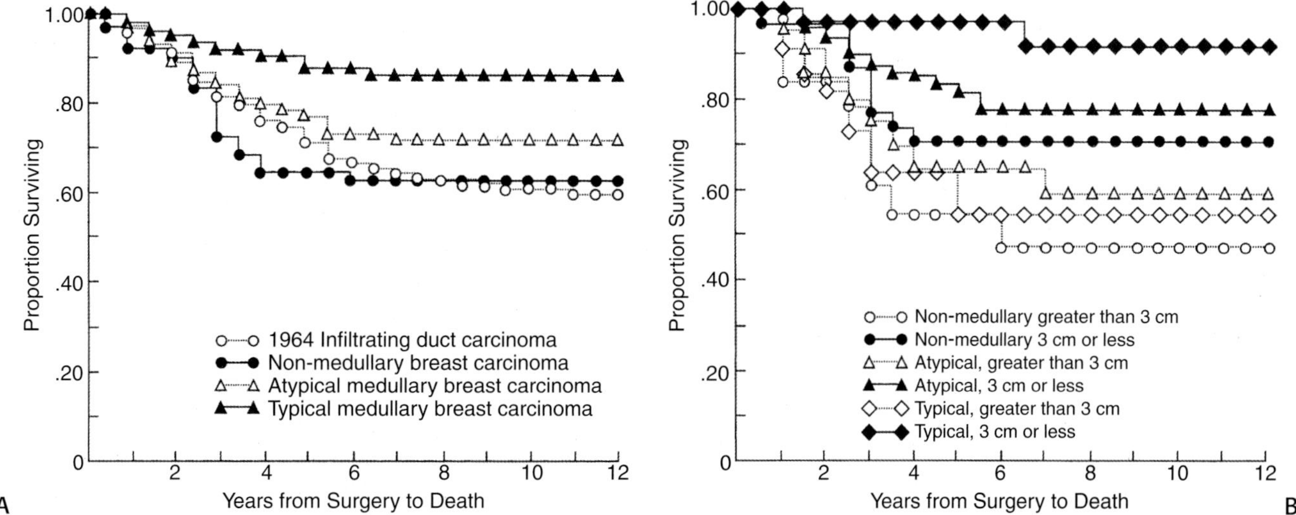

FIG. 15.33. ***Medullary carcinoma, survival analysis.*** **A:** The prognosis of patients with typical medullary carcinoma was significantly better than that of patients with three categories of non-medullary carcinoma. **B:** Patients with medullary carcinomas 3 cm or less in diameter had the best prognosis.

The major contribution of the term *invasive ductal carcinoma with medullary features* has been to draw attention to the existence of a subset of invasive ductal carcinomas that may be misdiagnosed as medullary carcinoma. Failure to distinguish medullary carcinoma from invasive ductal carcinoma with medullary features by not applying rigorous diagnostic criteria undoubtedly has been a factor in the several studies that have not observed a favorable prognosis in medullary carcinoma patients overall or in those with stage II disease.[6,121] The term "circumscribed carcinoma" is particularly misleading in this respect, because it suggests that gross circumscription is the most important diagnostic feature without putting sufficient emphasis on microscopic criteria.[122]

Recurrences tend to occur early in the clinical course of patients with medullary carcinoma, with very few women having recurrences or dying 5 years or more after diagnosis.[15,28,30,32] This phenomenon is observed equally in stage I and stage II patients. Most initial recurrences are systemic, but local recurrence has been observed in patients treated by modified or radical mastectomy. Survival after systemic recurrence tends to be brief, regardless of the site of the initial metastasis,[32] although an occasional patient may benefit from resection of a solitary metastasis.[28]

TREATMENT

There is presently little reported experience with breast-conserving surgery and radiotherapy of medullary carcinoma. It has been suggested that medullary carcinoma may be particularly radiosensitive.[123] One group of 39 patients said to have medullary carcinoma was treated by radiotherapy to the breast after carcinoma was diagnosed only by needle biopsy.[124] This series is not representative of medullary carcinomas in general, since virtually all of the patients had tumors larger than 3 cm, and more than half were considered to have positive ALNs on the basis of clinical examination. In addition, needle biopsy specimens do not provide adequate material to distinguish between medullary carcinoma and invasive ductal carcinoma with medullary features accurately. Twenty-four had radiation alone, whereas 15 others also received adjuvant chemotherapy after radiation was given. Thirty-one patients were considered to have had complete regression of their tumors, and eight had persistent disease that was treated with surgery. Follow-up revealed two patients dead of disease 3 and 31 months after recurrence, and four women alive 6 to 30 months after recurrence. Overall, eight patients (20%) in this series died of metastatic carcinoma.

Combined data from two institutions included 27 women with medullary carcinoma treated by breast-conserving surgery and radiotherapy.[125] The mammary recurrence rate was 4%, the 5-year OS was 90%, and RFS was 92% at 5 years. A series of 1,008 patients treated by breast conservation with radiotherapy at Yale University included 17 women with medullary carcinoma.[126] No patient developed a systemic recurrence, but there were five local breast recurrences (29%) after a median follow-up of nearly 17 years with the longest interval to recurrence of 18 years. In this study, the 10-year actuarial breast recurrence-free survival was lower for medullary carcinoma (75%) than for usual IDC (85%) but this difference is not statistically significant.

Presently, breast conservation with lumpectomy and radiotherapy appears to be a reasonable form of therapy for patients with true medullary carcinoma and especially for tumors 3 cm or smaller. Sentinel lymph node mapping is an appropriate procedure for staging the ALNs. Indications for systemic adjuvant therapy are similar to those for non-medullary invasive duct carcinoma, including tumor size, nodal status, and the presence of lymphatic tumor emboli. In some instances, adjuvant chemotherapy may be omitted in patients with T1N0M0 medullary carcinomas.

REFERENCES

1. Geschickter CF. *Diseases of the breast: diagnosis, pathology, treatment.* 2nd ed. Philadelphia: JB Lippincott, 1945:565–575.
2. Foote FW Jr, Stewart FW. A histologic classification of carcinoma of the breast. *Surgery* 1946;19:74–99.
3. Moore OS Jr, Foote FW Jr. The relatively favorable prognosis of medullary carcinoma of the breast. *Cancer* 1949;2:635–642.
4. Fisher ER, Gregorio RM, Fisher B, et al. The pathology of invasive breast cancer. A syllabus derived from findings of the National Surgical Adjuvant Breast Project (protocol no. 4). *Cancer* 1975;36:1–85.
5. Jacquemier J, Reis-Filho JS, Lakhani SR, et al. Carcinomas with medullary features. In: Lakhani SR, Ellis IO, Schnitt SJ, et al., eds. *WHO classification of tumours of the breast.* (*WHO Classification of Tumors,* vol. 4). 4th edn. Lyon: World Health Organization- IARC, 2012.
6. Maier WP, Rosemond GP, Goldman LI, et al. A ten year study of medullary carcinoma of the breast. *Surg Gynecol Obstet* 1977;144: 695–698.
7. Markovitz P, Contesso G, Sarrazin D, et al. Le carcinome medullaire du sein. Étude clinicque et anatomo-radiologique a propos de 56 observations. *Bull du Cancer* 1970;57:517–526.
8. Rapin V, Contesso G, Mouriesse H, et al. Medullary breast carcinoma. A reevaluation of 95 cases of breast cancer with inflammatory stroma. *Cancer* 1988;61:2503–2510.
9. Mitze M, Goepel E. Prognostiche faktoren beim medullären mammakarzinom. *Geburtsh Frauenheilk* 1989;49:635–641.
10. Ellis IO, Galea M, Broughton N, et al. Pathological prognostic factors in breast cancer. II. Histological type. Relationship with survival in a large study with long-term follow-up. *Histopathology* 1992;20:479–489.
11. Li CI, Uribe DJ, Daling JR. Clinical characteristics of different histologic types of breast cancer. *Br J Cancer* 2005;93:1046–1052.
12. Bässler R, Dittmann AM, Dittrich M. Mononuclear stromal reactions in mammary carcinoma, with special reference to medullary carcinomas with a lymphoid infiltrate. Analysis of 108 cases. *Virchows Arch A Pathol Anat Histol* 1981;393:75–91.
13. Richardson WW. Medullary carcinoma of the breast; a distinctive tumour type with a relatively good prognosis following radical mastectomy. *Br J Cancer* 1956;10:415–423.
14. Rosen PP. The pathological classification of human mammary carcinoma: past, present and future. *Ann Clin Lab Sci* 1979;9:144–156.
15. Bloom HJ, Richardson WW, Field JR. Host resistance and survival in carcinoma of breast: a study of 104 cases of medullary carcinoma in a series of 1,411 cases of breast cancer followed for 20 years. *Br Med J* 1970;3:181–188.
16. Rosen PP, Saigo PE, Braun DW Jr, et al. Predictors of recurrence in stage I (T1N0M0) breast carcinoma. *Ann Surg* 1981;193:15–25.
17. Rosen PP, Saigo PE, Braun DW, et al. Prognosis in stage II (T1N1M0) breast cancer. *Ann Surg* 1981;194:576–584.
18. Morrison AS, Black MM, Lowe CR, et al. Some international differences in histology and survival in breast cancer. *Int J Cancer* 1973;11:261–267.
19. Rosen PP, Ashikari R, Thaler H, et al. A comparative study of some pathologic features of mammary carcinoma in Tokyo, Japan and New York, USA. *Cancer* 1977;39:429–434.
20. Wynder EL, Kajitani T, Kuno J, et al. A comparison of survival rates between American and Japanese patients with breast cancer. *Surg Gynecol Obstet* 1963;117:196–200.
21. Berg JW, Robbins GF. The histologic epidemiology of breast cancer. In: *Breast cancer early and late. Proceedings of the Annual Clinical Conference of the MD Anderson Hospital and Tumor Institute.* Chicago: Year Book Medical Publishers, 1970:19–26.
22. Mittra NK, Rush BF Jr, Verner E. A comparative study of breast cancer in the black and white populations of two inner-city hospitals. *J Surg Oncol* 1980;15:11–17.
23. Natarajan N, Nemoto T, Mettlin C, et al. Race-related differences in breast cancer patients. Results of the 1982 national survey of breast cancer by the American College of Surgeons. *Cancer* 1985;56:1704–1709.
24. Ownby HE, Frederick J, Russo J, et al. Racial differences in breast cancer patients. *J Natl Cancer Inst* 1985;75:55–60.
25. Li CI, Malone KE, Daling JR. Differences in breast cancer hormone receptor status and histology by race and ethnicity among women 50 years of age and older. *Cancer Epidemiol Biomarkers Prev* 2002;11:601–607.
26. Rosen PP, Lesser ML, Senie RT, et al. Epidemiology of breast carcinoma III: relationship of family history to tumor type. *Cancer* 1982;50:171–179.
27. Burki N, Buser M, Emmons LR, et al. Malignancies in families of women with medullary, tubular and invasive ductal breast cancer. *Eur J Cancer* 1990;26:295–303.
28. Wargotz ES, Silverberg SG. Medullary carcinoma of the breast: a clinicopathologic study with appraisal of current diagnostic criteria. *Hum Pathol* 1988;19:1340–1346.
29. Rosen PP, Lesser ML, Senie RT, et al. Epidemiology of breast carcinoma IV: age and histologic tumor type. *J Surg Oncol* 1982;19:44–51.
30. Ridolfi RL, Rosen PP, Port A, et al. Medullary carcinoma of the breast: a clinicopathologic study with 10 year follow-up. *Cancer* 1977;40:1365–1385.
31. Flucke U, Flucke MT, Hoy L, et al. Distinguishing medullary carcinoma of the breast from high-grade hormone receptor-negative invasive ductal carcinoma: an immunohistochemical approach. *Histopathology* 2010;56:852–859.
32. Reinfuss M, Stelmach A, Mitus J, et al. Typical medullary carcinoma of the breast: a clinical and pathological analysis of 52 cases. *J Surg Oncol* 1995;60:89–94.
33. Anderson WF, Chu KC, Chang S, et al. Comparison of age-specific incidence rate patterns for different histopathologic types of breast carcinoma. *Cancer Epidemiol Biomarkers Prev* 2004;13:1128–1135.
34. Rosen PP, Lesser ML, Kinne DW, et al. Breast carcinoma in women 35 years of age or younger. *Ann Surg* 1984;199:133–142.
35. Rosen PP, Lesser ML, Kinne DW. Breast carcinoma at the extremes of age: a comparison of patients younger than 35 years and older than 75 years. *J Surg Oncol* 1985;28:90–96.
36. Lesser ML, Rosen PP, Kinne DW. Multicentricity and bilaterality in invasive breast carcinoma. *Surgery* 1982;91:234–240.
37. Haupt HM, Rosen PP, Kinne DW. Breast carcinoma presenting with axillary lymph node metastases. An analysis of specific histopathologic features. *Am J Surg Pathol* 1985;9:165–175.
38. Neuman ML, Homer MJ. Association of medullary carcinoma with reactive axillary adenopathy. *AJR Am J Roentgenol* 1996;167:185–186.
39. Rosen PP, Lesser ML, Kinne DW, et al. Discontinuous or "skip" metastases in breast carcinoma. Analysis of 1228 axillary dissections. *Ann Surg* 1983;197:276–283.
40. Jeong SJ, Lim HS, Lee JS, et al. Medullary carcinoma of the breast: MRI findings. *AJR Am J Roentgenol* 2012;198:W482–W487.
41. Meyer JE, Amin E, Lindfors KK, et al. Medullary carcinoma of the breast: mammographic and US appearance. *Radiology* 1989;170:79–82.
42. Cheung YC, Chen SC, Lee KF, et al. Sonographic and pathologic findings in typical and atypical medullary carcinomas of the breast. *J Clin Ultrasound* 2000;28:325–331.
43. Tominaga J, Hama H, Kimura N, et al. MR imaging of medullary carcinoma of the breast. *Eur J Radiol* 2009;70:525–529.
44. Kopans DB, Rubens J. Medullary carcinoma of the breast. *Radiology* 1989;171:876.
45. Pedersen L, Holck S, Schiodt T, et al. Inter- and intraobserver variability in the histopathological diagnosis of medullary carcinoma of the breast, and its prognostic implications. *Breast Cancer Res Treat* 1989;14:91–99.
46. Rubens JR, Lewandrowski KB, Kopans DB, et al. Medullary carcinoma of the breast. Overdiagnosis of a prognostically favorable neoplasm. *Arch Surg* 1990;125:601–604.
47. Rigaud C, Theobald S, Noel P, et al. Medullary carcinoma of the breast. A multicenter study of its diagnostic consistency. *Arch Pathol Lab Med* 1993;117:1005–1008.
48. Gaffey MJ, Mills SE, Frierson HF Jr, et al. Medullary carcinoma of the breast: interobserver variability in histopathologic diagnosis. *Mod Pathol* 1995;8:31–38.
49. Pedersen L, Zedeler K, Holck S, et al. Medullary carcinoma of the breast, proposal for a new simplified histopathological definition. Based on prognostic observations and observations on inter- and intraobserver variability of 11 histopathological characteristics in 131 breast carcinomas with medullary features. *Br J Cancer* 1991;63:591–595.
50. Jensen ML, Kiaer H, Andersen J, et al. Prognostic comparison of three classifications for medullary carcinomas of the breast. *Histopathology* 1997;30:523–532.
51. Tavassoli FA. Infiltrating carcinomas, common and familiar special types: medullary carcinoma. In: *Pathology of the breast.* Norwalk: Appleton & Lange, 1992:333–339.
52. Marginean F, Rakha EA, Ho BC, et al. Histological features of medullary carcinoma and prognosis in triple-negative basal-like carcinomas of the breast. *Mod Pathol* 2010;23:1357–1363.
53. Pedersen L, Schiodt T, Holck S, et al. The prognostic importance of syncytial growth pattern in medullary carcinoma of the breast. *APMIS* 1990;98:921–926.

54. McDivitt RW, Stewart FW, Berg JW. *Tumors of the breast.* (*AFIP Atlas of Tumor Pathology*, 2nd series, vol. 2). Bethesda: American Registry of Pathology, 1968.
55. Kline TS, Kannan V, Kline IK. Appraisal and cytomorphologic analysis of common carcinomas of the breast. *Diagn Cytopathol* 1985;1:188–193.
56. Howell LP, Kline TS. Medullary carcinoma of the breast. An unusual cytologic finding in cyst fluid aspirates. *Cancer* 1990;65:277–282.
57. Jacquemier J, Padovani L, Rabayrol L, et al. Typical medullary breast carcinomas have a basal/myoepithelial phenotype. *J Pathol* 2005;207:260–268.
58. Tot T. The cytokeratin profile of medullary carcinoma of the breast. *Histopathology* 2000;37:175–181.
59. Vincent-Salomon A, Gruel N, Lucchesi C, et al. Identification of typical medullary breast carcinoma as a genomic sub-group of basal-like carcinomas, a heterogeneous new molecular entity. *Breast Cancer Res* 2007;9:R24.
60. Larsimont D, Lespagnard L, Degeyter M, et al. Medullary carcinoma of the breast: a tumour lacking keratin 19. *Histopathology* 1994;24:549–552.
61. Dalal P, Shousha S. Keratin 19 in paraffin sections of medullary carcinoma and other benign and malignant breast lesions. *Mod Pathol* 1995;8:413–416.
62. Jensen ML, Kiaer H, Melsen F. Medullary breast carcinoma vs. poorly differentiated ductal carcinoma: an immunohistochemical study with keratin 19 and oestrogen receptor staining. *Histopathology* 1996;29:241–245.
63. Holck S, Pedersen L, Schiodt T, et al. Vimentin expression in 98 breast cancers with medullary features and its prognostic significance. *Virchows Arch A Pathol Anat Histopathol* 1993;422:475–479.
64. Domagala W, Harezga B, Szadowska A, et al. Nuclear p53 protein accumulates preferentially in medullary and high-grade ductal but rarely in lobular breast carcinomas. *Am J Pathol* 1993;142:669–674.
65. Reyes C, Gomez-Fernandez C, Nadji M. Metaplastic and medullary mammary carcinomas do not express mammaglobin. *Am J Clin Pathol* 2012;137:747–752.
66. Rosen PP, Menendez-Botet CJ, Nisselbaum JS, et al. Pathological review of breast lesions analyzed for estrogen receptor protein. *Cancer Res* 1975;35:3187–3194.
67. Reiner A, Reiner G, Spona J, et al. Histopathologic characterization of human breast cancer in correlation with estrogen receptor status. A comparison of immunocytochemical and biochemical analysis. *Cancer* 1988;61:1149–1154.
68. Stegner H, Jonat W, Maass H. Immunhistochemischer nachweis nuklearer ostrogenrezeptoren mit monoclonalen antikorpern in verschiedenen typen des mammakarzinoms. *Pathologe* 1986;7:156–163.
69. Patel JK, Nemoto T, Dao TL. Is medullary carcinoma of the breast hormone dependent? *J Surg Oncol* 1983;24:290–291.
70. Rosen PP, Lesser ML, Arroyo CD, et al. Immunohistochemical detection of HER2/neu in patients with axillary lymph node negative breast carcinoma. A study of epidemiologic risk factors, histologic features, and prognosis. *Cancer* 1995;75:1320–1326.
71. Bertucci F, Finetti P, Cervera N, et al. Gene expression profiling shows medullary breast cancer is a subgroup of basal breast cancers. *Cancer Res* 2006;66:4636–4644.
72. Rodríguez-Pinilla SM, Rodríguez-Gil Y, Moreno-Bueno G, et al. Sporadic invasive breast carcinomas with medullary features display a basal-like phenotype: an immunohistochemical and gene amplification study. *Am J Surg Pathol* 2007;31:501–508.
73. de Cremoux P, Salomon AV, Liva S, et al. p53 mutation as a genetic trait of typical medullary breast carcinoma. *J Natl Cancer Inst* 1999;91:641–643.
74. Dendale R, Vincent-Salomon A, Mouret-Fourme E, et al. Medullary breast carcinoma: prognostic implications of p53 expression. *Int J Biol Markers* 2003;18:99–105.
75. Rosen PP, Lesser ML, Arroyo CD, et al. p53 in node-negative breast carcinoma: an immunohistochemical study of epidemiologic risk factors, histologic features, and prognosis. *J Clin Oncol* 1995;13: 821–830.
76. Davidoff AM, Herndon JE II, Glover NS, et al. Relation between p53 overexpression and established prognostic factors in breast cancer. *Surgery* 1991;110:259–264.
77. Marchetti A, Buttitta F, Pellegrini S, et al. p53 mutations and histological type of invasive breast carcinoma. *Cancer Res* 1993;53:4665–4669.
78. Kajiwara M, Toyoshima S, Yao T, et al. Apoptosis and cell proliferation in medullary carcinoma of the breast: a comparative study between medullary and non-medullary carcinoma using the TUNEL method and immunohistochemistry. *J Surg Oncol* 1999;70:209–216.
79. Meyer JS, Friedman E, McCrate MM, et al. Prediction of early course of breast carcinoma by thymidine labeling. *Cancer* 1983;51 :1879–1886.
80. Kallioniemi OP, Blanco G, Alavaikko M, et al. Tumour DNA ploidy as an independent prognostic factor in breast cancer. *Br J Cancer* 1987;56:637–642.
81. Meyer JS, Bauer WC, Rao BR. Subpopulations of breast carcinoma defined by S-phase fraction, morphology, and estrogen receptor content. *Lab Invest* 1978;39:225–235.
82. Berglund P, Stighall M, Jirstrom K, et al. Cyclin E overexpression obstructs infiltrative behavior in breast cancer: a novel role reflected in the growth pattern of medullary breast cancers. *Cancer Res* 2005;65:9727–9734.
83. Rakha EA, Aleskandarany M, El-Sayed ME, et al. The prognostic significance of inflammation and medullary histological type in invasive carcinoma of the breast. *Eur J Cancer* 2009;45:1780–1787.
84. Ben-Ezra J, Sheibani K. Antigenic phenotype of the lymphocytic component of medullary carcinoma of the breast. *Cancer* 1987;59:2037–2041.
85. Ito T, Saga S, Nagayoshi S, et al. Class distribution of immunoglobulin-containing plasma cells in the stroma of medullary carcinoma of breast. *Breast Cancer Res Treat* 1986;7:97–103.
86. Kuroda H, Tamaru J, Sakamoto G, et al. Immunophenotype of lymphocytic infiltration in medullary carcinoma of the breast. *Virchows Arch* 2005;446:10–14.
87. Jacquemier J, Robert-Vague D, Torrente M, et al. Mise en evidence des immunoglobulines lymphoplasmocytaires et epitheliales dans les carcinomes infiltrants a stroma lymphoide et les carcinomes medullaires du sein. *Arch Anat Cytol Pathol* 1983;31:296–300.
88. Sieinski W. Immunohistological patterns of immunoglobulins in dysplasias, benign neoplasms and carcinomas of the breast. *Tumori* 1980;66:699–711.
89. Gaffey MJ, Frierson HF Jr, Mills SE, et al. Medullary carcinoma of the breast. Identification of lymphocyte subpopulations and their significance. *Mod Pathol* 1993;6:721–728.
90. Yakirevich E, Izhak OB, Rennert G, et al. Cytotoxic phenotype of tumor infiltrating lymphocytes in medullary carcinoma of the breast. *Mod Pathol* 1999;12:1050–1056.
91. Yazawa T, Hioshi K, Ogata T. Frequent expression of HLA-DR antigen in medullary carcinoma of the breast. A possible reason for its prominenet lymphocytic infiltration and favorable prognosis. *App Immunohistochem* 1993;1:289–296.
92. Lazzaro B, Anderson AE, Kajdacsy-Balla A, et al. Antigenic characterization of medullary carcinoma of the breast: HLA-DR expression in lymph node positive cases. *Appl Immunohistochem Mol Morphol* 2001;9:234–241.
93. Naidoo P, Chetty R. Lymphoepithelioma-like carcinoma of the breast with associated sclerosing lymphocytic lobulitis. *Arch Pathol Lab Med* 2001;125:669–672.
94. Lespagnard L, Cochaux P, Larsimont D, et al. Absence of Epstein-Barr virus in medullary carcinoma of the breast as demonstrated by immunophenotyping, in situ hybridization and polymerase chain reaction. *Am J Clin Pathol* 1995;103:449–452.
95. Ahmed A. The ultrastructure of medullary carcinoma of the breast. *Virchows Arch A Pathol Anat Histol* 1980;388:175–186.
96. Harris M, Lessells AM. The ultrastructure of medullary, atypical medullary and non-medullary carcinomas of the breast. *Histopathology* 1986;10:405–414.
97. Murad TM, Scharpelli DG. The ultrastructure of medullary and scirrhous mammary duct carcinoma. *Am J Pathol* 1967;50:335–360.
98. Gould VE, Miller J, Jao W. Ultrastructure of medullary, intraductal, tubular and adenocystic breast carcinomas: comparative patterns of myoepithelial differentiation and basal lamina deposition. *Am J Pathol* 1975;78:401–408.
99. Fisher ER. Ultrastructure of the human breast and its disorders. *Am J Clin Pathol* 1975;66:291–375.
100. McDivitt RW, Stone KR, Craig RB, et al. A proposed classification of breast cancer based on kinetic information: derived from a comparison of risk factors in 168 primary operable breast cancers. *Cancer* 1986;57:269–276.
101. Bullerdiek J, Bonk U, Staats B, et al. Trisomy 18 as the first chromosome abnormality in a medullary breast cancer. *Cancer Genet Cytogenet* 1994;73:75–78.
102. Geleick D, Muller H, Matter A, et al. Cytogenetics of breast cancer. *Cancer Genet Cytogenet* 1990;46:217–229.

103. Pandis N, Heim S, Bardi G, et al. Chromosome analysis of 20 breast carcinomas: cytogenetic multiclonality and karyotypic-pathologic correlations. *Genes Chromosomes Cancer* 1993;6:51–57.
104. Osin P, Lu YJ, Stone J, et al. Distinct genetic and epigenetic changes in medullary breast cancer. *Int J Surg Pathol* 2003;11:153–158.
105. Schmitt FC, Soares R, Gobbi H, et al. Microsatellite instability in medullary breast carcinomas. *Int J Cancer* 1999;82:644–647.
106. Lee SC, Berg KD, Sherman ME, et al. Microsatellite instability is infrequent in medullary breast cancer. *Am J Clin Pathol* 2001;115: 823–827.
107. Eisinger F, Jacquemier J, Charpin C, et al. Mutations at BRCA1: the medullary breast carcinoma revisited. *Cancer Res* 1998;58: 1588–1592.
108. Marcus JN, Page DL, Watson P, et al. BRAC1 and BRAC2 hereditary breast carcinoma phenotypes. *Cancer* 1997;80:543–556.
109. Lakhani SR, Gusterson BA, Jacquemier J, et al. The pathology of familial breast cancer: histological features of cancers in families not attributable to mutations in BRCA1 or BRCA2. *Clin Cancer Res* 2000;6:782–789.
110. Consortium BCL. Pathology of familial breast cancer: differences between breast cancers in carriers of BRCA1 or BRCA2 mutations and sporadic cases. Breast Cancer Linkage Consortium. *Lancet* 1997;349:1505–1510.
111. Robson M, Gilewski T, Haas B, et al. BRCA-associated breast cancer in young women. *J Clin Oncol* 1998;16:1642–1649.
112. Verhoog LC, Brekelmans CT, Seynaeve C, et al. Survival and tumour characteristics of breast-cancer patients with germline mutations of BRCA1. *Lancet* 1998;351:316–321.
113. Malone KB, Daling JR, Ostrander EA. BRAC1 and medullary breast cancer [reply to letter]. *JAMA* 1998;280:1227–1228.
114. Osin P, Crook T, Kote J, et al. Analysis of BRCA1 gene function in medullary breast cancer. *Mod Pathol* 2000;13:43A.
115. Iau PT, Marafie M, Ali A, et al. Are medullary breast cancers an indication for BRCA1 mutation screening? A mutation analysis of 42 cases of medullary breast cancer. *Breast Cancer Res Treat* 2004;85:81–88.
116. Eisinger F, Nogues C, Birnbaum D, et al. BRCA1 and medullary breast cancer. *JAMA* 1998;280:1227–1228.
117. Esteller M, Silva JM, Dominguez G, et al. Promoter hypermethylation and BRCA1 inactivation in sporadic breast and ovarian tumors. *J Natl Cancer Inst* 2000;92:564–569.
118. Sabatier R, Finetti P, Cervera N, et al. A gene expression signature identifies two prognostic subgroups of basal breast cancer. *Breast Cancer Res Treat* 2011;126:407–420.
119. Gamel JW, Meyer JS, Feuer E, et al. The impact of stage and histology on the long-term clinical course of 163,808 patients with breast carcinoma. *Cancer* 1996;77:1459–1464.
120. Fisher ER, Kenny JP, Sass R, et al. Medullary cancer of the breast revisited. *Breast Cancer Res Treat* 1990;16:215–229.
121. Black CL, Morris DM, Goldman LI, et al. The significance of lymph node involvement in patients with medullary carcinoma of the breast. *Surg Gynecol Obstet* 1983;157:497–499.
122. Lane N, Goksel H, Salerno RA, et al. Clinico-pathologic analysis of the surgical curability of breast cancers: a minimum ten-year study of a personal series. *Ann Surg* 1961;153:483–498.
123. Vilcoq JR, Calle R, Ghossein NA. Radiosensitivity and radiocurability of medullary carcinoma of the breast (Abstract). *Inter J Radiat Oncol Biol Phys* 1980;6:1343–1344.
124. Fourquet A, Vilcoq JR, Zafrani B, et al. Medullary breast carcinoma: the role of radiotherapy as primary treatment. *Radiother Oncol* 1987;10:1–6.
125. Kurtz JM, Jacquemier J, Torhorst J, et al. Conservation therapy for breast cancers other than infiltrating ductal carcinoma. *Cancer* 1989;63:1630–1635.
126. Haffty BG, Perrotta PL, Ward B, et al. Conservatively treated breast cancer: outcome by histologic subtype. *Breast J* 1997;3:7–14.

CHAPTER 16

Carcinoma with Metaplasia and Low-Grade Adenosquamous Carcinoma

EDI BROGI

CARCINOMA WITH METAPLASIA

Because carcinoma of the breast arises from the mammary glandular epithelium, it usually exhibits the features of adenocarcinoma. However, in less than 5% of mammary carcinomas, some or all of the neoplastic cells acquire nonglandular morphology and growth pattern, evidence of a process known as metaplasia (from the Greek verb *metaplasein* = *to mold into a new form*), meaning the change of one cell type into another. Lecene[1] provided the first description of a carcinoma resembling metaplastic carcinoma in 1906. One of the earliest studies of mammary metaplastic carcinoma was published by Huvos et al.[2] in 1973.

Benign Metaplasia

Apocrine change is by far the most common forms of metaplastic change involving the mammary glandular epithelium. Squamous metaplasia can be present in the glandular epithelium of benign breast neoplasms such as papillomas and fibroadenomas, and may occur in nonneoplastic epithelial proliferations, as in benign cysts and gynecomastia. Raju[3] described squamous metaplasia that arose in hyperplastic myoepithelial cells in a fibroadenoma. Immunoreactivity for actin and vimentin was present in myoepithelial and squamous metaplastic cells, but not in normal epithelial cells. Illustrations in this case report provide convincing evidence of transition from myoepithelial to squamous cells in a benign lesion. Reparative epithelium in ducts or lobules may undergo squamous metaplasia at a healing site (Fig. 16.1).

Heterologous osseous or chondroid metaplasia may be found in radial sclerosing lesions, adenomyoepitheliomas (AMEs), sites of old fat necrosis, and, rarely, in apparently normal fatty breast tissue.[4] Chondroid and osseous metaplasia occurring in a sclerosing papilloma results in a lesion that resembles mixed tumor of the salivary glands. Chondroid, adipose, or osseous metaplasia is also very rarely encountered in the stroma of fibroadenomas.

Malignant Metaplasia

Among malignant mammary neoplasms, the term "metaplasia" has traditionally been reserved for tumors that exhibit microscopic structural changes that diverge from glandular differentiation, such as squamous, spindle cell, chondroid, and osseous morphology. These phenotypic alterations are the expression of genotypic properties that are not typical of normal mammary epithelial and myoepithelial cells, but result from a process of genetic dedifferentiation. The scientific term used for this phenomenon is "epithelial to mesenchymal transition" (EMT). (See subsequent section on genetics and molecular studies.)

The extent of metaplastic changes in breast carcinomas varies from isolated microscopic foci in an otherwise typical mammary carcinoma, to complete replacement of glandular growth by the metaplastic phenotype. The frequency of metaplastic change in mammary carcinoma is probably underreported because inconspicuous foci are easily overlooked or

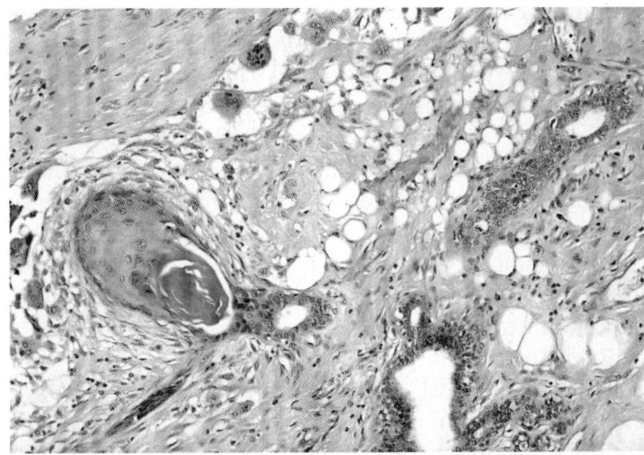

FIG. 16.1. ***Squamous metaplasia in reparative epithelium.*** Squamous metaplasia is present in the duct on the *left* in this healing biopsy site.

ignored. This limitation applies especially to spindle and squamous metaplasia. Heterologous components such as bone and cartilage seem to engender greater interest and are more likely to be noted. Fisher et al.[5] found squamous metaplasia in 3.6% of invasive carcinomas. Kaufman et al.[6] detected heterologous metaplasia in 26 (0.2%) of 12,045 breast carcinomas. Carcinomas with large central acellular zones of necrosis (also known as centrally necrotizing carcinoma) have an area of myxoid/chondroid metaplasia interposed between the necrotic/fibrotic center and the peripheral hypercellular ring of viable high-grade carcinoma.[7,8] Metaplastic changes occur more often in poorly differentiated duct carcinomas, but they may be found rarely in other types of carcinoma, including invasive lobular carcinoma and papillary tumors.

The confusing terminology used in the past to describe metaplastic carcinomas reflects the uncertainty about their histogenesis. Some lesions have been described as "mixed tumors," an unfortunate reference to tumors of the salivary glands that are predominantly benign.[9] Others have referred to metaplastic carcinomas as carcinosarcomas.[10] This term should be reserved for malignant neoplasms in which the carcinomatous and sarcomatous elements can be traced separately to epithelial and mesenchymal origins. True carcinosarcomas are extremely rare, if indeed they truly exist. In at least one case of invasive ductal carcinoma arising in a high-grade malignant phyllodes tumor (PT), the malignant epithelial and stromal components shared loss of heterozygosity (LOH) in the same regions of chromosomes 4, 11, 13, 17, and 21, in addition to other individual alterations, suggesting origin from a common precursor.[11] It has also been suggested that metaplastic carcinomas with minimal or no invasive carcinomatous component should be classified and managed as sarcomas or pseudosarcomas,[12] but this concept is not supported by histogenetic or immunohistochemical evidence.

There are no established criteria regarding the extent of metaplasia required to diagnose metaplastic carcinoma, and the extent of metaplastic component can range from about 10% to 100% of the tumor mass. Whether a carcinoma is classified as metaplastic or only as having metaplastic features, it is very important to always mention the presence and type of any metaplasia, independent of its extent.

The term "myoepithelial carcinoma" has been used for mammary spindle cell carcinomas showing myoepithelial differentiation.[13] Evidence discussed later in this chapter indicates that metaplastic spindle cell carcinomas display the myoepithelial or basal cell-like immunophenotype seen in the so-called myoepithelial carcinoma, making use of the latter term confusing and unnecessary.

Evidence of epithelial differentiation in a tumor with entirely or almost entirely metaplastic morphology includes identification of ductal carcinoma *in situ* (DCIS) and/or focal invasive carcinoma with usual morphology, and/or positive immunoreactivity for keratin and/or myoepithelial markers. Precise subclassification of carcinomas with metaplasia is rendered impractical by the extreme morphologic heterogeneity of these lesions and by the difficulty in quantifying the different morphologic components present in each tumor. A broad distinction is usually drawn between carcinomas with squamous and/or spindle cell metaplasia and carcinomas with heterologous component, such as chondromyxoid and/or osseous matrix. Metaplastic low-grade adenosquamous carcinoma (LGASC), however, shows characteristic morphology and clinical behavior and needs to be distinguished from all other metaplastic carcinomas. LGASC is discussed separately at the end of this chapter.

Clinical Presentation

Metaplastic breast carcinomas are rare tumors. Although the precise incidence is difficult to establish, 892 metaplastic carcinomas identified in the National Cancer Data Base[14] amounted to 0.24% of 365,464 breast malignant tumors diagnosed during a 3-year period (2001 to 2003), compared with 69.8% invasive ductal carcinomas.

Metaplastic carcinoma typically affects women. To the best of our knowledge, only one series has documented a case of metaplastic carcinoma in a male patient.[15] A tumor reported as triple negative metaplastic mammary carcinoma in a Pakistani male likely did not primarily arise in the breast parenchyma, as the main tumor mass appears to be too lateral in the chest wall in the image that was provided.[16]

The age range at diagnosis is similar to that of nonmetaplastic carcinomas, but women of perior postmenopausal age tend to be affected more commonly.[2,6,12,14,15,17–38] The mean age at diagnosis of metaplastic carcinoma was 61.1 years in one study,[14] with 13.5% of cases occurring in women older than 80 years and 7.8% in women younger than 40 years. About 72% to 81%[14,26] of metaplastic carcinomas occur in White women, 12% to 14% in women of African American ethnicity,[14,26] and 5%[14,32] to 11%[26] in women of Hispanic descent. Rare cases of metaplastic carcinoma have been reported in BRCA1 germline mutation carriers, including two cases with biphasic epithelial and sarcomatoid morphology[39,40] and two with chondroid metaplasia.[31] Chondroid metaplasia was also present in an atypical medullary carcinoma in a woman with BRCA1 germline mutation.[41]

The initial clinical presentation of a metaplastic carcinoma is typically as a palpable mass showing rapid growth over a short period of time.[18] Large lesions can be complicated by fixation to the skin or chest wall and skin ulceration.[20,42] Most tumors are unilateral, but one patient with bilateral metaplastic carcinoma has been described.[6] Reports of nipple discharge associated with a mass lesion are exceedingly rare.[43]

Imaging Studies

Choi and Shu[36] conducted a detailed radiologic analysis of 33 metaplastic carcinomas. The most common mammographic findings included high density (74%), circumscribed margins (59%), and oval shape (37%). Microcalcifications were present in 7 of 33 (23%) cases and were pleomorphic in 5 cases and linear or round in one case each. In some instances, calcifications may be present in DCIS rather than in the invasive metaplastic carcinoma. Mammography can also detect calcified areas in tumors with chondroid and osseous metaplasia[42,44,45] (Fig. 16.2). On sonographic examination, metaplastic carcinomas had a parallel orientation (97%),

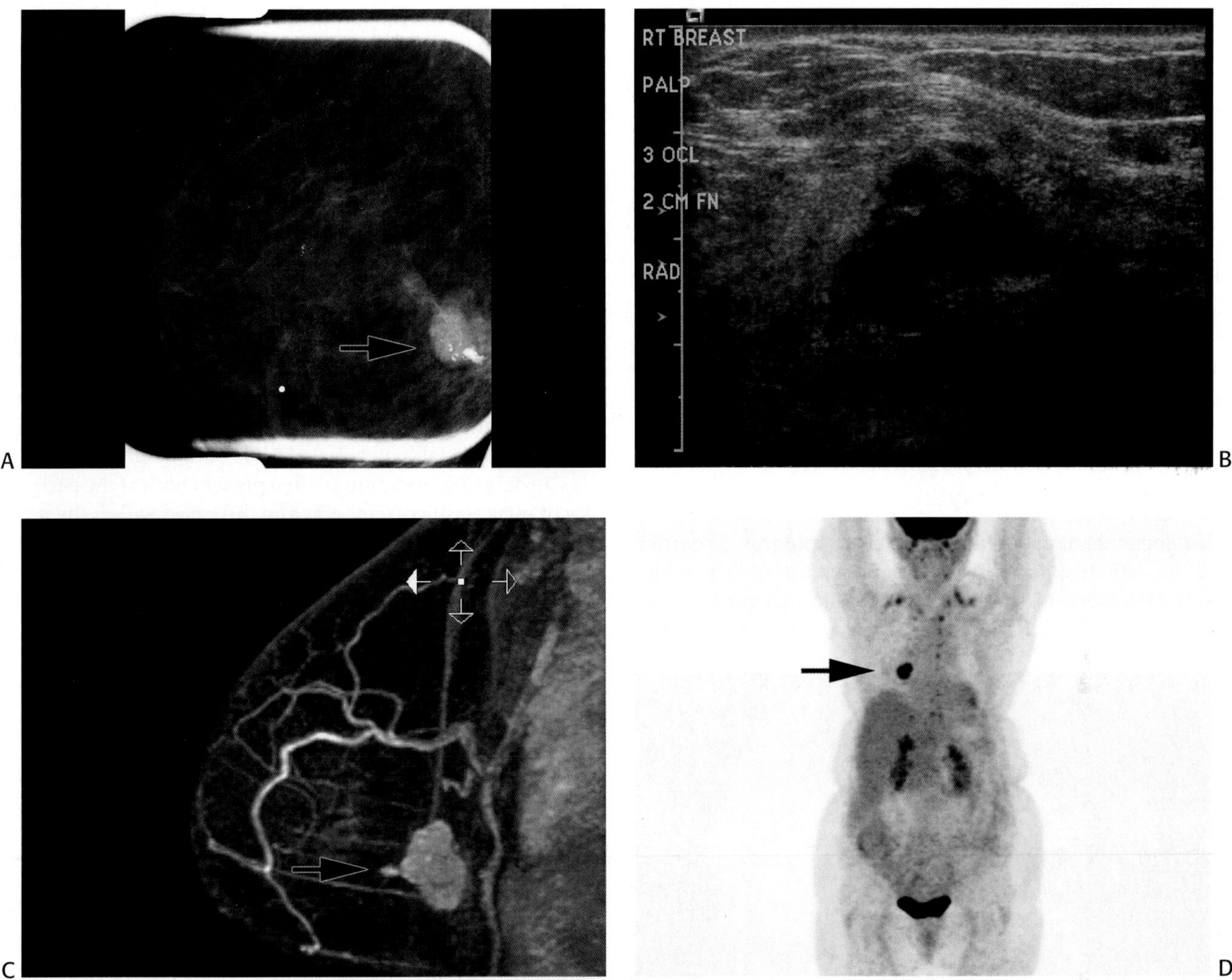

FIG. 16.2. ***Metaplastic carcinoma, imaging studies.*** All images are of the same metaplastic carcinoma in the right breast of a 66-year-old woman with history of ipsilateral invasive ductal carcinoma 20 years earlier treated with conservation therapy and contralateral invasive ductal carcinoma diagnosed 1 year earlier. Metaplastic carcinoma was a new independent primary carcinoma in the right breast. **A:** Spot compression mammographic view in the mediolateral oblique projection demonstrates a 2.6-cm high-density, irregular mass with coarse and pleomorphic calcifications in the posterior right breast. **B:** The sonogram shows an irregular, indistinct, and hypoechoic mass in the right breast with internal echogenic foci representing calcifications. **C:** The subtracted T1-weighted contrast-enhanced MRI demonstrates an irregular heterogeneously enhancing mass in the posterior breast near the chest wall. **D:** A maximal intensity projection image from F^{18}-fluorodeoxyglucose PET scan reveals intense hypermetabolism in the tumor (*arrow*) and an otherwise normal physiologic distribution of radiotracer. (All images courtesy of Kimberly Feigin M.D., Memorial Sloan-Kettering Cancer Center.)

complex echogenicity (81%), irregular shape (59.4%), posterior acoustic enhancement (50%), and a microlobulated margin (41%)[36] (Fig. 16.2). The most common magnetic resonance imaging (MRI) findings included an irregular heterogeneous enhancing mass (Fig. 16.2), with irregular shape (52.4%) and margin (57%), and high T2-weighted signal intensity (57%).[36] The latter feature has been correlated with the presence of necrosis[44] and with chondroid areas.[45] Choi and Shu[36] found heterogeneous internal enhancement in 71% of cases of metaplastic carcinoma, with delayed washout pattern on kinetic curve analysis in 67% of cases. Intense uptake of technetium 99m-methylene diphosphonate was observed in mammary carcinomas with osseous sarcomatoid metaplasia.[45–47] The tumors are highly metabolic on F^{18}-fluorodeoxyglucose positron emission tomography (PET) (Fig. 16.2).

Gross Pathology

The reported size of metaplastic mammary carcinomas ranges from 0.5 to 24 cm.[2,6,12,14,18–25,27,28,31,34,48] The mean or median sizes (3 to 4 cm) in various series tend to be greater than those of ordinary carcinomas, including triple negative breast carcinomas.[35] In one study, the median size of metaplastic spindle cell carcinomas and of carcinomas with areas of spindle cell metaplasia were 5.2 and 5.5 cm, respectively, and both measurements were substantially larger than the median size of all metaplastic carcinomas combined (3.7 cm).[23] In the study by Pezzi et al.,[14] 29.5% of 892 metaplastic carcinomas were T1 tumors, 49.6% T2 tumors, and 20.4% were T4 tumors. The majority of tumors are described as firm to hard, nodular, and circumscribed, but some lesions have infiltrative borders (Fig. 16.3). Degenerated cystic areas can be encountered, especially in tumors with squamous metaplasia.[18,49] Hemorrhagic areas can be seen in metaplastic carcinomas with choriocarcinomatous morphology, as well as in tumors with abnormal vascularity (Fig. 16.4).

Microscopic Pathology

Histologic examination of the excised tumor is required for the definitive diagnosis of metaplastic carcinoma. It has been customary to subdivide metaplastic carcinomas into two categories: *carcinomas with squamous and/or spindle cell metaplasia* and *carcinomas with heterologous metaplasia* that have a mesenchymal phenotype, including chondroid and osseous metaplasia. This distinction is not applicable to all metaplastic carcinomas because some tumors exhibit more than one type of growth. The most common combined configuration includes squamous and undifferentiated spindle cell areas, sometimes with a storiform pattern.[20,50,51] Chondroid or osseous metaplasia rarely coexists with squamous metaplasia.[52]

DCIS is present adjacent to metaplastic carcinoma in 11%[6] to 65%[17] of cases and usually, but not always, has high or intermediate nuclear grade (Figs. 16.4 and 16.5). The presence of DCIS strongly supports the diagnosis of metaplastic carcinoma. Rarely, lobular carcinoma *in situ* (LCIS) or atypical ductal hyperplasia (ADH) can be present.

Chronic inflammation is often present both at the periphery of metaplastic carcinomas and dispersed within the neoplasm (Fig. 16.6). A moderate inflammatory cell infiltrate consisting of mature lymphocytes is especially common in carcinomas with squamous and spindle cell metaplasia, but

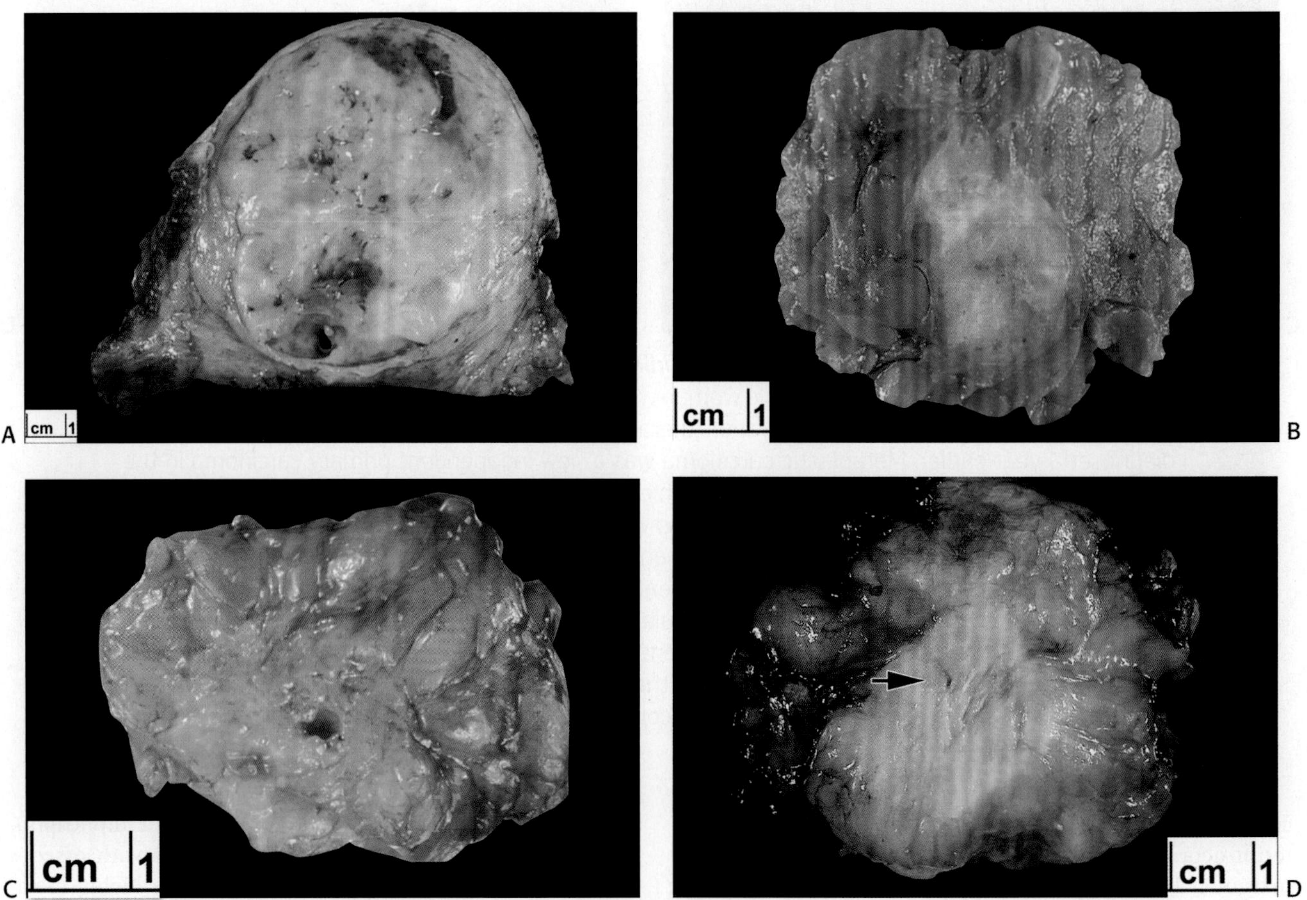

FIG. 16.3. ***Metaplastic carcinoma, gross appearance.*** **A:** The circumscribed fleshy tumor has a cystic area and hemorrhagic foci of angiosarcomatous metaplasia. **B:** A circumscribed carcinoma with spindle cell and squamous metaplasia has a dense, fibrous-appearing cut surface. **C:** Metaplastic carcinoma, spindle cell, and squamous type with cyst formation. **D:** The cut surface of a metaplastic spindle cell carcinoma is densely fibrous and relatively well circumscribed from the adjacent tissue. A hemorrhagic focus marks a prior biopsy site (*arrow*).

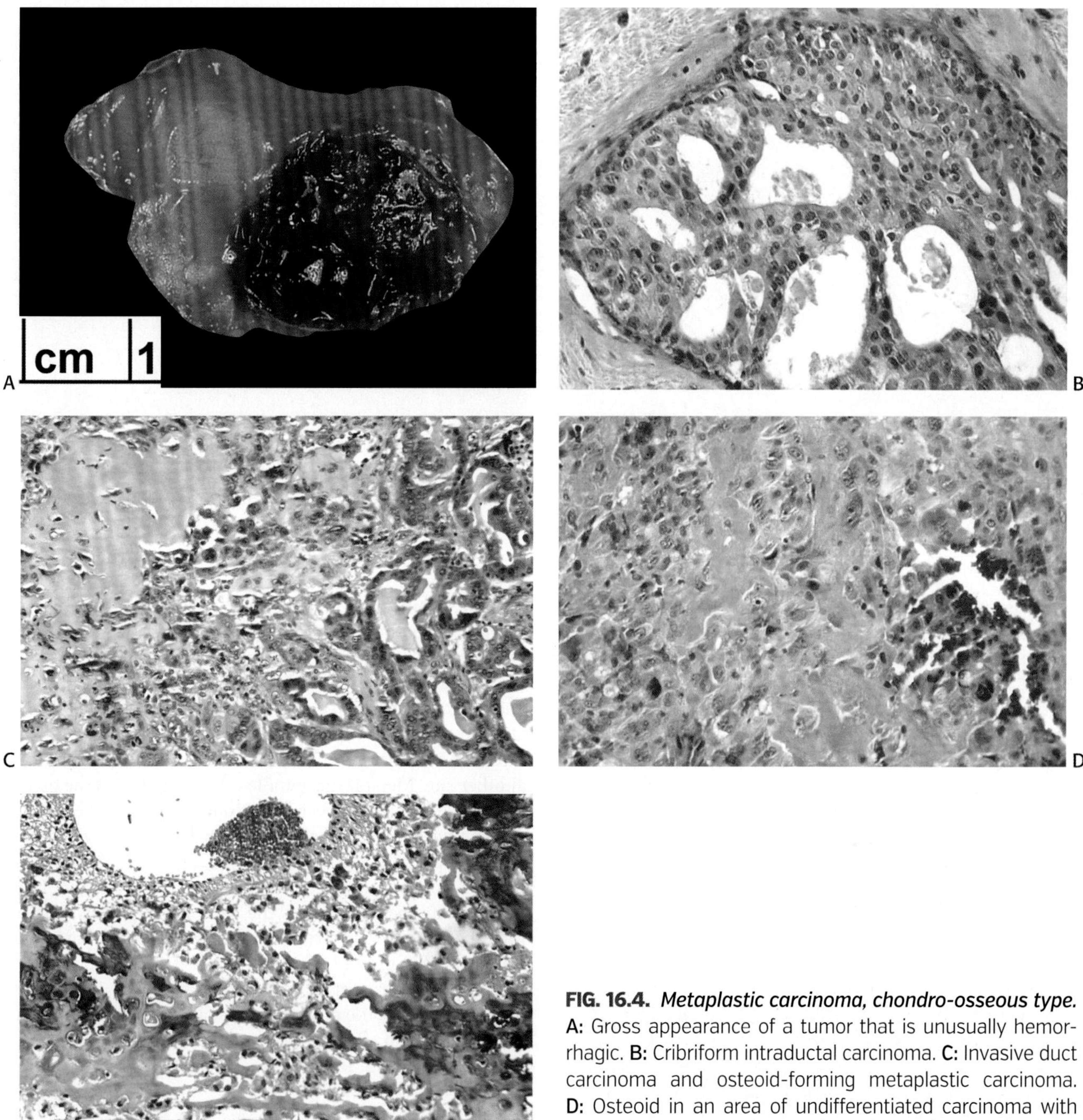

FIG. 16.4. ***Metaplastic carcinoma, chondro-osseous type.*** **A:** Gross appearance of a tumor that is unusually hemorrhagic. **B:** Cribriform intraductal carcinoma. **C:** Invasive duct carcinoma and osteoid-forming metaplastic carcinoma. **D:** Osteoid in an area of undifferentiated carcinoma with hemorrhage. **E:** Neoplastic ossified cartilage and a dilated vascular space suggestive of telangiectatic osteosarcoma.

is also found in carcinomas with heterologous elements. This is such a frequent feature that a diagnosis of metaplastic carcinoma should rarely be made when little or no inflammation is present.

Spindle Cell Metaplastic Carcinomas (with or without Squamous Metaplasia)

Metaplastic carcinomas with spindle cell (with or without squamous metaplasia) may show a variety of histologic appearances, depending on the proportions of the spindle cell and squamous components. The terminology used here to refer to these tumors is purely descriptive, but it is helpful to summarize their morphologic features. Metaplastic carcinomas consisting entirely of squamous metaplasia are discussed in Chapter 17.

Metaplastic Carcinoma with Spindle Cell Metaplasia (Intermediate or High Grade)

These tumors are a subset of carcinomas in which most or all of the neoplasm has assumed a pseudosarcomatous, spindle cell growth pattern that resembles fibrosarcoma.[18,51,53] In the

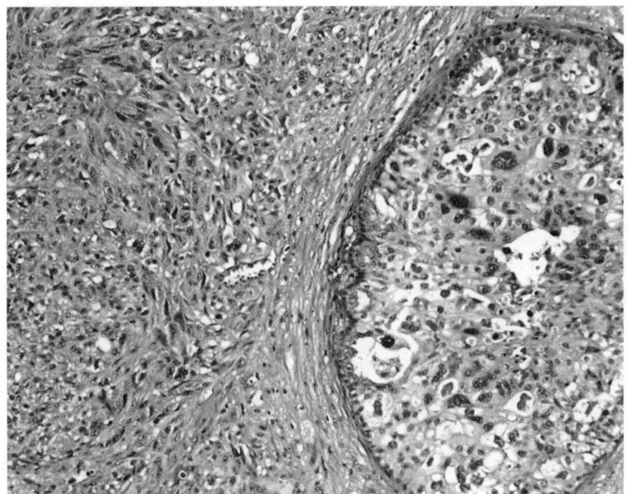

FIG. 16.5. ***Metaplastic spindle cell carcinoma and DCIS.*** High-grade metaplastic sarcomatoid spindle cell carcinoma is adjacent to a duct involved by solid DCIS with high nuclear grade and focal necrosis.

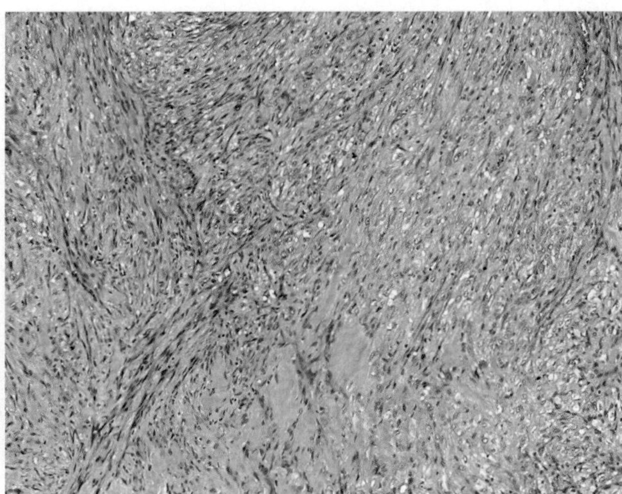

FIG. 16.7. ***Metaplastic carcinoma, spindle cell type.*** The tumor is composed of a dense proliferation of atypical spindle cells. A sclerotic focus is present (*lower center*).

latter instance, the distinction between spindle cell carcinoma and primary sarcoma of the breast can be difficult, and the neoplasm might be mistaken for fibrosarcoma or malignant fibrous histiocytoma (MFH) because of the minimal epithelial component and a storiform growth pattern (Fig. 16.7).[20,52] The tumor border can be infiltrative or pushing (Fig. 16.8). These lesions usually show moderate to high cellularity. The neoplastic spindle cells have moderate- to high-grade nuclear atypia. Mitoses are easily identified and usually numerous. Large areas of necrosis may be present, especially in cellular tumors with high nuclear grade (Fig. 16.9). Extensive sampling sometimes identifies focal areas of squamous differentiation (Fig. 16.10) or foci of DCIS (Figs. 16.4 and 16.5) or invasive adenocarcinoma not otherwise specified (NOS), but in most cases the invasive tumor shows no obvious epithelial elements. If present, squamous foci tend to be located at the tumor periphery. All histologic, immunohistochemical, and clinical features of a lesion must be taken into consideration to distinguish spindle cell metaplastic carcinoma from sarcoma, whether primary in the breast or metastatic from another site. Metaplastic spindle cell carcinoma of the breast typically grows in between nonneoplastic ducts and lobules, entrapping native mammary epithelial elements within the tumor, especially at its periphery (Fig. 16.11). This growth pattern differs from that of a metastatic spindle cell neoplasm of extramammary origin, as the latter typically destroys the mammary epithelial structures, without entrapping them. Rarely DCIS is present admixed with metaplastic spindle cell carcinoma.[54] Carter et al.[54] found DCIS in 4/29 (14%) cases. More commonly, the residual mammary ducts at the periphery of the lesion show gynecomastoid ductal hyperplasia of the usual type (Fig. 16.11).

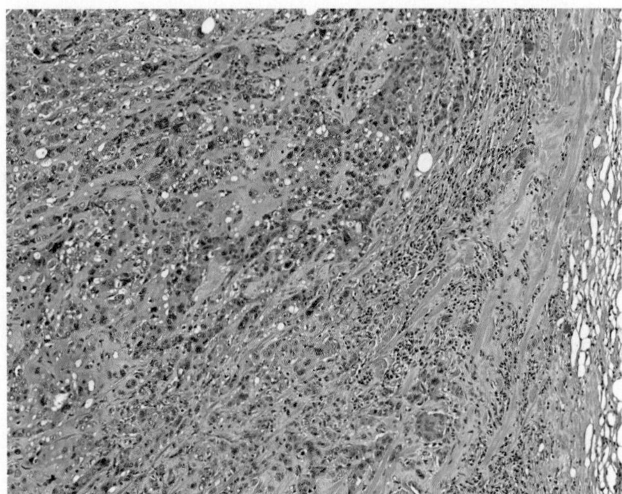

FIG. 16.6. ***Inflammation around metaplastic carcinoma.*** Many lymphocytes are clustered at the periphery of this metaplastic carcinoma with chondroid matrix. A few small lymphocytes are also sprinkled throughout the tumor.

Metaplastic Spindle Cell Carcinoma with "Low-Grade" or "Fibromatosis-Like" Pattern

Some metaplastic spindle cell carcinomas have dense, keloid-like areas of fibrosis in which the spindle cells display a storiform pattern (Fig. 16.12). Tumor cellularity is heterogeneous. Closely juxtaposed hypercellular and hypocellular areas are admixed with areas of collagenous fibrosis that can be extensive and deceivingly hypocellular or nearly acellular, especially in the center of the tumor. The neoplastic cells are organized in short interlacing fascicles with haphazard arrangement (Fig. 16.13). The cells tend to be inconspicuous and have ill-defined cell borders, no obvious cytoplasm, and elongated nuclei. Focally, the spindle cells display epithelioid morphology and have slightly more abundant and/or denser cytoplasm. The cells often line up, forming short arrays and chords that may superficially resemble small blood vessels,

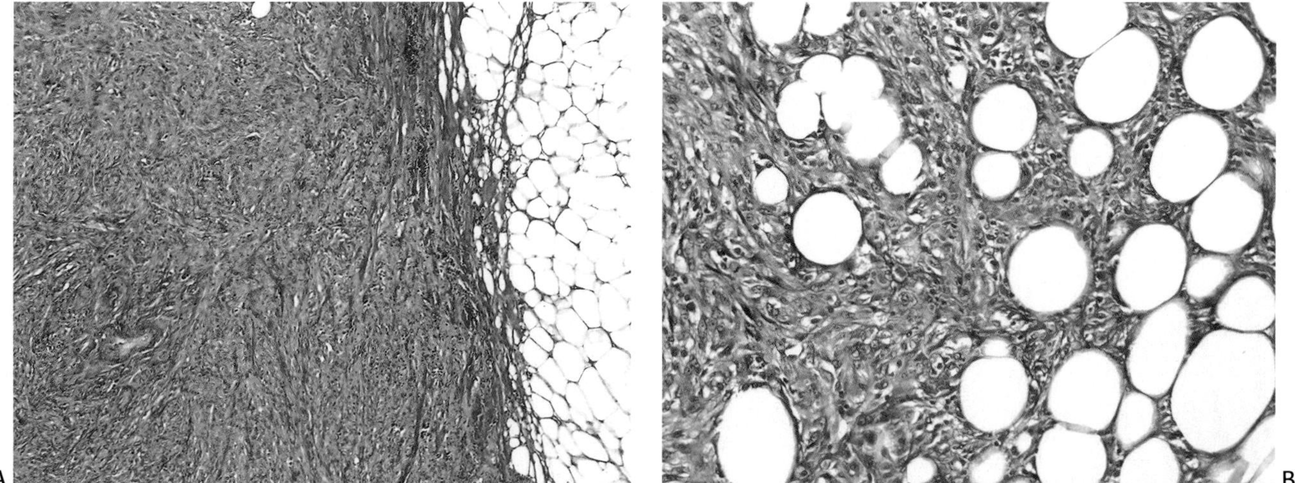

FIG. 16.8. ***Metaplastic spindle cell carcinoma, lesion border.*** **A:**The tumor has a relatively well-circumscribed interface with the surrounding tissue. **B:** Invasion of fat at the border of a metaplastic spindle cell mammary carcinoma.

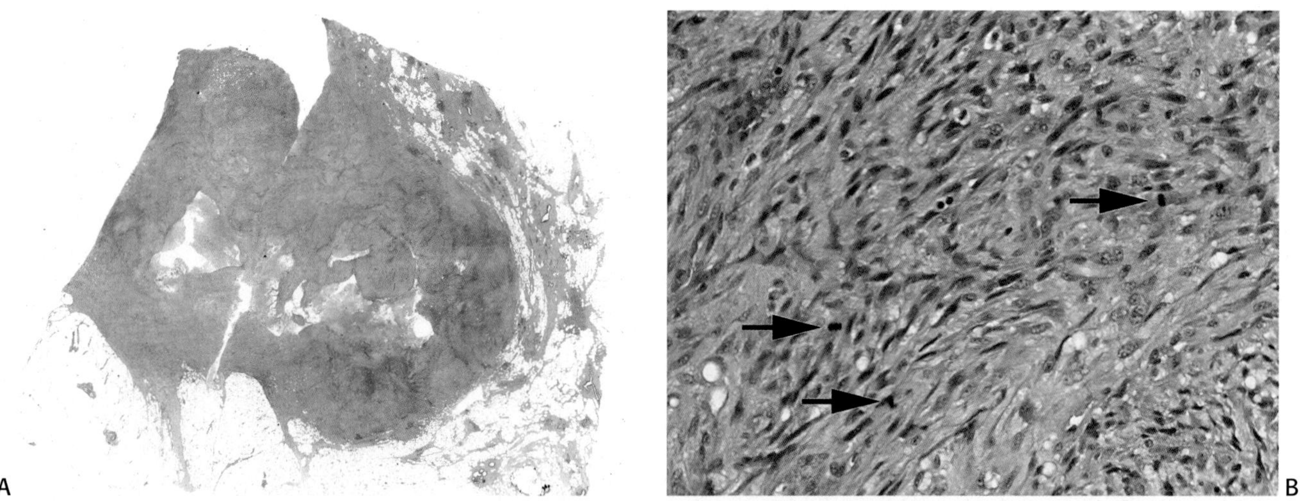

FIG. 16.9. ***Metaplastic spindle cell carcinoma, necrosis and cavitation.*** **A:**The carcinoma forms a discrete nodular mass that is well circumscribed. The center of the tumor is necrotic and partially cystic. **B:** Closer inspection reveals a solid cellular proliferation of neoplastic spindle cells with intermediate to high nuclear atypia. Mitoses are easily identified (*arrows*).

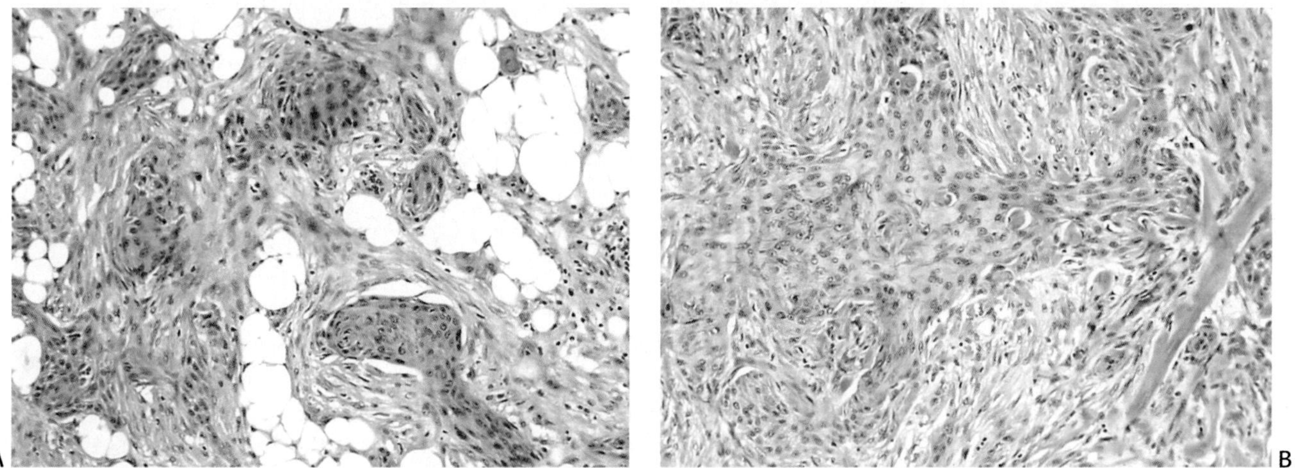

FIG. 16.10. ***Metaplastic carcinoma, spindle and squamous.*** **A:** Infiltrating carcinoma in fat showing transition from squamous to spindle cell metaplasia. **B:** The central stellate squamous area, less well differentiated than in **(A)**, blends imperceptibly with the surrounding spindle cell element.

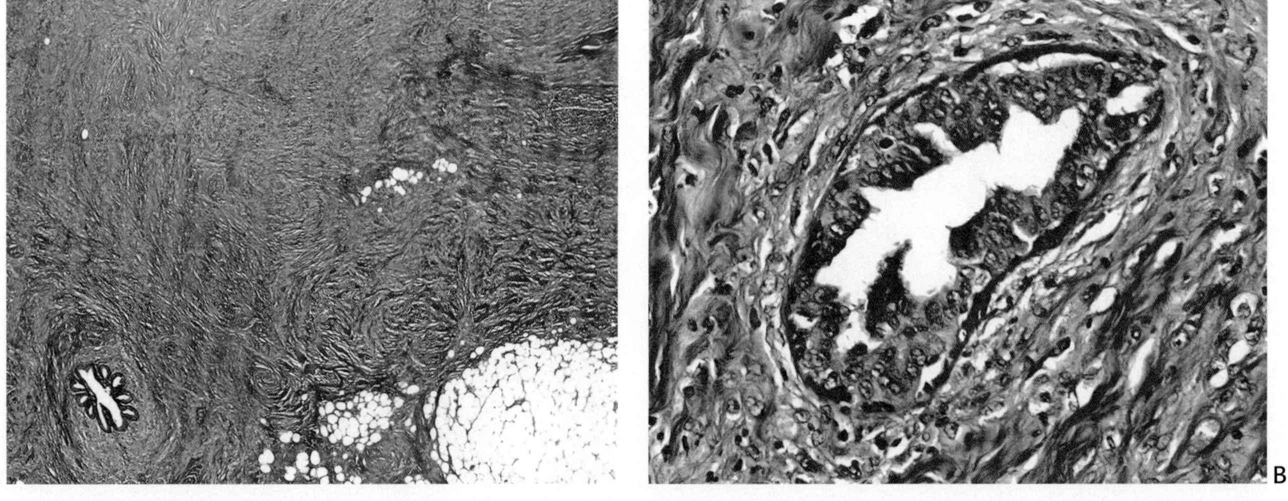

FIG. 16.11. ***Metaplastic spindle cell carcinoma, with ducts entrapped at the tumor periphery.*** **A:** A residual benign duct is present at the periphery of a metaplastic spindle cell carcinoma, a feature usually not found in metastatic sarcoma. Note storiform tumor growth on the *right*. **B:** A benign duct at the periphery of the tumor exhibits usual ductal hyperplasia with gynecomastoid morphology.

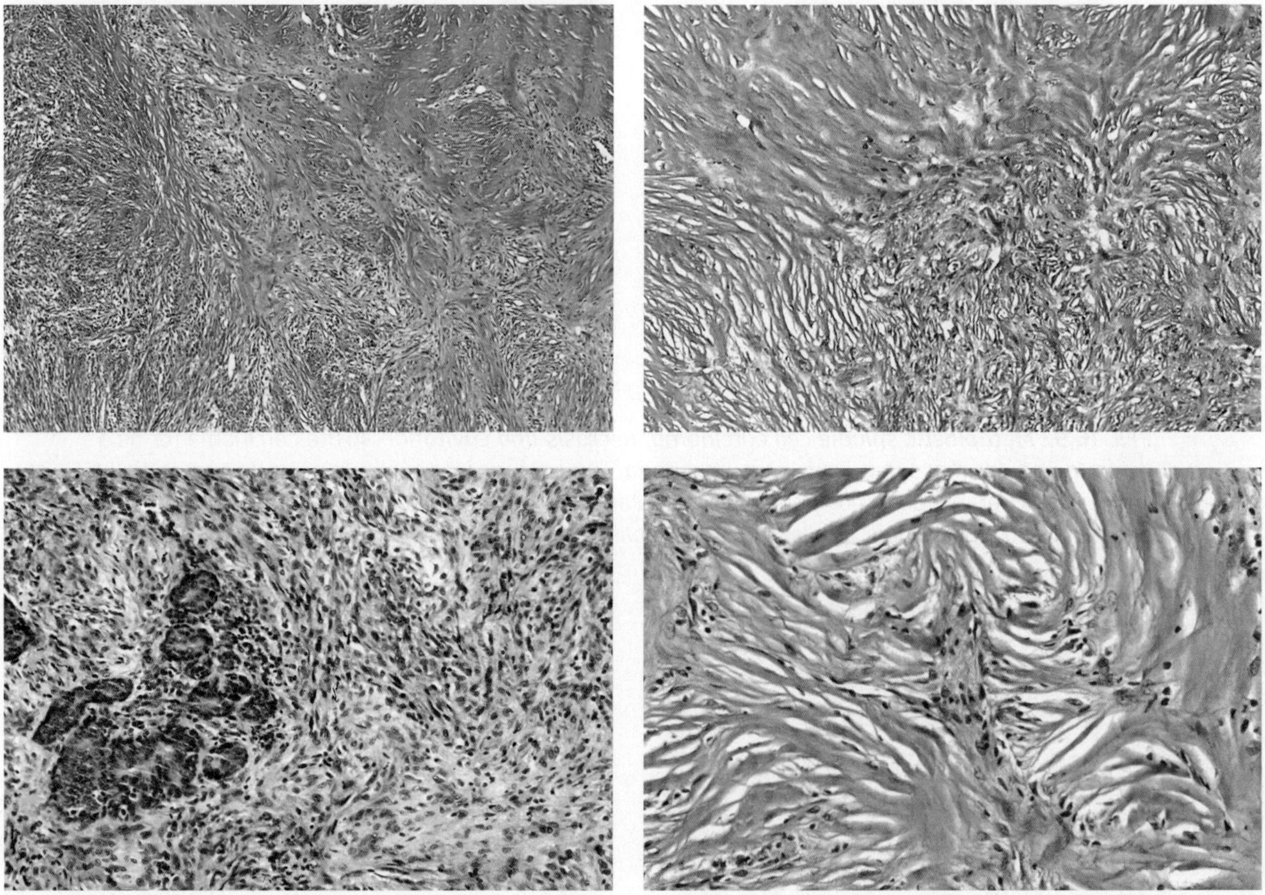

FIG. 16.12. ***Metaplastic carcinoma, spindle cell keloidal type.*** **A:** Cellular spindle cell growth with scattered lymphocytes merges with a collagenized keloidal area on the *right*. **B:** Magnified view of the junction between the cellular storiform and keloidal components. **C:** Magnified view of the spindle cell storiform component next to a lobule. **D:** Storiform structure in the keloidal area is shown. **E:** The immunostain for 34βE12 (K903) shows strong reactivity in the cellular region. A small squamous nodule is stained in the keloidal area (*arrow*). **F:** Closely juxtaposed hypercellular and hypocellular areas characterize this needle core biopsy sample from a metaplastic spindle cell carcinoma with "low-grade" "fibromatosis-like" morphology.

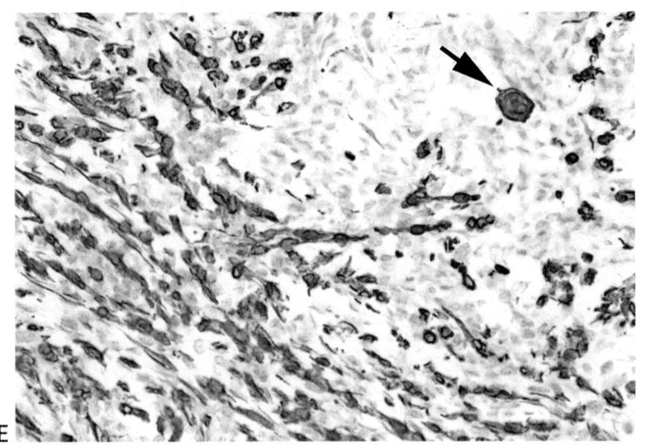

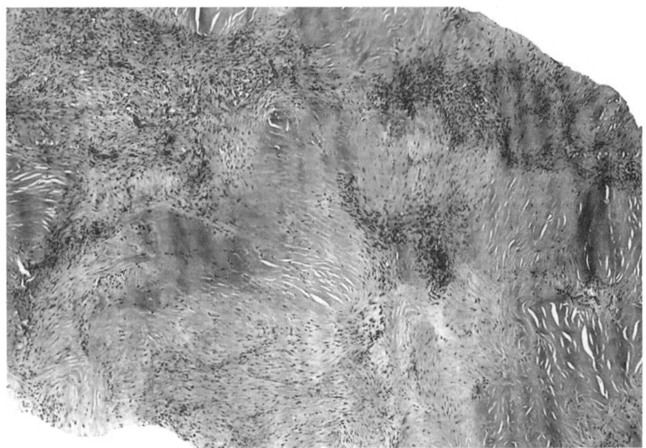

FIG. 16.12. *(Continued)*

but are not associated with red blood cells. These epithelioid foci usually display positive immunoreactivity for cytokeratins (CKs). Tissue sections containing these areas should be actively selected for immunohistochemical analysis, as CK positivity can be focal (Fig. 16.13). Closer examination discloses atypical cells characterized by nuclear enlargement and hyperchromasia. The nuclear atypia is usually focal and never of high grade. Mitotic activity tends to be low, ranging from

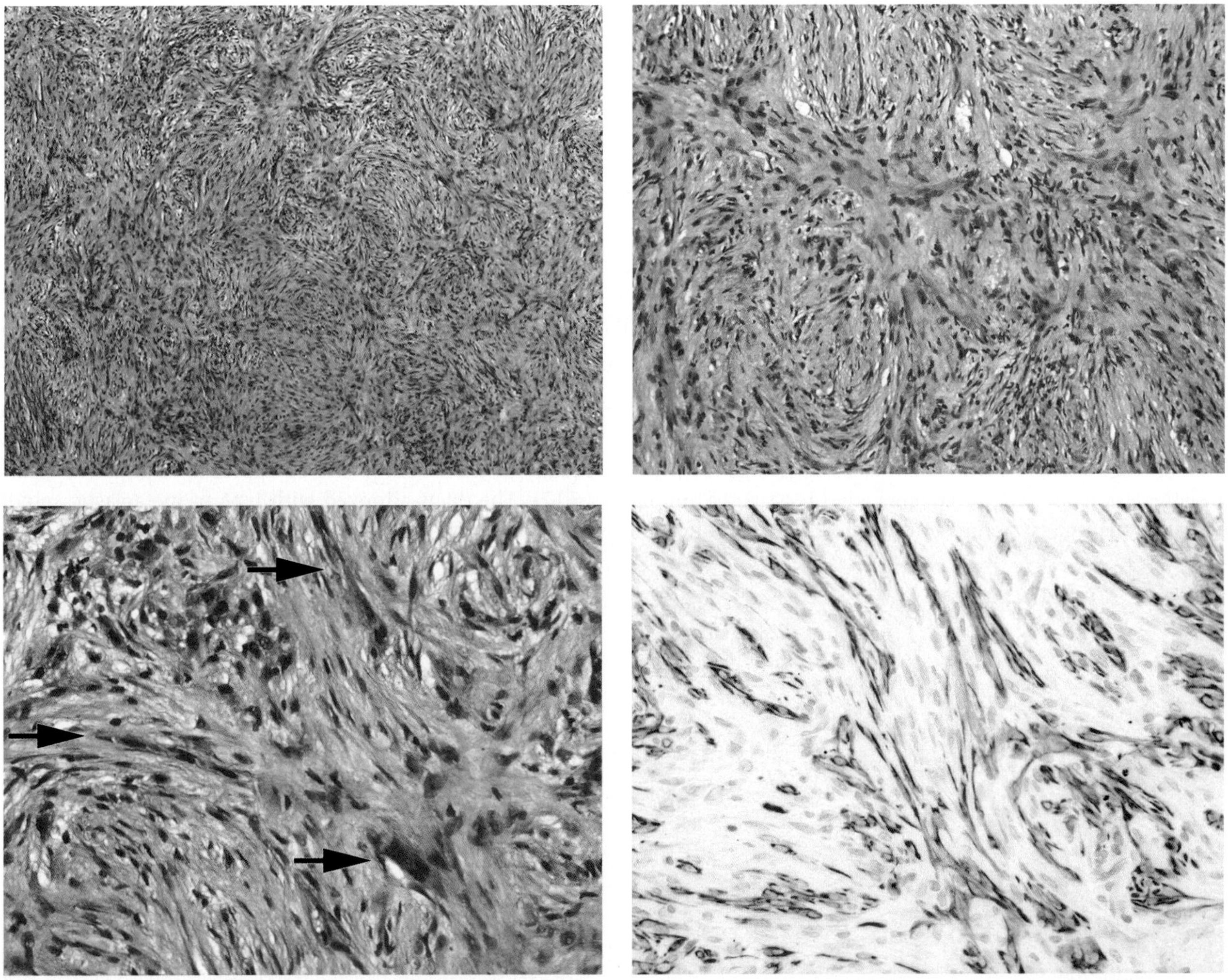

FIG. 16.13. ***Metaplastic spindle cell carcinoma, "low-grade" "fibromatosis-like" type.*** **A:** The tumor consists of short fascicles of atypical spindle cells with a storiform arrangement. **B,C:** Tumor cells focally acquire denser and more eosinophilic cytoplasm and are arranged in a storiform pattern with "epithelioid clusters" (*arrows*). **D:** The neoplastic spindle cells are immunoreactive for keratin 34βE12.

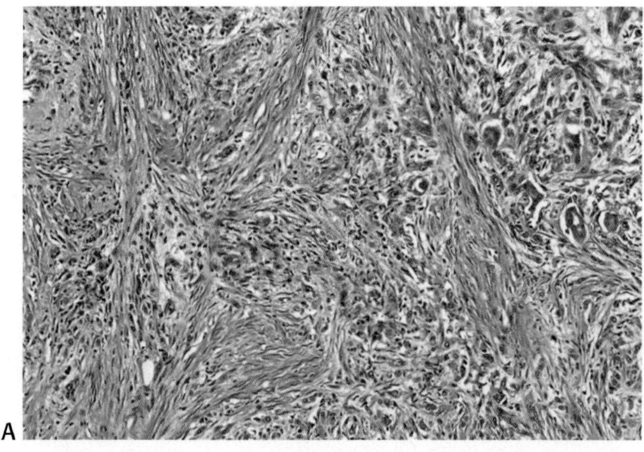

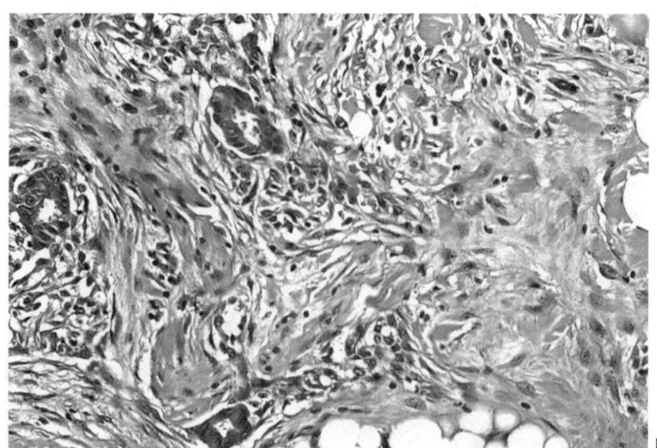

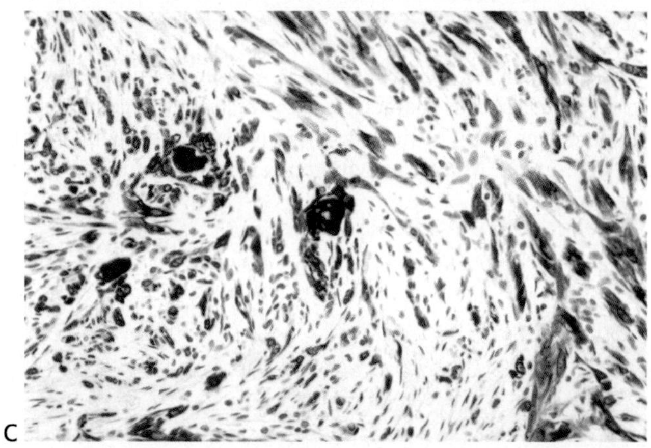

FIG. 16.14. ***Metaplastic carcinoma, spindle cell type with adenocarcinoma.*** **A:** The spindle cell neoplasm has a storiform pattern. Small carcinomatous glands are present (*upper right*). **B:** Well-differentiated adenocarcinoma in the spindle cell metaplastic carcinoma. **C:** CK7 reactivity is shown in glandular and spindle cells.

less than two mitoses per 10 high-power fields (HPFs) in most cases to three to five mitoses per 10 HPFs.[50,55] Atypia and mitoses are more obvious in the cellular areas. Foci of chronic inflammation are scattered throughout the carcinoma and at its periphery. In some cases, inflammation can be extensive and nearly mask the true nature of the tumor, raising the differential diagnosis of inflammatory pseudotumor or fasciitis. The latter lesions are very infrequent in the breast, and a tumor suggesting mammary fasciitis or inflammatory pseudotumor almost invariably proves to be metaplastic carcinoma. If invasive carcinoma with epithelial morphology is present, this should not represent more than 5% of the tumor mass.[50,55] Associated invasive epithelial carcinoma needs to have low-grade cytologic atypia[50,55] (Fig. 16.14) and can consist of invasive lobular carcinoma[22] (Fig. 16.15). Rarely, focal low-grade squamous morphology can be appreciated (Figs. 16.16 and 16.17). The ducts admixed with type of metaplastic spindle cell carcinoma may harbor low-grade DCIS,[50,55] LCIS,[55]

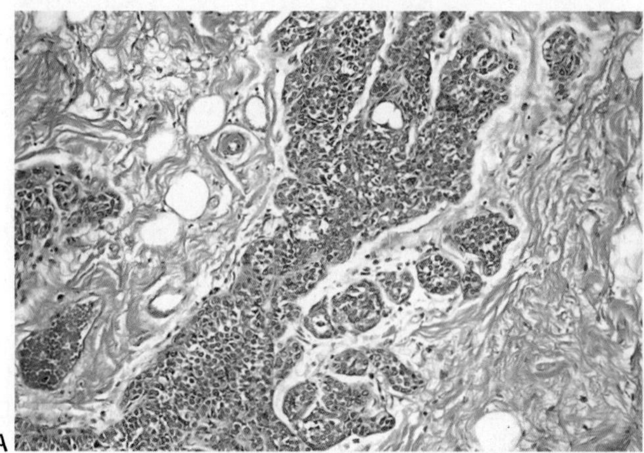

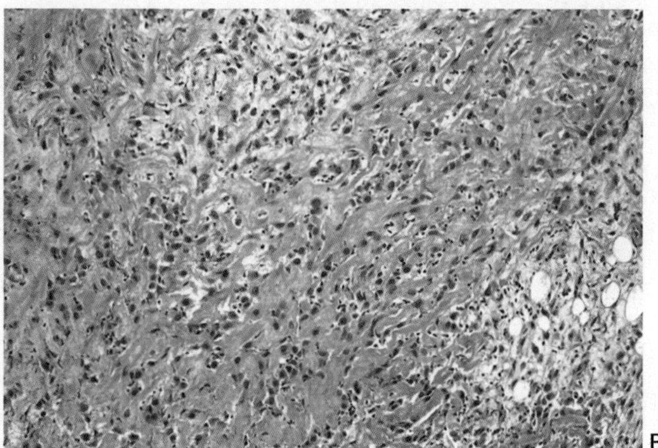

FIG. 16.15. ***Metaplastic carcinoma, spindle cell type with invasive lobular carcinoma.*** All images are from the same specimen. **A:**LCIS in a duct and lobular glands. **B:** Invasive lobular carcinoma, classical type. **C:** Spindle cell metaplastic carcinoma with focal squamous differentiation. **D:** Pseudoangiomatous metaplastic growth pattern.

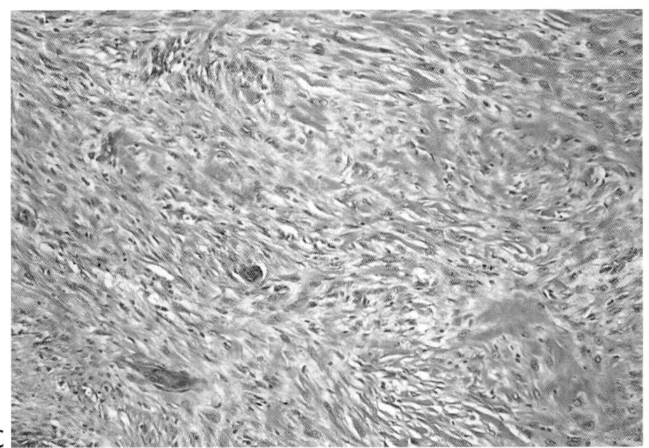

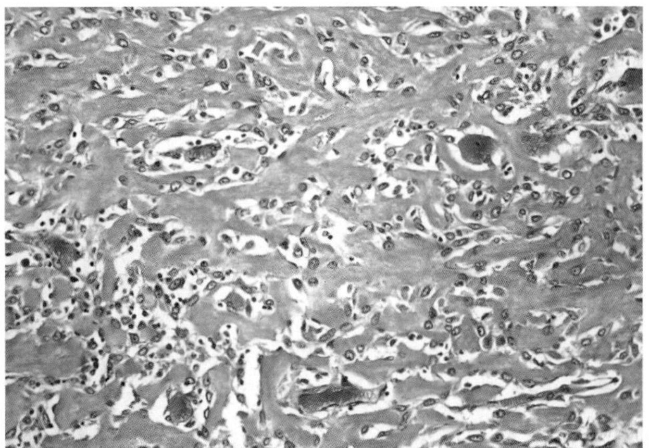

FIG. 16.15. *[Continued]*

(Fig. 16.15), or ADH,[22,50] but often show mild ductal hyperplasia of the gynecomastoid type, devoid of atypia.

Metaplastic spindle cell carcinomas with deceptively bland morphology have been described in association with papillomas[55,56] (Fig. 16.18), complex sclerosing lesions (CSLs), and nipple adenomas.[57,58] In these cases, presenting symptoms may include a mass lesion and/or nipple discharge.[57] Metaplastic spindle cell carcinomas with this morphology are referred to as "fibromatosis-like"[50] or "low-grade."[55] Despite having relatively bland morphology, these neoplasms are malignant and can metastasize to distant sites, especially to the lungs, and few patients have died of disease.[22,54,55] Nonetheless, metaplastic spindle cell carcinomas with "low-grade" "fibromatosis-like" morphology seem to be not as rapidly aggressive as metaplastic spindle cell carcinomas with intermediate- or high-grade morphology.

Metaplastic Carcinoma with Pseudoangiomatous/ Acantholytic Pattern

An unusual variant of mammary carcinoma with spindle and squamous metaplasia has been characterized as pseudoangiomatous or acantholytic carcinoma.[59–61] The acantholytic

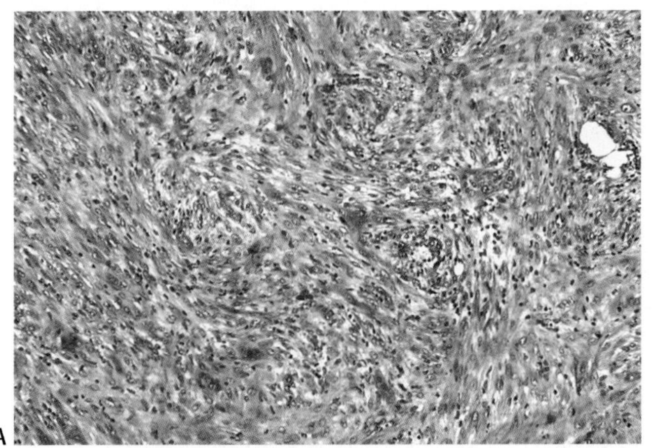

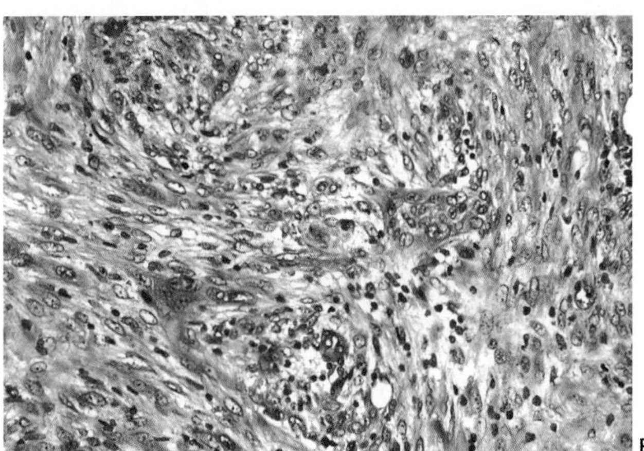

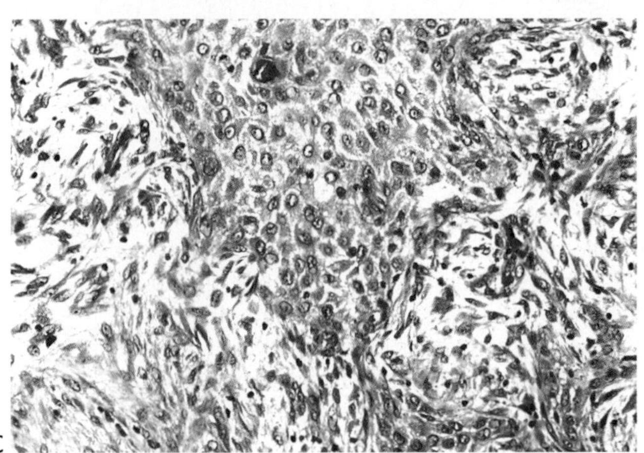

FIG. 16.16. ***Metaplastic carcinoma, spindle and squamous type.*** This specimen is from a subareolar tumor that caused nipple retraction in an 84-year-old woman. **A,B:** The malignant spindle cell neoplasm has a storiform pattern and a sprinkling of lymphocytes. **C:** Squamous differentiation in the carcinoma.

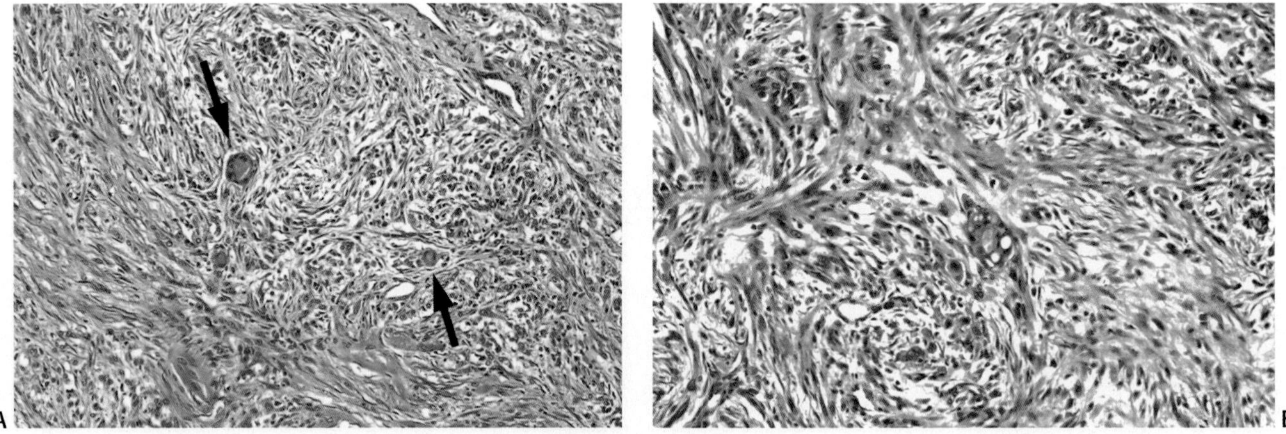

FIG. 16.17. ***Metaplastic carcinoma, spindle and squamous type.*** **A:** Small round groups of squamous cells (*arrows*) are the only evidence of epithelial differentiation in this spindle cell storiform neoplasm. Lymphocytes are scattered throughout the tumor (*lower center*). **B:** Magnified view of a squamous cell cluster blending with spindle cells.

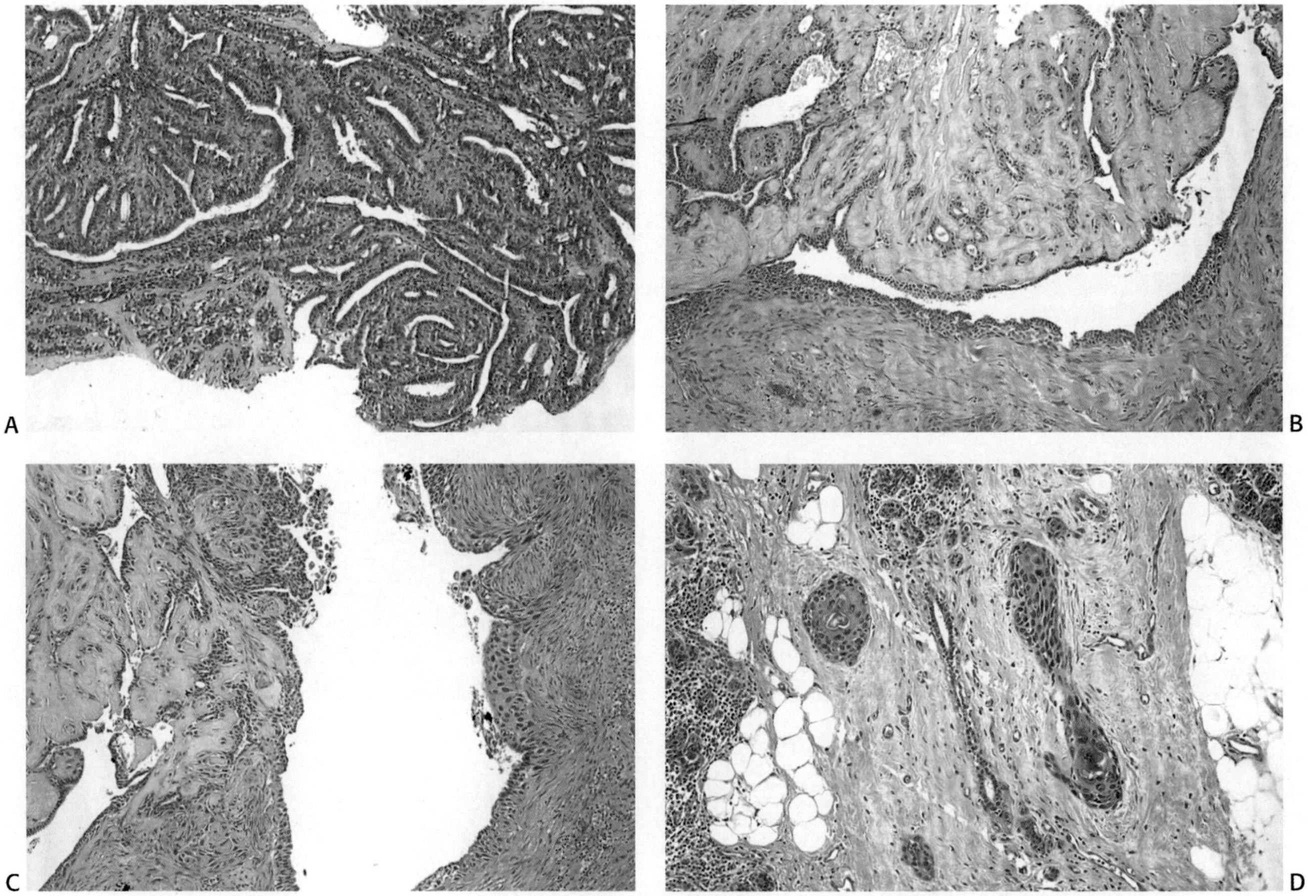

FIG. 16.18. ***Metaplastic carcinoma arising in cystic papilloma.*** All images are from the same patient. **A:** This needle core biopsy sample shows a papilloma at the site of an 8-mm mass. Surgical excision was not performed. Follow-up mammography revealed an enlarging lesion at the same site about 1 year later. **B:** The excised specimen contained a sclerotic cystic papilloma. **C:** Spindle and squamous metaplastic carcinoma appeared to arise from squamous differentiation of the surface epithelium of the cyst (*right*), shown here with the underlying spindle cell carcinoma. **D:** Invasive squamous carcinoma surrounding the papillary lesion.

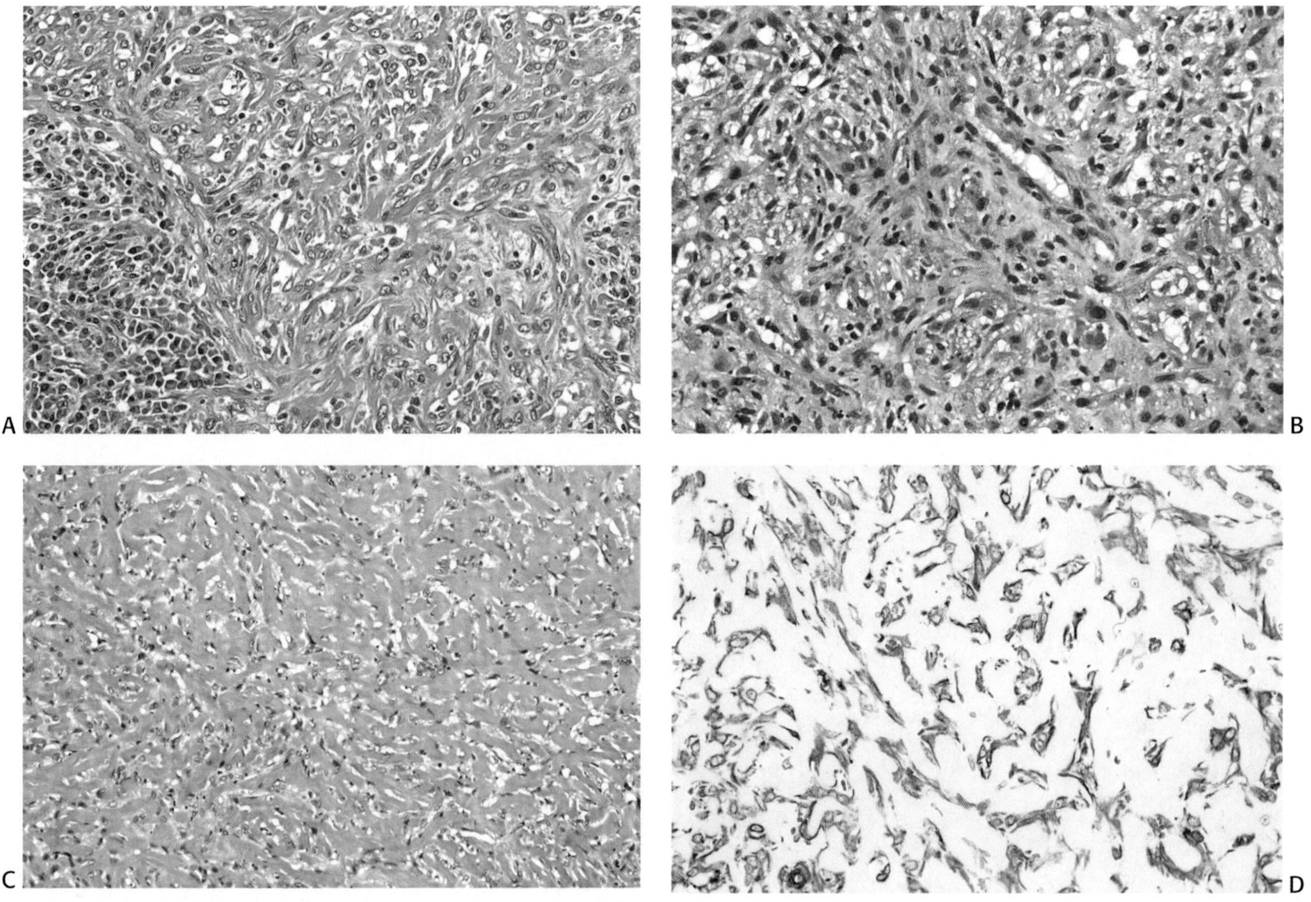

FIG. 16.19. ***Metaplastic carcinoma, acantholytic.*** **A,B:** Ill-defined spaces are formed in this relatively compact tumor. Note the collection of plasma cells (*left*) in **(A)**. **C:** A more fully developed pseudoangiomatous tumor. **D:** The immunostain for 34βE12 (K903) highlights the pseudoangiomatous structure.

appearance is due to degeneration of the neoplastic epithelial component embedded in abundant spindle cell stroma (Fig. 16.19), resulting in a pattern of complex anastomosing pseudovascular spaces[62] (Fig. 16.20). The cells lining these spaces are immunoreactive for CKs and do not stain for factor VIII or CD34. Spindle cell and acantholytic variants of metaplastic carcinoma are almost always immunoreactive with the high molecular weight CK 34βE12 (K903) (Figs. 16.19 and 16.20), even when other CK markers are negative. Positive reactivity for CK5, a basal CK, has also been reported.[61]

Metaplastic High-Grade Adenosquamous Carcinoma

A common pattern of metaplastic carcinoma is focal squamous metaplasia in an otherwise typical invasive ductal carcinoma (Fig. 16.21). When squamous metaplasia is the predominant pattern, a spectrum of differentiation may be found. Mature keratinizing epithelium, sometimes with keratohyaline granules, as well as adenocarcinoma can be associated with transitions to spindle cell, pseudosarcomatous areas. In unusual instances, the adenocarcinomatous component mingles with the metaplastic carcinomatous epithelium, sometimes with a pagetoid distribution. The term "high-grade adenosquamous carcinoma" is often used for tumors showing both squamous and glandular components with moderate to high cellularity and nuclear atypia (Fig. 16.22), in contrast to LGASC that is described at the end of this chapter. Mitotic activity is usually moderate to high, and areas of necrosis may be present.

Differential Diagnosis of Metaplastic Carcinoma with Spindle Cells (with or without Squamous Morphology)

The differential diagnosis of metaplastic carcinoma with spindle cells (with or without squamous morphology) includes PT, fibrosarcoma, and high-grade pleomorphic sarcoma. The differential diagnosis of "low-grade" metaplastic spindle cell carcinoma includes fibromatosis and nodular fasciitis.

The presence of leaf-like fronds lined by glandular epithelium is characteristic of PT. Occasionally, stromal cells in PT may show focal positivity for CK,[63] and this finding can be misleading, especially when only limited material is available for diagnosis. Even in the presence of focal CK staining in needle core biopsy material, a malignant lesion with exclusively spindle cell morphology and no overt epithelial component or frond-like architecture should always be classified with caution, including metaplastic spindle cell carcinoma and high-grade malignant PT in the differential diagnosis. The identification of a rare stromal frond focally

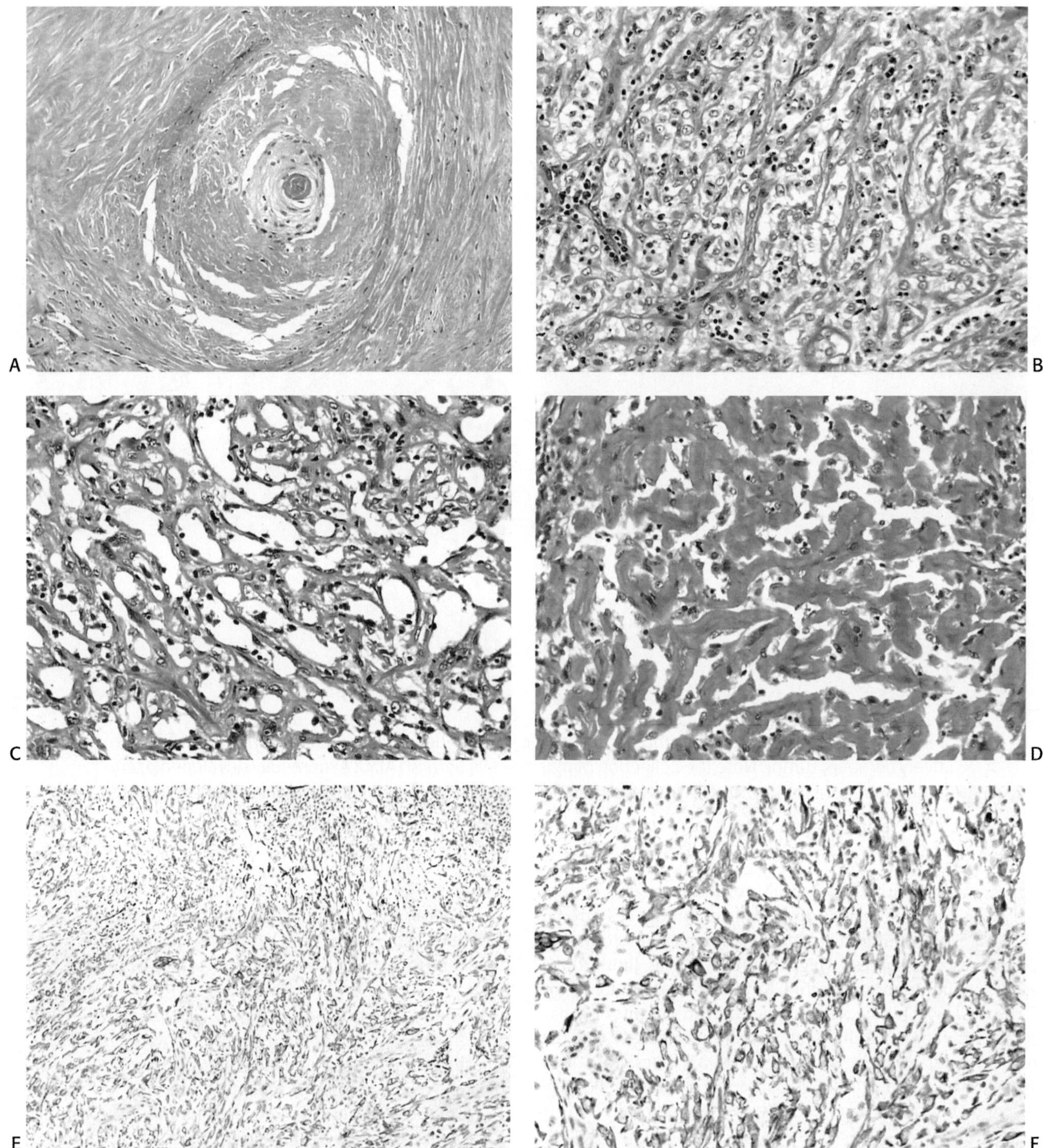

FIG. 16.20. ***Metaplastic carcinoma, acantholytic.*** **A:** Well-differentiated metaplastic squamous carcinoma surrounded by densely collagenous tissue that is part of the neoplastic process. **B:** Part of the tumor in which the carcinoma forms a trabecular pattern. There is a sparse infiltrate of lymphocytes, and scattered degenerating tumor cells are represented by pyknotic nuclei. **C:** Extensive degeneration of the carcinoma resulting in an angiomatous appearance. **D:** Dense stroma in angiomatous metaplastic carcinoma. **E:** Diffuse immunoreactivity for CK AE1:3. **F:** Diffuse immunoreactivity for 34βE12.

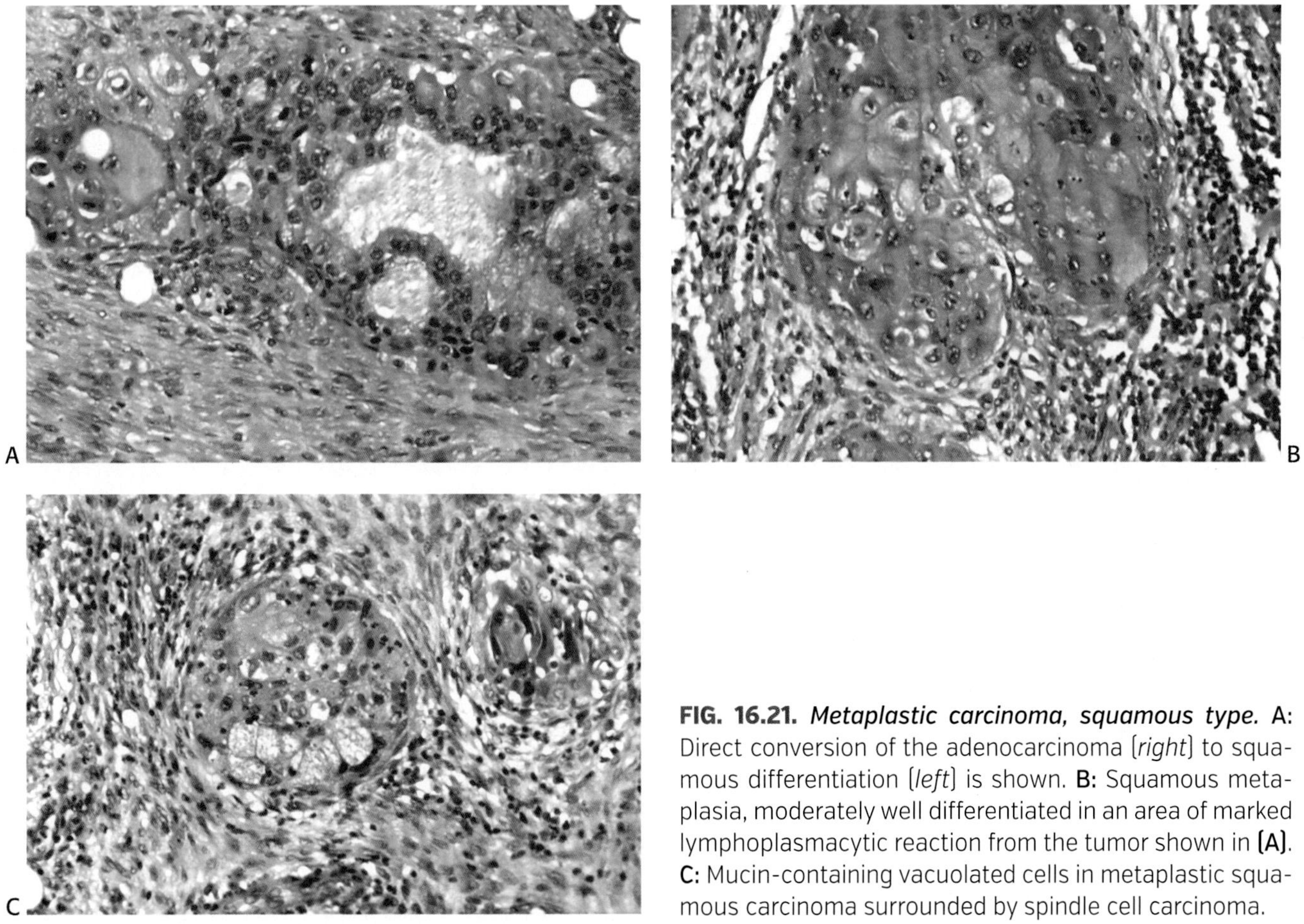

FIG. 16.21. ***Metaplastic carcinoma, squamous type.*** **A:** Direct conversion of the adenocarcinoma (*right*) to squamous differentiation (*left*) is shown. **B:** Squamous metaplasia, moderately well differentiated in an area of marked lymphoplasmacytic reaction from the tumor shown in **(A)**. **C:** Mucin-containing vacuolated cells in metaplastic squamous carcinoma surrounded by spindle cell carcinoma.

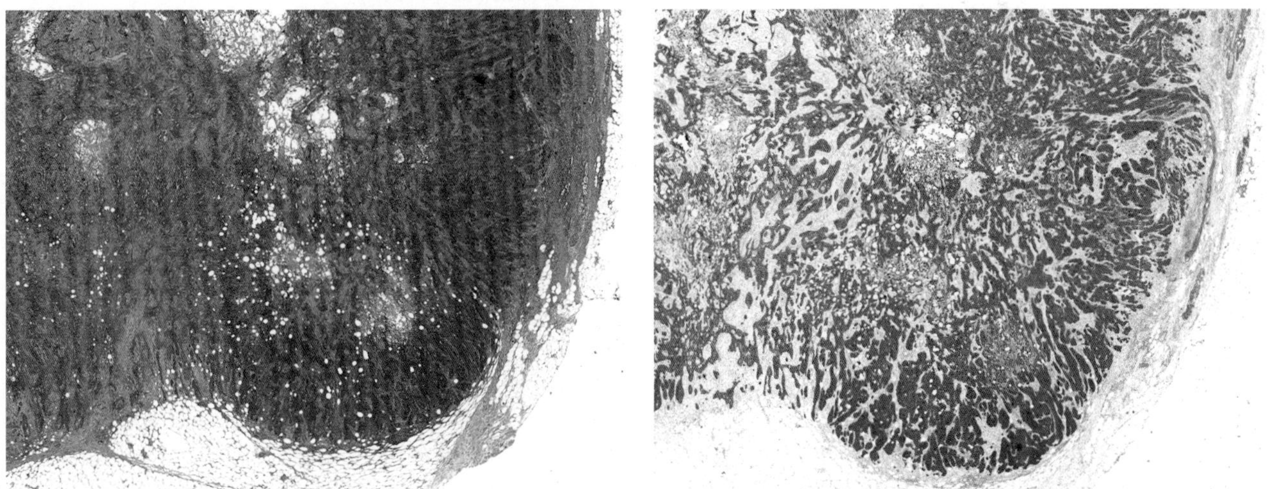

FIG. 16.22. ***Metaplastic carcinoma, high-grade adenosquamous type.*** **A:** This tumor has a nodular growth pattern. **B:** Strong immunoreactivity for 34βE12, a basal CK, highlights the carcinoma. Foci of necrosis have lighter and irregular staining. **C:** Bands of carcinoma in sclerotic stroma. **D:** Staining for CK7 highlights the glandular component. **E:** The myoepithelial/squamous component shows nuclear reactivity for p63.

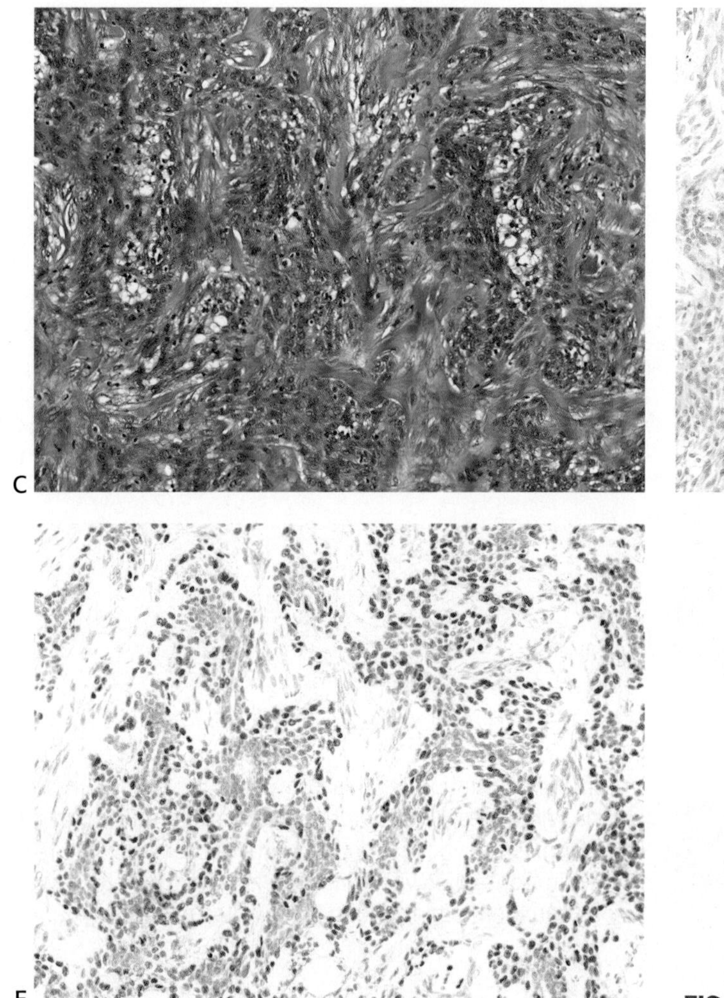

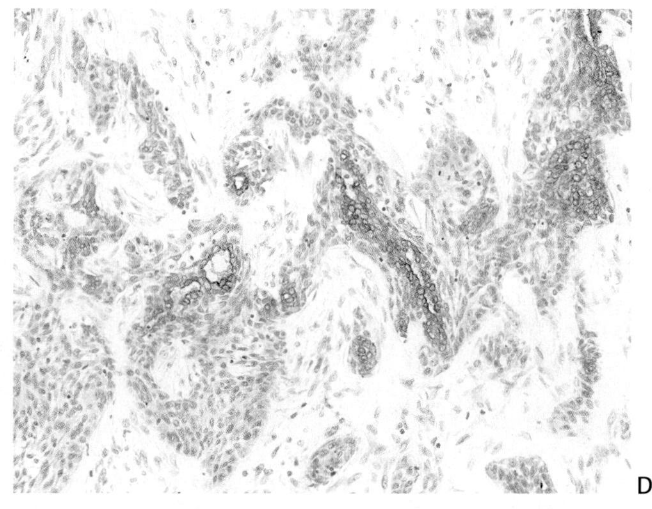

FIG. 16.22. *(Continued)*

lined by epithelium can be the only evidence differentiating a high-grade malignant PT from a metaplastic spindle cell carcinoma. The differential diagnosis of these two lesions has important implications for clinical management, and patient prognosis also varies greatly, depending on the diagnosis.

In contrast to metaplastic carcinoma, a malignant tumor common in peri- and postmenopausal women, fibromatosis tends to occur in women of fertile age, but this difference is not absolute. The spindle cells of fibromatosis are myofibroblasts arranged in broad sweeping fascicles and show no cytologic atypia. Mitoses are extremely infrequent. Positive nuclear staining for β-catenin in a spindle cell lesion involving the breast is not sufficient to diagnose fibromatosis. Lacroix-Triki et al.[64] documented nuclear staining for β-catenin in 94% of benign and 57% of malignant PTs, and in 23% of metaplastic carcinomas. The same authors found no mutations of the *β-catenin* gene in a subset of PTs and metaplastic carcinomas showing nuclear positivity for β-catenin.[64] Nuclear β-catenin staining occurring in a metaplastic breast carcinoma is regarded as a manifestation of EMT.

Metaplastic carcinoma with spindle cell morphology must be considered in the differential diagnosis of any spindle lesion encountered in a needle core biopsy specimen, including proliferations with bland cytology. Immunohistochemistry (IHC) should always be employed in an effort to detect CK expression or p63 reactivity (see Immunohistochemistry section in this chapter). Even if no keratin positivity is documented in the core biopsy material, the final report of a spindle cell lesion should mention metaplastic spindle cell carcinoma in the differential diagnosis and indicate the need to evaluate the excised tumor.

Heterologous Metaplastic Carcinoma

Heterologous metaplastic carcinoma is characterized by differentiation into elements with a mesenchymal phenotype such as cartilage or bone (Fig. 16.4). Zones of spindle cell metaplasia usually intervene between the adenocarcinomatous and heterologous elements. Metaplastic carcinomas with heterologous rhabdomyosarcomatous, liposarcomatous, and angiosarcomatous metaplasia can also occur, but they are much less frequent. One case of metaplastic carcinoma with neuroectodermal metaplasia has been reported.[65] In general, carcinomas with heterologous metaplasia tend to retain an epithelial component, which may be glandular and/or squamous (Figs. 16.23 and 16.24). In a few cases, the lesion is composed largely of undifferentiated spindle cell elements with scant heterologous components and tends to resemble

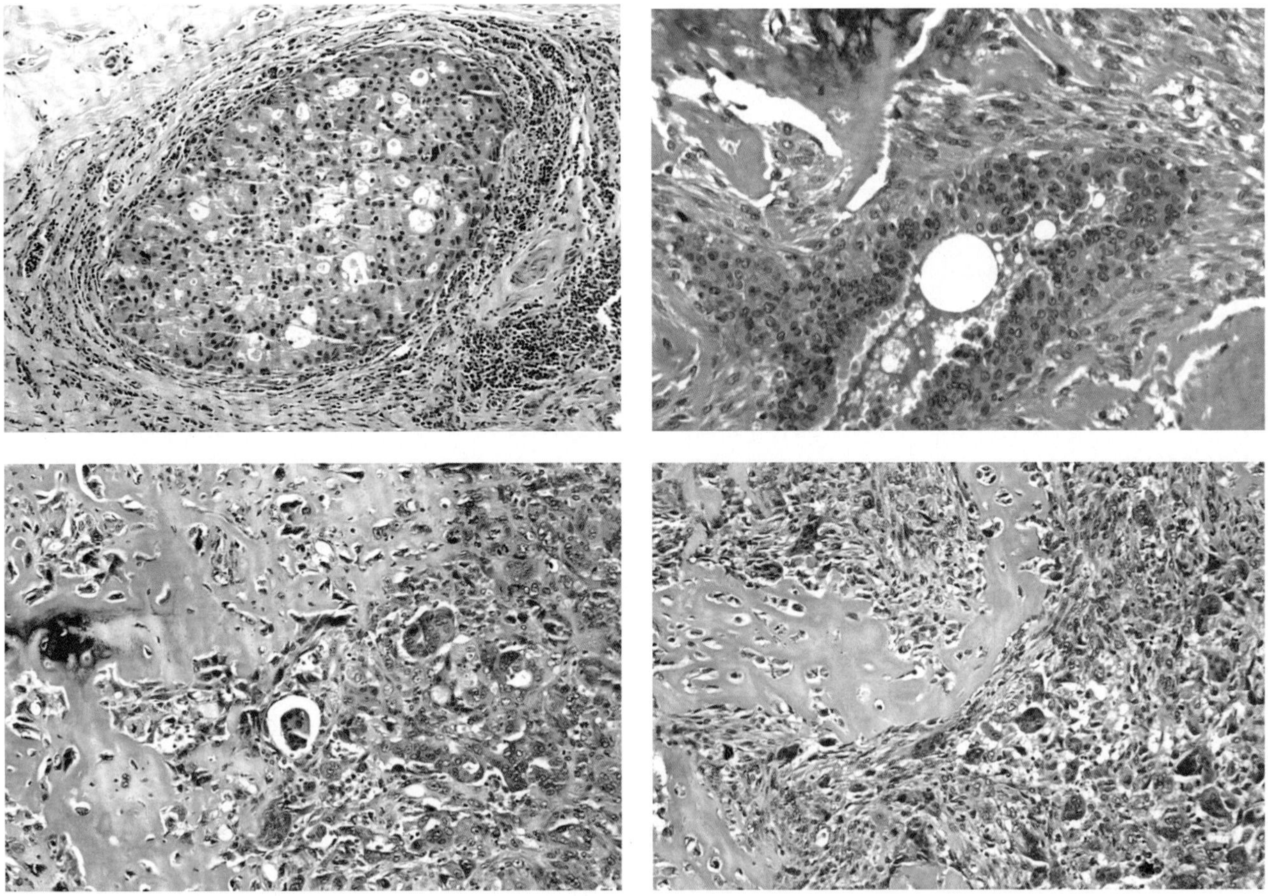

FIG. 16.23. ***Metaplastic carcinoma, osseous type.*** **A:** Intraductal carcinoma, apocrine cribriform type with low nuclear grade. **B:** Adenocarcinoma with spindle cell and osseous metaplastic carcinoma. **C:** Osseous metaplasia (*left*) and poorly differentiated adenocarcinoma with undifferentiated spindle cell carcinoma. **D:** Osseous metaplasia in spindle cell carcinoma with osteoclastic giant cells. All images are from the same tumor in a 53-year-old woman.

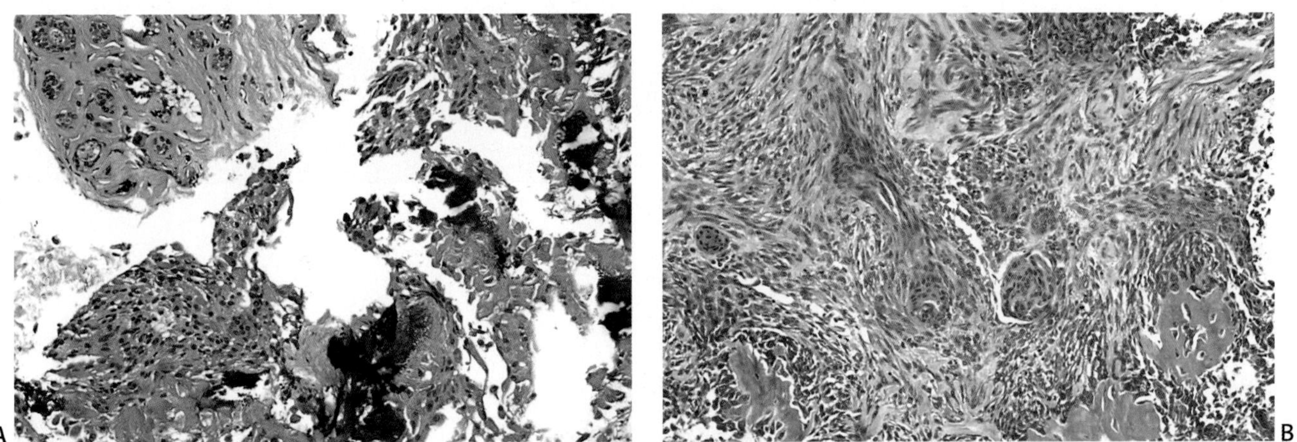

FIG. 16.24. ***Metaplastic carcinoma, chondro-osseous type.*** **A:** This needle core biopsy sample shows fragments of osseous tissue and breast parenchyma. **B:** Spindle and squamous metaplasia were found at the core biopsy site in the excised specimen. Osteoid formation is present (*below*). **C:** The bulk of the tumor consisted of ossifying osteoid with abundant osteoblasts and scattered osteoclastic cells. **D:** Isolated foci of adenosquamous differentiation were present in the osseous tissue.

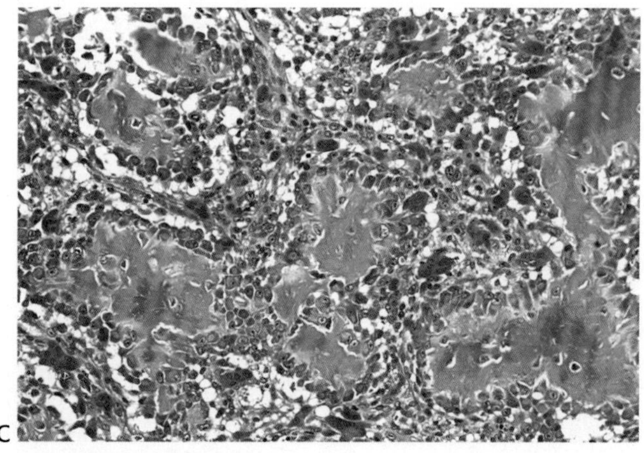

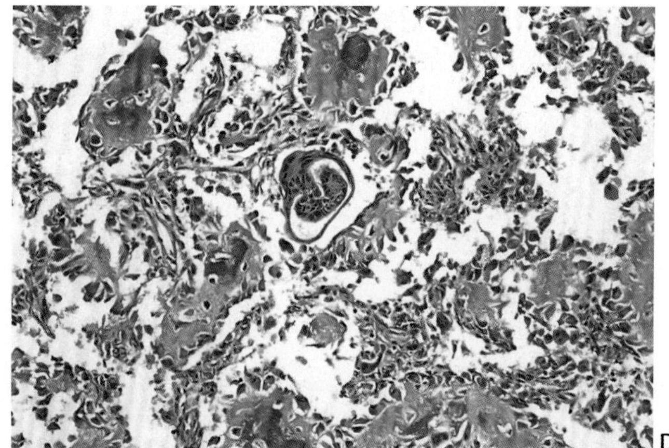

FIG. 16.24. *(Continued)*

a high-grade undifferentiated sarcoma[52] (Fig. 16.25). Myxoid change, a common feature of these undifferentiated elements, may also be found in transitional zones between adenocarcinoma and chondroid metaplasia. Highly cellular areas resembling fibrosarcoma were described in nearly half of the cases in one series.[6]

Metaplastic Carcinoma with Matrix Production (with or without Cartilaginous and/or Osteoid Matrix)

Matrix-producing carcinoma is a variant of heterologous metaplastic carcinoma composed of "overt carcinoma with direct transition to a cartilaginous and/or osseous stromal matrix without an intervening spindle cell zone or osteoclastic cells"[66] (Fig. 16.26). Well-formed cartilage and bone are absent. The majority of these tumors are circumscribed or nodular, but occasional lesions have infiltrative borders. Sonographic examination in one case revealed a well-circumscribed nodular hypoechoic tumor that exhibited marginal enhancement on contrast-enhanced computed tomography.[67]

Microscopically, the carcinomatous element in matrix-producing tumors is usually moderately to poorly differentiated

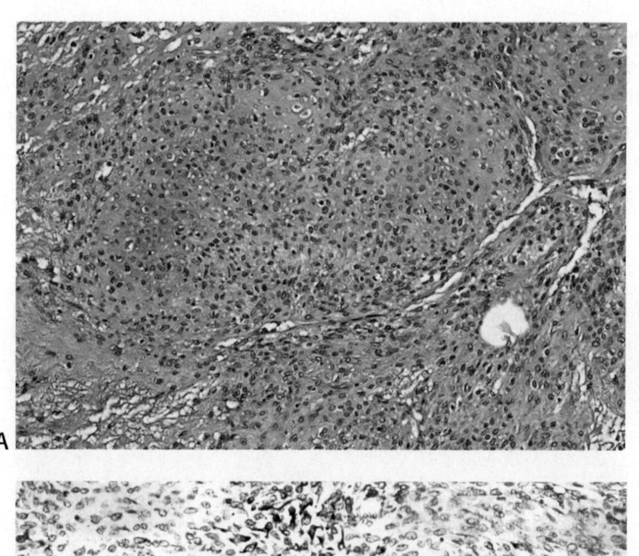

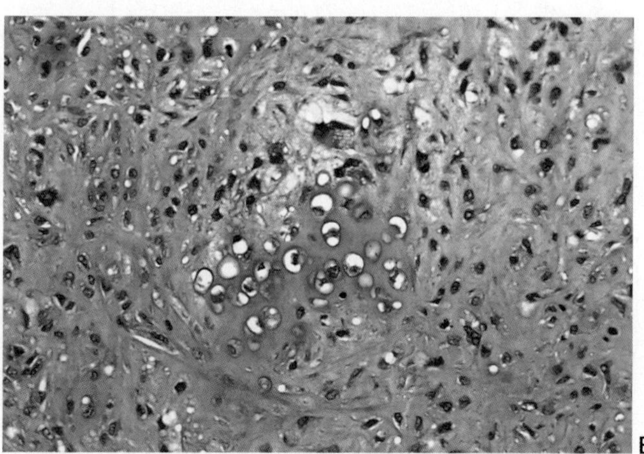

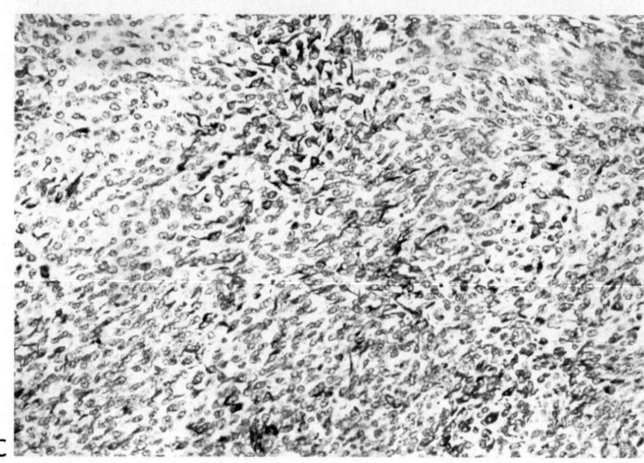

FIG. 16.25. ***Metaplastic carcinoma, spindle cell with chondroid differentiation.*** **A:** Focal chondroid differentiation in a spindle cell carcinoma. **B:** Magnified view of a well-developed cartilaginous focus. **C:** The spindle cell areas were immunoreactive for CK 34βE12.

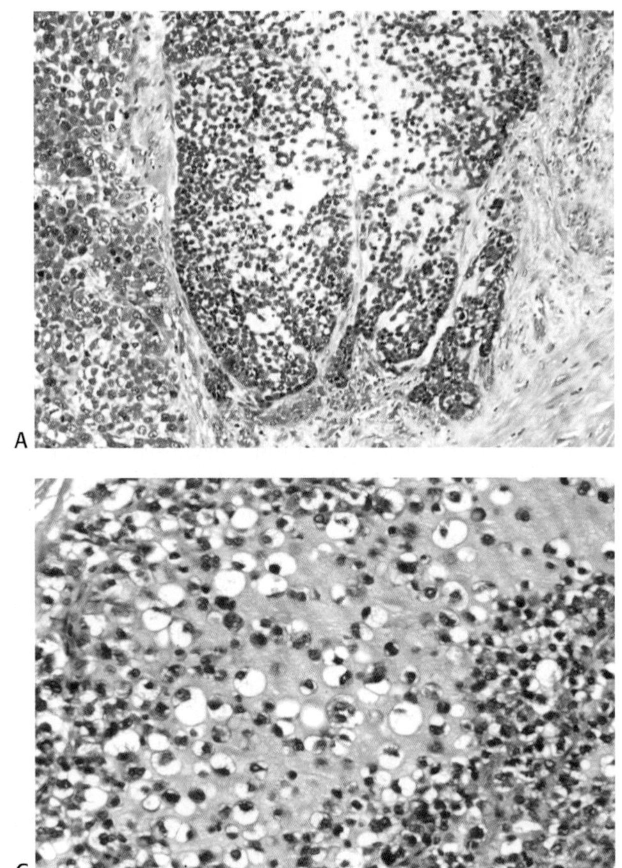

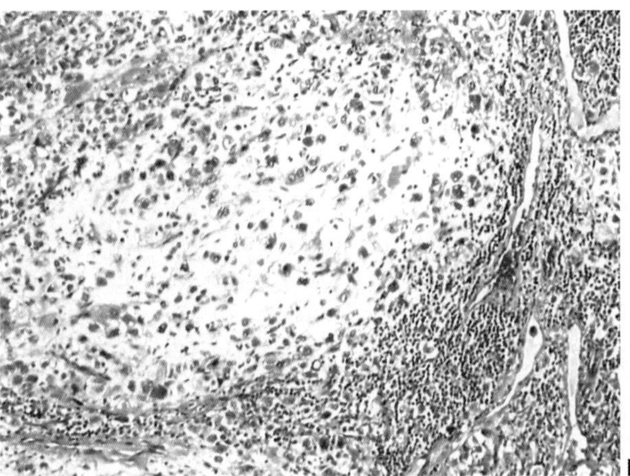

FIG. 16.26. ***Metaplastic carcinoma, matrix-producing type.*** **A:** A small focus of matrix formation emerging from poorly differentiated small cell carcinoma. **B:** Metastatic matrix-producing carcinoma in an ALN from the tumor shown in (A). **C:** Magnified view of matrix-producing carcinoma.

adenocarcinoma, often with small cell features and infrequent foci of squamous or apocrine metaplasia (Fig. 16.27). In some tumors, the mucoid matrix may superficially resemble mucinous carcinoma, especially if only limited material is available for review (Figs. 16.28 and 16.29). Mucin positivity is demonstrated in the stroma, but chondroid forming cells do not contain intracellular mucin. Areas that resemble pleomorphic adenoma can be found in some tumors.[68] The chondroid matrix has histochemical properties of a sulfated acid mucopolysaccharide consistent with chondroitin sulfate. The carcinoma cells stain positively for CK, epithelial membrane antigen (EMA), and S-100 in adenocarcinoma areas (Fig. 16.30).

In published series,[38,42,66,69–73] the patient mean age was 56 years, ranging from 50[38,42,70] to 58 years.[66] The mean tumor size ranged between 2.4[42] and 3.9 cm.[69] The smallest tumor spanned 0.7 cm[42] and the largest 11.0 cm.[70]

Downs-Kelly et al.[38] studied 32 cases of matrix-producing metaplastic carcinomas. Chondromyxoid or chondroid matrix constituted more than 40% of the tumor mass in 9 (28%) cases, between 10% and 40% of the tumor in another 9 (28%), and

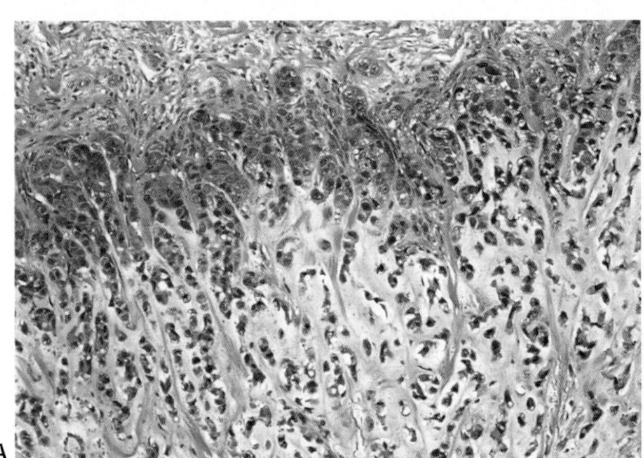

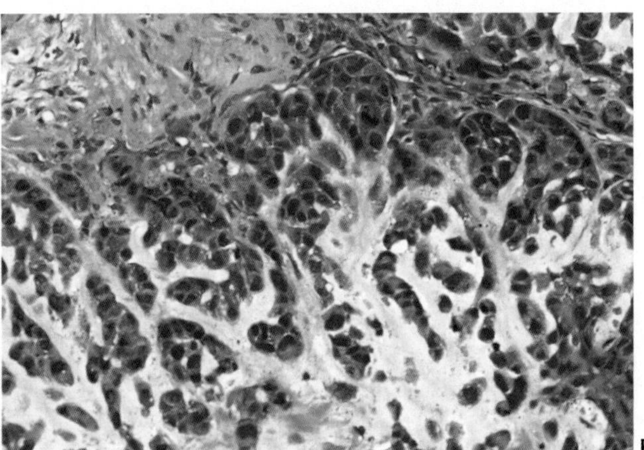

FIG. 16.27. ***Metaplastic carcinoma, matrix-producing type.*** **A,B:** Matrix-producing carcinoma with poorly differentiated carcinoma at the periphery. **C:** Another region in the tumor composed of small cell carcinoma with focal necrosis.

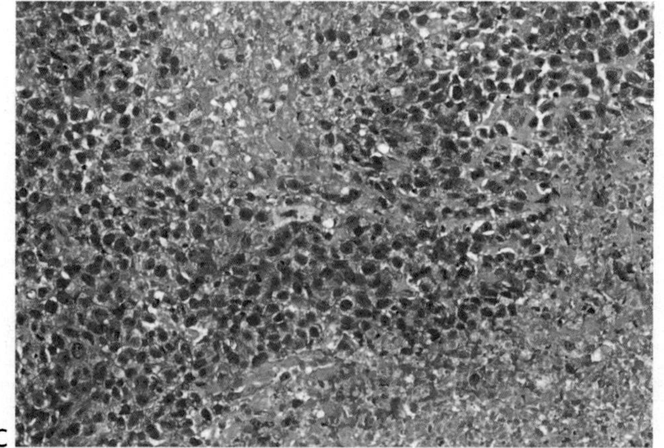

FIG. 16.27. *(Continued)*

comprised less than 10% of the tumor in the remaining 14/32 (44%) cases. The neoplastic cells in the matrix had low-grade morphology in 23/34 (72%) cases. One tumor also contained focal (less than 5%) osseous matrix. The tumor was minimally invasive in 50% of the cases, multinodular with pushing border in 33% and had a peripheral infiltrative pattern in 17% of the cases. The invasive NOS component associated with the carcinomas had high-grade morphology in 30/32 (94%) tumors, and central necrosis was present in 19/32 (59%). Lymphovascular invasion has been detected in up to 25% of tumors.[38]

Lymph node metastases were present in 5.8%,[66] 22%,[38] 23%,[69] and 45.5%[42] of cases (Figs. 16.26 and 16.31). The morphology of the lymph node metastases was chondroid in 60% of cases in one series.[42] In another study,[38] the lymph node metastases were purely carcinomatous in four of six cases available for review, consisted of matrix-producing carcinoma in one case and of carcinoma with focal (1 mm) chondromyxoid matrix in the remaining case. Distant metastases usually have the same matrix-producing pattern as the primary tumor.

In the series of 21 chondroid metaplastic carcinomas reported by Gwin et al.,[42] 38% of the lesions also had foci of squamous differentiation. All tumors were estrogen receptor (ER), progesterone receptor (PR), androgen receptor (AR), and HER2 negative, and 88% overexpressed epidermal growth factor receptor (EGFR). Positive staining for S-100, p63, and calponin was also identified. A similar pattern of immunoreactivity has been reported by Shui et al.,[70] who also observed low positivity for ER (one case) and PR (three cases).

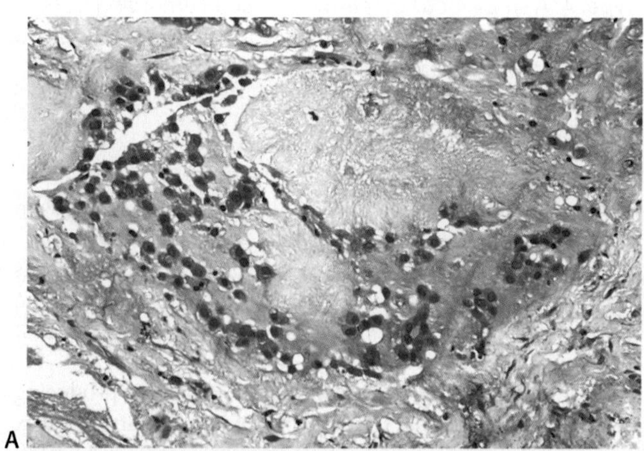

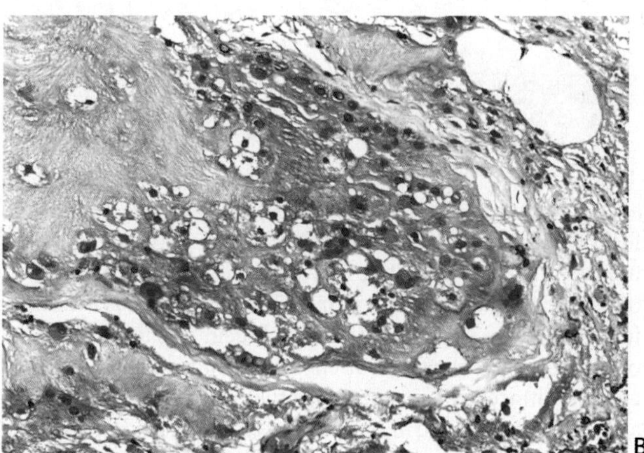

FIG. 16.28. ***Matrix-producing carcinoma with mucinous appearance.*** **A,B:** These areas lack a distinct rim of carcinoma cells and resemble invasive mucinous carcinoma.

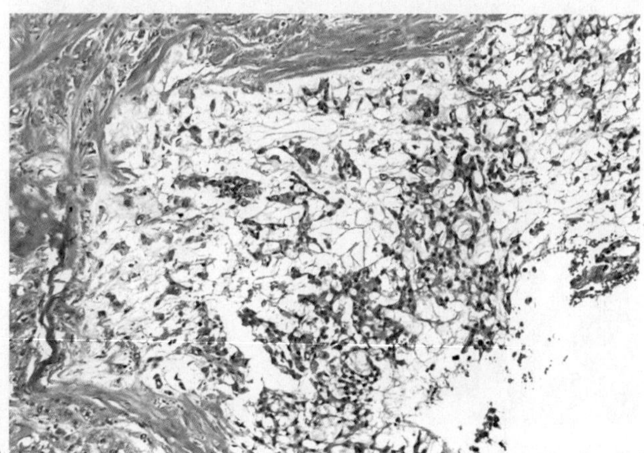

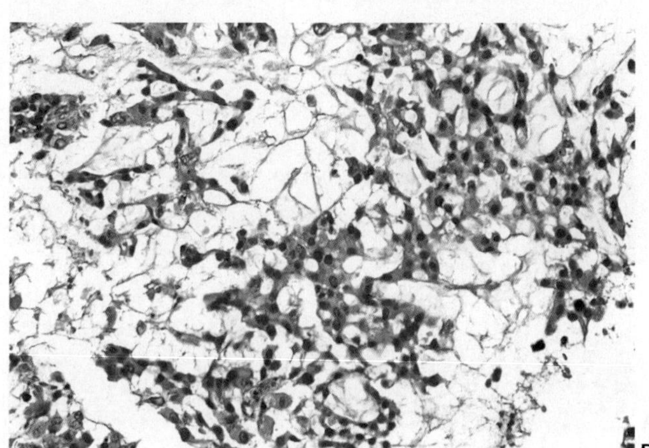

FIG. 16.29. ***Matrix-producing carcinoma, chest wall recurrence.*** **A,B:** The matrix-producing pattern resembles mucinous carcinoma.

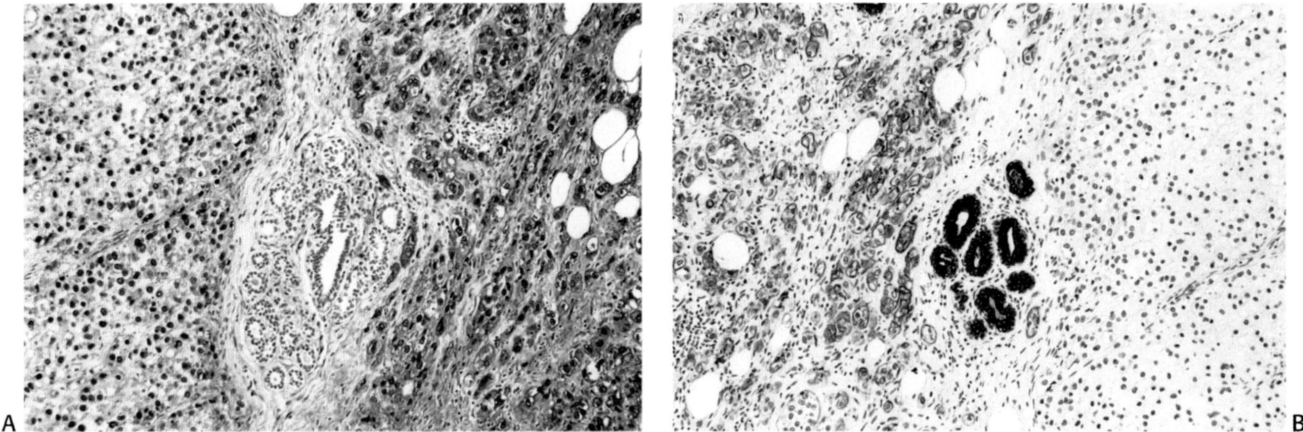

FIG. 16.30. ***Matrix-producing carcinoma immunoreactivity.*** **A:** Nuclear reactivity for S-100 protein is shown in adenocarcinoma (*right*) and matrix-producing carcinoma (*left*). Cytoplasmic reactivity is stronger in the adenocarcinoma area. **B:** Immunoreactivity for CK AE1:3 is limited to adenocarcinoma (*left*) and a normal lobule (*center*).

Tsuda et al.[7,8] described carcinomas with central acellular necrosis/fibrosis occupying at least 30% of the tumor mass (Fig. 16.32) that are characterized by myoepithelial differentiation and a propensity to develop lung and brain metastases. Tumors with similar morphology have also been reported by other authors, sometimes under different designations. In these carcinomas, myxoid matrix is sometimes present at the interface between the central area of acellular necrosis/fibrosis and the peripheral hypercellular rim of high-grade carcinoma, raising the differential diagnosis

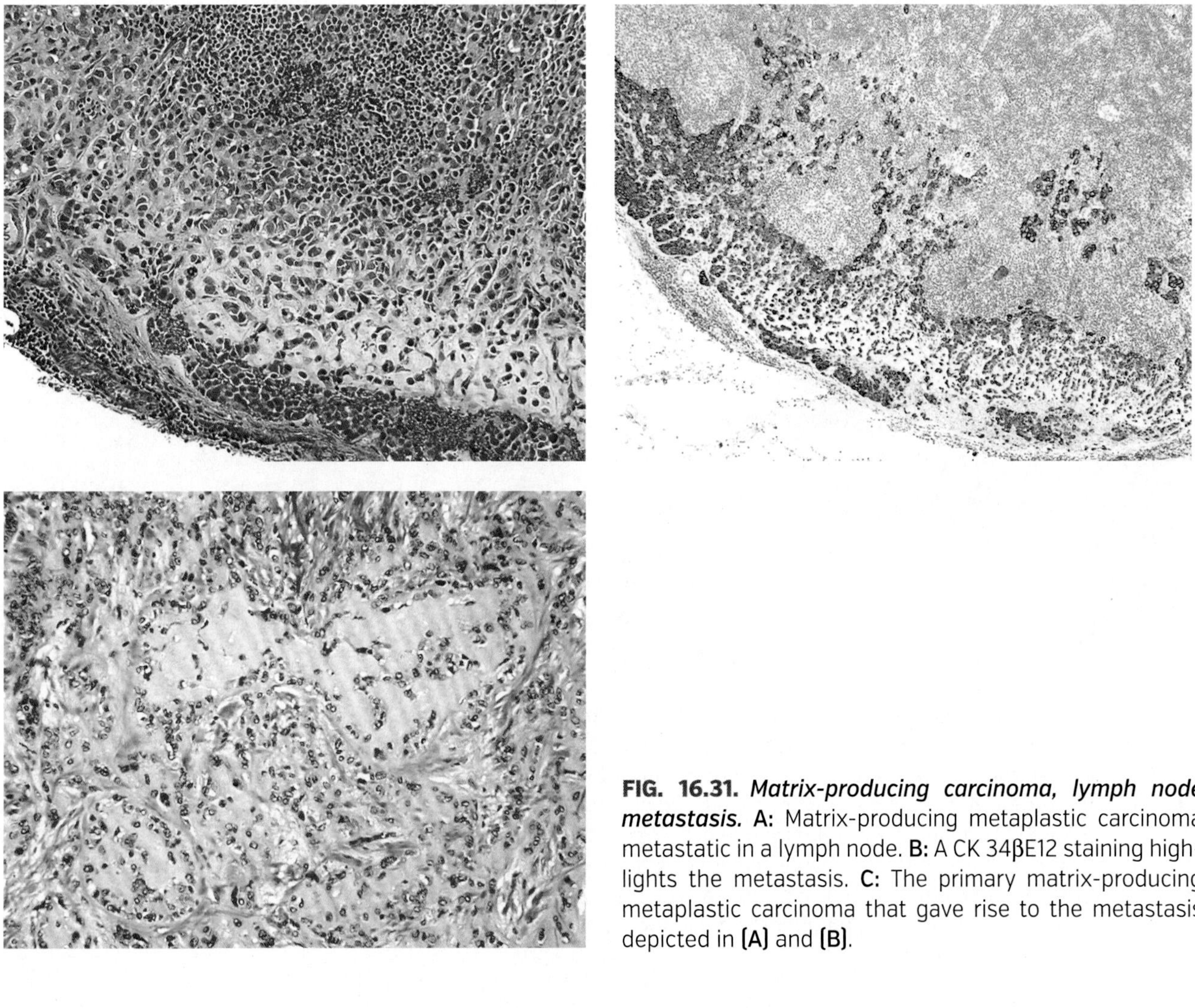

FIG. 16.31. ***Matrix-producing carcinoma, lymph node metastasis.*** **A:** Matrix-producing metaplastic carcinoma metastatic in a lymph node. **B:** A CK 34βE12 staining highlights the metastasis. **C:** The primary matrix-producing metaplastic carcinoma that gave rise to the metastasis depicted in **(A)** and **(B)**.

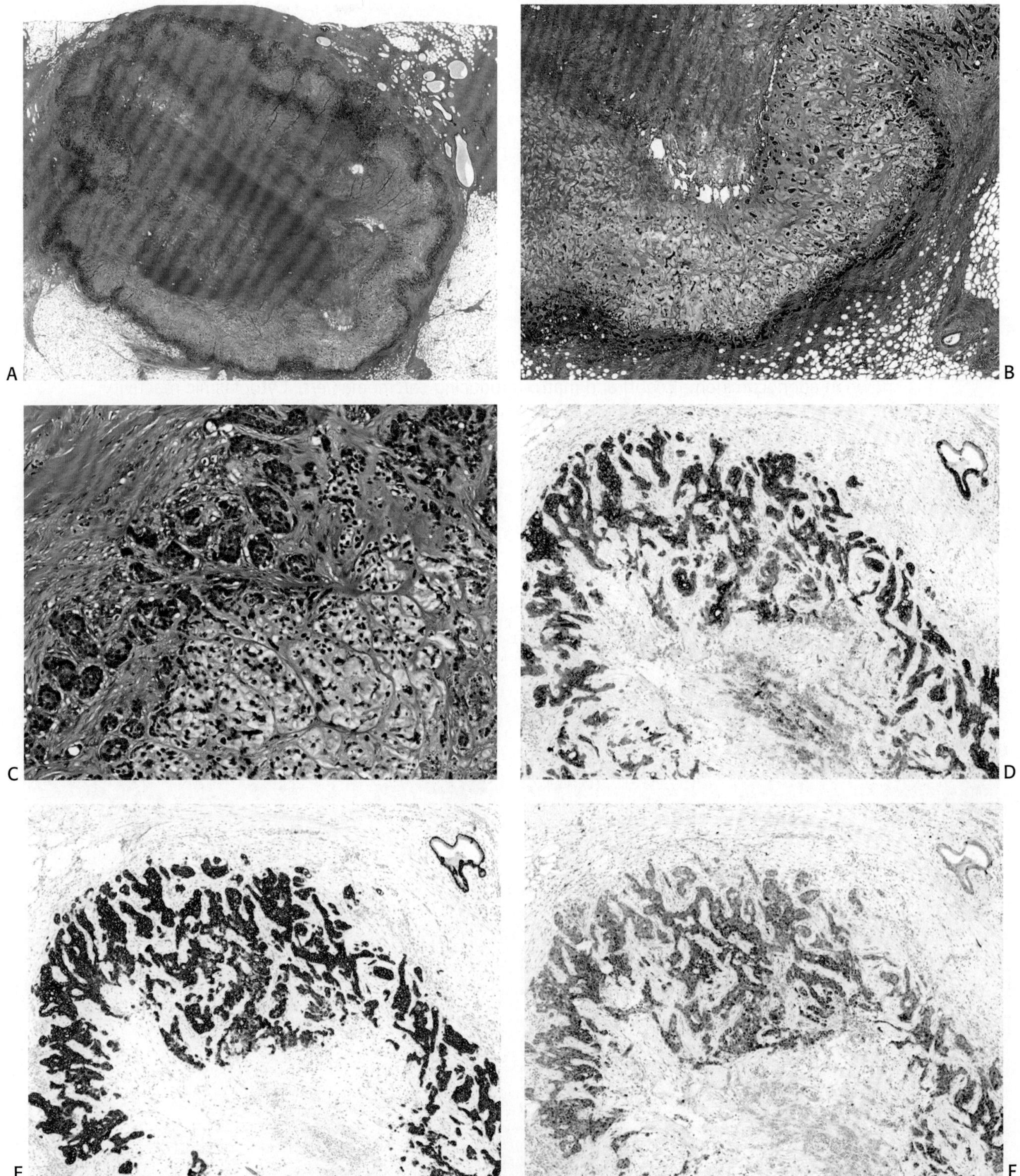

FIG. 16.32. ***Carcinoma with large central acellular zone of necrosis/fibrosis.*** **A:** The tumor forms a discrete nodule with a characteristic concentric arrangement. In this case, the necrotic/fibrotic center appears hemorrhagic because of a prior biopsy. This area represents more than a third of the tumor mass. It is surrounded by a band of gray hypocellular matrix, rimmed by a hypercellular area. **B:** Magnified view of the matrix-rich tissue band around the area of central necrosis/fibrosis. **C:** The matrix is relatively hypocellular compared with the hypercellular rim of basaloid cells at the periphery of the tumor. **D:** The tumor cells display strong immunoreactivity for CK 34βE12. **E:** Immunoreactivity for CK14. **F:** Immunoreactivity for S-100. There was no reactivity for p63 in this tumor.

with metaplastic carcinoma. There is debate on the classification of these carcinomas, as they have overtly epithelial morphology and only focal myxoid matrix. However, immunohistochemical studies have demonstrated some similarities between these tumors and matrix-producing metaplastic carcinomas, as both display the basal immunoprofile and frequently have myoepithelial differentiation[74] (Fig. 16.32).

DCIS associated with matrix-producing metaplastic carcinoma was identified in 28%[38] and 43%[42] of cases in two series. Gwin et al.[42] specified that the DCIS was solid, cribriform, micropapillary, or comedo type, with intermediate or high nuclear grade. The DCIS rarely has areas of matrix formation. In one series,[66] DCIS was identified in 7/26 cases and was matrix producing in 2 cases. Some cases of matrix-producing metaplastic carcinomas arise in association with microglandular adenosis.[70,75,76] One study[42] found no microcalcifications in DCIS and in the invasive component.

Metaplastic Carcinomas with Multinucleated Giant Cells Resembling Osteoclasts

These tumors often exhibit osseous or cartilaginous metaplasia,[6,18,77] but multinucleated giant cells can also occur admixed with malignant spindle cells without chondro-osseous metaplasia[17] (Fig. 16.33). Metaplastic carcinomas with this morphology usually do not display the degree of stromal hemorrhage and prominent adenocarcinoma typically found in carcinomas with osteoclast-like cells described in Chapter 23. Osteoclast-like giant cells may be found clustered around thin-walled vascular spaces in the primary tumor and in metastatic foci involving axillary lymph nodes (ALNs) and distant sites. Lee et al.[78] studied the *p53* gene in a metaplastic carcinoma with osteoclast-like giant cells. They found strong p53 reactivity and the same *p53* gene point mutation in the intraductal carcinoma and in the sarcomatoid component, but not in the osteoclast-like giant cells. Based on these findings, the authors concluded that the carcinomatous and sarcomatoid elements arose from a common progenitor cell, and that the giant cells were reactive constituents. DCIS is frequently found near these tumors.

Metastases of Metaplastic Breast Carcinoma

Metastases derived from a metaplastic carcinoma can consist entirely of adenocarcinoma, entirely of metaplastic elements, or they may contain a mixture of both components (Figs. 16.26, 16.31, 16.34, and 16.35). Tumors with squamous metaplasia often give rise to metastases with squamous differentiation in ALNs and other sites. On the other hand, ALN metastases from some tumors with heterologous metaplasia can consist entirely of adenocarcinoma, or only of heterologous elements. It is more common to find heterologous elements in local tumor recurrences on the chest wall and in visceral sites than in nodal metastases[6,18] (Fig. 16.29). Various combinations of epithelial and heterologous constituents have been described in separate metastases from one patient.[6] There does not appear to be a consistent relationship between the type and the amount of heterologous elements in the primary tumor and their representation in metastases. In one case, cutaneous metastases from a mammary carcinoma with chondroid metaplasia were indistinguishable from chondrosarcoma.[79]

Bone metastases of metaplastic carcinoma with chondroid or osseous metaplasia can be especially difficult to differentiate from a primary cartilaginous or osseous sarcoma. This is exemplified by one case studied by this author. It involved a metaplastic mammary carcinoma with chondroid matrix that gave rise to a single, large metastasis in an ischial bone. The mass mimicked a primary osseous chondrosarcoma clinically and radiologically, but the fine-needle aspiration (FNA) material yielded spindle and epithelioid cells admixed with matrix and positive for CK 34βE12 (Fig. 16.36). Immunohistochemical workup of additional tissue obtained from the tumor mass supported the diagnosis of metastatic metaplastic carcinoma. In similar cases, it is critical that the pathologist be informed of the patient's prior history of metaplastic breast carcinoma, so that appropriate

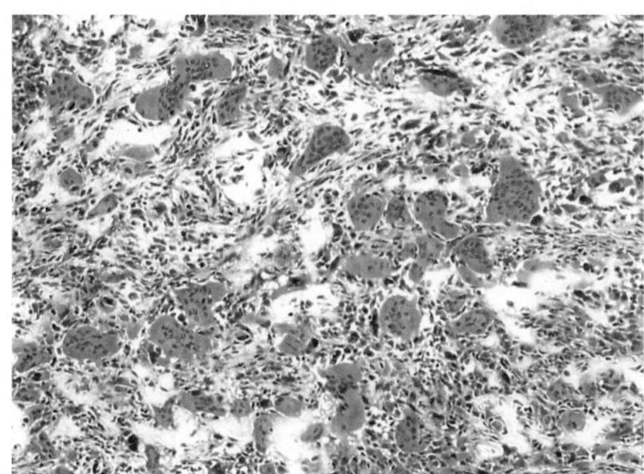

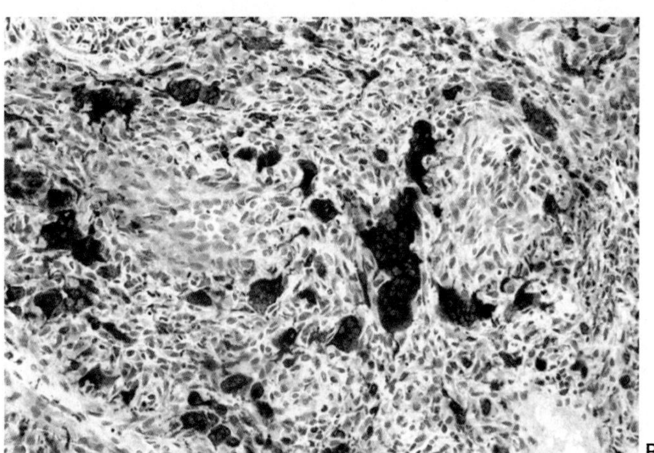

FIG. 16.33. ***Metaplastic carcinoma with osteoclast-like giant cells.*** **A:** The tumor did not exhibit cartilaginous and osseous differentiation. **B:** The giant cells and some stromal cells are immunoreactive for KP-1, a histiocytic marker.

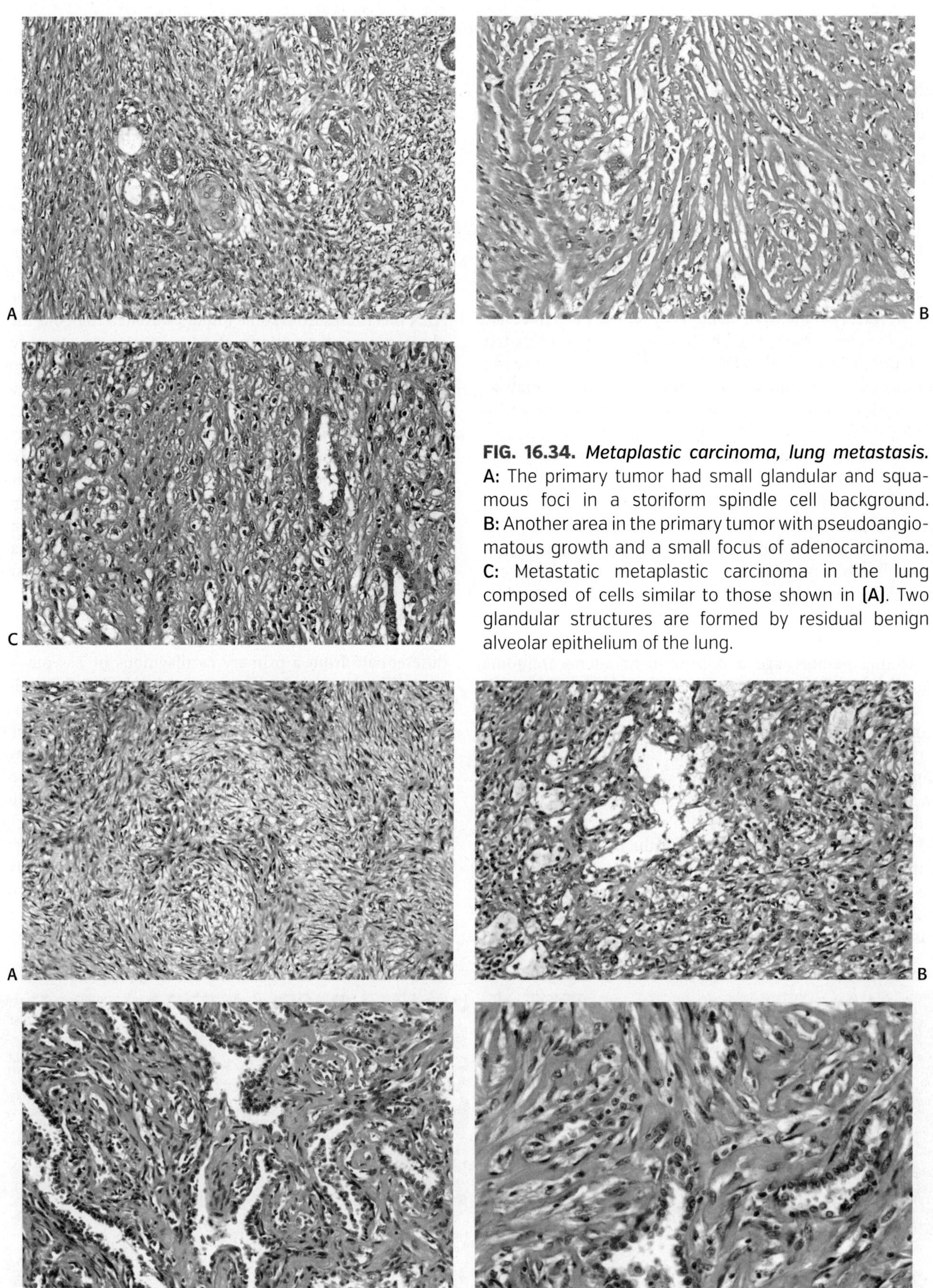

FIG. 16.34. ***Metaplastic carcinoma, lung metastasis.*** **A:** The primary tumor had small glandular and squamous foci in a storiform spindle cell background. **B:** Another area in the primary tumor with pseudoangiomatous growth and a small focus of adenocarcinoma. **C:** Metastatic metaplastic carcinoma in the lung composed of cells similar to those shown in **(A)**. Two glandular structures are formed by residual benign alveolar epithelium of the lung.

FIG. 16.35. ***Metastatic spindle cell metaplastic carcinoma in the lung.*** **A:** Typical primary mammary spindle cell metaplastic carcinoma with storiform structure. **B:** An angiomatous area in the primary tumor. **C,D:** Metastatic spindle cell metaplastic mammary carcinoma in the lung. Glandular structures formed by pulmonary alveolar epithelium trapped in the carcinoma mingle with pseudoangiomatoid components of the carcinoma.

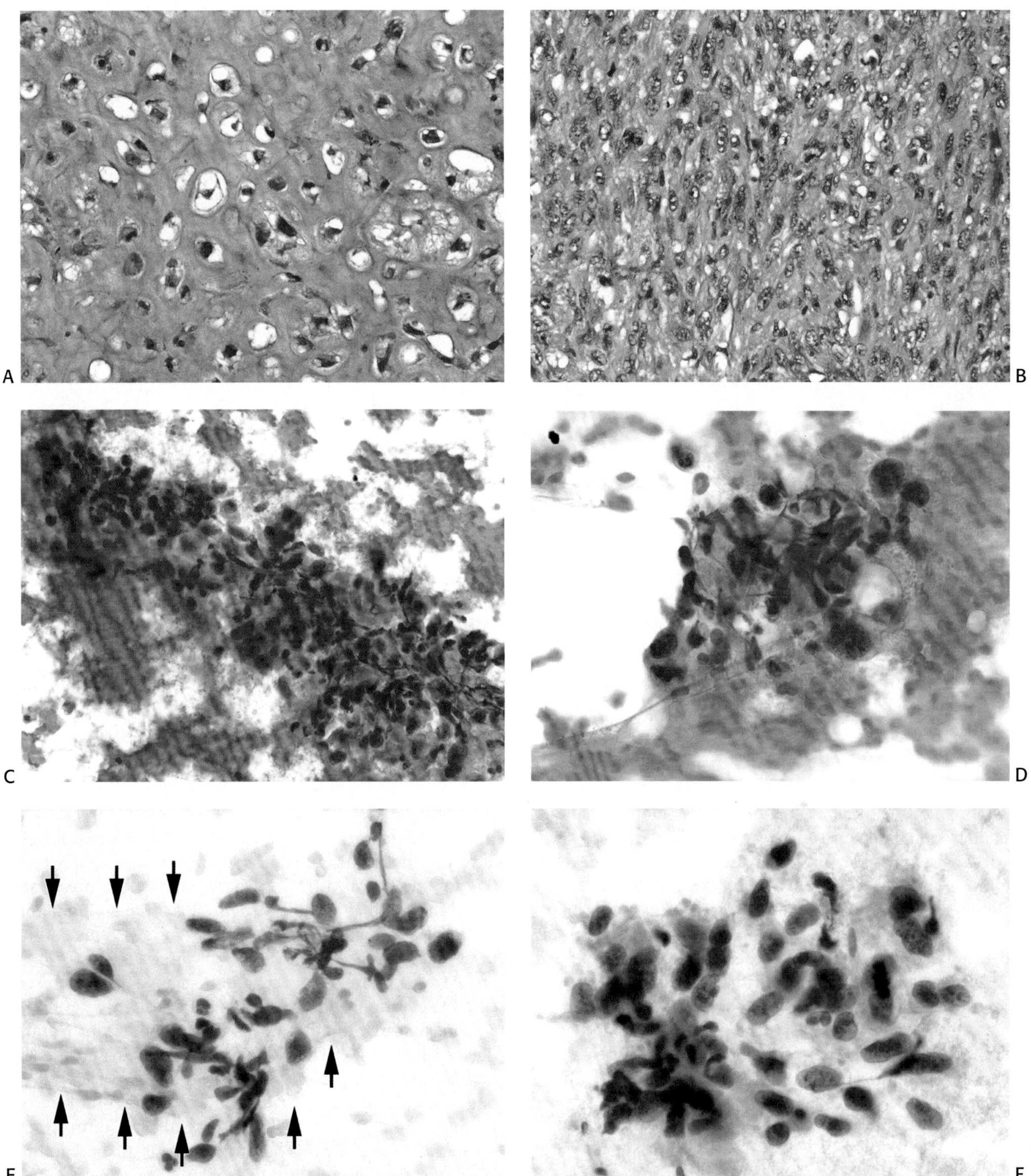

FIG. 16.36. ***Metastatic chondroid and spindle cell carcinoma in the bone.*** **A:** A chondroid area in the primary metaplastic mammary carcinoma. **B:** The primary tumor also showed spindle morphology, with high nuclear grade. **C,D:** This FNA specimen from a 5-cm lytic lesion in the ischial bone yielded loose clusters of spindle and epithelioid cells with high-grade atypia. **E:** Subtle evidence of gray mucoid matrix-like material was evident in a smear (*arrows*). **F:** This CK 34βE12 stain, performed on a destained smear, was interpreted as weakly positive. **G,H:** A subsequently obtained tissue sample from the lytic bone mass had chondroid (**G**) and spindle cell (**H**) areas, closely resembling the morphology of the primary metaplastic mammary carcinoma **I,J:** The bone metastasis was reactive for EMA (**I**) and calponin (**J**), supporting epithelial origin.

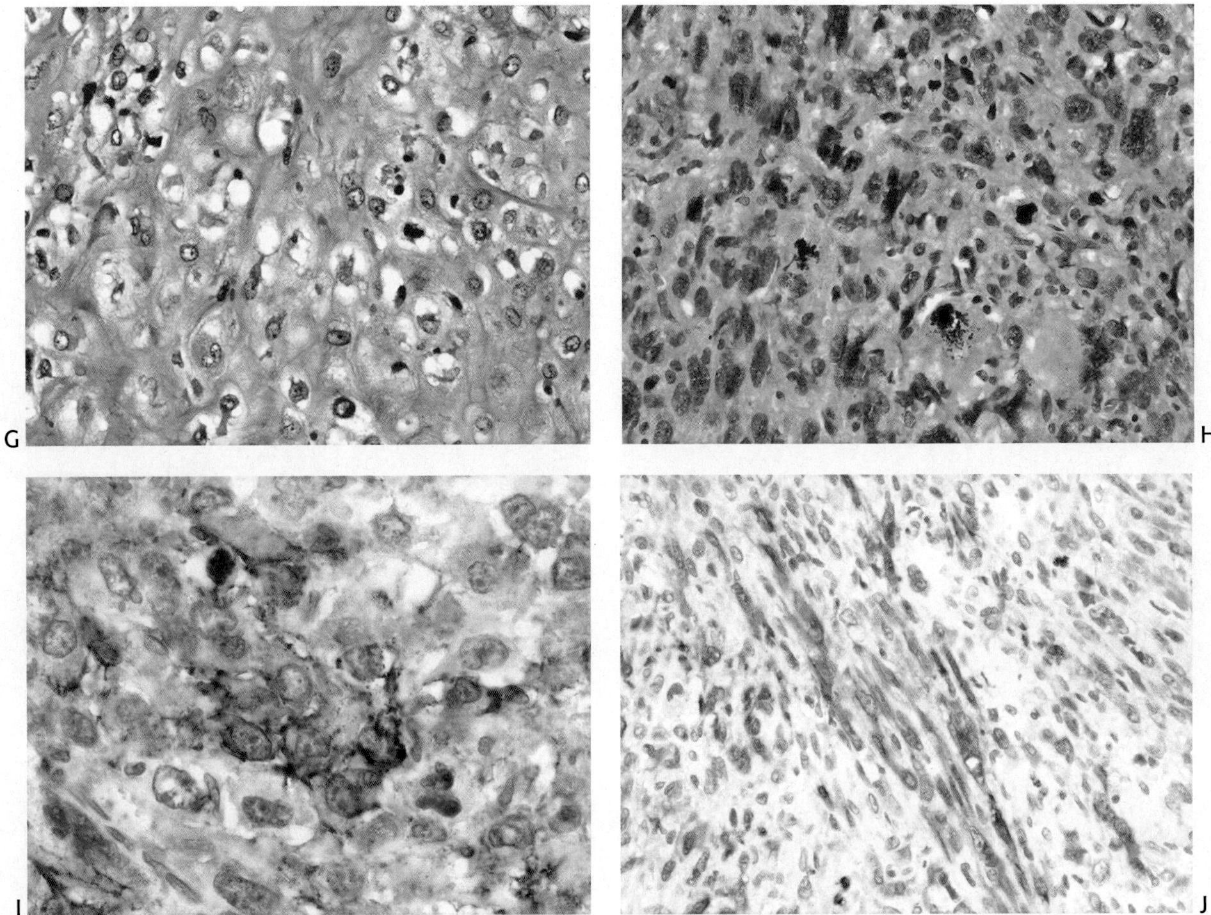

FIG. 16.36. *(Continued)*

immunohistochemical evaluation of the biopsy material obtained from the bone tumor can be performed.

It is also possible for metaplastic changes to develop within a metastasis or local recurrence, although corresponding metaplasia may not be detected in the primary tumor, even after generous sampling. This phenomenon was observed in a case reported by Chell et al.[80] The patient had a 2.2-cm primary carcinoma with chondroid metaplasia. Metastases in two ALNs showed chondroid differentiation and focal squamous metaplasia that was not seen in the primary tumor. This case is also of interest because the patient developed a pulmonary metastasis with chondroid features.

Metaplastic Carcinomas with Choriocarcinomatous Morphology

In some mammary carcinomas, metaplastic changes may be manifested by the formation of ectopic substances in quantity sufficient for detection by immunostains or histochemistry. Rarely, these substances are physiologically active. Corresponding structural metaplasia may be manifested in phenotypic morphologic patterns that, for example, resemble choriocarcinoma (Fig. 16.37). Metaplastic carcinomas with choriocarcinomatous areas have been described[81] and can be associated with production of human chorionic gonadotropin (HCG) and/or human placental lactogen. In these mammary carcinomas, areas that microscopically have the appearance of choriocarcinoma are strongly reactive for the β-unit of HCG. Carcinomas of the breast and other organs that exhibit structural choriocarcinomatous metaplasia have an aggressive clinical course, often resulting in early recurrence and death from disease. These tumors are extremely rare, can occur at any age, and have no specific presenting features. One patient reportedly developed a primary breast tumor with choriocarcinomatous features during pregnancy.[82] The pregnancy was terminated and "no evidence of gestational trophoblastic disease" was identified, but no details of the procedure and pathology studies were given. In similar cases, the possibility of metastases from a pregnancy-related choriocarcinoma needs to be carefully ruled out clinically and radiologically.

Most cases of metaplastic carcinoma with choriocarcinomatous differentiation have presented as a breast mass.[81–85] The carcinoma is typically soft and hemorrhagic. Histologically, the tumor is poorly differentiated and can show sarcomatoid areas. The choriocarcinomatous component consists of large cells with high nuclear-to-cytoplasmic ratio, coarse nuclear chromatin, and prominent, often irregular nucleoli. Multinucleated giant cells are often present. The identification of associated invasive carcinoma NOS type, metaplastic

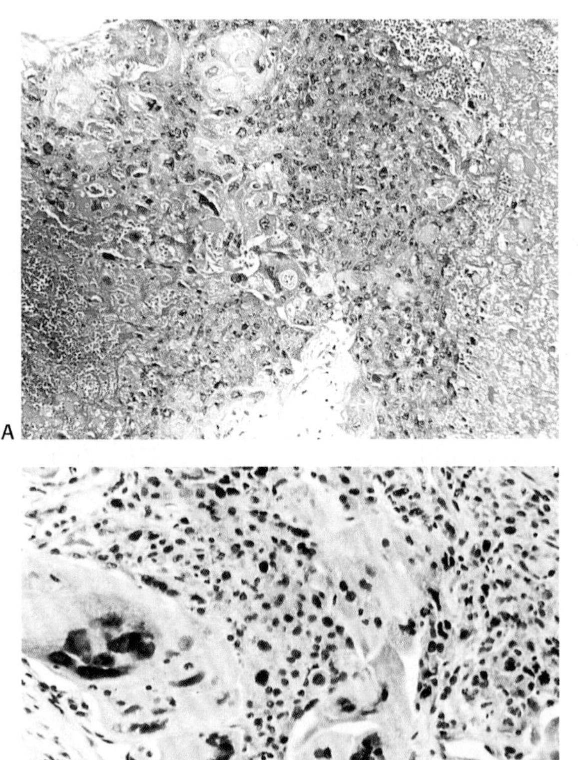

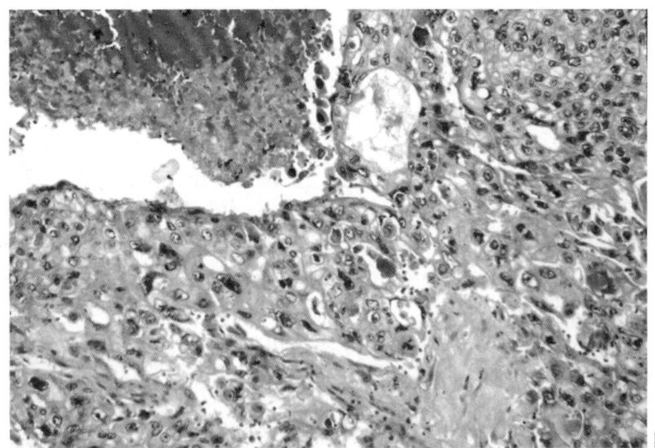

FIG. 16.37. *Metaplastic carcinoma, choriocarcinoma type.* **A,B:** High-grade metaplastic carcinoma with hemorrhagic necrosis. **C:** Giant cells that resemble syncytiotrophoblast. The tumor was focally immunoreactive for HCG, and the serum HCG level was markedly elevated.

carcinoma with nonchoriocarcinomatous morphology, or of mammary carcinoma *in situ* supports primary breast origin.

The differential diagnosis includes metastatic choriocarcinoma. In these cases, it is important to rule out concurrent or recent pregnancy and obtain clinical information about prior history of hydatidiform mole or choriocarcinoma. Because choriocarcinoma, though aggressive, is characterized by excellent response to chemotherapy, prompt diagnosis of metastatic disease is critical to avoid unnecessary surgery and ensure timely delivery of the appropriate treatment.

Isolated carcinoma cells that are reactive immunohistologically for α- and β-HCG can be found in 5% to 21% of ordinary infiltrating duct carcinomas that do not exhibit choriocarcinomatous metaplasia.[86] The reactive cells are otherwise morphologically indistinguishable microscopically from surrounding carcinoma cells that are not immunoreactive for HCG. The presence of these occasional HCG-positive cells does not appear to have prognostic significance, and no functional effects have been described.[86]

Cytology

Metaplastic carcinoma may be suspected in material obtained by FNA of a breast mass if epithelial and metaplastic elements are present.[68,87–91] When epithelial elements are not apparent in the aspirate, the material is likely to suggest a mesenchymal or fibroepithelial neoplasm.[92–96] The diagnosis of metaplastic carcinoma is entertained with greater confidence when distinct adenocarcinoma and either squamous or heterologous components are identified. Lui et al.[97] evaluated the FNA findings in a series of 19 metaplastic carcinomas. Morphologic overlap between the various metaplastic components was observed. The identification of dual morphology, unequivocal neoplastic squamous cells, chondroid stroma, and carcinoma with focal spindle cell morphology raised the possibility of metaplastic carcinoma, but these findings were uncommon and often difficult to detect with certainty. The differential diagnosis includes a variety of benign and malignant lesions, such as papilloma with squamous metaplasia possibly secondary to infarction, PT with epithelial hyperplasia, primary mammary sarcoma, and metastatic neoplasms. Joshi et al.[43] reported similar findings in a series of 10 metaplastic carcinomas initially sampled by FNA. Only 1 of 10 tumors was correctly diagnosed based on review of the FNA material. The cytologic diagnosis for the remaining nine cases included ductal carcinoma (five cases), poorly differentiated carcinoma (two cases), apocrine carcinoma, and PT (one case each). Osteoclastic-like giant cells may be found in the aspirate from a metaplastic carcinoma with heterologous metaplasia.[98]

FNA of a matrix-producing metaplastic carcinoma reveals cuboidal to oval tumor cells in a myxoid background.[67,99] The matrix material stains pale green in the Papanicolaou stain and purple red with the May–Giemsa stain. Tumor cells may be embedded in the matrix material.

Cytologic sampling of a metastasis of metaplastic carcinoma shows similar morphologic features (Fig. 16.36). Awareness of the prior history of metaplastic breast carcinoma is fundamental to avoid possible misdiagnosis. Whenever possible, the prior material should be reviewed, and immunoperoxidase stains for a panel of CKs should be performed if sufficient material is available. In questionable cases, it is prudent to request more tissue for diagnosis, such as a core biopsy sample, before a definitive surgical procedure is performed.

Immunohistochemistry

The specific cell type that gives rise to metaplastic carcinoma remains uncertain. Some investigators suggest that metaplastic carcinomas arise directly from a population of pluripotent mammary cancer stem cells. Another hypothesis involves origin from myoepithelial cells with stem cell properties. A third possibility is that metaplastic carcinomas might develop through a process of dedifferentiation secondary to EMT in nonmetaplastic breast carcinomas. Data relating to these hypotheses are presented in this and subsequent sections.

Metaplastic carcinomas demonstrate heterogeneous patterns of immunoreactivity for epithelial and mesenchymal markers that most likely reflect different genetic alterations in individual tumors. Coexpression of epithelial (CKs and EMA), myoepithelial (p63 and calponin), and mesenchymal (vimentin) antigens in cells with epithelial and/or mesenchymal phenotype has been reported in a number of studies of metaplastic carcinoma.[20,52,74,100–104] These observations support epithelial derivation of these tumors (Figs. 16.38 to 16.40).

Experimental studies have revealed the capacity of epithelial cells to undergo metaplastic change and assume a mesenchymal phenotype.[105,106] The process by which epithelial cells acquire the morphologic phenotype and functional properties of mesenchymal cells is known as EMT.[107] EMT occurs physiologically during embryogenesis and tissue repair.[108] Similar changes have been induced experimentally in mature epithelium, including mammary cells lines and in murine models of breast carcinoma.[105,106,109] EMT results in substantial changes in the cytoskeleton of metaplastic cells and in the extracellular matrix. These changes are consistent

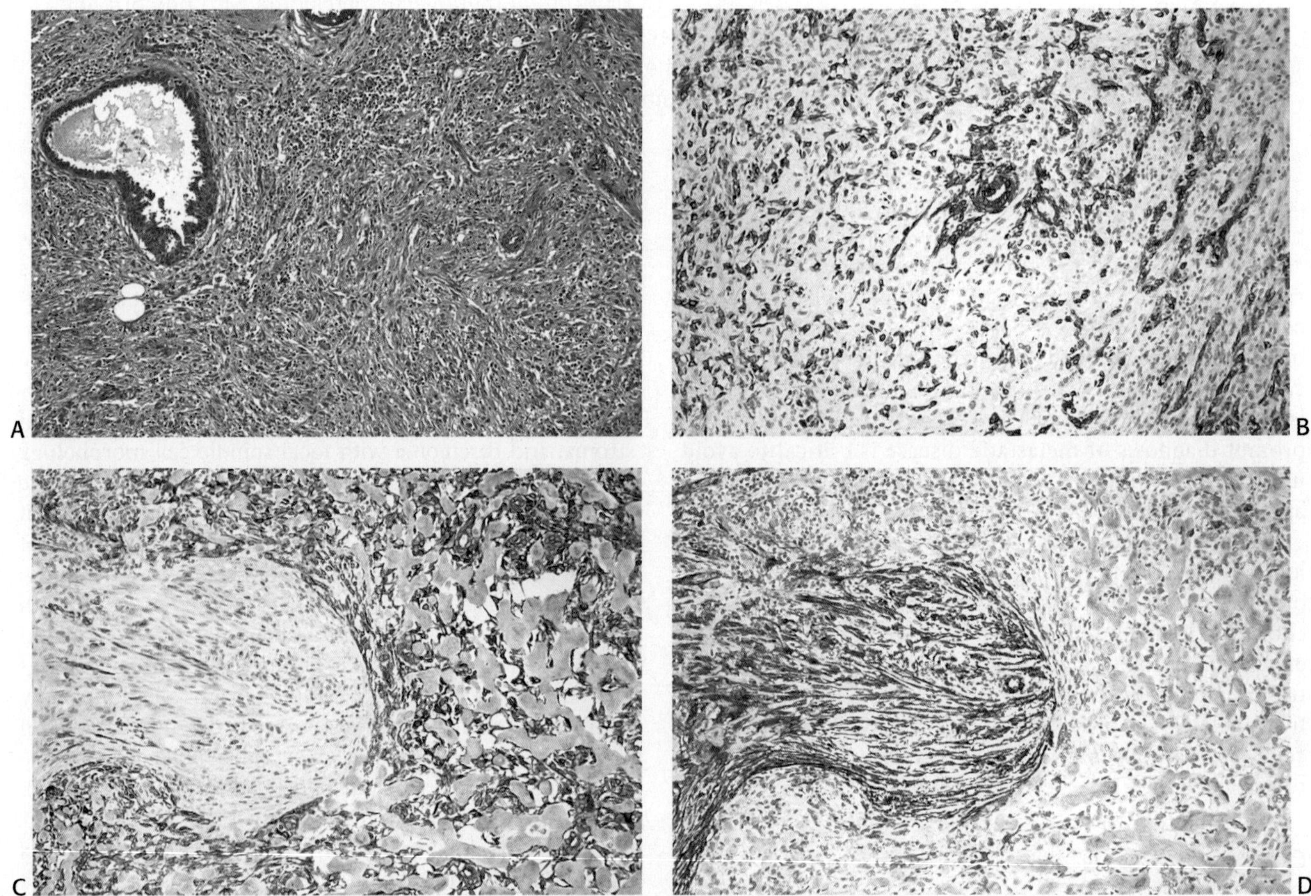

FIG. 16.38. ***Metaplastic carcinoma, immunoreactivity.*** **A:** A hyperplastic duct is surrounded by spindle cell metaplastic carcinoma. **B:** Immunoreactivity for CK AE1:3 is present in some but not all cells. **C:** Immunoreactivity for SMA is shown surrounding a discrete nonreactive zone. **D:** A section parallel to (C) showing immunoreactivity for CK AE1:3 limited to the region that was not reactive for actin (C).

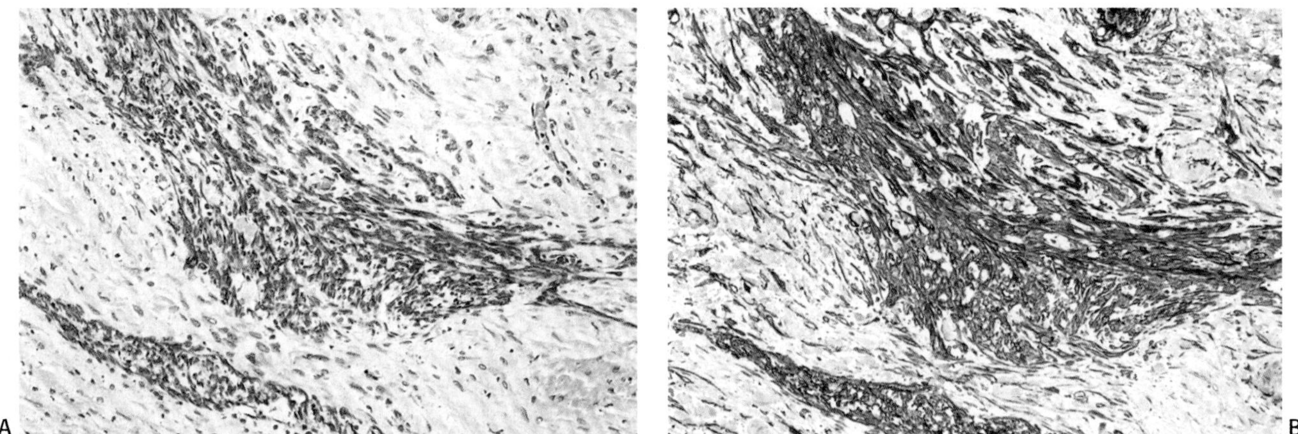

FIG. 16.39. ***Metaplastic carcinoma, immunoreactivity.*** Coexpression of CK and actin is demonstrated in parallel sections of a spindle cell metaplastic carcinoma. **A:** CK AE1:3 reactivity. **B:** Reactivity for SMA in the same region as **(A)**.

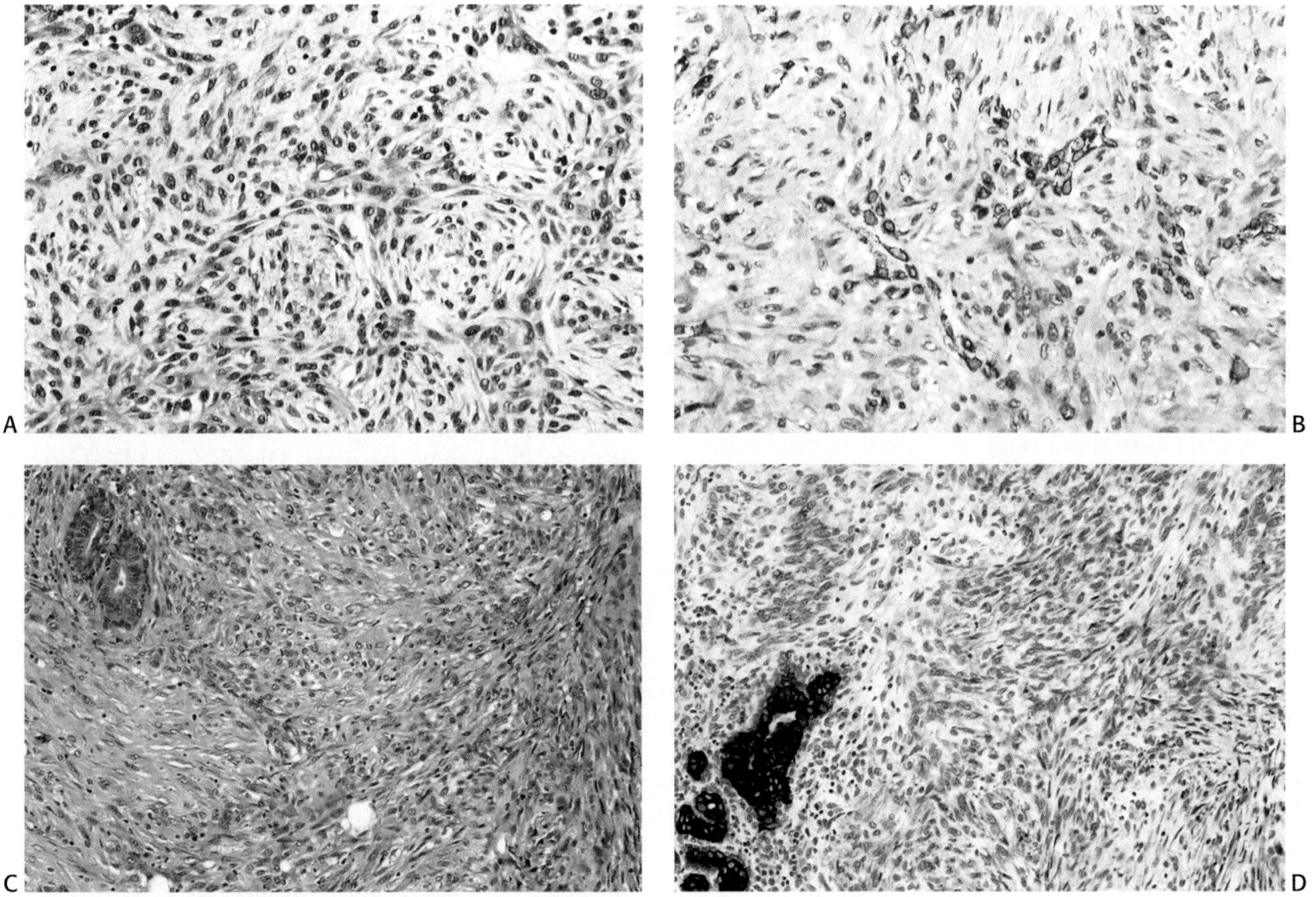

FIG. 16.40. ***Metaplastic carcinoma, immunoreactivity.*** **A:** The tumor has a storiform structure and a hint of angiomatous growth. **B:** The CK immunostain highlights angiomatous foci. **C:** Small ducts are surrounded by spindle cell metaplastic carcinoma. **D:** Immunoreactivity for CK7 is stronger in the ducts than in the metaplastic carcinoma.

with the combined epithelial and mesenchymal phenotypes displayed by metaplastic carcinomas. Genetic evidence supports EMT as the means by which metaplastic changes occur in mammary carcinomas, as described in the subsequent section on genetic and molecular studies. Morphologic evidence also suggests that metaplastic carcinomas arise from invasive ductal carcinomas through a process of dedifferentiation consistent with EMT.[110]

Cytokeratins

The diagnostic workup of a mammary tumor suspected to be metaplastic carcinoma requires testing for a panel of epithelial antigens inclusive of high molecular weight CKs. Rather than a single pattern of CK expression, metaplastic mammary carcinomas display a range of reactivity for different CKs because of the presence of differing types and proportions of cytoskeletal proteins even in morphologically similar tumors. Positive staining for CK in mesenchymal-appearing cells of a metaplastic carcinoma is especially useful for diagnostic classification. Because of the varied CK immunoreactivity in metaplastic carcinomas, the use of a CK panel is recommended.[54,111] The pancytokeratin cocktail MNF116, keratin 34βE12 (K903), CK5/6, CK14, and CK17 can all be very useful to document epithelial differentiation. CK5/6, CK14, CK17, and 34βE12 are high molecular weight CKs, also known as basal CKs, because they are expressed in the basal layer of multistratified epithelia. Normal mammary myoepithelial cells also express basal CKs. The pancytokeratin cocktail MNF116 reacts with basal CK5, CK6, and CK17, with low molecular weight CK8, and probably with CK19.

Carter et al.[54] reported that pancytokeratin MNF116 was positive in 27 of 29 (93%) metaplastic carcinomas with spindle cell morphology. CK14 was the second most sensitive marker, with positivity in 9 of 10 cases (90%). Dunne et al.[103] found positive staining for keratin 34βE12 in the sarcomatous areas of 11 of 18 (61%) metaplastic carcinomas, and detected CK5 in 7 of 18 (39%) cases and CK14 in 6 of 18 (33%). In a study by Reis-Filho et al.,[112] 56/65 (86.1%) metaplastic carcinomas were positive for CK5/6 and 53/65 (81.5%) for CK14. Carpenter et al.[113] documented CK5/6 positivity in 9/18 (50%) cases of metaplastic carcinoma, including three with chondroid matrix, three with squamous and sarcomatous morphology, two with only sarcomatous morphology, and one metaplastic "fibromatosis-like" carcinoma. None of the cases consisted of metaplastic carcinoma showing only squamous metaplasia. Keratin AE1:3 stained only 28% of metaplastic spindle cell carcinomas in one study[103] and 41% in another.[54] Similarly, positivity for CAM5.2 was only 28% in one study[103] and 40% in another.[54] EMA, another epithelial marker, was positive in 43% of metaplastic spindle cell carcinomas[54] Other CKs show less frequent reactivity in metaplastic carcinomas. Dunne et al.[103] documented positivity for CK7 in only 3 of 18 (16%) cases of metaplastic carcinomas; CK19 also stained only 3/18 (16%) tumors. In a study of 21 breast carcinomas with chondroid differentiation, Gwin et al.[42] observed positivity for keratin AE1:3 in 38% of cases.

In most metaplastic carcinomas, one CK may be more readily detectable and diffusely positive, but careful inspection of slides immunostained for other CKs may reveal isolated positive cells or small foci of reactivity in samples that appear to be not immunoreactive on cursory examination. This is an important corroborating observation (Figs. 16.38 to 16.40). Osteoclast-like giant cells in metaplastic carcinomas are immunoreactive for vimentin and sometimes for histiocytic markers, but not for EMA or CKs. On the other hand, CK immunoreactivity was found in the spindle cell mesenchymal component of 63% of these tumors.[17]

Myoepithelial Markers

The diagnosis of metaplastic carcinoma is most challenging if the tumor lacks a distinct epithelial component, as the differential diagnosis includes sarcoma. This scenario presents most commonly for tumors with pure spindle cell morphology and intermediate or high nuclear grade. Most metaplastic carcinomas, however, show some positive immunoreactivity for myoepithelial markers, especially for p63, supporting myoepithelial differentiation.[54,104,113] p63 is a p53 homolog found in the nuclei of myoepithelial and squamous cells, and only rarely in glandular epithelial cells.[114,115] It is often expressed in sarcomatoid metaplastic carcinomas of the breast.[54,104,113,115,116]

Koker and Kleer[104] assessed p63 reactivity in 189 invasive breast carcinomas, including 15 tumors with metaplastic morphology. Strong p63 staining was present in 13 of 15 (86.7%) metaplastic carcinomas, including all carcinomas with spindle cell and/or squamous differentiation and one of three metaplastic carcinomas with cartilaginous foci. Only one of 174 (0.6%) nonmetaplastic invasive carcinomas was positive for p63. In the same study, there was no p63 reactivity in 14 PTs and 5 primary breast sarcomas. The sensitivity and specificity of p63 for the diagnosis of metaplastic carcinoma were 86.7% and 99.4%, respectively.[104] Other studies have reported p63 positivity in 57%,[54] 68%,[113] and 70%[117] of metaplastic spindle cell carcinomas. When neither intraductal nor invasive adenocarcinoma is evident and the tumor is diffusely p63 positive, myoepithelial differentiation is likely.

Positive staining for p63 has been reported to occur occasionally in some sarcomas. One of four (25%) breast sarcomas in a series that included two undifferentiated sarcomas, a PT and an angiosarcoma (AS)[113] showed focal p63 staining, but the authors did not specify which tumors were positive.[113] Kallen et al.[118] reported p63 staining in some nonmammary osteoblastic tumors, including osteosarcomas. The same authors[119] also documented positive p63 staining in 5 of 21 (23.8%) malignant vascular tumors. In their series, a hemangioendothelioma showed p63 staining in more than 75% of the tumor cells and another in more than 60%; a third hemangioendothelioma and two ASs showed p63 positivity in less than 10% of the tumor cells. Focal CK and/or EMA expression has been occasionally observed in vascular tumors, in particular epithelioid AS and in hemangioendothelioma,[120] as well as in other sarcomas. CD10 positivity has also been described in vascular tumors.[121] Therefore, the use of vascular markers, such as CD34, CD31, or FLI1, should be considered in the diagnostic workup of p63-positive spindle cell lesions of the breast suspected to be metaplastic carcinoma if the tumor appears hemorrhagic.

In a comprehensive study, Jo and Fletcher[122] assessed p63 expression using IHC on whole tissue sections of 650 nonmammary soft tissue tumors and found it to be very limited. Most soft tissue tumors were negative for p63, including all their cases of AS, lipomatous neoplasms, dermatofibrosarcoma protuberans, solitary fibrous tumor, schwannoma, neurofibroma, gastrointestinal stromal tumor, and leiomyosarcoma. Nuclear reactivity for p63 was present in myoepithelioma and myoepithelial carcinoma of soft tissue, and in a subset of cellular neurothekeoma, soft tissue perineurioma, Ewing sarcoma/peripheral neuroectodermal tumor, diffuse-type giant cell tumor, and giant cell tumor of soft parts. Rare, weak, or focal staining for p63 was observed in low-grade fibromyxoid sarcoma, malignant peripheral nerve sheath tumor, extraskeletal myxoid chondrosarcoma, myxofibrosarcoma, proximal-type epithelioid sarcoma, synovial sarcoma, embryonal rhabdomyosarcoma, desmoplastic small round cell tumor, atypical fibroxanthoma, and spindle cell melanoma. Overall, these soft tissue tumors are extremely rare in the breast, but they could potentially arise primarily in the extralobular stroma or metastasize to the breast from an extramammary site. In general, p63 expression is usually much more widespread in metaplastic mammary carcinomas than in sarcomas, and, with rare exceptions, metaplastic carcinomas display much more CK reactivity. Nonetheless, ambiguous tumors with sparse p63 and CK expression can be encountered, and thorough analysis of all histologic and immunohistochemical features may be necessary to distinguish between metaplastic carcinoma and sarcoma.

Myoepithelial markers such as CD10, myosin, maspin, and smooth muscle actin (SMA) are also expressed in the sarcomatoid component of many metaplastic carcinomas, although less consistently than p63.[103,117,123] Immunoreactivity for SMA has been reported in 65%[117] and 71%[54] of metaplastic spindle cell carcinomas. Desmin positivity was noted in one case with a rhabdomyosarcomatous component.[54]

In 2006, Leibl and Moinfar[124] reported seven mammary tumors that they classified as "NOS-type sarcomas." All seven tumors were negative for CK, but positive for CD10 and vimentin. Three tumors expressed CD29 and SMA, and two had reactivity for p63 and calponin. Five of seven (71%) lesions had strong membranous positivity for EGFR. Local lymph nodes were negative in all three patients who underwent ALN evaluation. One patient with the largest (11 cm) tumor and negative ALNs had lung metastases, and five were known to be disease free. CD29 is a cell adhesion receptor, also known as integrin-β1. Although this marker was initially regarded as specific for myoepithelial cells, recent evidence suggests that CD29/integrin-β identifies a population of epithelial/myoepithelial stem cells located in the basal layer of mammary ducts and lobules.[125] The tumors reported by Leibl and Moinfar[124] most likely originated from the myoepithelium or from mammary stem cells admixed with it. Therefore, the designation of sarcomas does not appear to be appropriate for these lesions, as they likely represent metaplastic carcinomas with no detectable CK expression.

Metaplastic Carcinomas Are Usually Triple Negative

Metaplastic carcinomas are usually triple negative, although occasional tumors with focal positivity for ER and/or HER2 are encountered. In an epidemiologic study based on data collected by the National Cancer Data Base (study period: January 2001 to December 2003),[14] 72 of 892 (11.7%) metaplastic carcinomas were ER positive. Hennessy et al.[26] reported ER positivity in 6 of 100 (6%) metaplastic carcinomas, and Lester et al.[34] in 3 of 37 (8%). Two of 100 (2%) metaplastic carcinomas in the series by Hennessy et al.[26] were HER2- positive. In these studies, information about ER and HER2 status was based on clinical reports, and the extent and cellular distribution of the positive reactivity was not provided.

In the series described by Carpenter et al.,[113] one metaplastic carcinoma with squamous and sarcomatoid metaplasia was ER- positive in 10% of the cells, and a carcinoma with sarcomatoid morphology showed equivocal (2+) HER2 staining. Reis-Filho et al.[102] found some HER2 staining in two metaplastic carcinomas using two different antibodies. A carcinoma with squamous metaplasia displayed 1+ staining with only one of the two antibodies. The other carcinoma had spindle cell metaplasia: it showed 2+ staining with one antibody and 1+ with the other. In a subsequent study, Reis-Filho et al.[112] detailed the patterns of ER, PR, and HER staining in a series of 65 metaplastic carcinomas, including 26 tumors with squamous metaplasia. ER was detected in two carcinomas and decorated the mesenchymal-appearing cells in a metaplastic carcinoma with spindle cell morphology, but only the NOS component of a carcinoma with squamous metaplasia. Four of 19 (21%) carcinomas with squamous metaplasia, and 1 of 7 (14.3%) carcinomas with heterologous metaplasia showed positivity for PR, in most cases limited to the squamous foci. Some immunoreactivity for HER2 was present in three tumors, all with squamous metaplasia, with staining intensity of 1+ (negative), 2+ (equivocal), and 3+ (positive). The HER2- equivocal case showed no gene amplification by fluorescence *in situ* hybridization (FISH). Lee et al.[35] reported that 58 of 67 metaplastic carcinomas in their series were triple negative, whereas 9/67 (13.4%) showed some positivity for ER, PR, or HER2. Three tumors were ER- and/or PR- positive, five were HER2 positive, and one was positive for ER and HER2. In this study, the authors scored HER2 immunoreactivity according to the American Society of Clinical Oncology (ASCO)/College of American Pathologists (CAP) 2007 recommendations. Gwin et al.[42] reported 21 cases of metaplastic carcinomas with chondroid metaplasia, all of which were triple negative.

The foregoing results indicate that the non-epithelial component of metaplastic carcinoma is generally negative for ER, PR, and HER2, but focal positivity for one or more of these antigens may occasionally be present, usually confined to the neoplastic epithelial component. Even though the majority of metaplastic mammary carcinomas are triple negative, ER, PR, and HER2 testing is routinely assessed in these tumors, just as in any other type of mammary carcinoma.

Nielsen et al.[126] reported that the triple negative, EGFR- and/or CK5/6-positive immunoprofile identifies breast carcinomas characterized by basal gene array expression profile with 100% specificity and 76% sensitivity. Reis-Filho et al.[112] documented the triple negative, CK5/6- and/or EGFR-positive basal immunoprofile in 59 of 65 (91%) metaplastic breast carcinomas, supporting their classification among basal breast carcinomas. Recent genetic and immunohistochemical data have shown that metaplastic carcinomas constitute a specific subset of carcinomas characterized by basal immunophenotype and low expression of claudin-related genes and proteins (see section on genetics and molecular studies).

Epidermal Growth Factor Receptor

EGFR is a transmembrane tyrosine kinase receptor member of the ErbB receptor family. Activation of EGFR triggers downstream signal pathways that regulate cell proliferation, differentiation, motility, angiogenesis, and survival. Overexpression of EGFR secondary to gene amplification or to EGFR-activating mutations has been identified in a number of human malignant neoplasms and is associated with poor clinical outcome. Conversely, carcinomas with tyrosine kinase–activating mutations in the *EGFR* gene can be successfully treated using protein kinase inhibitors. In the breast, *EGFR* is overexpressed in the majority of metaplastic carcinomas with squamous differentiation,[61,127,128] and EGFR immunoreactivity is detected in the epithelial and spindle cell components of these tumors.[128] In one study,[127] EGFR was documented in ALN and bone metastases that exhibited squamous differentiation. Reis-Filho et al.[102] demonstrated *EGFR* gene amplification by chromogenic *in situ* hybridization in 37% of metaplastic carcinomas that were positive for EGFR by IHC. The same group of investigators reported EGFR amplification in 11 of 47 (23%) cases of metaplastic carcinoma in a subsequent study.[129] All EGFR-amplified carcinomas had either spindle cell morphology or squamous differentiation. Other authors have also reported EGFR expression in matrix-producing and heterologous metaplastic carcinomas.[128] In one study,[130] EGFR copy number analysis was performed in 27 metaplastic carcinomas. Eight tumors displayed high *EGFR* copy number by FISH analysis. This finding was secondary to *EGFR* gene amplification in one case and to chromosome 7 aneusomy, most frequently detected in the spindle cell component, in the remaining seven cases.

It has been suggested that EGFR-targeted treatment might be suitable for EGFR-positive metaplastic breast carcinomas[127,128]; however, at least three separate studies found no *EGFR*-activating mutations in metaplastic carcinomas.[129–131] Teng et al.[132] detected *EGFR*-activating mutations in 8 of 70 (11.8%) triple negative breast carcinomas. One of the cases in their series was a metaplastic carcinoma, but the authors did not specify whether it had an EGFR-activating mutation. Immunoreactivity for EGFR, as it is detected with most available antibodies, does not correlate with *EGFR* mutation status.[129,132] Recently, two antibodies specific for the E746-A750del and L858R *EGFR*-activating mutations have become available. Using these antibodies for IHC, Wen et al.[133] detected neither of the two activating mutations in 303 triple negative breast carcinomas, including four metaplastic carcinomas. In the same study, DNA sequencing of a triple negative breast carcinoma that showed 2+ staining intensity for L858R revealed no corresponding *EGFR*-activating mutation. Therefore, at present, there is no genetic evidence supporting the use of agents targeting specific *EGFR* tyrosine kinase–activating mutations for the treatment of metaplastic breast carcinomas, at least in most cases.

Vimentin

The intermediate filaments of vimentin are expressed in mesenchymal cells. In the adult breast, the myoepithelium also expresses vimentin, whereas the glandular/luminal cells are negative. Most mammary invasive carcinomas are vimentin negative, consistent with glandular/luminal genotype and phenotype, but vimentin positivity is found in most basal-like carcinomas[134] and in metaplastic carcinomas. The process of EMT accounts for vimentin positivity in metaplastic carcinomas. This marker, however, has no practical role in the diagnostic workup of a mammary lesion thought to be metaplastic carcinoma because it is highly expressed in normal and neoplastic mesenchymal cells.

Breast Carcinoma Stem Cells

According to some investigators, cancer stem cells are neoplastic cells able to renew themselves indefinitely, a property characteristic of all stem cells. The existence of cancer stem cells in the breast is controversial. Few studies have concluded that the breast contains stem cells that may be essential to tumor initiation, maintenance, renewal, and metastasis,[135] and might be involved in the process of EMT occurring in the breast. Different marker profiles have been used to identify breast cancer stem cells.[125,135] One of the recognized stem cell markers is aldehyde dehydrogenase-1 (ALDH1), a detoxifying enzyme responsible for the oxidation of intracellular aldehydes.[135] An enriched population of ALDH1-positive breast carcinoma stem cells has been demonstrated in metaplastic breast carcinomas using IHC.[136,137] In one study,[136] ALDH1-positive cells were found in 16 of 27 (59%) metaplastic carcinomas, including 71% of spindle cell tumors, 39% of squamous, 83% of chondroid, and 100% of carcinomas with osseous component. In another study,[137] ALDH1 was positive in 4 of 13 metaplastic carcinomas (30.8%) where it decorated the neoplastic epithelial cells in one case and tumor spindle cells in the remaining three.

CD44 is a cell adhesion receptor involved in cell–cell and cell–matrix interactions. It is strongly expressed in the basal layer of the squamous epithelium and also in the normal glandular epithelium in various organs, including the breast. Expression of CD44 has been observed in carcinomas of the breast[138] and other organs. The $CD44^{+}/CD24^{-/low}$ phenotype reportedly identifies breast cancer stem cells.[135] In a study by Gerhardt et al.,[137] $CD44^{+}/CD24^{-/low}$ cells represented more than 10% of neoplastic cells in 13 metaplastic breast carcinomas. The $CD44^{+}/CD24^{-/low}$ immunoprofile was found in all types of neoplastic cells, including glandular and squamous epithelial cells, as well as spindle and chondroid cells. The presence of breast carcinoma stem cells in metaplastic carcinomas is thought to account, at least in part, for the chemotherapy resistance characteristic of these tumors.

Snail and Other EMT-Related Proteins

Snail proteins are a family of transcription factors involved in embryonic development and in EMT.[107,139] Snail reduces cell adhesion, thereby promoting invasion, and contributes to the acquisition of a spindle cell phenotype through downregulation of the E-cadherin promoter. Snail also prolongs the cell cycle, a property that confers resistance to cell death that enhances the ability of malignant cells to form metastatic deposits.[139] Gwin et al.[31] documented nuclear and/or cytoplasmic staining for Snail by IHC in 91.6% of 12 cases of metaplastic carcinomas with chondroid matrix, and found that the expression of Snail was inversely correlated with membranous immunoreactivity for E-cadherin. Snail was present in cells with chondroid morphology, as well as in the malignant epithelium. One tumor displayed nuclear and cytoplasmic staining for Snail in chondroid cells, but only cytoplasmic positivity in the neoplastic epithelial cells. Nassar et al.,[28] however, reported that the specificity of Snail for the diagnosis of metaplastic carcinoma is only 3.8%, even though this marker had high (100%) sensitivity for metaplastic carcinomas, because it was also positive in 4 of 4 (100%) myofibroblastomas, in 14 of 14 (100%) PTs, and in 7 of 8 (87.5%) examples of pseudoangiomatous stromal hyperplasia.

Laminin 5

Laminin 5[140] is a heterotrimeric protein consisting of the α3, β3, and χ2 chains. The β3 and χ2 chains are specific for laminin 5, as they are not expressed in any other type of laminin. Laminin 5 is involved in binding of epithelial cells to the basement membrane through the formation of hemidesmosomes and in the migration of epithelial cells during wound repair. Carpenter et al.[113] evaluated the distribution of the β3 and χ2 chains of laminin 5 in 25 metaplastic breast carcinomas, including 7 carcinomas showing only squamous metaplasia. Both chains decorated 5% to 100% of the cells in 24/25 (96%) cases. Positivity was present in all metaplastic elements, including squamous, chondroid and sarcomatoid foci; glandular neoplastic cells, if present, were also positive. The pattern of immunoreactivity for both chains was similar in 21 of 24 positive cases, whereas the distribution of the χ2 chain was considerably greater in two cases and that of the β3 chain in one. Laminin 5 staining was more obvious at the tumor–stroma interface and absent from the extracellular matrix. Positivity for both β3 and χ2 chains was present in the cytoplasm of normal myoepithelial cells and sometimes in the stroma underneath the basement membrane. Laminin 5 had sensitivity comparable to p63 and CK5/6 for the detection of carcinoma with squamous metaplasia, but showed greater sensitivity than either marker for the detection of matrix-producing carcinomas. Laminin 5 also showed moderately increased sensitivity compared with p63 or CK5/6 for the detection of metaplastic sarcomatoid carcinoma. The authors also reported positivity for laminin 5 in 12 high-grade triple negative nonmetaplastic breast carcinomas, and negative staining in four sarcomas, including two undifferentiated sarcomas, one metastatic malignant PT, and one AS. These results suggest that laminin 5 might be a sensitive and specific novel marker for the diagnosis of metaplastic carcinoma. However, the diagnostic utility of laminin 5, especially in limited core biopsy material, requires further validation.

αB-crystallin

αB-crystallin is a heat shock protein encoded by the *CRYAB* gene located on chromosome 11q22.3 to q23.1. It is a component of the vertebrate eye crystallin. αB-crystallin has a cytoprotective effect, at least in part due to inhibition of apoptosis. Oxidative stress and heat shock induce its expression. In breast carcinomas, αB-crystallin is induced by neoadjuvant chemotherapy and is associated with chemotherapy resistance.[141] Moyano et al.[142] detected expression of αB-crystallin in 45% of basal carcinomas compared with only 6% of nonbasal carcinomas, and documented its association with poor outcome in multivariate analysis, independent of tumor grade, lymph node involvement, and ER and HER2 status. Sitterding et al.[143] demonstrated αB-crystallin expression in 86% of 29 metaplastic carcinomas. Reactivity was predominantly observed in the carcinomatous component of metaplastic carcinomas, but a positive reaction was also noted in the sarcomatous spindle cell component of five cases. This marker showed 86% sensitivity and 100% specificity for the basal-like carcinomas in the same study. Tsang et al.,[144] however, found positive αB-crystallin only in one of five metaplastic carcinomas in their series.

Other Markers

GATA3 is expressed in most ER-positive breast carcinomas. In a study evaluating primary carcinoma in different organs,[145] GATA3 decorated 91% of invasive ductal carcinomas and 100% of invasive lobular carcinomas, in addition to 86% of urothelial carcinomas and 2% of endometrial adenocarcinomas. Cimino-Mathews et al.[146] detected GATA3 in 7/13 (54%) metaplastic carcinomas and suggested that positivity for this antigen may be useful to document mammary origin of distant metastases of metaplastic carcinomas. GATA3 reactivity, however, has recently been documented also in 50% of salivary gland carcinomas.[147] Cimino-Matthews et al.[148] also reported positive reactivity for SOX10, a neural crest transcription factor regarded as highly specific for melanoma, in 46% of 13 metaplastic carcinomas, including 5 of 6 matrix-producing metaplastic carcinomas and 1 of 3 spindle and squamous metaplastic carcinomas. Awareness of the above staining patterns is important in the diagnostic workup of malignant neoplasms of unknown origin.

Electron Microscopy

Electron microscopy has usually supported the epithelial origin of heterologous elements in metaplastic carcinoma by revealing that many ultrastructural characteristics are shared by the various cell types in the tumor. In most,[6,149–153] but not all studies,[154] the authors reported finding cells that had ultrastructural features intermediate between the epithelial and heterologous elements. Myoepithelial cells were present to a variable extent, occasionally constituting a significant part of the lesion.[20,66]

Genetics and Molecular Studies

Basal Gene Profile

Gene array technology has identified distinct intrinsic gene expression profiles of breast carcinoma, namely luminal, *HER2*-overexpressing, and basal types.[155] With only few exceptions, basal carcinomas show no expression of ER- and HER2-related genes, but overexpress proliferation-related and basal genes. Basal genes, such as the genes encoding basal CK5, CK6, CK14, and CK17, are expressed by cells in the basal layer of multistratified epithelia. Most basal genes are also expressed in breast myoepithelial cells. Metaplastic breast carcinomas usually have the triple negative, CK5/6- and/or EGFR-positive phenotype[112] that has been found to have 100% specificity and 76% sensitivity for breast carcinomas with a basal gene array profile.[126] Reis-Filho et al.[112] documented the basal immunophenotype in 91% of metaplastic carcinomas. Weigelt et al.[156] demonstrated the presence of the basal gene expression profile in 19 of 20 (95%) metaplastic carcinomas, supporting the classification of metaplastic carcinomas among basal carcinomas.

Claudin-Low Carcinomas

Using unsupervised clustering to evaluate the gene expression profiles of murine and human mammary tumors, Herschkowitz et al.[157] identified an additional molecular subgroup of breast carcinomas that has been designated as "claudin-low." Claudins are a family of proteins involved in cell-to-cell adhesion, and they are highly expressed in carcinomas with epithelial morphology. Claudin-low tumors are characterized by low to absent expression of markers of luminal/glandular differentiation, such as E-cadherin, and by upregulation of mesenchymal antigens, such as vimentin, and they are rich in cancer stem cells.[137,158] These tumors, thought to constitute about 5% to 10% of all breast carcinomas, are triple negative and have basal-like phenotype.[159] Although they may still be regarded in a broad sense as "basal"-like carcinomas, claudin-low carcinomas cluster together as a distinct subgroup rich in stem cells.[159,160] Most claudin-low carcinomas are poorly differentiated, have high-grade morphology, and are rich in inflammatory cells.[157] Carcinomas with similar features have high metastatic potential and poor prognosis.[160–162] The morphologic, immunophenotypic, and genetic characteristics of metaplastic carcinomas are consistent with those of claudin-low tumors.[137,158]

Epithelial to Mesenchymal Transition

EMT is a multistep and reversible process.[107] Through loss of cell-to-cell junctions, modified cell matrix adhesion, and reorganization of the cytoskeleton, epithelial cells lose their glandular morphology and gain mesenchymal properties, such as spindle cell morphology, mesenchymal phenotype, enhanced migration, resistance to apoptosis, and the ability to produce extracellular matrix components. This process occurs physiologically during embryogenesis and is part of the regenerative changes that take place after tissue injury. It is also believed that EMT occurs transiently in all carcinomas, enabling stromal invasion, lymphatic and hematogenous spread, and seeding at distant sites. The reverse process, known as "mesenchymal to epithelial transition," is thought to occur once neoplastic cells have successfully seeded at a metastatic site.

A number of developmental transcription factors and activation pathways are involved in orchestrating EMT in adult tissues. Snail, Slug, Zinc finger E-box Binding homeobox-1 (ZEB1), Twist, Goosecoid, and FOXC2 are among the transcription factors that contribute to the initiation of EMT. These factors act, at least in part, through transcriptional repression of multiple epithelial-related antigens, such as the E-cadherin/β-catenin complex that participates in the maintenance of epithelial cell morphology. Accumulation of β-catenin in the nucleus is often associated with the functional loss of membranous E-cadherin and leads to increased susceptibility to EMT.[163] Loss of E-cadherin facilitates rearrangement of the cytoskeleton and the acquisition of a back-to-front polarity, both of which are associated with cell motility. TGF-β released by the extracellular matrix near the tumor usually acts as a tumor suppressor, but in some cases it could promote EMT through the induction of Smad3/4 and activation of activin receptor–like kinase 5 (ALK-5).[107]

Multiple lines of evidence demonstrate that EMT occurs in metaplastic breast carcinomas. Taube et al.[164] showed increased expression of genes involved in EMT, including Goosecoid, Snail, Twist, and TGFβ1, and downregulation of the E-cadherin-/β-catenin-associated signaling pathway in metaplastic carcinomas. The expression of the EMT regulators ZEB1[136] and Snail[28,31] is also increased in these tumors. Overexpression of Snail has been shown to downregulate the expression of the cell cycle protein cyclin D2, conferring resistance to cell death.[139]

Lien et al.[165] used gene array technology to evaluate the genomic profile of 34 ductal carcinomas and 4 metaplastic breast carcinomas with sarcomatous or osteochondroid metaplasia. Unsupervised clustering separated the two tumor types, also further separating metaplastic carcinomas with different morphology. Supervised analysis identified distinctive gene profiles. Metaplastic carcinomas were characterized by increased expression of genes involved in cell/cell matrix adhesion and remodeling/synthesis of extracellular matrix (*ADAMT5, HTRA3, MXRA8, TIPM3*), adhesion (*AGC1, EDIL3, PKD2*), and matrix proteins (*COL16A1, COL18A1, LUM, P4H8, SPARC, THB1, THB2*). Other genes were related to development, including cartilage development (*HOXA7, MSX1, POSTN, AGC1, PRRX1, SFRP2, SFRP4, TBX2*). Several of the discriminator genes were also upregulated in MCF7 cells transfected with Snail and exhibiting EMT *in vitro*, supporting a crucial role for EMT in the pathogenesis of metaplastic breast carcinomas.[165]

Mani et al.[166] reported that induction of EMT in immortalized breast epithelial cells resulted in the acquisition not only of mesenchymal features, but also of properties of breast cancer–initiating cells/tumor stem cells. The authors documented the presence of cells with similar properties in metaplastic carcinomas, where they also found increased levels of ALDH1-positive and $CD44^{+}/CD24^{-/low}$ breast carcinoma stem cells. Other studies have documented the presence of breast cancer stem/tumor-initiating cells in metaplastic carcinomas.[136,137,164] These data suggest that breast cancer stem cells may be involved in the process of EMT. No exon 3 mutation of the *CTNNB1* (β-catenin) gene was detected in metaplastic breast carcinomas in one study.[158]

Chromosomal Alterations

Metaplastic carcinomas show patterns of chromosomal gains and losses that differ from all other mammary epithelial tumors. Hennessy et al.[158] evaluated the genomic and mRNA array profiles of 28 metaplastic breast carcinomas, including 19 with sarcomatoid morphology and 9 with squamous metaplasia, and compared the results with those of nearly 500 breast carcinomas. The investigators found that metaplastic carcinomas have a pattern of chromosomal gains and losses different from those of nonmetaplastic breast carcinomas, including non-metaplastic basal carcinomas. In particular, metaplastic breast carcinomas showed gains of distal chromosome 1p and 5p and loss of 3q, alterations that are rarely observed in other types of breast carcinomas. Chromosome 1q gain and loss of 16q, typically found in low-grade breast carcinomas, were uncommon in metaplastic tumors.

Metaplastic carcinomas also demonstrated more frequent amplification of 1p, 11q, 12q, 14q, 19p, 19q, and 22q and increased frequency of 1q, 2p, 3q, and 8q losses than basal carcinomas. Retention of 5q, 9q, 15q, 16p, 17p, 17q, 19p, 19q, 20q, and 22q was also greater in metaplastic carcinomas than in basal carcinomas. Overall, the patterns of chromosomal alterations observed in metaplastic breast carcinomas did not resemble those found in either usual or basal carcinomas, suggesting that metaplastic breast carcinomas represent a genetically distinct subgroup of breast tumors.

Other Mutations

In a study by Hennessy et al.,[158] *p53* mutations were detected in 6 of 19 (32%) metaplastic carcinomas. The same investigators also found that phosphatidylinositol 3-kinase (*PIK3CA*) gene mutations, some of which may lead to constitutive activation of the PIK3CA pathway, were significantly more frequent in metaplastic carcinomas (9 of 19 cases, 47.4%) than in hormone receptor–positive carcinomas (80 of 232, 34.5%) ($p = 0.32$), *HER2*-amplified carcinomas (17 of 75, 22.7%) ($p = 0.04$), and triple negative carcinomas (20 of 240, 8.3%) ($p < 0.0001$). A metaplastic carcinoma with wild-type *PIK3CA* gene showed a *PTEN* mutation. Genomic aberrations in the *PI3K/AKT* pathway, including *AKT1* (chromosome 14), *AKT2* (chromosome 19), and *RPS6KB2* (p70S6K, chromosome 11) genes were also more common in metaplastic carcinomas, suggesting that alterations in the *PI3K/AKT* pathway may play a major role in the biology of these tumors.

McCarthy et al.[167] described the creation of a mouse model of basal-like spindle cell and squamous metaplastic carcinoma by inducing *BRCA1* and *p53* gene mutations. Only rare cases of metaplastic breast carcinoma occurring in patients with germline *BRCA1* gene mutation have been described,[39,40,42] and there are no reports of metaplastic breast carcinomas with somatic mutation of the *BRCA1* gene. Downregulation of the *BRCA1* gene, however, can also result from other mechanisms besides gene mutation. Turner et al.[168] documented downregulation of the *BRCA1* gene secondary to promoter methylation in 17 of 27 (63%) metaplastic breast carcinomas with basal immunoprofile. Weigelt et al.[156] found downregulation of *BRCA1*-mediated DNA damage response and of the G2/M DNA damage checkpoint regulation in 20 metaplastic breast carcinomas. *BRCA1*-induced growth arrest is dependent on phosphorylation of the retinoblastoma (*RB*) gene protein that is involved in the control of p53. In individuals that are not *BRCA1* germline mutation carriers, DNA alterations may result from partial inactivation of both *RB*- and *BRCA1*-controlled pathways of DNA repair. *In vitro* studies have shown that overexpression of *TWIST* and *ZEB1*, both powerful inducers of EMT, can functionally inhibit *p53*- and *RB*-dependent pathways in mammary cell lines and prevent cells from undergoing oncogene-induced senescence and apoptosis.[169] Weigelt et al.[156] also reported significant downregulation of *PTEN* and *TOP2A* in metaplastic carcinomas. These observations may account in part for the relative resistance to chemotherapy that characterizes metaplastic carcinomas compared with nonmetaplastic tumors.

MicroRNAs

MicroRNAs are short posttranslational RNA regulators. By binding to complementary mRNA sequences, they result in gene silencing through translational repression or degradation of the target mRNA. A number of studies have revealed that microRNAs are dysregulated in human malignant neoplasms, including breast carcinomas. In normal mammary epithelial cells, microRNA-200 family members suppress EMT drivers such as *ZEB1* and *ZEB2* and maintain E-cadherin expression.[170] Gregory et al.[171] found downregulation of five members of the microRNA-200 family in cells undergoing EMT *in vitro* and reported that the same microRNAs were low to absent in the mesenchymal-appearing component of metaplastic carcinomas. Shimono et al.[172] reported that members of the microRNA-200 family were downregulated in human and mouse mammary stem cells as well as in human breast carcinoma stem cells. These findings, as well as data by Mani et al.,[166] demonstrate a close relationship between mammary cells undergoing EMT and breast cancer stem cells.

Morel et al.[109] have recently shown that overexpression of the EMT-promoting factors Twist and ZEB in the mammary epithelium of transgenic mice with activated *K-ras* oncogene promotes the development of the murine equivalent of claudin-low breast carcinomas. Overexpression of an

EMT inducer in mammary glandular epithelial cells *in vitro* prompted acquisition of EMT features, including significant positivity for mesenchymal markers such as vimentin, and decreased expression of markers of epithelial differentiation such as E-cadherin. The type and level of expression of the EMT inducer determined the extent of epithelial to mesenchymal transdifferentiation. Overexpression of *ZEB1* was sufficient to promote EMT with acquisition of spindle cell morphology and complete loss of E-cadherin, even in the absence of a mitogenic factor. In contrast, glandular epithelial cells overexpressing *ZEB2* or *TWIST1* acquired intermediate phenotypes, maintaining E-cadherin expression and epithelial morphology, even if they acquired vimentin positivity. Gene array analysis of *ZEB1* ± *RAS* overexpressing mammary glandular epithelial cells yielded a profile similar to that of claudin-low tumors, whereas the gene expression profile of cells overexpressing *TWIST1* or *ZEB2* ± *RAS* resembled more than that of basal-like tumors. Twist and ZEB proteins can inhibit p53- and RB-dependent pathways.

Some or all of the above mechanisms may be involved in the pathogenesis of metaplastic carcinomas. The wide range of possible genetic alterations encountered in metaplastic carcinomas likely accounts for the extremely heterogeneous morphology that characterizes these tumors.

Prognosis

Because of the rarity of metaplastic carcinomas, all reported series are retrospective and include relatively limited numbers of cases. In addition, most studies provide only minimal information on tumor morphology, and the morphologic heterogeneity of these tumors complicates their classification and analysis. Other than perhaps rare cases included in large studies that are usually not specifically identified as metaplastic carcinomas, no prospective data are available.

Two epidemiologic series[14,26] include information about over a thousand patients, but provide no detailed information on tumor subtypes. Lymph node involvement was present in 20%[26] and 21.9%[14] of patients. The overall frequency of positive ALNs associated with heterologous metaplastic carcinoma, including matrix-producing tumors, ranges from 3%[21] to 45%.[42] At presentation, patients had stage I in 22%[14,26] of cases, stage II in 55%[14] and 59%,[26] and stage III in 10%[14] and 13.5%,[26] respectively. Surgical treatment consisted of mastectomy in 55.6% of cases and breast-conserving surgery in 44%.[14] Radiotherapy was administered to 42.5% of patients, including 11 who did not undergo surgery.[14] Over half of the patients (53.4%) received chemotherapy, and 6.4% hormonal therapy.[14] Based on Surveillance Epidemiology and End Results (SEER) data,[26] overall survival (OS) at 5 years was 81% for stage I, 59% for stage II, 67% for stage III, and 18% for stage IV. Disease-specific survival at 5 years was 93% for patients with stage I disease, 67% for stage II, 71% for stage III, and 20% for stage IV.

Sarcomatoid Metaplastic Carcinoma

Disease-free survival (DFS) of sarcomatoid metaplastic carcinomas, generally reported for 5 or more years of follow-up, ranges from 29%[12] to 83%.[54] Hennessy et al.[26] reported the findings in 100 patients with biphasic sarcomatoid carcinoma of the breast treated at one institution between 1985 and 2001. Of 94 patients with localized disease at diagnosis, 64% were treated by mastectomy and 29% by breast-conserving surgery. Lymph node metastases were found in 28% of patients who underwent lymph node evaluation. Adjuvant radiotherapy was administered to 54% of patients, including 26 treated by mastectomy (5 of 6 with positive/close margins) and 23 treated with breast-conserving surgery (3 of 4 with positive/close margins). Follow-up information was available for 89 patients, and 34 died of disease. The 5-year OS was 64%. There was no statistically significant difference in survival between patients who did or did not receive chemotherapy or radiotherapy. The risk of death due to disease was greater for patients with lymph node involvement (hazard ratio [HR] 2.51) and with T4 tumors (HR 18.33) compared with the risk of patients with T1 tumors. Forty-four of 91 (48.3%) patients with follow-up information about tumor recurrence developed disease, including 22 patients with distant recurrence, 6 with local and distant recurrence, and 16 with only local recurrence. The median time of recurrence-free survival (RFS) was 74 months, and the median survival following any disease recurrence was 14 months. Eighty-two patients received chemotherapy, including neoadjuvant treatment in 21. Overall, patients with metaplastic sarcomatoid carcinoma had a poor prognosis, slightly but not significantly worse than that of high-grade hormone receptor–negative ductal carcinomas. Information on HER2 status was not available. In the same series, radiotherapy did not seem to reduce the incidence of local recurrence in patients treated by breast conservation, but the data are inconclusive.

Other series report similar results. The 5-year OS ranged from 53% to 58.4% in two studies[25,26] and was 53.2% at 10 years in another study.[32] The rates of death due to metaplastic carcinoma in other recent series were 12.5%,[24] 23.9%,[29] 29.7%,[27] 32%,[25] 32.8%,[35] and 33%.[22] Nearly all patients who died of disease developed distant metastases, most often in the lungs and bones.

Metaplastic Carcinoma with Chondroid and/or Osteoid Matrix

Few published series are restricted to specific types of metaplastic carcinoma with chondroid and/or osteoid matrix. Chhieng et al.[69] reported the clinicopathologic features of 32 patients. Each neoplasm consisted of invasive adenocarcinoma accompanied by a cartilaginous and/or osseous component. In 10 neoplasms, the heterologous element consisted of cartilage, and in 2 it was osteoid or bone exclusively. The remaining 20 neoplasms contained a mixture of cartilaginous and osseous components. Twenty-four patients were treated by mastectomy and eight by local excision. Lymph node metastases were detected in 23% of the 26 patients who had an axillary dissection. Clinical follow-up was available for 29 of the 32 patients (91%). Six patients (21%) developed a local recurrence or distant metastases within 2 years of initial treatment, and four of them died of metastatic carcinoma.

The 5-year OS rate was 60%. When compared with control patients with infiltrating ductal carcinoma, the group with osteo/cartilaginous metaplastic carcinoma tended to have a more favorable prognosis after adjustment for nodal status and tumor size, although the difference was not statistically significant (Fig. 16.41).

Gwin et al.[42] studied 21 patients with metaplastic carcinoma with chondroid differentiation. Of 10 patients with available surgical information, 4 underwent mastectomy, and 6 had breast-conserving surgery. Lymph node involvement was present in 5/11 (45.5%) patients who had lymph node evaluation; the metastases were purely chondroid in 3/5 cases (60%). All 8 (100%) patients with available clinical information received adjuvant chemotherapy, and 7/8 (87.5%) had radiotherapy. Follow-up information was available for 8 patients, all of whom had received adjuvant chemotherapy, 7/8 (87.5%) had also received radiotherapy. Median patient survival was 38.6 months (range 2 to 156). Five of the eight patients developed distant metastases, and three died of disease. Two patients were alive with metastatic disease at 11 and 12 months, one was alive with locally recurrent disease at 35 months, and two patients were alive without disease at 2 and 156 months. Multiple sites of recurrent carcinoma were recorded, including the contralateral breast in two cases.

Downs-Kelly et al.[38] studied 32 cases of matrix-producing mammary carcinomas. Osteoid matrix was present in one tumor, and six cases had focal cartilage formation. Lymphovascular invasion was identified in 8/32 (25%) cases, and 8/32 (25%) also showed lymph node metastases. It is unclear how many tumors showed both lymphovascular invasion and lymph node involvement. Surgical treatment consisted of mastectomy in 14/32 (43.7%) cases and was followed by postmastectomy radiotherapy in 6/14 (43%) cases. Eighteen patients (56.3%) underwent breast-conserving surgery with uninvolved margins (at least 2 mm clearance), followed by radiotherapy in 16/18 (89%) cases. Three of 32 (9%) patients received neoadjuvant chemotherapy, 17/32 (53%) adjuvant chemotherapy, and 9/32 (28%) had neoadjuvant and adjuvant chemotherapy. Eight of 32 (25%) patients died of disease at a median follow-up time of 29 months

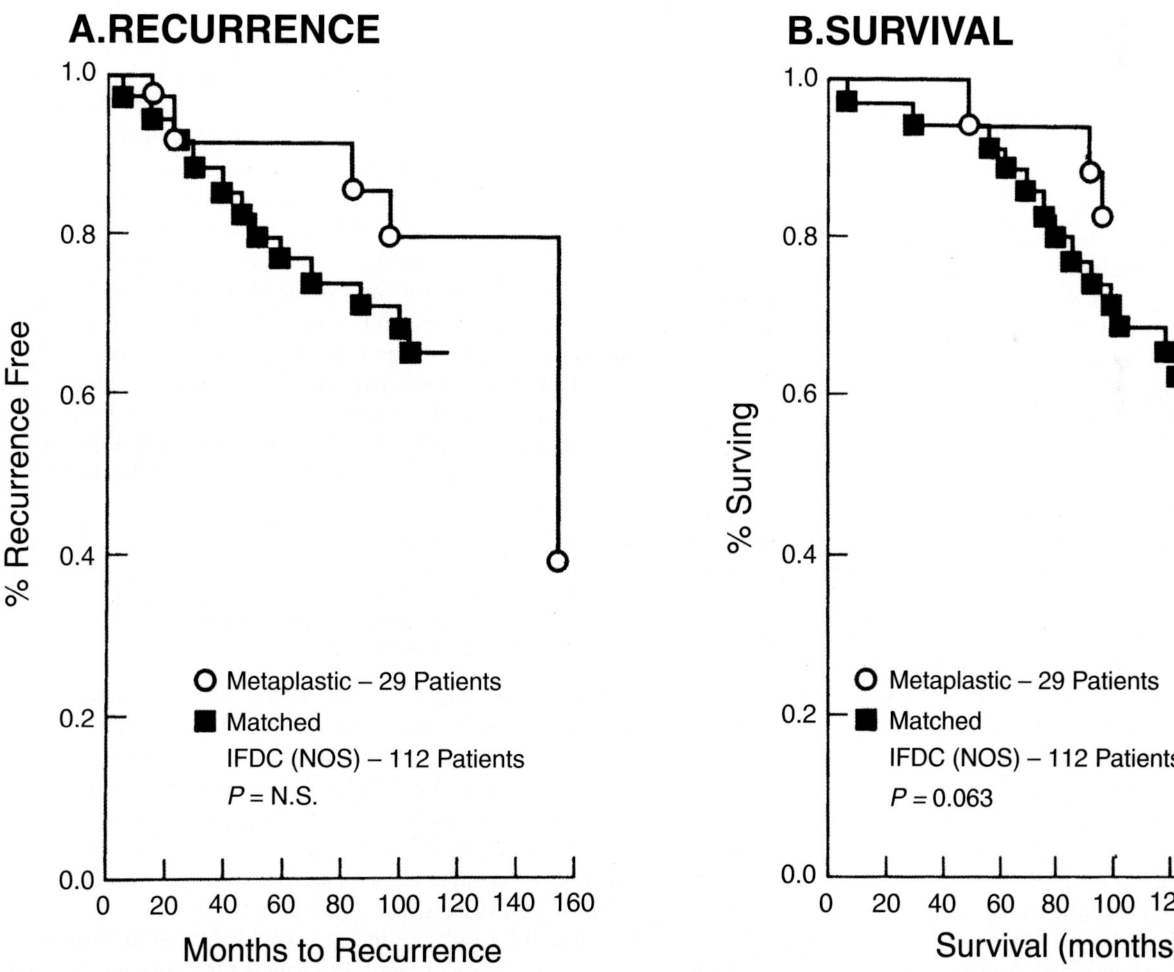

FIG. 16.41. ***Survival analysis for patients with osteocartilaginous metaplastic carcinoma.*** Patients with metaplastic carcinoma were compared with a cohort with invasive duct carcinoma matched for tumor stage. The two groups did not differ significantly in recurrence-free and OS. [From Chhieng C, Cranor M, Lesser ME, et al. Metaplastic carcinoma of the breast with osteocartilaginous heterologous elements. *Am J Surg Pathol* 1998;22:188–194, with permission.]

(range 11 to 50 months). Seven (22%) patients developed locoregional recurrence 1 to 56 months after surgery (median 25 months), including four patients who had not received radiotherapy at the time of initial treatment. Ten (31%) patients developed distant metastases 1 to 40 months after the initial surgery (median 28 months). Six had been treated initially by mastectomy and four with breast-conserving surgery. Metastatic sites included lung and/or pleural fluid (six cases), liver (two cases), and buttocks and leptomeninges in one case each. In univariate analysis, features associated with reduced local RFS included lymphovascular invasion ($p = 0.003$) and stage IV disease ($p < 0.001$). In multivariate analysis, lymphovascular invasion was significantly associated with local RFS (HR 6.54; 95% confidence interval [CI] 1.06 to 40.4; $p = 0.043$). Factors independently associated with disease RFS included lymphovascular invasion (HR 4.76; 95% CI, 1.19 to 19; $p = 0.027$) and stage IV disease (HR 60.1; 95% CI, 5.07 to 712; $p = 0.001$). When compared with a control group of 64 patients with invasive ductal carcinoma NOS matched by age, stage, and tumor grade, patients with matrix-producing metaplastic carcinoma had significantly lower 9-year actuarial local RFS (57% ± 16% vs. 88% ± 8%; $p = 0.001$) and distant RFS (56% ± 11% vs. 84% ± 8%; $p = 0.001$).

Spindle Cell Metaplastic Carcinoma

Spindle cell metaplastic carcinomas are characterized by a poor prognosis. Davis et al.[12] studied 22 cases of spindle cell metaplastic carcinomas with sarcomatoid morphology. The patient average age was 60 years (range 32 to 79). Metaplastic carcinomas with "low-grade" "fibromatosis-like" morphology and those treated with neoadjuvant chemotherapy were excluded. The tumors consisted entirely of spindle cells (16 cases) or had spindle cell and osseous areas (2 cases), spindle cells with chondroid and osseous areas (1 case), pleomorphic cells (2 cases, including one with osseous metaplasia and osteoclast-like giant cells), and MFH-like morphology (1 case). The sarcomatoid areas were intermediate grade in 5 cases and high grade in 17. Tumor size was known in 18 cases and ranged from 1.5 to 5.0 cm. Eleven patients underwent mastectomy, and an equal number had breast-conserving surgery. Seventeen patients had lymph node evaluation, but only 1/17 had lymph node involvement (3.5 mm metastasis in a sentinel lymph node [SLN] sampling). Twenty-one patients received chemotherapy, including four that were treated with chemotherapy only after local recurrence. Twelve patients had radiotherapy, three after breast-conserving surgery, four after primary mastectomy, and five after tumor relapse. The median follow-up time was 36 months (range 4 to 155). Ten of 21 patients developed a local recurrence, including 8 of 14 patients who did not receive primary radiotherapy. Only one of six patients treated with radiotherapy after initial surgery developed a local recurrence. Three patients treated with breast-conserving surgery followed by irradiation did not develop in-breast recurrence, but one developed lung metastases. In-breast recurrence occurred in seven women who did not receive breast irradiation after breast-conserving surgery. Nine patients who had breast-conserving surgery received postoperative chemotherapy according to a protocol for carcinoma in eight and for sarcoma in one. Six of 22 patients (27%) died of disease at 4, 6, 30, 34, 36, 37, and 91 months after treatment, and 2 were alive with disease 9 and 87 months later. One additional patient also developed a distant recurrence, but her status was unknown.

Lester et al.[34] published a series of 47 patients with spindle cell metaplastic carcinoma, using the same inclusion criteria as specified by Davis et al.[12] They compared patients with metaplastic carcinoma with a control group of patients with triple negative breast carcinoma matched by age, stage tumor grade, chemotherapy, and radiotherapy. The metaplastic component was entirely composed of neoplastic spindle cells in 72% of cases, and had MFH-like morphology in two cases, pleomorphic sarcomatoid component in one case, and osseous component with osteoclast-like giant cells in another case. Breast conservation was the primary surgical treatment for 22% (47%) patients, and 25 (53%) underwent mastectomy. Lymph node macrometastases were present in 8/36 (22%) patients who had lymph node evaluation; one patient had a micrometastasis and one isolated tumor cells. Thirty-eight patients received chemotherapy, 32 radiotherapy, and 5 hormonal therapy. Clinical follow-up was available for 43 patients. Twelve patients (28%) developed a locoregional recurrence, 17 (40%) distant metastases, and 9 (21%) had both local and distal recurrent disease. Seventeen patients (40%) died of disease. The 5-year DFS was 45%. Factors associated with significantly decreased DFS in patients with stage I to III were age older than 50 years and nodal macrometastases. A metaplastic component representing more than 95% of the tumor was associated with decreased DFS in stage I to II patients. Tumor size was the only independent factor associated with poor prognosis in stage I patients. For any stage at diagnosis, patients with metaplastic carcinoma had a decreased DFS compared with the control group. For patients with stage I to III, the 5-year DFS was 45% versus 74% in the control group, and for patients with stage I to II disease, the 5-year DFS was 53% versus 87% in the control group.

Summary of Prognosis for High-Grade Metaplastic Carcinoma

Results from other recent series[29,30,35,72,173] with fewer patients, often without a carefully matched control group, document unfavorable prognosis of patients with high-grade metaplastic breast carcinomas, even when compared with patients with high-grade triple negative breast carcinomas. The presence of an extensive high-grade spindle cell (or squamous) component consistently emerges as associated with a worse prognosis.

Only the results of the series by Beatty et al.[24] seem to differ from those of all other series, as the authors reported comparable outcome for patients with metaplastic and nonmetaplastic carcinomas. The authors described 18 patients with diverse forms of metaplastic carcinoma who were treated surgically by partial mastectomy. Axillary dissection was performed in 12 cases, and 6 had SLN sampling. All

18 patients received postoperative breast irradiation. Postoperative chemotherapy of diverse types, most often consisting of adriamycin–cytoxan–taxane, was administered in 13 cases. During the course of follow-up, three (17%) patients died of metastatic carcinoma. One patient (6%) was alive after having had a local recurrence and lung metastasis resected, and 14 (78%) patients were alive without recurrence. These authors reported survival analysis in which the metaplastic carcinoma patients were compared with a matched cohort of nonmetaplastic carcinoma patients. There was no significant difference in the frequency with which breast-conserving surgery was used in the two groups, and there was no statistically significant difference between the two groups with respect to local and distant recurrences, DFS, and OS. The 5-year estimates for RFS were 84% and 93% for the metaplastic and nonmetaplastic cases, respectively. Possible explanations for the different results of this study compared with other studies include the relatively small number and heterogeneous morphology of the cases in this series that included only two cases of metaplastic spindle cell carcinomas.

The foregoing information indicates that the prognosis of metaplastic carcinoma is influenced in part by the stage at diagnosis. Although metaplastic carcinomas have a lower frequency of ALN metastases compared with nonmetaplastic high-grade carcinomas, the prognosis of high-grade metaplastic carcinomas appears to be significantly worse than that of patients with nonmetaplastic carcinomas. In particular, extensive high-grade spindle cell metaplasia has a negative impact on prognosis. Patients with small metaplastic carcinomas are candidates for breast-conserving surgery that should always be followed by breast irradiation to reduce the risk of local recurrence. Postoperative adjuvant chemotherapy is standard practice, but there is no information on the most effective regimen. Overall, the response to neoadjuvant chemotherapy used in most breast protocols appears negligible, and new treatment options are needed.

Low-Grade Spindle Cell Metaplastic Carcinoma

Metaplastic carcinomas described as "low-grade" or "fibromatosis-like" are characterized by sparsely cellular spindle cell areas, an epithelial component comprising less than 5% of the tumor, low nuclear grade, low mitotic activity, and a tendency to local recurrence. In 1999, Gobbi et al.[50] reported the pathologic findings in 30 tumors with this morphology. Eight of 18 (44%) tumors recurred locally 6 to 88 months after the initial surgery. One of the eight patients recurred twice: the first recurrence was 88 months after the initial surgery, and the second followed 9 months later. Histologically, the recurrences were described as more cellular than the primary tumor. In this series, none of the 18 patients with follow-up information developed distant metastases or died of disease. Sneige et al.[55] reported a series of 24 tumors with similar morphology. Initial surgical treatment consisted of local excision (7 cases) or mastectomy (13 cases), and was unknown in 4 cases. No lymph node metastases were found in 15 patients who underwent ALN dissection. Information was available for 16 patients with a median follow-up of 33 months (range 8 to 90). Two of the six patients treated by excision developed local recurrences at 5 and 32 months later. Two patients, both initially treated with mastectomy, developed lung metastases within 2 years after the initial diagnosis. The metastatic tumors were histologically similar to the primary tumors.

Kurian and Al-Nafussi[22] reported the clinicopathologic features of five metaplastic carcinomas that morphologically resembled fibromatosis/nodular fasciitis. The tumors ranged in size from 2.2 to 5.8 cm and occurred in women ranging from 46 to 69 years of age. One of the tumors was associated with invasive lobular carcinoma, and another with ADH. Four of the five patients underwent mastectomy, and one had a wide excision. One of the five patients had lymph node metastasis. Two of the five (40%) patients developed lung metastases and died of disease. Carter et al.[54] also reported a series of 29 spindle cell metaplastic carcinomas, including 7 characterized as having low nuclear grade. Four of the seven patients with low-grade carcinoma developed recurrent disease: two died of disease at 12 and 21 months after initial surgery, and two were alive with disease at 35 and 42 months of follow-up. Therefore, review of the literature documents that these tumors are indeed carcinomas capable of both local recurrence and distant metastases, and need to be treated accordingly, although these tumors appear to be somewhat less aggressive than metaplastic spindle cell carcinomas with high-grade or intermediate-grade morphology.

Treatment

Patients in earlier series of metaplastic carcinoma were treated by mastectomy, usually with an axillary dissection, but in the past two decades, breast conservation therapy has also been used for treatment of this type of breast carcinoma.

Radiotherapy

Tseng and Martinez[32] used SEER data to estimate the benefit of irradiation in the treatment of patients with metaplastic carcinoma. Their study group consisted of 1,501 patients treated between 1988 and 2006. The tumors were classified as metaplastic carcinomas (57.3%) (68.7% having high-grade morphology), adenosquamous carcinomas (18.1%), and carcinosarcomas (11.7%). Tumor size was greater than 2 cm in 68.7% of patients, and 22.5% of patients had lymph node metastases. Most patients (55.5%) underwent mastectomy, 41% breast conserving surgery, and 2.9% did not have tumor resection. Overall, 580 (38.6%) patients received radiotherapy. The 10-year OS and disease-specific survival for all patients were 53.2% and 68.3%, respectively. Radiotherapy improved OS (60.3%) and overall disease-specific survival (71.7%) and was associated with a reduced risk of disease-related death on multivariate analysis.

Chemotherapy

Chemotherapy is routinely used in the treatment of patients with metaplastic carcinoma. The same chemotherapy regimen used for usual breast carcinomas is usually employed for these tumors, but some patients have been treated with sarcoma-specific chemotherapy. It is unclear which chemotherapy regimen is more effective.

Some of the recent series include information on the use of neoadjuvant chemotherapy for the treatment of metaplastic breast carcinoma.[24,26,27,29,35,174] Hennessy et al.[26] described 21 women with metaplastic breast carcinoma who were treated with anthracycline-based neoadjuvant chemotherapy; 5 also received a taxane, and 1 ifosfamide. There were two pathologic complete responses (10%), one complete clinical response (5%), and four clinical partial responses (20%). Nagao et al.[174] studied the response to neoadjuvant chemotherapy in relation to histologic subtypes in a series of patients with breast carcinoma, including nine women with metaplastic carcinoma (four spindle cell, four matrix producing, and one with cartilaginous/osseous metaplasia) and five carcinomas with squamous metaplasia. They reported that, in contrast to usual breast carcinomas, carcinomas with spindle cell or squamous metaplasia increased in size despite neoadjuvant treatment. These findings were consistent with those reported by Rayson et al.[21] in patients treated with conventional neoadjuvant chemotherapy regimens for breast carcinomas. The clinical response of carcinomas with metaplasia was significantly poorer than for usual carcinomas, and half of the metaplastic cases developed progressive disease. The incidence of recurrence or death was significantly higher in the metaplastic group. One example of metaplastic mammary carcinoma that was responsive to neoadjuvant chemotherapy regimen used for sarcomas has been reported.[175]

The chemoresistance displayed by metaplastic carcinomas finds explanation in the process of EMT that is associated with increased cell survival and resistance to apoptosis, as well as in the enriched population of breast cancer stem cells that characterizes these tumors. (see the prior section on genetics and molecular alterations.)

Four of nine patients with stage IV metaplastic carcinoma treated with the mTOR-/hypoxia-inducible factor inhibitor temsirolimus combined with liposomal doxorubicin in the phase I study by Moroney et al.[176] had a *PIK3CA* mutation, and two had *PTEN* loss/mutation. Two patients achieved complete remission. One patient was treated for 8 months with resolution of perihepatic implants, retrocrural lymphadenopathy, nodular pleural disease, and right subcarinal adenopathy. The other patient was treated for 12 months with complete resolution of a biopsy-proven single pulmonary metastasis. Presently, the use of targeted therapy remains limited to clinical trials.

LOW-GRADE ADENOSQUAMOUS CARCINOMA

LGASC is an unusual variant of metaplastic mammary carcinoma that is morphologically similar to adenosquamous carcinoma of the skin. Since its first description published in 1987 by Rosen and Ernsberger,[150] more than 100 examples of this tumor have been reported in a few series[57,58,177–182] and case reports.[178,183–187] Four examples of mammary LGASC have been reported under the diagnosis of syringomatous squamous tumors.[188] A woman with LGASC was a *BRCA1* germline mutation carrier,[184] and two patients with this tumor had a family history of breast carcinoma,[182] but no other association with familial cancer has been reported. Two patients with LGASC in the series by Kawaguchi and Shin[182] had personal histories of ipsilateral breast carcinoma.

Clinical Presentation

All reported cases of LGASC have occurred in women, usually of peri- or postmenopausal age, but patients as young as 19 years old[187] and 20 years old[182] have been reported. Most carcinomas present as a palpable mass, and some tumors are detected by mammography. The tumor arises in the breast parenchyma, but it can originate in the retroareolar area in some cases. Two patients presented with nipple discharge.[182] In the series by Kawaguchi and Shin,[182] a patient had bilateral florid papillomatosis of the nipple, and another developed a CSL in the contralateral breast. Two patients were pregnant at the time of diagnosis.

Mammography can detect LGASC, but the findings are nonspecific (Fig. 16.42). Ultrasound examination of a 5-cm tumor was reported as inconclusive.[187]

Gross Pathology

LGASCs are typically smaller than other varieties of metaplastic carcinoma (0.5 to 5.0 cm, average about 2.0 cm). On gross examination, they consist of hard, yellow-tan nodules with grossly ill-defined borders.

Microscopic Pathology

Microscopically, some tumors have a highly invasive, stellate growth pattern (Fig. 16.43), whereas others are partly or entirely circumscribed (Fig. 16.44). The invasive carcinoma exhibits variable amounts of epidermoid differentiation in collagenous stroma (Figs. 16.44 to 16.46). A tendency to grow between ducts and within lobules is seen throughout the tumor (Figs. 16.43 and 16.47). The identification of epithelial elements surrounded by desmoplastic stroma infiltrating between normal and undistorted lobules is characteristic of LGASC (Fig. 16.47). This feature also helps to differentiate LGASC from nonneoplastic CSLs. However, LGASCs sometimes have a central area of radial sclerosing proliferation such as a papilloma, a radial scar, or sclerosing adenosis from which the neoplasm appears to have arisen (Figs. 16.43 and 16.48). Association with adenomyoepitheliomatous proliferation has also been reported[181,189] (Fig. 16.49).

Squamous metaplasia is found in varying patterns including extensive epidermoid growth, syringoma-like differentiation, and isolated inconspicuous squamous foci in predominantly glandular lesions (Figs. 16.44 to 16.46). Large keratinizing cysts are uncommon, but microcysts that may contain keratotic debris with calcification are sometimes present. Osteocartilaginous foci have been encountered in primary tumors and in the chest wall recurrence of a tumor that did not have this component

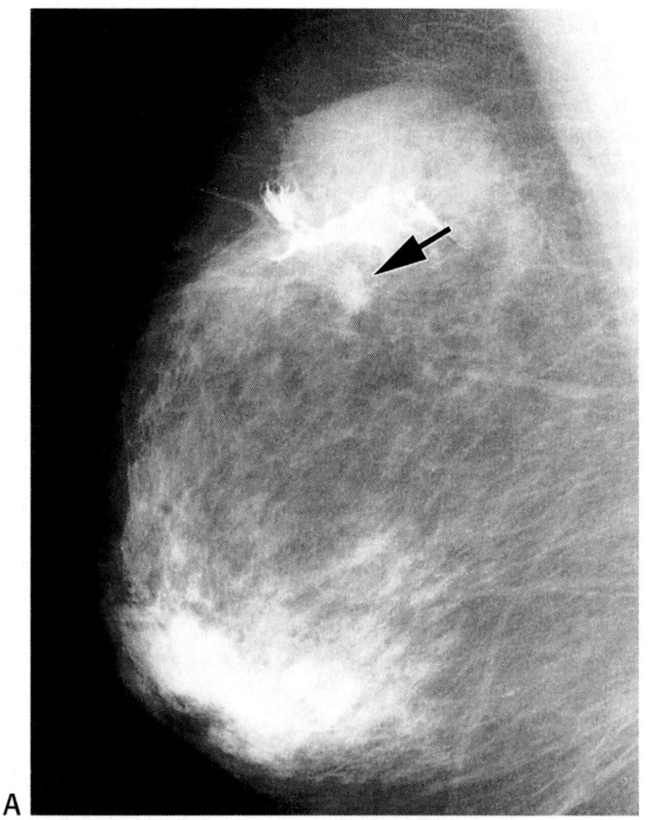

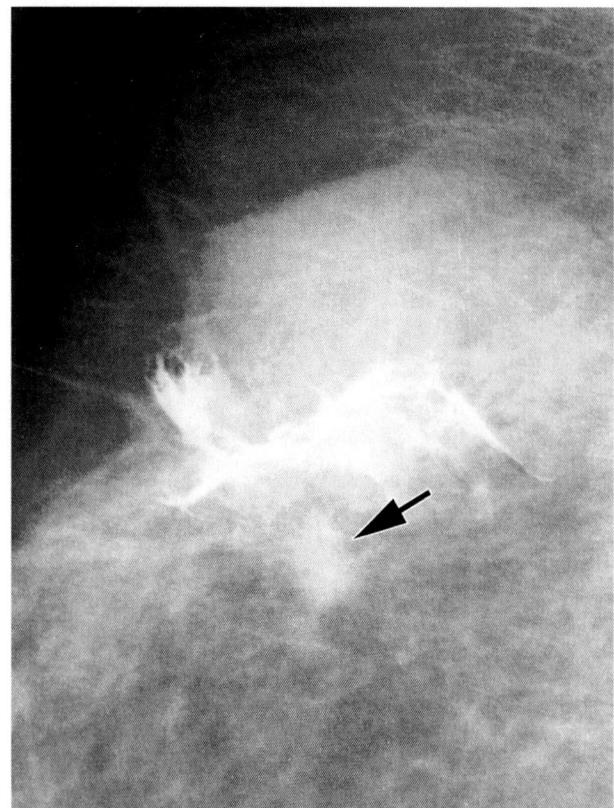

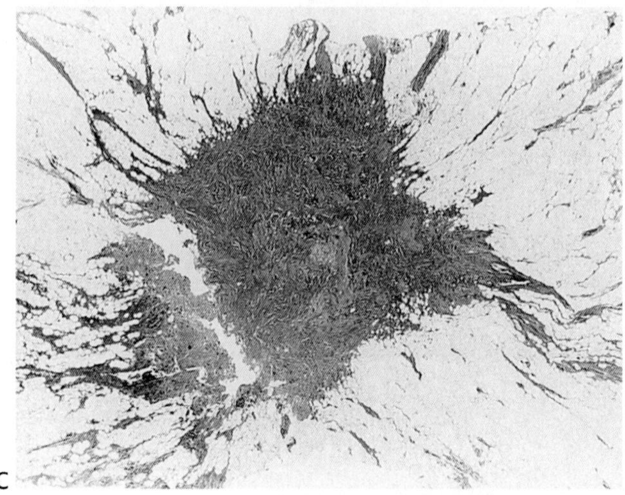

FIG. 16.42. *Low-grade adenosquamous carcinoma.* **A,B:** The tumor forms an oval stellate density (*arrow*) with ill-defined borders in the upper half of the breast below the site of dye injected to localize the lesion. **C:** Whole-mount histologic section of the LGASC shown in the mammogram. The tumor has infiltrating border.

in the primary lesion (Fig. 16.50). The tissue immediately around squamous foci often has a distinctive lamellar arrangement of spindle cells that merges with the epithelium (Figs. 16.44, 16.45 and 16.47). Rarely, LGASC shows transitions to conventional high-grade spindle cell and squamous sarcomatoid metaplastic carcinoma.[179,180,188] Intraductal carcinoma can be present, sometimes with apocrine features, but it may be difficult to distinguish from infiltrative areas.

Needle Core Biopsy Diagnosis

The diagnosis of LGASC can be extremely challenging in needle core biopsy samples because of the tumor's subtle morphology and to the difficulty in appreciating its infiltrative nature in limited material.[180] Occasionally, disorganized syringomatous squamous cords and duct-like structures surrounded by spindle cells in a lamellar arrangement suggest this diagnosis (Fig. 16.51). In some cases, however, the neoplastic epithelial clusters in the core biopsy material consist of only a few (two to five) cells showing densely eosinophilic and nearly refractile cytoplasm, admixed with fibrohyalinized or elastotic stroma, raising the differential diagnosis of a CSL. In general, it is good practice to entertain the differential diagnosis of LGASC when evaluating a sclerosing lesion that has unusual features in a needle core biopsy sample. The lamellar quality of the stroma is a very important diagnostic clue leading one to suspect LGASC.

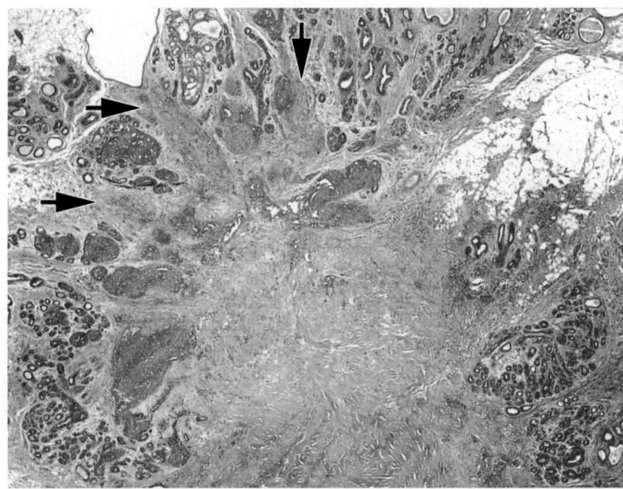

FIG. 16.43. ***Low-grade adenosquamous carcinoma.*** The tumor simulates a radial scar, but the scleroelastotic center consists of homogeneous stroma with no obvious entrapped tubules. In addition, the carcinoma has stellate branches that infiltrate between normal glandular structures at the periphery of the tumor (*arrows*).

Cytology

Because of the rarity of LGASC, the cytologic features of this lesion have been described only in single case reports or small series.[178,183,185,186] A definitive diagnosis of LGASC is rarely rendered on the basis of FNA material. Smears from LGASC typically have low to moderate cellularity, but one case with a hypercellular smear has been reported.[186] The epithelial clusters have varied morphology. Small cohesive angulated clusters shaped as commas or tadpoles are present, sometimes with squamous metaplasia. Other clusters contain uniform cells of small to medium size that tend to be oriented around a minute glandular lumen. In these clusters, the outer layer of cells is flattened or cuboidal and inconspicuous. Bipolar spindle cells, usually indicative of a benign lesion, are present in the background. Elongated cells are also present singly or in small clumps.[178] The biphasic nature of the FNA material may raise the possibility of LGASC. Immunohistochemical stains may also help to confirm squamous differentiation if material is available for immunohistochemical studies.[178,186]

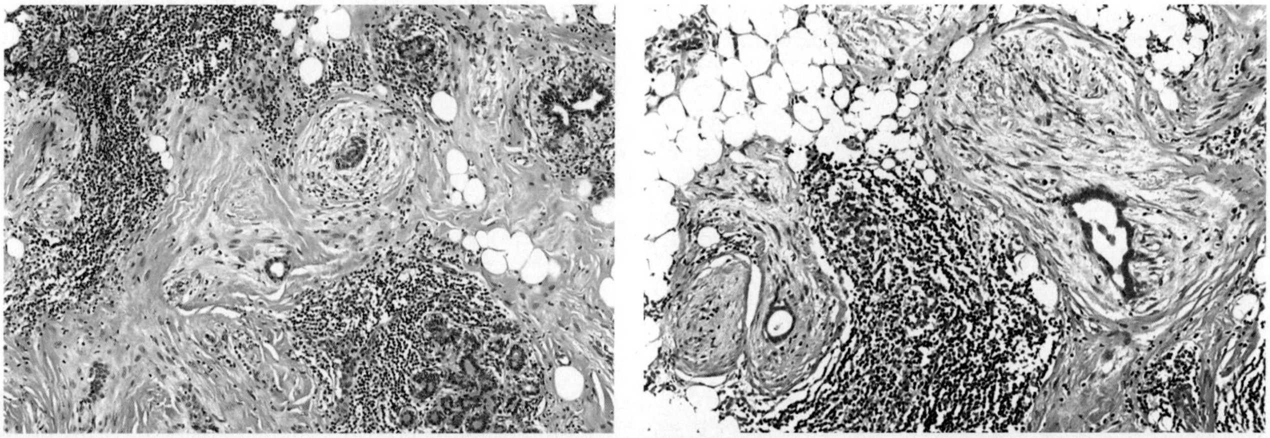

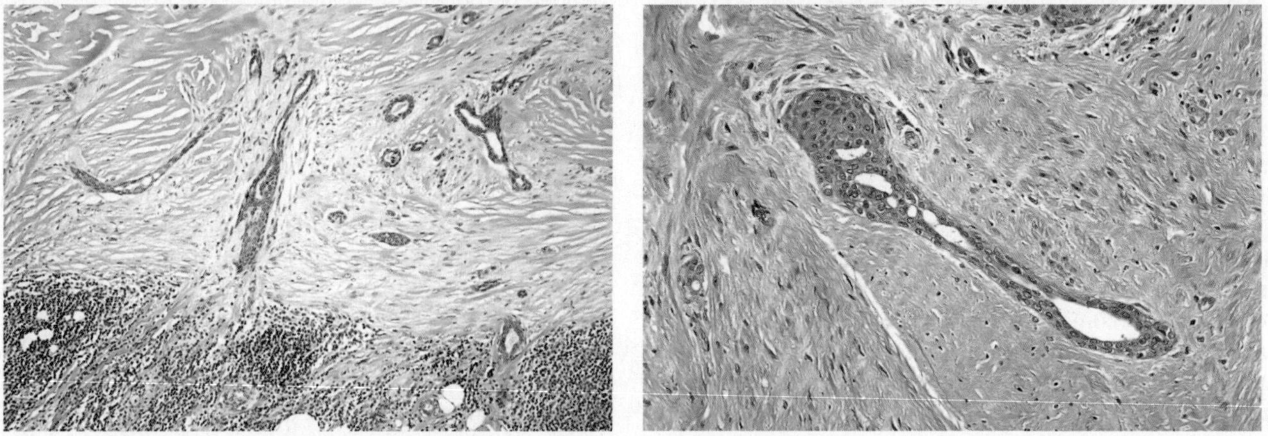

FIG. 16.44. ***Low-grade adenosquamous carcinoma.*** **A:** Tumor infiltrating breast stroma near a lobule (*below*) and duct (*upper right*). Note the character of the stroma around the neoplastic epithelium and the lymphocytic reaction. **B:** Carcinoma invading fat. **C:** A circumscribed LGASC with dense collagenous stroma and peripheral lymphocytic reaction. **D:** Adenosquamous differentiation in the tumor shown in **(C)**.

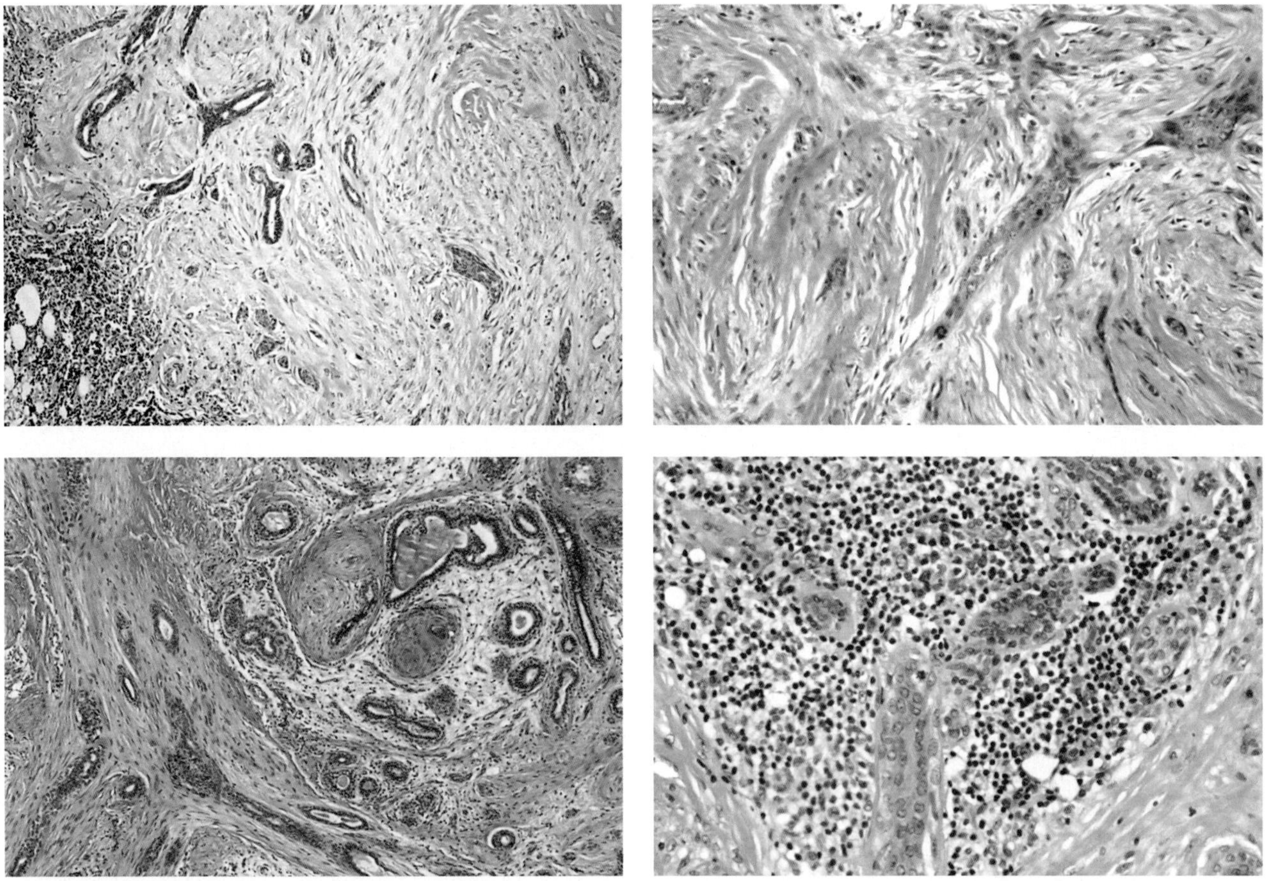

FIG. 16.45. ***Low-grade adenosquamous carcinoma.*** **A:** Prominent collagenized component typical of some of these tumors. Note the lymphocytic infiltrate at the border (*lower left*). **B:** Blending of spindle cell and epithelial elements resembles spindle cell metaplastic carcinoma. **C:** Appearance of the tumor invading in and around a lobule. This focus is predominantly glandular with one squamous nodule. **D:** Magnified view of LGASC invading a lobule. The upper end of the neoplastic gland oriented vertically in the six o'clock position contains a mitotic figure.

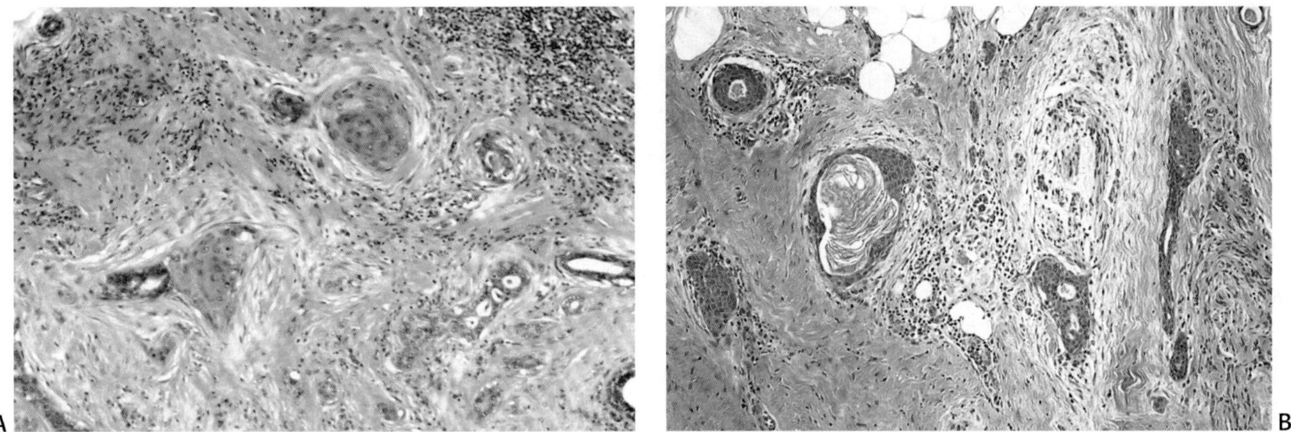

FIG. 16.46. ***Low-grade adenosquamous carcinoma.*** Various patterns of squamous differentiation are shown. **A:** Solid squamous foci. **B,C:** Keratin-forming foci with cystic degeneration. **D:** Keratin pearl formation. **E:** Marked cystic dilation of squamous epithelium with a dense lymphocytic reaction. **F:** Sebaceous metaplasia in the squamous epithelium. **G:** Foreign body giant cell reaction to keratin material in the stroma around foci of LGASC.

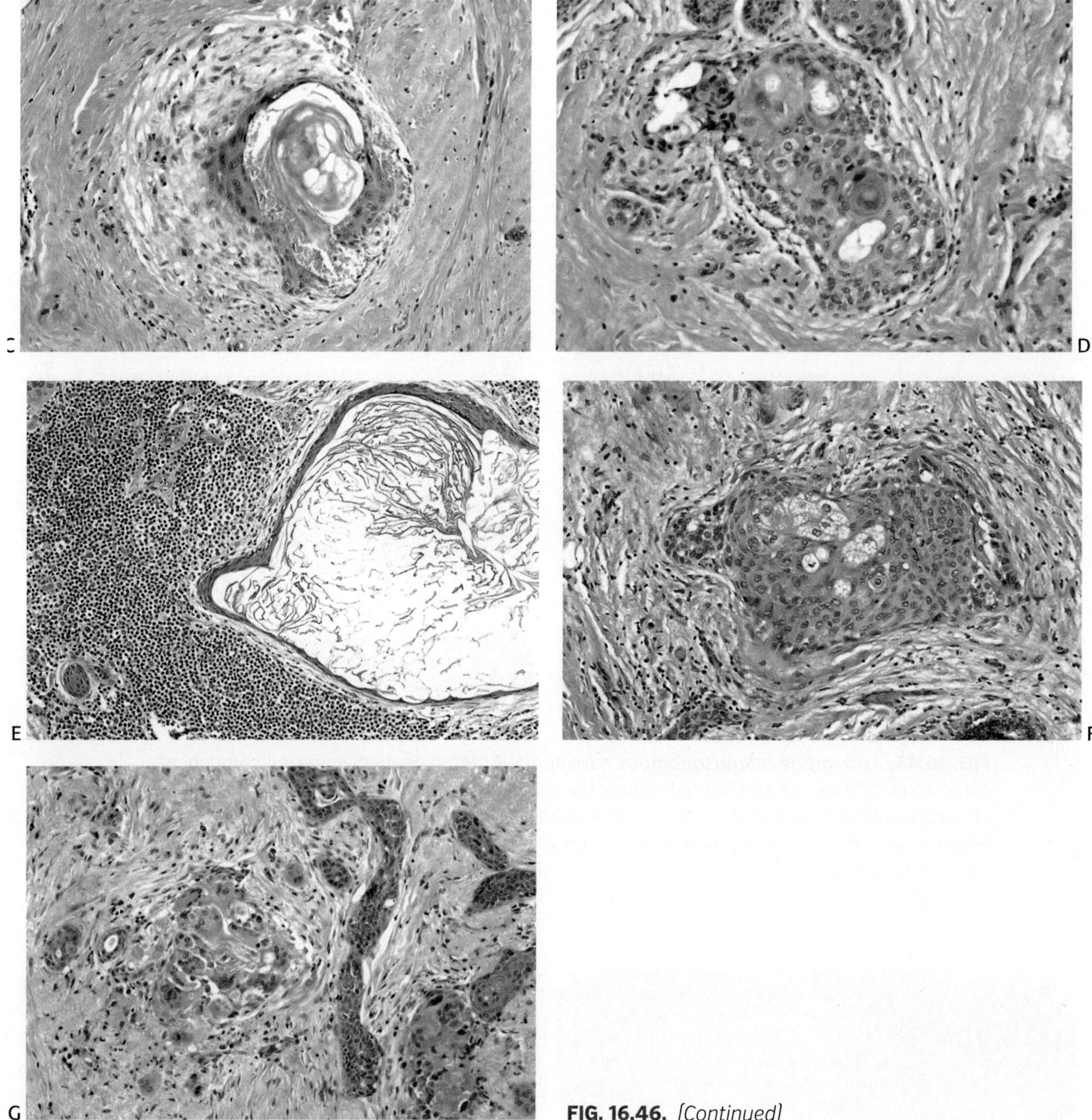

FIG. 16.46. *(Continued)*

Immunoreactivity

Kawaguchi and Shin[182] characterized the pattern of immunoreactivity for epithelial and myoepithelial markers in 30 LGASCs. Four tumors that arose in the retroareolar region, one that had been initially misdiagnosed as a syringomatous adenoma, and three with coexistent metaplastic spindle cell carcinoma. The epithelial clusters of 25 tumors stained for at least one CK (Fig. 16.52), including AE1:3, CK5/6, 34βE12, and CAM5.2. Some of the epithelial clusters in each tumor were negative for CK, although no single keratin was consistently negative in all the epithelial clusters of a case. Keratin AE1:3, CK5/6, and CK7 stained the core of the epithelial clusters in 57%, 58%, and 50% of cases, respectively, but core staining was less commonly seen with keratin 34βE12 (35%) and CAM5.2 (10%). Excluding the three cases with associated metaplastic spindle cell carcinoma, one case also showed positivity for CK7 in lesional stromal cells that was not attributable to the presence of epithelial cells. The same focus was negative for AE1:3, CK5/6, and 34βE12. In three other cases, epithelioid stromal cells were positive for CK7, including one case in which the spindle cells were also positive for 34βE12 and SMA. Another group also found strong positive reactivity for the basal CK5/6, CK14, and CK17 in five tumors.[179] The spindle cell stroma of LGASCs usually exhibits little or no CK reactivity (Fig. 16.52).

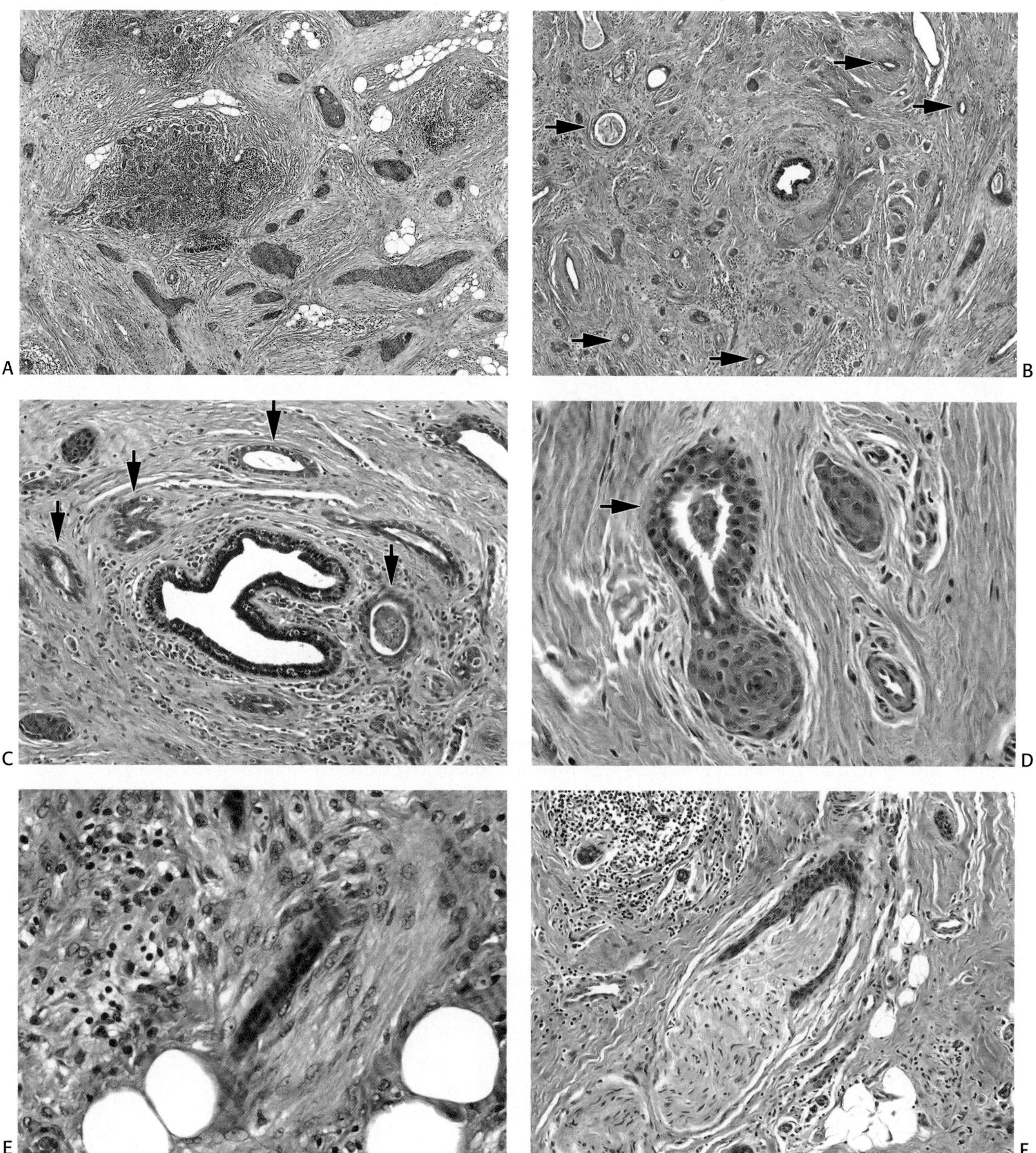

FIG. 16.47. ***Low-grade adenosquamous carcinoma, infiltrative pattern, and associated stroma.*** **A:** The nests of this LGASC surround a normal lobule that features a lymphocytic infiltrate. The stroma is characteristically moderately cellular with fibrotic bands and a sprinkling of lymphocytes. **B,C:** Small glands and squamoid nests surround normal ducts. Some of the neoplastic epithelium forms duct-like structures with lumens (*arrows*). Focal collections of lymphocytes are present. **D:** Squamoid and glandular differentiation. A myoepithelial layer is evident (*arrow*). **E:** Hypercellular stromal cells have a lamellar arrangement parallel to the densely eosinophilic squamoid/myoepithelial component. **F:** A rare example of perineural invasion by LGASC.

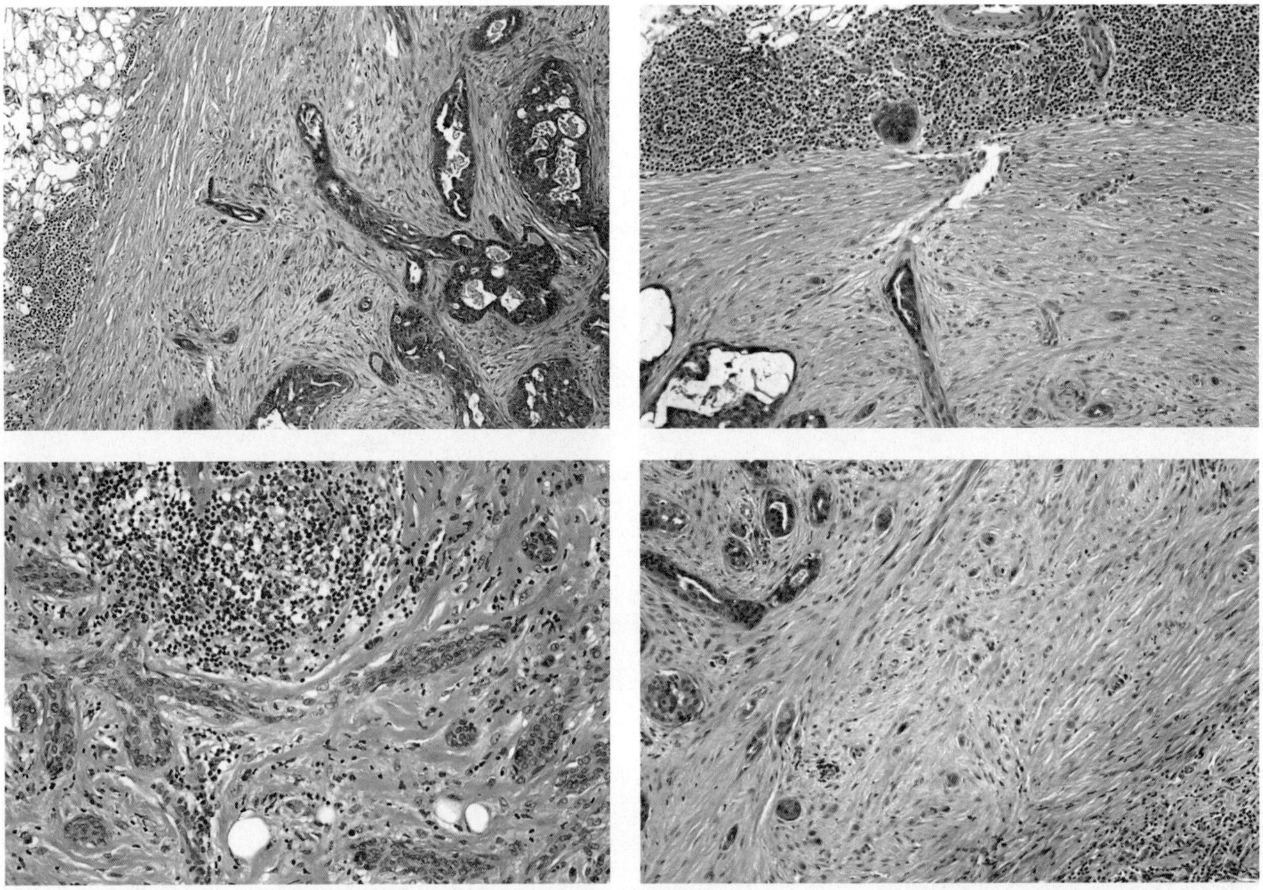

FIG. 16.48. ***Low-grade adenosquamous carcinoma arising in a sclerosing papilloma.*** **A:** Florid duct hyperplasia surrounded by low-grade invasive adenosquamous carcinoma. Note the peripheral lymphocytic infiltrate. **B:** Magnified view of the tumor showing a nest of carcinoma cells in the lymphoid infiltrate. **C:** The invasive tumor. **D:** This portion of the tumor has a prominent spindle cell element.

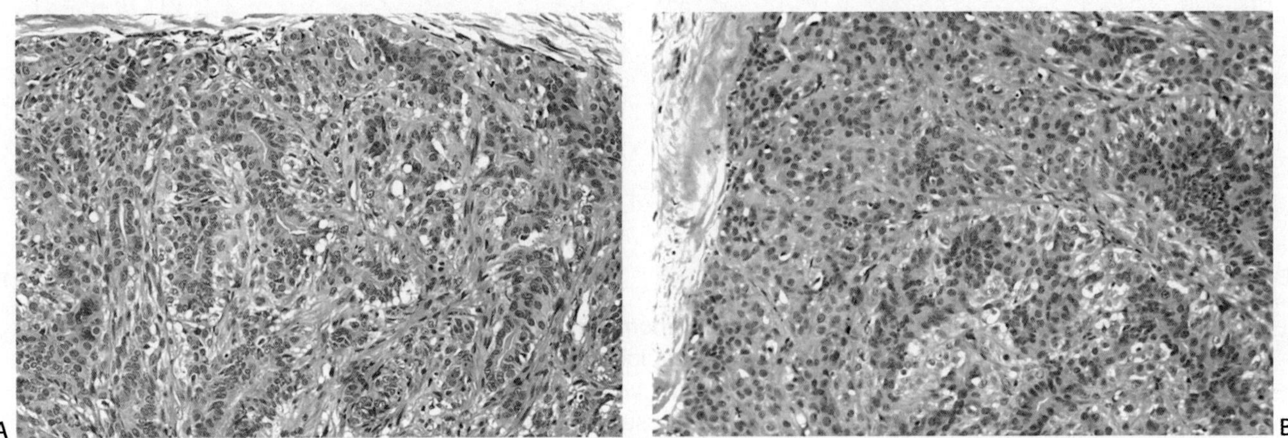

FIG. 16.49. ***Low-grade adenosquamous carcinoma arising in adenomyoepithelioma.*** **A,B:** AME with florid epithelial and myoepithelial elements in an excisional biopsy. **C:** Recurrent tumor 2 years later at the site of the AME. The glandular elements (*arrow*) are probably remnants of the AME surrounded by dense collagenized tissue representing part of the LGASC. **D:** Invasive LGASC at the periphery of the lesion. **E:** Two mitotic figures are present (*arrows*).

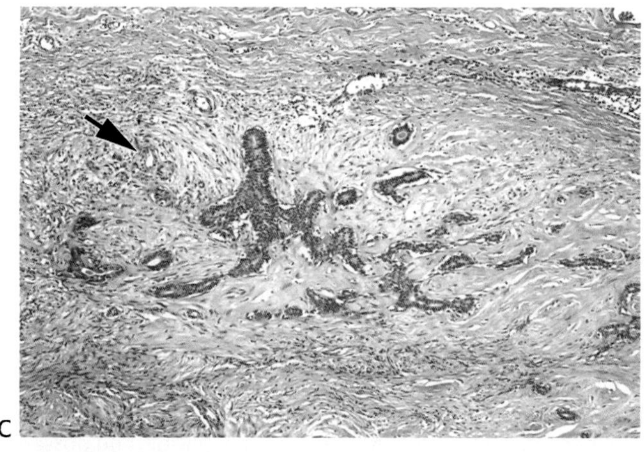

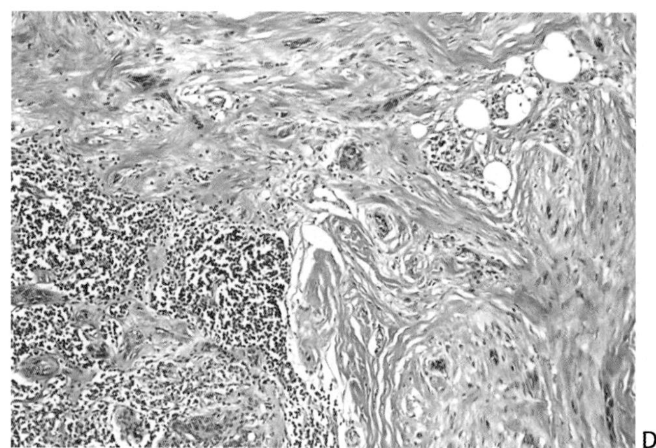

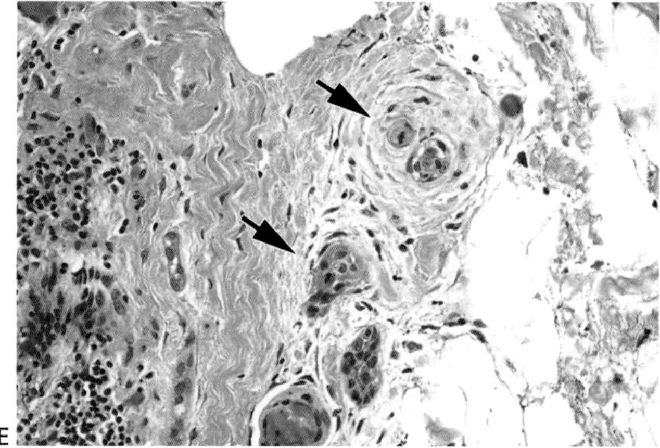

FIG. 16.49. *(Continued)*

Kawaguchi and Shin[182] detected complete circumferential staining for the myoepithelial markers p63, smooth muscle myosin heavy chain, SMA, CD10, and calponin around all epithelial nests in only 3 of 28 cases (11%). Ten of 28 (36%) cases showed coexistent complete, discontinuous and absent circumferential staining for myoepithelial markers, and only CD10 displayed immunoreactivity in all cases. The pattern of immunoreactivity for myoepithelial markers in five tumors involving the nipple and retroareolar

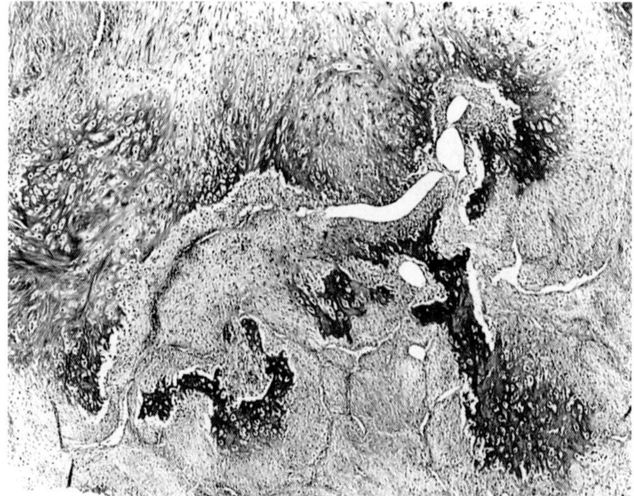

FIG. 16.50. ***Low-grade adenosquamous carcinoma, recurrent.*** Osteocartilaginous metaplasia in a tumor recurrent in the chest wall. The tumor was limited to soft tissue and had typical areas of LGASC.

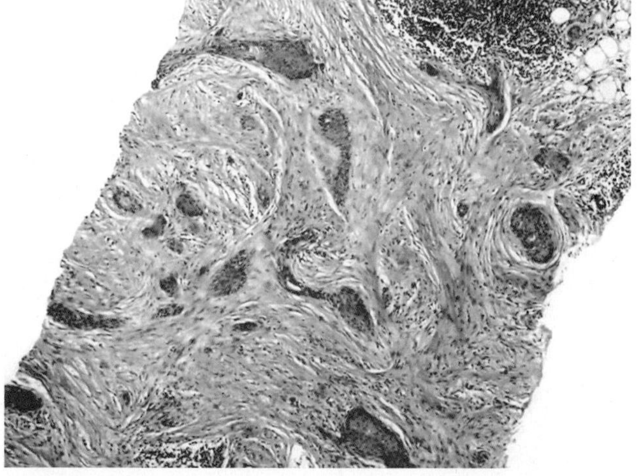

FIG. 16.51. ***Low-grade adenosquamous carcinoma, needle core biopsy.*** The typical features of LGASC are evident in this needle core biopsy sample. Note the lobular lymphocytic infiltrate at the *upper border*.

region was also inconsistent. Excluding the three tumors with coexisting spindle cell carcinoma, no lesion had p63 reactivity in the stromal cells. Lamellar stromal staining for smooth muscle myosin was noted in 10 of 19 cases (53%), and for calponin in 4 of 7 (57%). Reactivity for SMA was found occasionally. SMA stained epithelioid stromal cells in one case, and the same cells were also positive for CK7 and 34βE12. Glandular luminal staining was seen in 17 of 23 (74%) of the tumors evaluated for p63, but none of the other myoepithelial markers had a similar staining pattern, suggesting that p63 positivity is related to squamous and not to myoepithelial differentiation. LGASC is negative for ER, PR, and HER2. One study[179] reported EGFR staining in the epithelium of four of five cases. EGFR staining intensity was 3+ in the epithelium of two cases, and one tumor also displayed 3+ positivity in the stromal component. The latter case, however, had areas of transition from low-grade to high-grade adenosquamous carcinoma.

In summary, using currently available reagents, LGASCs do not have a consistent pattern of immunoreactivity for epithelial and myoepithelial markers. Familiarity with the morphologic features of this tumor and with its different patterns of immunoreactivity is necessary for accurate diagnosis of this rare carcinoma.

Genetics and Molecular Studies

Geyer et al.[179] analyzed two LGASCs using comparative genomic hybridization (CGH). One pure LGASC displayed chromosomal gains of 6p, 7pq, and 8q and losses of 1p, 6p, 6q, 8p, and 9q, and showed no gene amplifications. Results of chromogenic *in situ* hybridization of the *EGFR* gene and of CEP7 were consistent with an extra copy of chromosome 7 in the neoplastic epithelial clusters and in the surrounding stromal tumor cells. The other tumor had areas of low-grade and high-grade adenosquamous morphology and more complex genetic alterations, with a "firestorm" pattern and two amplification peaks on chromosome 7. Chromosomal gains were found in 1q, 5q, 7p, 8q, 12p, 14q, 16p, 16q, and 18pq; chromosomal losses were detected in 1p, 3q, 8p, 9p, 12q, 17p, 17q, 22q, and Xpq with high-level amplification of the 7p11.2 locus, encompassing the *EGFR* gene, and of 7q11.2. The neoplastic epithelial cells and a minor component of the adjacent stromal cells displayed *EGFR* amplification by chromogenic *in situ* hybridization. In particular, *EGFR* amplification was detected focally in the spindle cells associated with the high-grade carcinoma, but also in the spindle cells associated with the low-grade component.[179] Simultaneous IHC for SMA and chromogenic *in situ* hybridization for EGFR mRNA showed EGFR mRNA in the neoplastic epithelial clusters and coexpression of large gene clusters and SMA in a minority of the stromal spindle cells. These findings suggest that some of the spindle stromal cells associated with LGASC are also neoplastic, and possibly a product of EMT of the epithelial component.

Prognosis and Treatment

Lymph node involvement by LGASC is extremely rare, with only one documented case.[190] In the study by Kawaguchi and Shin,[182] one of two patients with SLN biopsy had dispersed epithelial clusters in four lymph nodes that were interpreted as secondary to artifactual displacement; the other patient had no SLN involvement.

There is only one documented report of systemic disease due to LGASC in a 33-year-old woman with an 8.0-cm tumor metastatic to the lung at presentation.[190] LGASC, however, tends to recur locally. Four of eight women treated initially by excisional biopsy had an ipsilateral in-breast recurrence 1 to 3.5 years after the initial treatment, and required mastectomy.[190] A tumor initially misdiagnosed as syringomatous adenoma of the nipple in a needle core biopsy sample had a recurrence after 5 years in the form of a 4- to 5-cm mass that required mastectomy.[182] It is unclear whether local recurrence has occurred only in patients whose tumors had been incompletely excised. The current management of LGASC is similar to that of other types of invasive breast carcinomas. Radiotherapy is used in patients treated with

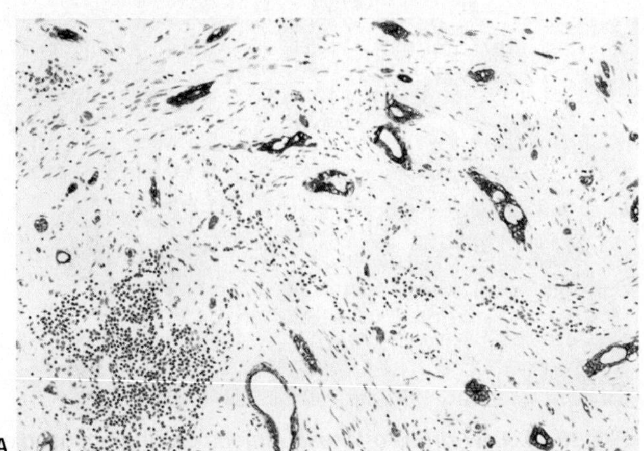

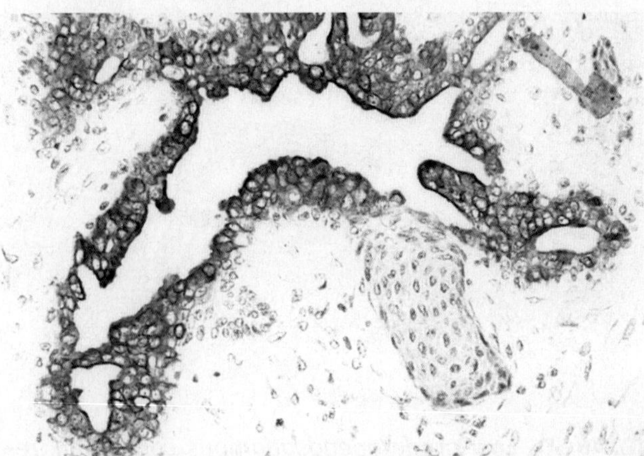

FIG. 16.52. ***Low-grade adenosquamous carcinoma, immunoreactivity.*** **A:** Staining for CK 34βE12 is limited to glandular elements with no reactivity in the spindle cell areas. **B:** Immunoreactivity for CK7 is present in glandular but not in squamous epithelium.

breast-conserving surgery. The role of chemotherapy in patients with LGASC remains indeterminate.

REFERENCES

1. Lecene P. Les tumeurs mixtes du sein. *Rev de chir Paris* 1906;33:434–439.
2. Huvos AG, Lucas JC Jr, Foote FW Jr. Metaplastic breast carcinoma. Rare form of mammary cancer. *N Y State J Med* 1973;73:1078–1082.
3. Raju GC. The histological and immunohistochemical evidence of squamous metaplasia from the myoepithelial cells in the breast. *Histopathology* 1990;17:272–275.
4. Gal-Gombos EC, Esserman LE, Poniecka AW, et al. Osseous metaplasia of the breast: diagnosis with stereotactic core biopsy. *Breast J* 2002;8:50–52.
5. Fisher ER, Gregorio RM, Fisher B, et al. The pathology of invasive breast cancer. A syllabus derived from findings of the National Surgical Adjuvant Breast Project (protocol no. 4). *Cancer* 1975;36:1–85.
6. Kaufman MW, Marti JR, Gallager S, et al. Carcinoma of the breast with pseudosarcomatous metaplasia. *Cancer* 1984;53:1908–1917.
7. Tsuda H, Takarabe T, Hasegawa T, et al. Myoepithelial differentiation in high-grade invasive ductal carcinomas with large central acellular zones. *Hum Pathol* 1999;30:1134–1139.
8. Tsuda H, Takarabe T, Hasegawa F, et al. Large, central acellular zones indicating myoepithelial tumor differentiation in high-grade invasive ductal carcinomas as markers of predisposition to lung and brain metastases. *Am J Surg Pathol* 2000;24:197–202.
9. Rottino A, Wilson K. Osseous, cartilaginous and mixed tumors of the human breast: a review of the literature. *Arch Surg* 1945;50:184–193.
10. Wargotz ES, Norris HJ. Metaplastic carcinomas of the breast. III. Carcinosarcoma. *Cancer* 1989;64:1490–1499.
11. Wang ZC, Buraimoh A, Iglehart JD, et al. Genome-wide analysis for loss of heterozygosity in primary and recurrent phyllodes tumor and fibroadenoma of breast using single nucleotide polymorphism arrays. *Breast Cancer Res Treat* 2006;97:301–309.
12. Davis WG, Hennessy B, Babiera G, et al. Metaplastic sarcomatoid carcinoma of the breast with absent or minimal overt invasive carcinomatous component: a misnomer. *Am J Surg Pathol* 2005;29:1456–1463.
13. Tavassoli FA. Myoepithelial lesions of the breast. Myoepitheliosis, adenomyoepithelioma, and myoepithelial carcinoma. *Am J Surg Pathol* 1991;15:554–568.
14. Pezzi CM, Patel-Parekh L, Cole K, et al. Characteristics and treatment of metaplastic breast cancer: analysis of 892 cases from the National Cancer Data Base. *Ann Surg Oncol* 2007;14:166–173.
15. Chen IC, Lin CH, Huang CS, et al. Lack of efficacy to systemic chemotherapy for treatment of metaplastic carcinoma of the breast in the modern era. *Breast Cancer Res Treat* 2011;130:345–351.
16. Rehman A. Triple-negative phenotype of poorly-differentiated metaplastic breast carcinoma in a male: an oncological rarity. *J Coll Physicians Surg Pak* 2013;23:370–372.
17. Wargotz ES, Norris HJ. Metaplastic carcinomas of the breast. 5. Metaplastic carcinoma with osteoclastic giant-cells. *Hum Pathol* 1990;21:1142–1150.
18. Oberman HA. Metaplastic carcinoma of the breast. A clinicopathologic study of 29 patients. *Am J Surg Pathol* 1987;11:918–929.
19. Smith BH, Taylor HB. The occurrence of bone and cartilage in mammary tumors. *Am J Clin Pathol* 1969;51:610–618.
20. Wargotz ES, Deos PH, Norris HJ. Metaplastic carcinomas of the breast. II. Spindle cell carcinoma. *Hum Pathol* 1989;20:732–740.
21. Rayson D, Adjei AA, Suman VJ, et al. Metaplastic breast cancer: prognosis and response to systemic therapy. *Ann Oncol* 1999;10:413–419.
22. Kurian KM, Al-Nafussi A. Sarcomatoid/metaplastic carcinoma of the breast: a clinicopathological study of 12 cases. *Histopathology* 2002;40:58–64.
23. Barnes PJ, Boutilier R, Chiasson D, et al. Metaplastic breast carcinoma: clinical-pathologic characteristics and HER2/neu expression. *Breast Cancer Res Treat* 2005;91:173–178.
24. Beatty JD, Atwood M, Tickman R, et al. Metaplastic breast cancer: clinical significance. *Am J Surg* 2006;191:657–664.
25. Dave G, Cosmatos H, Do T, et al. Metaplastic carcinoma of the breast: a retrospective review. *Int J Radiat Oncol Biol Phys* 2006;64:771–775.
26. Hennessy BT, Giordano S, Broglio K, et al. Biphasic metaplastic sarcomatoid carcinoma of the breast. *Ann Oncol* 2006;17:605–613.
27. Luini A, Aguilar M, Gatti G, et al. Metaplastic carcinoma of the breast, an unusual disease with worse prognosis: the experience of the European Institute of Oncology and review of the literature. *Breast Cancer Res Treat* 2007;101:349–353.
28. Nassar A, Sookhan N, Santisteban M, et al. Diagnostic utility of snail in metaplastic breast carcinoma. *Diagn Pathol* 2010;5:76.
29. Okada N, Hasebe T, Iwasaki M, et al. Metaplastic carcinoma of the breast. *Hum Pathol* 2010;41:960–970.
30. Park HS, Park S, Kim JH, et al. Clinicopathologic features and outcomes of metaplastic breast carcinoma: comparison with invasive ductal carcinoma of the breast. *Yonsei Med J* 2010;51:864–869.
31. Gwin K, Buell-Gutbrod R, Tretiakova M, et al. Epithelial-to-mesenchymal transition in metaplastic breast carcinomas with chondroid differentiation: expression of the E-cadherin repressor Snail. *Appl Immunohistochem Mol Morphol* 2010;18:526–531.
32. Tseng WH, Martinez SR. Metaplastic breast cancer: to radiate or not to radiate? *Ann Surg Oncol* 2011;18:94–103.
33. Bae SY, Lee SK, Koo MY, et al. The prognoses of metaplastic breast cancer patients compared to those of triple-negative breast cancer patients. *Breast Cancer Res Treat* 2011;126:471–478.
34. Lester TR, Hunt KK, Nayeemuddin KM, et al. Metaplastic sarcomatoid carcinoma of the breast appears more aggressive than other triple receptor-negative breast cancers. *Breast Cancer Res Treat* 2012;131:41–48.
35. Lee H, Jung SY, Ro JY, et al. Metaplastic breast cancer: clinicopathological features and its prognosis. *J Clin Pathol* 2012;65:441–446.
36. Choi BB, Shu KS. Metaplastic carcinoma of the breast: multimodality imaging and histopathologic assessment. *Acta Radiol* 2012;53:5–11.
37. Alvarenga CA, Paravidino PI, Alvarenga M, et al. Reappraisal of immunohistochemical profiling of special histological types of breast carcinomas: a study of 121 cases of eight different subtypes. *J Clin Pathol* 2012;65:1066–1071.
38. Downs-Kelly E, Nayeemuddin KM, Albarracin C, et al. Matrix-producing carcinoma of the breast: an aggressive subtype of metaplastic carcinoma. *Am J Surg Pathol* 2009;33:534–541.
39. Rashid MU, Shah MA, Azhar R, et al. A deleterious BRCA1 mutation in a young Pakistani woman with metaplastic breast carcinoma. *Pathol Res Pract* 2011;207:583–586.
40. Suspitsin EN, Sokolenko AP, Voskresenskiy DA, et al. Mixed epithelial/mesenchymal metaplastic carcinoma (carcinosarcoma) of the breast in BRCA1 carrier. *Breast Cancer* 2011;18:137–140.
41. Ashida A, Fukutomi T, Tsuda H, et al. Atypical medullary carcinoma of the breast with cartilaginous metaplasia in a patient with a BRCA1 germline mutation. *Jpn J Clin Oncol* 2000;30:30–32.
42. Gwin K, Wheeler DT, Bossuyt V, et al. Breast carcinoma with chondroid differentiation: a clinicopathologic study of 21 triple negative (ER-, PR-, Her2/neu-) cases. *Int J Surg Pathol* 2010;18:27–35.
43. Joshi D, Singh P, Zonunfawni Y, et al. Metaplastic carcinoma of the breast: cytological diagnosis and diagnostic pitfalls. *Acta Cytol* 2011;55:313–318.
44. Velasco M, Santamaria G, Ganau S, et al. MRI of metaplastic carcinoma of the breast. *AJR Am J Roentgenol* 2005;184:1274–1278.
45. Shin HJ, Kim HH, Kim SM, et al. Imaging features of metaplastic carcinoma with chondroid differentiation of the breast. *AJR Am J Roentgenol* 2007;188:691–696.
46. Evans HA, Shaughnessy EA, Nikiforov YE. Infiltrating ductal carcinoma of the breast with osseous metaplasia: imaging findings with pathologic correlation. *AJR Am J Roentgenol* 1999;172:1420–1422.
47. Pickhardt PJ, McDermott M. Intense uptake of technetium-99m-MDP in primary breast adenocarcinoma with sarcomatoid metaplasia. *J Nucl Med* 1997;38:528–530.
48. Chao TC, Wang CS, Chen SC, et al. Metaplastic carcinomas of the breast. *J Surg Oncol* 1999;71:220–225.
49. Wargotz ES, Norris HJ. Metaplastic carcinomas of the breast. IV. Squamous-cell carcinoma of ductal origin. *Cancer* 1990;65:272–276.
50. Gobbi H, Simpson JF, Borowsky A, et al. Metaplastic breast tumors with a dominant fibromatosis-like phenotype have a high risk of local recurrence. *Cancer* 1999;85:2170–2182.
51. Gersell DJ, Katzenstein AL. Spindle cell carcinoma of the breast. A clinocopathologic and ultrastructural study. *Hum Pathol* 1981;12:550–561.
52. Pitts WC, Rojas VA, Gaffey MJ, et al. Carcinomas with metaplasia and sarcomas of the breast. *Am J Clin Pathol* 1991;95:623–632.

53. Bauer TW, Rostock RA, Eggleston JC, et al. Spindle cell carcinoma of the breast: four cases and review of the literature. *Hum Pathol* 1984;15:147–152.
54. Carter MR, Hornick JL, Lester S, et al. Spindle cell (sarcomatoid) carcinoma of the breast: a clinicopathologic and immunohistochemical analysis of 29 cases. *Am J Surg Pathol* 2006;30:300–309.
55. Sneige N, Yaziji H, Mandavilli SR, et al. Low-grade (fibromatosis-like) spindle cell carcinoma of the breast. *Am J Surg Pathol* 2001;25:1009–1016.
56. Rekhi B, Shet TM, Badwe RA, et al. Fibromatosis-like carcinoma—an unusual phenotype of a metaplastic breast tumor associated with a micropapilloma. *World J Surg Oncol* 2007;5:24.
57. Gobbi H, Simpson JF, Jensen RA, et al. Metaplastic spindle cell breast tumors arising within papillomas, complex sclerosing lesions, and nipple adenomas. *Mod Pathol* 2003;16:893–901.
58. Denley H, Pinder SE, Tan PH, et al. Metaplastic carcinoma of the breast arising within complex sclerosing lesion: a report of five cases. *Histopathology* 2000;36:203–209.
59. Banerjee SS, Eyden BP, Wells S, et al. Pseudoangiosarcomatous carcinoma: a clinicopathological study of seven cases. *Histopathology* 1992;21:13–23.
60. Eusebi V, Lamovec J, Cattani MG, et al. Acantholytic variant of squamous-cell carcinoma of the breast. *Am J Surg Pathol* 1986;10: 855–861.
61. Aulmann S, Schnabel PA, Helmchen B, et al. Immunohistochemical and cytogenetic characterization of acantholytic squamous cell carcinoma of the breast. *Virchows Arch* 2005;446:305–309.
62. Lamovec J, Kloboves-Prevodnik V. Teleangiectatic sarcomatoid carcinoma of the breast. *Tumori* 1992;78:283–286.
63. Chia Y, Thike AA, Cheok PY, et al. Stromal keratin expression in phyllodes tumours of the breast: a comparison with other spindle cell breast lesions. *J Clin Pathol* 2012;65:339–347.
64. Lacroix-Triki M, Geyer FC, Lambros MB, et al. Beta-catenin/Wnt signalling pathway in fibromatosis, metaplastic carcinomas and phyllodes tumours of the breast. *Mod Pathol* 2010;23:1438–1448.
65. Tot T, Badani De La Parra JJ, Bergkvist L. Metaplastic carcinoma of the breast with neuroectodermal stromal component. *Patholog Res Int* 2011;2011:191–274.
66. Wargotz ES, Norris HJ. Metaplastic carcinomas of the breast. I. Matrix-producing carcinoma. *Human Pathology* 1989;20:628–635.
67. Murata T, Ihara S, Kato H, et al. Matrix-producing carcinoma of the breast: case report with radiographical and cytopathological features. *Pathol Int* 1998;48:824–828.
68. Hayes MM, Lesack D, Girardet C, et al. Carcinoma ex-pleomorphic adenoma of the breast. Report of three cases suggesting a relationship to metaplastic carcinoma of matrix-producing type. *Virchows Arch* 2005;446:142–149.
69. Chhieng C, Cranor M, Lesser ME, et al. Metaplastic carcinoma of the breast with osteocartilaginous heterologous elements. *Am J Surg Pathol* 1998;22:188–194.
70. Shui R, Bi R, Cheng Y, et al. Matrix-producing carcinoma of the breast in the Chinese population: a clinicopathological study of 13 cases. *Pathol Int* 2011;61:415–422.
71. Kinkor Z, Boudova L, Ryska A, et al. [Matrix-producing breast carcinoma with myoepithelial differentiation—description of 11 cases and review of literature aimed at histogenesis and differential diagnosis]. *Ceska Gynekol* 2004;69:229–236.
72. Yamaguchi R, Horii R, Maeda I, et al. Clinicopathologic study of 53 metaplastic breast carcinomas: their elements and prognostic implications. *Hum Pathol* 2010;41:679–685.
73. Rakha EA, Tan PH, Shaaban A, et al. Do primary mammary osteosarcoma and chondrosarcoma exist? A review of a large multi-institutional series of malignant matrix-producing breast tumours. *Breast* 2013;22:13–18.
74. Yamaguchi R, Tanaka M, Kondo K, et al. Immunohistochemical study of metaplastic carcinoma and central acellular carcinoma of the breast: central acellular carcinoma is related to metaplastic carcinoma. *Med Mol Morphol* 2012;45:14–21.
75. Rosenblum MK, Purrazzella R, Rosen PP. Is microglandular adenosis a precancerous disease? A study of carcinoma arising therein. *Am J Surg Pathol* 1986;10:237–245.
76. Geyer FC, Lacroix-Triki M, Colombo PE, et al. Molecular evidence in support of the neoplastic and precursor nature of microglandular adenosis. *Histopathology* 2012;60:E115–E130.
77. Wang X, Mori I, Tang W, et al. Metaplastic carcinoma of the breast: p53 analysis identified the same point mutation in the three histologic components. *Mod Pathol* 2001;14:1183–1186.
78. Lee JS, Kim YB, Min KW. Metaplastic mammary carcinoma with osteoclast-like giant cells: identical point mutation of p53 gene only identified in both the intraductal and sarcomatous components. *Virchows Arch* 2004;444:194–197.
79. Sexton CW, White WL. Chondrosarcomatous cutaneous metastasis. A unique manifestation of sarcomatoid (metaplastic) breast carcinoma. *Am J Dermatopathol* 1996;18:538–542.
80. Chell SE, Nayar R, De Frias DV, et al. Metaplastic breast carcinoma metastatic to the lung mimicking a primary chondroid lesion: report of a case with cytohistologic correlation. *Ann Diagn Pathol* 1998;2:173–180.
81. Saigo PE, Rosen PP. Mammary carcinoma with "choriocarcinomatous" features. *Am J Surg Pathol* 1981;5:773–778.
82. Resetkova E, Sahin A, Ayala AG, et al. Breast carcinoma with choriocarcinomatous features. *Ann Diagn Pathol* 2004;8:74–79.
83. Canbay E, Bozkurt B, Ergul G, et al. Breast carcinoma with choriocarcinomatous features. *Breast J* 2010;16:202–203.
84. Siddiqui NH, Cabay RJ, Salem F. Fine-needle aspiration biopsy of a case of breast carcinoma with choriocarcinomatous features. *Diagn Cytopathol* 2006;34:694–697.
85. Akbulut M, Zekioglu O, Ozdemir N, et al. Fine needle aspiration cytology of mammary carcinoma with choriocarcinomatous features: a report of 2 cases. *Acta Cytol* 2008;52:99–104.
86. Lee AK, Rosen PP, DeLellis RA, et al. Tumor marker expression in breast carcinomas and relationship to prognosis. An immunohistochemical study. *Am J Clin Pathol* 1985;84:687–696.
87. Cook SS, DeMay R. Adenocarcinoma of the breast with osseous metaplasia. Report of a case with needle aspiration cytology. *Acta Cytol* 1984;28:317–320.
88. Gal R, Gukovsky-Oren S, Lehman JM, et al. Cytodiagnosis of a spindle-cell tumor of the breast using antisera to epithelial membrane antigen. *Acta Cytol* 1987;31:317–321.
89. Stanley MW, Tani EM, Skoog L. Metaplastic carcinoma of the breast: fine-needle aspiration cytology of seven cases. *Diagn Cytopathol* 1989;5:22–28.
90. Kline TS, Kline IK. Metaplastic carcinoma of the breast—diagnosis by aspiration biopsy cytology: report of two cases and literature review. *Diagn Cytopathol* 1990;6:63–67.
91. Castella E, Gomez-Plaza MC, Urban A, et al. Fine-needle aspiration biopsy of metaplastic carcinoma of the breast: report of a case with abundant myxoid ground substance. *Diagn Cytopathol* 1996;14: 325–327.
92. Jebsen PW, Hagmar BM, Nesland JM. Metaplastic breast carcinoma. A diagnostic problem in fine needle aspiration biopsy. *Acta Cytol* 1991;35:396–402.
93. Pettinato G, Manivel JC, Petrella G, et al. Primary osteogenic sarcoma and osteogenic metaplastic carcinoma of the breast. Immunocytochemical identification in fine needle aspirates. *Acta Cytol* 1989;33:620–626.
94. Nogueira M, Andre S, Mendonca E. Metaplastic carcinomas of the breast—fine needle aspiration (FNA) cytology findings. *Cytopathology* 1998;9:291–300.
95. Johnson TL, Kini SR. Metaplastic breast carcinoma: a cytohistologic and clinical study of 10 cases. *Diagn Cytopathol* 1996;14:226–232.
96. Gupta RK. Cytodiagnostic patterns of metaplastic breast carcinoma in aspiration samples: a study of 14 cases. *Diagn Cytopathol* 1999;20:10–12.
97. Lui PC, Tse GM, Tan PH, et al. Fine-needle aspiration cytology of metaplastic carcinoma of the breast. *J Clin Pathol* 2007;60:529–533.
98. Boccato P, Briani G, d'Atri C, et al. Spindle cell and cartilaginous metaplasia in a breast carcinoma with osteoclastlike stromal cells. A difficult fine needle aspiration diagnosis. *Acta Cytol* 1988;32:75–78.
99. Fulciniti F, Mansueto G, Vetrani A, et al. Metaplastic breast carcinoma on fine-needle cytology samples: a report of three cases. *Diagn Cytopathol* 2005;33:205–209.
100. Ellis IO, Bell J, Ronan JE, et al. Immunocytochemical investigation of intermediate filament proteins and epithelial membrane antigen in spindle cell tumours of the breast. *J Pathol* 1988;154:157–165.
101. Santeusanio G, Pascal RR, Bisceglia M, et al. Metaplastic breast carcinoma with epithelial phenotype of pseudosarcomatous components. *Arch Pathol Lab Med* 1988;112:82–85.

102. Reis-Filho JS, Milanezi F, Carvalho S, et al. Metaplastic breast carcinomas exhibit EGFR, but not HER2, gene amplification and overexpression: immunohistochemical and chromogenic in situ hybridization analysis. *Breast Cancer Res* 2005;7:R1028–R1035.
103. Dunne B, Lee AH, Pinder SE, et al. An immunohistochemical study of metaplastic spindle cell carcinoma, phyllodes tumor and fibromatosis of the breast. *Human Pathology* 2003;34:1009–1015.
104. Koker MM, Kleer CG. p63 expression in breast cancer: a highly sensitive and specific marker of metaplastic carcinoma. *Am J Surg Pathol* 2004;28:1506–1512.
105. Sanchez-Tillo E, Lazaro A, Torrent R, et al. ZEB1 represses E-cadherin and induces an EMT by recruiting the SWI/SNF chromatin-remodeling protein BRG1. *Oncogene* 2010;29:3490–3500.
106. Cheng GZ, Chan J, Wang Q, et al. Twist transcriptionally up-regulates AKT2 in breast cancer cells leading to increased migration, invasion, and resistance to paclitaxel. *Cancer Res* 2007;67:1979–1987.
107. Kalluri R, Weinberg RA. The basics of epithelial-mesenchymal transition. *J Clin Invest* 2009;119:1420–1428.
108. Hay ED. Extracellular-matrix, cell skeletons, and embryonic-development. *Am J Med Genet* 1989;34:14–29.
109. Morel AP, Hinkal GW, Thomas C, et al. EMT inducers catalyze malignant transformation of mammary epithelial cells and drive tumorigenesis towards claudin-low tumors in transgenic mice. *PLoS Genet* 2012;8:e1002723.
110. van Deurzen CH, Lee AH, Gill MS, et al. Metaplastic breast carcinoma: tumour histogenesis or dedifferentiation? *J Pathol* 2011;224:434–437.
111. Adem C, Reynolds C, Adlakha H, et al. Wide spectrum screening keratin as a marker of metaplastic spindle cell carcinoma of the breast: an immunohistochemical study of 24 patients. *Histopathology* 2002;40:556–562.
112. Reis-Filho JS, Milanezi F, Steele D, et al. Metaplastic breast carcinomas are basal-like tumours. *Histopathology* 2006;49:10–21.
113. Carpenter PM, Wang-Rodriguez J, Chan OT, et al. Laminin 5 expression in metaplastic breast carcinomas. *Am J Surg Pathol* 2008;32:345–353.
114. Reis-Filho JS, Schmitt FC. Taking advantage of basic research: p63 is a reliable myoepithelial and stem cell marker. *Adv Anat Pathol* 2002;9:280–289.
115. Barbareschi M, Pecciarini L, Cangi MG, et al. p63, a p53 homologue, is a selective nuclear marker of myoepithelial cells of the human breast. *Am J Surg Pathol* 2001;25:1054–1060.
116. Reis-Filho JS, Schmitt FC. p63 expression in sarcomatoid/metaplastic carcinomas of the breast. *Histopathology* 2003;42:94–95.
117. Leibl S, Gogg-Kammerer M, Sommersacher A, et al. Metaplastic breast carcinomas: are they of myoepithelial differentiation?: immunohistochemical profile of the sarcomatoid subtype using novel myoepithelial markers. *Am J Surg Pathol* 2005;29:347–353.
118. Kallen ME, Sanders ME, Gonzalez AL, et al. Nuclear p63 expression in osteoblastic tumors. *Tumour Biol* 2012.
119. Kallen ME, Nunes Rosado FG, Gonzalez AL, et al. Occasional staining for p63 in malignant vascular tumors: a potential diagnostic pitfall. *Pathol Oncol Res* 2012;18:97–100.
120. Miettinen M, Fetsch JF. Distribution of keratins in normal endothelial cells and a spectrum of vascular tumors: implications in tumor diagnosis. *Hum Pathol* 2000;31:1062–1067.
121. Weinreb I, Cunningham KS, Perez-Ordonez B, et al. CD10 is expressed in most epithelioid hemangioendotheliomas: a potential diagnostic pitfall. *Arch Pathol Lab Med* 2009;133:1965–1968.
122. Jo VY, Fletcher CD. p63 immunohistochemical staining is limited in soft tissue tumors. *Am J Clin Pathol* 2011;136:762–766.
123. Popnikolov NK, Ayala AG, Graves K, et al. Benign myoepithelial tumors of the breast have immunophenotypic characteristics similar to metaplastic matrix-producing and spindle cell carcinomas. *Am J Clin Pathol* 2003;120:161–167.
124. Leibl S, Moinfar F. Mammary NOS-type sarcoma with CD10 expression: a rare entity with features of myoepithelial differentiation. *Am J Surg Pathol* 2006;30:450–456.
125. Kaimala S, Bisana S, Kumar S. Mammary gland stem cells: more puzzles than explanations. *J Biosci* 2012;37:349–358.
126. Nielsen TO, Hsu FD, Jensen K, et al. Immunohistochemical and clinical characterization of the basal-like subtype of invasive breast carcinoma. *Clin Cancer Res* 2004;10:5367–5374.
127. Bossuyt V, Fadare O, Martel M, et al. Remarkably high frequency of EGFR expression in breast carcinomas with squamous differentiation. *Int J Surg Pathol* 2005;13:319–327.
128. Leibl S, Moinfar F. Metaplastic breast carcinomas are negative for Her-2 but frequently express EGFR (Her-1): potential relevance to adjuvant treatment with EGFR tyrosine kinase inhibitors? *J Clin Pathol* 2005;58:700–704.
129. Reis-Filho JS, Pinheiro C, Lambros MB, et al. EGFR amplification and lack of activating mutations in metaplastic breast carcinomas. *J Pathol* 2006;209:445–453.
130. Gilbert JA, Goetz MP, Reynolds CA, et al. Molecular analysis of metaplastic breast carcinoma: high EGFR copy number via aneusomy. *Mol Cancer Ther* 2008;7:944–951.
131. Jacot W, Lopez-Crapez E, Thezenas S, et al. Lack of EGFR-activating mutations in European patients with triple-negative breast cancer could emphasise geographic and ethnic variations in breast cancer mutation profiles. *Breast Cancer Res* 2011;13:R133.
132. Teng YH, Tan WJ, Thike AA, et al. Mutations in the epidermal growth factor receptor (EGFR) gene in triple negative breast cancer: possible implications for targeted therapy. *Breast Cancer Res* 2011;13:R35.
133. Wen YH, Brogi E, Hasanovic A, et al. Immunohistochemical staining with EGFR mutation-specific antibodies: high specificity as a diagnostic marker for lung adenocarcinoma. *Mod Pathol* 2013;26:1197–1203.
134. Livasy CA, Karaca G, Nanda R, et al. Phenotypic evaluation of the basal-like subtype of invasive breast carcinoma. *Mod Pathol* 2006;19:264–271.
135. Charafe-Jauffret E, Monville F, Ginestier C, et al. Cancer stem cells in breast: current opinion and future challenges. *Pathobiology* 2008;75:75–84.
136. Zhang Y, Toy KA, Kleer CG. Metaplastic breast carcinomas are enriched in markers of tumor-initiating cells and epithelial to mesenchymal transition. *Mod Pathol* 2012;25:178–184.
137. Gerhard R, Ricardo S, Albergaria A, et al. Immunohistochemical features of claudin-low intrinsic subtype in metaplastic breast carcinomas. *Breast* 2012;21:354–360.
138. Kaufmann M, Heider KH, Sinn HP, et al. CD44 isoforms in prognosis of breast cancer. *Lancet* 1995;346:502.
139. Vega S, Morales AV, Ocana OH, et al. Snail blocks the cell cycle and confers resistance to cell death. *Genes Dev* 2004;18:1131–1143.
140. Patarroyo M, Tryggvason K, Virtanen I. Laminin isoforms in tumor invasion, angiogenesis and metastasis. *Semin Cancer Biol* 2002;12:197–207.
141. Ivanov O, Chen F, Wiley EL, et al. AlphaB-crystallin is a novel predictor of resistance to neoadjuvant chemotherapy in breast cancer. *Breast Cancer Res Treat* 2008;111:411–417.
142. Moyano JV, Evans JR, Chen F, et al. AlphaB-crystallin is a novel oncoprotein that predicts poor clinical outcome in breast cancer. *J Clin Invest* 2006;116:261–270.
143. Sitterding SM, Wiseman WR, Schiller CL, et al. AlphaB-crystallin: a novel marker of invasive basal-like and metaplastic breast carcinomas. *Ann Diagn Pathol* 2008;12:33–40.
144. Tsang JY, Lai MW, Wong KH, et al. AlphaB-crystallin is a useful marker for triple negative and basal breast cancers. *Histopathology* 2012;61:378–386.
145. Liu H, Shi J, Wilkerson ML, Lin F. Immunohistochemical evaluation of GATA3 expression in tumors and normal tissues: a useful immunomarker for breast and urothelial carcinomas. *Am J Clin Pathol* 2012;138:57–64.
146. Cimino-Mathews A, Subhawong AP, Illei PB, et al. GATA3 expression in breast carcinoma: utility in triple-negative, sarcomatoid, and metastatic carcinomas. *Hum Pathol* 2013;44:1341–1349.
147. Schwartz LE, Begum S, Westra WH, et al. GATA3 immunohistochemical expression in salivary gland neoplasms. *Head Neck Pathol* 2013.
148. Cimino-Mathews A, Subhawong AP, Elwood H, et al. Neural crest transcription factor Sox10 is preferentially expressed in triple-negative and metaplastic breast carcinomas. *Hum Pathol* 2013;44:959–965.
149. Fisher ER, Palekar AS, Gregorio RM, et al. Mucoepidermoid and squamous cell carcinomas of breast with reference to squamous metaplasia and giant cell tumors. *Am J Surg Pathol* 1983;7:15–27.
150. Battifora H. Spindle cell carcinoma: ultrastructural evidence of squamous origin and collagen production by the tumor cells. *Cancer* 1976;37:2275–2282.
151. Gonzalez-Licea A, Yardley JH, Hartmann WH. Malignant tumor of the breast with bone formation. Studies by light and electron microscopy. *Cancer* 1967;20:1234–1247.
152. Kahn LB, Uys CJ, Dale J, et al. Carcinoma of the breast with metaplasia to chondrosarcoma: a light and electron microscopic study. *Histopathology* 1978;2:93–106.

153. Llombart-Bosch A, Peydro A. Malignant mixed osteogenic tumours of the breast. An ultrastructural study of two cases. *Virchows Arch A Pathol Anat Histol* 1975;366:1–14.
154. An T, Grathwohl M, Frable WJ. Breast carcinoma with osseous metaplasia: an electron microscopic study. *Am J Clin Pathol* 1984;81:127–132.
155. Perou CM, Sorlie T, Eisen MB, et al. Molecular portraits of human breast tumours. *Nature* 2000;406:747–752.
156. Weigelt B, Kreike B, Reis-Filho JS. Metaplastic breast carcinomas are basal-like breast cancers: a genomic profiling analysis. *Breast Cancer Res Treat* 2009;117:273–280.
157. Herschkowitz JI, Simin K, Weigman VJ, et al. Identification of conserved gene expression features between murine mammary carcinoma models and human breast tumors. *Genome Biol* 2007;8:R76.
158. Hennessy BT, Gonzalez-Angulo AM, Stemke-Hale K, et al. Characterization of a naturally occurring breast cancer subset enriched in epithelial-to-mesenchymal transition and stem cell characteristics. *Cancer Res* 2009;69:4116–4124.
159. Prat A, Parker JS, Karginova O, et al. Phenotypic and molecular characterization of the claudin-low intrinsic subtype of breast cancer. *Breast Cancer Res* 2010;12:R68.
160. Perou CM. Molecular stratification of triple-negative breast cancers. *Oncologist* 2011;16(Suppl. 1):61–70.
161. Gordon LA, Mulligan KT, Maxwell-Jones H, et al. Breast cell invasive potential relates to the myoepithelial phenotype. *Int J Cancer* 2003;106:8–16.
162. Jones C, Mackay A, Grigoriadis A, et al. Expression profiling of purified normal human luminal and myoepithelial breast cells: identification of novel prognostic markers for breast cancer. *Cancer Res* 2004;64:3037–3045.
163. Kim K, Lu Z, Hay ED. Direct evidence for a role of beta-catenin/LEF-1 signaling pathway in induction of EMT. *Cell Biol Int* 2002;26:463–476.
164. Taube JH, Herschkowitz JI, Komurov K, et al. Core epithelial-to-mesenchymal transition interactome gene-expression signature is associated with claudin-low and metaplastic breast cancer subtypes. *Proc Natl Acad Sci U S A* 2010;107:15449–15454.
165. Lien HC, Hsiao YH, Lin YS, et al. Molecular signatures of metaplastic carcinoma of the breast by large-scale transcriptional profiling: identification of genes potentially related to epithelial-mesenchymal transition. *Oncogene* 2007;26:7859–7871.
166. Mani SA, Guo W, Liao MJ, et al. The epithelial-mesenchymal transition generates cells with properties of stem cells. *Cell* 2008;133:704–715.
167. McCarthy A, Savage K, Gabriel A, et al. A mouse model of basal-like breast carcinoma with metaplastic elements. *J Pathol* 2007;211:389–398.
168. Turner NC, Reis-Filho JS, Russell AM, et al. BRCA1 dysfunction in sporadic basal-like breast cancer. *Oncogene* 2007;26:2126–2132.
169. Jiang Z, Jones R, Liu JC, et al. RB1 and p53 at the crossroad of EMT and triple-negative breast cancer. *Cell Cycle* 2011;10:1563–1570.
170. Guttilla IK, Adams BD, White BA. ERalpha, microRNAs, and the epithelial-mesenchymal transition in breast cancer. *Trends Endocrinol Metab* 2012;23:73–82.
171. Gregory PA, Bert AG, Paterson EL, et al. The miR-200 family and miR-205 regulate epithelial to mesenchymal transition by targeting ZEB1 and SIP1. *Nat Cell Biol* 2008;10:593–601.
172. Shimono Y, Zabala M, Cho RW, et al. Downregulation of miRNA-200c links breast cancer stem cells with normal stem cells. *Cell* 2009;138:592–603.
173. Jung SY, Kim HY, Nam BH, et al. Worse prognosis of metaplastic breast cancer patients than other patients with triple-negative breast cancer. *Breast Cancer Res Treat* 2010;120:627–637.
174. Nagao T, Kinoshita T, Hojo T, et al. The differences in the histological types of breast cancer and the response to neoadjuvant chemotherapy: the relationship between the outcome and the clinicopathological characteristics. *Breast* 2012;21:289–295.
175. Brown-Glaberman U, Graham A, Stopeck A. A case of metaplastic carcinoma of the breast responsive to chemotherapy with Ifosfamide and Etoposide: improved antitumor response by targeting sarcomatous features. *Breast J* 2010;16:663–665.
176. Moroney JW, Schlumbrecht MP, Helgason T, et al. A phase I trial of liposomal doxorubicin, bevacizumab, and temsirolimus in patients with advanced gynecologic and breast malignancies. *Clin Cancer Res* 2011;17:6840–6846.
177. Drudis T, Arroyo C, Van Hoeven K, et al. The pathology of low-grade adenosquamous carcinoma of the breast. An immunohistochemical study. *Pathol Annu* 1994;29(Pt. 2):181–197.
178. Ferrara G, Nappi O, Wick MR. Fine-needle aspiration cytology and immunohistology of low-grade adenosquamous carcinoma of the breast. *Diagn Cytopathol* 1999;20:13–18.
179. Geyer FC, Lambros MB, Natrajan R, et al. Genomic and immunohistochemical analysis of adenosquamous carcinoma of the breast. *Mod Pathol* 2010;23:951–960.
180. Ho BC, Tan HW, Lee VK, Tan PH. Preoperative and intraoperative diagnosis of low-grade adenosquamous carcinoma of the breast: potential diagnostic pitfalls. *Histopathology* 2006;49:603–611.
181. Van Hoeven KH, Drudis T, Cranor ML, et al. Low-grade adenosquamous carcinoma of the breast. A clinocopathologic study of 32 cases with ultrastructural analysis. *Am J Surg Pathol* 1993;17:248–258.
182. Kawaguchi K, Shin SJ. Immunohistochemical staining characteristics of low-grade adenosquamous carcinoma of the breast. *Am J Surg Pathol* 2012;36:1009–1020.
183. Krigman HR, Iglehart JD, Coogan AC, et al. Fine-needle aspiration of low grade adenosquamous carcinoma of the breast. *Diagn Cytopathol* 1996;14:321–324.
184. Noel JC, Buxant F, Engohan-Aloghe C. Low-grade adenosquamous carcinoma of the breast—a case report with a BRCA1 germline mutation. *Pathol Res Pract* 2010;206:511–513.
185. Shizawa S, Sasano H, Suzuki T, et al. Low-grade adenosquamous carcinoma of the breast: a case report with cytologic findings and review of the literature. *Pathol Int* 1997;47:264–267.
186. Sironi M, Lanata S, Pollone M, et al. Fine-needle aspiration cytology of low-grade adenosquamous carcinoma of the breast. *Diagn Cytopathol* 2011;40:713–715.
187. Agrawal A, Saha S, Ellis IO, et al. Adenosquamous carcinoma of breast in a 19 years old woman: a case report. *World J Surg Oncol* 2010;8:44.
188. Suster S, Moran CA, Hurt MA. Syringomatous squamous tumors of the breast. *Cancer* 1991;67:2350–2355.
189. Foschini MP, Pizzicannella G, Peterse JL, et al. Adenomyoepithelioma of the breast associated with low-grade adenosquamous and sarcomatoid carcinomas. *Virchows Arch* 1995;427:243–250.
190. Rosen PP, Ernsberger D. Low-grade adenosquamous carcinoma. A variant of metaplastic mammary carcinoma. *Am J Surg Pathol* 1987;11:351–358.

CHAPTER 17

Squamous Carcinoma

EDI BROGI

Squamous carcinoma (SQC) of the breast is a form of metaplastic carcinoma. Because of its distinctive pathologic and clinical features, SQC is discussed here separately from all other metaplastic mammary carcinomas, including those with spindle cell and squamous differentiation, which are described in Chapter 16. The diagnosis of SQC is used for tumors in which 90% or more of the lesion consists of keratinizing SQC. By definition, a primary SQC of the breast has to be centered in the breast parenchyma. It may involve the skin only peripherally, thus excluding any primary cutaneous neoplasm that extends into the breast secondarily. Metastasis of SQC from an extramammary site should be ruled out clinically when carcinoma with squamous differentiation is encountered in the breast. The earliest examples of SQC were reported nearly a century ago.[1–3]

ORIGIN OF MAMMARY SQC

The origin of SQC of the breast remains uncertain. Cases of pure squamous ductal carcinoma *in situ* (DCIS) have been described, including one associated with an invasive carcinoma showing focal squamous differentiation,[4] but squamous DCIS is rarely found in association with invasive SQC. It is commonly believed that the majority of pure squamous mammary carcinomas probably originate from *benign squamous metaplasia*[5] that can occur in the epithelium of cysts,[6] in hyperplastic ducts and lobules (Figs. 17.1 and 17.2), and in papillomas.[7] Rarely the epithelium of multiple ducts in one portion of the breast can be extensively altered by squamous metaplasia.[7,8] Squamous metaplasia is also sometimes present in fibroepithelial lesions[9,10] and in gynecomastia where it is typically found as isolated foci involving part of the epithelium of ducts that also exhibit epithelial hyperplasia.[11] Reddick et al.[8] studied squamous metaplasia in a papilloma by using immunohistochemistry and electron microscopy and concluded that the metaplastic change originated in myoepithelial cells. Diffuse squamous metaplasia of duct and lobular epithelium in an area of fat necrosis has been described[12]; the patient remained well at follow-up 3 years after the biopsy. Squamous metaplasia can also be found in other inflammatory or necrotizing lesions such as infarcted adenomas,[13] in inflamed cysts or other forms of mastitis, in infarcted papillomas[14] and adenomyoepitheliomas (Fig. 17.3), and in healing biopsy sites (Fig. 17.4). Atypical cells obtained by fine-needle aspiration (FNA) or core biopsy from an irradiated biopsy site where there is squamous metaplasia may suggest carcinoma.[15]

Shousha[16] described a $2 \times 2 \times 1$ cm^3 multiloculated cyst lined largely by keratinizing stratified squamous epithelium in the breast of a 70-year-old woman. Mucin-containing glandular cells were also present in the squamous epithelium, individually and in small groups (Fig. 17.5). Metaplastic squamous epithelium may become embedded in the wall of an inflamed cyst, resulting in a pattern that is difficult to distinguish from invasive carcinoma. The diagnosis usually hinges on a careful evaluation of the cytologic appearance of the squamous epithelium.

Cutaneous squamous epithelium displaced into the breast by a needle core biopsy procedure may persist in the healed tissues, resulting in the formation of an epidermal inclusion cyst.[17] Squamous metaplasia of lactiferous ducts is important in the pathogenesis of subareolar abscesses.[18] Chronic inflammation resulting in benign squamous metaplasia likely represents a predisposing factor to SQC.

Insulin enhances the development of squamous metaplasia in organ cultures of human mammary tissue.[19,20] Chemical carcinogens cause keratinizing metaplasia *in vitro* in murine mammary[21] and prostate glands.[22] In one study, tissues obtained from patients in the early part of the menstrual cycle were less susceptible to the induction of squamous metaplasia than specimens taken later in the cycle, an observation suggesting that progesterone or estrogen, or both, may influence the process.[23]

CLINICAL PRESENTATION

SQC typically presents as a palpable mass. No clinical features are specific for SQC of the breast, but a substantial number of the reported cases have presented with clinical features of an abscess.[24–33] Behranwala et al.[34] described SQC that arose within a recurrent or long-standing breast cyst, in a chronic sinus, and in the capsule of a breast implant. Rare cases were associated with nipple discharge[34,35] or Paget disease.[32]

All reported examples of primary mammary SQC have been in female patients. There are no documented reports in men. The mean age at diagnosis of SQC was 64 years according to California Cancer Registry data pertaining to breast carcinomas diagnosed between 1988 and 2005.[36] Other

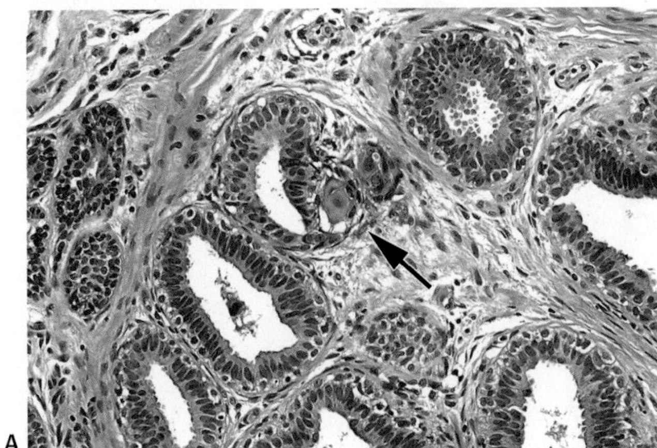

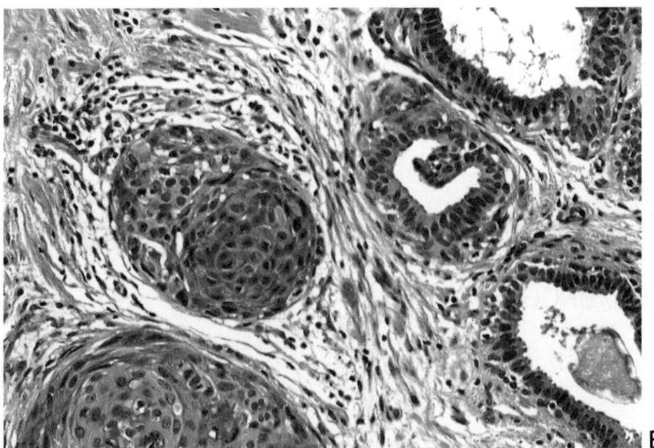

FIG. 17.1. ***Squamous metaplasia in normal breast.*** **A:** A small focus of squamous differentiation is shown in one of several ducts (*arrow*). **B:** Two ducts are fully involved by benign squamous epithelium.

studies have reported a median age at diagnosis of 52,[37] 54,[38] and 55,[39,40] years with a range of 24 to 91 years.[34,37,40–42] Sixty-four percent of patients diagnosed with SQC in a study from the M.D. Anderson Cancer Center were White/Caucasian, 21% African American, and 15% were of Hispanic ethnicity.[37] No association of primary SQC of the breast with familial cancer syndromes has been reported. Immunosuppressive treatment with azathioprine has been associated with increased incidence of squamous cell carcinoma (SQC) of the skin and oral mucosa. One case of SQC of the breast has been reported in a 35-year-old woman treated with azathioprine for Crohn disease.[43] A study found that primary mammary SQC is more common in the left breast,[41] but predominant breast laterality is not mentioned in other studies.

Fixation to the chest wall and invasion of the skin may complicate large tumors. Extension to and ulceration of the skin can make it difficult to distinguish between cutaneous origin and secondary skin involvement by a primary mammary lesion.[44] When the bulk of the tumor is in the breast and the clinical history indicates that a breast mass preceded a skin lesion, the lesion may be considered a mammary carcinoma. SQC of the breast typically presents as a mass lesion. It has indistinct or partially distinct margins on mammography, but no specific mammographic finding has been described.[45,46] Calcifications in necrotic squamous tissue may be detected radiographically. The cystic nature of the tumor is usually apparent on ultrasonography.[5] SQC that is cystic due to central necrosis has low T1 and high T2 signal intensity on magnetic resonance imaging (MRI).[47]

GROSS PATHOLOGY

SQC tend to be somewhat larger than other types of breast carcinoma. Reported sizes vary from 1 to 12.5 cm, with about 20%[39] to 40%[48] of the tumors measuring 5 cm or greater in

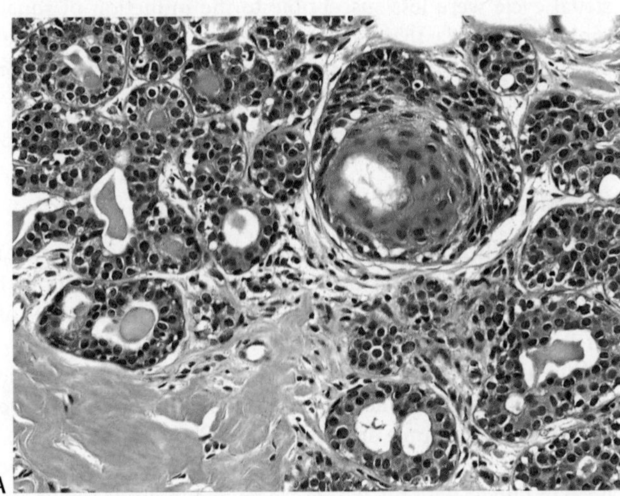

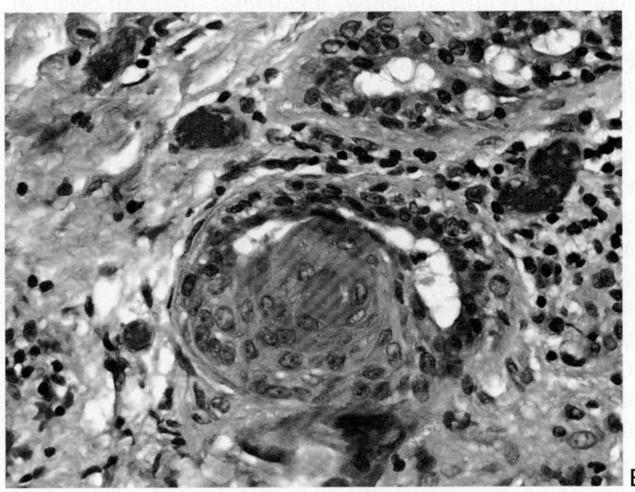

FIG. 17.2. ***Squamous metaplasia in mammary acini.*** **A,B:** Squamous differentiation in mammary acini.

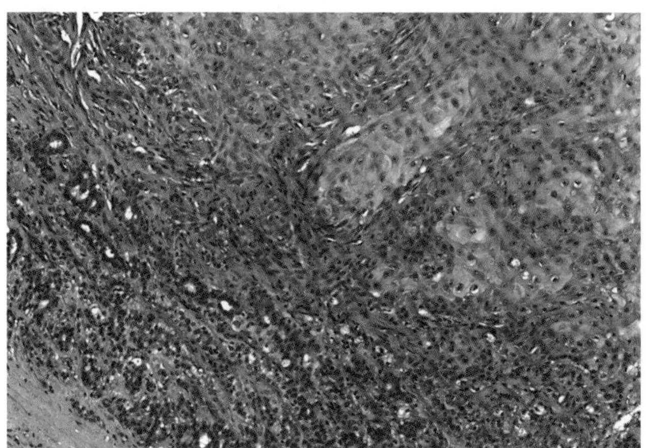

FIG. 17.3. *Squamous metaplasia in an adenomyoepithelioma.*

diameter. In one series, 61% of 31 pure SQC had T2 size at presentation, and 12% had T3 size.[37]

It is not unusual for the lesions to undergo cystic degeneration centrally (Fig. 17.6). This alteration is especially common in tumors larger than 2 cm, the cavity being filled with necrotic squamous and inflammatory debris.[49,50] The tumor tends to be softer and more granular when the lesion is composed largely of keratinizing epithelium, whereas spindle cell metaplasia produces a firmer lesion.

MICROSCOPIC PATHOLOGY

Before establishing a diagnosis of primary SQC of the breast, it is necessary to exclude a metastasis from an extramammary primary carcinoma.[40,50,51] The most common sources of metastatic SQC in the breast are the lung, uterine cervix, urinary bladder, and carcinomas of the head and neck regions.[52] Although clinically the patient may be known to have an extramammary primary malignancy, this information is sometimes not communicated to the pathologist, especially if the other lesion was not treated recently and no active tumor is apparent at the primary site. Cystic degeneration is not unusual in foci of SQC metastatic from extramammary sites.

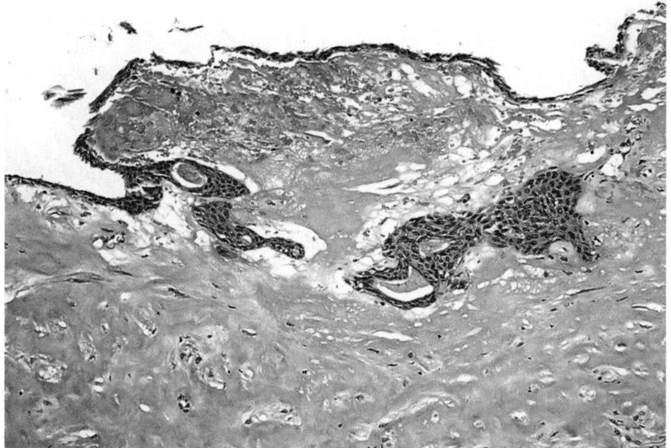

FIG. 17.4. *Squamous metaplasia in biopsy cavity.* A thin layer of squamous epithelium lines the surface of this partially healed biopsy cavity and a duct in the underlying tissue.

Mammary SQC are distinguished from the diverse group of metaplastic carcinomas by origin from *in situ* SQC in a cyst, ducts, or both, and by predominant squamous differentiation. Microscopically, they resemble SQC that arise in other sites (Fig. 17.7). Cytoplasmic clearing is present in some tumors (Fig. 17.8). Focal conversion of the squamous epithelial pattern to spindle cell pseudosarcomatous and acantholytic growth may occur[53,54] (Figs. 17.9 to 17.11). Spindle cell components may be obscured by the reactive stroma, but they can be highlighted with immunostains such as 34βE12 (K903), cytokeratin (CK) 14, CK5/6, and p63. An inflammatory infiltrate rich in granulocytes and lymphocytes is often present in association with SQC, especially in necrotic and/or keratinized areas (Figs. 17.7 and 17.12), accounting for the common clinical impression of an abscess.

The DCIS associated with SQC sometimes is differentiated sufficiently to keratinize,[4] and keratohyalin granules may be seen in the neoplastic epithelium, especially in the wall of a cystic carcinoma (Fig. 17.13). In most cases, however, the DCIS associated with mammary SQC intermediate or high nuclear grade, and squamous cytomorphology may be less obvious (Fig. 17.14). Invasive SQC is rarely associated with squamous DCIS. Rarely SQC *in situ* can arise in the epithelium of malignant phyllodes tumors (MPT) (Fig. 17.15).[55]

CYTOLOGY

Surgical biopsy is recommended to establish the diagnosis of mammary SQC, but it is often possible to recognize squamous differentiation in an aspiration cytology specimen from the breast.[5,49,50,56] The specimen obtained by FNA usually does not present a diagnostic problem when abundant malignant squamous cells are identified.[57] Anucleated and granular squamous cells are suggestive of an epidermal inclusion cyst, but they may be present in the aspirate from a well-differentiated mammary SQC. Isolated foci within a SQC may be so well differentiated that they are not distinguishable from benign squamous epithelium in a limited needle core biopsy specimen or in a fine-needle aspirate.

The distinction between a primary tumor and metastatic SQC cannot be made in an aspiration cytology specimen, and it is also unlikely to be resolved by a needle core biopsy sample unless intraductal carcinoma is also fortuitously sampled.

Atypical squamous metaplasia in seromas from irradiated lumpectomy sites can simulate a SQC in FNA material, although the atypical squamous cells tend to be less abundant than in a carcinoma. A cautious approach is imperative in these cases, and additional material is required for definitive evaluation.[15]

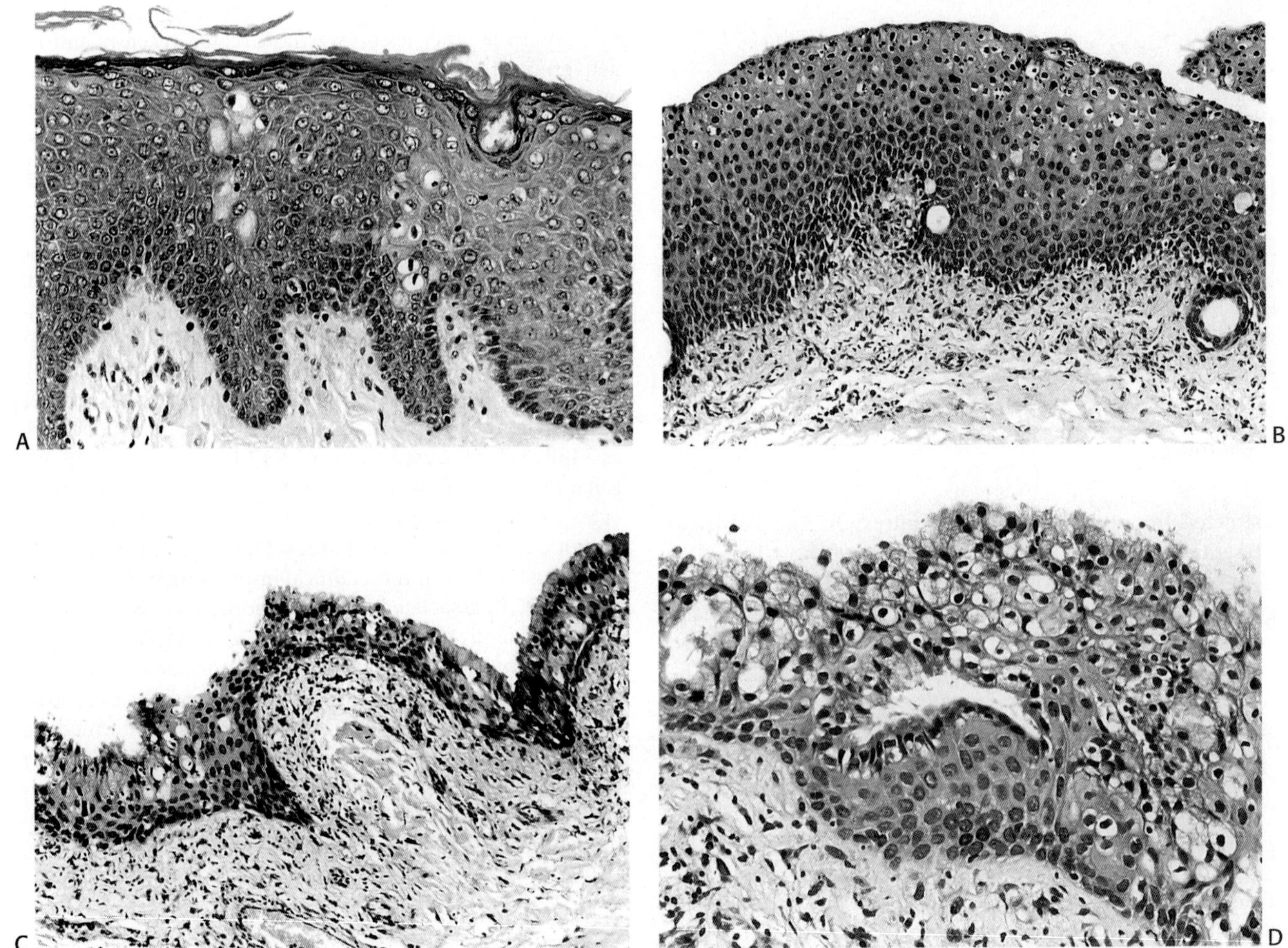

FIG. 17.5. ***Squamous metaplasia in cysts.*** **A:** Superficial keratinizing cells in this benign metaplastic epithelium have keratohyaline granules. **B:** Squamous metaplasia and one residual gland on the *right*. **C:** Benign metaplastic squamous epithelium beneath residual glandular ductal epithelium. **D:** Glandular and squamous epithelia are seen merging. (Courtesy of S. Shousha, MD.)

IMMUNOHISTOCHEMISTRY

A CK stain is useful for detecting superficial invasion in cystic lesions. Because squamous epithelium is p63-positive in about 70% of cases,[39] this stain is not helpful for identifying myoepithelium in intraductal SQC. p40 (ΔNp63) is an aminoterminal-truncated isoform of p63. It was found to be superior to p63 in detecting squamous differentiation in lung carcinomas,[58] but its utility in the diagnosis of breast lesions, especially in the detection of squamous differentiation in breast carcinomas, has not been fully assessed.

SQC is usually negative for estrogen receptor (ER) and progesterone receptor (PR).[5,37,39–41,59] One lesion that was positive for ER and PR had a diploid DNA content and a high S-phase fraction.[49] Human epidermal growth factor (HER2)/*neu* 3+ positivity has been reported in less than 10% of pure SQC.[37,39]

SQC often display reactivity for epidermal growth factor receptor (EGFR).[37,39,59] In one study, 5 of 30 cases of pure SQC showed strong (3+) reactivity for EGFR, and 87% of carcinomas with squamous differentiation showed less EGFR immunostaining.[59] Grenier et al.[39] reported that 81% of 11 pure SQC had EGFR reactivity in more than 10% of the cells compared with only 12% of invasive ductal carcinomas of no special type (NST). The extent to which EGFR immunoreactivity correlates with gene amplification and/or activating mutations has not been determined.

CK5/6 is expressed in 63%[39] to 89%[59] of pure SQC, and high-molecular-weight CK 34βE12 shows a similar staining pattern.

Hayes et al.[4] detailed the immunoprofile of three cases of squamous DCIS, including one associated with invasive carcinoma with squamous foci. All three DCIS were positive for EGFR and negative for ER, PR, and HER2/*neu*. They were also all positive for p63, although one case showed only focal staining. CK14 was strongly positive in one case, and the other two cases showed patchy CK14 reactivity.

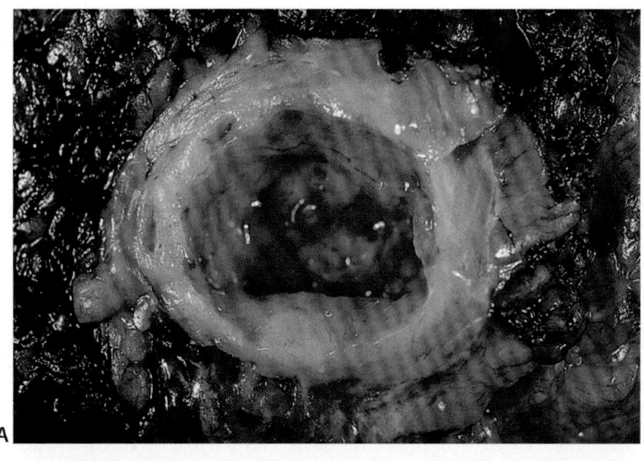

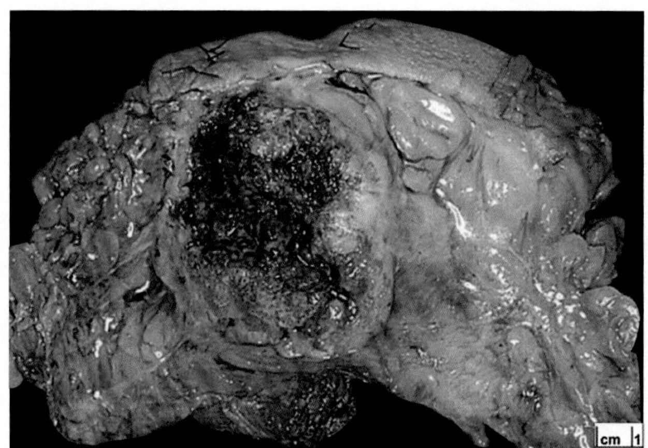

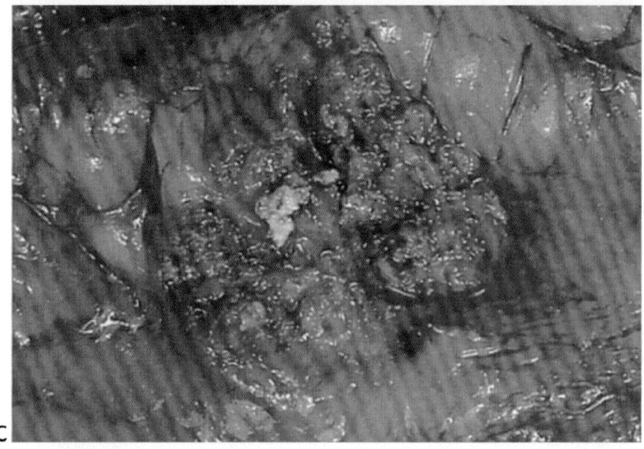

FIG. 17.6. ***Squamous carcinoma, gross appearance.*** **A:** Cystic tumor. The outer surface of the tissue has been colored with ink to demarcate the resection margin. **B:** Nodular foci of Squamous carcinoma protrude into the lumen of this partly cystic tumor. (Courtesy of Roger Adlesberg, MD.) **C:** A solid tumor with white foci of degenerated keratin.

Some reactivity for actin, epithelial membrane antigen (EMA), and CK7 was detected in two of the three examples of squamous DCIS, but the distribution of reactivity in the three cases showed no specific pattern. Reactivity for p53 was absent in one squamous DCIS and positive in more than 80% of the cells in another. Although the number of squamous DCIS cases studied is extremely limited, the immunoprofile suggests dual epithelial and myoepithelial differentiation, an observation that suggests possible myoepithelial origin of mammary SQC.

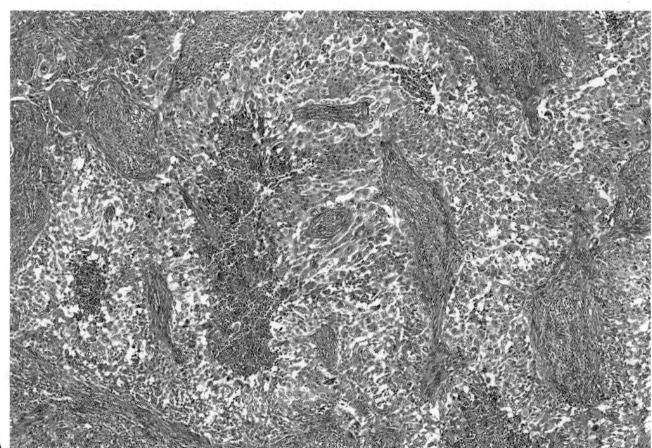

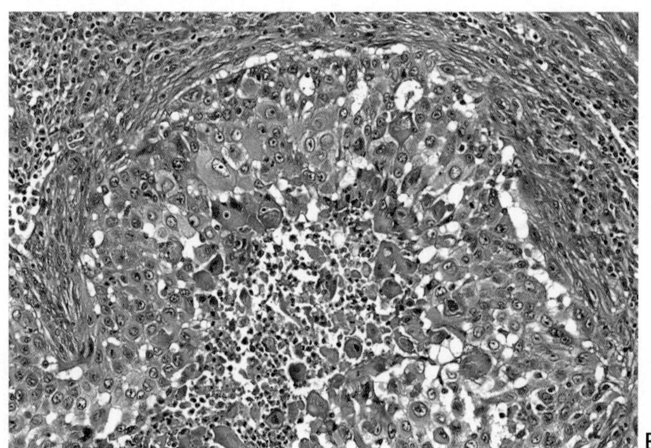

FIG. 17.7. ***Squamous carcinoma.*** The images are from the same tumor. **A:** The carcinoma consists of broad bands and ribbons of keratinizing cells, with central necrosis and admixed inflammation. **B:** The tumor cells have abundant eosinophilic cytoplasm. Dense hyperchromasia is evident in the necrotic cells.

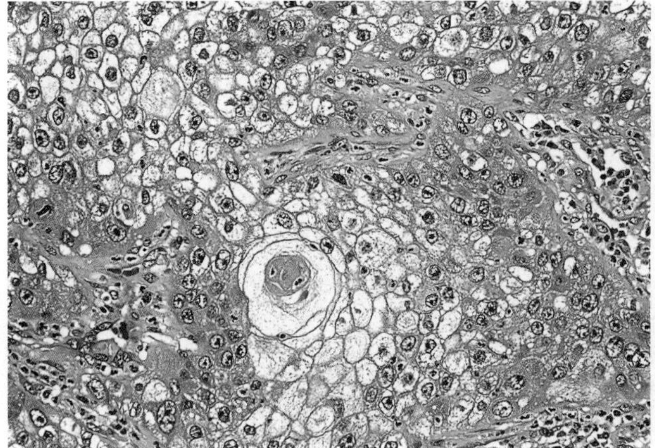

FIG. 17.8. *Invasive squamous carcinoma, clear cell.*

ELECTRON MICROSCOPY

Ultrastructural and immunohistochemical studies have confirmed the squamous character of the tissue,[53] but intracellular canaliculi seen in some cells are evidence that glandular features may persist in some of these tumors. Stevenson et al.[60] analyzed the ultrastructural findings in SQC. They reported that separate squamous and glandular cells were present in the same tumor or both histologic features coexisted in the same cells, suggesting that SQC of the breast may represent a morphologic continuum characterized by variable extent of squamous metaplasia that is most extensive in pure SQC.

GENETICS AND MOLECULAR STUDIES

Although pure SQC of the breast is frequently immunoreactive for EGFR, the extent of EGFR gene amplification in this type of tumor remains to be determined. In one study, the mean *EGFR* gene copy number in two SQC was 2.35. One of these tumors had trisomy of chromosome 7 in 50% of the cells.[61] *EGFR* gene amplification was detected by chromogenic *in situ* hybridization in the squamous component of 53% of 23 metaplastic carcinomas with mixed spindle cell and squamous morphology, but no EGFR-activating mutation was identified.[62] Results obtained by *in vitro* experiments using a human cell line established

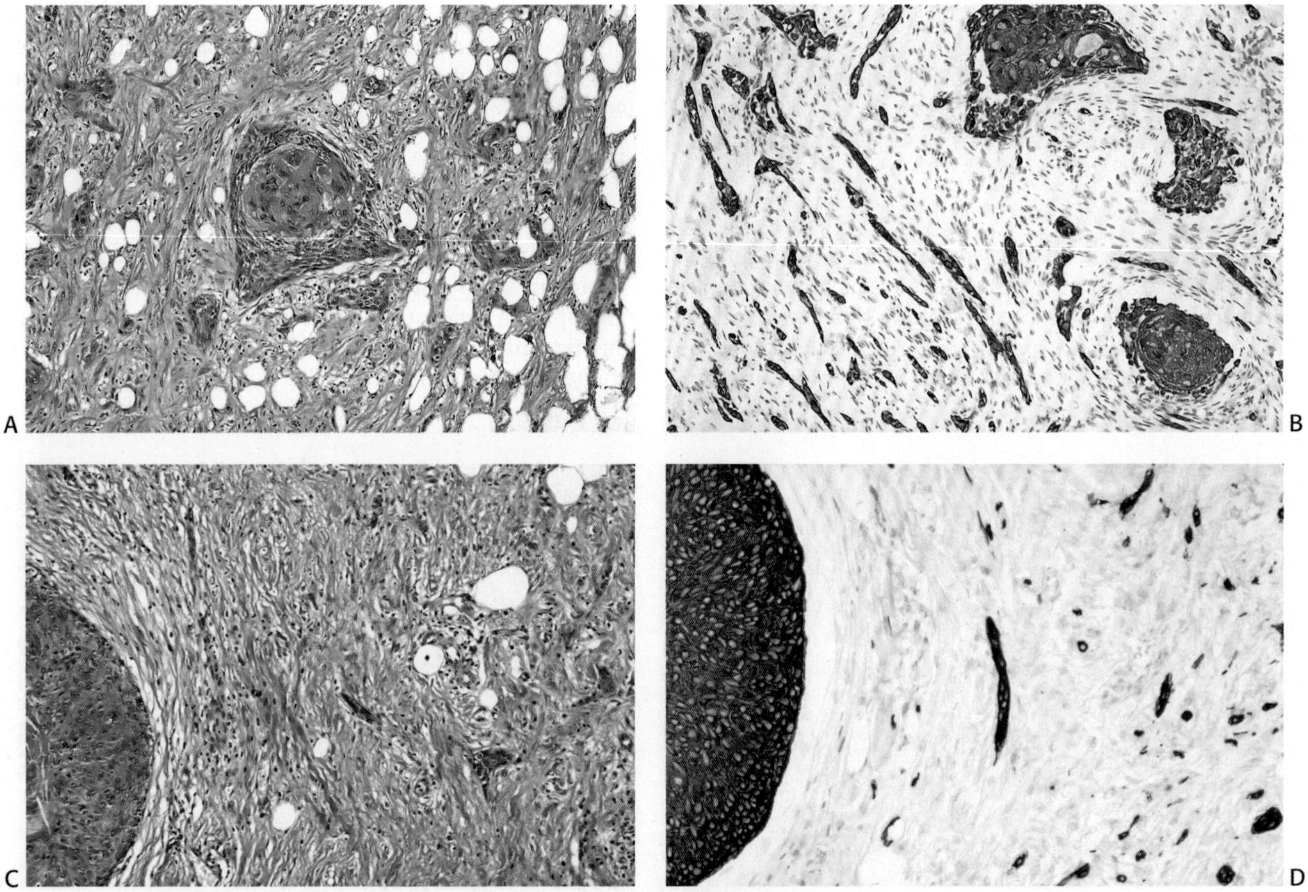

FIG. 17.9. ***Invasive squamous carcinoma, spindle cell.*** **A:** Invasive keratinizing carcinoma surrounded by small nests of carcinoma cells in a spindle cell proliferation. **B:** Cytokeratin reactivity is demonstrated in spindle cells with the antibody K903 (34βE12). **C:** A few inconspicuous foci of invasive Squamous carcinoma are seen in spindle cell stroma next to intraductal Squamous carcinoma. **D:** The K903 immunostain for cytokeratin highlights invasive carcinoma near the intraductal carcinoma.

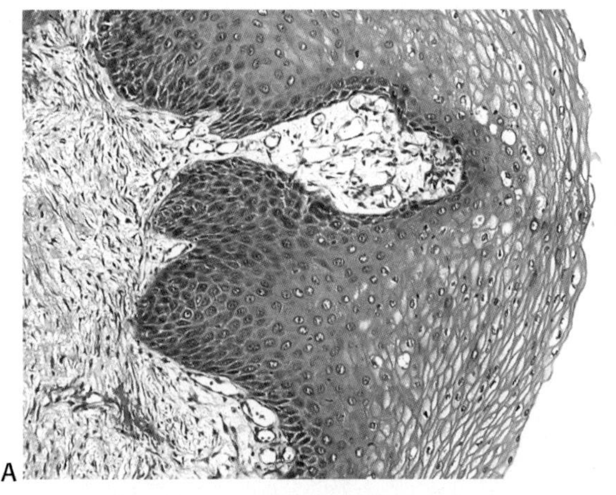

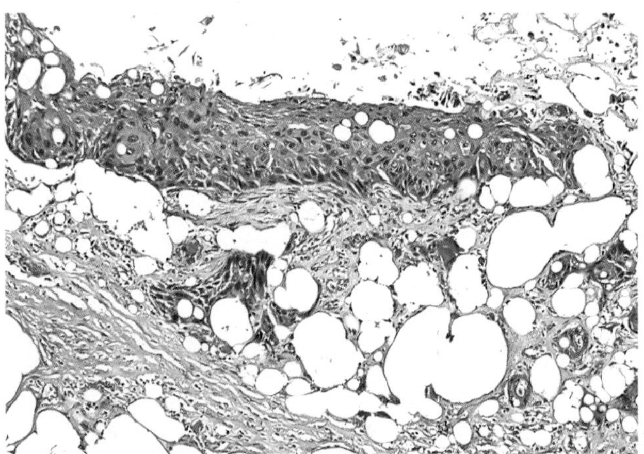

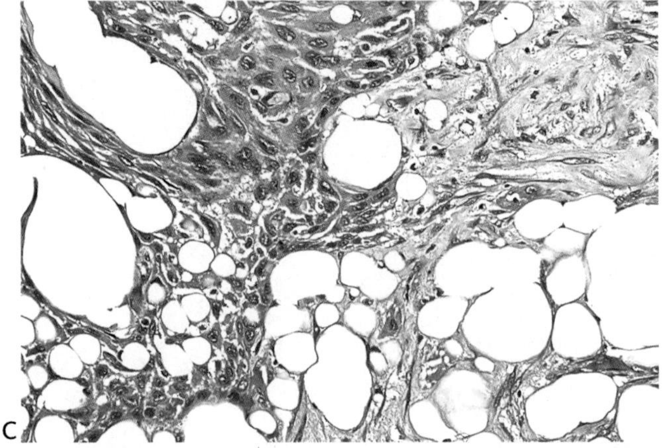

FIG. 17.10. ***Invasive squamous carcinoma arising at the site of a prosthetic breast implant.*** **A:** Mature metaplastic squamous epithelium such as this lined much of the implant site. **B:** *In situ* Squamous carcinoma overlying invasive carcinoma in fat necrosis. **C:** Acantholytic change is shown in the invasive carcinoma.

from a lymph node metastasis of SQC of the breast have demonstrated EGF-dependent enhancement of cell motility, which may correlate with increased invasiveness of the tumor.[63]

Genetic material from human papilloma virus was detected by polymerase chain reaction (PCR) analysis in 14% of mammary SQC in one study.[39] This result is consistent with the overall prevalence of this type of virus in breast carcinomas of no special type.[64]

Further discussion of pathogenesis and genetic alterations associated with mammary metaplastic carcinomas is found in Chapter 16.

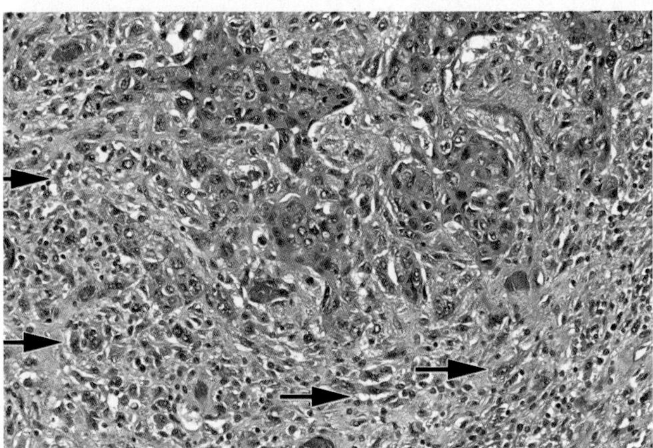

FIG. 17.11. ***Invasive squamous carcinoma, spindle cell.*** The neoplastic cells in the clusters of a high-grade invasive Squamous carcinoma transition into high-grade metaplastic spindle cells (*arrows*).

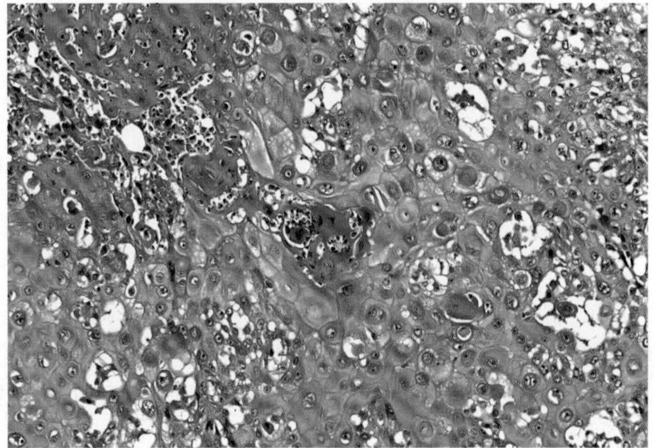

FIG. 17.12. ***Invasive squamous carcinoma with inflammation in keratinized necrotic cells.*** Acute inflammation and apoptotic debris are associated with pycnotic keratinized cells in areas of focal tumor necrosis.

TREATMENT AND PROGNOSIS

Information about the prognosis and follow-up of patients with primary mammary SQC tends to be variable or incomplete in reported cases. Many of the published reports do not distinguish clearly between metaplastic carcinoma with spindle and squamous differentiation and pure SQC or do not provide detailed clinical follow-up information.

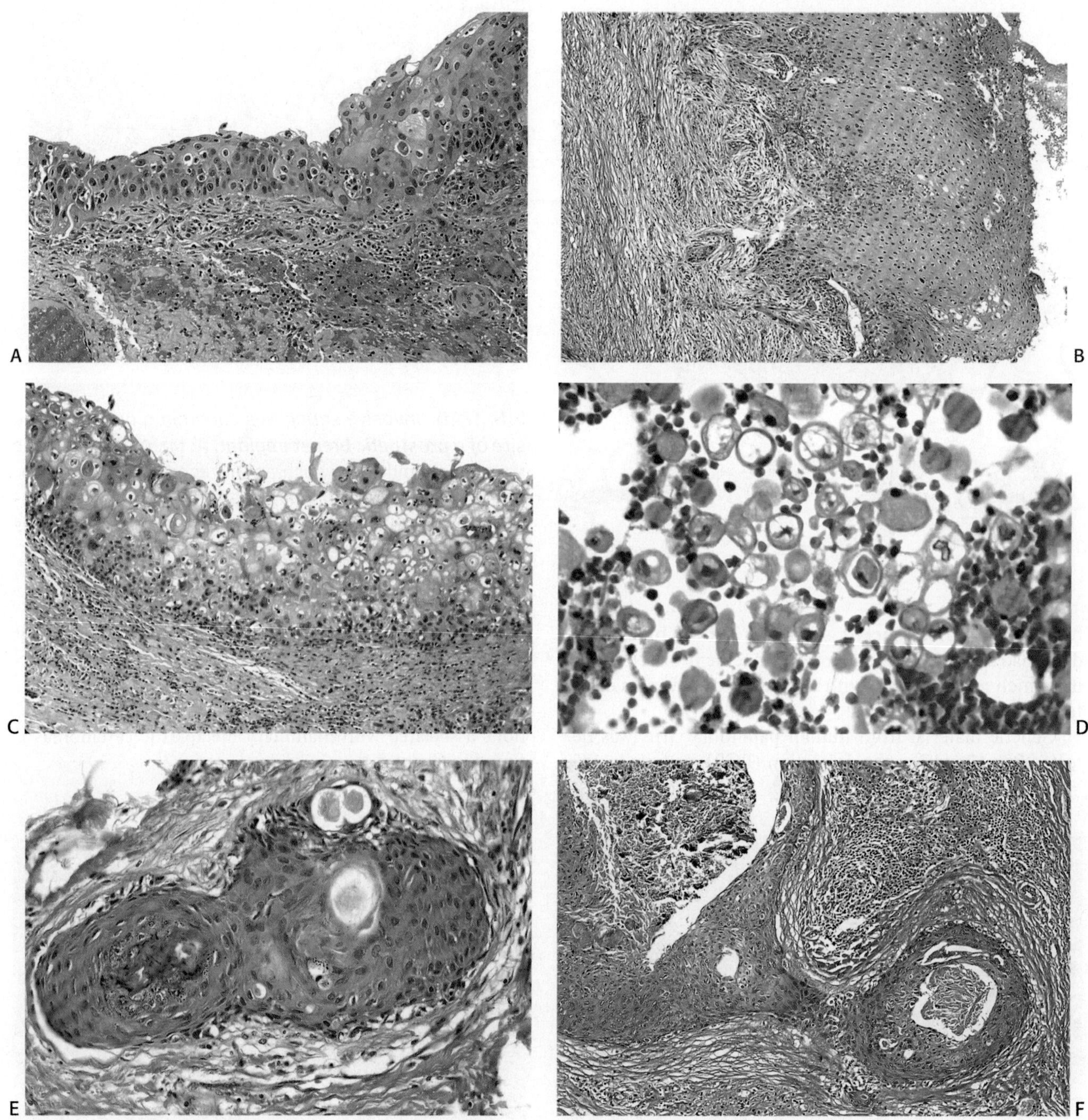

FIG. 17.13. ***Squamous carcinoma in situ.*** **A,B:** Carcinoma lining two cystic lesions. Superficial invasion is present at the deep surface of the epithelium in **(B)**. **C:** Keratinizing intracystic *in situ* Squamous carcinoma with high nuclear grade. **D:** Degenerated squamous cells in the cystic center of the tumor shown in **(C)**. **E:** Intraductal carcinoma with keratohyalin granules. A small remnant of the duct lumen can be seen near the *upper border*. **F:** Cystic degeneration of intraductal carcinoma with calcified keratotic debris.

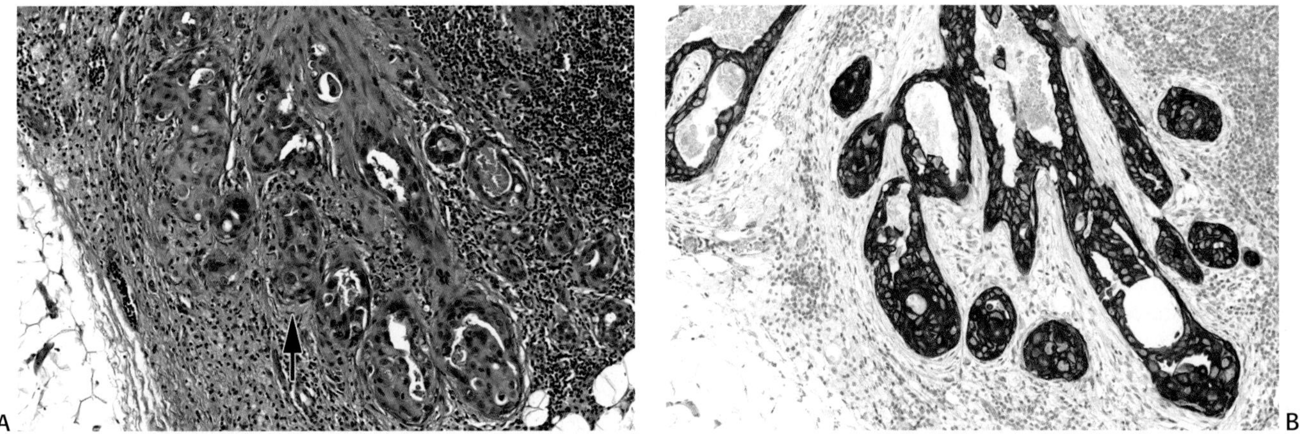

FIG. 17.14. ***Squamous carcinoma in situ.*** **A:** The DCIS in this case has traces of squamous differentiation (*arrow*). **B:** Squamous differentiation is highlighted by the positive reactivity for the basal keratins CK5 and CK14 (*brown*), whereas the remaining DCIS is positive only for the luminal CK7 and CK18 (*red*). This pattern of reactivity and the tumor morphology indicate focal squamous differentiation. No nuclear p63 reactivity is identified. (Multiplex staining with a CK5/14, p63, and CK7/18 antibody cocktail.)

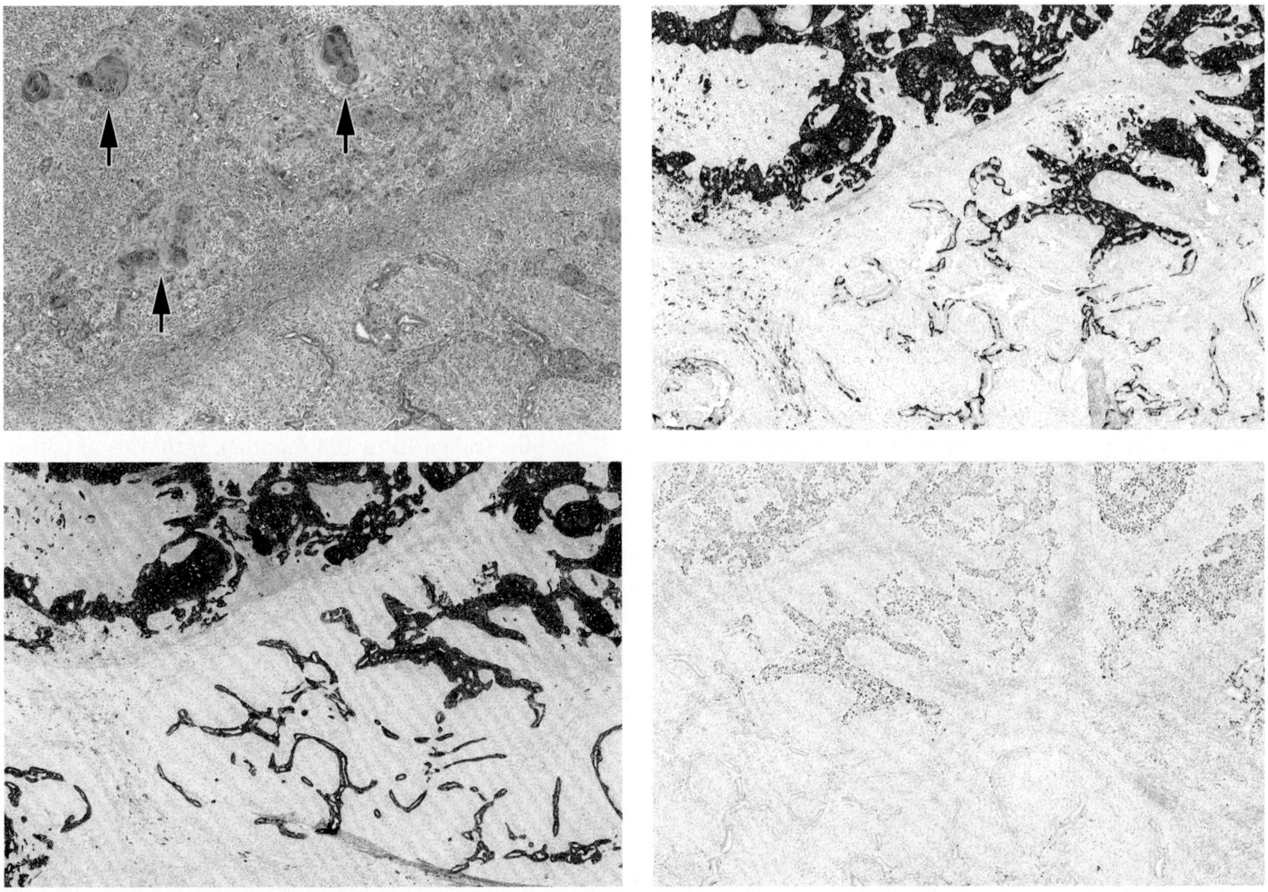

FIG. 17.15. ***Squamous carcinoma in a high-grade malignant phyllodes tumors.*** **A:** SQC is present in a high-grade malignant phyllodes tumor. Foci of keratin accumulation are noted (*arrows*). **B–D:** Immunohistochemical stains for CK14 **(B)**, keratin 34βE12 **(C)**, and p63 **(D)** highlight the *in situ* and invasive Squamous carcinoma.

Axillary Lymph Nodes

Axillary lymph node (ALN) dissection has been performed in nearly all cases, independent of the clinical and radiologic lymph node status.[34,37] No specific information is available regarding the use of sentinel lymph node biopsy in patients with SQC, but there is no apparent reason against its feasibility. In two large population-based studies, 20%[37] and 31.6%[36] of patients had lymph node metastases, and 9% had distant metastases at the time of diagnosis.[36,37] Lymph node metastases were present in 50% of patients in each of the three institution-based series that comprised a total of 90 cases,[37,39,59] but none of the 10 patients in another series had lymph metastases at presentation.[42] ALN metastases typically exhibit squamous differentiation[53] (Fig. 17.16). Benign squamous inclusions that sometimes occur in ALNs can usually be distinguished from metastatic carcinoma because they lack cytologic atypia (Fig. 17.17).

Therapy

Because of their relatively large size, most mammary SQC carcinomas have been treated surgically by mastectomy,[34,37,42] but breast conservation by wide excision or segmental mastectomy with adjuvant radiotherapy was adopted in about a third of patients in three series.[34,37,40]

In the past 10 to 20 years, adjuvant radiotherapy has been used in one-third[34] to two-thirds of patients.[37,38] In one patient with pure SQC who received neoadjuvant docetaxel, doxorubicin, and cyclophosphamide, the tumor shrank from 2 to 0.5 cm.[59] Five patients in one series received anthracycline-based neoadjuvant chemotherapy, with or without followed by radiotherapy in two cases. One of the two patients experienced progression of disease during treatment.[37] A patient with SQC received neoadjuvant 5-fluorouracil, epirubicin, and cyclophosphamide, but it is unclear whether the tumor was purely squamous, and no information on tumor response was provided.[38] A patient reported by Tsung[65] was treated with the same chemotherapy regimen, but experienced locally recurrent disease 3 weeks after mastectomy. At that point, she received taxotere and cisplatin chemotherapy and the tumor resolved completely. Another patient treated with cisplatin and 5-fluorouracil was also disease-free 28 months after surgery.[66] These anecdotal cases raise the possibility that cisplatin may be a useful agent for the treatment of mammary SQC, but no definitive data are available.

Prognosis

The 10-year cumulative survival rate in a Surveillance Epidemiology and End Results (SEER) population-based study was 81% for 93 patients with no regional or distant metastases at initial presentation and 46.9% for patients who presented with regional or distant metastases.[36] These survival figures were significantly lower than in patients with nonsquamous carcinomas and similar stage at diagnosis.

Some older studies suggested that the prognosis of patients with mammary SQC did not differ appreciably from that of patients with mammary adenocarcinoma of equal stage.[48,52] However, current data suggest that pure SQC has a lower recurrence-free survival (RFS) and worse prognosis than stage-matched invasive ductal carcinoma of no special type. Visceral metastases involving the lungs and/or liver were present in 6%[37] to 10%[59] of patients with mammary SQC at two institutions.

Nearly 40% of 31 patients with pure mammary SQC in a series from the M.D. Anderson Cancer Center experienced a locoregional recurrence that involved the ipsilateral breast in 4/12 (33%) patients, the chest in 6/12 (50%), and the ipsilateral axilla and contralateral supraclavicular fossa, respectively, in 1 case each (8%).[37] The median RFS was 20 months (range 1 to 108 months), and only 26% of patients had not experienced recurrent disease 5 years after the initial diagnosis. After a median follow-up of 50 months, 22/31 (71%) patients with initially localized disease had developed either recurrent or metastatic carcinoma. The median survival time was 37 months (range 12 to 108 months), with 40% of patients

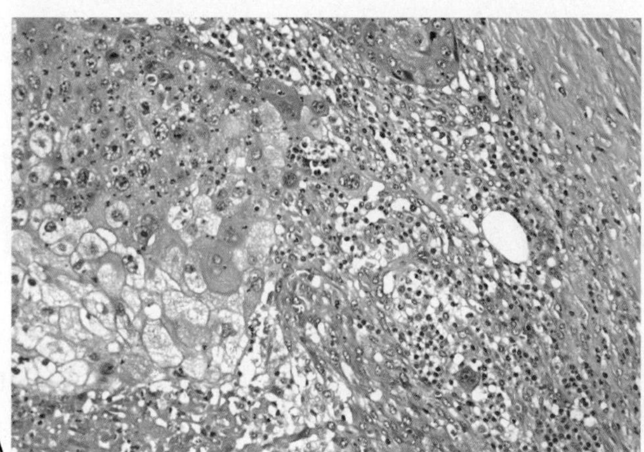

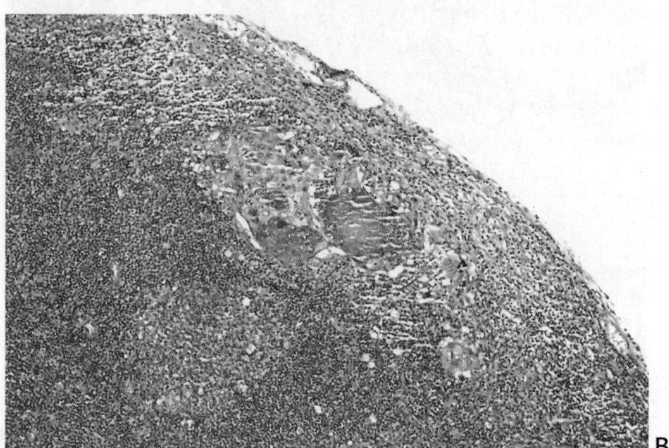

FIG. 17.16. ***Metastatic squamous carcinoma.*** **A:** Invasive carcinoma with high nuclear grade and necrosis. **B:** Metastatic carcinoma from the tumor in (A) involves an ALN.

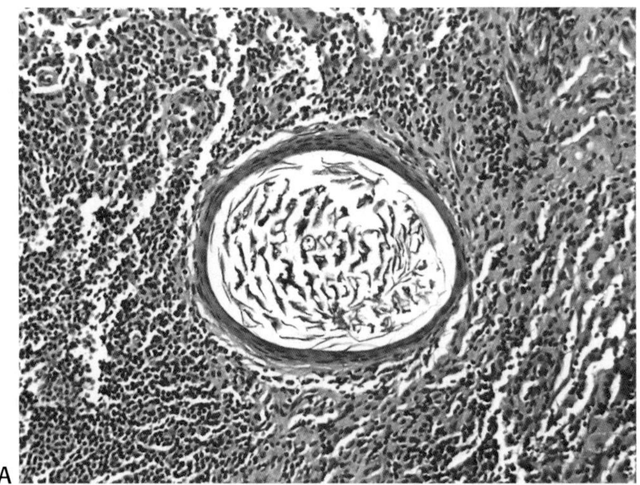

A

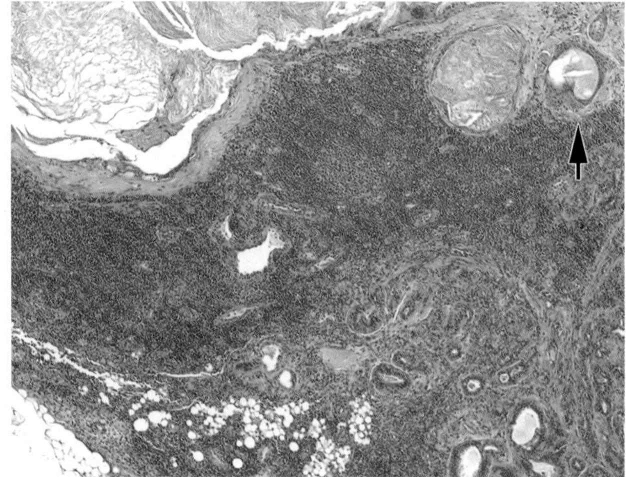

B

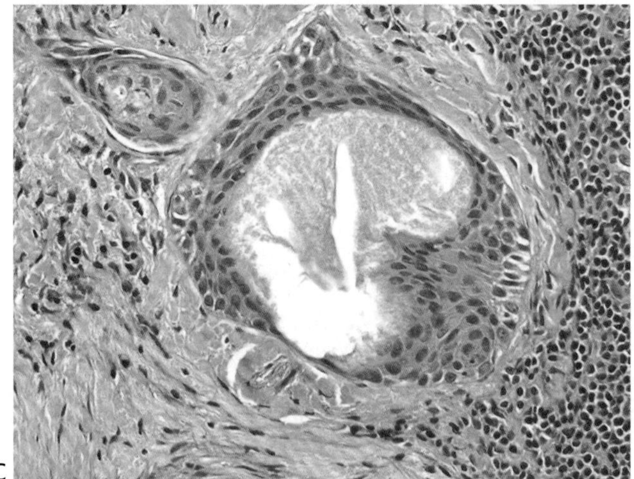

C

FIG. 17.17. ***Benign squamous structures in lymph nodes.*** **A:** A benign squamous cyst is present in a lymph node. **B:** The ectopic breast parenchyma in this lymph node shows focal squamous metaplasia (*arrow*). A collection of foamy histiocytes indicative of silicone adenopathy is also evident near the *lower edge* of the picture. **C:** Magnified view of the mammary cyst with squamous metaplasia in **(B)**.

alive at 5 years and projected 10-year overall survival (OS) rate of 26%. Higher stage at initial diagnosis was associated with worse OS, but the study found no association with age at diagnosis, race, and type of initial surgery.[37] In other studies, the 5-year survival rate for SQC was 63%[67] and 52%.[39] Yamaguchi et al.[68] reported that 8/22 (36%) of patients with pure SQC developed distant metastases. Metastatic site include the lungs, liver, adrenal glands, uterus, and skin.[40]

In a series of 20 patients with stage I to III was predictive of an increased 5-year OS,[40] but the relationship of the growth pattern and degree of differentiation in SQC to prognosis is uncertain. Although some fatal lesions have had a prominent spindle cell component or necrosis and acantholytic features,[54] metastases occur also in the absence of these features.

REFERENCES

1. Troell A. Zwei Falle von Palttenepithelcarcinom. *Nord Med Ark* 1908;1:1–11.
2. Harrington S, Miller J. Intramammary squamous-cell carcinoma. *Mayo Clin Proc* 1939;14:484–487.
3. Dalla Palma P, Parenti A. Squamous breast cancer: report of two cases and review of the literature. *Appl Pathol* 1983;1:14–24.
4. Hayes MM, Peterse JL, Yavuz E, et al. Squamous cell carcinoma *in situ* of the breast: a light microscopic and immunohistochemical study of a previously undescribed lesion. *Am J Surg Pathol* 2007;31:1414–1419.
5. Kokufu II, Yamamoto M, Fukuda K, et al. Squamous cell carcinoma of the breast: three case reports. *Breast Cancer* 1999;6:63–68.
6. Kwak JY, Park HL, Kim JY, et al. Imaging findings in a case of epidermal inclusion cyst arising within the breast parenchyma. *J Clin Ultrasound* 2004;32:141–143.
7. Soderstrom KO, Toikkanen S. Extensive squamous metaplasia simulating squamous cell carcinoma in benign breast papillomatosis. *Hum Pathol* 1983;14:1081–1082.
8. Reddick RL, Jennette JC, Askin FB. Squamous metaplasia of the breast. An ultrastructural and immunologic evaluation. *Am J Clin Pathol* 1985;84:530–533.
9. Salm R. Epidermoid metaplasia in mammary fibro-adenoma with formation of keratin cysts. *J Pathol Bacteriol* 1957;74:221–223.
10. Devi PM, Singh LR, Gatphoh ED. Fibroadenoma with squamous metaplasia. *Singapore Med J* 2007;48:682–683.
11. Gottfried MR. Extensive squamous metaplasia in gynecomastia. *Arch Pathol Lab Med* 1986;110:971–973.
12. Hurt MA, Diaz-Arias AA, Rosenholtz MJ, et al. Posttraumatic lobular squamous metaplasia of breast. An unusual pseudocarcinomatous metaplasia resembling squamous (necrotizing) sialometaplasia of the salivary gland. *Mod Pathol* 1988;1:385–390.
13. Lucey JJ. Spontaneous infarction of the breast. *J Clin Pathol* 1975;28:937–943.
14. Flint A, Oberman HA. Infarction and squamous metaplasia of intraductal papilloma: a benign breast lesion that may simulate carcinoma. *Hum Pathol* 1984;15:764–767.

15. Saad RS, Silverman JF, Julian T, et al. Atypical squamous metaplasia of seromas in breast needle aspirates from irradiated lumpectomy sites: a potential pitfall for false-positive diagnoses of carcinoma. *Diagn Cytopathol* 2002;26:104–108.
16. Shousha S. An unusual breast cyst. *Histopathology* 1989;14:423–425.
17. Davies JD, Nonni A, D'Costa HF. Mammary epidermoid inclusion cysts after wide-core needle biopsies. *Histopathology* 1997;31:549–551.
18. Habif DV, Perzin KH, Lipton R, et al. Subareolar abscess associated with squamous metaplasia of lactiferous ducts. *Am J Surg* 1970;119:523–526.
19. Van Bogaert L. Squamous metaplasia in human mammary epithelium in long-term organ culture. *Experientia (Basel)* 1977;33:1450–1451.
20. Elias JJ, Armstrong RC. Brief communication: hyperplastic and metaplastic responses of human mammary fibroadenomas and dysplasias in organ culture. *J Natl Cancer Inst* 1973;51:1341–1343.
21. Tonelli QJ, Custer RP, Sorof S. Transformation of cultured mouse mammary glands by aromatic amines and amides and their derivatives. *Cancer Res* 1979;39:1784–1792.
22. Lasnitzki I. Precancerous changes induced by 20-methylcholanthrene in mouse prostates grown *in vitro*. *Br J Cancer* 1951;5:345–352.
23. Schaefer FV, Custer RP, Sorof S. Squamous metaplasia in human breast culture: induction by cyclic adenine nucleotide and prostaglandins, and influence of menstrual cycle. *Cancer Res* 1983;43:279–286.
24. Cappellani A, Di Vita M, Zanghi A, et al. A pure primary squamous cell breast carcinoma presenting as a breast abscess: case report and review of literature. *Ann Ital Chir* 2004;75:259–262; discussion 262–253.
25. Comellas N, Marin Gutzke M. Primary pure squamous cell carcinoma of the breast presenting as a breast abscess. *J Plast Reconstr Aesthet Surg* 2009;62:e178–e179.
26. Damin AP, Nascimento FC, Andreola JB, et al. Primary epidermoid carcinoma of the breast presenting as a breast abscess and sepsis. *Sao Paulo Med J* 2011;129:424–427.
27. Gupta S, Usha O. Primary squamous cell carcinoma of the breast arising within an abscess. *J Indian Med Assoc* 1982;79:12–13.
28. Gupta C, Malani AK. Abscess as initial presentation of pure primary squamous cell carcinoma of the breast. *Clin Breast Cancer* 2006;7:180.
29. Melamed JB, Schein M, Decker GA. Squamous carcinoma of the breast presenting as an abscess. A case report. *S Afr Med J* 1986;69:771–772.
30. Nair VJ, Kaushal V, Atri R. Pure squamous cell carcinoma of the breast presenting as a pyogenic abscess: a case report. *Clin Breast Cancer* 2007;7:713–715.
31. Tan YM, Yeo A, Chia KH, et al. Breast abscess as the initial presentation of squamous cell carcinoma of the breast. *Eur J Surg Oncol* 2002;28:91–93.
32. Wong C, Wright C, Colclough A, et al. Case report: metaplastic carcinoma presenting as a breast abscess. *Int Semin Surg Oncol* 2006;3:23.
33. Wrightson WR, Edwards MJ, McMasters KM. Primary squamous cell carcinoma of the breast presenting as a breast abscess. *Am Surg* 1999;65:1153–1155.
34. Behranwala KA, Nasiri N, Abdullah N, et al. Squamous cell carcinoma of the breast: clinico-pathologic implications and outcome. *Eur J Surg Oncol* 2003;29:386–389.
35. Uzoaru I, Adeyanju M, Ray VH, et al. Primary squamous cell carcinoma of the breast presenting as a nipple discharge. *Acta Cytol* 1994;38:112–113.
36. Grabowski J, Saltzstein SL, Sadler G, et al. Squamous cell carcinoma of the breast: a review of 177 cases. *Am Surg* 2009;75:914–917.
37. Hennessy BT, Krishnamurthy S, Giordano S, et al. Squamous cell carcinoma of the breast. *J Clin Oncol* 2005;23:7827–7835.
38. Honda M, Saji S, Horiguchi S, et al. Clinicopathological analysis of ten patients with metaplastic squamous cell carcinoma of the breast. *Surg Today* 2011;41:328–332.
39. Grenier J, Soria JC, Mathieu MC, et al. Differential immunohistochemical and biological profile of squamous cell carcinoma of the breast. *Anticancer Res* 2007;27:547–555.
40. Nayak A, Wu Y, Gilcrease MZ. Primary squamous cell carcinoma of the breast: predictors of locoregional recurrence and overall survival. *Am J Surg Pathol* 2013;37:867–873.
41. Shousha S, James AH, Fernandez MD, et al. Squamous cell carcinoma of the breast. *Arch Pathol Lab Med* 1984;108:893–896.
42. Cardoso F, Leal C, Meira A, et al. Squamous cell carcinoma of the breast. *Breast* 2000;9:315–319.
43. Park KC, Ju DU, Heo SW, et al. [A case of squamous cell carcinoma of the breast in a patient with Crohn's disease taking azathioprine]. *Korean J Gastroenterol* 2012;60:373–376.
44. Cornog JL, Mobini J, Steiger E, et al. Squamous carcinoma of the breast. *Am J Clin Pathol* 1971;55:410–417.
45. Tashjian J, Kuni CC, Bohn LE. Primary squamous cell carcinoma of the breast: mammographic findings. *Can Assoc Radiol J* 1989;40: 228–229.
46. Samuels TH, Miller NA, Manchul LA, et al. Squamous cell carcinoma of the breast. *Can Assoc Radiol J* 1996;47:177–182.
47. Dash N, Sharma P, Lupetin AR, et al. Magnetic resonance imaging appearance of primary squamous cell carcinoma of the breast. *J Comput Tomogr* 1987;11:359–363.
48. Eggers JW, Chesney TM. Squamous cell carcinoma of the breast: a clinicopathologic analysis of eight cases and review of the literature. *Hum Pathol* 1984;15:526–531.
49. Chen KT. Fine needle aspiration cytology of squamous cell carcinoma of the breast. *Acta Cytol* 1990;34:664–668.
50. Leiman G. Squamous carcinoma of the breast: diagnosis by aspiration cytology. *Acta Cytol* 1982;26:201–209.
51. Farrand R, Lavigne R, Lokich J, et al. Epidermoid carcinoma of the breast. *J Surg Oncol* 1979;12:207–211.
52. DeLair DF, Corben AD, Catalano JP, et al. Non-mammary metastases to the breast and axilla: a study of 85 cases. *Mod Pathol* 2013;26:343–349.
53. Toikkanen S. Primary squamous cell carcinoma of the breast. *Cancer* 1981;48:1629–1632.
54. Eusebi V, Lamovec J, Cattani MG, et al. Acantholytic variant of squamous-cell carcinoma of the breast. *Am J Surg Pathol* 1986;10:855–861.
55. Sugie T, Takeuchi E, Kunishima F, et al. A case of ductal carcinoma with squamous differentiation in malignant phyllodes tumor. *Breast Cancer* 2007;14:327–332.
56. Lazarevic B, Katatikarn V, Marks RA. Primary squamous-cell carcinoma of the breast. Diagnosis by fine needle aspiration cytology. *Acta Cytol* 1984;28:321–324.
57. Motoyama T, Watanabe H. Extremely well differentiated squamous cell carcinoma of the breast. Report of a case with a comparative study of an epidermal cyst. *Acta Cytol* 1996;40:729–733.
58. Bishop JA, Teruya-Feldstein J, Westra WH, et al. p40 (DeltaNp63) is superior to p63 for the diagnosis of pulmonary squamous cell carcinoma. *Mod Pathol* 2012;25:405–415.
59. Bossuyt V, Fadare O, Martel M, et al. Remarkably high frequency of EGFR expression in breast carcinomas with squamous differentiation. *Int J Surg Pathol* 2005;13:319–327.
60. Stevenson JT, Graham DJ, Khiyami A, et al. Squamous cell carcinoma of the breast: a clinical approach. *Ann Surg Oncol* 1996;3:367–374.
61. Gwin K, Lezon-Geyda K, Harris L, et al. Chromosome 7 aneusomy in metaplastic breast carcinomas with chondroid, squamous, and spindle-cell differentiation. *Int J Surg Pathol* 2011;19:20–25.
62. Reis-Filho JS, Pinheiro C, Lambros MB, et al. EGFR amplification and lack of activating mutations in metaplastic breast carcinomas. *J Pathol* 2006;209:445–453.
63. Kimura F, Iwaya K, Kawaguchi T, et al. Epidermal growth factor-dependent enhancement of invasiveness of squamous cell carcinoma of the breast. *Cancer Sci* 2010;101:1133–1140.
64. Simoes PW, Medeiros LR, Simoes Pires PD, et al. Prevalence of human papillomavirus in breast cancer: a systematic review. *Int J Gynecol Cancer* 2012;22:343–347.
65. Tsung SH. Primary pure squamous cell carcinoma of the breast might be sensitive to Cisplatin-based chemotherapy. *Case Rep Oncol* 2012;5:561–565.
66. Murialdo R, Boy D, Musizzano Y, et al. Squamous cell carcinoma of the breast: a case report. *Cases J* 2009;2:7336.
67. Wargotz ES, Norris HJ. Metaplastic carcinomas of the breast. IV. Squamous cell carcinoma of ductal origin. *Cancer* 1990;65:272–276.
68. Yamaguchi R, Horii R, Maeda I, et al. Clinicopathologic study of 53 metaplastic breast carcinomas: their elements and prognostic implications. *Hum Pathol* 2010;41:679–685.

CHAPTER 18

Mucinous Carcinoma

ADRIANA D. CORBEN • EDI BROGI

Mucinous carcinoma is characterized by abundant production of extracellular mucin with admixed clusters of tumor cells. Other terms used to identify this tumor include gelatinous, colloid, mucous, and mucoid carcinoma.

The specific histologic appearance of mucinous carcinoma has been appreciated for more than 150 years.[1–3] Some of the earliest descriptions commented on the slow growth rate and favorable prognosis of these tumors. The importance of distinguishing between pure mucinous tumors and those with a nonmucinous component was emphasized by Geschickter[4] in 1938. He noted that prognosis varied "with the amount of mucoid substance found" in the tumor. Various criteria have been used to distinguish mucinous carcinoma from infiltrating duct carcinoma with mucinous differentiation. Pure mucinous carcinomas have been described as tumors that have no nonmucinous infiltrating duct carcinoma,[5] tumors which were "virtually pure,"[6] tumors with at least 50% growing in a mucinous pattern,[7] tumors in which extracellular mucin constituted at least 33% of the lesion,[8] and tumors with at least 90% mucinous component.[9] One author indicated that "these proportions were arbitrarily selected."[8] At present, the designation of pure mucinous carcinoma is best applied to tumors with at least a 90% mucinous component. The term "mixed mucinous carcinoma" should be used for tumors in which the mucinous component represents between 50% and 90% of the lesion. Invasive duct carcinomas with less than 50% mucinous component are best referred to as having focal mucinous differentiation. It is important that carcinomas with mixed histologic patterns be distinguished from pure mucinous carcinomas. Even though recent genetic evidence (discussed later in this chapter) shows that mixed mucinous carcinomas are closely related to pure mucinous carcinomas, mixed mucinous tumors are still best managed as infiltrating duct carcinomas not otherwise specified (NOS).

CLINICAL PRESENTATION

Incidence

When the diagnosis of mucinous carcinoma is restricted to tumors consisting of pure or nearly pure mucinous carcinoma, their incidence ranges from 1% to 2% of all breast carcinomas in most series.[8,10–16] Interestingly, mucinous carcinomas constituted 5.2% of breast carcinomas treated at one center in Tanzania.[17]

Focal mucinous differentiation may be found in up to 2% of other carcinomas. If this latter group is considered, the reported frequency of tumors with some degree of mucinous differentiation may be as high as 3.6%.[14,18]

Age

Mucinous carcinoma occurs throughout most of the age range of breast carcinoma. Most studies have reported the mean age of women with mucinous carcinoma to be older than that of patients with nonmucinous tumors.[11,14,15,19–23] Di Saverio et al.[21] evaluated Surveillance Epidemiology and End Results (SEER) data for 11,422 patients with pure mucinous carcinomas. The median and the mean age at diagnosis were 71 and 68.3 years (range 25 to 85), respectively, both significantly greater than for patients with invasive ductal carcinoma NOS (median and mean age, 61 years) ($p < 0.01$). Most patients with mucinous carcinoma (66.3%) were 65 years or older, 15.5% were between 55 and 65 years old, and 18.2% under age 55 years. In the Netherland Cancer Registry study,[11] the age of patients with mucinous carcinoma was 70 years or greater in 2,053/3,482 (59%) cases, and between 50 and 69 years in 971/3,482 (28%) cases. Only 458/3,482 (13%) patients were younger than 50 years old. Komenaka et al.[9] identified 65 patients (0.8%) with pure mucinous carcinoma among 7,676 women with breast carcinoma treated at a single institution. The age range at diagnosis was 13 to 93 years (mean, 67 years), and 85% of the patients were postmenopausal. Scopsi et al.[14] reported that a significantly greater proportion of women with mucinous carcinoma were older than 50 years than was the case among patients with carcinoma having focal mucinous differentiation or nonmucinous carcinoma. Analysis of patients at the extremes of the age distribution for breast carcinoma revealed a striking difference because mucinous carcinoma constituted about 7% of carcinomas in women 75 years or older and only 1% among those younger than 35 years.[24] No significant difference in the age distribution and median age of women with pure and mixed mucinous carcinoma has been found in a few studies,[25–27] but in a series by Paramo et al.[23] the mean age of patients with pure mucinous carcinoma was 75 years (range 59 to 90), whereas the mean age of patients with mixed mucinous carcinoma was 65 years (range 35 to 89). This difference was reported to be statistically significant ($p = 0.02$).

Compared with series of mucinous carcinoma in Western countries, a series from Tanzania[17] and two from South Korea[27,28] have reported relatively younger mean age at diagnosis of mucinous carcinoma than for nonmucinous tumors, namely age 55 years for Tanzanian women and 44[27] and 45[28] years for Korean women.

As might be expected from the age distribution, most patients in the United States with mucinous carcinoma are postmenopausal.[10,29] Two studies[29,30] found that about 78% of postmenopausal patients with mucinous carcinoma never used hormone replacement therapy, and less than 30% reported using hormone replacement therapy prior to or at diagnosis. A decreased incidence of mucinous carcinoma was observed in women taking combined estrogen and progesterone replacement therapy,[31] but there was no change in the incidence in women taking only estrogen-based replacement therapy. Work et al.[30] documented an inverse association of mucinous carcinoma with the use of oral contraceptives, late age of menarche, and parity, but a positive association with late age at first birth.

Inflammation in the adipose tissue of women with high body mass index (BMI) has been linked to increased aromatase levels that may play a role in the pathogenesis of breast carcinoma.[32] In one study,[29] 46.4% of women with mucinous carcinoma had a BMI greater than 26.6 kg/m^2 versus 33.4% of women with invasive ductal carcinoma NOS, but the authors did not evaluate whether this result was significantly associated with mucinous carcinoma. Li et al.[33] found no correlation between BMI and mucinous carcinoma, but they reported that height greater than 160 cm correlated with 2.5-fold increase in the relative risk (RR) of developing this tumor. In a Korean series,[27] a family history of breast carcinoma was reported in 9% of patients with pure mucinous carcinoma and 6.1% of patients with mixed mucinous carcinoma. Another study[33] found no association between mucinous carcinoma and having a first degree relative with breast carcinoma. No association of mucinous carcinoma and *BRCA1* germline mutation has been documented.[30] Lacroix-Triki et al.[34] found no evidence of microsatellite instability (MSI) that is associated with Lynch syndrome in mammary mucinous carcinomas.

Ethnicity

Mucinous carcinoma is most frequent among Caucasian women.[12,21,30,35] An analysis of 1973 to 2002 SEER data by Di Saverio et al.[21] found that 85.2% women with mucinous carcinoma were White, 7% were African American, and 7.8% of other or unknown ethnicity. A subsequent analysis of 1992 to 2007 SEER data by Li et al.[12] documented that 78.5% of women with mucinous carcinoma were non-Hispanic Whites, 7.1% African Americans, 9.1% Asian/Pacific Islanders, 4.1% Hispanic Whites, 0.7% American Indian/Alaska Native, and 0.4% of other ethnicity. Similar percentages were reported by Barkley et al.[35] In a population-based study[30] with data from California (United States), Ontario (Canada), and Melbourne (Australia), 54% of mucinous carcinomas occurred in Whites, 11% in Blacks, 11% in Hispanics, 19% in Asians, and 4% in other ethnic groups.

Mucinous carcinoma can also occur in men. Based on SEER data, the incidence of mucinous carcinoma in men was 0.5% between 1973 and 2002,[21] but rose to 2% between 1985 and 2000.[36] Burga et al.[37] found 21 (2.8%) pure mucinous carcinomas and 26 (3.4%) mixed mucinous carcinomas in a series of 759 primary invasive carcinoma in men.

Clinical Presentation

The initial symptom of a pure mucinous carcinoma usually is a soft breast mass, but, since the introduction of widespread screening mammography, a substantial proportion of patients present with nonpalpable mammographic lesions.[22,38,39] In one study,[29] 44.6% of 56 mucinous carcinomas were self-detected, 37.5% were detected at mammographic screening, and 17.9% were first identified at clinical examination. In another series,[40] a palpable mass was the presenting symptom in 87% cases. Nipple discharge,[22,40] Paget disease,[41] and pain are uncommon. Fixation to the skin and chest wall occurs with large lesions. Palpation reveals a soft to moderately firm lesion. On reviewing patient records one rarely finds the "swish sign" mentioned. About half of mucinous carcinomas occur in the upper outer quadrant, and the other half is distributed in the remaining quadrants,[21] with anatomic distribution not significantly different from that of other types of breast carcinoma. Mucinous carcinoma can arise in ectopic breast tissue at superficial sites such as the axilla or vulva that might be subject to needle biopsy.[42,43] The differential diagnosis in these unusual locations will involve metastatic carcinoma from an extrinsic primary or mucinous carcinoma arising from sweat glands. It is necessary to document the presence of benign mammary glands to consider a diagnosis of mucinous carcinoma originating in ectopic breast tissue. The presence of ductal carcinoma *in situ* (DCIS) in this tissue will firmly establish the diagnosis of primary mucinous carcinoma in an ectopic site.

Imaging

Tumors with a high proportion of mucin production tend to be mammographically (Fig. 18.1A) and sonographically (Fig. 18.1B) lobulated or circumscribed.[39,44–47] These lesions are likely to have a slow growth rate, determined by comparing serial mammograms and also low frequency of axillary nodal metastases. Only 37.5% of mucinous carcinomas in one series[29] were first detected at mammographic screening. In another study,[28] the sensitivity of mammogram for the detection of pure mucinous carcinoma was only 76.5% versus 100% for mixed mucinous carcinomas. In the series by Li et al.,[12] 31/39 (79.5%) pure mucinous carcinomas and 6/7 (86%) mixed mucinous carcinoma formed mammographically detected masses that were circumscribed and indistinct, respectively, in 36% and 28% of pure mucinous carcinomas, but showed equivalent features only in 14%

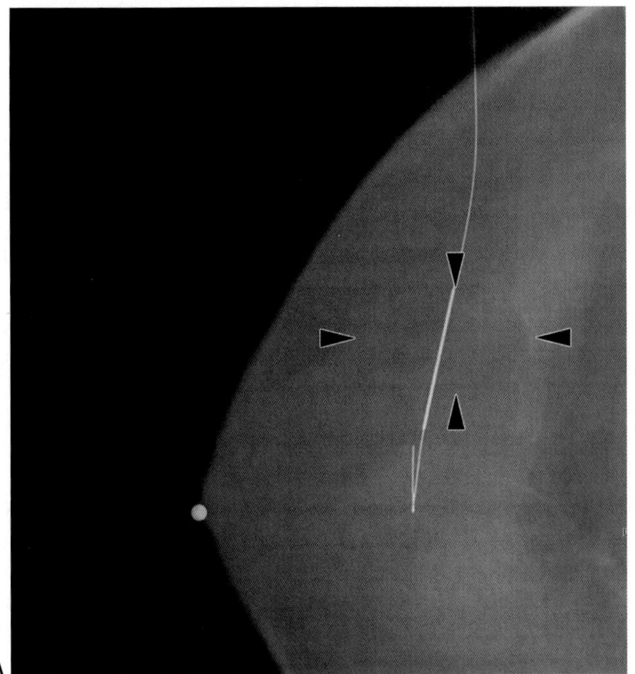

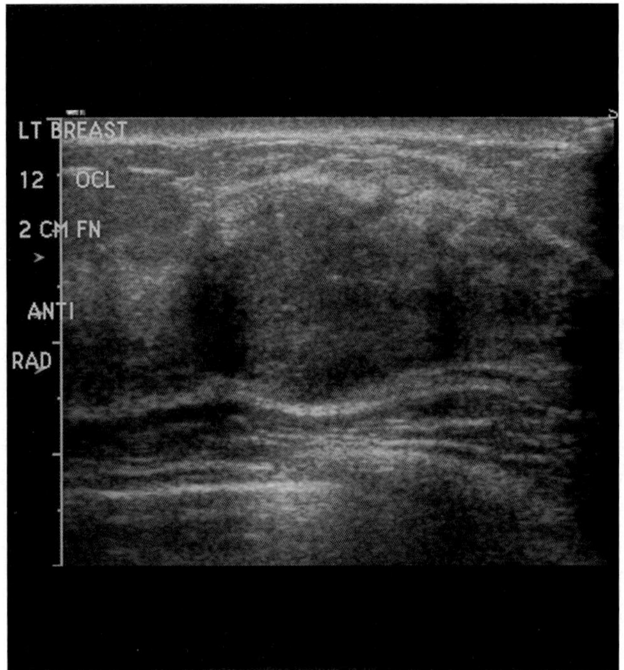

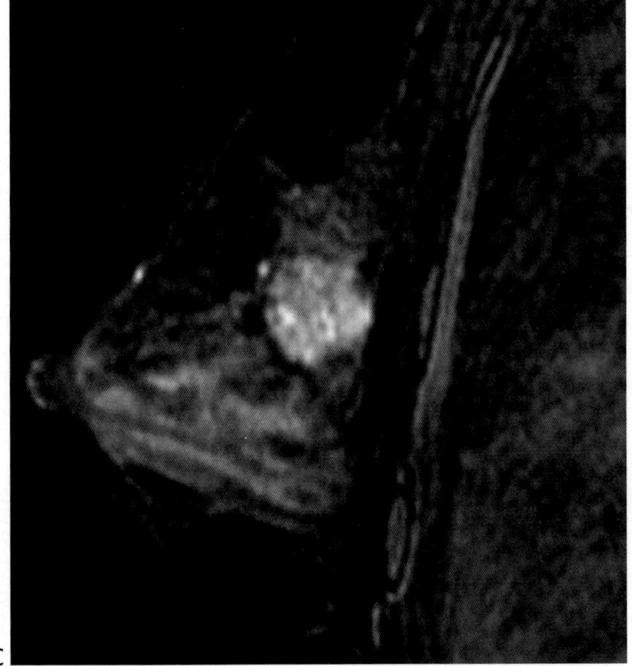

FIG. 18.1. ***Mucinous carcinoma, radiologic appearances.*** **A:** This mammographic image, postneedle localization, shows an irregular and heterogeneous 3 cm solid mass (*arrows*). The mass is localized by the thick portion of the wire. **B:** The sonographic image reveals an oval-shaped hypoechoic solid 1.5 cm mass with irregular borders. **C:** An MRI sagittal fat-suppressed T2-weighted image shows a lobulated T2-hyperintense rim-enhancing 2.3-cm mass. The surrounding breast is dense with moderate background enhancement.

of mixed mucinous tumors. Two pure mucinous and one mixed mucinous carcinoma were mammographically occult. Mixed mucinous carcinomas typically have irregular margins mammographically because of fibrosis and an infiltrative growth pattern.[48] A spiculated contour is associated with a lesser mucinous component and a higher frequency of lymph node metastases. Mammographically detected calcifications can occur in up to 40% of the tumors and involve the invasive portion of mucinous carcinomas in approximately 20% of cases.[22,40,46–49] Calcifications constituted the only mammographic evidence of a pure mucinous carcinoma in only a handful of cases,[40,45,50] and may be limited to associated DCIS or to a concurrent mucocele-like lesion (MLL).[51]

On ultrasound examination (Fig. 18.1B) mucinous carcinoma is isoechogenic to the breast fat,[52] and may be difficult to detect. In one study,[28] the sensitivity of ultrasound for the detection of pure mucinous carcinoma was 94.7%, whereas it was 100% for mixed mucinous carcinomas. In a series by Dhillon et al.,[47] 11/28 (39%) mammographically evident pure mucinous carcinomas were not seen on ultrasound. The tumor size ranged from 5 to 20 mm, with an average of 11 mm. A total of 13/34 (38%) pure mucinous carcinomas were not recognized as abnormal when first encountered in a mammogram or at ultrasound examination, with a consequent delay in diagnosis. The authors, however, specified that the delayed diagnosis did not have clinical impact, as none of the patients had lymph node metastases at the time of surgical excision. On ultrasound, myxoid fibroadenoma and benign cystic lesions, as well as high-grade matrix-producing carcinoma and high-grade carcinoma with central acellular zone, sometimes resemble pure mucinous carcinoma.[53]

In MRI imaging (Fig. 18.1C), pure mucinous carcinoma has a gradually enhancing contrast pattern and very high signal intensity on T2-weighted images.[54,55] In a study by Monzawa et al.,[56] pure mucinous carcinomas and mixed mucinous carcinomas had high signal intensity on T2-weighted images and the pattern of early phase enhancement varied with tumor cellularity and was more gradual in hypocellular tumors. The MRI characteristics of mucinous carcinomas and fibroadenomas are not distinctively different.[57,58]

Symptoms

The average duration of symptoms prior to biopsy and diagnosis tends to be 3 months or less, but some elderly patients who have large lesions may delay seeking treatment for considerably longer.[7] One group of investigators observed that the majority of patients with tumors 4 cm or larger were older than 70 years.[5]

GROSS PATHOLOGY

Size

Mucinous carcinomas can range in size from less than 1 cm to more than 20 cm in diameter. Studies published prior to 1975 stressed the relatively large size of mucinous carcinomas,[7,59,60] but this has not been observed in more recent reports.

In the study by Di Saverio et al.,[21] mucinous carcinoma had a mean size 2.2 cm and median size 1.6 cm, with 83.2% of tumors measuring 3.0 cm or less. The size of the mucinous carcinoma was significantly smaller than the size of invasive ductal carcinoma NOS in the same period, and the same trend applied to nodal involvement.

Mucinous carcinomas were slightly smaller than invasive ductal carcinomas also in a study by Cao et al.[22] Over half (56%) of the tumors measured 2 cm or less, 37.5% measured between 2 and 5 cm, and 4.9% were larger than 5 cm. The average size of mucinous carcinoma was 1.6 cm (range 0.1 to 6.0) in the series by Barkely et al.,[35] and larger tumor size significantly correlated with lymph node involvement. The average size of pure mucinous carcinomas with no lymph node metastases was 1.5 cm versus 2.6 cm for tumors with nodal involvement. In the series by Bae et al.,[27] pure mucinous carcinomas were T1 tumors in 55.6% of cases, T2 in 41.1%, T3 in 2.8%, and T4 in 0.5% of cases, compared with 45.3% T1, 47.2% T2, and 7.5% T3 mixed mucinous carcinomas.

A nationwide study of Danish patients with breast carcinoma found that only 16% of mucinous carcinomas were larger than 5 cm.[8] In a series from Finland, a greater proportion of mixed (48%) than of pure (22%) mucinous carcinomas was larger than 5 cm,[15] and a study from Japan stated that 53.6% of mucinous tumors measured 2.0 cm or less (T1) and 37.8% were 2.1 to 5.0 cm (T2).[18] Fentiman et al.[25] reported that pure mucinous tumors were significantly smaller (mean, 2.17 cm) than mixed mucinous tumors (mean, 3.25 cm). Ranade et al.[26] also found that the mean tumor size of pure mucinous carcinomas was 1.65 cm and 2.5 cm for mixed mucinous tumors,[26] but Diab et al.[20] did not find a significant difference in size between mucinous and nonmucinous carcinomas.

Out of 19 patients with pure mucinous carcinoma reported by Paramo et al.,[23] 6 (31%) had T1b tumors, 8 (42%) were T1c, 2 (11%) with tumors spanning between 2 and 3 cm, and 3 (16%) had tumors larger than 3 cm. In the group of 41 mixed mucinous carcinomas, 20% were T1b, 42% were T1c, 27% were T2 tumors spanning between 2 and 3 cm, 3 (7%) were T2 tumors larger than 3 cm, and 2 were T3 tumors. The size differences were not statistically significant.

Gross Characteristics

On palpation of the excised tumor, the consistency of mucinous carcinoma varies depending upon the amount of fibrous stroma in the lesion. When stroma is sparse, the tumor feels soft and gelatinous. The cut surface is typically moist and glistening, even in relatively fibrotic tumors (Fig. 18.2). Most mucinous carcinomas have a circumscribed gross margin, which may be accentuated by a peripheral red-to-purple zone of congested parenchyma. Cystic degeneration has been reported in relatively large tumors.

MICROSCOPIC PATHOLOGY

The hallmark of mucinous carcinomas is the accumulation of abundant extracellular mucin around the invasive tumor cells (Fig. 18.3). The relative proportions of mucin and neoplastic epithelium vary from one case to another, but the distribution in any one tumor is fairly constant (Figs. 18.3 and 18.4). Multiple sections may be required to detect carcinoma cells in a tumor composed almost entirely of extracellular mucin (Fig. 18.5). In one study, the proportion of extracellular mucin in tumors classified as pure mucinous carcinomas varied from slightly less than 70% to nearly 100%, with a mean percentage of 83.5 ± 14.3.[18] Infiltrating duct carcinomas with a mucinous component had a lower mean proportion of extracellular mucin (68.3% ± 16.6%), with the distribution ranging from 32% to 97%. In practice, the diagnosis of pure mucinous carcinoma is reserved for tumors in which more of 90% of the invasive component is admixed with stromal mucin. Any tumor with stromal mucin in 50% to 90% of the lesion is best classified as mixed mucinous carcinoma (Figs. 18.6 and 18.7). If stromal mucin

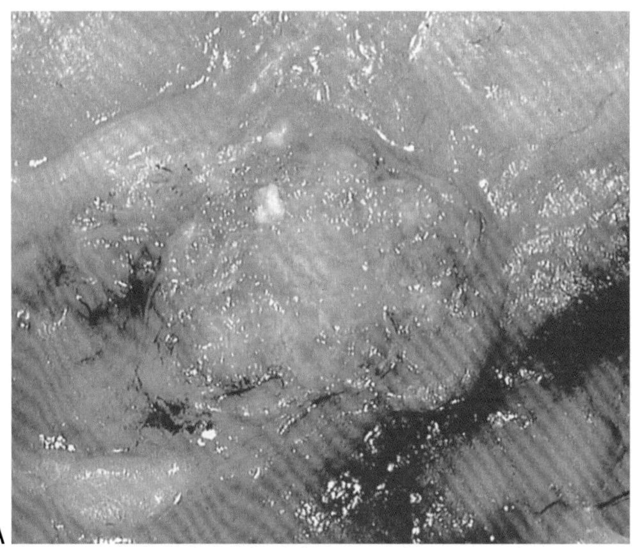

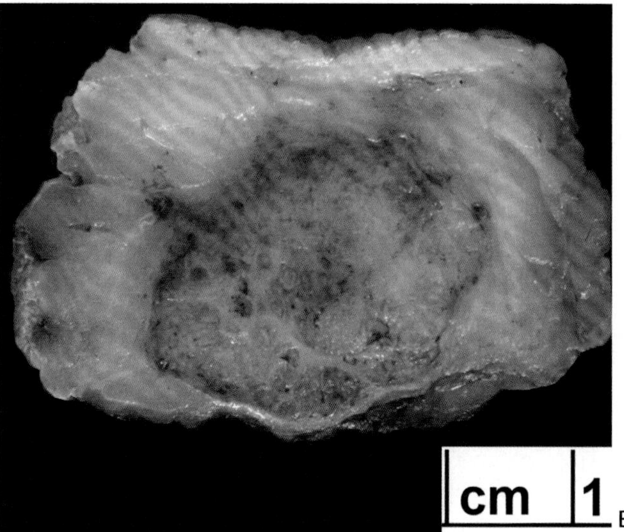

FIG. 18.2. ***Mucinous carcinoma, gross appearance.*** **A:** A homogeneous tumor with a circumscribed lobulated contour. **B:** This 2.5 cm mucinous carcinoma was located just beneath the skin. It formed a discrete nodular mass with a rounded outline. The cut surface is glistening and mucoid, with small focal cysts.

represents less than 50% of the tumor mass, the component should be mentioned in the diagnosis, but no specific designation applies. The abundant extracellular mucin in pure mucinous carcinomas may constitute an obstacle to tumor vascularization, lymphovascular permeation, and lymph node metastasis,[61] and account for the relatively good prognosis of these tumors. The majority of pure mucinous carcinomas are well to moderately differentiated. It is extremely rare for a mucinous carcinoma to have high nuclear grade,[26] and in such cases, this information should be clearly stated and emphasized in the diagnostic report, as the clinical behavior may not be as indolent as for usual pure mucinous carcinomas. In the SEER data–based series (11,422 cases) by Di Saverio et al.,[21] 53% of the tumors were well differentiated, 38% were moderately differentiated, and the remaining 9% were poorly differentiated or anaplastic.

In mucinous carcinomas, the tumor cells are arranged in a variety of patterns (Figs. 18.4 and 18.8). Usually the epithelial pattern duplicates the structure of the associated DCIS. These configurations include tumor cells in strands, alveolar

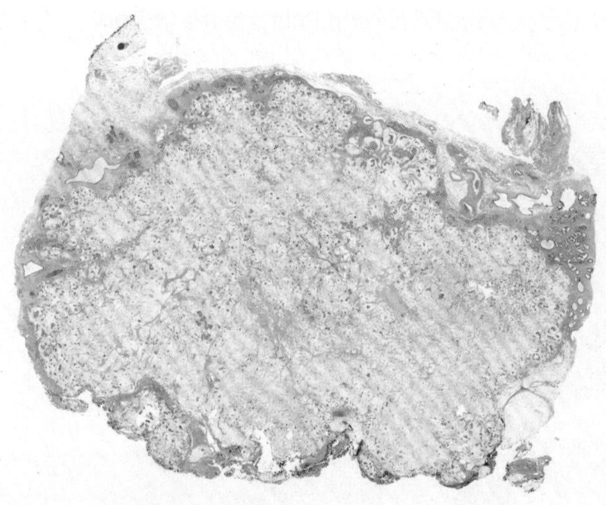

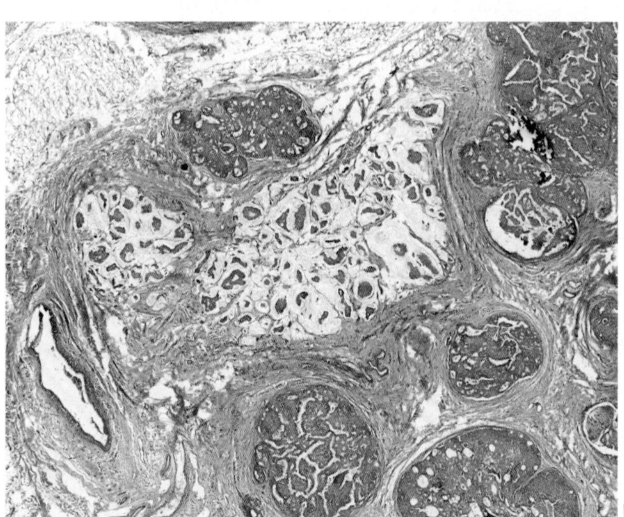

FIG. 18.3. ***Pure mucinous carcinoma.*** **A:** Low-power view of a pure mucinous carcinoma. The carcinoma is relatively hypocellular, and the neoplastic epithelial clusters are admixed with mucin throughout. **B:** This 3 mm pure mucinous carcinoma consists of clusters of neoplastic epithelial cells within mucin pools. Cribriform and papillary DCIS with intermediate nuclear grade and calcifications are present. Note the absence of extracellular mucin in the DCIS.

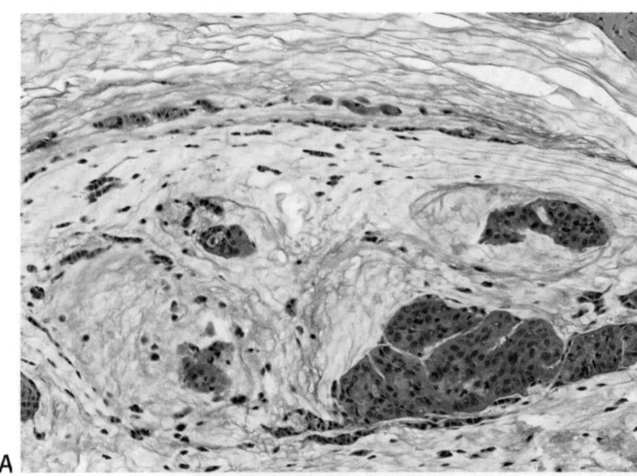

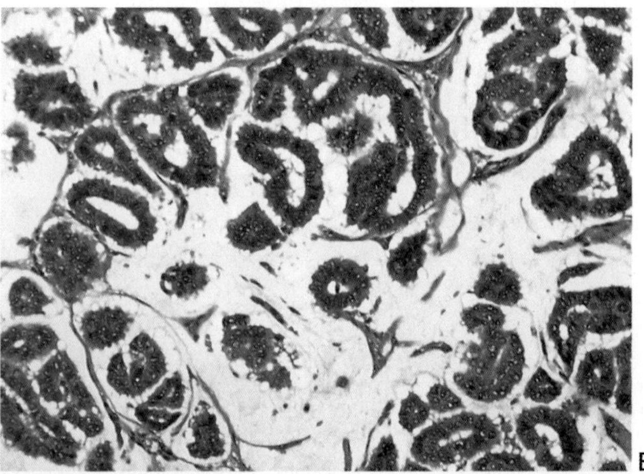

FIG. 18.4. ***Mucinous carcinoma.*** **A:** A moderately cellular carcinoma. Note the presence of capillaries in the mucin. **B:** A very cellular carcinoma with a glandular pattern.

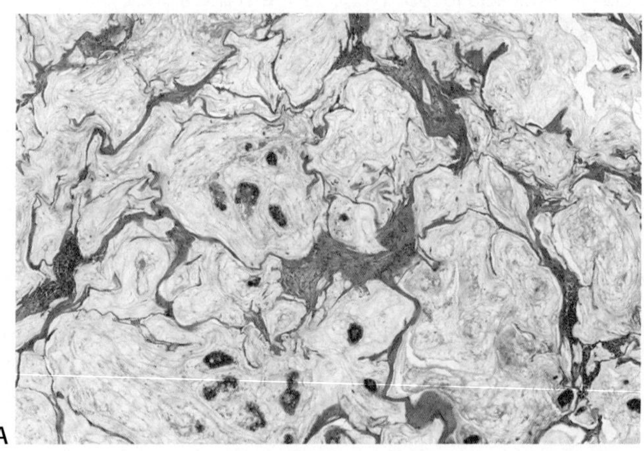

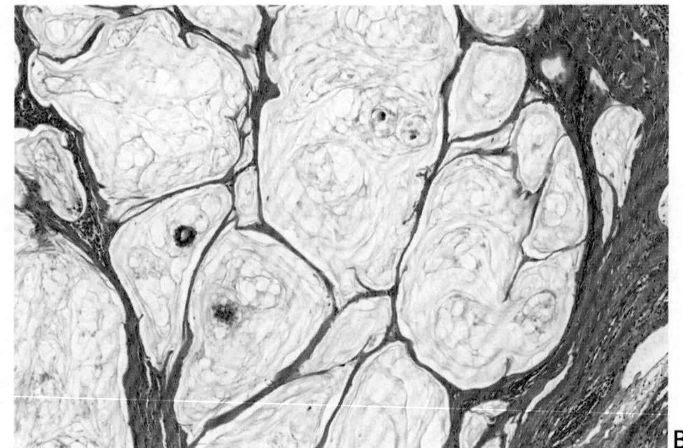

FIG. 18.5. ***Mucinous carcinoma.*** **A:** Part of this carcinoma consists of mucin devoid of neoplastic epithelium. Clusters of carcinoma cells are present in the *central* and *lower* portions of the image. **B:** An instance of virtually acellular mucinous carcinoma with only rare clusters of tumor cells.

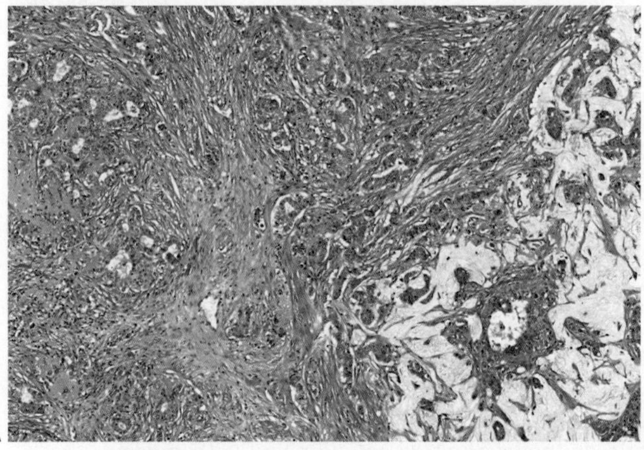

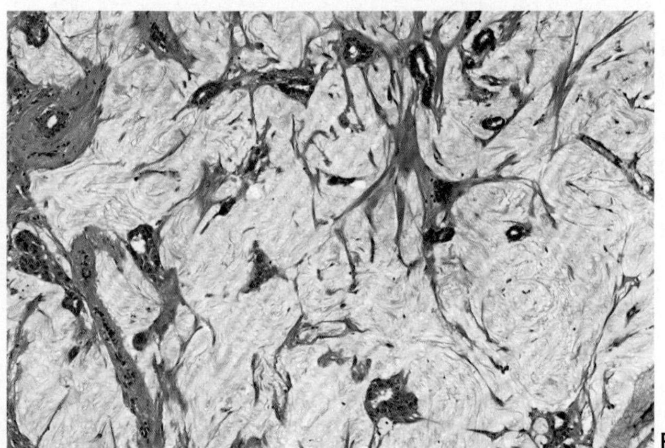

FIG. 18.6. ***Infiltrating ductal carcinoma with mucinous features.*** **A:** Poorly differentiated infiltrating ductal carcinoma (*left*) merging with carcinoma with focal stromal mucin (*right*). **B:** A more conventional focus of mucinous carcinoma in the same tumor.

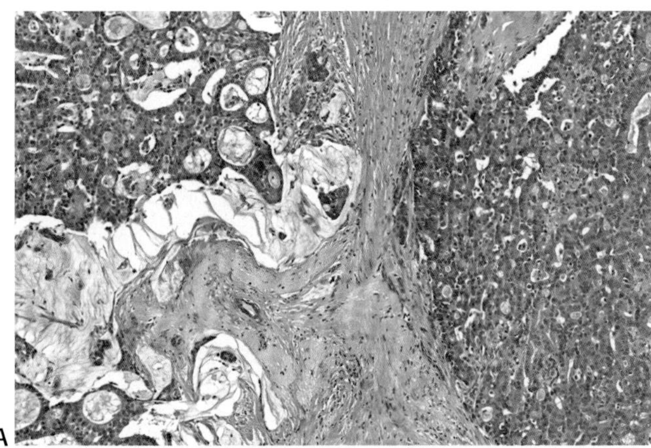

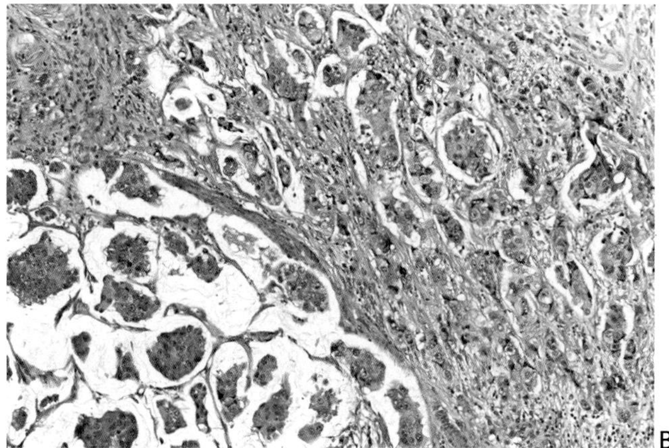

FIG. 18.7. ***Infiltrating ductal carcinoma with mucinous features.*** **A,B:** Two infiltrating ductal carcinomas that have limited, discrete areas of mucinous growth.

nests, and papillary clusters, as well as larger sheets of cells that may have cribriform areas or focal comedonecrosis. Tubule and gland formation are uncommon.

The margin of a mucinous carcinoma is determined by the extent of the mucinous component, even if no epithelial cells are seen in it. The periphery of the tumor is characterized by a pushing border in more than 70% of cases[45] (Figs. 18.3, 18.9, and 18.10). Some of these tumors have irregular or knobby contours formed by protrusions of the neoplasm into the breast parenchyma (Fig. 18.10). When assessing the margins of excision, it is important to look for transected protrusions that may be obscured by cautery artifact or blend with fat. When evaluating the margin status of a surgical specimen from a patient with known mucinous carcinoma, the presence of mucin at ink should be interpreted as tumor at margin, even if the transected mucin is devoid of neoplastic cells, as long as artifactual contamination can be excluded.

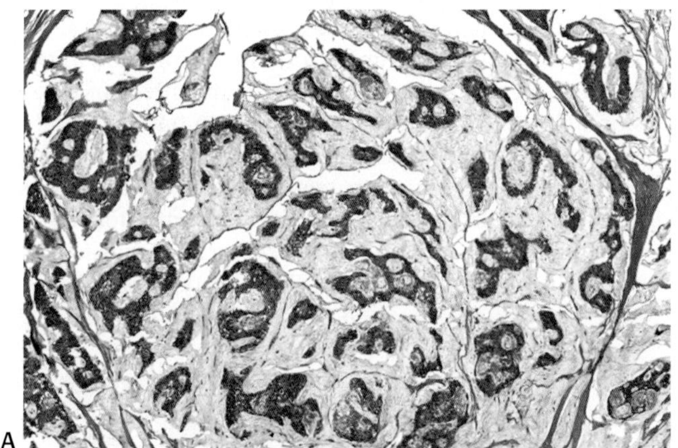

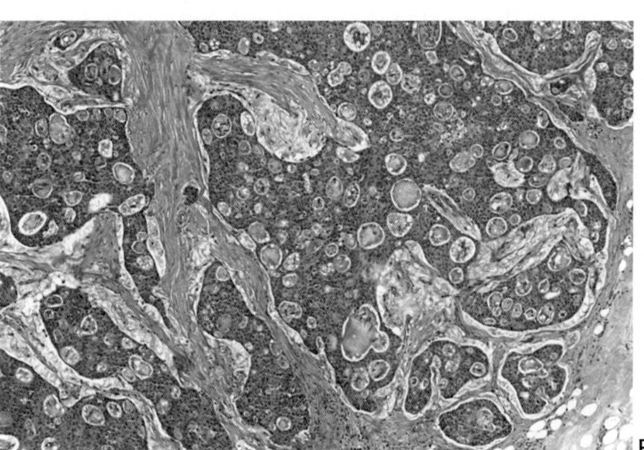

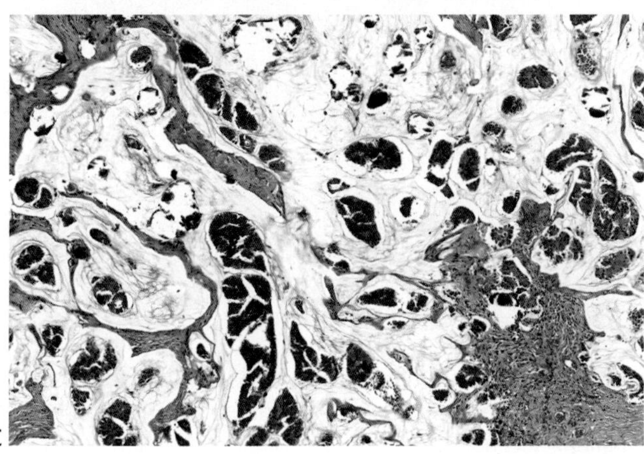

FIG. 18.8. ***Mucinous carcinoma, different patterns.*** **A:** Trabecular and cribriform patterns. **B:** Solid and cribriform patterns. **C:** Papillary mucinous carcinoma with calcifications.

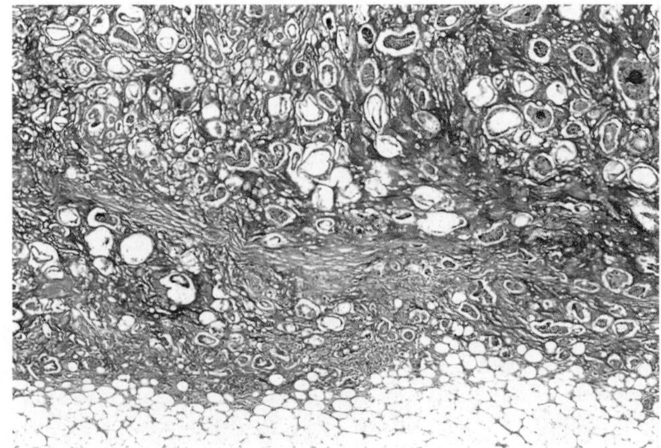

FIG. 18.9. *Mucinous carcinoma.* The mucin stained a rose color has a distinct and pushing border. Clusters of carcinoma cells are present in the mucin (mucicarmine stain).

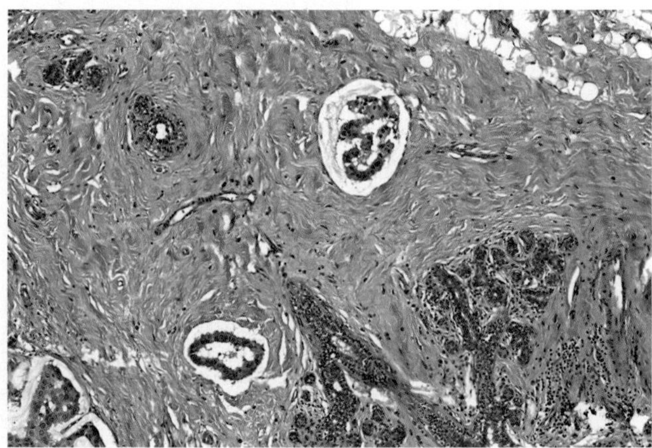

FIG. 18.11. *Mucinous carcinoma.* These discrete, sharply defined foci of invasive mucinous carcinoma resemble tumor in vascular spaces.

It is very difficult to recognize lymphatic tumor emboli in mucinous carcinoma. Clusters of carcinoma cells suspended in mucin often have an appearance that resembles intralymphatic carcinoma (Fig. 18.11). When the diagnosis of such foci is uncertain, a stain for mucin may be helpful, because the material surrounding the carcinoma cells will be clearly stained in mucinous carcinoma but it tends to be weakly reactive in lymphatic tumor emboli. However, this finding is not definitive, as mucin sometimes can be found admixed with clusters of carcinoma within vascular spaces (Fig. 18.12). Immunostains for vascular endothelial markers such as CD31, CD34, factor VIII, and D2-40 may also be helpful.

Among mucinous carcinomas of the breast, calcifications are most often found in tumors with papillary (Fig. 18.8C) or comedo epithelial patterns. The calcifications tend to be coarse and irregular. Mucinous carcinoma with micropapillary morphology often contains psammomatous calcifications.[48,50,62–65]

Type A, Type B, and Type AB Mucinous Carcinomas

Capella et al.[66] presented criteria for the subclassification of mucinous carcinoma on the basis of the epithelial growth pattern and some associated features. They described two principal types (A and B) and an intermediate category (AB). By definition, at least 33% of each tumor consisted of extracellular mucin, but, overall, mucin was more abundant in type A (Fig. 18.13A) than in type B lesions (Fig. 18.13B). Type A tumors had epithelium distributed in "trabeculae and ribbons or festoons." "Clumps" of cells, uncommon in type A tumors, were the characteristic growth pattern of type B lesions. Cribriform areas were seen in both tumor types. Intracytoplasmic mucin was more abundant in type B lesions, and the cells in these tumors tended to have more granular cytoplasm than in type A carcinomas. Cells with "foamy" cytoplasm were detected in a minority of type A tumors and in none of the type B group. Ten of 14 type B tumors contained

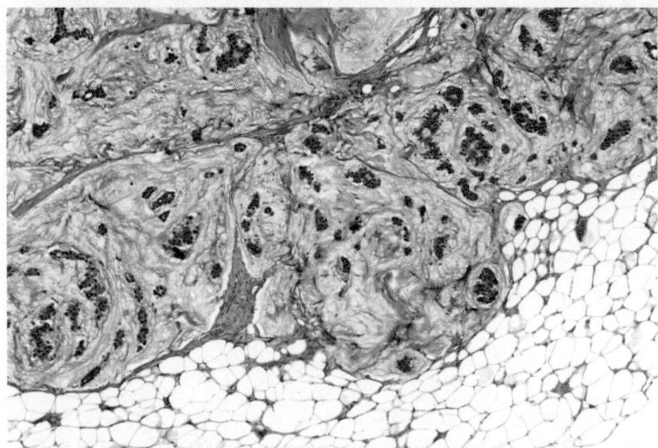

FIG. 18.10. *Mucinous carcinoma.* This is a mucinous carcinoma with peripheral knobby protrusions in the adjacent fatty breast tissue.

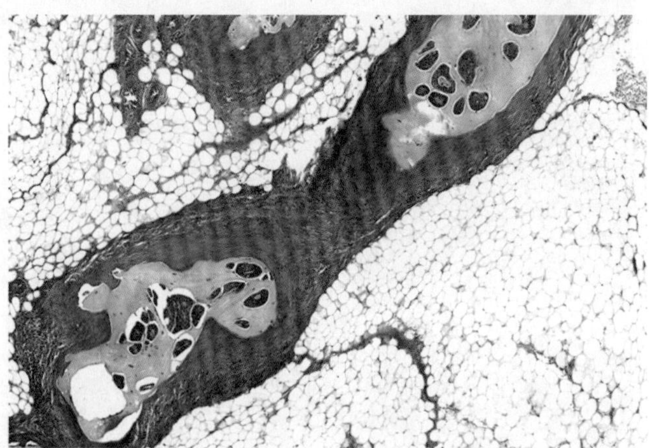

FIG. 18.12. *Mucinous carcinoma in vascular spaces.* Mucin is admixed with tumor emboli in vascular spaces of axillary soft tissue.

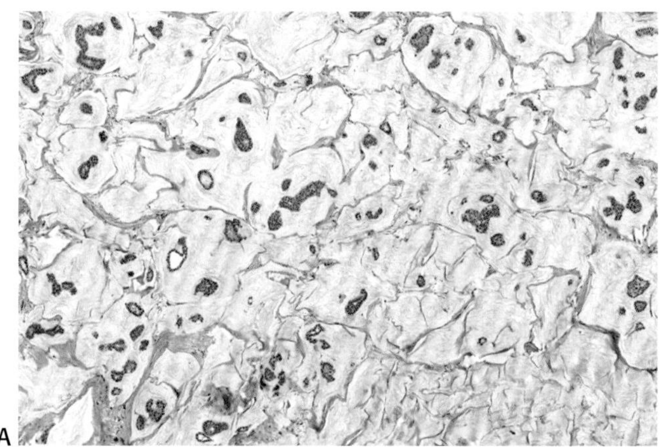

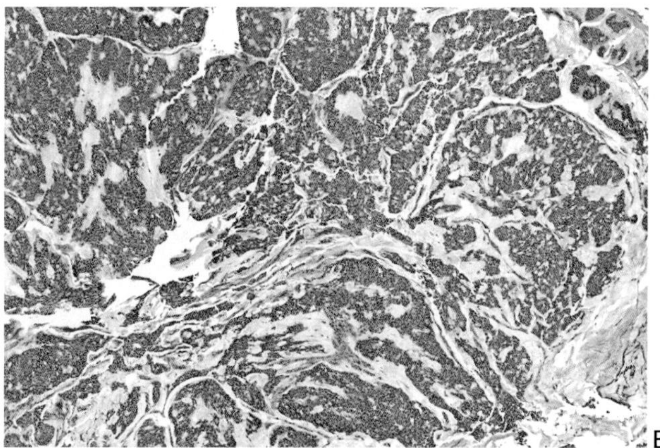

FIG. 18.13. *Mucinous carcinoma, types A and B.* **A:** Type A tumors such as this have abundant extracellular mucin. **B:** Type B tumors are hypercellular.

argyrophilic granules detected with Grimelius and Bodian stains, whereas all 15 type A tumors had no detectable argyrophilic granules (Fig. 18.14). A statistically significant difference was found in the age distribution of patients with type A and B lesions, with the former group tending to be younger at diagnosis. Type AB tumors constituted 20% of the cases studied and were described as having "indeterminate" features or features "indicative of transitional forms between the two major groups," but little information was given about these cases. The authors concluded that the type A lesions corresponded to carcinomas that were ordinarily regarded as classical pure mucinous carcinoma. It was recommended that type B tumors be regarded as a variant of mucinous carcinoma with endocrine differentiation.

Scopsi et al.[14] confirmed the common occurrence of argyrophilic granules in type B carcinomas. The presence or absence of argyrophilia was not significantly related to age, menstrual status, tumor size, or axillary nodal status. Classification as type A or type B did not prove to be prognostically significant.

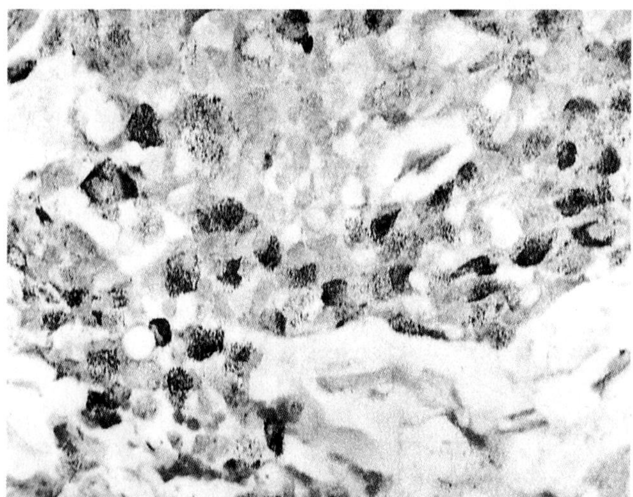

FIG. 18.14. *Mucinous carcinoma.* Clusters of fine black argyrophilic granules are demonstrated with the Grimelius stain in this island of solid carcinoma.

Ranade et al.[26] compared the characteristics of 37 type A and 8 type B pure mucinous carcinomas. The mean age of patients with type A tumors was 75 years. Type A mucinous carcinomas had a mean size 1.4 cm. Histologically, 65% of type A tumors were well differentiated, 35% were moderately differentiated, and none had high-grade morphology. Lymphovascular invasion was detected in 1/37 (3%) cases. One of three patients with type A carcinoma and lymph node metastases was 44 years old and the other two were 46 years old. Two of the three tumors with lymph node involvement had a micropapillary pattern. Two of 37 (5.5%) type A tumors were human epidermal growth factor 2 (HER2) positive. The mean age of patients with type B carcinoma was 55 years. Type B mucinous carcinomas had a mean size of 1.9 cm. Histologically, 50% type B tumors were moderately differentiated, 25% well differentiated, and 25% poorly differentiated. Lymphovascular invasion and lymph node involvement were detected in 2/8 (25%) patients, one of whom was 44 years old and the other 82 years old. Two of eight (25%) type B tumors were HER2 positive. These findings suggest that type A tumors may have more favorable characteristics than type B tumors, but this hypothesis needs confirmation in larger studies.

The morphologic distinction between type A and B mucinous carcinoma has a strong correlation with genetic subtype (see section on genetics and molecular alterations in this chapter), but at present, the designation of type A or B morphology has no clinical implications, and is rarely mentioned in routine diagnostic reports.

Micropapillary Variant of Pure Mucinous Carcinoma

A micropapillary variant of pure mucinous carcinoma has been described (Fig. 18.15).[26,62,67,69] The micropapillae are arranged in small clusters that are tightly cohesive or have

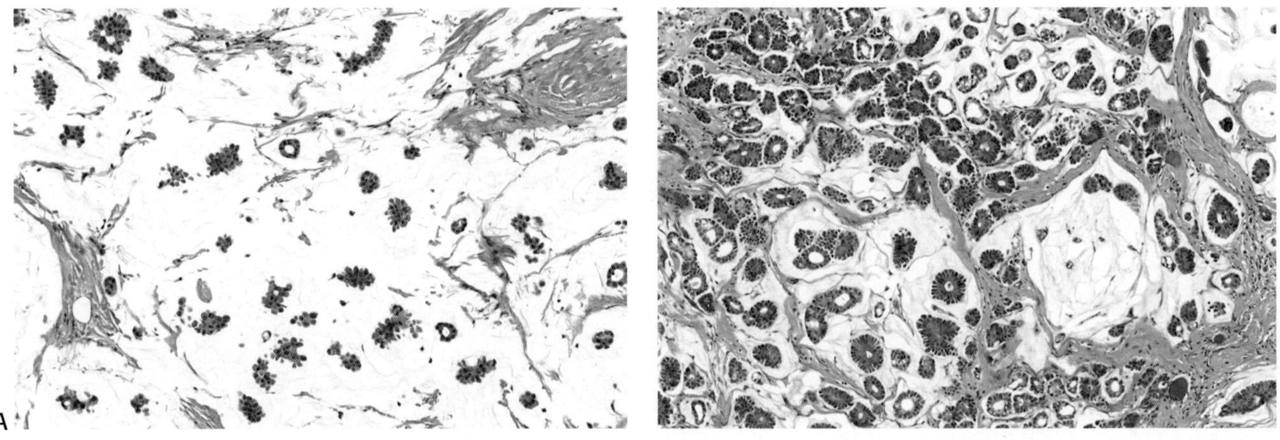

FIG. 18.15. ***Mucinous carcinoma, micropapillary variant.*** **A,B:** Tumor cells in small micropapillary clusters are admixed with mucin.

a central open space with a resulting ring-like configuration. The tumor clusters are surrounded by a clear space filled with mucin. Epithelial membrane antigen (EMA) decorates the outer surface of the micropapillae, confirming the everted polarity of the epithelium,[26,67,68] akin to invasive micropapillary carcinoma. A micropapillary component was recognized in 66.6%,[68] 35%,[67] and 20%[26] of pure mucinous carcinomas in three separate series. In a series of 102 pure mucinous carcinomas, Shet and Chinoy[68] had 20 cases in which a mucinous micropapillary component coexisted with invasive micropapillary carcinoma. In the series by Ranade et al.,[26] pure mucinous carcinomas with and without micropapillary component had similar average size (1.7 and 1.65 cm, respectively), but patients with a micropapillary component were younger than those without (47 vs. 60 years, respectively). Three of the five (60%) carcinomas with lymph node metastases in this series had a micropapillary component, whereas only 14% of pure mucinous carcinomas without lymph node involvement showed micropapillary foci.[26] In another series,[69] lymphovascular invasion was present in 9/15 (60%) mucinous micropapillary carcinomas. Lymph node metastases were found in 33% of all cases. One of 13 patients with follow-up information developed a chest wall recurrence 9 months after mastectomy.

Signet Ring Variant of Pure Mucinous Carcinoma

The pathognomonic feature of signet ring cells is abundant intracytoplasmic mucin, either concentrated within an intracytoplasmic vacuole or uniformly dispersed throughout the cytoplasm, resulting in indentation of the nucleus and displacement to one side of the cell. Carcinomas with abundant extracellular mucin rarely also have signet ring cell morphology (Fig. 18.16). On the other hand, the signet ring cell variant of infiltrating lobular carcinoma rarely has an extracellular mucinous component, and it is best considered as a mucinous variant of infiltrating lobular carcinoma,[70] not as a mucinous carcinoma. Signet ring cells admixed with mucin are often found in pure mucinous carcinomas with neuroendocrine features (type B), and can consist of single cells or, more commonly, large solid clusters. In their series of 102 pure mucinous carcinomas, Shet and Chinoy[68] identified seven solid and papillary carcinomas composed of signet ring cells arranged in solid epithelial clusters admixed with mucin. An example of this lesion is probably the case reported by Kuroda et al.[71]

Mucinous Carcinoma Associated with Solid and Papillary Carcinoma

Mucinous carcinoma may also arise from solid papillary carcinoma (Fig. 18.17). These tumors usually are pure mucinous carcinomas with type B morphology and show neuroendocrine differentiation or have neuroendocrine features. They overlap morphologically with carcinomas with neuroendocrine differentiation (see Chapter 20). Genetic evidence also supports a close relationship between the two entities.[72,73]

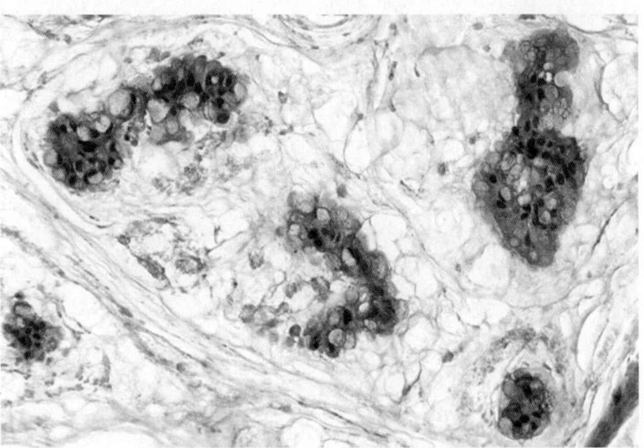

FIG. 18.16. ***Mucinous carcinoma, signet ring variant.*** Abundant intracytoplasmic mucin results in indentation of the tumor cell nucleus and nuclear displacement to one side of the cell.

Cystic Papillary Mucinous Carcinoma (Mucinous Cystadenocarcinoma)

One of the most infrequent variants of mucin-producing carcinoma is a cystic type of papillary mucinous carcinoma (Fig. 18.18). It is composed of multiple cysts distended by mucinous secretion and lined by micropapillary, papillary, and cribriform carcinoma. The mucinous epithelium can have blandly atypical nuclei or show more nuclear atypia, often accompanied by intracytoplasmic mucin depletion.[74–82] All reported cases have occurred in women, ranging in age from 41[83] to 96 years old.[75] Many of the case reports have involved women in Asian countries.[75,76,78,80,81,83,84] Lack of myoepithelial lining around the mucin-filled cysts of cystic papillary mucinous carcinoma has been documented,[74,78,82] a finding that supports an invasive process. Rarely, areas of invasive ductal carcinoma NOS[76,78] as well as foci of sarcomatoid metaplasia[74] have been observed admixed with these tumors, but the usual morphology of pure mucinous carcinoma has not been documented in this setting. Focal DCIS has also been found.[74,76,78,82] Squamoid differentiation has been reported in a few cases.[74,75]

Because cystic papillary mucinous carcinomas of the breast are estrogen receptor (ER) and progesterone receptor (PR) negative[74–78,80,81,83,84] (see section on immunohistochemistry [IHC]), whenever the differential diagnosis of cystic papillary mucinous carcinoma is considered and no adjacent DCIS and/or invasive mammary carcinoma NOS are identified, careful clinical and radiologic correlation and thorough review of the patient's prior medical history are recommended to rule out metastasis from an ovarian or colorectal mucinous carcinoma. Eleven patients with cystic papillary mucinous carcinoma described by Komaki et al.[85] had a relatively lower average age at diagnosis (41 years) than is typical for mucinous carcinoma. None of the patients had axillary nodal metastases when treated by mastectomy, and they remained disease-free for an average of nearly 10 years. Mucinous cystadenocarcinoma might be derived from a metaplasia of ordinary DCIS, but its pathogenesis and biologic behavior remain unclear. Despite their invasive nature and large size

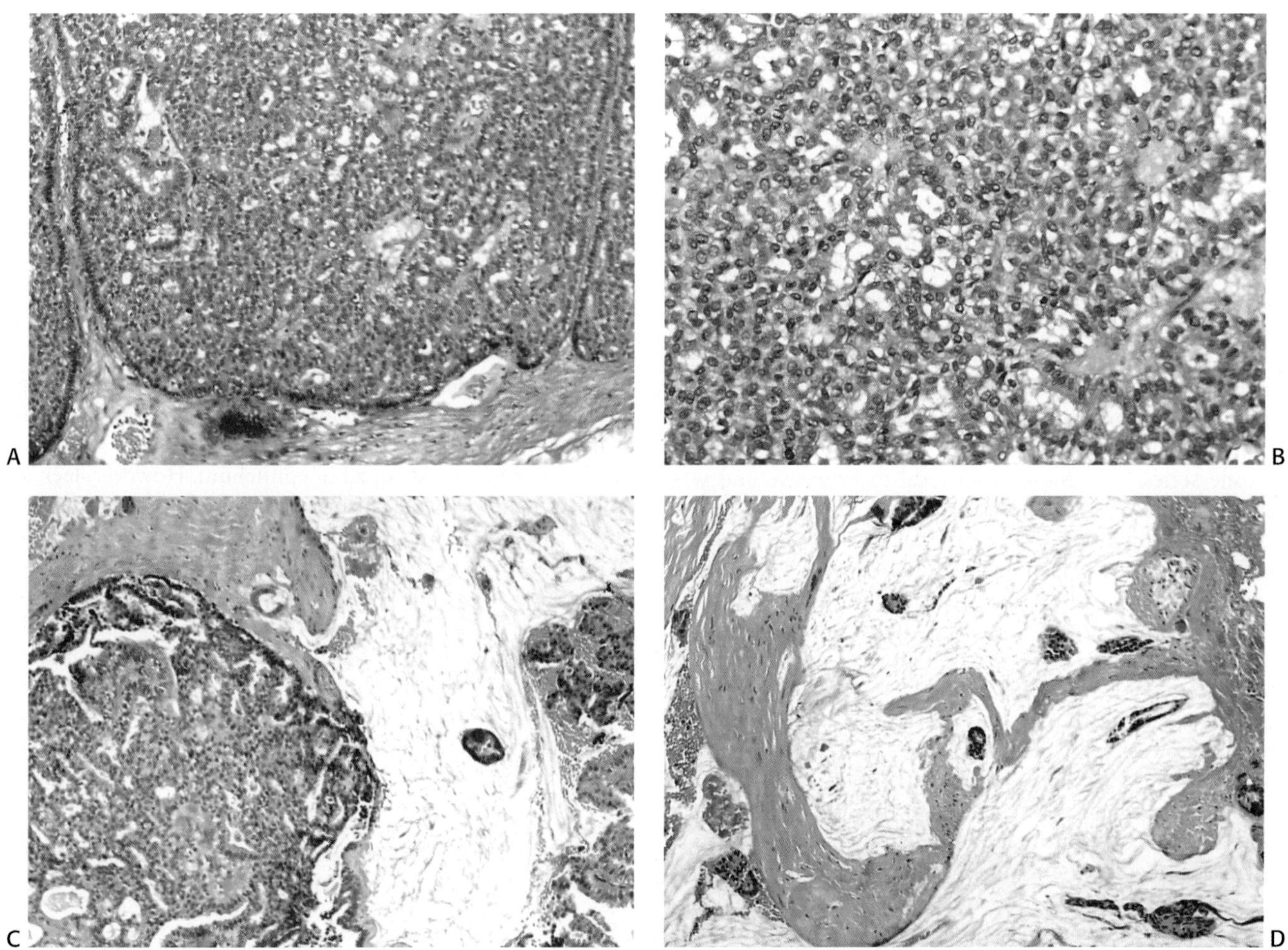

FIG. 18.17. ***Mucinous carcinoma, arising in solid papillary carcinoma.*** **A:** Solid papillary intraductal carcinoma. **B:** Mucin is present in microlumens in the intraductal carcinoma. **C:** The transition between intraductal *(left)* and infiltrating *(right)* mucinous carcinoma is shown here. **D:** Mucinous carcinoma.

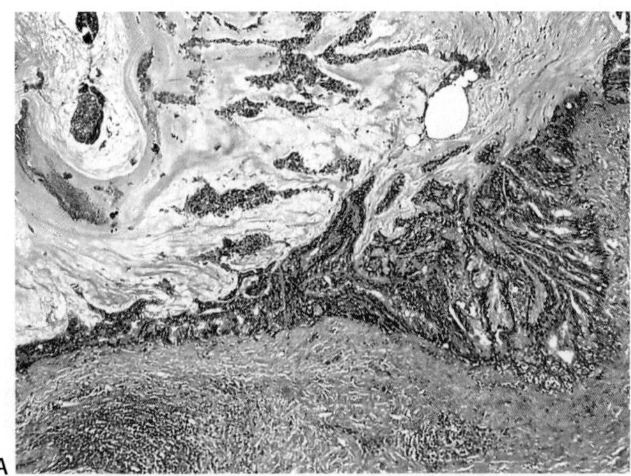
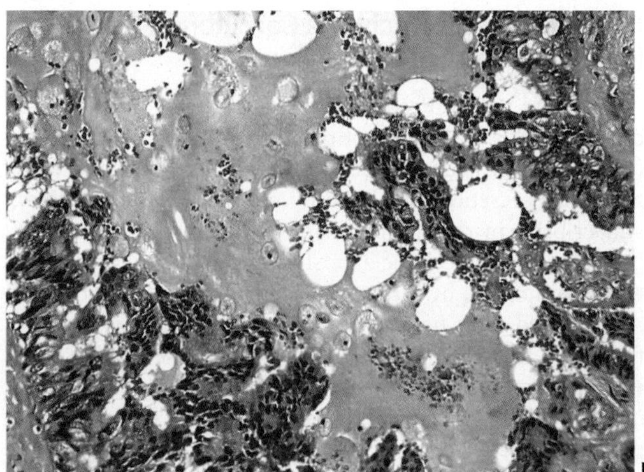

FIG. 18.18. *Mucinous carcinoma, cystic papillary type.* A,B: Fronds of papillary carcinoma surround the cyst filled with mucinous carcinoma.

at presentation, cystic papillary mucinous carcinomas of the breast appear to be associated with a relatively good prognosis, and only few patients had lymph node involvement.[74,75,83] Metastatic carcinoma arising from these tumors usually has morphology similar to that of the primary tumor.

Ductal Carcinoma *In Situ*

DCIS is found associated with 60% to 75% of the lesions, and is generally located at the tumor periphery.[25] The intraductal component has any of the conventional patterns of DCIS (cribriform, papillary, micropapillary, and solid patterns). Marked zonal necrosis is present rarely. Occasionally, prominent mucin is present in the lumen of the intraductal component (Fig. 18.19), and one can find transitions from intraductal to invasive mucinous carcinoma (Fig. 18.19). DCIS was present in 37/40 (92.5%) mucinous carcinomas in one series.[86] It ranged from focal to extensive and was cribriform in 24/37 (65%) cases, solid in 20/37 (54%), micropapillary in 11/37 (30%), and flat in 4/37 (11%). DCIS with necrosis was present in 11/37 (30%) cases. The nuclear grade was low in 12/37 (32%) cases, intermediate in 21/37 (57%), and high in 4/37 (11%) cases. Intraluminal mucin was identified in 32/37 (86%) DCIS cases and contained blood vessels in 26/37 (70%). The DCIS patterns most frequently associated with neovascularization of the intraluminal mucin were solid and cribriform. The high frequency of mucin neovascularization in the DCIS associated with mucinous carcinoma led the authors of the study to speculate that it might constitute an intermediate step toward stromal invasion, whereby the tumor cells first invade into the mucinous and vascularized stroma that they have induced and then into the surrounding fibroconnective tissue. However, in the absence of overt invasion, neovascularization of the mucin associated with DCIS should not be interpreted as evidence of tumor invasion (Fig. 18.20). A minority of mucinous carcinomas do not have detectable DCIS. These tend to be larger tumors, but rarely one encounters a pure mucinous carcinoma smaller than 2 cm with no apparent DCIS, sometimes arising in a MLL.

A diagnostic problem arises in patients who have only DCIS when extravasated mucin is present in the adjacent stroma. Extravasation of mucin from DCIS can be caused by a prior procedure or trauma or it may occur spontaneously. Mucin might also artifactually be extruded into the stroma during handling of a tissue specimen. For these reasons, the finding of extravasated mucin devoid of carcinoma cells does not necessarily always represent evidence of an invasive mucinous carcinoma. In these cases, it is necessary to obtain multiple recuts, and it is advisable to do a cytokeratin (CK) stain to determine whether epithelial cells are present in the mucin and to distinguish them from histiocytes. Immunoperoxidase stains for myoepithelial markers, such as calponin or p63, may highlight myoepithelial cells admixed with the detached clusters or present along the wall of ducts or lobules stripped of epithelium. However, lack of myoepithelium is not sufficient evidence of stromal invasion, especially if mucin and epithelial clusters are admixed with stromal changes secondary to a prior procedure. If carcinoma cells are found in the mucin, a diagnosis of invasive mucinous carcinoma is appropriate, unless there is compelling evidence to consider the alternative possibility of epithelial displacement, possibly secondary to a prior procedure. Most of the time, the mucin admixed with invasive carcinoma will also have a rounded to bulbous outline, neovascularization, and admixed inflammatory cells and fibroblasts.

Morphology of Metastases of Pure Mucinous and Mixed Mucinous Carcinoma

Axillary or systemic metastases (Fig. 18.21) that arise from mucinous carcinoma of the breast usually have the histologic characteristics of the primary tumor. Axillary metastases from tumors with mixed histology often resemble the nonmucinous component. Pure mucinous carcinomas occasionally can also have nonmucinous metastases.[25] The

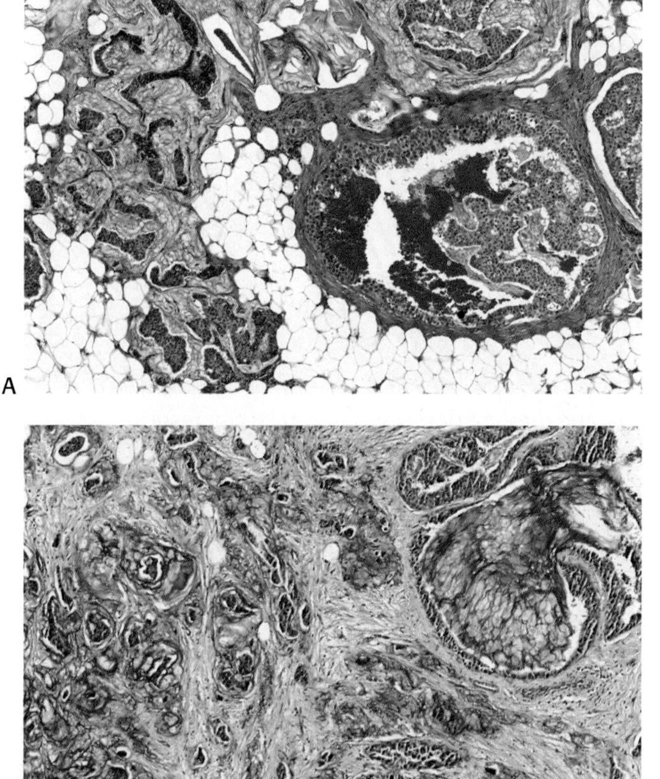

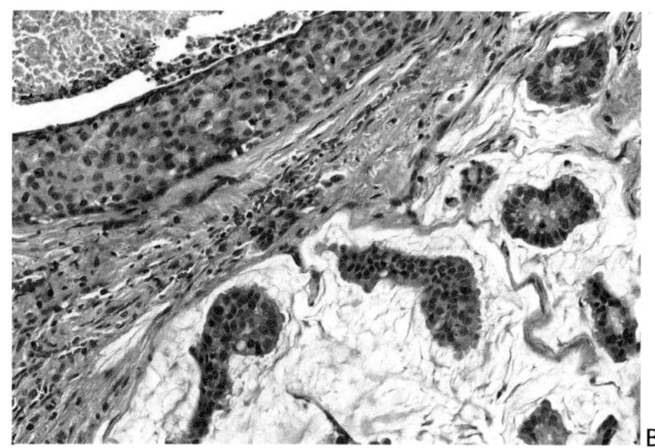

FIG. 18.19. *Intraductal carcinoma in mucinous carcinoma.* A: A duct containing DCIS and mucin (*lower right*) is present next to invasive mucinous carcinoma. B: DCIS with central necrosis (*upper left*) near invasive mucinous carcinoma. Intracellular mucin is evident in the DCIS cells C: Mucin stained pink is present in the lumen of the DCIS (*upper right corner*) and in the invasive carcinoma (mucicarmine stain).

distribution of sites of disseminated metastases does not differ from that of other types of ductal carcinoma, but an unusual fatal complication is cerebral infarction caused by mucin embolism.[87,88] The lymph node metastases of pure mucinous and micropapillary mucinous carcinoma are histologically similar to the primary tumor[62], but pure micropapillary metastases occur[69].

MUCOCELE-LIKE LESIONS

MLL, an entity first described and named by Rosen in 1986,[51] is composed of mucin-containing cysts that tend to rupture and discharge the secretion into the adjacent stroma (Fig. 18.22). The resultant picture resembles the mucocele of minor salivary gland origin found in the oral cavity. It is

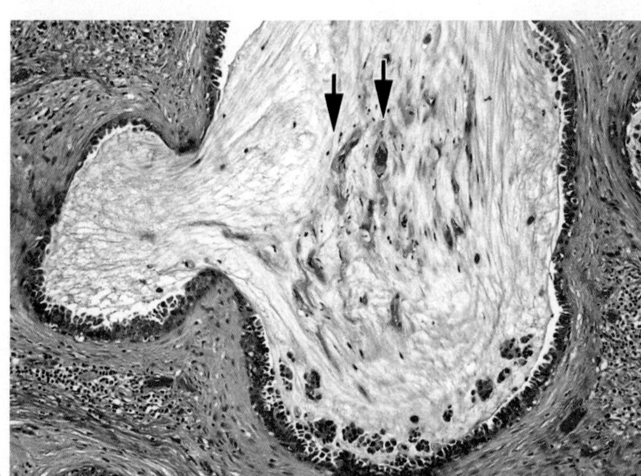

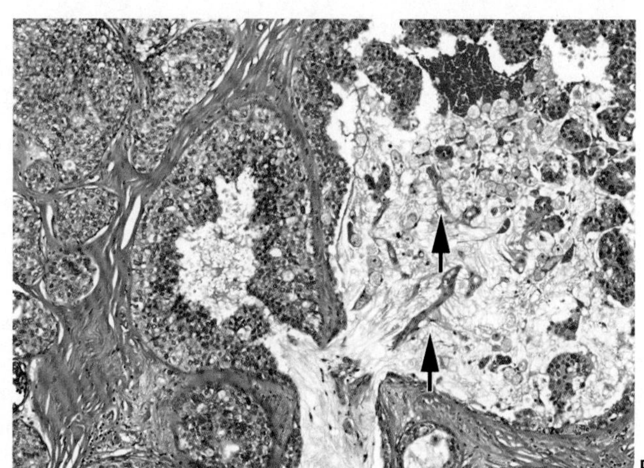

FIG. 18.20. *Intraductal mucinous carcinoma.* A,B: Neovascularization (*arrows*) of the mucin is present within the lumen of the DCIS. Papillary clusters of carcinoma cells are present in the mucin.

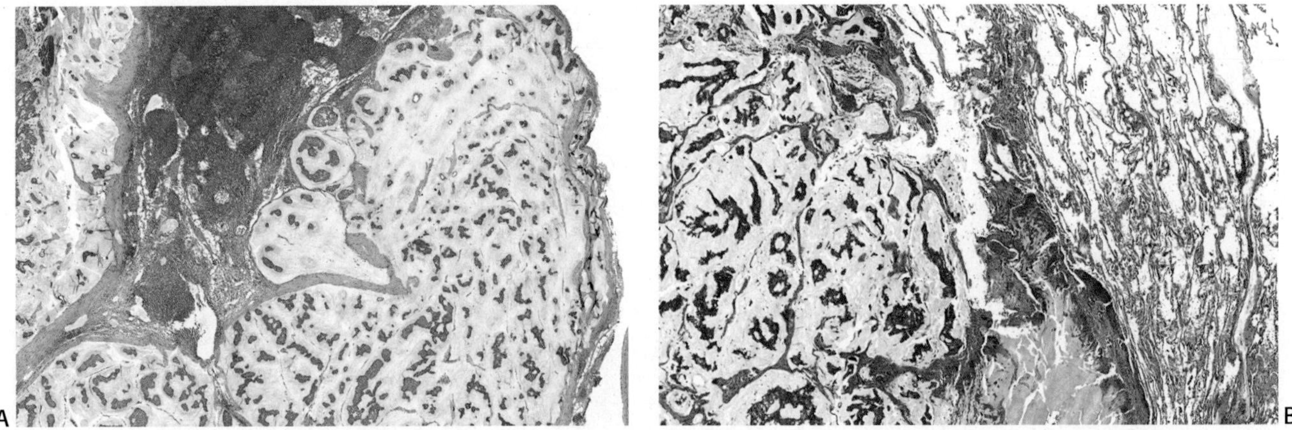

FIG. 18.21. ***Mucinous carcinoma, metastases.*** Metastatic mammary mucinous carcinoma resembles the primary tumor. **A:** Metastatic mucinous carcinoma in a lymph node. **B:** Metastatic mucinous carcinoma in the lung.

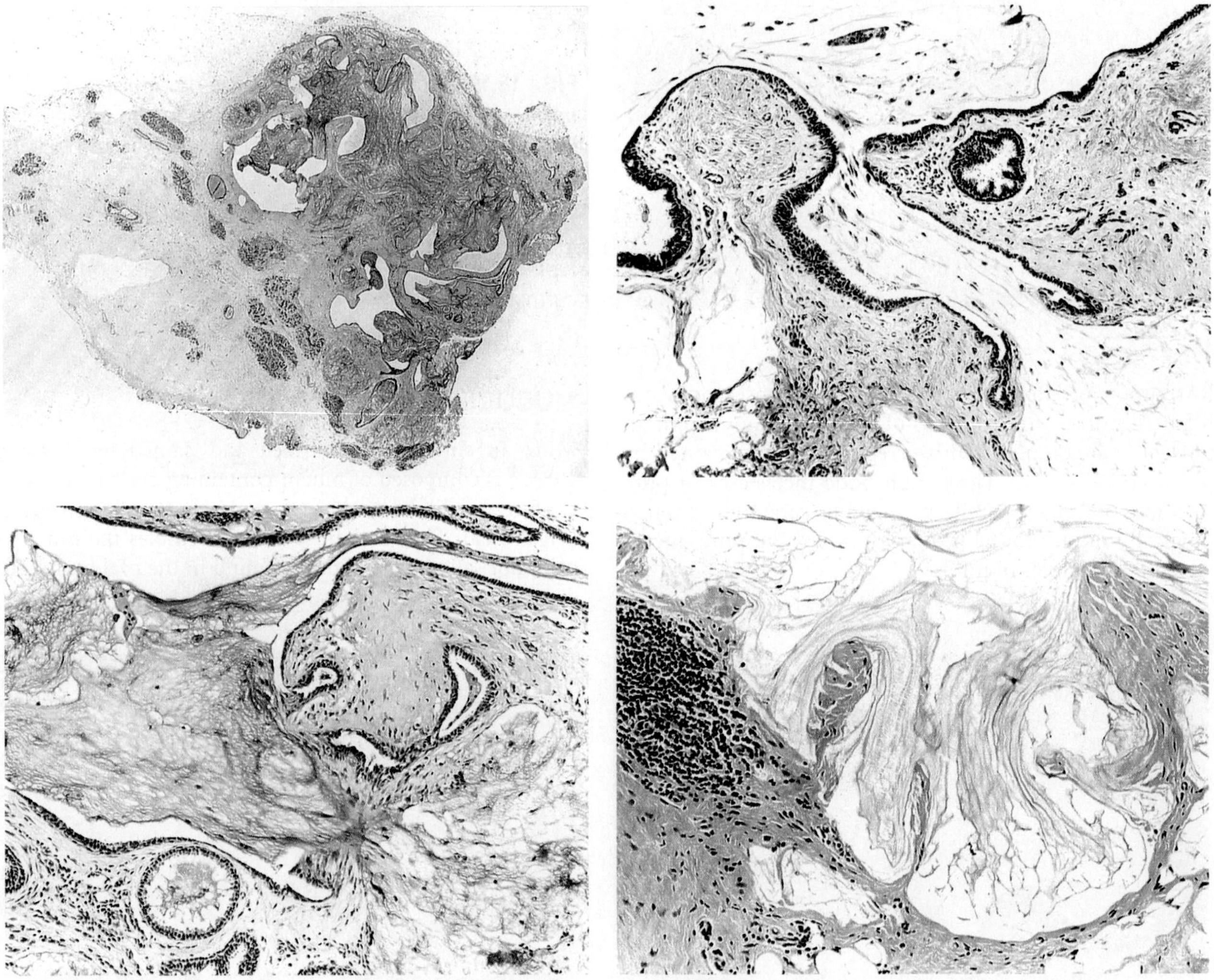

FIG. 18.22. ***Mucocele-like lesion.*** **A:** A whole-mount histologic section of a relatively small MLL. The dark oval foci to the *left* of the lesion are normal lobules. **B,C:** Two examples of ruptured cysts with mucin extruded into the surrounding stroma. Hyperplasia is evident in small ducts. Folding of epithelium toward the cyst of origin rather than into the stroma at the point of rupture is a typical finding. **D:** Pools of extruded mucin in fibrous stroma with a focal lymphocytic reaction. (Reproduced from Rosen PP. Mucocele-like tumors of the breast. *Am J Surg Pathol* 1986;10:464–469.)

important to note that the term "mucocele-like lesion" is descriptive and does not have specific implications regarding the biology of the lesion, which is dictated by the nature of the epithelium lining the cyst wall. Therefore, the final diagnostic report of a MLL needs to indicate whether the epithelium is benign, atypical, or frankly neoplastic. Some MLLs of the breast present as palpable tumors that are well circumscribed, lobulated lesions on mammography (Fig. 18.23), whereas others constitute incidental microscopic findings in excision specimen for a different lesion. An increasing number of small, nonpalpable, MLLs are detected by mammography alone. Mammography reveals a nodular lesion with or without calcifications, or clustered calcifications without a mass.[89–91] Ultrasonography shows a hypoechoic, round or lobulated, solid or cystic tumor, sometimes with an ill-defined margin.[92,93] Multiple aggregated cysts are evident grossly containing viscous, often transparent, mucinous material (Fig. 18.24).

The epithelium lining the ducts in the typical mammary MLL is largely flat, attenuated or low cuboidal (Fig. 18.25), but low columnar and minor papillary elements may be present or the epithelium may show a spectrum of proliferative changes ranging from hyperplasia to atypical ductal hyperplasia (ADH) (Fig. 18.26) to DCIS.[51,94,95] The distinction between mucinous carcinoma and MLL can sometimes be a challenging clinical, radiologic, and pathologic problem.[44]

In some cases, strips or clusters of epithelial cells detached from the duct walls are present in the mucin pools. The distinction from mucinous carcinoma can be difficult, particularly if the detached epithelium derives from ADH. The presence of epithelial ribbons and strips of cytologically bland and columnar epithelium in the mucin pools supports artifactual detachment. The immunohistochemical identification of myoepithelial cells within the epithelial clusters admixed with mucin also supports artifactual detachment. Nonetheless, particularly if the epithelium is atypical or frankly neoplastic, it may not be possible to distinguish definitively between artifactual detachment and (micro)invasive mucinous carcinoma in some cases.

Histiocytes and inflammatory cells may be present in the extruded mucin. Distinctive large and granular calcifications are formed in many MLLs (Fig. 18.27). The finding of this type of calcification in a needle core biopsy specimen suggests the diagnosis of a MLL.

Evidence that may link MLLs to mucinous carcinoma was obtained by Weaver et al.[96] A review of 23 mucinous carcinomas revealed mucin-filled ducts without hyperplastic epithelium in 15 cases (65%), ductal hyperplasia in mucin-filled ducts in 9 (39%), and ADH in mucin-filled ducts in 5 cases (22%). The authors did not comment on the presence or absence of extravasated mucin in areas of mucin-filled ducts.

Kikuchi et al.[97] reported a case of MLL that was diagnosed as a fibroadenoma by mammography and ultrasound, and as mucinous carcinoma by fine-needle aspiration (FNA). Leibman et al.[98] reported that 30 nonpalpable MLLs were identified by screening mammography over a 4-year period at an urban academic medical center. Twenty-five lesions were detected as calcifications, three as a mass lesion, and two as a mass lesion with calcifications. Twenty-two cases were diagnosed by needle core biopsy, seven by excisional biopsy, and one by FNA. Seventeen MLLs were classified as benign, eight had atypical hyperplasia, and five were accompanied by DCIS.

Ro et al.[94] described MLLs that contained areas of ADH, DCIS, and focal invasive mucinous carcinoma. In several of the cases, calcifications detected mammographically were localized to the mucinous content of cysts in histologic sections. Identical results were obtained when the secretion in mucinous carcinomas and in various MLLs was studied immunohistochemically. The mucin in cysts and in the stroma was largely composed of neutral and nonsulfated acid mucin (strongly positive with periodic acid–Schiff [PAS]/diastase, mucicarmine, and Alcian blue at pH 2.7; weakly negative with Alcian blue at pH 0.9).

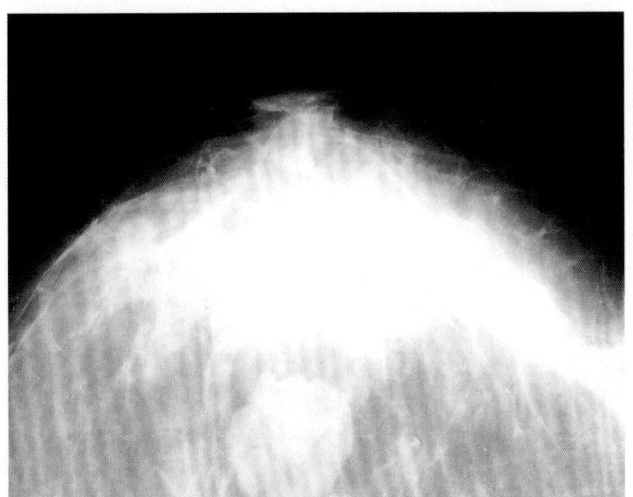

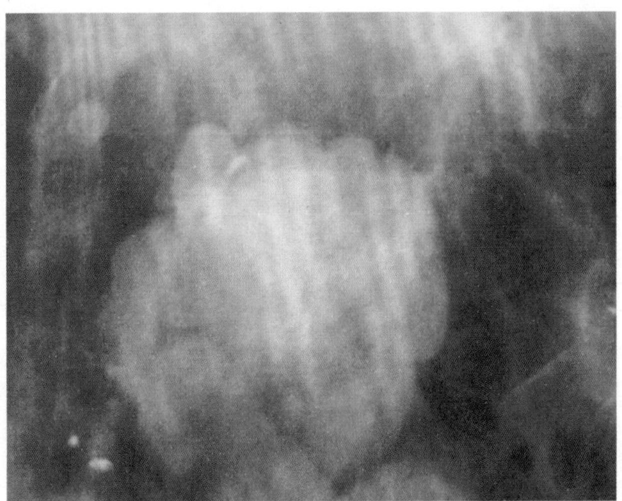

FIG. 18.23. ***Mucocele-like lesion, mammographic appearance.*** **A:** The lesion is a large, circumscribed, multinodular mass deep in the breast. **B:** The MLL is inhomogeneous.

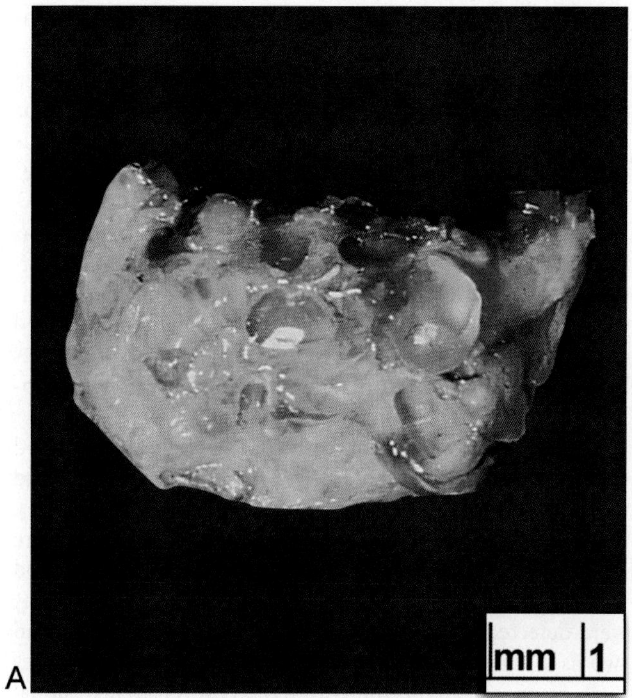

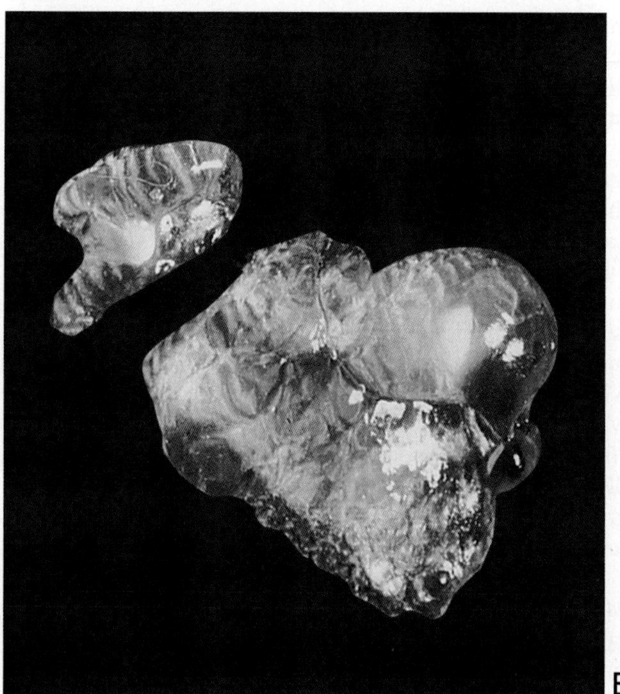

FIG. 18.24. *Mucocele-like lesion, gross appearance.* **A:** The tumor consists of many cysts. **B:** Masses of transparent gelatinous material from the tumor.

A MLL that originated in a cystic papilloma has been described[44] (Fig. 18.28). A MLL may also be present as an incidental finding in a specimen obtained for an unrelated lesion (Fig. 18.29), or it can be the source of a clinically detected tumor when multiple lobular foci become confluent (Fig. 18.30).

Small MLLs can also arise from lobules. Following earlier descriptions by Coyne and Irion[77] and Fadare and Mariappan,[99] Verschuur-Maes and Van Diest[100] have characterized a mucinous variant of columnar cell lesions, in which the involved acini are variably dilated and filled with mucin. The authors identified 20 needle core biopsies in which mucin was present in terminal duct lobular units (TDLUs) involved by columnar cell change: 17 had no epithelial atypia and 3 had ADH. The 20 mucinous columnar cell lesions with or without atypia constituted 0.5% of 4,164 core biopsies in the study. Stromal mucin was detected in 18/20 (90%) of the core biopsies with mucinous columnar cells. Nineteen core biopsies targeted mammographic microcalcifications, and a mammographic density with calcifications was the radiologic target in the remaining case. No evidence of carcinoma was found at surgical excision of 3/20 lesions (two with ADH and one without atypia).

Kulka and Davies[101] described two MLLs with ADH. In one case, the same breast harbored a separate nonmucinous

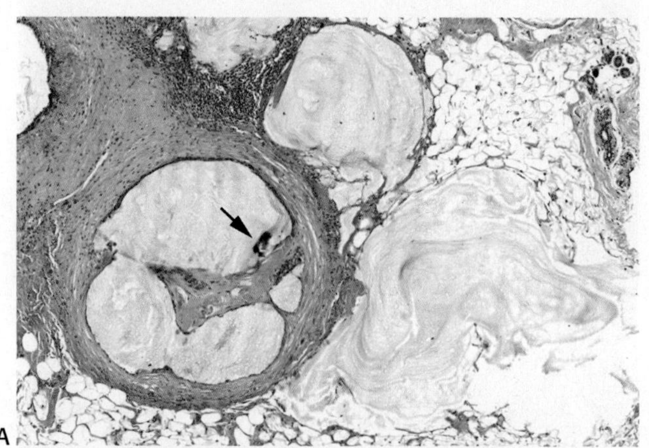

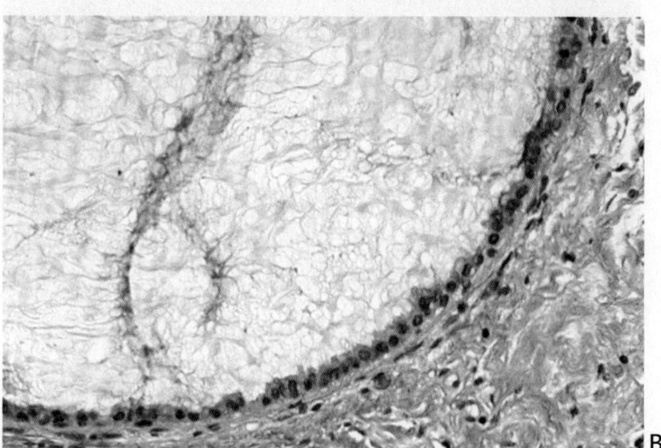

FIG. 18.25. *Mucocele-like lesion.* **A:** Cysts containing mucinous secretion and rare calcifications [*arrow*] are lined by a thin epithelial layer. Acellular mucin is present in the fat. **B:** Orderly, flat and low cuboidal epithelium in a MLL.

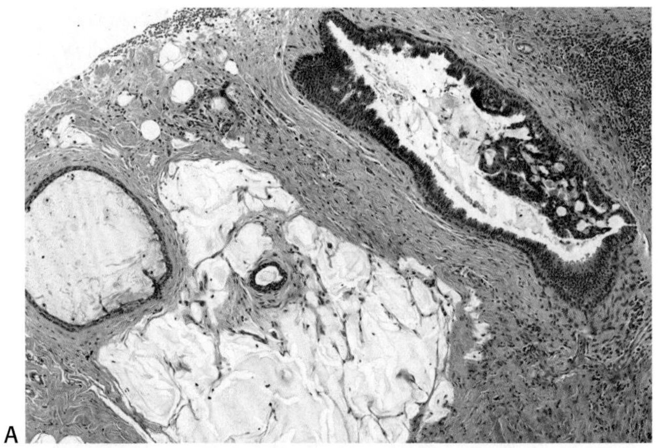

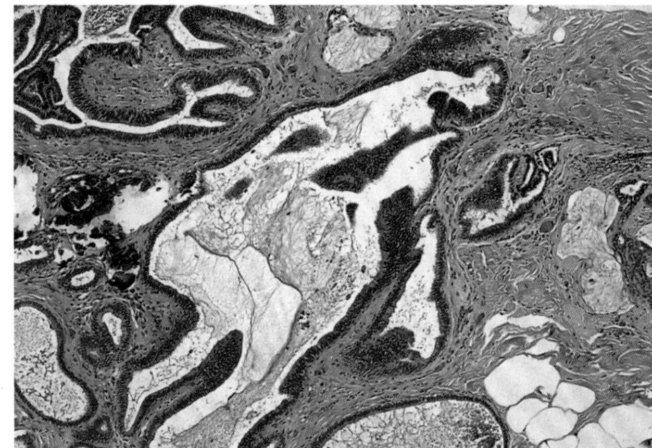

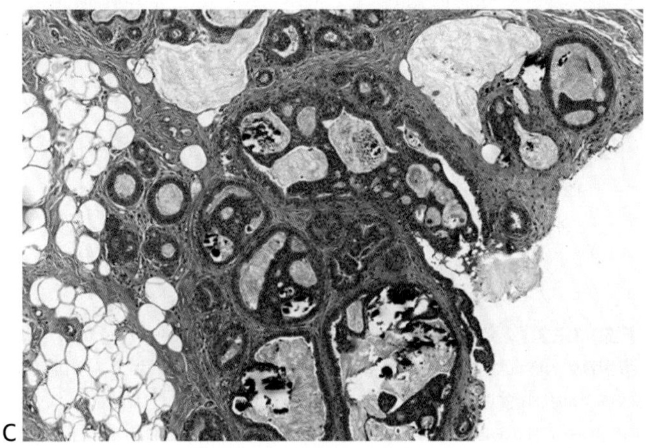

FIG. 18.26. ***Mucocele-like lesions with ductal hyperplasia.*** **A:** Atypical micropapillary and cribriform ductal hyperplasia near extravasated mucin. **B:** Columnar cell hyperplasia (CCH) with calcifications (*left*) and extravasated mucin (*right*). **C:** Ducts with ADH and calcifications, near extravasated mucin.

invasive duct carcinoma. Fisher and Millis[102] reported finding DCIS and mucinous carcinoma 1 year after excision of a MLL with ADH. Yeoh et al.[93] summarized 13 patients with MLLs, including 7 with ADH. No recurrences were recorded with follow-up of 1 month to 3.8 years.

Hamele-Bena et al.[95] reviewed 49 examples of MLLs. The age range for the entire group was 24 to 79 years (mean, 48 years), without significant differences in the age distribution of patients with benign and malignant lesions. Malignant MLLs tended to have coarse calcifications more often than the benign tumors (Figs. 18.31 and 18.32) and were, therefore, more frequently detected by mammography. Four patients had bilateral tumors that were benign in two cases and carcinomatous in the other two. Overall, 25 of the

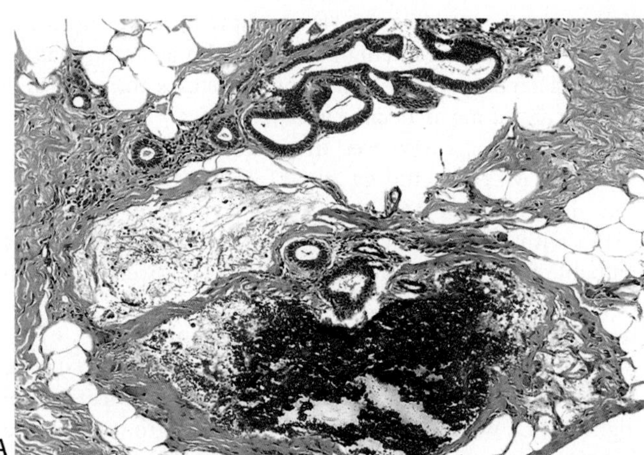

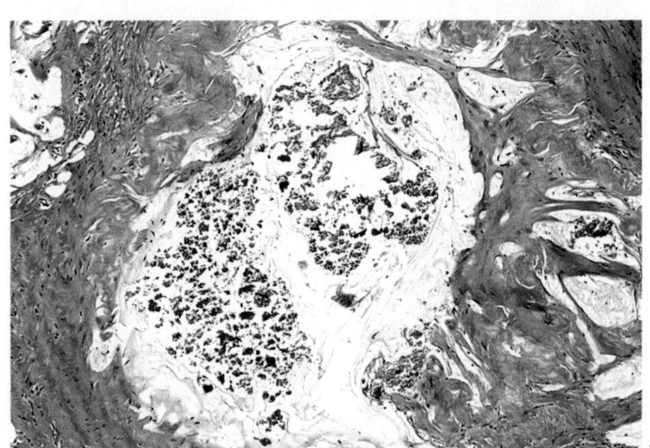

FIG. 18.27. ***Mucocele-like lesion with calcifications.*** Two different specimens are depicted. **A:** Coarse calcification in extravasated mucin associated with columnar cell change. **B:** Loosely granular calcification in extravasated mucin.

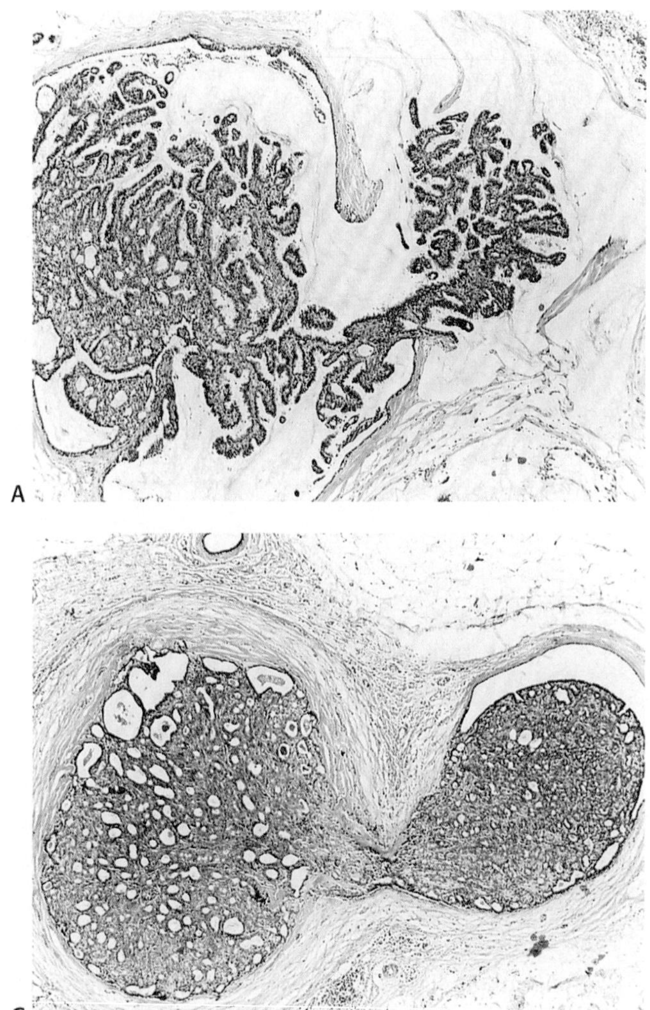

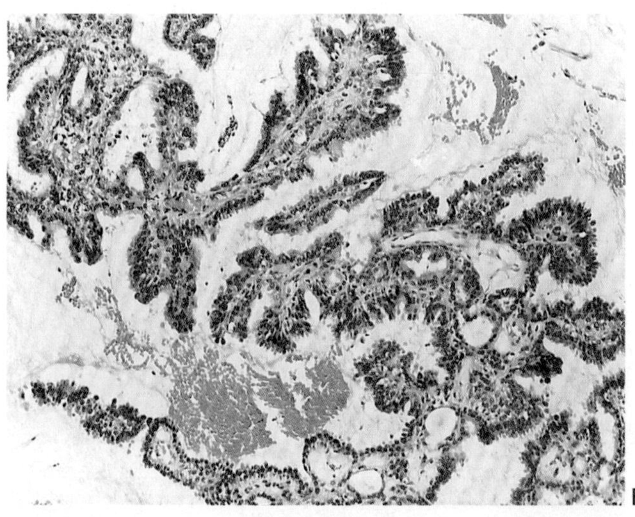

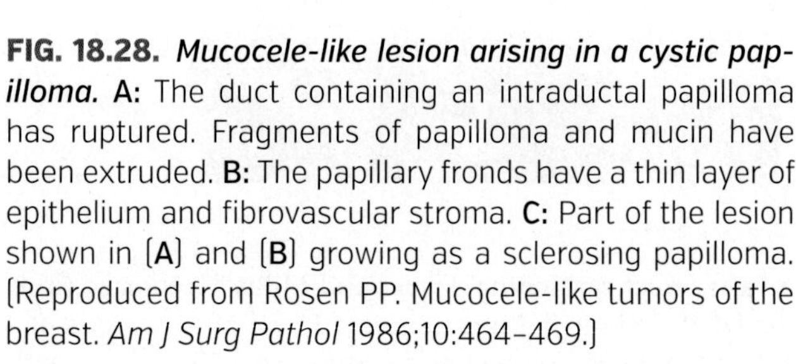

FIG. 18.28. ***Mucocele-like lesion arising in a cystic papilloma.*** **A:** The duct containing an intraductal papilloma has ruptured. Fragments of papilloma and mucin have been extruded. **B:** The papillary fronds have a thin layer of epithelium and fibrovascular stroma. **C:** Part of the lesion shown in (**A**) and (**B**) growing as a sclerosing papilloma. (Reproduced from Rosen PP. Mucocele-like tumors of the breast. *Am J Surg Pathol* 1986;10:464–469.)

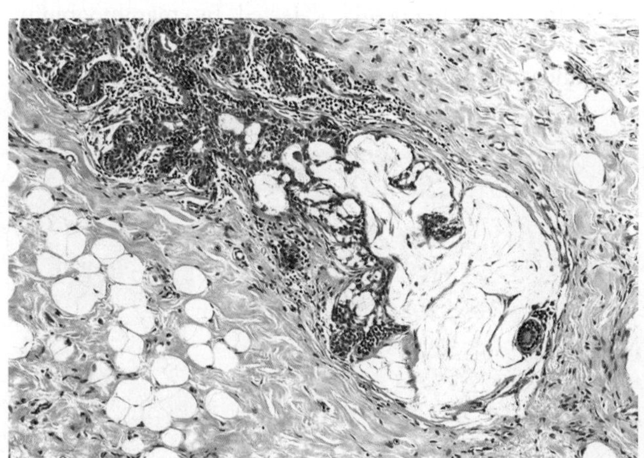

FIG. 18.29. ***Mucocele-like lesion arising in a lobule.*** Extravasated mucin arising from a TDLU. This was an incidental finding in a biopsy performed for an unrelated lesion.

lesions were classified as benign and 28 as carcinomatous. In 13 tumors, the carcinoma consisted of DCIS with predominant micropapillary (Fig. 18.33) and focally cribriform architecture. Twenty-five tumors had invasive carcinoma of the mucinous type (Fig. 18.34). Breast recurrences occurred in one patient with a benign and one with a carcinomatous lesion. There were no instances of metastases and no deaths due to carcinoma associated with a MLL.

Carkaci et al.[103] reviewed the radiologic findings in a series of 44 MLLs, including 29/44 (66%) MLLs without epithelial atypia, 7/44 (16%) MLLs with atypia, and 8/44 (18%) MLLs with DCIS. Most patients were asymptomatic, and a palpable breast mass was detected only in three (two with DCIS and one with ADH). At mammography, calcifications constituted the most common finding (27/44, 61%), 8/44 (18%) lesions presented as a mass, and 7/44 (16%) were masses associated with calcifications. The calcifications in eight MLLs with DCIS were all clustered/grouped coarse heterogeneous, those associated with MLLs with atypia

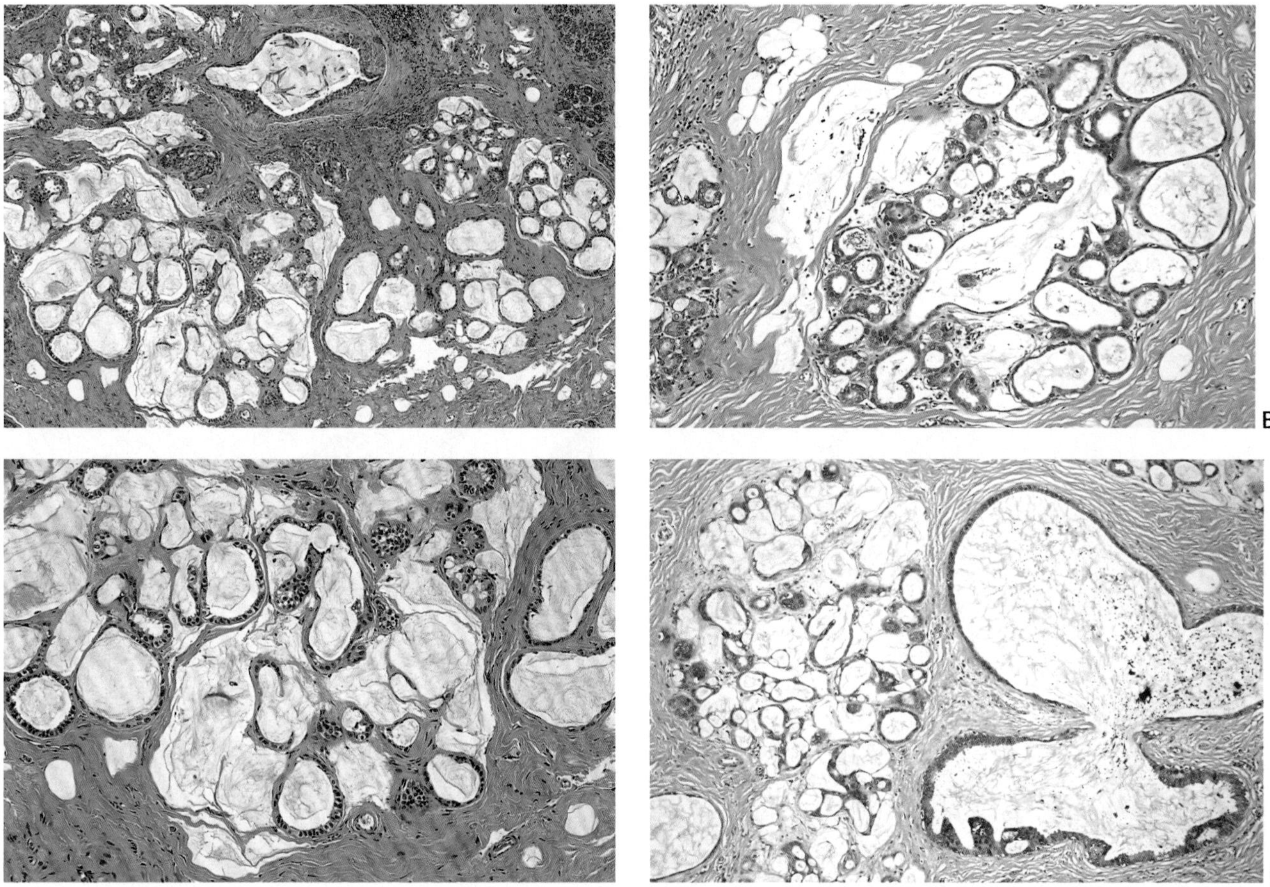

FIG. 18.30. ***Mucocele-like lesion arising in lobules.*** Four images from one specimen. **A:** A low-magnification view showing numerous lobular glands distended with mucin and extravasated mucin in the stroma. **B:** An early stage in the process. Mucin is present in lobular glands, an intralobular duct, and in adjacent stroma. **C,D:** The lobular architecture is substantially disrupted, and there is extensive mucin extravasation. Note micropapillary ADH in the cyst (*right*) in (**D**).

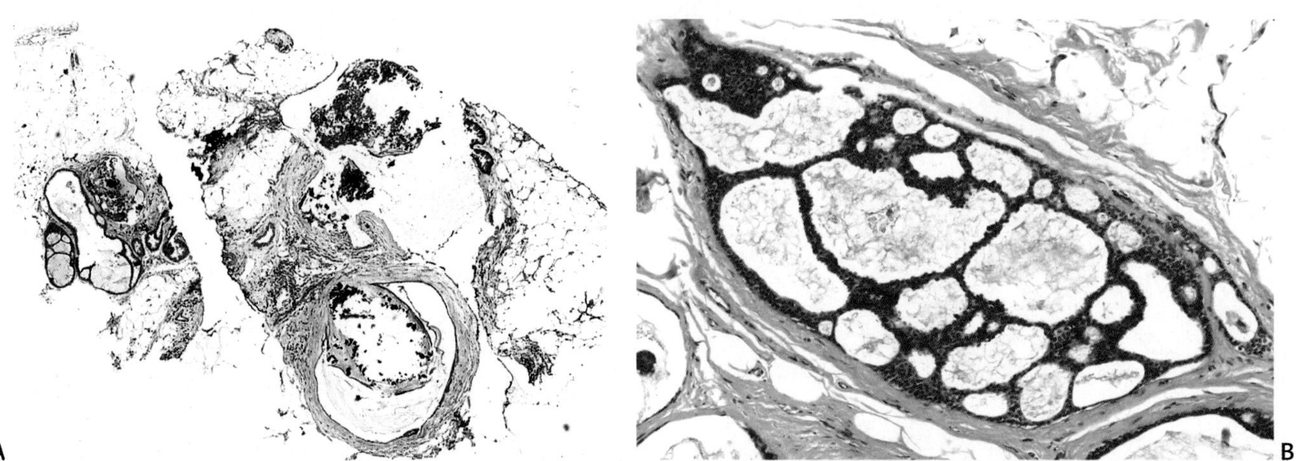

FIG. 18.31. ***Mucocele-like lesion with intraductal carcinoma and calcifications.*** **A:** A needle core biopsy specimen showing coarse calcifications (hematoxylin-phloxine-safranin stain). **B:** Cribriform DCIS in the same specimen in a H&E-stained section. Extravasated mucin is present in the upper right corner and mucocele cysts are evident below the DCIS.

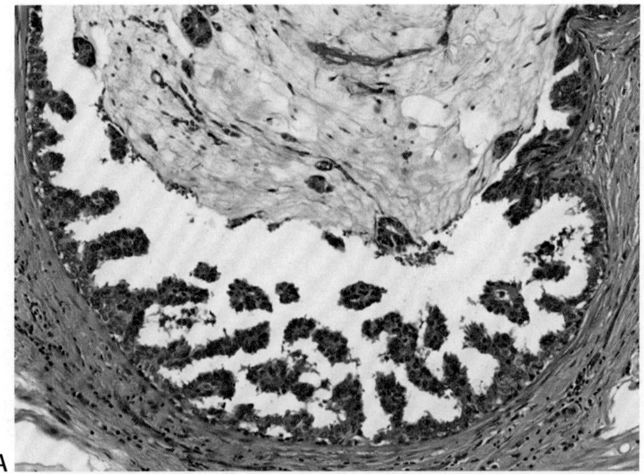

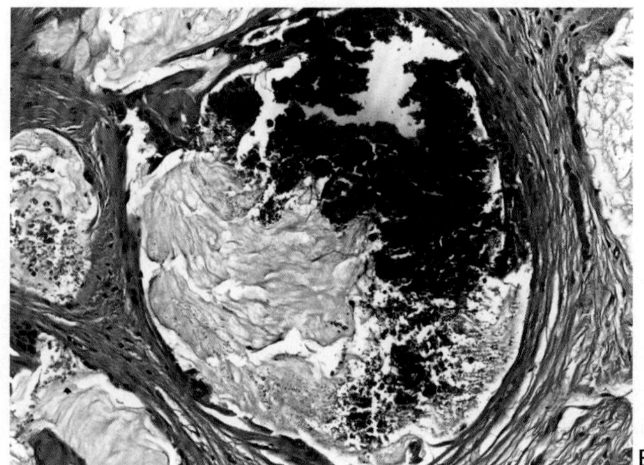

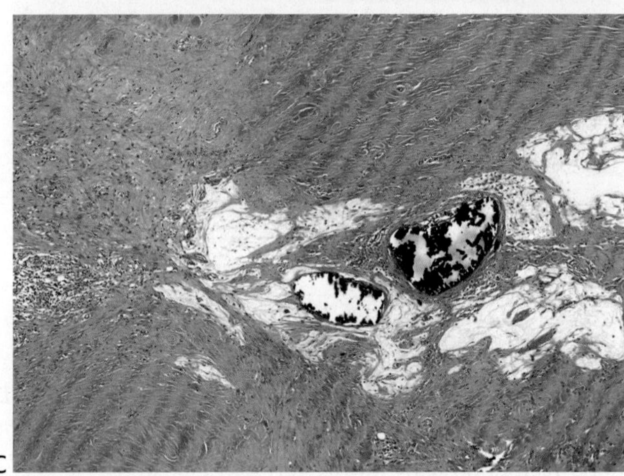

FIG. 18.32. ***Mucocele-like lesion with intraductal carcinoma.*** **A:** Micropapillary DCIS. Note neovascularity in the intraductal mucin. **B:** A large, coarse calcification in a cyst next to extruded mucin. Granular calcifications are present in extruded mucin on the *left*. Images **(A)** and **(B)** are from the same case. **C:** Mucin extravasation containing calcifications near biopsy site changes.

were clustered/grouped fine pleomorphic in 67% of cases, and those in MLLs without atypia were clustered/grouped coarse heterogeneous in 53% of cases. Seventeen MLLs underwent sonographic examination, including 3 with DCIS, 4 with ADH, and 10 without atypia. A sonographic mass was detected in 7/17 (41%) patients, and 6/17 (36%) appeared as complex cysts. Excision was performed in 26 cases, including all cases with preoperative diagnosis of DCIS or ADH at core biopsy, and 3 cases were upgraded from ADH to DCIS. Excision of 9/29 MLLs without epithelial atypia at core biopsy yielded no evidence of malignancy. The remaining 18/29 (62%) MLLs with no atypia at needle core biopsy were followed by clinical exam and imaging, and showed no evidence of malignancy at mean follow-up of 2.5 years (range 1 to 8 years).

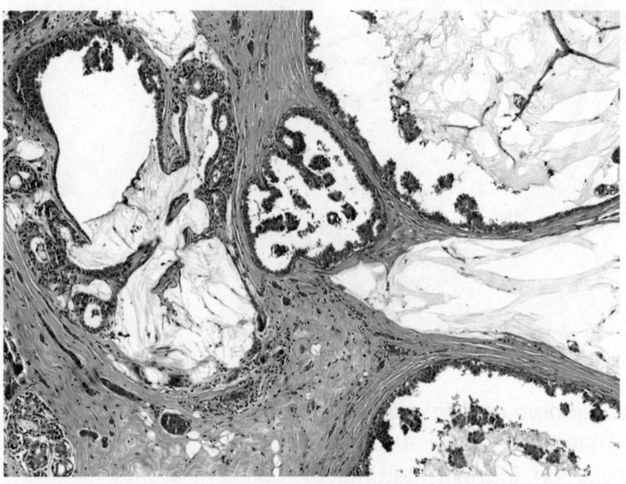

FIG. 18.33. ***Mucocele-like lesion with intraductal carcinoma.*** Micropapillary DCIS with mucin extravasation. Carcinoma cells were not present in the extravasated mucin.

MLL and Needle Core Biopsy

Benign (Fig. 18.25) and malignant (Fig. 18.31) mucinous tumors of the breast can usually be diagnosed by needle core biopsy sampling.[104,105] The diagnosis of mucinous carcinoma in a needle core biopsy specimen is usually straightforward if the sample consists of neoplastic epithelial cells surrounded by mucin. However, the distinction between pure and mixed mucinous carcinoma requires examination of the excised tumor to ensure adequate sampling.

A MLL can usually be suspected in a needle core biopsy sample, especially if epithelium is sparse or absent, and characteristic calcifications are present in the mucin. The risk of coexisting DCIS is increased when the core biopsy

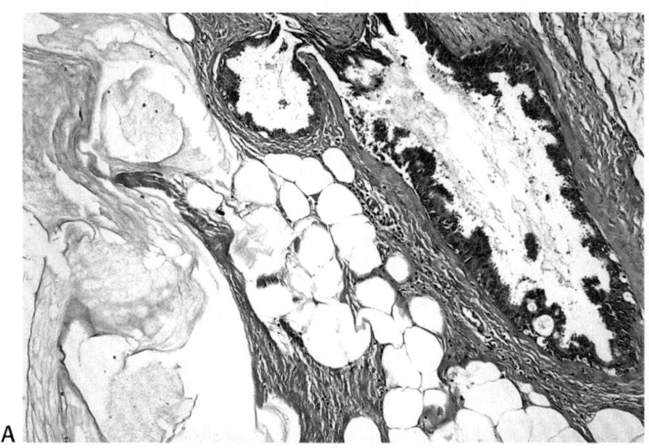

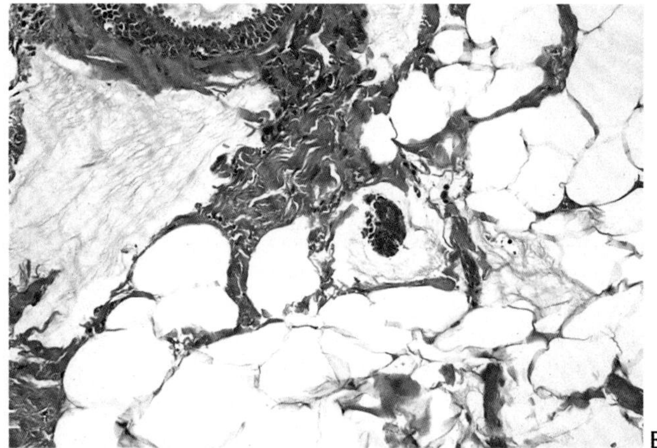

FIG. 18.34. ***Mucocele-like lesion with mucinous carcinoma.*** Both images are from the same specimen. **A:** Mucin in fat *(left)* and micropapillary intraductal carcinoma *(right)*. **B:** A cluster of carcinoma cells in mucin surrounded by fat, representing invasive mucinous carcinoma.

specimen shows ADH, or if the presenting signs include a mass lesion.[89] In a series reported by Carder et al.,[89] a total of 10 lesions with a core biopsy diagnosis of MML underwent surgical excision. Excision of atypical MMLs yielded one case of mucinous carcinoma, two DCIS, and one case of ADH. Excision of the nonatypical MMLs yielded two cases of ADH, one nonatypical MML, two cases with benign mucin cysts, and one case with stromal mucin. In a series by Leibman et al.,[98] 15 patients had a needle core biopsy diagnosis of benign MLL, including five patients with an atypical MML. Follow-up surgical excision was performed in four of six patients with a presurgical diagnosis of MML with atypia (five diagnosed at core biopsy and one at FNA). The surgical excision yielded DCIS in 3/4 (75%) of cases. On the basis of these findings, the authors concluded that surgical excision is recommended for all patients with benign MML at needle core biopsy. However, in this study, surgical excision was performed only for lesions with presurgical diagnosis of atypia, and clinical and radiologic follow-up was recommended for the seven patients with MML lacking atypia in the needle core biopsy material.

In the series by Ramsaroop et al.,[90] 5/12 MLLs diagnosed by needle core biopsy yielded carcinoma (four DCIS and one invasive carcinoma). The DCIS had low to intermediate nuclear grade and one was described as hypersecretory. However, the authors did not specify if the cases with upgrade were radiologically and pathologically concordant, and if the findings in the needle core biopsy material from cases with upgrade were atypical.

Needle core biopsy sampling of a nonatypical MLL usually yields variable amounts of clean mucin and a few benign cysts lined by flat epithelium. Sparse, histologically benign epithelial strips may be admixed with the mucin, as well as granular, powdery or coarse calcifications.

In some cases, it can be difficult to distinguish between a paucicellular mucinous carcinoma and stromal mucin because of artifactual disruption of a benign mucinous cyst in a needle core biopsy specimen. Before a diagnosis of MML can be rendered, it is recommended to evaluate deeper sections and even perform immunoperoxidase stains with CK AE1:3 to rule out the presence of epithelial cells admixed with mucin. If stromal mucin devoid of cells is present in a surgical excision specimen, it is recommended that additional tissue or the entire specimen be examined microscopically.

Stromal mucin devoid of cells is an exceedingly rare finding in a needle core biopsy, being found in only 0.32% of 4,297 breast needle core biopsy specimens in one retrospective series.[104] Few series[89,98,103,105–109] investigated the upgrade rate at surgical excision of MMLs at needle core biopsy, but only a few[104–108] have also assessed the radiologic–pathologic concordance of the target lesions, or correlated the surgical findings with the presence of atypia in the needle core biopsy material (Table 18.1).

In a series by Jaffer et al.,[109] 1/45 (2.2%) MLLs diagnosed by surgical excision contained DCIS and 7/45 (15.5%) had ADH. The authors reviewed the needle core biopsies of these cases, but did not specify how many showed epithelial atypia. Without this information, one cannot specifically assess the upgrade rate at surgical excision of needle core biopsy with or without epithelial atypia. Furthermore, the authors acknowledged that the pathologic findings at needle core biopsy of the only lesion with upgrade to DCIS "did not entirely correlate with the finding of suspicious calcifications."[106]

Renshaw[104] evaluated the findings at excision of 15 breast lesions with stromal mucin in a needle core biopsy. All of the seven lesions with a benign diagnosis at core biopsy were found to be benign in the surgical excision specimen, whereas each of the eight lesions with carcinoma in the core biopsy was confirmed as malignant in the excision. Wang et al.[105] conducted a similar study on 32 cases with diagnosis of a mucinous lesion at core biopsy. The index diagnosis was confirmed on review of the follow-up excision

TABLE 18.1 Findings at Surgical Excision of Lesions with Radiology-Pathology Concordance Yielding Mucin with or without Epithelial Atypia in a Needle Core Biopsy

		CBX without Atypia			CBX with Atypia			
Study	Total CBX with EXC	Cases	ADH at EXC/Cases (%)	Carcinoma at EXC/Cases (%)	Cases	Carcinoma at EXC/Cases (%)	Carcinoma at EXC/Total CBX	Total Patients with Carcinoma or ADH
Renshaw[104]	8	3	1/3 (33%)	0/3	5	0/5	0/8	6/8 (75%)
Wang[105]	11	7	0/7	0/7	4	0/4	0/11	4/11 (36%)
Begum[106]	23	10	0/10	1[a]/10 ([a]10%)	13	1/13 (7.6%)	2/23 (8.6%)	2[a]/23 (8.6%)
Sutton[108]	38	22	Not specified	0/22	16	5/16 (31%)	5/38 (13%)	5/38 (13%)
Edelweiss[107]	28	10	4/10 (40%)	0/10	18	4/18 (22%)	4/28 (14%)	8/28 (28%)
Total	108	52	5/30 (16.6%)	1[a]/52 (1.9%)	56	10/56 (17.3%)	11/100 (11%)	25/108 (23%)

[a]One case with discordant radiologic-pathologic findings.
CBX, core biopsy; EXC, surgical excision.

material in 29/32 patients (91%), and no residual mucinous lesion was present in the excision specimens from the remaining three patients (9%). None of the 7 lesions that yielded a benign or atypical diagnosis at needle core biopsy was upgraded to carcinoma. The authors concluded that "core biopsy is highly reliable for accurate diagnosis of mucinous lesions of the breast," and follow-up excision of lesions with stromal mucin and no atypia was not always necessary. Similar results were obtained by Begum et al.,[106] who analyzed 27 lesions with stromal mucin at needle core biopsy and follow-up surgical excision. The only case with upgrade in this series was radiologic–pathologic discordant. Edelweiss et al.[107] and Sutton et al.[108] also reported no upgrade to carcinoma at excision of radiologic–pathologic concordant lesions that had yielded stromal mucin but no cytologic atypia at needle core biopsy. The results of these studies emphasize the need for close clinical, radiologic, and pathologic correlation in the evaluation of any breast lesion undergoing needle core biopsy, and the value of surgical excision for any case with discordant imaging and pathologic findings.

These data demonstrate that either ADH or carcinoma, most often in the form of DCIS, is associated with a MLL in about 23% of cases (Table 18.1). The risk of upgrade to DCIS or invasive carcinoma for a MLL with atypia at needle core biopsy is about 17.8% (Table 18.1), consistent with the upgrade rate of ADH diagnosed in a needle core biopsy. Based on review of the recent literature, excision of lesions diagnosed as nonatypical MLL in a needle core biopsy with radiologic–pathologic concordant findings yielded ADH in 5/30 (16.6%) cases,[89,104–107] but there was no upgrade to carcinoma[89,103–108] (Table 18.1). Overall, these results demonstrate that excision of a MLL that shows no atypia in a needle core biopsy can be safely omitted if the radiologic and pathologic findings are concordant[104–108] (Table 18.1). Excisional biopsy is recommended for MLLs diagnosed by needle core biopsy, if the sample exhibits atypical hyperplasia or the radiologic and pathologic findings are discordant.[89,103,105–108]

DIFFERENTIAL DIAGNOSIS OF MUCINOUS LESIONS

Cystic Hypersecretory Lesions

Cystic hypersecretory lesions of the breast, encompassing cystic hypersecretory change, cystic hypersecretory hyperplasia (CHH), and cystic hypersecretory carcinoma, (see Chapter 24) may bear superficial similarity to MLLs because of the presence of cystically dilated duct spaces containing secretion, but the luminal contents are different. In histologic sections, mucin is pale gray to blue and translucent, whereas the secretion found in cystic hypersecretory lesions consists of uniformly gelatinous and eosinophilic material resembling thyroid colloid.[110–112] The dense hypersecretory material often has parallel lines of fracture, resulting in the characteristic pattern referred to as "Venetian blinds" shattering effect.

Secretory Carcinoma

Secretory carcinoma is an unusual distinct variant of breast carcinoma in which luminal and sometimes intracellular secretion is found[113,114] (see Chapter 22). It may sometimes be considered in the differential diagnosis of mucinous carcinoma. The latter is characterized by neoplastic epithelial clusters admixed with mucin pools, while the glands of secretory carcinoma contain intraluminal secretion that is amphophilic or pale to eosinophilic, and often bubbly in appearance.

Other Lesions

Several other breast lesions may also enter into the differential diagnosis of mucinous carcinoma. The mammary stroma can occasionally acquire a myxoid–mucoid quality, referred to as mucinosis. Nodular mucinosis of the breast is an extremely rare entity, usually presenting in young women in the subareolar region, and characterized pathologically as a myxoid mass composed microscopically of loosely placed spindle cells.[115] Myxoid stroma closely resembling mucin can occur in lesions such as a myxoid fibroadenoma, myxoma, and neurofibroma with prominent myxoid change. All these lesions, and especially myxoid fibroadenoma, can mimic mucinous carcinoma when only limited material is available for evaluation, such as a needle core biopsy or FNA material.[116,117] Mucoid stroma can also be encountered in phyllodes tumor, pleomorphic adenoma,[118] adenoid cystic carcinoma (AdCC), and metaplastic carcinoma. AdCC additionally demonstrates stromal acid mucopolysaccharide in the ductal lumina of cribriform epithelial islands.[119,120] Metaplastic breast carcinoma with myxoid matrix can focally resemble mucinous carcinoma, but usually has a greater degree of nuclear atypia. Squamous cell carcinoma (SQC) with prominent myxoid stroma is another extremely rare malignant breast tumor in which the stroma can be rich in sulfated mucopolysaccharides and mimic mucinous carcinoma.[121] Mucoepidermoid carcinoma features both mucinous cells and extracellular mucin, resembling its commoner counterpart in the salivary glands.[122]

Metastases in the breast can infrequently include tumors with mucinous elements. Tot[123] reported a unique case of metastatic chordoma that mimicked a primary mucinous breast carcinoma. Metastatic mucinous carcinoma in the breast from various extramammary sites has been reported (see Chapter 34).

Foreign material may also resemble extracellular mucin. Clues to the correct diagnosis include slightly different tinctorial quality, evidence of focal light refraction, and especially the presence of foreign-body-type giant-cell reaction,[124] but reactive changes are not always conspicuous. In such cases, obtaining complete and accurate clinical history is of foremost importance.

CYTOLOGY

The diagnosis of mucinous carcinoma may be suspected in material obtained by FNA.[125] Cytologic features diagnostic of mucinous breast carcinoma include high cellularity, numerous single cells or small clusters with mild to moderate nuclear atypia, and abundant background mucin (Figs. 18.35 and 18.36A). Although mucin is better detected by Romanovsky-type stain, it was also recognized in the Papanicolaou-stained aspirate.[64] Attention must be given to distinguishing mucin from lysed blood, interstitial fluid, necrotic debris, gel used during ultrasonographic examination, or protein such as albumin used to coat slides. However, the presence of mucin alone is not pathognomonic of mucinous carcinoma. There are numerous examples of benign mucin-producing lesions of the breast that would present with mucin on FNA, including MLLs, papillomas, and rarely fibroadenomas and papillary neoplasms.[51,126] Occasionally, myxoid material from an edematous fibroadenoma results in an aspirate that resembles mucinous carcinoma.[125,127] In one case, the FNA of a pleomorphic adenoma was erroneously interpreted as diagnostic of mucinous carcinoma.[118] The finding of spindly stromal cell nuclei in the myxoid material is suggestive of a fibroadenoma. However, stromal cells and capillaries may be found in mucin aspirated from a pure mucinous carcinoma (Fig. 18.36). A mucicarmine stain may be useful to confirm the presence of true mucin. Mucinous material can also be present in cysts within fibroepithelial lesions, and the aspirated material that is mucicarmine positive may simulate mucinous carcinoma.[116] Myxoid stroma associated with an inflammatory lesion such as a suture granuloma can also be confused with mucin in an aspiration cytology specimen.[128] Mucin may be found in the aspirate from an infiltrating duct carcinoma with mucinous differentiation.[129]

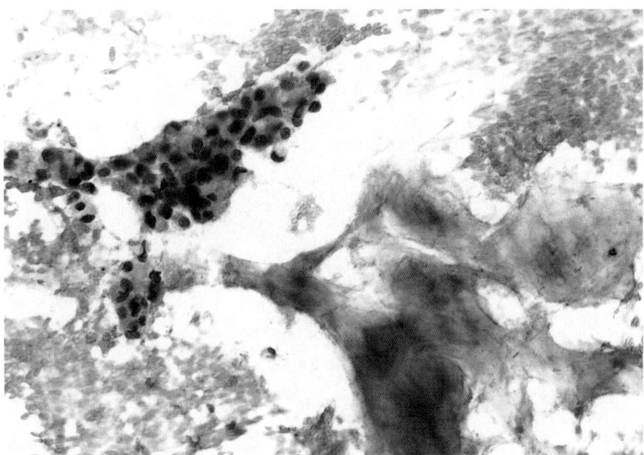

FIG. 18.35. ***Mucinous carcinoma, cytologic appearance.*** An irregular, cohesive cluster of carcinoma cells [*left*] and mucin [*right*] surrounded by red blood cells.

Difficulty is also encountered in the distinction between benign MLL and hypocellular mucinous carcinoma in FNA samples[18,130] (Fig. 18.37), as abundant extracellular mucin can be present in the aspirate from both lesions. Several studies have pointed out the lower cellular content, cellular cohesion, and lack of cytologic atypia in specimens from benign MLLs.[91,93,130] Because the cytologic atypia of mucinous lesions can be very subtle, it can be difficult to assess in an FNA sample. In contrast to needle core biopsy, any breast lesion that yields mucin in an FNA sample should be excised, even in the absence of epithelial atypia.

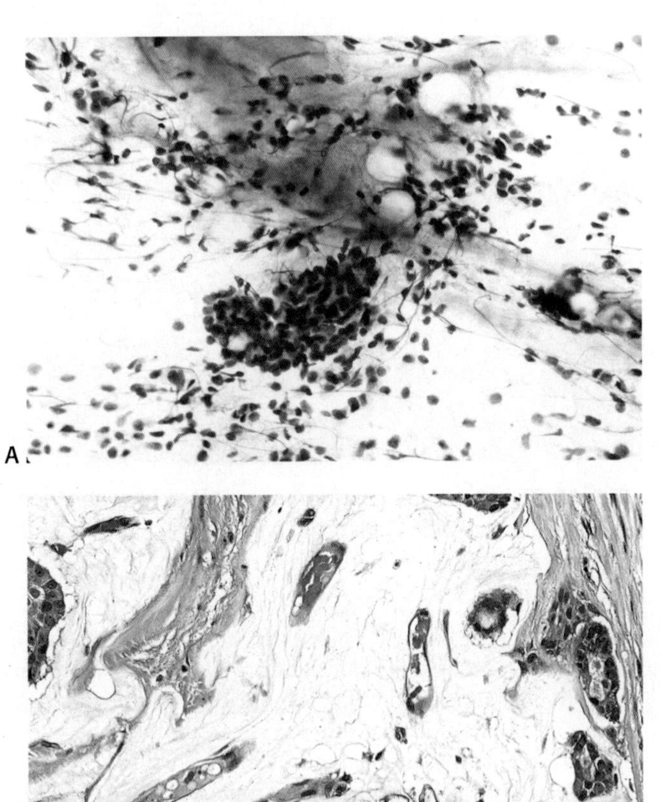

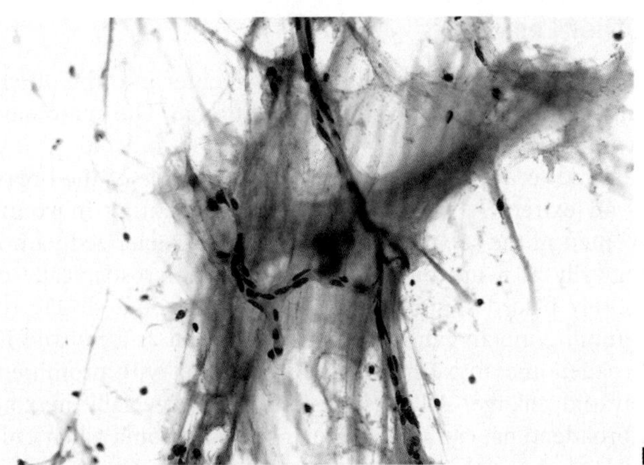

FIG. 18.36. *Mucinous carcinoma, cytologic appearance.* **A:** A FNA sample showing cohesive and disaggregated tumor cells associated with mucin. **B:** Another cytology specimen showing capillaries in the mucin from a mucinous carcinoma. Carcinomatous epithelium is absent in this region of the specimen. **C:** Note the presence of capillaries in the midst of mucin in this histological section from a pure mucinous carcinoma.

Rare cases of mucinous carcinoma associated with psammoma bodies in an FNA sample have been reported.[63,64] Jayaram et al.[63] and Pillai et al.[64] each encountered one case of pure mucinous carcinoma with psammoma bodies in FNA material.

In FNA material, mucinous carcinoma consists of tumor clusters admixed with mucin that can be vascularized. The background mucin shows metachromasia in air-dried Diff-Quick-stained smears. A FNA sample from a mucinous carcinoma is recognized as positive or suspicious for

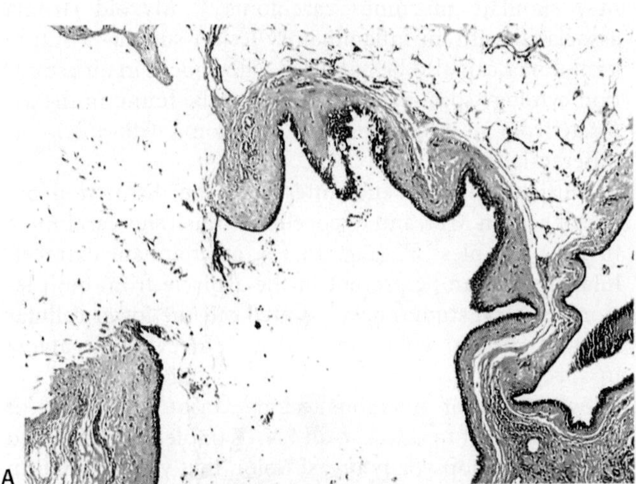

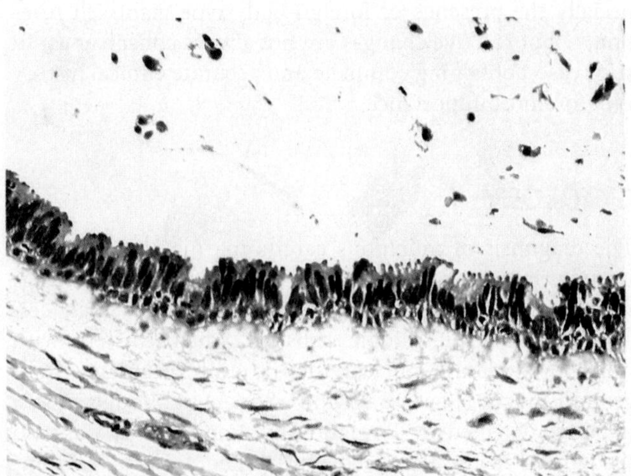

FIG. 18.37. *Mucocele-like lesion, cytologic appearance.* **A:** A ruptured cyst with extruded mucin (*upper left*). **B:** Columnar cell epithelium in the cyst with a myoepithelial cell layer. **C,D:** The FNA specimen with flat sheets of cytologically benign epithelial cells surrounded by mucin.

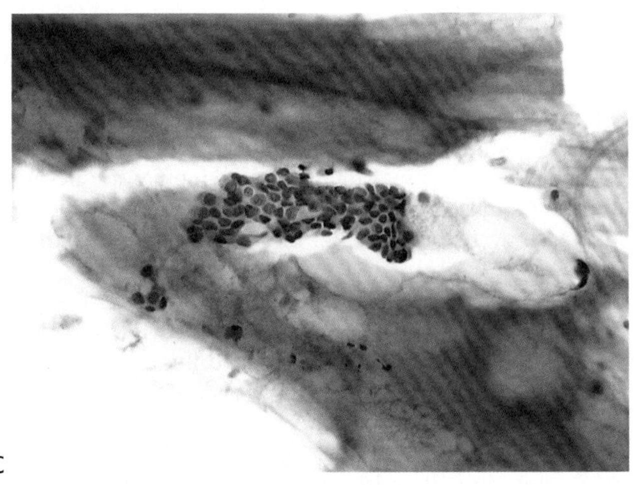
C

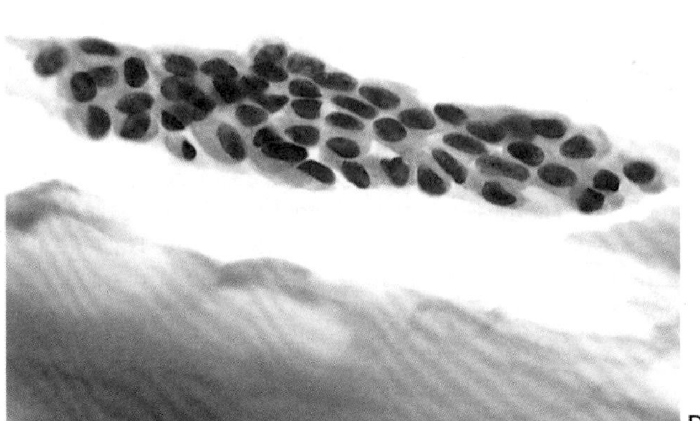
D

FIG. 18.37. *(Continued)*

malignant cells in 84.4% of cases,[131] but the reported accuracy in diagnosis ranges from 27.2%[131] to 56%[132] of cases. In contrast, the reported sensitivity and accuracy of core biopsy in the diagnosis of mucinous carcinoma are nearly 100%.[104,132]

HISTOCHEMISTRY AND IMMUNOHISTOCHEMISTRY

The amount of intracellular mucin in mucinous carcinomas is variable. Although some mucinous carcinomas have prominent signet ring cells (Fig. 18.16), often only a small proportion of the tumor cells can be shown to contain mucin by histochemical procedures. Mucinous carcinomas contain acid and neutral mucopolysaccharides.[133–135] Despite the abundant mucin present in mucocele-like tumors, intracellular mucin is not demonstrable unless there is associated carcinoma (Fig. 18.38).

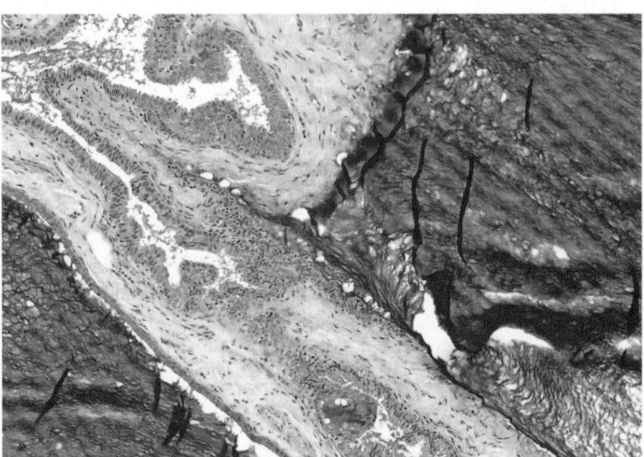

FIG. 18.38. ***Mucocele-like lesion, mucicarmine stain.*** Strong staining of mucin is seen in a cyst (*left*) and in extravasated mucin (*right*).

Mucins

Mucins are high-molecular-weight glycoproteins that can be cell membrane bound with a transmembrane location (including MUC1, MUC4, MUC16) or secreted (including MUC2, MUC5AC, MUC5B, MUC6). The expression of mucin genes and their corresponding mucin glycoproteins differs in mucinous and nonmucinous carcinomas.[136] Using IHC and *in situ* hybridization, O'Connell et al.[137] found that mucinous carcinomas were characterized by increased MUC2 and MUC5 protein expression and decreased MUC1, whereas nonmucinous carcinomas featured increased MUC1 but no increases in MUC2 and MUC5. Tumors with mucinous and nonmucinous components exhibited MUC patterns corresponding to these respective elements. Hyperplasia and intraductal carcinoma from breasts with mucinous carcinoma also showed increased MUC2 and MUC5 expression, an observation interpreted as evidence of a field effect in these patients. Subsequent studies have documented that mucinous breast carcinoma expresses MUC2 in over 80% of cases.[138–140] In the study by Kato et al.,[141] intracytoplasmic MUC2 was present in 100% pure mucinous carcinomas, as well as in 70% of the associated DCIS.

Intracytoplasmic MUC2 was also found in the mucinous and nonmucinous component of all cases of mixed mucinous carcinoma. MUC2 is a gel-forming intestinal-type secretory mucin. It is part of the extracellular mucin that surrounds the malignant clusters of mucinous carcinoma. It possibly interferes with tumor infiltration, thereby contributing to the indolent behavior of mucinous carcinoma.[139,142] Additional theories for the excellent prognosis of pure mucinous carcinomas include decreased tumor cell burden particularly in the paucicellular variant, diminished angiogenesis, and increased cytotoxic T-lymphocyte activity induced by extracellular MUC2-positive mucin.[137] Positivity for MUC2 has also been identified in 12/15 (80%) mucinous columnar cell lesions.[100]

In addition to MUC2, MUC6, a gastric, pyloric gland-type secretory mucin, is also expressed in over 50% of mucinous carcinoma.[61,137,138,140]

MUC1 is a membrane bound mucin detected in most epithelial cells. An early study by Yonezawa and Matsukita[143] found that MUC1 was widely expressed in mucinous as well as in nonmucinous carcinomas.[143] Kato et al.[141] found MUC1 on the free surface of 23/26 (88%) pure mucinous carcinomas, and in 60% of associated DCIS. In 7 mixed mucinous carcinomas, MUC1 was present on the free surface of the mucinous component in 5/7 (71%) cases and of the ductal NOS component in 2/7 (28%) cases.

MUC1/CORE is a nonglycosylated form of MUC1, and MUC1/HMFG-1 is a fully glycosylated form. These glycoforms have been correlated with a worse prognosis in gastric[144] and colorectal carcinomas.[145] A study by Matsukita et al.[139] has reported that MUC1/CORE and MUC1/HMFG-1 are significantly lower in mucinous than in nonmucinous carcinomas. In particular, mucinous carcinomas showed MUC1/CORE staining of moderate intensity in 24% of cases and weak in 52%, whereas 48% nonmucinous carcinomas had moderate staining and 50% weak staining. Staining for MUC1/HMFG-1 was moderate in 18% of mucinous carcinomas and weak in 47%, whereas it was moderate in 78% and weak in 20% of nonmucinous carcinomas. The low expression of these two MUC1 glycoforms might contribute to the relatively indolent behavior of mucinous carcinomas. Schmitt et al.[146] developed a monoclonal antibody to MUC5, which was reactive with 4 (6%) of 66 nonmucinous ductal carcinomas, an observation that suggested that MUC5 expression is not entirely specific for the mucinous type of mammary carcinoma. In a study by Matsukita et al.,[139] the expression of MUC5AC, a gastric, surface-type secretory mucin, was low in both mucinous and nonmucinous carcinomas.

External lamina and basement membrane were not detected around tumor clusters of mucinous carcinoma,[142] a result that is consistent with everted polarity of the tumor cells.

ER, PR, Androgen Receptor, HER2, and Ki67

About 60% of pure mucinous carcinomas were ER positive when studied biochemically,[147,148] but immunohistochemical studies have shown receptor activity in nearly all cases.[20,22,26,72,149] In a review of SEER data for 1992 to 2007,[12] information about ER and PR status was available for 6,561 mucinous carcinomas and 84% were ER+/PR+, 12.7% ER+/PR−, 0.5% ER−/PR+, and 2.8% ER−/PR−. Diab et al.[20] found nuclear reactivity for ER in 92% of pure mucinous carcinomas and for PR in 68%. Cao et al.[22] found ER positivity in 73.4% cases, and PR positivity in 65.4%. The rate of hormone positivity was significantly higher in mucinous carcinoma than in control tumors ($p < 0.001$).

Ranade et al.[26] reported that 95% of pure mucinous carcinomas were ER positive, 84% were PR positive, and 9% were HER2 positive. In the same series, 91% of mixed mucinous carcinomas showed positivity for ER, 87% for PR, and 33% for HER2. Lacroix-Triki et al.[34] documented ER in 100% of 36 pure mucinous carcinomas, and PR in 85.7%. Similar patterns of ER immunoreactivity were observed in nonargyrophilic and argyrophilic mucinous carcinomas, in mixed mucinous carcinomas, and in type A and type B mucinous carcinomas. One case had equivocal HER2 (2+) staining and was found to be HER2 amplified by chromogenic ISH. Overall the majority of mucinous carcinomas are negative for HER2, but a small proportion of mucinous carcinomas may also overexpress HER2. In a series of pure mucinous carcinomas in women 40 years old or younger,[150] 21/21 (100%) tumors with available information were ER positive, 17/21 (81%) were PR positive, and 1/21 (5%) was HER2 equivocal, with HER2 2+ staining and fluorescence *in situ* hybridization (FISH) *HER2/CEP17* gene ratio of 2. Diab et al.[20] reported immunoreactivity for HER2 in less than 5% of pure mucinous carcinomas.

In one study,[151] androgen receptor (AR) was positive in 5/301 (1.7%) mucinous carcinomas. Cho and Hsu[152] documented significantly lower expression of AR in mucinous carcinomas than in invasive ductal carcinomas NOS (21.7% vs. 51.4%, respectively; $p = 0.01$). Honma et al.[75] found that 3/6 (50%) mucinous carcinomas were AR positive. Sapino et al.[153] noted that AR showed diffuse positivity in all (9/9) mucinous carcinomas with neuroendocrine and apocrine differentiation, whereas only 3/16 (19%) cases of neuroendocrine mucinous carcinomas without apocrine differentiation were AR positive, and had weak staining limited to fewer than 5% of the cells.

Ki67 staining was reported to be as low in 20/26 (77%) and moderate in 6/26 (23%) pure mucinous carcinomas studied by Kato et al.[141] In another study, Lacroix-Triki et al.[72] reported that Ki67 was low (<10%) in 91.4% (32/35) cases, intermediate in 5.7% (2/35), and high (>30%) in only one case (2.9%). The mean and median percentages of Ki67-positive tumor cells were 16.8 and 15, respectively, in a study by Alvarenga et al.[154]

WT1

Nuclear staining for WT1, a marker associated with serous ovarian carcinoma, has been detected in mammary mucinous carcinomas. In a series by Domfeh et al.,[155] WT1 was present in 22/34 (65%) pure mucinous carcinomas and 11/33 (33%) mixed mucinous carcinomas. WT1 reactivity was weak in 7 (33%) pure mucinous carcinomas, moderate in 13 (62%), and strong in 1 (5%). WT1 expression was similar in the mucinous and the nonmucinous components. WT1 staining was significantly associated with low tumor grade ($p = 0.01$) and low cellularity ($p = 0.01$). Another study[72] found WT1 staining in 21/33 (63.7%) pure mucinous carcinomas.

Other Markers

Lacroix-Triki et al.[72] reported that cyclin D1 had a low or intermediate staining score in 8/34 pure mucinous carcinomas (23.5%) and that it was high in 18/34 (53%). Cortactin, a protein that promotes actin polymerization and branching, showed intermediate positivity in 22/32 (68.8%) cases, low positivity in 6/32 (18.7%), and high positivity in 4/32 (12.5%). Bcl-2 was positive in 32/34 (97.1%) cases. Most tumors (32/35, 94.1%) were p53 negative. All cases had membranous reactivity for E-cadherin and were negative for the basal markers CK5/6, CK14, and CK17 and epidermal growth factor receptors (EGFRs). Others reported immunoreactivity for basal cytokerating.[156,157] Lacroix-Triki et al[72] also observed positivity for smooth muscle actin (SMA) in 5/23 (22%) cases. Only rare cases of pure mucinous carcinomas are positive for p53.[72] Diab et al.[20] reported immunoreactivity for EGFR in less than 5% of pure mucinous carcinomas. Although carcinomas that arise because of alterations in DNA mismatch repair secondary to MSI in organs such as colon and ovary often show mucinous features, Lacroix-Triki et al.[72] found no evidence of MSI in 35 mucinous breast carcinomas and 35 histologic grade- and ER-matched invasive ductal carcinomas NOS using immunohistochemical stains for four MSI markers (MSH2, MSH6, MLH1, and PMS2). These results were further confirmed by polymerase chain reaction (PCR) analysis of a subset of nine mammary mucinous carcinomas.

Neuroendocrine Differentiation

The presence of argyrophilic Grimelius-positive granules in mucinous carcinoma cells has been noted in several repo rts.[14,15,66,159,160] These cytoplasmic particles with the ultrastructural features of endocrine secretory granules have been detected in 25% to 50% of mucinous carcinomas. Mucinous carcinomas that contain these granules tend to occur more frequently in elderly women, and the tumor cells often grow in clumps, sheets, or trabeculae, which sometimes suggest an endocrine growth pattern. Fentiman et al.[25] found Grimelius-positive staining more frequently in pure (25%) than in mixed mucinous carcinomas. The granules of some mucinous carcinomas contain immunohistochemically detectable serotonin[161] as well as somatostatin and gastrin.[161] The tumors are also positive for neuron-specific enolase (NSE).[14,161] Scopsi et al.[14] reported finding NSE, synaptophysin, and chromogranins A and B in all of the argyrophilic mucinous carcinomas in their series. In the same study, they detected NSE reactivity in 75% and synaptophysin reactivity in 39% of nonargyrophilic, granin-negative tumors.

Immunoreactivity for S-100 and carcinoembryonic antigen (CEA) was found in almost all argyrophilic mucinous carcinomas by Coady et al.[133] About half of duct carcinomas with mixed mucinous differentiation were CEA positive, but they were almost devoid of S-100. Nonargyrophilic pure mucinous carcinomas all lacked S-100 and only one was positive for CEA. These authors also found abundant elastic fibers in the stroma of argyrophilic mucinous carcinomas, whereas these fibers were sparse or absent in the stroma of nonargyrophilic mucinous tumors. In three studies, the presence of argyrophilic granules was not prognostically significant in pure mucinous tumors or in infiltrating duct carcinomas with focal mucinous differentiation.[8,14,133]

Immunoprofile of Cystic Papillary Mucinous Carcinoma

Cystic papillary mucinous carcinomas have a very different immunoprofile from all other mammary mucinous carcinomas, as they are typically ER and PR negative,[74–78,80,81,83,84] Only one ER-positive case has been reported.[79] One tumor tested for both ER-alpha and ER-beta showed no expression of either receptor.[75] HER2 is also negative in this type of carcinoma, except for one case with immunoreactivity for HER2 and *HER2* gene amplification by FISH analysis.[81] Cystic papillary mucinous carcinomas have no immunoreactivity for chromogranin and synaptophysin, CDX2 and CK20. Positivity for CK5/6 has been described in two cases,[83,84] and one case was also positive for EGFR.[83] p53 staining has been assessed in a handful of cases and has been reported as positive by some authors[75,76] and negative by others.[78,83]

ELECTRON MICROSCOPY

Intracellular mucin can be demonstrated by electron microscopy.[162–165] Several types of cytoplasmic granules have been described ultrastructurally in mucinous carcinomas.[163] Small (100 to 500 nm) and large (0.5 to 1.5 μm) dense core granules were found in tumors that contained argyrophilic granules, and they were absent in almost all nonargyrophilic lesions. This observation appears to confirm the findings of Capella et al.[66] Tumor cells in mucinous carcinoma reportedly contain abundant cytoplasmic filaments with a perinuclear distribution.[66,164] They may also exhibit luminal differentiation characterized by microvilli and well-formed intercellular junctions.[163,164] Basal lamina and myoepithelial cells are absent.[164]

GENETICS AND MOLECULAR STUDIES

The ploidy of mucinous carcinoma has been studied by flow cytometry. Pure mucinous carcinomas were reported to be diploid in 96% and 78% of cases, respectively.[20,166] Only 42% (8 of 19) of duct carcinomas with mucinous differentiation were diploid, with the majority described as aneuploid.[166] Diab et al.[20] reported that 83% of mucinous carcinomas had low S-phase, 10% were intermediate, and 7% were high.

Lacroix-Triki et al.[72] investigated the genomic profiles of pure and mixed mucinous carcinomas of the breast and found that these tumors have genetic aberrations distinct from those of grade- and ER-matched invasive ductal carcinoma NOS. These investigators used high-resolution microarray-based comparative genomic hybridization (CGH) to study microdissected samples from 15 pure mucinous carcinomas, 7 mixed mucinous breast carcinomas, and 30 grade- and ER-matched invasive ductal carcinomas NOS. The mucinous and nonmucinous components of mixed mucinous carcinomas were microdissected and analyzed separately. Pure mucinous carcinomas had a relatively low level of genetic instability, with a median of 19.5% chromosomal alterations that were similar in type A and type B tumors. Most tumors (60%) had a "simplex" pattern of genomic alteration, and 40% showed a "firestorm" pattern. Recurrent amplifications at 11q13.2–q13.4 (two cases) and 20q13.2 (two cases) were validated by FISH using probes specific for genes found at these loci, including *CTTN* (cortactin), *CCND1* (cyclin D1), and *ZNF217* (zinc-finger protein 217). Unsupervised hierarchical cluster analysis revealed that pure mucinous carcinomas were homogeneous and preferentially clustered together, separately from invasive ductal carcinomas NOS, with the exception of three tumors (one *CCND1*-amplified Type A carcinoma, one type B carcinoma, and one type AB carcinoma. Gains of 1q and 16p and losses of 16q and 22q were less common in mucinous carcinomas than grade- and ER-matched invasive ductal carcinoma NOS, and this difference was most striking in low-grade tumors. In particular, 14 cases of grade I and grade II pure mucinous carcinomas consistently lacked concurrent 1q+ and 16q−, whereas 16/28 (57%) invasive ductal carcinomas NOS of similar histologic grade had both chromosomal alterations ($p < 0.001$). The mucinous and nonmucinous components of mixed mucinous carcinomas clustered together in all but two cases, and both components clustered with mucinous carcinomas, suggesting that mixed mucinous carcinomas are genetically more similar to pure mucinous carcinomas than to invasive ductal carcinomas NOS. No characteristic pattern of genomic amplification was identified: *HER2* and *FGFR1* gene amplification were each encountered in one pure and two mixed mucinous carcinomas, *CCND1* amplification in two pure and two mixed mucinous carcinomas, and *ZNF217* amplification in two pure and one mixed mucinous carcinomas.

Weigelt et al.[73] used genome-wide oligonucleotide microarray analysis to study 10 type A and 8 type B pure mucinous carcinomas, 6 neuroendocrine carcinomas (defined as tumors positive for a neuroendocrine marker in >50% of tumor cells), and 91 grade-matched invasive ductal carcinomas NOS. Except for three type A mucinous tumors, all mucinous and neuroendocrine carcinomas clustered together and separately from invasive ductal carcinomas NOS when analyzed by unsupervised hierarchical clustering. In particular, type B mucinous carcinomas and neuroendocrine carcinomas were closely intermingled, whereas type A mucinous carcinomas formed a tighter cluster ($p < 10^{-6}$). Compared with invasive carcinomas NOS, mucinous carcinomas and neuroendocrine carcinomas exhibited upregulation of *ESR1*, *BCL2*, *ERBB4*, *TFF3*, keratin 18, and *CDKN1A* (p21) and downregulation of genes encoding matrix metalloproteinases, insulin-like growth factor–binding proteins, laminins, *HER2/ERB2*, and basal keratins 5 and 14. Further transcript analysis revealed differential expression of some genes in mucinous A versus mucinous B and neuroendocrine carcinomas, with upregulation of genes for extracellular matrix (i.e., collagens and fibulins), *TGFB1*, keratin 7 and of genes part of the "integrin signalling" canonical pathway in type A tumors.

Phosphatidylinositol-4,5-bisphosphate 3-kinase, catalytic subunit alpha (PIK3CA) is a key molecule in epithelial cell signal transduction, and alterations of the PIK3CA pathway secondary to mutations of the corresponding gene are common in breast carcinoma. Kehr et al.[167] performed PIK3CA genotyping for a panel of point mutations (>321 mutations in 30 genes) in 29 pure invasive mucinous carcinomas and 9 invasive ductal carcinomas with mucinous differentiation using a multiplex PCR panel with mass spectroscopy readout.[167] When available, they also studied the associated DCIS, hyperplasia, or columnar cell lesions (25 lesions in total). PIK3CA hotspot mutations were tested by direct sequencing of 3 invasive cases and 15 DCIS/proliferative lesions. The authors found PIK3CA point mutations in 35% of invasive ductal carcinomas NOS, but not in mucinous breast carcinoma, a finding that suggests a unique pathogenesis for mucinous carcinomas. PIK3CA hotspot point mutations were detected in 3/14 DCIS, in 2/3 cases each of ADH and usual ductal hyperplasia (UDH), and in 1/5 cases of columnar cell change associated with mucinous carcinoma. The authors speculated that PIK3CA mutations may play a role in the pathogenesis of intraductal epithelial proliferations associated with mucinous carcinoma, even though such alterations are not present in the invasive component.

TREATMENT AND PROGNOSIS

The relatively favorable prognosis commonly ascribed to mucinous carcinoma is supported by numerous studies.[4,6,7,11,12,14,15,21,22,27,28,35,59,60,166,168,169] Because the tumor is infrequent, few investigators have been able to assemble substantial numbers of patients, and even fewer studies have used a uniform definition for the diagnosis of pure mucinous carcinomas. Pure mucinous carcinomas tend to be smaller than tumors with a mixed pattern, and these patients have a lower frequency of axillary lymph node (ALN) metastases.[6–8,14,15,23,85,160,170] In a review of SEER data for T1a and T1b breast carcinomas, Maibenco et al.[171] found that the rate of lymph node involvement for small (<1 cm) mucinous carcinomas was 2.9%, with no lymph node metastases among 58 T1a tumors and only 3.5% in 256 T1b mucinous carcinoma. Larger tumor size correlates significantly with lymph node involvement.[21,35] The reported frequencies of negative ALNs in patients with pure mucinous carcinoma are 71%,[7] 74%,[35] 76%,[169] 81%,[27] 81.5%,[26] 81.7%,[28] 82.8%,[22] 83%,[35] 97%,[160] and 100%.[45] Most series of patients with duct carcinoma with a mucinous component have had at least 50% node-negative patients.[7,14,85,159,170] In an exceptional study, only 28% of patients with these lesions had negative nodes.[15] Overall, patients with pure mucinous carcinoma are candidates for axillary staging by sentinel lymph node mapping, but it is unclear in which situations nodal evaluation may be deferred. In the series by Barkley et al.,[35] node-positive patients had a mean tumor size of 2.7 cm compared with 1.5 cm for node-negative patients ($p = 0.0003$), and none of the 31 patients with tumor size smaller than 1 cm had known lymph node metastasis.

Micro- or macrometastases were present in sentinel lymph nodes from 7% of patients with mucinous carcinoma treated at different European centers,[172] although the protocols of sentinel lymph node histologic analysis were not uniform among the different institutions. Ranade et al.[26] reported that 18.5% of pure mucinous carcinomas had sentinel lymph node metastases versus 16% of mixed mucinous carcinomas. In this study, level sections and CK stains were obtained for all sentinel lymph nodes negative in the initial hematoxylin–eosin (H&E)-stained slides. Nonsentinel lymph nodes were positive in 14% of pure mucinous tumors versus 39% of mixed mucinous carcinomas.

In older series, most patients with pure mucinous carcinoma have been treated by mastectomy. Some very elderly women were treated by local excision or simple mastectomy.[20] In more recent series, the surgical treatment of mucinous carcinomas has consisted of breast-conserving surgery in 15.4%,[28] 20.7%,[22] 53.4%,[27] 67%,[35] and 81.1%[169] cases, whereas mastectomy was performed in 18.8%,[169] 33%,[35] 46.6%,[27] 72.1%,[28] and 79.3%[22] cases.

A few patients have done well after partial mastectomy alone,[5] but most patients treated with breast-conserving surgery also received radiation therapy.[9] In recent series, adjuvant radiotherapy was administered in 35.4%,[28] 64%,[35] 64.4%,[27] 74.8%,[169] and 90%[168] of cases. Overall, recent studies have confirmed that breast conservation therapy is an appropriate treatment for the majority of patients with early-stage mucinous carcinomas.[168]

Hormonal therapy was administered to 41%,[168] 66%,[28] 75.1%,[22] 75.5%,[169] and 86.6%[27] of patients with pure mucinous carcinomas, as well as to 96.1% of patients with mixed mucinous carcinoma.[27] Barkely et al.[35] specified that hormonal therapy alone was used in 54% of cases, and in combination with chemotherapy in 30%. Follow-up analysis of pure mucinous carcinomas in one series found that systemic adjuvant therapy is not necessarily indicated for node-negative pure mucinous carcinomas 3 cm or less in diameter.[173] The use of adjuvant chemotherapy for treatment of mucinous carcinomas has been reported in only 13%,[168] 10.5%,[169] and 3%[35] of patients in three series from Western countries, but appears to be more common in Asia, where three series reported its use in 40.8%,[27] 62.5%,[22] and 63.7%[28] of patients. Nonetheless, patients with pure mucinous carcinomas still received chemotherapy significantly less frequently than patients with mixed mucinous carcinomas (40.8% vs. 75%, $p < 0.001$).[27] In a study by Nagao et al.,[174] the clinical response in 12 mucinous carcinomas treated with neoadjuvant chemotherapy was significantly poorer than for invasive ductal carcinomas NOS. In contrast to invasive carcinomas NOS, the mean tumor size of mucinous carcinoma was only minimally reduced when compared with the size before treatment, and there were no cases of pathologic complete response. The correlation of poor response to neoadjuvant treatment with mucinous subtype was confirmed on multivariate analysis. Baretta et al.[175] reported the case of woman with an ER-, PR-, and HER2-positive mixed mucinous carcinoma of the breast with liver metastases at presentation. Treatment with chemotherapy and HER2-targeted therapy led to resolution of the hepatic disease, but extensive residual invasive ductal carcinoma with abundant stromal mucin was present in the mastectomy specimen obtained post chemotherapy. As stated by Nagao et al.,[174] because of the reported good prognosis of mucinous carcinoma and poor response to neoadjuvant chemotherapy, the latter is probably not needed.

When compared with patients who have infiltrating duct carcinoma with a mucinous component and with those who have infiltrating duct carcinoma, women with pure mucinous carcinoma have had a better relapse-free survival (RFS) 5 and 10 years after mastectomy.[6,7,14,19,59,60,170,176]

In a series of 61 patients treated by lumpectomy,[168] 90% received radiotherapy, 41% hormonal therapy, and 13% chemotherapy. Local recurrence and locoregional recurrence rates were both 5%, significantly lower than 8% and 10%, respectively, for invasive ductal carcinoma NOS, and also lower than for tubular carcinoma (both 13%). The disease-free survival (DFS) was 91.6% at 5 years and 75.3% at 10 years. The overall survival (OS) rate was 91.8% at 5 years and 74.5% at 10 years. In this study, the authors found no benefit of chemotherapy in patients with mucinous carcinoma. In a study based on SEER data by Di Saverio et al.,[21] adjuvant radiotherapy was associated with a small survival advantage on univariate analysis, but was not found to be significant on multivariate analysis.

In older series, 5-year survival after the treatment of pure mucinous carcinoma by mastectomy has been 84% disease-free,[8] 86% alive,[7] and 87% disease-free.[6] Norris and Taylor[5] reported an 80% 10-year survival. In their series, two of six patients with pure mucinous carcinoma who died of disease had a nonmucinous carcinoma of their opposite breast, which might have been responsible for the fatal outcome. Komaki et al.[85] described a 90% 10-year survival for pure mucinous carcinoma. The 10-year survival for corresponding patients with infiltrating duct carcinoma with a mucinous component was 60%. In another series, the 15-year DFS for pure mucinous and infiltrating duct carcinoma with a mucinous component was 85% and 63%, respectively.[15] The "20-year cumulative corrected survival rate" for pure mucinous carcinoma was 79% ± 11%.[15] An analysis of SEER data between 1973 and 2002[21] showed that 10-, 15-, and 20-year survival for 11,422 patients with pure mucinous carcinoma was 89%, 85%, and 81%, respectively, compared with 82% (5 year), 72% (10 year), 66% (15 year), and 62% (20 year) for 338,479 patients with invasive ductal carcinoma NOS. In this epidemiologic study, there were no significant differences in OS. Scopsi et al.[14] reported no deaths due to disease among 25 patients with node-negative pure mucinous carcinoma. In the same study, "there were no significant differences in OS rate" when node-positive patients with pure mucinous and nonmucinous carcinomas were compared. In a series of patients treated at a European center between 1997 and 2005,[177] 143 patients with mucinous carcinoma had 93% 5-year DFS and 96.3% OS. The DFS of mucinous and invasive ductal carcinomas of similar ER, PR, and HER2 status were not significantly different, but in this study mucinous carcinomas had a worse OS compared with ER+/PR+ and HER2− invasive ductal carcinomas (hazard ratio = 2.96; 95% confidence interval, 1.26 to 6.95; $p = 0.01$).

Major prognostic factors that are relevant for most types of breast carcinoma also apply to pure mucinous carcinoma.[6,15] Di Saverio et al.[21] found that nodal status was the most significant prognostic factor on multivariate analysis. Other significant parameters included age at diagnosis, tumor size, PR status, and nuclear grade. Recurrence is least likely with smaller tumors and the absence of lymph node metastases.[35] The presence of microcalcifications was associated with a relatively favorable outcome by Norris and Taylor.[5] The prognostic significance of endocrine differentiation in mucinous carcinomas has not been sufficiently investigated to be considered a standard prognostic feature.

In an analysis of factors affecting breast cancer lethality by Chen et al.,[178] only 8.2% of patients with mucinous carcinoma had lymph node involvement, and mucinous subtype was an independent factor significantly associated with reduced patient mortality ($p < 0.0001$). Based on mathematical analysis of comparative data for mucinous carcinoma and other subtypes of breast carcinoma, the authors concluded that ". . . cancer cells in patients with mucinous carcinoma have approximately half the chance of spreading to the periphery and causing death as the cancer cells in patients with ductal carcinoma."[178] Late systemic recurrences have been described after mastectomy in patients with mucinous carcinoma.[4,19,59,60,173,179] Geschickter[4] stated that "a period of 5 to 10 years of freedom from symptoms after treatment does not necessarily indicate permanent cure." He found that 14 of 59 patients had recurrences 6 to 18 years after diagnosis. In another series with a mean follow-up of 16 years, 27% of 41 patients with pure colloid carcinoma died of breast carcinoma, with 42% of the deaths occurring 12 years or more after diagnosis[19] (Fig. 18.39). Clayton[179] found that the median survival of patients who died of colloid carcinoma was 11.3 years after mastectomy. Some of the longest intervals to recurrence have been 25[180] and 30 years.[181] However, some studies have not observed a predilection for late recurrence[18,182] or late death due to disease[15] in women with small, pure mucinous carcinoma.

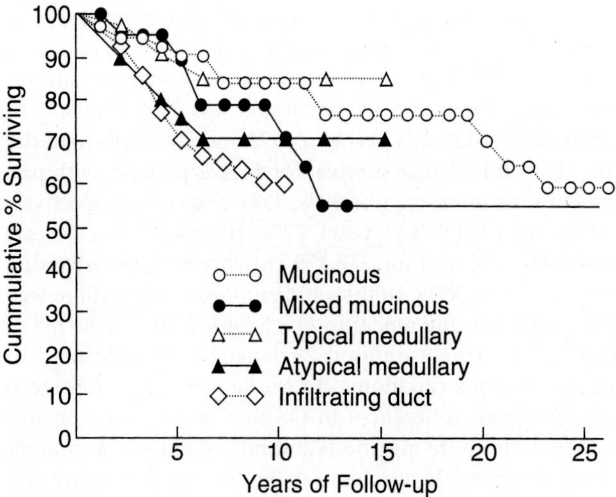

FIG. 18.39. ***Mucinous carcinoma, survival analysis.*** Life table analysis of survival comparing patients with mucinous, medullary, and duct carcinoma, not stratified by stage at diagnosis. Patients with mucinous and medullary carcinoma had equally favorable survival rates for 10 years of follow-up. Note the progressive decline in survival for mucinous carcinoma patients after 10 years.

Combined data from two institutions include 10 patients with mucinous carcinoma who remained disease-free after excision and radiotherapy with a median follow-up of 79 months.[183] A series of 1,008 women treated by breast conservation with radiotherapy at Yale University from 1970 to 1990 included 16 patients with mucinous carcinoma.[184] After a median follow-up of 11.2 years, there were no breast recurrences, and one patient developed a systemic recurrence 11 years after initial therapy.

A review of 111 patients with mucinous carcinoma was performed by Barkley et al.[35] Most patients (64%) underwent breast conservation therapy with adjuvant radiotherapy. Fourteen of 96 (13%) patients with lymph node evaluation had lymph node metastasis. After a median follow-up time of 63 months (range 2 to 116), there were no known breast cancer–related deaths. One patient had a local recurrence, three patients had distant recurrences, and one had both local and distant recurrent disease. In this study, patients with or without recurrent disease did not differ significantly in terms of tumor size; node involvement; ER, PR, and HER2 status; adjuvant chemotherapy; radiotherapy; or endocrine therapy.[35] In the studies by Diab et al.[20] and Vo et al.,[168] patients with node-positive mucinous carcinoma of the breast were significantly more likely to develop recurrent disease. Komenaka et al.[9] showed that the number of involved ALNs was the only significant predictor of patient death ($p = 0.02$). These results were also confirmed by Di Saverio et al.,[21] who identified in his large retrospective analysis of 11,422 pure mucinous carcinoma patients that positive nodal status appeared to be the most significant predictor of worse prognosis within the 20 years follow-up.

Even though the short-term prognosis of pure mucinous carcinoma is said to be better, a few studies have reported that long-term outcomes in pure and mixed mucinous carcinomas are comparable.[15,170]

REFERENCES

1. Lange F. Der Gallertkrebs der Brustdruse. *Beiitr z klin Chir* 1896;16:1–60.
2. Larey M. Tumeur gelatiniforme ou colloide de la mamelle. *Bull Soc Chir Paris* 1853;3:545
3. Robinson R. Gelatinous cancer of the breast. *Trans Pathol Soc London* 1852;4:275
4. Geschickter CF. Gelatinous carcinoma of the breast. *Arch Surg* 1938;20:568–590.
5. Norris HJ, Taylor HB. Prognosis of mucinous (Gelatinous) carcinoma of the breast. *Cancer* 1965;18:879–885.
6. Melamed MR, Robbins GF, Foote FW Jr. Prognostic significance of gelatinous mammary carcinoma. *Cancer* 1961;14:699–704.
7. Silverberg SG, Kay S, Chitale AR, et al. Colloid carcinoma of the breast. *Am J Clin Pathol* 1971;55:355–363.
8. Rasmussen BB, Rose C, Christensen IB. Prognostic factors in primary mucinous breast carcinoma. *Am J Clin Pathol* 1987;87:155–160.

9. Komenaka IK, El-Tamer MB, Troxel A, et al. Pure mucinous carcinoma of the breast. *Am J Surg* 2004;187:528–532.
10. Reeves GK, Pirie K, Green J, et al. Reproductive factors and specific histological types of breast cancer: prospective study and meta-analysis. *Br J Cancer* 2009;100:538–544.
11. Louwman MW, Vriezen M, van Beek MW, et al. Uncommon breast tumors in perspective: incidence, treatment and survival in the Netherlands. *Int J Cancer* 2007;121:127–135.
12. Li CI. Risk of mortality by histologic type of breast cancer in the United States. *Horm Cancer* 2010;1:156–165.
13. Albrektsen G, Heuch I, Thoresen SO. Histological type and grade of breast cancer tumors by parity, age at birth, and time since birth: a register-based study in Norway. *BMC Cancer* 2010;10:226
14. Scopsi L, Andreola S, Pilotti S, et al. Mucinous carcinoma of the breast. A clinicopathologic, histochemical, and immunocytochemical study with special reference to neuroendocrine differentiation. *Am J Surg Pathol* 1994;18:702–711.
15. Toikkanen S, Kujari H. Pure and mixed mucinous carcinomas of the breast: a clinicopathologic analysis of 61 cases with long-term follow-up. *Hum Pathol* 1989;20:758–764.
16. Avisar E, Khan MA, Axelrod D, et al. Pure mucinous carcinoma of the breast: a clinicopathologic correlation study. *Ann Surg Oncol* 1998;5:447–451.
17. Rambau PF, Chalya PL, Manyama MM, et al. Pathological features of breast cancer seen in Northwestern Tanzania: a nine years retrospective study. *BMC Res Notes* 2011;4:214.
18. Komaki K, Sakamoto G, Sugano H, et al. Mucinous carcinoma of the breast in Japan. A prognostic analysis based on morphologic features. *Cancer* 1988;61:989–996.
19. Rosen PP, Wang T-Y. Colloid carcinoma of the breast. Analysis of 64 patients with long-term follow-up. *Am J Clin Pathol* 1980;73:30.
20. Diab SG, Clark GM, Osborne CK, et al. Tumor characteristics and clinical outcome of tubular and mucinous breast carcinomas. *J Clin Oncol* 1999;17:1442–1448.
21. Di Saverio S, Gutierrez J, Avisar E. A retrospective review with long term follow up of 11,400 cases of pure mucinous breast carcinoma. *Breast Cancer Res Treat* 2008;111:541–547.
22. Cao AY, He M, Liu ZB, et al. Outcome of pure mucinous breast carcinoma compared to infiltrating ductal carcinoma: a population-based study from China. *Ann Surg Oncol* 2012;19:3019–3027.
23. Paramo JC, Wilson C, Velarde D, et al. Pure mucinous carcinoma of the breast: is axillary staging necessary? *Ann Surg Oncol* 2002;9:161–164.
24. Rosen PP, Lesser ML, Kinne DW. Breast carcinoma at the extremes of age: a comparison of patients younger than 35 years and older than 75 years. *J Surg Oncol* 1985;28:90–96.
25. Fentiman IS, Millis RR, Smith P, et al. Mucoid breast carcinomas: histology and prognosis. *Br J Cancer* 1997;75:1061–1065.
26. Ranade A, Batra R, Sandhu G, et al. Clinicopathological evaluation of 100 cases of mucinous carcinoma of breast with emphasis on axillary staging and special reference to a micropapillary pattern. *J Clin Pathol* 2010;63:1043–1047.
27. Bae SY, Choi MY, Cho DH, et al. Mucinous carcinoma of the breast in comparison with invasive ductal carcinoma: clinicopathologic characteristics and prognosis. *J Breast Cancer* 2011;14:308–313.
28. Park S, Koo J, Kim JH, et al. Clinicopathological characteristics of mucinous carcinoma of the breast in Korea: comparison with invasive ductal carcinoma—not otherwise specified. *J Korean Med Sci* 2010;25:361–368.
29. Newcomer LM, Newcomb PA, Trentham-Dietz A, et al. Detection method and breast carcinoma histology. *Cancer* 2002;95: 470–477.
30. Work ME, Andrulis IL, John EM, et al. Risk factors for uncommon histologic subtypes of breast cancer using centralized pathology review in the Breast Cancer Family Registry. *Breast Cancer Res Treat* 2012;134:1209–1220.
31. Reeves GK, Beral V, Green J, et al. Hormonal therapy for menopause and breast-cancer risk by histological type: a cohort study and meta-analysis. *Lancet Oncol* 2006;7:910–918.
32. Morris PG, Hudis CA, Giri D, et al. Inflammation and increased aromatase expression occur in the breast tissue of obese women with breast cancer. *Cancer Prev Res (Phila)* 2011;4:1021–1029.
33. Li CI, Daling JR, Malone KE, et al. Relationship between established breast cancer risk factors and risk of seven different histologic types of invasive breast cancer. *Cancer Epidemiol Biomarkers Prev* 2006;15:946–954.
34. Lacroix-Triki M, Lambros MB, Geyer FC, et al. Absence of microsatellite instability in mucinous carcinomas of the breast. *Int J Clin Exp Pathol* 2010;4:22–31.
35. Barkley CR, Ligibel JA, Wong JS, et al. Mucinous breast carcinoma: a large contemporary series. *Am J Surg* 2008;196:549–551.
36. Hodgson NC, Button JH, Franceschi D, et al. Male breast cancer: is the incidence increasing? *Ann Surg Oncol* 2004;11:751–755.
37. Burga AM, Fadare O, Lininger RA, et al. Invasive carcinomas of the male breast: a morphologic study of the distribution of histologic subtypes and metastatic patterns in 778 cases. *Virchows Arch* 2006;449:507–512.
38. Cardenosa G, Doudna C, Eklund GW. Mucinous (colloid) breast cancer: clinical and mammographic findings in 10 patients. *AJR Am J Roentgenol* 1994;162:1077–1079.
39. Lam WW, Chu WC, Tse GM, et al. Sonographic appearance of mucinous carcinoma of the breast. *AJR Am J Roentgenol* 2004;182:1069–1074.
40. Liu H, Tan H, Cheng Y, et al. Imaging findings in mucinous breast carcinoma and correlating factors. *Eur J Radiol* 2011;80:706–712.
41. Peschos D, Tsanou E, Dallas P, et al. Mucinous breast carcinoma presenting as Paget's disease of the nipple in a man: a case report. *Diagn Pathol* 2008;3:42.
42. Chung-Park M, Zheng LC, Giampoli EJ, et al. Mucinous adenocarcinoma of ectopic breast tissue of the vulva. *Arch Pathol Lab Med* 2002;126:1216–1218.
43. Yin C, Chapman J, Tawfik O. Invasive mucinous (colloid) adenocarcinoma of ectopic breast tissue in the vulva: a case report. *Breast J* 2003;9:113–115.
44. Conant EF, Dillon RL, Palazzo J, et al. Imaging findings in mucin-containing carcinomas of the breast: correlation with pathologic features. *AJR Am J Roentgenol* 1994;163:821–824.
45. Goodman DN, Boutross-Tadross O, Jong RA. Mammographic features of pure mucinous carcinoma of the breast with pathological correlation. *Can Assoc Radiol J* 1995;46:296–301.
46. Matsuda M, Yoshimoto M, Iwase T, et al. Mammographic and clinicopathological features of mucinous carcinoma of the breast. *Breast Cancer* 2000;7:65–70.
47. Dhillon R, Depree P, Metcalf C, et al. Screen-detected mucinous breast carcinoma: potential for delayed diagnosis. *Clin Radiol* 2006;61:423–430.
48. Wilson TE, Helvie MA, Oberman HA, et al. Pure and mixed mucinous carcinoma of the breast: pathologic basis for differences in mammographic appearance. *AJR Am J Roentgenol* 1995;165:285–289.
49. Ruggieri A, Scola F, Schepps B. Mucinous carcinoma of the breast: mammographic findings. *Breast Dis* 1995;8:353–361.
50. Pina Insausti LJ, Soga Garcia E. Mucinous breast carcinoma showing as a cluster of suspicious microcalcifications on mammography. *Eur Radiol* 1998;8:1666–1668.
51. Rosen PP. Mucocele-like tumors of the breast. *Am J Surg Pathol* 1986;10:464–469.
52. Memis A, Ozdemir N, Parildar M, et al. Mucinous (colloid) breast cancer: mammographic and US features with histologic correlation. *Eur J Radiol* 2000;35:39–43.
53. Yamaguchi R, Tanaka M, Mizushima Y, et al. "High-grade" central acellular carcinoma and matrix-producing carcinoma of the breast: correlation between ultrasonographic findings and pathological features. *Med Mol Morphol* 2011;44:151–157.
54. Kawashima M, Tamaki Y, Nonaka T, et al. MR imaging of mucinous carcinoma of the breast. *AJR Am J Roentgenol* 2002;179:179–183.
55. Okafuji T, Yabuuchi H, Sakai S, et al. MR imaging features of pure mucinous carcinoma of the breast. *Eur J Radiol* 2006;60:405–413.
56. Monzawa S, Yokokawa M, Sakuma T, et al. Mucinous carcinoma of the breast: MRI features of pure and mixed forms with histopathologic correlation. *AJR Am J Roentgenol* 2009;192:W125–W131.
57. Miller RW, Harms S, Alvarez A. Mucinous carcinoma of the breast: potential false-negative MR imaging interpretation. *AJR Am J Roentgenol* 1996;167:539–540.
58. Orel SG, Schnall MD, LiVolsi VA, et al. Suspicious breast lesions: MR imaging with radiologic-pathologic correlation. *Radiology* 1994;190:485–493.
59. Lee B, Hauser H, Pack G. Gelatinous carcinoma of the breast. *Surg Gynecol Obstet* 1934;59:841–857.

60. Wulsin JH, Schreiber JT. Improved prognosis in certain patterns of carcinoma of the breast. Colloid, medullary with lymphoid stroma, and intraductal. *Arch Surg* 1962;85:791–800.
61. Walsh MD, McGuckin MA, Devine PL, et al. Expression of MUC2 epithelial mucin in breast carcinoma. *J Clin Pathol* 1993;46:922–925.
62. Ng WK. Fine-needle aspiration cytology findings of an uncommon micropapillary variant of pure mucinous carcinoma of the breast: review of patients over an 8-year period. *Cancer* 2002;96:280–288.
63. Jayaram G, Swain M, Chew MT, et al. Cytology of mucinous carcinoma of breast: a report of 28 cases with histological correlation. *Malays J Pathol* 2000;22:65–71.
64. Pillai KR, Jayasree K, Jayalal KS, et al. Mucinous carcinoma of breast with abundant psammoma bodies in fine-needle aspiration cytology: a case report. *Diagn Cytopathol* 2007;35:230–233.
65. Rao P, Lyons B. Pure mucinous carcinoma of the breast with extensive psammomatous calcification. *Histopathology* 2008;52:650–652.
66. Capella C, Eusebi V, Mann B, et al. Endocrine differentiation in mucoid carcinoma of the breast. *Histopathology* 1980;4:613–630.
67. Bal A, Joshi K, Sharma SC, et al. Prognostic significance of micropapillary pattern in pure mucinous carcinoma of the breast. *Int J Surg Pathol* 2008;16:251–256.
68. Shet T, Chinoy R. Presence of a micropapillary pattern in mucinous carcinomas of the breast and its impact on the clinical behavior. *Breast J* 2008;14:412–420.
69. Barbashina V, Corben AD, Akram M, et al. Mucinous micropapillary carcinoma of the breast: an aggressive counterpart to conventional pure mucinous tumors. *Hum Pathol* 2013;44:1577–85.
70. Steinbrecher JS, Silverberg SG. Signet-ring cell carcinoma of the breast. The mucinous variant of infiltrating lobular carcinoma? *Cancer* 1976;37:828–840.
71. Kuroda N, Fujishima N, Ohara M, et al. Invasive ductal carcinoma of the breast with signet-ring cell and mucinous carcinoma components: diagnostic utility of immunocytochemistry of signet-ring cells in aspiration cytology materials. *Diagn Cytopathol* 2007;35:171–173.
72. Lacroix-Triki M, Suarez PH, MacKay A, et al. Mucinous carcinoma of the breast is genomically distinct from invasive ductal carcinomas of no special type. *J Pathol* 2010;222:282–298.
73. Weigelt B, Geyer FC, Horlings HM, et al. Mucinous and neuroendocrine breast carcinomas are transcriptionally distinct from invasive ductal carcinomas of no special type. *Mod Pathol* 2009;22:1401–1414.
74. Koenig C, Tavassoli FA. Mucinous cystadenocarcinoma of the breast. *Am J Surg Pathol* 1998;22:698–703.
75. Honma N, Sakamoto G, Ikenaga M, et al. Mucinous cystadenocarcinoma of the breast: a case report and review of the literature. *Arch Pathol Lab Med* 2003;127:1031–1033.
76. Chen WY, Chen CS, Chen HC, et al. Mucinous cystadenocarcinoma of the breast coexisting with infiltrating ductal carcinoma. *Pathol Int* 2004;54:781–786.
77. Coyne JD, Irion L. Mammary mucinous cystadenocarcinoma. *Histopathology* 2006;49:659–660.
78. Lee SH, Chaung CR. Mucinous metaplasia of breast carcinoma with macrocystic transformation resembling ovarian mucinous cystadenocarcinoma in a case of synchronous bilateral infiltrating ductal carcinoma. *Pathol Int* 2008;58:601–605.
79. Rakici S, Gonullu G, Gursel SB, et al. Mucinous cystadenocarcinoma of the breast with estrogen receptor expression: a case report and review of the literature. *Case Rep Oncol* 2009;2:210–216.
80. Gulwani H, Bhalla S. Mucinous cystadenocarcinoma: a rare primary malignant tumor of the breast. *Indian J Pathol Microbiol* 2010;53:200–202.
81. Petersson F, Pang B, Thamboo TP, et al. Mucinous cystadenocarcinoma of the breast with amplification of the HER2-gene confirmed by FISH: the first case reported. *Hum Pathol* 2010;41:910–913.
82. Sentani K, Tashiro T, Uraoka N, et al. Primary mammary mucinous cystadenocarcinoma: cytological and histological findings. *Diagn Cytopathol* 2012;40:624–628.
83. Deng Y, Xue D, Wang X, et al. Mucinous cystadenocarcinoma of the breast with a basal-like immunophenotype. *Pathol Int* 2012;62:429–432.
84. Li X, Peng J, Zhang Z, et al. Mammary mucinous cystadenocarcinoma. *Breast J* 2012;18:282–283.
85. Komaki K, Sakamoto G, Sugano H, et al. The morphologic feature of mucus leakage appearing in low papillary carcinoma of the breast. *Hum Pathol* 1991;22:231–236.
86. Gadre SA, Perkins GH, Sahin AA, et al. Neovascularization in mucinous ductal carcinoma *in situ* suggests an alternative pathway for invasion. *Histopathology* 2008;53:545–553.
87. Deck JH, Lee MA. Mucin embolism to cerebral arteries: a fatal complication of carcinoma of the breast. *Can J Neurol Sci* 1978;5:327–330.
88. Towfighi J, Simmonds MA, Davidson EA. Mucin and fat emboli in mucinous carcinomas. Cause of hemorrhagic cerebral infarcts. *Arch Pathol Lab Med* 1983;107:646–649.
89. Carder PJ, Murphy CE, Liston JC. Surgical excision is warranted following a core biopsy diagnosis of mucoele-like lesion of the breast. *Histopathology* 2004;45:148–154.
90. Ramsaroop R, Greenberg D, Tracey N, et al. Mucocele-like lesions of the breast: an audit of 2 years at BreastScreen Auckland (New Zealand). *Breast J* 2005;11:321–325.
91. Kim JY, Han BK, Choe YH, et al. Benign and malignant mucocele-like tumors of the breast: mammographic and sonographic appearances. *AJR Am J Roentgenol* 2005;185:1310–1316.
92. Kim Y, Takatsuka Y, Morino H. Mucocele-like tumor of the breast: a case report and assessment of aspirated cytological specimens. *Breast Cancer* 1998;5:317–320.
93. Yeoh GP, Cheung PS, Chan KW. Fine-needle aspiration cytology of mucocelelike tumors of the breast. *Am J Surg Pathol* 1999;23:552–559.
94. Ro JY, Sneige N, Sahin AA, et al. Mucocelelike tumor of the breast associated with atypical ductal hyperplasia or mucinous carcinoma. A clinicopathologic study of seven cases. *Arch Pathol Lab Med* 1991;115:137–140.
95. Hamele-Bena D, Cranor ML, Rosen PP. Mammary mucocele-like lesions. Benign and malignant. *Am J Surg Pathol* 1996;20:1081–1085.
96. Weaver MG, Abdul-Karim FW, al-Kaisi N. Mucinous lesions of the breast. A pathological continuum. *Pathol Res Pract* 1993;189:873–876.
97. Kikuchi S, Nishimura R, Osako T, et al. Mucocele-like tumor associated with ductal carcinoma *in situ* diagnosed as mucinous carcinoma by fine-needle aspiration cytology: report of a case. *Surg Today* 2012;42:280–284.
98. Leibman AJ, Staeger CN, Charney DA. Mucocelelike lesions of the breast: mammographic findings with pathologic correlation. *AJR Am J Roentgenol* 2006;186:1356–1360.
99. Fadare O, Mariappan MR. Mucocele-like tumor and columnar cell hyperplasia of the breast occurring in a morphologic continuum. *J Med Case Rep* 2008;2:138
100. Verschuur-Maes AH, Van Diest PJ. The mucinous variant of columnar cell lesions. *Histopathology* 2011;58:847–853.
101. Kulka J, Davies JD. Mucocoele-like tumours: more associations and possibly ductal carcinoma *in situ*? *Histopathology* 1993;22:511–512.
102. Fisher CJ, Millis RR. A mucocoele-like tumour of the breast associated with both atypical ductal hyperplasia and mucoid carcinoma. *Histopathology* 1992;21:69–71.
103. Carkaci S, Lane DL, Gilcrease MZ, et al. Do all mucocele-like lesions of the breast require surgery? *Clin Imaging* 2011;35:94–101.
104. Renshaw AA. Can mucinous lesions of the breast be reliably diagnosed by core needle biopsy? *Am J Clin Pathol* 2002;118:82–84.
105. Wang J, Simsir A, Mercado C, et al. Can core biopsy reliably diagnose mucinous lesions of the breast? *Am J Clin Pathol* 2007;127:124–127.
106. Begum SM, Jara-Lazaro AR, Thike AA, et al. Mucin extravasation in breast core biopsies—clinical significance and outcome correlation. *Histopathology* 2009;55:609–617.
107. Edelweiss M, Corben AD, Liberman L, et al. Focal extravasated mucin in breast core biopsies: is surgical excision always necessary? *Breast J* 2013;19:302–309.
108. Sutton B, Davion S, Feldman M, et al. Mucocele-like lesions diagnosed on breast core biopsy: assessment of upgrade rate and need for surgical excision. *Am J Clin Pathol* 2012;138:783–788.
109. Jaffer S, Bleiweiss IJ, Nagi CS. Benign mucocele-like lesions of the breast: revisited. *Mod Pathol* 2011;24:683–687.
110. Ellis IO. *Ductal carcinoma in situ*. 3rd ed. Edinburgh: Churchill Livingstone; 1998.
111. Guerry P, Erlandson RA, Rosen PP. Cystic hypersecretory hyperplasia and cystic hypersecretory duct carcinoma of the breast. Pathology, therapy, and follow-up of 39 patients. *Cancer* 1988;61:1611–1620.
112. Shin SJ, Rosen PP. Carcinoma arising from preexisting pregnancy-like and cystic hypersecretory hyperplasia lesions of the

breast: a clinicopathologic study of 9 patients. *Am J Surg Pathol* 2004;28:789–793.
113. Diallo R, Schaefer KL, Bankfalvi A, et al. Secretory carcinoma of the breast: a distinct variant of invasive ductal carcinoma assessed by comparative genomic hybridization and immunohistochemistry. *Hum Pathol* 2003;34:1299–1305.
114. Rosen PP, Cranor ML. Secretory carcinoma of the breast. *Arch Pathol Lab Med* 1991;115:141–144.
115. Sanati S, Leonard M, Khamapirad T, et al. Nodular mucinosis of the breast: a case report with pathologic, ultrasonographic, and clinical findings and review of the literature. *Arch Pathol Lab Med* 2005;129:e58–e61.
116. Simsir A, Tsang P, Greenebaum E. Additional mimics of mucinous mammary carcinoma: fibroepithelial lesions. *Am J Clin Pathol* 1998;109:169–172.
117. Ventura K, Cangiarella J, Lee I, et al. Aspiration biopsy of mammary lesions with abundant extracellular mucinous material. Review of 43 cases with surgical follow-up. *Am J Clin Pathol* 2003;120:194–202.
118. Iyengar P, Cody HS 3rd, Brogi E. Pleomorphic adenoma of the breast: case report and review of the literature. *Diagn Cytopathol* 2005;33:416–420.
119. Anthony PP, James PD. Adenoid cystic carcinoma of the breast: prevalence, diagnostic criteria, and histogenesis. *J Clin Pathol* 1975;28:647–655.
120. Bloom GD, Carlsoo B, Gustafsson H, et al. Distribution of mucosubstances in adenoid cystic carcinoma. *Virchows Arch A Pathol Anat Histol* 1977;375:1–12.
121. Foschini MP, Fulcheri E, Baracchini P, et al. Squamous cell carcinoma with prominent myxoid stroma. *Hum Pathol* 1990;21:859–865.
122. Di Tommaso L, Foschini MP, Ragazzini T, et al. Mucoepidermoid carcinoma of the breast. *Virchows Arch* 2004;444:13–19.
123. Tot T. Metastatic chordoma of the breast: an extremely rare lesion mimicking mucinous cancer. *APMIS* 2006;114:726–729.
124. Tan PH, Tse GM, Bay BH. Mucinous breast lesions: diagnostic challenges. *J Clin Pathol* 2008;61:11–19.
125. Gupta RK, McHutchison AG, Simpson JS, et al. Value of fine needle aspiration cytology of the breast, with an emphasis on the cytodiagnosis of colloid carcinoma. *Acta Cytol* 1991;35:703–709.
126. Dawson AE, Mulford DK. Benign versus malignant papillary neoplasms of the breast. Diagnostic clues in fine needle aspiration cytology. *Acta Cytol* 1994;38:23–28.
127. Matsuda M, Wada A, Nagumo S, et al. Pitfalls in fine needle aspiration cytology of breast tumors. A report of two cases. *Acta Cytol* 1993;37:247–251.
128. Maygarden SJ, Novotny DB, Johnson DE, et al. Fine-needle aspiration cytology of suture granulomas of the breast: a potential pitfall in the cytologic diagnosis of recurrent breast cancer. *Diagn Cytopathol* 1994;10:175–179.
129. Stanley MW, Tani EM, Skoog L. Mucinous breast carcinoma and mixed mucinous-infiltrating ductal carcinoma: a comparative cytologic study. *Diagn Cytopathol* 1989;5:134–138.
130. Bhargava V, Miller TR, Cohen MB. Mucocele-like tumors of the breast. Cytologic findings in two cases. *Am J Clin Pathol* 1991;95:875–877.
131. Young NA, Mody DR, Davey DD. Diagnosis and subclassification of breast carcinoma by fine-needle aspiration biopsy: results of the interlaboratory comparison program in non-gynecologic cytopathology. *Arch Pathol Lab Med* 2002;126:1453–1457.
132. Lam WW, Chu WC, Tse GM, et al. Role of fine needle aspiration and tru cut biopsy in diagnosis of mucinous carcinoma of breast—from a radiologist's perspective. *Clin Imaging* 2006;30:6–10.
133. Coady AT, Shousha S, Dawson PM, et al. Mucinous carcinoma of the breast: further characterization of its three subtypes. *Histopathology* 1989;15:617–626.
134. Tellem M, Nedwich A, Amenta PS, et al. Mucin-producing carcinoma of the breast. Tissue culture, histochemical and electron microscopic study. *Cancer* 1966;19:573–584.
135. Walker RA. Mucoid carcinomas of the breast: a study using mucin histochemistry and peanut lectin. *Histopathology* 1982;6:571–579.
136. Mukhopadhyay P, Chakraborty S, Ponnusamy MP, et al. Mucins in the pathogenesis of breast cancer: implications in diagnosis, prognosis and therapy. *Biochim Biophys Acta* 2011;1815:224–240.
137. O'Connell JT, Shao ZM, Drori E, et al. Altered mucin expression is a field change that accompanies mucinous (colloid) breast carcinoma histogenesis. *Hum Pathol* 1998;29:1517–1523.
138. Rakha EA, Boyce RW, Abd El-Rehim D, et al. Expression of mucins (MUC1, MUC2, MUC3, MUC4, MUC5AC and MUC6) and their prognostic significance in human breast cancer. *Mod Pathol* 2005;18:1295–1304.
139. Matsukita S, Nomoto M, Kitajima S, et al. Expression of mucins (MUC1, MUC2, MUC5AC and MUC6) in mucinous carcinoma of the breast: comparison with invasive ductal carcinoma. *Histopathology* 2003;42:26–36.
140. Baldus SE, Wienand JR, Werner JP, et al. Expression of MUC1, MUC2 and oligosaccharide epitopes in breast cancer: prognostic significance of a sialylated MUC1 epitope. *Int J Oncol* 2005;27:1289–1297.
141. Kato N, Endo Y, Tamura G, et al. Mucinous carcinoma of the breast: a multifaceted study with special reference to histogenesis and neuroendocrine differentiation. *Pathol Int* 1999;49:947–955.
142. Adsay NV, Merati K, Nassar H, et al. Pathogenesis of colloid (pure mucinous) carcinoma of exocrine organs: coupling of gel-forming mucin (MUC2) production with altered cell polarity and abnormal cell-stroma interaction may be the key factor in the morphogenesis and indolent behavior of colloid carcinoma in the breast and pancreas. *Am J Surg Pathol* 2003;27:571–578.
143. Yonezawa SNM, Matsukita S. et al. Expression of MUC2 gene product in mucinous carcinoma of the breast: comparison with invasive ductal carcinoma. *Acta Histochem Cytochem* 1995;28:239–246.
144. Utsunomiya T, Yonezawa S, Sakamoto H, et al. Expression of MUC1 and MUC2 mucins in gastric carcinomas: its relationship with the prognosis of the patients. *Clin Cancer Res* 1998;4:2605–2614.
145. Nakamori S, Ota DM, Cleary KR, et al. MUC1 mucin expression as a marker of progression and metastasis of human colorectal carcinoma. *Gastroenterology* 1994;106:353–361.
146. Schmitt FC, Pereira MB, Reis CA. MUC 5 expression in breast carcinomas. *Hum Pathol* 1999;30:1270–1271.
147. Lesser ML, Rosen PP, Senie RT, et al. Estrogen and progesterone receptors in breast carcinoma: correlations with epidemiology and pathology. *Cancer* 1981;48:299–309.
148. Rosen PP M-BC, Senie RT, et al. *Estrogen in receptor protein (ERP) and the histopathology of human mammary carcinoma*. New York: Raven Press; 1978.
149. Shousha S, Coady AT, Stamp T, et al. Oestrogen receptors in mucinous carcinoma of the breast: an immunohistological study using paraffin wax sections. *J Clin Pathol* 1989;42:902–905.
150. Slodkowska E, Corben AD, Catalano JP, et al. Pure mucinous carcinoma in women 40 years old or younger: clinico-pathological and follow-up study. 2012; USCAP Meeting Vancouver Canada, March 2012.
151. Park S, Koo J, Park HS, et al. Expression of androgen receptors in primary breast cancer. *Ann Oncol* 2010;21:488–492.
152. Cho LC, Hsu YH. Expression of androgen, estrogen and progesterone receptors in mucinous carcinoma of the breast. *Kaohsiung J Med Sci* 2008;24:227–232.
153. Sapino A, Righi L, Cassoni P, et al. Expression of apocrine differentiation markers in neuroendocrine breast carcinomas of aged women. *Mod Pathol* 2001;14:768–776.
154. Alvarenga CA, Paravidino PI, Alvarenga M, et al. Reappraisal of immunohistochemical profiling of special histological types of breast carcinomas: a study of 121 cases of eight different subtypes. *J Clin Pathol* 2012;65:1066–1071.
155. Domfeh AB, Carley AL, Striebel JM, et al. WT1 immunoreactivity in breast carcinoma: selective expression in pure and mixed mucinous subtypes. *Mod Pathol* 2008;21:1217–1223.
156. Shao MM, Chan SK, Yu AM, et al. Keratin expression in breast cancers. *Virchows Arch* 2012;461:313–322.
157. Abd El-Rehim DM, Pinder SE, Paish CE, et al. Expression of luminal and basal cytokeratins in human breast carcinoma. *J Pathol* 2004;203:661–671.
158. Skoog L, Macias A, Azavedo E, et al. Receptors for EGF and oestradiol and thymidine kinase activity in different histological subgroups of human mammary carcinomas. *Br J Cancer* 1986;54:271–276.
159. Fetissof F, Dubois MP, Arbeille-Brassart B, et al. Argyrophilic cells in mammary carcinoma. *Hum Pathol* 1983;14:127–134.
160. Rasmussen BB, Rose C, Thorpe SM, et al. Argyrophilic cells in 202 human mucinous breast carcinomas. Relation to histopathologic and clinical factors. *Am J Clin Pathol* 1985;84:737–740.
161. Hull MT, Warfel KA. Mucinous breast carcinomas with abundant intracytoplasmic mucin and neuroendocrine features: light microscopic,

immunohistochemical, and ultrastructural study. *Ultrastruct Pathol* 1987;11:29–38.
162. Ahmed A. Electron-microscopic observations of scirrhous and mucin-producing carcinomas of the breast. *J Pathol* 1974;112:177–181.
163. Ferguson DJ, Anderson TJ, Wells CA, et al. An ultrastructural study of mucoid carcinoma of the breast: variability of cytoplasmic features. *Histopathology* 1986;10:1219–1230.
164. Jao W, Lao IO, Chowdhury LN, et al. Ultrastructural aspects of mucinous (colloid) breast carcinoma. *Diagn Gynecol Obstet* 1980;2:83–92.
165. Harris M, Vasudev KS, Anfield C, et al. Mucin-producing carcinomas of the breast: ultrastructural observations. *Histopathology* 1978;2:177–188.
166. Toikkanen S, Eerola E, Ekfors TO. Pure and mixed mucinous breast carcinomas: DNA stemline and prognosis. *J Clin Pathol* 1988;41:300–303.
167. Kehr EL, Jorns JM, Ang D, et al. Mucinous breast carcinomas lack PIK3CA and AKT1 mutations. *Hum Pathol* 2012;43:2207–2212.
168. Vo T, Xing Y, Meric-Bernstam F, et al. Long-term outcomes in patients with mucinous, medullary, tubular, and invasive ductal carcinomas after lumpectomy. *Am J Surg* 2007;194:527–531.
169. Colleoni M, Rotmensz N, Maisonneuve P, et al. Outcome of special types of luminal breast cancer. *Ann Oncol* 2011;22:1736–1747
170. Andre S, Cunha F, Bernardo M, et al. Mucinous carcinoma of the breast: a pathologic study of 82 cases. *J Surg Oncol* 1995;58:162–167.
171. Maibenco DC, Weiss LK, Pawlish KS, et al. Axillary lymph node metastases associated with small invasive breast carcinomas. *Cancer* 1999;85:1530–1536.
172. Cserni G, Bianchi S, Vezzosi V, et al. Sentinel lymph node biopsy and non-sentinel node involvement in special type breast carcinomas with a good prognosis. *Eur J Cancer* 2007;43:1407–1414.
173. Rosen PP, Groshen S, Kinne DW. Survival and prognostic factors in node-negative breast cancer: results of long-term follow-up studies. *J Natl Cancer Inst Monogr* 1992;11:159–162.
174. Nagao T, Kinoshita T, Hojo T, et al. The differences in the histological types of breast cancer and the response to neoadjuvant chemotherapy: the relationship between the outcome and the clinicopathological characteristics. *Breast* 2012;21:289–295.
175. Baretta Z, Guindalini RS, Khramtsova G, et al. Resistance to Trastuzumab in HER2-positive mucinous invasive ductal breast carcinoma. *Clin Breast Cancer* 2013;13:156–158.
176. Veronesi U, Gennari L. Il carcinoma gelatinoso della mammella. *Tumori* 1960;46:119–155.
177. Colleoni M, Rotmensz N, Maisonneuve P, et al. Outcome of special types of luminal breast cancer. *Ann Oncol* 2012;23:1428–1436.
178. Chen LL, Nolan ME, Silverstein MJ, et al. The impact of primary tumor size, lymph node status, and other prognostic factors on the risk of cancer death. *Cancer* 2009;115:5071–5083.
179. Clayton F. Pure mucinous carcinomas of breast: morphologic features and prognostic correlates. *Hum Pathol* 1986;17:34–38.
180. Lee YT, Terry R. Surgical treatment of carcinoma of the breast. I. Pathological finding and pattern of relapse. *J Surg Oncol* 1983;23:11–15.
181. Scharnhorst D, Huntrakoon M. Mucinous carcinoma of the breast: recurrence 30 years after mastectomy. *South Med J* 1988;81:656–657.
182. Rosen PR, Groshen S, Saigo PE, et al. A long-term follow-up study of survival in stage I (T1N0M0) and stage II (T1N1M0) breast carcinoma. *J Clin Oncol* 1989;7:355–366.
183. Kurtz JM, Jacquemier J, Torhorst J, et al. Conservation therapy for breast cancers other than infiltrating ductal carcinoma. *Cancer* 1989;63:1630–1635.
184. Haffty BG, Perrotta P, Ward B, et al. Conservatively treated breast cancer: outcome by histologic subtype. *Breast J* 1997;3:7–14.

CHAPTER 19

Apocrine Carcinoma

EDI BROGI

Apocrine glands are normal appendages of the skin in the axilla, anogenital region, and eyelids, where they may give rise to cutaneous apocrine carcinoma.[1–3] Benign and malignant apocrine lesions can also occur in the breast.

The origin of the apocrine cells in the breast is a subject of long-standing debate. The term "apocrine metaplasia" that is used for benign apocrine cells commonly found in the breast implies that they develop from benign mammary epithelial cells through a metaplastic process.[4] Some authors have proposed that apocrine cells are degenerated[5] or terminally differentiated epithelial cells.[6,7] Cells with functional apocrine characteristics have been detected in fetal breast tissue.[8] This observation suggests that apocrine differentiation occurs in a subset of normal mammary glandular cells and that apocrine proliferative lesions found in the adult breast may arise by expansion of this constituent rather than through metaplastic alteration of nonapocrine cells.[9]

Recent molecular studies suggest that mammary carcinomas with apocrine differentiation constitute a distinct subset of estrogen receptor (ER)–negative, androgen receptor (AR)–positive mammary neoplasm.[10,11]

Apocrine cells are characterized by abundant cytoplasm that can be densely eosinophilic, granular, or vacuolated, and by large nuclei with prominent nucleoli. These morphologic features are present to some degree in a substantial proportion of mammary carcinomas, but the term "apocrine carcinoma" should be reserved for neoplasms in which all or nearly all of the epithelium has apocrine morphology. Apocrine carcinomas have the same ER-negative and AR-positive immunophenotype as apocrine metaplasia.[10,12] Further refinement of the diagnostic criteria is needed to achieve a more consistent definition of mammary apocrine lesions that integrates morphologic, immunophenotypical, and genetic data.

In this chapter, we review the literature on mammary apocrine carcinomas, specifying whether the data that are presented pertain to case series selected based on morphologic and/or immunohistochemical criteria.

CLINICAL PRESENTATION

Incidence, Age, and Gender

The frequency of apocrine carcinoma ranges from less than 1%[13,14] to about 4%.[9,15] This variability is probably the result of inconsistent diagnostic criteria and variations in the way cases were identified. When the diagnosis is limited to carcinomas that have apocrine morphology throughout or in most of the tumor, no more than 1% of breast carcinomas can be classified as apocrine carcinomas. In a series by Dellapasqua et al.,[16] 72 women with invasive carcinomas with apocrine morphology represented 1% of 6,971 patients with invasive carcinoma surgically treated at one Italian institution between 1997 and 2005. Tanaka et al.[15] identified 61 patients with apocrine breast carcinomas (57 invasive and 4 ductal carcinoma *in situ* [DCIS]) (2.9%) among 2,055 patients with breast carcinoma treated surgically at their center over a period of 10 years.

The reported age at diagnosis of apocrine carcinoma ranges from 19 to 90 years. Most patients tend to be postmenopausal and 5 to 10 years older than patients with nonapocrine ductal carcinomas.[13,16–20] Tanaka et al.[15] reported that the mean age of 57 patients with invasive apocrine carcinoma was 58.5 ± 10.9 years, significantly higher than the mean age of 54.4 ± 11 years for 1,583 women with invasive nonapocrine ductal carcinoma treated consecutively at a Japanese institution during the same period.

Apocrine carcinoma of the male breast has been described, but it is very uncommon. In one instance, the tumor had a glandular architecture and psammoma bodies.[21] In one series,[22] 17/643 (2.6%) primary invasive ductal carcinomas occurring in men had apocrine morphology in less than 50% of the tumor.

Genetic Predisposition

Data on risk factors for breast carcinoma such as family history are very limited in women with apocrine carcinoma. Six patients in one series gave a negative family history for breast carcinoma.[13] Breast lesions that occur in patients with Cowden syndrome often have apocrine morphology.[23,24] Banneau et al.[25] reported that the molecular signature of carcinomas in patients with *PTEN* germline mutation (Cowden disease) had significant overlap with that of molecular apocrine carcinoma. The apocrine Cowden carcinomas included 4/15 (27%) carcinomas with apocrine morphology, 2 (13%) invasive ductal carcinomas with apocrine features, and 1 (6.6%) invasive micropapillary apocrine carcinoma. The nonapocrine Cowden carcinomas included 6/15 (40%) invasive ductal carcinomas not otherwise specified (NOS), 1 (6.6%) invasive lobular carcinoma, and 1 (6.6%) DCIS. Apocrine carcinoma is not specifically linked to Cowden syndrome.

Symptoms and Imaging

There are no striking differences in the clinical or mammographic features of patients with apocrine and nonapocrine duct carcinomas.[26] Most patients with invasive apocrine carcinoma present with a mass. Pain, Paget disease, nipple discharge, and other symptoms are relatively uncommon initial manifestations of invasive or *in situ* apocrine carcinoma. Occasionally, apocrine DCIS is sufficiently abundant to form a mass lesion,[27] but more often it is detected by mammography. When compared with other types of breast carcinoma, the distribution of sites of apocrine carcinoma does not differ from that of most breast carcinomas, with the majority of the lesions located in the upper outer quadrant. The stage at diagnosis of apocrine carcinoma is also not appreciably different from that of nonapocrine carcinomas.

Twenty-eight of 29 triple negative apocrine carcinomas in one series[20] were unifocal. Patients with apocrine breast carcinoma sometimes have a contralateral nonapocrine carcinoma.[28] One study[16] found that patients with morphologically and immunophenotypically pure apocrine carcinomas had an increased risk of contralateral breast carcinoma (hazard ratio [HR], 4.12; 95% confidence interval [CI], 1.22 to 14) ($p = 0.02$). Bilateral apocrine carcinomas are very uncommon.[14] Schmitt et al.[29] studied simultaneous bilateral apocrine carcinomas found in a 74-year-old patient and demonstrated that they were independent primary tumors. The right breast invasive apocrine carcinoma was human epidermal growth factor 2 (HER2)-negative and p53-positive and exhibited a p53 mutation. The left breast invasive apocrine carcinoma was HER2-positive and showed no p53 reactivity or gene mutation. Moritani et al.[30] evaluated the relationship of DCIS and sclerosing adenosis (SA) in a series of 24 cases. They encountered one patient with high-grade apocrine DCIS secondarily involving apocrine SA in one breast and non-apocrine DCIS and SA separately located in the contralateral breast.

GROSS PATHOLOGY

Apocrine carcinoma has no specific gross morphologic features. Invasive carcinomas are firm-to-hard tumors that usually have infiltrating borders. The bisected tumor is generally gray or white. The tan-to-brown color found in some cellular benign apocrine lesions is generally not evident in apocrine carcinomas. Exceptional tumors are grossly cystic or have a medullary appearance (Fig. 19.1). Comedo necrosis can occur in apocrine DCIS.

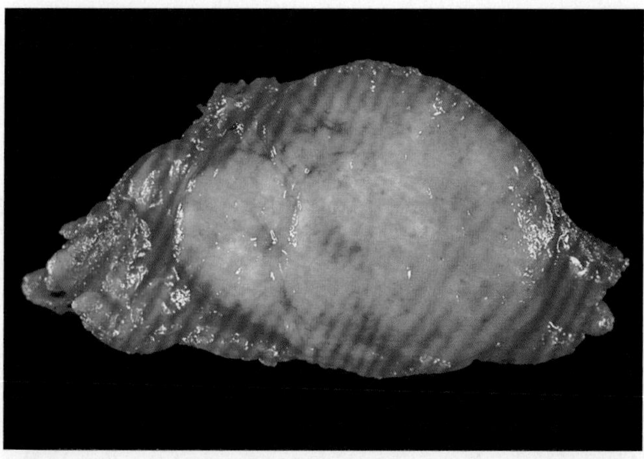

FIG. 19.1. ***Apocrine carcinoma, gross appearance.*** This invasive carcinoma has a well-defined border and a fleshy or medullary-appearing cut surface.

MICROSCOPIC PATHOLOGY

Malignant Apocrine Histology

The distinguishing feature of apocrine carcinoma is the cytologic appearance of the tumor cells. More than 80 years ago, Lee et al.[31] pointed out that apocrine carcinomas "have much the same structure as other mammary carcinomata; for example, we find that the bulky adenocarcinomata, the comedocarcinomata, the papillary, intraductal and intracystic carcinomata, the carcinoma simplex, and even scirrhous carcinomata of the breast are represented in this group." Apocrine cytomorphology has also been noted in mucinous carcinoma,[9] in duct carcinomas with tubular features,[13,32] in medullary carcinoma,[33] and in invasive lobular carcinoma.[9,34] Lin et al.[35] studied a series of HER2-positive invasive breast carcinomas and identified apocrine features in 67/96 (69.8%) invasive ductal carcinomas NOS, in 2/3 (66.7%) mucinous carcinomas, in 1/2 (50%) signet ring cell carcinomas, and in 1 (100%) invasive pleomorphic lobular carcinoma.

Cytologic features that characterize intraductal and invasive apocrine carcinomas are manifested in the nuclei and in the cytoplasm. The nuclei are enlarged and pleomorphic when compared with the nuclei of benign apocrine cells (Fig. 19.2). Nuclear membranes tend to be hyperchromatic and irregular. Nuclear grade can be determined within the spectrum of cytologic features found in apocrine carcinoma. Low-grade nuclei are usually slightly larger than nuclei in apocrine metaplasia and also darker due to denser chromatin. Nucleoli are usually present but inconspicuous

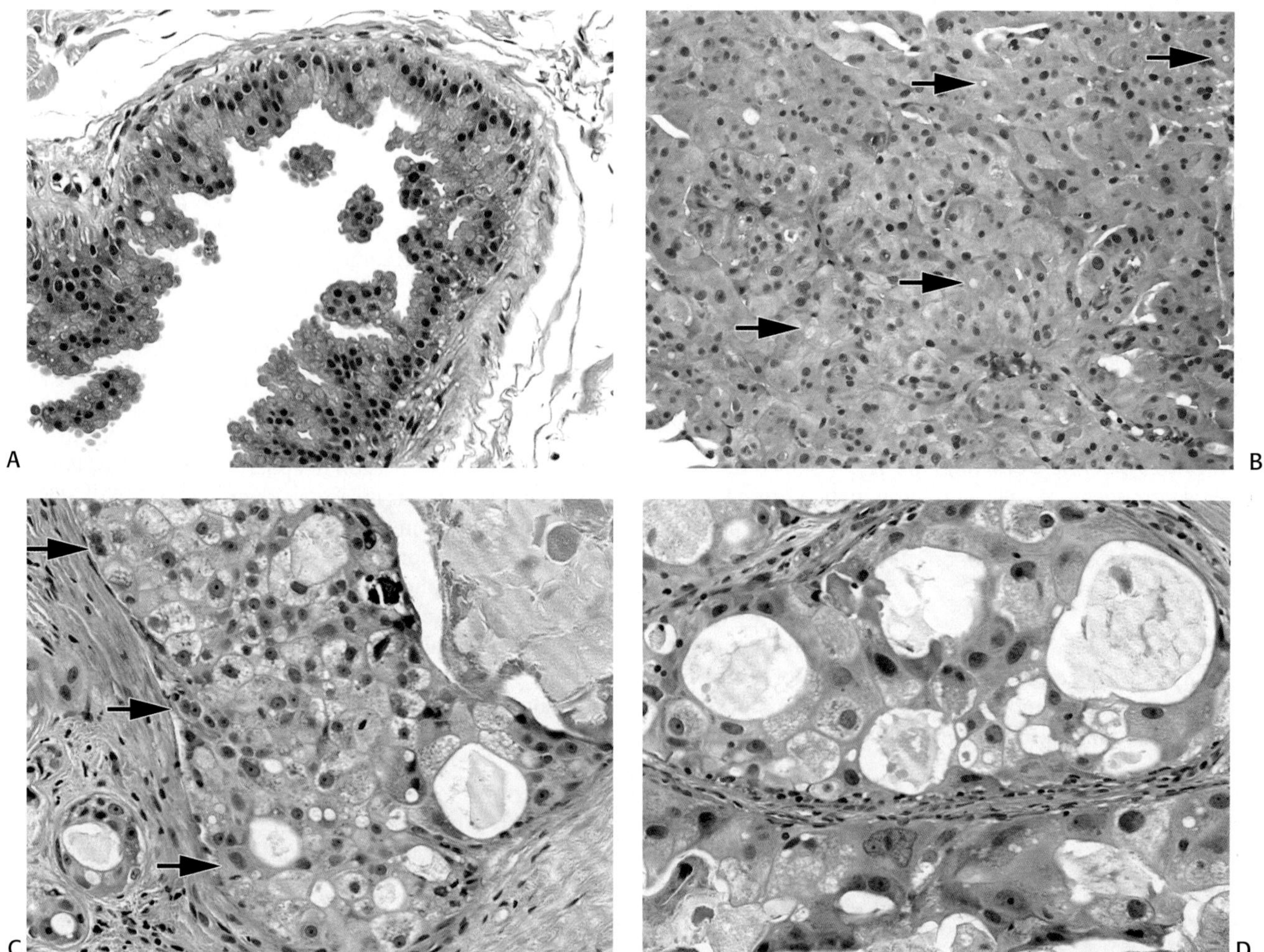

FIG. 19.2. ***Apocrine nuclei.*** All images were taken at the same magnification. **A:** The nuclei of apocrine metaplasia are round and uniform, with small nucleoli that are obscured by the dark chromatin. Note the abundant eosinophilic cytoplasm. **B:** Apocrine carcinoma with low nuclear grade. The nuclei vary slightly in size and shape and are larger than those of apocrine metaplasia. Note a few scattered intracytoplasmic vacuoles (*arrows*). **C:** Apocrine carcinoma with intermediate nuclear grade. The nuclei are enlarged and show greater variation in size and focal binucleation (*arrows*). The cytoplasm is pale focally, and intracytoplasmic vacuoles are evident. **D:** Apocrine carcinoma with high nuclear grade. More than threefold variation in nuclear size is evident. Some of the neoplastic cells have abundant vacuolated pale cytoplasm, and glandular lumens are evident.

(Fig. 19.2). High-grade nuclei feature diverse appearances (Figs. 19.2 and 19.3). Some nuclei are strikingly enlarged and pleomorphic with one or more macronucleoli that can be round, oval, or teardrop shaped. Other high-grade apocrine nuclei have deeply basophilic and smudged chromatin in which little or no internal structure can be discerned. In other instances, the chromatin is coarse and obscures the nucleoli. Binucleation is common. Variation in nuclear size is frequently observed, with adjacent nuclei showing threefold or greater difference in diameter.

In most cases, the cytoplasm exhibits eosinophilia that is densely homogeneous or slightly granular. Cytoplasmic vacuolization or clearing is a feature associated with atypical apocrine proliferations, and it is usually most prominent in apocrine carcinomas. The cytoplasm of some tumor cells occasionally has a light blue mucoid quality, and focal mucinous secretion may be present in the lumen of the neoplastic glands, but not in the stroma. Cell borders tend to be well defined (Fig. 19.4). Some apocrine carcinomas, especially the clear cell variant, attract an intense lymphocytic or lymphoplasmacytic reaction.

Invasive Apocrine Carcinoma

Invasive apocrine carcinomas can have any of the usual growth patterns of infiltrating duct carcinoma, but they tend to be structurally poorly differentiated (Figs. 19.4 and 19.5). In two studies, 40%[16] and 83%[18] of invasive carcinomas with

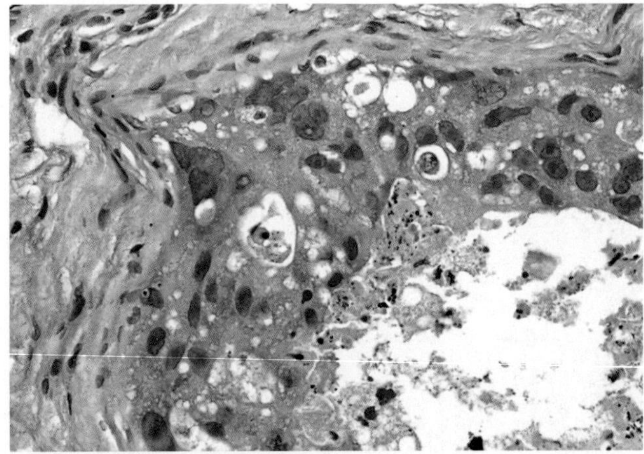

FIG. 19.3. ***Apocrine DCIS, high grade.*** This solid apocrine DCIS is composed of cells with large, hyperchromatic nuclei and nucleoli. Few binucleate cells are evident. Degenerated cells and necrotic debris are present in the duct lumen.

apocrine morphology were high grade. Apocrine carcinomas typically consist of medium-sized to small tumor nests. Stromal desmoplasia and moderate to abundant lymphocytic infiltrates are common in high-grade tumors. An uncommon variant of invasive apocrine carcinoma is composed of large polygonal cells with abundant foamy or eosinophilic cytoplasm and histiocytoid morphology (Fig. 19.6).[36] The presence of gross cystic disease fluid protein 15 (GCDFP-15), a marker of apocrine differentiation (see section on immunohistochemistry), has been demonstrated in these lesions by immunohistochemistry (IHC) and by *in situ* hybridization.[36] These carcinomas can be distinguished from invasive pleomorphic lobular carcinoma by being E-cadherin positive. At present, there is insufficient follow-up information to define the prognosis of the histiocytoid type of apocrine carcinoma.

Tanaka et al.[15] documented lymphatic invasion in 10/57 (17.5%) apocrine carcinomas compared with 502/1,583 (31.7%) invasive nonapocrine ductal carcinomas ($p = 0.02$); however, other investigators have reported high incidence of lymphovascular invasion in apocrine carcinomas. Peritumoral lymphovascular invasion was present in 35%,[16] 38%,[14] and 56%[37] of cases in three series. D'Amore et al.[38] encountered dermal invasion in 7/34 (21%) of their cases, including 4 (12%) with lymphatic invasion within the breast. A review of mammary carcinomas that recurred in an inflammatory pattern revealed that 33% of the primary tumors were apocrine carcinomas.[39] When examined retrospectively, the majority of the primary lesions had peritumoral lymphatic tumor emboli. It is notable that apocrine carcinoma,

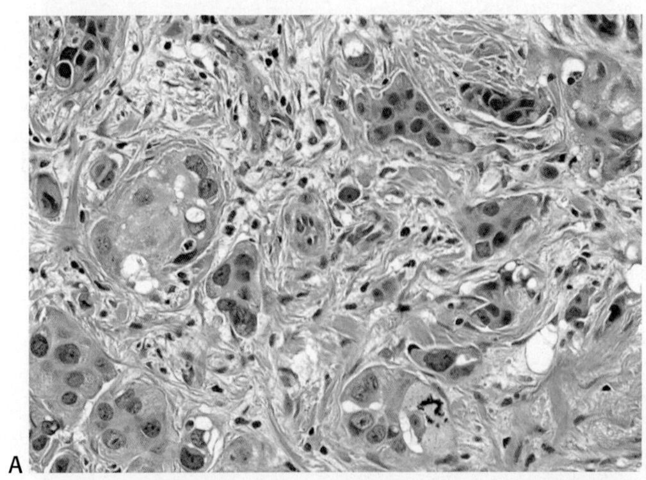

A

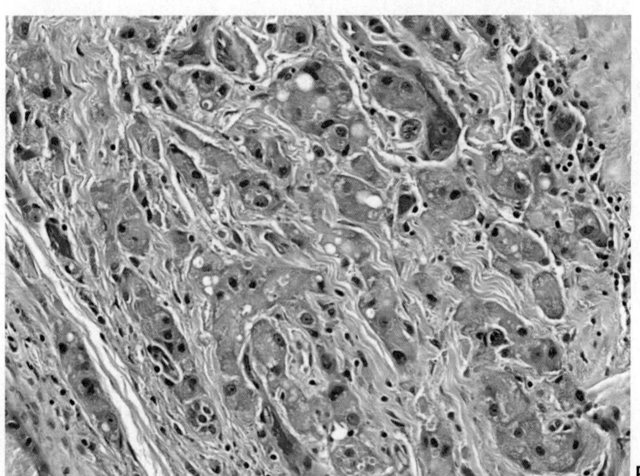

B

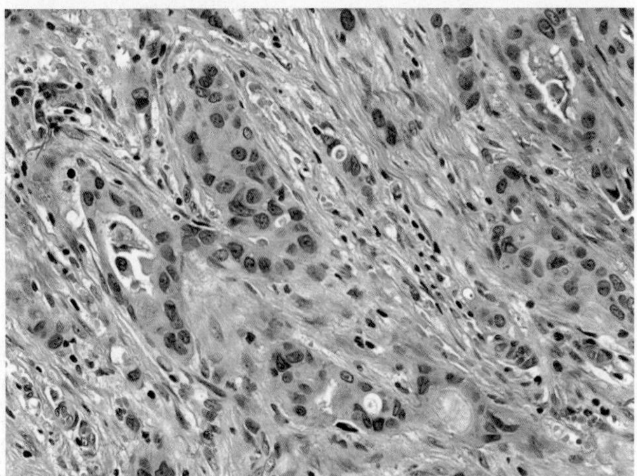

C

FIG. 19.4. ***Apocrine carcinoma, cytoplasmic and glandular features.*** **A:** Some of neoplastic nests composing this high-grade invasive apocrine carcinoma consist of cells with ample pale cytoplasm. Other nests consist of smaller cells with less conspicuous, but denser cytoplasm that is well demarcated from the surrounding stroma. An atypical mitotic figure is present [*lower right*]. **B:** Some of the invasive neoplastic cells have distinct cytoplasmic vacuoles. **C:** A few of the invasive glands contain pale blue intraluminal mucin, but no stromal mucin is identified.

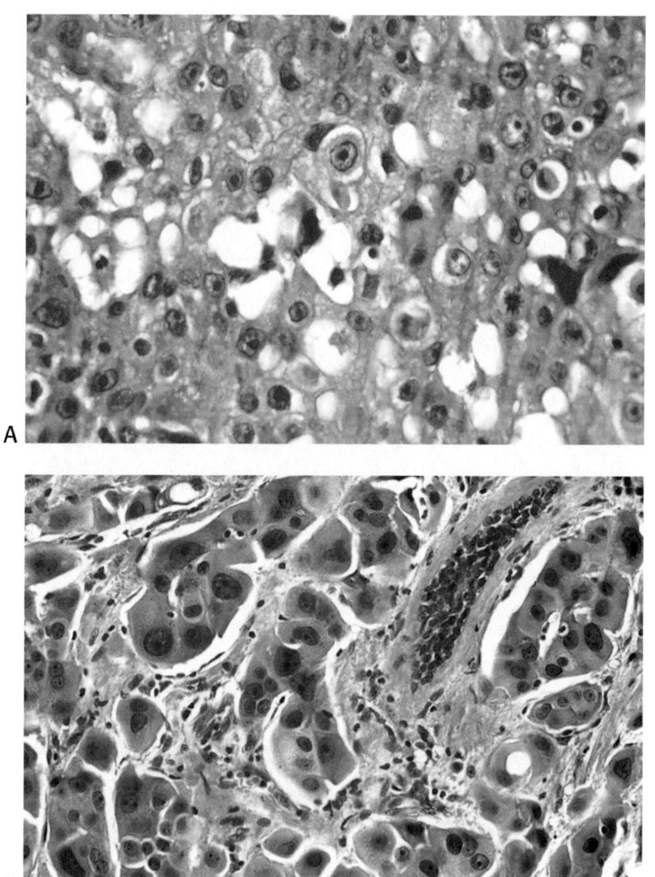
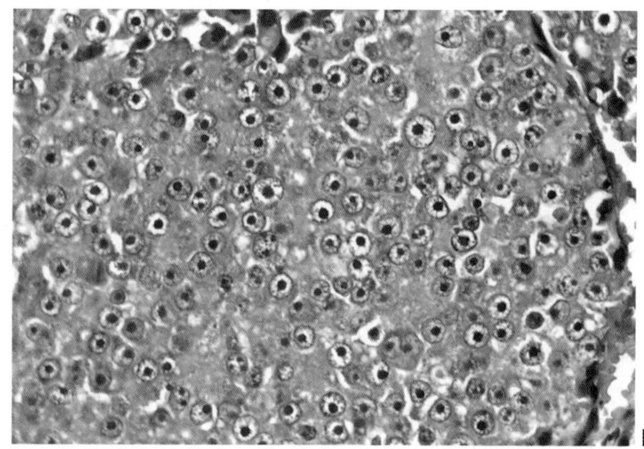

FIG. 19.5. ***Invasive apocrine carcinoma, nuclear grade.*** **A:** Low and intermediate nuclear grade. Nuclei and nucleoli are generally round and variable in size. **B,C:** High nuclear grade. Dense chromatin obscures the nucleoli in **(C)**.

an uncommon tumor, was relatively more frequent than expected among patients who experienced recurrent carcinoma with an inflammatory pattern.

Apocrine Ductal Carcinoma *In Situ*

The architecture of apocrine DCIS is similar to that commonly found in nonapocrine intraductal carcinomas including comedo, micropapillary (Fig. 19.7), solid (Fig. 19.8), cribriform (Fig. 19.9), and papillary (Fig. 19.10) patterns. Apocrine DCIS with low nuclear grade can sometimes be difficult to differentiate from apocrine metaplasia. Although the cytologic atypia of low-grade apocrine DCIS can be minimal, the carcinoma shows expansive solid growth and/or complex and rigid architectural patterns characteristic of other forms of low-grade DCIS. At the other end of the spectrum, apocrine DCIS with high nuclear grade has marked nuclear pleomorphism, prominent and often irregular or multiple nucleoli, and usually shows necrosis. High-grade apocrine DCIS closely resembles nonapocrine DCIS of the same grade, but differs from the latter because it has more abundant eosinophilic, granular, or vacuolated cytoplasm. Apocrine DCIS with dense cytoplasmic eosinophilia may resemble squamous DCIS, but lacks keratin formation. Apocrine DCIS with intermediate nuclear grade usually shows obvious apocrine cytology.

Calcifications may be seen in the affected ducts. They are typically small and punctate in low-grade DCIS, but coarse, heterogeneous, and often associated with necrosis in high-grade DCIS. Periductal fibrosis and inflammation are common reactive changes around the ducts involved by apocrine DCIS with intermediate or high nuclear grade. Foamy histiocytes may be a prominent feature of the reactive changes in the stroma around apocrine DCIS[40] and should not be mistaken for invasive carcinoma cells. In some cases, apocrine DCIS arises in complex papillary lesions in which there is also a benign hyperplastic component (Fig. 19.11).

Extension of apocrine DCIS into the epithelium of lobules is frequently present (Fig. 19.12).

Apocrine atypia often occurs in SA. Moritani et al.[30] studied the topographic, morphologic, and immunophenotypical features of DCIS confined to SA (type A), or involving SA as well as the adjacent breast parenchyma (type B). One of 13 (7%) type A DCIS was a high-grade solid and comedo-type apocrine carcinoma, with ER-negative, progesterone receptor (PR)–negative, and HER2-positive immunoprofile. The DCIS spanned 1.6 cm and was contained in a 4.5-cm focus of SA. In contrast, 5/11 (45%) type B DCIS had apocrine morphology. All five apocrine DCIS had high nuclear grade, and at least focal cribriform architecture. The second most common architectural pattern was solid in three cases.

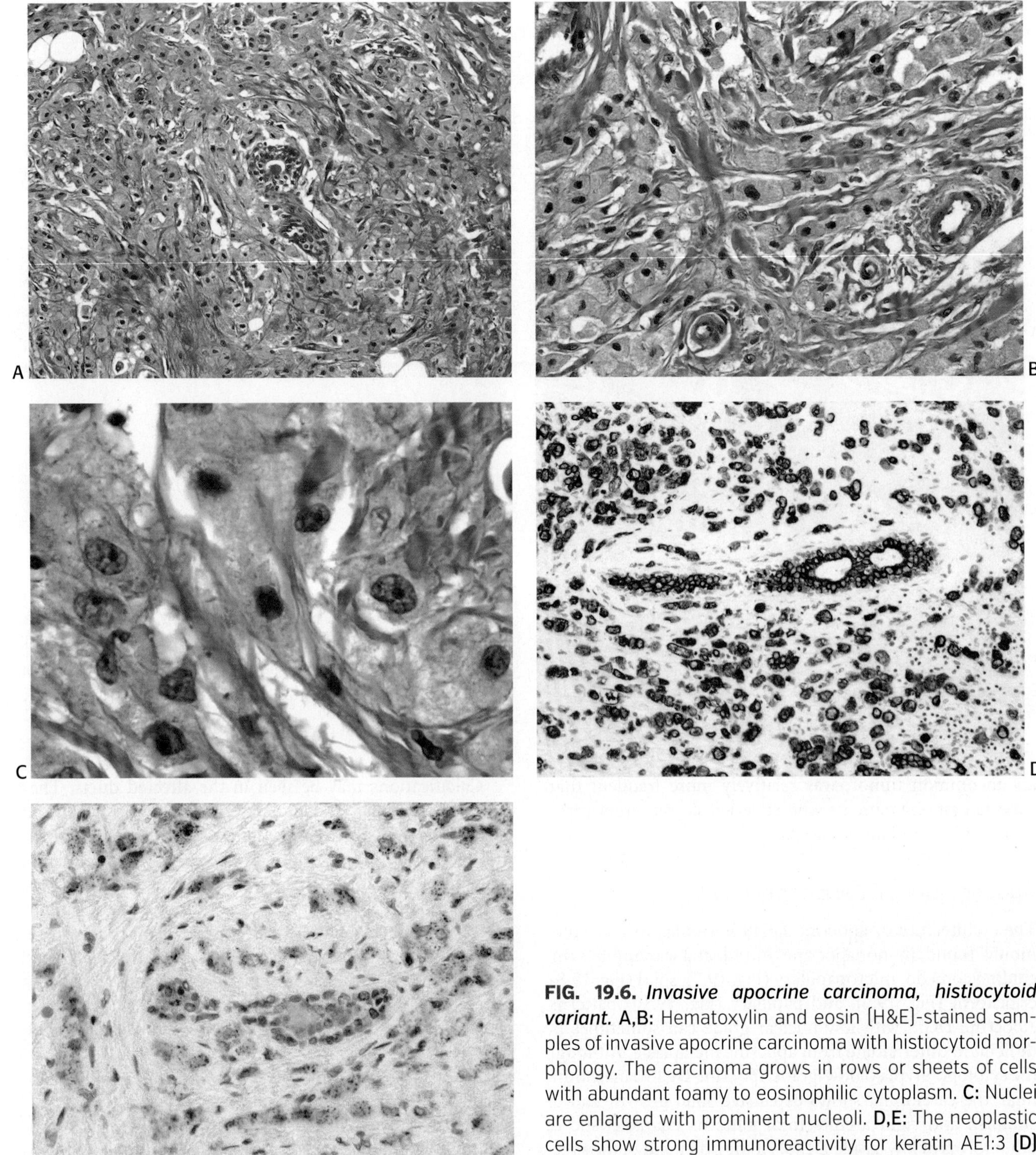

FIG. 19.6. ***Invasive apocrine carcinoma, histiocytoid variant.*** **A,B:** Hematoxylin and eosin (H&E)-stained samples of invasive apocrine carcinoma with histiocytoid morphology. The carcinoma grows in rows or sheets of cells with abundant foamy to eosinophilic cytoplasm. **C:** Nuclei are enlarged with prominent nucleoli. **D,E:** The neoplastic cells show strong immunoreactivity for keratin AE1:3 **(D)** and weak, granular reactivity for GCDFP-15 **(E)**.

The size of type B apocrine DCIS ranged from 2.7 to 4.2 cm, whereas the associated SA measured from 0.6 to 4.0 cm. All five type B apocrine DCIS were ER- and PR-negative; two cases were HER2-positive and two HER2-negative; the remaining DCIS had 2+ HER2 staining.

Fibrosis and chronic inflammation are often present around ducts and lobules involved by apocrine DCIS to a much greater degree than in benign apocrine lesions, especially when the DCIS has intermediate or high nuclear grade. Immunostains for myoepithelial markers and cytokeratin performed individually or in combination are usually helpful for detecting microinvasion in diagnostically difficult cases, or when apocrine DCIS involving a sclerosing lesion mimics invasive carcinoma.

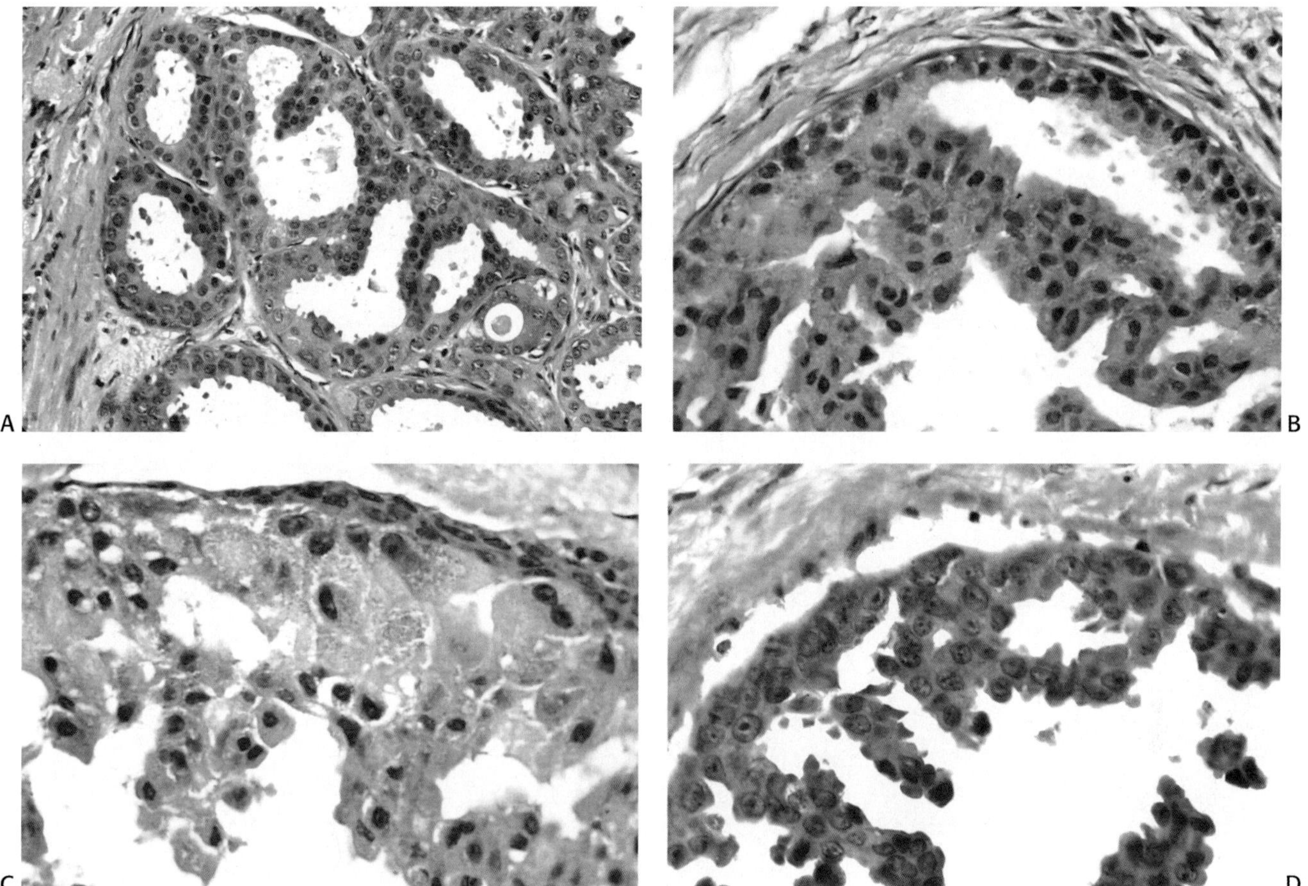

FIG. 19.7. ***Apocrine DCIS, micropapillary type.*** **A,B:** Low nuclear grade with slight nuclear pleomorphism and no nucleoli. **C:** Intermediate nuclear grade with moderate nuclear pleomorphism. The cells have variable amounts of cytoplasm. **D:** Micropapillary intraductal carcinoma with nucleoli in intermediate-grade nuclei.

The absence of inmmunoreactive myoepithelium in an apocrine lesion devoid of cytologic atypia is not an absolute criterion for the diagnosis of carcinoma. Histologically and cytologically benign cystic and papillary apocrine lesions with little or no detectable myoepithelium have been described by few investigators.[41–43] Cserni[41] described two apocrine papillary lesions with no detectable myoepithelium, and Tramm et al.[43] found large gaps in p63-positive myoepithelium surrounding apocrine metaplasia, especially papillary lesions, in the absence of cytologic atypia (Fig. 19.13). Immunoreactivity for calponin was more reliable for detecting myoepithelial cells in apocrine metaplasia, although some lesions were calponin-negative and p63-positive. Immunoreactive myoepithelium, however, is usually detectable in ducts involved by apocrine DCIS.

Despite using a panel of multiple myoepithelial markers, Seal et al.[44] were unable to detect immunoreactive myoepithelium in the fibrovascular cores and at the periphery of five apocrine papillary tumors ranging in size from 1.2 to 4.5 cm. These findings and the presence of cytologic atypia and/or mitotic activity led the authors to classify the lesions as encapsulated papillary variants of apocrine carcinoma.

Awareness of these findings is important, as they could potentially be misleading in some cases. When evaluating an apocrine lesion, and especially a papillary apocrine lesion, it is critical to determine whether the apocrine epithelial proliferation shows cytologic and architectural atypia, and these parameters need to guide the diagnostic interpretation. In addition, when ruling out invasive carcinoma, it is important to use a panel of myoepithelial markers.

Atypical Apocrine Lesions

Atypical apocrine proliferations often occur in sclerosing lesions, such as papilloma, radial scar, and SA (Figs. 19.14 and 19.15). The cytomorphology of the atypical apocrine cells is similar to that of low-grade or intermediate-grade apocrine DCIS, but the proliferation lacks evidence of expansive growth, complex architecture, and/or necrosis that would qualify the lesion as DCIS. An important consideration in establishing a diagnosis of apocrine DCIS is the determination that the lesion has a structural growth pattern customarily associated with a nonapocrine form of DCIS. This is

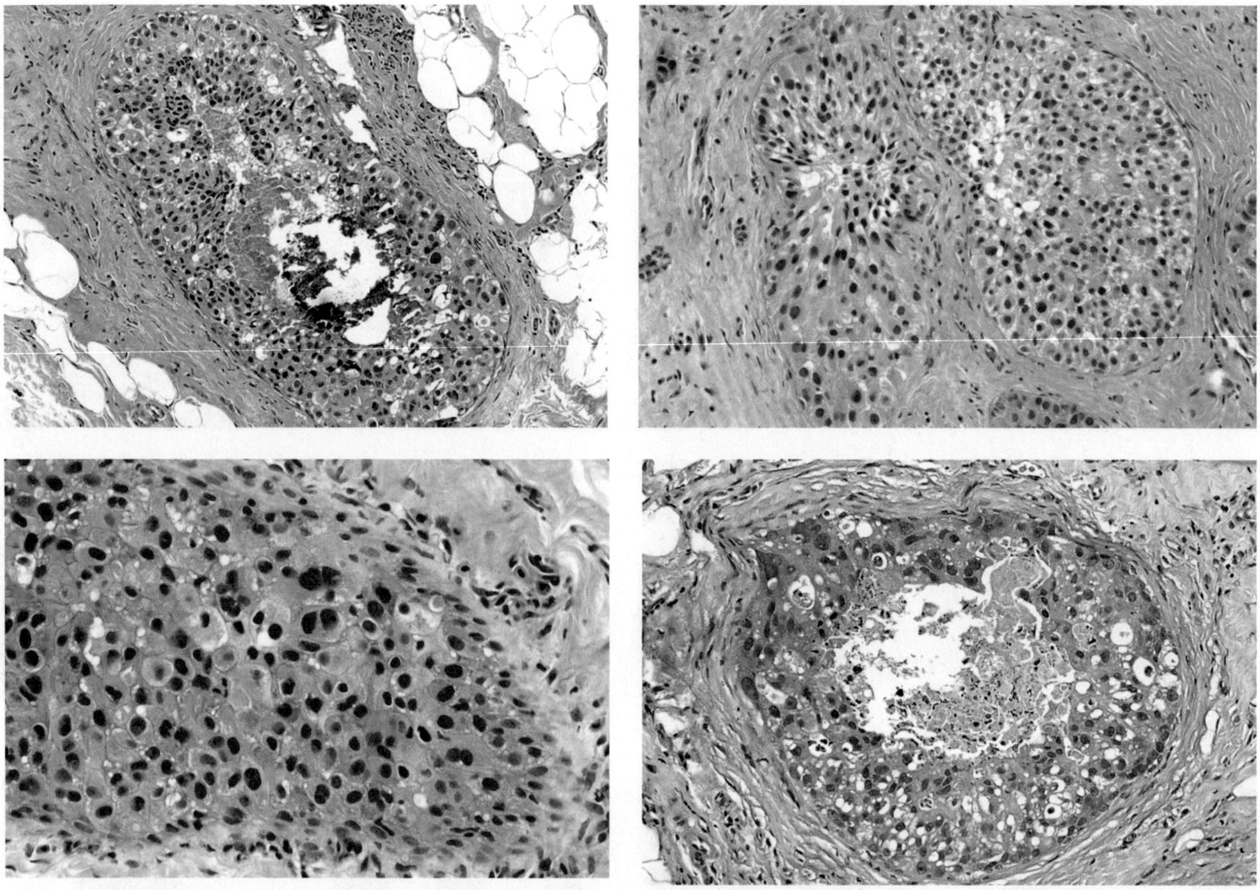

FIG. 19.8. ***Apocrine DCIS, solid type.*** **A:** Central necrosis, calcification, and intermediate nuclear grade. **B:** Low and intermediate nuclear grade. **C:** Low to high nuclear grade. **D:** Central necrosis, calcification, and pleomorphic nuclei.

a particularly significant factor when evaluating cytologically atypical apocrine components in lesions such as SA or radial scar. Carter and Rosen[45] described sclerosing breast lesions with atypical apocrine epithelium, which were characterized by nuclear atypia, varying degrees of cytoplasmic clearing, and rare mitoses. The distinction from DCIS was based in most cases on the absence of sufficient epithelial proliferation to produce the characteristic growth patterns of intraductal carcinoma. Seidman et al.[46] subsequently used similar criteria to define atypical apocrine adenosis. Rarely,

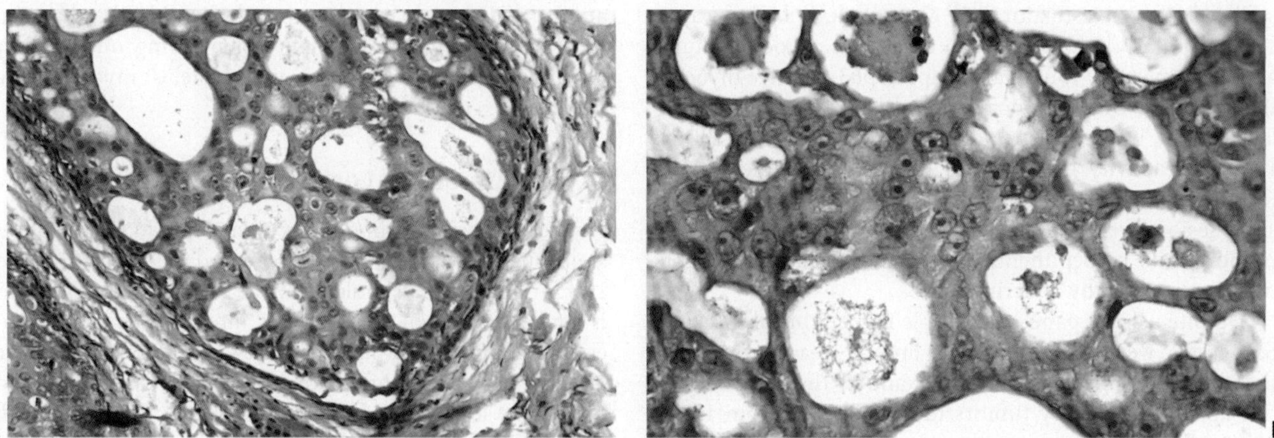

FIG. 19.9. ***Apocrine DCIS, cribriform type.*** **A–C:** Intermediate nuclear grade. Some nuclei have prominent nucleoli. **D:** Cystic ducts involved by cribriform DCIS.

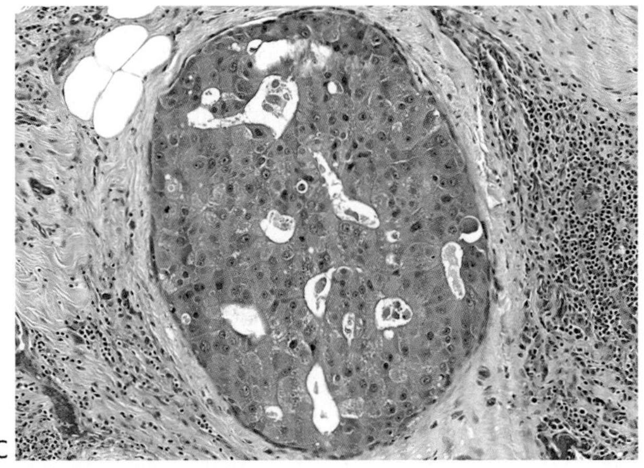

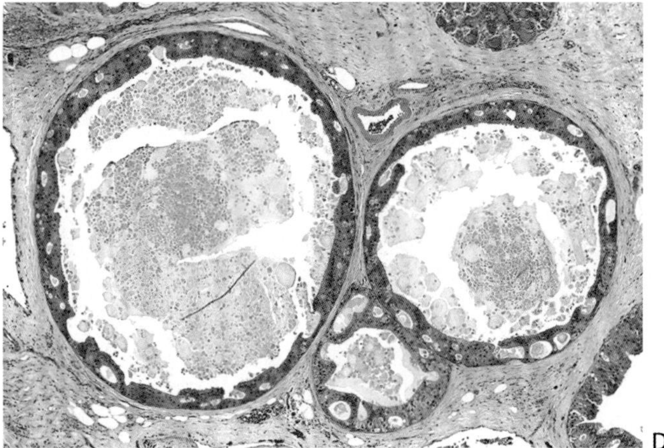

FIG. 19.9. *(Continued)*

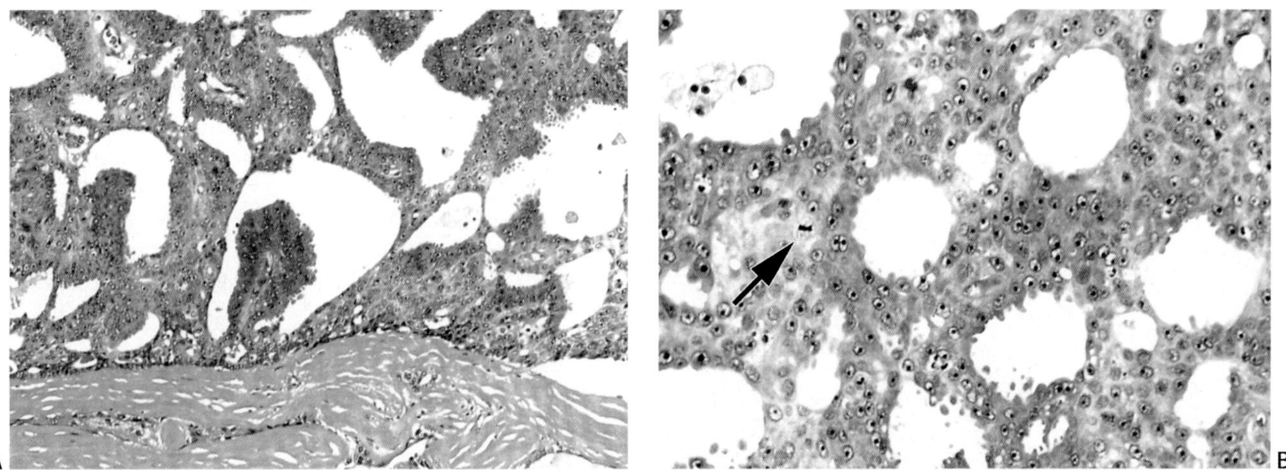

FIG. 19.10. ***Apocrine carcinoma, papillary type.*** **A:** Papillary fronds of apocrine carcinoma are shown. **B:** A cribriform area in the papillary carcinoma. The *arrow* indicates a mitotic figure. Note the prominent nucleoli.

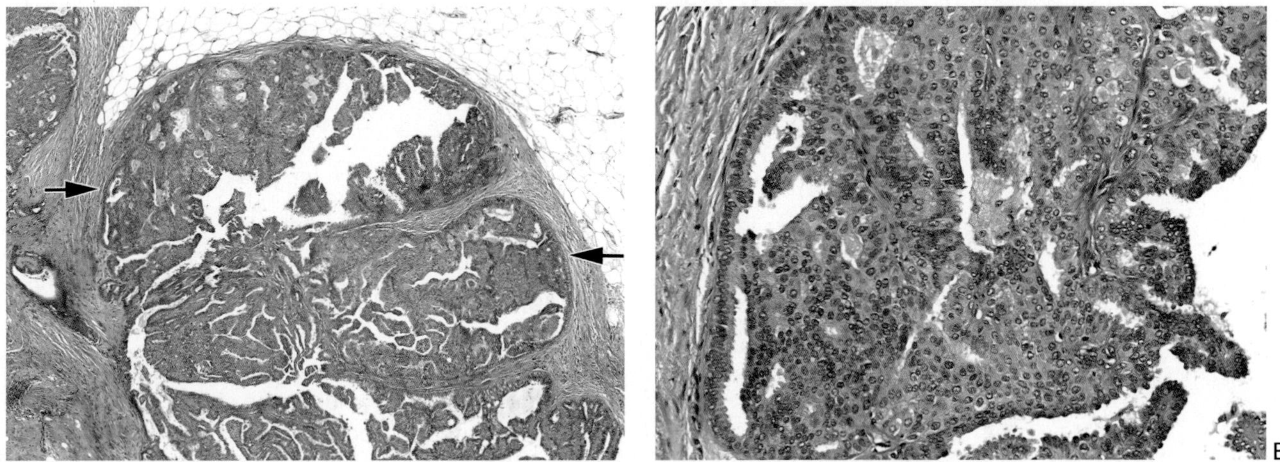

FIG. 19.11. ***Apocrine DCIS involving a sclerosing papilloma.*** **A:** Some of the fronds of a sclerosing papilloma are involved by apocrine DCIS (*arrows*). **B:** Magnified view of one area of DCIS indicated by an *arrow* in **(A)**.

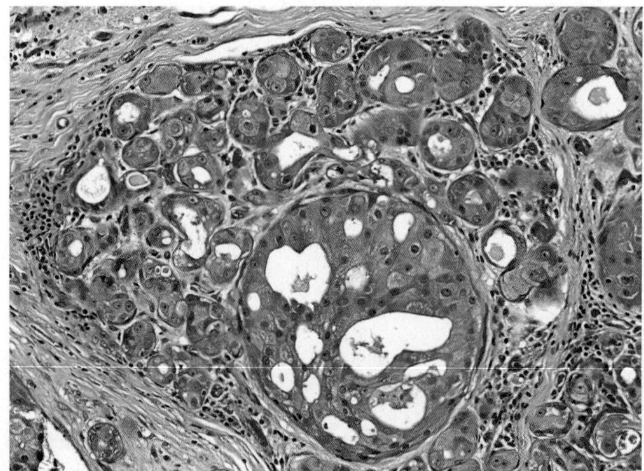

FIG. 19.12. ***Apocrine intraductal carcinoma with lobular extension.*** Apocrine DCIS with low nuclear grade and cribriform structure fills an enlarged intralobular ductule and extends into the acini.

the cytologic features are so abnormal in such lesions that a diagnosis of carcinoma *in situ* is indicated in the absence of a characteristic *in situ* carcinomatous structure.

Others have attempted to distinguish atypical apocrine lesions on the basis of extent as well as cytologic and structural criteria. Tavassoli and Norris[47] considered apocrine ductal lesions that occupied an area of less than 2 mm, regardless of cytologic and structural features, to be atypical apocrine hyperplasia. Larger, histologically identical foci qualified as apocrine DCIS. O'Malley et al.[48] used a combination of cytologic criteria and lesional diameter to define a "borderline" group of apocrine lesions. Foci with "borderline" cytologic features were considered to be apocrine DCIS if larger than 8 mm. Lesions with cytologic features of carcinoma were termed apocrine DCIS regardless of size, but those smaller than 4 mm were referred to as "limited." "Borderline" or atypical apocrine hyperplasias were proliferative foci smaller than 8 mm with nuclear atypia lacking the characteristic irregular nuclear membranes, coarse chromatin, and large, often multiple, nucleoli of apocrine carcinoma. For additional discussion of atypical apocrine hyperplasia and apocrine DCIS, see Chapters 9 and 11.

Apocrine Metaplasia

Benign apocrine change can be found in lobules and is especially common in cysts where it frequently has a papillary

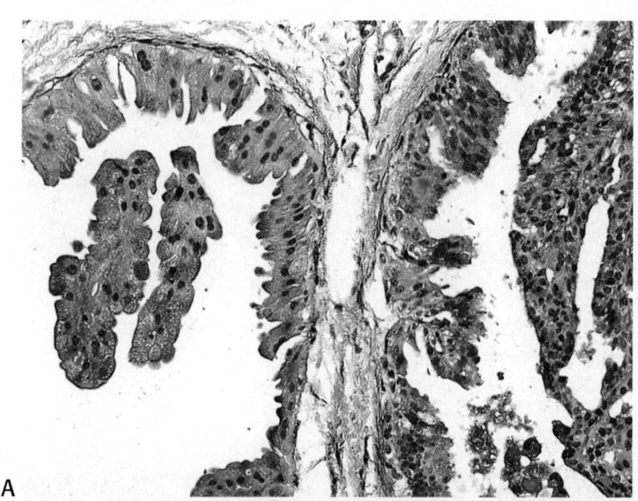

A

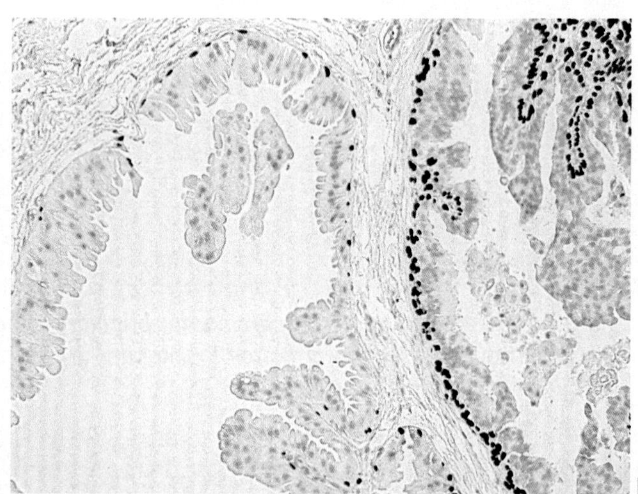

B

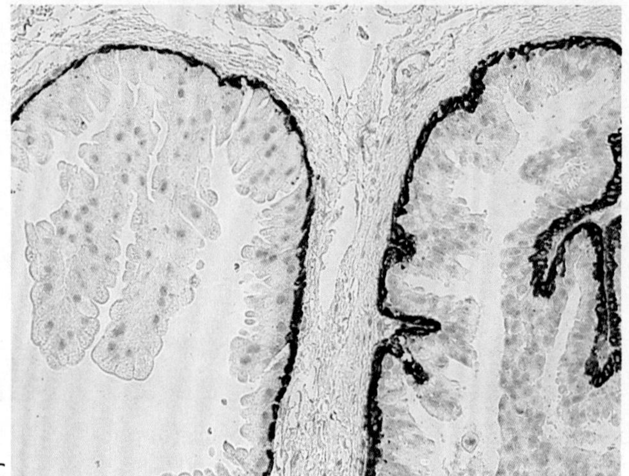

C

FIG. 19.13. ***Apocrine metaplasia and myoepithelium.*** **A:** Two glands with apocrine metaplasia. The gland on the right has atypical hyperplasia and appears to have myoepithelium. **B:** A p63 immunostain shows many fewer reactive myoepithelial nuclei around the ordinary apocrine gland (*left*) than around the atypical apocrine gland (*right*). **C:** A calponin immunostain shows a continuous layer of myoepithelium around both apocrine glands.

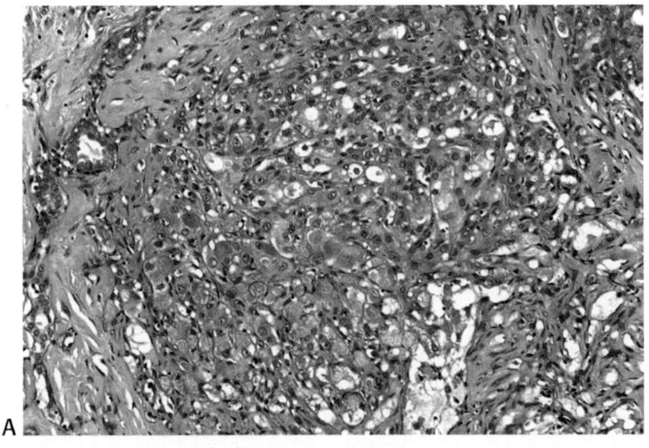

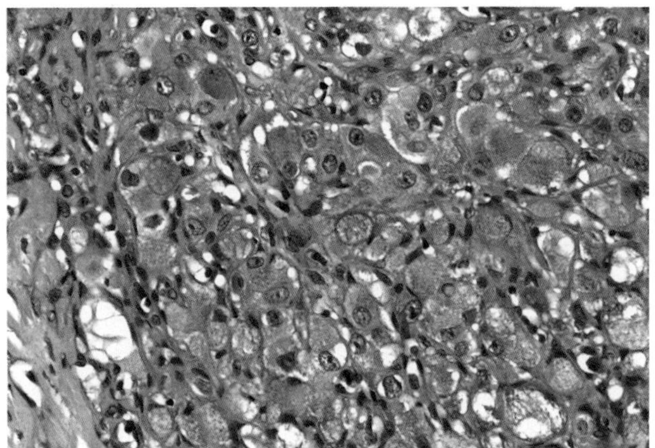

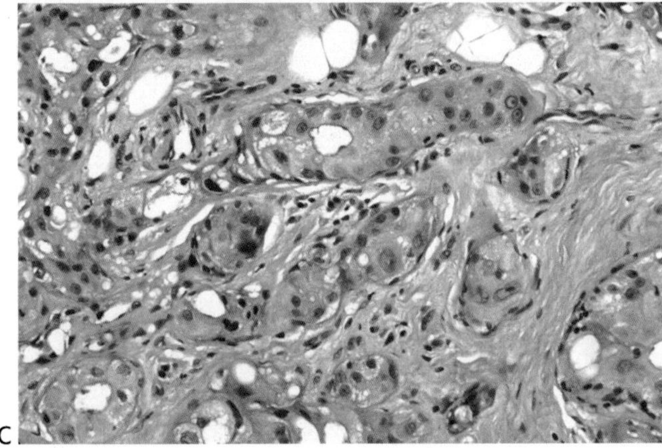

FIG. 19.14. ***Atypical apocrine adenosis bordering on apocrine DCIS.*** **A,B:** This unusual lesion features large cells with pleomorphic nuclei and basophilic intracytoplasmic mucin vacuoles. **C:** Pleomorphic cells with focal cytoplasmic vacuolization and clearing, but only minimal epithelial expansion.

or micropapillary configuration (Figs. 19.13 and 19.16). Apocrine metaplasia is prone to develop mammographically detectable calcium oxalate calcifications (Fig. 19.17). Calcium oxalate deposits are associated with benign apocrine lesions and only rarely occur in apocrine carcinoma.[49] Chapter 5 contains a detailed description of benign apocrine metaplasia.

It is possible that some apocrine carcinomas may arise from preexisting benign apocrine epithelium rather than *de novo*, but transitions from atypical hyperplastic apocrine lesions to carcinoma are evident only in rare examples of apocrine carcinoma.[50–52]

CYTOLOGY

The finding of atypical apocrine cells in fine-needle aspiration (FNA) material may suggest a diagnosis of apocrine carcinoma.[53] Cytology specimens obtained from apocrine carcinomas tend to be highly cellular, with marked nuclear pleomorphism, large nucleoli, and cellular debris.[54] The neoplastic cells are often binucleated and have distinct cytoplasmic borders. Caution should be exercised in the evaluation of such findings, especially when the aspirate is obtained from a mammographically detected nonpalpable lesion. FNA of atypical apocrine metaplasia in SA and radial scars,[45] which are likely to be identified in this fashion, closely simulates apocrine carcinoma cytologically, but it usually yields specimens of limited cellularity with admixed nonatypical epithelial cells and myoepithelium. The FNA material from three mass-forming lesions containing atypical apocrine adenosis was interpreted as benign in one case, diagnostic of fibroadenoma in another, and suspicious for carcinoma in the remaining case.[55]

The cytologic differential diagnosis of high-grade apocrine carcinoma includes squamous cell carcinoma, a keratin-producing tumor. Ductal carcinoma with neuroendocrine differentiation can enter the differential diagnosis of low-grade apocrine carcinoma. An FNA sample with degenerated apocrine metaplastic cells exfoliated from the lining of a benign cyst may be misinterpreted as suspicious for carcinoma. The differential diagnosis of granular cell tumor should also be considered.

ELECTRON MICROSCOPY

At the ultrastructural level, the cells of apocrine carcinoma contain abundant organelles, including mitochondria of different size[56] and often with incomplete cristae, as well

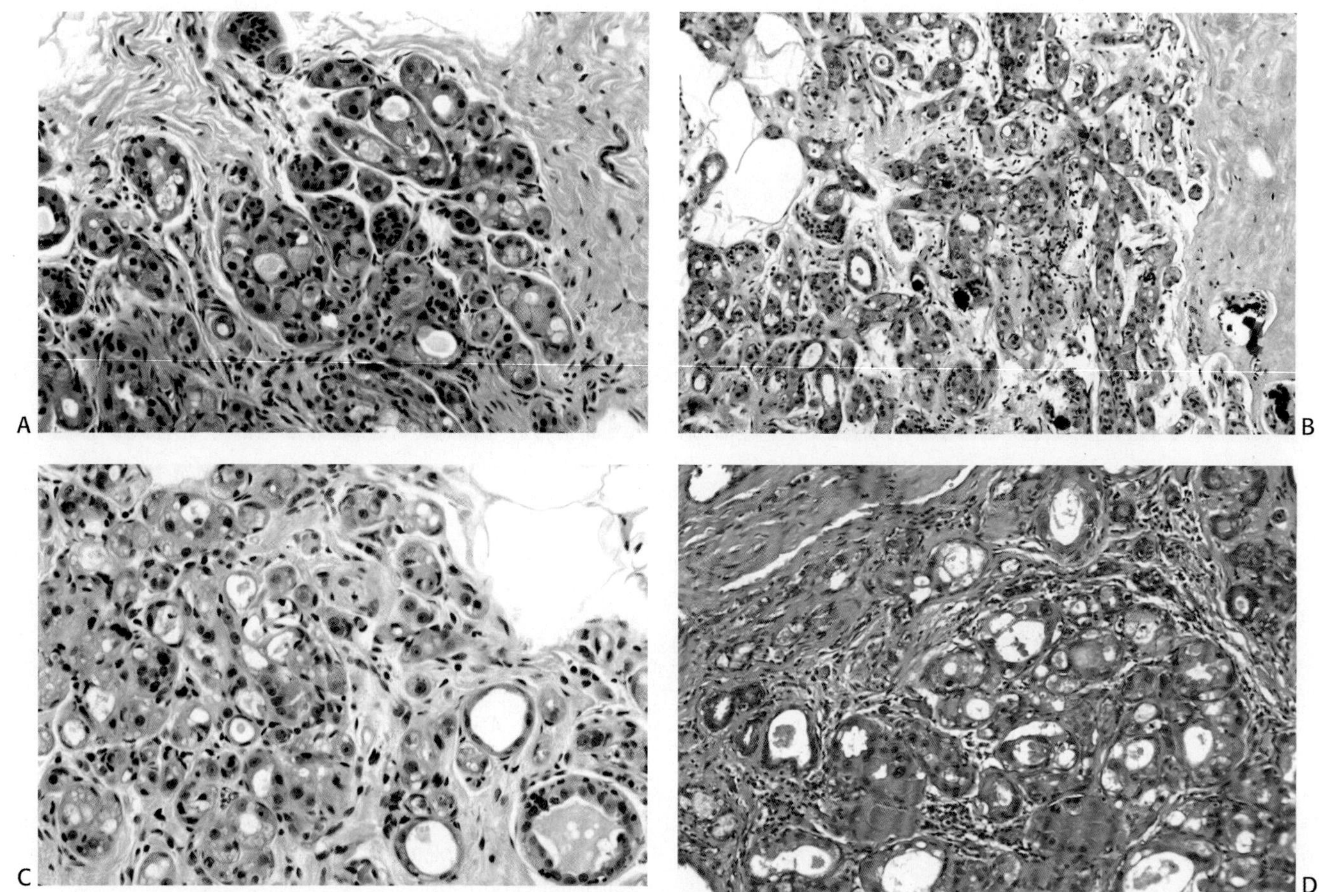

FIG. 19.15. ***Apocrine adenosis.*** **A:** Apocrine adenosis. **B:** Apocrine adenosis and calcifications. **C,D:** Atypia with glandular expansion.

as variable numbers of osmiophilic cytoplasmic secretory granules.[9,13,52] Many of the tumor cells also contain empty vesicles of about the same size as the osmiophilic granules.

IMMUNOHISTOCHEMISTRY

ER, PR, AR, HER2, and Ki67

Most intraductal and invasive apocrine carcinomas are negative for ER and PR.[9,13,27,47,57] More detailed analysis has shown that the low frequency of ER reactivity applies to ER-α and that nearly 75% of apocrine carcinomas express ER-β, as determined by IHC and ER-β mRNA analysis.[58] ER-β expression was equally frequent in intraductal and invasive apocrine carcinomas. Vranic et al.[59] found expression of ER-α36, a novel isoform of ER-α, in 18/19 (94.7%) pure apocrine carcinomas negative for ER-α66, the most common isoform of ER-α, as well as for PR. Of note, ER-α36 is reported to have cytoplasmic and membranous localization immunohistochemically.

AR is expressed in apocrine carcinomas[27,57,60] as well as in benign apocrine lesions.[60] *In vitro* studies have demonstrated enhanced metabolism of testosterone precursors by apocrine carcinomas when compared with other types of breast carcinoma.[47] Testosterone enhances the proliferation of apocrine breast cell lines *in vitro*, an effect that is inhibited by the antiandrogen flutamide.[61] It has been observed that the growth of cutaneous apocrine glands can be stimulated by androgens,[62] and that some androgen metabolites are concentrated in apocrine secretions.[63] In general, most ER-positive breast carcinomas also express AR, whereas about half of ER-negative breast carcinomas are also AR-negative.[64] In one study,[65] breast carcinomas with apocrine morphology were highly represented among ER-negative/AR-positive breast carcinomas, including 4/5 ER-negative/HER2-positive carcinomas and 2/3 triple negative/AR-positive tumors.

Some authors regard as "pure apocrine carcinomas" only tumors having apocrine morphology and the ER- and PR-negative, AR-positive immunoprofile characteristic of apocrine metaplasia. At least two groups[16,66] subdivided tumors with apocrine histology based on ER and AR immunoprofile into pure apocrine carcinomas (ER-negative and AR-positive) and apocrine-like carcinomas. The latter tumors were for most part ER- and AR-positive, but also ER-positive and AR-negative or ER- and AR-negative. About half of pure apocrine carcinomas were HER2-negative and half HER2-positive, with a slightly greater percentage of the latter.[16,66] Alvarenga et al.[18] found that 15/24 (62.5%) carcinomas with apocrine morphology were HER2-positive, including 8 that were also ER- and PR-positive with Ki67 index greater than 14% (luminal B-subtype by IHC). Tsutsumi[19] reported that 23/44 (52%) morphologically and immunophenotypically apocrine carcinomas overexpressed HER2.

In a study of 24 apocrine carcinomas by Alvarenga et al.,[18] the mean and median percentages of Ki67-positive cells were 48.4% and 42.5%, respectively. The Ki67 index was

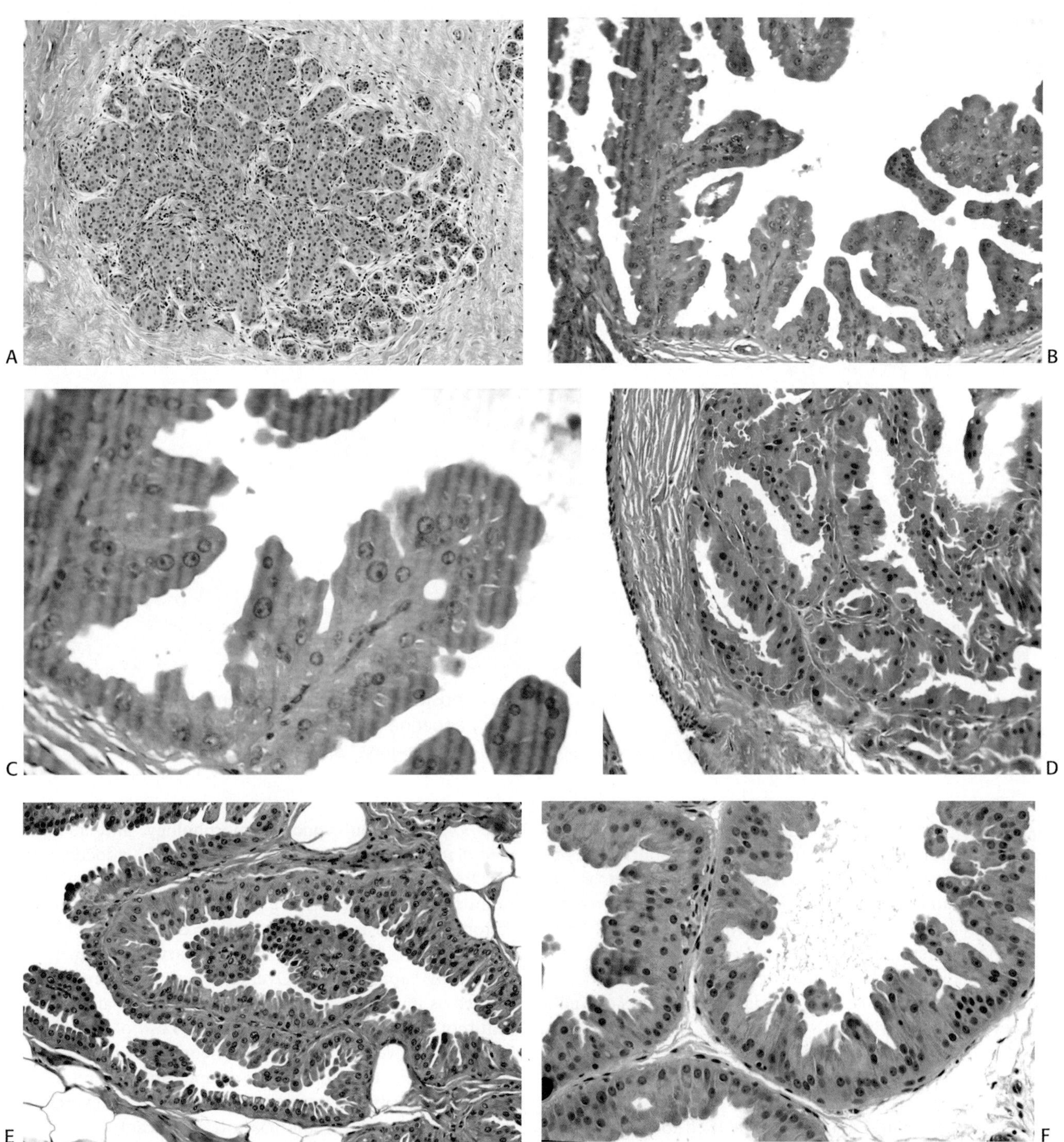

FIG. 19.16. ***Apocrine metaplasia.*** **A:** Apocrine metaplasia in a lobule that could be mistaken for lobular carcinoma *in situ* (LCIS). **B,C:** Cystic papillary apocrine metaplasia. Fibrovascular stroma is present in the papillary structures. Nuclei tend to be basally oriented and relatively evenly spaced. **D:** Complex papillary apocrine metaplasia. **E:** Papillary apocrine metaplasia. **F:** Micropapillary apocrine hyperplasia. **G,H:** Atypical micropapillary apocrine hyperplasia with a disorderly distribution of nuclei.

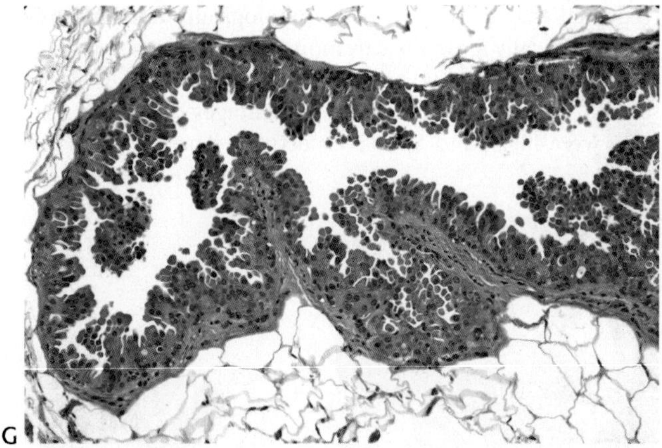

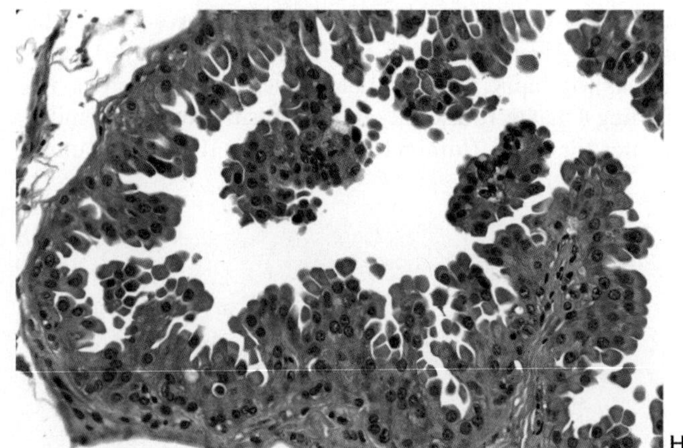

FIG. 19.16. *(Continued)*

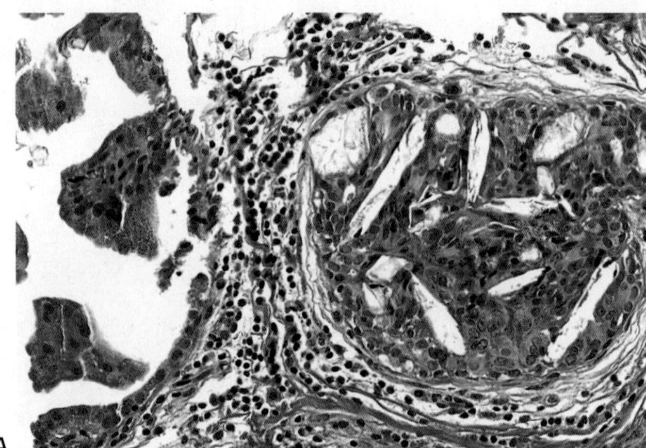

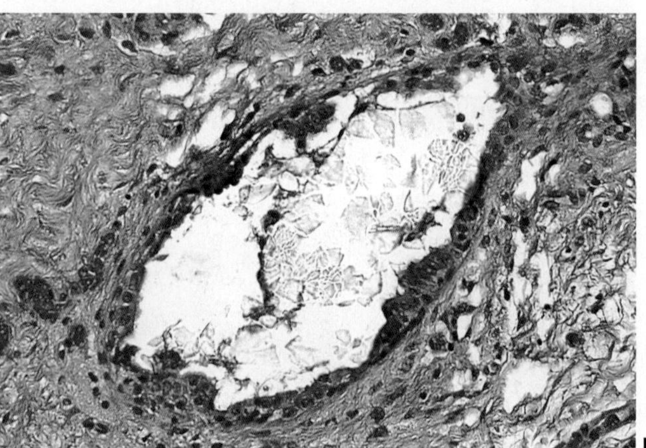

FIG. 19.17. ***Apocrine metaplasia with calcium oxalate deposits.*** **A:** Crystalline calcium oxalate deposits are shown in a hyperplastic duct next to papillary apocrine metaplasia. **B:** Translucent oxalate crystals in an apocrine cyst have the characteristic "broken glass" appearance.

higher than 14% in 81.8% of the tumors and 14% or lower in the remaining 18.2%. The mean Ki67 proliferative rate of 41 ER-negative/HER2-positive/AR-positive carcinomas in a study by Lin et al.[35] was 44.7% ± 23.71%. Thirty-three of the 41 carcinomas (80.5%) had apocrine morphology. Leal et al.[27] found that the Ki67 index increased significantly between low-, intermediate-, and high-grade apocrine DCIS, although there was substantial overlap in the ranges of Ki67 indices among the groups.

Apocrine Antigens

Immunohistochemical studies may be used to confirm the diagnostic impression of apocrine differentiation in some cases, but they are not essential to establish the morphologic diagnosis of apocrine carcinoma. GCDFP-15 was detected in a high percentage of intraductal and invasive carcinomas with apocrine cytology,[9,13] but only in only 23% of ductal carcinomas without apocrine morphology, and in 5% of medullary carcinomas. Kasashima et al.[37] documented GCDFP-15 positivity in 46/48 (96%) apocrine carcinomas. Immunostaining for GCDFP-15 has not been a useful predictor of prognosis.[67] The coexistence of apocrine and neuroendocrine differentiation in mammary carcinomas was studied by Sapino et al.[68] Overall, apocrine differentiation, defined as immunoreactivity for GCDFP-15 in at least 50% of tumor cells, was detected in 21/50 (42%) of carcinomas immunoreactive for at least one neuroendocrine marker, although the cytologic features of apocrine differentiation were not described. The presence of GCDFP-15 expression in neuroendocrine carcinomas was significantly associated with older age at diagnosis, coincidental immunoreactivity for AR, and a more favorable prognosis after 5 years of follow-up.

Recent studies have found few additional antigens with increased expression in apocrine lesions. Using proteomic analysis, Danish investigators identified 15-hydroxy-prostaglandin dehydrogenase (15-PGDH),[69] hydroxylethyl-glutaryl-coenzyme A reductase (HMG-CoA reductase),[69] and acyl-CoA synthetase medium chain family member 1[70] as biomarkers of apocrine cells. These antigens are expressed in benign as well as in malignant apocrine lesions, linking the two epithelial proliferations. The same investigators also found that psoriasin, S-100A9, and p53[69] are upregulated in apocrine breast carcinomas. In a subsequent study from the same investigators, apocrine cells were reported to be negative for ER and PR, as well as for bcl-2 and GATA3.[71]

In a study evaluating breast carcinomas in patients with Cowden syndrome[25] (see also section on genetics and molecular alterations), positive immunoreactivity for γ-glutamyltransferase 1 (GGT1) was strongly associated with apocrine morphology and apocrine molecular subtype. All (15/15; 100%) Cowden breast carcinomas were AR-positive, but only 27% were also ER-negative. Based on these findings, it can be concluded that not all breast carcinomas occurring in patients with Cowden syndrome are pure apocrine carcinomas immunohistochemically.

About half of apocrine carcinomas are triple negative. In a study by Choi et al.,[72] 19/122 (16%) triple negative carcinomas showed apocrine morphology. Twelve tumors (9.8%) had the apocrine profile defined as positive for AR and/or GGT1, but only eight of these carcinomas (66.7%) had apocrine morphology. In this series, 23/122 (18.9%) triple negative tumors were GGT1-positive and 7/122 (5.7%) were AR-positive. Triple negative carcinomas with apocrine subtype (AR- and/or GGT1-positive) showed lower Ki67 labeling ($p = 0.004$), lower histologic grade ($p = 0.109$), and relatively good prognosis ($p = 0.147$) with longer disease-free survival (DFS) and overall survival (OS) compared with nonapocrine triple negative carcinomas.

5α-reductase catalyzes the conversion of testosterone into biologically active androgen. Kasashima et al.[37] found expression of this antigen in 30/48 (62.5%) invasive carcinomas with apocrine morphology. 5α-Reductase-positive apocrine carcinomas were significantly larger and had higher histologic grade, more frequent lymphatic and vascular invasion, as well as shorter relapse-free survival (RFS) time than 5α-reductase-negative apocrine carcinomas. No evidence of 5α-reductase reactivity was detected in five apocrine DCIS that were not associated with invasion.

Bundred et al.[73] found reactivity for zinc alpha-2-glycoprotein, a protein present in breast cyst fluid, in benign apocrine cells, and in 36% of invasive breast carcinomas, but did not indicate if the tumors had apocrine morphology. Immunoreactivity for this antigen was not significantly correlated with tumor size, nodal status, grade, or hormone receptor expression in the carcinoma. However, carcinomas with zinc alpha-2-glycoprotein expression had a significantly reduced survival and disease-free interval. Nonetheless, none of the novel apocrine antigens mentioned above has practical diagnostic applications.

Non-apocrine Antigens

Apocrine carcinomas tend to be immunoreactive for carcinoembryonic antigen (CEA).[40] They are usually negative or only focally positive for S-100 protein and are always reactive for cytokeratins. Shao et al.[74] reported that 8/8 (100%) invasive ductal carcinomas with apocrine features were positive for CK7, CK8, and CK18, and 7/8 (87.5%) were positive for CK19. Notably, 4/8 (50%) invasive carcinoma with apocrine features were CK20-positive, in sharp contrast to no CK20 reactivity in nonapocrine carcinomas. None of the carcinomas with apocrine features in this study were positive for the basal cytokeratins CK5/6 and CK14. Alvarenga et al.[75] also documented CK19 positivity in all 21 apocrine carcinomas in their series.

Reactivity for p53 has been demonstrated in 38% to 68% of apocrine carcinomas, but not in benign apocrine proliferations.[27,76] Moriya et al.[76] reported that apocrine carcinomas with poorly differentiated nuclear grade were more likely to be p53-positive, and there was a lower frequency of p53 reactivity in invasive than in intraductal apocrine carcinomas. They also detected reactivity for p21 and p27, respectively, in 36.8% and 66.7% benign apocrine lesions and in 63.6% and 52.4% apocrine carcinomas. In a study by Tsutsumi,[19] p53 overexpression was more frequent in histologically defined apocrine carcinomas (33/44,75%) than in nonapocrine carcinomas (22/47, 47%).

Vranic et al.[66] detected epidermal growth factor receptor (EGFR) protein in 62% of apocrine carcinomas, with higher expression in pure apocrine (76%) than in apocrine-like carcinomas (29%) ($p = 0.006$). They observed an inverse correlation between the expression of EGFR and HER2 proteins in pure apocrine carcinomas ($p = 0.006$, $r = -0.499$).

Cutaneous and mammary apocrine carcinomas have similar immunohistochemical features. In most cases, the tumor cells contain diastase-resistant periodic acid–Schiff (PAS)-positive granules that are also stained with toluidine blue and appear red with the trichrome stain. Cytoplasmic iron granules, a feature of benign apocrine cells, are variably present in apocrine carcinomas. Occasional cells may contain mucicarmine-positive secretion, but most are negative for mucin and α-lactalbumin.[77,78] In exceptional cases, there can be extensive intracytoplasmic mucin accumulation, resulting in numerous signet ring–type cells that sometimes are substantially enlarged (Fig. 19.18).

DIFFERENTIAL DIAGNOSIS OF APOCRINE LESIONS

Metastatic Renal Cell Carcinoma

The presence of an abundant lymphocytic infiltrate and the cytologic features of invasive apocrine carcinoma with clear cell morphology occasionally may suggest that the tumor is metastatic from a conventional renal cell carcinoma and possibly involves a lymph node (Fig. 19.19). Immunoperoxidase

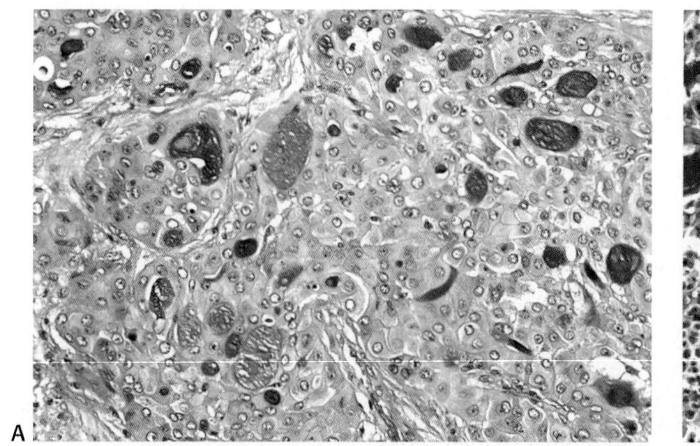

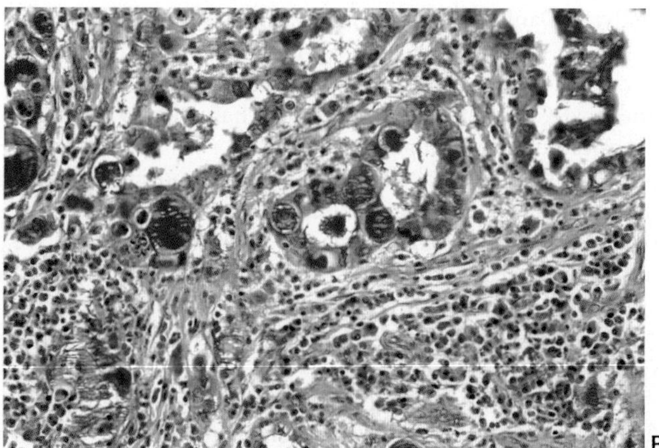

FIG. 19.18. ***Invasive apocrine carcinoma with mucin.*** **A:** Prominent basophilic mucin is present in glandular spaces and in tumor cells. **B:** Intracytoplasmic mucin is stained magenta with the mucicarmine stain in this gland-forming invasive apocrine carcinoma.

stains for CK7, AR, and GCDFP-15 highlight apocrine carcinoma but are negative in conventional (clear cell) renal cell carcinoma. Rarely, the mononuclear infiltrate may obscure the carcinoma especially when there is an accompanying granulomatous reaction. An immunohistochemical stain for cytokeratin can be used to highlight the presence of epithelial elements in such tumors. In most instances, the presence of DCIS can be documented morphologically or with immunoperoxidase stains for myoepithelial markers, supporting mammary origin.

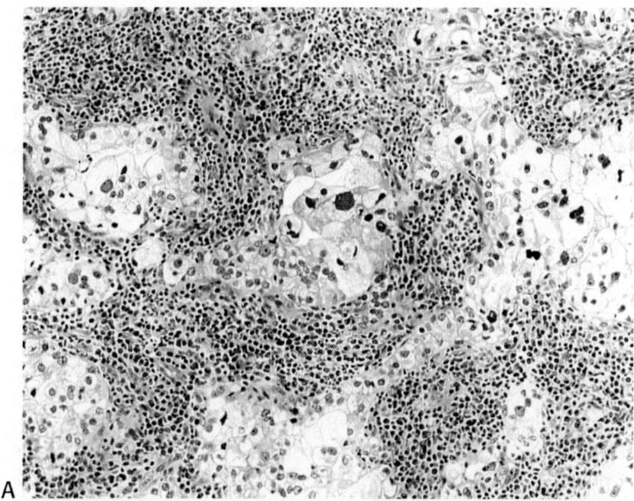

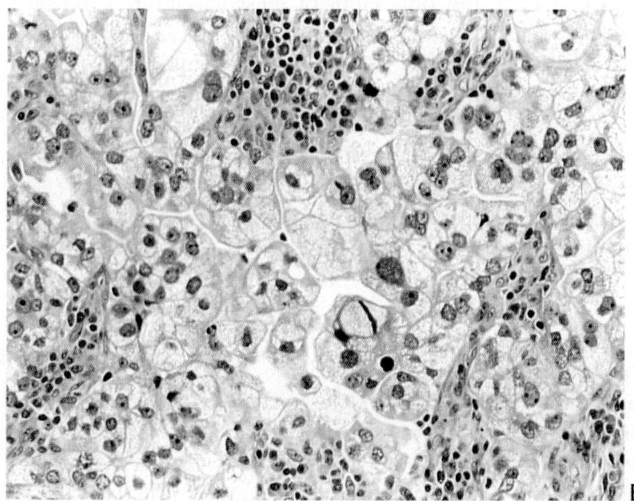

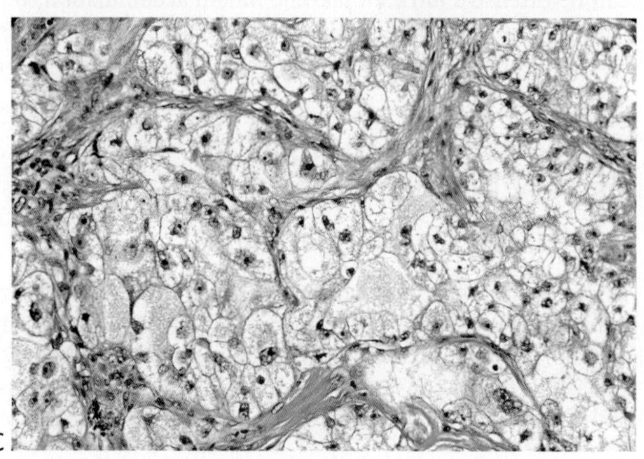

FIG. 19.19. ***Invasive apocrine carcinoma with clear cells.*** **A:** Islands of infiltrating apocrine carcinoma are surrounded by a lymphoplasmacytic infiltrate. **B,C:** The carcinoma cells have pleomorphic nuclei and abundant finely granular or clear cytoplasm, and closely mimic metastatic renal cell carcinoma.

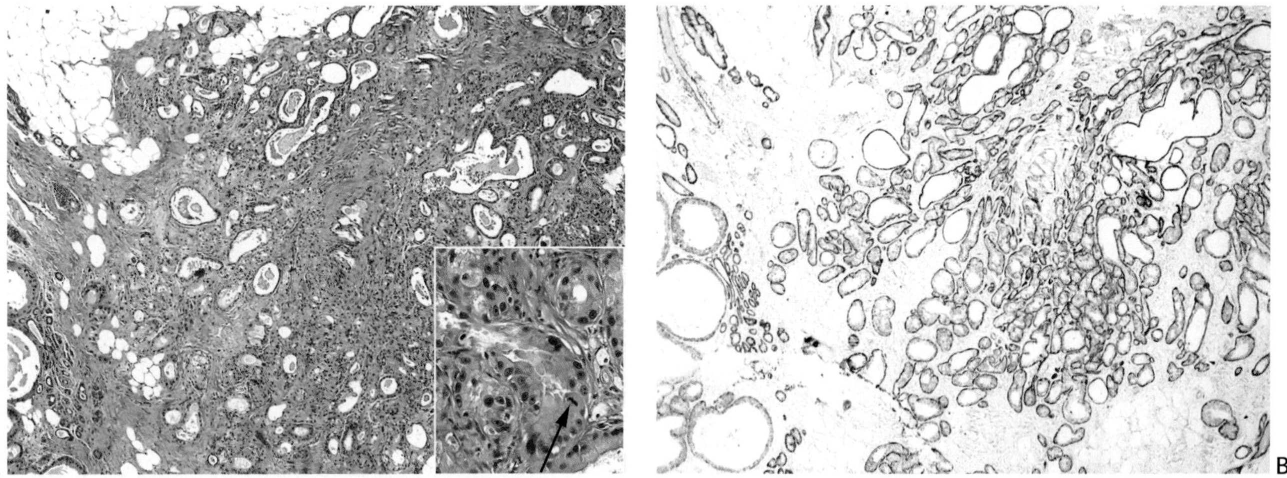

FIG. 19.20. *Apocrine DCIS involving sclerosing adenosis.* **A:** Apocrine DCIS involves the glands and tubules of SA. A detail view of the carcinoma (*inset*) shows a mitotic figure (*arrow*). **B:** A calponin immunostain highlights the myoepithelium lining the glands.

Carcinoma with Intralobular and Pagetoid Spread

Extension of apocrine DCIS into the epithelium of lobules is frequently present (Fig. 19.12). Apocrine DCIS growing extensively in SA may simulate an invasive carcinoma. The lobulocentric and swirling pattern of the glandular proliferation and the nonreactive eosinophilic quality of the stroma around SA are usually sufficient for correct interpretation (Fig. 19.20). Myoepithelial stains can be helpful in some cases.

Apocrine DCIS that is predominantly distributed in a pagetoid manner in small ducts and lobules can resemble lobular carcinoma *in situ* (LCIS). In this setting, the E-cadherin stain reveals diffuse membranous reactivity in the neoplastic apocrine cells as well as in the native epithelial cells. By contrast, E-cadherin reactivity is fragmented or absent from classical and pleomorphic LCIS.

Radiation Effect in Apocrine Lesions

Biopsies of the conserved breast after radiotherapy are difficult to interpret in women with apocrine carcinoma because the irradiation causes severe cytologic changes in nonneoplastic apocrine epithelium that can closely resemble apocrine carcinoma. In these cases, it is very helpful to have slides of the pretreatment carcinoma available for comparison with the posttreatment specimen (see Chapter 41).

Oncocytic Neoplasms

Rarely, tumors conventionally classified as apocrine are probably true oncocytic neoplasms characterized by very abundant mitochondria at the ultrastructural level. Damiani et al.[79] described three oncocytic carcinomas of the breast that were strongly immunoreactive with an antimitochondrial antibody but not for GCDFP-15, which is positive in most apocrine carcinomas. The term "oncocytic carcinoma" should be reserved for lesions demonstrated to have appropriate immunohistochemical and/or ultrastructural characteristics.

Granular Cell Tumor

The clinical, radiologic and microscopic differential diagnosis of invasive apocrine carcinoma includes granular cell tumor (Fig. 19.21). Occasionally, it can be very difficult to differentiate the latter from invasive apocrine carcinoma in dense collagenous stroma or from the histiocytoid variant of apocrine carcinoma (Fig. 19.6). The cells of granular cell tumor have abundant cytoplasm that is characteristically granular because of the presence of abundant lysosomes. The nuclei are relatively small and lack atypia. Immunoperoxidase stains can be used to resolve the differential diagnosis in problematic cases. Granular cell tumor is strongly CD68-positive and keratin AE1:3-negative, whereas apocrine carcinoma is keratin AE1:3-positive and CD68-negative. Granular cell tumor and apocrine carcinoma are both negative for ER and PR. S-100 is uniformly and diffusely positive in granular cell tumor, and can also show some reactivity in apocrine carcinoma, albeit usually focal and less intense.

GENETICS AND MOLECULAR ALTERATIONS

Ploidy has been evaluated in apocrine lesions by image analysis in Feulgen-stained sections. A diploid DNA content was found in benign apocrine metaplasia, atypical apocrine metaplasia, and orderly, low-grade forms of apocrine DCIS.[6,80] Ploidy correlated with grade, and almost all poorly differentiated apocrine carcinomas were aneuploid.[6] Apocrine lesions with an aneuploid DNA content are most likely to be carcinoma, but a diploid content does not distinguish between apocrine metaplasia, atypical apocrine metaplasia and apocrine carcinoma.

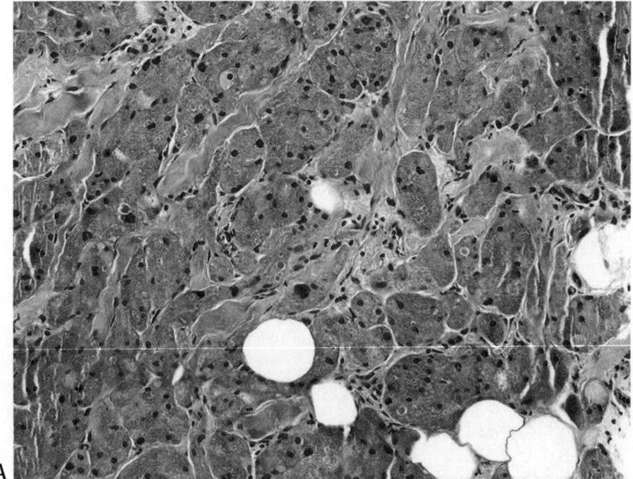

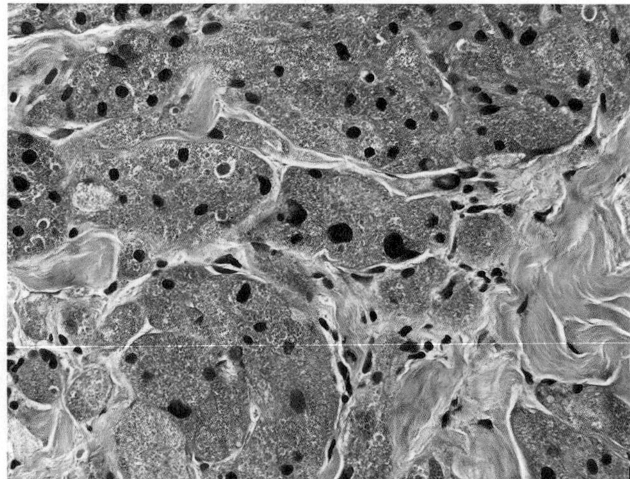

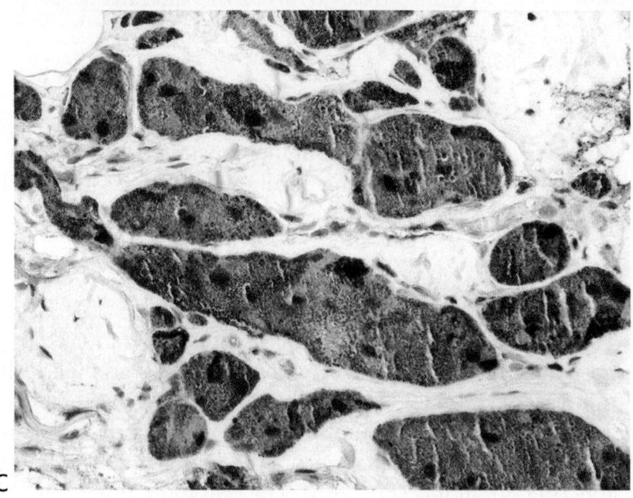

FIG. 19.21. ***Granular cell tumor simulating invasive apocrine carcinoma.*** **A,B:** Granular cell tumor consists of large cells with abundant granular cytoplasm. The cytoplasm and granules may be basophilic as shown here or eosinophilic. Note variation in nuclear size. **C:** An S-100 immunostain decorates the nuclei and cytoplasm of the cells.

Loss of heterozygosity (LOH) has been detected in benign and carcinomatous apocrine lesions.[11,81,82] Based on these observations, the investigators suggested that some benign apocrine proliferations may be clonal and that in some cases they may be precancerous. Jones et al.[11] compared the pattern of chromosomal alterations of apocrine metaplasia to those of apocrine DCIS and invasive carcinoma using comparative genomic hybridization (CGH). They found that benign and malignant apocrine lesions shared some similar genetic alterations, including losses of 1p, 16q, 17q, and 22q and gains of 1p and 2q. These provocative data raise the possibility that apocrine metaplasia may be a nonobligate precursor of some apocrine carcinomas.

Using gene array analysis, Farmer et al.[10] identified a molecular subtype of apocrine carcinoma that also encompasses invasive pleomorphic lobular carcinoma. Tumors in this group showed apocrine morphology ($p = 0.0002$), albeit with no perfect overlap with morphologically apocrine carcinomas, and were all AR-positive and ER-negative. Molecular apocrine carcinomas include tumors classified as HER2 overexpressing (ER- and PR-negative and HER2-positive) as well as some triple negative (ER-, PR-, and HER2-negative) carcinomas. Doane et al.[83] identified a subset of ER-negative and PR-negative breast carcinomas characterized by paradoxical expression of ER-dependent genes, and demonstrated that these findings were attributable to activation of the AR. The authors did not comment whether the carcinomas had apocrine morphology.

Guedj et al.[12] used unsupervised clustering to analyze data obtained from microarray analysis and transcriptome profiling of 355 breast carcinomas. They identified six classes of tumors that were also later reproduced by an analysis of publicly available data sets. One of the six groups consisted of AR-positive and ER-negative carcinomas showing some genetic similarities with the molecular apocrine carcinomas identified by Farmer et al.[10] Molecular apocrine tumors overexpressed *ERBB2/HER2* in 72% of cases and 70% of the tumors had 17q12 amplification. They also had the lowest rate of nondiploid cells of all molecular tumor subgroups. The molecular signature was characterized by activation of pathways involved in cell-to-cell adhesion and communication, lipid metabolism, and endocrine activation, including insulin signaling pathway and AR, HER2, and ER signaling. Activation of the phosphatidylinositide 3-kinase signaling pathway was also demonstrated. Clinically, molecular apocrine carcinomas had fewer bone metastases (57%) than luminal carcinomas (70% to 78%), but were more likely to metastasize to the brain (21% vs. 0%). They showed early relapse (18 to 60 months), but had stable metastases-free survival at longer follow-up. In an analysis of available genetic data from tumors treated with neoadjuvant therapy, the molecular apocrine subtype showed complete response in 37% of cases. In this study, however, it was not established whether molecular apocrine carcinomas had apocrine morphology. On the basis of proteomics data, Celis et al.[71] have also postulated the existence of a molecular apocrine subtype of breast carcinoma.

Banneau et al.[25] found that the gene array profile of three breast carcinomas from patients with *PTEN* germline mutation (Cowden syndrome) overlapped significantly with the molecular profile of apocrine carcinoma identified by Farmer et al.,[10] with 54 genes present in both signatures. Of note, all four Cowden patients with apocrine carcinoma carried the same *PTEN* germline mutation (c.209+5G>A). Although showing strong similarities, the gene profiles of Cowden breast carcinomas and of apocrine carcinomas do not overlap exactly.

In a study by Vranic et al.,[66] 20/37 (54%) pure apocrine carcinomas overexpressed *HER2* by fluorescence *in situ* hybridization (FISH), but only 2/35 (6%) overexpressed *EGFR*. Chromosome 7 polysomy was detected in 20/33 (61%) pure apocrine carcinomas and was significantly more frequent than in nonapocrine carcinomas (3/11; 27%) ($p = 0.083$). In this study, polysomy of chromosome 7 accounted for the increased levels of immunohistochemically detectable EGFR protein in pure apocrine carcinomas.

Some investigators dispute the existence of a specific molecular subtype of apocrine carcinoma because genetic evidence is very limited and its correlation with apocrine morphology is inconsistent. Furthermore, apocrine morphology can occur in many genetically distinct subtypes of breast carcinomas such as mucinous, micropapillary, tubular and lobular carcinoma.[84] Patani et al.[85] identified distinct genomic alterations in apocrine foci of invasive triple negative carcinomas showing intratumoral morphologic heterogeneity. In this study, the foci of carcinoma with apocrine morphology had the same immunoprofile as the nonapocrine areas of the tumors, except that they were AR-positive. Nonetheless, the apocrine foci had lower AR positivity than usually seen in apocrine carcinomas and were not immunoreactive for GCDFP-15. The morphologically apocrine component displayed low-level gain of chromosome 9p24.3–24.1 and 9p21.1–p11.1, and low-level loss of chromosome 9q21.13–q33.3. These alterations were not identified in nonapocrine regions of the same tumors. Based on these findings, the authors speculated that apocrine differentiation in these tumors constituted a late epiphenomenon, as the apocrine and nonapocrine components shared common genetic alterations. FISH analysis demonstrated an average of three to four copies of the 9p21 locus in 85% of the tumor cells, versus only two copies in nonapocrine regions. Of note, in the study by Jones et al.,[11] 9p gains were detected only in 2 of 14 (14%) cases (one DCIS and one invasive carcinoma), and 9q losses in 6/14 (43%) cases (four DCIS and two invasive carcinomas).

The triple negative AR-positive MDA-MB-453 cell line has been used by some investigators as *in vitro* model of apocrine carcinoma.[61,86] Comparative analysis of the genetic alterations in this cell line and in eight apocrine breast carcinomas (seven invasive and one DCIS) found substantial differences between the two cell populations, suggesting that the results obtained from the study of this cell line *in vitro* are not applicable to apocrine carcinoma.[87]

TREATMENT AND PROGNOSIS

Atypical Lesions

Atypical apocrine change in sclerosing lesions may be a risk factor for the subsequent development of carcinoma. Carter and Rosen[45] evaluated 51 patients with atypical sclerosing apocrine lesions and reported that no carcinomas were detected after a mean follow-up of 35 months. However, with a mean follow-up of 8.7 years, Seidman et al.[46] found that 4 of 37 (10.8%) women with apocrine adenosis developed carcinoma (3 ipsilateral, 1 contralateral). The overall relative risk of developing carcinoma was 5.5 when compared with a reference population. In this study, all patients who developed carcinoma were more than 60 years old when atypical adenosis was diagnosed, and the mean age for the diagnosis of carcinoma was 70 years. All carcinomas were detected 4 or more years after apocrine adenosis was diagnosed. The relative risk for developing carcinoma in women 60 years or older with atypical apocrine adenosis was 14.

In a series of 37 cases of atypical apocrine adenosis treated at the Mayo clinic[88] with long-term follow-up (median follow-up of 14 years), 3/37 (8%) patients developed recurrent disease, including ipsilateral invasive carcinoma at 4 and 18 years of follow-up. One patient developed contralateral DCIS at 12 years follow-up. None of the recurrent carcinomas had apocrine morphology.

On the basis of current data, patients with atypical apocrine lesions should be managed clinically with the same follow-up regimen as those with nonapocrine atypical proliferative lesions. The effectiveness of selective estrogen receptor modulators (SERMs) on atypical apocrine lesions that are typically ER-negative has not been determined.

Apocrine DCIS

Patients with apocrine DCIS have generally had the same clinical course as women with nonapocrine DCIS. In one study,[32] 33 (60%) of 55 patients were treated by mastectomy, whereas 22 (40%) had only an excisional biopsy. Recurrences occurred in the breast in 3 (15%) of 20 who had excisional biopsies alone but not in two others who had excision and radiotherapy. When treated by mastectomy, one patient whose index lesion appeared to be entirely intraductal had axillary metastases at the time of mastectomy and later died of systemic disease. All other patients with apocrine DCIS remained disease free at last follow-up. Follow-up information was available for 17 patients with apocrine DCIS in the series by Leal et al.,[27] and none developed recurrent disease after a median time of 37 months.

Invasive Apocrine Carcinoma

Several investigators have examined the prognosis of invasive apocrine mammary carcinoma. Lee et al.[31] reviewed 81 patients treated for "sweat gland" carcinoma and concluded that they did not differ clinically or in prognosis from "the general group of mammary cancers." Frable and Kay[28] compared 18 apocrine carcinoma patients with 34 matched controls and found no significant differences in survival between the two groups after treatment by mastectomy. A similar approach was used by d'Amore et al.[38] in an analysis of 34 cases and by Abati et al.,[32] who investigated 17 women with invasive apocrine carcinoma. Both of the latter series revealed no statistically significant differences between apocrine and nonapocrine carcinomas in recurrence-free survival or in OS after treatment by mastectomy (Fig. 19.22). Tanaka et al.[15] found no significant difference in relapse-free and OS between 57 patients with invasive apocrine carcinoma and 1,583 patients with nonapocrine carcinoma. Montagna et al.[20] studied 29 triple negative apocrine carcinomas. Lymphovascular invasion was present in 24% of the cases, and 45% of the patients had lymph node metastases. The 5-year OS of patients with triple negative apocrine carcinoma was 92%. The RFS was 83.7% at 5 years and 67% at 10 years. In this study and in the study by Dreyer et al.,[89] the outcome of triple negative apocrine carcinomas was similar to that of triple negative invasive ductal carcinomas of no special type. On the other hand, when considering all carcinomas with apocrine morphology, Dellapasqua et al.[16] found that pure invasive apocrine carcinomas had worse disease-free survival (DFS) than nonapocrine carcinomas (HR, 1.7; 95% CI, 1.01 to 2.86), whereas apocrine-like carcinomas and nonapocrine carcinomas had similar DFS and OS.

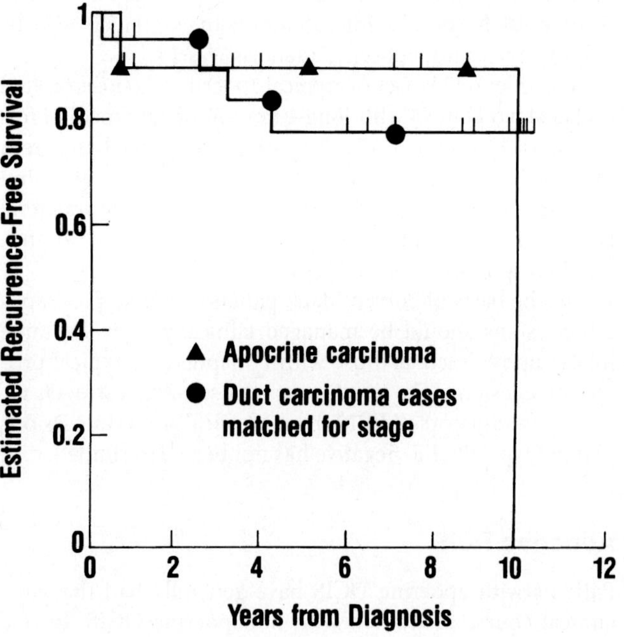

FIG. 19.22. *Apocrine carcinoma, survival analysis.* When compared with patients with nonapocrine duct carcinomas matched for stage, women with apocrine carcinoma do not have a significantly different recurrence-free survival. [From Abati AD, Kimmel M, Rosen PP. Apocrine mammary carcinoma: a clinicopathologic study of 72 patients. *Am J Clin Pathol* 1990;94:371–377, with permission.]

Five invasive apocrine carcinomas treated by neoadjuvant chemotherapy were part of a series studied by Nagao et al.[90] After treatment, the tumors showed only minimal reduction in size, and no clinical or pathologic complete response was observed in any of the cases. In this study, none of the patients with apocrine carcinoma developed a recurrence or died of disease at 10-year follow-up, but the number of cases is too small for any conclusion.

The prognosis of invasive apocrine carcinoma is determined mainly by conventional prognostic factors such as grade, tumor size, and nodal status.[28,31–33] Carcinomas with apocrine differentiation are usually strongly and diffusely AR-positive. AR expression in breast carcinoma appears to be related to tumor morphology and prognosis, but the relationship is quite complex. Rakha et al.[91] reported that AR-positive triple negative breast carcinomas had higher nuclear grade, and higher rate of recurrent disease and distant metastases. In a cohort of postmenopausal patients with ER-positive breast carcinoma, AR expression was associated with significantly reduced breast cancer–specific mortality (HR, 0.68; 95% CI, 0.47 to 0.99) and overall mortality (HR, 0.70; 95% CI, 0.53 to 0.91) by multivariate analysis.[92] In the same study, however, postmenopausal women with ER-negative and AR-positive breast carcinoma, such as apocrine carcinomas, had increased breast cancer–specific mortality (HR, 1.59; 95% CI, 0.94 to 2.68; $p = 0.08$). At present, patients with triple negative AR-positive metastatic breast carcinomas can be treated with flutamide, an AR antagonist, in the context of a clinical trial.

REFERENCES

1. Nishikawa Y, Tokusashi Y, Saito Y, et al. A case of apocrine adenocarcinoma associated with hamartomatous apocrine gland hyperplasia of both axillae. *Am J Surg Pathol* 1994;18:832–836.
2. Paties C, Taccagni GL, Papotti M, et al. Apocrine carcinoma of the skin. A clinicopathologic, immunocytochemical, and ultrastructural study. *Cancer* 1993;71:375–381.
3. Pelosi G, Martignoni G, Bonetti F. Intraductal carcinoma of mammary-type apocrine epithelium arising within a papillary hydradenoma of the vulva. Report of a case and review of the literature. *Arch Pathol Lab Med* 1991;115:1249–1254.
4. Tremblay G. Histochemical studies of oxidative enzymes in apocrine-like cells of the breast and in axillary apocrine glands. *J Invest Dermatol* 1968;50:238–243.
5. Wellings SR, Jensen HM, Marcum RG. An atlas of subgross pathology of the human breast with special reference to possible precancerous lesions. *J Natl Cancer Inst* 1975;55:231–273.
6. Raju U, Zarbo RJ, Kubus J, et al. The histologic spectrum of apocrine breast proliferations: a comparative study of morphology and DNA content by image analysis. *Hum Pathol* 1993;24:173–181.

7. Bussolati G, Sapino A, Gugliotta P, et al. Cytological analysis of benign breast disease. *Cancer Detect Prev* 1992;16:89–92.
8. Viacava P, Naccarato AG, Bevilacqua G. Apocrine epithelium of the breast: does it result from metaplasia? *Virchows Arch* 1997;431:205–209.
9. Eusebi V, Betts C, Haagensen DE Jr, et al. Apocrine differentiation in lobular carcinoma of the breast: a morphologic, immunologic, and ultrastructural study. *Hum Pathol* 1984;15:134–140.
10. Farmer P, Bonnefoi H, Becette V, et al. Identification of molecular apocrine breast tumours by microarray analysis. *Oncogene* 2005;24:4660–4671.
11. Jones C, Damiani S, Wells D, et al. Molecular cytogenetic comparison of apocrine hyperplasia and apocrine carcinoma of the breast. *Am J Pathol* 2001;158:207–214.
12. Guedj M, Marisa L, de Reynies A, et al. A refined molecular taxonomy of breast cancer. *Oncogene* 2012;31:1196–1206.
13. Mossler JA, Barton TK, Brinkhous AD, et al. Apocrine differentiation in human mammary carcinoma. *Cancer* 1980;46:2463–2471.
14. Matsuo K, Fukutomi T, Tsuda H, et al. Apocrine carcinoma of the breast: clinicopathological analysis and histological subclassification of 12 cases. *Breast Cancer* 1998;5:279–284.
15. Tanaka K, Imoto S, Wada N, et al. Invasive apocrine carcinoma of the breast: clinicopathologic features of 57 patients. *Breast J* 2008;14: 164–168.
16. Dellapasqua S, Maisonneuve P, Viale G, et al. Immunohistochemically defined subtypes and outcome of apocrine breast cancer. *Clin Breast Cancer* 2013;13:95–102.
17. Ogiya A, Horii R, Osako T, et al. Apocrine metaplasia of breast cancer: clinicopathological features and predicting response. *Breast Cancer* 2010;17:290–297.
18. Alvarenga CA, Paravidino PI, Alvarenga M, et al. Reappraisal of immunohistochemical profiling of special histological types of breast carcinomas: a study of 121 cases of eight different subtypes. *J Clin Pathol* 2012;65:1066–1071.
19. Tsutsumi Y. Apocrine carcinoma as triple-negative breast cancer: novel definition of apocrine-type carcinoma as estrogen/progesterone receptor-negative and androgen receptor-positive invasive ductal carcinoma. *Jpn J Clin Oncol* 2012;42:375–386.
20. Montagna E, Maisonneuve P, Rotmensz N, et al. Heterogeneity of triple-negative breast cancer: histologic subtyping to inform the outcome. *Clin Breast Cancer* 2013;13:31–39.
21. Bryant J. Male breast cancer: a case of apocrine carcinoma with psammoma bodies. *Hum Pathol* 1981;12:751–753.
22. Burga AM, Fadare O, Lininger RA, et al. Invasive carcinomas of the male breast: a morphologic study of the distribution of histologic subtypes and metastatic patterns in 778 cases. *Virchows Arch* 2006;449:507–512.
23. Schrager CA, Schneider D, Gruener AC, et al. Similarities of cutaneous and breast pathology in Cowden's Syndrome. *Exp Dermatol* 1998;7:380–390.
24. Schrager CA, Schneider D, Gruener AC, et al. Clinical and pathological features of breast disease in Cowden's syndrome: an underrecognized syndrome with an increased risk of breast cancer. *Hum Pathol* 1998;29:47–53.
25. Banneau G, Guedj M, MacGrogan G, et al. Molecular apocrine differentiation is a common feature of breast cancer in patients with germline PTEN mutations. *Breast Cancer Res* 2010;12:R63.
26. Gilles R, Lesnik A, Guinebretiere JM, et al. Apocrine carcinoma: clinical and mammographic features. *Radiology* 1994;190:495–497.
27. Leal C, Henrique R, Monteiro P, et al. Apocrine ductal carcinoma in situ of the breast: histologic classification and expression of biologic markers. *Hum Pathol* 2001;32:487–493.
28. Frable WJ, Kay S. Carcinoma of the breast. Histologic and clinical features of apocrine tumors. *Cancer* 1968;21:756–763.
29. Schmitt FC, Soares R, Seruca R. Bilateral apocrine carcinoma of the breast. Molecular and immunocytochemical evidence for two independent primary tumours. *Virchows Arch* 1998;433:505–509.
30. Moritani S, Ichihara S, Hasegawa M, et al. Topographical, morphological and immunohistochemical characteristics of carcinoma in situ of the breast involving sclerosing adenosis. Two distinct topographical patterns and histological types of carcinoma in situ. *Histopathology* 2011;58:835–846.
31. Lee B, Pack G, Scharnagel I. Sweat gland cancer of the breast. *Surg Gynecol Obstet* 1933;54:975–996.
32. Abati AD, Kimmel M, Rosen PP. Apocrine mammary carcinoma. A clinicopathologic study of 72 cases. *Am J Clin Pathol* 1990;94:371–377.
33. Burt AD, Seywright MM, George WD. Mixed apocrine-medullary carcinoma of the breast. Report of a case with fine needle aspiration cytology. *Acta Cytol* 1987;31:322–324.
34. Eusebi V, Magalhaes F, Azzopardi JG. Pleomorphic lobular carcinoma of the breast: an aggressive tumor showing apocrine differentiation. *Hum Pathol* 1992;23:655–662.
35. Lin Fde M, Pincerato KM, Bacchi CE, et al. Coordinated expression of oestrogen and androgen receptors in HER2-positive breast carcinomas: impact on proliferative activity. *J Clin Pathol* 2012;65:64–68.
36. Eusebi V, Foschini MP, Bussolati G, et al. Myoblastomatoid (histiocytoid) carcinoma of the breast. A type of apocrine carcinoma. *Am J Surg Pathol* 1995;19:553–562.
37. Kasashima S, Kawashima A, Ozaki S, et al. Expression of 5alpha-reductase in apocrine carcinoma of the breast and its correlation with clinicopathological aggressiveness. *Histopathology* 2012;60:E51–E57.
38. d'Amore ES, Terrier-Lacombe MJ, Travagli JP, et al. Invasive apocrine carcinoma of the breast: a long term follow-up study of 34 cases. *Breast Cancer Res Treat* 1988;12:37–44.
39. Robbins GF, Shah J, Rosen P, et al. Inflammatory carcinoma of the breast. *Surg Clin North Am* 1974;54:801–810.
40. Shousha S, Bull TB, Southall PJ, et al. Apocrine carcinoma of the breast containing foam cells. An electron microscopic and immunohistological study. *Histopathology* 1987;11:611–620.
41. Cserni G. Benign apocrine papillary lesions of the breast lacking or virtually lacking myoepithelial cells-potential pitfalls in diagnosing malignancy. *APMIS* 2012;120:249–252.
42. Cserni G. Lack of myoepithelium in apocrine glands of the breast does not necessarily imply malignancy. *Histopathology* 2008;52:253–255.
43. Tramm T, Kim JY, Tavassoli FA. Diminished number or complete loss of myoepithelial cells associated with metaplastic and neoplastic apocrine lesions of the breast. *Am J Surg Pathol* 2011;35:202–211.
44. Seal M, Wilson C, Naus GJ, et al. Encapsulated apocrine papillary carcinoma of the breast--a tumour of uncertain malignant potential: report of five cases. *Virchows Arch* 2009;455:477–483.
45. Carter DJ, Rosen PP. Atypical apocrine metaplasia in sclerosing lesions of the breast: a study of 51 patients. *Mod Pathol* 1991;4:1–5.
46. Seidman JD, Ashton M, Lefkowitz M. Atypical apocrine adenosis of the breast: a clinicopathologic study of 37 patients with 8.7-year follow-up. *Cancer* 1996;77:2529–2537.
47. Tavassoli FA, Norris HJ. Intraductal apocrine carcinoma: a clinicopathologic study of 37 cases. *Mod Pathol* 1994;7:813–818.
48. O'Malley FP, Page DL, Nelson EH, et al. Ductal carcinoma in situ of the breast with apocrine cytology: definition of a borderline category. *Hum Pathol* 1994;25:164–168.
49. Going JJ, Anderson TJ, Crocker PR, et al. Weddellite calcification in the breast: eighteen cases with implications for breast cancer screening. *Histopathology* 1990;16:119–124.
50. Foote FW Jr, Stewart FW. A histologic classification of carcinoma of the breast. *Surgery* 1946;19:74–99.
51. Higginson JF, Mc DJ. Apocrine tissue, chronic cystic mastitis and sweat gland carcinoma of the breast. *Surg Gynecol Obstet* 1949;88:1–10.
52. Yates AJ, Ahmed A. Apocrine carcinoma and apocrine metaplasia. *Histopathology* 1988;13:228–231.
53. Johnson TL, Kini SR. The significance of atypical apocrine cells in fine-needle aspirates of the breast. *Diagn Cytopathol* 1989;5:248–254.
54. Yoshida K, Inoue M, Furuta S, et al. Apocrine carcinoma vs. apocrine metaplasia with atypia of the breast. Use of aspiration biopsy cytology. *Acta Cytol* 1996;40:247–251.
55. Watanabe K, Nomura M, Hashimoto Y, et al. Fine-needle aspiration cytology of apocrine adenosis of the breast: report on three cases. *Diagn Cytopathol* 2007;35:296–299.
56. Roddy HJ, Silverberg SG. Ultrastructural analysis of apocrine carcinoma of the human breast. *Ultrastruct Pathol* 1980;1:385–393.
57. Bratthauer GL, Lininger RA, Man YG, et al. Androgen and estrogen receptor mRNA status in apocrine carcinomas. *Diagn Mol Pathol* 2002;11:113–118.
58. Honma N, Takubo K, Akiyama F, et al. Expression of oestrogen receptor-beta in apocrine carcinomas of the breast. *Histopathology* 2007;50:425–433.
59. Vranic S, Gatalica Z, Deng H, et al. ER-alpha36, a novel isoform of ER-alpha66, is commonly over-expressed in apocrine and adenoid cystic carcinomas of the breast. *J Clin Pathol* 2011;64:54–57.

60. Miller WR, Telford J, Dixon JM, et al. Androgen metabolism and apocrine differentiation in human breast cancer. *Breast Cancer Res Treat* 1985;5:67–73.
61. Naderi A, Hughes-Davies L. A functionally significant cross-talk between androgen receptor and ErbB2 pathways in estrogen receptor negative breast cancer. *Neoplasia* 2008;10:542–548.
62. Wales NA, Ebling FJ. The control of the apocrine glands of the rabbit by steroid hormones. *J Endocrinol* 1971;51:763–770.
63. Labows JN, Preti G, Hoelzle E, et al. Steroid analysis of human apocrine secretion. *Steroids* 1979;34:249–258.
64. Collins LC, Cole KS, Marotti JD, et al. Androgen receptor expression in breast cancer in relation to molecular phenotype: results from the Nurses' Health Study. *Mod Pathol* 2011;24:924–931.
65. Niemeier LA, Dabbs DJ, Beriwal S, et al. Androgen receptor in breast cancer: expression in estrogen receptor-positive tumors and in estrogen receptor-negative tumors with apocrine differentiation. *Mod Pathol* 2010;23:205–212.
66. Vranic S, Tawfik O, Palazzo J, et al. EGFR and HER-2/neu expression in invasive apocrine carcinoma of the breast. *Mod Pathol* 2010;23:644–653.
67. Mazoujian G, Bodian C, Haagensen DE Jr, et al. Expression of GCDFP-15 in breast carcinomas. Relationship to pathologic and clinical factors. *Cancer* 1989;63:2156–2161.
68. Sapino A, Righi L, Cassoni P, et al. Expression of apocrine differentiation markers in neuroendocrine breast carcinomas of aged women. *Mod Pathol* 2001;14:768–776.
69. Celis JE, Gromova I, Gromov P, et al. Molecular pathology of breast apocrine carcinomas: a protein expression signature specific for benign apocrine metaplasia. *FEBS Lett* 2006;580:2935–2944.
70. Celis JE, Gromov P, Cabezon T, et al. 15-Prostaglandin dehydrogenase expression alone or in combination with ACSM1 defines a subgroup of the apocrine molecular subtype of breast carcinoma. *Mol Cell Proteomics* 2008;7:1795–1809.
71. Celis JE, Cabezon T, Moreira JM, et al. Molecular characterization of apocrine carcinoma of the breast: validation of an apocrine protein signature in a well-defined cohort. *Mol Oncol* 2009;3:220–237.
72. Choi J, Jung WH, Koo JS. Clinicopathologic features of molecular subtypes of triple negative breast cancer based on immunohistochemical markers. *Histol Histopathol* 2012;27:1481–1493.
73. Bundred NJ, Walker RA, Everington D, et al. Is apocrine differentiation in breast carcinoma of prognostic significance? *Br J Cancer* 1990;62:113–117.
74. Shao MM, Chan SK, Yu AM, et al. Keratin expression in breast cancers. *Virchows Arch* 2012;461:313–322.
75. Alvarenga CA, Paravidino PI, Alvarenga M, et al. Expression of CK19 in invasive breast carcinomas of special histological types: implications for the use of one-step nucleic acid amplification. *J Clin Pathol* 2011;64:493–497.
76. Moriya T, Sakamoto K, Sasano H, et al. Immunohistochemical analysis of Ki-67, p53, p21, and p27 in benign and malignant apocrine lesions of the breast: its correlation to histologic findings in 43 cases. *Mod Pathol* 2000;13:13–18.
77. Bussolati G, Cattani MG, Gugliotta P, et al. Morphologic and functional aspects of apocrine metaplasia in dysplastic and neoplastic breast tissue. *Ann N Y Acad Sci* 1986;464:262–274.
78. Eisenberg BL, Bagnall JW, Harding CT 3rd. Histiocytoid carcinoma: a variant of breast cancer. *J Surg Oncol* 1986;31:271–274.
79. Damiani S, Eusebi V, Losi L, et al. Oncocytic carcinoma (malignant oncocytoma) of the breast. *Am J Surg Pathol* 1998;22:221–230.
80. De Potter CR, Praet MM, Slavin RE, et al. Feulgen DNA content and mitotic activity in proliferative breast disease. A comparison with ductal carcinoma in situ. *Histopathology* 1987;11:1307–1319.
81. Lininger RA, Zhuang Z, Man Y, et al. Loss of heterozygosity is detected at chromosomes 1p35-36 (NB), 3p25 (VHL), 16p13 (TSC2/PKD1), and 17p13 (TP53) in microdissected apocrine carcinomas of the breast. *Mod Pathol* 1999;12:1083–1089.
82. Selim AG, Ryan A, El-Ayat G, et al. Loss of heterozygosity and allelic imbalance in apocrine metaplasia of the breast: microdissection microsatellite analysis. *J Pathol* 2002;196:287–291.
83. Doane AS, Danso M, Lal P, et al. An estrogen receptor-negative breast cancer subset characterized by a hormonally regulated transcriptional program and response to androgen. *Oncogene* 2006;25:3994–4008.
84. Weigelt B, Horlings HM, Kreike B, et al. Refinement of breast cancer classification by molecular characterization of histological special types. *J Pathol* 2008;216:141–150.
85. Patani N, Barbashina V, Lambros MB, et al. Direct evidence for concurrent morphological and genetic heterogeneity in an invasive ductal carcinoma of triple-negative phenotype. *J Clin Pathol* 2011;64:822–828.
86. Chia KM, Liu J, Francis GD, et al. A feedback loop between androgen receptor and ERK signaling in estrogen receptor-negative breast cancer. *Neoplasia* 2011;13:154–166.
87. Vranic S, Gatalica Z, Wang ZY. Update on the molecular profile of the MDA-MB-453 cell line as a model for apocrine breast carcinoma studies. *Oncol Lett* 2011;2:1131–1137.
88. Fuehrer N, Hartmann L, Degnim A, et al. Atypical apocrine adenosis of the breast: long-term follow-up in 37 patients. *Arch Pathol Lab Med* 2012;136:179–182.
89. Dreyer G, Vandorpe T, Smeets A, et al. Triple negative breast cancer: clinical characteristics in the different histological subtypes. *Breast* 2013;22:761–6.
90. Nagao T, Kinoshita T, Hojo T, et al. The differences in the histological types of breast cancer and the response to neoadjuvant chemotherapy: the relationship between the outcome and the clinicopathological characteristics. *Breast* 2012;21:289–295.
91. Rakha EA, El-Sayed ME, Green AR, et al. Prognostic markers in triple-negative breast cancer. *Cancer* 2007;109:25–32.
92. Hu R, Dawood S, Holmes MD, et al. Androgen receptor expression and breast cancer survival in postmenopausal women. *Clin Cancer Res* 2011;17:1867–1874.

CHAPTER 20

Mammary Carcinomas with Endocrine Features

EDI BROGI

Some mammary carcinomas are able to synthesize hormones not considered to be normal products of the breast. The capacity to produce ectopic hormones may be considered endocrine or biochemical metaplasia. Such tumors have been found to contain peptide hormones including human chorionic gonadotropin (hCG),[1] calcitonin,[2] adrenocorticotropic hormone (ACTH),[3] parathormone,[4] as well as norepinephrine.[5] These substances are detectable not only by biochemical analysis, but also by immunohistochemical study of the tumor tissue, and rarely do they produce clinical symptoms.

In a few unusual instances, the microscopic growth pattern of the carcinoma simulates the structure of nonmammary neoplasms that commonly contain the ectopic substance, resulting in coincidence of the biochemical and structural phenotypes. A striking example of this phenomenon is mammary carcinoma with choriocarcinomatous differentiation.[1,6] Most breast carcinomas with endocrine features have neuroendocrine (NE) morphology or differentiation.

CARCINOMAS WITH NEUROENDOCRINE DIFFERENTIATION

Breast carcinomas with neuroendocrine differentiation (NE-BCs) are relatively uncommon. In this chapter, we describe NE-BCs of low- to intermediate-grade morphology. High-grade NE carcinomas/small cell carcinomas are discussed in Chapter 21.

In 1977, Cubilla and Woodruff[7] described breast carcinomas rich in argyrophilic granules and morphologically similar to carcinoid tumors that occur in other organs. The authors could not demonstrate argyrophilic granules in normal breast epithelium, but nonetheless suggested that these tumors were NE mammary neoplasms derived from argyrophilic cells of neural crest origin, presumed to have migrated to mammary ducts. This hypothesis has not found supportive evidence. Although it might be argued that NE-BCs could be referred to as "primary carcinoid tumors of the breast," this terminology is inappropriate, as these tumors are true carcinomas.

The origin of NE-BCs and their relationship with invasive ductal carcinomas of the usual type have been extensively investigated. Albeit limited, recent evidence suggests that NE-BCs constitute a genetically distinct group of breast carcinomas, and that they are unrelated to invasive ductal carcinomas of no special type (see section on genetics and molecular studies).

At present, positivity for one NE marker, either chromogranin A or synaptophysin, in at least 50% of the tumor cells is required for the diagnosis of invasive NE-BC. Breast carcinomas with NE morphology and positive reactivity for chromogranin and/or synaptophysin in less than 50% of the cells are referred to as breast carcinomas with NE morphology. NE morphology sometimes can be subtle, adding to the difficulties in achieving reproducible diagnosis.

Clinical Presentation

Incidence, Age, and Ethnicity

It is estimated that NE-BCs represent about 1% to 2% of all breast carcinomas, but definitive information on the incidence of this type of tumors is lacking.

The mean age at diagnosis of NE-BC was 54,[8] 47.8,[9] and 63 years[10] in three recent series. Most studies and case reports document the highest incidence in postmenopausal patients older than 60 years.[11–13] Few cases have been described in young women, many of them in Asian countries.[7,14,15] In one series from the M.D. Anderson Cancer Center,[10] 80% of patients were Caucasian, 11% Hispanic, 7% African American, 1% Asian, and 1% of unknown ethnicity. A patient developed an NE-BC during pregnancy.[16] NE-BCs can also occur in men.[10,13,17]

Clinical Findings

An NE-BC usually presents as a palpable mass[8] in the central and retroareolar region of the breast or in the upper outer quadrant. Nipple discharge, often bloody, is a relatively common presenting symptom. Kawasaki et al.[9] reported that 24/89 (27%) patients with bloody nipple discharge had a carcinoma with NE differentiation, including eight invasive carcinomas. Bilateral synchronous tumors have also been reported.[5,14] At present, there are no documented reports of NE-BCs occurring in patients with a known (neuro)endocrine syndrome.

Radiology

Gunhan-Bilgen et al.[18] evaluated the radiologic features of five NE-BCs. One of the tumors was detected at mammographic screening, and the other four presented as palpable masses, which were soft and mobile in two patients and firm and immobile in the other two. In all five cases, mammographic examination detected a high-density mass with no calcifications. The tumor mass was round in four of five cases and irregular in one. The margins were spiculated in two cases, and indistinct, microlobulated, and partially lobulated to partially obscured in one case each. At ultrasound examination, four of five masses had heterogeneous hypoechoic signal with mild posterior acoustic enhancement. The masses were round or irregular, and the margins appeared irregular, microlobulated, or well circumscribed. Magnetic resonance imaging (MRI) of one tumor revealed a round mass with irregular margins and homogeneous contrast enhancement. After gadolinium–injection, the tumor exhibited early enhancement, followed by signal plateau, consistent with a malignant neoplasm. Just as NE epithelial neoplasms occurring at other sites, NE-BCs may have a positive signal when examined by indium^{111}-octreotide radionuclide scanning.[19]

Gross Pathology

NE-BCs and breast carcinomas with NE features usually are grossly circumscribed and somewhat hemorrhagic (Fig. 20.1), with a white gray to tan cut surface. They often have a soft, delicate, even friable consistency. Rarely multiple foci of carcinoma were described in the breast.

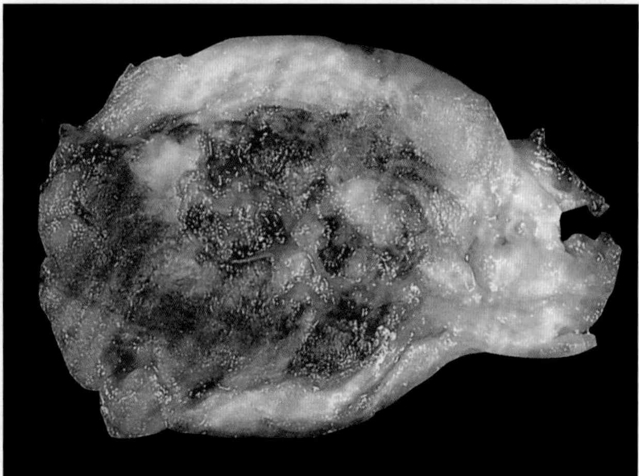

FIG. 20.1. ***Carcinoma with endocrine features, gross appearance.*** The carcinoma forms a circumscribed mass with a hemorrhagic cut surface.

The invasive tumors generally measure 1 to 5 cm in diameter, with most spanning between 1.5 and 3.0 cm. In one recent series,[8] the mean and the median tumor size were 2.7 and 2.2 cm, respectively, with a range from 0.8 to 13.5 cm.

Microscopic Pathology

Invasive Carcinomas with NE Differentiation and/or Features

NE-BCs and breast carcinomas with NE features commonly have a nested (Fig. 20.2) and/or solid–papillary (Fig. 20.3) growth pattern. The tumor nests are with a smooth or irregular outline and vary in size, ranging from large and cohesive to small and scattered. The nests are often distributed haphazardly like pieces of a jigsaw puzzle. Tumor rosettes and trabecular arrangement are commonly present, at least focally. Focal infiltration into the adipose tissue is usually evident. The papillae of papillary NE-BC are often large, typically solid, and have inconspicuous and delicate fibrovascular cores containing thin capillaries (Fig. 20.3). The nested and solid–papillary invasive variant of NE-BC can be difficult to recognize, as it can closely resemble ductal carcinoma *in situ* (DCIS)[13,20,21] (Figs. 20.2 and 20.3). Compared with the latter, invasive papillary NE-BC consists of nests and solid papillae of varying size and shape that are devoid of a myoepithelial layer (Fig. 20.3). In a series of solid and papillary carcinomas reported by Maluf and Koerner,[22] no smooth muscle actin (SMA) reactivity was present in the fibrovascular cores and at the periphery of 11/12 tumors, raising the possibility that most of the tumors were invasive. Righi et al.[12] studied a series of 89 NE-BCs. After excluding 11 "small cell" carcinomas, 35/78 (45%) cases had solid and cohesive architecture, 20/78 (25%) were solid and papillary, 13/78 (17%) cellular mucinous (Fig. 20.4), and 10/78 (13%) alveolar. The NE-BCs reported by Tang et al.[11] were papillary in 80% of cases; nested in 64%; and cellular mucinous, trabecular, or micropapillary in 3% of cases each. A glandular pattern of no special type was present in 18% of cases, and mixed architectural patterns were observed in 59% of tumors. Mucinous differentiation is not uncommon in NE-BC, often in the form of type B/cellular mucinous carcinoma or of mucinous carcinoma with type A and B morphology (see also Chapter 18). Any papillary epithelial proliferation with associated mucin should be regarded as at least atypical or suspicious for carcinoma and worked up accordingly. The tumor papillae have delicate filiform fibrovascular cores that are often apparent as cross sections of capillaries. Some papillae consist of abundant hyalinized and amorphous, nearly acellular stroma.

The tumor cells have relatively abundant cytoplasm (Fig. 20.5), which is often eosinophilic or granular, but can occasionally have a gray-blue hue because of intracytoplasmic mucin, or appear clear and almost vacuolated. The neoplastic cells are polygonal or plasmacytoid, but sometimes acquire signet cell morphology because of abundant intracytoplasmic mucin. Other shapes include ovoid, round, or spindled.

The nuclear features of NE-BC are also quite variable. Most often the nuclei are round to ovoid, located at the base

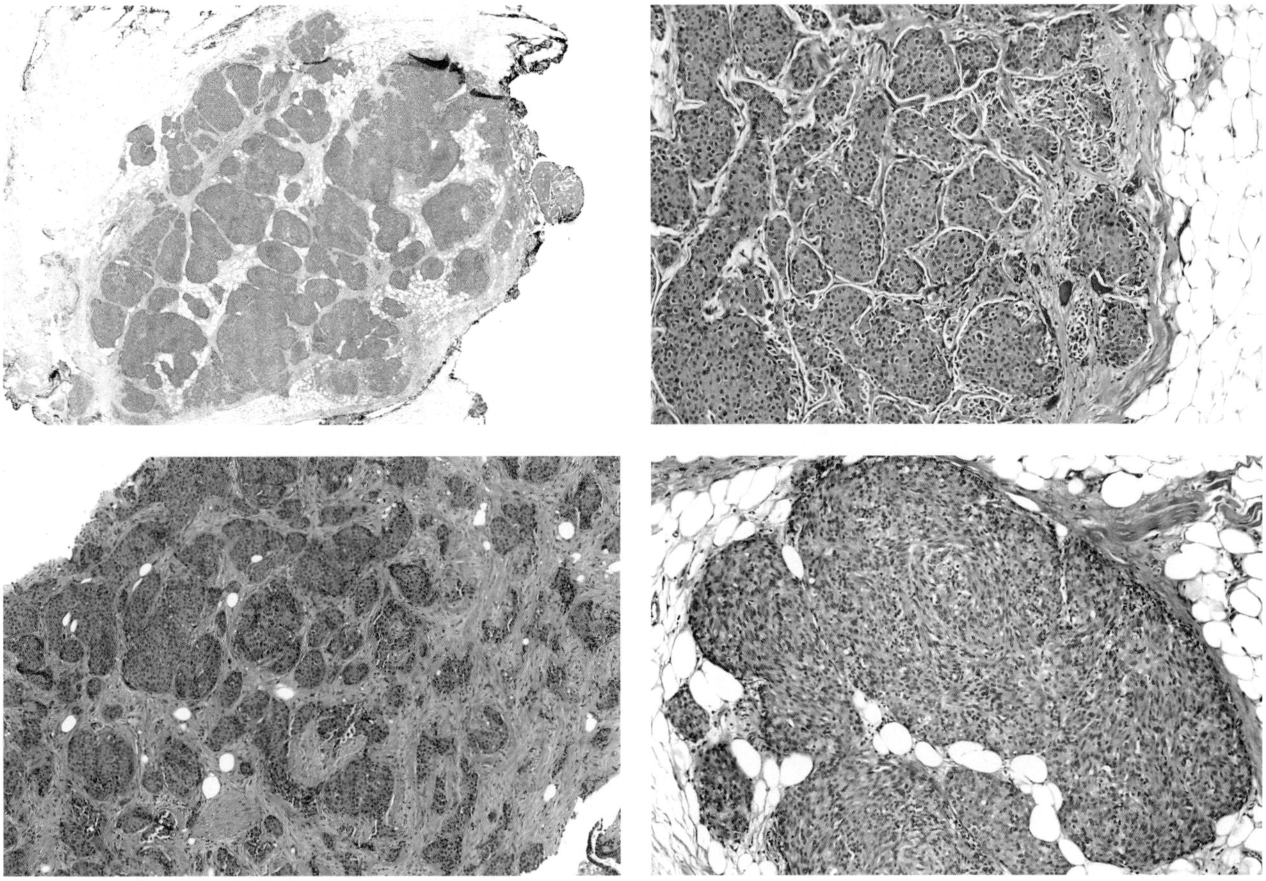

FIG. 20.2. ***Invasive carcinoma with neuroendocrine features, nested pattern.*** **A:** This whole-slide scanning magnification view shows that the neoplastic nests vary in size and shape, with slightly irregular outlines. **B:** At higher magnification, a delicate network of capillaries is evident around the tumor nests. **C:** In this needle core biopsy material, the nests of neoplastic cells abut on adipocytes. **D:** The large cohesive nests are scalloped, consistent with infiltration of the adipose tissue. The neoplastic cells have spindle cell morphology.

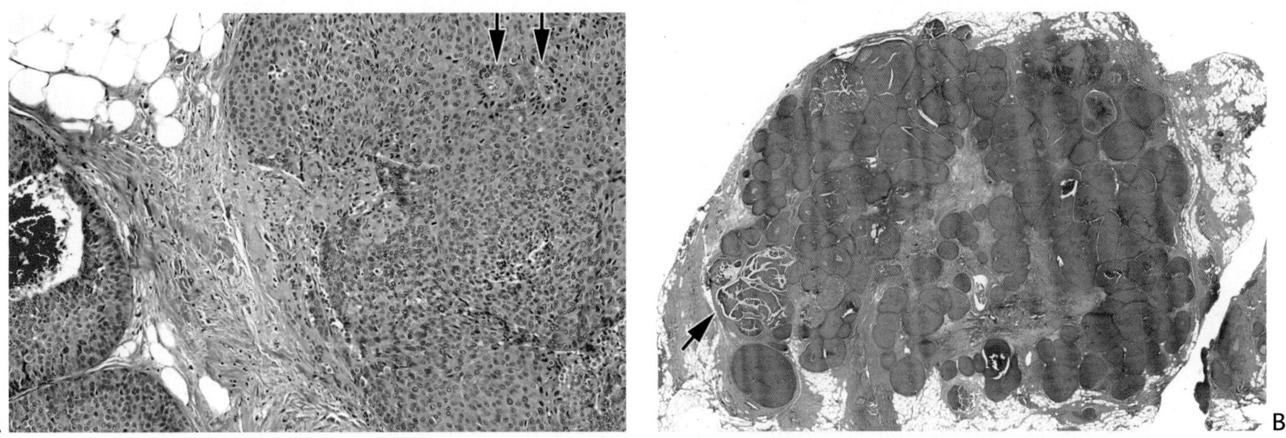

FIG. 20.3. ***Invasive carcinoma with neuroendocrine features, solid and papillary pattern.*** **A:** The solid and papillary invasive carcinoma on the *right* has an irregular edge. Rare delicate fibrovascular cores are noted (*arrows*). Two ducts involved by DCIS are present on the *left*. **B:** Whole-slide magnification of a mass-forming solid and papillary carcinoma. Most of the tumor has solid and papillary growth, but focal mucin production is evident (*arrow*). **C:** Large solid and papillary nodules of carcinoma with NE morphology in the tumor shown in **(B)**. **D:** The section stained for calponin reveals myoepithelium in normal ducts. The absence of staining in and around the tumor is not definitive evidence of invasion because myoepithelium may be lost in DCIS.

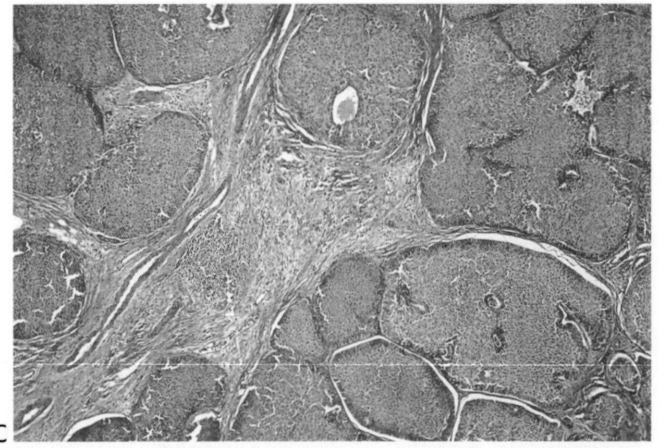

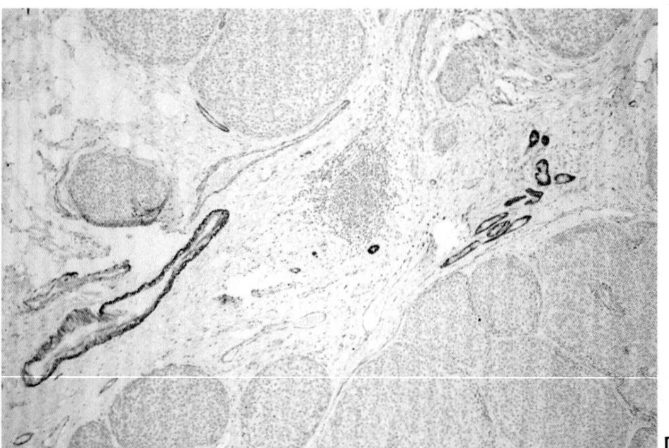

FIG. 20.3. *[Continued]*

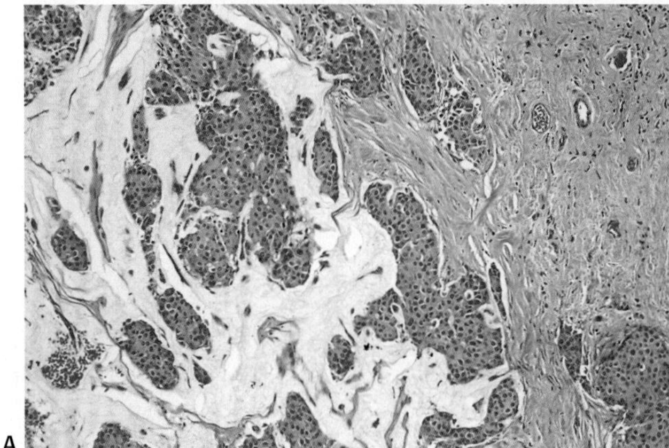

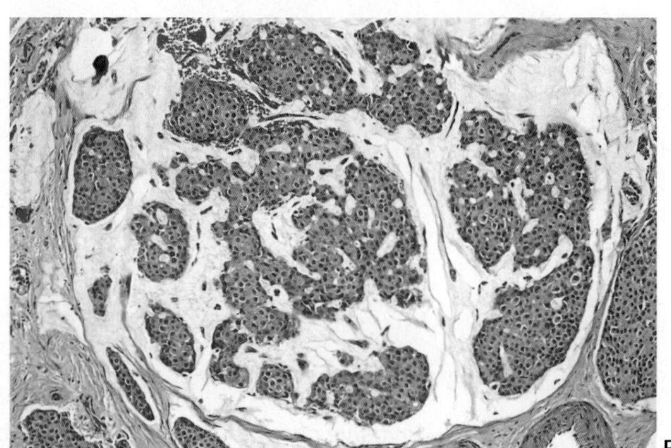

FIG. 20.4. ***Invasive carcinoma, with neuroendocrine and mucinous morphology.*** **A:** Invasive NE carcinoma with nested and mucinous morphology. **B:** Invasive carcinoma with predominantly mucinous type B morphology and cells with NE cytology.

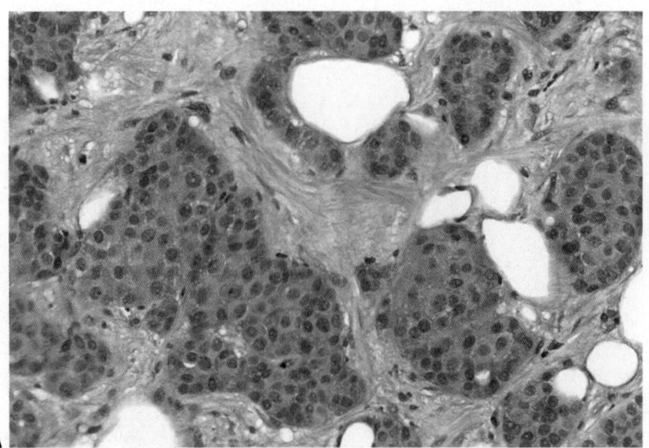

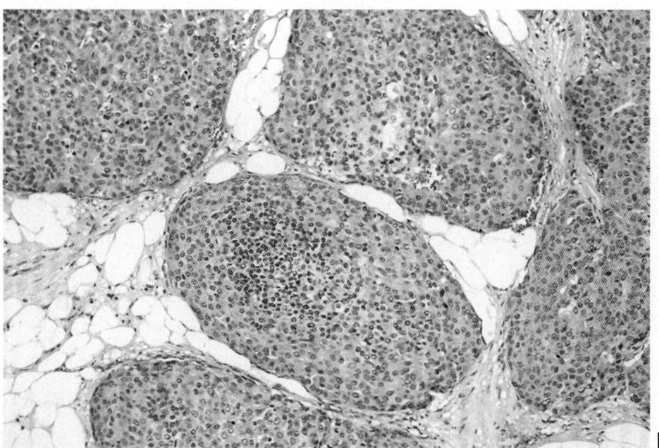

FIG. 20.5. ***Neuroendocrine carcinoma, cytomorphology.*** **A:** The neoplastic cells have plasmacytoid features and relatively abundant cytoplasm, focally granular and eosinophilic. **B:** The neoplastic cells are small and have inconspicuous nuclei.

or at one pole of the cell. They have smooth, fine, or "salt-and-pepper" chromatin. Nucleoli are usually absent or inconspicuous. The differential diagnosis of small cell carcinoma should be considered whenever an NE-BC has high-grade, basaloid nuclei and a high nuclear-to-cytoplasmic ratio.

Stromal desmoplasia tends to be rare, but a slight increase of stromal myofibroblasts admixed with inflammatory cells is a frequent finding around invasive tumor nests, at least focally. Focal peritumoral retraction and absence of basement membrane are easily detected. In some tumors, the stroma is

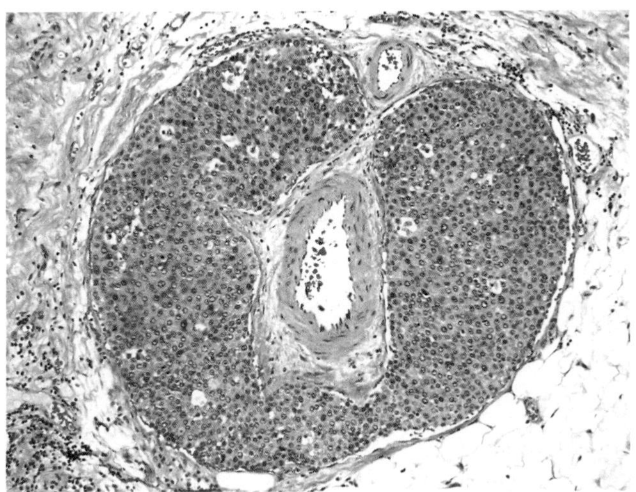

FIG. 20.6. ***Vascular invasion.*** A large solid embolus of NE carcinoma occludes a vascular space surrounding a small artery.

hyalinized, hypocellular, and nearly sclerotic. The tumors show prominent vascularity, with easily identifiable sinusoids and small feeding vessels. Blood lakes, extravasated red blood cells, hemosiderin deposits, and hemosiderin-laden macrophages are also frequently encountered. In one series,[11] lymphovascular invasion was present in 38% of 74 NE-BCs (Fig. 20.6).

Ductal Carcinoma In Situ

DCIS with NE features can occur alone or in association with invasive NE carcinoma. The largest series consisting of 34 cases of NE-DCIS, including 14/34 (41%) pure DCIS, was reported by Tsang and Chan.[23] Kawasaki et al.[24] identified NE differentiation in 20/294 (6.8%) consecutive cases of DCIS. Bloody nipple discharge is a common symptom.[23] It constituted the presenting sign in 13/20 (65%) cases in one series,[24] whereas only one NE-DCIS (6%) manifested as a mass lesion. Compared with non-NE-DCIS, DCIS with NE differentiation is rarely detected by mammographic screening. In a study by Kawasaki et al.,[24] the rate of mammographically detected NE-DCIS was 11% versus 54% for non-NE-DCIS ($p < 0.01$). Cases of bilateral NE-DCIS have been reported.[23,25,26]

Akin to NE-BCs, DCIS with NE features is also more common in postmenopausal women,[23] and often involves the central retroareolar region or the upper outer quadrant of the breast. It usually forms a circumscribed, tan-pink mass, with soft and friable consistency.

Morphologically NE-DCIS is often solid and/or papillary, with expansive growth. At least one case of solid papillary DCIS with SMA-positive myoepithelium lining the fibrovascular cores and the periphery of the tumor was part of the series by Maluf and Koerner.[22] The solid epithelial proliferation contains scattered small inconspicuous acini lined by polarized cells. A palisading "picket fence" arrangement along the fibrovascular cores is common (Fig. 20.7). The neoplastic cells are monotonous, small to medium sized, with columnar to ovoid, or sometimes spindle cell morphology (Fig. 20.8). Farshid et al.[27] reported that all eight cases of solid DCIS with spindle cell morphology in their series were positive for neuron-specific enolase (NSE) and synaptophysin, and four of eight (50%) cases were reactive for chromogranin in over 10% of the cells. The nuclear atypia of DCIS with NE differentiation is usually low, the nuclear chromatin is finely dispersed, and nucleoli are absent or inconspicuous.

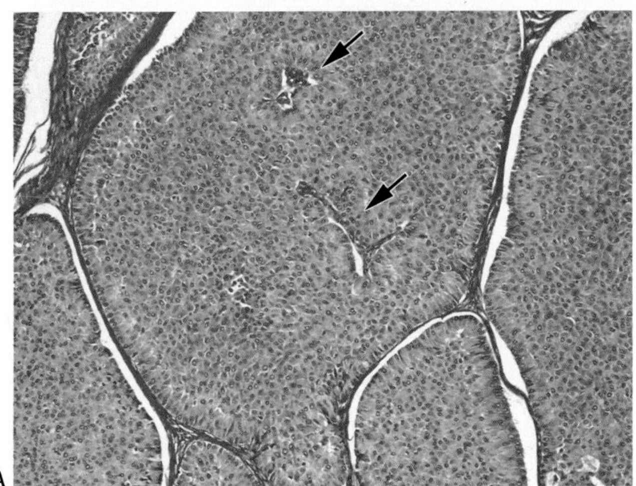

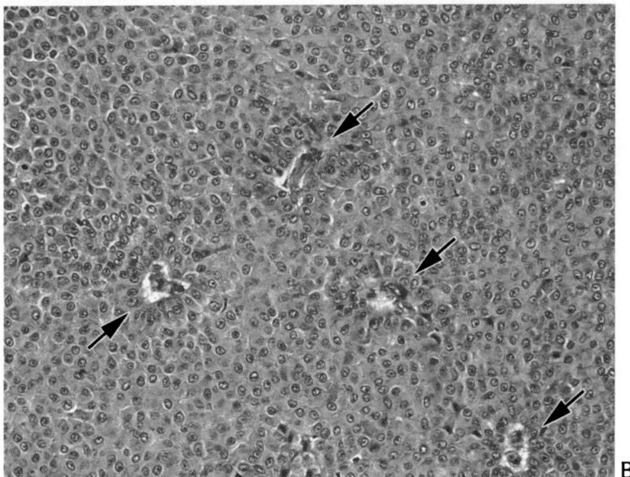

FIG. 20.7. ***Ductal carcinoma in situ, solid and papillary type.*** **A:** The carcinoma consists of large, solid nests of monotonous and orderly epithelial cells. Two fibrovascular cores are identified [*arrows*], evidence of papillary architecture. **B:** The solid neoplastic proliferation contains inconspicuous blood vessels [*arrows*]. The epithelial cells are elongated to plasmacytoid, and some have granular eosinophilic cytoplasm. The nuclei are small with fine chromatin. **C:** The neoplastic cells have a regular palisading arrangement around a thin fibrovascular core. Many of the cells have relatively abundant pale to clear cytoplasm. **D:** The presence of a nearly continuous layer of myoepithelium along the papillae and at the periphery of this solid and papillary carcinoma is demonstrated in a section immunostained for calponin. This finding confirms the diagnosis of DCIS.

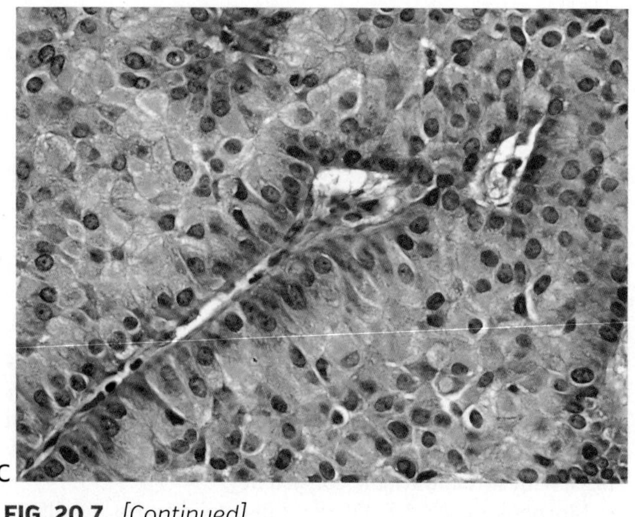

FIG. 20.7. *[Continued]*

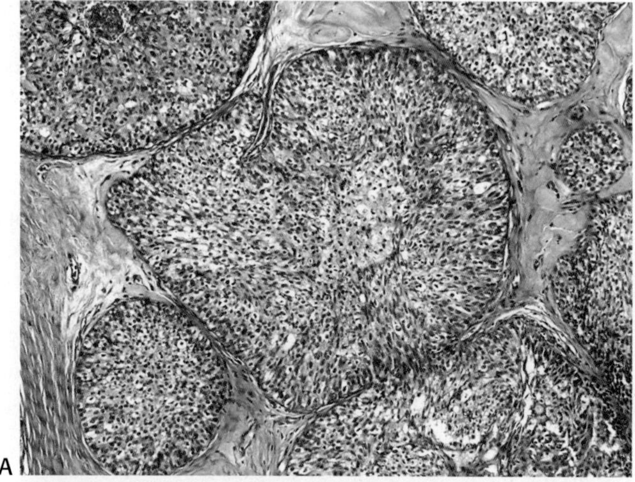

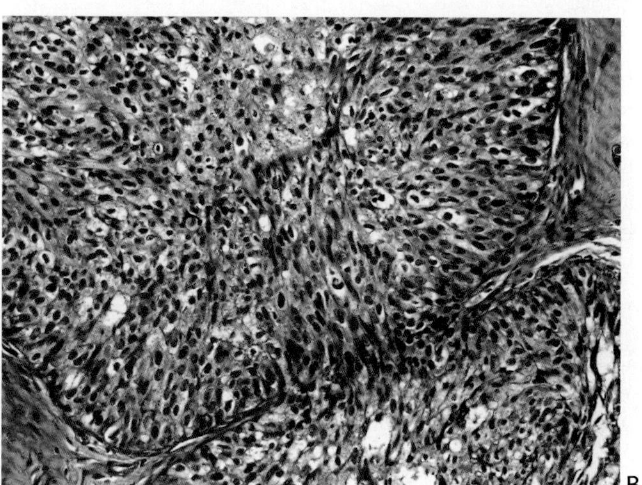

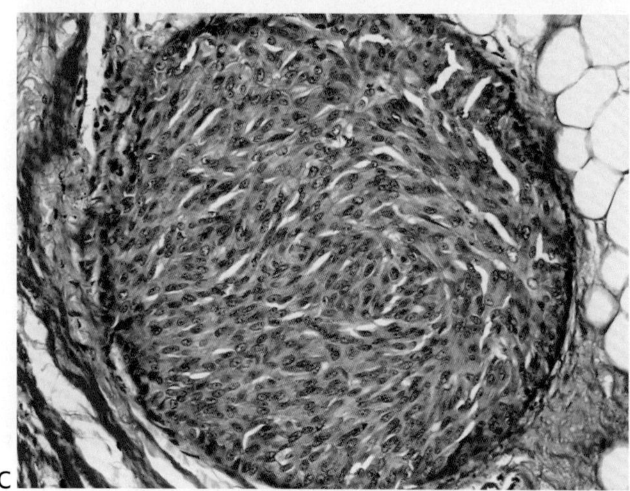

FIG. 20.8. ***Solid ductal carcinoma in situ, spindle cell type.*** **A,B:** DCIS with spindle cell morphology and low nuclear grade. The cells are uniform and show minimal cytologic atypia. Central necrosis is evident in ducts. **C:** A uniform population of neoplastic spindle cells with low-grade nuclear atypia. Myoepithelium is evident at the perimeter of the duct.

The neoplastic cells often contain intracytoplasmic mucin that at times displaces the nucleus to one side of the cell, resulting in signet ring cell morphology. Focal mucin can also be present in between the cells or in the stroma, and associated mucinous carcinoma can occur, with type A or, more often, type B morphology (see also Chapter 18). A mucicarmine stain will demonstrate the presence of intracytoplasmic mucin.

Calcifications are uncommon in DCIS with NE differentiation. In one study of 20 cases,[24] calcifications were abundant in 1 tumor (5%), sparse in 4 (20%), and absent in the remaining 15/20 (75%) cases. Tsang and Chan[23] observed the frequent presence of small papillomas in the breast parenchyma adjacent to NE-DCIS, often showing pagetoid involvement by carcinoma. Stromal hemorrhage, hemosiderin-laden macrophages, and reactive fibrosis are also common.

NE Mammary Epithelial Cells

Despite the efforts of many investigators to find progenitor argyrophilic/NE cells in normal mammary duct epithelium, such cells have rarely been detected and then only in very small numbers, leaving doubt as to the specificity of these observations.[28,29] In one study, no NE cells were detected in human fetal and adult breasts studied by immunohistochemistry (IHC) and electron microscopy.[30] Bussolati et al.[31] found scattered chromogranin-positive cells in normal breast epithelium. Kawasaki et al.[15] identified scattered cells positive for NE markers (chromogranin A and/or synaptophysin) in the benign breast parenchyma of mastectomy specimens from three women 21, 31, and 38 years old who had DCIS or invasive carcinoma with NE differentiation. Similar findings were detected in the mastectomy specimen from a 72-year-old woman with bilateral DCIS with NE differentiation.[26] Because carcinoma with NE differentiation was present in these four cases,[15,26] one cannot exclude the possibility that the scattered NE cells admixed with the benign appearing breast epithelium could represent minute clusters of carcinoma with pagetoid growth. At present, the evidence supporting the existence of NE mammary epithelial cells that could give rise to mammary carcinomas with NE differentiation remains very limited and is not compelling.

Cytology

The fine-needle aspiration (FNA) samples obtained from NE-BCs usually have moderate to high cellularity. Sapino et al.[32] studied the cytologic features of mammary carcinomas with NE differentiation. The tumors were characterized by cell clusters with rigid borders, isolated cells with a plasmacytoid appearance and peripheral chromogranin-positive cytoplasmic granules, which were demonstrated with the Giemsa stain. NE carcinomas with mucinous differentiation exhibited less cytoplasmic granularity.

In cytology preparations, the neoplastic cells have plasmacytoid, spindle cell, or signet ring cell morphology and low to intermediate nuclear grade. Mucoid material can be present in the background.[32] Loss of cell cohesion is also a useful diagnostic feature.[33]

Histochemistry

An uncommon form of biochemical and structural metaplasia in mammary carcinomas is the presence of argyrophilic cytoplasmic granules detected by light microscopy (Fig. 20.9). This alteration is not diagnostic of NE differentiation, but it is often associated with it, or at least with NE morphology. The procedures most commonly used to demonstrate argyrophilic granules rely on reactions in which ammoniacal silver is reduced to particulate metallic silver that can be visualized with the light microscope.[34] Argentaffin granules, typically found in midgut carcinoid tumors, contain endogenous reducing substances. In the argyrophilic reaction (e.g., Grimelius stain), an exogenous reducing agent is added, as some granules do not contain endogenous reducing substances. Because most cells with either argentaffin or argyrophilic granules are visualized with the argyrophilic reaction, this is the preferable procedure. Breast neoplasms that contain argyrophilic granules have been argentaffin-negative.[35,36] The reported frequency of argyrophilia in female mammary carcinomas varies from 3% to 25%.[37] Argyrophilia has been identified in breast carcinomas throughout the age distribution of the disease, ranging from patients in their early 30s to women in their late 80s.[7,35,38] No systematic study of the frequency of argyrophilic granules in male breast carcinomas has been reported, but a description of argyrophil-positive

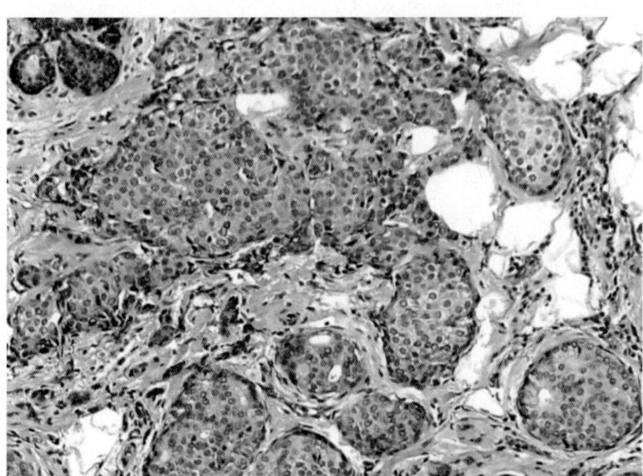

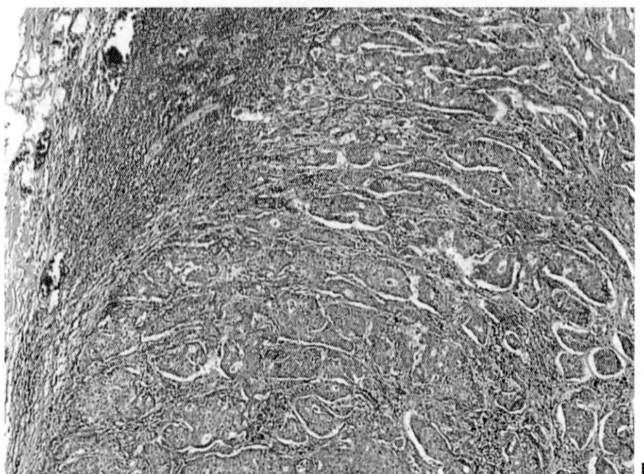

FIG. 20.9. ***Carcinoma with endocrine features, histochemistry.*** **A:** Moderately differentiated invasive duct carcinoma with small round nuclei and characteristic deeply staining cytoplasm. **B:** Metastatic carcinoma in an axillary lymph node with an endocrine growth pattern and stroma with hemosiderin. **C:** A positive Grimelius reaction in the carcinoma shown in **(A)**.

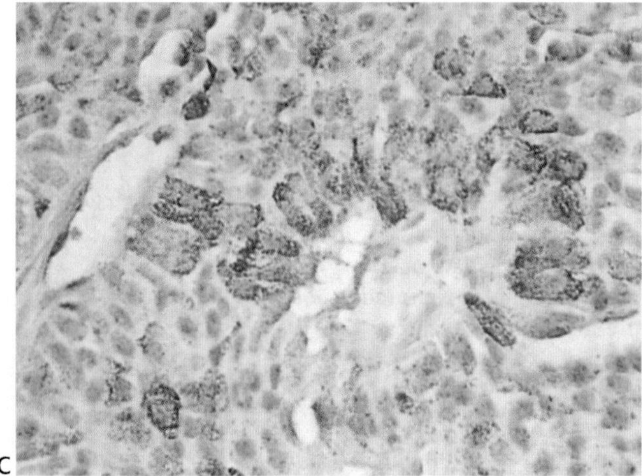

C

FIG. 20.9. *[Continued]*

tumors in men has been published.[39] Men with argyrophilic carcinomas have been 71 to 83 years old. Argyrophilic cells can be found in the intraductal, as well as in the invasive component of these tumors,[7,36] and in metastatic deposits originating from such tumors. Argyrophilic DCIS tend to have a distinctive solid–papillary or organoid growth pattern,[36,40] whereas conventional cribriform and comedo DCIS are typically nonargyrophilic.[40]

In several studies, the proportion of invasive mucinous carcinomas with argyrophilia ranged from 8% to 80%.[28,35,41] The reported frequency of argyrophilic infiltrating duct carcinomas varied from 15%[35] to 71%.[37] Among infiltrating lobular carcinomas, 50%[35] to 100%[37] have reportedly been argyrophilic.

In 1982, Clayton et al.[42] reported that the majority of argyrophilic carcinomas they studied were also reactive for lactalbumin. Intracytoplasmic localization of argyrophilia and lactalbumin showed a similar tendency to apical cytoplasmic staining in carcinomas as well as in lactating breast tissue. They concluded that argyrophilia might be evidence of lactational differentiation because "the secretory granules appear to contain milk secretory product rather than neuroendocrine polypeptides." This assumption was later rejected by Bussolati et al.,[43] who reported that the apparent immunoreactivity for α-lactalbumin found in argyrophilic carcinomas by Clayton et al.[42] was the result of a contaminant in the antibody preparation that had an affinity for endocrine cells.

Immunohistochemistry

Immunohistochemical evidence of NE marker expression has been detected in nearly 20% of mammary carcinomas, the majority of which do not resemble NE/carcinoid tumors structurally.[45,46] The diagnosis of NE-BCs is reserved for invasive carcinomas that show immunoreactivity for at least one NE marker in more than 50% of the tumor cells (Fig. 20.10). There is no definitive consensus on the most appropriate markers to identify NE tumors, but chromogranin A and synaptophysin are regarded as the most sensitive and specific in the breast as well as in other organs. In an analysis of 78 NE-BCs with different morphologic growth patterns (not inclusive of small cell breast carcinomas),[12] positivity for chromogranin A was highest (85%) in cellular mucinous carcinomas and lowest (60%) in NE-BCs with alveolar growth. In the same series, the finding of synaptophysin positivity and absence of chromogranin A reactivity varied in tumors with different morphology and architecture, ranging from 15% in cellular mucinous carcinomas to 40% in alveolar-type NE-BCs. Additional but less specific NE markers include NSE and CD56.

NE-BCs are usually strongly and diffusely positive for estrogen receptor (ER) (Fig. 20.11) and progesterone receptor (PR).[12] Wei et al.[10] reported that ER was positive in at least 10% of the tumor cells in 94.59% of 72 tumors in their series, and PR in 79.73%. Up to 45% NE-BCs are positive for androgen receptor (AR).[12] No human epidermal growth

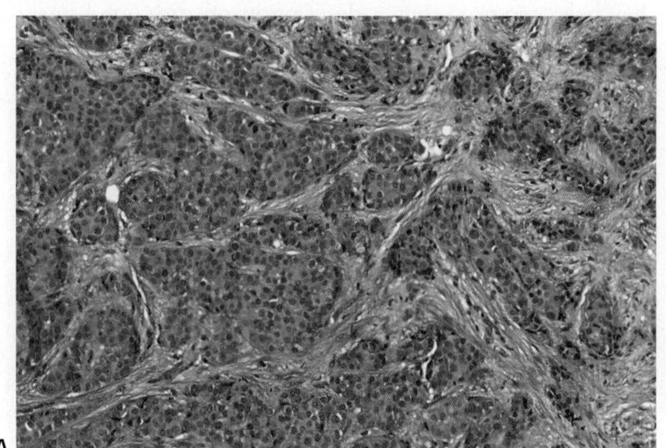

A

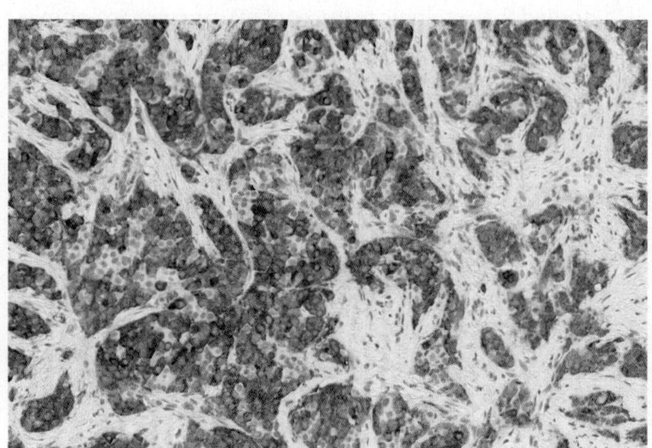

B

FIG. 20.10. ***Immunoreactivity for neuroendocrine markers.*** **A:** Invasive NE carcinoma. **B:** The invasive carcinoma in **(A)** shows strong and diffuse cytoplasmic immunoreactivity for synaptophysin in more than 50% of the tumor cells. **C:** This solid and papillary carcinoma shows strong immunoreactivity for synaptophysin. **D:** A solid papillary carcinoma with strong, focal immunoreactivity for synaptophysin, but some parts of the tumor are not reactive for the same marker. **E:** This carcinoma shows strong and diffuse immunoreactivity for chromogranin. **F,G:** This cellular mucinous carcinoma **(F)** has strong and diffuse immunoreactivity for chromogranin **(G)**.

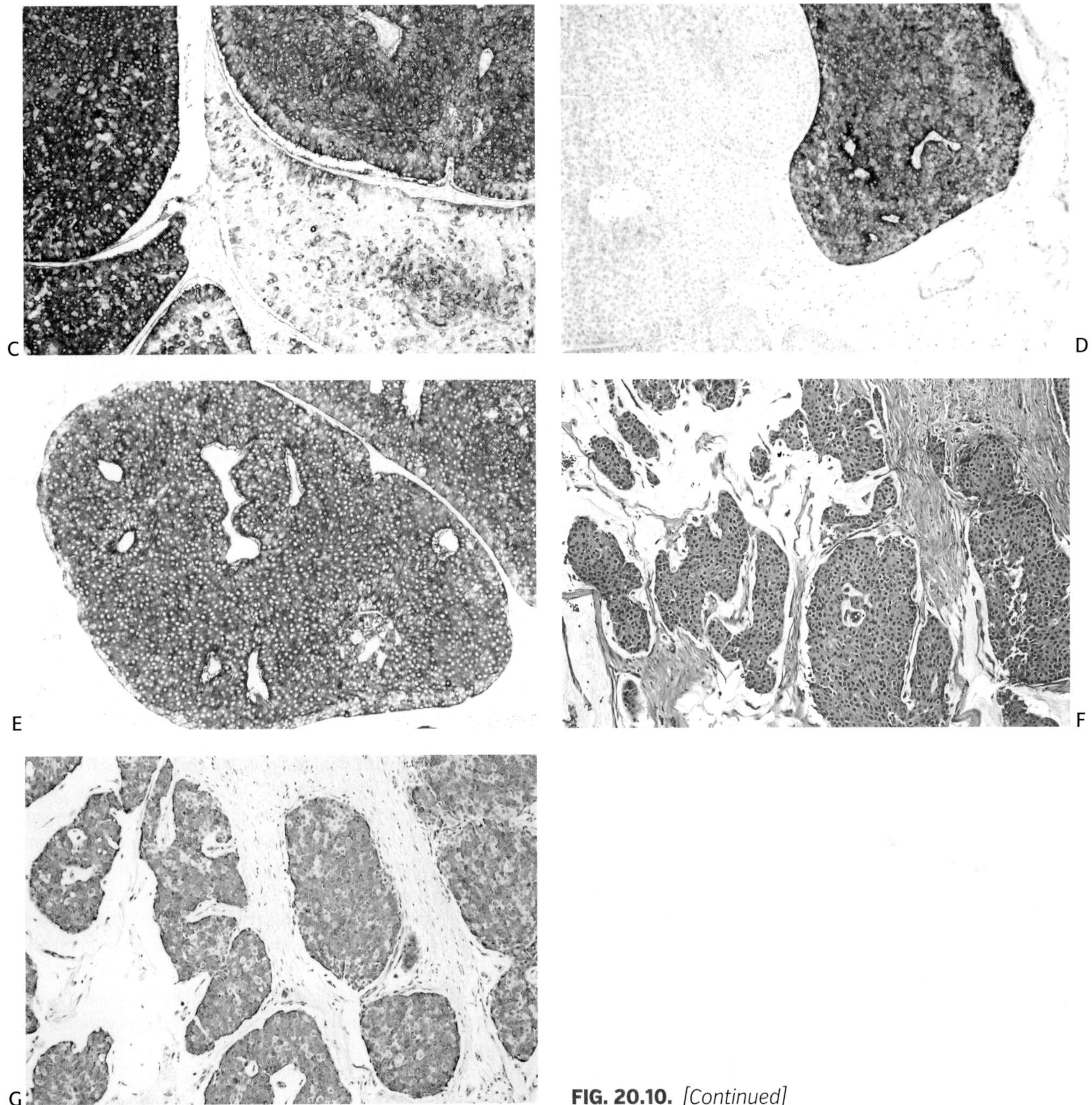

FIG. 20.10. *[Continued]*

factor 2 (HER2)–positive tumors were identified in a series by Righi et al.[12] Using IHC, Wei et al.[10] found only two HER2-positive cases (2.7%) and one with equivocal reactivity (1.35%). In a study by Kawasaki et al.,[9] 6/20 NE-BCs had equivocal (2+) HER2 staining and none had 3+ staining. Neither of the latter two studies provided HER2 fluorescence *in situ* hybridization (FISH) data. Horiguchi et al.[46] suggested that cytoplasmic reactivity for HER2 correlates with NE differentiation, but no other group has confirmed this finding.

Tse et al.[47] used IHC for NE markers to study 38 mucinous carcinomas. Twenty-four of 38 (63%) tumors were positive for NSE, 10/38 (26%) for chromogranin, and 10/38 (26%) for synaptophysin. All together, 28/38 (74%) tumors were positive for at least one NE marker, 11/38 (29%) for two, and 6/38 (16%) for all three. In this study, patients whose tumor had NE differentiation were older than patients whose tumor did not express NE markers. In particular, the age difference was statistically significant when patients with NSE-positive tumors were compared with those with NSE-negative tumors (71 vs. 58 years, respectively), and patients with tumors positive for at least two NE markers were compared with those with carcinomas showing lesser reactivity (77 vs. 62 years, respectively). Carcinomas with NE differentiation had lower nuclear grade than those without, and the difference in nuclear grade between tumors positive for at least two NE markers versus those with lesser reactivity (low nuclear grade in 91% vs. 59%, respectively) was statistically significant. Tumors with NE differentiation had a lower rate of lymph node metastases, and the difference was

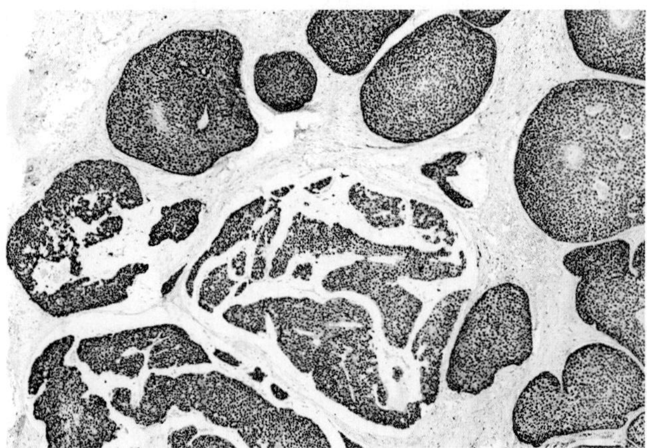

FIG. 20.11. *ER positivity in neuroendocrine carcinoma.* This solid papillary carcinoma with mucinous differentiation shows strong and diffuse immunoreactivity for ER.

statistically significant when comparing NSE-positive versus NSE-negative carcinomas (lymph node negative in 96% vs. 64% of cases, respectively). A study by Makretsov et al.[45] correlated the expression of NE antigens with long-term clinical follow-up data and found that the expression of chromogranin A, synaptophysin, as well as coexpression of multiple NE markers carried no prognostic significance. NSE demonstrated a statistically significant correlation with improved disease-specific survival (DFS) ($p = 0.043$) and overall survival ($p = 0.03$) in univariate analysis, but not in multivariate analysis.

NE-BCs can also express apocrine markers. In a series by Sapino et al.,[48] 19/43 (45%) tumors expressed gross cystic disease fluid protein-15 (GCDFP-15) and NE markers in more than 50% of the cells, including 5/19 cases with NE apocrine and mucinous morphology. NE-BCs do not express high molecular weight cytokeratin (CK) 34βE12.[12] The neoplastic epithelium of solid–papillary DCIS shows no immunoreactivity for CK5/6, and this marker can be helpful in the differential diagnosis with usual ductal hyperplasia involving a papilloma, as the latter is CK5/6 positive.[49] A mucicarmine stain usually demonstrates intracytoplasmic mucin in this tumor.

Human achaete-scute homolog-1 (hASH-1) is a basic helix-loop-helix transcription factor involved in the regulation of mammalian neural and NE cell development. Using IHC, Righi et al.[50] documented the expression of hASH-1 in 53/84 (63%) carcinomas with NE morphology and staining for NE markers in more than 50% of the cells, and in 8/21 (38%) breast carcinomas with NE morphology and reactivity for NE markers in less than 50% of the tumor cells. hASH-1 immunoreactivity did not correlate with any specific NE marker or clinical parameter, but was significantly correlated to a low mitotic count (less than 20 mitoses per 10 high-power fields [HPFs]) and low Ki67 proliferative index (less than 20% positive nuclei). None of the non-NE invasive breast carcinomas showed reactivity for hASH-1.

Comparison with Metastatic Extramammary NE Tumors in the Breast

Metastases in the breast from a carcinoid that arose at another site may be mistaken for a primary mammary NE tumor.[51,52] In these cases, the finding of an *in situ* component provides convincing evidence of breast origin. Knowledge of the patient's prior clinical history is also of fundamental importance. This topic is also discussed in Chapter 34.

Perry et al.[53] reported a series of 18 NE tumors metastatic in the breast from extramammary organs. The site of origin of the tumors was the gastrointestinal tract in 11/18 (62%) cases or the lungs in 5/18 (28%); the primary site was unknown in two cases. Five patients presented with unilateral breast involvement, and two had no prior diagnosis of an NE tumor. One of the metastases was discovered incidentally in a needle core biopsy specimen that targeted mammographic calcifications. In 8/18 (44%) cases, the tumor was initially misdiagnosed as primary breast carcinoma. In this series, all gastrointestinal NE tumors were caudal-type homeobox 2 (CDX2) positive, and three of five (60%) pulmonary NE tumors were thyroid transcription factor 1 (TTF-1)–positive. Weak positivity for ER was detected in 2/18 (11%) metastatic lesions.

Additional work-up should be considered when a tumor involving the breast has NE morphology and a nodular configuration and no DCIS is present. The diagnostic work-up should include immunoperoxidase stains for ER, PR, as well as for CDX2, and TTF-1, although not all primary gastrointestinal and pulmonary carcinoid tumors are positive for the relevant marker.[54] Whenever present, ER and/or PR positivity in metastases of an extramammary NE tumor is usually weak and very focal. This finding in a presumed NE mammary carcinoma with low to intermediate nuclear grade should always raise suspicion for extramammary origin. Primary mammary NE carcinomas with this morphology are usually strongly and diffusely ER- and PR-positive.[55] In the appropriate clinical setting, immunoreactivity for calcitonin should also be evaluated to rule out metastasis of a medullary thyroid carcinoma. GCDFP-15 and mammaglobin are useful in establishing mammary origin,[55] although some positivity can also occur in extramammary tumors. Wang et al.[56] identified positive reactivity for GCDFP-15 in some primary pulmonary epithelial tumors, including 1 of 23 pulmonary carcinoids. GATA-3 is a zinc finger transcription factor expressed in benign and malignant mammary epithelium,[57] as well as in benign and neoplastic urothelium,[57] in salivary gland carcinomas,[58] and in rare endometrial adenocarcinomas.[57] Recent data[59] indicate that reactivity for GATA-3 can be used to distinguish NE tumors of mammary origin from those originating at other sites.

NE tumors involving the lung in a patient with prior history of breast carcinoma should also be thoroughly evaluated. In particular, carcinoid tumorlets of the lung are often multiple and bilateral, and can mimic metastatic spread of a mammary NE-BC both radiologically and histologically.[60]

Electron Microscopy

Capella et al.[61] studied the ultrastructural characteristics of 24 breast carcinoma with morphologic, histochemical, and immunohistochemical features of NE-BCs. They identified five types of dense-core granules of neurosecretory type (confirmed by the ultrastructural localization of chromogranin A) as well as five different cell types. Some cells were found to contain mucin-containing vesicles as well as neurosecretory granules, supporting coexisting endocrine and exocrine differentiation (amphicrine cells). Chromogranin A and synaptophysin are usually regarded as the most sensitive and specific NE markers in the breast as well as in other organs. Ultrastructurally they have been associated with dense-core granules (chromogranin A and B) and presynaptic clear vesicles (synaptophysin) found in NE cells.[61] Dickersin et al.[62] reported that the cells of mammary NE carcinomas with solid and papillary morphology were ultrastructurally similar to those of other types of mammary carcinoma, and that they formed extracellular microlumens. Only rare cells had intracellular lumens. The tumor cells, however, contained a variety of granules, including "bull's-eye" mucinous granules, large serous-like granules, and small dense-core granules. Dense-core granules with albuminal or juxtavascular location were consistent with NE granules, whereas apical and subluminal granules appeared mucinous in type. Neurosecretory granules can be detected in some tumors by electron microscopy.[35,37,41]

Genetics and Molecular Studies

Few studies have assessed the genetics and molecular alterations of NE-BCs. Weigelt et al.[63] evaluated the genetic profile of 18 mucinous carcinomas and 6 NE-BCs using CGH. They found that the tumors clustered closely together and had profiles different from those of grade- and subtype-matched invasive ductal carcinomas not otherwise specified (NOS). In particular, the genetic profile of mucinous type B carcinomas and that of NE-BCs were nearly indistinguishable from one another, and differed slightly from that of type A mucinous carcinomas. In a subsequent study focused on mucinous carcinomas, Lacroix-Triki et al.[64] documented that mucinous type B carcinomas have significantly more frequently gains of 2q37 and 11q13 and less frequently loss of 16p11 than mucinous type A carcinomas. Mucinous tumors showed no concurrent loss of 16q and gain of 1q,[64] the hallmark genetic alterations of low-grade mammary epithelial neoplasia.[65] Taken together, these findings suggest that mucinous and NE carcinomas are genetically related, and their pathogenesis differs from that of low-grade ductal carcinomas of no special type.

Prognosis and Treatment

Data on the clinical follow-up of patients with NE-BCs are limited. Tse et al.[47] reported that mucinous carcinomas with NE differentiation had lower nuclear grade, a lower rate of lymph node involvement, and an overall better prognosis than non-NE mucinous carcinomas. NE-BCs with low nuclear grade seem to have a very good prognosis, with survival longer than 10 years in one series.[66]

In contrast to these results, Wei et al.[10] recently reported that NE-BCs are relatively aggressive tumors. Thirty-one of 74 (42%) patients with NE-BC in their series had lymph node involvement and 6 (8%) presented with distant metastases. The authors compared clinical follow-up of patients with stage I to III NE-BC with that of 142 control patients matched for gender, age, tumor stage, ER and HER2 receptor status, and treatment modalities. The study group median follow-up time was 29 months (range 6 to 260) versus 67 months (range 9 to 125) for the control group. In this study, patients with NE-BC had a significantly higher rate of local recurrence (10% vs. 3%, respectively; $p = 0.001$) and distant metastases (22% vs. 4%, respectively; $p < 0.0001$) than control subjects. Eleven patients (15%) with NE-BC died of disease between 25 and 260 months after the initial diagnosis, in contrast to only 5.6% patients with non-NE tumors. Distant metastases of NE-BC most frequently involved bone and liver. Other metastatic sites included the lungs, brain, pleura, mediastinal lymph nodes, adrenal glands, ovaries, fallopian tubes, colon, ileum, and pancreas. Another group[67] also reported a worse overall prognosis for 107 Chinese patients with invasive NE-BC than for a control group of 475 patients treated at the same center.

Overall, management of NE-BCs does not differ from that of other breast carcinomas and is based on tumor stage and receptor status. The relationship of immunohistochemically detected NE markers to prognosis is discussed in the section on IHC in this chapter.

REFERENCES

1. Saigo PE, Rosen PP. Mammary carcinoma with "choriocarcinomatous" features. *Am J Surg Pathol* 1981;5:773–778.
2. Coombes RC, Easty GC, Detre SI, et al. Secretion of immunoreactive calcitonin by human breast carcinomas. *Br Med J* 1975;4:197–199.
3. Woodard BH, Eisenbarth G, Wallace NR, et al. Adrenocorticotropin production by a mammary carcinoma. *Cancer* 1981;47:1823–1827.
4. Mavligit GM, Cohen JL, Sherwood LM. Ectopic production of parathyroid hormone by carcinoma of the breast. *N Engl J Med* 1971;285:154–156.
5. Kaneko H, Hojo H, Ishikawa S, et al. Norepinephrine-producing tumors of bilateral breasts: a case report. *Cancer* 1978;41:2002–2007.
6. Green DM. Mucoid carcinoma of the breast with choriocarcinoma in its metastases. *Histopathology* 1990;16:504–506.
7. Cubilla A, Woodruff J. Primary carcinoid tumor of the breast: a report of eight patients. *Am J Surg Pathol* 1977;1:283–292.
8. Tian Z, Wei B, Tang F, et al. Prognostic significance of tumor grading and staging in mammary carcinomas with neuroendocrine differentiation. *Hum Pathol* 2011;42:1169–1177.
9. Kawasaki T, Mochizuki K, Yamauchi H, et al. High prevalence of neuroendocrine carcinoma in breast lesions detected by the clinical symptom of bloody nipple discharge. *Breast* 2012;21:652–656.
10. Wei B, Ding T, Xing Y, et al. Invasive neuroendocrine carcinoma of the breast: a distinctive subtype of aggressive mammary carcinoma. *Cancer* 2010;116:4463–4473.
11. Tang F, Wei B, Tian Z, et al. Invasive mammary carcinoma with neuroendocrine differentiation: histological features and diagnostic challenges. *Histopathology* 2011;59:106–115.
12. Righi L, Sapino A, Marchio C, et al. Neuroendocrine differentiation in breast cancer: established facts and unresolved problems. *Semin Diagn Pathol* 2010;27:69–76.
13. Nassar H, Qureshi H, Adsay NV, et al. Clinicopathologic analysis of solid papillary carcinoma of the breast and associated invasive carcinomas. *Am J Surg Pathol* 2006;30:501–507.
14. Zhang JY, Chen WJ. Bilateral primary breast neuroendocrine carcinoma in a young woman: report of a case. *Surg Today* 2011;41:1575–1578.
15. Kawasaki T, Mochizuki K, Yamauchi H, et al. Neuroendocrine cells associated with neuroendocrine carcinoma of the breast: nature and significance. *J Clin Pathol* 2012;65:699–703.
16. Jach R, Piskorz T, Przeszlakowski D, et al. Solid papillary carcinoma of the breast with neuroendocrine features in a pregnant woman: a case report. *Neuro Endocrinol Lett* 2011;32:405–407.
17. Burga AM, Fadare O, Lininger RA, et al. Invasive carcinomas of the male breast: a morphologic study of the distribution of histologic subtypes and metastatic patterns in 778 cases. *Virchows Arch* 2006;449:507–512.
18. Gunhan-Bilgen I, Zekioglu O, Ustun EE, et al. Neuroendocrine differentiated breast carcinoma: imaging features correlated with clinical and histopathological findings. *Eur Radiol* 2003;13:788–793.

19. Suchak AA, Millo N, MacEwan R, et al. Neuroendocrine differentiated breast carcinoma with pleural metastases using indium-111 octreotide. *Clin Nucl Med* 2009;34:74–75.
20. Rakha EA, Gandhi N, Climent F, et al. Encapsulated papillary carcinoma of the breast: an invasive tumor with excellent prognosis. *Am J Surg Pathol* 2011;35:1093–1103.
21. Nicolas MM, Wu Y, Middleton LP, et al. Loss of myoepithelium is variable in solid papillary carcinoma of the breast. *Histopathology* 2007;51:657–665.
22. Maluf HM, Koerner FC. Solid papillary carcinoma of the breast. A form of intraductal carcinoma with endocrine differentiation frequently associated with mucinous carcinoma. *Am J Surg Pathol* 1995;19:1237–1244.
23. Tsang WY, Chan JK. Endocrine ductal carcinoma *in situ* (E-DCIS) of the breast: a form of low-grade DCIS with distinctive clinicopathologic and biologic characteristics. *Am J Surg Pathol* 1996;20: 921–943.
24. Kawasaki T, Nakamura S, Sakamoto G, et al. Neuroendocrine ductal carcinoma *in situ* (NE-DCIS) of the breast—comparative clinicopathological study of 20 NE-DCIS cases and 274 non-NE-DCIS cases. *Histopathology* 2008;53:288–298.
25. Honami H, Sotome K, Sakamoto G, et al. Synchronous bilateral neuroendocrine ductal carcinoma *in situ*. *Breast Cancer* 2011 Jul 7. DOI 10.1007/s12282-011-0278-1
26. Miura K, Nasu H, Ogura H. Double neuroendocrine ductal carcinomas *in situ* coexisting with a background of diffuse idiopathic neuroendocrine cell hyperplasia of breast: a case report and hypothesis of neuroendocrine tumor development. *Pathol Int* 2012;62:331–334.
27. Farshid G, Moinfar F, Meredith DJ, et al. Spindle cell ductal carcinoma *in situ*. An unusual variant of ductal intra-epithelial neoplasia that simulates ductal hyperplasia or a myoepithelial proliferation. *Virchows Arch* 2001;439:70–77.
28. Fisher ER, Palekar AS. Solid and mucinous varieties of so-called mammary carcinoid tumors. *Am J Clin Pathol* 1979;72:909–916.
29. Feyrter F, Hartmann G. [On the carcinoid growth form of the carcinoma mammae, especially the carcinoma solidum (Gelatinosum) mammae]. *Frankf Z Pathol* 1963;73:24–39.
30. Viacava P, Castagna M, Bevilacqua G. Absence of neuroendocrine cells in fetal and adult mammary gland. Are neuroendocrine breast tumours real neuroendocrine tumours? *Breast* 1995;4:143–146.
31. Bussolati G, Gugliotta P, Sapino A, et al. Chromogranin-reactive endocrine cells in argyrophilic carcinomas ("carcinoids") and normal tissue of the breast. *Am J Pathol* 1985;120:186–192.
32. Sapino A, Papotti M, Pietribiasi F, et al. Diagnostic cytological features of neuroendocrine differentiated carcinoma of the breast. *Virchows Arch* 1998;433:217–222.
33. Tang W, Taniguchi E, Wang X, et al. Loss of cell cohesion in breast cytology as a characteristic of neuroendocrine carcinoma. *Acta Cytol* 2002;46:835–840.
34. Smith DM Jr, Haggitt RC. A comparative study of generic stains for carcinoid secretory granules. *Am J Surg Pathol* 1983;7:61–68.
35. Fetissof F, Dubois MP, Arbeille-Brassart B, et al. Argyrophilic cells in mammary carcinoma. *Hum Pathol* 1983;14:127–134.
36. Partanen S, Syrjanen K. Argyrophilic cells in carcinoma of the female breast. *Virchows Arch A Pathol Anat Histol* 1981;391:45–51.
37. Nesland JM, Holm R, Johannessen JV. A study of different markers for neuroendocrine differentiation in breast carcinomas. *Pathol Res Pract* 1986;181:524–530.
38. Azzopardi JG, Muretto P, Goddeeris P, et al. 'Carcinoid' tumours of the breast: the morphological spectrum of argyrophil carcinomas. *Histopathology* 1982;6:549–569.
39. Gill IS. Carcinoid tumour of the male breast. *J R Soc Med* 1990;83:401.
40. Cross AS, Azzopardi JG, Krausz T, et al. A morphological and immunocytochemical study of a distinctive variant of ductal carcinoma *in-situ* of the breast. *Histopathology* 1985;9:21–37.
41. Min K-W. Argyrophilia in breast carcinomas: histochemical, ultrastructural and immunocytochemical study. *Lab Invest* 1983;48:58A–59A.
42. Clayton F, Sibley RK, Ordonez NG, et al. Argyrophilic breast carcinomas: evidence of lactational differentiation. *Am J Surg Pathol* 1982;6:323–333.
43. Bussolati G, Papotti M, Sapino A, et al. Endocrine markers in argyrophilic carcinomas of the breast. *Am J Surg Pathol* 1987;11:248–256.
44. Miremadi A, Pinder SE, Lee AH, et al. Neuroendocrine differentiation and prognosis in breast adenocarcinoma. *Histopathology* 2002;40:215–222.
45. Makretsov N, Gilks CB, Coldman AJ, et al. Tissue microarray analysis of neuroendocrine differentiation and its prognostic significance in breast cancer. *Hum Pathol* 2003;34:1001–1008.
46. Horiguchi S, Hishima T, Hayashi Y, et al. HER-2/neu cytoplasmic staining is correlated with neuroendocrine differentiation in breast carcinoma. *J Med Dent Sci* 2010;57:155–163.
47. Tse GM, Ma TK, Chu WC, et al. Neuroendocrine differentiation in pure type mammary mucinous carcinoma is associated with favorable histologic and immunohistochemical parameters. *Mod Pathol* 2004;17:568–572.
48. Sapino A, Righi L, Cassoni P, et al. Expression of apocrine differentiation markers in neuroendocrine breast carcinomas of aged women. *Mod Pathol* 2001;14:768–776.
49. Rabban JT, Koerner FC, Lerwill MF. Solid papillary ductal carcinoma *in situ* versus usual ductal hyperplasia in the breast: a potentially difficult distinction resolved by cytokeratin 5/6. *Hum Pathol* 2006;37:787–793.
50. Righi L, Rapa I, Votta A, et al. Human achaete-scute homolog-1 expression in neuroendocrine breast carcinoma. *Virchows Arch* 2012;460:415–421.
51. Kashlan RB, Powell RW, Nolting SF. Carcinoid and other tumors metastatic to the breast. *J Surg Oncol* 1982;20:25–30.
52. Ordonez NG, Manning JT Jr, Raymond AK. Argentaffin endocrine carcinoma (carcinoid) of the pancreas with concomitant breast metastasis: an immunohistochemical and electron microscopic study. *Hum Pathol* 1985;16:746–751.
53. Perry KD, Reynolds C, Rosen DG, et al. Metastatic neuroendocrine tumour in the breast: a potential mimic of *in-situ* and invasive mammary carcinoma. *Histopathology* 2011;59:619–630.
54. Lin X, Saad RS, Luckasevic TM, et al. Diagnostic value of CDX-2 and TTF-1 expressions in separating metastatic neuroendocrine neoplasms of unknown origin. *Appl Immunohistochem Mol Morphol* 2007;15:407–414.
55. Richter-Ehrenstein C, Arndt J, Buckendahl AC, et al. Solid neuroendocrine carcinomas of the breast: metastases or primary tumors? *Breast Cancer Res Treat* 2010;124:413–417.
56. Wang LJ, Greaves WO, Sabo E, et al. GCDFP-15 positive and TTF-1 negative primary lung neoplasms: a tissue microarray study of 381 primary lung tumors. *Appl Immunohistochem Mol Morphol* 2009;17:505–511.
57. Liu H, Shi J, Wilkerson ML, et al. Immunohistochemical evaluation of GATA3 expression in tumors and normal tissues: a useful immunomarker for breast and urothelial carcinomas. *Am J Clin Pathol* 2012;138:57–64.
58. Schwartz LE, Begum S, Westra WH, Bishop JA. GATA3 immunohistochemical expression in salivary gland neoplasms. *Head and Neck Pathol.* 2013 Apr 20. [Epub ahead of print] DOI 10.1007/s12105-013-0442-3
59. Chopra S, Kim S, Bose S, et al. GATA-3 is helpful in differentiating primary mammary neuroendocrine carcinomas from metastatic neuroendocrine tumors. *Modern Pathol* 2013 (Suppl. 2):130A.
60. Darvishian F, Ginsberg MS, Klimstra DS, et al. Carcinoid tumorlets simulate pulmonary metastases in women with breast cancer. *Hum Pathol* 2006;37:839–844.
61. Capella C, Usellini L, Papotti M, et al. Ultrastructural features of neuroendocrine differentiated carcinomas of the breast. *Ultrastruct Pathol* 1990;14:321–334.
62. Dickersin GR, Maluf HM, Koerner FC. Solid papillary carcinoma of breast: an ultrastructural study. *Ultrastruct Pathol* 1997;21:153–161.
63. Weigelt B, Geyer FC, Horlings HM, et al. Mucinous and neuroendocrine breast carcinomas are transcriptionally distinct from invasive ductal carcinomas of no special type. *Mod Pathol* 2009;22:1401–1414.
64. Lacroix-Triki M, Suarez PH, MacKay A, et al. Mucinous carcinoma of the breast is genomically distinct from invasive ductal carcinomas of no special type. *J Pathol* 2010;222:282–298.
65. Abdel-Fatah TM, Powe DG, Hodi Z, et al. Morphologic and molecular evolutionary pathways of low nuclear grade invasive breast cancers and their putative precursor lesions: further evidence to support the concept of low nuclear grade breast neoplasia family. *Am J Surg Pathol* 2008;32:513–523.
66. Sapino A, Papotti M, Righi L, et al. Clinical significance of neuroendocrine carcinoma of the breast. *Ann Oncol* 2001;12(Suppl. 2):S115–S117.
67. Zhang Y, Chen Z, Bao Y, Du Z, Li Q, Zhao Y, Tang F. Invasive neuroendocrine carcinoma of the breast: a prognostic research of 107 Chinese patients. *Neoplasma* 2012 Nov 25. [Epub ahead of print] DOI:10.4149/NEO_2013_029.

CHAPTER 21

Small Cell Carcinoma

FREDERICK C. KOERNER

Carcinomas that resemble small cell carcinoma (SCC, oat cell carcinoma) of the lung can occur in many extrapulmonary sites,[1] including the mammary gland, which gives rise to this type of carcinoma on rare occasions. In 1992, Papotti et al.[2] reported the first well-established cases of mammary neuroendocrine carcinoma displaying features similar to those of pulmonary SCC. Since the time of this publication, approximately 50 additional cases have been described.[3–26]

The diagnosis of primary mammary SCC can be made only if a nonmammary site is excluded as a source of metastasis to the breast or an *in situ* component is demonstrated histologically. Several reports fail to meet these criteria, and a few others do not provide sufficient details to substantiate the diagnosis of mammary SCC.[3,27–34] For example, one report described a 52-year-old woman with a large mammary tumor, clinically involved axillary lymph nodes (ALNs), and metastases in the liver and bones.[31] A modified Grimelius staining was negative for argyrophilic granules, but scattered neurosecretory granules were detected by electron microscopy. *In situ* carcinoma was not identified, and an autopsy was not performed to exclude the presence of a nonmammary primary site. Another report documents a 68-year-old woman with a 4-cm tumor that was classified as a SCC.[33] The tumor was negative with the Grimelius stain but was immunoreactive for chromogranin and neuron-specific enolase (NSE) and weakly immunoreactive for cytokeratin (CK). An *in situ* component was not detected. The patient died 21 months after diagnosis with widespread metastases, and a nonmammary primary site could not be excluded.

At times, pathologists have used the diagnosis of "small cell carcinoma" to describe a mammary carcinoma composed of small cells rather than to identify a carcinoma showing specific neuroendocrine attributes. For example, several papers described "small cell carcinoma" of the male breast.[35–37] On the basis of the illustrations and histologic descriptions provided, most of these appear to be examples of other types of carcinoma, possibly infiltrating lobular carcinoma. This confusion may have arisen because for a short time certain pathologists used the diagnosis of "small cell carcinoma" to refer to an invasive mammary carcinoma showing features of invasive lobular carcinoma but lacking an *in situ* component.[35] Contemporary usage classifies such carcinomas as invasive lobular carcinomas. Along similar lines, Fiorella et al.[38] described the cytologic features of a group of well-differentiated invasive ductal carcinoma, which the authors termed "small cell duct carcinoma." These carcinomas probably do not represent genuine SCC of the neuroendocrine type.

CLINICAL PRESENTATION

The age of patients with mammary SCC ranges from 29[11] to 81 years[15] with a mean of 53 years. A family history of breast carcinoma or evidence of breast cancer (BRCA)–associated carcinoma was only rarely mentioned in reports of mammary SCC. One patient had solid non–small cell ductal carcinoma *in situ* (DCIS) in her contralateral breast.[27] With the exception of one possible case,[10] all patients have been women. Jundt et al.[10] described a 52-year-old man with small cell (oat cell) carcinoma in the breast and ALNs. The histologic appearance was that of an oat cell carcinoma and the tumor cells were immunoreactive for NSE. Electron microscopy revealed desmosomes and cytoplasmic granules with neuroendocrine features. *In situ* carcinoma was not detected, but a nonmammary primary site was not evident by clinical evaluation.

SCC arises in all regions of the breast. It typically forms a single mass, but one patient had two masses in different quadrants of the same breast.[9] Another patient had multiple superficial nodules on the breast, a solitary breast mass, and matted ALNs.[15] Mammograms of SCC revealed well-defined or irregular masses with borders often described as microlobulated.[2,8,10,13,14,18,21,24] Sonography showed the masses to be solid, exhibiting low homogeneous echoes and mild posterior acoustic enhancement.[8,13,14,21] Magnetic resonance imaging (MRI) displayed early enhancement of the masses,[8,13,14,21,39] a hyperintense heterogeneous signal on T2-weighted images, and a hypointense signal on T1-weighted images.[13,39] In one case,[39] the tumor was isointense with normal tissue, and the images showed segmental non–mass-like enhancement. Positron emission tomogram-computerized tomogram (PET-CT) scans showed that the carcinomas demonstrate marked avidity for fluorodeoxyglucose.[5,24] The tumor doubling time based on imaging studies in one case was 12 days.[12] The pattern of enhancement on CT and MRI scans may be indicative of extensive DCIS.[39]

GROSS PATHOLOGY

The macroscopic appearance of SCC does not differ substantially from that of commonplace breast carcinomas. SCC has ranged from 1[3] to 14.5 cm[7] in greatest dimension; the average size was 4.1 cm. Pathologists usually described the tumors as firm and irregular. A "fleshy" consistency, a lobulated or nodular structure, and a mucoid quality were noted in individual cases.[40] The neoplastic tissue appears white, gray, or tan or variations of these colors, and shades of yellow or pink have been noted in a few cases. One group of observers[5] described a SCC as "pink to pale fawn."

MICROSCOPIC PATHOLOGY

The histologic characteristics of mammary SCC resemble those of SCC arising in other organs. The noninvasive component usually consists of small cells with scant cytoplasm and hyperchromatic nuclei. These cells may constitute the entire noninvasive neoplastic population (Fig. 21.1A, B) as they did in the four cases described by Papotti et al.[2] and five of the nine cases reported by Shin et al.,[19] or the small cells may represent only one component of an *in situ* carcinoma with mixed features. For example, Figure 21.2 illustrates a DCIS in which SCC coexists with large malignant cells showing traces of squamous metaplasia. The small tumor cells were CK-positive (CAM5.2) and variably stained with 34βE12, whereas the large tumor cells were negative for CAM5.2 and strongly stained with 34βE12. Figure 21.3A, B illustrates an intraductal carcinoma composed of cells with poorly differentiated nuclear grade merging with others showing features of SCC.

The invasive component typically consists of patternless sheets and clusters of cells that often contain zones of coagulative necrosis and foci of hemorrhage (Figs. 21.1C, D and 21.4A, B). Regions sometimes display architectural patterns of a neuroendocrine nature: organoid groups, trabeculae, or rosette-like structures surrounded by delicate blood vessels and stroma (Fig. 21.4C, D). The neoplastic cells appear small and round, polygonal, or spindly. They contain round to oval nuclei, homogeneous dark chromatin, inconspicuous nucleoli, and scant eosinophilic cytoplasm. The nuclear-to-cytoplasmic ratio is high. Nuclear molding can be seen, but it usually does not appear as prominent in tissue sections as it does in cytologic specimens.[19] Mitotic figures abound in most examples, and mitotic counts as high as 10 per high-power field have been recorded.[13] Disruption of nuclei occasionally leads to deposition of the nuclear material around blood vessels (the "Azzopardi" effect).[7,10] Vascular invasion often appears prominent. Staining with the Grimelius method produces variable results,[6,22,25,26] but pathologists no longer use this technique commonly and instead rely on immunostains, as discussed later.

Invasive SCC sometimes coexists with noninvasive carcinomas of conventional types. In two carcinomas in the series of Shin et al.,[19] the noninvasive carcinoma grew as solid DCIS with high nuclear grade. One SCC reported by Hoang et al.[7] coexisted with cribriform and comedo DCIS, and another arose in a woman who had had pleomorphic lobular carcinoma *in situ* (LCIS) in a specimen resected from the same breast 10 years earlier.

Certain invasive SCC, termed "dimorphic small cell carcinoma," display an abrupt juxtaposition of carcinoma cells of the small cell type with carcinoma cells displaying different characteristics without transitional forms. The second population can have lobular or tubulolobular (Fig. 21.5), squamous (Fig. 21.6), or glandular features (Fig. 21.7). Fukunaga and Ushigome[6] described an example of a dimorphic SCC from a 56-year-old woman with a 10.5-cm ulcerating tumor, 90% of which was small cell type. The authors reported that the "small cell and ductal carcinomatous lesions were mixed but there was no transition from the ordinary ductal to small cell carcinoma." The small cells contained argyrophilic granules, but these granules were not detected in the larger, conventional ductal carcinoma cells. The single lymph node metastasis was small cell type. Four of the nine carcinomas in the series by Shin et al.,[19] the largest in the literature, displayed dimorphic histologic patterns: two carcinomas had glandular elements, one showed foci of squamous differentiation, and the fourth consisted of a mixture of SCC and invasive lobular carcinoma. In tumors like the latter case, the SCC will stain for E-cadherin and lack hormone receptors, whereas the lobular component will not stain for E-cadherin or neuroendocrine markers but usually will express hormone receptors. In case 4 of the series of Papotti et al.,[2] "the small cell component constituted about 40% of the neoplastic population, while the remaining tumour consisted of spindled or round cells with eosinophilic cytoplasm. These cells formed alveolar structures reminiscent of the alveolar variant of invasive lobular carcinoma." Finally, the SCC described by Kinoshita et al.[12] contained conventional ductal carcinoma in both the *in situ* and the invasive portions, and the ones described by Salman et al.[16] and Sridhar et al.[20] contained invasive duct carcinoma of the usual type.

The malignant cells of SCC can involve the epidermis in a pagetoid pattern,[5,19] but the clinical manifestations of Paget disease of the nipple have not been reported.

Differential Diagnosis

The differential diagnosis of mammary SCC includes lymphomas and related neoplasms, certain sarcomas, and metastatic carcinomas. Evaluation of the growth pattern and cellular features of the malignant cells, the presence of noninvasive carcinoma, and the results of commonly employed immunohistochemical stains for epithelial and lymphoid makers should allow one to exclude the diagnosis of a lymphoproliferative malignancy. Sarcomas like Ewing sarcoma, osteosarcoma, mesenchymal chondrosarcoma, and synovial sarcoma would belong in the differential diagnosis in certain cases.[41,42] Evaluation of problematic tumors with immunohistochemical staining and genetic studies allows one to exclude these possibilities. Pathologists must keep in

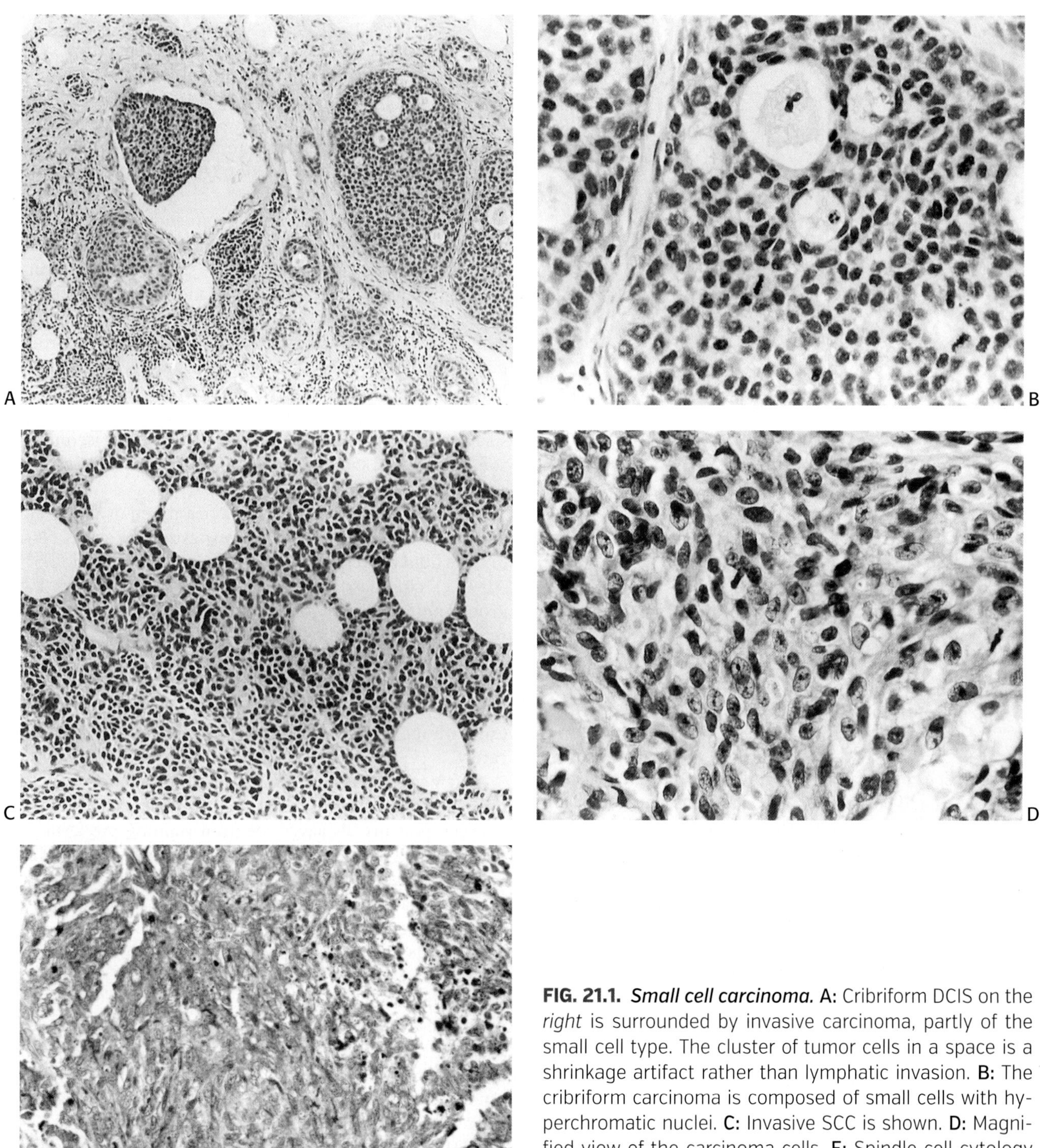

FIG. 21.1. ***Small cell carcinoma.*** **A:** Cribriform DCIS on the *right* is surrounded by invasive carcinoma, partly of the small cell type. The cluster of tumor cells in a space is a shrinkage artifact rather than lymphatic invasion. **B:** The cribriform carcinoma is composed of small cells with hyperchromatic nuclei. **C:** Invasive SCC is shown. **D:** Magnified view of the carcinoma cells. **E:** Spindle cell cytology with chromogranin reactivity is shown.

mind that mammary SCC can stain for CD99,[4,7] a protein that is usually present in the aforementioned mesenchymal tumors. To exclude the possibility of a metastatic lesion of any type, the pathologist should sample the specimen extensively to detect an *in situ* component. When the primary site is in doubt, clinicians should undertake a careful search for evidence of a primary carcinoma in another organ.

SCC of the lung stands out as the most likely primary source for metastatic neuroendocrine carcinoma in the breast. The literature contains several reports of metastatic nonmammary SCC in the breast.[16,43–45] In most cases, the existence of an extramammary primary carcinoma was previously documented in the lung or another site such as the uterine cervix.[43] Rarely, the mammary metastasis may be

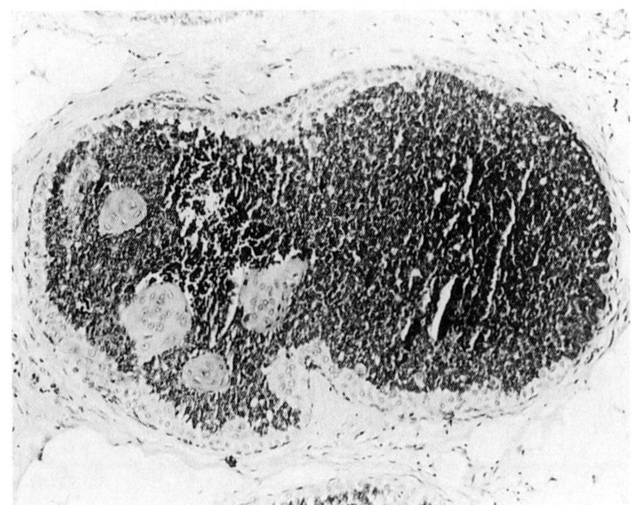

FIG. 21.2. ***Small cell carcinoma in situ.*** This dimorphic *in situ* carcinoma has clusters of large cells with squamous metaplasia.

the first manifestation of an occult pulmonary SCC. Spread from a Merkel cell carcinoma of the skin represents another possibility that can be excluded using the results of staining for CK20 and neurofilaments.[3,46]

CYTOLOGY

Cytologic specimens from SCC tend to be cellular, consisting of dispersed and clustered small cells with scant cytoplasm. The cells are approximately twice the size of small lymphocytes.[17,18,26,43] The cells exhibit high nuclear-to-cytoplasmic ratios, and they contain uniform round to oval nuclei with finely dispersed chromatin and inconspicuous nucleoli. Nuclear molding is a conspicuous feature.[43] The cytologic specimens exhibit the "squash" artifact typically found in SCC, which results from disruption of the nuclei.[24] Primary and metastatic lesions are not distinguishable cytologically.[43]

IMMUNOHISTOCHEMISTRY

As part of their studies of SCC, investigators have carried out immunohistochemical staining for many proteins, and most reports document the properties of the invasive cells. Shin et al.[19,40] carried out the most comprehensive study. Considering their findings in conjunction with other published results, one finds that no commonly used marker yielded identical results when applied to more than a handful of cases. Nevertheless, several generalizations emerge from this accumulated experience. Almost all cases were immunoreactive with AE1/3, but staining of cytologic smears by Sebenik et al.[18] did not yield a positive reaction, nor did staining of tissue sections in one case reported by Hoang et al.[7] and another by Kitakata et al.[13] The cells usually expressed CK7 or CK19 and they typically stained for CAM5.2, whereas most failed to stain for CK20. Exceptions were noted by Salmo and Connolly,[25] who described a tumor that did not stain for CAM5.2, and by Christie et al.,[5] who described a carcinoma that expressed CK20. Expression of CK8 has been observed in the few cases studied[21,22]; the results of staining for CK5/6 have varied,[21,47] while staining for 34βE12 has been variable or negative.[8,21,22]

Among proteins suggestive of neuroendocrine differentiation, expression of NSE represents the most consistent finding, although one carcinoma did not stain for the protein.[25] Staining for chromogranins (A, B, and C), synaptophysin, CD56, and leu 7 has produced variable results, but almost all mammary SCC have expressed at least one of these neuroendocrine molecules (Fig. 21.1E). Three carcinomas expressed PGP5.2.[3,25] Investigators have also tested a few tumors for expression of other proteins associated with endocrine cells such as gastrin-releasing peptide (bombesin), serotonin, somatostatin, calcitonin, and ACTH[2,19,22] but have not observed consistent results.

Staining for epithelial membrane antigen usually yields a positive reaction,[4,13,22,26] whereas testing for gross cystic disease fluid protein 15 (GCDFP-15) usually does not.[5,24,47] All 16 carcinomas tested expressed bcl-2.[4,8,13,19,20,22,26] Two groups noted staining for CD99,[4,7] and one group observed reactivity for epidermal growth factor receptor (EGFR).[47] With the exception of two examples,[4,22] SCC have expressed E-cadherin.[5,40] This observation suggests that the majority of mammary SCC are ductal in their histogenesis, although they may have a lobular immunophenotype rarely.

A few investigators have reported the staining results of both the noninvasive and invasive components of SCC. The two components displayed identical staining properties in two tumors,[3,5] but in two instances, the noninvasive and invasive cells exhibited different staining reactions.[16,47]

Because a SCC in the breast sometimes represents a metastasis rather than a primary carcinoma, investigators have studied the expression of thyroid transcription factor-1 (TTF-1) and CD117 in *bona fide* mammary SCC. Seven of 18 mammary SCC stained for TTF-1,[5,13,14,16,22,24,40,47] and researchers detected CD117 in three of four tumors.[4,8,21,26] In some cases, TTF-1 was expressed in the *in situ* as well as the invasive carcinoma,[5,16] whereas in others, TTF-1 was not detected in the *in situ* component.[47] These findings make clear that one cannot rely on the presence of either TTF-1 or CD117 to distinguish a mammary SCC from a metastasis from a SCC arising in the lung or another site.

SCC demonstrates variable immunoreactivity for estrogen receptor (ER) and progesterone receptor (PR) (Figs. 21.5B and 21.8). About 25% of cases have expressed ER and slightly more have stained for PR.[29] With two exceptions,[22,23] the carcinomas have not expressed human epidermal growth factor 2 (HER2). One tumor studied by Fukunaga and Ushigome[6] showed an aneuploid DNA content and an S-phase fraction (SPF) of 34.9%. Amano et al.[39] reported Ki67 indices of 33.4% and 8% in two cases, and indices as high as 95% have been reported in other examples.[7,21]

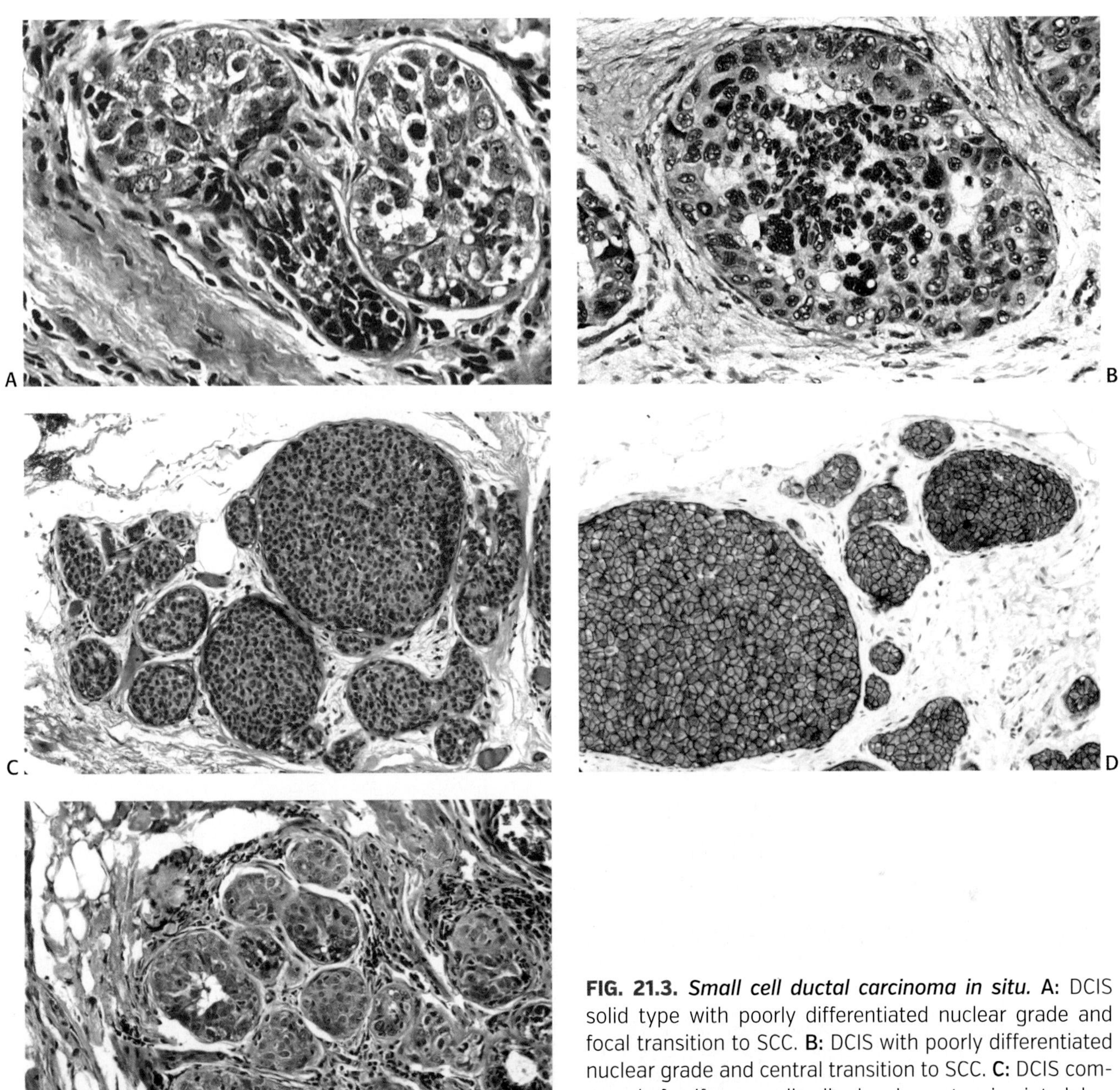

FIG. 21.3. ***Small cell ductal carcinoma in situ.*** **A:** DCIS solid type with poorly differentiated nuclear grade and focal transition to SCC. **B:** DCIS with poorly differentiated nuclear grade and central transition to SCC. **C:** DCIS composed of uniform small cells showing extension into lobular glands. **D:** The carcinoma in (C) is E-cadherin-positive. **E:** Lobular extension of small cell DCIS.

ELECTRON MICROSCOPY

Based on the study of just a few cases,[2,10,26] it seems that mammary SCC displays the ultrastructural features expected for neuroendocrine carcinomas seen in other organs. The cells possess scant cytoplasm containing dense core granules that vary from 80 to 250 nm in diameter, free ribosomes, mitochondria, rough endoplasmic reticulum, and Golgi complexes. The nuclei can exhibit irregularities in size and shape. They contain irregularly clumped chromatin deposited along the nuclear membrane and small nucleoli. Neighboring carcinoma cells occasionally display poorly formed cell junctions or desmosomes.

GENETIC STUDIES

Loss of heterozygosity (LOH) analysis of two examples of primary mammary SCC revealed multiple molecular alterations.[7] In one case, the intraductal and invasive components displayed the same alterations.

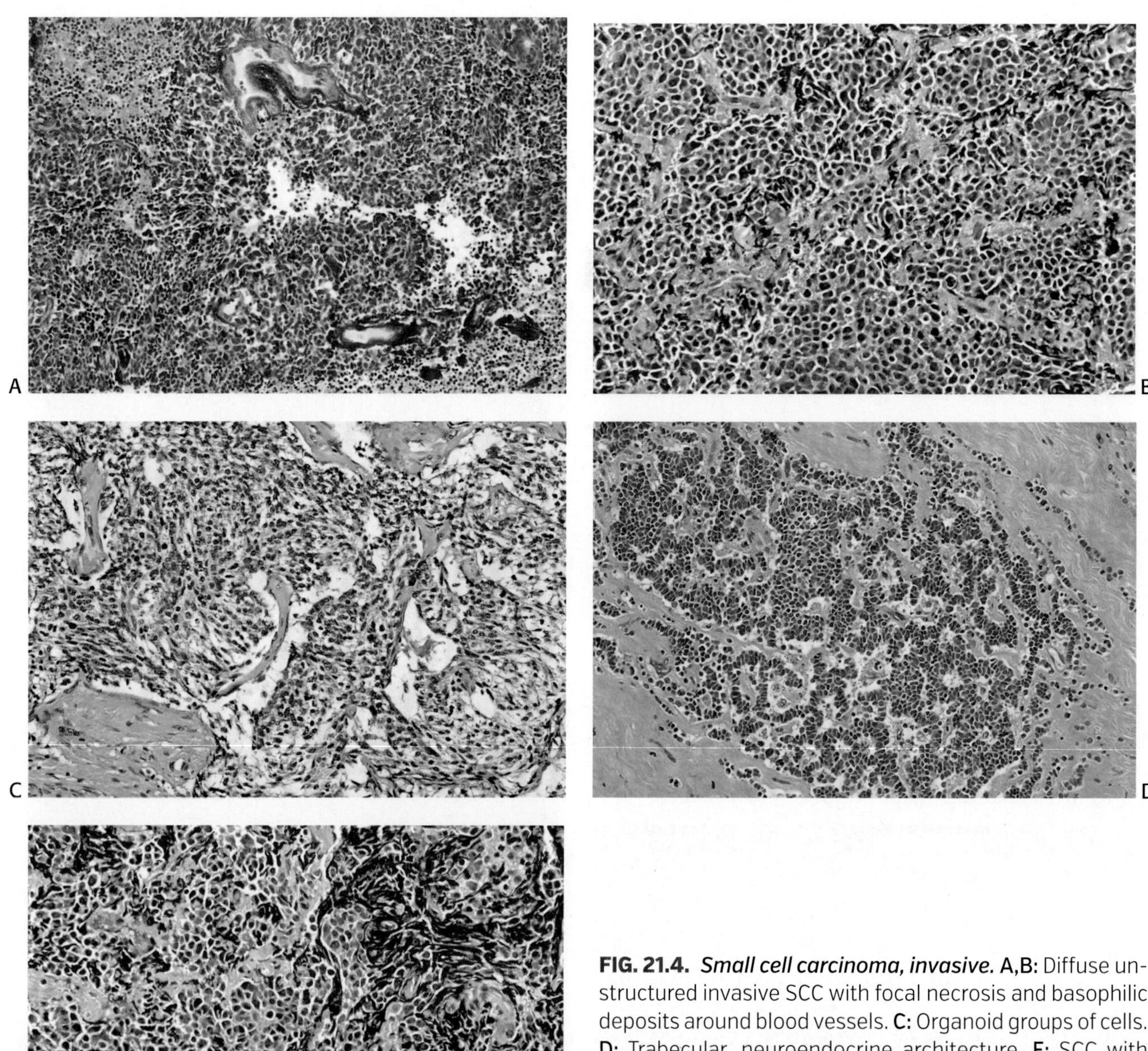

FIG. 21.4. ***Small cell carcinoma, invasive.*** **A,B:** Diffuse unstructured invasive SCC with focal necrosis and basophilic deposits around blood vessels. **C:** Organoid groups of cells. **D:** Trabecular, neuroendocrine architecture. **E:** SCC with crush artifact (*right*). (**D:** Reproduced from Shin SJ, DeLellis RA, Ying L, et al. Small cell carcinoma of the breast: a clinicopathologic and immunohistochemical study of nine patients. *Am J Surg Pathol* 2000;24:1231–1238, with permission).

TREATMENT AND PROGNOSIS

The small number of cases, the variation in the treatment, and the short duration of the follow-up prevent one from drawing secure conclusions regarding either the prognosis of patients with mammary SCC or its optimum treatment. Nevertheless, the published experience permits a few generalizations.[29] First, about two-thirds of patients had involvement of regional lymph nodes at the time of presentation. Second, approximately 20% of patients succumbed to carcinoma during intervals from 3 months[5] to approximately 2 years.[8] Third, approximately 20% of patients developed recurrences during the same interval, yet remained alive with disease. Finally, about one-half of patients followed for 3[19] to 48 months[6] remained free of carcinoma. The latter patient had a 10-cm tumor and a single ALN metastasis yet was well 4 years after treatment by mastectomy alone.[6] Follow-up intervals greater than 4 years have not been recorded.

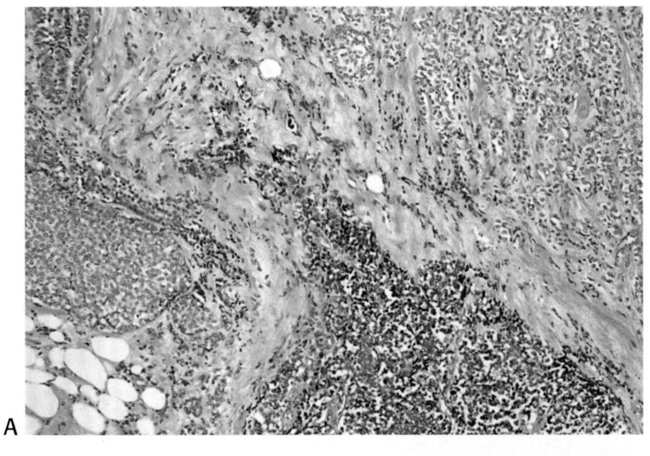

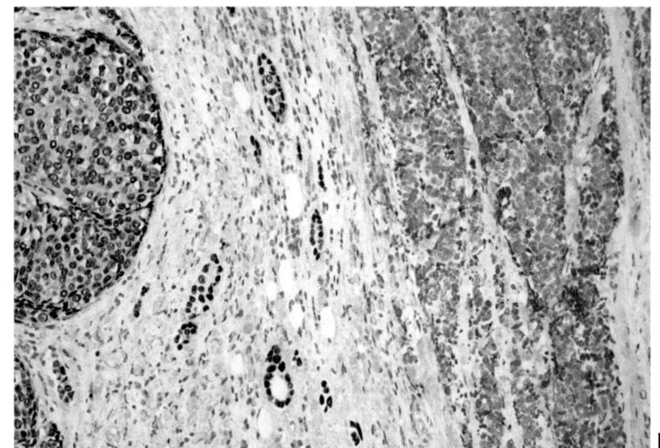

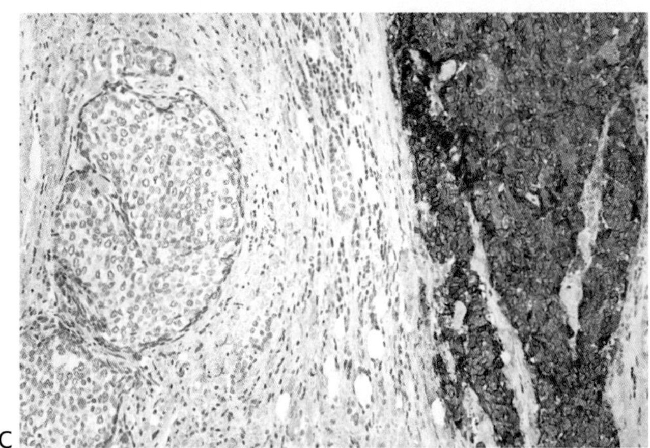

FIG. 21.5. ***Small cell carcinoma with invasive tubulolobular carcinoma.*** **A:** SCC in the *lower center* is surrounded by *in situ* (*left*) and invasive (*right*) lobular carcinoma. **B:** *In situ* lobular carcinoma (*left*) and invasive tubulolobular carcinoma (*center*) display nuclear immunoreactivity for ER. SCC (*right*) is nonreactive. **C:** Chromogranin immunoreactivity is diffusely present in SCC (*right*) and absent in lobular carcinoma (*left*).

In their review, Shin et al.[19] compared the pathologic features and outcome of the nine carcinomas in their study group with those of nine patients previously reported in the literature. The authors found that their patients had smaller carcinomas, presented with disease limited to the breast, and did not die of their carcinomas, whereas those patients in the earlier reports did not fare as well. The authors concluded that the prognosis for relatively early stage SCC may be more favorable than suggested by the early reports of patients with more advanced disease at presentation and that chemotherapy and radiotherapy may improve local and systemic control of mammary SCC.

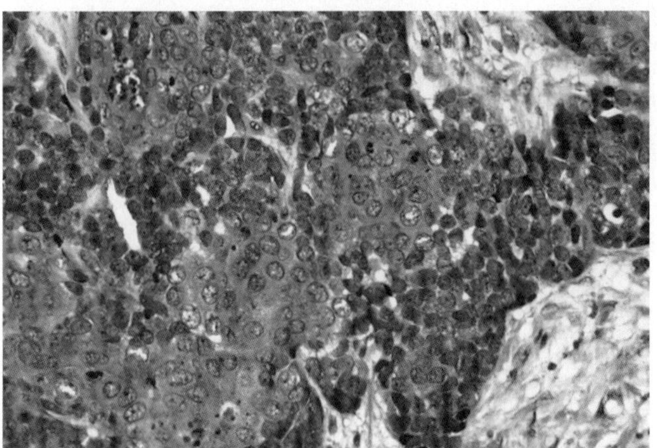

FIG. 21.6. ***Small cell carcinoma, squamoid dimorphic structure.*** Discrete clusters of cells with poorly differentiated squamous appearance surrounded by SCC.

The treatment of patients with mammary SCC has varied.[29] Surgical removal of the mass represents the primary treatment for most. However, one patient received only radiotherapy,[10] and one patient received only chemotherapy and radiotherapy.[15] In approximately two-thirds of patients, the surgical procedure consisted of a mastectomy, and the remaining patients had breast-conserving surgery, often followed by radiotherapy. Chemotherapy was typically administered following surgery, but adjuvant chemotherapy was administered to a substantial number of patients.[11,14,17–19,24,30,39] Oncologists have used several types of antineoplastic drugs: alkylating agents such as cisplatin and cyclophosphamide, topoisomerase inhibitors such as irinotecan and etoposide, and anthracyclines such as epirubicin and doxorubicin, as well as other agents commonly used in patients with conventional breast carcinomas and antiestrogens.

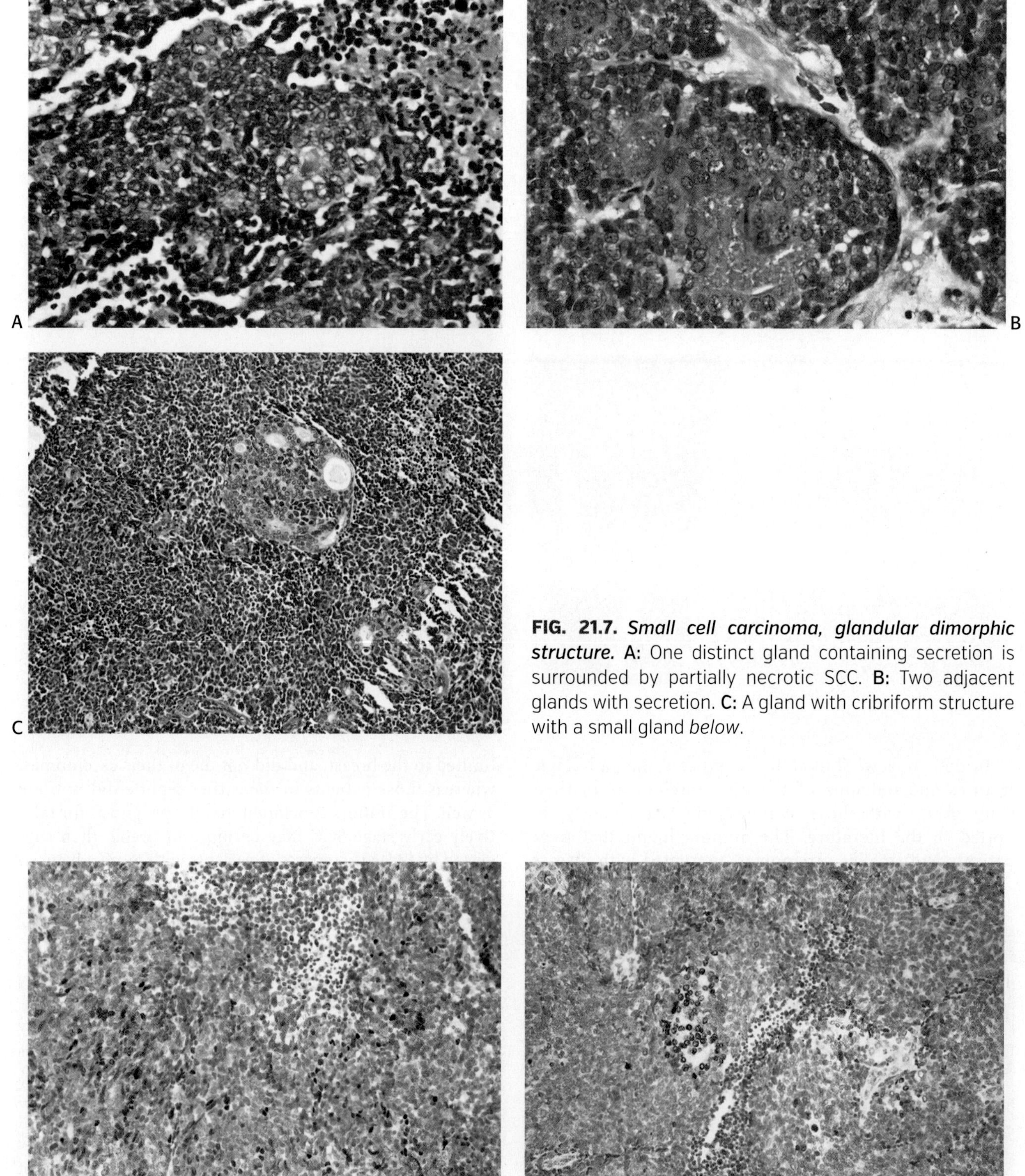

FIG. 21.7. ***Small cell carcinoma, glandular dimorphic structure.*** **A:** One distinct gland containing secretion is surrounded by partially necrotic SCC. **B:** Two adjacent glands with secretion. **C:** A gland with cribriform structure with a small gland *below*.

FIG. 21.8. ***Small cell carcinoma, hormone receptors.*** **A:** The tumor displays heterogeneous nuclear reactivity for PR. **B:** Nuclear reactivity for ER is limited to the glandular dimorphic component. Some tumors also display nuclear reactivity for ER in small cell areas. (*not shown here*).

REFERENCES

1. Levenson RM Jr, Ihde DC, Matthews MJ, et al. Small cell carcinoma presenting as an extrapulmonary neoplasm: sites of origin and response to chemotherapy. *J Natl Cancer Inst* 1981;67:607–612.
2. Papotti M, Gherardi G, Eusebi V, et al. Primary oat cell (neuroendocrine) carcinoma of the breast. Report of four cases. *Virchows Arch A Pathol Anat Histopathol* 1992;420:103–108.
3. Adegbola T, Connolly CE, Mortimer G. Small cell neuroendocrine carcinoma of the breast: a report of three cases and review of the literature. *J Clin Pathol* 2005;58:775–778.
4. Bergman S, Hoda SA, Geisinger KR, et al. E-cadherin-negative primary small cell carcinoma of the breast. Report of a case and review of the literature. *Am J Clin Pathol* 2004;121:117–121.
5. Christie M, Chin-Lenn L, Watts MM, et al. Primary small cell carcinoma of the breast with TTF-1 and neuroendocrine marker expressing carcinoma *in situ*. *Int J Clin Exp Pathol* 2010;3:629–633.
6. Fukunaga M, Ushigome S. Small cell (oat cell) carcinoma of the breast. *Pathol Int* 1998;48:744–748.
7. Hoang MP, Maitra A, Gazdar AF, et al. Primary mammary small-cell carcinoma: a molecular analysis of 2 cases. *Hum Pathol* 2001;32:753–757.
8. Hojo T, Kinoshita T, Shien T, et al. Primary small cell carcinoma of the breast. *Breast Cancer* 2009;16:68–71.
9. Jochems L, Tjalma WA. Primary small cell neuroendocrine tumour of the breast. *Eur J Obstet Gynecol Reprod Biol* 2004;115:231–233.
10. Jundt G, Schulz A, Heitz PU, et al. Small cell neuroendocrine (oat cell) carcinoma of the male breast. Immunocytochemical and ultrastructural investigations. *Virchows Arch A Pathol Anat Histopathol* 1984;404:213–221.
11. Kanat O, Kilickap S, Korkmaz T, et al. Primary small cell carcinoma of the breast: report of seven cases and review of the literature. *Tumori* 2011;97:473–478.
12. Kinoshita S, Hirano A, Komine K, et al. Primary small-cell neuroendocrine carcinoma of the breast: report of a case. *Surg Today* 2008;38:734–738.
13. Kitakata H, Yasumoto K, Sudo Y, et al. A case of primary small cell carcinoma of the breast. *Breast Cancer* 2007;14:414–419.
14. Mariscal A, Balliu E, Diaz R, et al. Primary oat cell carcinoma of the breast: imaging features. *AJR Am J Roentgenol* 2004;183:1169–1171.
15. Rineer J, Choi K, Sanmugarajah J. Small cell carcinoma of the breast. *J Natl Med Assoc* 2009;101:1061–1064.
16. Salman WD, Harrison JA, Howat AJ. Small-cell neuroendocrine carcinoma of the breast. *J Clin Pathol* 2006;59:888.
17. Samli B, Celik S, Evrensel T, et al. Primary neuroendocrine small cell carcinoma of the breast. *Arch Pathol Lab Med* 2000;124:296–298.
18. Sebenik M, Nair SG, Hamati HF. Primary small cell anaplastic carcinoma of the breast diagnosed by fine needle aspiration cytology: a case report. *Acta Cytol* 1998;42:1199–1203.
19. Shin SJ, DeLellis RA, Ying L, et al. Small cell carcinoma of the breast: a clinicopathologic and immunohistochemical study of nine patients. *Am J Surg Pathol* 2000;24:1231–1238.
20. Sridhar P, Matey P, Aluwihare N. Primary carcinoma of breast with small-cell differentiation. *Breast* 2004;13:149–151.
21. Yamaguchi R, Tanaka M, Otsuka H, et al. Neuroendocrine small cell carcinoma of the breast: report of a case. *Med Mol Morphol* 2009;42:58–61.
22. Yamamoto J, Ohshima K, Nabeshima K, et al. Comparative study of primary mammary small cell carcinoma, carcinoma with endocrine features and invasive ductal carcinoma. *Oncol Rep* 2004;11:825–831.
23. An JK, Woo JJ, Kang JH, et al. Small-cell neuroendocrine carcinoma of the breast. *J Korean Surg Soc* 2012;82:116–119.
24. Latif N, Rosa M, Samian L, et al. An unusual case of primary small cell neuroendocrine carcinoma of the breast. *Breast J* 2010;16:647–651.
25. Salmo EN, Connolly CE. Primary small cell carcinoma of the breast: report of a case and review of the literature. *Histopathology* 2001;38:277–278.
26. Yamasaki T, Shimazaki H, Aida S, et al. Primary small cell (oat cell) carcinoma of the breast: report of a case and review of the literature. *Pathol Int* 2000;50:914–918.
27. Bigotti G, Coli A, Butti A, et al. Primary small cell neuroendocrine carcinoma of the breast. *J Exp Clin Cancer Res* 2004;23:691–696.
28. Haji AG, Sharma S, Vijaykumar DK, et al. Primary mammary small-cell carcinoma: a case report and review of the literature. *Indian J Med Paediatr Oncol* 2009;30:31–34.
29. Sadanaga N, Okada S, Shiotani S, et al. Clinical characteristics of small cell carcinoma of the breast. *Oncol Rep* 2008;19:981–985.
30. Stein ME, Gershuny A, Abdach L, et al. Primary small-cell carcinoma of the breast. *Clin Oncol (R Coll Radiol)* 2005;17:201–202.
31. Wade PM Jr, Mills SE, Read M, et al. Small cell neuroendocrine (oat cell) carcinoma of the breast. *Cancer* 1983;52:121–125.
32. Chua RS, Torno RB, Vuletin JC. Fine needle aspiration cytology of small cell neuroendocrine carcinoma of the breast. A case report. *Acta Cytol* 1997;41:1341–1344.
33. Francois A, Chatikhine VA, Chevallier B, et al. Neuroendocrine primary small cell carcinoma of the breast. Report of a case and review of the literature. *Am J Clin Oncol* 1995;18:133–138.
34. Quirós Rivero J, Muños García JL, Cabrera Rodriguez JJ, et al. Extrapulmonary small cell carcinoma in the breast and prostate. *Clin Transl Oncol* 2009;11:698–700.
35. Giffler RF, Kay S. Small-cell carcinoma of the male mammary gland. A tumor resembling infiltrating lobular carcinoma. *Am J Clin Pathol* 1976;66:715–722.
36. Yogore MG III, Sahgal S. Small cell carcinoma of the male breast: report of a case. *Cancer* 1977;39:1748–1751.
37. Wolff M, Reinis MS. Breast cancer in the male: clinicopathological study of 40 patients and review of the literature. In: Fenoglio CM, Wolff M, eds. *Progress in surgical pathology*. New York: Masson Publishing USA, 1981:77–109.
38. Fiorella RM, Kragel PJ, Shariff A, et al. Fine-needle aspiration of well differentiated small-cell duct carcinoma of the breast. *Diagn Cytopathol* 1997;16:226–229.
39. Amano M, Ogura K, Ozaki Y, et al. Two cases of primary small cell carcinoma of the breast showing non-mass-like pattern on diagnostic imaging and histopathology. *Breast Cancer* Sept 12, 2012, doi:10.1007/s12282-012-0397-3.
40. Shin SJ, DeLellis RA, Rosen PP. Small cell carcinoma of the breast—additional immunohistochemical studies. *Am J Surg Pathol* 2001;25:831–832.
41. Kwak JY, Kim EK, You JK, et al. Metastasis of primitive neuroectodermal tumor to the breast. *J Clin Ultrasound* 2002;30:374–377.
42. Sezer O, Jugovic D, Blohmer JU, et al. CD99 positivity and EWS-FLI1 gene rearrangement identify a breast tumor in a 60-year-old patient with attributes of the Ewing family of neoplasms. *Diagn Mol Pathol* 1999;8:120–124.
43. Ali SZ, Miller BT. Small cell neuroendocrine carcinoma: cytologic findings in a breast aspirate. *Acta Cytol* 1997;41:1237–1240.
44. Deeley TJ. Secondary deposits in the breast. *Br J Cancer* 1965;19:738–743.
45. Hajdu SI, Urban JA. Cancers metastatic to the breast. *Cancer* 1972;29:1691–1696.
46. Bobos M, Hytiroglou P, Kostopoulos I, et al. Immunohistochemical distinction between merkel cell carcinoma and small cell carcinoma of the lung. *Am J Dermatopathol* 2006;28:99–104.
47. Ersahin C, Bandyopadhyay S, Bhargava R. Thyroid transcription factor-1 and "basal marker"—expressing small cell carcinoma of the breast. *Int J Surg Pathol* 2009;17:368–372.

CHAPTER 22

Secretory Carcinoma

FREDERICK C. KOERNER

Many of the histologic patterns of breast carcinoma that occur in adults have also been reported in patients younger than 20 years.[1] Secretory, or juvenile, carcinoma is often found in children, but the majority of cases have been reported in adults[2] (Fig. 22.1). Consequently, the term "secretory" is preferable to "juvenile" when referring to these neoplasms. The cellular characteristics of the lesion are identical in patients of all ages.

CLINICAL PRESENTATION

Age

Secretory carcinoma was first fully described in 1966 by McDivitt and Stewart[3] in a report on seven patients, whose ages ranged from 3 to 15 years and averaged 9 years. Six years later, Oberman and Stephens[4] reported the occurrence of secretory carcinomas in two women 25 and 56 years old, and Oberman[5] subsequently described four more examples in adult women 22 to 73 years old. Descriptions of many additional cases in both children and adults have been published since, mostly as single case reports or series composed of just a few patients. It has become clear that secretory carcinoma affects individuals throughout life. The reported ages of women with secretory carcinoma range from 3 to 91 years.[3,6,7] Several reports document carcinomas in girls aged 5 years or younger.[8–12] Male patients exhibited a similar age range (3 to 79 years)[13–15] and included a tumor in a 6-year-old boy.[16] The pediatric and adolescent age groups seem to account for a greater proportion of the secretory carcinomas seen in males. About one-half of the patients were beyond the age of 20 years, with a substantial number between 50 and 69 years (Fig. 22.1). Young patients are approximately evenly divided among children and those in their teens, but there seems to be a dearth of reports of individuals between the ages of 10 and 15 years.

Clinical Findings

Secretory carcinoma may occur in any part of the breast. Subareolar lesions have been associated with nipple discharge, but in most cases the patient describes a painless, circumscribed mass that may have been present for 1 or more years.[5,8–10] A subareolar tumor is most common in prepubertal girls and males because their breast tissue is localized in this region, but even among women, the central region of the breast stands out as a favored location. Secretory carcinoma usually grows as a single mass. Rare carcinomas present as two or more nodules evident on radiologic studies or macroscopic examination.[8,17–19]

Imaging Studies

Mammography typically reveals a discrete tumor with smooth or irregular borders.[2,10,17,19–23] A secretory carcinoma with a rounded contour can be mistaken for a fibroadenoma (FA) or a papilloma on imaging studies, especially in a young patient. Mammograms exhibit calcifications in rare cases only.[2] Sonography discloses a solid, hypoechoic to isoechoic mass, which may have a microlobulated border.[10,17,20,24–27] Mun et al.[28] described and illustrated the sonographic features of six secretory carcinomas in adult women. Radiologic studies are not commonly used in the evaluation of breast tumors in children; so the literature does not offer secure information regarding the imaging features of secretory carcinoma in this age range.

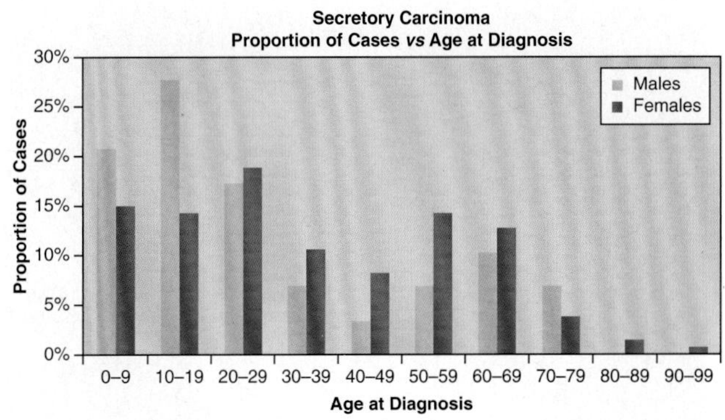

FIG. 22.1. ***Secretory carcinoma, age distribution.*** This chart based on a review of published cases shows the age distribution of secretory carcinoma in male and female patients. Represented are 133 females and 29 males. One male-to-female transgender person was classified as male. Note the relative abundance of female patients between the ages of 30 and 69 years and the preponderance of male patients 29 years of age or younger.

Unusual Clinical Presentations

Several cases of secretory carcinoma involve unusual clinical circumstances. For example, Paeng et al.[24] reported a 31-year-old woman with a history of acute myelogenous leukemia who developed secretory carcinoma while in complete remission after treatment with bone marrow transplantation and chemotherapy. Shin et al.[29] described a 46-year-old woman who developed secretory carcinoma in axillary breast tissue. The mass, which occasionally secreted fluid, had been present for 8 years before the carcinoma was diagnosed. Brandt et al.[30] recounted the case of a 13-year-old girl with a secretory carcinoma in the axilla. This example seemed to have arisen from cutaneous adnexal glands rather than from axillary breast tissue. Secretory carcinoma developed in the breast of a male-to-female transgender individual, who had undergone "long-term cross-sex hormone treatment" of an unspecified nature.[31] The tumor expressed the *ETV6–NTRK3* fusion gene that has been detected in most mammary secretory carcinomas.

No clinical evidence of a hormonal abnormality has been described that would explain the secretory properties of the tumor. Pregnancy has not been implicated in the development of secretory carcinoma. One pregnant patient noted a tumor that proved to be secretory carcinoma when excised 4 years later.[32] Associated breast conditions have been described in a few cases. Gynecomastia accompanied a minority of the secretory carcinomas in male patients. A 23-year-old man with secretory carcinoma reported that a small breast nodule present since the age of 2 years had been ascribed to gynecomastia.[33]

The coexistence of juvenile papillomatosis and secretory carcinoma has been described,[9,34–36] but the evidence presented to substantiate the diagnosis of juvenile papillomatosis is not convincing in all instances. For example, Tokunaga et al.[36] described a 13-year-old girl who succumbed to secretory carcinoma arising in the left breast. At autopsy, a proliferative lesion was found in the right breast. The diagnosis given to the proliferation in the right breast was "juvenile cystic papillomatosis," but the illustration provided shows a ductal epithelial proliferation more appropriately termed "juvenile papillary duct hyperplasia." A second case presented by these authors as secretory carcinoma in "juvenile papillomatosis" appears from the illustrations to be cystic transformation of secretory carcinoma.

GROSS PATHOLOGY

On gross examination, secretory carcinoma usually forms a circumscribed, firm mass, which may be lobulated (Fig. 22.2). The tumors tend to be 3 cm or less in diameter, although a carcinoma spanning 12.5 cm was reported in a man.[37] Among six women in one report, the mean tumor size was 1.7 cm (range 0.5 to 4.0 cm)[38]; in another publication,[39] it was 5.5 cm (range 2.5 to 10 cm) in seven female patients and one male patient 17 to 60 years old. Rarely the tumor has infiltrative margins. Various colors have been mentioned, usually shades of white to gray or tan to yellow. Observers noted that one secretory carcinoma appeared ". . . grayish-white to tan in color and had a center that varied between a spongy consistency and a microcystic nature. The margin of the lesion was ill defined. During sectioning, a colorless viscous secretion emerged from the central tissue compartment."[31]

MICROSCOPIC PATHOLOGY

Like other forms of ductal carcinoma, secretory carcinoma often has an intraductal component. All six secretory carcinomas reported by Lae et al.[38] had accompanying ductal carcinoma *in situ* (DCIS), and Kameyama et al.[22] described

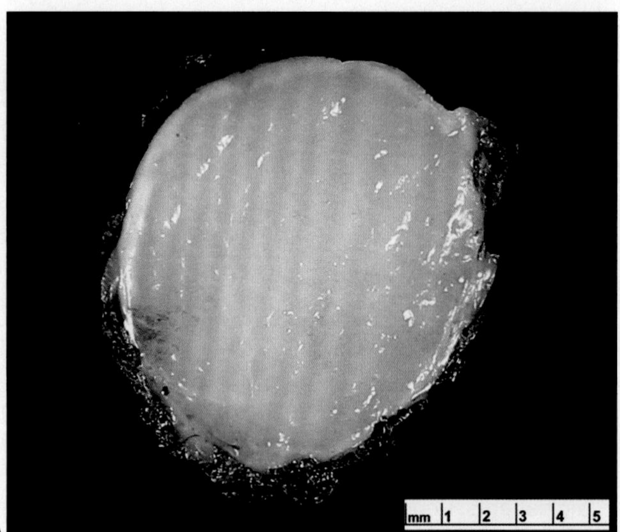

A

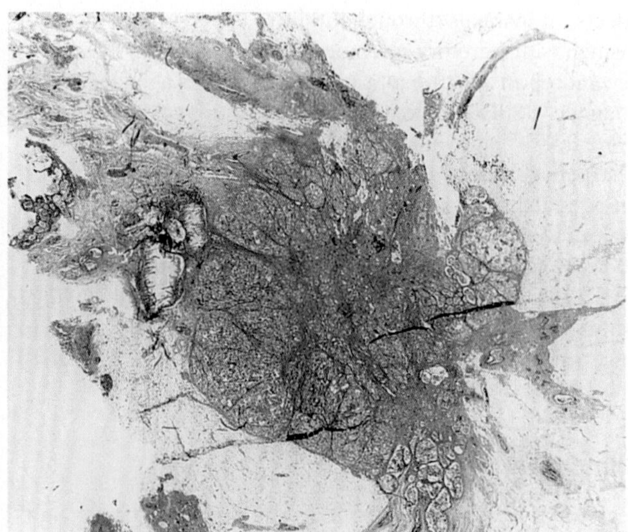
B

FIG. 22.2. ***Secretory carcinoma.*** **A:** The carcinoma has a well-defined smooth contour. **B:** This whole-mount histologic section demonstrates the lobulated and partly stellate structure of a tumor that had varied histologic patterns. **C:** Microlumens and "bubbly" cytoplasm with signet ring cells (*arrows*). **D:** Markedly vacuolated cells. **E:** An unusual mucinous pattern.

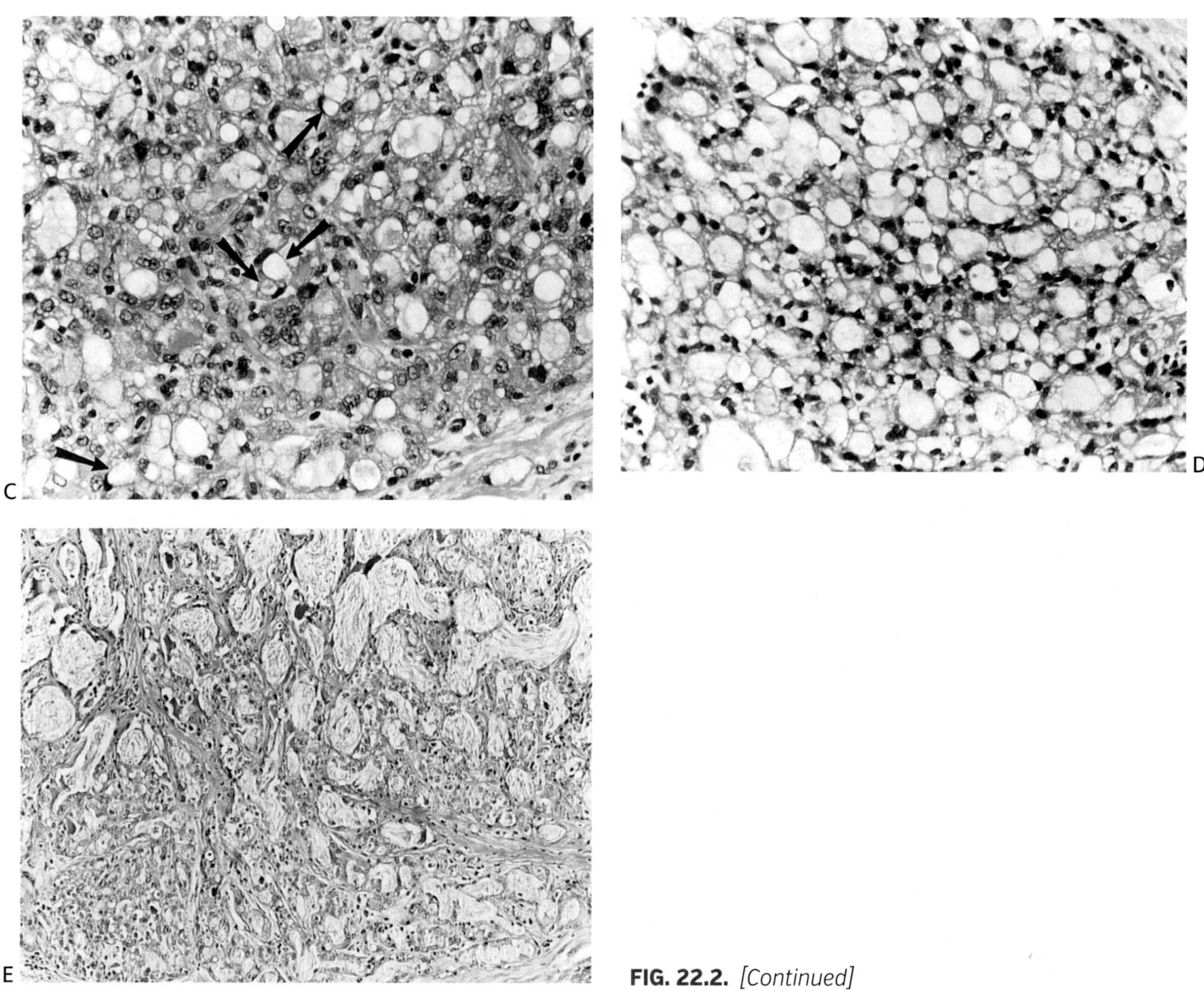

FIG. 22.2. *[Continued]*

a purely noninvasive form of secretory carcinoma. The *in situ* component of secretory carcinoma can exhibit certain of the growth patterns seen in the conventional types of ductal carcinoma. Most commonly, the DCIS is papillary (Fig. 22.3A) or cribriform,[22] but solid foci (Fig. 22.3B, C) and, rarely, comedonecrosis may also be found. These features are seen in the invasive components, which tend to be relatively compact with papillary, microcystic, and glandular patterns (Fig. 22.4). Lobulation evident on macroscopic examination usually results from fibrous septa within the mass (Fig. 22.5). The borders of the carcinoma are usually circumscribed microscopically, but overtly infiltrative growth is sometimes present (Fig. 22.6). Microcalcifications are rarely seen in the neoplastic glands or in the stroma. The tumor cells vary from secretory to apocrine in their features. Cells of a secretory nature possess pale to clear, pink or amphophilic cytoplasm that contains abundant secretion. The nuclei appear low-grade, and they vary from small to modest in size. The chromatin ranges from dark and finely dispersed to pale and granular. Nuclei with pale chromatin usually contain small, uniform nucleoli (Fig. 22.7). Cells with apocrine features contain granular eosinophilic cytoplasm and nuclei characteristic of apocrine cells[40,41] (Fig. 22.8). One usually finds both types of cell in a carcinoma, although one type or the other can predominate. On occasion, cells with apocrine features growing in a solid pattern comprise most of the tumor and thereby obscure the secretory nature of the carcinoma (Fig. 22.9). The cells do not display noticeable mitotic activity or necrosis.

Secretion accumulates in the tumor cells, in the glands formed by the tumor cells, and in the microcystic spaces associated with the tumor cells. The secretory material appears pale pink or amphophilic with hematoxylin and eosin (H&E) staining, and it often contains lacunae, which create a "bubbly" appearance. The secretion stains with the periodic acid–Schiff (PAS) and Alcian blue methods. PAS staining persists after diastase digestion (Fig. 22.10A), and Alcian blue staining persists after sialidase digestion. The secretory material stains with toluidine blue at pH 1.5 and reacts variably for mucin. These findings indicate that the secretory material contains sulfated mucopolysaccharides and sialomucin.[42] The material displays a purple or violet color with the crystal violet stain. The secretion in microcystic areas (Fig. 22.4B) resembles the material that accumulates in cystic hypersecretory lesions.

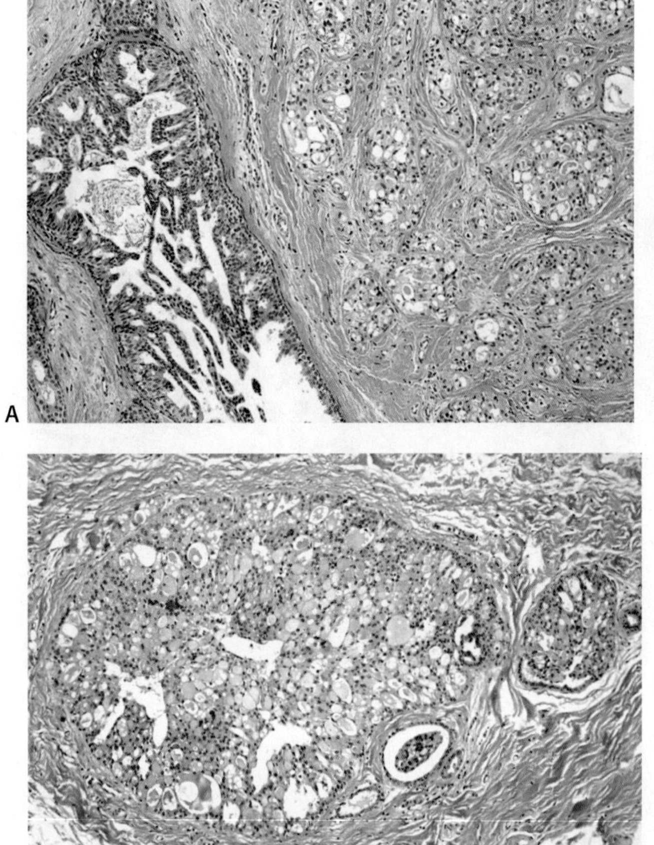

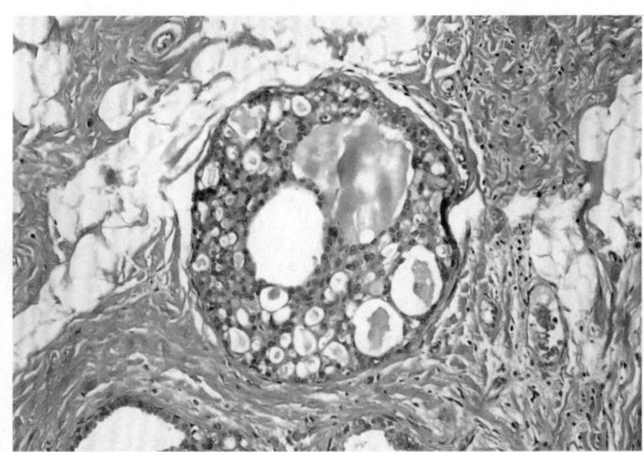

FIG. 22.3. ***Secretory carcinoma, intraductal.*** **A:** Papillary and micropapillary DCIS next to invasive secretory carcinoma. **B:** Solid growth with secretory carcinoma structure. **C:** Solid growth with irregular microlumens.

Pathologists should not have difficulty recognizing secretory carcinoma when they have sufficient material to study. It may require an excision of the mass to provide an adequate sample, but the diagnosis can be suspected in a needle aspiration or core biopsy specimen. Most examples demonstrate the characteristic histopathologic features. If cells with apocrine qualities predominate, the diagnosis of apocrine carcinoma could come to mind (see Chapter 19).

The recently described mammary acinic cell carcinoma[43] shares some clinical, morphologic, and immunohistochemical features with secretory carcinoma. The cells in so-called mammary acinic cell carcinoma are reportedly immunoreactive for lysozyme and salivary-type amylase,[43] molecules also detected in three examples of mammary secretory carcinoma.[44] This observation led the latter investigators to speculate that the two types of carcinoma might be closely related

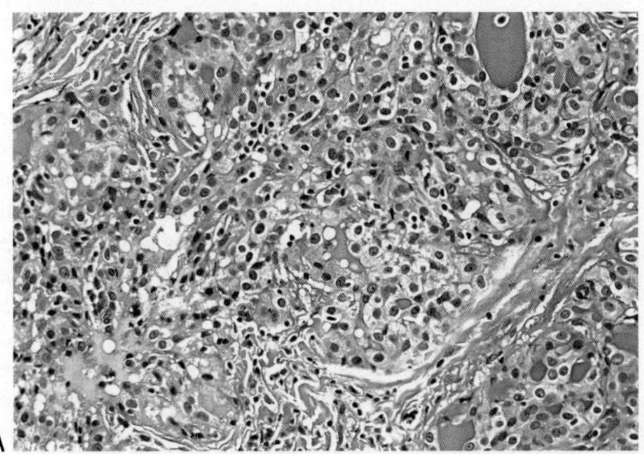

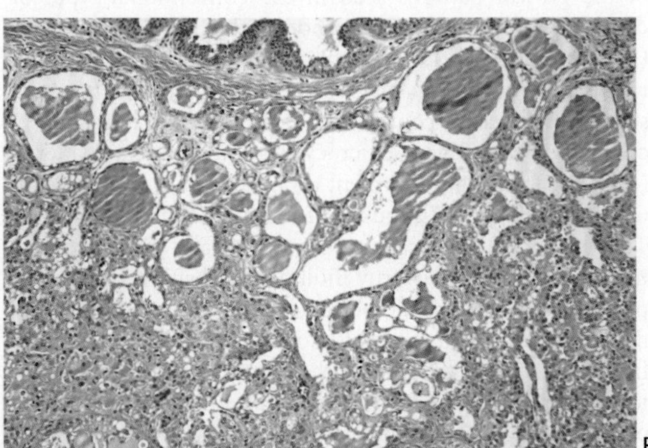

FIG. 22.4. ***Secretory carcinoma, growth patterns.*** Samples shown in **(A–C)** are from a 20-year-old woman. **A:** Solid growth. **B:** A microcystic area. **C:** Part of this tumor has a tubular structure. Atypical apocrine duct hyperplasia is also present (*left*). **D:** Papillary growth (**D:** Reproduced from Rosen PP, Cranor ML. Secretory carcinoma of the breast. *Arch Pathol Lab Med* 1991;115:141–144, with permission).

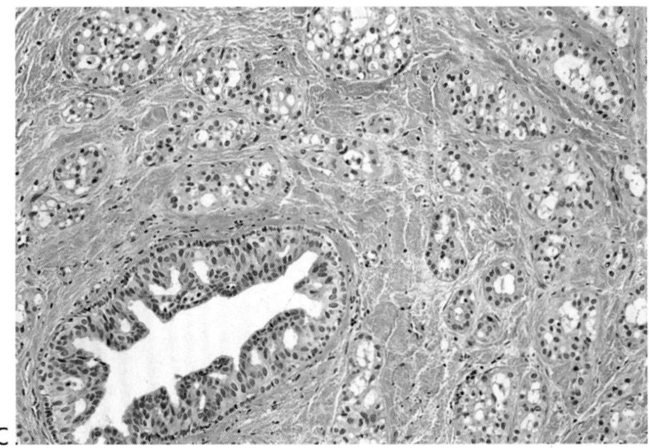
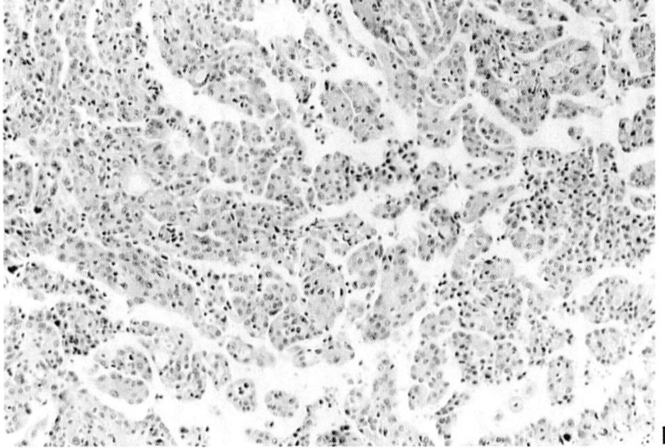

FIG. 22.4. *[Continued]*

and possibly variants of a single entity.[44] Reis-Filho et al.[45] studied six tumors that they identified as mammary acinic cell carcinomas and were unable to find evidence of the *ETV6* gene rearrangement (typically found in secretory carcinoma) in any of the neoplasms. However, this study may be flawed because two of the lesions depicted as acinic cell carcinoma most closely resemble atypical microglandular adenosis (see Chapter 7). In Figure 2A provided by Reis-Filho et al.,[45] the neoplastic glands appear to be encircled by basement membranes, a characteristic feature of microglandular adenosis. Because the cells in atypical microglandular adenosis can have oncocytic and acinic cell features, it is understandable that such a misclassification might occur. The relationship between these two lesions remains open to study.

CYTOLOGY

Needle aspiration specimens from secretory carcinomas typically yield hypercellular smears containing uniform cells forming large branching cohesive sheets, loosely cohesive groups, and intact single cells. The background often appears clean, but it can demonstrate erythrocytes and cellular debris[40,46–48] or colloid-like secretory material.[13] Most of the tumor cells appear uniform and only slightly atypical. They contain one or two round to oval nuclei,[46,49] homogeneous chromatin, nucleoli of varying size, and abundant cytoplasm. In most cases, a few cells demonstrate features indicative of more advanced atypia such as large nuclei or dark or clumped chromatin. The cytoplasmic borders can appear frayed. Cells with granular cytoplasm and prominent nuclei can also be encountered in carcinomas with apocrine differentiation. Secretory vacuoles of variable sizes occupy the cytoplasm, and they can create signet ring cells.[13,46,48–50] The vacuoles sometimes enclose large, round, dense bodies thought to represent inspissated secretory material.[47,48,51] When the vacuoles appear especially small, the cytoplasm takes on a lacy quality. Besides containing vacuoles of secretory material, the cytoplasm can also contain intracytoplasmic lumens,[48] which are evident during ultrastructural examination.[52,53] At times, the secretory material can also be seen in the background of the smears.[49,54]

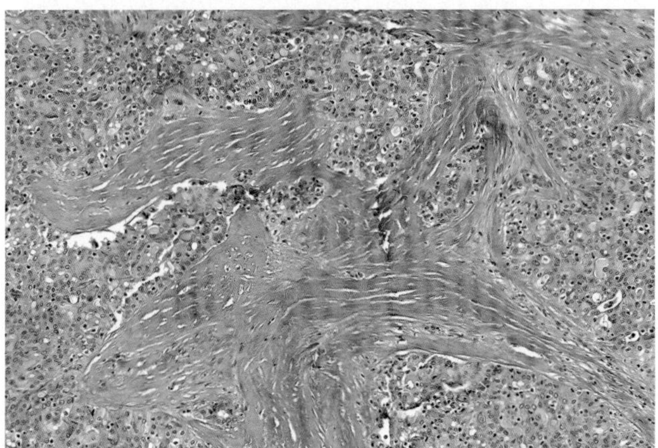

FIG. 22.5. ***Secretory carcinoma, stromal fibrosis.*** Bands of fibrous connective tissue traverse the center of the invasive carcinoma.

Shinagawa et al.[48,55] described "grapelike clusters of mucous globular structures," MGSs, which consist of "a small amount of centrally located, mucoid material and covering epithelia, usually composed of two or three and occasionally more cells." These groups displayed a uniform size. The cells composing them contained oval or crescentic bland nuclei and round, semilunar, or irregular collections of mucus. The cells did not display division figures. The individual "unit structures" probably represent the acini that are seen in histologic sections. Shinagawa et al.[55] stated: "We are firmly convinced that the presence of structures resembling a bunch of grapes and related forms, such as MGSs, is the most characteristic feature of secretory carcinoma and is essential to the cytological differential diagnosis of breast cancer." Three other reports describe or illustrate these structures.[7,34,56]

The distinction of secretory carcinoma from other types of breast carcinoma in a cytologic specimen should not usually cause difficulty. The vacuoles in conventional ductal, lobular, and mucinous carcinomas appear fewer and smaller, and the mucus produced in mucinous carcinomas stains pale blue with the Giemsa stain in contrast to the pink color of the secretory material in secretory carcinomas. If lipid-rich and glycogen-rich carcinomas enter the

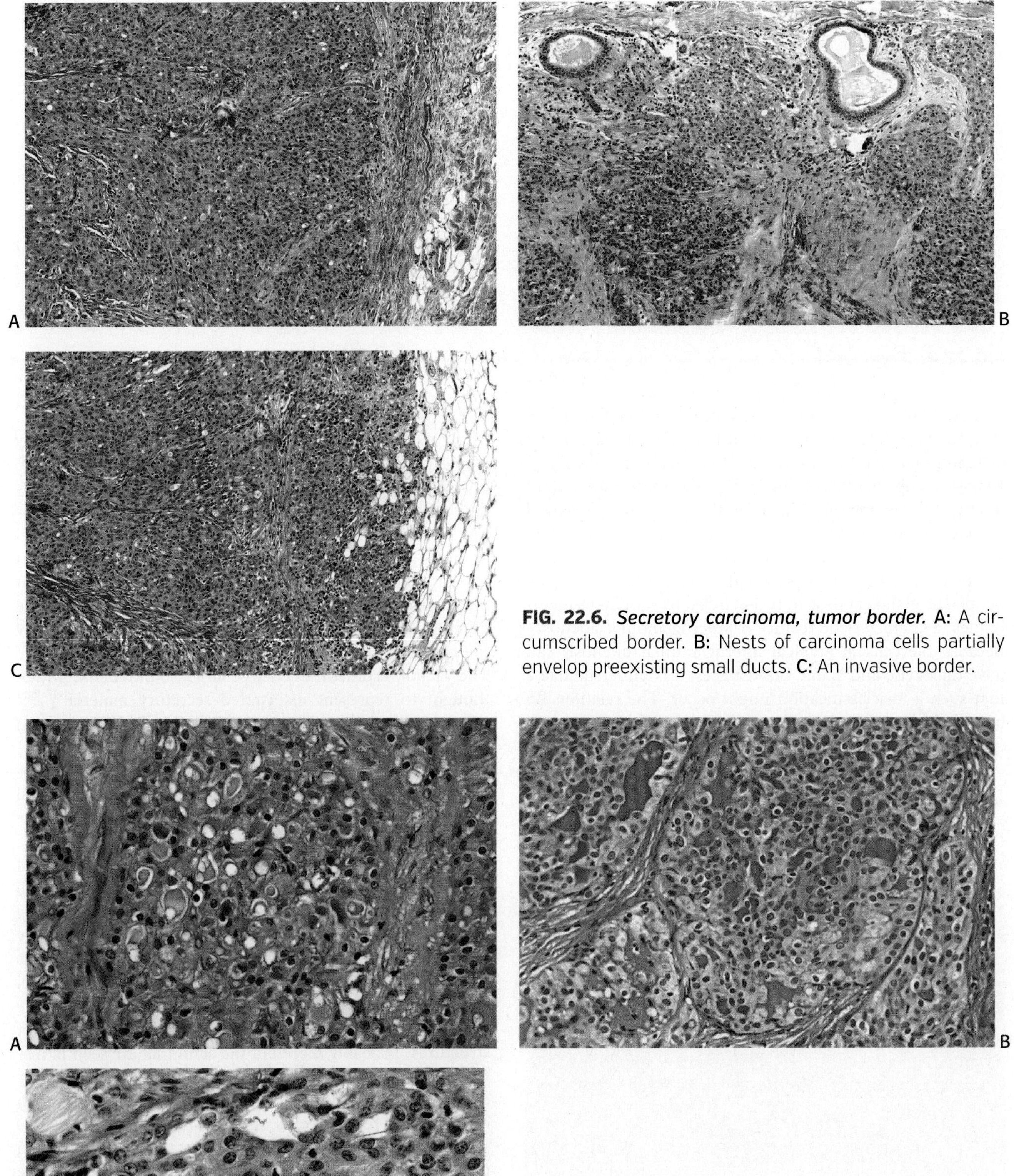

FIG. 22.6. ***Secretory carcinoma, tumor border.*** **A:** A circumscribed border. **B:** Nests of carcinoma cells partially envelop preexisting small ducts. **C:** An invasive border.

FIG. 22.7. ***Secretory carcinoma, variable structures.*** **A:** This tumor from a 69-year-old woman has a solid structure with small microlumens and dense secretion. Nuclei are small, round, and uniform without visible nucleoli. **B:** This tumor from a 5-year-old girl has a fenestrated structure. Nuclei are round to oval. **C:** This carcinoma from a 10-year-old girl has a microcystic structure. The nuclei possess pale granular chromatin and uniform small nucleoli.

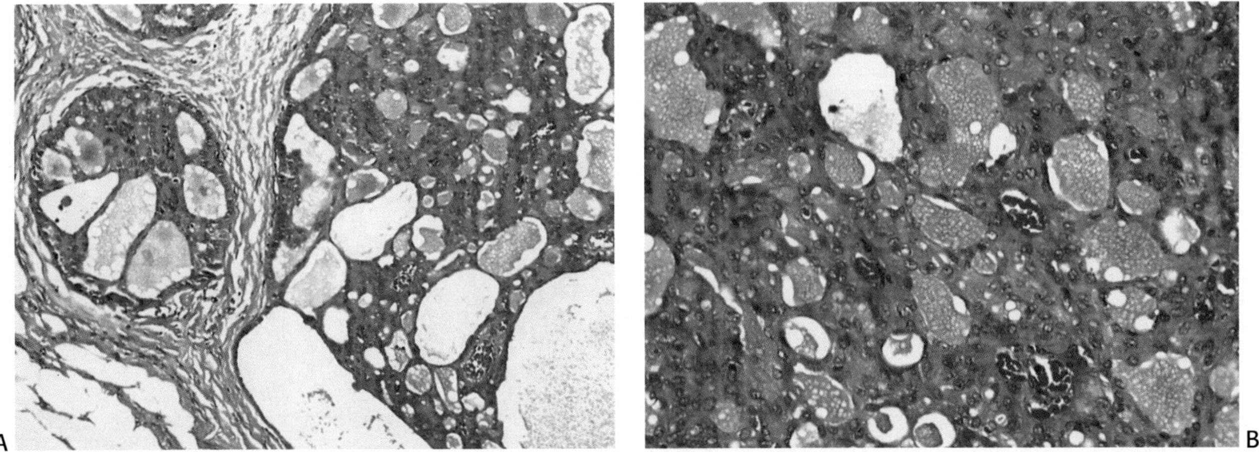

FIG. 22.8. ***Secretory carcinoma, apocrine.*** This tumor is from a 64-year-old woman. **A:** Intraductal carcinoma is present on the *left*. **B:** The tumor cells have apocrine features.

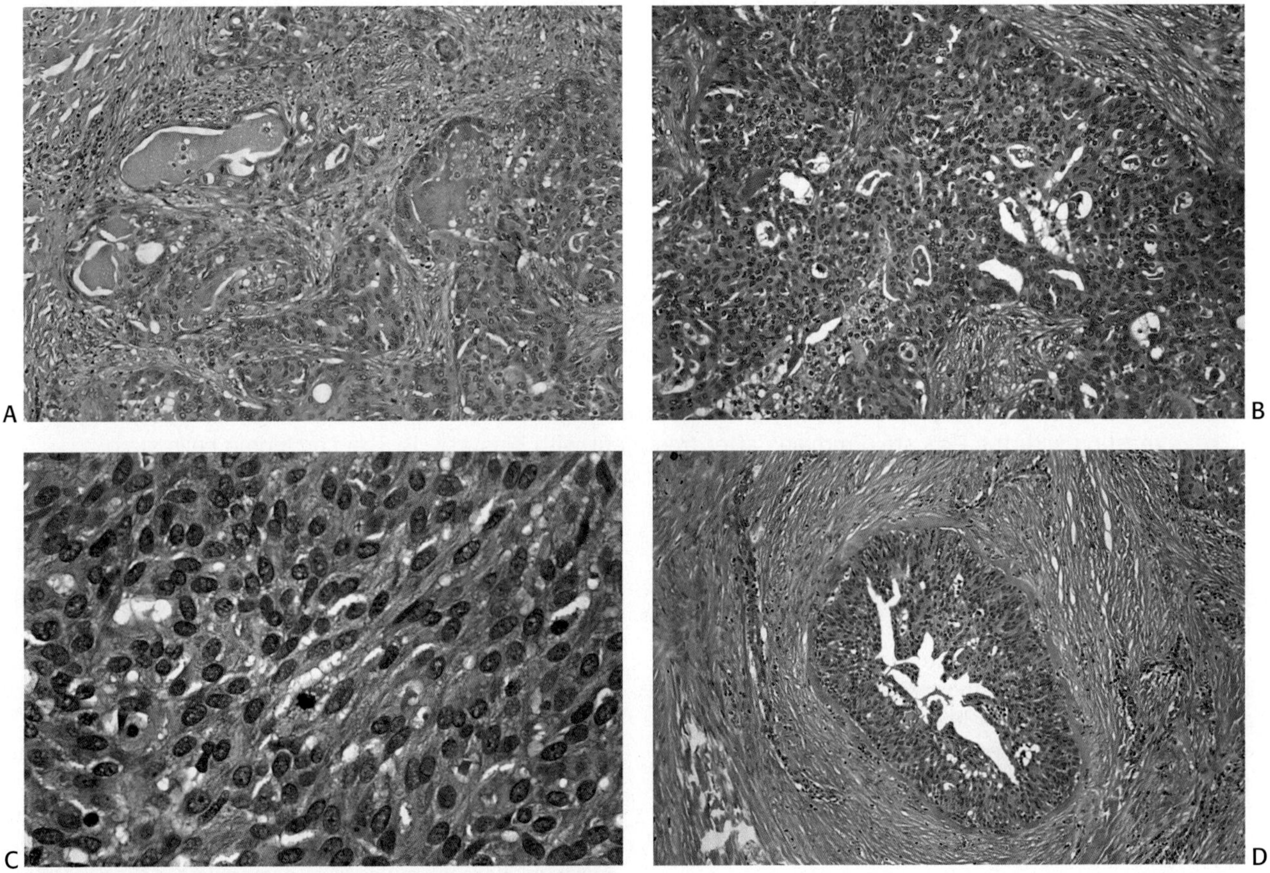

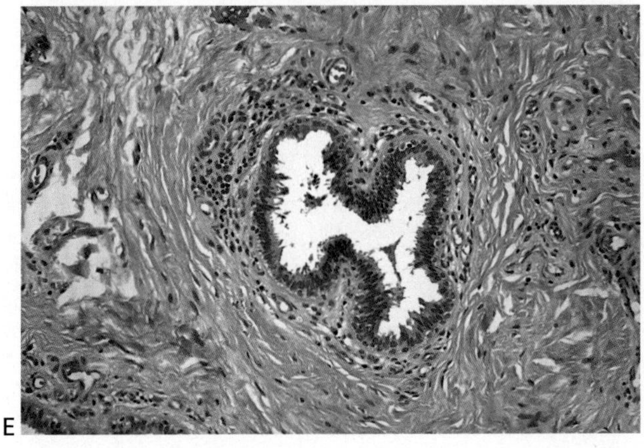

FIG. 22.9. ***Secretory carcinoma, apocrine and solid.*** This tumor from a 16-year-old boy produced an ALN metastasis. **A:** Secretory activity is seen at the invasive tumor border. **B:** A solid area with apocrine cytoplasm and irregular microlumens containing sparse secretion. **C:** Magnified view of carcinoma cells exhibiting moderate pleomorphism and a mitosis in the center. **D:** Intraductal carcinoma with scant secretory differentiation. Invasive carcinoma is present on the right. **E:** Mild columnar cell hyperplasia in the surrounding gynecomastia.

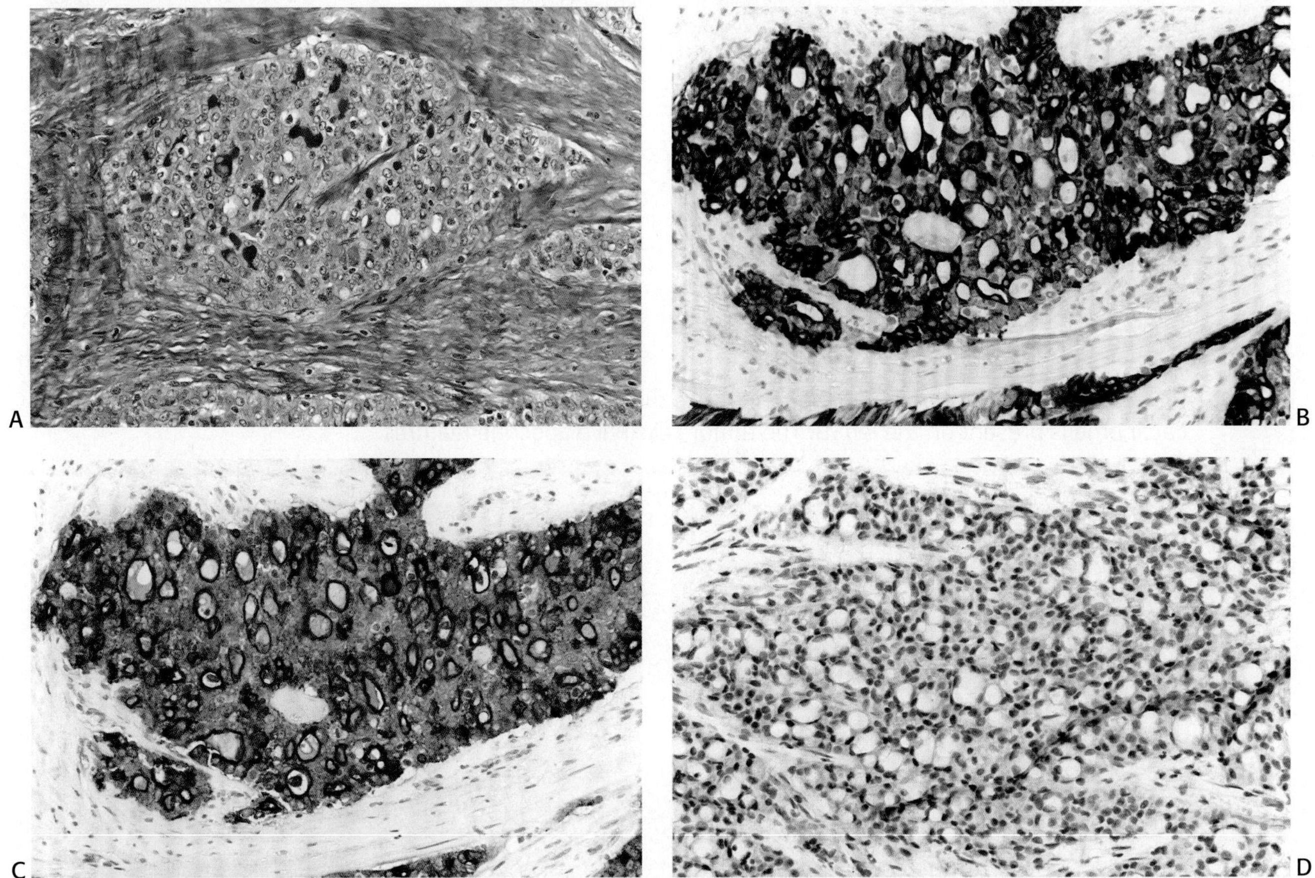

FIG. 22.10. *Secretory carcinoma, cytochemical and immunohistochemical staining.* **A:** A positive reaction with the PAS stain remains after treatment with diastase. **B:** The carcinoma cells stain intensely for CK5/6. **C:** The carcinoma cells react with a polyclonal CEA antiserum. **D:** The nuclei of many carcinoma cells stain weakly for ER.

differential diagnosis, staining for the appropriate molecules will allow one to evaluate these possibilities. Some of the findings seen in the aspirates from secretory carcinomas are difficult to distinguish from those seen in specimens showing lactational or pregnancy-like changes.[57] Consequently, the cytologic diagnosis of secretory carcinoma in the setting of pregnancy or lactation is especially difficult.

IMMUNOHISTOCHEMISTRY

To the extent that it can be determined from the reported data, the results of staining for cellular markers do not differ among tumors from females and males and among tumors from children and adults. Strong positive staining has been reported for α-lactalbumin.[22,33,49,58–61] The carcinoma cells stain for epithelial membrane antigen (EMA)[49,57,62] and E-cadherin,[38,63] and with rare exceptions[38,52] they have stained for S-100 protein.[13,24,30,38,44,57,58,60–62,64–67] Three reports document staining for epidermal growth factor receptor (EGFR).[38,66,68] The cells stain for one type of cytokeratin (CK) or another: positive or variable staining for CK8/18, CK5/6 (Fig. 22.10B), CK14, AE1, AE3, an unspecified CK antiserum, and a CK cocktail have been reported.[38,49,57,62,66,67,68] The results of staining for carcinoembryonic antigen (CEA) also have varied[13,30,31,33,44,49,53,57–61,65] (Fig. 22.10C). Tumors have not stained with monoclonal antibodies to CEA in the few cases tested.[60,61] Variable reactivity was observed for gross cystic disease fluid protein-15 (GCDFP-15).[13,30,44,49,57,58,60] Staining for proteins indicative of endocrine, muscle, and melanocytic differentiation has been negative.[62]

Most secretory carcinomas lack hormone receptors when studied with either biochemical or immunohistochemical methods. Rare examples have demonstrated the presence of estrogen receptor (ER) or progesterone receptor (PR), using the dextran-coated charcoal method[19,47,49,58,61,69] or immunohistochemical staining[18,22,44,57,70] (Fig. 22.10D), and a few have displayed borderline levels of the receptors.[30,38,68,71] Three carcinomas did not express the androgen receptor (AR).[13,31,66] Strong expression of human epidermal growth factor 2 (HER2) protein has been detected in only one secretory carcinoma.[13,18,24,30,38,66,68,72] In one study, staining for Ki67 yielded results that varied from less than 1% to 34%, with a mean value of 11.4%.[18] A value of 1% was recorded in the case examined by Alenda et al.,[13] and the Ki67 scores in the three carcinomas reported by Hirokawa et al.[44] ranged from 1.7% to 8.7%. Tumors studied by flow cytometry were diploid or near diploid with a low S-phase fraction (SPF).[49,57,58,62,63,73]

ELECTRON MICROSCOPY

The ultrastructural features of secretory carcinoma vary somewhat according to the histologic patterns created by the carcinoma cells.[42,55] Common cellular features include membrane-bound intracytoplasmic secretory vacuoles, intracytoplasmic lumens, intercellular lumens, and secretory material in extracellular spaces. The frequency of these findings differs according to the pattern of growth. Intracytoplasmic lumens abound in cells showing the microcytic pattern, but one does not find them as frequently when the cells grow in solid or glandular formations.[53] The cells often form well-defined clusters, and interdigitations of the cell membranes and desmosomes bind the cells within the groups to each other. The neoplastic cells vary in size and shape according to the amount of secretory material within their cytoplasm.[42,55] The secretory vacuoles often appear empty, but they can contain small round bodies interpreted as inspissated secretion.[42] The cells display intracytoplasmic lumens, which contain diffusely dispersed granular material and into which microvilli protrude. The cytoplasm also contains prominent empty dilated cisternae, Golgi apparatus, rough endoplasmic reticulum, mitochondria, and rare lipid droplets.[42,53,55] The nuclei appear round or oval, they may have indentations, and they possess nucleoli. Large, extracellular lumens occupy many cell clusters and communicate with the extracellular spaces. These extracellular lumens contain dispersed electron-dense granular material and round, electron-dense bodies, and microvilli protrude from the surface of the plasma membranes into these lumens.[6,32,34,49,74,75] Basal lamina partially surrounds cell clusters.[34]

MOLECULAR STUDIES

Chromosomal Abnormalities

A small number of studies have explored the genetic abnormalities in secretory carcinoma. One group[75] observed monosomy for chromosome 22 in one example of secretory carcinoma, but others have not reported this abnormality. Diallo et al.[18] used comparative genomic hybridization to examine eight secretory carcinomas, and they observed that these carcinomas displayed fewer genetic alterations than are found in conventional invasive breast carcinomas. The alterations included gains of chromosomes 8q and 1q and loss of chromosome 22q. Using the same method, Lambros et al.[66] also detected only a few genetic alterations and concluded that secretory carcinoma has a "simplex" genomic profile.

Maitra et al.[71] carried out genetic studies using 10 secretory carcinomas and 20 conventional ductal carcinomas. The two groups of carcinomas did not differ in their fractional regional loss index, fractional allelic loss index, or frequency of microsatellite alterations, but they did differ in the frequency of loss of heterozygosity (LOH) at 17p13 (the locus of the *p53* gene). The investigators did not detect LOH in any secretory carcinomas, but they observed it in 47% of typical invasive ductal carcinomas. The other 12 regions studied did not differ in their frequency of LOH. One of the 10 secretory carcinomas (10%) had a mutation in its *p53* gene. This frequency falls below the 25% to 40% rate of *p53* gene mutation reported for conventional invasive ductal carcinomas.

Human Papilloma Virus E6 Sequences

Aceto et al.[67] studied breast carcinomas from five female patients who were 25 years of age or younger for evidence of human papilloma virus (HPV) 16/18 *E6* sequences. They detected HPV 16 *E6* sequences in the secretory carcinoma from a 12-year-old girl and in an invasive ductal carcinoma from a 25-year-old woman. The primary invasive ductal carcinoma and a metastasis from the tumor in another case had HPV 16 and HPV 18 *E6* sequences. These tumors all showed immunostaining of p16INK4A, which is a marker for HPV-associated neoplasms. These observations led the investigators to speculate that HPV infection might play a role in the development of some mammary carcinomas in young patients, including secretory carcinoma.

ETV6–NTRK3 Fusion Gene

An abstract published in 1997 noted alterations in chromosomes 16, 8, 12, and 15 using the fluorescence *in situ* hybridization (FISH) technique in a case of secretory carcinoma.[76] Cytogenetic studies of a tumor from a 6-year-old girl revealed a reciprocal translocation between chromosomes 12p and 15q about which the authors stated, "We can make no conclusions regarding this information."[27] These observations presage the study by Tognon et al.[77] in which the investigators described the presence of the *ETV6–NTRK3* fusion gene, a gene previously detected in congenital fibrosarcoma and congenital cellular mesoblastic nephroma, in secretory carcinomas. The *ETV6* gene, located on chromosome 12, codes for an E26 transformation–specific transcription factor expressed in normal mammary epithelial cells, and the *NTRK3* gene, situated on chromosome 15, encodes a membrane receptor tyrosine kinase. Fusion of the two genes results in a chimeric tyrosine kinase protein that displays potent transforming activity for fibroblasts and mammary ductal epithelial cells (Fig. 22.11). Using FISH, sequencing of reverse transcription–polymerase chain reaction (RT–PCR) products, and immunoprecipitation, evidence of this oncoprotein was found in 12 of 13 (92%) secretory carcinomas and in only 1 of 50 (2%) of invasive ductal carcinomas studied by Tongon et al.[77] The single conventional invasive carcinoma that demonstrated fusion transcripts contained regions with features suggestive of secretory carcinoma. Testing of other cases of secretory carcinoma and of commonplace breast carcinomas has confirmed the presence of this fusion gene in most secretory carcinomas[31,64,66,78,79] and the absence of the gene in conventional breast carcinomas.[78] In one exceptionally unusual case, cells of the secretory carcinoma contained a duplication of the fusion gene.[66] A type of salivary gland carcinoma that demonstrates many features in common with mammary secretory carcinoma also contains an identical fusion gene.[80] Further study is needed to establish the role of this fusion gene in the carcinogenesis of mammary secretory carcinoma.

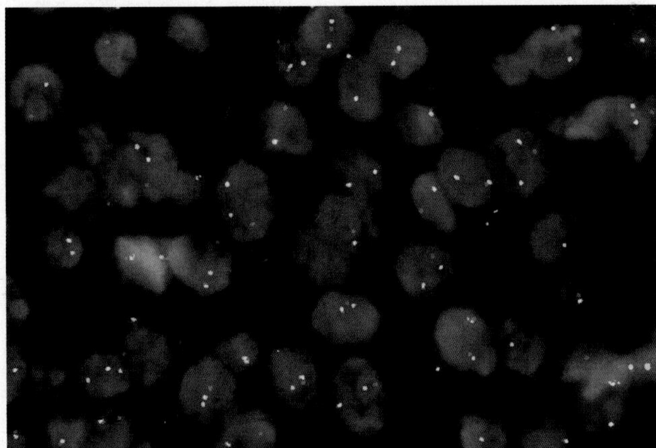

FIG. 22.11. ***Secretory carcinoma,* fluorescence *in situ* hybridization *study for the NTRK3 gene.*** In this "split apart" preparation, the 3′-end of the *NTRK3* gene is labeled with a *red* probe and the 5′-end with a *green* probe. Side-by-side signals indicate an intact *NTRK3* gene, whereas separated signals highlight a disrupted gene. (Courtesy of Dr. A. John Iafrate and Ms. Clarice Bo-Moon Chang.)

Overexpression of STAT5a

STAT5a, mammary growth factor, is one of several molecules involved in the transcription of differentiation proteins. Activation of STAT5a in the breast occurs largely as a result of the binding of prolactin to its receptor.[81] STAT5a expression is present in the majority of normal mammary gland cells and largely absent in atypical duct hyperplasia and carcinoma.[82] Overexpression of STAT5a occurs in secretory carcinoma as well as secretory change, usual ductal hyperplasia, and lactating mammary epithelium.[83] Activity of this growth factor might explain the secretory properties of the carcinoma cells. Strauss et al.[83] point out that unregulated tyrosine kinase activity of the fusion gene could lead to phosphorylation of STAT5a and consequent activation of its downstream pathways.

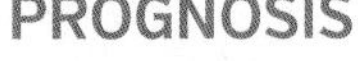

PROGNOSIS

In the majority of patients, secretory carcinoma has an indolent clinical course, resulting in an exceptionally favorable prognosis. Most patients treated by mastectomy remained free of disease, but a few developed recurrences. For example, two small lumps appeared 3 months after local excision in a 19-year-old boy.[84] A 4-year-old girl developed a local recurrence in the scar of a mastectomy 8 months postoperatively.[10] Irradiation was given to the region after excision, and the patient was reportedly free of disease 11 years after the initial diagnosis. Recurrence in residual breast tissue on the chest wall has been reported 8 years after modified radical mastectomy.[73] Most patients treated with excision alone have also remained free of disease during follow-up periods as long as 15 years,[3,5,42,62,85] but recurrences have developed in this setting, also.[2–4,8,59,61,74,79,86] Two patients who received radiation treatments following an excision remain free of disease.[69,71]

Although most recurrences emerge within a few years from the time of diagnosis and involve only the local site, long delayed recurrences and systemic metastases have been reported. Tixier et al.[79] recounted the case of a 30-year-old woman who developed a local recurrence of secretory carcinoma 16 years after the excision of the primary mass, and Oberman and Stephens[4] detailed the story of a 25-year-old woman who experienced recurrence of a secretory carcinoma in the scar of a mastectomy that had been performed 17 years previously. In five patients, recurrence took the form of disseminated disease.[37,41,64,72,86]

Axillary lymph node (ALN) metastases have been described, but they rarely involve more than three lymph nodes[2,14,15,28,29,32,34,39,58–60,63,86–90] (Fig. 22.12). Multiple matted lymph nodes involved by secretory carcinoma were found in the ipsilateral axilla of a 20-year-old man with a 12.5-cm tumor[37] and in the ipsilateral axilla of a 61-year-old woman with an 8-cm fungating secretory carcinoma. A 17-year-old boy with locally recurrent secretory carcinoma was found to have metastatic carcinoma in 10 ALNs,[91] and a 19-year-old boy developed axillary metastases 4 months after a mastectomy for a 2-cm carcinoma.[70]

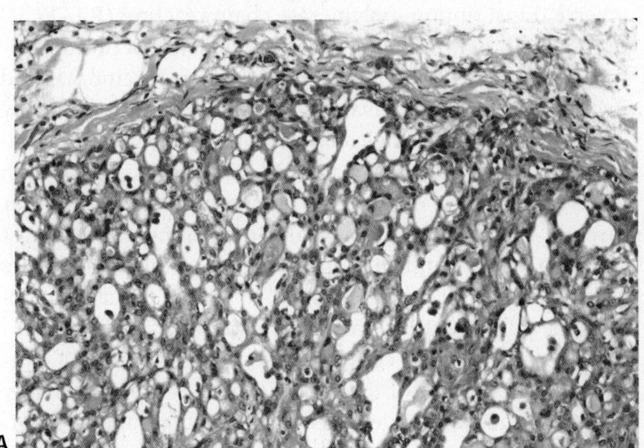

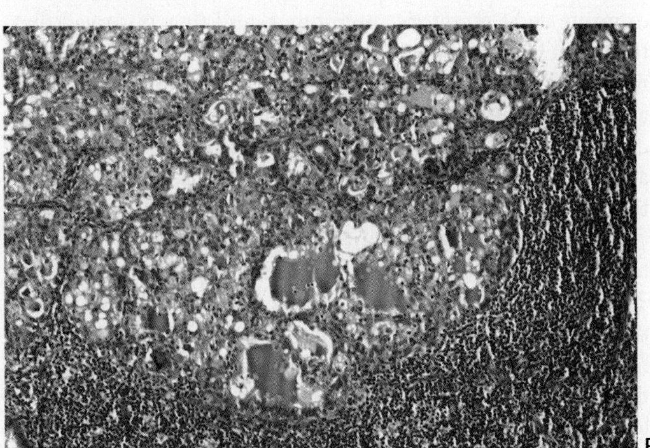

FIG. 22.12. ***Secretory carcinoma, metastasis.*** **A:** Primary secretory carcinoma. **B:** Metastatic secretory carcinoma in the same patient.

Some of the patients with positive lymph nodes have been more than 20 years of age,[2,14,29,32,58,60,61,63,86] but the risk of nodal involvement is at least as great in children. A literature review found that of the six children in whom lymph nodes were examined, three (50%) had positive nodes.[14] Richard et al.[19] reported that 9 of 33 (27%) adult women with secretory carcinoma had axillary nodal metastases. In another report, axillary metastases were first evident when a local recurrence was found 7 years after local excision of the primary mass from a 19-year-old woman.[59] Patients with axillary metastases have been reported to be well as long as 6 years after primary therapy, but the finding of multiple involved lymph nodes may be a harbinger of systemic metastases.[41,42] Metastatic deposits and recurrences of secretory carcinoma display the morphologic features characteristic of primary carcinomas.[42]

Although most patients with secretory carcinoma do not succumb to their disease, the literature contains reports of five cases in which the carcinoma proved lethal.[37,40,42,72,86] Krausz et al.[86] described the case of a 24-year-old man in whom secretory carcinoma was treated by simple mastectomy and axillary radiation. Twenty years later, the patient developed an axillary mass regarded as recurrent carcinoma and died of systemic metastases within a year. A biopsy of a metastatic lesion confirmed that it was secretory carcinoma.

TREATMENT

Local excision is the preferred initial treatment in children found to have secretory carcinoma.[61] Consideration should be given to preserving the breast bud in prepubertal patients. Unfortunately, this cannot always be accomplished, and breast development may be impaired or abolished in this circumstance. In postmenarchal girls and women, wide local excision may suffice for small lesions, but quadrantectomy can be necessary to obtain negative margins around larger tumors. Because of the small size of the male breast, surgical excision usually constitutes a mastectomy. Clinical examination is not always a good guide to the appropriateness of axillary dissection in children because most lymph node metastases in these patients have not been palpable. Sentinel lymph node mapping can be an effective method for assessing the axilla in patients with secretory carcinoma.[62,63]

It remains to be determined if adjuvant radiation therapy is beneficial in adults after excision. Because radiotherapy is likely to inhibit normal breast development if it is administered to the premenarchal or adolescent breast and it increases the risk of developing a new carcinoma in the treated breast at a later date, it is almost never indicated in this age group.

Because very few patients have received systemic adjuvant chemotherapy and various treatment regimens have been used,[29,41,52,63,72,86,88] it is not possible to judge the effectiveness of this treatment in children or adults with secretory carcinoma. Data on the effectiveness of radiotherapy and chemotherapy for the treatment of recurrent and metastatic secretory carcinoma are inconclusive for similar reasons.[41,64,72]

REFERENCES

1. Ashikari H, Jun MY, Farrow JH, et al. Breast carcinoma in children and adolescents. *Clin Bull* 1977;7:55–62.
2. Tournemaine N, Audouin AF, Anguill C, et al. Le carcinome secretoire juvenile. Cinq nouveaux cas chez des femmes d'age adulte. *Arch Anat Cytol Pathol* 1986;34:146–151.
3. McDivitt RW, Stewart FW. Breast carcinoma in children. *JAMA* 1966;195:388–390.
4. Oberman HA, Stephens PJ. Carcinoma of the breast in childhood. *Cancer* 1972;30:470–474.
5. Oberman HA. Secretory carcinoma of the breast in adults. *Am J Surg Pathol* 1980;4:465–470.
6. Gupta K, Lallu SD, Fauck R, et al. Needle aspiration cytology, immunocytochemistry, and electron microscopy in a rare case of secretory carcinoma of the breast in an elderly woman. *Diagn Cytopathol* 1992;8:388–391.
7. Noh WC, Paik NS, Cho KJ, et al. Breast mass in a 3-year-old girl: differentiation of secretory carcinoma versus abnormal thelarche by fine needle aspiration biopsy. *Surgery* 2005;137:109–110.
8. Ben Romdhane K, Ben Ayed M, Labbane N, et al. Carcinome sécrétant juvénile du sein. A propos d'une observation chez une fille de 4 ans. *Ann Pathol* 1987;7:227–230.
9. Ferguson TB Jr, McCarty KS Jr, Filston HC. Juvenile secretory carcinoma and juvenile papillomatosis: diagnosis and treatment. *J Pediatr Surg* 1987;22:637–639.
10. Longo OA, Mosto A, Moran JC, et al. Breast carcinoma in childhood and adolescence: case report and review of the literature. *Breast J* 1999;5:65–69.
11. Simpson JS, Barson AJ. Breast tumours in infants and children: a 40 year review of cases at a children's hospital. *Can Med Assoc J* 1969;101:100–102.
12. Tanimura A, Konaka K. Carcinoma of the breast in a 5 years old girl. *Acta Pathol Jpn* 1980;30:157–160.
13. Alenda C, Aranda FI, Segui FJ, et al. Secretory carcinoma of the male breast: correlation of aspiration cytology and pathology. *Diagn Cytopathol* 2005;32:47–50.
14. Karl SR, Ballantine TV, Zaino R. Juvenile secretory carcinoma of the breast. *J Pediatr Surg* 1985;20:368–371.
15. Cabello C, Alvarenga M, Alvarenga C, et al. Case report and review of the literature: secretory breast cancer in a 13-year-old boy—10 years of follow up. *Breast Cancer Res Treat* 2012;133:813–820.
16. Hartman AW, Magrish P. Carcinoma of breast in children; case report: six-year-old boy with adenocarcinoma. *Ann Surg* 1955;141:792–798.
17. Beatty SM, Orel SG, Kim P, et al. Multicentric secretory carcinoma of the breast in a 35-year-old woman: mammographic appearance and the use of core biopsy in preoperative management. *Breast J* 1998;4:200–203.
18. Diallo R, Schaefer KL, Bankfalvi A, et al. Secretory carcinoma of the breast: a distinct variant of invasive ductal carcinoma assessed by comparative genomic hybridization and immunohistochemistry. *Hum Pathol* 2003;34:1299–1305.
19. Richard G, Hawk JC III, Baker AS Jr, et al. Multicentric adult secretory breast carcinoma: DNA flow cytometric findings, prognostic features, and review of the world literature. *J Surg Oncol* 1990;44:238–244.
20. Siegel JR, Karcnik TJ, Hertz MB, et al. Secretory carcinoma of the breast. *Breast J* 1999;5:204–207.
21. de Bree E, Askoxylakis J, Giannikaki E, et al. Secretory carcinoma of the male breast. *Ann Surg Oncol* 2002;9:663–667.
22. Kameyama K, Mukai M, Iri H, et al. Secretory carcinoma of the breast in a 51-year-old male. *Pathol Int* 1998;48:994–997.
23. Amott DH, Masters R, Moore S. Secretory carcinoma of the breast. *Breast J* 2006;12:183.
24. Paeng MH, Choi HY, Sung SH, et al. Secretory carcinoma of the breast. *J Clin Ultrasound* 2003;31:425–429.
25. Titus J, Sillar RW, Fenton LE. Secretory breast carcinoma in a 9-year-old boy. *Aust N Z J Surg* 2000;70:144–146.
26. Vasudev P, Onuma K. Secretory breast carcinoma: unique, triple-negative carcinoma with a favorable prognosis and characteristic molecular expression. *Arch Pathol Lab Med* 2011;135:1606–1610.
27. Murphy JJ, Morzaria S, Gow KW, et al. Breast cancer in a 6-year-old child. *J Pediatr Surg* 2000;35:765–767.
28. Mun SH, Ko EY, Han BK, et al. Secretory carcinoma of the breast: sonographic features. *J Ultrasound Med* 2008;27:947–954.
29. Shin SJ, Sheikh FS, Allenby PA, et al. Invasive secretory (juvenile) carcinoma arising in ectopic breast tissue of the axilla. *Arch Pathol Lab Med* 2001;125:1372–1374.

30. Brandt SM, Swistel AJ, Rosen PP. Secretory carcinoma in the axilla: probable origin from axillary skin appendage glands in a young girl. *Am J Surg Pathol* 2009;33:950–953.
31. Grabellus F, Worm K, Willruth A, et al. ETV6-NTRK3 gene fusion in a secretory carcinoma of the breast of a male-to-female transsexual. *Breast* 2005;14:71–74.
32. Abe R, Masuda T. Secretory carcinoma of the breast in a Japanese woman. *Jpn J Surg* 1986;16:52–55.
33. Roth JA, Discafani C, O'Malley M. Secretory breast carcinoma in a man. *Am J Surg Pathol* 1988;12:150–154.
34. Nonomura A, Kimura A, Mizukami Y, et al. Secretory carcinoma of the breast associated with juvenile papillomatosis in a 12-year-old girl. A case report. *Acta Cytol* 1995;39:569–576.
35. Rosen PP, Holmes G, Lesser ML, et al. Juvenile papillomatosis and breast carcinoma. *Cancer* 1985;55:1345–1352.
36. Tokunaga M, Wakimoto J, Muramoto Y, et al. Juvenile secretory carcinoma and juvenile papillomatosis. *Jpn J Clin Oncol* 1985;15: 457–465.
37. Woto-Gaye G, Kasse AA, Dieye Y, et al. Carcinome sécrétoire du sein chez l' hommme. A propos d'un cas d'évolution rapide. *Ann Pathol* 2004;24:432–435; quiz 393.
38. Lae M, Freneaux P, Birolini M, et al. Secretory breast carcinoma: a low grade basal-like carcinoma associated with translocation. *Mod Pathol* 2008;21(Suppl. 1):42A.
39. Din NU, Idrees R, Fatima S, et al. Secretory carcinoma of breast: clinicopathologic study of 8 cases. *Ann Diagn Pathol* 2013;17:54–57.
40. Nguyen GK, Neifer R. Aspiration biopsy cytology of secretory carcinoma of the breast. *Diagn Cytopathol* 1987;3:234–237.
41. Anderson P, Albarracin CT, Resetkova E. A large, fungating breast mass. Secretory carcinoma with apocrine differentiation. *Arch Pathol Lab Med* 2006;130:e50–e52.
42. Tavassoli FA, Norris HJ. Secretory carcinoma of the breast. *Cancer* 1980;45:2404–2413.
43. Roncaroli F, Lamovec J, Zidar A, et al. Acinic cell-like carcinoma of the breast. *Virchows Arch* 1996;429:69–74.
44. Hirokawa M, Sugihara K, Sai T, et al. Secretory carcinoma of the breast: a tumour analogous to salivary gland acinic cell carcinoma? *Histopathology* 2002;40:223–229.
45. Reis-Filho JS, Natrajan R, Vatcheva R, et al. Is acinic cell carcinoma a variant of secretory carcinoma? A FISH study using ETV6 'split apart' probes. *Histopathology* 2008;52:840–846.
46. d'Amore ES, Maisto L, Gatteschi MB, et al. Secretory carcinoma of the breast. Report of a case with fine needle aspiration biopsy. *Acta Cytol* 1986;30:309–312.
47. Dominguez F, Riera JR, Junco P, et al. Secretory carcinoma of the breast. Report of a case with diagnosis by fine needle aspiration. *Acta Cytol* 1992;36:507–510.
48. Shinagawa T, Tadokoro M, Kitamura H, et al. Secretory carcinoma of the breast. Correlation of aspiration cytology and histology. *Acta Cytol* 1994;38:909–914.
49. Pohar-Marinsek Z, Golouh R. Secretory breast carcinoma in a man diagnosed by fine needle aspiration biopsy. A case report. *Acta Cytol* 1994;38:446–450.
50. Buchino JJ, Moore GD, Bond SJ. Secretory carcinoma in a 9-year-old girl. *Diagn Cytopathol* 2004;31:430–431.
51. Craig JP. Secretory carcinoma of the breast in an adult. Correlation of aspiration cytology and histology on the biopsy specimen. *Acta Cytol* 1985;29:589–592.
52. Yildirim E, Turhan N, Pak I, et al. Secretory breast carcinoma in a boy. *Eur J Surg Oncol* 1999;25:98–99.
53. Akhtar M, Robinson C, Ali MA, et al. Secretory carcinoma of the breast in adults. Light and electron microscopic study of three cases with review of the literature. *Cancer* 1983;51:2245–2254.
54. de la Cruz Mera A, de la Cruz Mera E, Leston JS, et al. Secretory carcinoma of the breast [Letter to the Editors]. *Acta Cytol* 1994;38: 968–969.
55. Shinagawa T, Tadokoro M, Takeuchi E, et al. Aspiration biopsy cytology of secretory carcinoma of the breast. A case report. *Acta Cytol* 1992;36:189–193.
56. Oh YH, Jang KS, Song YS, et al. Secretory carcinoma of the breast diagnosed by fine needle aspiration. *Acta Cytol* 2005;49:343–344.
57. Vesoulis Z, Kashkari S. Fine needle aspiration of secretory breast carcinoma resembling lactational changes. A case report. *Acta Cytol* 1998;42:1032–1036.
58. Lamovec J, Bracko M. Secretory carcinoma of the breast: light microscopical, immunohistochemical and flow cytometric study. *Mod Pathol* 1994;7:475–479.
59. Botta G, Fessia L, Ghiringhello B. Juvenile milk protein secreting carcinoma. *Virchows Arch A Pathol Anat Histol* 1982;395:145–152.
60. Kuwabara H, Yamane M, Okada S. Secretory breast carcinoma in a 66 year old man. *J Clin Pathol* 1998;51:545–547.
61. Rosen PP, Cranor ML. Secretory carcinoma of the breast. *Arch Pathol Lab Med* 1991;115:141–144.
62. Szanto J, Andras C, Tsakiris J, et al. Secretory breast cancer in a 7.5-year old boy. *Breast* 2004;13:439–442.
63. Vieni S, Cabibi D, Cipolla C, et al. Secretory breast carcinoma with metastatic sentinel lymph node. *World J Surg Oncol* 2006;4:88.
64. Arce C, Cortes-Padilla D, Huntsman DG, et al. Secretory carcinoma of the breast containing the ETV6-NTRK3 fusion gene in a male: case report and review of the literature. *World J Surg Oncol* 2005;3:35.
65. Bhagwandeen BS, Fenton L. Secretory carcinoma of the breast in a nine year old boy. *Pathology* 1999;31:166–168.
66. Lambros MB, Tan DS, Jones RL, et al. Genomic profile of a secretory breast cancer with an ETV6-NTRK3 duplication. *J Clin Pathol* 2009;62:604–612.
67. Aceto GM, Solano AR, Neuman MI, et al. High-risk human papilloma virus infection, tumor pathophenotypes, and BRCA1/2 and TP53 status in juvenile breast cancer. *Breast Cancer Res Treat* 2010;122:671–683.
68. Yorozuya K, Takahashi E, Kousaka J, et al. A case of estrogen receptor positive secretory carcinoma in a 9-Year-old girl with ETV6-NTRK3 fusion gene. *Jpn J Clin Oncol* 2012;42:208–211.
69. Serour F, Gilad A, Kopolovic J, et al. Secretory breast cancer in childhood and adolescence: report of a case and review of the literature. *Med Pediatr Oncol* 1992;20:341–344.
70. Gabal S, Talaat S. Secretory carcinoma of male breast: case report and review of the literature. *Int J Breast Cancer* 2011;2011:704657.
71. Maitra A, Tavassoli FA, Albores-Saavedra J, et al. Molecular abnormalities associated with secretory carcinomas of the breast. *Hum Pathol* 1999;30:1435–1440.
72. Herz H, Cooke B, Goldstein D. Metastatic secretory breast cancer. Non-responsiveness to chemotherapy: case report and review of the literature. *Ann Oncol* 2000;11:1343–1347.
73. Mies C. Recurrent secretory carcinoma in residual mammary tissue after mastectomy. *Am J Surg Pathol* 1993;17:715–721.
74. Sullivan JJ, Magee HR, Donald KJ. Secretory (juvenile) carcinoma of the breast. *Pathology* 1977;9:341–346.
75. Chevallier A, Boissy C, Rampal A, et al. Le carcinome sécrétoire du sein. A propos d'une observation chez un garçon de 9 ans. *Clin Exp Pathol* 1999;47:88–91.
76. Boman F, Gregorie MJ, Perrier ML, et al. Carcinome sécrétoire du sein: un cas pédiatrique étudié en cytogénetique et FISH. *Ann Pathol* 1997;17:220.
77. Tognon C, Knezevich SR, Huntsman D, et al. Expression of the ETV6-NTRK3 gene fusion as a primary event in human secretory breast carcinoma. *Cancer Cell* 2002;2:367–376.
78. Makretsov N, He M, Hayes M, et al. A fluorescence *in situ* hybridization study of ETV6-NTRK3 fusion gene in secretory breast carcinoma. *Genes Chromosomes Cancer* 2004;40:152–157.
79. Tixier H, Picard A, Guiu S, et al. Long-term recurrence of secretory breast carcinoma with metastatic sentinel lymph nodes. *Arch Gynecol Obstet* 2011;283(Suppl. 1):S77–S78.
80. Skálová A, Vanecek T, Sima R, et al. Mammary analogue secretory carcinoma of salivary glands, containing the ETV6-NTRK3 fusion gene: a hitherto undescribed salivary gland tumor entity. *Am J Surg Pathol* 2010;34:599–608.
81. Nevalainen MT, Xie J, Bubendorf L, et al. Basal activation of transcription factor signal transducer and activator of transcription (Stat5) in nonpregnant mouse and human breast epithelium. *Mol Endocrinol* 2002;16:1108–1124.
82. Bratthauer GL, Strauss BL, Tavassoli FA. STAT 5a expression in various lesions of the breast. *Virchows Arch* 2006;448:165–171.
83. Strauss BL, Bratthauer GL, Tavassoli FA. STAT 5a expression in the breast is maintained in secretory carcinoma, in contrast to other histologic types. *Hum Pathol* 2006;37:586–592.
84. Niveditha SR, Bajaj P, Nangia A. Secretory carcinoma of the male breast. *J Clin Pathol* 2004;57:894.
85. Masse SR, Rioux A, Beauchesne C. Juvenile carcinoma of the breast. *Hum Pathol* 1981;12:1044–1046.

86. Krausz T, Jenkins D, Grontoft O, et al. Secretory carcinoma of the breast in adults: emphasis on late recurrence and metastasis. *Histopathology* 1989;14:25–36.
87. Byrne MP, Fahey MM, Gooselaw JG. Breast cancer with axillary metastasis in an eight and one-half-year-old girl. *Cancer* 1973;31:726–728.
88. Costa NM, Rodrigues H, Pereira H, et al. Secretory breast carcinoma—case report and review of the medical literature. *Breast* 2004;13:353–355.
89. Heydenrych JJ, Villet WT, von der Heyden U. Carcinoma of the breast in children: a case report and review of the literature. *S Afr Med J* 1980;57:1005–1008.
90. Iglesias B, Monteagudo B, Rouco JS, et al. Secretory breast carcinoma in a 63-year-old man. *J Cutan Pathol* 2009;36 (Suppl. 1):86–88.
91. Kavalakat AJ, Covilakam RK, Culas TB. Secretory carcinoma of breast in a 17-year-old male. *World J Surg Oncol* 2004;2:17.

CHAPTER 23

Mammary Carcinoma with Osteoclast-like Giant Cells

FREDERICK C. KOERNER

Carcinomas containing osteoclast-like multinucleated giant cells arise in many organs, including the breast, lung, pancreas, small intestine, and thyroid gland. Similar giant cells have also been found in noncarcinomatous tumors such as uterine leiomyosarcoma[1] and intestinal carcinoid.[2] In 1979, Agnantis and Rosen[3] first documented the presence of osteoclast-like giant cells in mammary carcinomas, and since then approximately 200 examples of this type of mammary carcinoma have been reported.

CLINICAL PRESENTATION

Despite the unusual histologic properties of these tumors, the clinical features are similar to those of breast carcinoma generally. Patients' age ranged from 28 to 88 years, and the average age at diagnosis was approximately 50 years.[3–6] Typically, the patient presented with a palpable tumor in the upper outer quadrant, but the lesion has been found in all quadrants. Multifocal lesions were described clinically in two cases.[7,8] Bilateral primary carcinomas with osteoclast-like giant cells are exceedingly rare.[9] On mammography and ultrasonography, the well-circumscribed margin of most tumors may suggest a benign lesion such as a cyst or a fibroadenoma (FA).[5,10] Masses with irregular margins and inhomogeneous internal echoes have been reported.[8] Magnetic resonance imaging (MRI) of one carcinoma exhibited "rich vascularity, especially in the periphery."[11]

GROSS PATHOLOGY

The tumors are usually well defined, fleshy, and firm. Reported diameters range from 0.5 to 10 cm, with most carcinomas measuring 3 cm or less. The macroscopic appearance of most tumors is quite striking: when bisected, the dark brown or red-brown tumor tends to bulge slightly above the surrounding parenchyma from which it may be separated by a rounded, discrete margin (Fig. 23.1). Tumors with ill-defined margins and multinodules have been described.[7,12] The deep mahogany color may suggest heavily pigmented, metastatic malignant melanoma, but the color of carcinomas with osteoclast-like giant cells tends to be brown rather than black. Tumors with relatively few osteoclast-like giant cells or with little hemorrhage may appear tan or white. These unusual features are not specific for this neoplasm because some solid papillary or nonmedullary circumscribed carcinomas that lack giant cells microscopically are grossly indistinguishable from carcinomas with osteoclast-like giant cells (Fig. 23.2).

MICROSCOPIC PATHOLOGY

Most of these lesions are moderately or poorly differentiated invasive duct carcinomas (Fig. 23.3). A cribriform growth pattern is present relatively more often than occurs among duct carcinomas generally (Fig. 23.4). Uncommon examples of well-differentiated or tubular[4,12] (Fig. 23.5), lobular[3,9,10,13] (Fig. 23.6), squamous,[14] papillary[3] (Fig. 23.7), apocrine (Fig. 23.8), mucinous[6] (Fig. 23.9), metaplastic,[12] and neuroendocrine[15] carcinomas with osteoclast-like giant cells have been described. Rarely, the carcinoma has a glandular pattern reminiscent of that of infiltrating colonic carcinoma (Fig. 23.10). Osteoclast-like giant cells can be encountered in anaplastic carcinomas that are probably variants of metaplastic carcinoma (Fig. 23.11). When present, the ductal carcinoma *in situ* (DCIS) has the appearance of one of the conventional variants, usually cribriform, solid, or papillary. Osteoclast-like giant cells are not always present in the associated DCIS (Fig. 23.11). It is very uncommon to find osteoclast-like giant cells in DCIS in the absence of an invasive lesion (Fig. 23.12).[16]

The osteoclast-like giant cells range from 20 to 180 μm in diameter.[17] They contain abundant cytoplasm and many evenly distributed and usually centrally located oval nuclei, some of which contain small nucleoli. The giant cells tend to cluster close to the edges of carcinomatous glands or in intervening stroma, and they may be found in the glandular lumens (Figs. 23.7, 23.9, and 23.10). The stroma typically contains mononuclear histiocytes whose cytological features resemble those of the multinuclear giant cells.

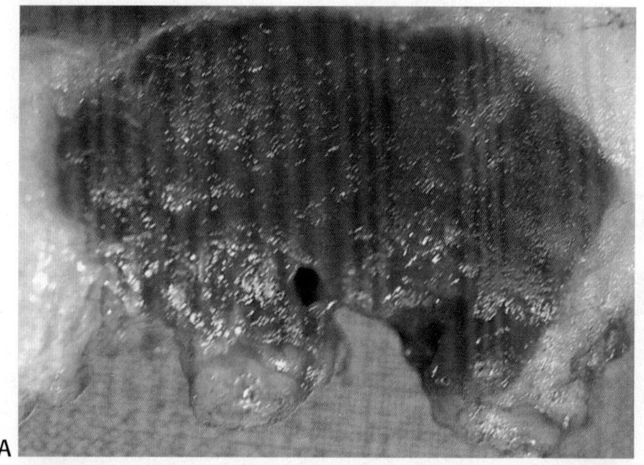

A

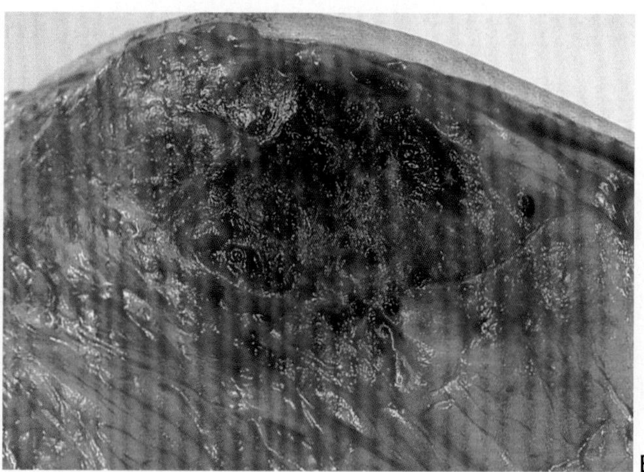

B

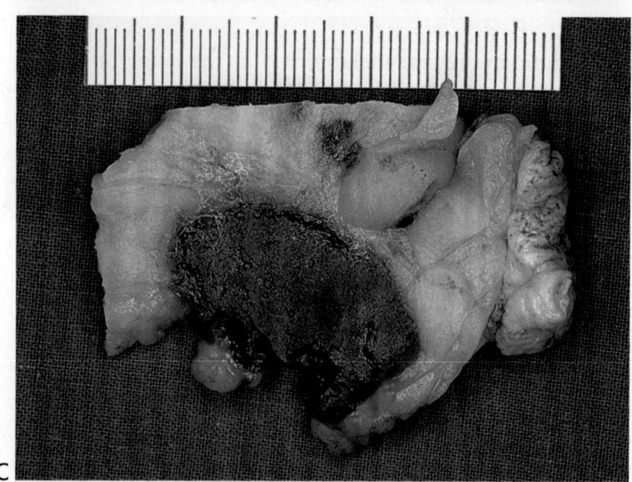

C

FIG. 23.1. ***Mammary carcinoma with osteoclast-like giant cells, gross.*** **A,B:** The tumors are usually well circumscribed and chocolate-brown or red-brown. **C:** The tumor shown in (A) retained the dark brown color after fixation in formalin.

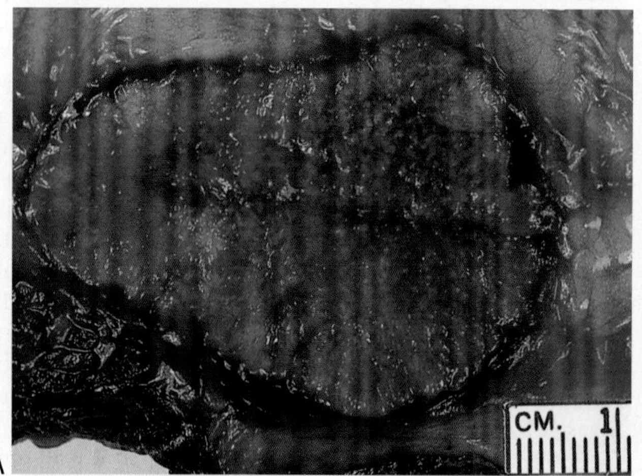

A

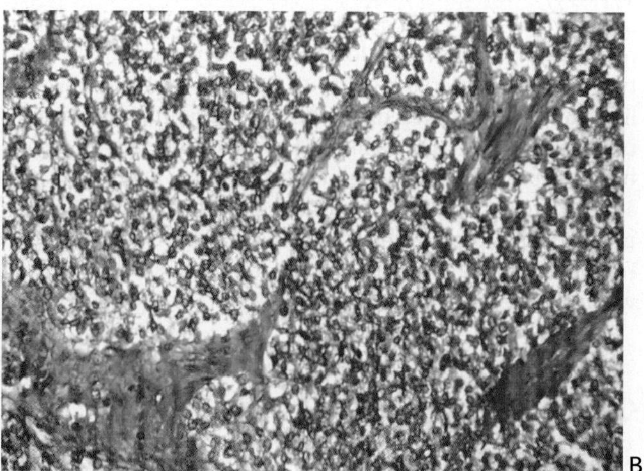

B

FIG. 23.2. ***Mammary carcinomas that grossly resemble carcinoma with osteoclast-like giant cells.*** **A:** A circumscribed, bulging tumor with a hyperemic border and red mottled surface. **B:** The tumor in (A) was a poorly differentiated carcinoma with stromal hemorrhage and no giant cells. **C:** The gross appearance of a bisected, circumscribed, dark red carcinoma. **D:** Histologic examination of the tumor in (C) revealed a solid papillary carcinoma lacking giant cells with stromal hemorrhage. Endocrine differentiation was evidenced by positive Grimelius and chromogranin stains and confirmed by electron microscopy.

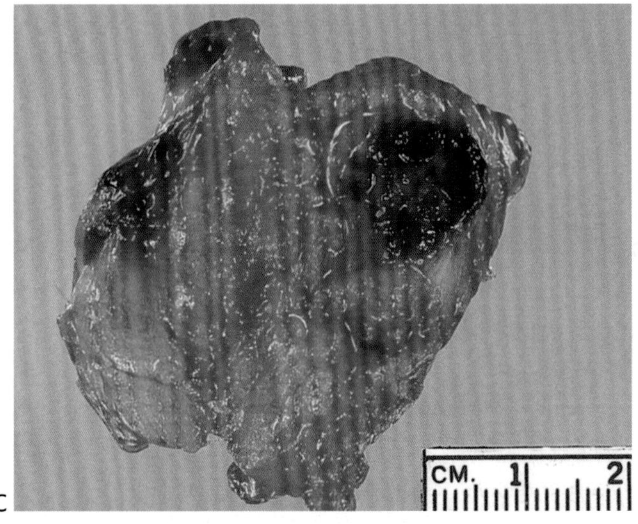

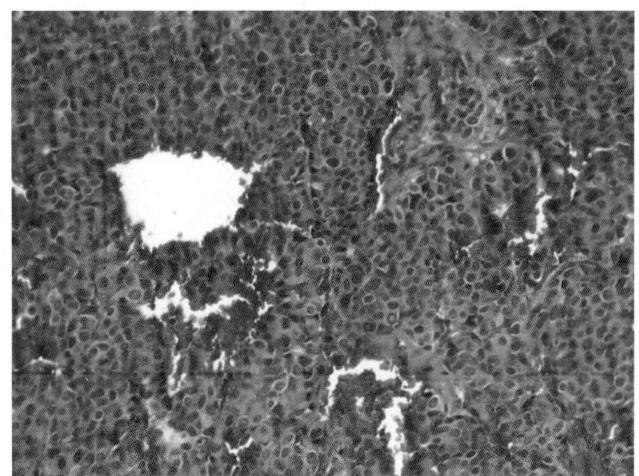

FIG. 23.2. *(Continued)*

The presence of extravasated erythrocytes and hemosiderin, which one finds in the vascular stroma in most cases, reflects recent and older episodes of hemorrhage (Figs. 23.3, 23.5, and 23.6). Erythrophagocytosis by the giant cells is uncommon, and they contain little hemosiderin detectable by light microscopy. Fibroblastic reaction, collagenization, angiogenesis, and lymphocytic infiltration are variably present in the stroma (Figs. 23.3, 23.4, and 23.13).

Osteoclast-like giant cells are found in examples of metaplastic carcinoma that contain areas of osseous and cartilaginous differentiation[18,19]; conversely, inconspicuous and infrequent metaplastic foci with spindle cells and squamous

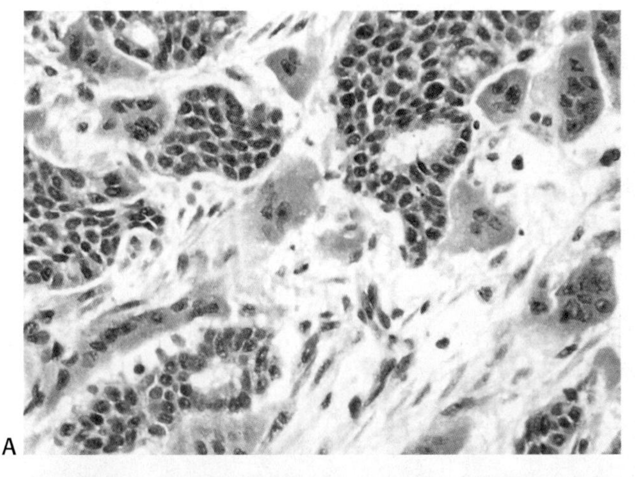

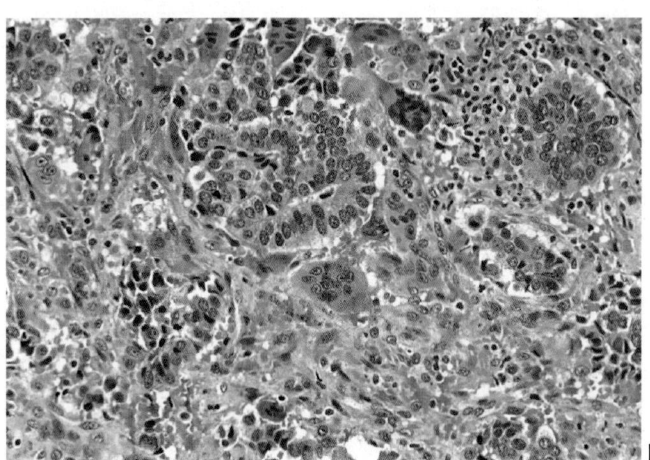

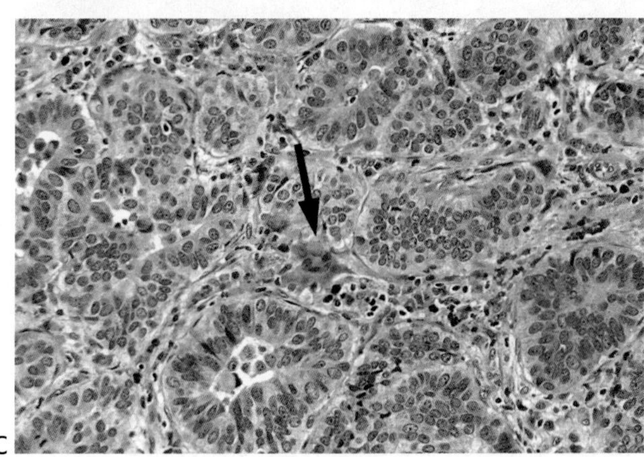

FIG. 23.3. ***Mammary carcinoma with osteoclast-like giant cells.*** **A:** Multinucleated giant cells in proximity to carcinomatous glands. The absence of stromal hemorrhage is unusual. **B:** Large multinucleated giant cells in the stroma mingle with lymphocytes, red blood cells, and stromal cells. **C:** One stellate osteoclast-like giant cell is shown (*arrow*). The stroma contains hemosiderin, lymphocytes, and plasma cells.

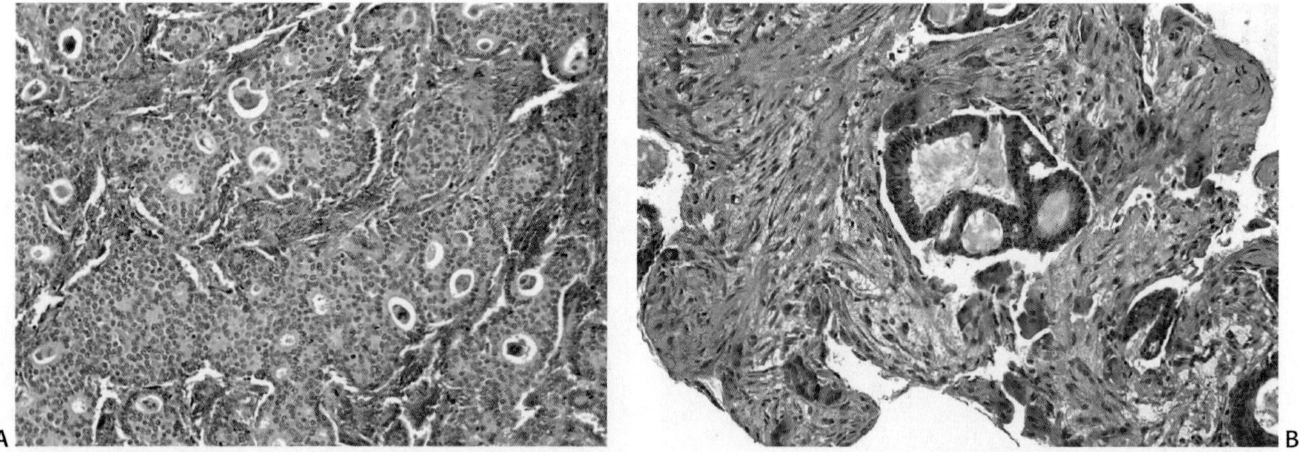

FIG. 23.4. ***Mammary carcinoma with osteoclast-like giant cells, cribriform.*** **A:** Diffuse stromal hemorrhage with hemosiderin obscures the osteoclast-like giant cells. **B:** A needle core biopsy sample with numerous osteoclast-like giant cells and cribriform duct carcinoma.

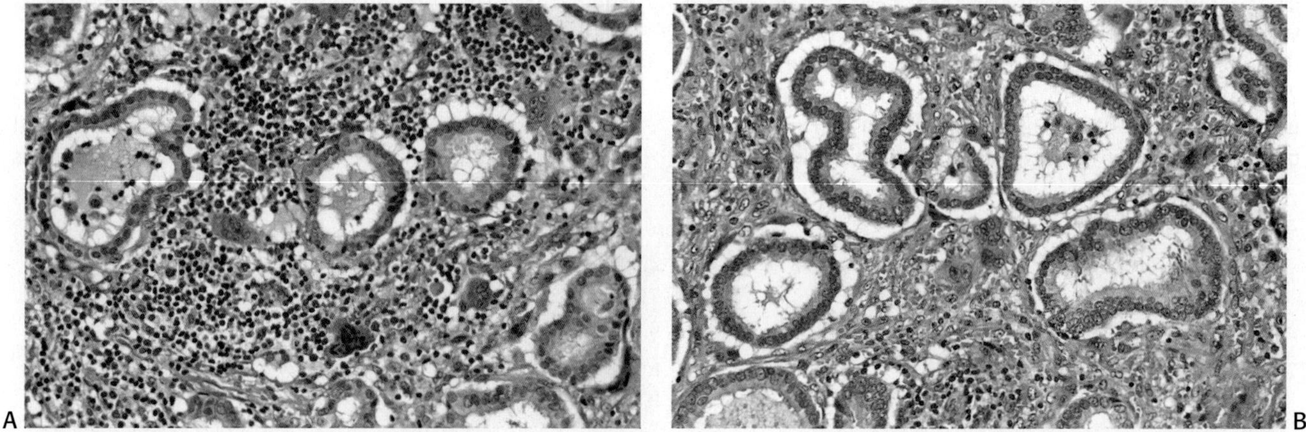

FIG. 23.5. ***Mammary carcinoma with osteoclast-like giant cells, well differentiated.*** **A,B:** The stroma in this tumor contains many lymphocytes and red blood cells.

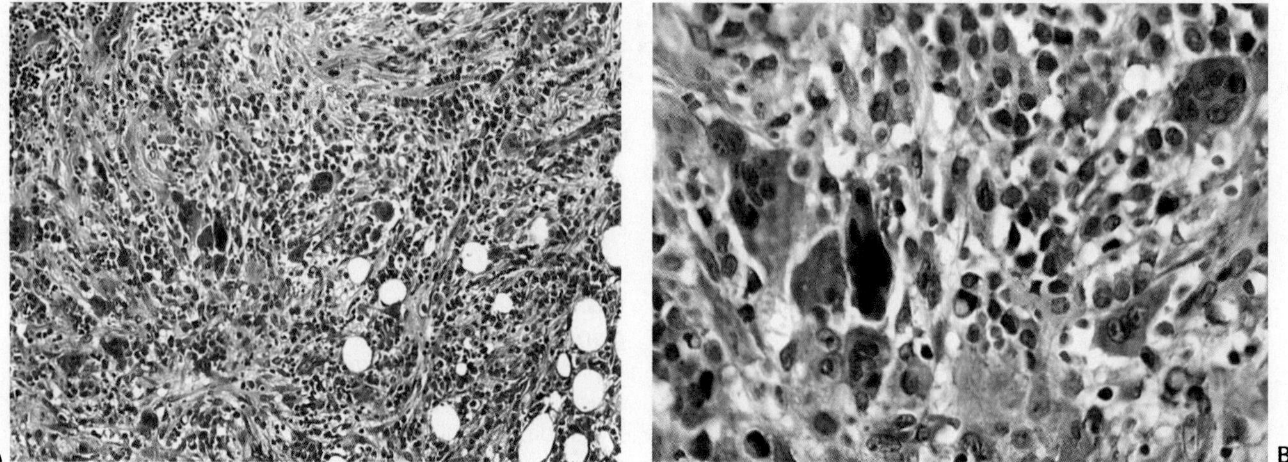

FIG. 23.6. ***Mammary carcinoma with osteoclast-like giant cells, infiltrating lobular.*** **A:** Multinucleated giant cells mingle with the carcinoma cells. **B:** Extravasated red blood cells, signet ring carcinoma cells, and giant cells are present, also.

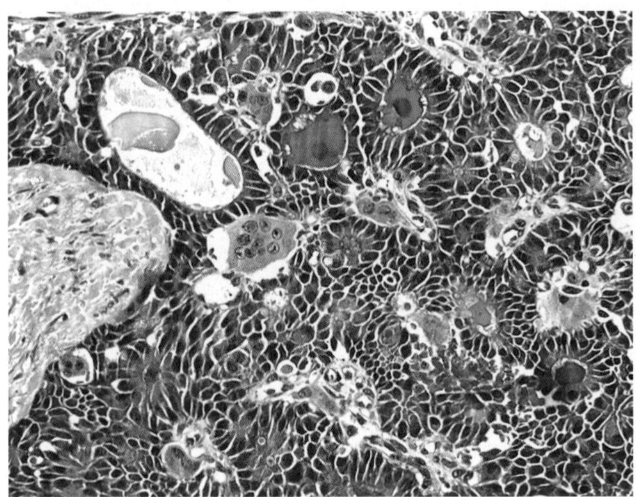

FIG. 23.7. ***Mammary carcinoma with osteoclast-like giant cells, solid papillary.***

or osseous features have been described in tumors that otherwise were typical examples of mammary carcinoma with osteoclast-like giant cells.[3,12] Mammary carcinoma with osteoclast-like giant cells may be a variant of metaplastic mammary carcinoma, but it seems appropriate to separate these tumors until investigators have better defined the clinicopathologic characteristics of these two types of mammary carcinoma.

Differential Diagnosis

The differential diagnosis includes certain noncarcinomatous lesions.[20] Megakaryocytes in myeloid metaplasia in the breast might be mistaken for osteoclast-like giant cells, but these lesions have abundant myeloid elements in various stages of maturation, a feature not found in carcinomas with osteoclast-like giant cells.[21] Granulomatous foci in inflammatory conditions such as sarcoidosis or coexistent with carcinoma also contain giant cells that differ histologically from those with osteoclast-like features[22,23] (Fig. 23.14). Because mammary carcinoma with osteoclast-like giant cells does not have a granulomatous pattern, the distinction from sarcoid or tuberculoid reactions can be made without difficulty in histologic sections (see Chapter 4). The osteoclast-like giant cells found in mammary carcinoma do not resemble the multinucleated stromal giant cells that are an incidental finding in breast tissue from patients with benign conditions or carcinoma (Fig. 23.15). Multinucleated stromal giant cells may also be found in the stroma of fibroepithelial tumors (see Chapter 8). They lack the relatively abundant cytoplasm seen in osteoclast-like giant cells.

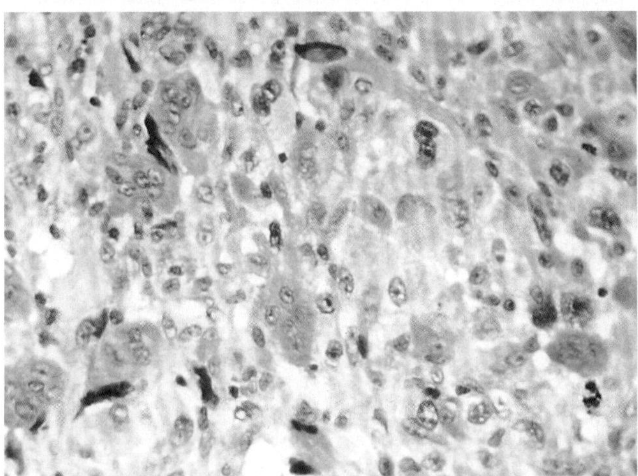

FIG. 23.8. ***Mammary carcinoma with osteoclast-like giant cells, apocrine.*** The giant cells mingle with apocrine carcinoma cells, which have prominent nucleoli.

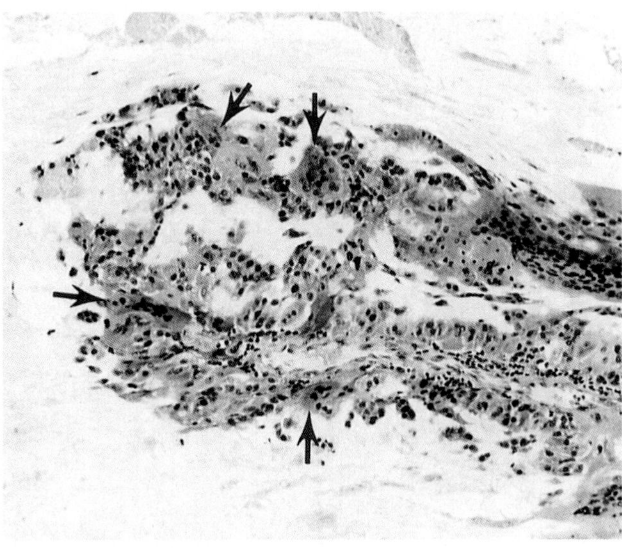

FIG. 23.9. ***Mammary carcinoma with osteoclast-like giant cells, mucinous.*** Giant cells (*arrows*) are hidden in this island of carcinoma surrounded by mucin.

Formation of Osteoclast-like Giant Cells

The mechanism by which osteoclast-like giant cells are formed in breast carcinoma is not known. It has been postulated that one or more substances produced by the neoplastic cells in these tumors induce the formation of the giant cells and that the same process is responsible for the accompanying angiogenesis and hemorrhage.[3,6] In experimental studies, the angiogenesis associated with mammary carcinoma has not been accompanied by osteoclast-like giant cells.[24] The formation of giant cells from blood monocytes incubated *in vitro* with human breast carcinoma cells has been ascribed to viruses presumably carried by the monocytes.[25] Jimi et al.[26] demonstrated *in vitro* that multinucleation and functional osteoclastic differentiation of stromal cells could be induced by interleukin-1. In a case study, Sano et al.[27] reported that the carcinoma cells in one such tumor secreted excess vascular endothelial growth factor (VEGF). The authors hypothesized that VEGF "promotes tumor angiogenesis and migration of macrophages," which "fuse with each other," giving rise to osteoclast-like giant cells. This conclusion is supported by observations made by Shishido-Hara et

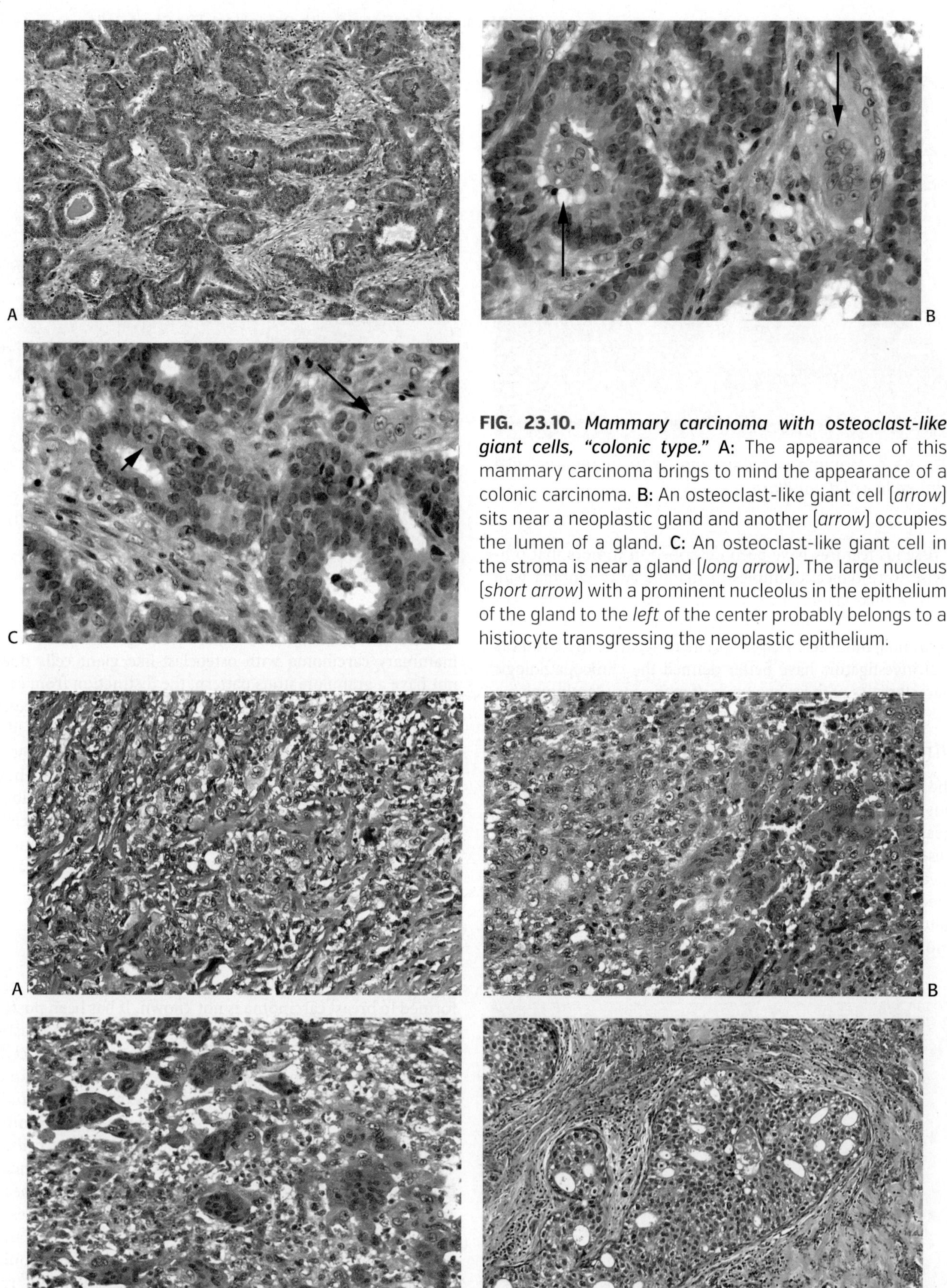

FIG. 23.10. ***Mammary carcinoma with osteoclast-like giant cells, "colonic type."*** **A:** The appearance of this mammary carcinoma brings to mind the appearance of a colonic carcinoma. **B:** An osteoclast-like giant cell [*arrow*] sits near a neoplastic gland and another [*arrow*] occupies the lumen of a gland. **C:** An osteoclast-like giant cell in the stroma is near a gland [*long arrow*]. The large nucleus [*short arrow*] with a prominent nucleolus in the epithelium of the gland to the *left* of the center probably belongs to a histiocyte transgressing the neoplastic epithelium.

FIG. 23.11. ***Mammary carcinoma with osteoclast-like giant cells, anaplastic.*** All images are from a single tumor. **A:** Giant cells are not evident in this part of the tumor. **B:** Osteoclast-like giant cells are difficult to distinguish from carcinoma cells in this region. **C:** Numerous osteoclast-like giant cells where carcinoma is inconspicuous. **D:** Cribriform DCIS without osteoclast-like giant cells.

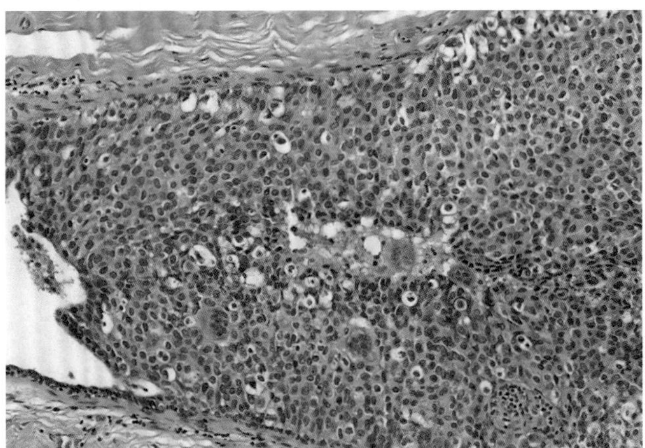

FIG. 23.12. *Osteoclast-like giant cells in DCIS.*

al.,[11] who studied lesions from two patients. Osteoclast-like giant cells were found to express markers associated with osseous osteoclasts (matrix metalloproteinase-9, tartrate-resistant acid phosphatase, and cathepsin K), as well as the histiocytic marker CD68, but they did not express HLA-DR. Additional studies are needed to evaluate this interesting observation.

CYTOLOGY

The diagnosis of mammary carcinoma with osteoclast-like giant cells may be suggested by the findings in a fine-needle aspiration (FNA) specimen.[7,10,18,28–33] The smears show a cellular aspirate containing a mixed population of carcinoma cells and multinucleate giant cells. The background may contain blood and/or hemosiderin-laden macrophages, as well as other inflammatory cells. The glandular clusters appear intermediate to large, they have irregular contours, and they form flat sheets and three-dimensional groups. The epithelial cells within the groups appear uniform, and they possess small round nuclei, smooth chromatin, inconspicuous nucleoli, and well-defined cytoplasm. One also finds scattered intact single cells displaying hyperchromatic nucleoli and a high nuclear-to-cytoplasmic ratio. Osteoclast-like giant cells vary in number, and densities as high as 30 per high-power field (HPF) have been reported.[34] The cells tend to sit between the epithelial groups, sometimes intimately associated with them, but the giant cells can also populate the periphery of the smear. The osteoclast-like cells possess abundant cytoplasm with branching processes, centrally located regular round to oval nuclei approximately three times the size of a small lymphocyte, and nucleoli variably described as small and prominent. The number of nuclei per cell ranges from 5 to 40. The aspirate often contains small numbers of mononuclear or binucleate cells with features similar to those of the giant cells. The distinction between osteoclast-like giant cells and multinucleated tumor giant cells may be difficult in an aspiration specimen.[35,36] Infiltrating lobular carcinoma with osteoclast-like giant cells can be recognized in a cytological preparation if the giant cells are found among small disaggregated tumor cells with signet ring features[10] (Fig. 23.16).

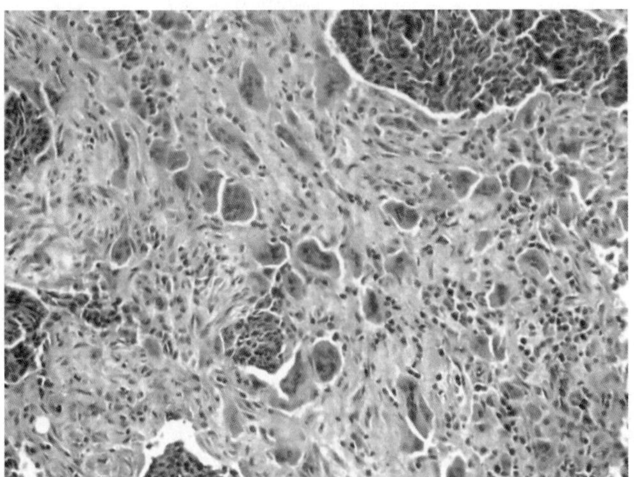

FIG. 23.13. ***Mammary carcinoma with osteoclast-like giant cells.*** This amount of stromal fibrosis is unusual. A lymphoplasmacytic infiltrate is present, but hemorrhage and hemosiderin are lacking.

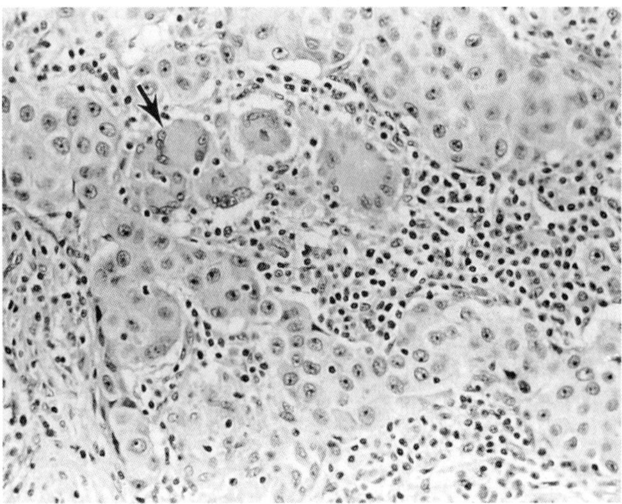

FIG. 23.14. ***Mammary carcinoma with a granulomatous reaction.*** Langhans-type giant cells (*arrow*) and a lymphocytic infiltrate distinguish this pattern from mammary carcinoma with osteoclast-like giant cells. Epithelioid granulomas, which are usually present, are not shown here.

IMMUNOHISTOCHEMISTRY

The carcinoma cells in these tumors are immunoreactive with various cytokeratins (CKs) (CK7, AE1/3, CAM5.2)[8–10,13,27,33,37] (Fig. 23.17) and epithelial membrane antigen

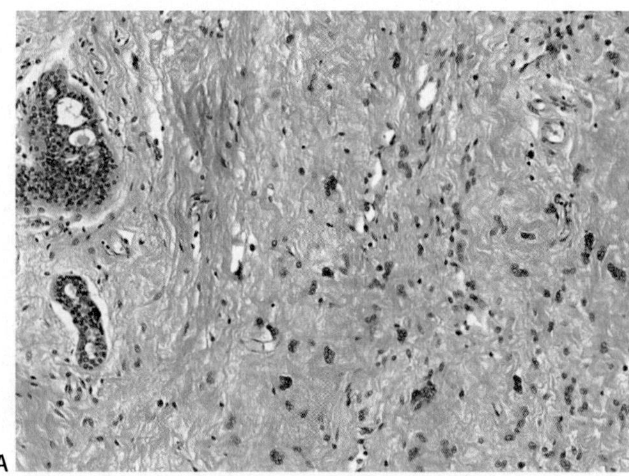

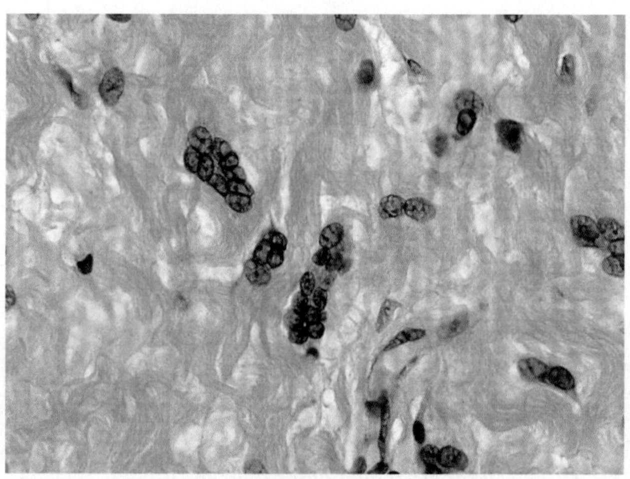

FIG. 23.15. ***Multinucleated stromal giant cells.*** **A:** These giant cells are localized in the stroma unassociated with epithelial components. **B:** Multiple overlapping nuclei and inconspicuous cytoplasm are characteristic features.

(EMA).[9,10,13,27,37,38] Staining for carcinoembryonic antigen (CEA), estrogen receptor (ER), progesterone receptor (PR), gross cystic disease fluid protein 15 (GCDFP-15), and human epidermal growth factor 2 (HER2) has yielded variable results.[6,8–10,13,20,33] The reactivity for these antigens probably depends on the nature of the carcinomatous component. Most tumors had low levels of ER, but many contained remarkably high levels of PR.[5,12,28] Immunohistochemical studies have shown conclusively that the giant cells lack epithelial features and that they are of mesenchymal origin (Fig. 23.17). The absence of factor VIII and *Ulex* activity in the osteoclast-like giant cells suggests that they are not of endothelial origin.[6,9,38,39] Staining of these cells for markers such as α_1-antitrypsin,[9] CD68[8–11,20,27,30,33,40] (Fig. 23.18), lysozyme or leucocyte common antigen in some[9,13,30,37] but not all[10,39] tumors, and several other proteins found in histiocytes[37] favors a histiocytic origin for the giant cells. Furthermore, the presence of acid phosphatase reactivity[4,12,41,42] and especially tartrate-resistant acid phosphatase reactivity,[11,27] matrix metalloproteinase-9,[11] and cathepsin K[11] suggests that the giant cells represent a specific type of histiocyte with osteoclastic functional capabilities.[41] The giant cells in two tumors did not stain for HLA-DR.[11] Lack of staining for Ki67[20] indicates that the giant cells do not replicate.

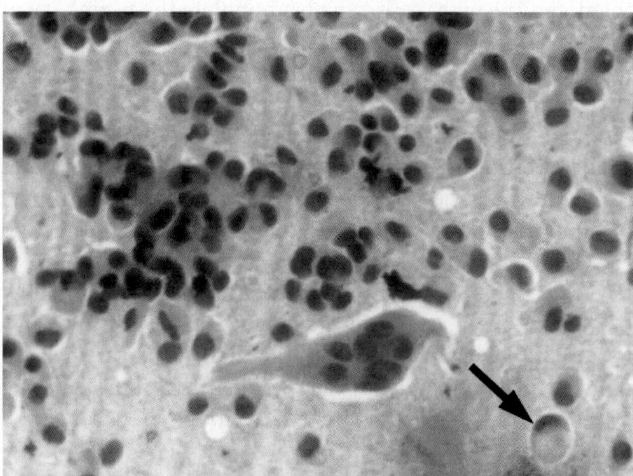

FIG. 23.16. ***Mammary carcinoma with osteoclast-like giant cells, cytology.*** An FNA smear showing infiltrating lobular carcinoma with an osteoclast-like giant cell. Note the signet ring cell in the *lower right* corner (*arrow*).

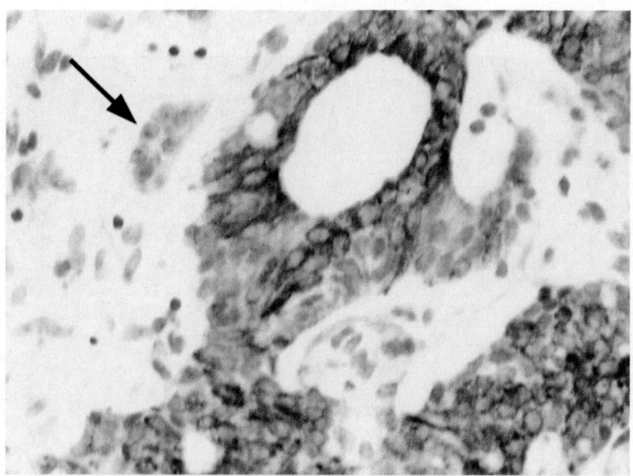

FIG. 23.17. ***Mammary carcinoma with osteoclast-like giant cells.*** The carcinoma cells are immunoreactive for AE1/3, but the osteoclast-like giant cell (*arrow*) is not stained.

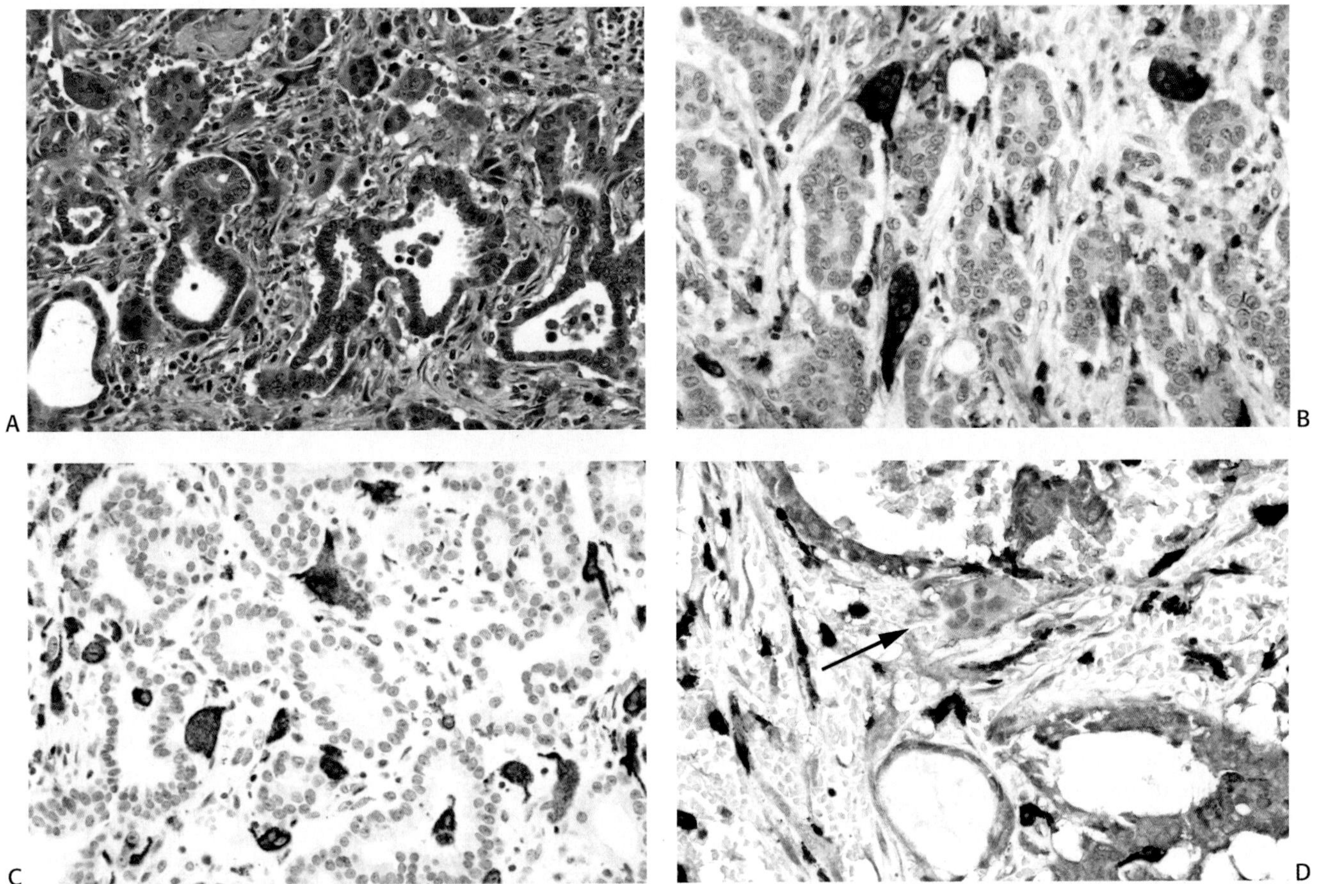

FIG. 23.18. ***Mammary carcinoma with osteoclast-like giant cells.*** **A:** A primary tumor with a well-differentiated glandular pattern. **B,C:** Immunoreactivity for KP1 (CD68) **(B)** and phosphoglycerate mutase 1 (PGM1) **(C)** is localized to the osteoclast-like giant cells. **D:** The osteoclast-like giant cell (*arrow*) does not stain for the histiocytic protein, CD163.

ELECTRON MICROSCOPY

Ultrastructural examination reveals that the carcinoma cells exhibit features characteristic of epithelial cells such as desmosomes and luminal microvilli. The osteoclast-like giant cells, on the other hand, differ substantially from the carcinoma cells and more closely resemble the accompanying mononuclear histiocytes.[4–6,9,12,13,17,36–39,43,44] The nuclei of the osteoclast-like giant cells have irregular outlines and deep invaginations. Dense chromatin coats the nuclear membrane, and the nuclei contain several prominent nucleoli. The cytoplasm appears electron dense and packed with organelles including mitochondria, free polyribosomes, and rough endoplasmic reticulum. The cells sometimes contain a few lysosomes or hemosiderin granules. The plasma membrane often appears ruffled and forms pseudopodia that enwrap nests of carcinoma cells.[5,43] The osteoclast-like giant cells occasionally form interdigitations with each other or with carcinoma cells, but they do not form cell junction when they do so. Mononuclear histiocytes display many of these features, but they usually contain numerous lysosomes.

OSTEOCLAST-LIKE GIANT CELLS IN METASTASES

Osteoclast-like giant cells are found in some but not all metastases in axillary lymph nodes (ALNs) or other sites[3,5,9,12,45,46] (Fig. 23.19). The presence of osteoclast-like giant cells within intralymphatic carcinomatous emboli[5] (Fig. 23.20) suggests that these stromal cells can be transported to regional lymph nodes and to distant metastases.

TREATMENT AND PROGNOSIS

ALN metastases have been reported in approximately one-third of cases. Local recurrences[5,12] and systemic metastases in the eye, liver, and other organs have been

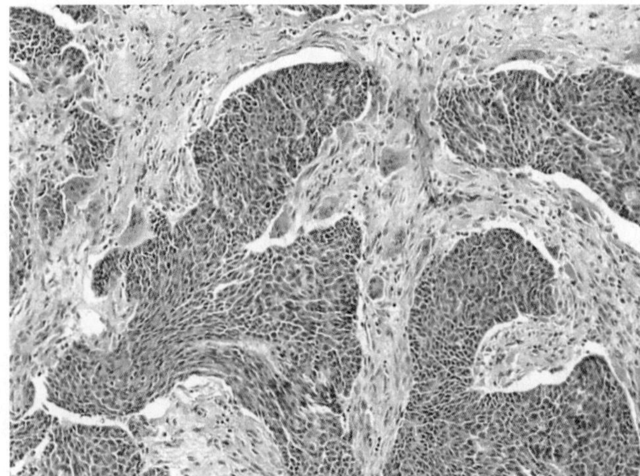

FIG. 23.19. ***Mammary carcinoma with osteoclast-like giant cells, metastatic.*** Osteoclast-like giant cells are present in the stroma of metastatic carcinoma in the liver.

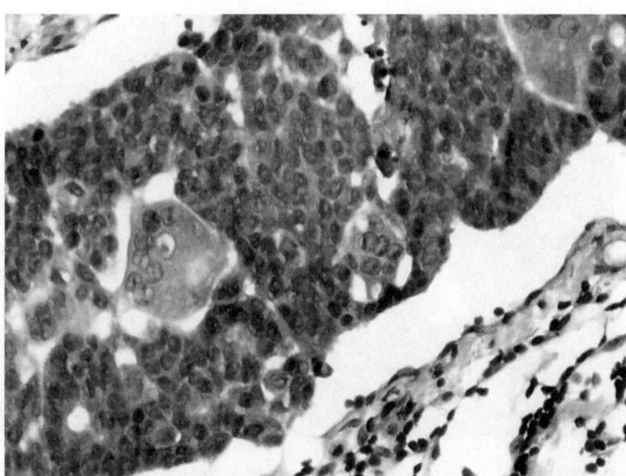

FIG. 23.20. ***Mammary carcinoma with osteoclast-like giant cells.*** Carcinoma with giant cells in a dilated lymphatic channel.

described.[3,12] Primary treatment in many reports was mastectomy with axillary dissection. Data on breast conservation with radiotherapy and adjuvant systemic therapy for this neoplasm are only anecdotal. Presently, it appears appropriate to employ the same criteria for breast conservation treatment as for invasive mammary carcinoma generally. Nearly two-thirds of patients have been reported to be alive and well, but the follow-up rarely extends beyond 5 years.[4,12,47]

REFERENCES

1. Darby AJ, Papadaki L, Beilby JO. An unusual leiomyosarcoma of the uterus containing osteoclast-like giant cells. *Cancer* 1975;36:495–504.
2. Alpers CE, Beckstead JH. Malignant neuroendocrine tumor of the jejunum with osteoclast-like giant cells. Enzyme histochemistry distinguishes tumor cells from giant cells. *Am J Surg Pathol* 1985;9:57–64.
3. Agnantis NT, Rosen PP. Mammary carcinoma with osteoclast-like giant cells. A study of eight cases with follow-up data. *Am J Clin Pathol* 1979;72:383–389.
4. Ichijima K, Kobashi Y, Ueda Y, et al. Breast cancer with reactive multinucleated giant cells: report of three cases. *Acta Pathol Jpn* 1986;36:449–457.
5. Holland R, van Haelst UJ. Mammary carcinoma with osteoclast-like giant cells. Additional observations on six cases. *Cancer* 1984;53:1963–1973.
6. Nielsen BB, Kiaer HW. Carcinoma of the breast with stromal multinucleated giant cells. *Histopathology* 1985;9:183–193.
7. Shabb NS, Tawil A, Mufarrij A, et al. Mammary carcinoma with osteoclastlike giant cells cytologically mimicking benign breast disease. A case report. *Acta Cytol* 1997;41:1284–1288.
8. Richter G, Uleer C, Noesselt T. Multifocal invasive ductal breast cancer with osteoclast-like giant cells: a case report. *J Med Case Rep* 2011;5:85.
9. Iacocca MV, Maia DM. Bilateral infiltrating lobular carcinoma of the breast with osteoclast-like giant cells. *Breast J* 2001;7:60–65.
10. Takahashi T, Moriki T, Hiroi M, et al. Invasive lobular carcinoma of the breast with osteoclast-like giant cells. A case report. *Acta Cytol* 1998;42:734–741.
11. Shishido-Hara Y, Kurata A, Fujiwara M, et al. Two cases of breast carcinoma with osteoclastic giant cells: are the osteoclastic giant cells protumoural differentiation of macrophages? *Diagn Pathol* 2010;5:55.
12. Tavassoli FA, Norris HJ. Breast carcinoma with osteoclastlike giant cells. *Arch Pathol Lab Med* 1986;110:636–639.
13. Pettinato G, Manivel JC, Picone A, et al. Alveolar variant of infiltrating lobular carcinoma of the breast with stromal osteoclast-like giant cells. *Pathol Res Pract* 1989;185:388–394; discussion 394–386.
14. Fisher ER, Palekar AS, Gregorio RM, et al. Mucoepidermoid and squamous cell carcinomas of breast with reference to squamous metaplasia and giant cell tumors. *Am J Surg Pathol* 1983;7:15–27.
15. Fadare O, Gill SA. Solid neuroendocrine carcinoma of the breast with osteoclast-like giant cells. *Breast J* 2009;15:205–206.
16. Krishnan C, Longacre TA. Ductal carcinoma *in situ* of the breast with osteoclast-like giant cells. *Hum Pathol* 2006;37:369–372.
17. Sugano I, Nagao K, Kondo Y, et al. Cytologic and ultrastructural studies of a rare breast carcinoma with osteoclast-like giant cells. *Cancer* 1983;52:74–78.
18. Boccato P, Briani G, d'Atri C, et al. Spindle cell and cartilaginous metaplasia in a breast carcinoma with osteoclast-like stromal cells. A difficult fine needle aspiration diagnosis. *Acta Cytol* 1988;32:75–78.
19. Wargotz ES, Norris HJ. Metaplastic carcinomas of the breast: V. Metaplastic carcinoma with osteoclastic giant cells. *Hum Pathol* 1990;21:1142–1150.
20. Cai G, Simsir A, Cangiarella J. Invasive mammary carcinoma with osteoclast-like giant cells diagnosed by fine-needle aspiration biopsy: review of the cytologic literature and distinction from other mammary lesions containing giant cells. *Diagn Cytopathol* 2004;30:396–400.
21. Brooks JJ, Krugman DT, Damjanov I. Myeloid metaplasia presenting as a breast mass. *Am J Surg Pathol* 1980;4:281–285.
22. Bassler R, Birke F. Histopathology of tumour associated sarcoid-like stromal reaction in breast cancer. An analysis of 5 cases with immunohistochemical investigations. *Virchows Arch A Pathol Anat Histopathol* 1988;412:231–239.
23. Oberman HA. Invasive carcinoma of the breast with granulomatous response. *Am J Clin Pathol* 1987;88:718–721.
24. Gullino PM. Natural history of breast cancer. Progression from hyperplasia to neoplasia as predicted by angiogenesis. *Cancer* 1977;39:2697–2703.
25. Al-Sumidaie AM, Leinster SJ, Jenkins SA. Transformation of blood monocytes to giant cells *in vitro* from patients with breast cancer. *Br J Surg* 1986;73:839–842.
26. Jimi E, Nakamura I, Duong LT, et al. Interleukin 1 induces multinucleation and bone-resorbing activity of osteoclasts in the absence of osteoblasts/stromal cells. *Exp Cell Res* 1999;247:84–93.

27. Sano M, Kikuchi K, Zhao C, et al. Osteoclastogenesis in human breast carcinoma. *Virchows Arch* 2004;444:470–472.
28. Bertrand G, Bidabe MC, Bertrand AF. Le carcinome mammaire a stroma reaction giganto-cellulaire. *Arch Anat Cytol Pathol* 1982;30:5–9.
29. Volpe R, Carbone A, Nicolo G, et al. Cytology of a breast carcinoma with osteoclastlike giant cells. *Acta Cytol* 1983;27:184–187.
30. Phillipson J, Ostrzega N. Fine needle aspiration of invasive cribriform carcinoma with benign osteoclast-like giant cells of histiocytic origin. A case report. *Acta Cytol* 1994;38:479–482.
31. Cai N, Koizumi J, Vazquez M. Mammary carcinoma with osteoclast-like giant cells: a study of four cases and a review of literature. *Diagn Cytopathol* 2005;33:246–251.
32. Ng WK. Fine needle aspiration cytology of invasive cribriform carcinoma of the breast with osteoclastlike giant cells: a case report. *Acta Cytol* 2001;45:593–598.
33. Neelam S, Sanjay G. Invasive duct carcinoma of the breast with multinucleated osteoclast-like giant cells: a rare case diagnosed on fine needle aspiration cytology. *Breast J* 2012;18:596–597.
34. Jacquet SF, Balleyguier C, Garbay JR, et al. Fine-needle aspiration cytopathology—an accurate diagnostic modality in mammary carcinoma with osteoclast-like giant cells: a study of 8 consecutive cases. *Cancer Cytopathol* 2010;118:468–473.
35. Douglas-Jones AG, Barr WT. Breast carcinoma with tumor giant cells. Report of a case with fine needle aspiration cytology. *Acta Cytol* 1989;33:109–114.
36. Gupta RK, Holloway LJ, Wakefield SJ, et al. Fine needle aspiration cytology, immunocytochemistry and electron microscopy in a rare case of carcinoma of the breast with malignant epithelial giant cells. *Acta Cytol* 1991;35:412–416.
37. Athanasou NA, Wells CA, Quinn J, et al. The origin and nature of stromal osteoclast-like multinucleated giant cells in breast carcinoma: implications for tumour osteolysis and macrophage biology. *Br J Cancer* 1989;59:491–498.
38. McMahon RF, Ahmed A, Connolly CE. Breast carcinoma with stromal multinucleated giant cells—a light microscopic, histochemical and ultrastructural study. *J Pathol* 1986;150:175–179.
39. Viacava P, Naccarato AG, Nardini V, et al. Breast carcinoma with osteoclast-like giant cells: immunohistochemical and ultrastructural study of a case and review of the literature. *Tumori* 1995;81:135–141.
40. Perez-Alonso P. Breast carcinoma with osteoclast-like giant cells diagnosed by fine-needle aspiration cytology. *Diagn Cytopathol* 2012;40:148–149.
41. Chilosi M, Bonetti F, Menestrina F, et al. Breast carcinoma with stromal multinucleated giant cells. *J Pathol* 1987;152:55–56.
42. Gupta RK, Wakefield SJ, Holloway LJ, et al. Immunocytochemical and ultrastructural study of the rare osteoclast-type carcinoma of the breast in a fine needle aspirate. *Acta Cytol* 1988;32:79–82.
43. Factor SM, Biempica L, Ratner I, et al. Carcinoma of the breast with multinucleated reactive stromal giant cells. A light and electron microscopic study of two cases. *Virchows Arch A Pathol Anat Histol* 1977;374:1–12.
44. Gjerdrum LM, Lauridsen MC, Sorensen FB. Breast carcinoma with osteoclast-like giant cells: morphological and ultrastructural studies of a case with review of the literature. *Breast* 2001;10:231–236.
45. Levin A, Rywlin AM, Tachmes P. Carcinoma of the breast with stromal epulis-like giant cells. *South Med J* 1981;74:889–891.
46. Vicandi B, Jimenez-Heffernan JA, Lopez-Ferrer P, et al. Fine needle aspiration cytology of mammary carcinoma with osteoclast-like giant cells. *Cytopathology* 2004;15:321–325.
47. Saimura M, Fukutomi T, Tsuda H, et al. Breast carcinoma with osteoclast-like giant cells: a case report and review of the Japanese literature. *Breast Cancer* 1999;6:121–126.

CHAPTER 24

Cystic Hypersecretory Carcinoma and Cystic Hypersecretory Hyperplasia

EDI BROGI

This variant of duct carcinoma first described in 1984 by Rosen and Scott[1,2] deserves separate discussion because of its unusual pathologic features. The majority of cases have been intraductal carcinomas. A benign proliferative lesion that resembles cystic hypersecretory carcinoma has been termed "cystic hypersecretory hyperplasia" (CHH).[2] At present, no study has evaluated the genetics and molecular alterations of cystic hypersecretory lesions.

CLINICAL PRESENTATION

Incidence, Age, and Imaging

Information about the incidence of cystic hypersecretory carcinoma is very limited because of its rarity and possible underreporting and/or misclassification as a benign lesion or ductal carcinoma *in situ* (DCIS) of no special type. The age distribution of cystic hypersecretory carcinoma is similar to that of breast carcinoma in general[3] with the youngest patient being 34 years old and the oldest thus far reported at 79 years.[2] The mean age in the largest series was 56 years.[2] All patients have been women, including a 40-year-old African American.[4] There are no reported familial genetic alterations or syndromes associated with cystic hypersecretory carcinoma, and no association with oral contraceptives or hormone replacement therapy has been described.

The presenting symptom has usually been a mass or other palpable abnormality. Nipple discharge is uncommon, but can be hemorrhagic.[5] A 48-year-old woman with a history of serous nipple discharge and a cystic mass was found to have cystic hypersecretory DCIS and Paget disease of the nipple.[6]

In cases of cystic hypersecretory carcinoma, mammography has yielded different findings. In one case with associated invasive carcinoma, it revealed "no discrete mass, but a 10-cm area of increased density with trabecular thickening that corresponded to the area of palpable concern."[4] Another lesion with associated invasive carcinoma appeared as a spiculated mass with multiple amorphous, rounded, or lucent-centered calcifications of variable size.[7] Similar calcifications were also noted in a 2.5-cm high-density mass that consisted mainly of cystic hypersecretory DCIS.[7] A "large tumor filling the upper outer quadrant" in a 50-year-old woman had "massive calcification" on mammography.[8] The mammography in a patient with cystic hypersecretory DCIS revealed "heterogeneous dense breast tissue with no definite abnormally increased density or microcalcifications" and sonography revealed "multiple small aggregated, anechoic cysts with good through transmission."[9] In one case, sonographic examination detected a decrease in the size of the cystic component of a complex cystic mass in the breast of a woman with cystic hypersecretory DCIS, but the lesion later grew in size, prompting excision.[10] The sonographic findings can be deceivingly benign appearing and simulate fibrocystic changes or intraductal papilloma.[9] Two patients with invasive cystic hypersecretory carcinoma were reported to have spiculated masses with calcifications on mammography.[11] No information on the magnetic resonance imaging (MRI) findings is available.

GROSS PATHOLOGY

The tumors have measured from 1 to 10 cm in diameter. Usually the lesion is firm, but not hard. It is visibly distinct from the surrounding breast parenchyma, but not sharply demarcated. The distinctive gross feature of cystic hypersecretory carcinoma is the presence of numerous cysts within the lesion (Fig. 24.1). Many of these tumors are a shade of brown or gray-brown that reflects the cyst contents. The cysts vary considerably in size, with the largest measuring up to 1.5 cm. Secretion within cysts has been described as sticky, mucinous, gelatinous, or as resembling thyroid colloid.

Although cystic hypersecretory lesions have a distinctive gross appearance, it is usually not possible to distinguish intraductal cystic hypersecretory carcinoma from CHH on gross inspection. An invasive component associated with cystic hypersecretory carcinoma typically produces a distinct, solid mass.

MICROSCOPIC PATHOLOGY

Microscopically, all cystic hypersecretory lesions have cysts containing eosinophilic secretion that bears a striking resemblance to thyroid colloid (Fig. 24.2). The secretion is homogeneous and usually virtually acellular. It often retracts from

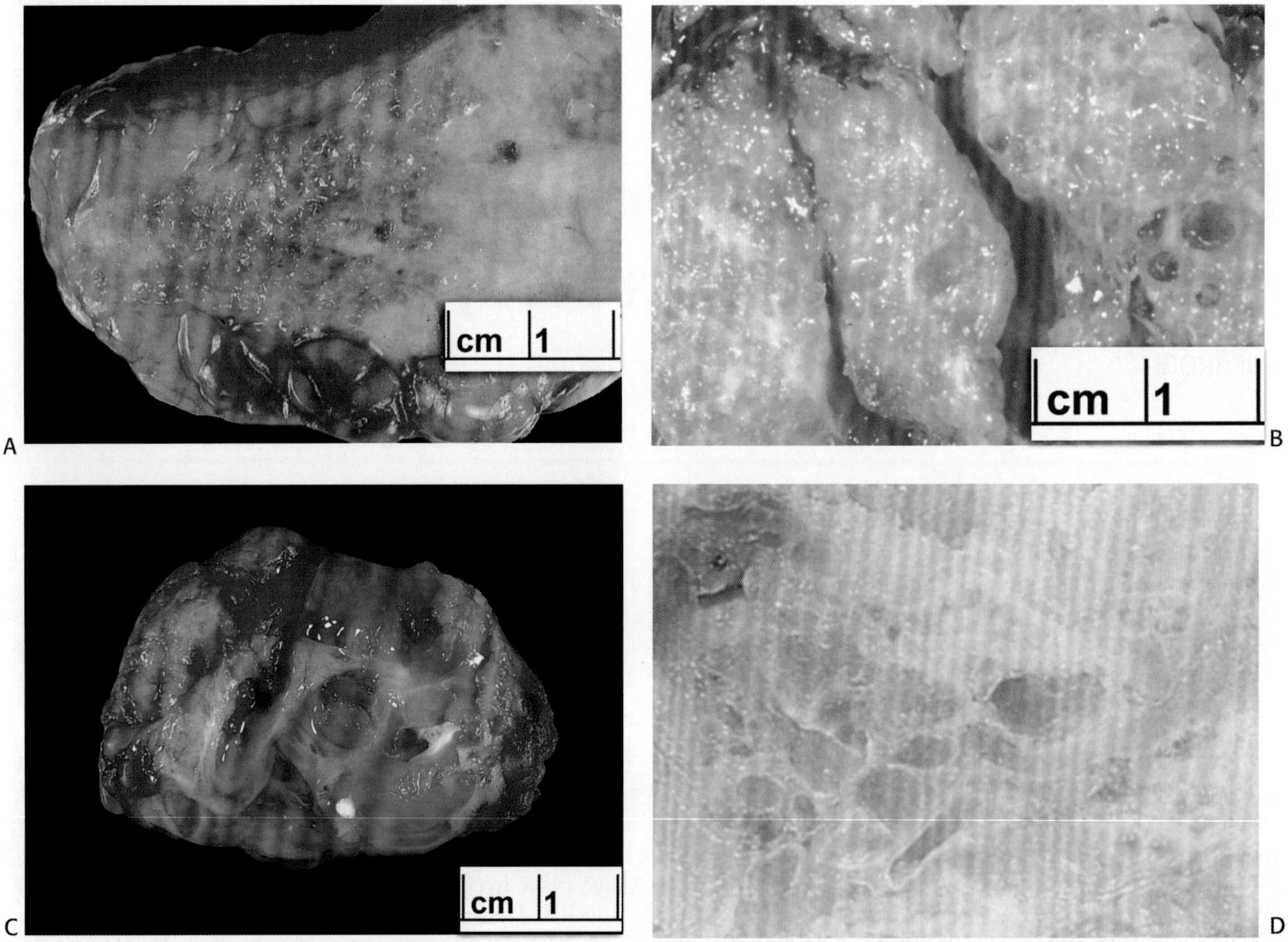

FIG. 24.1. ***Cystic hypersecretory carcinoma.*** **A:** The lesion is a discrete but not circumscribed mass with many cysts. **B:** Cysts filled with tan secretion that resembles thyroid colloid. **C:** Some of the cysts are larger than 1.0 cm. **D:** A fixed specimen that has been dissected to reveal numerous cysts.

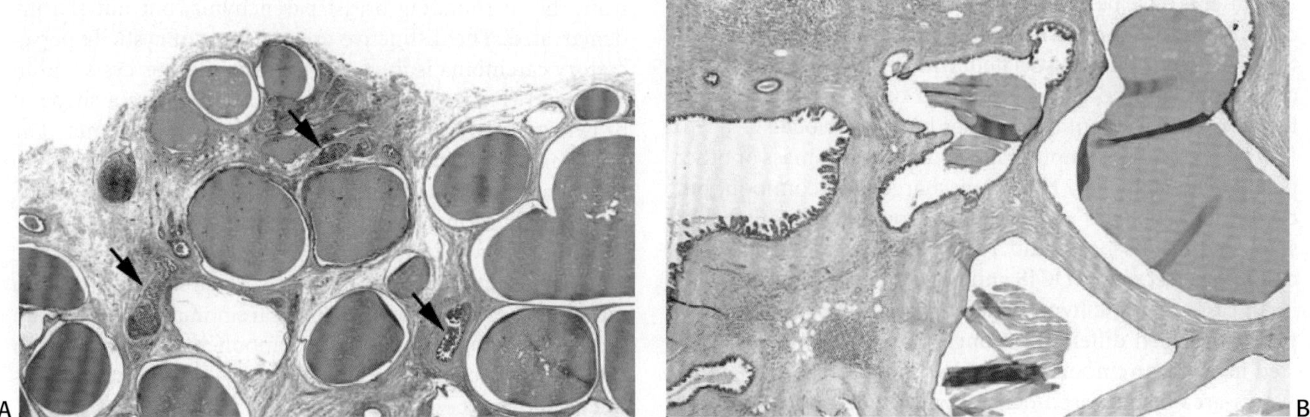

FIG. 24.2. ***Cystic hypersecretory carcinoma in a background of cystic hypersecretory change.*** **A:** Most of the lesion in this photograph is composed of cysts lined by flat epithelium characteristic of cystic hypersecretory change. The secretion closely resembles thyroid colloid. A few ducts with micropapillary DCIS are present (*arrows*). **B:** Micropapillary DCIS is present on the *left*.

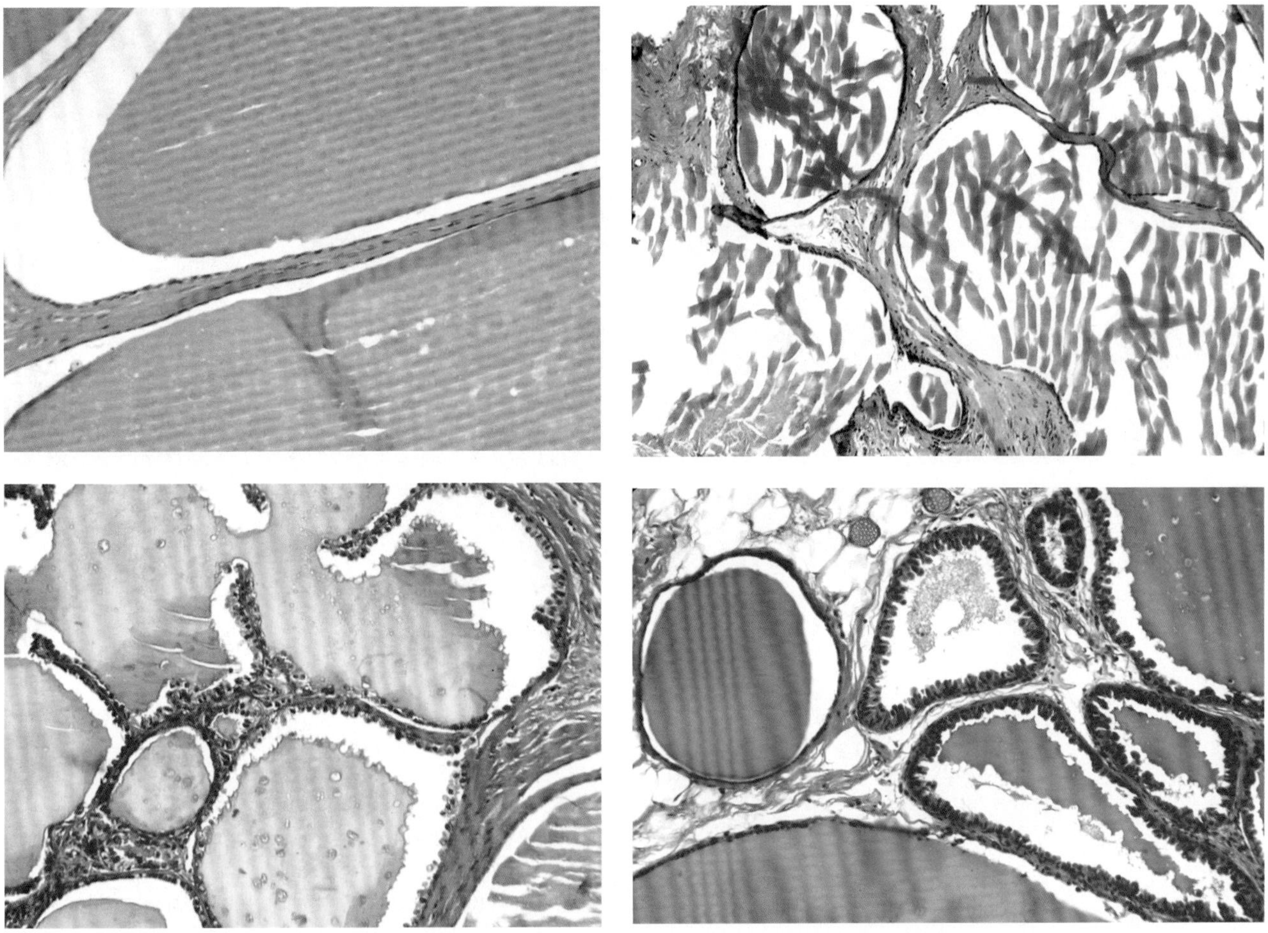

FIG. 24.3. ***Secretion in cystic hypersecretory lesions.*** **A:** These cysts are lined by flat epithelium. Note the wavy appearance and retraction of the secretion. **B:** This secretion displays exaggerated cracks as a result of fragmentation during histologic preparation. **C:** The hyperplastic epithelium has a hobnail appearance. Note the scalloped edges of the retracted and pockmarked secretion. **D:** Hyperplastic columnar epithelium lines a few cysts. The colloid-like secretion is homogeneous and densely eosinophilic.

the surrounding epithelium to create a smooth or scalloped margin that reflects the extent of epithelial proliferation. Defects in the secretion sometimes consist of folds, linear cracks, or small punched-out holes (Fig. 24.3). Necrosis and calcifications are not seen, but histiocytes are occasionally present in the secretion (Fig. 24.4). There are no appreciable differences in the character of the secretion between cystic hypersecretory carcinoma and CHH. Disruption of cysts results in spillage of cyst contents, eliciting an intense inflammatory reaction consisting of lymphocytes and histiocytes.

Cystic Hypersecretory Intraductal Carcinoma

In cystic hypersecretory DCIS, the epithelium of involved cysts and ducts grows as micropapillary intraductal carcinoma (Fig. 24.5). In any one case, a spectrum of epithelial patterns is encountered, ranging from short, knobby epithelial tufts to complex branching fronds that may extend across the duct lumen (Fig. 24.6). However, the so-called Roman arch, or bridging pattern, frequently seen in other forms of micropapillary DCIS, is uncommon in these lesions. DCIS with a solid pattern can also occur (Fig. 24.6). Ducts with DCIS may not contain the characteristic colloid-like secretion.

Cytologically, the cells that comprise this type of DCIS usually have crowded and overlapping hyperchromatic

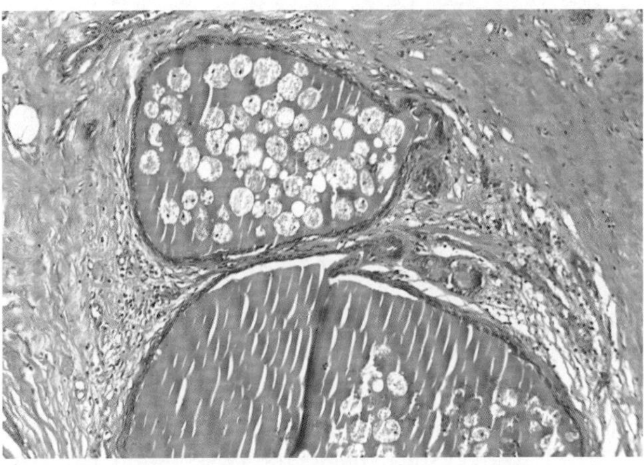

FIG. 24.4. ***Cystic hypersecretory change with histiocytes.***

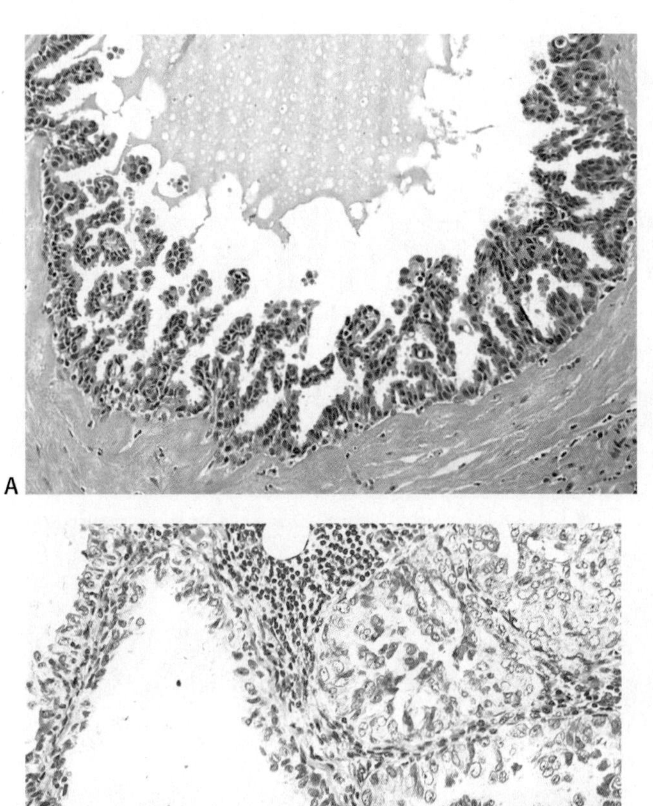

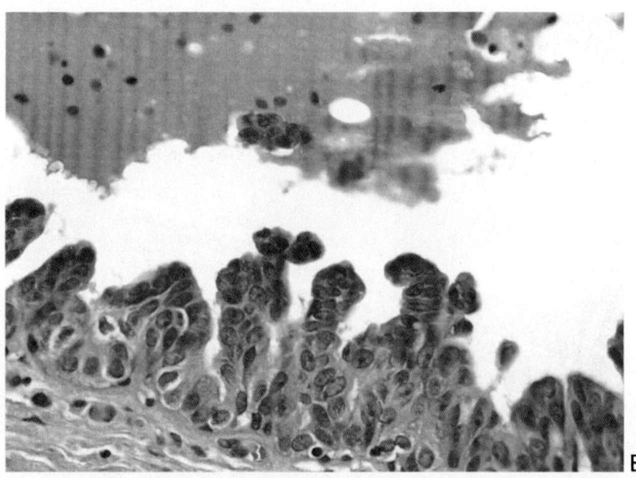

FIG. 24.5. *Cystic hypersecretory ductal carcinoma in situ.* **A,B:** Cystic hypersecretory DCIS, micropapillary. **C:** Cystic hypersecretory micropapillary carcinoma with vesicular nuclei.

nuclei and scant cytoplasm. In a series of 10 cases,[12] the nuclear grade was intermediate in half and high in the other half, and the microscopic tumor size ranged from 0.2 to 2.7 cm. Intranuclear inclusions and nuclear grooves may be observed. High-grade lesions exhibit more pronounced mitotic activity. There is no secretion within the cytoplasm, but frayed, irregular cell borders and apical cytoplasmic blebs are consistent with some degree of secretory activity in most foci of cystic hypersecretory DCIS. Calcifications were present in 7/10 (70%) cases in one series.[12]

Cystic Hypersecretory Change and Hyperplasia

Many of the cysts in cystic hypersecretory lesions are lined by inconspicuous flat cells or a single layer of cuboidal to columnar cells (Figs. 24.3 and 24.4). When this is the only

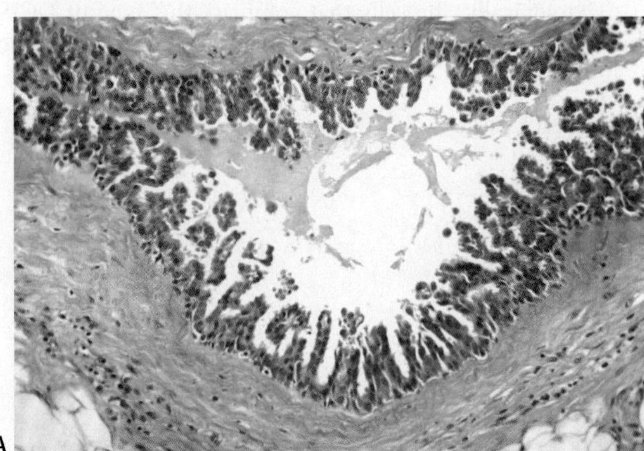

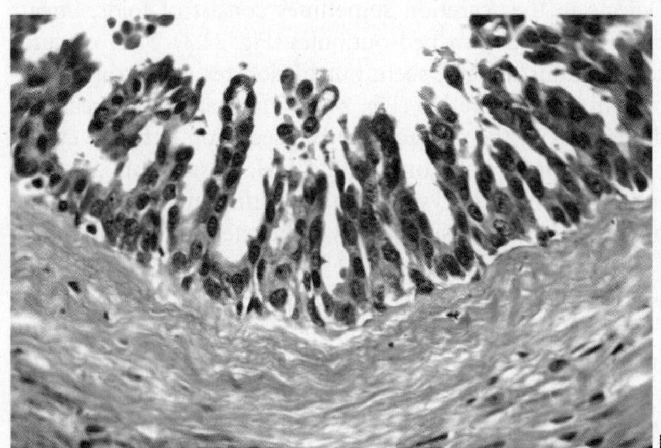

FIG. 24.6. *Cystic hypersecretory intraductal carcinoma.* **A,B:** Tall micropapillary fronds with intermediate nuclear grade. **C:** Micropapillary DCIS with high nuclear grade. **D,E:** Clear cell lesions with cystic hypersecretory secretion. **F,G:** Two examples of solid DCIS with cystic hypersecretory secretion.

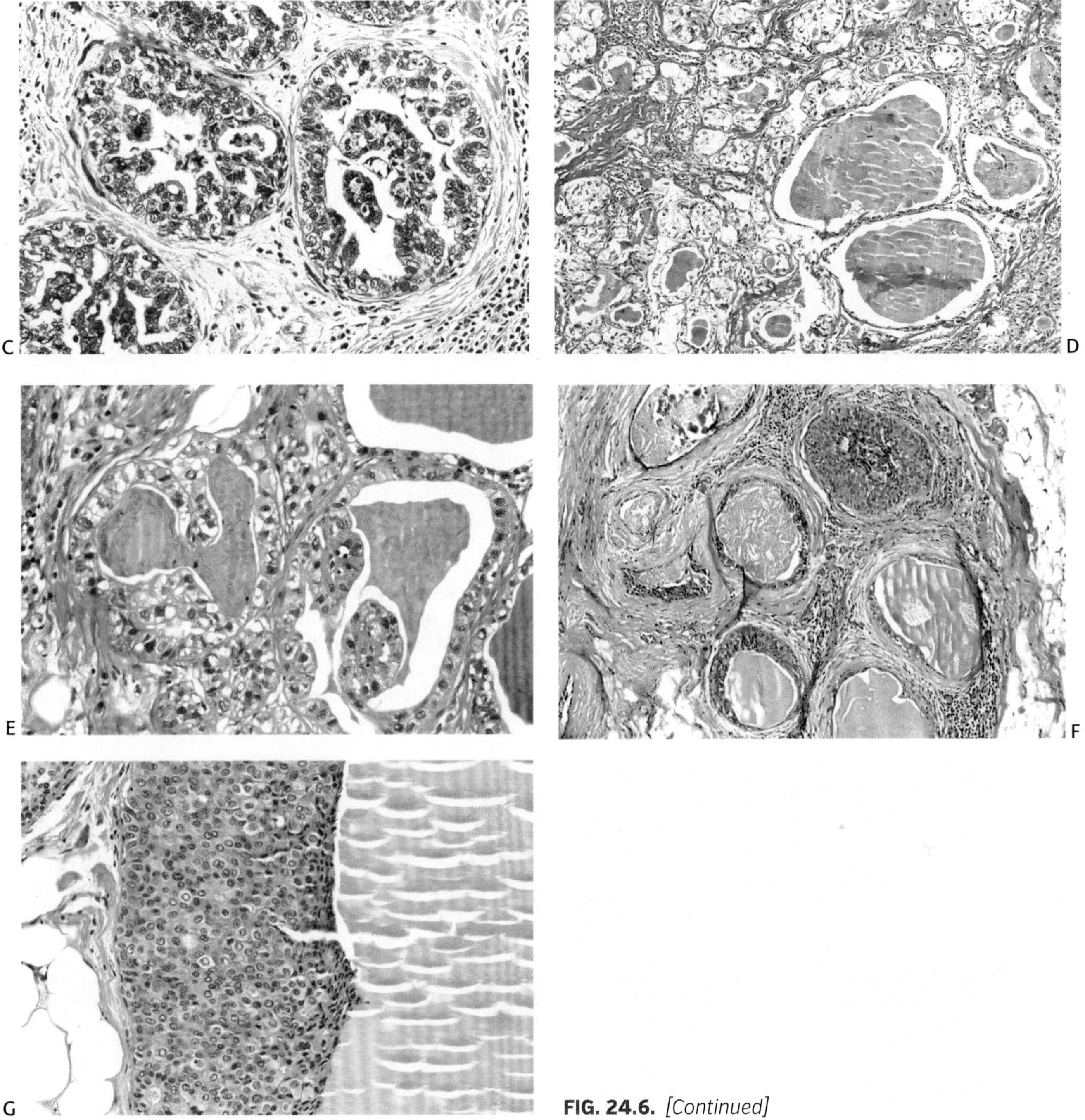

FIG. 24.6. *[Continued]*

epithelial pattern, the lesion is referred to as "cystic hypersecretory change." Generally, the cells in such lesions have uniform cytologically bland nuclei and inconspicuous cytoplasm. In CHH, the cells are columnar, often with apical blebs, but no atypia. CHH and cystic hypersecretory change are usually intimately admixed[2] (Fig. 24.3). Atypical features in this setting include epithelial crowding, hyperchromasia, rare mitotic figures, and enlarged nuclei with few nucleoli. Crowding of epithelial cells in CHH is an indication of atypical hyperplasia (Fig. 24.7).

The mammary lobules adjacent to cystic hypersecretory lesions often exhibit hypersecretory change with accumulation of intraluminal secretion (Fig. 24.8). This lobular abnormality may occur as an isolated finding in the absence of a fully developed cystic hypersecretory lesion, an observation that suggests that the process may originate in such foci.

Cystic hypersecretory change and hyperplasia can sometimes be subtle. On more than one occasion, an incompletely excised lesion has been misclassified as cystic disease,[1,2] with the true nature of the process becoming apparent when the lesion recurred.

Associated Invasive Carcinoma

An invasive carcinoma adjacent to cystic hypersecretory DCIS can also have hypersecretory features, although the

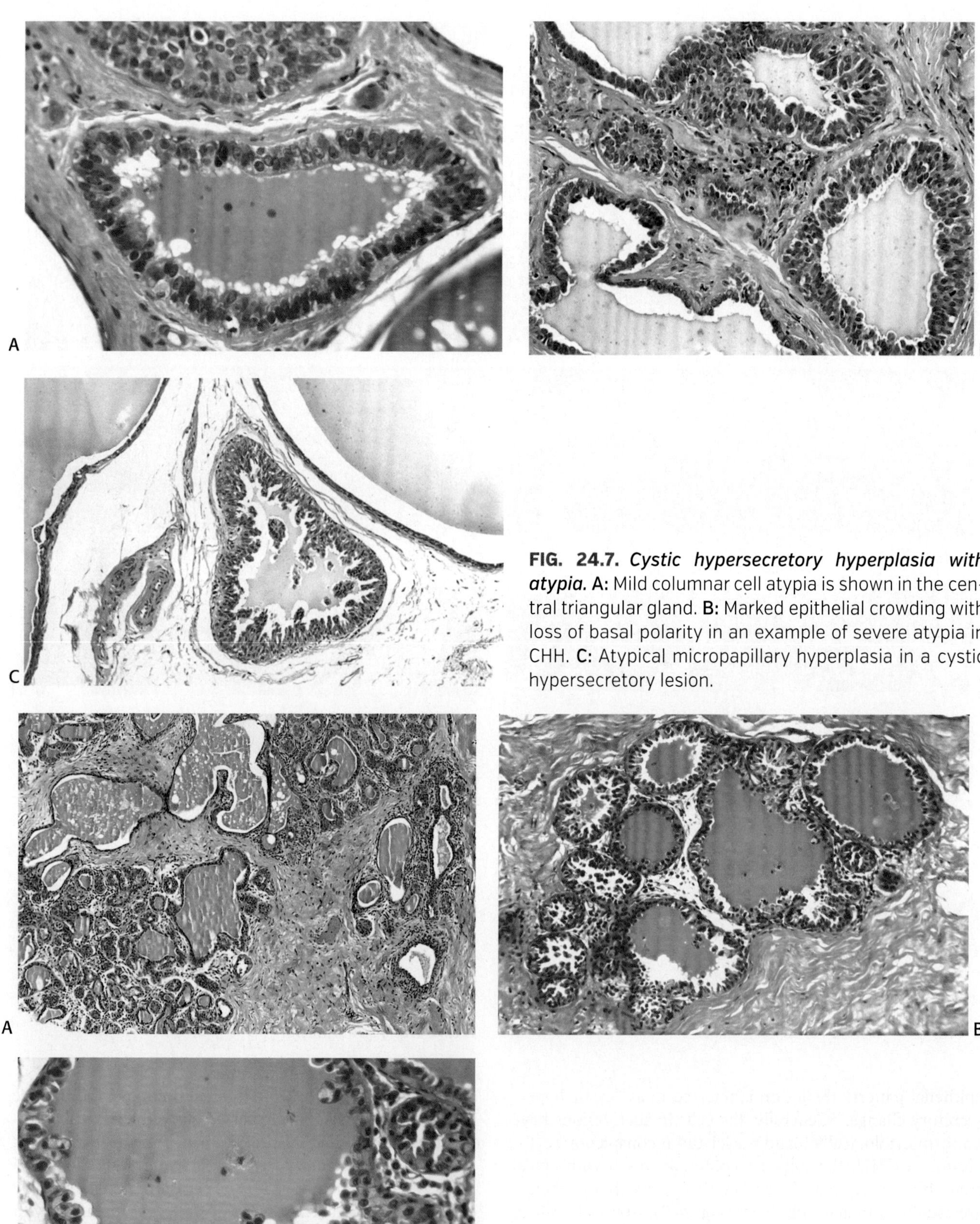

FIG. 24.7. ***Cystic hypersecretory hyperplasia with atypia.*** **A:** Mild columnar cell atypia is shown in the central triangular gland. **B:** Marked epithelial crowding with loss of basal polarity in an example of severe atypia in CHH. **C:** Atypical micropapillary hyperplasia in a cystic hypersecretory lesion.

FIG. 24.8. ***Hypersecretory change in lobules.*** The illustrations present lobular changes in patients with cystic hypersecretory carcinoma. **A:** Lobular glands and ducts dilated with secretion that exhibits typical pockmarks and parallel cracks. **B,C:** Atypical CHH extending into lobules.

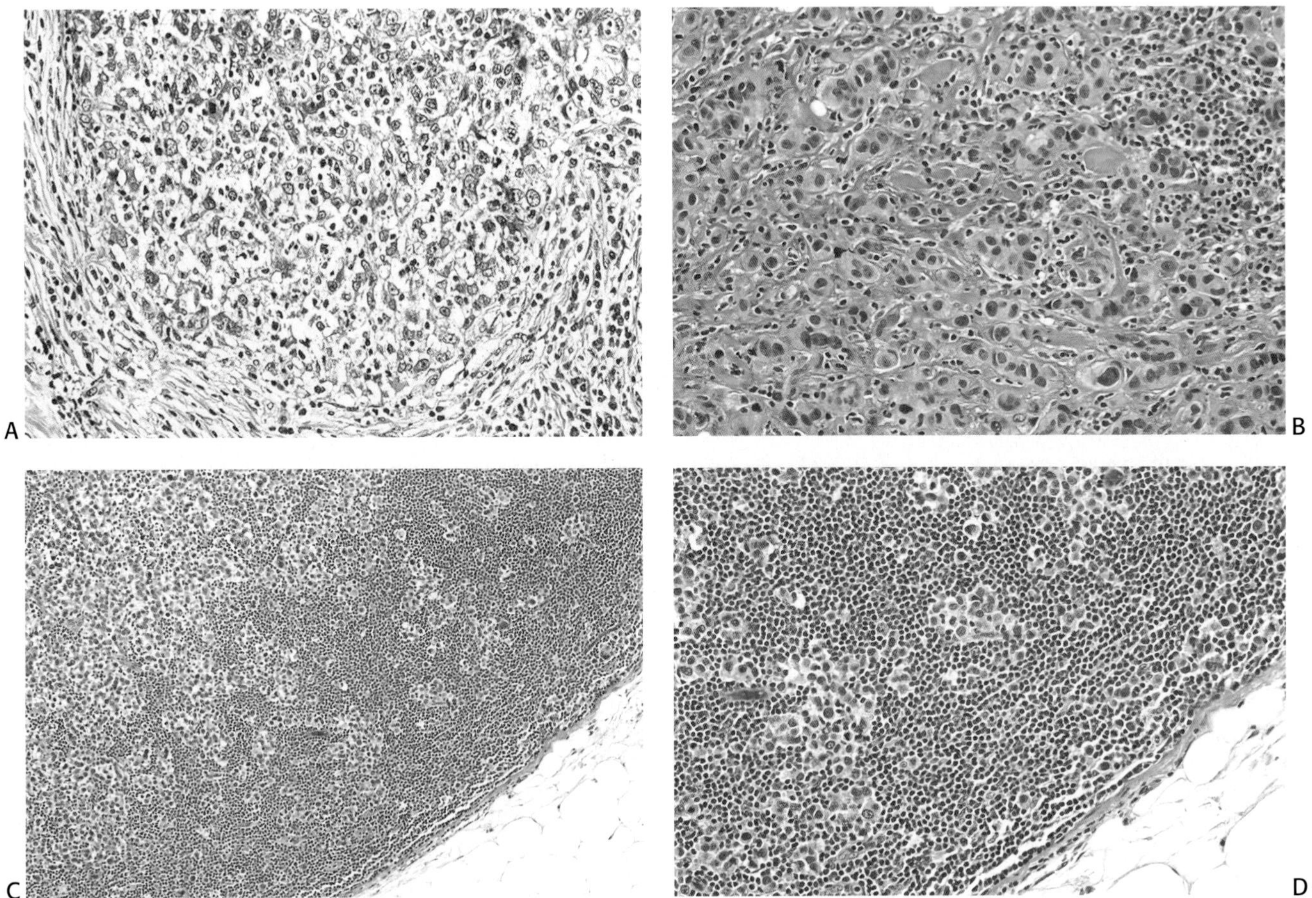

FIG. 24.9. ***Cystic hypersecretory carcinoma, invasive.*** **A:** Poorly differentiated invasive duct carcinoma with a lymphocytic infiltrate in the stroma. **B:** Magnified view of the invasive component in another case showing hyperchromatic and smudgy nuclei. A limited lymphocytic infiltrate is also noted. **C,D:** The ALN metastasis from the carcinoma shown in (**B**).

cytomorphology is rarely distinctive. Almost all invasive carcinomas thus far encountered in this setting have been poorly differentiated ductal type with a solid growth pattern[5,9] (Fig. 24.9). Nuclei of invasive carcinoma cells may have a clear vacuolated appearance, similar to the nuclei observed in papillary thyroid carcinoma. Lymphatic tumor emboli may be present in the vicinity of the invasive tumor.[5,13] Scattered lymphocytes are often admixed with invasive carcinoma[5] (Fig. 24.9). Light microscopy has disclosed little or no secretory activity within the carcinoma cells. Metastatic foci in the axillary lymph nodes (ALNs) of two patients had cystic elements that contained eosinophilic secretion.[2]

Rosen encountered a patient with invasive lobular carcinoma in a breast that also harbored cystic hypersecretory DCIS (Fig. 24.10). Takeuchi et al.[14] have reported a case with coexisting invasive lobular carcinoma and CHH. Another patient developed invasive lobular carcinoma of the contralateral breast 10 years after ipsilateral mastectomy for invasive cystic hypersecretory carcinoma.[3]

Associated Benign Epithelial Lesions

Pregnancy-like hyperplasia (PLH) (Fig. 24.11) sometimes coexists with CHH, and aspects of the two conditions seem to overlap when this occurs.[14–17] Secretion found in a cystic hypersecretory lesion may be found in glands formed by epithelium with the appearance of PLH. This convergence is usually marked by cytologic and structural atypia that may be severe. Rarely, the proliferative and cytologic abnormalities warrant a diagnosis of cystic hypersecretory DCIS that has features of pregnancy-like change with especially pronounced cytoplasmic vacuolization. Takeuchi et al.[14] found PLH merging with CHH in the breast of a woman with coexisting invasive lobular carcinoma. The relationship between PLH and cystic hypersecretory alterations has not been fully elucidated (see Chapter 1 for additional information about PLH).

ELECTRON MICROSCOPY

Electron microscopy has been performed in three cases.[2,5,8] The involved ductules were lined by epithelial cells surrounded by myoepithelial cells. Ductular epithelial cells were largely devoid of surface microvilli. No polarization of secretory vesicles or inclusions was seen. Large secretory granules that contained sparse, fine granular material were limited to the basal cytoplasm. Ductular lumens contained amorphous or finely granular material. These ultrastructural findings

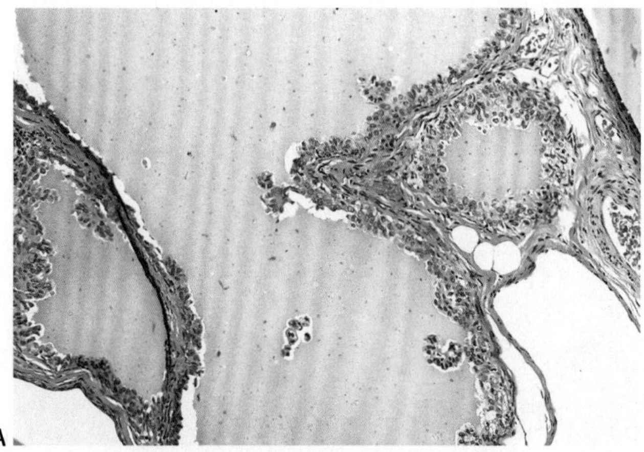

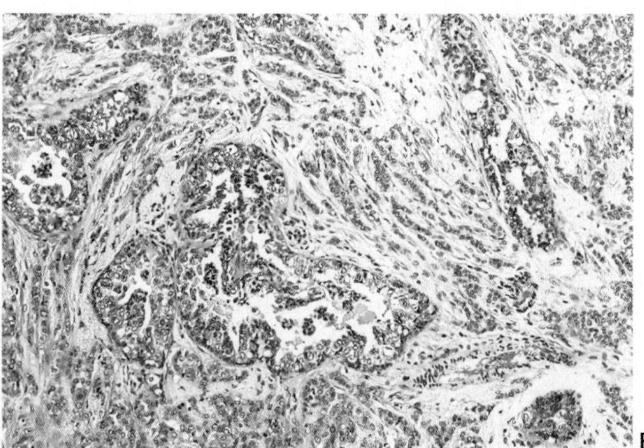

FIG. 24.10. ***Cystic hypersecretory carcinoma and invasive lobular carcinoma.*** **A:** Cystic hypersecretory micropapillary intraductal carcinoma. **B:** Another area in the tumor where papillary intraductal carcinoma is surrounded and partly overgrown by invasive lobular carcinoma.

differ appreciably from those seen in secretory carcinoma that features abundant intracytoplasmic secretory granules as well as intracytoplasmic glandular lumens. Mucinous carcinoma also differs ultrastructurally from cystic hypersecretory carcinoma in having abundant extracellular mucin and intracytoplasmic mucinogen granules.

CYTOLOGY

Cystic hypersecretory lesions can be diagnosed in a fine-needle aspiration (FNA) specimen if the characteristic secretion is recognized.[11,13,18] The secretory material forms dense masses that duplicate the appearance of this material in histologic sections (Fig. 24.12). Epithelial cells in clusters and individually may be found amidst the secretory material. Lesions with DCIS usually produce papillary clusters of tumor cells in an FNA specimen. The differential diagnosis includes mucinous carcinoma and mucocele-like lesions (MLLs).

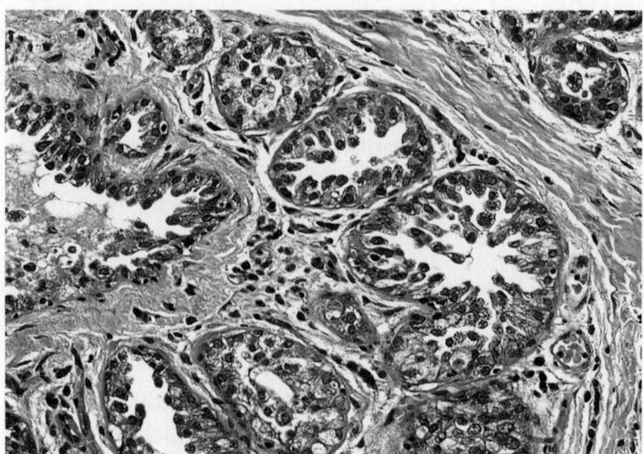

FIG. 24.11. ***Pregnancy-like hyperplasia.*** This intralobular lesion lacks cystic hypersecretory secretion. Note the vacuolated cytoplasm and apical nuclear extrusion. The florid micropapillary structure seen here is atypical and may coexist with cystic hypersecretory intraductal carcinoma.

IMMUNOHISTOCHEMISTRY

Estrogen receptor (ER) and progesterone receptor (PR) expression in cystic hypersecretory DCIS and associated invasive carcinoma is variable. In a series of 10 DCIS studied by D'Alfonso et al.,[12] 4/10 cases were ER and PR positive, 4/10 were ER positive but PR negative, and 2/10 were ER and PR negative. All DCIS cases were human epidermal growth factor 2 (HER2) negative. Another series and a case report also found a variable receptor profile.[4,5] In particular, three of five cases reported by Skalova et al.[5] were HER2 positive. In the same series,[5] 4/5 carcinomas were reactive for androgen receptor (AR), but only 3/10 (30%) cases studied by D'Alfonso et al.[12] were AR-positive. Positivity for p53 varies.[5] The basal markers cytokeratin (CK) 5, CK14, and epidermal growth factor receptor (EGFR) were negative in 8/10 cases in one series,[12] and only two tumors showed positive immunoreactivity for either CK5 or EGFR. Positive reactions for carcinoembryonic antigen (CEA), α-lactalbumin, and periodic acid–Schiff (PAS) (Fig. 24.13) have been observed in the cyst contents that are

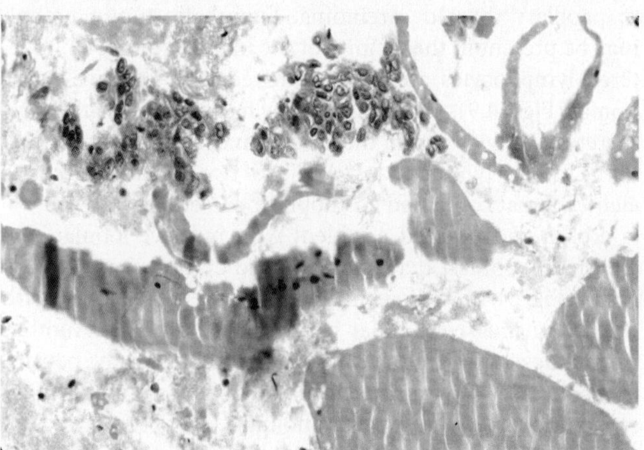

FIG. 24.12. ***Cystic hypersecretory carcinoma, fine-needle aspiration.*** The specimen consists of dislodged secretion with characteristic cracks and fragments of papillary carcinomatous epithelium.

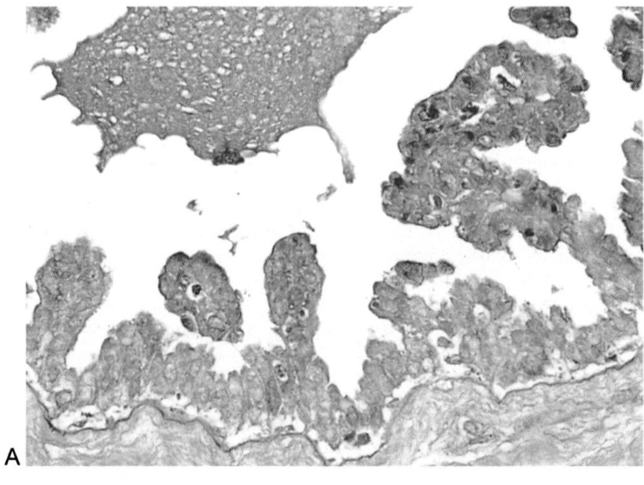

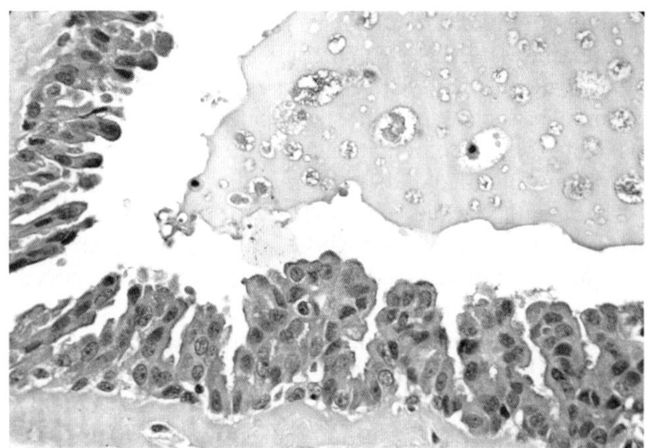

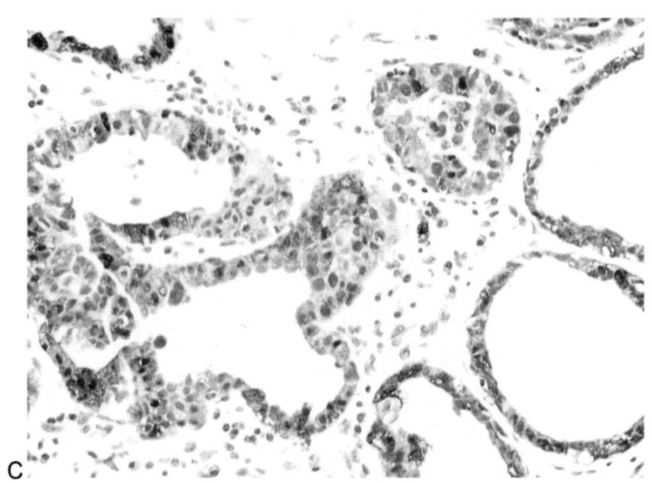

FIG. 24.13. ***Cystic hypersecretory lesions, histochemistry and immunoreactivity.*** **A:** A positive reaction with the PAS reagent that persisted after diastase treatment in cystic hypersecretory carcinoma (PAS-diastase). **B:** Faint mucicarmine staining is shown in the cells. Stronger staining is evident in vacuoles in the secretion. **C:** Immunoreactivity for S-100 decorates the nuclei and cytoplasm of cystic hypersecretory hyperplastic cells.

consistently negative for thyroglobulin. The DCIS may also exhibit focal diastase-resistant PAS reactivity and faint mucicarmine staining (Fig. 24.13). Immunoreactivity for S-100 (Fig. 24.13) and α-lactalbumin has been observed.

NEEDLE CORE BIOPSY

Excisional biopsy is required if CHH is present in a needle core biopsy specimen, even in the absence of cytologic atypia, because it is not possible to exclude adjacent carcinoma on the basis of such a limited sample. In a series of 67 benign needle core biopsies with diagnosis of secretory and/or hypersecretory changes, Galman et al.[17] found three cases with cystic hypersecretory changes and/or hyperplasia. Atypia was present in the needle core biopsy specimen obtained from an area of indeterminate calcifications in the breast of a *BRCA2* germline mutation carrier. Another needle core biopsy sampled mammographic calcifications in a woman with strong family history of breast carcinoma. In the latter case, cystic hypersecretory alterations merged with PLH with no evidence of atypia. In both of the foregoing cases, the target calcifications were associated with cystic hypersecretory changes and/or hyperplasia. The third needle core biopsy targeted a palpable mass, and the specimen contained focal cystic hypersecretory change adjacent to stromal fibrosis. CHH without atypia was present in the risk-reducing mastectomy specimen from the *BRCA2* germline mutation carrier; no follow-up information was available for the other two women. Shin and Rosen[15] identified CHH merging with PLH in the needle core biopsies from four women 40 to 52 years old. In three women, the needle core biopsy sampled a mass lesion. Galactorrhea was reported as the reason for biopsy in the fourth patient. CHH was atypical in three cases, two of which also contained calcifications. One of the women with epithelial atypia underwent bilateral mastectomy that showed similar findings. The other three women had no additional procedures.

TREATMENT AND PROGNOSIS

The clinical course of cystic hypersecretory DCIS has thus far not differed from that of other forms of DCIS. There have been only rare recurrences in women treated by mastectomy after a mean follow-up of 8 years, extending in one case to 23 years.[2,5] All had negative lymph nodes. One patient who was treated by mastectomy for DCIS developed invasive carcinoma in the surgical scar 18 months later,[5] and breast recurrences have been reported after lumpectomy. Several women with invasive cystic hypersecretory carcinoma have had metastases in ALNs.[2,5] In the series by Guerry et al.,[2] one patient presented with bone metastases and locally advanced carcinoma associated with cystic hypersecretory DCIS. She was treated with a combination of chemotherapy and radiation therapy but died of disease 9 months after diagnosis.

Therapeutic options for patients with cystic hypersecretory carcinoma are similar to those available to women with other forms of ductal carcinoma. Mastectomy has proved to be curative for most women with cystic hypersecretory DCIS. Follow-up information on the rare patients with cystic hypersecretory DCIS treated by lumpectomy with or without adjuvant radiotherapy[2,5,16] is very limited. Few patients have received adjuvant hormonal therapy.[16] A 78-year-old patient with cystic hypersecretory DCIS treated by surgical excision developed recurrent disease at 3 years of follow-up.[5] When invasive carcinoma is present, sentinel lymph node (SLN) mapping should be performed. Adjuvant chemotherapy should also be considered in view of the poorly differentiated character of the invasive tumors thus far encountered.

The finding of areas of CHH, sometimes with atypia, associated with cystic hypersecretory DCIS suggests that these processes are related, but definitive evidence of progression through these stages has not yet been presented. Review of prior biopsies from women later found to have cystic hypersecretory DCIS has disclosed various lesions, including seemingly unrelated common proliferative changes, CHH, and cystic hypersecretory carcinoma. Follow-up of eight patients with CHH revealed subsequent breast carcinoma in two cases.[2] One woman developed a fatal contralateral invasive duct carcinoma that lacked cystic hypersecretory features. The other patient had DCIS separate from CHH in a biopsy, and residual CHH in the mastectomy specimen. Bogomoletz[19] described a 55-year-old woman with no evidence of disease 6 years after excisional biopsy of a 7-cm example of CHH.

REFERENCES

1. Rosen PP, Scott M. Cystic hypersecretory duct carcinoma of the breast. *Am J Surg Pathol* 1984;8:31–41.
2. Guerry P, Erlandson RA, Rosen PP. Cystic hypersecretory hyperplasia and cystic hypersecretory duct carcinoma of the breast. Pathology, therapy, and follow-up of 39 patients. *Cancer* 1988;61:1611–1620.
3. Herrmann ME, McClatchey KD, Siziopikou KP. Invasive cystic hypersecretory ductal carcinoma of breast: a case report and review of the literature. *Arch Pathol Lab Med* 1999;123:1108–1110.
4. Resetkova E, Padula A, Albarraccin CT, et al. Pathologic quiz case: a large, ill-defined cystic breast mass. Invasive cystic hypersecretory duct carcinoma. *Arch Pathol Lab Med* 2005;129:e79–e80.
5. Skalova A, Ryska A, Kajo K, et al. Cystic hypersecretory carcinoma: rare and poorly recognized variant of intraductal carcinoma of the breast. Report of five cases. *Histopathology* 2005;46:43–49.
6. Sahoo S, Gopal P, Roland L, et al. Cystic hypersecretory carcinoma of the breast with paget disease of the nipple: a diagnostic challenge. *Int J Surg Pathol* 2008;16:208–212.
7. Park JM, Seo MR. Cystic hypersecretory duct carcinoma of the breast: report of two cases. *Clin Radiol* 2002;57:312–315.
8. Cserni G, Viragh S. Immunohistochemical and ultrastructural analysis of a mammary cystic hypersecretory carcinoma. *Pathol Oncol Res* 1997;3:287–292.
9. Park C, Jung JI, Lee AW, et al. Sonographic findings in a patient with cystic hypersecretory duct carcinoma of the breast. *J Clin Ultrasound* 2004;32:29–32.
10. Song SW, Whang IY, Chang ED. Cystic hypersecretory ductal carcinoma of the breast: a rare cause of cystic breast mass. *Jpn J Radiol* 2011;29:660–662.
11. Kim MK, Kwon GY, Gong GY. Fine needle aspiration cytology of cystic hypersecretory carcinoma of the breast. A case report. *Acta Cytol* 1997;41:892–896.
12. D'Alfonso TM, Liu Y-F, Shin SJ. Immunohistochemical characterization of cystic hypersecretory carcinoma. *Mod Pathol* 2013;26:35A.
13. Lee WY, Cheng L, Chang TW. Diagnosing invasive cystic hypersecretory duct carcinoma of the breast with fine needle aspiration cytology. A case report. *Acta Cytol* 1999;43:273–276.
14. Takeuchi T, Tsuzuki H, Numoto S, et al. Coexistence of pregnancy-like and cystic hypersecretory hyperplasia with invasive lobular carcinoma. *Onkologie* 2011;34:448–450.
15. Shin SJ, Rosen PP. Pregnancy-like (pseudolactational) hyperplasia: a primary diagnosis in mammographically detected lesions of the breast and its relationship to cystic hypersecretory hyperplasia. *Am J Surg Pathol* 2000;24:1670–1674.
16. Shin SJ, Rosen PP. Carcinoma arising from preexisting pregnancy-like and cystic hypersecretory hyperplasia lesions of the breast: a clinicopathologic study of 9 patients. *Am J Surg Pathol* 2004;28:789–793.
17. Galman L, Catalano J, Cordero A, et al. Secretory and cystic hypersecretory changes at breast core needle biopsy: clinical, radiologic and pathologic findings in 67 cases. *Mod Pathol* 2013;26:41A.
18. Colandrea JM, Shmookler BM, O'Dowd GJ, et al. Cystic hypersecretory duct carcinoma of the breast. Report of a case with fine-needle aspiration. *Arch Pathol Lab Med* 1988;112:560–563.
19. Bogomoletz WV. Cystic hypersecretory hyperplasia of the breast. A rare diagnosis in breast pathology. *Ann Pathol* 1994;14:131–132.

CHAPTER 25

Adenoid Cystic Carcinoma

EDI BROGI

The term "cylindroma," used interchangeably with "adenoid cystic carcinoma" (AdCC), was proposed by Billroth,[1] who concluded that the tumor was composed of entwined cylinders of stroma and epithelial cells. Ewing[2] mentioned AdCC of the salivary glands, and this term was applied in 1945 to tumors of the breast by Geschickter,[3] referring to lesions he classified as "adenocystic basal cell carcinoma." Three examples of mammary AdCC were cited by Foote and Stewart[4] in 1946. Two decades later, Galloway et al.[5] at the Mayo Clinic described the first series of mammary AdCCs and reviewed 12 others previously reported.

CLINICAL PRESENTATION

Incidence

AdCC can arise in many organs. It is most commonly found in major and minor salivary glands, and is one of the least frequent forms of primary mammary carcinoma. Only 22 cases of AdCC were recorded among nearly 28,000 patients with breast carcinoma included in the Kaiser Permanente Northern California Registry database.[6] The California Cancer Registry from 1988 to 2006[7] included 244 cases of mammary AdCC, representing 0.058% of all breast carcinomas in the same period. Review of data from nine registry areas in the Surveillance Epidemiology and End Results (SEER) program for 1977 to 2006 yielded 338 women with AdCC with an incidence rate of 0.92 per one million person-years.[8] The incidence rate was constant during the 30-year period.

Age, Gender, and Ethnicity

AdCC occurs in adult women throughout the age distribution of mammary carcinoma, with patient age ranging between 19 and 97 years.[7–17] The mean or median age varies from 50 to 63 years in various studies. In a series of 61 cases treated between 1980 and 2007 at 16 centers that are part of the Rare Cancer Network Study,[18] the median age at diagnosis was 59 years (range 28 to 94). In three studies, 70%,[18] 82.5%,[8] and 96%[19] of patients with AdCC were postmenopausal women. Most (82% to 87%) women with AdCC are White.[7,16,18] Two studies[7,18] found that 6% of women with AdCC were Black. In the study by Thompson et al.,[7] 5.7% of AdCC occurred in Asian/Pacific Islanders and 4.4% in Hispanic women. Isolated examples have been encountered in men[20–22] and in adolescents[17] (Fig. 25.1). Eight AdCCs constituted 1% of 759 primary carcinomas of the male breast in one series.[23] Cutaneous AdCC has been reported in the periareolar region of a 35-year-old man.[24] No specific association with familial syndromes, including familial cylindromatosis and multiple familial trichoepitheliomas (Brooke–Spiegler syndrome), has been described.

Presenting Symptoms

AdCC presents as a palpable, discrete, firm mass in about 80% of cases.[18] Pain[18,25,26] or tenderness[26] is described in some cases. These symptoms have not been specifically correlated with the histologic finding of perineural invasion. Pain in the affected breast was reported by 14% of patients in one series.[18] Skin dimpling, ulceration, and peau d'orange have been reported in patients with superficial or large lesions. Nipple discharge is rarely a presenting symptom[14] despite the fact that AdCC occurs with notable frequency centrally or in the subareolar part of the breast.[8,27] Rarely, AdCC arising in the nipple can be associated with Paget disease (Fig. 25.2). The most frequent sites of AdCC are the upper outer quadrant of the breast[8] and the retroareolar region.[8,27,28]

Most patients report that their tumor was detected shortly before seeking medical attention, but intervals of 9,[14,27] 10,[29,30] and 15[9] years have been described. The median duration in one series was 24 months, and six tumors were present for a year or more before diagnosis.[14]

The left and right breasts are equally affected,[8] but there is no predilection for AdCC to develop bilaterally.[8] Most tumors are unifocal, and only rare tumors consist of two[18,31] or more distinct foci.[18] In patients with AdCC, the frequency of subsequent carcinoma in either breast or of a solid malignant tumor at a nonmammary site is not greater than expected in the general population.[8]

Radiology

Mammography of clinically palpable tumors reveals a well-defined lobulated mass or an ill-defined lesion.[27,32,33] A mammographic spiculated mass can also be observed.[26] Only 18% of cases in the series by Khanfir et al.[18] were detected by mammography. The mammograms of 8 of the 10 cases studied by Glazebrook et al.[33] were abnormal. The AdCC

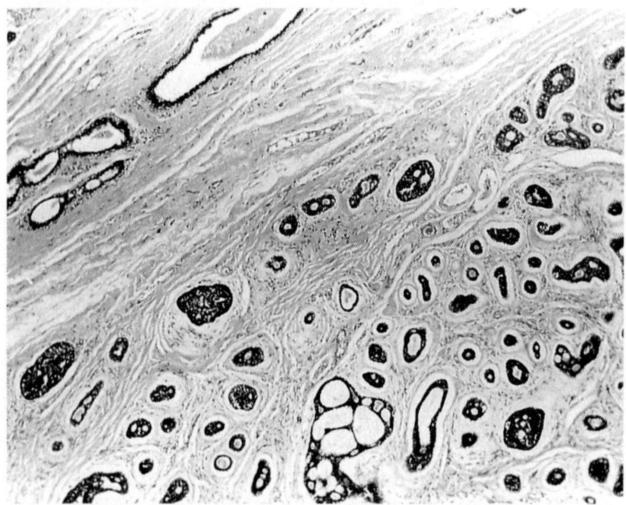

FIG. 25.1. ***Adenoid cystic carcinoma, child.*** This tumor arose in the breast of a 13-year-old boy. Juvenile breast ducts are visible in the *upper left corner*.

appeared as an irregular or lobular mass with microlobulated or indistinct margins in four of eight (50%) cases, a subtle architectural distortion in two of eight (12.5%), and as an asymmetric density in another two of eight (12.5%) cases. Two of the 10 (12.5%) AdCCs were mammographically undetected. None of the tumors had calcifications, a rare finding in AdCC. In some instances, the mammogram was reportedly negative.[14,27] The sonographic appearance is that of a heterogeneous or hypoechoic mass.[26,33] One tumor presented as an 8-mm hypoechoic nodule suggestive of an intramammary lymph node.[34] Eight of nine tumors studied sonographically by Glazebrook et al.[33] appeared as irregularly shaped hypoechoic or heterogeneous masses, oriented parallel to the skin, with no echogenic halo or posterior shadowing. Doppler sonography detected only minimal flow signal

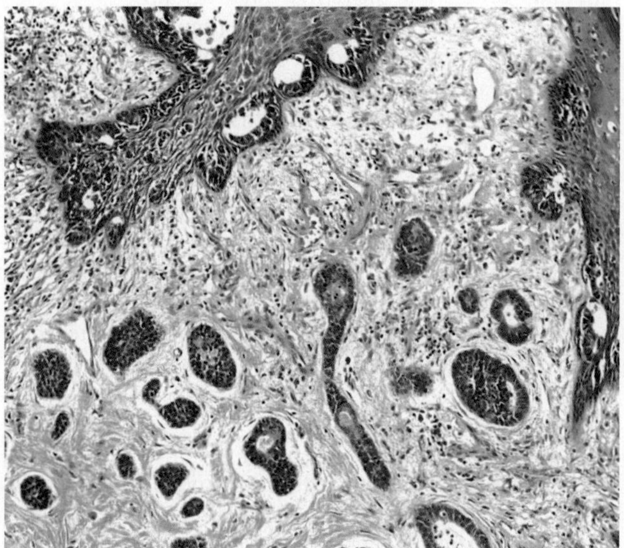

FIG. 25.2. ***Paget disease and adenoid cystic carcinoma.*** Carcinoma glands are apparent in the epidermis overlying AdCC, which was confined to the nipple.

around and within the tumor. In the same study, a palpable tumor was not detected by either mammographic or sonographic examination.

Magnetic resonance imaging (MRI) is helpful for defining the extent of the AdCC, especially in a dense breast.[33] An unusual pattern of rapid but somewhat zonal enhancement from the tumor periphery to the center has been described on T1-weighted images.[35] The lesions are irregular or lobulated, with rapid and heterogeneous enhancement after injection of gadolinium and have persistent or plateau kinetic.[33] T2-weighted images showed isointensity with the adjacent breast parenchyma or extensive high T2-weighted signal.

GROSS PATHOLOGY

The reported gross size of the tumors ranges from 2 mm to 25 cm.[9,14,15] Most lesions measure between 1 and 3 cm. Tumors with low-grade histologic features tend to be smaller (0.5 to 2.8 cm; mean, 1.6 cm) than high-grade tumors (1.5 to 8.0 cm; mean, 3.5 cm).

Most AdCCs are circumscribed or nodular grossly, despite a microscopically invasive growth pattern. Small cystic areas are not unusual, especially in lesions smaller than 5 cm. Larger tumors may have areas of gross cystic degeneration[5,9,14] (Fig. 25.3). The lesions have been variously described as gray, pale yellow, tan, and pink (Fig. 25.4).

MICROSCOPIC PATHOLOGY

AdCC consists of a mixture of proliferating glands (adenoid component) and basaloid/myoepithelial cells producing abundant basement membrane material ("pseudoglandular" or cylindromatous component) (Fig. 25.5). These components are rarely distributed homogeneously in a given tumor (Fig. 25.6). Some areas consist predominantly of the glandular or adenoid structures, creating a close resemblance to cribriform carcinoma, either *in situ* or invasive (Fig. 25.5).[36] Abundant basement membrane material in other parts of the tumor produces a cylindromatous pattern that, when extreme, may be mistaken for scirrhous carcinoma (Fig. 25.7).

Despite a fairly circumscribed and nodular gross appearance, many AdCCs have an invasive growth pattern microscopically, in which the tumor infiltrates the surrounding breast parenchyma beyond a grossly apparent central nodule[14] (Fig. 25.8). Microcystic areas formed by the coalescent spaces in dilated glands are seen in about 25% of tumors. When they are sufficiently large, these spaces can be appreciated grossly as well as microscopically (Figs. 25.8 and 25.9). Areas of nearly confluent solid growth as well as typical adenoid cystic components may be present in a single tumor (Fig. 25.10). Prominent basaloid features are seen in some instances, a pattern that is referred to as the solid variant of AdCC with basaloid features[37] (Figs. 25.11 to 25.13). Slodkowska et al.[21] reported that 9/41 (22%) AdCCs in their series had basaloid morphology. Ro et al.[38] suggested that AdCC be stratified into three grades on the basis of the proportion of

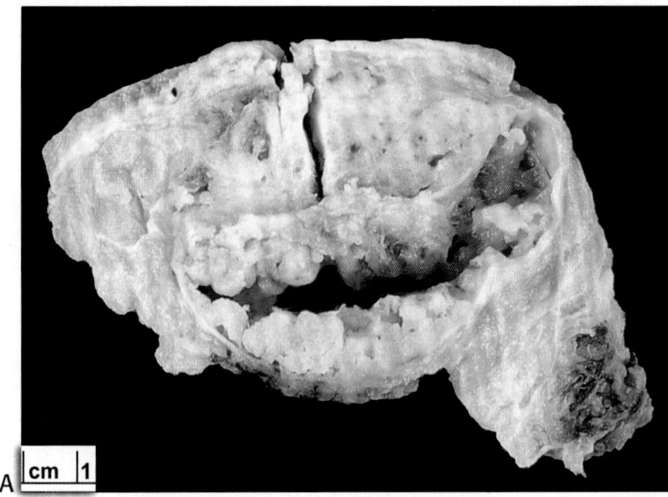

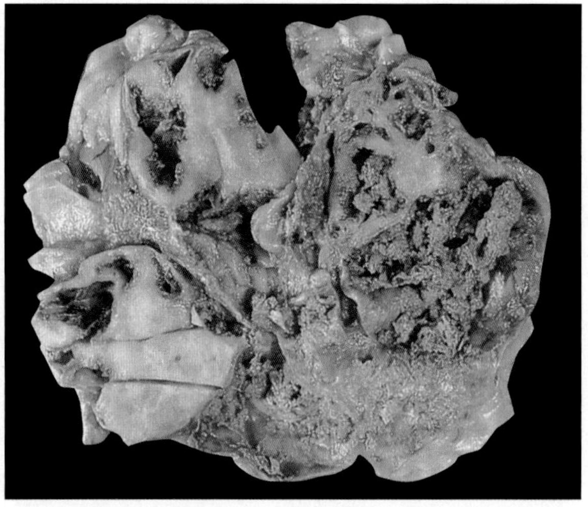

FIG. 25.3. ***Adenoid cystic carcinoma, cystic gross appearance.*** **A:** Mastectomy specimen with a large partly cystic tumor that occupied most of the breast. **B:** Extensive cystic degeneration developed in this tumor. Some solid areas remain.

solid growth within the lesion: grade I, no solid elements; grade II, less than 30% solid growth; and grade III, solid areas composing more than 30% of the tumor. In high-grade lesions, tumor cells are poorly differentiated and have sparse cytoplasm, relatively large, hyperchromatic nuclei, and frequent mitoses (Figs. 25.11 to 25.14). High-grade AdCCs do not seem to differ from low-grade AdCCs in regard to patient age, laterality, duration before treatment, hormone receptors, or in the likelihood of finding residual tumor in a mastectomy specimen.[14] Ro et al.[38] found that tumors with a solid component (grades II and III) tended to be larger and were more likely to have recurrences than those without a solid element (grade I). In their series, none of five patients with a grade I AdCC developed distant metastases, whereas two of six patients with grade II AdCC recurred distally; the only patient with a grade III AdCC also developed distant metastases. In the three cases with distant disease, the morphology of the metastatic carcinoma was similar to that of the primary tumor. A patient with solid AdCC in the series by Santamaria et al.[27] did not have axillary nodal metastases. The grading scheme proposed by Ro et al.[38] was not prognostically significant in one study.[28] In a follow-up study from the M. D. Anderson Cancer Center, Zhu et al.[15] reported that “patients with grade III tumors were more likely to have lower overall survival (OS) and recurrence-free survival (RFS) rates than patients with grade I or II tumors, although the differences were not statistically significant.”

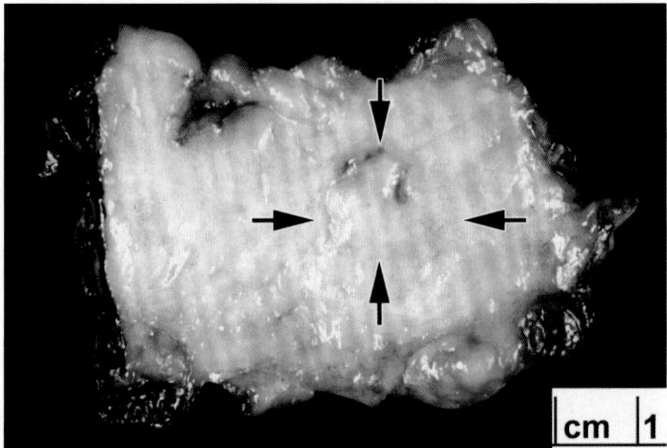

FIG. 25.4. ***Adenoid cystic carcinoma, gross appearance.*** A subtle ill-defined white-pink area (*arrows*) representing an infiltrating focus of AdCC is barely visible on the cut surface of a breast excision specimen. This is consistent with the grossly inconspicuous pattern of infiltration characteristic of AdCC. Two hemorrhagic lines in the center of the tumor constitute evidence of prior needle core biopsy.

A variety of microscopic growth patterns found in AdCC of the salivary glands[39] may also be present when this type of tumor occurs in the breast.[14,38,40,41] These configurations have been described as cribriform (Fig. 25.5), tubular (Fig. 25.15), reticular (trabecular) (Fig. 25.10), solid (Fig 25.10), and basaloid (Figs. 25.11 to 25.14). Sebaceous metaplasia is found in 14% of AdCC (Fig. 25.16), and a substantial number of the tumors have foci of squamous differentiation (Figs. 25.9 and 25.17).[42] Adenomyoepitheliomatous areas with ductular structures that resemble the intercalated ducts in salivary glands and salivary gland tumors (Fig. 25.18) and syringomatous areas (Fig. 25.19) are further evidence of structural diversity.[42]

Rarely, adipose differentiation and myofibroblastic hyperplasia can occur in the stroma of AdCC (Fig. 25.20). Noske et al.[43] described a high-grade basaloid AdCC that gave rise to a metaplastic spindle cell and glandular adenocarcinoma with melanomatous differentiation.

Perineural invasion (Figs. 25.14C and 25.21), a very common feature in AdCC of the oropharynx, was present in 8%[18] and 15%[21] of cases in two studies. It tends to be more frequent in tumors with basaloid morphology. Lymphovascular

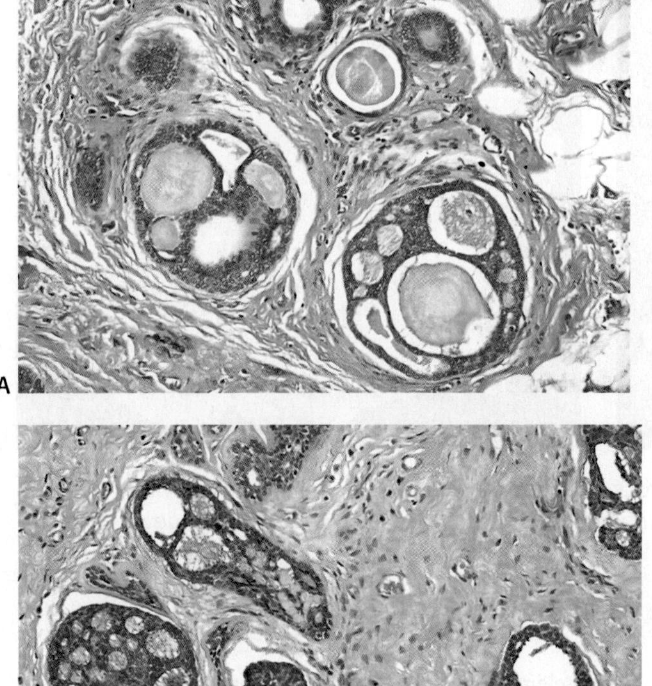

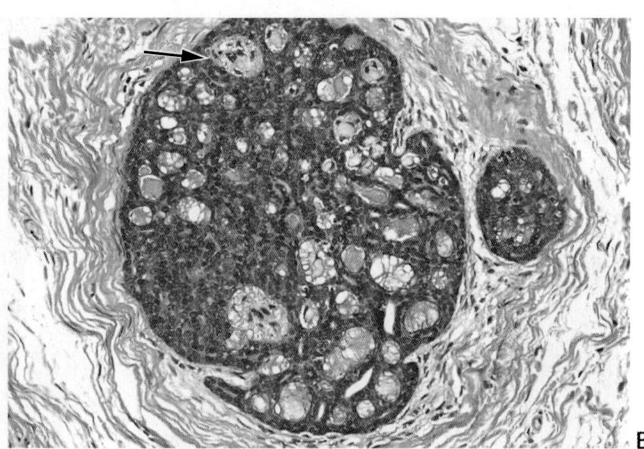

FIG. 25.5. *Adenoid cystic carcinoma.* **A:** Invasive tumor with conspicuous solid pink cylindromatous nodules and glandular spaces with basophilic secretion. **B:** Isolated nuclei of myoepithelial cells are attached to cylindromatous nodules *in the upper center* (*arrow*). Note the basophilic degeneration of some cylindromatous nodules that resembles collagenous spherulosis. **C:** This focus is predominantly cribriform with a minor cylindromatous component in the *upper left* gland.

invasion is extremely uncommon.[14] Shrinkage artifacts occur relatively often in AdCC, especially in fibrotic portions of the tumor (Fig. 25.22) and should not be mistaken for lymphatic tumor emboli. The pseudovascular spaces are not lined by endothelium.

Ductal Carcinoma *In Situ*

It is usually difficult to detect an *in situ* component, but in a minority of low-grade AdCCs there may be conspicuous lobular and duct involvement (Fig. 25.23). This type

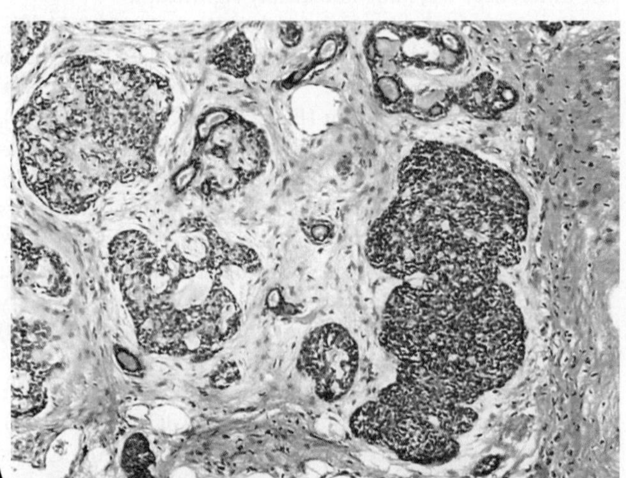

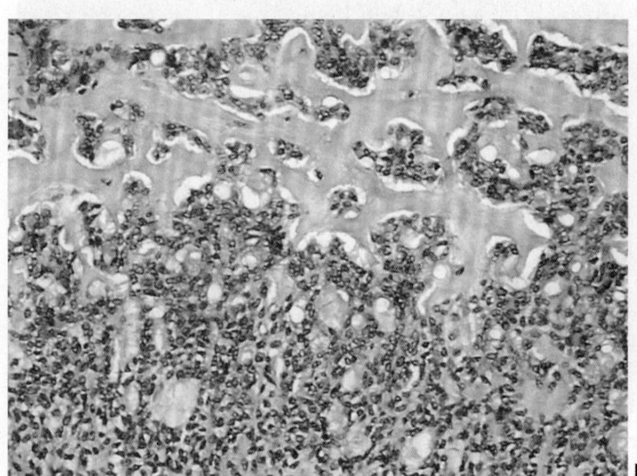

FIG. 25.6. *Adenoid cystic carcinoma, structural heterogeneity.* **A:** This microscopic field displays typical (*left*) and solid (*right*) growth patterns. **B:** An area of solid growth *below* and a striking cylindromatous component *above*. **C:** Dense amyloid-like stroma. The cellular constituent is almost entirely myoepithelial. **D:** A prominent cribriform element and, *at the upper border*, a more conventional adenoid cystic element.

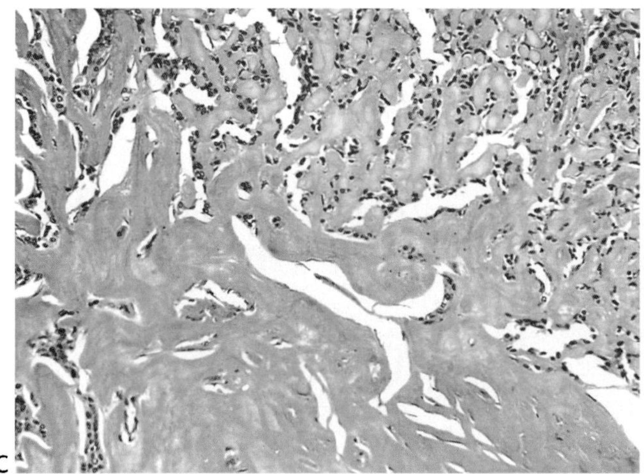

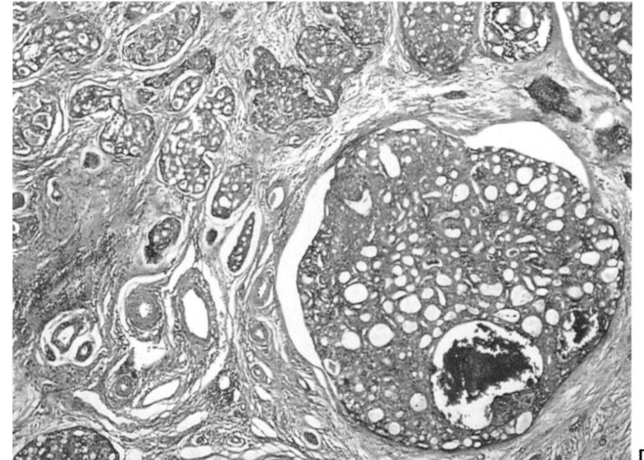

FIG. 25.6. *[Continued]*

of ductal carcinoma *in situ* (DCIS) cannot be appreciated grossly at surgery and may be responsible for local recurrence in some cases. Intraductal AdCC with lobular extension is sometimes seen in high-grade tumors. Compared with the invasive component with cribriform morphology, the DCIS lacks the distinctive periductal cuff of cellular myxoid stroma that typically surrounds the nests of invasive AdCC. Lobules and ducts adjacent to AdCC can display adenoid cystic traits, with small cylindromatous areas (Fig. 25.24).

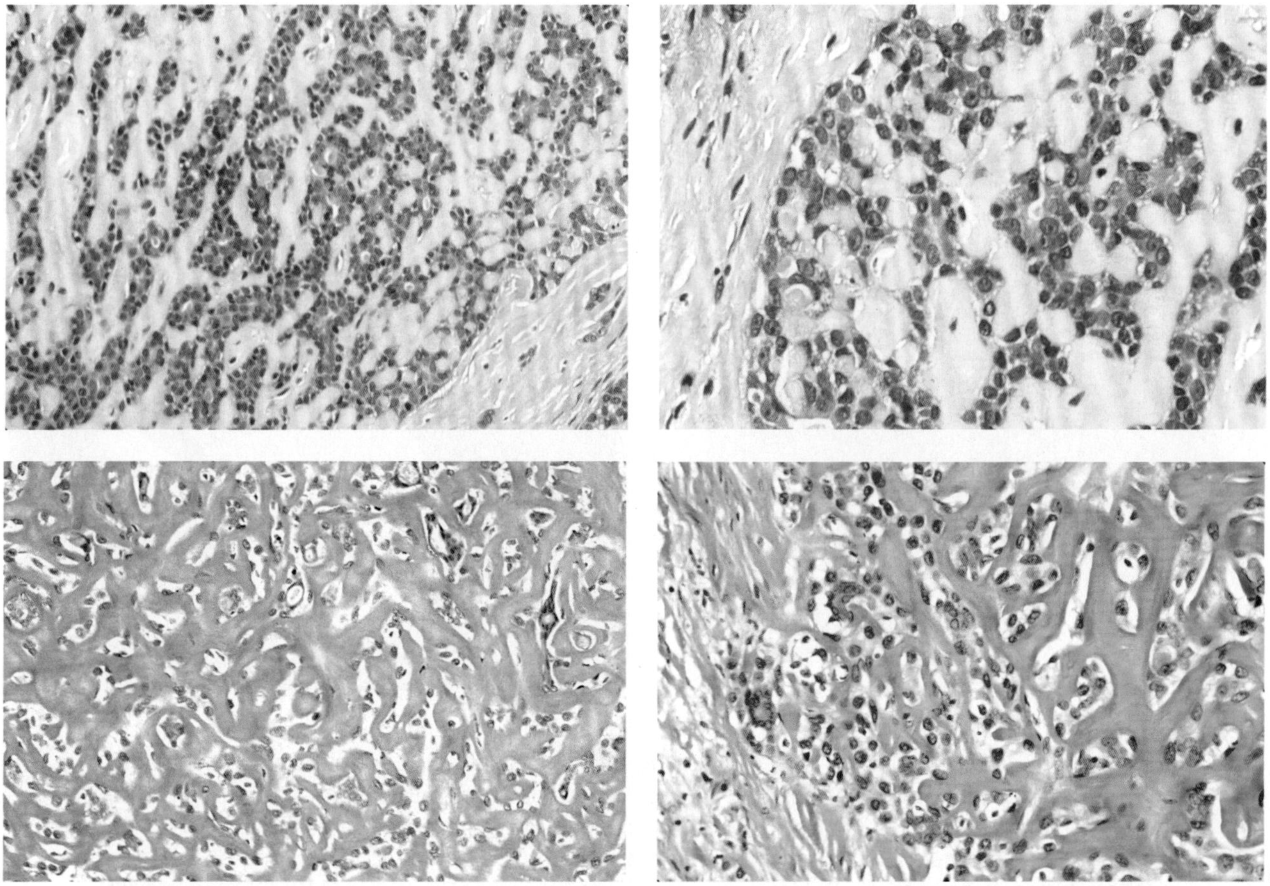

FIG. 25.7. ***Adenoid cystic carcinoma.*** **A,B:** Overgrowth of cylindromatous material compresses the glandular elements. A needle core biopsy sample could be mistaken for invasive lobular or scirrhous carcinoma. **C,D:** This tumor with abundant cylindromatous material resembles pseudoangiomatous stromal hyperplasia.

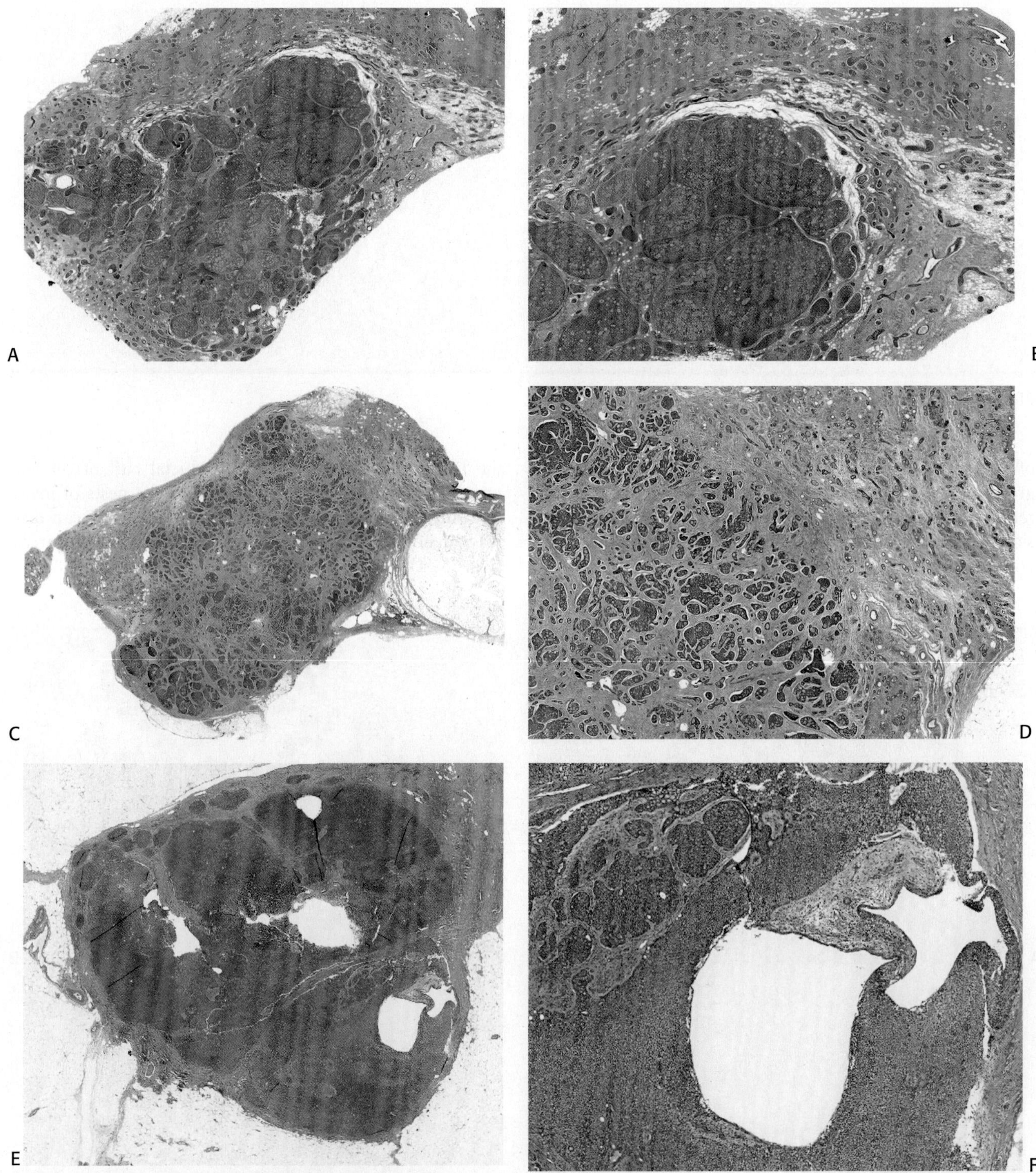

FIG. 25.8. ***Adenoid cystic carcinoma.*** **A:** A histologic section of an AdCC consisting of a fairly circumscribed central nodule with less conspicuous infiltration in all of the surrounding breast parenchyma. **B:** Magnified view of the tumor in **(A)** showing the nodular and solid growth in the center of the lesion and a more subtly infiltrative pattern at the tumor periphery. **C:** This histologic section demonstrates a circumscribed central tumor mass surrounded by small nests with an invasive pattern (*upper right and left*). **D:** Medium-power magnification of the tumor in **(C)**. **E,F:** In contrast to the two carcinomas shown in **(A–D)**, this solid and focally cystic tumor forms a discrete, circumscribed mass with no evidence of peripheral infiltration. **F:** Two cystic spaces in the tumor shown in **(E)**.

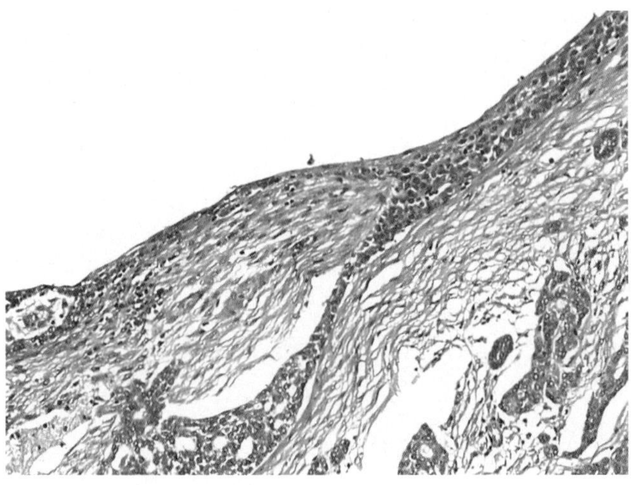

FIG. 25.9. ***Adenoid cystic carcinoma, cystic.*** The cyst cavity is lined by neoplastic epithelium with superficial squamous differentiation.

Associated Carcinomas

Other types of carcinoma may develop in the contralateral breast,[10,13,14,27] or in rare instances another type of carcinoma may be found in the same breast. One patient had separate, concurrent tubular carcinoma (Fig. 25.25) and lobular carcinoma *in situ* (LCIS). Another case of AdCC merged with a well-differentiated estrogen receptor (ER)–positive invasive ductal carcinoma (Fig. 25.26).

CYTOLOGY

Cytologic preparations of AdCC consist of small hyperchromatic epithelial cells with very scant cytoplasm that surround globules and cylinders of basement membrane–like material.[34,44–46] The latter has a bright magenta color in Diff-Quik- or Giemsa-stained slides (Fig. 25.27) or a pale blue hyaline quality in Papanicolau-stained preparations. In

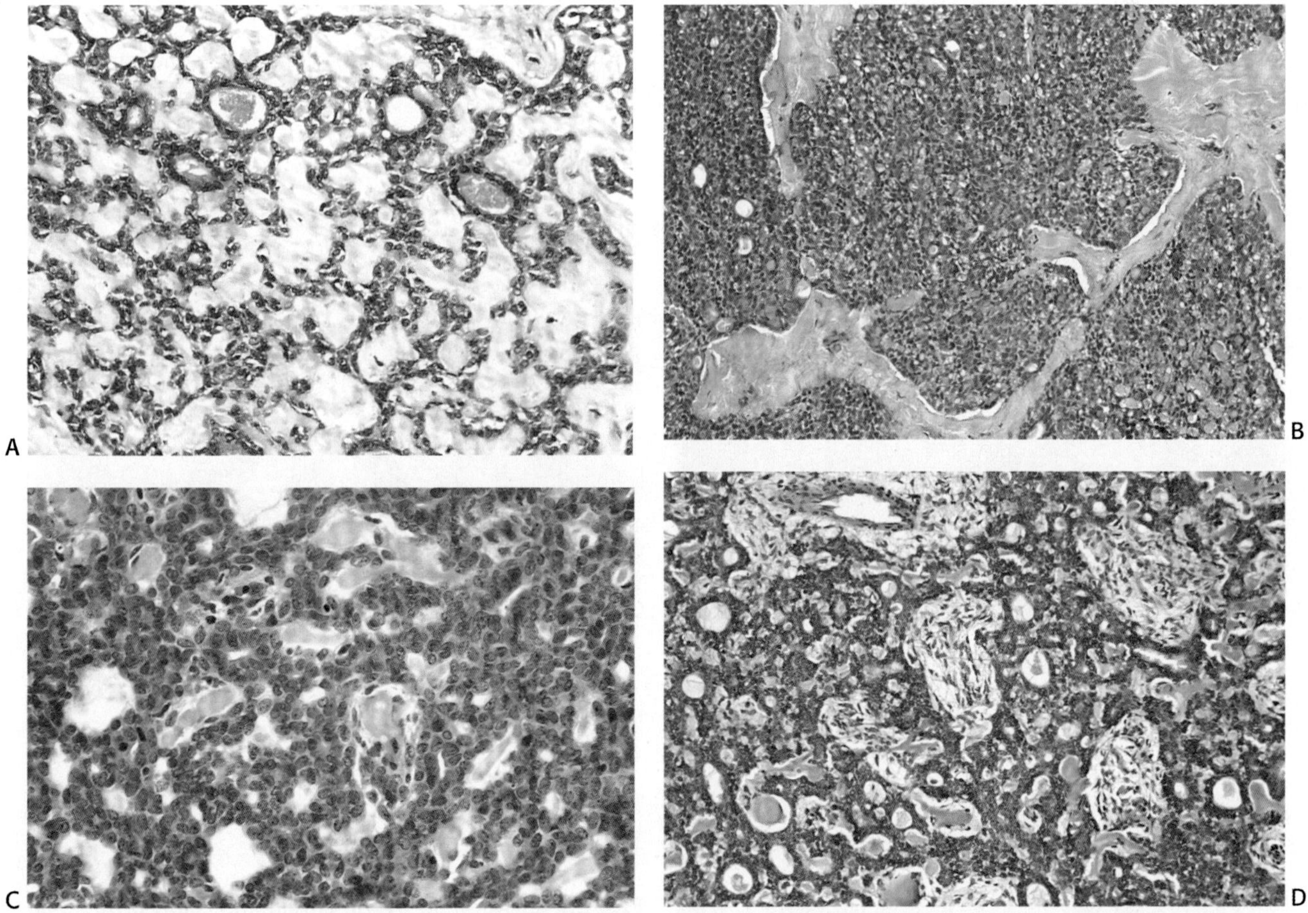

FIG. 25.10. ***Adenoid cystic carcinoma, reticular and solid patterns.*** **A:** Small glands remain in this predominantly reticular proliferation. **B:** Solid growth. **C:** Magnified view of solid lesion showing numerous cylindromatous nodules. **D:** Solid growth pattern with fibrovascular stroma. This appearance resembles solid papillary carcinoma.

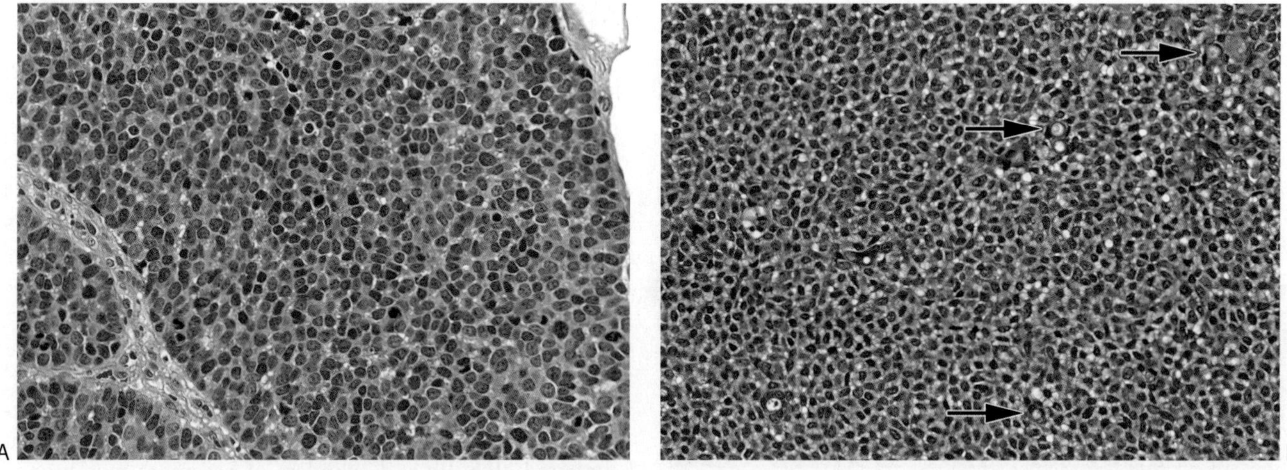

FIG. 25.11. ***Adenoid cystic carcinoma, high grade with basaloid growth pattern.*** **A:** A high-grade solid proliferation of basaloid cells. **B:** Another tumor with solid growth of basaloid cells. Minute cylindromatous deposits are present (*arrows*).

contrast to pleomorphic adenoma, the neoplastic cells surround the deposits of matrix material, but are not present within it. The differential diagnosis of a cytologic preparation from an AdCC includes invasive cribriform carcinoma, cribriform DCIS, collagenous spherulosis,[46] and pleomorphic adenoma of the breast.

IMMUNOHISTOCHEMISTRY

AdCC is a biphasic neoplasm composed of epithelial (luminal) and myoepithelial (basaloid) cells. The structural polarity of the glandular (luminal) cells can be demonstrated with immunostains for fodrin, E-cadherin, and β-catenin.[47] The

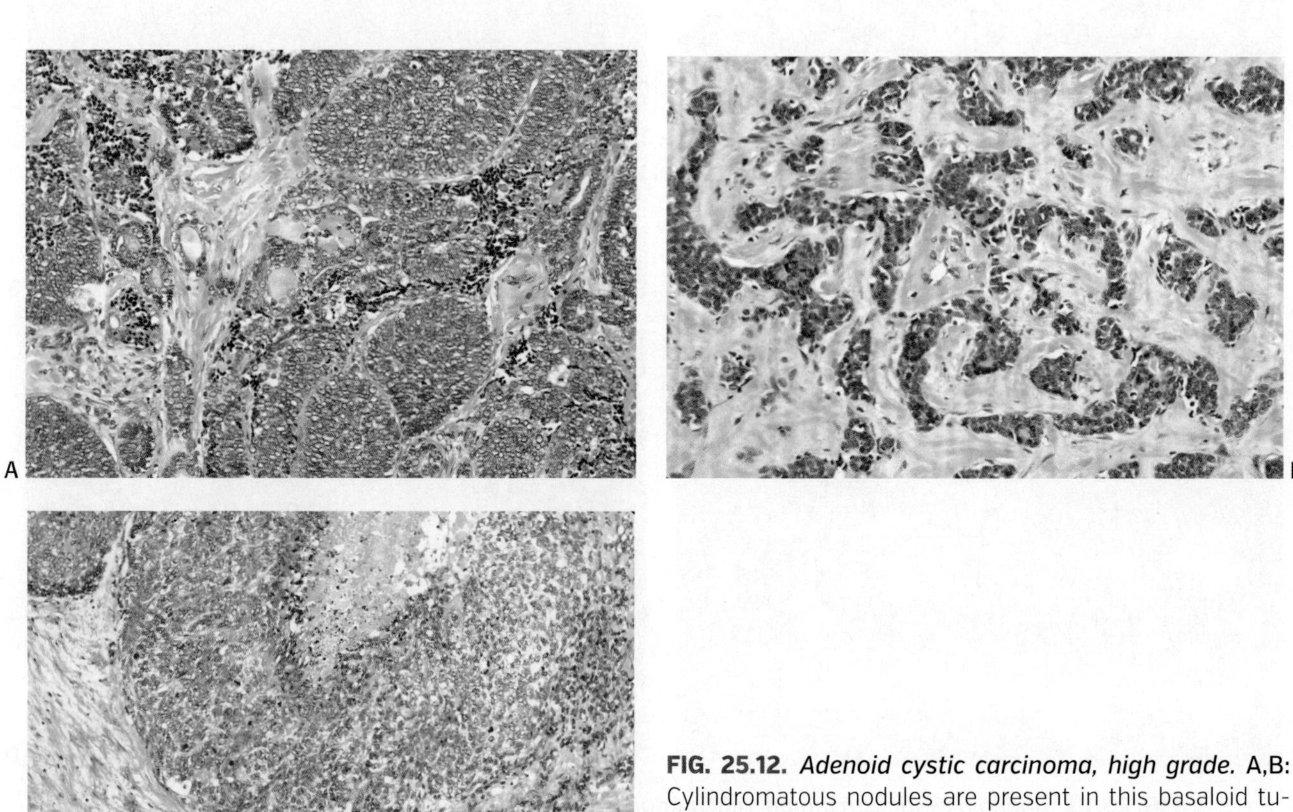

FIG. 25.12. ***Adenoid cystic carcinoma, high grade.*** **A,B:** Cylindromatous nodules are present in this basaloid tumor. Note zones of tumor disruption with darkly staining cells and nuclear debris. A limited sample of this tumor could be interpreted as SCC with "crush artifact." **C:** This tumor displays solid growth and necrosis.

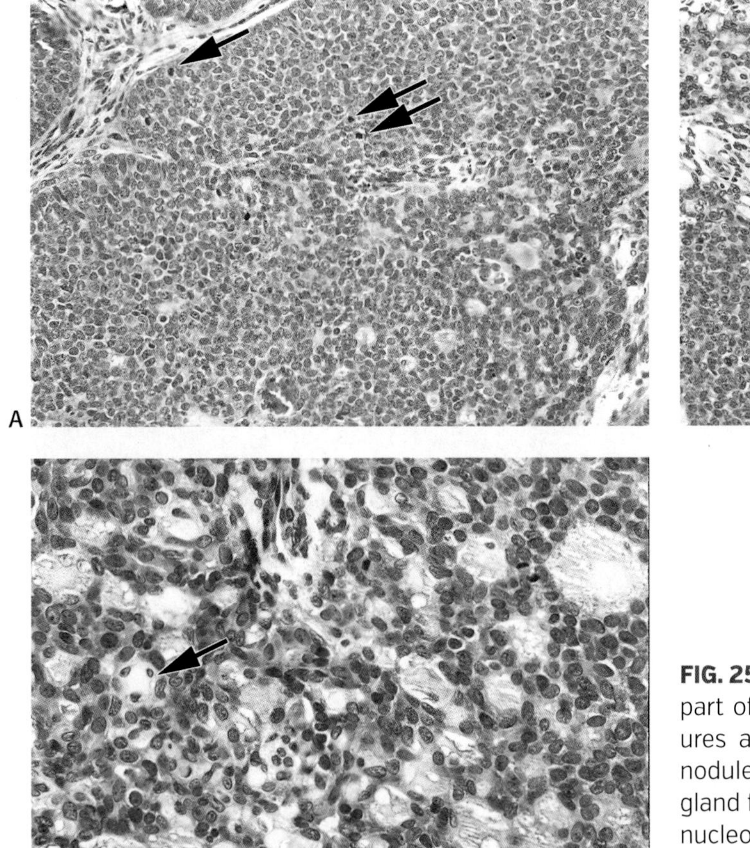

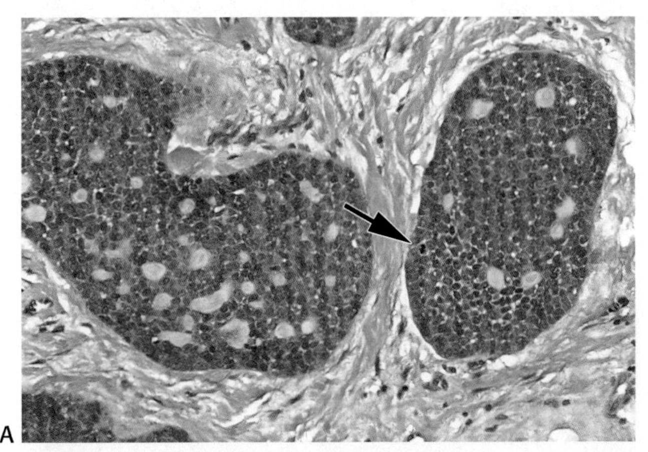

FIG. 25.13. ***Adenoid cystic carcinoma, high grade.*** **A:** This part of the tumor is almost completely solid. Mitotic figures are present (*arrows*). **B:** One pale cylindromatous nodule (*arrow*), surrounded by myoepithelial cells, and gland formation are shown. **C:** The tumor cells have small nucleoli. One cylindromatous nodule encircled by myoepithelial cells is evident (*arrow*).

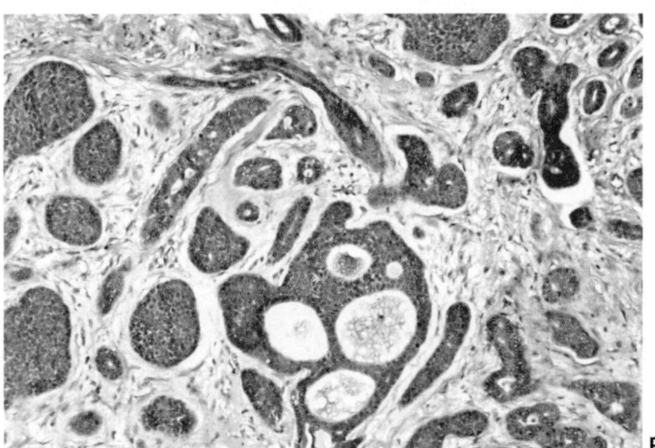

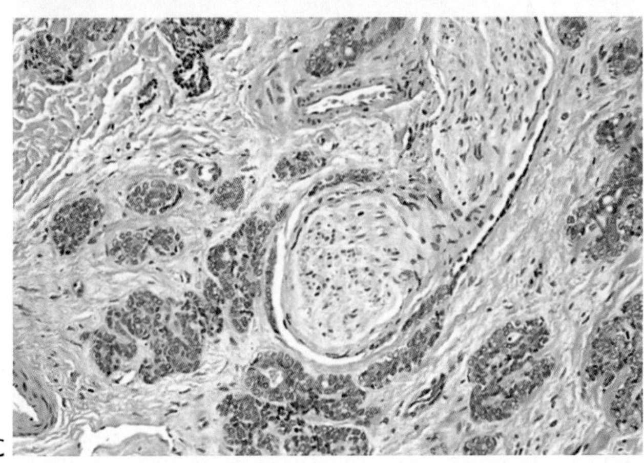

FIG. 25.14. ***Adenoid cystic carcinoma, high grade.*** **A:** Solid tumor nests containing cylindromatous nodules and mitotic activity (*arrow*). **B:** Cribriform and syringomatous elements in the tumor shown in (**A**). **C:** Perineural invasion.

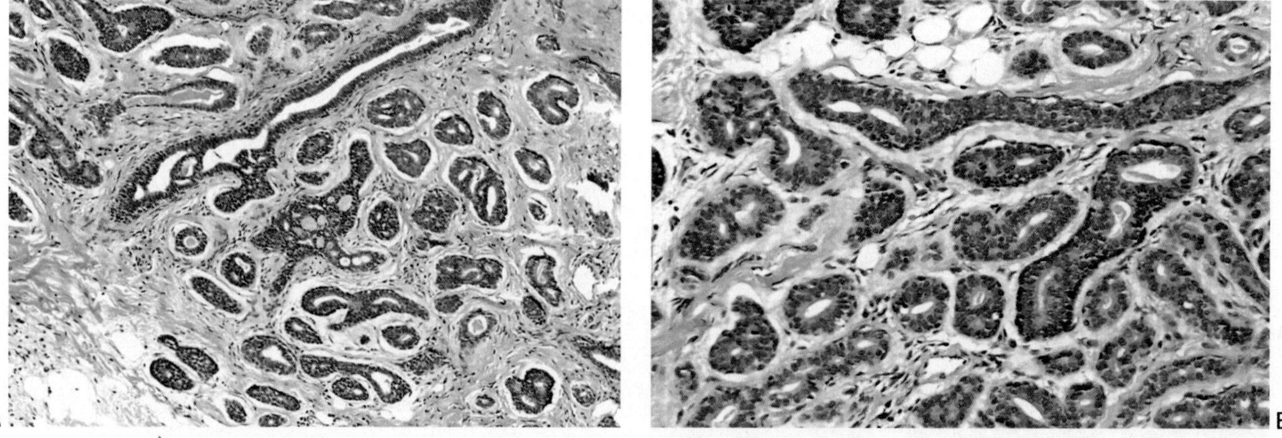

FIG. 25.15. ***Adenoid cystic carcinoma, tubular.*** **A:** Tubular growth surrounds a central tumor focus with cylindromatous nodules and a long benign duct. **B:** Pure tubular growth in the same tumor.

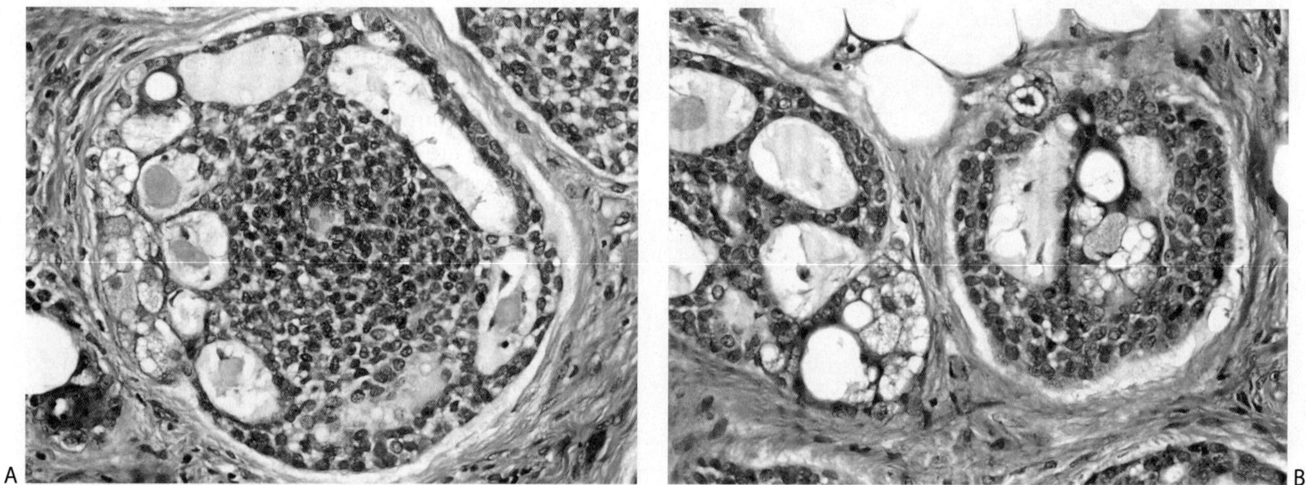

FIG. 25.16. ***Adenoid cystic carcinoma with sebaceous metaplasia.*** **A,B:** Two examples of sebaceous metaplasia.

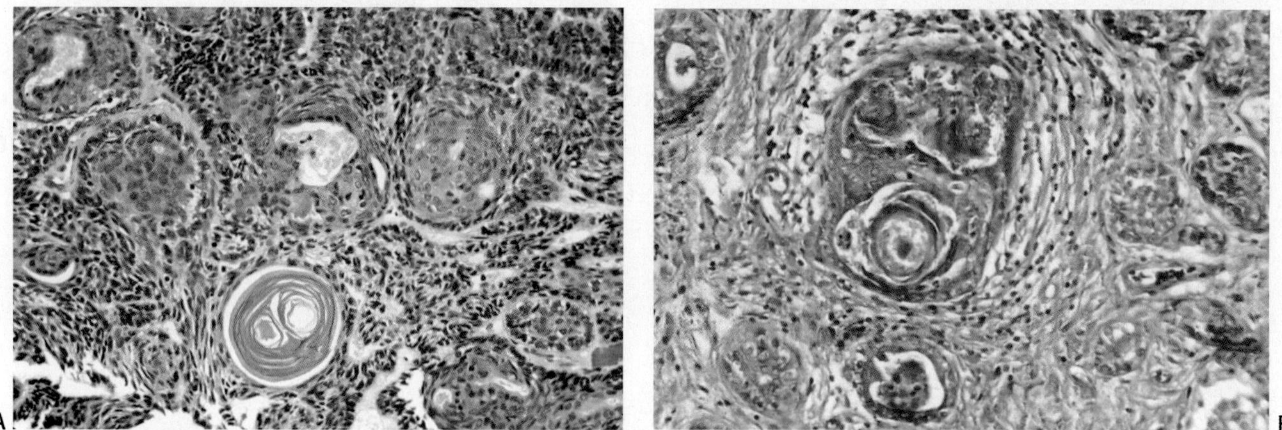

FIG. 25.17. ***Adenoid cystic carcinoma, squamous differentiation.*** **A:** Squamous metaplasia. **B:** A tumor nest with focal squamous differentiation.

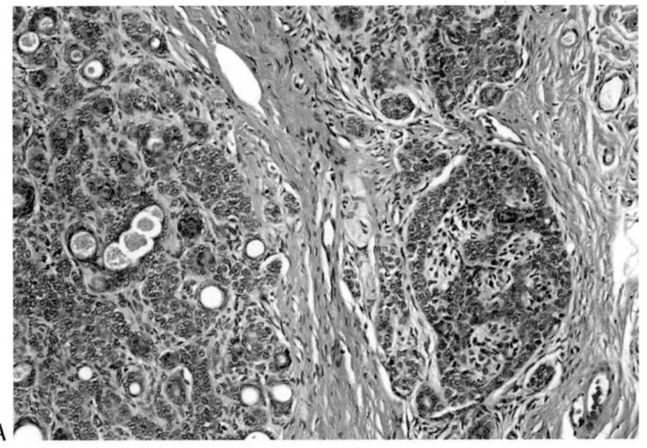

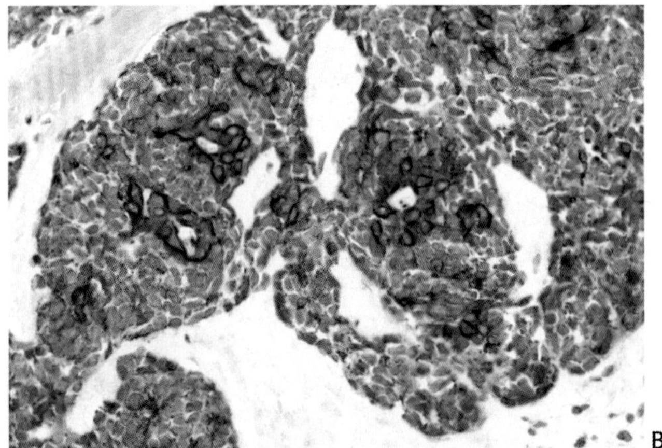

FIG. 25.18. ***Adenoid cystic carcinoma, ductular differentiation.*** **A:** Ductular structures that resemble intercalated salivary gland ducts with darkly stained cytoplasm and nuclei are present in this tumor. **B:** Ductules are immunoreactive with the antibody 34βE12 (K903).

glandular epithelial cells are immunoreactive for cytokeratin (CK) 7 (Figs. 25.28 and 25.29), carcinoembryogenic antigen (CEA), epithelial membrane antigen (EMA), CK5/6, CK8/18, and CD117/c-kit (Fig. 25.30).[48] A minority of luminal cells coexpress CK5/6 and CK8/18 on double immunostaining.[48] Using triple immunofluorescence, Boecker at al.[49] found reactivity for CK7/CK8/CK18 in the glandular epithelium of six mammary AdCCs.

The basaloid cells surrounding the globules of basement lamina material variably express the myoepithelial markers p63,[48,50] smooth muscle actin (SMA)[47,50] (Figs. 25.28 and 25.29), and maspin[51] as well as the basal keratins CK14 and CK17[52] and vimentin.[47] Some authors have reported no reactivity for calponin,[50] smooth muscle myosin heavy-chain (SMM-HC),[37,50] and CD10[53] in the basaloid/myoepithelial cells. Azoulay et al.[48] found no evidence of basaloid cells showing simultaneous positivity for CK5/6 and p63. Using a triple immunofluorescence technique to study six mammary AdCCs, Boecker et al.[49] observed that these tumors are composed for most part of the cells with myoepithelial differentiation (CK5-, CK14-, SMA-, and p63-positive), focally admixed with glandular cells (CK7-, CK8-, and CK18-positive) and sparse CK5- and CK14-positive progenitor cells.

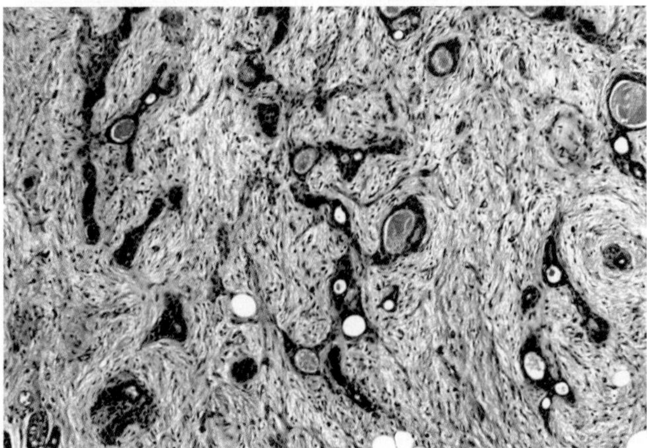

FIG. 25.19. ***Adenoid cystic carcinoma, syringomatous differentiation.*** Syringomatous glands in an AdCC.

The cylindromatous component of AdCC is composed of basal lamina material. Histochemical stains such as mucicarmine or Alcian blue ordinarily react with the secretion within glands. Laminin and fibronectin, noncollagenous glycoproteins associated with basal lamina, and type IV collagen can be demonstrated by immunohistochemistry in the cylindromatous elements.[47,54,55] The spherules that occur in collagenous spherulosis have staining properties similar to those of the cylindromatous nodules in AdCC.

Cheng et al.[56] examined the distribution of type IV collagen, laminin, heparin sulfate proteoglycan, and entactin, components of normal basement membrane, in AdCC. The cylindromatous component within nests of carcinoma cells and basement membrane surrounding these groups of cells was strongly reactive for each of these molecules. The authors concluded that the cells of AdCC produce, have an affinity for, and may require basement membrane components. They also speculated that this characteristic provides an explanation for the ability of AdCC to invade around nerves and blood vessels that are basement membrane–rich tissues.

The Ki67 proliferative index of AdCC is quite variable, ranging from 4% to 70%, with a trend to a higher index in high-grade tumors.[57] In one study,[58] three AdCC tumors with a low proliferative rate and no expression of p53 protein occurred in women with negative axillary lymph nodes (ALNs), whereas a fourth tumor with a high proliferative rate and p53 expression had axillary nodal metastases. Others have found that the Ki67 labeling index was not significantly related to prognosis.[28] Slodkowska et al.[21] reported that the average Ki67 index of basaloid AdCC was 22% (range 3 to 60) versus 9% (range 1 to 40) in nonbasaloid AdCC. The Ki67 proliferative index of 10 AdCCs with classic morphology in one study[31] was less than 14% in four cases, between 15% and 30% in five cases, and greater than 30% in one case.

Kit, a transmembrane tyrosine kinase receptor encoded by the protooncogene *c-KIT* located on chromosome

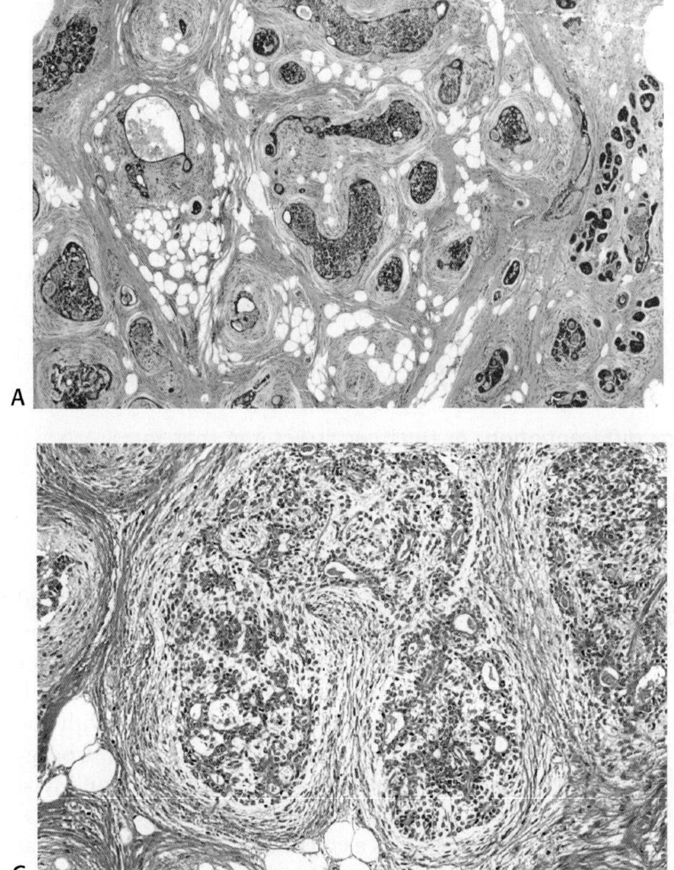

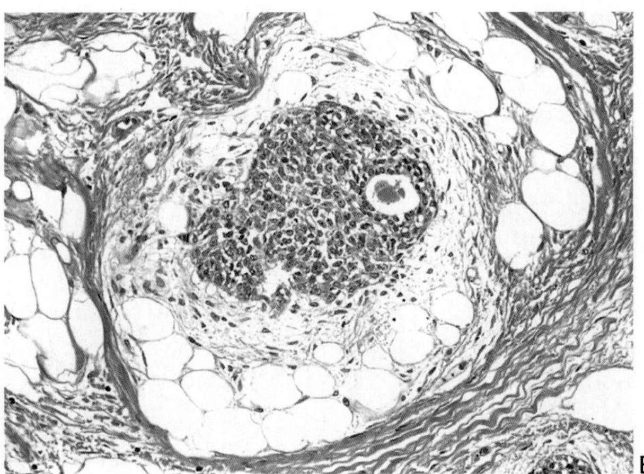

FIG. 25.20. ***Adenoid cystic carcinoma with unusual stromal differentiation.*** **A:** Nodular foci of AdCC surrounded by spindle cells and fat. **B:** A lobulated nest of tumor in an organoid structure bounded by fat and collagen. **C:** Organoid tumor clusters showing glandular differentiation. The circumscribed gross appearance of the tumor and internal organoid structure composed of adipose tissue and collagen suggests that these are intrinsic constituents of the tumor.

4(q11–12), is involved in the regulation of cell growth. Although kit is not detectable by immunohistochemistry in normal salivary glands, a study of 30 AdCCs of the salivary glands revealed expression in 90% of the tumors.[59] Kit is found in virtually all mammary AdCCs,[48,50,52,57,60] with positivity in 50% or more of the cells. It has strong membranous and weaker cytoplasmic positivity. Reportedly, reactivity for kit is limited to the epithelial component of cribriform AdCC, whereas it decorates nearly all cells in basaloid tumors[60] (Fig. 25.30). Kit immunoreactivity is absent from collagenous spherulosis[50] as well as cribriform mammary carcinomas.

Insulin-like growth factor-II mRNA-binding protein 3 (IMP3), a member of the insulin-like growth factor-II

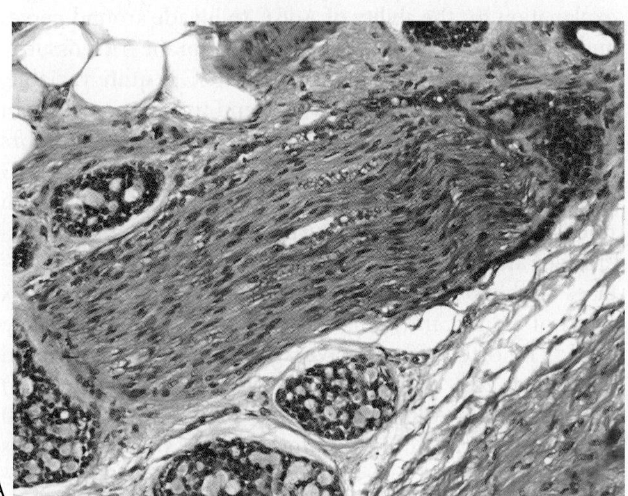

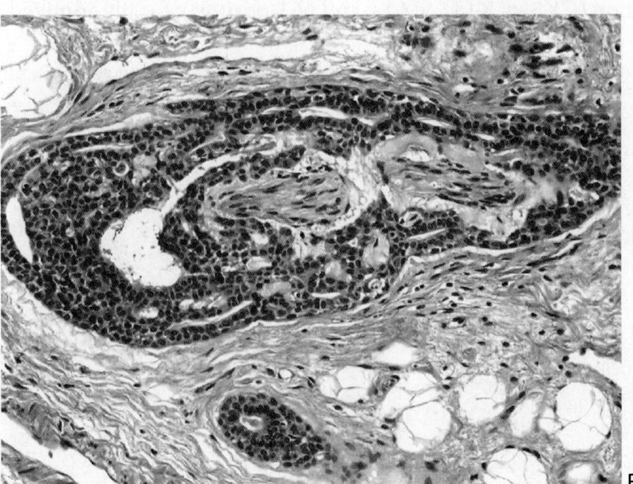

FIG. 25.21. ***Perineural invasion.*** **A,B:** Examples of perineural invasion in two different examples of AdCC.

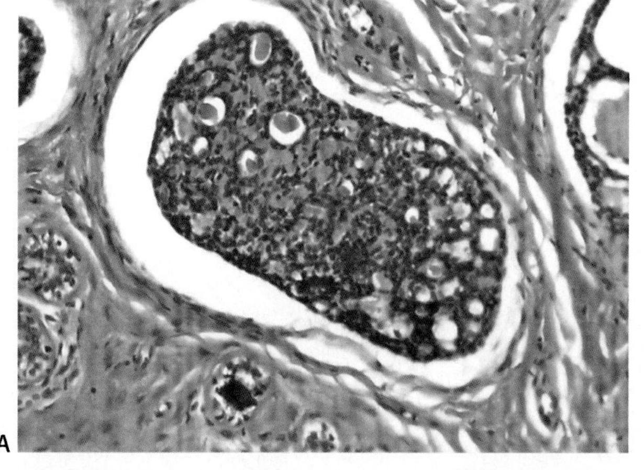

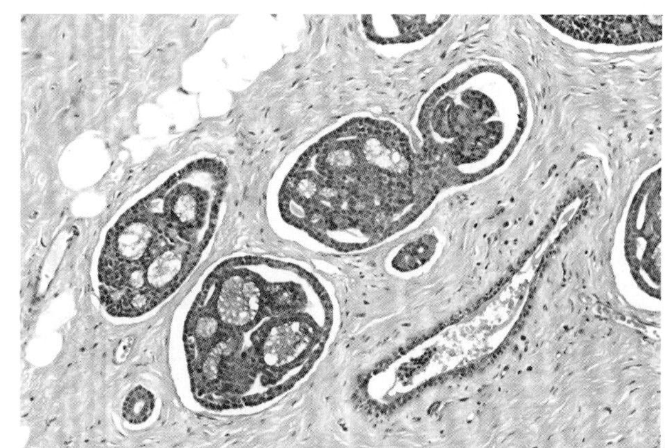

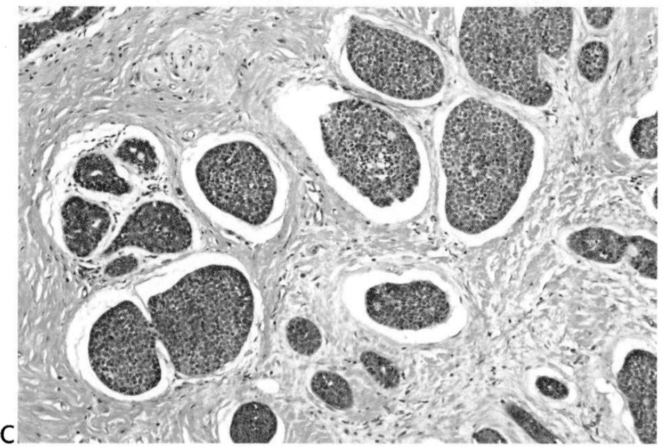

FIG. 25.22. ***Adenoid cystic carcinoma, shrinkage artifact.*** Carcinoma in such spaces may be mistaken for lymphatic tumor emboli. **A:** Classical growth pattern with cylindromatous and glandular elements. **B:** Cribriform growth. **C:** Solid high-grade lesion.

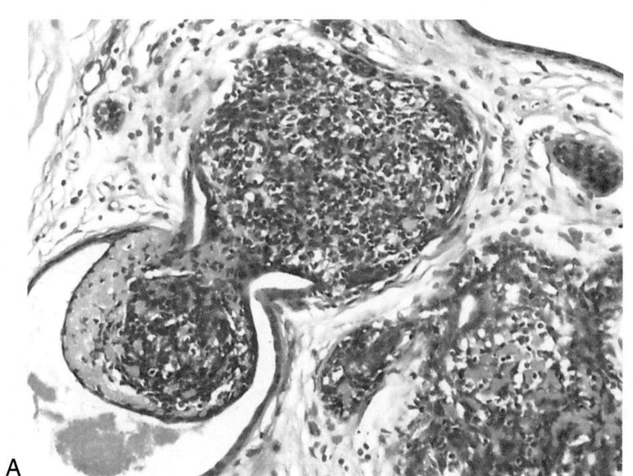

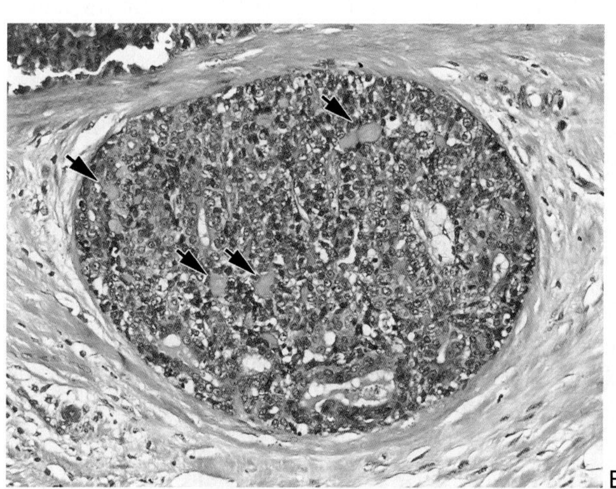

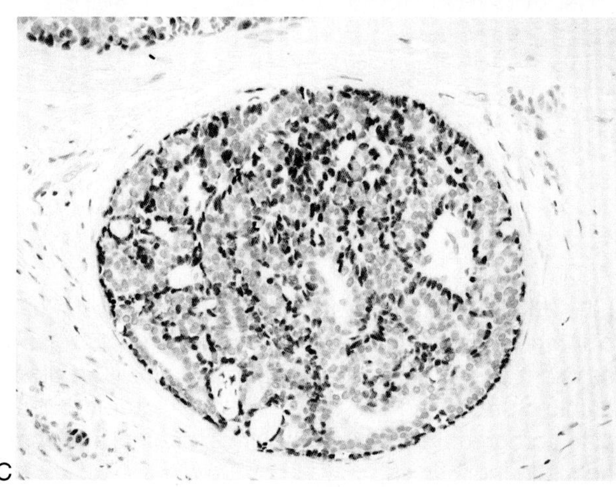

FIG. 25.23. ***Adenoid cystic DCIS.*** **A:** This small focus of DCIS was present in a reexcision specimen. It consists of an intraductal adenomyoepitheliomatous proliferation. The periductal stroma shows no reactive changes, a feature that helps to differentiate it from invasive AdCC. **B:** A focus of adenoid cystic DCIS with scattered small cylinders of basement lamina material (*arrows*). **C:** A p63 immunostain of the DCIS in **(B)** highlights myoepithelial cells around the cylinders and along the circumference of the duct. No desmoplasia is present in the stroma around adenoid cystic DCIS, in contrast to invasive AdCC.

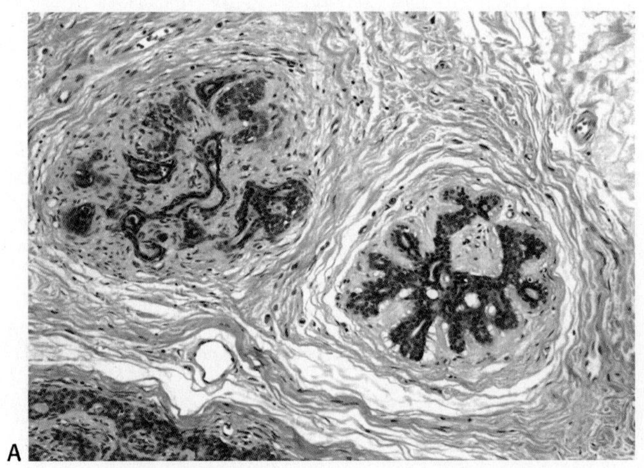

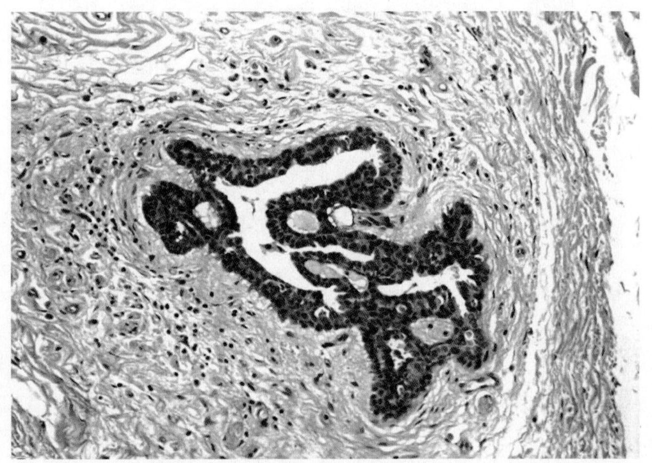

FIG. 25.24. ***Adenoid cystic features in lobules.*** **A:** Slight ductal hyperplasia with adenoid cystic traits (*right*) in a patient with AdCC (*below*). **B:** Micropapillary hyperplasia with cylindromatous nodules.

signaling pathway, is involved in tumor cell proliferation and invasion and is highly expressed in mammary basal-like carcinomas.[61] Vranic et al.[62] have documented membranous positivity for IMP3 in 81.3% of 16 primary AdCCs and in 2 metastatic AdCCs.

Many AdCCs are characterized by a chromosomal translocation that produces a *MYB–NFIB* fusion gene, with consequent overexpression of the *MYB* protooncogene (see also section on genetics and molecular alterations in this chapter). Brill et al.[63] detected overexpression of MYB protein by immunohistochemistry in 56 of 68 (82%) AdCCs from various sites, including four mammary AdCCs (Fig. 25.31). By contrast, MYB overexpression was identified in only 14% of 113 non-AdCC salivary gland tumors. At present, the finding of MYB immunoreactivity in a mammary carcinoma supports a diagnosis

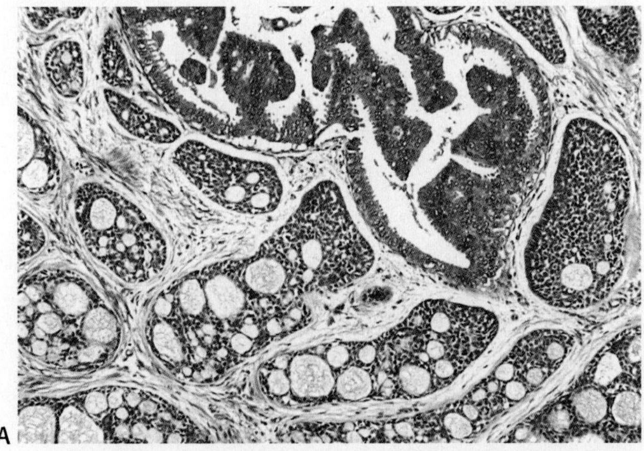

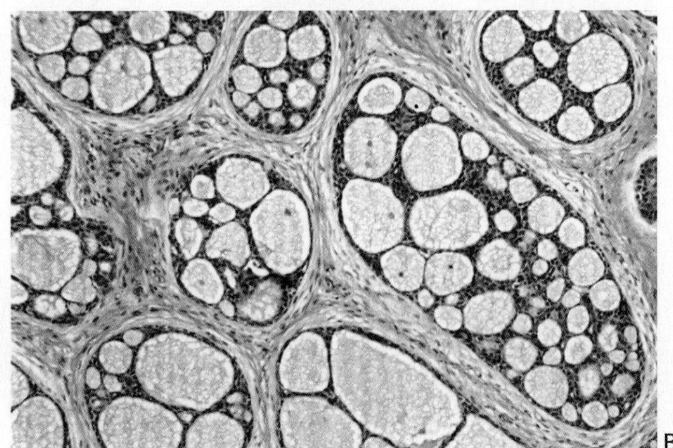

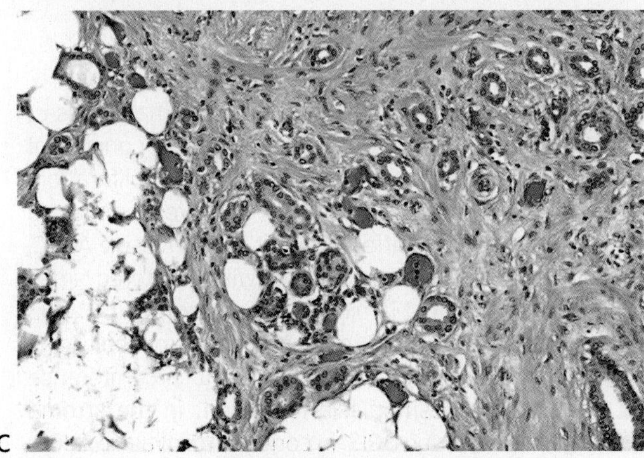

FIG. 25.25. ***Adenoid cystic carcinoma and tubular carcinoma.*** **A:** The primary tumor in this patient was AdCC adjacent to papillary intraductal carcinoma. **B:** Cribriform architecture in the AdCC. **C:** The mastectomy specimen also harbored a separate tubular carcinoma, shown here, and LCIS (not shown).

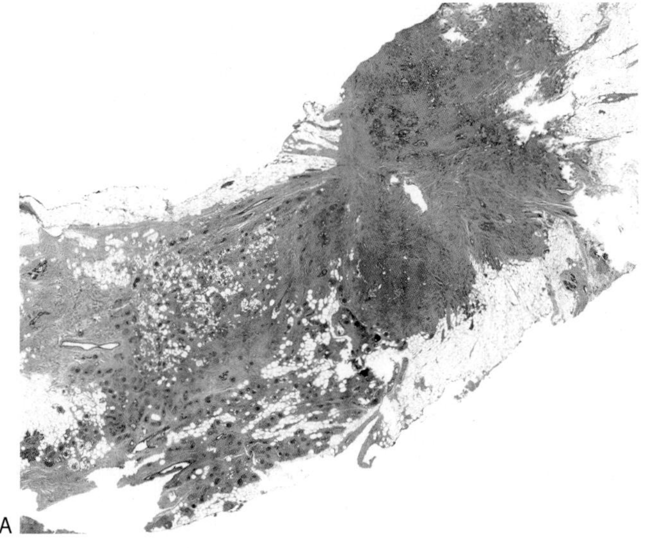

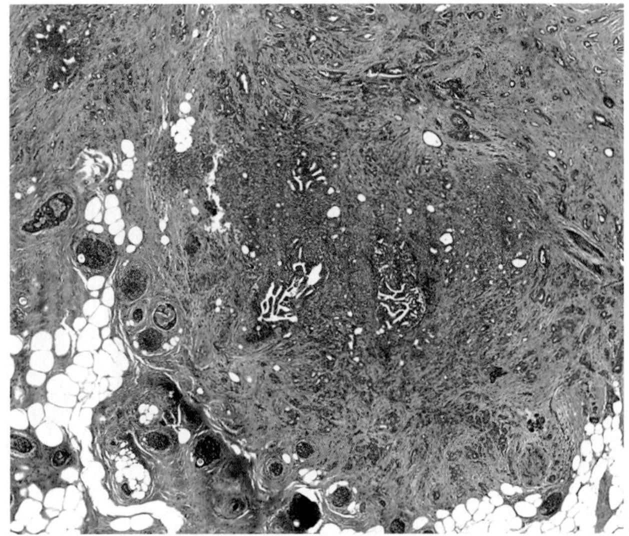

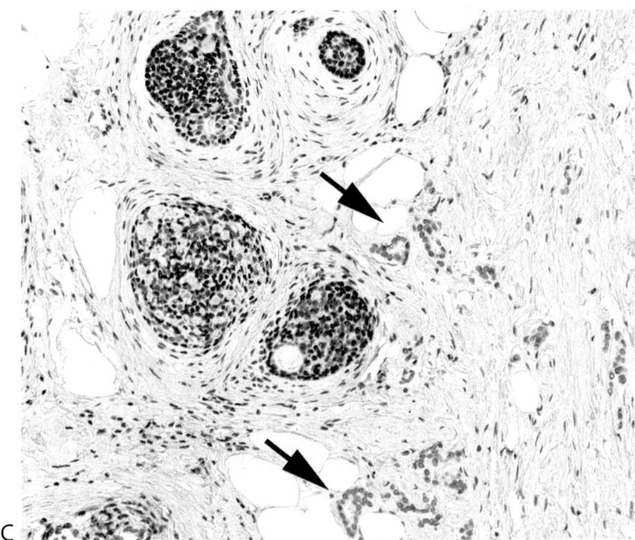

FIG. 25.26. ***Adenoid cystic carcinoma merging with tubular carcinoma.*** **A:** The primary tumor in this patient consisted of an invasive tumor with AdCC (*left*) and tubular carcinoma (*right*). **B:** The biphasic morphology of the tumor is evident at medium-power magnification. **C:** A p63 staining highlights the myoepithelial component in the AdCC. No p63-positive myoepithelium is present around the glands of the tubular carcinoma (*arrows*).

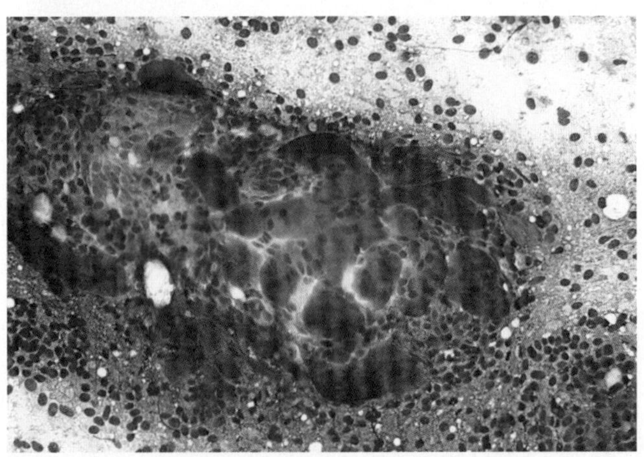

FIG. 25.27. ***Adenoid cystic carcinoma, aspiration cytology.*** This fine-needle aspiration (FNA) specimen shows eosinophilic nodules of cylindromatous material surrounded by neoplastic myoepithelial cells (Giemsa stain).

of AdCC, but definitive classification cannot be based on this finding alone. It is notable that immunohistochemical evidence of MYB overexpression is found in both *MYB–NFIB* fusion-positive and fusion-negative tumors, suggesting that mechanisms other than *MYB–NFIB* gene fusion can lead to activation of the *MYB* protooncogene.

Most AdCCs lack expression of ER,[41,48,52] progesterone receptor (PR), and androgen receptor (AR).[64] Very limited positivity for ER has been identified rarely in AdCCs.[18,33,37,57] Vranic et al.[64] have reported membranous and cytoplasmic positivity for ER-a36 protein, a novel isoform of ER-α36, in 8/11 (72.7%) cases of AdCC. Human epidermal growth factor/*neu* receptor (HER2/*neu*) staining is consistently negative.[18,33,37,41,48,52,57] Based on positive immunoreactivity for the basal CK5/6 and CK14, as well as for CK17,[52] AdCC can be classified as a basal-like triple negative carcinoma. Nonetheless, mammary AdCC differs from other basal-like carcinomas because it shows a distinctive pattern of genetic alterations (see section on

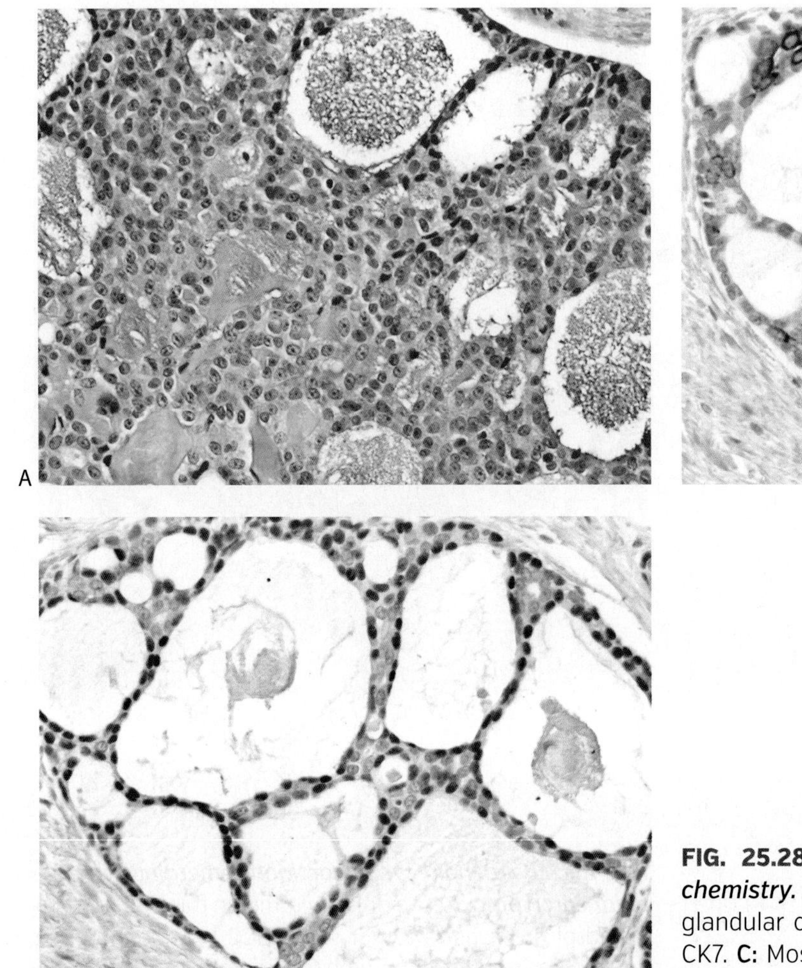

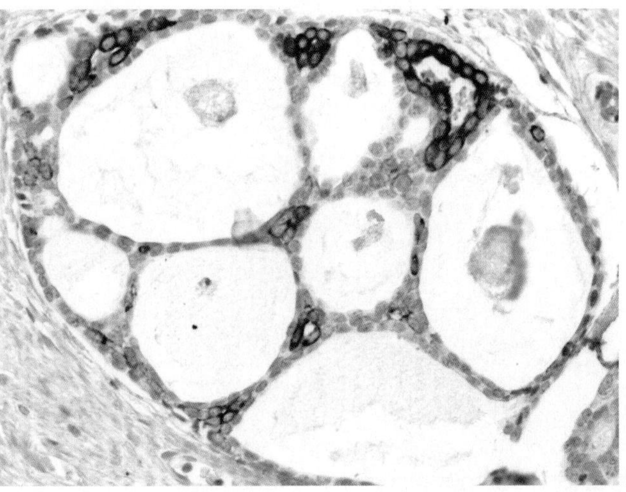

FIG. 25.28. ***Adenoid cystic carcinoma, immunohistochemistry.*** **A:** This AdCC has cribriform morphology. **B:** The glandular cells composing the tumor show reactivity for CK7. **C:** Most of the tumor cells are p63-positive, consistent with myoepithelial differentiation.

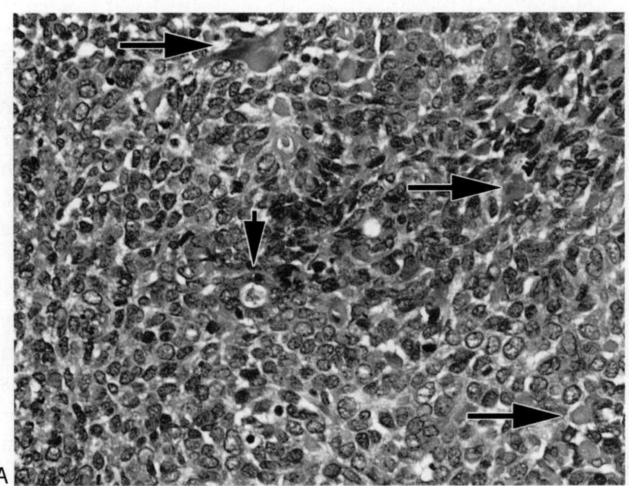

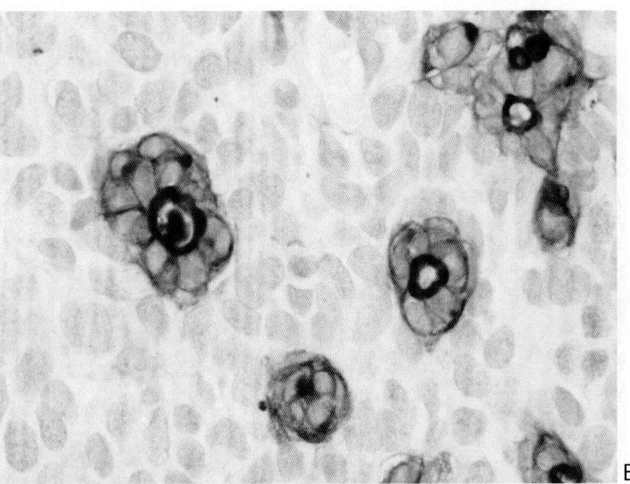

FIG. 25.29. ***Adenoid cystic carcinoma, immunohistochemistry.*** **A:** This AdCC has basaloid morphology. An inconspicuous glandular space is evident [*short arrow*]. Small deposits of cylindromatous material are present [*long arrows*]. **B:** The epithelial cells lining the small glands are highlighted with a CK7 stain. **C:** Most of the tumor is composed of p63-positive basaloid cells. Note lack of p63 reactivity in the glandular component.

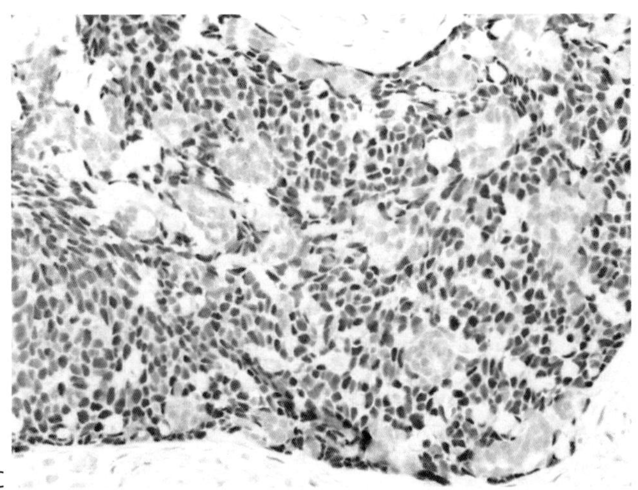

FIG. 25.29. *[Continued]*

genetics and molecular alterations).[52] This observation is consistent with the growing appreciation that triple negative breast carcinomas are a heterogeneous group of neoplasms with respect to their immunophenotype and patterns of molecular alterations, prognosis, and response to therapy.[65]

ELECTRON MICROSCOPY

Electron microscopic studies have revealed the same diverse cell types in mammary AdCC that are encountered in AdCC arising from salivary glands and other organs.[66] In addition to populations of epithelial and myoepithelial cells,[11,29,38,67] the tumors contain varying numbers of basaloid cells[67,68] as well as cells exhibiting sebaceous and adenosquamous differentiation.[68]

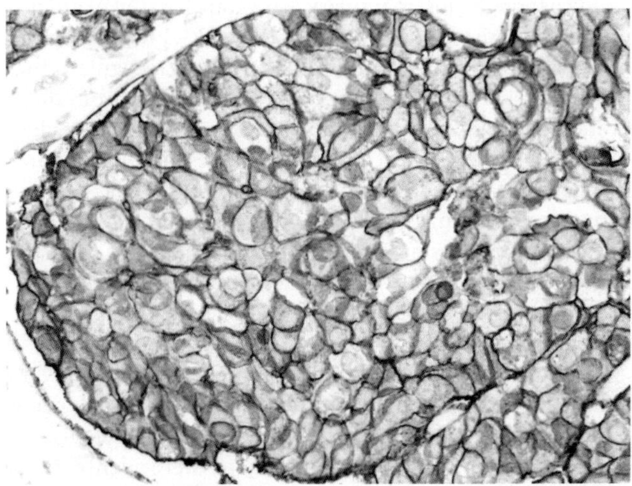

FIG. 25.30. ***Adenoid cystic carcinoma, immunohistochemistry.*** All tumor cells in this basaloid AdCC show reactivity for kit/CD117 protein.

DIFFERENTIAL DIAGNOSIS OF AdCC

Collagenous spherulosis combines gland formation and spherules of basement membrane components surrounded by myoepithelial cells in a pattern that mimics AdCC (Fig. 25.32). An important clinical distinction between the two lesions is that AdCC almost always presents as a palpable mass and/or is evident on imaging studies, whereas collagenous spherulosis typically presents as nonpalpable, mammographically detected calcifications.[69] However, collagenous spherulosis is sometimes part of a mass lesion consisting of fibrocystic changes and it may be present in a papilloma. The spherules of collagenous spherulosis contain elastin, periodic acid–Schiff (PAS)–positive material, and type IV collagen.[70,71] A distinct myoepithelial layer surrounding the spherules can be highlighted with p63, CD10, and actin immunostains. Immunohistochemical expression of kit is found in almost all AdCCs, but not in collagenous spherulosis,[35–37,48,50,57] whereas the reverse is true for calponin and SMM-HC.[50]

Some conventional forms of mammary carcinoma may be incorrectly diagnosed as AdCC.[9,36,72] In one review,[72] about half of the cases recorded by the Connecticut Tumor Registry as AdCC were misclassified. Most of the errors resulted from including duct carcinomas with a prominent cribriform component. Invasive cribriform carcinoma is a monophasic adenocarcinoma with no myoepithelial component and no obvious matrix deposits. Cribriform areas may be found in an AdCC, and their presence does not exclude the diagnosis if other diagnostic components are present. Occasional problems are encountered in distinguishing AdCC from solid papillary DCIS or papillomas with solid ductal hyperplasia, especially when collagenous spherulosis is present.

High-grade carcinoma arising in microglandular adenosis (MGA) resembles the solid, basaloid variant of AdCC with the exception that the former typically has a very high mitotic rate.[73,74] In addition, myoepithelial cells are absent in MGA and MGA-associated carcinomas, and a p63 immunostaining will not decorate these tumors.

High-grade AdCC with sparse glandular and cylindromatous areas might be mistaken for small cell carcinoma (SCC) (Fig. 25.24), but does not show neuroendocrine differentiation. A study of basaloid, small cell, and AdCCs of the oropharynx revealed some immunophenotypical differences.[75] Immunoreactivity for high-molecular-weight keratin detected with the 34βE12 antibody was present in virtually all basaloid carcinomas and AdCCs and absent from SCCs. Other CK antibodies were equally immunoreactive in the three types of tumor. SMA was detected in 75% of AdCCs, but it was absent from basaloid carcinomas and SCCs. Neuroendocrine markers were undetectable in virtually all basaloid carcinomas and AdCCs and variably expressed in SCCs. Vimentin was detected in 93% of AdCCs, 80% of SCCs, and 35% of basaloid carcinomas (see also Chapter 21). Cabibi et al.[76] have reported one case of AdCC merging with SCC.

The differential diagnosis of AdCC in the nipple includes syringomatous adenoma, a benign lesion that does not produce Paget disease. A cylindroma of the skin overlying the

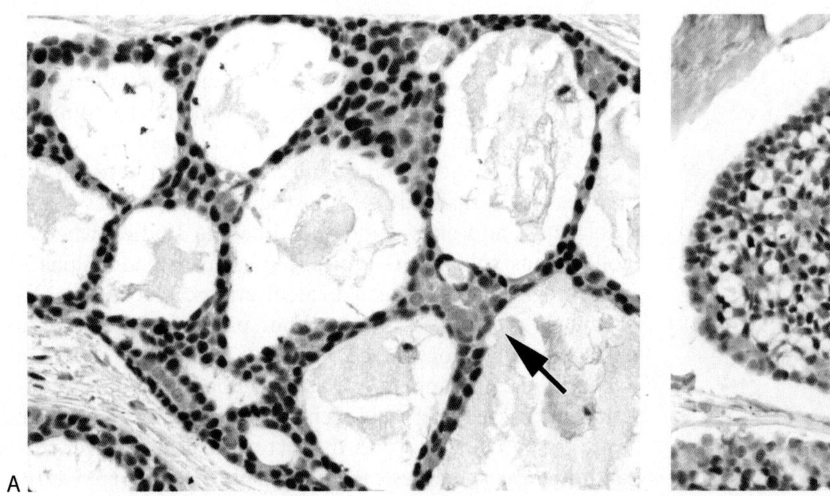

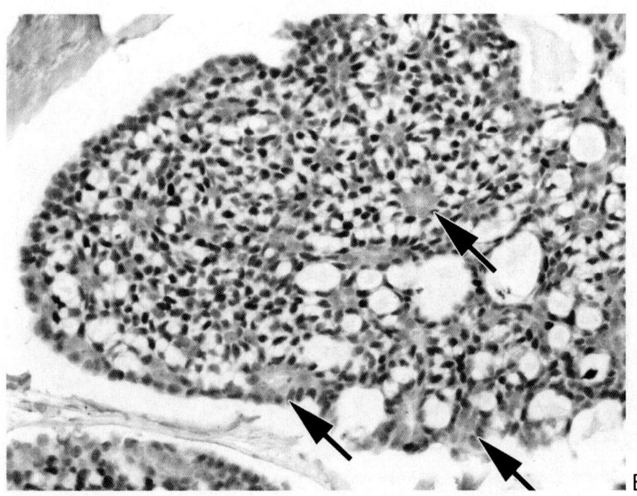

FIG. 25.31. ***Adenoid cystic carcinoma, immunohistochemistry.*** **A,B:** The myoepithelial/basaloid cells from two different AdCCs show reactivity for MYB protein. The glandular component (*arrows*) is MYB-negative.

breast can also be misdiagnosed as a mammary AdCC if one overlooks its superficial location and cutaneous origin.

Because of the intratumoral heterogeneity characteristic of AdCC, this tumor may be difficult to recognize in a needle biopsy specimen unless a characteristic sample has been obtained. In some cases, the cylindromatous material compresses the glandular elements, and a needle core biopsy sample could be mistaken for invasive lobular or scirrhous carcinoma (Fig. 25.7). Alternatively, inspissated secretion and stromal fragments from benign lesions or other forms of carcinoma may resemble cylindromatous material.

GENETICS AND MOLECULAR ALTERATIONS

A high percentage of AdCC of the breast, salivary glands, and other sites carry the *MYB–NFIB* fusion gene resulting from a t(6:9)(q22–23;p23–24) translocation.[52,63,77] Detection of the *MYB–NFIB* fusion product by fluorescence *in situ* hybridization (FISH) and reverse transcription-polymerase chain reaction (RT–PCR) analysis is strong evidence in favor of the diagnosis of AdCC, but a negative result does not completely rule out AdCC.[52,63] Immunohistochemical evidence of *MYB* overexpression is found in *MYB–NFIB* fusion-negative and fusion-positive tumors, suggesting that other mechanisms can lead to activation of the *MYB* protooncogene in AdCC.[63] At present, the only other histologically distinct subtype of mammary carcinoma harboring a characteristic chromosomal translocation is secretory carcinoma, another basal-like carcinoma, with the *ETV6–NTRK3* fusion found in more than 90% of cases.[78,79] It is interesting to note that in AdCC and secretory carcinoma, the same genetic alterations characterize mammary and extramammary tumors, as the *ETV6–NTRK3* fusion gene has been identified recently in the mammary secretory analog carcinoma of the salivary glands.[80] Mutations of the *p53* gene occur more frequently in high grade than in non-high-grade foci of mammary AdCC.[81]

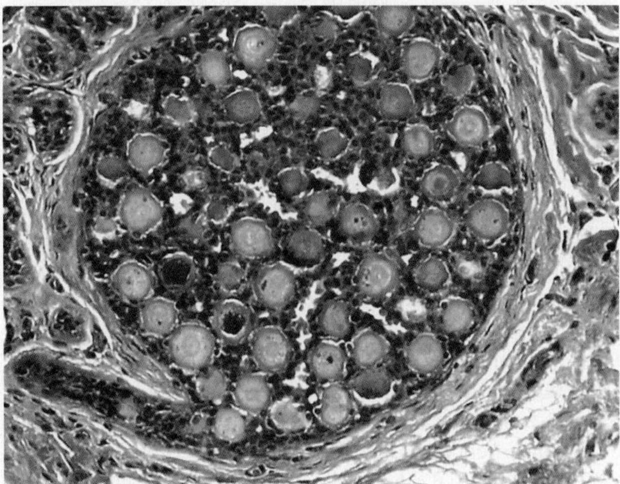

FIG. 25.32. ***Collagenous spherulosis.*** Note the concentric layers and central rings in some spherules.

Even though most mammary AdCCs are basal-like carcinomas, as they are immunohistochemically ER-, PR-, and HER2-negative and CK5/6- and CK14-positive, it is recognized that the patterns of genetic alterations of AdCC differ from those of more conventional triple negative basal-like invasive duct carcinomas.[52] Da Silva et al.[82] used high-resolution comparative genomic hybridization (CGH) to assess whole-genome copy number changes in a predominantly solid AdCC, tubular adenosis, and a small adenomyoepithelioma that coexisted in the breast of a 50-year-old woman. The three lesions had no common genomic alterations. The AdCC harbored deletion of small regions on chromosomes 16p and 17q.

Wetterskog et al.[83] used Sequenom analysis to study 13 mammary AdCCs. They detected no mutations in genes known to be implicated in breast carcinoma, namely *AKT1*, *ERBB2*, and *PIK3CA*. *BRAF* mutations were identified in 2/13 (15%) mammary AdCCs, including *BRAF* V600E, a high-activity mutant, and *BRAF* G464E, an intermediate-activity mutant. These *BRAF* mutations were also detected and validated using Sanger sequencing analysis. The investigators identified a *BRAF* D594G kinase–dead hotspot mutation in another breast AdCC, and an *HRAS* Q61K hotspot mutation in one salivary gland AdCC, adding to a true prevalence of mutation rate of at least 4% for *BRAF* and 1% for *HRAS* in a total of 65 AdCCs of mammary and extramammary origin. Another group of investigators has identified a *KRAS* mutation in one of 25 AdCCs of the salivary glands.[84] These findings suggest that *BRAF* may play a role in the pathogenesis of AdCC. None of the 13 mammary and 68 extramammary AdCCs studied by Wetterskog et al.[83] had activating *KIT* mutations. These observations document that *KIT* mutations are substantially absent in AdCC, despite strong and diffuse positive immunoreactivity for kit/CD177 protein in these tumors. Other studies have also found no activating *KIT*[85] and platelet-derived growth factor receptor α (*PDGFR-α*)[86] gene mutations in AdCC. Consistent with the absence of *KIT* mutations is also the observation that treatment with imatinib mesylate, a tyrosine kinase inhibitor active in tumors with *KIT* gene mutation, was ineffective in patients with unresectable or metastatic AdCC of the salivary glands.[86,87]

One of the four cylindromas of the breast reported by Nonaka et al.[88] occurred in a woman with Brooke–Spiegler syndrome, a genetic disease characterized by multiple familial trichoepitheliomas and familial cylindromas secondary to inherited autosomal mutation of the *CYLD* gene. A group of investigators[89] found two silent *CYLD* mutations but no missense *CYLD* mutations in 34 extramammary AdCCs. None of these mutations has been evaluated in mammary AdCCs.

When studied by flow cytometry, 22/24 (91.4%) AdCCs were diploid.[19]

TREATMENT AND PROGNOSIS

Until the last quarter of the 20th century, data on the prognosis of AdCC were based mainly on patients treated primarily by mastectomy, which was curative in virtually all cases.[9–14,18–20,22,25,26,29,38,67,72] Chest wall recurrence was reported after simple mastectomy in only rare cases, and there have been isolated instances of systemic metastases.[13,90–93]

Presently, breast-conserving surgery is the preferred primary therapy for mammary AdCC,[18,19,22,48,94] except for large tumors that require a mastectomy to achieve a negative margin.[18] Between 1980 and 2007, breast-conserving surgery was employed in 41/61 (67%) patients and mastectomy in 20/61 cases treated at a consortium of institutions constituting the Rare Cancer Network.[18] Surgical margin status was close or positive in 10 (16%) patients, negative in 50 (82%), and unknown in 1. None of the patients with close margins underwent reexcision. In one institution experience detailed by Sarnaik et al.,[26] microscopic examination revealed invasive growth that required further excision in four patients treated initially by partial mastectomy, even if the tumors appeared to be well circumscribed grossly. Three of these patients subsequently received radiotherapy. Kleer and Oberman[28] and Hodgson et al.[25] recommended obtaining wide-excision margins, as 50% or more of the surgical resection specimens in their series had tumor at ink.

The role of adjuvant radiotherapy in patients treated with breast-conserving surgery for mammary AdCC was investigated by Coates et al.[94] who studied 376 women with mammary AdCC recorded in the SEER data base for the years 1988 through 2005. Primary surgery consisted of lumpectomy in 227 patients (60%), and the remainder had a mastectomy. Adjuvant radiotherapy was given to 53% (120/227) of the lumpectomy patients and to 6% (9/149) of the patients treated by mastectomy. The OS of patients treated with surgery and radiotherapy was substantially better than the survival of patients treated with surgery alone, with a survival benefit of 12.4% at 5 years and 19.7% at 10 years in favor of patients who received radiotherapy. This study has limitations, including lack of information about margin status and sites of recurrence (local or systemic), as well as incomplete data for nodal status.

Radiotherapy was administered to 40/61 patients studied by Khanfir et al.,[18] including 35 who received whole-breast irradiation after breast-conserving surgery, and 5 who received postmastectomy chest wall irradiation. One patient was treated with partial breast brachytherapy. Eleven patients also had ALN irradiation. Indications for radiotherapy included T4 tumor size, positive margins, and tumor location in the internal quadrants of the breast. After a median follow-up of 79 months, local recurrence developed in 2/35 (5.7%) patients treated by local excision and radiotherapy and in 2/6 (33%) patients treated by lumpectomy alone. Two of the 61 (3.2%) patients died of disease, and four had died of other causes. A study by Arpino et al.[19] documented no local recurrences in six patients treated by lumpectomy, including five who received local radiotherapy. However, one of the patients who received radiotherapy had presented with metastatic disease, and another developed distant metastases 72 months after diagnosis.

Axillary nodal metastases of AdCC are uncommon. ALNs were examined in 51 of 61 patients with AdCC in the Rare Cancer Network,[18] including 10 of 51 who underwent sentinel lymph node (SLN) biopsy. None of the patients had lymph node involvement. The necessity of axillary staging in patients with mammary AdCC was studied by Thompson et al.[7] in the population-based California Cancer Registry. In the years 1988 to 2006, 244 women were listed as having AdCC of the breast. Among 144 patients with data for tumor size and nodal status, only 8 (5.5%) had axillary nodal metastases. The mean tumor size in patients with nodal metastases was 3.7 cm (range 1.4 to 7.7 cm) and of those without nodal metastases was 2.2 cm (range 0.1 to 8 cm). Although not statistically significant ($p = 0.06$), there appeared to be a direct relationship between tumor size and the likelihood of nodal involvement. Lymph node metastases were identified in 9 of 235 (3.8%) patients who underwent ALN dissection or SLN biopsy in nine combined series.[15,18,19,21,22,28,31,33,48] Two (2/235; 0.8%) additional patients had a lymph node with isolated tumor cells. Axillary involvement is more frequent in patients with basaloid AdCC. Shin and Rosen[37] documented lymph node metastases in two of six basaloid AdCCs in their series.

ALN involvement usually carries a negative prognosis, even though distant metastases can occur independent of any involvement of the ALNs. Two patients with lymph node metastases at the time of mastectomy[30,38] developed pulmonary metastases and died of disease. Zhu et al.[15] studied 33 patients with AdCC. After a median follow-up of 72 months, distant recurrences were detected in 12/33 (36%) patients. In this study, axillary nodal metastases were associated with a significantly reduced disease-free survival (DFS).

Adjuvant chemotherapy is rarely administered to patients with AdCC. Kulkarni et al.[16] reported that only 11.3% of 933 patients with AdCC in the 1998–2008 National Cancer Data Base received chemotherapy versus 45.4% of all patients with breast carcinoma treated in the same period ($p < 0.0001$). Only 15/61 (24.5%) patients studied by Khanfir et al.[18] received adjuvant chemotherapy.

None of the 18 women studied by Azoulay et al.[48] received chemotherapy. One patient whose tumor had been treated only by radiotherapy died of disease at 2 years. Two patients initially treated with breast-conserving surgery developed locally recurrent disease at 11 and 13 years. They were treated surgically and were alive 16 and 19 years after treatment. None of the patients in this study developed distant metastases.

Information about systemic adjuvant therapy was available for 23 patients in the series by Arpino et al.[19] Most (16/23; 70%) received no adjuvant therapy, 6 of 23 (26%) had hormonal therapy, and only 1 (4%) was treated with chemotherapy.

According to the National Cancer Data Base registry,[16] hormonal therapy was used in 8.9% in patients with AdCC versus 39.8% of patients with non-AdCCs ($p < 0.0001$). Only 7/61 (11.5%) patients in the series by Khanfir et al.[18] were prescribed tamoxifen. In this series,[18] local recurrences developed in 2 of 35 (5%) patients treated by lumpectomy and radiotherapy and in 2 of 6 (33%) patients treated by lumpectomy alone. No recurrences occurred in patients who had a mastectomy. The interval to recurrence ranged from 21 to 99 months. Local recurrences were treated by mastectomy after which the four patients remained disease free. Four local recurrences in the breast were also found among patients who had negative lumpectomy margins. All eight patients who had positive lumpectomy margins had postoperative radiotherapy, and none developed locally recurrent disease. Four of the 61 (6.5%) patients developed systemic metastases that were fatal at the time of last follow-up in two cases.

The OS of 61 patients with AdCC part of the Rare Cancer Network[18] was 94% and 86% at 5 and 10 years, respectively, and the corresponding DFS was 82% and 74%. In the series by Thompson et al.,[7] women with AdCC had a relative cumulative survival advantage of approximately 20% after 10 years of follow-up when compared with women with breast carcinoma in general.

Hodgson et al.[25] described 12 women treated for mammary AdCC with a median tumor size of 3.5 cm (range 1.0 to 7.0). Three patients (25%) underwent mastectomy and the remainder partial mastectomy. Positive margins were detected in 5 of 10 cases with documented margin status, including 4 who had breast-conserving surgery and 1 treated by mastectomy. Patients with positive margins had additional surgery consisting of lumpectomy or mastectomy, resulting in negative margins in four cases. Incomplete follow-up information in this series revealed local recurrences in three patients but did not correlate disease recurrence with the type of primary surgery or margin status.

A series of seven patients reported by Sarnaik et al.[26] should also be noted. The median tumor size was 1.8 cm (range 1.3 to 5.0 cm). The only local recurrence developed in a patient who had a total mastectomy for a 5-cm tumor with unknown margin status followed by immediate breast reconstruction. The patient did not have postoperative radiotherapy. Four years later, she developed a recurrence that was treated by excision and radiotherapy.

Follow-up data for 38 of 41 patients reported by Slodkowska et al.[21] documented local recurrences in 4 (10%) patients and distant metastases in 3 (7%). The median tumor size of patients with recurrent disease was 2.8 cm. Two patients with lung metastases were alive with disease 71 and 84 months after diagnosis. Zhu et al.[15] identified distant recurrences in 12/33 (36%) patients with AdCC and a median follow-up of 72 months. In this study, older age and axillary nodal metastases were associated with poor OS and reduced DFS, but the risk of recurrence was not significantly related to tumor grade. The relatively high recurrence rate is probably influenced by the fact that follow-up information was not available for 41% of the study patients. If there had been no recurrences in any of the patients with no follow-up information, the recurrence rate would have been 21% (12/56), only slightly higher than that reported by Slodkowska et al.[21] The higher rate of metastases in these two recent series is probably secondary to a relatively higher number of basaloid AdCCs than in older studies.

All patients with metastases have had pulmonary involvement (Fig. 25.33), with recurrences in the lung being detected as late as 6,[90] 8,[93] 9,[92] 10,[13] and 12 years[90,91] after initial treatment. All of these patients had negative ALNs. In addition to the lung, other sites of distant metastases include bone,[38] liver,[38] brain,[91,95] and kidneys.[90]

Imatinib mesylate, a selective inhibitor of the tyrosine kinases encoded by *ABL*, *PDGFR*, and *KIT* that has been successfully used to treat neoplasms with *KIT* mutation, has been ineffective in the treatment of metastatic AdCC of the salivary glands.[86,87] This finding is consistent with the absence of *KIT* mutations in these tumors. Data are lacking for the use of this medication for treating mammary AdCC.

In summary, patients with mammary AdCC have a very good prognosis with a low risk of systemic metastases and death because of AdCC. It is important to note that more recent series report a slightly worse prognosis, probably because of the inclusion of a higher numbers of cases of AdCC with basaloid morphology. As with other forms of breast carcinoma, breast-conserving surgery is recommended if a cosmetically satisfactory result can be achieved with negative margins. Because of the tendency to grossly imperceptible peripheral growth that increases the risk of incomplete excision that can lead to local recurrence, careful attention should be given to evaluating resection margins at the time of initial surgery. In most cases, the finding of a positive margin should lead to a wider excision or a mastectomy, depending on the circumstances in a particular case.

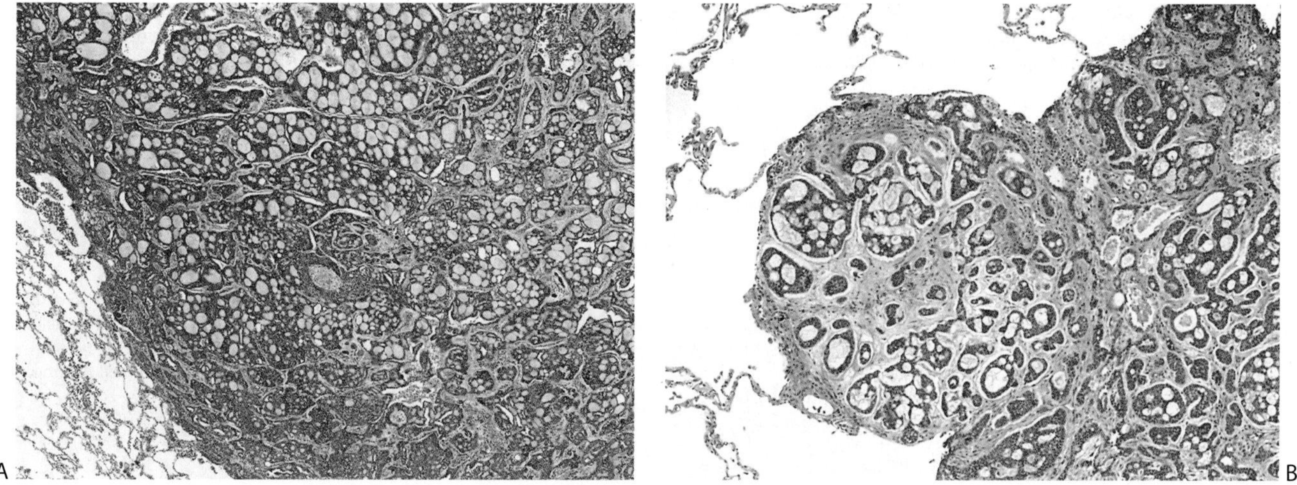

FIG. 25.33. ***Adenoid cystic carcinoma, metastatic.*** **A,B:** Two examples of metastatic AdCC in the lung.

Recurrences in the breast have been reported after treatment by local excision only[13,29,38] with the interval to recurrence ranging from less than 1 year to more than 20 years. Available data suggest that the addition of adjuvant radiotherapy in the setting of breast-conserving surgery reduces the likelihood of local recurrence and improves OS, especially for patients with a positive margin in the initial surgical procedure. It is not clear that radiotherapy alone is sufficient treatment for the patient with a positive margin, but it might be considered when reexcision would necessitate a mastectomy.

The overall likelihood of regional nodal and distant metastases is low and directly related to tumor size. In the absence of clinically abnormal lymph nodes, staging of the ipsilateral axilla can be accomplished by SLN sampling. Mapping of the SLN is always indicated when another form of invasive carcinoma is present with AdCC, for AdCC tumors larger than 3 cm, and high-grade AdCC. Although biopsy of the SLN might be omitted for T1a and T1b tumors, it should be noted that image-based measurements of tumor size may underestimate the full extent of AdCC because of grossly inapparent invasion beyond the palpable tumor in a substantial number of cases.[25,28] The decision to perform an axillary dissection after SLN sampling will depend on the size of the primary tumor, the findings in the SLN, and the surgical evaluation of the axilla.

Systemic adjuvant therapy is recommended for patients with nodal metastases larger than micrometastases and may be considered for patients with tumors larger than 3 cm or with high-grade lesions, regardless of nodal status.

REFERENCES

1. Billroth T. Beobachtungen uber Geschwulste der Speicheldrusen. *Virchows Arch B Cell Pathol Incl Mol Pathol* 1859;17:357–375.
2. Ewing J. Epithelial tumors of the salivary gland. In: *Neoplastic diseases: a treatise on tumors.* 3rd ed. Philadelphia: WB Saunders, 1919:780.
3. Geschickter CF. *Diseases of the breast: diagnosis, pathology, treament.* 2nd ed. Philadelphia: JB Lippincott, 1945.
4. Foote FW Jr, Stewart FW. A histologic classification of carcinoma of the breast. *Surgery* 1946;19:74–99.
5. Galloway JR, Woolner LB, Clagett OT. Adenoid cystic carcinoma of the breast. *Surg Gynecol Obstet* 1966;122:1289–1294.
6. McClenathan JH, de la Roza G. Adenoid cystic breast cancer. *Am J Surg* 2002;183:646–649.
7. Thompson K, Grabowski J, Saltzstein SL, et al. Adenoid cystic breast carcinoma: is axillary staging necessary in all cases? Results from the California Cancer Registry. *Breast J* 2011;17:485–489.
8. Ghabach B, Anderson WF, Curtis RE, et al. Adenoid cystic carcinoma of the breast in the United States (1977 to 2006): a population-based cohort study. *Breast Cancer Res* 2010;12:R54.
9. Cavanzo FJ, Taylor HB. Adenoid cystic carcinoma of the breast. An analysis of 21 cases. *Cancer* 1969;24:740–745.
10. Friedman BA, Oberman HA. Adenoid cystic carcinoma of the breast. *Am J Clin Pathol* 1970;54:1–14.
11. Koss LG, Brannan CD, Ashikari R. Histologic and ultrastructural features of adenoid cystic carcinoma of the breast. *Cancer* 1970;26:1271–1279.
12. Lerner AG, Molnar JJ, Adam YG. Adenoid cystic carcinoma of the breast. *Am J Surg* 1974;127:585–587.
13. Peters GN, Wolff M. Adenoid cystic carcinoma of the breast. Report of 11 new cases: review of the literature and discussion of biological behavior. *Cancer* 1983;52:680–686.
14. Rosen PP. Adenoid cystic carcinoma of the breast. A morphologically heterogeneous neoplasm. *Pathol Annu* 1989;24 (Pt. 2):237–254.
15. Zhu X, Chen J, Xing Y, et al. Adenoid cystic carcinoma of the breast: clinicopathologic and molecular analysis of 56 cases. *Mod Pathol* 2012;25(Suppl. 2):76A.
16. Kulkarni N, Pezzi CM, Greif JM, et al. Rare breast cancer: 933 adenoid cystic carcinomas from the National Cancer Data Base. *Ann Surg Oncol* 2013;20:2236–2241.
17. Delanote S, Van den Broecke R, Schelfhout VR, et al. Adenoid cystic carcinoma of the breast in a 19-year-old girl. *Breast* 2003;12:75–77.
18. Khanfir K, Kallel A, Villette S, et al. Management of adenoid cystic carcinoma of the breast: a Rare Cancer Network study. *Int J Radiat Oncol Biol Phys* 2012;82:2118–2124.
19. Arpino G, Clark GM, Mohsin S, et al. Adenoid cystic carcinoma of the breast: molecular markers, treatment, and clinical outcome. *Cancer* 2002;94:2119–2127.
20. Hjorth S, Magnusson PH, Blomquist P. Adenoid cystic carcinoma of the breast. Report of a case in a male and review of the literature. *Acta Chir Scand* 1977;143:155–158.
21. Slodkowska EA, Sahoo S, Akram M, et al. Adenoid cystic carcinoma of the breast: a morphologic study of 41 cases. *Mod Pathol* 2012;25(Suppl. 2):67A.
22. Millar BA, Kerba M, Youngson B, et al. The potential role of breast conservation surgery and adjuvant breast radiation for adenoid cystic carcinoma of the breast. *Breast Cancer Res Treat* 2004;87:225–232.

23. Burga AM, Fadare O, Lininger RA, et al. Invasive carcinomas of the male breast: a morphologic study of the distribution of histologic subtypes and metastatic patterns in 778 cases. *Virchows Arch* 2006;449:507–512.
24. Hollingsworth A, Iezzoni JC. Primary cutaneous adenoid cystic carcinoma of the male breast: a case report and review of the literature. *Breast Dis* 1994;7:213–218.
25. Hodgson NC, Lytwyn A, Bacopulos S, et al. Adenoid cystic breast carcinoma: high rates of margin positivity after breast conserving surgery. *Am J Clin Oncol* 2010;33:28–31.
26. Sarnaik AA, Meade T, King J, et al. Adenoid cystic carcinoma of the breast: a review of a single institution's experience. *Breast J* 2010;16:208–210.
27. Santamaria G, Velasco M, Zanon G, et al. Adenoid cystic carcinoma of the breast: mammographic appearance and pathologic correlation. *AJR Am J Roentgenol* 1998;171:1679–1683.
28. Kleer CG, Oberman HA. Adenoid cystic carcinoma of the breast: value of histologic grading and proliferative activity. *Am J Surg Pathol* 1998;22:569–575.
29. Qizilbash AH, Patterson MC, Oliveira KF. Adenoid cystic carcinoma of the breast. Light and electron microscopy and a brief review of the literature. *Arch Pathol Lab Med* 1977;101:302–306.
30. Wells CA, Nicoll S, Ferguson DJ. Adenoid cystic carcinoma of the breast: a case with axillary lymph node metastasis. *Histopathology* 1986;10:415–424.
31. Montagna E, Maisonneuve P, Rotmensz N, et al. Heterogeneity of triple-negative breast cancer: histologic subtyping to inform the outcome. *Clin Breast Cancer* 2013;13:31–39.
32. Bourke AG, Metcalf C, Wylie EJ. Mammographic features of adenoid cystic carcinoma. *Australas Radiol* 1994;38:324–325.
33. Glazebrook KN, Reynolds C, Smith RL, et al. Adenoid cystic carcinoma of the breast. *AJR Am J Roentgenol* 2010;194:1391–1396.
34. Saqi A, Mercado CL, Hamele-Bena D. Adenoid cystic carcinoma of the breast diagnosed by fine-needle aspiration. *Diagn Cytopathol* 2004;30:271–274.
35. Tsuboi N, Ogawa Y, Inomata T, et al. Dynamic MR appearance of adenoid cystic carcinoma of the breast in a 67-year-old female. *Radiat Med* 1998;16:225–228.
36. Harris M. Pseudoadenoid cystic carcinoma of the breast. *Arch Pathol Lab Med* 1977;101:307–309.
37. Shin SJ, Rosen PP. Solid variant of mammary adenoid cystic carcinoma with basaloid features: a study of nine cases. *Am J Surg Pathol* 2002;26:413–420.
38. Ro JY, Silva EG, Gallager HS. Adenoid cystic carcinoma of the breast. *Hum Pathol* 1987;18:1276–1281.
39. Azumi N, Battifora H. The cellular composition of adenoid cystic carcinoma. An immunohistochemical study. *Cancer* 1987;60:1589–1598.
40. Orenstein JM, Dardick I, van Nostrand AW. Ultrastructural similarities of adenoid cystic carcinoma and pleomorphic adenoma. *Histopathology* 1985;9:623–638.
41. Marchio C, Weigelt B, Reis-Filho JS. Adenoid cystic carcinomas of the breast and salivary glands (or 'The strange case of Dr Jekyll and Mr Hyde' of exocrine gland carcinomas). *J Clin Pathol* 2010;63:220–228.
42. Van Dorpe J, De Pauw A, Moerman P. Adenoid cystic carcinoma arising in an adenomyoepithelioma of the breast. *Virchows Arch* 1998;432:119–122.
43. Noske A, Schwabe M, Pahl S, et al. Report of a metaplastic carcinoma of the breast with multi-directional differentiation: an adenoid cystic carcinoma, a spindle cell carcinoma and melanoma. *Virchows Arch* 2008;452:575–579.
44. Gupta RK, Green C, Naran S, et al. Fine-needle aspiration cytology of adenoid cystic carcinoma of the breast. *Diagn Cytopathol* 1999;20:82–84.
45. Kasagawa T, Suzuki M, Doki T, et al. Two cases of adenoid cystic carcinoma: preoperative cytological findings were useful in determining treatment strategy. *Breast Cancer* 2006;13:112–116.
46. Pandya AN, Shah P, Patel R, et al. Adenoid cystic carcinoma of breast and the importance of differentiation from collagenous spherulosis by FNAC. *J Cytol* 2010;27:69–70.
47. Kasami M, Olson SJ, Simpson JF, et al. Maintenance of polarity and a dual cell population in adenoid cystic carcinoma of the breast: an immunohistochemical study. *Histopathology* 1998;32:232–238.
48. Azoulay S, Lae M, Freneaux P, et al. KIT is highly expressed in adenoid cystic carcinoma of the breast, a basal-like carcinoma associated with a favorable outcome. *Mod Pathol* 2005;18:1623–1631.
49. Boecker W, Stenman G, Loening T, et al. K5/K14-positive cells contribute to salivary gland-like breast tumors with myoepithelial differentiation. *Mod Pathol* 2013;1–15.
50. Rabban JT, Swain RS, Zaloudek CJ, et al. Immunophenotypic overlap between adenoid cystic carcinoma and collagenous spherulosis of the breast: potential diagnostic pitfalls using myoepithelial markers. *Mod Pathol* 2006;19:1351–1357.
51. Reis-Filho JS, Milanezi F, Silva P, et al. Maspin expression in myoepithelial tumors of the breast. *Pathol Res Pract* 2001;197:817–821.
52. Wetterskog D, Lopez-Garcia MA, Lambros MB, et al. Adenoid cystic carcinomas constitute a genomically distinct subgroup of triple-negative and basal-like breast cancers. *J Pathol* 2012;226:84–96.
53. Cabibi D, Giannone AG, Belmonte B, et al. CD10 and HHF35 actin in the differential diagnosis between collagenous spherulosis and adenoid-cystic carcinoma of the breast. *Pathol Res Pract* 2012;208:405–409.
54. d'Ardenne AJ, Kirkpatrick P, Wells CA, et al. Laminin and fibronectin in adenoid cystic carcinoma. *J Clin Pathol* 1986;39:138–144.
55. Due W, Herbst WD, Loy V, et al. Characterisation of adenoid cystic carcinoma of the breast by immunohistology. *J Clin Pathol* 1989;42:470–476.
56. Cheng J, Saku T, Okabe H, et al. Basement membranes in adenoid cystic carcinoma. An immunohistochemical study. *Cancer* 1992;69:2631–2640.
57. Mastropasqua MG, Maiorano E, Pruneri G, et al. Immunoreactivity for c-kit and p63 as an adjunct in the diagnosis of adenoid cystic carcinoma of the breast. *Mod Pathol* 2005;18:1277–1282.
58. Pastolero G, Hanna W, Zbieranowski I, et al. Proliferative activity and p53 expression in adenoid cystic carcinoma of the breast. *Mod Pathol* 1996;9:215–219.
59. Holst VA, Marshall CE, Moskaluk CA, et al. KIT protein expression and analysis of c-kit gene mutation in adenoid cystic carcinoma. *Mod Pathol* 1999;12:956–960.
60. Crisi GM, Marconi SA, Makari-Judson G, et al. Expression of c-kit in adenoid cystic carcinoma of the breast. *Am J Clin Pathol* 2005;124:733–739.
61. Walter O, Prasad M, Lu S, et al. IMP3 is a novel biomarker for triple negative invasive mammary carcinoma associated with a more aggressive phenotype. *Hum Pathol* 2009;40:1528–1533.
62. Vranic S, Gurjeva O, Frkovic-Grazio S, et al. IMP3, a proposed novel basal phenotype marker, is commonly overexpressed in adenoid cystic carcinomas but not in apocrine carcinomas of the breast. *Appl Immunohistochem Mol Morphol* 2011;19:413–416.
63. Brill LB II, Kanner WA, Fehr A, et al. Analysis of MYB expression and MYB-NFIB gene fusions in adenoid cystic carcinoma and other salivary neoplasms. *Mod Pathol* 2011;24:1169–1176.
64. Vranic S, Gatalica Z, Deng H, et al. ER-alpha36, a novel isoform of ER-alpha66, is commonly over-expressed in apocrine and adenoid cystic carcinomas of the breast. *J Clin Pathol* 2011;64:54–57.
65. Constantinidou A, Jones RL, Reis-Filho JS. Beyond triple-negative breast cancer: the need to define new subtypes. *Expert Rev Anticancer Ther* 2010;10:1197–1213.
66. Lawrence JB, Mazur MT. Adenoid cystic carcinoma: a comparative pathologic study of tumors in salivary gland, breast, lung, and cervix. *Hum Pathol* 1982;13:916–924.
67. Zaloudek C, Oertel YC, Orenstein JM. Adenoid cystic carcinoma of the breast. *Am J Clin Pathol* 1984;81:297–307.
68. Tavassoli FA, Norris HJ. Mammary adenoid cystic carcinoma with sebaceous differentiation. A morphologic study of the cell types. *Arch Pathol Lab Med* 1986;110:1045–1053.
69. Resetkova E, Albarracin C, Sneige N. Collagenous spherulosis of breast: morphologic study of 59 cases and review of the literature. *Am J Surg Pathol* 2006;30:20–27.
70. Clement PB, Young RH, Azzopardi JG. Collagenous spherulosis of the breast. *Am J Surg Pathol* 1987;11:411–417.
71. Grignon DJ, Ro JY, Mackay BN, et al. Collagenous spherulosis of the breast. Immunohistochemical and ultrastructural studies. *Am J Clin Pathol* 1989;91:386–392.
72. Sumpio BE, Jennings TA, Merino MJ, et al. Adenoid cystic carcinoma of the breast. Data from the Connecticut Tumor Registry and a review of the literature. *Ann Surg* 1987;205:295–301.
73. Khalifeh IM, Albarracin C, Diaz LK, et al. Clinical, histopathologic, and immunohistochemical features of microglandular adenosis and transition into *in situ* and invasive carcinoma. *Am J Surg Pathol* 2008;32:544–552.
74. James BA, Cranor ML, Rosen PP. Carcinoma of the breast arising in microglandular adenosis. *Am J Clin Pathol* 1993;100:507–513.

75. Morice WG, Ferreiro JA. Distinction of basaloid squamous cell carcinoma from adenoid cystic and small cell undifferentiated carcinoma by immunohistochemistry. *Hum Pathol* 1998;29:609–612.
76. Cabibi D, Cipolla C, Maria Florena A, et al. Solid variant of mammary "adenoid cystic carcinoma with basaloid features" merging with "small cell carcinoma". *Pathol Res Pract* 2005;201:705–711.
77. Persson M, Andren Y, Mark J, et al. Recurrent fusion of MYB and NFIB transcription factor genes in carcinomas of the breast and head and neck. *Proc Natl Acad Sci U S A* 2009;106:18740–18744.
78. Tognon C, Knezevich SR, Huntsman D, et al. Expression of the ETV6-NTRK3 gene fusion as a primary event in human secretory breast carcinoma. *Cancer Cell* 2002;2:367–376.
79. Lae M, Freneaux P, Sastre-Garau X, et al. Secretory breast carcinomas with ETV6-NTRK3 fusion gene belong to the basal-like carcinoma spectrum. *Mod Pathol* 2009;22:291–298.
80. Skalova A, Vanecek T, Sima R, et al. Mammary analogue secretory carcinoma of salivary glands, containing the ETV6-NTRK3 fusion gene: a hitherto undescribed salivary gland tumor entity. *Am J Surg Pathol* 2010;34:599–608.
81. Yamamoto Y, Wistuba II, Kishimoto Y, et al. DNA analysis at p53 locus in adenoid cystic carcinoma: comparison of molecular study and p53 immunostaining. *Pathol Int* 1998;48:273–280.
82. Da Silva L, Buck L, Simpson PT, et al. Molecular and morphological analysis of adenoid cystic carcinoma of the breast with synchronous tubular adenosis. *Virchows Arch* 2009;454:107–114.
83. Wetterskog D, Wilkerson PM, Rodrigues DN, et al. Mutation profiling of adenoid cystic carcinomas from multiple anatomical sites identifies mutations in the RAS pathway, but no KIT mutations. *Histopathology* 2013;62:543–550.
84. Dahse R, Driemel O, Schwarz S, et al. KRAS status and epidermal growth factor receptor expression as determinants for anti-EGFR therapies in salivary gland carcinomas. *Oral Oncol* 2009;45:826–829.
85. Aubry MC, Heinrich MC, Molina J, et al. Primary adenoid cystic carcinoma of the lung: absence of KIT mutations. *Cancer* 2007;110:2507–2510.
86. Lin CH, Yen RF, Jeng YM, et al. Unexpected rapid progression of metastatic adenoid cystic carcinoma during treatment with imatinib mesylate. *Head Neck* 2005;27:1022–1027.
87. Hotte SJ, Winquist EW, Lamont E, et al. Imatinib mesylate in patients with adenoid cystic cancers of the salivary glands expressing c-kit: a Princess Margaret Hospital phase II consortium study. *J Clin Oncol* 2005;23:585–590.
88. Nonaka D, Rosai J, Spagnolo D, et al. Cylindroma of the breast of skin adnexal type: a study of 4 cases. *Am J Surg Pathol* 2004;28:1070–1075.
89. Daa T, Nakamura I, Yada N, et al. PLAG1 and CYLD do not play a role in the tumorigenesis of adenoid cystic carcinoma. *Mol Med Rep* 2013;7:1086–1090.
90. Herzberg AJ, Bossen EH, Walther PJ. Adenoid cystic carcinoma of the breast metastatic to the kidney. A clinically symptomatic lesion requiring surgical management. *Cancer* 1991;68:1015–1020.
91. Koller M, Ram Z, Findler G, et al. Brain metastasis: a rare manifestation of adenoid cystic carcinoma of the breast. *Surg Neurol* 1986;26:470–472.
92. Lim SK, Kovi J, Warner OG. Adenoid cystic carcinoma of breast with metastasis: a case report and review of the literature. *J Natl Med Assoc* 1979;71:329–330.
93. Nayer HR. Case report section; cylindroma of the breast with pulmonary metastases. *Dis Chest* 1957;31:324–327.
94. Coates JM, Martinez SR, Bold RJ, et al. Adjuvant radiation therapy is associated with improved survival for adenoid cystic carcinoma of the breast. *J Surg Oncol* 2010;102:342–347.
95. Silva I, Tome V, Oliveira J. Adenoid cystic carcinoma of the breast with cerebral metastisation: a clinical novelty. *BMJ Case Rep* 2011;Oct 4,2011. doi: 10.1136/bcr.08.2011.4692.

CHAPTER 26

Invasive Cribriform Carcinoma

FREDERICK C. KOERNER

Cribriform carcinoma is a well-differentiated variant of invasive duct carcinoma. Many of these tumors are probably classified as low-grade invasive duct carcinomas without acknowledging the cribriform growth pattern. Because the information thus far available is limited, it has not been possible to determine whether invasive cribriform carcinoma represents a low-grade variant of invasive duct carcinoma or a specific subtype of carcinoma. For the present, it seems appropriate to employ a diagnosis of "invasive duct carcinoma, cribriform type" to identify these lesions for further study. Those tumors in which the majority of the invasive carcinoma exhibits a cribriform pattern are termed "classical invasive cribriform carcinomas." Some of these tumors have cribriform and tubular components. Tumors in which less than 50% of the lesion has an invasive cribriform pattern and in which the majority displays neither cribriform nor tubular patterns are designated "mixed invasive cribriform carcinoma."

Three major studies of invasive cribriform carcinoma have been published. Among 1,003 invasive breast carcinomas treated at the University of Edinburgh in a 10-year period, Page et al.[1] found 35 classical (4%) and 16 mixed (2%) invasive cribriform carcinomas. Venable et al.[2] reviewed 1,087 primary breast carcinomas at the George Washington University and reported that 32 (3%) were pure or largely invasive cribriform carcinomas and that 30 (3%) were mixed invasive cribriform carcinomas. Marzullo et al.[3] found three pure and two mixed cases in a series of 1,759 infiltrating carcinomas, representing 0.3% of the entire group.

CLINICAL PRESENTATION

The ages of the female patients ranged from 7 to 91 years. Page et al.[1] found that women with classical invasive cribriform carcinoma tended to be younger and to have smaller tumors than women with mixed lesions. Marzullo et al.[3] described three women with pure tumors who were between the ages of 70 and 90 years. Two reported patients were men.[2,4] Choi et al.[5] described a 6-cm invasive cribriform carcinoma occupying a 10-cm malignant phyllodes tumor (PT) in a 62-year-old woman. In a study of eight cases, mammograms revealed spiculated masses measuring 20 to 35 mm in four patients.[6] Two of these lesions contained a few punctate calcifications, and so did the case described by Nishimura et al.[4] Invasive cribriform carcinomas do not have consistent sonographic finding.[4,6,7] Magnetic resonance imaging (MRI) performed on one tumor displayed homogeneous early enhancement with a delayed wash-out kinetic pattern compatible with a carcinoma.[7]

GROSS PATHOLOGY

No specific gross pathologic features have been noted. Data from two studies suggested that a small but distinct proportion of invasive cribriform carcinomas occur as multifocal masses.[1,3] In one study, 7 of 35 (20%) patients with classical and 1 of 16 (6%) patients with mixed invasive cribriform carcinoma had macroscopically evident multifocal invasive foci in the affected breast.[1] One patient studied by Marzullo et al.[3] had two masses spanning 1.6 and 0.4 cm in the same breast.

MICROSCOPIC PATHOLOGY

The invasive component of cribriform carcinoma exhibits the same sieve-like growth pattern that characterizes conventional cribriform ductal carcinoma *in situ* (DCIS) (Fig. 26.1). The rounded and angular masses of uniform, well-differentiated tumor cells are embedded in variable amounts of collagenous stroma. Sharply outlined, round, or oval glandular spaces are distributed throughout these tumor aggregates, creating a fenestrated appearance. Mucin-positive secretion is present in varying amounts within the lumens,[8] which may also contain microcalcifications.[9] Specimens obtained by needle aspiration demonstrate bland ductal cells arranged in monolayered sheets or in cohesive three-dimensional clumps. Myoepithelial cells and naked nuclei do not appear obvious.[10] The tumor cells do not contain argyrophilic granules when examined with the Grimelius stain,[1] and myoepithelial cells are not demonstrable by actin immunostaining. The *in situ* component has a cribriform pattern in most but not all classical invasive cribriform carcinomas. Perineural invasion is rarely found in this type of low-grade carcinoma (Fig. 26.2). Nodal metastases from classical tumors also usually have a cribriform structure, whereas metastases derived from mixed tumors are more likely to lack a cribriform pattern (Fig. 26.3).[1,2]

In addition to the cribriform structure, a minority of tumors have areas of tubular growth, which can comprise as

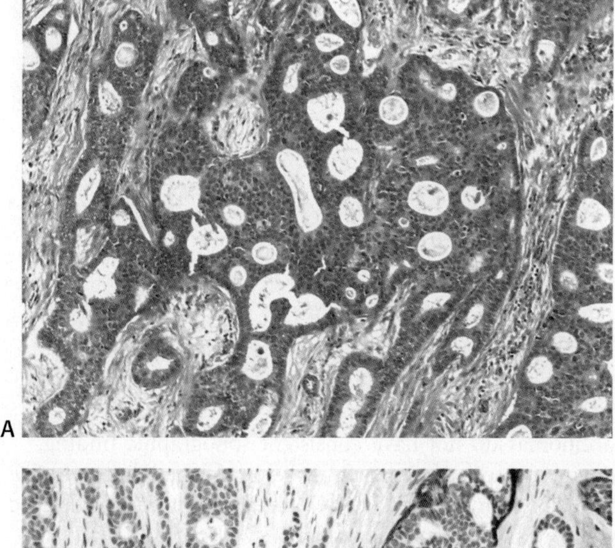

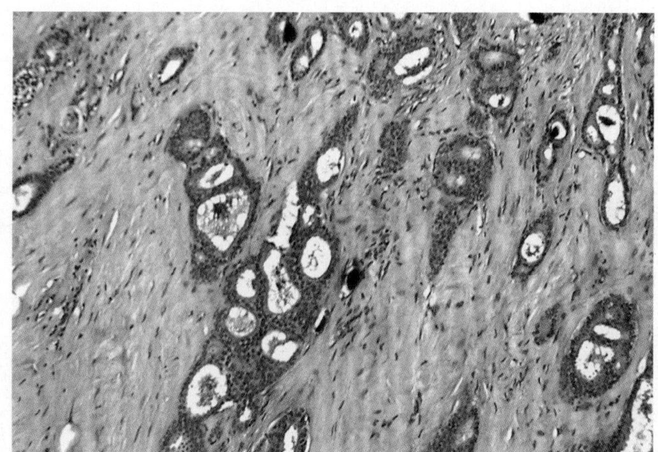

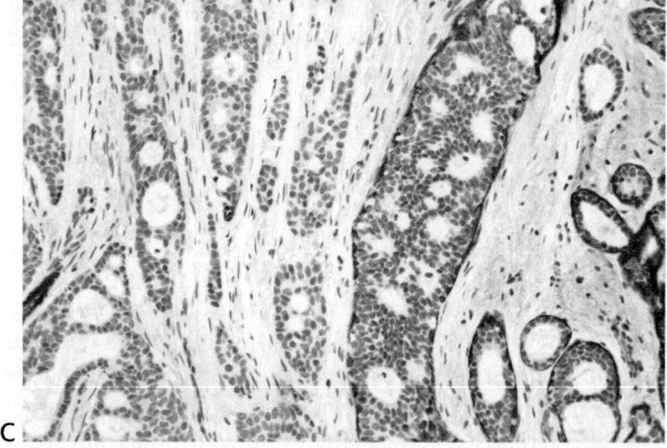

FIG. 26.1. ***Invasive cribriform carcinoma.*** **A:** Invasive carcinoma with a cribriform growth pattern. **B:** This tumor displays stromal fibrosis and some tubular glands. Calcifications are present. **C:** The smooth muscle myosin-heavy chain (SMM-HC) immunostain demonstrates myoepithelium around cribriform DCIS (*right center*) and benign glands (*right*). Myoepithelium is absent from the invasive cribriform carcinoma (*left*).

much as 50% of the lesion.[1,2] Page et al.[1] found tubular areas in 6 of 35 (17%) classical tumors. The presence of such foci does not justify the use of the diagnosis of tubular carcinoma for these cases. Tumors in which the invasive cribriform pattern accounts for 25% or more of the mass should be classified as invasive cribriform carcinomas rather than tubular carcinomas. When the tubular pattern represents at least 75% of the mass, one could consider the diagnosis of tubular carcinoma if the cytologic and architectural features of the tubules seem appropriate (see Chapter 13).

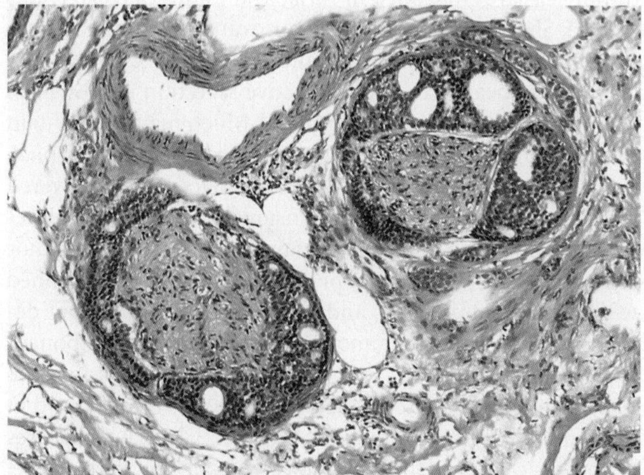

FIG. 26.2. ***Invasive cribriform carcinoma, perineural invasion.***

Invasive cribriform carcinoma should be distinguished from adenoid cystic carcinoma (AdCC). Cribriform growth of an invasive cribriform carcinoma produces a fenestrated structural pattern that lacks the cylindromatous components composed of basal lamina material characteristic of AdCC. AdCC, on the other hand, can contain regions showing prominent cribriform gland formation. Although the term "adenocystic" has been applied to the growth pattern of such regions,[11] they constitute part of the spectrum of AdCC[12] (see Chapter 25), and their presence need not suggest the diagnosis of invasive cribriform carcinoma.

IMMUNOHISTOCHEMISTRY

Venable et al.[2] reported that 16 classical and mixed invasive cribriform carcinomas were estrogen receptor (ER) positive and that 11 of the tumors (69%) were progesterone receptor (PR) positive. There was not an appreciable difference in PR positivity between classical and mixed cribriform tumors. Marzullo et al.[3] reported that one of two pure and two of two

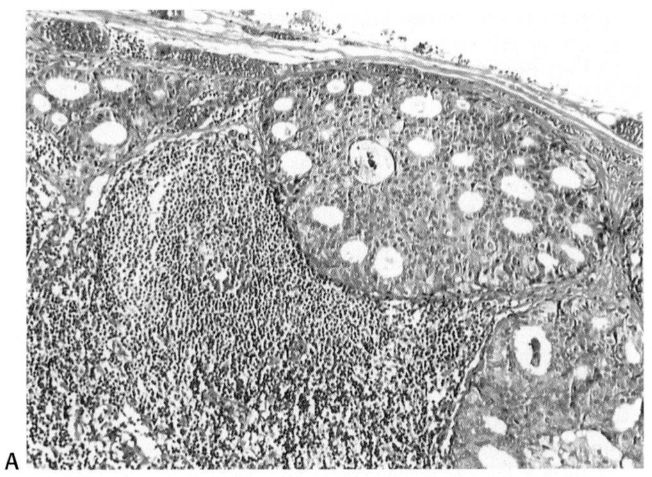

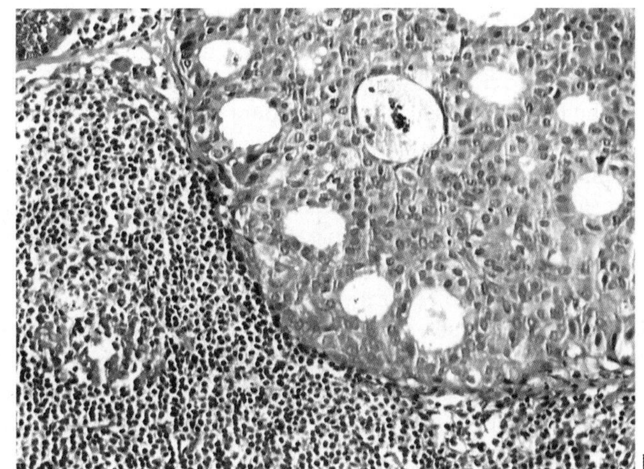

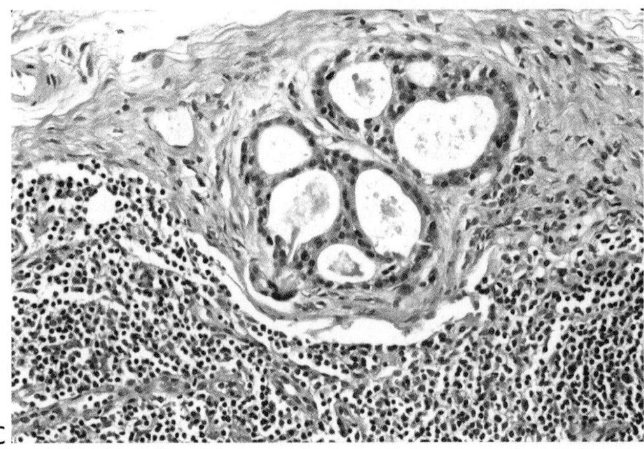

FIG. 26.3. ***Invasive cribriform carcinoma, metastatic.*** **A:** Metastatic cribriform carcinoma in an ALN. **B:** The rigid growth pattern resembles cribriform DCIS. **C:** Metastatic cribriform carcinoma in a lymph node capsule.

mixed tumors were positive for ER. Only one of the two pure tumors was positive for PR, and neither of the mixed tumors stained for PR. Other case reports describe positive staining for ER, variable staining for PR, and lack of staining for human epidermal growth factor 2 (HER2).[4,10,13]

ELECTRON MICROSCOPY

Electron microscopy reveals luminal differentiation of tumor cells that have microvilli and that are joined by tight junctions.[8–10] The cells can have mucin-containing vacuoles of variable electron density concentrated in the apical cytoplasm. Only a few scattered remnants of basal lamina are present, and neurosecretory-type granules have not been observed.[2,8]

TREATMENT AND PROGNOSIS

The majority of patients described in published reports were treated by mastectomy and axillary dissection.[1,2] One case report[13] documents spread to an internal mammary lymph node without involvement of axillary sentinel lymph nodes (SLNs). The authors of two studies concluded that patients with classical invasive cribriform carcinoma were less likely to develop axillary lymph node (ALN) metastases than women with mixed invasive cribriform carcinoma[1] or ordinary invasive duct carcinoma.[2] The data are not definitive because the groups compared were not standardized for tumor size or type of surgical treatment. Page et al.[1] reported that patients with mixed invasive cribriform carcinomas had nodal metastases more often (4 of 16, [25%]) than patients with classical tumors. However, the average size of classical tumors (3.1 cm) was substantially less than that of tumors with a mixed invasive cribriform pattern (4.2 cm). Venable et al.[2] also did not stratify their invasive cribriform and noncribriform cases for nodal status and tumor size, and their analysis apparently included patients treated without axillary dissection and patients for whom surgical therapy was unknown.

Deaths attributable to classical invasive cribriform carcinoma did not occur among 34 patients studied by Page et al.[1] with follow-up intervals of 10 to 21 years. One patient was alive with recurrent classical invasive cribriform carcinoma, and another died of metastases from a contralateral carcinoma. Among 16 women with mixed invasive cribriform carcinoma followed for an average of 12.5 years, there were six deaths resulting from the breast carcinoma. Venable et al.[2] reported a disease-free survival (DFS) of 100% among 45 patients with classical invasive cribriform carcinoma followed for 1 to 5 years. In this series, follow-up information was unavailable for 17 other patients. With follow-up of 6 years or less, Marzullo et al.[3] reported that three patients with pure and two with mixed tumors were free from disease.

The foregoing data suggest that pure invasive cribriform carcinoma has a favorable prognosis and a low frequency of axillary nodal metastases. If adequate excision can be performed, breast conservation therapy would appear feasible, although published prognostic data are presently largely based on mastectomy. The possibility of encountering multifocal lesions should be borne in mind. In the absence of axillary nodal metastases, systemic adjuvant therapy is probably not warranted for tumors 1 cm or smaller unless specific unfavorable findings such as lymphatic tumor emboli indicate otherwise. Axillary staging by SLN mapping is appropriate.

REFERENCES

1. Page DL, Dixon JM, Anderson TJ, et al. Invasive cribriform carcinoma of the breast. *Histopathology* 1983;7:525–536.
2. Venable JG, Schwartz AM, Silverberg SG. Infiltrating cribriform carcinoma of the breast: a distinctive clinicopathologic entity. *Hum Pathol* 1990;21:333–338.
3. Marzullo F, Zito FA, Marzullo A, et al. Infiltrating cribriform carcinoma of the breast. A clinicopathologic and immunohistochemical study of 5 cases. *Eur J Gynaecol Oncol* 1996;17:228–231.
4. Nishimura R, Ohsumi S, Teramoto N, et al. Invasive cribriform carcinoma with extensive microcalcifications in the male breast. *Breast Cancer* 2005;12:145–148.
5. Choi Y, Lee KY, Jang MH, et al. Invasive cribriform carcinoma arising in malignant phyllodes tumor of breast: a case report. *Korean J Pathol* 2012;46:205–209.
6. Stutz JA, Evans AJ, Pinder S, et al. The radiological appearances of invasive cribriform carcinoma of the breast. Nottingham Breast Team. *Clin Radiol* 1994;49:693–695.
7. Lim HS, Jeong SJ, Lee JS, et al. Sonographic findings of invasive cribriform carcinoma of the breast. *J Ultrasound Med* 2011;30:701–705.
8. Wells CA, Ferguson DJ. Ultrastructural and immunocytochemical study of a case of invasive cribriform breast carcinoma. *J Clin Pathol* 1988;41:17–20.
9. Shousha S, Schoenfeld A, Moss J, et al. Light and electron microscopic study of an invasive cribriform carcinoma with extensive microcalcification developing in a breast with silicone augmentation. *Ultrastruct Pathol* 1994;18:519–523.
10. Ng WK. Fine needle aspiration cytology of invasive cribriform carcinoma of the breast with osteoclastlike giant cells: a case report. *Acta Cytol* 2001;45:593–598.
11. Fisher ER, Gregorio RM, Fisher B, et al. The pathology of invasive breast cancer. A syllabus derived from findings of the National Surgical Adjuvant Breast Project (protocol no. 4). *Cancer* 1975; 36:1–85.
12. Rosen PP. Adenoid cystic carcinoma of the breast. A morphologically heterogeneous neoplasm. *Pathol Annu* 1989;24(Pt. 2):237–254.
13. Gatti G, Pruneri G, Gilardi D, et al. Report on a case of pure cribriform carcinoma of the breast with internal mammary node metastasis: description of the case and review of the literature. *Tumori* 2006;92: 241–243.

CHAPTER 27

Lipid-Rich Carcinoma

FREDERICK C. KOERNER

This rare variant of infiltrating ductal carcinoma features large cells with abundant cytoplasmic lipid that imparts a vacuolated or foamy appearance to the cytoplasm. The tumor was first described as "lipid-secreting carcinoma" by Aboumrad et al.[1] in a case report. Subsequently, these authors found one other example among 100 breast carcinomas and estimated the frequency of lipid-rich carcinoma to be 1%, but it is clearly less frequent. Ramos and Taylor,[2] who coined the less committal term, "lipid-rich carcinoma," described 13 cases collected during a retrospective review of more than 900 mammary carcinomas. The authors demonstrated lipid only in the four cases available as unfixed specimens; the histologic pattern alone established the diagnosis in the other nine cases. Since the time of these reports, only a few additional examples have been described.[3–21]

CLINICAL PRESENTATION

With one exception,[6] all adult patients have been women, whose ages ranged from 22 to 81 years. One patient was a 10-year-old girl.[17] Most patients presented with a distinct palpable mass, usually in the upper outer quadrant. Attachment to the skin or areola with dimpling, retraction, and redness has been reported[1,6,10,19] with ulceration and *peau d'orange* in some instances.[11,14] Lipid-rich carcinoma involved the overlying skin and chest wall in a child.[17] In one patient,[21] the lipid-rich carcinoma coexisted with a conventional high-grade non-lipid-rich invasive ductal carcinoma.

Radiologic imaging has been described in only a few cases.[3,9,10,15,20] Mammography revealed spiculated masses in three patients, and three tumors contained calcifications. Ultrasonography in one patient[20] demonstrated an irregular hypoechoic mass with indistinct borders and heterogeneous internal echoes. Using magnetic resonance imaging (MRI), the same mass displayed rapid enhancement to a high intensity with a peak-and-plateau pattern of the time–intensity curve. A hypoechoic mass was seen in one other patient.[3]

GROSS PATHOLOGY

The reported tumor size ranged from 1.2 cm (detected by screening mammography) to 15 cm,[11] with many tumors measuring 2 to 3 cm[11–13,15,16,18] and a few 5 cm or more.[10,11,14,19] Pathologists usually describe the masses as lobulated, firm, and white to yellow.

MICROSCOPIC PATHOLOGY

Histologic sections demonstrate a predominantly invasive carcinoma composed of sheets, nests, and cords of large, polygonal cells, which may have poorly defined borders. Malignant cells sometimes occupy ducts and lobules associated with the invasive component, and one case seems to represent an entirely noninvasive (*in situ*) form of lipid-rich carcinoma.[20] van Bogaert and Maldague[8] described three histopathologic patterns created by the malignant cells. The "histiocytoid" pattern, which represents the most common variety, consists of large cells with pale foamy cytoplasm and small dark nuclei that lack pleomorphism (Fig. 27.1). Cells with large irregular and bubbly vacuoles, pleomorphic nuclei, and prominent nucleoli characterize the "sebaceous" pattern of lipid-rich carcinoma. The third pattern consists of cells with apocrine qualities, which possess abundant, finely granular, eosinophilic cytoplasm and nuclei with coarse chromatin and prominent nucleoli. Cells with these different appearances sometimes mingle in a single carcinoma. One can usually detect mitotic figures without difficulty,[12,15] and the carcinomas usually fall in the category of histologic grade 2 or 3. Scalloping of the nuclei by the cytoplasmic vacuoles can bring to mind the appearance of sebaceous cells or brown fat. The foamy or vesicular quality of the cytoplasm arises because processing of the sample for histologic sectioning extracts the cytoplasmic lipid, a phenomenon that occurs in certain apocrine carcinomas.[4] To document the presence of lipid, one can employ oil red O or Sudan III stains using frozen sections of fresh tissue or sections of tissue processed in a fashion that preserves cytoplasmic lipids, or one can carry out ultrastructural studies. The carcinomas do not stain with periodic acid–Schiff (PAS), Alcian blue, toluidine blue, or mucicarmine stain.[10,13,15,20]

Differential Diagnosis

The diagnosis of lipid-rich carcinoma requires the presence of evidence of two types: appropriate cellular features, including clear, pale, or vacuolated cytoplasm seen in hematoxylin and eosin (H&E) stain, and intracytoplasmic lipid

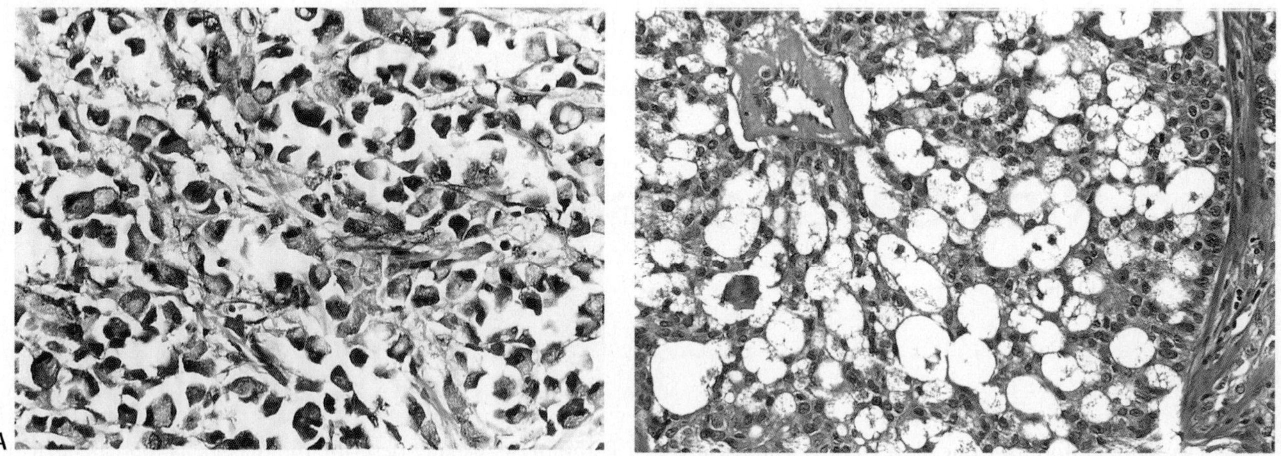

FIG. 27.1. ***Lipid-rich carcinoma.*** **A:** Marked cytoplasmic clearing is evident. The tumor cells were strongly sudanophilic in frozen sections. **B:** Intraductal carcinoma (case courtesy of Frank Brazza, MD).

demonstrated by special stains. Neither type of evidence alone can establish the diagnosis of lipid-rich carcinoma. Cells with clear, vacuolated cytoplasm have been found in benign breast lesions[22] and in occult conventional mammary carcinomas that present with axillary lymph node (ALN) metastases.[23] Using the oil red O stain, Fisher et al.[24] observed lipid in more than 75% of breast carcinomas; the staining appeared moderate or strong in approximately one-third of cases. These observations indicate that the intracytoplasmic lipid must be present in cells with the appropriate morphologic features to render a diagnosis of lipid-rich carcinoma.

The most commonly encountered carcinomas that superficially resemble lipid-rich carcinoma include glycogen-rich carcinoma, apocrine carcinoma, and secretory carcinoma; rare malignancies such as myoepithelial carcinoma and liposarcoma might enter into consideration, also. The cytoplasm of glycogen-rich carcinomas appears clear rather than foamy, and it contains diastase-sensitive, PAS-positive glycogen, some of which usually persists even after conventional processing, rather than lipid. Apocrine carcinomas often possess cytoplasm that appears pale or vacuolated, but the cells typically stain strongly for gross cystic disease fluid protein 15 (GCDFP-15), whereas lipid-rich carcinomas show only focal staining for this molecule. PAS-positive, Alcian blue–positive acid mucopolysaccharides form vacuoles in the cytoplasm of secretory carcinomas, and genetic studies demonstrate the characteristic translocation t(12;15)(p13;q25) affecting the *ETV6* and *NTRK3* genes. Myoepithelial carcinomas express characteristic proteins (HMWCK, p63, smooth muscle myosin-heavy chain [SMM-HC], etc.) not seen in lipid-rich carcinomas. The cells of liposarcoma do not commonly express keratin.

Unusual Patterns

A few cases of lipid-rich carcinomas have presented unusual features. One such carcinoma, which arose in the breast of a 55-year-old man, had high levels of estrogen receptor (ER) and progesterone receptor (PR). Varga et al.[9] described a lipid-rich carcinoma with focal chondroid metaplasia. Tsubura et al.[7] described two examples of an unusual variant of lipid-rich carcinoma in patients treated with neuroleptic drugs for severe psychiatric disorders. The *in situ* components of the carcinomas displayed growth patterns similar to that of pregnancy-like change. Large, pleomorphic carcinoma cells arranged in an alveolar pattern demonstrated a "hobnail" appearance, and the luminal borders of the cells exhibited apocrine-type cytoplasmic blebs and extrusion of hyperchromatic pleomorphic nuclei. Cytoplasmic clearing was more evident in the solid, diffusely invasive component, which showed little gland formation. Both carcinomas were strongly immunoreactive for α-lactalbumin, a finding not exhibited by the other carcinomas in the study group. Both patients had ALN metastases. Kimura et al.[16] reported a similar carcinoma in a patient who also received similar medications for many years. Indirect evidence suggests that these drugs might play a role in the lipid accumulation by the neoplastic cells in these cases. The drugs cause the release of prolactin, which increases the activity of fatty acid synthetase and other enzymes involved in the synthesis of milk proteins; consequently, patients treated with these medications often develop galactorrhea. The malignant cells in the carcinoma described by Kimura et al.[16] expressed prolactin receptors. Benign, focal, pregnancy-like changes have been attributed to neuroleptic drugs, also.[25]

CYTOLOGY

In cytologic specimens, the tumor cells have vacuolated, foamy, or clear cytoplasm.[3,5,13,18] The nuclei appear round or slightly oval, and they contain finely granular chromatin and easily seen nucleoli. When present in axillary nodal metastases, the carcinoma cells can grow in a dispersed pattern that might be mistaken for the cells of metastatic malignant melanoma or histiocytic lymphoma.[23]

IMMUNOHISTOCHEMISTRY

Lipid-rich carcinomas do not stain for cytokeratin (CK) 5/6, CK14, S-100 protein, smooth muscle actin (SMA), or p63 using immunohistochemical techniques.[12,13,15,16] Staining for α-lactalbumin and GCDFP-15 has yielded inconsistent results.[7,10,11] The results of studies of ER and PR expressions vary somewhat; most investigators report little or no detection of ER but modest expression of PR.[6,9,11–13,15,16] Many cases showed strong membrane staining for human epidermal growth factor 2 (HER2) and amplification of the *HER2* gene.[10,12,16,21] Staining for E-cadherin, CK7, mammaglobin, and carcinoembryogenic antigen (CEA) was observed in one case.[21] A Ki67 index of one tumor exceeded 20%.[21] One tumor studied by the Senior Editor was positive for PR but negative for ER and contained abundant sudanophilic cytoplasmic lipid. The cells were immunoreactive for epithelial membrane antigen (EMA), CK, and α-lactalbumin. Membrane-bound cytoplasmic lipid droplets were seen by electron microscopy. One carcinoma was aneuploid and demonstrated an S-phase fraction (SPF) of 10.8%.[6]

ELECTRON MICROSCOPY

The cases studied using electron microscopy have consistently demonstrated the presence of membrane-bound intracytoplasmic droplets, but other ultrastructural findings have varied.[2,3,9,11,12,14,19] Ramos and Taylor[2] and other workers[3,19] observed abundant rough endoplasmic reticulum and a well-developed Golgi apparatus, whereas Wrba et al.[11] failed to detect these structures. Ramos and Taylor[2] noted dark, needle-like crystalloid material within mitochondria; Lim-Co and Gisser[14] also reported intramitochondrial crystals in one unusual example of lipid-rich carcinoma. Other investigators did not record the presence of crystals within mitochondria.

TREATMENT AND PROGNOSIS

Patients with lipid-rich carcinoma reported in the literature have been treated by mastectomy and axillary dissection in almost all cases. Because there does not appear to be a proclivity for multifocality or multicentricity, breast-conserving surgery would currently be an alternative to mastectomy for patients with tumors that are amenable to this approach. Axillary nodal metastases have been found predominantly when the primary tumor measured more than 3 cm in diameter. In the series of 13 cases reported by Ramos and Taylor,[2] 11 of the 12 patients treated by radical mastectomy had axillary nodal metastases. Seventeen patients studied by Guan et al.[12] underwent axillary dissection with the finding of nodal metastases in all cases. Sentinel lymph node (SLN) sampling could be considered for small tumors and those in which clinical examination does not suggest the presence of nodal metastases. Because some patients with tumors larger than 3 cm have presented with systemic spread as well as axillary nodal metastases, an evaluation to determine the extent of the disease is indicated if the tumor is 3 cm or larger and may be considered for patients with even smaller tumors.

Of the 13 cases reported by Ramos and Taylor,[2] 6 patients died of metastatic carcinoma and 2 were alive with recurrent carcinoma. The remaining patients were alive and recurrence-free with the majority followed for less than 2 years. Guan et al.[12] described the outcomes of 17 patients but did not provide details of their therapy. The primary surgical treatment is presumed to have been mastectomy since none of the patients received radiotherapy or hormonal treatment. Adjuvant chemotherapy consisted of taxotere, adriamycin, and cyclophosphamide (TAC). The authors noted that at "about 25 months the survival rate was almost 0" and that 82% of the tumor spanned 2 to 4 cm.

Although patients with nodal metastases at the time of diagnosis have a poor prognosis, those with negative lymph nodes have survived for 5,[17] 8,[20] and 20 years.[16]

The accumulated information notwithstanding, the nature of lipid-rich carcinoma remains undefined. Lipids accumulate in carcinomas classified as ductal, lobular, and apocrine[26] among others, and carcinomas classified as lipid-rich might simply represent conventional types of carcinoma with especially abundant lipid production. Additional studies of more patients will be required to determine whether lipid-rich tumors constitute a morphologically and clinically distinctive type of carcinoma.

REFERENCES

1. Aboumrad MH, Horn RC Jr, Fine G. Lipid-secreting mammary carcinoma. Report of a case associated with Paget's disease of the nipple. *Cancer* 1963;16:521–525.
2. Ramos CV, Taylor HB. Lipid-rich carcinoma of the breast. A clinicopathologic analysis of 13 examples. *Cancer* 1974;33:812–819.
3. Aida Y, Takeuchi E, Shinagawa T, et al. Fine needle aspiration cytology of lipid-secreting carcinoma of the breast. A case report. *Acta Cytol* 1993;37:547–551.
4. Dina R, Eusebi V. Clear cell tumors of the breast. *Semin Diagn Pathol* 1997;14:175–182.
5. Lapey JD. Lipid-rich mammary carcinoma—diagnosis by cytology. Case report. *Acta Cytol* 1977;21:120–122.
6. Mazzella FM, Sieber SC, Braza F. Ductal carcinoma of male breast with prominent lipid-rich component. *Pathology* 1995;27:280–283.
7. Tsubura A, Hatano T, Murata A, et al. Breast carcinoma in patients receiving neuroleptic therapy. Morphologic and clinicopathologic features of thirteen cases. *Acta Pathol Jpn* 1992;42:494–499.
8. van Bogaert L-J, Maldague P. Histologic variants of lipid-secreting carcinoma of the breast. *Virchows Arch A Pathol Anat Histol* 1977;375:345–353.
9. Varga Z, Robl C, Spycher M, et al. Metaplastic lipid-rich carcinoma of the breast. *Pathol Int* 1998;48:912–916.
10. Umekita Y, Yoshida A, Sagara Y, et al. Lipid-secreting carcinoma of the breast: a case report and review of the literature. *Breast Cancer* 1998;5:171–173.
11. Wrba F, Ellinger A, Reiner G, et al. Ultrastructural and immunohistochemical characteristics of lipid-rich carcinoma of the breast. *Virchows Arch A Pathol Anat Histopathol* 1988;413:381–385.
12. Guan B, Wang H, Cao S, et al. Lipid-rich carcinoma of the breast clinicopathologic analysis of 17 cases. *Ann Diagn Pathol* 2011;15:225–232.
13. Catalina-Fernandez I, Saenz-Santamaria J. Lipid-rich carcinoma of breast: a case report with fine needle aspiration cytology. *Diagn Cytopathol* 2009;37:935–936.

14. Lim-Co RY, Gisser SD. Unusual variant of lipid-rich mammary carcinoma. *Arch Pathol Lab Med* 1978;102:193–195.
15. Shi P, Ma R, Gao HD, et al. Lipid-rich carcinoma of the breast: a case report. *Acta Chir Belg* 2008;108:115–118.
16. Kimura A, Miki H, Yuri T, et al. A case report of lipid-rich carcinoma of the breast including histological characteristics and intrinsic subtype profile. *Case Rep Oncol* 2011;4:275–280.
17. Balik E, Taneli C, Cetinkursun S, et al. Lipid secreting breast carcinoma in childhood: a case report. *Eur J Pediatr Surg* 1993;3:48–49.
18. Insabato L, Russo R, Cascone AM, et al. Fine needle aspiration cytology of lipid-secreting breast carcinoma. A case report. *Acta Cytol* 1993;37:752–755.
19. Vera-Sempere F, Llombart-Bosch A. Lipid-rich versus lipid-secreting carcinoma of the mammary gland. *Pathol Res Pract* 1985;180:553–558.
20. Nagata Y, Hanagiri T, Ono K, et al. A non-invasive form of lipid-secreting carcinoma of the breast. *Breast Cancer* 2012;19:83–87.
21. Machalekova K, Kajo K, Bencat M. Unusual occurrence of rare lipid-rich carcinoma and conventional invasive carcinoma in the one breast: case report. *Case Reports Pathol* 2012;2012:4.
22. Barwick KW, Kashgarian M, Rosen PP. "Clear-cell" change within duct and lobular epithelium of the human breast. *Pathol Annu* 1982; 17(Pt. 1):319–328.
23. Haupt HM, Rosen PP, Kinne DW. Breast carcinoma presenting with axillary lymph node metastases. An analysis of specific histopathologic features. *Am J Surg Pathol* 1985;9:165–175.
24. Fisher ER, Gregorio R, Kim WS, et al. Lipid in invasive cancer of the breast. *Am J Clin Pathol* 1977;68:558–561.
25. Kiaer HW, Andersen JA. Focal pregnancy-like changes in the breast. *Acta Pathol Microbiol Scand A* 1977;85:931–941.
26. Moritani S, Ichihara S, Hasegawa M, et al. Intracytoplasmic lipid accumulation in apocrine carcinoma of the breast evaluated with adipophilin immunoreactivity: a possible link between apocrine carcinoma and lipid-rich carcinoma. *Am J Surg Pathol* 2011;35:861–867.

CHAPTER 28

Glycogen-Rich Carcinoma

FREDERICK C. KOERNER

Carcinomas that accumulate abundant glycogen arise in many organs, including the lungs, endometrium, cervix, ovary, and salivary glands.[1] Extraction of the water-soluble glycogen during histologic processing causes the cytoplasm to become vacuolated or completely clear in conventional hematoxylin and eosin (H&E)–stained sections, and this phenomenon has led pathologists to designate such tumors as clear cell carcinomas. In 1981, Hull et al.[2] described an *in situ* and invasive mammary carcinoma composed of cells with clear cytoplasm and proposed the diagnosis of glycogen-rich clear cell carcinoma of the breast for this variant of mammary duct carcinoma. These writers did not establish criteria for this diagnosis, nor did they estimate the frequency of the lesion; however, subsequent observers have commented on both points. Fisher et al.[3] required that 50% or more of the cells contain "optically clear cytoplasm and, usually, centrally placed nuclei" to make the diagnosis of glycogen-rich clear cell carcinoma. Having done so, the authors classified 45 of 1,555 breast carcinomas (3%) as glycogen-rich clear cell carcinoma. Kuroda et al.[4] used the same threshold and discovered 20 glycogen-rich clear cell carcinomas in a group of 723 primary breast carcinomas (2.7%). Toikkanen and Joensuu[5] required that 90% of the carcinoma cells contain clear cytoplasm to make the diagnosis of glycogen-rich clear cell carcinoma. They found 6 of 439 breast carcinomas (1.4%) met their criteria for this diagnosis. Hull and Warfel[6] did not specify their diagnostic criteria, but they regarded only 9 of 936 breast carcinomas (1%) as glycogen-rich clear cell carcinomas. These findings indicate that glycogen-rich clear cell carcinoma is an exceedingly rare form of primary breast carcinoma. Fewer than 150 well-documented examples have been described since the first case was reported in 1981.

CLINICAL PRESENTATION

The patients, whose ages ranged from 32 to 81 years,[7] presented with a mass accompanied by skin dimpling, nipple retraction, or pain in some cases. Both *in situ* and invasive lesions may be detected by mammography[2,8–12] and sonography.[2,11] The imaging studies reveal an irregular spiculated mass[8,10,11,13] that may contain calcifications.[10,11,13]

GROSS PATHOLOGY

Glycogen-rich carcinomas resemble conventional breast carcinomas to the unaided eye. Distinctive macroscopic features have not been recorded. Most tumors measured between 2 and 5 cm; the largest spanned "about 15 cm."[13] In one series, the mean size was 3 cm.[7] Observers have described the masses as "brownish pink-gray or whitish-gray."[7] The carcinoma can form multifocal or multicentric masses, and macroscopically evident involvement of the skin occurred in several cases.[7,14] The seminal authors could appreciate an *in situ* papillary component during macroscopic examination.[2]

MICROSCOPIC PATHOLOGY

Glycogen-rich clear cell carcinomas have basic structural features of ductal carcinoma *in situ* (DCIS) alone or of DCIS and infiltrating duct carcinoma. The intraductal component can grow in papillary, solid, cribriform, micropapillary, and "intracystic" patterns. Cytoplasmic clearing appears most evident in solid areas that also exhibit moderate nuclear atypia (Fig. 28.1). The cells in cribriform and micropapillary regions usually have low-grade atypia and less often appear water-clear. The neoplastic cells can undergo focal necrosis, but abundant, comedo-like necrosis associated with high-grade nuclear atypia does not occur commonly.[9] In most cases, one can detect small regions in which the cells contain eosinophilic and granular cytoplasm or exhibit other clear-cut apocrine features. The invasive component usually exhibits the histologic growth pattern of a conventional invasive duct carcinoma, but it can also display the patterns seen in lobular, medullary, and tubular carcinomas.[3] The tumor cells typically form cords, solid nests, or papillary structures (Fig. 28.2). The formation of ductular or tubular structures occurs only rarely. The cells exhibit sharply defined borders and polygonal rather than rounded contours. The cytoplasm is clear or, less often, finely granular or foamy. Like the noninvasive component, the invasive carcinoma sometimes contains foci in which the cells have eosinophilic and granular cytoplasm that suggests an apocrine nature, and these cells often form a continuum with the clear cells. Observers have noted PAS-positive, diastase-resistant, intracytoplasmic hyalin droplets in rare cases.[9] The nuclei appear hyperchromatic and

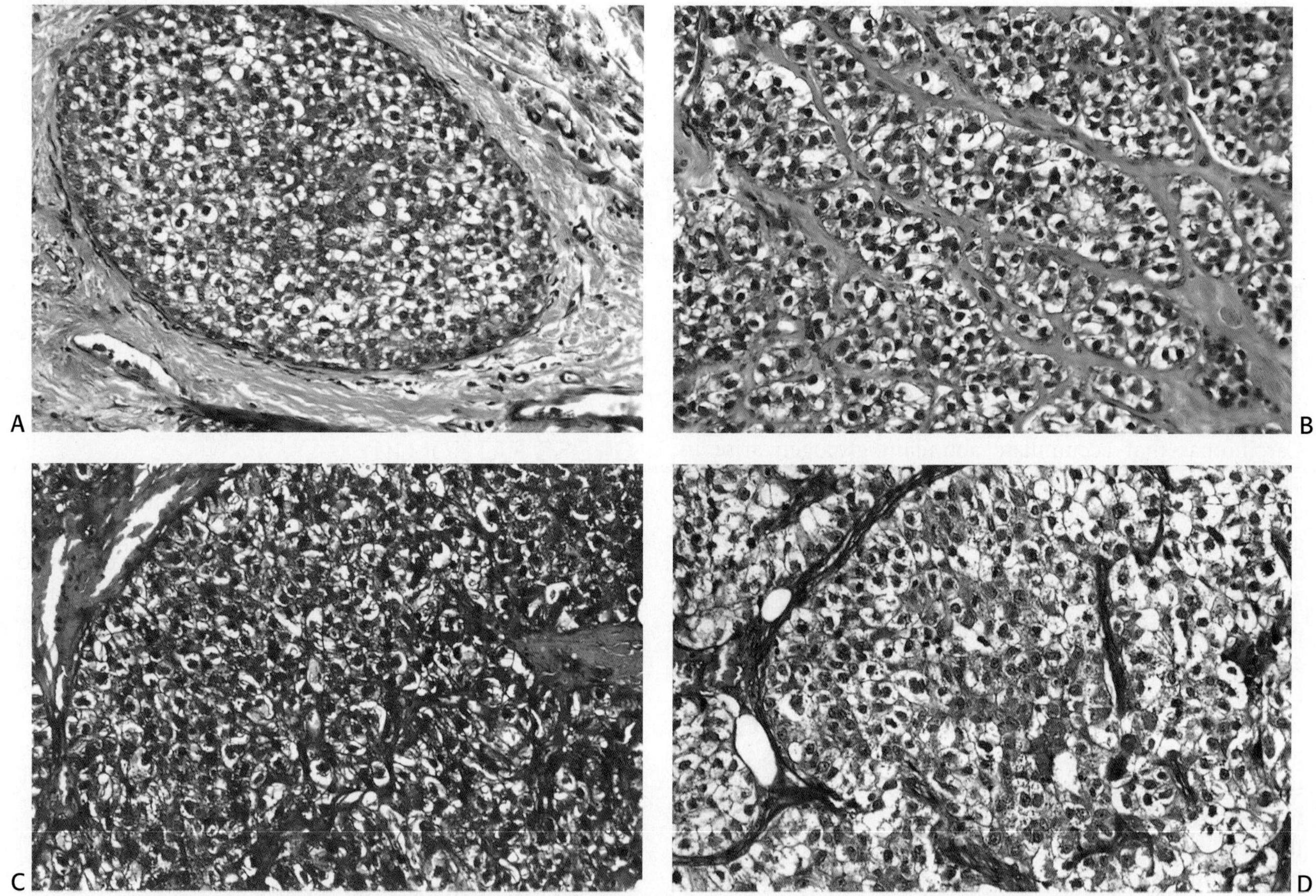

FIG. 28.1. ***Glycogen-rich carcinoma.*** **A,B:** DCIS and invasive carcinoma composed of cells with clear cytoplasm and small, dark, punctate nuclei. **C:** The tumor is strongly positive with the PAS reaction. **D:** After treatment with diastase, PAS reactivity is almost entirely abolished. The same pattern of PAS staining occurred in the intraductal carcinoma.

sometimes contain clumped chromatin and nucleoli. Mitotic figures are easily identified in most cases. One group[15] found as many as 70 mitotic figures per 10 high-power fields. Patches of necrosis often occur in large tumors. A linear pattern consisting of strands of cells resembling invasive lobular carcinoma may be seen, and glycogen-rich variants of tubular, medullary, and endocrine carcinomas have been described.[3,7,16,17] The carcinoma cells can invade lymphatic vessels and nerves. The histologic appearance of the primary tumor is duplicated in the metastases, which also contain abundant glycogen.[6]

Differential Diagnosis

The differential diagnosis of glycogen-rich carcinoma includes benign and malignant mammary and extramammary neoplasms. The clear cell type of hidradenoma (eccrine acrospiroma) shares the presence of many glycogen-laden clear cells with glycogen-rich carcinoma. However, hidradenomas are centered in the dermis, they have well-defined, smooth contours, and they consist of uniform bland cells. Atypical and malignant hidradenomas pose greater challenges in differential diagnosis (see Chapter 42). Myoepithelial cells with clear cytoplasm can dominate uncommon examples of mammary adenomyoepithelioma. Detection of a second population consisting of glandular cells and immunohistochemical demonstration of proteins characteristic of myoepithelial cells will distinguish this tumor from glycogen-rich carcinoma.

The detection of glycogen in a mammary carcinoma does not establish the diagnosis of glycogen-rich clear cell carcinoma, for Fisher et al.[3] found that 58% of breast carcinoma lacking clear cells contained intracytoplasmic glycogen. Among the types of primary mammary carcinomas, lipid-rich, secretory, histiocytoid lobular, and apocrine carcinomas exhibit certain features that may bring to mind the appearance of glycogen-rich carcinoma, but one can usually distinguish these tumors without difficulty. Lipid-rich carcinomas contain lipid rather than glycogen (see Chapter 27). Secretory carcinomas feature microcystic spaces containing eosinophilic secretions (see Chapter 22). Invasive lobular carcinomas of the histiocytoid type possess intracytoplasmic mucin rather than glycogen. Apocrine carcinomas can contain clear cells (see Chapter 19), and focal apocrine features are identified in the majority of glycogen-rich carcinoma. This association

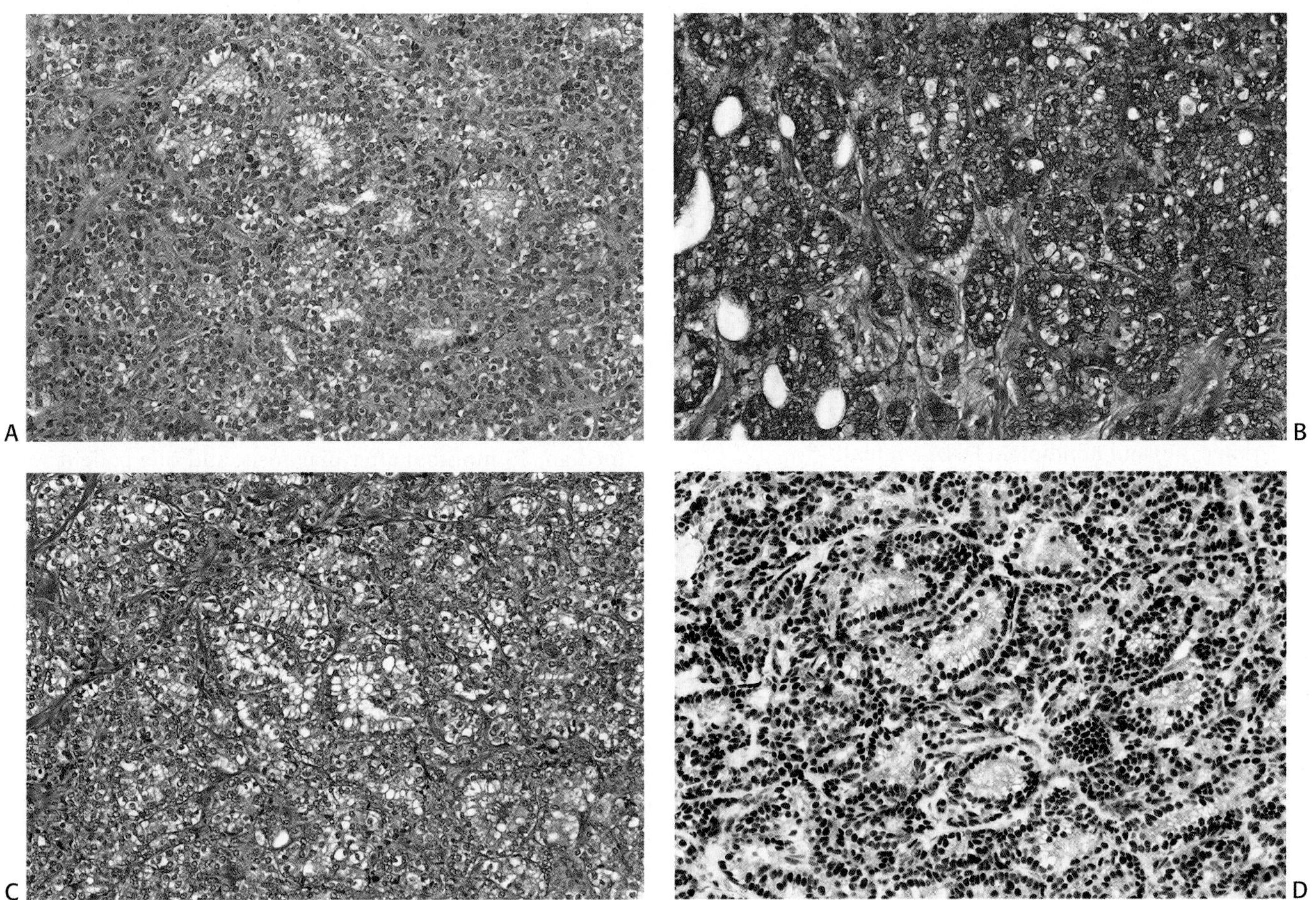

FIG. 28.2. *Glycogen-rich carcinoma.* **A:** This tumor has moderate cytoplasmic clearing and a gland-forming structure. **B:** PAS reactivity is strong. **C:** PAS reactivity is abolished by diastase treatment. **D:** Strong nuclear reactivity for ER is present.

suggests that that glycogen-rich carcinoma might constitute a variant of apocrine carcinoma.[9] These overlapping findings and the possibility of an etiological relationship notwithstanding, the usual apocrine carcinoma contains intracytoplasmic, diastase-resistant eosinophilic granules or droplets, a finding that does not characterize glycogen-rich carcinomas.

Metastatic clear cell carcinomas can mimic the appearance of glycogen-rich carcinoma. Carcinoma of the kidney is the most notable culprit in this regard (see Chapter 34).

CYTOLOGY

Descriptions of the cytological characteristics of specimens obtained by fine-needle aspiration vary somewhat from case to case depending on the attributes of the carcinoma.[7,11,14,15,18,19] Most authors report that the smears appear cellular and that the carcinoma cells form loosely cohesive groups. The aggregates sometimes display a branching architecture, and papillary formations can occur. At least a few intact dissociated cells can be seen in the background of the smears in most cases. The cells typically exhibit distinct cell membranes, but syncytial groups can be seen. The cytoplasm usually appears finely granular and eosinophilic or vacuolated; however, the degree of vacuolization and clearing of the cytoplasm varies and it sometimes represents only an inconspicuous cellular feature. The oval or round nuclei vary in size. They have irregular membranes and prominent nucleoli. In many cases, the nuclei demonstrate obvious pleomorphism and anaplasia. One can sometimes appreciate occasional mitotic figures.

IMMUNOHISTOCHEMISTRY

The cytoplasm gives a positive, diastase-labile reaction with the periodic acid–Schiff (PAS) stain (Figs. 28.1 and 28.2). The cells stain only focally or not at all with Alcian blue, mucicarmine, and colloidal iron stains,[6,8,10,11,14,15] and the oil red O and Sudan black B stains for lipid are negative.[8,11] The tumor cells are reactive for CK7, AE1/AE3, CK8/18, CAM5.2, and E-cadherin,[10,13,15,16,19] variably or weakly reactive for carcinoembryogenic antigen (CEA)[15,19] CK19, CK34βE12, and epithelial membrane antigen (EMA),[8,11,16,18] and only weakly reactive or unreactive for actin, smooth muscle actin (SMA), desmin, vimentin, S-100, α-lactalbumin, CK5/6,

CK14, CK20, CD31, and CD34.[8,10,16,19,20] Several case reports document staining for gross cystic disease fluid protein-15 (GCDFP-15).[10,11,20] Glycogen-rich carcinomas do not display a consistent pattern of staining for hormone receptors.[4,7,9,11,13–16,20,21] About one-half of the tumors express estrogen receptor (ER) (Fig. 28.2 D); the reported frequency varies from 35%[4] to 62%.[7] Most authors report the absence of progesterone receptor (PR)[9,14,16,21]; however, Satoh et al.[11] observed staining for PR in their single case, and Akbulut et al.[7] detected PR in 43% of their cases. Researchers have observed staining for human epidermal growth factor 2 (HER2) in 20% to 43% of cases.[4,7,15] The mean Ki67 score was 20% in one series,[7] and a value of 48% was recorded in a single case.[11] Observers have noted an elevated S-phase fraction (SPF) and nondiploid DNA content.[5,14]

ELECTRON MICROSCOPY

At the ultrastructural level, the cells have polygonal to columnar shapes.[2,6,8,11,17,19] The cytoplasmic borders can appear smooth or form complex interdigitations harboring junctional complexes and desmosomes. The cytoplasm contains intracytoplasmic lakes of non–membrane-bound glycogen and abundant small aggregates of glycogen intermixed with rough endoplasmic reticulum, mitochondria, ribosomes, lysosomes, and Golgi apparatus. In certain cases, the cytoplasm becomes distinctly segregated into two compartments: one containing the organelles and the other containing the glycogen. The nuclei appear oval to rectangular. Most exhibit smooth borders, but others have deep clefts. They contain moderate amounts of heterochromatin and nucleoli that vary from small to prominent, depending on the case. Lumens sometimes form among clusters of cells or within individual cells (intracytoplasmic lumens). The cells forming these primitive glands have short, broad microvilli on their luminal borders, and one can observe tight junctions and desmosomes between the cells.

TREATMENT AND PROGNOSIS

With rare exceptions, reported examples of invasive glycogen-rich carcinoma have been treated by mastectomy and axillary dissection. In one case,[13] neoadjuvant chemotherapy resulted in the reduction of the cellularity of the infiltrating tumor by 30% or less. Approximately 30% of the patients had metastatic tumor in their axillary lymph nodes. In one series, 50% of the patients treated by mastectomy died of metastatic mammary carcinoma 1 to 175 months (median, 15 months) after diagnosis, and one patient was alive with recurrent carcinoma 36 months after local excision and lymph node dissection.[6] Except for one woman who underwent simple mastectomy without axillary dissection, all patients with recurrent or fatal carcinoma had axillary nodal metastases. Toikkanen and Joensuu[5] found axillary nodal metastases in five of six cases. All five of these patients died of metastatic carcinoma within 7 years from the time of diagnosis, and the single woman with negative lymph nodes died of intercurrent disease without recurrence. Among the group described by Kuroda et al.,[4] 5 of 15 patients followed for 1 to 72 months died within 5 years of the time of diagnosis. Hayes et al.[9] reported that three of eight patients with follow-up information died of metastatic carcinoma. The length of follow-up was not reported. These data suggest that the prognosis of patients with glycogen-rich mammary carcinoma is not particularly favorable and that it may be similar to ordinary invasive duct carcinoma when analyzed on a stage- and grade-matched basis.[3,9]

The Senior Editor has examined slides from an unusual instance of glycogen-rich DCIS detected when calcifications

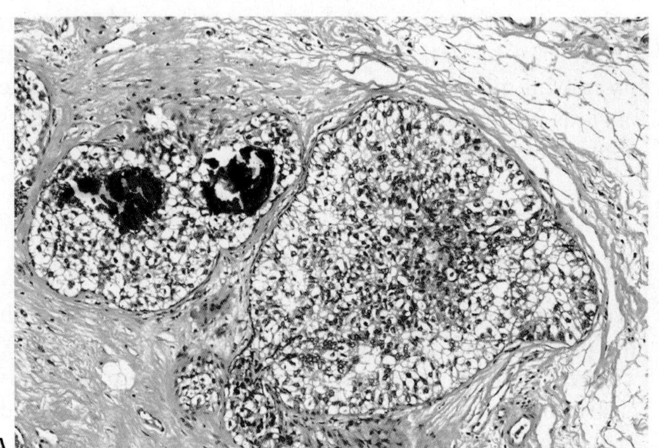

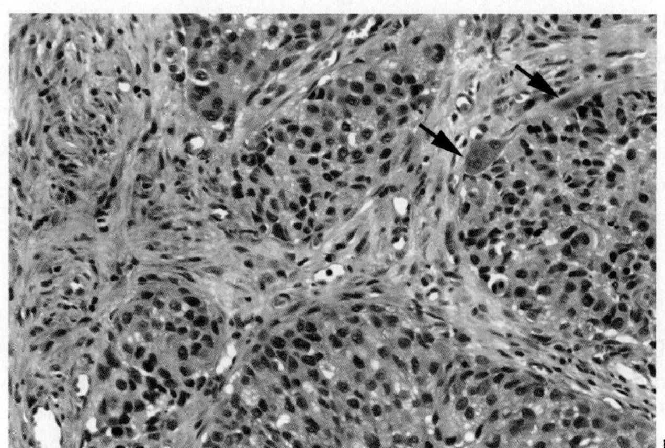

FIG. 28.3. *Glycogen-rich carcinoma.* **A:** DCIS with calcifications, which were detected by mammography. **B:** DCIS and invasive duct carcinoma with osteoclast-like giant cells (*arrows*) found in the breast 9 years after breast conservation treatment of the glycogen-rich DCIS shown in **(A)**.

were found by mammography (Fig. 28.3). Nine years after breast conservation therapy with radiotherapy, the patient developed recurrent DCIS and invasive duct carcinoma with osteoclast-like giant cells in the same breast. The recurrent carcinoma was not glycogen rich.

REFERENCES

1. Mohamed AH, Cherrick HM. Glycogen-rich adenocarcinoma of minor salivary glands. A light and electron microscopic study. *Cancer* 1975;36:1057–1066.
2. Hull MT, Priest JB, Broadie TA, et al. Glycogen-rich clear cell carcinoma of the breast: a light and electron microscopic study. *Cancer* 1981;48:2003–2009.
3. Fisher ER, Tavares J, Bulatao IS, et al. Glycogen-rich, clear cell breast cancer: with comments concerning other clear cell variants. *Hum Pathol* 1985;16:1085–1090.
4. Kuroda H, Sakamoto G, Ohnisi K, et al. Clinical and pathological features of glycogen-rich clear cell carcinoma of the breast. *Breast Cancer* 2005;12:189–195.
5. Toikkanen S, Joensuu H. Glycogen-rich clear-cell carcinoma of the breast: a clinicopathologic and flow cytometric study. *Hum Pathol* 1991;22:81–83.
6. Hull MT, Warfel KA. Glycogen-rich clear cell carcinomas of the breast: a clinicopathologic and ultrastructural study. *Am J Surg Pathol* 1986;10:553–559.
7. Akbulut M, Zekioglu O, Kapkac M, et al. Fine needle aspiration cytology of glycogen-rich clear cell carcinoma of the breast: review of 37 cases with histologic correlation. *Acta Cytol* 2008;52:65–71.
8. Sorensen FB, Paulsen SM. Glycogen-rich clear cell carcinoma of the breast: a solid variant with mucus. A light microscopic, immunohistochemical and ultrastructural study of a case. *Histopathology* 1987;11:857–869.
9. Hayes MM, Seidman JD, Ashton MA. Glycogen-rich clear cell carcinoma of the breast. A clinicopathologic study of 21 cases. *Am J Surg Pathol* 1995;19:904–911.
10. Trupiano JK, Ogrodowczyk E, Bergman S. Pathologic quiz case: mass in the right breast. Glycogen-rich clear cell carcinoma of the breast. *Arch Pathol Lab Med* 2003;127:1629–1630.
11. Satoh F, Umemura S, Itoh H, et al. Fine needle aspiration cytology of glycogen-rich clear cell carcinoma of the breast. A case report. *Acta Cytol* 1998;42:413–418.
12. Pak I, Kutun S, Celik A, et al. Glycogen-rich "clear cell" carcinoma of the breast. *Breast J* 2005;11:288.
13. Martíin-Martíin B, Berná-Serna JD, Sánchez-Henarejos P, et al. An unusual case of locally advanced glycogen-rich clear cell carcinoma of the breast. *Case Rep Oncol* 2011;4:452–457.
14. Kern SB, Andera L. Cytology of glycogen-rich (clear cell) carcinoma of the breast: a report of two cases. *Acta Cytol* 1997;41:556–560.
15. Satake N, Uehara H, Sano N, et al. Cytological analysis of glycogen-rich carcinoma of the breast: report of two cases. *J Med Invest* 2002;49:193–196.
16. Gurbuz Y, Ozkara SK. Clear cell carcinoma of the breast with solid papillary pattern: a case report with immunohistochemical profile. *J Clin Pathol* 2003;56:552–554.
17. di Tommaso L, Pasquinelli G, Portincasa G, et al. Carcinoma della mammella a cellule chiare ricche in glicogeno con aspetti di differenziazione neuroendocrina. *Pathologica* 2001;93:676–680.
18. Das AK, Verma K, Aron M. Fine-needle aspiration cytology of glycogen-rich carcinoma of breast: report of a case and review of literature. *Diagn Cytopathol* 2005;33:263–267.
19. Alexiev BA. Glycogen-rich clear cell carcinoma of the breast: report of a case with fine-needle aspiration cytology and immunocytochemical and ultrastructural studies. *Diagn Cytopathol* 1995;12:62–66.
20. Shirley SE, Escoffery CT, Titus IP, et al. Clear cell carcinoma of the breast with immunohistochemical evidence of divergent differentiation. *Ann Diagn Pathol* 2002;6:250–256.
21. Benisch B, Peison B, Newman R, et al. Solid glycogen-rich clear cell carcinoma of the breast (a light and ultrastructural study). *Am J Clin Pathol* 1983;79:243–245.

CHAPTER 29

Invasive Micropapillary Carcinoma

ADRIANA D. CORBEN • EDI BROGI

Invasive micropapillary carcinoma is a morphologically distinctive form of mammary carcinoma in which tumor cells are arranged in morule-like clusters devoid of fibrovascular cores and situated within empty stromal spaces. Fisher et al.[1] referred to this configuration as an "exfoliative appearance." This growth pattern may be found throughout the lesion (pure invasive micropapillary carcinoma) or as part of an otherwise conventional invasive duct carcinoma (mixed invasive micropapillary carcinoma). Criteria for distinguishing between mixed and "pure" invasive micropapillary carcinoma remain imprecise. Some authors have used the term "micropapillary" for lesions with micropapillary growth in at least 50% of the tumor. Others restrict the term to tumors that consist entirely of this pattern, an exceedingly rare occurrence. In practical terms, to be considered in the "pure" category, at least 75% of the invasive tumor should be micropapillary. Some mucin-producing carcinomas can also have this growth pattern, but there is no consensus on whether these tumors are variants of invasive micropapillary or mucinous carcinomas.

CLINICAL PRESENTATION

Age and Gender

The reported age at diagnosis ranges from 25 to 89 years.[2–9] The median ages in several studies were 46,[8] 48.9,[9] 50,[6] 57,[2,10] and 62[4] years. The mean ages in four series were 50,[5] 52.3,[11] 53.5,[7] and 58[12] years. Luna-Moré et al.[13] observed that patients whose tumors contained more than 50% micropapillary carcinoma tended to be older than patients with focal micropapillae. Rare cases of invasive micropapillary carcinoma have been described in male patients.[2,9,14–16] No specific genetic or ethnic association has been identified.

Clinical Examination

Most patients present with a palpable breast mass, but occasional lesions are detected mammographically as a density or because of microcalcifications.[4,5,7,9] One tumor clinically mimicked a hematoma because of extensive cystic degeneration and intratumoral hemorrhage.[7] Yun et al.[9] described nipple retraction, a hematoma, and diffuse skin thickening in one patient each. Two patients had nipple discharge.[9] Presentation as an "axillary mass" was described in one patient and in the subareolar region in another three.[5] The distribution of tumors in terms of laterality and location in the breast does not differ significantly from that of ordinary invasive ductal carcinomas.[4,5,12,13]

Radiology

The imaging features of invasive micropapillary carcinomas are highly suggestive of carcinoma. Yun et al.[9] evaluated the radiologic findings in a series of 29 patients. Nineteen of 29 (65.5%) carcinomas presented as a palpable mass, 7/29 (24.1%) with a screening abnormality, 1/29 (3.4%) with nipple discharge, and 1/29 (3.4%) as a mass and nipple discharge. One tumor was detected during follow-up of prior breast surgery. A mammogram that was available for 24/29 patients showed a mass (54.2%), an area of asymmetry (20.8%), and calcifications without mass or asymmetry (20.8%). One patient had no mammographic abnormalities. Calcifications were detected in 16 cases (66.7%), and most were the fine pleomorphic type (56.3%). Their distribution was often segmental (50%) or clustered (37.5%). By ultrasound, it was found that the tumor mass had an irregular shape (25/29; 86.2%), parallel orientation (25/29; 86.2%), a spiculated margin (17/29; 58.6%), an abrupt interface with the surrounding tissue (22/29; 75.9%), and a hypoechoic pattern (27/29; 93.1%). Magnetic resonance imaging (MRI) detected a mass with enhancement in 11/18 (61.1%) cases and non–mass-like enhancement in 7/18 (38.9%) cases. Kamitani et al.[17] reported the ultrasonographic findings of six invasive micropapillary carcinomas. Half of the tumors had uniform echogenicity compared with subcutaneous fat tissue. The authors speculated that the presence of a central lumen in the tumor clusters might have contributed to the relatively high internal echogenicity of these carcinomas.

GROSS PATHOLOGY

Tumor size in several reports ranged from 0.1 to 11 cm, with medians of 1.5,[4] 2.3,[18] 2.8,[2] 3.38,[6] and 3.9 cm[11] in five different series. The mean size of eight tumors in a series studied by Uddin et al.[7] was 2.9 cm (1.7 to 4.5 cm). Another study described larger lesions with a mean size of 4.9 cm, with only

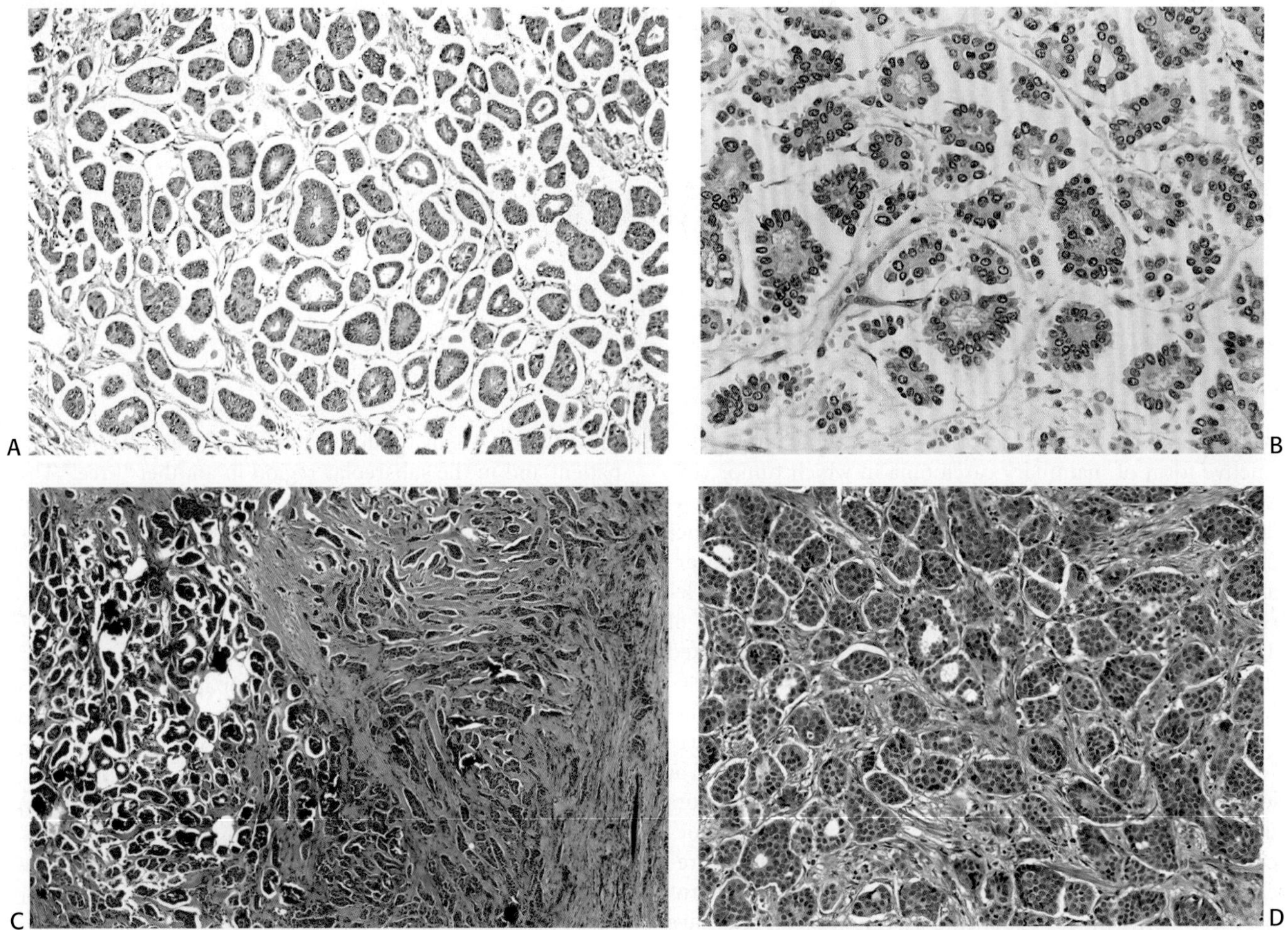

FIG. 29.1. ***Invasive micropapillary carcinoma.*** **A:** Morule-like clusters of tumor cells within spaces defined by a network of loose fibrocollagenous stroma. **B:** The micropapillary clusters have serrated outer borders. **C:** Mixed invasive micropapillary carcinoma showing papillary growth with calcifications and poorly differentiated invasive duct carcinoma. **D:** Most of the micropapillary clusters in this tumor have smooth outlines and are surrounded by a tight clear halo.

14.8% of T1 lesions, in contrast to 51.8% of T2, and 33.3% of T3 tumors.[2] In the same series, tumors with more than 50% of micropapillary growth tended to be larger (mean, 6 cm) than those with a lesser amount of this pattern (mean, 3.5 cm). Chen et al.[6] observed a similar trend in a study comparing 100 invasive carcinomas with micropapillary features and 100 invasive ductal carcinoma not otherwise specified (NOS) (3.38 vs. 2.39 cm; $p < 0.001$). The lesions may be multifocal grossly.[2]

MICROSCOPIC PATHOLOGY

Invasive micropapillary carcinoma consists of small clusters of neoplastic epithelial cells suspended in tight clear spaces, in a growth pattern that closely mimics lymphovascular invasion (Fig. 29.1). The clusters often have a serrated outer border. They are devoid of fibrovascular cores and display an "inside-out" arrangement with the luminal aspect of the cell present on the outer surface of the cluster. A central clear space is usually present, but solid groups may also occur (Fig. 29.1). Uncommon variants feature microcystic dilation of lumens within cell clusters (Fig. 29.2) or apocrine differentiation (Fig. 29.3). The neoplastic epithelial cells are cuboidal to columnar and display finely granular or dense eosinophilic cytoplasm. Nuclear grade is usually intermediate to high,[11] and mitotic activity is greater in higher grade lesions. Paterakos et al.[12] reported that invasive micropapillary carcinomas had a significantly increased proportion of high-grade features and a high mitotic rate. Chen et al.[6] observed that 32% of invasive carcinomas with micropapillary features were histologic grade III/III, 37% grade II/III, and 31% histologic grade I/III. Kim et al.[16] compared the nuclear grade of 38 invasive micropapillary carcinomas and 217 nonmicropapillary invasive duct carcinomas and found no significant differences, but the invasive micropapillary carcinomas were significantly larger (mean tumor size 3.8 vs. 2.5 cm; $p = 0.001$) and more often had lymphovascular

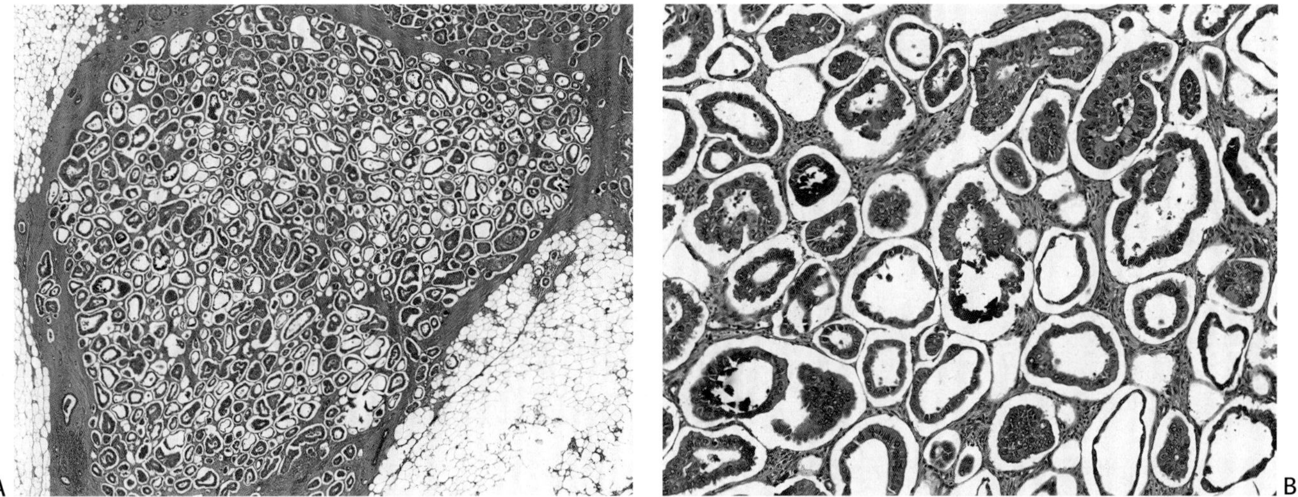

FIG. 29.2. ***Invasive micropapillary carcinoma.*** **A:** This aggregate of carcinomatous glands bears a superficial resemblance to adenosis. Tight clear spaces are present around the glands. **B:** Clear spaces are evident within the clusters. A few psammomatous calcifications are also present.

invasion (60.5% vs. 18.6%; $p < 0.001$). On the other hand, Yu et al.[8] observed significantly higher nuclear grade in 72 invasive micropapillary carcinomas than in 144 control tumors matched for age, size, and stage (52.8% vs. 37.5%; $p = 0.0387$). Lymphovascular invasion (Fig. 29.4) (68.1% vs. 38.2%; $p < 0.0001$) and lymph node metastases with extracapsular extension (Fig. 29.4) (40.3% vs. 28.9%; $p = 0.001$) were also significantly more common in invasive micropapillary carcinomas than in control tumors. Intracytoplasmic mucin may be present rarely in the tumor cells. Perineural invasion occurs occasionally. Necrosis[5] and a lymphocytic infiltrate[4] are not typical features of invasive micropapillary carcinoma, but in some instances a lymphoid infiltrate may permeate the stroma.

A clear space defined by intervening stroma consisting of dense fibrocollagenous tissue or a more delicate network of reticular tissue surrounds each tumor cell cluster. The resulting sponge-like pattern of spaces filled by tumor clusters characterizes primary tumors as well as metastatic lesions (Fig. 29.4). The clear spaces are not lined by endothelium,[4] and they are usually attributed to artifactual shrinkage of stromal elements secondary to formalin fixation. Although some authors reported that clearing around the clusters is not observed in frozen sections,[4] Acs et al.[19] documented clear spaces around tumor clusters in the frozen section from at least one case of invasive micropapillary carcinoma. These authors suggested that the clear spaces are points of weaker stromal density that facilitate tissue infiltration by the neoplastic cells.

The spaces generally appear to be empty, but in some instances mucinous material has been demonstrated with special stains.[13] Rare examples of invasive carcinoma composed

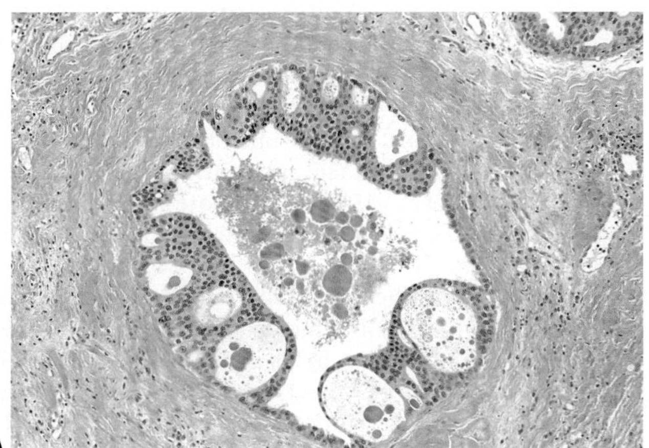

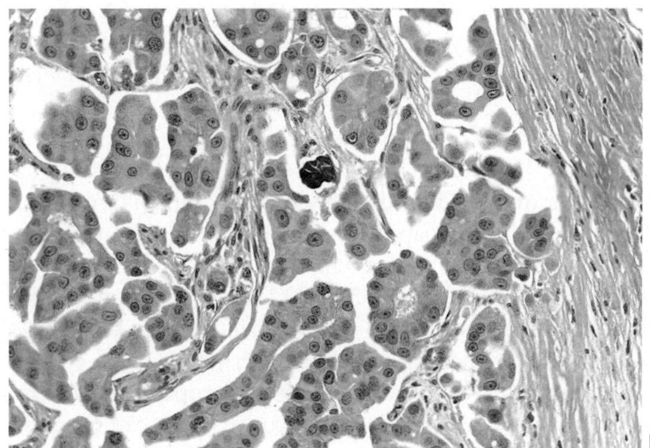

FIG. 29.3. ***Invasive micropapillary carcinoma, apocrine.*** **A:** Intraductal apocrine carcinoma with peripheral arcades. **B:** Invasive micropapillary apocrine carcinoma with a calcification.

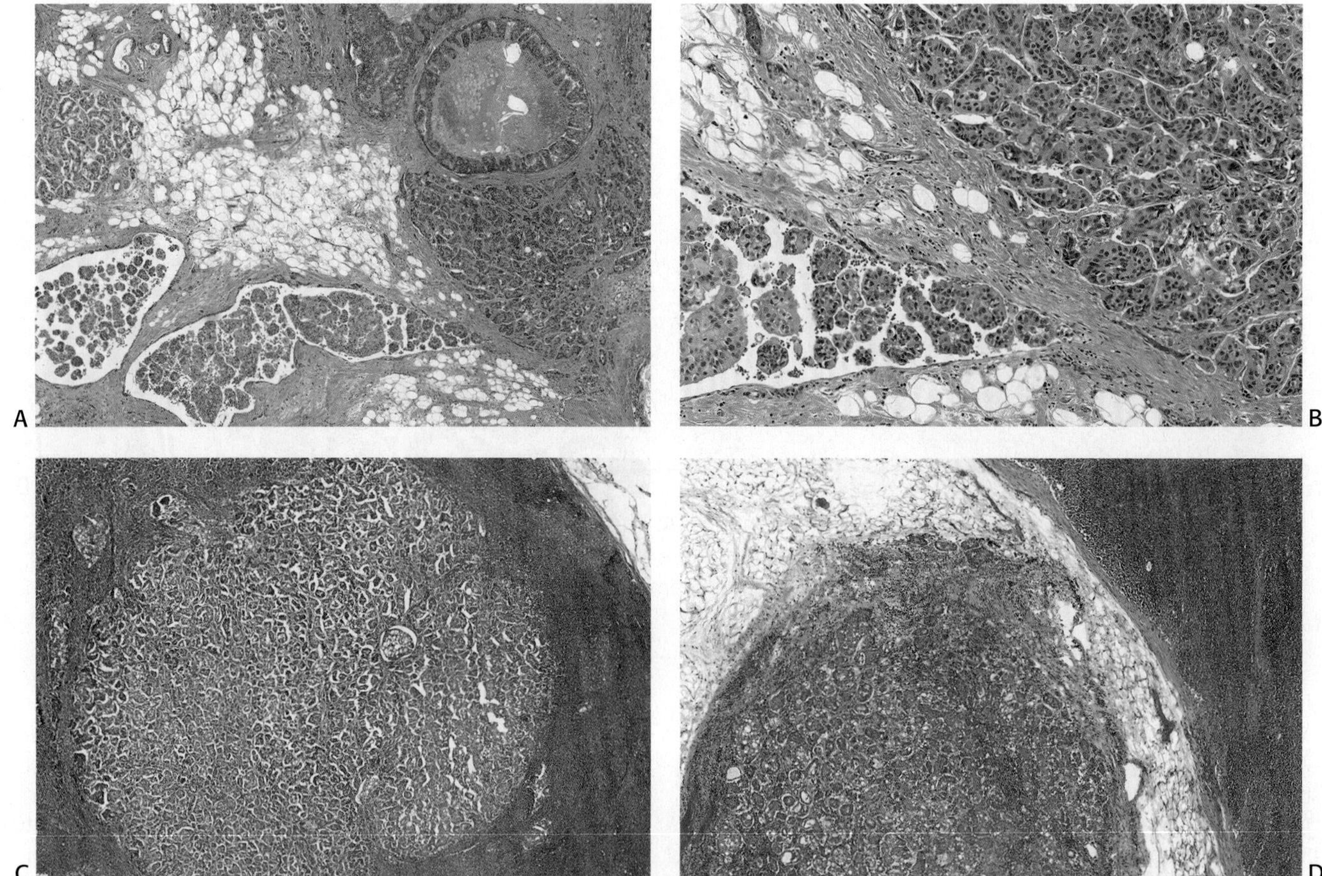

FIG. 29.4. ***Invasive micropapillary carcinoma, lymphovascular invasion and lymph node metastases.*** **A:** Dilated lymphatic channels adjacent to invasive micropapillary carcinoma are filled with tumor emboli. Micropapillary DCIS is also present. **B:** The intravascular tumor emboli are morphologically indistinguishable from the micropapillary clusters invading the stroma (same tumor as in image **A**). **C:** A lymph node metastasis shows the characteristic micropapillary arrangement. **D:** Lymph node metastasis of micropapillary carcinoma with extracapsular extension.

entirely of micropapillary clusters in mucin-filled spaces have been reported[20,21] (Fig. 29.5). There is no agreement on whether these tumors constitute a variant of mucinous or invasive micropapillary carcinoma. Myxoid stroma has been noted in a minority of cases.[4] Microcalcifications, which can be psammomatous, are variably present in the tumor cell clusters (Figs. 29.2 and 29.3).

Pure invasive micropapillary carcinomas are rare. In one series,[11] 4.83% of 1,056 consecutive cases reviewed at one center over a 9-month period had micropapillary areas. The invasive micropapillary component represented less than 25% of the tumor mass in 9 cases (18%), 25% to 49% in 11 cases (22%), 50% to 75% in 12 cases (24%), and more than 75% in 19 cases (37%). The last group comprised 1.80% of all breast carcinomas in the study period.

Luna-Moré et al.[13] found invasive micropapillary differentiation in 27 (2.7%) of 986 consecutive breast carcinomas. In 15 of the tumors, the invasive micropapillary component occupied more than 50% of the lesion. Pure invasive micropapillary carcinoma was present in 21 (1.7%) of 1,287 tumors reviewed by Paterakos et al.[12] Pettinato et al.[2] found an invasive micropapillary component in 62 (3.8%) of 1,635 carcinomas. The micropapillary pattern comprised 50% to 100% of 40 tumors (64.5%), 25% to 50% of 12 tumors (19.4%), and less than 25% of 10 (16.1%). About 4% of invasive ductal carcinomas studied by Kuroda et al.[3] were either pure or mixed forms of invasive micropapillary carcinoma. Out of 100 carcinomas with invasive micropapillary features reported by Chen et al.,[6] 45 (45%) had more than 75% micropapillary morphology, 26 (26%) had micropapillae in 50% to 75% of the tumor, 15 (15%) in 25% to 49%, and 14 (14%) in less than 25%. In the same study, the type of carcinoma associated with the invasive micropapillary component was ductal NOS in 68 cases, mucinous in 2, and invasive lobular in 1 case. In the study by Yun et al.,[9] the nonmicropapillary components coexisting with areas of invasive micropapillary carcinoma included conventional invasive ductal carcinoma (18 cases), invasive cribriform carcinoma (4 cases),

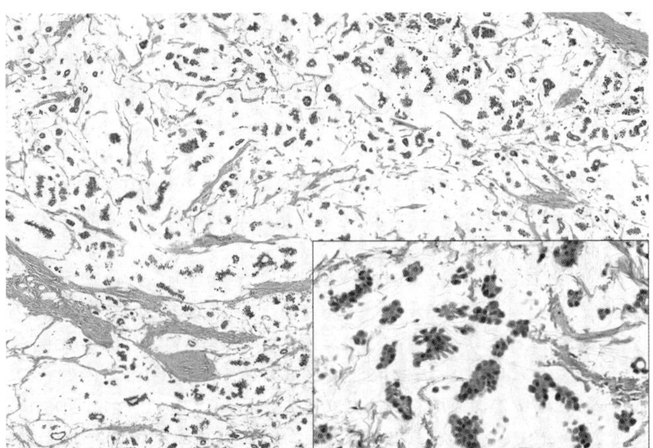

FIG. 29.5. ***Invasive micropapillary and mucinous carcinoma.*** In this case, the entire tumor consisted of micropapillary clusters suspended in abundant mucin. The tumor clusters are smaller than usually seen in mucinous carcinoma and have serrated outer borders [*inset image*]. It is unclear whether tumors with this morphology should be classified as invasive micropapillary or mucinous carcinomas.

mucinous carcinoma (2 cases), tubular carcinoma (1 case), and microinvasive ductal carcinoma (1 case).

Mixed micropapillary carcinomas usually show a sharp demarcation between the micropapillary and NOS components (Fig. 29.1).

Ductal carcinoma *in situ* (DCIS) is detected in most cases.[5] In pure invasive micropapillary carcinoma, the DCIS tends to be micropapillary or cribriform, with intermediate nuclear grade[22] (Figs. 29.3, 29.4, and 29.6). DCIS with marked necrosis is more common in tumors with only a focal invasive micropapillary pattern. The DCIS cells tend to have high-grade hyperchromatic nuclei rather than the bland nuclear cytology commonly found in micropapillary DCIS. Necrosis and calcifications are often present in the intraductal foci.

CYTOLOGY

The diagnosis of invasive micropapillary carcinoma may be suggested when fine-needle aspiration (FNA) material contains round to oval, three-dimensional and angular clusters of neoplastic cells lacking fibrovascular cores.[23] Dispersed, discohesive clusters of tumor cells may also be present. This cytologic pattern is likely to be duplicated in a specimen from metastatic invasive micropapillary carcinoma (Fig. 29.4).

IMMUNOHISTOCHEMISTRY

Even though the distribution of several prognostic markers varied considerably in some earlier reports,[2,5,12,13,16] more recent studies consistently show that most invasive micropapillary carcinomas are positive for estrogen receptor (ER) and progesterone receptor (PR).[7,10,15,18,22] Yamaguchi et al.[18] reported ER positivity in 11/15 (73%) cases (5/8 pure and 6/7 mixed micropapillary) and PR positivity in 10/15 (66%) (5/8 pure and 5/7 mixed micropapillary). All 24 pure invasive micropapillary carcinomas evaluated by Marchió et al.[15] were ER positive, and 20 (83.3%) were also PR positive. The same authors observed human epidermal growth factor 2 (HER2) 3+ positive staining in 1/24 (4.2%) pure invasive micropapillary carcinomas and HER2 2+ equivocal staining in two tumors (8.3%). *HER2* gene amplification was detected in 2/24 (8.3%) pure invasive micropapillary tumors. In a subsequent series of 40 invasive carcinomas with mixed micropapillary morphology, the investigators[24] observed HER2 3+ staining in the micropapillary component of six cases (15%) and in the nonmicropapillary component of

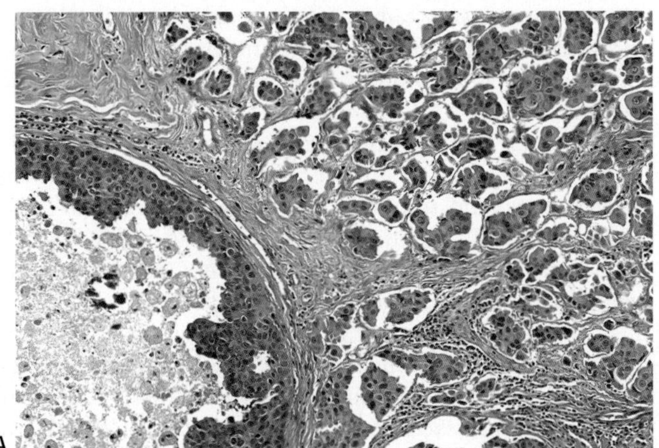

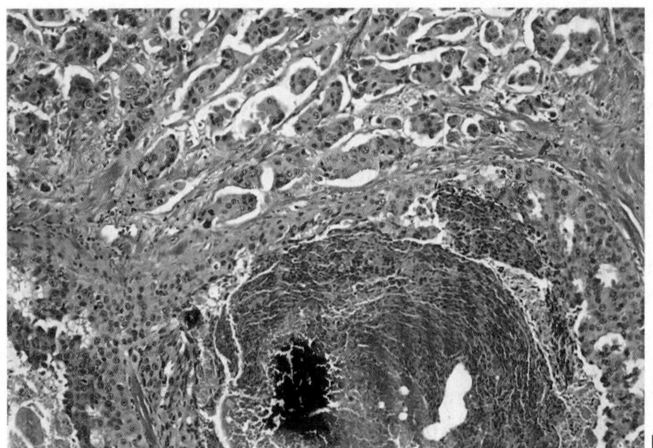

FIG. 29.6. ***Invasive micropapillary carcinoma, intraductal carcinoma.*** **A:** DCIS associated with invasive micropapillary carcinoma is often micropapillary as well, with intermediate or high nuclear grade. **B:** In this instance, the DCIS shows necrosis and calcifications.

five (14.3%). Equivocal HER2 2+ staining was present in the micropapillary component of five (12.5%) cases. Five cases (12.5%) had equivocal HER2 2+ staining in the nonmicropapillary component. The *HER2* gene was amplified in the micropapillary and nonmicropapillary components of seven (17.5%) cases with mixed morphology. In a series of cases studied by Yamaguchi et al.,[18] 5/15 (33%) cases were HER2 positive, including 2/8 pure micropapillary and 3/7 mixed micropapillary.

Ki67 positivity is usually substantial. Ki67 decorated 10% to 30% of cells in 54.2% of 24 pure invasive micropapillary carcinomas and more than 30% of cells in the remaining 45.8% of cases.[15] In a series of 15 patients with either the pure or mixed invasive micropapillary pattern,[18] the Ki67 labeling index was significantly higher in pure than in mixed micropapillary carcinomas (28.7% vs. 16.7%, respectively; $p = 0.02$) and in tumors with lymph node metastases than in those without ($p = 0.0029$).

Positive reactivity for p53 was detected in six of eight cases of pure invasive micropapillary carcinoma, in which it decorated between 20% and 50% of the tumor nuclei.[5] Another study[15] found positive p53 staining in 10/24 (41.7%) cases.

Marchió et al.[15] studied 24 pure invasive micropapillary carcinomas and 48 grade and ER-matched invasive ductal carcinomas available in tissue microarrays and found higher cyclin-D1 expression and proliferation rates in the invasive micropapillary tumors. Mixed invasive micropapillary carcinomas also displayed higher proliferative rates than grade- and ER-matched invasive ductal carcinomas NOS.[24]

The basal markers epidermal growth factor receptor (EGFR),[16] CK5/6, and CK14[24] have consistently been reported as negative, except for three cases found to be CK5/6 positive by Yamaguchi et al.[18] Only one of the three cases was a pure invasive micropapillary carcinoma. The other two tumors were mixed micropapillary carcinomas, and CK5/6 reactivity localized predominantly in the nonmicropapillary component. C-kit is also consistently negative in these tumors.[16,24] Overexpression of N-cadherin, which has been associated with tumor invasiveness, is also found frequently in invasive micropapillary carcinomas.[25]

The tumor cells are immunoreactive for epithelial membrane antigen (EMA), which stains the cell membranes at the periphery of the neoplastic clusters.[13] Complete linear EMA reactivity on the outer surface of the micropapillary clusters supports complete reversal of cell polarity. MUC-1 expression within ordinary gland-forming carcinomas is localized to the apical cell surface where the glycoprotein is involved in lumen formation. In invasive micropapillary carcinoma, MUC-1, just like EMA, is localized on the external surfaces of the tumor cell clusters, adjacent to the surrounding stroma.[2,26] A similar pattern of staining has also been reported for KL-6,[27] a glycoprotein normally expressed on the surface of polarized epithelial cells, such as in alveolar, intestinal, and ductal epithelium. Reversal of cell polarity is also a feature of lymphovascular tumor emboli.[28] Pettinato et al.[2] reported that E-cadherin reactivity was present between carcinoma cells but not on the contiguous surfaces of these cells. Marchió et al.[15] observed reduced E-cadherin staining in 2/24 cases (8.3%) and no reactivity in another two tumors (8.3%). On the other hand, Gong et al.[29] found strong expression of E-cadherin in 23/23 tumors and noted that immunoreactivity for CD44, a cell surface glycoprotein that acts as a receptor for hyaluronan, was present in 61% of cases.

Artifactual retraction of the stroma around nests of invasive ductal carcinoma NOS can produce an appearance that focally resembles invasive micropapillary carcinoma. In such cases, the tumor cells generally do not display the complete reverse polarity characteristic of invasive micropapillary carcinoma, and the nests of invasive ductal carcinoma usually show EMA staining only on the inner surfaces of the cells. However, Acs et al.[30] observed linear EMA reactivity on at least part of the outer surfaces of tumor clusters surrounded by a clear halo in 7% of 1,323 invasive ductal carcinomas with focal peritumoral retraction but no clear-cut micropapillary pattern. Based on these findings, the authors suggested that partial reverse cell polarity may occur focally in invasive nonmicropapillary carcinomas, and this phenomenon may play a role in initiating lymphovascular invasion. Kuba et al.[31] observed focal (less than 5% of tumor area) incomplete reverse cell polarity with the inside-out EMA staining pattern in 88/166 (53%) invasive ductal carcinomas NOS. Tumors with these features were larger and showed more often lymphovascular invasion and lymph node metastases than tumors lacking these features. These tumors also had poorer recurrence-free survival (RFS) by univariate analysis.

In a series of cases studied with endothelial markers (factor VIII, CD31), Pettinato et al.[2] identified vascular invasion in 63% of tumors examined. Lymphovascular permeation may be a function of the high lymphatic vessel density and increased vascular epidermal growth factor (VEGF)-C expression in invasive micropapillary carcinomas.[8] When convincing evidence of lymphatic emboli is encountered, the intravascular tumor cell clusters are arranged in micropapillary clusters similar to those that compose the invasive component present in the stroma. Lymphovascular invasion constitutes an independent adverse prognostic factor.[16,22]

Cui et al.[32] found that the expression of tumor necrosis factor (TNF) alpha (a critical modulator of inflammation, angiogenesis, and tumor proliferation), TNF-RII (a TNF-alpha receptor), and tumor microvessel density were all higher in invasive micropapillary carcinomas than in conventional invasive ductal carcinomas ($p < 0.05$). Similarly, Li et al.[33] observed higher microvessel density in 82 invasive micropapillary carcinomas than in 137 invasive ductal carcinomas NOS. The same authors reported that mRNA levels and immunoreactivity for CD146, a molecule associated with angiogenesis, were upregulated in invasive micropapillary carcinomas. CD146 was significantly associated with histologic grade, ER and PR status, p53 expression, and with tumor progression.

DIFFERENTIAL DIAGNOSIS

The differential diagnosis of invasive micropapillary carcinoma includes mucinous carcinoma. The clusters of cells in mucinous carcinoma have smooth outlines and are located in spaces filled with abundant mucin that can be highlighted with the help of special stains.[22] Nonetheless, rare carcinomas with serrated micropapillary clusters in mucin-filled spaces have been reported (Fig. 29.5). Classification of these tumors remains uncertain.

The differential diagnosis of invasive micropapillary carcinoma also includes carcinomas with micropapillary morphology that are metastatic from extramammary sites, such as papillary serous ovarian carcinoma,[34] and carcinomas of the lungs, colon, and urinary bladder. The identification of DCIS is a strong evidence in support of primary breast origin. In some cases, however, it may be necessary to use immunohistochemical markers to determine tumor origin. Serous ovarian carcinoma is usually strongly reactive for Wilms' tumor 1 (WT-1), a marker very infrequently found in invasive micropapillary breast carcinoma[21] and for PAX8, which is expressed in thyroid, renal, thymic, and müllerian tumors.[35] Lee et al.[36] reported that 21% invasive micropapillary carcinomas of the breast expressed CA125, whereas this marker decorated over 90% of serous papillary ovarian carcinomas, usually in 80% to 100% of cells. Nuclear expression of WT-1 was found in 26% of invasive micropapillary carcinomas, typically confined to fewer than 10% of cells. Very weak WT-1 cytoplasmic staining of uncertain significance was also noted in 59% of the tumors. Only 1 of 34 invasive micropapillary breast carcinomas displayed nuclear reactivity for WT-1 and cytoplasmic reactivity for CA125. In a series by Domfeh et al.,[21] only 2/20 invasive breast carcinomas with micropapillary morphology showed positive nuclear staining for WT-1, and stromal mucin was present around the tumor clusters of both cases. Among the remaining primary breast tumors in the study, WT-1 decorated 64% of 33 pure mucinous carcinomas, 29% of 31 mixed mucinous carcinomas, and 2% of 60 consecutive invasive breast carcinomas.

Lotan et al.[37] studied the utility of an immunohistochemical panel to assess the origin of 47 carcinomas with micropapillary morphology from different sites (13 bladder, 6 lung, 16 breast, and 12 ovarian). They found that uroplakin, CK20, thyroid transcription factor 1 (TTF-1), ER, mammaglobin, WT-1, and/or PAX8 were the most useful markers. Uroplakin and CK20 were the most sensitive markers of urothelial differentiation. Pulmonary invasive micropapillary carcinomas were uniformly TTF-1 positive. Invasive micropapillary carcinomas of the breast were positive for ER and mammaglobin, and negative for PAX8 and WT-1, whereas primary ovarian carcinomas were ER, WT-1, and PAX8 positive, but mammaglobin negative. Chivukula et al.[38] also reported that PAX2 is a highly sensitive and specific müllerian antigen. PAX2 decorated each of 5 mammary metastases of ovarian serous carcinoma but was not expressed in any of 89 primary breast carcinomas, including 26 with micropapillary morphology.

CORE BIOPSY

Micropapillae characteristic of invasive micropapillary carcinoma can be recognized in a needle core biopsy specimen, but the excised tumor must be examined before a definitive diagnosis of micropapillary carcinoma can be rendered.

Acs et al.[19] evaluated micropapillary features and retraction artifact (defined as "separation of tumor cells, glands, and nests from the surrounding stroma by a clear space without endothelial lining") in needle core biopsy specimens from 47 invasive micropapillary carcinomas and 424 invasive nonmicropapillary carcinomas and correlated the findings with lymph node involvement. Micropapillary features were present in 28/47 (59.5%) needle core biopsies of invasive micropapillary carcinomas, and lymph node metastases were subsequently found in 35/47 (74.5%) patients. Although the percentage of retraction artifact present in core biopsy material was significantly higher in micropapillary carcinomas than in nonmicropapillary carcinomas (median percentage of retraction artifact 30 vs. 10; $p < 0.0001$), some degree of peritumoral retraction artifact was identified in 293/471 (62.2%) core biopsies of nonmicropapillary carcinomas. Retraction artifact in core biopsies was significantly higher in invasive carcinomas associated with lymphovascular invasion and lymph node metastases than in tumors without these features. Based on these results, the authors concluded that retraction artifact in core biopsy material of nonmicropapillary carcinomas is a good predictor of lymphovascular invasion and lymph node metastases.

ELECTRON MICROSCOPY

Micropapillary breast carcinomas consist of small neoplastic epithelial clusters with a micropapillary arrangement, devoid of fibrovascular cores, and seemingly suspended in clear spaces. By electron microscopy, the cells composing the micropapillary clusters have microvilli on their cell membranes lining the outer surfaces of the cell clusters. This pattern suggests that the clear spaces are in fact tubular lumina.[13] This peculiar arrangement of cells within the clusters with their apical surfaces polarized to the outside has been referred to as an "inside-out growth pattern."[39]

GENETICS AND MOLECULAR STUDIES

Middleton et al.[5] documented loss of heterozygosity (LOH) at the p53 locus 17p13.1 in four of five (80%) tumors.

Using high-resolution microarray comparative genomic hybridization (CGH), Marchió et al.[15] found that chromosomal gains of 1q, 2q, 4p, 6p, 6q23.2–q27, 7p, 7q, 8p, 8q, 9p, 10p, 11q, 12p, 12q, 16p, 17p, 17q, 19p, 20p, 20q, and 21q and losses of 1p, 2p, 6q11.1–q16.3, 6q21–q22.1, 9p, 11p, 15q, and 19q were more common in a series of 12 pure invasive micropapillary carcinomas than in 20 grade- and ER-matched invasive ductal carcinomas NOS. In particular, high-level gains/amplifications of 8p12–p11, 8q12, 8q13, 8q21, 8q23, 8q24, 17q21, 17q23, and 20q13 as well as *MYC* (8q24) amplification were significantly associated with pure invasive micropapillary carcinoma, corroborating the morphologic impression that these tumors represent a distinct pathologic entity. *MYC* gene amplification was detected in 8/23 (34.8%) pure micropapillary carcinomas tested by chromogenic *in situ* hybridization. In a subsequent study, Marchió et al.[24] compared the genomic alterations of pure invasive micropapillary carcinomas and grade- and ER-matched invasive ductal carcinomas NOS to those of 10 carcinomas with mixed invasive micropapillary morphology. The pattern of genomic aberrations found in mixed invasive micropapillary carcinomas resembled that of pure invasive micropapillary carcinomas. Mixed invasive micropapillary carcinomas also frequently harbored amplifications of multiple regions on chromosome 8q ($p < 0.05$). In particular, pairwise comparison of the genomic profiles of pure invasive micropapillary carcinomas and of the micropapillary component of mixed invasive micropapillary tumors demonstrated striking similarities. The authors concluded that micropapillary differentiation in breast cancer identifies a subgroup of more aggressive, ER-positive breast carcinomas, which includes tumors with mixed micropapillary histology, and that mixed invasive micropapillary carcinomas are more closely related to pure invasive micropapillary carcinomas than to invasive ductal carcinomas NOS.

Flatley et al.[40] studied 20 invasive micropapillary carcinomas (4 with 100% invasive micropapillary component, 7 with greater than 75% invasive micropapillary component, and 9 invasive mixed micropapillary carcinomas) using a multiplexed polymerase chain reaction (PCR) mass spectroscopy–based technique, which encompassed 643 point mutations in a total of 53 genes. In this study, invasive micropapillary and NOS components of invasive mixed micropapillary carcinomas were microdissected and analyzed separately. The authors also analyzed microdissected samples of intraductal epithelial proliferations (11 DCIS, 1 lobular carcinoma *in situ* [LCIS], and 8 other proliferative lesions, including usual ductal hyperplasia [UDH]) adjacent to the tumors. Hotspot point mutations were found in the micropapillary component of 7/20 (35%) carcinomas. More specifically, four cases showed activating mutations in the phosphatidylinositol-3-kinase catalytic subunit A (*PIK3CA*) (*PIK3CA*-E545K and *PIK3CA*-H1047R) gene, two in the *AKT1* (*E17H* plekstrin homology domain) gene, one in the *KRAS* (*KRAS*-G12V) gene, and one in the *TP53* (*TP53*-R175H) gene. Six of 11 (55%) carcinomas with more than 75% micropapillary component had mutations, including two of three invasive micropapillary carcinomas with apocrine cytology. The mutation profiles were independent of ER and HER2 status. Micropapillary and nonmicropapillary components of mixed carcinomas showed concordant mutation profile in five of six cases (83%). Similarly, concordance was documented in invasive carcinomas and adjacent DCIS in 10/11 (91%) cases. These results demonstrate a high rate of *PIK3CA* mutations in invasive micropapillary carcinomas, which is similar to the rate of *PIK3CA* mutations in invasive ductal carcinomas NOS. In contrast, *AKT1*- and *KRAS*-activating mutations were relatively high in invasive micropapillary carcinomas, whereas they are present in only 1% to 2% of invasive ductal carcinomas NOS.

Using next generation sequencing to analyze formalin-fixed paraffin-embedded tumor samples, Li et al.[41] found substantial differences in the expression of microRNA species between five pure invasive micropapillary carcinomas and five invasive ductal carcinomas NOS. In the same study, using microRNA-specific reverse transcription (RT)–PCR to analyze RNA isolated from formalin-fixed paraffin-embedded samples, the authors documented significantly higher levels of let-7b, miR-30C, miR-148a, miR-181a, miR-181a*, and miR-181b in 22 pure micropapillary carcinomas than in 24 invasive ductal carcinomas NOS. MiR-30C expression is associated with response to tamoxifen treatment in advanced ER-positive tumors.[42] MiR-181 family members are involved in transforming growth factor (TGF)-beta-induced modulation of the stem cell-like features of mammospheres *in vitro*.[43] The altered microRNA profile of invasive micropapillary carcinoma could contribute to the characteristic arrangement of the tumor cells and to its invasive growth.

TREATMENT AND PROGNOSIS

Peritumoral lymphovascular invasion is present in 50% to 70% of invasive micropapillary carcinomas.[5,13,22,29] A high proportion of patients (72% to 77%) have axillary lymph node (ALN) metastases at the time of presentation.[13,22] Involvement of more than three lymph nodes is common. Six of seven cases with lymph node sampling in Uddin's[7] series had positive ALNs. Included in this group was also a mammographically detected nonpalpable primary tumor. Lymph node metastases were present in 9/10 patients with pure invasive micropapillary carcinoma in the series by De la Cruz et al.[44] Extranodal extension is not uncommon.[45] Occasionally, however, mammographically detected nonpalpable invasive micropapillary carcinoma can present with no axillary nodal metastases. Chen et al.[6] observed that compared with invasive carcinomas NOS, carcinomas with invasive micropapillary features had more frequent lymphovascular invasion (69% vs. 26%; $p < 0.001$) and more lymph node metastases (84.45% vs. 50%; $p < 0.001$) and involved a greater number of lymph nodes (14% vs. 3%; $p < 0.001$).

Information about the clinical course of invasive micropapillary carcinoma is limited, but most studies suggest that breast carcinomas with micropapillary features are more aggressive and have poorer prognosis than nonmicropapillary tumors. In the past, most patients were treated by mastectomy and axillary dissection, but currently patients with small invasive micropapillary carcinomas can be managed with breast conservation and whole-breast radiotherapy.

Fowler et al.[46] reported the case of a 67-year-old woman who developed local recurrence of invasive micropapillary breast carcinoma 5 years after breast-conserving surgery and partial-breast irradiation. The patient's primary tumor had prognostically favorable features except for the histology of invasive micropapillary carcinoma. Although this is a single case report, partial-breast irradiation should not be used in patients with invasive micropapillary carcinoma until its utility is validated in clinical trials.

Postmastectomy chest wall irradiation should be considered in patients with large tumors in view of the apparent proclivity for local recurrence after mastectomy. Middleton et al.[5] reported that 9/14 patients developed recurrences in the skin and chest wall following mastectomy, with a mean time to recurrence of 24 months. Among 10 patients with follow-up, 5 died of breast carcinoma 3 to 12 years after diagnosis and 5 were alive for 1 to 8 years. When compared with patients with nonmicropapillary invasive carcinoma, patients with invasive micropapillary carcinoma had a significantly shorter disease-free survival (DFS) and overall survival (OS) after a median follow-up of 13.8 years.[12] However, when stratified for the number of lymph nodes involved and other prognostic factors in multivariate analysis, patients with invasive micropapillary carcinoma had survival rates similar to patients with nonmicropapillary invasive duct carcinoma.

Pettinato et al.[2] reported that 71% of the patients in their study developed local recurrence in the chest wall or skin and that 49% died of metastatic tumor after a mean interval of 5.2 years. Kuroda et al.[47] reported a significantly less favorable prognosis for invasive micropapillary carcinoma when compared with nonmicropapillary tumors.

The treatment of choice for large invasive micropapillary carcinomas is mastectomy and axillary clearance with adjuvant hormonal therapy and chemotherapy added in cases having positive lymph nodes or tumor size larger than 1 cm. Yu et al.[8] compared prognostic factors and patterns of failure in 72 patients with invasive micropapillary carcinomas and 144 patients with age, size, stage, and treatment-matched nonmicropapillary tumors treated at one center between 1999 and 2007. Invasive micropapillary carcinomas were more commonly associated with lymphovascular invasion (68% vs. 38.2%; $p < 0.0001$), extracapsular extension from lymph nodes (40.3% vs. 28.9%; $p = 0.001$), and high nuclear grade (52.8% vs. 37.5%; $p = 0.0387$). Forty-seven (65.3%) patients with micropapillary carcinoma underwent mastectomy and 25 (34.7%) breast-conserving surgery. All patients treated with breast-conserving surgery or those with tumors larger than 5 cm and/or 4 or more involved lymph nodes received postoperative radiotherapy. Fifteen of the 72 patients (20.8%) developed recurrent disease after a median follow-up time of 26 months (range 3 to 115). Ten patients (13.9%) had distant metastases. Eleven (15.3%) patients had local recurrences that occurred in the postoperative scar or chest wall in seven (9.7%) cases, in the axillary tissue in eight (11.1%), in supraclavicular lymph nodes in four (5.6%), and in the internal mammary nodes in one (1.4%). Seven of the 57 patients (12.3%) with lymph node metastases at initial diagnosis developed axillary or supraclavicular recurrence. On the basis of these findings, the authors suggested that axillary and supraclavicular radiation therapy be considered in patients with axillary node metastases. In this study, patients with invasive micropapillary carcinomas had a 5-year OS of 86.0% and 5-year RFS of 68.2%. Locoregional RFS was significantly lower in patients with micropapillary carcinomas than in patients with nonmicropapillary tumors ($p = 0.0024$), but distant metastasis-free survival (78.1% vs. 79.3% at 5 years) did not differ between the two groups.

Chen et al.[6] studied 100 invasive breast carcinomas with an invasive micropapillary component treated at one center between 1989 and 2001. At the time of diagnosis, three patients had metastases to the supraclavicular lymph nodes, and each one had bone and liver metastases. Radical mastectomy was performed in 52 patients, modified radical mastectomy in 47, and simple mastectomy in 1. Forty patients received neoadjuvant and adjuvant chemotherapy, and 49 had adjuvant chemotherapy. Fifty-two patients received tamoxifen. Follow-up information was available for 98 patients, with a median time interval of 60.1 months (range 4 to 199). Eleven (11.2%) patients developed local recurrence with a median interval of 26.4 months (range 4 to 85). Thirty-eight (38.3%) patients developed distant metastases after a mean interval of 36 months. Thirty-six patients (36.7%) died of disease. The cumulative survival of 59% at 5 years and 48% at 10 years was significantly lower than in the control group ($p = 0.004$). On univariate analysis, only lymphovascular invasion was significantly associated with worse prognosis ($p = 0.026$), whereas tumor size, extent of micropapillary component, histologic grade, and lymph node metastases did not show a significant correlation. Multivariate survival analysis confirmed that lymphovascular invasion conferred an increased risk of death, whereas tamoxifen therapy was associated with improved survival. The combination of neoadjuvant chemotherapy and chemotherapy did not appear to provide a survival advantage.

Alvarado-Cabrero et al.[48] observed no change in tumor size and no histologic evidence of treatment effect in 29 pure invasive micropapillary carcinomas that underwent mastectomy and ALN dissection after anthracycline-based neoadjuvant chemotherapy (5-fluorouracil, epirubicin, cyclofosfamide or epirubicin and cyclofosfamide). Extensive residual and multifocal disease was observed in most cases (Fig. 29.7). Residual tumor cells were present in the axillary nodes of all 28/29 patients who had clinically involved lymph nodes at the time of diagnosis. These patients were also more likely to have at least six lymph node metastases than patients with invasive ductal, lobular, or mucinous carcinoma in the same study ($p < 0.01$).

One case of HER2-positive advanced inflammatory breast carcinoma with an invasive micropapillary component showing a clinically complete response to trastuzumab-containing treatment has been reported by Shigematsu et al.[49]

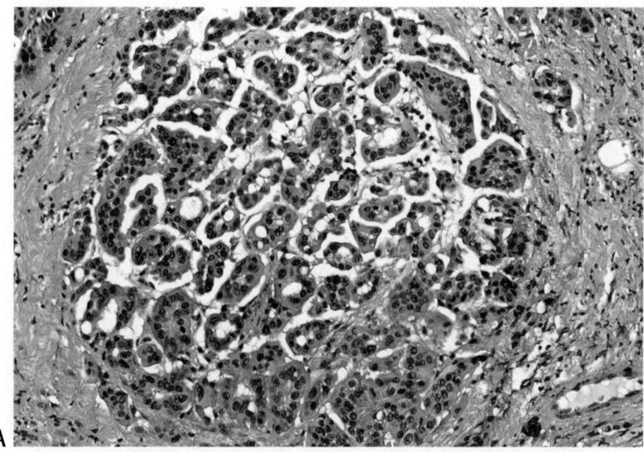

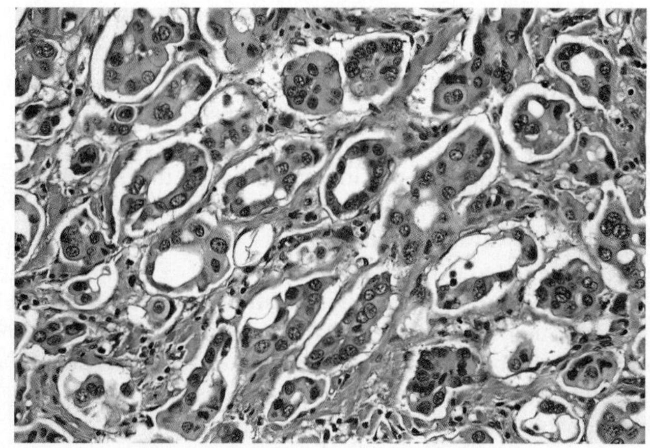

FIG. 29.7. ***Invasive micropapillary carcinoma and neoadjuvant chemotherapy.*** **A:** Invasive micropapillary carcinoma in core biopsy material, before neoadjuvant treatment. **B:** Same tumor after neoadjuvant chemotherapy. The neoplastic cells show minimal treatment effect.

REFERENCES

1. Fisher ER, Palekar AS, Redmond C, et al. Pathologic findings from the National Surgical Adjuvant Breast Project (protocol no. 4). VI. Invasive papillary cancer. *Am J Clin Pathol* 1980;73:313–322.
2. Pettinato G, Manivel CJ, Panico L, et al. Invasive micropapillary carcinoma of the breast: clinicopathologic study of 62 cases of a poorly recognized variant with highly aggressive behavior. *Am J Clin Pathol* 2004;121:857–866.
3. Kuroda H, Sakamoto G, Ohnisi K, et al. Clinical and pathologic features of invasive micropapillary carcinoma. *Breast Cancer* 2004;11:169–174.
4. Siriaunkgul S, Tavassoli FA. Invasive micropapillary carcinoma of the breast. *Mod Pathol* 1993;6:660–662.
5. Middleton LP, Tressera F, Sobel ME, et al. Infiltrating micropapillary carcinoma of the breast. *Mod Pathol* 1999;12:499–504.
6. Chen L, Fan Y, Lang RG, et al. Breast carcinoma with micropapillary features: clinicopathologic study and long-term follow-up of 100 cases. *Int J Surg Pathol* 2008;16:155–163.
7. Uddin Z, Idrees R, Aftab K, et al. Invasive micropapillary carcinoma of breast: an under-recognized entity. a series of eight cases. *Breast J* 2012;18:267–271.
8. Yu JI, Choi DH, Park W, et al. Differences in prognostic factors and patterns of failure between invasive micropapillary carcinoma and invasive ductal carcinoma of the breast: matched case-control study. *Breast* 2010;19:231–237.
9. Yun SU, Choi BB, Shu KS, et al. Imaging findings of invasive micropapillary carcinoma of the breast. *J Breast Cancer* 2012;15:57–64.
10. Luna-Moré S, de los Santos F, Breton JJ, et al. Estrogen and progesterone receptors, c-erbB-2, p53, and Bcl-2 in thirty-three invasive micropapillary breast carcinomas. *Pathol Res Pract* 1996;192:27–32.
11. Guo X, Chen L, Lang R, et al. Invasive micropapillary carcinoma of the breast: association of pathologic features with lymph node metastasis. *Am J Clin Pathol* 2006;126:740–746.
12. Paterakos M, Watkin WG, Edgerton SM, et al. Invasive micropapillary carcinoma of the breast: a prognostic study. *Hum Pathol* 1999;30:1459–1463.
13. Luna-Moré S, Gonzalez B, Acedo C, et al. Invasive micropapillary carcinoma of the breast. A new special type of invasive mammary carcinoma. *Pathol Res Pract* 1994;190:668–674.
14. Erhan Y, Zekioglu O. Pure invasive micropapillary carcinoma of the male breast: report of a rare case. *Can J Surg* 2005;48:156–157.
15. Marchió C, Iravani M, Natrajan R, et al. Genomic and immunophenotypical characterization of pure micropapillary carcinomas of the breast. *J Pathol* 2008;215:398–410.
16. Kim MJ, Gong G, Joo HJ, et al. Immunohistochemical and clinicopathologic characteristics of invasive ductal carcinoma of breast with micropapillary carcinoma component. *Arch Pathol Lab Med* 2005;129:1277–1282.
17. Kamitani K, Kamitani T, Ono M, et al. Ultrasonographic findings of invasive micropapillary carcinoma of the breast: correlation between internal echogenicity and histological findings. *Breast Cancer* 2012;19:349–352.
18. Yamaguchi R, Tanaka M, Kondo K, et al. Characteristic morphology of invasive micropapillary carcinoma of the breast: an immunohistochemical analysis. *Jpn J Clin Oncol* 2010;40:781–787.
19. Acs G, Paragh G, Chuang ST, et al. The presence of micropapillary features and retraction artifact in core needle biopsy material predicts lymph node metastasis in breast carcinoma. *Am J Surg Pathol* 2009;33:202–210.
20. Ng WK. Fine-needle aspiration cytology findings of an uncommon micropapillary variant of pure mucinous carcinoma of the breast: review of patients over an 8-year period. *Cancer* 2002;96:280–288.
21. Domfeh AB, Carley AL, Striebel JM, et al. WT1 immunoreactivity in breast carcinoma: selective expression in pure and mixed mucinous subtypes. *Mod Pathol* 2008;21:1217–1223.
22. Walsh MM, Bleiweiss IJ. Invasive micropapillary carcinoma of the breast: eighty cases of an under recognized entity. *Human Pathol* 2001;32:583–589.
23. Khurana KK, Wilbur D, Dawson AE. Fine needle aspiration cytology of invasive micropapillary carcinoma of the breast. A report of two cases. *Acta Cytol* 1997;41:1394–1398.
24. Marchió C, Iravani M, Natrajan R, et al. Mixed micropapillary-ductal carcinomas of the breast: a genomic and immunohistochemical analysis of morphologically distinct components. *J Pathol* 2009;218:301–315.
25. Nagi C, Guttman M, Jaffer S, et al. N-cadherin expression in breast cancer: correlation with an aggressive histologic variant––invasive micropapillary carcinoma. *Breast Cancer Res Treat* 2005;94:225–235.
26. Nassar H, Pansare V, Zhang H, et al. Pathogenesis of invasive micropapillary carcinoma: role of MUC1 glycoprotein. *Mod Pathol* 2004;17:1045–1050.
27. Ohtsuki Y, Kuroda N, Umeoka T, et al. KL-6 is another useful marker in assessing a micropapillary pattern in carcinomas of the breast and urinary bladder, but not the colon. *Med Mol Morphol* 2009;42:123–127.
28. Adams SA, Smith ME, Cowley GP, et al. Reversal of glandular polarity in the lymphovascular compartment of breast cancer. *J Clin Pathol* 2004;57:1114–1117.
29. Gong Y, Sun X, Huo L, et al. Expression of cell adhesion molecules, CD44s and E-cadherin, and microvessel density in invasive micropapillary carcinoma of the breast. *Histopathology* 2005;46:24–30.
30. Acs G, Esposito NN, Rakosy Z, et al. Invasive ductal carcinomas of the breast showing partial reversed cell polarity are associated with lymphatic tumor spread and may represent part of a spectrum of invasive micropapillary carcinoma. *Am J Surg Pathol* 2010;34:1637–1646.
31. Kuba S, Ohtani H, Yamaguchi J, et al. Incomplete inside-out growth pattern in invasive breast carcinoma: association with lymph

vessel invasion and recurrence-free survival. *Virchows Arch* 2011;458: 159–169.

32. Cui LF, Guo XJ, Wei J, et al. Overexpression of TNF-alpha and TNFRII in invasive micropapillary carcinoma of the breast: clinicopathological correlations. *Histopathology* 2008;53:381–388.
33. Li W, Yang D, Wang S, et al. Increased expression of CD146 and microvessel density (MVD) in invasive micropapillary carcinoma of the breast: comparative study with invasive ductal carcinoma-not otherwise specified. *Pathol Res Pract* 2011;207:739–746.
34. DeLair DF Corben AD, Catalano JP, et al. Non-mammary metastases to the breast and axilla: a study of 85 cases. *Mod Pathol* 2013;26(3):343–9.
35. Laury AR, Perets R, Piao H, et al. A comprehensive analysis of PAX8 expression in human epithelial tumors. *Am J Surg Pathol* 2011;35:816–826.
36. Lee AH, Paish EC, Marchio C, et al. The expression of Wilms' tumour-1 and Ca125 in invasive micropapillary carcinoma of the breast. *Histopathology* 2007;51:824–828.
37. Lotan TL, Ye H, Melamed J, et al. Immunohistochemical panel to identify the primary site of invasive micropapillary carcinoma. *Am J Surg Pathol* 2009;33:1037–1041.
38. Chivukula M, Dabbs DJ, O'Connor S, et al. PAX 2: a novel müllerian marker for serous papillary carcinomas to differentiate from micropapillary breast carcinoma. *Int J Gynecol Pathol* 2009;28:570–578.
39. Petersen JL. Breast carcinoma with an unexpected inside out growth pattern, rotation of polarisation associated with angioinvasion. *Pathol Res Pract* 1993;189:780.
40. Flatley E, Ang D, Warrick A, et al. PIK3CA-AKT pathway mutations in micropapillary breast carcinoma. *Hum Pathol* 2013;44(7):1320–7.
41. Li S, Yang C, Zhai L, et al. Deep sequencing reveals small RNA characterization of invasive micropapillary carcinomas of the breast. *Breast Cancer Res Treat* 2012;136:77–87.
42. Rodriguez-Gonzalez FG, Sieuwerts AM, Smid M, et al. MicroRNA-30c expression level is an independent predictor of clinical benefit of endocrine therapy in advanced estrogen receptor positive breast cancer. *Breast Cancer Res Treat* 2011;127:43–51.
43. Wang Y, Yu Y, Tsuyada A, et al. Transforming growth factor-beta regulates the sphere-initiating stem cell-like feature in breast cancer through miRNA-181 and ATM. *Oncogene* 2011;30:1470–1480.
44. De la Cruz C, Moriya T, Endoh M, et al. Invasive micropapillary carcinoma of the breast: clinicopathological and immunohistochemical study. *Pathol Int* 2004;54:90–96.
45. Zekioglu O, Erhan Y, Ciris M, et al. Invasive micropapillary carcinoma of the breast: high incidence of lymph node metastasis with extranodal extension and its immunohistochemical profile compared with invasive ductal carcinoma. *Histopathology* 2004;44:18–23.
46. Fowler AM, Andersen JJ, Conway PD. Local recurrence of invasive micropapillary breast cancer after MammoSite brachytherapy: a case report and literature review. *Clin Breast Cancer* 2009;9:253–257.
47. Kuroda H, Sakamoto G, Ohnisi K, et al. Overexpression of Her2/neu, estrogen and progesterone receptors in invasive micropapillary carcinoma of the breast. *Breast Cancer* 2004;11:301–306.
48. Alvarado-Cabrero I, Alderete-Vazquez G, Quintal-Ramirez M, et al. Incidence of pathologic complete response in women treated with preoperative chemotherapy for locally advanced breast cancer: correlation of histology, hormone receptor status, Her2/Neu, and gross pathologic findings. *Ann Diagn Pathol* 2009;13:151–157.
49. Shigematsu H, Nakamura Y, Tanaka K, et al. A case of HER-2-positive advanced inflammatory breast cancer with invasive micropapillary component showing a clinically complete response to concurrent trastuzumab and paclitaxel treatment. *Int J Clin Oncol* 2010;15:615–620.

CHAPTER 30

Paget Disease of the Nipple

ELENA BRACHTEL • FREDERICK C. KOERNER

In 1874, Sir James Paget[1] described "an eruption on the nipple and areola" with characteristics of "ordinary chronic eczema" or "psoriasis." He observed that "cancer of the mammary gland has followed within at the most two years" and that "the formation of cancer has not in any case taken place first in the diseased part of the skin. It has always been in the substance of the mammary gland." The carcinomas that occurred in these patients followed the clinical course of other cases without Paget disease and showed "nothing which might not be written in the ordinary history of cancer of the breast."

Paget did not describe the histopathology of this condition. However, he inferred from his clinical observations that "a superficial disease induces in the structures beneath it, in the course of many months, such degeneracy as makes them apt to become the seats of cancer." To support this conclusion, he referred to the development of carcinoma of the penis, tongue, and lip after "chronic soreness or irritation."

The existence of extramammary Paget disease was recognized before the end of the 19th century, by which time the characteristic histologic features of the disease had been reported.[2,3] Thin[3] studied a series of specimens in the pathologic museum of the British Medical Association and concluded that "this malignant dermatitis has neither the symptoms nor the pathologic anatomy of any known skin disease." He described the histopathologic features of breast carcinoma in Paget disease and illustrated the "blocking up of the lactiferous ducts in the affection by newly formed cancerous epithelium [which] may break through the wall of the duct into the connective tissue of the nipple." Thin interpreted his observations as indicating that secretions emerging from the mammary ducts injured the epidermis and that this process induced the underlying carcinoma. Although histologic, electron microscopic, and immunohistochemical data have been put forward to support the view that Paget disease is a neoplasm derived from altered epidermal keratinocytes,[4,5] this mechanism is no longer considered to be the histogenesis of the condition.

The concept that Paget disease represents the spread of carcinoma cells into the epidermis from an underlying mammary adenocarcinoma was first advanced in 1904 by Jacobaeus[6] on the basis of a histologic study of three cases (Fig. 30.1). He concluded that "Paget disease is a carcinoma from its inception, derived from the glandular epithelium of the lactiferous ducts." He also noted that extension through the duct system provided a mechanism for the development of Paget disease in association with a carcinoma located deep within the breast. These observations were confirmed in 1927 by Muir,[7] who also described the phenomenon of "secondary" Paget disease, which occurs when an invasive primary carcinoma of the breast extending directly into the epidermis is accompanied by the intraepidermal spread of Paget cells. Secondary Paget disease has also been described in the skin at sites of adenocarcinoma metastatic from the breast.[8]

Considerable data from anatomic, histopathologic, and molecular studies support the evidence that Paget cells are derived from an underlying adenocarcinoma. In particular, the distribution of carcinoembryogenic antigen (CEA),[9–11] casein,[12] milk-fat globule membrane antigens,[13,14] gross cystic disease fluid protein 15 (GCDFP-15),[15] MUC proteins,[16,17] cytokeratins (CKs),[18–20] estrogen receptor (ER),[21] and human epidermal growth factor 2 (HER2)[22] indicates a glandular origin.

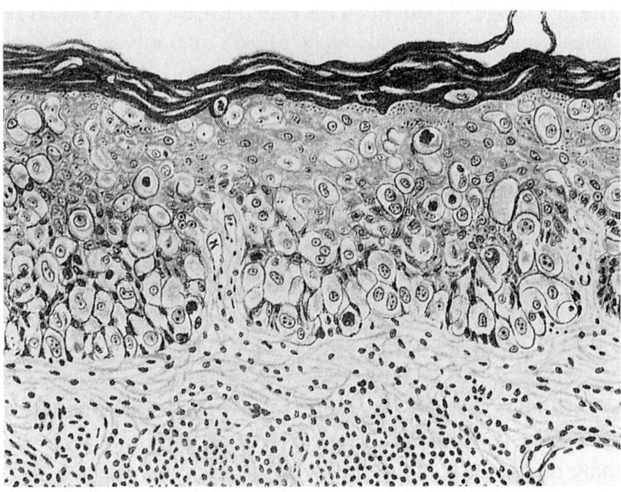

FIG. 30.1. *Paget disease.* The lesion illustrated by Jacobaeus showing characteristic features including a dermal lymphocytic infiltrate. Paget cells aggregated in the deep epidermis and scattered in the superficial epidermis. The cells have abundant pale cytoplasm and nucleoli are evident in the nuclei. [Reproduced from Jacobaeus HC. Pagets disease und sein Verhältnis zum Milchdrüsenkarzinom. *Virchows Arch* 1904;178:124–142.]

CLINICAL PRESENTATION

Frequency

Paget disease is an uncommon manifestation of mammary carcinoma that affects 1% to 3% of patients with breast carcinoma.[23] The majority of these women have a clinically evident nipple lesion. Ten percent to 28% of cases of Paget disease are detected only in histologic sections of the nipple removed at mastectomy, having caused no clinical abnormality. After reviewing incidence data recorded by nine registries in the Surveillance Epidemiology and End Results (SEER) program, Chen et al.[23] reported a 45% decline in the incidence of reported Paget disease between 1988 (age-adjusted incidence/100,000, 1.31) and 2002 (age-adjusted incidence/100,000, 0.64). The decline in incidence was limited to patients who had documented DCIS or invasive duct carcinoma (IDC). The incidence of Paget disease without associated clinical ductal carcinoma remained stable during this period. As a consequence, the relative portion of Paget disease without associated clinical ductal carcinoma increased from 12% to 15%. The authors did not discriminate between clinically apparent Paget disease and occult Paget disease discovered in routine sections of the nipple from mastectomy specimens. It is likely that the shift to breast-conserving surgery during this period contributed to the apparent decline in the incidence of Paget disease because fewer nipple samples were available for histologic examination. The fact that the incidence of Paget disease without underlying carcinoma, which is only detectable clinically, remained stable during this interval appears to support this interpretation.

Age

The age range of patients with Paget disease in several large series consisting cumulatively of 508 patients was 26 to 88 years,[18,24–26] and the average age at diagnosis in one series of 1,738 women was 62.5 years.[23] In this group, the mean age for women with Paget disease and IDC was 63.8 years, for women with Paget disease and ductal carcinoma *in situ* (DCIS) 66.2 years, and for women with Paget disease without underlying carcinoma 66.2 years.[23] Paget disease arose in the ectopic nipple of a 13-year-old girl[27] and in the nipple of a 90-year-old woman.[28]

Male Breast

One might expect Paget disease to occur more frequently in men than in women because almost all carcinomas of the male breast involve the subareolar region,[29] but fewer than 1% of reported cases of Paget disease have been found in men.[30] It occurred in 2.8% of 229 patients in one series of men with breast carcinoma.[31] About one-half of the early reports of Paget disease of the male breast lack histologic confirmation, so the literature contains fewer than 50 *bona fide* cases of Paget disease in men. Desai et al.[32] tabulated details of 33 convincing cases described before 1996, and several well-documented case descriptions have been published since.[33–46] In the series by Goss et al.,[31] men with Paget disease spanned 23 to 97 years in age, essentially the range seen in women with the disease.

Laterality

Paget disease typically involves only one breast, but both synchronous involvement in women[47–52] and men[43] and metachronous development[53–55] have occurred rarely.

Risk Factors

Researchers have not identified factors that specifically predispose to the development of Paget disease, but a few reports mention factors that generally predispose patients to the development of breast carcinomas. Loizou et al.[56] described a 36-year-old woman who underwent "extensive cardiac fluoroscopy" at birth and again at the age of 7 years who developed Paget disease at the age of 36 years. Paget disease has been found associated with breast carcinoma developing in men with Klinefelter syndrome.[53,57]

Unusual Presentation

Several cases of Paget disease have presented in unusual clinical settings. Kawawa et al.[58] detailed the case of a 66-year-old woman with Paget disease and neurofibromatosis, and Holloway et al.[38] described a similar case in a man. Fouad[59] reported a case of a man with Paget disease and lymphomatoid papulosis. A 35-year-old woman who had systemic scleroderma involving the skin of the breast with coexistent Paget disease has been described.[60] Kao et al.[61] observed DCIS and Paget disease in ectopic breast tissue on the chest of a 58-year-old woman, and two reports document Paget disease in accessory nipples.[27,62] Two women developed Paget disease confined to the areola.[63,64] Mendez-Fernandez et al.[65] detected Paget disease in the nipple of a woman 8 years after subcutaneous mastectomy for fibrocystic disease. Two cases of axillary Paget disease associated with mammary carcinoma have been described.[66,67]

Recurrent Carcinoma as Paget Disease

Recurrences of conventional breast carcinomas sometimes take the form of Paget disease. It developed in the nipple of a woman treated with excision alone[68] and those of 15 women treated with breast-conserving excision and irradiation,[69–76] 3 women treated with subcutaneous mastectomy,[77] 1 woman treated with an areola-sparing mastectomy,[78] and 7 women treated with a nipple-sparing mastectomy.[79] Basu et al.[80] reported an especially unusual case of a 64-year-old woman who underwent a left mastectomy and subsequent transverse rectus abdominus muscle (TRAM) flap reconstruction for carcinoma. During that procedure, the left nipple was reconstructed by means of the nipple-sharing technique using tissue from the right nipple. Six years later, Paget disease developed in the right nipple, and 7 years after that it arose in the reconstructed left nipple.

Symptoms and Clinical Appearance

Pain and itching are frequent complaints. Physical examination typically reveals a thickened, erythematous, scaling papule or plaque with irregular borders involving the nipple. The changes may be limited to the nipple or extend to the areola, and in advanced cases the lesion also involves the skin surrounding the areola (Fig. 30.2). Haagensen[81] wrote that "erosions that involve the areola or the skin of the adjacent breast leaving the nipple uninvolved are not Paget disease"; however, examples confined to the areola have been described.[63,64] Advanced cases often demonstrate ulceration, crusting, serous or bloody discharge from the nipple, and nipple retraction or inversion.[82] In one exceptional case, the alterations extended to the skin of the abdomen,[83] and in another, they involved the skin of the back and the proximal one-third of the arm.[84]

Because of the nonspecific nature of the clinical signs of Paget disease, a delay of 6 to 12 months prior to biopsy during which the symptoms are treated topically is not uncommon. In the series of Ascensão et al.,[85] the symptomatic intervals from 1 week to 20 years were recorded, and the average period of delay was 2.25 years.

Lesions that Mimic Paget Disease

The findings in Paget disease can be mistaken for eczema[86] or other inflammatory conditions such as seborrheic dermatitis, contact dermatitis, postirradiation dermatitis, psoriasis, and pagetoid dyskeratosis.[87] Pennell et al.[88] reported a case of cutaneous para-areolar schistosomiasis that mimicked Paget disease. Minute vesicles sometimes erupt and seem to heal, and this phenomenon may bring to mind the presence of a bullous disease such as pemphigus. Guyton et al.[89] described a case of pemphigus vulgaris initially thought to represent Paget disease and cited other examples of confusion of these two entities.[90,91] Rae et al.[92] described a 63-year-old woman in whom both pemphigus vulgaris and Paget disease involved the right nipple. Neoplastic lesions clinically confused with Paget disease include adult Langerhans cell histiocytosis,[93] intraepidermal squamous carcinoma (Bowen disease), and unusual examples of basal cell carcinoma[94] and melanoma.[95]

Pigmented Paget Disease

In an uncommon variant of Paget disease known as pigmented Paget disease, accumulation of melanin imparts

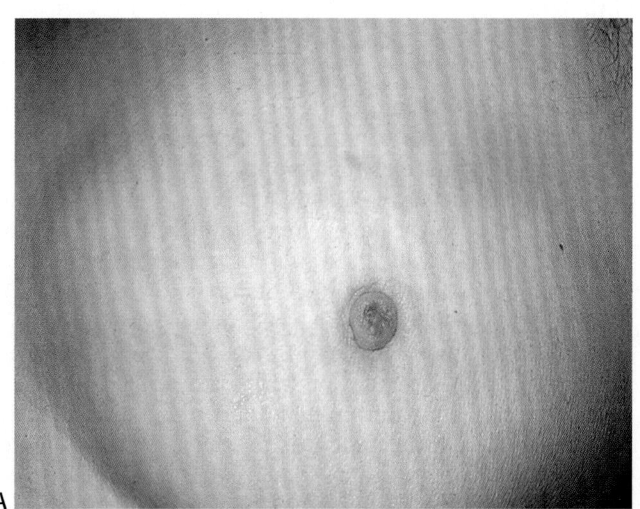

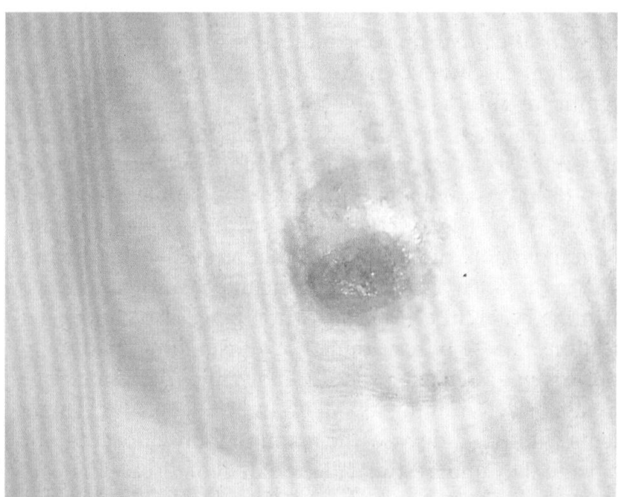

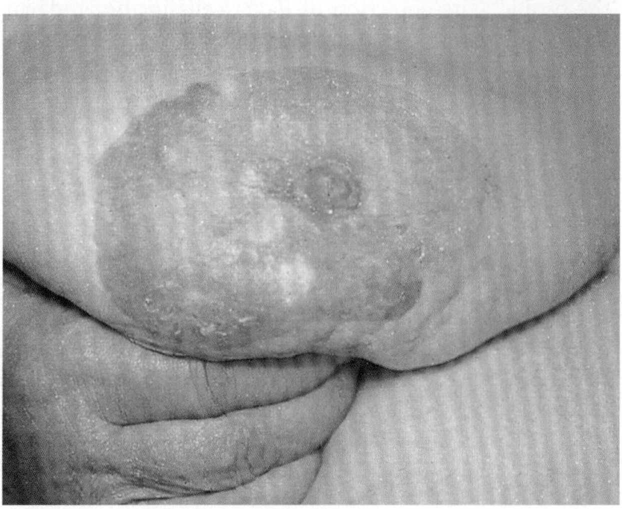

FIG. 30.2. ***Paget disease, clinical.*** **A:** The appearance of a lesion limited to the nipple surface. **B:** Paget disease extending to the areola. Note skin dimpling in the 6 o'clock radius. **C:** Paget disease extending to the skin of the breast. Skin dimpling is present in the 5 o'clock radius.

a brown color to the affected region. The publication by Soler et al.[96] lists details of 17 published cases, and other reports describe 7 additional examples.[39,42,45,97–100] One notes that a disproportionately high number of cases occurred in men.[37,39,42,44–46,101] For additional information regarding pigmented Paget disease, see Chapter 42.

Palpable Breast Tumor

Fifty percent to 60% of patients have a palpable tumor in the breast that exhibits Paget disease. In one study, the mean age of women with a tumor (49 years) was significantly less than that of women without a tumor (58 years).[25] An invasive carcinoma was detected in more than 75% to 90% of women who had Paget disease accompanied by a tumor,[18,24,102] and 45% to 66% of them reportedly had axillary lymph node (ALN) metastases.[18,24,25,102] In the absence of a clinically apparent tumor, invasive carcinoma occurs in no more than 40% of cases, and axillary metastases have been reported in 5% to 13% of cases.[18,24,25,102]

Imaging Studies

A number of mammographic abnormalities may be found in the breast underlying Paget disease.[103,104] Lesions anywhere in the breast may be indicative of a separate distant coexistent carcinoma. In the nipple–subareolar region, the significant findings include thickening of the nipple, an underlying mass, possibly with nipple retraction, and calcifications. Patients with clinically apparent Paget disease tend to have radiologic findings in the nipple–subareolar region. When Paget disease is not evident clinically, mammography more often discloses lesions away from the nipple region. Such abnormalities include a suspicious mass, asymmetry, architectural distortion, and suspicious calcifications. These observations notwithstanding, mammography is not a reliable procedure for either detecting Paget disease or determining its extent. In 22%[105] to 50%[103] of patients with Paget disease, the mammograms appeared normal and they underestimated the extent of disease in nearly one-half of the patients.[103,105–108] In a study of 25 breasts that proved to have Paget disease on pathologic examination, only three cases (12%) had nipple abnormalities on mammography.[109] Fourteen patients with clinical evidence of Paget disease in this series had underlying carcinomas. Among these 14 patients, mammography identified the underlying tumor in 6 (43%). Ultrasonography can sometimes reveal calcifications, dilatation of ducts, or flattening, asymmetry, or thickening of the nipple–areolar complex. The frequency of detection of abnormalities is similar to that of mammography.[106,110] Magnetic resonance imaging (MRI) of patients with Paget disease can disclose abnormal nipple enhancement, thickening and enhancement of the nipple–areolar complex, and coexisting enhancing DCIS or suspicious masses.[111,112] In both individual case reports[113–115] and small series,[112,116] this modality improved the detection of associated carcinomas in patients with clinical signs of Paget disease and negative mammography and ultrasonography.

GROSS PATHOLOGY

The macroscopic pathologic changes of Paget disease on the surface of the resected nipple are those observed clinically. Occasionally, enlarged lactiferous ducts can be detected if the nipple and underlying breast are examined carefully.

Most studies of Paget disease give little information about the distribution of underlying carcinoma in the breast. It can usually be found in at least one lactiferous duct. An invasive tumor, if present, tends to be central, but instances of peripherally placed tumors have been recorded.[117] Chaudary et al.[18] reported that 45% of palpable invasive carcinomas associated with Paget disease in their series were located in the upper outer quadrant. Clinically palpable tumors have no specific gross pathologic features. A small percentage of women who present with Paget disease and have no tumor detected on clinical examination are found to have a grossly evident invasive carcinoma in the resected breast.[24,117]

MICROSCOPIC PATHOLOGY

Biopsy Diagnosis

The diagnosis of Paget disease can be made from specimens obtained by a wedge biopsy, a superficial "shave" biopsy of epidermis, or punch biopsy. The wedge biopsy is most likely to yield a diagnostic specimen because the epidermis is adequately represented, and this type of specimen is likely to include a section of lactiferous duct. The shave biopsy is less likely to contain a sufficient number of Paget cells, because these specimens sometimes consist largely of superficial keratinized debris or inflammatory exudate. Although a punch biopsy will include the underlying stroma and possibly part of a duct, there is frequently very little epidermis to study. However, none of these procedures is always successful, and it is sometimes necessary to perform a second biopsy or to excise the nipple. The detection of Paget cells in the epidermis in a biopsy sample that appears to contain a florid papillomatosis is indicative of an associated carcinoma, even if the portion of the underlying lesion seen in the biopsy specimen appears benign.[118]

Paget Cells

The characteristic histopathologic feature of this condition is the presence of adenocarcinoma cells (Paget cells) in the keratinizing epithelium of the nipple epidermis (Fig. 30.3). These cells occur singly in superficial epidermal layers. In rare instances, they extend into eccrine ducts[36] and hair follicles.[119] Paget cells are more likely to form clusters in the basal portions of the epidermis and to have a distribution similar to that of junctional melanocytes. The resemblance to melanoma is enhanced if the carcinoma cells take up melanin pigment released by epidermal cells.[120,121] Isolated Paget cells appear to lie in vacuoles within the epidermis. The cytoplasm is usually pale or clear, and it may contain mucin secretion vacuoles. Nuclei of Paget cells tend to have prominent nucleoli. Rarely, Paget disease forms glands within the epidermis of the nipple[122,123] (Fig. 30.3F).

Other microscopic aspects of Paget disease sometimes obscure the lesion, and they may interfere with the diagnosis. Hyperplasia and hyperkeratosis of the epidermis occur to some degree, and they are occasionally severe enough to suggest pseudoepitheliomatous hyperplasia (Fig. 30.4). The superficial, dermal stroma of the nipple is usually infiltrated by a moderate-to-marked lymphocytic reaction. When ulceration denudes the affected epithelium, a biopsy of the exposed stroma will reveal only the underlying inflammatory reaction. Unless this misleading appearance is recognized, the biopsy findings may reinforce

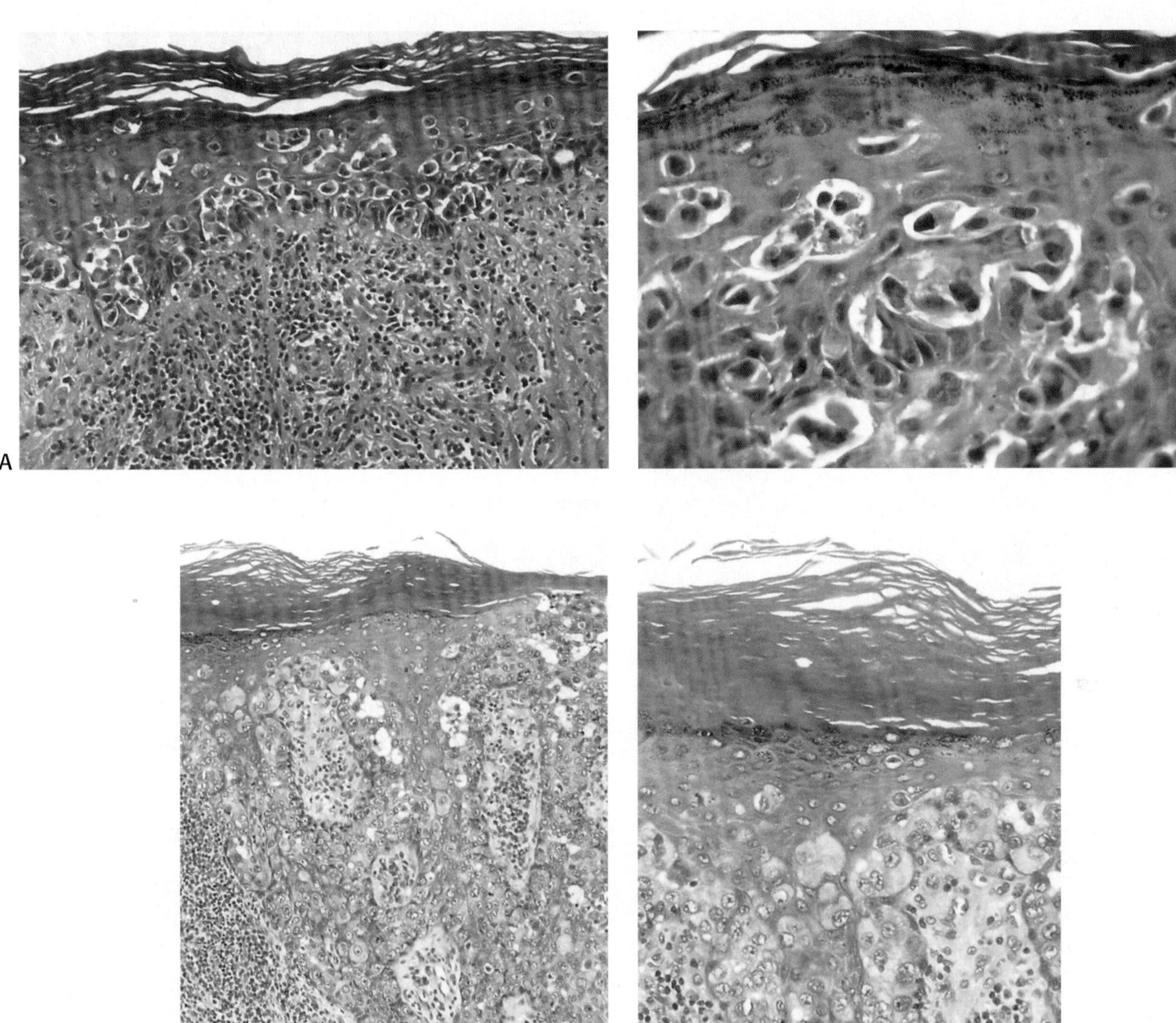

FIG. 30.3. ***Paget disease.*** **A:** Carcinoma cells form a band in the deep epidermis, and they are scattered individually throughout the squamous epithelium. **B:** A lacunar arrangement of carcinoma cells is commonly seen in Paget disease. **C:** A very extensive infiltrate with involvement largely concentrated in the deep epidermis. Lacunae are not conspicuous in this instance. **D:** The tumor cells have distinct borders, abundant pale cytoplasm, pleomorphic nuclei, and prominent nucleoli. **E:** Solid zonal replacement of the epidermis is evident on the *right*. **F:** Florid Paget disease with intraepidermal gland formation. **G:** Granules of dark brown melanin pigment are present in some Paget cells (*arrow*).

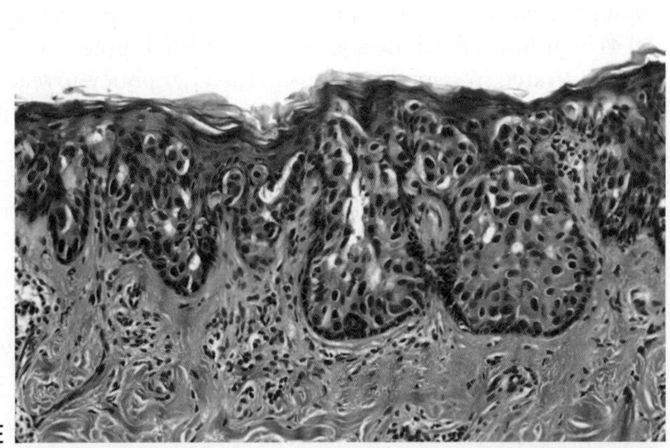
E

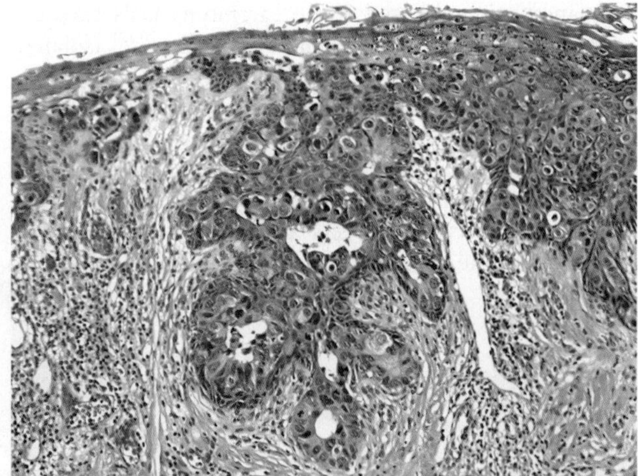
F

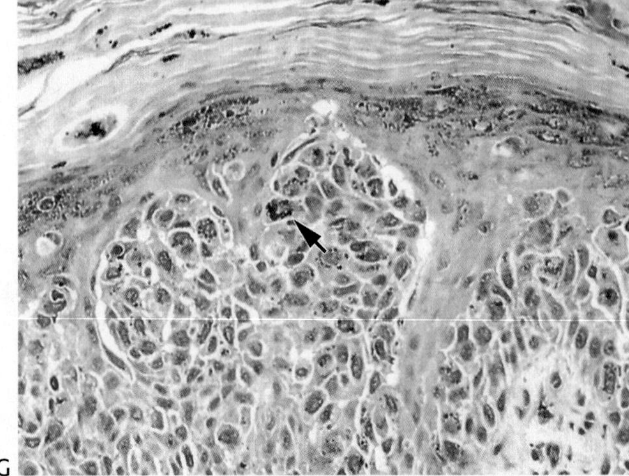
G

FIG. 30.3. *(Continued)*

an erroneous clinical diagnosis of an inflammatory condition. It is, therefore, important to state in the pathologic report whether epidermal tissue is present. Absence of epidermis is an indication for rebiopsy when Paget disease is suspected clinically.

An associated carcinoma has been found in the breast and/or the nipple in more than 95% of the hundreds of cases of Paget disease described in the literature. Virtually all have been duct carcinomas, with or without an invasive component. Rarely, these have been specialized forms of duct carcinoma (e.g., papillary or medullary)[24] or duct carcinoma arising in florid papillomatosis (adenoma) of the nipple.[118] Although the extension of cells from lobular carcinoma *in situ* (LCIS) to the epithelium of ducts within the breast, referred to as "pagetoid spread," may resemble Paget disease, this process does not often involve the major lactiferous ducts and only rarely spreads to the epidermis of the nipple (Fig. 30.5).[51]

Secondary Paget Disease

Paget disease can be encountered at sites of ductal squamous metaplasia in the breast (Fig. 30.6). Secondary Paget disease is the involvement of the epidermis over cutaneous metastases anywhere on the body or extension of a primary carcinoma to the skin (Fig. 30.7). Secondary Paget disease at sites of metastatic carcinoma is not specific for mammary carcinoma, because metastases from other carcinomas can produce this phenomenon. A case described by Paone and Baker[124] defies

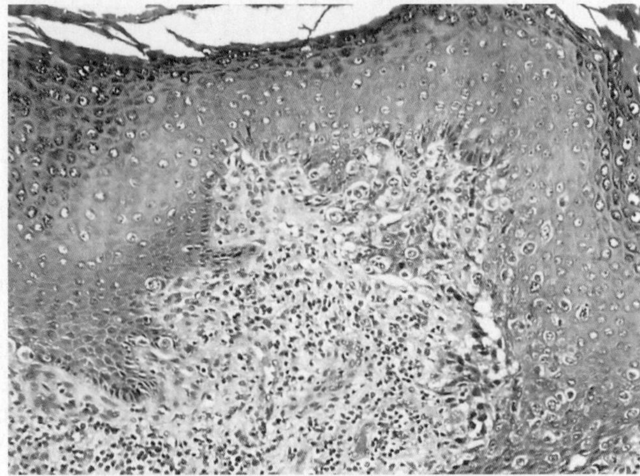

FIG. 30.4. ***Paget disease.*** Paget cells are obscured in this somewhat tangential section of hyperplastic epidermis. Note the dermal lymphocytic infiltrate, which is often present.

classification. The authors described the occurrence of Paget disease in the skin of the center of the breast of a woman who suffered from complete congenital absence of the nipple and areola. They noted, "[A]n underlying intraductal and infiltrating duct carcinoma was present, but there were no ducts leading to the affected area of the overlying skin."

Associated Carcinomas

DCIS associated with Paget disease characteristically has a comedo or solid growth pattern. Foci of cribriform and papillary duct carcinoma may also be found as part of the process somewhere in the breast, but the lactiferous ducts directly connected to Paget disease contain comedocarcinoma in most cases. Cribriform or papillary carcinoma is found in about 10% of cases, and about 40% have mixed types of DCIS.[125] Because comedocarcinoma frequently contains calcifications, the underlying DCIS may be detectable by mammography. In a series reported by Chaudary et al.,[18] 25 (78%) of 32 mastectomy specimens had DCIS beyond the subareolar area, and in 8 of these patients multicentric invasive foci were found. DCIS was limited to subareolar ducts in only two cases.

Invasive carcinoma associated with Paget disease does not have a specific histopathologic pattern. It is typically a poorly differentiated, solid, invasive carcinoma that arises from affected ducts within the underlying breast parenchyma. Rarely, invasive carcinoma may develop from a superficial or terminal portion of a lactiferous duct close to the site of Paget disease. In exceptional cases, invasion appears to arise directly from Paget disease in the epidermis growing downward into the nipple, there being no other invasive carcinoma elsewhere in the nipple and breast (Fig. 30.8). Three reports document 14 additional examples of this phenomenon.[34,126,127] In one case,[126] the microinvasive carcinoma originating from the Paget disease

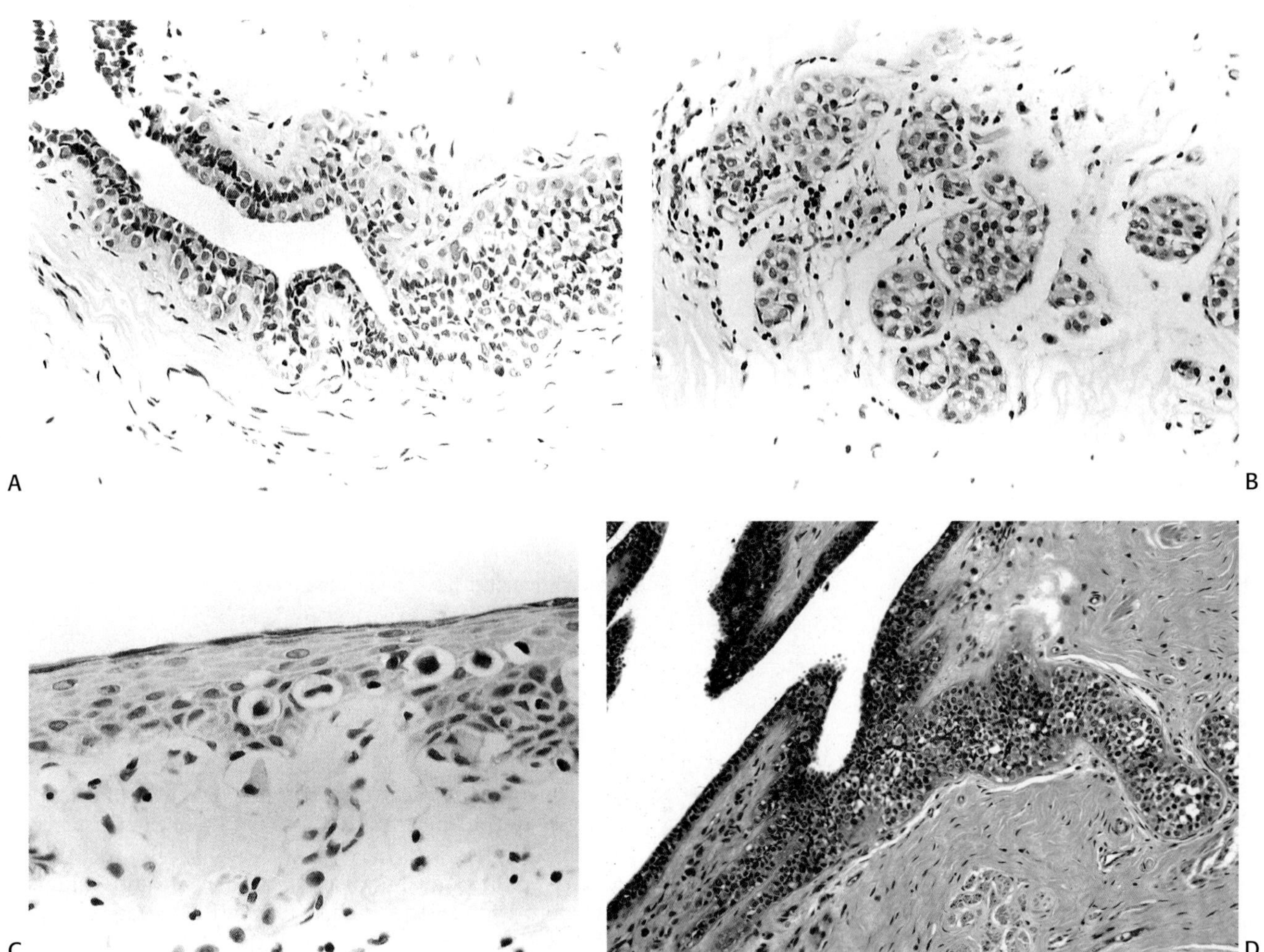

FIG. 30.5. ***Paget disease associated with lobular carcinoma*** **in situ. A:** *In situ* carcinoma with pagetoid spread in a large lactiferous duct. **B:** LCIS in a lobule. **C:** Paget disease of the nipple epidermis in the same specimen as **(A)** and **(B)**. **D–H:** Another case showing LCIS in a lactiferous duct **(D)**, negative E-cadherin stain in the *in situ* carcinoma **(E)**, Paget cells in the nipple epidermis **(F)**, CK7 reactivity in Paget cells **(G)**, and absence of E-cadherin reactivity between two Paget cells in the epidermis **(H)**.

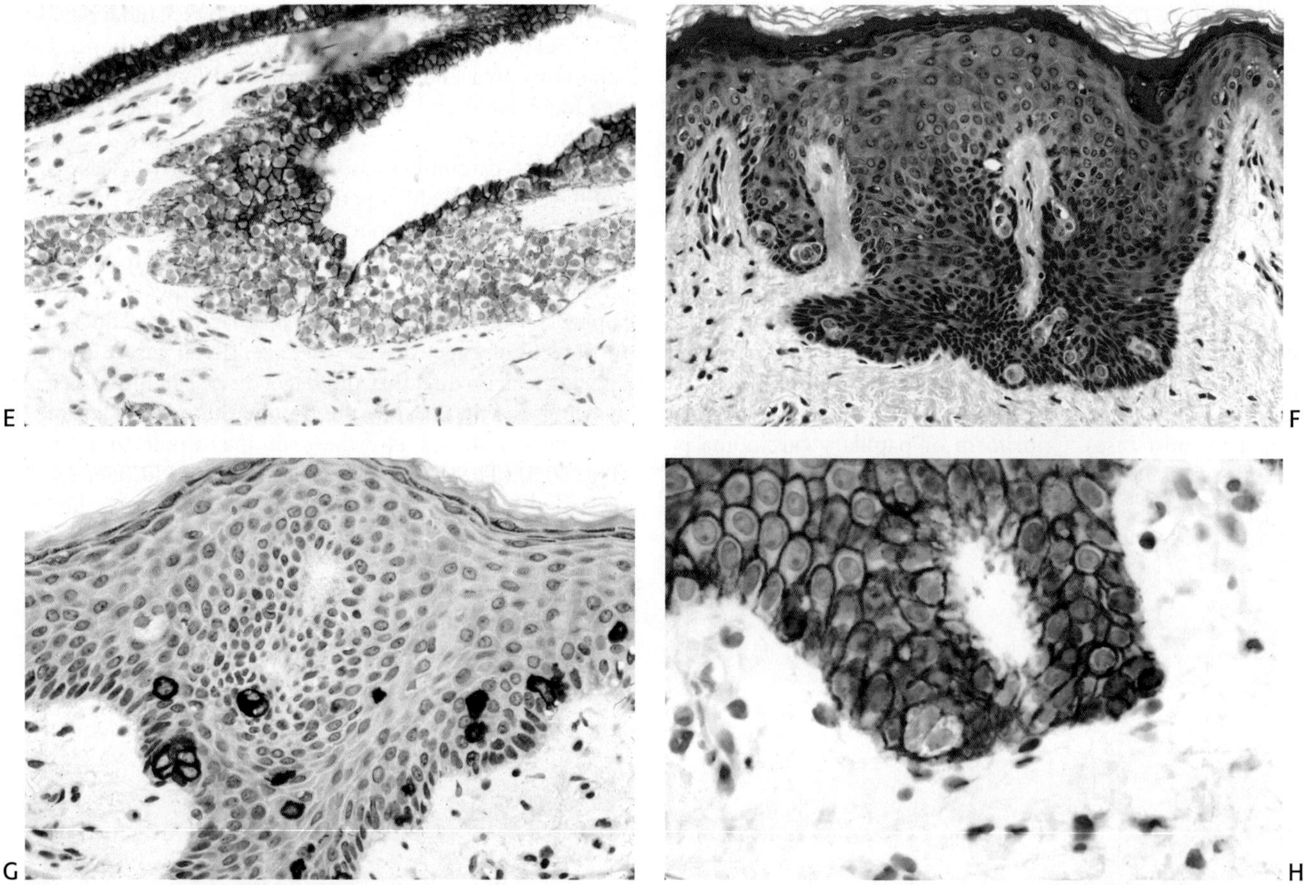

FIG. 30.5. *(Continued)*

apparently gave rise to isolated carcinoma cells in one of three axillary sentinel lymph nodes (SLNs). Although the clinical significance of this form of invasion has not been determined, limited evidence suggests that it may not signify the poor prognosis indicated by other forms of skin invasion. In the group studied by Sanders et al.,[127] five patients were treated with breast conservation and irradiation. During follow-up intervals ranging from 4 to 66 months (median, 20 months), the patients did not experience recurrences of their carcinomas. Similar examples of microinvasion have been observed in Paget disease of the vulva.[128]

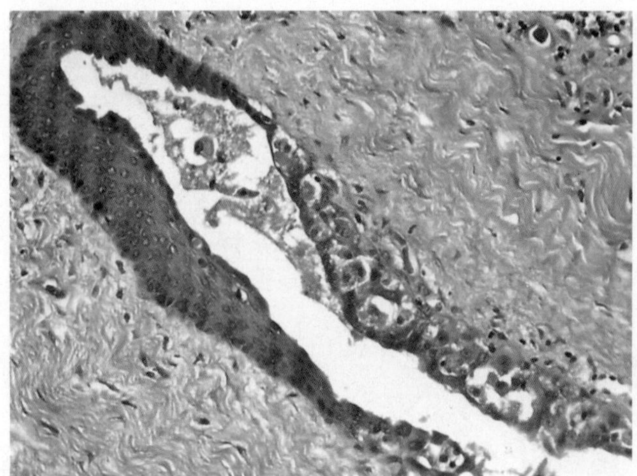

FIG. 30.6. ***Paget disease in squamous metaplasia.*** Paget disease extending from nearby DCIS involves the metaplastic squamous epithelium of this cyst within the breast parenchyma.

Absence of Associated Carcinoma

Failure to detect an underlying carcinoma in a very small number of cases has been used as an argument to support the concept that Paget disease arises directly from keratinocytes of the epidermis. In most of these rare instances, the carcinomas associated with Paget disease arise from ductal epithelium at or very near the squamocolumnar junction, with growth limited to upward spread as Paget disease (Fig. 30.9).[129] Origin of Paget disease from carcinoma of adnexal glands in the nipple is theoretically possible (Fig. 30.10). The claim that no underlying carcinoma was detectable in the breasts of patients treated only by excisional biopsy of the nipple is unwarranted, because the entire breast was not examined.[130]

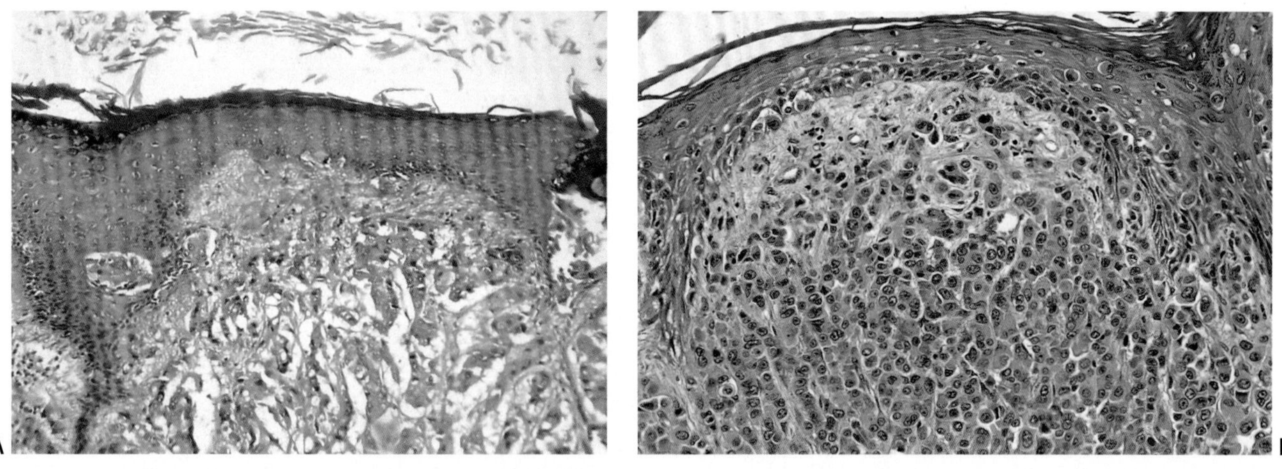

FIG. 30.7. ***Paget disease, secondary.*** **A:** IDC, apocrine-type, invading the skin from the underlying breast with Paget disease in the epidermis. **B:** Invasive pleomorphic lobular carcinoma in the nipple with overlying secondary Paget disease.

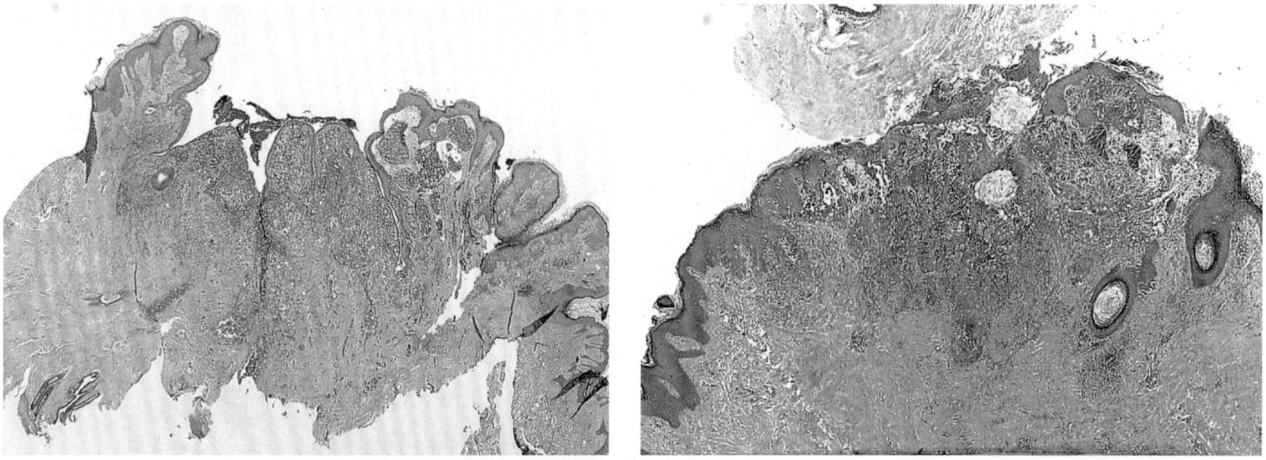

FIG. 30.8. ***Paget disease giving rise to invasive carcinoma of nipple.*** **A,B:** Specimens from two different patients showing IDC arising from lactiferous ducts near the surface of the nipple with Paget disease at the lateral borders. No carcinoma was found in the remainder of either breast. **C:** Florid Paget disease above gives rise to invasive carcinoma below in **(B)**.

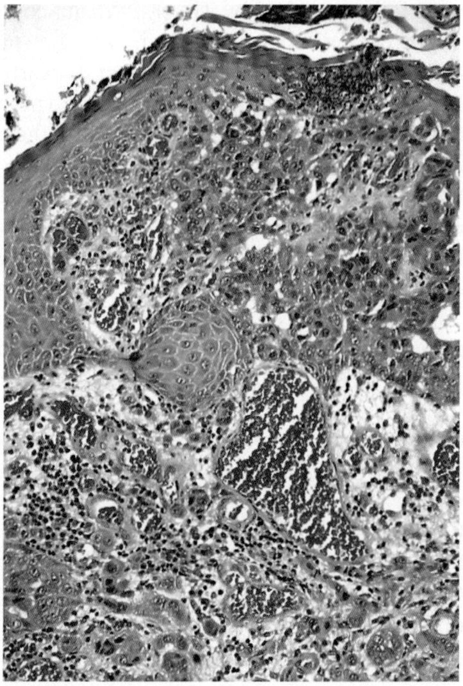

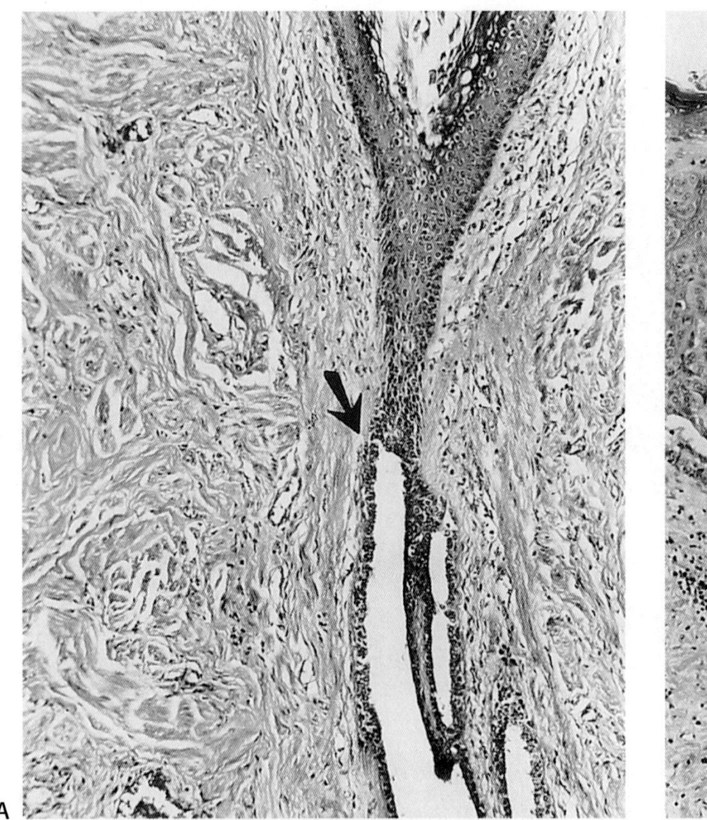

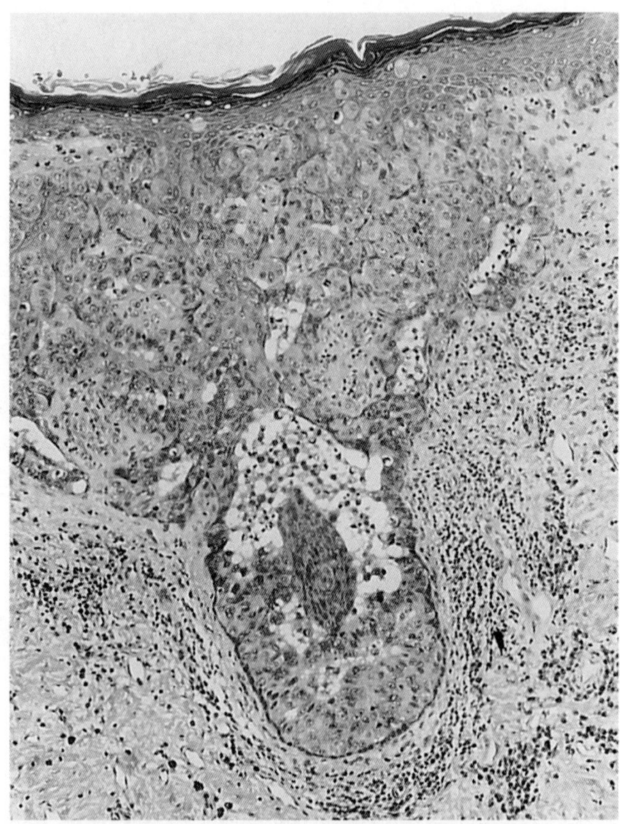

FIG. 30.9. ***Paget disease and DCIS of a terminal lactiferous duct.*** **A:** A section of a terminal lactiferous duct in which there is squamous metaplasia of the distal duct epithelium. Clear cell change is present in squamous cells. The *arrow* points to the squamocolumnar junction. **B:** DCIS in a terminal lactiferous duct in continuity with overlying Paget disease. The primary carcinoma in this case was limited to the superficial part of the nipple. **C:** Paget cells in the epidermis in (**B**).

Differential Diagnosis

The histologic differential diagnosis in a biopsy specimen obtained for suspected Paget disease includes inflammatory conditions of the skin, clear cell change in epidermal cells, florid papillomatosis of nipple ducts or nipple adenoma,[118] syringomatous adenoma[131] (see Chapter 5), and such extremely uncommon lesions as malignant melanoma[132] and squamous or basal cell carcinoma[133] (see Chapter 42). With an adequate sample, most of these lesions can be readily distinguished from Paget disease.[134]

One can observe two types of clear cells in the epidermis. Most commonly, they constitute a nonneoplastic alteration of keratinocytes (Fig. 30.11). The change tends to occur more extensively near or in the mid-epidermis with isolated cells also distributed in more superficial and deeper layers (Fig. 30.12). These cells have small, inconspicuous nuclei and, in extreme cases, consist largely of a vacuole that appears empty on routine sections (Fig. 30.13). The cells do not contain mucin or other secretory substances detectable in Paget cells.[134]

The second type of epidermal clear cells, so-called Toker cells, represents a normal constituent of the skin of the nipple and areola. First illustrated by Orr and Parish,[135] these cells were fully described by Toker.[136] Using conventional stains, one can observe them in approximately 10% of nipples,[87,136–138] but staining for CK7 revealed them in nearly 90% of nipples in a series of mastectomy specimens.[139] These cells tend to sit at the tip of the nipple near the orifices of the lactiferous sinus, but one can also find them in the areola and the ampullae of the lactiferous ducts. Most frequent in the basal region of the epidermis but not restricted to it, the cells appear larger than the keratinocytes. They have oval or polygonal shapes, abundant pale or slightly eosinophilic cytoplasm, nuclei that vary only slightly in size and shape, and nucleoli of small or modest sizes. Toker cells often contain small amounts of intracytoplasmic melanin. They appear as single cells or small clusters, which sometimes form glands or abortive tubules. Like Paget cells, Toker cells typically stain for CK7 and CAM5.2. Staining for ER and progesterone receptor (PR) has given variable results[137,139] and so has staining for epithelial membrane antigen (EMA).[138,140] The cells do not show significant staining for HER2,[87,137,139,140] and in small series they did not stain for CK20, GCDFP-15, S-100, 34βE12,[138,140] CD138, p53, p63,[137] or CEA using a polyclonal antiserum.[87] Toker cells can appear especially numerous, a situation referred to as "Toker

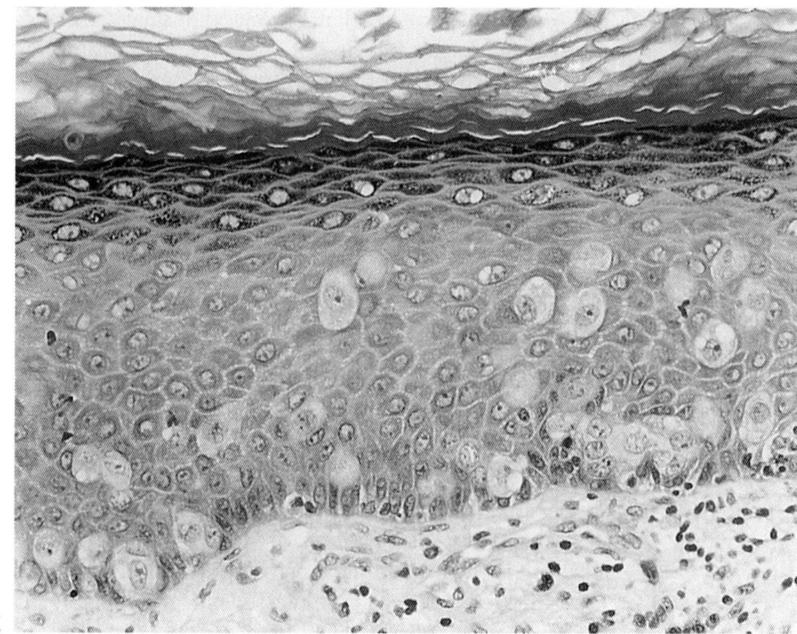

FIG. 30.9. *(Continued)*

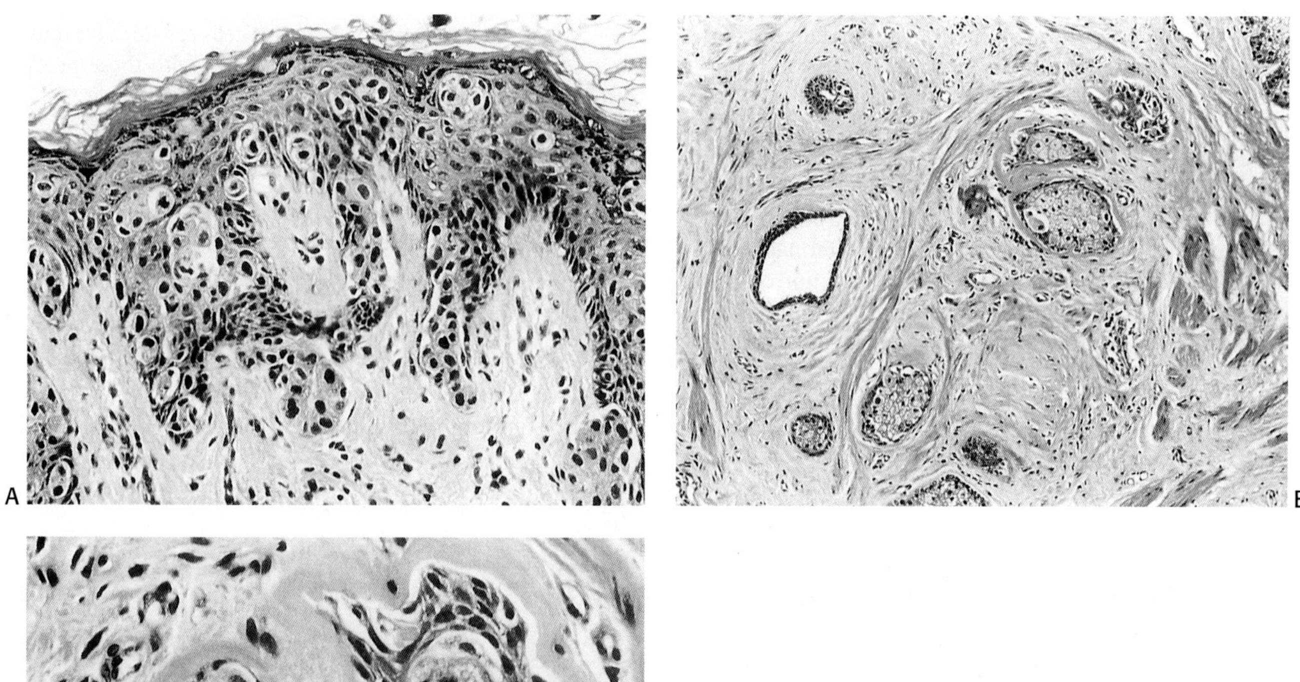

FIG. 30.10. ***Paget disease involving adnexal glands in the nipple.*** **A:** Paget disease with slight pseudoepitheliomatous hyperplasia of the epidermis. **B:** Paget cells are present in the epithelium of sebaceous glands. Also present are the dilated duct of a gland of Montgomery and bundles of subareolar smooth-muscle cells. **C:** A magnified view of a sebaceous gland with Paget cells.

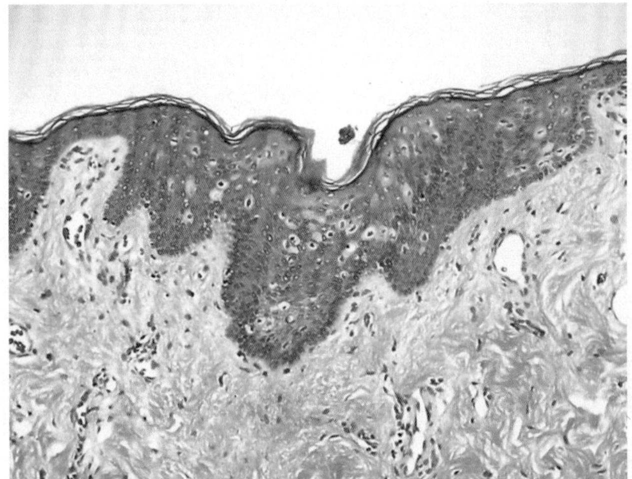

FIG. 30.11. *Clear cell change in the nipple epidermis.* Modified squamous cells with clear cytoplasm are distributed mainly in the mid-epidermis.

cell hyperplasia" by Di Tommaso et al.,[137] and even somewhat atypical. Although certain cellular features of Toker cells bring to mind the appearance of Paget cells, attention to the lack of pleomorphism and cytologic atypia in most cases and to the results of immunohistochemical staining allows one to distinguish usual Toker cells from Paget cells.

Malignant melanoma has been found to arise in the areola, but melanoma of the epidermis of the nipple proper, and especially the surface of the nipple, is exceedingly rare (Fig. 30.14).[95,132,141] The histopathologic distinction between malignant melanoma and Paget disease may be difficult in hematoxylin and eosin (H&E) sections of limited biopsy material. Routine cytologic features of the tumor cells and their distribution in the epidermis may be identical. One cannot rely on the presence of melanin in the malignant cells to establish the diagnosis of melanoma or the presence of mucin in the cells to establish the diagnosis of Paget disease. Some melanomas are devoid of pigment, whereas Paget cells can incorporate melanin from epidermal cells, and, in many cases, Paget cells do not contain mucin. Immunohistochemical staining for CKs, proteins found in melanomas, and HER2 may be necessary. In one study,[142] the results of staining for claudins distinguished Paget disease from melanoma and certain other skin tumors.

The distinction of Paget disease from intraepithelial squamous carcinoma (Bowen disease) also poses problems, especially when the cells of Paget disease appear unusually anaplastic.[143] In this situation, the cells appear moderately to marked pleomorphic, and they contain hyperchromatic nuclei and prominent nucleoli. Apoptotic bodies mimic the dyskeratotic cells of Bowen disease. The cells involve the entire thickness of the epidermis and do not display the nesting pattern expected in cases of conventional Paget disease. Keeping in mind the rare occurrence of Bowen disease in the nipple and using immunohistochemical staining for keratin molecules will prevent confusion of these two entities.

Prior to the availability of monoclonal antibodies, it was necessary to rely on routine histochemical stains for mucin to assist in diagnosing Paget disease. These procedures, especially mucicarmine and Alcian blue–periodic acid–Schiff (Ab-PAS) staining, are still useful, because they are readily available, rapid, and easy to perform (Fig. 30.15). Because few examples of Paget disease have numerous mucin-positive cells and because mucin-positive cells are not detectable in at least 25% of cases, a negative result with these procedures does not exclude the diagnosis of Paget disease.

CYTOLOGY

It may be possible to recognize carcinoma cells cytologically in an imprint or scraping from the nipple surface,[144–147] but this material is not suitable for the specific diagnosis of Paget disease. A case of pemphigus vulgaris was misinterpreted as Paget disease,[91] and the distinction of Paget disease from melanoma and squamous carcinoma may require the study of immunohistochemical stains for proteins found

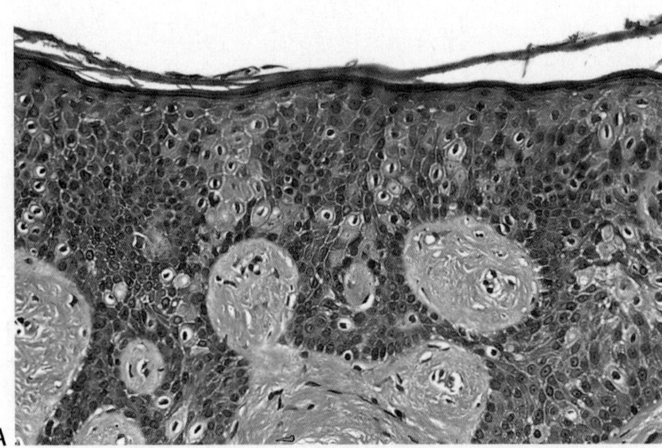

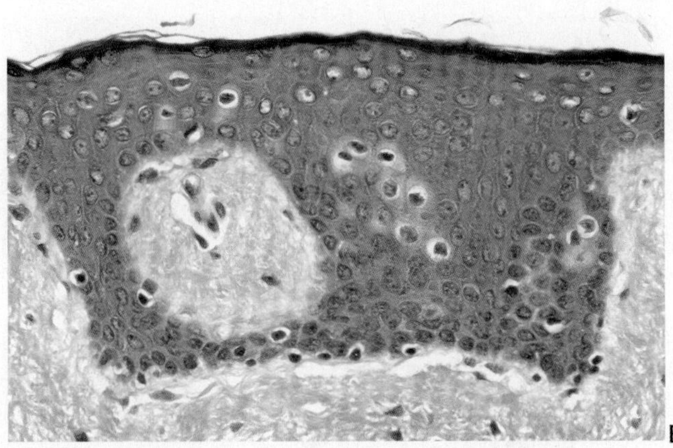

FIG. 30.12. *Clear cell change.* **A:** Alterations in squamous cells leading to clear cell change are evident. The process has a patchy distribution. Many of the cells in the affected areas display cytoplasmic pallor. **B:** Clear cell change appears to arise in cells with cytoplasmic pallor.

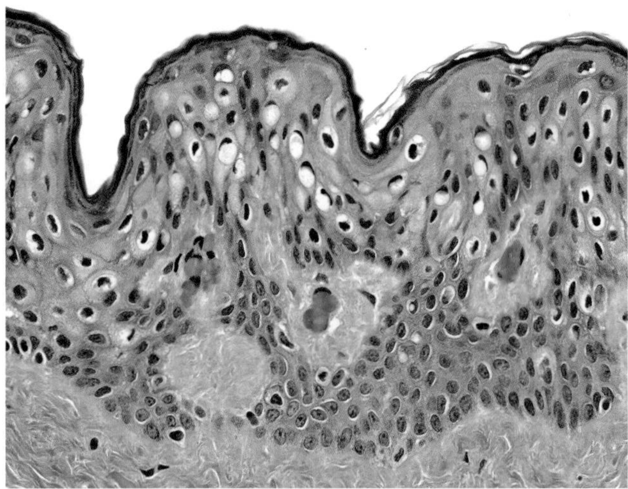

FIG. 30.13. ***Clear cell change, vacuolated.*** Marked vacuolization is evident in the mid-epidermis, largely sparing the deep layer. Vacuolated epidermal cells with eccentric nuclei resemble signet ring cells.

in melanoma cells, CKs, and HER2. Reactivity for ER has been demonstrated in Paget cells in cytologic specimens obtained by scraping the nipple with a scalpel.[21] Immunohistochemical staining for ER is not by itself a reliable basis for the diagnosis of Paget disease because the underlying carcinomas tend to be poorly differentiated and hormone receptor negative.

IMMUNOHISTOCHEMISTRY AND MARKERS

The neoplastic cells in Paget disease have histochemical and immunohistochemical properties in common with those of adenocarcinomas originating within the breast. Paget cells are reactive with monoclonal antibodies against low-molecular-weight CK[11,18,20,148–150] (Fig. 30.16), and they typically do not react with the antibodies to high-molecular-weight CKs, which stain the neoplastic cells of epidermoid carcinoma or Bowen disease.[11,20] Paget cells are immunoreactive for CK7 in nearly all cases and are not reactive for CK20.[138,151] This pattern differs from that of extramammary Paget disease, which exhibits immunoreactivity for CK20 as well as CK7.[138] Merkel cells and some epidermal clear cells have also been reported to be CK7-positive.[138] In one series,[152] only rare cases stained for CK5/6 or CK17. Paget cells are positive for EMA, human milk-fat globule (HMFG),[11,14,15,148] and mammary-type apomucin MUC1.[16] Approximately one-half of the cases stain for GCDFP-15.[15] The finding of immunoreactive CEA has proved to be a widely available useful procedure, because the protein is present in many mammary carcinomas. Paget cells were reportedly positive with a polyclonal anti-CEA, but negative with a monoclonal anti-CEA, in one study.[14] Ordóñez et al.,[11] using a different commercially available monoclonal anti-CEA reagent, reported that all eight examples of Paget disease that they studied were immunoreactive. Guarner et al.[15] detected CEA in 35% of cases. Reactivity for lysozyme, casein, and lactalbumin is seen in fewer than 10% of cases.[15]

Staining for S-100 protein has yielded variable results. Paget cells were reportedly negative for S-100 in two studies,[11,153] but positive for S-100 in 18% to 60% of lesions in other series.[15,154,155] Paget cells do not usually stain for HMB45,[155] whereas those of melanomas stain for the protein in virtually all cases. By using a panel of these markers (Table 30.1), it is possible to distinguish Paget disease from malignant melanoma and Bowen disease, but one must bear in mind that exceptions do occur. To cite a few examples, squamous carcinomas can stain for EMA[156]; Park et al.[99] reported a case in which the Paget cells stained for HMB45; and Williamson et al.[157] described two cases of pagetoid

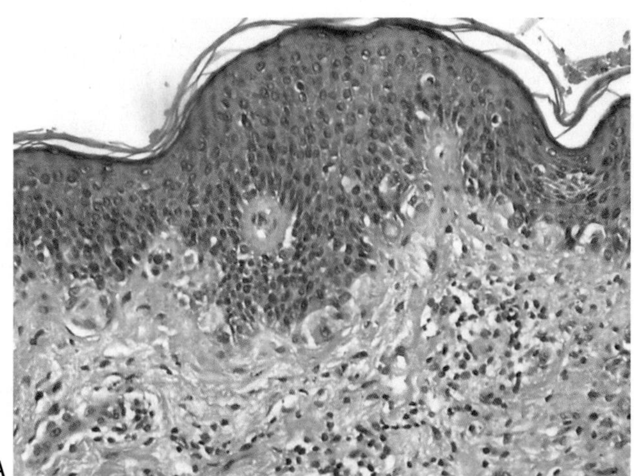

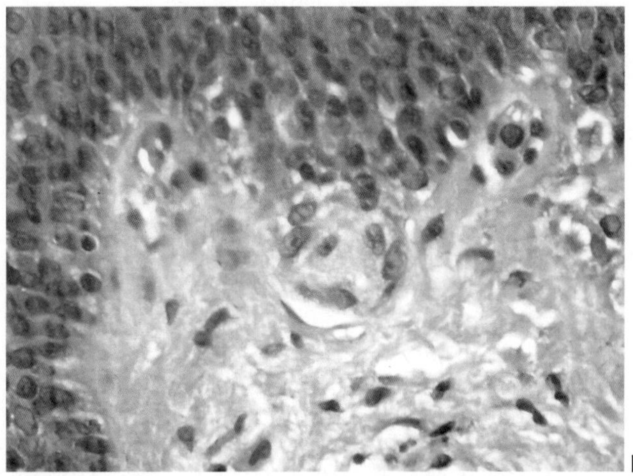

FIG. 30.14. ***Malignant melanoma of the nipple.*** **A:** The neoplastic junctional melanocytes resemble Paget cells. There is a mild dermal lymphocytic infiltrate. **B:** A nest of junctional cells. **C:** Junctional cells with nuclear vacuoles, a feature of malignant melanoma not typically seen in Paget disease. **D:** Melanoma cells are highlighted in the epidermis and dermis by this immunostain for S-100. **E:** Nuclear vacuoles can be seen in S-100-positive cells.

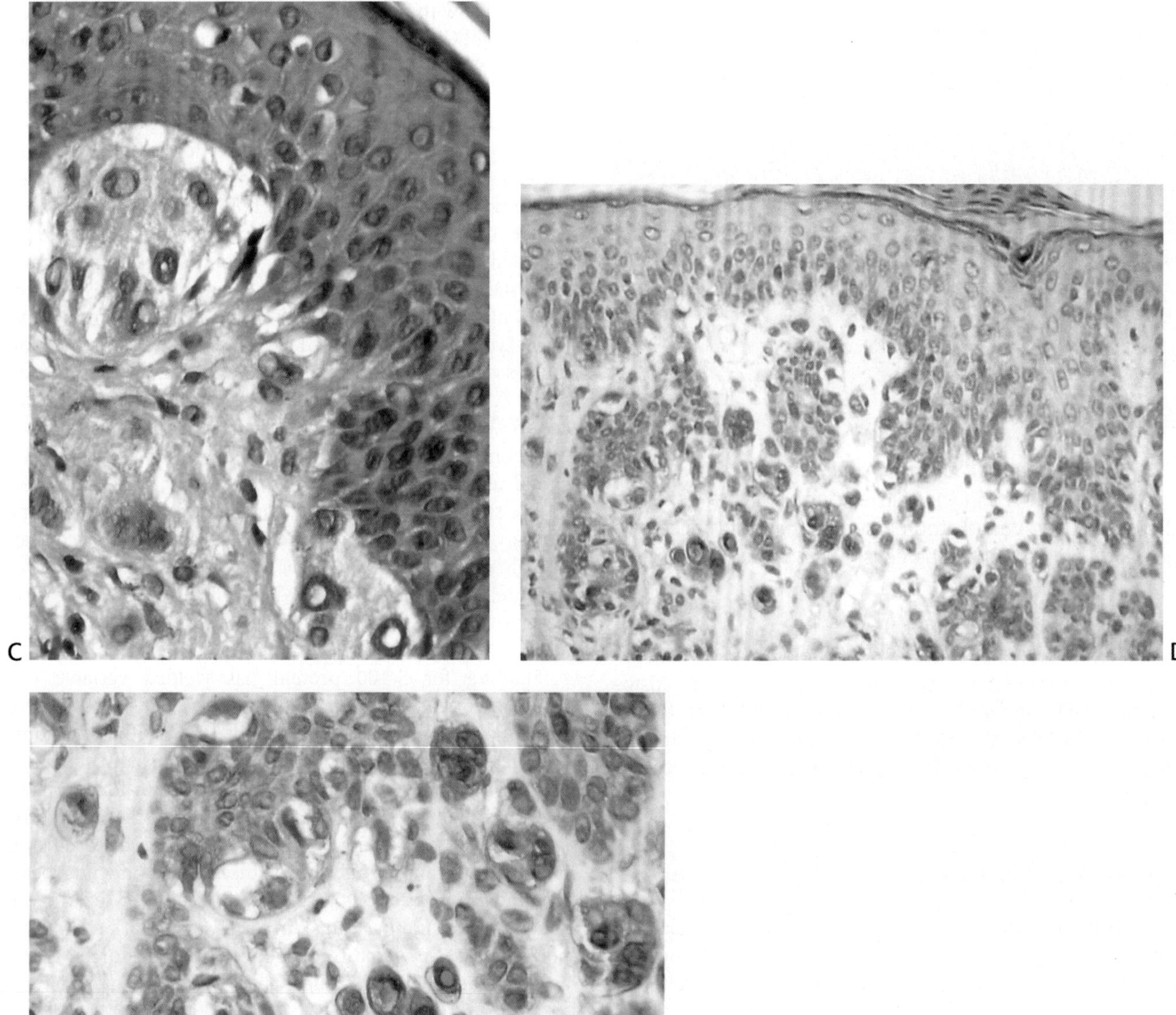

FIG. 30.14. *(Continued)*

Bowen disease in which the neoplastic cells stained for CK7. As always, one must interpret the results of immunohistochemical staining with the findings present in H&E-stained sections and the clinical details.

Androgen receptors (ARs) have been found in the majority of Paget disease cases, whereas ER and PR are present in approximately10%[152,158] to 30%[159–162] of cases, respectively.

Because Paget cells are, by their nature, entrapped among nonneoplastic squamous cells in the epidermis, it is difficult to determine the flow cytometry features of this neoplastic population. In one study of 10 cases,[163] the mean Ki67 index of the carcinoma cells in the epidermis was 26%, and the index of the intraductal component was 23%. Another investigation[164] revealed a Ki67 index of 11%. Analysis of one case[32] yielded an S-phase fraction (SPF) of 12.5%.

Immunoreactivity for the *ras* oncogene protein product, p21, has been demonstrated in mammary and extramammary Paget disease.[165] Immunohistochemical staining for p53 protein has been detected in 13%,[164] 33%,[166] and 50%[159,167] of cases in small series. Other studies comprising just a few examples reported the expression of p16,[168] Cox-2,[169] E-cadherin,[170] and the breast differentiation antigen NY-BR-1[171] and the absence of retinoblastoma protein[172] and plakoglobin[170] in most cases. Overexpression of cyclin D1[172] or Bcl-2[159] is seen in a small number of cases.

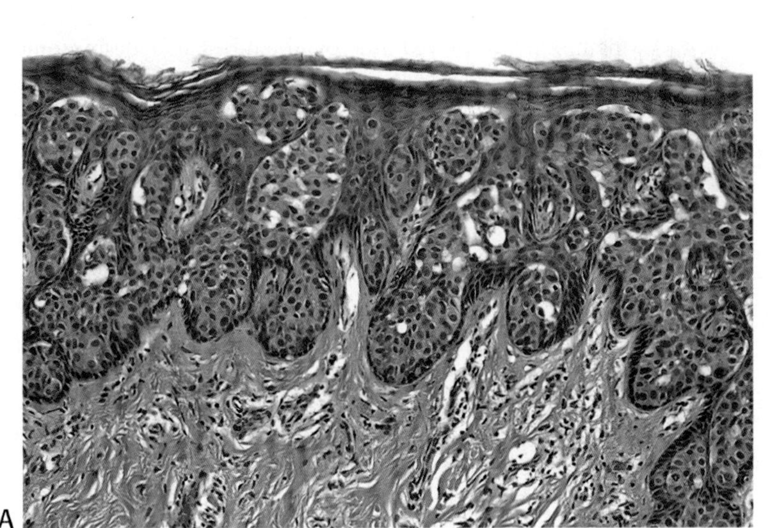

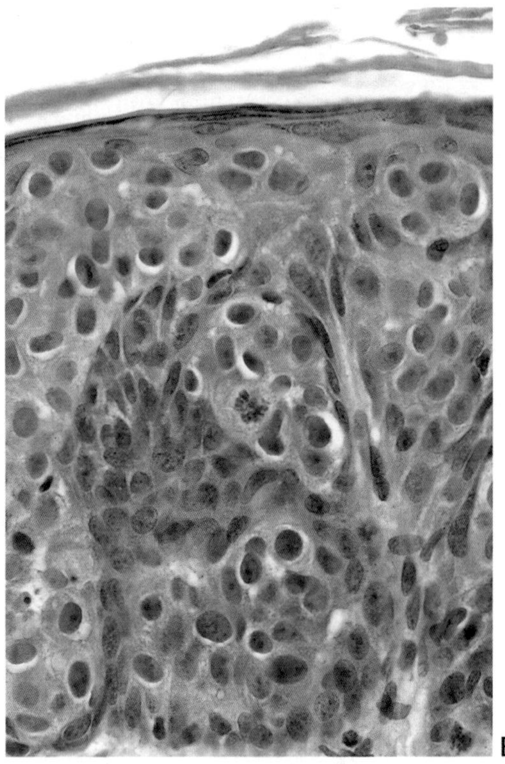

FIG. 30.15. ***Paget disease, mucin-positive.*** **A:** Paget disease fills most of the epidermis. **B:** Intracytoplasmic mucin appears pink with the mucicarmine stain. This relatively weak and sparse pattern of staining is typical.

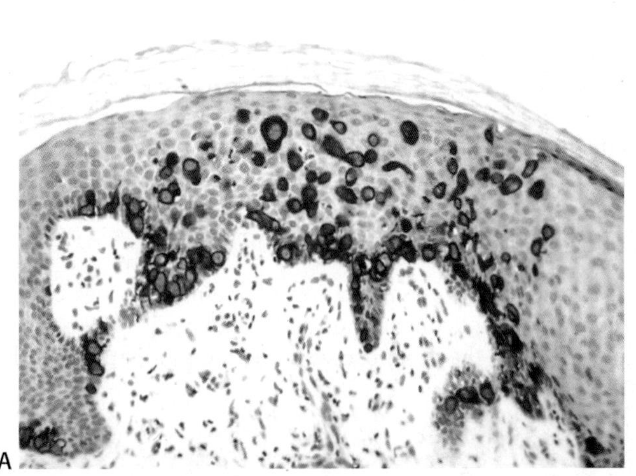

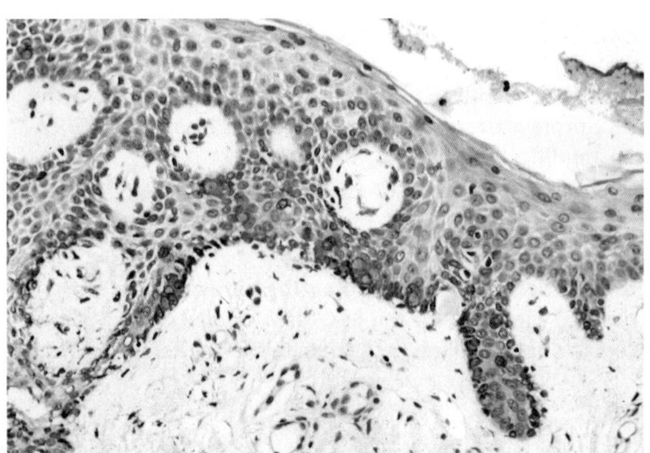

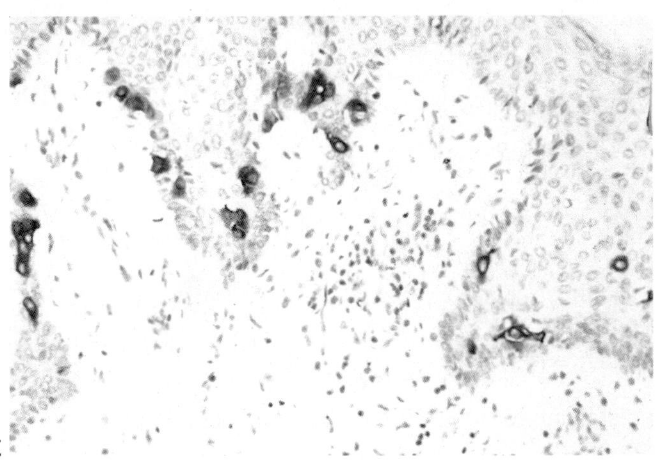

FIG. 30.16. ***Paget disease, cytokeratin reactivity.*** **A:** Many Paget cells are highlighted by the CAM5.2 immunostain. **B:** Isolated Paget cells are CAM5.2 reactive. **C:** Paget cells are CK7-positive.

TABLE 30.1 Reactivity of Antibodies in the Differential Diagnosis of Paget Disease

Monoclonal Antibody	Paget Disease	Bowen Disease	Malignant Melanoma
S-100	±	−	+
HMB45	−	−	+
CEA	±	−	−
EMA	+	−	−
CAM5.2	+	−	−
CK7	+	−	−
CK20	−	+	−
ER	±	−	−
HER2	+	−	−
AR	±	−	−
GCDFP-15	±	−	−

Strong immunoreactivity for the HER2 oncoprotein has been detected in 79% to 100% of mammary Paget disease samples[159,173–175] and 0% to 40% of cases of extramammary Paget disease[174–176] (Fig. 30.17). The majority of the breast lesions have underlying comedo or solid forms of DCIS, which is frequently HER2-positive.[173,177] Concordant with HER2 protein overexpression, Paget cells also show *HER2* gene amplification.[47,178]

ELECTRON MICROSCOPY

Little has been written regarding the ultrastructural properties of Paget cells. In the few cases studied,[11,28,130,179] the cytoplasm appeared less dense than that of the keratinocytes, and it contained free ribosomes, smooth and rough endoplasmic reticulum, and mitochondria. Lysosome-like bodies, Golgi apparatus, and smooth endoplasmic reticulum varied in amount. Melanin in the form of free particles, fully melanized melanosomes, and premelanosomes could be seen within the cytoplasm in some examples. The plasma membrane displayed microvilli and sparse desmosomes joining the Paget cells to each other and to keratinocytes. Abutting carcinoma cells formed intercellular lumens, and others housed intracytoplasmic canaliculi. The presence of microvilli distinguishes Paget cells from Toker cells at the ultrastructural level.[140]

GENETIC STUDIES

One group of investigators has described a method for isolating Paget cells from the epidermis in a biopsy of the nipple.[180] The tumor cells obtained from a patient with a 7-year history of Paget disease had a normal ploidy distribution. The case described by Desai et al.[32] showed a DNA index of 1.73. These results have limited applicability to most examples of Paget disease, which arise from high-grade DCIS.

Genetic analysis of 10 cases of Paget disease with associated carcinomas revealed genetic similarity between the intraepidermal carcinoma cells and those of the associated carcinoma in 1 case, minor genetic differences in 7 cases, and substantial genetic differences in 2 cases.[181] The minor genetic differences seen in most cases could arise from heterogeneity within a single neoplastic population, but the substantial differences observed in two cases suggest that the Paget cells represent an independent population originating in the nipple.

TREATMENT AND PROGNOSIS

Paget disease is a manifestation of mammary duct carcinoma; it does not constitute an independent disease process. Consequently, the prognosis and treatment of patients with

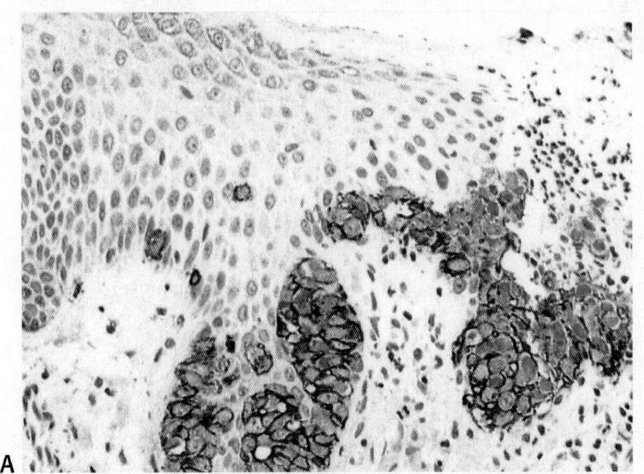

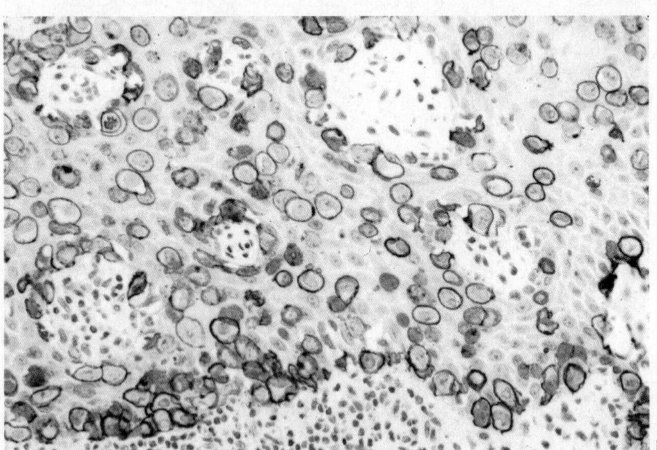

FIG. 30.17. ***Paget disease, HER2.*** **A,B:** Membrane staining for the HER2 protein highlights Paget cells in the epidermis.

Paget disease are determined by the features of the associated carcinoma.[24–26,102,182] One publication[183] suggests that the presence of Paget disease has an adverse effect on patient survival; however, the study has a mean follow-up interval of only 47 months, and the cases in the study and control groups were not matched according to the grade of the carcinomas. It seems that consideration of the usual radiologic and pathologic data will allow physicians to estimate the patient's prognosis according to the principles used in cases of carcinomas lacking Paget disease.

Mastectomy has long been considered the appropriate treatment for patients with Paget disease. The demonstration of the efficacy of breast-conserving surgery with irradiation in conventional breast carcinomas and the recognition of cases of Paget disease apparently confined to the nipple have called into question this traditional thinking. Several studies[162,184–186] provide evidence that breast-conserving surgery and irradiation offer a safe and effective alternative to mastectomy for certain patients with Paget disease even in the presence of an underlying carcinoma. On the other hand, the presence of extensive DCIS, multifocal carcinoma, or a peripheral carcinoma in a patient with Paget disease would usually indicate the need for a mastectomy.

Some patients with Paget disease, especially those without a palpable tumor or extensive disease demonstrated by mammography, may be candidates for breast-conserving therapy. Oncologists have tried several conservative approaches: limited surgery alone, irradiation alone, and a combination of the two modalities. In four series using limited surgery, it consisted of an excision of the nipple–areolar complex[130] or an excision of the nipple–areolar complex and a cone of underlying breast tissue.[124,187,188] One of the five patients (20%) treated by Lagios et al.[130] developed a recurrence of Paget disease during the first year after surgery, 40% of the patients in the investigation by Dixon et al.[187] suffered local recurrences within a mean follow-up period of 56 months, and 33% of the patients studied by Polgár et al.[188] suffered the same fate within a mean follow-up of 72 months. Blakeley et al.[189] reported a patient who developed a 9-mm invasive recurrent carcinoma at the site of a wide nipple excision performed 8 months previously for Paget disease. The initial mammogram showed no evidence of a parenchymal lesion. In contrast, the 19 patients followed up by Paone and Baker[124] did not die of breast carcinoma, although further details were not provided, and only 1 of the 19 women treated with limited surgery alone studied by Siponen et al.[190] developed a recurrence. Onoe et al.[161] estimated that it would require an excision with a radius of 4 cm to remove the entire carcinoma in 85% of patients.

Three studies[191–193] of a small number of patients described the results of treatment by means of irradiation only. Three of 17 patients treated in this fashion by Fourquet et al.[192] developed local recurrences within 23 to 49 months. Following mastectomy, all three remained free of disease for an additional 2 to 8 years. In the series of Stockdale et al.,[193] 3 of 19 patients developed recurrences in the form of invasive carcinoma 4 to 6 years after treatment, but the others remained well from 1 to 13 years later. Mastectomy apparently cured two of the three patients with recurrent carcinoma, but the third died of metastatic breast carcinoma. Bulens et al.[191] did not observe any recurrences among 13 patients followed for a mean of 58.6 months. Verniers et al.[194] describe the apparently successful treatment of a man with Paget disease confined to the nipple with irradiation alone.

Four publications[182,184,195,196] described the results of limited surgery combined with irradiation in the treatment of Paget disease associated with carcinoma confined to the region of the nipple. In 1969, Rissanen and Holsti[182] described the outcome of eight patients treated in this way. Three of the eight developed recurrences, and one woman died of breast carcinoma; however, the irradiation protocol may not have conformed to current practices. Three recent investigations[184,195,196] described better survival with this combined approach. Pierce et al.[196] reported 5- and 8-year local control rates with the breast as the only site of first recurrence of 91% and 84%, respectively, and 8-year cause-specific survival rate of 100%. The study by Marshall et al.[195] extends these favorable results to longer periods. The authors observed local control rates of 87% at 10 and 15 years, cause-specific survival rates of 97% at 10 and 15 years, and overall survival (OS) rates of 90% at 10 and 15 years. The study of Bijker et al.[184] contains the greatest number of patients. At a median follow-up of 6.4 years, the 5-year recurrence rate was 5.2%. Four of 61 patients suffered recurrences in the treated breasts. One patient developed DCIS, three patients developed IDC, and one woman succumbed to her carcinoma. These results seem to indicate that limited surgery and irradiation offers an acceptable alternative to mastectomy for patients with Paget disease in the setting of a carcinoma of limited extent.

Careful clinical and radiologic evaluation plays an especially important role when conservative surgery is considered in cases of Paget disease. A study[197] of 40 women with Paget disease who did not have palpable masses and whose mammograms did not display suspicious findings revealed that only 11 (27%) had disease confined to the region of the nipple. Twenty-seven of the 40 women (68%) had DCIS extending beyond the subareolar area, and 2 (5%) had invasive carcinoma. The authors warn, "[A] benign mammogram and the lack of a palpable mass do not exclude underlying cancer. . . . This observation calls into question the optimal treatment for [Paget disease]."

Examination of ALNs has been recommended for patients with Paget disease,[102,198] but certain authors believe it unnecessary for carefully evaluated patients with limited noninvasive carcinoma.[190]

REFERENCES

1. Paget J. On disease of the mammary areola preceding cancer of the mammary gland. *St. Bartholomew's Hosp Rep* 1874;10:87–89.
2. Darier J, Couillaud P. Sur un cas de maladie Paget de la region perioanale et scrotale. *Ann Dermatol Syph* 1893;4:25–31.

3. Thin G. Malignant papillary dermatitis of the nipple and the breast-tumours with which it is found associated. *Br Med J* 1881;1:760–763.
4. Nagle RB, Lucas DO, McDaniel KM, et al. Paget's cells. New evidence linking mammary and extramammary Paget cells to a common cell phenotype. *Am J Clin Pathol* 1985;83:431–438.
5. Willis RA. *Pathology of tumors*. 3rd ed. Washington: Butterworth, 1960:247.
6. Jacobaeus H. Pagets disease und sein Verhältnis zum Milchdrüsenkarzinom. *Virchows Arch* 1904;178:124–142.
7. Muir R. Paget's disease of the nipple and its relationships. *J Pathol Bacteriol* 1927;30:451–471.
8. Greenwood SM, Minkowitz S. Paget's disease in metastatic breast carcinoma. *Arch Dermatol* 1971;104:312–315.
9. Kuhajda FP, Offutt LE, Mendelsohn G. The distribution of carcinoembryonic antigen in breast carcinoma. Diagnostic and prognostic implications. *Cancer* 1983;52:1257–1264.
10. Mariani-Costantini R, Andreola S, Rilke F. Tumour-associated antigens in mammary and extramammary Paget's disease. *Virchows Arch A Pathol Anat Histopathol* 1985;405:333–340.
11. Ordóñez NG, Awalt H, Mackay B. Mammary and extramammary Paget's disease. An immunocytochemical and ultrastructural study. *Cancer* 1987;59:1173–1183.
12. Bussolati G, Pich A, Alfani V. Immunofluorescence detection of casein in human mammary dysplastic and neoplastic tissues. *Virchows Arch A Pathol Anat Histol* 1975;365:15–21.
13. Imam A, Yoshida SO, Taylor CR. Distinguishing tumour cells of mammary from extramammary Paget's disease using antibodies to two different glycoproteins from human milk-fat-globule membrane. *Br J Cancer* 1988;58:373–378.
14. Vanstapel MJ, Gatter KC, De Wolf-Peeters C, et al. Immunohistochemical study of mammary and extra-mammary Paget's disease. *Histopathology* 1984;8:1013–1023.
15. Guarner J, Cohen C, DeRose PB. Histogenesis of extramammary and mammary Paget cells. An immunohistochemical study. *Am J Dermatopathol* 1989;11:313–318.
16. Kondo Y, Kashima K, Daa T, et al. The ectopic expression of gastric mucin in extramammary and mammary Paget's disease. *Am J Surg Pathol* 2002;26:617–623.
17. Kuan SF, Montag AG, Hart J, et al. Differential expression of mucin genes in mammary and extramammary Paget's disease. *Am J Surg Pathol* 2001;25:1469–1477.
18. Chaudary MA, Millis RR, Lane EB, et al. Paget's disease of the nipple: a ten year review including clinical, pathological, and immunohistochemical findings. *Breast Cancer Res Treat* 1986;8:139–146.
19. Kariniemi AL, Ramaekers F, Lehto VP, et al. Paget cells express cytokeratins typical of glandular epithelia. *Br J Dermatol* 1985;112:179–183.
20. Shah KD, Tabibzadeh SS, Gerber MA. Immunohistochemical distinction of Paget's disease from Bowen's disease and superficial spreading melanoma with the use of monoclonal cytokeratin antibodies. *Am J Clin Pathol* 1987;88:689–695.
21. Tani EM, Skoog L. Immunocytochemical detection of estrogen receptors in mammary Paget cells. *Acta Cytol* 1988;32:825–828.
22. Lammie GA, Barnes DM, Millis RR, et al. An immunohistochemical study of the presence of c-erbB-2 protein in Paget's disease of the nipple. *Histopathology* 1989;15:505–514.
23. Chen CY, Sun LM, Anderson BO. Paget disease of the breast: changing patterns of incidence, clinical presentation, and treatment in the U.S. *Cancer* 2006;107:1448–1458.
24. Ashikari R, Park K, Huvos AG, et al. Paget's disease of the breast. *Cancer* 1970;26:680–685.
25. Kister SJ, Haagensen CD. Paget's disease of the breast. *Am J Surg* 1970;119:606–609.
26. Salvadori B, Fariselli G, Saccozzi R. Analysis of 100 cases of Paget's disease of the breast. *Tumori* 1976;62:529–535.
27. Martin VG, Pellettiere EV, Gress D, et al. Paget's disease in an adolescent arising in a supernumerary nipple. *J Cutan Pathol* 1994;21:283–286.
28. Jahn H, Osther PJ, Nielsen EH, et al. An electron microscopic study of clinical Paget's disease of the nipple. *APMIS* 1995;103:628–634.
29. Heller KS, Rosen PP, Schottenfeld D, et al. Male breast cancer: a clinicopathologic study of 97 cases. *Ann Surg* 1978;188:60–65.
30. Gupta S, Khanna NN, Khanna S, et al. Paget's disease of the male breast: a clinicopathologic study and a collective review. *J Surg Oncol* 1983;22:151–156.
31. Goss PE, Reid C, Pintilie M, et al. Male breast carcinoma: a review of 229 patients who presented to the Princess Margaret Hospital during 40 years: 1955–1996. *Cancer* 1999;85:629–639.
32. Desai DC, Brennan EJ Jr, Carp NZ. Paget's disease of the male breast. *Am Surg* 1996;62:1068–1072.
33. Bodnar M, Miller OF III, Tyler W. Paget's disease of the male breast associated with intraductal carcinoma. *J Am Acad Dermatol* 1999;40:829–831.
34. Chao C, Edwards MJ, Wolfson S, et al. Paget's disease of the male breast: an unusual case of dermal invasion. *Breast J* 2003;9:254.
35. El Harroudi T, Tijami F, El Otmany A, et al. Paget disease of the male nipple. *J Cancer Res Ther* 2010;6:95–96.
36. Hayes R, Cummings B, Miller RA, et al. Male Paget's disease of the breast. *J Cutan Med Surg* 2000;4:208–212.
37. Ho TC, St Jacques M, Schopflocher P. Pigmented Paget's disease of the male breast. *J Am Acad Dermatol* 1990;23:338–341.
38. Holloway KB, Ramos-Caro FA, Flowers FP. Paget's disease of the breast in a man with neurofibromatosis. *Int J Dermatol* 1997;36:609–611.
39. Menet E, Vabres P, Brecheteau P, et al. Maladie de Paget pigmentée du mamelon chez l'homme. *Ann Dermatol Venereol* 2001;128:649–652.
40. O'Sullivan ST, McGreal GT, Lyons A, et al. Paget's disease of the breast in a man without underlying breast carcinoma. *J Clin Pathol* 1994;47:851–852.
41. Piekarski J, Kubiak R, Jeziorski A. Clinically silent Paget disease of male nipple. *J Exp Clin Cancer Res* 2003;22:495–496.
42. Pimentel CL, Barnadas MA, Dalmau J, et al. Pigmented Paget's disease in a man previously treated with mammaplasty reduction for gynecomastia. *J Am Acad Dermatol* 2006;55:S62–S63.
43. Ucar AE, Korukluoglu B, Ergul E, et al. Bilateral Paget disease of the male nipple: first report. *Breast* 2008;17:317–318.
44. Stretch JR, Denton KJ, Millard PR, et al. Paget's disease of the male breast clinically and histopathologically mimicking melanoma. *Histopathology* 1991;19:470–472.
45. Kutzner H, Hugel H, Embacher G. Pigmentierter Morbus Paget und pigmentierte Mammakarziommetastase. *Hautarzt* 1992;43:28–31.
46. Nakamura S, Ishida-Yamamoto A, Takahashi H, et al. Pigmented Paget's disease of the male breast: report of a case. *Dermatology* 2001;202:134–137.
47. Anderson WR. Bilateral Paget's disease of the nipple: case report. *Am J Obstet Gynecol* 1979;134:877–878.
48. Fernandes FJ, Costa MM, Bernardo M. Rarities in breast pathology. Bilateral Paget's disease of the breast—a case report. *Eur J Surg Oncol* 1990;16:172–174.
49. Franceschini G, Masetti R, D'Ugo D, et al. Synchronous bilateral Paget's disease of the nipple associated with bilateral breast carcinoma. *Breast J* 2005;11:355–356.
50. Kijima Y, Owaki T, Yoshinaka H, et al. Synchronous bilateral breast cancer with Paget's disease and invasive ductal carcinoma: report of a case. *Surg Today* 2003;33:606–608.
51. Sahoo S, Green I, Rosen PP. Bilateral paget disease of the nipple associated with lobular carcinoma *in situ*. *Arch Pathol Lab Med* 2002;126:90–92.
52. Xie B, Zheng H, Lan H, et al. Synchronous bilateral Paget's disease of the breast: a case report. *Oncol Lett* 2012;4:83–85.
53. Coley GM, Kuehn PG. Paget's disease of the male breast. *Am J Surg* 1972;123:444–450.
54. Gubitosi A, Moccia G, Malinconico FA, et al. Metachronous Paget's disease of the breast: case report. *G Chir* 2009;30:153–155.
55. Markopoulos C, Gogas H, Sampalis F, et al. Bilateral Paget's disease of the breast. *Eur J Gynaecol Oncol* 1997;18:495–496.
56. Loizou CL, Garner D, Purushotham AD. Fluoroscopy and Paget's disease of the breast. *J BUON* 2005;10:123–126.
57. Moshakis V, Fordyce MJ, Griffiths JD. Klinefelter's syndrome associated with breast carcinoma and Paget's disease of the nipple. *Clin Oncol* 1983;9:257–261.
58. Kawawa Y, Okamoto Y, Oharaseki T, et al. Paget's disease of the breast in a woman with neurofibromatosis. *Clin Imaging* 2007;31:127–130.
59. Fouad D. Paget's disease of the breast in a male with lymphomatoid papulosis: a case report. *J Med Case Rep* 2011;5:43.
60. Suster S, Ronnen M, Huszar M, et al. Paget's disease of the breast with underlying carcinoma arising in systemic scleroderma. *J Dermatol Surg Oncol* 1988;14:648–650.
61. Kao GF, Graham JH, Helwig EB. Paget's disease of the ectopic breast with an underlying intraductal carcinoma: report of a case. *J Cutan Pathol* 1986;13:59–66.

62. Decaussin M, Laville M, Mathevet P, et al. Paget's disease versus Toker cell hyperplasia in a supernumerary nipple. *Virchows Arch* 1998;432:289–291.
63. Mitchell S, Lachica R, Randall MB, et al. Paget's disease of the breast areola mimicking cutaneous melanoma. *Breast J* 2006;12:233–236.
64. van der Putte SC, Toonstra J, Hennipman A. Mammary Paget's disease confined to the areola and associated with multifocal Toker cell hyperplasia. *Am J Dermatopathol* 1995;17:487–493.
65. Mendez-Fernandez MA, Henly WS, Geis RC, et al. Paget's disease of the breast after subcutaneous mastectomy and reconstruction with a silicone prosthesis. *Plast Reconstr Surg* 1980;65:683–685.
66. Oliveira A, Sanches M, Selores M. Axillary Paget's disease associated with breast carcinoma in an elderly patient. *Eur J Dermatol* 2011;21:102–103.
67. Castelli E, Wollina U, Anzarone A, et al. Extramammary Paget disease of the axilla associated with comedo-like apocrine carcinoma *in situ*. *Am J Dermatopathol* 2002;24:351–357.
68. Plowman PN, Gilmore OJ, Curling M, et al. Paget's disease of the nipple occurring after conservation management of early infiltrating breast cancer. *Br J Surg* 1986;73:45.
69. Joshi MG, Crosson AW, Tahan SR. Paget's disease of the nipple and angiosarcoma of the breast following excision and radiation therapy for carcinoma of the breast. *Mod Pathol* 1995;8:1–4.
70. Menzies D, Barr L, Ellis H. Paget's disease of the nipple occurring after wide local excision and radiotherapy for carcinoma of the breast. *Eur J Surg Oncol* 1989;15:271–273.
71. Peterse JL, van Dongen JA, Bartelink H. Recurrence of breast carcinoma after breast conserving treatment. *Eur J Surg Oncol* 1988;14:123–126.
72. Pizzichetta MA, Canzonieri V, Massarut S, et al. Pigmented mammary Paget's disease mimicking melanoma. *Melanoma Res* 2004;14:S13–S15.
73. Plastaras JP, Harris EE, Solin LJ. Paget's disease of the nipple as local recurrence after breast-conservation treatment for early-stage breast cancer. *Clin Breast Cancer* 2005;6:349–353.
74. Schnitt SJ, Connolly JL, Recht A, et al. Breast relapse following primary radiation therapy for early breast cancer. II. Detection, pathologic features and prognostic significance. *Int J Radiat Oncol Biol Phys* 1985;11:1277–1284.
75. Markopoulos C, Gazet JC. Paget's disease of the nipple occurring after conservative management of early breast cancer. *Eur J Surg Oncol* 1988;14:77–78.
76. Shousha S, Tisdall M, Sinnett HD. Paget's disease of the nipple occurring after conservative surgery for ductal carcinoma *in situ* of the breast. *Histopathology* 2004;45:416–418.
77. Shearman CP, Watts GT. Paget's disease of the nipple after subcutaneous mastectomy for cancer with primary reconstruction. *Ann R Coll Surg Engl* 1986;68:17–18.
78. Harness JK, Vetter TS, Salibian AH. Areola and nipple-areola-sparing mastectomy for breast cancer treatment and risk reduction: report of an initial experience in a community hospital setting. *Ann Surg Oncol* 2011;18:917–922.
79. Lohsiriwat V, Martella S, Rietjens M, et al. Paget's disease as a local recurrence after nipple-sparing mastectomy: clinical presentation, treatment, outcome, and risk factor analysis. *Ann Surg Oncol* 2012;19:1850–1855.
80. Basu CB, Wahba M, Bullocks JM, et al. Paget disease of a nipple graft following completion of a breast reconstruction with a nipple-sharing technique. *Ann Plast Surg* 2008;60:144–145.
81. Haagensen CD. Paget's carcionoma of the breast. In: *Diseases of the breast*. 3rd ed. Philadelphia: W.B. Saunders, 1986.
82. Valdes EK, Feldman SM. Paget's disease of the breast. *Breast J* 2006;12:83.
83. Taylor KE, Ormsby HM, Havercroft JM, et al. An unusually extensive case of Paget's disease of the nipple. *Breast* 2001;10:442–446.
84. Nicoletti G, Scevola S, Ruggiero R, et al. Gigantic Paget disease of the breast. *Breast* 2004;13:425–427.
85. Ascensão AC, Marques MS, Capitão-Mor M. Paget's disease of the nipple. Clinical and pathological review of 109 female patients. *Dermatologica* 1985;170:170–179.
86. Singla V, Virmani V, Nahar U, et al. Paget's disease of breast masquerading as chronic benign eczema. *Indian J Cancer* 2009;46:344–347.
87. Garijo MF, Val D, Val-Bernal JF. Pagetoid dyskeratosis of the nipple epidermis: an incidental finding mimicking Paget's disease of the nipple. *APMIS* 2008;116:139–146.
88. Pennell L, Seddon I, Anwar I. Cutaneous schistosomiasis mimicking Paget's disease of the breast. *Breast J* 2011;17:99–100.
89. Guyton DP, Sloan Stakleff K, Regula E. Pemphigus vulgaris mimicking Paget's disease of the breast. *Breast J* 2003;9:319–322.
90. Wolf R, Bernstein-Lipschitz L, Rothem A. Paget's disease of the nipple resembling an acantholytic disease on microscopic examination. *Dermatologica* 1989;179:42–44.
91. Kobayashi TK, ueda M, Nishino T, et al. Scrape cytology of Pemphigus vulgaris of the nipple, a mimicker of Paget's disease. *Diagn Cytopathol* 1996;16:156–159.
92. Rae V, Gould E, Ibe MJ, et al. Coexistent pemphigus vulgaris and Paget's disease of the nipple. An immunohistochemical study. *J Am Acad Dermatol* 1987;16:235–237.
93. Ansari B, Purdie CA, Brown DC. Adult Langerhans cell histiocytosis mimicking Paget's disease of the nipple. *Breast J* 2005;11:281–282.
94. Mikhaimer NC, Kahler KC, Schwarz T, et al. Giant basal cell carcinoma of the breast mimicking paget's disease: complete remission after photodynamic therapy. *Onkologie* 2010;33:613–615.
95. Lin CH, Lee HS, Yu JC. Melanoma of the nipple mimicking Paget's disease. *Dermatol Online J* 2007;13:18.
96. Soler T, Lerin A, Serrano T, et al. Pigmented paget disease of the breast nipple with underlying infiltrating carcinoma: a case report and review of the literature. *Am J Dermatopathol* 2011;33:e54–e57.
97. Oiso N, Kawara S, Inui H, et al. Pigmented spots as a sign of mammary Paget's disease. *Clin Exp Dermatol* 2009;34:36–38.
98. Meyer-Gonzalez T, Alcaide-Martin A, Contreras-Steyls M, et al. Pigmented mammary Paget disease mimicking cutaneous melanoma. *Int J Dermatol* 2010;49:59–61.
99. Park JS, Lee MJ, Chung H, et al. Pigmented mammary Paget disease positive for melanocytic markers. *J Am Acad Dermatol* 2011;65:247–249.
100. Yanagishita T, Tamada Y, Tanaka M, et al. Pigmented mammary Paget disease mimicking melanoma on dermatoscopy. *J Am Acad Dermatol* 2011;64:e114–e116.
101. Petersson F, Ivan D, Kazakov DV, et al. Pigmented Paget disease—a diagnostic pitfall mimicking melanoma. *Am J Dermatopathol* 2009;31:223–226.
102. Kollmorgen DR, Varanasi JS, Edge SB, et al. Paget's disease of the breast: a 33-year experience. *J Am Coll Surg* 1998;187:171–177.
103. Ikeda DM, Helvie MA, Frank TS, et al. Paget disease of the nipple: radiologic–pathologic correlation. *Radiology* 1993;189:89–94.
104. Lim HS, Jeong SJ, Lee JS, et al. Paget disease of the breast: mammographic, US, and MR imaging findings with pathologic correlation. *Radiographics* 2011;31:1973–1987.
105. Kothari AS, Beechey-Newman N, Hamed H, et al. Paget disease of the nipple: a multifocal manifestation of higher-risk disease. *Cancer* 2002;95:1–7.
106. Günhan-Bilgen I, Oktay A. Paget's disease of the breast: clinical, mammographic, sonographic and pathologic findings in 52 cases. *Eur J Radiol* 2006;60:256–263.
107. Sawyer RH, Asbury DL. Mammographic appearances in Paget's disease of the breast. *Clin Radiol* 1994;49:185–188.
108. Ceccherini AF, Evans AJ, Pinder SE, et al. Is ipsilateral mammography worthwhile in Paget's disease of the breast? *Clin Radiol* 1996;51:35–38.
109. Stomper P, Penetrante D, Carson W. Sensitivity of mammography on patients with Paget's disease of the nipple. *Breast Dis* 1995;8:173–178.
110. Kim HS, Seok JH, Cha ES, et al. Significance of nipple enhancement of Paget's disease in contrast enhanced breast MRI. *Arch Gynecol Obstet* 2010;282:157–162.
111. Frei KA, Bonel HM, Pelte MF, et al. Paget disease of the breast: findings at magnetic resonance imaging and histopathologic correlation. *Invest Radiol* 2005;40:363–367.
112. Echevarria JJ, Lopez-Ruiz JA, Martin D, et al. Usefulness of MRI in detecting occult breast cancer associated with Paget's disease of the nipple–areolar complex. *Br J Radiol* 2004;77:1036–1039.
113. Amano G, Yajima M, Moroboshi Y, et al. MRI accurately depicts underlying DCIS in a patient with Paget's disease of the breast without palpable mass and mammography findings. *Jpn J Clin Oncol* 2005;35:149–153.
114. Capobianco G, Spaliviero B, Dessole S, et al. Paget's disease of the nipple diagnosed by MRI. *Arch Gynecol Obstet* 2006;274:316–318.
115. Corsi F, Sartani A, Galli D, et al. Usefulness of preoperative diagnosis with magnetic resonance imaging for conservative surgery in Paget's disease of the breast. *Breast Care (Basel)* 2010;5:26–28.

116. Morrogh M, Morris EA, Liberman L, et al. MRI identifies otherwise occult disease in select patients with Paget disease of the nipple. *J Am Coll Surg* 2008;206:316–321.
117. Sievers D, Huvos A, Beattie EJ Jr, et al. Paget's disease of the nipple. *Mem Hosp Clin Bull* 1973;3:141–145.
118. Rosen PP, Caicco JA. Florid papillomatosis of the nipple. A study of 51 patients, including nine with mammary carcinoma. *Am J Surg Pathol* 1986;10:87–101.
119. Requena L, Sangueza M, Sangueza OP, et al. Pigmented mammary Paget disease and pigmented epidermotropic metastases from breast carcinoma. *Am J Dermatopathol* 2002;24:189–198.
120. Azzopardi JG, Eusebi V. Melanocyte colonization and pigmentation of breast carcinoma. *Histopathology* 1977;1:21–30.
121. Culberson JD, Horn RC Jr. Paget's disease of the nipple: review of twenty-five cases with special reference to melanin pigmentation of Paget cells. *AMA Arch Surg* 1956;72:224–231.
122. Barnes PJ, Dumont RJ, Higgins HG. Acinar pattern of mammary Paget's disease: a case report. *Breast J* 2007;13:520–526.
123. Shousha S. Glandular Paget's disease of the nipple. *Histopathology* 2007;50:812–814.
124. Paone JF, Baker RR. Pathogenesis and treatment of Paget's disease of the breast. *Cancer* 1981;48:825–829.
125. Vielh P, Validire P, Kheirallah S, et al. Paget's disease of the nipple without clinically and radiologically detectable breast tumor. Histochemical and immunohistochemical study of 44 cases. *Pathol Res Pract* 1993;189:150–155.
126. Duan X, Sneige N, Gullett AE, et al. Invasive paget disease of the breast: clinicopathologic study of an underrecognized entity in the breast. *Am J Surg Pathol* 2012;36:1353–1358.
127. Sanders MA, Dominici L, Denison C, et al. Paget disease of the breast with invasion from nipple skin into the dermis: an unusual type of skin invasion not associated with an adverse outcome. *Arch Pathol Lab Med* 2013;137:72–76.
128. Evans AT, Neven P. Invasive adenocarcinoma arising in extramammary Paget's disease of the vulva. *Histopathology* 1991;18:355–360.
129. Mai KT, Yazdi HM, Perkins DG. Mammary Paget's disease: evidence of diverse origin of the disease with a subgroup of Paget's disease developing from the superficial portion of lactiferous duct and a discontinuous pattern of tumor spread. *Pathol Int* 1999;49:956–961.
130. Lagios MD, Westdahl PR, Rose MR, et al. Paget's disease of the nipple. alternative management in cases without or with minimal extent of underlying breast carcinoma. *Cancer* 1984;54:545–551.
131. Rosen PP. Syringomatous adenoma of the nipple. *Am J Surg Pathol* 1983;7:739–745.
132. Papachristou DN, Kinne DW, Rosen PP, et al. Cutaneous melanoma of the breast. *Surgery* 1979;85:322–328.
133. Sauven P, Roberts A. Basal cell carcinoma of the nipple. *J R Soc Med* 1983;76:699–701.
134. Kohler S, Rouse RV, Smoller BR. The differential diagnosis of pagetoid cells in the epidermis. *Mod Pathol* 1998;11:79–92.
135. Orr JW, Parish DJ. The nature of the nipple changes in Paget's disease. *J Pathol Bacteriol* 1962;84:201–208.
136. Toker C. Clear cells of the nipple epidermis. *Cancer* 1970;25:601–610.
137. Di Tommaso L, Franchi G, Destro A, et al. Toker cells of the breast. Morphological and immunohistochemical characterization of 40 cases. *Hum Pathol* 2008;39:1295–1300.
138. Lundquist K, Kohler S, Rouse RV. Intraepidermal cytokeratin 7 expression is not restricted to Paget cells but is also seen in Toker cells and Merkel cells. *Am J Surg Pathol* 1999;23:212–219.
139. Nofech-Mozes S, Hanna W. Toker cells revisited. *Breast J* 2009;15:394–398.
140. Marucci G, Betts CM, Golouh R, et al. Toker cells are probably precursors of Paget cell carcinoma: a morphological and ultrastructural description. *Virchows Arch* 2002;441:117–123.
141. Kinoshita S, Yoshimoto K, Kyoda S, et al. Malignant melanoma originating on the female nipple: a case report. *Breast Cancer* 2007;14:105–108.
142. Soini Y. Claudins 2, 3, 4, and 5 in Paget's disease and breast carcinoma. *Hum Pathol* 2004;35:1531–1536.
143. Rayne SC, Santa Cruz DJ. Anaplastic Paget's disease. *Am J Surg Pathol* 1992;16:1085–1091.
144. Bhadani PP, Sharma MC, Sah SP, et al. Paget's disease of the nipple diagnosed on cytology: a case report. *Indian J Pathol Microbiol* 2004;47:246–248.
145. Gupta RK, Simpson J, Dowle C. The role of cytology in the diagnosis of Paget's disease of the nipple. *Pathology* 1996;28:248–250.
146. Lucarotti ME, Dunn JM, Webb AJ. Scrape cytology in the diagnosis of Paget's disease of the breast. *Cytopathology* 1994;5:301–305.
147. Samarasinghe D, Frost F, Sterrett G, et al. Cytologic diagnosis of Paget's disease of the nipple by scrape smears: a report of five cases. *Diagn Cytopathol* 1992;9:291–295.
148. Jones RR, Spaull J, Gusterson B. The histogenesis of mammary and extramammary Paget's disease. *Histopathology* 1989;14:409–416.
149. Reed W, Oppedal BR, Eeg Larsen T. Immunohistology is valuable in distinguishing between Paget's disease, Bowen's disease and superficial spreading malignant melanoma. *Histopathology* 1990;16:583–588.
150. Lau J, Kohler S. Keratin profile of intraepidermal cells in Paget's disease, extramammary Paget's disease, and pagetoid squamous cell carcinoma *in situ*. *J Cutan Pathol* 2003;30:449–454.
151. Smith KJ, Tuur S, Corvette D, et al. Cytokeratin 7 staining in mammary and extramammary Paget's disease. *Mod Pathol* 1997;10:1069–1074.
152. Sek P, Zawrocki A, Biernat W, et al. HER2 molecular subtype is a dominant subtype of mammary Paget's cells. An immunohistochemical study. *Histopathology* 2010;57:564–571.
153. Wood WS, Hegedus C. Mammary Paget's disease and intraductal carcinoma. Histologic, histochemical, and immunocytochemical comparison. *Am J Dermatopathol* 1988;10:183–188.
154. Gillett CE, Bobrow LG, Millis RR. S100 protein in human mammary tissue—immunoreactivity in breast carcinoma, including Paget's disease of the nipple, and value as a marker of myoepithelial cells. *J Pathol* 1990;160:19–24.
155. Ramachandra S, Gillett CE, Millis RR. A comparative immunohistochemical study of mammary and extramammary Paget's disease and superficial spreading melanoma, with particular emphasis on melanocytic markers. *Virchows Arch* 1996;429:371–376.
156. Hitchcock A, Topham S, Bell J, et al. Routine diagnosis of mammary Paget's disease. A modern approach. *Am J Surg Pathol* 1992;16:58–61.
157. Williamson JD, Colome MI, Sahin A, et al. Pagetoid bowen disease: a report of 2 cases that express cytokeratin 7. *Arch Pathol Lab Med* 2000;124:427–430.
158. Liegl B, Horn LC, Moinfar F. Androgen receptors are frequently expressed in mammary and extramammary Paget's disease. *Mod Pathol* 2005;18:1283–1288.
159. Fu W, Lobocki CA, Silberberg BK, et al. Molecular markers in Paget disease of the breast. *J Surg Oncol* 2001;77:171–178.
160. Lester T, Wang J, Bourne P, et al. Different panels of markers should be used to predict mammary Paget's disease associated with in situ or invasive ductal carcinoma of the breast. *Ann Clin Lab Sci* 2009;39:17–24.
161. Onoe S, Kinoshita T, Tamura N, et al. Feasibility of breast conserving surgery for Paget's disease. *Breast* 2011;20:515–518.
162. Dalberg K, Hellborg H, Warnberg F. Paget's disease of the nipple in a population based cohort. *Breast Cancer Res Treat* 2008;111:313–319.
163. Buxant F, Fayt I, Noel JC. Assessment of proliferating activity in Paget's disease of the nipple by double stain immunohistochemistry. *Eur J Gynaecol Oncol* 2009;30:500–502.
164. Ellis PE, Fong LF, Rolfe KJ, et al. The role of p53 and Ki67 in Paget's disease of the vulva and the breast. *Gynecol Oncol* 2002;86:150–156.
165. Mori O, Hachisuka H, Nakano S, et al. Expression of ras p21 in mammary and extramammary Paget's disease. *Arch Pathol Lab Med* 1990;114:858–861.
166. Kanitakis J, Thivolet J, Claudy A. p53 protein expression in mammary and extramammary Paget's disease. *Anticancer Res* 1993;13:2429–2433.
167. Nakamura G, Shikata N, Shoji T, et al. Immunohistochemical study of mammary and extramammary Paget's disease. *Anticancer Res* 1995;15:467–470.
168. Buxant F, Noel JC. p16 expressionin Paget's disease of the breast. *Eur J Gynaecol Oncol* 2008;29:441–443.
169. Horn LC, Purz S, Krumpe C, et al. COX-2 and Her-2/neu are overexpressed in Paget's disease of the vulva and the breast: results of a preliminary study. *Arch Gynecol Obstet* 2008;277:135–138.
170. Ellis PE, Cano SD, Fear M, et al. Reduced E-cadherin expression correlates with disease progression in Paget's disease of the vulva but not Paget's disease of the breast. *Mod Pathol* 2008;21:1192–1199.

171. Giger O, Caduff R, O'Meara A, et al. Frequent expression of the breast differentiation antigen NY-BR-1 in mammary and extramammary Paget's disease. *Pathol Int* 2010;60:726–734.
172. Ellis PE, Maclean AB, Crow JC, et al. Expression of cyclin D1 and retinoblastoma protein in Paget's disease of the vulva and breast: an immunohistochemical study of 108 cases. *Histopathology* 2009;55:709–715.
173. Gusterson BA, Machin LG, Gullick WJ, et al. Immunohistochemical distribution of c-erbB-2 in infiltrating and *in situ* breast cancer. *Int J Cancer* 1988;42:842–845.
174. Meissner K, Riviere A, Haupt G, et al. Study of neu-prexpression in mammary Paget's disease with and without underlying breast carcinoma and in extramammary Paget's disease. *Am J Pathol* 1990;137:1305–1309.
175. Wolber RA, Dupuis BA, Wick MR. Expression of c-erbB-2 oncoprotein in mammary and extramammary Paget's disease. *Am J Clin Pathol* 1991;96:243–247.
176. Keatings L, Sinclair J, Wright C, et al. c-erbB-2 oncoprotein expression in mammary and extramammary Paget's disease: an immunohistochemical study. *Histopathology* 1990;17:243–247.
177. van de Vijver MJ, Peterse JL, Mooi WJ, et al. Neu-protein overexpression in breast cancer. Association with comedo-type ductal carcinoma *in situ* and limited prognostic value in stage II breast cancer. *N Engl J Med* 1988;319:1239–1245.
178. Bianco MK, Vasef MA. HER-2 gene amplification in Paget disease of the nipple and extramammary site: a chromogenic *in situ* hybridization study. *Diagn Mol Pathol* 2006;15:131–135.
179. Sagebiel RW. Ultrastructural observations on epidermal cells in Paget's disease of the breast. *Am J Pathol* 1969;57:49–64.
180. Mori O, Hachisuka H, Nakano S, et al. A case of mammary Paget's disease without an underlying carcinoma: microscopic analysis of the DNA content in Paget cells. *J Dermatol* 1994;21:160–165.
181. Morandi L, Pession A, Marucci GL, et al. Intraepidermal cells of Paget's carcinoma of the breast can be genetically different from those of the underlying carcinoma. *Hum Pathol* 2003;34:1321–1330.
182. Rissanen PM, Holsti P. Paget's disease of the breast: the influence of the presence or absence of an underlying palpable tumor on the prognosis and on the choice of treatment. *Oncology* 1969;23:209–216.
183. Ortiz-Pagan S, Cunto-Amesty G, Narayan S, et al. Effect of Paget's disease on survival in breast cancer: an exploratory study. *Arch Surg* 2011;146:1267–1270.
184. Bijker N, Rutgers EJ, Duchateau L, et al. Breast-conserving therapy for Paget disease of the nipple: a prospective European Organization for Research and Treatment of Cancer study of 61 patients. *Cancer* 2001;91:472–477.
185. Caliskan M, Gatti G, Sosnovskikh I, et al. Paget's disease of the breast: the experience of the European Institute of Oncology and review of the literature. *Breast Cancer Res Treat* 2008;112:513–521.
186. Kawase K, Dimaio DJ, Tucker SL, et al. Paget's disease of the breast: there is a role for breast-conserving therapy. *Ann Surg Oncol* 2005;12:391–397.
187. Dixon AR, Galea MH, Ellis IO, et al. Paget's disease of the nipple. *Br J Surg* 1991;78:722–723.
188. Polgár C, Orosz Z, Kovacs T, et al. Breast-conserving therapy for Paget disease of the nipple: a prospective European Organization for Research and Treatment of Cancer study of 61 patients. *Cancer* 2002;94:1904–1905.
189. Blakeley S, Fornage B, Rapini R, et al. Ductal carcinoma after conservative management of Paget's disease of the breast: a case report. *Breast Dis* 1994;7:361–366.
190. Siponen E, Hukkinen K, Heikkila P, et al. Surgical treatment in Paget's disease of the breast. *Am J Surg* 2010;200:241–246.
191. Bulens P, Vanuytsel L, Rijnders A, et al. Breast conserving treatment of Paget's disease. *Radiother Oncol* 1990;17:305–309.
192. Fourquet A, Campana F, Vielh P, et al. Paget's disease of the nipple without detectable breast tumor: conservative management with radiation therapy. *Int J Radiat Oncol Biol Phys* 1987;13:1463–1465.
193. Stockdale AD, Brierley JD, White WF, et al. Radiotherapy for Paget's disease of the nipple: a conservative alternative. *Lancet* 1989;2:664–666.
194. Verniers D, Van den Bogaert W, van der Schueren E, et al. Paget's disease of the male breast treated by radiotherapy. *Br J Radiol* 1991;64:1062–1064.
195. Marshall JK, Griffith KA, Haffty BG, et al. Conservative management of Paget disease of the breast with radiotherapy: 10- and 15-year results. *Cancer* 2003;97:2142–2149.
196. Pierce LJ, Haffty BG, Solin LJ, et al. The conservative management of Paget's disease of the breast with radiotherapy. *Cancer* 1997;80:1065–1072.
197. Zakaria S, Pantvaidya G, Ghosh K, et al. Paget's disease of the breast: accuracy of preoperative assessment. *Breast Cancer Res Treat* 2007;102:137–142.
198. Sukumvanich P, Bentrem DJ, Cody HS III, et al. The role of sentinel lymph node biopsy in Paget's disease of the breast. *Ann Surg Oncol* 2006;14:1020–1023.

CHAPTER 31

Lobular Carcinoma *In Situ* and Atypical Lobular Hyperplasia

SYED A. HODA

LOBULAR CARCINOMA *IN SITU*

Although the distinction between classical lobular carcinoma *in situ* (LCIS) and pleomorphic lobular carcinoma *in situ* (PLCIS) variants was noted almost 30 years ago, the specificity of PLCIS as a variant of LCIS could not be determined until the relatively recent availability of immunostains for E-cadherin and catenin made it possible to consistently distinguish PLCIS from some forms of intraductal carcinoma (ductal carcinoma *in situ* [DCIS]). In the past two decades, there has been growing recognition of PLCIS as a distinct histologic entity and an appreciation of the relative rarity of PLCIS when compared with the frequency of LCIS. For these reasons and also the fact that many examples of PLCIS were probably diagnosed as DCIS, it is likely that studies of LCIS published before the year 2000 dealt almost exclusively with the classical variant.

Historical Note

Two papers published in 1941 established LCIS as a distinct morphologic entity. The description by Muir[1] appeared in an overview of the earliest stages of mammary carcinoma. Lesions were subdivided according to whether carcinoma appeared to originate in ducts or lobules ("acini"). Muir found that it may be difficult to prove origin from the lobular epithelium in some cases:

> "The question is complicated by the fact that when malignant cells are present within them they may not have developed *in situ*. Intra-acinous carcinoma is often merely the result of the spread of cancer cells from terminal ducts in which the malignant process has started."[1]

Among Muir's illustrations of "intra-acinous" carcinoma are some with histologic patterns that might be regarded today as ductal in type, thus constituting a condition now recognized as extension of duct carcinoma into lobules. One picture showed the typical features of LCIS.

Foote and Stewart[2] introduced the term "lobular carcinoma *in situ*" to describe "a disease of small lobular ducts and lobules." They described and commented on almost all of the important clinical and pathologic features of the disease:

1. The inconspicuous character of LCIS that cannot be detected by palpation or gross pathologic examination: "There is no way in which a clinical diagnosis of lobular carcinoma *in situ* can be made. There is no way by which it can be recognized grossly."
2. Multicentricity: "This lesion occurs in multiple lobules. It is always a disease of multiple foci."
3. Origin from the terminal duct–lobular complex or from terminal ducts.
4. Pagetoid extension in ducts and the rarity of true Paget disease: "Isolated cells or groups of cells in the terminal lobular duct recall certain features of Paget disease and we have designated them *pagetoid* cells. The clinical entity, Paget disease, has not been encountered in this group of cases."
5. Signet ring cells as a feature of LCIS: "the formation of central mucoid globules."
6. Association with a distinctive type of infiltrating carcinoma: "When the tumor infiltrates, it is apt to do so in a peculiar fashion which permits one, after some experience, to recognize the high probability of such origin."
7. Coexistence of LCIS with other patterns of carcinoma, including association with ordinary duct carcinoma and tubular carcinoma.
8. The tendency of infiltrating lobular carcinoma to grow around ducts and lobules, sometimes described as a targetoid growth pattern.
9. The desmoplastic stromal reaction in infiltrating lobular carcinoma.

Frequency and Epidemiology

Because LCIS is a microscopic lesion that does not form a palpable tumor, the incidence of the disease is unknown among asymptomatic women. When it occurs alone in biopsied patients, LCIS constitutes 1% to 6% of mammary carcinomas and 30% to 50% of noninvasive carcinomas.[3,4]

In retrospective reviews, each involving several thousand "benign" breast specimens, the frequency of LCIS was 1.5%,[5] 1.4%,[6] 0.6%,[7] and 0.5%.[8] A review of nearly 10,000 breast biopsies without other neoplastic lesions performed from 1960 through 1979 revealed that the annual frequency of LCIS or lobular neoplasia (LN) ranged from 1.2% to 4.3%, averaging 2.7%.[9]

An autopsy study of breasts from 83 elderly hospitalized women revealed LCIS in 3, or 3.6%.[10] This relatively small series, which included six women previously known to have breast carcinoma, cannot be regarded as generally representative. Nielsen et al.[11] examined breasts from young women, many of whom died unexpectedly, including only one with previously diagnosed breast carcinoma, and they found LCIS in 4 (3.6%) of 110 cases. Three other autopsy studies including more than 300 women failed to detect any examples of LCIS.[12–14]

Analysis of population-based data from 1978 to 1998 in the United States revealed an increase in the incidence of LCIS from 0.90/100,000 person-years to 3.19/100,000 person-years.[15] Incidence increased continuously throughout the study period among postmenopausal women, with the highest rate among women 50 to 59 years of age in 1996 to 1998 (11.47/100,000 person-years). Analysis of data from the Surveillance Epidemiology and End Results (SEER) program for 1999 to 2004 revealed that the age-related incidence of LCIS, not otherwise specified, rose from 0.9 per 100,000 women in the 30- to 39-year age group to a peak of 10.2 per 100,000 in the 50- to 59-year age group and then declined to 2.4 per 100,000 among women 80 or more years of age.[16] By contrast, the age-related incidence of DCIS peaked among women 70 to 79 years of age. The incidence of LCIS among White women (3.6 per 100,000) was nearly twice that of Black women (1.9 per 100,000), whereas the incidence of DCIS among White women (23.3 per 100,000) was only slightly greater than the incidence of DCIS among Black women (20.2 per 100,000). The annual incidence of LCIS remained relatively stable between 1999 and 2004, with a low rate of 3.2 per 100,000 women in 1999 and a high rate of 3.6 per 100,000 in 2002. The annual incidence of DCIS exhibited greater variation, rising from 22.1 per 100,000 in 1999 to 23.8 per 100,000 in 2001 and 2004.

The increasing use of mammography leading to more frequent biopsies is probably the most important factor responsible for the increased incidence of LCIS. In particular, columnar cell hyperplasia (CCH), a condition predisposed to develop calcifications, so often coexists with LCIS that this association is probably not coincidental. CCH is a frequent benign abnormality responsible for mammographically detected calcifications in the absence of a palpable lesion (see Chapter 9).

Clinical Presentation

LCIS is typically discovered coincidentally in breast tissue removed for proliferative lesions that cause a mass, or in apparently normal tissue surrounding a benign tumor such as a fibroadenoma (FA). Mammography has not been an effective method for detecting LCIS in most cases and cannot be depended upon to assess the multicentricity or bilaterality of the disease.[17,18] Only 4 of 50 patients with LCIS described in a report on the Breast Cancer Diagnosis Demonstration Projects had calcifications in LCIS seen on pathologic examination.[19] Proliferative fibrocystic changes are usually the site of mammographic abnormalities that lead to a biopsy in which LCIS is detected. Calcifications are infrequently formed by LCIS. They occur more commonly in coexisting lesions such as sclerosing adenosis (SA) and CCH,[20] atrophic lobules and ducts,[21–23] and collagenous spherulosis. In a retrospective study of LCIS-associated lesions in 31 patients with imaging abnormalities, calcifications were the most common mammographic abnormalities seen in 25 (80%) lesions.[21] In this series, "grouped amorphous" calcifications on mammography; a "shadowing, avascular, irregular, hypoechoic mass on ultrasound"; and "heterogeneous non–mass-like enhancement with persistent enhancement kinetics" on magnetic resonance imaging (MRI) were the most common imaging abnormalities.

An exceptional situation exists in infrequent instances of florid LCIS (FLCIS), which can cause marked expansion of ducts and lobules. This condition may be extensive, and it sometimes partially involves SA. Necrosis and calcification frequently occur in FLCIS, with a pattern and distribution more commonly encountered in DCIS.[24] The resultant appearance on mammography is likely to suggest DCIS. The histologic diagnosis of these lesions is sometimes controversial. As discussed later in this chapter, the most compelling evidence supporting classification of these cases as LCIS is the cytologic appearance that is typical of LCIS, association with invasive lobular carcinoma of the classical type, and lack of reactivity for E-cadherin.

Age and Estrogen Exposure

Haagensen et al.[25,26] reported that LCIS was largely a disease of premenopausal women, and they speculated that spontaneous regression of the disease occurred during the menopause. Later, Haagensen et al.[9,27] noted that 10% to 12% of LCIS patients were postmenopausal, and Gump[28] urged caution in concluding that LCIS regresses after menopause. Rosen et al.[29] have reported that up to 25% of LCIS patients were postmenopausal.

The relationship of LCIS with exogenous estrogens was studied in a consecutive series of 59 patients with LCIS and 190 "controls" treated consecutively for duct carcinoma.[29] Exogenous estrogen use was reported by 29% of LCIS patients and 35% of women with duct carcinoma. Most exogenous estrogen usage occurred more than 1 year before diagnosis. Among the postmenopausal women in the series with only LCIS, five had been postmenopausal for 11 to 29 years. Only one of these five women had used exogenous hormones. Documented use of exogenous hormones was slightly more frequent in postmenopausal patients with duct carcinoma than it was among those with LCIS. These data confirmed prior studies indicating that LCIS occurred in postmenopausal women and that the presence of LCIS was not related to the use of exogenous estrogenic hormones in most women found to have this lesion after the menopause.[30–32]

The age distribution of LCIS is similar to that of most other forms of mammary carcinoma. It occurs infrequently as an isolated lesion in women younger than 35 years or older than 75 years. LCIS arising in bilateral mammary "hypertrophy" has been reported in a 15-year-old girl.[33] In different studies, the average age at diagnosis of LCIS ranged from 44 to 54 years. In a consecutive series of more than 1,000 patients treated for breast carcinoma, the mean age of women with LCIS (53 years) was less than but not significantly different from the mean age of patients who had infiltrating ductal carcinoma (IFDC) (57 years).[34]

Bilaterality

The extent of bilaterality in many reported series is uncertain because few surgeons have routinely biopsied the contralateral breast or performed bilateral mastectomy for this disease. Involvement of both breasts by LCIS was described in 1959 by Barnes,[35] who documented two patients treated by bilateral mastectomy. Newman[36] found that 6 (23%) of 26 patients with LCIS had bilateral disease. Bilaterality among 18 women who actually had a contralateral biopsy was 33%. Lewison and Finney[31] found bilateral disease in 7 (46%) of 15 women who had tissue from both breasts examined, and bilateral LCIS was found in 25 of 84 LCIS patients (30%) with specimens from both breasts studied by Haagensen.[9]

Urban[37] systematically performed contralateral biopsies for all types of breast carcinoma and reported finding concurrent contralateral LCIS in 9 of 22 biopsied patients (40%). In addition, one woman had concurrent contralateral invasive carcinoma. Subsequently, Erdreich et al.[38] reported bilaterality in 12 (39%) of 31 women who had LCIS in one breast, but they did not specify the histologic type of contralateral disease. Sunshine et al.[39] reported that 21 (67%) of 36 women with LCIS treated by bilateral mastectomy had LCIS in their opposite breast.

Data on bilaterality in women with LCIS in one breast are presented in Table 31.1. The 59 women with LCIS represent 4.5% of patients with breast carcinoma treated at Memorial Hospital in New York from mid-1976 to early 1979.[29] Coincidental contralateral pathologic breast status was known for 43 patients (73%), a proportion substantially greater than for women with intraductal carcinoma. This difference reflects the tendency at the time to perform contralateral biopsies more often in patients with LCIS. Among the 43 women with LCIS in one breast for whom the status of the opposite breast was known, the distribution of contralateral findings was as follows: benign, 18 of 43 (42%); previous contralateral carcinoma treated by mastectomy, 9 of 43 (21%); and concurrent contralateral carcinoma, 16 of 43 (37%). Concurrent biopsy of the opposite breast was performed in the 34 women with an intact contralateral breast, revealing carcinoma in 16 (47%).

The foregoing data provide compelling evidence that women with LCIS have a significant risk of having carcinoma in the opposite breast, often at the same time, but it has not been shown that all women with LCIS always have bilateral disease. When the ipsilateral breast contains only LCIS, contralateral LCIS will be found in approximately 40% of breasts biopsied.[37] It seems likely that there are some women with LCIS in one breast may never have both breasts affected by LCIS or any other form of mammary carcinoma.

The finding of LCIS coexisting with invasive duct carcinoma (IDC) also implies a substantial risk of bilaterality. Data shown in Table 31.2 are drawn from a study of the relationship of bilaterality and multicentricity.[40] An IFDC was found in 420 patients, including 53 (13%) who had coexistent LCIS in the same breast. Bilaterality was found in 57% of women with both lesions, in 22% with IFDC alone, and in 28% with infiltrating lobular carcinoma ($p < 0.01$). Because coexistent LCIS was usually not detected in a frozen section (FS) at the time of operation for the ipsilateral carcinoma, the presence of LCIS in the ipsilateral breast was not a factor in the selection of patients for contralateral biopsy. Medullary carcinoma and carcinomas with medullary features were rarely associated with bilaterality.

Table 31.3 summarizes the relationship between the histologic types of invasive carcinoma in the ipsilateral and contralateral breasts. Lobular carcinoma, most often LCIS, was more likely to be found in the contralateral breast when the ipsilateral breast also had lobular carcinoma.

TABLE 31.1 Bilaterality in Patients with *In Situ* Carcinoma[a]

Benign Primary Diagnosis in One Breast[d]	Status of Opposite Breast[b]									
	Carcinoma[c]		No Biopsy		Total Cases		Prior		Concurrent	
	No. pts.	[%]	No. pts.	[%]	No. pts.	[%]	No. pts.	[%]	No. pts.	[%]
DCIS	25	[39]	5	[8]	4	[6]	30	[47]	64	[52]
LCIS	18	[31]	9	[15]	16	[27]	16	[27]	59	[48]
Total	43	[35]	14	[11]	20	[16]	46	[37]	123	

[a]$p < 0.004$ for entire table. $p < 0.02$ when cases not biopsied were excluded.
[b]Status of opposite breast determined by biopsy or mastectomy.
[c]Includes LCIS.
[d]Primary diagnosis based on pathologic examination of a mastectomy specimen.[29]

TABLE 31.2 Frequency of Bilaterality Associated with Selected Histologic Types of Invasive Breast Carcinoma

	Bilaterality					
	Yes		No		Total	
Histologic Type of Tumor[a]	No. pts.	(%)	No. pts.	(%)	No. pts.	(%)
Infiltrating duct	82	(22)	285	(78)	367	(72)
Infiltrating duct and LCIS	30	(57)	23	(43)	53	(10)
Infiltrating lobular	12	(28)	31	(72)	43	(8)
Medullary	3	(12)	23	(88)	26	(5)
Atypical medullary	2	(10)	19	(90)	21	(4)
Total	129	(25)	381	(75)	510[b]	

[a]Based on 880 women treated for invasive carcinoma of one breast.[40] The tumor type listed describes the dominant (ipsilateral) lesion. If bilateral carcinomas were simultaneously detected, criteria to assign one lesion as ipsilateral were as follows: (a) With bilateral invasive carcinoma, the larger tumor was considered ipsilateral; (b) With invasive disease in one breast and contralateral *in situ*, the breast with invasion was considered ipsilateral.

[b]The 510 patients shown in this table were all women with one of the five histologic types of ipsilateral tumor listed. All had a confirmed contralateral biopsy or mastectomy. Contralateral diagnoses subsequent to treatment of the ipsilateral tumor are not included.

Multicentricity

Multicentricity and bilaterality are interrelated characteristics of mammary carcinoma. Types of carcinoma associated with a high frequency of bilaterality are also more likely to occur as multicentric foci in the affected breast. The reported frequency of multicentricity is influenced by sampling techniques, but virtually all investigators have come to the conclusion about LCIS reached by Foote and Stewart[2] that "this lesion occurs in multiple lobules." Multicentric foci of LCIS have been found in 60% to 85% of patients undergoing mastectomy for LCIS.[29,31,41–43] A retrospective review of mastectomy specimens by Shah et al.[44] revealed that 26 (65%) of 40 breasts removed for LCIS had multicentric *in situ* carcinoma that was LCIS in 93% and intraductal in 7%. Carter and Smith[45] found *in situ* carcinoma in 31 (63%) of 49 mastectomies performed for LCIS. Occult, clinically unsuspected invasive carcinoma has been detected in 4% to 6% of breasts removed after a biopsy showed only LCIS.[29,44,45] Invasive carcinoma was present in 4 of 38 mastectomy and mammoplasty specimens (11%) obtained 2 years after a biopsy diagnosis of LCIS, and intraductal carcinoma was found in a fifth specimen.[46]

Gross Pathology

LCIS does not, by itself, result in a grossly apparent pathologic alteration in breast tissue, but the tissue that harbors LCIS is sometimes abnormal as a result of coexisting proliferative changes. The gross description often records nodular lesions such as FAs, areas of firm or hard tissue, or cysts.

TABLE 31.3 Relationship between Ipsilateral Tumor Type and Type of Carcinoma in the Contralateral Breast[a-c]

	Contralateral Breast					
	Ductal		Lobular		Total	
Type of Invasive Ipsilateral Carcinoma	No. pts.	(%)	No. pts.	(%)	No. pts.	(%)
Infiltrating duct	58	(81)	14	(19)	72	(62)
Infiltrating duct and LCIS	10	(37)	17	(63)	27	(23)
Infiltrating lobular	2	(17)	10	(83)	12	(10)
Medullary and atypical medullary	4	(80)	1	(20)	5	(4)
Total	74	(64)	42	(36)	116	

% CA, percent subsequent carcinoma; RR, relative risk of subsequent carcinoma when compared with specified age-matched controls.

[a]$p < 0.001$ (Fisher exact test) for infiltrating duct vs. infiltrating duct and LCIS vs. infiltrating lobular. Based on Lesser et al.[40]

[b]Based on 84 cases with follow-up.

[c]Diagnosis of LN included unspecified proportions of LCIS and of ALH.

None of these visible or palpable abnormalities is attributable to LCIS. In patients with extensive LCIS, FLCIS, or PLCIS, the cut surface of the breast tissue may have a faintly granular appearance when viewed with tangential light because the affected lobules are sufficiently enlarged to be visible.

Microscopic Pathology of Classical LCIS and PLCIS

The microscopic anatomic distribution of LCIS and PLCIS in lobules and ducts and alterations in the morphology of these structures influence the histopathologic appearance of LCIS in any given case. Foote and Stewart[2] observed that LCIS resides largely in the terminal ducts of the postmenopausal atrophic breast, whereas in premenopausal women LCIS is mainly distributed in the terminal duct–lobular complex.

Lobular Enlargement

In the typical lobular form of LCIS, a population of neoplastic cells replaces the normal epithelium of acini and intralobular ductules (Fig. 31.1). The abnormal cells may be sufficiently numerous to cause expansion of these structures as well as enlargement of the entire lobule in comparison with uninvolved lobules in the adjacent breast tissue, especially in FLCIS and PLCIS (Figs. 31.2 and 31.3). However, lobular enlargement is not an absolute diagnostic criterion (Fig. 31.4). Foote and Stewart[2] found that, "large lobules, small lobules, and hyalinized lobules may all assume this pattern. Occasionally, only part of a lobule is involved and a sharp line of division between normal epithelium and carcinoma *in situ* is seen. Distension of the lobule does not assume marked proportions prior to infiltration" (Figs. 31.5 and 31.6). Myoepithelial cells may persist in LCIS, especially when there is relatively little glandular enlargement (Fig. 31.5). They are less likely to be present in FLCIS or PLCIS.

There is no universal yardstick that permits accurate evaluation of what constitutes lobular distension. Comparison of adjacent involved and uninvolved lobules in a given case is a recommended approach, but in practice it becomes readily apparent that lobular diameters vary considerably within a given breast and from case to case. In one study, there was a slight, but not statistically significant, trend for a greater risk of subsequent carcinoma when distension of

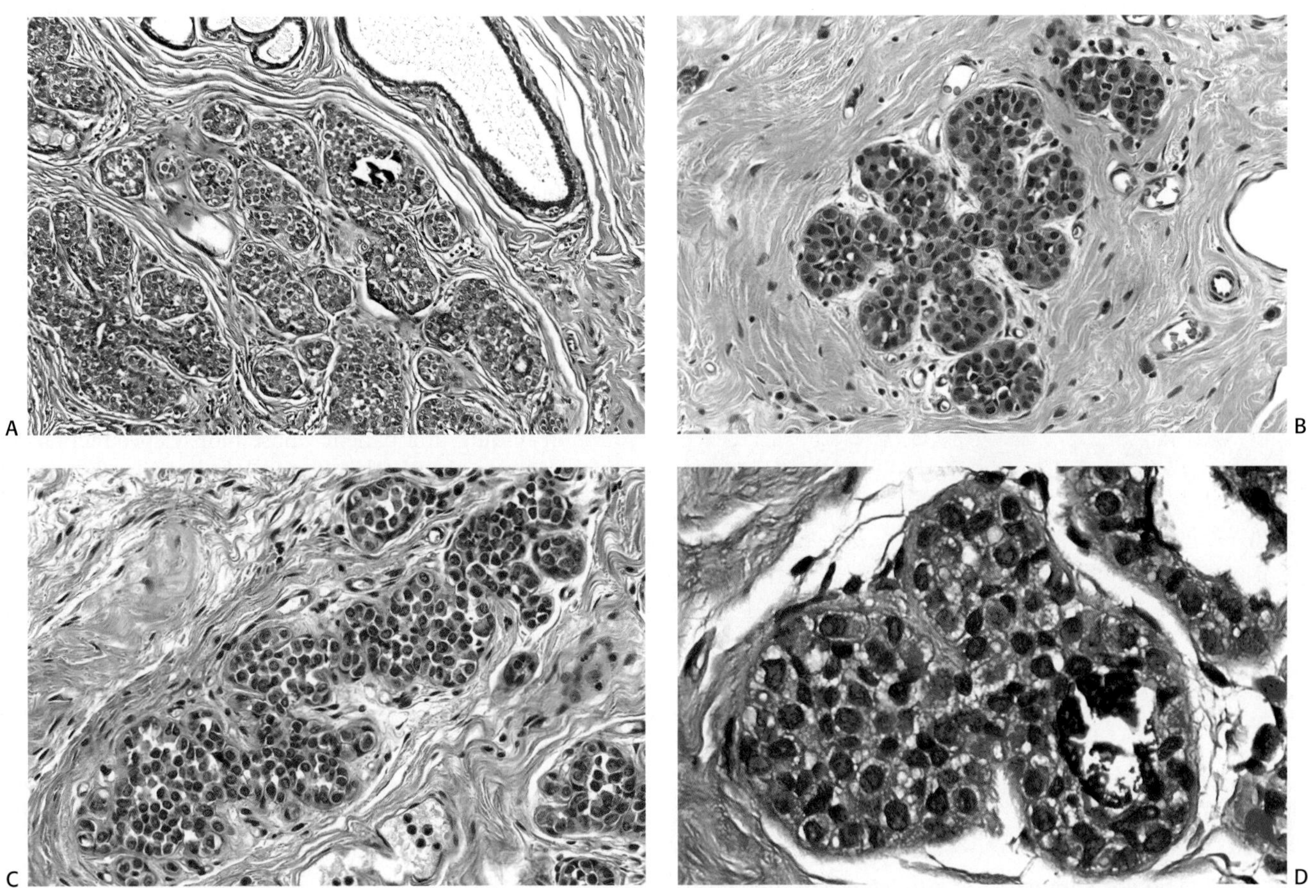

FIG. 31.1. ***Lobular carcinoma in situ, classical type.*** **A–E:** Five examples of classical type of LCIS are shown. Note the calcification in LCIS in **(A)**. **F:** E-cadherin reactivity is absent or fragmented and discontinuous in LCIS cells (seen in **E**), whereas the normal ductal epithelium (*upper right*) is strongly E-cadherin positive

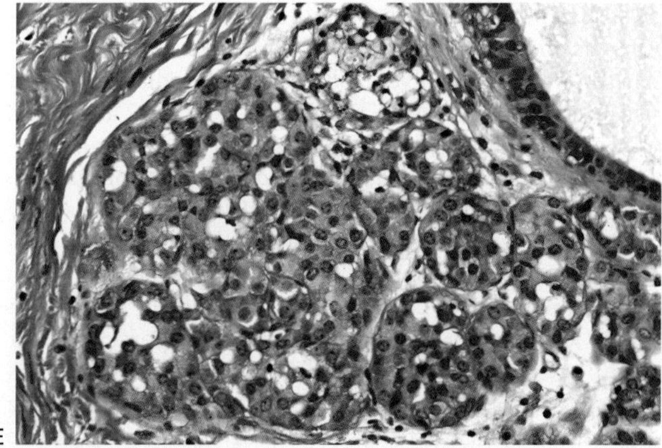

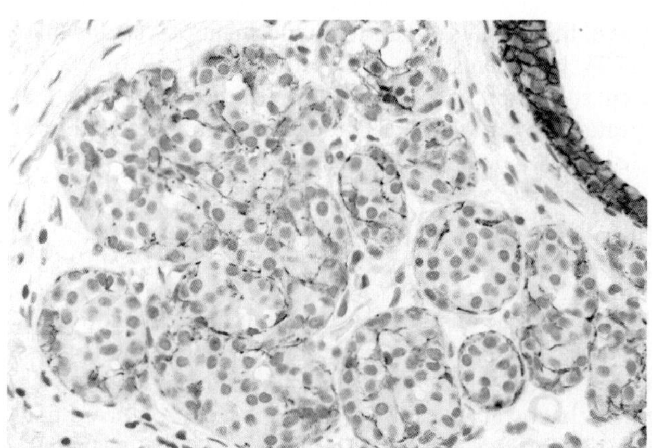

FIG. 31.1. *(Continued)*

lobular glands caused by LCIS was minimal.[6] Others found a slight increase in the risk of subsequent carcinoma in patients with maximal distention but did not regard the difference as significant.[9] The tendency to lobular atrophy in postmenopausal women makes expansion of lobular glands an unreliable diagnostic criterion on this group of patients. If the diagnosis of LCIS is to be meaningful because it identifies a lesion associated with a substantial risk of later invasive carcinoma, then lobular distension cannot be regarded as a decisive diagnostic criterion in lesions that have reached an acceptable qualitative level of cytologic abnormality. Important exceptions to this circumstance are FLCIS and PLCIS, in which extreme ductal and lobular enlargement occurs, sometimes with necrosis and calcification (Fig. 31.7). These cases should be examined very carefully for evidence of microinvasion that can be obscured by the stromal reaction.

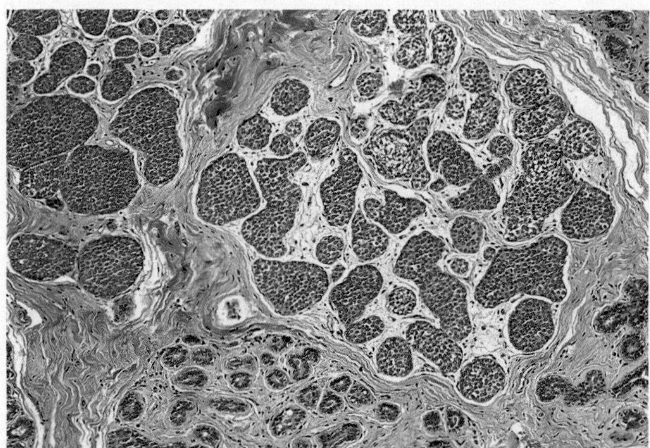

FIG. 31.2. *Lobular carcinoma in situ, classical type with marked glandular distension.* The enlarged lobular glands have filled most of the intralobular stroma. Note the variable size of glands with LCIS and the uninvolved lobule *below*.

Quantitative Factors

Quantitative factors have been included by some investigators among the diagnostic criteria for LCIS. The question of how much lobular involvement is necessary for the diagnosis of LCIS as a marker of risk remains unanswered. Some authors required that there be at least two lobules exhibiting diagnostic features.[47] Others concluded that one fully affected lobule was sufficient evidence for the diagnosis.[6,27] The latter position was based on the observation that the number of affected lobules in a biopsy did not prove to be related to the risk of subsequent carcinoma among patients not treated by mastectomy.[6] In particular, there was not a significant difference in risk between patients with one or with two lobules affected. As a consequence, there appears to be no logical reason for drawing a distinction between one and two involved lobules as the basis for a diagnosis of LCIS. The number of affected lobules is of questionable relevance for the diagnosis of needle core biopsy specimens that provide limited tissue samples.

Partial involvement of one or more lobules is not an uncommon finding in a patient whose biopsy specimen also contains many completely affected lobules. Glandular lumens persist in unaffected portions of a partially involved lobule, or the lumen may remain when glandular cells have been displaced but not destroyed as a consequence of pagetoid spread of LCIS cells within a lobule (Figs. 31.5 and 31.6). In some biopsy specimens, the only evidence of a neoplastic lobular proliferation is one lobule in which some, but not all, of the acini are involved. The significance of such minimal evidence has not been determined. It has been suggested arbitrarily that at least 50%[48] or 75%[4] of one lobule in a biopsy specimen needs to be involved to establish a diagnosis of LCIS and that specimens with lesser lesions be included in the category of atypical lobular hyperplasia (ALH).

Absence of Lobular Lumens

Complete absence of spaces or lumens is not necessary for the diagnosis of LCIS (Fig. 31.8). Loss of cohesion is a characteristic of neoplastic cells in LCIS, although this is not

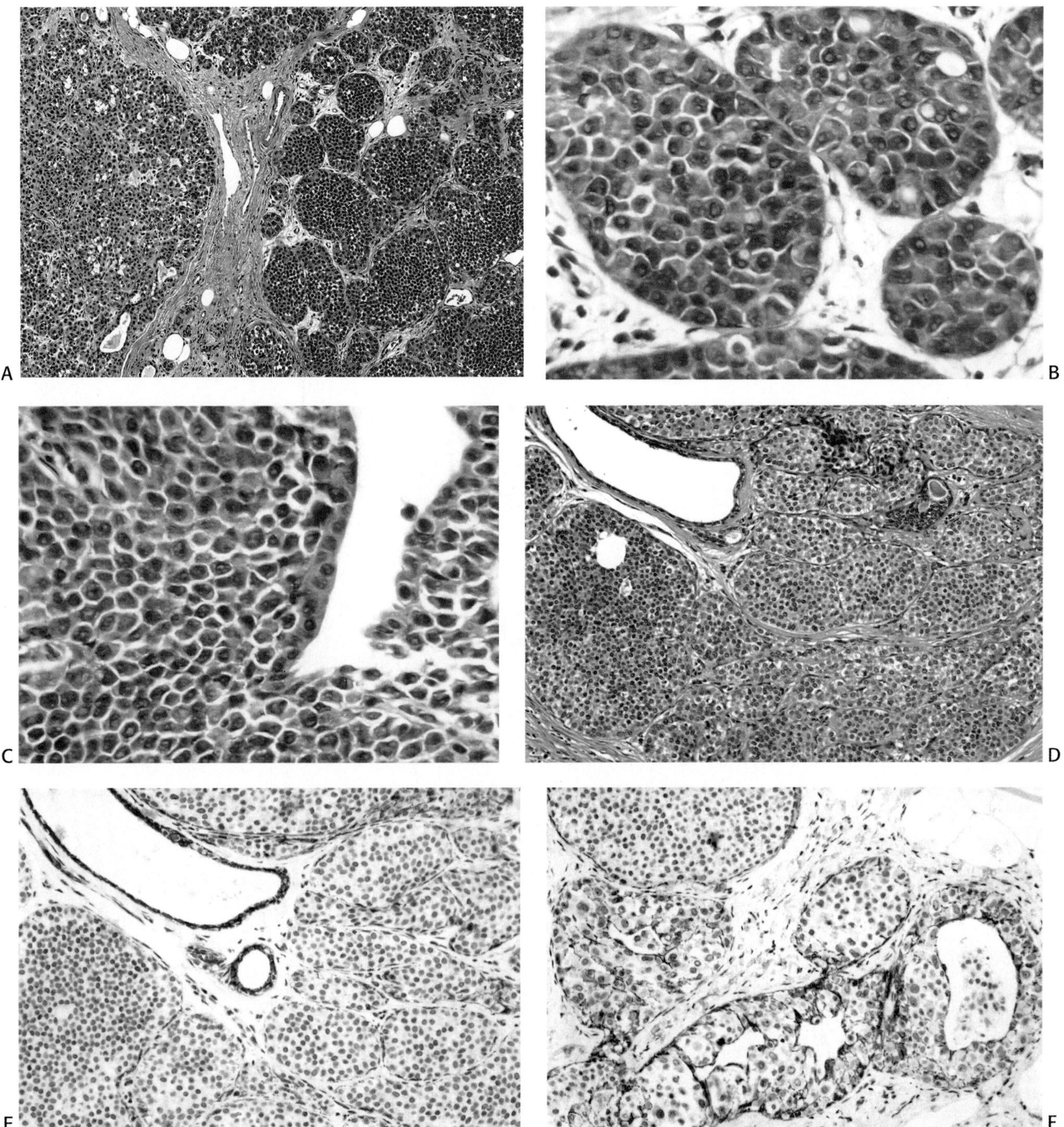

FIG. 31.3. ***Lobular carcinoma in situ, classical type with marked glandular distension.*** **A:** FLCIS involving almost all contiguous lobular glands seen in this field. **B:** Carcinoma in lobular glands with loss of cohesion. Some cells have intracytoplasmic lumens. **C:** LCIS in a duct beneath benign epithelium around the duct lumen. Loss of cohesion is evident. **D:** Lobular glands filled with carcinoma cells have effaced the intralobular stroma. **E:** E-cadherin reactivity is lost in the LCIS and preserved in uninvolved ducts. **F:** E-cadherin reactivity persists in residual myoepithelial and ductal epithelial cells around E-cadherin–negative LCIS cells in enlarged lobular glands with pagetoid ductal extension of LCIS.

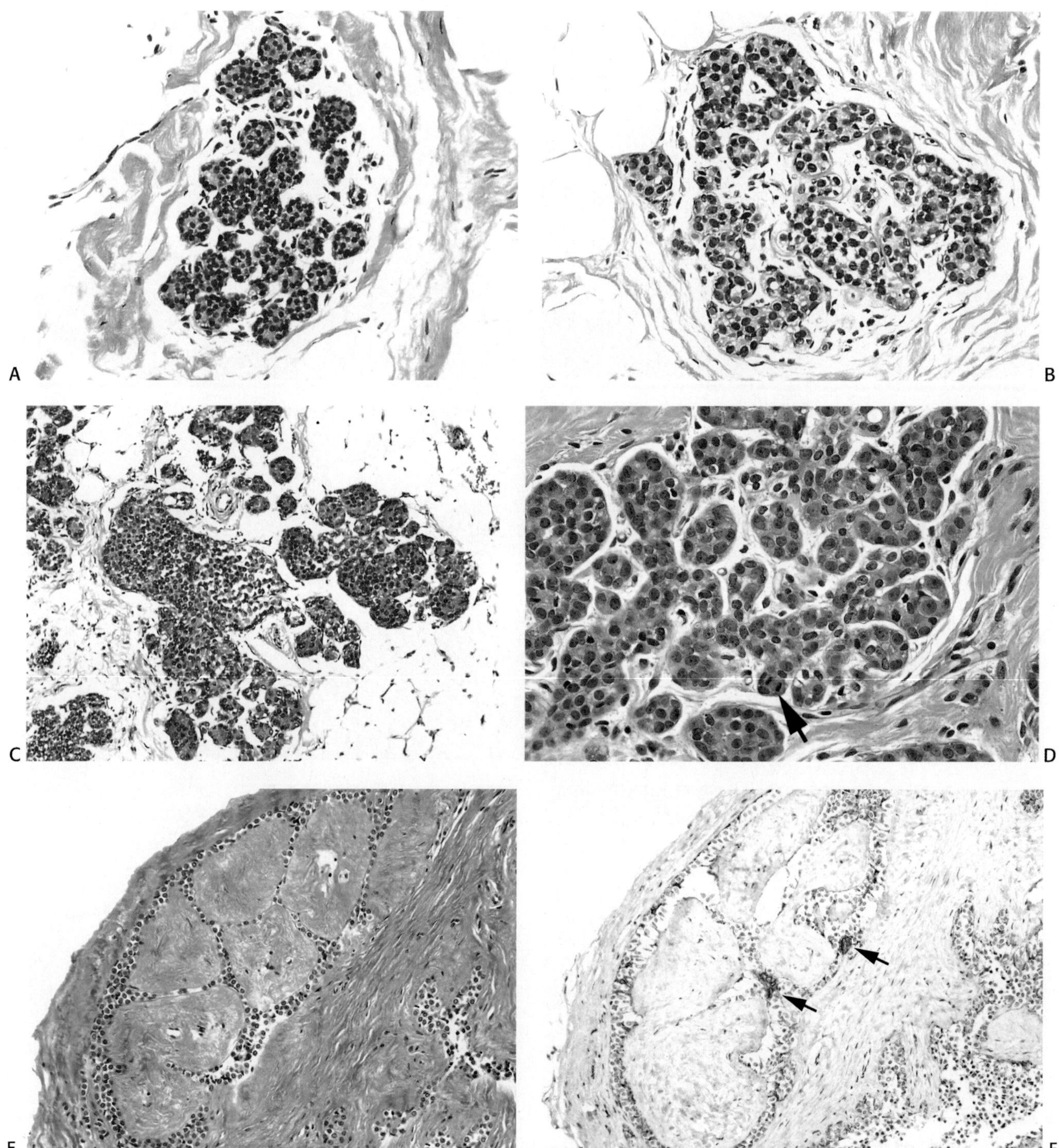

FIG. 31.4. ***Lobular carcinoma in situ, classical type without glandular distension.*** **A,B:** Two examples of *LCIS* in which the lobular glands are not enlarged. **C,D:** *In situ* carcinoma fills the terminal duct and adjacent lobular glands. A mitotic figure is present in the neoplastic epithelium (*arrow*). **E:** LCIS involving an FA. The epithelial clefts are populated by dyscohesive LCIS cells. **F:** E-cadherin is negative in LCIS cells (seen in **E**) with some staining in residual ductal cells and in myoepithelial cells (*arrows*).

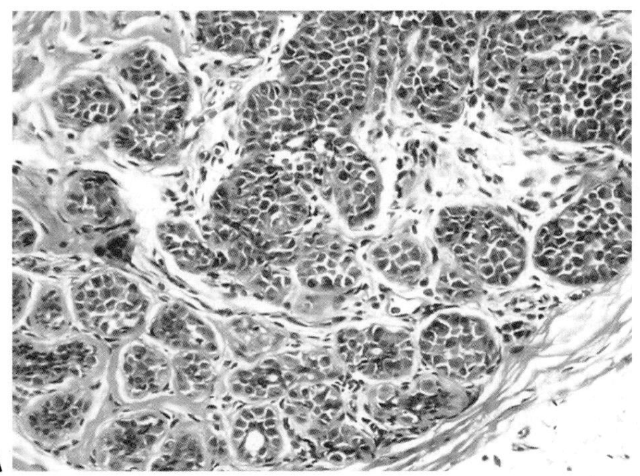

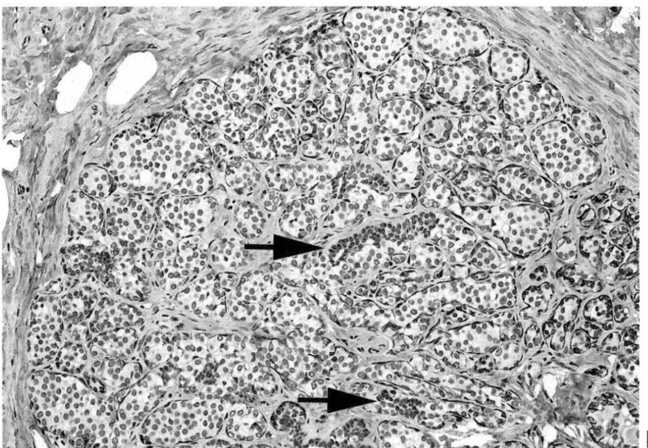

FIG. 31.5. ***Lobular carcinoma in situ, classical type.*** **A:** *In situ* carcinoma involves lobular glands on the *right* but spares the glands in the *lower left* corner. **B:** The immunostain for smooth muscle myosin-heavy chain (SMM-HC) highlights inconspicuous, attenuated myoepithelial cells in this lesion. Clusters of dark cells are residual nonneoplastic lobular epithelium (*arrows*).

always readily apparent in acini filled and expanded by the process. When loss of cohesion is prominent and the neoplastic cells have a dissociated distribution, spaces may be created between them that can be mistaken for glandular lumina. Degenerative changes may also disrupt the cellular composition of LCIS (Fig. 31.9). In these situations, the neoplastic cells are not arranged in the polarized fashion that characterizes nonneoplastic cells persisting around true glandular lumina.

Cytologic Characteristics of LCIS and PLCIS Cells

The neoplastic cells in LCIS have been described as having scant cytoplasm and small, round, cytologically bland nuclei that lack nucleoli (Fig. 31.10). In some instances, cytologic pleomorphism may be encountered, and the more varied cells have been classified as PLCIS (Fig. 31.11). LCIS cells tend to have a diploid DNA content, whereas PLCIS cells are largely hyperdiploid.[49] PLCIS cells have more abundant cytoplasm than cells classified as classical type, and larger more pleomorphic nuclei that sometimes have nucleoli. The nucleus in a PLCIS cell is usually lobulated or indented and eccentrically placed.

The cytologic features of PLCIS cells in some instances resemble those of ductal carcinoma. When the lesion is composed entirely of PLCIS cells, the distinction from intralobular extension of DCIS may be difficult to establish. The E-cadherin immunostain is very useful in this situation because absence of reactivity is diagnostic of LCIS or PLCIS.[50–52]

Sullivan et al.[53] reviewed 75 cases of solid DCIS diagnosed in needle core biopsy samples. Using the E-cadherin immunostain, they reclassified 10 (13.3%) as variants of LCIS, including 5 PLCIS, 4 FLCIS, and 1 LCIS. Some examples of LCIS display classical and pleomorphic cell types, both of which are E-cadherin negative (Fig. 31.12).

The presence of intracytoplasmic mucin secretion favors a diagnosis of LCIS. Intracytoplasmic mucinous secretion is often present in at least some cells in LCIS and PLCIS.[54,55] Mucin can be an inconspicuous feature that must be demonstrated and highlighted with a stain such as mucicarmine or Alcian blue–periodic acid–Schiff (PAS)[55] (Fig. 31.13). The mucin may be present diffusely in the cytoplasm, but more often it is limited to vacuoles that contain condensed globules of secretion, resulting in a targetoid appearance. An extreme manifestation of this phenomenon is the formation of signet ring cells in which a distended cytoplasmic vacuole causes the nucleus to be eccentric and indented into a crescentic shape[56] (Figs. 31.14 and 31.15). The signet ring cells in LCIS and infiltrating lobular carcinoma are cytologically similar (Fig. 31.16). Signet ring cells occur more often in LCIS than in PLCIS, but they can be a prominent feature of PLCIS.[57]

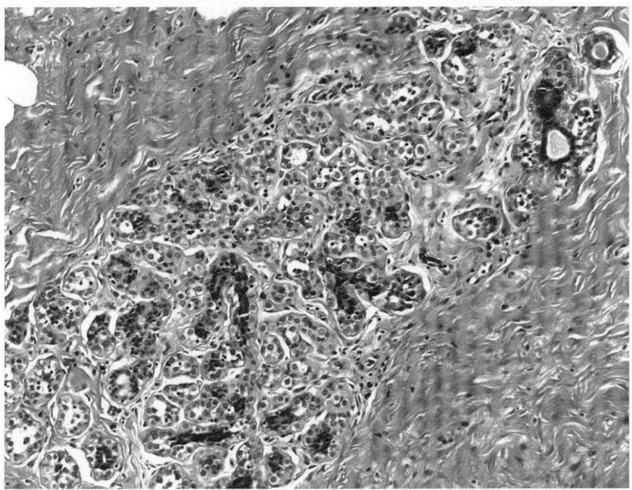

FIG. 31.6. ***Lobular carcinoma in situ, classical type with partial lobular involvement.*** LCIS involves most lobular glands.

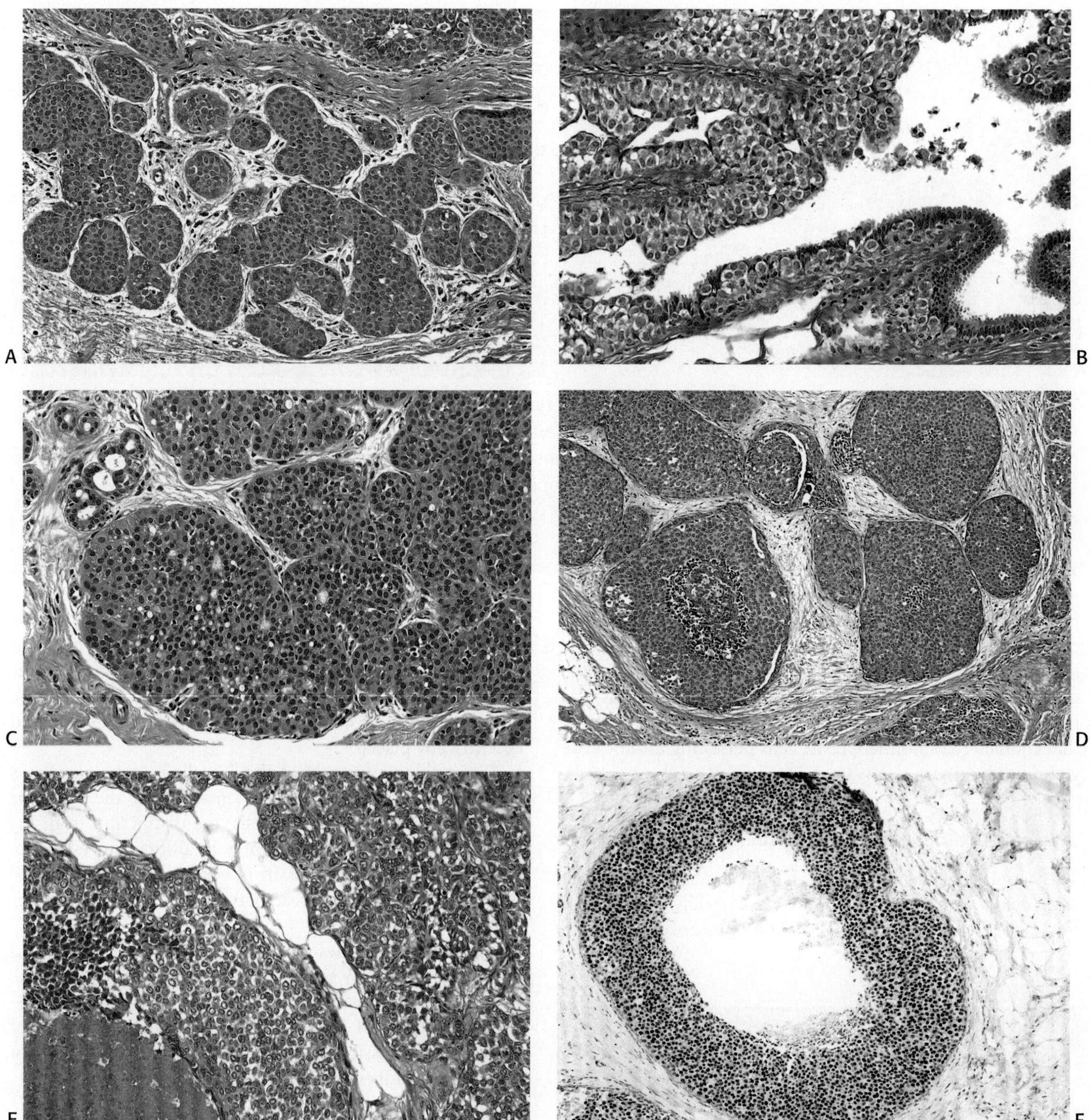

FIG. 31.7. ***Lobular carcinoma in situ, classical and pleomorphic types, florid with focal necrosis.*** Images **(A–I)** are from a single specimen. **A:** Well-developed LCIS. **B:** Pagetoid intraductal spread of LCIS. **C:** Severe enlargement of lobular glands. **D:** Florid enlargement of lobular glands with focal necrosis and small calcifications (*upper center*). Note persistence of lobular stroma around the *in situ* carcinoma. **E:** Magnified view showing identical dyscohesive cells in a lobule (*right*) and a duct with necrosis. **F:** LCIS around the necrotic center in a duct shows strong nuclear immunoreactivity for ER. **G:** The intact basement membrane of a duct with LCIS is demonstrated with the immunostain for laminin. **H:** Preserved myoepithelial cells are highlighted in a lobule comparable to **(C)** by the immunostain for SMM-HC. **I:** The duct is expanded by LCIS with necrosis. **J:** Myoepithelial cells are highlighted by the smooth muscle actin (SMA) immunostain. The duct is expanded by LCIS with necrosis. **K:** E-cadherin immunoreactivity is present in the normal lobule but not in the LCIS cells. **L:** Classical (*left*) and pleomorphic (*right*) dyscohesive LCIS cell types. *Inset*: E-cadherin reactivity is not present in either carcinoma cell type.

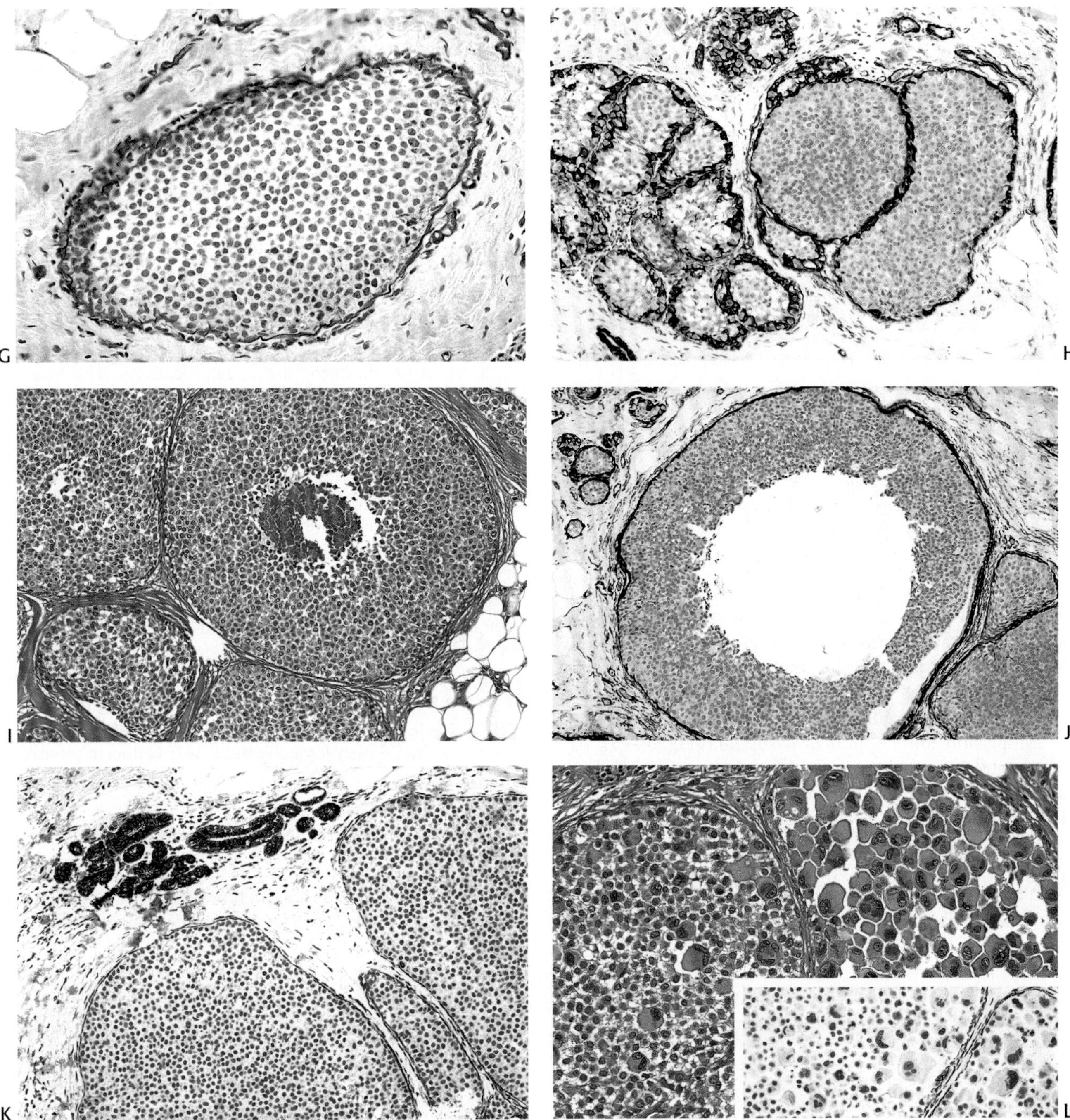

FIG. 31.7. *(Continued)*

Degenerative changes in the cytoplasm of LCIS cells and in the epithelium of hyperplastic lobules may produce cytoplasmic defects that resemble vacuoles, but intracytoplasmic mucin is not detectable in these cells (Figs. 31.9 and 31.11). Intracytoplasmic mucin is not demonstrable in the epithelial cells of a normal lobule, but it may be present in the glandular lumen (Fig. 31.17). It is important to distinguish between mucin in true intracytoplasmic vacuoles and mucin demonstrated in small pockets of the lobular lumen that reside between epithelial cells in hyperplastic lobules. Casein and other secretory products such as carcinoembryonic antigen (CEA) are also concentrated in the lobular secretion.[58] Because intracytoplasmic mucin vacuoles are uncommon in the cells of ductal carcinoma and are virtually absent in hyperplastic lesions of duct or lobular epithelium, their presence is an important but not a necessary criterion for the diagnosis of LCIS or PLCIS.[54–56]

Several uncommon cytologic features may also be found in LCIS. Cytoplasmic pallor or clear-cell change, more often encountered in nonneoplastic, hyperplastic lobules, occurs

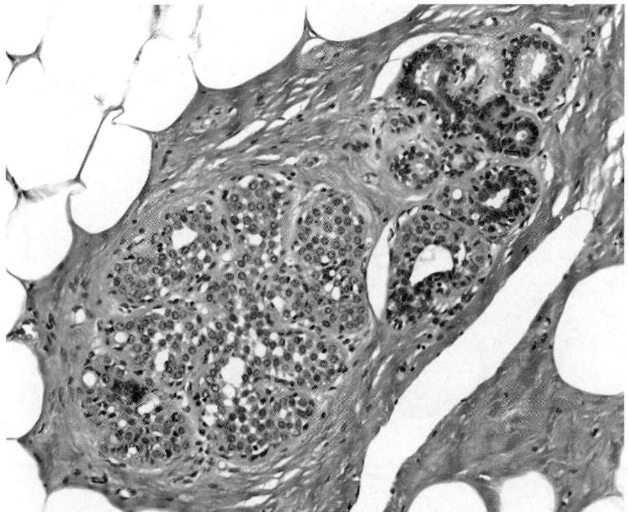

FIG. 31.8. ***Lobular carcinoma in situ, classical type with partial lobular involvement.*** *In situ* carcinoma involves about 75% of the lobular gland. A calcification is present in the lobule on the *left*.

rarely in LCIS.[59] Clear-cell LCIS is composed of cells with abundant intracytoplasmic mucin (Fig. 31.18). Apocrine differentiation has been described in LCIS and PLCIS, the latter being referred to as "apocrine PLCIS."[60] Mucin within LCIS cells that have undergone apocrine change is usually evident as cytoplasmic amphophilia or basophilia (Fig. 31.15). Another cytologic appearance, seen largely in atrophic lobules and terminal ducts of postmenopausal women, features PLCIS cells with dark eosinophilic to basophilic cytoplasm and deeply basophilic eccentric nuclei. This appearance is probably the result of cytoplasmic condensation associated with loss of cohesion and shrinkage of cells. These cells resemble myoblasts and have been referred to as the "myoid" form of PLCIS (Fig. 31.19). Similar cells are found in the corresponding infiltrating pleomorphic lobular carcinoma (Fig. 31.20). Myoid lobular carcinoma cells frequently have intracytoplasmic mucin. In another variant, the cells of LCIS have a "mosaic" or "fried egg" appearance that results from the presence of distinct cell borders between the cells and prominent, round, centrally placed nuclei surrounded by pale cytoplasm (Fig. 31.21). Intracytoplasmic mucin vacuoles can usually be found in this type of LCIS.

Chen et al.[61] described 10 examples of LCIS that they termed "pleomorphic apocrine lobular carcinoma *in situ*" (PALCIS). Cytologically, these cases exhibited features described in the foregoing paragraph pertaining to PLCIS with apocrine and myoid cytology. The patients ranged in age from 40 to 86 years (median, 58) and were identified as a result of mammographic calcifications. The lesions consisted of FLCIS with PLCIS cytology, signet ring cells, and necrosis. Immunoreactivity was as follows: E-cadherin (−) 100%; estrogen receptor (ER) (+) 50%; progesterone receptor (PR) (+) 45%; HER2/*neu* (+) 40%; cytokeratin (CK) 5/6 (+) 78%; Ki67 78% greater than 10%; and gross cystic disease fluid protein 15 (GCDFP-15) (+) 100%. Two lesions examined by comparative genomic hybridization had losses of 16q and gains at 1q, changes that are typically associated with LCIS and PLCIS. These data provide additional characterization of PLCIS and serve as a reminder of the prominence of apocrine differentiation encountered in some examples of PLCIS. Conversely, it is important to be aware of the fact that apocrine intraductal carcinoma has a predilection for lobular involvement. This entity can closely resemble PLCIS histologically but it is E-cadherin positive.

Patterns of Ductal Involvement by LCIS and PLCIS

LCIS and PLCIS typically involve intralobular and extralobular or terminal ductules as well as acinar units within the lobule. Extralobular LCIS in the epithelium of ducts and ductules occurs in 65% to 75% of patients[9,60,62,63] (Fig. 31.22).

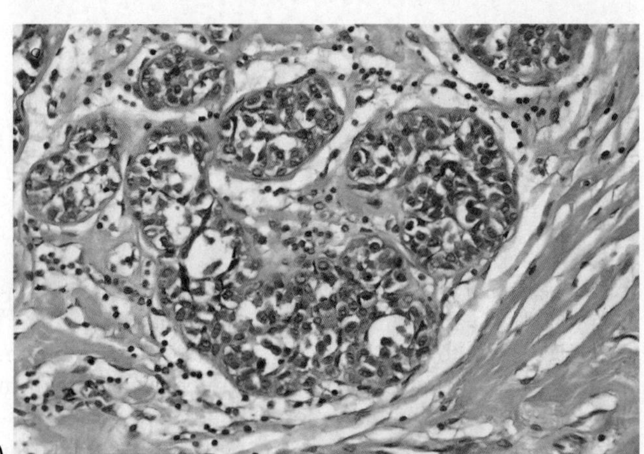

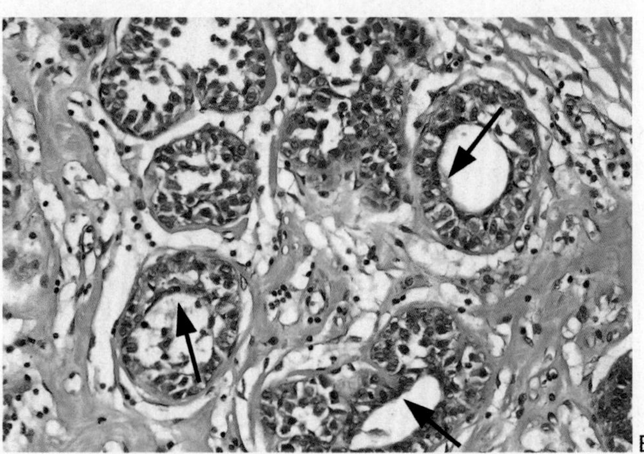

FIG. 31.9. ***Lobular carcinoma in situ, classical type.*** **A:** Spaces created among carcinoma cells shown here due to loss of cohesion should not be mistaken for glandular lumens. **B:** Flattened residual epithelial cells (*arrows*) encircle persisting true lumens in glands involved by pagetoid *in situ* carcinoma. Spaces in other glands (*upper center*) are the result of cellular dyscohesion.

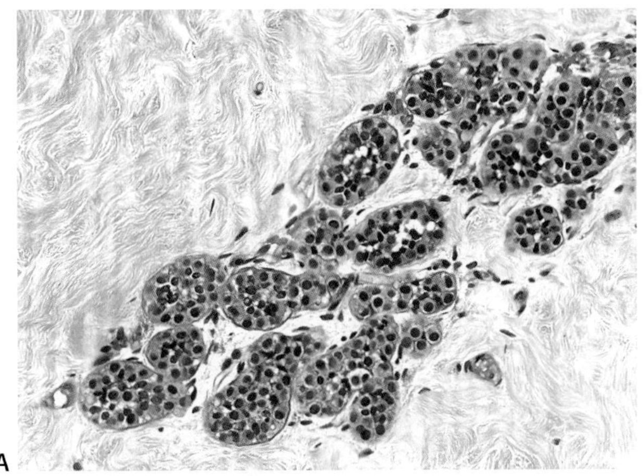

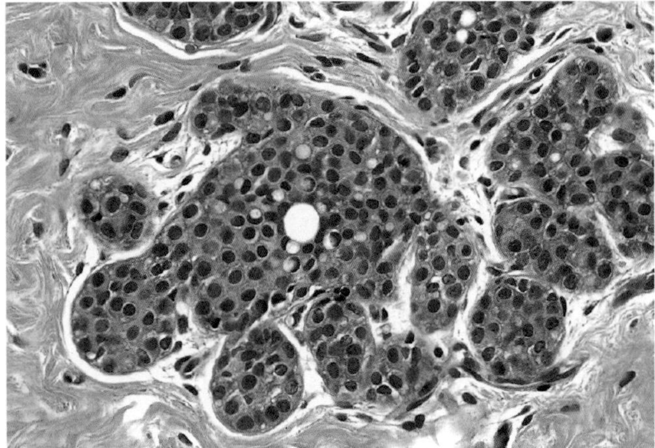

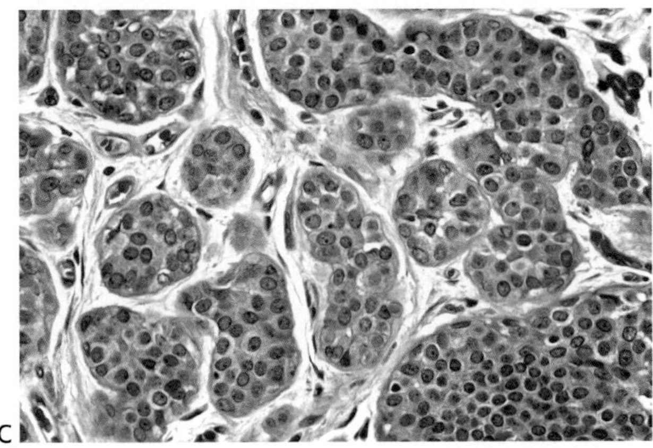

FIG. 31.10. ***Lobular carcinoma in situ, small cell classical type.*** **A–C:** *LCIS*, classical type. Classical LCIS with signet ring cells **(B)**.

In postmenopausal patients with atrophic lobules, duct involvement may be the only manifestation of LCIS[9,26] (Fig. 31.23). Haagensen[9] reported that the lobular phase, alone or in combination with ductal LCIS, was found in 95% of premenopausal and 53% of postmenopausal women. Quantitatively, there was not a significant difference between premenopausal and postmenopausal women with respect to the average amount of duct or lobular LCIS.

The irregular configuration of some ductules affected by LCIS has been described as saw-toothed or as resembling a cloverleaf. In such cases, there are clusters of LCIS cells that lie beneath the nonneoplastic ductal epithelium and form buds which protrude around the periphery (Fig. 31.24). The neoplastic cells are distributed continuously or discontinuously along the ductal system, undermining and ultimately displacing the normal ductal epithelium. When this occurs, the normal glandular epithelium sometimes persists, having been elevated and pushed toward the lumen (Fig. 31.25). The myoepithelial layer is preserved to a variable extent, and it may require an immunostain for actin, calponin, or p63 to confirm that it is present.

Pagetoid LCIS and PLCIS

In some instances, isolated LCIS cells may also be found singly or in small groups within the epithelium of lobules and ducts in a pattern that resembles Paget disease of the nipple (Figs. 31.26 and 31.27). This intraepithelial growth pattern has been referred to as *pagetoid spread* because of presumed growth of the neoplastic cells, originating in lobules, into the ductal epithelium. In postmenopausal women, the cloverleaf pattern sometimes appears to arise *de novo* in ducts rather than by pagetoid spread from lobules. The occurrence of this microscopic structural alteration in isolated large ducts, including those in the subareolar region, suggests that the ducts retain the capacity for lobular differentiation.[64] This provides an explanation for finding LCIS or ALH in breast biopsies without a classic lobular component. Paget disease of the squamous surface of the nipple is not a feature of LCIS, except in very rare instances when there is florid pagetoid involvement of lactiferous ducts.[65]

Two abnormalities in benign epithelium must be considered in the differential diagnosis of pagetoid spread of LCIS and PLCIS: histiocytes in the epithelium and epithelioid myoepithelial cell hyperplasia. When examined at high magnification, intraepithelial histiocytes are found to have abundant foamy cytoplasm, sometimes with lipofuscin or hemosiderin pigment, and small dark nuclei. Intracytoplasmic mucin is absent from intraepithelial histiocytes, and they are immunoreactive for histiocytic markers but not for CK. The overlying nonneoplastic epithelium is attenuated and flattened over intraepithelial histiocytes as well as over pagetoid spread of LCIS. Intraepithelial histiocytes may be relatively sparse or they may form a continuous layer one or more cells thick.

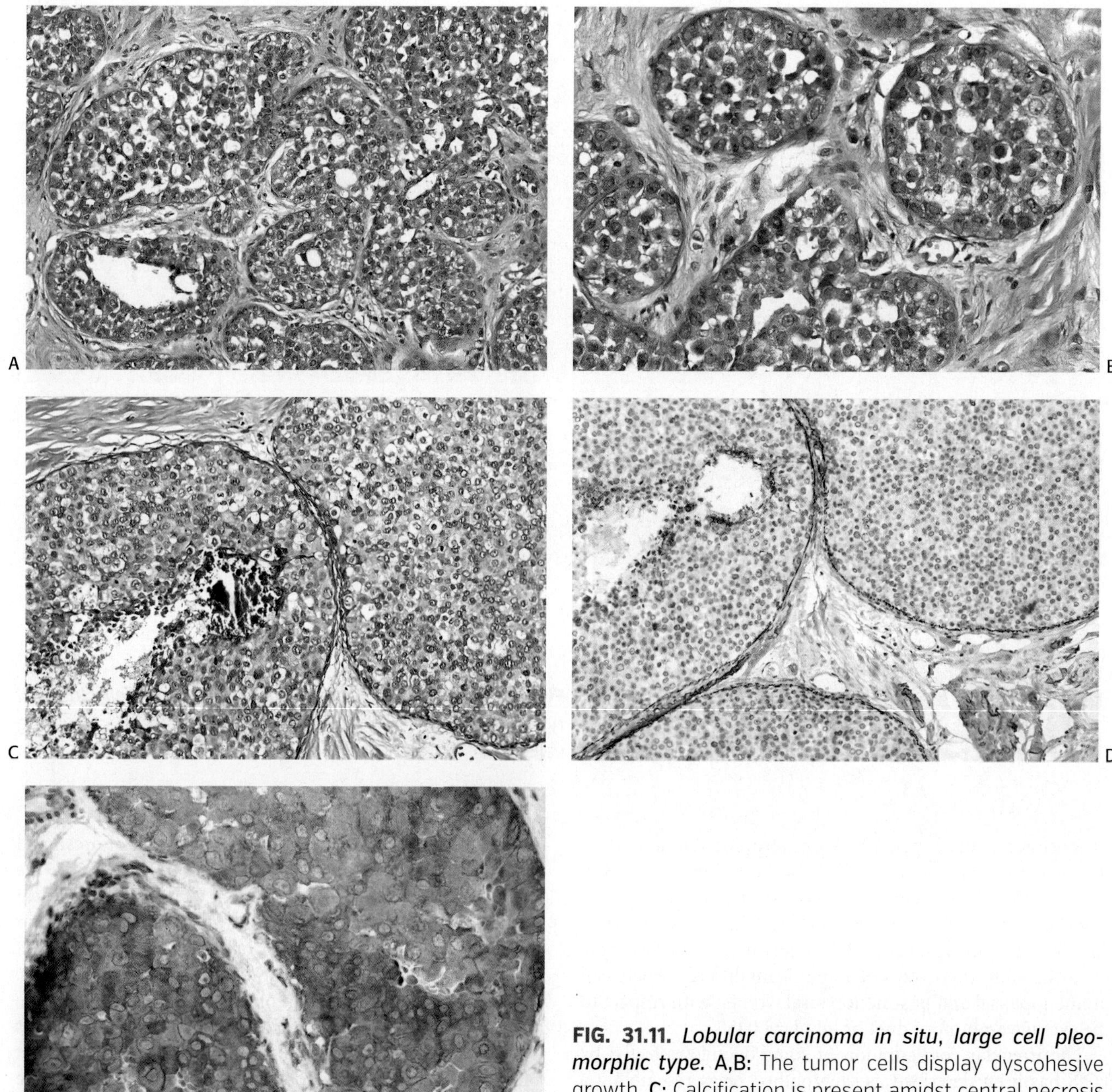

FIG. 31.11. ***Lobular carcinoma in situ, large cell pleomorphic type.*** **A,B:** The tumor cells display dyscohesive growth. **C:** Calcification is present amidst central necrosis in PLCIS. The PLCIS cells are negative for E-cadherin **(D)** and show cytoplasmic reactivity with p120 **(E)**.

Epithelioid myoepithelial hyperplasia is more likely to be mistaken for pagetoid spread of LCIS than is the presence of intraepithelial histiocytes. Epithelioid myoepithelial cells have abundant clear vesicular cytoplasm. Except in papillomas, hyperplastic myoepithelial cells tend to be distributed in a single layer, causing less attenuation of the overlying epithelium than pagetoid LCIS. Some myoid immunohistochemical properties are usually retained in epithelioid myoepithelial hyperplasia, but occasionally these cells entirely lack myoid cytoplasmic reactivity. The p63 immunostain is most reliable in this circumstance because nuclear reactivity as retained in epithelioid myoepithelial cells, whereas LCIS cells are p63 negative.

An uncommon growth pattern manifested by apocrine intraductal carcinoma is extension into ductules and terminal duct–lobular units. The neoplastic cells may displace the normal epithelium and fill the affected structures, or they may undermine the epithelium in a pagetoid fashion. This histologic appearance is an especially vexing problem when it is encountered in a needle core biopsy specimen or near the margins of a lumpectomy specimen. The E-cadherin immunostain is very useful in this situation, since a positive result establishes the diagnosis of pagetoid apocrine ductal carcinoma and a negative result is indicative of LCIS or PLCIS. When interpreting the E-cadherin immunostaining in

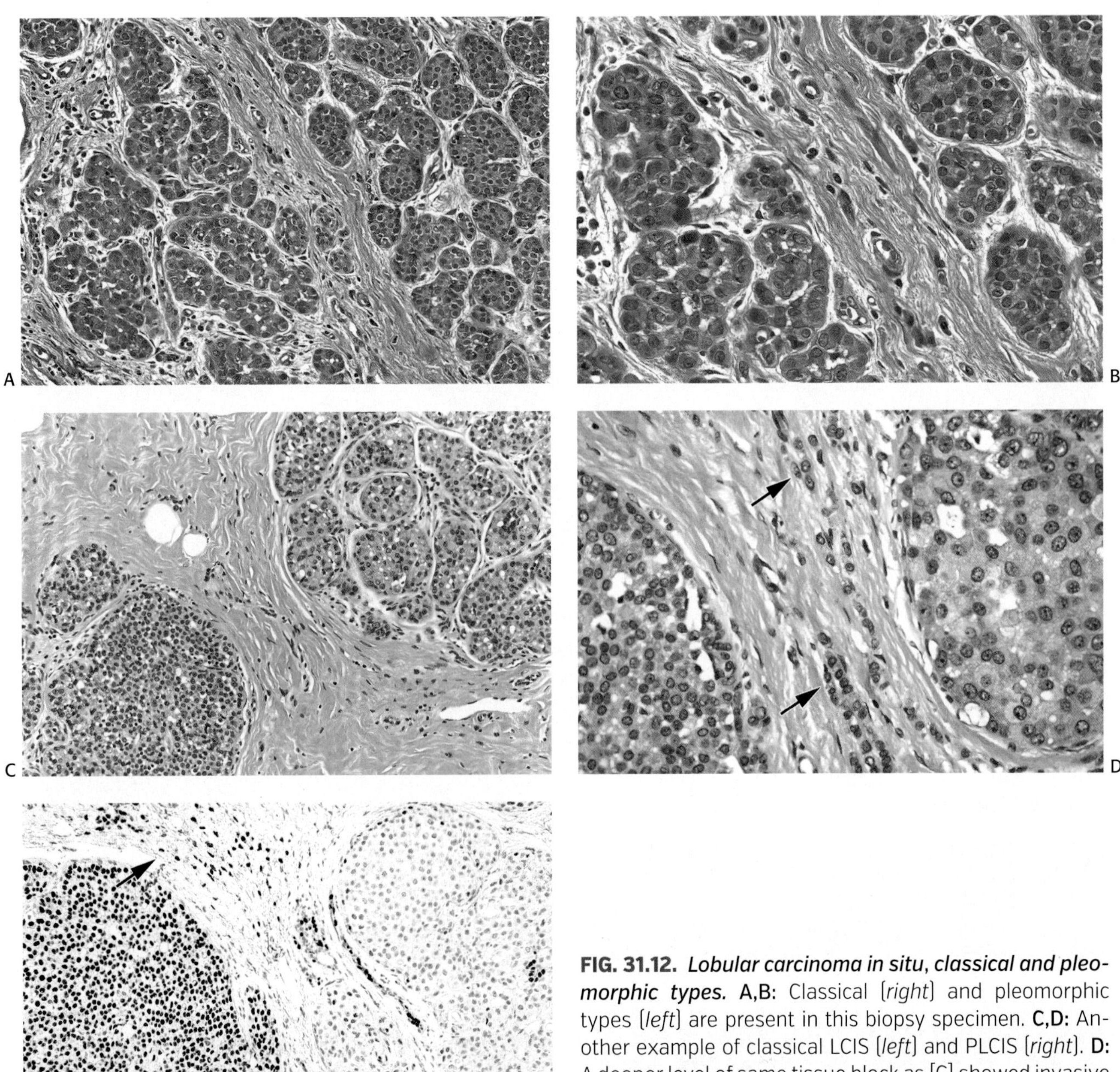

FIG. 31.12. ***Lobular carcinoma in situ, classical and pleomorphic types.*** **A,B:** Classical (*right*) and pleomorphic types (*left*) are present in this biopsy specimen. **C,D:** Another example of classical LCIS (*left*) and PLCIS (*right*). **D:** A deeper level of same tissue block as [C] showed invasive lobular carcinoma (*arrows*) **E:** Classical LCIS cells are ER (+), PLCIS cells are ER (−). Invasive lobular carcinoma cells (*arrow*) are ER (+).

such a case, it is important to distinguish reactivity in residual nonneoplastic epithelial and myoepithelial cells from reactivity in the neoplastic cells.

Coexisting LCIS and DCIS in a Single Duct

An unusual neoplastic proliferation is the coexistence of LCIS and intraductal carcinoma in a single duct. Such foci may have LCIS with a saw-toothed or cloverleaf configuration at the periphery of a duct in which ductal epithelium is carcinomatous and fills the lumen with a cytologically different population of cells growing as cribriform, papillary, or comedo intraductal carcinoma (Fig. 31.28). LCIS involving ducts that harbor apocrine intraductal carcinoma is another variant of such a combined lesion (Fig. 31.29).

Florid LCIS

In the most flagrant type of ductal involvement, LCIS proliferates to form a solid mass of tumor cells that fill and expand the duct lumen (Fig. 31.11). Foci such as these, termed FLCIS, can develop central necrosis and calcifications that are detectable on mammograms (see Fig. 31.7). Because of its tendency to involve and expand ducts with the development

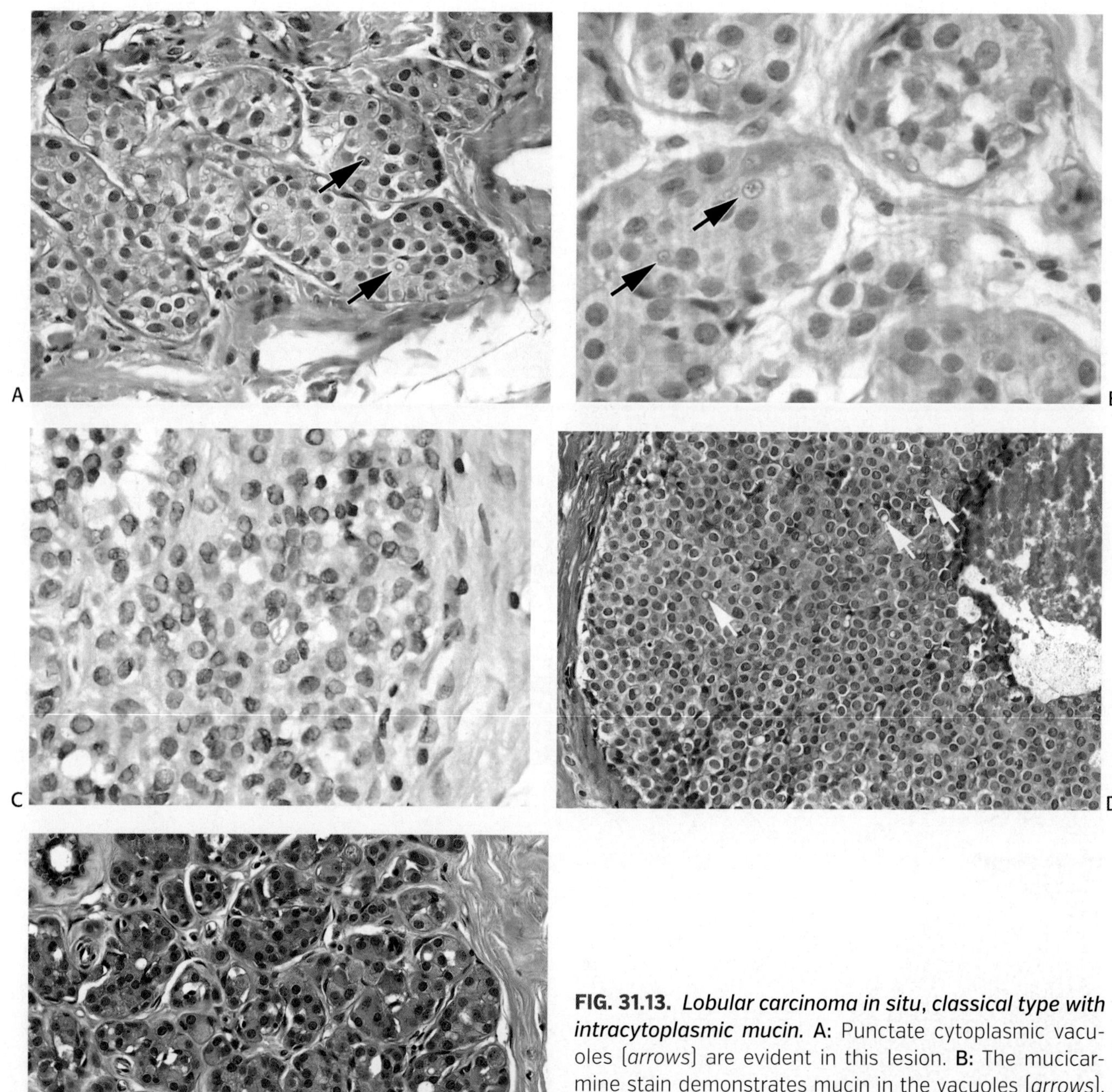

FIG. 31.13. ***Lobular carcinoma in situ, classical type with intracytoplasmic mucin.*** **A:** Punctate cytoplasmic vacuoles (*arrows*) are evident in this lesion. **B:** The mucicarmine stain demonstrates mucin in the vacuoles (*arrows*). **C:** Intracytoplasmic mucin stains blue with the Alcian blue reaction. **D:** Signet ring cells (*arrows*) in FLCIS with necrosis. **E:** Basophilia is evidence of diffuse cytoplasmic mucin in this example of LCIS.

of necrosis and calcification, FLCIS may be misdiagnosed as DCIS, especially when the cytology of the lesion corresponds to PLCIS.[66] A negative E-cadherin immunostaining distinguishes this FLCIS from E-cadherin–positive comedo intraductal carcinoma.[50] FLCIS with necrosis may consist of classical, pleomorphic, or both cell types. Signet ring cells may be present in FLCIS and rarely these are the predominant cell type.[67] The cells in FLCIS display the same predominant pattern of immunoreactivity that is found in LCIS and PLCIS [ER (+); PR (+); HER2/*neu* (−); 34βE12 (+)].[67] In some instances, the abundant cytoplasm of FLCIS cells has apocrine traits. FLCIS is so often associated with invasive lobular carcinoma that specimens found to have this lesion should be studied carefully for microinvasion when no overt invasive carcinoma is detected.

Fadare et al.[24] reviewed 18 patients with FLCIS whose ages ranged from 41 to 85 years (mean, 61.3 years). Twelve patients (67%) had associated invasive carcinoma,

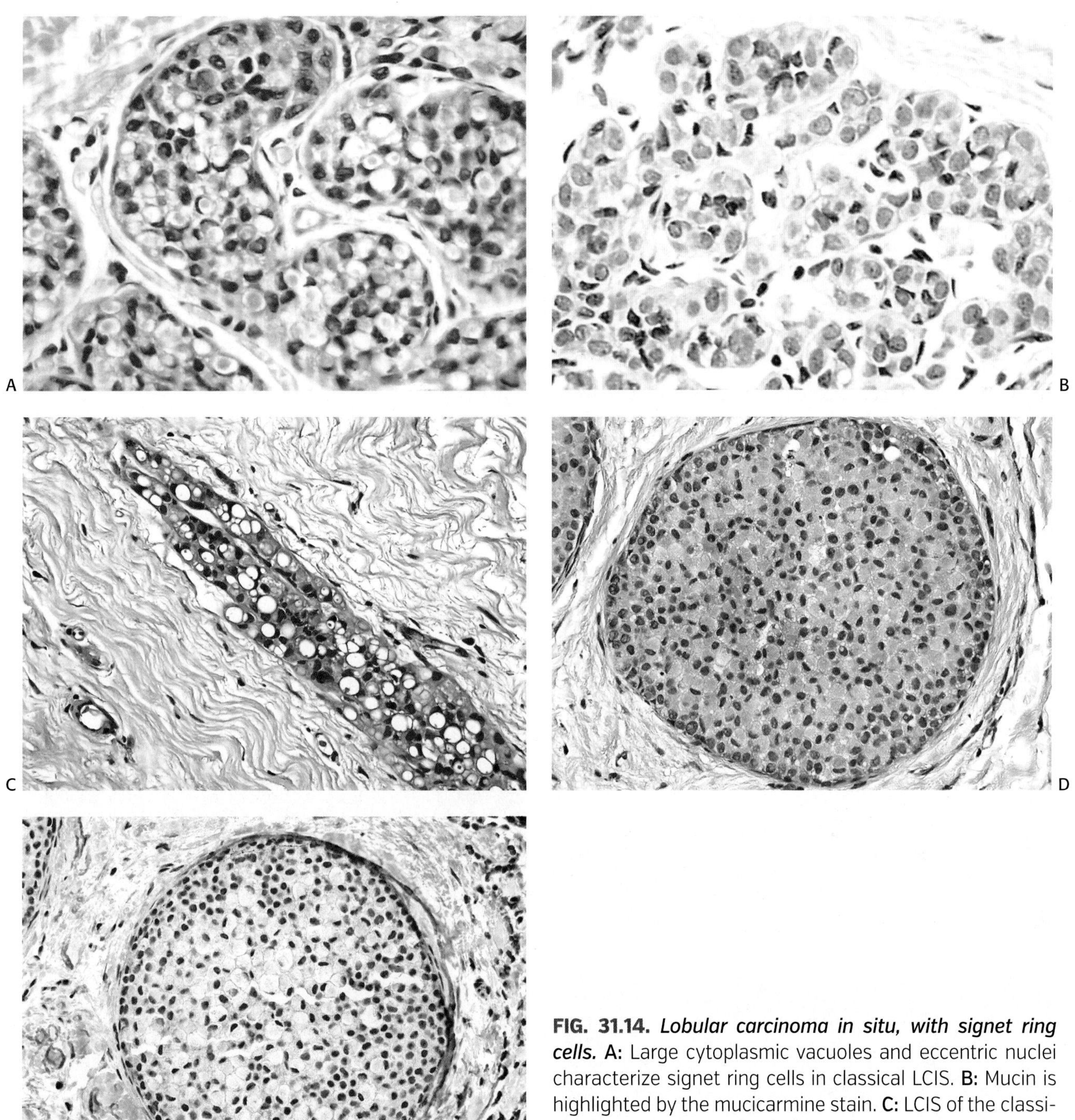

FIG. 31.14. ***Lobular carcinoma in situ, with signet ring cells.*** **A:** Large cytoplasmic vacuoles and eccentric nuclei characterize signet ring cells in classical LCIS. **B:** Mucin is highlighted by the mucicarmine stain. **C:** LCIS of the classical type with signet ring cells involves a terminal duct. **D,E:** LCIS of the florid type with diffuse cytoplasmic mucin. The neoplastic cells lack membranous E-cadherin reactivity **(E)**.

including seven classical lobular, one pleomorphic lobular, and four that were ductal or had a ductal component. Immunoreactivity was as follows: ER 94% (+); HER2 100% (−) in 15 cases; and high-molecular-weight keratin 94% (+). Excluded from this series were four E-cadherin–positive cases, which were histologically "not notably different from their E-cadherin–negative counterparts, with the exception that intracytoplasmic lumens were absent in all 4 cases." The latter four cases would be classified as intraductal carcinoma as a result of the presence of E-cadherin expression.

Bagaria et al.[68] studied 210 specimens containing LCIS, including 171 (81%) with a nonflorid growth pattern and 39 (19%) that were classified as florid. Non-FLCIS tended to be diffusely distributed in the specimen, whereas FLCIS was typically localized near invasive lobular carcinoma. Invasive

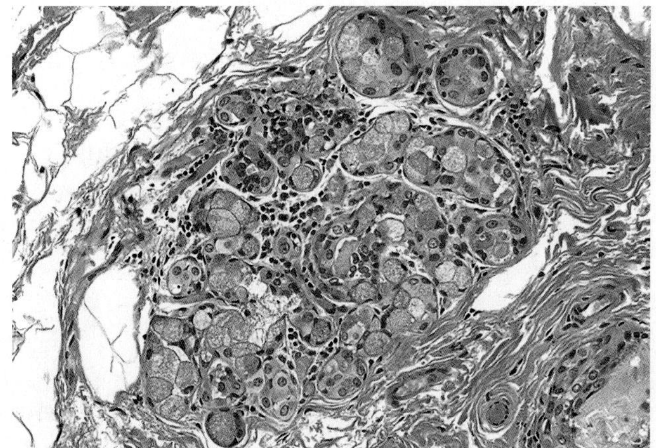

FIG. 31.15. ***Lobular carcinoma in situ, classical type with signet ring cells.*** An example of extreme signet ring cell formation in which the cytoplasm of LCIS cells is filled with basophilic mucin.

carcinoma was present more often (87%) with FLCIS than with non-FLCIS (73%). All invasive carcinomas associated with FLCIS were lobular type, whereas 18% of invasive carcinomas associated with non-FLCIS were classified as ductal. Invasive lobular carcinomas in patients with FLCIS always reflected the cytology of the *in situ* carcinoma, with 23 (68%) classical types (LCIS) and 11 (32%) pleomorphic types (PLCIS). Among those with non-FLCIS, 12/111 (10.8%) patients with classical cytology had pleomorphic invasive lobular carcinoma and 7/18 (28%) of patients with pleomorphic cytology had classical invasive lobular carcinoma. These data suggest that PLCIS, whether florid or not, is largely committed to evolve into pleomorphic invasive lobular carcinoma, whereas LCIS may retain the classical phenotype when it becomes invasive or evolve into pleomorphic invasive lobular carcinoma.

Since it is composed of LCIS or PLCIS cells, it is not surprising that FLCIS would exhibit the same chromosomal alterations as these entities in non-FLCIS, especially losses at 16q and gains at 1q. However, as reported by Boldt et al.,[69] the alterations in FLCIS are significantly more numerous

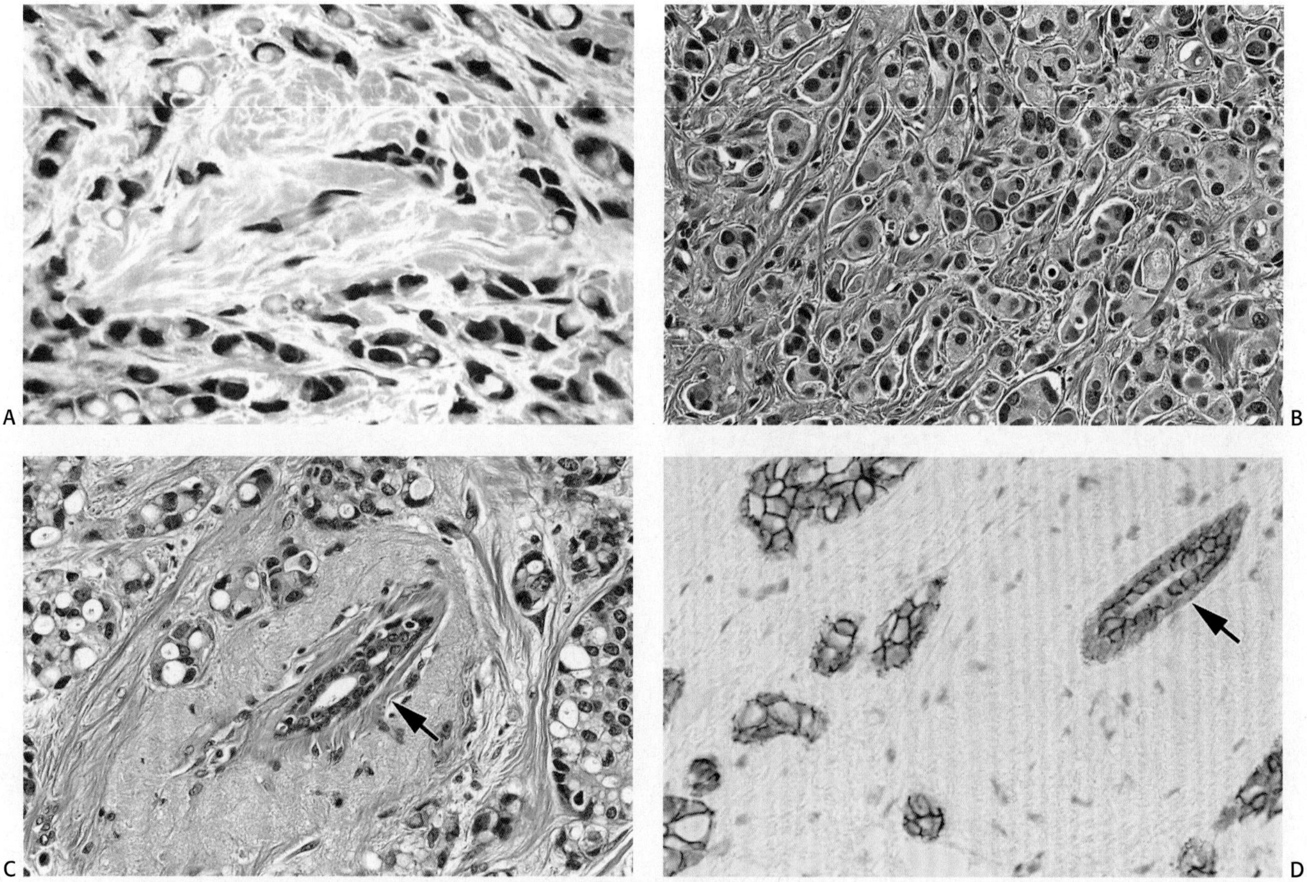

FIG. 31.16. ***Invasive lobular and duct carcinoma with signet ring cells.*** **A:** Invasive lobular carcinoma classical type with signet ring cells. **B:** Invasive pleomorphic lobular carcinoma with intracytoplasmic mucin and signet ring cells. **C,D:** Invasive ductal carcinoma with signet ring cells simulating invasive lobular carcinoma. The invasive carcinoma and normal ductal cells are positive for E-cadherin **(D)**. *Arrows* point to normal ducts **(C,D)**.

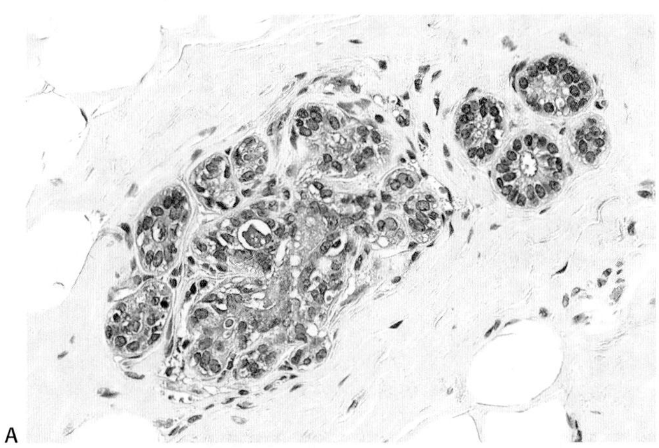

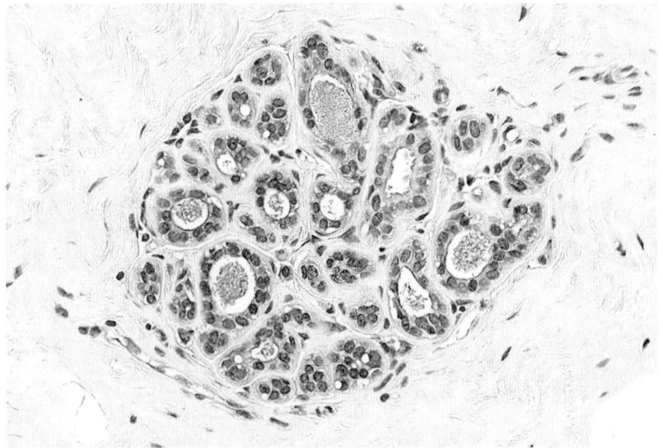

FIG. 31.17. ***Normal lobules, mucicarmine stain.*** **A,B:** Mucin in the glandular lumens is stained. There is no intracytoplasmic mucin.

and more complex than those in non-FLCIS. This finding suggests a heightened propensity to progress to invasion, a hypothesis that is supported by the relatively frequent occurrence of microinvasion or frank invasion associated with FLCIS.

LCIS and PLCIS in Benign Proliferative Lesions

Lobular tissue previously altered by various benign proliferative processes can harbor LCIS or rarely, PLCIS. LCIS has been encountered in FAs, papillomas (Fig. 31.30), radial sclerosing lesions (Fig. 31.31), and SA (Fig. 31.32). The diagnosis of LCIS under these circumstances rests largely on the identification of the appropriate cytologic features. The demonstration of intracytoplasmic mucin droplets is helpful for distinguishing florid adenosis from adenosis with LCIS (Figs. 31.33 and 31.34). LCIS in tubular adenosis has a striking histologic appearance (Fig. 31.35). In all of the foregoing circumstances, the most reliable means of confirming the presence of LCIS is the demonstration of loss of E-cadherin reactivity.

The lobular configuration is radically distorted in sclerosing lesions, and as a result it is difficult to exclude invasion when LCIS or PLCIS occurs in such foci[70,71] (Figs. 31.36 to 31.38). However, careful inspection usually reveals the underlying adenosis pattern in which glandular units are surrounded by a basement membrane, myoepithelial cells, and stroma (Fig. 31.42). These elements can be highlighted with the reticulin stain and by the immunohistochemical demonstration of basement membrane proteins (laminin and type IV collagen) and myoepithelium (Fig. 31.39). Attenuated, spindle-shaped myoepithelial cells persist in SA and may be accentuated when the lesion is colonized by LCIS.[72] Myofibroblastic proliferation in the stroma can obscure myoepithelial cells in SA. Cross-reactivity with stromal myofibroblasts that occurs with actin and calponin immunostains can be avoided by using the p63 immunostain to highlight the nuclei of myoepithelial cells. Invasion is very difficult to identify when the neoplastic cells remain confined to the configuration of SA. The diagnosis of invasion when there is LCIS in a sclerosing lesion is based on the finding of carcinoma cells in the stroma in the absence of immunoreactive myoepithelial cells (Fig. 31.39). CK stains are especially useful in this situation to highlight the distribution of invasive epithelial cells. The appearance of invasive foci outside SA is not different from that of invasive lobular carcinoma in the absence of a sclerosing lesion (Fig. 31.40). For additional discussion of LCIS in SA, see Chapter 7.

Most lobules are surrounded by fibrous stroma, but infrequently lobules are distributed in mammary adipose tissue. Lobules in fat are subject to the same pathologic alterations that occur in parenchymal lobules, including the development of SA and LCIS. These conditions may resemble invasive carcinoma. Important distinguishing features of LCIS in fat are the presence of well-circumscribed glands containing LCIS, basement membrane components, and myoepithelial cells (Figs. 31.41 and 31.42). Basement membrane can be highlighted with the reticulin stain and by the immunohistochemical demonstration of laminin and type IV collagen. Immunostains for p63, CD10, calponin, and actin identify myoepithelium. Myoepithelium and basement membranes are absent when infiltrating lobular carcinoma involves fat (Fig. 31.43).

An unusual pattern of ductal involvement occurs when LCIS develops in ducts altered by collagenous spherulosis[73] (Fig. 31.44). This configuration mimics cribriform intraductal carcinoma (Fig. 31.45). However, myoepithelial cells outline spherule material composed of basement membrane constituents that should be distinguished from the true microlumens of cribriform carcinoma. The carcinoma cells in such foci display loss of cohesion and intracytoplasmic vacuoles characteristic of lobular carcinoma. When LCIS involves collagenous spherulosis, myoepithelium can be highlighted with immunostains such as p63 and calponin. The LCIS will be E-cadherin negative. Pronounced myoepithelial cell proliferation rarely accompanies LCIS in collagenous spherulosis and radial scar lesions.[74] PLCIS is exceedingly rare in collagenous spherulosis.

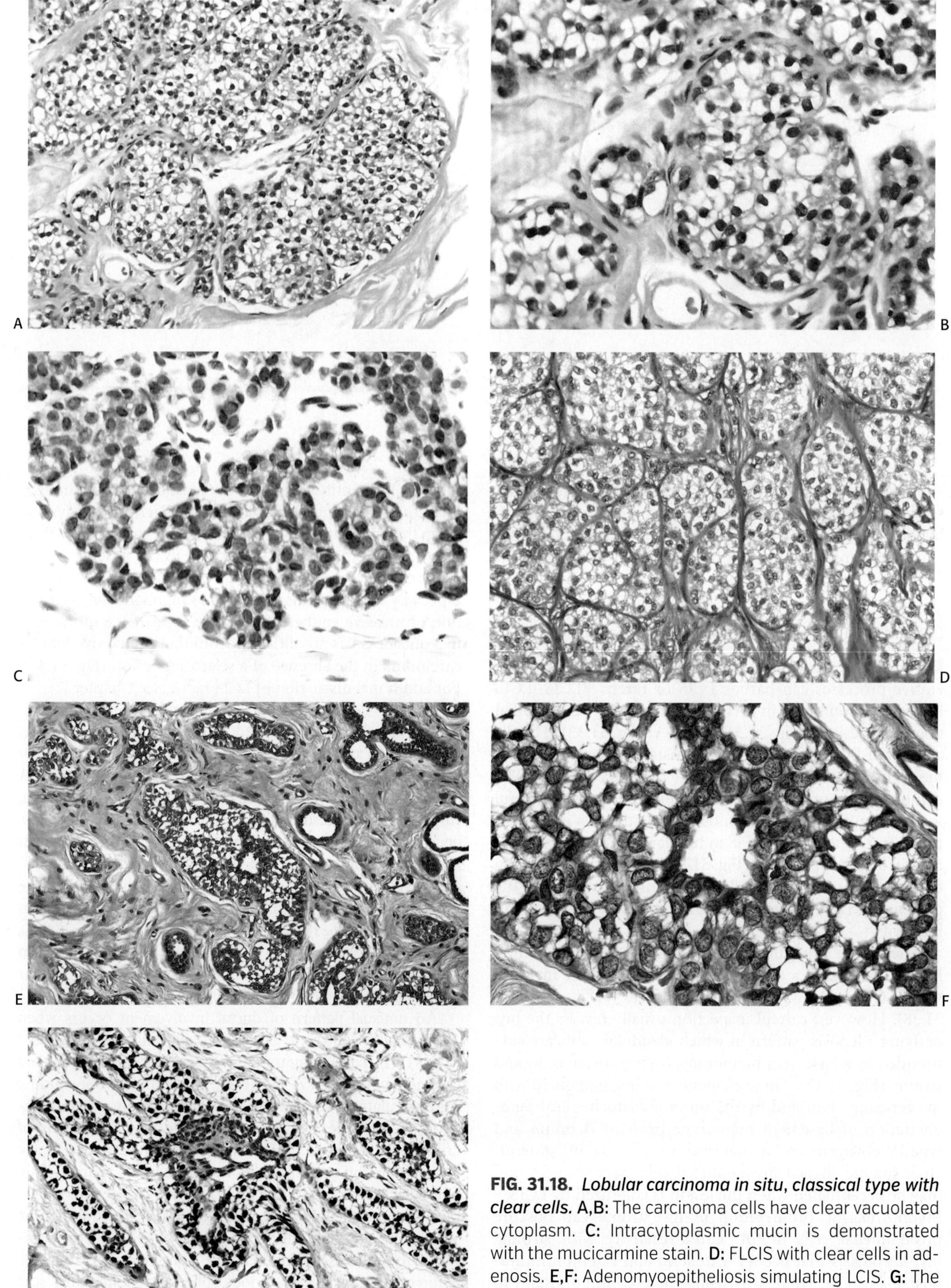

FIG. 31.18. ***Lobular carcinoma in situ, classical type with clear cells.*** **A,B:** The carcinoma cells have clear vacuolated cytoplasm. **C:** Intracytoplasmic mucin is demonstrated with the mucicarmine stain. **D:** FLCIS with clear cells in adenosis. **E,F:** Adenomyoepitheliosis simulating LCIS. **G:** The p63 immunostain highlights the nuclei of myoepithelial cells in adenomyoepitheliosis.

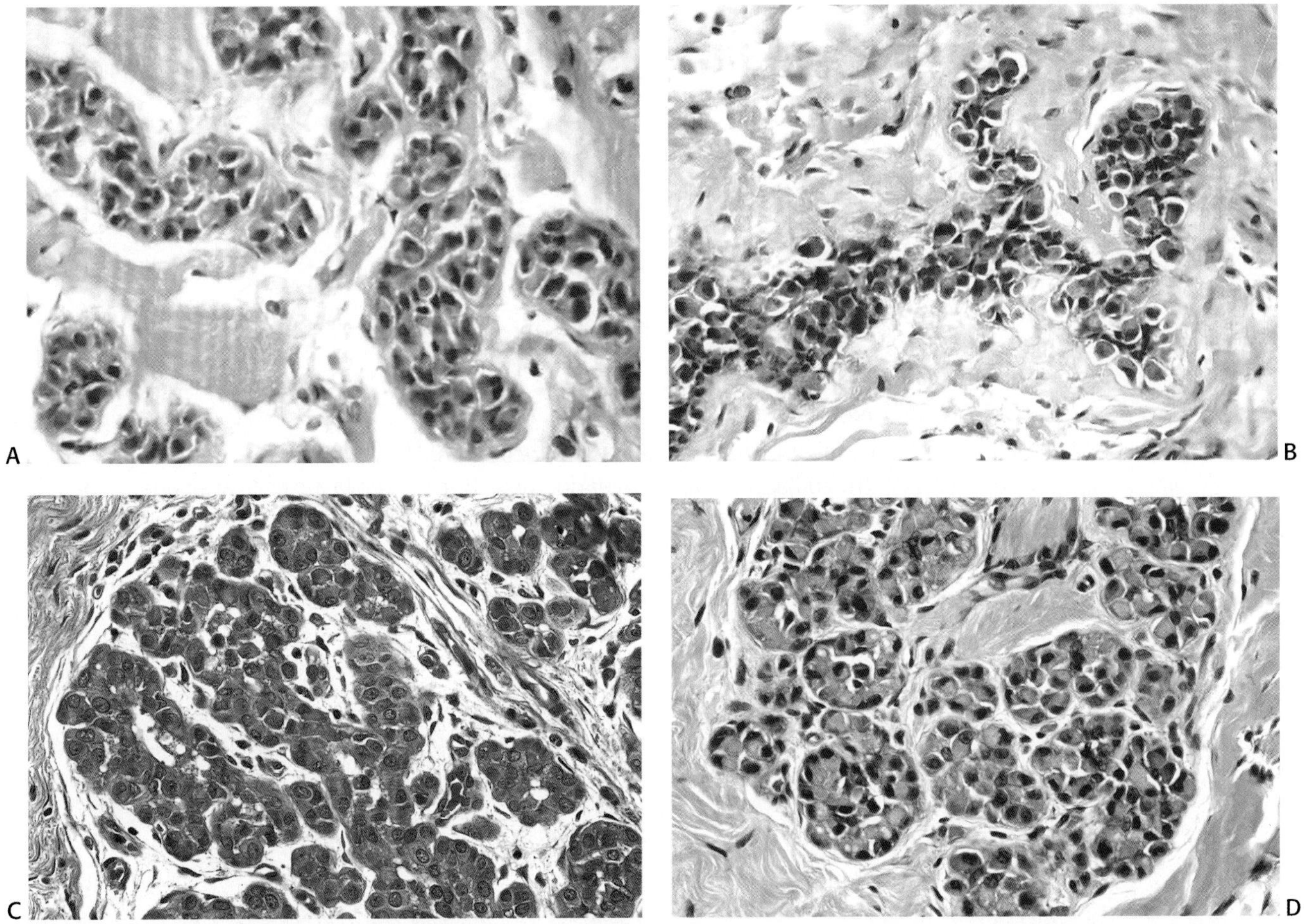

A B C D

FIG. 31.19. ***Lobular carcinoma in situ with myoid pleomorphic cells.*** **A,B:** The dyscohesive carcinoma cells have deeply stained, dense cytoplasm and irregular contours. **C,D:** Other examples of myoid PLCIS.

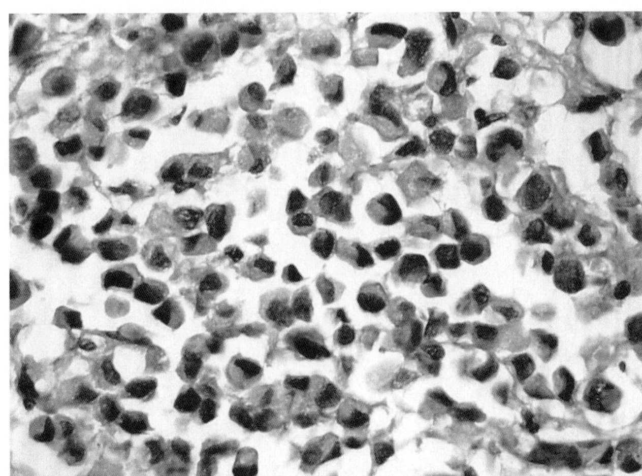

FIG. 31.20. ***Invasive lobular carcinoma with myoid pleomorphic cells.*** Many cells have eccentric nuclei. It is usually possible to demonstrate intracytoplasmic mucin in such cells.

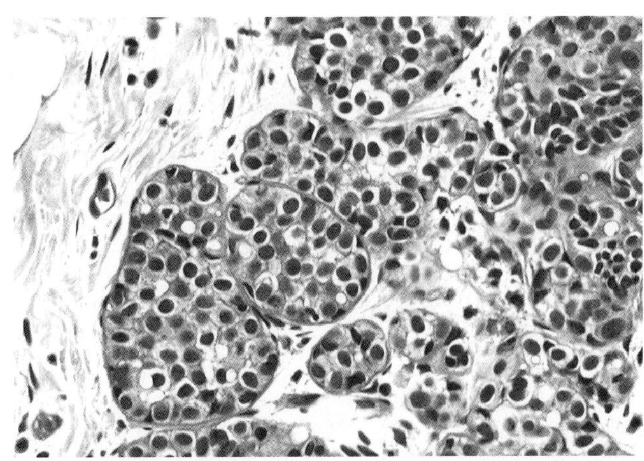

FIG. 31.21. ***Lobular carcinoma in situ, classical type with mosaic features.*** The cohesive cells have distinct cell borders and central nuclei. A few signet ring cells are present.

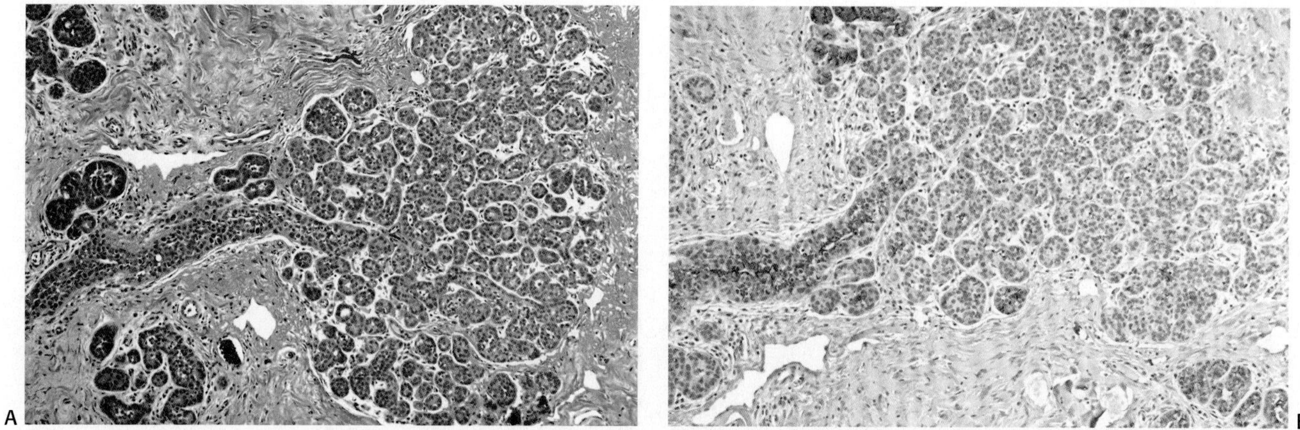

FIG. 31.22. ***Lobular carcinoma in situ, classical type with duct extension.*** **A:** *In situ* carcinoma involving a lobule as well as extralobular and intralobular ductules. **B:** The neoplastic cells are negative for E-cadherin. Residual ductal cells (*at the periphery of the lobule*) are positive for E-cadherin.

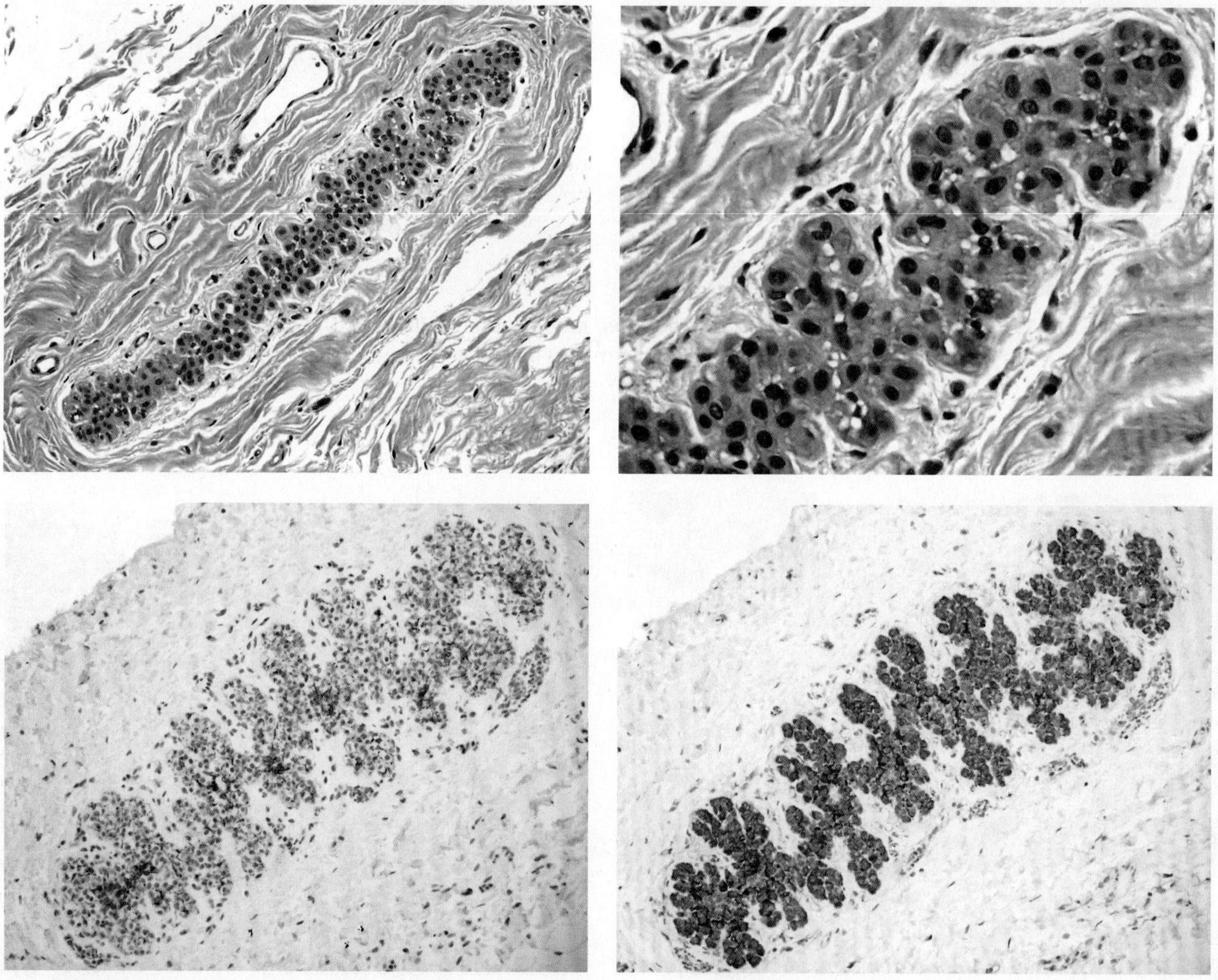

FIG. 31.23. ***Lobular carcinoma in situ, postmenopausal.*** **A,B:** *In situ* carcinoma fills an atrophic lobular ductule. **C,D:** The carcinoma cells are E-cadherin negative **(C)** and show cytoplasmic reactivity for p120 **(D)**.

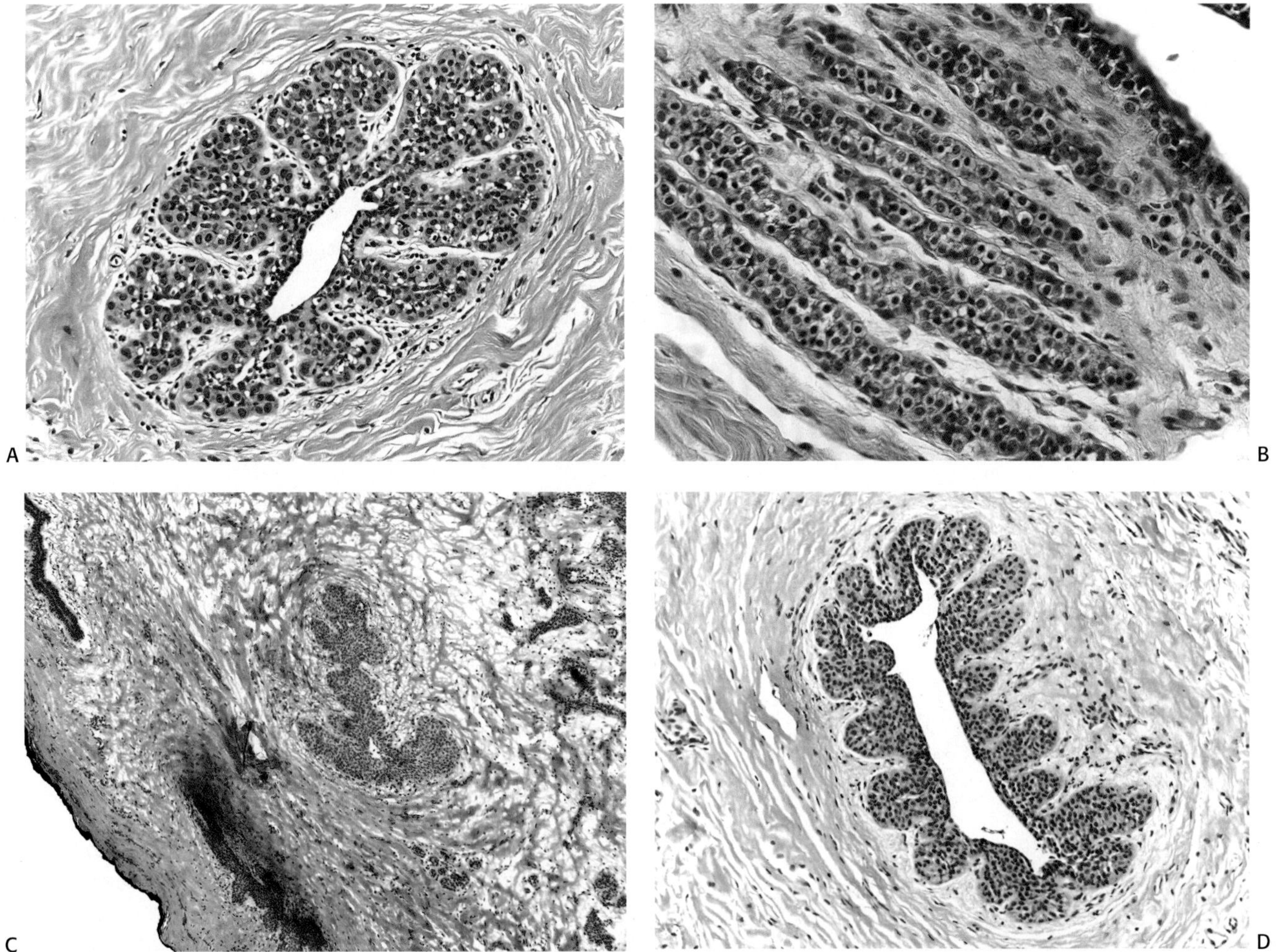

FIG. 31.24. ***Lobular carcinoma in situ, classical type with cloverleaf ductal pattern.*** **A:** *In situ* carcinoma bulges outward forming protruding buds around a duct. **B:** LCIS in glands around a duct, cut longitudinally, produces a complex serrated appearance. **C,D:** LCIS of classical type in an FS of the nipple margin in a nipple-sparing mastectomy. The corresponding paraffin-embedded permanent FS control is seen in **(D)**. Both preparations display LCIS with the cloverleaf pattern.

Cytology

Lobular carcinoma may be suspected in a fine-needle aspiration (FNA) specimen if signet ring cells are identified associated with detached fragments of lobular epithelium, so-called lobular casts. The samples are usually so sparsely cellular that a positive diagnosis is rarely possible.[75] The distinction between LCIS or PLCIS and invasive lobular carcinoma of either type cannot be made with certainty in an aspiration specimen.[72] The diagnosis of PLCIS in a ductal lavage sample has been reported.[76]

Microinvasion

The term "microinvasion" is applied to invasive carcinoma measuring less than 1 mm (T1mic). Invasive foci that are 1 mm or larger are described by the extent measured in a histologic section or in the gross specimen. This definition of microinvasion is the same as has been recommended for ductal carcinoma (Chapter 12). Microinvasive lobular carcinoma is a rare entity. Ross and Hoda[77] were able to document only 16 examples among 75,250 breast carcinomas (0.02%) recorded at the New York Presbyterian-Weill Cornell Medical Center between 1991 and 2009.

Microinvasive foci are characterized by carcinoma cells distributed singly or in slender cords within the stroma (Figs. 31.40 and 31.46).[78] One clue to the possible presence of these obscure invasive foci is slightly increased stromal cellularity that may contain activated myofibroblasts and lymphocytes as well as carcinoma cells.

Microinvasion should be looked for, especially when the specimen contains FLCIS with marked enlargement of duct–lobular structures accompanied by necrosis and calcification. Subtle irregularities of lobular gland borders suggesting disruption of the basement membrane are also of particular concern in FLCIS. Most if not all paraffin blocks

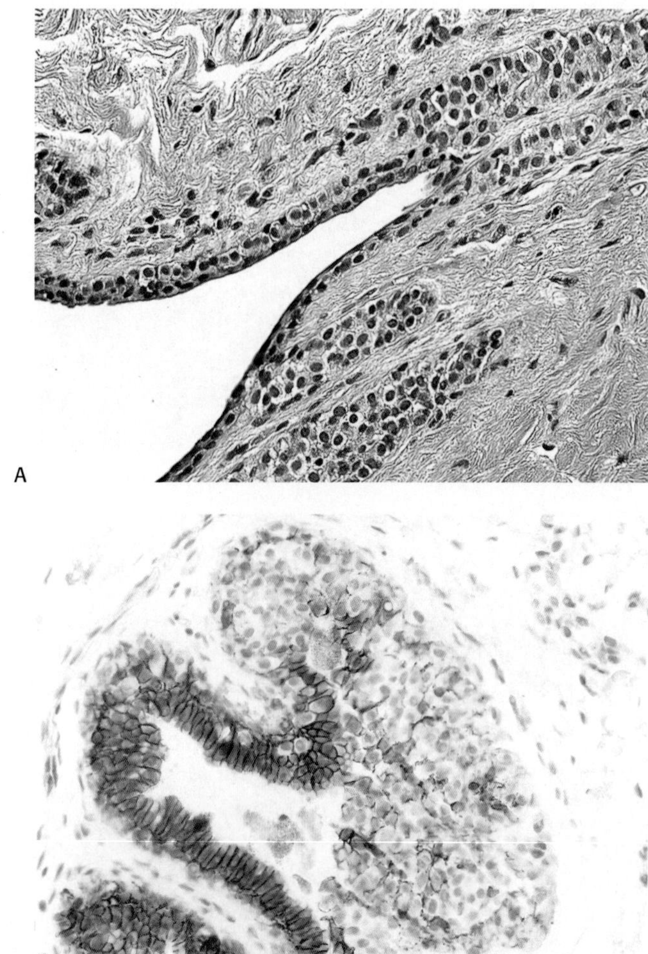

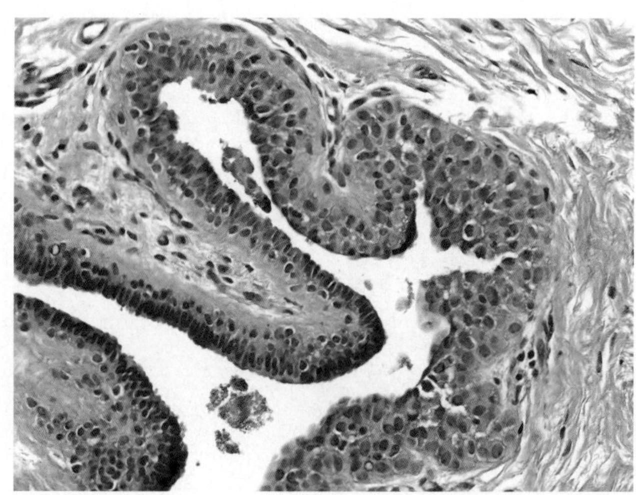

FIG. 31.25. ***Lobular carcinoma in situ, classical type with pagetoid ductal involvement.*** **A:** Pagetoid involvement of a duct by LCIS. **B,C:** Pagetoid ductal involvement of LCIS. The neoplastic cells are negative for E-cadherin **(C)**.

of tissue involved by FLCIS should be examined with a CK immunostain accompanied by a contemporaneous hematoxylin and eosin (H&E) recut slide.

Because of the limited sampling provided by needle core biopsy specimens, the diagnosis of microinvasive lobular carcinoma cannot be made on the basis of this sample alone until an excisional biopsy has been performed to establish that there is no further evidence of invasive carcinoma. More than one microinvasive focus may be present in a biopsy specimen.[78] Microinvasion is usually detected close

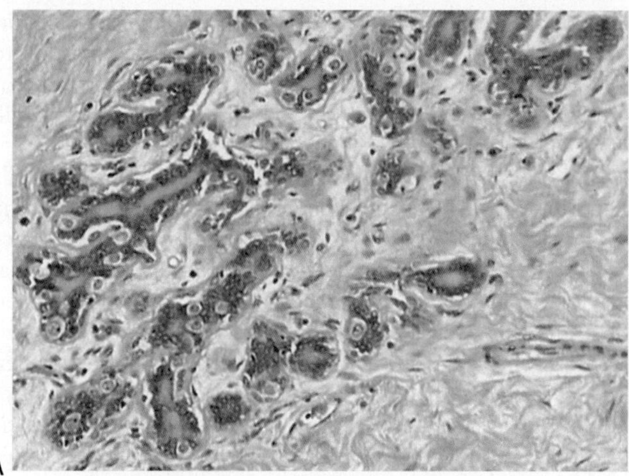

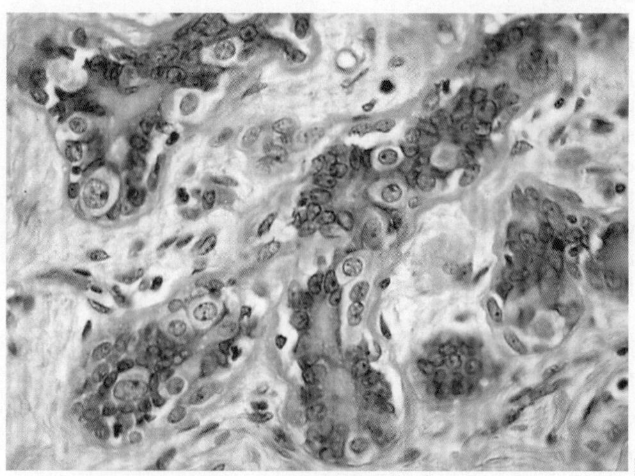

FIG. 31.26. *A,B: Lobular carcinoma in situ, classical type with pagetoid intralobular ductal involvement.*

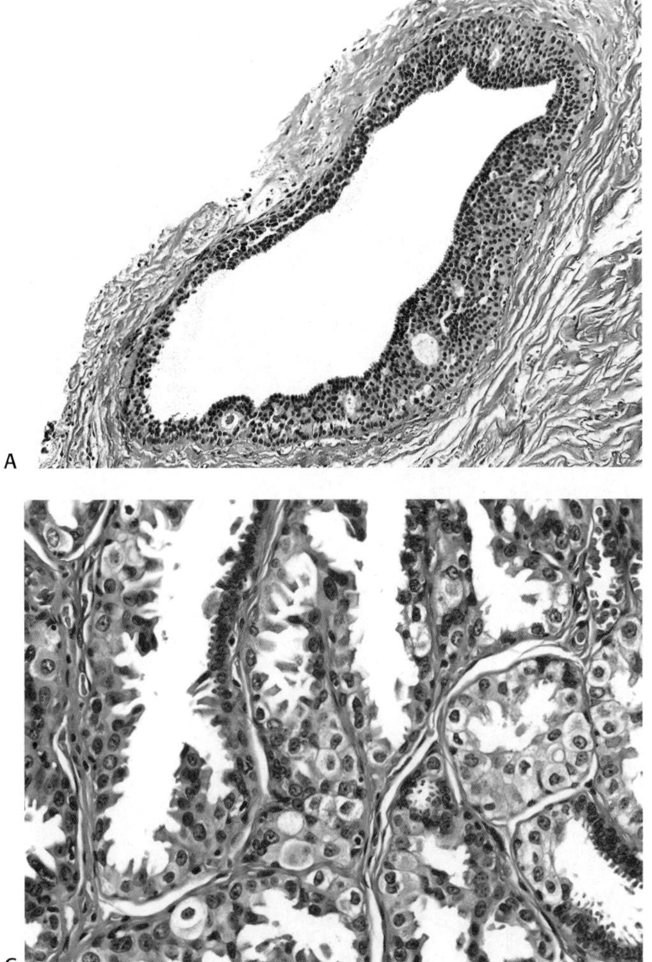

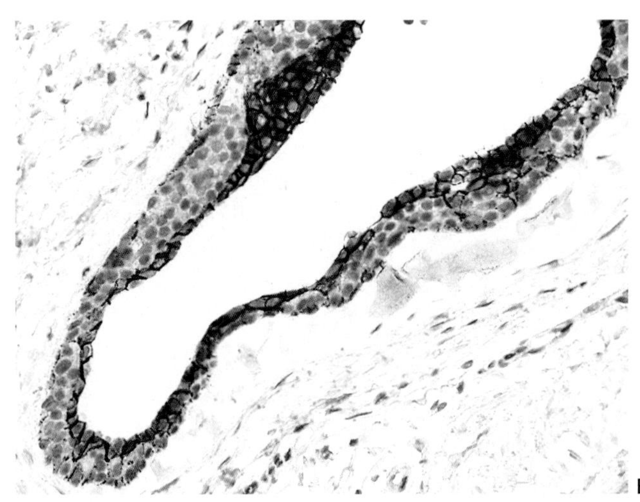

FIG. 31.27. ***Lobular carcinoma in situ, classical type with pagetoid ductal involvement.*** **A,B:** An attenuated layer of nonneoplastic cuboidal ductal cells overlies pagetoid LCIS in these two examples. E-cadherin immunoreactivity in the residual ductal cells on the luminal aspect of the duct is shown in **(B)**. **C:** Pagetoid LCIS cells are shown undermining columnar epithelial cells.

to a focus of LCIS, but rarely there is no contiguous *in situ* carcinoma. When LCIS, PLCIS, or ALH is identified in a needle core or surgical breast biopsy, the tissue should be thoroughly and carefully examined for inconspicuous foci of invasive lobular carcinoma.

Because small numbers of classical invasive lobular carcinoma cells may be difficult to distinguish from inflammatory or stromal cells, immunohistochemistry (IHC) is often helpful in these cases. CK immunostains such as CK7, 34βE12, and AE1/3 are especially useful to highlight carcinoma cells in the stroma. A new, contemporaneous H&E recut slide should be made whenever recuts are made to investigate microinvasion by CK IHC. Double immunostaining for actin as well as CK has been recommended to detect small or microinvasive foci of lobular carcinoma in sclerosing lesions (Fig. 31.39).[79] See Chapter 32 for additional information about microinvasive and invasive lobular carcinoma.

Electron Microscopy

Electron microscopic studies have documented the origin of LCIS from lobular epithelial cells.[80,81] Intracytoplasmic lumina lined by microvilli are seen ultrastructurally in the typical case. Residual myoepithelial cells have been demonstrated in LCIS by electron microscopy and by IHC.[82] The distribution of these cells tends to be disordered in LCIS, and they are less numerous or absent when LCIS is associated with invasive lobular carcinoma.[82] Protrusion of LCIS cells through the basement membrane, a phenomenon described by Ozzello,[80] seems to be uncommon. Discontinuity of basement membranes in LCIS was demonstrated histochemically by Andersen,[83] who noted that gaps could be detected not only in the basement membranes of lobules with LCIS but also in normal lobules.

IHC and Molecular Genetics

LCIS and PLCIS exhibit strong reactivity for the low-molecular-weight CK 34βE12 that is typically absent or weakly present in DCIS.[84] Immunoreactivity for ER and PR is found in virtually all examples of LCIS[85–88] but in only about 66% of PLCIS and in less than 25% of PLCIS with apocrine features.[88] Green et al.[89] found significantly more immunoreactivity for ER-α and ER-β in LCIS than in normal lobules. There was no significant difference in the expression of ER-α and ER-β subtypes between LCIS alone and LCIS associated with invasive lobular carcinoma. On the other hand, the immunoexpression of PR was significantly reduced in

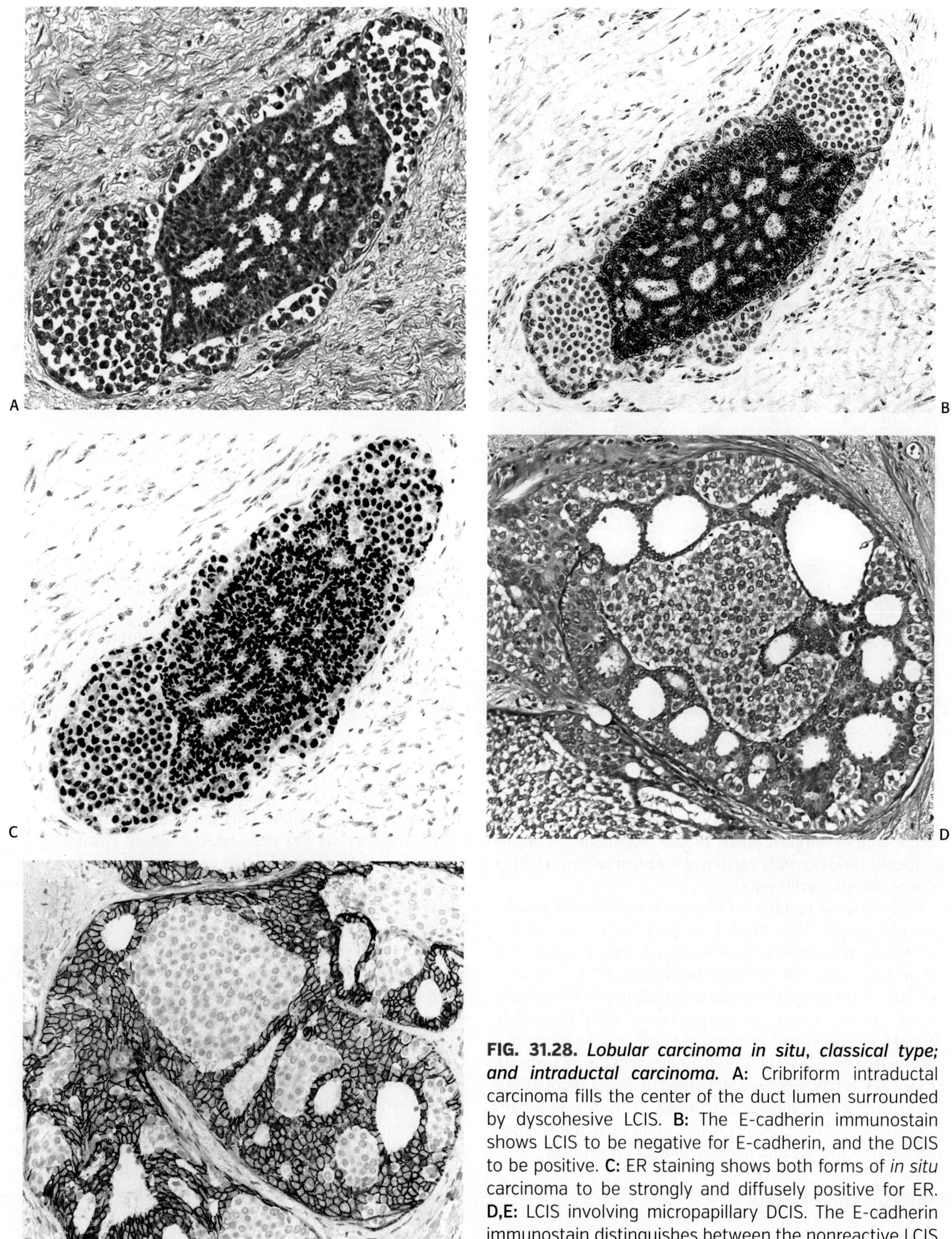

FIG. 31.28. ***Lobular carcinoma in situ, classical type; and intraductal carcinoma.*** **A:** Cribriform intraductal carcinoma fills the center of the duct lumen surrounded by dyscohesive LCIS. **B:** The E-cadherin immunostain shows LCIS to be negative for E-cadherin, and the DCIS to be positive. **C:** ER staining shows both forms of *in situ* carcinoma to be strongly and diffusely positive for ER. **D,E:** LCIS involving micropapillary DCIS. The E-cadherin immunostain distinguishes between the nonreactive LCIS and the reactive DCIS **(E)**.

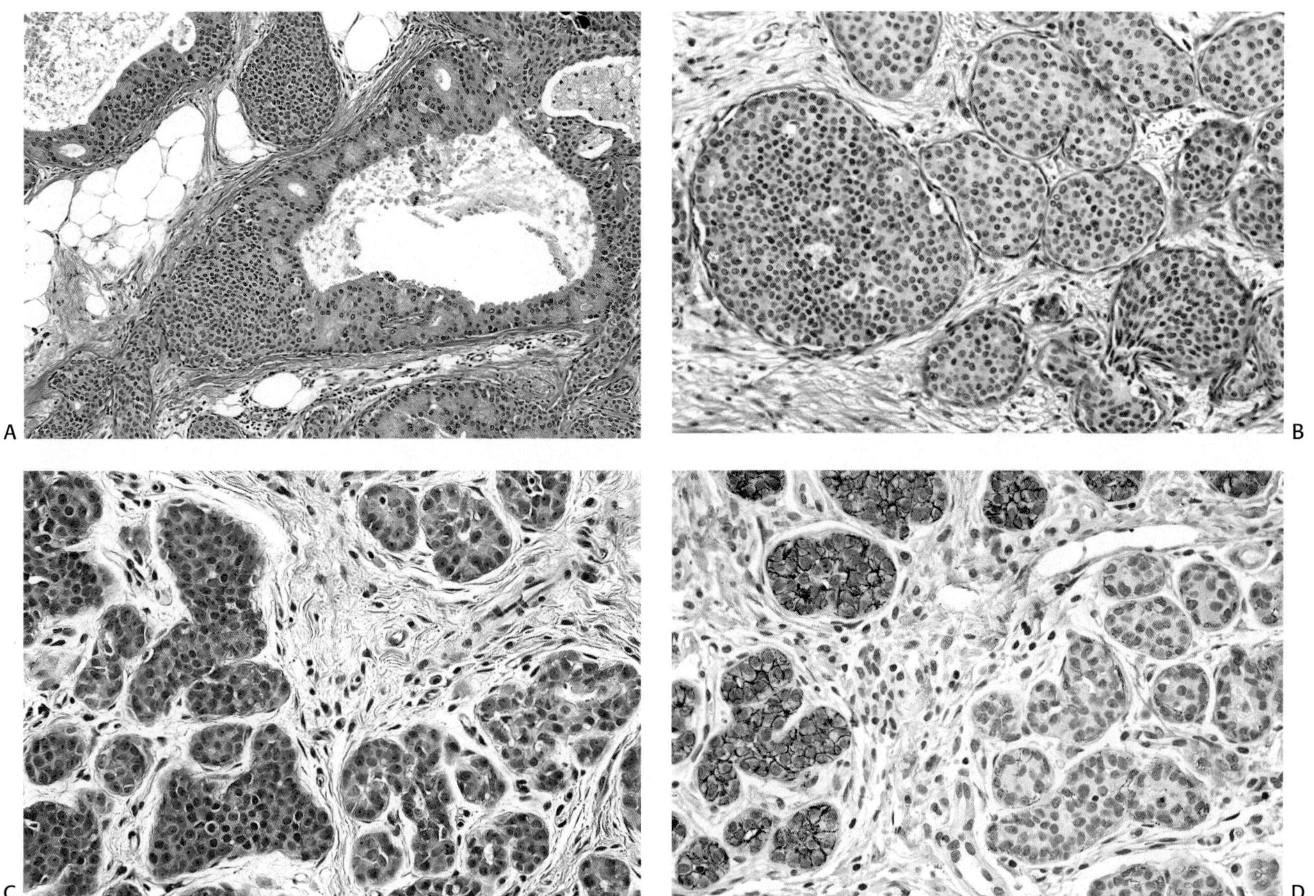

FIG. 31.29. ***Lobular carcinoma in situ, classical type associated with cribriform intraductal carcinoma.*** **A,B:** LCIS classical type, coexists with apocrine intraductal carcinoma. Classical LCIS in expanded lobular glands **(B)**. **C,D:** LCIS, classical type associated with lobular involvement by solid type of intraductal carcinoma. The LCIS cells are negative for E-cadherin (*lower right*), and the DCIS is positive **(D)**.

LCIS associated with invasive lobular carcinoma than in pure LCIS. When compared with the invasive carcinoma in a particular case, ER-α expression tended to be higher in the corresponding LCIS.

Membrane immunoreactivity for HER2/*neu* is very rarely detected in LCIS, and when present, it is associated with PLCIS.[61,85,88,90,91] Expression of GCDFP-15 is found in apocrine PLCIS.[88] Overexpression of p53 is not detectable by IHC in LCIS, and it is infrequently present in PLCIS.[92] Proliferative activity, as estimated by Ki67 nuclear reactivity, is typically low in classical LCIS. A higher risk of invasive relapse has been associated with a higher (greater than 10%) proliferation rate in classical LCIS, as measured by Ki67.[85] The relative risk (RR) of invasive relapse in the high-Ki67 LCIS group when compared with the low-Ki67 LCIS group was 10.42. PLCIS is characterized by a Ki67 index greater than 10%.[88]

The normal E-cadherin complex consists of the transmembrane E-cadherin protein that is anchored to the cell's actin cytoskeleton through α- and β-catenins localized to the inner cell membrane region. The E-cadherin immunostain is strongly positive in nonneoplastic ductal epithelium and in lesions derived from it, including intraductal carcinoma. Normal and nonneoplastic hyperplastic lobular epithelium is strongly E-cadherin positive. Almost all neoplastic lobular lesions are characterized by the absence of E-cadherin reactivity. Disruption of the E-cadherin complex in lobular neoplastic cells is reflected in loss of membranous reactivity for E-cadherin and p120 catenin and the appearance of cytoplasmic p120 catenin staining.[92,93] This phenomenon occurs early in the development of neoplastic lobular lesions, including ALH. Data presented by Morrogh et al.[94] suggest that the extent of E-cadherin expression is progressively downregulated in a stepwise fashion from normal lobules to LCIS and to invasive lobular carcinoma. Complete loss of α- and β-catenin immunoreactivity was observed more often in LCIS associated with invasive lobular carcinoma than in LCIS not accompanied by invasive lobular carcinoma. This is also illustrated by the finding that complete dissociation of the cadherin–catenin complex was found in 2/11 (18%) pure LCIS lesions, 11/18 (61%) of LCIS associated with invasive lobular carcinoma, and in 16/18 (89%) of invasive lobular carcinomas.

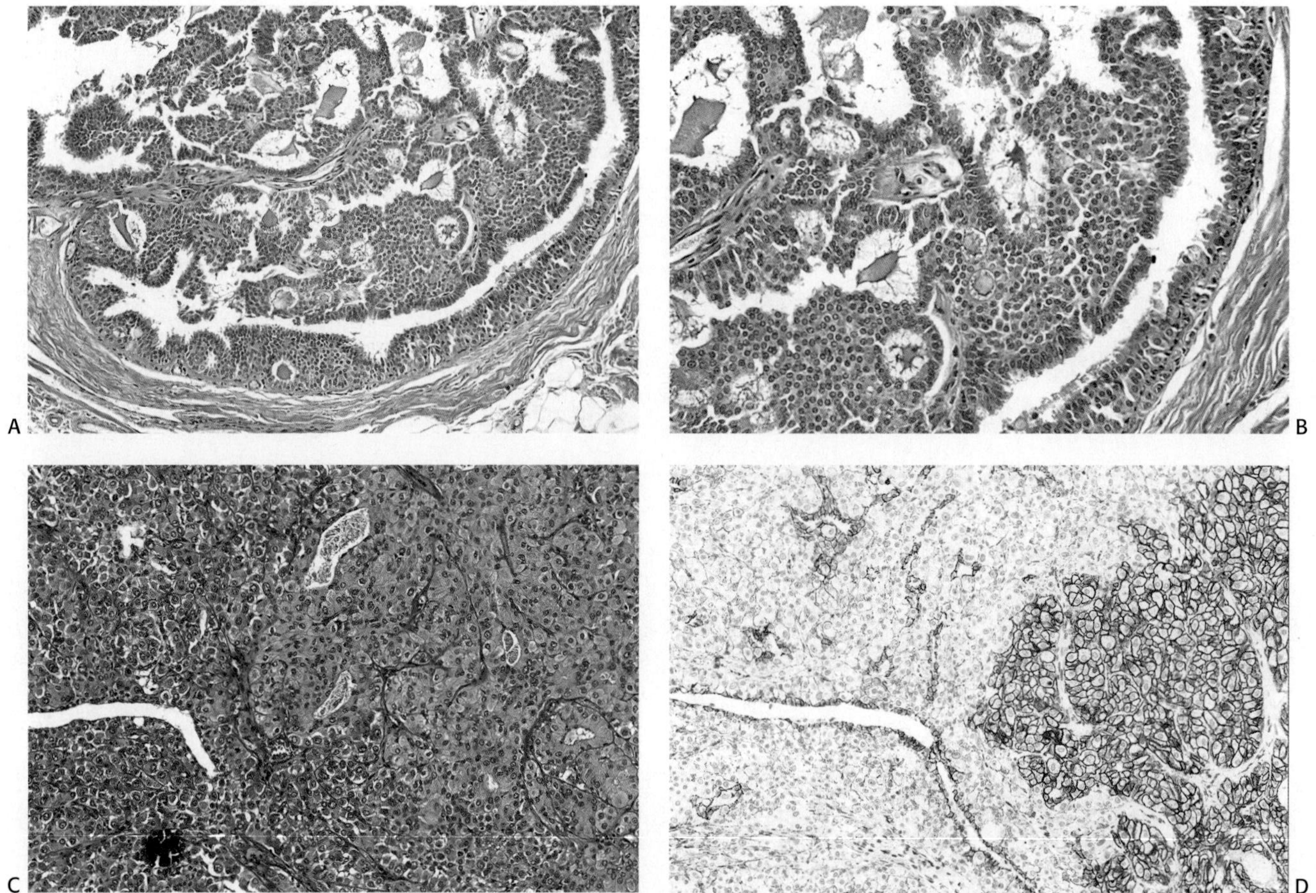

FIG. 31.30. ***Lobular carcinoma in situ, classical type, in papillary neoplasms.*** **A,B:** LCIS has a pagetoid distribution in this papilloma. **C,D:** LCIS involves a solid papillary carcinoma. The E-cadherin immunostain shows the characteristic reactivity pattern of the two neoplastic processes: positive in DCIS, negative in LCIS **(D)**.

In a minority of instances, lobular neoplastic cells display fragmented and discontinuous E-cadherin reactivity that is weaker than reactivity in ductal epithelium.[51,95] There are also exceedingly infrequent cases in which *in situ* carcinoma that is morphologically indistinguishable from LCIS displays strong E-cadherin membrane reactivity, sometimes coexisting with adjacent foci of LCIS that are E-cadherin negative. In these cases, the E-cadherin–positive *in situ* carcinoma has been interpreted as LCIS with "aberrant" E-cadherin reactivity.

Similar observations have been made in extremely rare examples of invasive lobular carcinoma where E-cadherin–positive and E-cadherin–negative foci coexist in a single tumor.[96] More extensive investigation of instances of "aberrant" E-cadherin reactivity is needed to determine the proper classification of these lesions. For the present, if the histologic appearance is that of LCIS, PLCIS, or invasive lobular carcinoma of the classical or pleomorphic type with E-cadherin expression, the lesion should be classified as lobular carcinoma with "aberrant" E-cadherin expression.

Loss of cell cohesion in lobular neoplastic lesions is largely attributable to genetic alterations in the *E-cadherin* gene. Losses in chromosome 16q 22.1, the site of the *E-cadherin* gene, are a common abnormality found in LCIS and PLCIS.[97] Despite the high frequency of somatic *E-cadherin* mutations in LCIS, germ line *E-cadherin* mutations are rarely detected in these patients.[97–99] Molecular analysis has been carried out to detect loss of heterozygosity (LOH) in samples of LCIS and ALH isolated by microdissection.[100] The investigators found LOH at chromosome 11q13 in 33% of evaluable cases. The frequency of LOH was higher (50%) in LCIS associated with infiltrating lobular carcinoma than in LCIS without an invasive component (11%). LOH at 11q13 was detected in 2 (10%) of 19 samples of ALHs and in 9 (41%) of 22 infiltrating lobular carcinomas. The authors concluded that LOH at 11q13 in LCIS might be a marker for increased risk of developing invasive carcinoma subsequently. Chen et al.[88] found loss in 16q and gains in 1q in most of the samples of LCIS and PLCIS that they studied. Genomic alterations were significantly more numerous in apocrine PLCIS than in LCIS or nonapocrine PLCIS.

Mastracci et al.[101] reported that all 12 examples of LCIS without invasive lobular carcinoma subjected to detailed immunohistochemical and molecular study were not

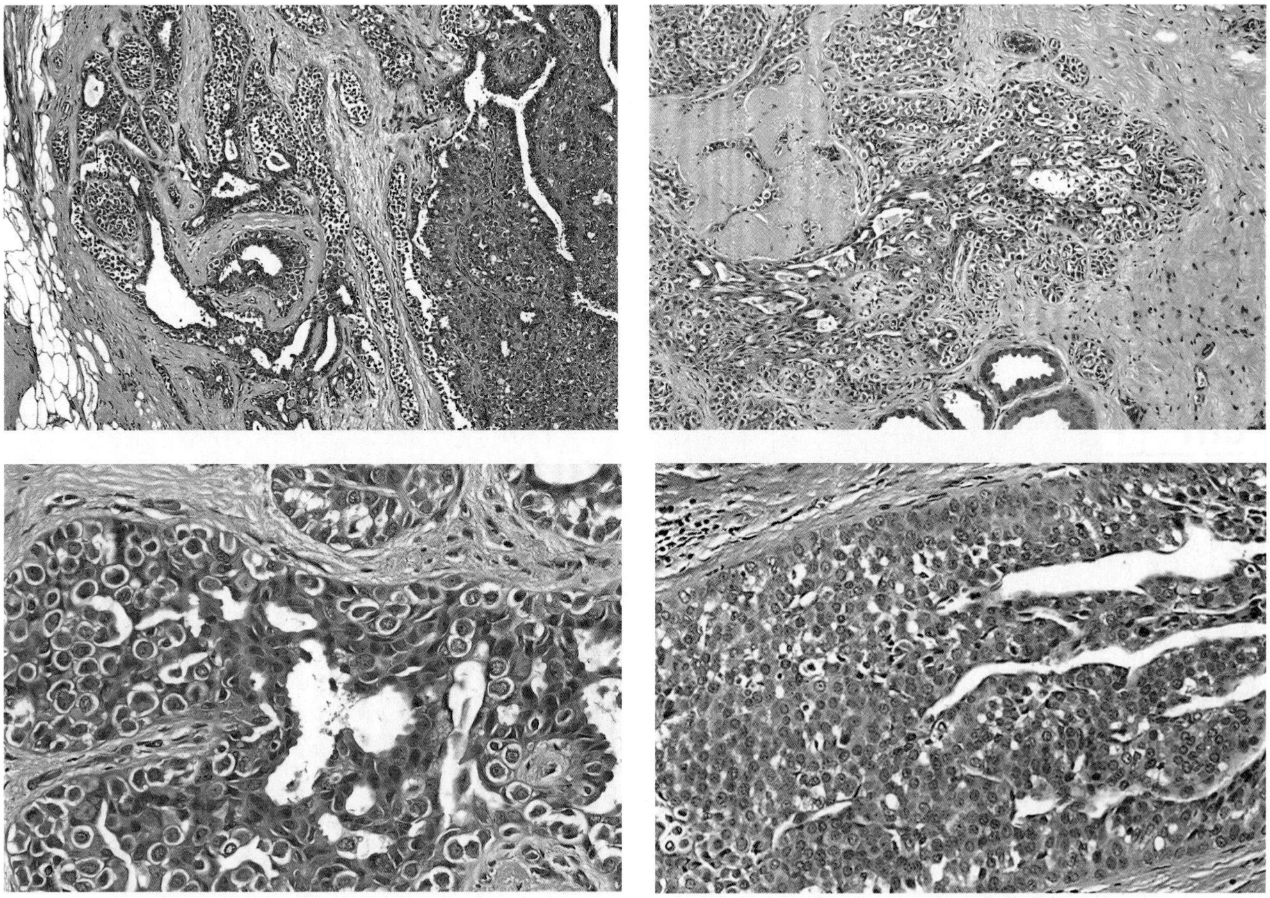

FIG. 31.31. ***Lobular carcinoma in situ, classical type, in complex sclerosing papillary lesions.*** **A:** Part of a sclerosing lesion with florid adenosis involved by LCIS. Marked dyscohesion of LCIS cells is apparent (*left*). **B,C:** Pagetoid LCIS. **D:** Part of the lesion where the ductal epithelium has been reduced to a thin layer of cells that outline slender remnants of the duct lumen and overlie LCIS.

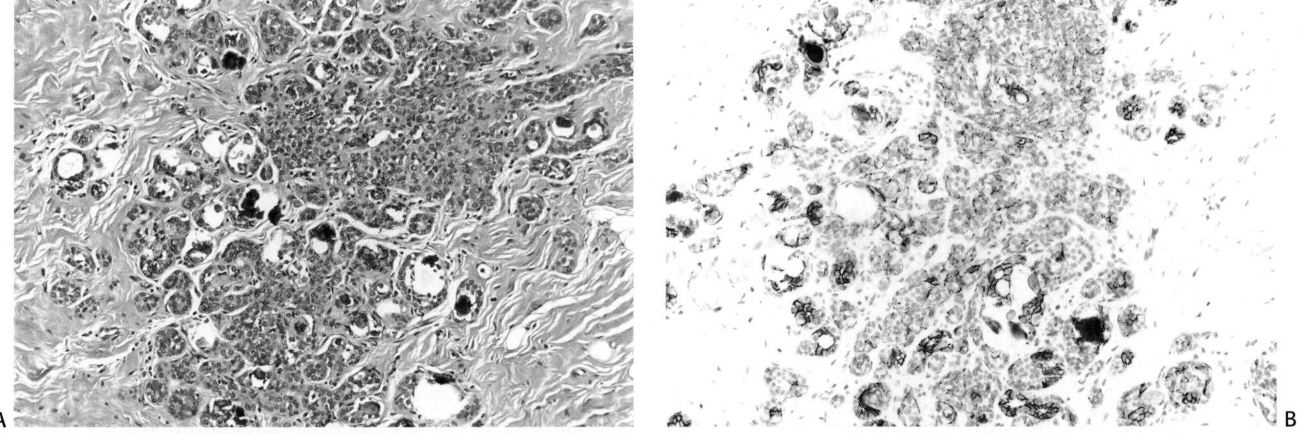

FIG. 31.32. ***Lobular carcinoma in situ, classical type in sclerosing adenosis.*** **A:** LCIS of the classical type involving SA with calcifications. LCIS cells are negative for E-cadherin **(B)**.

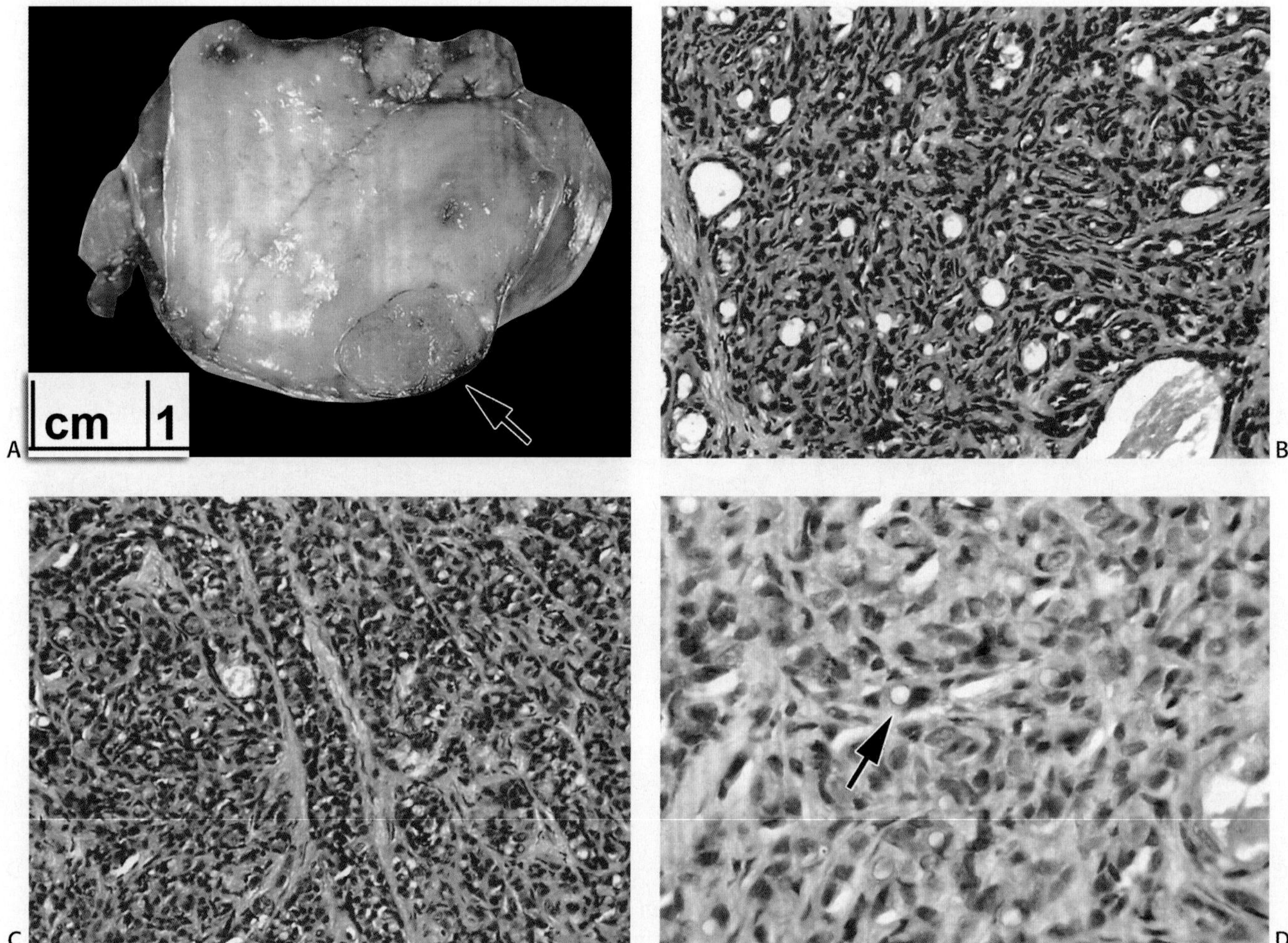

FIG. 31.33. ***Lobular carcinoma in situ, classical type in sclerosing adenosis.*** **A:** The gross appearance of the tan, oval, adenosis tumor at the lower edge of the specimen (*arrow*) gave no indication that it harbored LCIS. **B:** SA in the tumor shown in **(A)**. **C:** LCIS in the SA. **D:** Intracytoplasmic mucin in the LCIS (*arrow*).

reactive for E-cadherin and β-catenin. Ten of these lesions were negative for α-catenin and one was α-catenin positive. E-cadherin, α-catenin, and β-catenin reactivities were absent from all but one of a series of ALH lesions examined by the same investigators. These results suggest that loss of E-cadherin and catenin reactivity is an early event in the development of lobular neoplastic lesions. Keller et al.[102] described an exceptional instance of germ line mutations in the *E-cadherin* gene in a patient with familial diffuse gastric carcinoma and lobular carcinoma of the breast, but data presented by Rahman et al.[98] appear to indicate that LCIS is not caused by constitutional mutations in the *E-cadherin* gene.

Evidence that the prolactin receptor gene (*PRLr*) located on chromosome 5p is amplified in LCIS and invasive lobular carcinoma was presented by Tran-Thanh et al.[103] When compared with intraductal carcinoma and IDCs, LCIS and invasive lobular carcinoma exhibited significantly greater amplification of PRLr. IHC showed that PRLr expression was mainly localized in the cytoplasm, with expression found in the cytoplasm in 29/40 (73%) of *in situ* lobular lesions and 14/40 (35%) of DCIS. There was no significant difference in the expression of PRLr between ALH, LCIS, and PLCIS. Expression of PRLr was not increased when invasive lobular carcinoma was present with LCIS.

Differential Diagnosis

The differential diagnosis of LCIS encompasses a number of proliferative changes affecting terminal ducts and lobules. These include pregnancy-like or "pseudolactational" hyperplasia, clear-cell change, apocrine metaplasia, and ALH. The epithelium in all of these conditions, except ALH, is E-cadherin positive. Pregnancy-like hyperplasia occurs in premenopausal women who are not pregnant and in postmenopausal women. The cells may have vacuolated cytoplasm, apical apocrine tufts, and hyperchromatic, atypical nuclei. Psammoma-like calcifications that develop in this lesion lead to detection by mammography and needle core biopsy procedures. Clear-cell change that can be found in pre- and postmenopausal women may be a variant of apocrine metaplasia because the

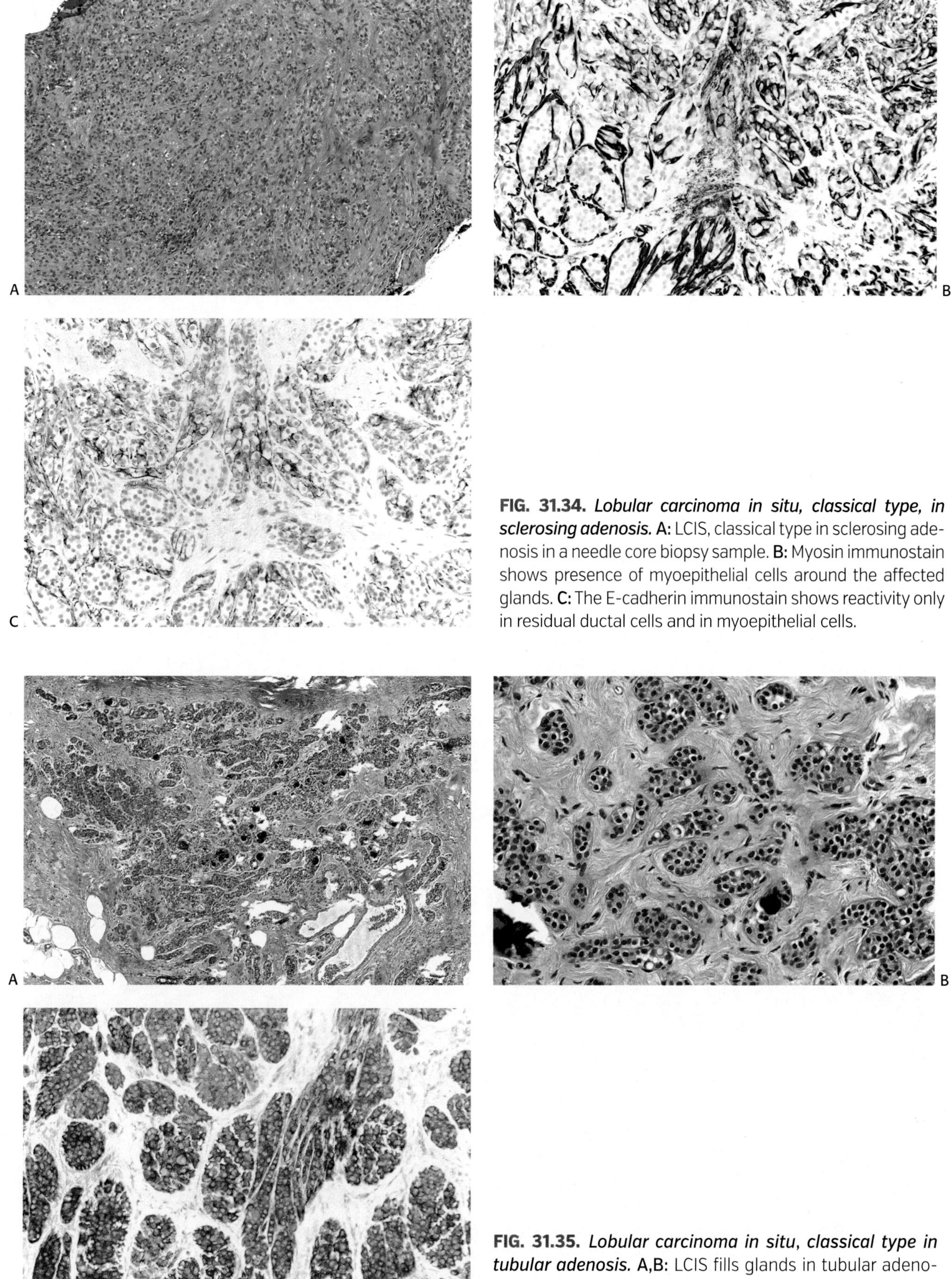

FIG. 31.34. ***Lobular carcinoma in situ, classical type, in sclerosing adenosis.*** **A:** LCIS, classical type in sclerosing adenosis in a needle core biopsy sample. **B:** Myosin immunostain shows presence of myoepithelial cells around the affected glands. **C:** The E-cadherin immunostain shows reactivity only in residual ductal cells and in myoepithelial cells.

FIG. 31.35. ***Lobular carcinoma in situ, classical type in tubular adenosis.*** **A,B:** LCIS fills glands in tubular adenosis. **C:** The p120 immunostain shows cytoplasmic reactivity in neoplastic cells (C).

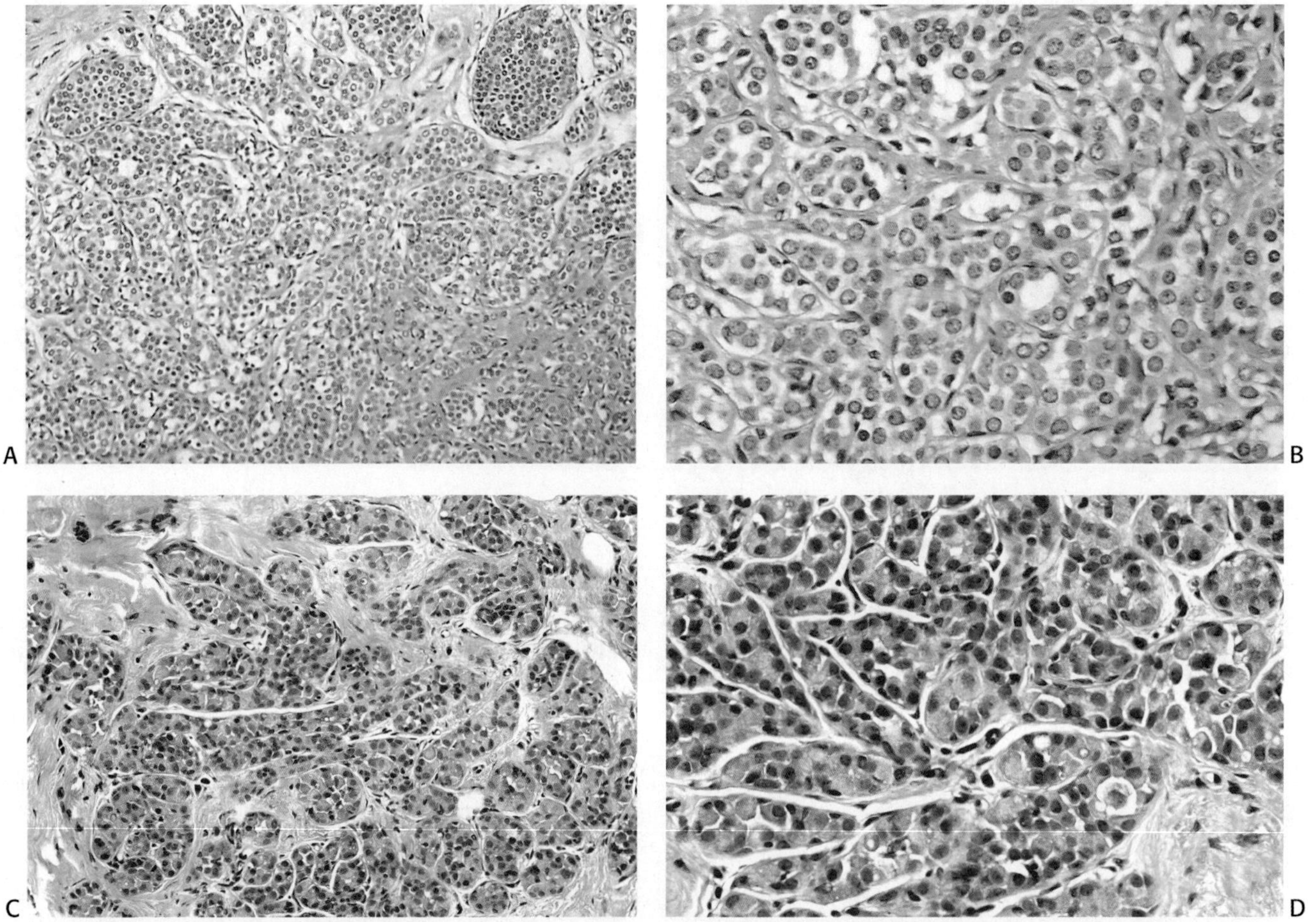

FIG. 31.36. ***Lobular carcinoma in situ, classical type in florid sclerosing adenosis.*** **A:** The underlying adenosis structure is obscured. **B:** At higher magnification, closely approximated adenosis glands appear to be outlined by basement membranes and myoepithelial cells. **C,D:** FLCIS, classical type, in another example of SA.

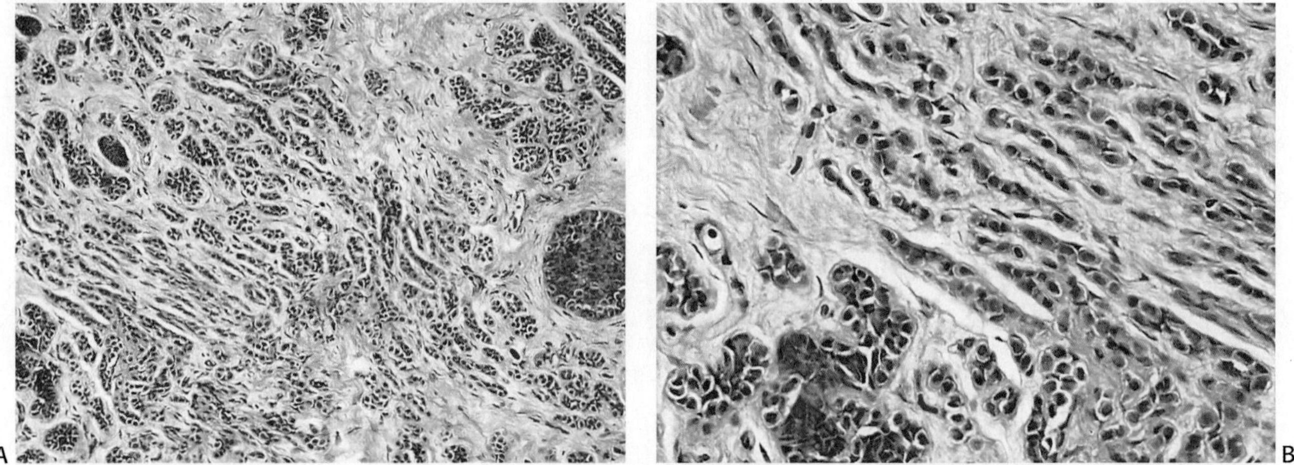

FIG. 31.37. ***Lobular carcinoma in situ in sclerosing adenosis with a tubular pattern.*** **A,B:** Pagetoid spread is evident in the lobule in the *upper right* (hematoxylin–phloxine–safranin).

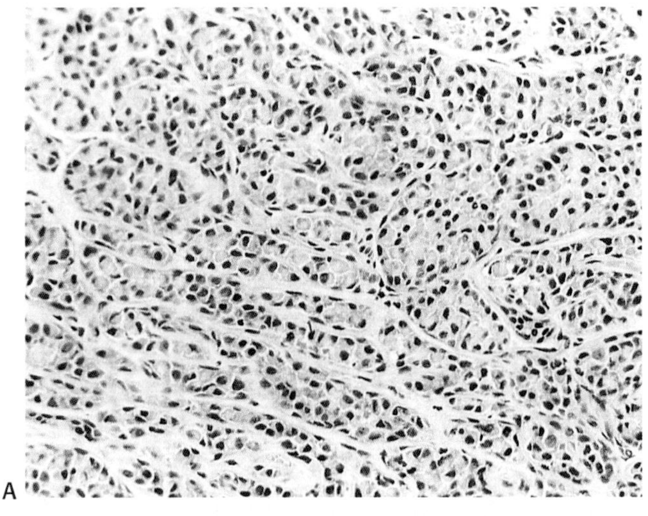

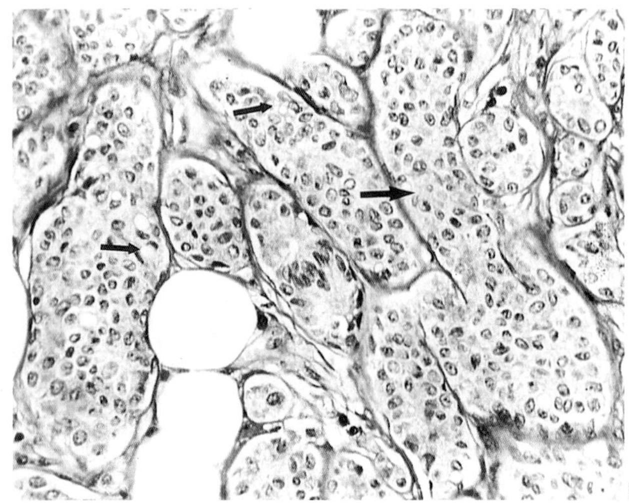

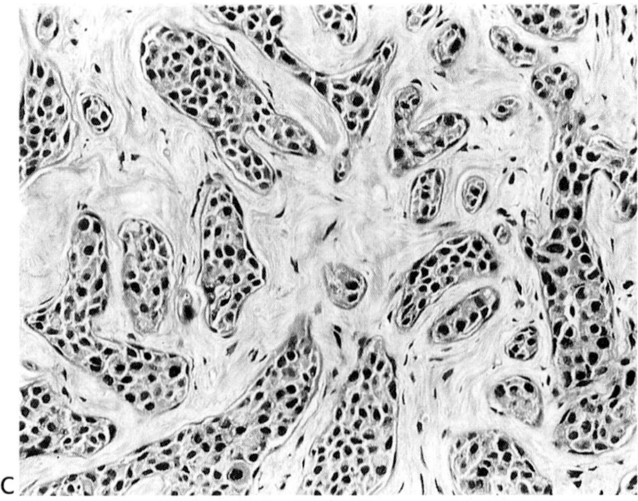

FIG. 31.38. ***Lobular carcinoma in situ in sclerosing adenosis.*** Four different structural patterns are represented. **A:** A compact lesion with fully developed classical LCIS in the round glands. **B:** LCIS with conspicuous signet ring cells (*arrows*). **C:** The adenosis glands are separated by distinct basement membranes. Note the loss of cohesion among the carcinoma cells.

two are sometimes combined in a single lobule (Fig. 31.47). Clear-cell change usually does not form calcifications and is often an incidental finding in a surgical or needle core biopsy specimen. These lobular proliferative changes are discussed and illustrated in Chapter 1.

Apocrine metaplasia in lobular hyperplasia is manifested by cytoplasmic eosinophilia (Fig. 31.48). The orderly cellular distribution of this alteration is usually distinguishable from LCIS with cytoplasmic eosinophilia, lobular involvement by apocrine PLCIS, and lobular extension of apocrine intraductal carcinoma (Fig. 31.49). Difficulty making these distinctions may be encountered in limited needle core biopsy samples. As previously noted, the cells in apocrine lobular hyperplasia are immunoreactive for E-cadherin.

ATYPICAL LOBULAR HYPERPLASIA

Clinical Presentation

There are no specific clinical features associated with the diagnosis of ALH. The clinical indications for a biopsy procedure are the same as those that lead to the detection of LCIS—a palpable lesion or a mammographic abnormality. ALH is usually an incidental finding, not specifically associated with the abnormality that prompted the diagnostic procedure. In one series of atypical lesions discovered in mammography-directed biopsy specimens, only 1 of 11 instances (9%) of ALH was at the site of the radiographic abnormality.[104] On the other hand, 20 of 42 instances (48%) of atypical duct hyperplasia in this series were at the site of the mammographic lesion.

Microscopic Pathology

The glandular proliferation in ALH has some features of LCIS, but they are not sufficiently developed to qualify for the latter diagnosis. As is the case with atypical duct hyperplasia and intraductal carcinoma, there are no universally accepted criteria for the precise distinction between ALH and LCIS. Qualitative and quantitative factors must be considered.

Quantitative criteria for the diagnosis of LCIS discussed in the foregoing section influence the distribution of cases classified as ALH. Most authors have recommended that

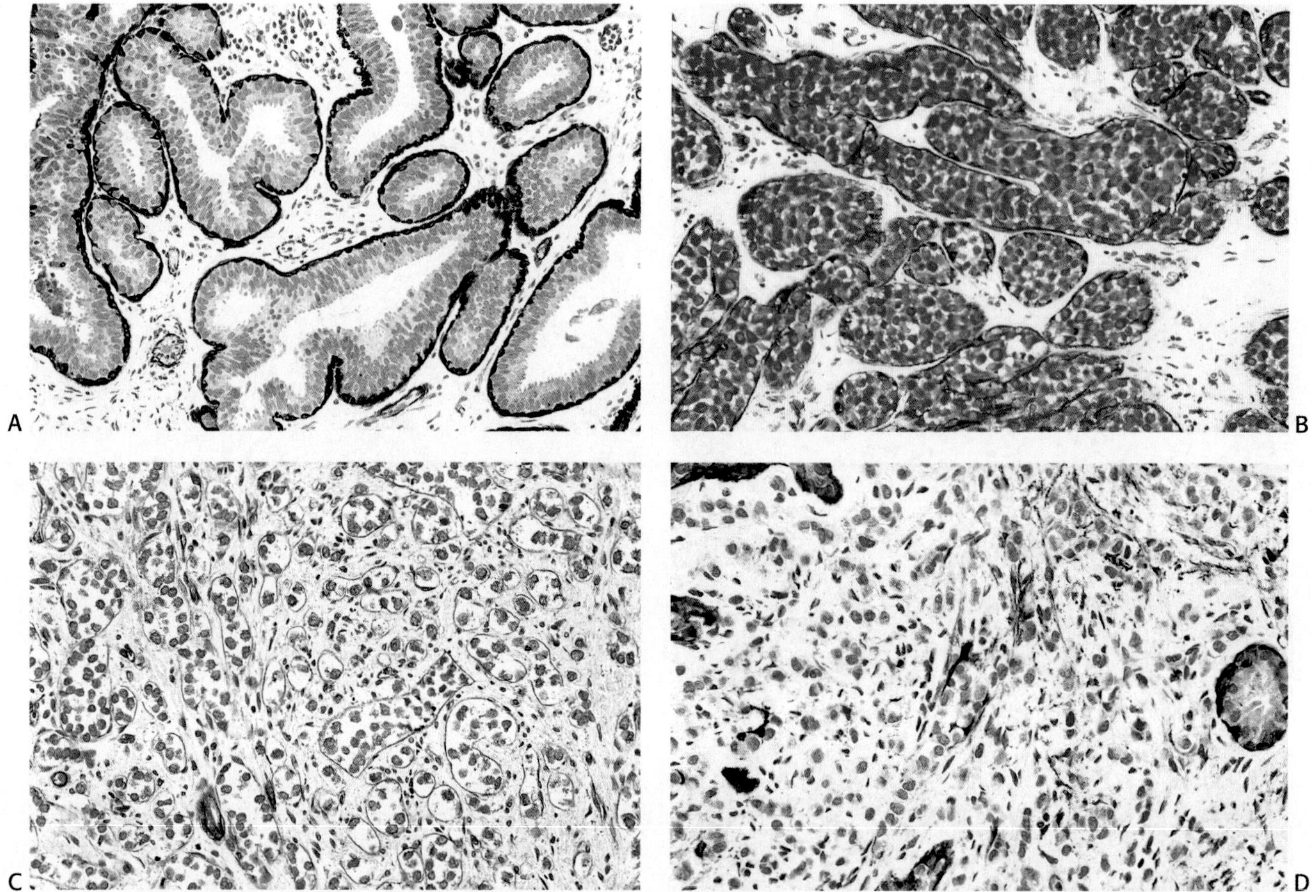

FIG. 31.39. ***Lobular carcinoma in situ, classical type in sclerosing adenosis, immunohistochemistry.*** **A:** Myoepithelial cells in florid SA are highlighted with the SMM-HC immunostain. **B:** Double immunolabeling demonstrates CK AE1/3-positive LCIS (*red*) and SMA-positive myoepithelial cells (*brown*). The LCIS is confined within the boundaries of the myoepithelial cells. **C:** An immunostain for laminin demonstrates attenuated basement membranes surrounding the LCIS cells. **D:** Immunoreactivity for SMM-HC was incomplete or absent in the lesion shown in **(C)**, but invasion was not diagnosed because of persistent basement membranes.

lesions that are quantitatively below the level of LCIS be classified as ALH. As previously discussed, some authors have diagnosed ALH if the lobular change involved less than 50% of one lobule or if less than one complete lobule was affected. The distinction proposed here, which is admittedly arbitrary, is to render a diagnosis of ALH if less than 75% of a lobule shows the features of LCIS (Figs. 31.50 and 31.51). Rarely, the distinction may be made solely on this quantitative basis. More often, qualitative criteria are also considered.

Qualitatively, ALH is characterized by the presence, within one or more lobules or ductules, of abnormal cells similar to those found in LCIS. In the least conspicuous configuration, these cells replace a portion of the normal lobular glandular epithelium, effacing the lumina (Fig. 31.52). Acinar units are not enlarged at this proliferative level (Fig. 31.53). As the process evolves, the accumulation of a greater number of these cells causes progressive acinar expansion, but the borders of individual acinar units and intralobular ductules remain indistinct (Fig. 31.54). Clear delineation of intralobular acinar units filled by the abnormal cell population is an important feature that distinguishes LCIS from ALH. This phenomenon reflects the accumulation in the acinar units of enough homogeneous neoplastic cells to cause the individual glands to have a distinct round or oval configuration (Fig. 31.55). The cells in ALH almost always lack intracytoplasmic mucin, and loss of cohesion is not prominent, but immunoreactivity for catenins and E-cadherin is absent.

Similar criteria apply to the diagnosis of some lobular proliferations that involve the terminal duct structures. These alterations tend to occur around rather than in the duct lumen, creating the cloverleaf pattern (Fig. 31.56). The lumen of such a duct is usually clearly defined by a distinct layer of cuboidal or flat ductal cells. Protruding outward from the lumen are circumferential pockets or outpouchings that may be open in continuity with the main duct lumen, or be filled to a variable degree by neoplastic cells

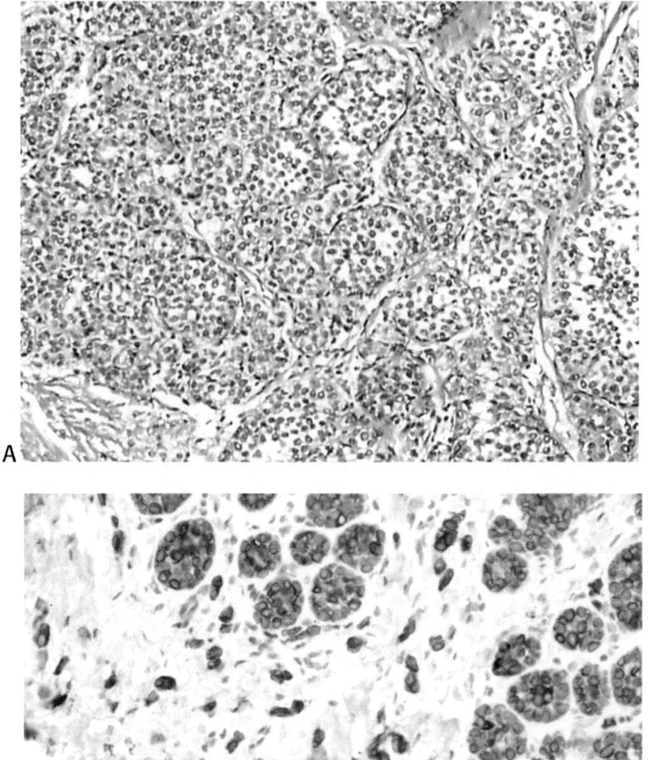

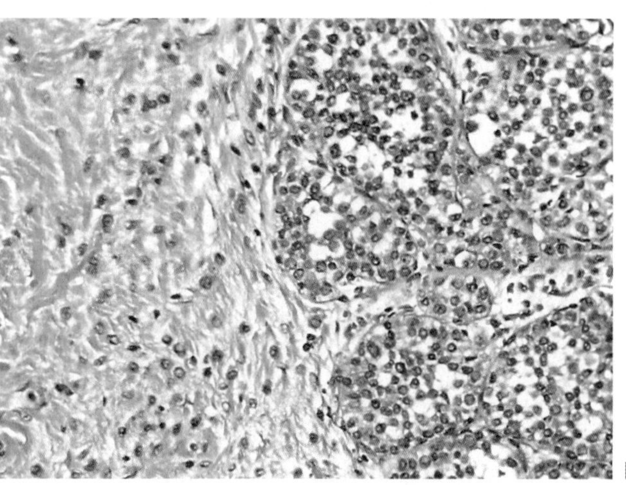

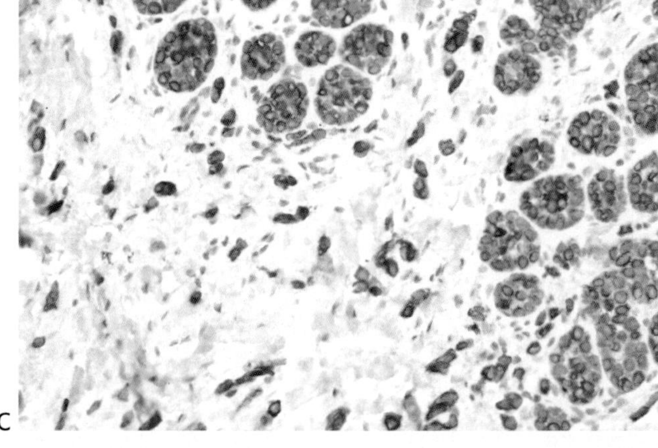

FIG. 31.40. ***Lobular carcinoma in situ, classical type in sclerosing adenosis with microinvasion.*** **A:** FLCIS lesion in SA. **B:** Individual carcinoma cells are shown in the stroma adjacent to the LCIS shown in **(A)**. **C:** Invasive carcinoma cells in the stroma are highlighted by the AE1/3 CK immunostain.

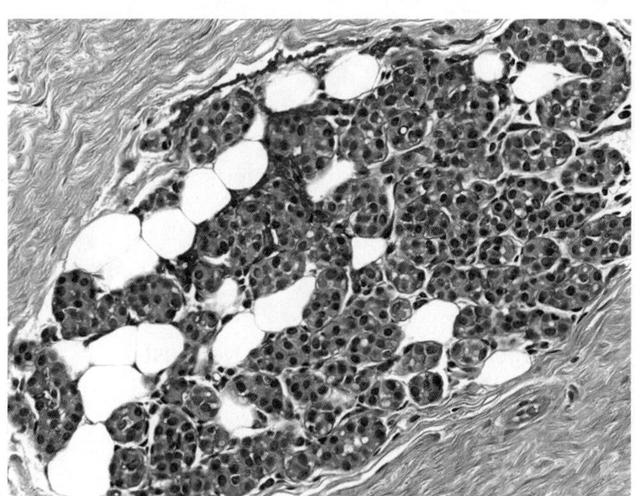

FIG. 31.41. ***Lobular carcinoma in situ, classical type in fat.*** No fibrous stroma separates the LCIS from fat.

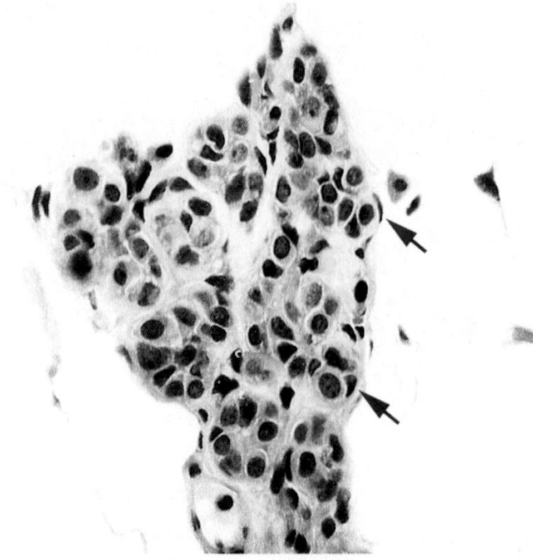

FIG. 31.42. ***Lobular carcinoma in situ, classical type in fat.*** A basement membrane and myoepithelial cells with crescentic nuclei (*arrows*) are present around most groups of carcinoma cells.

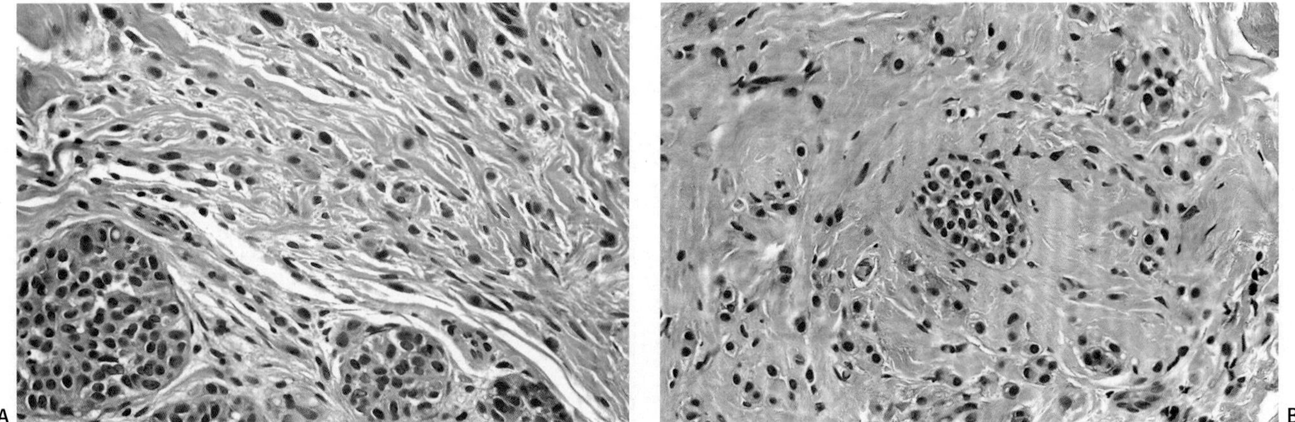

FIG. 31.43. ***Invasive lobular carcinoma associated with LCIS.*** **A,B:** Note desmoplastic reaction around the invasive carcinoma and stromal elastosis in [B].

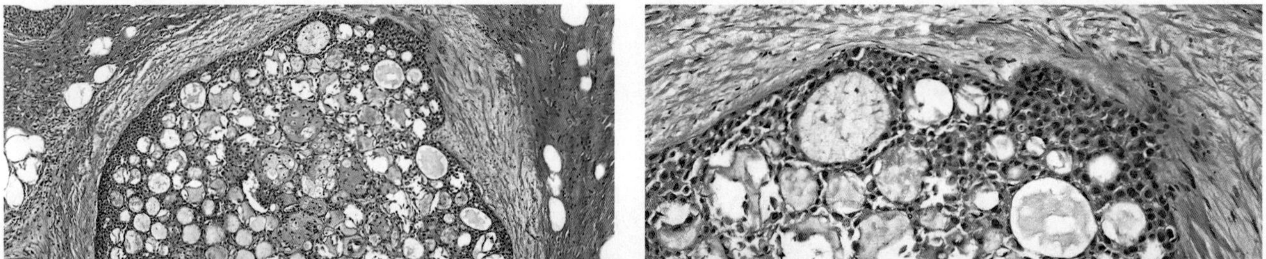

FIG. 31.44. ***Lobular carcinoma in situ, classical type in collagenous spherulosis.*** **A,B:** Neoplastic cells outline the degenerative spherules in this example of collagenous spherulosis in an intraductal papilloma. Fibrovascular stroma containing histiocytes (*arrows*) of the papilloma is shown in the *lower left* corner of **(B)**. **C:** Intracytoplasmic mucin is demonstrated with the mucicarmine stain. Fibrillar material in spherules is also weakly stained. **D:** The distribution of LCIS cells in the collagenous spherulosis is highlighted by the CK7 immunostain. **E:** FLCIS, classical type was also present in the specimen. **F:** Another example of *LCIS*, classical type in collagenous spherulosis. Basement membrane–like material ("spherules") within the cribriform-type luminal spaces is highlighted by the laminin immunostain **(G)**. Myoepithelial cells with nuclei stained for p63 are present around and within the affected glands **(H)**. **I:** LCIS cells are strongly and diffusely positive for ER.

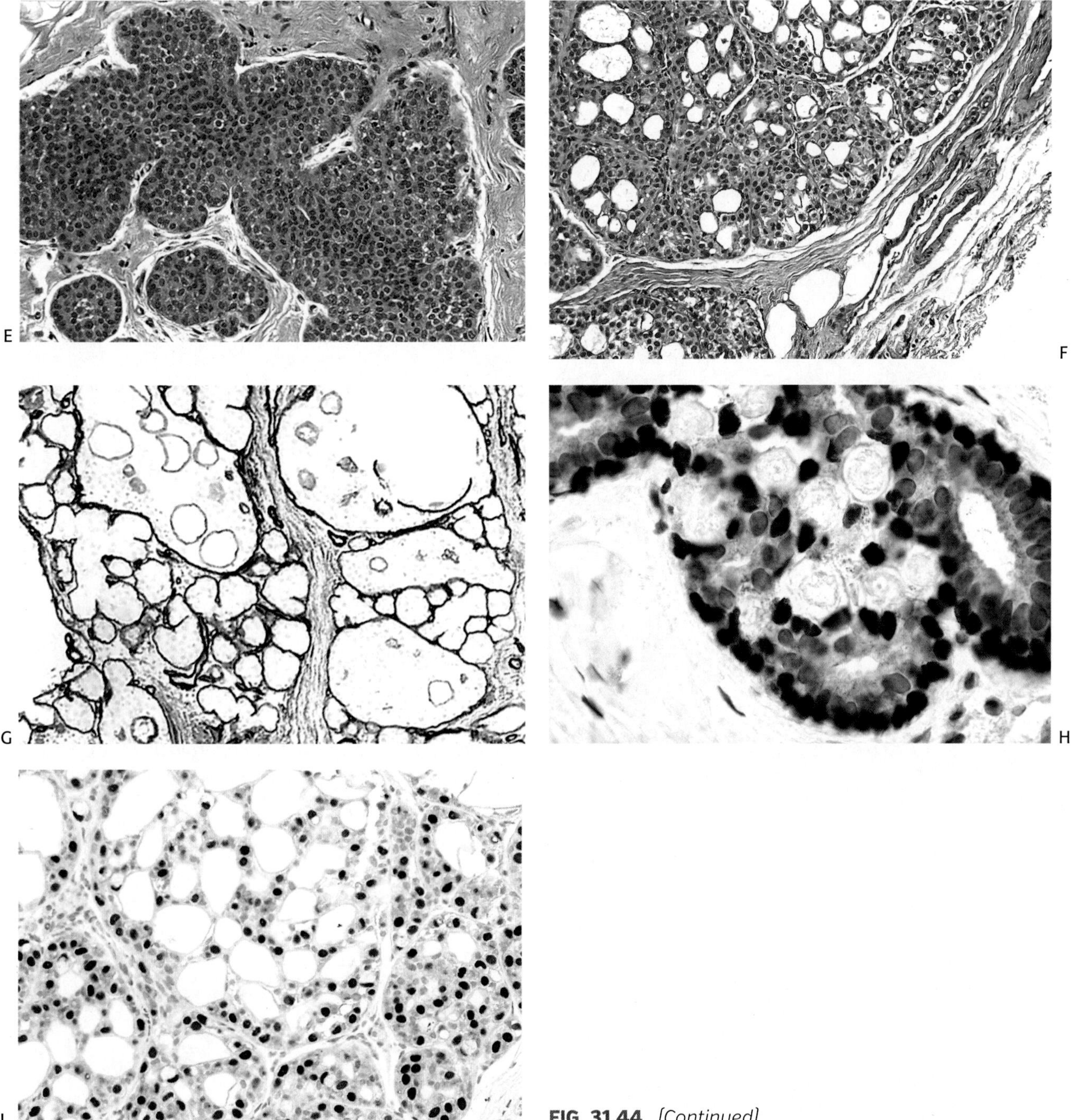

FIG. 31.44. *(Continued)*

(Fig. 31.57). When such ducts are cut transversely or tangentially, the outpouchings have a symmetrical distribution described as a saw-toothed appearance. ALH of ductules is diagnosed when the cellular proliferation in the outpouchings is insufficient to cause them to appear as individual, distinct knobs protruding around the duct. In this situation, the outpouchings are sometimes inhabited by a mixture of normal and neoplastic cells. ALH of terminal ducts may also occur in solid and flat forms that develop when the neoplastic growth is distributed in a continuous layer or around the duct lumen (Fig. 31.58). The flat form of ALH in ducts arises as a consequence of pagetoid spread of lesional cells between the basement membrane and ductal epithelial cells, forming a layer one cell to two cells deep. The solid form is usually composed of a mixture of hyperplastic duct epithelial and atypical lobular cells. ALH in ducts should be distinguished from duct hyperplasia involving terminal ducts or uncoiled lobules (Fig. 31.59) and duct hyperplasia extending into terminal duct lobular units sometimes referred to as "blunt duct adenosis" (Fig. 31.60).

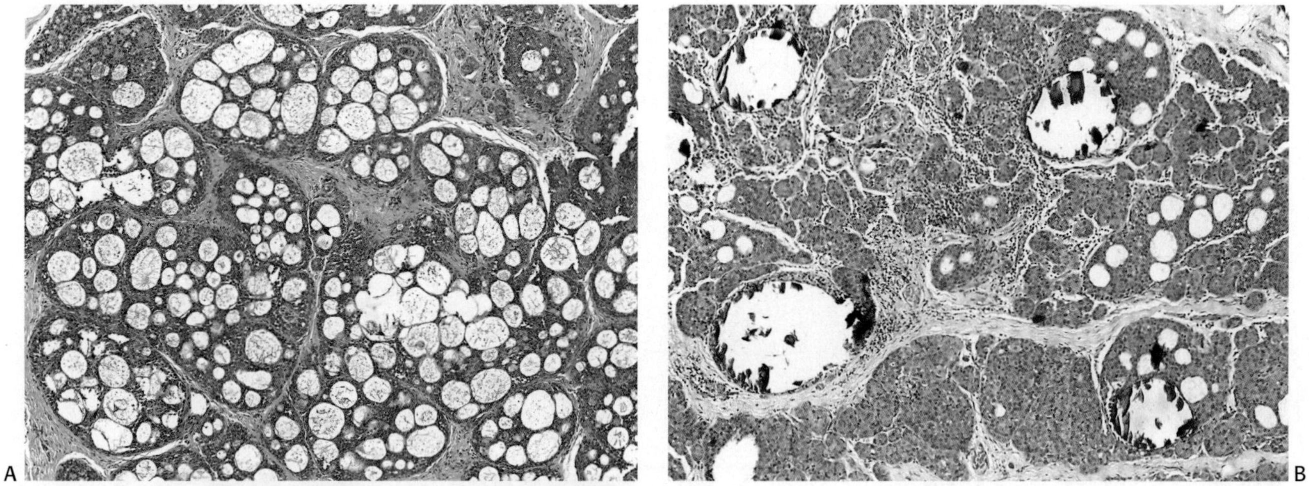

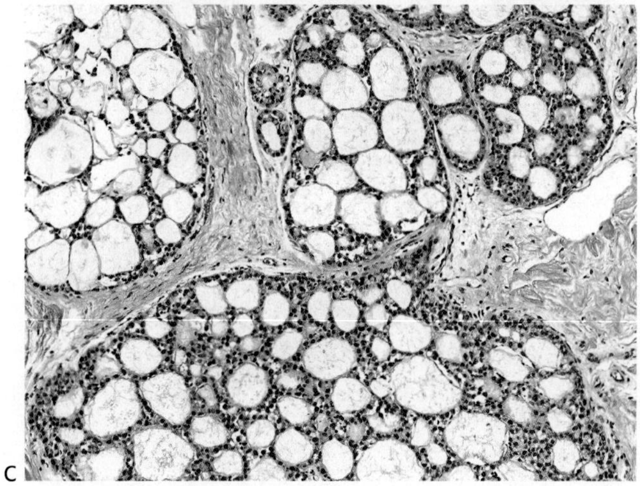

FIG. 31.45. ***Three examples of lobular carcinoma in situ, classical type in collagenous spherulosis*** **(A–C)**. Each of these specimens was mistakenly diagnosed as cribriform DCIS.

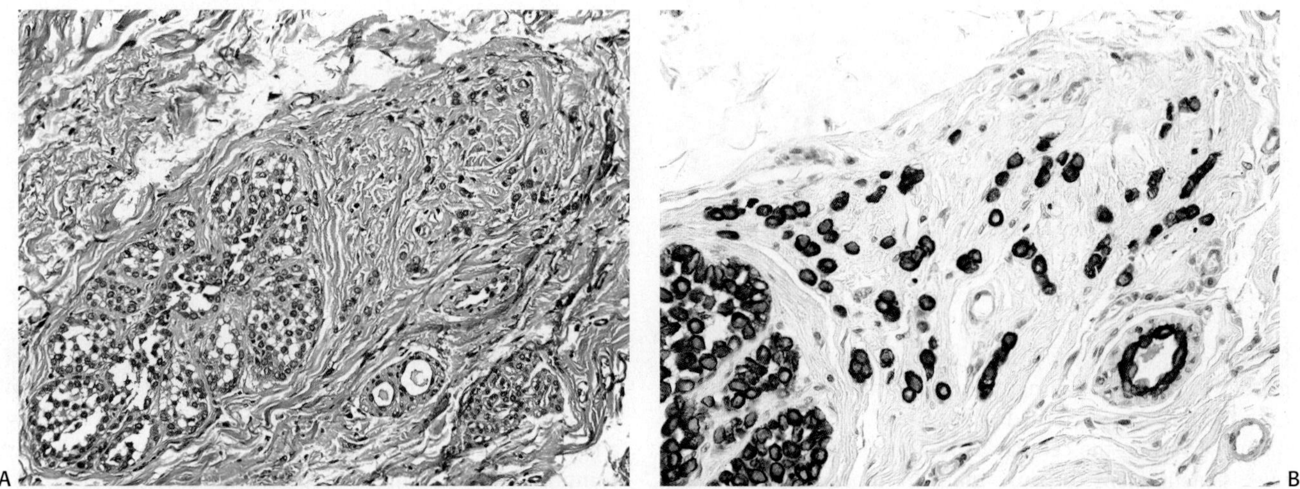

FIG. 31.46. ***Lobular carcinoma in situ and microinvasive lobular carcinoma, classical type.*** **A:** LCIS with adjacent microinvasive classical lobular carcinoma. **B:** The invasive carcinoma cells are highlighted by the CK immunostain (CK AE1/3).

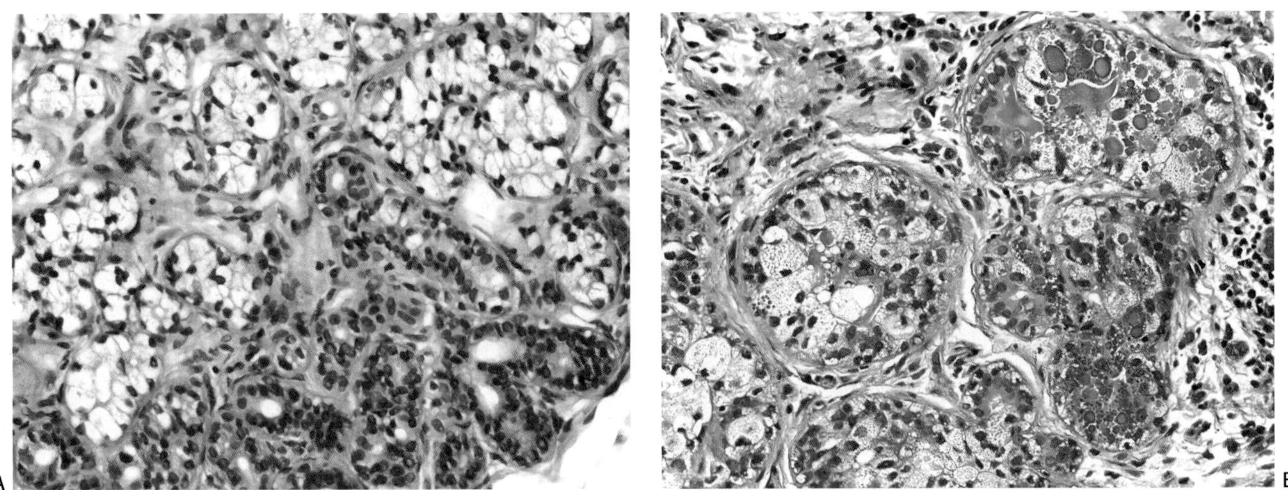

FIG. 31.47. ***Clear-cell change and apocrine metaplasia in lobules.*** **A:** Cells of the lobular glands show clear-cell change. **B:** Apocrine metaplasia is manifested by the presence of the variably sized apocrine cytoplasmic granules.

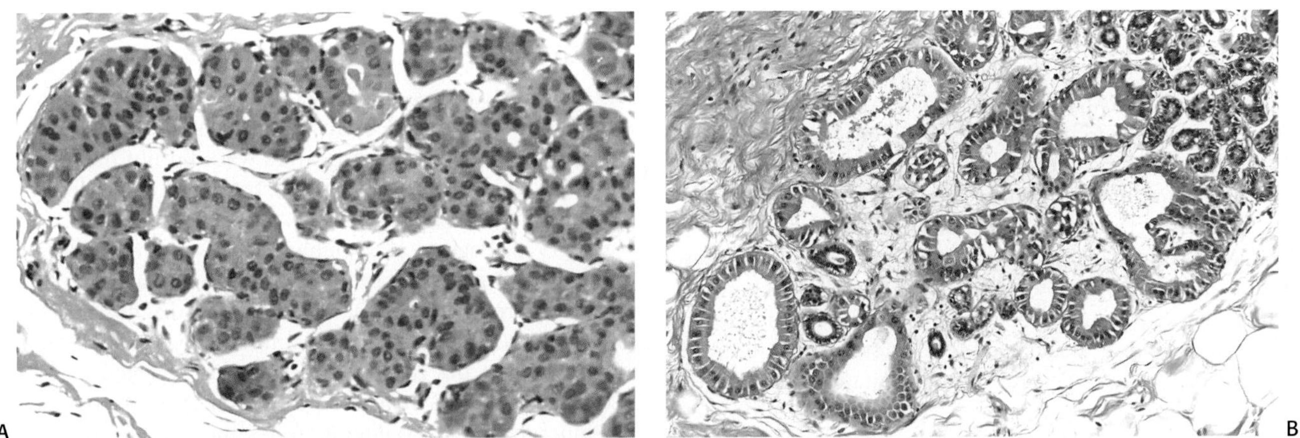

FIG. 31.48. ***Apocrine metaplasia in lobules.*** **A:** Note the small punctate nuclei that are distributed in a fairly regular pattern around the periphery of the glands. **B:** Cystic apocrine metaplasia in a lobule.

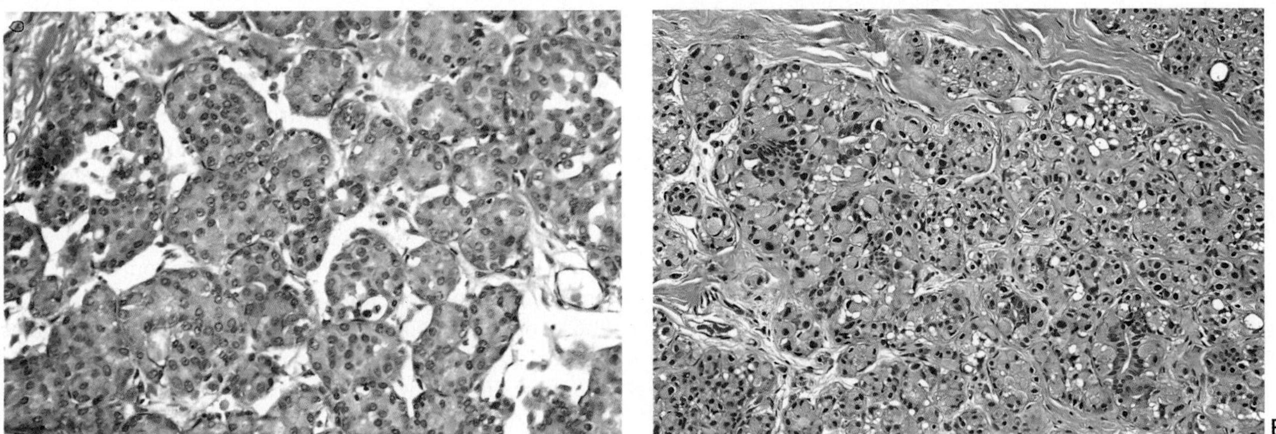

FIG. 31.49. ***Carcinoma with apocrine differentiation in lobules.*** **A:** LCIS with apocrine features. **B:** PLCIS. Note nuclear pleomorphism. Many cells have abundant diffuse intracytoplasmic mucin, resulting in eccentric, crescentic nuclei and intracytoplasmic vacuoles.

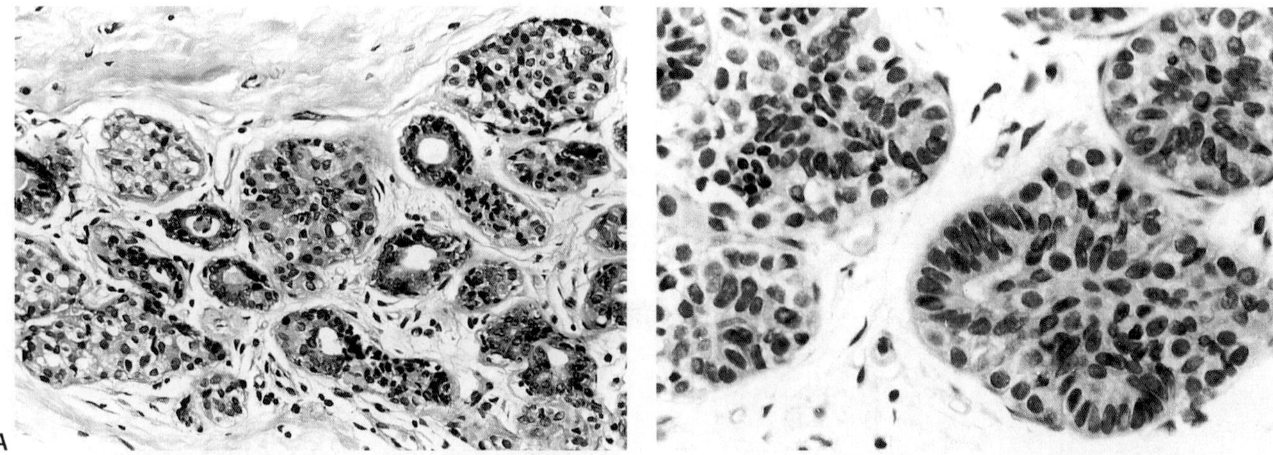

FIG. 31.50. ***Atypical lobular hyperplasia.*** **A:** Partial lobular involvement with evidence of pagetoid spread. This was the only affected lobule in the specimen, and less than 75% of the lobule was involved. **B:** Pagetoid spread of atypical cells in lobular glands in another case. Residual nonneoplastic lobular epithelium composed of columnar cells is evident.

ALH is E-cadherin negative,[101,105] a property it shares with LCIS. Both lesions also lack reactivity for α- and β-catenin and they both have an LOH at 16q.[101] Although mutations were consistently found at the *E-cadherin* gene locus CDH1 in LCIS by Mastracci et al.,[101] comparable mutations were rarely present in ALH lesions. The observation that reactivity for E-cadherin and α- and β-catenin is lost in both LCIS and ALH, but that mutations in the *E-cadherin* gene were found almost exclusively in LCIS, suggests that mechanisms other than mutations can be responsible for inactivation of E-cadherin and its associated proteins. It remains to be determined whether the acquisition of mutations in CDH1 is necessary for the evolution of ALH to LCIS and ultimately to the development of invasive lobular carcinoma.

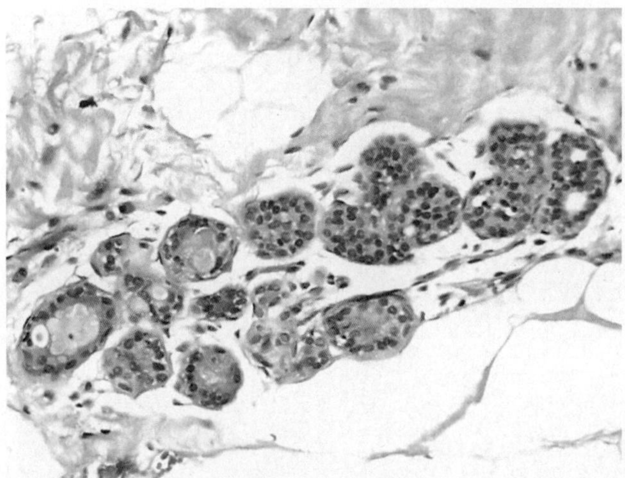

FIG. 31.51. ***Atypical lobular hyperplasia.*** A lobule in which less than 50% of the glandular epithelium is replaced by atypical cells.

Prognosis of ALH

Estimates of the risk of subsequent carcinoma in women with ALH are clouded by the absence of a clear definition for this lesion. Some investigators who did not distinguish between ALH and LCIS have reported RR estimates for both lesions under the heading of LN.[27,106]

In 1978, Page et al.[107] published a long-term follow-up study of patients with proliferative lesions identified in a retrospective review that included ALH. The diagnosis of ALH was "reserved for atypical epithelium involving lobular units which approaches in appearance that is accepted as LCIS. Loss of evidence of a two-cell population above the basement membrane and near obliteration of lumens in 50% of the involved structures, and modest distention of the ductules are necessary criteria. The cells have a small-to-moderate amount of clear cytoplasm and tend to have a regular relationship to each other. Nuclei are rounded similar to each other, and hyperchromatic."[93] On the basis of this definition, ALH was diagnosed in 33 (3.6%) of 925 women, 4 of whom later developed carcinoma. The RR of subsequent carcinoma was 4.0 when compared with the expected frequency of subsequent carcinoma in age-matched controls. The RR was significantly higher (6.06) among women 31 to 45 years of age than in those older than 45 years of age (3.17) when ALH was diagnosed.

A second follow-up study by Page et al.[108] of patients with ALH detected in a retrospective review of benign breast biopsies was published in 1985. The definition of ALH was similar to the one put forth in 1978. ALH was found in 126 (1.6%) of 10,542 biopsies examined, and 16 (12.6%) of these women later developed invasive breast carcinoma. Subsequent carcinomas were ipsilateral in 69% of the cases. The interval to subsequent carcinoma averaged 11.9 years (4.6 to 21.9 years). When compared with age-matched controls in the Third National Cancer Survey, the overall RR of subsequent carcinoma in women with ALH was 4.2 (95% confidence interval [CI], 2.6 to 6.9). The risk was higher in those

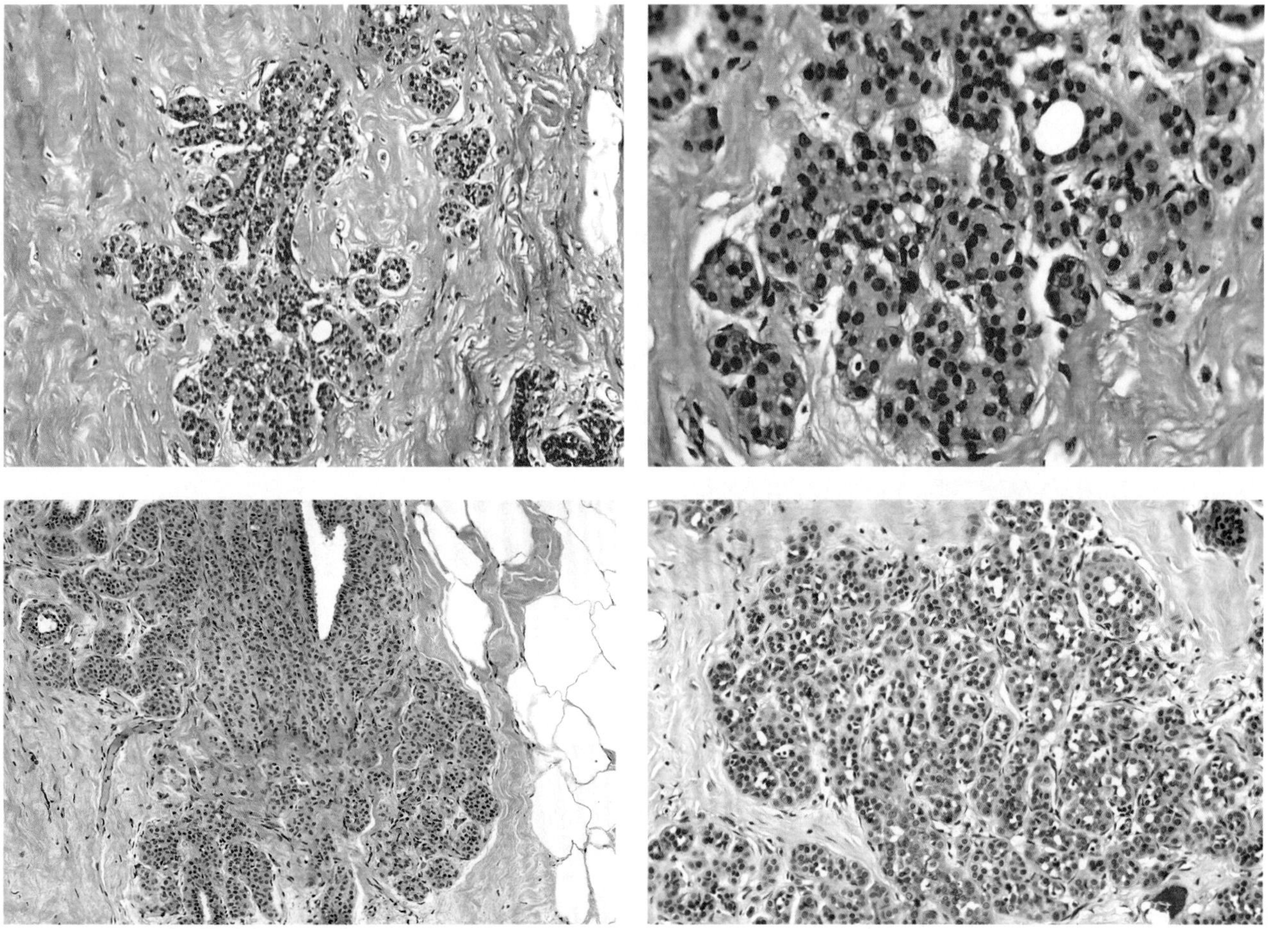

FIG. 31.52. ***Atypical lobular hyperplasia.*** **A,B:** An inconspicuous lobular lesion in which individual lobular glands are indistinct. **C:** Lobules clustered around a duct are involved by ALH. The lobule closest to the duct is altered by SA. **D:** ALH in an enlarged lobule.

with a family history of breast carcinoma in a female, first-degree relative (RR, 8.4; 95% CI, 3.5 to 20) than in those with no affected first-degree relatives (RR, 3.5; 95% CI, 1.9 to 6.2). Eighty-seven percent of patients with ALH were 31 to 55 years of age, and all subsequent carcinomas occurred in women initially identified in this age range. The RR was

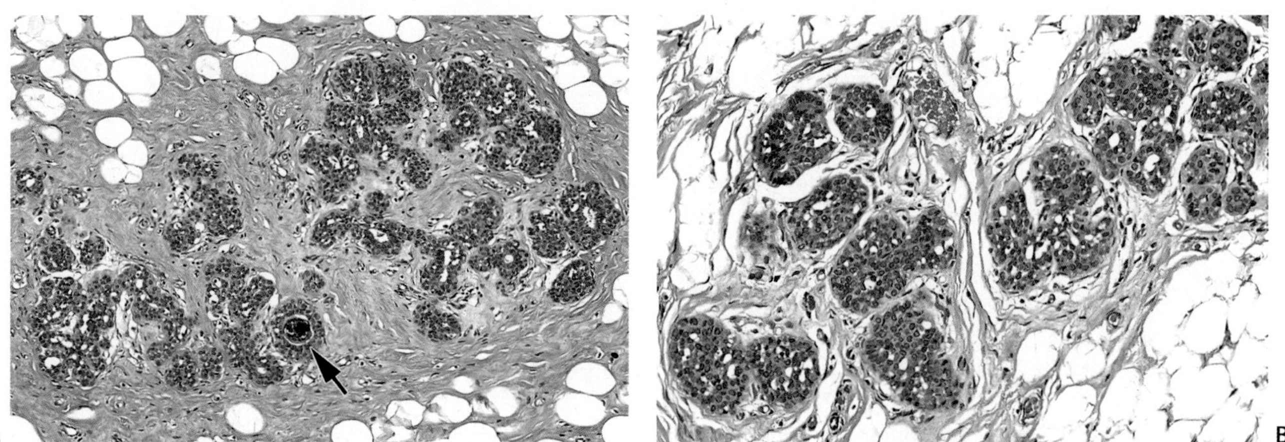

FIG. 31.53. ***Atypical lobular hyperplasia.*** **A,B:** The acinar glands are small. Patchy loss of cohesion is evident. *Arrow* in **(A)** indicates a calcification.

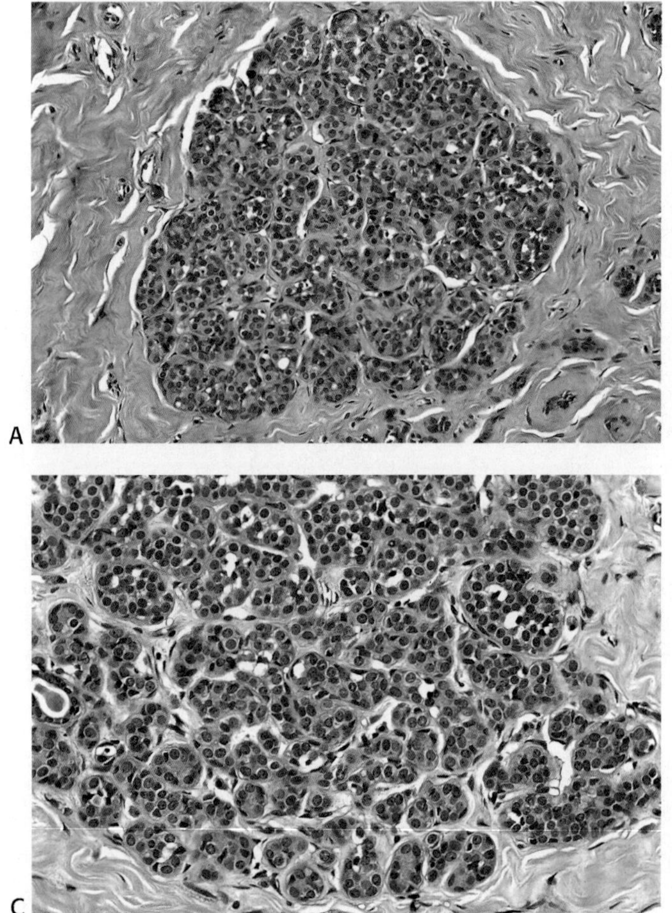

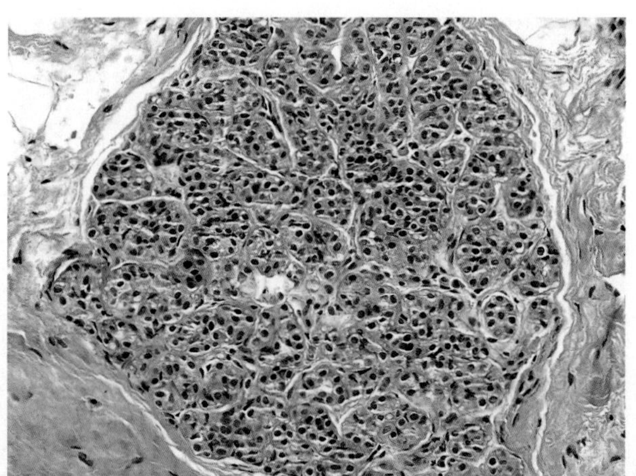

FIG. 31.54. ***Atypical lobular hyperplasia, borderline.*** **A:** There is minimal glandular expansion. **B:** Lobular expansion is more advanced than in (**A**), but individual glands are not distinct. **C:** The upper half of this lobule is composed of glands filled with small uniform cells compatible with LCIS, classical type.

higher (RR, 6.4; 95% CI, 3.6 to 11) among those who were 46 to 55 years old when ALH was diagnosed than among women 31 to 45 years old (RR, 2.7; 95% CI, 1.0 to 7.2). The overall RR for women with ALH as well as the RRs with or without a positive family history of breast carcinoma was similar to the RRs associated with atypical ductal hyperplasia (ADH) among women stratified in similar categories.

In an analysis that included age-matched controls, Page et al.[109] reported that the risk of developing carcinoma in women with ALH was increased when there was concomitant

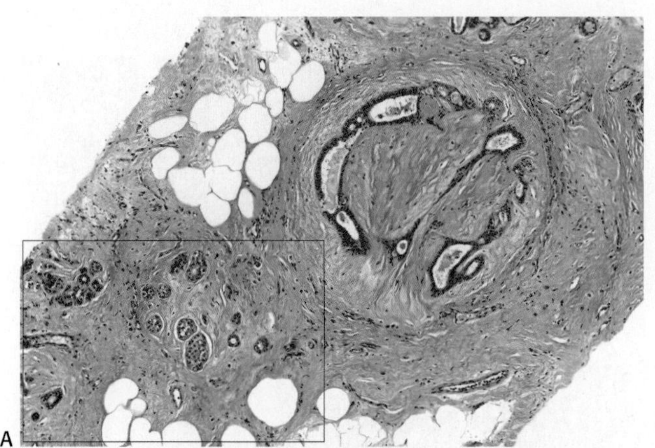

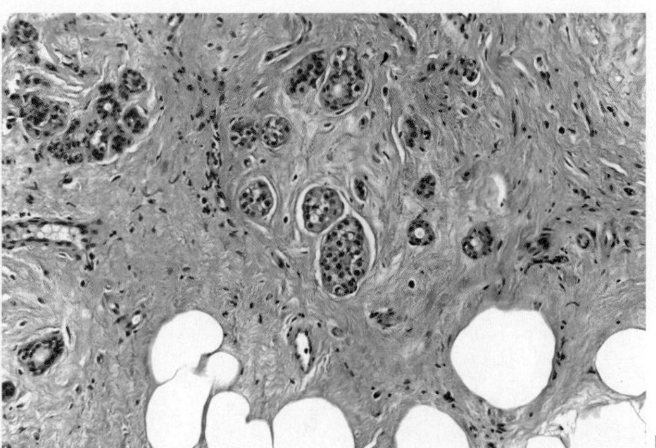

FIG. 31.55. ***Atypical lobular hyperplasia, adjacent to a fibroadenoma in a needle core biopsy specimen.*** This is a subtle lesion at low-power microscopy. *Boxed area* in (**A**) is shown at higher magnification in (**B**).

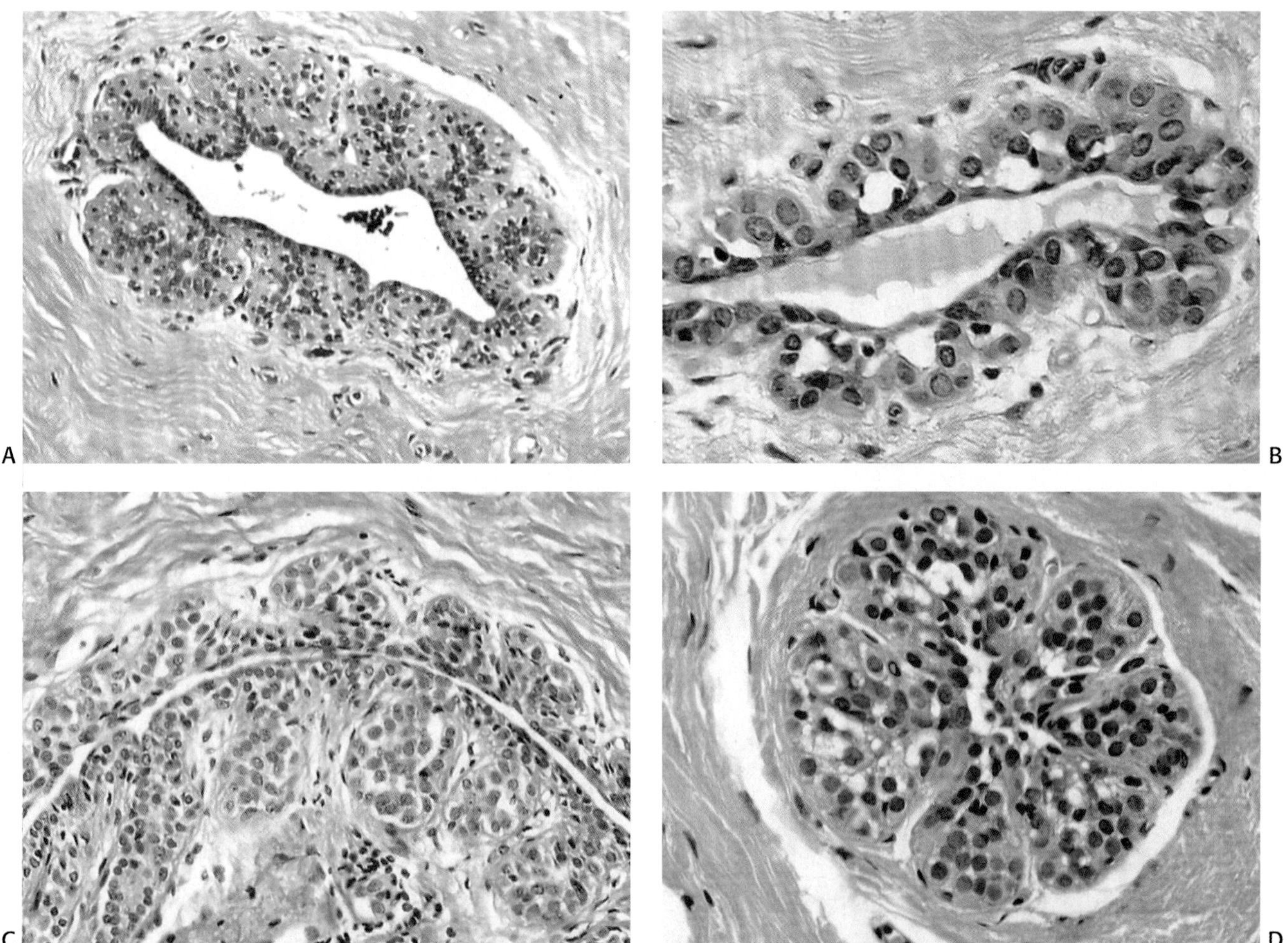

FIG. 31.56. ***Atypical lobular hyperplasia in ducts, cloverleaf pattern.*** **A:** A normal duct with a serrated contour created by abortive ductule formation. The resultant saccular structures have a lobular phenotype. **B:** Minimal ALH in a duct. **C:** More complex ALH involving a duct cut longitudinally. **D:** The cloverleaf pattern in a duct cut transversely.

atypical duct hyperplasia. Among the 250 women with ALH, 50 (20%) later developed invasive breast carcinoma. Thirty-four (68%) of subsequent carcinomas were in the ipsilateral breast. Data from a case-control study of women enrolled in the Nurses' Health Study revealed an adjusted odds ratio (OR) of 5.2 (95% CI, 3.0 to 9.1) for the subsequent development of breast carcinoma in women with ALH.[110]

McLaren et al.[111] described 252 women with ALH who had a median follow-up of 17 years. Subsequent invasive carcinoma was diagnosed in 48 (19%) of these women after a median interval of 17 years. The authors emphasized the relatively high frequency of "special types or variant types with a good prognosis," including infiltrating lobular, tubular, tubulolobular, "medullary variant," and "no special type carcinomas with lobular features." After an average follow-up of 13 years following the diagnosis of invasive carcinoma, 2 of the 20 patients (10%) with "special types" of carcinomas died of disease. This was significantly fewer breast carcinoma deaths than among the 28 control women with carcinomas of unknown or no special type (9%; 32%). These data indicate that a subset of patients with ALH is predisposed to develop relatively more favorable types of invasive carcinoma. No markers have been identified to assign an individual patient to this favorable risk group.

LCIS OR LN

The term "lobular neoplasia" was introduced largely to alter the treatment of LCIS by removing the word "carcinoma" from the diagnosis.[9] This may have been a useful strategy in an era when breast conservation therapy was not common for any form of breast carcinoma. Breast conservation therapy is now widely accepted for most types of carcinoma, and, therefore, this rationale for employing LN as a diagnostic term no longer exists.

LN refers to the spectrum of lobular proliferative lesions, including mild atypia, atypical hyperplasia with partial lobular involvement, fully developed LCIS involving one or more lobules, and sometimes to PLCIS. Advocates of the term

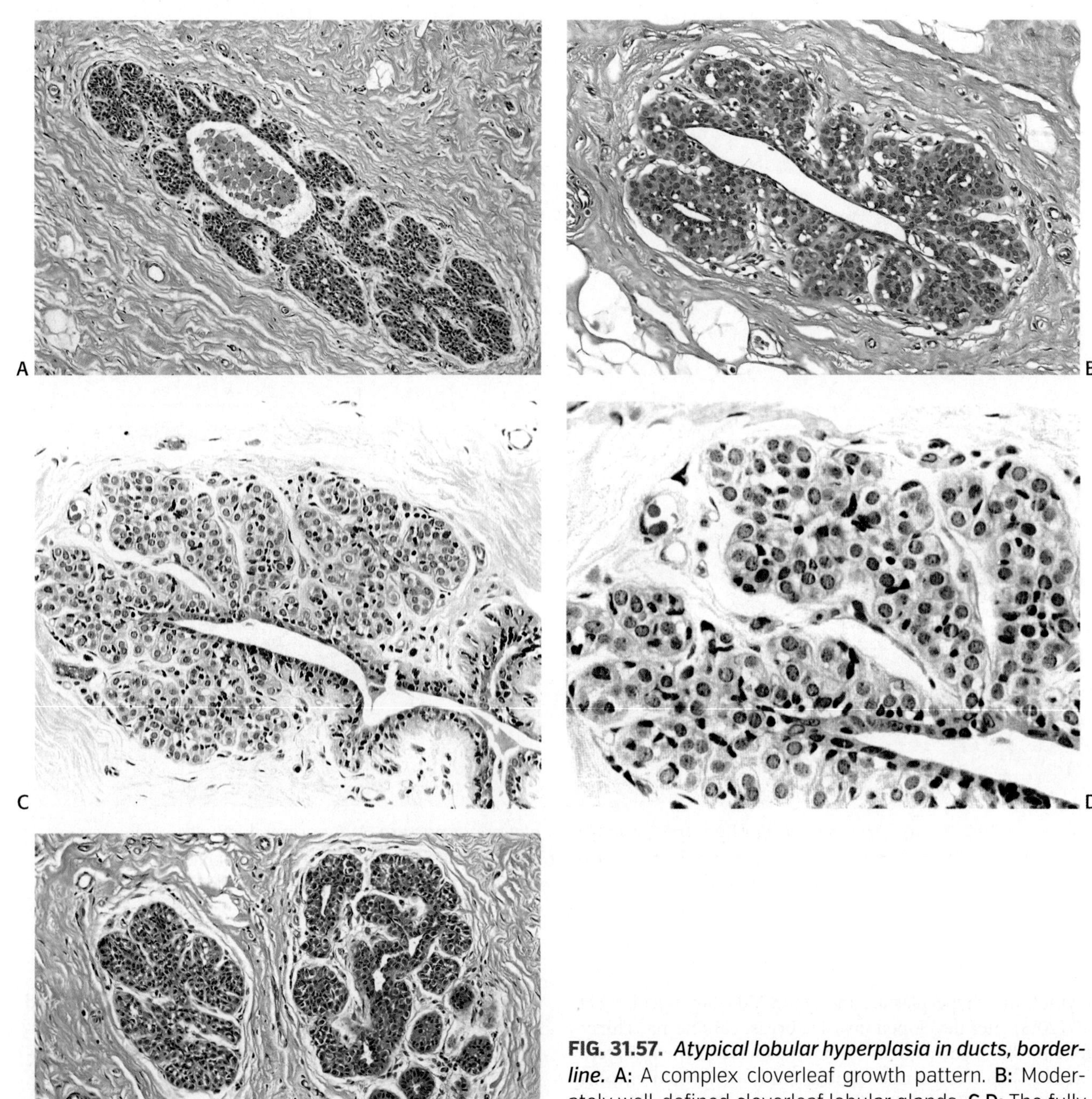

FIG. 31.57. ***Atypical lobular hyperplasia in ducts, borderline.*** **A:** A complex cloverleaf growth pattern. **B:** Moderately well-defined cloverleaf lobular glands. **C,D:** The fully developed cloverleaf pattern of ALH. **E:** ALH is present in the duct on the *left*, with pagetoid involvement of the terminal duct–lobular unit on the *right*.

"LN" point to differing criteria for the diagnosis of LCIS. An additional argument put forth in favor of using the diagnosis of LN is that both ALH and LCIS are associated with an increased risk of subsequent breast carcinoma.

The spectrum of lesions encompassed by LN is so broad as to render it a misleading and useless diagnostic term. In clinical practice, the use of this term creates a situation in which a single diagnosis does not discriminate between the patient with a minimal proliferative lesion that might only be mildly atypical hyperplasia and a patient who has fully developed FLCIS or PLCIS. The argument that it is sometimes difficult to classify borderline cases, or that there is no consensus on diagnostic criteria, does not justify a failure to distinguish between patients with lesions that are identifiable histologically in the majority of cases. Furthermore, this line of reasoning does not provide a clear-cut definition of lesions to be included in the LN category at the level of an ALH. Consequently, the term "LN" suffers from one

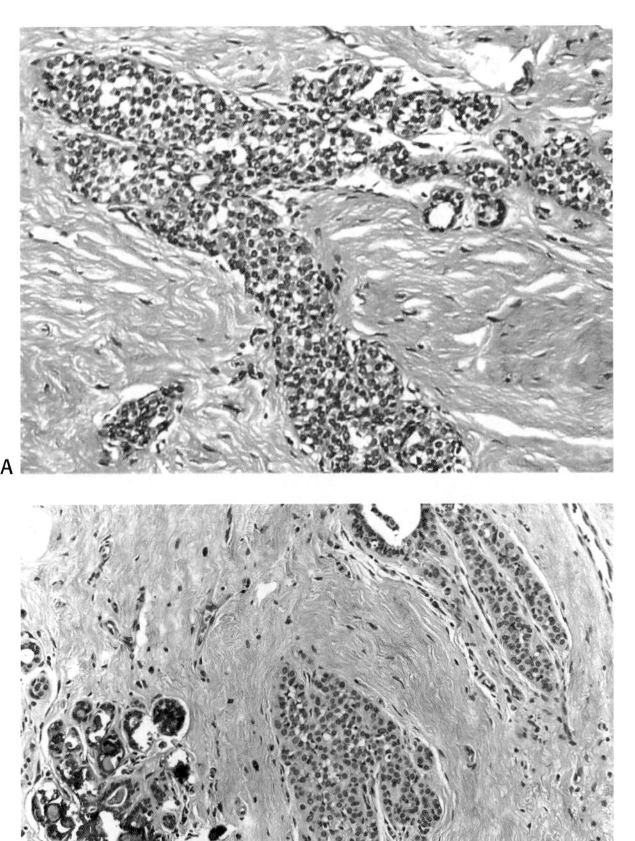

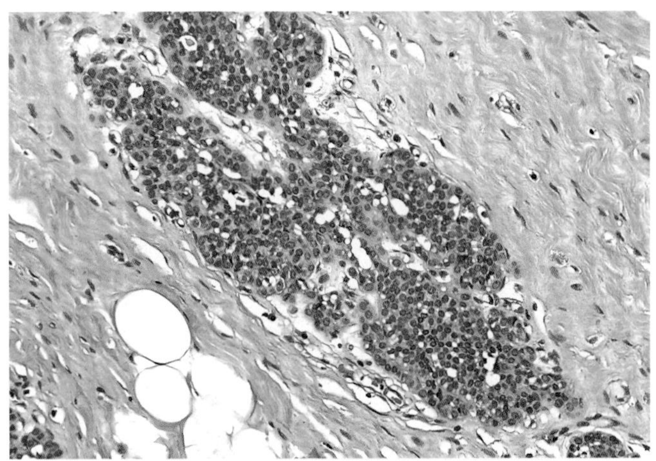

FIG. 31.58. ***Atypical lobular hyperplasia in ducts, borderline.*** **A:** Growth in this duct does not have a cloverleaf pattern. **B:** The cloverleaf pattern is obscured by cells that fill the duct lumen. The lesions in (**A**) and (**B**) border on LCIS. **C:** ALH adjacent to an atrophic lobule with dense calcific deposits. ALH extends into a terminal duct at the *top right*.

of the very flaws it was intended to address. Although it obviates the need to make a distinction between ALH and LCIS, the diagnosis of LN still requires separating ordinary lobular hyperplasia from a neoplastic proliferation in lobules. Although the term "lobular neoplasia" applies to all proliferative lesions that lack E-cadherin reactivity, an effort should be made to distinguish between ALH and LCIS on the basis of conventional histopathologic criteria.

The foregoing discussion provides a rationale for continuing to discriminate between ALH and LCIS and to

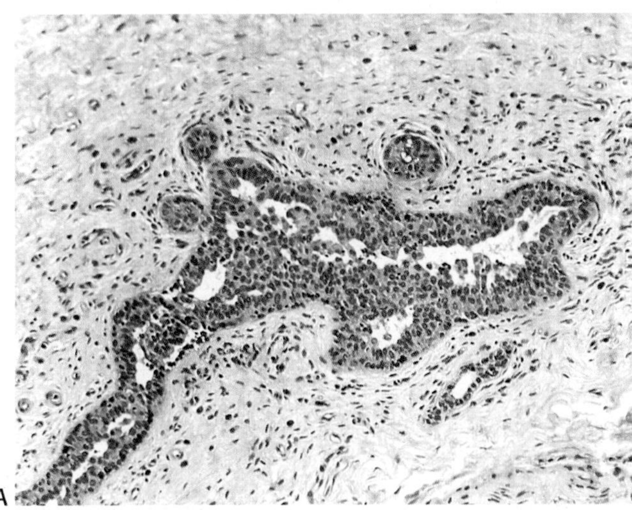

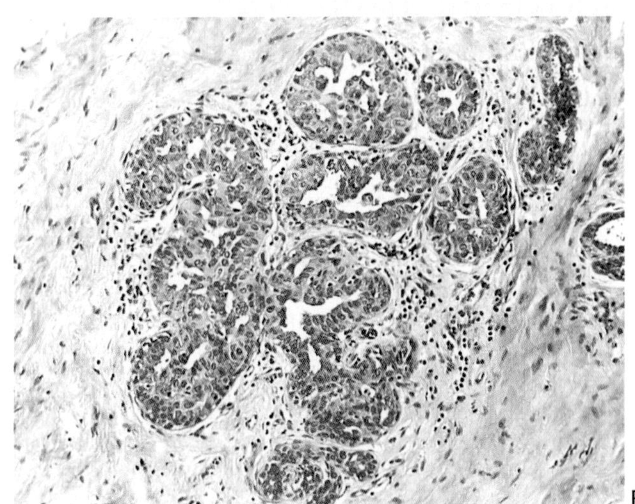

FIG. 31.59. ***Ductal hyperplasia with lobular extension.*** **A:** Hyperplasia with a papillary pattern in a duct. **B:** Papillary ductal hyperplasia in an uncoiled lobule from the same patient as (**A**).

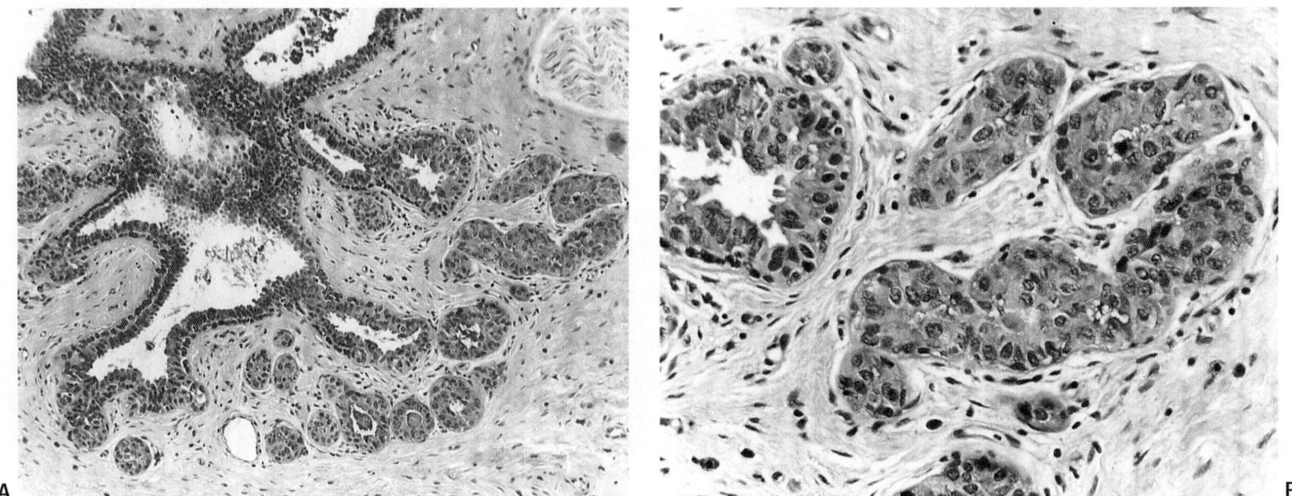

FIG. 31.60. ***Ductal hyperplasia with lobular extension.*** **A,B:** Columnar cell hyperplastic epithelium forms a thin layer around the duct and extends into contiguous lobular glands.

eschew the term "lobular neoplasia" whenever possible in clinical practice. Although this distinction may be difficult in individual cases, most often the diagnosis can be made by adhering to an established set of criteria such as those set forth in this chapter. Further studies that employ IHC and molecular biologic techniques may help in refining the diagnostic criteria by relating these properties to breast carcinoma risk. The term "lobular neoplasia" disguises our limitations and creates a false sense of specificity for the patient and clinician. The range of morphologic changes covered by LN is so broad that it is one of the least specific diagnoses in breast pathology and one that is not recommended.

FOLLOW-UP OF UNTREATED LCIS

Risk of Developing Invasive Carcinoma after LCIS–Retrospective Studies

In their original paper, Foote and Stewart[2] anticipated the most controversial aspect of LCIS, the risk that subsequent invasive carcinoma might develop if the breast harboring LCIS were not removed at the time of initial diagnosis. They commented:

> "It has been forcibly impressed upon us that a breast in which this process occurs in the slightest degree constitutes an extreme hazard. Whereas it is not clinical cancer until infiltration occurs, it is always a disease of multiple foci. In our first case, local excision revealed this process and we were unfortunately not aware of its significance. Within the space of a few months the patient had infiltrating cancer with axillary metastases and now has skeletal dissemination. It is our feeling that simple mastectomy is essential, with further procedure dependent on finding the least evidence of infiltration."[2]

The rapid clinical progression of disease in this case suggests that invasion had probably occurred when LCIS was diagnosed and that it was not represented in the biopsy specimen.

Several case reports followed more than a decade later. Godwin[112] described a patient who died of ipsilateral invasive lobular carcinoma that developed 12 years after a biopsy that contained LCIS had been interpreted as "cystic disease." Two additional reports described the development of carcinoma in the ipsilateral[113] and contralateral[25,113] breast after a biopsy specimen contained LCIS. The risk associated with residual breast tissue after mastectomy was documented by Newman[32] in a report that described a patient treated for LCIS. Four years after a mastectomy, a mass in the inferior aspect of the scar was found to contain residual breast tissue with *in situ* and infiltrating lobular carcinoma. Giordano and Klopp[114] traced 19 patients who did not undergo mastectomy for LCIS. Two had invasive carcinomas in the ipsilateral breast, 3 and 5 years subsequently treated by mastectomy. Thirteen patients remained well an average of 11.7 years (7 to 21 years) after biopsy.

Retrospective pathology studies were undertaken in the 1970s and 1980s to identify consecutive series of patients with LCIS not treated by mastectomy. In a study from Denmark, Andersen[5] reviewed the slides from 3,299 breast specimens obtained from 1942 to 1961, yielding 52 patients who had had LCIS. Five had been treated previously for contralateral invasive breast carcinoma. Ipsilateral mastectomy was performed for LCIS in six cases. After an average follow-up of 15 years, invasive carcinoma was detected in 8 (17.4%) of 46 patients with an ipsilateral breast available for study. The average interval to subsequent ipsilateral carcinoma was 9 years (range, 1 to 22 years). Four contralateral carcinomas (4 of 47, or 8.5%) were found an average of 13 years (range, 7 to 24 years) after biopsy. The total burden of contralateral carcinoma (9 of 25, or 17.3%) was essentially the same as for ipsilateral disease.

Another large series consisted of 48 patients with LCIS found in a retrospective review of 10,542 benign breast biopsies, an incidence of 0.5%.[8] Follow-up averaging 19 years was available for 39 patients, 9 (23%) of whom had subsequent invasive breast carcinoma. When compared with a control population, the overall RR of subsequent invasive breast carcinoma was 6.9, and the RR was 10.8 when compared with women who had nonproliferative changes in a breast biopsy. After 15 years of follow-up, the RR was 8.0 and the absolute risk was 17%. In this study, the risk of developing subsequent carcinoma was not affected by a family history of invasive breast carcinoma.

Two comprehensive follow-up investigations of LCIS that were undertaken at the Columbia-Presbyterian Medical Center (CPMC) and Memorial Sloan-Kettering Cancer Center (MSKCC) appeared in 1978. The studies from both institutions were based on retrospective reviews of histologic sections of breast biopsies that had been reported originally as benign.

CPMC Studies

The first report from CPMC was based on a review of 5,560 breast biopsies performed from 1930 to 1972.[27] A total of 211 patients were found to have lesions diagnosed as "LN" unassociated with invasive carcinoma, resulting in an incidence of 3.8% for LN. The term "LN" is used here with specific reference to data from CPMC series. This distinction is made because "LN" as used by these authors included lesions ordinarily diagnosed as ALH as well as LCIS. None of the patients was treated by mastectomy. Follow-up was obtained for 210 women, averaging 14 years (range, 1 to 42 years). Prior or subsequent carcinoma exclusive of LCIS was identified in 36, or 17.1%, of the patients in the CPMC series, including 3 with bilateral carcinoma. The number of carcinomas in the contralateral breast was nearly the same as in the ipsilateral breast. The incidence of breast carcinoma was seven times more than expected when compared with Connecticut State Cancer Registry data. After 15 years of follow-up, the cumulative probabilities for subsequent carcinoma were 10% and 9% in the ipsilateral and contralateral breasts, respectively. During the follow-up interval of 16 to 25 years, the risk of ipsilateral carcinoma reached 22%. For the contralateral breast, the risk increased to 15% by 25 years. It was recommended that patients with "LN" enter into follow-up by palpation every 4 months, rather than have treatment by mastectomy.

Data from CPMC were updated by Haagensen,[9] who extended the series to 1977, thereby including 297 patients with "LN." The average follow-up was 16.3 years, including 82 patients (27.6%) followed for more than 20 years. Subsequent carcinoma was found in 53 (18.6%) of 285 patients. When compared with data from the State of Connecticut, the ratio of observed to expected, or RR, for developing subsequent carcinoma was 5.9. The cumulative probability of subsequent ipsilateral carcinoma increased with longer follow-up from 8% at 6 to 10 years, to 12% at 11 to 15 years, and to 19% at 25 years. A similar trend was observed for contralateral carcinoma, which increased in frequency from 7% at 6 to 10 years, to 8% at 11 to 15 years, to 14% at 25 years, and to 23% at 35 years. Axillary dissection was performed in the treatment of 54 subsequent carcinomas. Lymph node metastases were found in 26% of these cases. Eleven (20.8%) of 53 patients with subsequent carcinoma died of metastatic carcinoma, and at last follow-up 2 others (3.7%) were alive with systemic metastases.

A third retrospective analysis of cases from CPMC was reported by Bodian et al.[106] in 1993. This series, based entirely on patients treated by Haagensen, included 99 women with lesions classified on review as LN/LCIS among 1,799 women analyzed in a follow-up study of proliferative breast disease. LCIS was not distinguished from ALH in reporting the results of the follow-up. After an average follow-up of 21 years, 24 women (24%) developed subsequent breast carcinoma other than LCIS. When compared with controls from the Connecticut Tumor Registry, the RR of subsequent carcinoma was 5.7 expected (95% CI, 3.8 to 8.5), similar to that in the 1986 report from the same institution.

A further analysis of the CPMC series published in 1996 consisted of 236 women with a median follow-up of 18 years.[115] The probability of developing subsequent carcinoma was 1 in 3 or 5.4 times the rate in the general population (95% CI, 4.2 to 7.0). The RR was elevated for more than 20 years after the diagnosis of LCIS and increased from 4.9 (95% CI, 3.7 to 6.4) for women with LCIS in one biopsy to 16.1 (95% CI, 6.9 to 31.8) for women with LCIS in a second biopsy.

MSKCC Stuvdy

The MSKCC study was based on a systematic review of 8,609 breast biopsy specimens obtained between 1940 and 1950.[6] Included were all specimens in which there was a diagnosis other than carcinoma. Sixty-four examples of previously unrecognized LCIS were found. During the same period, there were also 53 cases in which the original diagnosis had been LCIS. The incidence of LCIS was, therefore, 1.3% among biopsies that did not contain intraductal or invasive carcinoma. Eighteen patients with LCIS were excluded from subsequent analysis because incomplete identifying information precluded follow-up.

Follow-up averaging 24 years was obtained for 84 of the 99 study patients with LCIS, and it was found that 32 patients (38%) were treated at some time for mammary carcinoma other than the LCIS diagnosed in the biopsy under consideration. Subsequent ipsilateral carcinoma was diagnosed in 12 patients (14%), and 7 other patients (8%) had bilateral carcinomas. Twelve patients (14%) had only contralateral carcinoma, including three who had had treatment of contralateral carcinoma prior to the biopsy in which LCIS was found. Laterality was not known for one subsequent carcinoma. Thirty-nine patients (46%) who remained alive had had no breast carcinoma other than the original LCIS. Thirteen other patients (25%) with no evidence of breast carcinoma died of other causes.

In the MSKCC study, the average age at the diagnosis of subsequent ipsilateral carcinoma was 59 years, and for contralateral carcinoma it was 62 years. The intervals between the diagnosis of LCIS and carcinoma of the ipsilateral breast varied from 2 to 31 years, and from 3 to 30 years in the contralateral breast. In the ipsilateral breast, 6 (32%) of 19 subsequent carcinomas were diagnosed 20 or more years after LCIS. Forty-four percent of subsequent contralateral carcinomas (7 of 16) were not detected for at least 20 years after diagnosis of LCIS. Thirty-eight percent of all patients with subsequent carcinoma did not have evidence of the disease until at least 20 years after LCIS was found. The hazard rate for the subsequent development of carcinoma increased annually over a period of 25 years after the diagnosis of LCIS.

IFDC was the most common type of carcinoma to develop after LCIS in the MSKCC study (Fig. 31.61). Infiltrating lobular carcinoma was encountered in eight ipsilateral and five contralateral breasts. Subsequent carcinomas were treated by mastectomy. Lymph node status was known for 13 ipsilateral and 15 contralateral breasts with carcinoma. Axillary metastases were found in seven ipsilateral (54%) and in seven contralateral (47%) axillary dissections. Sixteen of the 32 patients (50%) with subsequent breast carcinoma died of their disease. Six of these women died of carcinoma of the ipsilateral breast and five died of carcinoma in the contralateral breast. Among the four patients with bilateral carcinoma, the fatal lesion was judged on the basis of size and nodal status to be ipsilateral in two and contralateral in one. In one case of bilateral carcinoma, it was not possible to ascertain which breast was primarily involved, and the fatal lesion was recorded as bilateral. In an additional case, laterality of the fatal primary carcinoma was not known.

The average length of survival of patients who died of breast carcinoma was 4 years following the diagnosis of subsequent invasive carcinoma. In 10 (77%) of 13 fatal cases for which nodal status could be determined, there were axillary metastases. When compared with an age-matched control population identified in the Connecticut State Tumor Registry, LCIS patients had nine times the expected frequency of subsequent carcinoma ($p < 0.001$). Deaths due to breast carcinoma, of which there were 16, were 10.7 times more frequent than expected.

In summary, the foregoing retrospective follow-up studies of LCIS have consisted of patients who were biopsied

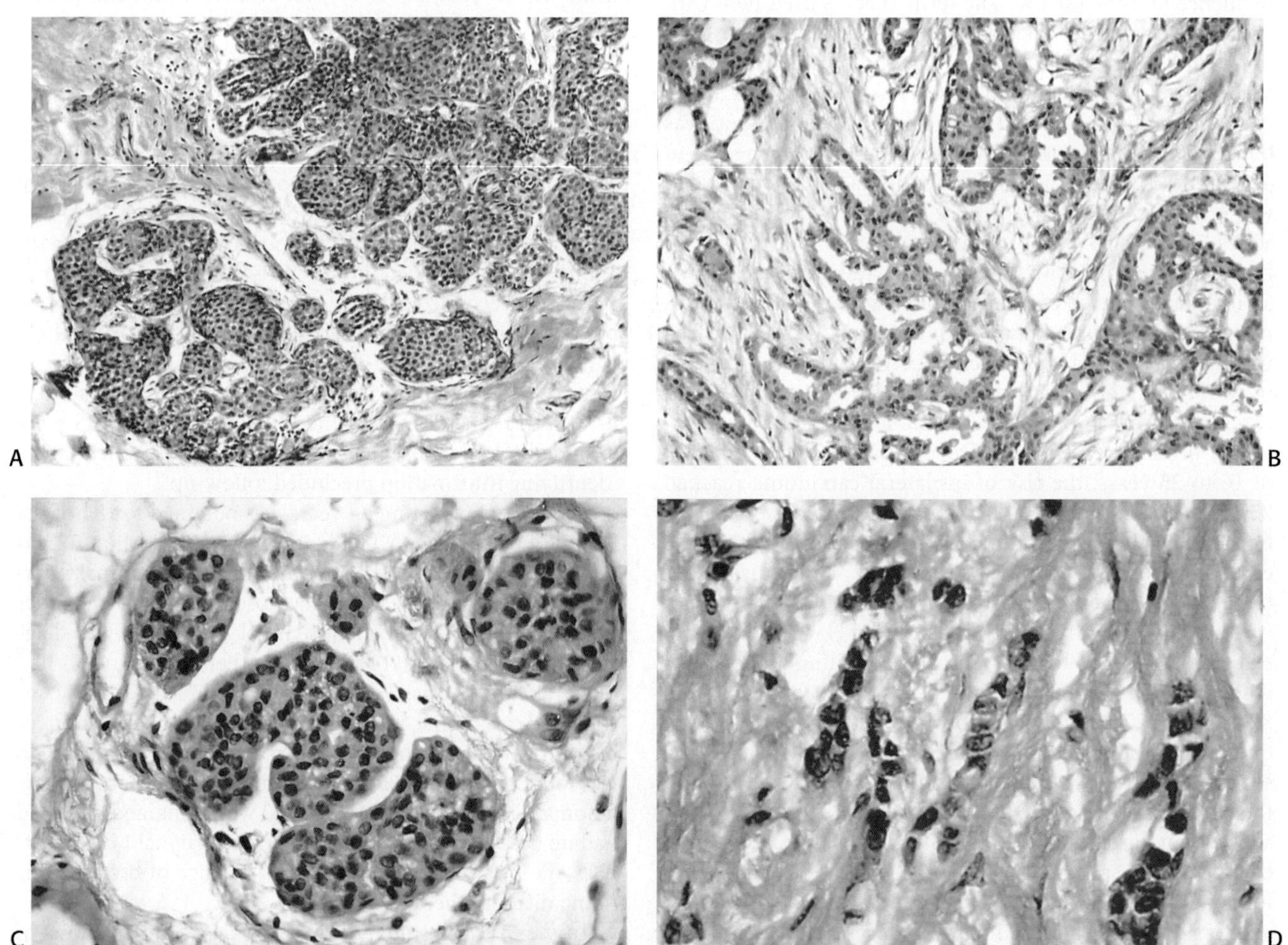

FIG. 31.61. ***Infiltrating ductal carcinoma subsequent to lobular carcinoma in situ.*** **A:** LCIS of the right breast in biopsy performed in 1948. No other treatment was given. **B:** IDC detected as a palpable tumor in the right breast in 1977. **C,D:** The mastectomy specimen in 1977 also had *in situ* **(C)** and invasive **(D)** lobular carcinoma.

for palpable clinical abnormalities in which LCIS was an incidental finding. The frequency of subsequent carcinoma varied from 17.4% to 24%.[1,19,116] Studies with longer follow-up tended to report a higher frequency of subsequent carcinoma. When compared with control populations, the RR to LCIS patients for the development of carcinoma was 4.0 to 12.0. In most studies, the risk of subsequent carcinoma was slightly higher in the ipsilateral than in the contralateral breast, although the difference was not great.

Risk of Developing Invasive Carcinoma after LCIS–Prospective Studies

Ciatto et al.[117] described the status of 60 women with an average follow-up of 5.3 years. Ipsilateral invasive carcinoma was detected subsequently in 5 (14%) of 37 who did not have mastectomy, and 2 others were found to have persistent LCIS. The intervals to subsequent invasive carcinoma were 5, 13, 20, 49, and 63 months. Three of the five invasive carcinomas were of the lobular variety. The RR of subsequent carcinoma based on age-specific incidence and years of follow-up for the 37 patients was 36 (95% CI, 11.6 to 83.3). Three of the five patients with subsequent invasive ipsilateral carcinoma developed metastases and died 6, 7, and 8 years after the initial diagnosis of LCIS. Two patients had metachronous contralateral carcinoma. On the basis of these results, the authors concluded that "the present study does not provide definitive evidence to recommend total mastectomy as the standard treatment of LCIS . . . [but] . . . when limited surgery is adopted as the standard treatment of LCIS, careful follow-up of the ipsilateral and contralateral breast is mandatory."[117]

The National Surgical Adjuvant Breast Project Protocol B-17 (NSABP B-17) randomized patients to receive or not receive radiotherapy after lumpectomy.[118] Included were 182 patients with LCIS whose only treatment was the diagnostic lumpectomy with a standardized follow-up program of mammography and clinical examination. Follow-up to 12 years revealed subsequent ipsilateral carcinoma in 26 (14%) and contralateral carcinoma in 14 (8%).[119] Nine of the ipsilateral and 10 contralateral carcinomas were invasive, with the majority in both groups classified as lobular type. All subsequent ipsilateral intraductal carcinomas occurred in the same quadrant as the initial LCIS. LCIS cases were "graded" on the extent of lobular distention: LCIS 1 included lesions with little or no distension, including "some lesions designated as ALH"; LCIS 2 lesions exhibited "modest" distension; LCIS 3 displayed "overt ductular and lobular distension with areas that exhibit little or no intraductular stroma." These three grades equate roughly to ALH, LCIS, and FLCIS, as described in this chapter. The average annual rates per 100 patient-years for developing subsequent ipsilateral invasive or intraductal carcinoma were LCIS 1, 0.14; LCIS 2, 1.22; and LCIS 3, 1.32 ($p < 0.04$). When LCIS 1 cases were compared with combined LCIS 2 and LCIS 3 cases, the difference in average annual ipsilateral carcinoma rates was highly significant ($p = 0.01$). These results confirm the lower risk of subsequent carcinoma after the diagnosis of ALH when compared with LCIS. The risk associated with FLCIS was marginally greater than for conventional LCIS. The authors also drew attention to a subset of six cases, which they designated as "ductolobular carcinoma *in situ*." These lesions "were characterized by the presence of classic DCIS in large ducts and LCIS in the distal portion of the same ductolobular unit." Because the investigators did not obtain E-cadherin staining in these cases, it is uncertain how many were true intraductal carcinomas and how many were PLCIS. These cases were excluded from the study because the authors had recommended breast irradiation for these patients.

Risk of Developing Invasive Carcinoma after LCIS–Population-Based Studies

Two population-based follow-up reports of LCIS are available. One prospective study has been provided by the Danish Breast Cancer Cooperative Group.[120] The series included 69 women with LCIS and 19 with LCIS and intraductal carcinoma entered into a nationwide program from 1982 to 1987. All patients underwent excisional biopsy, including two diagnosed in reduction mammoplasty specimens. After a median follow-up of 61 months, 15 patients (17%) were found to have subsequent intraductal or invasive carcinoma in the ipsilateral breast. Eight invasive, one intraductal, and four combined LCIS–intraductal carcinomas occurred in breasts with prior LCIS. Two subsequent carcinomas in patients with initial LCIS–intraductal carcinoma were of the same type. The median interval to detection of all subsequent carcinomas was 18 months (range, 6 to 42) and for invasive carcinomas 22.5 months (range, 7 to 42). The frequency of subsequent carcinomas was significantly higher (12 of 50, 24%) when there were 10 or more lobules with LCIS in the initial biopsy than if fewer than 10 lobules were affected (3 of 38, 8%). Nuclear size also proved to be a significant predictor, there being subsequent carcinoma in 8 (31%) of 26 with large nuclei and in 7 (11%) of 62 with small nuclei. No distinction was made between LCIS and PLCIS. The median size of invasive carcinomas was 10 mm. Axillary metastases were found in two patients with subsequent invasive carcinoma. At the time of the report, no patient had a systemic recurrence, and there were no deaths due to breast carcinoma. Compared with a reference control population, the frequency of subsequent invasive carcinoma was 11 times greater than expected (95% CI, 4.8 to 21.7). Despite careful surveillance, the authors noted that all eight subsequent invasive carcinomas presented as palpable tumors.

Li et al.[121] undertook a retrospective analysis of patients with intraductal carcinoma and LCIS recorded in the United States SEER database. Follow-up revealed that patients with LCIS had incidence of subsequent invasive carcinoma of 7.3/1,000 person-years and 5.2/1,000 person-years in the ipsilateral and contralateral breasts, respectively. LCIS patients had a 5.3 times greater likelihood of developing invasive lobular carcinoma than those with intraductal carcinoma.

Pathologic Predictors of Increased Risk Due to LCIS

Reliable pathologic predictors of increased risk of the subsequent development of carcinoma after LCIS was diagnosed by needle core or surgical biopsy remain elusive. Three studies reported a greater risk in patients with LCIS that contained both classical and pleomorphic cells in comparison with patients who had LCIS with either cell type alone.[6,27,118] Increased risk has also been associated with marked lobular distension.[118] Lesions with marked ductal distension (FLCIS), necrosis, and calcification with or without pleomorphic cytology are cause for special concern because they harbor an unexpectedly high frequency of microinvasion at the time of diagnosis. Specimens with these features should be examined carefully for microinvasion with CK and E-cadherin immunostains accompanied by contemporaneous H&E recuts.

Goldstein et al.[95] conducted a retrospective study of 82 patients with LCIS who did not undergo mastectomy. The actuarial rates for subsequent carcinoma were 7.8% after 10 years of follow-up and 15.4% after 20 years. Six of the subsequent 21 carcinomas (29%) developed 20 or more years after diagnosis. No E-cadherin reactivity was present in 73 LCIS lesions (89%), and 9 had focal weak and discontinuous reactivity. When compared with patients with E-cadherin–negative LCIS, the presence of focal E-cadherin reactivity was associated with a higher risk of developing subsequent carcinoma, earlier onset of carcinoma, and more frequent ductal carcinoma. This observation based on a small number of cases with focal E-cadherin reactivity remains to be confirmed by other investigators.

As noted earlier, the risk of invasive recurrence for patients with classical LCIS is substantially higher when the LCIS has a proliferation rate greater than 10% as measured by Ki67 IHC than if the proliferation rate is less than 10%.[85]

CLINICAL MANAGEMENT OF LCIS IN A NEEDLE CORE BIOPSY SPECIMEN

Although ALH and LCIS usually do not form calcifications, they often occur in conjunction with columnar cell lesions, proliferative lesions of terminal ducts and lobular units that are also variously referred to as columnar cell alterations, columnar cell change, flat epithelial atypia, and other terms (see Chapter 11). A common feature of columnar cell lesions is the presence of cystic, dilated duct–lobular structures that tend to develop calcifications.[122] Tubular carcinoma is often found to be associated with columnar cell lesions, ALH or LCIS, a complex that has been referred to as the "Rosen triad" by Brandt et al.[123] who found columnar cell lesions in each of the 86 examples of tubular carcinoma that they studied and 46 (53%) also had LCIS.

Mammographically detected calcifications in columnar cell lesions are frequently a target that leads to the discovery of ALH and LCIS. Calcifications formed in PLCIS have the characteristics of calcifications found in comedo intraductal carcinoma. The management of patients with LCIS in a mammographically directed needle core biopsy is a relatively recent concern. Liberman et al.[124] found LCIS as the only neoplastic lesion in 16 (1.2%) of 1,315 consecutive needle core biopsy procedures. Other significant proliferative lesions in the core biopsy specimens with LCIS included "radial scar" in three cases and ADH in two cases. Subsequent excision revealed intraductal carcinoma in the region of the LCIS in two cases and infiltrating carcinoma in a third. FLCIS involving markedly expanded ducts was present in two core biopsy specimens, after which surgery revealed intraductal carcinoma in one case and invasive carcinoma in the other. ADH accompanied LCIS in another core biopsy that was followed by intraductal carcinoma at surgery. The authors concluded that surgical biopsy should be performed when a core biopsy contains LCIS accompanied by a "high-risk" proliferative lesion, when florid LCIS is present resembling intraductal carcinoma, or if there is discordance between histologic and imaging findings.

A larger series included patients with either LCIS or ALH diagnosed in needle core biopsies performed for mammographic indications was reported by Lechner et al.[125] This multi-institutional study of 32,424 biopsies revealed 89 (0.3%) examples of LCIS and 154 (0.5%) instances of ALH. Surgical biopsies were performed on 58 (65%) of the LCIS lesions yielding invasive lobular carcinoma in 8 (14%), IDC in 2 (3%), tubular carcinoma in 8 (14%), and intraductal carcinoma in 2 (3%). Therefore, 20 (22.5%) of the 89 patients with LCIS in a core biopsy specimen had intraductal or invasive carcinoma in a subsequent surgical biopsy. Foster et al.[126] described 12 patients with LCIS in a core biopsy specimen who had a surgical excision performed. Four patients (25%) were found to have invasive or intraductal carcinoma. Crisi et al.[127] found invasive carcinoma in two (22%) of nine surgical specimens after a needle core biopsy specimen showed LCIS.

A summary of the foregoing reports and other studies, including a total of 140 patients with LCIS diagnosed in a needle core biopsy specimen who underwent surgical biopsy, was compiled by Arpino et al.[128] Carcinoma, either intraductal or invasive, was found in 40 (26%). A subsequent review of 15 reports by Hussain and Cunnick[129] included 241 patients with LCIS diagnosed in a needle core biopsy specimen. In the 61% of cases where surgical excision was performed the yield of DCIS detected ranged from 0% to 60%, averaging 32%. In 12 studies of "LN" in 246 needle core biopsy specimens summarized by Hussain and Cunnick, excisional biopsy was performed in 69% of cases, yielding intraductal or invasive carcinoma in 7% to 61% of the excisional biopsies, averaging 29%.

Data for PLCIS diagnosed in a needle core biopsy specimen have appeared in a few studies. Four reports summarized by Hussain and Cunnick[129] included 22 patients all of whom had an excisional biopsy. Nine invasive carcinomas detected in the 22 cases (41%) included eight invasive lobular carcinomas. Carder et al.[130] described 10 patients who had PLCIS in a needle core biopsy specimen, including 3 that were initially classified as high-grade DCIS. Two of these patients had microinvasive lobular carcinoma in the core biopsy specimen. Excisional biopsy revealed both PLCIS and LCIS in six cases, including one patient with microinvasive lobular carcinoma in the core biopsy specimen. Three other patients, including one with initial microinvasion had invasive lobular carcinoma in the excision and one had only LCIS.

Twelve additional patients with PLCIS in a needle core biopsy specimen were described by Chivukula et al.[131] Eleven of the needle biopsy procedures were performed for calcifications and one for a mass lesion. Subsequent surgery performed in all cases, ranging from excisional biopsy to mastectomy, revealed residual PLCIS in seven cases and LCIS in two cases. Three patients (25%) had invasive lobular carcinoma that was pleomorphic in one case, classical in another case, and both classical and pleomorphic in the third case.

These data support a recommendation to perform a surgical biopsy at the site where a previous needle core biopsy sample revealed PLCIS and in many patients with LCIS.[116] An important consideration in patients with LCIS is the degree to which the pathologic findings are concordant with imaging studies. Several investigators have reported that when there was concordance between the biopsy and imaging, the frequency of an upgraded diagnosis resulting from an excisional biopsy was so low that this procedure could be omitted in many cases.[132–134] On the other hand, they recommended that an excisional biopsy be performed when clinical and/or imaging findings are discordant with the needle biopsy results, or if the needle biopsy uncovers a lesion such as ADH. Menon et al.[132] found that discordant results most often occurred when the needle failed to provide an adequate sample from the target lesion. Hwang et al.[134] reported that when imaging and pathology were concordant in a patient found to have LCIS in a needle core biopsy sample, excisional biopsy yielded an upgrade rate of only 1%.

In their study of 100 patients with LCIS detected in a needle core biopsy specimen, Brem et al.[135] found that underdiagnosis was significantly more frequent when the biopsy target was a mass than if it was only calcifications, if the lesion was in a high Breast Imaging-Reporting and Data System (BI-RADS) category, and if a vacuum biopsy device was not used. They also reported that the average number of core biopsy samples was significantly lower (10) in discordant cases than in concordant cases (13.5). Nonetheless, it was concluded that sampling errors were sufficiently frequent that excisional biopsy was appropriate for patients with LCIS detected in a needle core biopsy sample even if imaging and pathology were concordant.

If a surgical excision is performed, further treatment will depend on the findings in the resultant specimen. Patients who do not undergo excision or whose only diagnosis remains LCIS after an excisional biopsy will be candidates for treatment as discussed elsewhere in this chapter.

CLINICAL MANAGEMENT OF ALH IN A NEEDLE CORE BIOPSY SPECIMEN

There is no consensus as to the optimal management of patients with ALH diagnosed by a needle core biopsy procedure. This uncertainty is due, in part, to variability in the diagnostic criteria for ALH. Lechner et al.[125] reported the results of a multi-institutional study that included 154 (0.5%) instances of ALH in 32,424 needle core biopsy specimens. Surgical biopsies performed in 84 cases of ALH (55%) revealed invasive lobular carcinoma in 3 (4%) and intraductal carcinoma in 4 (5%) for a total yield of 7 (8.3%) carcinomas in biopsied patients.

A review of 6,081 consecutive breast needle core biopsy procedures performed at two institutions uncovered 20 cases (0.3%) of ALH.[126] Surgical biopsies performed in 14 cases revealed intraductal carcinoma in 2 (14%). The six patients who did not have a surgical biopsy had not developed clinical evidence of carcinoma after a mean follow-up of 36 months.

Arpino et al.[128] reviewed 16 studies of patients with ALH diagnosed by needle core biopsy, including the foregoing reports. A total of 184 women had subsequent surgical excision that revealed either intraductal or invasive carcinoma in 30 (16%). The frequency of carcinoma detected in these excisions was somewhat lower than for LCIS, but not inconsequential.

Many additional studies of excisional biopsies performed after ALH was detected in a needle core biopsy sample have been published. Cangiarella et al.[136] reviewed 24 publications that described 393 patients with ALH among whom 51 (13%) were found to have DCIS or invasive carcinoma in a subsequent excisional biopsy specimen. A study reported by Brem et al.[135] included 178 patients with ALH in a needle core biopsy specimen. Excisional biopsies performed on 97 (54%) of the 178 patients yielded an upgraded diagnosis of DCI or invasive carcinoma in 21 (22%) of biopsied patients. A much lower yield was obtained by Hwang et al.[134] who reported an upgraded diagnosis in 1 of 48 (2%) women with ALH in a needle core biopsy specimen who had an excisional biopsy.

The foregoing data indicate that the yield from excisional biopsy in patients with ALH in a needle core biopsy specimen is substantially lower than among patients who have LCIS in a needle core biopsy specimen. If the pathology and imaging findings are concordant, most patients whose only significant finding in a needle core biopsy specimen is ALH can be managed by clinical follow-up alone. Whether the use of an antiestrogen would be beneficial in this situation remains to be determined. An excisional biopsy should be done in most cases if the pathology and imaging findings are discordant. The presence of other risks such as concurrent ADH or a family history of breast carcinoma can be indications for excisional biopsy.

CLINICAL FOLLOW-UP OF PATIENTS WITH ALH AND LCIS

The role of mammography as an adjunct to physical examination in the follow-up of ALH or LCIS is unresolved. Mammography is able to identify benign lesions such as SA that may coexist with LCIS, but it is much less effective for finding LCIS.[22] The most important role mammography plays in the follow-up of a patient with LCIS is to detect invasive carcinoma or intraductal carcinoma at a stage when they are most amenable to cure. As noted by Ottesen et al.,[120] mammography may be less reliable for the follow-up of premenopausal women with dense glandular breasts. Ultrasound examination is an important adjunct to mammography in this setting.

Recently reported data suggest that MRI can be helpful in the follow-up of women with LCIS. Sung et al.[137] studied 220 women with LCIS who had mammography and MRI studies. During the study period of approximately 5.5 years, 17 carcinomas were detected in 14 patients, including 9 invasive and 3 intraductal carcinomas identified by MRI alone. Two of five carcinomas detected by mammography alone were invasive and three were DCIS. Overall, MRI added substantially to the detection of subsequent carcinomas during the follow-up of women with LCIS.

When follow-up is recommended, it must be with the understanding that the patient accepts the responsibilities involved. Medical facilities must be provided for follow-up. An optimum practical schedule for repeated clinical examinations is yet to be devised.

Treatment Options for ALH and LCIS

Clinical Follow-up and Antiestrogens

Presently, clinical follow-up is recommended when the diagnosis is ALH and for most patients with LCIS. Biopsy of the opposite breast may be performed if there are clinical indications. The patient should be informed of the treatment options, and the potential benefits and risks of each. The clinical follow-up of patients with ALH and LCIS is a lifetime undertaking in view of the extended risk of late-occurring carcinomas.

The possibility that an antiestrogen, such as tamoxifen, might inhibit the evolution of ALH or LCIS was proposed in 1978.[6] It was later noted that patients receiving tamoxifen as adjuvant therapy following invasive carcinoma had a lower than expected frequency of contralateral carcinoma.[138–141] Clinical trials employed tamoxifen in patients with markers of a high breast carcinoma risk, including women with LCIS.[141,142] After 5 years of treatment with tamoxifen, women with LCIS had a 56% reduction in the risk of developing subsequent invasive carcinoma.[142] A subsequent randomized clinical trial compared the effects of tamoxifen and raloxifene in a total of nearly 20,000 postmenopausal women.[143] To be eligible for entry into the trial, women had to have a 1.66% 5-year risk of developing breast carcinoma as calculated by the Gail model. Most patients were eligible because of a family history of breast carcinoma. Only 9.2% had LCIS as the criterion for entry. Overall, each drug achieved about a 50% reduction in breast cancer risk. Both agents were equally effective in preventing invasive breast cancer in women with prior biopsies showing LCIS. The role of antiestrogens in women with ALH is yet to be determined.

It remains to be seen whether lifetime mortality due to subsequent invasive carcinoma can be reduced by close clinical surveillance and preventive intervention with antiestrogens. In the event that subsequent carcinomas were 1 cm or less in diameter when detected, data from the SEER Program[144] and other sources[145] indicate that axillary metastases would be found in 13% to 16% of cases. It is unlikely that even with the most careful clinical follow-up, all later invasive carcinomas would be found before axillary or systemic metastases had occurred.

Radiation Therapy

Although atrophy of radiated normal lobules is invariably seen in specimens from patients with recurrent carcinoma following lumpectomy and irradiation for DCIS or invasive carcinoma, LCIS that appears histologically unaffected by radiation has been observed in the same specimens. This observation suggests that LCIS is a relatively radiation-insensitive disease, but no systematic study of radiation therapy for classical LCIS alone has been undertaken. Data on the effects of radiotherapy on FLCIS and PLCIS are lacking. Cutuli et al.[146] described 25 women with LCIS that was not further classified who received whole-breast radiotherapy between 1980 and 1992. Surgery consisted of quadrantectomy (5 patients) or lumpectomy (20 patients). The median radiation dose was 52 Gy. In addition to biopsy and radiation, 12 patients received tamoxifen for 2 years (20 mg/day). During follow-up ranging from 58 to 240 months (median 153 months), one patient developed an ipsilateral IFDC 179 months after excision and radiotherapy, and one had contralateral IFDC 20 months after treatment for LCIS.

Mastectomy and Biopsy of the Contralateral Breast

Mastectomy may be considered in highly selected instances, such as a strong family history of breast carcinoma. Total mastectomy is the preferred operation if a mastectomy is to be performed. Subcutaneous mastectomy, whether unilateral or bilateral, may leave an appreciable amount of breast tissue, especially if the nipple is preserved, because lobules occur in the nipple.[64] In view of the fact that about 5% of breasts with LCIS diagnosed in a surgical biopsy specimen also harbor inapparent invasive carcinoma,[43,108] sentinel lymph node (SLN) mapping of the axilla should be considered at the time of a mastectomy. Imaging studies of both breasts, possibly including MRI, should be performed to minimize the likelihood of overlooking the presence of occult DCIS or invasive carcinoma before surgery.

Bilaterality of LCIS occurs frequently, but it is unproven that it occurs in every patient. Among patients with LCIS in one breast who underwent a contralateral biopsy, about 40% were found to have LCIS in the opposite breast. Biopsy of the opposite breast should be considered before performing an ipsilateral mastectomy for LCIS, especially if there are any palpable or imaging abnormalities in the other breast. The biopsy should be a substantial one to provide adequate material for histologic examination. Clinical features, genetic predisposition to breast carcinoma, and psychological factors must be weighed before unilateral or bilateral mastectomy is considered.[147]

Significance of LCIS in Breast Conservation Therapy for DCIS and Invasive Carcinoma

Controversy exists regarding the significance of LCIS in conjunction with DCIS and various types of invasive carcinoma in patients treated by breast-conserving therapy. In part, contradictory results reported in published studies reflect differences in patient groups, types of initial treatment, the use of adjuvant therapy, and the length of follow-up. No distinction was made between LCIS and PLCIS in most studies, but it is likely that the data relate mainly to LCIS because of the relative rarity of PLCIS.

LCIS and Invasive Lobular Carcinoma

One study of interest is a report by Stolier et al.[148] describing 40 patients who had breast-conserving treatment for invasive lobular carcinoma. With a mean follow-up of only 67 months, the authors found no local breast recurrences although 38% of the women had LCIS at or close to a margin. Despite the relatively short follow-up, these results led the authors to conclude that the presence of LCIS at a margin did not predispose patients with invasive lobular carcinoma to breast recurrence after breast-conserving treatment.

LCIS and DCIS

Rudloff et al.[149] investigated the risk of local recurrence in patients with DCIS associated with concurrent LCIS and proliferative lesions in 294 patients who had breast-conserving treatment. Breast recurrences occurred in 10 of 20 women (50%) who had coexisting LCIS and in 4 of 18 (22%) who had ALH. Breast recurrence was detected in 12 of 26 women (46%) who had "LN" (LCIS or ALH) at the surgical margin. Overall, patients with DCIS and "LN" had a significantly greater frequency of breast recurrences (15/41; 37%) than patients without "LN" (40/227; 18%). The cumulative incidence of breast recurrence was significantly higher in the DCIS–"LN" group at 5, 10, and 15 years of follow-up. The risk of breast recurrence was not significantly increased by the concurrent presence of ADH or columnar cell changes.

LCIS and Invasive Carcinoma

The majority of reports have assessed the impact of LCIS on breast recurrence in patients with IDC without distinguishing between ductal and lobular types. Generally, these studies concluded that the presence of LCIS in conjunction with invasive carcinoma did not significantly increase the risk of breast recurrence in women treated by breast-conserving surgery after a median follow-up of 45 to 161 months.[150–153] In the study with the longest follow-up,[151] the 8-year breast recurrence rate was 13% in 119 patients with LCIS and 12% among 1,062 patients without LCIS. The risk of recurrence in either the ipsilateral or the contralateral breast, or systemically, was not significantly related to the amount of LCIS in the treated breast. The study with the shortest follow-up by Ben-David et al.[152] revealed that local recurrence in the breast was not increased by the presence of LCIS at the margin of the surgical biopsy site or by the amount of LCIS.

Ciocca et al.[153] studied patients with DCIS as well as stage I or stage II invasive carcinoma with a median follow-up of 72 months after breast-conserving surgery and radiotherapy. LCIS was present in the lumpectomy from 290 patients, including 84 with LCIS at the margin. Another 2,604 patients had no LCIS. Among women with LCIS, 47.2% had invasive lobular carcinoma and the remainder had DCIS, or some form of IDC. When LCIS was absent, only 4.1% had invasive lobular carcinoma. The presence of LCIS, whether at the margin or not, was not a significant predictor for local recurrence in the breast. The 10-year actuarial local recurrence rate was 6% for patients with LCIS at the margin and also for patients with no LCIS. An important confounding factor in this study is the fact that adjuvant systemic therapy was administered significantly more often to patients with LCIS (chemotherapy 6.9%; tamoxifen 40.7%; both 22.8%) than to patients without LCIS (chemotherapy 14.5%; tamoxifen 29.8%; both 14.8%). In multivariate analysis, local recurrence was significantly reduced among women who received chemotherapy plus tamoxifen or tamoxifen alone.

A minority of studies yielded data that led investigators to conclude that the presence of LCIS predisposes patients to breast recurrence after breast-conserving therapy. Sason et al.[154] compared 65 patients who had LCIS coexisting with invasive carcinoma with 1,209 control patients without LCIS. After 5 years of follow-up, the two groups had similar rates of breast recurrence (LCIS 5%; control 3%), but the 10-year cumulative recurrence risk for LCIS patients (29%) was significantly higher than in the control group. However, the 10-year cumulative risks were not significantly different for women who received tamoxifen (LCIS 8%; control 6%), indicating that treatment with an antiestrogen could ameliorate the risk of recurrence associated with LCIS in patients who have breast-conserving treatment.

Jolly et al.[155] analyzed 607 patients who underwent breast-conserving treatment for invasive carcinoma with a median follow-up of 8.7 years. The 10-year breast recurrence rate (14%) was significantly higher when LCIS was present than when LCIS was absent (7%). LCIS significantly increased the risk of local recurrence whether it was present at the margin or not. Mechera et al.[156] also reported that LCIS significantly increased the risk of breast recurrence in a study of 335 consecutive patients with a median follow-up of 70.6 months.

Pleomorphic LCIS

Downs-Kelly et al.[157] evaluated the significance of PLCIS at or near resection margins in 26 patients treated by breast-conserving surgery. In the primary excision, 20 patients had only PLCIS, and 6 also had invasive foci that measured 3 mm or less. PLCIS was present at the margin of excision in six cases. Sixteen patients received chemoprevention, radiation, or both. With a mean follow-up of 46 months (range, 4 to 108 months), one patient with an initially positive margin treated with chemoprevention developed mammographically detected calcifications that were the sites of recurrent PLCIS 19 months after initial surgery.

Consideration of the foregoing studies suggests that the presence of LCIS in conjunction with invasive carcinoma or DCIS whether at the margin or not is not a contraindication to breast conservation with radiation therapy. If LCIS predisposes some patients to an increased risk of local recurrence after breast-conserving surgery and radiotherapy, the mechanisms by which this occurs remain obscure. To the extent that coexisting LCIS might contribute to local recurrence, this risk can be partially offset by adjuvant chemoprevention and antiestrogen therapy. Almost all reported studies failed to distinguish between classical LCIS and PLCIS in evaluating the impact of coexisting LCIS on the risk of local breast recurrence. Since PLCIS is relatively uncommon, they probably dealt with LCIS. One currently available study that specifically addressed PLCIS is inconclusive.

CONCLUDING COMMENTS

It is evident from the foregoing discussion that LCIS is a morphologically and clinically heterogeneous disease. The concept that LCIS is simply a "marker" lesion has been widely promulgated. The impression created by this idea is that LCIS is a proliferative abnormality associated with an increased risk of the development of breast carcinoma, but, in contrast to DCIS, LCIS is rarely, if ever, a direct precursor to invasive carcinoma. This unfortunate and oft-repeated misperception widely disseminated for more than two decades is now falling into disfavor. Data extensively set forth in three previous editions of this book that are amplified and updated in this chapter and in Chapter 32 on invasive lobular carcinoma support the conclusion that LCIS is a direct precursor to invasive lobular carcinoma, and possibly in a minority of instances to IDC (e.g., ductolobular, tubulolobular), although this progression is not observed in the lifetime of every patient with LCIS.

As detailed earlier in this chapter, data closely linking LCIS to invasive lobular carcinoma come from molecular studies of the two lesions when they coexist. For example, Vos et al.[92] demonstrated that LCIS and invasive lobular carcinomas had losses of the same alleles in 16q22.1 and the same *E-cadherin* mutations. Similar results were obtained by Sarrió et al.[158] who found that coincidental LCIS and invasive lobular carcinomas shared the same *E-cadherin* mutations and same distribution of LOH. Additional supporting studies were published by Nayar et al.[100] and Hwang et al.[159]

It appears that progression of LCIS to the invasive phenotype is less frequent, and that on average it takes longer than is the case for DCIS. When LCIS and DCIS coexist in a patient, it is not surprising that IDC might develop sooner and be the primary diagnosis more frequently than invasive lobular carcinoma, leading to treatment before the *in situ* lobular lesion has had an opportunity to evolve into invasive lobular carcinoma.

LCIS is a cytologically and structurally heterogeneous disease. The relationship of these differences to prognosis or to the risk of progression has not been well characterized. Until the disease is better characterized, its management will likely continue to be controversial. Indeed, even the preliminary decision on whether or not to perform an excisional biopsy following a needle core biopsy diagnosis of LCIS continues to be a contentious one with relatively divergent recommendations.[160–165]

Perhaps the greatest challenge to regarding LCIS as a "marker" lesion has come from the recent recognition of FLCIS and PLCIS that are characterized by marked gland expansion with a tendency to necrosis and calcification. Although LCIS is usually discovered as an incidental lesion when mammography detects another abnormality, FLCIS and PLCIS are likely to present with calcifications and a pattern that resembles DCIS. The paradigm of LCIS as an incidental "marker" lesion does not fit well with this clinical presentation and histopathologic findings. Additional study of FLCIS and PLCIS is needed, especially with long-term clinical correlation. In view of the relatively frequent instances of coincidental invasive lobular carcinoma, FLCIS and PLCIS might, in some cases, be treated as if they were DCIS, at least with respect to local surgical control in the conserved breast. The effectiveness of radiotherapy for treating FLCIS and PLCIS has not been determined.[166] The role of chemoprevention with tamoxifen or other agents also needs to be investigated in patients with FLCIS and PLCIS. Further molecular characterization of LCIS, and its variants, is likely to provide a basis in the future for the selective treatment of subgroups of patients with this heterogeneous disease.[167]

REFERENCES

1. Muir R. The evolution of carcinoma of the mamma. *J Pathol Bacteriol* 1941;52:155–172.
2. Foote FW Jr, Stewart FW. Lobular carcinoma *in situ*: a rare form of mammary cancer. *Am J Pathol* 1941;17:491–496.
3. Rosen PP. The pathological classification of human mammary carcinoma: past, present and future. *Ann Clin Lab Sci* 1979;9:144–156.
4. Rosen PP. Lobular carcinoma *in situ* and intraductal carcinoma of the breast. In: McDivitt RW, Oberman HA, Ozzello L, et al., eds. *The breast*. Baltimore: Williams and Wilkins, 1984:59–105.
5. Andersen J. Lobular carcinoma *in situ*: a long-term follow-up in 52 cases. *Acta Pathol Microbiol Scand (A)* 1974;82:519–533.
6. Rosen PP, Lieberman PH, Braun DW Jr, et al. Lobular carcinoma *in situ* of the breast. Detailed analysis of 99 patients with average follow-up of 24 years. *Am J Surg Pathol* 1978;2:225–251.
7. Wheeler JE, Enterline HT, Roseman J, et al. Lobular carcinoma *in situ* of the breast: long term follow-up. *Cancer* 1974;34:554–563.
8. Page DL, Kidd Jr TE, Dupont WD, et al. Lobular neoplasia of the breast: higher risk for subsequent invasive cancer predicted by more extensive disease. *Hum Pathol* 1991;22:1232–1239.
9. Haagensen CD. Lobular neoplasia (Lobular carcinoma *in situ*). In: *Diseases of the breast*. 3rd ed. Philadelphia: WB Saunders, 1986:192–781.
10. Nielsen M, Jensen J, Andersen J. Precancerous and cancerous breast lesions during lifetime and at autopsy. *Cancer* 1984;54:612–615.
11. Nielsen M, Thomsen JL, Primdahl L, et al. Breast Cancer and atypia among young and middle-aged women: a study of 110 medicolegal autopsies. *Br J Cancer* 1987;56:814–819.
12. Alpers CE, Wellings SR. The prevalence of carcinoma *in situ* in normal and cancer associated breasts. *Hum Pathol* 1985;16:796–807.

13. Frantz VK, Pickren JW, Melcher GW, et al. Incidence of chronic cystic disease in so-called normal breasts: a study based on 225 postmortem examinations. *Cancer* 1951;4:762–783.
14. Kramer WM, Rush BF Jr. Mammary duct proliferation in the elderly. *Cancer* 1973;31:130–137.
15. Li CI, Anderson BO, Daling JR, et al. Changing incidence of lobular carcinoma *in situ* of the breast. *Breast Cancer Res Treat* 2002;75:259–268.
16. Eheman CR, Shaw KM, Ryerson AB, et al. The changing incidence of *in situ* and invasive ductal and lobular breast carcinomas: United States, 1999–2004. *Cancer Epidemiol Biomarkers Prev* 2009;18:1763–1769.
17. Mackarem G, Yacoub LK, Lee AKC, et al. Effects of screening on detection of lobular carcinoma *in situ* of the breast: nonspecificity of mammography and physical examination. *Breast Dis* 1994;7:339–345.
18. Morris DM, Walker AP, Cocker DC. Lack of efficacy of xeromammography in preoperatively detecting lobular carcinoma *in situ* of the breast. *Breast Cancer Res Treat* 1982;1:365–368.
19. Beahrs O, Shapiro S, Smart C. Report of the working group to review the National Cancer Institute—American Cancer Society Breast Cancer Demonstration Projects. *J Natl Cancer Inst* 1979;62:640–708.
20. Rosen PP. Columnar cell hyperplasia is associated with lobular carcinoma *in situ* and tubular carcinoma. *Am J Surg Pathol* 1999;23:1561.
21. Scoggins M, Krishnamurthy S, Santiago L, et al. Lobular carcinoma *in situ* of the breast: clinical, radiological, and pathological correlation. *Acad Radiol* 2013;20:463–470.
22. Hutter RVP, Snyder RE, Lucas J, et al. Clinical and pathologic correlation with mammographic findings in lobular carcinoma *in situ*. *Cancer* 1969;23:826–839.
23. Pope TL Jr, Fechner RE, Wilhelm MC, et al. Lobular carcinoma *in situ* of the breast: mammographic features. *Radiology* 1988;168:63–66.
24. Fadare O, Dadmanesh F, Alvarado-Cabrero I, et al. Lobular intraepithelial neoplasia [lobular carcinoma *in situ*] with comedo-type necrosis. A clinicopathologic study of 18 cases. *Am J Surg Pathol* 2006;30:1445–1453.
25. Haagensen CD. Lobular carcinoma of the breast. A precancerous lesion? *Clin Obstet Gynecol* 1962;5:1093–1101.
26. Haagensen CD, Lane N, Lattes R. Neoplastic proliferation of the epithelium of the mammary lobules: adenosis, lobular neoplasia and small cell carcinoma. *Surg Clin North Am* 1972;52:497–524.
27. Haagensen CD, Lane N, Lattes R, et al. Lobular neoplasia (so-called lobular carcinoma *in situ*) of the breast. *Cancer* 1978;42:737–769.
28. Gump FE. Lobular carcinoma *in situ*. Pathology and treatment. *Surg Clin North Am* 1990;70:873–883.
29. Rosen PP, Senie R, Ashikari R, et al. Age, menstrual status, and exogenous hormone usage in patients with lobular carcinoma *in situ* (LCIS). *Surgery* 1979;85:219–224.
30. Dall'Olmo CA, Ponka JL, Horn RC Jr, et al. Lobular carcinoma *in situ*. Are we too radical in its treatment? *Arch Surg* 1975;110:537–542.
31. Lewison EF, Finney GG Jr. Lobular carcinoma *in situ* of the breast. *Surg Gynecol Obstet* 1968;126:1280–1286.
32. Newman W. Lobular carcinoma of the female breast. Report of 73 cases. *Ann Surg* 1966;164:305–314.
33. Ackerman BL, Otis C, Stueber K. Lobular carcinoma *in situ* in a 15-year-old girl: a case report and review of the literature. *Plast Reconst Surg* 1994;94:714–718.
34. Rosen PP, Lesser ML, Senie RT, et al. Epidemiology of breast carcinoma IV: age and histologic tumor type. *J Surg Oncol* 1982;19:44–47.
35. Barnes JP. Bilateral lobular carcinoma *in situ* of the breast. Report of two cases. *Texas State J Med* 1959;55:581–584.
36. Newman W. *In situ* lobular carcinoma of the breast. *Ann Surg* 1963;151:591–599.
37. Urban JA. Biopsy of the "normal" breast in treating breast cancer. *Surg Clin North Am* 1969;49:291–301.
38. Erdreich LS, Asal NR, Hoge AF. Morphologic types of breast cancer: age, bilaterality and family history. *Southern Med J* 1980;73:28–32.
39. Sunshine JA, Moseley HS, Fletcher WS, et al. Breast carcinoma *in situ*. A retrospective review of 112 cases with minimum 10 year follow-up. *Am J Surg* 1985;150:44–51.
40. Lesser ML, Rosen PP, Kinne DW. Multicentricity and bilaterality in invasive breast carcinoma. *Surgery* 1982;91:234–240.
41. Andersen JA. Multicentric and bilateral appearance of lobular carcinoma *in situ* of the breast. *Acta Pathol Microbiol Scand (A)* 1974;82:730–734.
42. Farrow JH. Current concepts in the detection and treatment of the earliest of the early breast cancers. *Cancer* 1970;25:458–479.
43. Warner NE. Lobular carcinoma of the breast. *Cancer* 1969;23:840–846.
44. Shah JP, Rosen PP, Robbins GF. Pitfalls of local excision in the treatment of carcinoma of the breast. *Surg Gynecol Obstet* 1973;136:721–725.
45. Carter D, Smith AL. Carcinoma *in situ* of the breast. *Cancer* 1977;40:1189–1193.
46. Tulusan AH, Egger H, Schneider ML, et al. A contribution to the natural history of breast cancer. IV. Lobular carcinoma *in situ* and its relation to breast cancer. *Arch Gynecol* 1982;231:219–226.
47. Hutter RVP, Foote FW Jr, Farrow JH. *In situ* lobular carcinoma of the female breast, 1939–1968. In: *Breast cancer, early and late*. Chicago: Year Book Medical Publishers, 1970:201–236.
48. Page DL, Anderson TJ. *Diagnostic histopathology of the breast*. New York: Churchill Livingstone, 1987.
49. Zippel HH, Hematsch HJ, Kunze WP. Morphometric and cytophotometric investigations of lobular neoplasia of the breast with ductal involvement. *J Cancer Res Clin Oncol* 1979;93:265–274.
50. Acs G, Lawton TJ, Rebbeck TR, et al. Differential expression of E-cadherin in lobular and ductal neoplasms of the breast and its biological and diagnostic implications. *Am J Clin Pathol* 2001;115:85–89.
51. Goldstein NS, Bassi D, Watts JC, et al. E-Cadherin reactivity of 95 noninvasive ductal and lobular lesions of the breast. Implications for the interpretation of problematic lesions. *Am J Clin Pathol* 2001;115:534–542.
52. Jacobs TW, Pliss N, Kouria G, et al. Carcinomas *in situ* of the breast with indeterminate features. Role of E-cadherin staining in categorization. *Am J Surg Pathol* 2001;25:229–236.
53. Sullivan ME, Khan SA, Sullu Y, et al. Lobular carcinoma *in situ* variants in breast cores. Potential for misdiagnosis, upgrade rates at surgical excision, and practical implications. *Arch Pathol Lab Med* 2010;134:1024–1028.
54. Andersen JA, Vendelhoe ML. Cytoplasmic mucous globules in lobular carcinoma *in situ*. Diagnosis and prognosis. *Am J Surg Pathol* 1981;5:251–255.
55. Gad A, Azzopardi JG. Lobular carcinoma of the breast: a special variant of mucin secreting carcinoma. *J Clin Pathol* 1975;28:711–716.
56. Breslow A, Brancaccio ME. Intracellular mucin production by lobular carcinoma cells. *Arch Pathol Lab Med* 1976;100:620–621.
57. Fadare O. Pleomorphic lobular carcinoma *in situ* of the breast composed almost entirely of signet ring cells. *Pathol Int* 2006;56:683–687.
58. Eusebi V, Pich A, Macchiorlatti E, et al. Morphofunctional differentiation in lobular carcinoma of the breast. *Histopathology* 1977;1:301–314.
59. Barwick K, Kashgarian M, Rosen PP. "Clear cell" change within duct and lobular epithelium of the human breast. *Pathol Annu* 1982;17 (Part 1):319–328.
60. Eusebi V, Betts C, Haagensen DE, et al. Apocrine differentiation in lobular carcinoma of the breast: a morphologic, immunologic and ultrastructural study. *Hum Pathol* 1984;15:134–140.
61. Chen Y, Fitzgibbons P, Jacobs T, et al. Pleomorphic apocrine lobular carcinoma *in situ* (PALCIS): phenotypic and genetic study of a distinct variant of lobular carcinoma *in situ* (LCIS). *Mod Pathol* 2005;18 (Suppl. 1):29A.
62. Andersen JA. Lobular carcinoma *in situ* of the breast with ductal involvement. Frequency and possible influence on prognosis. *Acta Pathol Microbiol Scand (A)* 1974;82:655–662.
63. Fechner RE. Epithelial alterations in extralobular ducts of breasts with lobular carcinoma. *Arch Pathol* 1972;93:164–171.
64. Rosen PP, Tench W. Lobules in the nipple. Frequency and significance for breast cancer treatment. *Pathol Annu* 1985;20 (Part 2):317–322.
65. Sahoo S, Green I, Rosen PP. Bilateral Paget disease of the nipple associated with lobular carcinoma *in situ*. Application of immunohistochemistry to a rare finding. *Arch Pathol Lab Med* 2002;126:90–92.
66. Rosa M, Mohammadi A, Masood S. Lobular neoplasia displaying central necrosis: a potential diagnostic pitfall. *Pathol Res and Pract* 2010;206:544–549.
67. Alvarado-Cabrero I, Coronel GP, Cedillo RV, et al. Florid lobular intraepithelial neoplasia with signet ring cells, central necrosis and calcifications: a clinicopathological and immunohistochemical analysis of ten cases associated with invasive lobular carcinoma. *Arch Med Research* 2010;41:436–441.
68. Bagaria SP, Shamonki J, Kinnaird M, et al. The florid subtype of lobular carcinoma *in situ*: marker or precursor for invasive lobular carcinoma? *Ann Surg Oncol* 2011;18:1845–1851.
69. Boldt V, Stacher E, Halbwedl I, et al. Positioning of necrotic lobular intraepithelial neoplasias (LIN, Grade 3) within the sequence

of breast carcinoma progression. *Genes, Chromosomes & Cancer* 2010;49:463–470.
70. Fechner RE. Lobular carcinoma *in situ* in sclerosing adenosis. A potential source of confusion with invasive carcinoma. *Am J Surg Pathol* 1981;5:233–239.
71. Oberman HA, Markey BA. Noninvasive carcinoma of the breast presenting in adenosis. *Mod Pathol* 1991;4:31–35.
72. Auger M, Huttner I. Fine-needle aspiration cytology of pleomorphic lobular carcinoma of the breast. *Cancer* 2008;36:657–661.
73. Sgroi D, Koerner FC. Involvement of collagenous spherulosis by lobular carcinoma *in situ*. Potential confusion with cribriform ductal carcinoma *in situ*. *Am J Surg Pathol* 1995;19:1366–1370.
74. Shousha S. *In situ* lobular neoplasia of the breast with marked myoepithelial proliferation. *Histopathology* 2011;58:1081–1085.
75. Salhany KE, Page DL. Fine-needle aspiration of mammary lobular carcinoma *in situ* and atypical lobular hyperplasia. *Am J Clin Pathol* 1989;92:22–26.
76. Miller MJ, Massimiliano C, Casadio C. Cytologic findings of breast ductal lavage and concurrent fine needle aspiration in pleomorphic lobular carcinoma *in situ*. *Acta Cytol* 2008;52:207–210.
77. Ross DS, Hoda SA. Microinvasive (T1mic) lobular carcinoma of the breast: clinicopathologic profile of 16 cases. *Am J Surg Pathol* 2011;35:750–756.
78. Nemoto T, Castillo N, Tsukada Y, et al. Lobular carcinoma *in situ* with microinvasion. *J Surg Oncol* 1998;67:41–46.
79. Prasad ML, Hyjek E, Giri DD, et al. Double immunolabeling with cytokeratin and smooth-muscle actin in confirming early invasive carcinoma of breast. *Am J Surg Pathol* 1999;23:176–181.
80. Ozzello L. Ultrastructure of intra-epithelial carcinomas of the breast. *Cancer* 1971;28:1508–1515.
81. Tobon H, Price HM. Lobular carcinoma *in situ*. Some ultrastructural observations. *Cancer* 1972;30:1082–1091.
82. Bussolati G. Actin-rich (myoepithelial) cells in lobular carcinoma *in situ* of the breast. *Virchows Arch [A]* 1980;32:165–176.
83. Andersen JA. The basement membrane and lobular carcinoma *in situ* of the breast. A light microscopical study. *Acta Pathol Microbiol Scand (A)* 1975;83:245–250.
84. de Deus Moura R, Wludarski SC, Carvalho FM, et al. Immunohistochemistry applied to the differential diagnosis between ductal and lobular carcinoma of the breast. *Appl Immunohistochem Mol Morphol* 2013;21:1–12.
85. Vincent-Salomon A, Hajage D, Rouquette A, et al. High Ki67 expression is a risk marker of invasive relapse for classical lobular carcinoma *in situ* patients. *Breast* 2012;21:380–383.
86. Bur ME, Zimarowski MJ, Schnitt SJ, et al. Estrogen receptor immunohistochemistry in carcinoma *in situ* of the breast. *Cancer* 1992;69:174–1181.
87. Pallis L, Wilking N, Cedermark B, et al. Receptors for estrogen and progesterone in breast carcinoma *in situ*. *Anticancer Res* 1992;12:2113–2115.
88. Chen Y-Y, Hwang E-SS, Roy R, et al. Genetic and phenotypic characteristics of pleomorphic lobular carcinoma *in situ* of the breast. *Am J Surg Pathol* 2009;33:1683–1694.
89. Green AR, Young P, Krivinskas S, et al. The expression of ERα, ERß, and PR in lobular carcinoma *in situ* of the breast determined using laser microdissection or real-time PCR. *Histopathology* 2009;54:419–427.
90. Ramachandra S, Machin L, Ashley S, et al. Immunohistochemical distribution of c-erbB-2 in *in situ* breast carcinoma—a detailed morphological analysis. *J Pathol* 1990;161:7–14.
91. Somerville JE, Clarke LA, Biggart JD. c-erbB-2 overexpression and histological type of *in situ* and invasive breast carcinoma. *J Clin Pathol* 1992;45:16–20.
92. Vos CB, Cleton-Jones AM, Berx G, et al. E-Cadherin in-activation in lobular carcinoma *in situ* of the breast: an early event in tumor genesis. *Br J Cancer* 1997;76:1131–1133.
93. Moll R, Mitze M, Frixen UH, et al. Differential loss of E-cadherin expression in infiltrating ductal and lobular carcinomas. *Am J Pathol* 1993;143:1737–1742.
94. Morrogh M, Andrade VP, Giri D, et al. Cadherin-catenin complex dissociation in lobular neoplasia of the breast. *Breast Cancer Res Treat* 2012;132:641–652.
95. Goldstein NS, Kestin LL, Vicini FA. Clinicopathologic implications of E-cadherin reactivity in patients with lobular carcinoma *in situ* of the breast. *Cancer* 2001;92:738–747.
96. DaSilva L, Parry S, Reid L, et al. Aberrant expression of E-cadherin in lobular carcinomas of the breast. *Am J Surg Pathol* 2008;32:773–783.
97. Etzell JE, DeVries S, Chew K, et al. Loss of chromosome 16q in lobular carcinoma *in situ*. *Hum Pathol* 2001;32:292–296.
98. Rahman N, Stone JG, Coleman G, et al. Lobular carcinoma *in situ* of the breast is not caused by constitutional mutations in the E-cadherin gene. *Br J Cancer* 2000;82:568–570.
99. Salahshor S, Haixin L, Huo H, et al. Low frequency of E-cadherin alterations in familial breast cancer. *Breast Cancer Res* 2001;3:199–207.
100. Nayar R, Zhuang Z, Merino MJ, et al. Loss of heterozygosity on chromosome 11q13 in lobular lesions of the breast using tissue microdissection and polymerase chain reaction. *Hum Pathol* 1997;28:277–282.
101. Mastracci TL, Tjan S, Ban AL, et al. E-Cadherin alterations in atypical lobular hyperplasia and lobular carcinoma *in situ* of the breast. *Mod Pathol* 2005;18:741–751.
102. Keller G, Vogelsang H, Becker I, et al. Diffuse-type gastric and lobular breast carcinoma in familial gastric cancer patients with E-cadherin germline mutation. *Am J Pathol* 1999;155:337–342.
103. Tran-Thanh D, Arneson NC, Pintilie M, et al. Amplification of the prolactin receptor gene in mammary lobular neoplasia. *Breast Cancer Res Treat* 2011;128:31–40.
104. Helvie MA, Hessler C, Frank TS, et al. Atypical hyperplasia of the breast: mammographic appearance and histologic correlation. *Radiology* 1991;179:759–764.
105. Ioffe O, Silverberg SG, Simsir A. Lobular lesions of the breast: immunohistochemical profile and comparison with ductal proliferations. *Mod Pathol* 2000;13:23A.
106. Bodian CA, Perzin KH, Lattes R, et al. Prognostic significance of benign proliferative breast disease. *Cancer* 1993;71:3896–3907.
107. Page DL, Van der Zwaag R, Rogers LW, et al. Relation between component parts of fibrocystic disease complex and breast cancer. *J Natl Cancer Inst* 1978;61:1055–1063.
108. Page DL, Dupont WD, Rogers LW, et al. Atypical hyperplastic lesions of the female breast. A long-term follow-up study. *Cancer* 1985;55:2698–2708.
109. Page DL, Schuyler PA, Dupont WD, et al. Atypical lobular hyperplasia as a unilateral predictor of breast cancer risk: a retrospective cohort study. *Lancet* 2003;361:125–129.
110. Collins L, Baer H, Tamimi R, et al. Magnitude and laterality of breast cancer risk in women with atypical hyperplasia of ductal and lobular types. *Mod Pathol* 2006;19 (Suppl.1):24A.
111. McLaren BK, Schuyler PA, Sanders ME, et al. Excellent survival, cancer type and Nottingham grade after atypical lobular hyperplasia in initial breast biopsy. *Cancer* 2006;107:1227–1233.
112. Godwin JT. Chronology of lobular carcinoma of the breast. *Cancer* 1952;5:259–266.
113. Miller HW Jr, Kay S. Infiltrating lobular carcinoma of the female mammary gland. *Surg Gynecol Obstet* 1956;102:661–667.
114. Giordano JM, Klopp CT. Lobular carcinoma *in situ*: incidence and treatment. *Cancer* 1973;31:105–109.
115. Bodian CA, Perzin KH, Lattes R. Lobular neoplasia. Long term risk of breast cancer and relation to other factors. *Cancer* 1996;78:1024–1034.
116. Cohen MA. Cancer upgrades at excisional biopsy after diagnosis of atypical lobular hyperplasia or lobular carcinoma *in situ* at core-needle core biopsy: some reasons why. *Radiology* 2004;231:671–621.
117. Ciatto S, Cataliotti C, Cardona G, et al. Risk of infiltrating breast cancer subsequent to lobular carcinoma *in situ*. *Tumori* 1992;78:244–246.
118. Fisher ER, Costantino J, Fisher B, et al., for the National Surgical Adjuvant Breast and Bowel Project Collaborating Investigators. Pathologic findings from the National Surgical Adjuvant Breast Project (NSABP) Protocol B-17. Five-year observations concerning lobular carcinoma *in situ*. *Cancer* 1996;78:1403–1416.
119. Fisher ER, Land SR, Fisher B, et al. Pathologic findings from the National Surgical Adjuvant Breast and Bowel Project. Twelve-year observations concerning lobular carcinoma *in situ*. *Cancer* 2004;100:238–244.
120. Ottesen GL, Graversen HP, Blichert-Toft M, et al. Lobular carcinoma *in situ* of the female breast. Short-term results of a prospective nationwide study. *Am J Surg Pathol* 1993;17:14–21.
121. Li CI, Malone KE, Saltzman BS, et al. Risk of invasive breast carcinoma among women diagnosed with ductal carcinoma *in situ* and lobular carcinoma *in situ* 1998–2001. *Cancer* 2006;106:2104–2112.
122. Carley AM, Chivukula M, Carter GJ, et al. Frequency and clinical significance of simultaneous association of lobular neoplasia and

columnar cell alterations in breast tissue. *Am J Clin Pathol* 2008;130:254–258.
123. Brandt, SM, Young GQ, Hoda SA. The "Rosen Triad': tubular carcinoma, lobular carcinoma *in situ*, and columnar cell lesions. *Adv Anat Pathol* 2008;15;140–146.
124. Liberman L, Sama M, Susnik B, et al. Lobular carcinoma *in situ* at percutaneous breast biopsy: surgical biopsy findings. *AJR Am J Roentgenol* 1999;173:291–299.
125. Lechner MD, Park SL, Jackman RJ, et al. Lobular carcinoma *in situ* and atypical lobular hyperplasia at percutaneous biopsy with surgical correlation: a multi-institutional study. *Radiology* 1999;213:106.
126. Foster MC, Helvie MA, Gregory NE, et al. Lobular carcinoma *in situ* or atypical lobular hyperplasia at core-needle biopsy: is excisional biopsy necessary? *Radiology* 2004;231:813–819.
127. Crisi GM, Mandavilli S, Cronin E, et al. Invasive mammary carcinoma after immediate and short-term follow-up for lobular neoplasia on core biopsy. *Am J Surg Pathol* 2003;27:325–333.
128. Arpino G, Allred DC, Mohsin SK, et al. Lobular neoplasia on core-needle biopsy—clinical significance. *Cancer* 2004;101:242–250.
129. Hussain M, Cunnick GH. Management of lobular carcinoma *in-situ* and atypical lobular hyperplasia of the breast—a review. *EJSO* 2011;37:279–289.
130. Carder PJ, Shaaban A, Alizadeh Y, et al. Screen-detected pleomorphic lobular carcinoma *in situ* (PLICS): risk of concurrent invasive malignancy following a core biopsy diagnosis. *Histopathology* 2010;57:472–478.
131. Chivukula M, Haynik DM, Brufsky A, et al. Pleomorphic lobular carcinoma *in situ* (PLCIS) on breast core needle biopsies. Clinical significance and immunoprofile. *Am J Surg Pathol* 2008;32:1721–1726.
132. Menon S, Porter GJR, Evans AJ, et al. The significance of lobular neoplasia on needle core biopsy of the breast. *Virchows Arch* 2008;452:473–479.
133. Murray MP, Luedtke C, Liberman L, et al. Classic lobular carcinoma *in situ* and atypical lobular hyperplasia at percutaneous breast core biopsy: outcomes of prospective excision. *Cancer* 2013;119:1073–1079.
134. Hwang H, Barke LD, Mendelson EB, et al. Atypical lobular hyperplasia and classic lobular carcinoma *in situ* in core biopsy specimens: routine excision is not necessary. *Mod Pathol* 2008;21:1208–1216.
135. Brem RF, Lechner MC, Jackman RJ, et al. Lobular neoplasia at percutaneous breast biopsy: variables associated with carcinoma at surgical excision. *AJR* 2008;190:637–641.
136. Cangiarella J, Guth A, Axelrod D, et al. Is surgical excision necessary for the management of atypical lobular hyperplasia and lobular carcinoma *in situ* diagnosed on needle core biopsy? *Arch Pathol Lab Med* 2008;132:979–983.
137. Sung JS, Malak SF, Bajaj P, et al. Screening breast MR imaging in women with a history of lobular carcinoma *in situ*. *Radiology* 2011;261:414–420.
138. Baum M, Brinkley DM, Dossett JA, et al. Control trial of tamoxifen and adjuvant agent in management of early breast cancer. *Lancet* 1983;1:257–269.
139. Nayfield SG, Karp JE, Ford LG, et al. Potential role of tamoxifen in prevention of breast cancer. *J Natl Cancer Inst* 1991;83:1450–1459.
140. Rutqvist LE, Cedermark B, Glas U, et al. Contralateral primary tumors in breast cancer patients in a randomized trial of adjuvant tamoxifen therapy. *J Natl Cancer Inst* 1991;83:1299–1306.
141. Powles TJ, Hardy JR, Ashley SE, et al. Chemoprevention of breast cancer. *Breast Cancer Res Treat* 1989;14:23–31.
142. Fisher B, Costantino JP, Wickerham DL, et al. Tamoxifen for prevention of breast cancer: report of the National Surgical Adjuvant Breast and Bowel Project P-1 Study. *J Natl Cancer Inst* 1998;90:1371–1388.
143. Wickerham DL, Constantino JP, Vogel V, et al. The study of tamoxifen and raloxifene (STAR): initial findings from the NSABP P-2 breast cancer prevention study [Meeting Abstracts]. *J Clin Oncol* 2006;24:LBA5.
144. Smart CR, Myers MH, Gloeckler LA. Implications from SEER data on breast cancer management. *Cancer* 1978;41:787–789.
145. Rosen PP, Saigo PE, Braun DW Jr. Predictors of recurrence in stage I (T1N0M0) breast carcinoma. *Ann Surg* 1981;193:15–31.
146. Cutuli B, Jaeck D, Renaud R, et al. Lobular carcinoma *in situ* of the breast: results of a radiosurgical conservative treatment. *Oncol Rep* 1998;5:1531–1533.
147. Osborne MP, Borgen PI. Atypical ductal and lobular hyperplasia and breast cancer risk. *Surg Oncol Clin N Am* 1993;2:1–11.
148. Stolier AJ, Barre G, Bolton JS, et al. Breast conservation therapy for invasive lobular carcinoma: the impact of lobular carcinoma *in situ* in the surgical specimen on local recurrence and axillary node status. *Ann Surg* 2004;70:818–821.
149. Rudloff U, Brogi E, Brockway JP, et al. Concurrent lobular neoplasia increases the risk of ipsilateral breast cancer recurrence in patients with ductal carcinoma *in situ* treated with breast-conserving therapy. *Cancer* 2009;115:1203–1214.
150. Moran M, Haffty BG. Lobular carcinoma *in situ* as a component of breast cancer: the long-term outcome in patients treated with breast-conservation therapy. *Int J Radiat Oncol Biol Phys* 1998;40:353–358.
151. Abner AL, Connolly JL, Recht A, et al. The relation between the presence and extent of lobular carcinoma *in situ* and the risk of local recurrence for patients with infiltrating carcinoma of the breast treated with conservative surgery and radiation therapy. *Cancer* 2000;88:1072–1077.
152. Ben-David MA, Kleer CG, Paramgul C, et al. Is lobular carcinoma *in situ* as a component of breast carcinoma a risk factor for local failure after breast-conserving therapy? Results of a matched pair analysis. *Cancer* 2006;106:28–34.
153. Ciocca RM, Li T, Freedman GM, et al. The presence of lobular carcinoma *in situ* does not increase local recurrence in patients treated with breast-conserving therapy. *Ann Surg Oncol* 2008;15:2263–2271.
154. Sasson AR, Fowble B, Hanlon AL, et al. Lobular carcinoma *in situ* increases the risk of local recurrence in selected patients with stages I and II breast carcinoma treated with conservative surgery and radiation. *Cancer* 2001;91:1862–1869.
155. Jolly S, Kestin LL, Goldstein NS, et al. The impact of lobular carcinoma *in situ* in association with invasive breast cancer on the rate of local recurrence in patients with early-stage breast cancer treated with breast-conserving therapy. *Int J Radiat Oncol Biol Phys* 2006;66:365–371.
156. Mechera R, Viehl CT, Oertli D. Factors predicting in-breast tumor recurrence after breast-conserving therapy. *Breast Cancer Res Treat* 2009;116:171–177.
157. Downs-Kelly E, Bell D, Perkins GH, et al. Clinical implications of margin involvement by pleomorphic lobular carcinoma *in situ*. *Arch Pathol Lab Med* 2011;135: 737–743.
158. Sarrió D, Moreno-Bueno G, Hardisson E, et al. Epigenetic and genetic alterations of APC and CDH1 genes in lobular breast cancer: relationships with abnormal E-cadherin and catenin expression and microsatellite instability. *Int J Cancer* 2003;106:208–215.
159. Hwang ES, Nyante SJ, Chen YY, et al. Clonality of lobular carcinoma *in situ* and synchronous invasive lobular carcinoma. *Cancer* 2004;100:2562–272.
160. Niell B, Specht M, Gerade B, et al. Is excisional biopsy required after a breast core biopsy yields lobular neoplasia? *AJR Am J Roentgenol* 2012;199:929–935.
161. Ibrahim N, Bessissow A, Lalonde L, et al. Surgical outcome of biopsy-proven lobular neoplasia: is there any difference between lobular carcinoma *in situ* and atypical lobular hyperplasia? *AJR Am J Roentgenol* 2012;198:288–291.
162. Zhao C, Desouki MM, Florea A, et al. Pathologic findings of follow-up surgical excision for lobular neoplasia on breast core biopsy performed for calcification. *Am J Clin Pathol* 2012;138:72–78.
163. Shah-Khan MG, Geiger XJ, Reynolds C, et al. Long-term follow-up of lobular neoplasia (atypical lobular hyperplasia/lobular carcinoma *in situ*) diagnosed on core needle biopsy. *Ann Surg Oncol* 2012;19:3131–3138.
164. Rendi MH, Dintzis SM, Lehman CD, et al. Lobular *in situ* neoplasia on breast core needle biopsy: imaging indication and pathologic extent can identify which patients require excisional biopsy. *Ann Surg Oncol* 2012;19:914–921.
165. Chaudhary S, Lawrence L, McGinty G, et al. Classic lobular neoplasia on core biopsy: a clinical and radio-pathologic correlation study with follow-up excision biopsy. *Mod Pathol* 2013;26:762–771.
166. Masannat YA, Bains SK, Pinder SE, et al. Challenges in the management of pleomorphic lobular carcinoma *in situ* of the breast. *Breast* 2013;22:194–196.
167. Monhollen L, Morrison C, Ademuyiwa FO, et al. Pleomorphic lobular carcinoma: a distinctive clinical and molecular breast cancer type. *Histopathology* 2012;61:365–377.

CHAPTER 32

Invasive Lobular Carcinoma

SYED A. HODA

The term "lobular carcinoma" became fully established in 1941 with the publication of the classic paper on lobular carcinoma *in situ* (LCIS) by Foote and Stewart.[1] They stated, "When the tumor infiltrates, it is apt to do so in a peculiar fashion which permits one, after some experience, to recognize the high probability of such origin." An associated desmoplastic stromal reaction, linear arrangement of the carcinoma cells, and their tendency to grow in a circumferential fashion around ducts and lobules (targetoid growth) were "peculiar" diagnostic features emphasized by Foote and Stewart. They also observed that although concurrent LCIS was not found in every case, the histologic pattern was sufficiently distinctive to be considered a specific histologic type of invasive carcinoma that arose from *in situ* carcinoma of the lobular and terminal duct epithelium.

Invasive lobular carcinoma (ILC), as it was described by Foote and Stewart, is now referred to as classical ILC. In the past 15 years or so, with the recognition that lobular carcinoma is characterized by loss of immunoreactivity for catenins and E-cadherin, classical type of ILC has been distinguished from pleomorphic type of ILC (PILC). Virtually all data about ILC published in the 20th century relate to classical ILC. In this chapter, the abbreviation ILC is used when referring to studies published before and after 2000, unless they refer specifically to PILC.

Less than 5% of invasive mammary carcinomas are composed of a mixture of ductal and lobular histologic features. These mixed carcinomas constituted 3.6% of 4,412 breast carcinomas described in a report by Rakha et al.[2] They consist of areas with solid or cohesive growth, sometimes with focal gland–forming elements, typical for invasive ductal carcinoma (IDC) and areas of dyscohesive cells distributed in linear arrays found in ILC. Varying proportions of these components may be present in an individual tumor. The histologic appearance of axillary nodal metastases usually corresponds to the predominant growth pattern of the primary tumors. *In situ* carcinoma consisting of IDC, ILC, or both is often present. After adjustment for grade, analysis of various markers revealed an expression profile that was intermediate between IDC and ILC but with no significant difference in survival between IDC and ILC.

INCIDENCE

When the diagnosis of ILC is based strictly on the criteria of Foote and Stewart, ILC usually constitutes 5% or less of the carcinomas in most series. Newman[3] reviewed 1,396 carcinomas treated over a 17-year period and found that 5% could be classified as ILC, and a review of more than 4,000 carcinomas treated at the Mayo Clinic revealed that 3.2% were ILC.[4] An analysis of more than 21,000 breast carcinomas diagnosed in the United States from 1969 to 1971 found 3% classified as infiltrating lobular type.[5]

A population-based study of women with invasive breast carcinoma diagnosed in the United States between 1987 and 1999 revealed that the incidence of lobular carcinoma increased during this period.[6] The increased incidence of ILC was greatest in women aged 50 years or older. On the other hand, the incidence of IDC was relatively constant. Subsequent analysis of data representing 92.1% of the women in the United States between 1999 and 2004 revealed that the age-adjusted incidence of ILC declined by 20.5%, whereas the age-adjusted incidence of IDC and all breast carcinomas were reduced by 14.2% and 11.6%, respectively.[7] The authors speculated that the decreased incidence of ILC could be "related to a reduced use of combined hormone replacement therapy." Chikman et al.[8] analyzed 2,175 consecutive patients with breast carcinoma in Israel between 1992 and 2009. During the entire period, 8.6% of the carcinomas were classified as ILC, rising from 4.6% in 1992 to 1994 to 10.9% in 2004 to 2006 and falling to 8.7% in 2007 to 2009. Estrogen-based hormone replacement therapy was used significantly more frequently by women aged 50 to 64 years diagnosed with ILC compared with women diagnosed with IDC.

Allen-Brady et al.[9] investigated the relationship between lobular breast carcinoma and the risk of familial breast carcinoma in the Utah Population Database. Among the 22,519 cases of breast carcinoma recorded, 1,453 (6.5%) were classified as lobular type, including *in situ* and invasive carcinomas. Female first-degree relatives of women with ILC had a significantly increased risk of breast carcinoma, specifically lobular carcinoma, when compared with the risk associated with a history of breast cancer of unspecified type.

CLINICAL PRESENTATION

Age and Sex

ILC occurs throughout virtually the entire age range of breast carcinoma in adult women (28 to 86 years). Most studies have placed the median age at diagnosis between 45 and 56 years.[3,4,10–15] At the extremes of the age distribution of breast carcinoma,[15] ILC is relatively more common among women older than 75 years (11%) than among women 35 years or younger. In an analysis of the age distribution of patients with various types of breast carcinoma, the mean age of women with both ILC and IDC was 57 years.[16]

Differences have been reported in the age distributions of the classical and variant forms of ILC. Three studies found that patients with classical ILC tended to be younger than those with variant types of ILC.[10,12] A fourth study reported that patients with variant tumors had a lower median age at diagnosis (47 years) than those with classical ILC (53 years).[14] Buchanan et al.[17] found no significant difference in the median age and range of age at diagnosis between patients with ILC (median 61 years; range 34 to 89 years) and those with PILC (median 59 years; range 36 to 86 years).

Because lobules and terminal ductules that are the sites where lobular carcinoma arises are not normally formed in the male breast, men rarely develop LCIS or ILC. When found in men, ILC is usually the classical type,[18–21] but isolated examples of PILC have been reported in men.[22,23]

Human Immunodeficiency Virus

An exceptional instance of ILC occurring in a woman seropositive for human immunodeficiency virus (HIV) has been reported.[24] In this case report, tumor progression was observed in the presence of a CD4 count greater than 500 mm^{-3}. Other case reports of breast carcinoma in HIV-positive women have described a variety of histologic tumor types. The evidence for an association between tumor type, clinical course, and immunodeficiency in these patients is inconclusive.[25–27]

Clinical Signs

The presenting symptom in most cases is a mass with ill-defined margins, but in some instances, the only evidence of the neoplasm is vague thickening or fine, diffuse nodularity. Large lesions are more likely to cause skin retraction or fixation, but these signs can be encountered with small superficial tumors. Paget disease of the nipple is not ordinarily caused by ILC, but it can develop secondarily when a centrally located tumor extends directly to the epidermis of the nipple.[28]

Mammography

Classical ILC is not prone to form calcifications, but calcifications may be present coincidentally in benign proliferative lesions such as sclerosing adenosis (SA)[29] or when there is florid LCIS (FLCIS) in ducts with necrosis and calcification. Several investigators have reported a much lower frequency of calcifications detected by mammography in ILC than in IDC.[30–33] Kim et al.[34] compared the mammographic findings in 27 patients with ILC with 85 patients with IDC. Calcifications were found in the lesion in three ILC cases (11.1%), all of which were associated with a mass. On the other hand, 27 (31.9%) of IDC presented with calcifications, including 14 (16.7%) in which calcifications were the only abnormality. False-negative mammograms were reported in four ILC cases (14.8%) and only one IDC case (1.1%). Brem et al.[35] reported negative imaging studies in 21%, 32%, and 17%, respectively, of patients with ILC who had mammography, sonography, and magnetic resonance imaging (MRI). The lowest frequency of false-negative imaging (7%) was obtained with breast-specific gamma imaging (BSGI) that detected six ILC that were not appreciated by mammography and two ILC that were missed by MRI.

In a screening situation, ILC was more likely to be diagnosed clinically during intervals between examinations than by the mammographic screening examination.[36] ILC was relatively more frequent among interval carcinomas recorded in a breast cancer–screening program than in the screening-detected group.[37] Retrospective analysis revealed that a disproportionate number of interval lesions had been "missed" in the screening process. The only mammographic abnormality in some cases is asymmetrical density or architectural distortion without a distinct mass.[34,38]

It has been reported that ILC has been associated with a decrease in breast size or volume on mammography, although no change in size was perceived clinically.[39] These patients tend to present with thickening rather than a discrete mass on clinical examination, corresponding to diffuse invasive carcinoma in the breast. Kim et al.[34] reported decreased breast volume in 22.2% of patients with ILC and 2.3% of those with IDC.

A comparison between mammograms of ILC and other types of carcinoma detected by mammography revealed that lobular carcinomas are more often spiculated and are more often associated with retraction of the nipple or skin.[32,40] The most common mammographic manifestations of ILC were asymmetrical, ill-defined, or irregular, spiculated masses.[30,32,41] Carcinomas with mixed lobular and duct features tended to have mammographic features intermediate between the groups. The absences of well-defined margins and, in some cases, a tendency to form multiple small nodules throughout the breast are features that may hinder the radiologic detection of ILC and lead to a false-negative diagnosis. Patients with a spiculated mass are less likely to have residual carcinoma when reexcision is performed than are those with ill-defined or asymmetric lesions.[41] A minority of ILC are round or oval tumors on mammography.[42]

Mendelson et al.[29] described five mammographic patterns that they found associated with ILC. These included asymmetric density without defined margins, dense spiculated mass, dense breast without a distinct tumor, microcalcifications, and a discrete round mass. Asymmetric, ill-defined density was the most common pattern. It was concluded that ILC did not produce a specific or characteristic mammographic appearance. Mitnick et al.[40] did not find a significant difference in average tumor size among lesions with differing mammographic appearances. The average size of the tumors was 1.2 cm.

Sonography

On sonography, Butler et al.[43] reported that 60.5% of ILC produced "a heterogeneous hypoechoic mass with angular or ill-defined margins and posterior acoustic shadowing." The remaining tumors had various other sonographic characteristics, including 12% that were "sonographically invisible." The sensitivity of sonography for tumors measuring less than 1 cm was 85.7%. Classical ILC tended to produce "focal shadowing without a discrete mass," whereas tumors with pleomorphic histology were seen as "a shadowing mass." Tumors of the alveolar, solid, and signet ring cell variety were most often manifested as a "lobulated, well-circumscribed mass."[43] According to Kim et al.,[34] posterior acoustic shadowing is seen significantly more frequently with ILC (59.2%) than with IDC. Selinko et al.[44] found that the sensitivity of sonography for detecting ILC was 98%, substantially higher than the sensitivity of mammography (65%). The most common sonographic presentation was as a hypoechoic mass, more often with (58%) than without (27%) an acoustic shadow. The authors were also able to use ultrasound to localize axillary lymph nodes (ALN) for fine-needle aspiration (FNA) examination and staging. Albayrak et al.[38] observed that sonography detected ILC in 9 of 11 (81.8%) patients with negative mammograms and that it was especially useful in women with mammographically dense breasts. However, sonography can also yield a false-negative result, as reported by Brem et al.[35] in 8 of 25 (32%) patients with ILC.

The mammographic estimate of tumor size tends to be less than the grossly measured size in a significant proportion of cases,[45] and MRI has been helpful for determining tumor size in these patients.[46] Rodenko et al.[47] found that MRI was more effective than mammography for determining the extent of the primary ILC in a significant proportion of cases, but the presence of metastatic carcinoma in ALN was not detected in four cases examined. Yeh et al.[48] reported that tumor morphology seen on MRI combined with quantitative measurement of gadolinium uptake was effective for detecting ILC in most cases. Ultrasonography has been useful for detecting multifocal and multicentric ILC.[49]

Magnetic Resonance Imaging

Studies that compared the sensitivity of mammography, sonography, and MRI have usually found MRI to be the most sensitive of the three imaging modalities.[34,35,50] The sensitivity of MRI is typically 90% or greater. One of the important advantages of MRI is its high sensitivity for detecting multicentric and multifocal ILC. Mann et al.[50] reported that MRI detected secondary foci of ipsilateral carcinoma that were not found by sonography or mammography in 32% of ILC and that occult contralateral carcinoma was detected in 7% of the patients studied only by MRI. Levrini et al.[51] described five MRI patterns for ILC, including the presence of multiple small enhancing foci and a dominant lesion surrounded by additional foci. These patterns correspond to multicentric and multifocal distributions. Tumor morphology as seen in the MRI image combined with quantitative measurement of gadolinium uptake was effective for detecting ILC in most cases. ILC is characterized by a slower rate of MRI enhancement than IDC, but peak enhancement is similar for both tumor types.[52]

Although MRI has not been adopted as a modality for population-based screening on the scale that mammography is used, the foregoing data indicate that it can play an important role in the follow-up of certain high-risk patient groups, including subsets of women with a greater than 20% lifetime risk of developing breast carcinoma such as those with a family history of breast and ovarian carcinoma or a history of mantle irradiation for Hodgkin disease.[53] Women with a history of biopsy-proven atypical lobular hyperplasia (ALH) or LCIS are more likely to develop ILC than any other patient group and should have MRI included in a follow-up regimen that also includes mammography and sonography. Because of the increased likelihood that a woman with ILC in one breast may have occult ILC in the opposite breast or develop it later, MRI should also be used in the management of these patients.

PILC cannot be differentiated from the classical type of ILC on imaging studies, although PILC is less often missed. In a study of 22 PILC cases, Jung et al.[54] found that one case (5%) was not detected on mammography, and no such case was missed on MRI. On the other hand, 7 (15%) of 46 cases of classical type of ILC were missed on mammography, and 2 (5%) of 40 cases were not detected on MRI. These authors found that 3 (23%) of 13 PILC and 9 (23%) of 40 classical ILC were occult on sonography.

Breast-Specific Gamma Imaging

BSGI has been used for the detection of breast carcinoma; and in one study, it proved to be superior to mammography, sonography, and MRI with a sensitivity of 93%.[35] BSGI uses a high-resolution gamma camera to detect differences in the uptake of technetium (Tc) 99m sestamibi between carcinoma cells and normal breast tissue. Brem et al.[35] reported that increased tracer uptake was detected in 26 of 28 ILC, including 6 lesions that were not found by mammography and 2 that were missed by MRI. The mean size of ILC detected by BSGI was 20.3 mm (range 2 to 77 mm). Two ILC missed by BSGI measured 5 and 90 mm.

Measuring the Size and Extent of ILC

Determining tumor size is important for preoperative staging of patients with breast carcinoma. Among those with ILC, the mammographic estimate of tumor size tends to be less than the gross measurement of the resected tumor in a significant proportion of cases.[45] MRI has proven to be more accurate than either mammography or sonography for measuring the size and extent of ILC when compared with gross measurement.[45–47,55] Nonetheless, when compared with histologic examination of the excised specimen, MRI may underestimate the size and extent of ILC in as many as 60% of cases because it is unable to detect microscopic foci of tumor.[56]

Microinvasive (T1mic) lobular carcinoma was found in 16 (0.02%) of 75,250 breast carcinomas recorded in one academic medical center over an 18-year period.[57] Microinvasion was defined as invasion that measured less than 1 mm. The number of microinvasive foci ranged from 1 to 5 with a mean of 1.5 per case. Eleven cases also had classical LCIS, four had FLCIS, and one had pleomorphic LCIS (PLCIS). When examined at low magnification, the first indication of microinvasive ILC in histologic sections was focal-increased stromal cellularity. Lymph nodes sampled in 13 cases were negative.

Assessment of Lumpectomy Margins

Close or positive margins are a significant issue in patients with ILC who undergo lumpectomy as their primary surgical procedure for ILC in anticipation of breast conservation. Dillon et al.[58] reported finding close or positive margins in 38 of 77 (49%) patients with ILC and in 143 of 588 (24%) patients treated for IDC. In this study, mammographic tumor size greater than 1.5 cm and multifocal or multicentric tumor were significant predictors of close or positive margins. A study by Fortunato et al.[59] revealed significantly more frequent positive margins at the time of initial tumor excision for ILC (21/171 or 12.3%) than for IDC (71/1,011 or 7%). Close or positive margins were reported in 50 of 101 (50%) patients by Silberfein et al.[60] and in 39% of cases studied by Sakr et al.[61] Patients whose diagnosis was established preoperatively on the basis of a needle-core biopsy were significantly less likely to have close or positive margins in a lumpectomy specimen, presumably because surgeons aware of the diagnosis of ILC anticipated the possibility of more extensive carcinoma and performed a wider excision.[60,62] This conclusion is supported by the data presented by Sakr et al.[61] that ascribed the relatively low frequency (39%) of close or positive margins in their series to wider excisions that they described as "full thickness excision" or "oncoplastic surgery" in 73 patients with ILC.

Preoperative MRI reduces the reexcision rate in patients with ILC who undergo breast-conserving surgery.[55,60,63] Mann et al.[63] found that 27% of women who did not have a preoperative MRI required reexcision because of close or positive margins, whereas reexcision was only done in 9% of cases where preoperative MRI was obtained. Although the data were based on a retrospective review of cases rather than a randomized prospective trial, there was no significant difference in tumor size or the frequency of multifocal tumor between patients who did and did not have preoperative breast MRI. In a prospective study of patients with known ILC who agreed to have preoperative MRI, Lau and Romero[64] reported that additional foci of carcinoma were found in 8 of 20 (40%) women with ILC, including 2 with occult contralateral carcinomas. The MRI results led to beneficial changes in surgery for 42% of the patients, and only one patient required reexcision because of a positive margin.

Bilaterality

Patients with ILC are generally considered to have a relatively high frequency of bilateral carcinoma when compared with women who have other types of carcinoma.[65] The reported relative risk (RR) of contralateral carcinoma in women with ILC when compared with women with breast carcinoma generally or with women with ductal carcinoma alone ranged from 1.6 (95% confidence interval [CI], 0.7 to 3.6) to 2.0 (95% CI, 0.8 to 8.4) in three studies.[65–68] The wide range of overall bilaterality that has been described (6% to 47%) has been influenced by how the data have been tabulated. Prior and concurrent contralateral carcinomas were present in 6% to 28% of cases.[3,4,12,13,69–71] The reported incidence of subsequent contralateral carcinoma ranged from 1.0[69,72] to 2.38[73] per 100 women per year or 0.7% per patient-year of follow-up.[74] Lee et al.[75] estimated the frequency of subsequent contralateral carcinoma to be 10% after 10 years of follow-up. There is some evidence that the frequency of bilaterality is higher in patients with classical ILC than in patients with variant subtypes.[73] Follow-up studies have described subsequent contralateral carcinoma in 4% to 14% of patients who had previously been treated for ILC.[11,69,71] A lobular component was present in the majority of the synchronous or metachronous contralateral carcinomas, and at least 50% of these were invasive.[13,69,70,72] Hislop et al.[72] found that patients with stage II infiltrating lobular carcinoma were more likely to develop contralateral carcinoma subsequently than those who have had negative lymph nodes.

In one series, random concurrent contralateral biopsies in 108 patients with ILC revealed ductal carcinoma *in situ* (DCIS) in 6% and invasive carcinoma in 10% of patients.[76] Biopsies performed for clinical indications in an additional 22 cases yielded DCIS in 5% and invasive carcinoma in 32% of patients. The probability of detecting contralateral invasive carcinoma was significantly greater in women who had multicentric ILC in the ipsilateral breast, or if there were ipsilateral lymph node metastases.

Routine biopsy of the contralateral breast is not indicated on the basis of currently available data for patients with ILC.[74] When LCIS is excluded, the overall yield of significant findings from this procedure is not greater than for patients with IDC. Contralateral biopsy is appropriate when indicated by imaging or clinical findings and possibly in patients with a strong family history or other evidence of a genetic predisposition to breast carcinoma. The issue of differences in the long-term risk of bilateral breast carcinoma (metachronous as well as synchronous) between patients with IDC and ILC in one breast is unresolved. Data based on patients studied before the use of tamoxifen and other treatments that inhibit the development of contralateral carcinoma may not be directly applicable after the introduction of this and other selective estrogen receptor–modulating drugs.

GROSS PATHOLOGY

Size

The size of ILC ranges from occult, grossly inapparent lesions of microscopic dimensions to tumors that diffusely involve the entire breast. The median and average sizes of measurable tumors are not significantly different from the dimensions of IDC in some studies, but Buchanan et al.[17] found that the median size of PILC was significantly greater than that of ILC and IDC (20 vs. 15 vs. 13 mm) in a study of 52 PILC, 356 ILC, and 3,978 IDC.

Typically, ILC forms a firm-to-hard tumor with irregular borders. The edges of the lesion may be more easily appreciated by palpation than by inspection, because the margin may blend imperceptibly with the surrounding parenchyma. Cyst formation, hemorrhage, necrosis, or grossly visible calcifications in the form of "chalky streaks" are generally not present. Most tumors are gray or white, with a scirrhous or fibrous appearance. Cellular variants of ILC are sometimes described as tan.

In some cases, the excised specimen may not be visibly abnormal and only slightly firm to palpation, although substantial involvement by tumor is evident microscopically. This situation was vividly described by Foote and Stewart[77]:

> On some occasions the gross specimens can be quite confusing and misleading. These episodes usually come about at the time of operation when a locally excised specimen of breast tissue is sent in for frozen section diagnosis. Such a specimen may present no distinctly visible lesion and yet contain a palpable area of peculiar induration, the precise limits of which are vague. Such lesions can cause difficulty in frozen section diagnosis. After the diagnosis of cancer is made it is well to be prepared for querulousness from the operating surgeon who understandably would like to be operating for something more finite than indistinct induration.

Another gross manifestation of ILC is the formation of numerous, fine, hard nodules that feel like tiny pebbles or grains of sand in the breast parenchyma. These foci mimic the appearance of SA grossly and microscopically. Indistinct foci of induration or minute nodules may be the only gross evidence of carcinoma in a contralateral breast biopsy specimen when the opposite breast was deemed not to be affected by clinical examination.

T Category

The T category of ILC may be underestimated if it is based solely on the dimension of a grossly apparent tumor because there can be additional grossly inapparent foci of invasive carcinoma. This phenomenon was demonstrated by Moatamed and Apple,[78] who compared gross tumor size with the aggregate tumor size of histologically identified ILC in 74 cases. All 26 tumors initially classified as T0 were upstaged (T1, 69%; T2, 19%; and T3, 12%). Among 26 tumors grossly staged as T1, 35% and 15% were restaged as T2 and T3, respectively. Half of the initial T2 tumors were restaged as T3. Overall, 40% to 50% of cases were upstaged when the microscopic extent of carcinoma was taken into consideration. The authors did not correlate gross and microscopic T category with prognostic data such as nodal status or with clinical follow-up. These findings suggest that current tumor (size), regional node (involvement), (distant) metastases (TNM) staging criteria based on the largest single tumor focus may significantly underestimate the primary tumor burden in a substantial number of patients with ILC.

MICROSCOPIC PATHOLOGY

Foote and Stewart[77] summarized their definition of the microscopic characteristics of ILC 5 years after they briefly mentioned the lesion in their paper on LCIS. On this second occasion, they emphasized the following:

> The infiltrating portions of lobular carcinoma typically reveal thread-like strands of tumor cells rather loosely dispersed throughout a fibrous stroma. After infiltration has occurred there is no tendency for the cells to simulate atypical lobules. Sheet-like growth is distinctly uncharacteristic. . . . Great cellularity in the primary tumor is unusual but there are occasional cases in which this does occur.

At the cytologic level, the tumor cells were described as "small- or medium-sized," "rather uniform in their staining properties," and as exhibiting relatively little "irregularity." Because of the small size of the carcinoma cells and the extremely dense cellularity sometimes encountered in lymph node metastases, Foote and Stewart cautioned against mistaking such metastases for lymphoma. They noted that the presence of "central mucoid globules" in the tumor cells was a helpful diagnostic feature.[1]

Classical Form

Foote and Stewart's[77] description of ILC has been widely accepted as defining the classical pattern of this type of carcinoma, and most subsequent clinicopathologic studies adhere closely to this definition. The study of Newman,[3] published in 1966, described the first large series of cases. After reviewing histologic sections of 142 tumors that had features of ILC, he determined that 73 could be regarded as "pure" because they exhibited largely or entirely a "single-cell pattern" of growth. He excluded cases in which there was a prominent duct-forming component or the growth pattern was not largely linear.

Several growth patterns may be encountered in lesions classified as classical ILC. The tumor cells exhibit a lack of cohesion. The most prominent manifestation of this property in the two-dimensional plane of a histologic section is a tendency to form slender strands of cells arranged in a linear fashion (Figs. 32.1 and 32.2). For the most part, the strands are no more than one or two cells across. Broader bands of cells constitute "trabecular" ILC (Fig. 32.3).

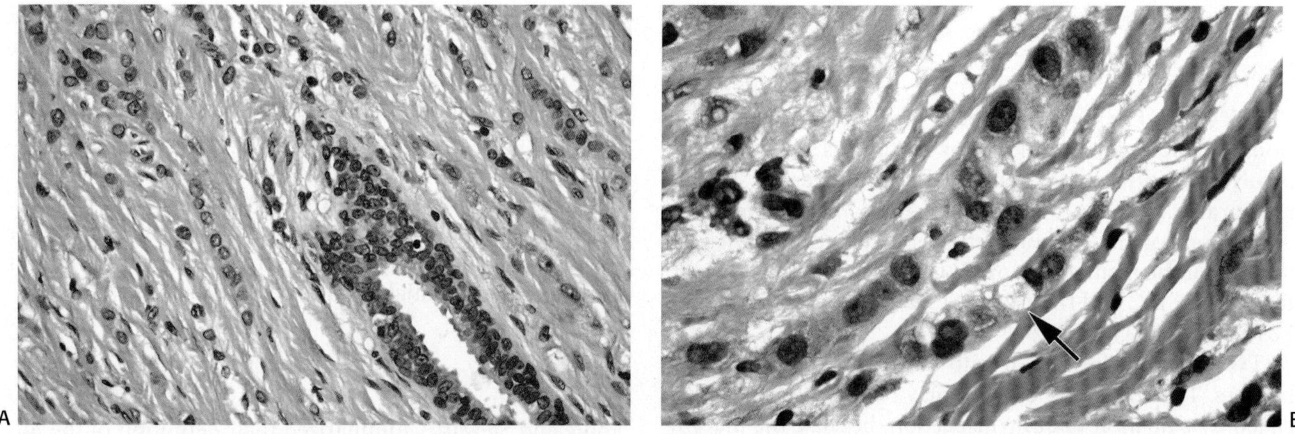

FIG. 32.1. ***Invasive lobular carcinoma, classical type.*** Linear growth and loss of cohesion are illustrated. **A:** Strands of carcinoma one cell across are shown. **B:** A cytoplasmic mucin vacuole is present (*arrow*).

Some tumors feature a growth pattern in which the tumor cells are arranged around ducts and lobules in a concentric fashion (Figs. 32.4 and 32.5). This distribution can have a bull's-eye or "targetoid" appearance. Inflammatory cells distributed around ducts may mimic the targetoid pattern of ILC, and this phenomenon can present a notable diagnostic problem, especially in a frozen section (FS) or in a needle-core biopsy specimen.[79]

ILC is only rarely accompanied by a lymphocytic reaction (Fig. 32.6). In exceptional cases, an intense lymphoid infiltrate with germinal centers is encountered, and this may suggest a diagnosis of coexistent lymphocytic mastitis[80] (Fig. 32.7). Lymphoplasmacytic reaction is found relatively more often in the solid and alveolar variants than in classical ILC. Granulomatous inflammation is very unusual in ILC (Fig. 32.8). The term "lymphoepithelial-like

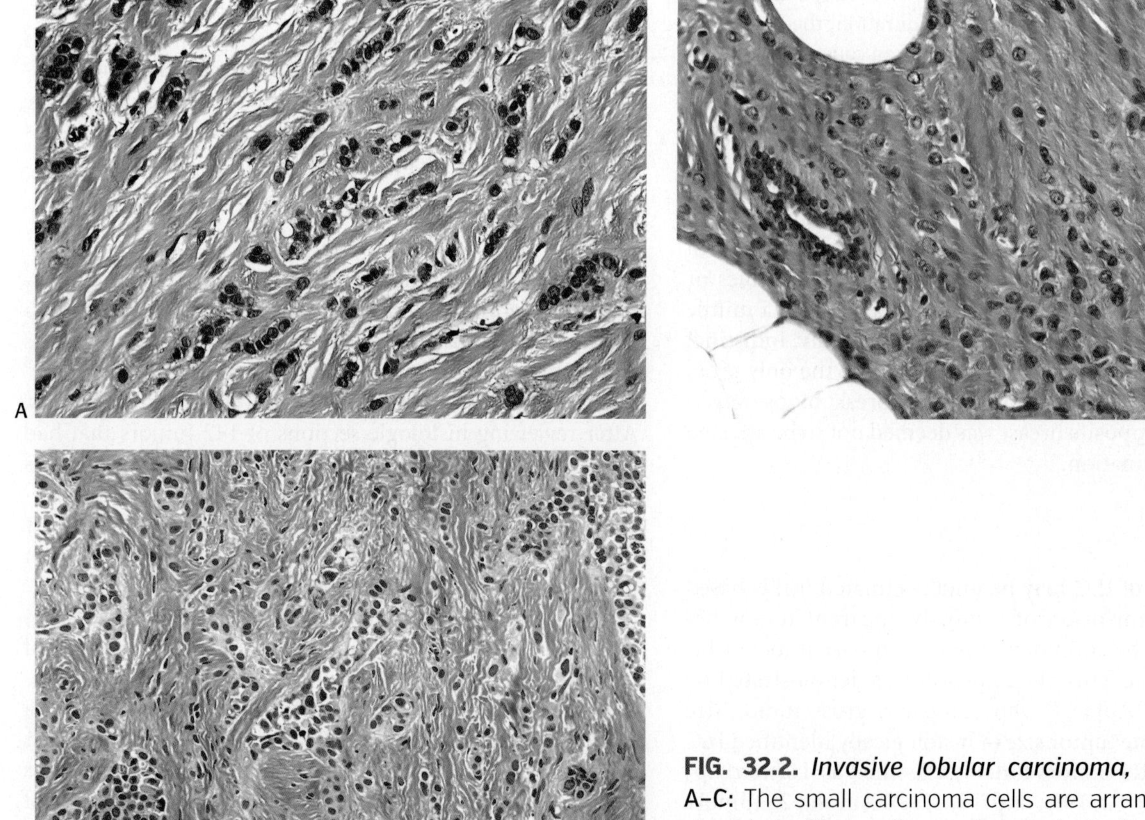

FIG. 32.2. ***Invasive lobular carcinoma, classical type.*** **A–C:** The small carcinoma cells are arranged in slender strands in fibrous tissue. Some clustering of carcinoma cells is evident in **(C)**.

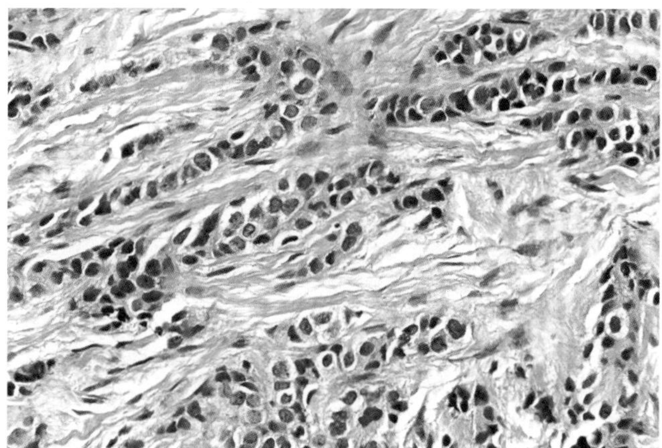

FIG. 32.3. ***Invasive lobular carcinoma, trabecular type.*** The classical structure on the *top left* contrasts with the trabecular pattern elsewhere.

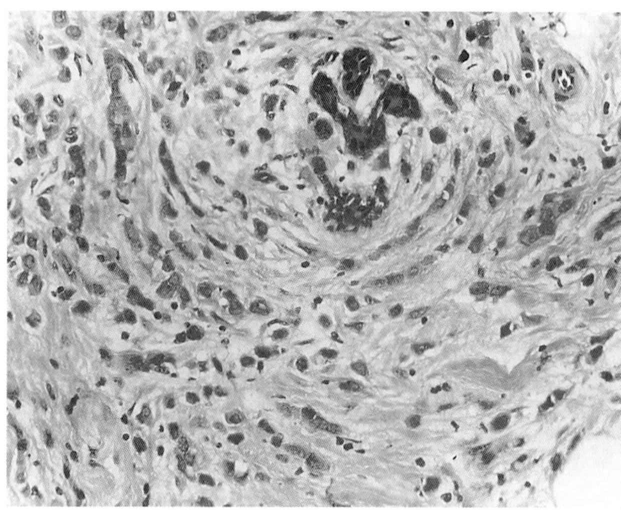

FIG. 32.4. ***Invasive lobular carcinoma.*** Circumferential infiltration around an atrophic lobule is shown.

carcinoma" has been applied to an ILC with a prominent lymphocytic reaction.[81] One such tumor was negative for the Epstein–Barr virus.

In a minority of cases, the linear strand-forming pattern is not conspicuous and the tumor cells tend to grow mainly in small dispersed, disorderly foci. This type of invasive growth does not produce a discrete mass and is largely found in patients with little or no gross evidence of invasive carcinoma. The small tumor cells in these invasive foci may be mistaken for lymphocytes or plasma cells in areas of fibrosis or fat when a section is examined at low magnification (Figs. 32.9 and 32.10). The interlobular stroma should be carefully studied for cryptic foci of invasion in biopsies from patients with LCIS (Figs. 32.10 to 32.12).

It is quite unusual to encounter an invasive carcinoma in which 100% of the microscopic fields fulfill the foregoing histologic criteria for classical ILC. Many of the tumors composed largely of classical ILC have minor components in which cytologically similar cells exhibit other growth patterns. This situation led Richter et al.[4] to limit the diagnosis of ILC to tumors in which at least 70% had a "single-file" growth pattern, and this quantitative criterion has been generally accepted. The diversity of growth patterns is a factor that contributes to problems in reproducible diagnosis reported with ILC.[82,83]

Variant Forms of Classical ILC

Tumors with the cytologic features of ILC in which there are substantial elements of nonlinear growth have been referred to as "variant" forms of ILC. Areas of classical ILC with a linear pattern are found in most variant forms. "Trabecular" (Fig. 32.3), "alveolar" (Fig. 32.13), and "solid" (Fig. 32.14) variants have been described, extending the diagnosis of ILC to a larger group of tumors. Fechner[14] described that six carcinomas in which the confluent growth pattern was characterized as "solid" were composed of cells typically found in classical ILC. The cells were "arranged in irregularly shaped solid nests . . . sometimes in continuity with a single-file pattern of cytologically identical cells." Sometimes, these

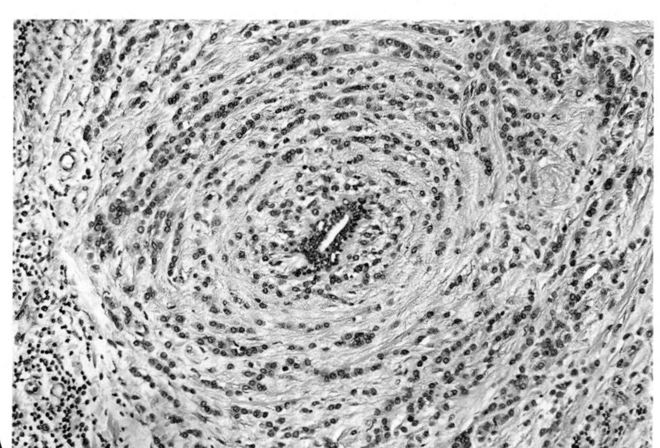

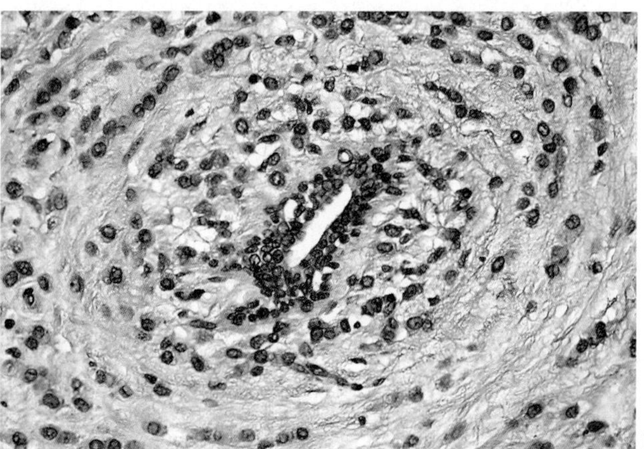

FIG. 32.5. ***Invasive lobular carcinoma, periductal.*** **A,B:** Concentric ("target-like") infiltration around an inactive duct is shown.

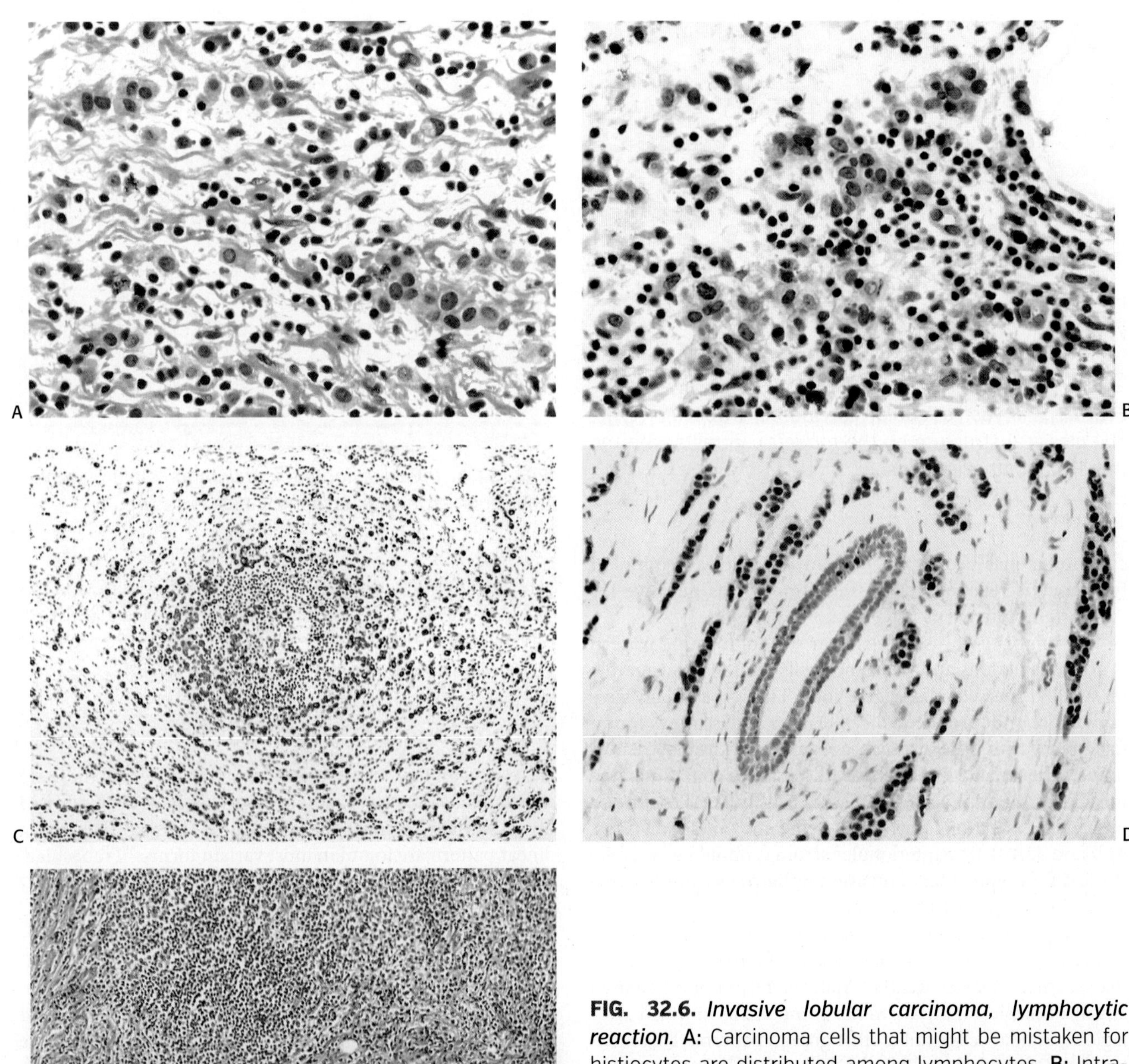

FIG. 32.6. ***Invasive lobular carcinoma, lymphocytic reaction.*** **A:** Carcinoma cells that might be mistaken for histiocytes are distributed among lymphocytes. **B:** Intracytoplasmic mucin within carcinoma cells is stained red with the mucicarmine stain. **C:** The carcinoma cells distributed circumferentially in the lymphocytic reaction around an atrophic duct are highlighted by a CK immunostain for AE1/3. **D:** Nuclear immunoreactivity for ER is shown. **E:** A nodular lymphocytic infiltrate [*above*], adjacent to invasive carcinoma.

confluent or solid groups of tumor cells were distributed in circumscribed rounded masses that could be appreciated not only microscopically, but also grossly. No significant differences were observed in age distribution or in tumor size between women with classical and those with the solid variant of ILC. Others found the solid pattern in 9 (41%) of 22 ILC.[64] Coexistent LCIS was detected in 10 (45%) of the 22 cases.

Twenty-four examples of "tubulolobular carcinoma" were found among 1,665 tumors in the National Surgical Adjuvant Breast Project (NSABP) series reviewed by Fisher et al.[85] These lesions, which constituted 1.4% of the series, were composed of small tubules as well as cords of tumor cells growing in the linear arrangement of classical ILC. Because it had many features intermediate between classical ILC and tubular carcinoma, including a less favorable

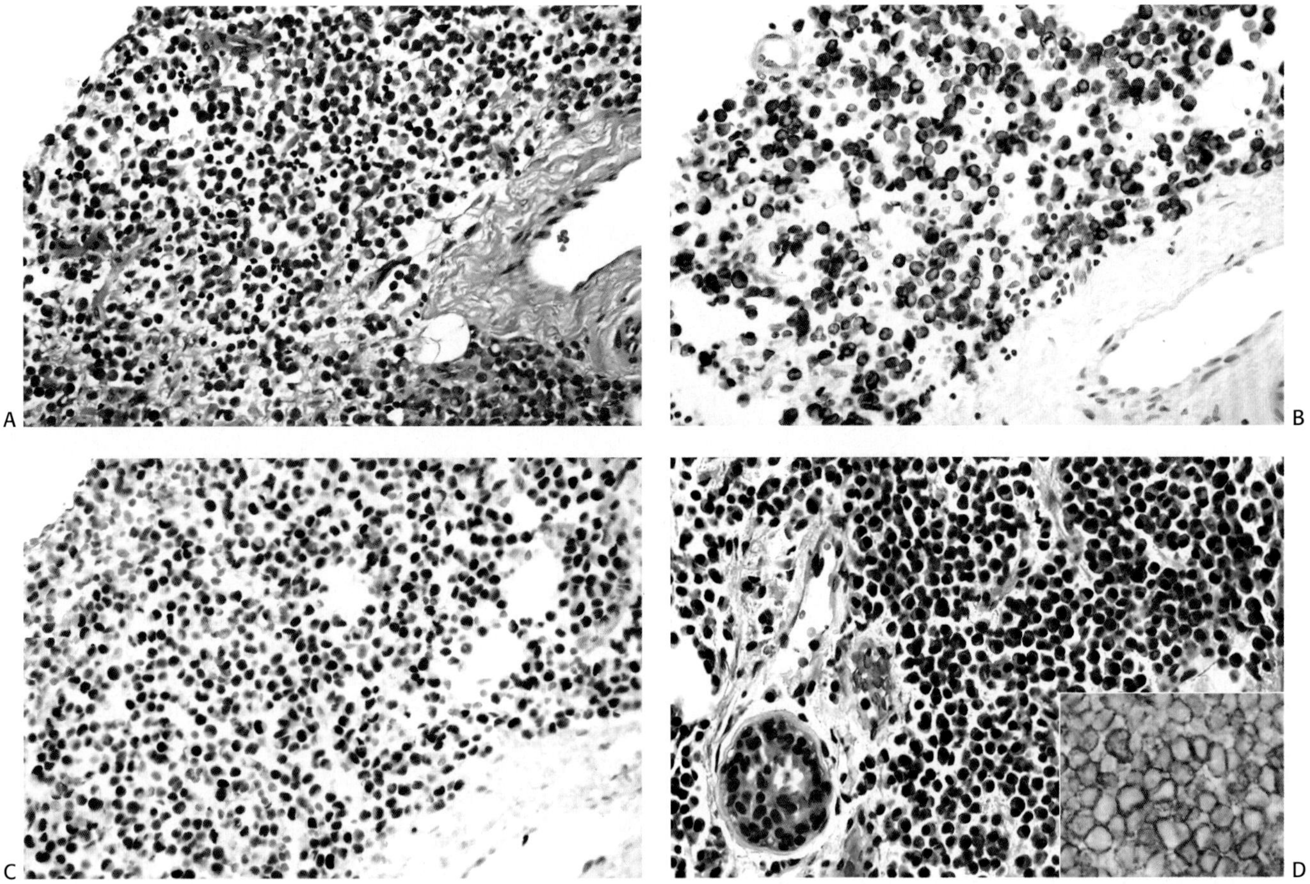

FIG. 32.7. ***Invasive lobular carcinoma, "plasmacytoid" type.*** **A–C:** ILC cells display plasma cell-type cytology **(A)**. The invasive carcinoma cells show cytoplasmic reactivity for CK AE1/3 **(B)** and nuclear immunoreactivity for ER **(C)**. Intramammary solitary plasmacytoma is shown for comparison **(D)**. *Inset* in **(D)** reveals reactivity for CD138 that typifies plasma cells.

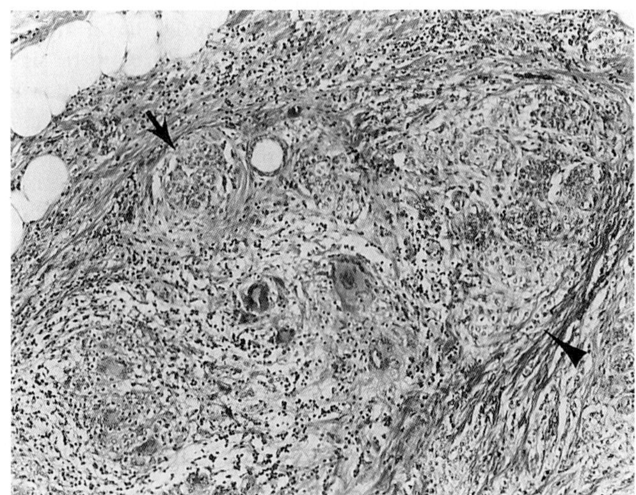

FIG. 32.8. ***Invasive lobular carcinoma, granulomatous reaction.*** Residual LCIS on the left (*arrow*) and ILC on the right (*arrowhead*) with intervening granulomatous inflammation.

prognosis than tubular carcinoma, the authors concluded that tubulolobular carcinoma should be regarded as a separate variant of ILC. Illustrations and a discussion of tubulolobular carcinoma can be found in Chapter 13.

The trabecular variant of ILC consists mainly of trabeculae that are one to three cells thick. To be meaningful, the term probably should be restricted to tumors with prominent bands, more than two cells broad. Usually, the trabecular pattern is found in association with other variants, and such tumors are classified as mixed ILC. The "alveolar" pattern is composed of globular aggregates of 20 or more cells, as seen in the plane of a histologic section. The fact that some examples of classical ILC have minor components of alveolar, tubular, trabecular, or solid growth provides evidence to support the classification of neoplasms in which these features are more prominent as variants of ILC. This conclusion is also supported by the fact that these variant forms are negative for E-cadherin.

A major problem in attempts to define and compare the variant forms of ILC has been the rarity of this entire group of tumors and the relatively small numbers of the several

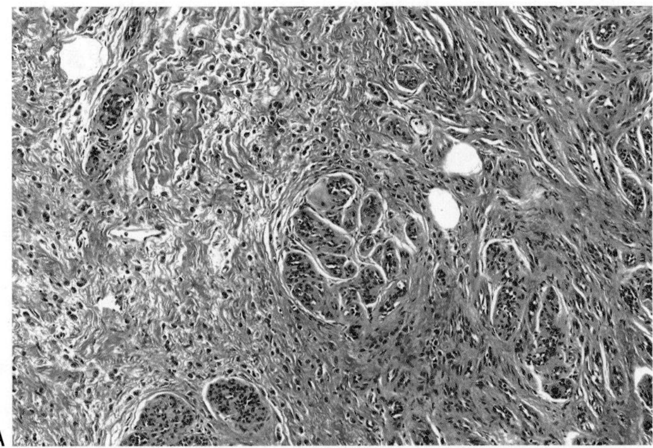

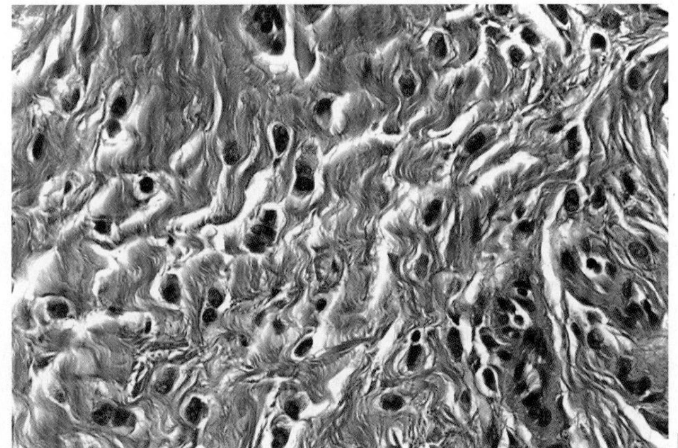

FIG. 32.9. ***Invasive lobular carcinoma.*** **A,B:** Inconspicuous strands of small cells in the stroma.

variant types. A series of 230 patients with stage I and stage II ILC included 176 women with classical lesions and 54 (23%) with variant growth patterns.[12] Except for a younger age at diagnosis of classical ILC, no clinical differences were found when patients with classical and variant lesions were compared. Women with classical ILC had significantly more frequent ductular extension, and they exhibited a stronger trend to multicentricity that was manifested by greater frequencies of bilaterality as well as gross and microscopic multifocality.

The reported frequency of finding LCIS in association with ILC of the classical type varies considerably. Newman[3] found LCIS in 72 (98%) of 73 cases. DiCostanzo et al.[12] detected LCIS associated with 65% of 176 examples of classical ILC and 57% of 54 variant tumors. In other smaller series of classical ILC, an LCIS component was found in 31%,[86] 45%,[84] and 87%[10] of the cases. In the latter series, proliferative lesions described as ALH and LCIS were grouped together. These authors also reported finding LCIS in association with 56% of 72 variant types of ILC.[10]

Classical and Pleomorphic Lobular Carcinoma Cells

The cytology of cells that comprise ILC has received considerable attention. All of the cytologic appearances found in LCIS and PLCIS may also be present in ILC. Classical ILC is composed of small, uniform cells with round nuclei and inconspicuous nucleoli. A variable proportion of cells have intracytoplasmic lumina containing sialomucins demonstrable with the mucicarmine and Alcian blue stains[87,88] (Fig. 32.15). When the secretion is prominent, the cells have a signet ring configuration (Figs. 32.15 and 32.16). With the aforementioned stains, it is often possible to demonstrate small amounts of secretion in non–signet ring cells. The majority of so-called signet ring cell carcinomas are forms of ILC,[12,87–90] but similar cells are also rarely found in IDC.[91–93]

Some ILC consist entirely or in part of cells with relatively abundant, eosinophilic cytoplasm that are larger than the cells in classical ILC (Fig. 32.17). The nucleus in some examples is hyperchromatic and eccentric with a distinct nucleolus creating a plasmacytoid appearance (Fig. 32.18). These cells have been referred to variously as myoid,[12] histiocytoid,[94–96] and PILC (Figs. 32.18 and 32.19). The hyperchromatic nuclei of PILC cells are typically three to four times larger than a mature lymphocyte. They are often eccentrically positioned in the cell and may be or lobated. One or more nucleoli are sometimes evident. The growth pattern resembles that of ILC, consisting of a diffuse infiltration of dissociated cells that have a linear arrangement and may encircle ducts and lobules. Other histologic evidence that PILC is a variant of lobular carcinoma includes *in situ* ductal involvement with a "cloverleaf" pattern, the presence of intracytoplasmic mucin and signet ring cells, as well as coexistent classical LCIS and ILC in some cases. This conclusion is supported by a study by Weigelt et al.[97] who used gene expression profiling to analyze a series of matched ILC, PILC, and IDC. There was less than a 0.1% difference in gene expression between ILC and PILC, whereas there was a 5.8% difference between ILC and IDC.

When compared with classical ILC, PILC has a higher mitotic rate—a finding that is potentially of prognostic significance.[98] In one study, the two types of lobular carcinoma did not differ significantly with respect to intratumoral vascular density.[99]

Eusebi et al.[100] emphasized the presence of apocrine differentiation in PILC and concluded that these patients have an especially aggressive clinical course because 9 of 10 patients in their series developed recurrences. Each of these nine patients had nodal metastases at the time of diagnosis. Apocrine differentiation was also noted by other authors who drew attention to transitions between classical and pleomorphic patterns cell types in the *in situ* components.[96,101] PILC is immunoreactive for gross cystic disease fluid protein 15 (GCDFP-15), a marker of apocrine differentiation.[102,103]

It should be borne in mind that an uncommon variant of invasive apocrine duct carcinoma is composed of dispersed pleomorphic tumor cells, sometimes with linear growth and intracytoplasmic mucin vacuoles. This growth pattern is the result of the growth of the carcinoma cells in stroma altered

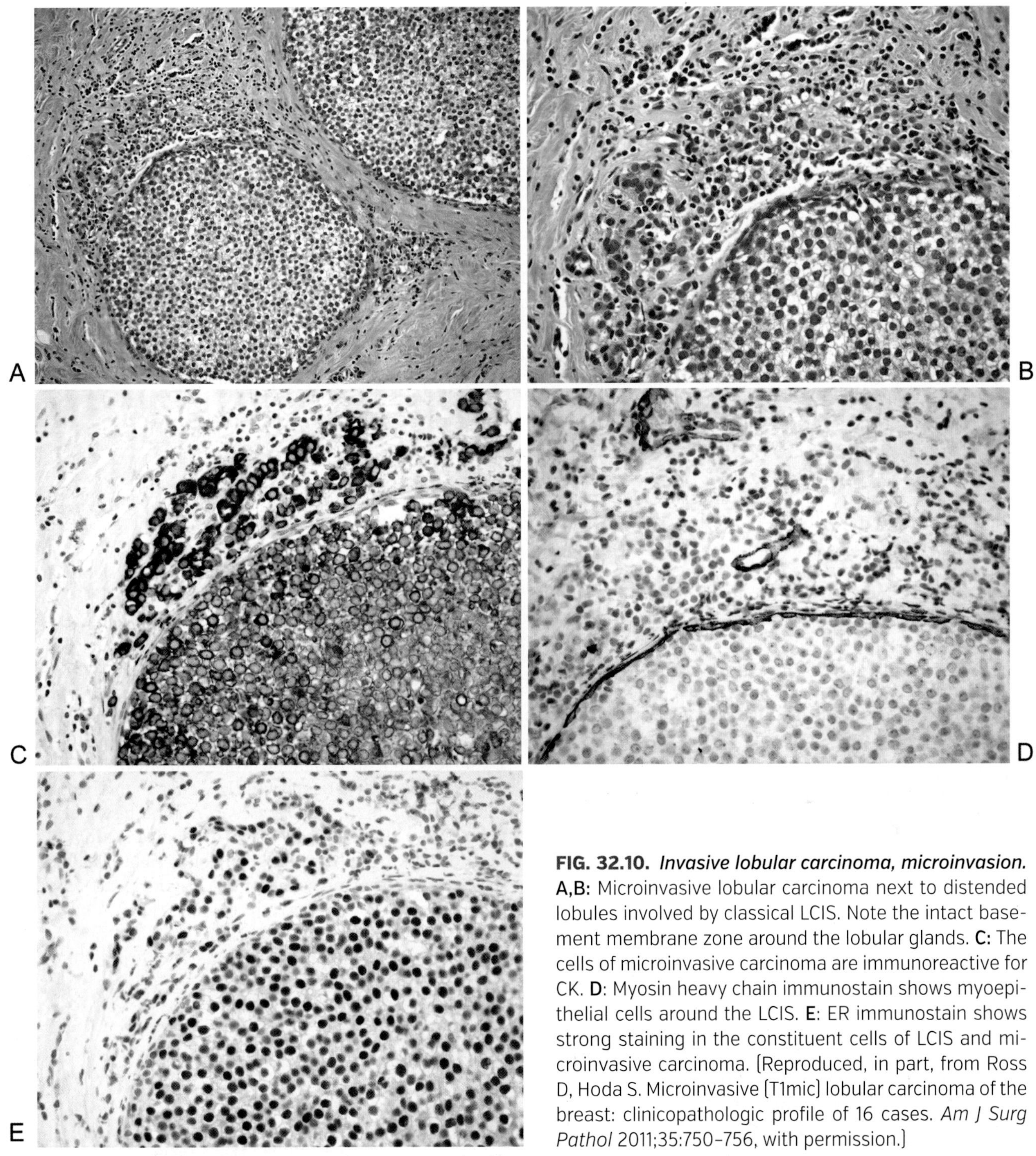

FIG. 32.10. ***Invasive lobular carcinoma, microinvasion.*** **A,B:** Microinvasive lobular carcinoma next to distended lobules involved by classical LCIS. Note the intact basement membrane zone around the lobular glands. **C:** The cells of microinvasive carcinoma are immunoreactive for CK. **D:** Myosin heavy chain immunostain shows myoepithelial cells around the LCIS. **E:** ER immunostain shows strong staining in the constituent cells of LCIS and microinvasive carcinoma. (Reproduced, in part, from Ross D, Hoda S. Microinvasive (T1mic) lobular carcinoma of the breast: clinicopathologic profile of 16 cases. *Am J Surg Pathol* 2011;35:750–756, with permission.)

by pseudoangiomatous stromal hyperplasia (PASH).[104] Intraductal carcinoma, typically solid with necrosis and lobular extension, is usually present. A low frequency of reactivity for estrogen receptor (ER) and progesterone receptor (PR) is found in PILC,[105] and apocrine carcinomas are also typically not reactive for these hormone receptors. Androgen receptors (AR) have been detected in PILC[106] and are typically present in apocrine carcinomas.

The available evidence suggests that mammary carcinomas classified as histiocytoid are a variant of lobular carcinoma with apocrine differentiation.[101,107,108] The tumors are composed of cells with pale, finely vacuolated or granular cytoplasm ("ground glass" appearance) and indistinct cell membranes. Nuclei are dark, and typically grade 1 or 2. The cells are arranged in clusters or strands, sometimes distributed around ducts or lobules. LCIS

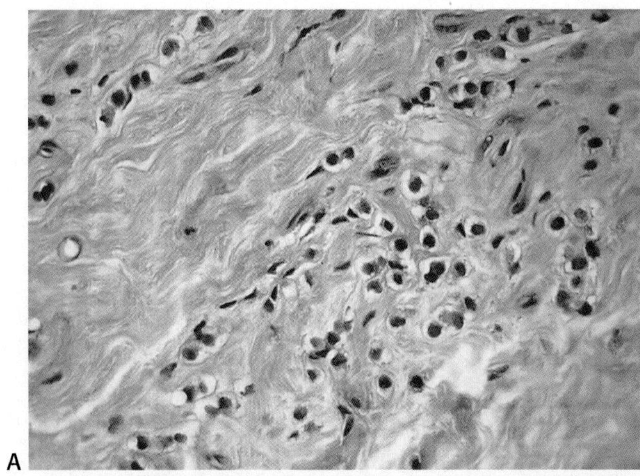

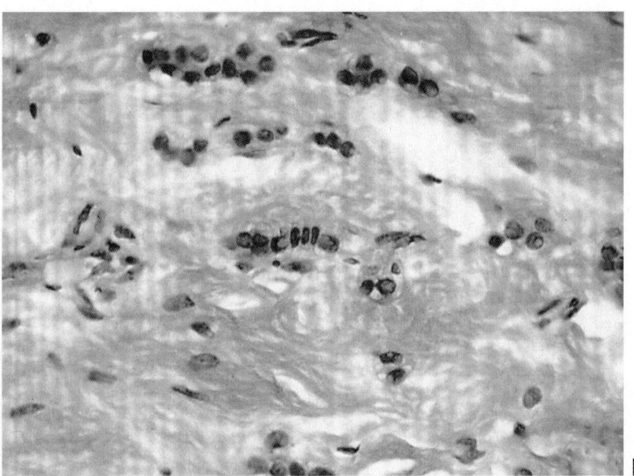

FIG. 32.11. ***Invasive lobular carcinoma, dispersed.*** **A,B:** These ill-defined foci of inconspicuous invasive carcinoma cells can be mistaken for inflammatory cells dispersed in collagenous stroma.

or ALH with similar cytologic features may be present. E-cadherin reactivity is absent in most cases, but incomplete staining that occurs in a minority of lobular carcinomas has been reported.[109] Expression of GCDFP-15 in most cases is consistent with apocrine differentiation that is displayed by the tumor cells. The differential diagnosis of histiocytoid ILC includes histiocytic inflammatory lesions, granular cell tumor, Rosai–Dorfman disease, lipid-rich and glycogen-rich carcinoma, true apocrine carcinoma, and metastatic neoplasms such as renal carcinoma and melanoma.

Perineural and Lymphatic Invasion

Perineural invasion is uncommon in ILC but may occur when the lesion is very extensive (Fig. 32.20). Lymphatic tumor emboli are also infrequently identified in routine sections of ILC. In some situations, shrinkage artifacts may simulate carcinoma in lymphatic spaces. True lymphatic tumor emboli usually consist of small clusters of tumor cells or isolated cells. Using routine histologic sections, Buchanan et al.[17] reported finding lymphatic tumor emboli significantly more often in PILC (10/52 or 19.2%) than in ILC (3/298 or 1%). The frequency of lymphatic tumor emboli was not significantly different between PILC and IDC (959/3,984 or 24.1%).

Antibodies such as D2-40, a novel marker for lymphatic endothelial cells, are useful for detecting lymphatic channels and lymphatic tumor emboli in ILC. Laser et al.[110] used D2-40 to search for lymphatic invasion in one histologic section each from 78 patients with ILC. They found lymphatic tumor emboli in 12 (15%) cases in routine histologic sections, and in 19 (24%) cases in D2-40–stained sections of the same tumors. Lymphatic tumor emboli in eight D2-40–positive cases had been missed in routine histologic sections. Axillary nodal metastases were present in 11/12 (92%) patients

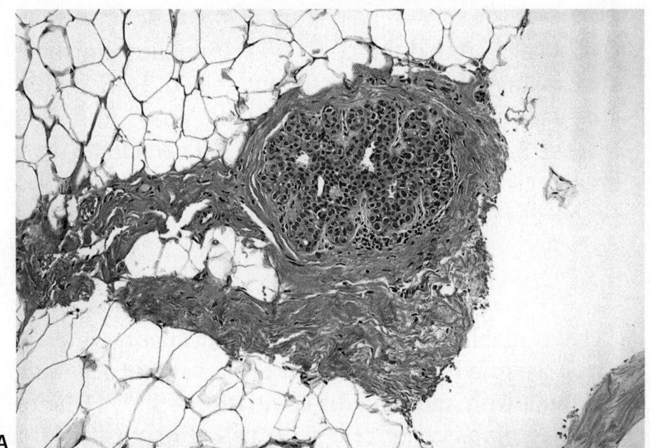

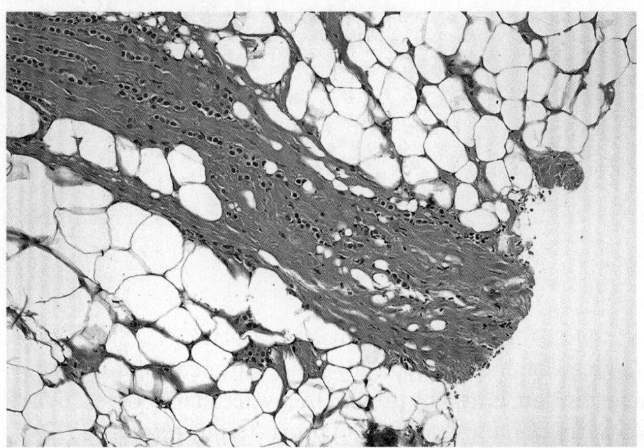

FIG. 32.12. ***Invasive lobular carcinoma, needle-core biopsy.*** **A:** LCIS in a small duct. **B:** The only evidence of invasive carcinoma was this small focus in collagenous stroma near the edge of one core biopsy sample.

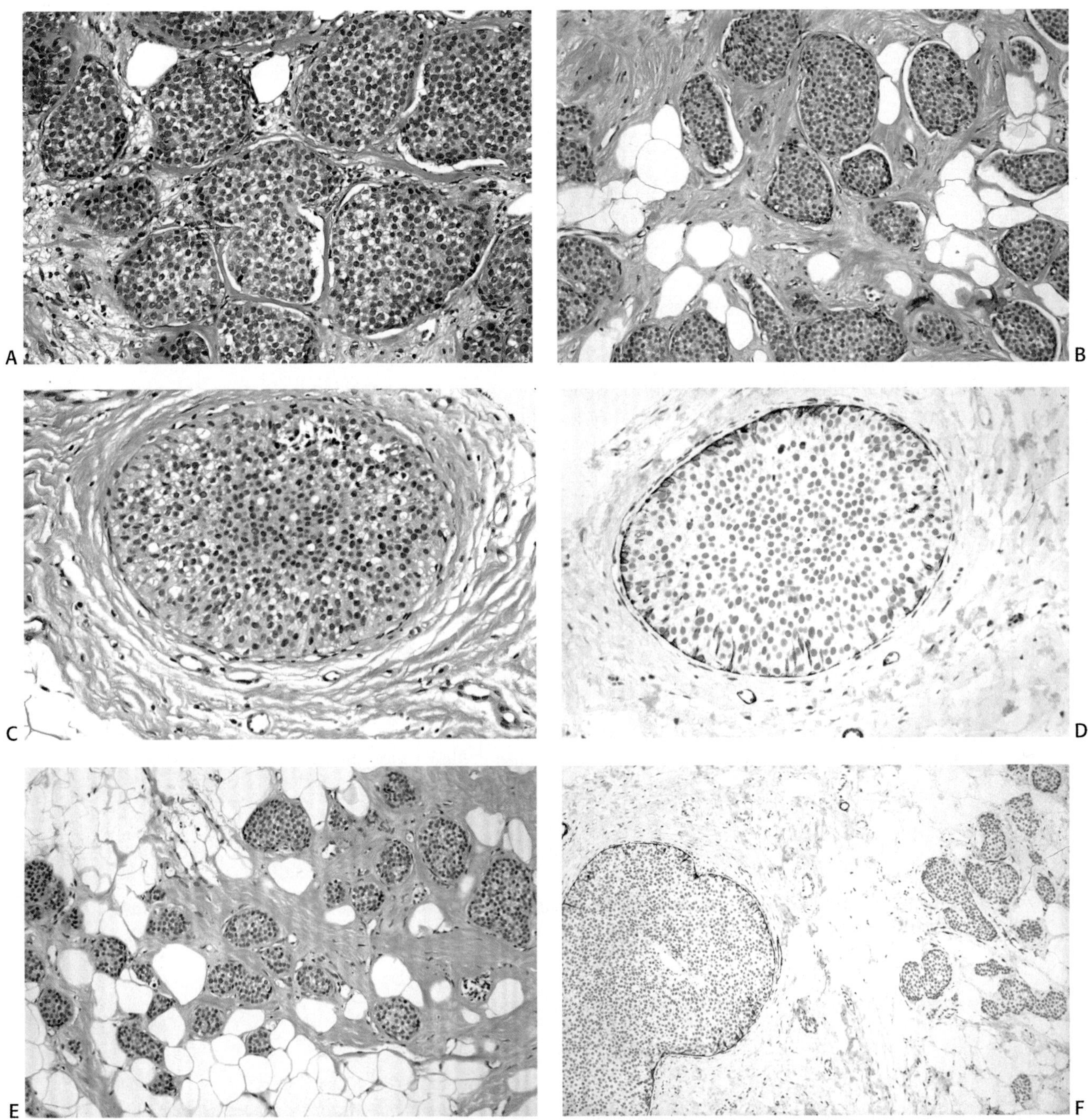

FIG. 32.13. ***Invasive lobular carcinoma, alveolar type.*** **A:** Discrete, alveolar groups of carcinoma cells are separated by thin bands of fibrous stroma. The cells have uniform, round central nuclei. **B:** Alveolar nests of invasive lobular carcinoma. Note the varied shapes and evidence of shrinkage artifact. **C–F:** Images are from a single case. LCIS in a duct (**C**) has persisting myoepithelium demonstrated by the smooth muscle actin (SMA) immunostain (**D**). **E:** Invasive alveolar lobular carcinoma. **F:** Myoepithelium is present in the duct involved by LCIS (*left*) but not in the invasive alveolar lobular carcinoma (*right*) (SMA).

with lymphatic tumor emboli detected in routine sections and in 14/19 (74%) cases studied with the D2-40 stain. When broken down by subtype of ILC, lymphatic invasion was found by routine histology in 6/69 (7%) classical ILC and in 6/9 (66%) PILC. The D2-40 antibody made it possible to find lymphatic invasion more frequently in classical ILC but did significantly increase the detection of lymphatic invasion in PILC.

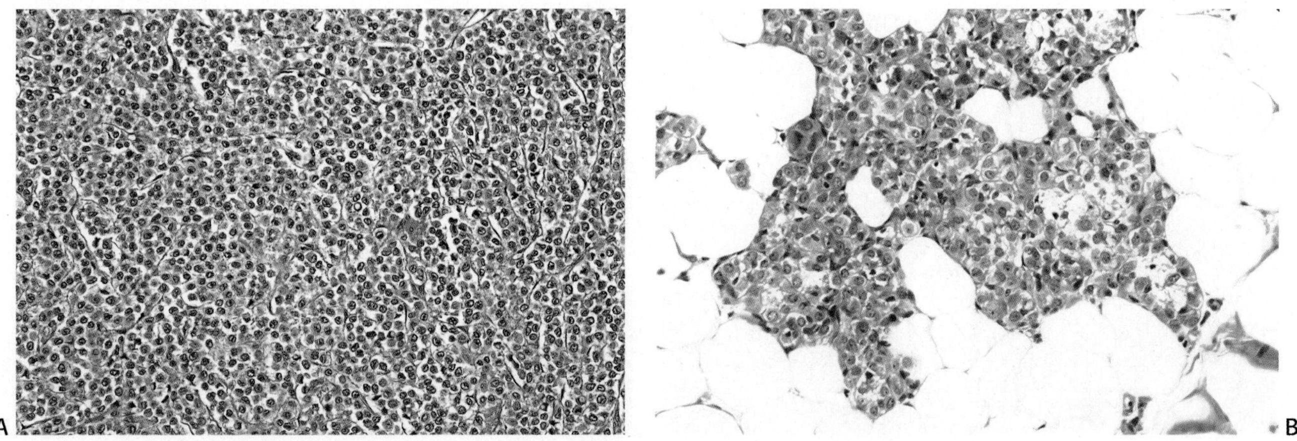

FIG. 32.14. ***Invasive lobular carcinoma, solid type.*** **A:** Loss of cohesion, a feature commonly present in ILC, is illustrated in this solid area. Slender strands of stroma are present. **B:** Solid growth in fat.

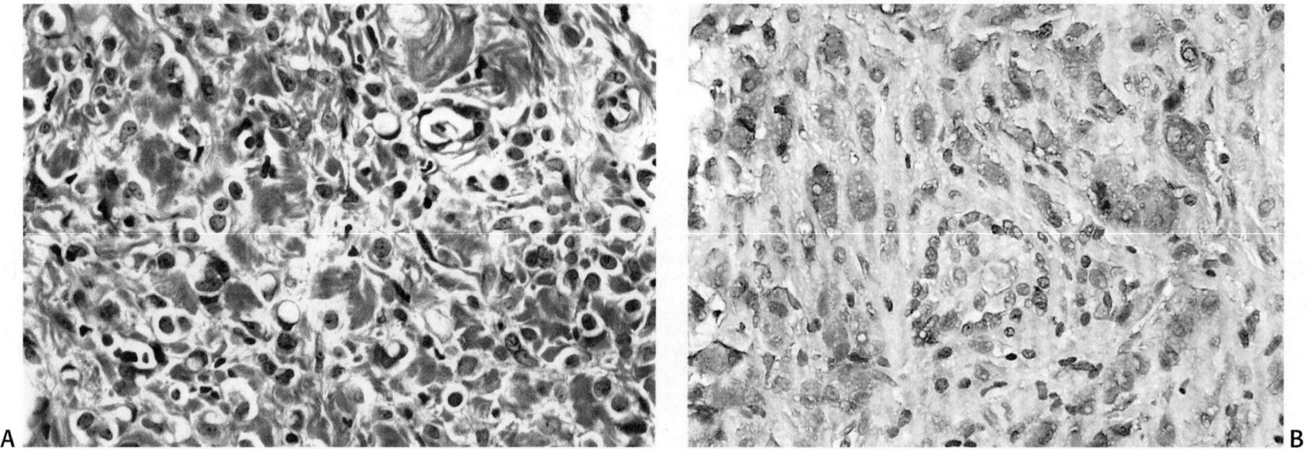

FIG. 32.15. ***Invasive lobular carcinoma with mucin secretion.*** **A:** Some of the carcinoma cells have large cytoplasmic vacuoles. **B:** The mucin is stained red with the mucicarmine stain.

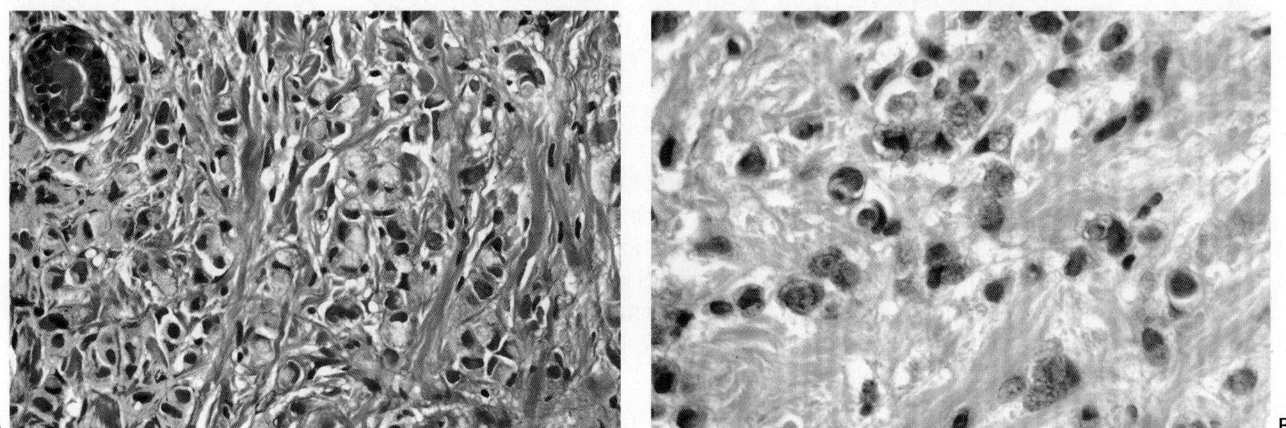

FIG. 32.16. ***Invasive lobular carcinoma, signet ring cells.*** **A:** The invasive carcinoma cells display signet ring cell appearance with eccentric, semilunar nuclei and transparent cytoplasmic vacuoles. The tumor cells were negative for E-cadherin immunostain. **B:** Mucin is demonstrated in signet ring cells with the mucicarmine stain.

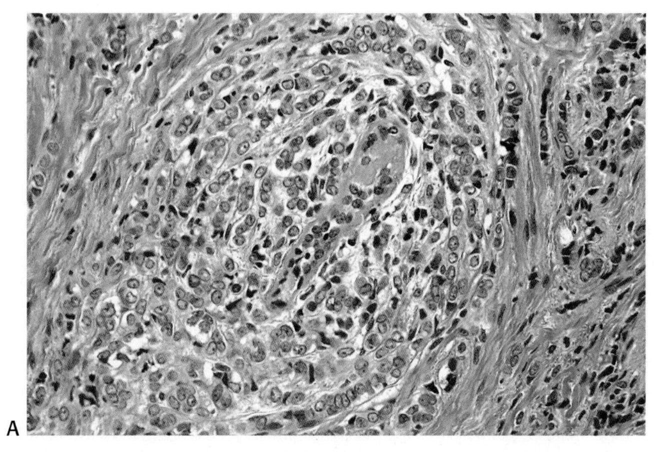

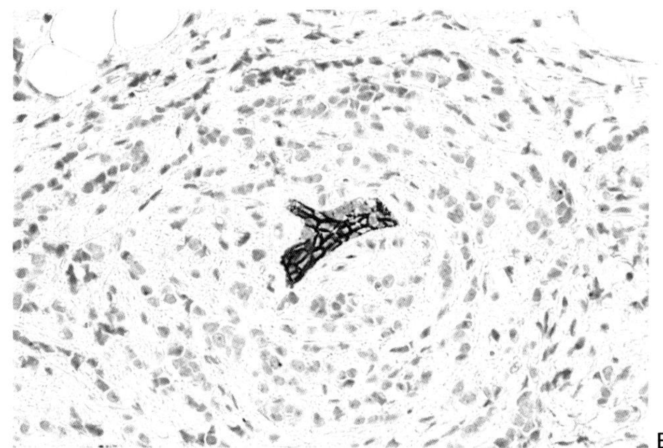

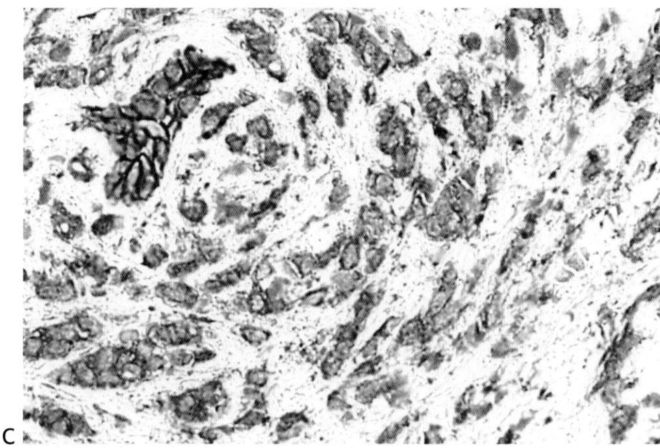

FIG. 32.17. *Invasive lobular carcinoma, pleomorphic.* **A–C**: The carcinoma cells with high-grade nuclei are arranged around an inactive duct in a "bull's-eye" appearance **(A)**. The invasive tumor cells are negative for E-cadherin **(B)**, and they show cytoplasmic reactivity with p120 **(C)**. Note membrane reactivity with p120 and E-cadherin in the centrally entrapped benign duct **(B,C)**.

Angiogenesis

Morphopoulos et al.[111] studied the extent of angiogenesis in ILC by immunohistochemistry (IHC) using the factor VIII–related antibody. Microvessel density (MVD) was not significantly related to age, menopausal status, tumor size, histologic subtype of the lesion, or lymph node involvement. MVD was not a predictor of overall survival (OS) or of relapse-free survival (RFS).

IMMUNOHISTOCHEMISTRY

Hormone Receptors

Early biochemical studies suggested that ILC was exceptionally ER rich,[112] but this was not substantiated in a subsequent analysis of a larger group of patients.[113] Particularly high levels of ER were found in the alveolar variant of ILC.[73,114] The majority of these lesions also had high levels of PR. Immunohistochemical methods have reportedly detected ER in the majority of ILC, including classical and variant types.[102] Heterogeneous immunoreactivity for ER can be present. Decreased or absent immunoreactivity for ER and PR has been reported in PILC.[102] However, Buchanan et al.[17] reported that there was no significant difference in the frequency of ER positivity between PILC (50/52 or 96.1%) and ILC (273/290 or 94.1%). ER was expressed significantly more often in PILC than in IDC (2,647/3,419 or 66.4%).

Riva et al.[115] found immunohistochemical expression of AR in 33 (87%) of 38 ILC and 118 (56%) of 212 IDC. AR was detected in 85% of ILC and 65% of PILC. AR-positive tumors tended to be ER-positive (87.5%) or PR-positive (75.0%). A small subset of ILC was ER (−), PR (−), and AR (+). These results are consistent with prior reports that drew attention to the coexpression of ER, PR, and AR in IDC[116,117] and in ILC.[117]

Carcinoembryonic Antigen

A substantial number of ILC have some reactivity for carcinoembryonic antigen (CEA).[118–120] The intensity of expression tends to be correlated with mucin secretion, being most pronounced in tumors with the most prominent signet ring cell features (Fig. 32.15). Variable reactivity for α-lactalbumin has also been reported in ILC, with the proportion of positive tumors varying from 19% to 100%.[118,119,121] Casein-positive cells have been found in the majority of lobular carcinomas, but reactivity may be limited to only a few cells.[88]

Gross Cystic Disease Fluid Protein 15

Immunoreactivity for GCDFP-15 occurs in ILC, predominantly those with pleomorphic and signet ring cytology.[58,100,122–124]

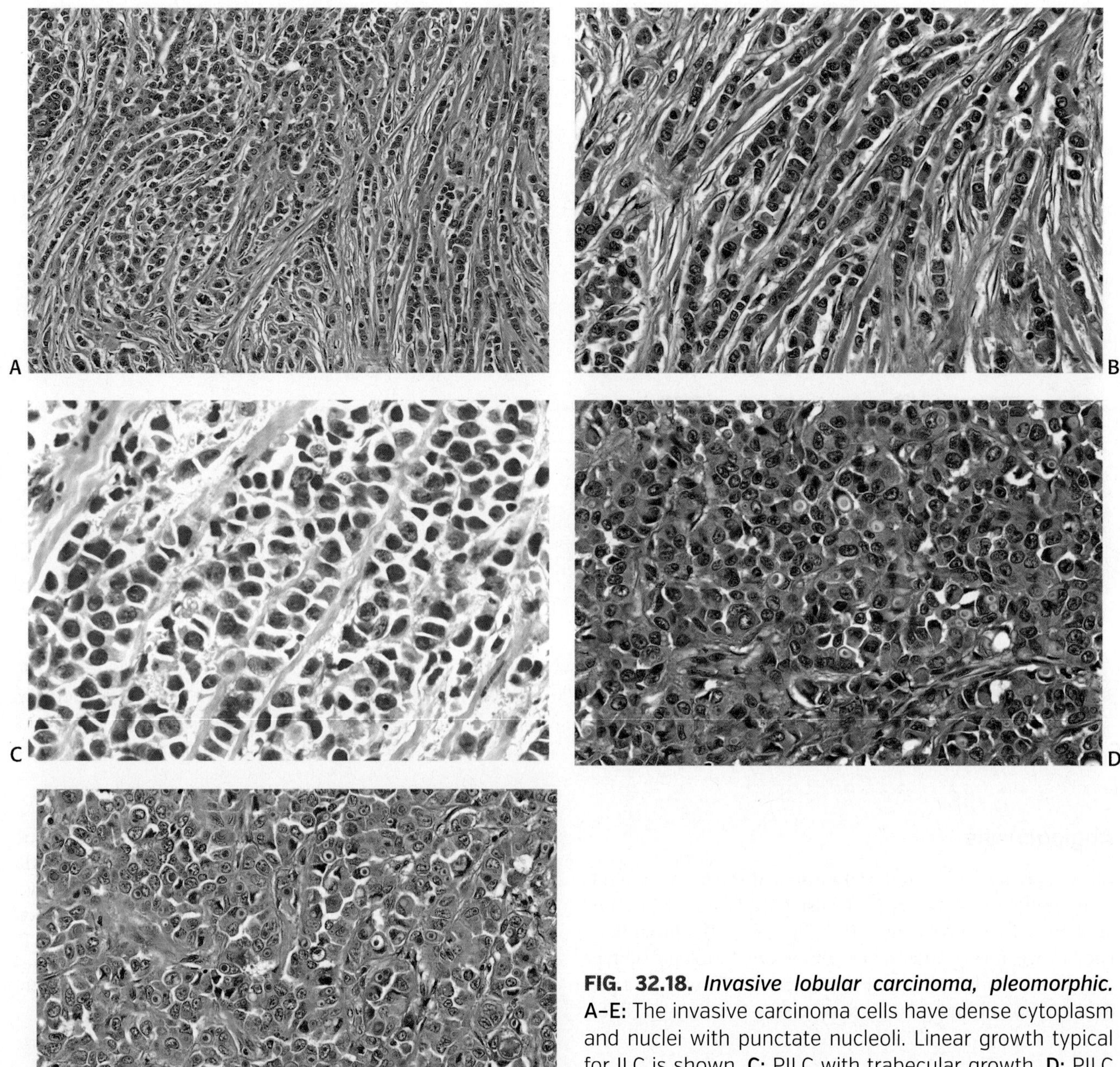

FIG. 32.18. ***Invasive lobular carcinoma, pleomorphic.*** **A–E:** The invasive carcinoma cells have dense cytoplasm and nuclei with punctate nucleoli. Linear growth typical for ILC is shown. **C:** PILC with trabecular growth. **D:** PILC with solid growth and signet ring cells. **E:** Intracytoplasmic mucin is demonstrated by the mucicarmine stain in the tumor shown in (**D**).

Human Epidermal Growth Factor 2

The human epidermal growth factor 2 (*HER2*) gene product is rarely detected by IHC in LCIS or ILC.[125] When present, it is more likely to be associated with PILC.[126–129] Monhollen et al.[129] detected *HER2* gene amplification in 14/38 (37%) examples of PILC.

Yu et al.[130] compared 12 HER2 (+) with 40 HER2 (−) ILC. There was no significant difference between the two groups in mean age, mean or median tumor size, frequency of multifocality, or stage at diagnosis. HER2 (+) cases had a higher average Ki67 index, were more likely to be PR (−), and had a higher mitotic count than HER2 (−) cases. Fluorescence *in situ* hybridization (FISH) studies revealed *HER2* gene amplification in the five HER2 (+) cases in which the study was done. LCIS, present in eight HER2 (+) cases, was strongly HER2 (+) in four and weakly positive in the other four cases. Histiocytoid histology was found in 4/12 (33%) of the HER2 (+) cases and in none of the HER2 (−) cases.

Cyclin-D1 Protein

The majority of classical ILC are reported to express cyclin-D1 protein.[131,132] Immunohistochemical study revealed expression of cyclin-D1 in 80% of ILC but very infrequent

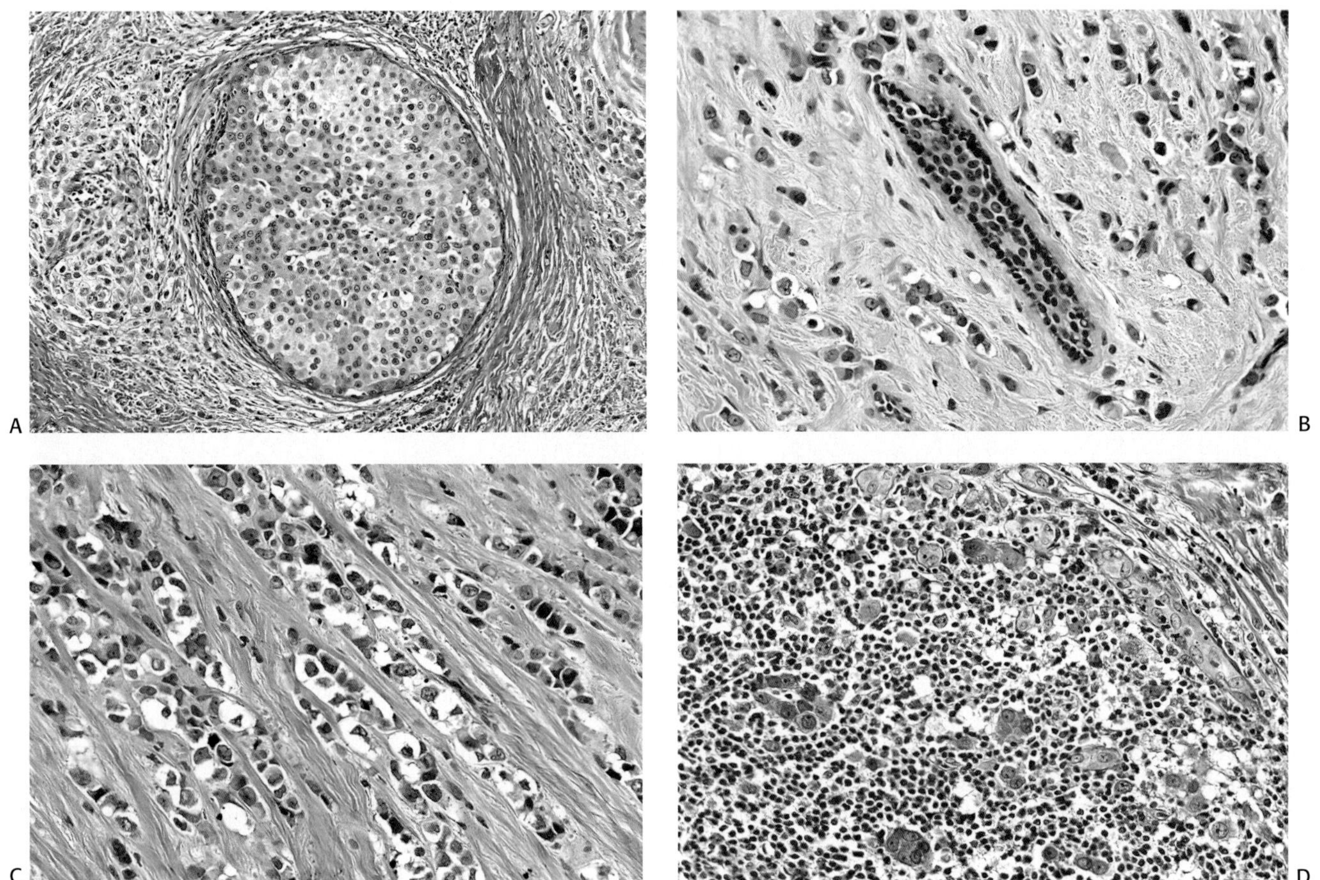

FIG. 32.19. ***Invasive lobular carcinoma, pleomorphic.*** **A–D:** The invasive carcinoma cells have variable amounts of cytoplasm and higher grade nuclei than classical ILC. The tumor cells have apocrine features in **(A)**. Linear ("single-file") growth pattern typical for ILC is shown in **(B)**. PILC with trabecular growth is evident in **(C)**. Pleomorphic lobular carcinoma cells are associated with a lymphoid infiltrate in **(D)**.

immunoreactivity in LCIS.[131] Most of the cyclin-D1 immunoreactive cells did not stain for Ki67, a protein expressed in proliferating cells. There was no correlation between cyclin-D1 and p27 expressions in ILC. These observations suggested that cyclin-D1 does not act to accelerate the rate of cell cycling in ILC. Overexpression of the *cyclin-D1* oncogene has been detected in a substantial proportion of ILC.[131]

Epidermal Growth Factor Receptor

Immunohistochemical analyses of the expression of epidermal growth factor receptor (EGFR) in ILC have not produced consistent results. One report stated that "EGFR-positive cases were much less common in invasive lobular than in invasive duct carcinoma," a difference that was statistically significant.[133] Others also reported a lower frequency of EGFR positivity in ILC than in IDC, but the difference was not statistically significant.[134] A third investigation stated that "no significant relationship was observed between EGFR tumor content and histologic type."[135] Monhollen et al.[129] reported EGFR reactivity in 1/26 (3.9%) PILC.

p53

Nuclear immunoreactivity for the p53 protein is usually absent from ILC.[136] When present, *p53* mutations are more frequently found in PILC than in ILC.[137]

Stromal Proteins

Immunohistochemical studies of the stroma in ILC have yielded some interesting observations. Fibronectin is a noncollagenous glycoprotein associated with basement membranes as well as interstitial collagen. Increased fibronectin is typically found in the stroma of most malignant tumors.[138,139] Coincidental with a decrease in other basement membrane constituents such as laminin and type IV collagen, loss of fibronectin has also been observed immediately around tumor cells.[140,141] Fibronectin is reportedly strikingly decreased in ILC, especially in tumors with the classical growth pattern.[140] Fibronectin staining is preserved in basement membranes around the LCIS associated with ILC. Because fibronectins have properties that contribute to cell adhesiveness,[142] the paucity of this glycoprotein in the stroma of ILC

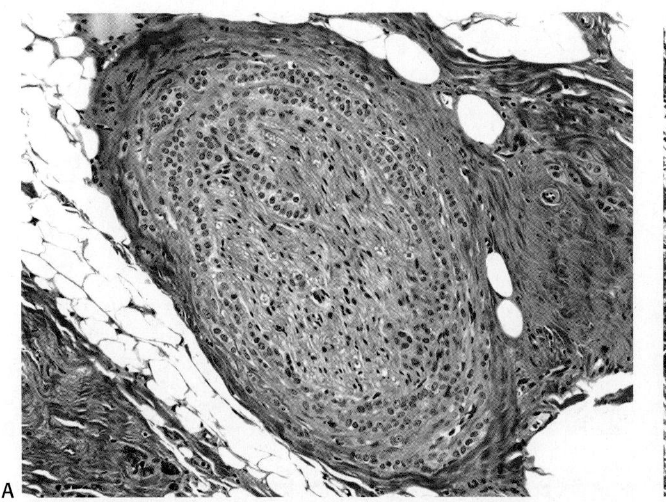
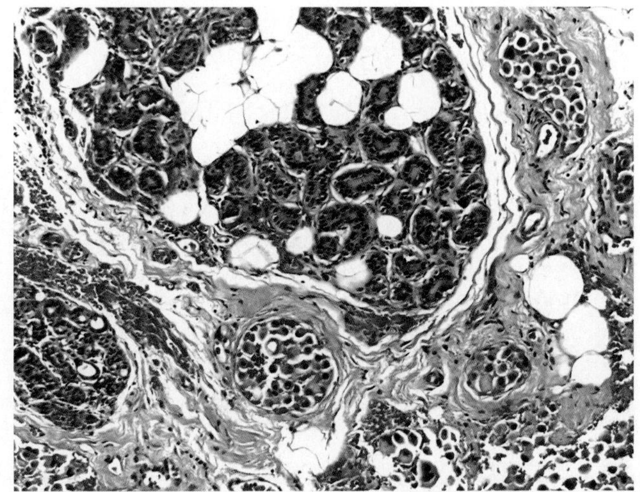

FIG. 32.20. ***Invasive lobular carcinoma, perineural and lymphovascular channel invasion.*** **A**: Classical type of ILC cells are distributed concentrically around and invade a nerve. **B:** PILC cells are present within multiple lymphatic channels around a lobule.

may contribute to its linear and dispersed growth pattern. In contrast to the consistent absence of stromal CD34 (+) fibrocytes in IDC, Ebrahimsade et al.[143] found that these cells were preserved in about one-third of ILC, present in reduced numbers in another third and absent from the remainder.

Extremely rare instances of coexisting amyloidosis and carcinoma of the breast have been reported.[144,145] Sabate et al.[146] described ILC in a 91-year-old woman in which the stroma contained immunoglobulin light chain amyloid that was demonstrated with the Congo red and thioflavin T stains. The patient had no clinical or laboratory evidence of systemic amyloidosis.

Another exceptional instance of ILC with unusual stroma is a tumor that had abundant extracellular stromal mucin. Centrally, the appearance was that of mucinous carcinoma, whereas at the periphery the growth pattern was that of ILC.[147] Foci of classical ILC were present in the surrounding breast tissue and there was a 2.5-mm focus of metastatic ILC without stromal mucin in an ALN. The carcinoma cells displayed no membrane reactivity for E-cadherin. They have strong cytoplasmic staining for p120, strong membrane reactivity for HER2, and amplified expression of the *HER2* gene. By contrast, 4/40 (10%) typical mucinous carcinomas displayed reduced E-cadherin reactivity, and these tumors lacked cytoplasmic p120 and membrane reactivity for HER2.

E-Cadherin

E-cadherin is an epithelium-specific molecule involved in cell-to-cell adhesion that acts as a tumor invasion suppressor gene. When compared with IDC, E-cadherin expression is markedly reduced or absent in the great majority of ILC when studied by IHC,[148–151] and there is also loss of reactivity for α-, β-, and γ-catenins.[149] Dissolution of the E-cadherin complex, characterized by the absence of membranous immunoreactivity of E-cadherin and α- and β-catenins, was found in 16/18 (89%) ILC by Morrogh et al.[152] who also reported an inverse relationship between membrane E-cadherin or catenin expression and nuclear expression of *TWIST*, a posttranscriptional regulator gene.

Qureshi et al.[151] found E-cadherin reactivity in 203 (99.5%) of 204 IDC. Among classical ILC, 44/49 (90%) were E-cadherin negative and 5 (10%) were E-cadherin positive. The frequency of E-cadherin negativity was slightly lower (8/10; 80%) among PILC. Rakha et al.[153] detected membranous E-cadherin reactivity in 16/149 (10.7%) classical ILC, 6/12 (50%) classical ILC with variant growth patterns, and none of the 5 examples of PILC. However, strong E-cadherin staining was found in only 3 of the 16 classical ILC and in 3 of 6 variant lesions that were considered to be E-cadherin positive.

Loss of E-cadherin reactivity in carcinomas that appear to be ductal by usual histologic criteria is seen more often in poorly differentiated tumors[148,151] with the basal-like and triple negative phenotype,[154] but can occur even in well-differentiated carcinomas.[155] Because the E-cadherin staining pattern is so highly associated with histologic tumor type, lesions that depart from expected E-cadherin reactivity are described as having "aberrant" E-cadherin staining patterns.[155] Instances of aberrant E-cadherin staining may be due to unusual molecular alterations that cause the E-cadherin protein to be present but nonfunctional in a lobular carcinoma[156,157] or absent from ductal carcinoma because of gene deletion or transcription defects.[158]

Mutations of the *E-cadherin* gene have been reported in classical ILC[159–162] and PILC.[163] In one study, a molecular abnormality was detected in 2 (10%) of 20 examples of ILC that were examined. Because only exons 5 to 8 were studied, the authors could not exclude the possibility of different point mutations in other cases.[159] They also found a protein truncating mutation in an E-cadherin exon in 21 (66%) of 32 ILC with loss of immunoreactivity for E-cadherin.[161] Loss of heterozygosity

(LOH) at 16q22.1, the location coding for the *E-cadherin* gene, was found with greater frequency in ILC than in IDC.[162]

Loss of E-cadherin immunoreactivity is consistently observed in LCIS and PLCIS in the presence of or absence of ILC.[162,163] When studied by comparative genomic hybridization (CGH), coexistent LCIS and ILC in an individual patient display similar patterns of genomic changes, suggestive of clonality and progression from *in situ* to invasive carcinoma.[164,165] In one study of paired LCIS and ILC samples from 24 patients, loss of the entire 16q arm was detected in all specimens, and it was concluded that "the striking similarity in genomic changes between the *in situ* and invasive components of these lesions clearly demonstrated the common clonality of the two lesions."[165]

Catenins are proteins involved in connecting the E-cadherin membrane complex to the intracellular actin cytoskeleton. It has been reported that lobular carcinomas of the classical and pleomorphic types exhibit absence of membrane catenin immunoreactivity, which parallels loss of E-cadherin reactivity in these carcinomas.[166,167] Strong diffuse cytoplasmic or punctate paranuclear p120 catenin staining is usually observed in lobular carcinoma cells.[166,167] By contrast, ductal carcinomas and normal mammary epithelium exhibit continuous membrane p120 catenin reactivity. As sometimes occurs with E-cadherin immunostaining, p120 catenin rarely has dot-like or beaded membrane staining in lobular carcinoma cells. However, weak membrane p120 catenin staining can rarely be observed in ductal carcinomas, and this subset of lesions might be misclassified as lobular carcinomas based on p120 catenin staining alone. Although the E-cadherin stain by itself is adequate to distinguish between lobular and ductal carcinomas in most instances, it may be helpful to employ stains for p120, as well as α- and β-catenins, in ambiguous cases. The use of the antibody 34βE12 to localize high-molecular-weight cytokeratin (CK) may also be useful as it typically shows strong staining in lobular carcinomas and displays little or no reactivity in ductal carcinomas.[168]

Cytokeratin 5/6

CK5/6 immunoreactivity has been used as a surrogate marker for the basal-like phenotype. It was detected in 3/26 (11.5%) ILC studies by Monhollen et al.[129] and in 14/82 (17%) ILC investigated by Fadare et al.[169] In the latter study, CK5/6 (+) cases were significantly more likely to be ER (−) than CK5/6 (−) cases, but the two groups did not differ in tumor size, nodal status, or in architectural and cytologic features.

Topoisomerase-11

Topoisomerase-11α gene has been used as a marker for responsiveness to anthracycline-based chemotherapy because tumors with this genetic alteration are more sensitive to these drugs.[170,171] Brunello et al.[172] reported that 44/46 (95%) ILC of various types lacked *topoisomerase-11α* gene amplification and that the *HER2* gene was not amplified in the same 44 tumors. Two tumors that displayed amplification for both genes were two of the four PILC in the study. These observations provide a basis for the observation discussed later in this chapter that ILC is generally not as responsive to neoadjuvant chemotherapy that often includes anthracycline drugs as IDC.

HISTOCHEMISTRY

Grimelius-positive cells have been described in a minority of ILC, generally in tumors with a variant growth pattern.[118] Chromogranin immunoreactivity has been detected in classical ILC and PILC, generally in 5% or less of the tumor cells.[102] Dense core granules of a "neurosecretory" type have also been detected by electron microscopy.[118,173] In view of this finding and coexistence of the two tumor types in some cases, it has been suggested that small cell (oat cell) neuroendocrine carcinoma of the breast may be a variant of ILC.[174,175] Some small cell mammary carcinomas have a component of ILC (see Chapter 21).

PLOIDY

When studied by flow cytometry, classical ILC were typically diploid and with a low S-phase fraction, and these factors played a minor role as predictors of prognosis.[176,177]

MOLECULAR GENETICS

Nayar et al.[178] studied LOH on chromosome 11q13 in ILC using the microsatellite markers INT-2 and PYGM. LOH was found in 9 (41%) of 22 informative cases. It has been postulated that LOH at the 11q13 region is associated with the loss of one or more tumor suppressor genes, an alteration that could contribute to mammary carcinogenesis.

Nishizaki et al.[179] compared the frequency of genetic alterations in IDC and ILC. Gains in DNA copy number were significantly lower in ILC. However, 79% (15 of 19) of ILC had increased copy number of 1q, and 12 (63%) exhibited loss of 16q. These genetic alterations were not significantly correlated with nodal status or classification as classical or pleomorphic subtype. The frequency of 16q loss was higher in ILC than in IDC, but a lower frequency of 8q and 20q gains was found in ILC.

ELECTRON MICROSCOPY

Electron microscopy has yielded variable ultrastructural findings in ILC.[118,180–182] In some cases, the cells of LCIS and ILC have pale or clear, organelle-poor cytoplasm. Intracytoplasmic lumina are often but not always present. Cells with darker, irregular nuclei and organelle-rich cytoplasm correspond to examples of "myoid" ILC. It has been found that neoplastic cells in the alveolar form of ILC have organelle-poor cytoplasm with oval, pale nuclei and inconspicuous nucleoli.[118,182]

CYTOLOGY

The diagnosis of ILC may be suggested by an FNA.[183,184] The sample is often sparsely cellular, a circumstance that can lead to false-negative reports.[185] In one series of 56 patients, only 29 FNAs (52%) from ILC yielded diagnostic cytology specimens.[186] Ten of the 27 patients with nondiagnostic FNA were subsequently diagnosed by needle-core biopsy.

Small cells with scanty, inconspicuous cytoplasm are dispersed singly or in small groups on the slide in the FNA sample from ILC.[187] Signet ring cell forms may be found, but they are conspicuous in a minority of cases. In one study, intracytoplasmic lumina were found in 58% of aspirates from ILC.[187] Some cytoplasmic lumina may contain a central globule of condensed secretion, which, if present, helps to distinguish true lumina from nonspecific vacuoles (Fig. 32.21).[188] Linear arrays of tumor cells are a characteristic feature in the aspirate from classic ILC. The FNA specimen obtained from invasive PILC is a "hybrid" between the appearances of ILC and IDC.[187] The specimens are more cellular than aspirates from classical ILC, the cells are larger, and the nuclei are more pleomorphic.[189] A "rosette-like" pattern may be found in the aspirate from the alveolar variant of ILC.[189] Intranuclear vacuoles are reported to be less frequent in variant forms than in classical ILC.[190]

PATTERNS OF METASTASES

ILC can metastasize via lymphatics or by hematogenous dissemination. Metastatic deposits of lobular carcinoma tend to duplicate the cytologic features of the primary tumor (Fig. 32.22). On occasion, signet ring cell formation is more conspicuous in metastases than in the primary lesion.[191]

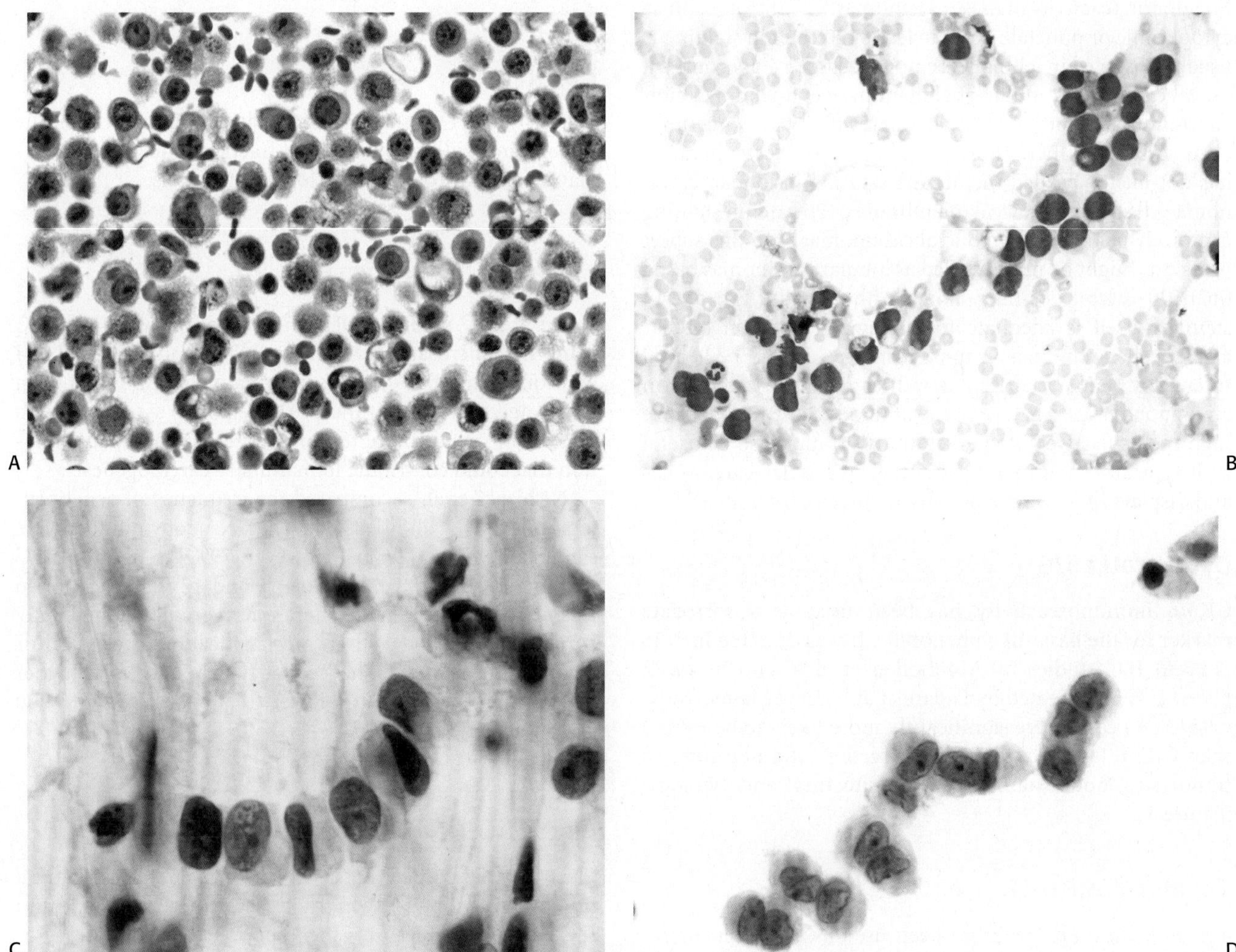

FIG. 32.21. ***Invasive lobular carcinoma, cytology.*** Invasive lobular carcinoma cells are shown in various preparations from FNA procedures of the breast. **A:** Signet ring cells are apparent in a cell block with the H&E stain. **B:** The direct smear with Diff-Quik stain shows signet ring cells. **C:** A conventional Papanicolaou-stained smear shows signet ring cells in a linear array. **D:** A linear array of carcinoma cells found in a monolayer ThinPrep.

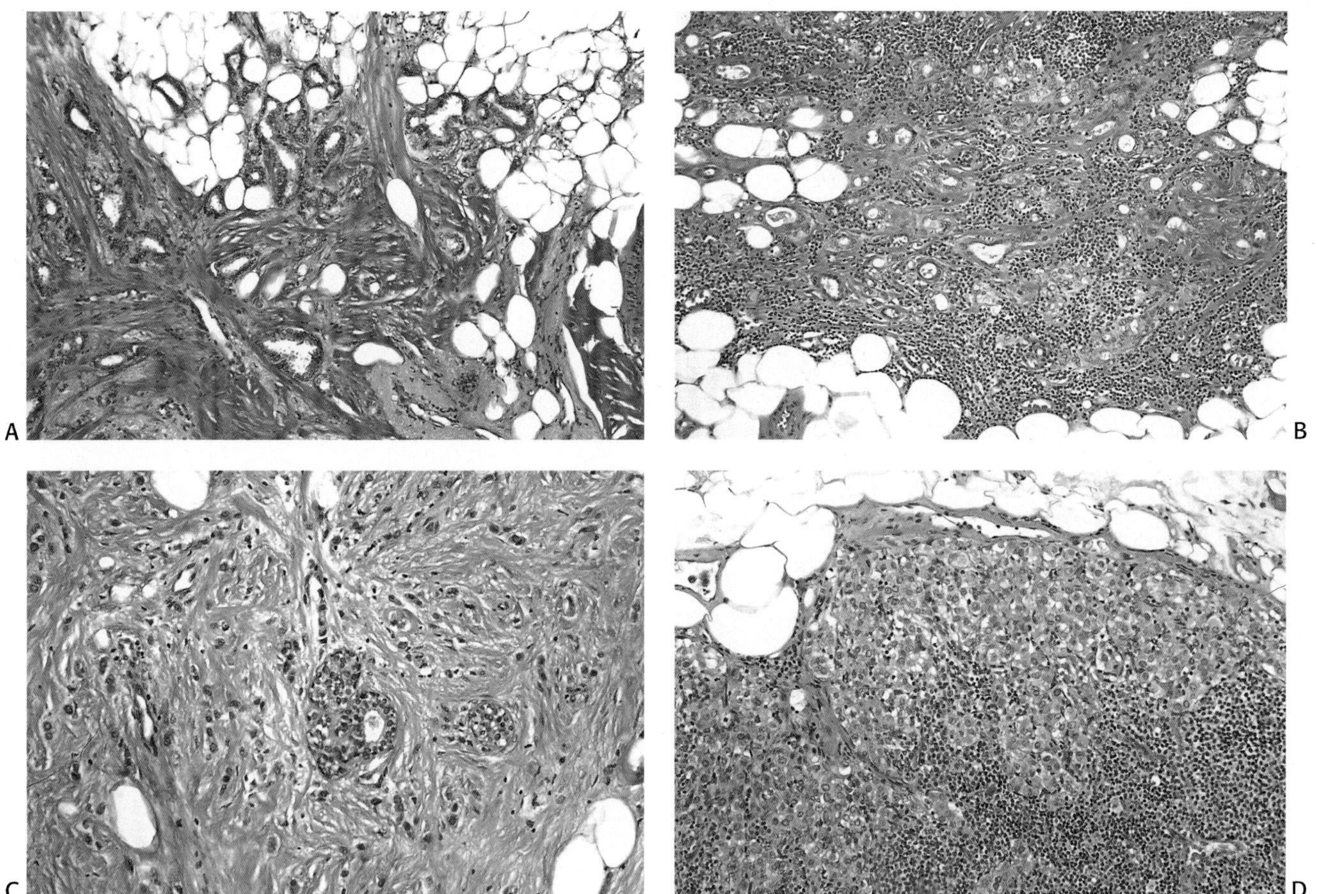

FIG. 32.22. ***Invasive lobular carcinoma with lymph node metastases.*** This patient had separate primary IDC and ILC in the same breast. **A:** Invasive duct carcinoma, well-differentiated tubular type, in the breast. **B:** Metastatic tubular carcinoma in an ALN and in perinodal fat. **C:** ILC, classical type in the breast. **D:** Metastatic lobular carcinoma fills the subcapsular sinuses in an ALN.

Lymph Nodes

ALN metastases derived from ILC of the classical type may be distributed largely in sinusoids, or they may involve sinusoids and lymphoid areas (Fig. 32.23). When lymph node involvement is sparse, the distinction between tumor cells and histiocytes can be difficult. Problems may also be encountered when there are extensive nodal metastases that are limited to sinusoids, because the appearance resembles severe sinus histiocytosis. This pattern of metastatic spread has been described as "sinus catarrh." In this setting, tumor cells are also sometimes distributed individually or in small groups in the lymphoid areas. On occasion, one may encounter lymph nodes in which metastatic lobular carcinomas are concentrated in sinusoids of the hilum. Fernández et al.[192] found significant differences between the "overall predominant pattern" of nodal metastases in patients with ILC and IDC, with diffuse growth more common in ILC. The analysis was limited to 246 patients with a single positive lymph node (219 IDC; 271 ILC). The growth patterns of metastases were classified as nodular (IDC 74%; ILC 66.7%), diffuse (IDC 6.8%; ILC 18.5%), nodular and diffuse (IDC 7.3%; ILC 18.5%), and sinusoidal (IDC 11.9%; ILC 0%).

Reactive changes in histiocytes in the sinusoids of lymph nodes may resemble metastatic lobular carcinoma. Vacuolated histiocytes associated with silicone mastitis resemble signet ring cells, but they are not ordinarily limited to the sinusoids, and a giant cell reaction is typically present. "Signet ring cell sinus histiocytosis," a rare nonneoplastic reactive change of unknown etiology, is especially difficult to distinguish from metastatic lobular carcinoma (Fig. 32.24).[193,194] Signet ring histiocytes resemble metastatic lobular carcinoma in routine hematoxylin and eosin (H&E) sections, necessitating the use of histochemical and immunohistochemical procedures. Cytoplasmic staining with periodic acid–Schiff (PAS) that is abolished with diastase, and a weakly to moderately positive mucicarmine reaction, can be found in signet ring cell histiocytes. These cells are not immunoreactive with markers associated with epithelial cells such as CK or GCDFP-15, and they are reactive for histiocytic markers, including lysozyme, CD68, and α_1-antitrypsin.[193] Electron microscopic examination reveals an open cytoplasmic vacuole or amorphous, electron-dense lipid in signet ring histiocytes.[193] The etiology of signet ring histiocytes is uncertain,

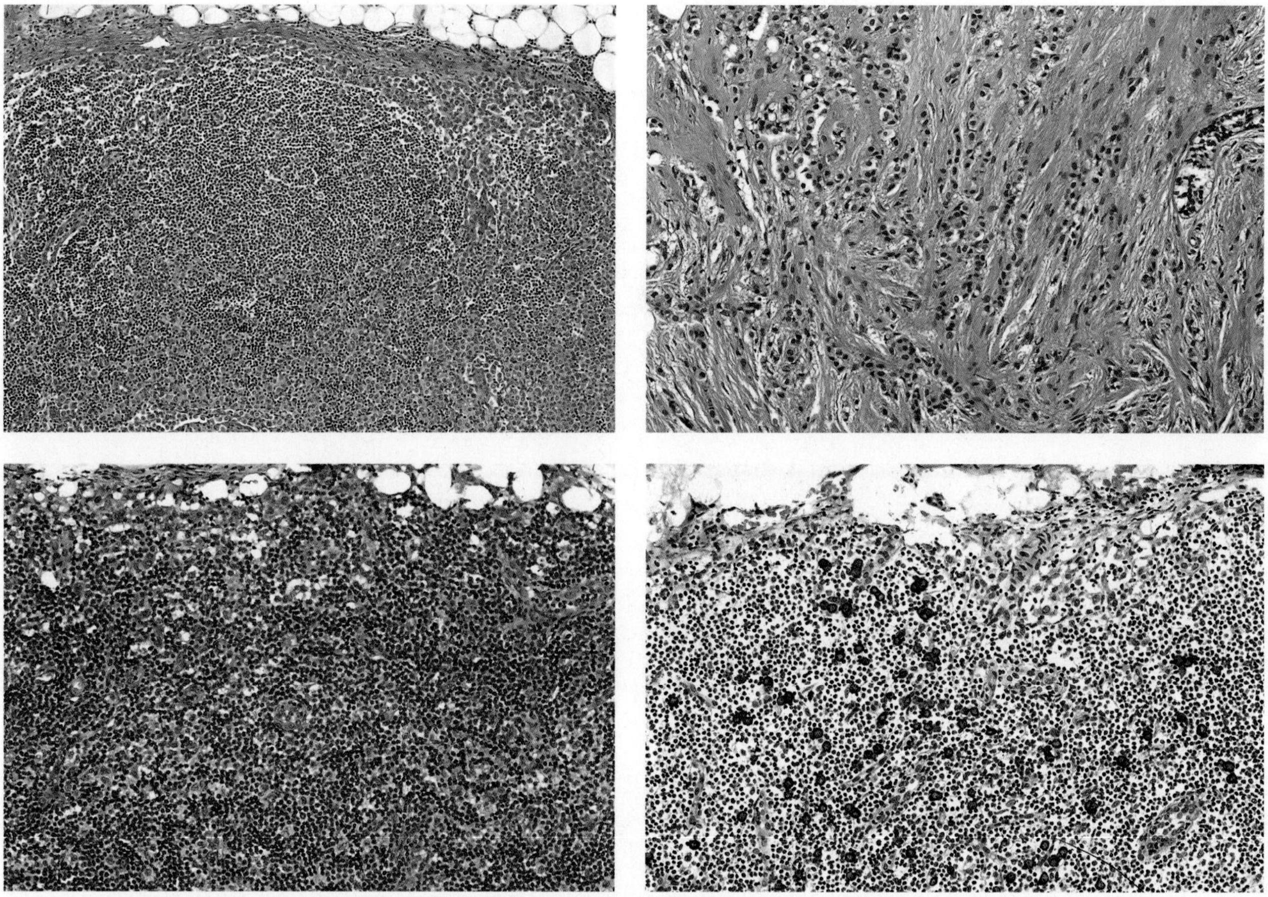

FIG. 32.23. ***Invasive lobular carcinoma, axillary lymph node metastasis.*** **A**: Metastatic carcinoma cells are present in the subcapsular sinuses and in lymphoid tissue. Images **(B–D)** are from another patient. **B:** ILC in the breast. **C:** A SLN with no apparent metastatic carcinoma. **D:** The same region of the SLN in **(C)** prepared with the CAM5.2 CK immunostain displays isolated metastatic carcinoma cells.

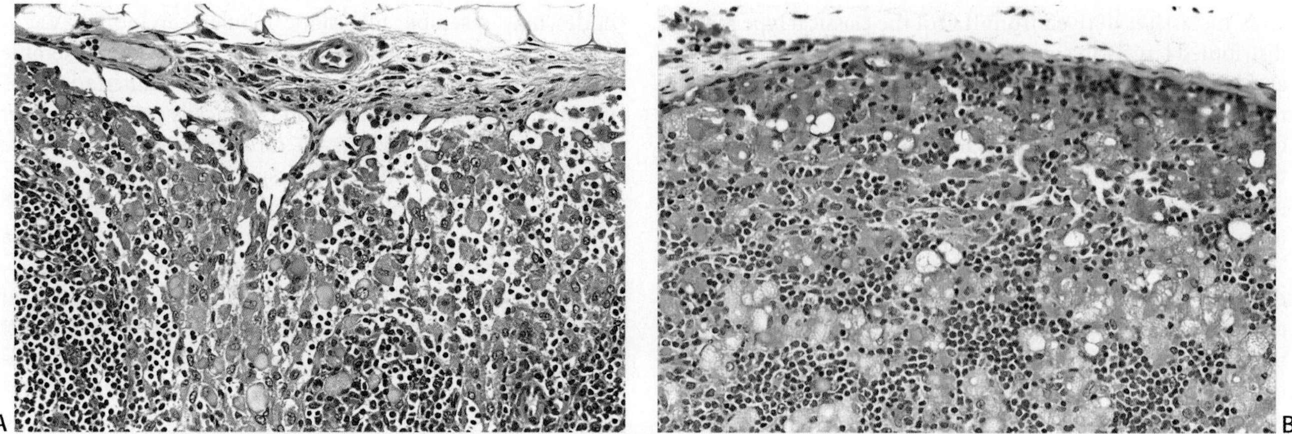

FIG. 32.24. ***Signet ring cell histiocytes.*** **A:** The subcapsular sinuses are filled with signet ring cell histiocytes. **B:** The cytoplasm of the histiocytes is tinted pink with the mucicarmine stain, but the cytoplasmic vacuoles are not mucicarminophilic.

but most reported patients have had prior surgery involving the chest wall for breast carcinoma or coronary artery disease.[193–195] The lipid present in these cells may derive from injury to fat caused by prior procedures.

When the presence of metastatic lobular carcinoma in lymph nodes cannot be determined with confidence in routine histologic sections, immunohistochemical studies for CK can be employed to detect inapparent micrometastases. There is not a consensus on the utility of routine immunohistochemical study of lymph nodes from patients with ILC for detecting micrometastases, but published data suggest that this is a useful procedure. Some authors reported finding occult micrometastases by this method in nearly one-third of cases.[196,197] Cote et al.[198] used additional H&E sections as well as CK IHC to detect metastatic carcinoma in ALN previously reported as negative in women with ILC or mixed ILC and IDC. Occult metastases were found in 39% of 64 cases by IHC and in 3% with H&E sections.

CK IHC is usually employed in the diagnosis of sentinel lymph nodes (SLNs) and should be considered for all lymph nodes from patients with ILC if the SLN is involved by metastatic carcinoma larger than a micrometastasis. A review of 449 patients with ILC staged by SLN mapping revealed that 189 (42%) had metastatic carcinoma in an SLN.[199] The frequency of nodal involvement was directly related to tumor size (less than or equal to 1 cm, 17%; 1.1 to 2 cm, 33%; 2.1 to 3.0 cm, 60%; 3.1 to 4.0 cm, 74%). Metastatic carcinoma was detected solely by IHC in 65 cases (34%), including 17 instances of isolated tumor cells, 40 micrometastases, and 8 macrometastases. Axillary dissection was performed in 161 (85%) of the 189 cases, with the discovery of metastatic carcinoma in non-SLNs in 66 (41%). None of the patients with isolated tumor cells in a SLN had a positive non-sentinel node. Overall, 12 (24%) of 50 patients with an immunohistochemically positive SLN had metastatic carcinoma in a non-SLN.

Khoury et al.[200] described a modified Alcian blue stain that could be applied to fresh imprints taken from an SLN that was superior to routine H&E or the Giemsa stains for the intraoperative detection of metastatic lobular carcinoma in an SLN. The modified Alcian blue method increased the sensitivity for detecting a positive lymph node from 55.6% to 83.3%.

Horvath et al.[201] reported that there was no significant difference in the sensitivity of FS analysis of SLN in patients with ILC and IDC. The study was based on 131 consecutive cases of ILC and 133 randomly selected cases of IDC. The results were as follows: sensitivity—ILC 67%, IDC 75%; specificity—ILC and IDC 100%; false-negative rate—ILC 33%, IDC 25%. Taras et al.[202] reached the same conclusion after a comparison of 66 women with ILC and 810 with IDC who each had an SLN examined intraoperatively by imprint cytology that was supplemented by FS in a minority of cases.

Differences between ILC and IDC in patterns of axillary nodal metastases suggested by recent studies need further investigation. Vandorpe et al.[203] studied 4,292 consecutive patients treated for breast carcinoma at a Belgian university hospital. The investigators observed that patients with ILC were significantly less likely to have axillary nodal metastases than those with IDC when adjusted for tumor size. A similar result was obtained when the analysis was limited to SLN. Fernández et al.[192] reported that among patients with positive lymph nodes, those with ILC had significantly more involved nodes than those with IDC. This was manifested in a higher ratio of positive to total nodes removed and a higher pN category for ILC patients (IDC: pN2 4.3%, pN3 0.2%; ILC: pN2 8.9%, pN3 4.2%).

Non-nodal Metastases

Difficulty in distinguishing metastatic lobular carcinoma from histiocytes has been described at sites other than lymph nodes.[77] Orbital metastases can be mistaken for malignant lymphoma or melanoma (Fig. 32.25). In the eyelid, the lesion may resemble a chalazion.[95,204] Isolated tumor cells in the bone marrow can resemble hematopoietic elements.[205] A retrospective review of bone marrow core biopsies, all proven to harbor metastatic breast carcinoma by CK IHC, revealed that metastatic lobular carcinoma was correctly identified in H&E sections from 39% of these cases.[205] In the same study, carcinoma was detected in 58% of H&E sections of bone marrow core biopsies from patients with IDC. It is recommended that immunostains for CK be included in the routine work-up of bone marrow biopsies from patients with mammary carcinoma, especially if they have ILC.

Distinctive patterns of systemic metastases are also associated with ILC. Investigators have compared the metastatic patterns of duct and lobular carcinoma at autopsy[206] or from clinical records.[207] Both approaches have revealed statistically significant greater frequencies of metastatic lobular carcinoma in the peritoneum and retroperitoneum, leptomeninges, gastrointestinal tract, and gynecologic organs, and a lower frequency of pulmonary or pleural metastases.[158] Bone is a common site of metastases from ILC. In one study, parenchymal metastases in the liver, lungs, and brain were detected less often clinically or at autopsy in patients with ILC than in those with IDC.[208] Others reported that hepatic metastases were significantly more frequent with ILC than with IDC,[209] or that there was no significant difference in the frequency of liver metastases.[206,207] No significant differences have been found in the distribution of metastases between patients with the classical and variant patterns of ILC.[12]

Central nervous system involvement usually takes the form of carcinomatous meningitis and consists of diffuse leptomeningeal infiltration.[206,208,210,211] Occult carcinoma presenting with symptoms attributable to leptomeningeal metastases has been described.[212] Jayson et al.[213] found that 67% of patients with carcinomatous meningitis had lobular or mixed lobular and duct carcinomas. The disease had a rapidly progressive course, with a median interval of 10.9 months from primary diagnosis to meningeal recurrence. Cerebral infarcts have been ascribed to mucin emboli in a patient with ILC that had prominent signet ring cell features.[214] Signet ring cells are typically present in the cerebrospinal fluid.[212]

Intra-abdominal metastases tend to involve the serosal surfaces and retroperitoneum,[206,208,209,215] or ovaries[206,216]

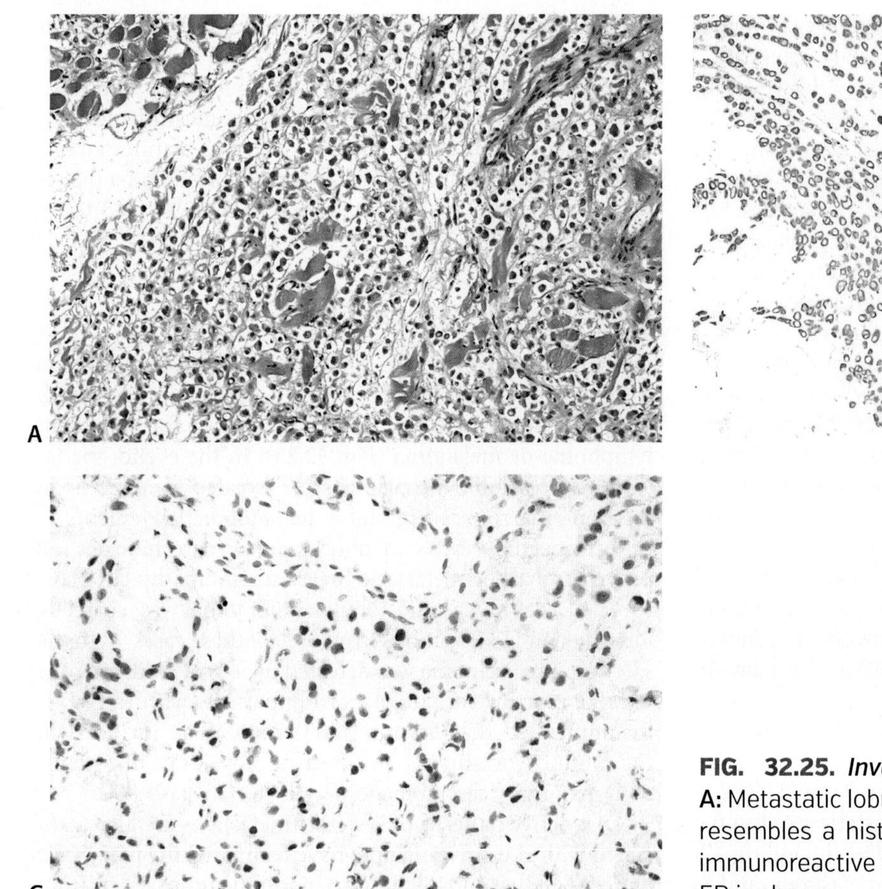

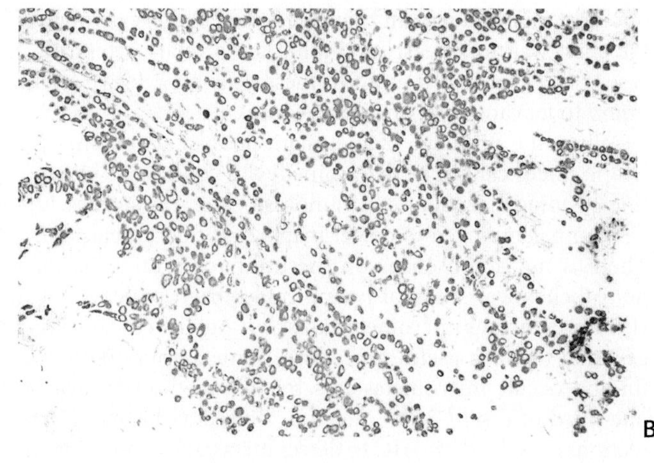

FIG. 32.25. ***Invasive lobular carcinoma, metastatic.*** **A:** Metastatic lobular carcinoma in the muscles of the orbit resembles a histiocytic infiltrate. **B:** The tumor cells are immunoreactive for CK7. **C:** Nuclear immunoreactivity for ER is shown.

(Fig. 32.26). Carcinoma cells from ILC and IDC in pleural and peritoneal effusions may resemble, and be difficult to distinguish from, reactive mesothelial cells.[217,218] A panel of immunostains such as CK7, hormone receptors, BerEp4, and CAM5.2 that will highlight carcinoma cells—and calretinin and mesothelin that decorate mesothelial cells—can be useful in this circumstance, especially if performed on a cell block preparation. At surgery, exploration sometimes reveals thickening of serosal, mesenteric, and retroperitoneal tissues, with no discrete mass. Ureteral obstruction can develop as a consequence of retroperitoneal metastases.[211] In other cases, there is diffuse spread to the uterus and ovaries with ovarian enlargement creating the features of Krukenberg tumor. Computed tomography (CT) scanning has proven especially useful for the detection of abdominal metastases of ILC.[219]

Metastatic lobular carcinoma in the uterus can also present a challenging diagnostic problem.[220] The carcinoma cells blend with normal endometrial stromal cells and may be overlooked in endometrial curettings obtained from a patient with vaginal bleeding (Fig. 32.27). The cells of metastatic lobular carcinoma in the endometrium may be detectable in a cervicovaginal smear.[221,222] Liebmann et al.[223] described a patient with a previously unrecognized ILC in the breast who had metastatic lobular carcinoma discovered in a uterine leiomyoma. Metastatic lobular carcinoma has been found in endometrial polyps associated with tamoxifen treatment.[224]

ILC can be a source of serosal, mural, and mucosal metastases involving the stomach (Fig. 32.28). This usually occurs in patients who have a known mammary primary and develop abdominal symptoms. Metastases are often present at other sites such as bone.[225] The clinical and pathologic findings may be indistinguishable from those of a primary gastric carcinoma.[191,208,226–228] In one remarkable case, a gastrectomy was performed for carcinoma involving the stomach that was thought to be primary at this site, 18 months before ILC that metastasized to the stomach was found in the breast.[229] An immunohistochemical stain for ER can be employed to distinguish between gastric and mammary carcinoma, but a weakly positive result does not rule out gastric carcinoma. ER has been detected in gastric adenocarcinoma by biochemical[230,231] and immunohistochemical[232,233] procedures, largely in Asian patients. In one study, ER was detected significantly more often in poorly differentiated than in well-differentiated gastric carcinomas, and immunoreactivity was not sex related.[233] Chaubert et al.[234] have reported that immunoreactivity was absent from gastric carcinoma in European patients. Metastatic mammary signet ring cell carcinoma involving the stomach and other

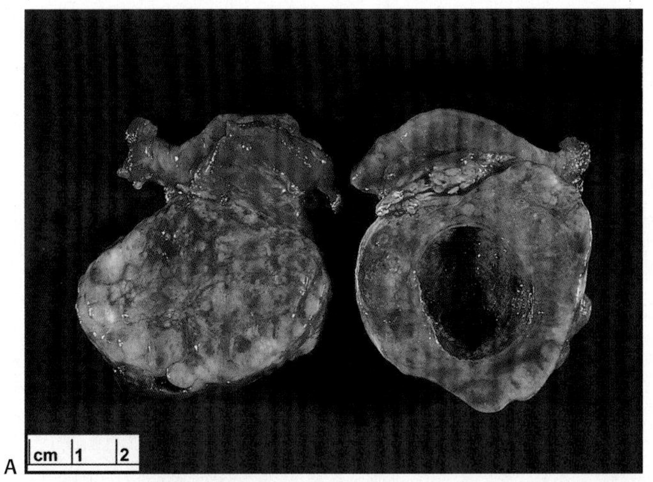

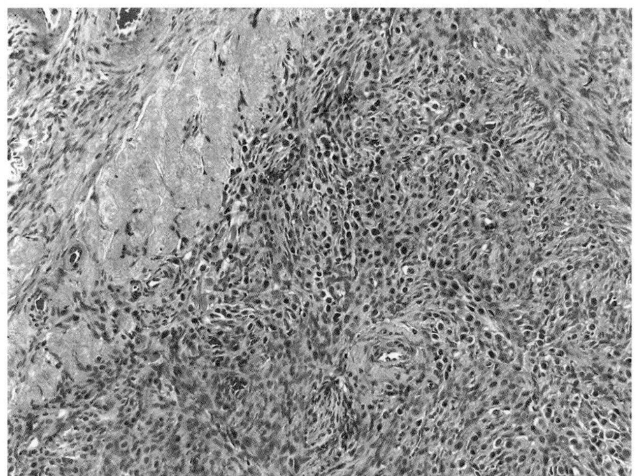

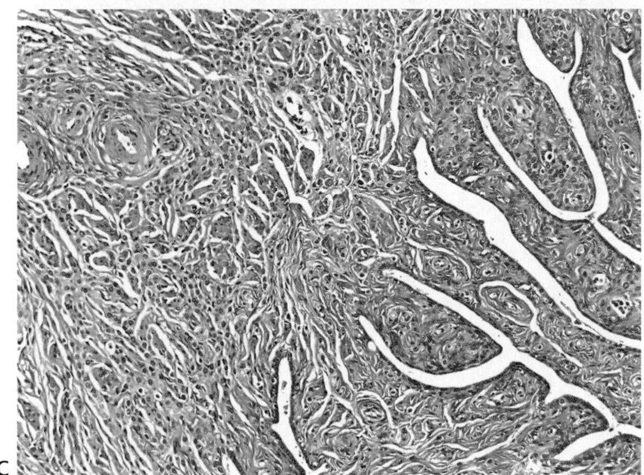

FIG. 32.26. ***Metastatic lobular carcinoma in the ovary and fallopian tube.*** **A:** The bisected ovary is diffusely involved by metastatic lobular carcinoma around a cyst. **B,C:** Carcinoma cells are difficult to recognize in the ovarian stroma next to a corpus albicans **(B)** and in the stroma of mucosal folds of the fallopian tube **(C)**.

sites is likely to be positive for GCDFP-15, whereas primary gastric carcinoma is rarely immunoreactive for GCDFP-15. Loss of E-cadherin expression has been found in gastric carcinomas, and familial gastric carcinoma has been associated with germline mutations of the *E-cadherin* gene.[235] Metastatic lobular carcinoma in the colon may mimic a primary colonic carcinoma.[236] The distinction between metastatic lobular carcinoma and some carcinoid tumors can present a challenging diagnostic problem (Fig. 32.29). An infiltrative epithelioid variant of myofibroblastoma can be mistaken for ILC, especially since this benign tumor can be ER-positive (Fig. 32.30).

PROGNOSIS

Classical ILC

A number of studies have reported on the prognosis of patients with ILC. Newman's[3] paper that described 72 patients with classical ILC treated by mastectomy was the first to provide substantial prognostic data. He found that 5 (14%) of 36 patients with stage I carcinoma and 17 (46%) of 37 patients with stage II carcinoma died of disease, with follow-up averaging nearly 8 years. Ashikari et al.[11] reported 5- and 10-year survivals of 86% and 74%, respectively, for patients with stage I ILC treated by mastectomy not further stratified on the basis of tumor size. There were no significant differences in survival when the patients were compared with women treated for IDC with similar nodal status.

A few series have included enough patients to compare the prognosis of patients treated by mastectomy for structurally classical and structurally variant types of classical ILC. Dixon et al.[10] studied 103 women with ILC. Overall, the combined group had a significantly more favorable prognosis than women with IDC. However, the groups of lobular and duct carcinoma patients were not specifically matched for stage and treatment and hence may not have been comparable. Dixon et al.[10] also found that patients with classical ILC had a more favorable prognosis than those with structurally variant forms of ILC when treated by mastectomy. Because the patients with classical ILC and variant forms of classical ILC were not stratified by stage, these results may also be misleading. For example, the frequency of cases with stage I carcinoma varied from 33% among those with a mixed histologic pattern to 74% in the group with alveolar variant tumors. Furthermore, most patients included in the study did not have an axillary dissection.

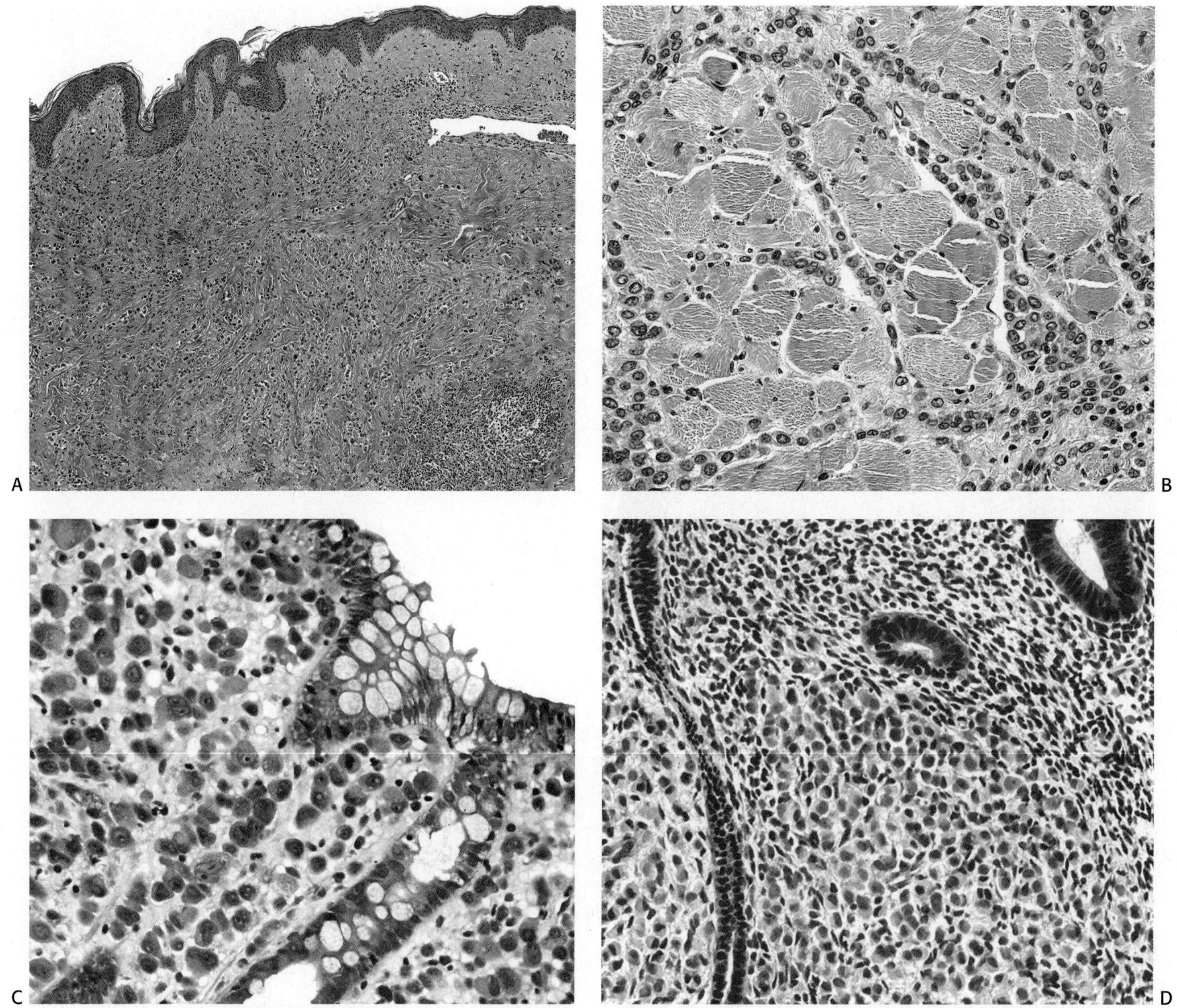

FIG. 32.27. ***Metastatic lobular carcinoma in various organs.*** **A:** Lobular carcinoma with negligible reactive changes in the dermis of the skin. **B:** Involvement of skeletal muscle. **C:** Diffuse involvement of the colonic mucosa. **D:** Lobular carcinoma blends with stromal cells in the endometrium.

Analysis of 171 patients with ILC by du Toit et al.[73] revealed that women with the classical subtype had a slightly better prognosis than those with alveolar and solid variants. The best prognosis, a 12-year actuarial survival of 100%, was observed in patients with tubulolobular carcinoma. Systemic recurrences were found in 44% of patients with classical ILC and in 40% to 57% of patients with variant forms. The results in this study are difficult to assess because patients were not stratified by stage and they were not treated in a consistent manner. Primary surgery consisted of "simple mastectomy, subcutaneous mastectomy, or a lumpectomy followed by whole-breast irradiation," and "lymph node status was determined by a triple-node biopsy technique" rather than by conventional axillary dissection.

Frost et al.[237] reviewed 92 patients with ILC subclassified by histologic growth pattern. There was no statistically significant relationship between the architecture of the ILC (classical, alveolar, solid, mixed) and prognosis. Variant lesions were similar in regard to age distribution, tumor size, nodal status, and hormone receptor expression.

Two hundred and thirty patients with stage I and stage II ILC treated by mastectomy and axillary dissection were studied by DiCostanzo et al.[12] They compared 176 women with classical ILC with 54 with variant histologic patterns of classical ILC (10 solid, 14 alveolar, 30 mixed). The classical group was significantly younger at diagnosis (52 vs. 57 years). The groups did not differ significantly in tumor size, nodal status, or TNM stage. OS and recurrence-free survival were similar in the two groups (Fig. 32.31). Although not statistically significant, the survival of patients with stage I and level I node-positive stage II classical ILC was better than that of patients with variant tumors of similar stage

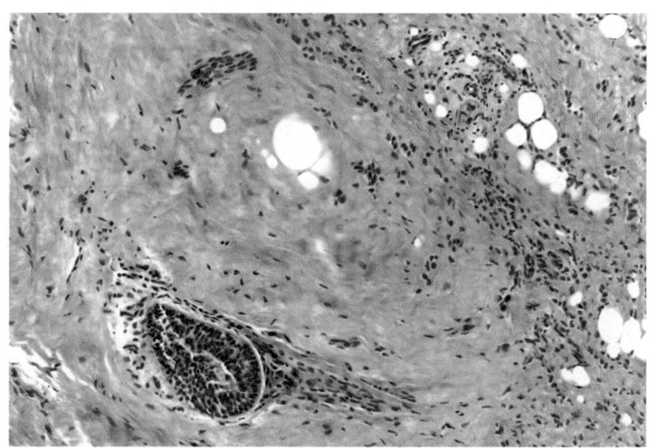

FIG. 32.28. ***Invasive lobular carcinoma on frozen section of the nipple margin in a nipple-sparing mastectomy.*** The invasive carcinoma is almost imperceptible in the FS.

(Fig. 32.32). When compared with patients with classical ILC, each of the variant subsets showed a trend to more frequent recurrence and death due to disease, but none of the differences was statistically significant (Fig. 32.33). Iorfida et al.[238] analyzed a larger series of 981 consecutive patients with ILC that included 541 (55.8%) classical lesions and 400 (44.2%) with variant forms of ILC. Patients with the solid and mixed variant forms of ILC had a poorer disease-free survival (DFS) and OS than patients with classical ILC, and there was a trend to a less favorable outcome in the solid ILC group when compared with other variant forms.

In a further analysis by DiCostanzo et al.,[12] women with classical ILC were compared with a series of patients treated for IDC, matched for age, tumor size, and nodal status[12] (Fig. 32.34). When stratified by stage, patients with stage I classical ILC had a significantly better recurrence-free survival than duct carcinoma patients (Fig. 32.35). No significant difference in survival was found when patients with stage II carcinoma were compared. In 2007, Jayasinghe et al.[239] reported the results of a population-based study of 307 women treated in 1992 for either ILC or IDC in part of Sydney, Australia. There was no significant difference in surgical treatment between the two groups, with mastectomy slightly more frequent in ILC patients. The overall 10-year survival of patients with ILC was higher (84%) than that of women with IDC (69%) ($p = 0.073$). The marginally more favorable overall prognosis of lobular carcinoma patients was also observed in patients with stage I and stage II carcinoma, but the differences were not statistically significant. This analysis did not consider the subtypes of lobular carcinoma.

Fortunato et al.[59] found no difference in OS, DFS, and locoregional control in an analysis of 171 patients with ILC and 1,011 patients with IDC who were treated by mastectomy

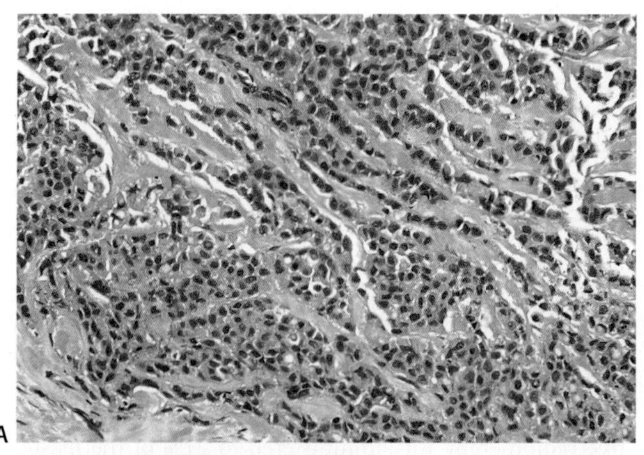

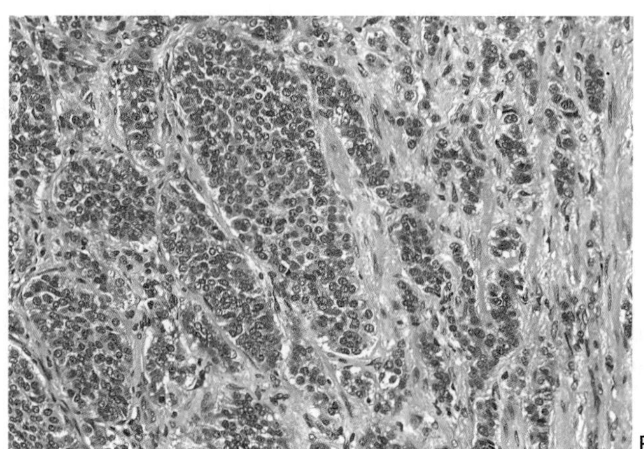

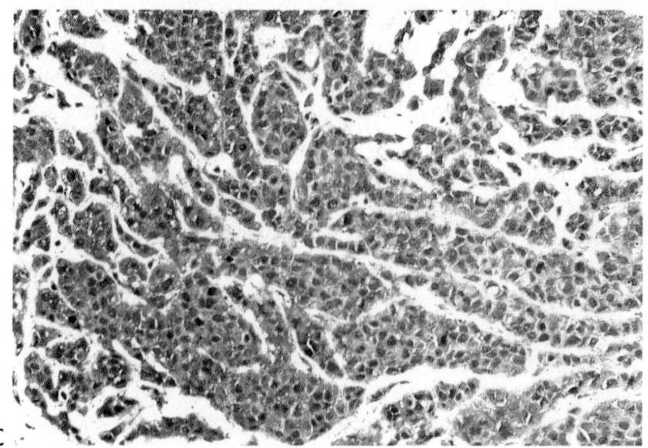

FIG. 32.29. ***Invasive lobular carcinoma and appendiceal carcinoid tumor.*** All images are from the same patient. **A:** ILC, classical type in the breast. **B:** Abdominal symptoms subsequently led to discovery of this tumor in the appendix, initially interpreted as metastatic lobular carcinoma. **C:** On further investigation, the tumor proved to be immunoreactive for neuron-specific enolase, shown here, and other neuroendocrine markers. There was no reactivity for ER. The lesion was an appendiceal carcinoid.

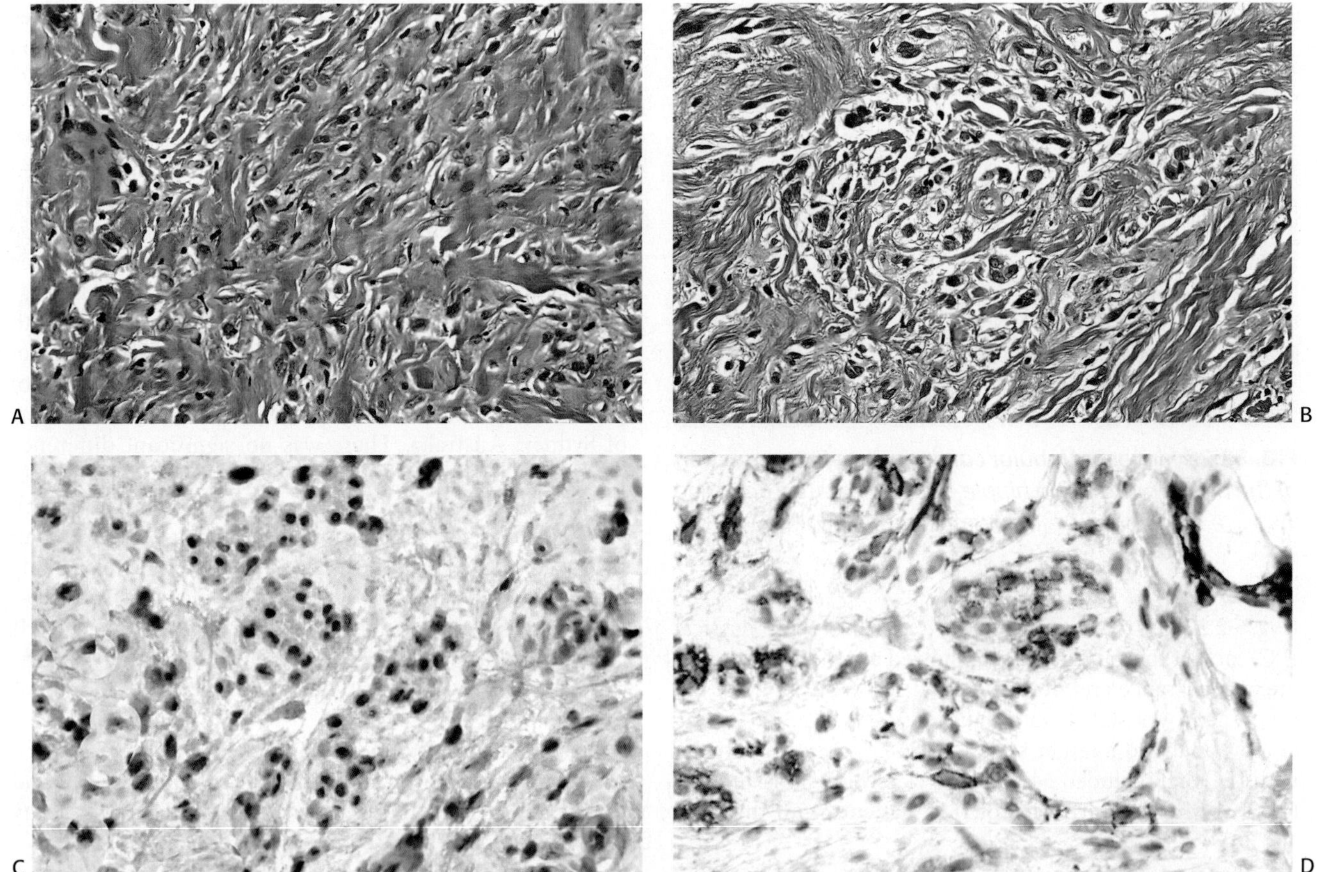

FIG. 32.30. ***Epithelioid myofibroblastoma mistaken for invasive lobular carcinoma on needle-core biopsy.*** **A,B:** This epithelioid myofibroblastoma had a single-cell infiltrative pattern that simulated the classical type of ILC. The tumor cells were diffusely and strongly ER-positive **(C)**, a result that seemingly corroborated the diagnosis of ILC, but myofibroblastomas are typically ER-positive as well as CD34-positive **(D)**.

and breast-conserving surgery. After 10 years of follow-up, Moran et al.[240] found no significant difference in the frequency of breast recurrence, distant metastases, and survival between patients with ILC and IDC who were treated by breast-conserving surgery and radiotherapy. A similar conclusion was reached by Peiro et al.[241] who studied 1,624 patients with stage I and stage II invasive carcinoma that were treated with breast-conserving surgery and radiotherapy. These investigators also reported that the outcome for patients whose tumors had mixed duct–lobular features was not significantly different from those with ILC and IDC. On the other hand, Bharat et al.[242] reported that patients with IDC had a significantly poorer 10-year survival (61%) than patients with IDC (68%) and those with mixed duct–lobular carcinomas. A stage-matched analysis of 263,408 women recorded in a National Cancer Institute database revealed a significantly better 5-year disease-specific survival for patients with ILC when compared with those with IDC.[243] In a multivariate analysis, patients with ILC had a 14% survival benefit.

Length of follow-up may be a crucial factor in the analysis of outcome for patients with ILC. In a study of 268 women with ILC, Anwar et al.[244] compared the time to recurrence in 79 women who had breast-conserving surgery and 156 who had a mastectomy. The nonrandomized nature of the study is manifested in the fact that mastectomy patients had significantly larger tumors than those treated by breast-conservation therapy (mean tumor size: 37 vs. 17 mm) and more frequent multifocal tumors (25% vs. 9%). Postoperative radiotherapy was administered to 21% of the mastectomy group and all breast-conservation patients. Despite the less favorable clinical presentation of patients who had a mastectomy and the less frequent use of adjuvant radiotherapy, local recurrences were found in 13.4% of mastectomy patients and 34% of those who had breast conservation. Overall, the mean time to local recurrence was 127 months (range 24 to 196 months). The mean time to local recurrence for patients treated by mastectomy (133.5 months) was significantly longer than the mean time to local recurrence after breast-conserving surgery (122 months). Despite the difference in frequency of and time to local recurrence, there was no significant difference in the length of OS between the two treatment groups. These data suggest that studies with follow-up of 5 years or less that use local recurrence as an

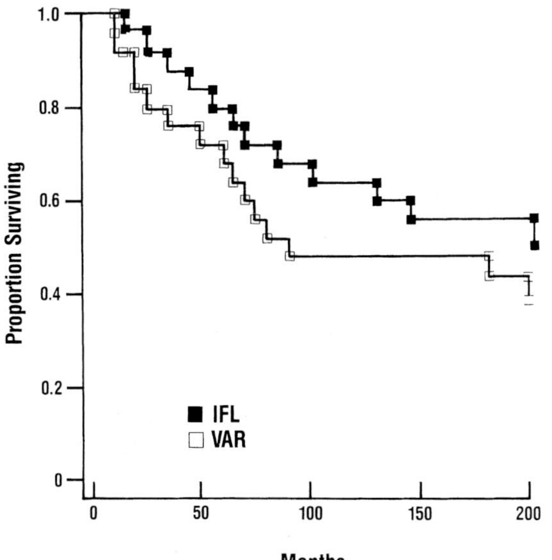

FIG. 32.31. ***Survival analysis comparing classical and variant forms of invasive lobular carcinoma.*** The difference in survival between patients with classical (IFL) and variant (VAR) forms of carcinoma was not statistically significant. (Reproduced from DiCostanzo D, Rosen PP, Gareen I, et al. Prognosis in infiltrating lobular carcinoma: an analysis of "classical" and variant tumors. *Am J Surg Pathol* 1990;14:12–23.)

endpoint could give an incomplete picture of the prognosis of patients with ILC.

Pleomorphic ILC

Weidner and Semple[245] found that patients who had the PILC had a significantly worse recurrence-free survival than those with ILC. The comparison was based on groups similar with respect to tumor size and nodal status. The RRs of recurrence were 4.13 for node-negative PILC, 7.35 for node-positive ILC, and 30.4 for node-positive PILC when compared with node-negative ILC patients. A subsequent comparative study from the same institution revealed a shorter RFS for patients with PILC but no significant difference from ILC for OS.[188] Bentz et al.[103] reported a fatal outcome in 9 (75%) of 12 patients with PILC with a median survival of 2.1 years after diagnosis. This outcome was significantly worse than for comparison groups of patients with IDC and ILC.

After a median follow-up of 42 months, Monhollen et al.[129] reported that 11/36 patients (30.6%) with PILC had a recurrence and/or died of disease. The median time to recurrence was 27.2 months, and the projected 5-year RFS was 54.9%. A detailed analysis of prognosis for PILC was reported by Buchanan et al.,[17] who compared 52 patients with PILC with 298 with ILC and 3,978 with IDC treated at a single institution. The cases were obtained from and limited to a database of patients who had an SLN biopsy dating from 1996. PILC tumors were significantly larger (median size: PILC 20 mm, ILC 15 mm, IDC 13 mm), were more likely to have a positive SLN, and more often required a mastectomy (PILC 63.5%, ILC 38.7%, IDC 28.8%). When compared with ILC patients, those with PILC had significantly more distant metastases (PILC 11.5%, ILC 3.7%).

Summary of Prognosis for Classical ILC and PILC

In summary, various studies of prognosis in patients with ILC have not shown a consistent difference from patients with IDC treated by mastectomy when stage at diagnosis is taken into consideration. Most studies indicated that patients with classical ILC had a better prognosis than those with variant forms of classical ILC as a group, but the differences have not been statistically significant. No reproducible differences in prognosis have been demonstrated among the

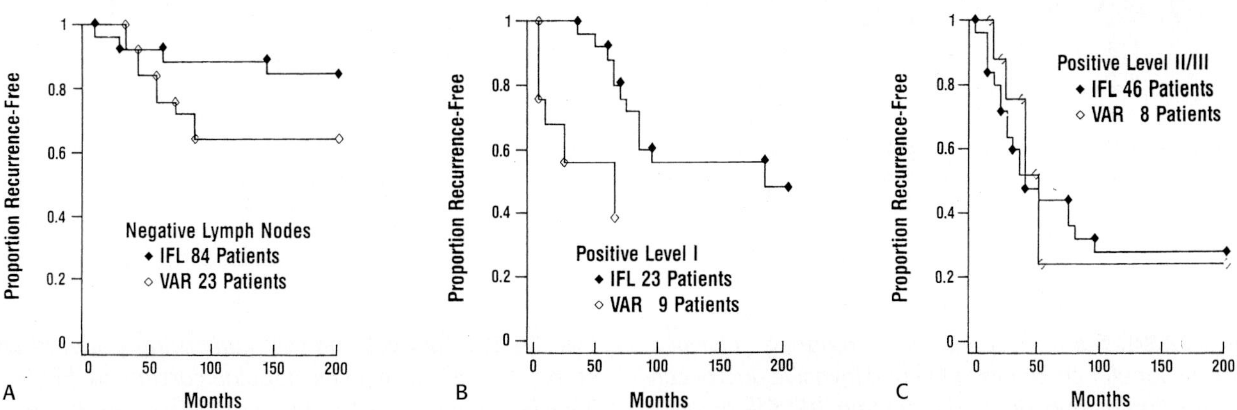

FIG. 32.32. ***Survival analysis comparing classical invasive lobular carcinoma (IFL) to variant forms (VAR) stratified by stage.*** Although patients with variant forms tend to have a lower recurrence-free survival in each subset, the differences are not statistically significant. (Reproduced from DiCostanzo D, Rosen PP, Gareen I, et al. Prognosis in infiltrating lobular carcinoma: an analysis of "classical" and variant tumors. *Am J Surg Pathol* 1990;14:12–23.)

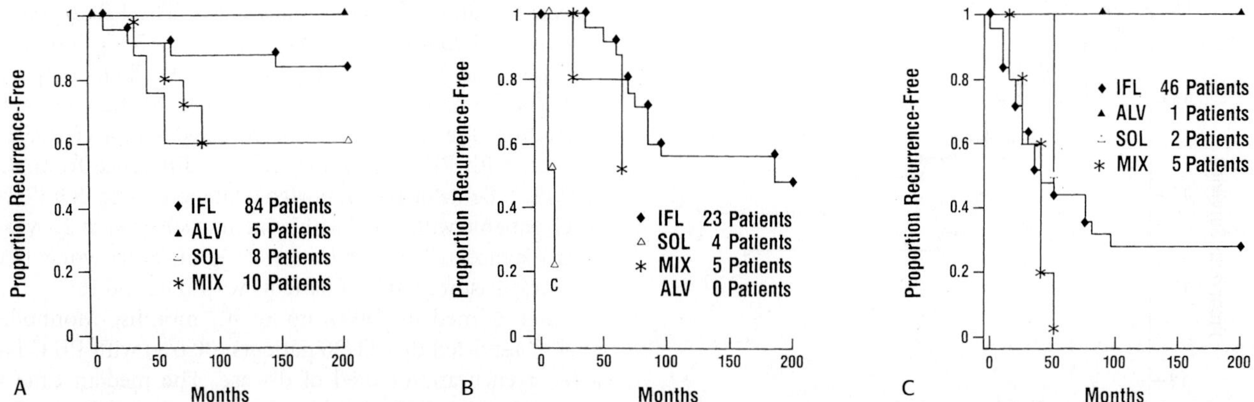

FIG. 32.33. ***Survival analysis comparing classical invasive lobular carcinoma (IFL) to subtypes of variant forms (VAR).*** The differences are not statistically significant in each stage grouping. **A:** Negative node patients. **B:** Patients with lymph node metastases at level I. **C:** Patients with lymph node metastases at levels II and III. ALV, alveolar; SOL, solid; MIX, mixed. (Reproduced from DiCostanzo D, Rosen PP, Gareen I, et al. Prognosis in infiltrating lobular carcinoma: an analysis of "classical" and variant tumors. *Am J Surg Pathol* 1990;14:12–23.)

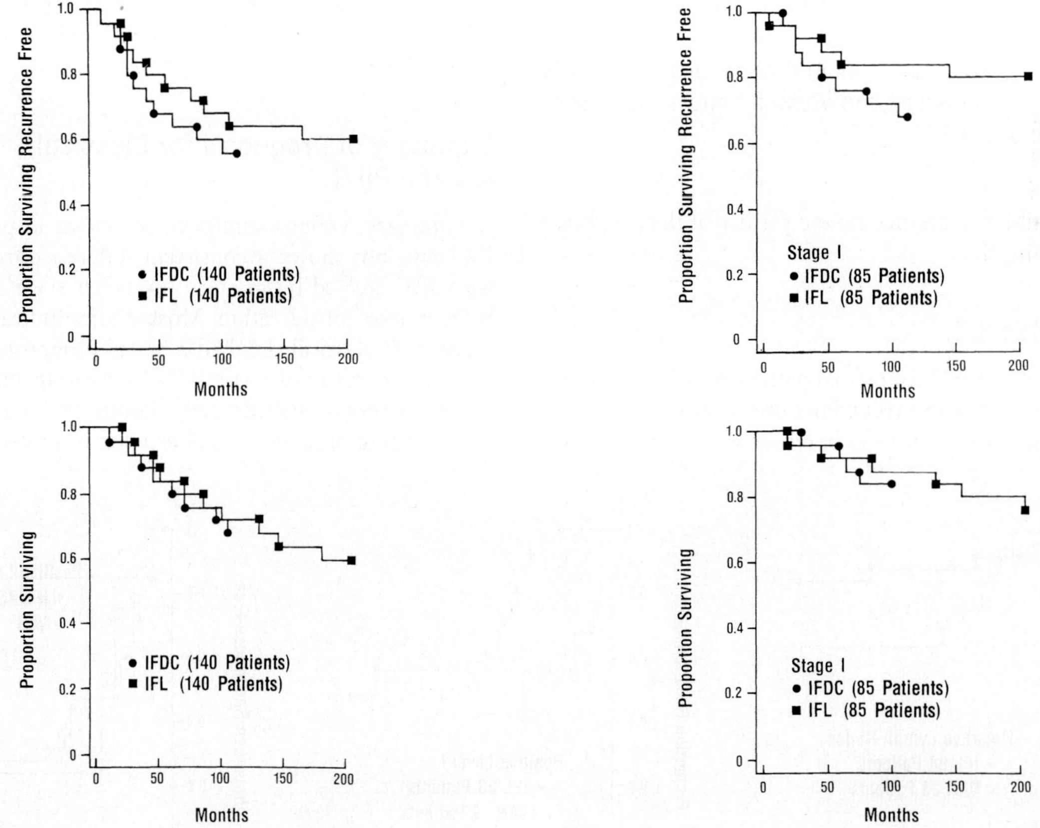

FIG. 32.34. ***Survival analysis comparing classical invasive lobular carcinoma (IFL) and invasive ductal carcinoma (infiltrating ductal carcinoma [IFDC]).*** Survival and recurrence-free survival were virtually the same for the two groups of patients matched for age and primary tumor stage. (Reproduced from DiCostanzo D, Rosen PP, Gareen I, et al. Prognosis in infiltrating lobular carcinoma: an analysis of "classical" and variant tumors. *Am J Surg Pathol* 1990;14:12–23.)

FIG. 32.35. ***Survival analysis comparing patients with stage I classical invasive lobular carcinoma (IFL) and invasive ductal carcinoma (IFDC).*** The difference between the two groups was statistically significant for recurrence-free survival rate ($p = 0.02$) but not for OS rate. (Reproduced from DiCostanzo D, Rosen PP, Gareen I, et al. Prognosis in infiltrating lobular carcinoma: an analysis of "classical" and variant tumors. *Am J Surg Pathol* 1990;14:12–23.)

variant subtypes of classical ILC, and it is evident that very large numbers of cases would be needed to document significant differences if they exist. Classical ILC has a more favorable prognosis than PILC.

The most important determinants of prognosis for patients with ILC are primary tumor size and nodal status.[246] Analysis of more than 15,000 patients in the Colorado Tumor Registry demonstrated that tumor size was the most significant indicator of ALN status.[247] The frequency of ALN metastases was nearly identical for patients with IDC and ILC when stratified by tumor size. Among women with tumors 2 cm or smaller, ALN were positive in 25% with ILC and 27% with IDC and for tumors 0.5 cm or smaller, the frequencies of axillary metastasis were 13% and 12%, respectively.[247] Additional information about prognosis can be found in the following section.

TREATMENT

Mastectomy and Breast-Conserving Surgery

Yeatman et al.[45] reported that mastectomy rather than lumpectomy with breast conservation was performed significantly more often in patients with ILC than with IDC. Conversion from lumpectomy to mastectomy because of positive margins after reexcision occurred more frequently among patients treated for ILC. If a mastectomy is performed, it should be a total mastectomy, in order to minimize the chance of leaving breast tissue at the surgical site. Subcutaneous mastectomy is not appropriate for these patients.

Singletary et al.[248] analyzed data from the National Cancer Data Base for 1989 to 2001 to examine trends in treatment for ILC. Among the 21,596 patients selected for the study, 8,108 (37.5%) had some form of breast-conservation treatment and the remainder (62.5%) underwent a mastectomy. The frequency of breast-conservation therapy was inversely related to TN category but increased from about 20% to 25% in 1998 to between 50% and 60% in 2001. There was also a doubling in the frequency of SLN mapping for staging from about 10% to 15% to between 20% and nearly 30% in the same time period. Substantial regional differences in the frequency of breast-conservation treatment for ILC were found with the percentages ranging from approximately 40% to 50% in New England, the middle Atlantic, and Pacific regions to around 25% in the south and central regions.

Many reports of the treatment of ILC by breast conservation with radiotherapy have appeared. The data obtained from nonrandomized studies indicate that local control and survival for patients with ILC treated by breast conservation are similar to the results obtained for IDC at 5 years of follow-up.[41,240,249–256] Most of these studies do not have comprehensive data for 10 years of follow-up, an important consideration because of the observed trend to later local recurrence of ILC in the breast described by some investigators.[71,244]

Warneke et al.[256] analyzed 111 patients treated for stage I and stage II ILC over a 10-year period at the University of Arizona. There was no difference in the frequency of local recurrence between the breast-conservation and mastectomy patients. When compared with the lumpectomy and radiotherapy patients, the mastectomy group was characterized by larger clinical tumor size (3.0 vs. 1.6 cm), larger pathologic tumor size (2.6 vs. 2.1 cm), and more frequent ALN metastases (44% vs. 27%). Among 34 (37%) who had lumpectomy with radiotherapy, there was one (3%) local recurrence. The remaining 59 patients (63%) underwent modified radical mastectomy after which there were two (3%) local recurrences.

Kurtz et al.[249] found that local failure in the breast after 5 years was more frequent in patients with ILC (13.5%) than after treatment of IDC (8.8%), but the difference was not statistically significant. Virtually all recurrences were at some distance from the primary tumor, or they were multifocal. The 5-year actuarial survival rates were 100% and 77% for node-negative and node-positive patients, respectively. Schnitt et al.[252] reported that the 5-year actuarial risk of local recurrence was nearly identical for patients with ILC (12%) and IDC (11%). The 12% local recurrence rate for ILC was greater than the recurrence rate of patients with IDC that lacked an extensive intraductal component (5%), but less than the 23% recurrence rate encountered for IDC with extensive intraductal carcinoma. In this series, all recurrences of ILC were in the vicinity of the initial primary tumor.

Poen et al.[251] studied 60 patients with ILC followed 2.5 to 10 years (mean, 5.5 years) after lumpectomy and radiation therapy. Two patients had recurrences in local nodal regions and one developed recurrent carcinoma in the affected breast. The 5-year actuarial locoregional control rate was 95%. During the same interval, 11 patients were found to have distant metastases leading to death in 6 cases. White et al.[41] reported 5-year local recurrence rates of 3.3% and 4.2%, respectively, for ILC and IDC.

Analysis of data from the state of Rhode Island tumor registry for the years 1984 to 1994 included 4,886 women diagnosed and treated for IDC and ILC.[254] Women with ILC had a significantly older mean age at diagnosis (lobular, 64.5 vs. ductal, 61.6 years) and larger tumor size (lobular, 28.6 vs. ductal, 23.9 mm), with nearly identical frequencies of axillary nodal metastases (lobular, 33.4% vs. ductal, 33.1%). There were no significant differences in 5-year survival (lobular, 68% vs. ductal, 71%), 5-year local recurrence after breast conservation (lobular, 2.8% vs. ductal, 2.5%), or in the incidence of contralateral carcinoma (lobular, 6.6% vs. ductal, 6.5%).

An important study by Santiago et al.[257] compared the results of breast-conservation therapy in 1,093 patients with stage I and stage II IDC and 55 patients with stage I and stage II ILC treated at the University of Pennsylvania between 1977 and 1995. The median follow-up was 8.7 and 10.2 years for the IDC and ILC patients, respectively. There were no significant differences in 10-year actuarial rates for OS, disease-specific survival, and distant DFS. Local recurrences were more frequent in patients with ILC (18%) than those with IDC (12%), but the difference was not statistically significant. It is interesting to note that the 10-year rates of contralateral carcinoma (lobular, 12% vs. duct, 8%) were not significantly different.

Summary of Surgical Treatment for ILC

The foregoing data suggest that ILC of the classical cytologic type, whether structurally classical or variant, can be effectively managed by breast-conservation therapy. Criteria to select patients for this treatment are essentially the same as for IDC. The presence of invasive carcinoma at a margin will usually require further excision. However, in contrast to the distribution of DCIS in patients with IDC, LCIS at the margin in a patient with ILC does not necessitate additional surgery. Lumpectomy should be supplemented by breast irradiation unless there are exceptional circumstances.

Limited information is available about the treatment of PILC by breast-conserving surgery. If this is done, it has been suggested that PLCIS be viewed as similar to intraductal carcinoma with respect to assessing margins.

Neoadjuvant Chemotherapy and Endocrine Therapy

Neoadjuvant chemotherapy is usually administered to a patient with potentially operable breast carcinoma in order to reduce tumor size and thereby increase the likelihood of successful breast-conserving surgery as well as to assess the response of the tumor to a particular form of therapy. A discussion of clinical and pathologic effects of neoadjuvant chemotherapy on breast carcinomas in general can be found in Chapter 41. The information here relates specifically to ILC.

A study by Sullivan and Apple[258] compared the response with an unspecified neoadjuvant chemotherapy regimen in 40 patients with IDC and 9 with ILC. Among seven evaluable cases of ILC, there were no complete responses and only one partial response (14%) on imaging and physical exam. When evaluated by physical examination or imaging, 11/37 (30%) evaluable patients with IDC had a complete response. In the IDC group, partial responses on imaging were recorded in 24% of cases and by physical exam in 43%. Histologic changes such as the accumulation of foam cells, nuclear degeneration, and cellular enlargement that characterize response to neoadjuvant chemotherapy were found less often in posttreatment ILC specimens than in IDC specimens after therapy. Additional evidence that ILC is less responsive than IDC to some forms of adjuvant chemotherapy was presented by Cristofanilli et al.,[259] Purushotham et al.,[260] and Nagao et al.[261]

One potential benefit from the use of neoadjuvant chemotherapy in patients with ILC would be to reduce the likelihood of having a positive margin at the time of lumpectomy in anticipation of breast conservation. To date, retrospective observational studies suggest that neoadjuvant chemotherapy regimens of various sorts do not significantly improve breast-conservation rates by reducing the frequency of positive margins. Wagner et al.[262] studied 93 patients with ILC who had neoadjuvant chemotherapy before lumpectomy and 218 who had surgery without neoadjuvant chemotherapy. There was no significant difference in the frequency of margin positivity, reoperation, or the finding of residual carcinoma between the two groups. After controlling for initial tumor size, Boughey et al.[263] found that neoadjuvant chemotherapy did not significantly increase the proportion of patients with ILC who were eligible for or underwent breast-conserving surgery when compared with patients with ILC who did not have neoadjuvant chemotherapy. With a mean follow-up of 47 months, the two groups had similar local recurrence rates. Others have also noted little or no significant improvement from the administration of neoadjuvant chemotherapy to patients with ILC with respect to reducing the frequency of positive lumpectomy margins or increasing the rate of breast conservation.[264,265]

Letrozole, a potent aromatase inhibitor, provided more effective neoadjuvant endocrine therapy than tamoxifen in a randomized trial of patients with ER (+) breast carcinoma.[266] Dixon et al.[267] investigated the effectiveness of neoadjuvant letrozole in ER (+) "large operable or locally advanced" ILC in postmenopausal women. The study included 61 patients with a total of 63 carcinomas. Among 60 tumors that were assessable after 3 months of letrozole treatment, the mean and median reductions in tumor volume were 66% and 75%, respectively. Nine (15%) of the patients were classified as having a complete response, 39 (65%) as having a partial response, and the remainder as having minimal response, stable or progressing. Successful breast conservation was achieved in 25/31 (81%) patients in whom it was attempted, including clear margins at the time of initial excision in more than 60% of the 31 patients.

Adjuvant Chemotherapy or Endocrine Therapy

After surgery or surgery with radiotherapy, adjuvant chemotherapy or endocrine therapy for patients with ILC is indicated largely on the basis of existing criteria used for IDC. Hormonal therapy with tamoxifen or letrozole is an important component of adjuvant treatment of patients with ILC.[268]

The pathologic response of ILC to various forms of chemotherapy and endocrine therapy may well be a function of the molecular characteristics of the tumor cells.[269,270] These characteristics can be expected to play an increasingly important role with wider adoption of "personalized" treatment directed toward specific molecular targets.

REFERENCES

1. Foote FW Jr, Stewart FW. Lobular carcinoma *in situ*: a rare form of mammary cancer. *Am J Pathol* 1941;17:491–496.
2. Rakha EA, Gill MS, El-Sayed ME, et al. The biological and clinical characteristics of breast carcinoma with mixed ductal and lobular morphology. *Breast Cancer Res Treat* 2009;114:243–250.
3. Newman W. Lobular carcinoma of the female breast. Report of 73 cases. *Ann Surg* 1966;164:305–314.

4. Richter GO, Dockerty MB, Clagett OT. Diffuse infiltrating scirrhous carcinoma of the breast. Special consideration of the single filing phenomenon. *Cancer* 1967;20:363–370.
5. Henson D, Tarone R. A study of lobular carcinoma of the breast based on the Third National Cancer Survey in the United States of America. *Tumori* 1979;65:133–142.
6. Li CL, Anderson BO, Daling JR, et al. Trends in incidence rates of invasive lobular and ductal breast carcinoma. *JAMA* 2003;289:1421–1424.
7. Eheman CR, Shaw KM, Ryerson AB, et al. The changing incidence of *in situ* and invasive ductal and lobular carcinomas: United States, 1999–2004 . *Cancer Epidemiol Biomarkers Prev* 2009;18:1763–1769.
8. Chikman B, Lavy R, Davidson T, et al. Factors affecting the rise in the incidence of infiltrating lobular carcinoma of the breast. *IMAJ* 2010;12:697–700.
9. Allen-Brady K, Cam NJ, Ward JH, et al. Lobular breast cancer: excess familiality observed in the Utah Population Database. *Int J Cancer* 2005;117:655–661.
10. Dixon JM, Anderson TJ, Page DL, et al. Infiltrating lobular carcinoma of the breast. *Histopathology* 1982;6:149–161.
11. Ashikari R, Huvos AG, Urban JA, et al. Infiltrating lobular carcinoma of the breast. *Cancer* 1973;31:110–116.
12. DiCostanzo D, Rosen PP, Gareen I, et al. Prognosis in infiltrating lobular carcinoma: an analysis of "classical" and variant tumors. *Am J Surg Pathol* 1990;14:12–23.
13. Fechner RE. Infiltrating lobular carcinoma without lobular carcinoma *in situ*. *Cancer* 1972;29:1539–1545.
14. Fechner RE. Histologic variants of infiltrating lobular carcinoma of the breast. *Hum Pathol* 1975;6:373–378.
15. Rosen PP, Lesser ML, Kinne DW. Breast carcinoma at the extremes of age: a comparison of patients younger than 35 years and older than 75 years. *J Surg Oncol* 1985;28:90–96.
16. Rosen PP, Lesser ML, Senie RT, et al. Epidemiology of breast carcinoma IV. Age and histologic tumor type. *J Surg Oncol* 1982;19:44–47.
17. Buchanan CL, Flynn LW, Murray MP, et al. Is pleomorphic lobular carcinoma really a distinct clinical entity? *J Surg Oncol* 2008;98:314–317.
18. Koc M, Oztas S, Erem MT, et al. Invasive lobular carcinoma of the male breast: a case report. *Jpn J Clin Oncol* 2001;31:444–446.
19. Yamac E, Osman Z, Yildiz E. Invasive lobular carcinoma of the male breast. *Can J Surg* 2006;49:365–366.
20. Spencer JT, Shutter J. Synchronous bilateral invasive lobular breast cancer presenting as carcinomatosis in a male. *Am J Surg Pathol* 2009;33:470–474.
21. Briest S, Vang R, Terrell K, et al. Invasive lobular carcinoma of the male breast: a rare histology in an uncommon disease. *Breast Care* 2009;4:36–38.
22. Rohini B, Singh PA, Vatsala M, et al. Pleomorphic lobular carcinoma in a male breast: a rare occurrence. *Pathol Res Int* 2010;2010:871369.
23. Maly B, Maly A, Pappo I, et al. Pleomorphic variant of invasive lobular carcinoma of the male breast. *Virchows Arch* 2005;446:344–345.
24. Monti F, Ravaioli A, Tassinari D, et al. Infiltrating lobular breast carcinoma in a woman with HIV infection. *Eur J Cancer* 1998;34:591.
25. Cuvier C, Espie M, Extra JM, et al. Breast cancer and HIV infection: two case reports. *Eur J Cancer* 1997;33:507–508.
26. Mayer AP, Greenberg ML. FNB diagnosis of breast carcinoma associated with HIV infection: a case report and review of HIV associated malignancy. *Pathology* 1996;28:90–95.
27. Spina M, Nasti G, Simonelli C, et al. Breast cancer in a woman with HIV infection: a case report. *Ann Oncol* 1994;5:661–662.
28. Erben Y, Ghosh K, Nassar A, et al. Invasive lobular carcinoma of the nipple. *Breast J* 2012;18:280–281.
29. Mendelson EB, Harris KM, Doshi N, et al. Infiltrating lobular carcinoma: mammographic patterns with pathologic correlation. *Am J Radiol* 1989;153:265–271.
30. Helvie MA, Paramagul C, Oberman HA, et al. Invasive lobular carcinoma imaging features and clinical detection. *Invest Radiol* 1993;28:202–207.
31. Krecke KN, Gisvold JJ. Invasive lobular carcinoma of the breast: mammographic findings and extent of disease at diagnosis in 184 patients. *Am J Roentgenol* 1993;161:957–960.
32. Le Gal M, Ollivier L, Asselain B, et al. Mammographic features of 455 invasive lobular carcinomas. *Radiology* 1992;185:705–708.
33. Newstead GM, Bante PB, Toth HK. Invasive lobular and ductal carcinoma: mammographic findings and stage at diagnosis. *Radiology* 1992;184:623–627.
34. Kim SH, Cha ES, Park CS, et al. Imaging features of invasive lobular carcinoma: comparison with invasive ductal carcinoma. *Jpn J Radiol* 2011;29:475–482.
35. Brem RF, Ioffe M, Rapelyea JA, et al. Invasive lobular carcinoma: detection with mammography, sonography, MRI, and breast-specific gamma imaging. *AJR* 2009;192:379–383.
36. Porter PL, El-Bastawissi AY, Mendelson MT, et al. Breast tumor characteristics as predictors of mammographic detection: comparison of interval- and screen-detected cancers. *J Natl Cancer Inst* 1999;91:2020–2028.
37. Peeters PHM, Verbeek ALM, Hendriks JHCL, et al. The occurrence of interval cancers in the Nijmegen screening programme. *Br J Cancer* 1989;59:929–932.
38. Albayrak ZK, Önay HK, Karatağ GY, et al. Invasive lobular carcinoma of the breast: mammographic and sonographic evaluation. *Diagn Interv Radiol* 2011;17:232–238.
39. Harvey JA, Fechner RE, Moore MM. Apparent ipsilateral decrease in breast size at mammography: a sign of infiltrating lobular carcinoma. *Radiology* 2000;214:883–889.
40. Mitnick JS, Gianutsos R, Pollack AH, et al. Comparative value of mammography, fine-needle aspiration biopsy, and core biopsy in the diagnosis of invasive lobular carcinoma. *Breast J* 1998;4:75–83.
41. White JR, Gustafson GS, Wimbish K, et al. Conservative surgery and radiation therapy for infiltrating lobular carcinoma of the breast. The role of preoperative mammograms in guiding treatment. *Cancer* 1994;74:640–647.
42. Evans WP, Burhenne LJW, Laurie L, et al. Invasive lobular carcinoma of the breast: mammographic characteristics and computer-aided detection. *Radiology* 2002;225:182–189.
43. Butler RS, Venta LA, Wiley EL, et al. Sonographic evaluation of infiltrating lobular carcinoma. *AJR Am J Roentgenol* 1999;172:325–330.
44. Selinko VL, Middleton LP, Dempsey PJ. Role of sonography in diagnosing and staging invasive lobular carcinoma. *J Clin Ultrasound* 2004;32:323–332.
45. Yeatman TJ, Cantor AB, Smith TJ, et al. Tumor biology of infiltrating lobular carcinoma. Implications for management. *Ann Surg* 1995;222:549–561.
46. Esserman L, Hylton N, Yassa L, et al. Utility of magnetic resonance imaging in the management of breast cancer: evidence for improved preoperative staging. *J Clin Oncol* 1999;17:110–119.
47. Rodenko GN, Harms SE, Pruneda JM, et al. MR imaging in the management before surgery of lobular carcinoma of the breast: correlation with pathology. *AJR Am J Roentgenol* 1996;167:1415–1419.
48. Yeh ED, Slanetz PJ, Edmister WB, et al. Invasive lobular carcinoma: spectrum of enhancement and morphology on magnetic resonance imaging. *Breast J* 2003;9:13–18.
49. Berg WA, Gilbreath PL. Multicentric and multifocal cancer: whole-breast US in preoperative evaluation. *Radiology* 2000;214:59–66.
50. Mann RM, Hoogeveen YL, Blickman JG, et al. MRI compared to conventional diagnostic work-up in the detection and evaluation of invasive lobular carcinoma of the breast: a review of existing literature. *Breast Cancer Res Treat* 2008;107:1–14.
51. Levrini G, Mori CA, Vacondio R, et al. MRI patterns of invasive lobular carcinoma: T1 and T2 features. *Radiol Med* 2008;113:1110–1125.
52. Mann RM, Veltman J, Huisman H, et al. Comparison of enhancement characteristics between invasive lobular carcinoma and invasive ductal carcinoma. *J Magn Reson Imaging* 2011;34:293–300.
53. Saslow D, Boetes C, Burke W, et al. American Cancer Society guidelines for breast cancer screening with MRI as an adjunct to mammography. *CA Cancer J Clin* 2007;57:75–89.
54. Jung HN, Shin JH, Han BK, et al. Are the imaging features of the pleomorphic variant of invasive lobular carcinoma different from classic ILC of the breast? *Breast* 2013;22:324–329.
55. McGhan LJ, Wasif N, Gray RJ, et al. Use of preoperative magnetic resonance imaging for invasive lobular cancer: good, better, but maybe not the best? *Ann Surg Oncol* 2010;17:S255–S262.
56. Behjatnia B, Sim J, Bassett LW, et al. Does size matter? Comparison study between MRI, gross, and microscopic tumor sizes in breast cancer lumpectomy specimens. *Int J Clin Exp Pathol* 2010;3:303–309.
57. Ross D, Hoda SA. Microinvasive (T1mic) lobular carcinoma of the breast: clinicopathologic profile of 16 cases. *Am J Surg Pathol* 2011;35:750–756.
58. Dillon ME, Hill AD, Fleming FJ, et al. Identifying patients at risk of compromised margins following breast conservation for lobular carcinoma. *Am J Surg* 2006;191:201–205.

59. Fortunato L, Mascaro A, Poccia I, et al. Lobular breast cancer: same survival and local control compared with ductal cancer, but should both be treated in the same way? Analysis of an institutional database over a 10-year period. *Ann Surg Oncol* 2012;19:1107–1114.
60. Silberfein EJ, Hunt KK, Broglio K, et al. Clinicopathologic factors associated with involved margins after breast-conserving surgery for invasive lobular carcinoma. *Clin Breast Cancer* 2010;10:52–58.
61. Sakr RA, Poulet B, Kaufman GJ, et al. Clear margins for invasive lobular carcinoma: a surgical challenge. *EJSO* 2011;37:350–356.
62. Smitt MC, Horst K. Association of clinical and pathological variable with lumpectomy surgical margin status after preoperative diagnosis or excisional biopsy of invasive breast cancer. *Ann Surg Oncol* 2007;14:1040–1044.
63. Mann RM, Loo CE, Wobbes T, et al. The impact of preoperative breast MRI in the re-excision rate in invasive lobular carcinoma of the breast. *Breast Cancer Res Treat* 2010;119:415–422.
64. Lau B, Romero LM. Does preoperative magnetic resonance imaging beneficially alter surgical management of invasive lobular carcinoma? *Am Surgeon* 2011;77:1368–1371.
65. Broët P, de la Rochefordière A, Scholl SM, et al. Contralateral breast cancer: annual incidence and risk parameters. *J Clin Oncol* 1995;13:1578–1583.
66. Bernstein JL, Thompson WD, Risch N, et al. Risk factors predicting the incidence of second primary breast cancer among women diagnosed with a first primary breast cancer. *Am J Epidemiol* 1992;136:925–936.
67. Horn PL, Thompson WD. Risk of contralateral breast cancer: associations with factors related to initial breast cancer. *Am J Epidemiol* 1988;128:309–323.
68. Kollias J, Ellis IO, Elston CW, et al. Clinical and histologic predictors of contralateral breast cancer. *Eur J Surg Oncol* 1999;25:584–589.
69. Dixon JM, Anderson TJ, Page DL, et al. Infiltrating lobular carcinoma of the breast: an evaluation of the incidence and consequence of bilateral disease. *Br J Surg* 1983;70:513–516.
70. Lesser ML, Rosen PP, Kinne DW. Multicentricity and bilaterality in invasive breast carcinoma. *Surgery* 1982;1:234–240.
71. Bouvet M, Ollila DW, Hunt KK, et al. Role of conservation therapy for invasive lobular carcinoma of the breast. *Ann Surg Oncol* 1997;4:650–654.
72. Hislop TG, Ng V, McBride ML, et al. Incidence and risk factors for second breast primaries in women with lobular breast carcinoma. *Breast Dis* 1990;3:95–105.
73. du Toit RS, Locker AP, Ellis IO, et al. Invasive lobular carcinomas of the breast—the prognosis of histopathological subtypes. *Br J Cancer* 1989;60:605–609.
74. Yeatman TJ, Lyman GH, Smith SK, et al. Bilaterality and recurrence rates for lobular breast cancer: considerations for treatment. *Ann Surg Oncol* 1997;4:198–202.
75. Lee JS, Grant CS, Donohue JH, et al. Arguments against routine contralateral mastectomy or undirected biopsy for invasive lobular breast cancer. *Surgery* 1995;118:640–647.
76. Simkovich AH, Sclafani LM, Masri M, et al. Role of contralateral breast biopsy in infiltrating lobular cancer. *Surgery* 1993;114:555–557.
77. Foote FW Jr, Stewart FW. A histologic classification of carcinoma of the breast. *Surgery* 1946;19:74–99.
78. Moatamed NA, Apple SK. Extensive sampling changes T-staging of infiltrating lobular carcinoma of breast: a comparative study of gross versus microscopic tumor sizes. *Breast J* 2006;12:511–517.
79. Underwood JCE, Parsons MA, Harris SC, et al. Frozen section appearances simulating invasive lobular carcinoma in breast tissue adjacent to inflammatory lesions and biopsy sites. *Histopathology* 1988;13:232–234.
80. Chetty R, Butler AE. Lymphocytic mastopathy associated with infiltrating lobular breast carcinoma. *J Clin Pathol* 1993;46:376–377.
81. Cristina S, Boldorini R, Brustia F, et al. Lymphoepithelioma-like carcinoma of the breast. An unusual pattern of infiltrating lobular carcinoma. *Virchows Arch* 2000;437:98–202.
82. Cserni G. Reproducibility of a diagnosis of invasive lobular carcinoma. *J Surg Oncol* 1999;70:217–221.
83. Kiaer H, Andersen JA, Rank F, et al. Quality control of patho-anatomical diagnosis of carcinoma of the breast. *Acta Oncol* 1988;27:745–747.
84. Van Bogaert L-J, Maldaque P. Infiltrating lobular carcinoma of the female breast. Deviations from the usual histopathologic appearance. *Cancer* 1980;45:979–984.
85. Fisher ER, Gregorio RM, Redmond C, et al. Tubulolobular invasive breast carcinoma: a variant of lobular invasive cancer. *Hum Pathol* 1977;8:679–683.
86. Davis RP, Nora PF, Kooy RG, et al. Experience with lobular carcinoma of the breast. Emphasis on recent aspects of management. *Arch Surg* 1979;114:485–488.
87. Breslow A, Brancaccio ME. Intracellular mucin production by lobular breast carcinoma cells. *Arch Pathol Lab Med* 1976;100:620–621.
88. Gad A, Azzopardi JG. Lobular carcinoma of the breast: a special variant of mucin secreting carcinoma. *J Clin Pathol* 1975;28:711–716.
89. Frost AR, Terahata S, Yeh I-T, et al. The significance of signet ring cells in infiltrating lobular carcinoma of the breast. *Arch Pathol Lab Med* 1995;119:64–68.
90. Merino MJ, LiVolsi VA. Signet ring carcinoma of the female breast: a clinicopathologic analysis of 24 cases. *Cancer* 1981;48:1830–1837.
91. Battifora H. Intracytoplasmic lumina in breast carcinoma. *Arch Pathol* 1975;99:614–617.
92. Erlandson RA, Carstens PHB. Ultrastructure of tubular carcinoma of the breast. *Cancer* 1972;29:987–995.
93. Hull MT, Seo IS, Battersby JS, et al. Signet-ring cell carcinoma of the breast: a clinicopathologic study of 24 cases. *Am J Clin Pathol* 1980;73:31–35.
94. Allenby PL, Chowdhury LN. Histiocytic appearance of metastatic lobular breast carcinoma. *Arch Pathol Lab Med* 1986;110:759–760.
95. Hood CI, Font RI, Zimmerman LE. Metastatic mammary carcinoma in the eyelid with histiocytoid appearance. *Cancer* 1973;31:793–800.
96. Shimizu S, Kitamura H, Ito T, et al. Histiocytoid breast carcinoma: histological, immunohistochemical, ultrastructural, cytological and clinicopathological studies. *Pathol Int* 1998;48:549–556.
97. Weigelt B, Geyer FC, Natrajan R, et al. The molecular underpinning of lobular histological growth pattern: a genome-wide transcriptional analysis of invasive lobular carcinomas and grade- and molecular subtype-matched invasive ductal carcinomas of no special type. *J Pathol* 2010;220:45–57.
98. Rakha EA, van Deurzen CH, Paish EC, et al. Pleomorphic lobular carcinoma of the breast: is it a prognostically significant pathological subtype independent of histological grade? *Mod Pathol* 2013;26:496–501.
99. Cha I, Weidner N. Correlation of prognostic factors and survival with classical and pleomorphic variants of invasive lobular carcinoma. *Breast J* 1996;2:385–393.
100. Eusebi V, Magalhaes F, Azzopardi JG. Pleomorphic lobular carcinoma of the breast: an aggressive tumor showing apocrine differentiation. *Hum Pathol* 1992;23:655–662.
101. Walford N, Ten Velden J. Histiocytoid breast carcinoma: an apocrine variant of lobular carcinoma. *Histopathology* 1989;14:515–522.
102. Radhi JM. Immunohistochemical analysis of pleomorphic lobular carcinoma: higher expression of p53 and chromogranin and lower expression of ER and PgR. *Histopathology* 2000;36:156–160.
103. Bentz JS, Yassa N, Clayton F. Pleomorphic lobular carcinoma of the breast: clinicopathologic features of 12 cases. *Mod Pathol* 1998;11:814–822.
104. Cameselle-Teijeiro J, Alfonsin-Barreiro N, Allegue F, et al. Apocrine carcinoma with signet ring cells and histiocytoid features. *Pathol Res Prac* 1997;193:713–720.
105. Shimzu S, Kitamura H, Nakamura T, et al. Histiocytoid breast carcinoma. Histological, immunohistochemical, ultrastructural, cytological and clinicopathological studies. *Pathol Int* 1998;48:849–856.
106. Augros M, Buenerd A, Decouassoux-Shisheboran M, et al. Infiltrating lobular carcinoma of the breast with histiocytoid features. *Ann Pathol* 2004;24:259–263.
107. Tan PH, Harada O, Thike AA, et al. Histiocytoid breast carcinoma: an enigmatic lobular entity. *J Clin Pathol* 2010;64:654–659.
108. Fujiwara M, Horiguchi M, Mori S, et al. Histiocytoid breast carcinoma: solid variant of invasive lobular carcinoma with decreased expression of both E-cadherin and CD44 epithelial variant. *Pathol Int* 2005;55:353–359.
109. Gupta D, Croitou CM, Ayala AG, et al. E-cadherin immunohistochemical analysis of histiocytoid carcinoma of the breast. *Ann Diag Pathol* 2002;6:141–147.
110. Laser J, Cangiarella J, Singh B, et al. Invasive lobular carcinoma of the breast: role of endothelial lymphatic marker D2-40. *Ann Clin Lab Sci* 2008;38:99–104.
111. Morphopoulos G, Pearson M, Ryder WDJ, et al. Tumour angiogenesis as a prognostic marker in infiltrating lobular carcinoma of the breast. *J Pathol* 1996;180:44–49.
112. Rosen PP, Menendez-Botet CJ, Senie RT, et al. Estrogen receptor protein (ERP) and histopathology of human mammary carcinoma. In: *Hormones, receptors and breast Cancer*. W.L. McGuire, ed. New York: Raven Press, 1978;71–83.

113. Lesser ML, Rosen PP, Senie RT, et al. Estrogen and progesterone receptors in breast carcinoma: correlations with epidemiology and pathology. *Cancer* 1981;48:299–309.
114. Shousha S, Backhous CM, Alaghband-Zadeh J, et al. Alveolar variant of invasive lobular carcinoma of the breast. *Am J Clin Pathol* 1986;85:1–5.
115. Riva C, Dainese E, Caprara C, et al. Immunohistochemical study of androgen receptors in breast carcinoma. Evidence of their frequent expression in lobular carcinoma. *Virchows Arch* 2005;447:695–700.
116. Ellis LM, Wittliff L, Bryant MS. Correlation of estrogen, progesterone and androgen receptors in breast cancer. *Am J Surg* 1989;157:557–581.
117. Kuenen-Boumeester V, Vanderkwast TH, VanPutten WLJ, et al. Immunohistochemical determination of androgen receptors in relation to oestrogen and progesterone receptors in female breast cancer. *Int J Cancer* 1992;52:581–584.
118. Nesland JM, Holm R, Johannessen JV. Ultrastructural and immunohistochemical features of lobular carcinoma of the breast. *J Pathol* 1985;145:39–52.
119. Lee AK, Rosen PP, DeLellis RA, et al. Tumor marker expression in breast carcinomas and relationship to prognosis. An immunohistochemical study. *Am J Clin Pathol* 1985;84:687–696.
120. Kuhajda FP, Offutt LE, Mendelsohn G. The distribution of carcinoembryonic antigen in breast carcinoma. Diagnostic and prognostic implications. *Cancer* 1983;52:1257–1264.
121. Lee AK, DeLellis RA, Rosen PP, et al. Alphalactalbumin as an immunohistochemical marker for metastatic breast carcinomas. *Am J Surg Pathol* 1984;8:93–100.
122. Mazoujian G, Pincus GS, Davis S, et al. Immunohistochemistry of a breast gross cystic disease fluid protein (GCDFP-15): a marker of apocrine epithelium and breast carcinomas with apocrine features. *Am J Pathol* 1983;110:105–111.
123. Mazoujian G, Bodian C, Haagensen DE Jr, et al. Expression of GCDFP-15 in breast carcinomas. Relationship to pathologic and clinical factors. *Cancer* 1989;63:2156–2161.
124. Eusebi V, Betts C, Haagensen DE Jr, et al. Apocrine differentiation in lobular carcinoma of the breast: a morphologic, immunologic, and ultrastructural study. *Hum Pathol* 1984;15:134–140.
125. Porter PL, Garcia R, Moe R, et al. C-erbB-2 oncogene protein in *in situ* and invasive lobular breast neoplasia. *Cancer* 1991;68:331–334.
126. Simpson PT, Reis-Filho JS, Lambros MBK, et al. Molecular profiling of pleomorphic lobular carcinomas of the breast: evidence for a common molecular genetic pathway with classic lobular carcinomas. *J Pathol* 2008;215:231–244.
127. Jacobs M, Fan F, Tawfik O. Clinicopathologic and biomarker analysis of invasive pleomorphic lobular carcinoma as compared with invasive classic lobular carcinoma: an experience in our institution and review of the literature. *Ann Diagn Pathol* 2012:16:185–189.
128. Reis-Filho JS, Simpson PT, Jones C, et al. Pleomorphic lobular carcinoma of the breast: role of comprehensive molecular pathology in characterization of an entity. *J Pathol* 2005;207:1–13.
129. Monhollen L, Morrison C, Ademuyiwa FO, et al. Pleomorphic lobular carcinoma: a distinctive clinical and molecular breast cancer type. *Histopathology* 2012;61:365–377.
130. Yu J, Dabbs DJ, Shuai Y, et al. Classical-type invasive lobular carcinoma with HER2 overexpression: clinical, histologic, and hormone receptor characteristics. *Am J Clin Pathol* 2011;136:88–97.
131. Oyama T, Kashiwabara K, Yoshimoto K, et al. Frequent overexpression of cyclin D1 oncogene in invasive lobular carcinoma of the breast. *Cancer Res* 1998;58:2876–2880.
132. Naidu R, Wahab NA, Yadav MM, et al. Expression and amplification of cyclin D1 in primary breast carcinomas: relationship with histopathological types and clinicopathological parameters. *Oncol Rep* 2002;9:409–416.
133. Martinazzi M, Crivelli F, Zampatti C, et al. Epidermal growth factor receptor immunohistochemistry in different histological types of infiltrating breast carcinoma. *J Clin Pathol* 1993;46:1009–1110.
134. Sainsbury JRC, Nicholson S, Angus B, et al. Epidermal growth factor receptor status of histological sub-types of breast cancer. *Br J Cancer* 1988;58:458–460.
135. Charpin C, Devictor B, Bonnier P, et al. Epidermal growth factor receptor in breast cancer: correlation of quantitative immunocytochemical assays to prognostic factors. *Breast Cancer Res Treat* 1993;25:203–210.
136. Domagala W, Markiewski M, Kubiak R, et al. Immunohistochemical profile of invasive lobular carcinoma of the breast: predominantly vimentin and p53 protein negative cathepsin D and oestrogen receptor positive. *Virchows Arch [A]* 1993;423:497–502.
137. Ercan C, van Diest PJ, van der Ende B, et al. p53 mutations in classic and pleomorphic invasive lobular carcinoma of the breast. *Cell Oncol* 2012;35:111–118.
138. d'Ardenne AJ, Burns J, Sykes BC, et al. Fibronectin and type III collagen in epithelial neoplasms of gastrointestinal tract and salivary gland. *J Clin Pathol* 1983;36:756–763.
139. Stenman S, Vaheri A. Fibronectin in human solid tumours. *Int J Cancer* 1981;27:427–435.
140. d'Ardenne AJ, Barnard NJ. Paucity of fibronectin in invasive lobular carcinoma of breast. *J Pathol* 1989;157:219–224.
141. Gusterson BA, Warburton MJ, Mitchell D, et al. Distribution of myoepithelial cells and basement membrane protein in the normal breast and in benign and malignant breast diseases. *Cancer Res* 1982;42:4763–4770.
142. Yamada KM, Olden K. Fibronectins-adhesive glycoproteins of cell surface and blood. *Nature* 1978;275:179–184.
143. Ebrahimsade S, Westhoff CC, Barth PJ. CD34+ fibrocytes are preserved in most invasive lobular carcinomas of the breast. *Pathol Res Pract* 2007;203:695–698.
144. White JD, Marshall DAS, Seywright MM, et al. Primary amyloidosis of the breast associated with invasive breast cancer. *Oncol Rep* 2004;11:761–763.
145. Santini D, Pasquinelli G, Alberghini M, et al. Invasive breast carcinoma with granulomatous response and deposition of unusual amyloid. *J Clin Pathol* 1992;45:885–888.
146. Sabate JM, Clotet M, Torrubia S, et al. Localized amyloidosis of the breast associated with invasive lobular carcinoma. *Brit J Radiol* 2008;81:e252–e254.
147. Yu J, Bhargava R, Dabbs DJ. Invasive lobular carcinoma with extracellular mucin production and HER-2 overexpression: a case report and further case studies. *Diagn Pathol* 2010;5:36.
148. Moll R, Mitze M, Frixen UH, et al. Differential loss of E-cadherin expression in infiltrating ductal and lobular breast carcinomas. *Am J Pathol* 1993;143:1731–1742.
149. De Leeuw WJ, Berx G, Vos CB, et al. Simultaneous loss of E-cadherin and catenins in invasive lobular breast cancer and lobular carcinoma *in situ*. *J Pathol* 1997;183:404–411.
150. Wahed A, Connelly J, Reese T. E-cadherin expression in pleomorphic lobular carcinoma: an aid to differentiation from ductal carcinoma. *Ann Diagn Pathol* 2002;6:349–351.
151. Qureshi HS, Linden MD, Divine G, et al. E-cadherin status in breast cancer correlates with histologic type but does not correlate with established prognostic parameters. *Am J Clin Pathol* 2006;125:377–385.
152. Morrogh M, Andrade VP, Giri D, et al. Cadherin–catenin complex dissociation in lobular neoplasia of the breast. *Breast Cancer Res Treat* 2012;132:641–652.
153. Rakha EA, Patel A, Powe DG, et al. Clinical and biological significance of E-cadherin protein expression in invasive lobular carcinoma of the breast. *Am J Surg Pathol* 2010;34:1472–1479.
154. Mahler-Araujo B, Savage K, Parry S, et al. Reduction of E-cadherin expression is associated with non-lobular breast carcinomas of basal-like and triple negative phenotype. *J Clin Pathol* 2008;61:615–620.
155. Harigopal M, Shin SJ, Murray MP, et al. Aberrant E-cadherin staining patterns in invasive mammary carcinoma. *World J Surg Oncol* 2005;3:73–83.
156. Simoyama Y, Nagafuchi A, Fujita S, et al. Cadherin dysfunction in a human cancer cell line: possible involvement of loss of alpha-catenin expression in reduced cell-cell adhesiveness. *Cancer Res* 1992;52:5770–5774.
157. Da Silva L, Parry S, Reid L, et al. Aberrant expression of E-cadherin in lobular carcinomas of the breast. *Am J Surg Pathol* 2008;32:773–783.
158. Hajra KM, Chen DY, Fearon ER. The SLUG zinc-finger protein represses E-cadherin in breast cancer. *Cancer Res* 2002;62:1613–1618.
159. Kanai Y, Oda T, Tsuda H, et al. Point mutation of the E-cadherin gene in invasive lobular carcinoma of the breast. *Jpn J Cancer Res* 1994;85:1035–1039.
160. Berx G, Cleton-Jansen AM, Nollet F, et al. E-cadherin is a tumour/invasion suppressor gene mutated in human lobular breast cancers. *EMBO J* 1995;14:6107–6115.
161. Berx G, Cleton-Jansen AM, Strumane K, et al. E-cadherin is inactivated in a majority of invasive human lobular breast cancers by truncation mutations throughout its extracellular domain. *Oncogene* 1996;13:1919–1925.

162. Huiping C, Sigurgeirsdottir JR, Jonasson JG, et al. Chromosome alterations and E-cadherin gene mutations in human lobular breast cancer. *Br J Cancer* 1999;81:1103–1110.
163. Palacios J, Sarrio D, Garcia-Macias MC, et al. Frequent E-cadherin gene inactivation by loss of heterozygosity in pleomorphic lobular carcinoma of the breast. *Mod Pathol* 2003;16:674–678.
164. Nyante SJ, Derries S, Chen YY, et al. Array-based comparative genomic hybridization of ductal carcinoma *in situ* and synchronous invasive lobular cancer. *Hum Pathol* 2004;35:759–763.
165. Hwang ES, Nyante SJ, Chen YY, et al. Clonality of lobular carcinoma *in situ* and synchronous invasive lobular carcinoma. *Cancer* 2004;100:2562–2572.
166. Dabbs DJ, Kaplai M, Chivukula M, et al. The spectrum of morphomolecular abnormalities of the E-cadherin/catenin complex in pleomorphic lobular carcinoma of the breast. *Appl Immunohistochem Mol Morphol* 2007;15:260–266.
167. Dabbs DJ, Bhargava R, Chivukula M. Lobular versus ductal breast neoplasms: the diagnostic utility of P120 catenin. *Am J Surg Pathol* 2007;31:427–437.
168. de Deus Moura R, Wludarski SC, Carvalho FM, et al. Immunohistochemistry applied to the differential diagnosis between ductal and lobular carcinoma of the breast. *Appl Immunohistochem Mol Morphol* 2013;21:1–12.
169. Fadare O, Wang SA, Hileeto D. The expression of cytokeratin 5/6 in invasive lobular carcinoma of the breast: evidence of a basal-like subset? *Hum Pathol* 2008;39:331–336.
170. Oakman C, Moretti E, Galardi F, et al. The role of topoisomerase II alpha and HER-2 in predicting sensitivity to anthracyclines in breast cancer patients. *Cancer Treat Rev* 2009;35:662–667.
171. Coon JS, Marcus E, Gupta-Burt S, et al. Amplification and overexpression of topoisomerase II alpha predict response to anthracycline-based therapy in locally advanced breast cancer. *Clin Cancer Res* 2002;8:1061–1067.
172. Brunello E, Brunelli M, Manfrin E, et al. Classical lobular breast carcinoma consistently lacks *topoisomerase-IIα* gene amplification: implications for the tailored use of anthracycline-based chemotherapies. *Histopathology* 2012;60:482–488.
173. Gould VE, Chejfec G. Lobular carcinoma of the breast with secretory features. *Ultrastruct Pathol* 1980;1:151–156.
174. Jundt G, Schulz A, Heitz PU, et al. Small cell neuroendocrine (oat cell) carcinoma of the male breast. *Virchows Arch [A]* 1984;404:213–221.
175. Wade PM, Mills SE, Read M, et al. Small cell neuroendocrine (oat cell) carcinoma of the breast. *Cancer* 1983;52:121–125.
176. Pandis N, Idvall I, Bardi G, et al. Correlation between karyotypic pattern and clinicopathologic features in 125 breast cancer cases. *Int J Cancer* 1996;66:191–196.
177. Frost AR, Karcher DS, Terahata S, et al. DNA analysis and S-phase fraction determination by flow cytometric analysis of infiltrating lobular carcinoma of the breast. *Mod Pathol* 1996;9:930–937.
178. Nayar R, Zhuang Z, Merino MJ, et al. Loss of heterozygosity on chromosome 11q13 in lobular lesions of the breast using tissue microdissection and polymerase chain reaction. *Hum Pathol* 1996;28:277–282.
179. Nishizaki T, Chew K, Chu L, et al. Genetic alterations in lobular breast cancer by comparative genomic hybridization. *Int J Cancer* 1997;74:513–517.
180. Eusebi V, Pich A, Macchiorlatti E, et al. Morphofunctional differentiation in lobular carcinoma of the breast. *Histopathology* 1977;1:301–314.
181. Shousha S, Bull TB, Burn I. Alveolar variant of invasive lobular carcinoma of the breast. *Ultrastruct Pathol* 1986;10:311–319.
182. Nesland JM, Holm R, Lunde S, et al. Diagnostic problems in breast pathology: the benefit of ultrastructural and immunocytochemical analysis. *Ultrastruct Pathol* 1987;11:293–311.
183. Kline TS, Kannan V, Kline IK. Appraisal and cytomorphologic analysis of common carcinomas of the breast. *Diagn Cytopathol* 1985;1:188–193.
184. Oertel YC. *Fine needle aspiration of the breast.* Stoneham: M.A. Butterworth, 1987:145–149.
185. Lerma E, Furmanal V, Carreras A, et al. Undetected invasive lobular breast cancer: review of false negative smears. *Mod Pathol* 2000;13:37A.
186. Sadler GP, McGee S, Dallimore NS, et al. Role of fine-needle aspiration cytology and needle-core biopsy in the diagnosis of lobular carcinoma of the breast. *Br J Surg* 1994;81:1315–1317.
187. Jayaram G, Swain M, Chew MT, et al. Cytologic appearances in invasive lobular carcinoma of the breast. A study of 21 cases. *Acta Cytol* 2000;44:169–174.
188. Robinson IA, McKee G, Jackson PA, et al. Lobular carcinoma of the breast: cytological features supporting the diagnosis of lobular cancer. *Diagn Cytopathol* 1995;13:196–201.
189. Auger M, Huttner I. Fine-needle aspiration cytology of pleomorphic lobular carcinoma of the breast. Comparison with the classic type. *Cancer (Cancer Cytopathol)* 1997;81:29–32.
190. Greeley CF, Frost AR. Cytologic features of ductal and lobular carcinoma in fine needle aspirates of the breast. *Acta Cytologica* 1997;41:333–340.
191. Raju UR, Ma CK, Shaw A. Signet ring variant of lobular carcinoma of the breast: a clinicopathologic and immunohistochemical study. *Mod Pathol* 1993;6:516–520.
192. Fernández B, Paish EC, Green AR, et al. Lymph-node metastases in invasive lobular carcinoma are different from those in ductal carcinoma of the breast. *J Clin Pathol* 2011;64:995–1000.
193. Frost AR, Shek YH, Lack EE. "Signet ring" sinus histiocytosis mimicking metastatic adenocarcinoma: report of two cases with immunohistochemical and ultrastructural study. *Mod Pathol* 1992;5:497–500.
194. Gould E, Perez J, Albores-Saavedra J, et al. Signet ring cell sinus histiocytosis. A previously unrecognized histologic condition mimicking metastatic adenocarcinoma in lymph nodes. *Am J Clin Pathol* 1989;92:509–512.
195. Cappellari J, Islander S, Woodruff R. Signet ring cell sinus histiocytosis. *Am J Clin Pathol* 1990;94:800–801.
196. Trojani M, de Mascarel I, Bonichon F, et al. Micrometastases to axillary lymph nodes from carcinoma of breast: detection by immunohistochemistry and prognostic significance. *Br J Cancer* 1987;55:303–306.
197. Wells CA, Heryet A, Brochier HJ, et al. The immunocytochemical detection of axillary micrometastases in breast cancer. *Br J Cancer* 1984;50:193–197.
198. Cote RJ, Peterson HF, Chaiwun B, et al. Role of immunohistochemical detection of lymph-node metastases in management of breast cancer. International Breast Cancer Study Group. *Lancet* 1999;354:896–900.
199. Cserni G, Bianchi S, Vezzosi V, et al. The value of cytokeratin immunohistochemistry in the evaluation of axillary sentinel lymph nodes in patients with lobular breast carcinoma. *J Clin Pathol* 2006;59:518–522.
200. Khoury T, Malik D, Fan C, et al. Modified Alcian blue enhances the intraoperative diagnosis of sentinel lymph node metastasis in invasive lobular carcinoma: a prospective study. *Arch Pathol Lab Med* 2010;134:1513–1519.
201. Horvath JW, Barnett GE, Jimenez RE, et al. Comparison of intraoperative frozen section analysis for sentinel lymph node biopsy during breast cancer surgery for invasive lobular carcinoma and invasive ductal carcinoma. *World J Surg Oncol* 2009;7:34.
202. Taras AR, Hendrickson NA, Pugliesse MS, et al. Intraoperative evaluation of sentinel lymph nodes in invasive lobular carcinoma of the breast. *Am J Surg* 2009;197:643–647.
203. Vandorpe T, Smeets A, Van Calster B, et al. Lobular and non-lobular breast cancers differ regarding axillary lymph node metastasis: a cross-sectional study on 4,292 consecutive patients. *Breast Cancer Res Treat* 2011;128:429–435.
204. Weinstein GW, Goldman JN. Metastatic adenocarcinoma of the breast masquerading as chalazion. *Am J Ophthalmol* 1970;69:259–264.
205. Bitter MA, Fiorito D, Corkell ME, et al. Bone marrow involvement by lobular carcinoma of the breast cannot be identified reliably by routine histological examination alone. *Hum Pathol* 1994;25:781–788.
206. Lamovec J, Bracko M. Metastatic pattern of infiltrating lobular carcinoma of the breast: an autopsy study. *J Surg Oncol* 1991;48:28–31.
207. Borst MJ, Ingold JA. Metastatic patterns of invasive lobular versus invasive ductal carcinoma of the breast. *Surgery* 1993;114:637–642.
208. Harris M, Howell A, Chrissohou M, et al. A comparison of the metastatic pattern of infiltrating lobular carcinoma and infiltrating duct carcinoma of the breast. *Br J Cancer* 1984;50:23–30.
209. Dixon AR, Ellis IO, Elston CW, et al. A comparison of the clinical metastatic patterns of invasive lobular and ductal carcinomas of the breast. *Br J Cancer* 1991;63:634–635.
210. Olsen ME, Chernik NL, Posner JB. Infiltration of the leptomeninges by systemic cancer. A clinical and pathologic study. *Arch Neurol* 1974;30:122–137.

211. Smith DB, Howell A, Harris M, et al. Carcinomatous meningitis associated with infiltrating lobular carcinoma of the breast. *Eur J Surg Oncol* 1985;11:33–36.
212. Heimann A, Merino MJ. Carcinomatous meningitis as the initial manifestation of breast cancer. *Acta Cytol* 1986;30:25–28.
213. Jayson GC, Howell A, Harris M, et al. Carcinomatous meningitis in patients with breast cancer. An aggressive disease variant. *Cancer* 1994;74:3135–3141.
214. Deck JHN, Lee MA. Mucin embolism to cerebral arteries: a fatal complication of carcinoma of the breast. *Can J Neurol Sci* 1978;5:327–330.
215. Feun L, Drelichman A, Singhakowinta A, et al. Ureteral obstruction secondary to metastatic breast carcinoma. *Cancer* 1979;44:1164–1171.
216. Gagnon Y, Tetu B. Ovarian metastases of breast carcinoma. A clinicopathologic study of 59 cases. *Cancer* 1989;64:892–898.
217. Antic T, Gong Y, Sneige N. Tumor type and single-cell/mesothelial-like cell pattern of breast carcinoma metastases in pleural and peritoneal effusions. *Diagn Cytopathol* 2012;40:311–315.
218. Monaco SE, Dabbs, DJ, Kanbour-Shakir A. Pleomorphic lobular carcinoma in pleural fluid: diagnostic pitfall for atypical mesothelial cells. *Diagn Cytopathol* 2008;36:657–661.
219. Kidney DD, Cohen AJ, Butler J. Abdominal metastases of infiltrating lobular breast carcinoma: CT and fluoroscopic imaging findings. *Abdom Imaging* 1997;22:156–159.
220. Kumar NB, Hart WR. Metastases to the uterine corpus from extragenital cancers. A clinicopathologic study of 63 cases. *Cancer* 1982;50:2163–2169.
221. Mallow DW, Humphrey PA, Soper JT, et al. Metastatic lobular carcinoma of the breast diagnosed in cervicovaginal samples. A case report. *Acta Cytol* 1997;41:549–555.
222. Vadmal M, Brones C, Hajdu SI. Metastatic lobular carcinoma of the breast in a cervical-vaginal smear [letter]. *Acta Cytol* 1997;41:1236–1237.
223. Liebmann RD, Jones KD, Hamid R, et al. Fortuitous diagnosis in a uterine leiomyoma of metastatic lobular carcinoma of the breast [letter]. *Histopathology* 1998;32:577–578.
224. Houghton JP, Ioffe OB, Silverberg SG, et al. Metastatic breast lobular carcinoma involving tamoxifen-associated endometrial polyps: report of two cases and review of tamoxifen-associated polypoid uterine lesions. *Mod Pathol* 2003;16:395–398.
225. Kolke K, Kitahara K, Higaki M, et al. Clinicopathological features of gastric metastasis from breast cancer in three cases. *Breast Cancer* 2011. PMID:21779814
226. Cormier WJ, Gaffey TA, Welch JM, et al. Linitis plastica caused by metastatic carcinoma of the breast. *Mayo Clin Proc* 1980;55:747–753.
227. Hartmann, WH, Sherlock P. Gastroduodenal metastases from carcinoma of the breast. An adrenal steroid induced phenomenon. *Cancer* 1961;14:426–431.
228. Yoshida Y. Metastases and primary neoplasms of the stomach in patients with breast cancer. *Surgery* 1973;125:738–743.
229. Kobayashi T, Shibata K, Matsuda Y, et al. A case of invasive lobular carcinoma of the breast first manifesting with duodenal obstruction. *Breast Cancer* 2004;11:306–308.
230. Matsui M, Kokima O, Uehara Y, et al. Characterization of estrogen receptor in human gastric cancer. *Cancer* 1991;68:305–308.
231. Tokunaga A, Nishi K, Matsukura N, et al. Estrogen and progesterone receptors in gastric cancer. *Cancer* 1986;57:1376–1379.
232. Harrison JD, Morris DL, Ellis IO, et al. The effect of tamoxifen and estrogen receptor status on survival in gastric carcinoma. *Cancer* 1989;64:1007–1010.
233. Yokozaki H, Takemura N, Takanashi A, et al. Estrogen receptors in gastric adenocarcinoma: a retrospective immunohistochemical analysis. *Virchows Arch [A]* 1988;413:297–302.
234. Chaubert P, Bouzourene H, Saraga E. Estrogen and progesterone receptors and pS2 and ERD5 antigens in gastric carcinomas from the European population. *Mod Pathol* 1996;9:189–193.
235. Keller G, Vogelsang H, Becker I, et al. Diffuse type gastric and lobular breast carcinoma in a familial gastric cancer patient with an E-cadherin germline mutation. *Am J Pathol* 1999;155:337–342.
236. Voravud N, El-Naggar AK, Balch CM, et al. Metastatic lobular breast carcinoma simulating primary colon cancer. *Am J Clin Oncol* 1992;15:365–369.
237. Frost AR, Terahata S, Siegel RS, et al. An analysis of prognostic features in infiltrating lobular carcinoma of the breast. *Mod Pathol* 1995;8:830–836.
238. Iorfida M, Maiorano E, Orvieto E, et al. Invasive lobular breast cancer: subtypes and outcome. *Breast Cancer Res Treat* 2012;133:713–723.
239. Jayasinghe UW, Bilous AM, Boyages J. Is survival from infiltrating lobular carcinoma different from that of infiltrating ductal carcinoma? *Breast J* 2007;13:479–485.
240. Moran MS, Yang Q, Haffty BG. The Yale University experience of early-stage invasive lobular carcinoma (ILC) and invasive ductal carcinoma (IDC) treated with breast-conservation treatment (BCT): analysis of clinical-pathologic features, long-term outcomes, and molecular expression of COX-2, Bcl-2, and p53 as a function of histology. *Breast J* 2009;15:571–578.
241. Peiro G, Bornstein BA, Connolly JL, et al. The influence of infiltrating lobular carcinoma on the outcome of patients treated with breast-conserving surgery and radiation therapy. *Breast Cancer Res Treat* 2000;59:49–54.
242. Bharat A, Gao F, Margenthaler JA. Tumor characteristics and patient outcomes are similar between invasive lobular and mixed invasive ductal/lobular breast cancers but differ from pure invasive ductal breast cancers. *Am J Surg* 2009;198:516–519.
243. Wasif N, Maggard MA, Ko CY, et al. Invasive lobular vs. ductal breast cancer: a stage-matched comparison of outcomes. *Ann Surg Oncol* 2010;17:1862–1869.
244. Anwar IF, Down SK, Rizvi S, et al. Invasive lobular carcinoma of the breast: should this be regarded as a chronic disease? *Int J Surg* 2010;8:346–352.
245. Weidner N, Semple JP. Pleomorphic variant of invasive lobular carcinoma of the breast. *Hum Pathol* 1992;23:1167–1171.
246. Moreno-Elola A, Aguilar A, Roman JM, et al. Prognostic factors in invasive lobular carcinoma of the breast: a multivariate analysis. A multicentre study after seventeen years of follow-up. *Ann Chir Gynaecol* 1999;88:252–258.
247. Leonard CE, Philpott P, Shapiro H, et al. Clinical observations of axillary involvement for tubular, lobular, and ductal carcinomas of the breast. *J Surg Oncol* 1999;70:13–20.
248. Singletary SE, Patel-Parekh L, Bland K. Treatment trends in early-stage invasive lobular carcinoma: a report from the National Cancer Data Base. *Ann Surg* 2005;242:281–289.
249. Kurtz JM, Jacquemier J, Torhorst J, et al. Conservation therapy for breast cancers other than infiltrating ductal carcinoma. *Cancer* 1989;63:1630–1635.
250. Biglia N, Maggiorotto F, Liberale V, et al. Clinical-pathologic features, long term-outcome and surgical treatment in a large series of patients with invasive lobular carcinoma (ILC) and invasive ductal carcinoma (IDC). *Eur J Surg Oncol* 2013;39:455–460.
251. Poen JC, Tran L, Juillard G, et al. Conservation therapy for invasive lobular carcinoma of the breast. *Cancer* 1992;69:2789–2795.
252. Schnitt SJ, Connolly JL, Recht A, et al. Influence of lobular histology on local tumor control in breast cancer patients treated with conservative surgery and radiotherapy. *Cancer* 1989;64:448–454.
253. Francis M, Cakir B, Bilous M, et al. Conservative surgery and radiation therapy for invasive lobular carcinoma of the breast. *Aust N Z J Surg* 1999;69:450–454.
254. Chung MA, Cole B, Wanebo HJ, et al. Optimal surgical treatment of invasive lobular carcinoma of the breast. *Ann Surg Oncol* 1997;4:545–550.
255. Morrow M, Keeney K, Scholtens D, et al. Selecting patients for breast-conserving therapy. The importance of lobular histology. *Cancer* 2006;106:2563–2568.
256. Warneke J, Berger R, Johnson C, et al. Lumpectomy and radiation treatment for invasive lobular carcinoma of the breast. *Am J Surg* 1996;172:496–500.
257. Santiago RJ, Harris EER, Quin L, et al. Similar long-term results of breast-conservation treatment for stage I and II invasive lobular carcinoma compared with invasive duct carcinoma of the breast. The University of Pennsylvania experience. *Cancer* 2006;103:2447–2454.
258. Sullivan PS, Apple SK. Should histologic type be taken into account when considering neoadjuvant chemotherapy in breast carcinoma? *Breast J* 2009;15:146–154.
259. Cristofanilli M, Gonzalez-Angulo A, Sneige N, et al. Invasive lobular carcinoma classic type: response to primary chemotherapy and survival outcomes. *J Clin Oncol* 2005;23:41–48.
260. Purushotham A, Pinder S, Cariati M, et al. Neoadjuvant chemotherapy: not the best option in estrogen receptor-positive, HER2-negative, invasive classical lobular carcinoma of the breast? *J Clin Oncol* 2010;28:3552–3554.

261. Nagao T, Kinoshita T, Hojo T, et al. The difference in the histological types of breast cancer and the response to neoadjuvant chemotherapy: the relationship between outcome and the clinicopathological characteristics. *Breast* 2012;21:289–295.
262. Wagner J, Boughey JC, Garrett B, et al. Margin assessment after neoadjuvant chemotherapy in invasive lobular cancer. *Am J Surg* 2009;198:387–391.
263. Boughey JC, Wagner J, Garrett BJ, et al. Neoadjuvant chemotherapy in invasive lobular carcinoma may not improve rates of breast conservation. *Ann Surg Oncol* 2009;16:1606–1611.
264. Tubiana-Hulin M, Stevens D, Lasry SW, et al. Response to neoadjuvant chemotherapy in lobular and ductal carcinomas: a retrospective study on 860 patients from one institution. *Ann Oncol* 2006;17:1228–1233.
265. Cocquyt VF, Blondeel PN, Depypere HT, et al. Different responses to preoperative chemotherapy in invasive lobular and invasive ductal breast carcinoma. *Eur J Surg Oncol* 2003;29:361–367.
266. Ellis MJ, Coop A, Singh B, et al. Letrozole is more effective neoadjuvant endocrine therapy than tamoxifen for ErbB-1- and/or ErbB-2 positive, estrogen receptor-positive primary breast cancer: evidence from a phase III randomized trial. *J Clin Oncol* 2001;19:3808–3816.
267. Dixon JM, Renshaw L, Dixon J, et al. Invasive lobular carcinomas: response to neoadjuvant letrozole therapy. *Breast Cancer Res Treat* 2011;130:871–877.
268. Rakha EA, El-Sayed ME, Powe DG, et al. Invasive lobular carcinoma of the breast: response to hormonal therapy and outcomes. *Eur J Cancer* 2008;44:73–83.
269. Joh JE, Esposito NN, Kiluk JV, et al. Pathologic tumor response of invasive lobular carcinoma to neo-adjuvant chemotherapy. *Breast J* 2012;18:569–574.
270. Lips EH, Mukhtar RA, Yau C, et al. Lobular histology and response to neoadjuvant chemotherapy in invasive breast cancer. *Breast Cancer Res Treat* 2012;136:35–43.

CHAPTER 33

Unusual Clinical Presentation of Carcinoma

SYED A. HODA

Breast carcinoma can have myriad clinical presentations. In this chapter, the salient clinical and pathologic aspects of breast carcinomas that present during pregnancy or lactation, in patients at relative extremes of ages, within fibroepithelial tumors, in ectopic breast tissue, with an "inflammatory" appearance, with axillary nodal involvement, or in transverse rectus abdominus muscle (TRAM) flaps, are presented.

CARCINOMA IN PREGNANCY AND LACTATION

Breast carcinoma is the most common malignant neoplasm encountered during pregnancy, afflicting one in 3,000 pregnancies.[1] The frequency of coincident pregnancy in women with breast carcinoma is 1% to 3%.[2] The average age of women who have breast cancer in pregnancy is in the mid- to late 30s.[2] About 6% of women with breast carcinoma diagnosed by age 35 are pregnant when the tumor is detected.[3] With the trend for women in some sociocultural groups to delay pregnancy to their late 30s and 40s, it is likely that coincident pregnancy and breast carcinoma will be increasingly encountered.[1] Breast carcinoma has been reported in pregnant teenage girls.[4,5] Data from one study suggest that women from BRCA1-positive families may be at increased risk of developing breast carcinoma during and after pregnancy.[6]

Clinical Presentation

The usual presenting symptom is a painless mass that may be obscured by pregnancy-associated physiologic changes in the breast. This factor can contribute to delay in seeking medical attention on the part of the patient, as well as physician delay in recognizing the presence of a neoplasm and obtaining a biopsy. In one study, more than 50% of patients with breast carcinoma diagnosed postpartum had a palpable mass detected and followed during pregnancy.[7]

With appropriate precautions, mammography can be performed during pregnancy.[8,9] The effectiveness of mammography may be reduced during pregnancy because of increased parenchymal density.[10] Liberman et al.[11] reported that the sensitivity of mammography for detecting carcinoma during pregnancy or within 1 year postpartum was 78%. In one study, ultrasound was 100% sensitive as a method for detecting solid tumors in a series of pregnant women, and is now regarded as the preferred initial diagnostic procedure in this setting.[12,13] Ultrasound is also essential for monitoring response to neoadjuvant chemotherapy during pregnancy and for evaluating axillary lymph nodes (ALNs).[14] Invasive carcinomas can be identified in lactating breast tissue by magnetic resonance imaging (MRI),[15] but uncertainty about the effects of gadolinium on the fetus and issues related to positioning the pregnant patient have raised concern about this diagnostic procedure.[16]

Pathology

A diagnosis of carcinoma during pregnancy and lactation can be made by fine-needle aspiration (FNA) biopsy.[17] However, caution should be exercised when interpreting cytology specimens in this setting, because physiologically altered non-neoplastic mammary epithelial cells can appear atypical in cytologic preparations in this setting, and the material often consists of abundant dyscohesive cells.[18] For these reasons, needle core biopsy or excisional biopsy are preferable for definitive diagnosis.

The histologic spectrum of pregnancy-associated breast carcinoma is not significantly different from breast carcinoma unrelated to pregnancy in women of a comparable age.[7,16,19–21] Invasive ductal carcinoma (IDC) is present in about 90% of both groups. There were small numbers of patients with invasive lobular, mucinous, medullary, and other types of carcinoma. Tumors are significantly larger, and vascular invasion as well as axillary nodal involvement is more frequent in the pregnancy group. In one case-control study, intraductal carcinoma was present in 4.8% of control patients and in 1.6% of women with pregnancy-related carcinoma.[19] ALN metastases are present in 60% to 70% of women with pregnancy-related breast carcinoma.[7,19,22]

Prognostic Markers

Estrogen receptors (ER) and progesterone receptors (PR) are significantly more often negative in carcinomas from pregnant and lactating women than in tumors from nonpregnant age-matched controls.[16,19,22–26] A substantial proportion of such carcinomas, ranging from 44% to 58%, are HER2-positive.[24–26]

Treatment and Prognosis

Although the primary treatment has generally been surgical, the use of adjuvant chemotherapy and breast conservation is an increasingly exercised option, depending on the circumstances in a particular case.[16] Surgery and chemotherapy are relatively safe treatment options after the fetal organogenesis period of the first 16 weeks has elapsed. Therapeutic irradiation ought to be delayed until after completion of pregnancy.[27] However, the use of chemotherapy at any time during pregnancy has been linked to underdevelopment of placenta.[28] The most significant obstetrical outcome in women who have received chemotherapy during pregnancy is low birth weight.[29] Although no long-term complications have been reported in children whose mothers received chemotherapy for hematologic neoplastic diseases during pregnancy, the effects of fetal *in utero* exposure to maternal chemotherapy for breast carcinoma have not been well studied.[30]

In the past, a modified radical mastectomy was performed in most cases for local control, in part to avoid radiation of the fetus during breast conservation therapy.[16,31–34] Radiation should be delayed until after pregnancy.[16] Results in 9 patients treated by breast conservation in pregnancy were reported by Kuerer et al.[35] The patients were all stage I and stage II, with a median fetal gestation of 7 months. After a median follow-up of 24 months, there were no recurrences in the breast, although three women had distant recurrences.

Thus far, no adverse effects have been reported with the use of either lymphoscintigraphy or methylene blue in pregnancy for the detection of sentinel lymph nodes (SLNs),[36–41] although the use of lymphoscintigraphy alone has been recommended in this setting.[16] In general, breast carcinoma in pregnancy can now be safely and effectively treated; however, management needs to be guided by duration of pregnancy and stage of breast cancer.[32]

The overall prognosis of women with breast carcinoma diagnosed in pregnancy and lactation is relatively poor owing to the high proportion of patients with nodal metastases.[31,42] In one study, axillary nodal metastases were present in 74% of patients younger than 40 years of age with breast carcinoma diagnosed during pregnancy, whereas 37% of nonpregnant patients in the same age group had positive nodes.[43] When stratified by stage, some investigators reported no significant difference in outcomes between pregnancy-related and non–pregnancy-related patients of comparable age.[7,20,22,44] In a number of reports, 75% to 80% of node-negative patients remained alive or recurrence free with follow-up of 5 to 10 years. In one case-control study, node-negative women in the pregnancy and lactation group had a poorer survival (85%) at 10 years than women with non–pregnancy-associated breast carcinoma (93%), but the outcomes for both groups were favorable.[19] The same series reported a greater discrepancy in node-positive cases, with survival of 62% and 37% in the nonpregnant and pregnant groups, respectively. Others also found the prognosis of pregnancy-associated breast carcinoma to be relatively unfavorable after adjustment for tumor size and nodal status.[45]

The impact of subsequent pregnancy on prognosis in women previously treated for breast carcinoma remains uncertain.[46] Most studies of this subject conducted retrospectively appear to indicate that the prognosis for such patients is the same as or better than for patients who do not become pregnant.[47,48] Women who have received chemotherapy are generally advised to delay pregnancy for at least 6 months before attempting to conceive.[49] One case-control study compared 53 women who became pregnant after treatment of breast carcinoma with a cohort without subsequent pregnancy, matched for stage of disease at diagnosis and a disease-free survival (DFS) at least as long as the interval to pregnancy in the study individual.[50] There were 5 deaths due to breast carcinoma among 53 women (9.6%) with subsequent pregnancies and 34 deaths among 265 controls (13%). The relative risk (RR) of death due to breast carcinoma in the subsequent pregnancy group was 0.8 (95% confidence interval [CI], 0.3 to 2.3), a result indicative of no increase in risk associated with subsequent pregnancy. A prospective study will be required to fully evaluate this issue, especially in the context of current management practices.

An unusual complication of pregnancy concurrent with or subsequent to the diagnosis of breast carcinoma is the development of placental metastases. This is most likely to occur in women who have disseminated metastatic tumors.[51–53] Gross evidence of metastatic carcinoma is usually apparent on the placental surface, and microscopic examination discloses tumor cells in the intervillous spaces, rarely with villous invasion (Fig. 33.1).

BREAST CARCINOMA IN "YOUNGER" AND "OLDER" WOMEN

The average age at diagnosis of patients with breast carcinoma is in the mid-50s. The ages of the majority of affected women are within two decades above or below this midpoint. Within this framework, the extremes of age may be considered younger than 35 years and older than 75 years.

Breast carcinoma is widely thought to have a relatively poor prognosis in women younger than 35 years of age, whereas in those older than 75 it has been described as an indolent disease. Many published studies of this issue are not easily compared because of differences in defining age extremes or in the treatment that patients received. These are important considerations, especially when comparing data from the era when therapy consisted of surgery alone with recent data including neoadjuvant and adjuvant therapy, breast conservation, and radiation therapy. Data obtained

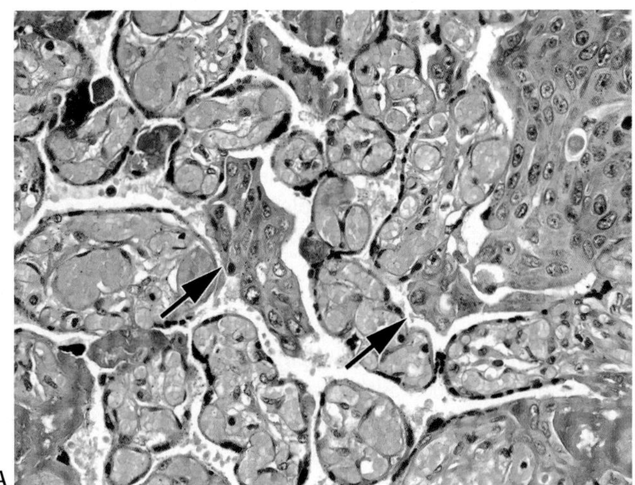

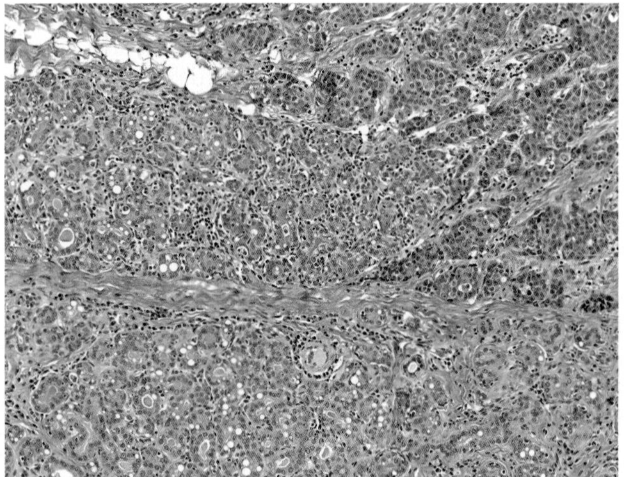

FIG. 33.1. ***Breast carcinoma in pregnancy.*** **A:** Metastatic breast carcinoma in the placenta. Clusters of metastatic carcinoma cells (*arrows*) are present in the intervillous spaces. **B:** The patient had a poorly differentiated invasive ductal breast carcinoma (*upper right*), late in the second trimester of pregnancy, with a partial pathologic response to chemotherapy.

from a statewide tumor registry for patients treated between 1985 and 1992 suggest that age-related differences in prognosis are influenced by the stage at diagnosis.[54]

Patients Younger Than 40 Years

Simmons et al.[55] investigated the incidence of breast carcinoma in women younger than 25 years of age by reviewing data from a Minnesota county between 1935 and 2005 for histologically confirmed cases. The four cases diagnosed over the 1,201,539 person-years yielded an annual age-adjusted incidence of 3.2 per million (95% CI, 0.1 to 6.2). Since all patients were in the 20- to 24-year age group, the age-specific incidence in this subset was 16.2 per million. The authors noted that delay in diagnosis was a common feature in these cases.

Kothari et al.[56] reported on 15 women 25 years or younger at the time of diagnosis. Two patients had intraductal carcinoma. None of the invasive carcinomas in 13 patients were low grade. Nine (69%) of the 13 women with invasive carcinoma died as a result of recurrent carcinoma—with a median DFS of 86 months. There was no statistically significant difference in overall survival (OS) between women 25 years or younger and those 26 to 35 years of age at the time of diagnosis.

Feldman and Welch[57] studied 29 women who were younger than 30 years when diagnosed and treated for breast carcinoma. The patients were identified between 1953 and 1983 in the records of an urban teaching hospital. Age at diagnosis ranged from 20 to 29 years. Seven patients (26%) were pregnant at the time of diagnosis. Delay in diagnosis was probably a factor in the prognosis of these patients since the stage at diagnosis was II or higher in 26 of 27 cases with documented data. Twenty-two patients (76%) died of breast carcinoma, including three who developed recurrences 12.7, 14.6, and 19.9 years after diagnosis. It should be noted that virtually all patients were treated by mastectomy and none received systemic adjuvant therapy.

A larger series of patients 30 years or younger at diagnosis, consisting of 185 women, was reported by Xiong et al.[58] The distribution of patients by stage was as follows: stage I, 11%; stage II, 45%; stage III, 38%; and stage IV, 6%. Treatment consisted of various combinations of mastectomy or breast-conserving surgery with adjuvant or neoadjuvant chemotherapy and radiotherapy. The 5-year OS rates by stage were stage I, 87%; stage II, 60%; stage III, 42%; and stage IV, 16%. When compared with control patients identified in the National Cancer Data Base, women diagnosed at age 30 or younger had poorer 5-year OS rates.

A retrospective case-controlled study by Peng et al.[59] concluded that diagnosis at or before 35 years of age was an independent negative prognostic risk factor. They compared 551 women 35 years or younger who had operable breast carcinoma to a cohort of women 36 to 50 years of age at diagnosis matched for year of diagnosis, family history, pathologic stage at diagnosis, hormone receptor status and adjuvant therapy. The younger women had a significantly shorter disease-free interval to first recurrence (median 23.2 vs. 28.4 months), a lower DFS (63.7% vs. 74.7%), and lesser OS (79.5% vs. 85.6%).

Liukkonen et al.[60] studied 212 Finnish women treated between 1997 and 2007 for breast carcinoma who were younger than 35 years. At diagnosis, 117 (55%) had axillary nodal metastases and 14 (7%) had distant metastases. One hundred and forty (65%) women were treated with mastectomy and 68 with breast conservation surgery. Postoperative treatment included chemotherapy, endocrine therapy, and radiation, singly or in combination. Local recurrence occurred in 10 (15%) of women treated with breast conservation surgery, and 8 (6%) of patients treated with mastectomy. The disease-free interval was shorter in patients with hormone receptor–positive carcinoma after a median follow-up of 78 months. The overall 5-year survival was 80%, suggesting that the prognosis of patients in this age group is improved by earlier diagnosis and the use of modern treatment modalities in addition to surgery.

Patients 40 to 49 Years of Age

Most studies of clinical issues in the diagnosis of breast carcinoma in younger women have focused on the relatively large group of patients 40 to 49 years of age. A report of 809 consecutive patients biopsied for nonpalpable, mammographically detected lesions revealed carcinoma in 5% of biopsies prior to age 40, in 15% of biopsies in the 40- to 49-year age group, and in 34% of biopsies from women older than 50 years.[61] Twenty-five percent of carcinomas in women 40 to 49 years old and 16% in women 50 years or older were noninvasive. Mean tumor size was the same in both groups (1.5 cm), but nodal metastases were present more often in the 40- to 49-year age group (25%) than in the group 50 years or older (17%).

McPherson et al.[62] investigated the relationship of method of tumor detection to prognosis in women 40 to 49 years of age using a database of patients diagnosed in North Dakota, South Dakota, and Minnesota. When compared with the risk of dying from carcinomas detected by mammography, the RRs of dying from carcinomas detected by breast self-examination (BSE) (2.5), clinical breast exam (CE) (2.7), or discovered by the patient incidentally (2.8) were significantly greater. The mean size of mammographically detected tumors (1.9 cm) was significantly smaller than those in the CE (2.3 cm), BSE (2.8 cm), and incidental (2.9 cm) groups. After adjusting for stage (tumor size and nodal status), the RRs of dying of carcinomas were greater when detected by BSE (1.5), CE (1.9), or incidentally (1.6), when compared with tumors detected by mammography. These results suggest that mammography makes a contribution to improving the prognosis of women with carcinoma 40 to 49 years of age. The implications of these observations for mammographic screening in this age group and in women younger than 40 years remain controversial.

Clinical problems encountered in the diagnosis of breast carcinoma in women 49 years and younger were detailed in a report by Lannin et al.[63] The authors analyzed the results of mammography and physical examination in a consecutive series of patients evaluated in a university hospital clinic in order to compare women 20 to 49 years of age with those 50 years or older. The positive predictive value (PPV) of mammography was 28% for women younger than 50 and 53% in those 50 years or older. The PPV of an abnormal physical examination resulting in biopsy was 11% and 57% in women younger than 50 years and 50 or older, respectively. There was also a statistically significant difference in the sensitivity of mammography between patients younger than and 50 years or older (68% and 91%, respectively). The sensitivity of physical examination did not differ significantly between the two groups. This discrepancy was not observed between nonpalpable and palpable tumors in women younger than 50 years (mean tumor size, 4.0 and 3.4 cm, respectively). These results led the authors to conclude that physical examination and mammography were less sensitive in women 20 to 49 years old when compared with women 50 years or older. They suggested that "tumors in young women are nonpalpable, not because they are small, but because of background density of the mammary tissue or because of the more diffuse growth pattern of tumors at this age. These are exactly the same reasons mammography is less sensitive in young women." The addition of FNA or needle core biopsy for abnormalities detected by mammography and clinical examination constitutes the "triple test" for the diagnosis of breast tumors, a method that improves diagnostic accuracy, especially in younger women.[64]

Pathology

Most pathologic features of breast carcinoma do not differ appreciably in adults who are relatively young or old.[65–68] Tumor size is not significantly different when young and elderly patients are compared.[67] Approximately 50% of patients have tumors 2 cm or smaller, 40% have tumors in the 2.1- to 5.0-cm range, and the rest have tumors larger than 5 cm. The left breast is more often affected than the right in both age extremes. The location of the tumor (lateral vs. medial-central), the overall frequency of bilaterality, and concurrent bilaterality are not significantly different at the extremes of the age distribution.

Several differences with respect to tumor type exist at the extremes of age.[66] Patients younger than 35 have a higher proportion of medullary carcinoma, and lower proportions of infiltrating lobular (2.0% vs. 11.0%) and of mucinous carcinoma (1.0% vs. 7.0%), in comparison with patients older than 75. A marked lymphocytic reaction occurs in a higher proportion of women younger than 35 than in the elderly group (34% vs. 12%).

Collins et al.[69] analyzed clinical and pathologic data for 657 patients with intraductal carcinoma (ductal carcinoma *in situ* [DCIS]) to identify features that might explain the greater risk for local recurrence in young women after breast-conserving therapy. Four age groups were compared, with the youngest consisting of 111 women less than 45 years of age at diagnosis, who proved to have significantly more extensive DCIS and more frequent lobular cancerization than women older than 45. DCIS was detected by mammography significantly less often in women younger than 45 years than in any of the older cohorts. There was no statistically significant relationship between age and the following features of DCIS: architectural type, nuclear grade, comedonecrosis, or the expression of receptors for ER, PR, or epidermal growth factor receptor 2 (EGFR2).

Prognostic and Predictive Markers in Invasive Carcinoma

Studies of growth rate and tumor cell kinetics suggest an inverse relationship between patient age at diagnosis and the proliferative activity in the invasive carcinoma.[70,71] Growth rate tends to be reduced in breast carcinomas that arise in elderly women.[71] Others have reported that the presence of ALN metastases in breast carcinoma patients 34 years or younger is significantly related to p53 positivity and high proliferative index.[72]

Walker et al.[73] found an inverse relationship between p53 immunopositivity and age, with positive staining in 67% and 37% of tumors from women 25 to 29 and 50 to 67 years of age, respectively. Proliferative rate, assessed by Ki67 immunostaining, was also inversely related to age, with 72% of tumors in patients 25 to 29 classified as "high" compared with 40% in the group 50 to 67 years of age.

The proportion of ER-positive invasive carcinomas is higher in postmenopausal than in premenopausal women, and there is evidence indicating that the growth rate and positive ER status of breast carcinomas are inversely related.[71] Although breast carcinomas in younger women are now more often detected before involving lymph nodes than 10 years ago, a larger percentage is triple-negative.[74] The proportion of ER- and PR-positive tumors does not increase significantly with advancing age in postmenopausal women 65 years or older.[75] Gennari et al.[76] reported that the frequency of estrogen and progesterone positivity was significantly higher in postmenopausal women 65 years of age or older when compared with postmenopausal women 50 to 64 years old. The older postmenopausal women had a significantly lower frequency of HER2-positive tumors. These observations appear to support the perception that breast carcinoma tends to have less aggressive biologic features and a more favorable clinical course in the elderly. Nonetheless, no significant differences in prognosis were observed when patients younger than 35 and older than 75 were matched on the basis of tumor stage.[66]

Breast Conservation Therapy

Women 40 years of age or younger are more likely than older patients to develop breast recurrences after breast-conserving surgery and radiotherapy for invasive carcinoma.[77–81] This phenomenon has been attributed to more frequent poorly differentiated carcinomas in this age group, difficulty in determining extent of carcinoma intraoperatively, and a high prevalence of carcinomas with an extensive intraductal component or lymphatic emboli in peritumoral tissue.[78] The addition of adjuvant chemotherapy appears to lower the risk of breast recurrence in women younger than 35 years who are treated by breast conservation.[79,82,83] Chest wall irradiation has been recommended if carcinoma is present at or close to (less than 5 mm) the deep margin of a mastectomy.[84] The risk of breast recurrence after breast conservation does not appear to be affected by a family history of breast cancer.[85]

Vicini et al.[86] reported that patients younger than 45 years of age had a significantly greater risk of breast recurrence after conservation therapy (excision and radiotherapy) for intraductal carcinoma than women who were 45 years or older. The frequency of invasive recurrence was substantially greater in the younger age group. When the volume of tissue was considered in the analysis, age at diagnosis proved not to be significantly related to recurrence risk, and it was concluded that the higher local failure rate in patients younger than 45 was related to smaller excision volumes in this age group.

Arvold et al.[87] studied 1,434 consecutive patients with invasive breast cancer who received breast conservation therapy over a 10-year period ending 2006. Ninety-one percent received adjuvant systemic therapy. The median follow-up was 85 months, and the overall 5-year cumulative incidence of local recurrence was 2.1%. The 5-year cumulative incidence of local recurrence was 5.0% for ages 23 to 46 years; 2.2% for ages 47 to 54 years; 0.9% for ages 55 to 63 years; and 0.6% for ages 64 to 88 years. On multivariable analysis, increasing age was associated with decreased risk of local recurrence.

Carcinoma in Elderly Women

The Cancer and Leukemia Group B (CALGB) trial 9343 examined the contribution of radiation after lumpectomy in women aged 70 and older with ER-positive node-negative breast carcinomas that were 2 cm or smaller.[88] After tumor excision, the patients were randomized to tamoxifen alone versus radiation plus tamoxifen. An update of this study with a 10.5-year median follow-up showed that 98% of the radiation plus tamoxifen group and 92% of the tamoxifen-only group were recurrence free.[89] Based on the 6% lower frequency of ipsilateral breast tumor recurrence for the radiation group, it was estimated that 300 women would have to be radiated to prevent 20 local recurrences. The fact that the two groups did not differ significantly in overall 10-year survival and breast-cancer–specific survival suggests that the small difference in the frequency of breast recurrence did not significantly affect survival 10 years after initial treatment.

Results of the ongoing Postoperative Radiation in Minimal Risk Elderly Patients (PRIME II) trial[90] in the United Kingdom may further define the effect of omission of radiation in elderly patients with hormone receptor node-negative invasive carcinomas. Until then, the advantages of radiation after breast conservation therapy in this subset of elderly patients should be weighed against its morbidities, and the decision to radiate should be individualized.

Genetic Considerations

Some special considerations are to be kept in mind regarding genetic abnormalities and breast carcinoma in young adult women.

"Secretory carcinoma" is the most common malignant epithelial neoplasm encountered in children. Its occurrence in younger patients accounts for the previously used term juvenile carcinoma, but it can be found in adult women of all ages. Because secretory carcinoma almost always has a balanced chromosomal translocation, t(12:15)(p13;q25) that leads to fusion of the *ETV6* and *NTRK3* genes,[91] it has been referred to as "a genetically defined carcinoma entity."[92]

More information about secretory carcinoma can be found in Chapter 22.

Among the 132 *BRCA-positive women* with breast carcinoma who participated in a high-risk protocol at The University of Texas M.D. Anderson Cancer Center, 106 second-generation women could be paired with a family member in the previous (first) generation who was diagnosed with a BRCA-related carcinoma in either breast or ovarian carcinoma.[93] The median age of carcinoma diagnosis in the first-generation patients was 48 years (range, 30 to 72 years) and in the second-generation patients, it was 42 years (range, 28 to 55 years). This trend was found in subgroups with either a *BRCA1* or *BRCA2* mutation. The statistically significant difference in age at diagnosis suggests that *BRCA*-mutation–related carcinomas in at least one subsequent generation occur at an earlier age after the first case is identified. The prognosis of breast carcinoma patients in *BRCA 1* and *BRCA 2* carriers has been controversial. In a large international population-based cohort study *BRCA1* and *BRCA2* mutation carriers were found to have no significant difference in outcome when compared with patients with sporadic breast carcinoma after adjusting for age, stage and grade of tumor, lymph node and hormone receptor status, and year of diagnosis.[94]

Li-Fraumeni syndrome is a rare autosomal dominant disorder that is linked to germline mutations of the *p53* tumor suppressor gene. The syndrome increases susceptibility to certain forms of cancer, including those of the breast, bone, and soft tissues. A cohort of eight breast carcinoma patients with a median age at diagnosis of 30 from Li-Fraumeni families with the associated germline *p53* mutations was studied in France.[95] Six of eight received radiation (including three after mastectomy). After a median follow-up of 6 years, an extraordinarily high incidence of subsequent events occurred in the six radiated patients consisting of three ipsilateral breast recurrences; three contralateral breast carcinomas; two radiation-associated sarcomas; one thyroid carcinoma in field. The data suggest that bilateral mastectomy is appropriate and that radiation therapy is contraindicated in this setting because the patients appear to have a genetic predisposition to develop radiation-associated malignant neoplasms.

CARCINOMA ARISING IN FIBROEPITHELIAL NEOPLASMS

Fibroepithelial neoplasms consist of proliferating epithelial and stromal mammary tissues. Fibroadenomas (FA) arise from the stroma and epithelium of lobular-terminal duct units, whereas phyllodes tumors (PT) are composed predominantly of periductal stroma and duct epithelium.

In 1931, Cheatle and Cutler[96] described carcinoma arising in a FA, and similar lesions were reported in 1940 by Harrington and Miller.[97] The first series, consisting of 26 patients, was published in 1967.[98] Numerous cases have been subsequently reported.[99–103] Carcinoma occurs in less than 0.5% of FA,[101,104] and in 1% to 2% of PT.[101,102]

Clinical Presentation

The age of patients with carcinoma arising in a FA ranges from 15 to 70 years, with a mean age of 42 to 44 years.[101,104] Women with *in situ* carcinoma have a mean age of 42 to 45 years, and the mean age for patients with invasive carcinoma in a FA is 47 to 52 years.[99] Because patients who have carcinoma in a FA tend to be somewhat older than those with FA that lack carcinoma, the possibility of encountering carcinoma should be anticipated when a FA is excised from a patient 35 years or older. The age distribution of women with carcinoma in or associated with a PT is not appreciably different from women with PT generally, reflecting the older age distribution of PT.

There are no specific clinical or radiologic clues to indicate the presence of *in situ* carcinoma within a FA or a PT. Invasive carcinoma in or associated with a FA may distort or blur the margin of the tumor in a mammogram.[105,106] Rarely, the pattern of calcifications in a FA can suggest intraductal carcinoma.[105,107] Carcinoma is more likely to be detected in a fine-needle aspirate from a FA if the carcinomatous component is extensive. The diagnosis depends upon recognizing neoplastic cells in the customary background of benign epithelium and stromal cells obtained from a typical FA.[108,109] If the lesion consists of *in situ* carcinoma limited to a small part of the tumor, there may not be sufficient material in a FNA or a needle core biopsy specimen to be diagnostic.[110] Because there are no good clinical indicators of the presence of carcinoma in a fibroepithelial tumor, the diagnosis is generally not suspected until a needle core biopsy has been obtained or the excised tumor has been examined pathologically.

Gross Pathology

When *in situ* carcinoma is present in a FA or PT, it will often not be apparent on gross inspection.[99] FA that harbor carcinoma may not be especially large and many do not exceed 2 cm. Unusual firmness may develop at the site of intraductal carcinoma, particularly in those which are of high-grade with necrosis and calcifications. Invasive carcinoma confined to a FA is generally inconspicuous grossly, but invasion into the adjacent breast tissue can distort the tumor enough to be evident.

Microscopic Pathology

The distinction between atypical hyperplasia and *in situ* carcinoma in a FA or PT is based on the same criteria that are used to assess epithelial proliferation in the mammary parenchyma. The characteristics of epithelial abnormalities within a FA or PT do not necessarily reflect the proliferative status of the surrounding breast tissue.

Fibroadenoma

The morphology of carcinomas that arise in FA is not peculiar to this setting, but the relative frequency of the types of carcinoma differs from that of carcinomas found in non-fibroepithelial breast parenchyma. In published reports, more than 50% of the affected FA had lobular carcinoma *in situ* (LCIS)[99,100] (Fig. 33.2). Among patients who were treated by mastectomy, LCIS was found in the surrounding

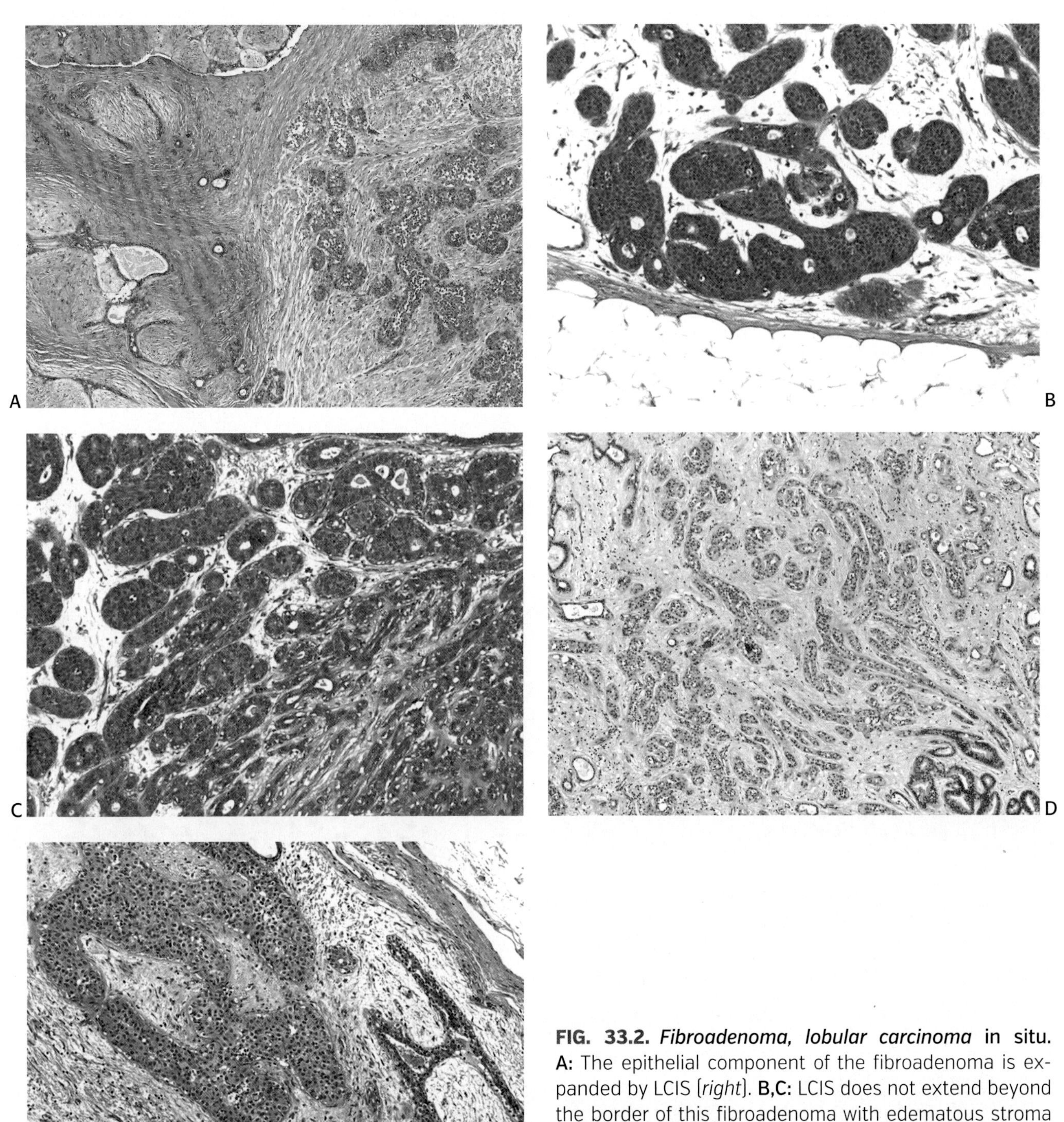

FIG. 33.2. ***Fibroadenoma, lobular carcinoma*** **in situ. A:** The epithelial component of the fibroadenoma is expanded by LCIS (*right*). **B,C:** LCIS does not extend beyond the border of this fibroadenoma with edematous stroma and sclerosing adenosis. **D:** LCIS involving an area of tubular adenosis in another complex fibroadenoma. **E:** Much of the epithelial element of this fibroadenoma is greatly expanded by LCIS.

breast tissue in about half of the cases. Nearly 20% had DCIS (Figs. 33.3 and 33.4). IDC accounted for 20% of the cases (Fig. 33.5), and about 10% had invasive lobular carcinoma (ILC) (Fig. 33.6). The IDCs have well-differentiated to moderately differentiated lesions. It is exceedingly unusual for special types of duct carcinoma to arise in a FA or PT. Atypical epithelial lesions in fibroepithelial tumors are prone to having a conspicuous myoepithelial component, and are associated with a variety of findings, including sclerosing adenosis (SA), cysts, apocrine metaplasia, and calcifications, which constitute the so-called complex FA. Petersson et al.[111] described a complex FA that gave rise to a low-grade *in situ* and invasive ductal carcinoma (IDC) associated with columnar cell change.

The probability of finding carcinoma in breast tissue outside a FA that is involved by carcinoma has been difficult to determine on the basis of published reports, because many patients were treated only by excisional biopsy. A literature review of 62 published cases found extra-fibroadenomatous carcinoma in 42% of patients.[104] Diaz et al.[99] reported that the type and amount of carcinoma in a FA and the age at diagnosis were not significant predictors of the likelihood of finding carcinoma in the surrounding breast tissue. Among women treated by mastectomy, carcinoma was limited to the FA in one-third to one-half of cases that had LCIS, DCIS, or ILC.[101,104] IDC that arose in a FA involved the surrounding breast tissue in at least 50% of cases. With rare exceptions, the same type of carcinoma has been found in the FA and in the breast tissue. LCIS may be detected in multiple FA in one breast or in bilateral FA.[100] ALN metastases have arisen from invasive carcinoma present *exclusively* within a FA in two cases.[97,112] Ten percent to 15% of patients with carcinoma in a FA have had contralateral carcinomas concurrently or previously treated.[96,100,101] The opposite breast contained IDC in the majority of these cases. Subsequent contralateral carcinoma has been described in about 6% of cases.[99]

Phyllodes Tumor

Florid hyperplasia involving epithelial and myoepithelial cells is often encountered in PT. The degree of atypia in the epithelial hyperplasia parallels that of the stromal component in some but not all cases. Mitoses may be seen in hyperplastic epithelial and myoepithelial cells.

Carcinomas arising in PT are histologically similar to carcinomas developing in FA. LCIS (Fig. 33.7) is less

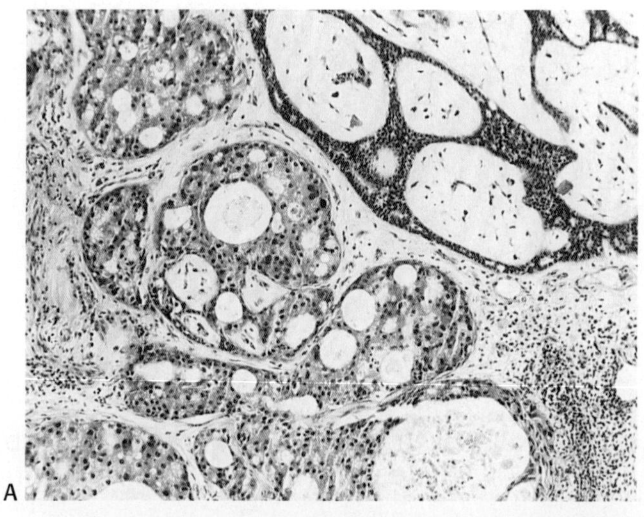
A

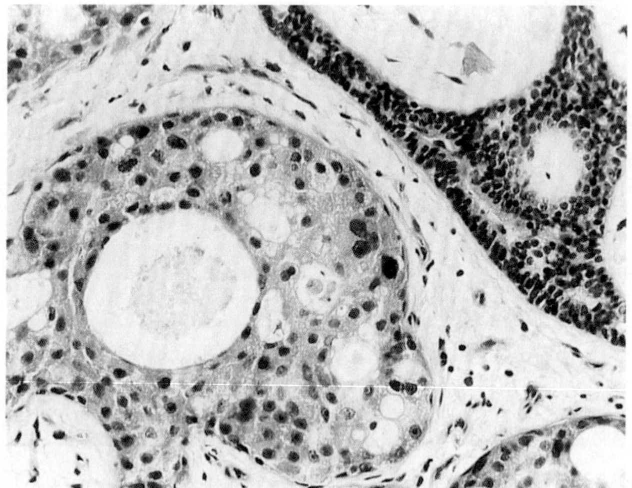
B

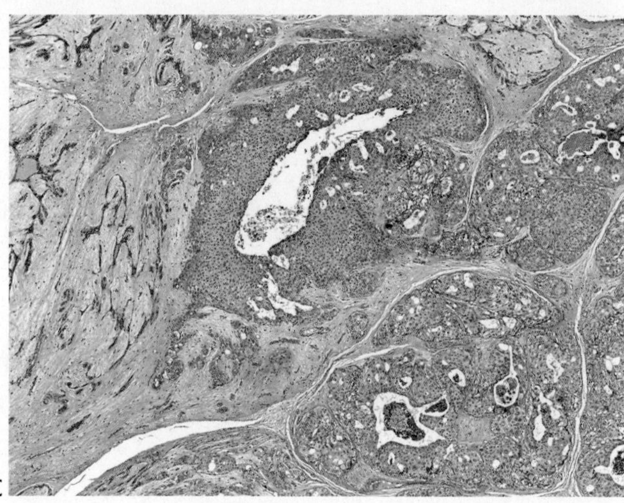
C

FIG. 33.3. ***Fibroadenoma, intraductal carcinoma.*** **A:** Cribriform growth pattern. **B:** Apocrine cytology. **C:** Cribriform and solid types of DCIS involving a FA and glands within its vicinity.

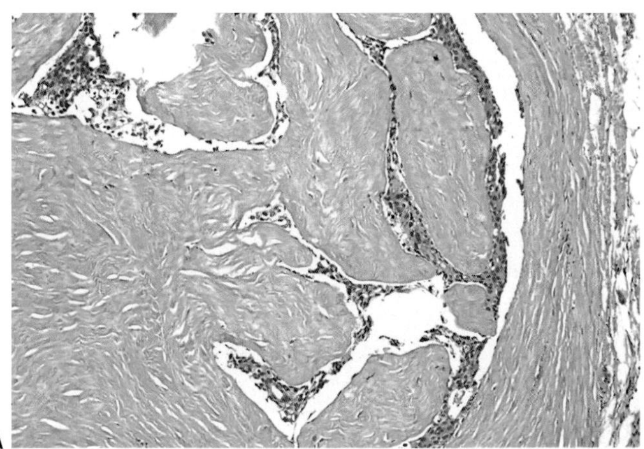
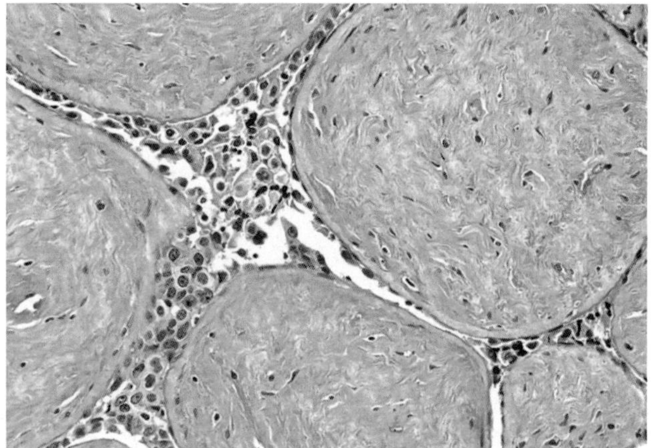

FIG. 33.4. ***Fibroadenoma, intraductal carcinoma.*** **A,B:** The usual epithelium in these two different sclerotic fibroadenomas has been replaced by high-grade DCIS.

frequent than DCIS (Fig. 33.8). Infiltrating duct carcinomas (Fig. 33.9) have also been described.[101,102,113–116] An IDC arising in a low-grade malignant PT in a 24-year-old woman was the source of isolated tumor cells in an ipsilateral SLN.[117] Korula et al.[118] described a 51-year-old woman who had DCIS in and around an malignant PT. Lymphatic tumor emboli were found in the PT, and metastatic carcinoma was present in two ALNs, but no invasive tumor was detected in the PT or in the breast. Microinvasive and ILC can also be found in this setting.[119] A high-grade malignant PT that contains carcinoma is a form of *carcinosarcoma*, because these lesions are, by definition, neoplasms that combine carcinomatous and sarcomatous elements derived from the mammary epithelium and stroma. Carcinoma has been found in the surrounding breast tissue concurrently with, or subsequent to, excision of a PT that contained carcinoma.[102,120,121]

Well-differentiated infiltrating duct carcinoma[122] and tubular carcinoma[115,123] have been described in PT. The latter case was unusual in that tubular carcinoma was found in the second recurrence of a benign PT. The first recurrence contained LCIS. In the case reported by Quinlan-Davidson,[115] LCIS and tubular carcinoma coexisted in a low-grade malignant PT.

Other unusual pathologic presentations have been coexistent DCIS and LCIS in a benign PT,[124] invasive carcinoma with ductal, secretory, and squamous components,[125] infiltrating duct carcinoma coincidental with but separate from benign PT[102] and malignant PT,[126] LCIS in a PT with liposarcomatous stroma,[127] and microinvasive lobular carcinoma in a benign PT.[119] PT that harbor carcinoma are usually benign or low-grade malignant tumors, whereas carcinoma is more often found in breast tissue outside an malignant PT.[114,121]

There are rare instances of PT with carcinoma that developed after treatment for another malignant neoplasm. Aziz et al.[121] described a 43-year-old woman who had carcinoma in a malignant liposarcomatous PT. Approximately 20 years earlier she had received chemotherapy for Hodgkin disease and radiotherapy to the lumbar region. Another woman who developed a liposarcomatous and chondrosarcomatous malignant PT associated with carcinoma when 26 years old had been treated by surgery and chemotherapy without radiotherapy for tibial osteosarcoma 11 years earlier.[120]

Molecular Analysis

Macher-Goeppinger et al.[128] described the results of the molecular analysis of an IDC within an malignant PT. DNA was isolated from the microdissected epithelial and stromal components of the PT, and from the high-grade IDC. Using the multiplex polymerase chain reaction (PCR), comparative allelotyping was performed with a panel of 11 microsatellite markers. Analysis of the data revealed that the stromal component of the PT showed loss of heterozygosity (LOH) at chromosome 16q23, 17q12, 17q25, and 22q13 and that the epithelial element of the tumor shared the loss of 16q23. The invasive carcinoma had lost divergent alleles at 16q23, 17q12, and 17q25. These findings were interpreted as demonstrating a lack of clonality between the malignant PT and the invasive carcinoma that arose within it.

Treatment and Prognosis

There have been very few deaths due to carcinoma arising in a FA, and these have been attributable to IDCs.[101,104] Recurrence in the breast following excisional biopsy of a FA that harbored *in situ* lobular or intraductal carcinoma has been uncommon and appears to be less frequent than when the same lesions that occur outside of FA have been treated only by excisional surgery.[99] There are virtually no published data on breast conservation therapy that employed radiation in addition to excisional surgery to treat intraductal carcinoma in a FA. The low frequency of subsequent carcinomas may reflect to some extent the relatively short follow-up, averaging less than 10 years, in most series of patients with carcinoma arising in a FA.

There are no systematic data on the treatment and prognosis of women who had carcinoma arising in a PT. The need to ensure adequate excision of the PT in some cases

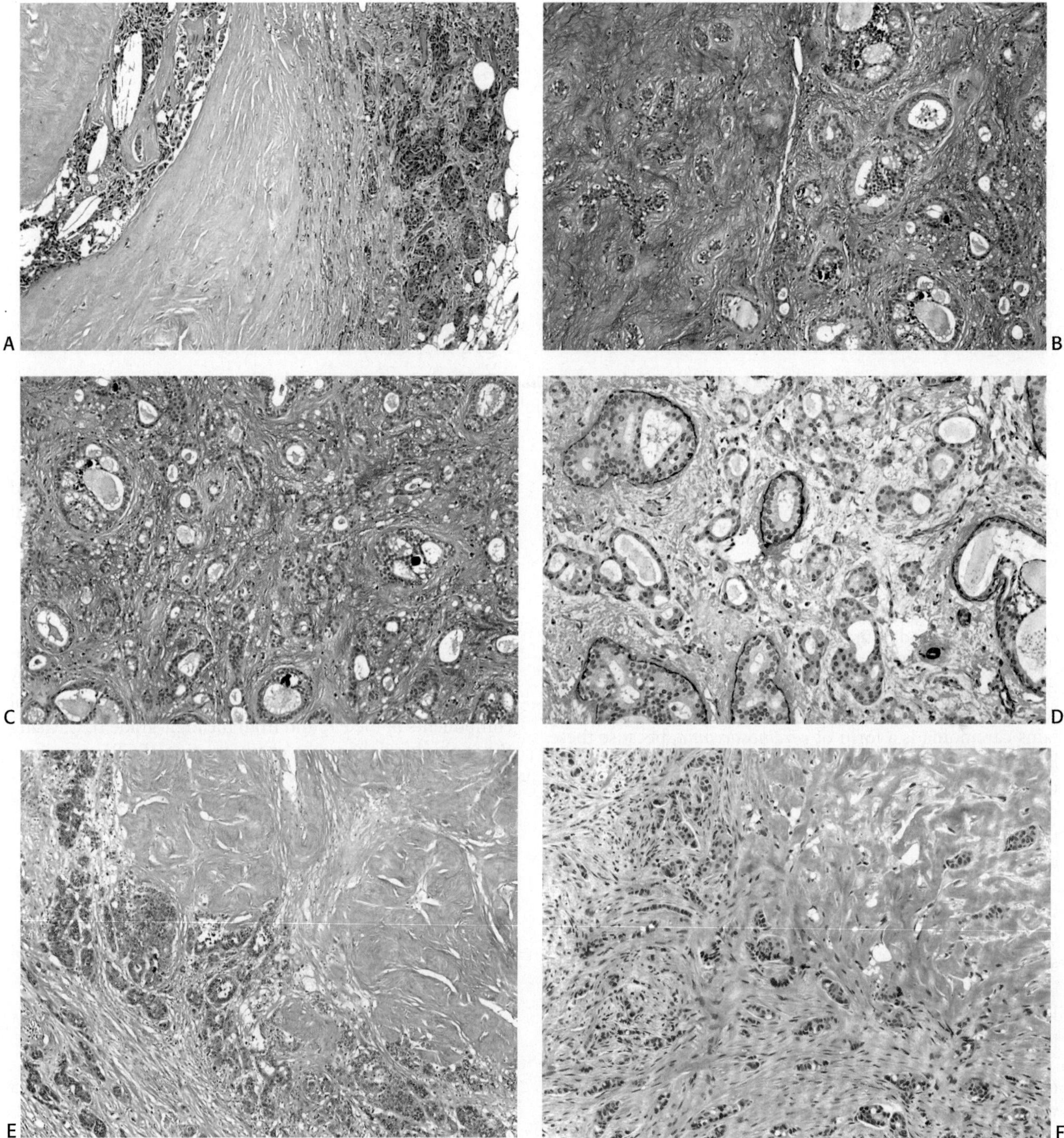

FIG. 33.5. ***Fibroadenoma, infiltrating ductal carcinoma.*** **A:** IDC involving the periphery of a sclerotic fibroadenoma. Intraductal carcinoma is shown on the *left*. **B-D:** Cribriform intraductal carcinoma with calcifications in a myxoid fibroadenoma from a 30-year-old woman. Non-carcinomatous epithelium is on the *left* and invasive carcinoma is on the *far right* (B). Several ducts with cribriform intraductal carcinoma and calcifications in the midst of invasive well-differentiated ductal carcinoma (c). Immunoreactivity for smooth muscle myosin heavy chains is shown around intraductal carcinoma. Staining is absent around invasive carcinoma (D). **E:** IDC secondarily extending into a sclerosed fibroadenoma. **F:** Another ductal carcinoma invading circumscribed pseudoangiomatous stromal hyperplasia. The tumor cells appear to occupy the "pseudoangiomatous" spaces (*upper right*).

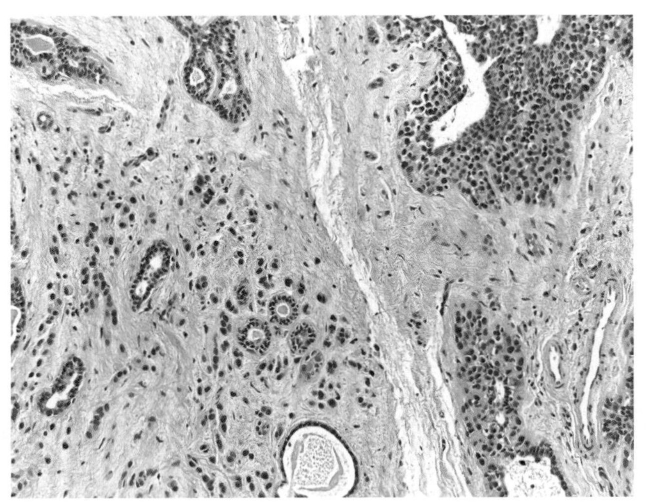

FIG. 33.6. ***Fibroadenoma, invasive lobular carcinoma.*** ILC in a FA with pagetoid LCIS in adjacent ducts.

necessitates a mastectomy even when the carcinoma would be adequately treated by breast conservation.

OCCULT CARCINOMA PRESENTING WITH ALN METASTASES

Fewer than 1% of patients who have mammary carcinoma present with an ALN metastasis as the first clinical manifestation of the disease.[129,130] Among 10,014 patients with primary operable breast carcinoma treated at one institution, 35 (0.35%) had occult carcinoma presenting with axillary metastases.

Clinical Presentation

This condition occurs throughout the entire age distribution of breast carcinoma,[129–135] with the mean and median age around 57 years.[136] The right axilla and breast were affected slightly more often (54%) than the left in one series,[94] but others have reported left predominance.[137–139] A positive family history of breast carcinoma has been reported in

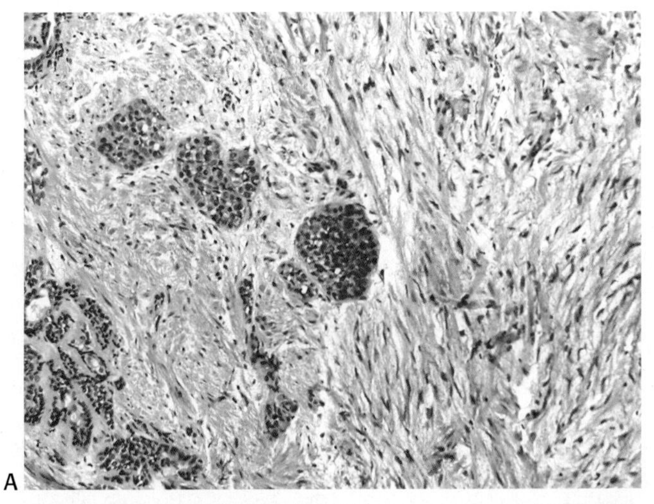

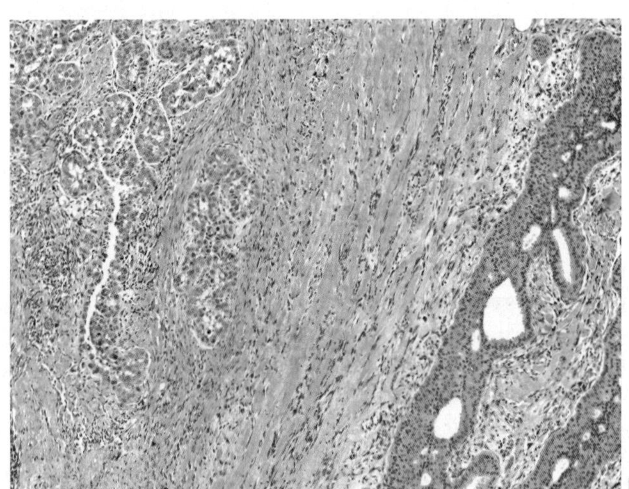

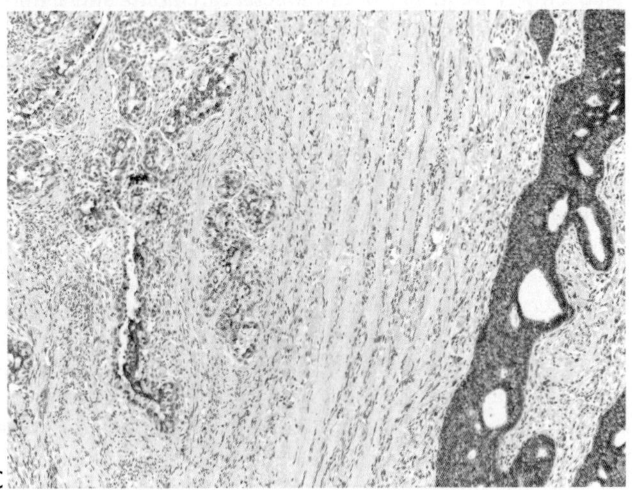

FIG. 33.7. ***Phyllodes tumor, benign, with lobular carcinoma*** **in situ. A:** Benign PT with LCIS. **B:** Benign PT with atypical ductal hyperplasia (bordering on DCIS) and LCIS (*left*). **C:** LCIS is negative for E-cadherin (*left*), whereas the ductal lesion is positive for E-cadherin (*right*).

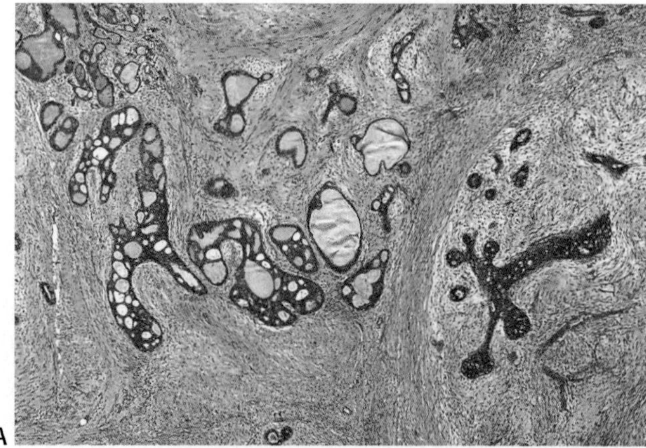

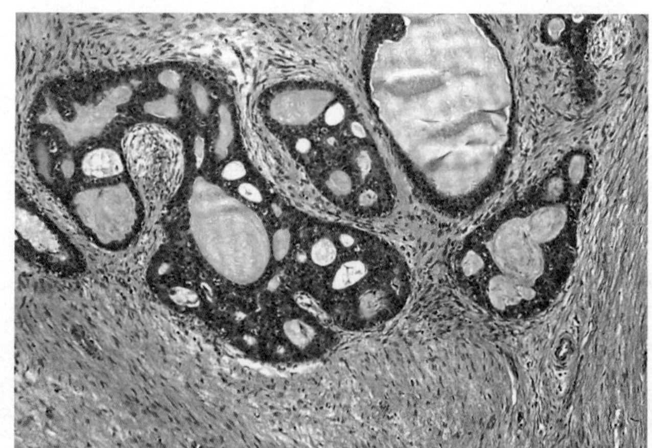

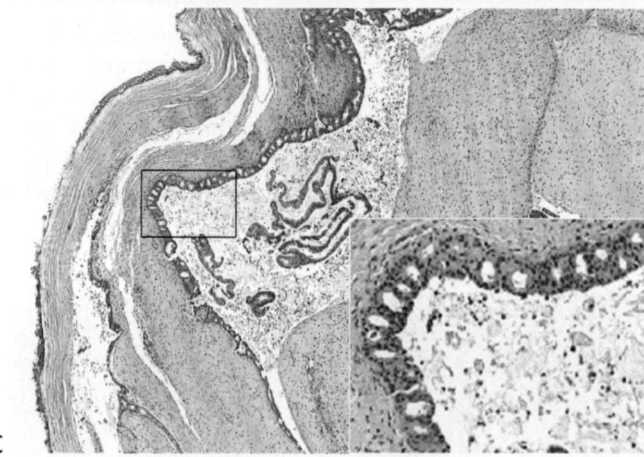

FIG. 33.8. ***Phyllodes tumor, benign, with intraductal carcinoma.*** **A,B:** Cribriform DCIS has replaced some of the epithelium. **C:** Another example of Benign PT with cribriform DCIS. Inset shows detail.

nearly 50% of patients,[133,135] with about 25% having a maternal first-degree relative affected.[129]

The initial clinical presentation is enlargement of one or more ALNs. An abnormality may be reported on clinical examination of the ipsilateral breast in 25% of patients, but it is often not regarded as suspicious, or on follow-up it may not correlate with the location in the breast where carcinoma is ultimately detected.[131,133,140] This observation is consistent with data compiled by Rosen et al.,[141] who studied nearly 3,500 patients with palpable breast lesions and were studied by mammography. Carcinoma was diagnosed in 64 women. The palpable lesion proved to be carcinoma in 54 of these cases, but in 10 women the palpable tumor was benign, and carcinoma was a nonpalpable lesion detected by mammography alone. In this series, none of the patients was initially examined because of axillary nodal involvement, but the study demonstrated the capacity of mammography to detect clinically occult carcinoma in the presence of a benign, palpable mass.

Clinical Evaluation

To rule out an extramammary tumor or other metastases, most women have been studied with a variety of techniques.[131,133,134] Marcantonio and Libshitz[142] demonstrated ALN enlargement by computed tomography (CT) in patients with pulmonary carcinoma and proved the presence of metastatic carcinoma by biopsy in six cases, confirming the lung as one of the alternate primary sites for an occult carcinoma that presents with axillary metastases.

Mammography has revealed abnormalities in12%,[131] 25%,[134] 26.5%,[129] 31%,[138] and 35%[133,140] of patients examined. Tartter et al.[143] compared women with false-negative and positive mammograms. The two groups were similar with respect to tumor differentiation, tumor size, and ER status. However, women with false-negative mammography had a lower frequency of intraductal carcinoma and significantly more frequent metastases in ALNs. Some investigators have excluded patients with significant mammographic abnormalities from the syndrome of subclinical carcinoma presenting with ALN metastases,[132,144] but others found no consistent correlation between the location of the radiologic abnormality and the site at which a carcinoma was ultimately located.[133] If mastectomy is delayed, repeat mammograms of patients who initially had negative studies may reveal new findings suggestive of carcinoma.[140] In one study, the interval until the detection of a breast abnormality clinically or by mammography was 6 to 39 months, with a mean of 15 months in women who did not undergo a mastectomy.[145] The presence of mammographically detectable calcifications in metastatic carcinoma in ALNs may be a clue to the diagnosis of a subclinical mammary carcinoma.[146,147]

MRI has proven to be an effective method for detecting occult carcinomas that are not evident mammographically. MRI detected occult carcinoma in 143 of 234 (61%) patients

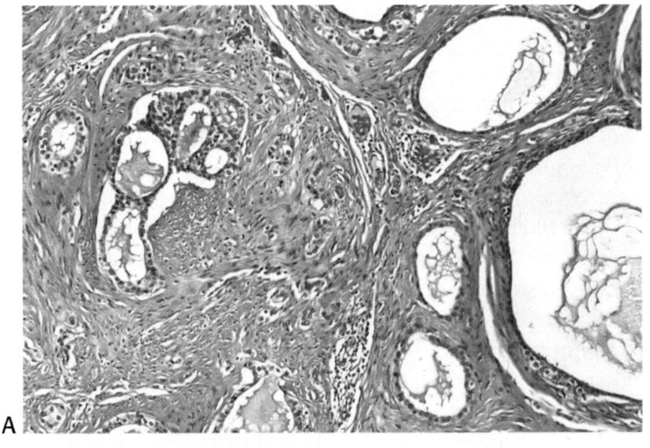

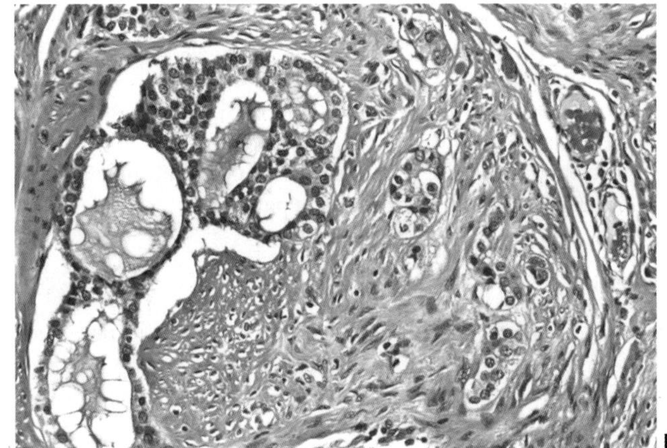

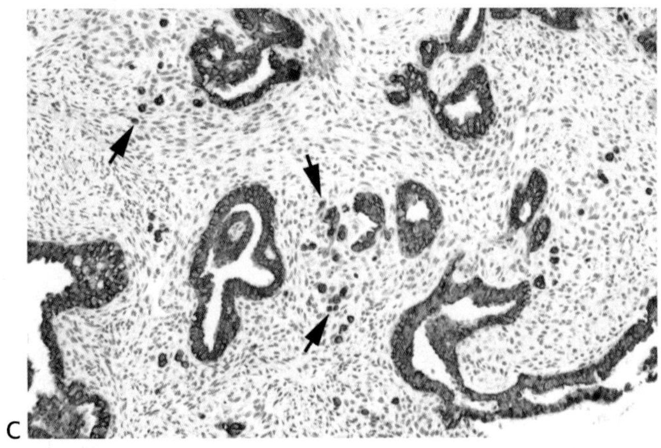

FIG. 33.9. ***Phyllodes tumor, benign, with intraductal and invasive ductal carcinoma.*** **A,B:** Cribriform intraductal carcinoma is next to IDC. **C:** Isolated cells (*arrows*) of IDC are highlighted by a CK immunostain in a benign PT. Glandular components of the PT are also cytokeratin positive (CK7).

in pooled results from 10 studies published until 2008.[148] In another pooled study published in 2010, the specificity of MRI was 31% on pooled data (range, 22% to 50%) from seven studies.[149] However, not all lesions detected by MRI in this setting prove to be carcinoma. Buchanan et al.[136] reported false-positive MRI studies in 15 of 69 patients, and in another series, MRI yielded a false-positive result in 2 of 15 cases.[150] The diagnostic yield is low in patients with a negative mammogram and a negative MRI,[136] a situation that led the European Society of Breast Cancer Specialists to recommend that surgical treatment be avoided if MRI of the breast is negative.[148] Positive MRI findings should be investigated by biopsy. In a high proportion of cases, lesions detected by mammography can be localized by sonography, making them amenable to sonographically directed needle core biopsy.[151]

Occasionally, nodal enlargement occurs in the contralateral axilla of a patient treated previously for mammary carcinoma.[139,152] This phenomenon was observed in 52 (3.6%) of 1,440 patients in one series.[153] Most of these patients were judged to have systemic disease. Six of the 52 patients (0.04%) were treated by contralateral mastectomy, and 2 had a primary tumor in the contralateral breast. Breslow[154] reported that 6 (0.39%) of 1,543 patients with unilateral breast carcinoma subsequently developed carcinoma in contralateral ALNs, and that a primary tumor was detected in four of the opposite breasts. In a series of patients presenting with axillary metastases from subclinical breast carcinoma, about 8% were previously treated for contralateral breast carcinoma[129,131] or developed subsequent carcinoma in the contralateral breast.[129,132] One patient had an augmentation prosthesis in the breast that harbored a subclinical carcinoma.[129] Huston et al.[155] studied seven women who developed contralateral axillary nodal metastases. The median interval between treatment of the initial carcinoma and subsequent contralateral axillary metastases was 71 months. All had adjuvant chemotherapy and five underwent axillary dissection. There were no axillary recurrences after a median follow-up of 35 months, at which time five women were alive, two with recurrent carcinoma, and two had died of metastatic carcinoma. It is possible that the prior contralateral carcinoma is the source of axillary metastases in many of these situations, but in some instances an occult primary may give rise to the newly apparent nodal metastases.[139]

Clonal analysis may be employed to evaluate metastatic carcinoma in contralateral ALNs if material from the ipsilateral tumor is available for comparison. In the majority of cases, clonal analysis of the carcinomas in both breasts of patients with bilateral tumors has demonstrated cytogenetic differences indicative of independent origin of the lesions.[156,157] Rarely, the pattern of the clonal abnormalities in both tumors suggests metastatic spread from one breast to the other.[157] A similar conclusion would be supported by finding that a primary carcinoma and a metastatic tumor at another site such as the chest wall or contralateral ALNs shared the same karyotypic abnormalities.[156]

Occult breast carcinoma presenting as an ALN metastasis is exceedingly unusual in men.[158-160] In some cases, axillary metastases from a nonmammary primary, such as carcinoma of the lung, have been documented in men, generally after treatment of the pulmonary primary.[145,161,162] There is insufficient experience with this presentation of male breast carcinoma to compare with female patients.

Gross Pathology

The frequency with which a primary tumor is detected pathologically in the ipsilateral breast varies from 55%[133] to 82%.[130,138] In most series, the proportion with a documented primary was about 75%.[129,131,133,135,140] Although not clinically palpable, the majority of carcinomas were found upon gross examination of a mastectomy or excisional biopsy specimen (Fig. 33.10). Rarely, the breast has contained two separate, grossly evident invasive primary carcinomas, each of which may be accompanied by an *in situ* component.[135,152] The lesions have measured up to 6.5 cm,[130,134,135] but most were 1 to 2 cm or less in diameter. In one series, the median size was 1.9 cm and the mean 1.5 cm, with 82% classified as T1, 14% as T2, and 4% as T3.[135] In a review of eight retrospective studies published in 2010, de Bresser et al.[149] reported that lesions detected by MRI measured between 5mm and 3cm and that the pathologically measured size of these lesions ranged from 1 mm to 5 cm. Smaller tumors were often discrete, with a stellate or circumscribed contour, but those larger than 2 cm more often had ill-defined margins and tended to blend grossly with the surrounding breast tissue. The majority of the primary lesions occur in the upper outer quadrant and less often in other quadrants.[131,133-135,137] The occult primary tumor has rarely been detected in the axillary tail.[151]

About 30% of the clinically occult primary carcinomas are not evident when a mastectomy specimen is examined grossly. These lesions are found by taking multiple random sections of breast tissue that appears grossly normal. Consequently, sampling should not be limited to grossly abnormal parenchyma. Radiography of breast biopsies and mastectomies has not been helpful for locating the primary and cannot be relied upon for guidance in the sampling of tissue for histologic study. This is not unexpected in view of the lack of success with clinical mammography in these patients.

The likelihood of finding a primary lesion in the breast is related to the thoroughness with which the available tissue has been studied. In some cases, the primary tumor remains undetected because a breast biopsy, or mastectomy, or both, was not performed. Despite careful and extensive gross and microscopic examination of a mastectomy, there are rare instances in which no primary is found. Patients not proven to have a primary breast carcinoma or a primary tumor at another site have a similar age distribution, similar lymph node findings, and comparable survival results as those with a pathologically demonstrated clinically occult breast carcinoma. In one series, none of the 12 patients without a documented primary breast lesion were later shown to have an extramammary primary.[133]

Axillary Lymph Nodes

Among patients subjected to axillary dissection, the number of lymph nodes found to be involved by metastatic carcinoma varies from one to as many as 65.[130,131,135,139] When numerous lymph nodes are involved, they rarely form a matted mass with extranodal extension. In one series, one-half of the 40 patients had one to three involved lymph nodes (1 to 3 positive), including 13 patients whose only positive lymph node was the one removed for diagnosis (Fig. 33.11). Among 15 women with carcinoma, in four or more lymph nodes the median number involved was 11.

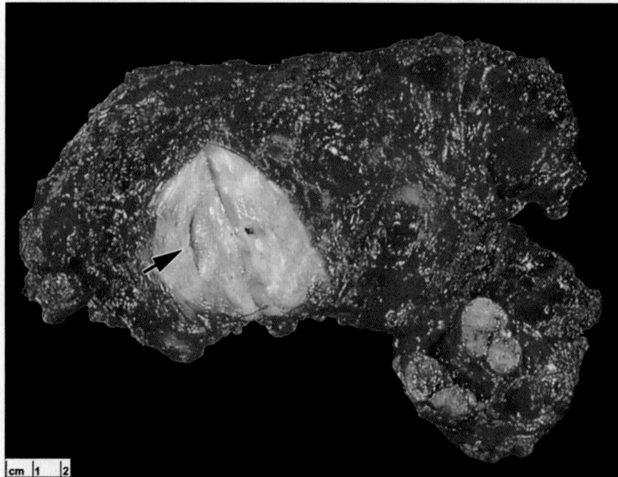

FIG. 33.10. ***Occult carcinoma, mastectomy.*** The *arrow* indicates a small IDC that was not palpable clinically. A bisected ALN with metastatic carcinoma is shown in the *lower right* portion of the specimen.

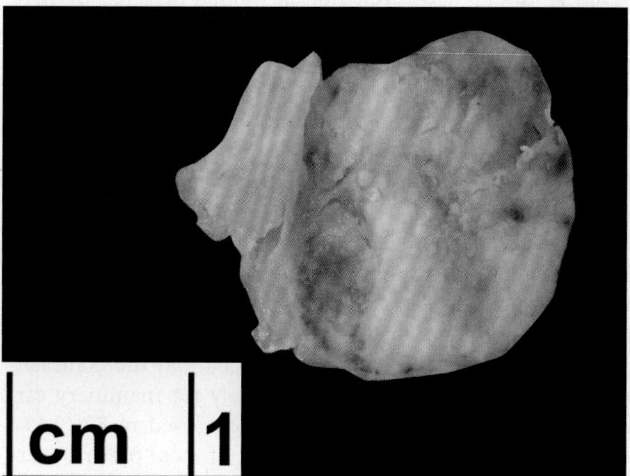

FIG. 33.11. ***Occult carcinoma.*** This solitary enlarged ALN containing metastatic papillary carcinoma is greater than 2 cm in diameter. No primary tumor was detected in either breast by clinical palpation or on radiological evaluation. The metastatic carcinoma in the lymph node was ER (+), CK7 (+), CK20 (−), WT-1 (+), and PAX8 (+). A 3.0-cm ovarian papillary serous carcinoma was subsequently resected.

TABLE 33.1 Lymph Node Pathology in Patients With and Without Primary Breast Carcinoma

	With Primary	Without Primary
	(N = 31)	(N = 12)
	No. (%)	No. (%)
Large apocrine cells	20 (65)	8 (67)
Mammary carcinoma pattern	7 (23)	1 (8)
Mixed pattern	4 (13)	3 (25)

Adapted from Haupt HM, Rosen PP, Kinne DW. Breast carcinoma presenting with axillary lymph node metastases. An analysis of specific histopathologic features. *Am J Surg Pathol* 1985;9:165–175.

Microscopic Pathology of ALNs

Metastatic adenocarcinoma found in the ALNs derived from an occult breast carcinoma usually has one of three patterns found in ductal carcinomas (Table 33.1). In about 65% of cases, the lymph nodes contain extensive infiltrates of large cells, often with apocrine features, diffusely distributed in the lymphoid tissue as well as in sinusoids (Figs. 33.12 and 33.13). Less often, the lymph nodes contain predominantly sinusoidal metastases. Apocrine features include substantial cytoplasmic eosinophilia in most instances, but in some metastases there is prominent cytoplasmic clearing (Fig. 33.14). Little or no gland formation is evident in these metastases, but mucicarmine-positive secretion can be demonstrated in at least a few cells in most cases. Nuclei tend to be large, round or oval, and to be vacuolated with prominent, frequently eosinophilic nucleoli. This cell type and distribution are sometimes suggestive of metastatic malignant melanoma (Fig. 33.15), and metastatic renal cell carcinoma may be considered if cytoplasmic clearing is prominent. When the tumor cells are dispersed singly or in small groups throughout a lymph node, the resulting pattern might be confused with diffuse malignant lymphoma (Fig. 33.16). Small well-differentiated glandular metastases in an otherwise hyperplastic lymph node may be the presenting manifestation of an occult tubular carcinoma (Fig. 33.17). In these cases, the lymph node is enlarged by lymphoid hyperplasia, possibly in response to the metastatic carcinoma. Metastatic tubular carcinoma should not be misinterpreted as benign glandular inclusions (see Chapter 43).

About 20% of ALN metastases consist of adenocarcinoma with growth patterns similar to those more commonly encountered in primary carcinomas in the breast. These include cribriform, papillary forms of invasive carcinoma (Fig. 33.18). A desmoplastic stromal reaction is rarely present in these nodal metastases. The remaining 15% of the lymph nodes contain mixtures of tumor with the conventional patterns and diffuse apocrine cells. Metastatic carcinoma from a nonmammary site such as the lung may be difficult to distinguish from these mixed types of breast carcinoma (Fig. 33.19).

Approximately 50% of the lymph nodes involved by each of the three patterns of metastases have some mucicarmine-positive cells. Among cases in which tissue blocks were available to cut fresh sections for the mucicarmine stain, 75% gave a positive reaction. A positive result with this simple procedure narrows the differential diagnosis substantially, especially when gland formation is not apparent. It is not unusual to find mucin-positive cells limited to isolated tumor cells in only one of several involved lymph nodes.

If a diagnosis of adenocarcinoma is not apparent from the growth pattern and mucin stain, other studies may be helpful. Immunohistochemical studies for cytokeratins, especially CK7 and CK20, hormone receptors, epithelial

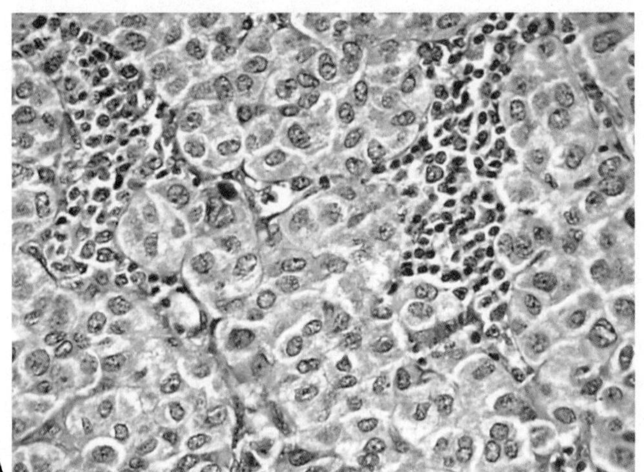

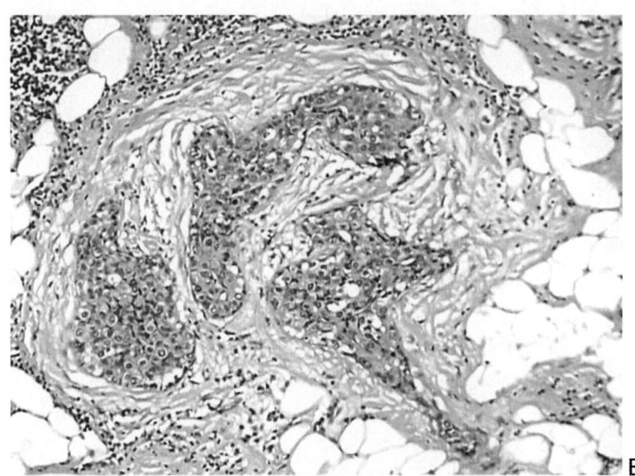

FIG. 33.12. ***Occult carcinoma.*** **A:** Metastatic adenocarcinoma in an ALN. The tumor cells have apocrine features consisting of abundant, finely granular eosinophilic cytoplasm, large open nuclei, and prominent nucleoli. **B:** This microscopic focus of intraductal carcinoma with periductal fibrosis and lymphocytic reaction was the only parenchymal lesion in the mastectomy specimen.

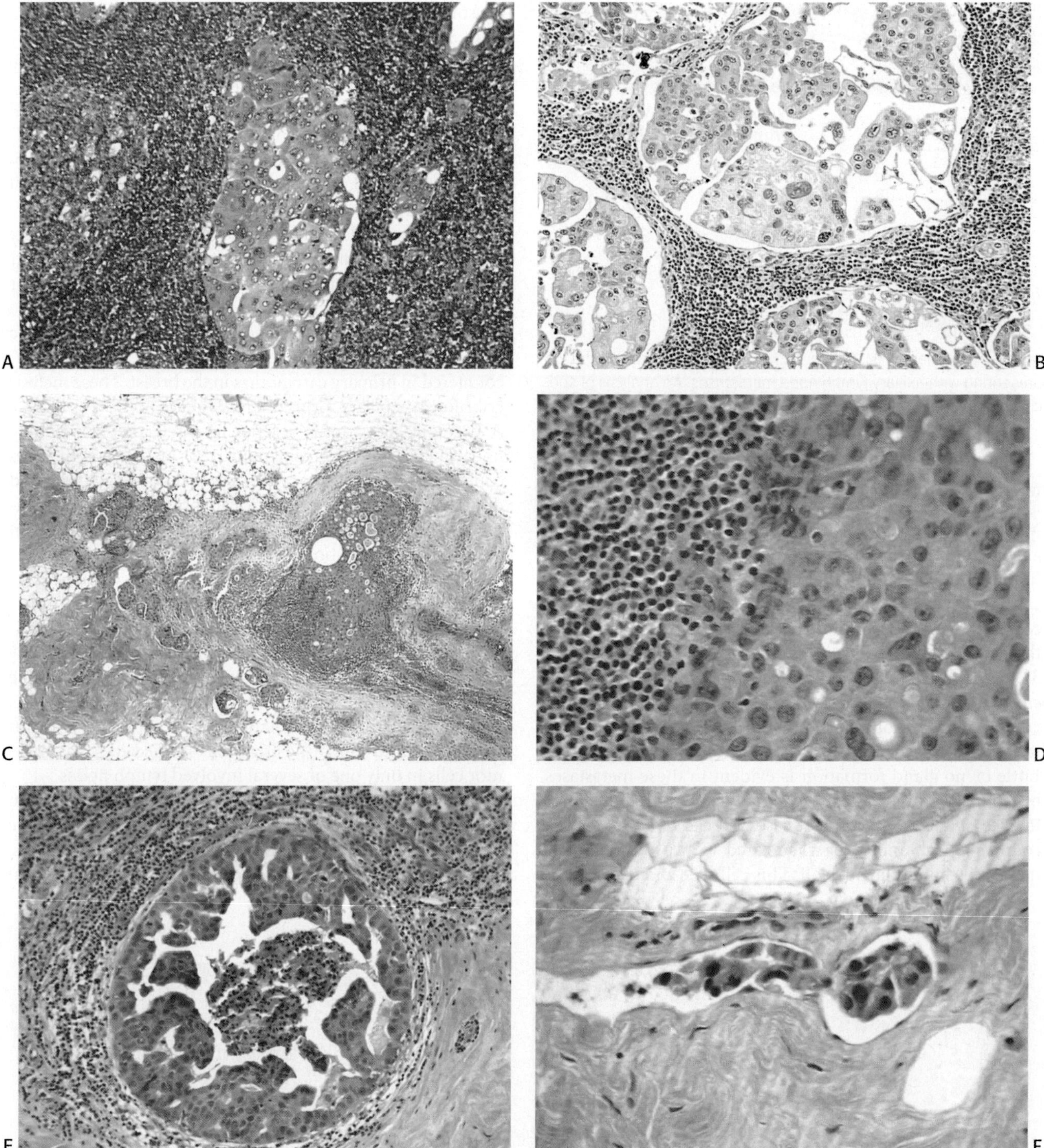

FIG. 33.13. ***Occult carcinoma, apocrine.*** **A:** Metastatic carcinoma, apocrine type, in a sinusoidal space of an ALN. **B:** Intracytoplasmic mucin is demonstrated with the mucicarmine stain. **C:** The nonpalpable intraductal and infiltrating primary ductal carcinoma in the breast has focal lymphocytic infiltrates. **D:** Apocrine differentiation in the primary carcinoma. **E:** Intraductal carcinoma, papillary, with necrosis. **F:** Lymphatic tumor emboli in the primary carcinoma. All images are from one case.

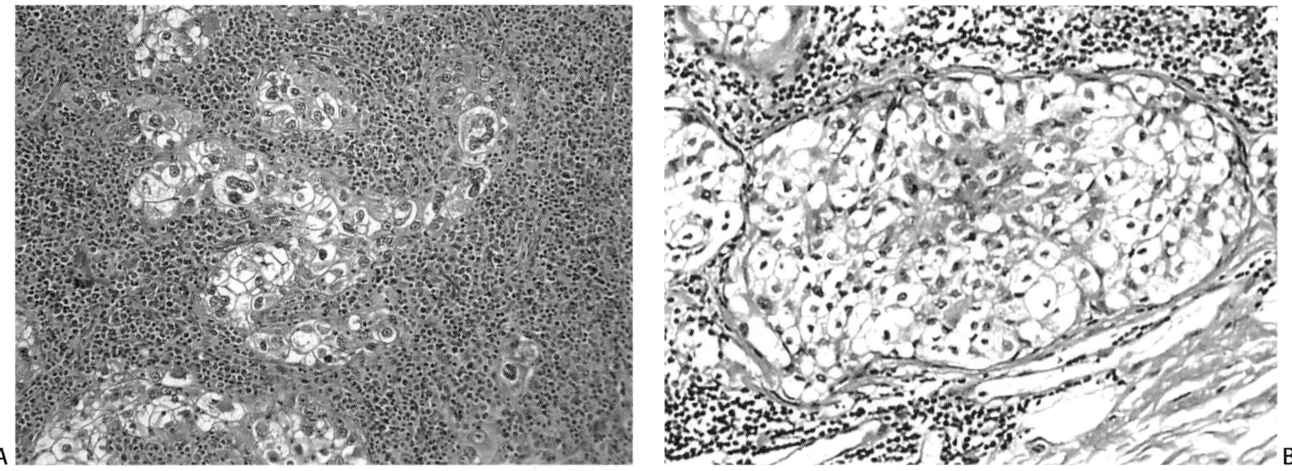

FIG. 33.14. ***Occult carcinoma, clear cell.*** **A:** This metastatic carcinoma in an ALN was the initial manifestation of breast carcinoma in this patient. **B:** A clinically unapparent focus of intraductal carcinoma, clear cell type, with a surrounding lymphocytic reaction was found in the breast.

membrane antigen (EMA), S-100 protein, carcinoembryonic antigen (CEA), lymphoid markers, and other markers usually resolve the differential diagnosis. Mammary carcinoma is typically immunoreactive for CK7 but not for CK20. Absence of reactivity for E-cadherin is helpful for identifying metastatic lobular carcinoma. In current practice, it is almost never necessary to employ electron microscopy.[163]

When adenocarcinoma has been diagnosed in tissue removed from an axillary mass, there may be uncertainty as to whether this represents a metastasis or a primary axillary tumor. Because this distinction cannot be made reliably on the basis of a needle biopsy sample, excisional biopsy is essential. Variation in the characteristics of tumor among affected lymph nodes can be helpful for diagnosis. Several sections of a mass of matted lymph nodes may be required to find a portion of uninvolved lymph node. The specimen should be examined for axillary breast tissue (see following discussion of Carcinoma in Ectopic Breast Tissue). An unusual, largely hypothetical, source for mammary carcinoma arising in the axilla is ectopic breast tissue in an ALN.[164,165] This phenomenon is not likely to be recognized in a case presenting with an enlarged lymph node, because the heterotopic tissue will probably have been overgrown by the carcinoma.

The distinction between medullary carcinoma and metastatic carcinoma in a lymph node can be a particularly vexing problem. A reticulin stain is useful in this situation to reveal the underlying architecture of ducts that may be present in a primary carcinoma or the structure of a

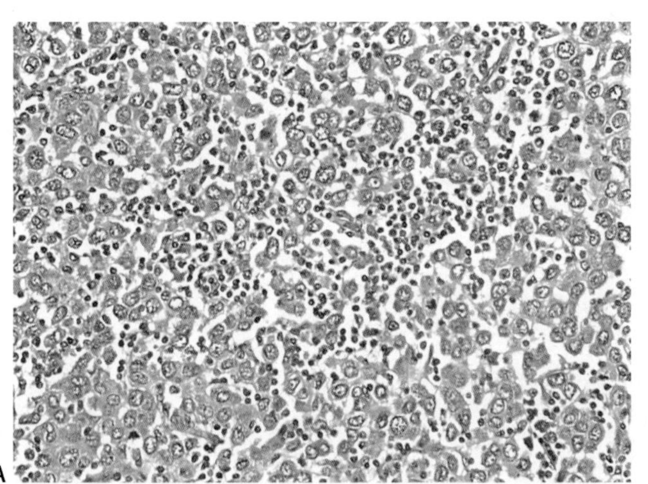

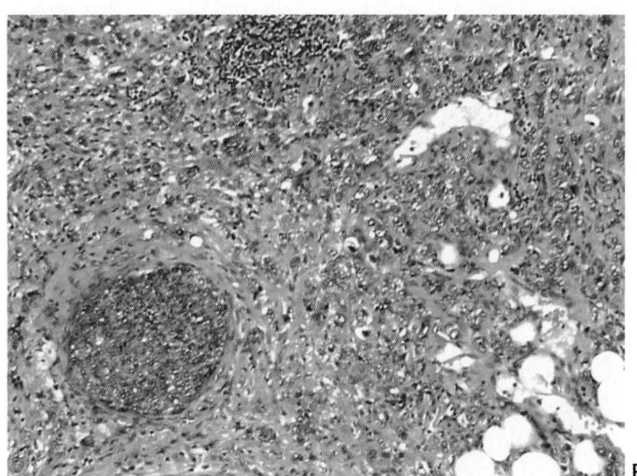

FIG. 33.15. ***Occult carcinoma, diffuse.*** **A:** The patient presented with this enlarged ALN found to contain malignant cells diffusely infiltrating the lymphoid tissue. The tumor cells were immunoreactive for cytokeratin (*not shown here*). **B:** Poorly differentiated infiltrating ductal carcinoma found in the breast.

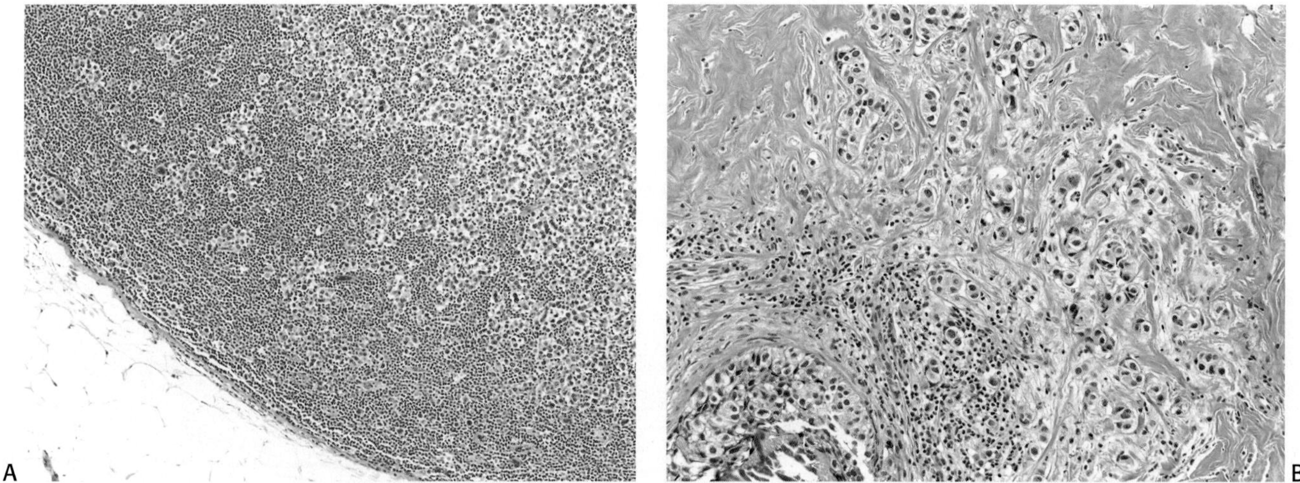

FIG. 33.16. ***Occult carcinoma, diffuse.*** **A:** An enlarged ALN in which poorly differentiated malignant cells, most prominent in the *upper right corner*, mingle with lymphocytes. The differential diagnosis for this pattern includes metastatic carcinoma, malignant lymphoma, and metastatic melanoma. The tumor cells in this case were immunoreactive for cytokeratin. **B:** An ipsilateral breast biopsy, targeting a minute focus of calcification, showed a focus of DCIS with calcification (*lower left*) and microinvasive ductal carcinoma.

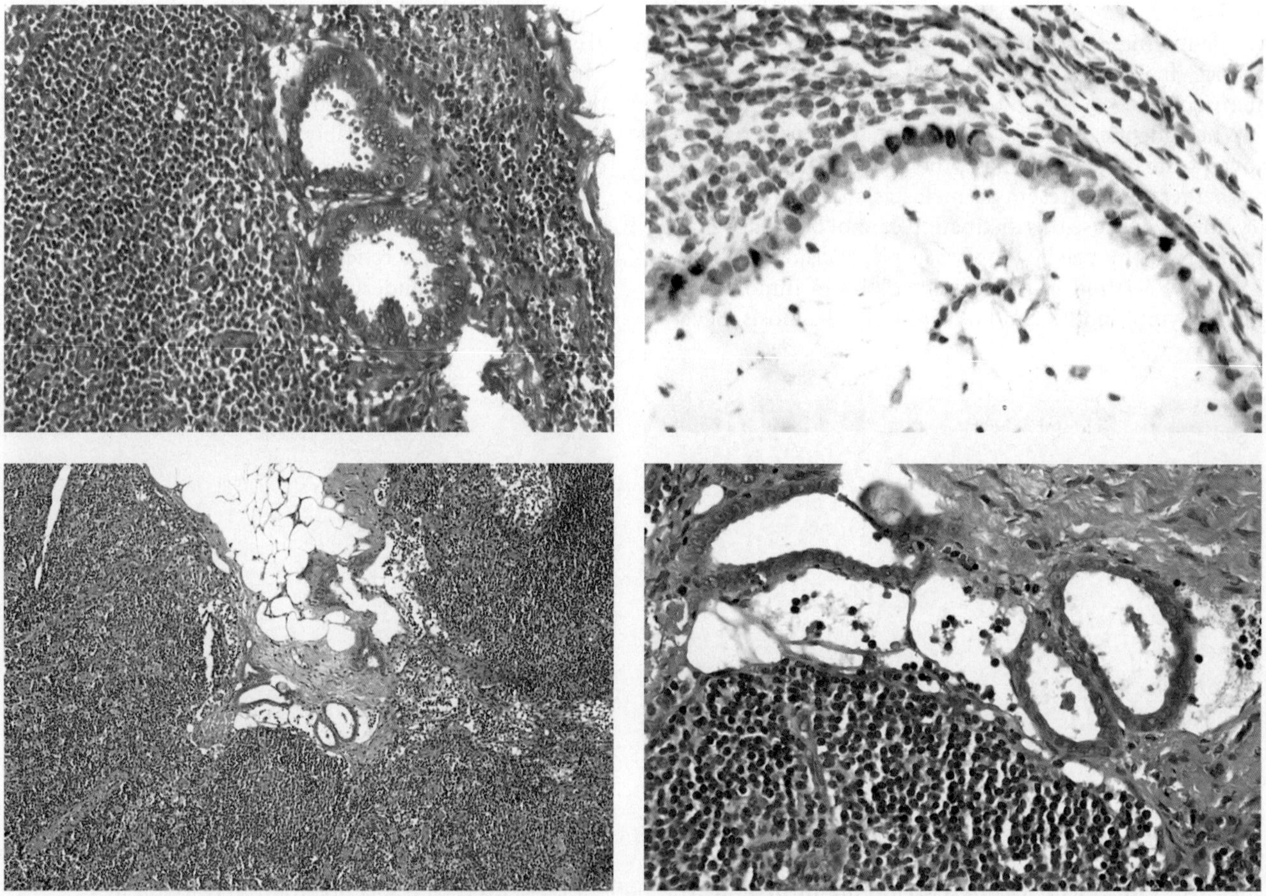

FIG. 33.17. ***Occult carcinoma, tubular type.*** **A:** Two glands of metastatic tubular carcinoma in lymph node tissue. **B:** Nuclear immunoreactivity for estrogen receptor is shown in one of the glands from (**A**). **C,D:** Metastatic tubular carcinoma in subcapsular sinusoids of a hyperplastic lymph node.

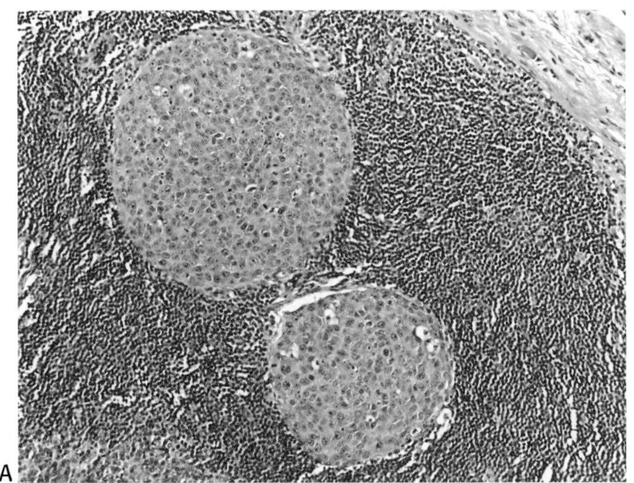

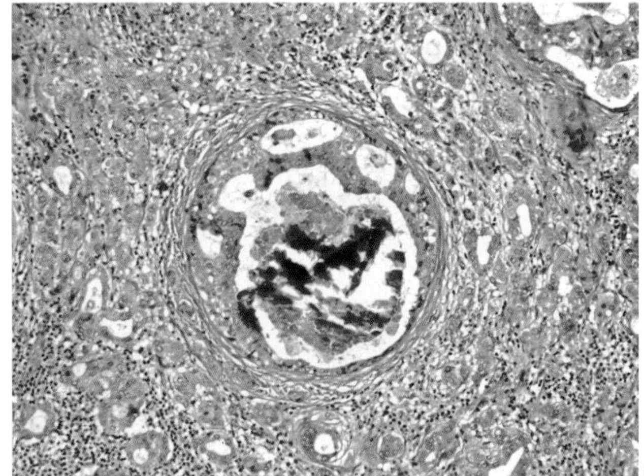

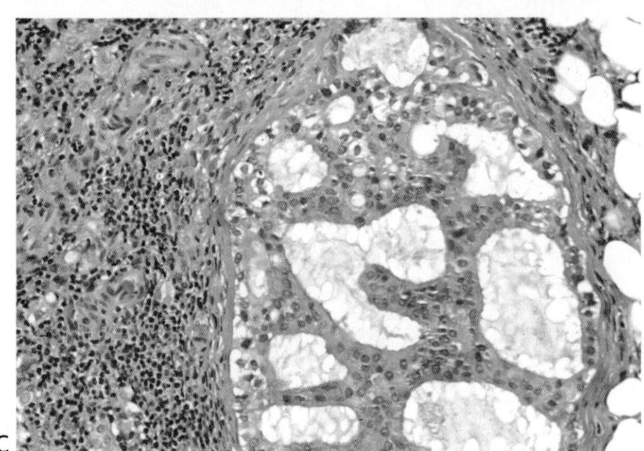

FIG. 33.18. ***Axillary nodal metastases that resemble intraductal carcinoma.*** All images are from cases of occult carcinoma presenting as axillary nodal metastases. **A:** Round, "solid" aggregates of metastatic ductal carcinoma. **B:** Necrosis and calcification in intraductal-like metastatic carcinoma. **C:** Metastatic apocrine cribriform carcinoma with peritumoral fibrosis that resembles a basement membrane.

lymph node obscured by metastatic tumor. Tissue around the tumor should be studied for evidence of axillary breast tissue. If found, this is presumptive evidence in support of an axillary primary, but it is necessary to find *in situ* carcinoma in conjunction with an invasive axillary lesion to establish a diagnosis of carcinoma arising in axillary breast tissue.

Benign lesions that may be associated with ALNs, such as nevus cell aggregates and heterotopic glands, should not be misinterpreted as metastatic carcinoma.[166] For further information about heterotopic mammary tissue in ALNs and nodal nevus cell aggregates, see Chapter 43.

ER and PR have been examined in axillary nodal metastases from patients with occult carcinoma.[129,135,163,167,168] The largest series presented similar results, with 32% to 35% of nodal metastases positive for ER and PR, 24% to 27% positive for ER and negative for PR, and 38% to 44% negative for both receptors.[129,135] Others have also reported that ER and PR were negative in the majority of ALNs analyzed.[136] Lu et al.[151] reported that about one-third of the metastatic carcinomas were triple-negative. The presence of ER is highly suggestive of, but not specific for, mammary carcinoma.

Pathology of the Occult Primary Carcinoma

The primary tumor in more than 90% of cases is a form of usual IDC that is accompanied by intraductal carcinoma in most instances.[149,151] The histologic characteristics of the primary tumor and nodal metastases are similar (Fig. 33.12). A striking characteristic of many of the primary lesions, particularly tumors too small to be palpable, is a prominent lymphocytic reaction in and around the lesion[133,138] (Figs. 33.13, 33.14, and 33.20). This is especially conspicuous when the primary lesion appeared to be largely or entirely *in situ*.

An exceptionally high proportion of the occult primary duct carcinomas have apocrine cytology, and there is a tendency for cytoplasmic clearing in the primary lesions as well as in the metastases (Figs. 33.12 and 33.13). The invasive carcinomas tend to be poorly differentiated histologically and cytologically. The data presented in Table 33.2 show some cases in which the only carcinoma detected in the breast appeared to be noninvasive. This phenomenon has been described in several studies.[131,140,167,169] It is thought that metastases in these cases arose from invasive carcinoma that was inapparent with the light microscope amid the *in situ*

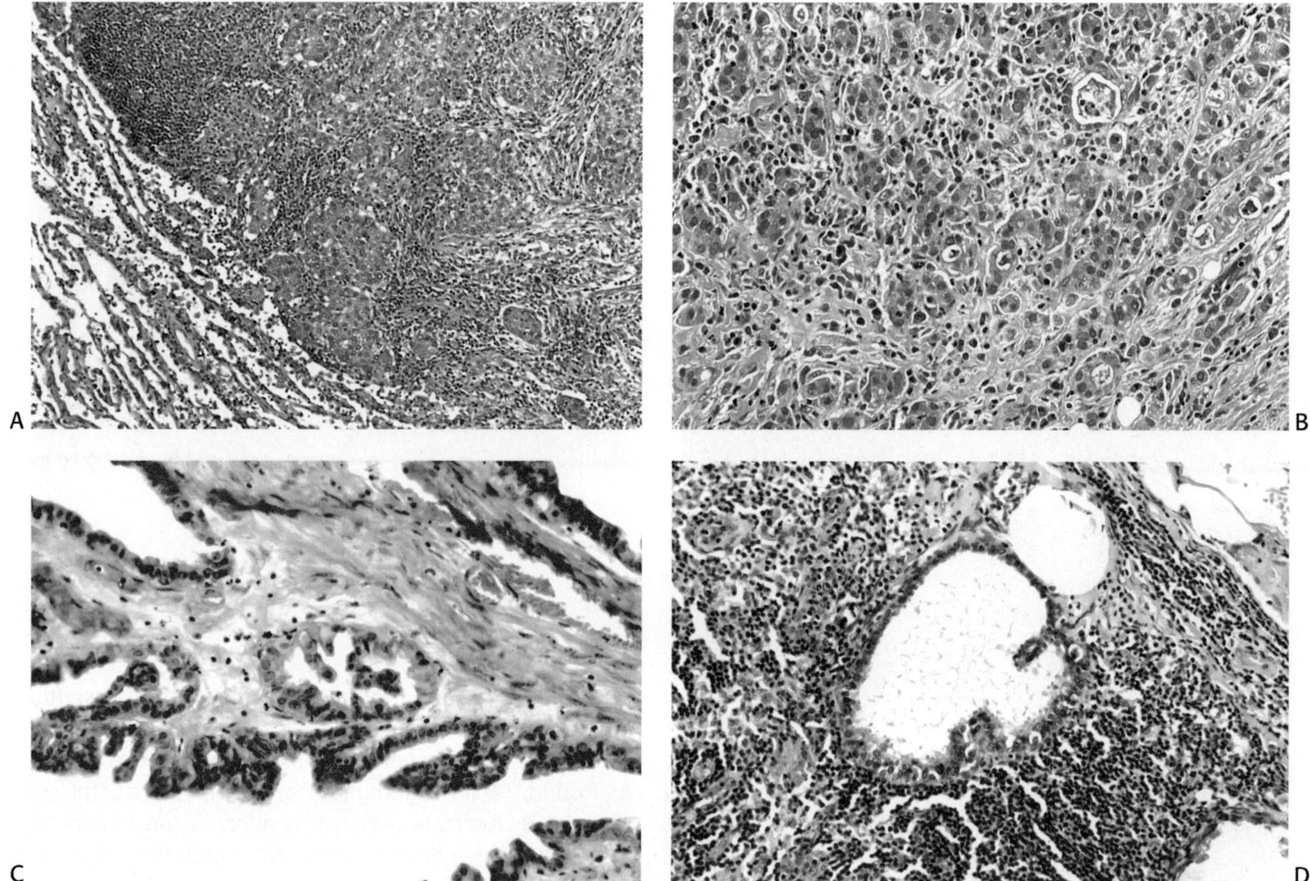

FIG. 33.19. *Metastatic nonmammary carcinoma.* **A:** Poorly differentiated adenocarcinoma of the lung. **B:** Metastatic pulmonary carcinoma in an ALN. **C,D:** Serous ovarian carcinoma (**C**) metastatic in an ALN (**D**).

lesion[130,131,138,168,169] or from foci of "healed" invasive carcinoma (Fig. 33.18). Infrequent examples of infiltrating lobular,[130,131] medullary,[138,154,163,170] mucinous,[130] tubular,[138,149] and papillary,[130] and invasive micropapillary[151] carcinoma have been described. Analysis of hormone receptors in one series of primary tumors revealed positive levels of ER in 4 (36%) of 11 cases and of PR in 4 (44%) of 9.[138]

Treatment

In 1907, Halsted reported that up to 2 years might elapse before a primary tumor became clinically apparent in the breast if the patient did not undergo a biopsy or mastectomy.[171] A more recent series included 17 patients with an untreated ipsilateral breast and a negative mammogram.[138] Nine (52%) developed a clinically apparent primary tumor within 2 to 34 months (mean, 13 months). Two of the remaining eight patients died of progressive systemic disease without manifesting a mammary primary, and six remained disease free, with an average follow-up of 6 years. Another report included 13 patients who did not have breast surgery or radiotherapy.[137] Seven women (54%) developed a clinically evident primary tumor in the ipsilateral breast 11 to 47 months after diagnosis of the axillary metastasis (average, 27 months). Three of the carcinomas were in the upper outer quadrant, and two were in the upper inner quadrant. One lesion was subareolar, and diffuse involvement was observed in the seventh woman. Others have observed a subsequent primary tumor in the untreated breast in 2 (13%) of 15,[171] 1 (20%) of 5,[172] and 7 (88%) of 8[173,174] patients after average follow-up of 7.7, 2.2, and 3.5 years, respectively.

Currently after it has been determined that an excised lymph node contains metastatic adenocarcinoma consistent with mammary origin in the absence of clinical evidence of a nonmammary tumor, treatment should be based on the assumption that there is an invasive primary carcinoma in the ipsilateral breast.

A survey of 776 members of the American Society of Breast Surgeons published in 2005 revealed the following preferred treatment options: mastectomy, 43%; whole-breast radiation, 37%; and other, 22%.[175] The "other" category included observation until a primary lesion became evident, deference to patient choice, or various combinations of treatment involving chemotherapy, axillary dissection, radiation, and mastectomy.

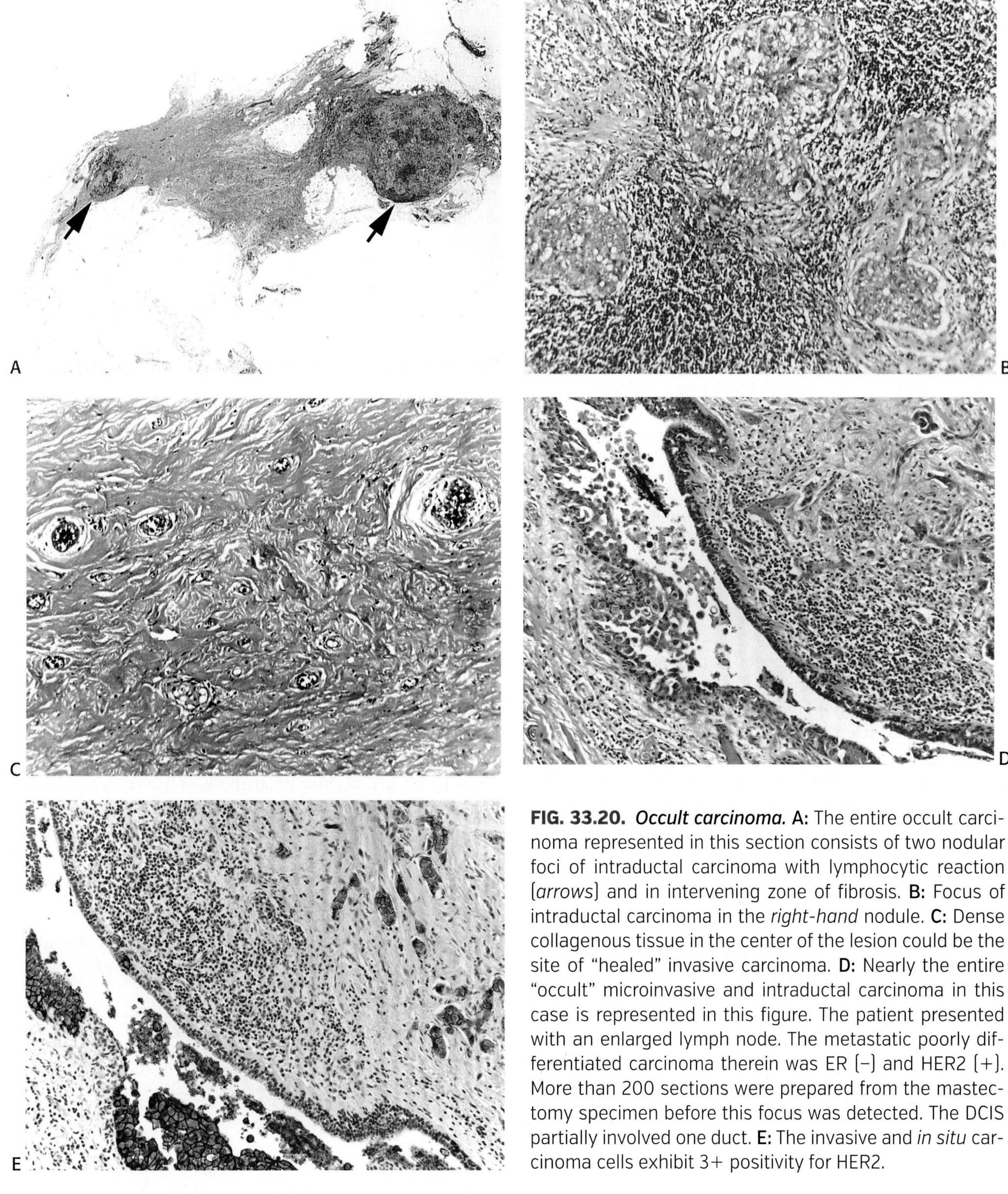

FIG. 33.20. ***Occult carcinoma.*** **A:** The entire occult carcinoma represented in this section consists of two nodular foci of intraductal carcinoma with lymphocytic reaction (*arrows*) and in intervening zone of fibrosis. **B:** Focus of intraductal carcinoma in the *right-hand* nodule. **C:** Dense collagenous tissue in the center of the lesion could be the site of "healed" invasive carcinoma. **D:** Nearly the entire "occult" microinvasive and intraductal carcinoma in this case is represented in this figure. The patient presented with an enlarged lymph node. The metastatic poorly differentiated carcinoma therein was ER (−) and HER2 (+). More than 200 sections were prepared from the mastectomy specimen before this focus was detected. The DCIS partially involved one duct. **E:** The invasive and *in situ* carcinoma cells exhibit 3+ positivity for HER2.

When a localized lesion has been detected and excised from the breast, the patient may be a candidate for breast conservation coupled with axillary dissection and breast irradiation.[129,144,148,176] Radiation may be given to the breast and axilla after the diagnosis of carcinoma was established by excisional or needle biopsy of an enlarged ALN if a primary lesion is not detected in the breast.[132,144,170] The 5-year DFS reported with the latter approach varied from 66% to

TABLE 33.2 Primary Carcinomas Found in Breast

	No. (%)*
Invasive	22 (79)
Invasive duct	(65)
Invasive lobular	(6)
Medullary	(6)
Colloid	(3)
Noninvasive	7 (21)
Intraductal	(12)
In situ lobular	(6)
Intraductal and *in situ* lobular	(3)

Adapted from Rosen PP, Kimmel M. Occult breast carcinoma presenting with axillary lymph node metastases: a follow-up study of 48 patients. *Hum Pathol* 1990;21:518–523. *Percentages rounded.

76%.[132,138,170,177,178] A primary tumor was detected clinically during follow-up in the ipsilateral breast of 7% to 33% of these patients.

Prognosis

The first large series of patients with occult breast carcinoma presenting as axillary nodal metastases with follow-up from a single institution, the Mayo Clinic, was published in 1954.[174] This article included the first reported example of this condition in a man. Follow-up of 25 patients revealed that 9 patients (36%) died of breast carcinoma, 3 (12%) died of other causes, and 13 (52%) remained well. The authors concluded that these patients had "a better prognosis than is observed for the average carcinoma of the breast with nodal metastasis."

Several later studies also described a relatively favorable clinical course for patients treated by mastectomy and axillary dissection. Patel et al.[134] reported that 29% of patients died of disease, suggesting that the "prognosis is as good as or better than it is for palpable breast cancer with axillary metastases." Two follow-up studies from Memorial Hospital in New York reported that 23%[129] and 25%[135] of patients died of breast carcinoma. In reports based on smaller series, 9%[131] and 12%[133] of patients had recurrent carcinoma and/or died of breast carcinoma.

Survival results for a series of 48 patients are shown in Table 33.3.[135] Follow-up ranged from 5 to 267 months (mean, 71; median, 60). Among patients alive and disease free, follow-up ranged from 33 to 367 months (median, 64 months; mean, 73 months). The intervals between diagnosis of breast carcinoma and the deaths of two patients of causes other than mammary carcinoma were 91 and 204 months. Two other patients surviving with recurrent carcinoma were alive 53 to 166 months after the original diagnosis of carcinoma in an ALN. Patients who died of metastatic carcinoma survived 5 to 68 months (median, 26 months; mean, 31 months). Overall, 29 of the 48 patients (60%) remained alive and disease free. Two women (4%) died of causes other than mammary carcinoma, and the status of 2 patients (4%) was unknown. Recurrences occurred in 15 cases (31%), including 12 patients (25%) who died of metastatic breast carcinoma. There was not a statistically significant difference in the frequency of recurrence or of death due to breast carcinoma between patients with one to three positive lymph nodes and those with four or more affected nodes, although the recurrence rate was higher in the latter group.

Twenty-two of the patients in the preceding study found to have a measurable primary tumor at mastectomy were chosen for a case-control analysis of survival.[135] Matching was based on tumor size (±0.5 cm in T category), total number of involved lymph nodes (one to three vs. four or more, selected for closest total count), tumor type, and age at diagnosis. All patients were treated by mastectomy, and

TABLE 33.3 Follow-up of Patients with Occult Breast Carcinoma

		Number of Involved Lymph Nodes[a]		
	Total Patients	One to Three	Four or More	Unknown
Status	# (%)*	# (%)	# (%)	# (%)
NED	29 (60)	12 (60)	14 (70)	3 (38)
AWD	3 (6)	1 (5)	1 (5)	1 (12)
DOD	12 (25)	5 (25)	4 (20)	3 (38)
DOC	2 (4)	1 (5)	1 (5)	0 0)
UNK	2 (4)	1 (5)	0 (0)	1 (12)
Total	48	20	20	8

NED, alive, no evidence of disease; AWD, alive with disease; DOC, dead of other causes; UNK, unknown; DOD, dead of disease.
[a]Includes lymph node(s) removed for diagnosis and those obtained by axillary dissection.*Percentages rounded.
Based on Rosen PP, Kimmel M. Occult breast carcinoma presenting with axillary lymph node metastases: a follow-up study of 48 patients. *Hum Pathol* 1990;21:518–523.

TABLE 33.4 Follow-up of Matched Patients with Occult and Palpable Breast Carcinomas

	Number of Lymph Nodes with Metastases					
	Total		One to Three		Four or More	
Patient Status	Occult (%)	Palpable (%)	Occult (%)	Palpable (%)	Occult (%)	Palpable (%)
NED	16 (73)	15 (36)	9 (75)	9 (38)	7 (70)	6 (33)
AWD	1 (5)	4 (10)	1 (8)	3 (13)	0 (0)	1 (6)
DOD	5 (23)	18 (43)	2 (17)	7 (29)	3 (30)	11 (61)
DOC	0 (0)	5 (12)	0 (0)	5 (21)	0 (0)	0 (0)
Total	22	42	12	24	10	18

From Rosen PP, Kimmel M. Occult breast carcinoma presenting with axillary lymph node metastases: a follow-up study of 48 patients. *Hum Pathol* 1990;21:518–523. Percentages rounded

almost all patients in both groups received systemic adjuvant chemotherapy. The distributions of primary tumor size and of axillary nodal involvement in the two groups were very similar. A comparison of follow-up results revealed a lower frequency of recurrence and death due to breast carcinoma among patients who presented with axillary metastases and an occult primary tumor (Table 33.4). Survival curve analysis for the two groups is shown in Figure 33.21. Although patients with occult lesions exhibited a more favorable prognosis overall, as well as when stratified by tumor size and nodal status, the differences were not statistically significant (Figs. 33.22 and 33.23). These survival results in stage II patients who presented with nodal metastases and an occult primary are striking. Although there was no statistically significantly difference, patients with palpable breast tumors had a less favorable outcome despite similar treatment, which included chemotherapy for both groups.

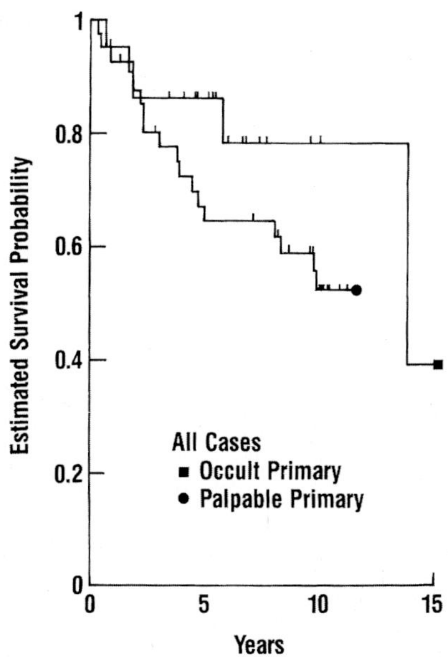

FIG. 33.21. ***Occult carcinoma, overall survival.*** Kaplan-Meier survival rate comparison of patients with clinically occult primary tumors to stage-matched patients who presented with a palpable breast tumor. Patients with clinically unapparent (occult) primary tumors had a more favorable survival, but the difference was not statistically significant. (Reproduced with permission from Rosen PP, Kimmel M. Occult breast carcinoma presenting with ALN metastases: a follow-up study of 48 patients. *Hum Pathol* 1990;21:518–523. Copyright W.B. Saunders Co.)

Four other studies also provided survival curve analyses of patients with occult stage II carcinoma.[129,134,137,138] In a series of 29 women, the 5- and 10-year DFS rates were 28% and 17%, respectively.[134] These authors reported similar results for a comparison group of 127 patients who presented with palpable mammary primary tumors, but gave no indication as to how patients with "known" breast carcinoma were chosen. Their patients with occult carcinoma did not have substantially larger primary tumors or more numerous involved lymph nodes than have been reported in other recent series, and the data provide no other obvious explanation for the unusually poor survival rate of stage II patients in both groups. Baron et al.[129] carried out a survival analysis of 35 patients and found that 63% were alive disease free. Their study did not include a matched series of women who presented with palpable breast tumors.

Ellerbroek et al.[137] reported an OS rate of 71.8% at 5 years and 65% at 10 years. This study included two features found to be significantly associated with 5-year survival: axillary dissection (performed, 88.9% survival; not performed, 46.7% survival) and gross residual tumor in axilla after surgery (absent, 79.9% survival; present, 20% survival). In this study, there was not a statistically significant difference in survival between patients treated by mastectomy and those treated by breast conservation. Although patients who received adjuvant chemotherapy had a better 5-year survival (92.9%) than those who did not receive systemic treatment (63.5%), the difference was not statistically significant.

Survival rates at 5 and 10 years reported by Merson et al.[138] were 76.6% and 58.3%, respectively. There was a trend to a more favorable prognosis if metastases involved not more than three ALNs when compared with women with four or more nodal metastases, but the difference was

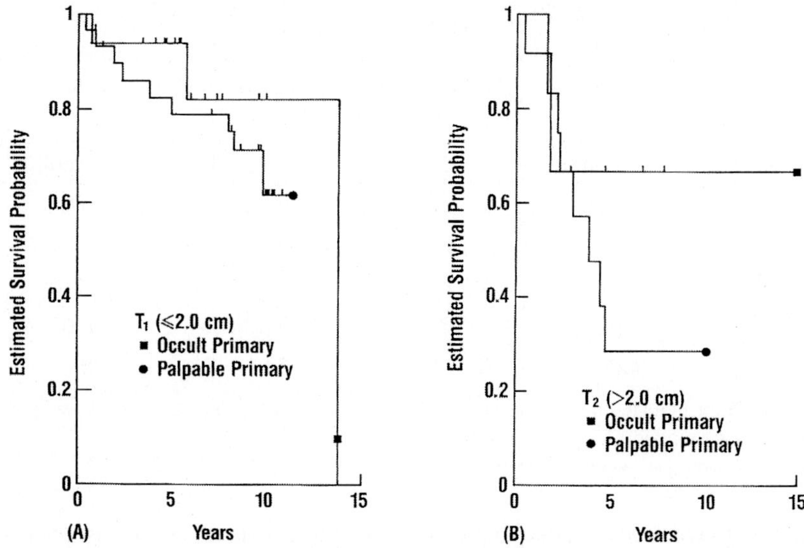

FIG. 33.22. ***Occult carcinoma, tumor size and survival.*** Kaplan–Meier survival rate comparison of matched patients stratified by primary tumor size. The differences are not statistically significant; (*left*) T1 tumors, (*right*) T2 tumors. (Reproduced with permission from Rosen PP, Kimmel M. Occult breast carcinoma presenting with ALN metastases: a follow-up study of 48 patients. *Hum Pathol* 1990;21:518–523. Copyright W.B. Saunders Co.)

not statistically significant. Prognosis also appeared to be better in the group that underwent mastectomy or breast irradiation when compared with patients who had no treatment of the breast ($p = 0.06$). Adjuvant systemic therapy did not significantly influence survival. Read et al.[170] also reported a lower frequency of local breast recurrence and a lower systemic recurrence rate in women with three or fewer nodal metastases after breast irradiation and axillary dissection. In this latter series, DFS was higher in the group that received systemic adjuvant therapy, but the difference from untreated patients was not statistically significant.

Several studies have compared the outcomes of patients with occult breast carcinoma treated by mastectomy with those who had breast preservation and radiation.[129,137,138] Survival rates did not differ significantly for the two treatment groups. Breast recurrences have been reported in 19% and 23% of patients treated with mammary radiation.[132,137] In one of these reports the intervals between the diagnosis of the axillary metastasis and the detection of the primary breast carcinoma were 8, 44, and 106 months.[137] In a recently published study, 31 occult breast carcinomas that were ER negative, PR-negative and HER2-negative (so-called "triple-negative" carcinomas) had the highest risk of recurrence and death in a series of 80 patients treated at the European Institute of Oncology.[179]

In conclusion, available data indicate that patients with stage II disease who present with an axillary nodal metastasis and an inapparent breast primary have a prognosis similar to and possibly better than that of patients with stage II disease who present with a palpable breast carcinoma. This probably reflects the fact that the majority of the stage II patients with clinically and, in some cases, radiographically occult carcinomas prove to have relatively small invasive tumors detected in their breast by imaging studies or on pathologic examination of a surgical specimen. The actual pathologically determined tumor (size), regional node (involvement), (distant) metastases (TNM) stage is probably a more important determinant of prognosis than the apparent clinical stage when the patient is first examined. MRI imaging is very useful for detecting an occult primary carcinoma in the breast if none is evident on mammography.

Two cases of occult breast carcinomas manifesting as ALN metastases in men have been reported.[180]

CARCINOMA IN ECTOPIC BREAST TISSUE

Ectopic breast tissue is subject to various proliferative and nonproliferative changes that occur in the mammary gland proper.[181,182] "Adenomas" have been described in ectopic breast tissue, most commonly in the axilla[183] and vulva.[184,185] These lesions develop for the most part during pregnancy or lactation, and represent nodules of lactational hyperplasia that assume an adenomatous form.[186] The tumors measured from 1.0 to 6.0 cm. Bilateral vulvar FA have been reported.[185] Patients with vulvar FA have generally been between 20 and 50 years of age. A benign PT that originated in vulvar mammary tissue has been described in a 20-year-old woman.[187] PT of anogenital mammary-like glands in a 41-year-old male, presenting with anal bleeding, has been described.[188] Breast tissue surrounding the tumor showed fibrocystic changes, including apocrine metaplasia and papillomatosis. The lesion recurred locally 8 months after excisional biopsy.

Carcinoma has been described arising in axillary[182,189–190] and vulvar[189–195] breast tissue. Intra et al.[195] described a woman with synchronous intraductal carcinoma in the breast and

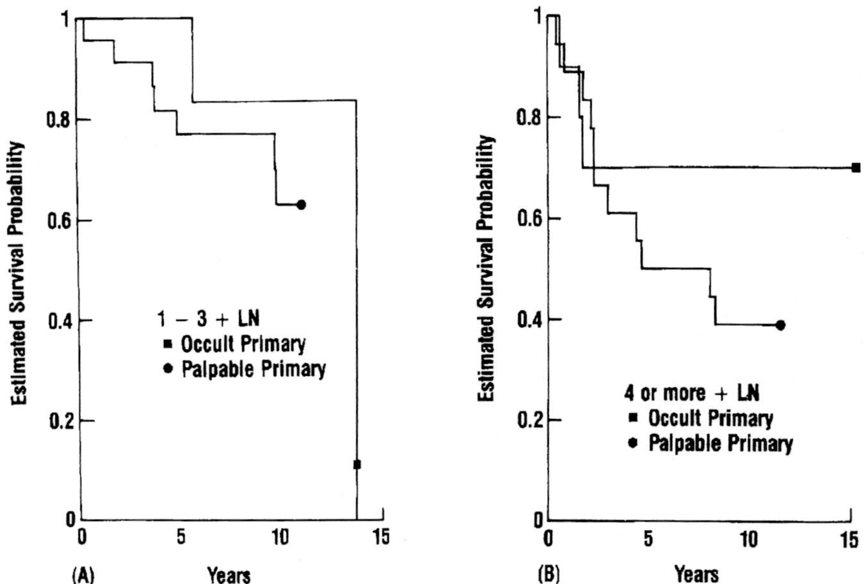

FIG. 33.23. *Occult carcinoma, lymph node status and survival.* Kaplan-Meier survival rate comparison of patients stratified for the number of involved lymph nodes. The differences are not statistically significant; (*left*) one to three positive nodes, (*right*) four or more positive nodes. (Reproduced with permission from Rosen PP, Kimmel M. Occult breast carcinoma presenting with ALN metastases: a follow-up study of 48 patients. *Hum Pathol* 1990;21:518–523. Copyright W.B. Saunders Co.)

IDC that arose in ectopic vulvar mammary tissue. A woman reported by Guerry et al.[193] had asynchronous bilateral mammary carcinomas and a separate primary mammary-type adenocarcinoma that arose in ectopic vulvar breast tissue. Goyal et al.[196] described a patient with a history of locally advanced disease because of an axillary mass thought clinically to be nodal metastases that proved to be benign axillary breast tissue. Breast carcinoma has been reported in a patient with a history of familial functional axillary breast tissue.[197]

The most frequent site of ectopic breast tissue is in the axilla, mainly affecting women 40 years of age or older (28 to 90 years).[198] Separate primary carcinomas arising concurrently in ectopic axillary breast tissue and in the ipsilateral breast are an extremely unusual coincidence.[199] Anterior chest wall locations include the parasternal, subclavicular, and inframammary locations.[199-201] In one case, a 46-year-old woman was found to have a 1.2-cm E-cadherin–negative ER-positive infiltrating pleomorphic lobular carcinoma that arose in ectopic breast tissue on the inframammary anterior chest wall.[201] ALN mapping yielded metastatic carcinoma in a SLN with extranodal extension. No carcinoma was clinically evident in either breast. Carcinoma originating in ectopic breast tissue has been described in the subclavicular and anterior axillary regions, over the sternum, and in the upper abdominal skin outside the distribution of the milk lines.[202-204]

Histologically, most adenocarcinomas arising in ectopic breast tissue have had a ductal growth pattern. Infrequent examples of medullary, papillary,[202] and infiltrating lobular carcinoma have been reported (Fig. 33.24).[199-201] The extraordinary occurrence of secretory carcinoma arising in ectopic breast tissue in an adult patient has been described.[205]

Ectopic breast tissue, especially when located in the axilla, may be distributed in subcutaneous tissue and the deep dermis of the skin (Fig. 33.25). The breast tissue may mingle with normal skin appendage glands rather than forming a discrete, independent structure. In this circumstance it can be difficult to distinguish between carcinoma of mammary and skin appendage gland origin.[206] The diagnosis of carcinoma arising in ectopic axillary breast tissue beyond the usual anatomic extent of the breast can be made if intraductal and/or invasive carcinoma are found in subcutaneous mammary glandular parenchyma beyond the normal extent of the breast.

The distinction between breast tissue remaining after mastectomy and ectopic breast tissue depends largely upon location. Residual breast tissue, not necessarily ectopic in its distribution, is a potential source for a new primary carcinoma on the chest wall after mastectomy.[207,208] The presence of noncarcinomatous breast tissue and/or an *in situ* component will distinguish such a new primary from a conventional cutaneous local recurrence. It is essential that a lesion labeled clinically as a "local recurrence" at the site of a prior mastectomy be carefully examined histologically for evidence of residual breast tissue and *in situ* carcinoma (Fig. 33.26). The presence of the latter features indicates that the tumor is probably a new primary carcinoma with a clinical course determined by its specific histologic and biologic properties. Rarely, there may be substantial differences in histologic features between the initial carcinoma

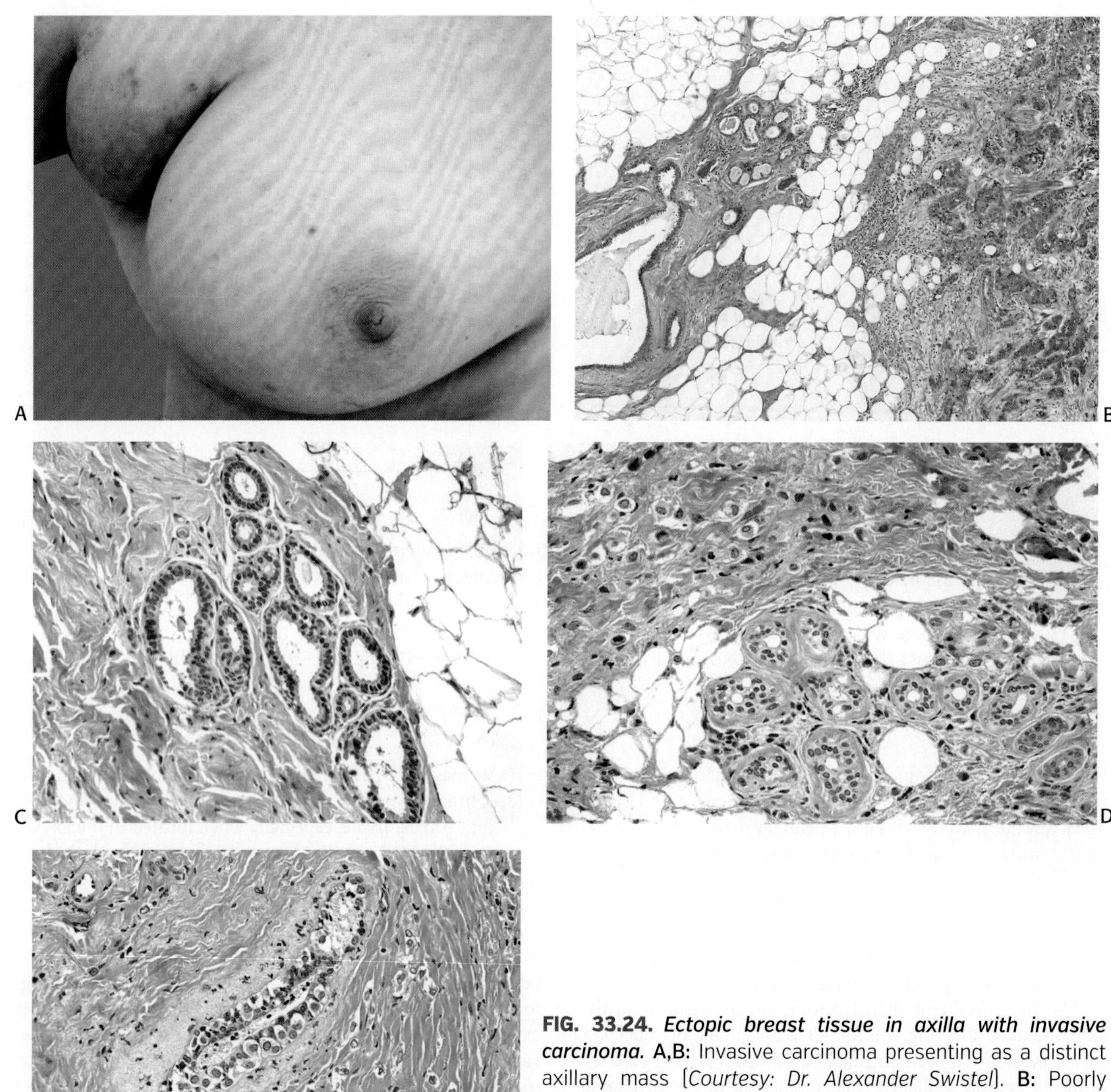

FIG. 33.24. ***Ectopic breast tissue in axilla with invasive carcinoma.*** **A,B:** Invasive carcinoma presenting as a distinct axillary mass (*Courtesy: Dr. Alexander Swistel*). **B:** Poorly differentiated ductal carcinoma in ectopic breast tissue in the axilla. **C–E:** These images are from a single axillary tumor. **C:** A normal lobule in axillary breast tissue. **D:** ILC in axillary tissue above a lobule. **E:** Pagetoid LCIS in a duct surrounded by ILC.

and the new primary tumor that arises in residual breast tissue (Fig. 33.27).

Surgical treatment for ectopic invasive mammary carcinomas is wide local excision and regional lymphadenectomy. Metastases from mammary-type carcinomas that arose in ectopic breast tissue have been reported in ipsilateral axillary[189] and groin lymph nodes.[192,195] SLN biopsy has been successfully performed in such situations.[201] The choice of the lymph node group most likely to be involved by metastases may be difficult if, for example, the lesion is located over the sternum or the upper abdomen.[209] Mastectomy is not indicated if origin in ectopic axillary breast tissue can be documented and there is no evidence of a separate primary tumor in the breast. Vulvar lesions are managed by partial vulvectomy with SLN sampling and/or ipsilateral groin dissection. Many of these tumors have had an aggressive clinical course, with systemic metastases reported to have arisen from axillary and vulvar lesions.[195] Adjuvant treatment with tamoxifen[191,192] or

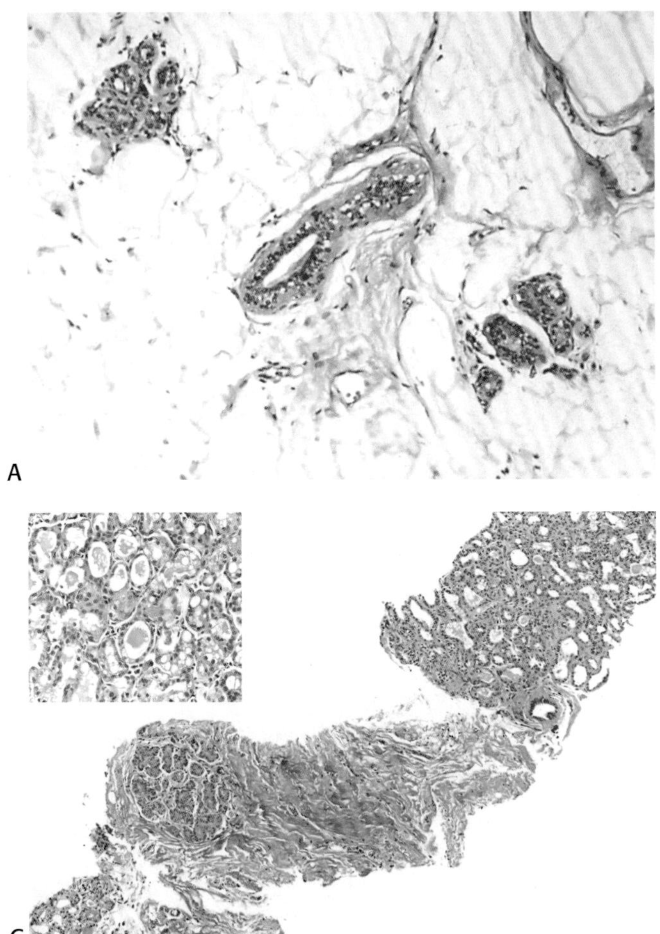

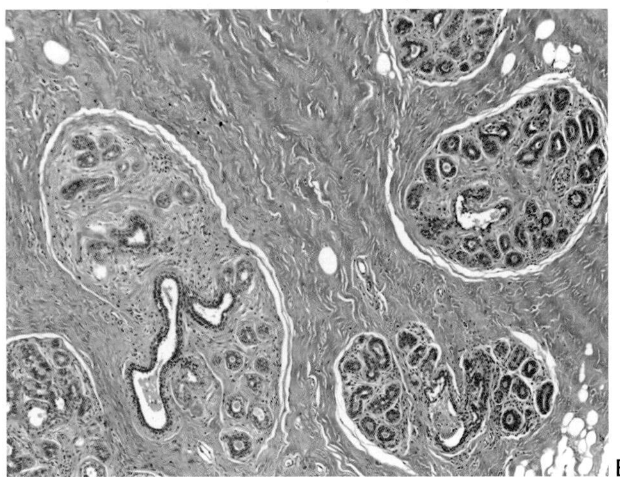

FIG. 33.25. ***Ectopic breast tissue in axilla.*** **A:** A mammary duct and lobular glands found in the adipose tissue of an ALN dissection. **B:** Sclerosing lobular hyperplasia involving ectopic axillary breast tissue. **C:** Lactational hyperplasia seen in a needle core biopsy of a "high" axillary mass in a woman in the second trimester of pregnancy. Lactational change is present (*inset*).

radiotherapy[201] has been reported. The use of chemotherapy will depend on the stage of the carcinoma.

Breast tissue in a teratoma is a potential site for occult mammary carcinoma (Fig. 33.28). Extramammary Paget disease has been described in ovarian and retroperitoneal teratomas,[210–212] including one with invasive carcinoma.[213]

The cytologic diagnosis of carcinoma arising in ectopic breast tissue has been reported[214–218]; however, the unequivocal diagnosis of a primary carcinoma arising in ectopic breast tissue can be made only if there is histologic confirmation of intraductal carcinoma and benign mammary glandular parenchyma beyond the normal extent of the breast

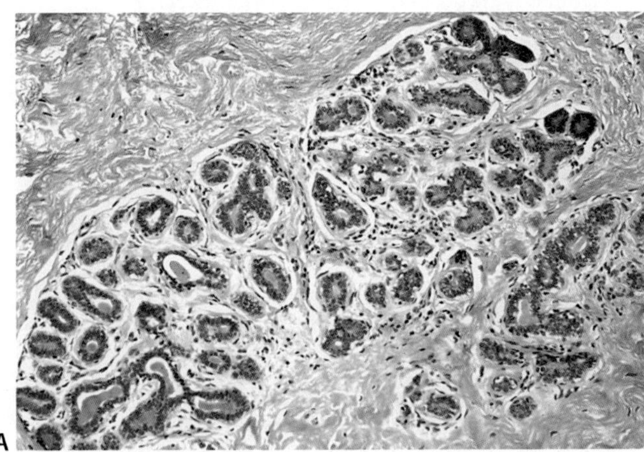

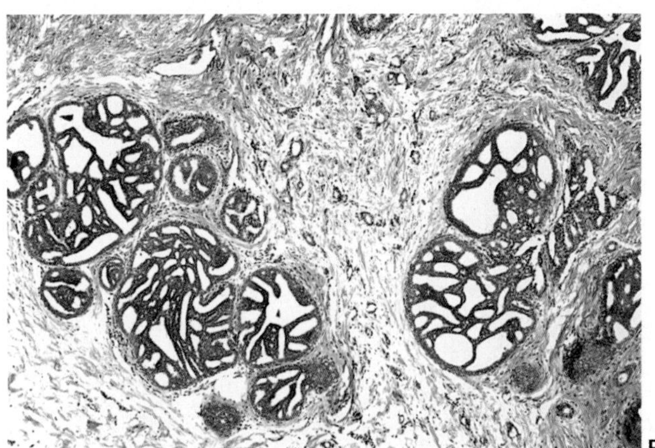

FIG. 33.26. ***Residual breast tissue with carcinoma after mastectomy.*** **A:** Residual breast tissue in the chest wall 8 years after a mastectomy. **B:** A mass at this site contained cribriform intraductal carcinoma and invasive well-differentiated ductal carcinoma.

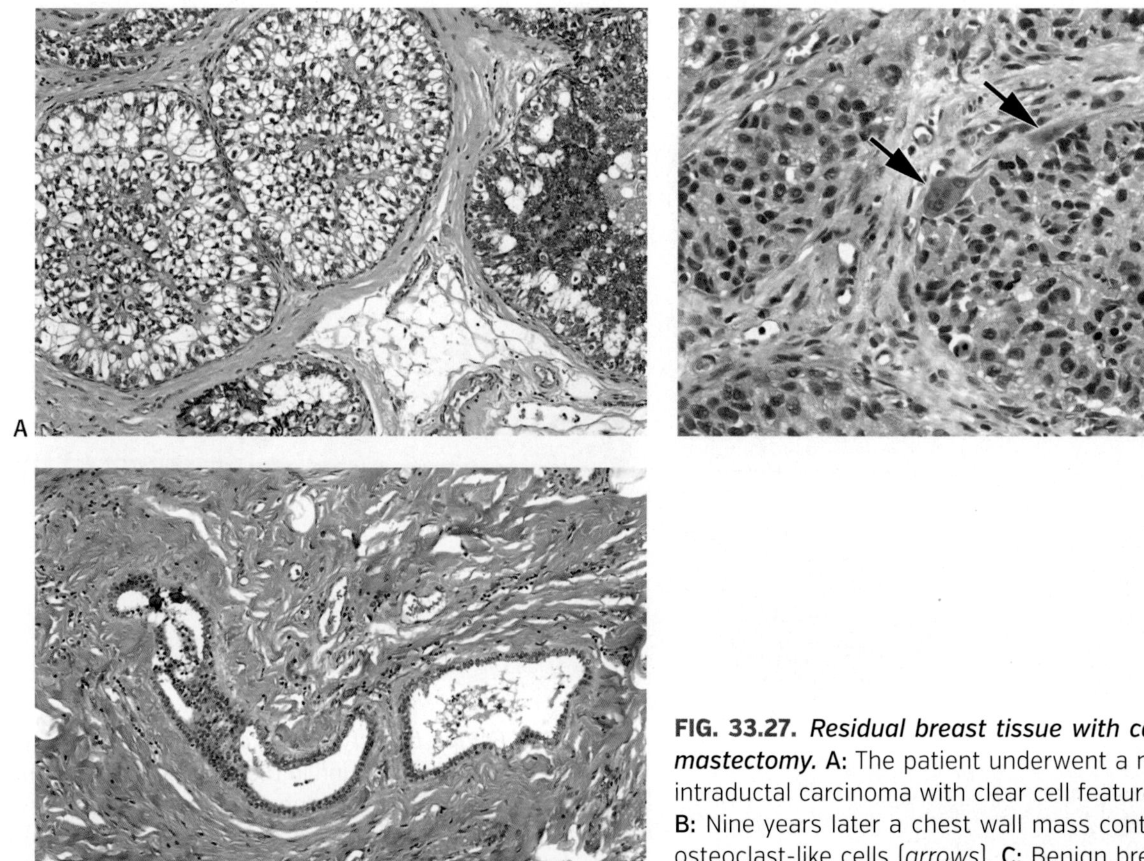

FIG. 33.27. ***Residual breast tissue with carcinoma after mastectomy.*** **A:** The patient underwent a mastectomy for intraductal carcinoma with clear cell features shown here. **B:** Nine years later a chest wall mass contained IDC with osteoclast-like cells (*arrows*). **C:** Benign breast tissue was also present.

(Fig. 33.29). In addition to carcinoma arising in ectopic breast tissue, the differential diagnosis of a FNA specimen containing atypical epithelial cells obtained from an axillary mass includes a proliferative lesion in ectopic breast and metastatic carcinoma. Proliferative epithelium is most likely to be encountered when ectopic breast tissue enlarges during pregnancy or in rare instances of fibroepithelial neoplasms arising from such tissue.[216] One unusual case in which the diagnosis was made by FNA involved a 45-year-old woman with a 3.0-cm subcutaneous lesion on the submammary

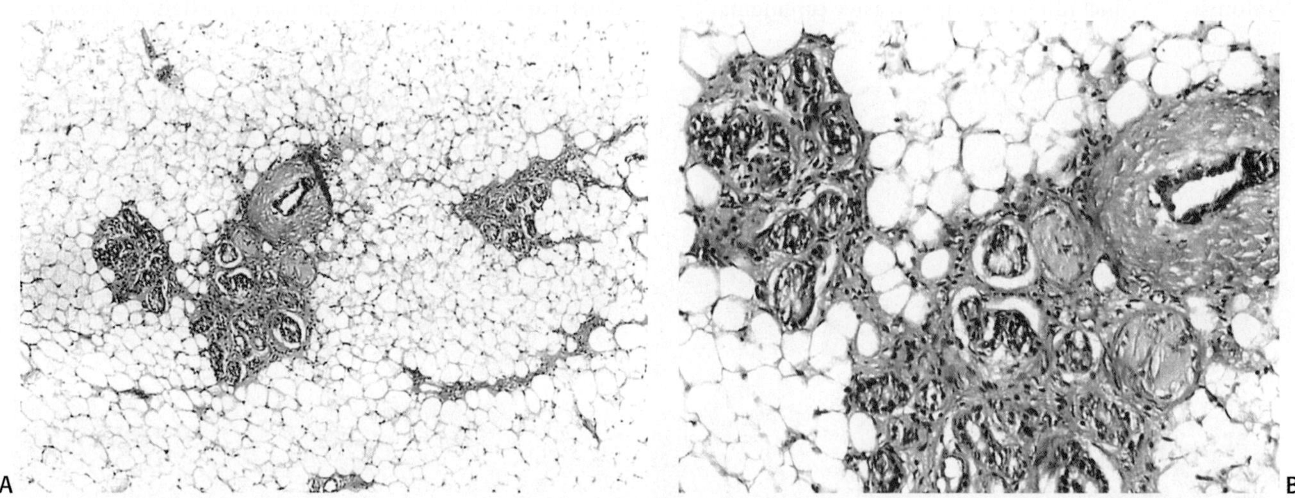

FIG. 33.28. ***Breast tissue in a mediastinal teratoma.*** **A:** A duct and atrophic lobular glands in fat. **B:** Magnified view of (**A**).

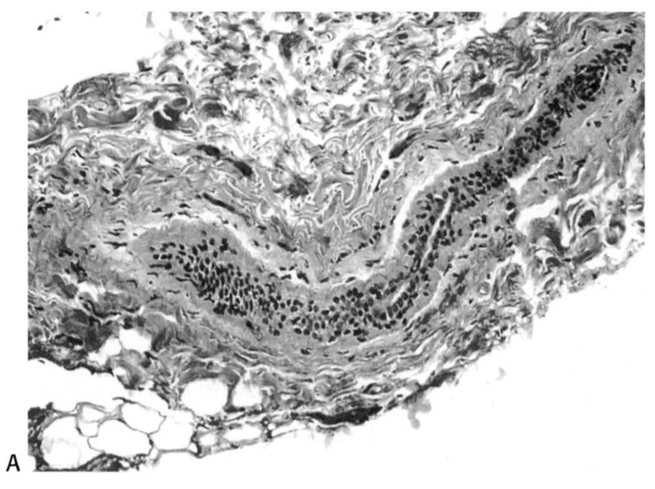

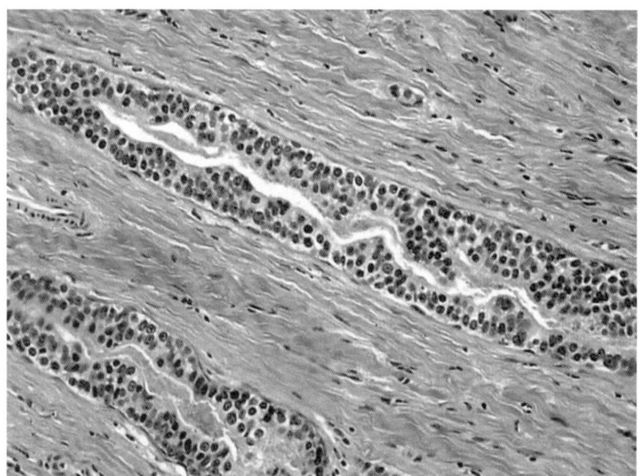

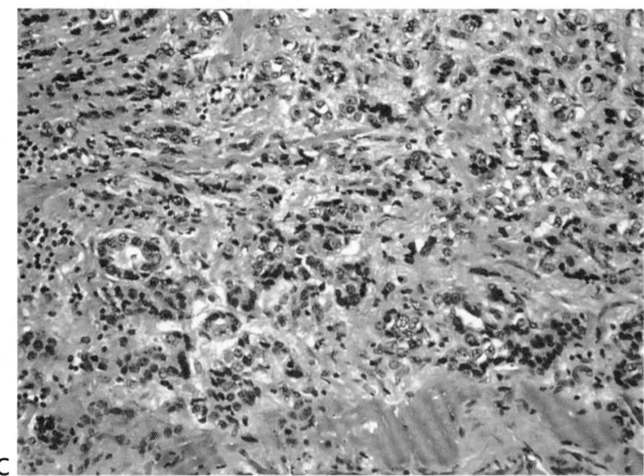

FIG. 33.29. ***Aberrant breast tissue.*** **A:** A mammary duct in the subcutaneous tissue around a carcinoma excised from the upper abdominal wall below the inframammary fold. **B:** Intraductal carcinoma in the same specimen. **C:** Infiltrating ductal carcinoma.

chest wall.[217] Excisional biopsy confirmed the presence of infiltrating duct carcinoma that arose in ectopic breast tissue.

Benign glandular inclusions in ALNs can mimic carcinoma. This topic is considered in detail in Chapter 43.

INFLAMMATORY CARCINOMA

In 1807, Charles Bell reported that "when a purple color is on the skin over the tumor it is a very unpropitious beginning."[219] This is said to be the first clinical reference to inflammatory carcinoma. Lee and Tannenbaum[220] proposed the currently used term *inflammatory carcinoma* in 1924. In the latest American Joint Committee on Cancer (AJCC) Staging System, inflammatory breast carcinoma (IBC) is defined as "a clinical and pathological entity characterized by erythema and edema involving a third or more of the skin of the breast," and is classified as T4d.[221] IBC is not a specific histologic subtype of mammary carcinoma. However, some investigators have included histopathologic findings among their diagnostic criteria.

An assessment of the frequency of this uncommon condition depends largely on clinical reporting, but IBC is generally thought to account for not more than 2.5% of all breast carcinoma cases.[222] In institutional series, the frequency of IBC reportedly varies from 1% to 10%, depending upon diagnostic criteria and also upon the nature of the institution. Patients with this condition are often referred to tertiary treatment centers where they constitute a relatively higher proportion of patients than would be encountered in general clinical practice. IBC has been reported to be more common in African Americans than in whites irrespective of whether clinical or histopathologic diagnostic criteria are used.[223-226] However, recent Surveillance, Epidemiology and End Results (SEER) data suggest that African American women are generally susceptible to more aggressive forms of breast carcinoma, but not to IBC.[227] The disease was originally thought to be prevalent in Tunisia until a review revealed that ulcerated breast carcinomas had been included in the category of IBC,[228] exemplifying the importance of applying appropriate diagnostic criteria to characterize this disease.

The age distribution of primary IBC is not significantly different from that of common infiltrating duct carcinoma, averaging about 55 years. It is only rarely encountered in children[229,230] and men.[231] Pregnancy and lactation do not predispose to the clinical presentation of IBC, although breast carcinomas that arise in this setting are prone to have lymphatic tumor emboli in the breast parenchyma.[232,233]

Clinical Features

IBC is primarily a clinical diagnosis characterized by erythema of the mammary skin (Fig. 33.30). Typically, the skin is thickened, especially at the edge of the erysipeloid area, with *peau d'orange* changes that are usually more conspicuous over dependent portions of the breast.[234–236] The cutaneous changes are due to lymphedema initiated by tumor emboli within dermal lymphatic channels. These changes may extend to the skin of the chest wall (Fig. 33.31). In advanced cases, the breast is diffusely indurated or a mass can be palpated centrally, but the lesion may not be palpable in earlier stages of the disease.[237] Mammography usually demonstrates skin thickening, and within the breast there may be a mass or diffusely increased parenchymal density.[238–241] However, cutaneous edema is not a specific radiologic feature of inflammatory carcinoma.[236,242] Calcifications may be present in the parenchymal tumor. Skin thickening, mass lesions, axillary lymphadenopathy, and other abnormalities may be evident on ultrasound examination of the patient with inflammatory carcinoma.[241] Positron emission tomography with computerized tomography (PET-CT) and MRI have proven to be particularly effective for the diagnosis of IBC.[243,244]

Cutaneous erythema is sometimes localized to the region overlying a palpable tumor. Detection of a mass may precede the appearance of the skin change. Despite Haagensen's original requirement that the lesion involve at least one-third of the mammary skin to qualify as IBC[232]—a definition still used in the latest AJCC-TNM guidelines[221]—it has been noted that the prognosis of patients with less extensive cutaneous changes may be just as grave as that of women with classical inflammatory carcinoma.[245] According to current guidelines, the "rare case that exhibits all the features of inflammatory breast carcinoma, but in which skin changes involve less than one-third of the skin, should be classified as T4b or T4c."[221] Patients with IBC tend to be younger than women with locally advanced carcinoma without an inflammatory component, and their tumors are more likely to be ER negative.[226,245–247] A substantial number of patients with IBC present with enlarged regional lymph nodes.[234] IBC may be mistaken for a non-neoplastic inflammatory condition because of its rapid onset and the main symptom of pain.[220] Diffuse leukemic or lymphomatous involvement of the breast may simulate inflammatory carcinoma.

Immunohistochemistry and Molecular Studies

The primary tumor of IBC has been negative for ER and PR in up to 83% of cases.[246,248–251] HER2 overexpression was found significantly more often in inflammatory (41%) than in noninflammatory (19%) breast carcinomas,[249] and there was a trend toward more frequent amplified expression of HER2/*neu* in cases with negative ER or with positive lymph nodes. In another study, all 22 samples of IBC were immunoreactive for HER2.[248] A transplantable xenograft model of human inflammatory carcinoma displayed the same absence of ER and PR and EGFR as the primary tumor used to develop the xenograft.[252]

Overexpression of p53 occurs in up to 84% of IBC.[253–255] Charafe-Jauffret et al.[256] reported that IBC was characterized by the following immunophenotype: high E-cadherin expression, ER negativity, high MIB1 proliferative index, cytoplasmic MUC-1 (mucin glycoprotein) expression, and HER2 overexpression. If all five features were present, there was a 90.5% chance that a tumor was inflammatory carcinoma. There was a 75% likelihood of this diagnosis when any four of five markers were found. The prognosis for patients with non-IBC that expressed four or five of these markers was not significantly different from the prognosis for patients with IBC.[256]

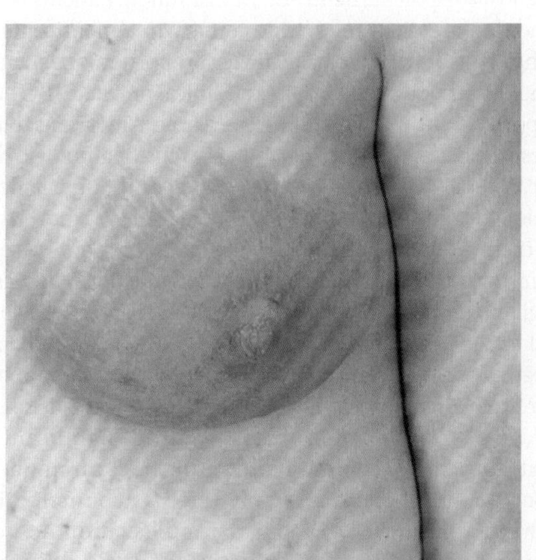

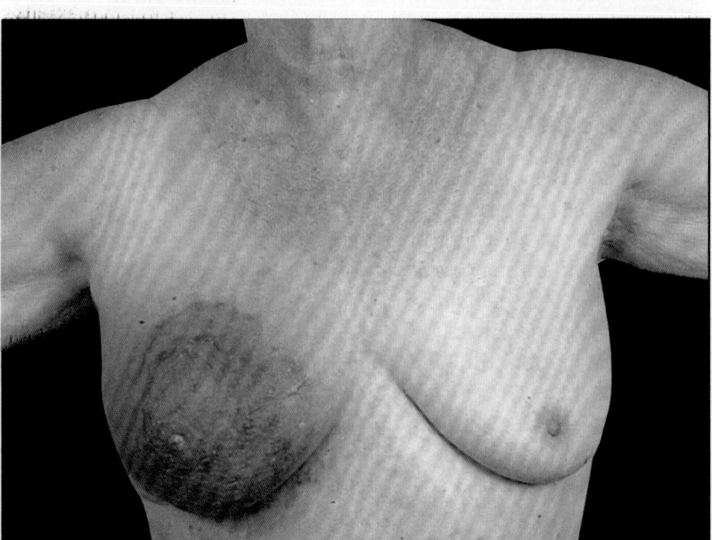

FIG. 33.30. ***Primary inflammatory carcinoma.*** **A:** Cutaneous erythema predominantly over the dependent part of the breast. **B:** Most of the swollen breast is involved, and there is desquamation of the skin.

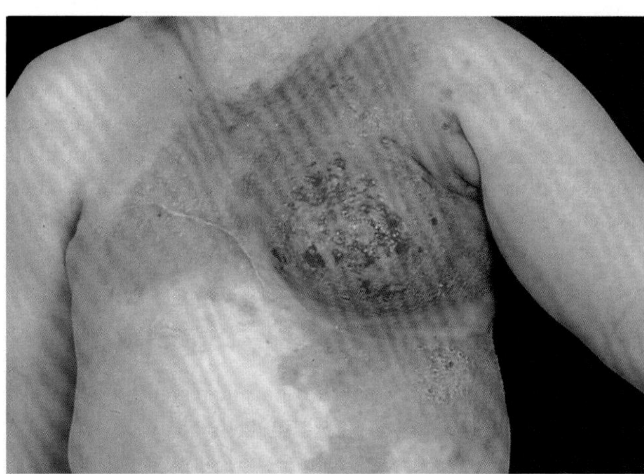

FIG. 33.31. ***Inflammatory carcinoma.*** Spread to the chest wall is evident.

In comparisons of samples from primary IBC before and after neoadjuvant chemotherapy, two groups of investigators found no significant difference in immunohistochemical HER2 expression.[257,258] Overexpression of HER2 was also maintained in metastatic carcinoma foci. Arens et al.[258] also documented the absence of changes in HER2 expression in pre- and posttreatment samples of the primary tumor by fluorescence *in situ* hybridization (FISH) analysis. There were no significant differences in the expression of ER and PR and p53 between pre- and posttreatment samples from primary carcinomas.

IBC exhibits prominent angiogenesis, as evidenced by high microvessel density (MVD)[259] and a high endothelial proliferation index.[260] It has been reported that a number of angiogenesis-related genes are upregulated in IBC[261] and that some angiogenic factors are overexpressed in these tumors.[262] Angiogenic factors are likely to be targeted as the treatment of IBC evolves. Wedam et al.[263] described the antiangiogenic effect of bevacizumab, a recombinant humanized monoclonal antibody to vascular endothelial growth factor (VEGF), which was given prior to and during anthracycline and taxane neoadjuvant treatment of 21 patients with inflammatory and locally advanced breast carcinoma. After anti-VEGF treatment alone, expression of the phosphorylated tyrosine kinase receptor VEGFR2 in tumor cells was reduced by a median of 66.7%, and apoptosis in the tumor increased by a mean of 128.9%, but there was no change in MVD or in VEGF-A expression. Dynamic contrast-enhanced MRI yielded results indicative of reduced angiogenesis. Antiangiogenic effects of bevacizumab were also observed when the monoclonal antibody was administered with combination chemotherapy.

Noninflammatory Cutaneous Involvement by Breast Carcinoma

The histopathologic finding of tumor emboli in dermal lymphatic channels without characteristic clinically evident cutaneous manifestations does not qualify as IBC. Staging in this group should be based on tumor size and axillary nodal status. Guth et al.[264] reported that the prognosis of patients with clinically evident noninflammatory cutaneous involvement by carcinoma was significantly less favorable than that of patients with skin involvement that was not clinically apparent. The 5-year distant DFS was 56.9% in the former group and 82.0% in the latter.

Secondary Inflammatory Carcinoma

The term "secondary IBC" refers to metastatic foci with inflammatory features in the skin of patients most of whom did not have primary inflammatory carcinoma. It more often develops on the chest wall at the site of prior mastectomy than at sites of distant cutaneous metastases.[265] Clinically, the inflammatory form of recurrent carcinoma is characterized by discoloration, edema, and *peau d'orange* appearance of the skin, similar to primary inflammatory carcinoma. Occasionally, secondary inflammatory carcinoma is limited to the treated region in patients who received postoperative radiotherapy, or it may occur only outside of an irradiated field (Fig. 33.32). Palpable tumor infiltrates are commonly found clinically in the skin.[265] Inflammatory changes are not specific for mammary carcinoma, since they have been reported in skin metastases from carcinoma of the pancreas, stomach, lung, and other sites.[266,267]

Gross Pathology

Patients with primary IBC have an underlying invasive mammary carcinoma. The primary tumor is typically indistinct—clinically, radiologically, and pathologically. If a mastectomy is performed, the size of the tumor may not be recorded because the gross margins cannot be defined (Fig. 33.33). Frequently, the breast is said to be diffusely involved, or a large tumor is described.[268] As a consequence, accurate data about the size distribution of the primary tumors are unavailable. In one series, localized tumors measured 2 to 12 cm (averaging

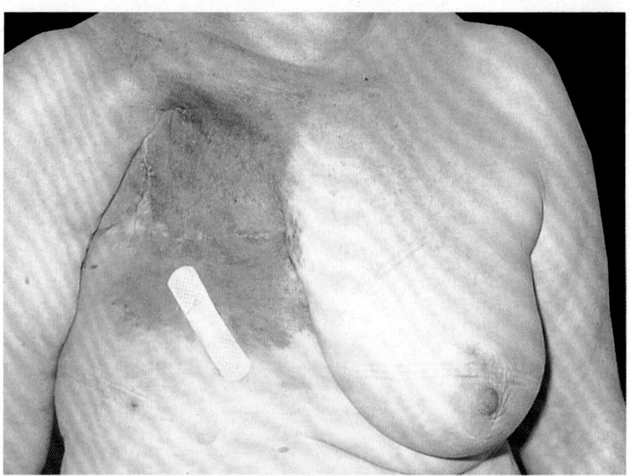

FIG. 33.32. ***Recurrent inflammatory carcinoma.*** Inflammatory carcinoma appears to be restricted to the area of radiation on the chest wall and clavicular region.

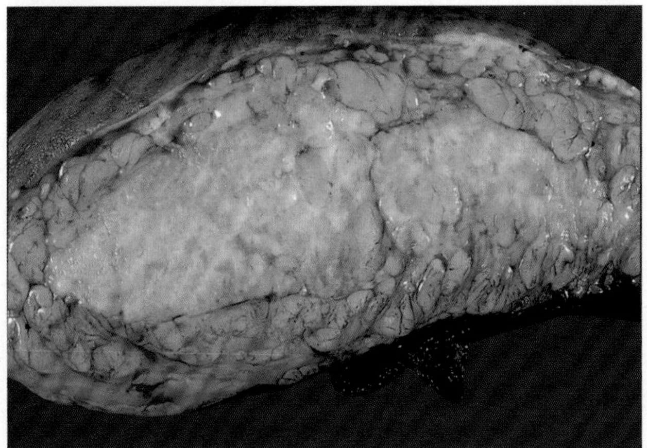

FIG. 33.33. ***Inflammatory carcinoma, mastectomy.*** Invasive carcinoma is present throughout the breast. There is *peau d'orange* change in the skin.

6 cm in greatest diameter).[268] The majority of the carcinomas were central, or they were large enough to occupy virtually the entire breast. Diffuse induration of the mammary parenchyma was palpable, and the skin was visibly thickened, measuring 2 to 8 mm thick (averaging 4 mm). This is substantially more than the normal thickness that varies from 1 ± 0.2 mm over the upper outer quadrant to 1.5 ± 0.4 mm over the areola.[269] Despite diffuse dermal involvement by tumor emboli, direct invasion into the skin with cutaneous ulceration is found only in advanced cases. Paget disease of the nipple is uncommon, although the nipple is often retracted.[269] When present, Paget disease is typically accompanied by intraductal carcinoma of major lactiferous ducts.

Microscopic Pathology

"Primary inflammatory carcinoma" is usually a manifestation of infiltrating duct carcinoma that is almost always poorly differentiated[268,269] (Fig. 33.34). Tumor emboli are usually encountered throughout the breast, but this may rarely be an inconspicuous feature. Many of the vascular spaces containing carcinoma are devoid of red blood cells and are considered to be lymphatics. However, channels of similar structure and caliber containing erythrocytes and tumor emboli are also encountered, especially in patients with extensive vascular and lymph node involvement. Hence, a distinction between blood vessel and lymphatic emboli is often difficult in hematoxylin and eosin (H& E) stained sections.

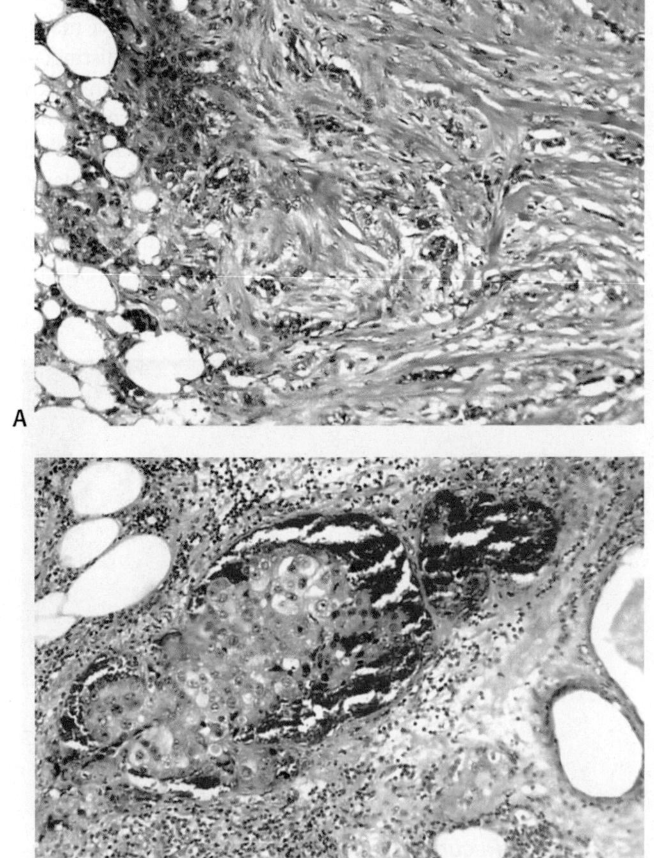

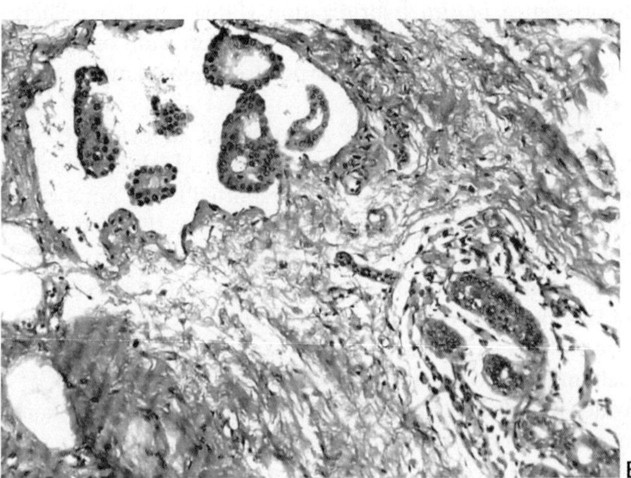

FIG. 33.34. ***Primary inflammatory carcinoma.*** **A:** The primary tumor is an infiltrating, poorly differentiated ductal carcinoma. **B:** Clusters of carcinoma cells lie in a dilated lymphatic channel. **C:** Carcinomatous emboli in a vascular channel with red blood cells.

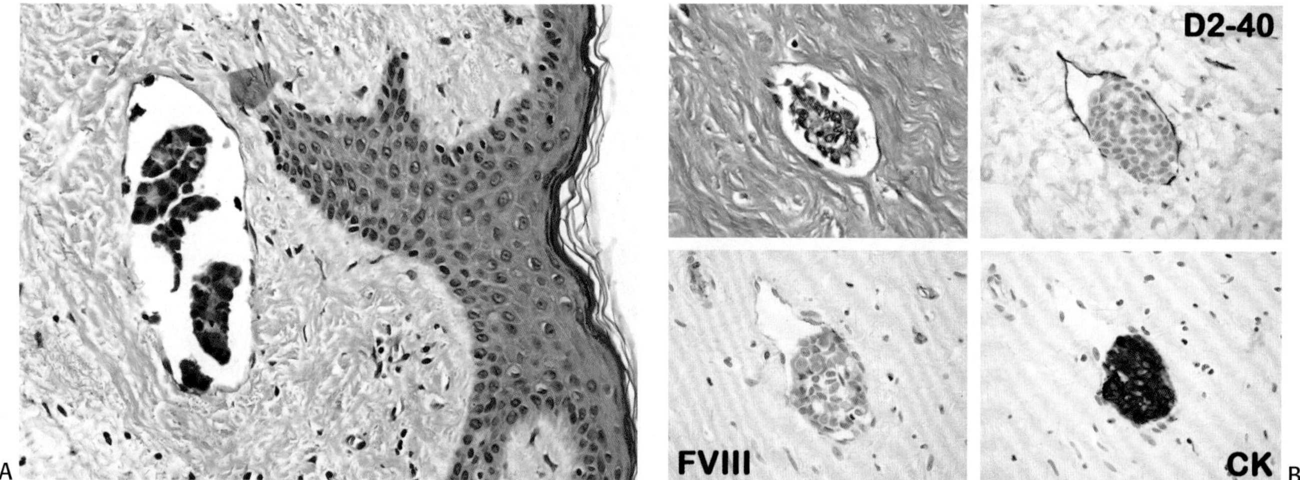

FIG. 33.35. ***Primary inflammatory carcinoma, cutaneous pathology.*** **A:** A cluster of carcinoma cells is present in a lymphatic space in the dermis. **B:** A solitary cluster of cells "suspicious for carcinoma" is seen in this punch biopsy of skin performed to rule out inflammatory carcinoma. The differential diagnosis includes carcinoma, histiocytes, and endothelial hyperplasia with "telescoping." The endothelial lining cells display immunoreactivity for D2-40 and factor VIII, and the "suspicious" cells are cytokeratin (ck) positive. These findings are diagnostic of dermal lymphatic involvement by carcinoma.

A lymphoplasmacytic reaction may be encountered in the carcinoma or in the surrounding breast, but it does not differ in intensity, pattern, or frequency from the findings in patients with noninflammatory carcinoma.[234,268,269] The intensity of the inflammatory reaction in the breast and skin is usually similar, but these reactive components have not been found to correlate with the severity and distribution of the clinical cutaneous manifestations of the disease. That is, patients with the most marked lymphoplasmacytic reaction do not necessarily have the most intense cutaneous erythema or the most severe edema. There is also no direct relationship between the number of lymphatic tumor emboli or the extent of vascular distension and the clinical findings. Neutrophils, eosinophils, or numerous mast cells are not a common feature of IBC.

Because the cutaneous manifestations of IBC are so clinically striking, there has been a great deal of interest in the microscopic pathology of the skin. An incisional biopsy of the skin is often performed for diagnostic purposes, but the diagnosis of carcinoma can be made easily by needle biopsy of the breast if there is an underlying palpable mass. It is not necessary to obtain a skin biopsy to establish the diagnosis of IBC when a patient presents with characteristic clinical findings and a biopsy-proven breast carcinoma.

The skin often displays a variety of histologic alterations associated with IBC (Fig. 33.35). The collagenous reticular dermal layer is broader than normal because of increased amounts of collagen and edema. Dilation of lymphatics tends to be prominent in the papillary and reticular dermis, and intralymphatic tumor emboli can be found at either level of the dermis. When present, a lymphoplasmacytic reaction is localized around dilated lymphatic channels.

The microscopic pathology of the skin varies greatly among patients with IBC. Histologic features of the skin may not correlate with the clinical findings. Samples of skin from within and outside the zone of erythema and edema may appear histologically similar, with lymphatic tumor emboli detectable in areas that appear clinically uninvolved. When carcinoma is found in the skin of a patient with primary IBC, it is usually limited to lymphatic emboli. Extralymphatic dermal tumor infiltrates are uncommon. FNA in suspected cases of IBC presenting without a palpable mass may be successful in establishing the diagnosis if samples taken from all four quadrants with "extra passes in the antigravity areas are attempted."[270]

In some patients with the classical clinical appearance of IBC, tumor may not be found in biopsy samples from the skin, even if serial sections of the specimen are prepared.[235,236,237,269] In one study, the skin biopsy specimen was reportedly negative in 50% of IBC patients.[236] Thus, no pattern of histologic findings is specifically associated with the clinical diagnosis of primary IBC.

"Inflammatory recurrent carcinoma" (secondary inflammatory carcinoma) is usually accompanied by nodules and plaques of invasive carcinoma in the dermis of the skin, as well as intralymphatic tumor emboli (Fig. 33.36). In some of these cases lymphatic tumor emboli are inconspicuous or not detectable. Clinically, erythema and edema occur equally in the skin over and around palpable dermal tumor infiltrates, regardless of the presence of dermal lymphatic tumor emboli.

A review of the primary lesions in patients who developed an inflammatory recurrence suggested some predisposing features.[234] All patients initially had primary infiltrating duct carcinomas, including a disproportionately high number with apocrine cytology. Inflammatory recurrence was rarely found following treatment of papillary, medullary, and mucinous carcinomas. Although these patients did not exhibit

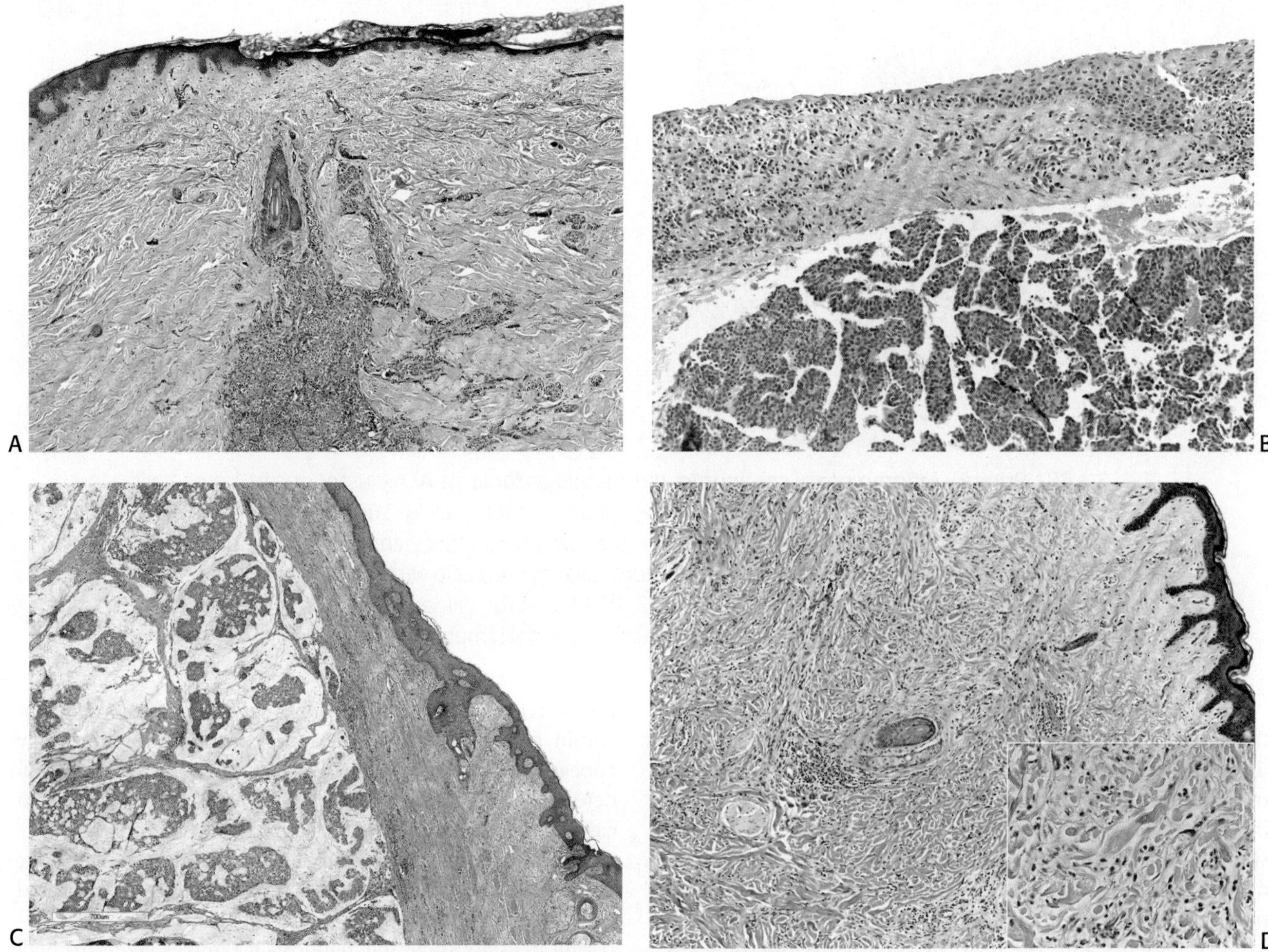

FIG. 33.36. ***Inflammatory recurrent carcinoma.*** Dermal infiltration with recurrent carcinomas on the chest wall and the clinical manifestations of inflammatory carcinoma. Shown here are poorly differentiated ductal carcinoma (**A**), papillary carcinoma (**B**), mucinous carcinoma (**C**), and ILC (**D**, *detail in inset*).

the clinical signs of inflammatory carcinoma when initially treated, parenchymal intralymphatic tumor emboli were seen in many of the mastectomy specimens. A number of these patients also had lymphatic tumor emboli in the nipple and/or the skin of the breast (Fig. 33.37). The majority of patients with an inflammatory recurrence initially have metastases involving many enlarged ALNs, but this type of recurrence can develop in a patient who did not have ALN metastases.

The term "occult inflammatory carcinoma" describes a group of patients who have cutaneous and parenchymal lymphatic tumor emboli associated with their primary tumor in the absence of cutaneous erythema and other clinical changes that typify IBC.[224,269] Occult inflammatory carcinoma occurs in 1% to 2% of patients with invasive carcinomas that are not clinically inflammatory.[269] The primary tumors tend to be central, larger than 4 cm, and often multicentric. The pathologic findings are not appreciably different from those in women with primary IBC, and these patients are predisposed to develop inflammatory recurrences.[234]

Treatment and Prognosis

Until the introduction of combined modality treatment, including intensive chemotherapy, fewer than 5% of patients with IBC survived 5 years.[234] In recent years, the management of this disease has evolved into a multimodality approach that combines chemotherapy, surgery, and radiotherapy.[271] In general, the currently favored therapeutic approach is preoperative chemotherapy to render the tumor operable, followed by mastectomy and radiation.[272]

Although one group of investigators suggested that IBC patients with no detectable dermal lymphatic tumor emboli had a more favorable prognosis,[223] others did not find this to be the case.[237,269,273] Patients with "occult" IBC may have a

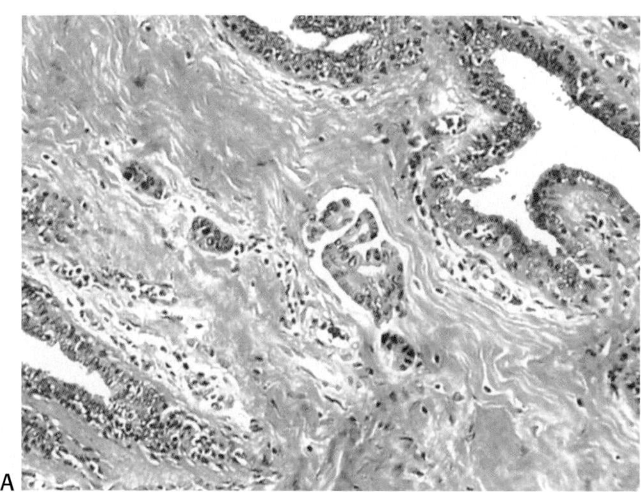

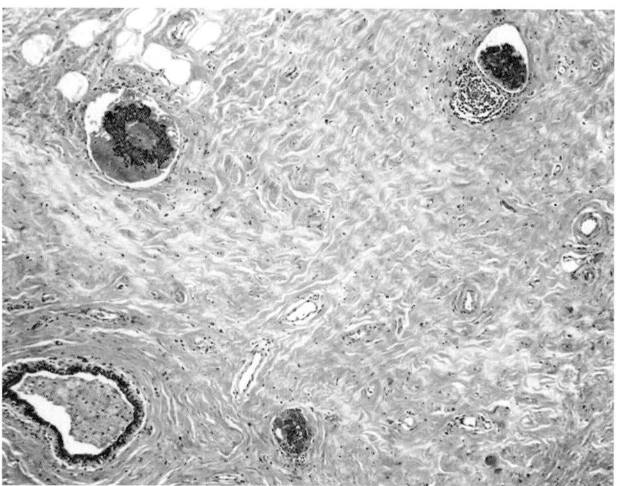

FIG. 33.37. ***Lymphatic tumor emboli in the nipple.*** **A,B:** Carcinoma cells in lymphatic channels in the stroma of nipples in patients who did not have clinical manifestations of inflammatory carcinoma. Recurrent carcinoma in such patients is likely to have inflammatory features clinically.

slightly less acute clinical course, but ultimately not a better survival, than women with classical primary IBC.

Reports in the 1980s and early 1990s described a substantial improvement in prognosis when compared with earlier data for primary IBC with 5-year survivals ranging from 25% to 48%[273–276] and 10-year survival of 32%.[276] Certain clinical features of the disease (including nodal metastases and chest wall adhesion) at presentation and stage at the time of diagnosis have an important influence on prognosis, with a better 5-year survival observed in those with localized than with regional disease.[274,276]

Mastectomy was shown in the past to be ineffective by itself and was rarely performed for IBC,[234] but it is now considered an integral part of the multimodality treatment program. Mastectomy has been relatively effective for obtaining local control of the primary tumor when preceded by combination chemotherapy followed by radiation.[250,277–281] Treatment with anthracycline-based neoadjuvant chemotherapy followed by surgery and/or radiotherapy can result in local control in at least 80% of patients and 5-year survival rates greater than 50%.[282]

Radiation and chemotherapy often cause a diminution in the clinical manifestations of IBC prior to a mastectomy. The effects of treatment include some or all of the following: decrease or elimination of erythema, reduction in breast size, loss of cutaneous edema, and decrease in the size of a palpable tumor if present. Enlarged ALNs may also become smaller. In a few patients, clinical signs disappeared entirely (clinical complete response), but residual carcinoma was found microscopically at mastectomy in virtually all cases.[250,275,278,280,281,283] Clinical complete response has been reported in 12% to 52% of patients, with pathologic complete response in 4% to 33%.[282] Various sequences of treatment have been shown to reliably improve local control and DFS. Amelioration of edema, erythema, breast enlargement, and tumor mass has been associated with a relatively longer DFS than has been achieved in patients who do not respond to neoadjuvant treatment.[273,278,284]

The clinical description of response to treatment does not always correlate well with the pathologic findings in the mastectomy specimen. Considerable residual tumor, often with substantial lymphatic tumor emboli, may persist despite what appears to be a complete clinical response. Alternatively, women reported to have partial or minimal clinical response may prove to have little or no microscopically demonstrable tumor. In the latter situation, one typically finds substantial alterations in the mammary parenchyma where the tumor has been destroyed (Fig. 33.38). These changes, varying from simple fibrosis to chronic granulomatous inflammation, are described in detail in Chapter 41. Similar effects have been observed in ALNs that were pathologically devoid of tumor after treatment although there appeared to be little response clinically.

It has been observed that pathologic findings in the mastectomy specimen predict prognosis more accurately than the clinical assessment of response to treatment.[284,285] In one study, "therapeutic response parameters" associated with the most favorable outcome were complete regression after induction therapy within 8 months of diagnosis and complete regression of inflammatory symptoms within 3 months of neoadjuvant therapy.[276] Patients who exhibit a good response clinically and pathologically appear to have the best prognosis.

The number of involved ALNs may be a particularly important prognostic factor, and for this reason surgical staging has been advocated.[285] However, pretreatment with chemotherapy may result in downstaging of axillary involvement in patients who have a response that destroys axillary metastases without leaving residual fibrosis in the nodes. A cytokeratin immunostain can be employed to detect microscopic residual carcinoma in ALNs or in the

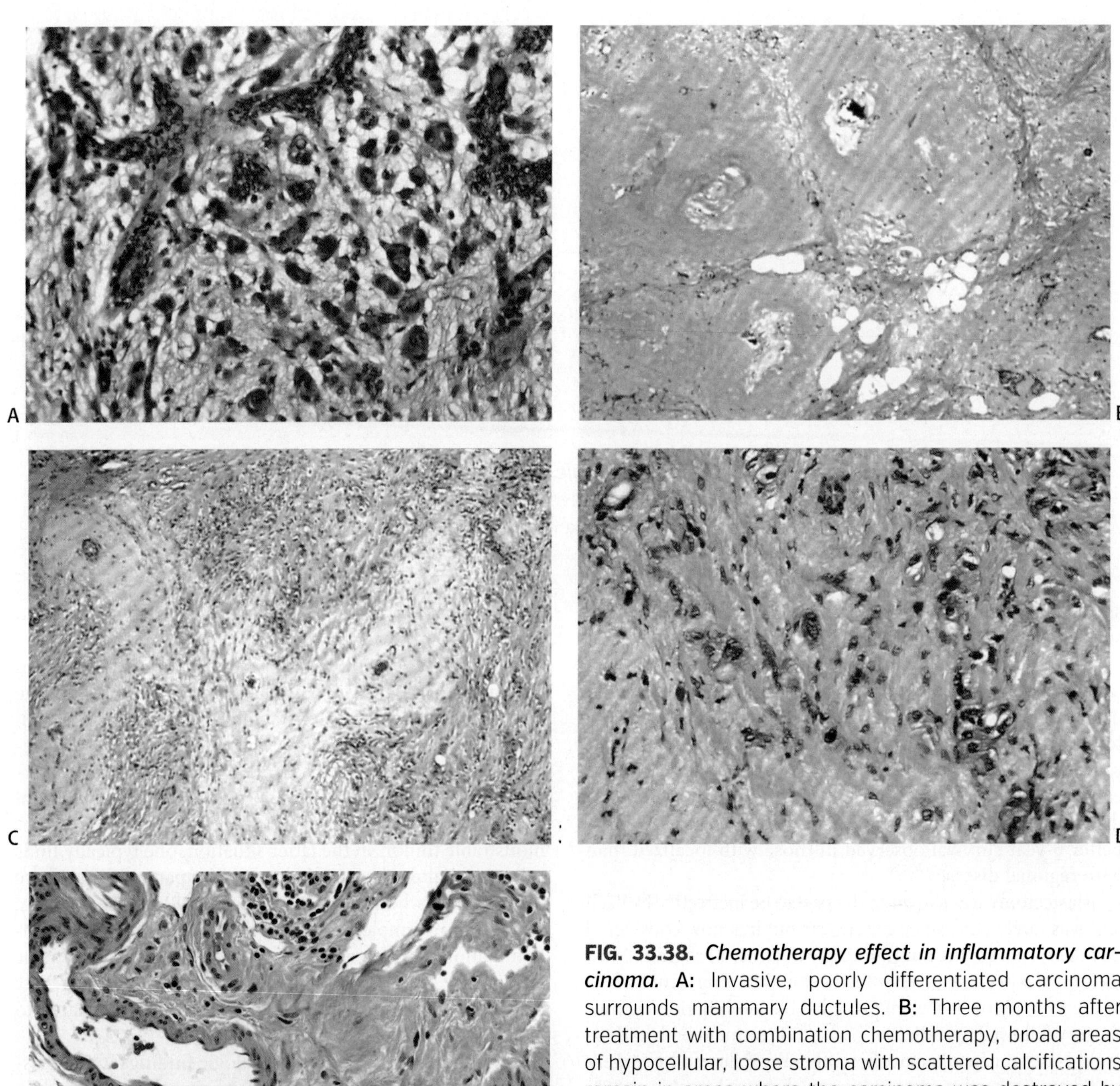

FIG. 33.38. ***Chemotherapy effect in inflammatory carcinoma.*** **A:** Invasive, poorly differentiated carcinoma surrounds mammary ductules. **B:** Three months after treatment with combination chemotherapy, broad areas of hypocellular, loose stroma with scattered calcifications remain in areas where the carcinoma was destroyed by treatment and resorbed. **C:** Fibrosis and mild chronic inflammation beginning to occupy an area of resorbed carcinoma. **D:** Microscopic foci of carcinoma remaining in the treated breast. **E:** Typical appearance of tumor cells in a lymphatic channel after chemotherapy. Note the cytoplasmic vacuolization in tumor cells.

breast after chemotherapy and radiation therapy. Nodal scarring after chemotherapy in the absence of demonstrable neoplastic cells in a patient with IBC can be attributed to tumor regression.

The presence of metastatic carcinoma in the ALNs of patients with IBC can be documented by FNA prior to primary chemotherapy. Hennesy et al.[286] reported that no carcinoma was detected in the posttreatment ALNs from 14 (23%) of 61 women with inflammatory carcinoma who had metastatic carcinoma in a pretreatment cytologic specimen. The 5-year recurrence-free survival for women with a pathologically documented complete axillary response to combined anthracycline and taxane–based primary chemotherapy was 78.6%, which was significantly better than that for women who had residual axillary nodal carcinoma (25.4%). Complete pathologic response in the ALNs of women with noninflammatory carcinoma has also been associated with a significantly higher relapse-free survival rate than in patients who do not have a complete response in their ALNs.[287] In both studies, patients who had complete regression of their axillary nodal metastases more often had less or no residual carcinoma in the breast. Among women with noninflammatory carcinoma, the presence of residual carcinoma in the breast did not have a negative effect on the relatively favorable prognosis associated with complete ALN response.

The outcome for IBC patients treated in the modern era of trastuzumab and taxane-based chemotherapy remains modest. A retrospective study of 104 patients with nonmetastatic IBC treated over a 10-year period (2000 to 2009) with a median follow-up time of 34 months showed that the 5-year OS for the entire cohort was 46%.[288] In this study, fifty-seven (55%) tumors were ER (−) and PR (−) negative, and 34 (33%) were HER2 (+). Seventy-five (72%) patients completed all intended therapy, of whom 67 (89%) received a taxane and 18/28 (64%) of HER2 (+) patients received trastuzumab. Despite the use of taxanes and trastuzumab, outcomes remain modest, particularly for those with ER (−) and PR (−) disease, and those without a pathologic complete response.

Lastly, it should be remembered that various forms of mastitis and other types of neoplastic processes including lymphoma and metastatic nonmammary carcinoma in the breast can mimic IBC.[289–291] Thus, it is crucial that the clinical diagnosis of IBC be documented by a biopsy of the skin or breast that demonstrates the presence of mammary carcinoma.

RECURRENT CARCINOMA IN TRAM FLAP

Approximately one in seven women in the United States who undergo mastectomy receive immediate breast reconstruction.[292] The latter procedure employs various techniques, including the TRAM flap. Women who are younger and are treated at tertiary settings are more likely to get immediate reconstruction, the advantages of which include less psychological consequences, more pleasing aesthetic results, and cost reductions. Thus, immediate breast reconstruction, including the use of the TRAM flap procedure, is likely to increase in popularity. TRAM flap reconstruction performed after a mastectomy employs skin and subcutaneous tissue and rectus muscle from the abdominal wall to recreate the breast. This procedure has been in use for more than three decades.[293]

Recurrent carcinoma may develop in the TRAM flap as an isolated event or as a manifestation of systemic spread. The reported TRAM recurrence rate ranges from 3.8% to 11.7%.[294–296] The latter series included patients who initially had stage III and stage IV tumors. Recurrent carcinoma in a TRAM flap usually presents as a palpable tumor,[296–298] but nonpalpable recurrences have been detected by mammography.[299,300] Mammographic indicators of recurrent carcinoma include mass lesions, sometimes with a spiculated contour, and calcifications. Dystrophic calcification amid fat necrosis associated with flap construction may simulate recurrent carcinoma.[301]

The primary carcinoma for which the mastectomy was performed has almost always been invasive ductal type, usually moderately to poorly differentiated. There have been infrequent instances in which the primary carcinoma was well-differentiated invasive ductal, or papillary, or giant papillary[298,300,302] carcinoma. Recurrent carcinoma in the TRAM flap tissue usually duplicates the histologic appearance of the primary tumor. Recurrent carcinoma concurrently involving the mastectomy bed, TRAM flap, abdominal donor site, and precostal tunnel has been reported.[303]

In a study of patients treated with postmastectomy radiotherapy to the chest wall or TRAM flap, Huang et al.[304] found no significant difference in the incidences of complications, local recurrence, and distant metastases between those who have had a TRAM flap and those who did not have a TRAM reconstruction. An angiosarcoma developed 6 years subsequent to mastectomy and immediate TRAM flap construction followed by radiation,[305] and a leiomyosarcoma developed 20 years after a mastectomy and radiation, and 10 years after a delayed TRAM flap construction.[306] Both sarcomas were attributed to radiation effect.

Until the mechanism of carcinomatous involvement of TRAM flaps is elucidated, it should be regarded as a form of local recurrence. Long-term follow-up data in these cases are not known at this time; however, anecdotal evidence suggests that TRAM flap recurrences may be a harbinger of systemic spread.

It should be understood that most local masses occurring after autologous breast reconstruction are benign. In an analysis of 66 such masses occurring after 365 autologous breast flap reconstructions in 272 patients, performed over a 10-year period, the majority of these were fat necrosis.[307] Fat necrosis occurred in 54 (15%) breasts and represented 54/66 (82%) of the tumors. Recurrent carcinoma was diagnosed in 13 (3.6%) of the post-TRAM flap breasts. In this study, factors associated with carcinoma in postreconstruction masses were closer (less than 1 cm) surgical margins and tumoral involvement of lymphovascular channels. Furthermore, 51/54 (94.4%) instances of fat necrosis were diagnosed in the first postsurgical year and none after 2 years, whereas the mean time to the detection of recurrent carcinoma in a TRAM flap was 24 months.

REFERENCES

Carcinoma in Pregnancy and Lactation

1. Rovera F, Frattini F, Coglitore A, et al. Breast cancer in pregnancy. *Breast J* 2010;16:S22–S25.
2. Wallack MK, Wolf JA Jr, Bedwenek J, et al. Gestational carcinoma of the female breast. *Curr Probl Cancer* 1983;7:1–58.
3. Rosen PP, Lesser ML, Kinne DW, et al. Breast carcinoma in women 35 years of age or younger. *Ann Surg* 1984;199:133–142.
4. Birks DM, Crawford GM, Ellison LG, et al. Carcinoma of the breast in women 30 years of age or less. *Surg Gynecol Obstet* 1973;137:21–25.
5. Richards SR, Chang F, Moynihan V, et al. Metastatic breast cancer complicating pregnancy. *J Reprod Med* 1984;29:211–213.
6. Johannsson O, Loman N, Borg A, et al. Pregnancy-associated breast cancer in BRCA1 and BRCA2 germline mutation carriers. *Lancet* 1998;352:1359–1360.

7. Petrek JA, Dukoff R, Rogatko A. Prognosis of pregnancy-associated breast cancer. *Cancer* 1991;67:869–872.
8. Ahn BY, Kim HH, Moon WK, et al. Pregnancy-and lactation-associated breast cancer: mammographic and sonographic findings. *J Ultrasound Med* 2003;22:491–497.
9. Mazonakis M, Varveris H, Damilakis J, et al. Radiation dose to conceptus resulting from tangential breast irradiation. *Int J Radiat Oncol Biol Phys* 2003;55:386–391.
10. Swinford AE, Adler DD, Garver KE. Mammographic appearance of the breasts during pregnancy and lactation: false assumptions. *Acad Radiol* 1998;5:467–472.
11. Liberman L, Geiss CS, Dershaw DD, et al. Imaging of pregnancy-associated breast cancer. *Radiology* 1994;191:245–248.
12. Hogge JP, Shaw de Paredes E, Magnant DM, et al. Imaging and management of breast masses during pregnancy and lactation. *Breast J* 1999;5:272–283.
13. Sabate JM, Clotet M, Torrubia S, et al. Radiologic evaluation of breast disorders related to pregnancy and lactation. *Radiographics* 2007;27:S101–S124.
14. Yang WT, Dryden MJ, Gwyn K, et al. Imaging of breast cancer diagnosed and treated with chemotherapy during pregnancy. *Radiology* 2006;239:52–60.
15. Espinosa LA, Daniel BL, Vidarsson L, et al. The lactating breast: contrast-enhanced MR images of normal tissue and cancer. *Radiology* 2005;237:429–436.
16. Loibl S, von Minckwitz G, Gwyn K, et al. Breast carcinoma during pregnancy. International recommendations from an expert meeting. *Cancer* 2006;106:237–246.
17. Bottles K, Taylor RN. Diagnosis of breast masses in pregnant and lactating women by aspiration cytology. *Obstet Gynecol* 1985;66:76S–78S.
18. Novotny DB, Maygarden SJ, Shermer RW, et al. Fine needle aspiration of benign and malignant breast masses associated with pregnancy. *Acta Cytol* 1991;35:676–686.
19. Ishida T, Yokoe T, Kasumi F, et al. Clinicopathologic characteristics and prognosis of breast cancer patients associated with pregnancy and lactation: analysis of case-control study in Japan. *Jpn J Cancer Res* 1992;83:1143–1149.
20. Tobon H, Horowitz LF. Breast cancer during pregnancy. *Breast Dis* 1993;6:127–134.
21. King RM, Welch JS, Martin Jr JK, et al. Carcinoma of the breast associated with pregnancy. *Surg Gynecol Obstet* 1985;160:228–232.
22. Ribeiro G, Jones DA, Jones M. Carcinoma of the breast associated with pregnancy. *Br J Surg* 1980;73:607–609.
23. Middleton LP, Amin M, Gwyn K, et al. Breast carcinoma in pregnant women: assessment of clinicopathologic and immunohistochemical features. *Cancer* 2003;98:1055–1060.
24. Reed W, Sandstad B, Holm R, et al. The prognostic impact of hormone receptors and c-erbB-2 in pregnancy-associated breast cancer and their correlation with BRCA1 and the cell cycle. *Int J Surg Pathol* 2003;11:65–74.
25. Elledge RM, Ciocca DR, Langone G, et al. Estrogen receptor, progesterone receptor, and HER-2/neu protein in breast cancers from pregnant patients. *Cancer* 1993;71:2499–2506.
26. Shousha S. Breast carcinoma presenting during or shortly after pregnancy and lactation. *Arch Pathol Lab Med* 2000;124:1053–1060.
27. García-Manero M, Royo MP, Espinos J, et al. Pregnancy associated breast cancer. *Eur J Surg Oncol* 2009;35:215–218.
28. Abellar RG, Pepperell JR, Greco D, et al. Effects of chemotherapy during pregnancy on the placenta. *Pediatr Dev Pathol* 2009;12:35–41.
29. Pavlidis N, Pentheroudakis G. The pregnant mother with breast cancer: diagnostic and therapeutic management. *Cancer Treat Rev* 2005;31:439–447.
30. Aviles A, Neri N. Hematological malignancies and pregnancy: a final report on 84 children who received chemotherapy in utero. *Clin Lymphoma* 2001;2:173–177.
31. Gemignani ML, Petrek JA. Pregnancy-associated breast cancer: diagnosis and treatment. *Breast J* 2000;6:68–73.
32. Colfry AJ III. Miscellaneous syndromes and their management: occult breast cancer, breast cancer in pregnancy, male breast cancer, surgery in stage IV disease. *Surg Clin North Am* 2013;93:519–531.
33. Daniilidis A, Giannoulis C, Sardeli C, et al. Pregnancy-associated breast cancer—a review analysis. *Eur J Gynaecol Oncol* 2010;31:485–490.
34. Molckovsky A, Madarnas Y. Breast cancer in pregnancy: a literature review. *Breast Cancer Res Treat* 2008;108:333–338.
35. Kuerer HM, Cunningham JD, Bleiweiss IJ, et al. Conservative surgery for breast carcinoma associated with pregnancy. *Breast J* 1999;4:171–176.
36. Gentilini O, Gremonesi M, Trifiro G, et al. Safety of sentinel node biopsy in pregnant patients with breast cancer. *Ann Oncol* 2004;15:1348–1351.
37. Keleher A, Wendt R III, Delpassand E, et al. The safety of lymphatic mapping in pregnant breast cancer patients using Tc-99 m sulfur colloid. *Breast J* 2004;10:492–495.
38. Mondi MM, Cuenca RE, Ollila DW, et al. Sentinel lymph node biopsy during pregnancy: initial clinical experience. *Ann Surg Oncol* 2007;14:218–221.
39. Khera SY, Kiluk JV, Hasson DM, et al. Pregnancy-associated breast cancer patients can safely undergo lymphatic mapping. *Breast J* 2008;14:25–254.
40. Pruthi S, Haakenson C, Brost BC, et al. Pharmacokinetics of methylene blue dye for lymphatic mapping in breast cancer-implications for use in pregnancy. *Am J Surg* 2011;201:70–75.
41. Spanheimer PM, Graham MM, Sugg SL, et al. Measurement of uterine radiation exposure from lymphoscintigraphy indicates safety of sentinel lymph node biopsy during pregnancy. *Ann Surg Oncol* 2009;16:1143–1147.
42. Anderson BO, Petre JA, Byrd DR, et al. Pregnancy influences breast cancer stage at diagnosis in women 30 years of age or younger. *Am J Obstet Gynecol* 1996;3:204–211.
43. Nugent P, O'Connell TX. Breast cancer in pregnancy. *Arch Surg* 1985;120:1221–1224.
44. Maggard MA, O'Connell JB, Lane KE, et al. Do young breast cancer patients have worse outcomes? *J Surg Res* 2003;113:109–113.
45. Guinee VF, Olsson H, Möller T, et al. Effect of pregnancy on prognosis for young women with breast cancer. *Lancet* 1994;343:1587–1589.
46. Surbone A, Petrek JA. Childbearing issues in breast carcinoma survivors. *Cancer* 1997;79:1271–1278.
47. Danforth DN. How subsequent pregnancy affects outcome in women with a prior breast cancer. *Oncology* 1991;11:23–29.
48. Petrek JA. Pregnancy safety after breast cancer. *Cancer* 1994;74:528–531.
49. Lawrenz B, Banys M, Henes M, et al. Pregnancy after breast cancer: case report and review of the literature. *Arch Gynecol Obstet* 2011; 283:837–843.
50. Velentgas P, Daling JR, Malone KE, et al. Pregnancy after breast carcinoma: outcomes and influence on mortality. *Cancer* 1999;85:2424–2432.
51. Salamon MA, Sherer DM, Saller DNJ, et al. Placental metastases in a patient with recurrent breast carcinoma. *Am J Obstet Gynecol* 1994;171:573–574.
52. Eltorky M, Khare VK, Osborne P, et al. Placental metastasis from maternal carcinoma. A report of three cases. *J Reprod Med* 1995;40:399–403.
53. Tan K, Sinclair E, Angus G, et al. Mucinous adenocarcinoma of the breast metastatic to the placenta. *Pathology* 2010;42:688–690.

Carcinoma in Young Adult Women

54. Chung M, Chang HR, Bland KI, et al. Younger women with breast carcinoma have a poorer prognosis than older women. *Cancer* 1996;77:97–103.
55. Simmons PS, Jayasinghe YL, Wold LE, et al. Breast carcinoma in young women. *Obstet Gynecol* 2011;118:529–536.
56. Kothari AS, Beechey-Newman N, D'Arrigo C, et al. Breast carcinoma in women age 25 years or less. *Cancer* 2002;94:606–614.
57. Feldman AL, Welch JP. Long-term outcome in women less than 30 years of age with breast cancer. *J Surg Oncol* 1998;68:193–198.
58. Xiong Q, Valero V, Kau V, et al. Female patients with breast carcinoma age 30 years and younger have a poor prognosis. The M.D. Anderson Cancer Center experience. *Cancer* 2001;92:2523–2528.
59. Peng R, Wang S, Shi Y, et al. Patients 35 years old or younger with operable breast cancer are more at risk for relapse and survival: a retrospective matched case-control study. *Breast* 2011;20:568–573.
60. Liukkonen S, Leidenius M, Saarto T, et al. Breast cancer in very young women. *Eur J Surg Oncol* 2011;37:1030–1037.
61. Lein BC, Alex WR, Zebley M, et al. Results of needle localized breast biopsy in women under age 50. *Am J Surg* 1996;171:356–359.

62. McPherson CP, Swenson KK, Jolitz G, et al. Survival of women ages 40–49 years with breast carcinoma according to method of detection. *Cancer* 1997;79:1923–1932.
63. Lannin DR, Harris RP, Swanson FH, et al. Difficulties in diagnosis of carcinoma of the breast in patients less than fifty years of age. *Surg Gynecol Obstet* 1993;177:457–462.
64. Vetto JT, Pommier RF, Schmidt WA, et al. Diagnosis of palpable breast lesions in younger women by the modified triple test is accurate and cost-effective. *Arch Surg* 1996;131:967–974.
65. Rosen PP, Lesser ML, Kinne DW, et al. Breast carcinoma in women 35 years of age or younger. *Ann Surg* 1984;199:133–142.
66. Rosen PP, Lesser ML, Kinne DW. Breast carcinoma at the extremes of age: a comparison of patients younger than 35 years and older than 75 years. *J Surg Oncol* 1985;28:90–96.
67. Schaefer G, Rosen PP, Lesser ML, et al. Breast carcinoma in elderly women: pathology, prognosis, and survival. *Pathol Annu* 1984;19 (Pt. 1):195–219.
68. Ashkanani F, Eremin O, Heys SD. The management of cancer of the breast in the elderly. *Eur J Surg Oncol* 1998;24:396–402.
69. Collins LC, Achacoso N, Nekhlyudov L, et al. Relationship between clinical and pathologic features of ductal carcinoma *in situ* and patient age: an analysis of 657 patients. *Am J Surg Pathol* 2009;33:1802–1808.
70. Meyer JS, Bauer WC, Rao BR. Subpopulations of breast carcinoma defined by S-phase fraction, morphology and estrogen receptor content. *Lab Invest* 1978;39:225–235.
71. Silvestrini R, Daidore MG, Gentili C. Biologic characteristics of breast cancer and their clinical relevance. *Commun Res Breast Dis* 1981;2:1–40.
72. Gattuso P, Bloom K, Yaremko L, et al. Prognostic predictors of lymph node metastasis in young patients with breast carcinoma. *Mod Pathol* 1997;10:19A.
73. Walker RA, Lees E, Webb MB, et al. Breast carcinomas occurring in young women (<35 years) are different. *Br J Cancer* 1996;74:1796–1800.
74. Banz-Jansen C, Heinrichs A, Hedderich M, et al. Are there changes in characteristics and therapy of young patients with early-onset breast cancer in Germany over the last decade? *Arch Gynecol Obstet* 2013;288:379–383.
75. Dhodapkar MV, Ingle JN, Cha SS, et al. Prognostic factors in elderly women with metastatic breast cancer treated with tamoxifen. An analysis of patients entered on four prospective clinical trials. *Cancer* 1996;77:683–690.
76. Gennari R, Curigliano G, Rotmensz N, et al. Breast carcinoma in elderly women. Features of disease presentation, choice of local and systemic treatments compared with younger post menopausal patients. *Cancer* 2004;101:1302–1310.
77. Recht A, Connolly JL, Schnitt SJ, et al. The effect of young age on tumor recurrence in the treated breast after conservative surgery and radiotherapy. *Int J Radiat Oncol Biol Phys* 1998;14:3–10.
78. Kurtz JM, Jacquemier J, Amalric R, et al. Why are local recurrences after breast-conserving therapy more frequent in younger patients? *J Clin Oncol* 1990;8:591–598.
79. Fowble BL, Schultz DJ, Overmoyer B, et al. The influence of young age on outcome and early stage breast cancer. *Int J Radiat Oncol Biol Phys* 1994;30:23–33.
80. Matthews RH, McNeese MD, Montague ED, et al. Prognostic implications of age in breast cancer patients treated with tumorectomy and irradiation or with mastectomy. *Int J Radiat Oncol Biol Phys* 1988;14:659–663.
81. Fourquet A, Campana F, Zafrani B, et al. Prognostic factors of breast recurrence in the conservative management of early breast cancer: a 25-year follow-up. *Int J Radiat Oncol Biol Phys* 1989;17:719–725.
82. Rose MA, Henderson IC, Gelman R, et al. Premenopausal breast cancer patients treated with conservative surgery, radiotherapy and adjuvant chemotherapy have a low risk of local failure. *Int J Radiat Oncol Biol Phys* 1989;17:711–717.
83. Haffty BG, Fischer D, Rose M, et al. Prognostic factors for local recurrence in the conservatively treated breast cancer patient: a cautious interpretation of the data. *J Clin Oncol* 1991;9:997–1003.
84. Freedman GM, Fowble BL, Hanlon AL, et al. A close or positive margin after mastectomy is not an indication for chest wall irradiation except in women aged fifty or younger. *Int J Radiat Oncol Biol Phys* 1998;41:599–605.
85. Chabner E, Nixon A, Gelman R, et al. Family history and treatment outcome in young women after breast-conserving surgery and radiation therapy for early-stage breast cancer. *J Clin Oncol* 1998;16:2045–2051.
86. Vicini FA, Kestin LL, Goldstein NS, et al. Impact of young age on outcome in patients with ductal carcinoma-in-situ treated with breast-conserving therapy. *J Clin Oncol* 2000;18:296–306.
87. Arvold ND, Taghian AG, Niemierko A, et al. Age, breast cancer subtype approximation, and local recurrence after breast-conserving therapy . *J Clin Oncol* 2011;29:3885–3891.
88. Hughes KS, Schnaper LA, Berry D, et al. Lumpectomy plus tamoxifen with or without irradiation in women 70 years of age or older with early breast cancer. *N Engl J Med* 2004;351:971–957.
89. Hughes KS. Lumpectomy plus tamoxifen with or without irradiation in women 70 or older with early breast cancer. ASCO Annual Meeting, June 4–8, 2010, Chicago, IL. Abstract 507.
90. http://homepages.ed.ac.uk/prime/prime2.html, accessed July 2013.
91. Tognon C, Knezevich SR, Huntsman D, et al. Expression of the ETV6-NTRK3 gene fusion as a primary event in human secretory breast carcinoma. *Cancer Cell* 2002;2:367–376.
92. Diallo R, Tognon C, Knezevich SR, et al. Secretory carcinoma of the breast: a genetically defined carcinoma entity. *Verh Dtsch Ges Pathol* 2003;87:193–203.
93. Litton JK, Ready K, Chen H, et al. Earlier age of onset of BRCA mutation-related cancers in subsequent generations. *Cancer* 2012;118:321–325.
94. Goodwin PJ, Phillips K-A, West DW, et al. Breast cancer prognosis in BRCA1 and BRCA2 mutation carriers: an International Prospective Breast Cancer Family Registry population-based cohort study. *J Clin Oncol* 2012;30:19–26.
95. Heymann S, Delaloge S, Rahal A, et al. Radio-induced malignancies after breast cancer postoperative radiotherapy in patients with Li-Fraumeni syndrome. *Radiat Oncol* 2010;5:104.

Carcinoma in Fibroepithelial Tumors

96. Cheatle GL, Cutler M. *Tumours of the breast. Their pathology, symptoms, diagnosis and treatment.* London: Edward Arnold & Co, 1931;483–484.
97. Harrington SW, Miller JM. Malignant changes in fibro-adenoma of the mammary gland. *Surg Gynecol Obstet* 1940;70:615–619.
98. McDivitt RW, Stewart FW, Farrow JH. Breast carcinoma arising in solitary fibroadenomas. *Surg Gynecol Obstet* 1967;125:572–576.
99. Diaz NM, Palmer JO, McDivitt RW. Carcinoma arising within fibroadenomas of the breast. A clinicopathologic study of 105 patients. *Am J Clin Pathol* 1991;95:614–622.
100. Fondo EY, Rosen PP, Fracchia AA, et al. The problem of carcinoma developing in a fibroadenoma. Recent experience at Memorial Hospital. *Cancer* 1979;43:563–567.
101. Ozzello L, Gump FE. The management of patients with carcinomas in fibroadenomatous tumors of the breast. *Surg Gynecol Obstet* 1985;160:99–103.
102. Rosen PP, Urban JA. Coexistent mammary carcinoma and cystosarcoma phyllodes. *Breast* 1975;1:9–15.
103. Yoshida Y, Takaoka M, Fukumoto M. Carcinoma arising in fibroadenoma. Case report and review of the world literature. *J Surg Oncol* 1985;29:132–140.
104. Pick PW, Iossifides IA. Occurrence of breast carcinoma within a fibroadenoma. A review. *Arch Pathol Lab Med* 1984;108:590–594.
105. Borecky N, Rickard M. Preoperative diagnosis of carcinoma within fibroadenoma on screening mammograms. *J Med Imaging Radiat Oncol* 2008;52:64–67.
106. Tajima S, Kanemaki Y, Kurihara Y, et al. A case of a fibroadenoma coexisting with an invasive lobular carcinoma in the breast. *Breast Cancer* 2011;18:319–323.
107. Baker KS, Monsees BS, Diaz NM, et al. Carcinoma within fibroadenomas: mammographic features. *Radiology* 1990;176:371–374.
108. Gupta RK. Fine needle aspiration (FNA) cytology of concurrent breast carcinoma in fibroadenoma. *Cytopathology* 1995;6:201–203.
109. Psarianos T, Kench JG, Ung OA, et al. Breast carcinoma in a fibroadenoma: diagnosis by fine needle aspiration cytology. *Pathology* 1998;30:419–421.

110. Ooe A, Takahara S, Sumiyoshi K, et al. Preoperative diagnosis of ductal carcinoma *in situ* arising within a mammary fibroadenoma: a case report. *Jpn J Clin Oncol* 2011;41:918–923.
111. Petersson F, Tan PH, Putti TC. Low-grade ductal carcinoma *in situ* and invasive mammary carcinoma with columnar cell morphology arising in a complex fibroadenoma in continuity with columnar cell change and flat epithelial atypia. *Int J Surg Pathol* 2010;18:352–357.
112. Goldman RL, Friedman NB. Carcinoma of the breast arising in fibroadenomas, with emphasis on lobular carcinoma. *Cancer* 1969;23:544–550.
113. Gittleman MA, Horstmann JP. Cystosarcoma phyllodes with concurrent infiltrating ductal carcinoma. *Breast* 1983;9:15–17.
114. Grimes MM. Cystosarcoma phyllodes of the breast: histologic features, flow cytometry analysis, and clinical correlations. *Mod Pathol* 1992;5:232–239.
115. Quinlan-Davidson S, Hodgson N, Elavathil L, et al. Borderline phyllodes tumor with an incidental invasive tubular carcinoma and lobular carcinoma *in situ* component: a case report. *J Breast Cancer* 2011;14:237–240.
116. Nomura M, Inoue Y, Fujita S, et al. A case of noninvasive ductal carcinoma arising in malignant phyllodes tumor. *Breast Cancer* 2006;13:89–94.
117. Kuo YJ, Ho DM, Tsai YF, et al. Invasive ductal carcinoma arising in phyllodes tumor with isolated tumor cells in sentinel lymph node. *J Chin Med Assoc* 2010;73:602–604.
118. Korula A, Varghese J, Thomas M, et al. Malignant phyllodes tumour with intraductal and invasive carcinoma and lymph node metastasis. *Singapore Med J* 2008;49:e318–e21.
119. Hayes BD, Quinn CM. Microinvasive lobular carcinoma arising in a fibroadenoma. *Int J Surg Pathol* 2013;21:419–421.
120. Kefeli M, Yildiz L, Akpolat I, et al. The coexistence of invasive ductal carcinoma and malignant phyllodes tumor with liposarcomatous and chondrosarcomatous differentiation in the same breast in a post-osteosarcoma case. *Pathol Res Pract* 2008;204:919–923.
121. Abdul Aziz M, Sullivan F, Kerin MJ, et al. Malignant phyllodes tumour with liposarcomatous differentiation, invasive tubular carcinoma, and ductal and lobular carcinoma *in situ*: case report and review of the literature. *Pathol Res Int* 2010; 2010:501274.
122. Klausner JM, Lelcuk S, Ilia B, et al. Breast carcinoma originating in cystosarcoma phyllodes. *Clin Oncol* 1983;9:71–74.
123. Leon AS-Y, Meredith DJ. Tubular carcinoma developing within a recurring cystosarcoma phyllodes of the breast. *Cancer* 1980;46:1863–1867.
124. Knudsen PJ, Ostergaard J. Cystosarcoma phyllodes with lobular and ductal carcinoma *in situ*. *Arch Pathol Lab Med* 1987;111:873–875.
125. Ramdass MJ, Dindyal S. Phyllodes breast tumour showing invasive squamous-cell carcinoma with invasive ductal, clear-cell, secretory, and squamous components. *Lancet Oncol* 2006;7:880.
126. Huntrakoon M. Malignant cystosarcoma phyllodes with simultaneous carcinoma in the ipsilateral breast. *S Med J* 1984;77:1176–1178.
127. Padmanabhan V, Dahlstrom JE, Chong GC, et al. Phyllodes tumor with lobular carcinoma *in situ* and liposarcomatous stroma. *Pathology* 1997;29:224–226.
128. Macher-Goeppinger S, Marme F, Goeppert B, et al. Invasive ductal breast cancer within a malignant phyllodes tumor: case report and assessment of clonality. *Hum Pathol* 2010;41:293–296.

Occult Carcinoma Presenting with Axillary Lymph Node Metastases

129. Baron PL, Moore MP, Kinne DW, et al. Occult breast cancer presenting with axillary metastases: updated management. *Arch Surg* 1990;125:210–215.
130. Fitts WT Jr, Steiner GC, Enterline HT. Prognosis of occult carcinoma of the breast. *Am J Surg* 1963;106:460–463.
131. Ashikari R, Rosen PP, Urban JA, et al. Breast cancer presenting as an axillary mass. *Ann Surg* 1976;183:415–417.
132. Campana F, Fourquet A, Ashby MA, et al. Presentation of axillary lymphadenopathy without detectable breast primary (T0N1b breast cancer): experience at Institut Curie. *Radiother Oncol* 1989;15:321–325.
133. Haupt HM, Rosen PP, Kinne DW. Breast carcinoma presenting with axillary lymph node metastases. An analysis of specific histopathologic features. *Am J Surg Pathol* 1985;9:165–175.
134. Patel J, Nemoto T, Rosner D, et al. Axillary lymph node metastasis from an occult breast cancer. *Cancer* 1981;47:2923–2927.
135. Rosen PP, Kimmel M. Occult breast carcinoma presenting with axillary lymph node metastases: a follow-up study of 48 patients. *Hum Pathol* 1990;21:518–523.
136. Buchanan CL, Morris EA, Dorn PL, et al. Utility of breast magnetic resonance imaging in patients with occult primary breast cancer. *Ann Surg Oncol* 2005;12:1045–1053.
137. Ellerbroek N, Holmes F, Singletary E, et al. Treatment of patients with isolated axillary nodal metastases from an occult primary carcinoma consistent with breast origin. *Cancer* 1990;66:1461–1467.
138. Merson M, Andreola S, Galimberti V, et al. Breast carcinoma presenting as axillary metastases without evidence of a primary tumor. *Cancer* 1992;70:504–508.
139. Lanitis S, Behranwala KA, Al-Mufti R, et al. Axillary metastatic disease as presentation of occult or contralateral breast cancer. *Breast* 2009;18:225–227.
140. Westbrook KC, Gallager HS. Breast carcinoma presenting as an axillary mass. *Am J Surg* 1971;122:607–611.
141. Rosen EL, Sickles E, Keating D. Ability of mammography to reveal nonpalpable breast cancer in women with palpable breast masses. *AJR Am J Roentgenol* 1999;172:309–312.
142. Marcantonio DR, Libshitz HI. Axillary lymph node metastases of bronchogenic carcinoma. *Cancer* 1995;76:803–806.
143. Tartter PI, Weiss S, Ahmed S, et al. Mammographically occult breast cancers. *Breast J* 1999;5:22–35.
144. Vilcoq JR, Calle R, Ferme F, et al. Conservative treatment of axillary adenopathy due to probable subclinical breast cancer. *Arch Surg* 1982;117:1136–1138.
145. Jackson B, Scott-Conner C, Moulder J. Axillary metastasis from occult breast carcinoma: diagnosis and management. *Am Surg* 1995;61:431–434.
146. Dunnington GL, Pearce J, Sherrod A, et al. Breast carcinoma presenting as mammographic microcalcifications in axillary lymph nodes. *Breast Dis* 1995;8:193–198.
147. Helvie MA, Rebner M, Sickles EA, et al. Calcifications in metastatic breast carcinoma in axillary lymph nodes. *Am J Radiol* 1988;151:921–922.
148. Sardanelli F, Boetes C, Borisch B, et al. Magnetic resonance imaging of the breast: recommendations from the EUSOMA working group. *Eur J Cancer* 2010;46:1296–1316.
149. de Bresser J, de Vos B, van der Ent F, et al. Breast MRI in clinically and mammographically occult breast cancer presenting with an axillary metastasis: a systematic review. *Eur J Surg Oncol* 2010;36:114–119.
150. Lieberman S, Sella T, Maly B, et al. Breast magnetic resonance imaging characteristics in women with occult primary breast carcinoma. *Isr Med Assoc J* 2008;10:448–152.
151. Lu H, Xu YL, Zhang SP, et al. Breast magnetic resonance imaging in patients with occult breast carcinoma: evaluation on feasibility and correlation with histopathological findings. *Chin Med J (Engl)* 2011;124:1790–1795.
152. Jaffer S, Goldfarb AB, Gold JE, et al. Contralateral axillary lymph node metastasis as the first evidence of locally recurrent breast carcinoma. *Cancer* 1995;75:2875–2878.
153. Devitt JE, Michalchuk AW. Significance of contralateral axillary metastases in carcinoma of the breast. *Can J Surg* 1969;12:178–180.
154. Breslow A. Occult carcinoma of second breast following mastectomy. *JAMA* 1973;226:1000–1001.
155. Huston TL, Pressman PI, Moore A, et al. The presentation of contralateral axillary lymph node metastases from breast carcinoma: a clinical management dilemma. *Breast J* 2007;13:158–164.
156. Noguchi S, Motomura K, Inaji H, et al. Differentiation of primary and secondary breast cancer with clonal analysis. *Surgery* 1994;115:458–462.
157. Pandis N, Teixeira MR, Gerdes A-M,et al. Chromosome abnormalities in bilateral breast carcinomas. Cytogenetic evaluation of the clonal origin of multiple primary tumors. *Cancer* 1995;76:250–258.
158. Axelsson J, Andersson A. Cancer of the male breast. *World J Surg* 1983;7:281–287.
159. Balish SM, Khandekhar JD, Sener SF. Cancer of the male breast presenting as an axillary mass. *J Surg Oncol* 1993;53:68–70.
160. Yap HY, Tashima CK, Blumenschein GR, et al. Male breast carcinoma—a natural history study. *Cancer* 1979;44:748–754.
161. Kemeny MM, Rivera DE, Terz JJ, et al. Occult primary adenocarcinoma with axillary metastases. *Am J Surg* 1986;152:43–47.

162. Riquet M, Le Pimpec-Barthes F, Danel C. Axillary lymph node metastases from bronchogenic carcinoma. *Ann Thorac Surg* 1998;66:920–922.
163. Inglehart JD, Ferguson BJ, Shingleton WW, et al. An ultrastructural analysis of breast carcinoma presenting as isolated axillary adenopathy. *Ann Surg* 1982;196:8–13.
164. Walker AN, Fechner RE. Papillary carcinoma arising from ectopic breast tissue in an axillary lymph node. *Diagn Gynecol Obstet* 1982;4:141–145.
165. Layfield LJ, Mooney E. Heterotopic epithelium in an intramammary lymph node. *Breast J* 2000;6:63–67.
166. Ridolfi R, Rosen PP, Thaler H. Nevus cell aggregates associated with lymph nodes: estimated frequency and clinical significance. *Cancer* 1977;39:164–171.
167. Bhatia SK, Saclarides TJ, Witt TR, et al. Hormone receptor studies in axillary metastases from occult breast cancers. *Cancer* 1987;59:1170–1172.
168. Grundfest S, Steiger E, Sebek B. Metastatic axillary adenopathy. Use of estrogen receptor protein as an aid in diagnosis. *Arch Surg* 1978;113:1108–1109.
169. Rosen PP. Axillary lymph node metastases in patients with occult noninvasive breast carcinoma. *Cancer* 1980;46:1298–1306.
170. Read NE, Strom EA, McNeese MD. Carcinoma in axillary nodes in women with unknown primary site—results of breast-conserving therapy. *Breast J* 1996;2:403–409.
171. Halsted WS. Results of radical operation for the cure of carcinoma of breast. *Ann Surg* 1907;46:1–19.
172. Jackson B, Scott-Conner C, Moulder J. Axillary metastasis from occult breast carcinoma: diagnosis and management. *Am Surg* 1995;61:431–434.
173. van de Weijer GH, van Ooijen B, Hesp WL, et al. [Expectant management concerning the breast in five patients with occult breast carcinoma]. *Ned Tijdschr Geneeskd* 1995;139:1648–1650.
174. Owen HW, Dockerty MB, Gray HK. Occult carcinoma of the breast. *Surg Gynecol Obstet* 1954;98:302–308.
175. Khandelwal A-K, Garguilo GA. Therapeutic options for occult breast cancer: a survey of the American Society of Breast Surgeons and review of the literature. *Am J Surg* 2005;190:609–613.
176. Barton SR, Smith IE, Kirby AM, et al. The role of ipsilateral breast radiotherapy in management of occult primary breast cancer presenting as axillary lymphadenopathy. *Eur J Cancer* 2011;47:2099–2106
177. Willis D, Brown PW, Rodger A. Adenocarcinoma from an unknown primary presenting in women with an axillary mass. *Clin Oncol (R Coll Radiol)* 1990;2:189–192.
178. van Ooijen B, Bontenbal M, Henzen-Logmans SC, et al. Axillary nodal metastases from an occult primary consistent with breast carcinoma. *Br J Surg* 1993;80:1299–1300.
179. Montagna E, Bagnardi V, Rotmensz N, et al. Immunohistochemically defined subtypes and outcome in occult breast carcinoma with axillary presentation. *Breast Cancer Res Treat* 2011;129:867–875.
180. Hur SM, Cho DH, Lee SK, et al. Occult breast cancers manifesting as axillary lymph node metastasis in men: a two-case report. *J Breast Cancer* 2012;15:359–363.

Carcinoma in Ectopic Breast Tissue

181. Rickert RR. Intraductal papilloma arising in supernumerary vulvar breast tissue. *Obstet Gynecol* 1980;55:84S–87S.
182. DeCholnoky T. Accessory breast tissue in the axilla. *NY State J Med* 1951;5:2245–2248.
183. O'Hara MF, Page DL. Adenomas of the breast and ectopic breast under lactational influences. *Hum Pathol* 1985;16:707–712.
184. Foushee JHS, Pruitt AB. Vulvar fibroadenoma from aberrant breast tissue—report of two cases. *Obstet Gynecol* 1967;29:819–823.
185. Hassim AM. Bilateral fibroadenoma in supernumerary breasts of the vulva. *Br J Obstet Gynecol* 1969;76:275–277.
186. Garcia JJ, Verkauf BS, Hochberg CJ, et al. Aberrant breast tissue of the vulva. A case report and review of the literature. *Obstet Gynecol* 1978;52:225–228.
187. Tabakhi A, Cowan DF, Kumor D, et al. Recurring phyllodes tumor in aberrant breast tissue of the vulva. *Am J Surg Pathol* 1993;17:946–950.
188. Ho SP, Tseng HH, King T, et al. Anal phyllodes tumor in a male patient: a unique case presentation and literature review. *Diagn Pathol* 2013;8:49.
189. Smith GMR, Greening WP. Carcinoma of aberrant breast tissue. A report of 3 cases. *Br J Surg* 1972;59:89–90.
190. Nihon-Yanagi Y, Ueda T, Kameda N, et al. A case of ectopic breast cancer with a literature review. *Surg Oncol* 2011;20:35–42.
191. Bailey CL, Sankey HZ, Donovan JT, et al. Case report. Primary breast cancer of the vulva. *Gynecol Oncol* 1993;50:379–383.
192. Cho D, Buscema J, Rosenshein NB, et al. Primary breast cancer of the vulva. *Obstet Gynecol* 1985;66:79–81.
193. Guerry RL, Pratt-Thomas HR. Carcinoma of supernumerary breast of vulva with bilateral mammary cancer. *Cancer* 1976;38:2570–2574.
194. Hoogerland DL, Buchler DA. Inflammatory carcinoma of the vulva. *Gynecol Oncol* 1979;8:240–245.
195. Intra M, Maggioni A, Sonzogni A, et al. A rare association of synchronous intraductal carcinoma of the breast and invasive carcinoma of ectopic breast tissue of the vulva: case report and literature review . *Int J Gynecol Cancer* 2006;16(suppl. 1):428–433.
196. Goyal S, Puri T, Gupta, R, et al. Accessory breast tissue in axilla masquerading as breast cancer recurrence. *J Cancer Res Ther* 2008;4:95–96.
197. Osswald SS, Osswald MB, Elston DM. Ectopic breast: familial functional axillary breasts and breast cancer arising in an axillary breast. *Cutis* 2011;87:300–304.
198. Visconti G, Eltahir Y, Van Ginkel RJ, et al. Approach and management of primary ectopic breast carcinoma in the axilla: where are we? A comprehensive historical literature review. *J Plast Reconstr Aesthet Surg* 2011;64:e1–e11.
199. Marshall MB, Moynihan JJ, Frost A, et al. Ectopic breast cancer: case report and literature review. *Surg Oncol* 1994;3:295–304.
200. da Silva BB, dos Santos AR, Pires CG, et al. Ectopic breast cancer in the anterior chest wall: a case report and literature review. *Eur J Gynaecol Oncol* 2008;29:653–635.
201. van Herwaarden-Lindebloom MYA, van Hillegersberg R, van Diest PJ. Ectopic lobular breast cancer on the anterior chest wall: a rare entity. *J Clin Pathol* 2007;60:940–941.
202. Finical S, Pennanen MF, Magnant CM, et al. Intracystic papillary carcinoma of aberrant breast tissue. Report of a case and review of the literature. *Breast Dis* 1993;6:295–301.
203. Dyes DL, Tucker JA, Ferrara JJ. Carcinoma in a supernumerary nipple/breast complex: case report and review of the literature. *Breast Dis* 1995;8:77–84.
204. Kao GF, Graham JG, Helwig EB. Paget's disease of the ectopic breast with an underlying intraductal carcinoma. *J Cutan Pathol* 1986;13:59–66.
205. Shin SJ, Sheikh FS, Allenby PA, et al. Invasive secretory (juvenile) carcinoma arising in ectopic breast tissue of the axilla. *Archiv Pathol Lab Med* 2001;25:1372–1374.
206. Sanguinetti A, Ragusa M, Calzolari F, et al. Invasive ductal carcinoma arising in ectopic breast tissue of axilla. Case report and review of the literature. *G Chir* 2010;31:383–383.
207. Miller LA, Khan SA. Second ipsilateral breast cancer after modified radical mastectomy: a case report and review of the literature. *Surgery* 1997;121:109–111.
208. Willemsen HW, Kaas R, Peterse JH, et al. Breast carcinoma in residual breast tissue after prophylactic bilateral subcutaneous mastectomy. *Eur J Surg Oncol* 1998;24:331–332.
209. Petrek J, Rosen PP, Robbins GF. Carcinoma of aberrant breast tissue. *Clin Bull* 1980;10:13–15.
210. Shimizu S, Kobayashi H, Suchi T, et al. Extramammary Paget's disease arising in mature cystic teratoma of the ovary. *Am J Surg Pathol* 1991;15:1002–1006.
211. Zaino RJ. Paget's disease in a retroperitoneal teratoma. *Hum Pathol* 1991;15:622–624.
212. Monteagudo C, Torres J-V, Llombart-Bosch A. Extramammary Paget's disease arising in a mature cystic teratoma of the ovary. *Histopathology* 1999;35:579–585.
213. Randall BJ, Hutchinson RC. Paget's disease and invasive undifferentiated carcinoma occurring in a mature cystic teratoma of the ovary. *Histopathology* 1991;18:469–470.
214. Bhambhani S, Rajwanshi A, Pant L, et al. Fine needle aspiration cytology of supernumerary breasts. Report of three cases. *Acta Cytol* 1987;31:311–312.
215. Youn SN, Kim YK, Park YL. A case report of infiltrating ductal carcinoma originating from aberrant breast tissue. *J Dermatol* 1994;21:960–964.

216. Velanovich V. Fine needle aspiration cytology in the diagnosis and management of ectopic breast tissue. *Am Surg* 1995;61:277–278.
217. Vargas J, Nevado M, Rodríguez-Peralto J, et al. Fine needle aspiration diagnosis of carcinoma arising in an ectopic breast. A case report. *Acta Cytol* 1995;39:941–944.
218. Paksoy N. Ectopic lesions as potential pitfalls in fine needle aspiration cytology: a report of 3 cases derived from the thyroid, endometrium and breast. *Acta Cytol* 2007;51:222–226.

Inflammatory Carcinoma

219. Bell C. *A system of operative surgery,* vol. 1. London: Longman, 1807:180.
220. Lee BJ, Tannenbaum E. Inflammatory carcinoma of the breast: a report of twenty-eight cases from the breast clinic of the Memorial Hospital. *Surg Gynecol Obstet* 1924;39:580–595.
221. Edge SB, Byrd DR, Compton CC, et al., eds. *AJCC Cancer Staging Manual.* 7th ed. New York: Springer, 2009:354–355.
222. Robertson FM, Bondy M, Yang W, et al. Inflammatory breast cancer: the disease, the biology, the treatment. *CA Cancer J Clin* 2010;60:351–375.
223. Ellis DL, Teitelbaum SL. Inflammatory carcinoma of the breast. A pathologic definition. *Cancer* 1974;33:1045–1047.
224. Saltzstein SL. Clinically occult inflammatory carcinoma of the breast. *Cancer* 1974;34:382–388.
225. Levine PH, Steinhorn SC, Ries LG, et al. Inflammatory breast cancer: the experience of the surveillance, epidemiology, and end results (SEER) program. *J Natl Cancer Inst* 1985;74:291–297.
226. Chang S, Parker SL, Pham T, et al. Inflammatory breast carcinoma incidence and survival: the surveillance, epidemiology, and end results program of the National Cancer Institute, 1975–1992. *Cancer* 1998;82:2366–2372.
227. Il'yasova D, Siamakpour-Reihani S, Akushevich I, et al. What can we learn from the age- and race/ethnicity- specific rates of inflammatory breast carcinoma? *Breast Cancer Res Treat* 2011;130:691–697.
228. Boussen H, Bouzaiene H, Ben Hassouna J, et al. Inflammatory breast cancer in Tunisia: epidemiological and clinical trends. *Cancer* 2010;116(11 Suppl.):2730–2735.
229. Chamadol W, Pesie M, Puapairoj A. Inflammatory carcinoma of the breast in a 12 year old Thai girl. *J Med Assoc Thai* 1987;70:543–547.
230. Nichini F, Holdman L, Lapayowker M, et al. Inflammatory carcinoma of the breast in a 12-year-old girl. *Arch Surg* 1972;105:505–508.
231. Treves N. Inflammatory carcinoma of the breast in a male patient. *Surgery* 1953;34:810–820.
232. Haagensen CD. Inflammatory carcinoma. In: *Diseases of the breast,* 2nd ed. Philadelphia: WB Saunders, 1971:576–584.
233. Stocks L, Patterson S. Inflammatory carcinoma of the breast. *Surg Gynecol Obstet* 1976;143:885–889.
234. Robbins GF, Shah J, Rosen P, et al. Inflammatory carcinoma of the breast. *Surg Clin N Am* 1974;54:801–810.
235. Barker JL, Nelson AJ III, Montague ED. Inflammatory carcinoma of the breast. *Radiology* 1976;121:173–176.
236. Droulias CA, Sewell CW, McSweeney MB, et al. Inflammatory carcinoma of the breast. A correlation of clinical radiologic and pathologic findings. *Ann Surg* 1976;184:217–222.
237. Nussbaum H, Kagan AR, Gilbert H, et al. Management of inflammatory breast carcinoma. *Breast* 1977;3:25–28.
238. Dershaw DD, Moore MP, Liberman L, et al. Inflammatory breast carcinoma: mammographic findings. *Radiology* 1994;190:831–834.
239. Tardivon AA, Viala J, Rudelli AC, et al. Mammographic patterns of inflammatory breast carcinoma: a retrospective study of 92 cases. *Eur J Radiol* 1997;24:124–130.
240. Kushwaha AC, Whitman GJ, Stelling CB, et al. Primary inflammatory carcinoma of the breast: retrospective review of mammographic findings. *AJR Am J Roentgenol* 2000;174:535–538.
241. Gunhan-Bilgen I, Ustun EE, Memis A. Inflammatory breast carcinoma: mammographic, ultrasonographic, clinical and pathologic findings in 142 cases. *Radiology* 2002;223:829–838.
242. Shukla HS, Hughes LE, Gravelle IH, et al. The significance of mammary skin edema in noninflammatory breast cancer. *Ann Surg* 1979;89:53–57.
243. Le-Petross CH, Bidaut L, Yang WT. Evolving role of imaging modalities in inflammatory breast cancer. *Semin Oncol* 2008;35:51–63.
244. Le-Petross HT, Cristofanilli M, Carkaci S, et al. MRI features of inflammatory breast cancer. *AJR Am J Roentgenol* 2011;197:W769–W776.
245. Piera JM, Alonso MC, Ojeda MB, et al. Locally advanced breast cancer with inflammatory component: a clinical entity with a poor prognosis. *Radiother Oncol* 1986;7:199–204.
246. Kokal WA, Hill RL, Porudominsky D, et al. Inflammatory breast carcinoma: a distinct entity? *J Surg Oncol* 1985;30:152–155.
247. Anderson WF, Chuk C, Chang S. Inflammatory breast carcinoma and noninflammatory locally advanced breast carcinoma: distinct clinicopathologic entities. *J Clin Oncol* 2003;21:2254–2259.
248. Charpin C, Bounier P, Khouzami A, et al. Inflammatory breast carcinoma: an immunohistochemical study using monoclonal anti-pHER-2/neu, pS2, cathepsin, ER and PR. *Anticancer Res* 1992;12:591–598.
249. Guerin M, Gabillot M, Mathieu M-C, et al. Structure and expression of c-erbB-2 and EGF receptor genes in inflammatory and non-inflammatory breast cancer: prognostic significance. *Int J Cancer* 1989;43:201–208.
250. Schäfer P, Alberto P, Forni M, et al. Surgery as part of a combined modality approach for inflammatory breast carcinoma. *Cancer* 1987;59:1063–1067.
251. Gong Y. Pathologic aspects of inflammatory breast cancer: part 2. Biologic insights of its aggressive phenotype. *Semin Oncol* 2008; 35:33–40.
252. Alpaugh ML, Tomlinson JS, Shao ZM, et al. A novel human xenograft model of inflammatory breast cancer. *Cancer Res* 1999;59:5079–5084.
253. Resetkova E, Gonzalez-Angulo AM, Sneige N, et al. Prognostic value of P53, MDM-2, and MUC-1 for patients with inflammatory breast carcinoma. *Cancer* 2004;101:913–917.
254. Riou G, Le MG, Travagli JP, et al. Poor prognosis of p53 gene mutation and nuclear overexpression of p53 protein in inflammatory breast carcinoma. *J Natl Cancer Inst* 1993;85:1765–1767.
255. Turpin E, Bieche I, Bertheau P, et al. Increased incidence of ERBB2 overexpression and TP53 mutation in inflammatory breast cancer. *Oncogene* 2002;21:7593–7597.
256. Charafe-Jauffret E, Tarpin C, Bardou V-J, et al. Immunophenotypic analysis of inflammatory breast cancers: identification of an inflammatory signature. *J Pathol* 2004;202:265–273.
257. Vincent-Salomon A, Jouve M, Genin P, et al. HER2 status in patients with breast carcinoma is not modified selectively by preoperative chemotherapy and is stable during the metastatic process. *Cancer* 2002;94:2169–2173.
258. Arens N, Bleyl U, Hildenbrand R. HER2/neu, p53, Ki67 and hormone receptors do not change during neoadjuvant chemotherapy in breast cancer. *Virchows Arch* 2005;446:489–496.
259. McCarthy NJ, Yang X, Linnoila IR, et al. Microvessel density, expression of estrogen receptor alpha, MIB-1, p53 and c-erbB-2 in inflammatory breast cancer. *Clin Cancer Res* 2002;8:3857–3862.
260. Colpaert CG, Vermeulen PB, Benou I, et al. Inflammatory breast cancer shows angiogenesis with high endothelial proliferation rate and strong E-cadherin expression. *Br J Cancer* 2003;88:718–725.
261. Bioche I, Lereboure F, Tozlu S, et al. Molecular profiling of inflammatory breast cancer" Identification of a poor-prognosis gene expression signature. *Clin Cancer Res* 2004;10:6789–6795.
262. Kleer CG, vanGolen KL, Merajver SD. Molecular biology of breast cancer metastasis. Inflammatory breast cancer: clinical syndrome and molecular determinants. *Breast Cancer Res* 2000;2:423–429.
263. Wedam SB, Low JA, Yang SX, et al. Antiangiogenic and antitumor effects of bevacizumab in patients with inflammatory and locally advanced breast cancer. *J Clin Oncol* 2006;24:769–777.
264. Guth U, Moch H, Herberich L, et al. Noninflammatory breast carcinoma with skin involvement. Clinical diagnosis is relevant to appropriate classification in the TNM system. *Cancer* 2004;1000:470–478.
265. Tschen EH, Apisarnthanarax P. Inflammatory metastatic carcinoma of the breast. *Arch Dermatol* 1981;177:120–121.
266. Brownstein MH, Helwig EB. Spread of tumors to the skin. *Arch Dermatol* 1973;107:80–86.
267. Hazelrigg DC, Rudolph AH. Inflammatory metastatic carcinoma. *Arch Dermatol* 1977;113:69–70.
268. Meyer AC, Dockerty MB, Harrington SW. Inflammatory carcinoma of the breast. *Surg Gynecol Obstet* 1948;87:417–424.
269. Lucas FV, Perez-Mesa C. Inflammatory carcinoma of the breast. *Cancer* 1978;41:1595–1605.
270. Kumar N, Sayed S, Moloo Z, et al. Fine-needle aspiration in suspected inflammatory breast cancer: case series with emphasis on approach to specimen adequacy. *Acta Cytol* 2011;55:239–244.

271. Dawood S, Merajver SD, Viens P, et al. International expert panel on inflammatory breast cancer: consensus statement for standardized diagnosis and treatment. *Ann Oncol* 2011;22:515–523.
272. Overmoyer BA, Lee JM, Lerwill MF. Case records of the Massachusetts General Hospital. Case 17-2011. A 49-year-old woman with a mass in the breast and overlying skin changes. *N Engl J Med* 2011;364:2246–2254.
273. Fastenberg NA, Buzdar AV, Montague ED, et al. Management of inflammatory carcinoma of the breast. A combined modality approach. *Am J Clin Oncol* 1985;8:134–141.
274. McBride CM, Hortobagyi GN. Primary inflammatory carcinoma of the female breast: staging and treatment possibilities. *Surgery* 1985;98:792–798.
275. Moore MP, Ihde JK, Crowe JP Jr, et al. Inflammatory breast cancer. *Arch Surg* 1991;126:304–306.
276. Palangie T, Mosseri V, Mihura J, et al. Prognostic factors in inflammatory breast cancer and therapeutic implications. *Eur J Cancer* 1994;30A:921–927.
277. Brun B, Otmezguine Y, Feuilhade F, et al. Treatment of inflammatory breast cancer with combination chemotherapy and mastectomy versus breast conservation. *Cancer* 1988;61:1096–1103.
278. Chevallier B, Asselain B, Kunlin A, et al. Inflammatory breast cancer. Determination of prognostic factors by univariate and multivariate analysis. *Cancer* 1987;60:897–902.
279. Jaiyesimi IA, Buzdar AU, Hortobagyi G. Inflammatory breast cancer: a review. *J Clin Oncol* 1992;10:1014–1024.
280. Knight CD Jr, Martin JK Jr, Welch JS, et al. Surgical considerations after radiation therapy for inflammatory breast cancer. *Surgery* 1986;99:385–391.
281. Picciocchi A, Masetti R, Terribile D, et al. Inflammatory breast carcinoma: contribution of surgery as part of a combined modality approach. *Breast Dis* 1994;7:143–149.
282. Carlson RW, Favret AM. Multidisciplinary management of locally advanced breast cancer. *Breast J* 1999;5:303–307.
283. Crowe J, Hakes T, Rosen PP, et al. Changing trends in the management of inflammatory breast cancer: a clinical-pathological review of 69 patients. *Am J Clin Oncol* 1985;8:21.
284. Feldman LD, Hortobagyi GN, Buzdar AW, et al. Pathological assessment of response to induction chemotherapy in breast cancer. *Cancer Res* 1986;46:2578–2581.
285. McCready DR, Hortobagyi GN, Kau SW, et al. The prognostic significance of lymph node metastases after preoperative chemotherapy for locally advanced breast cancer. *Arch Surg* 1989;124:21–25.
286. Hennessy BT, Gonzalez-Angulo AM, Hortobagyi GN, et al. Disease-free and overall survival after pathologic complete disease remission of cytologically proven inflammatory breast carcinoma axillary lymph node metastases after primary systemic chemotherapy. *Cancer* 2006;106:1000–1006.
287. Hennessy BT, Hortobagyi GN, Rouzier R, et al. Outcome after pathologic complete eradication of cytologically proven breast cancer axillary node metastases following chemotherapy. *J Clin Oncol* 2005;23:9304–9311.
288. Rehman S, Reddy CA, Tendulkar RD. Modern outcomes of inflammatory breast cancer. *Int J Radiat Oncol Biol Phys* 2012;84:619–624.
289. Krishnan C, Moline S, Anders K, et al. Intravascular ALK positive anaplastic large-cell lymphoma mimicking inflammatory breast carcinoma. *J Clin Oncol* 2009;27:2563–2565
290. Khalifeh I, Deavers MT, Cristofanilli M, et al. Primary peritoneal serous carcinoma presenting as inflammatory breast cancer. *Breast J* 2009;15:176–181.
291. Papakonstantinou K, Antoniou A, Palialexis K, et al. Fallopian tube cancer presenting as inflammatory breast carcinoma: report of a case and review of the literature. *Eur J Gynaecol Oncol* 2009;30:568–571.

Recurrent Carcinoma in Transverse Rectus Abdominis Myocutaneous (TRAM) Flap

292. Alderman AK, McMahon L Jr, Wilkins EG. The national utilization of immediate and early delayed breast reconstruction and the effect of sociodemographic factors. *Plast Reconstr Surg* 2003;111:695–703.
293. Hartrampf CR, Cheflan M, Black PW. Breast reconstruction with a transverse abdominal island flap. *Plast Reconstr Surg* 1982;69:216–224.
294. Singletary SE. Skin-sparring mastectomy with immediate breast reconstruction in the M.D. Anderson Cancer Center experience. *Ann Surg Oncol* 1996;3:411–416.
295. Slavin SA, Love SM, Goldwyn RM. Recurrent breast cancer following immediate reconstruction with myocutaneous flaps. *Plast Reconstr Surg* 1994;93:1191–1204.
296. Howard MA, Polo K, Pusic AL, et al. Breast cancer local recurrence after mastectomy and TRAM flap reconstruction: incidence and treatment options. *Plast Reconstr Surg* 2006;117:1381–1386.
297. Shaikh N, LaTrenta G, Swistel A, et al. Detection of recurrent breast cancer after TRAM flap reconstruction. *Ann Plast Surg* 2001;47:602–607.
298. Chung SM, Shin SJ, Chen X, et al. Recurrent breast carcinoma arising in a transverse rectus abdominis myocutaneous flap. *Arch Pathol Lab Med* 2004;128:1157–1160.
299. Helvie MA, Bailey JE, Roubidoux MA, et al. Mammographic screening of TRAM flap breast reconstructions for detection of nonpalpable recurrent cancer. *Radiology* 2002;224:211–216.
300. Mund DF, Wolfson P, Corczyca DP, et al. Mammographically detected recurrent nonpalpable carcinoma developing in a transverse rectus abdominis myocutaneous flap: a case report. *Cancer* 1994;74:2804–2807.
301. Hsu W, Sheen-Chen SM, Eng HL, et al. Mammographic microcalcification in an autogenously reconstructed breast simulating recurrent carcinoma. *Tumori* 2008;94:574–576.
302. Franceschini G, Salgarello M, Masetti R, et al. A giant papillary carcinoma of the breast treated with mastectomy and bipedicled TRAM flap. *Ann Ital Chir* 2006;77:341–344.
303. Kobraei EM, Kenady DE, Rogers WB III, et al. Cancer recurrence involving a TRAM flap and abdominal donor site following mastectomy and immediate breast reconstruction: a case report. *Ann Plast Surg* 2012;68:559–561.
304. Huang CJ, Hou MF, Lin SD, et al. Comparison of local recurrence and distant metastases between breast cancer patients after postmastectomy radiotherapy with and without immediate TRAM flap reconstruction. *Plast Reconstr Surg* 2006;118:1079–1086.
305. Hanasono MM, Osborne MP, Dielubanza EJ, et al. Radiation-induced angiosarcoma after mastectomy and TRAM flap breast reconstruction. *Ann Plast Surg* 2005;54:211–214.
306. Olcina M, Merck B, Giménez-Climent MJ, et al. Radiation-induced leiomyosarcoma after breast cancer treatment and TRAM flap reconstruction. *Sarcoma* 2008;2008:456950.
307. Casey WJ III, Rebecca AM, Silverman A, et al. Etiology of breast masses after autologous breast reconstruction. *Ann Surg Oncol* 2013;20:607–614.

CHAPTER 34

Metastases in the Breast from Nonmammary Neoplasms

SYED A. HODA

In 1936, Dawson[1] described a 25-year-old woman who had diffuse lymphatic channel involvement in both breasts from gastric signet ring cell adenocarcinoma. Her review of the literature revealed four patients with breast metastases from gastric carcinoma and two from ovarian carcinoma. All patients had generalized metastases, as did three women with breast metastases from uterine cervical carcinoma reported in 1947[2] and 1948.[3] A 43-year-old woman with metastatic intestinal carcinoid in the breast documented in 1952 presented with carcinoid syndrome, an enlarged liver, and multiple metastatic nodules in both breasts.[4] Autopsy disclosed a malignant ileal carcinoid.

Ten more patients with metastases in the breast were described by Charache[5] in 1953. This series included two men with malignant melanoma and individual men with carcinomas of the prostate gland and kidney. The man with prostatic carcinoma presented with a breast mass, and the primary site was not detected until autopsy. This is probably the first reported case of an occult nonmammary neoplasm presenting as a metastatic tumor in the breast in the absence of coincidental systemic metastases. Included in the article were two women who had metastatic ovarian carcinoma in the breast, and there were single instances of metastases of malignant melanoma, renal carcinoma, and carcinoma of the thyroid gland and endometrium. One of the patients with ovarian carcinoma developed a solitary breast mass 4 years after treatment of the ovarian primary.

A series of patients reported by Sandison[6] in 1959 included four women whose breast tumors were the initial manifestation of occult nonmammary neoplasms. The primary lesions were myeloid sarcoma, small cell carcinoma of the lung, and carcinomas of the stomach and kidney. Subsequent systemic metastases and a rapidly fatal course were described in the four cases. Also included in Sandison's report were patients who had breast involvement as part of systemic spread of the following neoplasms: malignant melanoma, lymphoma, leiomyosarcoma, and cutaneous squamous carcinoma.

Numerous publications, including those describing case series and individual case reports, of mammary metastases continue to appear regularly.[7–9] These reports have described a wide variety of primary sites that gave rise to metastatic carcinoma in the breast. In one large series covering cases from 1907 to 1999, metastatic nonmammary malignant neoplasms in the breast represented 3% of malignant breast tumors, with one-third derived from occult extramammary primary lesions.[7] However, the 60 cases listed as metastases in the breast included 32 instances (52%) of mammary involvement by lymphoma or leukemia. Williams et al.[10] studied 169 patients with metastatic breast involvement by nonmammary "solid organ primary tumors" recorded at the M.D. Anderson Cancer Center between 1983 and 1998. One hundred and forty-nine patients (88.2%) had a history of a previously treated primary tumor, and the primary was occult in 20 (11.8%). The breast lesion was a solitary metastasis in 68 (46.1%) cases. Cutaneous melanoma and pulmonary and gynecologic carcinomas accounted for 78.1% of the primary tumors.

Malignant lymphoma in the breast may be regarded as either a primary breast neoplasm or as part of a systemic lymphoproliferative disease. The inclusion of lymphomas from this category influences statistics on the frequency of metastases in the breast. Malignant lymphoma in the breast is discussed in Chapter 40.

CLINICAL PRESENTATION

It is important to consider metastatic tumor in the differential diagnosis when faced with any breast lesion that has unusual clinical, radiologic, gross, or microscopic features. This concern applies to routine biopsy and cytology specimens[11] and to mammography.[8,12] The pathologist, cytologist, or radiologist does not always have information about previously treated malignant tumors. Alternatively, the primary lesion may be a new, occult neoplasm. The preoperative clinical work-up of an apparently healthy patient with a breast mass is often perfunctory and unlikely to exclude an occult extramammary primary.

Radiographically, metastatic lesions are more often discrete, round shadows without spiculation than being stellate tumors.[8,12,13] They are usually not distinguishable from circumscribed primary breast carcinomas, which may be of the papillary, medullary, or colloid type (Fig. 34.1). Microcalcifications are uncommon but have been described in

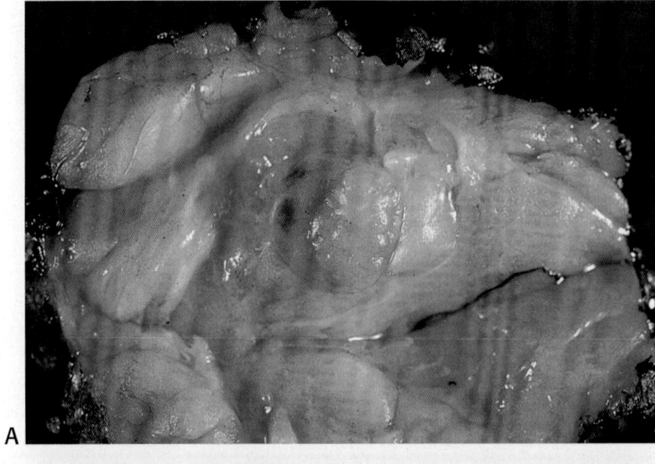

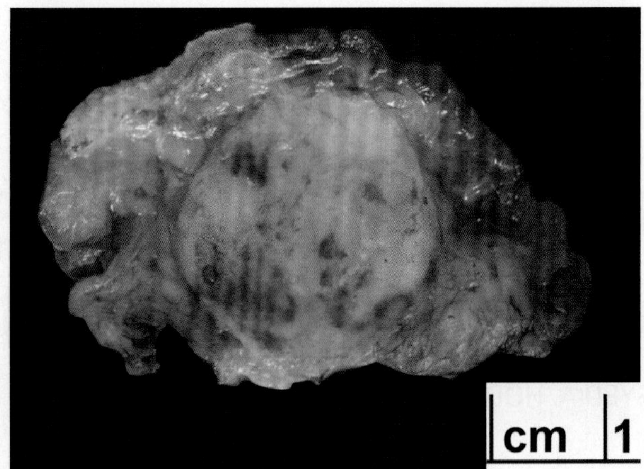

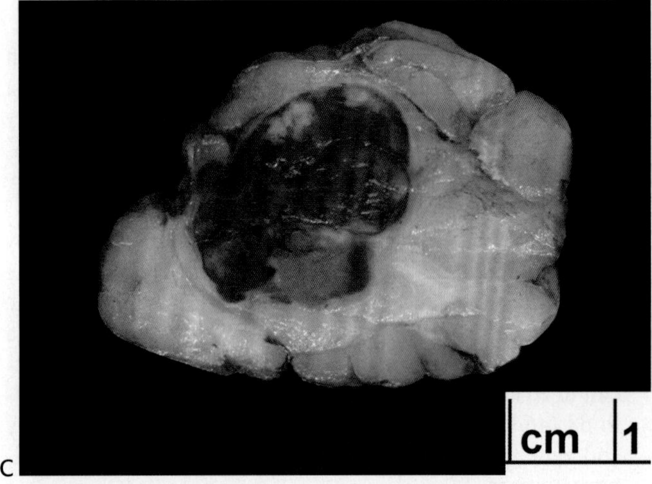

FIG. 34.1. ***Gross appearance of metastatic tumors in the breast.*** Bulging and circumscribed metastatic ovarian (**A**) and metastatic myofibroblastic sarcoma (**B**) lesions are indistinguishable from primary mammary neoplasms. **C:** Heavily pigmented metastatic malignant melanoma in a patient with disseminated metastases.

metastatic ovarian carcinoma[13–16] and in metastatic medullary thyroid carcinoma.[17] Metastatic foci are usually solitary initially, but they may become multiple and bilateral with progression of the patient's clinical course. In one case, metastatic renal carcinoma was detected as a solitary nodule in the breast 15 years after treatment of the primary tumor.[18] Squamous carcinoma of the uterine cervix metastatic to the breast studied by ultrasound appeared to be a solid tumor with hypoechoic areas.[19] In adolescent girls, metastatic rhabdomyosarcoma appeared as "heterogeneous nodules that were quite different from the usual benign lesions," although no consistent sonographic pattern was observed.[20] A study of various tumors in the breast including metastatic lesions and lymphoma led the authors to conclude that the "gray-scale" sonographic features of nonmammary malignancies of the breast are a hypoechoic mass with indistinct and occasionally irregular margins, frequently without a posterior acoustic phenomenon.[21] Breast metastasis of medullary carcinoma of thyroid detected by F-fluoro-2-deoxy-D-glucose positron emission tomography (FDG-PET) has been reported.[22]

Some clinical features are helpful in recognizing that a neoplasm in the breast is a metastatic tumor. The average interval to the development of a mammary metastasis is approximately 2 years for patients with previously treated cancer. Usually, there will already be metastases at other sites, or the metastases in the breast and other sites are detected coincidentally. Isolated initial metastases limited to the breast are uncommon.[23] However, when it occurs, metastatic tumor in the breast is at first a single lesion in about 85% of cases.[8] A minority of patients have multiple (10%) or diffuse (5%) involvement initially. With progression, multiple breast metastases may become evident, and bilateral breast metastases are eventually found in about 25% of patients. Metastases have been described in ipsilateral axillary lymph nodes (ALNs) in 25% to 48% of patients.[8] The frequency of ALN involvement tends to be higher in series that include malignant lymphomas. In patients with metastatic carcinoma or melanoma in the breast, involvement of the ipsilateral ALNs is generally a manifestation of systemic spread, and it is not unusual to also find metastatic tumor in the supraclavicular lymph nodes and at other sites, including the contralateral axilla.

A breast lesion is the initial manifestation of a nonmammary malignant neoplasm in 25% to 35% of patients who have metastatic tumor in the breast.[24] The primary tumor is usually a melanoma or carcinoma. One of the most common sites is the lungs, including a surprising number of small cell carcinomas.[25]

Other sites of occult, clinically inapparent neoplasms that have presented with metastases in the breast include the kidneys,[6,7,26,27] stomach,[1,6] intestinal carcinoid tumor,[28–32] ovarian carcinoma,[33–36] uterine cervix,[19] and thyroid gland.[37] Occult alveolar soft part sarcoma has also presented as a breast metastasis.[38] In an exceptional case, metastatic carcinoma in the breast was the first evidence of an occult renal primary in a woman who previously had mammary carcinoma in the ipsilateral breast treated by breast-conserving surgery.[26]

Previously diagnosed tumors that have given rise to metastases in the breast, sometimes rather late in the clinical course of disease, include melanoma[8,11,39] and sarcomas,[6,10,39–41] in addition to various carcinomas such as urothelial carcinoma of the bladder[42] and carcinomas of the lung[39,43] and ovary.[13] An uncommon cause of metastatic tumor in the postpartum breast is choriocarcinoma.[44,45]

MICROSCOPIC PATHOLOGY

An unusual histologic pattern and clinical information about a prior neoplasm are the best clues for identifying a metastatic nonmammary tumor in the breast. It is important to be sensitive to morphologic patterns that are not typical for breast carcinoma. Certain histologic patterns present especially difficult problems because tumors of similar or identical appearance arise in the breast as well as in other organs. Included in this group are squamous, mucinous, mucoepidermoid, and clear cell carcinomas, as well as spindle cell lesions such as malignant melanoma, renal carcinoma, sarcomatoid carcinoma,[46] and sarcomas.

When metastatic tumor is a consideration, a search should be made for *in situ* carcinoma to establish origin in the breast. Since *in situ* carcinoma cannot be found in all primary mammary carcinomas, this information is only definitive when *in situ* carcinoma is present. Absence of *in situ* carcinoma is not a conclusive evidence that a lesion is metastatic.

Metastatic tumor often surrounds and displaces normal-appearing breast parenchyma, which typically shows little or no hyperplasia. A peripheral lymphocytic infiltrate and stromal reaction are not unusual at the site of metastatic tumor in the breast as well as primary breast carcinomas. The finding of more than two grossly evident tumor nodules should lead one to consider metastatic tumor, especially if the histologic pattern is unusual. Lymphatic tumor emboli may result from metastases in the breast, as well as from primary breast carcinomas. Diffuse lymphatic spread of metastatic tumor within the breast can occur, rarely producing the clinical appearance of inflammatory carcinoma.[47]

The distinction between a primary breast tumor and a metastasis in the breast is critical for treatment. Some types of metastatic tumor in the breast can be accurately diagnosed by needle aspiration cytology or needle core biopsy, if the patient has a previously diagnosed nonmammary malignant neoplasm.[39,45,48,49] In some cases, excisional biopsy may be necessary to obtain an adequate sample for a complete immunohistochemical work-up.

Melanoma

Metastatic melanoma presenting clinically as a breast tumor may be difficult to recognize if the primary lesion is occult, if the pathologist is not informed that the patient received prior treatment for such a lesion, or if the primary site is clinically occult[45,50] (Figs. 34.2 to 34.5). Ravdel et al.[23] reviewed 27 patients with metastatic melanoma in the breast recorded in a single institution database. All patients were women, and all had a history of primary cutaneous malignant melanoma. Seventy percent were premenopausal. The majority (82.6%) of primary skin lesions were on the upper body. Melanoma was the most common metastatic neoplasm in the breast in a series of 169 cases of mammary metastases diagnosed at M.D. Anderson Cancer Center from 1983 to 1998.[10] Primary malignant melanoma arising in the breast is usually a form of metaplastic carcinoma, and these tumors may display focal reactivity for cytokeratin (CK) (see Chapter 42).

Melanoma can assume multiple histologic appearances and may not produce melanin. Consequently, it should be considered in the differential diagnosis of poorly differentiated carcinoma in the breast. Immunohistochemical studies are usually helpful in establishing the diagnosis. S-100 is a sensitive, but not specific, marker for melanoma. A103, HMB45, MART1 (melan-A), microphthalmia transcription factor (MITF), and tyrosinase are less sensitive, but more specific markers for melanoma.[51] A commercial cocktail preparation utilizing a combination of HMB45, MART1, and tyrosinase is useful in this respect.

Pulmonary Carcinoma and Mesothelioma

Carcinoma of the lung has diverse histologic appearances, some of which may resemble mammary carcinoma (Fig. 34.6). Papillary carcinoma of the lung can produce cystic papillary metastases, which mimic primary papillary carcinoma of the breast. Knowledge that carcinoma of the lung was previously diagnosed, or is currently present, and comparative review with histologic sections of the lung tumor are vital aides in this circumstance.

Immunostaining for the thyroid transcription factor 1 (TTF-1) is positive virtually in all pulmonary carcinomas and rarely in mammary carcinoma. Robens et al.[52] reported TTF-1 immunoexpression in 13 of 546 (2.4%) breast carcinomas, a result that emphasizes the need to employ a battery of markers, and the danger of relying on any one marker in such settings. Napsin A, a functional aspartic proteinase, is a sensitive marker for pulmonary adenocarcinoma that is useful in this setting.[53]

An exceedingly rare source of metastatic tumor in the breast is epithelioid mesothelioma. Immunoreactivity for D2-40, podoplanin, and calretinin strongly favors mesothelioma over carcinoma.[54]

Carcinoid Tumors

Carcinoid tumors, particularly those originating in the small intestine, are a surprisingly frequent source of breast metastases and can mimic primary breast carcinoma.[55] In some

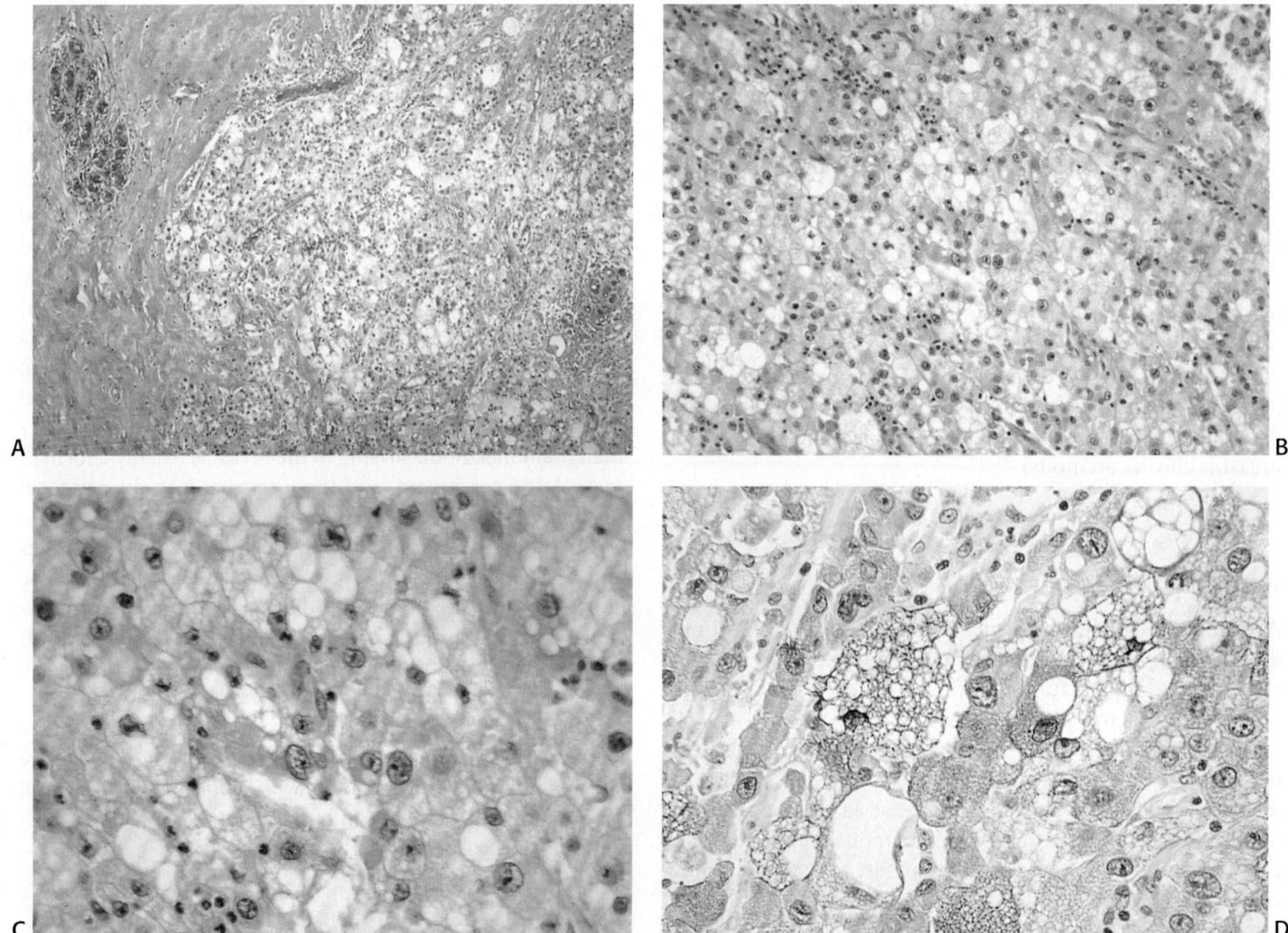

FIG. 34.2. ***Metastatic malignant melanoma, clear cell type.*** **A,B:** Metastatic tumor in the breast composed of epithelioid cells with pale-to-clear cytoplasm. **C:** The cytoplasmic features and prominent nucleoli suggest apocrine carcinoma. **D:** Melanin pigment was not seen in routine histologic sections. Melanosomes were demonstrated by electron microscopy. The tumor cells were immunoreactive for S-100 protein, but not for keratin, GCDFP-15, or epithelial membrane antigen (EMA). The only cutaneous lesion found was suggestive of a regressed melanoma (anti-S-100 protein).

of these cases, the breast metastasis was the first clinical finding.[29,32,56–58] In other instances, the breast metastasis occurred in patients who had a known carcinoid tumor and/or carcinoid syndrome.[4,29,32,56,59] The cytologic diagnosis of metastatic carcinoid in the breast by fine-needle aspiration (FNA) has been reported in a woman previously treated for an ileal carcinoid.[60] Without knowledge of an extramammary primary, metastatic carcinoid tumor in the breast is easily mistaken for a primary mammary tumor with neuroendocrine differentiation[29,56] (Fig. 34.7). Perry et al.[55] reviewed 18 cases of metastatic carcinoid involving the breast recorded by two hospitals over a 15-year period. Eleven (62%) of the metastases were derived from the gastrointestinal tract, five from the lungs, and two from unknown sites. All of the gastrointestinal carcinoids were immunoreactive for CDX2, a marker associated with intestinal neoplasms, and CK20. Three of the five (60%) metastatic pulmonary carcinoids expressed TTF-1. Thus, expression of CDX2 and CK20 favors origin in the gastrointestinal tract, whereas the presence of TTF-1 favors pulmonary origin.[61] Radionuclide imaging has been used to detect metastatic carcinoid tumors in the breast.[62] Fishman et al.[63] described a patient with a solitary breast metastasis from a clinically occult ovarian carcinoid tumor. The breast lesion was diagnosed and treated as lobular carcinoma 1 year before the ovarian primary was identified. One woman developed metastatic carcinoid in the breast from a bronchial primary.[32] The case report suggests that the lung tumor may have been present for 19 years prior to appearance of the breast metastasis, but resection of the lung tumor was performed only 4 years before the breast biopsy. In another case, a breast metastasis was detected 13 months after diagnosis of a primary bronchial carcinoid.[64]

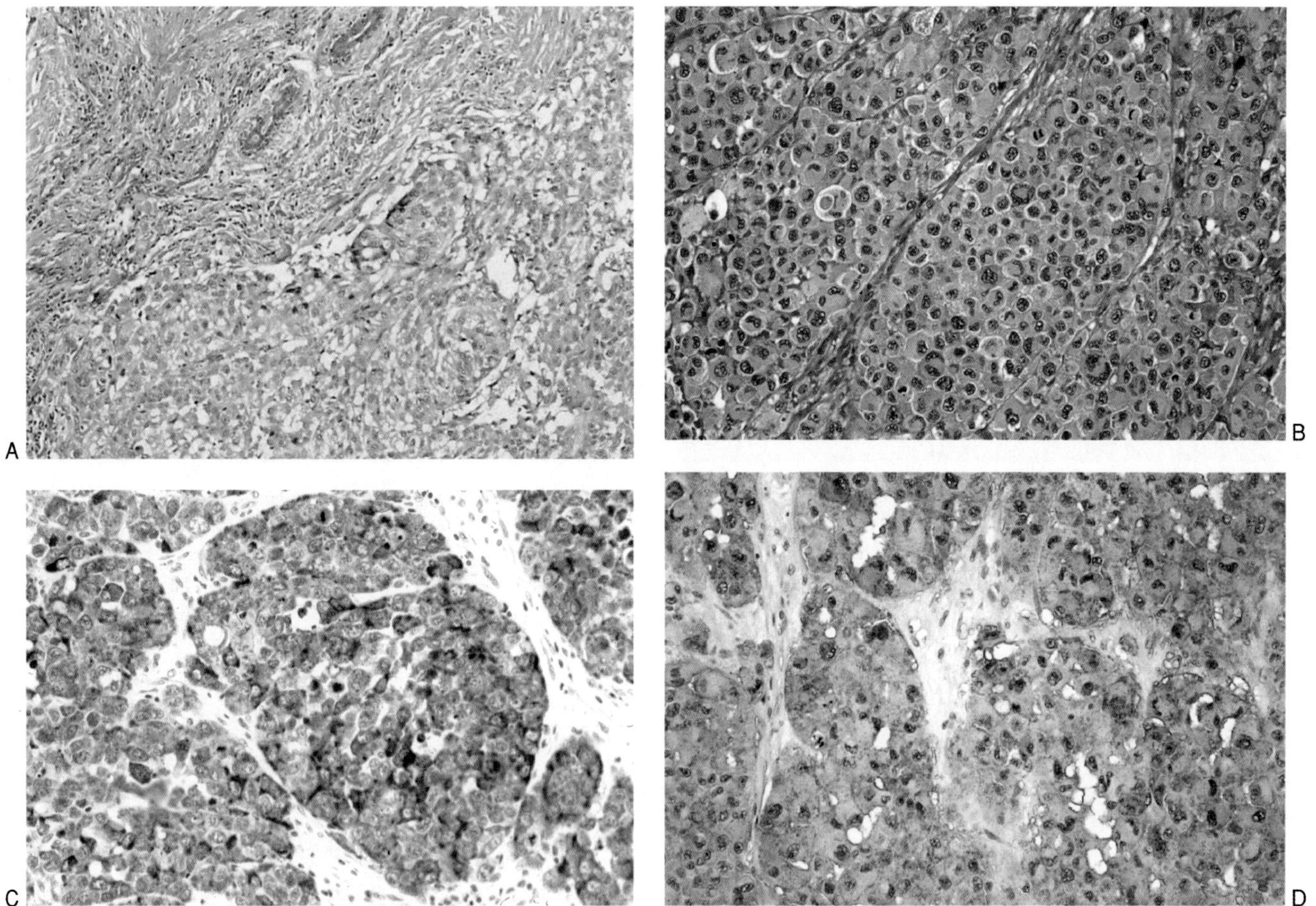

FIG. 34.3. ***Metastatic malignant melanoma, epithelioid.*** **A:** Sharp juxtaposition of the metastatic tumor and breast tissue is evident. **B:** Numerous intranuclear inclusions typically seen in malignant melanoma are shown. **C:** Immunoreactivity for HMB45 in the cytoplasm of tumor cells. **D:** Nuclear and cytoplasmic reactivity for S-100 protein.

Small Blue Round Cell Neoplasms

Mammary metastases from various small blue round cell neoplasms including medulloblastoma,[65,66] rhabdomyosarcoma[45,67–69] (Fig. 34.8), and neuroblastoma[11] have been reported in children and adults. In the appropriate clinical setting, immunoreactivity of tumor cell nuclei for MyoD1 is supportive of the diagnosis of metastatic rhabdomyosarcoma.[70,71] The distinction between, including other small blue round cell tumors metastatic small cell pulmonary carcinoma, lymphoma and Merkel cell carcinoma can present a diagnostic problem.[11,43] Merkel cell carcinoma[72] shows intense perinuclear "dot-like" cytoplasmic positivity with CK, particularly CK20.[73]

Carcinomas of the Ovaries and Endometrium

Metastatic ovarian carcinomas have generally been serous,[13] rather than mucinous or clear cell, and in the absence of a known ovarian primary may be mistaken for papillary mammary carcinoma (Fig. 34.9),[33,47] especially if there is also metastatic tumor in ALNs.[13] Immunostaining for Wilms tumor 1 (WT-1), a nuclear marker associated with ovarian and peritoneal serous papillary carcinomas, is nonreactive in mammary carcinomas,[13,74,75] with the exception of rare instances of invasive micropapillary breast carcinoma[76,77] and mucinous mammary carcinomas.[78,79] This is of interest because of the reported upregulation of the *WT-1* gene[80,81] in breast carcinomas and the observation that higher WT-1 mRNA levels were associated with a relatively poor prognosis in a series of 99 patients with a median follow-up of 48 months.[82] Focal cytoplasmic reactivity for WT-1 in breast carcinomas noted in one report[80] is not considered a positive result. Wilsher and Cheerala[83] found "nuclear, cytoplasmic and membranous expression" WT-1 immunoreactivity in malignant melanomas but did not specify the frequency of nuclear staining, and the illustrations in their report appear to depict cytoplasmic staining. Because the majority of ovarian carcinomas are CA125 positive, and this marker is negative in mammary carcinomas other than invasive micropapillary and mucinous carcinomas, nuclear reactivity for WT-1 and cytoplasmic reactivity for CA125 strongly favors

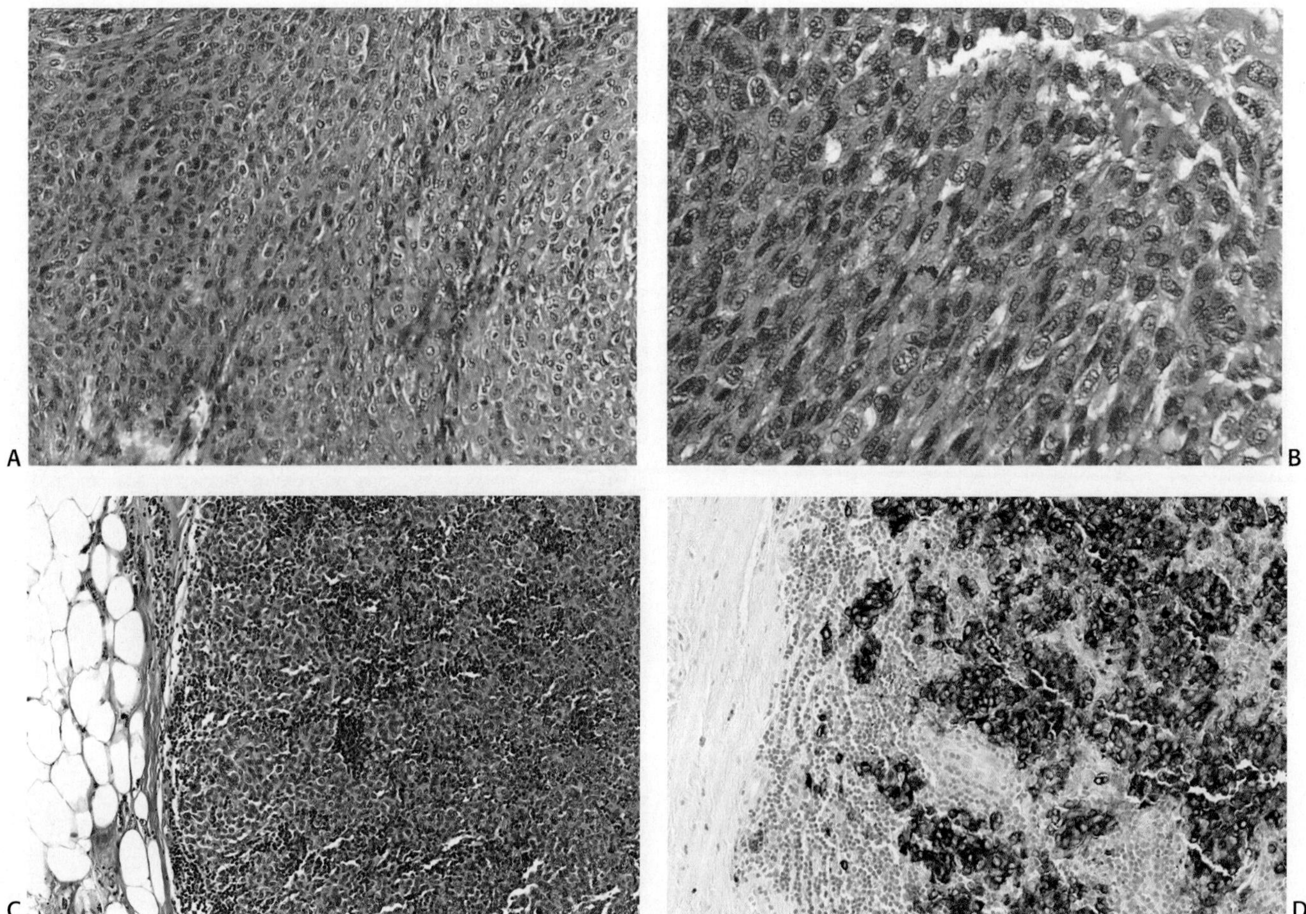

FIG. 34.4. ***Metastatic malignant melanoma.*** This metastasis had a mixture of spindle and epithelioid cells. **A:** A predominantly round cell component of the tumor. **B:** A spindle cell area in the tumor. **C:** Malignant melanoma metastatic to an intramammary lymph node. **D:** Immunoreactivity for HMB45 is shown.

metastatic ovarian carcinoma over primary mammary carcinoma.[75,77] PAX8 is a transcription factor operative in the genesis of thyroid, kidney, and the müllerian organs, and it has recently emerged as a specific and sensitive immunomarker for neoplasms of these organs.[51,84] PAX8 has, thus far, not been reported in mammary tumors. Metastatic endometrial carcinoma with a solid growth pattern may mimic poorly differentiated mammary carcinoma (Fig. 34.10).

Gastrointestinal Carcinoma

Adenocarcinomas of the gastrointestinal tract, especially of the colon and rectum, are rarely the source of metastatic carcinoma in the breast despite their relative frequency in the population at large.[85–88] Metastatic gastrointestinal mucinous carcinoma is histologically indistinguishable from primary mammary mucinous carcinoma (Figs. 34.11 and 34.12). Immunostaining for CDX2, a marker that is reportedly sensitive and specific for gastrointestinal neoplasms, can be helpful for distinguishing between mammary and colonic carcinoma.[89]

Boutis et al.[90] described a case of gastric signet ring cell carcinoma presenting with marked "left breast inflammation" that on needle core biopsy showed diffuse infiltration of intramammary lymphatic channels by neoplastic signet ring cells, reminiscent of the metastatic tumor described by Dawson[1] some 70 years earlier. CDX2 is found in up to 70% of gastric adenocarcinomas but not in mammary carcinomas.[61]

Thyroid Carcinoma

Papillary and follicular carcinoma of the thyroid may rarely metastasize to the breast[91] (Fig. 34.13). Metastatic Hurthle cell carcinoma has been reported in the breast and axilla,[92] where it could be mistaken for primary mammary carcinoma of the apocrine type. Thyroid carcinoma will be immunoreactive for TTF-1, a marker that is not usually expressed in mammary carcinoma, especially if the SPT24 clone (Leica/Novocastra, Buffalo Grove, IL), rather than 8G7G3/1 clone (Dako, Carpinteria, CA), is used.[93] PAX8 is expressed by the majority of papillary, follicular, and medullary carcinomas of the thyroid gland, but not expressed in mammary

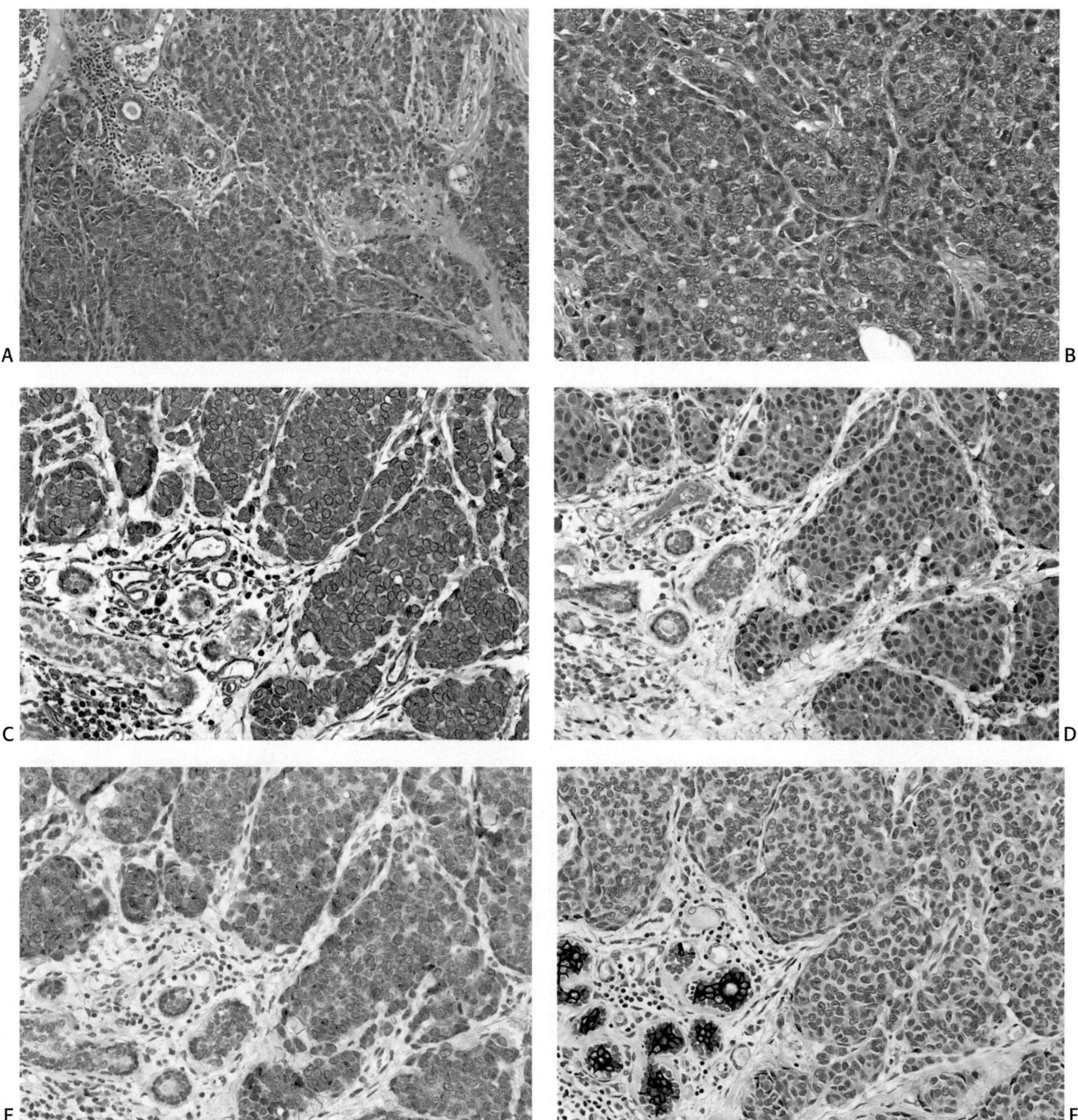

FIG. 34.5. ***Metastatic malignant melanoma, epithelioid.*** **A,B:** Metastatic tumor in the breast that was mistaken for alveolar lobular carcinoma. Subsequent metastases in the opposite breast led to further studies that established the diagnosis of metastatic melanoma, including reactivity for vimentin (**C**), S-100 (**D**), and MEL-A (**E**). **F:** The tumor was not reactive for any CK reagent tested (CK7 shown).

carcinomas.[51,84] Metastatic medullary carcinoma of the thyroid gland has been described growing in the breast with the pattern of infiltrating lobular carcinoma.[94,95] Nofech-Mozes et al.[22] described a 50-year-old woman with previously treated medullary thyroid carcinoma and elevated serum calcitonin who had occult metastatic medullary carcinoma in the breast and liver that was detected by FDG-PET.

Metastatic tumor in the breast from the tall-cell variant of papillary thyroid carcinoma[96] resembles the so-called tall-cell variant papillary mammary carcinoma.[97,98] A study

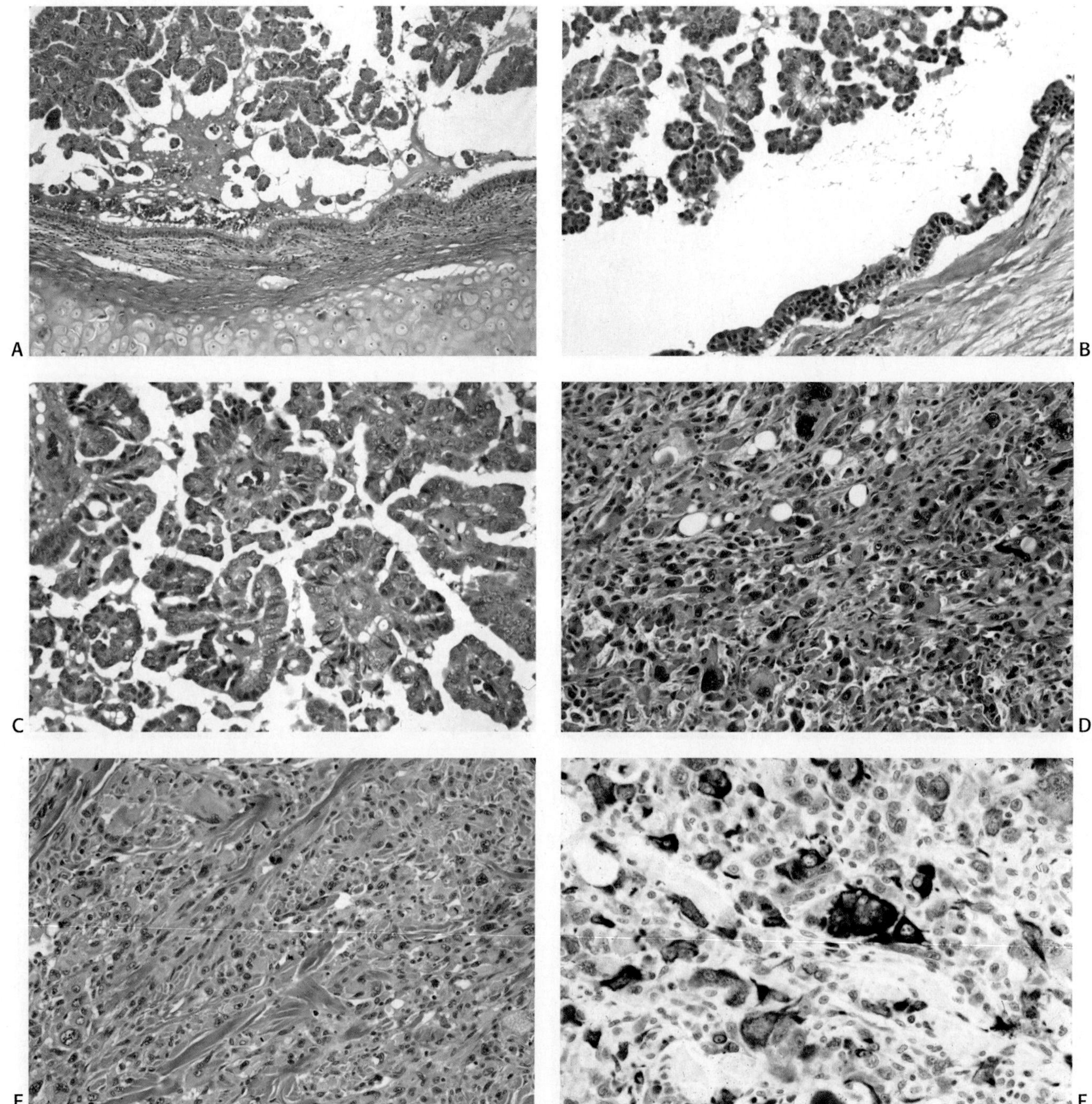

FIG. 34.6. ***Metastatic carcinoma of the lung.*** **A:** Primary papillary adenocarcinoma of the lung growing in a bronchus. **B,C:** Cystic papillary metastasis in the breast derived from the tumor shown in (A). **D:** Primary spindle and giant cell carcinoma of the lung. **E,F:** Metastatic tumor in the breast derived from the lung primary shown in (D). The tumor is immunoreactive for CK (F). **G,H:** Metastatic moderately differentiated gland-forming pulmonary adenocarcinoma in the breast. **I,J:** The metastatic carcinoma shown in (G,H) displays nuclear immunoreactivity for TTF-1 (I) and cytoplasmic reactivity for napsin (J).

of usual and solid papillary mammary carcinomas revealed cytoarchitectural features associated with thyroid papillary carcinomas in some lesion (nuclear grooves, 42%; nuclear clearing, 27%; tall-cell features, 6%; nuclear inclusions, 3%).[98] None of the 19 papillary mammary carcinomas tested by reverse transcription-polymerase chain reaction (RT-PCR) exhibited RET fusion transcripts that are frequently found in papillary thyroid carcinomas.[99]

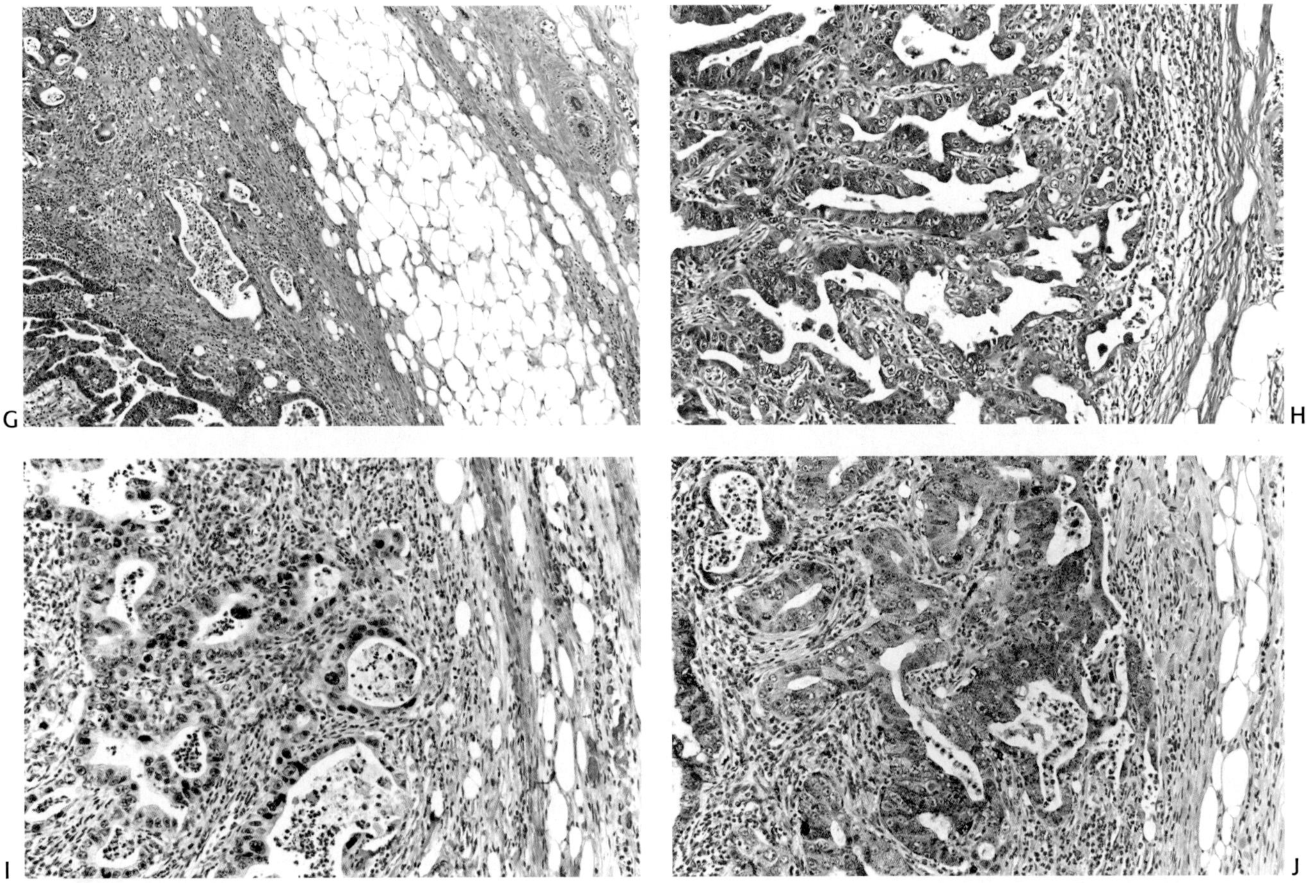

FIG. 34.6. *(Continued)*

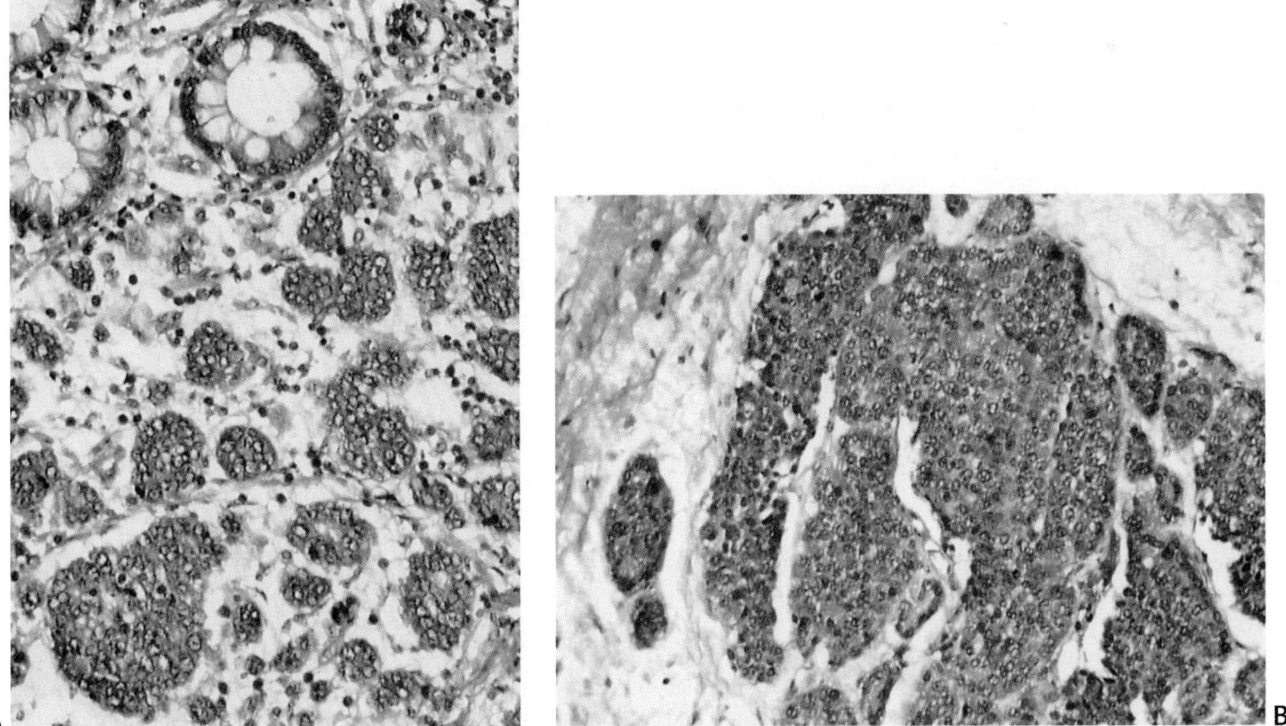

FIG. 34.7. ***Metastatic neuroendocrine neoplasms.*** **A:** A primary colonic carcinoid tumor. **B:** A metastasis in the breast from the tumor shown in **(A)**.

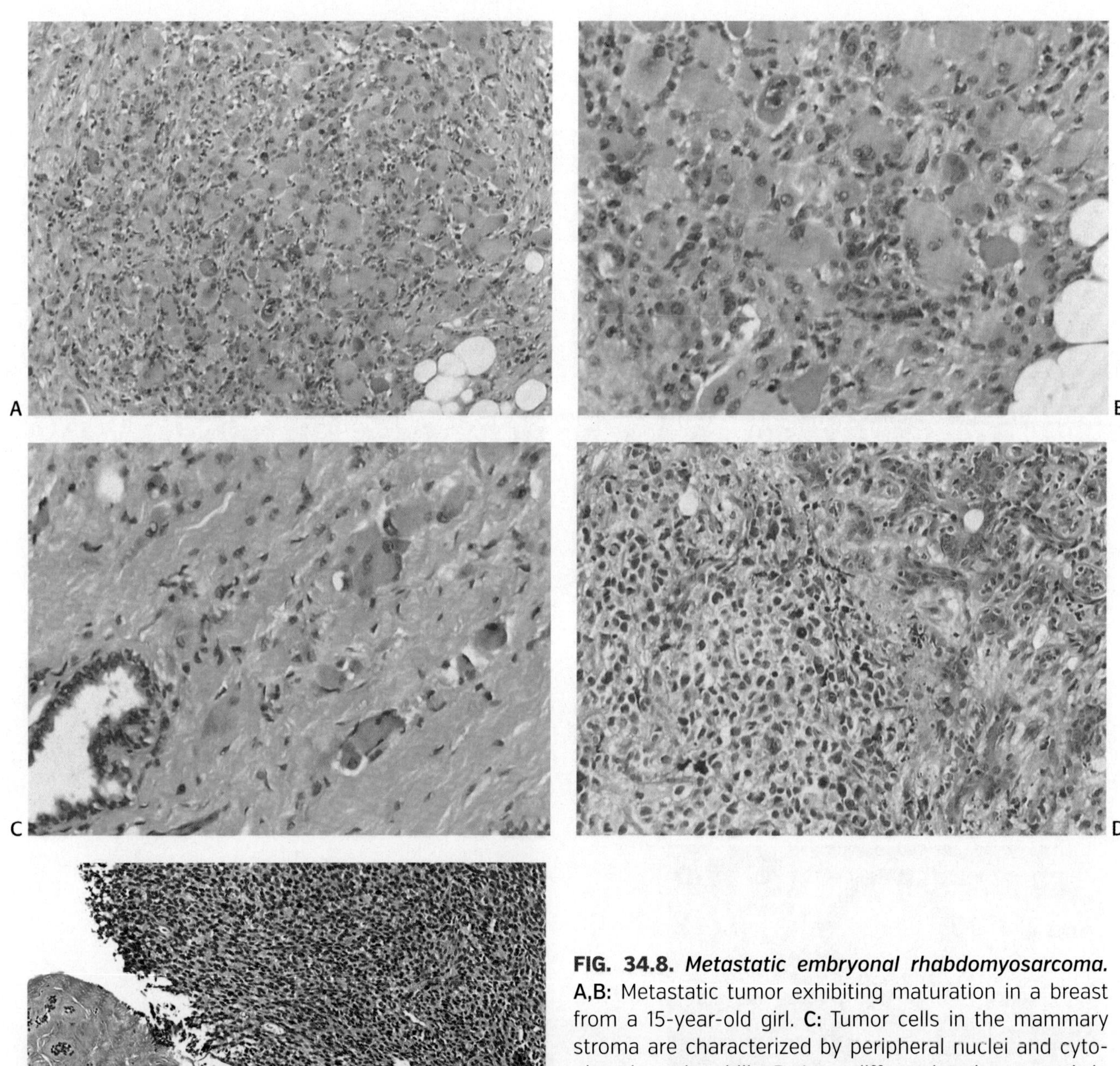

FIG. 34.8. ***Metastatic embryonal rhabdomyosarcoma.*** **A,B:** Metastatic tumor exhibiting maturation in a breast from a 15-year-old girl. **C:** Tumor cells in the mammary stroma are characterized by peripheral nuclei and cytoplasmic eosinophilia. **D:** An undifferentiated metastasis in the breast from a retroperitoneal primary in a 27-year-old patient. **E:** Metastatic tumor from a head and neck primary with spindle cell features in a needle core biopsy sample from the breast of a 16-year-old girl [*inset* shows a higher magnification view].

Salivary Gland Carcinoma

One series included two patients with metastatic mucoepidermoid carcinoma of the parotid gland, a lesion not often considered as a source of metastatic tumor in the breast.[12] Metastatic carcinoma that originated from mucoepidermoid carcinoma of the minor salivary glands in the floor of the mouth has also been reported (Fig. 34.14).[100] The primary tumor and the mammary metastasis were discovered coincidentally. In another patient, metastatic epidermoid carcinoma involved one breast and bone at the time that a primary tumor in the pharynx was identified.[101] The Senior Editor has also had the opportunity to examine an example of metastatic acinic cell carcinoma of salivary gland origin in the breast (Fig. 34.15).

Renal Carcinoma

Metastatic clear cell renal carcinoma resembles mammary carcinoma of the clear cell type (Fig. 34.16). Immunostaining for PAX2, PAX8, MUC1, CD10, and renal cell carcinoma monoclonal antibody (RCCma) is helpful in confirming renal origin in this situation.[51,84,102,103] Metastatic clear cell

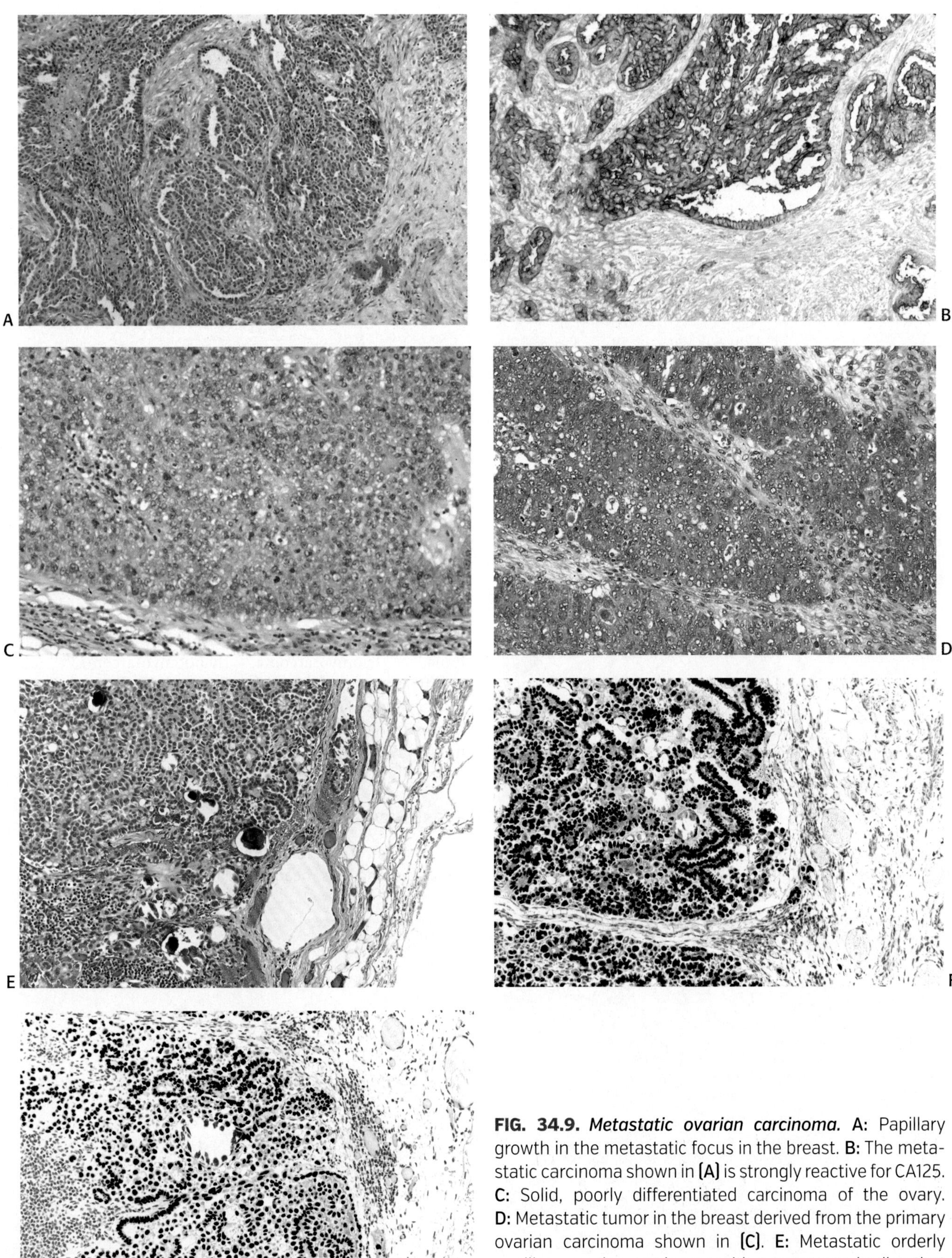

FIG. 34.9. ***Metastatic ovarian carcinoma.*** **A:** Papillary growth in the metastatic focus in the breast. **B:** The metastatic carcinoma shown in (**A**) is strongly reactive for CA125. **C:** Solid, poorly differentiated carcinoma of the ovary. **D:** Metastatic tumor in the breast derived from the primary ovarian carcinoma shown in (**C**). **E:** Metastatic orderly papillary ovarian carcinoma with psammoma bodies that involved an ALN in a 32-year-old woman. The tumor cells show nuclear reactivity with WT-1 (**F**) and PAX2 (**G**).

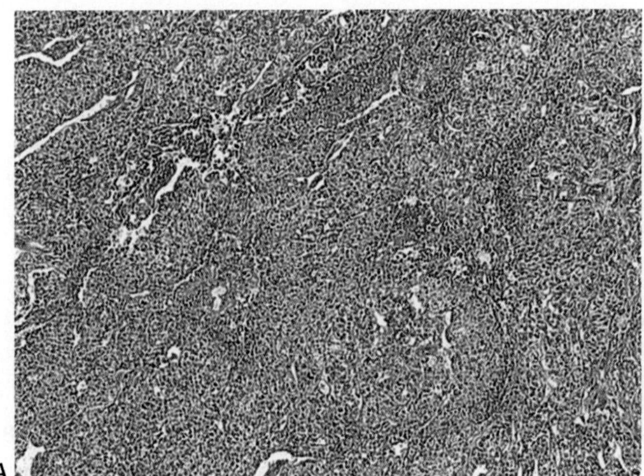

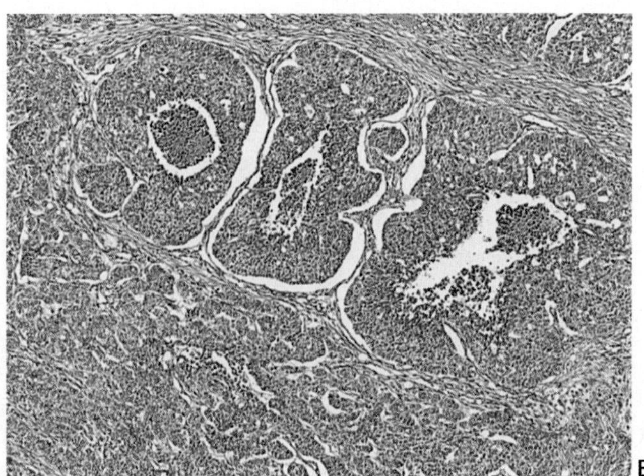

FIG. 34.10. ***Metastatic endometrial carcinoma.*** **A:** Solid, infiltrating, poorly differentiated carcinoma of the endometrium in the uterus. Note focal comedonecrosis in this primary tumor. **B:** Metastatic endometrial carcinoma in the breast with areas of comedonecrosis.

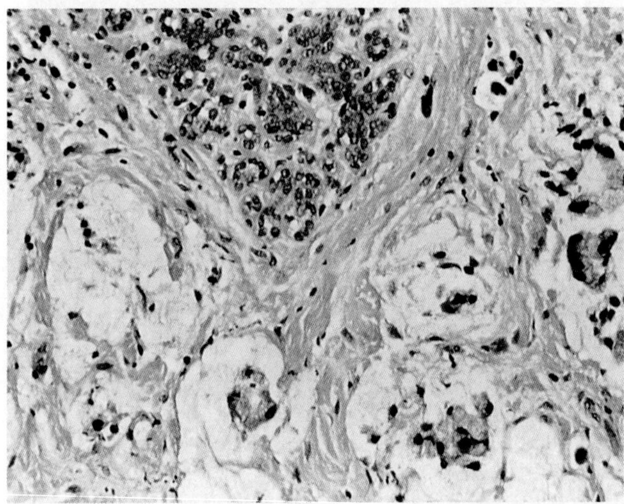

FIG. 34.11. ***Metastatic gastric carcinoma.*** The metastatic focus next to a lobule has mucinous differentiation.

renal carcinoma that originated in an occult primary has been described in a man.[104] Without knowledge of a renal primary, metastatic spindle cell renal carcinoma can easily be mistaken for a primary mammary sarcoma.[46]

Sarcoma

Among sarcomas metastatic in the breast hemangiopericytoma,[40,105] leiomyosarcoma,[45] rhabdomyosarcoma,[70,71] and undifferentiated pleomorphic sarcoma (malignant fibrous histiocytoma)[45] may be difficult to distinguish from primary mammary sarcomas and some metaplastic mammary carcinomas (Figs. 34.17 and 34.18).

Prostatic Carcinoma

Involvement of the male breast by metastatic prostatic adenocarcinoma has been a relatively frequent finding at

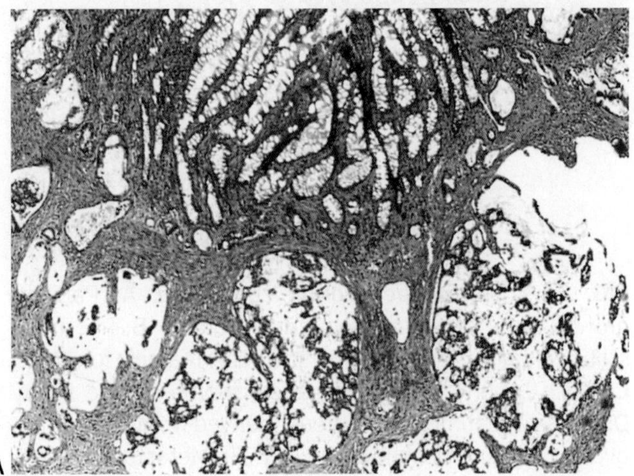

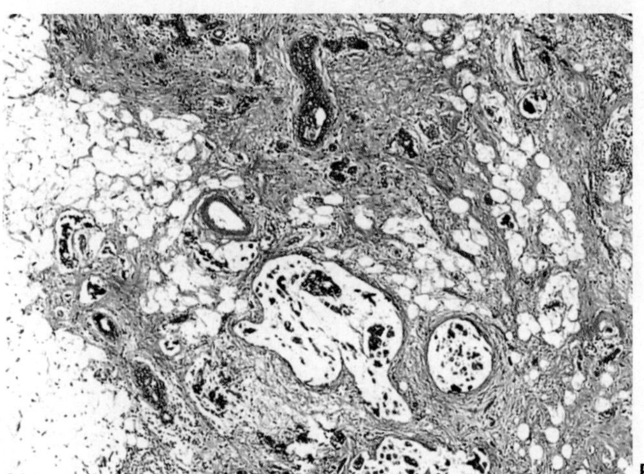

FIG. 34.12. ***Metastatic colonic carcinoma.*** **A:** Primary mucinous adenocarcinoma in the sigmoid colon of a 28-year-old woman. **B:** Two years later, this metastatic mucinous carcinoma was detected in one breast.

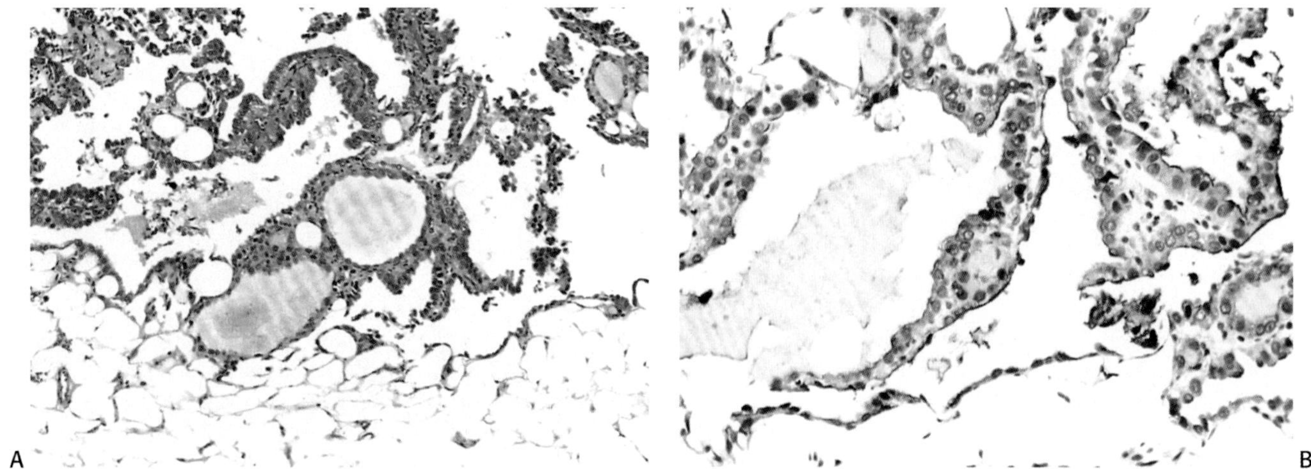

FIG. 34.13. ***Metastatic carcinoma of the thyroid gland.*** The patient had previously undergone a total thyroidectomy for "diffuse nodular hyperplasia." **A:** Metastatic, well-differentiated thyroid carcinoma with papillary and follicular features. **B:** The breast lesion was immunoreactive for thyroglobulin.

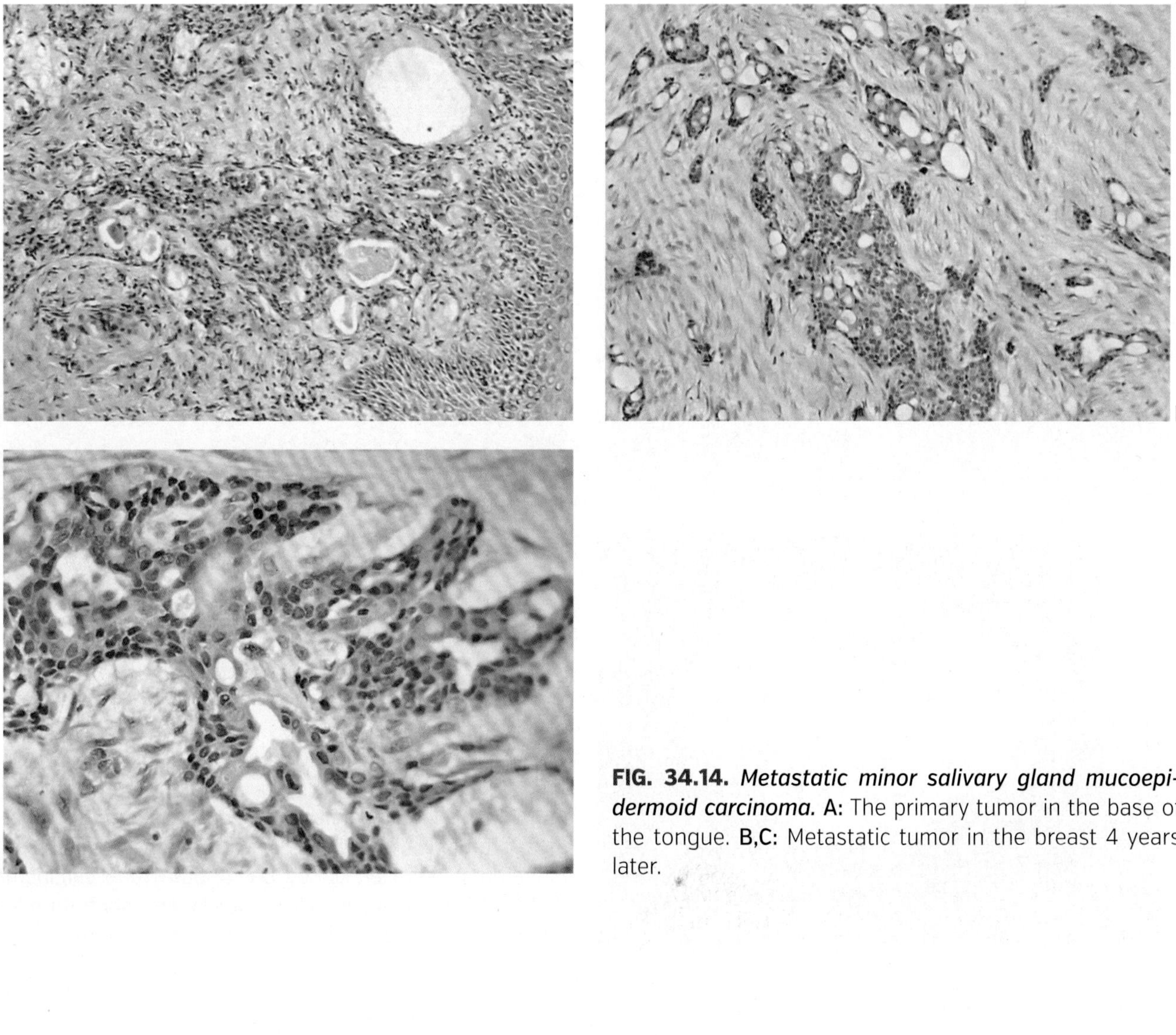

FIG. 34.14. ***Metastatic minor salivary gland mucoepidermoid carcinoma.*** **A:** The primary tumor in the base of the tongue. **B,C:** Metastatic tumor in the breast 4 years later.

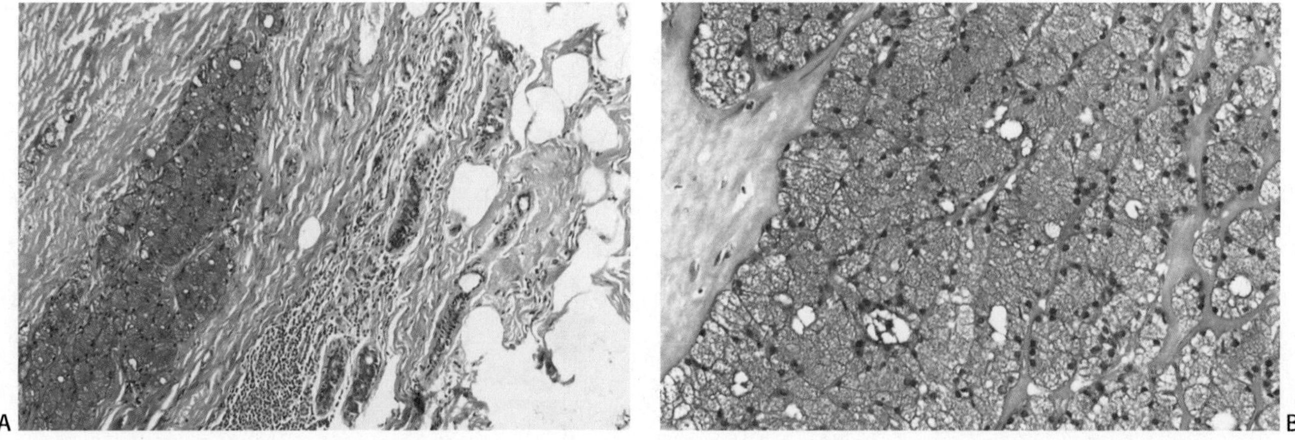

FIG. 34.15. ***Metastatic salivary gland acinic cell carcinoma.*** **A:** Metastatic acinic cell carcinoma in the breast. **B:** Typical vacuolated basophilic tumor cells.

autopsy. Microscopic breast involvement was found in 11 of the 46 men (26%) with breast tissue available in one series of 222 autopsied patients with prostatic carcinoma, although none had clinically apparent metastases.[106] With two exceptions, the men had gynecomastia, and all had been treated with estrogens. Several authors have described patients with bilateral breast metastases from prostatic carcinoma.[107–109] Although a breast mass in a man with prostatic carcinoma often proves to be metastatic from the prostatic tumor, there have been a few patients described who had independent

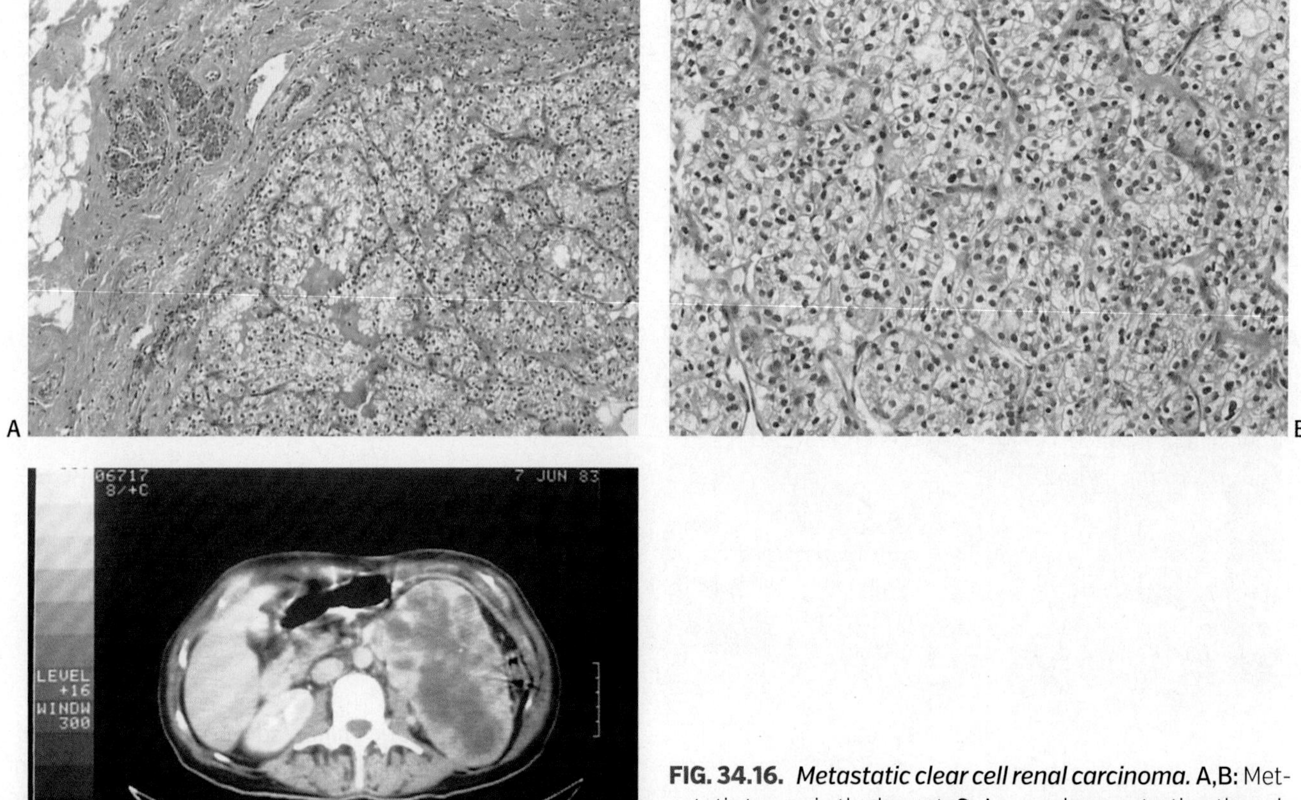

FIG. 34.16. ***Metastatic clear cell renal carcinoma.*** **A,B:** Metastatic tumor in the breast. **C:** A scan demonstrating the primary tumor in the left kidney. **D,E:** Another renal carcinoma metastatic in the breast. Note the circumscribed rounded edge of the metastatic tumor deposits in each case.

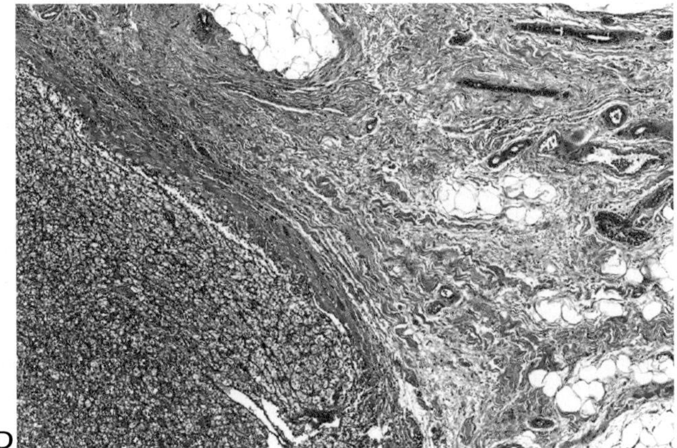

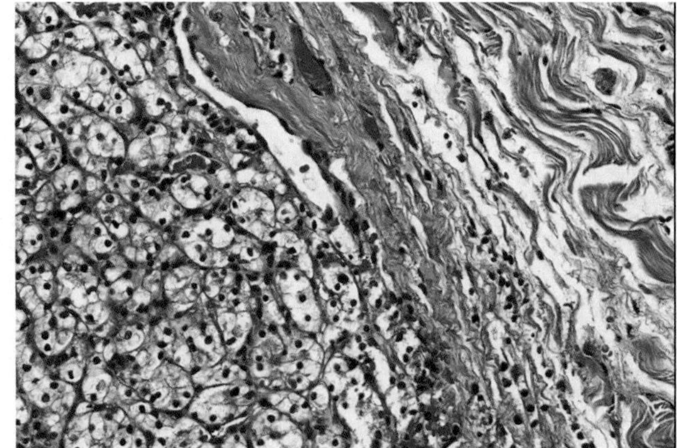

FIG. 34.16. *(Continued)*

synchronous or metachronous primary carcinomas of the prostate and breast.[110,111] On review, some purported examples of male mammary carcinoma that arose after estrogen therapy appear to be instances of metastatic prostatic carcinoma.[112] When a breast mass is discovered in a man known to have prostatic carcinoma, excisional biopsy is preferable to needle core biopsy or FNA, although the latter procedures may provide samples adequate for evaluation. In addition to routine histologic examination, immunostaining should be obtained for prostate-specific membrane antigen (PSMA), prostate-specific antigen (PSA), prostatic specific acid phosphatase (PSAP) and NKX3.1,[48,113,114] estrogen receptor (ER), progesterone receptor (PR), androgen receptor (AR), gross cystic disease fluid protein 15 (GCDFP-15), CK7, and CK20. PSA has been detected in breast carcinomas from men and women, and therefore a positive immunostaining is not specific for prostatic carcinoma.[115–117] The typical immunoprofile for prostatic carcinoma is as follows: ER and PR (−) or variably (+); CK7 (−); CK20 (−); GCDFP-15 (−); NKX 3.1 (+); and PSA (+) (Fig. 34.19). Mammary carcinoma in men typically has the following immunophenotypes: ER (+); PR variably (+); CK7 (+); CK20 (−); GCDFP-15 (+); NKX3.1 (−); and PSA (−) (see Chapter 36). Immunoreactivity for PSA has been detected in less than 5% of male and female primary mammary carcinomas that are virtually never reactive for PSAP.[118] The only nonprostate cancer case that was reactive for NKX3.1, which "seems to be a highly sensitive and specific tissue marker of metastatic prostatic adenocarcinoma," was an invasive lobular carcinoma of the breast.[114] A collision tumor consisting of metastatic prostatic carcinoma in a solid papillary carcinoma of the male breast has been described.[119]

TREATMENT AND PROGNOSIS

Metastatic involvement of the breast is a manifestation of generalized metastases in the great majority of cases. The prognosis depends on the clinical characteristics of the specific neoplasm.

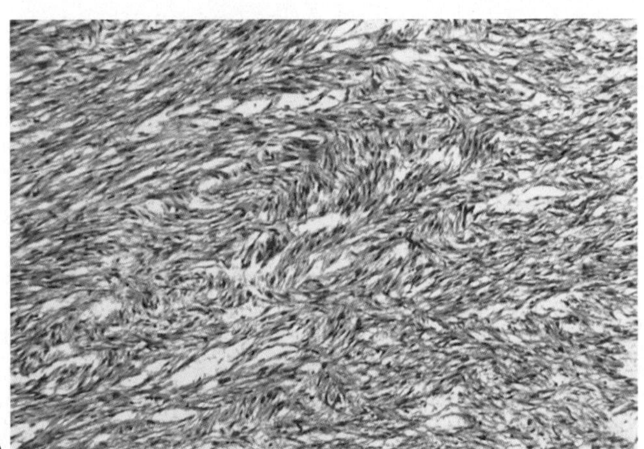

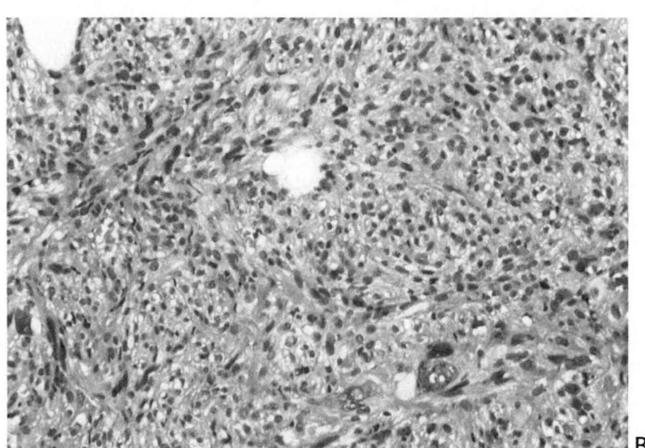

FIG. 34.17. ***Metastatic leiomyosarcoma.*** **A:** The primary tumor in the thigh. **B:** Metastatic lesion in the breast 1 year later showing spindle cells and pleomorphic giant cells.

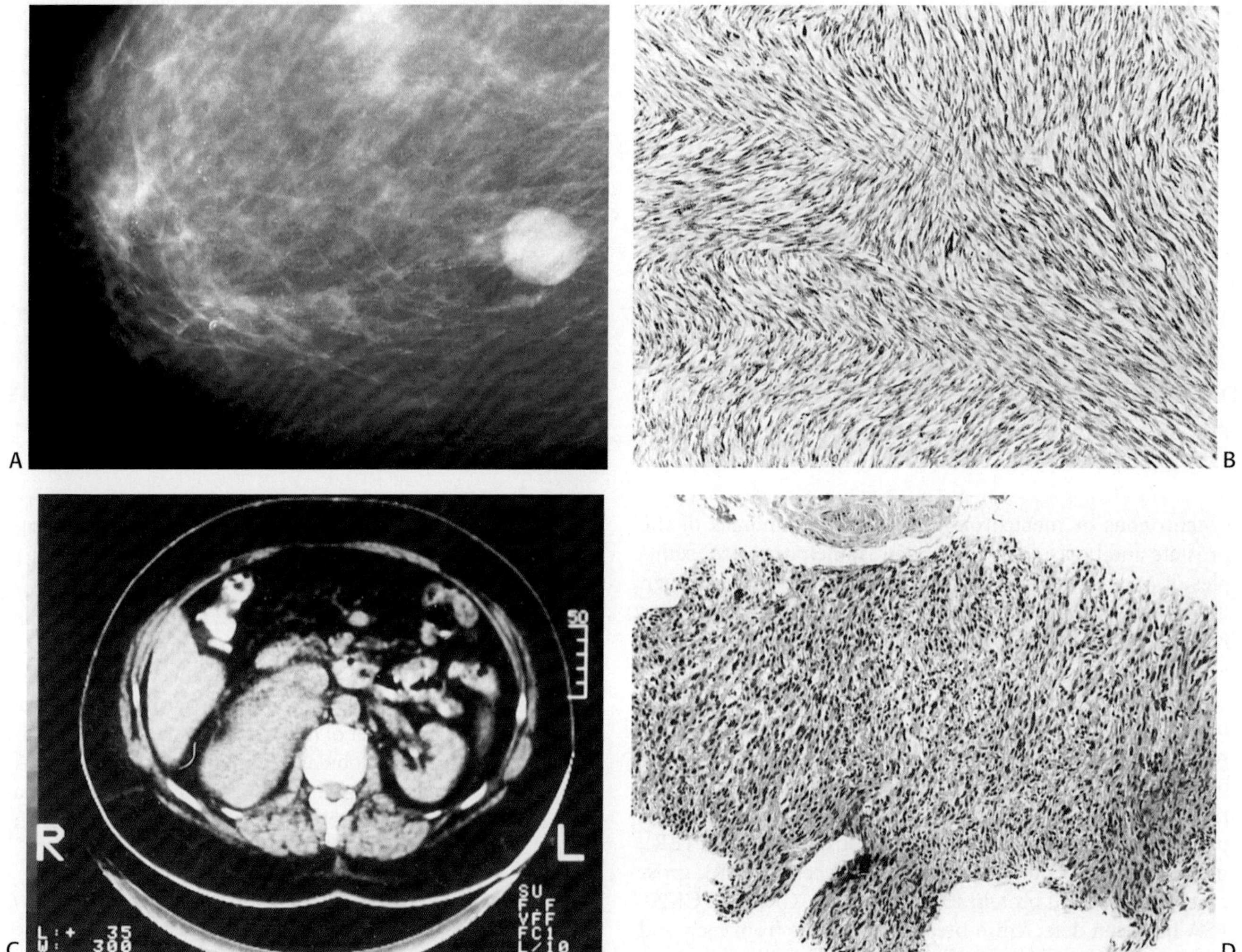

FIG. 34.18. ***Metastatic sarcomatoid renal carcinoma.*** **A:** The mammogram shows a dense, well-circumscribed tumor in the inferior part of the breast. **B:** Histologically, the breast tumor was composed of spindle cells arranged in a storiform pattern. **C:** A computed tomography (CT) scan demonstrated a tumor of the right kidney. **D:** A needle biopsy of the right renal mass revealed sarcomatoid carcinoma.

In a review of 169 patients with pathologically confirmed metastatic neoplasms in the breast, the median survival from the time the metastasis was diagnosed was 10 months, with a range of 0.4 to 192.7 months.[10] In this study, univariate analysis revealed that patients with no metastases other than in the breast had a significantly better survival, as did patients with neuroendocrine tumors and patients who underwent excision of metastasis. On multivariate analysis, patients who did not undergo resection of metastatic tumor in the breast were 88% more likely to die during the follow-up period than those who had metastatic tumor excised.

In a review of 85 patients with metastases from distant organs to the breast, axilla, or both, which appeared in 2013, 96% of the patients with follow-up were dead of disease with a median survival of 15 months after diagnosis.[120] Incidentally, in this set of cases, all managed at Memorial Sloan-Kettering Cancer Center in New York City, "the failure of the pathologist to recognize the metastatic nature of the lesion resulted most often because of the absence of a prior cancer history provided by the clinician at the time of initial interpretation."

Mastectomy is not appropriate for metastatic tumor in the breast in most cases, but it may be performed to obtain local control of bulky, ulcerated, necrotic, or otherwise symptomatic lesions. Wide excision can be supplemented by radiotherapy to the breast for radiosensitive neoplasms, and axillary dissection may be performed, especially if the lymph nodes seem grossly involved. Emphasis should necessarily be placed on systemic treatment appropriate to the primary lesion, and "local therapy should be tailored to each individual."[10] The overriding objective in the management of cases with metastases to the breast should be "to avoid unnecessary procedures and treatments."[120]

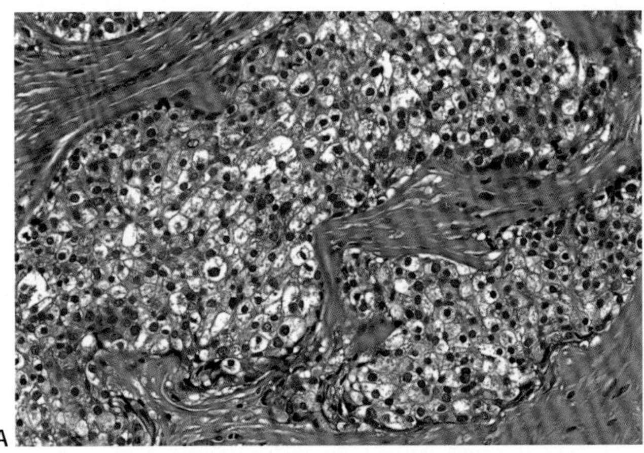
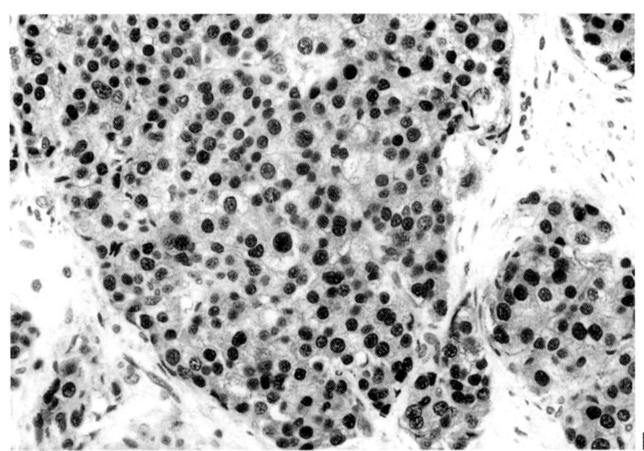

FIG. 34.19. ***Metastatic prostatic carcinoma.*** The primary tumor was diagnosed 1 year ago. The patient now presents with an elevated serum PSA, bone metastases, and a breast tumor shown here. **A:** The carcinoma had prominent clear cell features, which were present focally in the primary prostatic tumor. **B:** Strong diffuse nuclear immunoreactivity for ARs is shown. The carcinoma displayed cytoplasmic reactivity for PSA (not shown). There was no nuclear reactivity for ERs and PRs. Immunostaining for CK7 and CK20 was negative.

REFERENCES

1. Dawson EK. Metastatic tumour of the breast, with report of a case. *J Pathol Bacteriol* 1936;43:53–60.
2. de Alvarez PP, Russell P. Causes of death in cancer of the cervix uteri. *Am J Obstet Gynecol* 1947;54:91–96.
3. Speert H, Greeley AV. Cervical cancer with metastasis to breast. *Am J Obstet Gynecol* 1948;55:894–895.
4. Zetzel L, Scully RE. Case records of the Massachusetts General Hospital. *N Engl J Med* 1957;256:703–707.
5. Charache H. Metastatic tumors in the breast with a report of ten cases. *Surgery* 1953;33:385–390.
6. Sandison AT. Metastatic tumours in the breast. *Br J Surg* 1959;47:54–58.
7. Georgiannos SN, Chin J, Goode AW, et al. Secondary neoplasms of the breast. A survey of the 20th century. *Cancer* 2001;92:2259–2266.
8. Toombs BD, Kalisher L. Metastatic disease in the breast: clinical, pathologic and radiographic features. *AJR Am J Roentgenol* 1977;129:673–676.
9. Nielsen M, Andersen JA, Henriksen FW, et al. Metastases to the breast from extramammary carcinomas. *Acta Pathol Microbiol Scand (A)* 1981;89:251–256.
10. Williams SA, Ehlers RA II, Hunt KK, et al. Metastases to the breast from nonbreast solid neoplasms: presentation and determinants of survival. *Cancer* 2007;110:731–737.
11. Silverman JF, Feldman PS, Covell JL, et al. Fine needle aspiration cytology of neoplasms metastatic to the breast. *Acta Cytol* 1987;31:291–300.
12. Bohman L, Bassett LW, Gold RH, et al. Breast metastases from extramammary malignancies. *Radiology* 1982;144:309–312.
13. Recine MA, Deavers MT, Middleton LP, et al. Serous carcinoma of the ovarian and peritoneum with metastases to the breast and axillary lymph nodes. A potential pitfall. *Am J Surg Pathol* 2004;28:1646–1651.
14. Duda RB, August CZ, Schink JC. Ovarian carcinoma metastatic to the breast and axillary node. *Surgery* 1991;110:552–556.
15. Raptis S, Kanbour AI, Dusenbery D, et al. Fine-needle aspiration cytology of metastatic ovarian carcinoma to the breast. *Diagn Cytopathol* 1996;15:1–6.
16. Moncada R, Cooper RA, Garces M, et al. Calcified metastases from malignant ovarian neoplasm. *Radiology* 1974;113:31–35.
17. Soo MS, Williford ME, Elenberger CD. Medullary thyroid carcinoma metastatic to the breast: mammographic appearance. *AJR Am J Roentgenol* 1995;165:65–66.
18. Bowditch MG, Peck R, Shorthouse AJ. Metastatic renal adenocarcinoma presenting in a breast screening programme. *Eur J Surg Oncol* 1996;22:641–643.
19. Kelkar PS, Helbich TH, Becherer A, et al. Solitary breast metastasis as the first sign of a squamous cell carcinoma of the cervix: imaging findings. *Eur J Radiol* 1997;24:159–162.
20. Chateil JF, Arboucalot F, Pérel Y, et al. Breast metastases in adolescent girls: US findings. *Pediatr Radiol* 1998;28:832–835.
21. Yang WT, Metreweli C. Sonography of nonmammary malignancies of the breast. *AJR Am J Roentgenol* 1999;172:343–348.
22. Nofech-Mozes S, Mackenzie R, Kahn HJ, et al. Breast metastasis by medullary thyroid carcinoma detected by FDG positron emission tomography. *Ann Diagn Pathol* 2008;12:67–71.
23. Ravdel L, Robinson WA, Lewis K, et al. Metastatic melanoma in the breast: a report of 27 cases. *J Surg Oncol* 2006;94:101–104.
24. Hajdu SI, Urban JA. Cancers metastatic to the breast. *Cancer* 1972;29:1691–1696.
25. Kelly C, Henderson D, Corris P. Breast lumps: rare presentation of oat cell carcinoma of lung. *J Clin Pathol* 1988;41:171–172.
26. Chica GA, Johnson DE, Ayala AG. Renal cell carcinoma presenting as breast carcinoma. *J Urol* 1980;15:389–390.
27. Kannan V. Fine-needle aspiration of metastatic renal-cell carcinoma masquerading as primary breast carcinoma. *Diagn Cytopathol* 1998;18:343–345.
28. Silverman EM, Oberman HA. Metastatic neoplasms in the breast. *Surg Gynecol Obstet* 1974;138:26–28.
29. Mosunjac MB, Kochhar R, Monsunjac MI, et al. Primary small bowel carcinoid tumor with bilateral breast metastases. Report of 2 cases with different clinical presentations. *Arch Pathol Lab Med* 2004;128:292–297.
30. Harrist TJ, Kalisher L. Breast metastasis: an unusual manifestation of a malignant carcinoid tumor. *Cancer* 1977;40:3102–3106.
31. Hawley PP. A case of secondary carcinoid tumors in both breasts following excision of primary carcinoid of the duodenum. *Br J Surg* 1966;53:818–820.
32. Kashlan RB, Powell RW, Nolting SF. Carcinoid and other tumors metastatic to the breast. *J Surg Oncol* 1982;20:25–30.
33. Elit LM, Cunnane MF. Breast metastasis from ovarian carcinoma: report of two cases and literature review. *J Surg Pathol* 1995;1:69–74.
34. Frauenhoffer EE, Ro JY, Silva EG, et al. Well differentiated serous ovarian carcinoma presenting as a breast mass: a case report and flow cytometric DNA study. *Int J Gynecol Pathol* 1991;10:79–87.
35. Ron IG, Inbar M, Halpern M, et al. Endometrioid carcinoma of the ovary presenting as primary carcinoma of the breast. A case report and review of the literature. *Acta Obstet Gynecol Scand* 1992;71:81–83.

36. Yamasaki H, Saw D, Zdanowitz J, et al. Ovarian carcinoma metastasis to the breast. Case report and review of the literature. *Am J Surg Pathol* 1993;17:193–197.
37. Ascani S, Nati S, Liberati F, et al. Breast metastasis of thyroid follicular carcinoma. *Acta Oncol* 1994;33:71–73.
38. Hanna NN, O'Donnell K, Wolfe GRZ. Alveolar soft part sarcoma metastatic to the breast. *J Surg Oncol* 1996;61:159–162.
39. Sneige N, Zachariah S, Fanning TV, et al. Fine needle aspiration cytology of metastatic neoplasms in the breast. *Am J Clin Pathol* 1989;92:27–35.
40. Breitbart AS, Harris MN, Vazquez M, et al. Metastatic hemangiopericytoma of the breast. *NY State J Med* 1992;92:158–160.
41. Tulasi NR, Kurian S, Mathew G, et al. Breast metastases from primary leiomyosarcoma. *Aust NZ J Surg* 1997;67:71–72.
42. Belton AL, Stull MA, Grant T, et al. Mammographic and sonographic findings in metastatic transitional cell carcinoma of the breast. *AJR Am J Roentgenol* 1997;168:511–512.
43. Domanski HA. Metastases to the breast from extramammary neoplasms. A report of six cases with diagnosis by fine needle aspiration cytology. *Acta Cytol* 1996;40:1293–1300.
44. Fowler CA, Nicholson S, Lott M, et al. Choriocarcinoma presenting as a breast lump. *Eur J Surg Oncol* 1995;21:576–578.
45. Shukla R, Pooja B, Radhika S, et al. Fine-needle aspiration cytology of extramammary neoplasms metastatic to the breast. *Cytopathology* 2005;32:193–197.
46. Ding GTY, Hwang JS, Tan PH. Sarcomatoid renal cell carcinoma metastatic to the breast: report of a case with diagnosis on fine needle aspiration cytology. *Acta Cytol* 2007;51:451–455.
47. Moore DH, Wilson DK, Hurteau JA, et al. Gynecologic cancers metastatic to the breast. *J Am Coll Surg* 1998;187:178–181.
48. Green LK, Klima M. The use of immunohistochemistry in metastatic prostatic adenocarcinoma to the breast. *Hum Pathol* 1991;22:242–246.
49. Vazquez MF, Mitnick JS, Roses DF. Diagnosis of metastatic melanoma to the breast by aspiration biopsy. *Breast Dis* 1995;8:387–390.
50. Cangiarella J, Symmans WF, Cohen JM, et al. Malignant melanoma metastatic to the breast. A report of seven cases diagnosed by fine-needle aspiration cytology. *Cancer (Cancer Cytopathol)* 1998;84:160–162.
51. Laury AR, Perets R, Piao H, et al. A comprehensive analysis of PAX8 expression in human epithelial tumors. *Am J Surg Pathol* 2011;35:816–826.
52. Robens J, Goldstein L, Gown AM, et al. Thyroid transcription factor-expression in breast carcinomas. *Am J Surg Pathol* 2010;34:1881–1885.
53. Turner BM, Cagle PT, Sainz IM, et al. Napsin A, a new marker for lung adenocarcinoma, is complementary and more sensitive and specific than thyroid transcription factor 1 in the differential diagnosis of primary pulmonary carcinoma: evaluation of 1674 cases by tissue microarray. *Arch Pathol Lab Med* 2012;136:163–171.
54. Ordóñez NG. Immunohistochemical diagnosis of epithelioid mesothelioma. An update. *Arch Pathol Lab Med* 2005;129:1407–1414.
55. Perry KD, Reynolds C, Rosen DG, et al. Metastatic neuroendocrine tumour in the breast: a potential mimic of in-situ and invasive mammary carcinoma. *Histopathol* 2011;59:619–630.
56. Upalakalin JN, Collins LC, Tawa N, et al. Carcinoid tumors in the breast. *Am J Surg* 2006;191:799–805.
57. Schürch W, Lamoureux E, Lefebvre R, et al. Solitary breast metastasis: first manifestation of an occult carcinoid of the ileum. *Virchows Arch A Pathol Anat Histol* 1980;386:117–124.
58. Turner M, Gallager HS. Occult appendiceal carcinoid. Report of a case with fatal metastases. *Arch Pathol* 1959;88:188–190.
59. Chodoff RJ. Solitary breast metastasis from carcinoid of the ileum. *Am J Surg* 1965;109:814–815.
60. Lozowski MS, Faegenberg D, Mishriki Y, et al. Carcinoid tumor metastatic to breast diagnosed by fine needle aspiration. Case report and literature review. *Acta Cytol* 1989;33:191–194.
61. Lee AHS. The histological diagnosis of metastases to the breast from extramammary malignancies. *J Clin Pathol* 2007;60:1333–1341.
62. Kaltsas GA, Putignano P, Mukherjee JJ, et al. Carcinoid tumours presenting as breast cancer: the utility of radionuclide imaging with ^{123}I-MIBG and ^{111}In-DTPA pentetreotide. *Clin Endocrinol* 1998;49:685–689.
63. Fishman A, Kim HS, Girtanner RE, et al. Solitary breast metastasis as first manifestation of ovarian carcinoid tumor. *Gynecol Oncol* 1994;54:222–226.
64. Helvie MA, Frank TS. Enhancing breast metastases from bronchial neuroendocrine carcinoid carcinoma. *Breast Dis* 1993;6:233–236.
65. Baliga M, Holmquist ND, Espinoza CG. Medulloblastoma metastatic to breast diagnosed by fine-needle aspiration biopsy. *Diagn Cytopathol* 1994;10:33–36.
66. Kapila K, Sarkar C, Verma K. Detection of metastatic medulloblastoma in a fine needle breast aspirate. *Acta Cytol* 1996;40:384–385.
67. Howarth GB, Caces JN, Pratt CB. Breast metastases in children with rhabdomyosarcoma. *Cancer* 1980;46:2520–2524.
68. Hogge JP, Magnant CM, Lage JM, et al. Rhabdomyosarcoma metastatic to the breast. *Breast J* 1996;2:270–274.
69. Kwan WH, Choi PHK, Li CK, et al. Breast metastasis in adolescents with alveolar rhabdomyosarcoma of the extremities: report of two cases. *Pediatr Hemat Oncol* 1996;13:277–285.
70. Tan GC, Shiran MS, Hayati AR, et al. Alveolar rhabdomyosarcoma of the left hand with bilateral breast metastases in an adolescent female. *J Chin Med Assoc* 2008;71:639–642.
71. Yaren A, Guclu A, Sen N, et al. Breast metastasis in a pregnant woman with alveolar rhabdomyosarcoma of the upper extremity. *Eur J Obstet Gynecol Reprod Biol* 2008;140:131–133.
72. Schnabel T, Glag M. Breast metastases of Merkel cell carcinoma. *Eur J Cancer* 1996;32A:1617–1618.
73. Alzaraa A, Thomas GD, Vodovnik A, et al. Merkel cell carcinoma in a male breast: a case report. *Breast J* 2007;13:517–519.
74. Tornos C, Soslow R, Chen S, et al. Expression of WT1, CA 125, and GCDFP-15 as useful markers in the differential diagnosis of primary ovarian carcinomas versus metastatic breast cancer to the ovary. *Am J Surg Pathol* 2005;29:1482–1489.
75. Goldstein NS, Uzieblo A. WT1 immunoreactivity in uterine papillary serous carcinomas is different from ovarian serous carcinomas. *Am J Clin Pathol* 2002;117:541–545.
76. Karabakhtsian R, Bhargava R. WT-1 expression in primary invasive breast carcinomas: occasional expression in micropapillary and mucinous subtypes. *Mod Pathol* 2007;20(Suppl. 2):38A.
77. Lee AHS, Paish EC, Marchio C, et al. The expression of Wilms' tumour-1 and Ca125 in invasive micropapillary carcinoma of the breast. *Histopathology* 2007;51:824–828.
78. Domfeh AB, Carley AM, Striebel J, et al. WT-1 expression in primary mucinous carcinoma of the breast. *Mod Pathol* 2008;21(Suppl. 1):28A.
79. Rowsell C, Hanna WM, Kahn HJ. WT-1 expression in breast carcinomas with mucinous morphology. *Mod Pathol* 2008;21(Suppl. 1):52A.
80. Silberstein GB, Van Horn K, Strickland P, et al. Altered expression of the WT1 Wilms tumor suppressor gene in human breast cancer. *Proc Natl Acad Sci USA* 1997;94:8132–8137.
81. Loeb DM, Evron E, Patel CB, et al. Wilms' tumor suppressor gene (WT1) is expressed in primary breast tumors despite tumor-specific promoter methylation. *Cancer Res* 2001;61:921–925.
82. Miyoshi Y, Ando A, Egawa C, et al. High expression of Wilms' tumor suppressor gene predicts poor prognosis in breast cancer patients. *Clin Cancer Res* 2002;8:1167–1171.
83. Wilsher M, Cheerala B. WT1 as a complementary marker of malignant melanoma: an immunohistochemical study of whole sections. *Histopathology* 2007;51:605–610.
84. Tacha D, Zhou D, Cheng L. Expression of PAX8 in normal and neoplastic tissues: a comprehensive immunohistochemical study. *Appl Immunohistochem Mol Morphol* 2011;19:293–299.
85. Alexander HR, Turnbull AD, Rosen PP. Isolated breast metastases from gastrointestinal carcinomas. *J Surg Oncol* 1989;42:264–266.
86. Ho YY, Lee WK. Metastasis to the breast from an adenocarcinoma of the colon. *J Clin Ultrasound* 2009;37:239–241.
87. Selcukbiricik F, Tural D, Bay A, et al. A malignant mass in the breast is not always breast cancer. *Case Rep Oncol* 2011;4:521–525.
88. Noh KT, Oh B, Sung SH, et al. Metastasis to the breast from colonic adenocarcinoma. *J Korean Surg Soc* 2011;81:S43–S46.
89. Werling RW, Yazijii, Bacchi CE, et al. CDX2, a highly sensitive and specific marker for adenocarcinomas of intestinal origin: an immunohistochemical survey of 476 primary and metastatic carcinomas. *Am J Surg Pathol* 2003;27:303–310.
90. Boutis AL, Andreadis C, Patakiouta F, et al. Gastric signet-ring adenocarcinoma presenting with breast metastasis. *World J Gastroenterol* 2006;12:2958–2961.
91. Loureiro MM, Leite VH, Boavida JM, et al. An unusual case of papillary carcinoma of the thyroid with cutaneous and breast metastases only. *Eur J Endocrinol* 1997;137:267–269.

92. Al-Abed Y, Gray E, Wolfe K, et al. Metastatic Hurthle cell carcinoma of the thyroid presenting as a breast lump: a case report. *Int Semin Surg Oncol* 2008;5:14.
93. Bisceglia M, Galliani C, Rosai J. TTF-1 expression in breast carcinoma-the chosen clone matters. *Am J Surg Pathol* 2011;35:1087–1088.
94. Kiely N, Willimas N, Wilson G, et al. Medullary carcinoma of the thyroid metastatic to breast. *Postgrad Med J* 1995;71:744–754.
95. Ali SD, Teichberg S, Attie JN, et al. Medullary thyroid carcinoma metastatic to breast masquerading as infiltrating lobular carcinoma. *Ann Clin Lab Sci* 1994;24:441–447.
96. Fiche M, Cassagnau E, Aillet G, et al. Breast metastasis from a "tall cell variant" of papillary thyroid carcinoma. *Ann Pathol* 1998;18:130–132.
97. Tosi AL, Ragazzi M, Asioli S, et al. Breast tumor resembling the tall cell variant of papillary thyroid carcinoma: report of 4 cases with evidence of malignant potential. *Int J Surg Pathol* 2007;15:14–19.
98. Masood S, Davis C, Kubik MJ. Changing the term "breast tumor resembling the tall cell variant of papillary thyroid carcinoma" to "tall cell variant of papillary breast carcinoma." *Adv Anat Pathol* 2012;19:108–110.
99. Hameed O, Perry A, Banerjee R, et al. Papillary carcinoma of the breast lacks evidence of RET rearrangements despite morphological similarities to papillary thyroid carcinoma. *Mod Pathol* 2009;22:1236–1242.
100. Kirsch RLA, Rosen PP. An unusual well-circumscribed breast tumor. *Mem Hosp Bull* 1976;6:60–61.
101. Nunez DA, Sutherland CGC, Sood RK. Breast metastasis from a pharyngeal carcinoma. *J Laryngol Otol* 1989;103:227–228.
102. Gokden N, Gokden M, Phan DC, et al. The utility of PAX-2 in distinguishing metastatic clear cell renal cell carcinoma from its morphologic mimics: an immunohistochemical study with comparison to renal cell carcinoma marker. *Am J Surg Pathol* 2008;32:1462–1467.
103. Sangoi AR, Karamchandani J, Kim J, et al. The use of immunohistochemistry in the diagnosis of metastatic clear cell renal cell carcinoma: a review of PAX-8, PAX-2, hKIM-1, RCCma, and CD10. *Adv Anat Pathol* 2010;17:377–393.
104. Gibbons CER, Lewi HJE, Kashif KM. Breast lump—an unusual presentation of renal cell carcinoma. *Br J Urol* 1995;76:131.
105. Kindblom LG, Ullman A. Malignant hemangiopericytoma with admixed glandular structures in breast and lung metastases. *Appl Pathol* 1983;1:50–59.
106. Salyer WR, Salyer DC. Metastases of prostatic carcinoma to the breast. *J Urol* 1973;109:671–675.
107. Hartley LCJ, Little JH. Bilateral mammary metastases from carcinoma of the prostate during oestrogen therapy. *Med J Aust* 1971;1:434–436.
108. Malek GA, Madsen PO. Carcinoma of the prostate with unusual metastases. *Cancer* 1969;24:194–197.
109. Scott J, Robb-Smith AHT, Burns I. Bilateral breast metastases from carcinoma of the prostate. *Br J Urol* 1974;46:209–214.
110. Moldwin RM, Orihuela E. Breast masses associated with adenocarcinoma of the prostate. *Cancer* 1989;63:2229–2233.
111. Wilson SE, Hutchinson WB. Breast masses in males with carcinoma of the prostate. *J Surg Oncol* 1976;8:105–112.
112. Jakobsen AHI. Bilateral mammary carcinoma in the male following stilboestrol therapy. *Acta Path Microbiol Scand* 1952;31:61–66.
113. Choudhury M, DeRosas J, Papsidero L, et al. Metastatic prostatic carcinoma to the breast or primary breast carcinoma. *J Urol* 1982;19:297–299.
114. Gurel B, Ali TZ, Montgomery EA, et al. NKX3.1 as a marker of prostatic origin in metastatic tumors. *Am J Surg Pathol* 2010;34:1097–1105.
115. Gupta RK. Immunoreactivity of prostate-specific antigen in male breast carcinoma: two examples of a diagnostic pitfall in discriminating a primary breast cancer from metastatic prostatic carcinoma. *Diagn Cytopathol* 1999;21:167–169.
116. Bodey B, Bodey B Jr, Kaiser HE. Immunocytochemical detection of prostate specific antigen expression in human breast carcinoma cells. *Anticancer Res* 1997;17:2577–2581.
117. Yu H, Levesque MA, Clark GM, et al. Enhanced prediction of breast cancer prognosis by evaluating expression of p53 and prostate-specific antigen in combination. *Br J Cancer* 1999;81:490–495.
118. Kraus TS, Cohen C, Siddiqui MT. Prostate-specific antigen and hormone receptor expression in male and female breast carcinoma. *Diagn Pathol* 2010;5:63.
119. Sahoo S, Smith RE, Potz JL, et al. Metastatic prostatic adenocarcinoma within a primary solid papillary carcinoma of the male breast. Application of immunohistochemistry to a unique collision tumor. *Arch Pathol Lab Med* 2001;125:1101–1103.
120. Delair DF, Corben AD, Catalano JP, et al. Non-mammary metastases to the breast and axilla: a study of 85 cases. *Mod Pathol* 2013;26:343–349.

CHAPTER 35

Benign Proliferative Lesions of the Male Breast

MELISSA P. MURRAY • EDI BROGI

PAPILLOMA

Several examples of intraductal papilloma arising in the male breast have been reported[1–4] (Figs. 35.1 and 35.2). The patients have ranged in age from 3 months to 82 years. The usual presenting symptom is nipple discharge that is bloody or blood tinged. Cystic lesions may be palpable. The ultrasound appearance of benign cystic papillary tumors of the male breast has been documented.[5–7] One patient treated with phenothiazines for more than 10 years had a multiloculated cystic tumor measuring 7 × 6 × 3 cm that recurred as a 1 × 1 cm cystic lesion 6 months after initial excision.[3] Microscopic examination revealed an orderly benign papillary tumor composed of cells with apocrine features and prominent secretory activity. A cystic papilloma described by Shim et al.[6] also had apocrine features.

Local recurrence of a multiloculated cystic papilloma in an 82-year-old man was described by David.[8] Because of the relatively high proportion of papillary carcinomas of the adult male breast, all male papillary tumors should be carefully evaluated pathologically. It is useful to investigate low-grade orderly papillary lesions of the male breast that may be papillomas with immunostains for myoepithelial cells, such as smooth muscle actin (SMA), p63, CD10, and cytokeratin (CK) 5/6. The absence of myoepithelium supports the diagnosis of papillary carcinoma, whereas the presence of myoepithelium is consistent with papilloma or papillary DCIS. In the latter circumstance, structural and cytologic features of the epithelium must be relied upon (see Chapters 5 and 14).

Florid Papillomatosis of the Nipple

Less than 5% of the reported examples of florid papillomatosis of the nipple have been in men.[9–11] Some of these lesions have contained carcinoma.[9,11] The histologic features are identical to those of florid papillomatosis in women (see Chapter 5).

FIBROEPITHELIAL TUMORS

Fibroepithelial lesions in the male breast usually arise in patients with gynecomastia.[12–19] A number of these patients had been treated with estrogens or antiandrogen therapy, resulting in gynecomastia with lobular differentiation.[13,20–22] Rare examples of fibroadenoma (FA) have been reported in

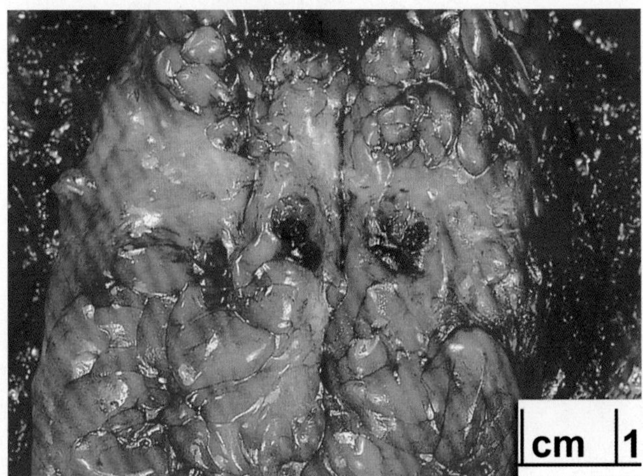

FIG. 35.1. ***Papilloma.*** An intracystic papilloma in the male breast.

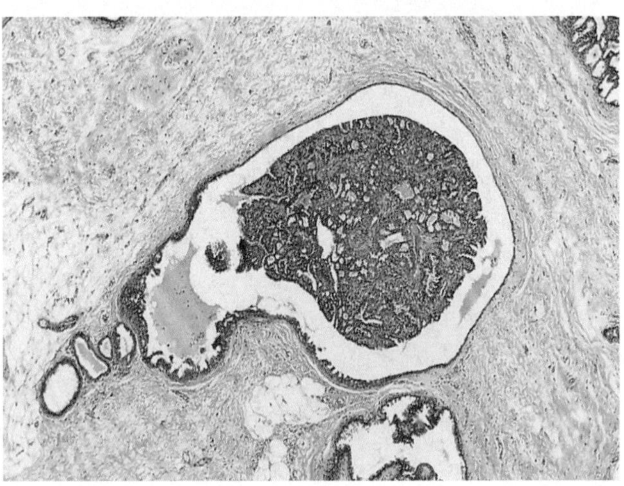

FIG. 35.2. ***Papilloma.*** A papilloma in a cystically dilated duct.

transsexual men.[17,18] Most PT in men have been histologically and clinically benign. In one case,[21] the stromal component of a 30-cm tumor was described as malignant, but the histologic appearance of the lesion was not illustrated.

FA occur in the male breast, but in retrospect, many of the lesions described in case reports were poorly documented or appear to have been nodular foci of gynecomastia (Fig. 35.3). Tumors measuring up to 5 cm have been described.[16] Four male patients with FA were reported from the Armed Forces Institute of Pathology (AFIP).[12] Age at diagnosis in this series ranged from 37 to 71 years. One patient had been treated with estrogens, and another had received methyldopa and chlordiazepoxide. Gynecomastia with lobular differentiation was present microscopically in each case. A particularly unusual patient was a 15-year-old boy with a 7-cm benign fibroepithelial tumor that arose in unilateral gynecomastia.[23] He had not received any medications. Gynecomastia was found histologically in the surrounding breast tissue, but there was no evidence of lobular differentiation.

Bilateral FA were described in a 66-year-old man under treatment with Lupron for prostatic carcinoma.[19] Cells in the stroma of one FA contained inclusion bodies identical to those found in infantile digital fibromas. A 75-year-old man under treatment for prostate cancer developed a 9-mm mass that increased in size on subsequent imaging. A core biopsy of the mass showed a FA.[13] In both cases, the FA arose in a background of gynecomastia.

Nielsen[15] documented a 16-cm fibroadenomatoid tumor that arose in one breast of a 69-year-old man with bilateral gynecomastia. The patient had chronic heart disease treated with digoxin and furosemide for 23 years, during which time his breasts appeared clinically normal. Breast enlargement and the appearance of the unilateral tumor began after spironolactone was added to his medication regimen, suggesting that this drug contributed to the mammary lesion. Gynecomastia has been associated with use of digitalis[24] and spironolactone.[25]

DUCT ECTASIA

Duct dilation or ectasia with periductal mastitis, a relatively common condition in the female breast, has also been rarely described in men.[1,26,27] Andersen and Gram[26] found duct ectasia in 9 (26%) of 35 "normal" breasts and in 19 (35%) of 55 breasts with gynecomastia examined at autopsy. Downs et al.[28] have reported a case of duct ectasia in a man with human immunodeficiency virus (HIV) infection, but it is unclear whether the lesion was due to the viral infection or may have been related to some form of estrogen treatment. The histologic appearance is similar in men and women, there being less inflammation and fibrosis in lesions that are clinically asymptomatic.

FIBROCYSTIC CHANGES

Proliferative fibrocystic changes (FCC) resembling those in women are only rarely encountered in the male breast. Several case reports document men who were under 50 years of age at the time of diagnosis.[29–32] Two of the men were described as karyotypically and phenotypically normal.[29,30] One patient reported having a swelling of the affected breast for 17 years, which doubled in size during the year prior to biopsy.[31] Grossly, each patient had a circumscribed multicystic tumor. The FCC include cysts with apocrine metaplasia, papillary apocrine metaplasia, duct hyperplasia, and duct stasis with mastitis. Gynecomastia was evident histologically in two cases. The gross and microscopic features in these lesions resemble juvenile papillomatosis.[31] Sanguinetti et al.[33] described a circumscribed, 1.5-cm grossly multicystic lesion with histologic features of juvenile papillomatosis that was excised from a 17-year-old boy. No images of the histopathology were provided.

Sclerosing adenosis (SA) arising in lobules was described as an incidental finding in the postmortem examination of a 41-year-old man with disseminated pulmonary oat cell

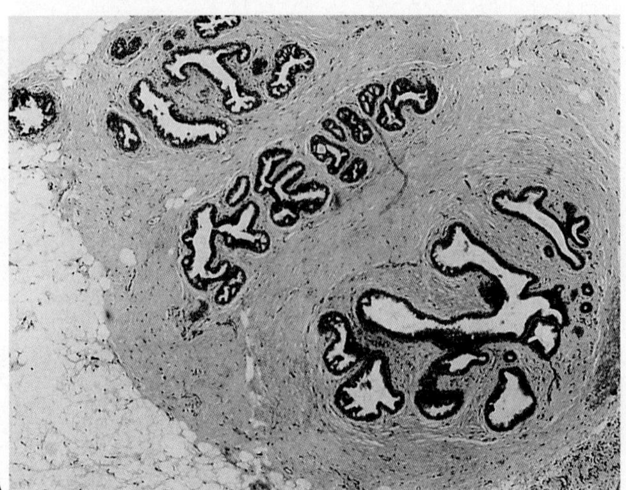
A

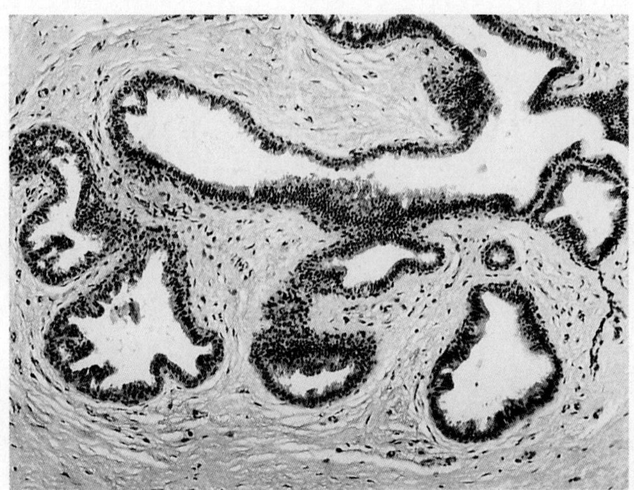
B

FIG. 35.3. ***Fibroadenomatoid gynecomastia.*** **A,B:** Nodular gynecomastia with early lobular differentiation. The patient was being treated with estrogen for prostatic carcinoma.

carcinoma.[34] Grossly, the lesion was a unilateral, firm, white 1.8 × 1.5 × 1.0 cm nodule. Ectopic hormone production was not documented in this case.

An unusual retroareolar mass in a 38-year-old man proved to be a 2.5-cm cyst lined by benign squamous epithelium.[35] There were no skin appendage glands in the cyst wall, and surrounding tissue contained mammary gland ducts.

GYNECOMASTIA

Clinical Presentation

Gynecomastia (*gynecain* = Greek word for female; *mastos* = Greek word for breast) is the most common clinical and pathologic abnormality of the male breast. The initial clinical signs of gynecomastia are breast enlargement and a palpable mass that may be accompanied by pain or tenderness in patients with more recent onset. Enlargement of the nipple and areola occurs in a minority of patients. Nipple retraction and discharge are rarely encountered. The palpable mass is located in the central subareolar region in all but a very small number of patients, who have eccentric or peripherally located lesions. On clinical examination, the mass may measure 10 cm or larger, but in most cases it spans 2 to 6 cm in diameter.

Both breasts are affected in the majority of patients with gynecomastia at all ages. Among those with unilateral gynecomastia, the left breast is involved more often than the right.[36] Bilateral involvement is usually synchronous, but it may be asynchronous. Patients with bilateral involvement tend to have diffuse lesions, whereas unilateral gynecomastia is more likely to produce a discrete mass. Some patients report pain associated with the mass. In one study,[37] administration of gamolenic acid was associated with reduced pain. Clinically, invasive carcinoma arising in gynecomastia can usually be detected as a localized, asymmetric area of firmness.

Radiology

Two mammographic patterns are associated with gynecomastia: a dendritic configuration featuring a retroareolar density with prominent radial extensions and a triangular subareolar density lacking radiating extensions. The triangular pattern is more common in gynecomastia of recent onset, whereas gynecomastia present for 6 months or longer tends to have the dendritic configuration. Mammography is helpful for distinguishing between gynecomastia and carcinoma, and it may identify carcinoma developing in gynecomastia.[38] Presently, the combined use of ultrasonography and mammography is considered the optimal approach for evaluating a patient who presents with clinical findings of gynecomastia in order to rule out carcinoma.[39–41]

Etiology

Idiopathic and/or physiologic gynecomastia accounts for the majority of cases. Gynecomastia is fairly common in newborn male infants, reflecting exposure to maternal estrogens. It usually regresses spontaneously in a few weeks. Gynecomastia in prepubertal boys is relatively infrequent,[42] but it has been reported in 30% to 40% of adolescent[43] and adult males.[44–46]

Numerous conditions have been associated with gynecomastia. Systemic diseases include hyperthyroidism, cirrhosis of the liver, chronic renal failure, chronic pulmonary disease, and hypogonadism. Gynecomastia has been related to the use of hormones such as estrogens, androgens, and many commonly used drugs, including digitalis, cimetidine, spironolactone, marijuana, and tricyclic antidepressants. There are reports of gynecomastia associated with the use of 3-hydroxy-3-methyl-glutaryl-CoAcetyl reductase inhibitors for the control of cholesterol level.[47,48] Androgen administered to develop muscular strength in athletes can cause gynecomastic breast enlargement and has rarely been associated with the development of male breast carcinoma. Gynecomastia is a frequent adverse side effect of finasteride administration to treat prostatic hyperplasia.[49]

Bilateral gynecomastia occurs in men treated with imatinib mesylate for chronic myeloid leukemia or gastrointestinal stromal tumor (GIST).[50,51] Liu et al.[52] found gynecomastia in 6 of 57 (10.5%) patients under treatment for GIST. Three patients with gynecomastia had elevated serum estradiol levels that did not change significantly after treatment with tamoxifen.

Neoplasms that are most likely to cause gynecomastia as a result of paraneoplastic hormone production are pulmonary carcinoma and testicular germ cell tumors.[46] Breast enlargement in HIV-positive men receiving antiretroviral therapy is usually due to true gynecomastia with dense stroma rather than fat accumulation or lipomastia.[53] Pantanowitz et al.[54] reported that gynecomastia was present in 7 of 12 (58%) HIV-positive patients and that all men with gynecomastia received antiretroviral therapy.

Gross Pathology

Gross examination reveals soft rubbery or firm, gray or white tissue that forms a discrete mass or an ill-defined area of induration. Rarely fat is admixed with the fibrous tissue.

Microscopic Pathology

Histopathologic studies show similar microscopic alterations regardless of etiologic factors.[36,42,46,55–57] Three phases of proliferative change have been described.

Florid Gynecomastia

Florid gynecomastia, ordinarily seen within 1 year of onset, is characterized by epithelial hyperplasia in ducts that have flat or micropapillary patterns or a combination of both forms (Figs. 35.4 and 35.5). Mitoses may be found in the epithelium. There is usually concomitant myoepithelial hyperplasia. Duct ectasia is not conspicuous during this phase. The increased amount and cellularity of periductal stroma are accompanied by prominent vascularity, edema, and a round cell infiltrate.

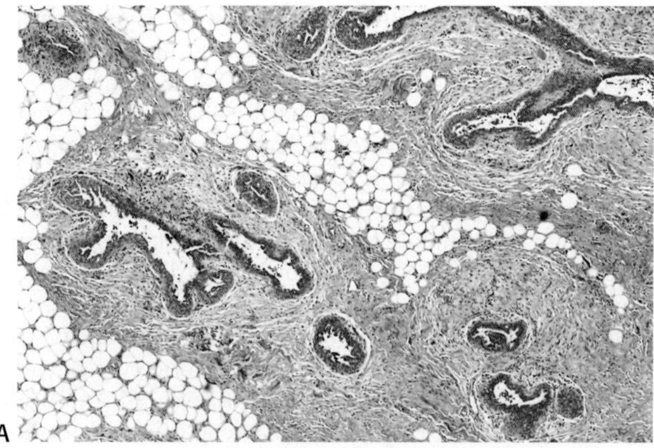
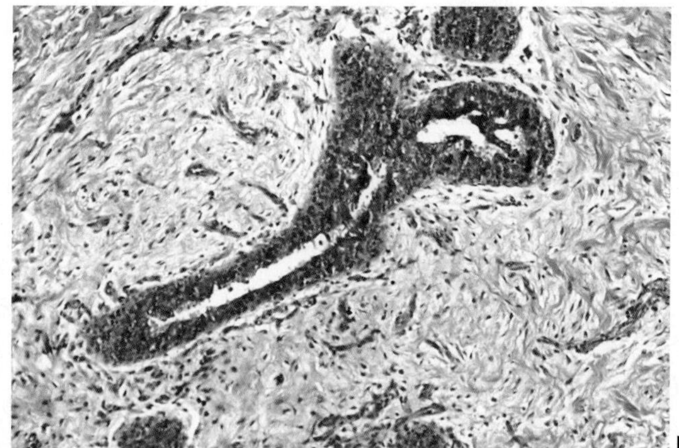

FIG. 35.4. ***Gynecomastia, florid.*** **A:** Periductal edema and cellular stroma with flat and micropapillary epithelial hyperplasia. **B:** Magnified view of a duct with predominantly flat epithelial hyperplasia and vascularized, edematous periductal stroma.

Intermediate Gynecomastia

Intermediate gynecomastia, which has florid and fibrous components, tends to be present for 6 months or less. It constitutes a transitional phase in the maturation of the lesion.

Fibrous (Inactive) Gynecomastia

Fibrous or inactive gynecomastia typically occurs after the lesion has been present for 12 months or longer. The epithelial proliferation is much less conspicuous than it is in the florid phase, the stroma is more collagenous, with less edema, and there is reduced vascularity (Fig. 35.6).

Pseudoangiomatous stromal hyperplasia (PASH) may be found in any phase of gynecomastia, but it is more pronounced in the active and intermediate stages (Fig. 35.7). Rarely, multinucleated giant cells are formed in PASH (Fig. 35.7).

Additional Epithelial Changes

A variety of other proliferative epithelial changes have been found in gynecomastia. Lobule formation, initially attributed to exogenous estrogen administration,[58] has been associated with diverse etiologies, including prepubertal gynecomastia,[59] spironolactone treatment (Fig. 35.8), and androgen administration (Fig. 35.9). Pseudolactational hyperplasia occurs rarely in lobules formed in gynecomastia (Fig. 35.10). Apocrine metaplasia occurs in all three phases (Fig. 35.11). Focal squamous metaplasia is most common in the florid stage (Fig. 35.12). Extensive squamous metaplasia is present in rare cases.[60]

The cytologic features and growth pattern of the epithelial proliferation in ducts may be atypical.[26,36,61] This occurs most often in the florid phase. Atypical features are the development of fenestrated and solid growth patterns, or an epithelial proliferation in which a cytologically atypical cell type appears to overgrow the usual dimorphic cell population that characterizes florid gynecomastia (Figs. 35.13 to 35.15). Mitotic activity is usually sparse, but it may be more abundant in ducts exhibiting severely atypical hyperplasia. Cytologic atypia in gynecomastia has also been associated with flutamide therapy for prostatic carcinoma[62] (Fig. 35.16) and for the treatment of alopecia.[63] Chemotherapy can cause secondary cytologic atypia in gynecomastia (Fig. 35.17).

Gynecomastia-like Hyperplasia in Women

Gynecomastia-like hyperplasia is a proliferative lesion of the female breast with the histologic features of florid gynecomastia, including three-layered ductal epithelium[64] (Fig. 35.18). It occurs as a discrete tumor or as incidental microscopic foci.[65] The lesion may appear on mammography as an asymmetric density or as a nodule, but the radiographic features are nonspecific.[65,66] The incidence of gynecomastia-like hyperplasia was 0.15%[65] and 0.56%[66] in two reports. Gynecomastia-like hyperplasia has been found in axillary breast tissue[66] and in various locations within the breast.

Cytology and Needle Core Biopsy

Fine-needle aspiration (FNA) is an effective method for the diagnosis of gynecomastia.[67–70] A review of FNAs of the breast performed in three US academic centers from 1990 to 2000 revealed that about 4% of 14,026 specimens had been obtained from men.[68] The most frequent diagnoses were gynecomastia and ductal carcinoma. Gynecomastia was diagnosed in 43/44 (97.8%) breast FNAs in men at a New Zealand institution[67] and in 86/119 (72.3%) at one hospital in India.[69] The cytologic features of gynecomastia are closely reminiscent of those in a FA. FNA of gynecomastia typically yields moderately cellular smears consisting of epithelial and stromal fragments. Naked bipolar to oval myoepithelial nuclei are present in the background. The epithelial fragments

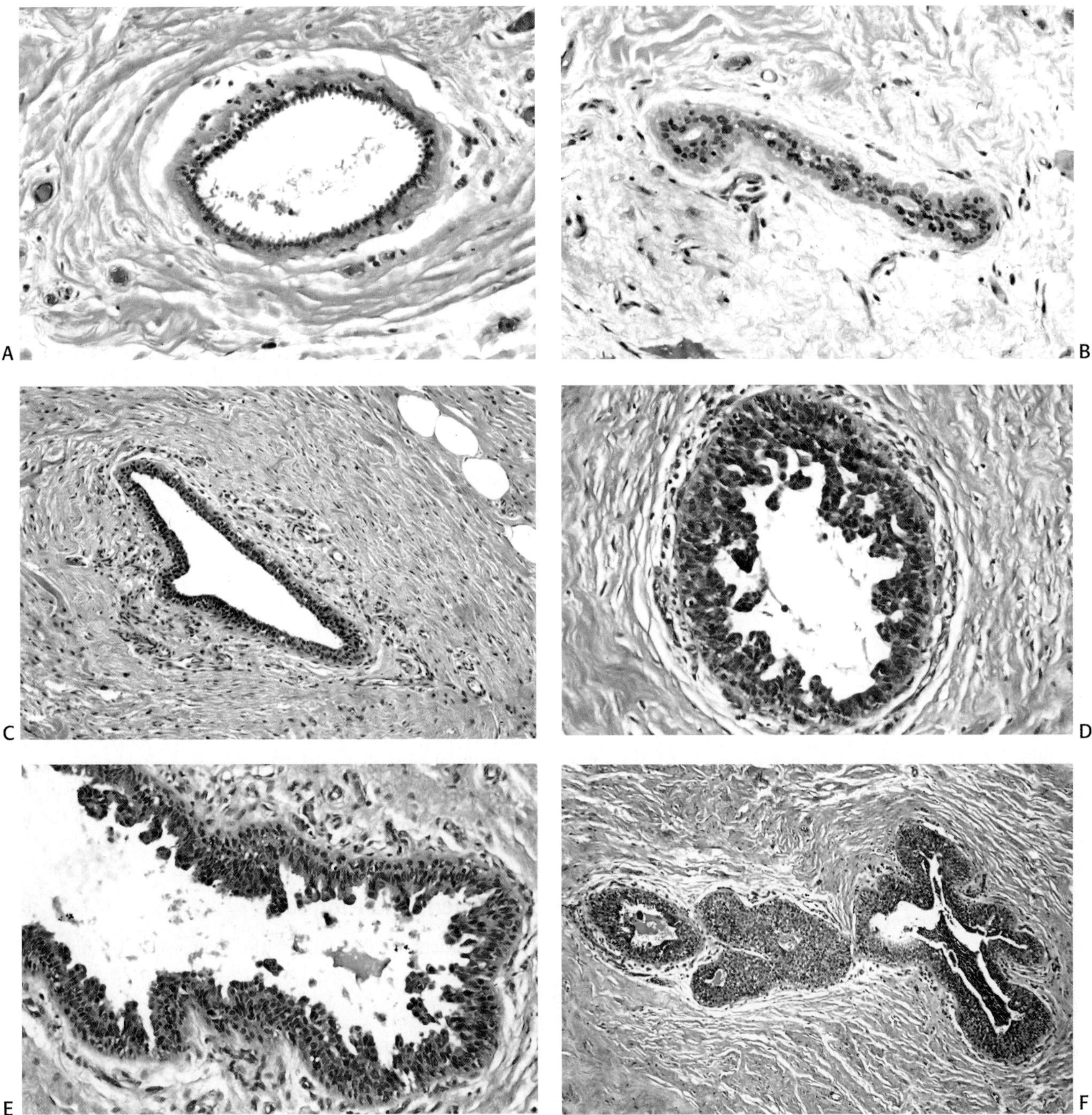

FIG. 35.5. ***Gynecomastia, ductal hyperplasia.*** **A:** Normal breast duct in a 43-year-old man. **B:** Normal atrophic breast duct in a 75-year-old man. **C:** Flat ductal hyperplasia in gynecomastia in a 54-year-old man Note increased periductal vascularity. **D:** Micropapillary hyperplasia in gynecomastia. **E:** Micropapillary hyperplasia with prominent myoepithelial cells. **F:** Florid ductal hyperplasia.

are usually large and tightly cohesive, and consist of flat monolayered sheets or show some crowding with nuclear overlap and indistinct cell borders. Occasional cell dyshesion and slight cytologic atypia may be noted, but the smears are usually not as cellular as one would see in a carcinoma. FNA sampling of fibrous lesions often yields insufficient material. Notably, FNA of gynecomastia may be associated with substantial discomfort, and the patient may refuse additional sampling. Apocrine cells are rarely present in FNA specimens from gynecomastia. Needle core biopsy is also widely used to diagnose gynecomastia. A pathology group servicing several community hospitals in the Netherlands received

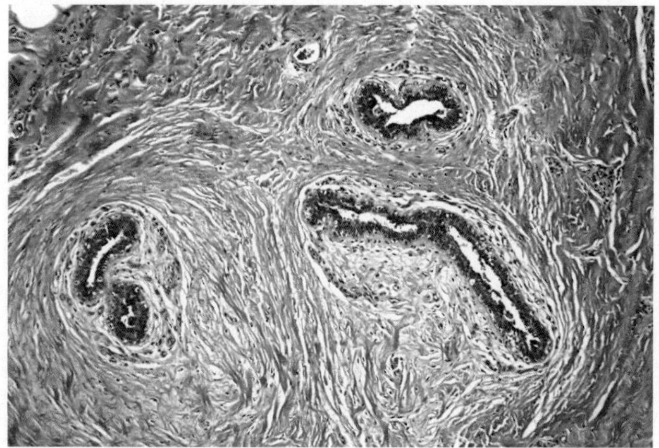

FIG. 35.6. ***Gynecomastia, inactive.*** Periductal edema is considerably reduced, and partly collagenized stroma surrounds the ducts.

26 core biopsy specimens of the male breast in a 10-year period, or 2.6 specimens per year.[71] Gynecomastia was diagnosed in 15 cases; 6 revealed carcinoma and 5 were "benign." Gynecomastia was diagnosed in 93% of 113 core biopsies for unilateral breast masses in men.[37] The remaining cases were two carcinomas, one lymphoma, and one mastitis.

Immunohistochemistry

Gynecomastic breast tissue contains receptors for estradiol (estrogen receptor [ER]),[72–75] dihydrotestosterone,[73] androgen (androgen receptor [AR]),[74] progesterone (progesterone receptor [PR]),[72–74] and glucocorticoids.[73,74] In one series, ER and dihydrotestosterone receptor were detected in about 75% of samples of gynecomastia.[73] Using an immunohistochemical procedure, Andersen et al.[76] demonstrated epithelial nuclear reactivity for ER in 89% of gynecomastia specimens examined. Strong, focal immunoreactivity for prostate-specific antigen (PSA) has been detected in nonhyperplastic and hyperplastic male ductal epithelium in gynecomastia.[77] The epithelium was not immunoreactive for prostatic acid phosphatase. Using a panel of immunohistochemical markers, Kornegoor et al.[78] demonstrated that the ductal epithelium in proliferative gynecomastia is composed of three layers of cells that are distinguishable histologically and on the basis of their immunoprofile. The peripheral myoepithelial cells were immunoreactive for CK5, CK14, and p63, but they were negative for ER, PR, AR, bcl-2, and cyclin D1. The two luminal cell layers had differing immunoprofiles. The intermediate layer, composed of vertically oriented cuboidal or columnar cells, was immunoreactive for ER, PR, AR, bcl-2, and cyclin D1, but it was almost always negative for CK5 and CK14. Flattened cells forming the inner luminal layer tended to be reactive for CK5, CK14, and bcl-2 with minimal weak reactivity for ER, PR, AR, and cyclin D1. Because the two epithelial cell types in proliferative gynecomastia are comparable to the epithelium seen in usual ductal hyperplasia in the female breast that is not considered to be precancerous, the authors concluded that "gynecomastia does not seem to be an obligate precursor lesion of male breast cancer."

Electron Microscopy

Electron microscopy of gynecomastia confirms the presence of proliferating myoepithelial and epithelial cells.[79] Splitting and duplication of the basement membrane is frequently seen, and may be interrupted by gaps formed by protruding epithelial cells. The stroma contains fibroblasts and myofibroblasts. The ultrastructural features are similar to those encountered in usual ductal hyperplasia of the female breast.

Treatment and Prognosis

No treatment is required for the majority of patients with gynecomastia, especially those with the senescent form of

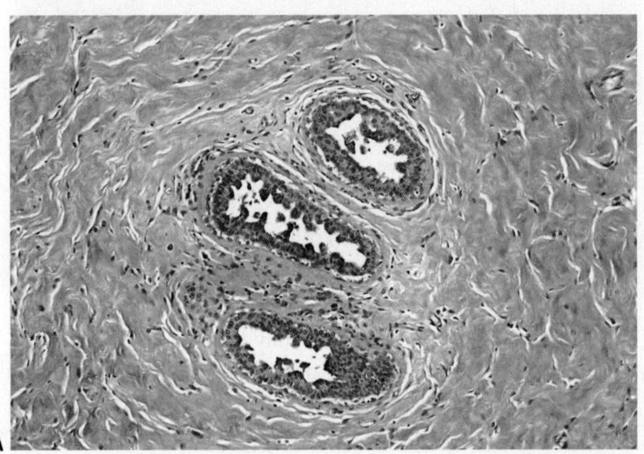

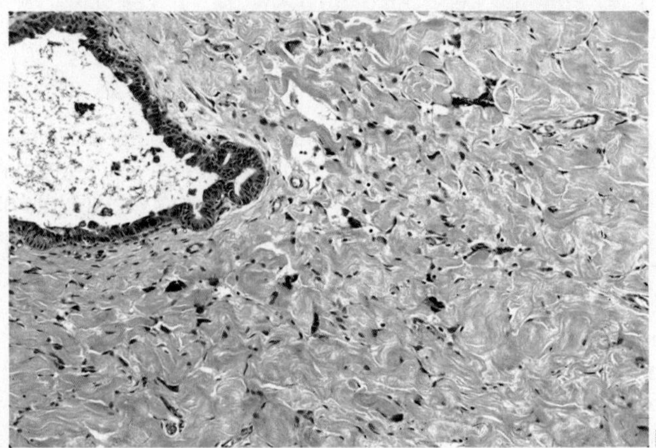

FIG. 35.7. ***Gynecomastia, pseudoangiomatous stromal hyperplasia.*** **A:** The typical pseudoangiomatous appearance is shown. **B:** Multinucleated giant cells are present in the stroma.

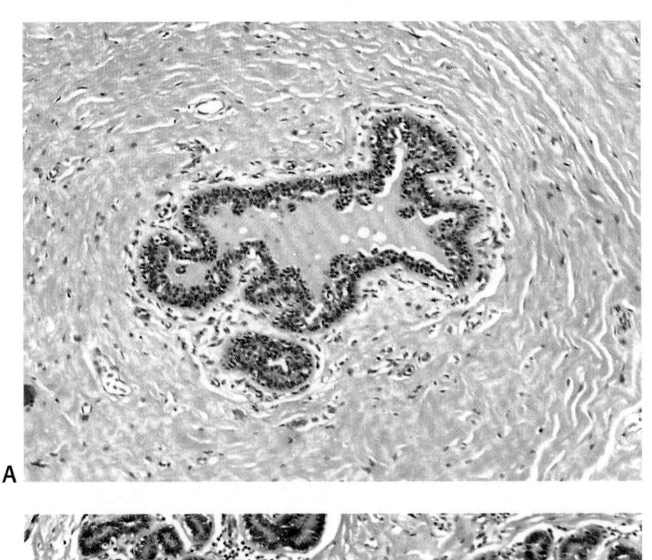
A

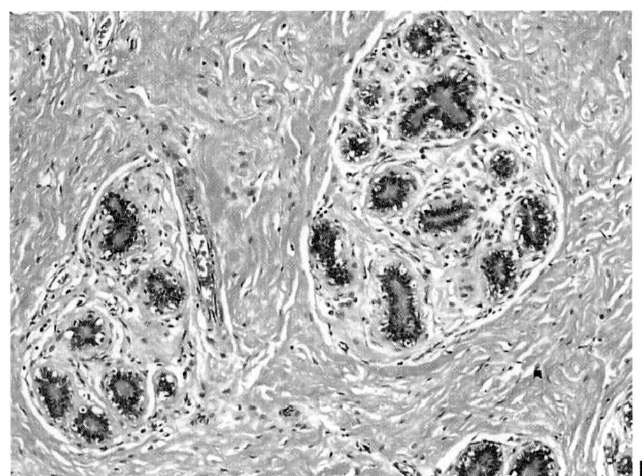
B

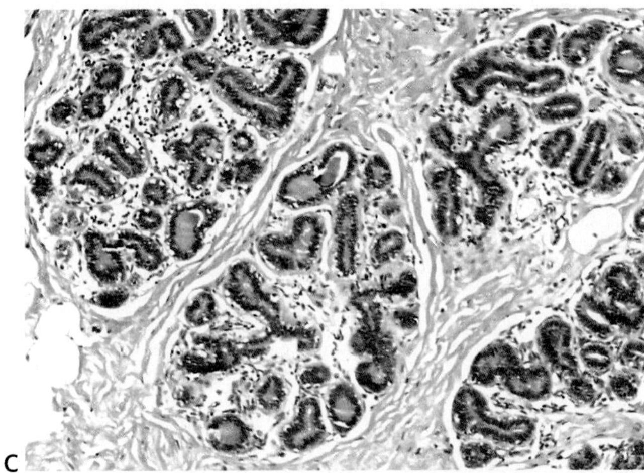
C

FIG. 35.8. *Gynecomastia, lobular differentiation.* The patient had hepatic cirrhosis and was being treated with spironolactone. **A:** A duct with micropapillary hyperplasia. **B:** Lobules with distinct epithelial and myoepithelial components. **C:** Lobules containing secretion.

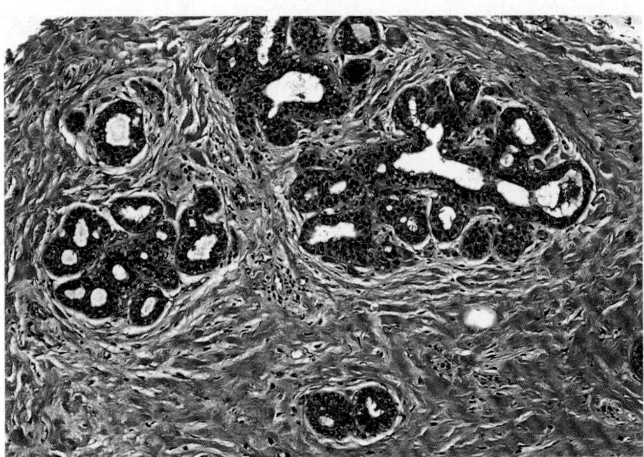

FIG. 35.9. *Gynecomastia, lobular differentiation.* Lobules were present in this biopsy of gynecomastia from a 27-year-old man who was using "over-the-counter" androgen supplements for body building.

the lesion that is often due to medications and/or underlying medical conditions.[80] Regression of gynecomastia has been described in patients with hyperthyroidism[56] and alcoholic liver disease[81] when the underlying conditions were treated, as well as after treatment with antiestrogens such as tamoxifen and danazol. Usually, however, breast enlargement persists. In the past, radiation has been effective in preventing gynecomastia in patients receiving exogenous estrogens to treat prostatic carcinoma,[82,83] but it is no longer used due to it's damaging side effects.

Excisional biopsy may be indicated to exclude primary or metastatic carcinoma. Surgical reduction by liposuction may be appropriate for fatty gynecomastia, whereas excision is indicated when the lesion consists predominantly of glandular tissue.[84] Liposuction can result in epithelial displacement that mimics invasive carcinoma, a phenomenon that is also associated with needle core biopsy sampling.[85]

Although carcinoma may arise in conjunction with gynecomastia, there is presently no evidence based on long-term follow-up studies that atypical proliferative changes in gynecomastia are associated with an increased risk of the subsequent development of carcinoma.[86]

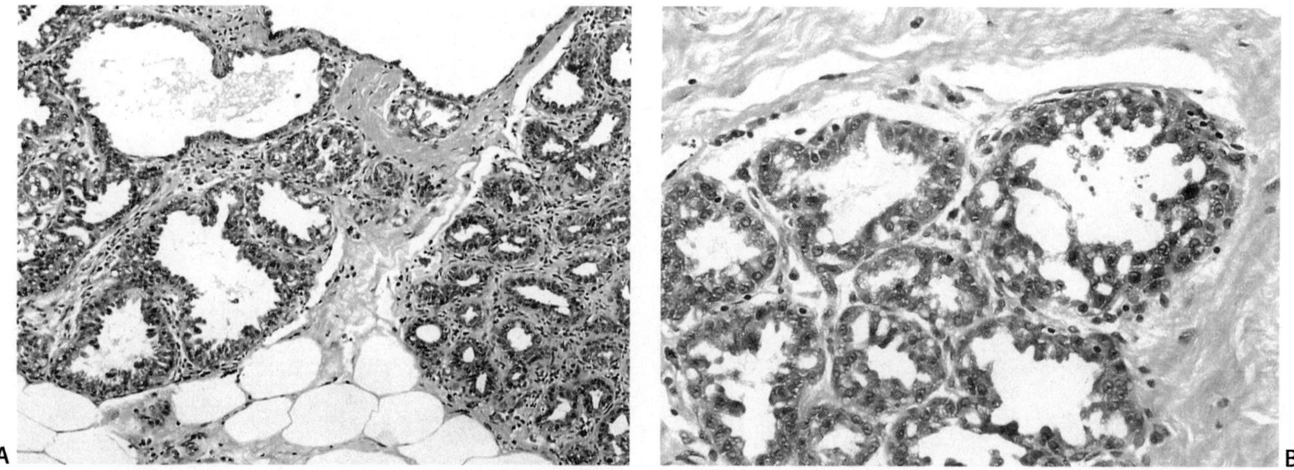

FIG. 35.10. ***Gynecomastia.*** **A,B:** Pseudolactational hyperplasia.

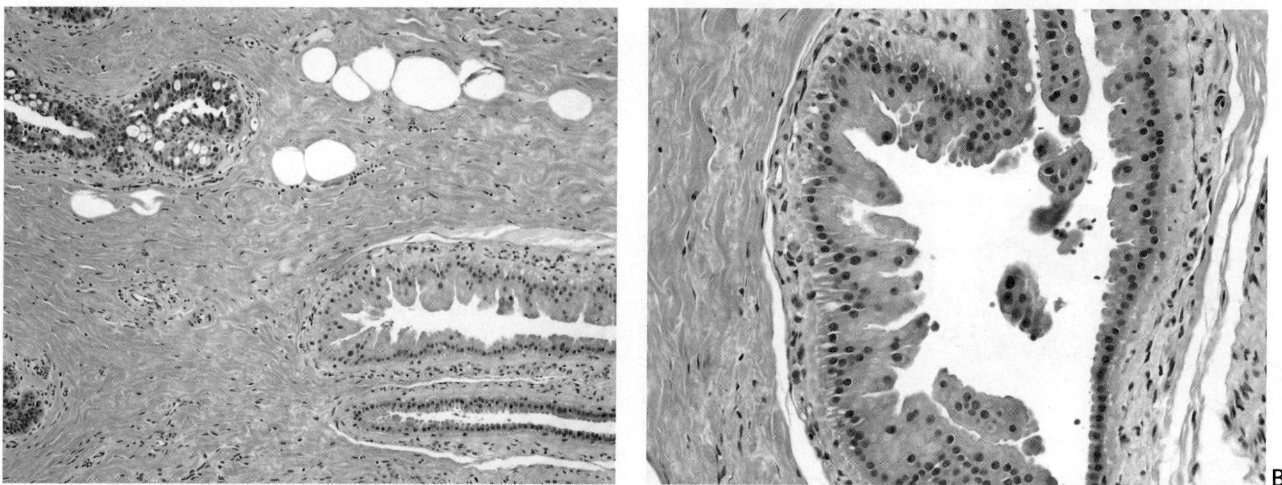

FIG. 35.11. ***Gynecomastia, apocrine metaplasia.*** **A:** Apocrine metaplasia is present (*lower right*). **B.** Columnar and micropapillary apocrine metaplasia is morphologically similar to that seen in the female breast.

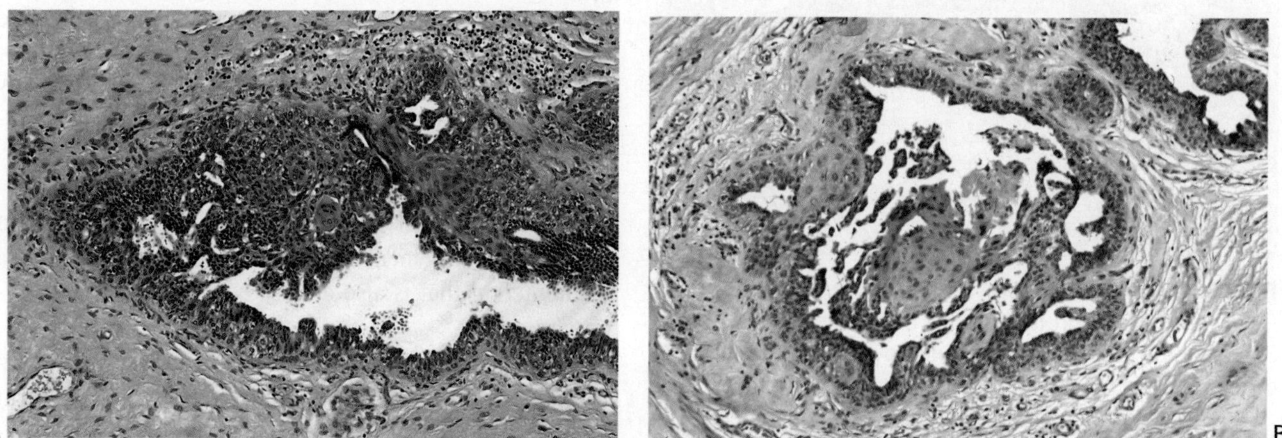

FIG. 35.12. ***Gynecomastia, squamous metaplasia.*** **A:** Inconspicuous foci of squamous metaplasia are present in the partly papillary epithelial hyperplasia. **B:** Prominent squamous metaplasia in papillary ductal hyperplasia.

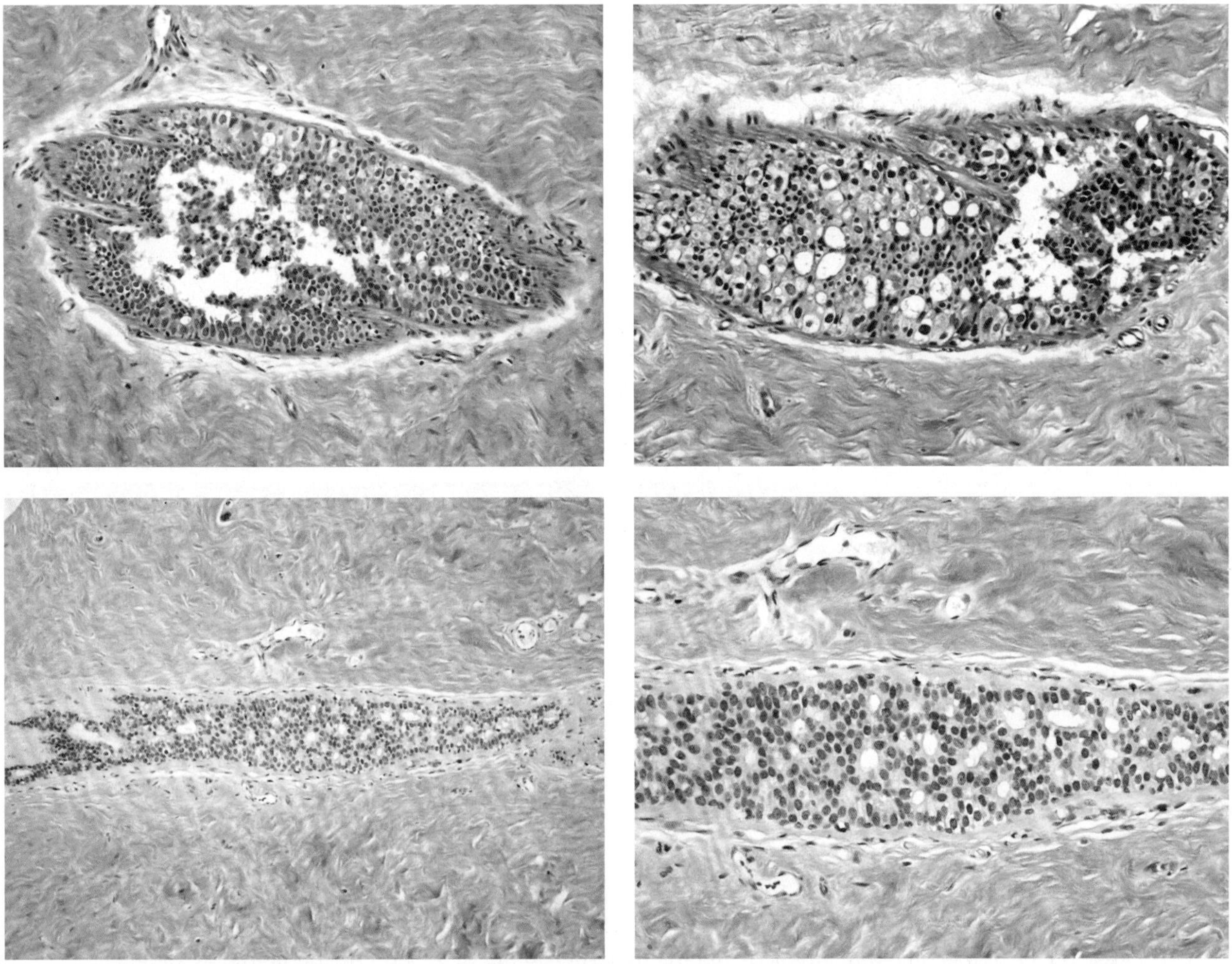

FIG. 35.13. ***Gynecomastia, atypical ductal hyperplasia.*** **A:** A mix of cells with small and enlarged nuclei. Myoepithelial cells are evident at the perimeter of the duct on the *left*, where the tissue has been sectioned tangentially. Some large cells with more abundant pale cytoplasm have apocrine features. **B:** A solid proliferation of atypical cells fills this duct. **C:** Atypical ductal hyperplasia (ADH) with a fenestrated (cribriform) growth pattern. **D:** Magnified view of the ADH shown in **(C)**.

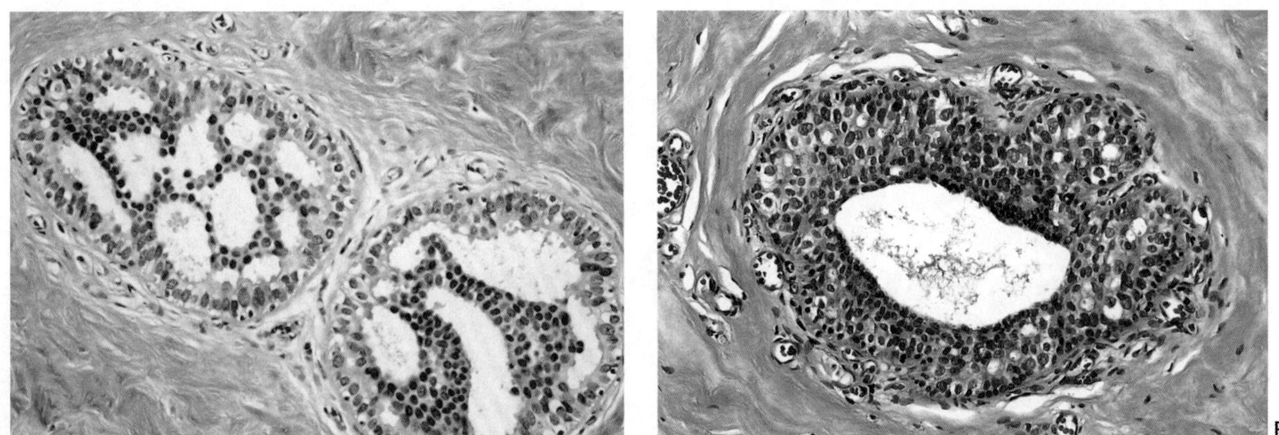

FIG. 35.14. ***Gynecomastia, atypical ductal hyperplasia.*** **A:** A monomorphic population of cells forms bridges across these ducts. **B:** Solid ADH.

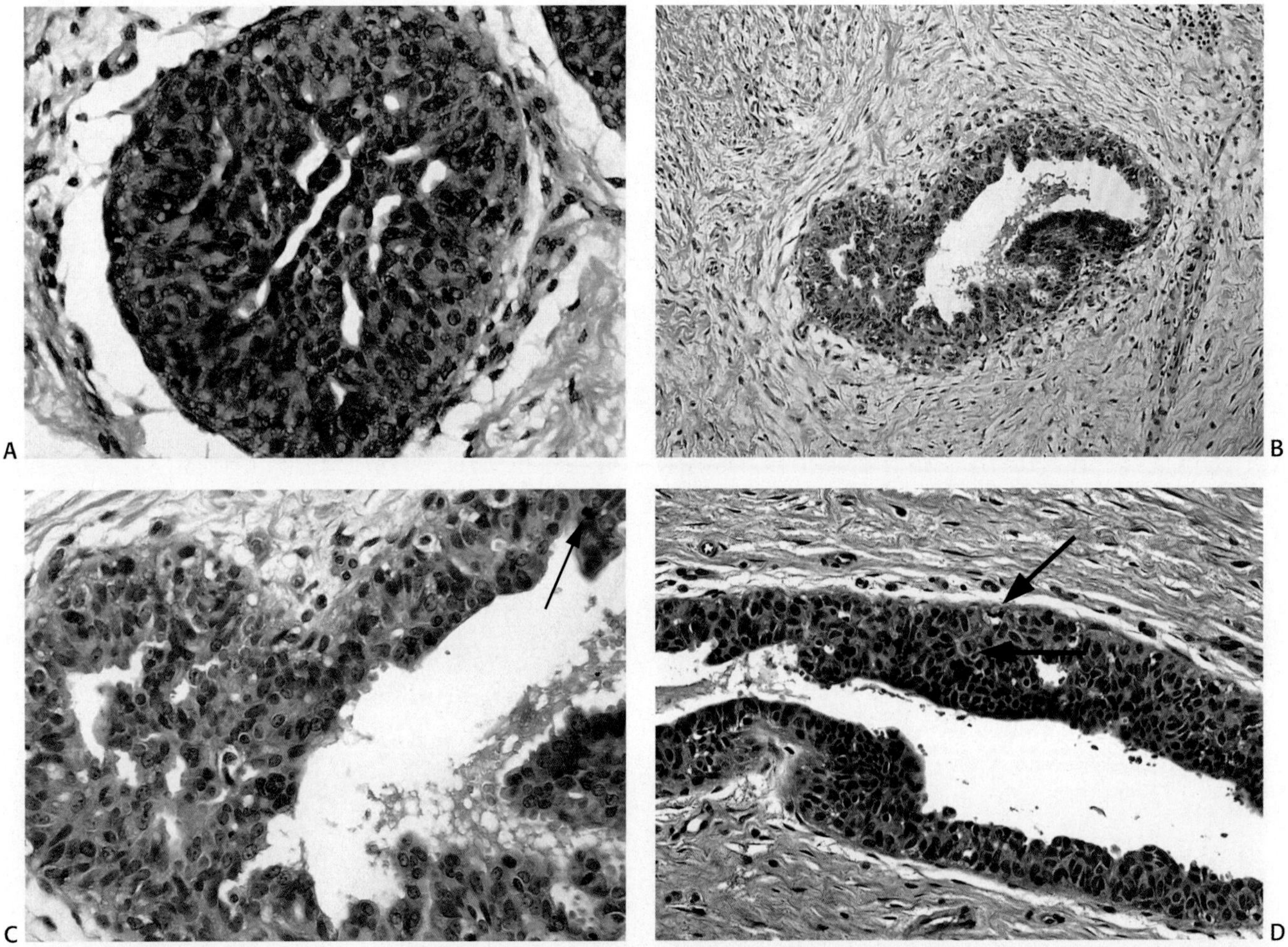

FIG. 35.15. ***Gynecomastia, atypical ductal hyperplasia.*** **A:** A disorderly proliferation of epithelial cells nearly fills the duct. Some cellular heterogeneity and slight streaming are evident. **B,C:** Focal micropapillary ductal hyperplasia in a patient with ductal carcinoma *in situ* elsewhere in the biopsy. A mitotic figure can be seen in the *upper right corner* of **(C)** (*arrow*). **D:** ADH lines this duct. The cells have a disorderly distribution. Note that nuclei become smaller and hyperchromatic near the lumen. Two mitotic figures are shown (*arrows*).

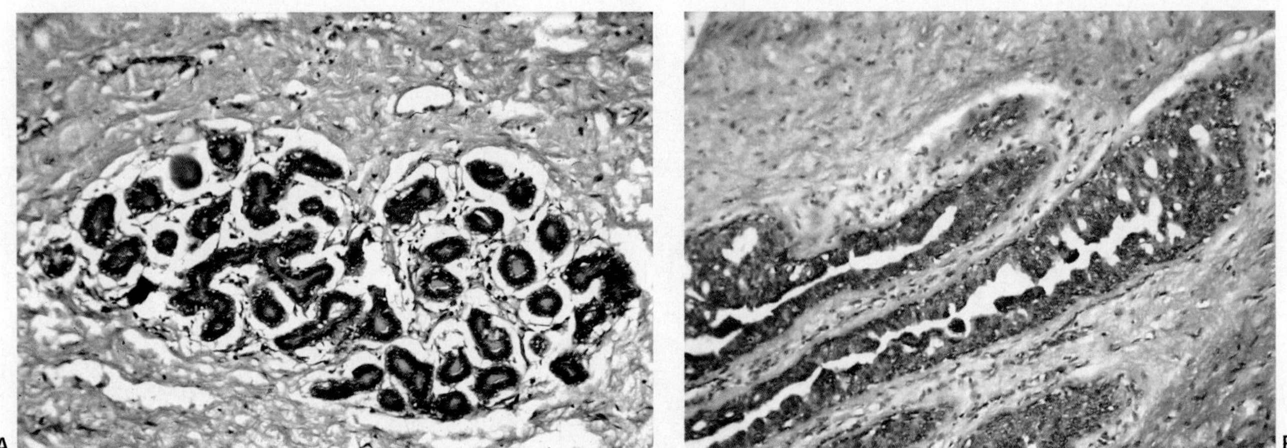

FIG. 35.16. ***Gynecomastia, atypical ductal hyperplasia.*** The patient was treated for prostatic carcinoma with flutamide. **A:** Lobular differentiation. **B:** Atypical micropapillary hyperplasia.

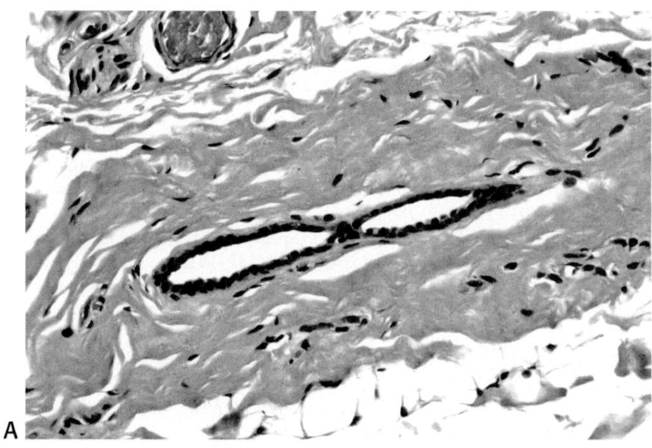
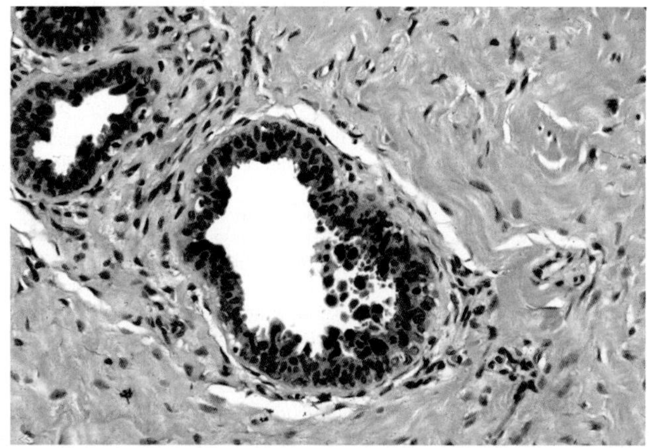

FIG. 35.17. ***Gynecomastia in a 24-year-old man after chemotherapy and bone marrow transplantation for acute myelogenous leukemia.*** **A:** A normal duct is shown. **B:** Micropapillary hyperplasia with cytologic atypia in gynecomastia. Note the increased stromal cellularity when compared with (**A**).

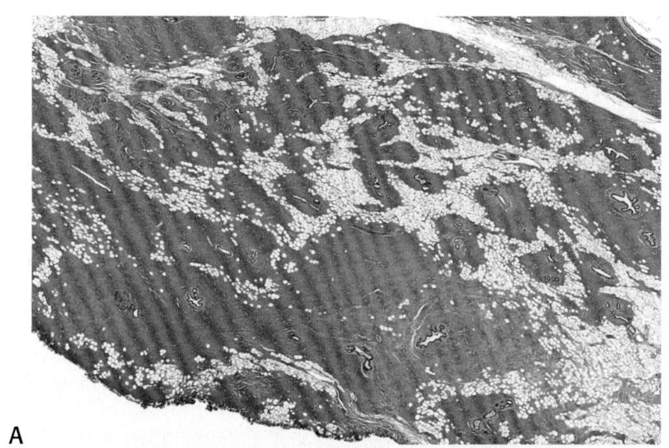
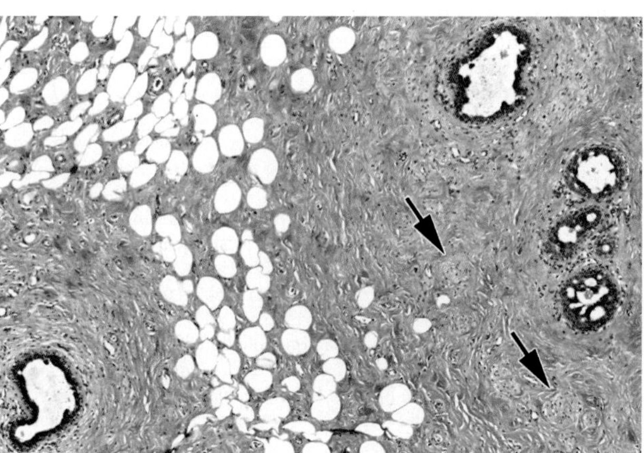
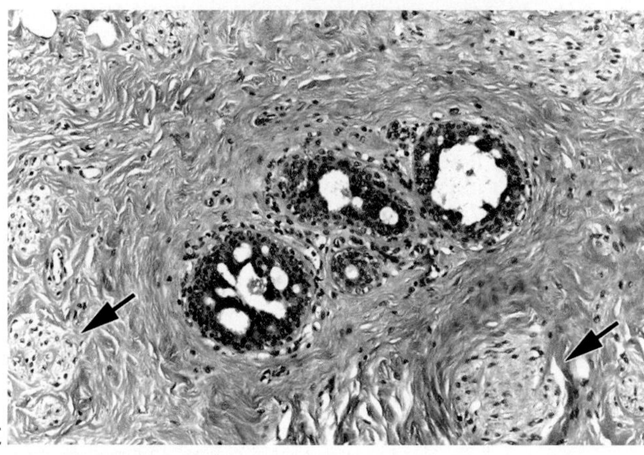

FIG. 35.18. ***Gynecomastia-like hyperplasia in the female breast.*** **A:** The mammary parenchyma of a 35-year-old woman shows periductal fibrosis and focal inconspicuous lobules. **B,C:** Periductal stromal proliferation with flat and micropapillary epithelial hyperplasia. Note the bundles of myoid myofibroblasts in the stroma (*arrows*).

REFERENCES

1. Detraux P, Benmussa M, Tristant H, et al. Breast disease in the male: galactographic evaluation. *Radiology* 1985;154:605–606.
2. Giltman LI. Solitary intraductal papilloma of the male breast. *South Med J* 1981;74:774.
3. Sara AS, Gottfried MR. Benign papilloma of the male breast following chronic phenothiazine therapy. *Am J Clin Pathol* 1987;87:649–650.
4. Simpson JS, Barson AJ. Breast tumours in infants and children: a 40-year review of cases at a children's hospital. *Can Med Assoc J* 1969;101:100–102.

5. Navas MDM, Povedano JLR, Mendivil EA, et al. Intracystic papilloma in male breast: ultrasonography and pneumocystography diagnosis. *J Clin Ultrasound* 1993;21:38–40.
6. Shim JH, Son EJ, Kim EK, et al. Benign intracystic papilloma of the male breast. *J Ultrasound Med* 2008;27:1397–1400.
7. Durkin ET, Warner TF, Nichol PF. Enlarging unilateral breast mass in an adolescent male: an unusual presentation of intraductal papilloma. *J Pediatr Surg* 2011;46:e33–e35.
8. David VC. Papillary cystadenoma of the male breast. *Ann Surg* 1922;75:652–657.
9. Burdick C, Rinehart RM, Matsumoto T, et al. Nipple adenoma and Paget's disease in a man. *Arch Surg* 1965;91:835–839.
10. Shapiro L, Karpas CM. Florid papillomatosis of the nipple. First reported case in a male. *Am J Clin Pathol* 1965;44:155–159.
11. Waldo ED, Sidhu GS, Hu AW. Florid papillomatosis of male nipple after diethylstilbestrol therapy. *Arch Pathol* 1975;99:364–366.
12. Ansah-Boateng Y, Tavassoli FA. Fibroadenoma and cystosarcoma phyllodes of the male breast. *Mod Pathol* 1992;5:114–116.
13. Gupta P, Foshee S, Garcia-Morales F, et al. Fibroadenoma in male breast: case report and literature review. *Breast Dis* 2011;33:45–48.
14. Vancil M, Locke W. Acromegaly, hyperparathyroidism, and probable mammary fibroadenoma in a man. *Am J Surg* 1965;110:495–497.
15. Nielsen BB. Fibroadenomatoid hyperplasia of the male breast. *Am J Surg Pathol* 1990;14:774–777.
16. Uchida T, Ishii M, Motomiya Y. Fibroadenoma associated with gynaecomastia in an adult man. Case report. *Scand J Plast Reconstr Surg Hand Surg* 1993;27:327–329.
17. Kanhai RC, Hage JJ, Bloemena E, et al. Mammary fibroadenoma in a male-to-female transsexual. *Histopathology* 1999;35:183–185.
18. Lemmo G, Garcea N, Corsello S, et al. Breast fibroadenoma in a male-to-female transsexual patient after hormonal treatment. *Eur J Surg Suppl* 2003;69–71.
19. Shin SJ, Rosen PP. Bilateral presentation of fibroadenoma with digital fibroma-like inclusions in the male breast. *Arch Pathol Lab Med* 2007;131:1126–1129.
20. Bartoli C, Zurrida SM, Clemente C. Phyllodes tumor in a male patient with bilateral gynaecomastia induced by oestrogen therapy for prostatic carcinoma. *Eur J Surg Oncol* 1991;17:215–217.
21. Pantoja E, Llobet RE, Lopez E. Gigantic cystosarcoma phyllodes in a man with gynecomastia. *Arch Surg* 1976;111:611.
22. Reingold IM, Ascher GS. Cystosarcoma phyllodes in a man with gynecomastia. *Am J Clin Pathol* 1970;53:852–856.
23. Hilton DA, Jameson JS, Furness PN. A cellular fibroadenoma resembling a benign phyllodes tumour in a young male with gynaecomastia. *Histopathology* 1991;18:476–477.
24. Lewinn EB. Gynecomastia during digitalis therapy; report of eight additional cases with liver-function studies. *N Engl J Med* 1953;248:316–320.
25. Mann N. Gynecomastia during therapy with spironolactone. *JAMA* 1963;184:778–780.
26. Andersen JA, Gram JB. Male breast at autopsy. *Acta Pathol Microbiol Immunol Scand A* 1982;90:191–197.
27. Tedeschi LG, McCarthy PE. Involutional mammary duct ectasia and periductal mastitis in a male. *Hum Pathol* 1974;5:232–236.
28. Downs AM, Fisher M, Tomlinson D, et al. Male duct ectasia associated with HIV infection. *Genitourin Med* 1996;72:65–66.
29. Banik S, Hale R. Fibrocystic disease in the male breast. *Histopathology* 1988;12:214–216.
30. McClure J, Banerjee SS, Sandilands DG. Female type cystic hyperplasia in a male breast. *Postgrad Med J* 1985;61:441–443.
31. Sund BS, Topstad TK, Nesland JM. A case of juvenile papillomatosis of the male breast. *Cancer* 1992;70:126–128.
32. Robertson KE, Kazmi SA, Jordan LB. Female-type fibrocystic disease with papillary hyperplasia in a male breast. *J Clin Pathol* 2010;63:88–89.
33. Sanguinetti A, Fioriti L, Brugia M, et al. Juvenile papillomatosis of the breast in young male: a case report. *G Chir* 2011;32:374–375.
34. Bigotti G, Kasznica J. Sclerosing adenosis in the breast of a man with pulmonary oat cell carcinoma: report of a case. *Hum Pathol* 1986;17:861–863.
35. Newcomer TA, Green AJ, Sutton J, et al. Epithelial inclusion cyst in a male breast. *Breast Dis* 1995;8:91–95.
36. Bannayan GA, Hajdu SI. Gynecomastia: clinicopathologic study of 351 cases. *Am J Clin Pathol* 1972;57:431–437.
37. Janes SE, Lengyel JA, Singh S, et al. Needle core biopsy for the assessment of unilateral breast masses in men. *Breast* 2006;15:273–275.
38. Michels LG, Gold RH, Arndt RD. Radiography of gynecomastia and other disorders of the male breast. *Radiology* 1977;122:117–122.
39. Munoz Carrasco R, Alvarez Benito M, Munoz Gomariz E, et al. Mammography and ultrasound in the evaluation of male breast disease. *Eur Radiol* 2010;20:2797–2805.
40. Iuanow E, Kettler M, Slanetz PJ. Spectrum of disease in the male breast. *AJR Am J Roentgenol* 2011;196:W247–W259.
41. Rahmani S, Turton P, Shaaban A, et al. Overview of gynecomastia in the modern era and the Leeds Gynaecomastia Investigation algorithm. *Breast J* 2011;17:246–255.
42. August GP, Chandra R, Hung W. Prepubertal male gynecomastia. *J Pediatr* 1972;80:259–263.
43. Nydick M, Bustos J, Dale JH Jr, et al. Gynecomastia in adolescent boys. *JAMA* 1961;178:449–454.
44. Carlson HE. Gynecomastia. *N Engl J Med* 1980;303:795–799.
45. Nuttall FQ. Gynecomastia as a physical finding in normal men. *J Clin Endocrinol Metab* 1979;48:338–340.
46. Williams MJ. Gynecomastia. Its incidence, recognition and host characterization in 447 autopsy cases. *Am J Med* 1963;34:103–112.
47. Roberto G, Biagi C, Montanaro N, et al. Statin-associated gynecomastia: evidence coming from the Italian spontaneous ADR reporting database and literature. *Eur J Clin Pharmacol* 2012;68:1007–1011.
48. Oteri A, Catania MA, Travaglini R, et al. Gynecomastia possibly induced by rosuvastatin. *Pharmacotherapy* 2008;28:549–551.
49. Green L, Wysowski DK, Fourcroy JL. Gynecomastia and breast cancer during finasteride therapy. *N Engl J Med* 1996;335:823.
50. Caocci G, Atzeni S, Orru N, et al. Gynecomastia in a male after dasatinib treatment for chronic myeloid leukemia. *Leukemia* 2008;22:2127-8.
51. Tanriverdi O, Unubol M, Taskin F, et al. Imatinib-associated bilateral gynecomastia and unilateral testicular hydrocele in male patient with metastatic gastrointestinal stromal tumor: a literature review. *J Oncol Pharm Pract* 2012;18:303–310.
52. Liu H, Liao G, Yan Z. Gynecomastia during imatinib mesylate treatment for gastrointestinal stromal tumor: a rare adverse event. *BMC Gastroenterol* 2011;11:116.
53. Schinina V, Busi Rizzi E, Zaccarelli M, et al. Gynecomastia in male HIV patients MRI and US findings. *Clin Imaging* 2002;26:309–313.
54. Pantanowitz L, Sen S, Crisi GM, et al. Spectrum of breast disease encountered in HIV-positive patients at a community teaching hospital. *Breast* 2011;20:303–308.
55. Andersen JA, Gram JB. Gynecomasty: histological aspects in a surgical material. *Acta Pathol Microbiol Immunol Scand A* 1982;90:185–190.
56. Becker KL, Matthews MJ, Higgins GA Jr, et al. Histologic evidence of gynecomastia in hyperthyroidism. *Arch Pathol* 1974;98:257–260.
57. Nicolis GL, Modlinger RS, Gabrilove JL. A study of the histopathology of human gynecomastia. *J Clin Endocrinol Metab* 1971;32:173–178.
58. Schwartz IS, Wilens SL. The formation of acinar tissue in gynecomastia. *Am J Pathol* 1963;43:797–807.
59. Haibach H, Rosenholtz MJ. Prepubertal gynecomastia with lobules and acini: a case report and review of the literature. *Am J Clin Pathol* 1983;80:252–255.
60. Gottfried MR. Extensive squamous metaplasia in gynecomastia. *Arch Pathol Lab Med* 1986;110:971–973.
61. Hamady ZZ, Carder PJ, Brennan TG. Atypical ductal hyperplasia in male breast tissue with gynaecomastia. *Histopathology* 2005;47:111–112.
62. Pinedo F, Vargas J, de Agustin P, et al. Epithelial atypia in gynecomastia induced by chemotherapeutic drugs. A possible pitfall in fine needle aspiration biopsy. *Acta Cytol* 1991;35:229–233.
63. Zimmerman RL, Fogt F, Cronin D, et al. Cytologic atypia in a 53-year-old man with finasteride-induced gynecomastia. *Arch Pathol Lab Med* 2000;124:625–627.
64. Cheuk W, Tsang WY, Chan JK. The 3-layered ductal epithelium in the female breast. *Am J Surg Pathol* 2012;36:1738–1740; author reply 1740–1731.
65. Kang Y, Wile M, Schinella R. Gynecomastia-like changes of the female breast. *Arch Pathol Lab Med* 2001;125:506–509.

66. Umlas J. Gynecomastia-like lesions in the female breast. *Arch Pathol Lab Med* 2000;124:844–847.
67. Gupta RK, Naran S, Simpson J. The role of fine needle aspiration cytology (FNAC) in the diagnosis of breast masses in males. *Eur J Surg Oncol* 1988;14:317–320.
68. Siddiqui MT, Zakowski MF, Ashfaq R, et al. Breast masses in males: multi-institutional experience on fine-needle aspiration. *Diagn Cytopathol* 2002;26:87–91.
69. Singh R, Anshu, Sharma SM, et al. Spectrum of male breast lesions diagnosed by fine needle aspiration cytology: a 5-year experience at a tertiary care rural hospital in central India. *Diagn Cytopathol* 2012;40:113–117.
70. Rosa M, Masood S. Cytomorphology of male breast lesions: diagnostic pitfalls and clinical implications. *Diagn Cytopathol* 2012;40:179–184.
71. Westenend PJ. Core needle biopsy in male breast lesions. *J Clin Pathol* 2003;56:863–865.
72. Contesso G, Delarue JC, Guerinot F, et al. [Estrogen and progresterone receptors in male breast diseases]. *Nouv Presse Med* 1977;6:1951–1953.
73. Grilli S, De Giovanni C, Galli MC, et al. The simultaneous occurrence of cytoplasmic receptors for various steroid hormones in male breast carcinoma and gynaecomastia. *J Steroid Biochem* 1980;13:813–820.
74. Pacheco MM, Oshima CF, Lopes MP, et al. Steroid hormone receptors in male breast diseases. *Anticancer Res* 1986;6:1013–1017.
75. Rosen PP, Menendez-Botet CJ, Nisselbaum JS, et al. Estrogen receptor protein in lesions of the male breast: a preliminary report. *Cancer* 1976;37:1866–1868.
76. Andersen J, Orntoft TF, Andersen JA, et al. Gynecomastia. Immunohistochemical demonstration of estrogen receptors. *Acta Pathol Microbiol Immunol Scand A* 1987;95:263–267.
77. Gatalica Z, Norris BA, Kovatich AJ. Immunohistochemical localization of prostate-specific antigen in ductal epithelium of male breast. Potential diagnostic pitfall in patients with gynecomastia. *Appl Immunohistochem Mol Morphol* 2000;8:158–161.
78. Kornegoor R, Verschuur-Maes AH, Buerger H, et al. The 3-layered ductal epithelium in gynecomastia. *Am J Surg Pathol* 2012.
79. Hassan MO, Olaizola MY. Ultrastructural observations on gynecomastia. *Arch Pathol Lab Med* 1979;103:624–630.
80. Ikard RW, Vavra D, Forbes RC, et al. Management of senescent gynecomastia in the Veterans Health Administration. *Breast J* 2011;17:160–166.
81. Becker KL, Matthews MJ, Winnacker J, et al. Sequential histological study of the regression of gynecomastia in a patient with alcoholic liver disease. *Am J Med Sci* 1967;254:685–691.
82. Waterfall NB, Glaser MG. A study of the effects of radiation on prevention of gynaecomastia due to oestrogen therapy. *Clin Oncol* 1979;5:257–260.
83. Wolf H, Madsen PO, Vermund H. Prevention of estrogen-induced gynecomastia by external irradiation. *J Urol* 1969;102:607–609.
84. Li CC, Fu JP, Chang SC, et al. Surgical treatment of gynecomastia: complications and outcomes. *Ann Plast Surg* 2012;69:510–515.
85. McLaughlin CS, Petrey C, Grant S, et al. Displaced epithelium after liposuction for gynecomastia. *Int J Surg Pathol* 2011;19:510–513.
86. Olsson H, Bladstrom A, Alm P. Male gynecomastia and risk for malignant tumours—a cohort study. *BMC Cancer* 2002;2:26.

CHAPTER 36

Carcinoma of the Male Breast

MELISSA P. MURRAY • EDI BROGI

EPIDEMIOLOGY

Incidence

Breast carcinoma is an uncommon neoplastic condition in men, accounting for not more than 1% of all breast carcinomas and for less than 0.1% of male cancer deaths.[1–5] Worldwide, the incidence is generally less than 1 case per 100,000 men per year.

Hodgson et al.[6] analyzed 1,396 cases of male breast carcinoma diagnosed in the state of Florida between 1985 and 2000. The age-adjusted incidence rose from 0.9 to 1.5 cases per 100,000 men between 1990 and 2000. The highest incidence (12.5 per 100,000) occurred in men aged 85 years or older. These results are consistent with a nationwide rise in incidence recorded by Giordano et al.,[7] who analyzed data from the Surveillance Epidemiology and End Results (SEER) program from 1973 to 1998. During this period, the incidence of male breast carcinoma rose from 0.86 to 1.08 per 100,000 ($p < 0.001$). In a California-based study,[8] the number of cases of male breast carcinoma diagnosed per year rose from 87 in 2005 to 139 in 2009. The rising incidence of male breast carcinoma is probably a function of overall aging of the population, but the contribution of other factors cannot be excluded. More recently, Anderson et al.[5] reported that breast carcinoma incidence and mortality rates for men and women in the United States decreased from 1996 to 2005, with a decline of 28% among men and 42% among women in the adjusted hazard rate for breast cancer death.

On the basis of data from the SEER program, Siegel et al.[9] estimated that there would be 2,190 new cases of male breast carcinoma and 410 deaths from the disease in 2012 in the United States. By comparison, the projected number of women diagnosed with breast carcinoma in 2012 was estimated to be 226,870, with 39,510 breast carcinoma deaths. An international population-based study using data for 459,846 women and 2,665 men with breast carcinoma from six countries reported standardized incidence of 66.7 and 0.4 per 100,000 person-years for women and men, respectively.[10]

Race and Ethnicity

Racial variations have been described, with the incidence reportedly lower among Japanese[11] and higher among Blacks in West Africa[12] and the United States[13] when compared with Whites in the United States. The average annual age-adjusted breast carcinoma death rate is higher among non-White men in the United States[4] and lower among Japanese men in Japan[11] than among White men in the United States, Canada, Europe, or Scandinavia. A higher incidence of breast carcinoma has been found in Israel[14] and among Jewish men when compared with other White ethnic subgroups.[2,4,15,16] The incidence and age-specific death rate for male breast carcinoma increase in a linear fashion with advancing age among different racial and ethnic groups.[1,4,11,15] This straight-line relationship between incidence and age among men differs from that of female breast carcinoma, which is characterized by a less steep slope after age 50 among postmenopausal women.[17] Ethnicity of men with breast carcinoma was evaluated in detail in a California-based population study.[8] Most (431/606; 71%) patients were non-Hispanic White men, 45/606 (7.4%) non-Hispanic Blacks, 67/606 (11.1%) Hispanics, and the remaining 63/606 (10.4%) were Asian/Pacific Islanders or of other ethnicities. Most (82.8%) non-Hispanic White men had hormone receptor–positive carcinomas, 14.6% had HER2–positive tumors, and only 2.6% were reported to have triple negative carcinomas. Among non-Hispanic Blacks, 73.3% of carcinomas were hormone receptor–positive, 17.8% HER2-positive, and 8.9% triple negative carcinomas. Among Hispanic men, 77.6% of the carcinomas were hormone receptor–positive, 16.4% HER2-positive, and 6% triple negative. Despite these differences, race and ethnicity did not affect patient survival.

Hormones and Testicular Dysfunction

Some investigators[18] have found increased levels of estradiol and other estrogenic hormones in men with breast carcinoma, but others have not detected increased or abnormal estrogen concentrations.[19,20] Case-control studies by Schottenfeld et al.[4] and Mabuchi et al.[2] found a relatively high frequency of antecedent mumps orchitis among men with breast carcinoma. It was suggested that testicular atrophy after orchitis causes relative hyperestrogenism. A follow-up study of 132 men who had mumps orchitis in one community revealed that the median age of patients with mumps was 8 years and that of patients with mumps orchitis was 29 years.[21] Follow-up of 20 years or more was obtained for 36% of the patients, revealing testicular neoplasms in two. The absence of subsequent male mammary carcinoma in this cohort may reflect the relative youth of the patients at follow-up and the lack of information about most of the men. Nicolis et al.[22] described a patient who developed breast carcinoma 30 years after mumps orchitis that resulted in testicular atrophy. Casagrande et al.[23] found no relationship between mumps in adulthood and male breast carcinoma, but they did not evaluate orchitis as a specific factor. An association with antecedent testicular trauma was observed by Mabuchi et al.[2] Further evidence that testicular dysfunction might contribute to male breast carcinoma risk was reported by Thomas et al.,[24] who studied 227 patients and 300 controls. The strongest association was detected for undescended testes, but orchitis, injury, late puberty, and infertility were also relevant factors.

Prostatic Carcinoma

An international comparison of age-standardized incidence for prostatic and male breast carcinomas revealed a direct relationship between the two diseases.[25] On the other hand, the actual reported frequency of both diseases in individual patients was quite low, occurring in less than 1% of 397 men with breast carcinoma in a 1995 report.[26]

Leibowitz et al.[27] found a prostatic carcinoma in 10 (6.2%) of 161 men with breast carcinoma treated at two centers in Boston between 1977 and 2000. In eight patients, breast carcinoma was diagnosed prior to prostatic carcinoma. The mean ages for the diagnosis of mammary and prostatic carcinomas were 65.7 years (47 to 72 years) and 68.0 years (51 to 76 years), respectively. Seven patients had a history of breast carcinoma in a first-degree female relative, and one had a family history of prostatic carcinoma. The fact that mammary carcinoma preceded prostatic carcinoma in most of the cases reported by Leibowitz et al.[27] makes it unlikely that prostate carcinoma treatment played a role in the development of breast carcinoma.

Among 62 male patients with breast carcinoma studied by Kiluk et al.,[28] 18 (29%) had a family history of breast, ovarian, or colon carcinoma. Seven (11.3%) of the patients had previously been treated for prostatic carcinoma.

There is limited evidence that the administration of exogenous estrogens to treat prostatic carcinoma might contribute to the development of male breast carcinoma. Epidemiologic studies have failed to demonstrate an excess frequency of subsequent breast carcinoma among men with prostatic carcinoma,[29] despite the fact that most patients treated for this disease with estrogens develop gynecomastia. The duration of treatment rarely exceeds 10 years, and the exposure may not be sufficient for mammary carcinogenesis to become apparent. Schlappack et al.[30] described two men who had breast carcinoma diagnosed after 12 years of estrogen therapy for prostatic carcinoma, Wilson and Hutchinson[31] described another man with a 7-year interval between estrogen therapy and diagnosis of breast carcinoma, and Carlsson et al.[32] reported four patients who developed carcinoma after estrogen therapy. Some case reports of breast carcinoma that developed in men with prostatic carcinoma are difficult to evaluate because of the well-known predilection of the latter to metastasize to the breast. The sporadic occurrence of primary concurrent prostatic and mammary carcinomas has been reported.[33] Breast carcinoma has been described in transsexuals after castration and prolonged estrogen treatment.[34–36] Benign histologic changes in the breast associated with this therapy include fully formed lobules, apocrine metaplasia, and pseudolactational hyperplasia.

Trauma

Traumatic injury of the breast has been cited in some older studies as a possible predisposing event.[4] The fact that most patients who have related their carcinoma to trauma report a single incident rather than sustained or repeated injury has led most investigators to discount this as a significant factor. In many instances, documentation that the carcinoma arose at the site of injury is not available. Occupational exposure as a potential source of injury has not been explored in most studies. An association with employment in steel works, blast furnaces, and rolling mills was noted by Mabuchi et al.[2] Other occupations reportedly associated with excess risk were work as a butcher and employment with exposure to high environmental temperatures.[37,38] Cocco et al.[39] carried out a case-control study that compared 178 male breast carcinoma patients with 1,041 controls. There was a significantly increased risk of breast carcinoma among men employed in occupations with exposure to blast furnaces, steel works, and rolling mills (odds ratio [OR], 3.4; 95% confidence interval [CI], 1.1 to 10.1) and in motor vehicle manufacturing (OR, 3.1; 95% CI, 1.2 to 8.2). Breast cancer risk was not significantly related to exposure to electromagnetic fields, herbicides, pesticides, high temperatures, and organic solvents.

Radiation

Radiation exposure has been implicated as a risk factor. In some instances, radiation was administered to the breast to treat gynecomastia or other local conditions, or for intrathoracic diseases.[17,40–43] Male breast carcinoma has also been associated with a source of radiation linked to increased breast carcinoma risk among women, multiple fluoroscopic examinations,[44] but not to atomic bomb explosions.[45] Although not statistically significant, Casagrande et al.[23] found a trend toward more frequent breast carcinoma in men who had the greatest thoracic radiation exposure by fluoroscopy or during therapeutic irradiation. One patient received radiotherapy for chondrosarcoma of a rib prior to developing breast carcinoma.[26]

Pituitary Gland Dysfunction

An excess risk of breast carcinoma has been reported among men treated with medications that cause hyperprolactinemia.[37] Bilateral breast carcinoma has been described in a man treated for a prolactin-secreting pituitary adenoma.[46] Olsson et al.[20] found that plasma prolactin levels in 15 male patients with breast carcinoma were elevated when compared with those in controls with other neoplasms. Concurrent breast carcinoma and pituitary prolactinoma were described in a 68-year-old man who did not have gynecomastia.[47] Lactational change was not evident in the carcinoma.

Klinefelter Syndrome

Klinefelter syndrome, a genetic abnormality that usually becomes evident during or after puberty, has been associated with an increased risk of the development of male breast carcinoma. The majority of patients with Klinefelter syndrome have at least two X chromosomes and a Y chromosome. Prominent clinical manifestations are gynecomastia and testicular atrophy. Abnormal hormonal findings include reduced testosterone production, low plasma testosterone, and a high estradiol-to-testosterone ratio, at least partially augmented by increased testicular estrogen secretion. Microscopic examination of the testes reveals hyalinization of spermatic tubules with disappearance of germ cells and Sertoli cells. Hyperplasia with pleomorphism of interstitial cells develops concurrently.[48] The extra X, or 47th, chromosome is identified cytologically as the nuclear Barr body.

Most papers relating male breast carcinoma to Klinefelter syndrome have been individual case reports in which the chromosomal abnormality has been documented by genetic studies.[48–51] The reported incidence of breast carcinoma among patients with Klinefelter syndrome varies from 1% to 3%.[52,53] Breast carcinoma has also been described in a phenotypic male with an XX genotype.[54]

It has been estimated that 1% to 3% of male breast carcinoma patients have Klinefelter syndrome.[55,56] Using fluorescence *in situ* hybridization (FISH) to examine tissues from men with breast carcinoma, Hultborn et al.[57] found the prevalence of Klinefelter syndrome to be 7.5%. The authors concluded that individuals with Klinefelter syndrome had a 50-fold increased risk of developing breast carcinoma when compared with men without this genetic syndrome. Klinefelter syndrome did not have a significant effect on the median age at diagnosis or on survival after diagnosis.

Family History of Breast Carcinoma

Cutuli et al.[26] found a positive family history of breast carcinoma in 5.6% of 397 men with breast carcinoma. A twofold increased risk of breast carcinoma among first-degree relatives of male breast carcinoma patients, largely due to an excess of carcinoma in sisters, was reported by Casagrande et al.[23] Rosenblatt et al.[58] reported that the increased risk associated with sisters having breast carcinoma was significantly greater among men with carcinoma diagnosed before age 60. The relative risk (RR) of male breast carcinoma among men with an affected sister was 3.93. The RR in men whose mothers had breast carcinoma was also increased (2.33). Gough et al.[59] found that a positive family history of breast carcinoma was associated with 27% of male breast carcinomas treated at the Mayo Clinic. Olsson et al.[60] have also reported a lower incidence of prostatic carcinoma among male relatives of men with breast carcinoma.

Several instances of the familial occurrence of male breast carcinoma have been described in which father and son,[58,61–63] brothers,[58,64,65] and other groups of male relatives[58,66–69] have been affected. Multiple female and male relatives have been affected in some kindreds.[66] One family included an individual with Klinefelter syndrome.[61] Genetic analysis of two brothers who developed breast carcinoma at ages 55 and 75, respectively, revealed a mutation consisting of a G-to-A substitution in exon 3 of the androgen receptor (*AR*) gene.[70] Both men were born with penoscrotal hypospadias and undescended testes. A study of DNA extracted from the tumor tissue of 12 male breast cancer patients who did not have clinical features of androgen insensitivity failed to reveal comparable mutations of the *AR* gene.[71]

Analysis of 22 families with at least one male and multiple female breast carcinomas revealed no linkage to the BRCA1 locus.[72] The carcinomas in approximately 16% of families with multiple women and one or more men affected are attributable to *BRCA1* mutation.[73] In the same study, analysis of 26 families with one or more male breast carcinomas revealed that 76% were associated with *BRCA2* mutations. Male carriers of *BRCA2* mutations were found to have a cumulative risk of 6.3% to develop breast carcinoma by age 70.[74] Analysis of 111 families with *BRCA2* mutations revealed that 11% of breast carcinomas diagnosed in these families occurred in men.[75] Among 18 Hungarian men with breast carcinoma, 6 (33%) had truncating mutations in the *BRCA2* gene.[76] None of the six patients with *BRCA2* mutations reported a family history of breast or ovarian carcinoma, but four other men without *BRCA2* mutations had such a history. A study of Icelandic men with breast carcinoma revealed that 40% had a *BRCA2* mutation.[77] Linkage to mutations in the BRCA2 region on chromosome 13q has been demonstrated in one family with multiple cases of male breast carcinoma.[78] Others have reported finding loss of heterozygosity (LOH) on chromosome 11q13 in 13 (68.4%) of 19 male breast carcinomas[79] and on chromosome 8 in 19 (83%) of 23 cases[80] studied. Data from a Danish cancer registry revealed that the RR of developing breast carcinoma in daughters of affected men was 16.4 (95% CI, 3.3 to 47.7).[81] Deb et al.[82] studied the clinical and pathologic characteristics of 60 patients with familial male breast carcinomas. Most patients (25/60; 41.7%) were *BRCA2* germline mutation carriers, only 3/60 (5%) were *BRCA1* mutation carriers, and the remaining 32/60 (53.3%) had no known *BRCA1* or *BRCA2* gene mutation. Ottini et al.[83] studied 382 breast carcinomas in Italian men, including 4 in *BRCA1* and 46 in *BRCA2* germline mutation carriers. Men with BRCA2-associated carcinoma were diagnosed at a mean age of 58.9 years, and 12 (26.1%)

had other carcinomas (prostate carcinoma and contralateral breast carcinoma). BRCA2-associated carcinomas were mostly grade 3 invasive ductal carcinomas 62.5% presented at stage I to II and 56.7% had positive lymph nodes. BRCA2-associated carcinomas were HER2-positive in 63.2% of cases and 56.2% had high Ki67. HER2 positivity in male breast carcinoma was significantly associated with *BRCA2* germline mutation carrier status ($p = 0.001$).

Other genes implicated in the etiology of male breast carcinoma include *RAD51B*[84] and *CHEK2*1100delC*,[85,86] both of which are involved in ensuring fidelity of DNA double-strand break repair, and the tumor suppressor *PTEN*, which is associated with Cowden syndrome.[87] An association with polymorphism in the *CYP17* gene encoding cytochrome p450, a key enzyme in the conversion of steroids in peripheral tissues, has also been described.[88]

Increased urinary estrogen excretion has been reported among male relatives of male patients with breast carcinoma. Many of these families have had relatives with other malignant neoplasms.[61,62,64,65,68] The incidence of breast carcinoma and other malignant neoplasms in wives of men with breast carcinoma is similar to that in the general population.[60]

Gynecomastia

The relationship between gynecomastia and the development of male breast carcinoma is not clear. A major factor that has contributed to the problem is differing definitions of gynecomastia, including the distinction between clinical and pathologic manifestations of the condition. Gynecomastia has florid or proliferative and quiescent phases, but the histologic diagnosis is sometimes limited to the former pattern. Nonetheless, clinical manifestations may be as prominent when the process is inactive. Evidence linking gynecomastia to the pathogenesis of male breast carcinoma includes epithelial atypia in gynecomastia, relatively lower mean age at diagnosis of breast carcinoma when associated with gynecomastia, the association of gynecomastia and carcinoma with Klinefelter syndrome, and the finding of microscopic gynecomastia associated with 5% to 40% of carcinomas.[89,90] Histologic transitions from usual or florid epithelial hyperplasia in gynecomastia to intraductal carcinoma have very rarely been described.[90,91] Satisfactory long-term follow-up studies of men who have gynecomastia with atypical ductal hyperplasia (ADH) are not available.

Finasteride, a medication employed since 1992 to treat prostatic hyperplasia, interferes with the conversion of testosterone to dihydrotestosterone by blocking AR, thereby causing an increase in the ratio of estrogen to androgen. Gynecomastia has been a frequent adverse side effect of finasteride therapy,[92] and there have been rare cases of breast carcinoma arising in finasteride-related gynecomastia.

Gynecomastia associated with breast carcinoma has been observed in young men who employed androgenic steroids to enhance muscle development. Staerkle et al.[93] reported the diagnosis of bilateral synchronous DCIS in a 30-year-old man who developed bilateral gynecomastia after the administration of an androgenic steroid for bodybuilding. It seems likely that the coexistence of male breast carcinoma and gynecomastia is due to the fact that both conditions are often related to one or more common predisposing factors. However, current evidence suggests that gynecomastia rarely serves as a precancerous condition and that the epithelial hyperplasia in gynecomastia is not usually an intermediate step in the development of carcinoma (See Chapter 35).

Other Associated Factors

Other factors that have been associated with the development of male breast carcinoma in various studies include liver disease, obesity, tuberculosis, and therapeutic use of digitalis, although the relationship has not been statistically significant in all instances.[23,37,94]

Prior Diagnosis of Breast Carcinoma

Men with a prior diagnosis of breast carcinoma have a 30-fold increased risk of developing a contralateral breast carcinoma,[95] a substantially higher risk compared with the fourfold increase in women with the same disease. The risk of contralateral breast carcinoma in men diagnosed with breast carcinoma before age 50 was increased 110-fold. The risk of contralateral breast carcinoma appears to be unrelated to the treatment modalities.

Nonmammary Malignant Neoplasms

Several authors have commented on the development of nonmammary malignant neoplasms (NMMNs) among men with mammary carcinoma.[17,26,90,96–98] The frequency of NMMNs in these patients ranges from 3.5%[24] to 13%.[98–100] The more common sites of NMMNs include the lungs, colon and rectum, stomach, pancreas, and prostate gland.[100] A study of 229 male patients with breast carcinoma diagnosed over a 40-year period in Canada revealed prior or subsequent NMMNs in 24.5%, including tumors of the skin and undocumented sites.[101] In view of the relatively advanced age of men with mammary carcinoma, the frequency of NMMNs in this population does not appear to be excessive, especially if one includes NMMNs diagnosed before and after the index breast carcinoma.

CLINICAL PRESENTATION

Location in the Breast

The majority of male breast carcinomas are located centrally in a retroareolar position (Fig. 36.1), but eccentric lesions, particularly in the upper outer quadrant, have been described.[3,102] Rarely, the tumor may arise in the nipple and invade the underlying breast (Fig. 36.2). Synchronous, clinically evident bilateral carcinoma is exceedingly unusual.[98,103,104] It has been

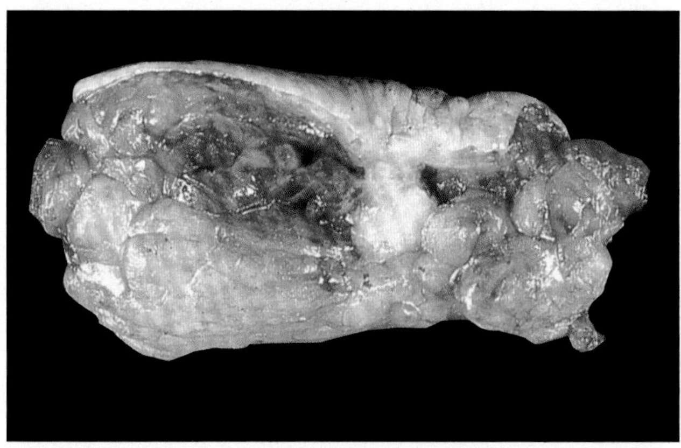

FIG. 36.1. ***Male breast carcinoma.*** In this gross specimen, a carcinoma in the central part of the breast has caused retraction of the nipple.

estimated that the cumulative risk of bilateral disease is 3% or less.[40,96]

Symptoms

About 75% of patients present with a painless mass. When a mass is absent, the lesion is invariably detected because of nipple ulceration, retraction, or discharge. Carcinoma is found in about 75% of male patients with a mass and bloody discharge. Approximately one-half of the patients with serous discharge and a mass prove to have carcinoma.[105] Serous discharge alone may indicate intraductal carcinoma.[106,107] The mean duration of symptoms prior to clinical consultation has been reported to be between 6 months[108] and nearly 1 year.[97] Patients with locally advanced lesions may have a periareolar mass with erosion of the overlying skin and nipple.[109]

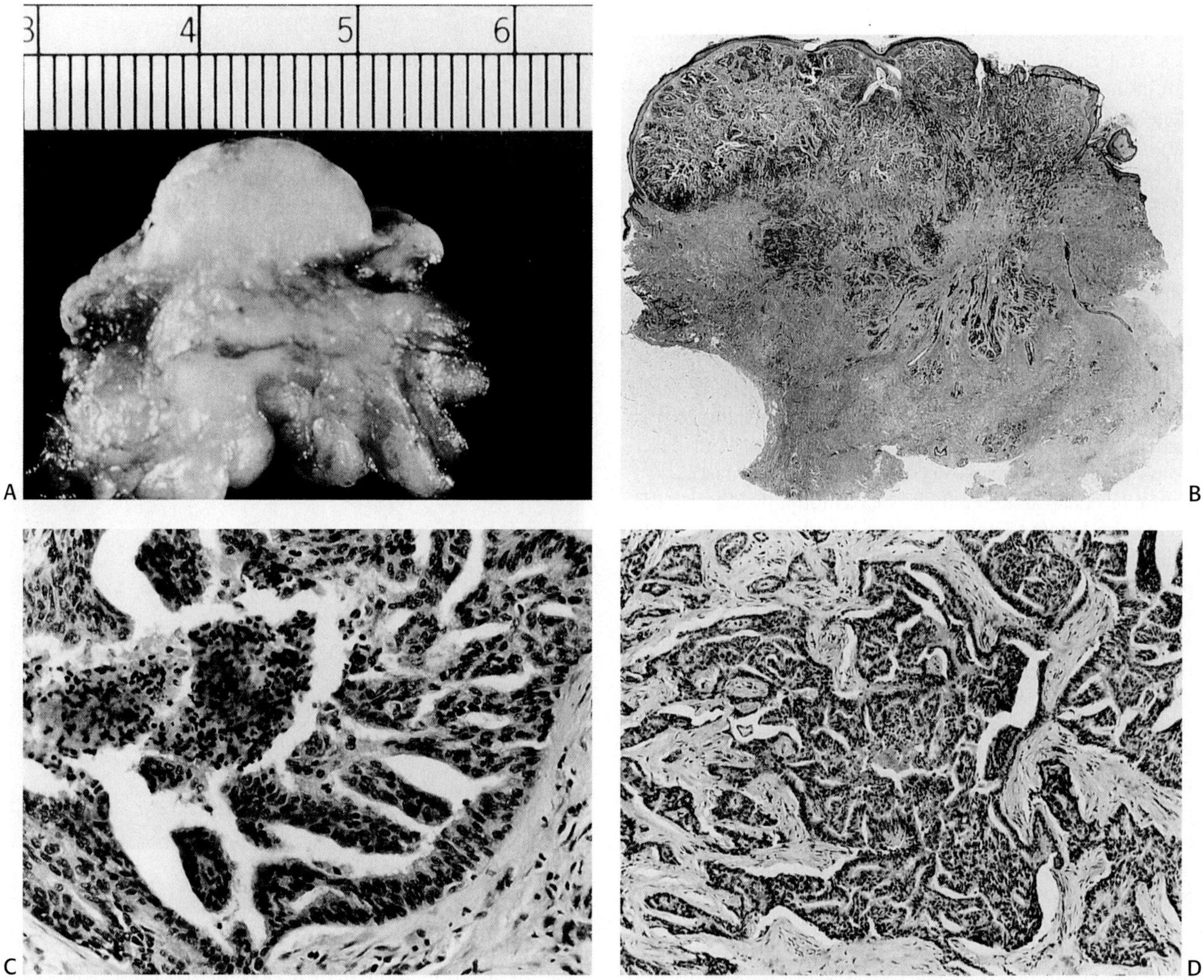

FIG. 36.2. ***Male breast carcinoma in the nipple.*** **A:** Gross hemisection of the nipple and underlying tissue with carcinoma in the nipple. **B:** Whole-mount histologic section of invasive carcinoma in the nipple. **C:** Papillary intraductal carcinoma in the tumor. **D:** Infiltrating papillary carcinoma in the nipple tumor.

Age

The average age at diagnosis is between 60 and 67 years, approximately 5 to 10 years greater than in women with the same disease.[5,7,110–113] However, breast carcinoma has been diagnosed in males at virtually all ages, including children and adults younger than 30 years.[99,111,114,115] In a population-based study of 606 cases by Chavez-MacGregor et al.,[8] the median age at diagnosis of breast carcinoma was 68 years. The authors observed a statistically significant difference in tumor subtype according to age ($p = 0.020$), with younger patients more likely to have HER2-positive tumors.

Breast carcinoma is very uncommon in men younger than 45 years, but may have a relatively unfavorable prognosis in this age group.[116] Patients older than 65 years may also have a worse prognosis,[7] although the data are inconclusive. In one study,[117] men older than 65 years tended to have larger tumors at diagnosis, but the tumors were most often estrogen receptor (ER)–positive. These patients had worse prognosis on univariate analysis, but age was not a statistically significant factor on multivariate analysis. Hill et al.[118] reported that a family history of breast carcinoma did not have a significant effect on the age and stage at diagnosis or on the prognosis of men with breast carcinoma.

Among men with intraductal carcinoma, 6 of 31 patients were younger than 40 years and the median age at diagnosis was 58 years.[26] Hittmair et al.[119] reported an age range of 25 to 94 years and a median age of 65 years in 84 men with ductal carcinoma *in situ* (DCIS).

Mammography and MRI

Mammograms of men with breast carcinoma typically reveal distinct lesions with invasive margins that contrast sharply with the surrounding fatty tissue,[120,121] but carcinoma may be obscured by concurrent gynecomastia.[122,123] Cystic or encapsulated papillary carcinoma produces a discrete round mass that may contain calcifications. The cystic character of such a lesion and the presence of an internal papillary component can be demonstrated by ultrasonography.[124,125] An irregular border around a cystic lesion may be an evidence of invasion.[126] Mammograms of gynecomastia typically reveal accentuated glandular tissue and ducts extending from the nipple. Ultrasonography is useful for distinguishing between gynecomastia and carcinoma.[67] The mammographic density associated with gynecomastia is usually symmetrical. It often has a triangular configuration at an early stage, but may develop a dendritic pattern in established lesions.[120,127]

Microcalcifications have been found in 9% to 30% of male breast carcinomas studied mammographically.[102,122,123] There are several reports of occult carcinoma detected by mammography in the contralateral breast of men previously treated for breast carcinoma.[120,123,128,129] The mammographic diagnosis was based on the detection of nonpalpable nodules in two cases and on the presence of microcalcifications in two other cases. Two of these patients were carriers of *BRCA2* mutations.[128,129] At present, there are no guidelines recommending mammographic screening for men, even in individuals with documented genetic predisposition.[129]

Magnetic resonance imaging (MRI) of breast carcinoma in men does not appear to differ from that of similar tumors in women, although the available information remains limited.[130]

Inflammatory carcinoma of the male breast produces diffuse enlargement of the affected breast and skin thickening,[131] which can be detected by MRI. Invasion of the skin and enlarged lymph nodes may be evident radiographically.[132]

GROSS PATHOLOGY

Carcinoma of the male breast appears identical grossly to carcinoma arising in the female breast. Cystic, encapsulated papillary carcinomas may present as striking tumors grossly (Fig. 36.3).

MICROSCOPIC PATHOLOGY

Invasive Carcinoma

Approximately 85% of infiltrating male mammary carcinomas are of the infiltrating ductal variety[133] (Fig. 36.4). In the study by Chavez-MacGregor et al.,[8] 85% of tumors were IDC not otherwise specified (NOS); 2% were invasive lobular carcinomas (ILC); and the remaining 13% had papillary, mixed, or other or unknown morphologies. The majority of the invasive tumors are moderately or poorly differentiated,[8,83,112,117,134,135] but low-grade and tubular carcinomas

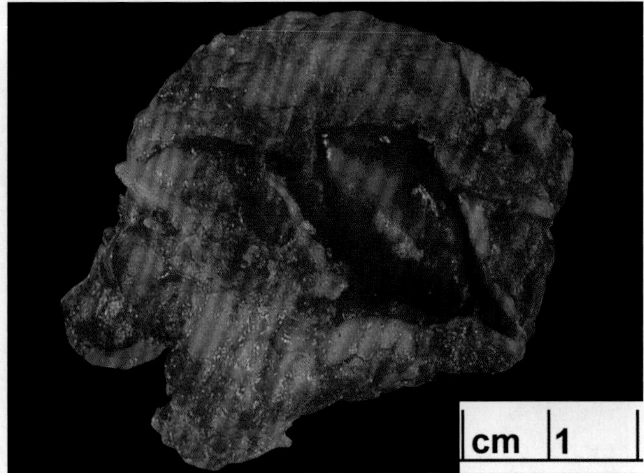

FIG. 36.3. ***Cystic papillary carcinoma.*** The specimen is from the right breast of a 72-year-old man. The cyst, shown here opened, measured 5.5 cm. On the *left*, there is an intracystic papillary tumor with an underlying nodule of invasive carcinoma. On the *right*, the inner surface of the cyst is smooth.

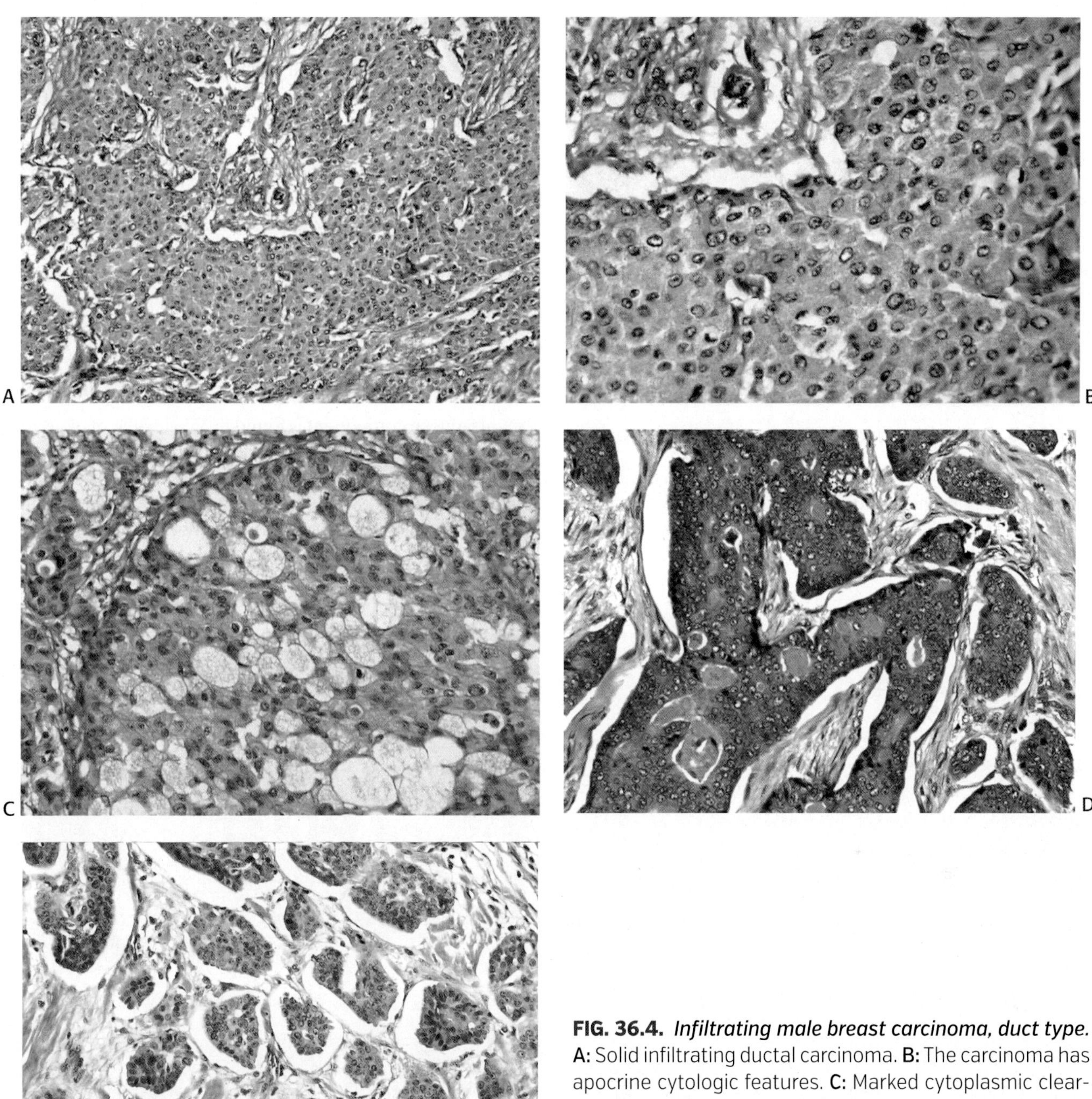

FIG. 36.4. ***Infiltrating male breast carcinoma, duct type.*** **A:** Solid infiltrating ductal carcinoma. **B:** The carcinoma has apocrine cytologic features. **C:** Marked cytoplasmic clearing and vacuolization. **D:** High-grade infiltrating ductal carcinoma. This histologic appearance resembles a pattern seen in prostatic carcinoma. **E:** Infiltrating papillary carcinoma.

have been described[89,135–147] (Fig. 36.5). The growth patterns seen in male infiltrating duct carcinomas duplicate those encountered in the female breast, including cribriform, comedo, papillary, solid, or gland-forming components (Fig. 36.6).

Periductal elastosis is found in some IDC.[148] Apocrine differentiation, which has rarely been described, may be present in intraductal as well as invasive lesions.[149,150]

Kornegoor et al.[151] have reported that 25% of male breast carcinomas in their series showed a fibrotic focus, often located near the center of the tumor, consisting mainly of collagen and fibroblasts. The fibrotic focus was significantly associated with high nuclear grade, high mitotic index, lymph node metastases, and overexpression of hypoxia inducible factor 1α (HIF-1α). HIF-1α-positive tumors were more often high grade and HER2 amplified. Overexpression

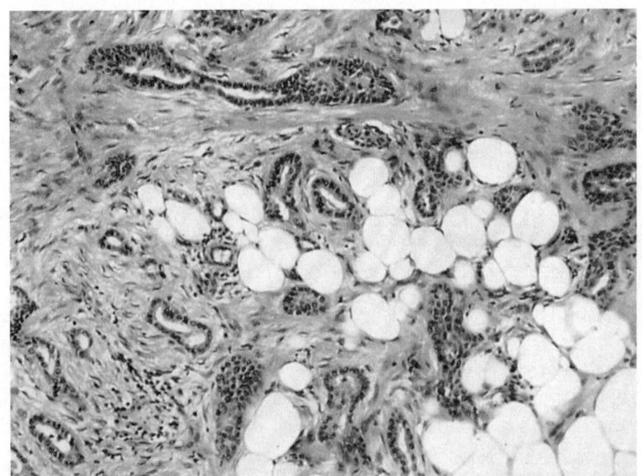

FIG. 36.5. ***Infiltrating ductal carcinoma, tubular type.***

of HIF-1α was an independent predictor of survival in multivariate analysis. These morphologic findings have not yet been verified by others.

Cystic, Encapsulated Papillary Carcinoma

Papillary carcinomas, often with a prominent cystic component, are relatively more common among men than among women, constituting 3% to 5% of male carcinomas[13,89,90,135,146] but only 1% to 2% of carcinomas in women. The majority of male papillary carcinomas are intracystic. A very orderly cystic, encapsulated papillary carcinoma may be mistaken for papillary hyperplasia or a papilloma (Fig. 36.7). The diagnosis of papillary lesions of the male breast in needle core biopsy samples relies on the histologic and immunohistochemical criteria that are applied to papillary tumors of the female breast (see Chapters 5 and 14).

Ductal Carcinoma *In Situ*

An intraductal component is found in 35% to 50% of male and 75% of female infiltrating ductal carcinomas.[89] Extensive DCIS constituting more than 25% of the invasive tumor and involving surrounding breast is uncommon in men.[107] The structure and cytology of associated DCIS usually resembles the invasive tumor, often growing as solid or comedocarcinoma.[119]

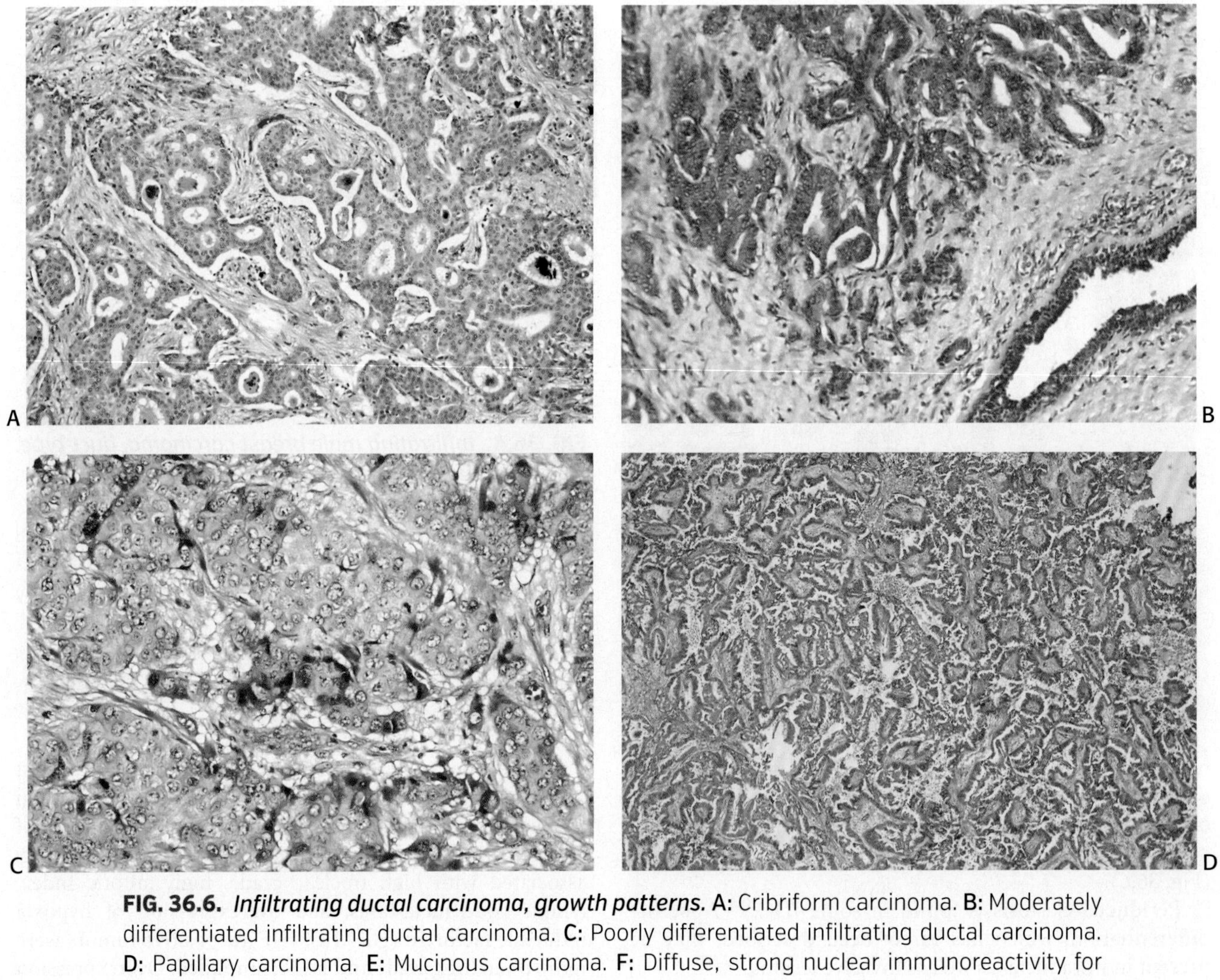

FIG. 36.6. ***Infiltrating ductal carcinoma, growth patterns.*** **A:** Cribriform carcinoma. **B:** Moderately differentiated infiltrating ductal carcinoma. **C:** Poorly differentiated infiltrating ductal carcinoma. **D:** Papillary carcinoma. **E:** Mucinous carcinoma. **F:** Diffuse, strong nuclear immunoreactivity for ER in IDC.

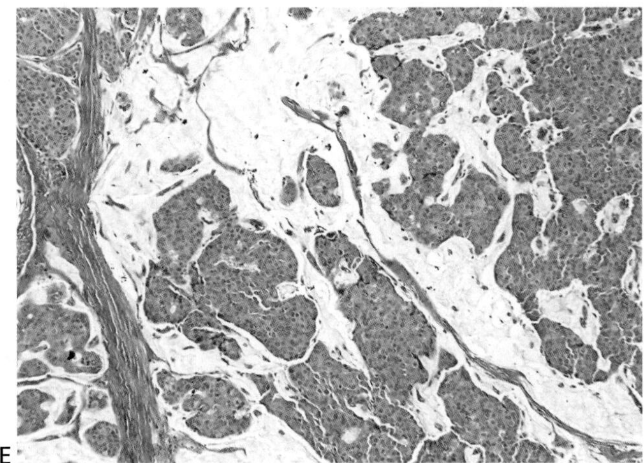

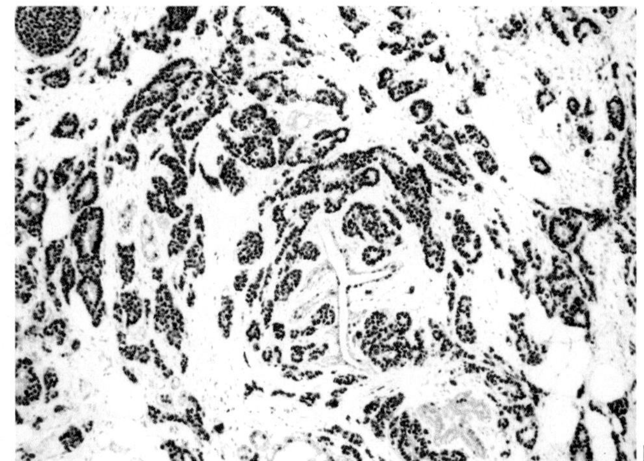

FIG. 36.6. *(Continued)*

About 5% of male breast carcinomas are entirely intraductal lesions.[13,89,91,92,99] In one series, 26% of the carcinomas were intraductal.[90] Others found 12%[107] and 17%[152] to be noninvasive. A review of 282 cases identified in 10 US population-based cancer registries revealed 10.4% to be intraductal.[138] Nahleh et al.[112] reported that 6.7% of 612 men with breast carcinoma in their series had only *in situ* disease, compared with 16.3% of 2,413 women with breast carcinoma. Patients with only DCIS constituted 13% of 77 men with breast carcinoma who had sentinel lymph node (SLN) biopsy at Memorial Hospital in New York City between 1996 and 2005, versus 9% of all women who underwent the same procedure.[113]

The histologic appearance of DCIS in men duplicates that of DCIS in women (Figs. 36.8 and 36.9). Male intraductal

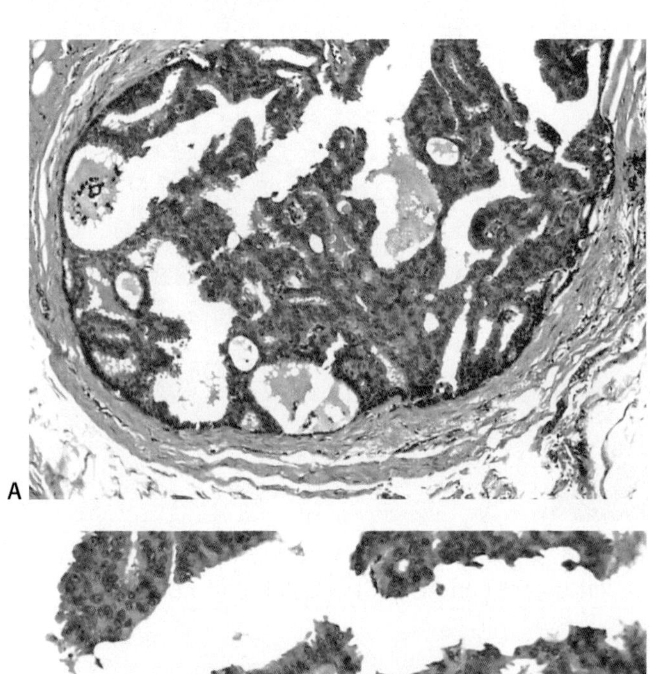

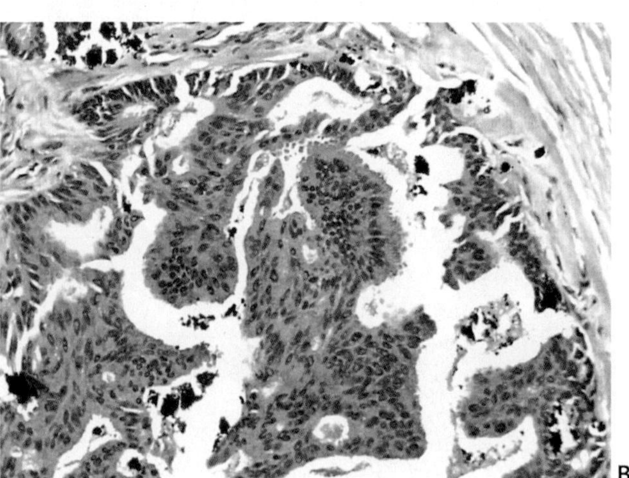

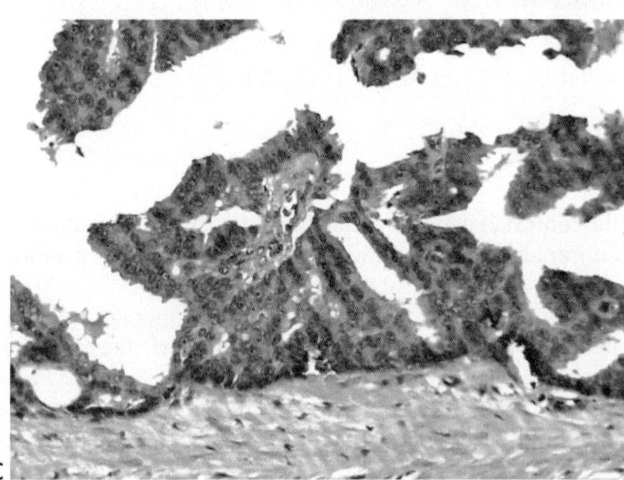

FIG. 36.7. ***Cystic papillary carcinoma.*** **A:** A cystic and papillary carcinoma with orderly architecture. **B,C:** The carcinoma has apocrine features and microcalcifications.

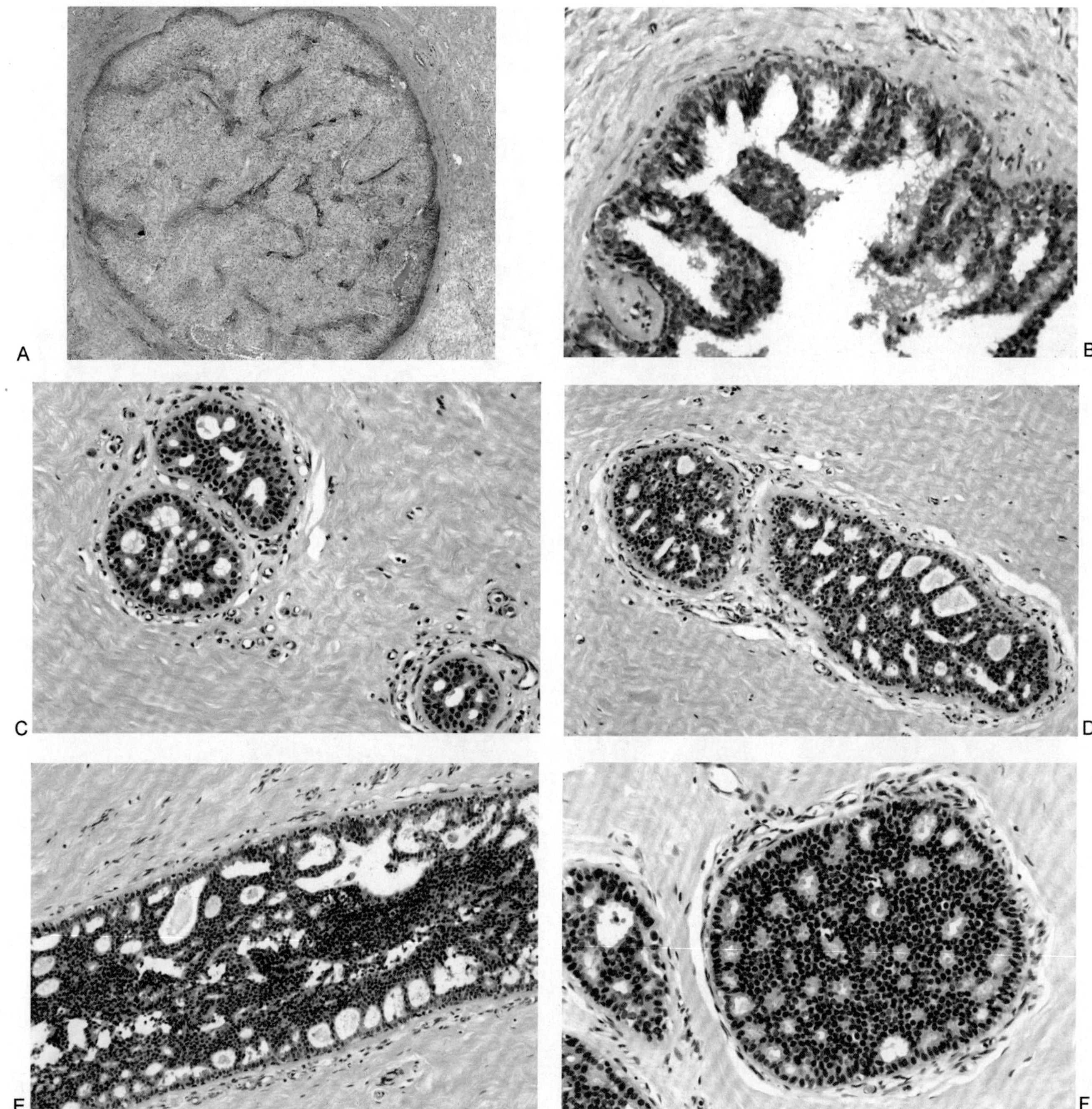

FIG. 36.8. ***Male breast carcinoma, intraductal.*** **A:** Solid papillary carcinoma. **B:** Micropapillary DCIS. **C–F:** Bilateral DCIS in a 44-year-old man. The left breast had ADH **(C)** and cribriform DCIS **(D,E)**. Cribriform DCIS in the right breast **(F)**.

carcinoma without invasion is papillary or cribriform in about 75% of patients, and infrequently solid with comedonecrosis[119] (Fig. 36.8). Myoepithelial cells usually persist and occasionally can become hyperplastic (Fig. 36.10). Many cribriform intraductal lesions in the male breast are intraductal carcinomas, especially if they contain calcifications. On the other hand, micropapillary intraductal lesions are most often hyperplastic rather than intraductal carcinoma, especially in the context of gynecomastia. The presence of calcifications in an intraductal proliferative lesion of the male breast should elicit a high index of suspicion for DCIS.

Approximately 2% of male breast carcinomas are complicated by Paget disease of the nipple, nearly the same frequency as Paget disease in women.[99,153–155] Bilateral Paget disease was reported in a patient with Klinefelter syndrome and multiple other malignant neoplasms.[50] Secondary Paget

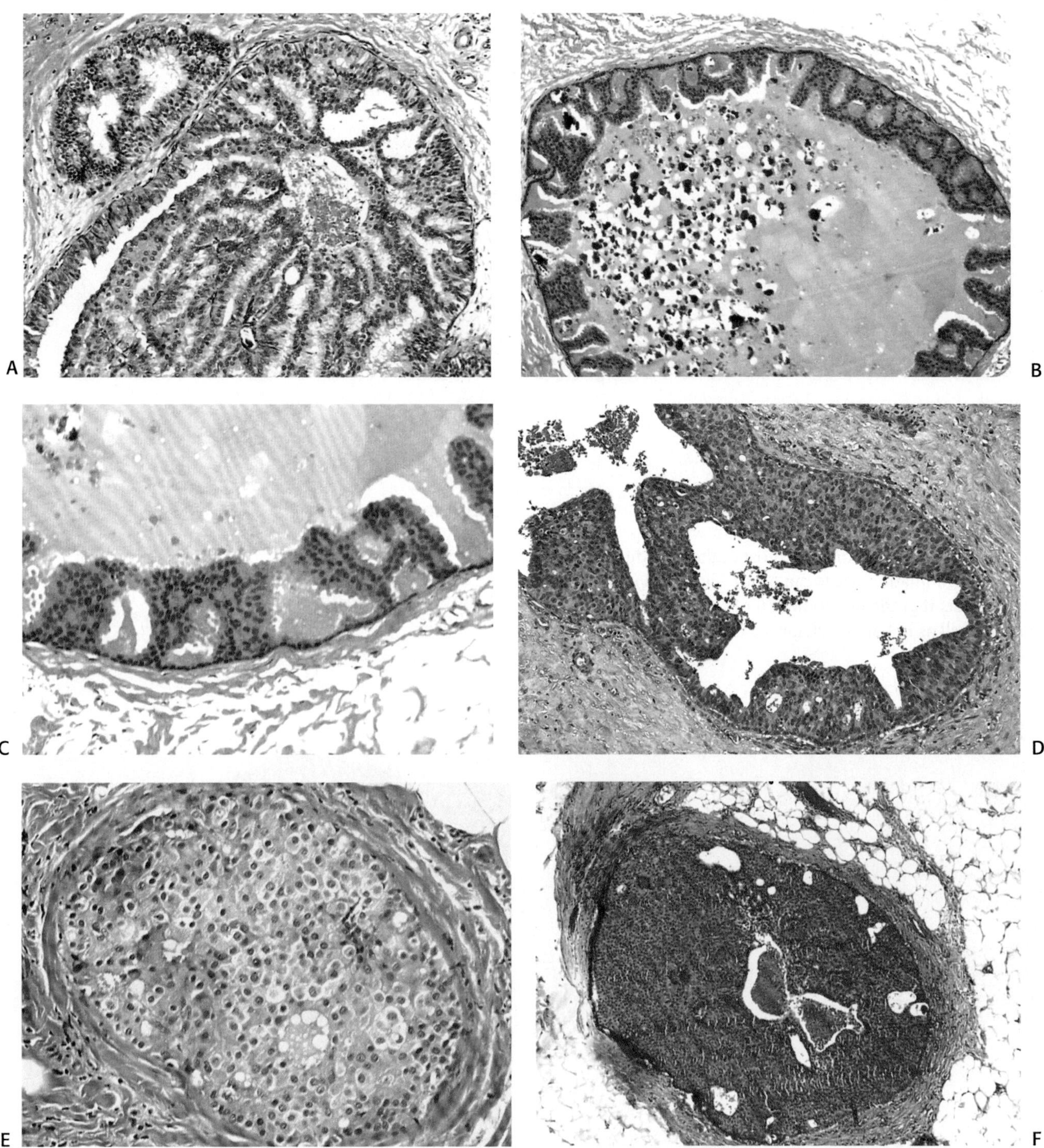

FIG. 36.9. ***Male breast carcinoma, intraductal.*** **A:** Papillary carcinoma with focal necrosis. **B,C:** Micropapillary carcinoma with calcifications. **D:** Solid type distributed at the periphery of a duct. Note the prominent myoepithelial cell layer. **E:** Solid apocrine type. **F:** Solid intraductal carcinoma with a few microlumens and central necrosis. **G,H:** Cribriform DCIS with microcalcifications and distinct cell borders.

disease occurs when an underlying invasive tumor extends into the epidermis of the nipple or adjacent skin.[109,156]

Associated clinically apparent abnormalities that may be responsible for the detection of DCIS include nipple erosion caused by Paget disease, bloody nipple discharge, and gynecomastia. When DCIS arises in gynecomastia, it is rarely possible to find transitions from atypical duct hyperplasia in gynecomastic ducts to carcinoma.[53] Comedonecrosis and

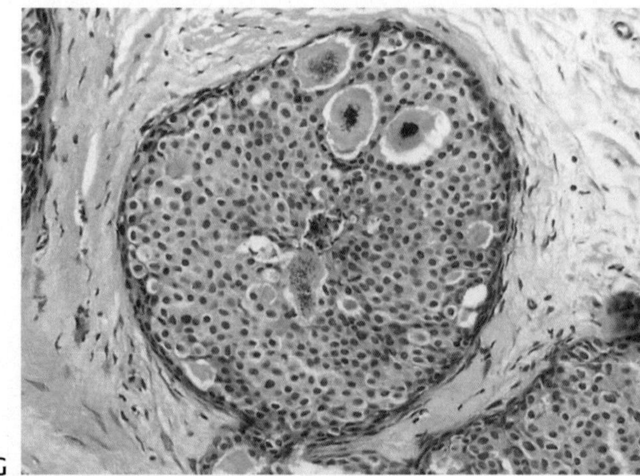

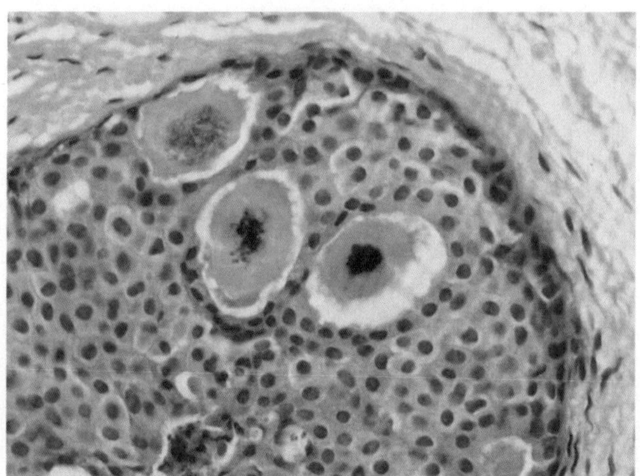

FIG. 36.9. *(Continued)*

epithelial clear cell change are features more strongly associated with intraductal carcinoma than with hyperplasia in gynecomastia. Replacement of most of the intraductal carcinoma by granulation tissue can occur (Fig. 36.11). This finding suggests that the phenomenon of "healing" can occur in male as well as in female DCIS (see Chapter 11).

Lobular Carcinoma

Because lobular differentiation is so rarely seen in the male breast, the existence of lobular carcinoma has been questioned in this setting. Isolated examples of "small cell carcinoma" or lobular carcinoma have been described,[37,90,146,157–160] but

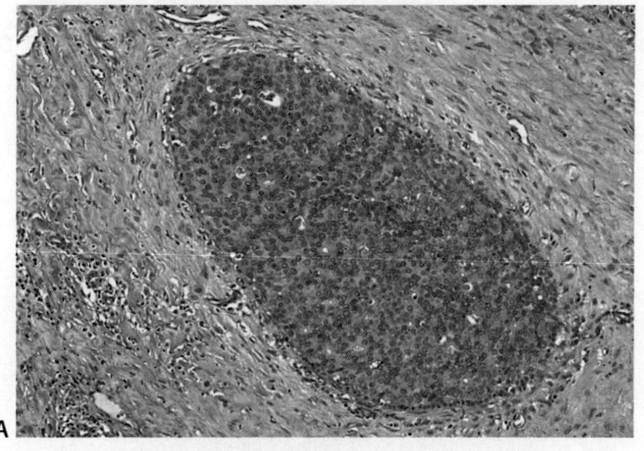

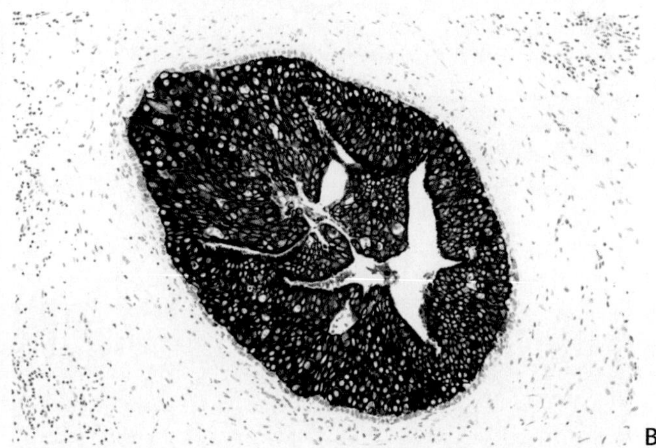

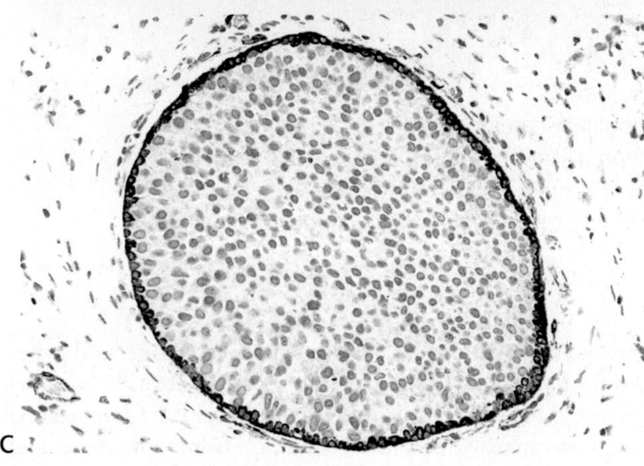

FIG. 36.10. ***Intraductal carcinoma, myoepithelial cells.*** **A:** A distinct band of myoepithelial cells surrounds this solid intraductal carcinoma. **B:** The carcinoma cells are intensely stained with an antibody to CK7. **C:** Myoepithelial cells are highlighted with the antibody to smooth muscle myosin heavy chain.

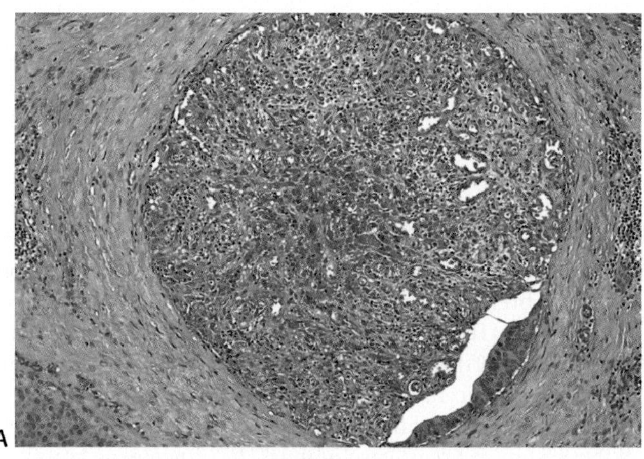
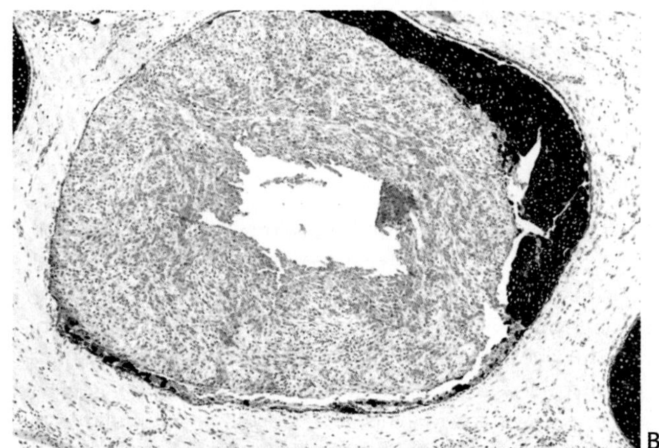

FIG. 36.11. ***Intraductal carcinoma with granulation tissue.*** **A:** Most of the duct lumens are filled with granulation tissue. **B:** Residual carcinoma displays reactivity with the antibody to CK7.

there was none in several larger series.[17,89,99,135] The microscopic appearance of the lesions depicted in several of the papers is consistent with ILC.[158–160]

Michaels et al.[161] described a 59-year-old man with infiltrating lobular carcinoma, no *in situ* lobular carcinoma, and a normal male karyotype. E-Cadherin–negative invasive pleomorphic lobular carcinoma in 44- and 55-year-old men was reported by Maly et al.[162] and Rohini et al.,[163] respectively. Invasive E-cadherin–negative histiocytoid lobular carcinoma in a 68-year-old man reported by Hutchinson and Geradts[164] was immunoreactive for ER, progesterone receptor (PR), and AR, as well as vimentin and pancytokeratin (weak). It was not reactive for several cytokeratin (CK) markers (CAM5.2, 34βE12, AE1/3, and CK7), gross cystic disease fluid protein 15 (GCDFP-15), and HER2/*neu*. A 58-year-old man described by Spencer and Shutter[165] presented with metastatic carcinoma of unknown origin and was found to have bilateral invasive E-cadherin–negative classical lobular carcinoma with a focus of lobular carcinoma *in situ* (LCIS) involving a duct. Other cases of ILC are also part of more recent series.[82,83,134,166–168] Sanchez et al.[159] have reported a case of ILC in a patient with Klinefelter syndrome.

Other Types of Breast Carcinoma

Deb et al.[82] encountered eight cases of invasive micropapillary carcinoma (Fig. 36.4E) in a series of male patients with familial breast carcinoma and documented a strong trend for association with *BRCA2* germline mutation status.

Other uncommon types of invasive carcinoma encountered in the male breast include "medullary,"[3,13,90,133,135,146] mucinous,[89,90,133,135,146,157,166,169] and adenoid cystic.[133,169,170] Carcinoma with osteoclast-like giant cells,[133] and several instances of secretory carcinoma[133,171–175] have been described in the adult male breast. The diagnosis of secretory carcinoma has been supported in some cases by demonstrating the presence of *ETV6–NTRK3* gene fusion,[172] including one male-to-female transsexual patient.[175]

DIFFERENTIAL DIAGNOSIS OF MALE BREAST CARCINOMA

Metastatic Prostatic Carcinoma in the Breast

Metastatic prostatic adenocarcinoma involving one or both breasts has been well documented.[31,176–178] On occasion, the distinction between a primary carcinoma of the breast and metastatic prostatic carcinoma may be difficult. Both types of carcinoma can express ER. Strong nuclear reactivity for AR is typically associated with prostatic carcinoma, but AR also occurs in mammary carcinomas, especially the apocrine type.

Patients with prostatic adenocarcinoma treated with estrogens invariably have gynecomastia, which may exhibit atypical papillary epithelial hyperplasia. In men with known prostatic carcinoma, the diagnosis of mammary carcinoma is relatively easy in the presence of convincing evidence of intraductal carcinoma, usually cribriform or comedo in type, or the finding of invasive growth patterns such as tubular, medullary, or mucinous carcinoma. Khalbuss et al.[179] reported that they were able to make a diagnosis of primary papillary carcinoma in a 67-year-old man with a history of prostatic carcinoma with the aid of the cell block of a fine-needle aspiration (FNA) specimen. The cells were positive for ER and mammaglobin and negative for prostate-specific antigen (PSA). Greater difficulty is encountered with poorly differentiated carcinomas that lack DCIS. The immunohistochemical demonstration of PSA favors a diagnosis of metastatic prostatic carcinoma, whereas finding intracellular mucin supports a diagnosis of mammary carcinoma. However, aberrant expression of PSA detected by immunohistochemistry (IHC) has been reported in breast carcinomas from men[180,181] and women.[182] The tissue concentration of PSA in breast carcinomas may be prognostically significant.[183] After long-standing hormonal treatment, prostatic carcinoma may acquire a poorly differentiated morphology and become negative or only focally positive for PSA. Therefore, a diagnosis of primary mammary carcinoma with triple negative immunophenotype in a man with long-standing history of prostatic carcinoma should be rendered with caution and only after careful clinical and radiologic correlation.

CYTOLOGY

FNA cytology is helpful for evaluating tumors of the male breast.[184,185] Joshi et al.[186] reviewed breast aspirates from 507 men. Satisfactory specimens were obtained from 393 (78%), among which 70 (13.8%) revealed carcinoma. Cellular aspirates may be obtained from carcinomas or from gynecomastia, but the specimens exhibit qualitative differences. The specimen from florid gynecomastia contains abundant epithelial cells, largely arranged in sheets and cohesive clusters, with only scattered isolated cells.[184,187] Dispersed epithelial cells are a prominent feature of most male carcinomas, but epithelioid cell clusters may be encountered in specimens from papillary tumors.[188,189] Considerable cytologic atypia that can occur in the epithelial hyperplasia of gynecomastia may present a diagnostic problem in an FNA specimen.[136,184] Mitotic figures may be found in aspirates from gynecomastia, but they are more frequent in carcinoma.[187] Myoepithelial cells with small, dark nuclei are seen in almost all aspirates from gynecomastia.[136] They are more numerous in material from florid lesions, and such specimens may also have a scattering of lymphocytes. The aspirate from mature, stable gynecomastia is ordinarily sparsely cellular, consisting of scanty epithelial elements, largely in loosely cohesive sheets, and connective tissue cells.

In FNA cytology specimens, samples from papillary carcinoma of the male breast feature greater cellularity than papillomas, and there are many three-dimensional cell clusters that sometimes contain fibrovascular stroma.[190]

IMMUNOHISTOCHEMISTRY

Hormone Receptors

A high frequency of ER-positive male breast carcinomas was first noted in 1976 by Rosen based on biochemical analysis.[137] Subsequent reports that employed biochemical and immunochemical tests confirmed this observation, revealing that 85% to 90% of male breast carcinomas are ER-positive and 85% are PR-positive[138–141,188,191] (Fig. 36.6F). The expression of ER in male breast carcinoma does not appear to be age-related.[138] Gynecomastic breast tissue also contains receptors for estradiol,[137,141,142] androgen,[141] and progesterone.[141]

Using IHC, Rayson et al.[192] detected AR in 95% of male breast carcinomas and bcl-2 in 94%. Most (90%) of the 80 cases studied by Jaggessarsingh et al.[191] expressed AR.

HER2/*neu* and p53

Some membrane immunoreactivity for HER2/*neu* has been found in 14%,[193] 17%,[194,195] 29%,[192] 35%,[196] 39%,[197] and 41%[198] of male breast carcinomas. In one series,[195] HER2/*neu* reactivity was present in 3 (17%) of 18 IDC, but it was absent from three examples of DCIS and 12 specimens of gynecomastia. Following the introduction of specific guidelines for the assessment of HER2 positivity,[199] the percentage of male breast carcinomas classified as HER2-positive based on a combination of immunoreactivity and/or gene amplification is substantially lower. Jaggerssarsingh et al.[191] and Sanchez-Munoz et al.[167] found no HER2-positive tumors in their series adding to a total of 132 male breast carcinomas. Kornegoor et al.[200] found some staining for HER2 in 88/130 (68%) breast carcinomas, but only 4/130 (3%) tumors showed *HER2* gene amplification by chromogenic *in situ* hybridization. Rudlowski et al.[201] detected HER2 3+ staining in 7/99 (7%) and 2+ staining in 8/99 (8%) male breast carcinomas. *HER2/neu* gene amplification was found in 11/99 (11%) cases, including all HER2 3+ tumors and 4/8 (50%) HER2 equivocal (2+) cases.[201] Fonseca et al.[193] found HER2 immunoreactivity in 7/50 (14%) male breast carcinomas (4/7 with 2+ staining and 3/7 with 3+ staining), but *HER2* gene amplification was confirmed in only four cases (8%), including only one of the four cases with HER2 equivocal staining. Nilsson et al.[134] found HER2 3+ positivity in 3/185 (1.6%) cases and 2+ HER2 in 19/185 (10%). They detected *HER2* gene amplification in 21 cases (11%), including 6 with negative HER2 staining. A recent study by Deb et al.[82] identified *HER2* gene amplification in 5/60 (9.1%) cases of familial male breast carcinoma. Arslan et al.,[166] however, have reported that 18/77 (23.4%) male breast carcinomas in their series showed either HER2 3+ immunoreactivity or equivocal (2+) staining and *HER2* gene amplification.

Nuclear immunoreactivity for p53 protein has been detected in 2%,[202] 14%,[203] 21%,[192] 25%,[204] 29%,[198] 31%,[194] and 53%[205] of male breast carcinomas.

Joshi et al.[198] reported that HER2/*neu* immunoreactivity was prognostically unfavorable, and Fonseca et al.[193] observed that HER2/*neu* overexpression and amplification were associated with decreased overall survival (OS). Pich et al.[206] found that p53 positivity was significantly associated with a poor prognosis in a multivariate analysis. Coexpression of p53 and HER2/*neu* was prognostically significant in one report that found no 5-year survivors among men whose tumors were immunoreactive for both oncoproteins, whereas all patients with nonreactive tumors survived for nearly 5 years.[207] Anti-HER2–targeted therapy is currently prescribed to all men whose carcinoma meets the current American Society of Clinical Oncology/College of American Pathology (ASCO/CAP) guidelines for HER2 positivity (See Chapter 12).

Other Antigens

Cyclin D1 was detected in 58% and MIB1 in 38% of 77 male breast carcinomas studied by Rayson et al.[192] Tumors classified as cyclin D1–positive had a significantly better disease-free survival (DFS), whereas MIB1-positive tumors had a decreased DFS. Nilsson et al.[208] evaluated 197 male breast cancers and found cyclin D1 expression to be a positive prognostic marker. Cyclin A and B expression and an elevated mitotic count resulted in a two- to threefold higher risk of breast cancer death.

Fox et al.[209] reported detecting membrane immunoreactivity for epidermal growth factor receptor (EGFR) in 76% of 21 male breast carcinomas, of which 86% were ER-positive. Others found EGFR expression in 12%[200] and 13.8% of male breast carcinomas.[194]

Bcl-2 expression was evident in 28 (82%) of 34 male breast carcinomas studied by Pich et al.[210] and was not significantly related to p53 expression, proliferative activity, or prognosis.

Analysis of CK expression in male breast carcinomas suggests that there may be small subset with a basal-like immunophenotype. Ciocca et al.[211] found that 4 (12.5%) of 32 male breast carcinomas expressed CK5/6 and CK14 and did not express HER2/*neu*. However, three of these tumors expressed ER. These tumors were not studied for EGFR expression. In a series of 130 male breast carcinomas, Kornegoor et al.[200] found that 91% were CK14-negative. Only four (3%) could be classified as basal-like (ER−, PR−, HER2/*neu*−, CK5/6+ and/or CK14+, and/or EGFR+), a frequency that is considerably lower than the approximately 15% occurrence of basal-like carcinomas in women. The majority of male carcinomas were classified as luminal type A (75%) (ER and/or PR+, HER2/*neu*−, and low Ki67) or as luminal type B (20%) (ER and/or PR+, HER2/*neu*+, and/or high Ki67). Shaaban et al.[212] studied biomarkers in 514 matched cases of male and female breast cancer and showed that luminal type A was the most common phenotype in both groups. In this study, luminal type B and HER2/*neu*-positive carcinomas were not seen in men, and basal phenotype was infrequent in both groups. AR-positive luminal type A male breast carcinomas had improved OS over female breast carcinomas at 5 but not at 10 years. Of the 89 male breast carcinomas studied by Jaggerssarsingh et al.,[191] 60% were classified as luminal type A and 40% as luminal type B. All carcinomas in this series were CK5/6- and CK14-negative, and none was basal-like. The authors found no association between outcome and immunoprofile, but this series has a relatively short follow-up (median 2.65 years).

Neurosecretory-type granules in one male papillary carcinoma[213] proved to be argyrophilic, and they were not reactive immunohistochemically for S-100 protein, lactalbumin, or a variety of endocrine substances. In another papillary carcinoma of the male breast, melanin was evident in routine sections and confirmed by histochemical stains.[214] Alm et al.[215] studied 51 consecutive male breast carcinomas for evidence of neuroendocrine differentiation. Chromogranin immunoreactivity was found in 23 (45%) neoplasms, including one example of intraductal carcinoma. Chromogranin immunoreactivity did not have a significant correlation with prognosis.

ELECTRON MICROSCOPY

The ultrastructural features of carcinoma in the male breast appear to be similar to those in the female breast.[216] Neurosecretory-type, electron-dense, membrane-bound cytoplasmic granules were found by electron microscopy in one male papillary carcinoma.[213] "Endocrine-like" granules were detected in the cytoplasm of six tumors studied by electron microscopy by Alm et al.[215]

GENETICS AND MOLECULAR STUDIES

Molecular analysis of DNA extracted from paraffin-embedded male breast carcinomas revealed *p53* mutations in 12 of 29 tumors (41.4%).[217] Only one of these tumors gave a positive reaction for the p53 protein by IHC. The presence or absence of *p53* mutations was not significantly related to prognosis, although it was observed that patients with altered p53 had shorter median DFS and OS.[217] Nayak et al.[218] reported that *p53* mutations occurred in exon 5 or 6 of the *p53* gene in 33% of female breast carcinomas studied with positive IHC in all cases. Mutations in *p53* were found in 90% of male breast carcinomas, all in exon 6, and 86% of these tumors were immunohistochemically positive for p53.

Knowledge of gene profiling in male breast carcinoma is sparse. Johansson et al.[219] performed gene expression analysis of 66 male breast carcinomas and compared the findings with those in female breast tumors. They identified two unique subgroups of male breast carcinomas that were different in biologic features and outcome. The larger group, termed by the authors as "luminal M1 group," contained 46/66 (70%) cases that exhibited expression of genes involved in cell proliferation, HER2-dependent pathways, stromal invasion and metastasis. The second group, referred as luminal M2 group, consisted of 20/66 (30%) tumors expressing ER-related genes, and also genes related to the class I histocompatibility complex, which is involved in immune response regulation. The authors did not indicate whether M2 tumors had a more prominent lymphocytic infiltrate than M1 tumors. These two subgroups of male breast carcinomas differed from the established gene expression subgroups of female breast carcinomas, and the authors suggested that these are novel subgroups of breast carcinoma occurring exclusively in men.

Kornegoor et al.[220] found that copy number gains of the genes *CCND1* (11q13), *TRAF4* (17q11), *CDC6* (17q21), and *MTDH* (8q22) were very common in male breast carcinomas (greater than 40%). Amplification of *CCND1*, the most important single alteration, correlated with poor survival and had independent prognostic value. *EGFR* ($p = 0.005$) and *CCND1* ($p = 0.041$) genes were more frequently amplified in male than in female breast carcinoma.

In a study of epigenetic changes in male breast carcinoma[220] using high-throughput methylation-specific multiplex ligation-dependent probe amplification, more than 50% of the tumors showed methylation in *MSH6*, Wilms tumor 1 (*WT-1*), *PAX5*, *CDH13*, *GATA5*, and *PAX6*. High methylation status correlated with a more aggressive phenotype and poor survival. Female and male breast carcinomas shared a set of commonly methylated genes, but many of the genes were less frequently methylated in male breast carcinoma, pointing toward possible differences between male and female breast carcinogenesis. Pinto et al.[221] evaluated promoter methylation of RARβ and of RASSF1A, which are known to downregulate the expression of ER-α, and the expression of microRNAs (miR17, miR21, miR124, and let-7a) in 56 familial breast carcinomas (27 men and 29 women) and 16 sporadic cases. They found that methylation of RASSF1A was more common in male than in female breast carcinomas (76% vs. 28%, respectively), resulting in inactivation of RASSF1A expression in methylated samples. In particular, RASSF1 was significantly more methylated (92% vs. 58%, respectively, $p = 0.06$) and underexpressed (100% vs. 33%, $p = 0.0001$) in ER-negative tumors than in ER-positive ones. Methylation of RARβ was also high and correlated with low RAR expression in both male and female breast carcinomas. MicroRNA analysis showed higher expression of miR17 and let-7a in ER-negative carcinomas, but the finding was significant only for female breast carcinomas. MicroRNAs miR17, miR21, and let-7a were significantly overexpressed in familial carcinomas than in sporadic ones. Overall, these results emphasize different patterns of regulation in male and female breast carcinomas, at least in the subgroup of men with familial disease. In particular, RASSF1 inactivation was observed in *BRCA1* germline mutation carriers, and RARβ methylation was found in *BRCA1* germline mutation carriers and in BRCA2 wild-type carriers.

TREATMENT AND PROGNOSIS

Most men with breast carcinoma have been treated by total mastectomy and ALN dissection. Total mastectomy alone has been employed mostly for patients with DCIS. In the past, mastectomy was followed by radiation of the chest wall in patients with large tumors for whom the risk of local recurrence was relatively high,[222,223] but it has not been demonstrated that postmastectomy adjuvant radiotherapy improves the overall prognosis.[224-226] Two men who underwent partial mastectomies without radiotherapy for DCIS developed recurrent DCIS in the conserved breasts 30 and 108 months after primary surgery.[152]

Lumpectomy and radiation therapy have only rarely been adopted, usually in elderly patients,[97] but they are not as infrequent in more recent years. In a series by Nilsson et al.,[134] 9% of 197 men with breast carcinomas underwent lumpectomy. The authors reported a local recurrence rate of 7%, but did not indicate whether and how many patients treated with breast-conserving surgery developed locally recurrent disease. Golshan et al.[227] reported breast-conserving treatment in seven men with mean age of 61 years. Six patients had invasive carcinoma (five IDC and one ILC) with mean size 1.7 cm, and all received radiotherapy. The seventh patient had only DCIS and received no radiation. None of the seven patients developed local recurrence at a median follow-up of 67 months. In one case, comedo DCIS treated only by excisional biopsy was followed 4 years later by the development of IDC in the same breast, leading to osseous metastases.[91]

Lymph node metastases are more common in men than in women. Based on an analysis of 1973–1998 SEER data, the rate of lymph node–positive carcinomas was 31.4% in men versus 22.7% in women. Nahleh et al.[112] reported that 41.8% of men in their series had lymph node involvement, compared with 28.2% in a control group of women. Staging of axillary nodal status in men can be effectively accomplished by SLN biopsy. Combined data from early studies using SLN biopsy in male patients[28,228–232] included 25 men, and SLNs were identified in 24 (96%). A SLN was positive in 9/24 (37.5%) cases, with 3 positive at the time of frozen section. In a subset of 21 men with a T1 tumor, 8 (38%) had a positive SLN. Kiluk et al.[28] reported that 10/34 (29.4%) men who had an SLN biopsy at a single institution had a positive SLN. Additional series[113,233] have confirmed the utility of SLN biopsy in male patients with breast carcinoma.

Numerous studies have described the prognosis of male breast carcinoma after treatment by mastectomy and ALN dissection. Prognosis was significantly related to stage at diagnosis as determined by tumor size and nodal status.[3,89,98,224,226,234–237] The presence of lymphatic tumor emboli negatively influences prognosis.[198] Most investigators have concluded that male and female patients with the same stage of disease have a similar prognosis,[96,98,212,225,236,238,239] but some studies have reported worse overall prognosis in men.[112] Heller et al.[89] reported that node-negative male and female patients had nearly identical survivals when compared 5 and 10 years after treatment. In the same study, node-positive male and female patients did not differ in survival at 5 years, but there were substantially fewer survivors among men 10 years after treatment. Survival at 5 and 10 years in pathologically node-negative patients was 70% to 84%.[89,98,224,225,235–237] Among node-positive patients, 5-year survival has been reported to be 59% ± 18%,[80] 57%,[235] and 37%.[224] Ten-year survival has been described as 25% ± 14%[237] and 11% ± 13%.[89] When stratified by the number of lymph nodes with metastases, survival was 73% at 5 years and 44% at 10 years for one to three positive nodes, and 55% at 5 years and 14% at 10 years for four or more nodal metastases.[236] Nahleh et al.[112] stratified OS by disease stage and found that the OS of stage I and stage II male patients was significantly lower than for women with same stage disease, but they found no significant difference in the median OS of men and women with stage III and IV disease. In the same study, the OS of men with lymph node-negative disease was also significantly lower than that of women (6.1 years vs. 14.6 years, $p < 0.005$), but the OS of patients with lymph node involvement was not different. In the study by Tural et al.,[117] 5- and 10-year cancer-specific survivals for all male breast carcinoma patients were 75.2% and 52.5%, respectively. On multivariate analysis, lymph node involvement and larger tumor size were statistically significant predictors of worse survival.[117] Many reports present data in terms of clinical rather than pathologic stage and are difficult to interpret because of the acknowledged inaccuracy of clinical staging. Unfavorable prognostic factors regardless of nodal status are tumor size larger than 2 cm[98,237] and poor histologic differentiation.[225,237]

Treatment recommendations for male patients with breast carcinoma are often based on guidelines established for female carcinoma such as those adopted by the National Comprehensive Cancer Network[240] according to tumor size, regional node involvement, distant metastases (TNM) staging. Surgical treatment usually consists of mastectomy to achieve local control because of concern over nipple or skin involvement by tumors that are typically subareolar in location. In some situations, breast-conserving surgery may be possible.[227] Postoperative adjuvant radiation is indicated for close or positive margins regardless of the surgical procedure, and for patients with large or locally advanced tumors.[241] Yu et al.[242] reported on the utility of postmastectomy radiotherapy in men with breast carcinoma by comparing 46 men who completed treatment with 29 who did not receive radiation. They observed no differences in OS, but a significantly improved local recurrence-free survival ($p < 0.001$) in men treated with radiation therapy.

Hormonal therapy is used for treatment of male breast carcinoma. Treves et al.[105] observed that bilateral orchiectomy could cause regression of the unresected primary tumor when performed in men who presented with systemic metastases. Estradiol and, to a lesser degree, estrone levels are reduced following orchiectomy,[243] and the procedure has proven effective in producing symptomatic relief as well as objective responses in metastatic disease, especially in bone.[244] Presently, orchiectomy is used very rarely, and it has been largely replaced by nonsurgical hormonal and chemotherapy. Tamoxifen is the most frequent adjuvant hormonal therapy.[245] Data from a limited number of patients suggest that this may be effective, but none of the studies has included a randomized control group for comparison.[97,226,246] Ribeiro[97] reported a 5-year survival of 55% among 23 stage II to III men given adjuvant tamoxifen. The 5-year survival in a prior period for men with equivalent stages was 28% without adjuvant tamoxifen. Selective aromatase inhibitors (AIs) are also used in the treatment of male breast carcinoma.[238] A study by Eggemann et al.[115] compared the use of tamoxifen ($n = 207$) or AI ($n = 50$) in a series of 257 German men of similar age and disease stage. The median follow-up time was 42.2 months. All patients were treated with radical mastectomy and axillary lymph node (ALN) dissection or SLN biopsy; 54.9% also received radiotherapy and 37.7% had adjuvant chemotherapy. There were 37 (17.9%) deaths in the tamoxifen-treated group compared with 16 (32%) in the AI group, and the OS of patients treated with tamoxifen was significantly higher than that of AI-treated patients ($p = 0.007$). On multivariate analysis, treatment with AI was associated with significantly increased mortality in men with stage I to III ER-positive carcinoma compared with treatment with tamoxifen. It is to be noted, however, that tamoxifen has some unpleasant side effects, and men are often even less compliant than women in taking this drug.

Chemotherapy is routinely used for the treatment of invasive male breast carcinoma. Patel et al.[246] described 11 men with stage II to III carcinoma treated with 5-fluorouracil and cyclophosphamide combined with either doxorubicin or methotrexate. After a median follow-up of 52 months, 7 were recurrence-free, and their estimated 5-year survival was greater than 85%. Spence et al.[226] were unable to detect benefit from adjuvant hormone therapy in seven patients or from adjuvant chemotherapy in another seven men. Donegan et al.[247] were not able to demonstrate an overall beneficial effect of adjuvant chemotherapy or hormonal therapy in a multi-institutional database. Subset analysis demonstrated a beneficial effect among patients with ER-positive and axillary node–positive tumors from both types of adjuvant treatment. Walshe et al.[248] reported data for stage II male breast carcinoma patients entered into a prospective adjuvant trial of cyclophosphamide, methotrexate, and fluorouracil (CMF). The OS probability after 20 years of follow-up was 42.4% (95% CI, 25.8% to 60.8%) and the median survival was 16.3 years. This trial did not include a control group of patients not treated with CMF.

REFERENCES

1. Ewertz M, Holmberg L, Karjalainen S, et al. Incidence of male breast cancer in Scandinavia, 1943–1982. *Int J Cancer* 1989;43:27–31.
2. Mabuchi K, Bross DS, Kessler II. Risk factors for male breast cancer. *J Natl Cancer Inst* 1985;74:371–375.
3. Ouriel K, Lotze MT, Hinshaw JR. Prognostic factors of carcinoma of the male breast. *Surg Gynecol Obstet* 1984;159:373–376.
4. Schottenfeld D, Lilienfeld AM, Diamond H. Some observations on the epidemiology of breast cancer among males. *Am J Public Health Nations Health* 1963;53:890–897.
5. Anderson WF, Jatoi I, Tse J, et al. Male breast cancer: a population-based comparison with female breast cancer. *J Clin Oncol* 2010;28:232–239.
6. Hodgson NC, Button JH, Franceschi D, et al. Male breast cancer: is the incidence increasing? *Ann Surg Oncol* 2004;11:751–755.
7. Giordano SH, Cohen DS, Buzdar AU, et al. Breast carcinoma in men: a population-based study. *Cancer* 2004;101:51–57.
8. Chavez-Macgregor M, Clarke CA, Lichtensztajn D, et al. Male breast cancer according to tumor subtype and race: a population-based study. *Cancer* 2013;119:1611–1617.
9. Siegel R, Naishadham D, Jemal A. Cancer statistics for Hispanics/Latinos, 2012. *CA Cancer J Clin* 2012;62:283–298.
10. Miao H, Verkooijen HM, Chia KS, et al. Incidence and outcome of male breast cancer: an International Population-Based Study. *J Clin Oncol* 2011;29:4381–4386.
11. Moolgavkar SH, Lee JA, Hade RD. Comparison of age-specific mortality from breast cancer in males in the United States and Japan. *J Natl Cancer Inst* 1978;60:1223–1225.
12. Ajayi DO, Osegbe DN, Ademiluyi SA. Carcinoma of the male breast in West Africans and a review of world literature. *Cancer* 1982;50:1664–1667.
13. Simon MS, McKnight E, Schwartz A, et al. Racial differences in cancer of the male breast—15 year experience in the Detroit metropolitan area. *Breast Cancer Res Treat* 1992;21:55–62.
14. Ly D, Forman D, Ferlay J, et al. An international comparison of male and female breast cancer incidence rates. *Int J Cancer.* 2013;132:1918–1926.
15. Steinitz R, Katz L, Ben-Hur M. Male breast cancer in Israel: selected epidemiological aspects. *Isr J Med Sci* 1981;17:816–821.
16. Newill VA. Distribution of cancer mortality among etimic subgroups of the white population of New York City, 1953–58. *J Natl Cancer Inst* 1961;26:405–417.
17. Hultborn R, Friberg S, Hultborn KA. Male breast carcinoma. I. A study of the total material reported to the Swedish Cancer Registry 1958–1967 with respect to clinical and histopathologic parameters. *Acta Oncol* 1987;26:241–256.
18. Nirmul D, Pegoraro RJ, Jialal I, et al. The sex hormone profile of male patients with breast cancer. *Br J Cancer* 1983;48:423–427.

19. Ballerini P, Recchione C, Cavalleri A, et al. Hormones in male breast cancer. *Tumori* 1990;76:26–28.
20. Olsson H, Alm P, Aspegren K, et al. Increased plasma prolactin levels in a group of men with breast cancer—a preliminary study. *Anticancer Res* 1990;10:59–62.
21. Beard CM, Benson RC Jr, Kelalis PP, et al. The incidence and outcome of mumps orchitis in Rochester, Minnesota, 1935 to 1974. *Mayo Clin Proc* 1977;52:3–7.
22. Nicolis GL, Sabetghadam R, Hsu CC, et al. Breast cancer after mumps orchitis. *JAMA* 1973;223:1032–1033.
23. Casagrande JT, Hanisch R, Pike MC, et al. A case-control study of male breast cancer. *Cancer Res* 1988;48:1326–1330.
24. Thomas DB, Jimenez LM, McTiernan A, et al. Breast cancer in men: risk factors with hormonal implications. *Am J Epidemiol* 1992;135:734–748.
25. Sobin LH, Sherif M. Relation between male breast cancer and prostate cancer. *Br J Cancer* 1980;42:787–790.
26. Cutuli B, Lacroze M, Dilhuydy JM, et al. Male breast cancer: results of the treatments and prognostic factors in 397 cases. *Eur J Cancer* 1995;31A:1960–1964.
27. Leibowitz SB, Garber JE, Fox EA et al. Male patients with diagnoses of both breast cancer and prostate cancer. *Breast J* 2003;9:208–212.
28. Kiluk JV, Lee MC, Park CK, et al. Male breast cancer: management and follow-up recommendations. *Breast J* 2011;17:503–509.
29. McClure JA, Higgins CC. Bilateral carcinoma of male breast after estrogen therapy. *J Am Med Assoc* 1951;146:7–9.
30. Schlappack OK, Braun O, Maier U. Report of two cases of male breast cancer after prolonged estrogen treatment for prostatic carcinoma. *Cancer Detect Prev* 1986;9:319–322.
31. Wilson SE, Hutchinson WB. Breast masses in males with carcinoma of the prostate. *J Surg Oncol* 1976;8:105–112.
32. Carlsson G, Hafstrom L, Jonsson PE. Male breast cancer. *Clin Oncol* 1981;7:149–155.
33. Tajika M, Tuchiya T, Yasuda M, et al. A male case of synchronous double cancers of the breast and prostate. *Intern Med* 1994;33:31–35.
34. Pritchard TJ, Pankowsky DA, Crowe JP, et al. Breast cancer in a male-to-female transsexual. A case report. *JAMA* 1988;259:2278–2280.
35. Symmers WS. Carcinoma of breast in trans-sexual individuals after surgical and hormonal interference with the primary and secondary sex characteristics. *Br Med J* 1968;2:83–85.
36. Ganly I, Taylor EW. Breast cancer in a trans-sexual man receiving hormone replacement therapy. *Br J Surg* 1995;82:341.
37. Lenfant-Pejovic MH, Mlika-Cabanne N, Bouchardy C, et al. Risk factors for male breast cancer: a Franco-Swiss case-control study. *Int J Cancer* 1990;45:661–665.
38. Rosenbaum PF, Vena JE, Zielezny MA, et al. Occupational exposures associated with male breast cancer. *Am J Epidemiol* 1994;139:30–36.
39. Cocco P, Figgs L, Dosemeci M, et al. Case-control study of occupational exposures and male breast cancer. *Occup Environ Med* 1998;55:599–604.
40. Crichlow RW. Carcinoma of the male breast. *Surg Gynecol Obstet* 1972;134:1011–1019.
41. Eldar S, Nash E, Abrahamson J. Radiation carcinogenesis in the male breast. *Eur J Surg Oncol* 1989;15:274–278.
42. Lowell DM, Martineau RG, Luria SB. Carcinoma of the male breast following radiation. Report of a case occurring 35 years after radiation therapy of unilateral prepubertal gynecomastia. *Cancer* 1968;22:585–586.
43. Young G, Wong J, Pezner R. Bilateral breast cancer in a male after radiation therapy for Hodgkin's diesease: a case report and review of the literature. *Breast Dis* 1995;8:185–191.
44. Boice JD Jr, Monson RR. Breast cancer in women after repeated fluoroscopic examinations of the chest. *J Natl Cancer Inst* 1977; 59:823–832.
45. Tokunaga M, Norman JE Jr, Asano M, et al. Malignant breast tumors among atomic bomb survivors, Hiroshima and Nagasaki, 1950–74. *J Natl Cancer Inst* 1979;62:1347–1359.
46. Olsson H, Alm P, Kristoffersson U, et al. Hypophyseal tumor and gynecomastia preceding bilateral breast cancer development in a man. *Cancer* 1984;53:1974–1977.
47. Haga S, Watanabe O, Shimizu T, et al. Breast cancer in a male patient with prolactinoma. *Surg Today* 1993;23:251–255.
48. Dodge OG, Jackson AW, Muldal S. Breast cancer and interstitial-cell tumor in a patient with Klinefelter's syndrome. *Cancer* 1969;24:1027–1032.
49. Brown PW, Terz JJ. Breast carcinoma associated with Klinefelter syndrome: a case report. *J Surg Oncol* 1978;10:413–415.
50. Coley GM, Otis RD, Clark WE IInd. Multiple primary tumors including bilateral breast cancers in a man with Klinefelter's syndrome. *Cancer* 1971;27:1476–1481.
51. Nadel M, Koss L. Klinefelter's syndrom and male breast cancer. *Lancet* 1967;2:366.
52. Evans DB, Crichlow RW. Carcinoma of the male breast and Klinefelter's syndrome: is there an association? *CA Cancer J Clin* 1987;37:246–251.
53. Scheike O, Visfeldt J. Male breast cancer. 4. Gynecomastia in patients with breast cancer. *Acta Pathol Microbiol Scand A* 1973;81:359–365.
54. Giammarini A, Rocchi M, Zennaro W, et al. XX male with breast cancer. *Clin Genet* 1980;18:103–108.
55. Harnden DG, Maclean N, Langlands AO. Carcinoma of the breast and Klinefelter's syndrome. *J Med Genet* 1971;8:460–461.
56. Scheike O, Visfeldt J, Petersen B. Male breast cancer. 3. Breast carcinoma in association with the Klinefelter syndrome. *Acta Pathol Microbiol Scand A* 1973;81:352–358.
57. Hultborn R, Hanson C, Kopf I, et al. Prevalence of Klinefelter's syndrome in male breast cancer patients. *Anticancer Res* 1997;17:4293–4297.
58. Rosenblatt KA, Thomas DB, McTiernan A, et al. Breast cancer in men: aspects of familial aggregation. *J Natl Cancer Inst* 1991;83:849–854.
59. Gough DB, Donohue JH, Evans MM, et al. A 50-year experience of male breast cancer: is outcome changing? *Surg Oncol* 1993;2:325–333.
60. Olsson H, Andersson H, Johansson O, et al. Population-based cohort investigations of the risk for malignant tumors in first-degree relatives and wives of men with breast cancer. *Cancer* 1993;71:1273–1278.
61. Lynch HT, Kaplan AR, Lynch JF. Klinefelter syndrome and cancer. A family study. *JAMA* 1974;229:809–811.
62. Manheimer L. Breast cancer in a father and son. *Breast* 1977;3:21–23.
63. Schwartz RM, Newell RB Jr, Hauch JF, et al. A study of familial male breast carcinoma and a second report. *Cancer* 1980;46:2697–2701.
64. Everson RB, Li FP, Fraumeni JF Jr, et al. Familial male breast cancer. *Lancet* 1976;1:9–12.
65. Marger D, Urdaneta N, Fischer JJ. Breast cancer in brothers: case reports and a review of 30 cases of male breast cancer. *Cancer* 1975;36:458–461.
66. Hauser AR, Lerner IJ, King RA. Familial male breast cancer. *Am J Med Genet* 1992;44:839–840.
67. Jackson VP, Gilmor RL. Male breast carcinoma and gynecomastia: comparison of mammography with sonography. *Radiology* 1983;149:533–536.
68. Kozak FK, Hall JG, Baird PA. Familial breast cancer in males. A case report and review of the literature. *Cancer* 1986;58:2736–2739.
69. Siddiqui T, Weiner R, Moreb J, et al. Cancer of the male breast with prolonged survival. *Cancer* 1988;62:1632–1636.
70. Wooster R, Mangion J, Eeles R, et al. A germline mutation in the androgen receptor gene in two brothers with breast cancer and Reifenstein syndrome. *Nat Genet* 1992;2:132–134.
71. Hiort O, Naber SP, Lehners A, et al. The role of androgen receptor gene mutations in male breast carcinoma. *J Clin Endocrinol Metab* 1996;81:3404–3407.
72. Stratton MR, Ford D, Neuhasen S, et al. Familial male breast cancer is not linked to the BRCA1 locus on chromosome 17q. *Nat Genet* 1994;7:103–107.
73. Ford D, Easton DF, Stratton M, et al. Genetic heterogeneity and penetrance analysis of the BRCA1 and BRCA2 genes in breast cancer families. The Breast Cancer Linkage Consortium. *Am J Hum Genet* 1998;62:676–689.
74. Easton DF, Steele L, Fields P, et al. Cancer risks in two large breast cancer families linked to BRCA2 on chromosome 13q12-13. *Am J Hum Genet* 1997;61:120–128.
75. Neuhausen SL, Godwin AK, Gershoni-Baruch R, et al. Haplotype and phenotype analysis of nine recurrent BRCA2 mutations in 111 families: results of an international study. *Am J Hum Genet* 1998;62: 1381–1388.
76. Csokay B, Udvarhelyi N, Sulyok Z, et al. High frequency of germ-line BRCA2 mutations among Hungarian male breast cancer patients without family history. *Cancer Res* 1999;59:995–998.
77. Thorlacius S, Sigurdsson S, Bjarnadottir H, et al. Study of a single BRCA2 mutation with high carrier frequency in a small population. *Am J Hum Genet* 1997;60:1079–1084.
78. Thorlacius S, Tryggvadottir L, Olafsdottir GH, et al. Linkage to BRCA2 region in hereditary male breast cancer. *Lancet* 1995;346:544–545.

79. Sanz-Ortega J, Chuaqui R, Zhuang Z, et al. Loss of heterozygosity on chromosome 11q13 in microdissected human male breast carcinomas. *J Natl Cancer Inst* 1995;87:1408–1410.
80. Chuaqui RF, Sanz-Ortega J, Vocke C, et al. Loss of heterozygosity on the short arm of chromosome 8 in male breast carcinomas. *Cancer Res* 1995;55:4995–4998.
81. Storm HH, Olsen J. Risk of breast cancer in offspring of male breast-cancer patients. *Lancet* 1999;353:209.
82. Deb S, Jene N, Investigators K, et al. Genotypic and phenotypic analysis of familial male breast cancer shows under representation of the HER2 and basal subtypes in BRCA-associated carcinomas. *BMC Cancer* 2012;12:510.
83. Ottini L, Silvestri V, Rizzolo P, et al. Clinical and pathologic characteristics of BRCA-positive and BRCA-negative male breast cancer patients: results from a collaborative multicenter study in Italy. *Breast Cancer Res Treat* 2012;134:411–418.
84. Orr N, Lemnrau A, Cooke R, et al. Genome-wide association study identifies a common variant in RAD51B associated with male breast cancer risk. *Nat Genet* 2012;44:1182–1184.
85. Wasielewski M, den Bakker MA, van den Ouweland A, et al. CHEK2 1100delC and male breast cancer in the Netherlands. *Breast Cancer Res Treat* 2009;116:397–400.
86. Meijers-Heijboer H, van den Ouweland A, Klijn J, et al. Low-penetrance susceptibility to breast cancer due to CHEK2(*)1100delC in noncarriers of BRCA1 or BRCA2 mutations. *Nat Genet* 2002;31:55–59.
87. Fackenthal JD, Marsh DJ, Richardson AL, et al. Male breast cancer in Cowden syndrome patients with germline PTEN mutations. *J Med Genet* 2001;38:159–164.
88. Young IE, Kurian KM, Annink C, et al. A polymorphism in the CYP17 gene is associated with male breast cancer. *Br J Cancer* 1999;81:141–143.
89. Heller KS, Rosen PP, Schottenfeld D, et al. Male breast cancer: a clinicopathologic study of 97 cases. *Ann Surg* 1978;188:60–65.
90. Wolff M, Reinis M. Breast cancer in the male: clinicopathologic study of 40 patients and review of the literature. In: Fenoglio M, Wolff M, eds. *Progress in surgical pathology*. New York: Masson Publishers; 1981.
91. Cole FM, Qizilbash AH. Carcinoma *in situ* of the male breast. *J Clin Pathol* 1979;32:1128–1134.
92. Green L, Wysowski DK, Fourcroy JL. Gynecomastia and breast cancer during finasteride therapy. *N Engl J Med* 1996;335:823.
93. Staerkle RF, Lenzlinger PM, Suter SL, et al. Synchronous bilateral ductal carcinoma *in situ* of the male breast associated with gynecomastia in a 30-year-old patient following repeated injections of stanozolol. *Breast Cancer Res Treat* 2006;97:173–176.
94. El-Gazayerli MM, Abdel-Aziz AS. On Bilharziasis and male breast cancer in Egypt: a preliminary report and review of the literature. *Br J Cancer* 1963;17:566–571.
95. Auvinen A, Curtis RE, Ron E. Risk of subsequent cancer following breast cancer in men. *J Natl Cancer Inst* 2002;94:1330–1332.
96. Langlands AO, Maclean N, Kerr GR. Carcinoma of the male breast: report of a series of 88 cases. *Clin Radiol* 1976;27:21–25.
97. Ribeiro G. Male breast carcinoma—a review of 301 cases from the Christie Hospital & Holt Radium Institute, Manchester. *Br J Cancer* 1985;51:115–119.
98. Yap HY, Tashima CK, Blumenschein GR, et al. Male breast cancer: a natural history study. *Cancer* 1979;44:748–754.
99. Gadenne C, Contesso G, Travagli JP, et al. [Male breast tumours. Anatomico-clinical study based on 73 cases (author's transl)]. *Nouv Presse Med* 1982;11:2331–2334.
100. Hemminki K, Scelo G, Boffetta P, et al. Second primary malignancies in patients with male breast cancer. *Br J Cancer* 2005;92:1288–1292.
101. Goss PE, Reid C, Pintilie M, et al. Male breast carcinoma: a review of 229 patients who presented to the Princess Margaret Hospital during 40 years: 1955–1996. *Cancer* 1999;85:629–639.
102. Ouimet-Oliva D, Hebert G, Ladouceur J. Radiographic characteristics of male breast cancer. *Radiology* 1978;129:37–40.
103. Brodie EM, King ER. Histologically different, synchronous, bilateral carcinoma of the male breast (a case report). *Cancer* 1974;34: 1276–1277.
104. Wolloch Y, Zer M, Dintsman M, et al. Simultaneous bilateral primary breast carcinoma in the male. *Isr J Med Sci* 1972;8:158–162.
105. Treves N, Abels JC, Woodard HQ, et al. The effects of orchiectomy on primary and metastatic carcinoma of the breast. *CA Cancer J Clin* 1978;28:182–190.
106. Ranieri E, D'Andrea MR, D'Alessio A, et al. Male breast carcinoma *in situ*. Report of a case diagnosed by nipple discharge cytology alone. *Anticancer Res* 1995;15:1589–1592.
107. Wang Y, Abreau M, Hoda S. Mammary duct carcinoma *in situ* in males: pathologic findings and clinical considerations. *Mod Pathol* 1997;10:27A.
108. Scheike O. Male breast cancer. 5. Clinical manifestations in 257 cases in Denmark. *Br J Cancer* 1973;28:552–561.
109. Hali F, Khadir K, Idhammou W, et al. [Cutaneous manifestations of male breast cancer]. *Presse Med* 2011;40:e483–e488.
110. Hill TD, Khamis HJ, Tyczynski JE, et al. Comparison of male and female breast cancer incidence trends, tumor characteristics, and survival. *Ann Epidemiol* 2005;15:773–780.
111. Vermeulen JF, Kornegoor R, van der Wall E, et al. Differential expression of growth factor receptors and membrane-bound tumor markers for imaging in male and female breast cancer. *PLoS One* 2013; 8:e53353.
112. Nahleh ZA, Srikantiah R, Safa M, et al. Male breast cancer in the veterans affairs population: a comparative analysis. *Cancer* 2007;109:1471–1477.
113. Flynn LW, Park J, Patil SM, et al. Sentinel lymph node biopsy is successful and accurate in male breast carcinoma. *J Am Coll Surg* 2008;206:616–621.
114. Saltzstein EC, Tavaf AM, Latorraca R. Breast carcinoma in a young man. *Arch Surg* 1978;113:880–881.
115. Eggemann H, Ignatov A, Smith BJ, et al. Adjuvant therapy with tamoxifen compared to aromatase inhibitors for 257 male breast cancer patients. *Breast Cancer Res Treat* 2013;137:465–470.
116. Mejias A, Sittler S, Mies C. Poor prognostic features are prevalent in young men with breast carcinoma. *Lab Invest* 1994;70:18A.
117. Tural D, Selcukbiricik F, Aydogan F, et al. Male breast cancers behave differently in elderly patients. *Jpn J Clin Oncol* 2013;43:22–27.
118. Hill A, Yagmur Y, Tran KN, et al. Localized male breast carcinoma and family history. An analysis of 142 patients. *Cancer* 1999;86:821–825.
119. Hittmair AP, Lininger RA, Tavassoli FA. Ductal carcinoma *in situ* (DCIS) in the male breast: a morphologic study of 84 cases of pure DCIS and 30 cases of DCIS associated with invasive carcinoma—a preliminary report. *Cancer* 1998;83:2139–2149.
120. Dershaw DD. Male mammography. *AJR Am J Roentgenol* 1986;146:127–131.
121. Chantra PK, So GJ, Wollman JS, et al. Mammography of the male breast. *AJR Am J Roentgenol* 1995;164:853–858.
122. Tukel S, Ozcan H. Mammography in men with breast cancer: review of the mammographic findings in five cases. *Australas Radiol* 1996;40:387–390.
123. Dershaw DD, Borgen PI, Deutch BM, et al. Mammographic findings in men with breast cancer. *AJR Am J Roentgenol* 1993;160:267–270.
124. Fallentin E, Rothman L. Intracystic carcinoma of the male breast. *J Clin Ultrasound* 1994;22:118–120.
125. Sonksen CJ, Michell M, Sundaresan M. Case report: intracystic papillary carcinoma of the breast in a male patient. *Clin Radiol* 1996;51:438–439.
126. Chinn K, Kalisher L, Rickert RR. Intracystic papillary breast carcinoma in a 55-year-old man: radiologic and pathologic correlation. *Can Assoc Radiol J* 1989;40:40–42.
127. Michels LG, Gold RH, Arndt RD. Radiography of gynecomastia and other disorders of the male breast. *Radiology* 1977;122:117–122.
128. Brenner RJ, Weitzel JN, Hansen N, et al. Screening-detected breast cancer in a man with BRCA2 mutation: case report. *Radiology* 2004;230:553–555.
129. Freedman BC, Keto J, Rosenbaum Smith SM. Screening mammography in men with BRCA mutations: is there a role? *Breast J* 2012;18:73–75.
130. Morakkabati-Spitz N, Schild HH, Leutner CC, et al. Dynamic contrast-enhanced breast MR imaging in men: preliminary results. *Radiology* 2006;238:438–445.
131. Weiss LM DL, Esposito MJ, et al. Mammographic appearance of inflammatory carcinoma in the male breast. *Breast Dis* 1987;1:33–36.
132. Kalisher L, Peyster RG. Xerographic manifestations of male breast disease. *Am J Roentgenol Radium Ther Nucl Med* 1975;125:656–661.
133. Burga AM, Fadare O, Lininger RA, et al. Invasive carcinomas of the male breast: a morphologic study of the distribution of histologic subtypes and metastatic patterns in 778 cases. *Virchows Arch* 2006;449:507–512.
134. Nilsson C, Johansson I, Ahlin C, et al. Molecular subtyping of male breast cancer using alternative definitions and its prognostic impact. *Acta Oncol* 2013;52:102–109.

135. Visfeldt J, Scheike O. Male breast cancer. I. Histologic typing and grading of 187 Danish cases. *Cancer* 1973;32:985–990.
136. Gupta RK, Naran S, Simpson J. The role of fine needle aspiration cytology (FNAC) in the diagnosis of breast masses in males. *Eur J Surg Oncol* 1988;14:317–320.
137. Rosen PP, Menendez-Botet CJ, Nisselbaum JS, et al. Estrogen receptor protein in lesions of the male breast: a preliminary report. *Cancer* 1976;37:1866–1868.
138. Stalsberg H, Thomas DB, Rosenblatt KA, et al. Histologic types and hormone receptors in breast cancer in men: a population-based study in 282 United States men. *Cancer Causes Control* 1993;4:143–151.
139. Thompson EB, Perlin E, Tormey D. Steroid-binding proteins in carcinoma of the human male breast. *Am J Clin Pathol* 1976;65:360–363.
140. Everson RB, Lippman ME, Thompson EB, et al. Clinical correlations of steroid receptors and male breast cancer. *Cancer Res* 1980;40:991–997.
141. Pacheco MM, Oshima CF, Lopes MP, et al. Steroid hormone receptors in male breast diseases. *Anticancer Res* 1986;6:1013–1017.
142. Rajendran KG, Shah PN, Bagli NP, et al. Oestradiol receptors in non-neoplastic gynaecomastic tissue of phenotypic males. *Horm Res* 1976;7:193–200.
143. Friedman MA, Hoffman PG Jr, Dandolos EM, et al. Estrogen receptors in male breast cancer: clinical and pathologic correlations. *Cancer* 1981;47:134–137.
144. Lopez M, Di Lauro L, Lazzaro B, et al. Hormonal treatment of disseminated male breast cancer. *Oncology* 1985;42:345–349.
145. Nomura Y, Kondo H, Yamagata J, et al. Detection of the estrogen receptor and response to endocrine therapy in male breast cancer patients. *Gann* 1977;68:333–336.
146. Norris HJ, Taylor HB. Carcinoma of the male breast. *Cancer* 1969;23:1428–1435.
147. Taxy JB. Tubular carcinoma of the male breast: report of a case. *Cancer* 1975;36:462–465.
148. Raju GC, Lee YS. Elastosis in the male breast. *Histopathology* 1988;12:203–209.
149. Bryant J. Male breast cancer: a case of apocrine carcinoma with psammoma bodies. *Hum Pathol* 1981;12:751–753.
150. Costa MJ, Silverberg SG. Oncocytic carcinoma of the male breast. *Arch Pathol Lab Med* 1989;113:1396–1399.
151. Kornegoor R, Verschuur-Maes AH, Buerger H, et al. Fibrotic focus and hypoxia in male breast cancer. *Mod Pathol* 2012;25:1397–1404.
152. Camus MG, Joshi MG, Mackarem G, et al. Ductal carcinoma *in situ* of the male breast. *Cancer* 1994;74:1289–1293.
153. Crichlow RW, Czernobilsky B. Paget's disease of the male breast. *Cancer* 1969;24:1033.
154. Serour F, Birkenfeld S, Amsterdam E, et al. Paget's disease of the male breast. *Cancer* 1988;62:601–605.
155. Coley GM, Kuehn PG. Paget's disease of the male breast. *Am J Surg* 1972;123:444–450.
156. Chao C, Edwards MJ, Wolfson S, et al. Paget's disease of the male breast: an unusual case of dermal invasion. *Breast J* 2003;9:254.
157. Giffler RF, Kay S. Small-cell carcinoma of the male mammary gland. A tumor resembling infiltrating lobular carcinoma. *Am J Clin Pathol* 1976;66:715–722.
158. Nance KV, Reddick RL. *In situ* and infiltrating lobular carcinoma of the male breast. *Hum Pathol* 1989;20:1220–1222.
159. Sanchez AG, Villanueva AG, Redondo C. Lobular carcinoma of the breast in a patient with Klinefelter's syndrome. A case with bilateral, synchronous, histologically different breast tumors. *Cancer* 1986;57:1181–1183.
160. Yogore MG IIIrd, Sahgal S. Small cell carcinoma of the male breast: report of a case. *Cancer* 1977;39:1748–1751.
161. Michaels BM, Nunn CR, Roses DF. Lobular carcinoma of the male breast. *Surgery* 1994;115:402–405.
162. Maly B, Maly A, Pappo I, et al. Pleomorphic variant of invasive lobular carcinoma of the male breast. *Virchows Arch* 2005;446:344–345.
163. Rohini B, Singh PA, Vatsala M, et al. Pleomorphic lobular carcinoma in a male breast: a rare occurrence. *Patholog Res Int* 2010;2010:871369.
164. Hutchinson CB, Geradts J. Histiocytoid carcinoma of the male breast. *Ann Diagn Pathol* 2011;15:190–193.
165. Spencer JT, Shutter J. Synchronous bilateral invasive lobular breast cancer presenting as carcinomatosis in a male. *Am J Surg Pathol* 2009;33:470–474.
166. Arslan UY, Oksuzoglu B, Ozdemir N, et al. Outcome of non-metastatic male breast cancer: 118 patients. *Med Oncol* 2012;29:554–560.
167. Sanchez-Munoz A, Roman-Jobacho A, Perez-Villa L, et al. Male breast cancer: immunohistochemical subtypes and clinical outcome characterization. *Oncology* 2012;83:228–233.
168. Tawil AN, Boulos FI, Chakhachiro ZI, et al. Clinicopathologic and immunohistochemical characteristics of male breast cancer: a single center experience. *Breast J* 2012;18:65-68.
169. Ottini L, Rizzolo P, Zanna I, et al. BRCA1/BRCA2 mutation status and clinical-pathologic features of 108 male breast cancer cases from Tuscany: a population-based study in central Italy. *Breast Cancer Res Treat* 2009;116:577–586.
170. Hjorth S, Magnusson PH, Blomquist P. Adenoid cystic carcinoma of the breast. Report of a case in a male and review of the literature. *Acta Chir Scand* 1977;143:155–158.
171. Krausz T, Jenkins D, Grontoft O, et al. Secretory carcinoma of the breast in adults: emphasis on late recurrence and metastasis. *Histopathology* 1989;14:25–36.
172. Diallo R, Schaefer KL, Bankfalvi A, et al. Secretory carcinoma of the breast: a distinct variant of invasive ductal carcinoma assessed by comparative genomic hybridization and immunohistochemistry. *Hum Pathol* 2003;34:1299–1305.
173. Kuwabara H, Yamane M, Okada S. Secretory breast carcinoma in a 66 year old man. *J Clin Pathol* 1998;51:545–547.
174. Alena C AF, Segui FJ, Laforga J. Secretory carcinoma of the male breast: correlation of aspiration cytology and pathology. *Diagn Cytopathol* 2005;32:47–50.
175. Grabellus F, Worm K, Willruth A, et al. ETV6-NTRK3 gene fusion in a secretory carcinoma of the breast of a male-to-female transsexual. *Breast* 2005;14:71–74.
176. Berge T. Metastases to the male breast. *Acta Pathol Microbiol Scand A* 1971;79:491–496.
177. Campbell J, Cummins S. Metastases simulating mammary cancer in prostatic carcinoma under estrogenic therapy. *Cancer* 1951;4:303–311.
178. Hartley LC, Little JH. Bilateral mammary metastases from carcinoma of the prostate during oestrogen therapy. *Med J Aust* 1971;1:434–436.
179. Khalbuss WE, Ambaye A, Goodison S, et al. Papillary carcinoma of the breast in a male patient with a treated prostatic carcinoma diagnosed by fine-needle aspiration biopsy: a case report and review of the literature. *Diagn Cytopathol* 2006;34:214–217.
180. Gupta RK. Immunoreactivity of prostate-specific antigen in male breast carcinomas: two examples of a diagnostic pitfall in discriminating a primary breast cancer from metastatic prostate carcinoma. *Diagn Cytopathol* 1999;21:167–169.
181. Carder PJ, Speirs V, Ramsdale J, et al. Expression of prostate specific antigen in male breast cancer. *J Clin Pathol* 2005;58:69–71.
182. Bodey B, Bodey B Jr, Kaiser HE. Immunocytochemical detection of prostate specific antigen expression in human breast carcinoma cells. *Anticancer Res* 1997;17:2577–2581.
183. Yu H, Levesque MA, Clark GM, et al. Enhanced prediction of breast cancer prognosis by evaluating expression of p53 and prostate-specific antigen in combination. *Br J Cancer* 1999;81:490–495.
184. Lilleng R, Paksoy N, Vural G, et al. Assessment of fine needle aspiration cytology and histopathology for diagnosing male breast masses. *Acta Cytol* 1995;39:877–881.
185. Rose M MS. Cytomorphology of male breast lesions: diagnostic pitfalls and clinical implications. *Diagn Cytopathol* 2012;40:179–184.
186. Joshi A, Kapila K, Verma K. Fine needle aspiration cytology in the management of male breast masses. Nineteen years of experience. *Acta Cytol* 1999;43:334–338.
187. Das DK, Junaid TA, Mathews SB, et al. Fine needle aspiration cytology diagnosis of male breast lesions. A study of 185 cases. *Acta Cytol* 1995;39:870–876.
188. Bhagat P, Kline TS. The male breast and malignant neoplasms. Diagnosis by aspiration biopsy cytology. *Cancer* 1990;65:2338–2341.
189. Russin VL, Lachowicz C, Kline TS. Male breast lesions: gynecomastia and its distinction from carcinoma by aspiration biopsy cytology. *Diagn Cytopathol* 1989;5:243–247.
190. Reid-Nicholson MD, Tong G, Cangiarella JF, et al. Cytomorphologic features of papillary lesions of the male breast: a study of 11 cases. *Cancer* 2006;108:222–230.
191. Jaggessarsingh J CJ, Akram A, Brogi E, et al. Male breast carcinoma: clinicopathologic and molecular analysis of 89 cases. *Mod Pathol* 2013;26:47A.
192. Rayson D, Erlichman C, Suman VJ, et al. Molecular markers in male breast carcinoma. *Cancer* 1998;83:1947–1955.

193. Fonseca RR, Tomas AR, Andre S, et al. Evaluation of ERBB2 gene status and chromosome 17 anomalies in male breast cancer. *Am J Surg Pathol* 2006;30:1292–1298.
194. Moore J, Friedman MI, Gansler T, et al. Prognostic indicators in male breast carcinoma. *Breast J* 1998;4:261–269.
195. Dawson PJ, Paine TM, Wolman SR. Immunocytochemical characterization of male breast cancer. *Mod Pathol* 1992;5:621–625.
196. Gattuso P, Reddy VB, Green L, et al. Prognostic significance of DNA ploidy in male breast carcinoma. A retrospective analysis of 32 cases. *Cancer* 1992;70:777–780.
197. Leach IH, Ellis IO, Elston CW. c-erb-B-2 expression in male breast carcinoma. *J Clin Pathol* 1992;45:942.
198. Joshi MG, Lee AK, Loda M, et al. Male breast carcinoma: an evaluation of prognostic factors contributing to a poorer outcome. *Cancer* 1996;77:490–498.
199. Wolff AC, Hammond ME, Schwartz JN, et al. American Society of Clinical Oncology/College of American Pathologists guideline recommendations for human epidermal growth factor receptor 2 testing in breast cancer. *Arch Pathol Lab Med* 2007;131:18–43.
200. Kornegoor R, Verschuur-Maes AH, Buerger H, et al. Molecular subtyping of male breast cancer by immunohistochemistry. *Mod Pathol* 2012;25:398–404.
201. Rudlowski C, Friedrichs N, Faridi A, et al. Her-2/neu gene amplification and protein expression in primary male breast cancer. *Breast Cancer Res Treat* 2004;84:215–223.
202. Hecht JR WJ, Ramos L, et al. Male breast cancers rarely overexpress p53 protein. *Lab Invest* 1994;35:214.
203. Weber-Chappuis K, Bieri-Burger S, Hurlimann J. Comparison of prognostic markers detected by immunohistochemistry in male and female breast carcinomas. *Eur J Cancer* 1996;32A:1686–1692.
204. Dawson PJ, Schroer KR, Wolman SR. ras and p53 genes in male breast cancer. *Mod Pathol* 1996;9:367–370.
205. Wieczorek R HP, Feiner H, et al. p53 protein overexpression in male breast cancer: clinicopathologic (CPC) correlation. *Lab Invest* 1994;70:24A.
206. Pich A, Margaria E, Chiusa L, et al. DNA ploidy and p53 expression correlate with survival and cell proliferative activity in male breast carcinoma. *Hum Pathol* 1996;27:676–682.
207. Pich A, Margaria E, Chiusa L. Oncogenes and male breast carcinoma: c-erbB-2 and p53 coexpression predicts a poor survival. *J Clin Oncol* 2000;18:2948–2956.
208. Nilsson C, Koliadi A, Johansson I, et al. High proliferation is associated with inferior outcome in male breast cancer patients. *Mod Pathol* 2013;26:87–94.
209. Fox SB, Rogers S, Day CA, et al. Oestrogen receptor and epidermal growth factor receptor expression in male breast carcinoma. *J Pathol* 1992;166:13–18.
210. Pich A, Margaria E, Chiusa L. Bcl-2 expression in male breast carcinoma. *Virchows Arch* 1998;433:229–235.
211. Ciocca V, Bombonati A, Gatalica Z, et al. Cytokeratin profiles of male breast cancers. *Histopathology* 2006;49:365–370.
212. Shaaban AM, Ball GR, Brannan RA, et al. A comparative biomarker study of 514 matched cases of male and female breast cancer reveals gender-specific biological differences. *Breast Cancer Res Treat* 2012;133:949–958.
213. Ramos CV, Boeshart C, Restrepo GL. Intracystic papillary carcinoma of the male breast. Immunohistochemical and ultrastructural study. *Arch Pathol Lab Med* 1985;109:858–861.
214. Romanelli R, Toncini C. Pigmented papillary carcinoma of the male breast. *Tumori* 1986;72:105–108.
215. Alm P, Alumets J, Bak-Jensen E, et al. Neuroendocrine differentiation in male breast carcinomas. *APMIS* 1992;100:720–726.
216. Hassan MO, Olaizola MY. Male breast carcinoma. An ultrastructural study. *Arch Pathol Lab Med* 1979;103:191–195.
217. Anelli A, Anelli TF, Youngson B, et al. Mutations of the p53 gene in male breast cancer. *Cancer* 1995;75:2233–2238.
218. Nayak BK, Baral RN, Das BR. p53 gene mutation in relation to p53 protein accumulation in male and female breast cancer. *Neoplasma* 1996;43:305–310.
219. Johansson I, Nilsson C, Berglund P, et al. Gene expression profiling of primary male breast cancers reveals two unique subgroups and identifies N-acetyltransferase-1 (NAT1) as a novel prognostic biomarker. *Breast Cancer Res* 2012;14:R31.
220. Kornegoor R, Moelans CB, Verschuur-Maes AH, et al. Promoter hypermethylation in male breast cancer: analysis by multiplex ligation-dependent probe amplification. *Breast Cancer Res* 2012; 14:R101.
221. Pinto R, Pilato B, Ottini L, et al. Different methylation and MicroRNA expression pattern in male and female familial breast cancer. *J Cell Physiol* 2013;228:1264–1269.
222. Robison R, Montague ED. Treatment results in males with breast cancer. *Cancer* 1982;49:403–406.
223. Schuchardt U, Seegenschmiedt MH, Kirschner MJ, et al. Adjuvant radiotherapy for breast carcinoma in men: a 20-year clinical experience. *Am J Clin Oncol* 1996;19:330–336.
224. Erlichman C, Murphy KC, Elhakim T. Male breast cancer: a 13-year review of 89 patients. *J Clin Oncol* 1984;2:903–909.
225. Scheike O. Male breast cancer. 6. Factors influencing prognosis. *Br J Cancer* 1974;30:261–271.
226. Spence RA, MacKenzie G, Anderson JR, et al. Long-term survival following cancer of the male breast in Northern Ireland. A report of 81 cases. *Cancer* 1985;55:648–652.
227. Golshan M, Rusby J, Dominguez F, et al. Breast conservation for male breast carcinoma. *Breast* 2007;16:653–656.
228. Cimmino VM, Degnim AC, Sabel MS, et al. Efficacy of sentinel lymph node biopsy in male breast cancer. *J Surg Oncol* 2004;86:74–77.
229. Port ER, Fey JV, Cody HS III, et al. Sentinel lymph node biopsy in patients with male breast carcinoma. *Cancer* 2001;91:319–323.
230. Mullan MH, Kissin MW. Positive sentinel node biopsy in male breast carcinoma. *ANZ J Surg* 2001;71:438–440.
231. Albo D, Ames FC, Hunt KK, et al. Evaluation of lymph node status in male breast cancer patients: a role for sentinel lymph node biopsy. *Breast Cancer Res Treat* 2003;77:9–14.
232. Kitada M, Ozawa K, Sato K, et al. Sentinel lymph node biopsy in patients with male breast carcinoma: report of two cases. *Surg Today* 2011;41:837–840.
233. Gentilini O, Chagas E, Zurrida S, et al. Sentinel lymph node biopsy in male patients with early breast cancer. *Oncologist* 2007;12: 512–515.
234. Adami HO, Hakulinen T, Ewertz M, et al. The survival pattern in male breast cancer. An analysis of 1429 patients from the Nordic countries. *Cancer* 1989;64:1177–1182.
235. Ciatto S, Iossa A, Bonardi R, et al. Male breast carcinoma: review of a multicenter series of 150 cases. Coordinating Center and Writing Committee of FONCAM (National Task Force for Breast Cancer), Italy. *Tumori* 1990;76:555–558.
236. Guinee VF, Olsson H, Moller T, et al. The prognosis of breast cancer in males. A report of 335 cases. *Cancer* 1993;71:154–161.
237. Hultborn R, Friberg S, Hultborn KA, et al. Male breast carcinoma. II. A study of the total material reported to the Swedish Cancer Registry 1958–1967 with respect to treatment, prognostic factors and survival. *Acta Oncol* 1987;26:327–341.
238. Borgen PI, Senie RT, McKinnon WM, et al. Carcinoma of the male breast: analysis of prognosis compared with matched female patients. *Ann Surg Oncol* 1997;4:385–388.
239. Anan K, Mitsuyama S, Nishihara K, et al. Breast cancer in Japanese men: does sex affect prognosis? *Breast Cancer* 2004;11:180–186.
240. Network NCC. NCCN Clinical Practice Guidelines in Oncology (NCCN Guidelines): Breast Cancer 2013 [02/01/2013]. Available from: http://www.nccn.org/professionals/physician_gls/pdf/breast.pdf.
241. Macdonald G, Paltiel C, Olivotto IA, et al. A comparative analysis of radiotherapy use and patient outcome in males and females with breast cancer. *Ann Oncol* 2005;16:1442–1448.
242. Yu E, Suzuki H, Younus J, et al. The impact of post-mastectomy radiation therapy on male breast cancer patients—a case series. *Int J Radiat Oncol Biol Phys* 2012;82:696–700.
243. Hellman L, Fishman J. Oestradiol production rates in men before and after orchiectomy for cancer. *J Endocrinol* 1970;40:113–114.
244. Kraybill WG, Kaufman R, Kinne D. Treatment of advanced male breast cancer. *Cancer* 1981;47:2185–2189.
245. Fentiman IS, Fourquet A, Hortobagyi GN. Male breast cancer. *Lancet* 2006;367:595–604.
246. Patel HZ II, Buzdar AU, Hortobagyi GN. Role of adjuvant chemotherapy in male breast cancer. *Cancer* 1989;64:1583–1585.
247. Donegan WL, Redlich PN, Lang PJ, et al. Carcinoma of the breast in males: a multiinstitutional survey. *Cancer* 1998;83:498–509.
248. Walshe JM, Berman AW, Vatas U, et al. A prospective study of adjuvant CMF in males with node positive breast cancer: 20-year follow-up. *Breast Cancer Res Treat* 2007;103:177–183.

CHAPTER 37

Breast Tumors in Children

EDI BROGI

Mass-forming breast lesions in children and adolescents are rare, and the majority are benign. The newborn breast may swell shortly after birth and during lactation because of hormones passing from the mother to the baby through the breast milk. This alteration is usually bilateral and transient. Persistent bilateral breast enlargement in a child typically indicates a hormonal imbalance due to genetic alteration or to a hormone-producing neoplasm and should be investigated accordingly.

Pettinato et al.[1] evaluated 113 breast lesions that presented as diffuse breast enlargement or a mass-forming lesion in children and adolescents 20 years old or younger at three hospitals in Minnesota and Alabama. Congenital and developmental abnormalities were found in 10 (9%) cases and consisted mainly of accessory breast tissue and supernumerary nipple in patients aged 10 to 15 years. A case of congenital hypertrophy was documented in a newborn. Inflammatory conditions, such as acute and chronic mastitis and fat necrosis, constituted 14% of all cases and also tended to occur in children aged 10 to 15 years. Nonneoplastic tumor-like lesions, including juvenile hypertrophy (20 cases) and juvenile papillomatosis (JP) (5 cases), comprised 22% of all cases. The remaining 40% of cases were primary mammary neoplasms, such as juvenile fibroadenoma (FA) (18 cases) and phyllodes tumors (2 cases), nipple duct adenoma (florid papillomatosis of the nipple) (2 cases), and lesions that are not exclusive of the breast parenchyma, including lipomas, vascular tumors (6 cases), metastatic extramammary malignant neoplasms (8 cases, all in teenage girls), rhabdomyosarcoma, and malignant lymphoma.

Most breast masses in children and adolescents develop around the time of puberty, but not all of them require immediate surgical intervention. During a 22-year period, 684 females aged 14 to 20 years were referred for evaluation of a breast mass at the University Hospital in Athens, Greece.[2] Most patients (442/684; 64.6%) were managed by observation alone, and only about a third (242/684; 35.4%) underwent surgical excision. The histologic findings were benign in 97.5% of cases, including FA in 72.9%, fibrocystic changes in 24.6%, and benign cysts in 2.5%. Only six (2.5%) cases were malignant.

The most frequent breast mass lesions in female adolescents are FA and juvenile macromastia.[2–7] A series from Nigeria[7] documents a similar prevalence of breast lesions in African female adolescents. Gynecomastia is the most common breast mass in boys under 20 years and typically develops during puberty.

Imaging

Ecographic examination is the preferred technique for evaluation of a mass in the breast of a child or adolescent, whereas mammography has limited to no value in these age groups. A search of the ecographic studies of breast masses in patients younger than 19 years treated between 2001 and 2009 at a pediatric hospital yielded a total of 332 exams.[8] Solid masses were identified in 91 (27.4%) girls. A tissue diagnosis was available for 49 (14.7%) lesions: 91% were FA, and the rest included one case each of hamartoma, non-Hodgkin lymphoma (NLH), tubular adenoma, pseudoangiomatous stromal hyperplasia (PASH), and lactation changes.

Risk of Subsequent Carcinoma

With the exception of JP, described later in this chapter, most benign mass-forming lesions occurring in the breast in the first two decades of life are not associated with an increased risk of developing subsequent breast carcinoma. Genetic testing for known germline mutations associated with high risk of breast carcinoma usually is not pursued in children or adolescents and should be considered only after the patient reaches the age of consent. At present, no other parameters are available that could help identify young individuals at high risk of developing breast carcinoma. A study by Wu et al.[9] found lower global methylation levels in white blood cells of girls aged between 6 and 17 years with a strong family history of breast carcinoma than in those without, suggesting that the effect of environmental factors resulting in epigenetic alterations of gene expression may have an impact quite early in life.

JUVENILE PAPILLOMATOSIS

Clinical Presentation

Age and Gender

The localized benign proliferative lesion known as JP usually occurs in women younger than 30 years. At the time of diagnosis, two-thirds of the patients are younger than 25 (Fig. 37.1). JP is uncommon prior to puberty and after the age of 40.[10,11] Rare cases of JP in infants with neurofibromatosis are not fully convincing.[12–14] On the basis of the

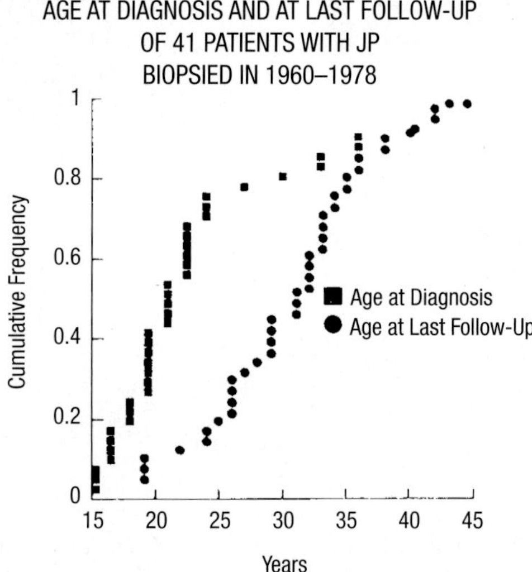

FIG. 37.1. *Juvenile papillomatosis, age distribution.* In this series of patients with relatively long-term follow-up, the mean and median ages at diagnosis were, respectively, 19 and 21 years. (Reproduced from Rosen PP, Kimmel M. Juvenile papillomatosis of the breast: a follow-up study of 41 patients having biopsies before 1979. *Am J Clin Pathol* 1990;93:599–603.)

illustrations provided, the lesion described by Tan et al.[12] appears to have been papillary duct hyperplasia rather than JP. Although it had "extensive microcysts" grossly, this feature is not evident in the published histologic picture. The cystic expansion of ducts that can occur in juvenile papillary duct hyperplasia lacks apocrine metaplasia and other features that are conspicuous in JP. Pacilli et al.[13] described a cystic mass "containing whitish milky fluid attached to the under-surface of the nipple" in a 13-month-old infant. The lesion illustrated appears to be stasis of secretion in dilated ducts, possibly a galactocele, in a fibrotic nodule. A report by Rice[14] describes two male infants with lesions purported to be JP. However, the single histologic picture provided shows only cystic duct ectasia without the characteristic proliferative changes of JP, leaving the diagnosis of JP in doubt.

No clinical data on the prevalence of JP are available. However, JP was found in 1 of 519 forensic autopsies of females 14 years or older performed over a 5-year interval by a state medical examiner.[15] Because JP was not formally characterized before 1980, it was not recognized as a specific lesion in earlier reports, which, in retrospect, described this condition.[16] Only few series of JP have been reported, and case reports are sporadic. Rare instances of JP have been described in boys,[17,18] including a 17-year-old boy who presented with 2- to 3-month-long history of intermittent nipple discharge,[18] but images of the histologic findings were not provided.

Presenting Symptoms

The typical clinical finding is a solitary, firm, discrete unilateral tumor that clinically mimics a FA. Very rarely the presenting symptoms of JP include pain[11] and/or nipple discharge, which rarely can be bloody.[11,18] Bilateral JP may be synchronous or metachronous. Very rare instances of multifocal tumors in one breast have been reported. A separate coexisting FA is not unusual.

It is not unusual for patients with JP to have had one or more biopsies of the ipsilateral or contralateral breast prior to the diagnosis of JP. Concurrent contralateral biopsies and subsequent biopsies of either breast have also been reported.[19] Most prior biopsies have been for FA or benign proliferative lesions other than JP. Similar findings have been reported in most concurrent contralateral biopsies, but rare patients have had carcinoma in the opposite breast.

Subsequent biopsies of one or both breasts are also not unusual. About one-third of subsequent ipsilateral biopsies revealed JP. Other lesions encountered subsequently included benign proliferative changes without the typical configuration of JP, such as FA, scar, and, rarely, carcinoma.

Imaging

Few descriptions of the mammographic findings in JP are available because mammography is not usually performed preoperatively in these young women. The mammograms reveal a localized area of increased density with a border that is generally not as well defined as that of a FA[11,20] (Fig. 37.2). The sonographic appearance of JP is that of an ill-defined or discrete inhomogeneous, hypoechoic mass with multiple cysts.[20–22] The magnetic resonance imaging (MRI) findings of JP in female patients 29, 24, and 13 years of age[23,24] have been reported. The lesions were mass forming with a complex solid and cystic pattern, multiple small cysts on T2-weighted images and continuous enhancement on kinetic evaluation.

Family History of Breast Carcinoma

At the time of diagnosis, patients with JP report a frequency of positive family history for breast carcinoma that is similar to that of patients who have mammary carcinoma.[25,26] With

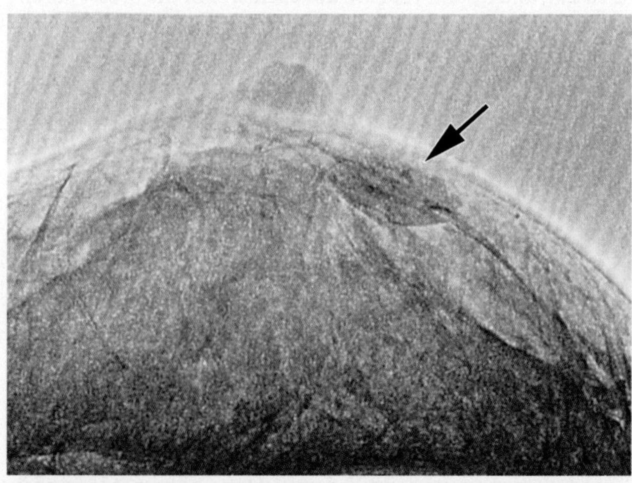

FIG. 37.2. *Juvenile papillomatosis, mammography.* The lesion forms the oval mass indicated by an *arrow* in this xeromammogram.

further follow-up, the frequency of positive family history exceeds 50%.[19] Because of the youth of JP patients, the high frequency of breast carcinoma in these families is particularly remarkable, since it may be assumed that female relatives of patients with JP tend to be younger than comparable relatives of breast carcinoma patients.

About 10% to 15% of patients with JP also have breast carcinoma.[11,19,26] Women with JP and coexistent carcinoma are usually in the upper quartile of the age distribution of JP. Virtually all of these women have had a positive family history for breast carcinoma, usually affecting their mother or a maternal aunt.[19,26] Breast carcinoma and other benign breast tumors, including JP, have only rarely been seen in the sisters of JP patients. The female relatives of patients with JP most likely to be affected by breast carcinoma are their mothers and maternal aunts. JP is not associated with an increased frequency of breast carcinoma in paternal female relatives, and there is no association with any type of nonmammary neoplasm. Given the rarity of JP in boys, it is unclear whether this lesion in males carries the same high association with familial breast carcinoma.

Genetic Alterations

The genetic alterations associated with JP have not been evaluated. In particular, no study has assessed *BRCA1* and *BRCA2* germline mutations in patients with JP or their relatives.

Gross Pathology

The excised tumor is a firm discrete mass that appears to be distinct from the surrounding breast on the cut surface but lacks the sharply circumscribed border typical of a FA. The lesions measure 1 to 8 cm in diameter and average 4 cm (Fig. 37.3). The most prominent gross feature is multiple cysts ranging from 1 mm to 2 cm in size. The larger cysts tend to be located in the center of the lesion. The intervening tissue often has white or yellow flecks that resemble comedonecrosis (Fig. 37.4).

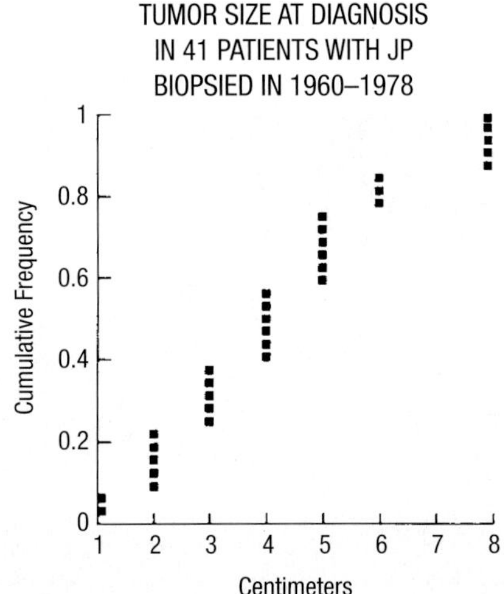

FIG. 37.3. ***Juvenile papillomatosis, tumor size.*** The median size was 4 cm (range, 1 to 8 cm). (Reproduced from Rosen PP, Kimmel M. Juvenile papillomatosis of the breast: a follow-up study of 41 patients having biopsies before 1979. *Am J Clin Pathol* 1990;93:599–603.)

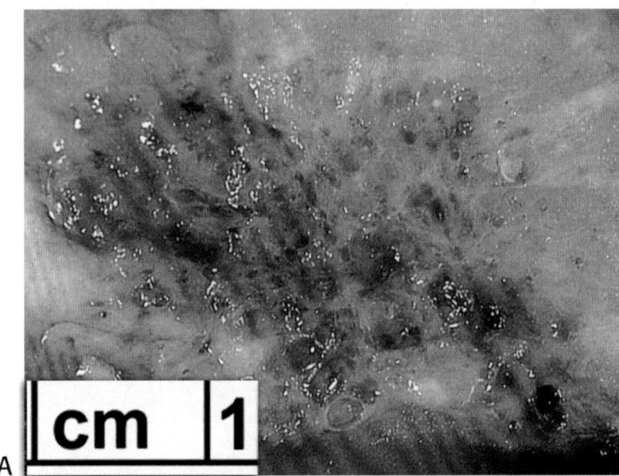

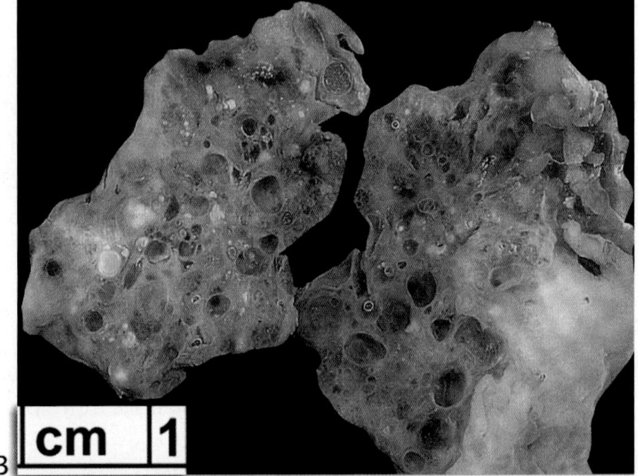

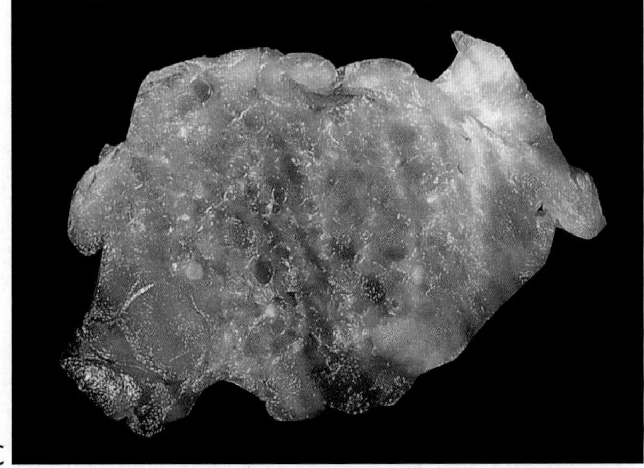

FIG. 37.4. ***Juvenile papillomatosis, gross appearance.*** **A–C:** Three different specimens that show localized lesions with multiple small cysts and white or yellow flecks.

Microscopic Pathology

Histologic examination reveals a spectrum of benign proliferative changes that are present in varying proportions in individual cases. The alterations tend to be localized. Cysts and duct hyperplasia are constant features (Figs. 37.5 to 37.7). The epithelium of cysts and duct hyperplasia frequently exhibits apocrine metaplasia (Fig. 37.8), which may be flat or papillary. Stasis of secretion in cysts and ducts manifested by collections of lipid-laden histiocytes is seen in most specimens (Fig. 37.9). These reactive alterations correspond to the yellow and white flecks observed grossly. Sclerosing adenosis (SA), lobular hyperplasia, and fibroadenomatoid hyperplasia are variably present.

In most cases, the ductal proliferative changes consist of usual hyperplasia. Sometimes ductal hyperplasia is accompanied by sclerosis that produces a radial scar pattern. Atypical changes in the ductal hyperplasia include cribriform or micropapillary growth patterns and intraductal necrosis (Fig. 37.10). In one series, there was significant atypia in 40% and intraductal necrosis in 15% of JP cases.[19] The stroma admixed with the epithelial alterations of JP tends to be dense and fibrous with a resulting "Swiss cheese" appearance on gross examination.

Differential Diagnosis

The diagnosis of JP should not be used for lesions that consist only of cysts, cystic papillomas, or papillomas. For example, illustrations of the lesion reported as "juvenile papillomatosis" by Talisman et al.[27] show cysts and intracystic papillomas rather than the typical features of JP. Specimens showing only a solitary papilloma, multiple dispersed papillomas, and sclerosing papillomas with a radial scar configuration

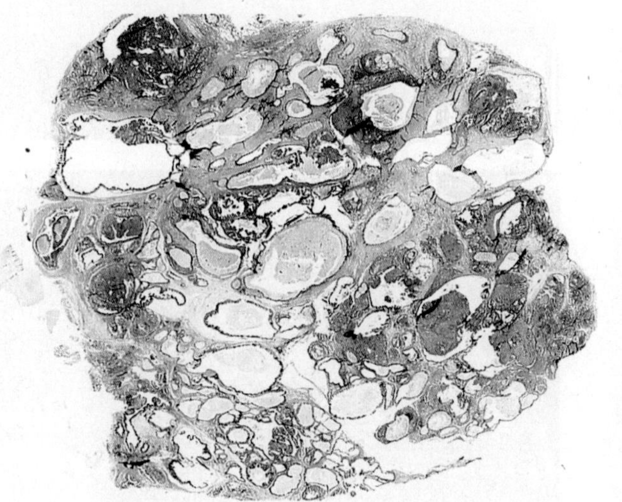
A

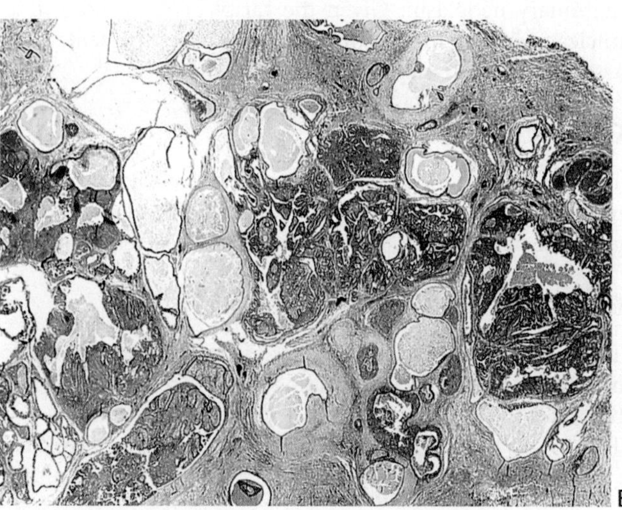
B

FIG. 37.5. ***Juvenile papillomatosis.*** **A,B:** Whole-mount photographs of histologic sections of two lesions. Papillary duct hyperplasia is more pronounced in **(B)**.

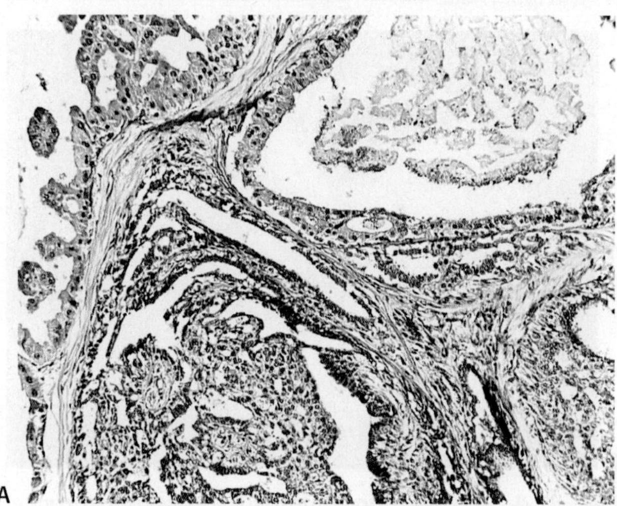
A

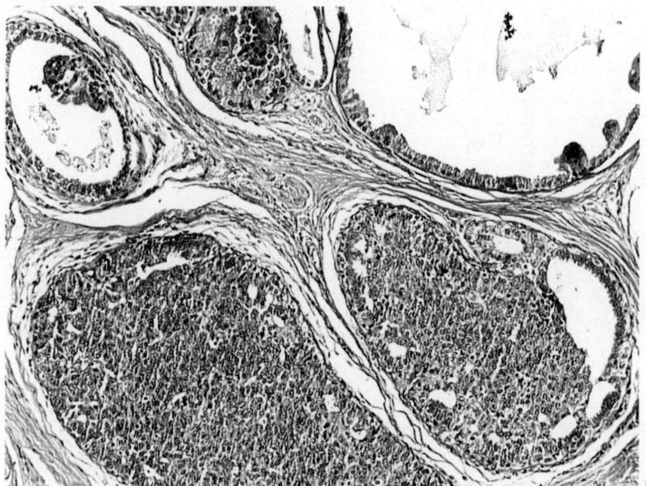
B

FIG. 37.6. ***Juvenile papillomatosis, cysts and duct hyperplasia.*** **A,B:** Two microscopic fields showing patterns of duct hyperplasia characteristic of JP.

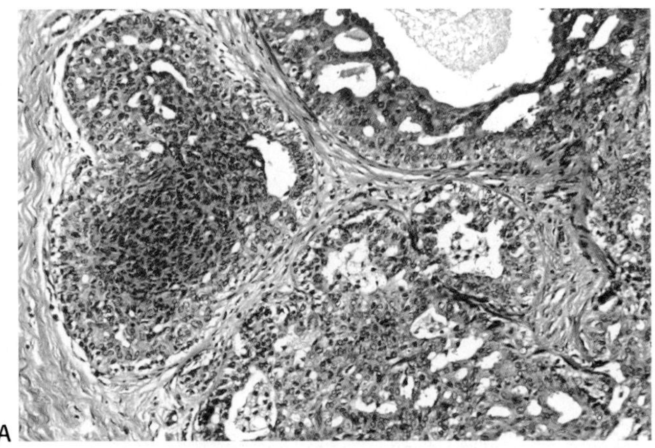

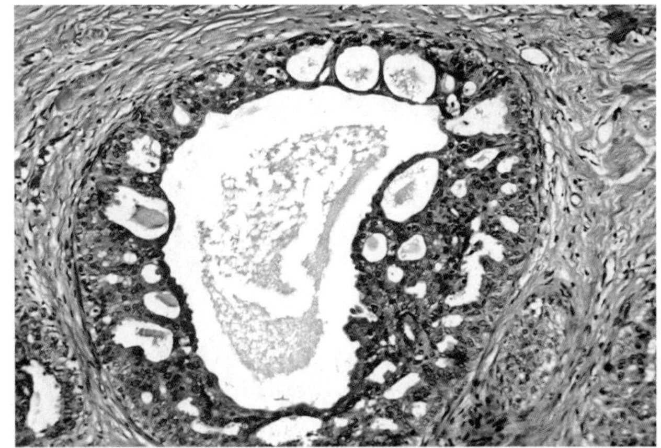

FIG. 37.7. ***Juvenile papillomatosis, duct hyperplasia.*** **A,B:** Solid and cribriform duct hyperplasia with apocrine metaplasia. This appearance is frequently found in JP.

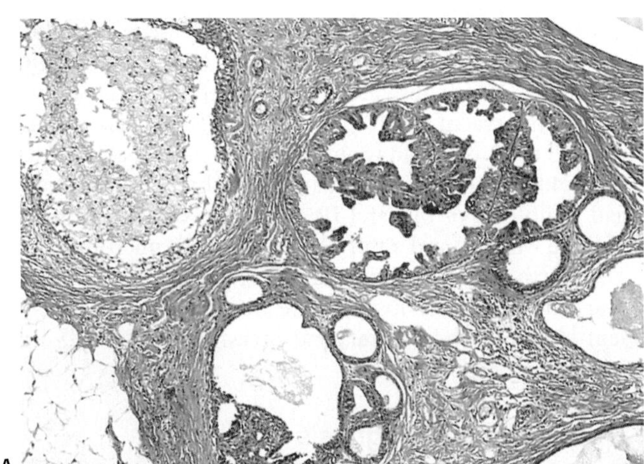

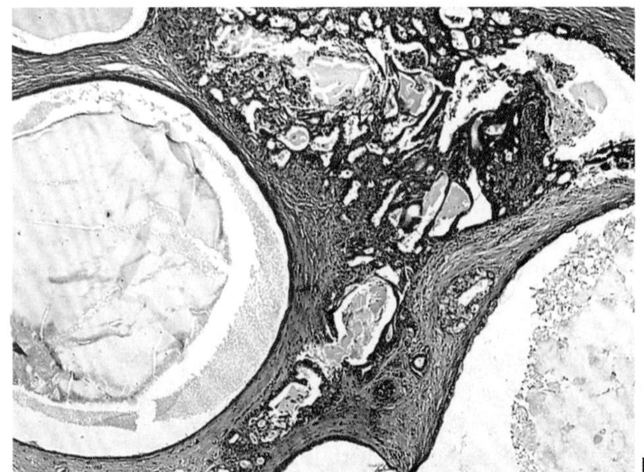

FIG. 37.8. ***Juvenile papillomatosis, apocrine metaplasia.*** **A:** Papillary apocrine metaplasia. **B:** Apocrine metaplasia of cyst epithelium and in papillary duct hyperplasia.

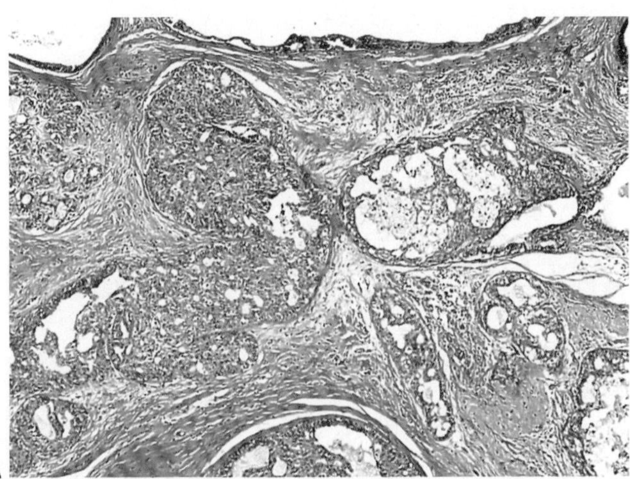

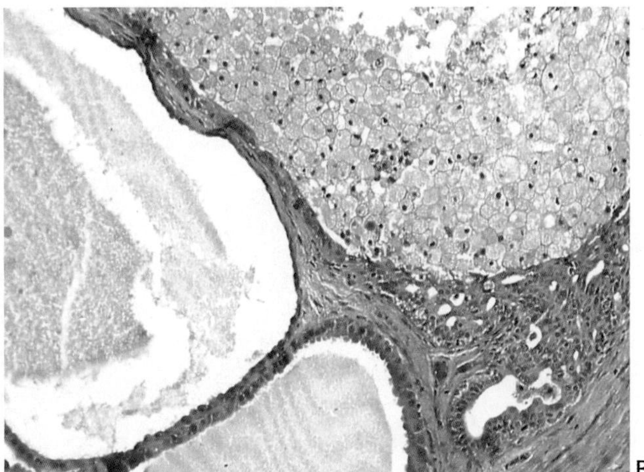

FIG. 37.9. ***Juvenile papillomatosis, histiocytes.*** **A:** Histiocytes in a focus of duct hyperplasia. **B:** One of three cysts lined by apocrine epithelium is filled with lipid histiocytes. Cysts like this are seen grossly as yellow flecks.

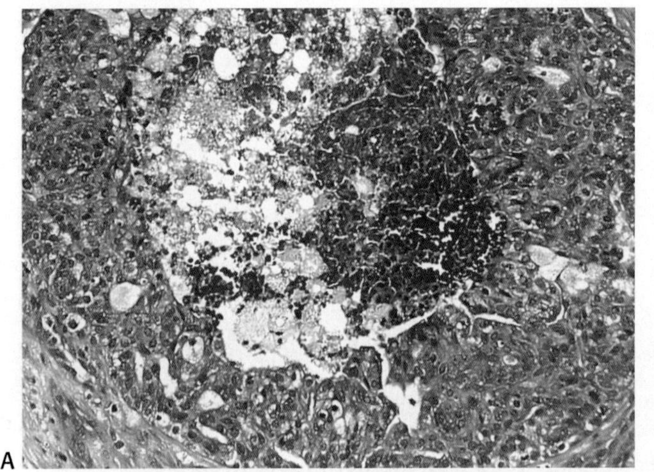

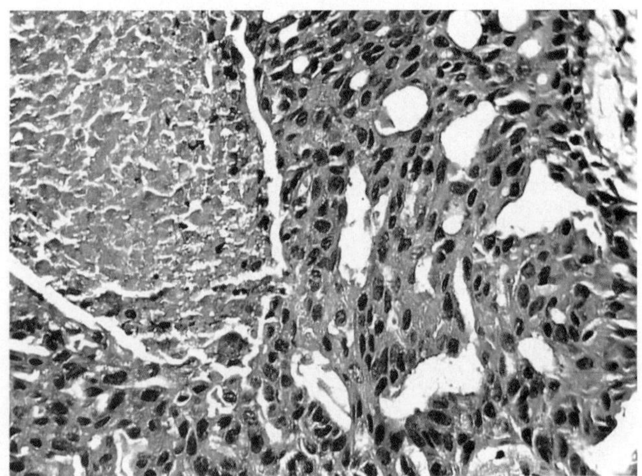

FIG. 37.10. ***Juvenile papillomatosis, epithelial necrosis.*** **A:** Necrosis, hemorrhage, and histiocytes in duct hyperplasia. **B:** Comedo-type necrosis in a focus of sclerosing papillary hyperplasia.

included in the group of lesions termed "papillary duct hyperplasia" are not part of the spectrum of JP.[28–31]

Breast Carcinomas Associated with JP

The types of breast carcinoma associated with JP include ductal carcinoma *in situ* (DCIS), lobular carcinoma *in situ* (LCIS), infiltrating duct carcinoma, infiltrating lobular carcinoma, and secretory (juvenile) carcinoma. Most patients have had carcinoma and JP diagnosed concurrently[19,26] (Figs. 37.11 and 37.12), typically at an age older than adolescence. With few exceptions, the carcinoma occurred within JP and appeared to arise from it. One exceptional patient had JP in one breast and concurrent contralateral secretory carcinoma not associated with JP.

Risk of Subsequent Breast Carcinoma

The risk of subsequent carcinoma in patients who had JP excised previously has been evaluated in one series.[19] A review of 41 patients with at least 10 years of follow-up after the diagnosis of JP (median 14 years) found that 4 patients (10%) subsequently developed breast carcinoma after an interval of 5 to 15 years[19] (Fig. 37.13). These patients were 25 to 42 years old when JP was diagnosed, and thus all were older than the mean age for JP. Three of the patients had multifocal or bilateral JP. DCIS was diagnosed in two of these women, and a third had DCIS with microinvasion. The fourth patient had unilateral JP at the age of 29. Thirteen years later, recurrent ipsilateral JP was found, and a concurrent biopsy of the contralateral breast revealed DCIS that was not associated with JP.

Treatment and Prognosis

JP is rarely considered as the preoperative diagnosis. In most instances, the clinical findings suggest a FA. Consequently, excisional biopsy is often performed with little margin. Incomplete excision probably predisposes to local recurrence, but this may occur even when the margins appear

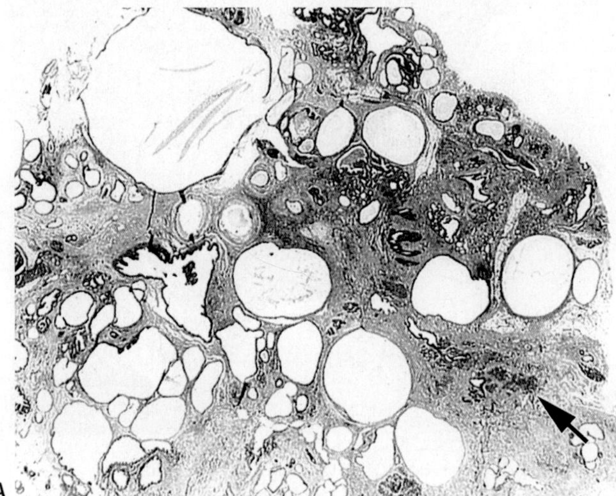

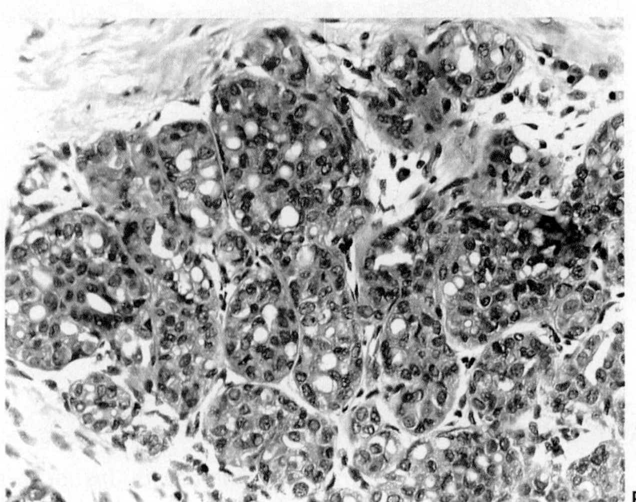

FIG. 37.11. ***Juvenile papillomatosis with lobular carcinoma in situ.*** **A:** The *arrow* indicates a focus of LCIS in this histologic section of JP. **B:** LCIS shown in **(A)**.

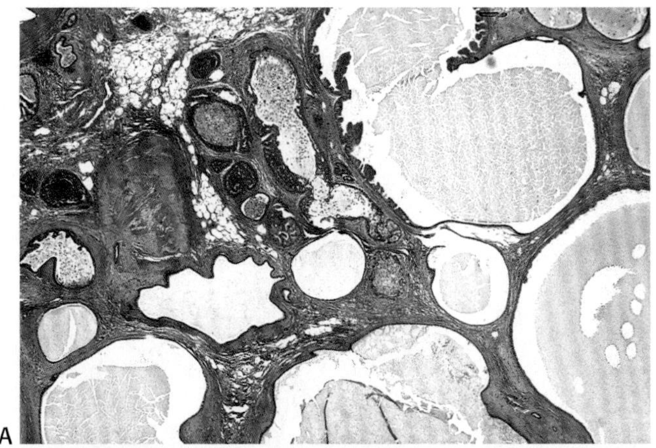

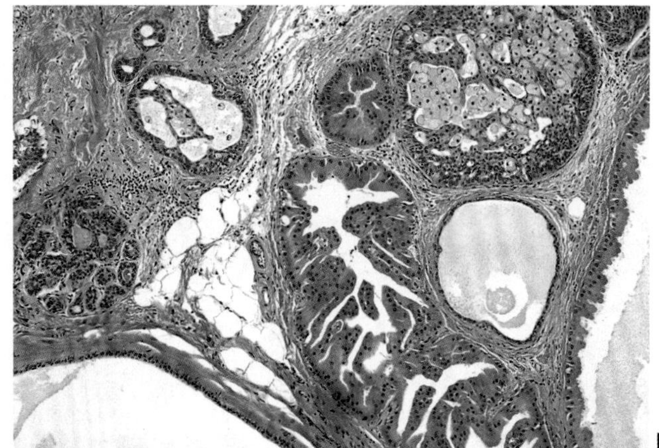

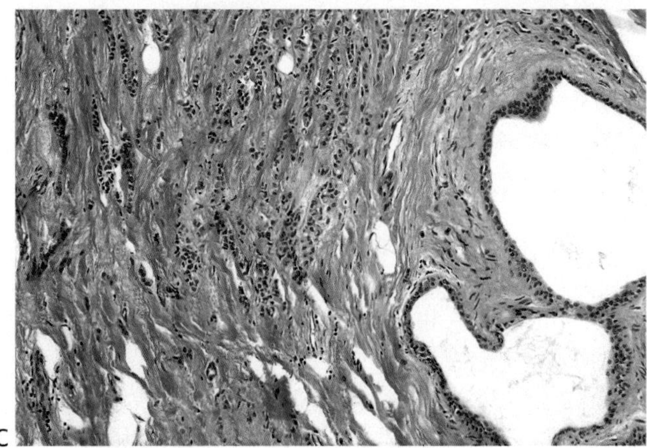

FIG. 37.12. ***Invasive lobular carcinoma in juvenile papillomatosis.*** The specimen is from a 46-year-old woman. **A,B:** Cysts, duct hyperplasia, and apocrine metaplasia in JP. **C:** Invasive lobular carcinoma adjacent to cysts in the tumor shown in **(A)** and **(B)**.

to be adequate histologically. It is the opinion of the Senior Editor that reexcision of the biopsy site would be prudent if the lesion has not been completely excised, and the reexcision will not cause a significant cosmetic defect. Reexcision is also recommended for incompletely excised JP with atypical hyperplasia, or if the lesion is a recurrence of JP and the margin remains involved.

Unless carcinoma is found in the tumor, no treatment is necessary after complete excisional biopsy. Follow-up examinations should be scheduled annually or more frequently for patients who have multifocal, bilateral, or recurrent JP, and if there are other risk factors such as a positive family history for breast carcinoma. Mammography should be employed judiciously during follow-up, especially for patients younger than 35 years of age, to minimize radiation exposure and because its sensitivity is limited in this age group. Ultrasonography is the preferred method for evaluation of breast masses in this young age group. MRI surveillance is also a possible consideration, but no data are available. Female relatives of JP patients, especially on the maternal side, should also be advised to have regular breast surveillance. No data are currently available regarding the prevalence of *BRCA* mutations in patients with JP or their relatives.

Presently, the frequency of carcinoma in patients with JP does not warrant considering this to be a precancerous condition. Care should be taken *not* to exaggerate the near-term risk of developing breast carcinoma in patients with JP. The importance of risk factors such as positive family history of breast carcinoma and pathologic atypia remains to be determined.

PAPILLOMA AND PAPILLARY DUCT HYPERPLASIA IN CHILDREN AND YOUNG WOMEN

Clinical Presentation

Age and Gender

Papillary duct hyperplasia and papillomas are infrequent breast lesions in patients younger than 30 years.[32] Other than exceptional male cases,[33] the patients have been female with a median age of 17 years.[31] The majority (70%) were 15 to 25 years of age, but a sizable group (24%) has been younger, including rare neonatal patients.

Symptoms

The most frequent presenting symptom is a mass, but some authors report nipple discharge that may be bloody or clear, as a presenting sign.[34,35] There is no predilection for either breast. Periareolar or subareolar lesions are most common.

Bloody nipple discharge is a rare phenomenon in infants and children under 4 years and is not always associated with a mass lesion. In these cases, mastitis should be ruled out. Harmsen et al.[36] reported instances of bloody nipple

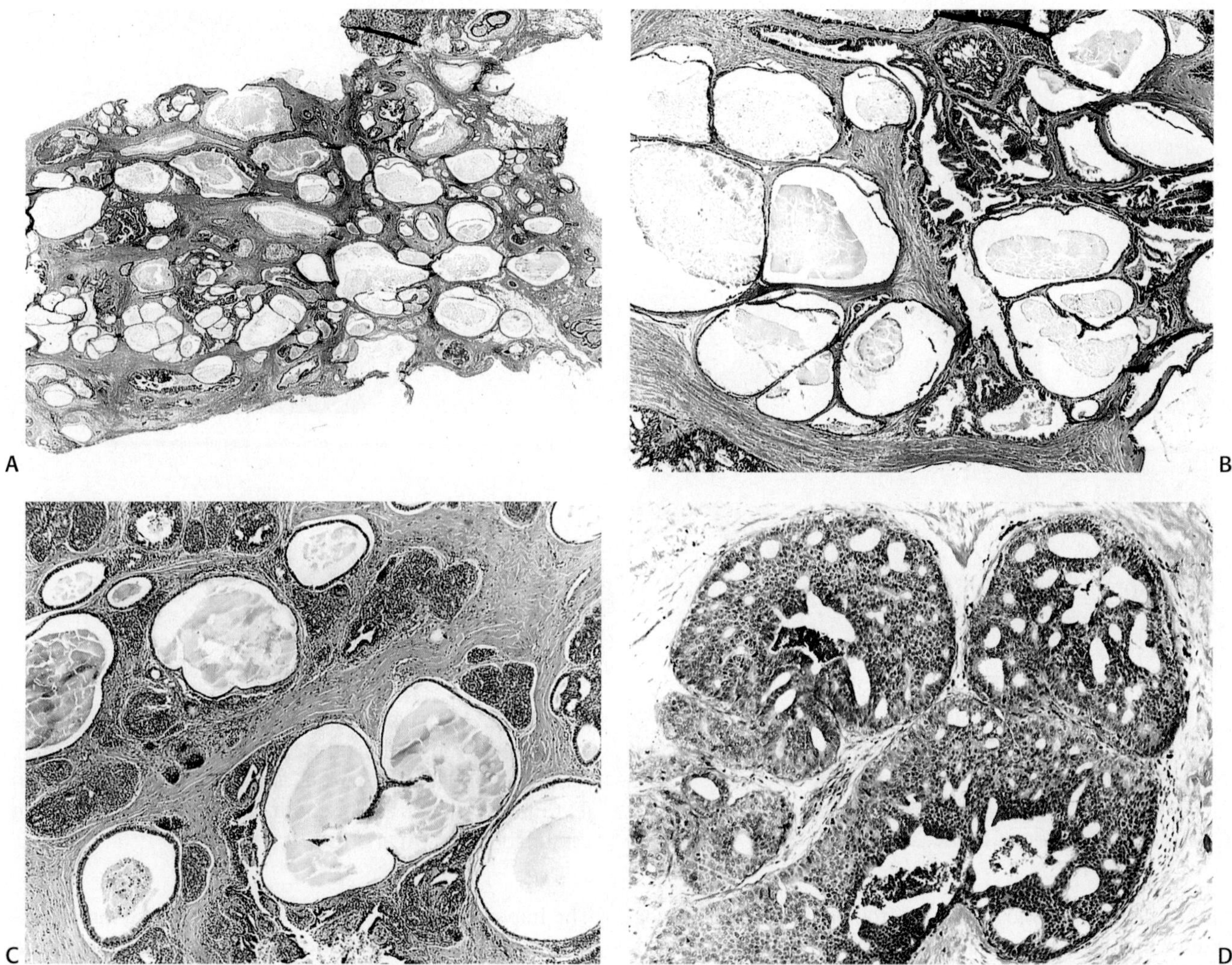

FIG. 37.13. ***Juvenile papillomatosis with subsequent carcinoma.*** **A:** JP of the right breast at age 20. **B:** JP of the left breast at age 24. **C:** Recurrent JP of the left breast at age 32. **D:** DCIS in the left breast in the recurrent JP. (**A,B,D:** From Rosen PP, Holmes G, Lesser ML, et al. Juvenile papillomatosis and breast carcinoma. *Cancer* 1985;55:1345–1352.)

discharge in two healthy infants, an 8-month-old female infant and a 9-month-old male infant, with no associated breast mass. The discharge resolved spontaneously in a few months, and reportedly had benign follow-up, albeit of short length. In a review of the literature published between 1956 and 2010 on this topic, the same authors[36] identified a total of 38 cases of bloody nipple discharge involving male and female infants and young children; however, the real incidence is likely to be higher. Except for four cases, all patients were 4 years old or younger. All reported cases were benign, and usually they were not associated with a mass lesion.

Imaging

Very few patients with papillary breast lesions have had mammography, and the results were reportedly nonspecific.[31] Microcalcifications have been found in a few cases. Sonographic examination is the preferred method of preoperative evaluation, and it usually shows a mass contained in an anechoic cystic cavity. These patients have a moderate frequency (13%) of breast carcinoma among family members, most often affecting maternal female relatives.

Gross Pathology

Lesions measuring up to 5 cm have been reported. The tumors have been well circumscribed or ill defined. Numerous 1- to 3-mm cysts that contain papillary excrescences may be present in papillomatosis. An 11-cm, complex, partly cystic papillary tumor from a 3-year-old girl has been recorded (Fig. 37.14).

Microscopic Pathology

The morphology of papillomas and papillary hyperplasia without atypia occurring in children and adolescents resembles that of equivalent lesions in adults (see Chapters 5 and 6). Three microscopic growth patterns have been described.

Sclerosing papillary duct hyperplasia is the most common type and is found in nearly 50% of cases (Figs. 37.15

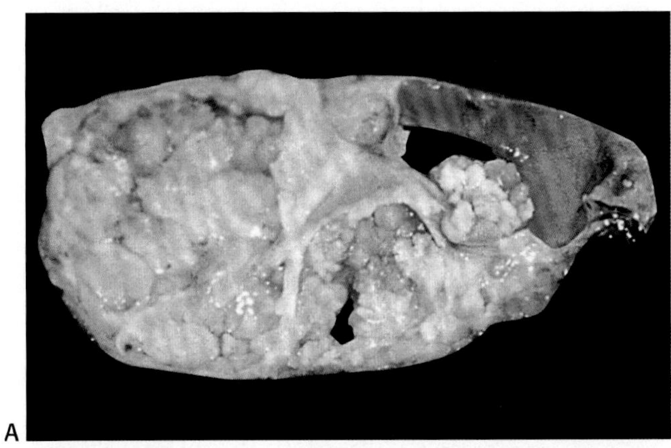

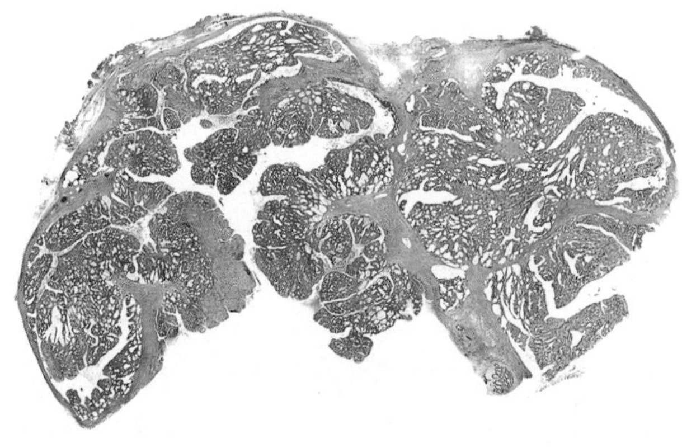

FIG. 37.14. ***Papilloma.*** **A,B:** An 11-cm tumor from a 3-year-old girl.

and 37.16). It consists of a papilloma that is distorted and disrupted by a desmoplastic proliferation of myoepithelial and stromal cells, resulting in a radial scar-like pattern of sclerosis. Small clusters of epithelial cells and lobules incorporated into the stromal proliferation may raise the differential diagnosis of invasive carcinoma. Use of a panel of myoepithelial markers (including calponin and p63) is helpful in the more challenging cases.

Papillomas limited to a single focus, with little or no sclerosis, comprise about one-third of the lesions. The papillomas consist of one or more contiguous dilated ducts that contain papillary fronds of epithelial cells in single or multiple layers, supported by fibrovascular stroma (Figs. 37.17 and 37.18). Infrequent mitoses may be encountered in the epithelium. Myoepithelial cell hyperplasia is variably present (Fig. 37.19).

Papillomatosis is a term used to describe papillary hyperplasia of the usual type involving multiple ducts. It occurs in about 25% of cases. Papillary fronds supported by fibrovascular stroma are seen in some foci, but the hyperplasia often has a solid or micropapillary pattern devoid of stroma (Fig. 37.20). In micropapillary areas, the nuclei of hyperplastic epithelial cells tend to become smaller and more hyperchromatic at the tips of individual papillae with characteristic "maturation" (see Chapter 6 for the differential diagnosis of atypical and nonatypical micropapillary ductal hyperplasia). Some lesions, however, occasionally exhibit cytologic atypia (Fig. 37.21) that may be severe. The clinical significance of this finding remains unclear at present. Myoepithelial cell hyperplasia may also be present.

Prominent cyst formation, extensive apocrine metaplasia, stasis, mastitis, and other benign proliferative changes that characterize JP are largely absent from these forms of papillary duct hyperplasia.[37]

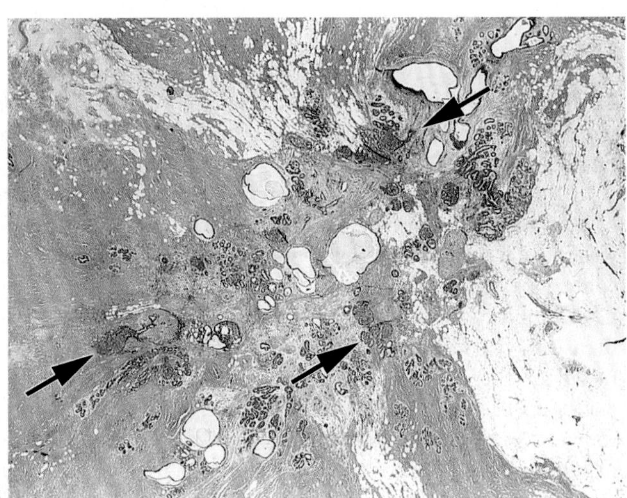

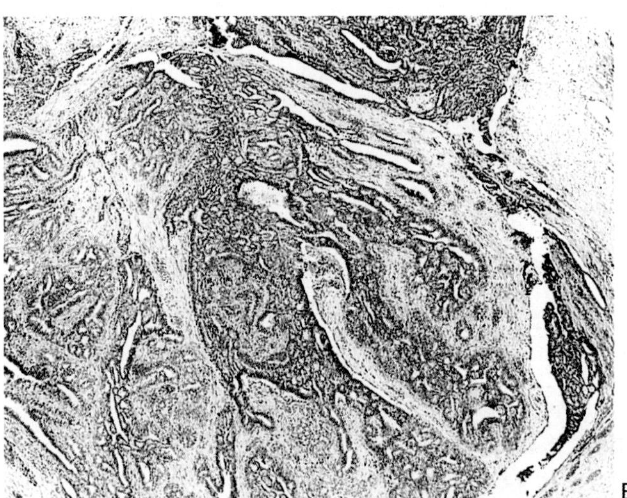

FIG. 37.15. ***Papillary duct hyperplasia, sclerosing type.*** **A,B:** The patient was a 15-year-old girl with a palpable tumor. **A:** The lesion has a radial scar configuration. Some papillary foci are indicated by *arrows*. **B:** Part of a sclerosing papilloma in the lesion is shown in **(B)**. **C,D:** This lesion was excised from a 16-year-old girl. Attenuated epithelium in the sclerotic stroma can be mistaken for invasive carcinoma when the plane of section results in isolated groups of epithelial cells in the stroma.

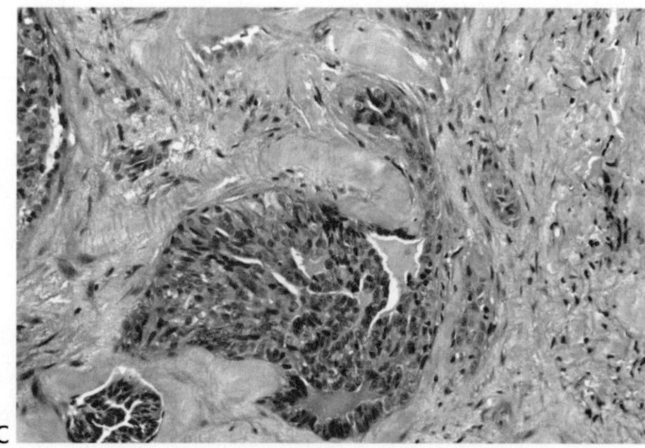

C D

FIG. 37.15. *(Continued)*

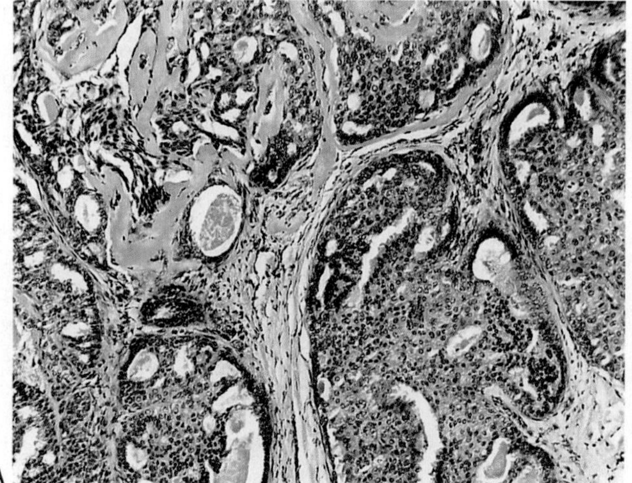

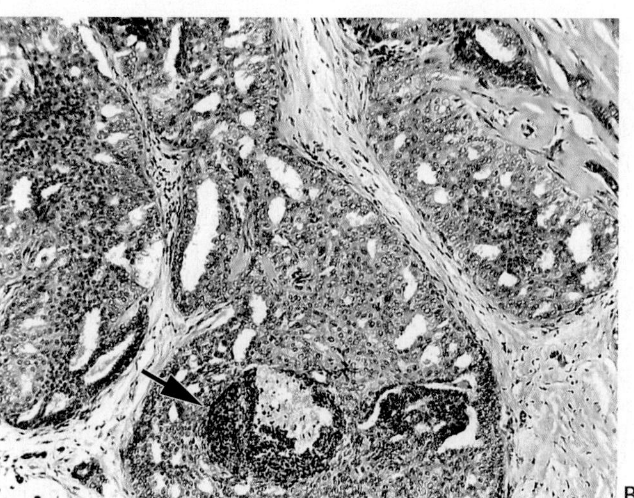

FIG. 37.16. ***Papillary duct hyperplasia, sclerosing type.*** The lesion was a palpable tumor in a 14-year-old girl. **A:** Sclerosing papilloma. **B:** Focal necrosis in the hyperplastic epithelium (*arrow*).

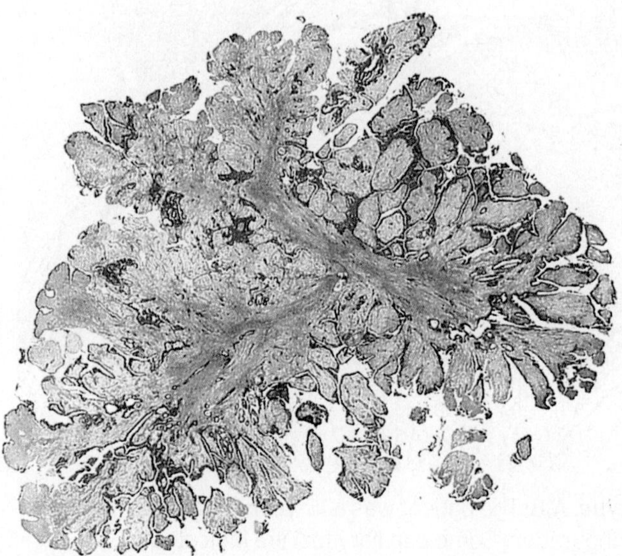

FIG. 37.17. ***Papilloma.*** A papilloma removed from the subareolar tissue of a 14-year-old girl who had bloody nipple discharge.

Treatment and Prognosis

Most patients with a papilloma or papillomatosis can be managed by excisional biopsy. Larger lesions may require quadrantectomy.

In one series, breast recurrences were detected in 16% of patients after a median interval of 3 years.[38] Recurrence was more frequent in patients with sclerosing papilloma and solitary papilloma than in those with papillomatosis.

A single patient developed invasive carcinoma in one breast 27 years after bilateral papillomatosis had been diagnosed at the age of 11.[39] However, follow-up rarely has exceeded 10 years. Information presently available supports the view that these patterns of papillary duct hyperplasia do not predispose children and young women to develop breast carcinoma at an early age. This conclusion is consistent with the observation that breast carcinoma detected in women 35 years of age or younger has not been associated with a history of antecedent papillary proliferative breast lesions.[40] Extended follow-up, perhaps with genetic studies, will be necessary to fully assess the precancerous potential of these proliferative conditions.

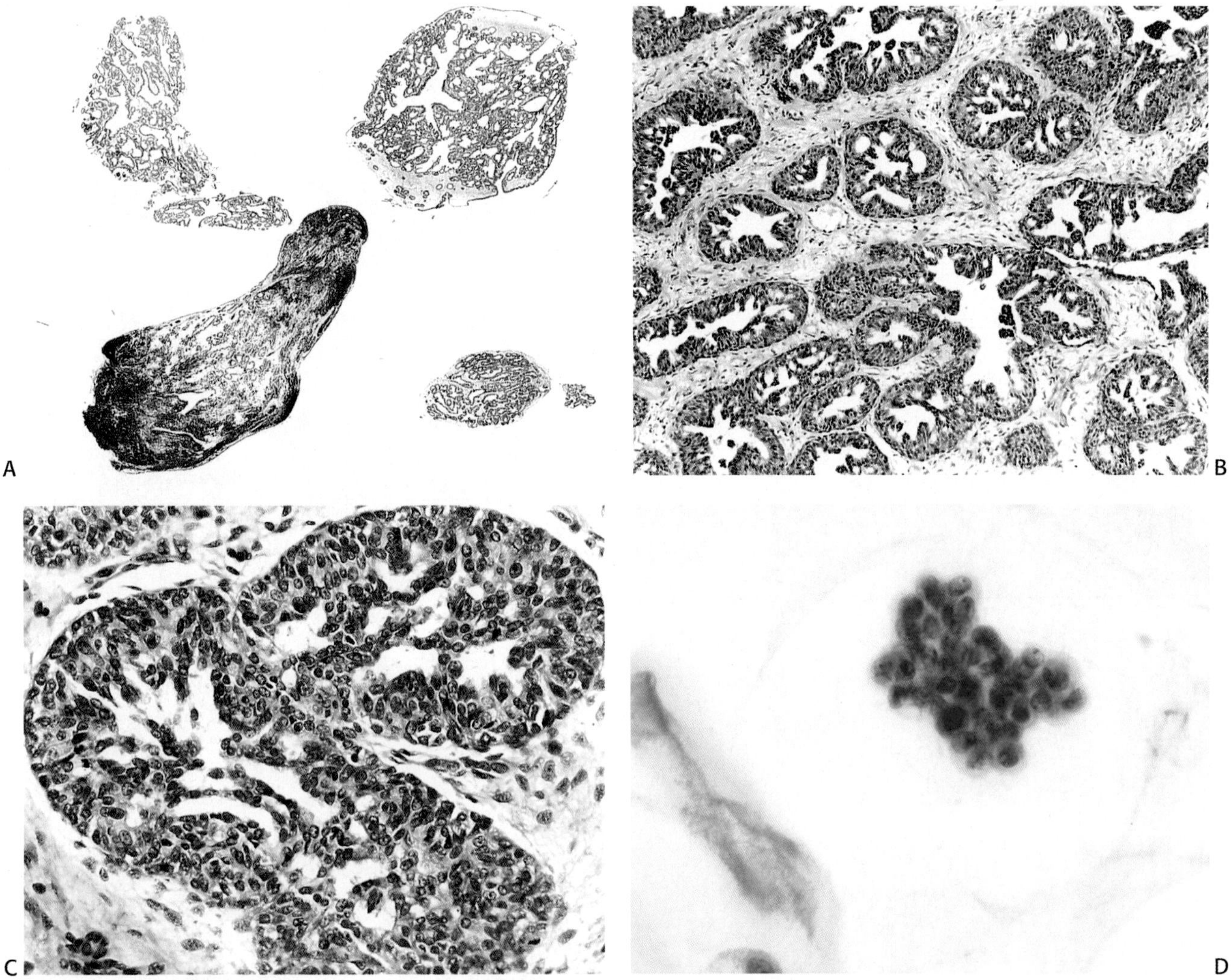

FIG. 37.18. ***Papilloma.*** The patient was a 13-year-old girl with a subareolar tumor. **A:** Multiple fragments of the papilloma in one histologic section. The darkened tissue in the *lower left* is hemorrhagic as a result of infarction. **B:** Magnified view of the papilloma demonstrating diffuse, epithelial hyperplasia. **C:** Micropapillary hyperplasia. **D:** The image shows a cytology specimen made from nipple discharge obtained from an 11-year-old girl whose biopsy specimen was similar to the one shown in (**A–C**).

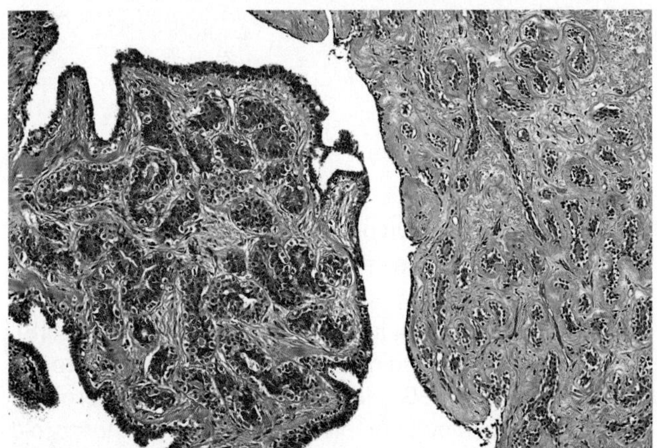

FIG. 37.19. ***Papilloma, myoepithelial hyperplasia.*** Myoepithelial hyperplasia is present around glands in proliferative (*left*) and sclerotic (*right*) portions of this papilloma from a 14-year-old girl.

JUVENILE ATYPICAL DUCT HYPERPLASIA

Juvenile atypical duct hyperplasia (juvenile ADH) is a microscopic ductal proliferative lesion found in young women that was first described in 1992.[41] The report included nine female patients aged 18 to 26 years, with a mean age of 21 years at diagnosis. Juvenile ADH was found in biopsies of breast "thickening" (four cases) or in specimens from patients who underwent reduction mammoplasty for "mammary hypertrophy" (five cases). Three (33%) of the patients reported a family history of breast carcinoma.

No specific gross features are indicative of juvenile ADH. The lesion usually presents as an incidental microscopic finding, and no discrete lesion is produced by the ductal proliferation. The specimens are generally described as fibrous breast tissue with variable amounts of fat.

Histologic examination reveals isolated ducts involved by ductal epithelial hyperplasia with micropapillary or

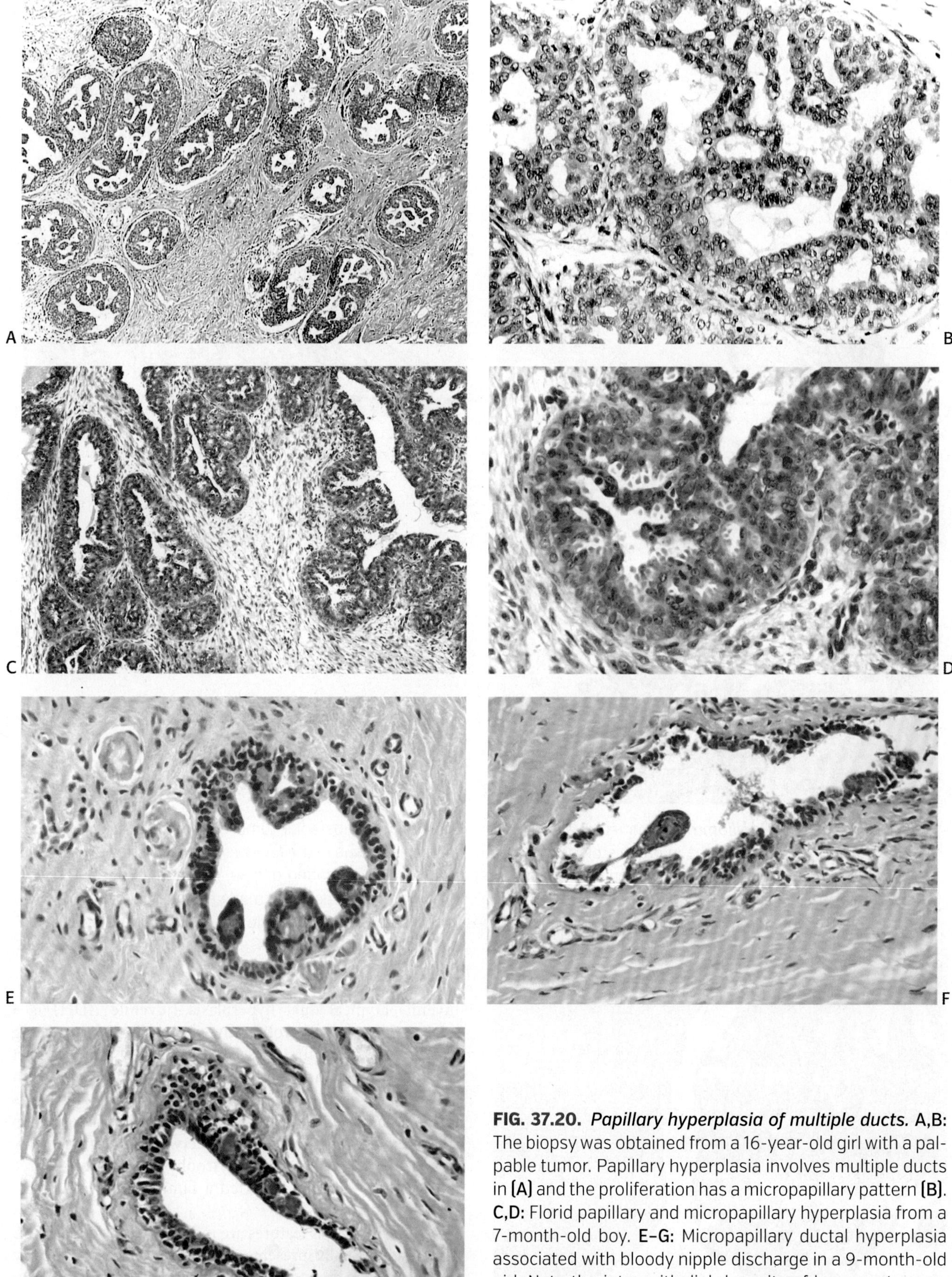

FIG. 37.20. ***Papillary hyperplasia of multiple ducts.*** **A,B:** The biopsy was obtained from a 16-year-old girl with a palpable tumor. Papillary hyperplasia involves multiple ducts in **(A)** and the proliferation has a micropapillary pattern **(B)**. **C,D:** Florid papillary and micropapillary hyperplasia from a 7-month-old boy. **E–G:** Micropapillary ductal hyperplasia associated with bloody nipple discharge in a 9-month-old girl. Note the intraepithelial deposits of basement membrane material which were periodic acid–PAS positive **(F,G)** and immunoreactive for laminin (not shown).

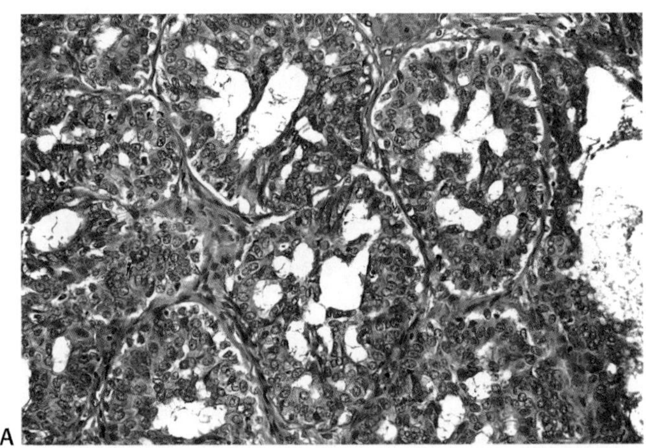

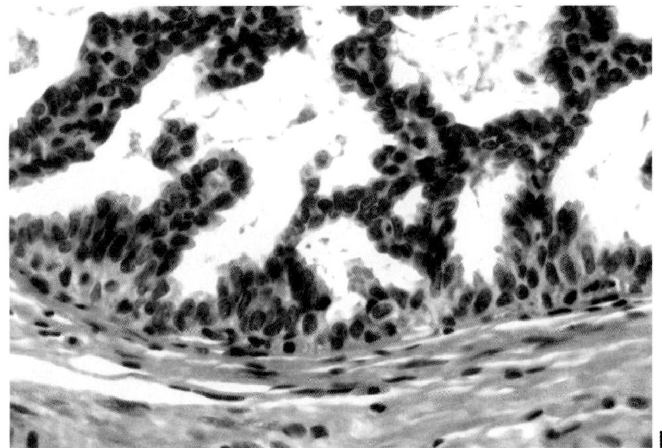

FIG. 37.21. ***Papillary hyperplasia of multiple ducts, with focal atypia.*** The specimen was obtained from an 11-year-old girl. **A:** Micropapillary hyperplasia and focal myoepithelial hyperplasia are identified. **B:** The ductal epithelium shows focal atypia.

cribriform architecture, morphologically similar to ADH occurring in older women (see Chapter 6). Usually, the area between the hyperplastic ducts is occupied by dense, collagenous stroma in which there are also sparse lobules and widely spaced ducts without hyperplasia (Fig. 37.22). The hyperplastic changes tend to develop focally rather than diffusely in the epithelium of an affected duct (Fig. 37.22). In some ducts, the hyperplastic epithelium forms a laciform or cribriform network in the lumen (Figs. 37.23 and 37.24). Myoepithelial cells are present in a continuous or discontinuous fashion (Fig. 37.25). Juxtaposition of duct cross sections showing juvenile ADH with ducts lacking hyperplasia is a characteristic feature (Figs. 37.26 and 37.27).

Follow-up at the time of the 1992 report averaged 39 months (range, 5 to 68 months) during which time rebiopsy in two cases revealed persistent ADH. Long-term follow-up will be necessary to assess the precancerous significance of this lesion.

GYNECOMASTIA

Age

Gynecomastia is encountered as a transient phenomenon postpartum in children of both genders, as a result of maternal estrogen crossing the placenta, and it resolves spontaneously a few weeks after birth. Slight bilateral or unilateral

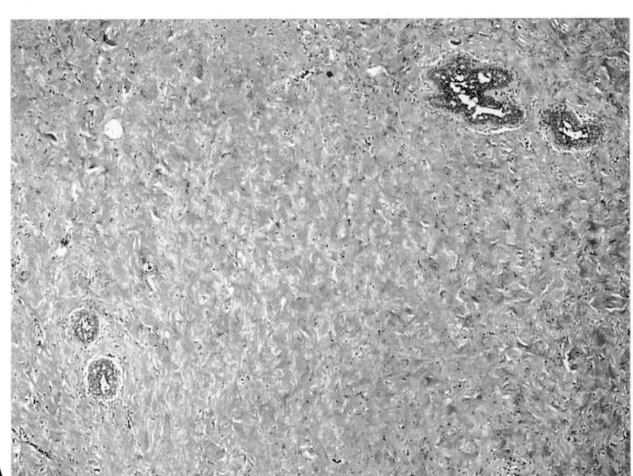

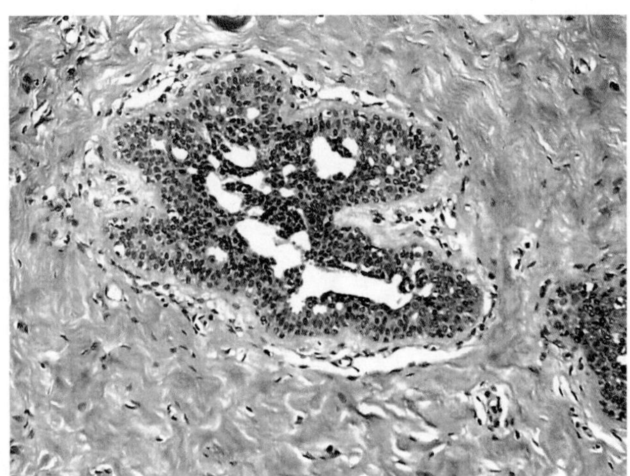

FIG. 37.22. ***Juvenile atypical duct hyperplasia.*** The patient was 18 years old. **A:** Ducts with hyperplastic epithelium in the *upper right* and *lower left* corners are separated by dense collagenized stroma. **B:** The hyperplastic epithelium has micropapillary features. Myoepithelial cells form a continuous layer around the duct.

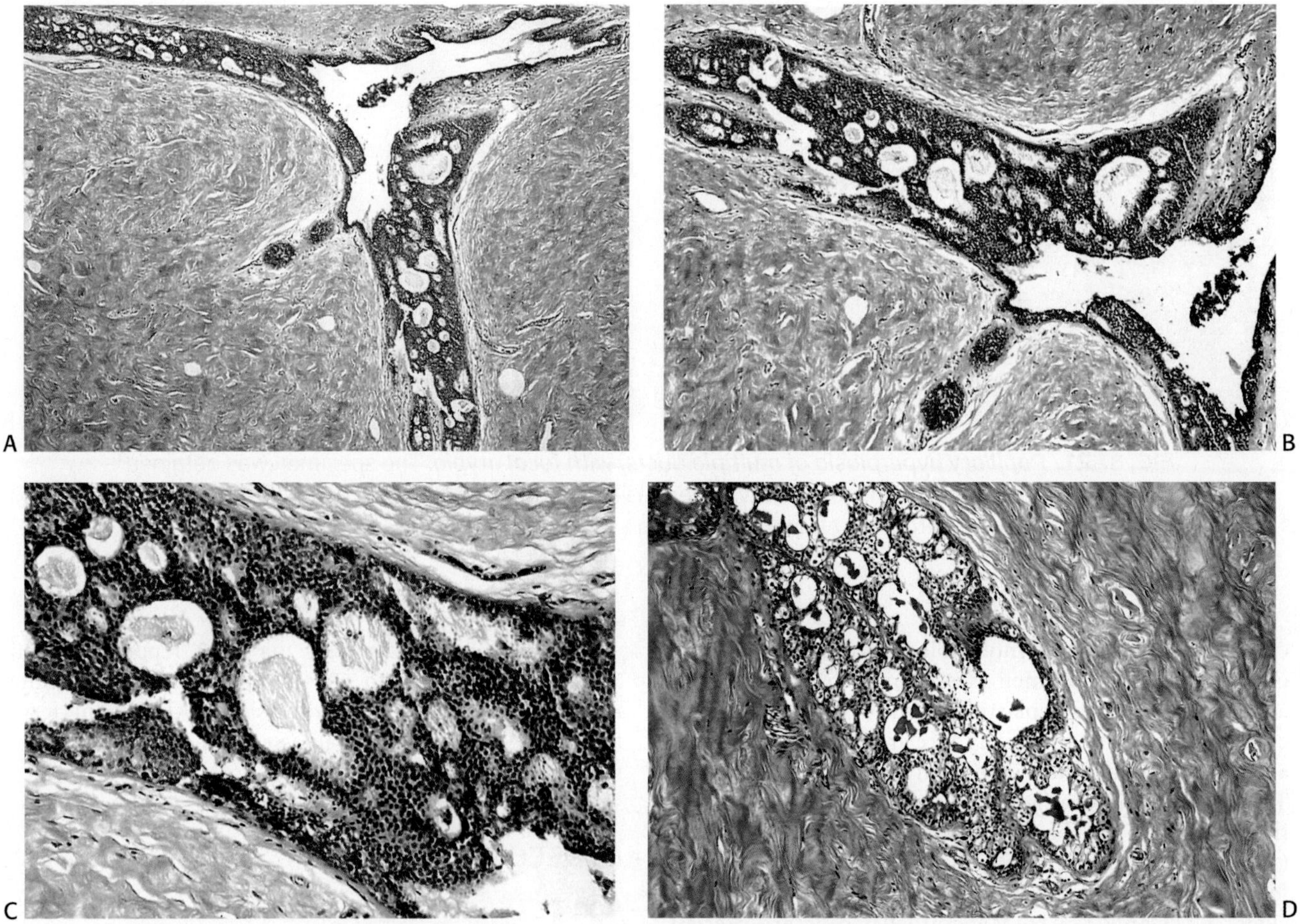

FIG. 37.23. ***Juvenile atypical duct hyperplasia.*** The specimens in (A–C) were obtained from a 20-year-old girl who had a reduction mammoplasty for mammary "hypertrophy." **A,B:** Epithelial hyperplasia is present focally in two of three branches of this duct system. **C:** The hyperplastic epithelium has a cribriform pattern. **D:** Atypical cribriform hyperplasia in another case.

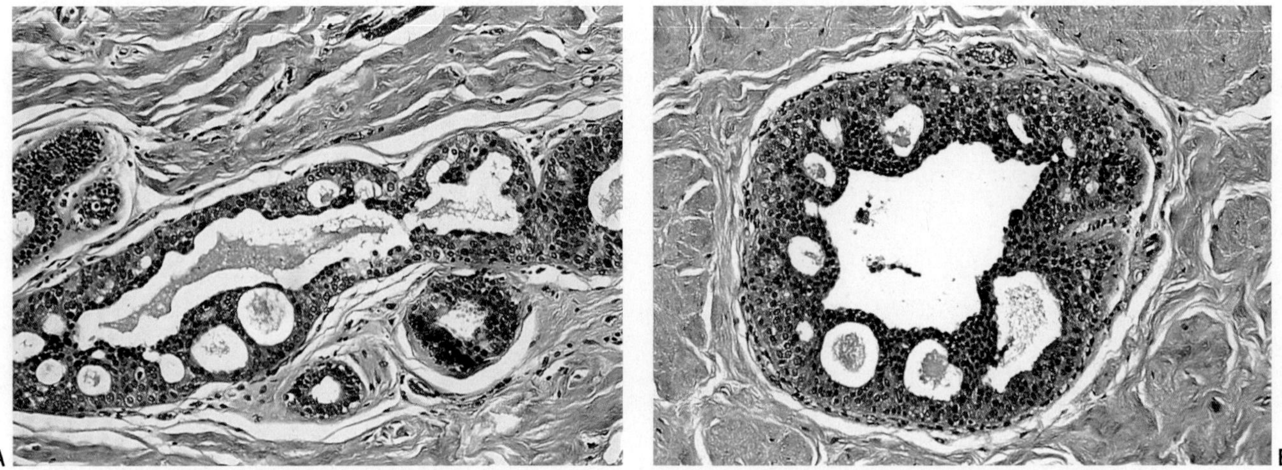

FIG. 37.24. ***Juvenile atypical duct hyperplasia.*** This 23-year-old patient had a breast biopsy for an area of "thickening." **A:** A terminal duct cut longitudinally as it enters an undeveloped lobule. The hyperplastic epithelium forms peripheral arcades. **B:** A transverse section of a duct similar to (A) in which the hyperplastic epithelium forms a circumferential arcade. **C:** Adjacent duct cross sections with cribriform hyperplasia. **D:** Cribriform structure seen in a longitudinal section of a specimen from a 17-year-old girl with macromastia.

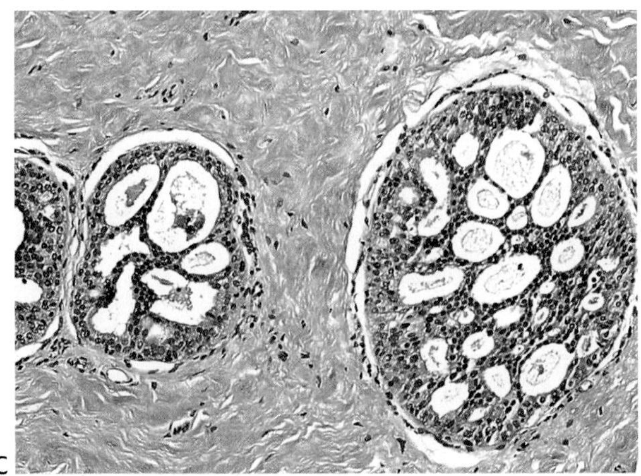

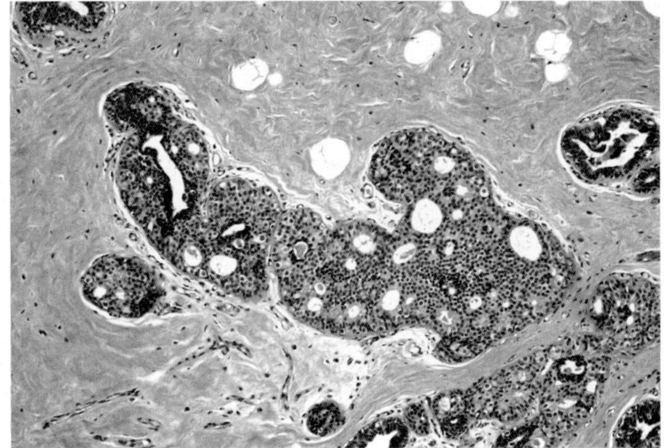

FIG. 37.24. *(Continued)*

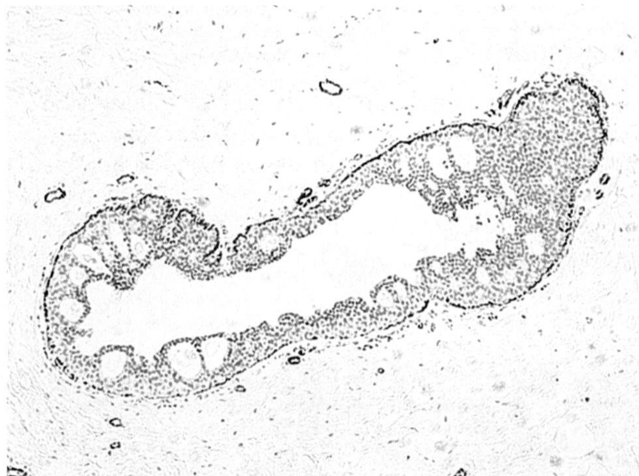

FIG. 37.25. ***Juvenile atypical duct hyperplasia.*** The peripheral myoepithelial layer is highlighted by the immunostain for smooth muscle actin.

gynecomastia limited to the subareolar breast bud often occurs as a physiologic phenomenon in 60% to 70% of boys during puberty. Breast enlargement peaks at 13 to 14 years of age and may persist for few months to a couple of years. This alteration has been attributed to a relative increase of estrogen over testosterone in pubertal boys. In particular, increased peripheral conversion of testosterone to estrogen by aromatase in adipocytes is regarded as a possible pathogenetic factor in overweight or obese boys. In addition to hormonal disorders, anabolic steroids, antidepressant and mood-regulating medications, as well as marijuana are other potential etiologic factors. Idiopathic gynecomastia tends to be more common in Caucasian boys. Association with Klinefelter syndrome was documented in 3/81 (3.7%) cases in one series.[42]

Presenting Symptoms

Gynecomastia generally produces ill-defined induration or thickening. Less often it forms a discrete mass that may

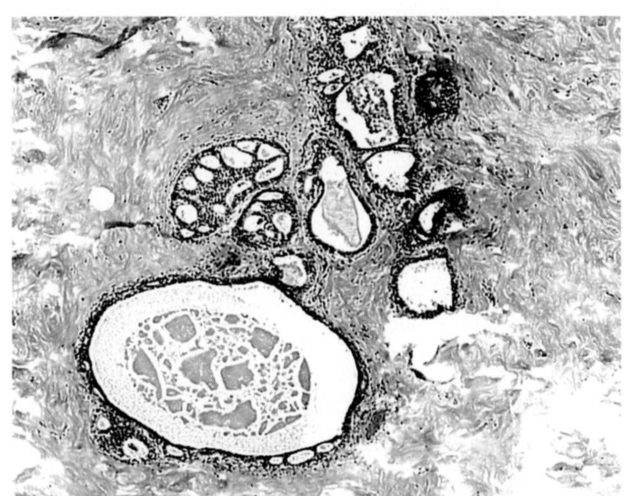

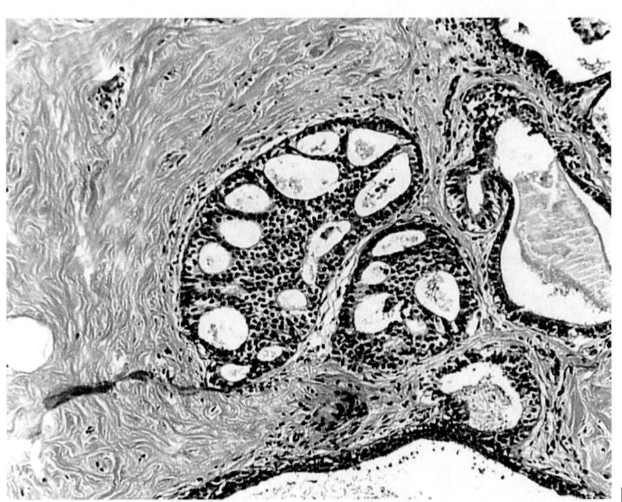

FIG. 37.26. ***Juvenile atypical duct hyperplasia.*** The specimen is from a 21-year-old woman. **A,B:** Two duct cross sections with cribriform hyperplasia are shown in proximity to dilated ducts without hyperplasia.

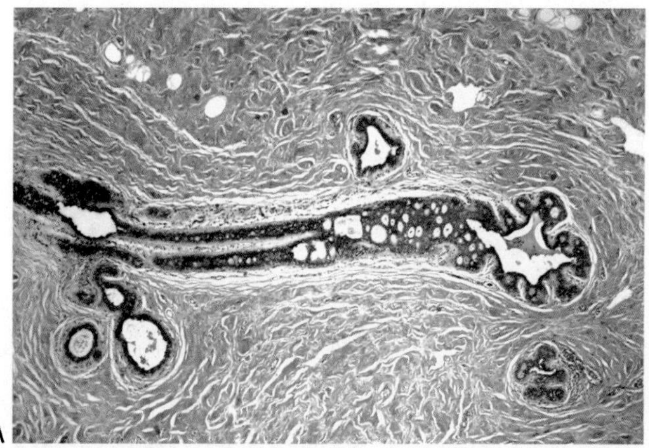

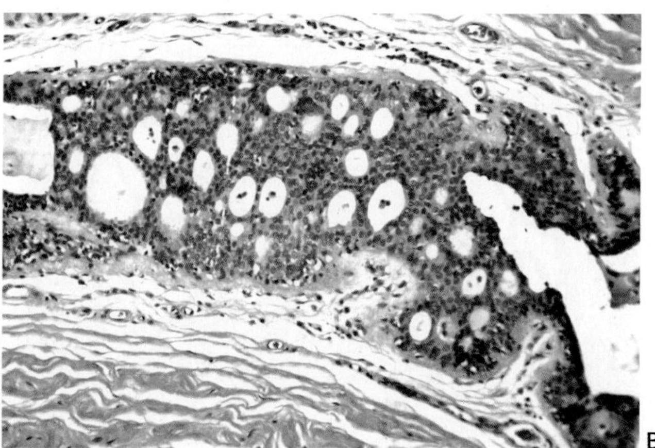

FIG. 37.27. ***Juvenile atypical duct hyperplasia.*** **A,B:** Focal atypical cribriform hyperplasia in a longitudinal section of a duct. The specimen is from a 21-year-old woman.

suggest a neoplasm for which an excision may be mistakenly performed (Fig. 37.28) (see also discussion of gynecomastia in Chapter 36). The alteration can be bilateral or unilateral. More substantial enlargement of the breast tends to occur in overweight or frankly obese boys. In these cases, it is difficult to distinguish true gynecomastia from diffuse adipocyte hyperplasia short of pursuing a tissue diagnosis.

Treatment

A conservative approach is usually adopted in most cases of gynecomastia in adolescent males, as it usually resolves physiologically without treatment. In cases of pseudogynecomastia occurring in overweight or obese boys, a combination of diet and exercise can be helpful. In a retrospective study including data from three hospitals in Texas,[42] 81 adolescents and

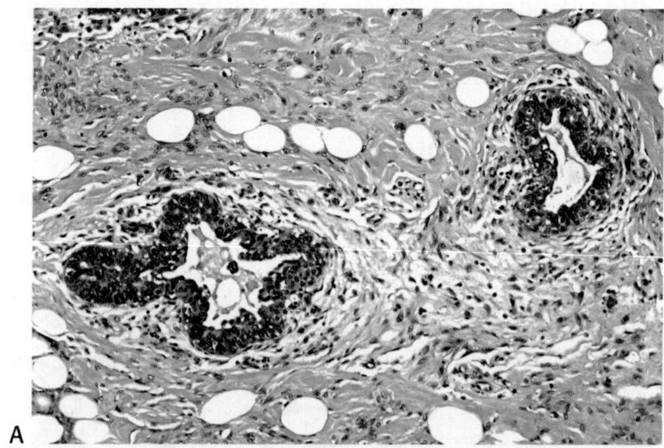

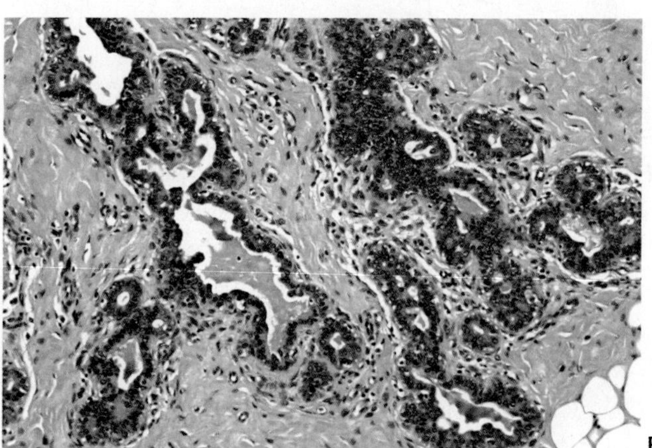

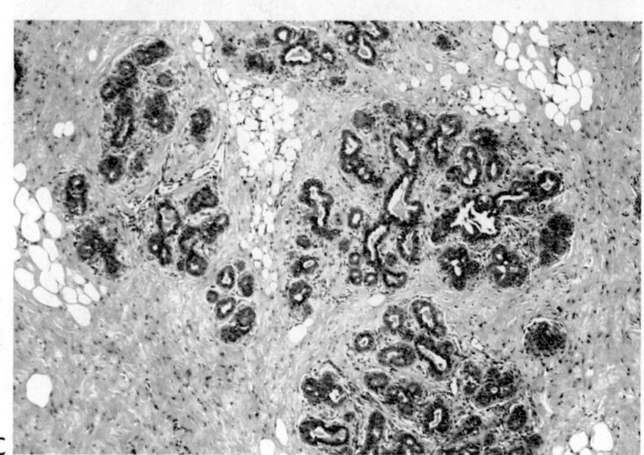

FIG. 37.28. ***Gynecomastia.*** **A:** The images show the histologic appearance of a localized mass from a 2-year-old boy. **A:** Typical active gynecomastia with stromal proliferation around ducts. **B:** Ductal proliferation and intraductal secretion. **C:** Lobules.

young males under age 21 years underwent breast reduction procedures over a 10-year period (between 1999 and 2010), and 79% had bilateral abnormalities. The average age at surgery was 16.2 years (range, 10 to 21). The average patient body mass index was 28.1 (range, 18.4 to 44.6), indicating that most of the patients undergoing surgical treatment were overweight or obese. The average weight of tissue removed was 170.2 g, ranging from 5 to 812 g. Only one case showed cytologic atypia. The authors concluded that pathologic examination of gynecomastic tissue from patients 21 years of age or younger was not necessary unless requested by the patient, his family, or the patient's physician.

Akgul et al.[43] reported that after tamoxifen treatment, only adipose tissue was present at surgical excision of gynecomastia in three boys 16 to 18 years of age, and interpreted this finding as an effect of the drug. This conclusion cannot be accepted, as the mass lesion could have been pseudogynecomastia secondary to adipocytic hyperplasia. Treatment with tamoxifen is not recommended in patients of such young age. In most instances, gynecomastia in adolescent boys tends to resolve spontaneously. Surgical excision is indicated infrequently and usually for cosmetic reasons.[44]

Neurofibromatosis and Gynecomastia

Cho et al.[45] reported six cases of unilateral gynecomastia in nonobese prepubertal boys affected by neurofibromatosis with no evidence of an endocrine abnormality. The mean age at the onset of symptoms was 7.5 years (range, 4 to 8). The age at surgical biopsy ranged from 6 to 11 years. Five of the six boys were African Americans. Gynecomastia was bilateral in four boys and unilateral in two. In four cases, it was limited to the subareolar area, whereas it diffusely involved the breast in another two. A few additional sporadic cases of prepubertal gynecomastia in boys with neurofibromatosis have also been reported,[46] for most part consisting of PASH with or without associated giant stromal cells.[47,48] In a few cases, neurofibromas were also present.[46,49]

Rarely, cystic hygromas involving the chest wall or the breast of a prepubertal or adolescent boy may simulate unilateral gynecomastia.[50–52]

Gynecomastia and ADH or Carcinoma

A recent review of the literature compiled by Koshy et al.[42] focused on the findings in breast surgical excision specimens from 615 adolescent boys. Most of the patients underwent surgical excision for gynecomastia. The authors documented only four instances of atypia and six carcinomas. The carcinomas included secretory carcinoma in a 17-year-old boy,[53] bilateral low-grade DCIS in an 18-year-old male patient with neurofibromatosis type 1,[54] focal low-grade DCIS in two patients of 20 and 16 years of age,[55,56] and intermediate nuclear grade DCIS in a 16-year-old boy.[57] The illustrations provided in two of these cases[56,57] reveal PASH in the tissue surrounding the DCIS. All foci of DCIS were very small and sometimes limited to one or two cross sections of small ducts.

FIBROEPITHELIAL TUMORS IN CHILDREN AND ADOLESCENTS

Age and Ethnicity

Fibroepithelial lesions are the most common tumors in adolescent girls. In a series of 54 cases studied by Ross et al.,[58] the mean and median ages at diagnosis were 15.4 and 16 years, respectively (range, 10 to 18 years). Fibroepithelial tumors are usually regarded as more common in African American adolescent girls,[59] but geographic factors may also play a role. In the series by Ross et al.,[58] race and/or ethnicity information was available for 45/54 patients treated at Memorial Hospital in New York City, and 67% of patients were Caucasians, 27% African Americans, 4% Hispanics, and 2% Asians.

Fibroadenoma

FA account for at least 75% of breast tumors in adolescent girls.[24–26] Sanchez et al.[60] identified 91 solid breast masses in female adolescents younger than 19 years who underwent ultrasound examination at a pediatric hospital. Pathologic diagnosis of 49 lesions from 38 patients identified 44 FA (90%). The other tumors were one example each of hamartoma, NLH, tubular adenoma, PASH, and lactation changes. The mean age was 16.6 years, ranging from 11.8 to 18.9 years. In this series, 11/38 girls were African Americans and 27 Caucasians. The mean and median age of patients with usual FA in the series by Ross et al.[58] was 17 years (range, 15 to 18) and that of patients with juvenile FA was 15 and 16 years, respectively (range, 11 to 18). The mean age at menarche was 12 years for either lesion, but the mean time from menarche to diagnosis was 72 months for usual FA and 36 months for juvenile FA.

Presenting Symptoms

A discrete, rubbery, ovoid and mobile mass lesion is the most common presenting symptom. In one series,[60] the mass was self-detected in 34/38 patients (89.5%) and constituted an incidental finding only in 4 cases (10.5%). Rarely the mass is painful. Bloody nipple discharge is exceedingly rare.[61] In one case, it was attributed to spontaneous infarction of the FA.[62]

Size

In the study by Ross et al.,[58] the mean tumor size of 34 FA was 2.9 cm (range, 0.5 to 7). Between 5% and 10% of FA in adolescent girls attain substantial size. Some of these tumors have been referred to as "giant fibroadenomas," but this term should be avoided, as it refers to the clinical presentation and has been used in the past for FA, as well as benign phyllodes tumors, and tumor-forming PASH. Despite their rapid growth, large FA have a benign clinical course.[63]

Microscopic Findings

Most of these FA are similar histologically to comparable tumors in young adult women.[64] Pericanalicular and intracanalicular growth patterns are encountered. Focal stromal

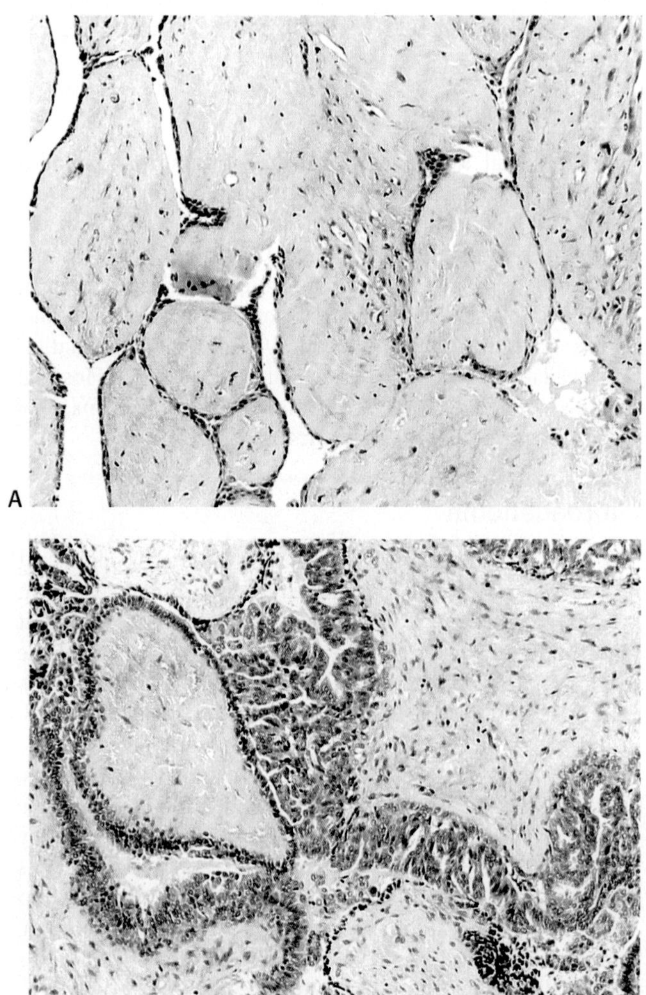

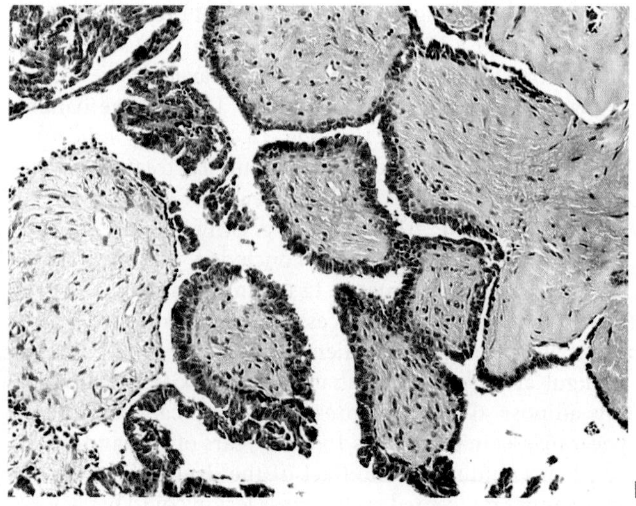

FIG. 37.29. ***Fibroadenoma with epithelial heterogeneity.*** The tumor was obtained from a 15-year-old girl. **A:** Part of the lesion with hyalinized stroma and flat epithelium. **B:** Mild epithelial hyperplasia. **C:** Moderate epithelial hyperplasia with some detached epithelial fragments.

hyalinization as well as epithelial hyperplasia can rarely occur in childhood FA[65] (Fig. 37.29). In the study by Ross et al.,[58] 11/34 FA had usual morphology and 23/34 were classified as juvenile FA. Epithelial hyperplasia was identified in 2/11 (18%) usual FA and in 7/23 (30%) juvenile FA. A more complete discussion of FA can be found in Chapter 8.

FA in children with multiple cysts may suggest JP grossly (Figs. 37.30 and 37.31). In some instances, histologic examination reveals the complex proliferative pattern of JP in fibroadenomatous stroma. The precise relationship of these infrequent lesions to the conventional presentation of JP remains to be determined. FA containing only cysts lined by flat or cuboidal epithelium are not considered to be part of JP.

Phyllodes Tumor

These tumors present clinically as mass lesions, often characterized by rapid growth. Tagaya et al.[66] described a benign cystic and papillary phyllodes tumor in an 11-year-old child who presented with nipple bleeding. Another phyllodes tumor with bloody nipple discharge reported by Martino et al.[67] in a 13-year-old girl was 4.5 cm in greatest dimension.

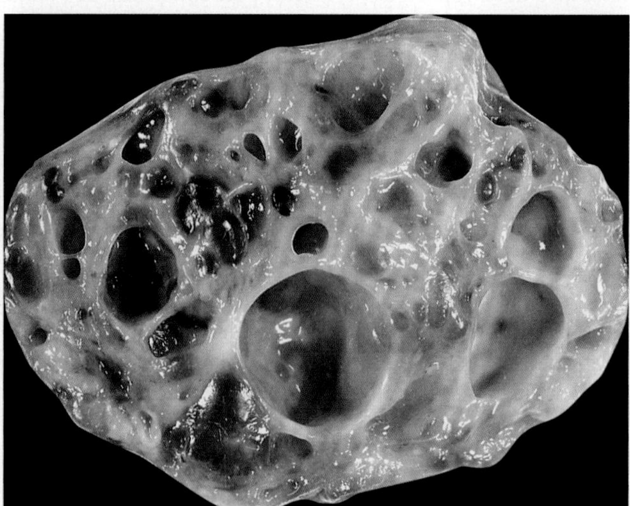

FIG. 37.30. ***Fibroadenoma with cysts.*** This tumor from a 20-year-old woman exhibits striking cyst formation reminiscent of JP but histologically the lesion lacked the characteristic proliferative components.

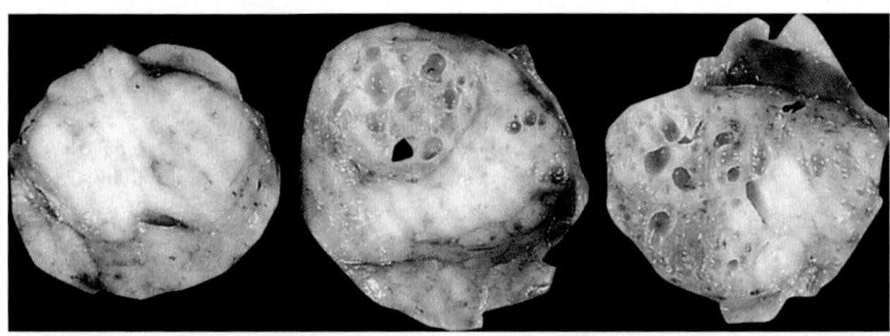

FIG. 37.31. ***Fibroadenoma with juvenile papillomatosis-like hyperplasia.*** Proliferative changes similar to JP were present in the localized cystic area within this complex FA.

Microscopic Findings

PT in this age group have the same histologic characteristics as comparable tumors in adults.[68] One or more features that distinguish phyllodes tumors from FA are present in an individual case. These include stromal overgrowth relative to the epithelium, a tendency for cellularity to be greatest in the subepithelial stroma, and, in some cases, an invasive border. Stromal mitoses may be present, especially in the subepithelial zone. In this age group, mitotic activity by itself is not always indicative of a phyllodes tumor when other features of this tumor type are absent since a modest mitotic rate can be found in some juvenile FA. Uncommon stromal differentiation includes adipose, leiomyomatous, and rhabdomyoid elements, as well as myofibroblastic proliferation that resemble myofibroblastoma (Fig. 37.32). Cystic papillary phyllodes tumors that may be benign or malignant can occur in children (Fig. 37.33). Although most phyllodes tumors in children follow a benign clinical course after excision, rare instances of local recurrence (Fig. 37.34) and malignant tumors with systemic metastases have been reported (Fig. 37.35).[68–72] Additional discussion of phyllodes tumors can be found in Chapter 8.

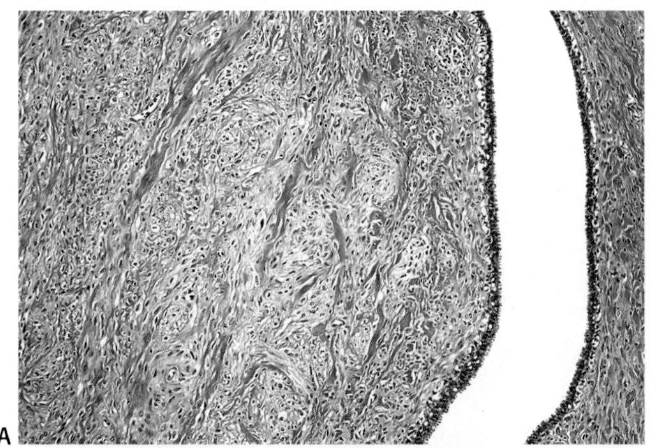

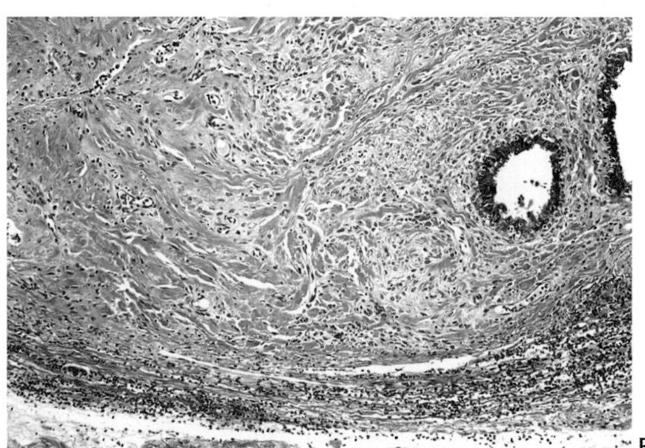

FIG. 37.32. ***Phyllodes tumor with myofibroblastoma-like stroma.*** **A:** The stroma in this benign tumor from a 12-year-old girl shows myofibroblastic hyperplasia and collagen bands. Note the phyllodes epithelial structure. **B:** The tumor has a circumscribed border. Traces of pseudoangiomatous architecture are present.

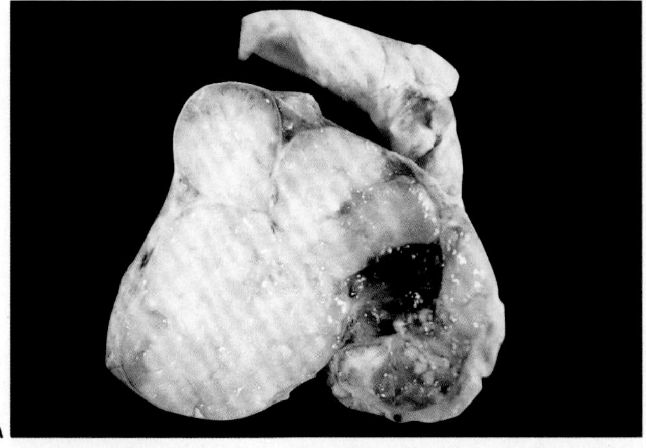

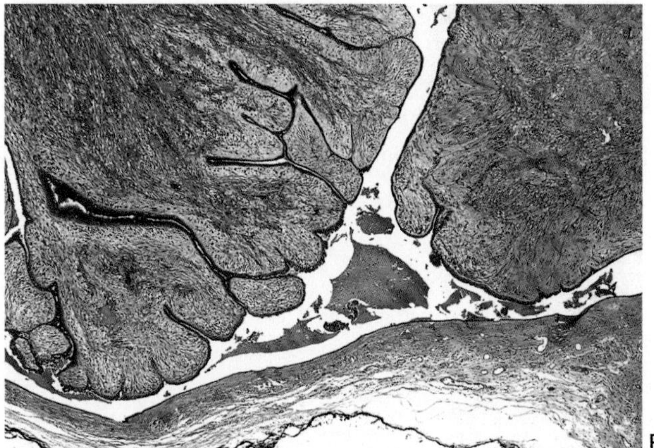

FIG. 37.33. ***Cystic papillary phyllodes tumor.*** **A:** Part of the cystic portion of this benign tumor from a 12-year-old girl contains clotted blood (*lower right*). **B:** A cystic papillary low-grade malignant phyllodes tumor from a 13-year-old girl. **C:** Moderate stromal cellularity and one atypical mitosis (*arrow*) in the same lesion as **(B)**. **D:** A focus with multiple mitoses (*arrows*) from the tumor in **(B)** and **(C)**.

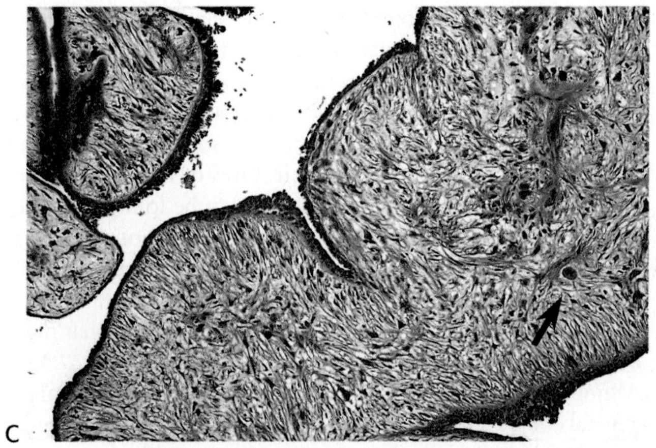

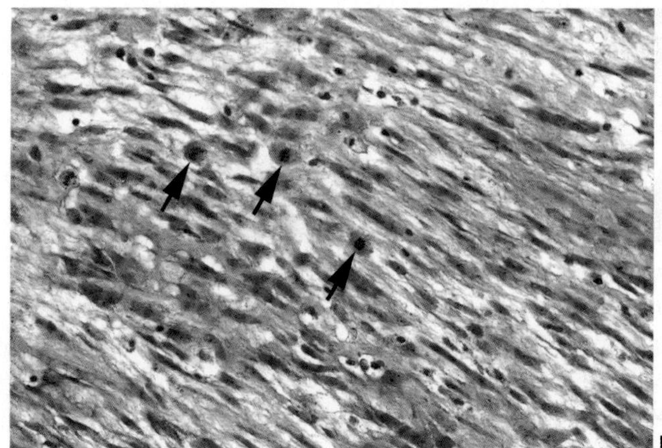

FIG. 37.33. *(Continued)*

PASH occurs as an incidental finding in the stroma of pediatric fibroepithelial tumors and in adolescent macromastia with juvenile ADH. It can also present rarely as a discrete tumor that is indistinguishable clinically from a FA in girls (Fig. 37.36).[73,74] PASH has also been found in the breasts of pubertal boys presenting clinically with gynecomastia. It has also been identified in the breast of boys with neurofibromatosis.[47,48,74] PASH also accounted for a well-circumscribed nodular mass evident for about a year and clinically suspected to be a hamartoma or a lipoma in the breast of a 3-year-old boy.[74]

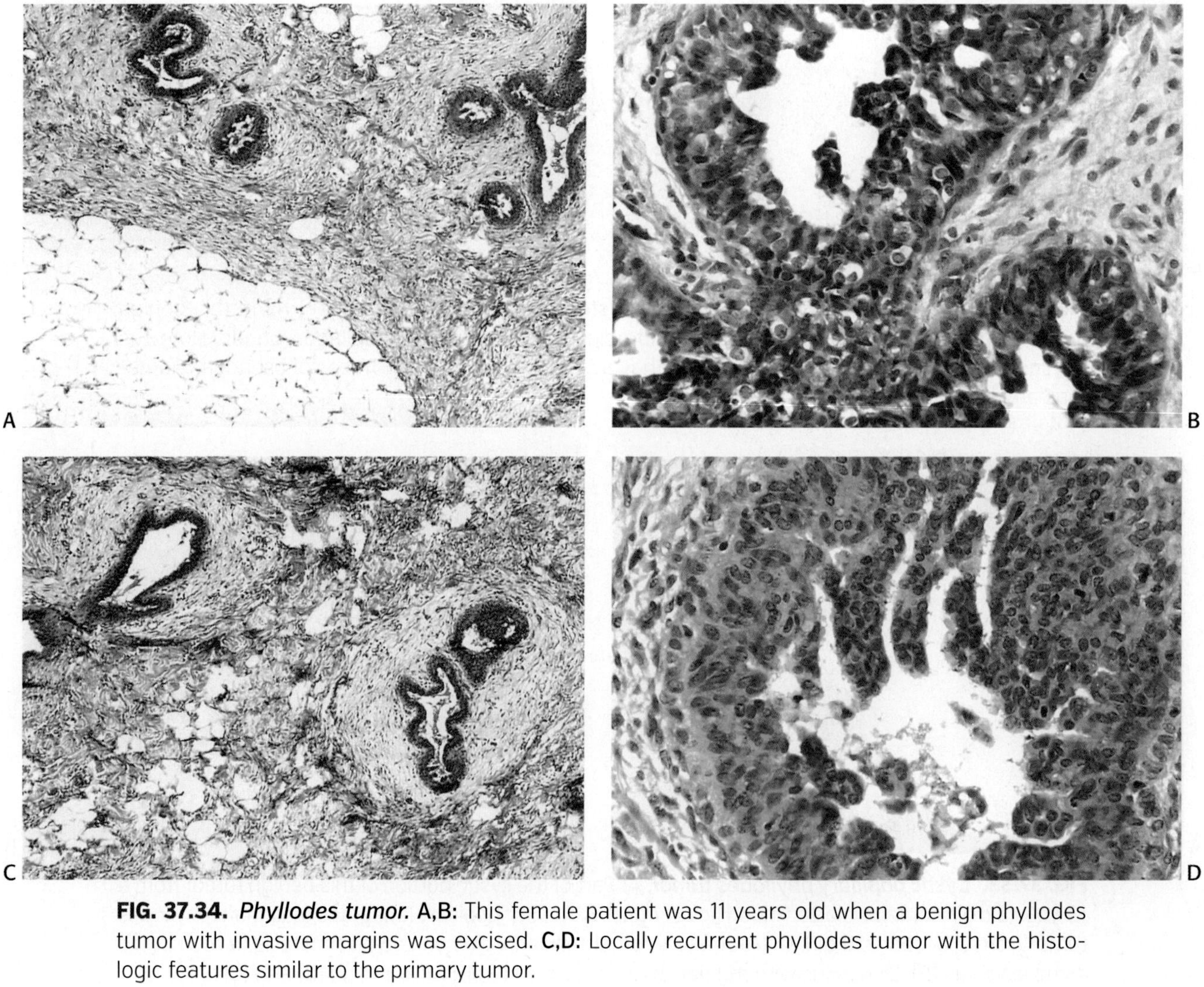

FIG. 37.34. ***Phyllodes tumor.*** **A,B:** This female patient was 11 years old when a benign phyllodes tumor with invasive margins was excised. **C,D:** Locally recurrent phyllodes tumor with the histologic features similar to the primary tumor.

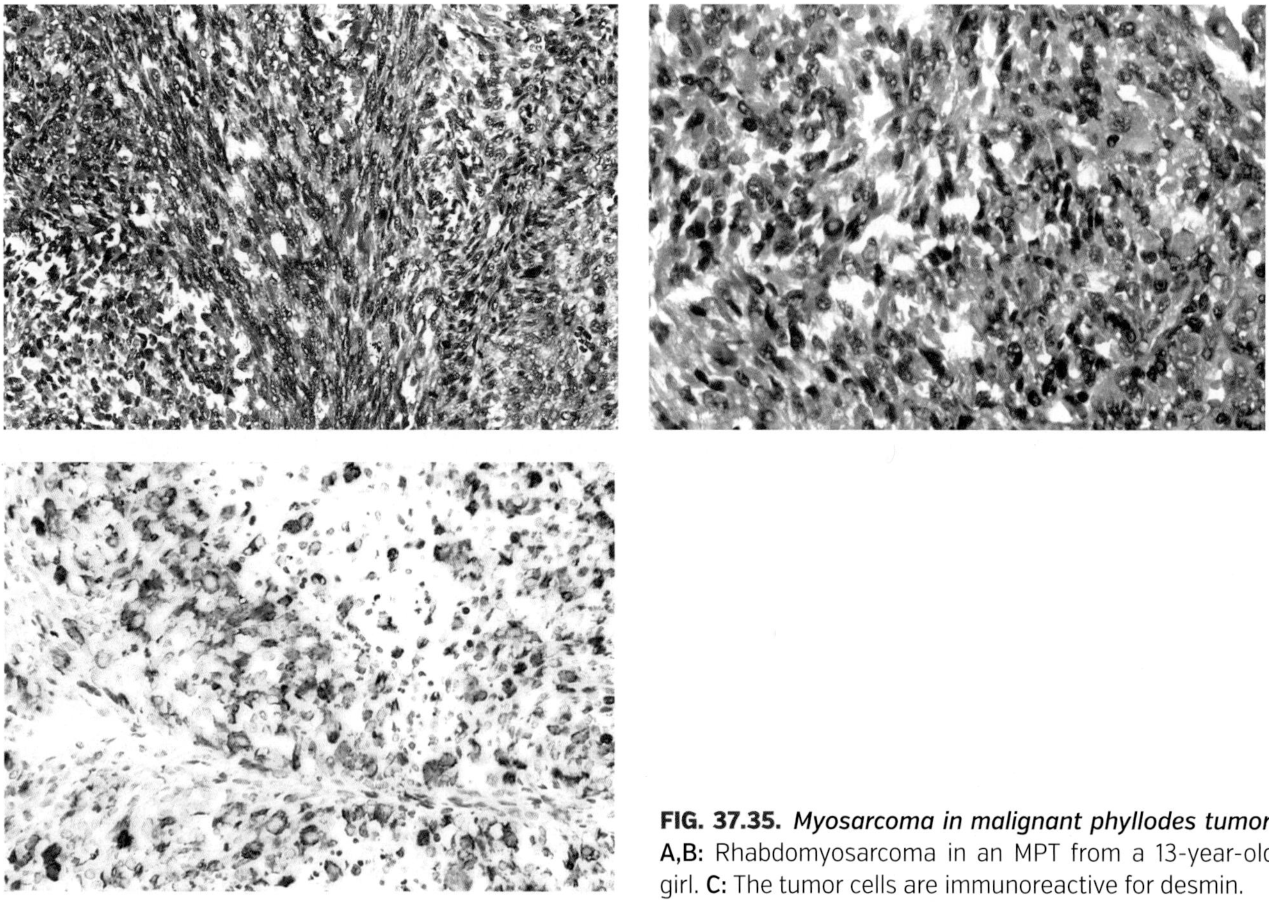

FIG. 37.35. ***Myosarcoma in malignant phyllodes tumor.*** **A,B:** Rhabdomyosarcoma in an MPT from a 13-year-old girl. **C:** The tumor cells are immunoreactive for desmin.

CARCINOMA IN CHILDREN AND ADOLESCENTS

Carcinoma of the breast is extremely unusual in this age group and accounts for less than 1% of all breast lesions.[75] A literature review published in 1977 listed 74 cases reported between 1888 and 1972.[76] A few case reports and series have since documented infiltrating ductal carcinomas,[59,72,77,78] pleomorphic carcinoma,[79] adenoid cystic carcinoma (AdCC),[80] and secretory carcinoma.[81–87]

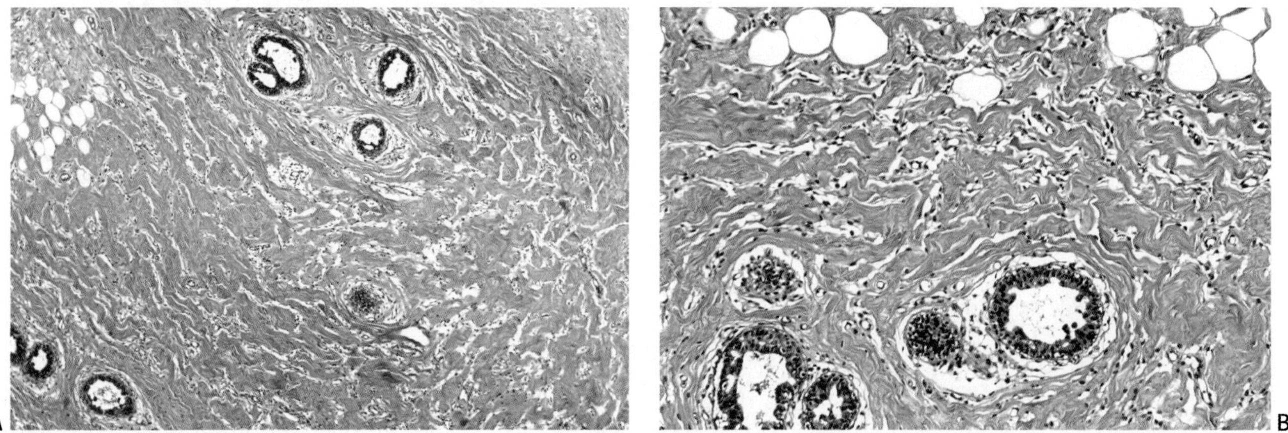

FIG. 37.36. ***Pseudoangiomatous stromal hyperplasia.*** The patient was a 15-year-old girl with a discrete breast tumor thought clinically to be a FA. **A,B:** Typical stromal clefts of PASH and minimal epithelial hyperplasia.

Predisposing Factors

Prior irradiation appears to be a predisposing factor in some instances. Close and Maximov[88] described a poorly differentiated carcinoma in the left breast of a 17-year-old girl who had received mediastinal irradiation for an enlarged thymus gland at 3 months of age. Carcinoma in the breast of an 18-year-old boy has also been reported after thymic irradiation during childhood.[89] Irradiation in the region of the breast in children and young adults has also been associated with breast carcinoma diagnosed in adulthood.[90–94]

Age and Presenting Symptoms

Most of the patients have been females, with an average age of about 13 years. With few exceptions, the presenting sign has been a mass. Nipple discharge and diffuse breast enlargement are uncommon. The carcinomas have ranged in size from 1 to 9 cm.

Microscopic Findings

A substantial number of the tumors are of the secretory (juvenile) type[81–87] (Figs. 37.37 and 37.38), an entity discussed in Chapter 22. Other types of carcinoma commonly found in adults have also been described.[1,76,95] Small cell carcinoma of the breast in children is a highly malignant neoplasm that is difficult to distinguish from lymphoma and embryonal rhabdomyosarcoma in routine sections[72,88,96,97] (Fig. 37.39). *In situ* carcinoma may not be found, and the tumor cells do not have the cytologic features of typical infiltrating lobular carcinoma such as mucin secretion. Immunoreactivity for cytokeratin (CK) is usually detectable, and the cells are not reactive with markers for lymphoma or myosarcoma. Cystic and papillary carcinoma is extremely rare in girls (Fig. 37.40). A case of AdCC in a 19-year-old girl has been reported.[80] A rare case of LCIS has also been described in a 15-year-old girl.[98]

Breast carcinoma in boys is usually the secretory type, but other types are rarely encountered (Fig. 37.41).

OTHER TUMORS

The juvenile breast may be involved by systemic diseases such as lymphoma or leukemia. Metastases from primary tumors arising at other sites, such as rhabdomyosarcoma (Fig. 37.42)

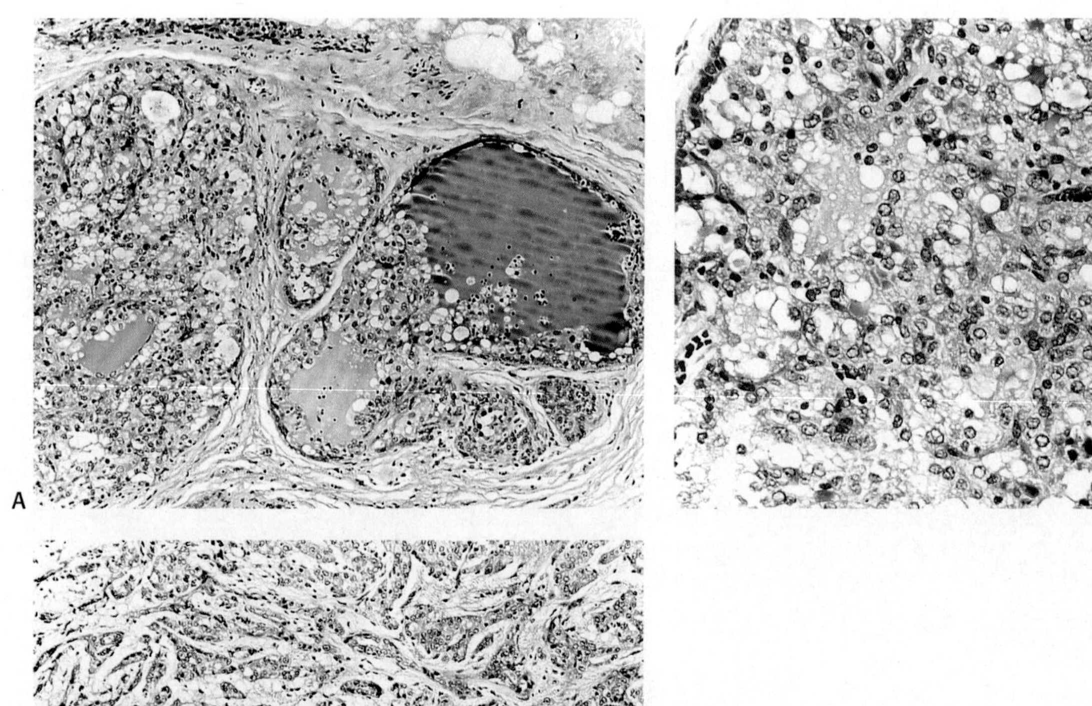

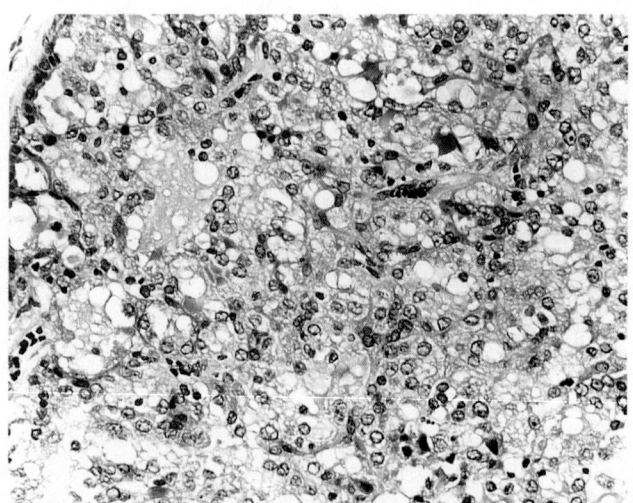

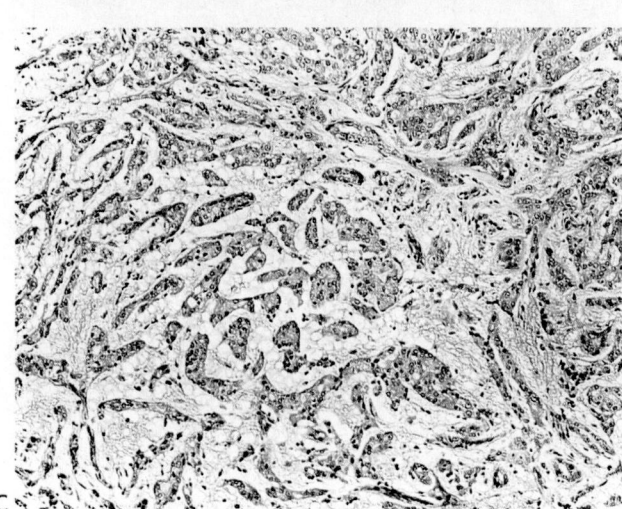

FIG. 37.37. ***Secretory and infiltrating duct carcinoma.*** **A,B:** The intraductal component of this lesion is secretory carcinoma. **C:** The infiltrating component lacks secretory features.

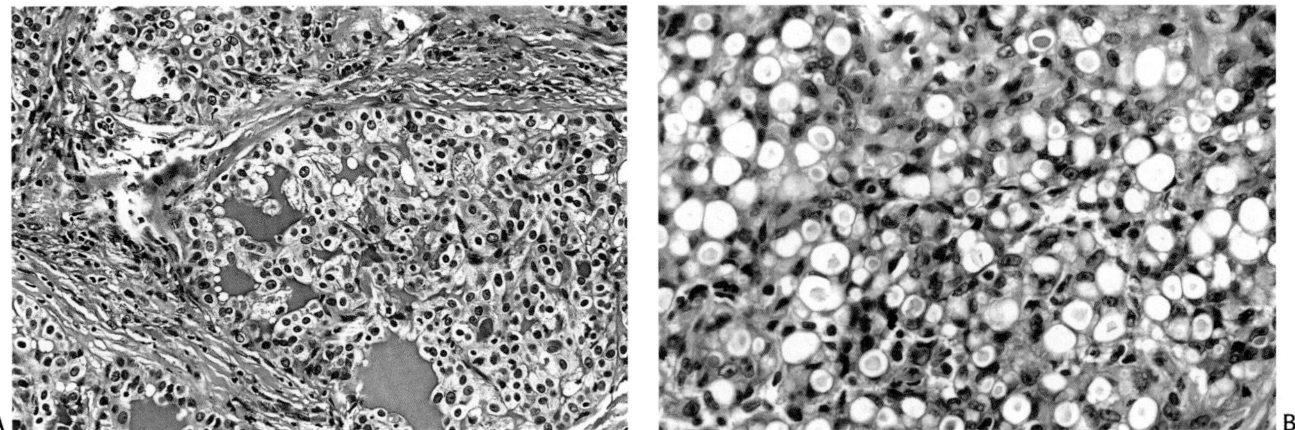

FIG. 37.38. ***Secretory carcinoma.*** This tumor is from a 5-year-old girl. **A:** DCIS. **B:** Infiltrating secretory carcinoma showing secretion in microlumens.

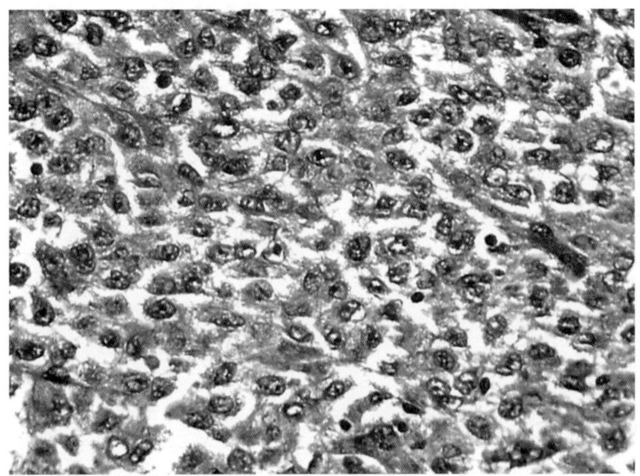

FIG. 37.39. ***Small cell carcinoma.*** The patient was a 17-year-old girl.

and medulloblastoma, have been reported. Howarth et al.[99] observed that even if rhabdomyosarcoma is more common in boys, breast metastases most frequently occur in girls. Rhabdomyosarcoma metastatic to the breast typically is of alveolar type,[99,100] with most tumors originating in the extremities or buttocks. Patient age ranges from 11 to 20 years. In a series of seven cases with breast metastases detected 3 to 12 months after initial diagnosis,[100] the primary tumor sites included a hand, a leg, retroperitoneum, and the vagina in one case each. One patient reportedly had primary mammary rhabdomyosarcoma in one breast and developed metastases in the contralateral breast. The site of origin was unknown in one case. Predilection for metastatic involvement of the breast in adolescent girls is attributed to the rapid growth, hormonal stimulation, and vascularization of the pre- and pubertal breast. Occasional examples of primary mammary rhabdomyosarcoma have also been reported.[1,91,100,101]

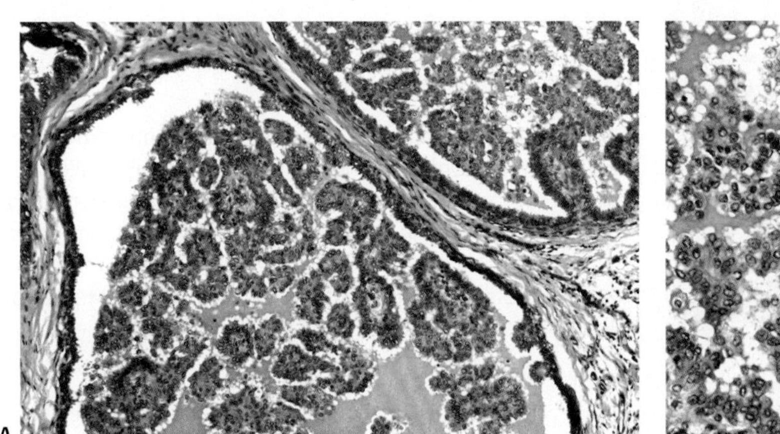

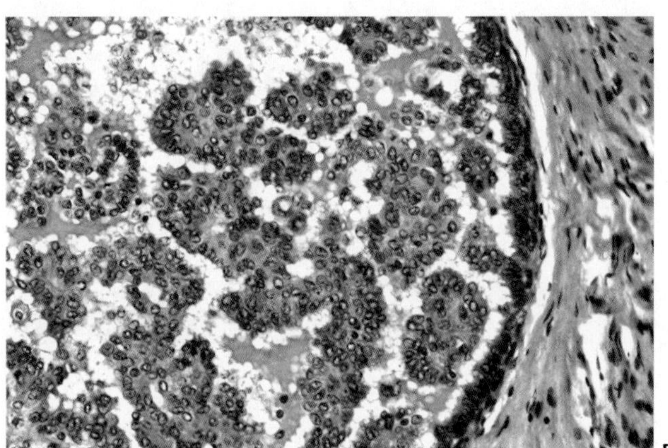

FIG. 37.40. ***Papillary carcinoma.*** **A,B:** Cystic papillary carcinoma in a 12-year-old girl. The epithelial proliferation lacks stroma and myoepithelial cells.

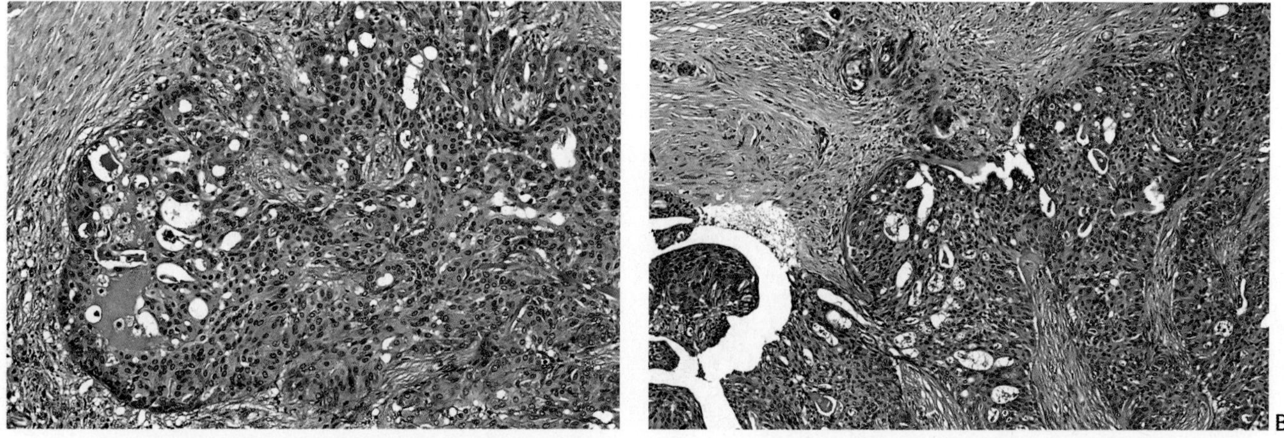

FIG. 37.41. ***Solid papillary carcinoma.*** This tumor is from a 16-year-old boy. Metastatic tumor was found in an axillary lymph node. **A:** Solid papillary growth with apocrine and secretory features. **B:** An area of stromal invasion is shown at the *upper border* of the tumor.

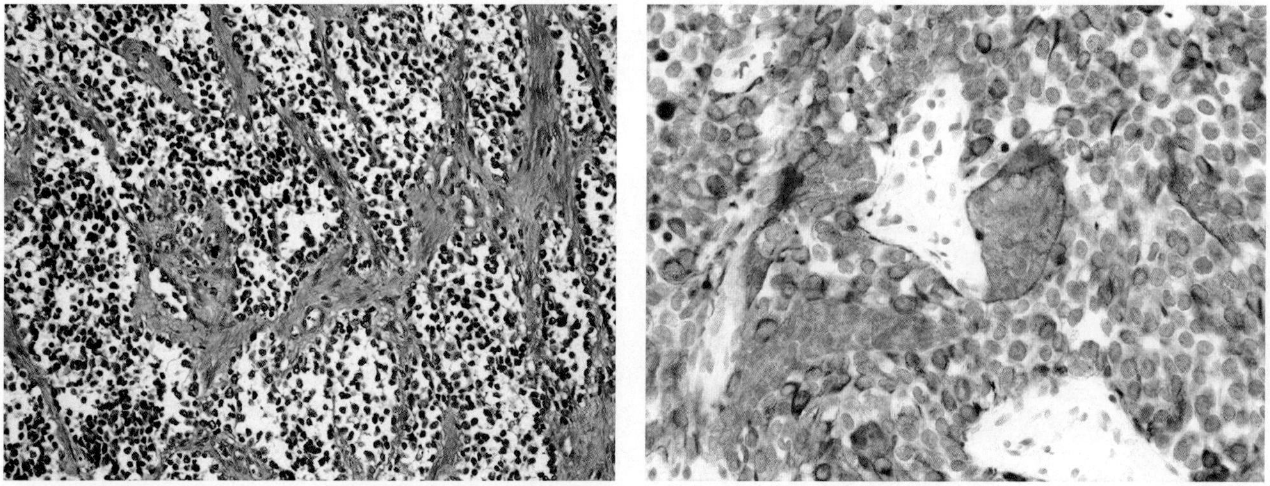

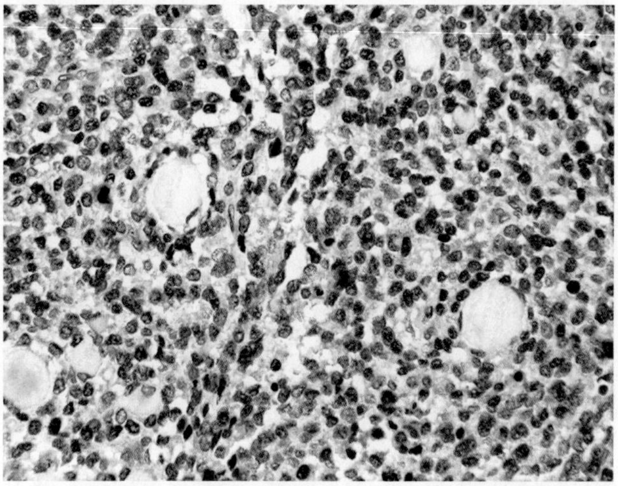

FIG. 37.42. ***Metastatic alveolar rhabdomyosarcoma.*** **A:** The tumor consists of loose nests of highly malignant round blue cells with alveolar arrangement, separated by broad bands of collagenous stroma. **B:** A desmin stain decorates the cytoplasm. **C:** Nuclear staining for myogenin. (Images courtesy of Dr. C. Antonescu, Memorial Sloan-Kettering Cancer Center).

Primary mammary sarcoma is exceedingly uncommon in this age group. Rare examples of primary mammary angiosarcoma have been reported in the second decade of life,[102] including a case of bilateral angiosarcoma in a 14-year-old child.[103] For further discussion of these topics, see relevant chapters elsewhere in this volume.

Hematologic neoplasms that may primarily or secondarily affect the breast are discussed in Chapter 40.

REFERENCES

1. Pettinato G, Manivel JC, Kelly DR, et al. Lesions of the breast in children exclusive of typical fibroadenoma and gynecomastia. A clinicopathologic study of 113 cases. *Pathol Annu* 1989;24(Pt. 2):296–328.
2. Elsheikh A, Keramopoulos A, Lazaris D, et al. Breast tumors during adolescence. *Eur J Gynaecol Oncol* 2000;21:408–410.
3. Bower R, Bell MJ, Ternberg JL. Management of breast lesions in children and adolescents. *J Pediatr Surg* 1976;11:337–346.
4. Simpson JS, Barson AJ. Breast tumours in infants and children: a 40-year review of cases at a children's hospital. *Can Med Assoc J* 1969;101:100–102.
5. Stone AM, Shenker IR, McCarthy K. Adolescent breast masses. *Am J Surg* 1977;134:275–277.
6. Tea MK, Asseryanis E, Kroiss R, et al. Surgical breast lesions in adolescent females. *Pediatr Surg Int* 2009;25:73–75.
7. Ozumba BC, Nzegwu MA, Anyikam A, et al. Breast disease in children and adolescents in eastern Nigeria—a five-year study. *J Pediatr Adolesc Gynecol* 2009;22:169–172.
8. Sanchez R, Ladino-Torres MF, Bernat JA, et al. Breast fibroadenomas in the pediatric population: common and uncommon sonographic findings. *Pediatr Radiol* 2010;40:1681–1689.
9. Wu HC, John EM, Ferris JS, et al. Global DNA methylation levels in girls with and without a family history of breast cancer. *Epigenetics* 2011;6:29–33.

Juvenile Papillomatosis

10. Rosen PP, Cantrell B, Mullen DL, et al. Juvenile papillomatosis (Swiss cheese disease) of the breast. *Am J Surg Pathol* 1980;4:3–12.
11. Rosen PP, Holmes G, Lesser ML, et al. Juvenile papillomatosis and breast carcinoma. *Cancer* 1985;55:1345–1352.
12. Tan TY, Amor DJ, Chow CW. Juvenile papillomatosis of the breast associated with neurofibromatosis 1. *Pediatr Blood Cancer* 2007;49:363–364.
13. Pacilli M, Sebire NJ, Thambapillai E, et al. Juvenile papillomatosis of the breast in a male infant with Noonan syndrome, cafe au lait spots, and family history of breast carcinoma. *Pediatr Blood Cancer* 2005;45:991–993.
14. Rice HE, Acosta A, Brown RL, et al. Juvenile papillomatosis of the breast in male infants: two case reports. *Pediatr Surg Int* 2000;16:104–106.
15. Bartow SA, Pathak DR, Black WC, et al. Prevalence of benign, atypical, and malignant breast lesions in populations at different risk for breast cancer. A forensic autopsy study. *Cancer* 1987;60:2751–2760.
16. Uriburu J, Mosta A, Gomez M. Displasia proliferative juvenil focalizada. *Prensa Medica Argentina* 1975;62:172–176.
17. Sund BS, Topstad TK, Nesland JM. A case of juvenile papillomatosis of the male breast. *Cancer* 1992;70:126–128.
18. Sanguinetti A, Fioriti L, Brugia M, et al. Juvenile papillomatosis of the breast in young male: a case report. *G Chir* 2011;32:374–375.
19. Rosen PP, Kimmel M. Juvenile papillomatosis of the breast. A follow-up study of 41 patients having biopsies before 1979. *Am J Clin Pathol* 1990;93:599–603.
20. Kersschot EA, Hermans ME, Pauwels C, et al. Juvenile papillomatosis of the breast: sonographic appearance. *Radiology* 1988;169:631–633.
21. Hidalgo F, Llano JM, Marhuenda A. Juvenile papillomatosis of the breast (Swiss cheese disease). *AJR Am J Roentgenol* 1997;169:912.
22. Sabate JM, Clotet M, Torrubia S, et al. Radiologic evaluation of breast disorders related to pregnancy and lactation. *Radiographics* 2007;27(Suppl. 1):S101–S124.
23. Mussurakis S, Carleton PJ, Turnbull LW. Case report: MR imaging of juvenile papillomatosis of the breast. *Br J Radiol* 1996;69:867–870.
24. Durur-Subasi I, Alper F, Akcay MN, et al. Magnetic resonance imaging findings of breast juvenile papillomatosis. *Jpn J Radiol* 2013;31:419–423.
25. Rosen PP, Lyngholm B, Kinne DW, et al. Juvenile papillomatosis of the breast and family history of breast carcinoma. *Cancer* 1982;49:2591–2595.
26. Bazzocchi F, Santini D, Martinelli G, et al. Juvenile papillomatosis (epitheliosis) of the breast. A clinical and pathologic study of 13 cases. *Am J Clin Pathol* 1986;86:745–748.
27. Talisman R, Nissim F, Rothstein H, et al. Juvenile papillomatosis of the breast. *Eur J Surg* 1993;159:317–319.
28. Batchelor JS, Farah G, Fisher C. Multiple breast papillomas in adolescence. *J Surg Oncol* 1993;54:64–66.
29. Kiaer HW, Kiaer WW, Linell F, et al. Extreme duct papillomatosis of the juvenile breast. *Acta Pathol Microbiol Scand A* 1979;87A:353–359.
30. Rosen PP. Papillary duct hyperplasia of the breast in children and young adults. *Cancer* 1985;56:1611–1617.
31. Wilson M, Cranor ML, Rosen PP. Papillary duct hyperplasia of the breast in children and young women. *Mod Pathol* 1993;6:570–574.

Papilloma and Papillary Duct Hyperplasia in Children and Young Women

32. Rosen PP. Papillary duct hyperplasia of the breast in children and young adults. *Cancer* 1985;56:1611–1617.
33. Hughes DE, Orr JD, Smith NM. Intraduct papillomatosis of the breast in a peripubertal male. *Pediatr Pathol* 1994;14:561–565.
34. Greydanus DE, Matytsina L, Gains M. Breast disorders in children and adolescents. *Prim Care* 2006;33:455–502.
35. Greydanus DE, Parks DS, Farrell EG. Breast disorders in children and adolescents. *Pediatr Clin North Am* 1989;36:601–638.
36. Harmsen S, Mayatepek E, Klee D, et al. Bloody nipple discharge (BND) in an 8 months old girl and a 9 months old male—rational diagnostic approach. *Klin Padiatr* 2010;222:79–83.
37. Rosen PP, Cantrell B, Mullen DL, et al. Juvenile papillomatosis (Swiss cheese disease) of the breast. *Am J Surg Pathol* 1980;4:3–12.
38. Wilson MP, Cranor ML, Rosen PP. Papillary duct hyperplasia of the breast in children and young women. *Mod Pathol* 1993;6:570–574.
39. Kiaer HW, Kiaer WW, Linell F, et al. Extreme duct papillomatosis of the juvenile breast. *Acta Pathol Microbiol Scand A* 1979;87A:353–359.
40. Rosen PP, Lesser ML, Kinne DW, et al. Breast carcinoma in women 35 years of age or younger. *Ann Surg* 1984;199:133–142.

Juvenile Atypical Ductal Hyperplasia

41. Eliasen CA, Cranor ML, Rosen PP. Atypical duct hyperplasia of the breast in young females. *Am J Surg Pathol* 1992;16:246–251.

Gynecomastia

42. Koshy JC, Goldberg JS, Wolfswinkel EM, et al. Breast cancer incidence in adolescent males undergoing subcutaneous mastectomy for gynecomastia: is pathologic examination justified? A retrospective and literature review. *Plast Reconstr Surg* 2011;127:1–7.
43. Akgul S, Kanbur N, Gucer S, et al. The histopathological effects of tamoxifen in the treatment of pubertal gynecomastia. *J Pediatr Endocrinol Metab* 2012;25:753–755.
44. Welch ST, Babcock DS, Ballard ET. Sonography of pediatric male breast masses: gynecomastia and beyond. *Pediatr Radiol* 2004;34:952–957.
45. Cho YR, Jones S, Gosain AK. Neurofibromatosis: a cause of prepubertal gynecomastia. *Plast Reconstr Surg* 2008;121:34e–40e.
46. Murat A, Kansiz F, Kabakus N, et al. Neurofibroma of the breast in a boy with neurofibromatosis type 1. *Clin Imaging* 2004;28:415–417.
47. Damiani S, Eusebi V. Gynecomastia in type-1 neurofibromatosis with features of pseudoangiomatous stromal hyperplasia with giant cells. Report of two cases. *Virchows Arch* 2001;438:513–516.
48. Zamecnik M, Michal M, Gogora M, et al. Gynecomastia with pseudoangiomatous stromal hyperplasia and multinucleated giant cells. Association with neurofibromatosis type 1. *Virchows Arch* 2002;441:85–87.
49. Curran JP, Coleman RO. Neurofibromata of the chest wall simulating prepubertal gynecomastia. *Clin Pediatr (Phila)* 1977;16:1064–1066.
50. Ekmez F, Pirgon O, Bilgin H, et al. Cystic hygroma of the breast in a 5 year old boy presenting as a gynecomastia. *Eur Rev Med Pharmacol Sci* 2012;16(Suppl. 4):55–57.
51. Singh O, Singh Gupta S, Upadhyaya VD, et al. Cystic lymphangioma of the breast in a 6-year-old boy. *J Pediatr Surg* 2009;44:2015–2018.
52. Gupta SS, Singh O. Cystic lymphangioma of the breast in an 8-year-old boy: report of a case with a review of the literature. *Surg Today* 2011;41:1314–1318.
53. Kavalakat AJ, Covilakam RK, Culas TB. Secretory carcinoma of breast in a 17-year-old male. *World J Surg Oncol* 2004;2:17.
54. Wilson CH, Griffith CD, Shrimankar J, et al. Gynaecomastia, neurofibromatosis and breast cancer. *Breast* 2004;13:77–79.
55. Fodor PB. Breast cancer in a patient with gynecomastia. *Plast Reconstr Surg* 1989;84:976–979.
56. Chang HL, Kish JB, Smith BL, et al. A 16-year-old male with gynecomastia and ductal carcinoma in situ. *Pediatr Surg Int* 2008;24:1251–1253.

57. Wadie GM, Banever GT, Moriarty KP, et al. Ductal carcinoma in situ in a 16-year-old adolescent boy with gynecomastia: a case report. *J Pediatr Surg* 2005;40:1349–1353.

Fibroepithelial Tumors in Children and Adolescents

58. Ross D, Giri D, Akram M, et al. Fibroepithelial lesions in the breast of adolescent females: a clinicopathological profile of 35 cases. *Modern Pathol* 2012;92(Suppl. 2):254A.
59. Bauer BS, Jones KM, Talbot CW. Mammary masses in the adolescent female. *Surg Gynecol Obstet* 1987;165:63–65.
60. Sanchez Rf, Ladino-Torres MF, Bernat JA, et al. Breast fibroadenomas in the pediatric population: common and uncommon sonographic findings. *Pediatr Radiol* 2010;40:1681–1689.
61. Liu H, Yeh ML, Lin KJ, et al. Bloody nipple discharge in an adolescent girl: unusual presentation of juvenile fibroadenoma. *Pediatr Neonatol* 2010;51:190–192.
62. Fowler CL. Spontaneous infarction of fibroadenoma in an adolescent girl. *Pediatr Radiol* 2004;34:988–990.
63. Raganoonan C, Fairbairn JK, Williams S, et al. Giant breast tumours of adolescence. *Aust N Z J Surg* 1987;57:243–247.
64. Ashikari R, Farrow JH, O'Hara J. Fibroadenomas in the breast of juveniles. *Surg Gynecol Obstet* 1971;132:259–262.
65. Kern WH, Clark RW. Retrogression of fibroadenomas of the breast. *Am J Surg* 1973;126:59–62.
66. Tagaya N, Kodaira H, Kogure H, et al. A Case of phyllodes tumor with bloody nipple discharge in juvenile patient. *Breast Cancer* 1999;6:207–210.
67. Martino A, Zamparelli M, Santinelli A, et al. Unusual clinical presentation of a rare case of phyllodes tumor of the breast in an adolescent girl. *J Pediatr Surg* 2001;36:941–943.
68. Rajan PB, Cranor ML, Rosen PP. Cystosarcoma phyllodes in adolescent girls and young women: a study of 45 patients. *Am J Surg Pathol* 1998;22:64–69.
69. Gibbs BF Jr, Roe RD, Thomas DF. Malignant cystosarcoma phyllodes in a pre-pubertal female. *Ann Surg* 1968;167:229–231.
70. Hoover HC, Trestioreanu A, Ketcham AS. Metastatic cystosarcoma phylloides in an adolescent girl: an unusually malignant tumor. *Ann Surg* 1975;181:279–282.
71. Leveque J, Meunier B, Wattier E, et al. Malignant cystosarcomas phyllodes of the breast in adolescent females. *Eur J Obstet Gynecol Reprod Biol* 1994;54:197–203.
72. Roisman I, BarakV, Robinson E, et al. Breast malignancies in adolescents in Israel (1967-1989). *Breast Dis* 1992;5:149–168.
73. Baker M, Chen H, Latchaw L, et al. Pseudoangiomatous stromal hyperplasia of the breast in a 10-year-old girl. *J Pediatr Surg* 2011;46:e27–e31.
74. Shehata BM, Fishman I, Collings MH, et al. Pseudoangiomatous stromal hyperplasia of the breast in pediatric patients: an underrecognized entity. *Pediatr Dev Pathol* 2009;12:450–454.

Carcinoma and Other Malignant Tumors in Children and Adolescents

75. Pettinato GC, Manivel JC, Kelly DR, et al. Lesions of the breast in children exclusive of typical fibroadenoma and gynecomastia. A clinicopathologic study of 113 cases. *Pathol Annu* 1989;24(Pt. 2):296–328.
76. Ashikari H, Jun MY, Farrow JH, et al. Breast carcinoma in children and adolescents. *Clin Bull* 1977;7:55–62.
77. Hammer B. Childhood breast carcinoma: a report of a case. *J Pediatr Surg* 1981;16:77–78.
78. Munoz F, Fernandez E, Varela De Urgarte A. Cancer de mama en una nina de 6 anos. *Rev Clin Esp* 1980;159:289–290.
79. Yamaguchi R, Tanaka M, Yamaguchi M, et al. Pleomorphic carcinoma of the breast in a 17-year-old woman. *Med Mol Morphol* 2010;43:43–47.
80. Delanote S, Van den Broecke R, Schelfhout VR, et al. Adenoid cystic carcinoma of the breast in a 19-year-old girl. *Breast* 2003;12:75–77.
81. Buchino JJ, Moore GD, Bond SJ. Secretory carcinoma in a 9-year-old girl. *Diagn Cytopathol* 2004;31:430–431.
82. Murphy JJ, Morzaria S, Gow KW, et al. Breast cancer in a 6-year-old child. *J Pediatr Surg* 2000;35:765–767.
83. Tadesse A, Tesfaye W, Hailemariam B. Breast carcinoma in a 7-years-old girl. *Ethiop Med J* 2012;50:89–94.
84. Yorozuya K, Takahashi E, Kousaka J, et al. A case of estrogen receptor positive secretory carcinoma in a 9-year-old girl with ETV6-NTRK3 fusion gene. *Jpn J Clin Oncol* 2012;42:208–211.
85. Vesoulis Z, Kashkari S. Fine needle aspiration of secretory breast carcinoma resembling lactational changes. A case report. *Acta Cytol* 1998;42:1032–1036.
86. Byrne MP, Fahey MM, Gooselaw JG. Breast cancer with axillary metastasis in an eight and one-half-year-old girl. *Cancer* 1973;31:726–728.
87. Longo OA, Mosto A, Moran JC, et al. Breast carcinoma in childhood and adolescence: case report and review of the literature. *Breast J* 1999;5:65–69.
88. Close MB, Maximov NG. Carcinoma of breast in young girls. *Arch Surg* 1965;91:386–389.
89. Deutsch M, Altomare FJ Jr, Mastrian AS, et al. Carcinoma of the male breast following thymic irradiation. *Radiology* 1975;116:413–414.
90. Lowell DM, Martineau RG, Luria SB. Carcinoma of the male breast following radiation. Report of a case occurring 35 years after radiation therapy of unilateral prepubertal gynecomastia. *Cancer* 1968;22:585–586.
91. Rogers DA, Lobe TE, Rao BN, et al. Breast malignancy in children. *J Pediatr Surg* 1994;29:48–51.
92. Tefft M, Vawter GF, Mitus A. Second primary neoplasms in children. *Am J Roentgenol Radium Ther Nucl Med* 1968;103:800–822.
93. Yahalom J, Petrek JA, Biddinger PW, et al. Breast cancer in patients irradiated for Hodgkin's disease: a clinical and pathologic analysis of 45 events in 37 patients. *J Clin Oncol* 1992;10:1674–1681.
94. Cutuli B, Borel C, Dhermain F, et al. Breast cancer occurred after treatment for Hodgkin's disease: analysis of 133 cases. *Radiother Oncol* 2001;59:247–255.
95. Corpron CA, Black CT, Singletary SE, et al. Breast cancer in adolescent females. *J Pediatr Surg* 1995;30:322–324.
96. Nichini FM, Goldman L, Lapayowker MS, et al. Inflammatory carcinoma of the breast in a 12-year-old girl. *Arch Surg* 1972;105:505–508.
97. Ramirez G, Ansfield FJ. Carcinoma of the breast in children. *Arch Surg* 1968;96:222–225.
98. Ackerman BL, Otis C, Stueber K. Lobular carcinoma in situ in a 15-year-old girl: a case report and review of the literature. *Plast Reconstr Surg* 1994;94:714–718.
99. Howarth CB, Caces JN, Pratt CB. Breast metastases in children with rhabdomyosarcoma. *Cancer* 1980;46:2520–2524.
100. D'Angelo P, Carli M, Ferrari A, et al. Breast metastases in children and adolescents with rhabdomyosarcoma: experience of the Italian Soft Tissue Sarcoma Committee. *Pediatr Blood Cancer* 2010;55:1306–1309.
101. Nogi H, Kobayashi T, Kawase K, et al. Primary rhabdomyosarcoma of the breast in a 13-year-old girl: report of a case. *Surg Today* 2007;37:38–42.
102. Yang WT, Hennessy BT, Dryden MJ, et al. Mammary angiosarcomas: imaging findings in 24 patients. *Radiology* 2007;242:725–734.
103. van Geel AN, den Bakker MA. Bilateral angiosarcoma of the breast in a fourteen-year-old child. *Rare Tumors* 2009;1:e38.

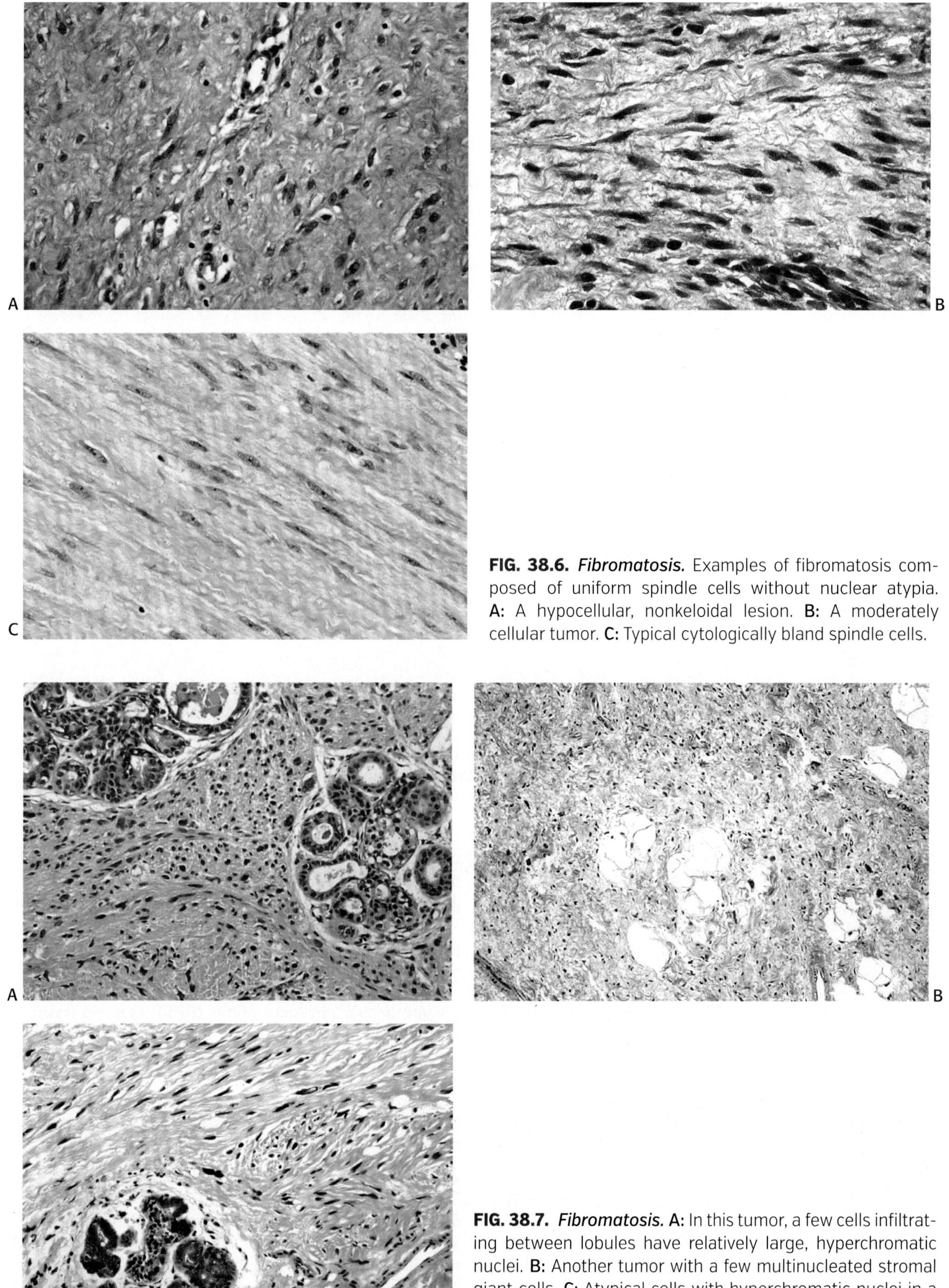

FIG. 38.6. ***Fibromatosis.*** Examples of fibromatosis composed of uniform spindle cells without nuclear atypia. **A:** A hypocellular, nonkeloidal lesion. **B:** A moderately cellular tumor. **C:** Typical cytologically bland spindle cells.

FIG. 38.7. ***Fibromatosis.*** **A:** In this tumor, a few cells infiltrating between lobules have relatively large, hyperchromatic nuclei. **B:** Another tumor with a few multinucleated stromal giant cells. **C:** Atypical cells with hyperchromatic nuclei in a specimen from a 17-year-old girl.

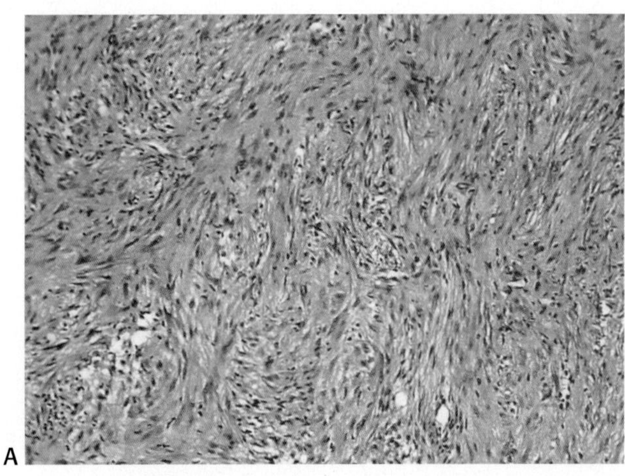

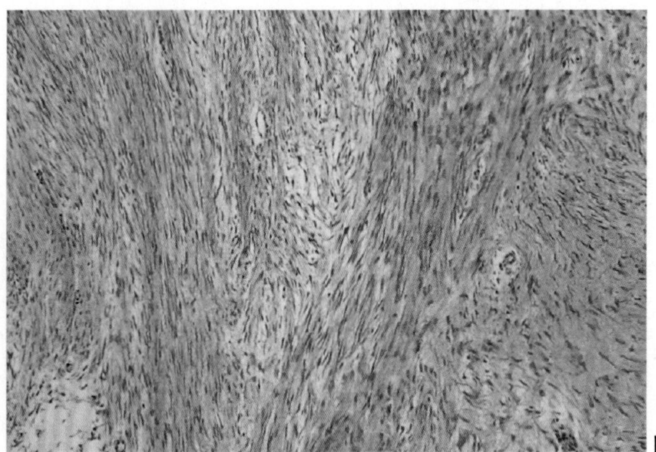

FIG. 38.8. ***Fibromatosis.*** **A:** Storiform pattern. **B:** Interlacing bundles of cells and collagen in a herringbone pattern.

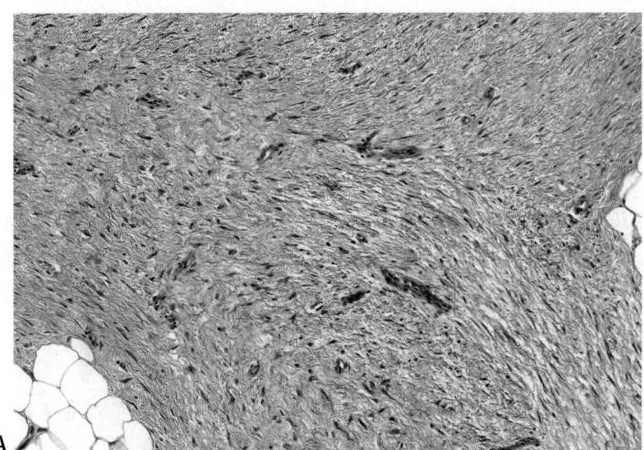

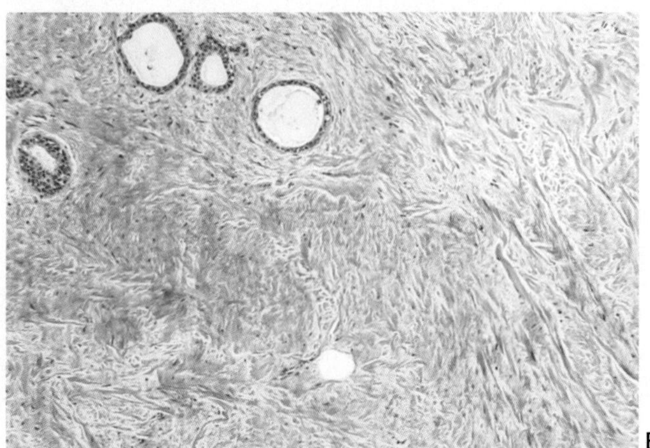

FIG. 38.9. ***Fibromatosis, myxoid.*** **A:** Fibromatosis with myxoid stroma. **B:** Basophilic stromal ground substance is unusually prominent in this example of fibromatosis, which surrounds cystic lobular glands.

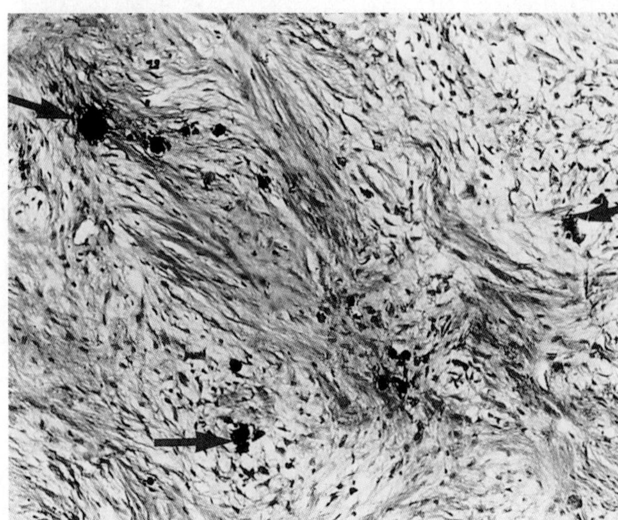

FIG. 38.10. ***Fibromatosis, myxoid with calcifications.*** The irregular *black* granular bodies (*arrows*) are calcifications present in myxoid and collagenous regions.

described as "limited in cellularity" or "scanty." The specimen consists of small uniform spindle cells dispersed singly or in groups, which may be clusters or relatively flat sheets. The spindle cells, largely devoid of cytoplasm, are represented by "naked" nuclei. Epithelial cells in groups and sheets and lymphocytes may be found in the background. The differential diagnosis of such an FNA specimen includes FA and benign phyllodes tumor (BPT). Features favoring the diagnosis of fibromatosis are a sparse or absent epithelial component relative to the number of stromal cells and the virtual absence of flat sheets of epithelium commonly found in a fibroepithelial tumor. In most instances, IHC and excisional biopsy are necessary to exclude other lesions such as metaplastic carcinoma.[35]

Differential Diagnosis

Several lesions must be considered in the differential diagnosis of mammary fibromatosis. Some examples of spindle cell metaplastic carcinoma have readily identified squamous or carcinomatous components, but others are virtually devoid

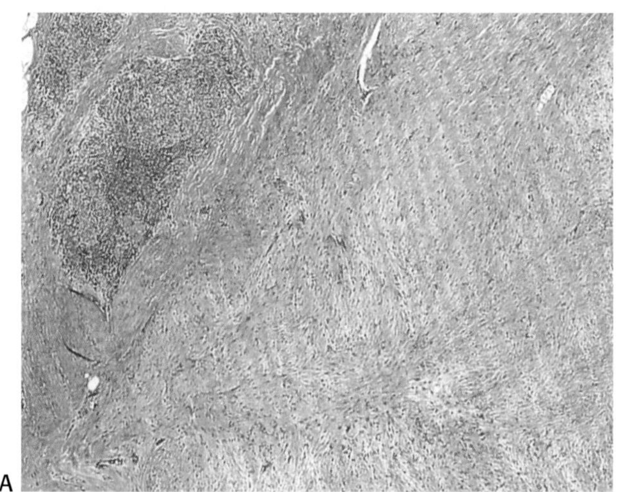

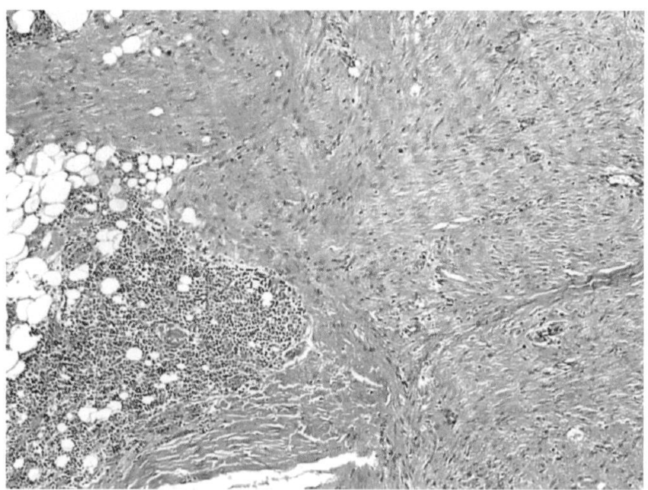

FIG. 38.11. ***Fibromatosis, lymphocytic aggregates.*** **A:** A circumscribed lymphocytic nodule with germinal center formation is present at the edge of the tumor. **B:** An ill-defined lymphocytic infiltrate.

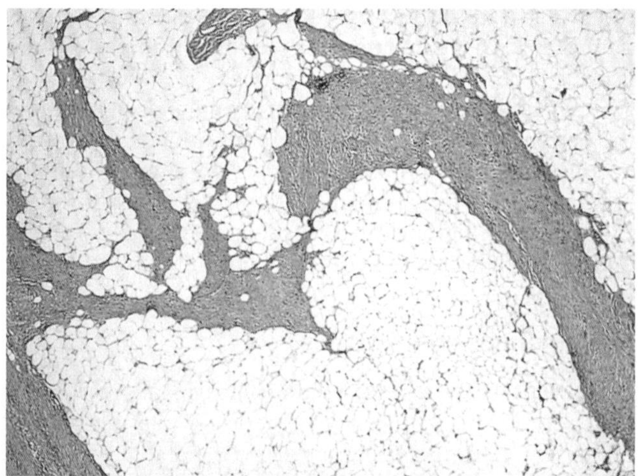

FIG. 38.12. ***Fibromatosis, invasive border.*** Slender tentacles of tumor extending into mammary fat are shown.

of epithelial elements. One feature favoring metaplastic carcinoma is a highly cellular and pleomorphic spindle cell component with mitoses, whereas desmoid-like foci and lymphoid aggregates suggest fibromatosis. An inflammatory reaction, which may be predominantly lymphocytic, occurs more diffusely in and around most metaplastic carcinomas than it does in fibromatosis. Immunoreactivity for proteins such as CK, p63, and CD10 characterizes metaplastic carcinoma, whereas current evidence suggests that nuclear reactivity for β-catenin favors, but is not specific for, fibromatosis. Conversely, absence of β-catenin reactivity does not exclude the diagnosis of fibromatosis.

The distinction between fibromatosis and high-grade fibrosarcoma, or undifferentiated "stromal sarcoma," is determined on the basis of cellularity, cytologic pleomorphism, and especially mitotic activity. Although a mitotic rate of 3 per 10 HPFs has been described in fibromatosis, this is exceptional and such a lesion is more likely to be a

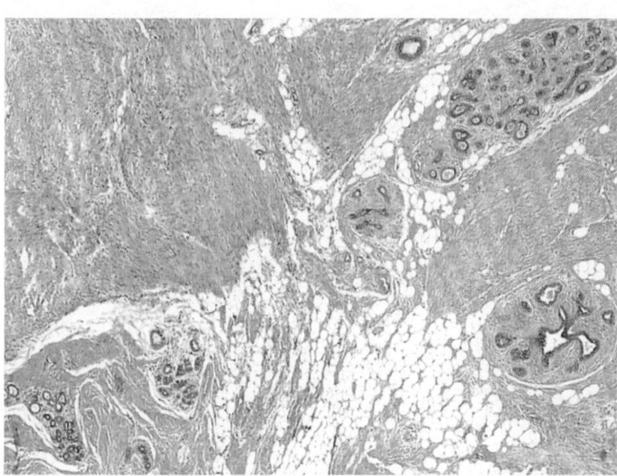

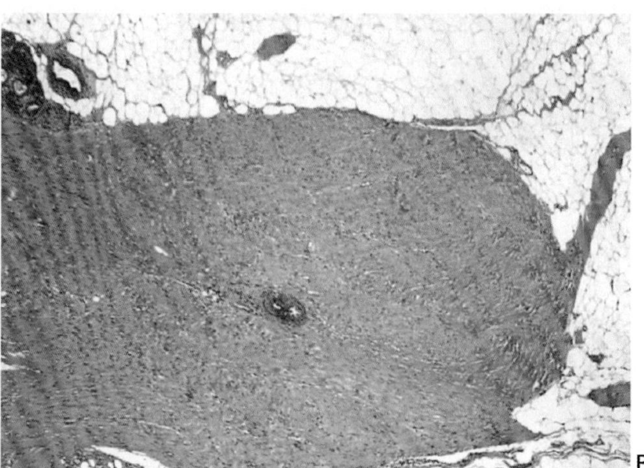

FIG. 38.13. ***Fibromatosis, invasive border.*** **A:** The tumor engulfs lobules and ducts. **B:** A small duct surrounded by fibromatosis. **C:** The tumor (*left*) blends with fibrous mammary stroma (*right*). There is no clear demarcation between the tumor and normal stroma. **D:** An atrophic lobule (*lower right*) is surrounded by fibromatosis.

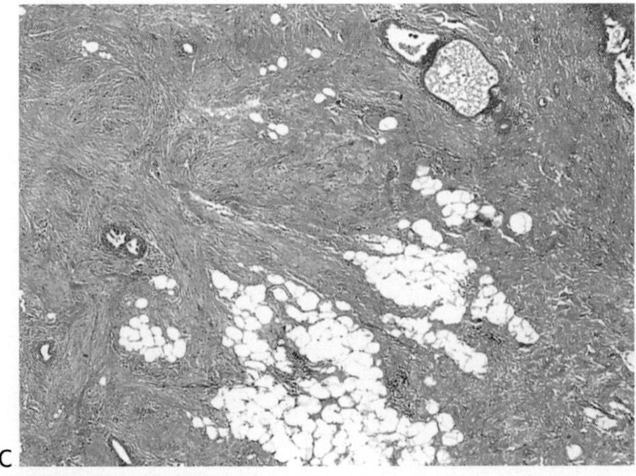

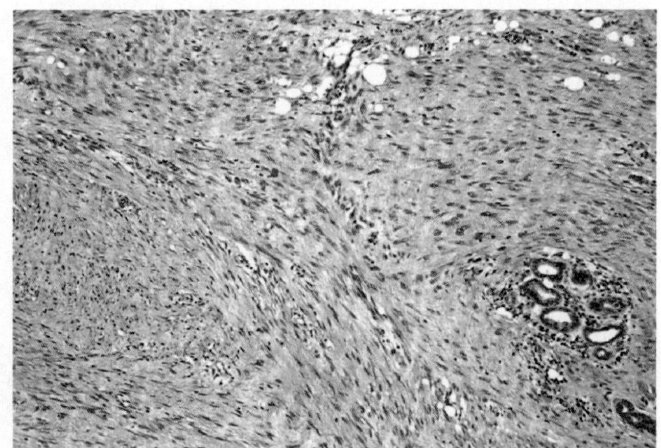

FIG. 38.13. *(Continued)*

low-grade sarcoma. Typically the mitotic rate does not exceed 1 per 10 HPFs, and usually no mitoses can be found. Nuclear reactivity for Ki67 is very much lower in fibromatosis than in spindle cell sarcoma or metaplastic carcinoma.

A lesion reported to be "the first described case of ossifying fibromatosis" in the breast was not well characterized and lacked follow-up.[37] The histologic appearance illustrated would be compatible with metaplastic carcinoma containing an osseous heterologous component.

Another neoplasm in the differential diagnosis is fibrous histiocytoma. Although mammary fibromatosis may have storiform areas, this is rarely a prominent pattern. Epithelioid, histiocytic, and multinucleated cells often found in fibrous histiocytoma are not features of fibromatosis.

Reparative and reactive processes can simulate the appearance of fibromatosis. Scars from healed fat necrosis, remote trauma, and surgery must be distinguished from fibromatosis. Calcifications are more likely to be associated with fat necrosis, but rarely they can occur in fibromatosis. Foreign body granulomas, sometimes with partly absorbed suture material, are an indication of prior surgery. If the patient has recurrent fibromatosis, reparative changes caused by an earlier operation may mingle with recurrent tumor, further complicating the diagnosis. Lymphoid infiltrates that commonly occur in fibromatosis should not lead to the erroneous diagnosis of an inflammatory condition such as nodular fasciitis. The inflammatory component of fibromatosis is typically limited to isolated separate lymphoid aggregates at the periphery of the lesion. In fasciitis, inflammatory cells are dispersed more diffusely at the periphery and within the lesion, although localized areas of inflammation also occur. "Myoid" and multinucleated cells characteristically found in nodular fasciitis are not a feature of fibromatosis.[38]

Immunohistochemistry

Nuclear localization of β-catenin is a surrogate marker for Wnt pathway activation and is seen in a high proportion of somatic fibromatosis tumors, both sporadic and those associated with FAP (Fig. 38.15). Bhattacharya et al.[39] found nuclear β-catenin reactivity in each of 21 examples of "deep"

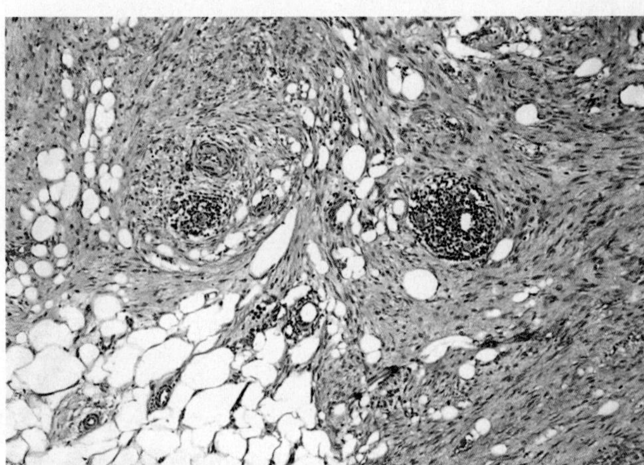

FIG. 38.14. ***Fibromatosis.*** The presence of focal lymphocytic infiltrates favors a diagnosis of fibromatosis over BPT.

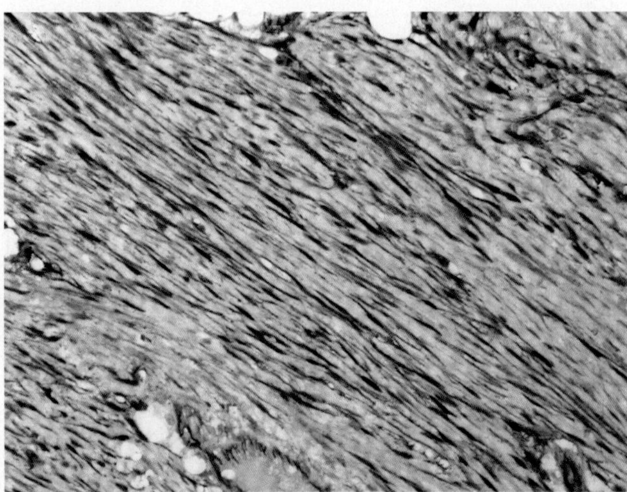

FIG. 38.15. ***Fibromatosis, β-catenin protein.*** Immunohistochemical staining demonstrates nuclear localization of β-catenin. Cytoplasmic reactivity is also present.

fibromatosis, none of which involved the breast, with the degree of positivity ranging from 10% to 90% of tumor cell nuclei. In contrast, 67 other spindle cell lesions that might be considered in the differential diagnosis showed variable cytoplasmic but no nuclear reactivity for β-catenin. Among 53 examples of mammary fibromatosis pooled from three series,[5,19,40] 83% demonstrated nuclear β-catenin reactivity.[5,19,40] The majority showed diffuse and intense nuclear staining, although occasional tumors demonstrated only focal reactivity.[5] β-Catenin accumulated in tumor cell nuclei but not in the nuclei of normal stromal cells or epithelial cells. Balzer and Weiss[24] found focal nuclear β-catenin reactivity in two examples of mammary fibromatosis associated with breast implants.

Others have questioned the specificity of β-catenin nuclear reactivity for the diagnosis of fibromatosis. Amary et al.[41] reported finding *β-catenin* mutations in 87% of 76 examples of desmoid-type fibromatosis and no comparable mutations in 39 fibromatosis-like spindle cell lesions, including low-grade fibromyxoid sarcoma, solitary fibrous tumor, and nodular fasciitis. When tested by IHC, all of the examples of fibromatosis exhibited nuclear reactivity for β-catenin but so did 72% of the fibromatosis-like lesions. Further evidence that β-catenin nuclear reactivity is not specific for fibromatosis was reported by Carlson and Fletcher,[42] who found β-catenin nuclear expression in 80% of sporadic fibromatosis tumors, 67% of examples of FAP-associated fibromatosis, 56% of superficial fibromatosis tumors, and in 5% to 30% of nonfibromatosis spindle cell tumors. In the breast, β-catenin nuclear reactivity has been observed in spindle cell metaplastic carcinomas and the stromal cells of phyllodes tumors and FAs. Twenty-three percent of spindle cell metaplastic carcinomas, 72% to 87% of phyllodes tumors, and 70% to 100% of FAs are reported to show nuclear localization of β-catenin.[19,40,43,44] The staining intensity is variable but can be moderate to strong, particularly in fibroepithelial tumors.

The spindle cells of fibromatosis are virtually never reactive for CD34. They are variably reactive for actin and desmin. Anecdotal observations suggest that actin and desmin reactivities may be more common in subcutaneous than in parenchymal fibromatosis. The tumor cells are negative for CK. Mammary fibromatosis is usually negative for ER-α and PR.[4,31]

Electron Microscopy

Electron microscopic studies of mammary fibromatosis have been reported.[9,32,36] Many cells contain bundles of microfilaments with dense bodies. The spindle cells are predominantly fibroblasts with lesser numbers of myofibroblasts.

Molecular Studies

In a study of 32 examples of sporadic mammary fibromatosis and one FAP-associated tumor, Abraham et al.[5] found mutations in exon 3 of the *β-catenin* gene in 15 tumors (45%). Somatic APC alterations (mutation, 5q allelic loss, or both) were identified in 11 of the remaining tumors (33%). Overall, 79% harbored alterations in either the β-catenin or *APC* gene. In another study, Kim et al.[19] found mutations in exon 3 of the *β-catenin* gene in 9 of 12 (75%) sporadic mammary fibromatosis tumors. In both studies, the most common alterations in the *β-catenin* gene were 1-bp missense mutations in codon 41, which encodes a GSK-3β phosphorylation site that is important for β-catenin protein degradation.

Treatment and Prognosis

Recommended treatment is wide local excision. Because of the ill-defined character of most lesions, it is difficult to judge the adequacy of margins intraoperatively by inspection or frozen section. The excision specimen should be inked and the margins sampled generously. When a tumor is adherent to fascia, muscle, or skin, the excision should be extended to include the affected area, and it may be necessary to perform a mastectomy to achieve adequate margins of resection for a bulky tumor. In many cases, the nature of the tumor has not been established prior to surgery, and the surgeon does not anticipate the need for a particularly generous margin. The frequency of local recurrence ranges from 21% to 29%.[1–3,6] Although the risk of recurrence is higher in patients with positive margins,[3,6] recurrences have been observed in cases with apparently negative margins. Not all patients with positive margins develop recurrences, and there have been unusual instances in which locally advanced lesions stabilized or regressed after incomplete excision.[1] Most recurrences occur within 3 years of diagnosis, but in a few instances they were not detected for nearly a decade. Multiple recurrences have been documented in some cases.[6] Histologic features such as cellularity, mitotic activity, and cellular pleomorphism are not helpful for predicting recurrence.

Immediate reexcision of the biopsy site should be considered if the initial biopsy was small and margins are positive, especially for lesions located deep in the breast or peripherally near the chest wall. Recurrences at these sites may be difficult to control and are best avoided (Fig. 38.16). On the other hand, follow-up is preferable to reexcision of relatively

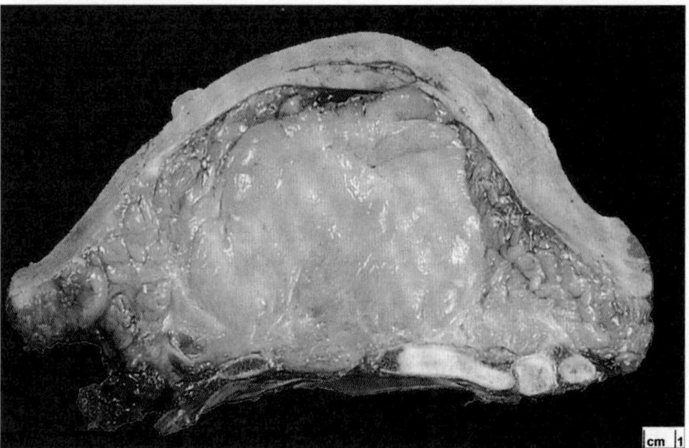

FIG. 38.16. ***Fibromatosis, chest wall invasion.*** Recurrent fibromatosis forming a distinct tumor that occupies most of the breast and invades the chest wall between the ribs.

superficial lesions or subareolar fibromatosis, which might require excision of the nipple. Radiotherapy has been useful as an adjunct to surgery for primary treatment or to control large or extensive recurrences in patients with nonmammary fibromatosis.[45] Radiotherapy is not an established modality for the treatment of mammary fibromatosis.

There are several reports of attempts to employ hormonal treatment for fibromatosis. Administration of an antiestrogen such as tamoxifen alone or in combination with an anti-inflammatory agent has resulted in remission in some patients with nonmammary fibromatosis.[46–50] One review found a complete or partial response rate of 50%, a disease stabilization rate of 30%, and a disease progression rate of 20% in 141 cases in the literature.[51] Response of nonmammary fibromatosis to tamoxifen is manifested as a slow reduction in tumor size, which may not become evident until after therapy has been stopped. The effect of tamoxifen on mammary fibromatosis has not been well-documented, although individual cases with marked reduction in tumor size or complete clinical response have been reported.[6,52]

Chemotherapy has been used successfully to treat "deep" nonmammary fibromatosis, which was unresectable or recurrent.[53,54] Gega et al.[55] reported complete responses in three patients and partial responses in four patients treated with doxorubicin-based combination chemotherapy for unresectable FAP–associated fibromatosis. Chemotherapy such as this might be considered for a patient with primary or recurrent mammary fibromatosis with demonstrated unresectable invasion of the chest wall, axilla, or supraclavicular region.

NODULAR FASCIITIS

Nodular fasciitis is a benign reactive fibroblastic and myofibroblastic proliferation. Although it is a common tumor-like lesion of the soft tissues, it only rarely occurs in the breast. It should be distinguished from spindle cell carcinoma with a fasciitis-like appearance, which is more common at this site, and from fibromatosis.

Clinical Presentation

Nodular fasciitis of the breast occurs in both females and males. Patients' ages range from 15 to 84 years.[56,57] Most present with a palpable firm mass of short duration, often with a history of rapid enlargement. Prior trauma is usually not reported.

The radiographic findings are often suspicious for carcinoma. Mammography demonstrates a high-density mass with spiculated or irregular margins, and ultrasonography reveals a hypoechoic mass with irregular borders.[58–60] Magnetic resonance imaging (MRI) performed in one case showed high contrast enhancement suggestive of malignancy.[61]

Gross Pathology

In a literature review by Squillaci et al.,[60] reported examples ranged from 1 to 7 cm, with an average size of 2.4 cm. The lesions are firm with white-gray cut surfaces. Gelatinous areas may be observed.

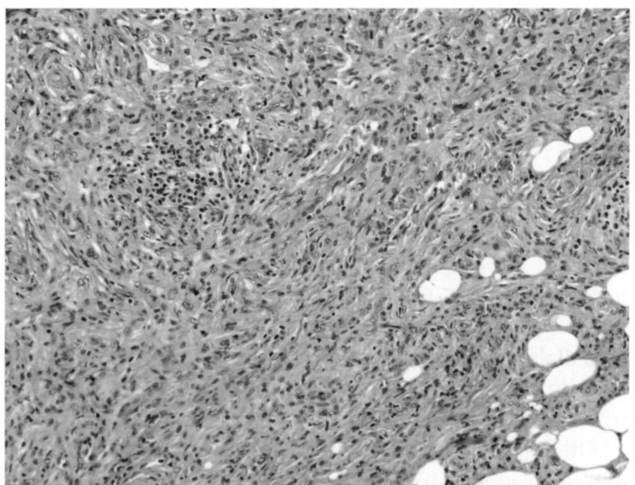

FIG. 38.17. ***Nodular fasciitis.*** Loose storiform proliferation of bland spindle cells with scattered inflammatory cells and extravasated red blood cells.

Microscopic Pathology

The proliferative spindle cells form short bundles and fascicles that are randomly dispersed in a loose myxoid background. The appearance is often described as having a feathery or tissue culture–like quality. Older lesions show greater collagenization. The spindle cells have bipolar to oval nuclei with delicate chromatin and small nucleoli; atypia is lacking. Cellularity is high in early lesions, and mitotic activity may be brisk. Inflammatory cells (Fig. 38.17), extravasated red blood cells, and prominent thin-walled vessels are present within the lesion. The borders are irregular, and benign ducts and lobules can become entrapped in the proliferation but are usually absent.

Cytology

FNA biopsy yields single cells, sheets, and stromal tissue fragments composed of uniform fusiform fibroblasts.[56,62] Nuclei are round to oval and have delicate chromatin with inconspicuous nuclei. Lymphocytes, red blood cells, multinucleated giant cells, and myxoid material are present in the background. Epithelial cells are usually absent.

Differential Diagnosis

Spindle cell carcinoma can closely mimic the appearance of nodular fasciitis. The presence of nuclear atypia, clustered cell aggregates, or *in situ* carcinoma favors a diagnosis of spindle cell carcinoma. Some spindle cell carcinomas, however, may appear cytologically bland or lack overt epithelial differentiation. IHC can be diagnostically helpful since spindle cell carcinoma usually demonstrates at least some reactivity for one or more CKs and p63. Fibromatosis is characterized by longer, sweeping fascicles and greater infiltration, and nuclear reactivity for β-catenin is present in most cases. Myofibroblastoma demonstrates more defined fascicles intermixed with conspicuous bands of bright eosinophilic collagen, is usually sharply circumscribed, and is positive for CD34. The absence of nuclear atypia and pleomorphism in nodular fasciitis helps to distinguish it from sarcoma.

Immunohistochemistry

The spindle cells in nodular fasciitis are positive for smooth muscle actin (SMA) and MSA.[63] They are negative for nuclear β-catenin[64] and CD34. The cells are typically negative for keratin,[63] but Barak et al.[65] observed rare keratin AE1/3-positive spindle cells in 3 of 35 (9%) examples of nodular fasciitis derived largely from the extremities; no staining for CK5 was observed.

Molecular Studies

Recurrent genomic rearrangements of the *USP6* locus were identified in 44 of 48 examples of nodular fasciitis from various sites studied by Erickson-Johnson et al.[66] In 31 of the lesions, the novel fusion gene *MYH9–USP6* was formed. Four lesions were negative for rearrangements of both *USP6* and *MYH9* loci, including the one case in the series of nodular fasciitis arising in the breast.

Treatment and Prognosis

Nodular fasciitis is a benign, self-limited process. Stanley et al.[67] reported a case of mammary nodular fasciitis with spontaneous regression after FNA. Brown and Carty[58] described a 7-cm breast mass in a 65-year-old woman, which markedly decreased in size after core biopsy and resolved within 6 months of presentation. Nevertheless, excision is recommended for lesions sampled by core biopsy or FNA because of the morphologic overlap with more clinically significant mammary tumors such as spindle cell carcinoma. Recurrence after surgical excision is rare.

FIBROUS TUMOR

This condition presents as a discrete breast mass composed of collagenized mammary stroma. It was first characterized by Haagensen[68] as fibrous disease. Other names that have been given to this entity include fibrous mastopathy,[69] fibrosis of the breast,[70] and focal fibrous disease.[71] Because of the clinical presentation as a distinct mass, the term "fibrous tumor" is preferable to distinguish it from more frequent nonspecific and involutional stromal changes.[72] A few tumors illustrated and described as focal fibrous disease[71] and fibrous tumor[72] appear to be examples of pseudoangiomatous stromal hyperplasia (PASH). Some lesions sampled by needle core biopsy that are diagnosed as "focal fibrosis" probably represent examples of fibrous tumor.[73]

Clinical Presentation

Fibrous tumor is a disease of premenopausal women. On palpation, it is a firm-to-hard, distinct tumor measuring 2 to 5 cm. Skin retraction and dimpling are not evident. Mammography reveals an area of density with borders varying from irregular to smooth. Calcifications are usually not a feature of fibrous tumor,[74] but they have been reported in one example.[75]

Harvey et al.[76] studied 14 patients with "fibrous nodules," which appear to correspond histologically to fibrous tumors. Ten patients (71%) were premenopausal. Three of the four postmenopausal women were receiving hormone replacement therapy. Twelve women had nonpalpable mammographically detected tumors. One woman had synchronous bilateral nonpalpable lesions. On mammograms, 11 of 13 nonpalpable tumors were round or oval, 6 of the 11 had circumscribed margins, and 5 had indistinct borders. Two tumors had irregular shapes and spiculated margins.

Revelon et al.[77] described the imaging findings in a series of patients with a histologic diagnosis of "focal fibrosis" of the breast. Seventeen with "mass-like" lesions appear to correspond most closely to fibrous tumor. Mammography revealed a mass in seven cases, six had an asymmetric density, one had architectural distortion, and three were not visualized. Ultrasound examination performed in 13 cases detected a mass in 9, shadowing without a mass in 2, and no lesion in 2.

Gross Pathology

Fibrous tumor forms a firm-to-hard mass (Fig. 38.18) ranging from 0.5 to 5 cm (mean, 2 to 3 cm).[69,72,74,76] The extent of the lesion can be appreciated on palpation by the operating surgeon, and the excised specimen typically has the appearance of a discrete tumor. The cut surface of the bisected tumor reveals white, homogeneous rubbery tissue.

Microscopic Pathology

Histologically, fibrous tumor consists of collagenous stroma that contains markedly decreased or absent ductal and lobular elements, which are atrophic (Fig. 38.18). Capillaries, other vascular structures, and nerves are very sparse; perivascular and perilobular inflammatory infiltrates are absent. Cysts, apocrine metaplasia, SA, and duct hyperplasia are not features of fibrous tumor. The diagnosis of fibrous tumor may be suggested if a needle core biopsy sample from a nonpalpable, relatively discrete mammographically detected lesion consists of hypocellular collagenous tissue devoid of glandular structures.

Molecular Studies

Cytogenetic analysis of a lesion reported to be a fibrous tumor in a 26-year-old woman revealed a clonal translocation in mesenchymal cells which was characterized as t(4;14)(q24–25;q24.3).[78] The histologic features illustrated in this report, however, are best interpreted as PASH.

Treatment and Prognosis

Fibrous tumor is a benign, self-limited stromal proliferation adequately treated by local excision.

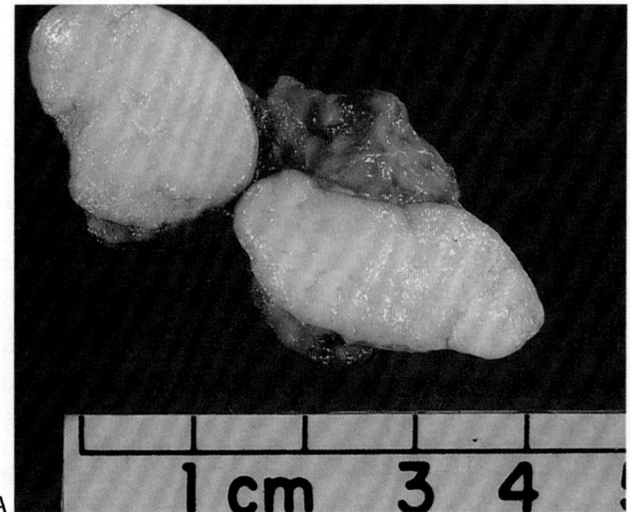

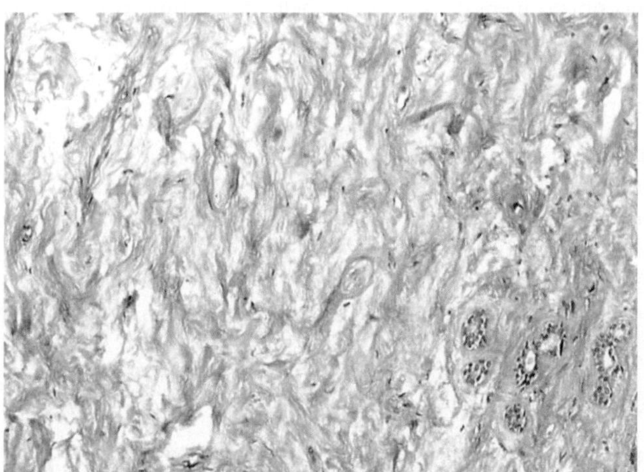

FIG. 38.18. *Fibrous tumor.* **A:** A circumscribed white tumor. **B:** An atrophic lobule is present in the collagenous stroma that contains scattered fibroblasts.

PSEUDOANGIOMATOUS HYPERPLASIA OF MAMMARY STROMA

PASH is a benign stromal proliferation characterized by the formation of slit-like spaces within dense collagenous stroma. It is a frequent incidental microscopic finding, but on occasion it can form a clinically or radiographically detected mass. The term "pseudoangiomatous" was proposed to emphasize the fact that the histologic pattern mimics, but does not actually constitute, a vasoformative proliferation. The presence of myoid differentiation in examples of PASH has led some authors to classify certain examples as hamartomas.[79,80] This is an inappropriate use of the term "hamartoma" defined as "a benign tumor or tumor-like lesion composed of one or more tissues, normal to the organ but abnormally mixed and overgrown."[81] PASH is a lesion formed by myofibroblasts with variable expression of myoid and fibroblastic features. Glandular hyperplasia is sometimes also present.

Clinical Presentation

With rare exceptions, reported examples of tumor-forming PASH have been in females. The age at diagnosis ranges from 3 to 86 years, and the mean age ranges from 37 to 51 years in several series.[82–92] The vast majority of patients are premenopausal women. Tumoral PASH is distinctly less common in postmenopausal women, and when it does occur, patients often have a history of hormone replacement therapy.[84,86,87] Rare examples of mass-forming PASH have been described in children and adolescents.[89,91,93] One of the youngest patients was 3-year-old male, who had a 5.5-cm right breast tumor.[89] Singh et al.[93] described a menarchal 12-year-old girl with marked bilateral breast enlargement due to PASH.

Most women have a palpable, painless, unilateral mass that is firm or rubbery. Any part of the breast can be affected, including the nipple–areolar complex,[94] although there is a predilection for the upper outer quadrant.[90] Rare examples are located in the axillary tail.[87] Occasional patients have had asynchronous or concurrent bilateral PASH. Diffuse breast enlargement is seen rarely, and rapid growth of the lesion may occur. One patient presented with unilateral mildly painful breast enlargement with *peau d'orange* change suggesting inflammatory carcinoma.[95] *Peau d'orange* change and skin necrosis have been observed in patients who have massive breast enlargement due to PASH during pregnancy (Fig. 38.19).

Although most women present with a clinically palpable mass, PASH has been detected by mammography in patients who are asymptomatic[96,97] Recent studies show an increasing number of radiographically detected examples

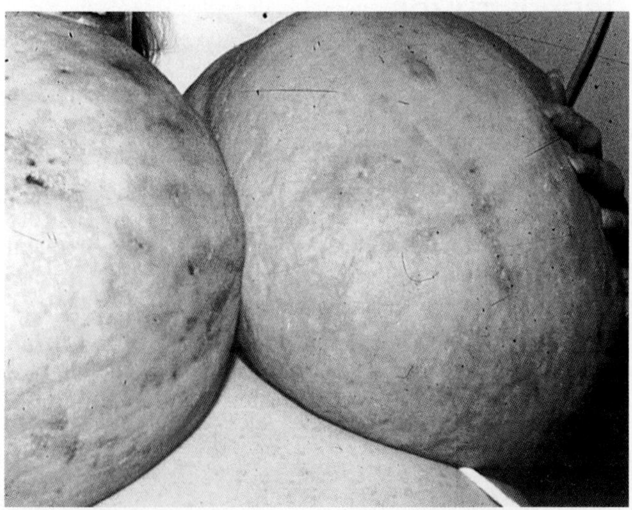

FIG. 38.19. *Pseudoangiomatous stromal hyperplasia.* This patient developed massive breast enlargement during pregnancy. A biopsy revealed diffuse PASH.

when compared to older series.[86,87,90,91] The lesion presents on mammography as a mass without calcification or, less frequently, as a focal asymmetric density.[91,98] The borders of the mass are usually smooth, but a minority of tumors have spiculated or ill-defined margins sometimes obscured by surrounding tissue. Ultrasound examination reveals a well-defined hypoechoic mass.[86,97] MRI often demonstrates focal or segmental clumped enhancement.[91] Clinically asymptomatic PASH detected by mammography may occur in postmenopausal patients, whereas palpable lesions are almost always found in premenopausal women or in postmenopausal women who have been treated with hormone replacement therapy.

PASH is a frequent incidental component of gynecomastia, having been found in 44 (47.4%) of 93 consecutive male breast biopsies, among which 43 of the 44 specimens with PASH exhibited gynecomastia.[99] Milanezi et al.[100] found PASH in 21 (23.8%) of 88 cases of gynecomastia. One exceptional case report described the finding of PASH in rapidly growing gynecomastia in the axillary breast tissue of a 39-year-old man.[101] Gynecomastia-like hyperplasia of the female breast has been described in a renal transplantation patient during cyclosporin treatment.[102] The published images suggest florid PASH, and the breast lesion regressed after cyclosporin was discontinued. Baildam et al.[103] described a series of patients who developed multiple, often bilateral, breast tumors while being treated with cyclosporin after renal transplantation. The lesions were described clinically as "fibroadenomas," but were not biopsied, and these might represent other examples of gynecomastia-like hyperplasia in this setting.

Gross Pathology

In patients with localized PASH, the excised tumors are well-demarcated, and the smooth external surfaces sometimes resemble capsules. The tumors measure less than 1 to 15 cm in greatest dimension and average about 5 cm (Fig. 38.20). Postmenopausal patients tend to have smaller tumors than premenopausal patients.[92] The cut surface usually consists of homogeneous fibrous tan, gray, or white tissue, occasionally containing cysts up to 1 cm in diameter. A small number of the tumors are grossly nodular (Fig. 38.20). Hemorrhage and necrosis are not seen except in tumors subjected to needle biopsy or aspiration.

Microscopic Pathology

In hematoxylin and eosin (H&E)–stained sections, the tumors are composed of intermixed stromal and epithelial

A

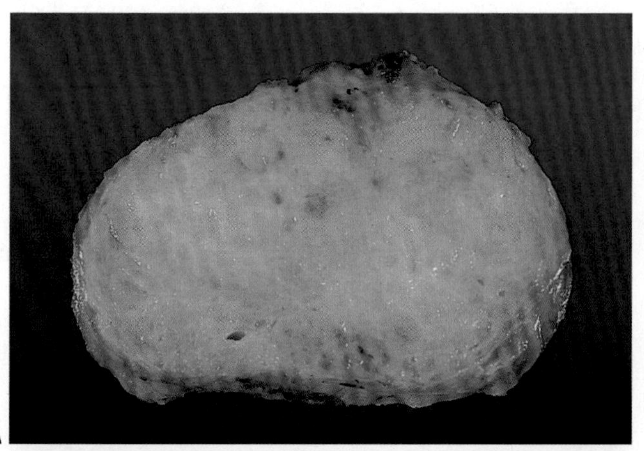

B

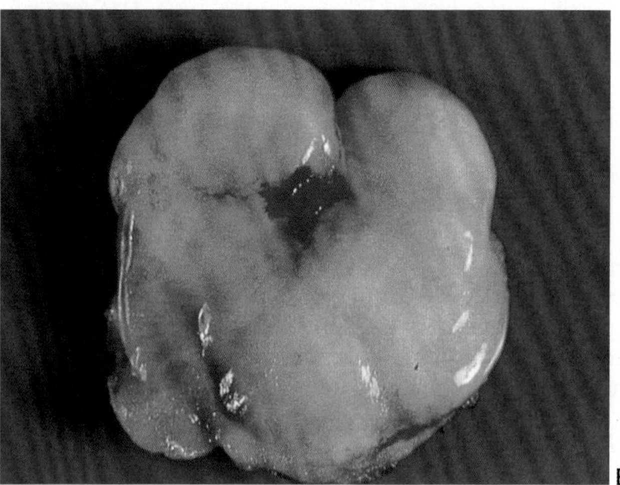

C

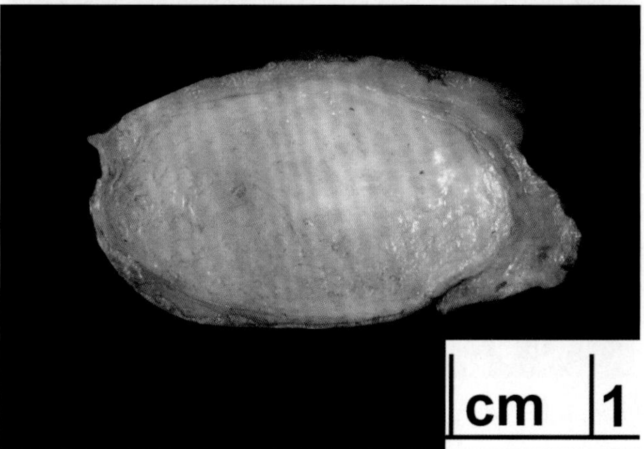

FIG. 38.20. ***Pseudoangiomatous stromal hyperplasia, gross appearance.*** **A:** The circumscribed oval tumor measured 5 cm in the long axis. **B:** This tumor is circumscribed and lobulated. The hemorrhagic focus is a biopsy site. **C:** A well-demarcated tumor with a fibrous cut surface.

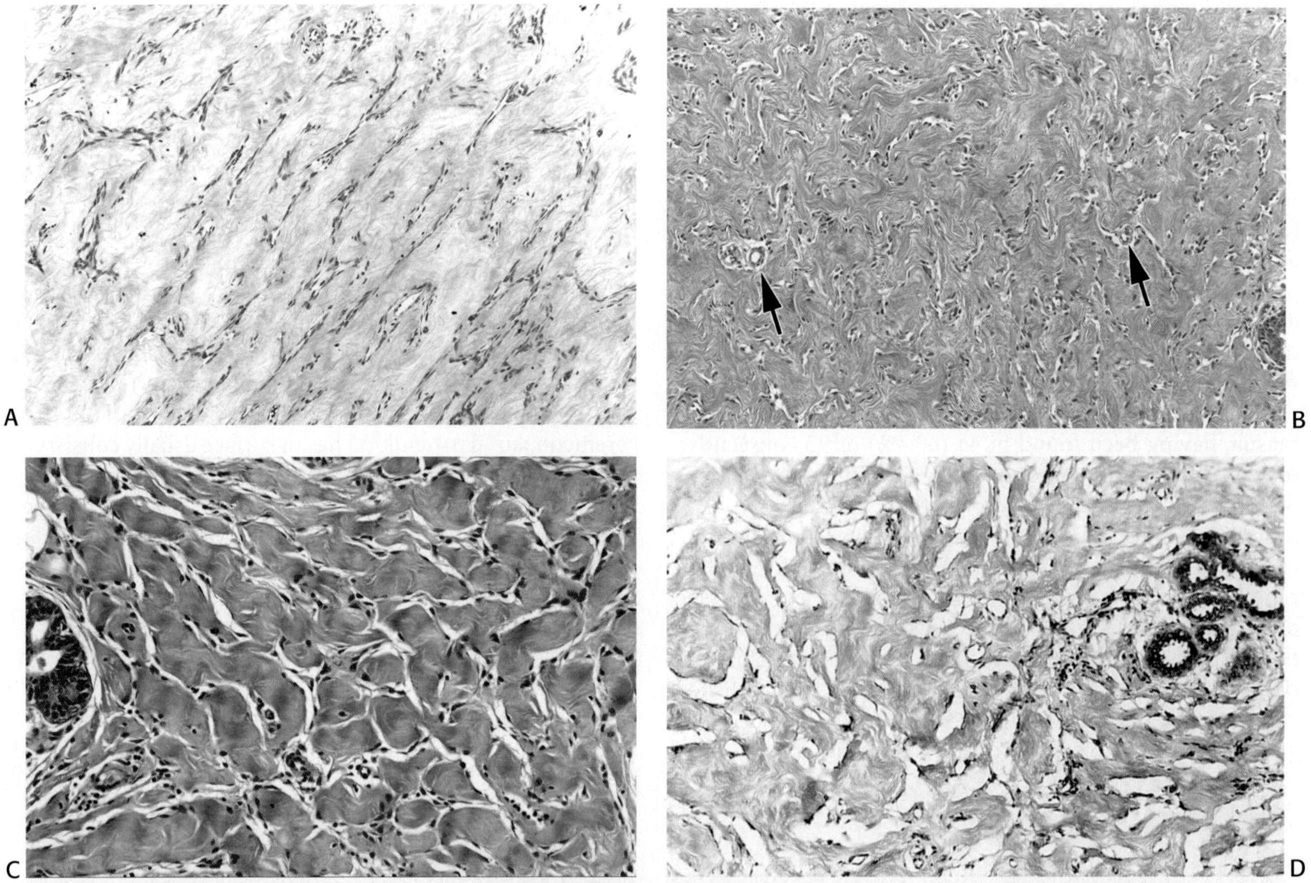

FIG. 38.21. ***Pseudoangiomatous stromal hyperplasia.*** Various histologic appearances are shown. **A:** Slender cords of myofibroblasts with almost no spaces between them. **B:** Inconspicuous spaces and true capillaries (*arrows*). **C:** Well-formed anastomosing spaces. **D:** Dilated spaces.

elements. The lobular and duct structures are usually separated by an increased amount of stroma. Collagenization of intralobular stroma and duct attenuation producing FA-like features are common. Nonspecific proliferative epithelial changes include mild hyperplasia of duct and lobular epithelium, often with some accentuation of myoepithelial cells, and apocrine metaplasia with or without cyst formation.

The most striking histologic finding is a complex pattern of largely empty, often anastomosing, spaces in the dense collagenous stroma (Figs. 38.21 and 38.22). These slits, sufficiently large to be identified at low magnification, are

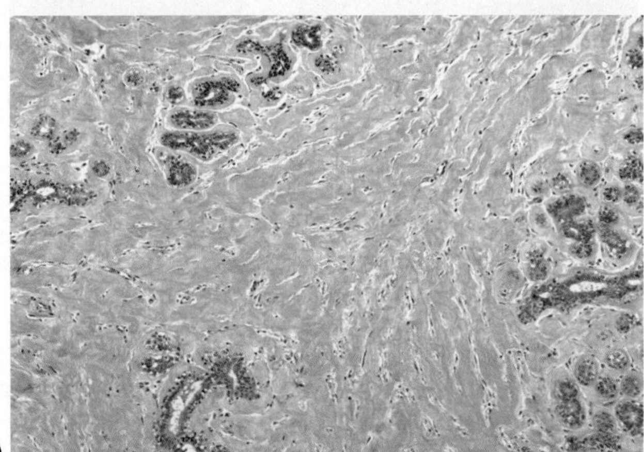

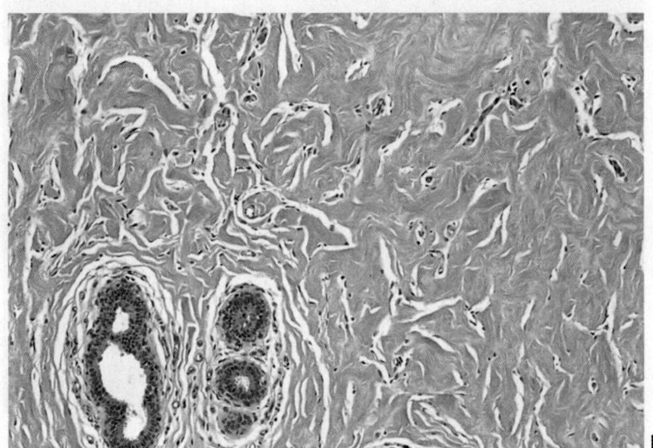

FIG. 38.22. ***Pseudoangiomatous stromal hyperplasia.*** **A,B:** A diffuse complex network of spaces is evident.

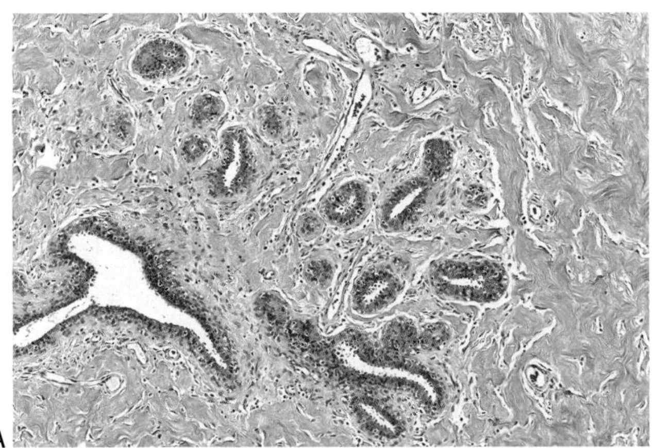
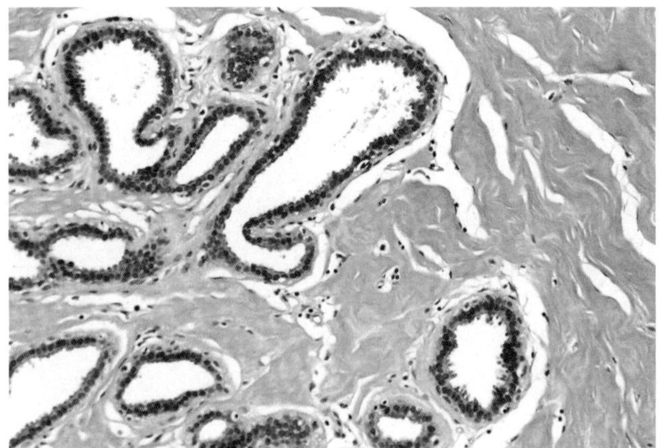

FIG. 38.23. ***Pseudoangiomatous stromal hyperplasia, lobular involvement.*** **A,B:** Pseudoangiomatous spaces involve perilobular and intralobular stroma.

often present in intralobular as well as interlobular stroma (Fig. 38.23). The spaces rarely contain a few red blood cells. Collagen fibrils may traverse the space. Myofibroblasts distributed singly and discontinuously at the margins of the spaces resemble endothelial cells (Fig. 38.24). The nuclei of the myofibroblasts are usually attenuated, lack atypia, and do not show mitotic activity, but some of these cells are enlarged and they have noticeably hyperchromatic nuclei (Fig. 38.24). Multinucleated cells may rarely line the slit-like spaces.[99] Stromal pseudoangiomatous spaces can be seen in frozen sections, indicating that they are not simply an artifact of formalin-fixed, paraffin-embedded tissue. Also present in the stroma are round or oval blood-containing true capillaries lined by endothelial cells.

The myofibroblasts may accumulate in distinct bundles or fascicles in a background of conventional PASH, forming "fascicular PASH" (Figs. 38.25 and 38.26). These groups of cells are evidence of a more pronounced proliferation of myofibroblasts. The most pronounced examples of this cellular form of PASH have a growth pattern reminiscent of a myofibroblastoma (Figs. 38.26 and 38.27). This is especially the case when the myofibroblasts have abundant cytoplasm and PASH occurs as a localized tumor rather than as a diffuse process (Fig. 38.28). Myofibroblastoma and PASH are related conditions, representing the extremes of a spectrum of lesions, sharing a common histogenesis in the myofibroblast. Myoid differentiation to a smooth muscle phenotype can occur in isolated cells, and rarely this is a diffuse process that resembles multiple ill-defined leiomyomas (Fig. 38.29).

An extremely unusual variant of PASH has cytoplasmic inclusion bodies of the type found in digital fibromas. The inclusions are immunoreactive for actin and desmin (Fig. 38.30).

Atypical PASH

Cytologic alterations of myofibroblasts are sometimes encountered in PASH. Pleomorphic nuclei are infrequent. They can be found in conventional and in fascicular PASH, sometimes accompanied by mitotic activity (Fig. 38.31). Several instances of tumor-forming PASH in teenage girls

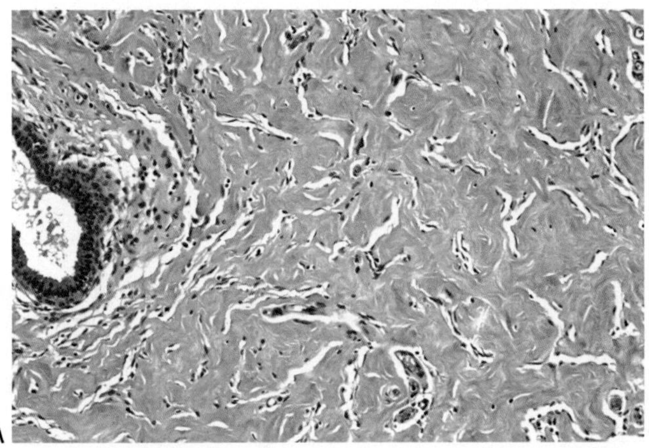
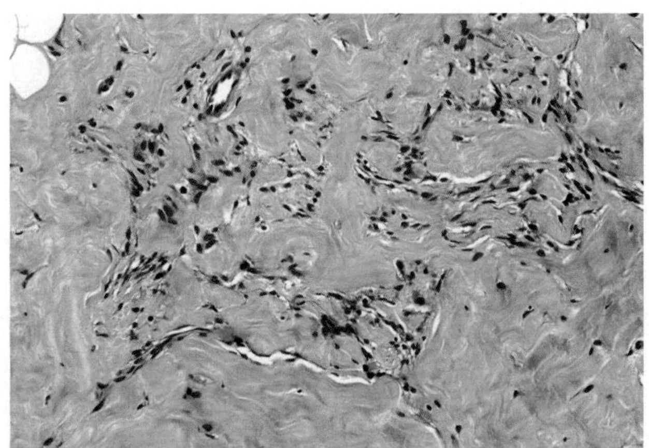

FIG. 38.24. ***Pseudoangiomatous stromal hyperplasia.*** **A:** Connected slits outlined by myofibroblasts with uniform, small flat nuclei. **B:** Focal myofibroblastic hyperplasia is shown.

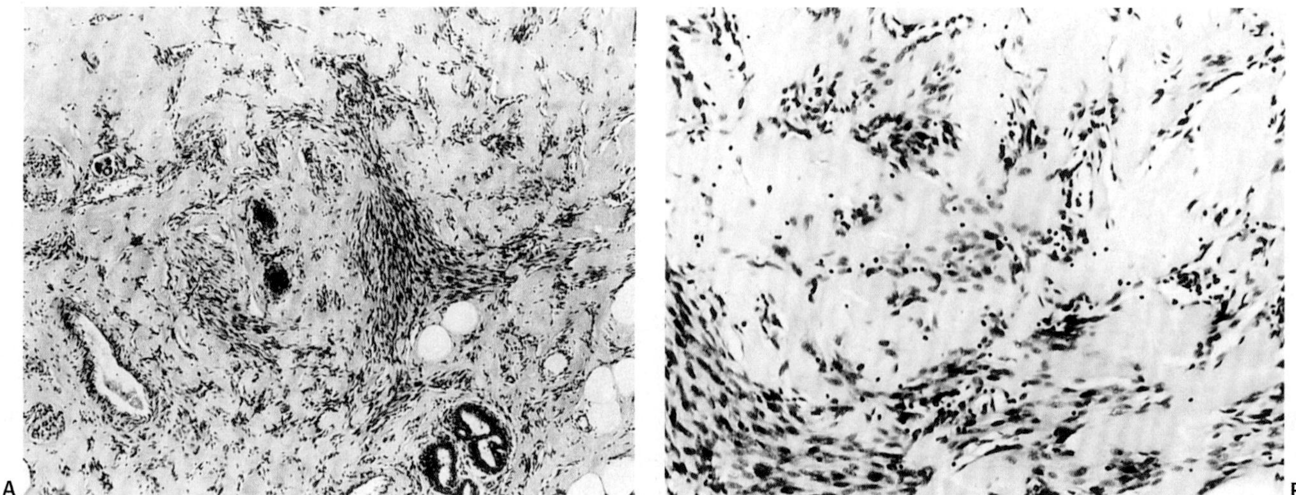

FIG. 38.25. ***Pseudoangiomatous stromal hyperplasia, fascicular.*** **A,B:** Bundles and sheets of myofibroblasts in a background of conventional PASH.

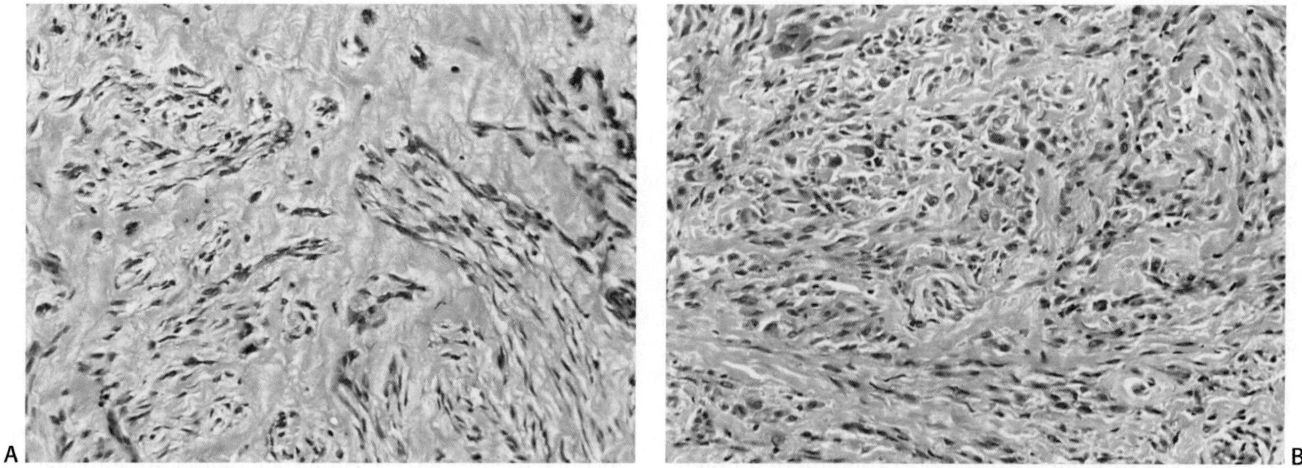

FIG. 38.26. ***Pseudoangiomatous stromal hyperplasia, fascicular.*** Bundles of myofibroblasts sectioned longitudinally (**A**) and transversely (**B**). Areas such as those shown here can occur in a myofibroblastoma.

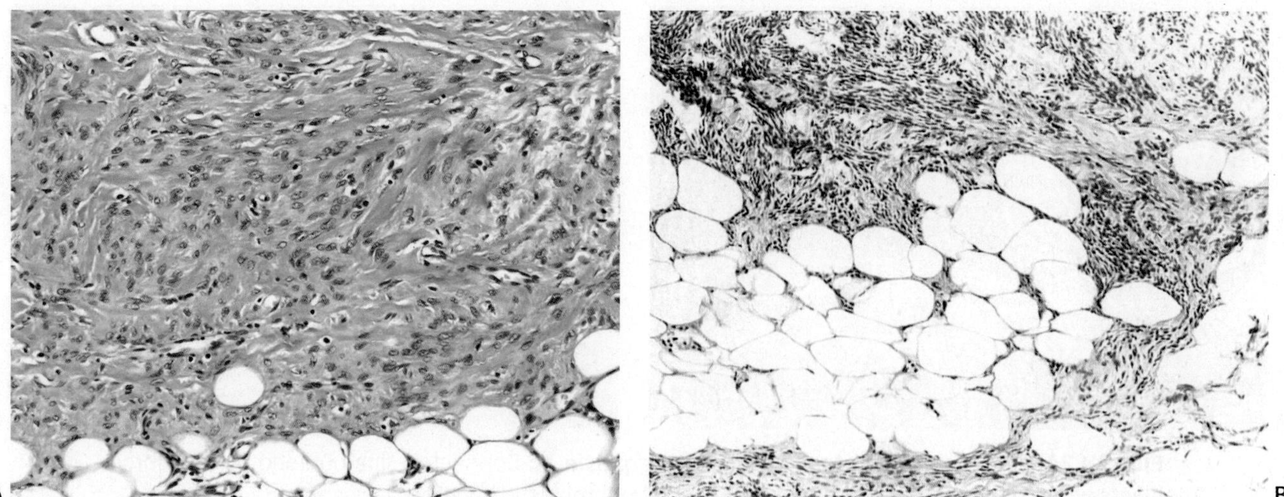

FIG. 38.27. ***Pseudoangiomatous stromal hyperplasia, fascicular.*** **A,B:** Pronounced fascicular growth that resembles a myofibroblastoma.

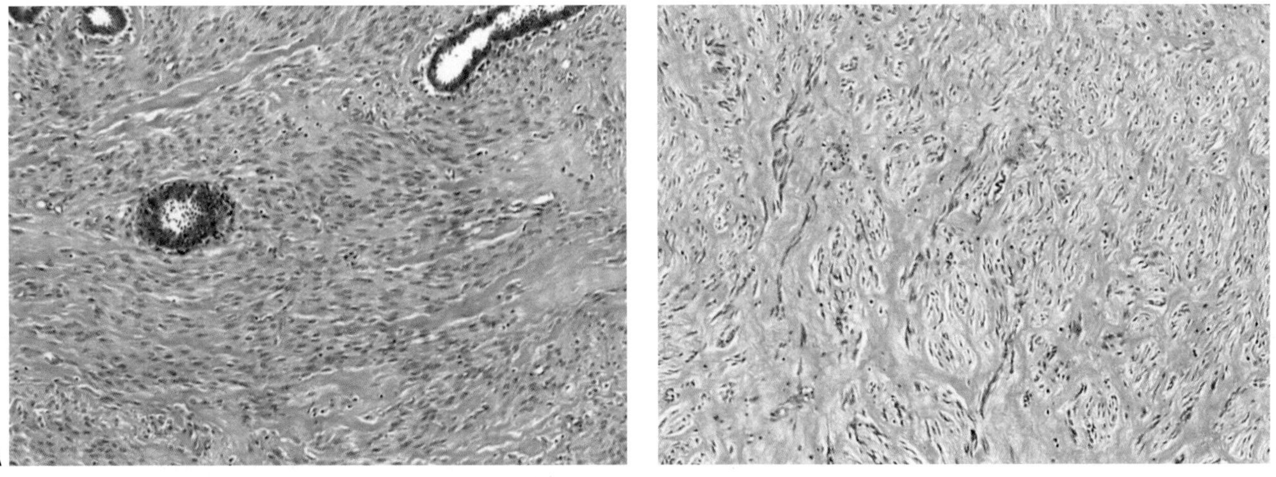

FIG. 38.28. ***Pseudoangiomatous stromal hyperplasia, fascicular.*** **A,B:** The collagen bands and fascicles of myofibroblasts with abundant cytoplasm separated by collagen bands resemble a classical myofibroblastoma.

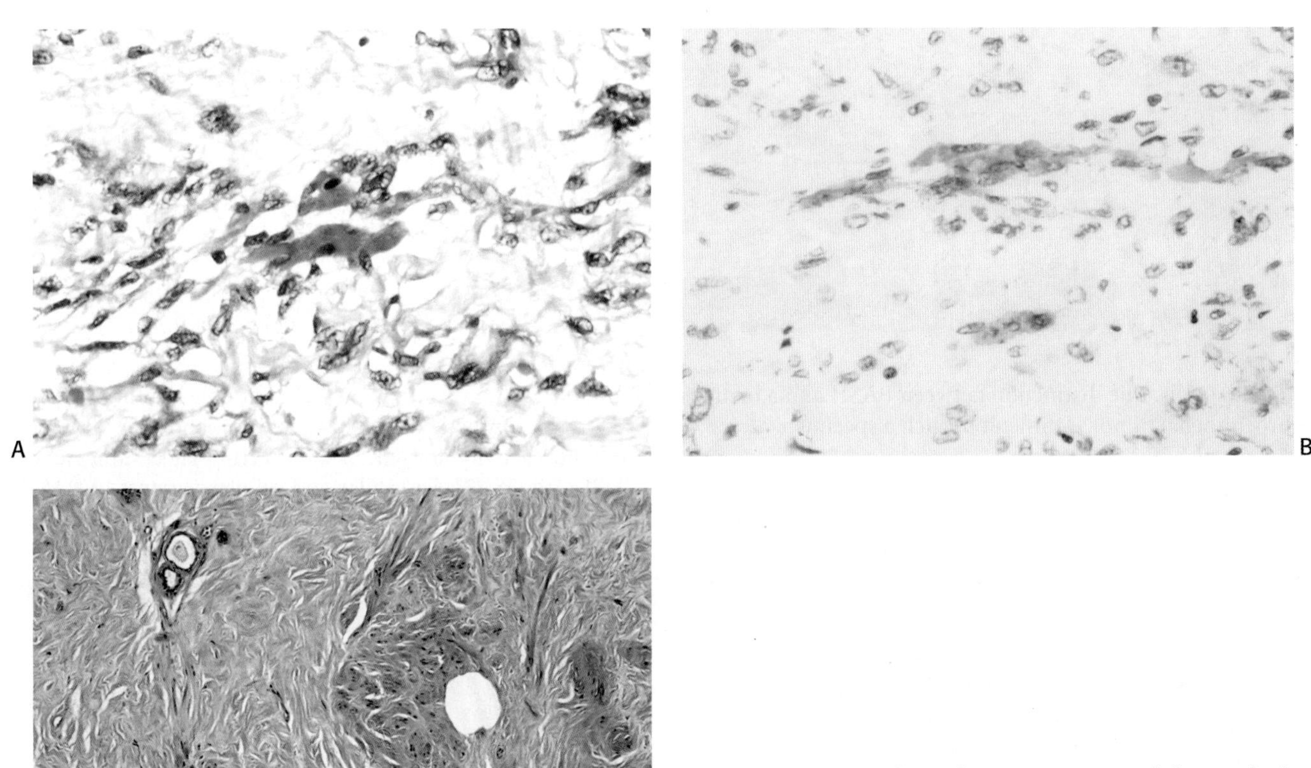

FIG. 38.29. ***Pseudoangiomatous stromal hyperplasia, myoid.*** **A:** An elongated myoid cell with eosinophilic cytoplasm in PASH. **B:** The same focus stained for SMA shows several immunoreactive cells. **C:** Myomatous myoid myofibroblasts.

characterized by marked cytologic atypia, multinucleated cells, and mitotic activity have been encountered (Fig. 38.32). These appear to be examples of myofibroblastic sarcoma arising in PASH. Insufficient information is available to characterize the clinical course of these tumors.

Cytology

The diagnosis of PASH by FNA has been reported.[104,105] The specimens are likely to be hypocellular with loosely connected or isolated bipolar spindle cells and clusters of benign

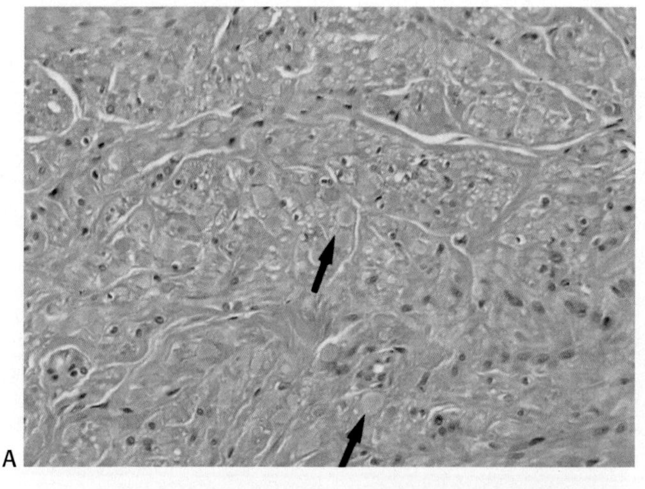

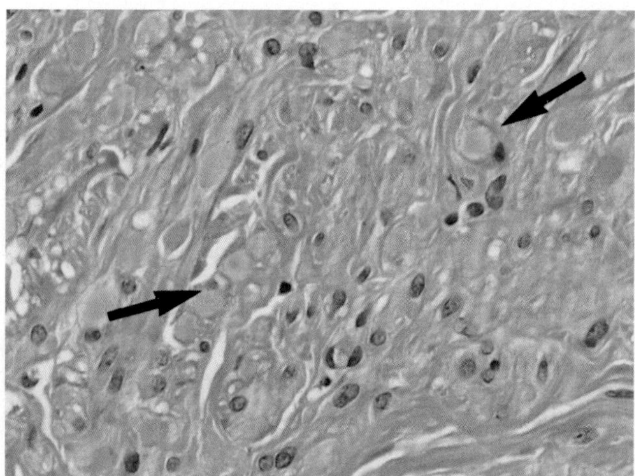

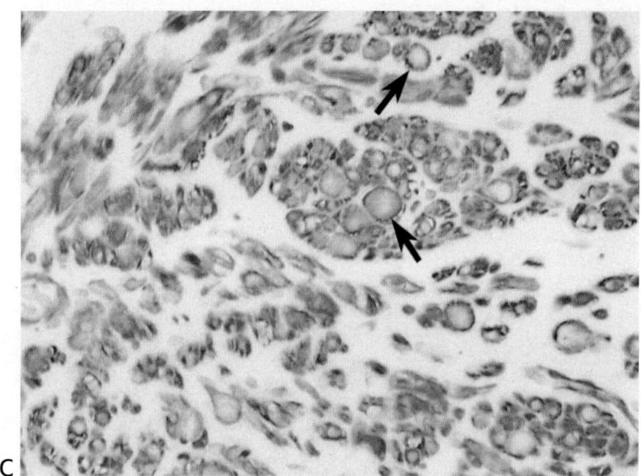

FIG. 38.30. ***Pseudoangiomatous stromal hyperplasia, digital fibroma-like inclusions.*** **A,B:** Round eosinophilic cytoplasmic inclusions (*arrows*) with dense centers in myofibroblasts in a lesion with a fascicular growth pattern. **C:** Immunoreactivity for actin in myofibroblasts is less intense in the cytoplasmic inclusions (*arrows*).

epithelial cells. The distinction between PASH and a benign fibroepithelial tumor is difficult in such a specimen.[105]

Immunohistochemistry

Myofibroblasts lining pseudoangiomatous spaces are usually CD34 immunoreactive (Fig. 38.33).[84,85,100] They exhibit strong immunoreactivity for vimentin and variable immunoreactivity for SMA, muscle actin, and calponin, and they show no immunoreactivity for CK, factor VIII–related antigen, or CD31 (Fig. 38.33). Fascicular and cellular variants of PASH retain immunoreactivity for CD34 and may be reactive for SMA, desmin, and calponin (Fig. 38.33). The presence of CD34 reactivity in cells staining for vimentin, desmin, and SMA in

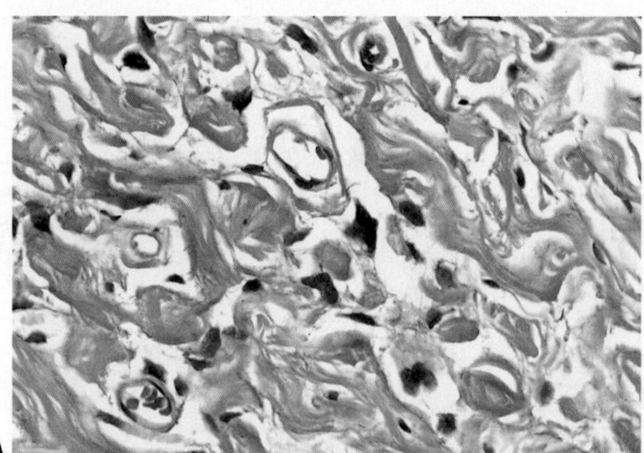

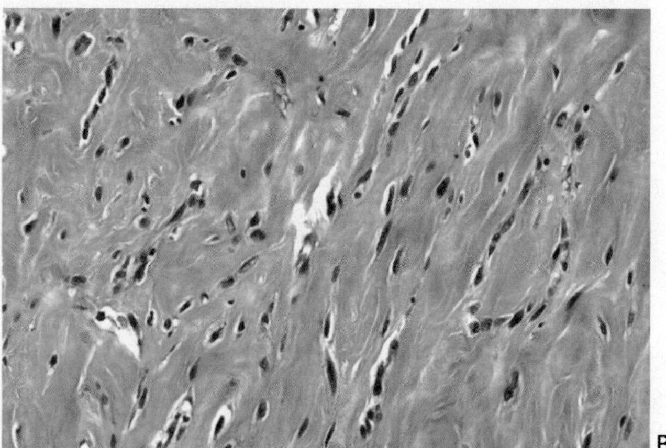

FIG. 38.31. ***Pseudoangiomatous stromal hyperplasia, atypia.*** **A:** Nuclei of myofibroblasts are hyperchromatic and pleomorphic. **B,C:** Myofibroblasts with hyperchromatic nuclei in PASH. **D:** Nuclear pleomorphism and two mitoses (*arrows*) are shown in fascicular PASH.

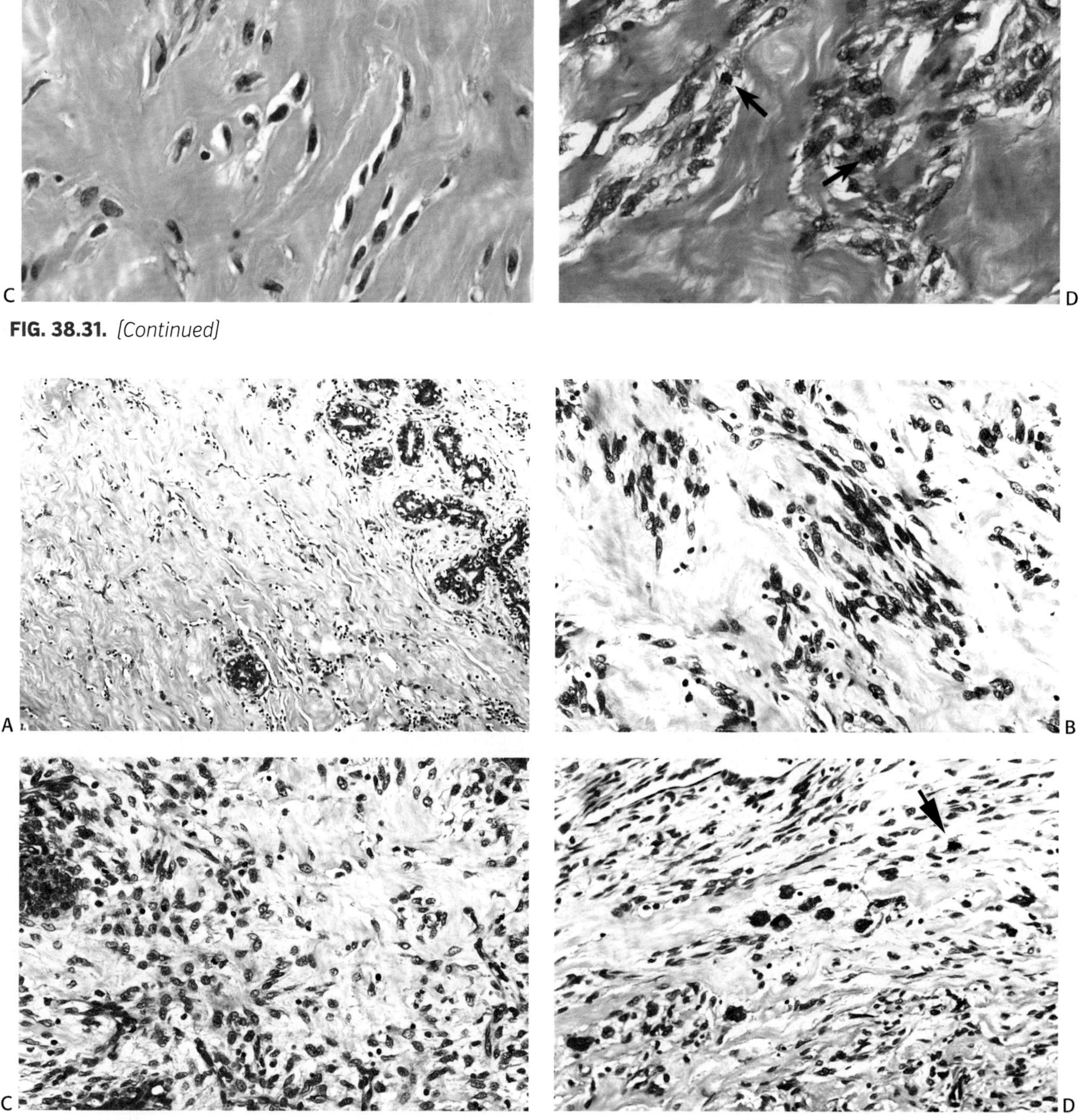

FIG. 38.31. *(Continued)*

FIG. 38.32. ***Pseudoangiomatous stromal hyperplasia, giant cells and atypia.*** All images are from a specimen obtained from an 18-year-old nonpregnant woman with a mass. **A:** A region showing conventional PASH. **B:** Fascicular growth with hyperchromatic nuclei. **C:** Cellular overgrowth obscures the PASH architecture in this region. **D:** Atypical multinucleated stromal cells. Note the mitotic figure (*arrow*).

PASH suggests that it is a marker for myofibroblastic differentiation. Basement membrane material is not demonstrable around the slit-like spaces. Alcian blue staining, demonstrable in the spaces, is removed by hyaluronidase treatment.

The nuclei of myofibroblasts in PASH are sometimes immunoreactive for PR.[83,84,92] In most reports, ER is absent or only weakly present when the tissues are studied by IHC.[79,83–85,100] In a recent study, Bowman et al.[92] found high rates of ER (79%) and PR (63%) immunoreactivity among their cases of PASH; the majority of the ER-positive cases showed only "occasional" positive cells. More sensitive antibodies and improved immunohistochemical techniques

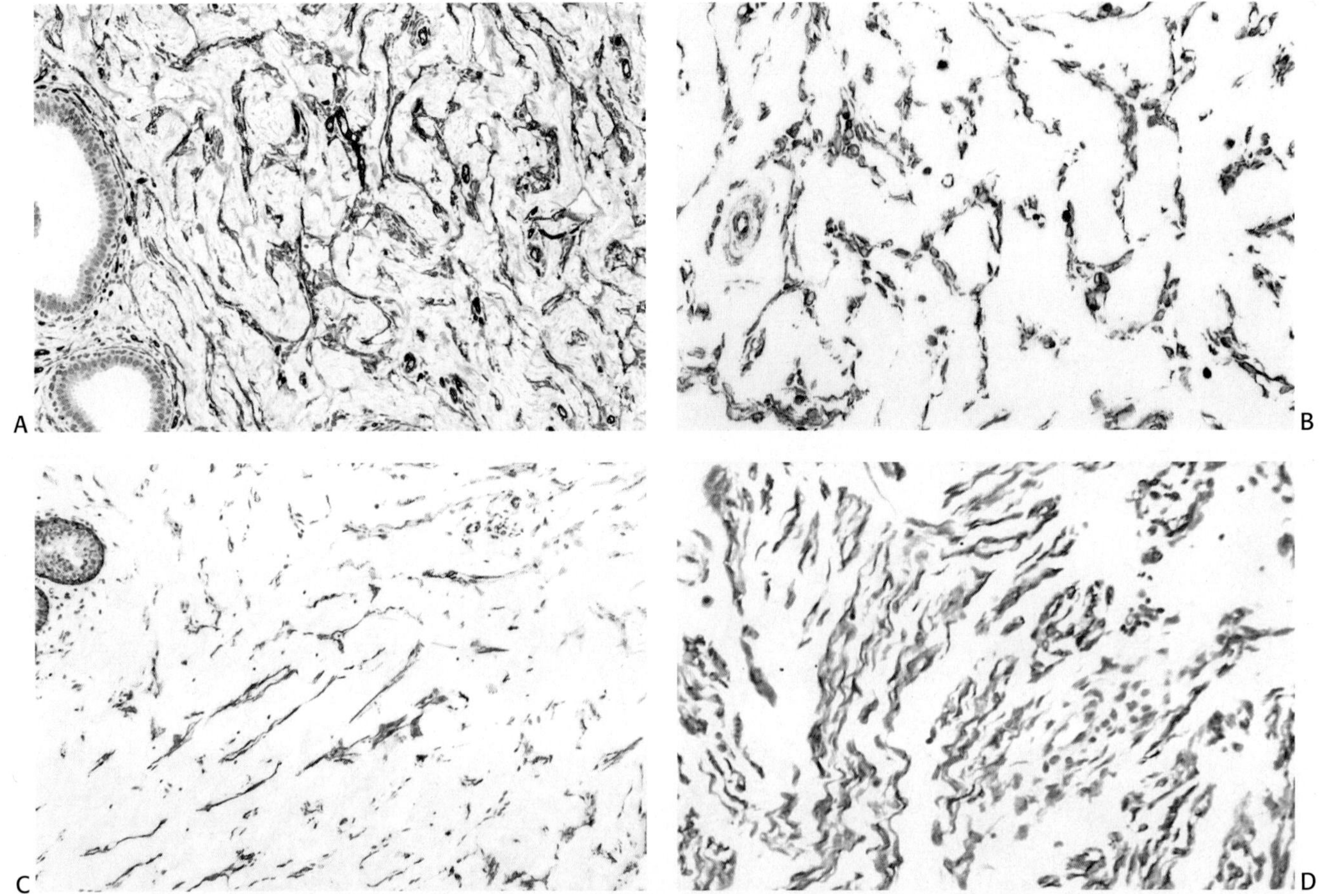

FIG. 38.33. *Pseudoangiomatous stromal hyperplasia, immunohistochemistry.* **A:** The myofibroblasts are strongly immunoreactive for CD34. **B:** Immunoreactivity for vimentin highlights the pseudoangiomatous structure. **C:** Immunoreactivity for SMA. **D:** A fascicular example showing immunoreactivity for CD34.

may have contributed to the higher rate of positivity in their study compared to prior ones.

Electron Microscopy

Samples from two tumors examined by electron microscopy revealed similar findings.[82,95] Well-formed vascular structures, usually capillaries, were readily distinguished from pseudoangiomatous spaces. True vessels were lined by endothelial cells joined by tight junctions, and they were surrounded by a basement membrane and pericytes. Pinocytotic vesicles, intermediate filaments, and Weibel–Palade bodies were evident in endothelial cells. On the other hand, pseudoangiomatous spaces were lined by an incomplete layer of fibroblastic cells that featured a fairly well-developed endoplasmic reticulum and prominent Golgi apparatus. Slender cytoplasmic processes extended along and around the spaces, sometimes joined by small rudimentary cell junctions, or they terminated in the collagenous stroma. The intervening stroma consisted of collagen fibrils and slender cells with longitudinally arranged, highly attenuated cytoplasmic processes joined by occasional tight or rudimentary cell junctions.

Treatment and Prognosis

PASH that forms a clinically palpable tumorous mass appears to be a highly exaggerated manifestation of physiologic changes commonly encountered microscopically. In the latter setting, PASH seems to be part of the proliferative process rather than a separate lesion. The diffuse form of PASH often contributes to the clinical impression of a mass when the histologic findings are described as fibrocystic changes.[85] Vogel et al.[106] described distinct alterations in mammary epithelium and stroma at various phases of the menstrual cycle. They found "loose, broken" stroma in the luteal phase (days 15 to 20) and a "loose, edematous" stroma in the secretory phase (days 21 to 27). The open clefts of PASH contain hyaluronidase-sensitive mucopolysaccharide and resemble physiologic changes depicted in Figures 4 and 5 of the report of Vogel et al.[106] Ibrahim et al.[95] found microscopic foci of PASH in 23% of 200 consecutive breast specimens obtained for benign or malignant conditions. Eighty-nine percent of the patients with PASH were younger than 50 years. The majority of these specimens exhibited epithelial hyperplasia, sometimes including secretory changes in lobules. Degnim et al.[107] found evidence of PASH in 6% of 9,065 consecutive benign breast surgical biopsies. Eighty-eight percent of their patients with PASH were younger than 45 years.

It appears that under as yet undefined conditions, microscopic and clinically inapparent PASH becomes capable of autonomous growth. The fact that the vast majority of patients with tumorous pseudoangiomatous stroma have been premenopausal underscores the probable importance of hormonal factors in the development of this lesion. Hormonal influence is further suggested by the frequent presence of PASH in gynecomastia and in fibroepithelial neoplasms.[85,100] Traces of PASH can be found in breast tissue from a postmenopausal woman, but well-developed PASH in this age group is often associated with hormone replacement therapy.

In several instances, biopsies of PASH have been misinterpreted as low-grade angiosarcoma, and this has led to treatment by mastectomy. Most patients have remained well after excisional biopsy of PASH, but ipsilateral recurrences have been reported in 2% to 13% of patients.[84,88,90,98,108] Higher recurrence rates of 22% and 30% were reported in two studies.[82,91] Rare patients have had multiple ipsilateral recurrences.[84] Incomplete excision of tumorous PASH probably predisposes to local recurrence, but it is also possible that residual breast stroma may become susceptible to the same unknown stimuli, even after apparently complete removal of the tumor. Lesions followed by recurrence are histologically indistinguishable from PASH in women who did not have recurrences. Recurrent lesions ordinarily exhibit no change in cellularity or other atypical features.

The recommended treatment is wide local excision. Mastectomy rarely may be considered to control multiple recurrent tumors.[93] A small number of patients have proceeded with clinical observation after a diagnosis of PASH by needle core biopsy or other percutaneous biopsy. Of 80 such cases with reported follow-up information, 78% had stable disease, 18% showed progression, and 5% had regression or resolution of the imaging findings.[86–88,91,108] Most lesions that progressed were subsequently excised, and pathologic evaluation revealed PASH with no atypical features. A few patients continued observation even after initial progression, and further follow-up demonstrated stable disease. Careful clinicopathologic correlation is required in such instances since PASH can be an incidental finding unrelated to the targeted abnormality.

Isolated case reports document response of PASH to selective ER modulators. Pruthi et al.[109] described a 39-year-old woman with bilateral symptomatic PASH who obtained relief after treatment with tamoxifen and raloxifene. Transient response to tamoxifen was reported in a 15-year-old boy who had a 13-cm unilateral gynecomastia tumor with histologically documented PASH.[110] Conversely, the administration of estrogenic hormone replacement therapy to a perimenopausal woman with a prior history of PASH, but no recently active lesions, resulted in the development of breast tumors consistent with PASH.

PASH is occasionally an incidental finding in breast specimens containing invasive or *in situ* carcinoma.[98,108,111] The malignancies and PASH are generally anatomically separate. In one unusual case, a 0.9-cm IDC was present within a 4-cm PASH tumor.[87] The area of invasive carcinoma had suspicious features on imaging that differed from those of the larger PASH nodule. PASH is not associated with an increased risk of subsequent breast carcinoma.[107]

MYOFIBROBLASTOMA

Mammary neoplasms derived largely or entirely from myofibroblasts are uncommon. Myofibroblasts are spindle-shaped or fusiform mesenchymal cells probably derived from fibroblasts.[112] They are present in small numbers in virtually all tissues outside the central nervous system. Proliferation of myofibroblasts triggered by cytokines is conspicuous in various inflammatory conditions such as healing wounds,[113] and they are a component of various benign mesenchymal tumors[114] and some sarcomas.[115,116] Soft tissue neoplasms of the breast thought to be composed of myofibroblasts have been classified as myofibroblastomas.[117] The structural and immunohistochemical characteristics of these tumors are similar to those of solitary fibrous tumor.[118,119] Some investigators have suggested that myofibroblastomas of the breast should be regarded as solitary fibrous tumors and diagnosed by this name.[119] Others have attempted to distinguish between the two entities on the basis of structural, cytologic, and immunohistochemical features.[120] The latter authors reserved the diagnosis of myofibroblastoma for lesions expressing actin and CD34, and they classified actin-negative, CD34-positive lesions as solitary fibrous tumors. These hair-splitting distinctions seem totally unwarranted in view of the "plasticity" of myofibroblastic phenotypic expression.[121] It is appropriate to employ the term "myofibroblastoma" for these tumors in the breast regardless of the expression of actin. If so-called solitary fibrous tumors at other sites take origin from myofibroblasts, perhaps they should also be designated as myofibroblastomas.

Myofibroblastic proliferation occurs in many mammary carcinomas, being most prominent in scirrhous, desmoplastic tumors.[122,123] The presence of myofibroblasts in scirrhous breast carcinomas has been confirmed by electron microscopy[122–124] and by IHC.[123,125] It has been possible to characterize myofibroblasts isolated *in vitro* from scirrhous carcinomas by electron microscopy and IHC.[126] In a study by Chauhan et al.,[127] myofibroblasts were positive for CD34 and mainly negative for SMA in the normal breast and in the presence of most proliferative lesions, whereas in invasive carcinoma they were negative for CD34 and positive for SMA. In the presence of ductal carcinoma *in situ* (DCIS), expression of CD34 and SMA in the surrounding stroma was related to the grade of the carcinoma, with loss of CD34 expression greatest in association with high-grade lesions.

Myofibroblasts are distinguished from spindled myoepithelial cells largely on the basis of their distribution, as well as their immunohistochemical and electron microscopic characteristics.[124] Ultrastructurally, both types of cells have cytoplasmic actin-like microfilaments measuring 5 to 7 nm in diameter, with focal dense bodies and pinocytotic vesicles (more numerous in myoepithelial cells). In contrast to myoepithelial cells, myofibroblasts lack prekeratin tonofilaments. Desmosomes are readily found between myoepithelial cells, whereas they are absent or poorly formed between myofibroblasts. Depending on their phenotypic state, both types of cells may be reactive for calponin and actin antibodies. Myoepithelial cells are immunoreactive for smooth muscle myosin heavy chain, which stains myofibroblasts weakly or not at all. Myoepithelial cells are variably positive for S-100 protein and CKs such as 34βE12 and CK5/6, but myofibroblasts are negative with these antibodies. Nuclear reactivity for p63 is found in myoepithelial cells but not in myofibroblasts.

Clinical Presentation

Myofibroblastoma is predominantly a tumor of middle-aged to elderly patients (age range, 41 to 87 years; mean, 7th decade).[120,128–131] It is only exceptionally seen in younger patients.[132] The initial description of mammary myofibroblastoma by Wargotz et al.[128] indicated a male predominance, but subsequent experience suggests that it is equally common in women.[129,133]

Most patients present with a solitary, slowly growing, painless, and mobile mass. Progressive enlargement of the tumor may occur over the course of years; in a case reported by Bégin,[134] a 77-year-old patient experienced progressive breast enlargement over 7 years, resulting in a $6.5 \times 6.0 \times 4.5$ cm^3 tumor. Very rare tumors demonstrate rapid enlargement, and associated *peau d'orange* change of the skin has been described in one such case in a 65-year-old man.[135] The vast majority of tumors are unilateral. Rare examples of bilateral myofibroblastoma have been reported in men. Two of the lesions described by Toker et al.[136] as "benign spindle cell breast tumors" in men were probably myofibroblastomas. One patient had two identical separate tumors in his left breast, which were treated by simple mastectomy, and 17 years later, he underwent a right mastectomy, which disclosed six foci of the same neoplastic process. In addition, a male patient with synchronous bilateral tumors was reported by Hamele-Bena et al.[129]

Radiographically, the tumors are homogeneous, lobulated, and well-circumscribed and lack microcalcifications.[134,137] Nonpalpable myofibroblastomas have been detected by mammography.[138] Ultrasonography suggests a FA.[138] MRI of a myofibroblastoma in the male breast revealed homogeneous enhancement with internal septations.[139]

Concurrent gynecomastia is reported in some male patients.[119,132,140,141] One woman developed a myofibroblastoma in a breast 4 years after ipsilateral lumpectomy and radiotherapy for DCIS.[142] In another woman, a myofibroblastoma developed in the surgical scar 1.5 years after excision of an IDC.[130] The Senior Editor has seen the specimen from a 76-year-old woman in which moderately differentiated IDC coexisted with and invaded a mammary myofibroblastoma. Two men with myofibroblastoma of the breast and coincidental primary carcinomas of the pancreas and kidney, respectively, have also been seen in consultation.

Gross Pathology

The average diameter of the tumors is approximately 2 cm, with most smaller than 4 cm. Size extremes include one lesion that measured 0.9 cm[129] and one 15-cm tumor.[135] The excised mass is firm and rubbery with a lobulated external surface. The cut surface consists of homogeneous, bulging gray-to-pink whorled or lobulated tissue (Fig. 38.34), which in one case had myxoid gelatinous areas.[134] Cystic degeneration, necrosis, and hemorrhage are absent.

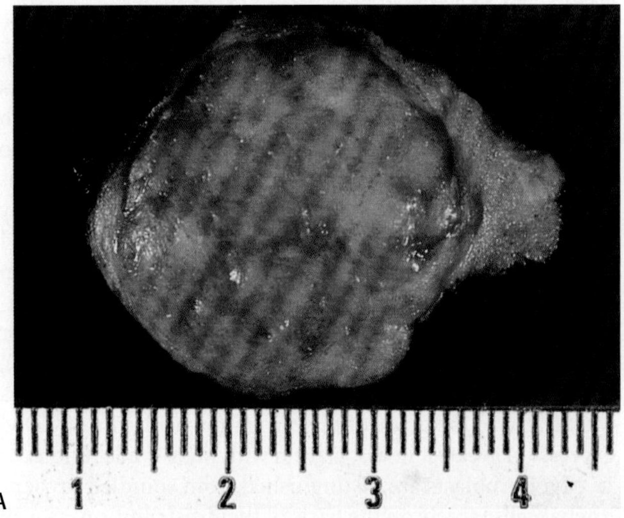

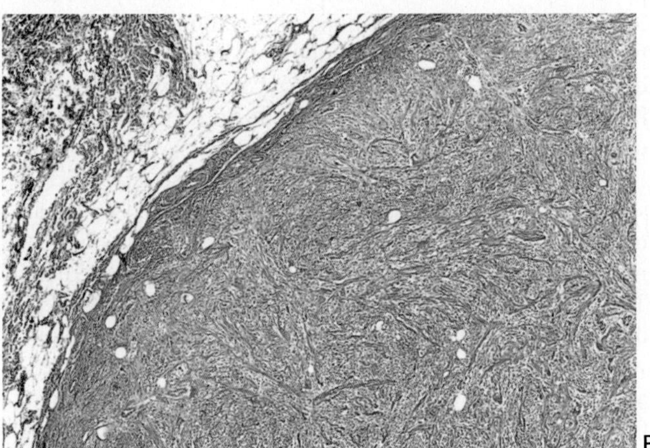

FIG. 38.34. ***Myofibroblastoma, gross appearance.*** **A:** The tumor is well-circumscribed, fleshy, and nodular. **B:** A whole-mount histologic section showing the circumscribed border and cellular solid growth. **C:** This well-circumscribed tumor contains abundant fat. **D:** The tumor is composed of closely apposed ovoid cells arranged in intersecting bundles. **E:** Collagen bands among the tumor cells.

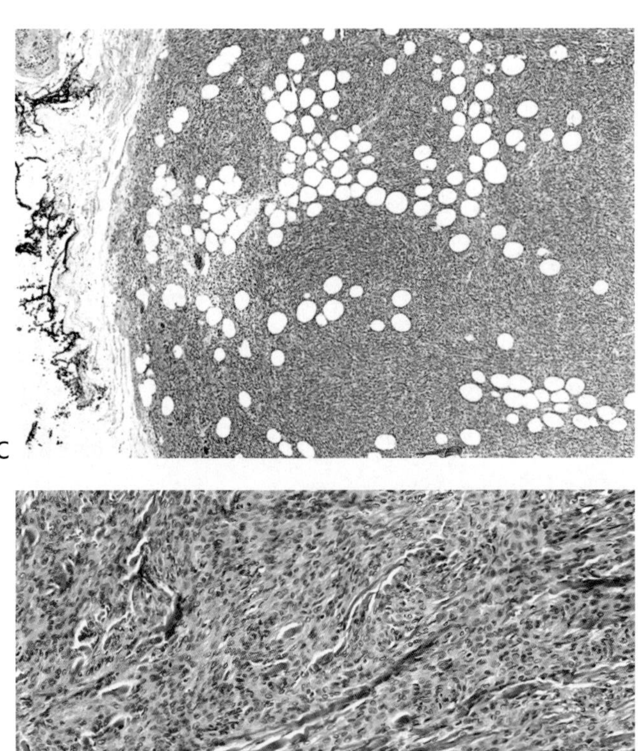

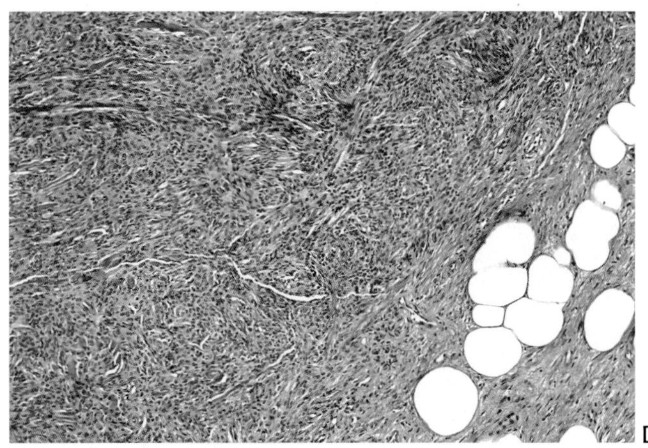

C D E

FIG. 38.34. *(Continued)*

Microscopic Pathology

Microscopically, the classic type of myofibroblastoma is devoid of mammary ducts and lobules with compressed breast parenchyma forming a peripheral pseudocapsule. The border of the tumor is usually circumscribed microscopically, but in a minority of cases the tumor has an invasive margin. Two distinctive histologic features are bundles of slender, bipolar, uniform spindle-shaped cells typically arranged in short fascicular clusters, and interspersed broad bands of hyalinized collagen distributed throughout the tumor (Figs. 38.34 and 38.35). The spindle cells have bland, ovoid to spindled nuclei with dispersed chromatin and small nucleoli. Nuclear grooves may be present. The cytoplasm is typically pale and eosinophilic, and cell borders are indistinct. Mitotic figures are sparse or undetectable. Multinucleated cells are uncommon, and pleomorphic nuclei that are believed to represent a degenerative phenomenon are encountered only rarely.[141,143,144] In a minority of lesions, fat cells or small amounts of glandular tissue are incorporated into the tumor, reflecting invasion of surrounding parenchyma. Rarely, fat cells are dispersed separately or in small groups throughout the tumor. Some myofibroblastomas have foci of leiomyomatous differentiation or cartilaginous differentiation (Fig. 38.36).[128,143] A perivascular lymphoplasmacytic infiltrate is sometimes identified.

Variant Forms

Variant forms of myofibroblastoma have received little attention. They exhibit a spectrum of histologic appearances between classical myofibroblastoma and PASH. A single variant pattern may dominate in a tumor, or different variant patterns may be mixed. Presently, the variant forms of myofibroblastoma have not been well characterized pathologically or clinically.

In a "collagenized" or "fibrous myofibroblastoma," the spindle cells are distributed in collagenous stroma (Fig. 38.37). The broad, deeply eosinophilic fibrous bands that are so prominent in a classical myofibroblastoma are absent or greatly reduced in number. Irregular slit-like spaces are formed between tumor cells. The stroma is reminiscent of PASH, and some of these tumors have a fascicular structure.

The "epithelioid variant" of myofibroblastoma features medium-sized to large polygonal or epithelioid cells arranged in alveolar groups (Fig. 38.38). Nuclei are round to oval and may be eccentrically located. Mild to moderate nuclear pleomorphism can be seen, and scattered bi- and multinucleated cells are not uncommon.[145] Mitotic activity is absent or minimal. Epithelioid areas may be mixed with more classical elements, or they can constitute the predominant growth pattern. The term "epithelioid variant" is used arbitrarily for tumors in which more than 50%

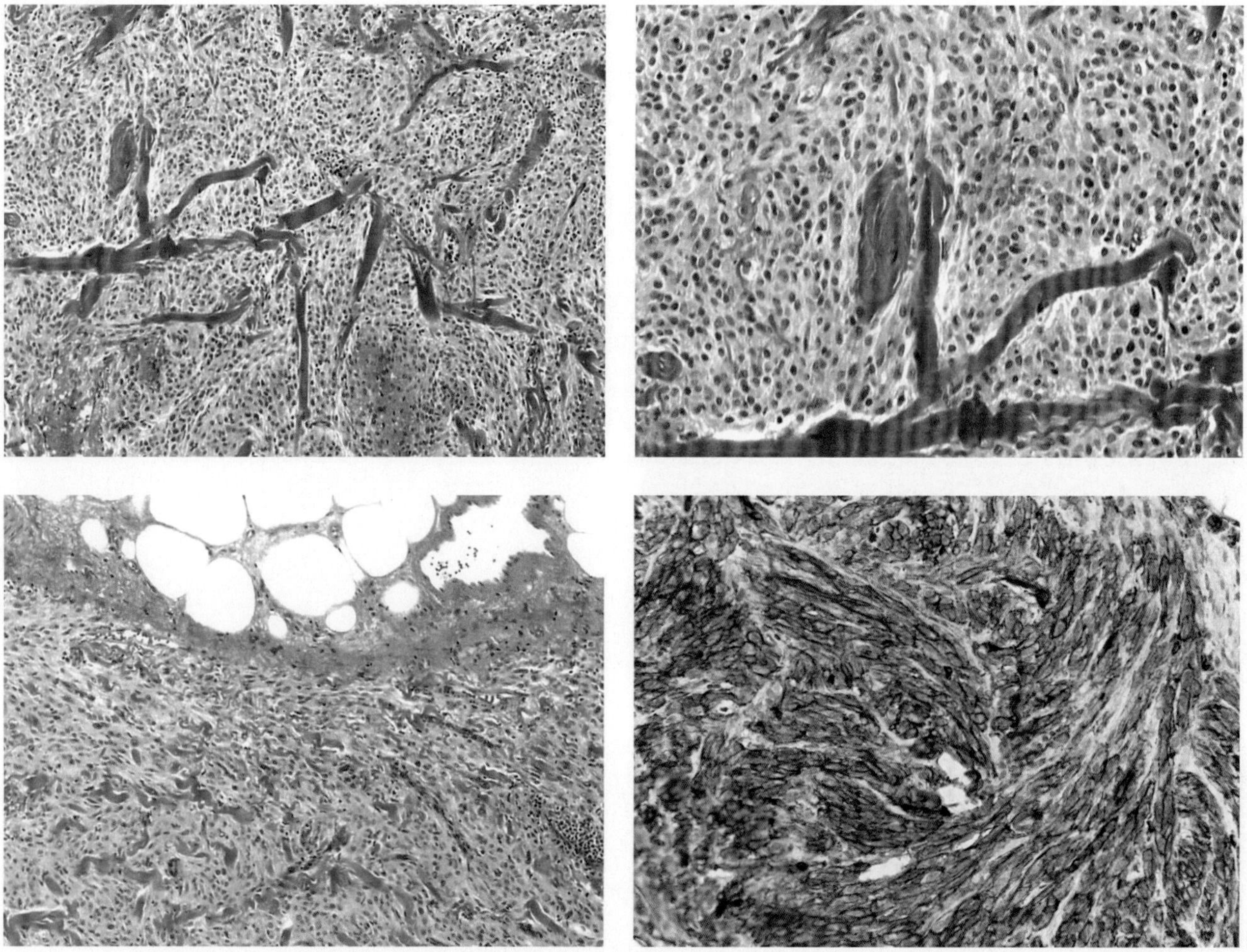

FIG. 38.35. ***Myofibroblastoma, classic type.*** **A,B:** The tumor is composed of a homogeneous population of predominately spindle-shaped cells with ovoid nuclei and pale cytoplasm. **C:** The sharply circumscribed border is shown. A small cluster of lymphocytes can be seen in the tumor on the *right*. **D:** Immunoreactivity for CD34 is present in the tumor cells.

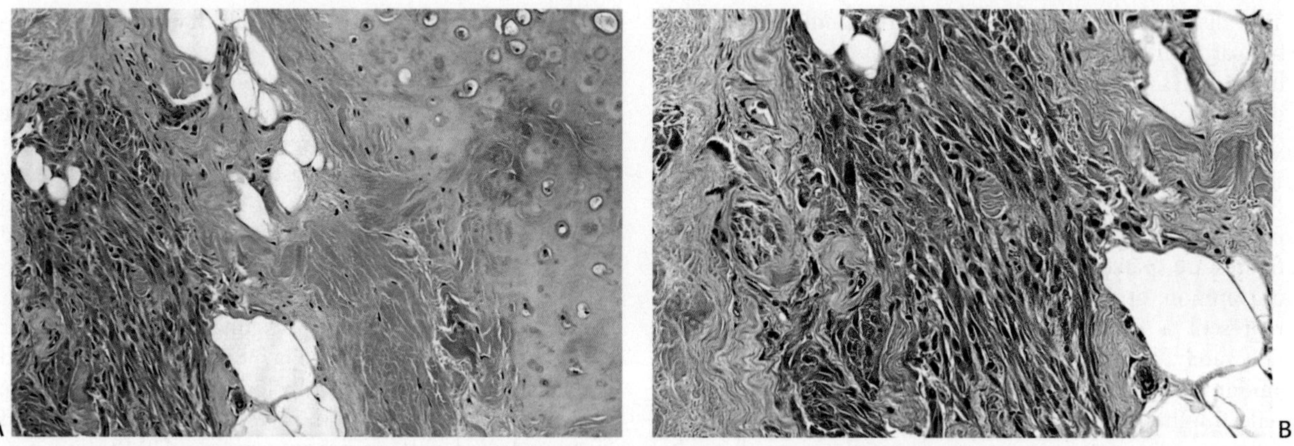

FIG. 38.36. ***Myofibroblastoma with myoid and cartilaginous differentiation.*** **A:** Myoid cells (*left*) and cartilage (*right*). **B:** Magnified view of the myoid focus.

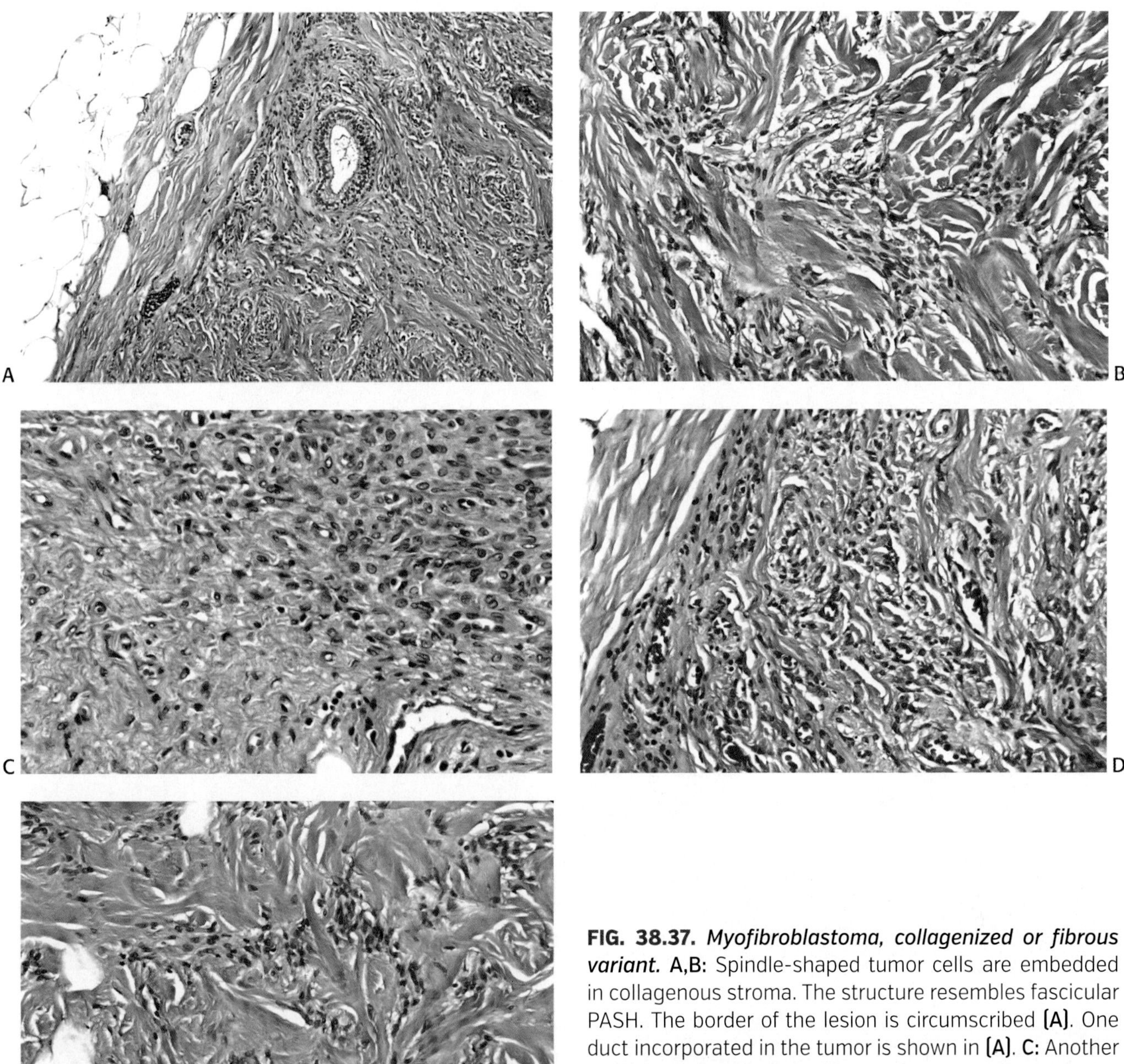

FIG. 38.37. ***Myofibroblastoma, collagenized or fibrous variant.*** **A,B:** Spindle-shaped tumor cells are embedded in collagenous stroma. The structure resembles fascicular PASH. The border of the lesion is circumscribed **(A)**. One duct incorporated in the tumor is shown in **(A)**. **C:** Another myofibroblastoma with fine collagen fibrils among the tumor cells and a fibrous region (*left*). **D,E:** The growth pattern in this fibrous myofibroblastoma resembles fascicular PASH.

of the lesion has this histologic pattern. The epithelioid cells in an epithelioid myofibroblastoma with sclerotic stroma can have a linear growth pattern that resembles invasive lobular carcinoma (ILC). In contrast to invasive carcinoma, however, epithelioid myofibroblastoma usually has well-circumscribed borders. Rare tumors contain large cells with abundant glassy cytoplasm and vesicular nuclei and have been referred to as a "deciduoid-like variant."[146]

A "cellular variant" of myofibroblastoma features a dense proliferation of spindle-shaped neoplastic myofibroblasts (Fig. 38.39). Collagenous bands may be absent in some parts of the lesion. These tumors tend to have infiltrative borders microscopically. Rarely, cellular and collagenous or fibrous growth patterns are combined in a single tumor (Fig. 38.40). The existence of these hybrid tumors supports the conclusion that breast tumors with the appearance of solitary fibrous tumor are myofibroblastomas.

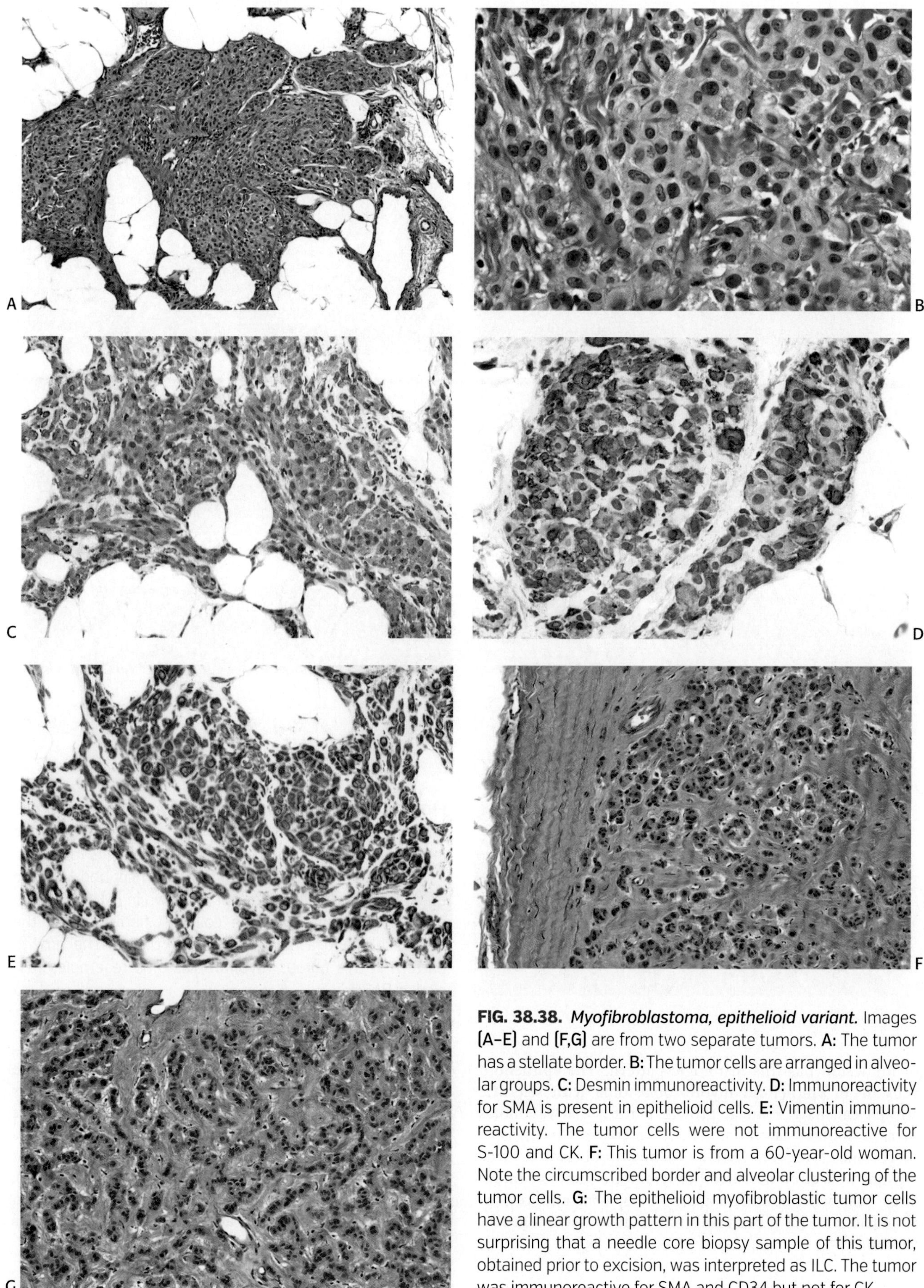

FIG. 38.38. ***Myofibroblastoma, epithelioid variant.*** Images (A–E) and (F,G) are from two separate tumors. **A:** The tumor has a stellate border. **B:** The tumor cells are arranged in alveolar groups. **C:** Desmin immunoreactivity. **D:** Immunoreactivity for SMA is present in epithelioid cells. **E:** Vimentin immunoreactivity. The tumor cells were not immunoreactive for S-100 and CK. **F:** This tumor is from a 60-year-old woman. Note the circumscribed border and alveolar clustering of the tumor cells. **G:** The epithelioid myofibroblastic tumor cells have a linear growth pattern in this part of the tumor. It is not surprising that a needle core biopsy sample of this tumor, obtained prior to excision, was interpreted as ILC. The tumor was immunoreactive for SMA and CD34 but not for CK.

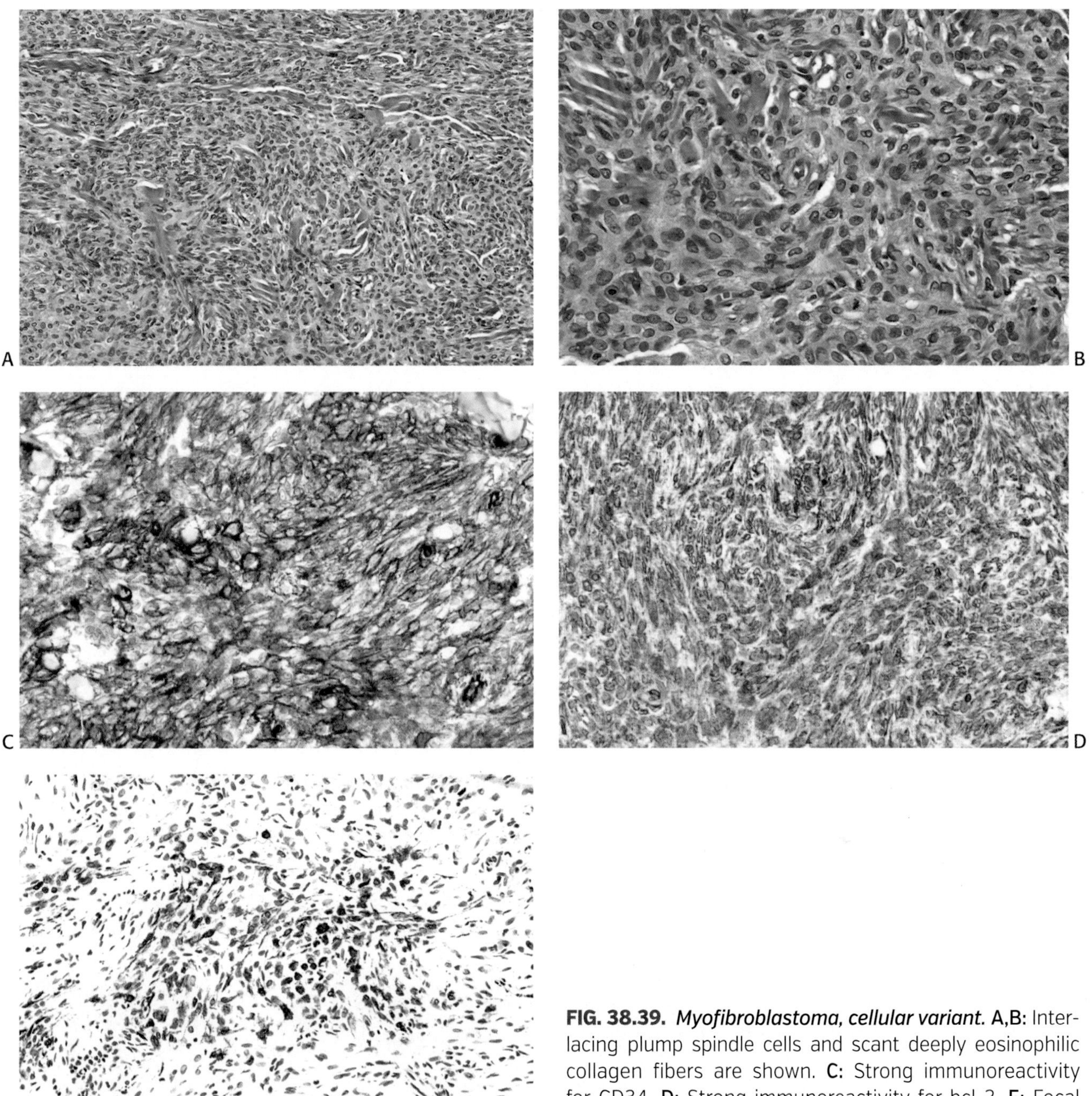

FIG. 38.39. ***Myofibroblastoma, cellular variant.*** **A,B:** Interlacing plump spindle cells and scant deeply eosinophilic collagen fibers are shown. **C:** Strong immunoreactivity for CD34. **D:** Strong immunoreactivity for bcl-2. **E:** Focal immunoreactivity for desmin.

The "infiltrative variant" of myofibroblastoma is characterized by invasive growth. These lesions form a tumor that consists of not only the lesional tissue but also fat, mammary stroma, ducts, and lobules (Fig. 38.41). This pattern differs from that of the classical and the other foregoing variants of myofibroblastoma, which incorporate fat, glandular tissue, or both into what is essentially a discrete tumor composed in large measure of the lesional tissue. The infiltrative variant of myofibroblastoma consists of bundles of relatively evenly dispersed spindle, ovoid, and epithelioid cells embedded in collagenous stroma. Some of these lesions exhibit a peculiar tendency for the neoplastic myofibroblasts to be oriented around blood vessels.

The Senior Editor has encountered several tumors that appear to be "myxoid myofibroblastomas" (Fig. 38.42). The sparse spindle cells distributed in the myxoid stroma of these lesions display immunoreactivity for CD34 and actin, consistent with myofibroblastic histogenesis. Some tumors classified as mucinosis (see subsequent text) may be myxoid myofibroblastomas.

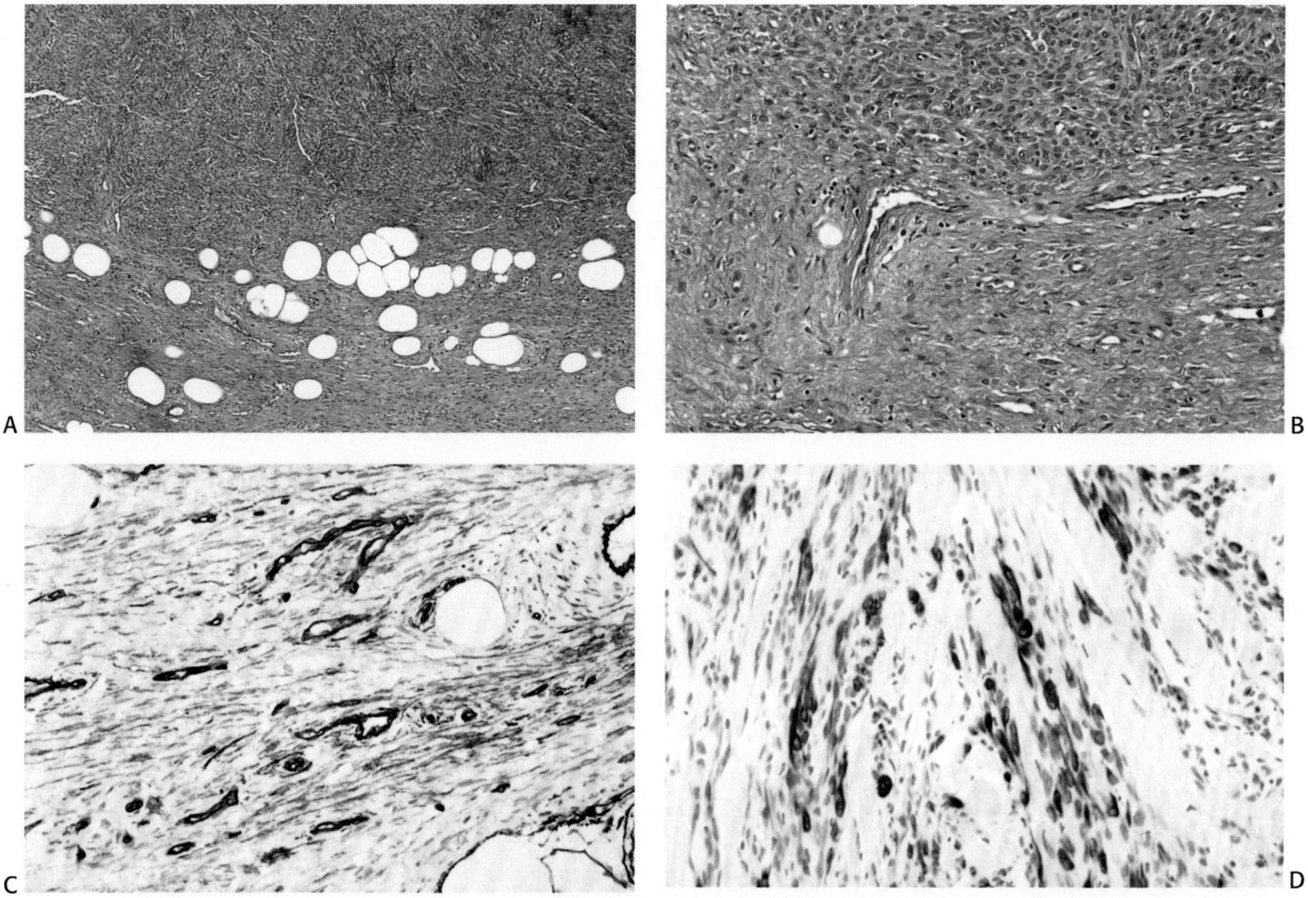

FIG. 38.40. ***Myofibroblastoma, combined cellular and fibrous variant.*** **A:** A low-magnification view showing the cellular component *above* and the peripheral fibrous component infiltrating fat *below*. **B:** Magnified view of the junction between the cellular and fibrous regions. **C:** Immunoreactivity for CD34 in the fibrous area. **D:** Immunoreactivity for desmin in a fibrous area.

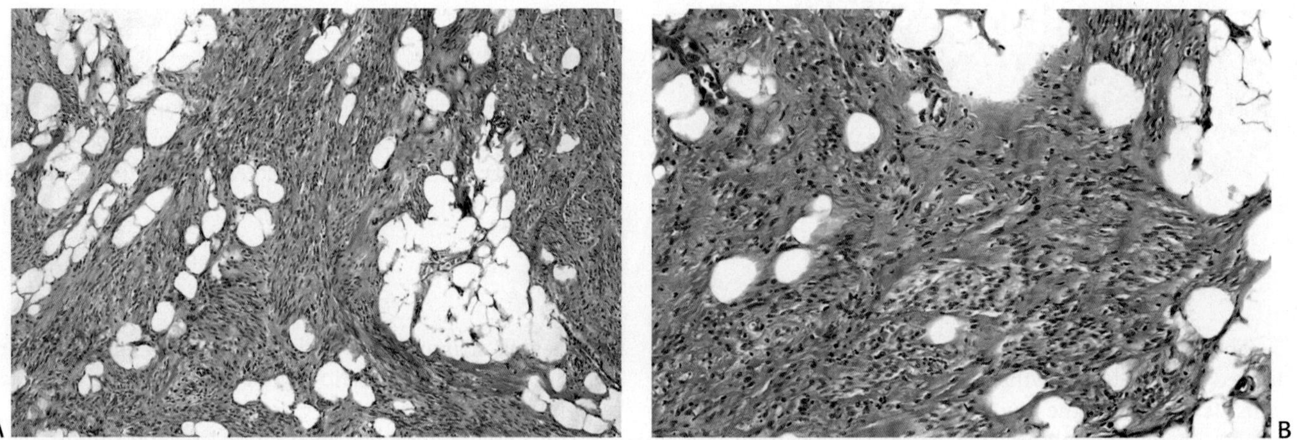

FIG. 38.41. ***Myofibroblastoma, infiltrative variant.*** **A–C:** The tumor infiltrates fat. **D:** Two benign ducts are surrounded by an infiltrative myofibroblastoma. **E:** Intense immunoreactivity for SMA.

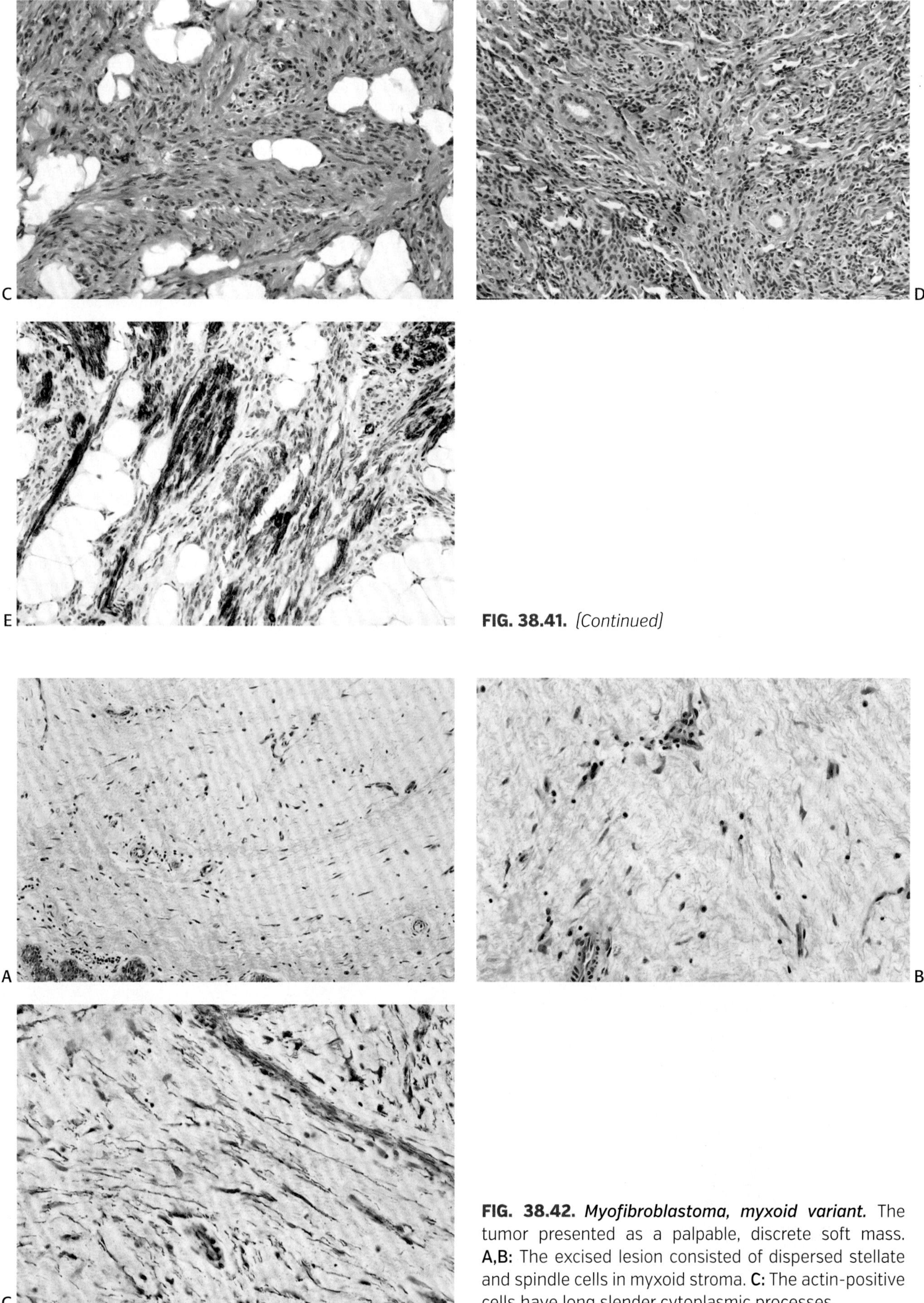

FIG. 38.41. *(Continued)*

FIG. 38.42. ***Myofibroblastoma, myxoid variant.*** The tumor presented as a palpable, discrete soft mass. **A,B:** The excised lesion consisted of dispersed stellate and spindle cells in myxoid stroma. **C:** The actin-positive cells have long slender cytoplasmic processes.

Rarely, myofibroblastomas contain abundant fat suggestive of a lipomatous element. The term "lipomatous myofibroblastoma" has been suggested for this group of lesions.[147]

Cytology

The FNA cytology specimen from a classical myofibroblastoma consists of spindle-shaped cells distributed singly or in clusters (Fig. 38.43).[148–152] A fascicular arrangement may be evident in cell clusters.[150] The oval nuclei have fine granular chromatin that may be divided by a "nuclear groove."[153] Nucleoli are small and inconspicuous.

Differential Diagnosis

Myofibroblastoma must be considered in the differential diagnosis of spindle cell mammary tumors. Sarcoma and metaplastic carcinoma are typically more cellular than myofibroblastomas, with greater atypia and frequent mitoses, and many have distinguishing histologic features (e.g., squamous metaplasia). Fasciitis and fibromatosis, which also contain myofibroblasts, tend to be stellate invasive lesions. Plump myoid cells and the inflammatory reaction of fasciitis are not seen in myofibroblastoma. Fibromatosis exhibits abundant collagen and spindle cells arranged in broad bands rather than in short fascicular clusters. Spindle cell lipomas are also commonly seen in men and sometimes may be well-circumscribed. They have more abundant adipose tissue than myofibroblastomas. However, the distinction between spindle cell lipoma and myofibroblastoma (particularly the lipomatous variant) by light microscopy can sometimes be difficult[136]; molecular analysis indicates that the two may represent related rather than distinct entities.[154]

The epithelioid variant of myofibroblastoma can mimic an invasive carcinoma such as pleomorphic lobular carcinoma or apocrine carcinoma.[145,155] The distinction can be particularly problematic in the core biopsy setting. Morphologic features that suggest the diagnosis of epithelioid myofibroblastoma include a well-circumscribed, pushing border; absent or minimal mitotic activity; associated spindle cells with more classical morphology; lack of glandular elements within the tumor; and dense collagenized stroma.

Immunohistochemistry

The majority of myofibroblastomas are immunoreactive for vimentin, desmin, calponin, SMA, muscle actin, CD10, CD34, bcl-2, and CD99.[120,129–131] Vimentin is usually diffusely positive, whereas the other markers can show variable reactivity. This immunoprofile is demonstrable in FNA specimens.[152] Focal positivity for H-caldesmon in 2% to 10% of lesional cells has been observed in a subset of cases.[156] The tumors are not immunoreactive for CK or factor VIII and only rarely weakly reactive for S-100 protein. They are usually positive for ER and PR by IHC.[131] Nuclear immunoreactivity for AR was detected in each of 5 myofibroblastomas studied by Morgan and Pitha[157] and in 6 of 11 tumors studied by Magro et al.[131]

Epithelioid cells in these tumors are strongly immunoreactive for vimentin and variably immunoreactive for desmin, SMA, CD10, CD34, bcl-2, and CD99.[145] All four cases of epithelioid myofibroblastoma reported by Magro[145] demonstrated positivity for ER, PR, and AR. There is no reactivity for CK in epithelioid myofibroblastoma.

Myofibroblasts exhibiting overt smooth muscle differentiation are strongly immunoreactive for actin and desmin but not for CD34.[158]

Molecular Studies

Mammary myofibroblastoma demonstrates recurrent monoallelic loss of the 13q14 chromosomal region, which includes

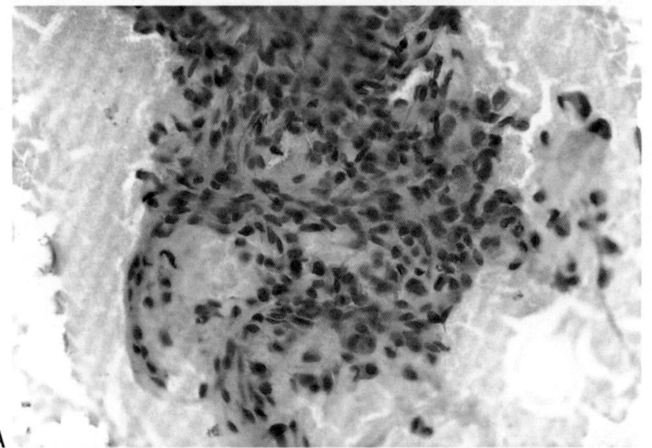

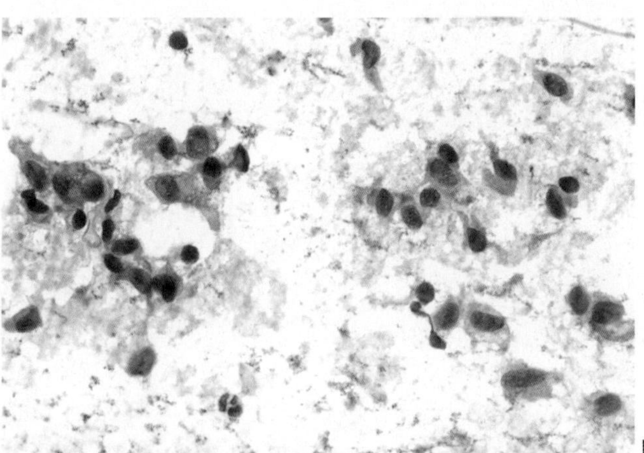

FIG. 38.43. ***Myofibroblastoma, cytology.*** **A:** Cohesive spindle cells with a few dyshesive epithelioid cells [*right*]. **B:** Dyshesive epithelioid cells from a myofibroblastoma. This sample could suggest carcinoma. Note the presence of oval nuclei and spindle cells.

RB1 and *FOXO1* loci.[154,159,160] Deletion of the 13q14 region is also seen in spindle cell lipoma, extramammary myofibroblastoma, and cellular angiofibroma,[154,160–163] supporting the hypothesis that these morphologically similar tumors are pathogenetically related. In contrast, solitary fibrous tumors do not show loss of 13q14 when assayed by fluorescence *in situ* hybridization (FISH) for the *RB1* gene locus.[154]

Treatment and Prognosis

No recurrences have been reported after follow-up periods of 3 to 126 months. Two patients were treated by mastectomy after an erroneous diagnosis of sarcoma,[128] and mastectomies have been performed for very large tumors occurring in men.[135,140] Virtually all patients are managed adequately by excisional biopsy.[128,134,145,148] Complete excision is recommended when a myofibroblastoma is identified in a needle core biopsy sample. Wider excision may be considered if a myofibroblastoma is present at the margin of an excision specimen, or the patient may be managed by clinical follow-up to detect a local recurrence early.

TUMORS WITH PERIVASCULAR MYOID DIFFERENTIATION

Tumors with perivascular myoid differentiation have been described under various names. Most involve the skin and subcutaneous tissue, commonly in the extremities. Breast involvement has rarely been cited in published reports, but the Senior Editor has encountered several mammary tumors with this appearance. A striking feature of these lesions is nodular fibrohistiocytic growth, predominantly with a perivascular localization (Fig. 38.44). Osteoclast-like giant cells are variably present (Fig. 38.45). Immunoreactivity for actin is present in the spindle cells, whereas the histiocytic elements are KP-1-positive.[164]

The terms "myofibromatosis-type perivascular myoma" and "myopericytoma" have been applied to an unusual and histologically distinctive group of neoplasms characterized by spindle cell perivascular proliferation.[165] Areas with hemangiopericytoma-like and glomangiopericytoma patterns may be encountered in these tumors. The spindle cells are consistently immunoreactive for actin.

Local recurrence in soft tissues at the primary site has been described in several reports of the various nonmammary lesions in this group of tumors. Occasional patients have had repeated recurrences over two or more decades, and metastases have rarely been reported.[166] No systematic study of these lesions in the breast has been published, but the Senior Editor has observed instances of local recurrence. Angioblastic sarcoma is discussed in Chapter 39.

GIANT CELL FIBROBLASTOMA

This uncommon soft tissue tumor of children has only rarely been encountered in the breast.[167] The lesion presents as a lobulated, circumscribed, firm, superficial mass that is composed of grossly homogeneous pale tissue. Microscopic examination reveals spindle and multinucleated giant cells, which often lie at the borders of clefts in the collagenous stroma. This pattern bears a close resemblance to PASH, although the latter usually lacks multinucleated stromal cells. Some giant cell fibroblastomas are immunoreactive for CD34. Electron microscopy reveals multisegmented nuclei and some cells with multiple nuclei. Numerous cytoplasmic microfilaments have been described,[167] and the ultrastructural findings suggest that the spindle cells are of fibroblastic or myofibroblastic origin. Local recurrence may occur after incomplete excision.

GRANULAR CELL TUMOR

The first report of this tumor attributed its origin to striated muscle cells; consequently, the lesion was termed a "myoblastoma."[168] Tissue culture studies of three granular cell

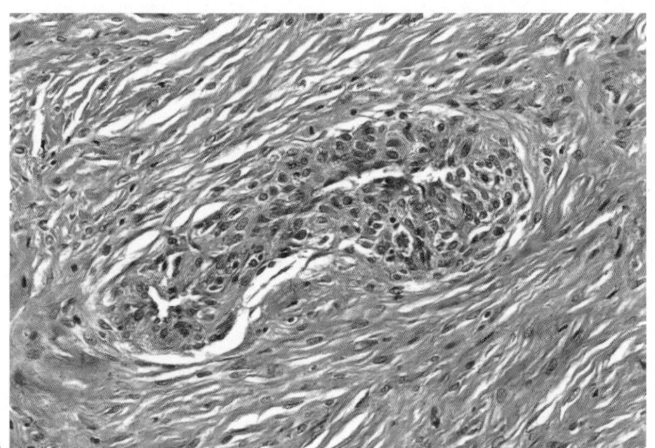
A

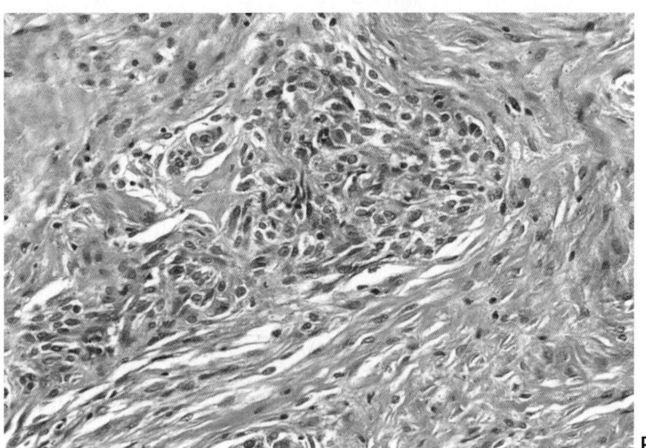
B

FIG. 38.44. ***Perivascular myocytic neoplasm.*** **A:** Epithelioid myocytic cells surround a slit-shaped vascular space. **B:** A nodular focus that contains inconspicuous vascular channels.

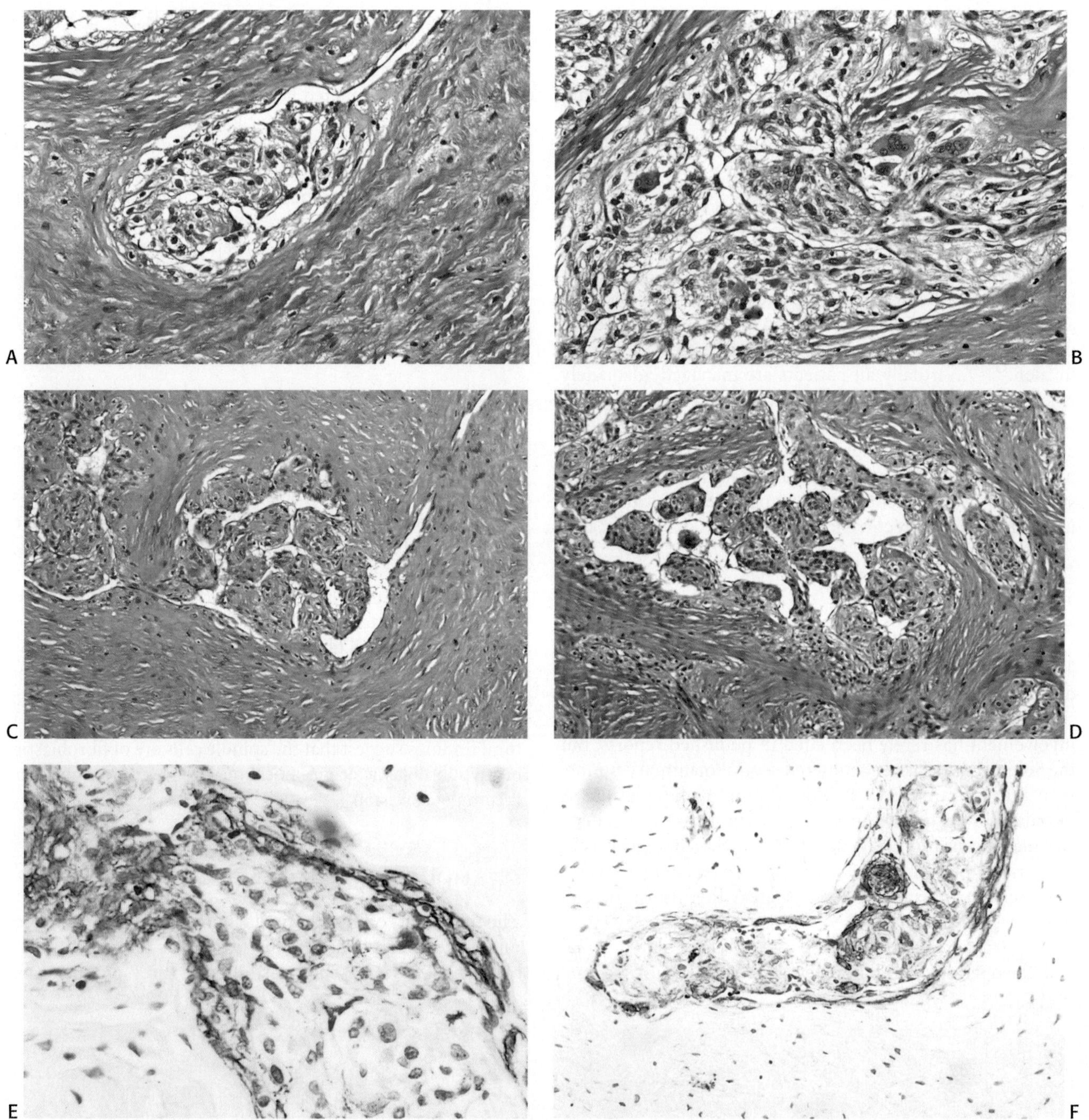

FIG. 38.45. ***Perivascular myocytic neoplasm.*** **A:** A small vascular channel extends from the *upper right* to *the center* of the image, where it is distorted by the perivascular myocytic proliferation. **B:** A more complex nodule from the same case with osteoclast-like giant cells. **C,D:** Expansion of vascular channels has caused the lesion to have a pseudopapillary or glomeruloid appearance. **E:** Reactivity for factor VIII is localized to endothelial cells. **F:** Immunoreactivity for SMA is shown.

tumors, including two from the breast, appeared to support this interpretation.[169] Subsequent evidence has shown that the tumors are derived from the Schwann cells of peripheral nerves. Granular cell tumors occur throughout the body with about 5% of them originating in the breast.[170] The first description of a mammary granular cell tumor was published in 1931.[171] In 1946, Haagensen and Stout[172] reported the first series of patients with mammary granular cell tumor and emphasized the importance of distinguishing this benign tumor from carcinoma.

Clinical Presentation

Granular cell tumor of the breast (GCTB) is most often encountered in women aged 30 to 50 years, but it has been described in adolescents and elderly women with an overall age range of 14 to 77 years[170,173–177] and a mean of 53.5 years.[178] About 7% to 10% of GCTB occurs in the male breast.[173–175,178,179] In several studies, the majority of patients have been African Americans.[176,180–183] Papalas et al.[176] reported a younger average age at presentation for African American patients (41 years) compared to Caucasian ones (54 years).

In most cases, the patient presents with a firm or hard, painless mass. The left and right breasts are affected with equal frequency. GCTB may arise in any part of the breast parenchyma, including the axillary tail, or in a subcutaneous location. The lesions tend to develop more often in the upper and medial quadrants. Superficial lesions may cause skin retraction, and nipple inversion has been reported when the tumor is in a subareolar location. Large tumors or those that arise deep in the breast may be adherent to the pectoral fascia. GCTB usually occurs as a solitary unilateral lesion, but rare instances of multiple and bilateral tumors have been reported.[180,181,183] Patients who have multiple granular cell tumors at various sites may have one or more lesions in the breast.[176,181–182,184,185] Unusual clinical presentations include nonpalpable GCTB detected by mammography,[186,187] coincidental GCTB and infiltrating duct carcinoma in the same[176,181,188] or opposite breast,[187] and GCTB in the contralateral breast of a patient with previously treated DCIS.[186]

On mammography, GCTB is difficult to distinguish from carcinoma.[189–191] It typically forms a stellate mass lacking calcifications with a dense core, but circumscribed lesions occasionally occur.[180,182,183,192–194] Ultrasound examination usually reveals a solid mass with indistinct margins and posterior shadowing suggestive of carcinoma,[180,182,183,186,192–195] but, rarely, the ultrasound pattern is hypoechoic with or without attenuation of the sound beam.[179,180,186,196] MRI findings can overlap with those of carcinoma.[197,198]

Gross Pathology

In the excised specimen, GCTB usually presents as a firm or hard mass. Many of the tumors appear well-circumscribed when bisected. Other examples have ill-defined infiltrative borders. The cut surface looks white, gray, yellow, or tan (Fig. 38.46). Lesions measuring up to 9 cm have been reported, but the tumors are generally 2 cm or smaller.

Microscopic Pathology

With very rare exceptions, GCTB is a benign neoplasm. The histologic, histochemical, and ultrastructural features of mammary GCTB are indistinguishable from those of granular cell tumors arising at other sites. The tumor is composed of compact nests or sheets of cells that contain eosinophilic cytoplasmic granules (Fig. 38.47). The granules are usually prominent and fill the cytoplasm, but in some lesions there is a tendency to cytoplasmic vacuolization and clearing. The cytoplasmic granules are PAS-positive and diastase-resistant. Cell borders are typically well-defined, and the cells vary from polygonal to spindly in shape. Nuclei are round to slightly oval with an open chromatin pattern. Nucleoli tend to be prominent. In some cases, a modest amount of nuclear pleomorphism, occasional multinucleated cells, and rare mitoses may be found, but these features should not be interpreted as evidence of a malignant neoplasm. Variable amounts of collagenous stroma are present. One group of investigators reported a direct correlation between the amount of stromal fibrosis and the presence of elastosis in the lesion.[199] Small nerve bundles are sometimes seen in the tumor or in close association with stellate peripheral extensions of the lesion. Cells that resemble those of granular cell tumor have been observed

A

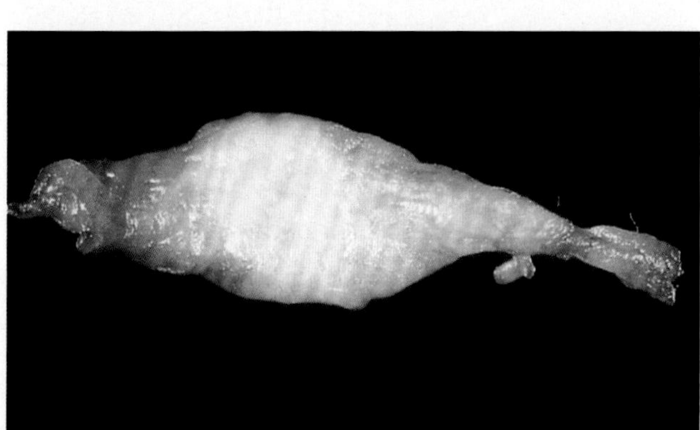

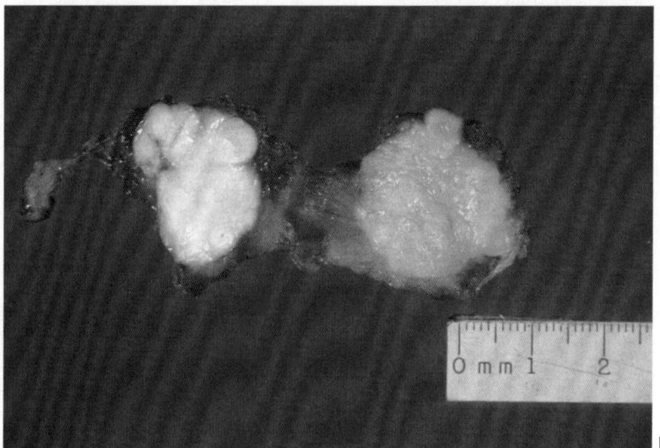

B

FIG. 38.46. ***Granular cell tumor, gross appearance.*** **A:** A pale yellow homogeneous tumor that blends with the fibrous parenchyma. **B:** This tumor is circumscribed and lobulated.

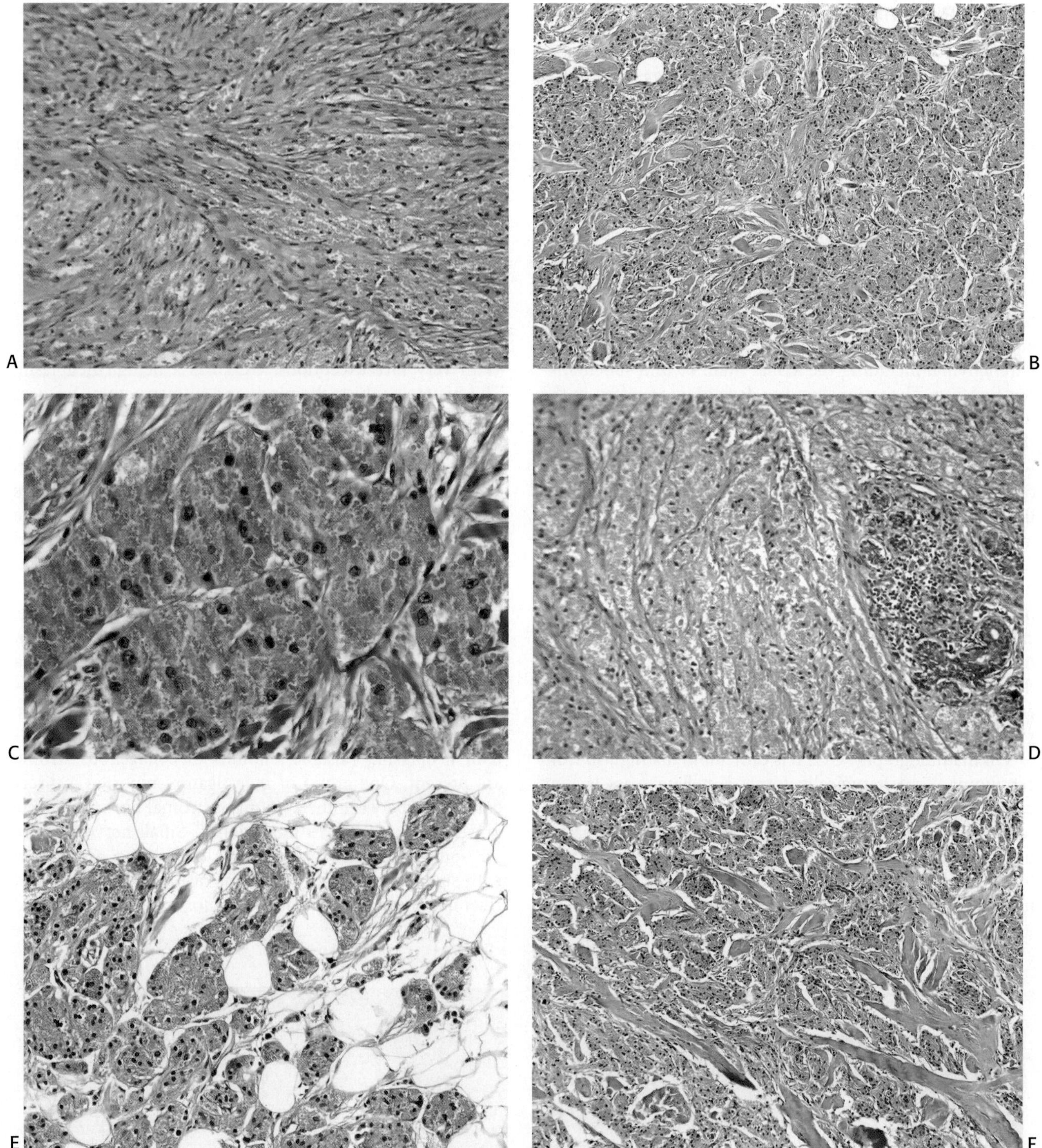

FIG. 38.47. ***Granular cell tumor.*** **A:** The tumor cells are arranged in a fascicular pattern. **B:** This tumor demonstrates a nested growth pattern. **C:** Tumor cells with small round nuclei and granular eosinophilic cytoplasm. **D:** Invasion around a lobule. **E:** Invasion of fat. **F:** Tumor cells distributed between thick bands of collagen.

in nerves close to but not directly involved by granular cell tumors.[200] Although many of the tumors appear grossly circumscribed, microscopic examination usually reveals an infiltrating growth pattern at the margins of the lesion (Fig. 38.47). Ducts and lobules are typically surrounded by the invasive tumor cells and incorporated into the lesion. Granular cell tumor cells may infiltrate into lobules and into the dermis of the skin.

Cytology

FNA of GCTB usually yields a cellular specimen, and the cells, which are dispersed separately or in irregular clusters, have mildly pleomorphic nuclei that often contain prominent nucleoli.[179] Numerous granules distributed throughout the background as well as in the cells stain blue with Romanovsky stain and red with the Papanicolaou and the H&E stain. The distinction between GCTB and mammary carcinoma, especially apocrine carcinoma, is particularly difficult in FNA specimens.[201–204] This difficulty can result in a false-positive diagnosis of carcinoma.[205,206]

Differential Diagnosis

Histologically, GCTB must be distinguished from mammary carcinoma, histiocytic lesions, and metastatic neoplasms. The infiltrative character of GCTB composed of cells with prominent nucleoli, especially when the lesion has collagenous stroma, results in a close resemblance to scirrhous carcinoma, particularly in frozen sections. The similarity between invasive apocrine carcinoma and GCTB is sometimes striking. The presence of DCIS, often with lobular extension as well as cytologic pleomorphism usually serve to identify invasive apocrine carcinoma. In some instances, the lesions can only be distinguished with confidence by immunohistochemical studies, especially if *in situ* carcinoma is not evident. Apocrine carcinomas are immunoreactive for CK and ARs, and usually for epithelial membrane antigen (EMA) and GCDFP-15. GCTB is not reactive for epithelial markers or GCDFP-15 and it does not contain mucin.

A superficial resemblance between the cells of GCTB and histiocytes can lead to confusion with a granulomatous inflammatory reaction or a histiocytic tumor. GCTB is immunohistochemically negative for histiocyte-associated antigens such as α_1-antitrypsin, α_1-antichymotrypsin, and muramidase,[191,207] but reactivity for CD68 (KP-1) has been described in GCTB.[208,209] Histiocytes and GCTB cells are immunoreactive for S-100.

GCTB must be distinguished from metastatic neoplasms in the breast that have oncocytic or clear cell features such as renal carcinoma and malignant melanoma. The differential diagnosis also includes alveolar soft part sarcoma. Granular cell tumors are not immunoreactive for myoglobin.[210] The cytoplasmic granules in these tumors are Luxol fast blue-positive, an observation that suggests that they contain myelin.[211]

Immunohistochemistry

GCTB is characterized by strong, diffuse immunoreactivity for S-100 protein (Fig. 38.48) and carcinoembryonic antigen (CEA). However, these results do not themselves distinguish GCTB from mammary carcinoma, since some carcinomas are also S-100- and CEA-positive.[191,201,202,207,210] A high proportion of granular cell tumors are reactive for vimentin, which is detectable in relatively few carcinomas.[207] GCTB is negative for CK, GCDFP-15,[212] ER, and PR.[181]

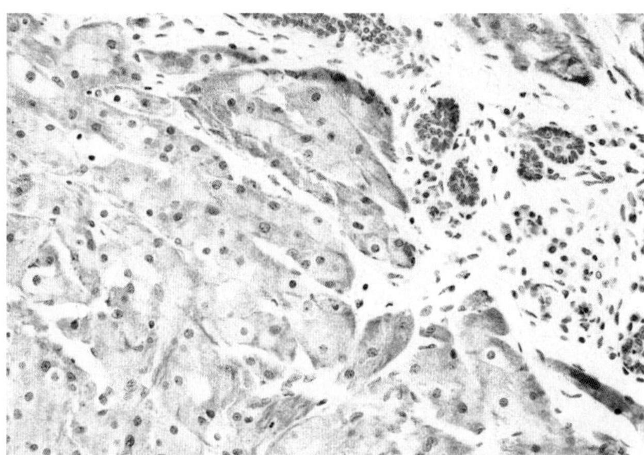

FIG. 38.48. ***Granular cell tumor, S-100 protein.*** The tumor cells invading around a lobule are immunoreactive for S-100 protein.

Electron Microscopy

Electron microscopy reveals myelin figures as well as numerous lysosomes in granular cell tumors.[175,191,207,210] Observations in one electron microscopic study suggested that the granules are formed by infolding of the cell membrane resulting in myelin figures phagocytosed by lysosomes.[211] The process appeared to be analogous to the mechanism by which myelin is formed around axons in nerves. Some cells also have angulate bodies, which are rounded triangular membrane-bound structures that contain microtubules and microfibrils.

Treatment and Prognosis

Benign GCTB is treated by wide excision. Local recurrence may occur after incomplete excision, but it is sometimes difficult to distinguish between recurrence and asynchronous multifocal lesions. Most patients with positive or close (less than 0.1 cm) margins do not experience recurrence of their tumors.[176,180] Direct invasion of an axillary lymph node (ALN) by a GCTB that arose in the axillary tail has been reported.[180] No recurrence was evident after 47 months of follow-up.

Fewer than 1% of all granular cell tumors, including mammary lesions, are malignant (Fig. 38.49). Both locoregional and distant metastatic spread from GCTB have been described.[213–215] Metastases in the breast and ALNs from extramammary granular cell tumors have also been reported.[216,217] In some instances, it may not be possible to distinguish between the clinical presentation of multifocal benign granular cell tumors, including breast lesions, and metastatic malignant granular cell tumor.

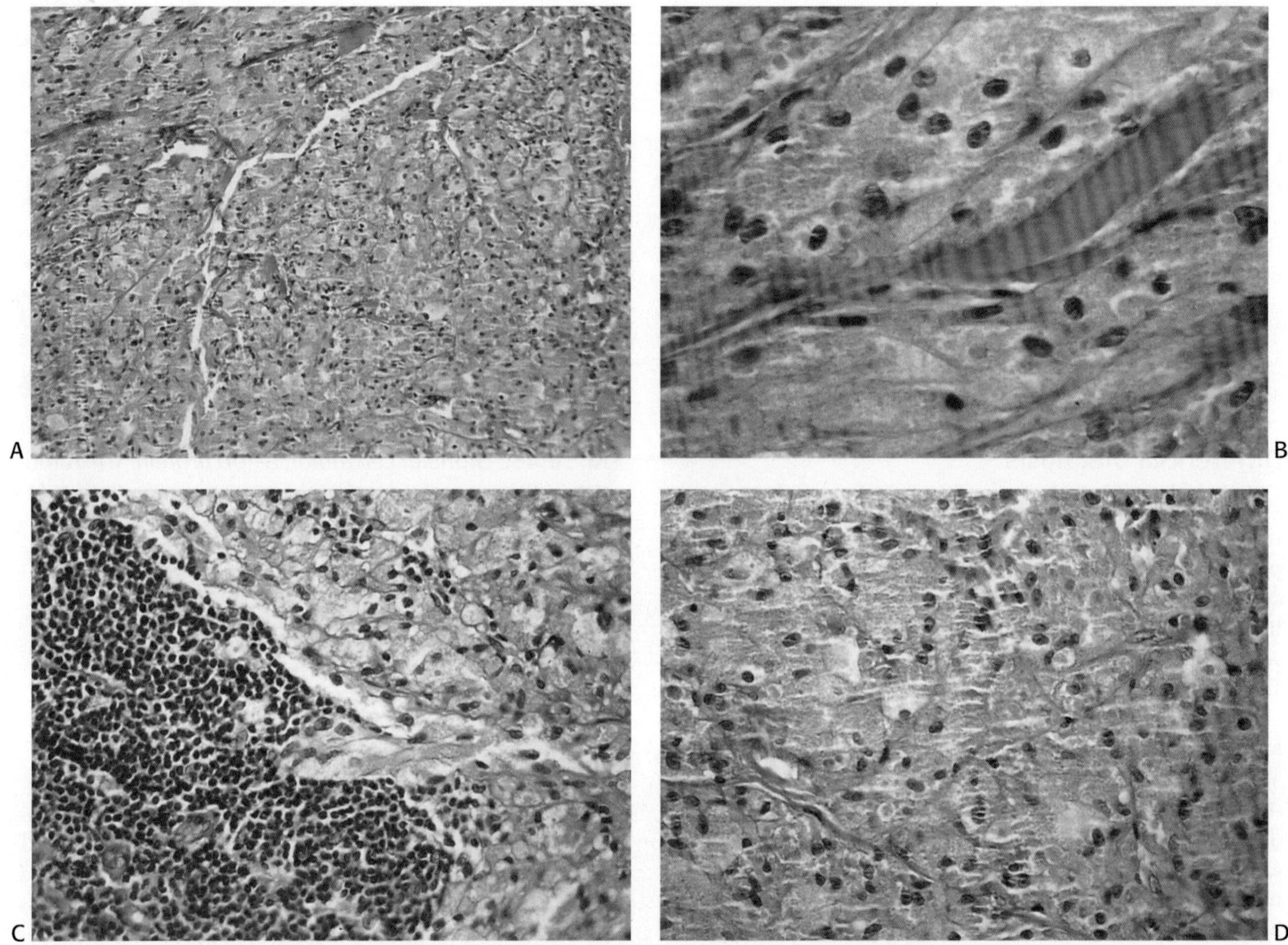

FIG. 38.49. *Granular cell tumor, malignant.* **A,B:** The histologic appearance of the cells in the primary tumor is not exceptional. **C,D:** Metastatic granular cell tumor that arose from the tumor shown in (**A**) and (**B**) is present in an ALN.

TUMORS OF NERVE AND NERVE SHEATH ORIGIN

Benign neural neoplasms commonly found in the soft tissues at various sites occur rarely in the breast. Benign nerve sheath tumors of the breast have been reported, usually diagnosed as "neurilemomas" or as schwannomas.[218–221] Many of these tumors arose in the mammary subcutaneous tissue, but parenchymal lesions were also described. Patients with von Recklinghausen disease develop neurofibromas in the subcutaneous tissues and the breast, but massive neurofibromatosis of the breast is uncommon.[222,223] A patient with von Recklinghausen disease can develop mammary carcinoma; therefore, the appearance of a new breast mass in this setting should prompt appropriate diagnostic evaluation.[224]

Clinical Presentation

The age range at diagnosis is 6 to 81 years, with most patients in their 30s to 50s. Although most patients have been female, benign neural neoplasms of the male breast have been described.[225–227] A schwannoma presents as a painless, well-defined mass that is clinically indistinguishable from a FA. Either breast may be involved, and there is no predilection for a specific site in the breast. Rare examples may be mammographically detected.[228] A patient with two schwannomas of one breast has been reported.[229]

Mammary neurofibroma in neurofibromatosis type 1 patients commonly involves the nipple–areolar region.[230,231] The cutaneous tumors range in appearance from large pedunculated masses to small appendages that mimic accessory nipples. Neurofibroma is less commonly situated within the breast parenchyma. Multiple parenchymal neurofibromas in a single breast have been reported.[232] Neurofibroma has also been reported as a cause of breast enlargement mimicking gynecomastia in prepubertal boys.[227]

Gross Pathology

The circumscribed tumor consists of dense, firm gray or white tissue, which may have soft mucoid regions (Fig. 38.50). One tumor measured 14.0 cm in greatest diameter,[233] but most are smaller, and one schwannoma was an asymptomatic 7-mm lesion detected by mammography.[228]

Microscopic Pathology

Microscopic examination of a schwannoma reveals the typical histologic features of a benign nerve sheath tumor, consisting of spindle cells in bundles, sometimes with nuclei arranged in

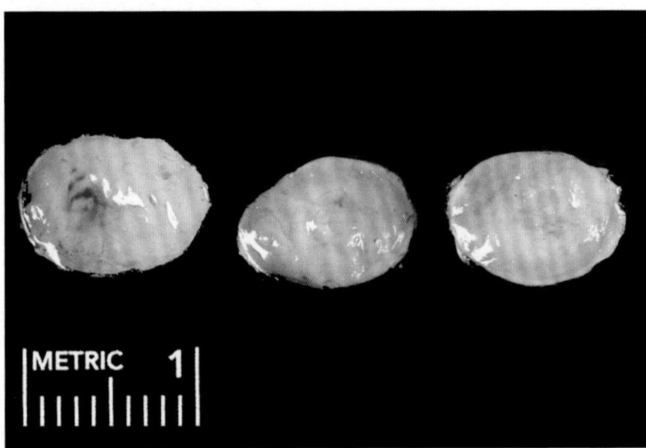

FIG. 38.50. ***Schwannoma, gross appearance.*** This well-circumscribed tumor consists of glistening, tan-yellow tissue.

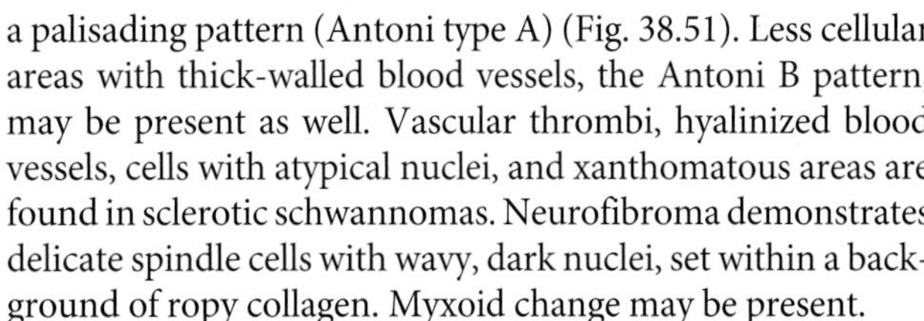

a palisading pattern (Antoni type A) (Fig. 38.51). Less cellular areas with thick-walled blood vessels, the Antoni B pattern, may be present as well. Vascular thrombi, hyalinized blood vessels, cells with atypical nuclei, and xanthomatous areas are found in sclerotic schwannomas. Neurofibroma demonstrates delicate spindle cells with wavy, dark nuclei, set within a background of ropy collagen. Myxoid change may be present.

The differential diagnosis includes other spindle cell tumors such as FAs, phyllodes tumor, fibromatosis, and metaplastic carcinoma. These lesions are usually readily distinguished in histologic sections, but difficulty may be encountered in material obtained by FNA.[226,229,234,235] The nuclei of cells seen in the aspirate from a benign neural tumor are typically spindly or oval with homogeneous fine chromatin. Palisaded cells may be evident in an FNA specimen.[218] Pleomorphic, irregular, hyperchromatic nuclei may be encountered, particularly in the lesions termed "ancient" nerve sheath tumors.[236]

The diagnosis of a benign peripheral nerve sheath tumor is supported by a positive immunohistochemical stain for S-100 protein, a negative immunostain for actin, and the absence of mitotic activity.

Immunohistochemistry

Schwannomas tend to demonstrate more diffuse expression of S-100 protein than neurofibromas; in the latter tumors, only a subset of cells usually is positive.

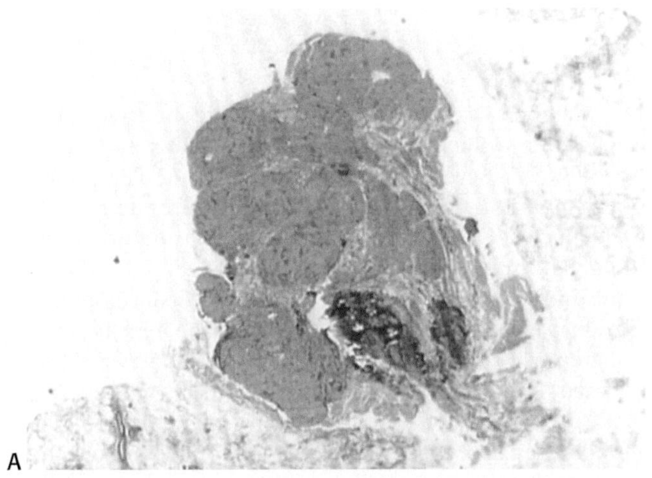

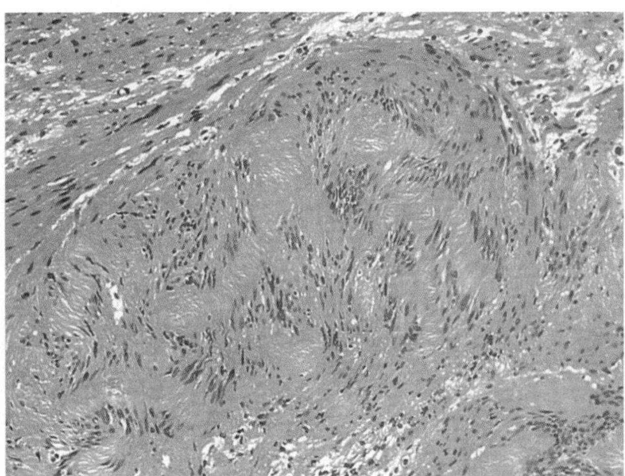

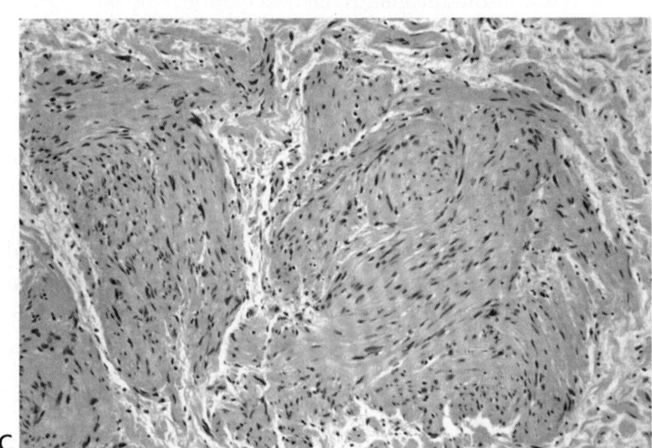

FIG. 38.51. ***Schwannoma.*** **A:** A whole-mount histologic section of a circumscribed, nodule that presented as a nonpalpable lesion detected by mammography. Hemorrhage in the lesion is the result of a needle core biopsy. **B:** Palisading of tumor cells. **C:** This part of the tumor resembles a reparative neuroma. (Courtesy of Dr S. Hoda.)

Treatment and Prognosis

Complete excision provides adequate therapy.

HAMARTOMA

Stedman's Medical Dictionary defines hamartoma as "a focal malformation that resembles a neoplasm, grossly and even microscopically, but results from faulty development in an organ; it is composed of an abnormal mixture of tissue elements, or an abnormal proportion of a single element normally present at that site."[237]

This term was first applied to lesions of the breast in 1971 by Arrigoni et al.,[238] who described 10 patients with encapsulated breast tumors that clinically and grossly resembled FAs. Microscopic examination revealed "mammary glandular tissue with a prominent lobular arrangement, fibrous stroma, and fat in variable proportions." Cystic and papillary apocrine metaplasia was evident in some lesions.

There has been a tendency among some authors to employ the diagnosis mammary hamartoma more broadly and to apply it to a variety of benign, circumscribed lesions such as PASH.[80,239,240] The fact that the radiologic appearances of these lesions are quite similar has reinforced this misconception, which obscures the definition of hamartoma by lumping together several pathologically distinct lesions. This is exemplified by one lesion diagnosed as mammary hamartoma that was reported twice with identical illustrations, but is an example of PASH.[241,242] Two tumors reported to be "multiple hamartomas" in the breast of a 20-year-old woman had a radiologic appearance consistent with this diagnosis, but in publication appear grossly and histologically to be FAs.[243] In another case report, a 14-cm mass with the radiologic appearance of a hamartoma proved to be "juvenile hypertrophy" histologically.[244]

Clinical Presentation

Tumors that best qualify as hamartoma of the breast occur most often in premenopausal women, but they have been described in teenagers and in women in their 60s. Association with pregnancy has been noted in a minority of cases.[245] Multiple and bilateral hamartomas and "hamartoma-like lesions" have been described in patients with Cowden syndrome[246,247]; however, most patients with mammary hamartoma do not appear to have the syndrome. Some patients report slow enlargement, whereas others describe rapid growth. The tumors have been as large as 17 cm, thereby resulting in substantial asymmetry. In some cases, large tumors responsible for macromastia may not be palpable as distinct lesions, although they are clearly evident in a mammogram. Mammography reveals a well-circumscribed, dense, round or oval mass surrounded by a narrow lucent zone.[245,248,249] Hamartomas were diagnosed in 16 of 10,000 mammography examinations reviewed by Hessler et al.[249] The ultrasound appearance of mammary hamartoma is reported to be variable and not specific, an observation that reflects intrinsic differences in the lesions and probably also the inclusion of assorted entities in this diagnostic category.[250] An example of hamartoma arising in axillary breast tissue has been reported.[251]

Gross Pathology

The size of the tumors ranges from less than 1 to 17 cm.[252] They are well-circumscribed with a firm to rubbery consistency. Most tumors are tan-pink to white, and islands of yellow adipose tissue are occasionally observed. Scattered cysts may be present.

Microscopic Pathology

Hamartomas are discrete masses composed of mammary glandular tissue, fibrous stroma, and fat mixed in various proportions. The glandular elements usually retain a lobular architecture, although the lobules may be larger or more disorganized than those in the surrounding normal breast tissue. Some hamartomas contain only a very minor to negligible amount of fat. In others, fat may comprise the majority of the lesion. Two common variants of mammary hamartoma are "adenolipoma" and "chondrolipoma."

Adenolipoma

Adenolipoma has a broad age distribution, having been reported in women in their 20s and 80s with a mean age in the 40s.[249,253] Several patients were pregnant. The presenting symptom is a painless mass that measures up to 13 cm in diameter. On clinical examination, the tumor forms a dominant mass, which may be well-defined and mobile or indistinct. In some cases, the lesion is difficult to appreciate on palpation, although it is readily apparent by mammography. Radiologic examination demonstrates a sharply defined round or oval tumor that appears encapsulated and surrounded by a radiolucent ring. Predominantly fatty tumors may have the lucent appearance of lipomas, whereas those with abundant glandular tissue appear dense.[249,253,254] Ultrasonography reveals a mixed pattern of echogenic and sonolucent regions.[255]

Gross examination discloses a soft, circumscribed, sometimes lobulated mass bordered by a thin fibrous pseudocapsule (Fig. 38.52). The cut surface has a variegated pattern of fat and fibrous breast parenchyma. Lesions with the most abundant fat resemble lipomas. Small cysts may be seen.

Microscopically, the tissue consists of mature fat and mammary parenchyma mixed in varying proportions and delimited by a pseudocapsule of compressed breast tissue (Fig. 38.53). Lobules and ducts present in the lesion appear structurally normal with little or no proliferative change.

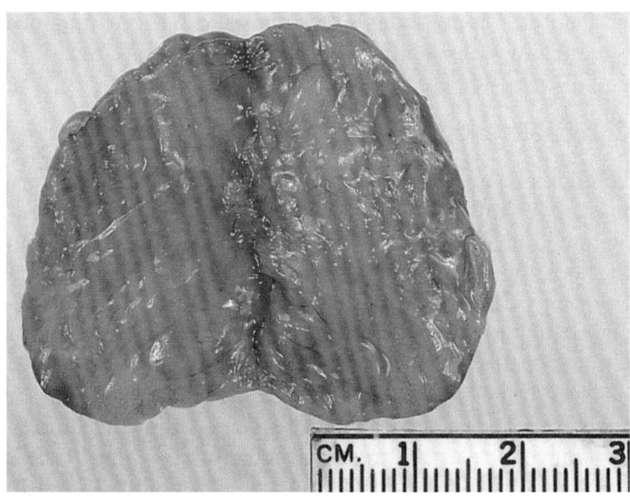

FIG. 38.52. *Hamartoma, gross appearance.*

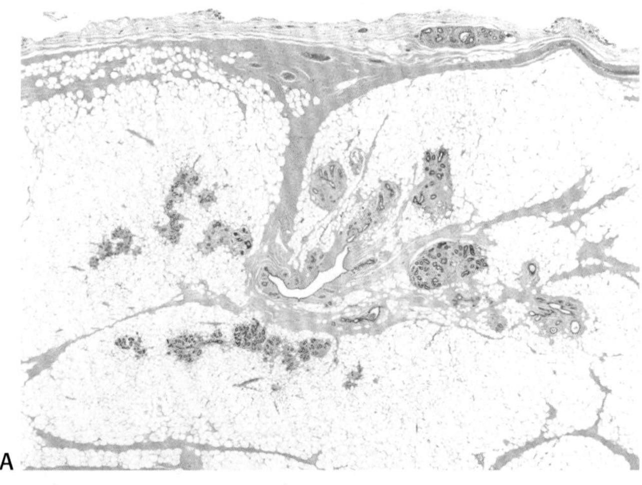

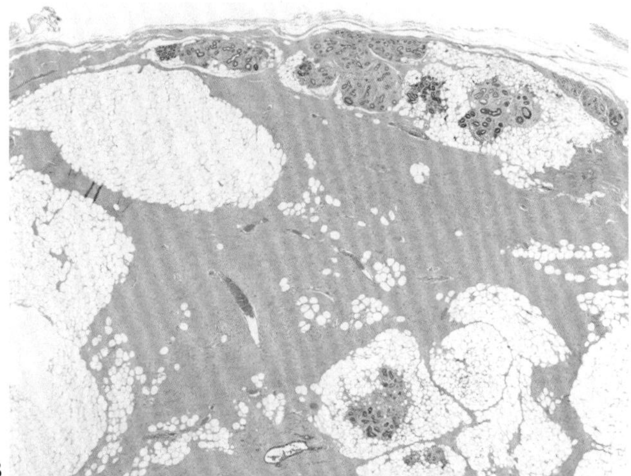

FIG. 38.53. *Hamartoma, adenolipoma type.* A,B: Nodular aggregates of lobular breast parenchyma in a circumscribed lipomatous tumor with focal fibrous areas in (B).

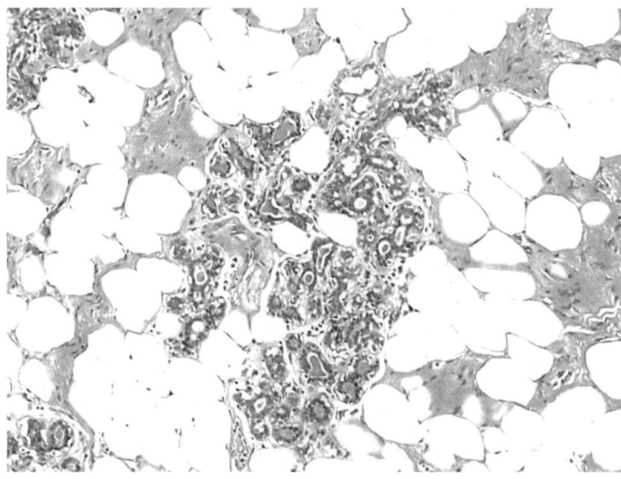

FIG. 38.54. *Hamartoma, adenolipoma type.* The lobular aggregates lack distinctive stroma and tend to blend with the fat.

The most significant abnormality is the unusual tissue distribution (Fig. 38.54). In this setting, the term "dysplastic" has been employed to describe the structural composition of the lesion rather than proliferative and cytologic abnormalities.[249] Rare examples containing brown fat have been described ("adenohibernoma").[256–258]

Adenolipoma differs structurally from other mammary lesions that contain fat. It lacks the adenomatous component seen in FAs with adipose metaplasia and does not exhibit the cytologic atypia seen in the stroma of phyllodes tumors with adipose differentiation.[259]

Adenolipoma should be treated by excisional biopsy. Good cosmetic results have been reported even when tumors larger than a quadrant were excised.[249]

Chondrolipomas

Chondrolipomas are composed of mature adipose tissue and hyaline cartilage.[235,260–262] The patients have been adult women aged 37 to 79 years who presented with palpable tumors. One tumor was present for several years, but most were noted no more than 2 months before diagnosis. Several chondrolipomas measured 2 cm in diameter and one lesion was 6 cm. Mammography revealed a well-circumscribed mass resembling a FA. In one case, the radiographic findings were described as "probably mammary dysplasia."[262]

The excised tumor is a soft or rubbery circumscribed lobulated mass composed of gray or pink-white tissue that is not obviously fat. Plate-like foci of cartilage and gritty areas may be evident grossly.[260] Microscopic examination reveals sharply defined islands of hyaline cartilage, sometimes with focal calcification, distributed in mature fat and fibrofatty glandular mammary parenchyma. Smooth muscle has been noted rarely, and these lesions are probably myofibroblastomas with chondroid and myoid differentiation.[263] The margin of the tumor is demarcated by compressed mammary tissue, resulting in an encapsulated appearance.[262] Glandular elements may be absent or scanty in some lesions.[262,264,265] The cytologic specimen obtained by FNA reveals benign hyaline cartilage and fat.[265]

Chondrolipoma is treated by excisional biopsy. Recurrences have not been reported.

LEIOMYOMA

Most leiomyomas of the breast arise from smooth muscle in the nipple and areola.[266] Parenchymal leiomyomas probably arise as a result of smooth muscle metaplasia of myoepithelial or myofibroblastic cells, or from blood vessels (Fig. 38.55). Myoid differentiation of myofibroblastic cells is discussed and illustrated in a preceding section of this chapter. The diagnosis of leiomyoma should be restricted to lesions composed entirely of smooth muscle. Fibroadenomas[267] and SA[268] with myomatous metaplasia should be excluded from this category. The so-called adenoleiomyoma described by Haagensen[269] is an example of adenosis with leiomyomatous hyperplasia of myoepithelial cells.

Clinical Presentation

Leiomyoma of the breast presents as a palpable, solitary mass. Pain and discomfort have been reported with parenchymal and nipple lesions. There is no predilection as to the location of parenchymal lesions. Patients' age ranges from 34 to 69 years. Radiologic examination of a parenchymal leiomyoma revealed a circumscribed 3-cm tumor without calcification.[270] A nonpalpable leiomyoma was detected during the course of routine follow-up mammography of a 50-year-old woman receiving adjuvant tamoxifen for contralateral invasive carcinoma.[271] The tumor formed a distinct, slightly lobulated oval nodule 9 mm in largest dimension. Leiomyomas of the male breast have been reported.[272,273] The mammographic appearance of a subareolar leiomyoma of the male breast was described by Velasco et al.[273]

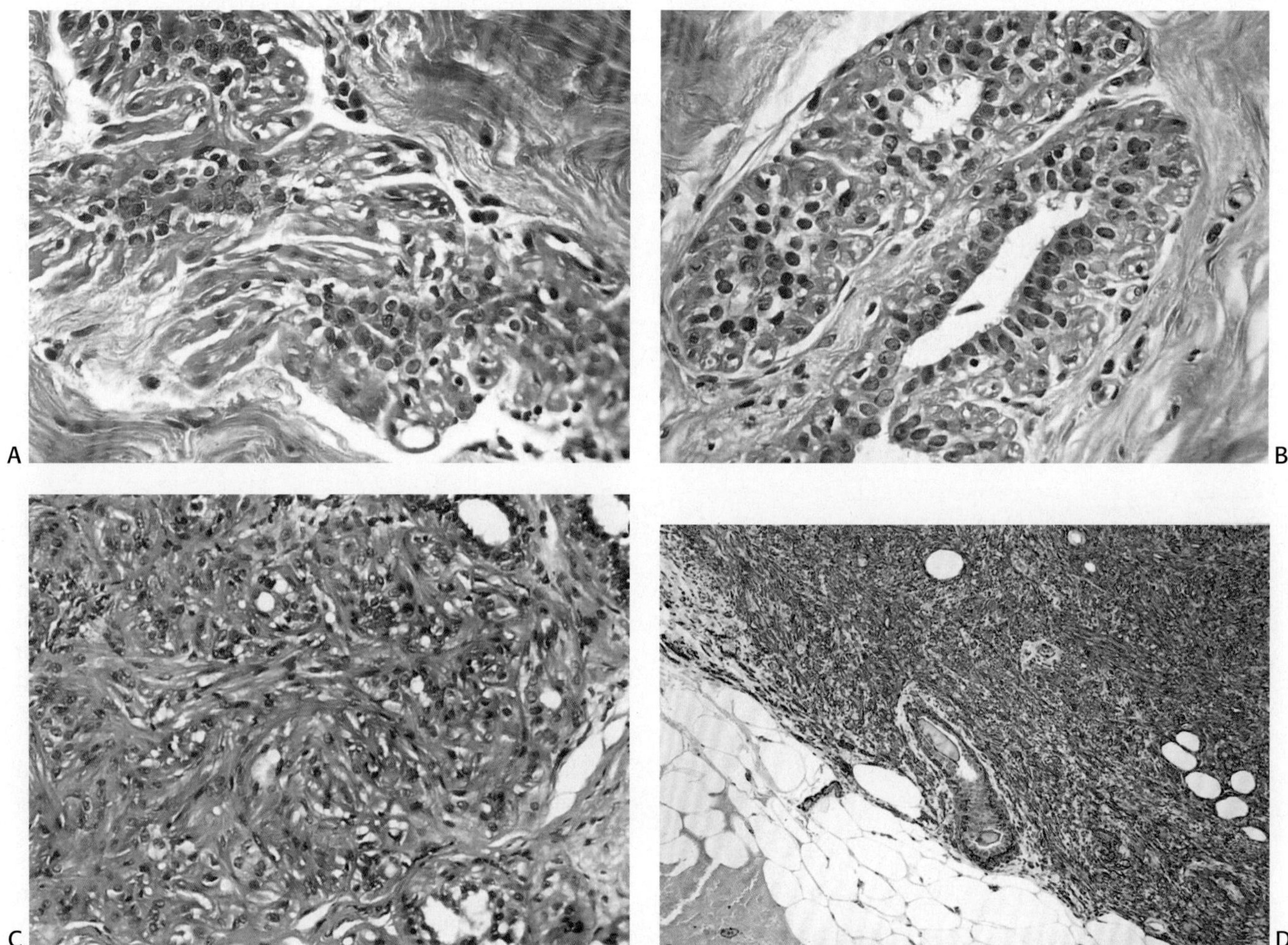

FIG. 38.55. ***Myoid metaplasia of myoepithelial cells.*** **A:** Myoepithelial cells with a myoid phenotype are cut longitudinally in this section of an atrophic terminal duct–lobular complex. **B:** Myoid myoepithelial cells are cut transversely in this section of a duct. **C:** Nodular myoid metaplasia in SA. **D:** An actin immunostain of a lesion similar to **(C)** showing abundant myoepithelial cells with a myoid phenotype.

Gross Pathology

The tumor forms a firm, circumscribed mass with a whorled cut surface. Tumors as large as 13 cm have been reported, but most are smaller than 5 cm.

Microscopic Pathology

Microscopically, circumscription is also evident. The growth pattern features interlacing fascicles of spindle cells with eosinophilic cytoplasm (Fig. 38.56). Cytologic atypia, mitoses, and necrosis, which characterize leiomyosarcoma, are absent. An epithelioid variant of mammary parenchymal leiomyoma was described by Roncaroli et al.[274] The tumor cells had fine granular cytoplasm and were immunoreactive for desmin and actin, but not for S-100 protein. Similar staining results are obtained in nonepithelioid variants of mammary leiomyoma.

Treatment and Prognosis

Complete excision is recommended. This may necessitate removing the nipple if the lesion is in the subareolar region or nipple. Local recurrence has been reported[275] rarely. One recurrence was treated by reexcision. Another recurrence growing as leiomyosarcoma with mitoses and necrosis was treated by mastectomy.[275]

MYOID "HAMARTOMA"

This tumor, also termed *muscular hamartoma*, is a benign proliferative lesion composed of ducts, lobules, stroma, and bands of smooth muscle cells. Most examples of this neoplasm are adenosis tumors with leiomyomatous myoid metaplasia of the myoepithelial cell component. Regrettably, the designation of these tumors as hamartomas is now well entrenched in the literature.

Clinical Presentation

Myoid "hamartoma" forms a circumscribed palpable tumor ranging from 1 to 11 cm in diameter.[276–278] A duration of 4 years or longer is sometimes reported.[279,280] The tumor is most often located in the upper outer quadrant. Mammography reveals a well-demarcated lesion of variable density, often with a radiolucent halo.[277,278,280,281] Cystic areas may be suggested by mammography or by sonography.[277,279]

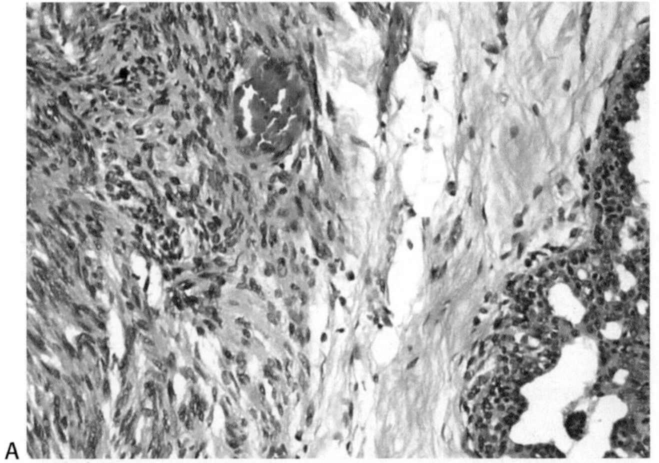
A

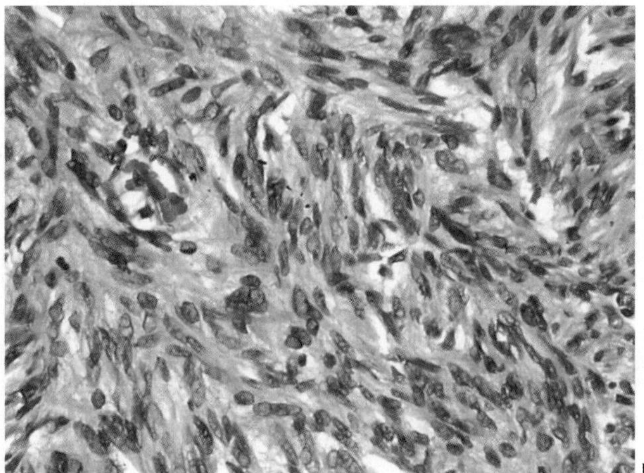
B

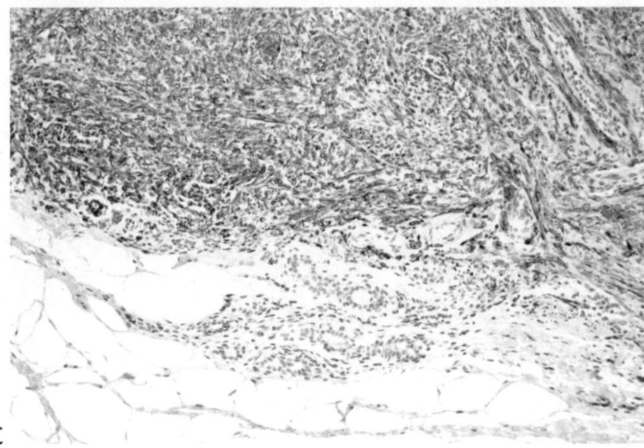
C

FIG. 38.56. *Leiomyoma.* **A:** Epithelial hyperplasia is evident in a duct next to the tumor. **B:** The interlacing spindle cells have oval nuclei. **C:** The cytoplasm is immunoreactive for desmin.

Gross Pathology

The tumor is a well-circumscribed, bosselated firm mass appearing fibrous on the cut surface. Adipose tissue is not usually evident in the lesion grossly. Cysts of varying size containing brown fluid have been described in a minority of cases.[277,279,280]

Microscopic Pathology

The histologic composition of myoid "hamartomas" is variable, depending on the relative proportions of glandular, cystic, myomatous, and fibrous elements. In most lesions, interlacing bundles of smooth muscle constitute focal leiomyoma formation, whereas in a minority of tumors, the myoid component mingles more diffusely with adipose and fibrous tissues. Epithelioid differentiation of myoepithelial cells can result in a pattern resembling infiltrating lobular carcinoma, especially in the limited sample of a needle core biopsy.[278] Adequate sampling reveals foci of SA in virtually all examples, and at these sites the origin of the myoid element can be traced to myoepithelial cells[282] (Figs. 38.55 and 38.57). Associated "fibrocystic changes" include cystic apocrine metaplasia and duct hyperplasia. The histologic features of myoid "hamartoma" have been found in a FA, a not unexpected observation, since SA develops occasionally in FAs.[280]

Electron microscopy and IHC confirm the myoid character of the spindle cell component of the lesion and support origin from myoepithelial cells.[276,279,280]

Treatment and Prognosis

Myoid "hamartoma" is adequately treated by excisional biopsy performed by "shelling out" the tumor. There is no tendency toward local recurrence, multifocality, or bilaterality.

MYELOID METAPLASIA

Tumorous extramedullary hematopoiesis (EMH) (myeloid metaplasia) may involve virtually any organ. The breast is one of the least frequent sites of this condition,[283–285] which is discussed in Chapter 40.

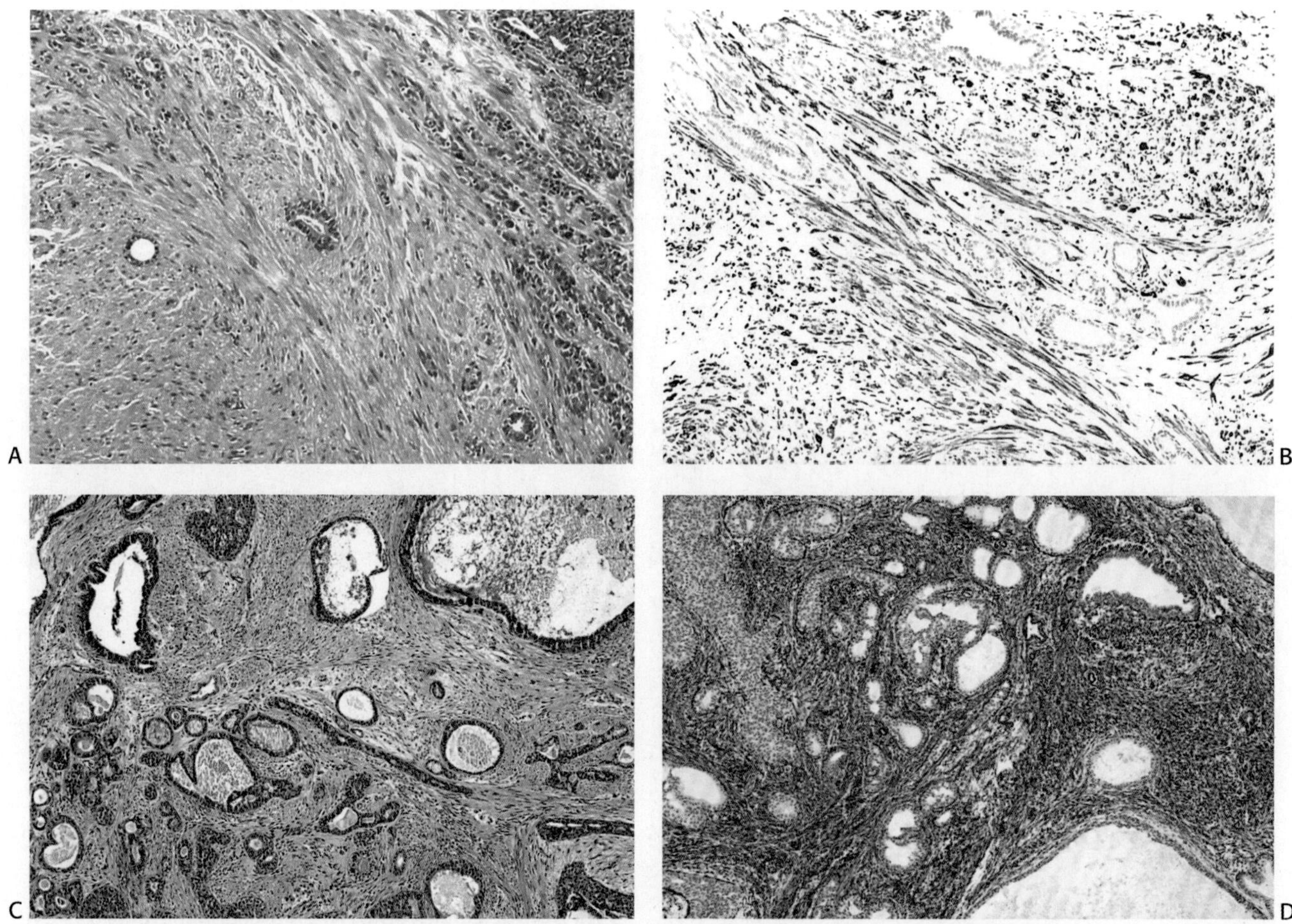

FIG. 38.57. *Myoid "hamartoma."* **A:** A myomatous nodule *(lower left)* in a tumor adjacent to SA. A few glands remain in the myomatous area. **B:** Desmin reactivity in the myomatous tissue around SA glands. **C:** Another lesion in which adenosis glands are surrounded by myomatous stroma. **D:** SMA immunoreactivity is shown in the stroma of the lesion depicted in **(C)**.

MYXOMA

Myxomas are discrete stromal tumors, which only rarely occur in the breast. Although they are commonly cited as part of the spectrum of myxoid breast lesions seen in Carney complex, the syndromic lesions are usually characterized by multifocal myxoid expansion of the intralobular stroma and contain residual lobular elements.[286]

Clinical Presentation

Myxomas have been reported over a broad age range (19 to 75 years).[287–289] Patients may present with a palpable breast mass, or the tumor may be initially detected by mammography. Occasional patients have a history of a slowly growing mass of several years' duration.[287] Tumors have been reported in both subareolar and parenchymal locations. Mammography demonstrates a mass or architectural distortion without associated calcifications. Ultrasound examination reveals an ovoid, hypoechoic or isoechoic mass that may be well-defined or have indistinct margins.[287,289,290]

Gross Pathology

Tumors range in size from 1.5 to 8 cm.[288,290] They are well-circumscribed with gray-white, gelatinous cut surfaces. Occasional tumors are multinodular.

Microscopic Pathology

Microscopic examination reveals hypocellular myxoid neoplastic tissue containing bland stellate and spindle-shaped undifferentiated mesenchymal cells without mitotic activity (Fig. 38.58). The myxoid material is positive with Alcian blue at pH 2.5, and positivity is lost after hyaluronidase digestion. The myxoid stroma is also positive for colloidal iron and negative with the PAS stain. Glandular elements are usually not identified within the tumor. Chondroid and lipoblastic differentiation have not been described.

Differential Diagnosis

The differential diagnosis of myxoma includes myxoid FA, myxoid stromal change (myxomatosis), myxoid neurofibroma, myxoid myofibroblastoma, and mucinosis. Myxoid FA and myxoid stromal change have been reported in breast tissue from patients with Carney complex and, in this setting, are the result of a specific genetic defect that results in the excessive production of proteoglycans by stromal cells.[286] The presence of epithelial elements and multiple myxoid nodules distinguishes these conditions from myxoma. Strong immunoreactivity with markers of neural differentiation such as S-100 serves to identify myxoid neurofibroma.[291] Some tumors reported to be mammary myxomas, which were not fully investigated by IHC, may have been examples of myxoid myofibroblastoma or mucinosis as discussed in the next section.

Immunohistochemistry

The tumor cells are positive for vimentin. They may demonstrate focal immunoreactivity for actin and calponin. Focal weak immunoreactivity for S-100 and α_1-antichymotrypsin has also been reported. The tumor cells are negative for CD34, CD99, CD117, CD10, α_1-antitrypsin, desmin, myogenin, EMA, CK, p63, ER, and PR.[287,289,290]

Electron Microscopy

Electron microscopy reveals abundant, dilated rough endoplasmic reticulum, scant secondary lysosomes, and no junctional complexes or basal lamina.[287]

Treatment and Prognosis

Myxoma is adequately treated by excisional biopsy. Although myxomas appear to be benign lesions, the reported follow-up has been brief. In a case examined by the Senior Editor, local recurrence and progression to high-grade sarcoma with

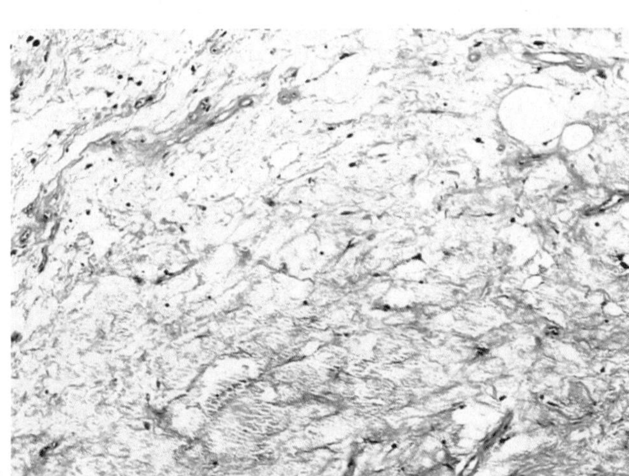

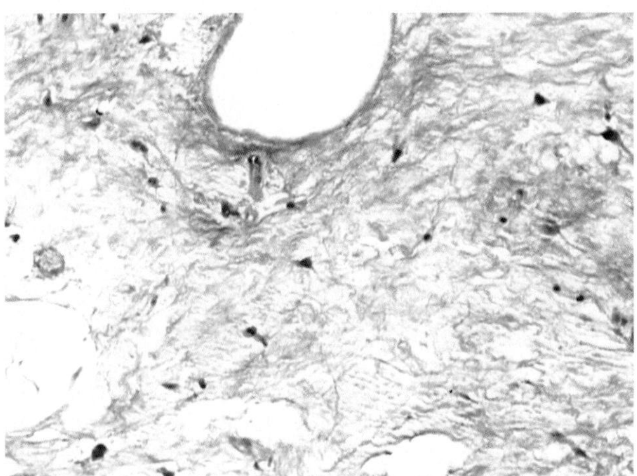

FIG. 38.58. *Myxoma.* **A,B:** The tumor is hypocellular and consists of cytologically benign, widely scattered cells with ill-defined cytoplasm suspended in myxoid stromal matrix.

features of malignant fibrous histiocytoma were observed. In retrospect, the initial lesion was the myxoid form of fibrous histiocytoma.

MUCINOSIS

Nodular mucinosis is an extremely rare stromal tumor. Its histogenesis has not been determined.

Clinical Presentation

Nodular mucinosis is typically a disease of young females (15 to 30 years old), but it also exceptionally occurs in elderly women and men.[292–296] Although most often located in the nipple or in a subareolar location,[297] nodular mucinosis may occur at other sites in the breast. In one case, nodular mucinosis was described in a supernumerary nipple near the areolar border.[296] Most patients present with complaints of a mass or swelling. Less commonly, associated pain, skin retraction, or oozing of the nipple lesion has been reported.[292,293,295] Ultrasonography demonstrates a circumscribed, hypoechoic or isoechoic mass; a thin echogenic rim or cystic component has been noted in individual cases.[293,294] None of the patients described in the literature reported symptoms of Carney complex.[292–296] One patient had an ipsilateral mucinous carcinoma treated by excision and radiation therapy 21 months prior.[295]

Gross Pathology

The tumors range in size from 0.9 to 2.9 cm.[293,295] They appear circumscribed with nodular, gray-pink to yellow-tan, glistening cut surfaces.

Microscopic Pathology

The lesion consists of myxoid material in fibrocollagenous stroma (Fig. 38.59), typically with a multinodular pattern. The basophilic myxoid substance forms distinct, irregular pools that contain scattered histiocytes, and it is also dispersed in the fibrocollagenous matrix from which it appears to arise. Sparse bland spindle cells can be identified. Epithelial elements are not evident in routine sections and they are not demonstrated with immunostains for CK. The stromal myxoid material stains intensely with the Alcian blue and colloidal iron stains.[292] The Alcian blue and colloidal iron stainings are diastase-resistant and eliminated by hyaluronidase treatment. It is imperative that a diagnosis of mucinous carcinoma or mucocele-like tumor be ruled out by carefully searching for epithelial elements.

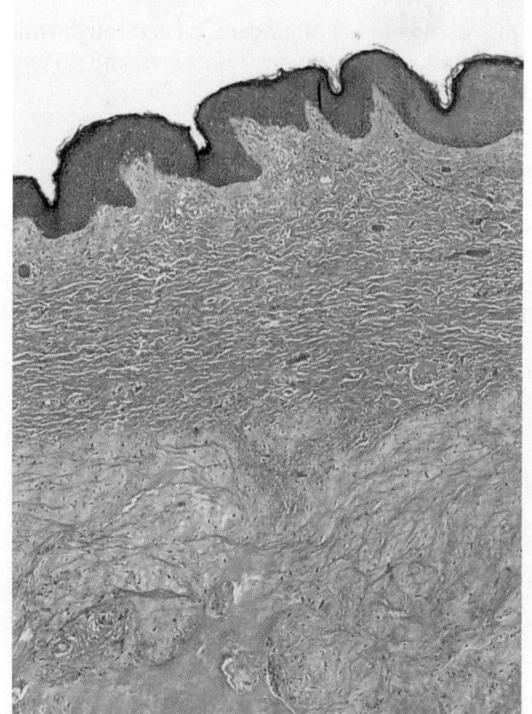

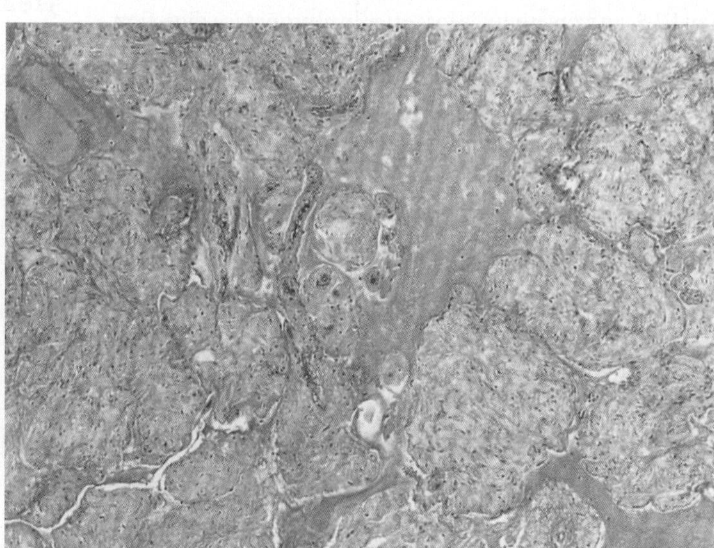

FIG. 38.59. ***Mucinosis.*** **A:** This lesion occurred in the nipple of a 16-year-old girl. No duct structures are evident in the basophilic myxoid stromal tumor. **B,C:** Serpiginous myxoid deposits in the vascularized stroma. A few large histiocytes are evident at this magnification. **D:** Basophilic material is present in the stroma. **E:** The few histiocytes scattered in the myxoid substance and at its interface with the collagenous stroma should not be mistaken for epithelial cells. **F:** Myxoid material in the stroma stains strongly with the mucicarmine stain. **G:** Intense staining with colloidal iron is shown.

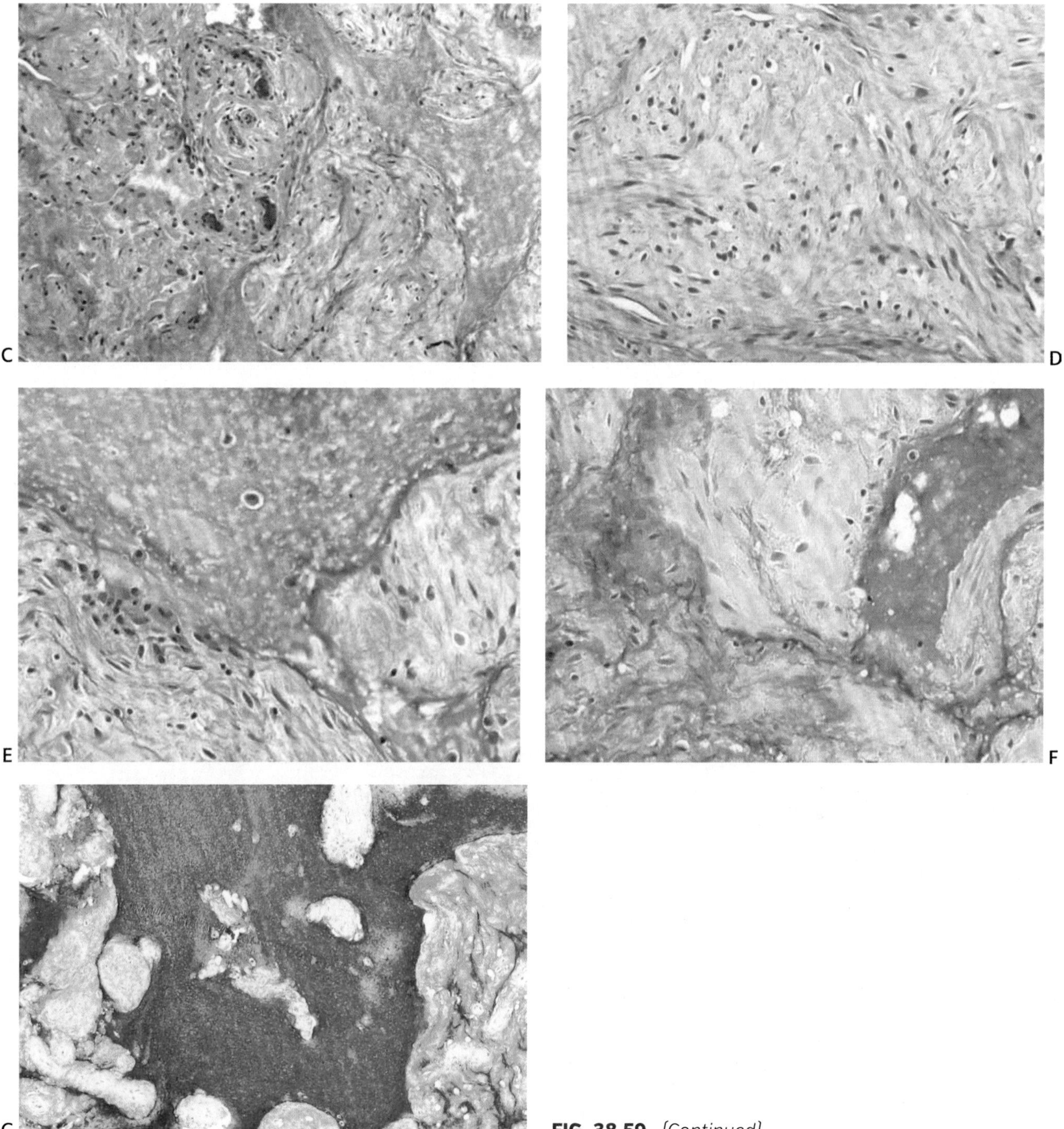

FIG. 38.59. *(Continued)*

Immunohistochemistry

The Senior Editor studied two lesions with the histologic appearance of mucinosis using a series of immunostains. The sparse spindle cells in the lesions had staining characteristics of myofibroblasts, raising the possibility that mucinosis is a variant of myofibroblastoma. This conclusion is supported by the findings in a 21-year-old woman with mucinosis of the nipple studied by Sanati et al.[294] The spindle cells in this lesion were positive for SMA but negative for smooth muscle myosin and S-100. Manglik et al.[296] demonstrated calponin positivity in an example of mucinosis. If further investigation establishes the myofibroblastic origin of mucinosis, these tumors will still be notable for their unusual clinical presentation in the nipple or nipple region in young women.

Treatment and Prognosis

Local excision is adequate therapy but may necessitate removal of the nipple. No recurrences have been reported from 1 month to 6 years after diagnosis, although follow-up in most cases has been short.[292,293,295,296] Further investigation will be needed to determine if mucinosis is related to pathologic changes in the breast that have been associated with Carney complex.[298]

LIPOMA

Lipomas of the breast are usually solitary tumors, but multiple lipomas may be encountered. Many of these lesions are located in the subcutaneous fat. A lipoma often presents mammographically as a radiolucent homogeneous mass with a distinct border or capsule.[299] Grossly, the tumors are typically circumscribed, well-defined masses of mature adipose tissue. In some instances, a clinically palpable lesion proves to be mature fat without the characteristic circumscription of lipoma. Fat necrosis within a lipoma may present as a spiculated lesion on mammography.[300]

"Hibernomas" are tumors composed of brown fat. In the mammary region, hibernomas occur in the axillary tail of the breast or in the axilla (Fig. 38.60). Rare tumors containing both brown fat and mammary glands have been described and are sometimes referred to as "adenohibernomas."[256–258]

"Fibrolipomas" are grossly well-circumscribed tumors composed of mature adipose tissue and collagenous stroma that contain prominent fibroblasts (Fig. 38.61). Microscopically the lesion may blend with glandular parenchyma. The stromal cells do not exhibit the myoid features of myofibroblasts.

"Spindle cell lipomas" rarely occur in the breast.[299–303] One lesion presented as an asymptomatic 2.1-cm well-circumscribed mass on mammography that was hyperechoic on ultrasonography.[303] Biopsy reveals lipomatous tissue mixed with spindly myofibroblasts and variably collagenous stroma (Fig. 38.62). CD10 and CD34 immunoreactivity can be demonstrated in the spindle cell myofibroblastic component,[304,305] features thought to link spindle cell lipoma histogenetically to myofibroblastoma. Recurrent loss of the 13q14 chromosomal region has been reported in both spindle cell lipomas and in myofibroblastomas.[154,160,306]

ANGIOMAS AND OTHER BENIGN VASCULAR LESIONS

The majority of the vascular lesions of the breast described in published reports have been angiosarcomas. Major textbooks of breast or surgical pathology emphasize the need for extreme caution in the interpretation of grossly evident vascular tumors,

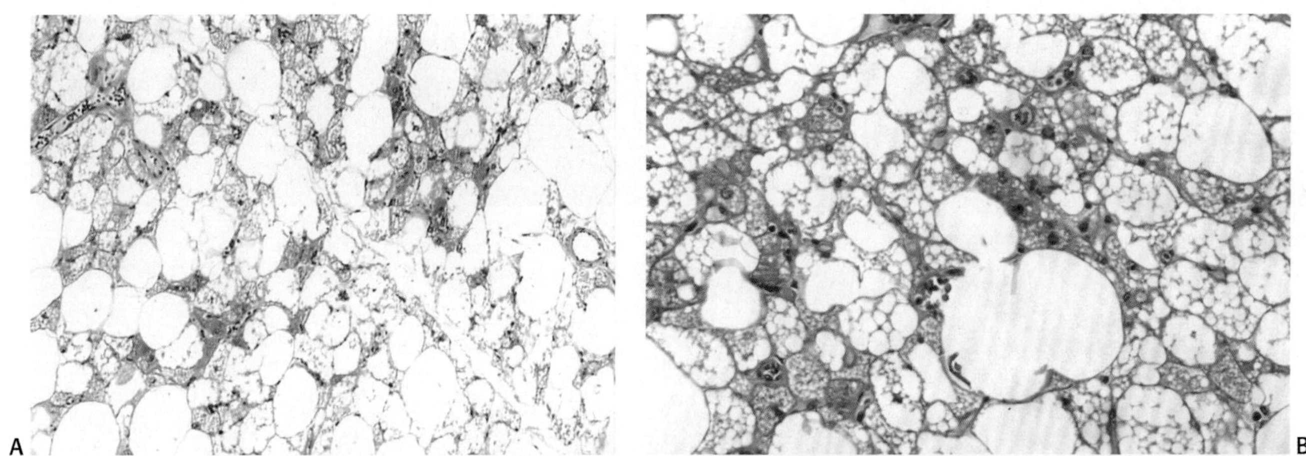

FIG. 38.60. *Hibernoma.* **A,B:** A tumor in the axilla of a 24-year-old woman.

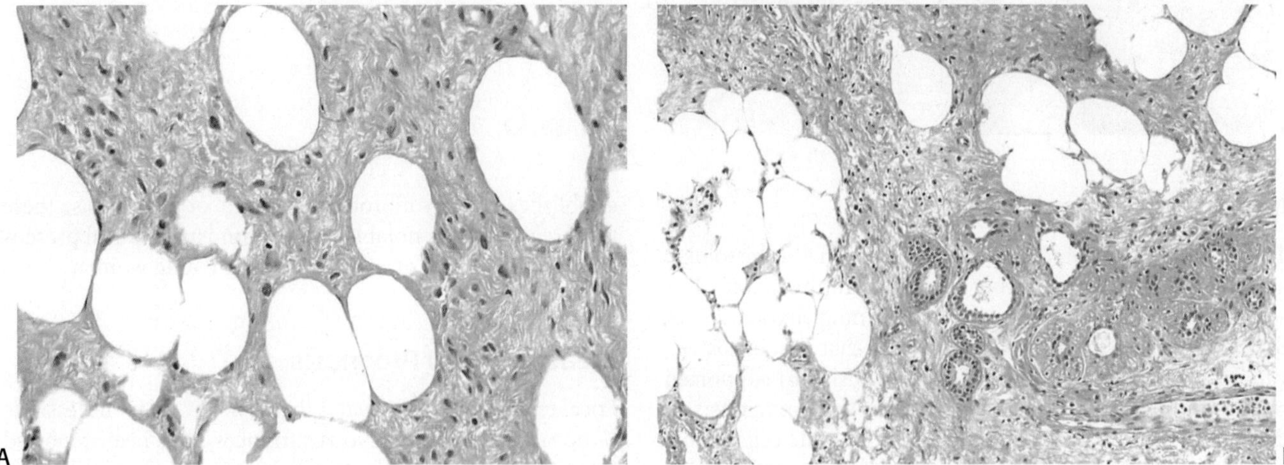

FIG. 38.61. *Fibrolipoma.* **A:** Cellular collagenous stroma and fat cells. **B:** Lobular glands are present in the lesion.

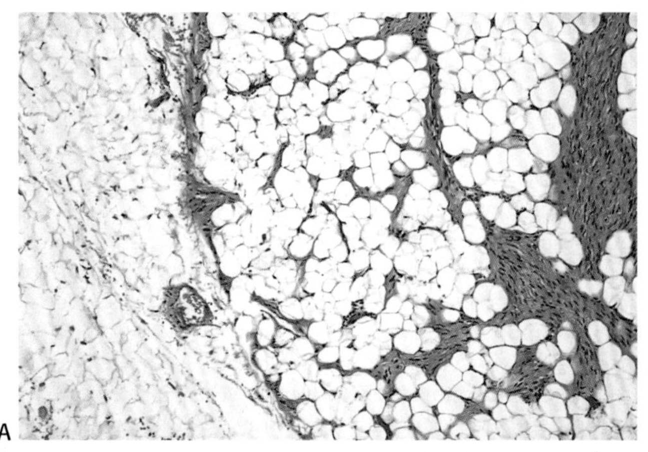

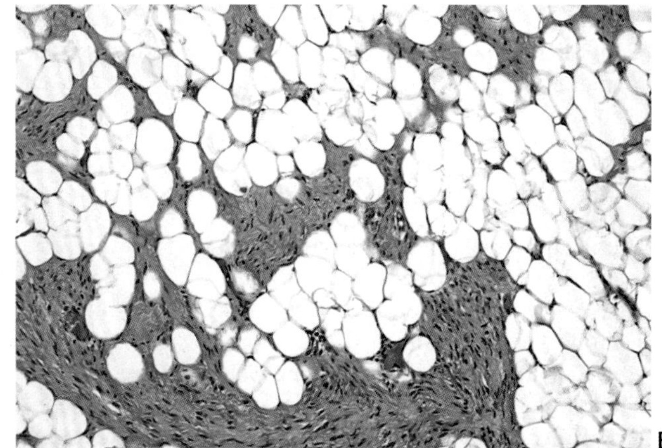

FIG. 38.62. ***Spindle cell lipoma.*** **A:** The tumor has a distinct border (*left*). **B:** Spindle cells in collagenous stroma course through the lipomatous fat.

TABLE 38.1 Benign Vascular Lesions of the Breast

Perilobular hemangioma
Hemangioma cavernous, capillary, or complex
Angiomatosis (lymphangiomatosis)
Venous hemangioma
Subcutaneous nonparenchymal hemangiomas
Angiolipoma
Cavernous
Capillary
Juvenile
Venous
Papillary endothelial hyperplasia
Aneurysm/AVF

because portions of angiosarcomas may appear deceptively bland histologically. Azzopardi[307] indicated that "a benign angioma has never to date constituted a palpable or symptom-producing breast tumor." McDivitt et al.[308] stated that "after the perilobular angiomas have been eliminated, it must be inferred that all the capillary tumors... [of the breast]... are malignant." Subsequent studies have proven these statements to be incorrect.

Pathologic analysis of hundreds of mammary vascular tumors studied by the Senior Editor revealed diverse, grossly evident angiomas and other nonmalignant vascular lesions of the breast, as well as nonparenchymal hemangiomas of the mammary subcutaneous fat (Table 38.1).

PERILOBULAR HEMANGIOMA

Clinical Presentation

The perilobular hemangioma is a microscopic benign vascular lesion detected in sections of breast tissue taken to evaluate various unrelated benign and malignant lesions.[309] Although a few have reportedly measured between 2 and 4 mm on a histologic section, none was grossly or mammographically apparent.[310,311] On macroscopic examination, these hemangiomas sometimes appear as pinpoint red spots.

Two studies (Table 38.2) evaluated the frequency and clinicopathologic features of perilobular hemangiomas.[310,311] They were found in 1.3% of mastectomies performed for carcinoma,[311] 4.5% of biopsies for benign breast lesions, and in 11% of women whose breast tissue was sampled in forensic

TABLE 38.2 Perilobular Hemangiomas

	Authors of Study	
Feature Evaluated	**Rosen and Ridolfi[311]**	**Lesueur et al.[310]**
Type of specimen	Surgical mastectomy	Forensic autopsy
Laterality	519 unilateral 18 bilateral	210 bilateral
Number of patients	537	210
Number of breasts	555	420
Number of patients with hemangioma	7	23
Percentage of patients with hemangioma	1.3	11

autopsies.[310] The age distribution apparently reflects the ages of the patients studied. Age of patients with perilobular hemangiomas found at autopsy ranged from 29 to 82 years (mean, 51.5 years).[310]

Microscopic Pathology

Multiple perilobular hemangiomas may be found in one breast, and a number of patients have had these lesions in both breasts.[310–312] Microscopically, perilobular hemangiomas are not limited to a perilobular distribution (Fig. 38.63). Many are partially or completely within the lobular stroma,[310,311,313] whereas others are located in extralobular stroma sometimes in proximity to ducts or apparently in no particular relationship to a duct or lobule[311] (Fig. 38.64). In a series studied by Lesueur et al.,[310] only 2 of 32 microscopic hemangiomas had a perilobular position. Although the term "perilobular" does not accurately describe the microanatomic distribution of many of these lesions, it is widely used, and there is no compelling reason to propose an alternative name.

Perilobular hemangiomas can often be identified histologically at low magnification because they usually contain red blood cells. In some instances, the contents lack erythrocytes and consist of fluid that may be lymph. The lesion is typically a defined collection of small, distinct vascular channels arranged in a meshwork fashion. Rarely it may have ill-defined borders with vessels that extend into the adjacent fatty and fibrous stroma. The vessels vary in caliber from capillary size to ectatic miniature cavernous channels. Anastomosing channels may be seen but are not conspicuous. The thin, delicate vessels consist of endothelial cells encased in inconspicuous stroma with little or no supporting smooth muscle coat. It is not unusual to find varying numbers of lymphocytes in the stroma regardless of the presence or absence of erythrocytes within the vascular spaces.

Some microscopic vascular lesions with the general features of perilobular hemangiomas have endothelial cells that appear cytologically atypical because they have prominent hyperchromatic nuclei.[309] Interconnected channels are often present, but endothelial papillary proliferation, mitotic activity, and extensive vascular anastomoses are not seen in these "atypical perilobular hemangiomas." Most atypical perilobular hemangiomas have rounded, circumscribed contours and are separated into aggregates of vessels or

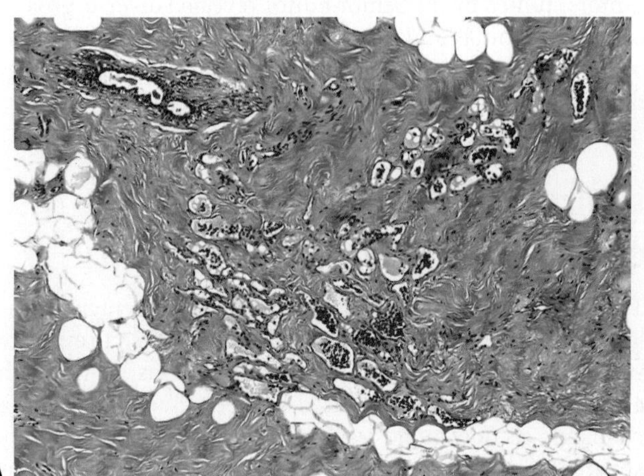

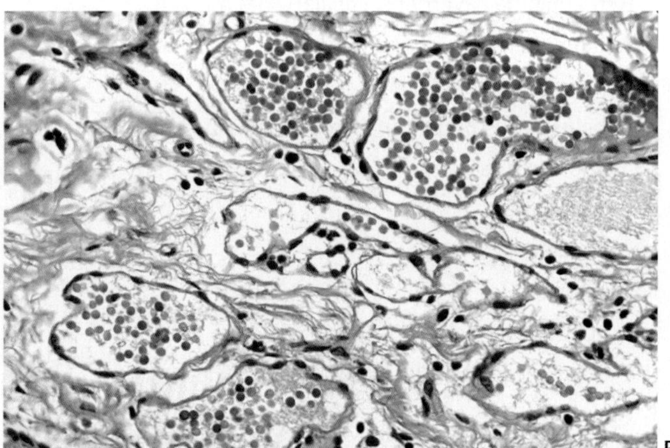

FIG. 38.63. ***Perilobular hemangioma.*** **A,B:** Hemangioma composed of congested capillaries in the extralobular stroma.

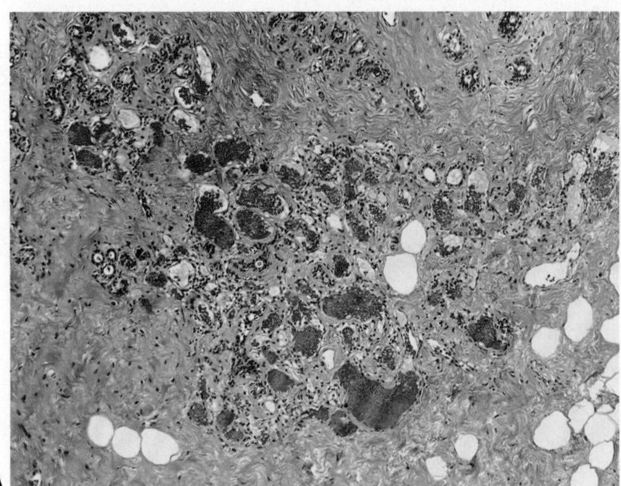

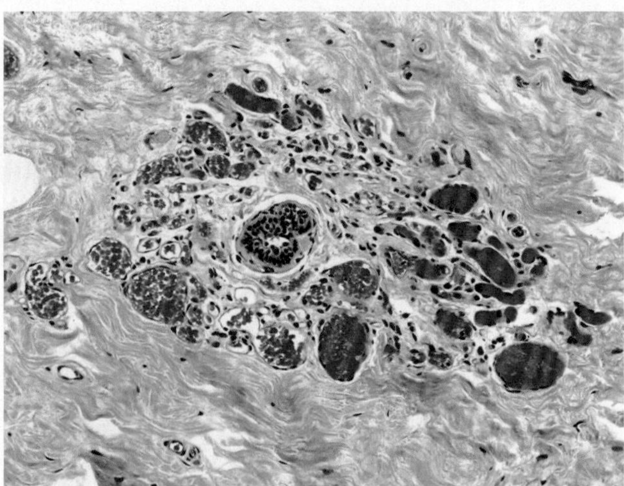

FIG. 38.64. ***Perilobular hemangioma.*** **A,B:** The capillary proliferation mingles with lobules **(A)** and surrounds a small duct **(B)**.

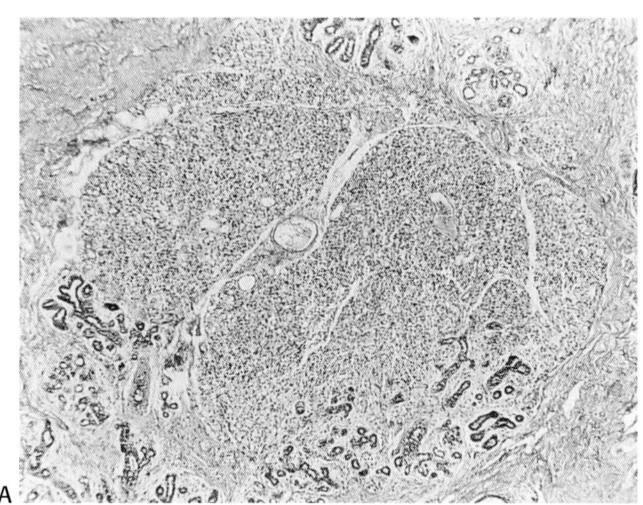

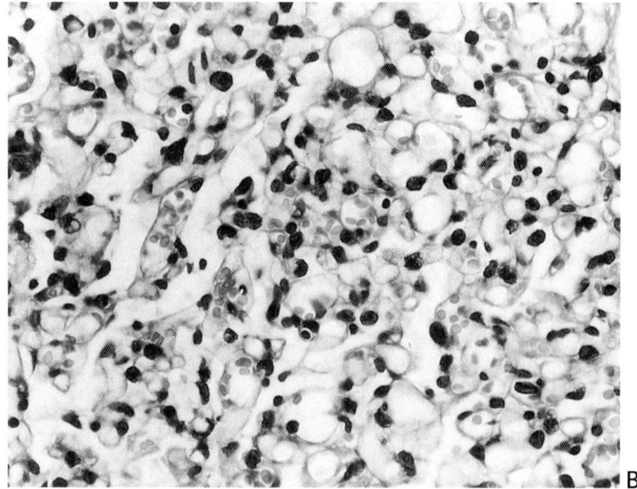

FIG. 38.65. *Atypical perilobular hemangioma.* This 2-mm lesion has been referred to as an "atypical" hemangioma because of its relatively large size and nuclear atypia. **A:** The compact circumscribed lesion involving intra- and perilobular stroma is subdivided by fibrous septa. The well-formed central vessel is probably a branch of the feeding vessel. **B:** Capillary channels, some anastomosing, with prominent hyperchromatic nuclei are present. (**A,B:** Reproduced from Jozefczyk MA, Rosen PP. Vascular tumors of the breast. II. Perilobular hemangiomas and hemangiomas. *Am J Surg Pathol* 1985;9:491–503, with permission.)

vascular lobules by slender fibrous septa (Fig. 38.65). A few lesions with irregular margins have been noted (Fig. 38.66).

Treatment and Prognosis

Perilobular hemangiomas, whether unifocal, multiple, or bilateral, are incidental pathologic findings, which do not require treatment. There is no evidence that angiosarcoma arises from these lesions, although the existence of cytologically atypical variants leaves this issue open to speculation. Given the rarity of mammary angiosarcoma and the relatively frequent detection of perilobular hemangiomas in "normal" breast tissue or in specimens examined for various unrelated conditions, malignant transformation of perilobular hemangiomas must be exceedingly uncommon, if it does occur.

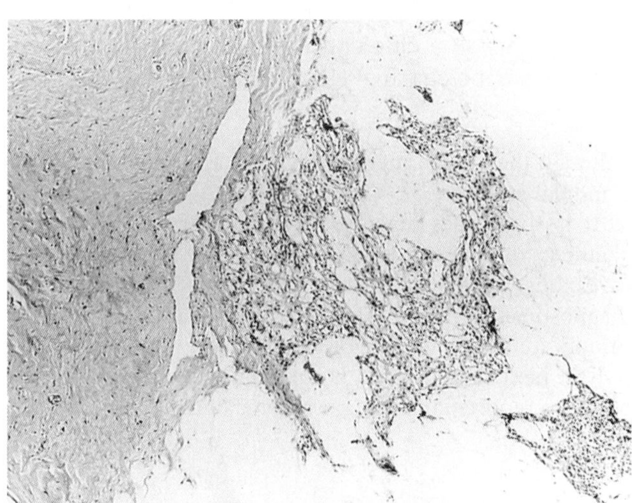

FIG. 38.66. *Perilobular hemangioma.* An irregularly shaped capillary proliferation in extralobular fibrofatty tissue previously characterized as atypical. A dilated feeder vessel is present at the *left border* of the lesion. (Reproduced from Jozefczyk MA, Rosen PP. Vascular tumors of the breast. II. Perilobular hemangiomas and hemangiomas. *Am J Surg Pathol* 1985;9:491–503, with permission.)

Whether treated by mastectomy in the management of mammary carcinoma or local excision, no patient with an atypical perilobular hemangioma is known to have experienced recurrence of the lesion or progression to angiosarcoma. No treatment other than local excision is recommended for atypical perilobular hemangiomas.

HEMANGIOMAS

Clinical Presentation

Hemangiomas are benign vascular tumors large enough to be clinically palpable or detected by mammography.[314] The lesions measure between 0.3 and 2.5 cm, and they occur in patients aged 18 months to 82 years.[314–316] MRI was used to assess the relationship of the hemangioma to the breast bud in the infantile and immature breasts of patients aged 5 months to 7 years.[317] Multiple mammary hemangiomas were demonstrated by MRI in the breast of a 41-year-old woman with Kasabach–Merritt syndrome.[318]

A substantial number of hemangiomas are currently detected by mammography in the absence of a clinically palpable tumor (Fig. 38.67) or by ultrasonography (Fig. 38.68). With increasing use of breast MRI, hemangiomas are occasionally detected by that modality as well.[319] Nonpalpable

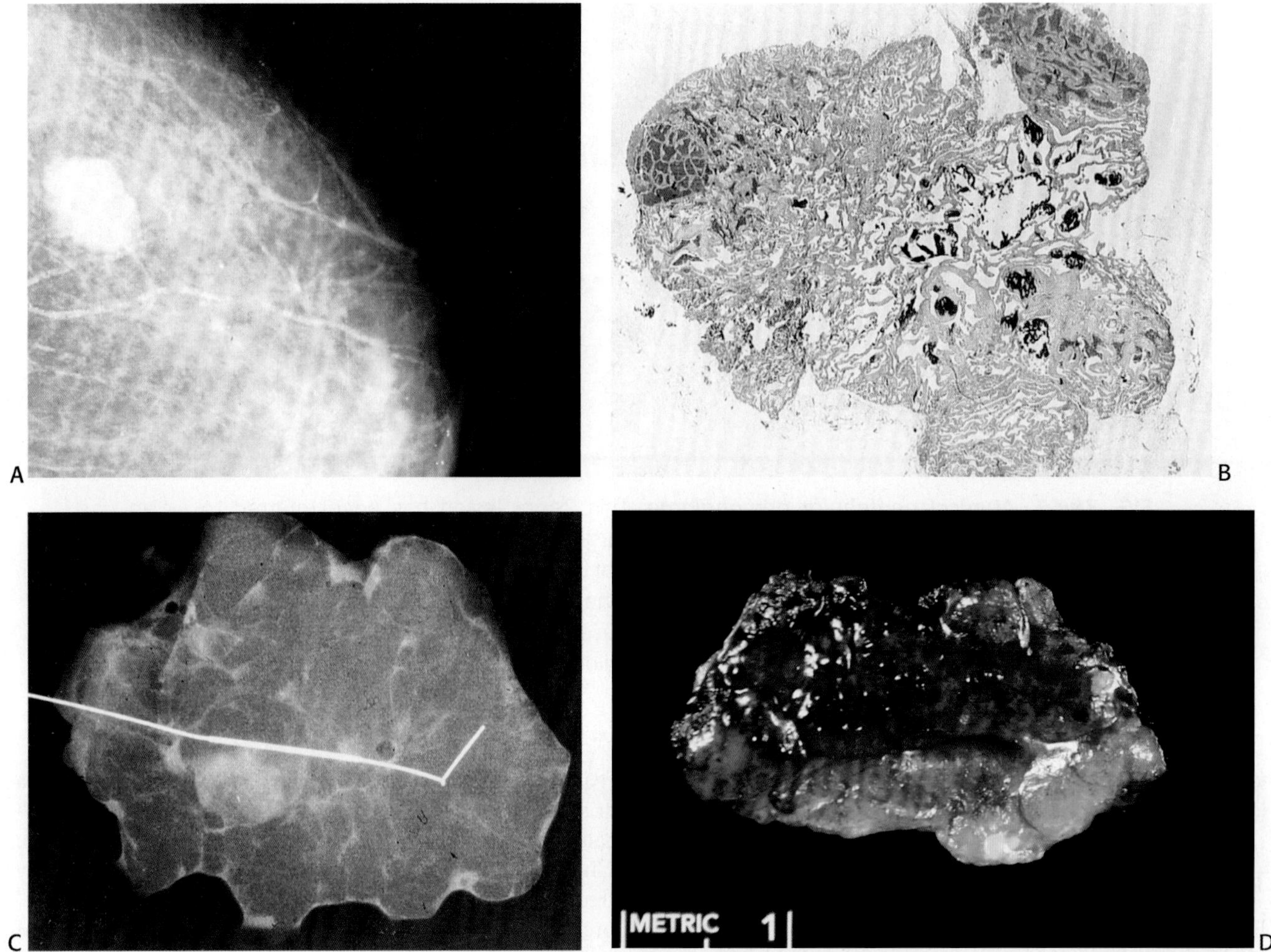

FIG. 38.67. *Hemangioma, mammogram and gross specimen.* **A:** The lesion appears as a well-circumscribed, lobulated oval mass on this mammogram. **B:** A whole-mount histologic section of the hemangioma shown in (A). **C:** The radiographic appearance of a different hemangioma in a biopsy specimen with a localization wire. **D:** The macroscopic appearance of a surgically resected cavernous hemangioma.

hemangiomas range in size from 0.4 to 2.0 cm with a mean diameter of 0.9 cm. The majority of patients have been women aged 19 to 82 years (mean 60 years). The mammographic appearance is usually that of a well-defined lobulated mass, which may have fine or coarse calcifications.[320–324] Almost all palpable vascular tumors of the male breast have been hemangiomas.[322]

Gross Pathology

Hemangiomas tend to be well-circumscribed. There is no predilection for any particular location in the breast. Palpable lesions are described as firm.

Microscopic Pathology

Most hemangiomas have well-circumscribed borders grossly, but microscopically the vascular channels may blend with the surrounding breast parenchyma. As part of this process, the vessels are infrequently seen within lobules, although they much more often grow around and displace glandular structures.

It is sometimes possible to find EMH in the vascular channels of a breast hemangioma, especially those with cavernous or capillary components. This is an important diagnostic clue. Among more than 500 mammary vascular tumors studied by the Senior Editor, EMH was encountered only in hemangiomas and not in angiosarcomas. EMH has not been reported in an angiosarcoma of the breast.

Cavernous Hemangiomas

Cavernous hemangiomas are one of the most common forms of mammary hemangioma. The lesion is typically described as a dark red or brown circumscribed mass that may grossly appear spongy.[314,315,325] Microscopic examination reveals dilated vessels congested with red blood cells (Fig. 38.69). Small vessels of capillary dimension may be seen in portions of a cavernous hemangioma. The individual channels appear to be independent, there being few if any anastomosing

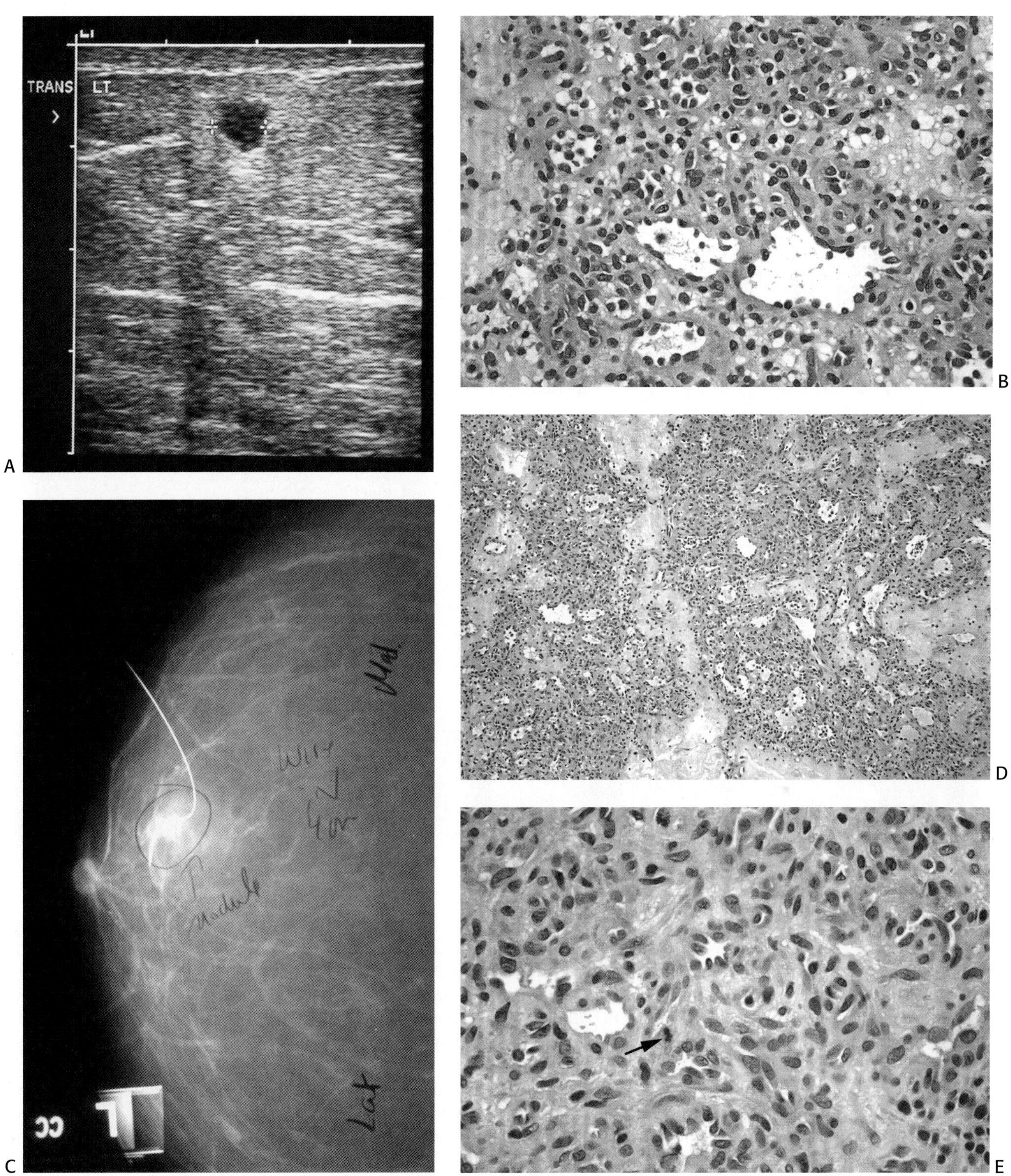

FIG. 38.68. ***Hemangioma, ultrasound study, mammogram, and histologic sections.*** **A:** The dark circumscribed nodule between the markers in this ultrasound image is a hemangioma. **B:** The lesion seen in **(A)** is a compact epithelioid capillary hemangioma. **C:** Mammogram in another case with a localization wire in an ill-defined tumor. **D,E:** The lesion seen in **(C)** is an atypical epithelioid hemangioma with infrequent mitoses (*arrow*) shown in **(E)**.

vessels (Fig. 38.70). Endothelial nuclei are inconspicuous and flat. The vessels are supported by fibrous stroma, which tends to be more prominent toward the center of the tumor. Calcification may occur in the stroma.[314,315] EMH in vascular channels should be distinguished from lymphocytic reaction, which occurs mainly in the stroma. Thrombosis

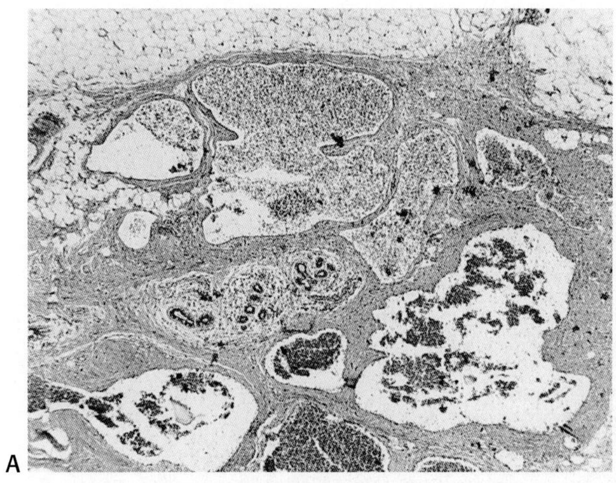

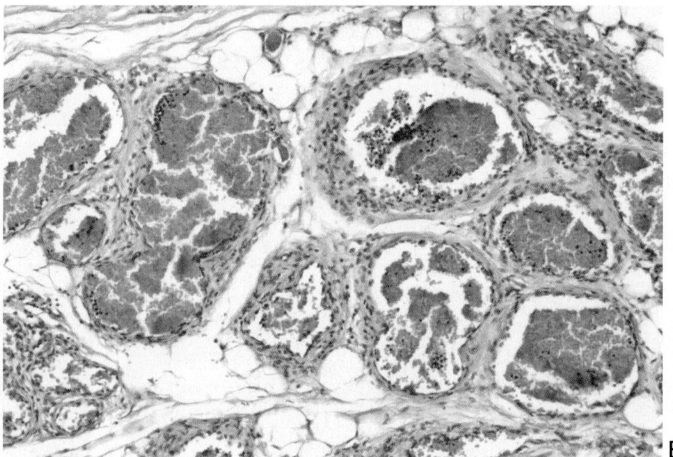

FIG. 38.69. ***Cavernous hemangioma.*** **A:** Dilated, congested vascular spaces surround a lobule. **B:** Blood-filled cavernous vascular channels.

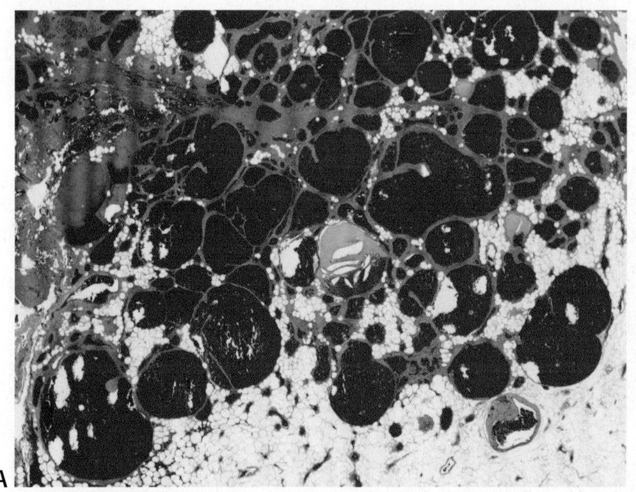

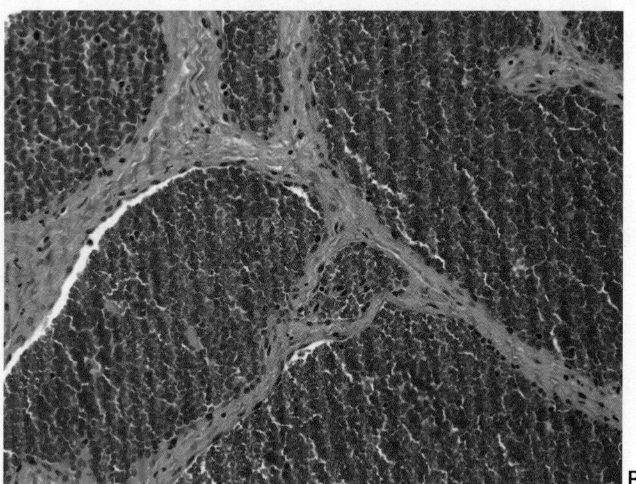

FIG. 38.70. ***Cavernous hemangioma.*** **A:** The lesion consists of a compact mass of separate distended, congested vascular channels. **B:** Fibrous septa extend between the vascular spaces lined by inconspicuous endothelium.

within cavernous channels sometimes elicits a lymphocytic reaction, and endothelial proliferation may be seen within the organizing clot. These alterations can result in papillary endothelial hyperplasia, which should not be mistaken for angiosarcoma (Fig. 38.71).

There is considerable variability in the degree of circumscription seen microscopically. In many cavernous hemangiomas, the vascular channels drift into the fatty parenchyma, becoming smaller at the periphery. This pattern duplicates the histologic appearance of peripheral parts of some well-differentiated angiosarcomas (Fig. 38.72).

Noncavernous Hemangiomas

Other types of hemangioma comprise a heterogeneous group of lesions. Because of their dimensions, atypical cytologic features in some instances, and concern that they might be precursors of angiosarcoma, some were initially characterized as "atypical" hemangiomas.[314] Additional follow-up has demonstrated that so-called atypical hemangiomas are not borderline or low-grade variants of angiosarcoma and has not provided evidence that they predispose to the development of angiosarcoma.[315] Consequently, they should simply be classified as types of "noncavernous hemangiomas" for which the designation "atypical" is no longer warranted in most cases. The designation "atypical" is now reserved for a small group of hemangiomas with cytologically atypical cells or evidence of proliferative activity manifested by rare mitoses or a Ki67-labeling index in the upper range for hemangiomas.[326]

Microscopically, slender fibrous septa frequently divide noncavernous hemangiomas into segments, resulting in a lobulated structure. Some of the tumors have prominent anastomosing vascular channels. Papillary endothelial hyperplasia may be present, usually at sites of organizing thrombi. Florid papillary endothelial hyperplasia can obscure the basic angiomatous character of the lesion or even suggest a well-differentiated angiosarcoma.[327] When present in the

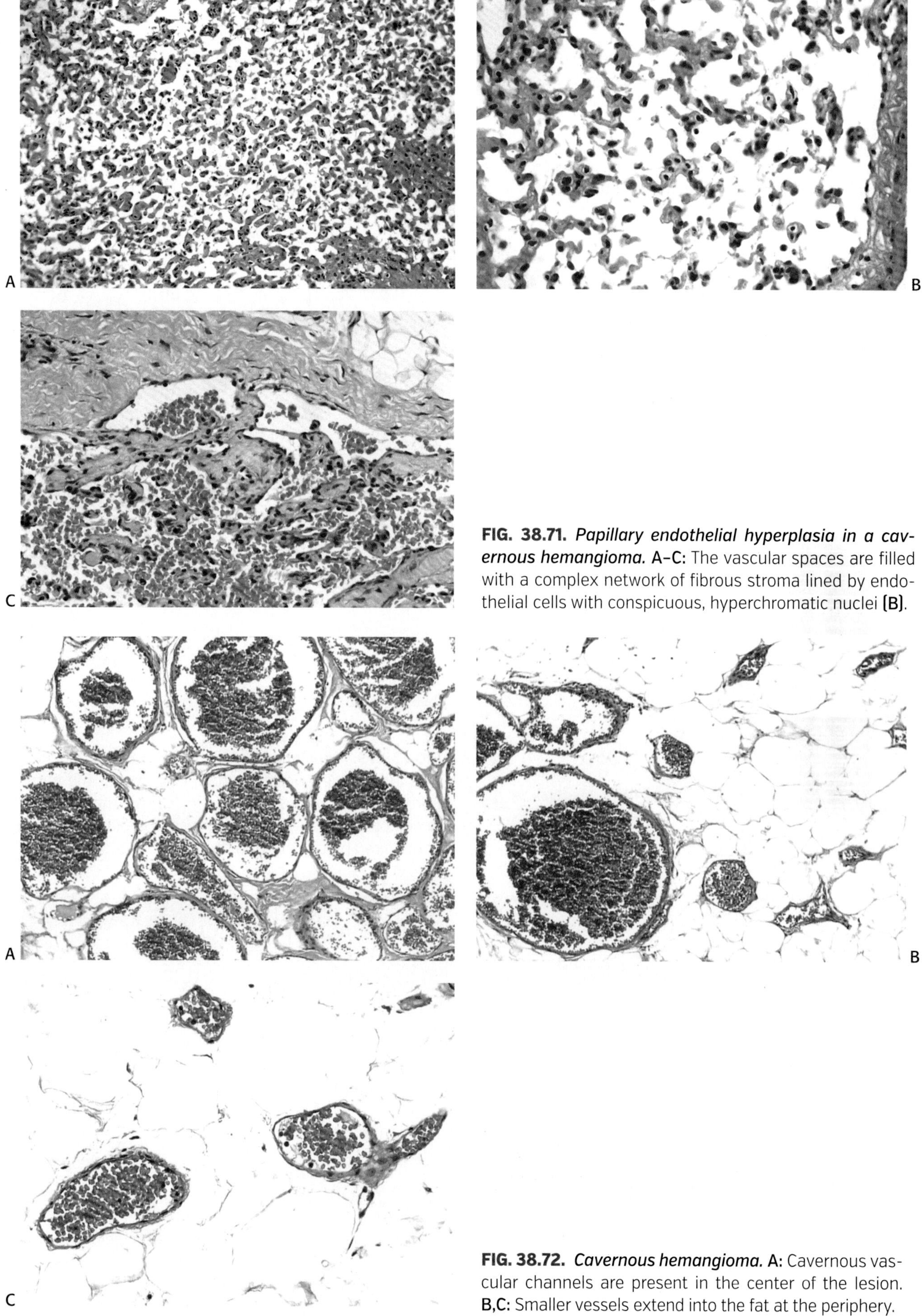

FIG. 38.71. ***Papillary endothelial hyperplasia in a cavernous hemangioma.*** **A–C:** The vascular spaces are filled with a complex network of fibrous stroma lined by endothelial cells with conspicuous, hyperchromatic nuclei **(B)**.

FIG. 38.72. ***Cavernous hemangioma.*** **A:** Cavernous vascular channels are present in the center of the lesion. **B,C:** Smaller vessels extend into the fat at the periphery.

breast, papillary endothelial hyperplasia invariably arises in a hemangioma and it does not indicate a specific category of breast tumor. Mast cells are frequently present individually or in small clusters in mammary hemangiomas.

Capillary hemangiomas tend to be cellular and to superficially resemble pyogenic granulomas. The mean gross size of these hemangiomas is 1.0 cm. Many of these lesions have been detected by mammography. Microscopically, capillary hemangiomas are composed of small vascular channels lined by endothelial cells that may have hyperchromatic nuclei (Fig. 38.73). Fibrous bands are variably present subdividing the lesion. Larger, muscular vessels may be found within and at the periphery of the tumor, apparently constituting branches of a feeding vessel or vessels (Fig. 38.74). These

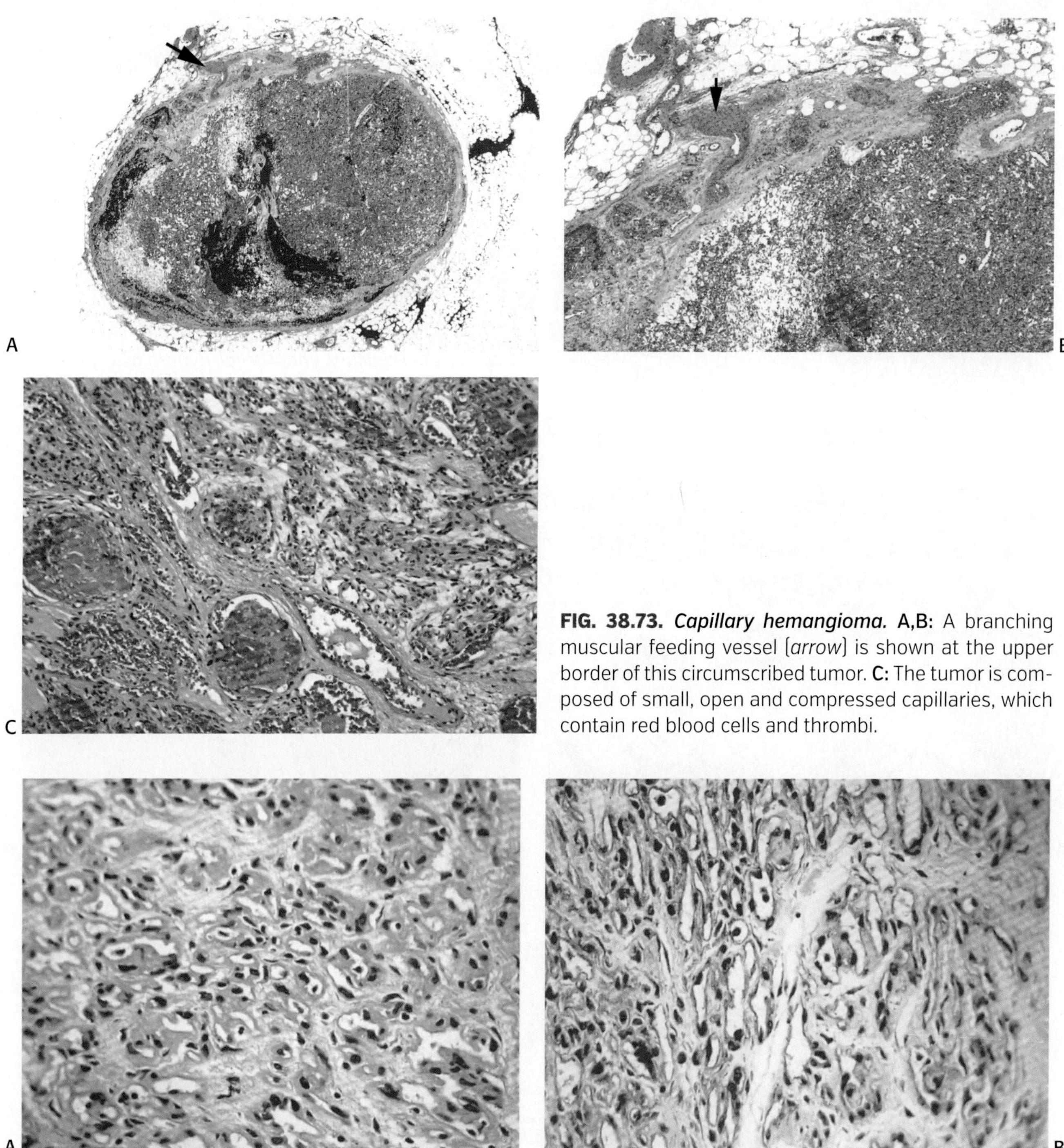

FIG. 38.73. ***Capillary hemangioma.*** **A,B:** A branching muscular feeding vessel (*arrow*) is shown at the upper border of this circumscribed tumor. **C:** The tumor is composed of small, open and compressed capillaries, which contain red blood cells and thrombi.

FIG. 38.74. ***Capillary hemangioma.*** **A:** Delicate clusters of capillaries that have prominent hyperchromatic nuclei are shown. **B:** Collagen between the capillaries is stained with a trichrome stain. **C:** A feeding vessel at the border of the tumor. **D:** Branches of the feeding vessel within a fibrous septum are highlighted by the trichrome stain.

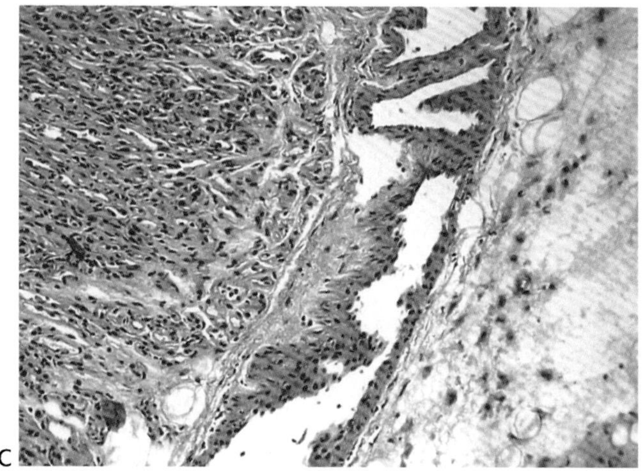

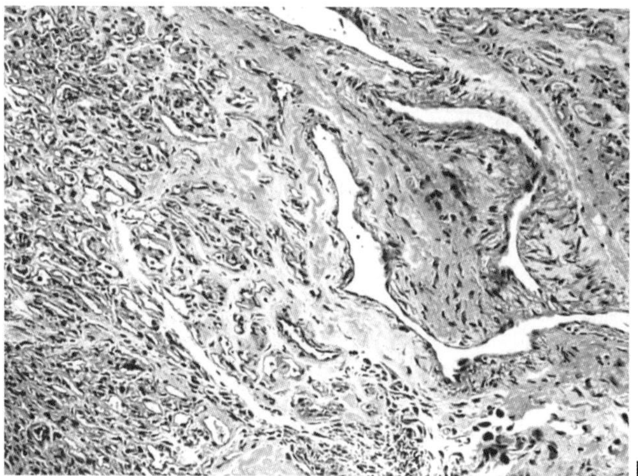

FIG. 38.74. *(Continued)*

are nonneoplastic muscular vessels with features of arteries and/or veins. Often, the muscular component of these vessels seems malformed or incomplete, and the vessels have a sinuous configuration. The resultant configuration suggests that the hemangioma arose from the feeding vessel. Capillary hemangiomas are usually well-circumscribed, but some lesions have irregular borders (Fig. 38.75).

Complex hemangiomas consist of dilated vascular channels of varying size as well as compact, dense aggregates of capillary structures (Fig. 38.76). Many complex

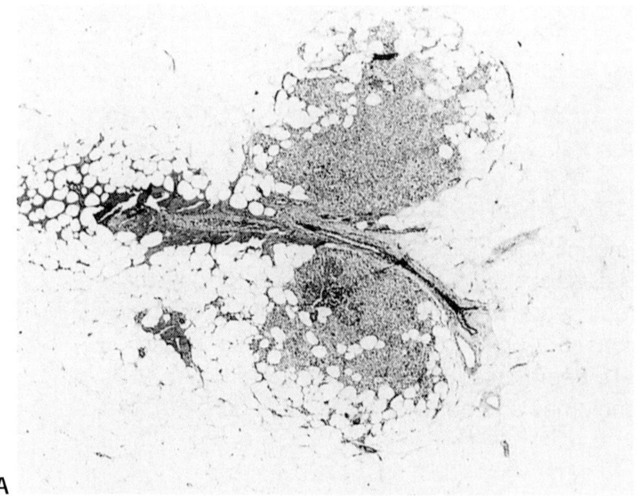

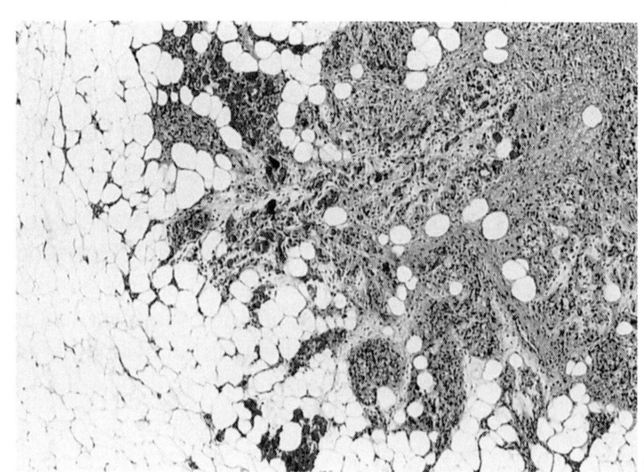

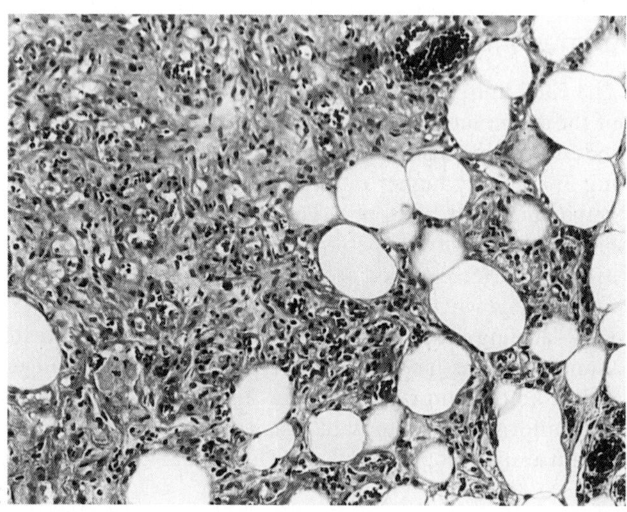

FIG. 38.75. ***Capillary hemangioma.*** **A:** A whole-mount histologic section showing a central feeding vessel. The lesion has the shape of a butterfly. **B,C:** Hemangiomatous capillaries blending with fat are illustrated. (**A–C:** Reproduced from Hoda SA, Cranor ML, Rosen PP. Hemangiomas of the breast with atypical histological features. Further analysis of histological subtypes confirming their benign character. *Am J Surg Pathol* 1992;16:553–560, with permission.)

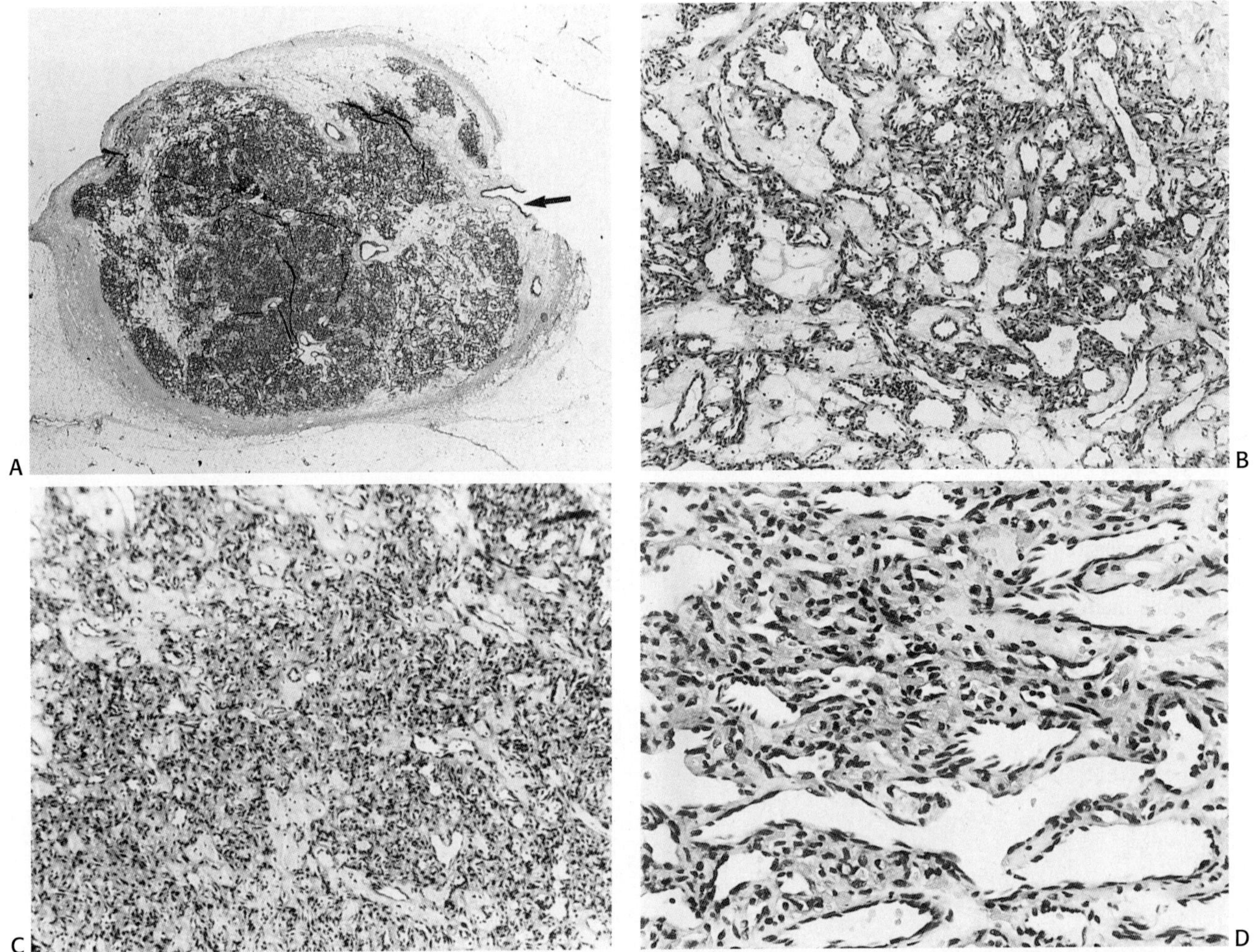

FIG. 38.76. *Complex hemangioma.* **A:** A whole-mount histologic section of a circumscribed, seemingly encapsulated tumor. Part of the feeding vessel is shown at the *right border* (*arrow*) and several branches of this vessel are present in fibrous septa within the hemangioma. **B:** Dilated, irregular, sometimes anastomosing vascular channels. **C:** Compressed capillaries. **D:** An anastomosing vascular channel with an avian shape. (**A–D:** Reproduced from Jozefczyk MA, Rosen PP. Vascular tumors of the breast. II. Perilobular hemangiomas and hemangiomas. *Am J Surg Pathol* 1985;9:491–503, with permission.)

hemangiomas that measure 1.0 cm or less, averaging 0.7 cm, have been detected by mammography. A feeding vessel may be evident at the periphery of the tumor. Some complex hemangiomas have conspicuous anastomosing vascular channels (Fig. 38.77).

Hemorrhage and infarction can occur in hemangiomas, especially lesions detected radiologically and subjected to needle core biopsy or needle localization excision (Fig. 38.78). This should not be confused with the pattern of hemorrhagic necrosis that results in the formation of "blood lakes" characteristically found in high-grade angiosarcomas. Calcification may occur in organized thrombi, sometimes associated with endothelial hyperplasia, or in fibrous septa between vascular spaces. Marked septal fibrosis is sometimes found in hemangiomas (Fig. 38.79).

Immunohistochemistry

The Ki67 immunostain is a useful adjunct in the diagnosis of the mammary hemangiomas. The nuclear Ki67-labeling index in mammary hemangiomas is very low, rarely exceeding 5%. Focally higher rates of labeling may be found in a hemangioma at sites of organizing thrombi or where a biopsy was previously performed. Therefore, it is important to have an H&E-stained section available to visualize structural details when the Ki67 stain is being interpreted. The Ki67-labeling index of mammary angiosarcomas is greater than that of hemangiomas and typically exceeds 20% even in low-grade tumors. Because the distribution of labeling is not uniform in an angiosarcoma, it is possible by chance to obtain a small biopsy sample with less than 5% labeling from

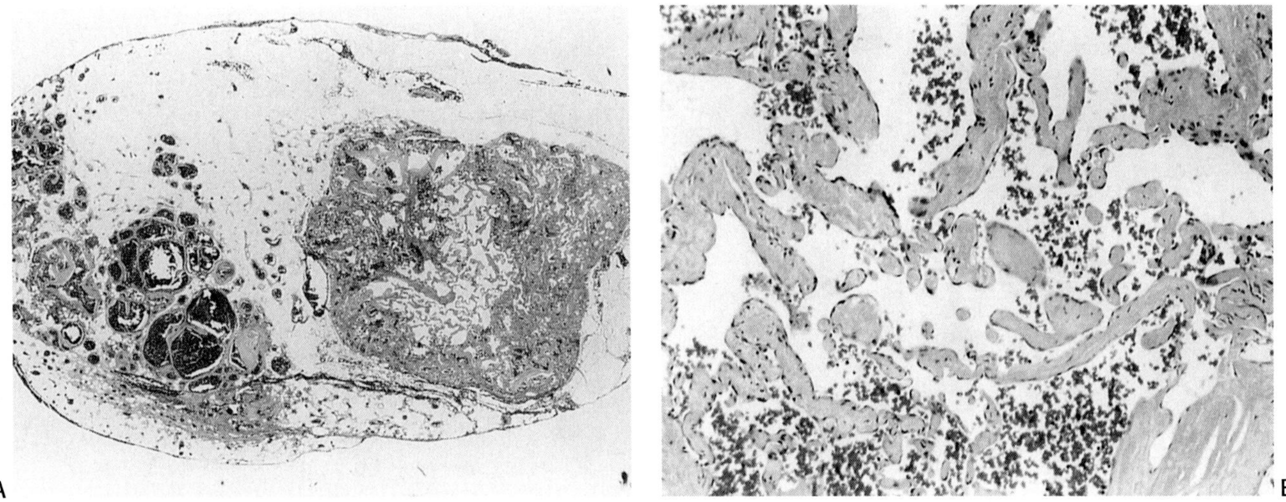

FIG. 38.77. ***Complex hemangioma.*** **A:** In this whole-mount histologic section, the area on the *left* has the diffuse pattern of a conventional cavernous hemangioma, whereas the circumscribed component on the *right* has numerous anastomosing vascular channels. **B:** The endothelium is flat and inconspicuous in this image from the right of the lesion. Red blood cells are present. [**A,B:** Reproduced from Rosen PP, Oberman HA. Tumors of the mammary gland. *AFIP Atlas of tumor pathology*, 3rd series, vol. 7. MA: American Registry of Pathology, 1993, with permission.]

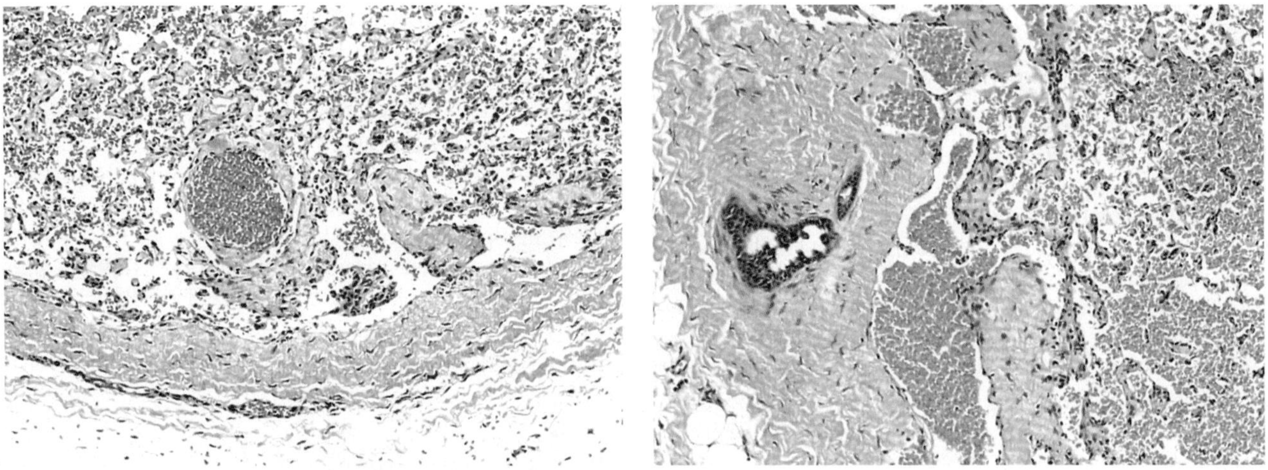

FIG. 38.78. ***Hemangioma with necrosis and papillary endothelial hyperplasia.*** **A:** The hemangioma has a circumscribed border. **B:** A duct in the outer wall of the hemangioma. **C:** The infarcted portion of the lesion is in the *lower half* of the picture.

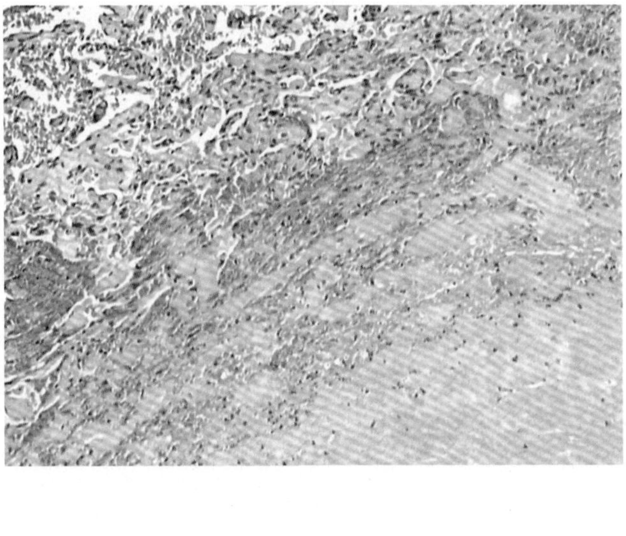

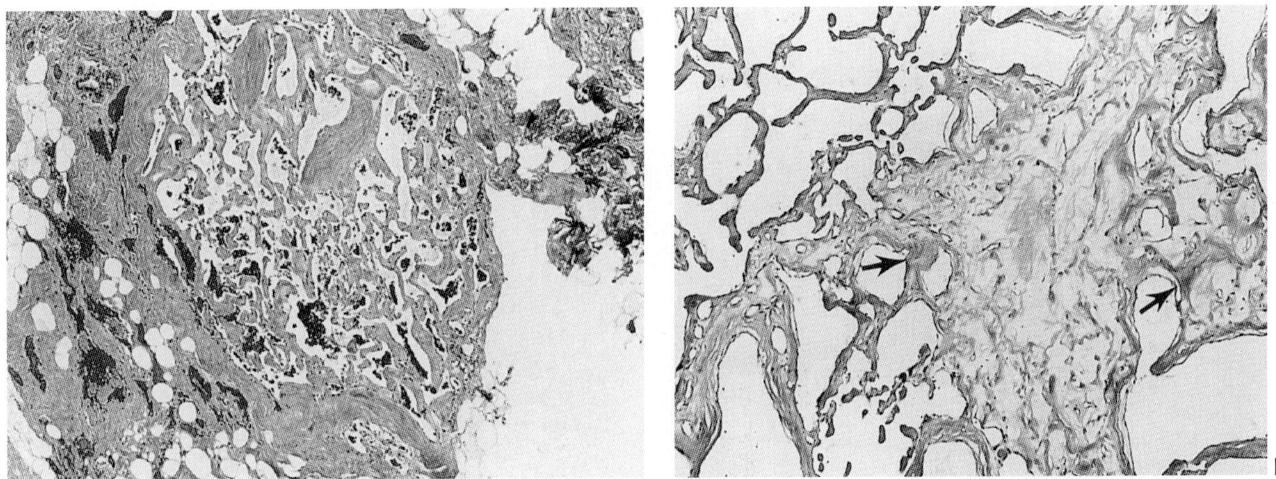

FIG. 38.79. ***Hemangioma.*** **A:** In this whole-mount histologic section, hemorrhage in the breast tissue (*left*) around the hemangioma was caused by needle localization of the mammographically detected lesion. Fibrosis of septa between anastomosing vascular channels is apparent. **B:** Dark zones within the fibrous septa represent delicate bands of calcification (*arrows*).

a low-grade angiosarcoma. A robust Ki67-labeling index on a needle core biopsy from a mammary vascular lesion would strongly favor angiosarcoma. Very sparse labeling in such a limited sample can assist in making a diagnosis of hemangioma when correlated with the H&E appearance of the lesion.

Treatment and Prognosis

Reexcision of the biopsy site may be indicated if it appears that a substantial portion of the lesion has not been extirpated. Further surgery is not necessary if only a few peripheral capillaries extend to the margin of excision. It is often not possible to recognize residual hemangioma in the granulation tissue of a healing biopsy site.

Complete excision of a hemangioma is necessary for accurate diagnosis. The material obtained with a needle core biopsy is rarely sufficient for this purpose (Fig. 38.80). Peripheral portions of a cavernous hemangioma may be indistinguishable from low-grade angiosarcoma. Hemangiomas usually do not exceed 2.0 cm in diameter, whereas few angiosarcomas are smaller than 3.0 cm; however, these generalizations are primarily based on observations from clinically palpable tumors. The current availability of needle core biopsy samples from small nonpalpable vascular tumors has created situations in which lesions smaller than 3 cm with the histologic characteristics of angiosarcoma can be encountered. As a consequence, it is prudent to perform an excision when a needle core biopsy reveals a vascular lesion. In cases in which postbiopsy imaging indicates that the procedure removed most or all of a histologically benign lesion and a clip has been left at the biopsy site, follow-up by mammography can be an alternative to excision.

Mastectomy is not indicated but has been performed in a few instances in which a lesion was incorrectly diagnosed as angiosarcoma. No patient with any of the foregoing types of hemangiomas has had a recurrence after excision with follow-up averaging 44 months but extending as long as 140 months.

ANGIOMATOSIS

The name angiomatosis is a descriptive compromise when applied to vascular tumors, which are often composed of hemangiomatous and lymphangiomatous channels. An example of angiomatosis in a 49-year-old woman with prominent lymphangiomatous features has been described as a "cystic hygroma of the breast."[328] Angiomatosis should be distinguished from "hemangiomatosis," the diagnosis recommended by Hamperl[329] for patients with several perilobular hemangiomas. It is preferable to refer to this latter condition as multiple perilobular hemangiomas, although rarely perilobular hemangiomas may be so numerous as to suggest a diffuse vascular proliferation. Multiple perilobular hemangiomas retain the localized capillary structure that typifies these lesions and thus are easily distinguished from the larger, irregularly shaped channels that characterize angiomatosis.

Clinical Presentation

Four female patients have been reported.[330,331] Three were adults, 19 to 40 years old, when the lesion was diagnosed, and the fourth had a congenital tumor. Each presented with a mass in the breast. Other examples described as "cystic lymphangioma" and "lymphangiomatosis" have also been reported, with symptoms of breast enlargement sometimes first occurring after pregnancy or breast feeding.[332,333]

Gross Pathology

The lesions are grossly cystic and spongy. Those lesions from the adult women measured 11.0, 9.3, and 9.0 cm in largest dimension. One tumor had a 15-cm blood-filled cyst.[330] When the vascular spaces contain blood, the tumor appears hemorrhagic and resembles an angiosarcoma (Fig. 38.81).

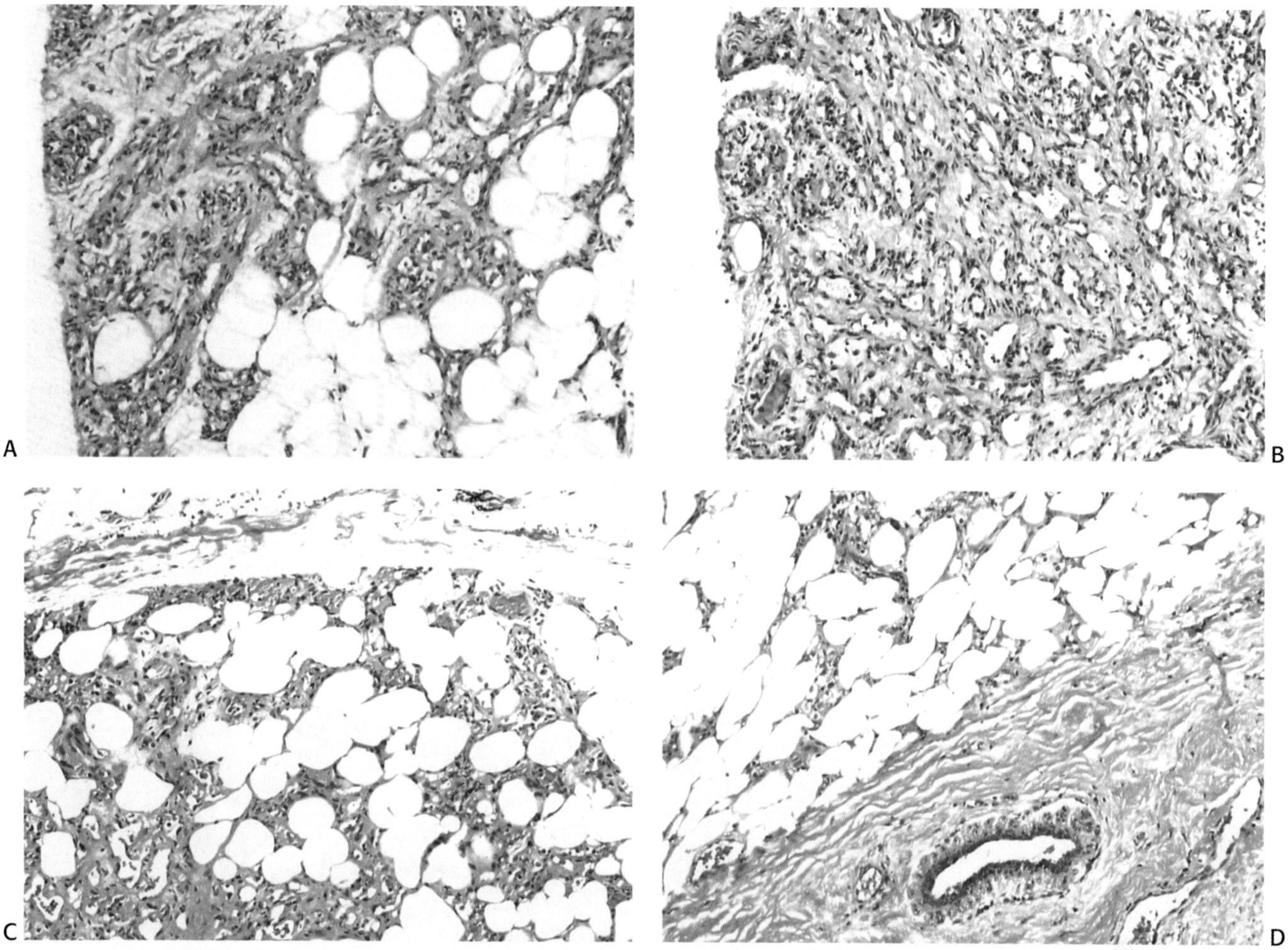

FIG. 38.80. ***Hemangioma, needle core biopsy specimen.*** The lesion was detected by mammography. **A,B:** Areas in the needle core biopsy samples showing varying cellularity and spread into the fat. **C,D:** The excised tumor was a capillary hemangioma.

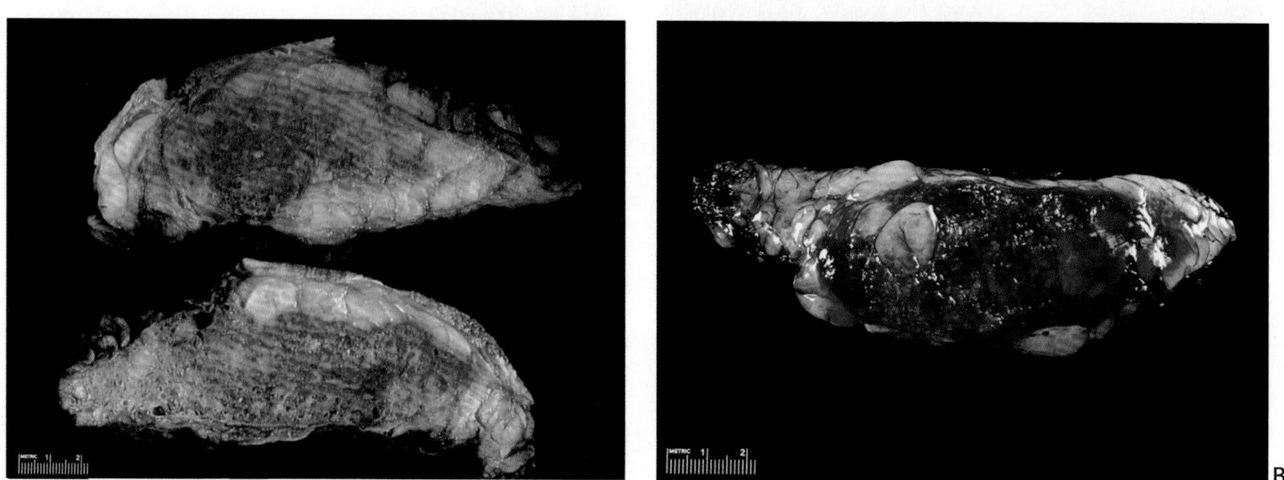

FIG. 38.81. ***Angiomatosis, gross appearance.*** **A,B:** Two mastectomy specimens demonstrating diffuse cystic hemorrhagic angiomatosis.

Microscopic Pathology

Although angiomatosis forms a mass clinically and on macroscopic pathologic examination, it does not have the microscopically circumscribed structure that typifies mammary hemangiomas. The lesion is composed of anastomosing, large vascular channels extending diffusely in the breast parenchyma (Fig. 38.82). They surround ducts and lobules but do not invade the lobular stroma. The vessels are lined by flat inconspicuous endothelium with sparse supporting mural tissue that is virtually devoid of smooth muscle. The vascular structures consist predominantly of hemangiomatous erythrocyte-containing channels, lymphangiomatous empty channels accompanied by lymphoid aggregates, or a mixture of the two types of vessels. This configuration is similar to that of somatic angiomatosis as described by Enzinger and Weiss[334]:

> ...a proliferation of small to medium-sized vessels of irregular shape that diffusely infiltrate skin, subcutis, muscle and even bone in a given area. The vessels are usually thin walled or at best contain a few poorly formed fascicles of smooth muscle. They may be blood filled or empty and are sometimes surrounded by foci of lymphocytes, features that raise the question of focal lymphangiomatosis differentiation.

Angiomatosis may occur in breast tissue involved by other conditions such as a FA (Fig. 38.83). An extremely unusual capillary variant of angiomatosis presents as a breast mass. The specimen consists of numerous clusters of histologically benign-appearing capillaries distributed throughout fibrous and fatty breast tissue (Fig. 38.84). Association with renal failure and dialysis in one case may be coincidental.

The microscopic distinction between angiomatosis and low-grade angiosarcoma may be difficult, especially in a small biopsy sample. Anastomosing channels that are "empty" or contain erythrocytes occur in both lesions. When multiple areas are sampled, significant differences become apparent. The vascular channels in angiomatosis are distributed uniformly throughout the tumor with very little variation. On the other hand, even the most well-differentiated

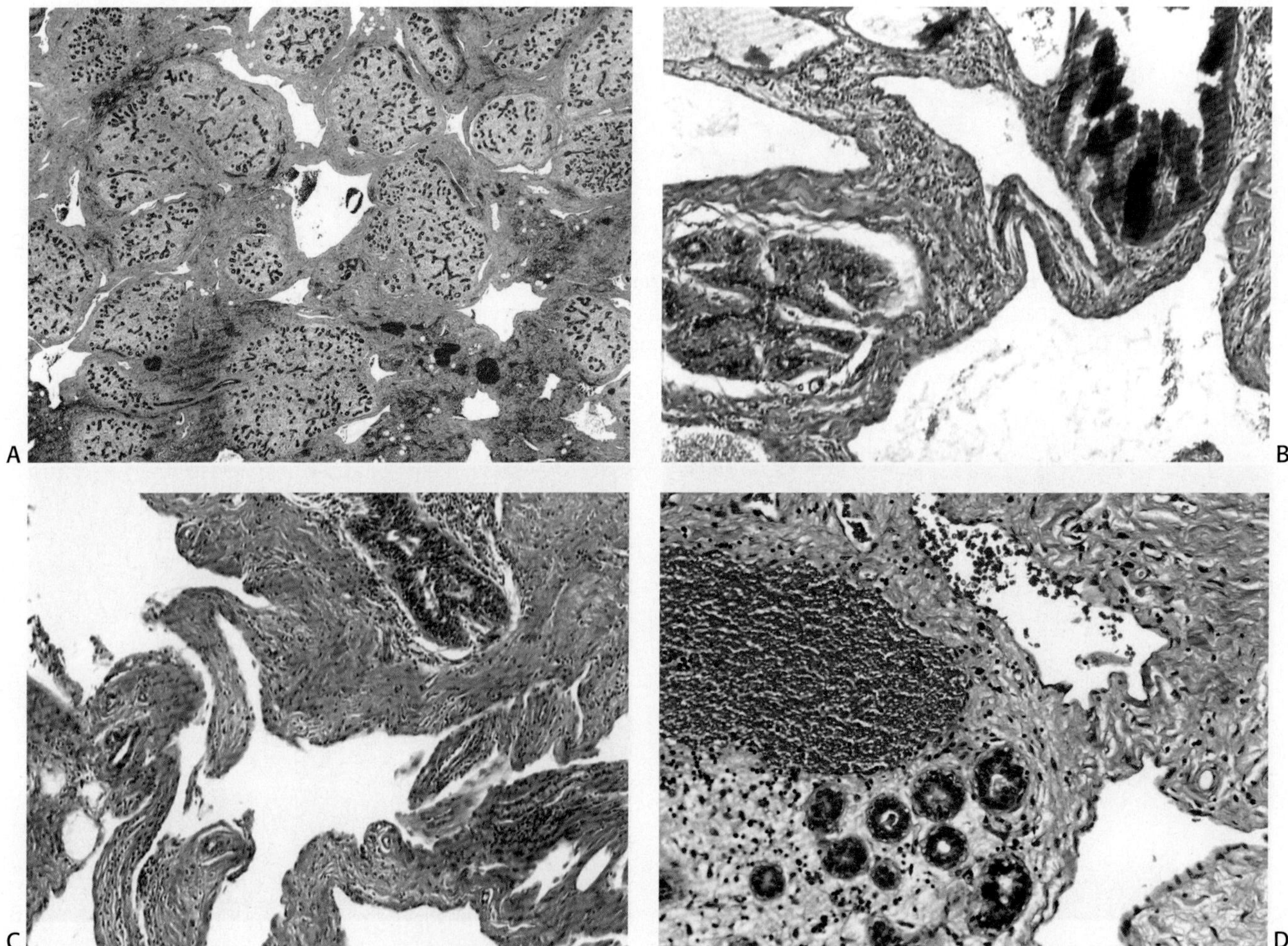

FIG. 38.82. *Angiomatosis.* **A:** Dilated blood-filled and empty vascular channels extending through the interlobular fibrous stroma with sparing of the lobules. **B,C:** Vascular channels that surround ducts. The stroma contains sparse smooth muscle cells and lymphocytes. **D:** The flat endothelium is inconspicuous.

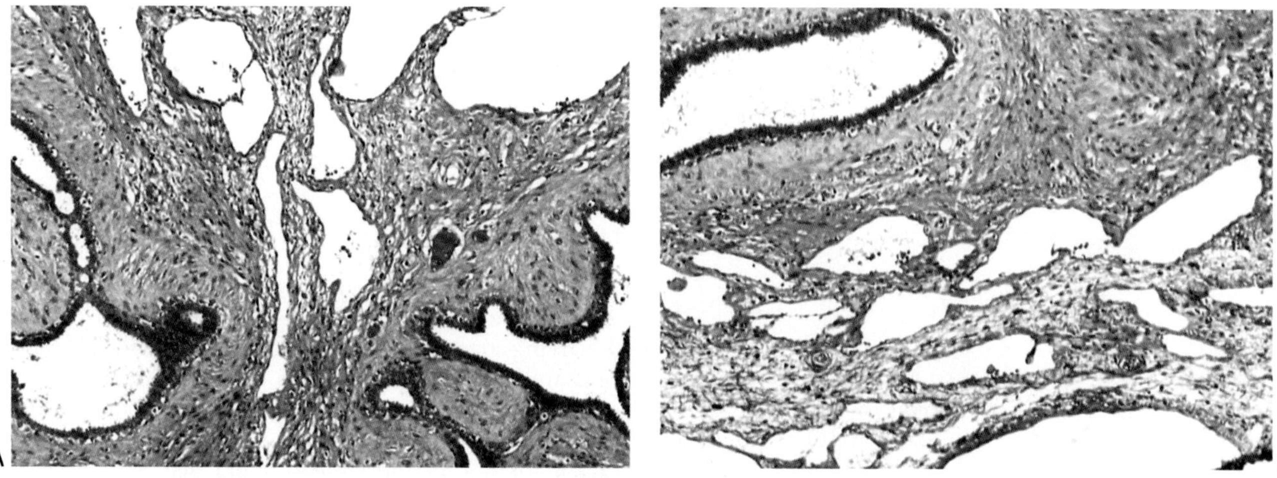

FIG. 38.83. ***Angiomatosis in a fibroadenoma.*** **A,B:** A lymphangiomatous vascular proliferation is present in a FA and in the surrounding breast tissue.

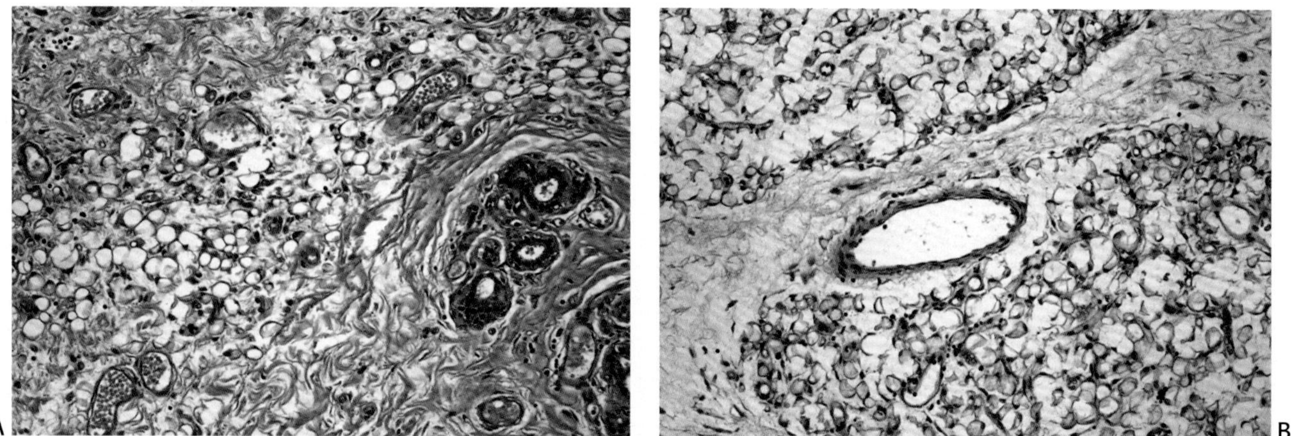

FIG. 38.84. ***Angiomatosis, capillary type.*** **A:** Small, uniform capillaries are distributed in the fat. **B:** Two discrete adjacent foci of capillary proliferation in fat.

angiosarcoma has a heterogeneous pattern of vessels that are numerous in some regions and more widely separated elsewhere. The vascular structures of angiomatosis tend not to diminish in caliber at the periphery, whereas neoplastic vessels of capillary size merge with the surrounding tissue at the periphery of angiosarcomas. The vascular proliferation in angiomatosis surrounds lobules but does not invade them; however, in angiosarcomas, the vascular channels grow into lobules, which are consequently destroyed. Finally, endothelial nuclei are histologically normal in angiomatosis, or they may be so attenuated that they may be difficult to find. More prominent, hyperchromatic endothelial nuclei are found in angiosarcomas, even when papillary endothelial proliferation is absent. Mitoses are not found in angiomatosis, which has a very low Ki67-labeling index.

Treatment and Prognosis

In their discussion of angiomatosis of the soft tissues, Enzinger and Weiss[334] noted that "the lesions are capable of repeated local recurrence. However, we are not aware that malignant degeneration of these lesions occurs or that acceptable cases have given rise to metastatic disease.... a conservative surgical approach seems advisable initially, and more extensive surgery should be reserved for persistently recurring lesions."

Angiomatosis of the breast is comparable to similar lesions that arise at other anatomic sites. The large size attained in the breast without the development of a histologically or clinically malignant component indicates that these are benign tumors. It may be necessary to perform a mastectomy to control a bulky lesion, but less extensive surgery is preferable whenever possible. Recurrence may occur, sometimes after a long interval, indicating that the lesion is a chronic condition in some patients.[331]

The clinical course of one patient with a congenital tumor is of particular interest. At birth, she had a cavernous hemangioma of the right anterior chest. It measured "3 × 4 inches" and was described as "not smooth but rolling as if enlarged vessels lie underneath." At surgery, a tumor was found "extending from beneath the right nipple upward... to the level of the clavicle and outward... to the

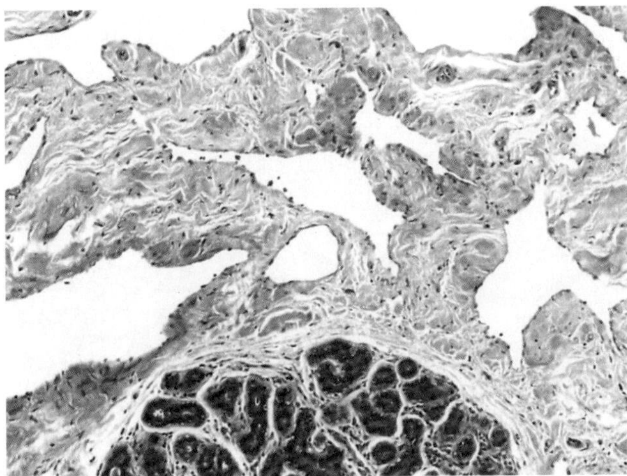

FIG. 38.85. *Angiomatosis.* A recurrent lymphangioma in the breast growing as angiomatosis.

anterior axillary fold." The specimen, resected when the patient was 11 weeks old, consisted of many empty channels of varying size lined by flat endothelium. Although no breast tissue was described histologically, the breast did not develop fully at puberty presumably because part of the breast bud had been removed. Twenty-eight years later, the patient underwent bilateral mammoplasty with insertion of a right breast prosthesis. Six years after this operation, when 34 years old, the patient had a mass resected from the right superior lateral chest wall, which proved to be angiomatosis in fat and skeletal muscle. Many of the vascular spaces were congested with red blood cells. At 39 years of age, the patient presented with two soft masses near the areola involving the upper and lower inner quadrants overlying the right breast implant. Microscopic examination revealed angiomatosis in the mammary parenchyma (Fig. 38.85).

VENOUS HEMANGIOMA

The microscopic appearance of these vascular tumors of the breast corresponds most closely to that of soft tissue[335] and bone[336] lesions that have been termed "venous hemangiomas" or "vascular anomalies." It is not known whether these are true neoplasms, but progressive enlargement of extramammary venous hemangiomas has been observed as a result of growth in fat, skeletal muscle, and bone. It is unlikely that trauma contributes to the development of venous hemangiomas, although antecedent injury was reported by one patient with a mammary venous hemangioma. Fat necrosis and hemosiderin-laden macrophages, which would be expected in a trauma-associated vascular lesion, have been largely absent from venous hemangiomas.

Clinical Presentation

Five cases have been reported.[337] The patients' ages range from 24 to 59 years (average 40 years). Each presented with a palpable tumor. One patient reported that the mass had been present for 13 years. Another patient became aware of the lesion after trauma to the breast.

Gross Pathology

The tumors have measured from 1.0 to 5.3 cm in greatest dimension (average 3.2 cm). They are well-circumscribed, firm, and darkly colored. Hemorrhagic cysts measuring 0.5 to 1.3 cm in diameter were noted in one lesion.

Microscopic Pathology

The lesions are characterized by some histologic diversity. All have dilated venous channels with smooth muscle walls of varying structural completeness (Fig. 38.86). Red blood cells are present in the lumens of some vascular spaces; other spaces are empty or contain lymph. Thick-walled arterial channels and capillaries are not conspicuous, except for one of the larger tumors that had capillary-forming areas. A large, well-formed muscular artery was found at the margin of one tumor (Fig. 38.87). A few lobules and ducts are sometimes distributed in the mammary stroma between the vascular channels that form the lesion (Fig. 38.88). Focal perivascular lymphocytic infiltrates are also present in the stroma often accompanied by congested capillaries. Lobular carcinoma *in situ* (LCIS) was present in breast tissue outside the venous hemangioma in one case.[337]

The dilated vascular channels are irregularly shaped and vary greatly in caliber. A smooth muscle layer is evident in the wall of some of the tumor vessels, but often it does not encompass the entire circumference (Fig. 38.89). In some areas, smooth muscle elements appear to be incompletely formed or absent in sections stained with H&E, an impression that is confirmed with a trichrome stain and with immunohistochemical stains for SMA.

Microscopic features most often associated with angiosarcoma are absent. These include pleomorphism and hyperchromasia of endothelial cell nuclei, papillary proliferation of endothelium, endothelial mitoses, hemorrhagic necrosis, and destructive invasion into glandular mammary parenchyma.

Treatment and Prognosis

One patient underwent a mastectomy because the lesion was thought to be adherent to the pectoral muscle at the time of surgery; however, the vascular tumor was later found to be confined to the breast. Another patient who had coincidental LCIS had no residual tumor in the specimen obtained when the original biopsy site was reexcised. Three other patients were treated by excision. With follow-up ranging from 6 months to 11 years, there were no recurrences of venous hemangiomas. Excisional biopsy is the recommended treatment for this benign vascular lesion.

NONPARENCHYMAL HEMANGIOMAS OF THE MAMMARY REGION

For many years, considerable emphasis was placed on the distinction between subcutaneous and intraparenchymal vascular lesions of the breast. The former virtually all proved

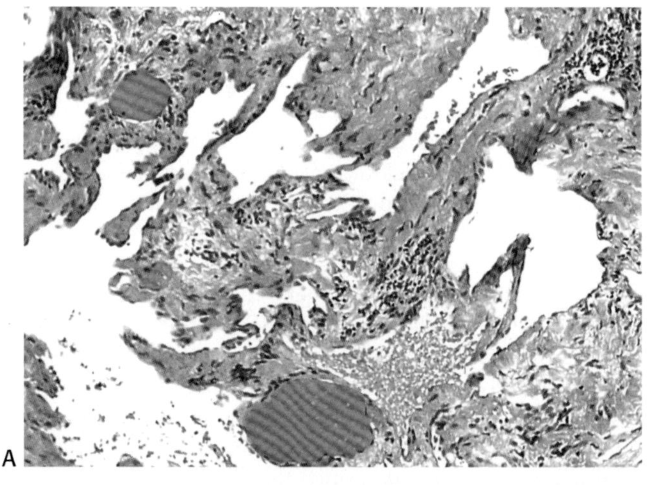

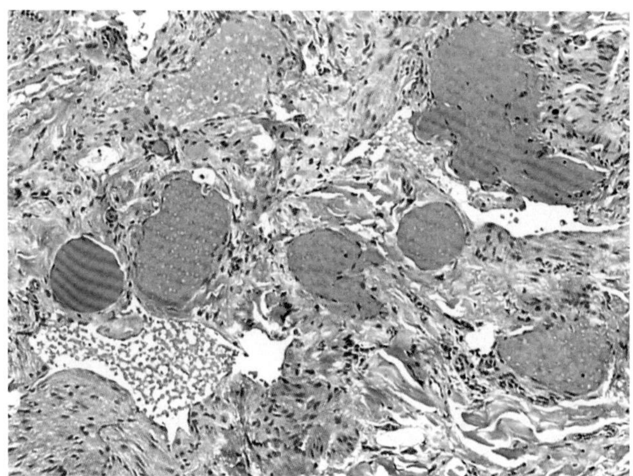

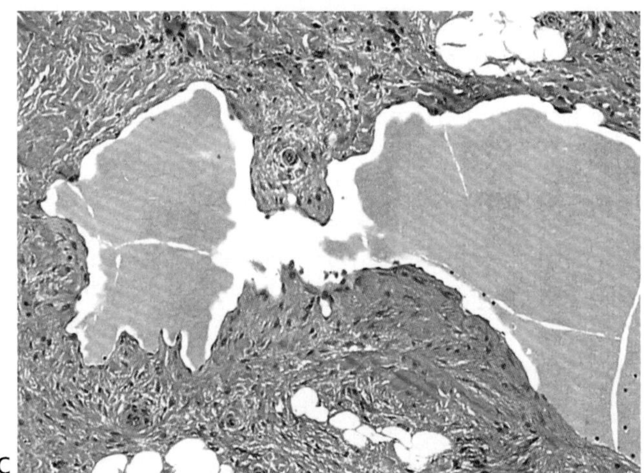

FIG. 38.86. ***Venous hemangioma.*** **A:** Some vascular spaces contain blood. **B:** Many congested vessels are present in this region. **C:** This vessel contains homogeneous pink fluid that is probably lymph.

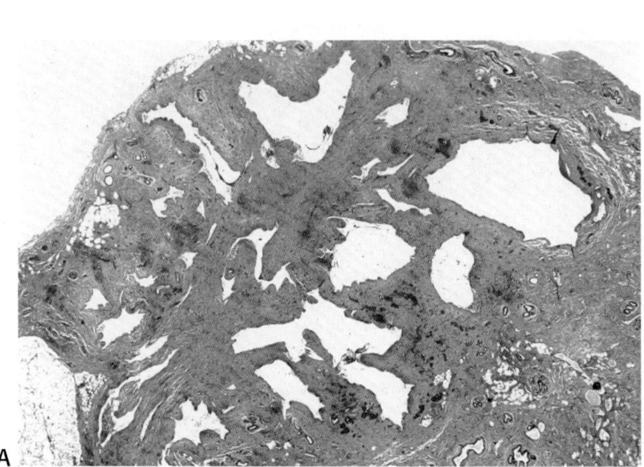

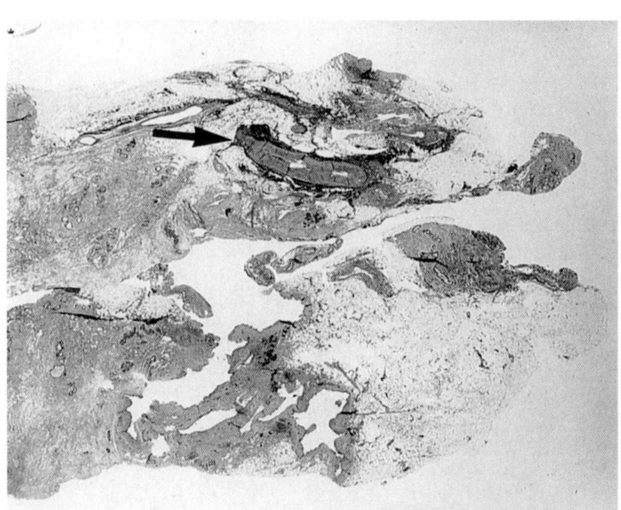

FIG. 38.87. ***Venous hemangioma.*** **A:** This whole-mount histologic section reveals a circumscribed group of irregular dilated vascular channels. **B:** In this whole-mount section from another patient, there is a large feeding artery (*arrow*) in the upper piece of tissue from the periphery of the tumor. The lower sample contains less well-formed, thin-walled vascular channels characteristic of a venous hemangioma. (**B:** Reproduced from Rosen PP, Jozefczyk MA, Boram LH. Vascular tumors of the breast. IV. The venous hemangioma. *Am J Surg Pathol* 1985;9:659–665, with permission.)

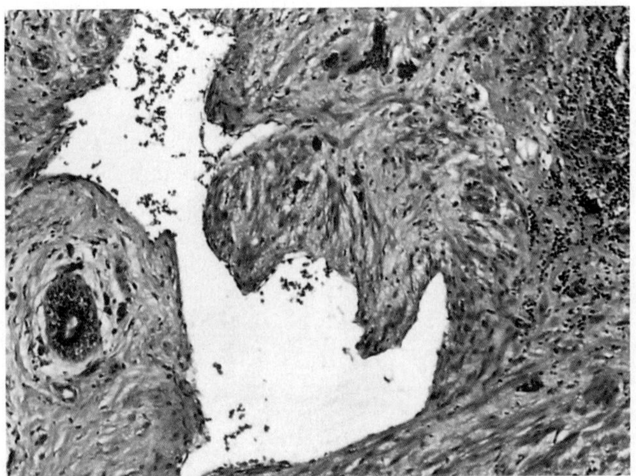

FIG. 38.88. *Venous hemangioma.* A small duct is shown on the *left* and a perivascular lymphocytic infiltrate on the *right*.

to be benign, whereas the majority of the latter were interpreted as angiosarcomas. However, location alone is not sufficient to determine the diagnosis, because the existence of intraparenchymal hemangiomas is now well-documented, and angiosarcoma may involve the mammary skin and subcutaneous tissue.

Little attention has been paid to the clinical and pathologic characteristics of nonparenchymal hemangiomas of the breast. In 1933, Menville and Bloodgood[338] reported several patients with mammary subcutaneous cavernous and capillary hemangiomas. They emphasized the difference between hemangiomas of the skin and of the subcutaneous tissue, noting that "subcutaneous lesions have no connection with the epidermis." Two of the seven hemangiomas in their series were misdiagnosed as angiosarcomas and treated by mastectomy. Madding and Hershberger[339] described a 23-year-old patient with a "birthmark" on her right breast, which was treated with radiation. Subsequent ulceration and persistent bleeding led to a mastectomy, which revealed an 8 × 7 × 6 cm vascular tumor of the subcutaneous tissue. Microscopically, "no breast ducts were observed admixed with the tumor." Although the authors described the vessels as "for the most part dilated capillaries," they noted that "few of the larger vessels showed scattered muscle fibers but no elastic tissue. These latter vessels were interpreted to be small venules." The pictures that accompany the report illustrate vascular channels typically associated with venous hemangiomas.

Clinical Presentation

A variety of nonparenchymal hemangiomas occur in the mammary region.[340] Dermal or cutaneous hemangiomas, the majority of which are capillary hemangiomas and do

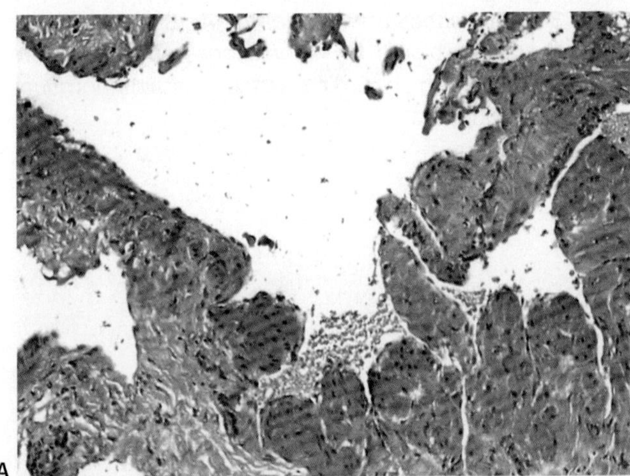

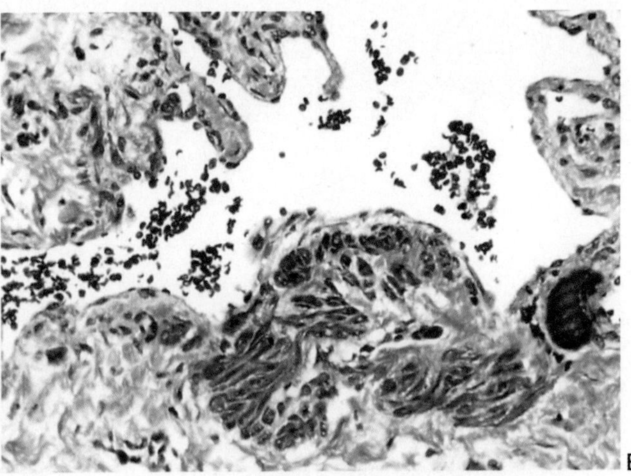

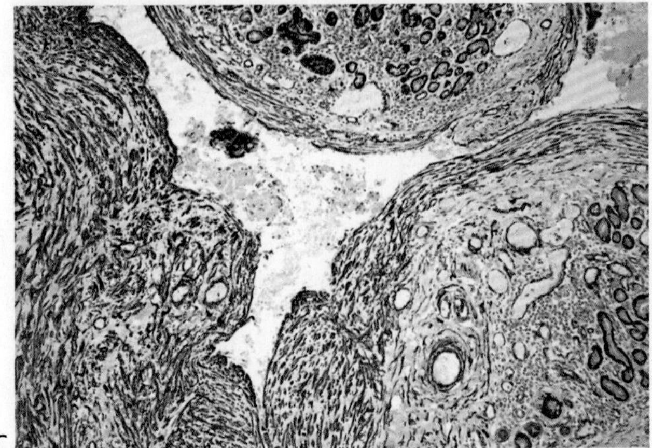

FIG. 38.89. *Venous hemangioma.* **A:** Bundles of smooth muscle cells are present around part of the vascular channel. **B:** The smooth muscle is *red* in this section stained with Masson trichrome. **C:** A vascular channel with abundant actin-positive mural smooth muscle.

not present a diagnostic problem, are excluded from this category. Almost all patients are women whose age ranges from 20 to 76 years, averaging 53 years. Nonparenchymal subcutaneous hemangiomas of the male breast have also been encountered.[341,342] The right and left breasts are involved with nearly equal frequency. Some lesions occur in the inframammary region, but the majority are distributed in various quadrants. The presenting symptom is a mass. A cavernous hemangioma of the pectoralis muscle presented as a 2.5-cm tumor deep in the breast on mammography.[343] At surgery, the lesion proved to be intramuscular. Siewert et al.[344] described a 42-year-old woman with a 5-mm subcutaneous complex capillary hemangioma. The lesion was palpable but not visualized by mammography. Sonography revealed a circumscribed, slightly hypoechoic mass with no acoustic shadowing. Sonography is a useful procedure for determining whether the lesion is in subcutaneous tissue or in the breast.[344,345]

Benign angiomatous lesions that occur in the skin after radiation therapy are discussed in Chapter 39.

Gross and Microscopic Pathology

Tumor sizes range from 0.8 to 3.2 cm, averaging 1.8 cm. Breast parenchyma may be included in the biopsy specimen. The lesion is classified as nonparenchymal if the neoplastic vessels do not involve the mammary glandular tissue.

The diagnosis of nonparenchymal vascular tumors is based on the descriptions and the classification of benign vascular tumors of soft tissues proposed by Enzinger and Weiss.[346] Several types of hemangiomas have been identified: angiolipoma (Figs. 38.90 and 38.91), cavernous hemangioma (Fig. 38.92), hemangioma with papillary endothelial hyperplasia (Fig. 38.93), capillary hemangioma (Fig. 38.94), and venous hemangioma. The frequencies of these types of hemangiomas correspond roughly to their relative occurrence in the soft tissues generally. This suggests that there is no strong predilection for a particular type of hemangioma to occur in the mammary subcutaneous tissue.

It is possible that selected regions of the breast are prone to develop certain types of hemangiomas. In one study, two angiolipomas were located in the upper inner quadrant and two cavernous hemangiomas were excised from the inframammary region.[340] Yu et al.[347] described a 2-cm "cellular" angiolipoma that was excised from the upper inner quadrant of the left breast of a 64-year-old woman. A study of angiolipomas noted that "many of the lesions were removed from sites subject to repeated pressure and irritation."[348] About 8% of the angiolipomas occurred on the anterior chest, but the frequency of the lesions in the female breast was not stated.

The histologic appearance of various types of hemangiomas in the mammary subcutaneous tissue does not differ from comparable lesions in other subcutaneous locations.

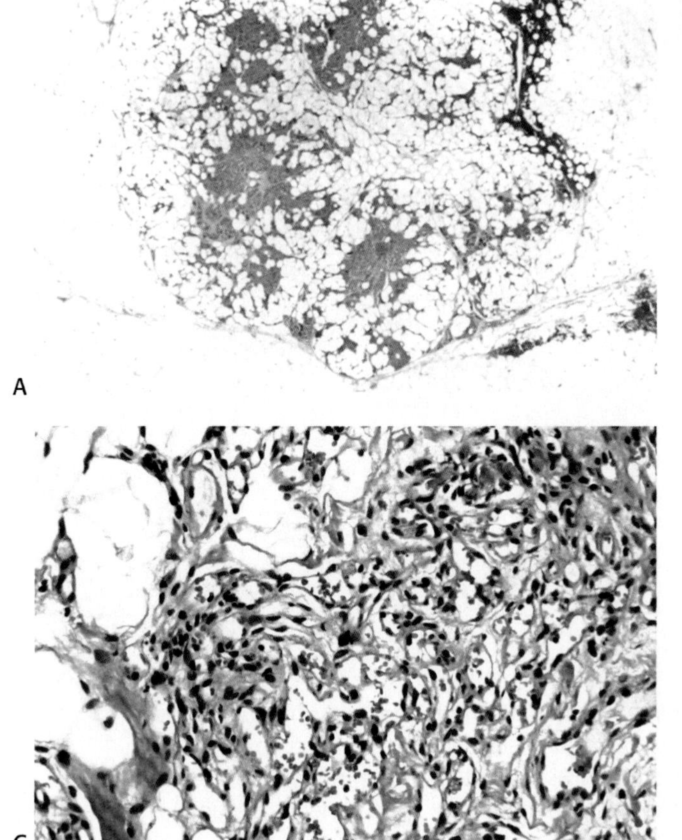

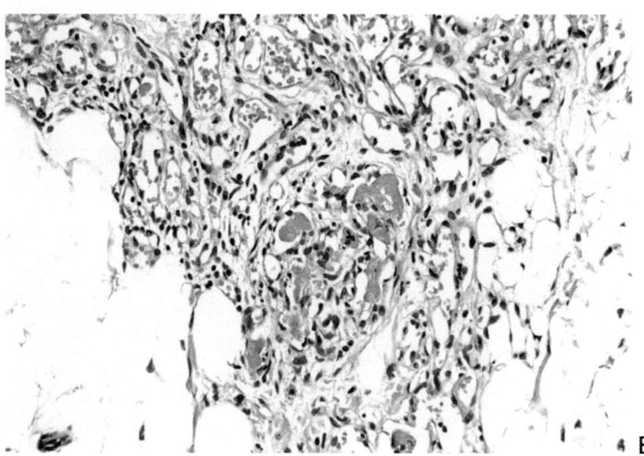

FIG. 38.90. ***Nonparenchymal angiolipoma.*** **A:** This whole-mount histologic section shows the capillary proliferation distributed in fat. **B,C:** Capillaries meshed in delicate fibrous stroma. Fibrin thrombi are present in **(B)**.

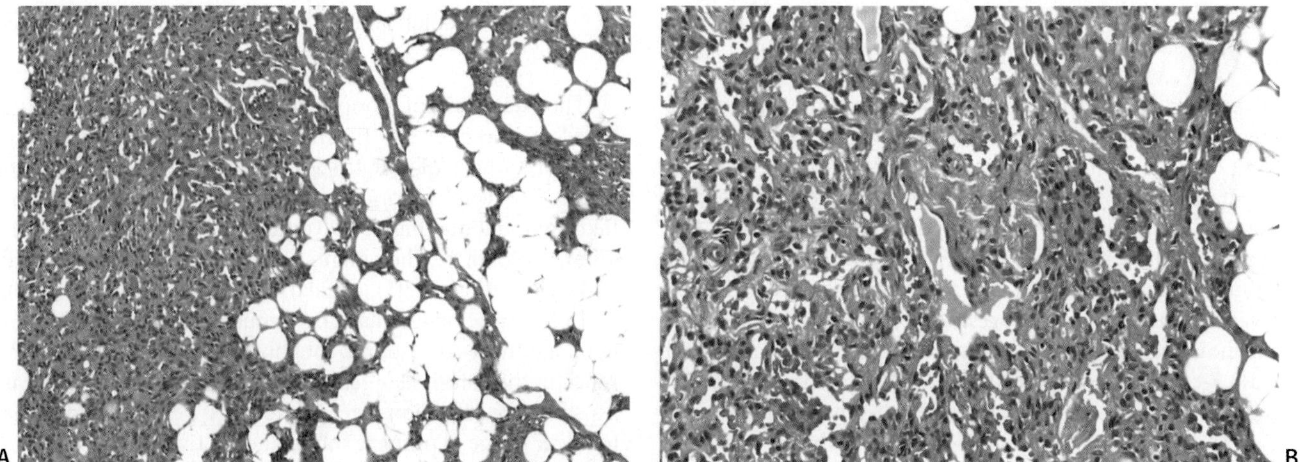

FIG. 38.91. ***Nonparenchymal angiolipoma.*** **A:** The capillary component of this tumor has a relatively solid growth pattern. **B:** The capillaries form a network of small anastomosing channels. Microthrombi are present.

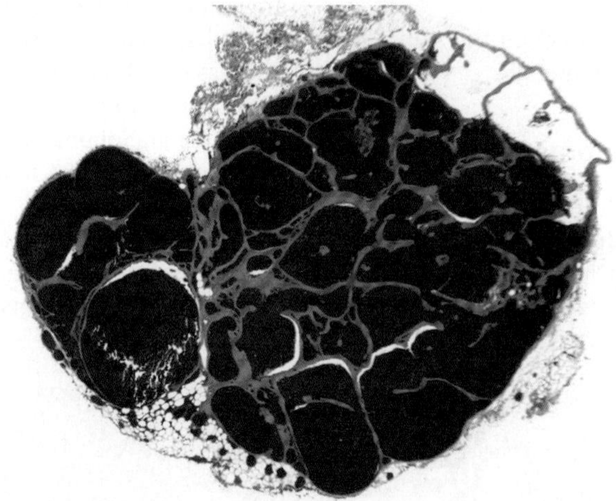

FIG. 38.92. ***Nonparenchymal cavernous hemangioma.*** The tumor is well-circumscribed.

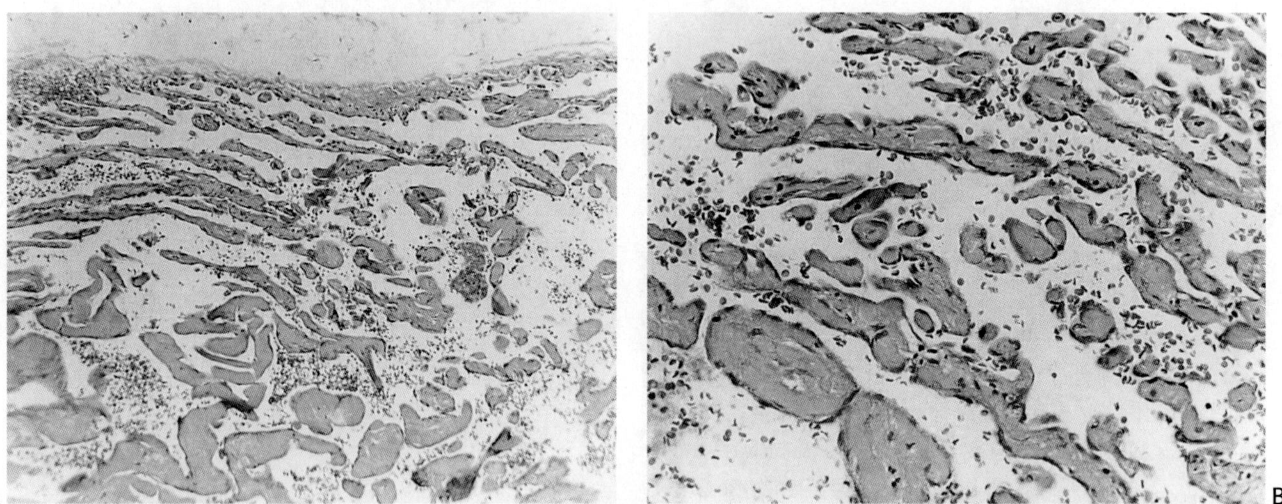

FIG. 38.93. ***Nonparenchymal hemangioma, papillary endothelial hyperplasia.*** **A:** The tumor has a well-circumscribed border. **B:** Widely anastomosing vascular spaces are distributed among branching, disrupted papillary fronds of collagenous stroma. (**A,B:** Reproduced from Rosen PP. Vascular tumors of the breast. V. Non-parenchymal hemangiomas of mammary subcutaneous tissue. *Am J Surg Pathol* 1985;9:723–729, with permission.)

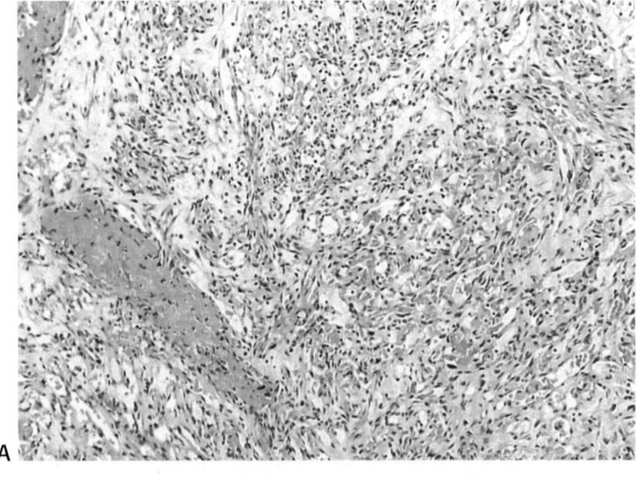

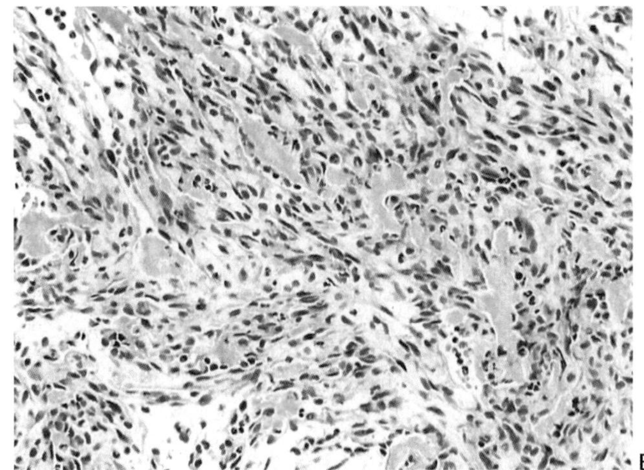

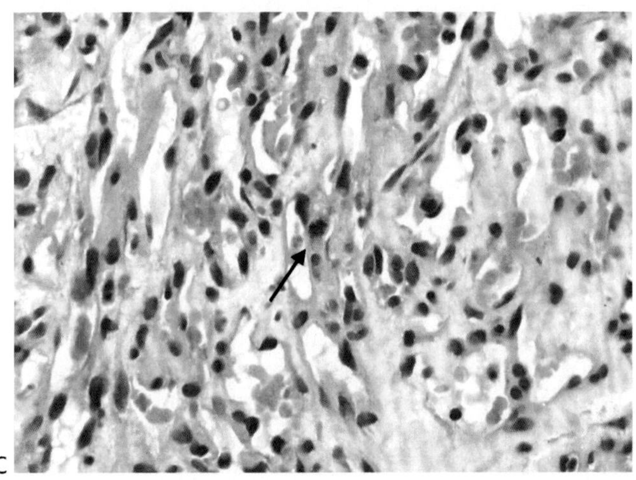

FIG. 38.94. ***Nonparenchymal capillary hemangioma.*** **A:** Most of the tumor is compact and the vascular spaces are compressed slits. **B:** A region with conspicuous stromal spindle cells. **C:** A mitotic figure (*arrow*) is present in the center between the capillaries.

Some hemangiomas found in mammary subcutaneous tissue feature interconnected vascular channels (Fig. 38.95). Areas in which these septa are disrupted have a pseudopapillary pattern (Fig. 38.93). The vascular spaces can be larger toward the center than at the periphery, where they tend to spread into the subcutaneous fat producing an ill-defined margin microscopically. Encapsulation of angiolipomas is often difficult to determine after the lesions have been dissected. Concern about the diagnosis often arises because of the abundant closely apposed vascular spaces with intervening spindle cell stroma[347] and uncertainty about whether the lesion is truly extraparenchymal.

Treatment and Prognosis

Nonparenchymal subcutaneous hemangiomas of the breast are adequately treated by local excision. Reexcision of the biopsy site may be indicated when the location of the lesion (subcutaneous vs. parenchymal) is in doubt or if there is uncertainty about the adequacy of the margins. Complete removal of the tumor also helps to exclude the possibility that a vascular lesion that appears benign in a small biopsy specimen is a subcutaneous extension from an underlying low-grade angiosarcoma.

ANEURYSM

Aneurysms occurring in and around the breast are very uncommon nonneoplastic vascular tumors (Fig. 38.96). Most are false aneurysms caused by medical intervention or blunt trauma. Iatrogenic pseudoaneurysms have been reported after stereotactic and vacuum-assisted core biopsies. They have been identified from 1 day to 9 months after the procedures and have ranged in size from 1 to 3 cm.[349–351] El Khoury et al.[352] described a pseudoaneurysm that presented as a 2-cm palpable, throbbing mass 3 weeks after a core biopsy had been performed for a BI-RADS (Breast Imaging-Reporting and Data System) category 4 lesion. Three weeks later, spontaneous complete thrombosis was evident sonographically. Other patients have developed pseudoaneurysms after falls associated with breast injury.[353,354]

An arteriovenous fistula (AVF) was identified 4 months after a needle core biopsy procedure with clip placement.[355] The AVF was manifested clinically by a palpable thrill and bruit. Ultrasound imaging demonstrated an AVF arising from the external mammary artery draining via venous connections to the internal mammary vein.

Two reports describe pseudoaneurysms in hypertensive patients. One was a 57-year-old woman with a 3-cm, smooth

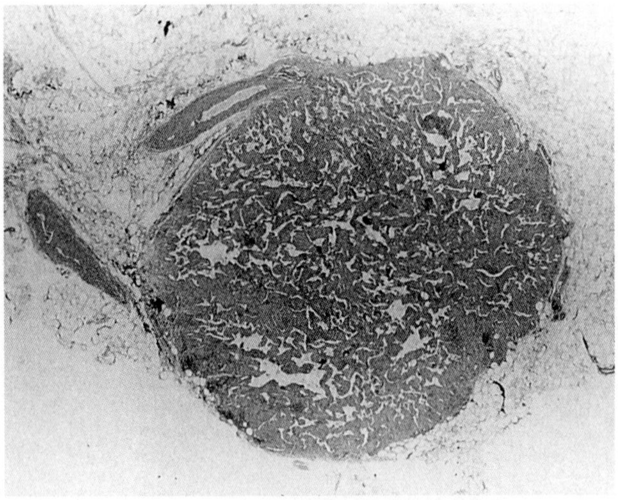

FIG. 38.95. ***Nonparenchymal hemangioma.*** **A:** This whole-mount histologic section shows a circumscribed vascular tumor in fat. Two segments of feeding vessel were captured on the *left* of this fortuitous section. The appearance suggests that they may be afferent and efferent portions of a single artery that gave rise to the hemangioma. **B:** A complex network of anastomosing vascular channels with intervening fibrous septa. **C:** A magnified view of the upper feeding vessel shown in **(A)**. The vascular proliferation involves the lumen of the artery.

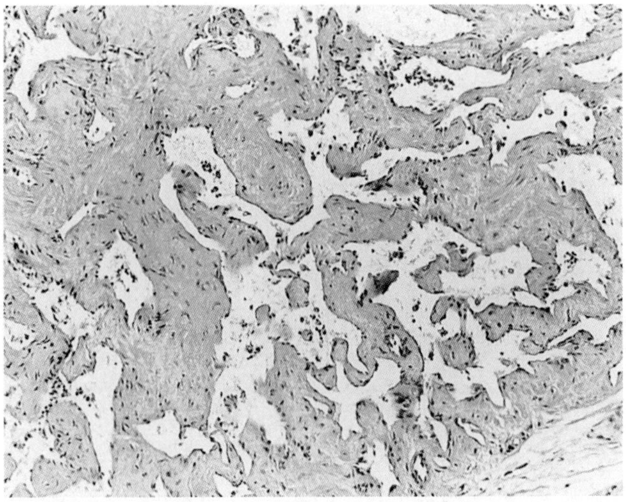

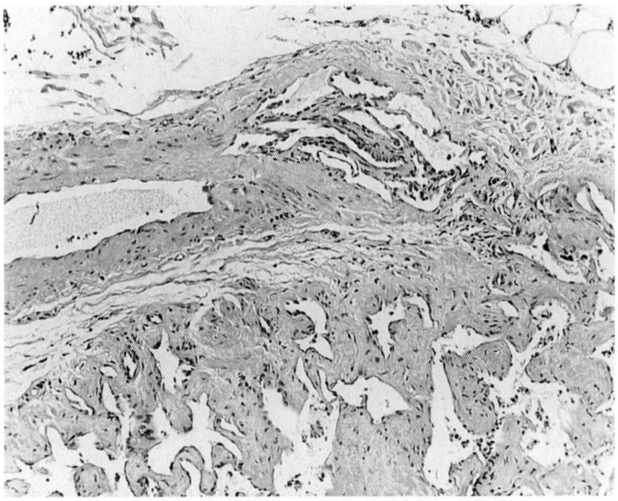

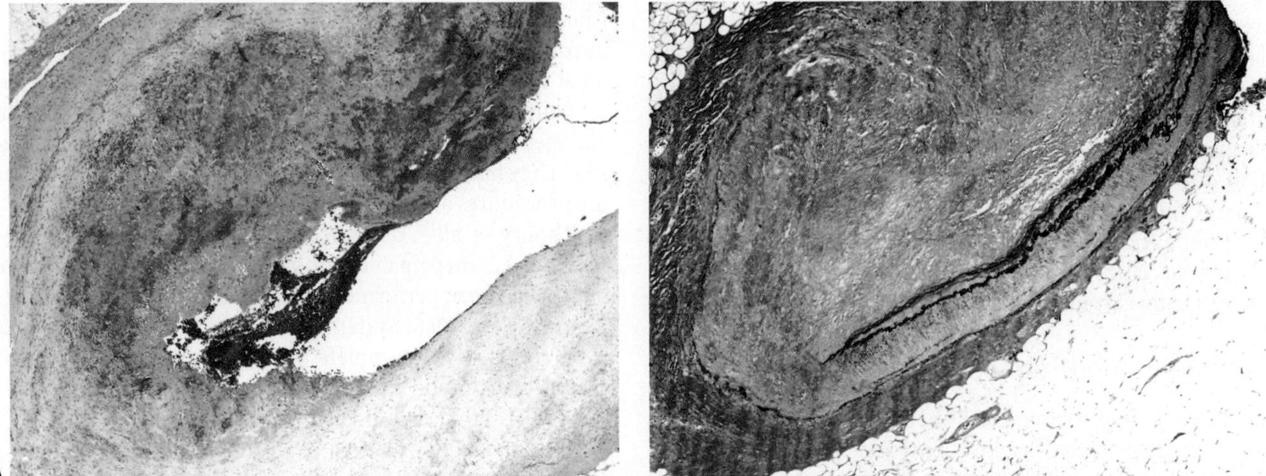

FIG. 38.96. ***Aneurysm.*** The specimen is from a 73-year-old woman with a palpable, pulsatile breast mass. She was not known to be hypertensive, and there was no history of trauma or prior surgery. **A:** Part of the resected aneurysmal artery showing blood clot. **B:** Mural elastic tissue is highlighted on the *right* by an elastin stain. Note the aneurysmal dilatation, absence of elastica, and clot on the *left* (Verhoeff Van Gieson elastic stain). **C:** Mural smooth muscle preserved in the artery wall appears as a *red* band (*right*). Smooth muscle is almost entirely absent from the aneurysmal region (*left*) (Masson trichrome stain).

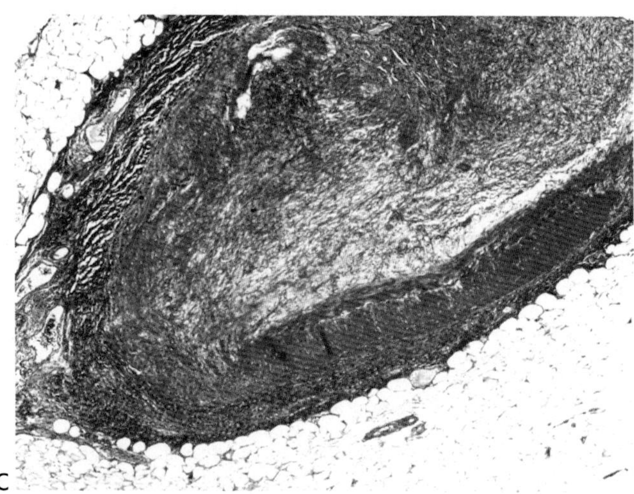

FIG. 38.96. *(Continued)*

mobile tumor in the upper outer quadrant of the right breast.[356] The lesion was brought to clinical attention because of sudden severe pain and ecchymosis in the area. Angiography revealed an aneurysmal AVF arising from the underlying intercostal artery. The excised specimen was described as "a false aneurysm filled with blood clot in continuity with the feeding artery" with no evidence of atherosclerotic, traumatic, or inflammatory etiology or of medial degeneration. The other hypertensive patient was a 55-year-old woman with a painful, pulsatile 1 × 1.5 cm tumor accompanied by ecchymosis involving the left medial breast and chest wall.[357] A diagnosis of pseudoaneurysm was made radiologically and successfully treated by percutaneous insertion of an occluding wire embolus. The specific artery affected was not identified.

In another instance, mammography demonstrated a bilobed 3.5-cm mass adjacent to arterial calcifications in the breast of a 57-year-old woman.[358] It was predominantly cystic on ultrasonography and appeared to be pulsatile. The patient had systemic lupus erythematosus in remission and was receiving anticoagulant therapy after replacement of a heart valve. Histologic examination revealed a false aneurysm arising in the wall of a medium-sized artery with medial calcification. No arteritis was evident.

Davies and Kulka[359] reviewed histologic sections of 107 surgically excised radial sclerosing lesions and reported finding false aneurysms in five cases. All of the radial sclerosing lesions in specimens that had aneurysms were 10 mm or larger. FNA had been performed in four cases 18 to 22 days previously. The interval was 121 days in the fifth case.

True aneurysms of the breast have been described only rarely. Cox et al.[360] reported a 50-year-old woman with multiple bilateral arterial aneurysms that were identified during evaluation of a spontaneous left breast hematoma. The patient was noted to have a history of chronic amphetamine abuse.

REFERENCES

Fibromatosis

1. Gump FE, Sternschein MJ, Wolff M. Fibromatosis of the breast. *Surg Gynecol Obstet* 1981;153:57–60.
2. Rosen PP, Ernsberger D. Mammary fibromatosis. A benign spindle-cell tumor with significant risk for local recurrence. *Cancer* 1989;63:1363–1369.
3. Wargotz ES, Norris HJ, Austin RM, et al. Fibromatosis of the breast. A clinical and pathological study of 28 cases. *Am J Surg Pathol* 1987;11:38–45.
4. Devouassoux-Shisheboran M, Schammel MD, Man YG, et al. Fibromatosis of the breast: age-correlated morphofunctional features of 33 cases. *Arch Pathol Lab Med* 2000;124:276–280.
5. Abraham SC, Reynolds C, Lee JH, et al. Fibromatosis of the breast and mutations involving the APC/beta-catenin pathway. *Hum Pathol* 2002;33:39–46.
6. Neuman HB, Brogi E, Ebrahim A, et al. Desmoid tumors (fibromatoses) of the breast: a 25-year experience. *Ann Surg Oncol* 2008;15:274–280.
7. Ali M, Fayemi AO, Braun EV, et al. Fibromatosis of the breast. *Am J Surg Pathol* 1979;3:501–505.
8. Cederlund CG, Gustavsson S, Linell F, et al. Fibromatosis of the breast mimicking carcinoma at mammography. *Br J Radiol* 1984;57:98–101.
9. el-Naggar A, Abdul-Karim FW, Marshalleck JJ, et al. Fine-needle aspiration of fibromatosis of the breast. *Diagn Cytopathol* 1987;3:320–322.
10. Haggitt RC, Booth JL. Bilateral fibromatosis of the breast in Gardner's syndrome. *Cancer* 1970;25:161–166.
11. Kalisher L, Long JA, Peyster RG. Extra-abdominal desmoid of the axillary tail mimicking breast carcinoma. *AJR Am J Roentgenol* 1976;126:903–906.
12. Jewett ST Jr, Mead JH. Extra-abdominal desmoid arising from a capsule around a silicone breast implant. *Plast Reconstr Surg* 1979;63:577–579.
13. Pierce VE Jr, Rives DA, Sisley JF, et al. Estradiol and progesterone receptors in a case of fibromatosis of the breast. *Arch Pathol Lab Med* 1987;111:870–872.
14. Tani EM, Stanley MW, Skoog L. Fine needle aspiration cytology presentation of bilateral mammary fibromatosis. Report of a case. *Acta Cytol* 1988;32:555–558.
15. Adair FE, Herrmann JB. Sarcoma of the breast with a report of thirty cases. *Surgery* 1946;19:55–73.
16. Norris HJ, Taylor HB. Sarcomas and related mesenchymal tumors of the breast. *Cancer* 1968;22:22–28.
17. Das Gupta TK, Brasfield RD, O'Hara J. Extra-abdominal desmoids: a clinicopathological study. *Ann Surg* 1969;170:109–121.
18. Simpson RD, Harrison EG Jr, Mayo CW. Mesenteric fibromatosis in familial polyposis. A variant of Gardner's Syndrome. *Cancer* 1964;17:526–534.
19. Kim T, Jung EA, Song JY, et al. Prevalence of the CTNNB1 mutation genotype in surgically resected fibromatosis of the breast. *Histopathology* 2012;60:347–356.
20. Needelman P, Leibman AJ, Capasse J. Fibromatosis of the axillary breast in a young patient. *Breast Dis* 1996;9:171–175.
21. Gupta AK, Atri SC, Naithani YP. Multiple pedunculated fibromatosis of breast. *J Indian Med Assoc* 1978;70:228–229.
22. Kalbhen CL, Cooper RA, Candel AG. Mammographic and stereotactic core biopsy findings in fibromatosis of the breast: case report. *Can Assoc Radiol J* 1998;49:229–231.
23. Bogomoletz WV, Boulenger E, Simatos A. Infiltrating fibromatosis of the breast. *J Clin Pathol* 1981;34:30–34.
24. Balzer BL, Weiss SW. Do biomaterials cause implant-associated mesenchymal tumors of the breast? Analysis of 8 new cases and review of the literature. *Hum Pathol* 2009;40:1564–1570.
25. Mátrai Z, Tóóth L, Gulyás G, et al. A desmoid tumor associated with a ruptured silicone breast implant. *Plast Reconstr Surg* 2011;127:1e–4e.
26. Zayid I, Dihmis C. Familial multicentric fibromatosis-desmoids. A report of three cases in a Jordanian family. *Cancer* 1969;24:786–795.
27. Barth AI, Nathke IS, Nelson WJ. Cadherins, catenins and APC protein: interplay between cytoskeletal complexes and signaling pathways. *Curr Opin Cell Biol* 1997;9:683–690.
28. Hayry P, Reitamo JJ, Vihko R, et al. The desmoid tumor. III. A biochemical and genetic analysis. *Am J Clin Pathol* 1982;77:681–685.
29. Leithner A, Gapp M, Radl R, et al. Immunohistochemical analysis of desmoid tumours. *J Clin Pathol* 2005;58:1152–1156.
30. Deyrup AT, Tretiakova M, Montag AG. Estrogen receptor-beta expression in extraabdominal fibromatoses: an analysis of 40 cases. *Cancer* 2006;106:208–213.
31. Rasbridge SA, Gillett CE, Millis RR. Oestrogen and progesterone receptor expression in mammary fibromatosis. *J Clin Pathol* 1993;46:349–351.
32. Pettinato G, Manivel JC, Gould EW, et al. Inclusion body fibromatosis of the breast. Two cases with immunohistochemical and ultrastructural findings. *Am J Clin Pathol* 1994;101:714–718.
33. Bittesini L, Dei Tos AP, Doglioni C, et al. Fibroepithelial tumor of the breast with digital fibroma-like inclusions in the stromal component.

Case report with immunocytochemical and ultrastructural analysis. *Am J Surg Pathol* 1994;18:296–301.
34. Shin SJ, Rosen PP. Bilateral presentation of fibroadenoma with digital fibroma-like inclusions in the male breast. *Arch Pathol Lab Med* 2007;131:1126–1129.
35. Shuler FJ, Cronin EB, Ricci A Jr, et al. Fibromatosis of the breast diagnosed by stereotaxic core biopsy. *AJR Am J Roentgenol* 1997;168:846–847.
36. Pettinato G, Manivel JC, Petrella G, et al. Fine needle aspiration cytology, immunocytochemistry and electron microscopy of fibromatosis of the breast. Report of two cases. *Acta Cytol* 1991;35:403–408.
37. Mayers MM, Evans P, MacVicar D. Case report: ossifying fibromatosis of the breast. *Clin Radiol* 1994;49:211–212.
38. Fritsches HG, Muller EA. Pseudosarcomatous fasciitis of the breast. Cytologic and histologic features. *Acta Cytol* 1983;27:73–75.
39. Bhattacharya B, Dilworth HP, Iacobuzio-Donahue C, et al. Nuclear beta-catenin expression distinguishes deep fibromatosis from other benign and malignant fibroblastic and myofibroblastic lesions. *Am J Surg Pathol* 2005;29:653–659.
40. Lacroix-Triki M, Geyer FC, Lambros MB, et al. Beta-catenin/Wnt signalling pathway in fibromatosis, metaplastic carcinomas and phyllodes tumours of the breast. *Mod Pathol* 2010;23:1438–1448.
41. Amary MF, Pauwels P, Meulemans E, et al. Detection of beta-catenin mutations in paraffin-embedded sporadic desmoid-type fibromatosis by mutation-specific restriction enzyme digestion (MSRED): an ancillary diagnostic tool. *Am J Surg Pathol* 2007;31:1299–1309.
42. Carlson JW, Fletcher CD. Immunohistochemistry for beta-catenin in the differential diagnosis of spindle cell lesions: analysis of a series and review of the literature. *Histopathology* 2007;51:509–514.
43. Sawyer EJ, Hanby AM, Rowan AJ, et al. The Wnt pathway, epithelial–stromal interactions, and malignant progression in phyllodes tumours. *J Pathol* 2002;196:437–444.
44. Sawyer EJ, Hanby AM, Poulsom R, et al. Beta-catenin abnormalities and associated insulin-like growth factor overexpression are important in phyllodes tumours and fibroadenomas of the breast. *J Pathol* 2003;200:627–632.
45. Ballo MT, Zagars GK, Pollack A, et al. Desmoid tumor: prognostic factors and outcome after surgery, radiation therapy, or combined surgery and radiation therapy. *J Clin Oncol* 1999;17:158–167.
46. Kinzbrunner B, Ritter S, Domingo J, et al. Remission of rapidly growing desmoid tumors after tamoxifen therapy. *Cancer* 1983;52:2201–2204.
47. Klein WA, Miller HH, Anderson M, et al. The use of indomethacin, sulindac, and tamoxifen for the treatment of desmoid tumors associated with familial polyposis. *Cancer* 1987;60:2863–2868.
48. Procter H, Singh L, Baum M, et al. Response of multicentric desmoid tumours to tamoxifen. *Br J Surg* 1987;74:401.
49. Sportiello DJ, Hoogerland DL. A recurrent pelvic desmoid tumor successfully treated with tamoxifen. *Cancer* 1991;67:1443–1446.
50. Hansmann A, Adolph C, Vogel T, et al. High-dose tamoxifen and sulindac as first-line treatment for desmoid tumors. *Cancer* 2004;100:612–620.
51. Bocale D, Rotelli MT, Cavallini A, et al. Anti-oestrogen therapy in the treatment of desmoid tumours: a systematic review. *Colorectal Dis* 2011;13:e388–e395.
52. Plaza MJ, Yepes M. Breast fibromatosis response to tamoxifen: dynamic MRI findings and review of the current treatment options. *J Radiol Case Rep* 2012;6:16–23.
53. Patel SR, Evans HL, Benjamin RS. Combination chemotherapy in adult desmoid tumors. *Cancer* 1993;72:3244–3247.
54. Okuno SH, Edmonson JH. Combination chemotherapy for desmoid tumors. *Cancer* 2003;97:1134–1135.
55. Gega M, Yanagi H, Yoshikawa R, et al. Successful chemotherapeutic modality of doxorubicin plus dacarbazine for the treatment of desmoid tumors in association with familial adenomatous polyposis. *J Clin Oncol* 2006;24:102–105.

Nodular Fasciitis

56. Maly B, Maly A. Nodular fasciitis of the breast: report of a case initially diagnosed by fine needle aspiration cytology. *Acta Cytol* 2001;45:794–796.
57. Birdsall SH, Shipley JM, Summersgill BM, et al. Cytogenetic findings in a case of nodular fasciitis of the breast. *Cancer Genet Cytogenet* 1995;81:166–168.
58. Brown V, Carty NJ. A case of nodular fasciitis of the breast and review of the literature. *Breast* 2005;14:384–387.
59. Hayashi H, Nishikawa M, Watanabe R, et al. Nodular fasciitis of the breast. *Breast Cancer* 2007;14:337–339.
60. Squillaci S, Tallarigo F, Patarino R, et al. Nodular fasciitis of the male breast: a case report. *Int J Surg Pathol* 2007;15:69–72.
61. Iwatani T, Kawabata H, Miura D, et al. Nodular fasciitis of the breast. *Breast Cancer* 2012;19:180–182.
62. Paker I, Kokenek TD, Kacar A, et al. Fine needle aspiration cytology of nodular fasciitis presenting as a mass in the male breast: report of an unusual case. *Cytopathology* 2013;24:201–203.
63. Montgomery EA, Meis JM. Nodular fasciitis. Its morphologic spectrum and immunohistochemical profile. *Am J Surg Pathol* 1991;15:942–948.
64. Bhattacharya B, Dilworth HP, Iacobuzio-Donahue C, et al. Nuclear beta-catenin expression distinguishes deep fibromatosis from other benign and malignant fibroblastic and myofibroblastic lesions. *Am J Surg Pathol* 2005;29:653–659.
65. Barak S, Wang Z, Miettinen M. Immunoreactivity for calretinin and keratins in desmoid fibromatosis and other myofibroblastic tumors: a diagnostic pitfall. *Am J Surg Pathol* 2012;36:1404–1409.
66. Erickson-Johnson MR, Chou MM, Evers BR, et al. Nodular fasciitis: a novel model of transient neoplasia induced by MYH9-USP6 gene fusion. *Lab Invest* 2011;91:1427–1433.
67. Stanley MW, Skoog L, Tani EM, et al. Nodular fasciitis: spontaneous resolution following diagnosis by fine-needle aspiration. *Diagn Cytopathol* 1993;9:322–324.

Fibrous Tumor

68. Haagensen CD. Fibrous disease of the breast. In: *Diseases of the breast*. Philadelphia: WB Saunders, 1971:185–190.
69. Minkowitz S, Hedayati H, Hiller S, et al. Fibrous mastopathy. A clinical histopathologic study. *Cancer* 1973;32:913–916.
70. Vassar PS, Culling CF. Fibrosis of the breast. *AMA Arch Pathol* 1959;67:128–133.
71. Rivera-Pomar JM, Vilanova JR, Burgos-Bretones JJ, et al. Focal fibrous disease of breast. A common entity in young women. *Virchows Arch A Pathol Anat Histol* 1980;386:59–64.
72. Puente JL, Potel J. Fibrous tumor of the breast. *Arch Surg* 1974;109:391–394.
73. Rosen EL, Soo MS, Bentley RC. Focal fibrosis: a common breast lesion diagnosed at imaging-guided core biopsy. *AJR Am J Roentgenol* 1999;173:1657–1662.
74. Venta LA, Wiley EL, Gabriel H, et al. Imaging features of focal breast fibrosis: mammographic–pathologic correlation of noncalcified breast lesions. *AJR Am J Roentgenol* 1999;173:309–316.
75. Chowdhury N, Bhat RV, Barman PP. Fibrous tumor of the breast: case report of an underrecognized entity. *Pathol Res Int* 2011; 2010:847594.
76. Harvey SC, Denison CM, Lester SC, et al. Fibrous nodules found at large-core needle biopsy of the breast: imaging features. *Radiology* 1999;211:535–540.
77. Revelon G, Sherman ME, Gatewood OM, et al. Focal fibrosis of the breast: imaging characteristics and histopathologic correlation. *Radiology* 2000;216:255–259.
78. Belda F, Lester SC, Pinkus JL, et al. Lineage-restricted chromosome translocation in a benign fibrous tumor of the breast. *Hum Pathol* 1993;24:923–927.

Pseudoangiomatous Hyperplasia of Mammary Stroma

79. Fisher CJ, Hanby AM, Robinson L, et al. Mammary hamartoma—a review of 35 cases. *Histopathology* 1992;20:99–106.
80. Tse GM, Law BK, Ma TK, et al. Hamartoma of the breast: a clinicopathological review. *J Clin Pathol* 2002;55:951–954.
81. *Churchill's Illustrated Medical Dictionary*. New York: Churchill-Livingstone, 1989.
82. Vuitch MF, Rosen PP, Erlandson RA. Pseudoangiomatous hyperplasia of mammary stroma. *Hum Pathol* 1986;17:185–191.
83. Anderson C, Ricci A Jr, Pedersen CA, et al. Immunocytochemical analysis of estrogen and progesterone receptors in benign stromal lesions of the breast. Evidence for hormonal etiology in pseudoangiomatous hyperplasia of mammary stroma. *Am J Surg Pathol* 1991;15:145–149.
84. Powell CM, Cranor ML, Rosen PP. Pseudoangiomatous stromal hyperplasia (PASH). A mammary stromal tumor with myofibroblastic differentiation. *Am J Surg Pathol* 1995;19:270–277.

85. Zanella M, Falconieri G, Lamovec J, et al. Pseudoangiomatous hyperplasia of the mammary stroma: true entity or phenotype? *Pathol Res Pract* 1998;194:535–540.
86. Mercado CL, Naidrich SA, Hamele-Bena D, et al. Pseudoangiomatous stromal hyperplasia of the breast: sonographic features with histopathologic correlation. *Breast J* 2004;10:427–432.
87. Ferreira M, Albarracin CT, Resetkova E. Pseudoangiomatous stromal hyperplasia tumor: a clinical, radiologic and pathologic study of 26 cases. *Mod Pathol* 2008;21:201–207.
88. Wieman SM, Landercasper J, Johnson JM, et al. Tumoral pseudoangiomatous stromal hyperplasia of the breast. *Am Surg* 2008;74:1211–1214.
89. Shehata BM, Fishman I, Collings MH, et al. Pseudoangiomatous stromal hyperplasia of the breast in pediatric patients: an underrecognized entity. *Pediatr Dev Pathol* 2009;12:450–454.
90. Celliers L, Wong DD, Bourke A. Pseudoangiomatous stromal hyperplasia: a study of the mammographic and sonographic features. *Clin Radiol* 2010;65:145–149.
91. Jones KN, Glazebrook KN, Reynolds C. Pseudoangiomatous stromal hyperplasia: imaging findings with pathologic and clinical correlation. *AJR Am J Roentgenol* 2010;195:1036–1042.
92. Bowman E, Oprea G, Okoli J, et al. Pseudoangiomatous stromal hyperplasia (PASH) of the breast: a series of 24 patients. *Breast J* 2012;18:242–247.
93. Singh KA, Lewis MM, Runge RL, et al. Pseudoangiomatous stromal hyperplasia. A case for bilateral mastectomy in a 12-year-old girl. *Breast J* 2007;13:603–606.
94. Iancu D, Nochomovitz LE. Pseudoangiomatous stromal hyperplasia: presentation as a mass in the female nipple. *Breast J* 2001;7:263–265.
95. Ibrahim RE, Sciotto CG, Weidner N. Pseudoangiomatous hyperplasia of mammary stroma. Some observations regarding its clinicopathologic spectrum. *Cancer* 1989;63:1154–1160.
96. Polger MR, Denison CM, Lester S, et al. Pseudoangiomatous stromal hyperplasia: mammographic and sonographic appearances. *AJR Am J Roentgenol* 1996;166:349–352.
97. Cohen MA, Morris EA, Rosen PP, et al. Pseudoangiomatous stromal hyperplasia: mammographic, sonographic, and clinical patterns. *Radiology* 1996;198:117–120.
98. Hargaden GC, Yeh ED, Georgian-Smith D, et al. Analysis of the mammographic and sonographic features of pseudoangiomatous stromal hyperplasia. *AJR Am J Roentgenol* 2008;191:359–363.
99. Badve S, Sloane JP. Pseudoangiomatous hyperplasia of male breast. *Histopathology* 1995;26:463–466.
100. Milanezi MF, Saggioro FP, Zanati SG, et al. Pseudoangiomatous hyperplasia of mammary stroma associated with gynaecomastia. *J Clin Pathol* 1998;51:204–206.
101. Seidman JD, Borkowski A, Aisner SC, et al. Rapid growth of pseudoangiomatous hyperplasia of mammary stroma in axillary gynecomastia in an immunosuppressed patient. *Arch Pathol Lab Med* 1993;117:736–738.
102. Kollias J, Gill PG, Leong AS, et al. Gynaecomastia presenting as fibroadenomatoid tumours of the breast in a renal transplant recipient associated with cyclosporin treatment. *Aust N Z J Surg* 1998;68:679–681.
103. Baildam AD, Higgins RM, Hurley E, et al. Cyclosporin A and multiple fibroadenomas of the breast. *Br J Surg* 1996;83:1755–1757.
104. McCluggage WG, Allen M, Anderson NH. Fine needle aspiration cytology of mammary pseudoangiomatous stromal hyperplasia. A case report. *Acta Cytol* 1999;43:1147–1149.
105. Levine PH, Nimeh D, Guth AA, et al. Aspiration biopsy of nodular pseudoangiomatous stromal hyperplasia of the breast: clinicopathologic correlates in 10 cases. *Diagn Cytopathol* 2005;32:345–350.
106. Vogel PM, Georgiade NG, Fetter BF, et al. The correlation of histologic changes in the human breast with the menstrual cycle. *Am J Pathol* 1981;104:23–34.
107. Degnim AC, Frost MH, Radisky DC, et al. Pseudoangiomatous stromal hyperplasia and breast cancer risk. *Ann Surg Oncol* 2010;17:3269–3277.
108. Gresik CM, Godellas C, Aranha GV, et al. Pseudoangiomatous stromal hyperplasia of the breast: a contemporary approach to its clinical and radiologic features and ideal management. *Surgery* 2010;148:752–757; discussion 757–758.
109. Pruthi S, Reynolds C, Johnson RE, et al. Tamoxifen in the management of pseudoangiomatous stromal hyperplasia. *Breast J* 2001;7:434–439.
110. Seltzer MH, Kintiroglou M. Pseudoangiomatous hyperplasia and response to tamoxifen therapy. *Breast J* 2003;9:344.
111. Drinka EK, Bargaje A, Erşahin CH, et al. Pseudoangiomatous stromal hyperplasia (PASH) of the breast: a clinicopathological study of 79 cases. *Int J Surg Pathol* 2012;20:54–58.

Myofibroblastoma

112. Schürch W, Seemayer TA, Gabbiani G. The myofibroblast: a quarter century after its discovery. *Am J Surg Pathol* 1998;22:141–147.
113. Majno G. The story of the myofibroblasts. *Am J Surg Pathol* 1979;3:535–542.
114. Nakanishi I, Kajikawa K, Okada Y, et al. Myofibroblasts in fibrous tumors and fibrosis in various organs. *Acta Pathol Jpn* 1981;31:423–437.
115. Lagacé R, Schürch W, Seemayer TA. Myofibroblasts in soft tissue sarcomas. *Virchows Arch A Pathol Anat Histol* 1980;389:1–11.
116. Vasudev KS, Harris M. A sarcoma of myofibroblasts: an ultrastructural study. *Arch Pathol Lab Med* 1978;102:185–188.
117. Herrera GA, Johnson WW, Lockard VG, et al. Soft tissue myofibroblastomas. *Mod Pathol* 1991;4:571–577.
118. Lee AH, Sworn MJ, Theaker JM, et al. Myofibroblastoma of breast: an immunohistochemical study. *Histopathology* 1993;22:75–78.
119. Damiani S, Miettinen M, Peterse JL, et al. Solitary fibrous tumour (myofibroblastoma) of the breast. *Virchows Arch* 1994;425:89–92.
120. Salomao DR, Crotty TB, Nascimento AG. Myofibroblastoma and solitary fibrous tumour of the breast: histopathologic and immunohistochemical studies. *Breast* 2001;10:49–54.
121. Schmitt-Graff A, Desmouliere A, Gabbiani G. Heterogeneity of myofibroblast phenotypic features: an example of fibroblastic cell plasticity. *Virchows Arch* 1994;425:3–24.
122. Seemayer TA, Lagace R, Schurch W, et al. Myofibroblasts in the stroma of invasive and metastatic carcinoma: a possible host response to neoplasia. *Am J Surg Pathol* 1979;3:525–533.
123. Schürch W, Lagace R, Seemayer TA. Myofibroblastic stromal reaction in retracted scirrhous carcinoma of the breast. *Surg Gynecol Obstet* 1982;154:351–358.
124. Ohtani H, Sasano N. Myofibroblasts and myoepithelial cells in human breast carcinoma. An ultrastructural study. *Virchows Arch A Pathol Anat Histol* 1980;385:247–261.
125. Bussolati G, Alfani V, Weber K, et al. Immunocytochemical detection of actin on fixed and embedded tissues: its potential use in routine pathology. *J Histochem Cytochem* 1980;28:169–173.
126. Barsky SH, Green WR, Grotendorst GR, et al. Desmoplastic breast carcinoma as a source of human myofibroblasts. *Am J Pathol* 1984;115:329–333.
127. Chauhan H, Abraham A, Phillips JR, et al. There is more than one kind of myofibroblast: analysis of CD34 expression in benign, *in situ*, and invasive breast lesions. *J Clin Pathol* 2003;56:271–276.
128. Wargotz ES, Weiss SW, Norris HJ. Myofibroblastoma of the breast. Sixteen cases of a distinctive benign mesenchymal tumor. *Am J Surg Pathol* 1987;11:493–502.
129. Hamele-Bena D, Cranor ML, Sciotto C, et al. Uncommon presentation of mammary myofibroblastoma. *Mod Pathol* 1996;9:786–790.
130. Gocht A, Bösmüller HC, Büssler R, et al. Breast tumors with myofibroblastic differentiation: clinico-pathological observations in myofibroblastoma and myofibrosarcoma. *Pathol Res Pract* 1999;195:1–10.
131. Magro G, Bisceglia M, Michal M, et al. Spindle cell lipoma-like tumor, solitary fibrous tumor and myofibroblastoma of the breast: a clinicopathological analysis of 13 cases in favor of a unifying histogenetic concept. *Virchows Arch* 2002;440:249–260.
132. Reis-Filho JS, Faoro LN, Gasparetto EL, et al. Mammary epithelioid myofibroblastoma arising in gynecomastia: case report with immunohistochemical profile. *Int J Surg Pathol* 2001;9:331–334.
133. Nucci MR, Fletcher CD. Myofibroblastoma of the breast: a distinctive benign stromal tumor. *Pathol Case Rev* 1999;4:214–219.
134. Bégin LR. Myogenic stromal tumor of the male breast (so-called myofibroblastoma). *Ultrastruct Pathol* 1991;15:613–622.
135. Abeysekara AM, Siriwardana HP, Abbas KF, et al. An unusually large myofibroblastoma in a male breast: a case report. *J Med Case Rep* 2008;2:157.
136. Toker C, Tang CK, Whitely JF, et al. Benign spindle cell breast tumor. *Cancer* 1981;48:1615–1622.
137. Rebner M, Raju U. Myofibroblastoma of the male breast. *Breast Dis* 1993;6:157–160.

138. Greenberg JS, Kaplan SS, Grady C. Myofibroblastoma of the breast in women: imaging appearances. *AJR Am J Roentgenol* 1998;171:71–72.
139. Vourtsi A, Kehagias D, Antoniou A, et al. Male breast myofibroblastoma and MR findings. *J Comput Assist Tomogr* 1999;23:414–416.
140. Ali S, Teichberg S, DeRisi DC, et al. Giant myofibroblastoma of the male breast. *Am J Surg Pathol* 1994;18:1170–1176.
141. Lázaro-Santander R, García-Prats MD, Nieto S, et al. Myofibroblastoma of the breast with diverse histological features. *Virchows Arch* 1999;434:547–550.
142. Yagmur Y, Prasad ML, Osborne MP. Myofibroblastoma in the irradiated breast. *Breast J* 1999;5:136–140.
143. Fukunaga M, Ushigome S. Myofibroblastoma of the breast with diverse differentiations. *Arch Pathol Lab Med* 1997;121:599–603.
144. Magro G, Amico P, Gurrera A. Myxoid myofibroblastoma of the breast with atypical cells: a potential diagnostic pitfall. *Virchows Arch* 2007;450:483–485.
145. Magro G. Epithelioid-cell myofibroblastoma of the breast: expanding the morphologic spectrum. *Am J Surg Pathol* 2009;33:1085–1092.
146. Magro G, Gangemi P, Greco P. Deciduoid-like myofibroblastoma of the breast: a potential pitfall of malignancy. *Histopathology* 2008;52: 652–654.
147. Magro G, Michal M, Vasquez E, et al. Lipomatous myofibroblastoma: a potential diagnostic pitfall in the spectrum of the spindle cell lesions of the breast. *Virchows Arch* 2000;437:540–544.
148. Ordi J, Riverola A, Sole M, et al. Fine needle aspiration of myofibroblastoma of the breast in a man. A report of two cases. *Acta Cytol* 1992;36:194–198.
149. Amin MB, Gottlieb CA, Fitzmaurice M, et al. Fine-needle aspiration cytologic study of myofibroblastoma of the breast. Immunohistochemical and ultrastructural findings. *Am J Clin Pathol* 1993;99:593–597.
150. Negri S, Bonzanini M, Togni R, et al. Fine needle aspiration of myofibroblastoma of the breast. Case report. *Pathologica* 1995;87:719–722.
151. Deligeorgi-Politi H, Kontozoglou T, Joseph M, et al. Myofibroblastoma of the breast: cytologic, histologic, immunohistochemical, and ultrastructural findings in two cases with differing cellularity. *Breast J* 1997;3:365–371.
152. Schmitt FC, AAC Mera. Fine needle aspiration cytology presentation of a cellular variant of breast myofibroblastoma. Report of a case with immunohistochemical studies. *Acta Cytol* 1998;42:721–724.
153. Odashiro AN, Odashiro Miiji LN, Odashiro DN, et al. Mammary myofibroblastoma: report of two cases with fine-needle aspiration cytology and review of the cytology literature. *Diagn Cytopathol* 2004;30:406–410.
154. Fritchie KJ, Carver P, Sun Y, et al. Solitary fibrous tumor: is there a molecular relationship with cellular angiofibroma, spindle cell lipoma, and mammary-type myofibroblastoma? *Am J Clin Pathol* 2012;137:963–970.
155. Wahbah MM, Gilcrease MZ, Wu Y. Lipomatous variant of myofibroblastoma with epithelioid features: a rare and diagnostically challenging breast lesion. *Ann Diagn Pathol* 2011;15:454–458.
156. Magro G, Gurrera A, Bisceglia M. H-caldesmon expression in myofibroblastoma of the breast: evidence supporting the distinction from leiomyoma. *Histopathology* 2003;42:233–238.
157. Morgan MB, Pitha JV. Myofibroblastoma of the breast revisited: an etiologic association with androgens? *Hum Pathol* 1998;29: 347–351.
158. Thomas TM, Myint A, Mak CK, et al. Mammary myofibroblastoma with leiomyomatous differentiation. *Am J Clin Pathol* 1997;107:52–55.
159. Pauwels P, Sciot R, Croiset F, et al. Myofibroblastoma of the breast: genetic link with spindle cell lipoma. *J Pathol* 2000;191:282–285.
160. Magro G, Righi A, Casorzo L, et al. Mammary and vaginal myofibroblastomas are genetically related lesions: fluorescence *in situ* hybridization analysis shows deletion of 13q14 region. *Hum Pathol* 2012;43:1887–1893.
161. Dal Cin P, Sciot R, Polito P, et al. Lesions of 13q may occur independently of deletion of 16q in spindle cell/pleomorphic lipomas. *Histopathology* 1997;31:222–225.
162. Maggiani F, Debiec-Rychter M, Verbeeck G, et al. Extramammary myofibroblastoma is genetically related to spindle cell lipoma. *Virchows Arch* 2006;449:244–247.
163. Flucke U, van Krieken JH, Mentzel T. Cellular angiofibroma: analysis of 25 cases emphasizing its relationship to spindle cell lipoma and mammary-type myofibroblastoma. *Mod Pathol* 2011;24:82–89.

Tumors with Perivascular Myoid Differentiation

164. Hollowood K, Holley MP, Fletcher CD. Plexiform fibrohistiocytic tumour: clinicopathological, immunohistochemical and ultrastructural analysis in favour of a myofibroblastic lesion. *Histopathology* 1991;19:503–513.
165. Granter SR, Badizadegan K, Fletcher CD. Myofibromatosis in adults, glomangiopericytoma, and myopericytoma: a spectrum of tumors showing perivascular myoid differentiation. *Am J Surg Pathol* 1998;22:513–525.
166. Dictor M, Elner A, Andersson T, et al. Myofibromatosis-like hemangiopericytoma metastasizing as differentiated vascular smooth-muscle and myosarcoma. Myopericytes as a subset of "myofibroblasts". *Am J Surg Pathol* 1992;16:1239–1247.

Giant Cell Fibroblastoma

167. Pinto A, Hwang WS, Wong AL, et al. Giant cell fibroblastoma in childhood immunohistochemical and ultrastructural study. *Mod Pathol* 1992;5:639–642.

Granular Cell Tumor

168. Abrikossoff AI. Über Myome, ausgehend von der quergestreiften willkürlichen Muskulatur. *Virchows Arch* 1926;260:215–233.
169. Murray MR. Cultural characteristics of three granular-cell myoblastomas. *Cancer* 1951;4:857–865.
170. Turnbull AD, Huvos AG, Ashikari R, et al. Granular-cell myoblastoma of breast. *N Y State J Med* 1971;71:436–438.
171. Abrikossoff AI. Weitere Untersuchungen über Myoblastenmyome. *Virchows Arch* 1931;280:723–740.
172. Haagensen CD, Stout AP. Granular cell myoblastoma of the mammary gland. *Ann Surg* 1946;124:218–227.
173. Weitzner S, Nascimento AG, Scanlon LJ. Intramammary granular cell myoblastoma. *Am Surg* 1979;45:34–37.
174. Boulat J, Mathoulin MP, Vacheret H, et al. Tumeurs à cellules granuleuses du sein. *Ann Pathol* 1994;14:93–100.
175. DeMay RM, Kay S. Granular cell tumor of the breast. *Pathol Annu* 1984;19 (Part 2):121–148.
176. Papalas JA, Wylie JD, Dash RC. Recurrence risk and margin status in granular cell tumors of the breast: a clinicopathologic study of 13 patients. *Arch Pathol Lab Med* 2011;135:890–895.
177. De Simone N, Aggon A, Christy C. Granular cell tumor of the breast: clinical and pathologic characteristics of a rare case in a 14-year-old girl. *J Clin Oncol* 2011;29:e656–e657.
178. Brown AC, Audisio RA, Regitnig P. Granular cell tumour of the breast. *Surg Oncol* 2011;20:97–105.
179. Placidi A, Aversa A, Foggi CM, et al. Granular cell tumour of breast in a young man preoperatively diagnosed by fine needle aspiration (FNA) cytology. *Cytopathology* 1995;6:343–348.
180. Gibbons D, Leitch M, Coscia J, et al. Fine needle aspiration cytology and histologic findings of granular cell tumor of the breast: review of 19 cases with clinical/radiologic correlation. *Breast J* 2000; 6:27–30.
181. Adeniran A, Al-Ahmadie H, Mahoney MC, et al. Granular cell tumor of the breast: a series of 17 cases and review of the literature. *Breast J* 2004;10:528–531.
182. Yang WT, Edeiken-Monroe B, Sneige N, et al. Sonographic and mammographic appearances of granular cell tumors of the breast with pathological correlation. *J Clin Ultrasound* 2006;34:153–160.
183. Irshad A, Pope TL, Ackerman SJ, et al. Characterization of sonographic and mammographic features of granular cell tumors of the breast and estimation of their incidence. *J Ultrasound Med* 2008;27: 467–475.
184. Moscovic EA, Azar HA. Multiple granular cell tumors ("myoblastomas"). Case report with electron microscopic observations and review of the literature. *Cancer* 1967;20:2032–2047.
185. Murray DE, Seaman E, Utzinger W. Granular cell myoblastomas in successive generations. *J Surg Oncol* 1969;1:193–197.
186. Loyer E, Sahin A, David C. Granular cell tumor of the breast: sonographic and histologic patterns. *Breast Dis* 1996;9:101–106.
187. Tai G, D'Costa H, Lee D, et al. Case report: coincident granular cell tumour of the breast with invasive ductal carcinoma. *Br J Radiol* 1995;68:1034–1036.

188. Tran TA, Kallakury BV, Carter J, et al. Coexistence of granular cell tumor and ipsilateral infiltrating ductal carcinoma of the breast. *South Med J* 1997;90:1149–1151.
189. Bassett LW, Cove HC. Myoblastoma of the breast. *AJR Am J Roentgenol* 1979;132:122–123.
190. D'Orsi CJ, Feldhaus L, Sonnenfeld M. Unusual lesions of the breast. *Radiol Clin North Am* 1983;21:67–80.
191. Willen R, Willen H, Balldin G, et al. Granular cell tumour of the mammary gland simulating malignancy. A report on two cases with light microscopy, transmission electron microscopy and immunohistochemical investigation. *Virchows Arch A Pathol Anat Histopathol* 1984;403:391–400.
192. Green DH, Clark AH. Case report: granular cell myoblastoma of the breast: a rare benign tumour mimicking breast carcinoma. *Clin Radiol* 1995;50:799.
193. Vos LD, Tjon ATRT, Vroegindeweij D, et al. Granular cell tumor of the breast: mammographic and histologic correlation. *Eur J Radiol* 1994;19:56–59.
194. Mátrai Z, Langmár Z, Szabó E, et al. Granular cell tumour of the breast: case series and review of the literature. *Eur J Gynaecol Oncol* 2010;31:636–640.
195. Scatarige JC, Hsiu JG, de la Torre R, et al. Acoustic shadowing in benign granular cell tumor (myoblastoma) of the breast. *J Ultrasound Med* 1987;6:545–547.
196. Baum JK, Robins JR, Schnitt S, et al. The ultrasound appearance of granular cell tumor of the breast: a case report. *Breast Dis* 1994;7:281–285.
197. Scaranelo AM, Bukhanov K, Crystal P, et al. Granular cell tumour of the breast: MRI findings and review of the literature. *Br J Radiol* 2007;80:970–974.
198. Maki DD, Horne D, Damore LJ IInd, et al. Magnetic resonance appearance of granular cell tumor of the breast. *Clin Imaging* 2009;33:395–397.
199. McMahon JN, Rigby HS, Davies JD. Elastosis in granular cell tumours: prevalence and distribution. *Histopathology* 1990;16:37–41.
200. Fust JA, Custer RP. On the neurogenesis of so-called granular cell myoblastoma. *Am J Clin Pathol* 1949;19:522–535.
201. Hahn HJ, Iglesias J, Flenker H, et al. Granular cell tumor in differential diagnosis of tumors of the breast. The role of fine needle aspiration cytology. *Pathol Res Pract* 1992;188:1091–1094.
202. Shousha S, Lyssiotis T. Granular cell myoblastoma: positive staining for carcinoembryonic antigen. *J Clin Pathol* 1979;32:219–224.
203. Franzen S, Stenkvist B. Diagnosis of granular cell myoblastoma by fine-needle aspiration biopsy. *Acta Pathol Microbiol Scand* 1968;72: 391–395.
204. Löwhagen T, Rubio CA. The cytology of the granular cell myoblastoma of the breast. Report of a case. *Acta Cytol* 1977;21:314–315.
205. Mitnick JS, Vazquez MF, Pressman PI, et al. Stereotactic fine-needle aspiration biopsy for the evaluation of nonpalpable breast lesions: report of an experience based on 2,988 cases. *Ann Surg Oncol* 1996;3:185–191.
206. Chhieng DC, Cangiarella JF, Waisman J, et al. Fine-needle aspiration cytology of spindle cell lesions of the breast. *Cancer* 1999;87:359–371.
207. Buley ID, Gatter KC, Kelly PM, et al. Granular cell tumours revisited. An immunohistological and ultrastructural study. *Histopathology* 1988;12:263–274.
208. Sirgi KE, Sneige N, Fanning TV, et al. Fine-needle aspirates of granular cell lesions of the breast: report of three cases, with emphasis on differential diagnosis and utility of immunostaining for CD68 (KP1). *Diagn Cytopathol* 1996;15:403–408.
209. Rekhi B, Jambhekar NA. Morphologic spectrum, immunohistochemical analysis, and clinical features of a series of granular cell tumors of soft tissues: a study from a tertiary referral cancer center. *Ann Diagn Pathol* 2010;14:162–167.
210. Ingram DL, Mossler JA, Snowhite J, et al. Granular cell tumors of the breast. Steroid receptor analysis and localization of carcinoembryonic antigen, myoglobin, and S100 protein. *Arch Pathol Lab Med* 1984;108:897–901.
211. Mittal KR, True LD. Origin of granules in granular cell tumor. Intracellular myelin formation with autodigestion. *Arch Pathol Lab Med* 1988;112:302–303.
212. Damiani S, Koerner FC, Dickersin GR, et al. Granular cell tumour of the breast. *Virchows Arch A Pathol Anat Histopathol* 1992;420:219–226.
213. Crawford ES, De Bakey ME. Granular-cell myoblastoma; two unusual cases. *Cancer* 1953;6:786–789.
214. Chetty R, Kalan MR. Malignant granular cell tumor of the breast. *J Surg Oncol* 1992;49:135–137.
215. Akahane K, Kato K, Ogiso S, et al. Malignant granular cell tumor of the breast: case report and literature review. *Breast Cancer* 2012. doi:10.1007/s12282-012-0362-1.
216. Uzoaru I, Firfer B, Ray V, et al. Malignant granular cell tumor. *Arch Pathol Lab Med* 1992;116:206–208.
217. Chen J, Wang L, Xu J, et al. Malignant granular cell tumor with breast metastasis: a case report and review of the literature. *Oncol Lett* 2012;4:63–66.

Tumors of Nerve and Nerve Sheath Origin

218. Bernardello F, Caneva A, Bresaola E, et al. Breast solitary schwannoma: fine-needle aspiration biopsy and immunocytochemical analysis. *Diagn Cytopathol* 1994;10:221–223.
219. Das Gupta TK, Brasfield RD, Strong EW, et al. Benign solitary Schwannomas (neurilemomas). *Cancer* 1969;24:355–366.
220. Fisher PE, Estabrook A, Cohen MB. Fine needle aspiration biopsy of intramammary neurilemoma. *Acta Cytol* 1990;34:35–37.
221. van der Walt JD, Reid HA, Shaw JH. Neurilemoma appearing as a lump in the breast. *Arch Pathol Lab Med* 1982;106:539–540.
222. Lipper S, Willson CF, Copeland KC. Pseudogynecomastia due to neurofibromatosis--a light microscopic and ultrastructural study. *Hum Pathol* 1981;12:755–759.
223. Sherman JE, Smith JW. Neurofibromas of the breast and nipple-areolar area. *Ann Plast Surg* 1981;7:302–307.
224. Murayama Y, Yamamoto Y, Shimojima N, et al. T1 breast cancer associated with von Recklinghausen's neurofibromatosis. *Breast Cancer* 1999;6:227–230.
225. Hock YL, Mohamid W. Myxoid neurofibroma of the male breast: fine needle aspiration cytodiagnosis. *Cytopathology* 1995;6:44–47.
226. Martinez-Onsurbe P, Fuentes-Vaamonde E, Gonzalez-Estecha A, et al. Neurilemoma of the breast in a man. A case report. *Acta Cytol* 1992;36:511–513.
227. Cho YR, Jones S, Gosain AK. Neurofibromatosis: a cause of prepubertal gynecomastia. *Plast Reconstr Surg* 2008;121:34e–40e.
228. Gultekin SH, Cody HS III, Hoda SA. Schwannoma of the breast. *South Med J* 1996;89:238–239.
229. Galant C, Mazy S, Berliere M, et al. Two schwannomas presenting as lumps in the same breast. *Diagn Cytopathol* 1997;16:281–284.
230. Bongiorno MR, Doukaki S, Arico M. Neurofibromatosis of the nipple-areolar area: a case series. *J Med Case Rep* 2010;4:22.
231. Friedrich RE, Hagel C. Appendices of the nipple and areola of the breast in Neurofibromatosis type 1 patients are neurofibromas. *Anticancer Res* 2010;30:1815–1817.
232. Gokalp G, Hakyemez B, Kizilkaya E, et al. Myxoid neurofibromas of the breast: mammographical, sonographical and MRI appearances. *Br J Radiol* 2007;80:e234–e237.
233. Cohen MB, Fisher PE. Schwann cell tumours of the breast and mammary region. *Surg Pathol* 1991;4:47–56.
234. Hood IC, Qizilbash AH, Young JE, et al. Needle aspiration cytology of a benign and a malignant schwannoma. *Acta Cytol* 1984;28:157–164.
235. Silverman JF, Geisinger KR, Frable WJ. Fine-needle aspiration cytology of mesenchymal tumors of the breast. *Diagn Cytopathol* 1988;4:50–58.
236. Ryd W, Mugal S, Ayyash K. Ancient neurilemmoma: a pitfall in the cytologic diagnosis of soft-tissue tumors. *Diagn Cytopathol* 1986;2:244–247.

Hamartoma

237. *Stedman's Medical Dictionary*, 24th ed. Baltimore: Williams and Wilkins, 1982.
238. Arrigoni MG, Dockerty MB, Judd ES. The identification and treatment of mammary hamartoma. *Surg Gynecol Obstet* 1971;133:577–582.
239. Daya D, Trus T, D'Souza TJ, et al. Hamartoma of the breast, an underrecognized breast lesion. A clinicopathologic and radiographic study of 25 cases. *Am J Clin Pathol* 1995;103:685–689.
240. Oberman HA. Hamartomas and hamartoma variants of the breast. *Semin Diagn Pathol* 1989;6:135–145.
241. Andersson I, Hildell J, Linell F, et al. Mammary hamartomas. *Acta Radiol Diagn (Stockh)* 1979;20:712–720.
242. Ljungqvist U, Andersson I, Hildell J, et al. Mammary hamartoma, a benign breast lesion. *Acta Chir Scand* 1979;145:227–230.

243. Altermatt HJ, Gebbers JO, Laissue JA. Multiple hamartomas of the breast. *Appl Pathol* 1989;7:145–148.
244. Cooper RA, Johnson MS. Juvenile hypertrophy presenting as a discrete breast mass. *Can Assoc Radiol J* 1992;43:218–220.
245. Linell F, Ostberg G, Soderstrom J, et al. Breast hamartomas. An important entity in mammary pathology. *Virchows Arch A Pathol Anat Histol* 1979;383:253–264.
246. Schrager CA, Schneider D, Gruener AC, et al. Clinical and pathological features of breast disease in Cowden's syndrome: an underrecognized syndrome with an increased risk of breast cancer. *Hum Pathol* 1998;29:47–53.
247. Sabaté JM, Gómez A, Torrubia S, et al. Evaluation of breast involvement in relation to Cowden syndrome: a radiological and clinicopathological study of patients with PTEN germ-line mutations. *Eur Radiol* 2006;16:702–706.
248. Evers K, Yeh I-T, Troupin RH, et al. Mammary hamartomas. The importance of radiologic-pathologic correlation. *Breast Dis* 1992;5: 35–43.
249. Hessler C, Schnyder P, Ozzello L. Hamartoma of the breast: diagnostic observation of 16 cases. *Radiology* 1978;126:95–98.
250. Adler DD, Jeffries DO, Helvie MA. Sonographic features of breast hamartomas. *J Ultrasound Med* 1990;9:85–90.
251. Desai A, Ramesar K, Allan S, et al. Breast hamartoma arising in axillary ectopic breast tissue. *Breast J* 2010;16:433–434.
252. Charpin C, Mathoulin MP, Andrac L, et al. Reappraisal of breast hamartomas. A morphological study of 41 cases. *Pathol Res Pract* 1994;190:362–371.
253. Borochovitz D. Adenolipoma of the breast: a variant of adenolipoma. *Breast* 1982;8:32–33.
254. Crothers JG, Butler NF, Fortt RW, et al. Fibroadenolipoma of the breast. *Br J Radiol* 1985;58:191–202.
255. Yasuda S, Kubota M, Noto T, et al. Two cases of adenolipoma of the breast. *Tokai J Exp Clin Med* 1992;17:139–144.
256. Damiani S, Panarelli M. Mammary adenohibernoma. *Histopathology* 1996;28:554–555.
257. Garijo MF, Torio B, Val-Bernal JF. Mammary hamartoma with brown adipose tissue. *Gen Diagn Pathol* 1997;143:243–246.
258. Kapucuoglu N, Percinel S, Angelone A. Adenohibernoma of the breast. *Virchows Arch* 2008;452:351–352.
259. Oberman HA, Nosanchuk JS, Finger JE. Periductal stromal tumors of breast with adipose metaplasia. *Arch Surg* 1969;98:384–387.
260. Kaplan L, Walts AE. Benign chondrolipomatous tumor of the human female breast. *Arch Pathol Lab Med* 1977;101:149–151.
261. Lugo M, Reyes JM, Putong PB. Benign chondrolipomatous tumors of the breast. *Arch Pathol Lab Med* 1982;106:691–692.
262. Marsh WL Jr, Lucas JG, Olsen J. Chondrolipoma of the breast. *Arch Pathol Lab Med* 1989;113:369–371.
263. Metcalf JS, Ellis B. Choristoma of the breast. *Hum Pathol* 1985;16: 739–740.
264. Peison B, Benisch B, Tonzola A. Case report: benign chondrolipoma of the female breast. *N J Med* 1994;91:401–402.
265. Fushimi H, Kotoh K, Nishihara K, et al. Chondrolipoma of the breast: a case report with cytological and histological examination. *Histopathology* 1999;35:478–479.

Leiomyoma

266. Nascimento AG, Karas M, Rosen PP, et al. Leiomyoma of the nipple. *Am J Surg Pathol* 1979;3:151–154.
267. Eusebi V, Cunsolo A, Fedeli F, et al. Benign smooth muscle cell metaplasia in breast. *Tumori* 1980;66:643–653.
268. Davies JD, Riddell RH. Muscular hamartomas of the breast. *J Pathol* 1973;111:209–211.
269. Haagensen CD. Non-epithelial neoplasms of the breast. In: *Diseases of the breast.* Philadelphia: WB Saunders, 1971:292–325.
270. Diaz-Arias AA, Hurt MA, Loy TS, et al. Leiomyoma of the breast. *Hum Pathol* 1989;20:396–399.
271. Son EJ, Oh KK, Kim EK, et al. Leiomyoma of the breast in a 50-year-old woman receiving tamoxifen. *AJR Am J Roentgenol* 1998;171:1684–1686.
272. Allison JG, Dodds HM. Leiomyoma of the male nipple. A case report and literature review. *Am Surg* 1989;55:501–502.
273. Velasco M, Ubeda B, Autonell F, et al. Leiomyoma of the male areola infiltrating the breast tissue. *AJR Am J Roentgenol* 1995;164:511–512.
274. Roncaroli F, Rossi R, Severi B, et al. Epithelioid leiomyoma of the breast with granular cell change: a case report. *Hum Pathol* 1993;24:1260–1263.
275. Boscaino A, Ferrara G, Orabona P, et al. Smooth muscle tumors of the breast: clinicopathologic features of two cases. *Tumori* 1994;80: 241–245.

Myoid "Hamartoma"

276. Daroca PJ Jr, Reed RJ, Love GL, et al. Myoid hamartomas of the breast. *Hum Pathol* 1985;16:212–219.
277. Huntrakoon M, Lin F. Muscular hamartoma of the breast. An electron microscopic study. *Virchows Arch A Pathol Anat Histopathol* 1984;403:307–312.
278. Garfein CF, Aulicino MR, Leytin A, et al. Epithelioid cells in myoid hamartoma of the breast: a potential diagnostic pitfall for core biopsies. *Arch Pathol Lab Med* 1996;120:676–680.
279. Shepstone BJ, Wells CA, Berry AR, et al. Mammographic appearance and histopathological description of a muscular hamartoma of the breast. *Br J Radiol* 1985;58:459–461.
280. Eusebi V, Cunsolo A, Fedeli F, et al. Benign smooth muscle cell metaplasia in breast. *Tumori* 1980;66:643–653.
281. Fiirgaard B, Kristensen S. Muscular hamartoma of the breast. A case report. *Acta Radiol* 1992;33:115–116.
282. Davies JD, Riddell RH. Muscular hamartomas of the breast. *J Pathol* 1973;111:209–211.

Myeloid Metaplasia

283. Brooks JJ, Krugman DT, Damjanov I. Myeloid metaplasia presenting as a breast mass. *Am J Surg Pathol* 1980;4:281–285.
284. Glew RH, Haese WH, McIntyre PA. Myeloid metaplasia with myelofibrosis. The clinical spectrum of extramedullary hematopoiesis and tumor formation. *Johns Hopkins Med J* 1973;132:253–270.
285. Martinelli G, Santini D, Bazzocchi F, et al. Myeloid metaplasia of the breast. A lesion which clinically mimics carcinoma. *Virchows Arch A Pathol Anat Histopathol* 1983;401:203–207.

Myxoma

286. Carney JA, Toorkey BC. Myxoid fibroadenoma and allied conditions (myxomatosis) of the breast. A heritable disorder with special associations including cardiac and cutaneous myxomas. *Am J Surg Pathol* 1991;15:713–721.
287. Arihiro K, Inai K, Kurihara K, et al. Myxoma of the breast: report of a case with unique histological and immunohistochemical appearances. *Acta Pathol Jpn* 1993;43:340–346.
288. Chan YF, Yeung HY, Ma L. Myxoma of the breast: report of a case and ultrastructural study. *Pathology* 1986;18:153–157.
289. Magro G, Cavanaugh B, Palazzo J. Clinico-pathological features of breast myxoma: report of a case with histogenetic considerations. *Virchows Arch* 2010;456:581–586.
290. Balci P, Kabakci N, Topcu I, et al. Breast myxoma: radiologic and histopathologic features. *Breast J* 2007;13:88–90.
291. Wee A, Tan CE, Raju GC. Nerve sheath myxoma of the breast. A light and electron microscopic, histochemical and immunohistochemical study. *Virchows Arch A Pathol Anat Histopathol* 1989;416:163–167.

Mucinosis

292. Michal M, Ludvikova M, Zamecnik M. Nodular mucinosis of the breast: report of three cases. *Pathol Int* 1998;48:542–544.
293. Koide N, Akashi-Tanaka S, Fukutomi T, et al. Nodular mucinosis of the breast: a case report with clinical and imaging findings. *Breast Cancer* 2002;9:261–264.
294. Sanati S, Leonard M, Khamapirad T, et al. Nodular mucinosis of the breast: a case report with pathologic, ultrasonographic, and clinical findings and review of the literature. *Arch Pathol Lab Med* 2005;129: e58–e61.
295. Chisholm C, Greene Jr JF. Nodular mucinosis of the breast: expanding our understanding with an unusual case. *Am J Dermatopathol* 2010;32:187–189.
296. Manglik N, Berlingeri-Ramos AC, Boroumand N, et al. Nodular mucinosis of the breast in a supernumerary nipple: case report and review of the literature. *J Cutan Pathol* 2010;37:1178–1181.

297. Tavassoli FA. Diseases of the nipple. In: *Pathology of the breast.* Norwalk, CT: Appleton & Lange, 1992:589.
298. Carney JA, Toorkey BC. Myxoid fibroadenoma and allied conditions (myxomatosis) of the breast. A heritable disorder with special associations including cardiac and cutaneous myxomas. *Am J Surg Pathol* 1991;15:713–721.

Lipoma

299. Pui MH, Movson IJ. Fatty tissue breast lesions. *Clin Imaging* 2003;27:150–155.
300. Hansen PE, Williamson EO. Lipoma with central fat necrosis: is core biopsy a good way to diagnose fat necrosis of the breast? *Breast J* 1999;5:202–203.
301. Chan KW, Ghadially FN, Alagaratnam TT. Benign spindle cell tumour of breast—a variant of spindled cell lipoma or fibroma of breast? *Pathology* 1984;16:331–336.
302. Lew WY. Spindle cell lipoma of the breast: a case report and literature review. *Diagn Cytopathol* 1993;9:434–437.
303. Smith DN, Denison CM, Lester SC. Spindle cell lipoma of the breast. A case report. *Acta Radiol* 1996;37:893–895.
304. Magro G, Caltabiano R, Di Cataldo A, et al. CD10 is expressed by mammary myofibroblastoma and spindle cell lipoma of soft tissue: an additional evidence of their histogenetic linking. *Virchows Arch* 2007;450:727–728.
305. Magro G, Bisceglia M, Pasquinelli G. Benign spindle cell tumor of the breast with prominent adipocytic component. *Ann Diagn Pathol* 1998;2:306–311.
306. Pauwels P, Sciot R, Croiset P, et al. Myofibroblastoma of the breast: genetic link with spindle cell lipoma. *J Pathol* 2000;191:282–285.

Angiomas and Other Benign Vascular Lesions

307. Azzopardi JG. Sarcomas of the breast. In: *Problems in breast pathology.* (Major problems in pathology, vol. 11). Philadelphia: WB Saunders, 1979.
308. McDivitt RW, Stewart FW, Berg JW. Tumors of the breast. (*AFIP Atlas of tumor pathology*, 2nd series, vol. 2). Bethesda: American Registry of Pathology, 1968.

Perilobular Hemangioma

309. Jozefczyk MA, Rosen PP. Vascular tumors of the breast. II. Perilobular hemangiomas and hemangiomas. *Am J Surg Pathol* 1985;9:491–503.
310. Lesueur GC, Brown RW, Bhathal PS. Incidence of perilobular hemangioma in the female breast. *Arch Pathol Lab Med* 1983;107:308–310.
311. Rosen PP, Ridolfi RL. The perilobular hemangioma. A benign microscopic vascular lesion of the breast. *Am J Clin Pathol* 1977;68:21–23.
312. Hamperl H. Hämangiome der menschlichen Mamma. Beiträge zur pathologischen Histologie der Mamma. VI. *Geburtshilfe Frauenheilkd* 1973;33:13–17.
313. Nielsen B. Haemangiomas of the breast. *Pathol Res Pract* 1983;176:253–257.

Hemangioma

314. Jozefczyk MA, Rosen PP. Vascular tumors of the breast. II. Perilobular hemangiomas and hemangiomas. *Am J Surg Pathol* 1985;9:491–503.
315. Hoda SA, Cranor ML, Rosen PP. Hemangiomas of the breast with atypical histological features. Further analysis of histological subtypes confirming their benign character. *Am J Surg Pathol* 1992;16:553–560.
316. Nagar H, Marmor S, Hammar B. Haemangiomas of the breast in children. *Eur J Surg* 1992;158:503–505.
317. Miaux Y, Lemarchand-Venencie F, Cyna-Gorse F, et al. MR imaging of breast hemangioma in female infants. *Pediatr Radiol* 1992;22:463–464.
318. Courcoutsakis NA, Hill SC, Chow CK, et al. Breast hemangiomas in a patient with Kasabach-Merritt syndrome: imaging findings. *AJR Am J Roentgenol* 1997;169:1397–1399.
319. Eliahou R, Sella T, Allweis T, et al. Magnetic resonance-guided interventional procedures of the breast: initial experience. *Isr Med Assoc J* 2009;11:275–279.
320. Webb LA, Young JR. Case report: haemangioma of the breast—appearances on mammography and ultrasound. *Clin Radiol* 1996;51:523–524.
321. Tabar L, Dean PB. *Teaching atlas of mammography.* New York: Thieme-Stratton, 1983.
322. Glazenbrook KN, Morton MJ, Reynolds C. Vascular tumors of the breast: mammographic, sonographic, and MRI appearances. *AJR Am J Roentgenol* 2005;184:331–338.
323. Shin SJ, Lesser M, Rosen PP. Hemangiomas and angiosarcomas of the breast: diagnostic utility of cell cycle markers with emphasis on Ki-67. *Arch Pathol Lab Med* 2007;131:538–544.
324. Mesurolle B, Sygal V, Lalonde L, et al. Sonographic and mammographic appearances of breast hemangioma. *AJR Am J Roentgenol* 2008;191:W17–W22.
325. Sebek BA. Cavernous hemangioma of the female breast. *Cleve Clin Q* 1984;51:471–474.
326. Galindo LM, Shienbaum AJ, Dwyer-Joyce L, et al. Atypical hemangioma of the breast: a diagnostic pitfall in breast fine-needle aspiration. *Diagn Cytopathol* 2001;24:215–218.
327. Branton PA, Lininger R, Tavassoli FA. Papillary endothelial hyperplasia of the breast: the great impostor for angiosarcoma: a clinicopathologic review of 17 cases. *Int J Surg Pathol* 2003;11:83–87.

Angiomatosis

328. Sieber PR, Sharkey FE. Cystic hygroma of the breast. *Arch Pathol Lab Med* 1986;110:353.
329. Hamperl H. Hamangiome der menschlichen mamma. Beitrage zur pathologischen histologie der mamma. V. *Geburtsh u Frauenheilk* 1973;33:13–17.
330. Morrow M, Berger D, Thelmo W. Diffuse cystic angiomatosis of the breast. *Cancer* 1988;62:2392–2396.
331. Rosen PP. Vascular tumors of the breast. III. Angiomatosis. *Am J Surg Pathol* 1985;9:652–658.
332. Kwon SS, Kim SJ, Kim L, et al. Huge cystic lymphangioma involving the entire breast. *Ann Plast Surg* 2009;62:18–21.
333. Hynes SO, McLaughlin R, Kerin M, et al. A unique cause of a rare disorder, unilateral macromastia due to lymphangiomatosis of the breast: a case report. *Breast J* 2012;18:367–370.
334. Enzinger FM, Weiss SW. Venous hemangioma. In: *Soft tissue tumors.* St. Louis: CV Mosby, 1983:391.

Venous Hemangioma

335. Enzinger FM, Weiss SW. Angiomatosis (diffuse hemangioma). In: *Soft tissue tumors.* St. Louis: CV Mosby, 1983:407–409.
336. Wold LE, Swee RG, Sim FH. Vascular lesions of bone. *Pathol Annu* 1985;20 (Part 2):101–137.
337. Rosen PP, Jozefczyk MA, Boram LH. Vascular tumors of the breast. IV. The venous hemangioma. *Am J Surg Pathol* 1985;9:659–665.

Nonparenchymal Hemangiomas of the Mammary Region

338. Menville JG, Bloodgood JC. Subcutaneous angiomas of the breast. *Ann Surg* 1933;97:401–413.
339. Madding GF, Hershberger LR. Hemangioma of the breast; report of case. *Surgery* 1949;26:685–687.
340. Rosen PP. Vascular tumors of the breast. V. Nonparenchymal hemangiomas of mammary subcutaneous tissues. *Am J Surg Pathol* 1985;9:723–729.
341. Franco RL, de Moraes Schenka NG, Schenka AA, et al. Cavernous hemangioma of the male breast. *Breast J* 2005;11:511–512.
342. Noel JC, Van Geertruyden J, Engohan-Aloghe C. Angiolipoma of the breast in a male: a case report and review of the literature. *Int J Surg Pathol* 2011;19:813–816.
343. Perugini G, Bonini G, Giardina C, et al. Cavernous hemangioma of the pectoralis muscle mimicking a breast tumor. *AJR Am J Roentgenol* 1994;162:1321–1322.
344. Siewert B, Jacobs T, Baum JK. Sonographic evaluation of subcutaneous hemangioma of the breast. *AJR Am J Roentgenol* 2002;178:1025–1027.
345. Webb LA, Young JR. Case report: haemangioma of the breast—appearances on mammography and ultrasound. *Clin Radiol* 1996;51:523–524.
346. Enzinger FM, Weiss SW. Benign tumors and tumorlike lesions of blood vessels. In: *Soft tissue tumors.* St. Louis: CV Mosby, 1983:379–421.
347. Yu GH, Fishman SJ, Brooks JS. Cellular angiolipoma of the breast. *Mod Pathol* 1993;6:497–499.
348. Howard WR, Helwig EB. Angiolipoma. *Arch Dermatol* 1960;82:924–931.

Aneurysm

349. Beres RA, Harrington DG, Wenzel MS. Percutaneous repair of breast pseudoaneurysm: sonographically guided embolization. *AJR Am J Roentgenol* 1997;169:425–427.
350. Smith SM. Breast pseudoaneurysm after core biopsy. *AJR Am J Roentgenol* 1996;167:817.
351. Sohn YM, Kim MJ, Kim EK, et al. Pseudoaneurysm of the breast during vacuum-assisted removal. *J Ultrasound Med* 2009;28:967–971.
352. El Khoury M, Mesurolle B, Kao E, et al. Spontaneous thrombosis of pseudoaneurysm of the breast related to core biopsy. *AJR Am J Roentgenol* 2007;189:W309–W311.
353. Al Hadidy AM, Al Najar MS, Farah GR, et al. Pseudoaneurysm of the breast after blunt trauma: successful treatment with ultrasound-guided compression. *J Clin Ultrasound* 2008;36:440–442.
354. Lee KH, Ko EY, Han BK, et al. Thrombosed pseudoaneurysm of the breast after blunt trauma. *J Ultrasound Med* 2009;28:233–238.
355. Joseph KA, Ditkoff BA, Komenaka I, et al. Acquired arteriovenous fistula of the breast. *Breast J* 2004;10:156–158.
356. Dehn TC, Lee EC. Aneurysm presenting as a breast mass. *Br Med J (Clin Res Ed)* 1986;292:1240.
357. Pettinger TW, Dublin AB, Lindfors KK. Percutaneous embolotherapy of an arterial pseudoaneurysm of the breast: a case report. *Breast Dis* 1995;97–101.
358. Daunt N. An intramammary pseudoaneurysm presenting as a breast mass. *Australas Radiol* 1995;39:71–72.
359. Davies JD, Kulka J. Traumatic arterial damage after fine-needle aspirational cytology in mammary complex sclerosing lesions. *Histopathology* 1996;28:65–70.
360. Cox J, Kaye B, Burn D, et al. Multiple aneurysms in the female breast: a case report. *Br J Radiol* 2007;80:e275–e277.

CHAPTER 39

Sarcoma

FREDERICK C. KOERNER

Mammary sarcomas are a heterogeneous group of malignant neoplasms that arise from the mammary stroma. Excluded from this chapter are malignant lymphomas and malignant phyllodes tumor (MPT), which are covered in other chapters. Lesions at the most low-grade end of the spectrum of fibroblastic tumors constitute the group of neoplasms discussed in Chapter 38 under the heading of "fibromatosis." Although mammary fibromatosis does not metastasize, it can pursue an inexorable course of local recurrence, resulting in extensive local destruction and even death as a consequence of visceral invasion. Neoplasms included in the category of mammary sarcoma, or stromal "sarcoma," are thought to arise from interlobular mesenchymal elements, which constitute the supporting mammary stroma.

A diagnosis of mammary sarcoma can be established only after metaplastic carcinoma is excluded. The distinction is important for treatment as well as for prognosis. The lesion should be sampled extensively for evidence of *in situ* or invasive carcinoma. Perhaps the most difficult distinction in this regard lies between fibrosarcoma and a metaplastic spindle cell carcinoma, which has no discernible epithelial component. Immunohistochemical studies for epithelial and myoepithelial markers are useful for detecting evidence of epithelial origin or inconspicuous foci of epithelial cells in a carcinoma that has undergone a virtually complete conversion to a spindle cell neoplasm (see Chapter 16).

The diagnosis of mammary sarcomas should be reported in the same histogenetic terms used for soft part sarcomas, which occur throughout the body. The relative frequency of specific types of breast sarcomas is difficult to determine from the literature because these lesions have sometimes been referred to by the general term "stromal sarcoma." However, some differences in frequency do appear to exist. For example, one of the most common forms of mammary sarcoma, angiosarcoma, is proportionately less common among somatic sarcomas. Other distinct mammary sarcomas include leiomyosarcoma, liposarcoma, sarcomas with bone and cartilage, malignant fibrous histiocytoma (MFH) and fibrosarcoma, rhabdomyosarcoma, and other rare types.

Mammary sarcomas arise only rarely. According to data from the Surveillance Epidemiology and End Results (SEER) database, the annual incidence is 4.6 cases per million women.[1] Several factors predispose patients to the development of mammary sarcomas. Women treated for breast carcinoma experience a slight increase in their risk of soft-tissue sarcomas,[2,3] and the use of irradiation further increases the risk of the development of angiosarcomas, pleomorphic undifferentiated carcinomas, and other rare types of sarcoma within the field of irradiation.[2–4] The risk of developing postirradiation sarcoma increases significantly 3 years after the diagnosis of carcinoma, peaks at approximately 10 years, and declines to approximately the risk seen in patients who did not receive irradiation after 23 years.[4] Rare mammary sarcomas have developed in association with cosmetic implants or foreign material,[5] but the evidence does not prove a causal relationship between the presence of these substances and the development of the sarcoma.

Women make up the vast majority of patients with mammary sarcomas, and they accounted for 98.5% of the cases of sarcoma in the 19 studies tabulated by Al-Benna et al.,[6] some of which included cases of MPTs and metaplastic carcinomas. These data may not account for all cases affecting men, because certain tumors in men may have been classified as sarcomas of the chest wall rather than of the breast. Females of all ages are affected. In the largest series,[7] the patients' ages range from 13 to 86 years, and the median age is 55 years. Using information from published studies, Al-Benna et al.[6] calculated a weighted mean age of 50.0 years.

As a group, mammary sarcomas vary greatly in size, ranging from less than 1 to 30 cm or more. In most studies, the mean and median sizes fall between 4 and 7 cm. The authors of one large series[7] reported a median tumor size of 4.45 cm. The gross appearance of the tumors is influenced in part by the specific histologic characteristics of the lesion, but the specimens typically consist of fleshy, moderately firm, pale tissue with varying amounts of hemorrhage and necrosis (Fig. 39.1). Most sarcomas appear well circumscribed grossly, even if the border is invasive histologically.

The prognosis for patients with mammary sarcomas varies somewhat depending on certain characteristics of the sarcoma. For example, high-grade angiosarcomas have an especially unfavorable prognosis, whereas the outcomes of patients with other histologic types of sarcoma do not differ significantly. The size of the sarcoma may also provide prognostic information, but the data regarding this relationship vary. In a group of 83 women with primary breast sarcomas studied by Zelek et al.,[1] with a median follow-up of 7.8 years, the 10-year overall survival (OS) and disease-free survival

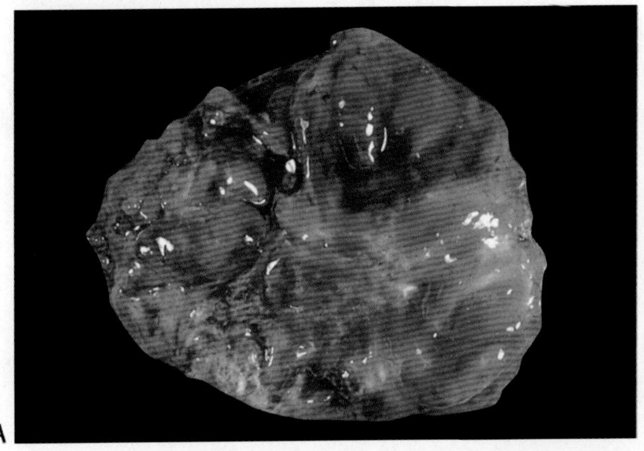

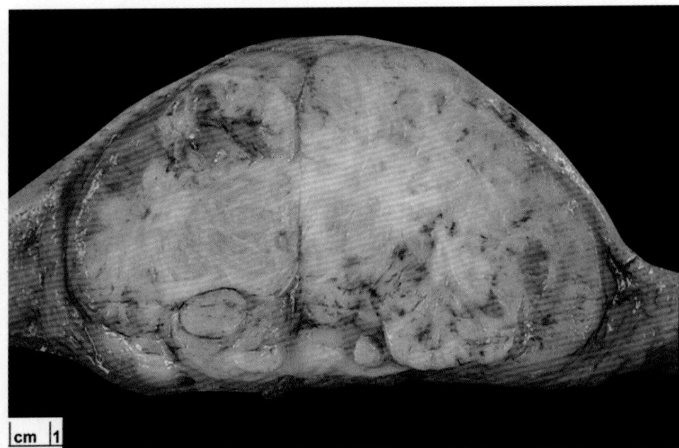

FIG. 39.1. ***Sarcoma, gross appearance.*** **A:** This tumor had areas of osteosarcoma and liposarcoma. **B:** Fibrosarcoma in a 42-year-old woman replaces much of the breast parenchyma in this mastectomy specimen. Necrosis imparts a pale yellow color centrally. Viable tumor forms a beige rim to the mass and deep secondary nodules [Courtesy of Hyunee Kim, MD].

(DFS) rates were 62% and 50%, respectively. Tumor size (less than 5 cm, 5 to 10 cm, or larger than 10 cm) was significantly related to 10-year DFS. Another series of 25 women with primary breast sarcomas and a mean follow-up of 10.5 years was reported by Adem et al.[8] Local recurrence occurred in 11 patients after a mean follow-up of 15 months, and 10 patients (40%) had systemic metastases. The 5-year DFS was 90% for tumors 5 cm or less and 50% for tumors larger than 5 cm. In the group of 59 cases studied by Barrow et al.,[9] the median OS for tumors 0 to 2.0 cm in size was 80 months, for tumors 2.1 to 4.9 cm 37 months, and for tumors 5.0 cm or more 20 months. In two other studies,[7,10] on the other hand, the size of the sarcoma did not correlate with the survival of the patients.

Although grading of mammary sarcomas is prognostically important for angiosarcoma, its significance for other types of sarcoma is unclear. Bousquet et al.[7] and Zelek et al.,[1] for example, found it significant for certain measures of survival, but three other investigations did not demonstrate prognostic significance for the grade of the sarcoma.[8,10,11] Hemangiopericytoma represents a special case, since all of these tumors reported thus far have pursued a benign clinical course regardless of size or histologic features.

The adequacy of the definitive treatment represents an influential factor in determining survival. If disease remained after the completion of initial treatment, the 10-year probability of local control and of DFS was 0% for both parameters in one study.[7] Several other studies[9–12] detected an adverse effect of positive margins on the chance of survival.

Complete excision of the sarcoma represents the crucial aspect of treatment of mammary sarcomas. The surgical procedure can consist of either a mastectomy or an excision depending on the size of the mass and other surgical and personal considerations. Five studies[7,9–11,13] have failed to demonstrate a relationship between the type of primary surgical procedure and the survival of the patient. Contemporary multimodal approaches, including irradiation and chemotherapy, may reduce the frequency of local and systemic recurrence in somatic sarcomas, but the results to date are inconclusive.[7,9–11,13–15]

Axillary lymph node (ALN) metastases are exceedingly uncommon at the time of primary therapy. In the series of Bousquet et al.,[7] metastatic sarcoma was found in 4 of 44 (9%) patients who underwent lymph node evaluation; three of these patients had angiosarcomas. Gutman et al.[13] reported that "[R]egional lymph node metastases were always and only in the context of disseminated disease." Blanchard et al.[10] discovered axillary metastases in 2 of 22 patients; both had distant metastases. Axillary dissection or sentinel lymph node (SLN) sampling are not ordinarily indicated in the absence of clinically involved lymph nodes.[7,8,10,13,16]

Radiation-induced sarcomas of the breast have attracted special interest. A publication by Sheth et al.[17] lists 124 original articles describing 1,831 cases of radiation-induced mammary sarcomas. The authors did not analyze the reported histologic features of the sarcomas, but they did note that both the size and the grade of the tumor had prognostic significance. On the basis of the accumulated published data, the authors concluded that "surgery with widely negative margins remains the primary treatment of [radiation-induced sarcomas]. Unfortunately, the role of adjuvant and neoadjuvant chemotherapy remains uncertain." These conclusions would seem to indicate that neither the nature nor the treatment of radiation-induced sarcomas of the breast differs significantly from those of spontaneously occurring mammary sarcomas.

STROMAL SARCOMA

The term "stromal sarcoma" was introduced in 1962 to describe 25 primary mammary sarcomas that did not qualify for a diagnosis of MPT or angiosarcoma.[18] The histologic appearance included "fibrous, myxoid, and fatty patterns." A liposarcomatous component was identified in six tumors, and others had elements that resembled leiomyosarcoma or "neurosarcoma." None of the tumors exhibited osseous or rhabdomyosarcomatous differentiation. The authors concluded that the neoplasms had a common "basic stromal-like structure" composed of elongated cells with an "off center" nucleus and, on this basis, chose the term "stromal sarcoma." The ages of 25 patients ranged from 25 to 64 years, averaging 48 years. All but one were women. Among 15 patients treated by local excision, 9 developed local recurrences within 5 years, and 5 of these patients died of disease. A sixth patient treated by local excision died of sarcoma without local recurrence. Local recurrence occurred in one patient treated by mastectomy whose tumor initially invaded the chest wall. No patient had ALN metastases. The actuarial 5-year survival rate was 60%. In retrospect, the illustrations and microscopic descriptions suggest that the majority of the tumors included in the report would be classified currently as liposarcoma, MFH, or fibrosarcoma. It is now considered preferable to subclassify mammary sarcomas according to their patterns of growth and differentiation using the same terminology as used for sarcomas at other anatomic sites.[19,20]

Despite the lack of diagnostic specificity, the diagnosis of stromal sarcoma is still sometimes used. The breast is composed of specialized, hormonally responsive stroma localized in lobules and around ducts as well as intervening fibrous, adipose, and other mesenchymal tissues. If the term "stromal sarcoma" were selected to designate any of the mesenchymal neoplasms of the breast, it should be applied to those derived from the hormonally responsive specialized stroma; however, most neoplasms arising from this type of stroma belong to the already well-established category of phyllodes tumor (see Chapter 8). The term "periductal stromal sarcoma" has been used for those tumors derived from specialized stroma that lack the leaf-like growth pattern characteristic of phyllodes tumors[21–23]; however, certain cases reported as periductal stromal sarcomas seem to represent phyllodes tumor with myxoid stroma,[23] phyllodes tumor with lipomatous stroma,[21] or other rare variants of phyllodes tumors.[22] Besides differing in the architecture of the stroma, phyllodes tumor and stromal sarcoma differ in the appearance of the glandular component. The glandular tissue within phyllodes tumors demonstrates evidence of proliferation, whereas the ducts and lobules entrapped within stromal sarcomas do not. Those exceptionally rare tumors in which specialized stromal fibroblasts constitute the only proliferative population can be classified as true stromal sarcomas of the breast[24] (Fig. 39.2).

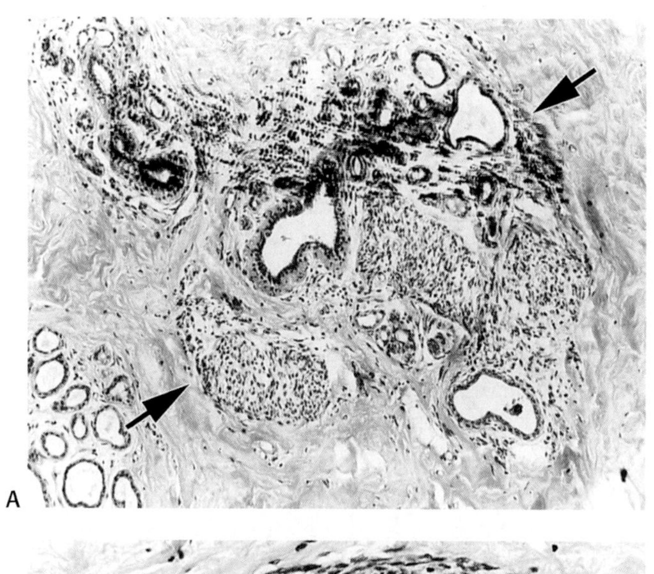

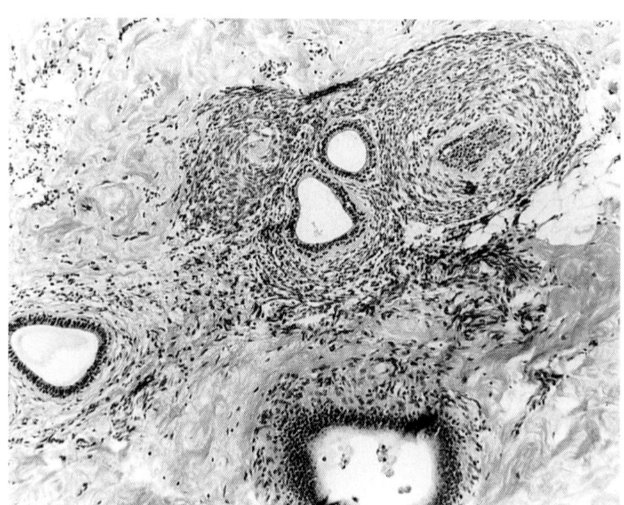

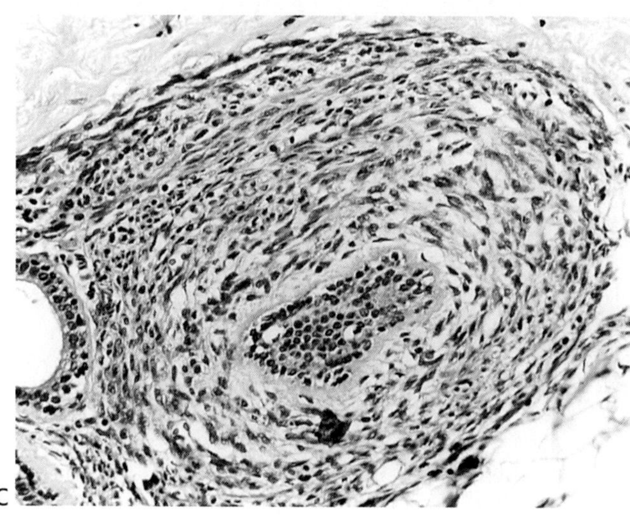

FIG. 39.2. ***True stromal sarcoma.*** **A:** Sarcoma limited to the intralobular stroma between the *arrows*. The interlobular stroma is normal. **B,C:** Sarcoma limited to periductal stroma in the same tumor as **(A)**. [**A,B:** Reproduced from Callery CD, Rosen PP, Kinne DW. Sarcoma of the breast. A study of 32 patients with reappraisal of classification and therapy. *Ann Surg* 1985;201:527–532, with permission.]

LEIOMYOSARCOMA

Leiomyosarcoma arises in the breast only very rarely and accounts for fewer than 5% of the reported sarcomas of the breast. Fujita et al.[25] tabulated clinical features of 46 cases reported as single examples or in small series, Adem et al.[26] listed 13 major series of mammary sarcomas, 6 of which contain a total of 9 leiomyosarcomas, and 6 later series of sarcomas of the breast[27–32] document 15 additional cases. This form of sarcoma probably originates from blood vessels, the smooth muscle of the nipple–areolar complex, or myofibroblasts. A predisposition of smooth muscle in the nipple to give rise to neoplasms is evidenced by reports of leiomyomata[33–35] and leiomyosarcomas[36,37] at this site. Myoid transformation of myoepithelial cells and myofibroblasts are other histogenetic mechanisms.[38,39] One leiomyosarcoma may have arisen in an ectopic areola.[40]

Clinical Presentation

Most patients have been women, but origin in the male breast has been reported.[36,41] The age at diagnosis ranges from 18[25] to 86 years,[42] and the mean age is approximately 53 years. Patients present with a mass measuring from 0.5[43] to 23 cm[44,45] and averaging approximately 5.5 cm. Pain is reported rarely.[46] Almost one-half of the tumors are in or near the nipple–areola complex, but any quadrant may be affected. The tumors are circumscribed and firm, and fixation to the skin and ulceration can occur.[45,46] A 50-year-old woman who reported a 10-year history of treatment with intermittent low-dose cyclophosphamide for systemic lupus erythematosus developed a 3.2-cm leiomyosarcoma in her left breast.[47]

Imaging Studies

Mammography reveals a dense, lobulated lesion with a defined border. Calcifications are seen only infrequently.[48] In one case,[49] pronounced lobulation created the impression of four discrete masses on sonography, and the radiologist described the lesion as "well-circumscribed, oval, and possibly a cluster of fibroadenomas." Sonograms of another case[50] revealed an irregular solid mass with a nonhomogeneous internal echo pattern and an increased anteroposterior dimension and acoustic shadowing. Calcifications were not seen. In one case studied with magnetic resonance imaging (MRI),[48] the mass appeared hypointense on T1 images and of heterogeneous intensity on T2 images.

Gross and Microscopic Pathology

Gross examination reveals a circumscribed, firm, lobulated pale tumor. Areas of necrosis may be apparent.

Microscopically, the neoplasm consists of interlacing bundles of fusiform cells with typical blunt-end nuclei characteristic of smooth muscle tumors (Fig. 39.3). Cells with an epithelioid phenotype are variably present. Malignant cytologic features reported in most cases have consisted of nuclear hyperchromasia, pleomorphism (sometimes with multinucleated giant cells), and readily identified mitoses ranging from 2[51] to 50[52] per 10 high-power fields (HPFs), with an average of 12 per 10 HPFs (Fig. 39.4). Focal areas of degeneration are characterized by nuclear pyknosis, necrosis, and lymphocytic infiltration. Areas of hyalinized stromal fibrosis with a pattern that resembles pseudoangiomatous stromal hyperplasia (PASH) may be present (Fig. 39.5). Mammary ducts and lobules, sometimes with proliferative changes, can be incorporated into the neoplasm, particularly at the periphery, a feature that may lead to considering alternative diagnoses such as metaplastic carcinoma and phyllodes tumor. One tumor classified as leiomyosarcoma contained areas of "benign" metaplastic bone and cartilage,[53] and another tumor had focal rhabdomyoblastic differentiation.[42] Two examples of leiomyosarcoma with osteoclast-like giant cells have been described[54,55] (Fig. 39.6). One tumor was classified as an epithelioid leiomyosarcoma.[56]

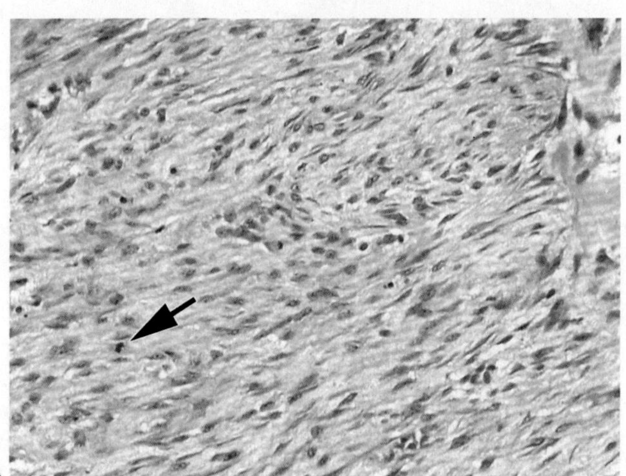

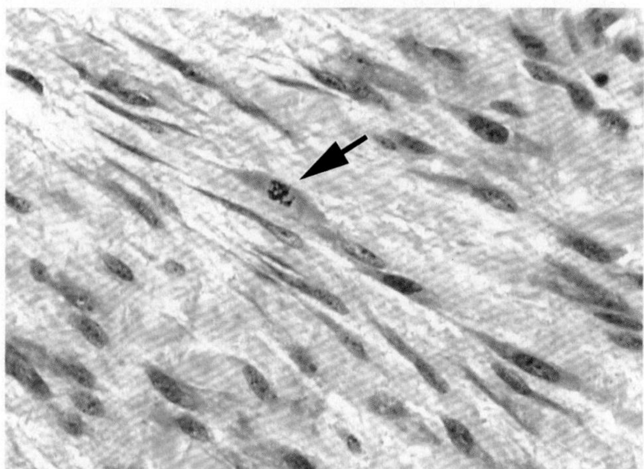

FIG. 39.3. ***Leiomyosarcoma.*** **A:** A moderately cellular tumor composed of fusiform tumor cells with blunt-end nuclei. One mitosis is evident (*arrow*). **B:** A mitotic figure is shown (*arrow*).

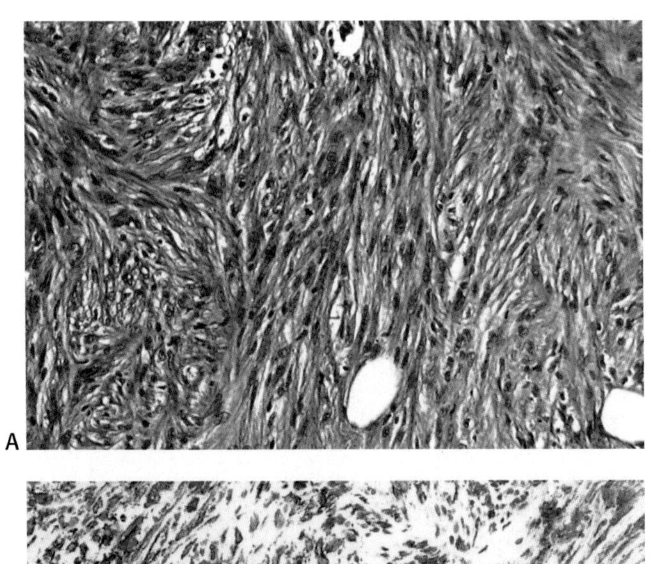

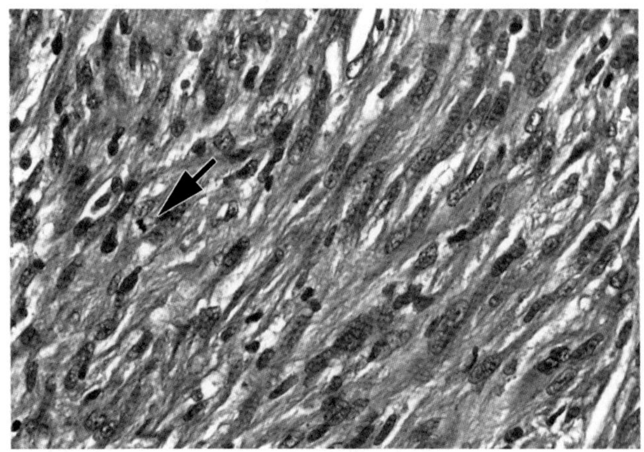

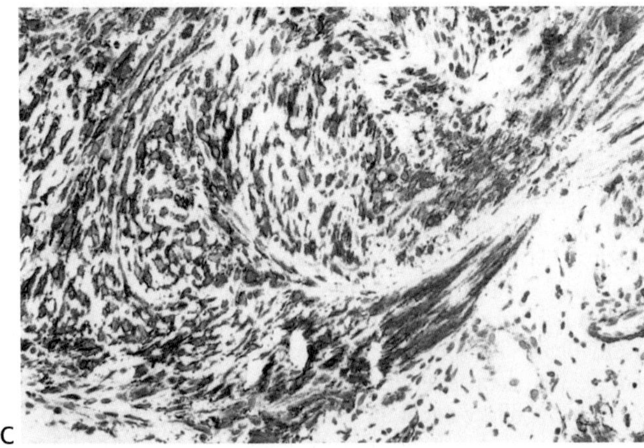

FIG. 39.4. *Leiomyosarcoma.* **A:** A highly cellular tumor composed of interlacing fascicles of spindle cells with hyperchromatic pleomorphic nuclei. **B:** A mitotic figure is shown (*arrow*). **C:** Immunoreactivity for SMA.

Cytology

Fine-needle aspiration (FNA) specimens demonstrate dissociated and poorly cohesive clusters of plump, spindle, or polygonal cells that vary in size and shape.[37,46,54,57–59] The cells contain moderate amounts of cytoplasm, which can contain small, round, and smooth vacuoles.[54] On occasion, the vacuoles appear sufficiently large to create signet ring cells. The nuclei measure 3 to 8 times the size of an erythrocyte, and they usually occupy an eccentric position. They appear pleomorphic and hyperchromatic and they display round, oval, or irregular shapes. The nuclei contain one or more nucleoli and occasional intranuclear cytoplasmic invaginations. Mitotic figures can be identified often. The extent of pleomorphism, hyperchromasia, and mitotic activity in the FNA specimen reflects the histologic appearance of the neoplasm.

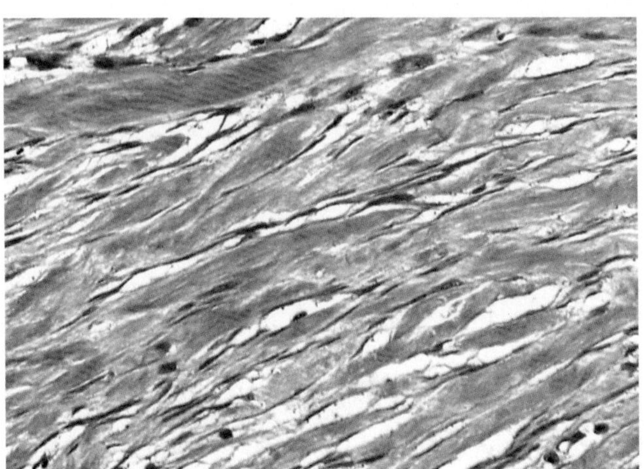

FIG. 39.5. *Leiomyosarcoma.* The collagenized stroma and clefts resemble PASH.

Immunohistochemistry

Immunohistochemical staining is usually at least focally positive for desmin, smooth muscle actin (SMA), and vimentin (Figs. 39.4 and 39.6), and reactivity for H-caldesmon[46] has been reported. Most examples were negative for cytokeratin (AE1/3, CAM5.2), S-100, and epithelial membrane antigen (EMA), but rare examples have been weakly positive for cytokeratin[37] and S-100[37,60,61] and focally positive for EMA.[60] The precise classification of the tumors with aberrant cytokeratin immunoreactivity remains uncertain. A few examples stained only weakly or not at all for actin, desmin, or SMA.[27,42,43,48,56,58,61] Weak reactivity for vimentin has been described.[37,61,62] One leiomyosarcoma did not stain for HMB45.[63] Weak or absent staining for CD34, CD68,

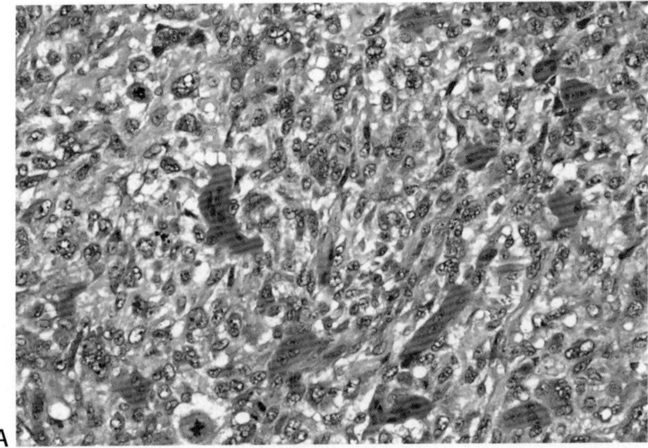

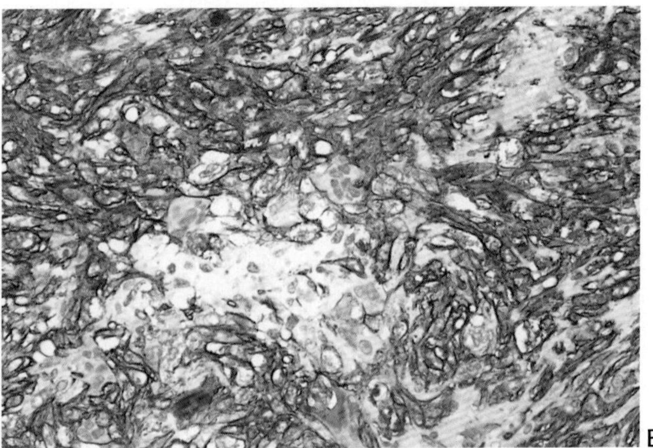

FIG. 39.6. ***Leiomyosarcoma, osteoclast-like giant cells.*** **A:** Osteoclast-like giant cells mingle with epithelioid leiomyosarcoma cells. Mitoses are present in sarcoma cells. **B:** Strong SMA immunoreactivity is limited to the sarcoma cells. The giant cells were immunoreactive for CD68, a histiocytic marker (not shown), and reactivity for cytokeratin was not present.

factor VIII, myoglobin, α_1-antichymotrypsin, neuron-specific enolase (NSE), and p53 was reported in isolated cases.[42,52,56,57]

In one case,[59] the Ki67 score was 5%, whereas in another,[43] the presenting tumor displayed a Ki67 score of 0% and the recurrence a score of 34%. Jun Wei et al.[54] reported staining for MIB-1 in 30% of the cells in one tumor.

Six tumors failed to stain for ER,[42,46,52,59] five did not stain for PR,[42,52,59] and one did not express human epidermal growth factor 2 (HER2).[59]

Electron Microscopy

Electron microscopy has been carried out on just a few cases.[36,43,51,56,57,60,64–66] The studies revealed spindle cells with nuclei, ribosomes, mitochondria, variably developed rough endoplasmic reticulum, thin basal lamina, and pinocytotic vesicles. The chromatin appeared randomly dispersed, and scattered condensations of chromatin could be seen at the periphery of the nuclear membrane. Myofilaments were described in eight cases.[51,56,64,66]

Genetic Studies

One tumor was aneuploid.[36] Comparative genomic hybridization (CGH) analysis of two leiomyosarcomas detected six chromosomal aberrations in one case and nine aberrations in the other.[63] The alterations consisted of losses located at 13q11–q21, 10q23–qter, and 17p and gains at 17p or 1q. Chromosome 13q and 10q deletions were observed in both examples, and these alterations have been seen in approximately 75% of leiomyosarcomas arising in the uterus and deep soft tissues.

Treatment and Prognosis

The publication by Rane et al.[67] lists the treatment and follow-up of most cases published in the English literature. Primary treatment consisted of total mastectomy in approximately 75% of the patients. Twelve patients[26,43,49,51,52,54,60,62,64,67,68] underwent excision alone. Of these, seven developed local recurrences[26,43,51,60,64,68] and two died.[26,51] Local recurrence on the chest wall after mastectomy has been reported.[37,46,69] The likelihood of local recurrence may depend on the amount of seemingly uninvolved surrounding tissue removed during the primary surgical procedure. Fujita et al.[25] suggested a margin of 3 cm or more. Axillary nodal metastases have not been reported.

Irradiation has been used in circumstances that did not permit excision with an adequate margin[44,45] and to treat recurrences on the chest wall.[37,46] Chemotherapy has been administered in just a few cases,[26,37,43,46] so its value cannot be assessed.

Among the nearly 50 reported cases of mammary leiomyosarcoma, 6 patients died of the disease.[26,29,37,51,56] Outcome has not correlated well with the mitotic rate in the primary tumor, because fatalities occurred in cases with 2 or 3 mitoses per 10 HPFs as well as in tumors with higher mitotic rates. Late recurrences and death from disease 15 and 20 years after initial diagnoses have been reported.[51,65]

LIPOSARCOMA

This malignant neoplasm may arise from periductal or perilobular stroma in the form of an MPT[70,71] or from interlobular stroma to present as a primary stromal sarcoma.[70] Liposarcoma arising in PTs is discussed in Chapter 8. Liposarcomas account for approximately 5% of mammary sarcomas reported in the literature.

Clinical Presentation

Patients' ages range from 16[72] to 90[73] years at the time of diagnosis with an average age of 49 years. Two male patients have been described.[70] The presenting symptom is a mass of variable duration occasionally accompanied by pain.[70,74]

Two instances of bilateral low-grade liposarcoma have been described,[74,75] and the patient described by Lifvendahl[76] had several nodules in both breasts. One patient was pregnant at the time of diagnosis,[70] and three came to attention during the postpartum period.[76–78] Radiation-related pleomorphic liposarcoma of the chest wall has been reported 17 months after excision and irradiation[79] and 10 years after mastectomy.[80]

On clinical examination, the tumor is typically firm and well circumscribed, but ill-defined lesions have been reported. The overlying skin is usually unaffected, but ulceration was observed associated with a 20-cm tumor[81] and another that spanned 28 cm.[73]

Imaging Studies

The mammographic features of mammary liposarcoma vary. Two examples[79,82] appeared well-defined and smoothly outlined, and these features suggested the diagnosis of fibroadenoma (FA). On the other hand, other examples had ill-defined margins,[83] and mammography in a patient with bilateral involvement revealed "a bizarre pattern of widespread density in the posterior and axillary region of each breast."[74] Sonography may demonstrate a mass with a complex echo pattern produced by the presence of cystic and solid components[77,83] or a lesion suggestive of a benign tumor such as a FA[78] or a "fibroadenolipoma."[79] MRI of one tumor revealed a hypodense mass with a distinct border on T1-weighted images, and two tumors appeared hyperdense on T2-weighted scans.[83,84]

Gross and Microscopic Pathology

The tumors have measured 2 to 40 cm, averaging about 8 cm. Some tumors looked well circumscribed or encapsulated, whereas others appeared multinodular or infiltrative. The tumors have been described as ". . . greasy, yellow-grey, bulky, circumscribed masses. When sectioned, the tumour appears to bulge from its cut surface. Some areas have a slimy gelatinous appearance; it is from these areas that a thick mucoid secretion may be expressed."[85] The gelatinous areas suggest the presence of a component of myxoid liposarcoma.[78] Necrosis and cavitation can occur.[73,77,86]

The histologic features of liposarcoma in the breast are identical to those of liposarcoma arising in the extremities or trunk. Among published reports, including 25 mammary tumors classified in the manner used for liposarcomas in other sites, 14 (41%) were myxoid (Fig. 39.7), 9 (26%) were well differentiated, 7 (21%) were pleomorphic, and 4 (12%) were poorly differentiated.[70,73,74,78,81–83,85–95] The well-differentiated liposarcomas include several examples of sclerosing or fibrous liposarcomas.[73,82,83] There was no apparent consistent relationship between tumor type, tumor size, and patient age at diagnosis.

Cytology

Specimens obtained by needle aspiration demonstrate variably cellular smears with atypical cells occurring singly and in small groups.[78,79,81] The shapes of the cells vary from spindly to round or polygonal. The nuclei appear hyperchromatic and contain coarse chromatin and occasional nucleoli. The pale cytoplasm contains vacuoles of varying size, which indent the nucleus. Oil red O stain demonstrates the presence of lipid in the vacuoles.[79] In one case, the vacuolated cells were mistaken for vacuolated neoplastic lobular cells.[74] Multinucleate large cells are sometimes seen.[81] The presence of a background branching capillary network and myxoid material would suggest the diagnosis of a myxoid liposarcoma.[78]

Immunohistochemistry

Immunohistochemical staining yields the results seen in liposarcomas of other sites. The malignant cells do not stain for epithelial markers in most cases,[81,84,86] but they typically stain for S-100.[78,82] The Ki67 score of one tumor was less than 5%.[84] One tumor did not stain for ER or PR.[81]

Electron Microscopy

Electron microscopy demonstrates pleomorphic tumor cells with eccentric, large, indented nuclei.[81] Ultrastructural study of a well-differentiated liposarcoma[96] revealed cells with small amounts of endoplasmic reticulum, rare mitochondria, and membrane-bound cytoplasmic droplets. Large, sometimes indented nuclei sat at the periphery of the cells, and the cell membranes lacked desmosomes. Basal lamina and granular extracellular material surrounded many cells.

Treatment and Prognosis

In many cases, treatment has consisted of simple or radical mastectomy.[70] Nandipati et al.[77] tabulated the treatment and outcome of many of the reported cases. Wide local excision constituted the primary surgical procedure in seven cases.[70,73,79,83,97] ALN metastases have not been reported. With follow-up ranging from less than a year to 20 years, approximately 70% of patients have remained recurrence-free, 6% were alive with systemic recurrence, and 24% died of metastatic liposarcoma.[70,74,87–89,92–94,98] Systemic recurrences and deaths due to disease usually occurred within 2 years of diagnosis and were limited to patients with pleomorphic or high-grade tumors. Tumor size by itself was not predictive of outcome. In isolated cases, systemic chemotherapy and irradiation have been used for palliative purposes.

OSTEOSARCOMA AND CHONDROSARCOMA

Malignant tumors displaying the features of extraskeletal osteosarcomas or chondrosarcomas occasionally arise in the breast. Publications by Silver and Tavassoli[99] and Trihia et al.[100] list many of the reported cases, and several cases have been published since.[84,101–116] Several authors point out that most mammary neoplasms with malignant osseous or cartilaginous differentiation are variants of heterologous metaplastic carcinoma or MPTs. Rakha et al.[117] adopt a more

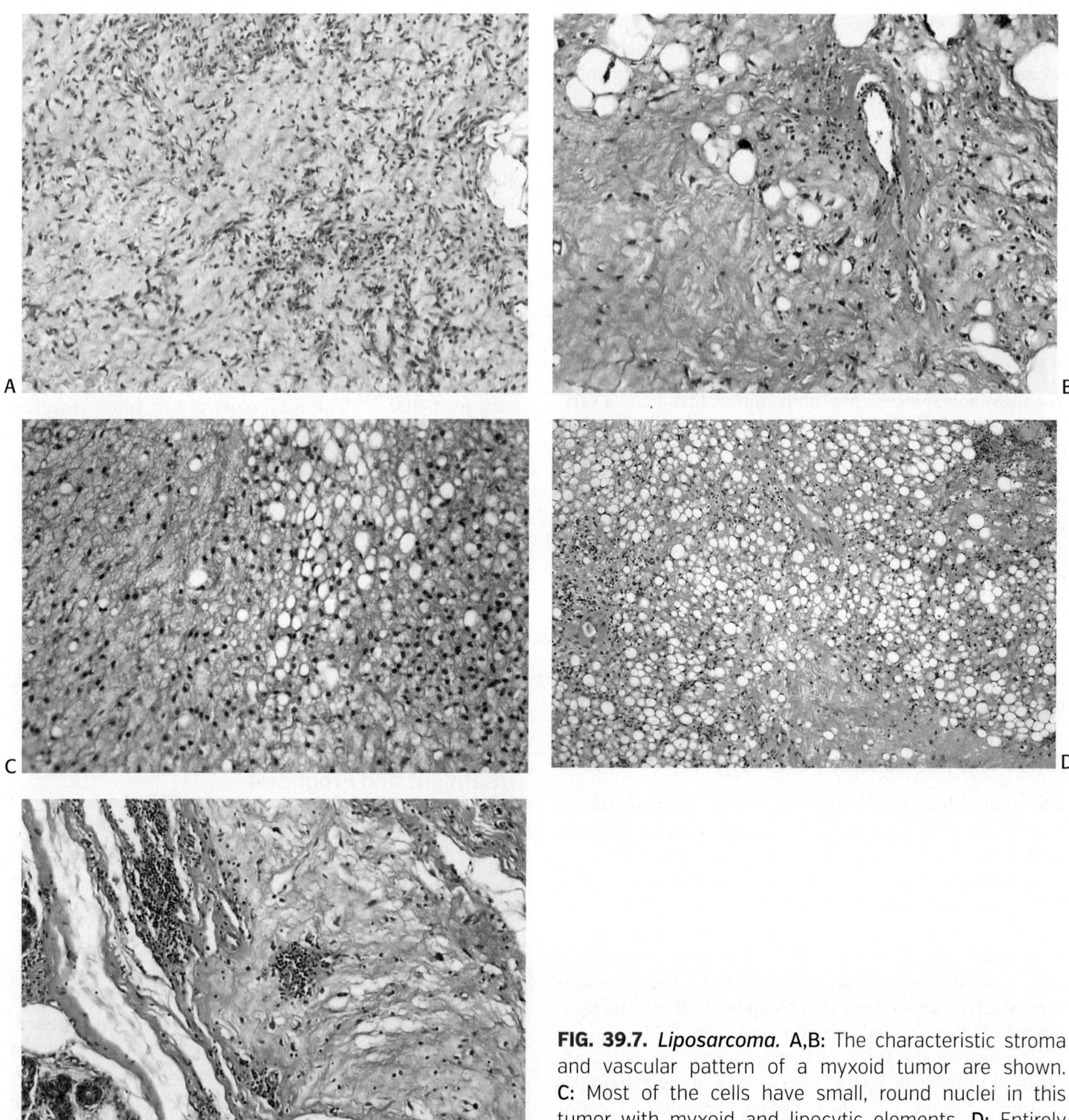

FIG. 39.7. ***Liposarcoma.*** **A,B:** The characteristic stroma and vascular pattern of a myxoid tumor are shown. **C:** Most of the cells have small, round nuclei in this tumor with myxoid and lipocytic elements. **D:** Entirely lipocytic growth. **E:** Myxoid liposarcoma invading breast parenchyma.

extreme position and suggest that essentially all mammary malignancies showing osseous or chondroid features represent either matrix-producing metaplastic carcinomas or phyllodes tumors with massive stromal overgrowth. Whatever the pathogenesis of these malignant tumors, a body of literature describes their clinical and pathologic features.

Clinical Presentation

The ages of the patients range from 16[112] to 96 years.[102] The mean age in the largest series of osteosarcomas was 64.2 years.[99] Origin in the male breast has been described rarely.[99] The presenting symptom is a mass typically described as circumscribed and freely movable. A minority of the tumors are irregular or multinodular. Fixation to the skin or the chest wall and ulceration of the skin occur in a minority of cases.[118] The ulceration may result from stretching of the skin rather than from infiltration by the malignant cells.[119] One osteosarcoma arose in the breast of a woman 9 years after excision and irradiation of a breast carcinoma in the same breast,[99] and radiation-associated postmastectomy osteosarcoma and chondrosarcoma of the chest wall have been reported.[120,121]

Imaging Studies

Mammography reveals a dense mass, which can appear either well-defined[102,108,109,122] or ill-defined.[104] The mammographic appearance sometimes suggests the diagnosis of FA.[99,105,113,123] Tumors in which the osteosarcomatous component dominates appear heavily calcified. The patterns of the calcifications seen in these tumors have varied. Certain calcifications have been described as "soft,"[108,124] and others as "a cluster of crushed stone-like calcifications, which gave the tumor a raw cotton-like appearance."[107] Several authors noted dense central calcifications and finer peripheral ones.[109,112] Coussy et al.[103] described the mammographic features of one mass as ". . . containing the following components: a large macrocalcification closely resembling bone, with lobulated borders; a peripheral soft-tissue mass with well-defined borders; and a transition zone between the two that was denser than the soft-tissue mass, had a striated aspect (resembling a perpendicular periosteal hair-on-end reaction) and contained small calcifications." Tumors of a chondrosarcomatous nature appear hyperdense,[122,125] and they may contain calcifications.[125] The sarcoma may appear hypoechoic by sonography. One example had heterogeneous echogenicity with an anterior halo and posterior shadowing and enhancement,[124] and another[101] demonstrated "a densely shadowing mass, compatible with the extensive calcification seen on mammography. Increased through transmission was also present." Sonograms of other cases showed complex masses with cystic and solid regions and posterior shadowing.[104,107,109,113,125] Marked surrounding vascularity was noted on Doppler evaluation in one case.[101] These tumors may be positive on a technetium-99 scan.[103,109,111,126–128] Computed tomography (CT) scans disclose the mass,[112] and findings suggestive of hemorrhage, necrosis, and bone formation can be seen on MRI studies in certain cases.[103,109]

Gross and Microscopic Pathology

The excised tumors have measured 5 to 25 cm in diameter, with an average size of 10 cm. A well-defined border is described in most cases. The cut surface usually has a variegated appearance with areas of softening or gelatinous degeneration and foci of necrosis distributed in firm gray or white tissue. A gritty sensation is encountered when cutting the tumor in areas of ossification. In addition, gross calcification may be visible and palpable.[129]

Histologic examination reveals a spectrum of microscopic patterns (Fig. 39.8). The tumors have in common a prominent component of high-grade spindle cell sarcoma with a variable mitotic rate. Mitotic counts as high as 52 per 10 HPFs have been noted.[101] Tumors with chondroid differentiation alone are less frequent than those with osseous differentiation in which there may be a chondroid element. Most of the former tumors have been reported as single case reports.[118,119,122,125,130–134] Beltaos and Banerjee[135] described two such cases, and Kennedy and Biggart[136] included one example in their group of mammary sarcomas. Multinucleate osteoclastic giant cells are usually present in areas of bone formation.[115] Rarely, giant cells constitute a conspicuous element, and they may be associated with hemorrhagic cysts with a telangiectatic appearance.[116,137]

Cytology

The findings in an FNA specimen depend on the composition of the lesion.[100,123,124,137–139] The smears usually appear cellular, but hypocellular aspirates sometimes occur. Large atypical cells lie singly and in loose clusters. The cells appear pleomorphic and possess one or two oval- or spindle-shaped nuclei, coarse chromatin, prominent nucleoli, and moderate amounts of dense cytoplasm, which was described as "filamentous" in one report.[139] Atypical mitotic figures can be seen, and osteoclast-like giant cells may be present. Small-or medium-sized plaques of osteoid, which stains red-purple with the May–Grünwald–Giemsa stain, may be seen in the background. The plaques have round, polyhedral, or bizarre shapes and are sometimes surrounded by malignant cells. If the predominant cellular elements consist of spindle and giant cells, the distinction between a primary sarcoma, an MPT, and a metaplastic carcinoma cannot be made with certainty.

Immunohistochemistry

Immunohistochemical staining for cytokeratins, myoepithelial proteins, and molecules found in muscle cells are negative. Lack of reactivity for cytokeratin and myoepithelial markers is essential to rule out an epithelial component and thereby to exclude the diagnosis of metaplastic carcinoma. Areas with cartilaginous differentiation can be immunoreactive for EMA,[99,102,140] and reactivity for S-100 is sometimes found in cartilaginous lesions.[99,102,130–132,139,140] Staining for SMA has varied in the few cases tested.[102,103,131,132] Most tumors in the series of Silver and Tavassoli[99] stained for α_1-antichymotrypsin and α_1-antitrypsin. The cells in isolated cases have failed to stain for polyclonal carcinoembryogenic antigen (CEA), c-kit, CD57, and CD34.[102,107,131] Osteoclastic giant cells were immunoreactive for KP-1 (CD68), a marker of histiocytic differentiation.[99,103,139,141] A Ki67 score of 20% was reported in one case.[103] None of the cases studied have expressed ER, PR, or HER2.[99,101–103,105,106,108,119,122]

Electron Microscopy

The electron microscopic features of six osteosarcomas[99,129,142] and one chondrosarcoma[130] have been reported. The malignant osteoblasts appeared elongated and possessed conspicuous and often dilated rough endoplasmic reticulum, conspicuous perinuclear Golgi, eccentric nuclei, and large nucleoli. Large osteoclast-like cells contained abundant mitochondria and nondilated rough endoplasmic reticulum. The cell borders of some of the osteoclast-like cells can appear "ruffled." Undifferentiated round or oval cells, myofibroblasts, and histiocytes may be present. The osteoid had typical long-spaced collagen fibers and hydroxyapatite crystal "puffs." Desmosomes have been observed linking undifferentiated cells in two osteosarcomas.[99,142]

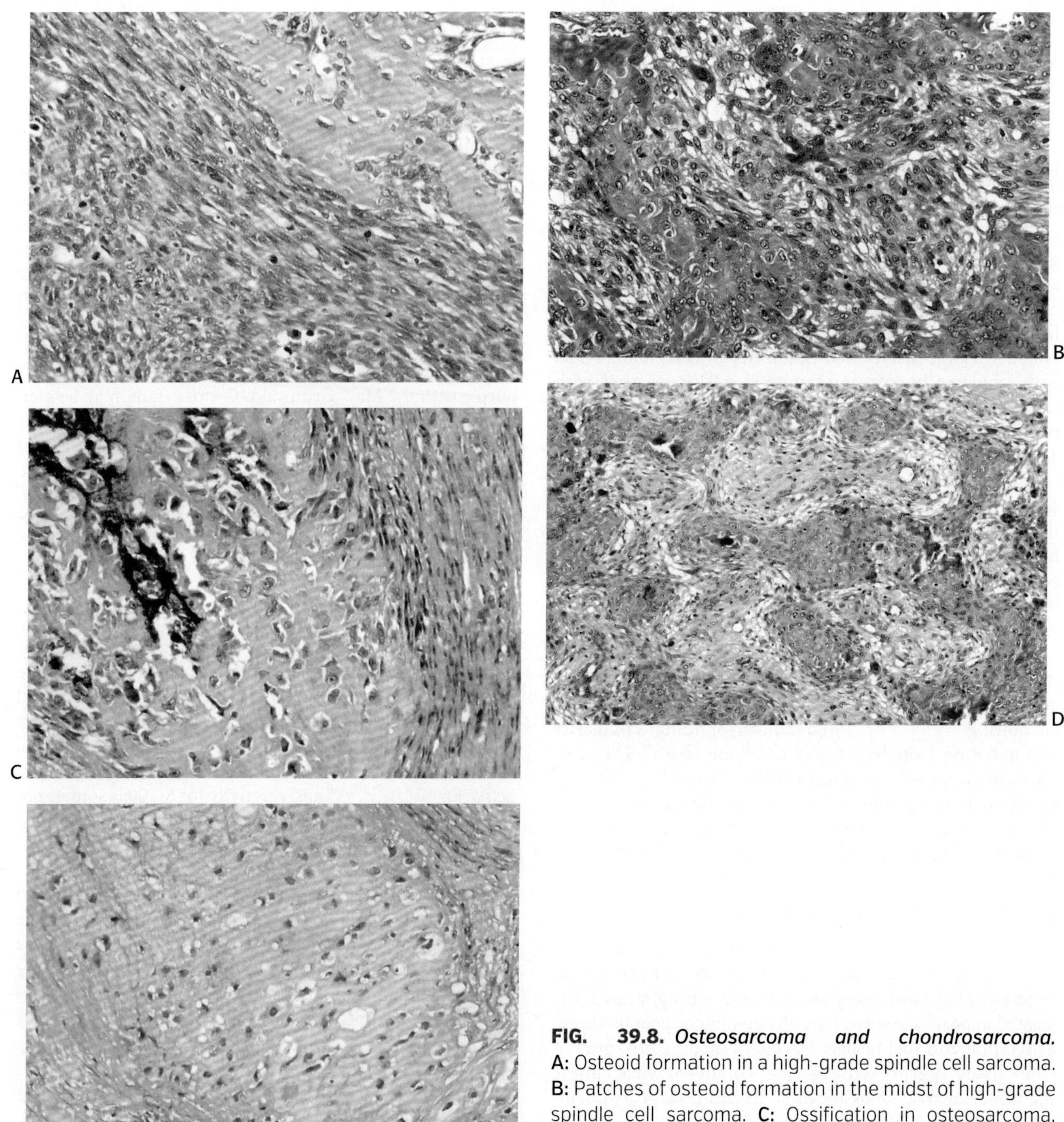

FIG. 39.8. *Osteosarcoma and chondrosarcoma.* **A:** Osteoid formation in a high-grade spindle cell sarcoma. **B:** Patches of osteoid formation in the midst of high-grade spindle cell sarcoma. **C:** Ossification in osteosarcoma. **D:** Ossification with an epithelioid appearance in osteosarcoma. **E:** Chondrosarcoma.

Treatment and Prognosis

The series of patients studied by Silver and Tavassoli[99] provides the most detailed analysis of the treatment and clinical outcome of patients with mammary osteosarcomas. Of the 50 patients in the study group, 18 were treated with limited surgery and 32 with a simple, modified, or radical mastectomy. Local recurrences developed in 67% of patients treated with limited surgery and 11% of those who underwent a mastectomy. Of the eight patients treated with limited surgery who developed local recurrences, seven had positive margins of their surgical specimens. Metastases were not detected in any of the 20 patients who underwent axillary staging. Metastases appeared in 41% of patients, usually within a year from the time of diagnosis. These patients all experienced rapid progression of their disease and died within 20 months. The median survival time was 2 months from the time of detection of the metastases. Using the Kaplan–Meier method, the probability of OS was 38% at 5 years and 10% at 10 years. Patients with osteosarcomas smaller than 4.6 cm had a higher likelihood for survival than patients with larger tumors, and patients with the fibroblastic type of osteosarcoma had a better prognosis than patients with the osteoclastic or osteoblastic subtypes. The status of the margins of the surgical specimen did not correlate with the likelihood of survival.

Only a few other reports provide follow-up information,[100,106,107,110,112,135,137,139,143,144] and the details given support the conclusions reached by Silver and Tavassoli.[99] Three publications confirm the absence of ALN metastases in five patients.[100,104,106] An 80-year-old woman developed a local recurrence 4 months after a simple mastectomy for osteosarcoma and pulmonary involvement and direct extension into the chest led to her death a few months later.[144] Another woman[143] developed pulmonary metastases 8 years after the time of diagnosis of a low-grade osteosarcoma; her death ensued 11 months later accompanied by other metastatic deposits.

Irradiation and systemic chemotherapy have been administered in several cases, but the variable nature of these treatments and conditions for which they were used preclude drawing secure conclusions regarding their efficacy.

MFH AND FIBROSARCOMA

Histologic descriptions of spindle cell sarcomas of the breast have not always clearly distinguished between fibrosarcoma and MFH. As noted by Jones et al.,[145] "these two tumors have many features in common; thus, classification of some into one or the other group can be arbitrary." Furthermore, changes in concepts regarding the nature of these tumors as well as their diagnostic criteria make it impossible to determine the nature of many cases reported in the literature. For example, MFH, once considered a specific type of histiocytic neoplasm showing facultative fibroblastic differentiation, now is seen simply as a poorly differentiated sarcoma, which can originate from any of a variety of types of mesenchymal cells. Reflecting this change in thinking, the diagnosis of "MFH" has given way to "undifferentiated pleomorphic sarcoma" when referring to such tumors arising in soft tissues. Pathologists continue to regard fibrosarcoma as specific type of sarcoma derived from cells of a fibroblastic nature; however, the recognition of several specific subtypes of fibrosarcomas has led to reclassification of many of these cases and thereby reduced the number of tumors that remain in the fibrosarcoma category. Bahrami and Folpe[146] re-examined 163 tumors of soft tissue classified as fibrosarcomas at the Mayo Clinic between 1960 and 2008 and confirmed the diagnosis in only 26 (16%) cases. The authors reclassified the remaining 137 tumors as 32 examples of MFH, 20 variants of fibrosarcoma, 78 mesenchymal tumors of other types, and 7 nonmesenchymal tumors. The authors concluded that "true [fibrosarcoma] is exceedingly rare . . . and should be diagnosed with great caution." Although the writers issued this warning in the context of tumors of soft tissues, it may apply equally well to sarcomas of the breast.

MFH (Undifferentiated Pleomorphic Sarcoma)

For the purposes of the discussion in this chapter, a breast tumor was accepted as MFH if this was the reported diagnosis and the growth pattern was predominantly storiform. Although rare, MFH represents one of the common types of mammary sarcomas. It accounted for 36% of the 240 breast sarcomas in the studies published after 1982 tabulated by Adem et al.[147] and 24% of the 25 cases from the Mayo Clinic discussed in this publication. Kijima et al.[148] list selected pathologic and clinical features of 31 cases, and 9 series[149–157] include mention of another 122 examples.

Clinical Presentation

The majority of patients have been women, but low-grade[145] and high-grade[149,158] MFH of the male breast has been reported. Jeong et al.[159] described the case of a 76-year-old man in whom a tumor classified as an "atypical spindle cell lesion" recurred after 1 year as an undifferentiated pleomorphic sarcoma. The age at diagnosis ranges from 24 to 93 years, averaging 52 years. In one series, patients with low-grade tumors tended to be younger (average age, 46 years) than those with high-grade tumors (average age, 64 years).[145] The initial symptom is a mass, which may be located in any portion of the breast. Symptomatic intervals from 1 month to 17 years have been reported.[145] The tumors are usually solitary, but patients with multiple tumors have been described.[145,160] The overlying skin can exhibit dimpling, induration, ecchymosis, or ulceration.[160–162] Antecedent trauma is occasionally reported.[145]

A number of case reports suggest an association between irradiation for breast carcinoma and the development of MFH.[163,164] In most of these instances, the sarcoma arose in the chest wall after mastectomy[165–168] or in sites of nodal irradiation such as the axilla.[166,169,170] Several patients with breast carcinoma treated with breast conservation and irradiation have developed MFH in the conserved breast. In one case, the sarcoma appeared 2 years after excision and radiotherapy[171]; in another case,[172] the interval between irradiation and the appearance of the sarcoma was 52 months. In one series,[166] an interval as long as 7 years between irradiation and the diagnosis of mammary sarcoma was reported.

Gross and Microscopic Pathology

The tumors have measured from 1.0 to 20 cm in size,[173] averaging 7.5 cm. In a patient with multiple nodules, the two largest were both 7.0 cm.[160] The mass may have a circumscribed or an ill-defined border. The neoplasm is fleshy, firm, or hard and composed of gray, tan, or white tissue. Hemorrhage, necrosis, mucoid change, and calcification are infrequent.

The microscopic hallmark of MFH is the storiform growth pattern in which the spindle cells are arranged in a pin-wheel pattern (Fig. 39.9). Capillaries or small blood vessels may be found at the center of the storiform complex. Giant cells, usually with multiple nuclei, myxoid change, and a chronic inflammatory cell infiltrate, are variably present

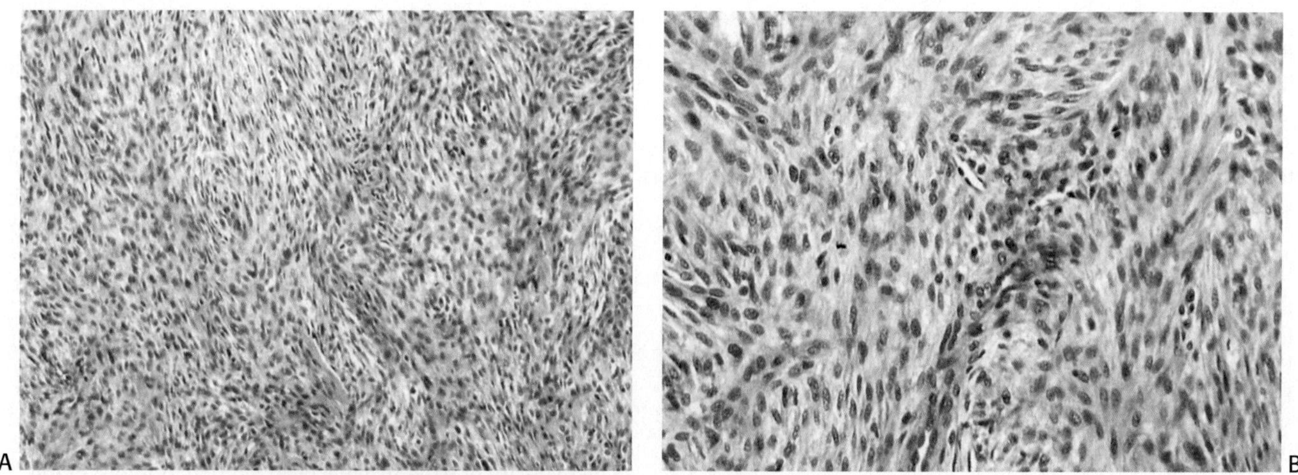

FIG. 39.9. *Malignant fibrous histiocytoma.* **A,B:** The characteristic storiform pattern is shown.

(Fig. 39.10). High-grade lesions are characterized by easily identified mitoses, generally numbering more than 3 per HPF, prominent cellular pleomorphism, and necrosis. Low-grade tumors have little mitotic activity, as well as minimal pleomorphism and necrosis. Cellularity alone is not a reliable criterion for distinguishing between low- and high-grade MFHs of the breast.

Cytology

Aspiration cytology yields cellular smears displaying spindle cells, giant cells, and conspicuous capillaries with fragments of collagen in the background.[174–176] The tumor cells have large, pleomorphic nuclei with irregular nuclear membranes and vacuolated cytoplasm. Both intact cells and naked

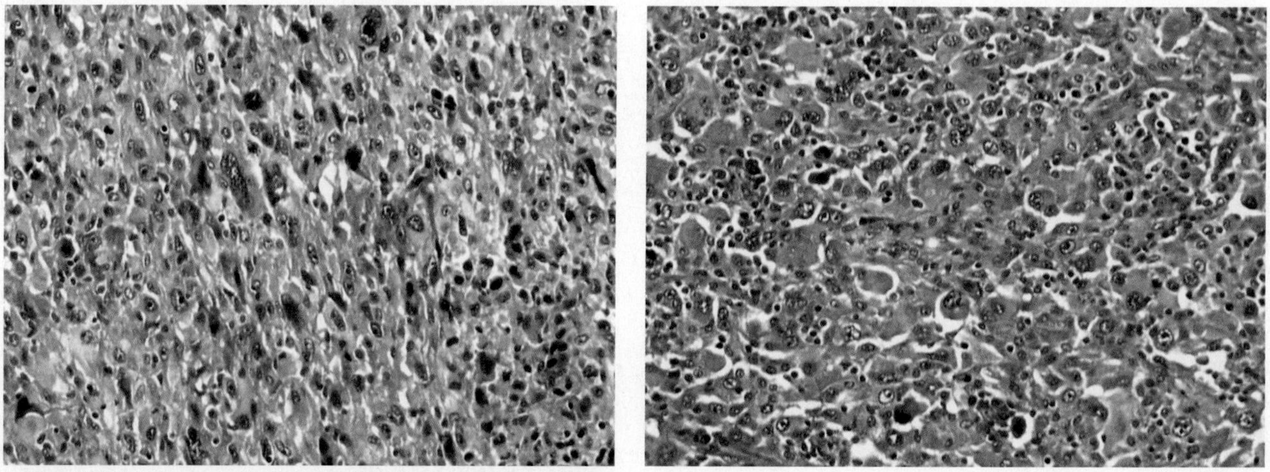

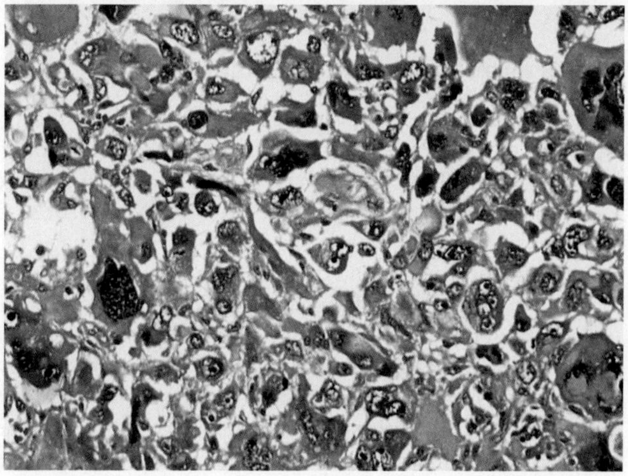

FIG. 39.10. *Malignant fibrous histiocytoma.* All images are from a single tumor. **A:** Epithelioid and spindle cells. **B:** Epithelioid cells with lymphocytes and plasma cells are present. **C:** Bizarre giant cells formed in a degenerated part of the tumor.

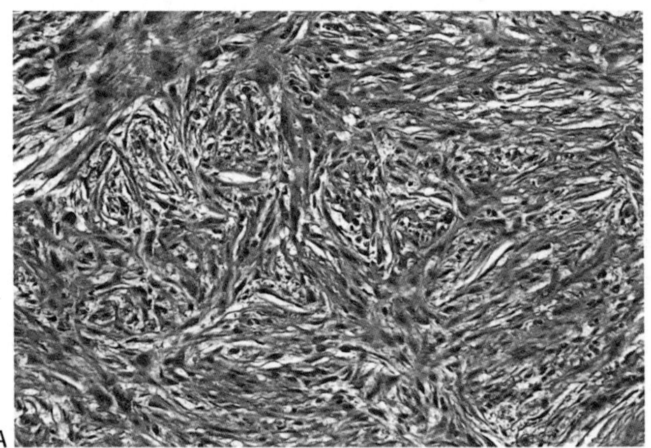
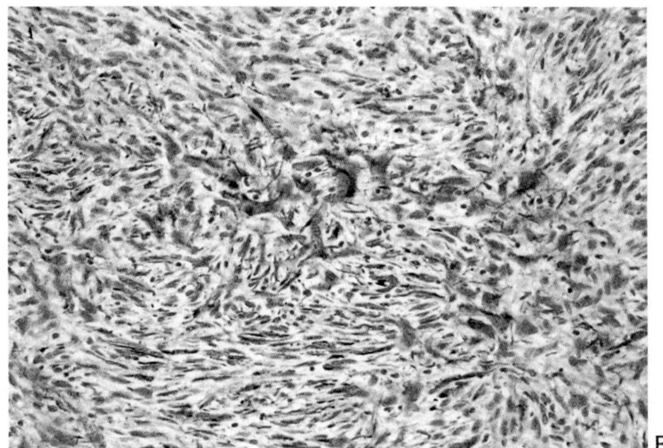

FIG. 39.11. *Malignant fibrous histiocytoma.* **A:** A low-grade tumor from a 22-year-old woman. Mitotic figures were infrequent. **B:** The tumor displayed focal immunoreactivity for CK7 (shown) and vimentin but not for actin.

nuclei can be seen. Mitotic figures are often numerous, and atypical mitotic figures can be found. Multinucleate tumor cells may be evident. The tumor cells can contain engulfed erythrocytes.[176]

Immunohistochemistry

Immunohistochemical stains are not specific. The malignant cells are reactive for vimentin, occasionally for actin,[145] and rarely for cytokeratin (Fig. 39.11). All pathologic and clinical features must be given careful consideration when a tumor with storiform growth displays cytokeratin reactivity, since these lesions are usually metaplastic carcinomas, but aberrant cytokeratin expression is present in sarcomas rarely. Immunoreactivity for α_1-antitrypsin has been reported in MFH of the breast[156] and MFH arising in other organs.[177,178]

Electron Microscopy

Several publications described the ultrastructural features of MFH.[160,167,168,175] The tumors contain a mixture of cell types. Fibroblast-like cells and histiocytic cells predominate. The former have spindly or polygonal shapes, oval nuclei, containing abundant euchromatin, frequent nucleoli, rough and smooth endoplasmic reticulum, abundant ribosomes, mitochondria, lysosomes, Golgi apparatus, and a few droplets of fat. Some fibroblast-like cells contained bundles of filaments resembling myofilaments. The histocytic cells have oval or stellate shapes, abundant cytoplasm containing ribosomes, lysosomes, smooth endoplasmic reticulum, and pleomorphic nuclei. Langerhans cell granules have been seen in histiocytic cells,[167] and occasional cells show intercellular junctions. Other types of cells present in smaller numbers include those with both fibroblastic and histiocytic features, multinucleate giant cells, and undifferentiated mesenchymal cells. The tumor cells sit in amorphous matrix containing sparse bands of collagen.

Treatment and Prognosis

With few exceptions, treatment has been by mastectomy with or without axillary dissection. A small minority of patients have been managed successfully by local excision alone. Local recurrence has been reported after both mastectomy and local excision. The choice between mastectomy and local excision depends on the individual clinical presentation and must include consideration of the likelihood of obtaining complete excision and a cosmetically satisfactory result. Rare examples of MFH have metastasized to ALNs,[160] but ALN dissection is not indicated unless needed to obtain an adequate margin or the clinical findings suggest the presence of nodal metastases.

Recurrence and death due to disease have been reported in approximately 40% of patients. The most frequent sites of metastases are the lungs and bones. Tumors that developed metastases have been high-grade histologically. Local recurrence is not infrequent among low-grade tumors. Systemic recurrences and deaths usually occurred within 3 years and rarely more than 5 years after diagnoses.[145,148,173,175]

FIBROSARCOMA

The series of mammary sarcomas listed by Adem et al.[147] include 94 tumors said to represent fibrosarcomas, and a few case reports and small series describe or mention several other sarcomas classified as mammary fibrosarcomas. Certain of these cases were phyllodes tumors with a fibrosarcomatous pattern,[179] fibrosarcomas arising from a dermatofibrosarcoma protuberans (DFSP),[180] or myofibroblastic tumors.[181] Most were examined without the benefit of the current understanding of the nature of sarcomas and the availability of ancillary studies such as electron microscopy, immunohistochemical staining, and genetic analysis. Because of these limitations, one has reason to question the validity of the diagnoses in nearly all the published cases.

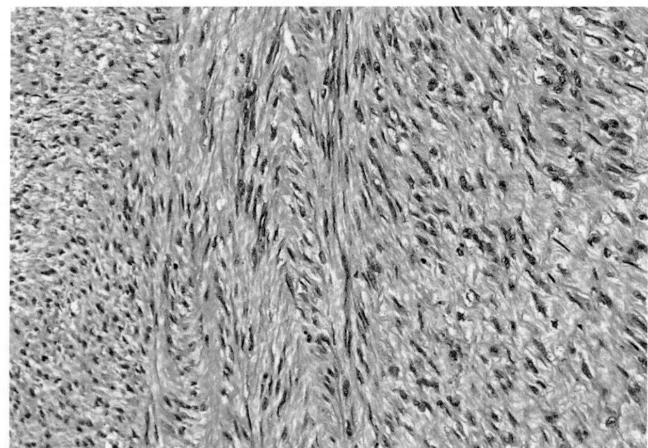

FIG. 39.12. *Fibrosarcoma.* The tumor consists of spindle cells with elongated nuclei arranged in interwoven bundles. The gross appearance of this tumor is shown in Figure 39.1B.

Currently proposed histologic criteria for the diagnosis of fibrosarcoma of soft tissue consist of hyperchromatic spindled cells showing no more than moderate pleomorphism, a fascicular, "herringbone" pattern of growth, the presence of interstitial collagen, the absence of morphologic features of all subtypes of fibrosarcomas (myxofibrosarcoma, low-grade fibromyxoid sarcoma, sclerosing epithelioid fibrosarcoma, and fibrosarcoma arising in DFSP), and lack of expression of all markers except vimentin and very minimal SMA.

It seems reasonable to apply these criteria to sarcomas arising in the breast. Thus, mammary sarcomas composed of elongated spindle cells with hyperchromatic spindly nuclei, variably prominent nucleoli, and scant cytoplasm predominantly arranged in broad interdigitating sheets, bands, or fascicles displaying the "herringbone" pattern would be classified as fibrosarcoma (Fig. 39.12). Mitotic figures are almost always evident. The amount of extracellular collagen varies from sparse delicate strands to broad keloidal bands. According to the French system for grading sarcomas (Fédération Nationale des Centres de Lutte Contre le Cancer [FNCLCC]), fibrosarcomas should fall in grade 1 or grade 2 categories. Deviations from these characteristics should prompt consideration of another diagnosis. For example, tumors showing more than a moderate degree of cellular pleomorphism usually merit the diagnosis of undifferentiated pleomorphic sarcoma (MFH). The presence of large areas showing a storiform growth pattern would bring up the diagnosis of fibrosarcoma arising from a DFSP, and the presence of focal adipocytic differentiation would suggest the diagnosis of dedifferentiated liposarcoma. Tumors showing a loosely structured growth pattern without the typical "herringbone" arrangement or showing foci of osteoid formation without osteoblastic differentiation (Fig. 39.13) may represent a specific subtype of fibrosarcoma such as low-grade fibromyxoid sarcoma or myxofibrosarcoma. Finally, detection of proteins characteristic of stromal cells other than fibroblasts would exclude a sarcoma from the fibrosarcoma category. Staining for CD34, for instance, would provoke consideration of the diagnosis of fibrosarcoma arising from either DFSP or solitary fibrous tumor.

One must not forget that other types of sarcomas such as synovial sarcoma, malignant peripheral nerve sheath tumor, solitary fibrous tumor, rhabdomyosarcoma, angiosarcoma, and epithelioid sarcoma and epithelial malignancies such as melanoma and spindle cell carcinoma sometimes display regions resembling fibrosarcomas. Immunohistochemical staining and testing for genetic alterations should allow one to exclude these possibilities in problematic cases.

These considerations suggest that one should probably consider the diagnosis of fibrosarcoma only after excluding all other possibilities. The limited information provided in published cases of mammary fibrosarcomas does not allow one to evaluate the nature of the sarcomas thoroughly; consequently, the diagnosis of fibrosarcoma remains open to question in almost every instance. The case reported by Lee et al.[182] may represent a *bona fide* mammary fibrosarcoma. A 47-year-old woman sought medical attention because of a 10-day history of a 3-cm painless breast mass. Radiologic imaging demonstrated the mass but did not allow for a specific diagnosis. The resected specimen displayed a "firm, fleshy, well-circumscribed, round mass that was gray-white." Uniform fusiform or spindle-shaped cells with scant cytoplasm and slightly to moderately atypical nuclei embedded in a scant collagenous matrix composed the mass. The mitotic rate was as high as 10 per HPF. The malignant cells failed to stain for cytokeratin, SMA, S-100, and EMA. The patient's treatment consisted of surgical excision, and she remained free of disease 10 months later.

Postirradiation fibrosarcomas affecting women treated for breast carcinoma have been reported. Most have developed in the chest wall after mastectomy, but rare examples of parenchymal origin after breast conservation and radiotherapy have been reported.[183] The authors of the latter publication[183] cited several reports of radiation-associated fibrosarcomas of the breast, but they cautioned that "some of these tumors would be classified differently today."

The lack of well-documented cases of fibrosarcoma makes it impossible to make secure statements about the clinical behavior and optimal treatment of this type of sarcoma. Lacking well-founded information, physicians should probably evaluate and treat patients with fibrosarcomas according to the principles used for other types of mammary sarcomas.

RHABDOMYOSARCOMA

Primary rhabdomyosarcoma of the breast is a very uncommon and poorly characterized neoplasm. Most tumors in the breast with rhabdomyosarcomatous features are variants of metaplastic carcinoma, or MPT,[184] or metastases from nonmammary primary sites.[185–188] Evidence for origin in the breast parenchyma or for myomatous differentiation is questionable in most published cases. For example, three rhabdomyosarcomas classified as mammary sarcomas in one report[189] "superficially infiltrated skeletal muscle but the tumors were centered in the breast." Striations were identified microscopically in only one of the three neoplasms. The

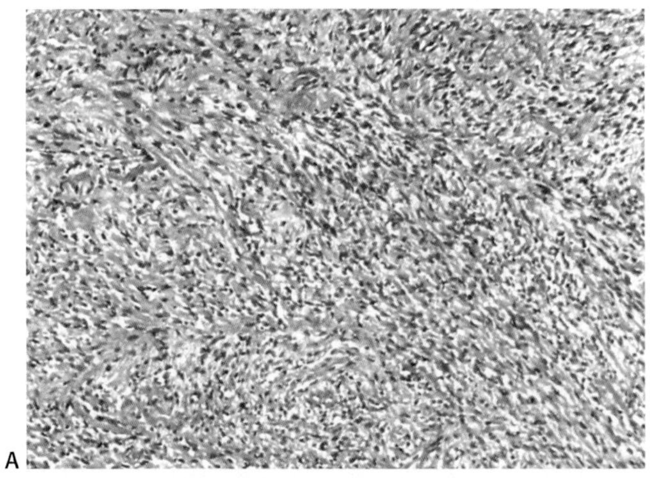

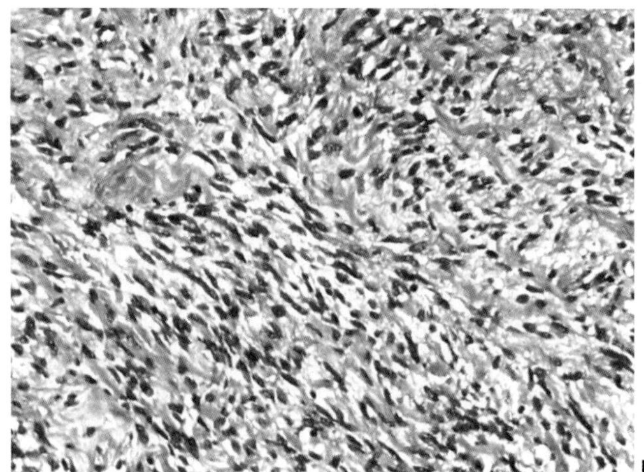

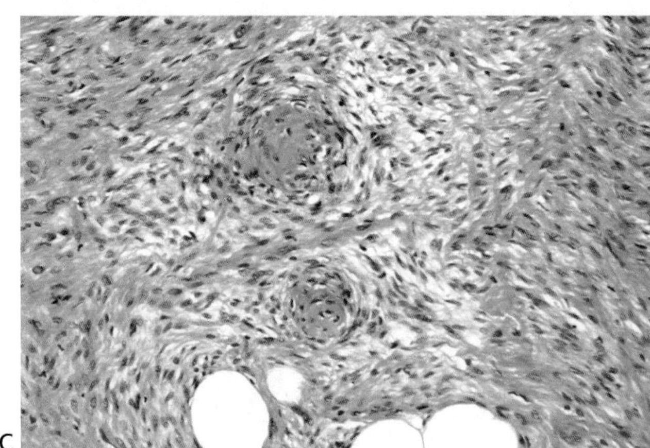

FIG. 39.13. *Fibrosarcoma, unusual findings.* **A,B:** Loosely organized groups of spindle cells are present in the collagenous stroma. **C:** The presence of focal ossification suggests that the tumor may represent a subtype of fibrosarcoma.

other two tumors had "racquet" and "strap" cells with peripherally placed nuclei. Two of the tumors recurred locally with chest wall invasion in one case. Striations were also absent from another sarcoma, which had "strap" and "racquet" cells.[184] None of these tumors was examined by electron microscopy, and the reports predate the general availability of immunohistochemistry (IHC).

Evans[190] described a 4 × 6 × 12 cm circumscribed tumor in the upper outer quadrant of a 41-year-old woman as a mammary rhabdomyosarcoma. "Primitive" cross striations were detected by special stains. The report predated the availability of IHC, and electron microscopy needed to confirm myogenous origin. Recurrence in the muscles of the ipsilateral upper arm, which occurred 32 months after mastectomy, was treated by forequarter amputation. The patient was alive 4 years after diagnosis with recurrent tumor in the supraclavicular region.

A mammary neoplasm with well-documented rhabdomyosarcomatous differentiation was reported by Woodard et al.[191] The tumor was a 5-cm mass in the central part of the breast of a 16-year-old girl. The patient remained well 11 years after mastectomy. Microscopic examination revealed rhabdomyosarcoma and a 2.3-cm FA "immediately adjacent without capsular separation." The FA was described as having "cell-poor stroma." Cross striations were seen in routine sections, and rhabdomyosarcomatous differentiation was confirmed by electron microscopy. In this instance, origin from the associated fibroepithelial neoplasm cannot be excluded.

Primary Rhabdomyosarcoma

A few primary sarcomas situated in the breast may represent genuine primary mammary rhabdomyosarcomas. The largest series comes from a group of more than 3,500 patients with rhabdomyosarcoma enrolled in the Intergroup Rhabdomyosarcoma Study.[188] Within this cohort were seven young women with apparently primary mammary rhabdomyosarcomas; they constitute less than 0.2% of the entire group. Details of the pathologic evaluation were not described in the publication. Nine other reports[192–200] give details of 10 additional cases. In seven, the rhabdomyomatous nature of the malignant cells was established using immunohistochemical staining for myoglobin, myogenin, or MyoD1. The tumor in one case[194] contained the *FKHR–PAX3* fusion gene, in another[196] the sarcoma contained the typical transcripts for the *FKHR–PAX3* fusion gene, and cells in the final case[195] demonstrated convincing cross striations. Clinical evaluations did not disclose sites of origin beyond the breasts.

All patients in these reports were female and 13 of 17 were between the ages of 13 and 17 years. Four women were 30, 45 or 46, 46, and 51 years old at the time of diagnosis. The patients usually recounted the presence of a growing mass. Physical examinations detected nontender masses, usually mobile, without alterations of the overlying skin or nipple. Clinical enlarged ALNs were noted in one patient.[199] Sonography of one tumor[194] revealed a well-demarcated mass with irregular internal echoes, and CT scanning revealed a huge mass with rich blood flow. In another case,[197] an ultrasound study demonstrated a "slightly lobulated, discretely inhomogeneous, hypoechoic tissue density mass." Using MRI, the mass had high signal intensity on the T2- and nonenhanced T1-weighted images, and dynamic studies showed early enhancement with the formation of a peripheral, strongly vascularized ring. On late dynamic scans, the mass filled completely, but the peripheral hyperintense ring persisted.

On macroscopic examination, the tumors in the adolescents ranged from 3 to 21 cm in size and those in the adults were smaller (2.5, 3.4, and 4.5 cm). Pathologists described the tumors as round to oval, soft or firm, unencapsulated masses composed of grayish yellow, gray, or white tissue. The presence of necrosis was recorded in one description.[195] Microscopical study showed the typical histologic features of rhabdomyosarcoma occurring in conventional sites. The sarcomas were categorized as embryonal in eight of these cases, and alveolar in the remaining nine. The embryonal rhabdomyosarcomas were composed of pleomorphic cells showing varying degrees of skeletal muscle differentiation (Figs. 39.14A, B), whereas tumors classified as alveolar featured small, round to oval cells with scant cytoplasm growing in nests separated by collagenous septa (Figs. 39.14C, D). Extensive involvement of ALNs was present in 6 of the 17 cases. Seven of the 14 patients for whom follow-up data were available succumbed to their rhabdomyosarcoma between 4 and 28 months following presentation.[188,193,194,196,199] The remaining seven patients were reportedly free of disease between 6 and 34 months from the time of diagnosis.[188,192,195,197]

Metastatic Rhabdomyosarcoma

Metastatic rhabdomyosarcoma in the breast is usually the alveolar type in children and young adults.[185,186,188,196,201–203] Mammary involvement is most often a manifestation of widespread metastases (see Chapter 34). Five patients with mammary metastases had primary tumors of the perineum.[185,187,201] A review of 19 patients whose initial site of metastases was the

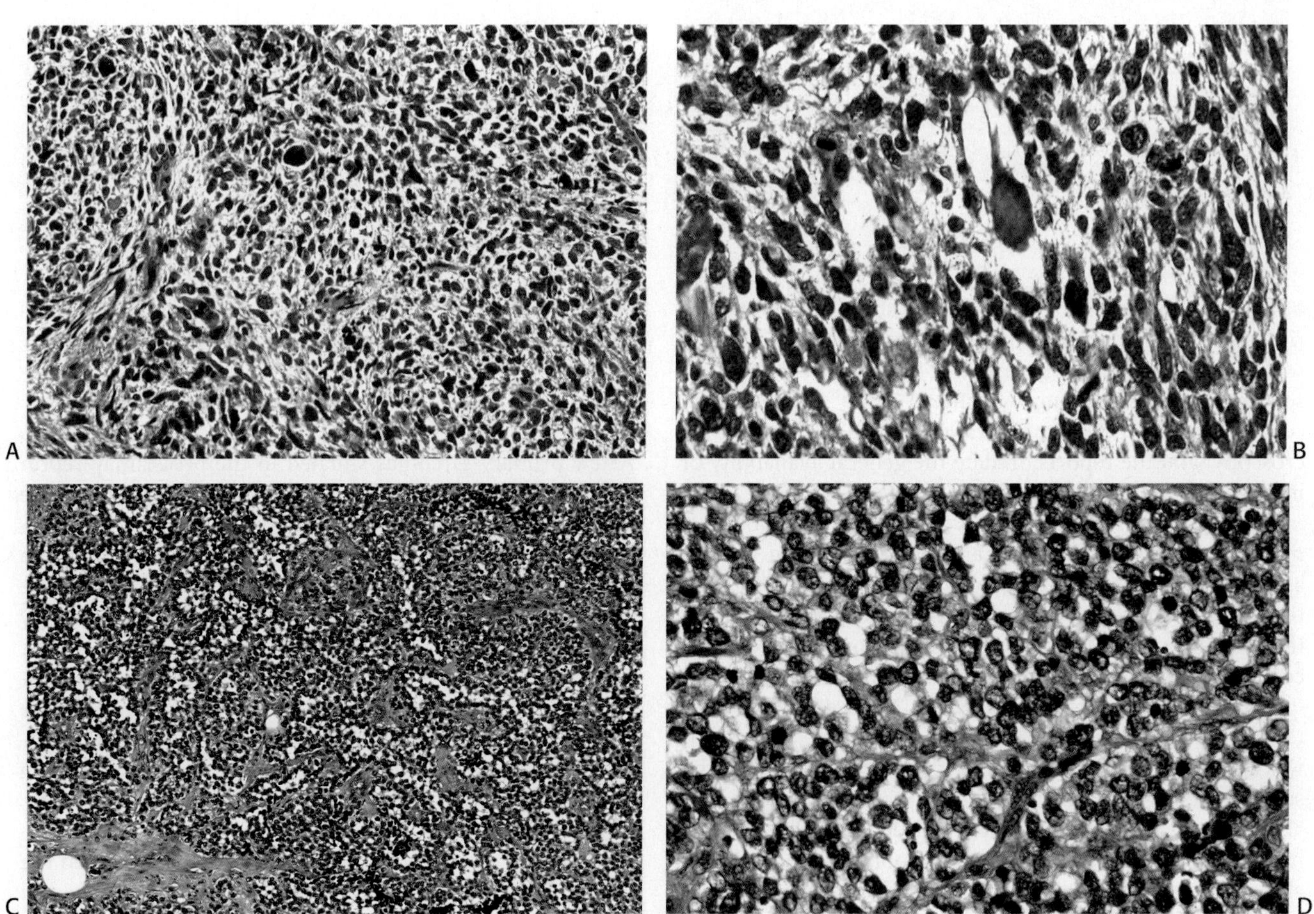

FIG. 39.14. ***Rhabdomyosarcoma, embryonal and alveolar.*** **A,B:** Strap cells with eosinophilic cytoplasm are distributed in this embryonal rhabdomyosarcoma. **C,D:** This primary alveolar rhabdomyosarcoma in the breast of a 13-year-old girl consists of nests of loosely cohesive small cells with scant cytoplasm. The cells stained for myogenin and myo D1 (not shown).

breast revealed the following distribution of initial primary tumors: extremity, 8 cases; nasopharynx/paranasal sinuses, 7 cases; and trunk, 4 cases.[188] The histologic subtype was alveolar in 18 determinate cases. The median age at diagnosis of the primary tumor was 15.0 years. Three patients were alive and disease-free after follow-up of 7.6, 15.7, and 17 years. In another series[196] of seven young women with metastatic rhabdomyosarcoma involving the breast at presentation, the primary site was an extremity in three patients, the retroperitoneum, vagina, and breast in one patient each, and unknown in one patient. Once again, the histologic subtype was exclusively alveolar. The mean age at diagnosis was 14.6 years. All the patients died of their disease with a median survival time of 20 months (range, 15 to 48 months). Rarely, the breast metastasis is the presenting manifestation of a previously undiagnosed nonmammary rhabdomyosarcoma.[203]

Histologically, metastatic alveolar rhabdomyosarcoma is composed of small round-to-oval cells that form poorly defined aggregates in the mammary parenchyma. Mitoses are easily identified. The differential diagnosis, which includes malignant lymphoma and invasive lobular carcinoma, can be readily resolved with immunohistochemical studies for myoid, epithelial, and lymphoid differentiation.

The cytologic appearance of rhabdomyosarcoma in the breast of an adolescent has been reported.[204] The smears contained two types of malignant cells. More numerous were small cells with irregular, hyperchromatic, and eccentric nuclei containing coarsely clumped chromatin and finely vacuolated cytoplasm. Isolated large cells resembling rhabdomyoblasts contained multiple nuclei, prominent nucleoli, and granular eosinophilic cytoplasm forming bipolar processes. Myoid differentiation was confirmed with a positive staining for myoglobin. The patient had bilateral mammary and axillary involvement as well as left inguinal metastases. This pattern of involvement suggests that the mammary tumors were metastatic in origin, and clinical work-up did not exclude a nonmammary primary.

In one report, two tumors with clinical and histologic features compatible with metastatic alveolar rhabdomyosarcoma in children were immunoreactive for vimentin and α-sarcomeric actin; negative for desmin, myoglobin, and α-SMA; and did not have "distinct crossbanding" when studied by electron microscopy.[203] The tumors from six patients with metastatic alveolar rhabdomyosarcoma in a recent series[196] had transcripts from the *FKHR–PAX3* fusion gene.

HEMANGIOPERICYTOMA (SOLITARY FIBROUS TUMOR)

Hemangiopericytoma, an uncommon mesenchymal neoplasm derived from the pericytes of blood vessels, was characterized in 1942 by Stout and Murray.[205] This type of tumor arises in the soft tissues throughout the body. The breast is an uncommon site, with fewer than 30 cases documented in published reports.[206–212] The report of Kanazawa et al.[212] lists clinical and pathologic features of 25 cases reported in the English and Japanese literature.

During the past decade, pathologists who specialize in diseases of the soft tissues have noted morphologic similarities between hemangiopericytomas and cellular regions of solitary fibrous tumors.[213] Citing these common features, these pathologists have come to believe that hemangiopericytomas represent examples of solitary fibrous tumors. This conceptual change has not taken hold for tumors arising in every tissue site, and publications still appear referring to tumors of the breast as hemangiopericytomas.

Clinical Presentation

With the exception of a 7-year-old girl and a 5-year-old boy,[214] the patients were adults. They include three men aged 24,[215] 40,[207] and 60 years[216] and women from 22 to 70 years.[212] The patients presented with enlarging painless masses, which occurred in the left and right breasts with equal frequency. The masses usually had been present for a few weeks or months, but symptomatic intervals as long as 1 year have been noted.[217] Examining physicians described the masses as irregular and firm. The overlying skin displayed "reddish discoloration" and erosion in one case,[212] and the vessels beneath the skin overlying the mass appeared prominent in another patient.[218]

Imaging Studies

Mammography reveals a well-circumscribed dense mass lacking calcifications.[219,220] In one case,[220] the radiologist could identify a vascular pedicle entering the tumor. Sonography demonstrates a solid hypoechogenic mass with heterogeneous internal echoes and posterior enhancement.[219,220] The borders have appeared well-defined in several cases and partly ill-defined in another.[221] Doppler sonography in one case showed a highly vascular tumor continuous with a large blood vessel within the mass.[220] Using MRI, one tumor had inhomogeneous low intensity and partial intermediate to high intensity on T1-weighted images and inhomogeneous high signal intensity on T2-weighted images.[217] The regions of high intensity correlated with foci of hemorrhage and those of intermediate intensity to areas of necrosis.

Hemangiopericytomas originating from the buttock,[222] retromastoid tentorium,[223] and eye[224] have metastasized to the breast after intervals from 10 months to 11 years, and one arising in the retroperitoneum has spread to both breasts 6 years after treatment of the primary tumor.[225]

Gross Pathology

These well-circumscribed round-to-oval tumors consist of firm to hard homogeneous pale yellow, gray, or white tissue. The cut surface may have a whorled texture with dilated vascular spaces and a nodular contour. The diameters ranged from 1[208] to 20 cm,[211] and the average size was 6.5 cm.

Microscopic Pathology

The histologic features are identical to those of hemangiopericytoma in other sites. The tumor is composed of round,

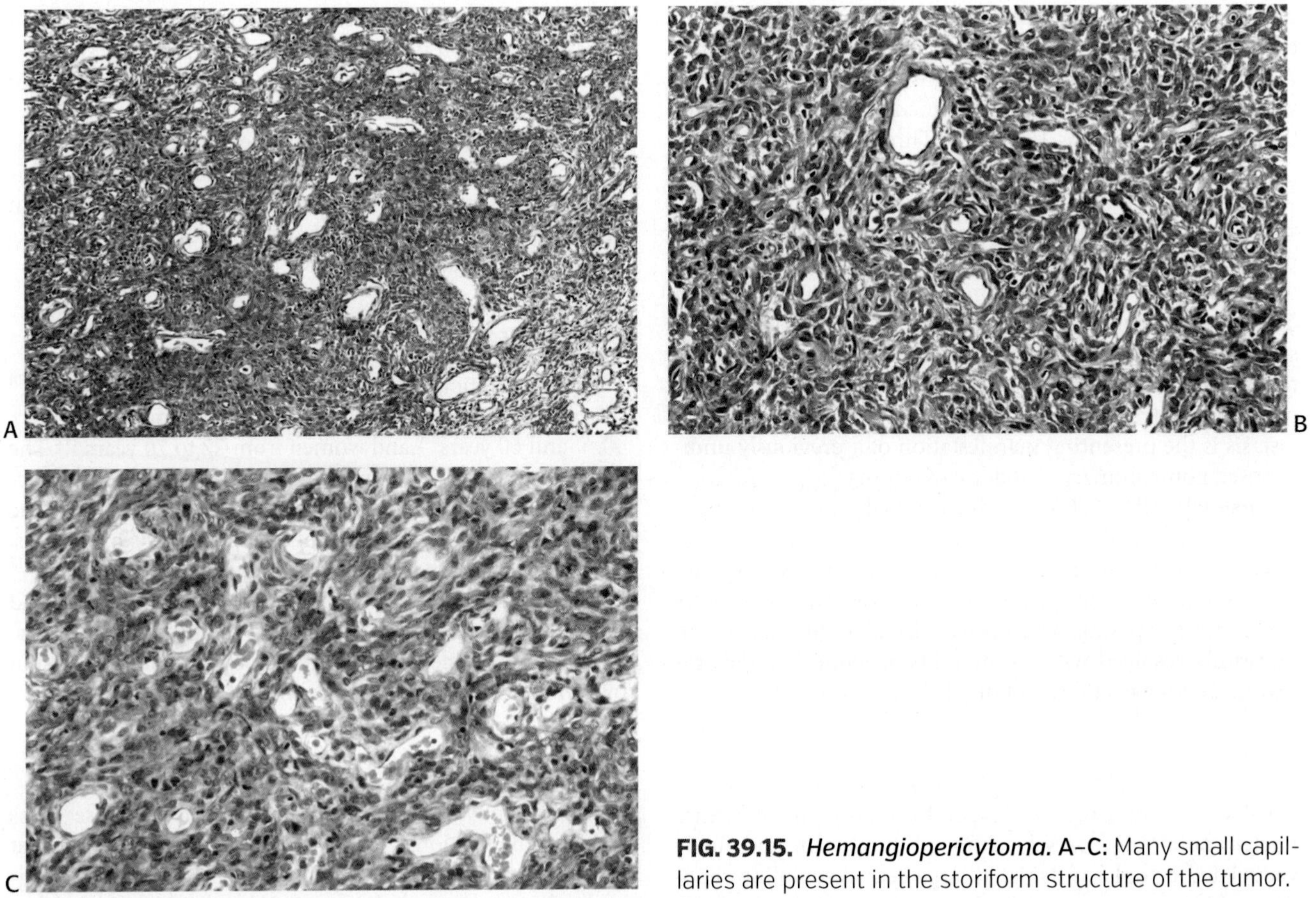

FIG. 39.15. *Hemangiopericytoma.* **A–C:** Many small capillaries are present in the storiform structure of the tumor.

plump, oval, and spindle cells oriented around vascular channels of varying caliber (Fig. 39.15). The vessels often have a branching or "staghorn" configuration. More compact zones have a spongiform appearance. The endothelium is supported by a reticulin stroma without appreciable collagen or actin-positive cells (Fig. 39.16). Focal fibrosis occurs in scattered patches and may be especially prominent at the tumor margin where atrophic breast tissue compressed by the expanding tumor tends to form a pseudocapsule. In one case,[225] preexisting mammary lobules became incorporated into nodules of metastatic hemangiopericytoma, and the presence of glandular spaces within the tumor created diagnostic confusion. Perivascular fibrosis is variably present (Fig. 39.17). Areas of necrosis rarely occur in mammary hemangiopericytomas.

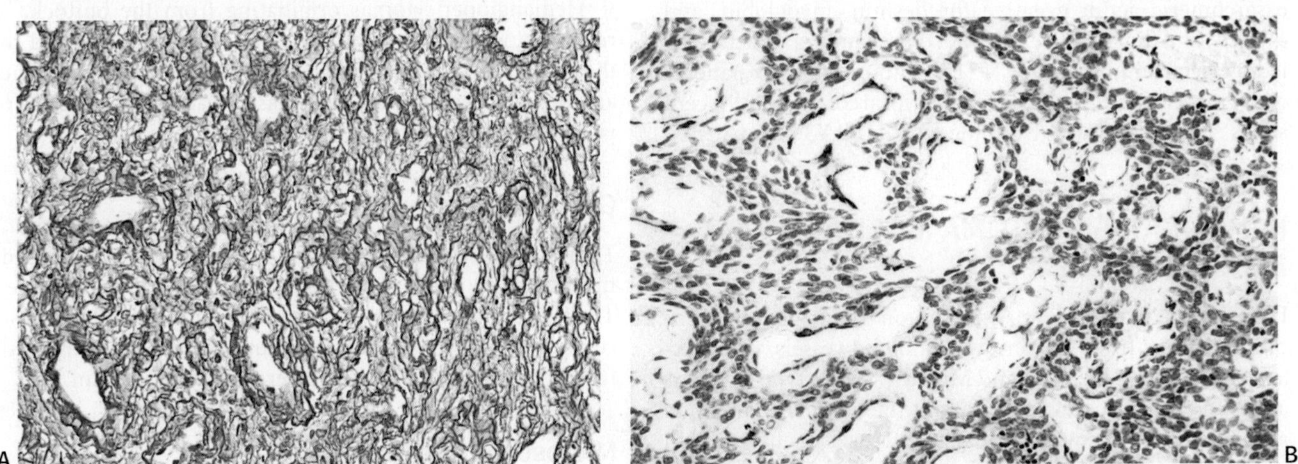

FIG. 39.16. *Hemangiopericytoma.* **A:** Cellular elements and vascular spaces are outlined by a network of reticulin fibers (reticulin stain). **B:** Scant SMA immunoreactivity is limited to cells lining small blood vessels.

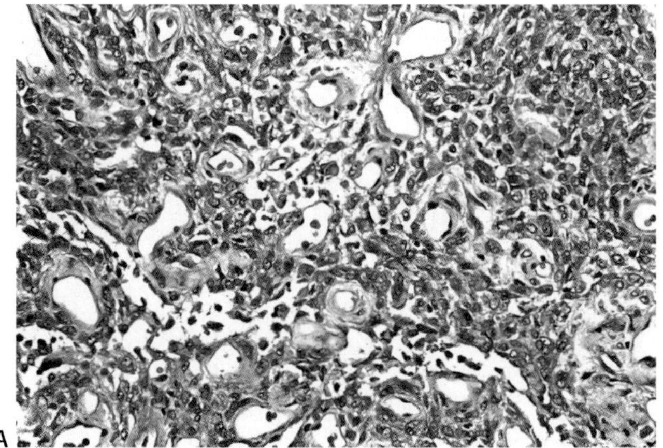

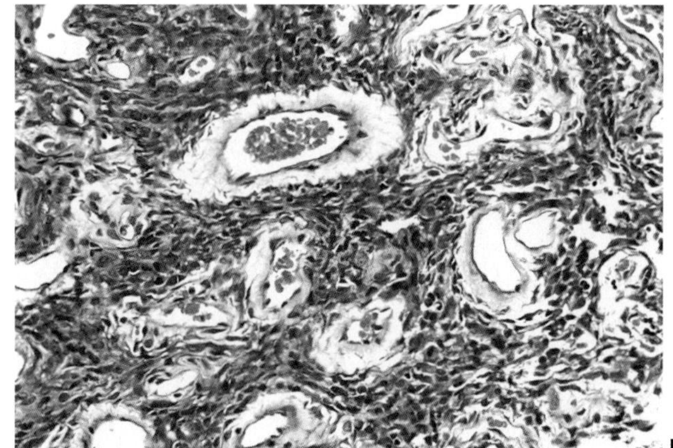

FIG. 39.17. *Hemangiopericytoma.* **A:** Thin bands of collagen outline some vascular structures. **B:** Conspicuous collagen bands surround the larger vascular channels.

The tumor cells are distributed in compact sheets, bands, and trabeculae around and between the vascular spaces. Mitoses are infrequent in most mammary hemangiopericytomas, and the cells lack other cytologic features of a high-grade sarcoma such as anaplasia and pleomorphism.

Cytology

Cytologic specimens obtained by FNA appear cellular and contain dispersed cells and clumps of tissue and dispersed single cells in a bloody background. The neoplastic cells exhibit spindle to oval shapes and possess ovoid hyperchromatic nuclei, inconspicuous nucleoli, and scant cytoplasm with indistinct cell borders. The smears also demonstrate abundant capillaries, some very large, lined by apparently normal endothelial cells. The appearance is suggestive of a mesenchymal neoplasm but is not specific for hemangiopericytoma.[207] Similar findings were reported in a metastatic hemangiopericytoma involving the right breast of a 48-year-old woman.[222]

Immunohistochemistry

Endothelial cells of the capillaries are immunoreactive for *Ulex europaeus* 1 lectin (UEA-1), factor VIII, CD34, and CD31, and CD34 reactivity has been found in the tumor cells. Reactivity for vimentin[206,208,217] has been observed in tumor cells, and in isolated cases, the tumor cells have stained for CD99, factor VIII, and SMA.[215] Variable staining for actin and CD117 has been reported.[206,208,215,221] In isolated cases, the tumor cells did not stain for factor VIII–related antigen, EMA, cytokeratin, S-100, HMB45, MART1, CD10, CD31, CD68, UEA-1, α_1-antitrypsin, SMA, and desmin.[212,215,217]

Electron Microscopy

Electron microscopy of two breast tumors revealed neoplastic pericytic cells closely apposed to the endothelial cells.[208,212] An incomplete basal lamina surrounded tumor cells, which were characterized by complex interdigitating cytoplasmic processes with pinocytotic vesicles and microvilli. Scattered nonspecific cellular junctions were identified. The cells contained oval nuclei, sparse organelles, and fine microfilaments. Dense bodies and plaques were absent. Myofibrils were seen in one case.[212] The electron microscopic appearance is the same as that of hemangiopericytoma at other sites,[226] and a metastatic hemangiopericytoma involving the breast demonstrated similar ultrastructural findings.[225]

Treatment and Prognosis

The diagnosis of hemangiopericytoma as a specific tumor in the breast is important because of the very favorable prognosis of this neoplasm. Other more malignant tumors may have vascular areas that resemble hemangiopericytoma. High-grade leiomyosarcoma and MFH have readily identifiable mitotic figures and structural features that distinguish these tumors from hemangiopericytoma. Metastatic sarcomatous renal carcinoma in the breast may mimic mammary hemangiopericytoma, and rarely hemangiopericytoma originating at another site may metastasize to the breast.[224]

Reported follow-up varies from less than 12 to 276 months. Approximately equal numbers of patients have been treated by mastectomy and local excision. No patient had metastases detected in an ALN dissection. None of the patients described in published reports has developed a local recurrence whether treated by local excision or mastectomy, with follow-up as long as 23 years and averaging 5 years. One patient treated with a modified radical mastectomy for a 5.5-cm malignant hemangiopericytoma apparently confined to the breast succumbed to disease involving the bones, brain, lungs, pleura, skin, and liver 14 months from the time of diagnosis.[227] The Senior Editor has seen an example of a mitotically active high-grade hemangiopericytoma of the breast that resulted in pulmonary metastases (Fig. 39.18). As a consequence, mammary hemangiopericytomas that lack high-grade features such as necrosis or numerous mitoses should be considered low-grade neoplasms. Treatment can be conservative, with emphasis on wide local

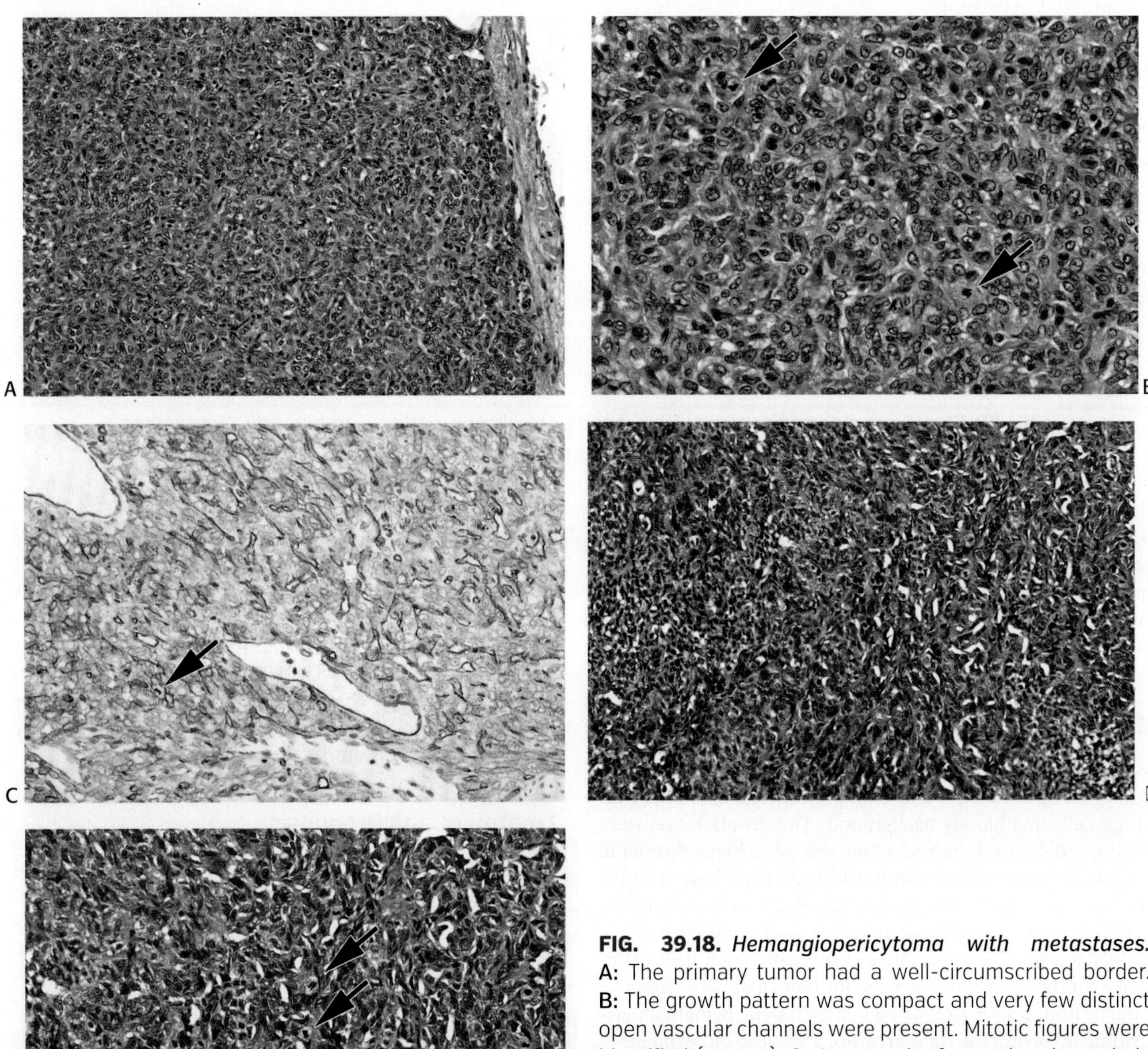

FIG. 39.18. *Hemangiopericytoma with metastases.* **A:** The primary tumor had a well-circumscribed border. **B:** The growth pattern was compact and very few distinct open vascular channels were present. Mitotic figures were identified (*arrows*). **C:** A network of vascular channels is highlighted in the primary tumor by the immunostain for CD34. The *arrow* indicates a mitotic figure. **D,E:** The appearance of a pulmonary metastasis approximately 2 years after excision of the breast tumor. Mitoses are present (*arrows*).

excision rather than mastectomy if an adequate margin can be achieved with an acceptable cosmetic result. Axillary dissection is not indicated for mammary hemangiopericytoma.

DERMATOFIBROSARCOMA PROTUBERANS

DFSP, a tumor that arises in the skin and subcutaneous tissue, is not a primary breast neoplasm. However, the distinction is not always readily apparent clinically and treatment may involve mastectomy. Histologic study of most examples reveals features indicating an origin in the skin, but rare cases apparently originated within the mammary parenchyma.

Clinical Presentation

DFSP arises throughout life. Ahmed et al.[228] described a case in a 2-year-old girl and postulated that it had been present since birth, and Cottier et al.[229] reported a tumor in a 75-year-old woman. The average age is approximately 40 years. Although most cases have afflicted women, a 41-year-old man developed a DFSP.[230] The tumor may arise more commonly in African Americans.[231]

Patients describe the presence of a mass, sometimes of long duration. In one case,[232] a 74-year-old woman presented with a mass that had existed for 20 years and may have represented a recurrence of a "benign" mass removed 50 years earlier. Patients sometimes describe recent increase in the size of the mass.[233–235] They usually do not complain of pain, although it can develop after several years.[231] One patient[236] was taking estrogen replacement therapy, and another[237] noted changes in the skin of the breast attributable to the tumor during pregnancy. In one case,[238] the tumor arose within a surgical scar, and in another[239] the mass appeared in the field of irradiation delivered 75 years before.

Physical examination demonstrates a firm, well-defined, usually mobile, nontender mass. In some cases, it formed a polypoid nodule protruding from the skin surface.[239–241] The overlying skin can appear normal, red, or ulcerated,[241,242] and sometime it is tethered to the mass.[243] In one case,[244] the lesion was described as a "red plaque with an irregularly shaped lustrous central nodule." The presence of two or more nodules has been noted.[230,238] The relatively superficial involvement of the breast may provide a clue to suggest the diagnosis of DFSP.

Imaging Studies

The imaging characteristics of DFSP have received much attention. Lee et al.[231] reported the radiologic findings of five cases and listed those reported in five earlier studies. Several later case reports add additional details.[229,230,238,241,243,245] Mammography has shown well-defined, dense masses without calcifications. Most lesions appear skin-based, but intraparenchymal lesions have been described.[231,246] On sonography, the masses typically appeared well-defined, oval, and parallel to the skin surface, although Liu et al.[245] and Lin et al.[235] illustrated examples with ill-defined margins. Several tumors displayed lobulations of the posterior or lateral borders. The internal echo pattern has been variable, and acoustic enhancement has been described.[231,238,247,248] Doppler studies demonstrated highly vascular masses.[229,238] MRI usually shows a signal isointense to breast parenchyma on T1-weighted images and a hyperintense signal on T2-weighted images,[231,241] but some variation in the signal intensity on T2-weighted images has been noted.[230,243] In one case,[243] multivoxel proton (hydrogen 1 [1H]) MR spectroscopy using a voxel size of 0.5 cm^3 did not disclose a choline peak.

Gross and Microscopic Pathology

The excised tumor consists of firm white to tan tissue with a grossly well-defined border. The sizes have ranged from 0.9[246] to 7.7 cm[234] and one multinodular mass measured 10 cm.[238] Microscopically, the neoplasm is composed of uniform spindle cells arranged in a very prominent storiform pattern (Fig. 39.19). Mitotic figures are not usually conspicuous, although Zee et al.[249] noted a "moderately high" mitotic rate, and Tsang et al.[250] counted 2 to 3 mitotic figures per 10 HPFs. Giant cells are not a characteristic feature of this neoplasm.

Cytology

Direct smears and cytospin preparations of needle aspiration specimens reveal numerous monomorphic spindle cells arranged in a vaguely storiform pattern.[249,250] The cells contain oval or spindly nuclei, fine chromatin, inconspicuous nucleoli, and pale cytoplasm with indistinct borders. Mitotic figures are not seen, and the background does not show myxoid material or evidence of inflammation or necrosis.

Immunohistochemistry

Immunohistochemical studies have reported positive reactions for CD34 in all cases, and the few tumors tested have all stained for vimentin. Staining for S-100,[229,230,234,236,237,239,246] actin,[246,250] SMA,[230,234,236,237,239,251] desmin,[230,239,246,251] and CD31[229,237,246] has been negative. Staining for miscellaneous proteins such as cytokeratin, factor XIII A, EMA, HMB45, ER, PR, brst-2, CD31, CD68, CD99, c-kit, and bcl-2 has been negative in isolated examples.[230,234,236,237,239,246,251]

Genetic Studies

Like DFSP arising at other sites, those involving the breast possess a characteristic translocation (t(17;22)(q22;q23)) in which the *COL1A1* and *PDGFB* genes form a fusion gene. It most commonly resides on a supernumerary ring chromosome with other genetic material from chromosomes 17, 22, and possibly others. One can detect the fusion gene by chromosome analysis[228] and fluorescence *in situ* hybridization (FISH) analysis,[228,234] and the products of the *COL1A1/PDGFB* fusion gene by reverse transcription–polymerase chain reaction (RT–PCR).[236]

Treatment and Prognosis

These tumors do not metastasize, but they frequently recur if not completely extirpated. The neoplastic stromal cells tend to penetrate deeply into surrounding tissue, and this phenomenon makes it imperative to remove wide margins of apparently uninvolved tissue. Mastectomy is usually necessary for large bulky tumors. Local excision, sometimes using special techniques,[252] may be attempted for smaller lesions. In rare cases, such as the one described by Kim et al.,[232] the tumor can evolve into a fibrosarcoma. Development of a "herringbone" pattern of growth, increased cellularity, increased mitotic activity, necrosis, and loss of reactivity for CD34 would indicate such an event.

Most recurrences occur within a few years, but they can come to attention in as little as 6 months,[245] and recurrences after long interval have been observed. Swan et al.[237] described a case in which the tumor recurred after 26 years, Dragoumis et al.[247] recounted a patient with a recurrence after 13 years, and one patient in the series published by Lee et al.[231] suffered recurrences 11 and 17 years from the time of diagnosis. Recurrence-free survival as long as 15 years has been reported.[242,253]

Except for the case in which a fibrosarcoma emerged from a DFSP,[232] adjuvant radiation treatment has not played a role in the treatment of this tumor. Imatinib mesylate, an inhibitor of the platelet-derived growth factor receptor-associated tyrosine kinase, has demonstrated clinical activity in the treatment of advanced cases of DFSP at other sites and might offer a therapeutic option for problematic tumors originating in the breast.

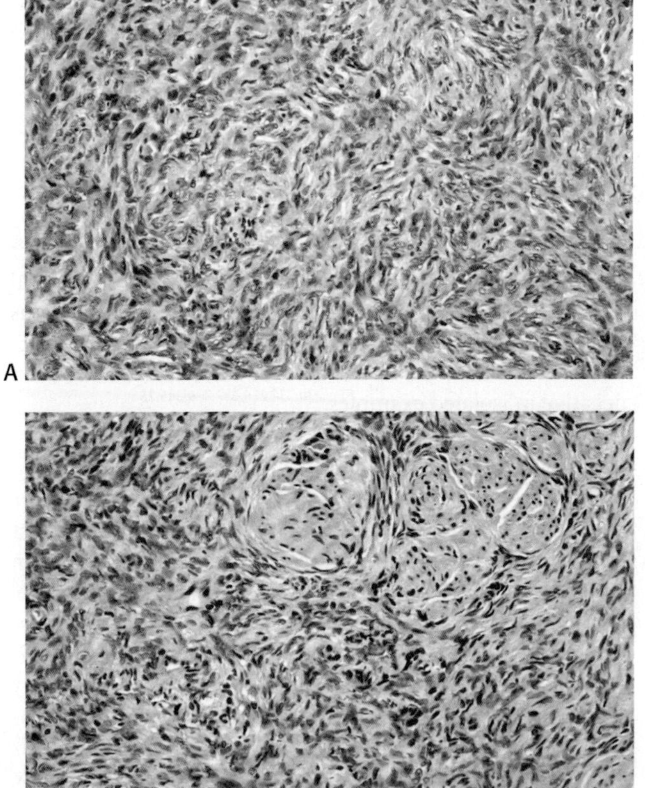

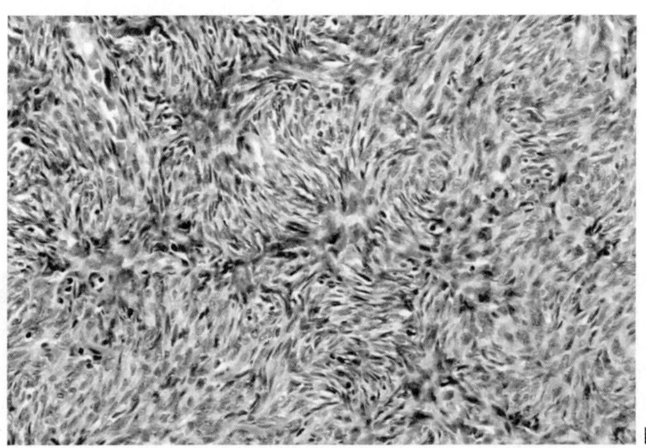

FIG. 39.19. *Dermatofibrosarcoma protuberans.* **A:** The tumor was located in subcutaneous tissue of the breast near the areola and invaded the nipple. **B:** The storiform pattern is shown. **C:** The tumor surrounds smooth muscle bundles in the nipple. An actin immunostain was not reactive in the tumor.

SARCOMAS OF PERIPHERAL NERVES

These sarcomas consist of cells whose morphologic features resemble those of the cells comprising the supporting sheath of peripheral nerves. In most tumors, the neoplastic cells exhibit characteristics of Schwann cells, but occasionally the tumor cells resemble perineurial fibroblasts. Mammary malignant peripheral nerve sheath tumors can arise in the setting of von Recklinghausen disease,[254,255] but they also develop in its absence. Six case reports[256–261] describe examples of malignant peripheral nerve sheath tumors in patients lacking stigmata of von Recklinghausen disease, and several series[262–265] list cases without providing details. The tumor described by Thanapaisal et al.[261] presented unusual features.

The patients' ages were between 19[261] and 65 years.[257] The latter patient was a man, and the series of Visfeldt and Scheike[264] includes a man with a "neurogenic sarcoma." One patient recounted a 15-year symptomatic interval.[259] Mammography demonstrated dense masses with lobulated[258] or mostly smooth borders.[259,260] Sonography revealed variable echo patterns with posterior enhancement.[258,260] The masses measured 1.2 to 6.5 cm in greatest dimension. To the unaided eye, they appeared "unencapsulated" and "grey white." A histologic and cytologic study[256] revealed malignant tumors composed of spindle cells with pleomorphic and hyperchromatic nuclei displaying numerous mitotic figures. One tumor[257] contained melanin and stained for HMB45. Immunohistochemical reactivity for vimentin and S-100 protein was described in three cases.[255–258] Two tumors stained for NSE,[256,261] and one expressed S-100 protein, neurofilaments, and glial fibrillary acidic protein.[261]

Treatment consists of complete excision without removal of ALNs. Adjuvant radiation may reduce the likelihood of recurrence.

MISCELLANEOUS SARCOMAS

The literature contains six reports of "primitive neuroectodermal tumor" (Ewing family of tumors) arising in the breast.[266–269b] The patients' ages range from 26[269b] to 60[268] years and the maximum dimension of tumors from 1.8[269] to 12 cm.[267] Radiologic studies of a tumor that came to attention 3 months after an episode of trauma were interpreted as showing a hematoma or cyst.[268] In another patient,[269b] the imaging studies suggested the diagnosis of fibroadenoma. One tumor was described as "well-circumscribed" and "brownish,"[269] and another[269a] as "grayish tan, fish flesh like, and slightly friable." Histologic study and cytologic examination[269] revealed neoplasms composed of small, round, undifferentiated cells. In all six cases,[266–269b] the diagnosis of primitive neuroectodermal tumor was confirmed by immunohistochemical staining for CD99 (MIC2), and three tumors[266,268,269] demonstrated the presence of the characteristic t(11;22)(q24;q12) translocation using FISH, RT–PCR, or karyotype analysis. Except in one case considered inoperable at presentation,[267] treatment consisted of complete surgical excision and chemotherapy. One tumor proved rapidly fatal,[266] one patient suffered a relapse 2 years after presentation,[267] and four patients were reportedly free of disease after intervals of 6 to 36 months.

A 49-year-old woman with a primitive neuroectodermal tumor of the back developed two metastatic foci in the upper outer region of the left breast and in ipsilateral ALNs.[270] Based on the radiologic findings, a diagnosis of breast carcinoma with axillary metastases was suggested, but core biopsy of the nodules and the lymph nodes revealed metastatic primitive neuroectodermal tumor. A 30-year-old woman developed multiple bilateral breast masses in the setting of disseminated primitive neuroectodermal tumor.[270a] The primary site was not established.

"Alveolar soft part sarcoma" involving the right breast of a 16-year-old girl was described by Luna Vega et al.[271] The patient presented with a 4-cm painless subareolar mass that was reportedly "present without change for years." The tumor involved the underlying pectoral muscle, necessitating total mastectomy and partial resection of the affected muscle. Wu et al.[272] reported another case in a woman aged 44 years. The recognition of the nature of this neoplasm was confounded by the presence of prominent xanthomatous features. Immunohistochemical staining demonstrated the presence of TFE3 protein. Bilateral pulmonary metastases were detected at the time of presentation, and a brain metastasis became evident 30 months from the time of diagnosis. One case is included in the series of Pollard et al.[273]

Metastatic alveolar soft part sarcoma in the breast has been described in four women between the ages of 18 and 29 years.[274–277] The primary sites were the left thigh (two cases), posterior left axilla, and left buttock. In one patient,[274] detection of the mass in the breast led to the discovery of the primary tumor in the thigh and of metastases in other organs. The other patients developed metastatic mammary masses between 7 months[275] and 7 years[277] from the time of diagnosis. In the latter instance, metastases appeared in both lungs prior to the detection of the breast mass.

A "malignant mesenchymoma" in a 61-year-old woman was treated by simple mastectomy, and the patient died of lung metastases 7 months after diagnosis.[278] Histologically, the tumor consisted of myxoid stroma; spindle cell sarcoma with osteoid, bone, and cartilage; and liposarcomatous elements.

Two cases of synovial sarcoma have been described.[279,280] A 36-year-old woman developed a huge, osteolytic pelvic lesion in the left ilium 2 years after a mastectomy for a "spindle cell" sarcoma. Both the primary sarcoma and the ilial mass

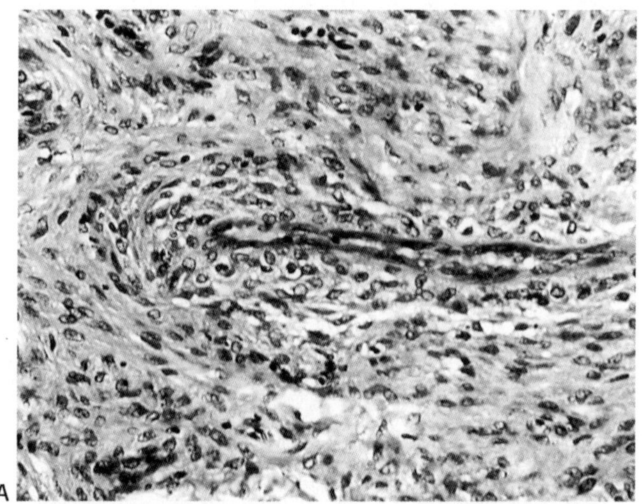

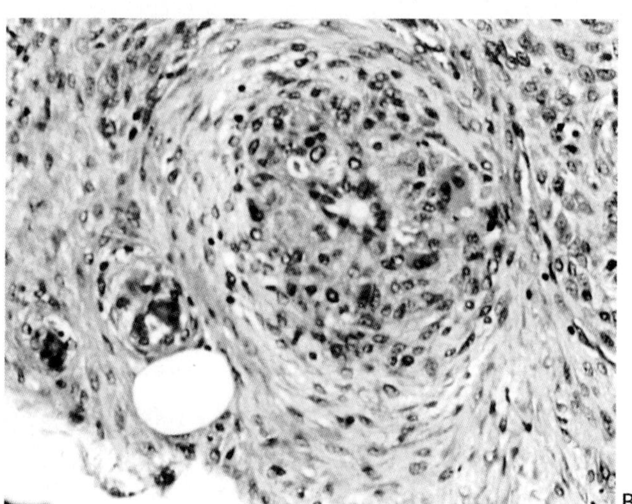

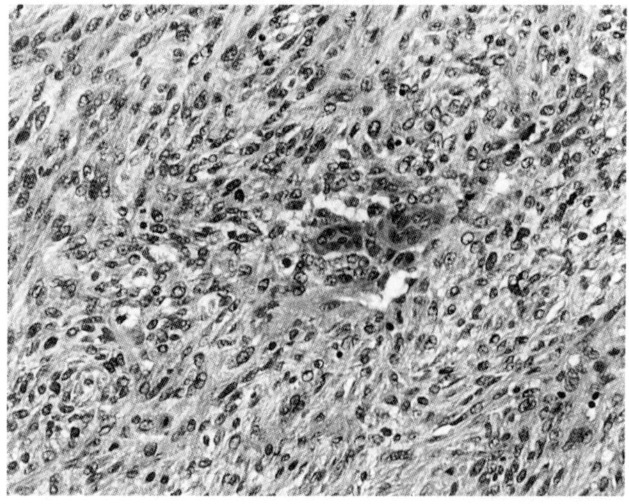

FIG. 39.20. ***Angioblastic sarcoma.*** **A:** A conspicuous feature of this sarcoma is the perivascular proliferation of atypical cells and the prominence of endothelial cells with hyperchromatic nuclei. **B:** A transverse section of a vessel similar to the one in (A) showing the circumferential orientation of neoplastic cells and small multinucleated cells. **C:** A capillary obscured by multinucleated histiocytoid cells is shown in the *center*.

demonstrated the t(X;18)(p11;q11) translocation characteristic of synovial sarcoma.[280]

Several tumors with a plexiform growth pattern and the histologic appearance of "angioblastic sarcoma" have been encountered in the breast (Fig. 39.20).

The literature contains several reports of sarcomas classified as "myofibroblastic sarcomas."[281–284] Low-grade myofibroblastic sarcoma features pleomorphic hyperchromatic invasive spindle cells associated with areas of pseudoangiomatous stromal growth and sparse mitoses (Fig. 39.21), whereas high-grade myofibroblastic sarcomas have more abundant mitoses and a less well-defined pseudoangiomatous structure. The tumors are variably immunoreactive for CD34, actin, calponin, and desmin. In the case reported by Taccagni et al.,[284] the diagnosis of myofibroblastic sarcoma was confirmed by electron microscopy and IHC. The patient died of metastatic tumor 11 months after diagnosis. A 60-year-old man with at 2.5-cm myofibroblastic sarcoma was described by González-Palacios et al.[281] Histologic examination revealed a spindle cell neoplasm in which the tumor cells had "faintly eosinophilic cytoplasm" and a mitotic rate of 10 per HPF. A mastectomy was performed. There were no nodal metastases. During the ensuing 10 years, the patient had five local recurrences, which were treated by excision. Invasion of skeletal muscle was documented in one recurrence.

Kaposi sarcoma is exceedingly uncommon as a primary tumor of the breast. Ng et al.[285] reported secondary involvement of the breast in a 33-year-old HIV-positive man, who initially presented with skin lesions on the abdomen and hip. The mammary lesions consisted of a cutaneous rash and an underlying 2-cm mass in the breast as well as two masses in the axilla. The diagnosis of Kaposi sarcoma in the breast was confirmed by biopsy.

A myxoid variant of follicular dendritic cell sarcoma originating in the breast has been described.[286]

ANGIOSARCOMA

Angiosarcoma arises in the breast more often than in any other organ. It occurs in two forms, sporadic angiosarcoma and postirradiation angiosarcoma. Although these two forms of angiosarcoma exhibit many common features, the tumors differ in certain clinical, histologic, immunohistochemical, and therapeutic respects.

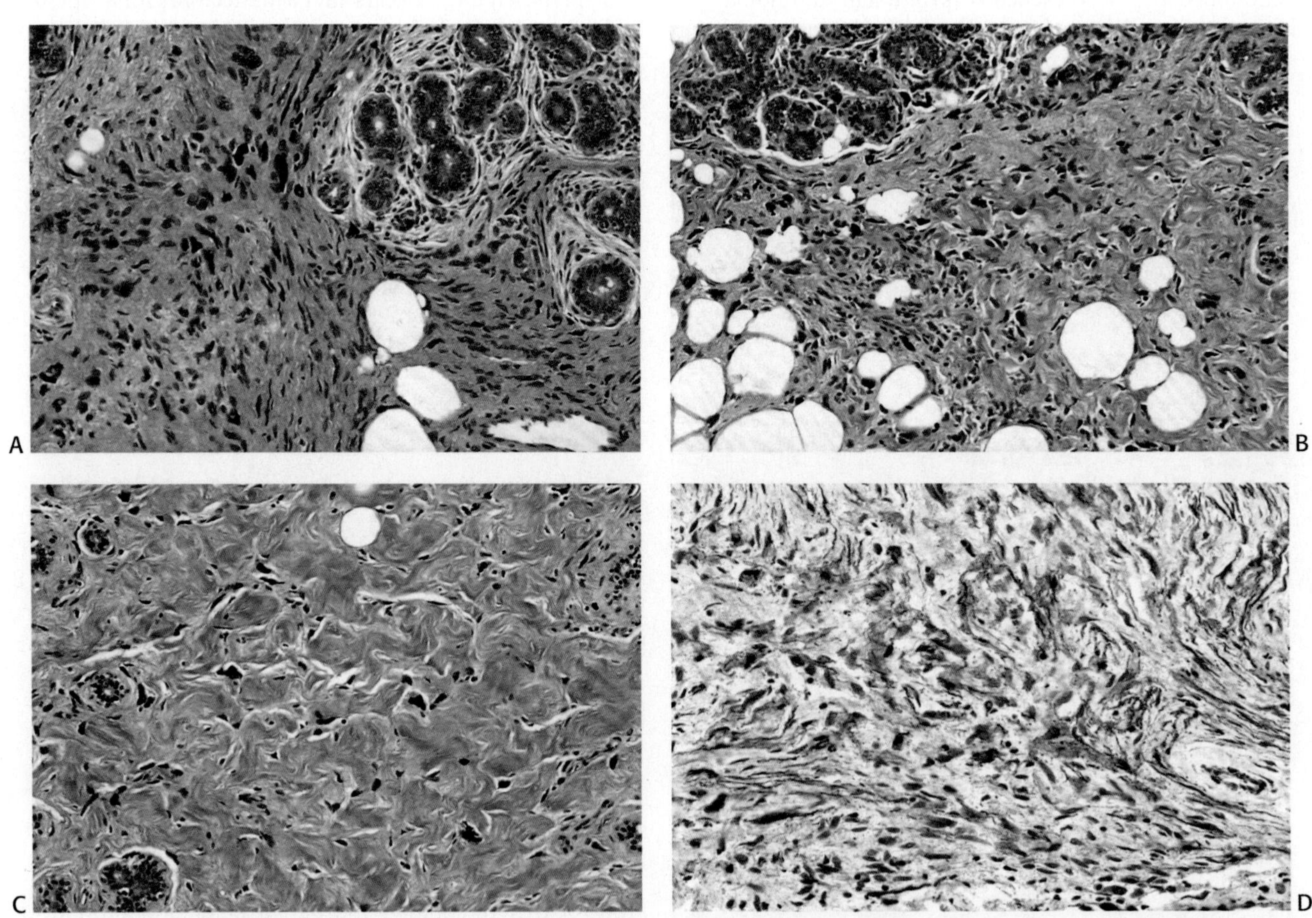

FIG. 39.21. *Myofibroblastic sarcoma.* **A,B:** Pleomorphic and hyperchromatic spindle cell tumor cells involve perilobular and intralobular stroma. Traces of pseudoangiomatous architecture are evident in perilobular stroma in **(B)**. **C:** Myofibroblastic sarcoma with pseudoangiomatous stromal growth pattern. **D:** The tumor cells are immunoreactive for SMA. **E:** Immunoreactivity for CD34 is shown in tumor surrounding a small duct. **F–H:** Another myofibroblastic sarcoma showing fascicular growth **(F,G)** and partially epithelioid cytology with a mitotic figure (*arrow*) in a tadpole-shaped cell **(H)**.

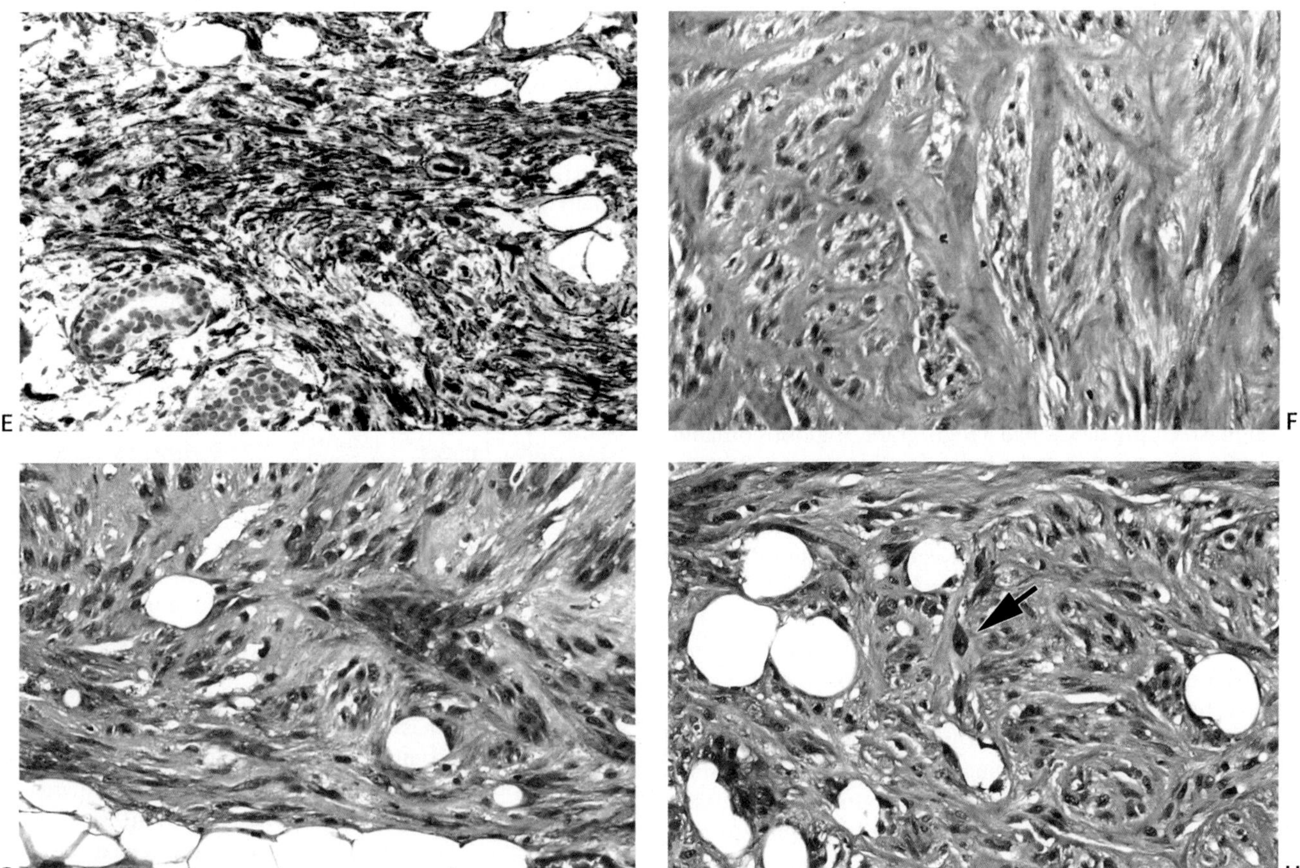

FIG. 39.21. *(Continued)*

Sporadic Angiosarcoma

Clinical Presentation

Sporadic angiosarcoma afflicts women almost exclusively. Only four well-documented instances of angiosarcoma in men have been reported.[287–290] A fifth case is questionable because the patient had systemic metastases at the time of presentation of the tumor in the breast, there was clinical evidence of bone metastases 2 years earlier, and photographic support for the diagnosis is not convincing.[291] The details provided in a putative sixth case[292] do not establish the diagnosis of angiosarcoma conclusively. Two publications[293,294] mention in passing seemingly the same man with angiosarcoma, but the papers do not describe either the clinical or the pathologic details of this case.

The age at diagnosis ranges from the teens[287,295–299] to 91 years[300] with a mean age of 34[296] and a median of 38 to 39 years.[287] In view of the relative youth of patients with sporadic mammary angiosarcoma, it is not unexpected that a number of the patients were also pregnant.[287,301–304] Coexistent pregnancy was present in 4 (6%) of 63 cases in one series.[287]

With rare exceptions, sporadic angiosarcoma presents as a painless mass. Patients usually report the presence of symptoms for only a short time, but symptomatic intervals as long as 5 years have been described.[288] Antecedent trauma has been noted by some authors,[305] but there is no convincing evidence to implicate injury as an etiologic factor. Trauma may draw attention to an already existing tumor, especially if hemorrhage in the lesion causes it to enlarge. Angiosarcomas at various somatic sites have been associated with foreign body material retained for many years.[306] Two reports[307,308] described angiosarcomas associated with breast implants, and a third case described an angiosarcoma that involved the site of silicone injection carried out many years previously for cosmetic purposes.[309]

The left and right breasts are involved with nearly equal frequency. Concurrent bilateral angiosarcomas are very uncommon.[296,310–314] Contralateral breast involvement is usually evidence of metastatic spread, often the first site of metastasis to be identified.[295,299,301,314–316]

Physical examination often discloses a mass or a region of swelling, but in some cases there are no external features to suggest angiosarcoma. Blue or purple discoloration of the skin reflecting hemorrhage or the vascularity of the lesion accompanies large or superficial tumors. Blistering was noted in one case,[317] and large angiosarcomas can present as fungating masses.[318]

The Kasabach–Merritt syndrome, a condition characterized by consumptive thrombocytopenia and typically seen as a complication of angiomas in infants and children, has been attributed to angiosarcoma of the breast in four case reports.[319–322] One series described nonneoplastic thyroid disease in 30% of patient with mammary angiosarcoma.[288]

Angiosarcoma and Other Neoplasms

Rarely, sporadic angiosarcoma and mammary carcinoma have coexisted in the same breast.[323] In one unusual case, mastectomy revealed coexistent, concurrent adenocarcinoma and angiosarcoma in a breast that had chronic lymphedema 4 years after segmental mastectomy without radiotherapy for carcinoma.[300] Coincidental angiosarcoma and infiltrating lobular carcinoma in the same breast were reported in a 59-year-old woman.[324] A 33-year-old woman with a high-grade invasive ductal carcinoma (IDC) treated with mastectomy developed a high-grade angiosarcoma in the operative site 8 months following the surgery. Review of the mastectomy specimen revealed a 0.5-cm focus of angiosarcoma identical to the recurrence close to the invasive carcinoma.[325] Ryan and Kealy[326] reported the case of a 43-year-old woman who underwent a mastectomy for an angiosarcoma and presented 5 months later with metastatic carcinoma in an ALN. Re-examination of the mastectomy specimen disclosed an overlooked poorly differentiated IDC. Asynchronous contralateral mammary carcinoma has been described in three women. Two patients had contralateral carcinoma treated by mastectomy prior to developing angiosarcoma.[287,327] In the third case, right breast carcinoma had been treated by lumpectomy and radiotherapy 5 years before angiosarcoma was detected in the left breast.[328] A 44-year-old woman with a germline *BRCA2* mutation developed an angiosarcoma at the site of a mastectomy performed 3 years before for an IDC. Postmastectomy irradiation had not been administered.[329] The Senior Editor has reviewed slides from a 17-year-old girl with concurrent low-grade angiosarcoma and MPT in one breast.

Malignant neoplasms at sites other than the breast have been found in patients with mammary angiosarcoma only rarely. These include malignant lymphoma,[287,288] Hodgkin lymphoma,[287] and pulmonary adenocarcinoma.[287]

Imaging Studies

Radiologic imaging studies often do not demonstrate distinctive findings. In one study,[330] mammography failed to demonstrate 7 (33%) of 21 lesions, and Yang et al. [331] reported that 3 (19%) of 16 angiosarcomas evident using ultrasonography and MRI were not detected by mammography. Angiosarcomas not evident on mammograms tend to display a low histologic grade.[330] When detected by mammography, the tumor can appear as only a focally asymmetric region or as a mass. Those forming a mass can have either ill-defined or circumscribed borders and round, oval, or lobulated shapes.[330,332] The masses usually lack spicules. Calcifications occur in approximately 10% of cases[330] Several authors have reported nonspecific mammographic alterations.[316,333–335] Rarely, nonpalpable angiosarcomas measuring less than 3 cm have been detected by mammography, but most small nonpalpable vascular lesions have proven to be hemangiomas.[336]

Ultrasonography demonstrates variable findings.[312,316,320,330,332,333,335,337] Sonograms usually disclose the tumor, which can appear as either a mass or a region of abnormal echogenicity. The lesion can display hypoechoic, hyperechoic, or mixed patterns, and the nature of posterior acoustic phenomena varies. Tumors that appear as masses usually do not produce posterior echo phenomena; however, lesions with other echo patterns can give rise to either posterior shadowing or posterior enhancement. The latter suggests the presence of dilated vascular spaces or cystic regions.[337] Color Doppler studies typically reveal the hypervascular nature of the mass.[320,331,332]

MRI reveals a mass characterized by heterogeneously hypointense T1-weighted images and heterogeneously hyperintense T2-weighted images.[300,312,316,330,331,335,338,339] Irregular areas of high signal intensity on T1-weighted images reflect the hemorrhagic nature and heterogeneous architecture of certain tumors. Following contrast administration, T1-weighted images may demonstrate regions of high signal intensity surrounding a central zone of low signal intensity.[339] The results of dynamic studies usually demonstrate rapid initial enhancement followed by variable washout patterns.[331,335,340,341] Large vessels associated with the masses were illustrated in three cases.[332,334,339] CT scans revealed the masses in two patients.[298,332] Positron emission tomography–computerized tomography (PET–CT) scans will demonstrate the hypermetabolic nature of certain angiosarcomas.[321,332,340,342] These scans demonstrated metastatic foci in one patient,[298] but failed to detect an osteoblastic metastasis of low-grade angiosarcoma.[338]

Because patients with angiosarcoma in one breast may develop asynchronous primary or metastatic contralateral angiosarcoma, imaging studies of the opposite breast should be obtained at the time of diagnosis and periodically during follow-up.

Gross Pathology

The tumors vary in size from 0.7 to 25 cm,[311] averaging between 5.5 and 7.0 cm.[311,343,344] Very few angiosarcomas are smaller than 2 cm. There is no significant difference in the average size of high- and low-grade lesions.[311]

In many cases, angiosarcoma forms a friable, firm or spongy hemorrhagic tumor (Fig. 39.22). Areas of cystic hemorrhagic necrosis are commonly evident in large, high-grade lesions. Focal hemorrhage or hemorrhagic discoloration in the surrounding breast is usually an indication of tumor extending beyond the grossly evident mass. Some angiosarcomas exhibit little or no hemorrhage grossly (Fig. 39.23). Angiosarcomas that do not appear to be vascular grossly are generally described as poorly defined areas of thickening or induration.

Microscopic Pathology

Angiosarcomas display a variety of microscopic patterns, a phenomenon recognized as early as 1942 by Hill and Stout,[345] who stated that "malignant hemangioendothelioma can be divided into three general classes." One group consisted of cases in which the primary tumor and its metastases resembled a "simple angioma." In the intermediate type, the

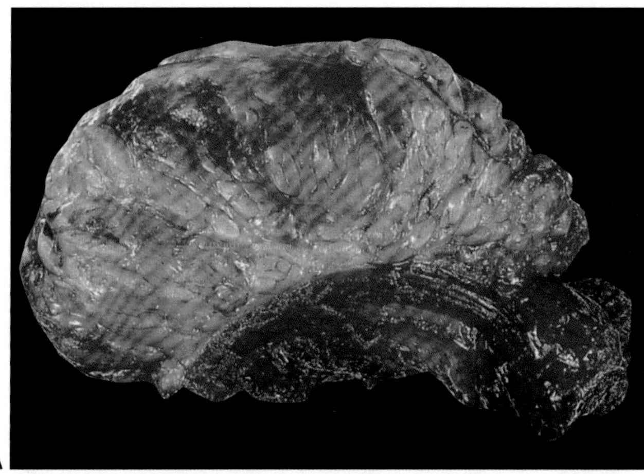

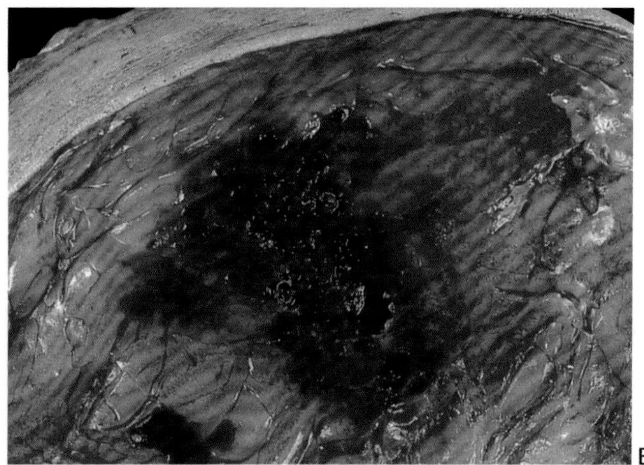

FIG. 39.22. ***Angiosarcoma, gross appearance.*** **A:** An ill-defined red mass occupies the center of the breast. **B:** A circumscribed tumor with cystic hemorrhagic foci is evident.

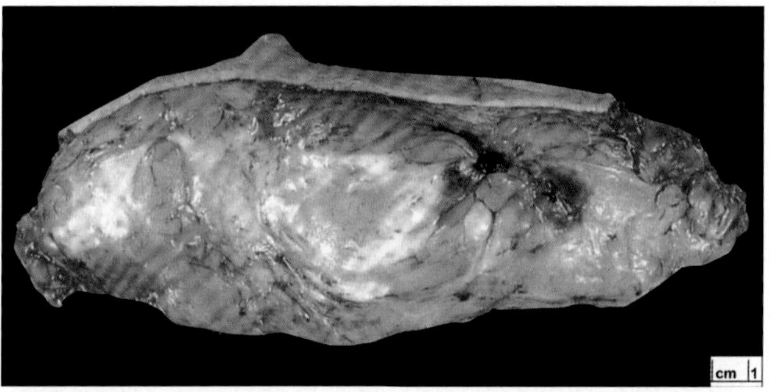

FIG. 39.23. ***Angiosarcoma, gross appearance.*** Punctate red foci of sarcoma are present throughout much of the pale fibrous and fatty breast tissue. The stellate hemorrhagic focus on the *right* is a biopsy site.

primary tumor appeared "well differentiated and innocent," but recurrent or metastatic lesions were clearly malignant. Tumors in the third group were "recognizable as malignant from the beginning."

Detailed characteristics of the three histologic patterns of growth in the primary tumor have been described (Table 39.1). These reflect the degree of differentiation and have proven to correlate with prognosis.[287,296,346]

Low-grade or type I tumors are composed of open, anastomosing vascular channels that proliferate diffusely in mammary glandular tissue and fat (Fig. 39.24). Infiltration into lobules is characterized by spread of the vascular channels within the intralobular stroma, a process that leads to separation and atrophy of the lobular glandular units (Fig. 39.25). Some prominent, hyperchromatic endothelial nuclei may be found, but the endothelial cells often have inconspicuous nuclei (Fig. 39.26). Endothelial cells are distributed in a flat single cell layer around the vascular spaces. Papillary formations are absent or at most very infrequent. Mitotic figures are rarely seen in the neoplastic endothelial cells of a low-grade tumor (Fig. 39.27). If mitotic figures are encountered with regularity in a low-grade area in a biopsy specimen, high-grade areas are likely to be present elsewhere in the tumor, the Ki67 labeling index will be greater than is

TABLE 39.1 Histologic Characteristics of Mammary Angiosarcoma

	Grade		
Histologic Features	**Low**	**Intermediate**	**High**
Lesions involving breast parenchyma	Present	Present	Present
Anastomosing vascular channels	Present	Present	Present
Hyperchromatic endothelial cells	Present	Present	Present
Endothelial tufting	Minimal	Present	Prominent
Papillary formations	Absent	Focally present	Present
Solid and spindle cell foci	Absent	Absent or minimal	Present
Mitoses	Rare or absent	Present in papillary areas	Numerous; present even in structurally low-grade areas
"Blood lakes"	Absent	Absent	Present
Necrosis	Absent	Absent	Present

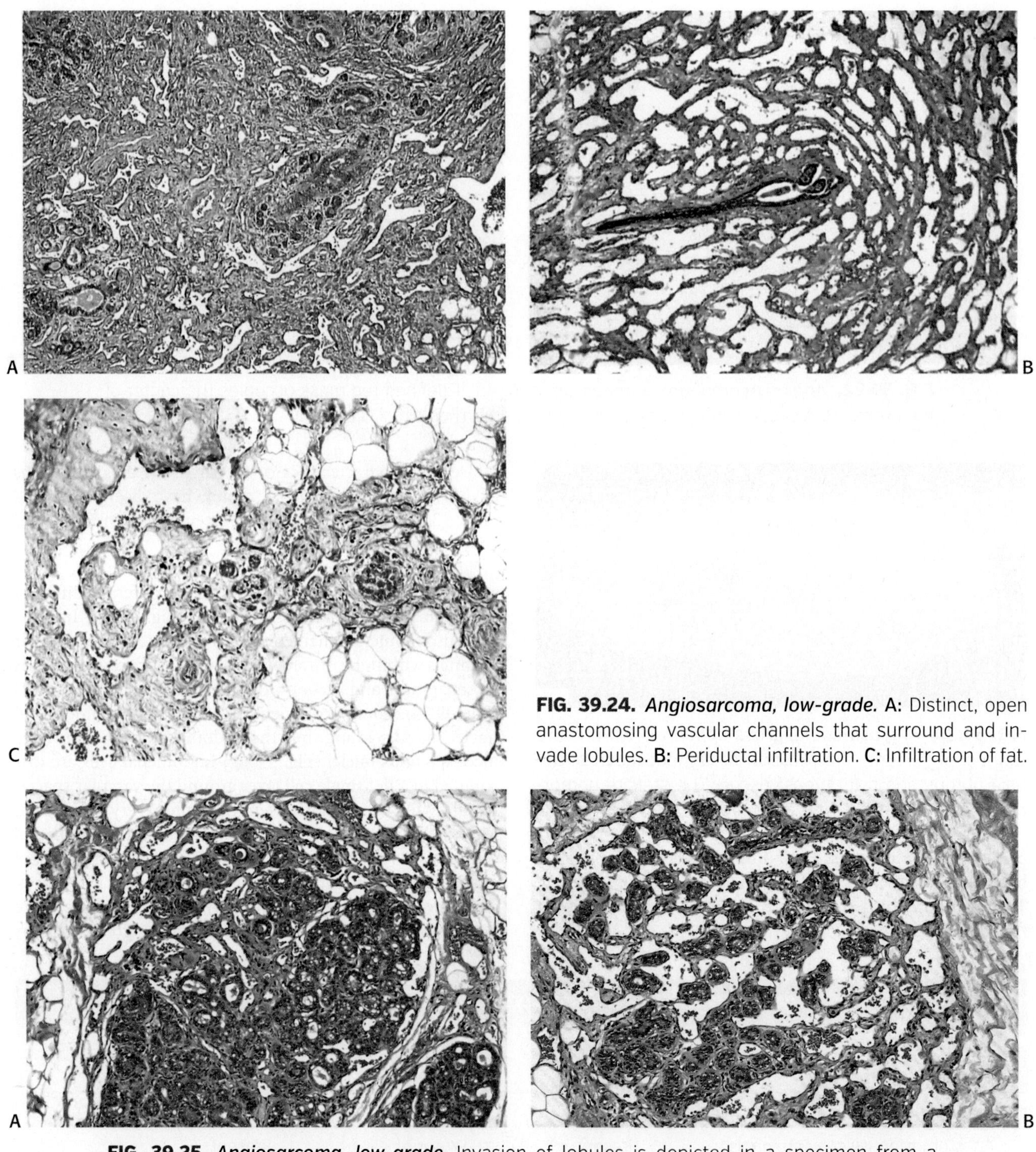

FIG. 39.24. *Angiosarcoma, low-grade.* A: Distinct, open anastomosing vascular channels that surround and invade lobules. B: Periductal infiltration. C: Infiltration of fat.

FIG. 39.25. *Angiosarcoma, low-grade.* Invasion of lobules is depicted in a specimen from a 41-year-old woman who was 6 months pregnant. A: Neoplastic capillaries in and around a lobule. Out of context, this image is indistinguishable from a perilobular hemangioma. B: Acinar units have been forced apart by the infiltrating neoplastic vessels. This appearance is not seen in perilobular hemangiomas. C: Lobular glands are dispersed in the neoplasm. D: The vascular pattern of angiosarcoma invading a lobule is highlighted by the factor VIII immunostain.

typical for low-grade angiosarcoma, and the tumor is likely to be high grade when it recurs (Fig. 39.27). The vascular lumens are usually large, open, and anastomosing in low-grade angiosarcomas. Red blood cells are typically present in small numbers, but the vessels in occasional lesions are congested.

Several unusual structural variants of low-grade angiosarcoma may be difficult to recognize. One of these is composed

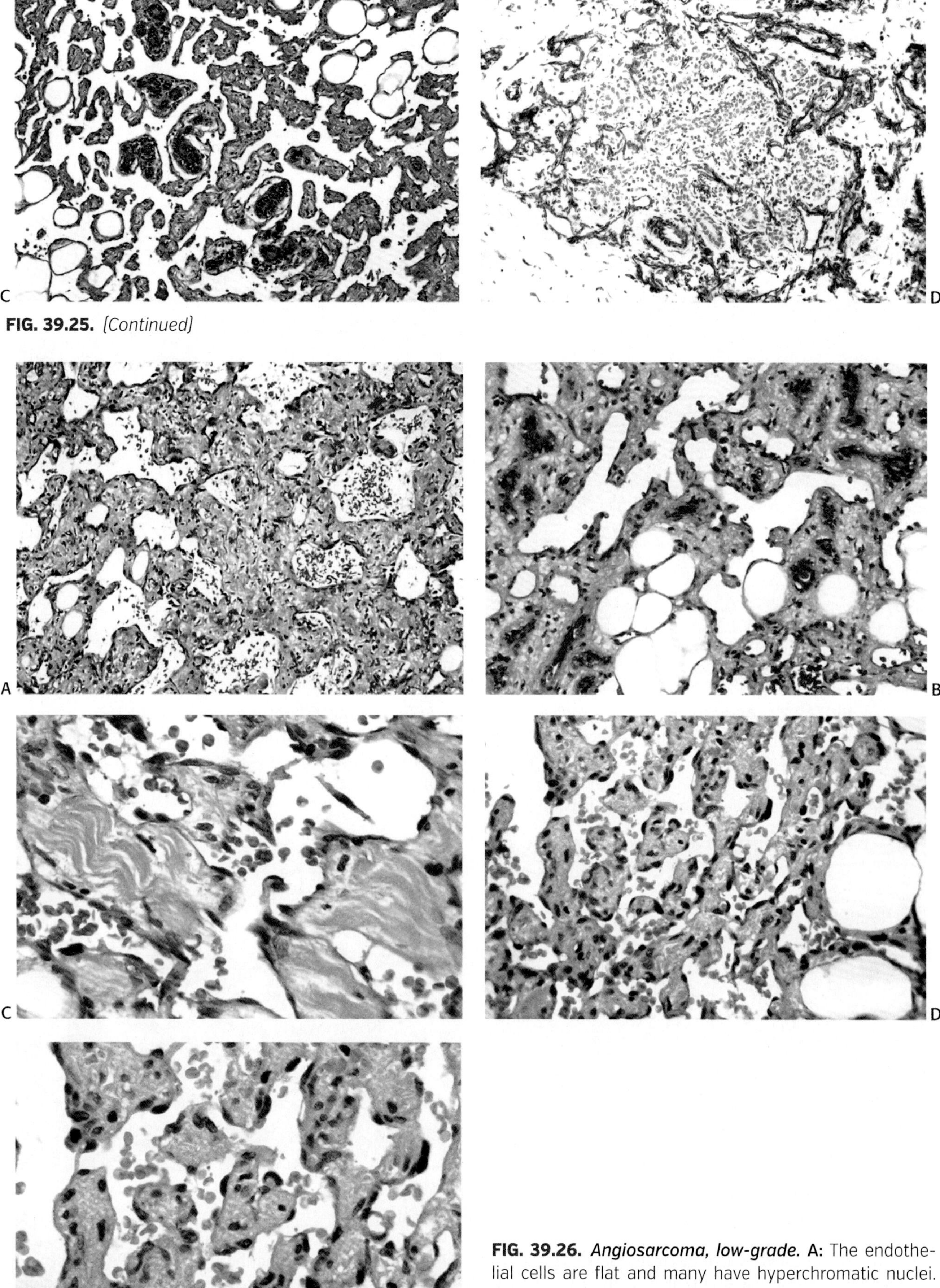

FIG. 39.25. *(Continued)*

FIG. 39.26. ***Angiosarcoma, low-grade.*** **A:** The endothelial cells are flat and many have hyperchromatic nuclei. **B:** The majority of the nuclei are pale and small. **C:** The endothelial cell nuclei are inconspicuous. **D,E:** Another tumor in which some endothelial cell nuclei are prominent.

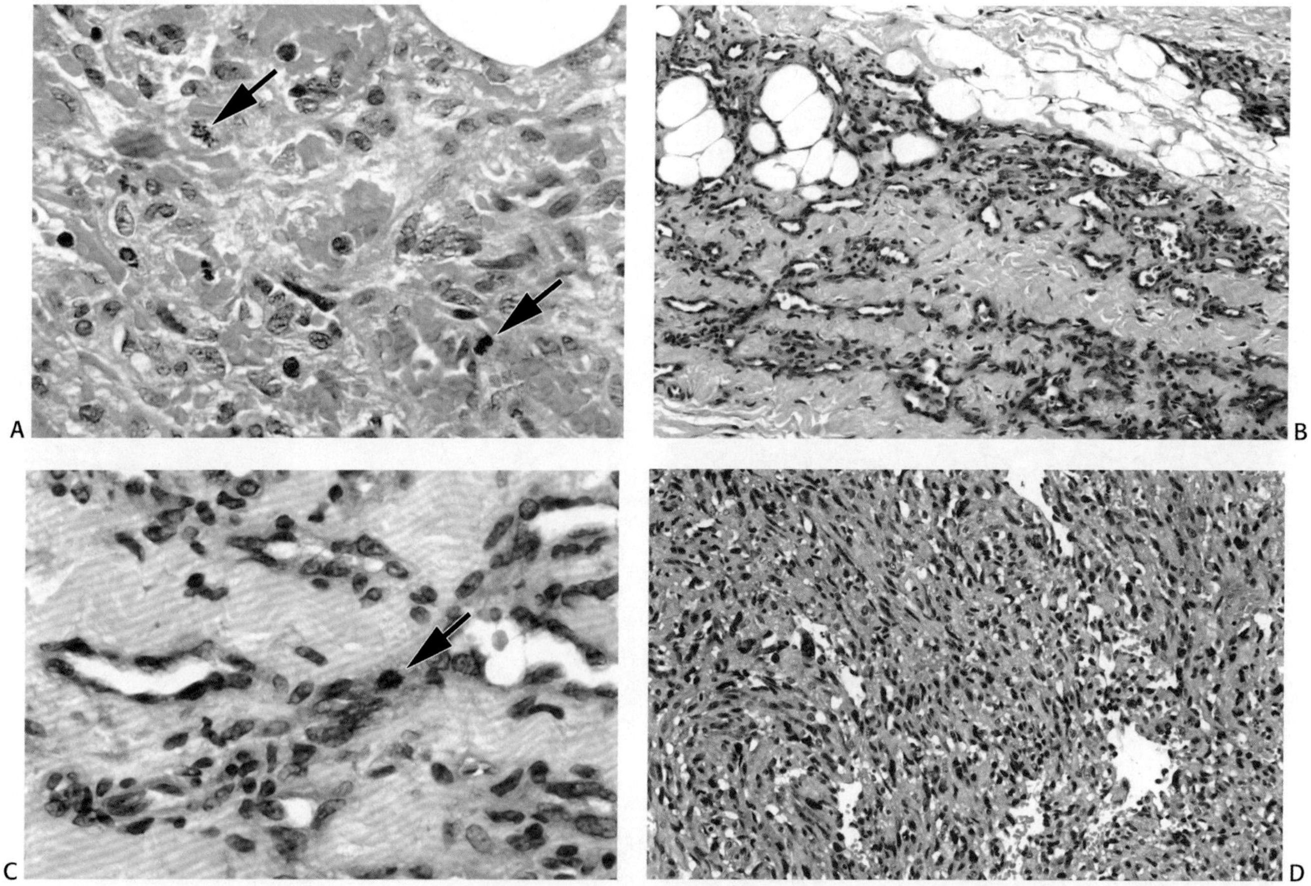

FIG. 39.27. ***Angiosarcoma, low-grade with mitoses.*** **A:** Two mitotic figures are shown in one HPF (*arrows*). The nuclei of the tumor cells are pleomorphic. This finding in a structurally low-grade appearing tumor is likely to be associated with high-grade foci elsewhere in the tumor. **B,C:** Structurally low-grade angiosarcoma with a mitosis in **(C)** (*arrow*). **D:** Metastatic high-grade angiosarcoma derived from the tumor shown in **(B)** and **(C)**.

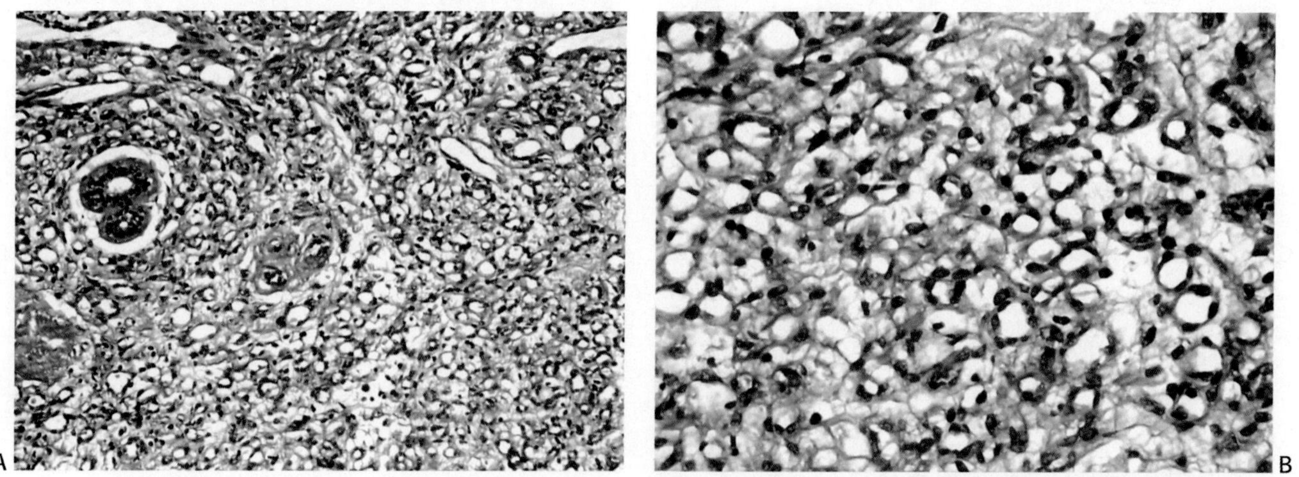

FIG. 39.28. ***Angiosarcoma, low-grade, capillary type.*** **A,B:** The neoplasm is composed of small, closely packed round capillaries, which have hyperchromatic nuclei.

predominantly of capillary-like vascular spaces (Fig. 39.28). Another type of lesion consists of small, often narrow, vascular channels without a conspicuous anastomosing structure (Fig. 39.29). The manner in which the neoplastic vessels are dispersed in the stroma may be mistaken for PASH. Diffusely infiltrating low-grade angiosarcoma composed predominantly of spindle cells may be mistaken for an angiolipoma if only a limited sample is available to examine (Fig. 39.30).

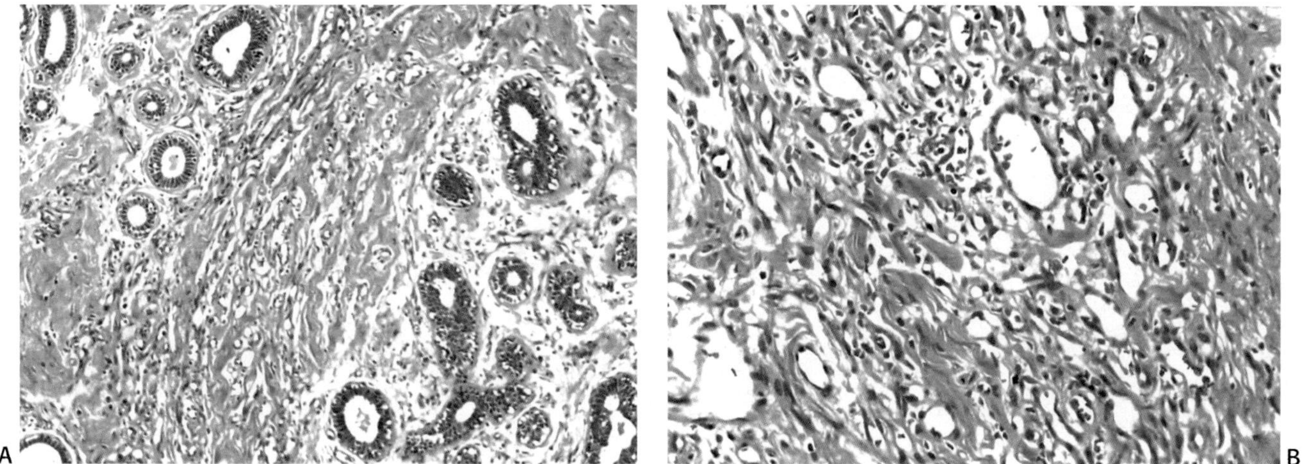

FIG. 39.29. ***Angiosarcoma, low-grade, resembling pseudoangiomatous stromal hyperplasia.*** **A:** Small round and elongated vascular structures infiltrating the collagenous stroma are shown. There is a tendency to spare lobules. **B:** The vascular spaces vary in size and shape. Anastomoses are not conspicuous.

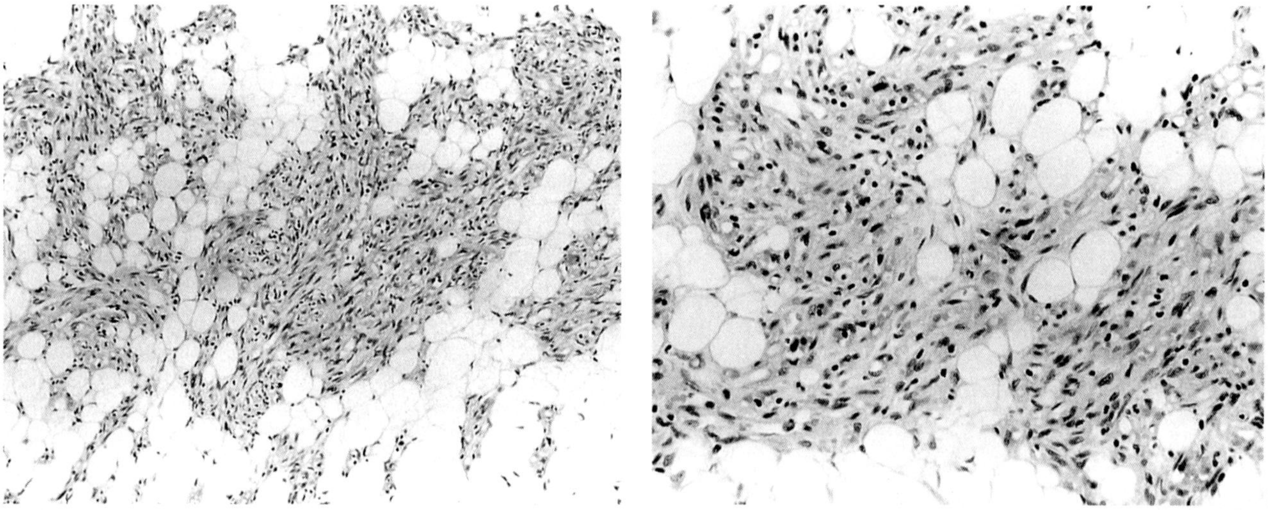

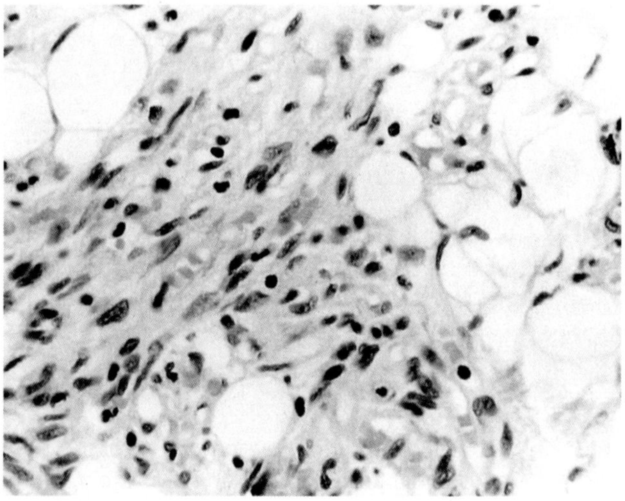

A B

C

FIG. 39.30. ***Angiosarcoma, low-grade, resembling angiolipoma.*** **A:** Irregular, interconnected sheets of small spindle cells infiltrating fat form the basic structure. **B,C:** Ill-defined small vascular lumens that contain red blood cells are present among the spindle cells. **D,E:** Low-grade angiosarcoma in fat with congested capillaries, which was mistakenly diagnosed as angiolipoma.

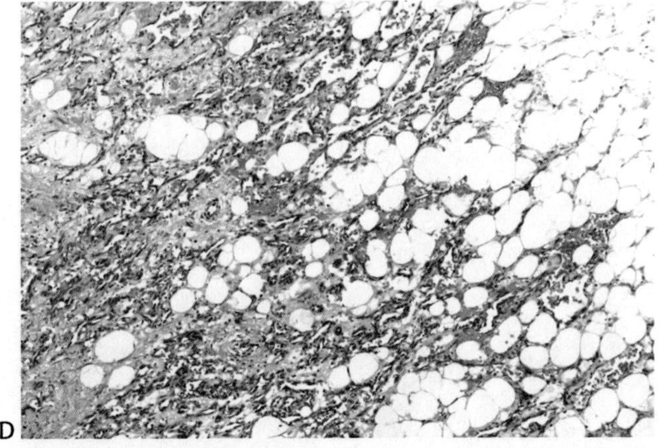

FIG. 39.30. *(Continued)*

The amount of stroma formed in low-grade angiosarcomas varies to a considerable degree. In most instances, little stroma is formed and the lesion consists largely of vascular channels permeating the mammary parenchyma. In a minority of low-grade angiosarcomas, there is focal or diffuse collagenous stroma (Fig. 39.31). Despite their more dense appearance, these lesions qualify as low-grade tumors if there is no endothelial proliferation and mitoses are sparse or not detectable.

Low-grade components are found in intermediate- and high-grade lesions, sometimes comprising the bulk of the tumor. This is particularly true for type II or intermediate-grade angiosarcomas, which are distinguished from low-grade tumors by having scattered focal areas of more cellular

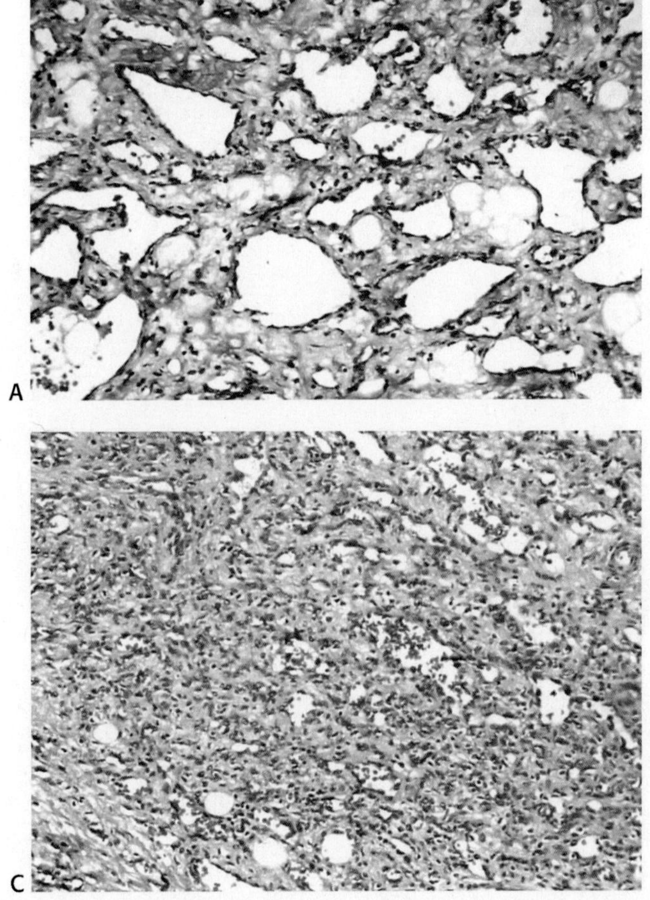

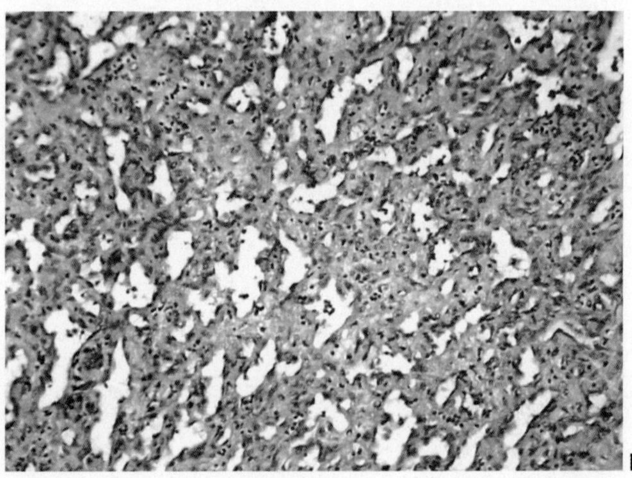

FIG. 39.31. ***Angiosarcoma, low-grade, stromal fibrosis.*** **A:** A few spindle cells are seen in the myxoid stroma. **B:** The moderately cellular stroma is composed of spindle cells. **C:** In some areas, the stroma tends to obscure the neoplastic vascular pattern.

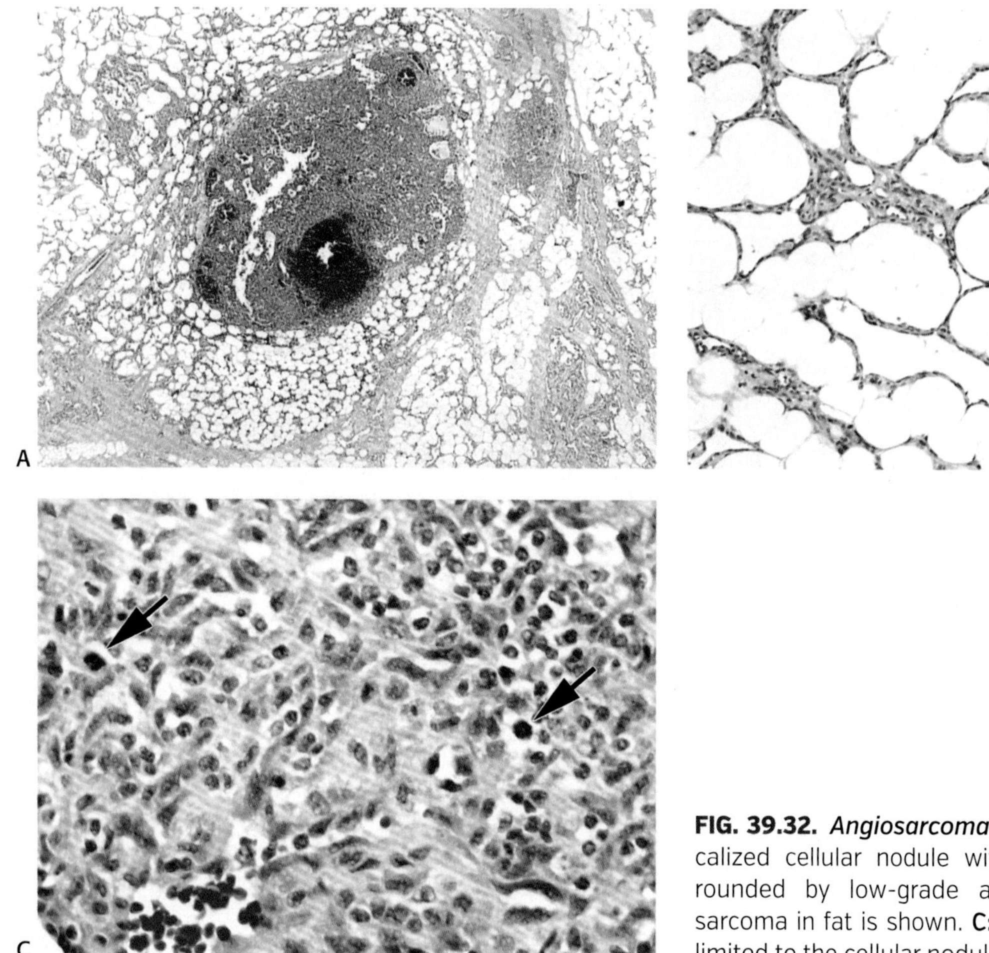

FIG. 39.32. ***Angiosarcoma, intermediate-grade.*** **A:** A localized cellular nodule with focal hemorrhage is surrounded by low-grade angiosarcoma. **B:** Low-grade sarcoma in fat is shown. **C:** Mitotic figures (*arrows*) were limited to the cellular nodule.

proliferation (Figs. 39.32 and 39.33). The latter usually consist of small buds or papillary fronds of endothelial cells that project into the vascular lumens (Figs. 39.34 and 39.35). Less often, the focally cellular areas feature polygonal and spindle cells, or there are foci that combine spindle cell and papillary elements. Infrequent mitoses may be found in papillary or spindle cell areas. Some spindle cell foci resemble lesions encountered in Kaposi sarcoma (Fig. 39.36). At least 75%

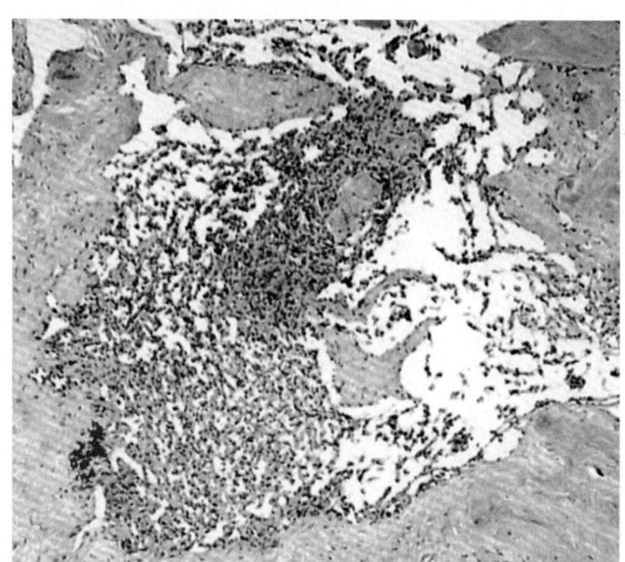

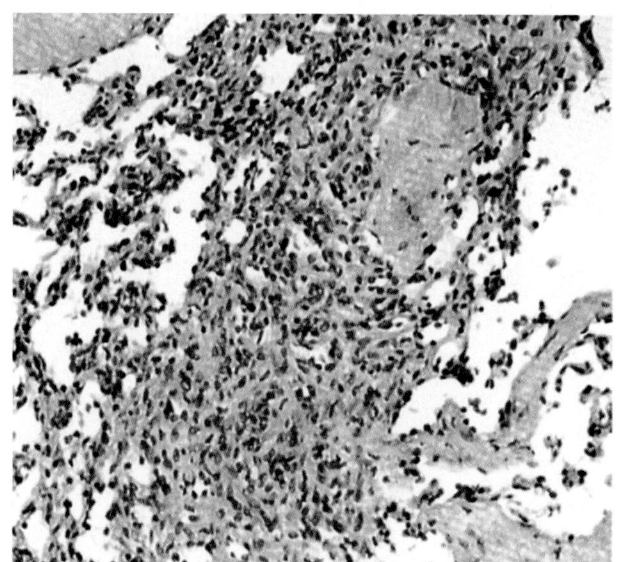

FIG. 39.33. ***Angiosarcoma, intermediate-grade.*** **A,B:** The pictures show a localized focus of papillary endothelial growth.

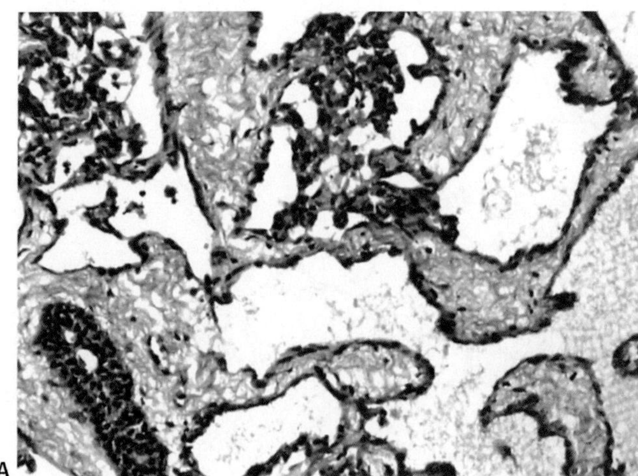

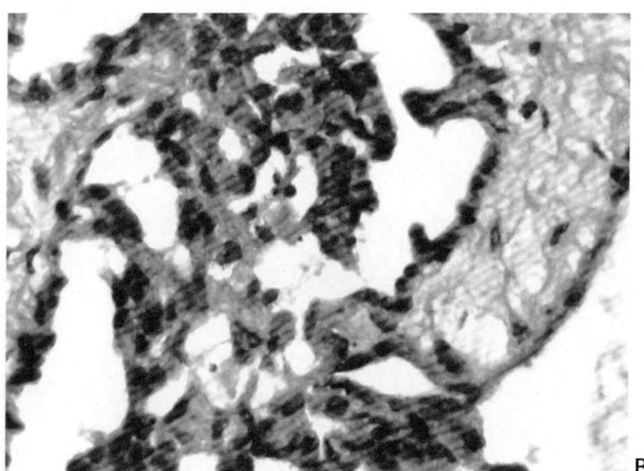

FIG. 39.34. ***Angiosarcoma, intermediate-grade.*** **A,B:** A focus of well-developed papillary endothelial proliferation is depicted.

of intermediate-grade angiosarcomas consist of low-grade elements with cellular foci scattered throughout the tumor. Transitions to cellular foci occur abruptly. An unusual variant of intermediate-grade angiosarcoma features numerous nodules composed of spindle cells with a swirling pattern (Fig. 39.37). The distribution of these nodules suggests a perithelial origin. Ki67 labeling is most evident in the focally cellular areas, whereas the remainder of the tumor exhibits labeling similar to that found in low-grade angiosarcoma. The mean Ki67 labeling index is about 40% in cellular areas.[347]

Type III or high-grade angiosarcoma exhibits the malignant histologic features usually attributed to angiosarcomas. Part of the lesion is composed of low- and intermediate-grade elements, but in many cases more than half of the tumor has high-grade malignant features. These consist of prominent endothelial tufting and solid papillary formations that contain cytologically malignant endothelial cells (Fig. 39.38). In some lesions, there are conspicuous solid and spindle cell areas with sparse vascular elements (Fig. 39.39). Mitoses are usually identified without difficulty in the cellular components. Typically, Ki67 labeling is found in 45% or more of the tumor cells in high-grade angiosarcoma. Areas of hemorrhage, often accompanied by necrosis, have been referred to as "blood lakes" (Figs. 39.40 and 39.41). Necrosis and "blood lakes" are seen only in high-grade angiosarcomas.

Epithelioid angiosarcoma is an uncommon high-grade variant with histologic features similar to angiosarcoma in the Stewart–Treves syndrome (STS).[290,311,348–351] The lesion consists predominantly or exclusively of large, polygonal or rounded epithelioid endothelial cells containing abundant amphophilic or eosinophilic cytoplasm, large vesicular nuclei, and lining slit-like spaces. Because of the epithelioid appearance of the cells, the tumor may be mistaken for mammary adenocarcinoma. The results of immunohistochemical stains will assist in distinguishing the two lesions.[348,351]

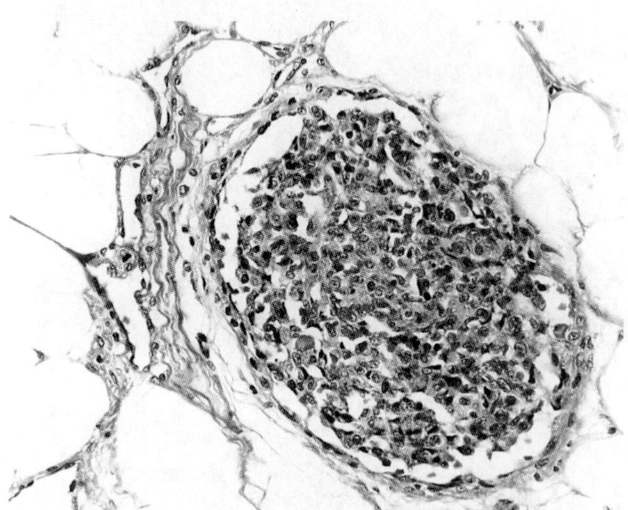

FIG. 39.35. ***Angiosarcoma, intermediate-grade.*** An intravascular papillary focus is illustrated.

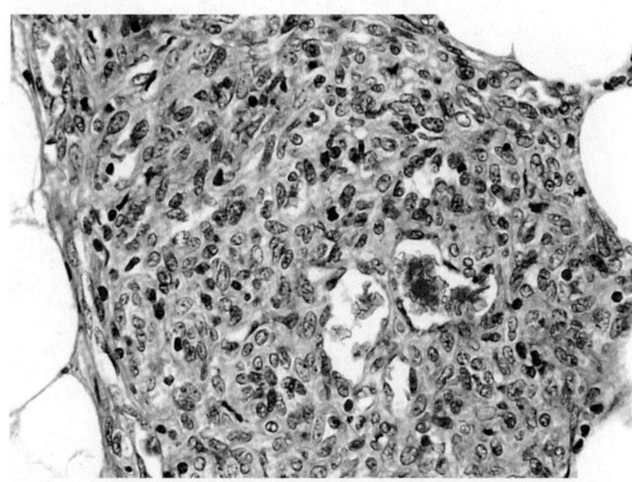

FIG. 39.36. ***Angiosarcoma, intermediate-grade.*** This nodule is composed of spindle cells with scattered red blood cells around small vascular spaces.

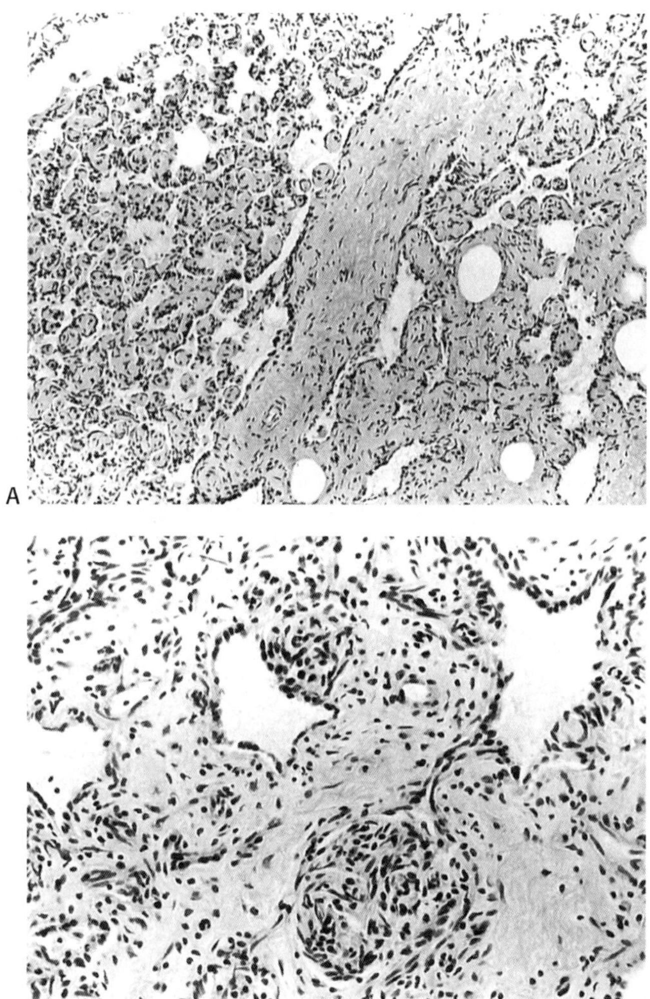

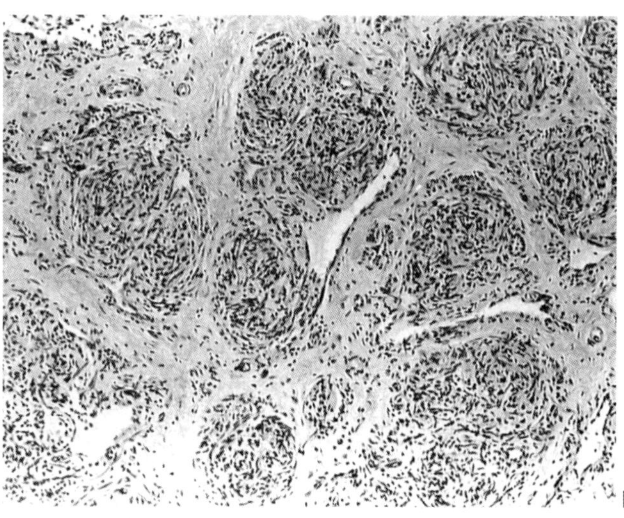

FIG. 39.37. ***Angiosarcoma, intermediate-grade.*** **A:** Papillary and low-grade parts of the lesion can be seen. **B,C:** Nodular spindle cell foci have a perithelial distribution.

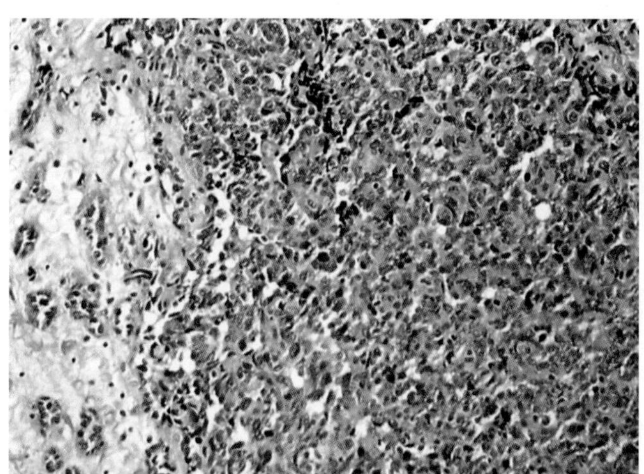

FIG. 39.38. ***Angiosarcoma, high-grade.*** The tumor had extensive densely cellular areas like the one shown here composed of cells with hyperchromatic pleomorphic nuclei.

With few exceptions, angiosarcomas have infiltrative borders that feature well-formed or low-grade vascular channels. In some cases, the peripheral vascular component is so orderly that the neoplastic vascular channels are either structurally indistinguishable from existing capillaries in the normal parenchyma or resemble an angiolipoma (Fig. 39.42).

Because of the varied microscopic structure of intermediate- and high-grade lesions, it is not possible to classify a tumor as low-grade angiosarcoma accurately unless it has been excised and generously sampled. The tendency for peripheral portions of an intermediate- or high-grade angiosarcoma to have a low-grade structure is likely to lead to an erroneous diagnosis if one examines only a superficial biopsy. This phenomenon may also lead to a mistaken diagnosis of hemangioma[287] and, in part, explains the clinical behavior of lesions classified as "metastasizing hemangiomas."[352,353]

It is not difficult to distinguish a high-grade angiosarcoma from a hemangioma, but problems may be encountered with low-grade and intermediate-grade tumors. Some general guidelines are helpful in these situations.[296,336]

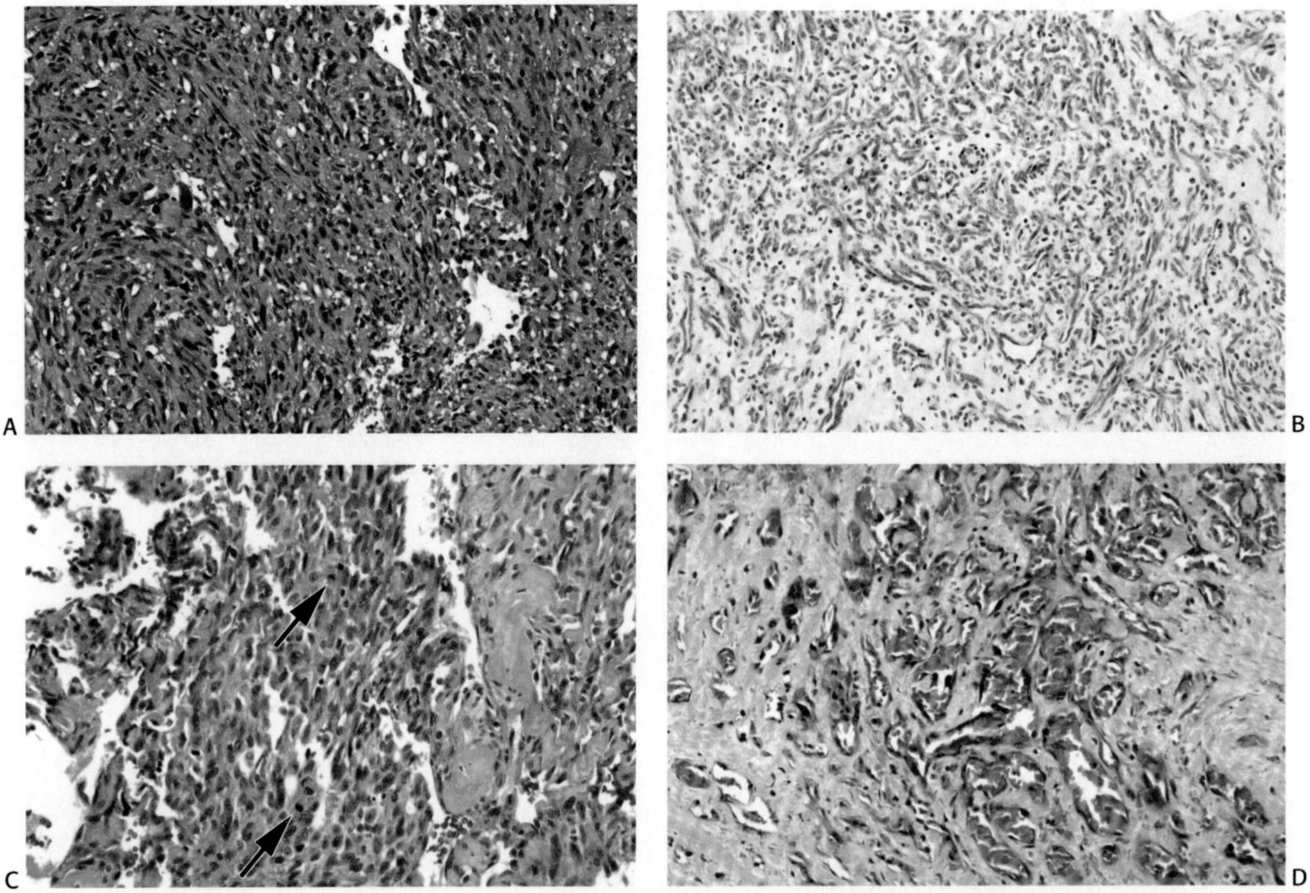

FIG. 39.39. ***Angiosarcoma, high-grade.*** **A:** A spindle cell area with few vascular spaces. **B:** Immunoreactivity for factor VIII is shown. **C:** Mitotic figures are present (*arrows*). **D:** A structurally low-grade area in the tumor.

Hemangiomas are rarely larger than 2 cm, and few angiosarcomas measure less than 2 cm. Most hemangiomas tend to have well-circumscribed borders grossly and microscopically, whereas angiosarcomas have invasive margins. Many angiomas are divided into lobules or nodules by fibrous septa, a feature not seen in angiosarcomas, which lack an internal structure. Angiomas usually consist of isolated largely unconnected vascular channels such as those typically seen

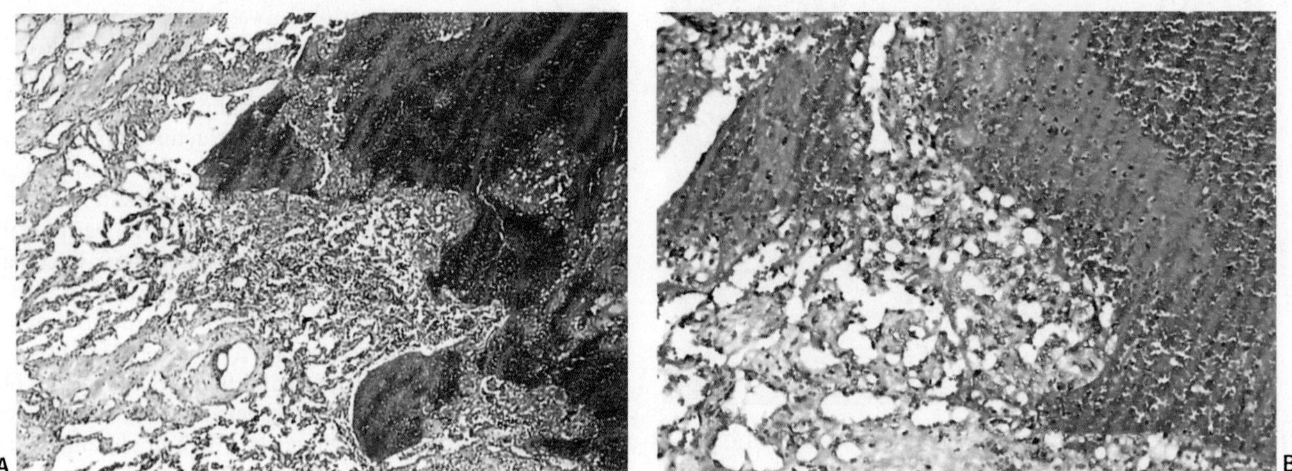

FIG. 39.40. ***Angiosarcoma, high-grade.*** **A,B:** Hemorrhagic foci referred to as "blood lakes" are shown.

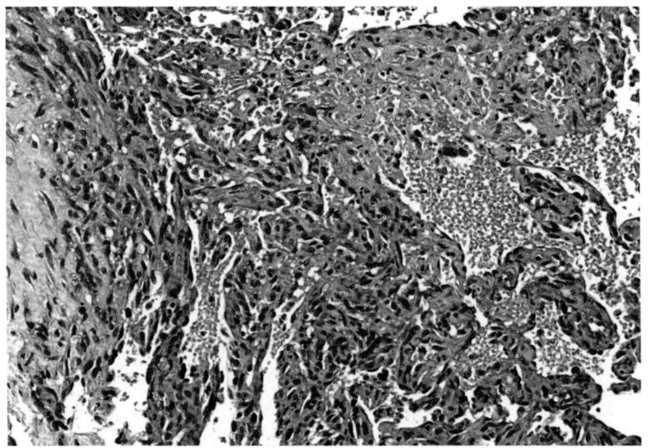

FIG. 39.41. ***Angiosarcoma, high-grade.*** Focal necrosis is shown in the *upper right* in a tumor with spindle cell growth.

in cavernous hemangiomas. Anastomosing vascular spaces may be found in angiomas; however, except in angiomatosis,[354] anastomoses are not as numerous or serpiginous as in angiosarcomas. In the mammary parenchyma, the vascular proliferation in angiosarcomas invades into and expands lobules, whereas angiomas other than perilobular hemangiomas tend to surround lobules and ducts.[355] A thick-walled nonneoplastic "feeding" blood vessel is sometimes found at the periphery of hemangiomas; this is not a finding seen in angiosarcomas.

Relationship with Hemangiomas

A few patients with mammary angiosarcoma have also had hemangiomas.[287] One patient with low-grade angiosarcoma had a hemangioma of her scalp diagnosed at the same time her breast tumor was detected. Since she was disease-free 5 years after mastectomy, the diagnosis of a coincidental cutaneous hemangioma was substantiated not only by differences in the histologic appearance of the lesions but also by clinical follow-up. Incidental perilobular hemangiomas have been found in mastectomy specimens from patients with mammary angiosarcoma. This association is probably coincidental, because perilobular hemangiomas are frequent in breast tissue from women with benign breast lesions and mammary carcinoma. A few perilobular hemangiomas and small nonpalpable hemangiomas with cytologically atypical endothelial cells and irregularly shaped margins have been described.[336] None of these patients developed angiosarcoma. It is unlikely that origin of angiosarcoma from a

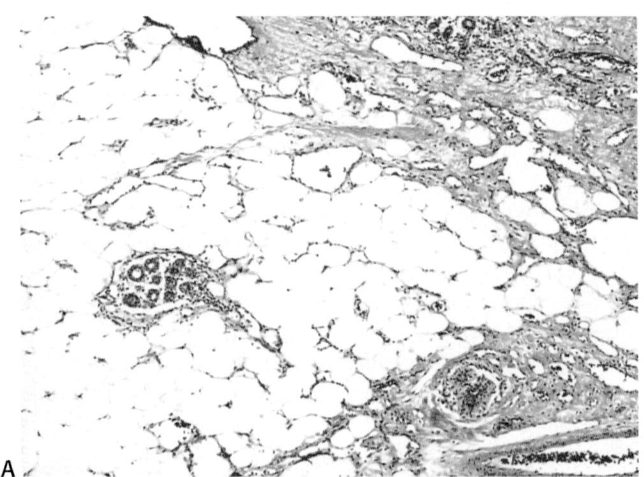

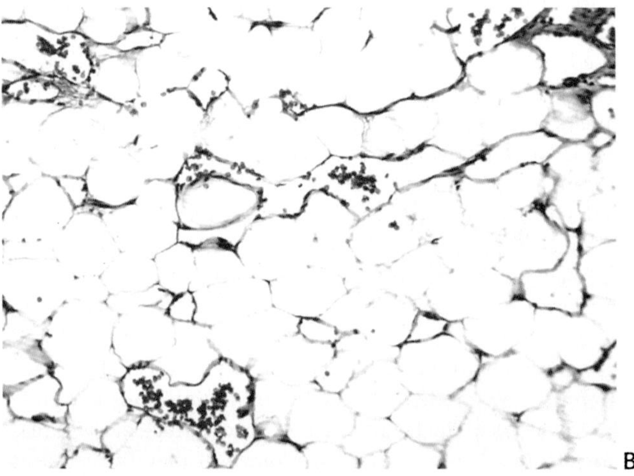

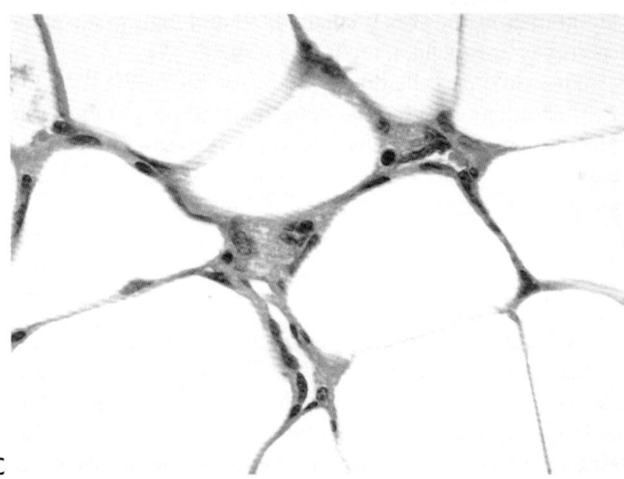

FIG. 39.42. ***Angiosarcoma, high-grade with low-grade component invading fat.*** All images are from a single tumor. **A:** Angiosarcoma involves glandular parenchyma and fat. **B:** Irregular dilated neoplastic vascular channels with an inconspicuous endothelium are shown. **C:** Capillaries in the fat that could be traced to the angiosarcomatous part of the lesion.

perilobular hemangioma or microscopic hemangioma will be demonstrable, because such a small precursor lesion would almost certainly be obliterated by the larger malignant neoplasm. Perilobular hemangiomas may be multifocal in one breast or involve both breasts[355] and should not be mistaken for metastatic angiosarcoma.

The relationship between grossly evident hemangiomas and angiosarcomas remains obscure. Hemangiomas with atypical cytologic and structural features resemble components of angiosarcomas, but all such lesions also retain at least some hemangiomatous elements such as circumscription, lobulation, or association with nonneoplastic vessels that have well-developed muscular walls. Atypical hemangiomas are rarely larger than 2 cm. Origin of an angiosarcoma from a hemangioma or atypical hemangioma has not been reported in the literature. The difficulty in establishing such a relationship is akin to that of proving origin of liposarcoma from a lipoma. The Senior Editor has seen only one case that may qualify as an angiosarcoma arising in a hemangioma.

Cytology

The cytologic findings of needle aspiration biopsy specimens vary according to the characteristics of angiosarcoma.[304,313,318,327,356,357] Because of this variability and the rarity of the lesion, cytologic criteria have not been established, and the diagnosis of angiosarcoma is rarely made based on cytologic material. Direct smears of aspirated specimens vary in the degree of their cellularity. Although the smears can appear hypocellular,[357] most appear moderately cellular or hypercellular. They usually exhibit a bloody background, which may also contain inflammatory cells, macrophages, and adipocytes. Atypical cells are present singly and in clusters. The cells have round, oval, or spindle shapes, and they possess eccentric, round- to spindle-shaped nuclei and scant cytoplasm. The degree of nuclear enlargement, hyperchromasia, and pleomorphism and the number and prominence of the nucleoli depend on the grade of the angiosarcoma. Low-grade tumors contain monotonous and only slightly atypical nuclei and inconspicuous nucleoli, whereas those from high-grade angiosarcomas display the features characteristic of poorly differentiated neoplasms. Cells identical to the dispersed cells form thick three-dimensional branching aggregates, loose collections, and papillary tufts. Careful inspection of the dense aggregates often reveals small arborizing thin-walled blood vessels. In the absence of vascular structures, the presence of loose tangles of collagen associated with atypical cells disposed in a parallel array, which probably represent disrupted neoplastic blood vessels, suggests the diagnosis of angiosarcoma.[357] The atypical cells also form acini-like structures.[357] The presence of these acini-like structures may represent a characteristic feature of angiosarcomas, but this finding is often especially subtle and may not be present in angiosarcomas of low grade. Mitotic figures usually are not numerous, and the presence of intracytoplasmic erythrocytes and intracytoplasmic lumens has been reported.

Immunohistochemistry

Immunoreactivity for factor VIII–related antigen (von Willebrand factor) has been detected in angiomas and angiosarcomas originating in the breast and in other organs[346,358–361] (Fig. 39.43). Two studies of mammary angiosarcomas reported more intense staining for factor VIII–related antigen in well-differentiated than in poorly differentiated portions of the tumor.[346,360] Sparse or absent reactivity for factor VIII–related antigen has been reported more commonly in nonmammary angiosarcomas.[359,361] Variable staining for UEA-1 has also been described in angiosarcomas.[361] In one series, the neoplastic endothelium in 6 of 14 angiosarcomas was reactive for factor VIII–related antigen, and 11 stained for UEA-1.[361] Angiosarcomas also exhibit reactivity for CD34 and CD31.[313,317,362] These markers are especially useful for distinguishing epithelioid forms of angiosarcoma from carcinoma and other neoplasms. Epithelioid angiosarcomas typically stain for CD31, but reactivity for CD34 varies.[290,350,351] Immunoreactivity for D2-40 has been detected in certain angiosarcomas,[299,358,363] but others have not stained for the protein.[315] The angiosarcomas studied in one report[315] demonstrated immunoreactivity for FLI-1, HIF-1α, vascular endothelial growth factor (VEGF), vascular endothelial growth factor receptor (VEGFR), and Wilms tumor 1 (WT-1). The tumor in another report expressed VEGFR-2,[321] and several low- and intermediate-grade angiosarcomas studied by Gennaro et al.[364] stained for VEGFR. Shet et al.[365] observed reactivity for WT-1 in 11 of 12 angiosarcomas. These workers also noted that 10 of 12 angiosarcomas did not stain for c-kit but that the remaining 2 showed weak staining. Isolated cases have failed to stain for EMA, S-100, CD68, desmin, and HHV-8.[290,305,318,325]

Although angiosarcomas usually do not stain for keratin, two reports,[290,311] including one describing an epithelioid angiosarcoma[290] have noted staining for keratin in two cases. In one report, 3 of 14 angiosarcomas arising at unspecified sites stained for p63.[366]

The Ki67 labeling index of angiosarcomas (mean, 38.1; median, 40.3) is substantially higher than the labeling index of hemangiomas (mean, 4.6; median, 1.7).[347] The labeling index of low-grade angiosarcomas (mean, 29.4; median, 24.5) is considerably less than the labeling indices for intermediate-grade (mean, 41.6; median, 42.9) and high-grade angiosarcomas (mean, 44.8; median, 43.5).

The sarcoma cells do not stain for ER or PR.[321,339] One epithelioid angiosarcoma demonstrated 2+ staining for HER2,[351] but another conventional angiosarcoma did not express the protein.[321] Biochemical assays for ER have yielded low[367] or negative[288,339,368,369] results.

Electron Microscopy

Several authors have described the ultrastructural features of mammary angiosarcoma.[328,346,370,371] Weibel–Palade bodies were described in neoplastic endothelial cells in most of the lesions, although they may be inconspicuous or absent in areas of solid growth. Neoplastic endothelial cells

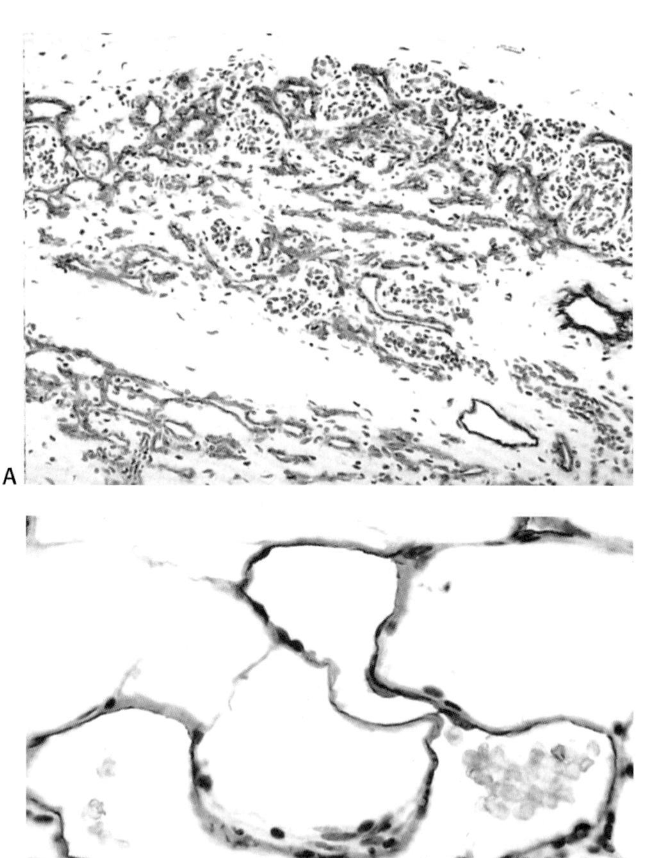

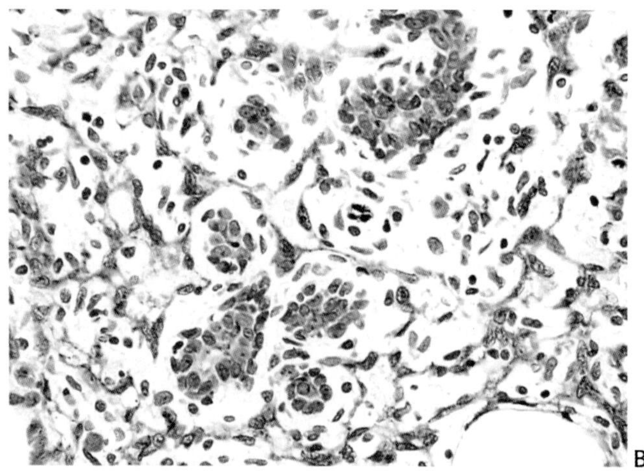

FIG. 39.43. ***Angiosarcoma, immunoreactivity with vascular markers.*** **A:** This low-grade angiosarcoma infiltrating lobules is immunoreactive for factor VIII–related antigen. **B,C:** Low-grade angiosarcoma immunoreactive for *Ulex europaeus* agglutinin-1 is shown in a lobule and in fat.

contain pinocytotic vesicles at the luminal and basal surfaces. Small cytoplasmic projections or papillae have been noted protruding into the vascular lumen. The neoplastic endothelium and basal lamina are frequently discontinuous. Pericytic cells have been found associated with endothelial cells in some of the tumors.

Scanning electron microscopy of mammary angiosarcomas revealed ultrastructural features similar to those found in chemically induced angiosarcoma of the murine liver.[371,372] When compared with normal vessels, endothelial cells in the sarcoma were oriented in an overlapping disorderly fashion, sometimes projecting into the vascular lumen to form bridges or cord-like structures. Along the vascular wall, these cells were arranged in a "spider-web" pattern. Although a disorderly and lace-like arrangement of endothelial cells was found in vessels in reactive lesions and in benign vascular tumors, none of these had clusters and cords of atypical endothelial cells protruding into the vascular lumen.

Genetic Studies

The results of cytogenetic analysis of three angiosarcomas demonstrated complex alterations involving 25 chromosomes: gains in 13 chromosomes and losses in 12.[373]

Prognosis

Until recently, angiosarcoma of the breast was regarded as almost always fatal.[295,374,375] In 1980, Chen[295] reviewed 87 published cases and reported that 14% of the patients were free from disease at 3 years and only 7% survived disease-free for 5 years or more. The report by Steingaszner et al.[375] includes two patients who survived more than 5 years. A patient treated initially by excision underwent a mastectomy 2 years later for a local recurrence and remained well 11 years after the mastectomy.[326] Other examples of patients who survived longer than 5 years were published during the same period,[310,376–379] and a recent study of nine women[380] revealed a 5-year OS of 42.9% and a median time of 46.8 months from diagnosis of angiosarcoma to death.

Because of the poor survival results in reports through 1980, little information could be obtained about prognostic factors. Steingaszner et al.[375] reviewed 10 cases from the Armed Forces Institute of Pathology and concluded that a high mitotic rate and relatively long pretreatment duration were associated with a poor prognosis. Subsequently, it was reported that patients who were aware of the tumor and delayed obtaining medical care had significantly ($p < 0.01$) larger tumors (median size, 6 cm) than those who sought treatment at first awareness (median size, 3 cm).[287] However, the size and duration of symptoms were not significantly correlated with the grade of the tumors, the likelihood of recurrence of the tumors, or the patients' survival.

In 1981, Donnell et al.[296] studied 40 patients with mammary angiosarcoma treated by mastectomy and found that the overall DFS was 41% at 3 years and 33% at 5 years. Tumor grade was the most important prognostic factor. The majority of patients with orderly or low-grade lesions remained disease-free, whereas virtually all women with high-grade tumors died of recurrent sarcoma within 5 years (Fig. 39.44).

An expanded series of 87 patients confirmed the statistically significant correlation between the grade of angiosarcoma and the patients' prognosis.[287] Twenty-five of the patients (40%) had low-grade lesions, 12 (19%) had intermediate-grade tumors, and 26 (41%) had high-grade angiosarcomas. The authors detected a statistically significant correlation between the patients' age at diagnosis and the grade of the tumor. The median ages of patients with low-, intermediate-, and high-grade tumors were 43, 34, and 29 years, respectively. Analysis of survival for these patients revealed the following estimated probabilities of DFS 5 years after treatment: low grade, 76%; intermediate grade, 70%; and high grade, 15%. The values did not change at the 10-year time point. The median duration of DFS was also correlated with tumor grade (low, more than 15 years; intermediate, more than 12 years; and high, 15 months). The longest survival in this series was 18 years with no evidence of disease in a patient who was 23 years old when she was treated for a high-grade mammary angiosarcoma.

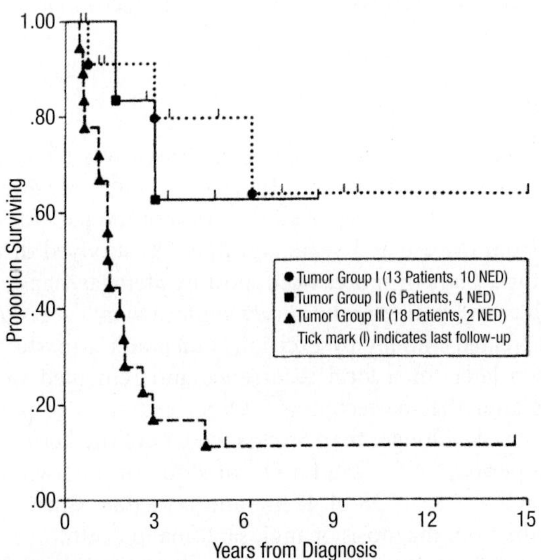

FIG. 39.44. ***Angiosarcoma, survival analysis.*** The patients were stratified by histologic group [grade]. Patients with high-grade sarcomas [group 3] had a significantly lower survival rate when compared to women with low-grade [group 1] and intermediate-grade [group 2] tumors. [Reproduced from Donnell RM, Rosen PP, Lieberman PH, et al. Angiosarcoma and other vascular tumors of the breast. Pathologic analysis as a guide to prognosis. *Am J Surg Pathol* 1981;5:629–642, with permission.]

Despite the relatively favorable prognosis of low-grade angiosarcoma, patients with these tumors can develop local and systemic recurrences.[287,296] A patient who initially has a low-grade angiosarcoma may develop intermediate- or high-grade areas in recurrent lesions, an observation that supports the concept that progression from low to high grade might occur over time at the primary site, also. Recurrences and metastases that originate from high-grade sarcomas can be composed in part or entirely of low-grade components.

The prognosis of intermediate-grade angiosarcoma is slightly less favorable than, but not significantly different from, that of low-grade angiosarcoma. It is interesting that the median age of these patients falls between the median ages of women with low- and high-grade lesions. These tumors are relatively infrequent, constituting 20% or fewer of mammary angiosarcomas. For the present, one should identify patients with intermediate-grade angiosarcomas in order to assemble a larger group that will make it possible to determine the prognosis of this category more accurately.

Vorburger et al.[297] reported the follow-up of 32 women with angiosarcoma. In this series, the size of the tumor, the grade of tumor, and age of the patient at diagnosis were not significantly related to DFS. Grade was described dichotomously as "low" or "high," with intermediate-grade tumors considered "high" grade. As previously noted, the prognosis of intermediate-grade primary mammary angiosarcomas is close to that of low-grade tumors. Inclusion of these cases in the "high"-grade category is likely to have biased the data in a way that would diminish differences between "low"- and "high"-grade cases, leading to failure to detect a significant difference in DFS. The investigation of mammary angiosarcomas carried out by Nascimento et al.[311] failed to detect a relationship between the grade of the angiosarcoma and the rate of local recurrence, distant metastasis, or death.

Patients with angiosarcoma diagnosed during pregnancy seem to have an especially poor prognosis, apparently because most have high-grade tumors. This probably reflects their youth rather than a particular association between high-grade angiosarcoma and pregnancy. One woman who reportedly had a 15-cm low-grade angiosarcoma during pregnancy developed a local recurrence 2 years later and remained well for 5 years following excision of the recurrence.[302] The earlier age at diagnosis of patients with high-grade lesions may also explain the relatively high frequency of bilateral involvement, since the contralateral breast lesions are usually metastases.[301,375] There is no evidence that these tumors are hormone-dependent.

The most frequent sites of metastases are the bones, the lungs, the liver, the contralateral breast, and the skin apart from the mastectomy site.[287] Spread to the opposite breast may be a manifestation of the apparent cutaneous tropism of these tumors. Three instances of metastases in the gingiva have been reported.[381–383] Metastatic angiosarcoma has been described in the ovary,[315,384] placenta,[385] and pituitary,[323] and rarely metastases may present in remote subcutaneous sites.[386,387]

The distinction between metastatic tumor in the contralateral breast and a new primary contralateral angiosarcoma is very difficult. To distinguish these two situations, one should make note of the interval between the detection of the two tumors and compare their morphologic features.

Treatment

A review by Kaklamanos et al.[388] summarizes information regarding treatment and survival culled from 10 major series that include cases of mammary angiosarcomas published prior to 2008. Total mastectomy is the recommended primary surgical therapy. Unless there is a clinically apparent nodal abnormality, axillary dissection is not indicated for mammary angiosarcoma because metastases involve these lymph nodes in fewer than 10% of cases.[287,295,343] Radical mastectomy is not appropriate unless the tumor is close to or involves the deep fascia. Rarely, a small lesion might be encompassed by quadrantectomy.

The role of radiation in the primary treatment of mammary angiosarcoma has not been determined. In one series, individual patients with low- and intermediate-grade lesions remained disease-free after excision and radiotherapy.[287] One patient with a high-grade tumor developed a mammary recurrence after breast-conserving surgery.

Following surgery, systemic adjuvant chemotherapy may be offered, but the effectiveness of this treatment remains uncertain. Donnell et al.[296] reported that 9 of 15 patients who remained disease-free had been treated with adjuvant chemotherapy after surgery (14 patients) or excisional biopsy (1 patient). Most of these patients were treated with actinomycin D.[296,389] It was also noted that nearly 50% of patients (8 of 14) who died of recurrent sarcoma had not had adjuvant therapy. Adjuvant therapy with cyclophosphamide and vincristine,[372] vinblastine,[378] doxorubicin-containing regimens,[368] and various other drugs[288] has also been reported in a few cases, without proving to be particularly effective.

Rosen et al.[287] compared the clinical course of 32 patients who received adjuvant chemotherapy with 31 women not so treated. The drugs most often used were doxorubicin or actinomycin D. Eleven patients also received chest wall radiation. Among patients not treated with adjuvant chemotherapy, four had chest wall irradiation. The median size of tumors among women given adjuvant chemotherapy (5 cm) was not significantly different from that of patients not so treated (4 cm). Recurrences developed in 14 (45%) of 31 patients who received adjuvant chemotherapy and in 18 (56%) of 32 not treated. When stratified by tumor grade, recurrences were consistently less frequent among women treated with adjuvant chemotherapy, although the differences were not statistically significant. Because high-grade lesions have such a poor prognosis and most of the few long-term survivors had adjuvant chemotherapy, this treatment should be considered for these patients.

Complete clinical response of liver and lung metastases to metronomic trofosfamide has been reported in one patient.[390]

Radiation and Angiosarcoma

Exposure to radiation represents the most important predisposing factor for the development of angiosarcoma of the breast. Rare angiosarcomas have arisen following irradiation for Hodgkin disease,[293,358,391] but radiation is most commonly administered to treat breast carcinoma, either following a mastectomy or as a component of breast conservation therapy. An analysis of SEER data[392] demonstrated that women with breast carcinoma who undergo irradiation experience a relative risk of 15.9 for the development of angiosarcoma at all sites compared to nonirradiated patients. When considering only angiosarcoma of the breast or chest wall, the comparable relative risk is 59.3.

Radiation-related angiosarcomas can arise in either the chest wall after a mastectomy[393–397] or the breast after partial mastectomy. Although certain publications focus on tumors occurring in one or the other situation, many reports include angiosarcomas developing in both clinical settings.

Angiosarcoma Following Breast Conservation Therapy

Angiosarcoma of the irradiated breast is an infrequent complication of breast conservation therapy. The incidence varies from 0.05%[398] to 1.11%[399] and averages approximately 0.1%. Most patients received radiation treatment as part of their initial therapy. The publication by Abbott and Palmieri[397] lists selected clinical details of 237 such cases published prior to 2008. In almost every case, radiation was delivered using an external beam, but an angiosarcoma arose in the breast of a 74-year-old woman 4 years after receiving MammoSite® balloon brachytherapy.[400]

Irradiation may not constitute the only component of breast conservation therapy that predisposes patients to the development of angiosarcoma. A study by Mery et al.[401] using data from 563,155 patients with breast carcinoma in the 1973 to 2003 SEER database seems to show that the use of partial mastectomy as the primary surgical procedure elevates the risk of the development of angiosarcoma. Patients treated with partial mastectomy had a sevenfold higher risk of developing angiosarcoma when compared with women treated with mastectomy even after accounting for the use of irradiation and lymph node dissection. These authors could only speculate about the explanation of this finding.

Clinical Presentation

The interval between irradiation and the diagnosis of angiosarcoma ranges from 12[358] to 291 months.[402] The median latency intervals in the five largest series were 59,[403] 73.5,[283] 74,[404] 84,[405] and 91[297] months. In the largest single institution study,[405] the latency ranged from 1.4 to 26 years. Most cases come to attention within 6 years after radiotherapy.[297,406] The latent period for the appearance of postirradiation angiosarcoma tends to be shorter than for other types of sarcoma,[407] and it appears inversely related to the patient's age at the time of treatment for breast carcinoma, decreasing with advancing age.[404] Billings et al.[403] reported that for each 1-year increase in the age of the patient, the latency period decreases by 0.5 month.

Published case reports have not shown a consistent relationship between cutaneous angiosarcoma of the breast and either mammary edema following radiation of the breast or chronic edema after treatment of the breast and axilla.[403,404,408–410] The amount of radiation and the use of a radiation boost have not been associated with a predilection for the development of postirradiation angiosarcoma of the breast or for the location of the tumor.[404,409] The median radiation dose in 137 published cases is 50 Gy.[397]

With few exceptions, women were older than 50 years when treated for mammary carcinoma.[403,406,411,412] In one study, the median age at diagnosis of postirradiation mammary angiosarcoma was 70.6 years, with a range of 46.2 to 87.2 years.[297] Other studies reported a mean age of 69[403] and median ages of 68,[404] 71,[405] and 71.3 years.[283] A meta-analysis of 184 published cases[397] yielded a median age of 70 years and a range of 36 to 92 years. A 98-year-old woman developed an epithelioid angiosarcoma 5 years after treatment of an IDC.[413] Several studies document a difference in the average age between women with sporadic and postirradiation angiosarcomas.[293,294,344,414,415] The differences in ages range from 13.9[414] to 30 years.[344]

Postirradiation angiosarcoma presents more frequently in the skin than within the conserved breast.[403,408,409,416–421] A review of the comprehensive national database of the Netherlands identified 21 patients with postirradiation angiosarcoma of the conserved breast diagnosed between 1987 and 1995.[404] The origin was described as cutaneous in 17 (81%). The tumors usually involve the skin overlying the site of the prior carcinoma or the scar from the excision.[297] They can present as palpable skin or subcutaneous nodules, but equally frequently they create plaques or papules described as shades of blue, purple, or red (Fig. 39.45A). One tumor was characterized as "an ivory-coloured plaque of fibrous consistency with a smooth and shiny surface."[422] Certain examples cause edema, the formation of vesicles, or *peau d'orange* change, and others mimic a hematoma.[423] Skin thickening and dimpling sometimes occur,[424,425] and multiple nodules are common.[293,405] They sometimes number so many that they cover the entire breast.[426,427] On the other hand, the skin changes may be especially subtle. In one case, "a little bit of purplish discoloration" was interpreted as postradiotherapy telangiectasia, and a later ecchymotic area was attributed to trauma.[428] The formation of an exophytic pedunculated mass has been described.[429] Many patients who present with angiosarcoma in the skin will have parenchymal involvement, also.

One patient had recurrent carcinoma as well as angiosarcoma in the same breast,[430] and in two cases, angiosarcoma developed in breasts reconstructed with silicone implants after breast-conserving surgery and radiotherapy.[411,431] Hanasono et al.[432] reported a case of a postirradiation angiosarcoma arising in a transverse rectus abdominus muscle (TRAM) flap. A 68-year-old woman developed synchronous angiosarcoma, melanoma, and morphea in the skin of the breast 14 years after irradiation and breast conservation therapy.[422] A 55-year-old woman who carried a duplication of exon 13 of the *BRCA1* gene and had undergone bilateral breast-conserving surgery with irradiation for bilateral breast carcinoma developed synchronous bilateral angiosarcomas within the fields of irradiation.[433] de Bree et al.[434] described a similar case of a 76-year-old woman with metachronous postirradiation angiosarcomas. Loss of heterozygosity (LOH) studies demonstrated that the two angiosarcomas were not related. The series of Lindford et al.[435] contains two patients with bilateral involvement by angiosarcoma.

Imaging Studies

Imaging studies in patients with postirradiation angiosarcomas do not demonstrate distinctive findings.[424,436] Mammograms sometime display thickening of the skin or enhancement of the trabecular pattern.[436] Skin thickening may also be apparent on CT scans.[436] In other respects, the imaging findings in patients with postirradiation angiosarcomas do not differ from those in patient with sporadic angiosarcomas. A PET/CT scan may disclose the hypermetabolic nature of the angiosarcoma.[342]

Gross Pathology

The macroscopic pathologic characteristics of skin-based angiosarcomas duplicate the findings evident on clinical examination. Larger nodules and those involving the mammary parenchyma display the macroscopic features seen in angiosarcomas arising *de novo*.

Microscopic Pathology

Low-grade,[404,412,418–421] intermediate-grade,[404,412,416] and high-grade[404,408,409] postirradiation angiosarcomas have been described. The high-grade examples constitute a greater proportion of the angiosarcomas in this setting compared with those arising spontaneously.[294] The high-grade lesions usually exhibit the same heterogeneous mixture of low- and high-grade components seen in sporadic parenchymal angiosarcomas, and they typically form multiple subcutaneous and dermal tumor nodules.

The histologic characteristics of postirradiation angiosarcoma of the skin, subcutaneous tissue, and breast differ in some details from primary parenchymal angiosarcoma not associated with radiotherapy.[408] High-grade areas, found in the majority of these cases, are composed of solid epithelioid,[283,403,436–439] or solid spindle cell foci, with variable numbers of slit-like spaces containing intraluminal or extravasated red blood cells (Figs. 39.45B–E). Hemorrhage resulting in the formation of blood lakes is typically distributed in these sarcomatous foci. Lesions with low- and intermediate-grade structural patterns exhibit variable vasoformative growth and papillary endothelial hyperplasia (Fig. 39.46). In contrast to sporadic parenchymal angiosarcomas in which nuclear grade frequently parallels structural differentiation regardless of the microscopic pattern, the malignant cells in postirradiation angiosarcoma typically have poorly differentiated nuclei, dark chromatin, prominent nucleoli, and

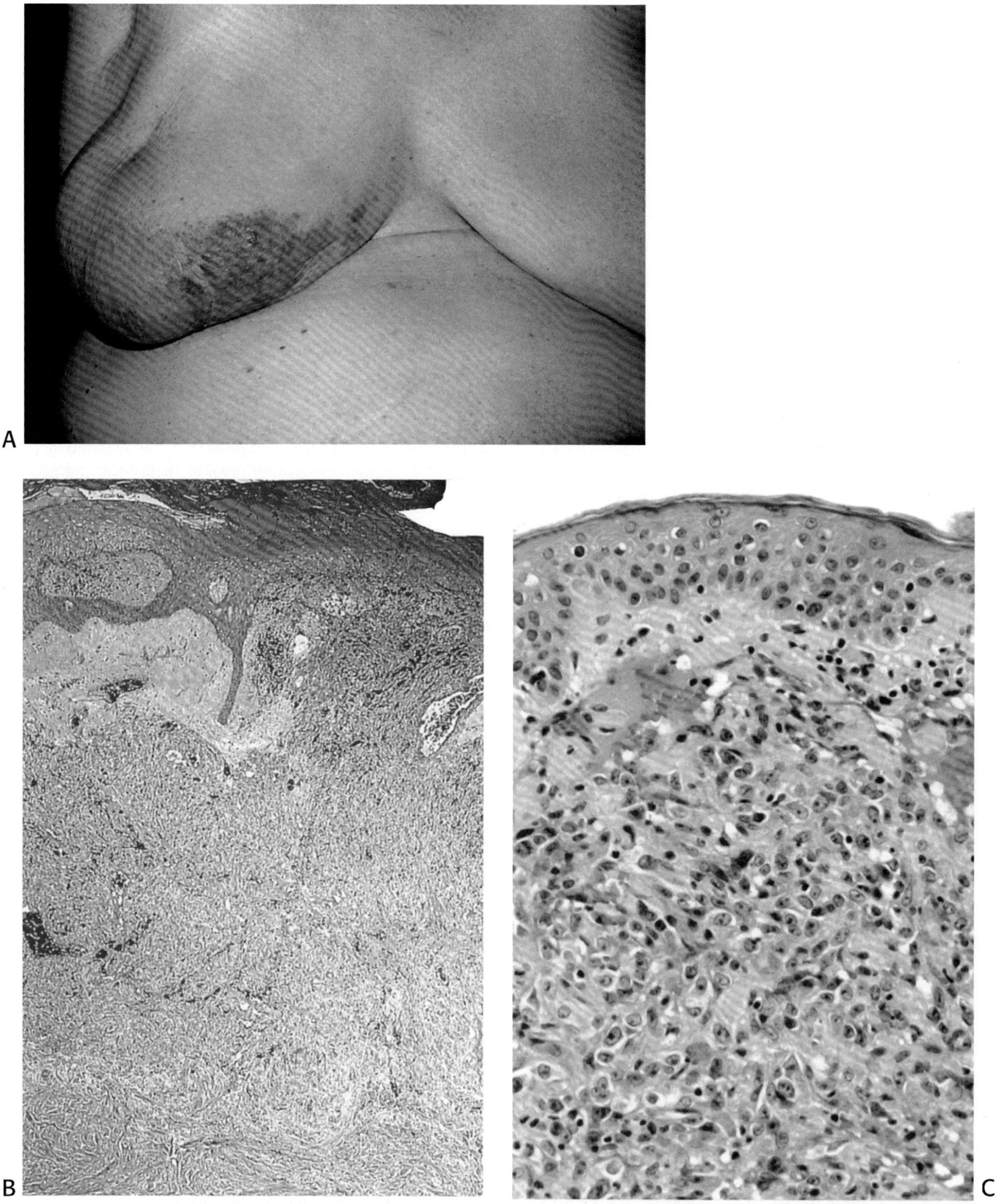

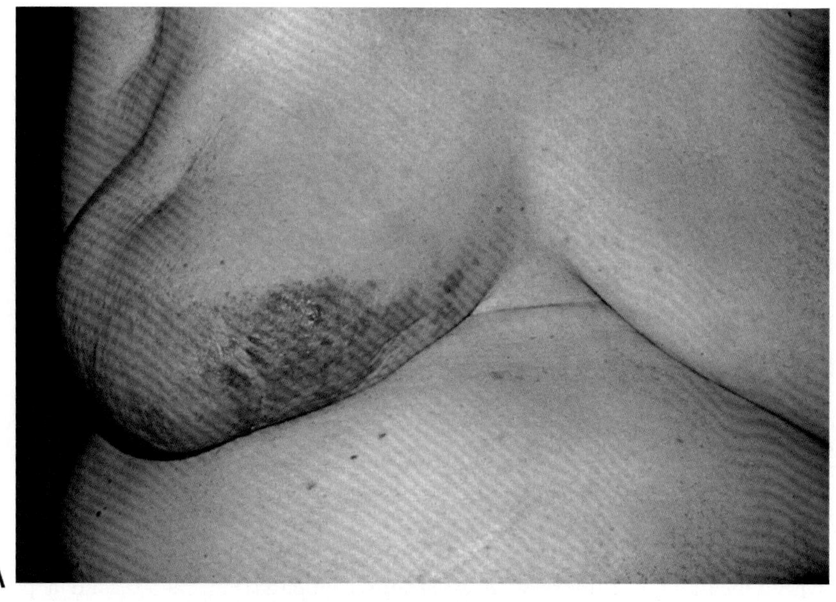

FIG. 39.45. ***Angiosarcoma of mammary skin after breast-conserving surgery and irradiation for carcinoma.*** **A:** Angiosarcoma involves the skin and much of the lower half of the breast. The retracted area in the *upper outer quadrant* is the site of a prior lumpectomy. **B:** Solid mass of high-grade angiosarcoma in the dermis. **C:** Epithelioid and spindle cells in a superficial part of the tumor. **D:** This part of the sarcoma is composed of spindle cells and dilated vascular channels lined by plump malignant endothelial cells. **E:** The nuclei have vesicular chromatin and one or more prominent nucleoli.

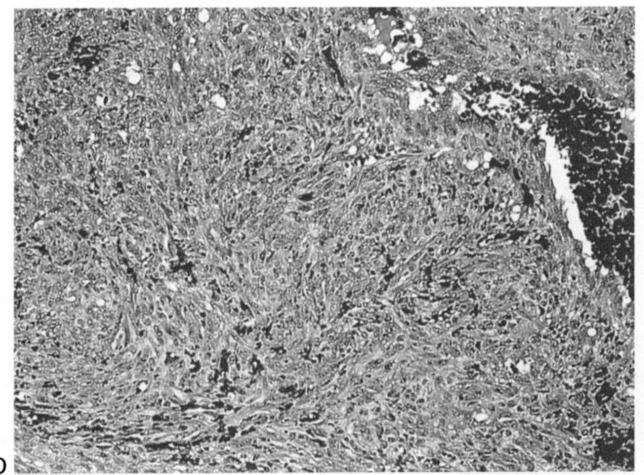

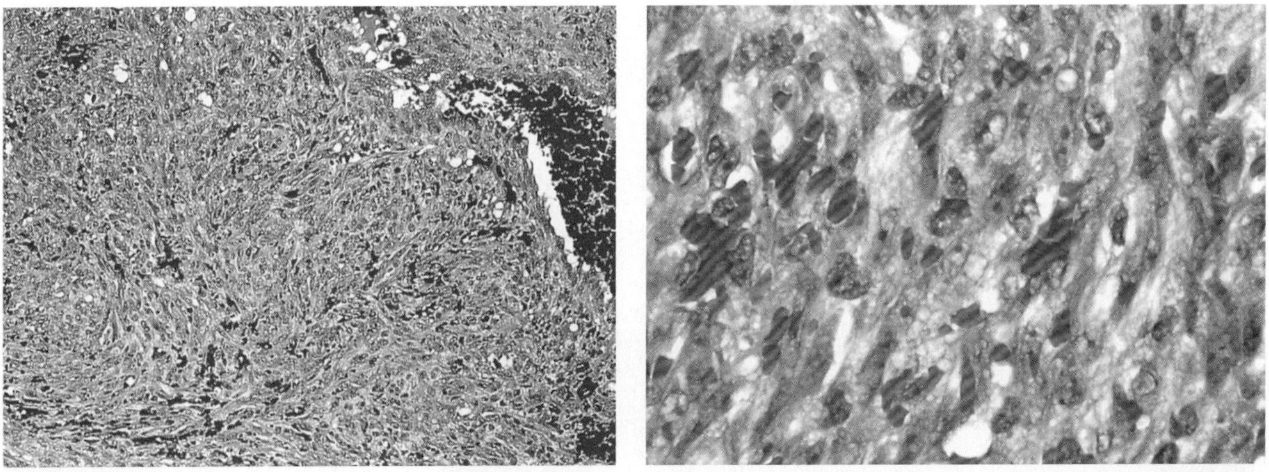

FIG. 39.45. *(Continued)*

mitotic figures[403] (Fig. 39.47). The mitotic rate varies from fewer than 1 to 35 mitotic figures per HPF with a mean of 9 per HPF.[403] Unusual histologic variants of cutaneous angiosarcoma include a perithelial arrangement of neoplastic cells (Fig. 39.48), storiform spindle cell growth (Fig. 39.49), tumors with cavernous elements (Fig. 39.50), and a pattern that mimicked epidermotropic metastatic mammary carcinoma.[440]

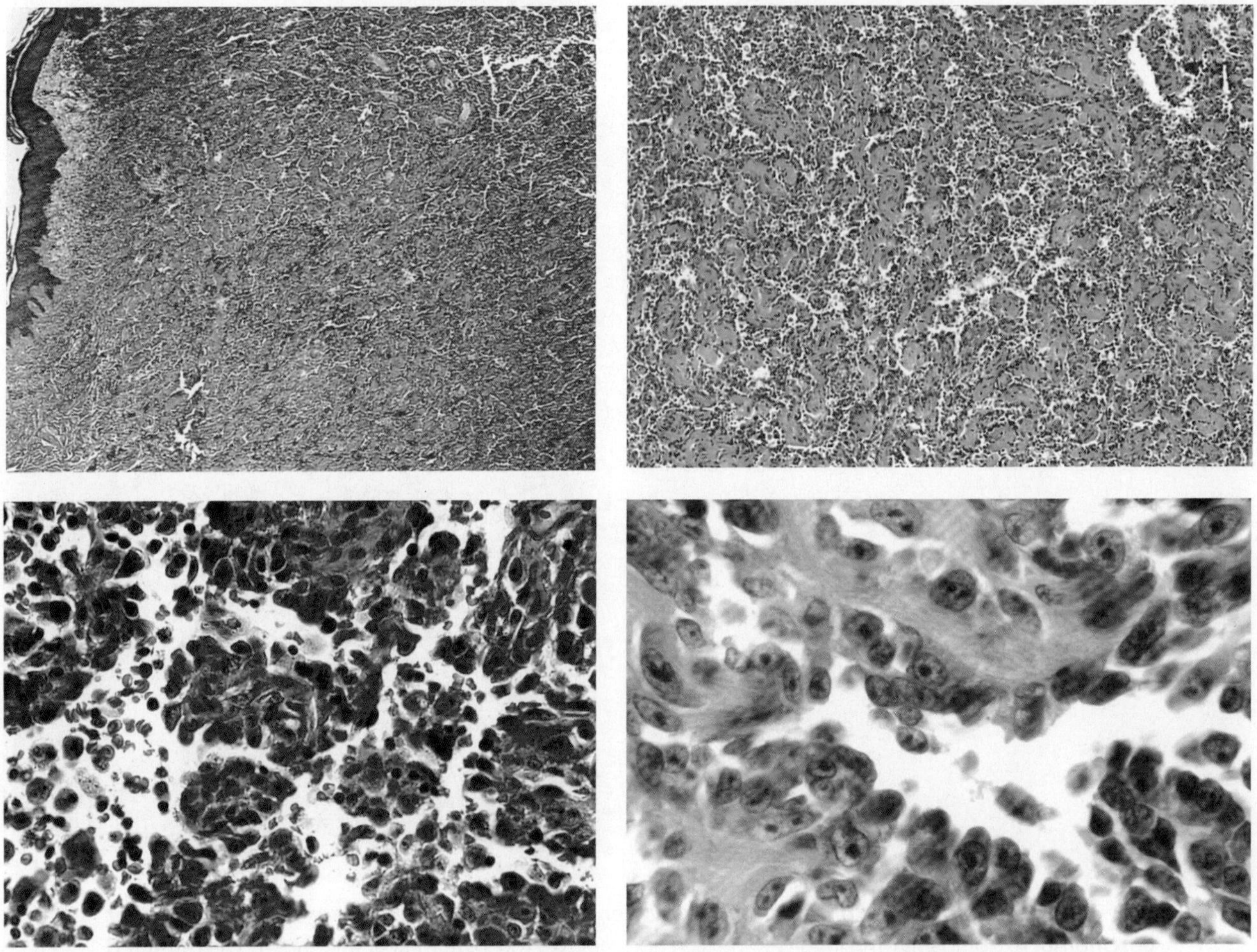

FIG. 39.46. ***Angiosarcoma of the mammary skin and breast after breast-conserving surgery and irradiation for carcinoma.*** **A:** This intermediate-grade sarcoma has extensive anastomosing vascular channels that create a papillary configuration in areas. **B,C:** The papillary structures are composed of malignant endothelial cells supported by slender cores of fibrovascular stroma. **D:** The nuclei have prominent nucleoli.

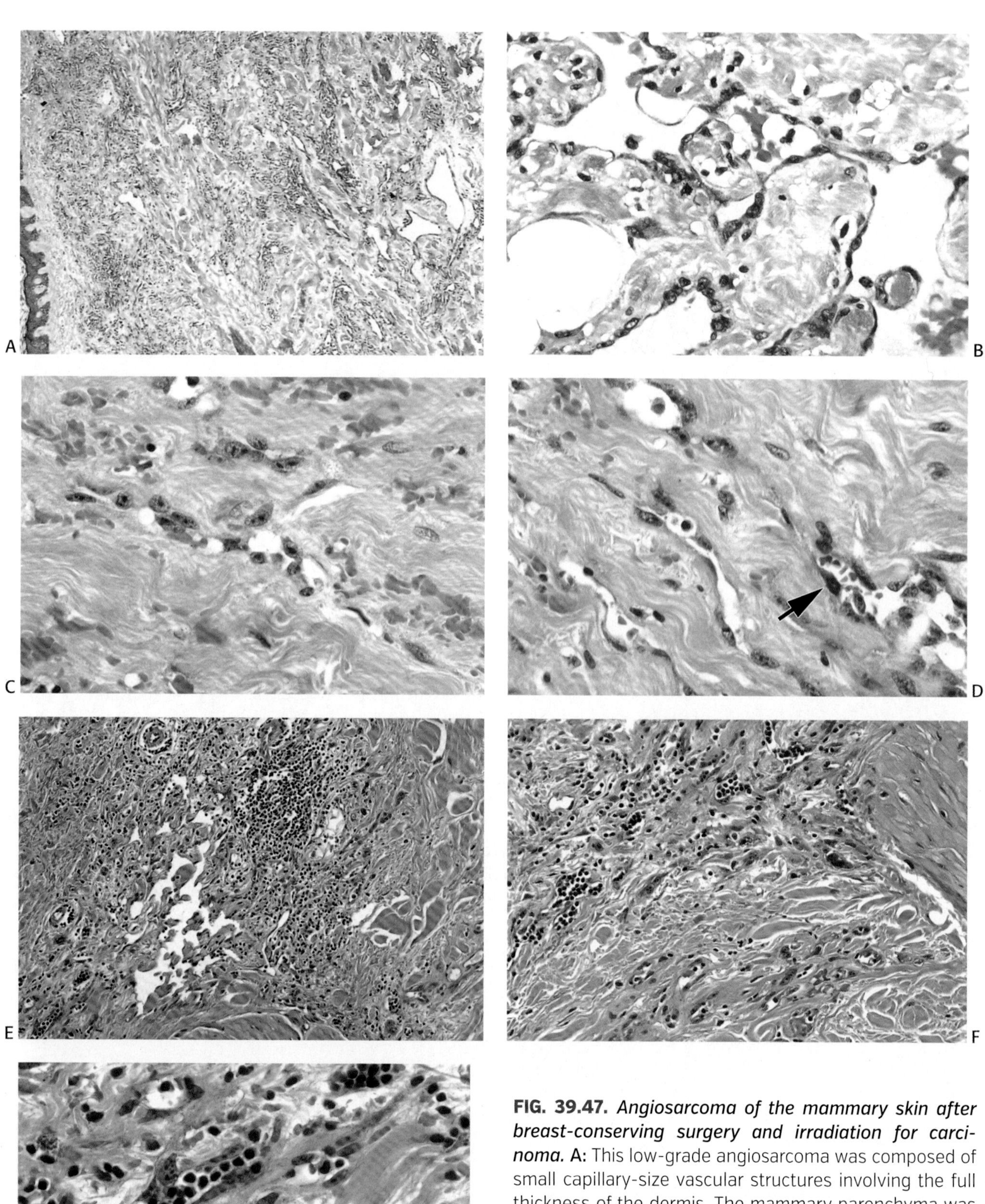

FIG. 39.47. ***Angiosarcoma of the mammary skin after breast-conserving surgery and irradiation for carcinoma.*** **A:** This low-grade angiosarcoma was composed of small capillary-size vascular structures involving the full thickness of the dermis. The mammary parenchyma was also involved. **B,C:** Nuclei are vesicular with punctate nucleoli. **D:** A mitosis in an endothelial cell is shown (*arrow*). **E–G:** These images are from another patient who developed cutaneous angiosarcoma 9 years after radiotherapy. Image **(E)** shows ectatic vascular channels and atypical cells in the stroma. Tumor cells with pleomorphic nuclei and multiple atypical nucleoli are shown in **(G)**.

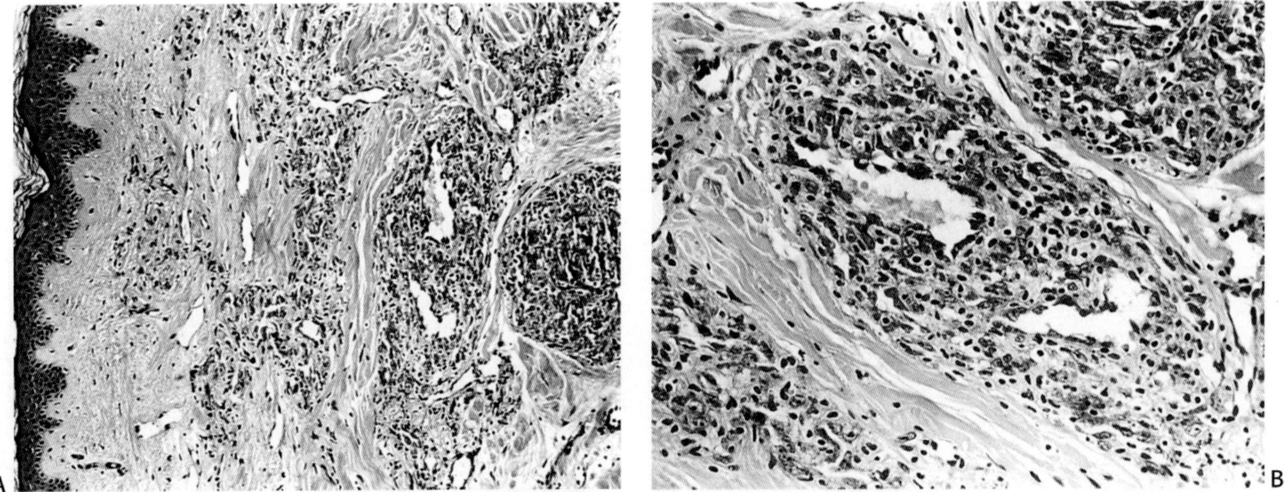

FIG. 39.48. ***Angiosarcoma of the mammary skin after breast-conserving surgery and irradiation for carcinoma.*** **A,B:** This sarcoma has an unusual nodular perithelial structure.

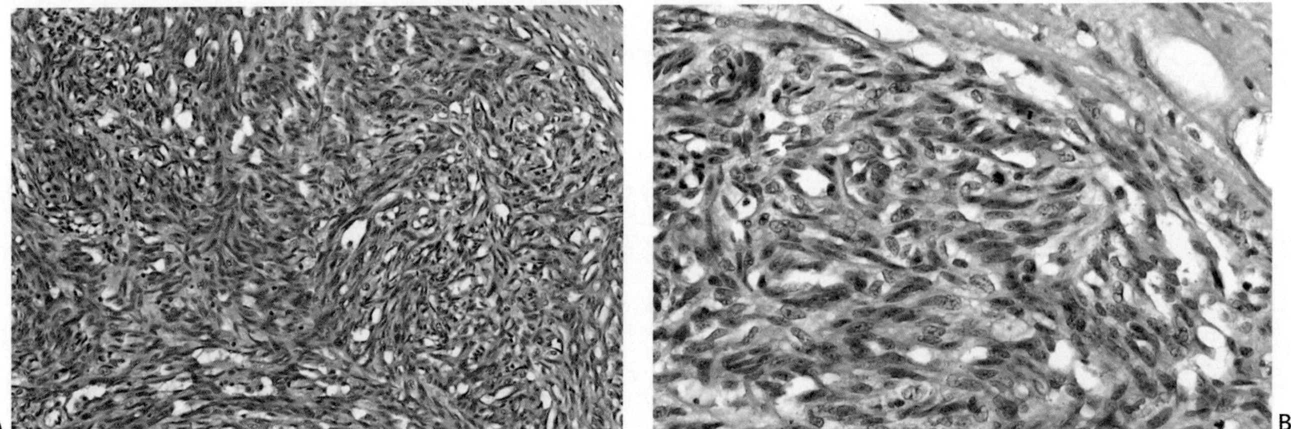

FIG. 39.49. ***Angiosarcoma of the mammary skin after breast-conserving surgery and irradiation for breast carcinoma.*** **A:** The tumor is composed of spindle cells with a swirling, storiform architecture. **B:** The malignant cells possess large, vesicular nuclei.

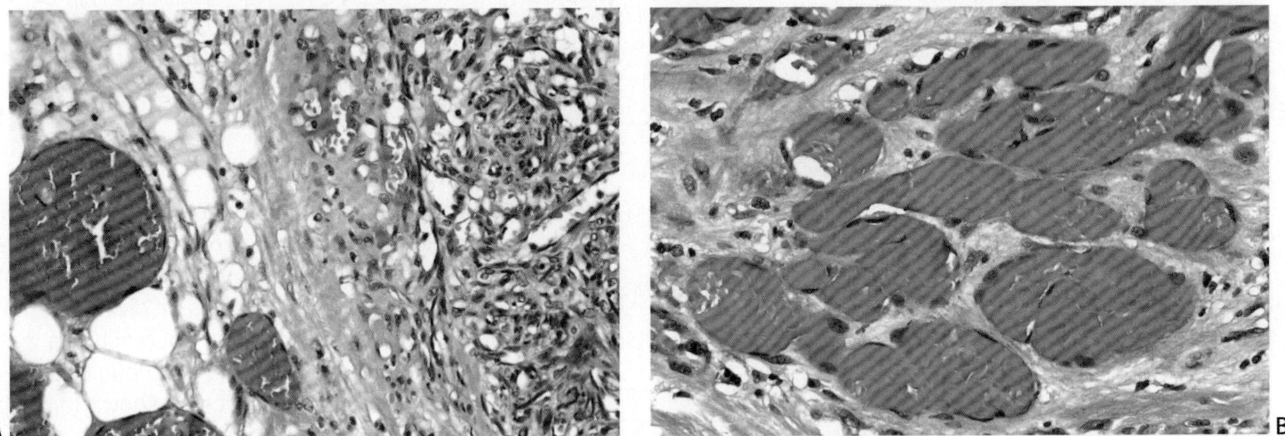

FIG. 39.50. ***Angiosarcoma of the mammary skin after breast-conserving surgery and irradiation for breast carcinoma.*** **A:** Dilated, cavernous vascular spaces are shown next to a portion of the tumor with a capillary structure. **B:** Note the prominent nuclei in this cavernous area.

Cytology

The diagnosis of postirradiation angiosarcoma can be suggested in a specimen obtained by FNA.[441] The findings of cytologic preparations resemble those observed in similar specimens obtained from patients with sporadic angiosarcomas. Epithelioid forms of angiosarcoma can resemble recurrent carcinoma in a cytologic specimen, and immunohistochemical studies may be required to distinguish these lesions.[437,442,443]

Immunohistochemistry

Like their sporadic counterparts, postirradiation angiosarcomas typically stain for vimentin and proteins found in endothelial cells such as CD31, CD34, and factor VIII. Strong reactivity for FLI-1, focal positivity for von Willebrand factor, and staining of one case for CD30 have been noted.[444] One abstract[363] reported reactivity for D2-40. Two epithelioid angiosarcomas stained for keratin.[413,438] Postirradiation angiosarcomas in case reports did not stain for HMB45,[437,439,445] "melanocytic markers,"[413] LCA,[438,445] S-100[437–439,442] CD20,[438,444] desmin, CD68, EMA, UCHL, Ki-1, and PAX5.[430,437,438,444] A Ki67 score of 83% was observed in the solid component of one case.[446] Immunohistochemical staining for ER and PR has been negative.[425,437,439]

Electron Microscopy

Seo and Min[438] described the ultrastructural features of one postirradiation epithelioid angiosarcoma. An external lamina enclosed groups of tumor cells. They contained sparse organelles, large nuclei, and prominent nucleoli. The cytoplasm harbored a loosely arranged fibrillary matrix and a few paranuclear aggregates of intermediate filaments. The cell membranes of closely apposed cells displayed rare primitive junctions. The cell clusters contained rudimentary lumens containing erythrocytes and platelets. Occasional membrane-bound granules highly suggestive of Weibel–Palade bodies were evident.

Genetic Studies

Cytogenetic studies of two postirradiation angiosarcomas revealed complex chromosomal alterations. The tumor in one case[373] showed gains in chromosomes 8q, 17q, and 22q and a loss in chromosome 3q. The second tumor[447] exhibited alteration involving 13 chromosomes: gains in 4q, 5q, 6q, 9q, 12p, 12q, and 20q and losses in 2p, 2q, 7p, 8q, 22q, and Xq.

Recent genetic studies implicate overexpression of *MYC* in the development of postirradiation angiosarcomas. Manner et al.[448] studied both sporadic angiosarcomas and those associated with irradiation or chronic lymphedema involving a variety of organs. Using array CGH, the workers detected high-level amplification of chromosome 8q24.21, and interphase FISH analysis identified *MYC* as the amplified gene in this locus. Amplification of *MYC* was detected in 18 of 33 angiosarcomas arising following irradiation or in the setting of chronic lymphedema but none of the 28 sporadic angiosarcomas. The investigation by Guo et al.[449] examined vascular lesions arising in several clinical settings and at several anatomic sites. Interphase FISH analysis demonstrated *MYC* amplification in 22 of 22 patients with postirradiation and lymphedema-associated angiosarcomas of the breast but not in atypical vascular lesions (AVLs) of the breast, sporadic angiosarcomas at various sites, and postirradiation sarcomas of other types. MYC protein was strongly expressed in those angiosarcomas associated with irradiation or chronic lymphedema, and MYC-II was the predominant isoform. This isoform was preferentially expressed in the radiation- or lymphedema-associated angiosarcomas but was not found in sporadic tumors. A subset of the former angiosarcomas also demonstrated amplification of *FLT4*, which codes for VEGFR3. Mentzel et al.[450] observed *MYC* amplification in 25 of 25 cases of postirradiation cutaneous angiosarcomas from women with breast carcinoma. The workers did not observe amplification of *MYC* in reactive or benign vascular proliferations, atypical vascular proliferations related to irradiation, and angiosarcomas unrelated to irradiation. Fernandez et al.[451] found that six of six postirradiation angiosarcomas of the breast showed *MYC* amplification and nuclear staining for C-Myc, whereas four AVLs did not demonstrate either finding. The findings of these four studies indicate that amplification of *MYC* represents an important alteration in the genesis of postirradiation angiosarcomas, including those arising following irradiation for breast carcinoma.

Prognosis

The prognosis of angiosarcoma arising in the breast after radiotherapy does not appear to differ substantially from that of angiosarcoma unassociated with radiotherapy. Vorburger et al.[297] compared survival data for 32 women with sporadic angiosarcomas of the breast with the outcome of 23 women with radiation-associated angiosarcomas. Patients with sporadic angiosarcoma presented with metastatic tumor significantly more often than those with postirradiation angiosarcoma (38% vs. 13%), but the two groups did not differ significantly in the distribution of tumor size or grade. The former group had a better DFS in the first 3 years of follow-up, but the differences were not statistically significant when plotted in Kaplan–Meier curves. The investigation of Scow et al.[344] included 27 cases of sporadic angiosarcoma and 14 cases of postirradiation angiosarcomas, and the median follow-up period was 2.3 years. The investigators did not detect a difference in the median time from diagnosis to death or the 5-year OS, and the Kaplan–Meier plots did not demonstrate a difference in survival between the two groups. Morgan et al.[283] discovered a 5-year OS of 43% in a group of 33 patients with postirradiation angiosarcoma and a 5-year OS of 55% for patients with sporadic angiosarcoma treated similarly. Hodgson et al.[414] did not detect a difference in mortality between patients with sporadic and postirradiation angiosarcomas, nor did Hui et al.[415] In one study[293] of 26 patients with a median follow-up of 23 months, patients with sporadic angiosarcomas demonstrated a better 5-year DFS compared to those with postirradiation angiosarcomas (68.6 vs. 22.0), although the 5-year OS did not differ significantly between the two groups.

A meta-analysis based on 151 cases[397] demonstrated a median OS of 18 months (range, 1 to 92 months) for patients with postirradiation angiosarcoma; however, studies from single institutions report higher median OS values of 35.5[297] and 48.5 months.[283] The largest single institution study[405] includes 95 patients followed for a median of 10.8 years. Local recurrences occurred in 48% of patients and distant metastases in 27%. The 1-, 2-, and 5-year OS values are 91%, 78%, and 54%, respectively, and the 1-, 2-, and 5-year disease-specific survival values are 94%, 84%, and 63%, respectively. Several other studies report information regarding the survival of patients with postirradiation angiosarcoma. Morgan et al.[283] studied 33 patients and reported median and 5-year local recurrence–free survivals of 18.2 months and 46.8%, respectively, and median and 5-year locoregional and distant metastasis–free survivals of 13.0 months and 39.2%, respectively. In the study of Strobbe et al.,[404] which included 21 patients followed for a median of 24 months, the 2- and 5-year OS rates were 72% and 55%, respectively, and the DFS rate was 35% at both points in time. Billings et al.[403] presented data for 22 patients with a median follow-up of 44 months (range, 12 to 91 months). The median time from diagnosis to death was 33.5 months.

Investigations of factors predicting the outcome of patients with postirradiation angiosarcoma have not yielded consistent findings. Torres et al.[405] found that tumor size larger than 10 cm represented the only adverse prognostic factor in multivariable analysis, and Morgan et al.[452] found that age greater than 70 years and presentation as an area of ecchymosis or violaceous discoloration indicated an adverse outcome in univariate analysis. Billings et al.[403] studied the predictive power of several histologic features: solitary versus multifocal disease, nuclear grades 1 and 2 versus nuclear grade 3, nuclear grade 1 versus nuclear grades 2 and 3, mitotic rate greater than 10 per HPF, and epithelioid morphology, but they did not correlate them with an adverse outcome. In other studies, the age of the patient, the length of the latent period, the clinical appearance at presentation, the grade of the tumor, the status of the margin of the specimen, and the size of the tumor have not consistently correlated with the patient's outcome.

Treatment

As is the case with sporadic angiosarcomas, surgery constitutes the primary treatment of postirradiation angiosarcomas. In 85% of the cases summarized by Abbott and Palmieri,[397] the surgical procedure was a mastectomy; wide excision was used in 12% and extensive surgery such as forequarter amputation or chest wall resection in 3% of cases. Surgical excision does not control the disease in most patients. Among the 75 patients with at least 1 year of follow-up culled from the literature by Monroe et al.,[410] 55 (73%) developed recurrences after surgery. Of them, 84% developed recurrences within a year of surgery, and only two patients experienced a recurrence more than 2 years after primary excision. Most of the recurrences arose in the bed of the tumor or the mastectomy scar, and the local disease represented the only site of recurrence in 82% of cases. In the investigation of Fraga-Guedes et al.,[293] which included both sporadic and postirradiation angiosarcomas, the choice of surgical procedure did not affect the survival of the patients.

Incomplete excision of the angiosarcoma leads to a high risk of recurrence and death from the tumor. In one study[453] of 14 patients with a median follow-up of 15 months, those with incomplete excision experienced 2- and 5-year OS rates of 0%. On the other hand, the absence of sarcoma at the margin of the specimen does not guarantee that the patient will not suffer a local recurrence. Six of seven patients in which the margin of excision was 1 cm or larger suffered recurrences with a median time of 12 months,[453] and Seinen et al.[454] observed local recurrences in 14 of 23 patients with negative margins after a median interval of just 6 months. Torres et al.[405] reported similar findings.

The high rate of local recurrence even in the face of seemingly complete excision has led several investigators to conclude that many postirradiation angiosarcomas involve the irradiated tissue in a discontinuous, multifocal manner. Torres et al.[405] wrote: "Angiosarcoma is a multifocal disease characterized by microsatellite lesions that may comprise occult sarcoma spread beyond apparent [negative] margins. . . ." On the basis of this belief, certain oncologists advocate excision of all irradiated skin. Two patients in the series of Seinen et al.[454] underwent mastectomy and excision of all irradiated tissue, and 12 of 33 patients in the study of Morgan et al.[452] were treated similarly. The authors of the latter study reported: "Although this did not universally prevent recurrence, we found that patients who did not undergo resection of all irradiated breast skin trended toward a worse median [local relapse-free survival] (10.0 vs. 80.8 months) and [OS] (29 months vs. not achieved)." Further studies will define the value of this approach.

Because angiosarcomas spread to lymph nodes uncommonly, lymph node excision is not usually carried out as a component of the primary therapy. Lymph node metastases have been detected both at the time of presentation[293,439,455] and in the setting of recurrences.[293,403,454–457] Fraga-Guedes et al.[293] described a patient whose presenting complaint was an enlarged ALN, and Cunha et al.[439] reported a case in which a contralateral ALN contained metastatic angiosarcoma at the time of presentation.

Radiation therapy has not usually played a role in the primary treatment of postirradiation angiosarcomas. It has been used, sometimes combined with hyperthermia,[420,456,458] both as an adjuvant to primary surgery[398,403,445,459,460] and as a treatment of recurrences.[445,456,458] A few patients have received hyperfractionated radiotherapy.[399,410,426,455] Palta et al.[455] reported the greatest experience with hyperfractionated and accelerated irradiation. Nine of the 14 patients treated with this form or radiotherapy and surgery remained continuously free of disease for a median of 61 months (range, 1 to 28 months). The progression-free survival rates at 2 and 5 years were 71% and 64%, respectively, and the overall and cause-specific survival rates at 2 and 5 years were 86% at both times.

Antineoplastic agents, including gemcitabine, docetaxel, paclitaxel, doxorubicin, ifosfamide, dacarbazine, and interferon, have been administered singly and in various combinations in both the adjuvant and neoadjuvant setting, but success has been limited. A few patients have shown responses to paclitaxel[427,446,461,462] and docetaxel,[463] agents that have demonstrated promising results in the treatment of angiosarcomas of the scalp and face. In one patient, the use of paclitaxel controlled the disease for 4 years,[462] and in another, it led to complete disappearance of a gingival metastasis from a postirradiation angiosarcoma.[461] Administration of oral thalidomide stabilized the disease in one patient[445] and was followed by a temporary complete clinical response in another.[459]

Targeted therapies may hold promise, but the literature contains only minimal information in this regard. The presence of VEGFR[315,364] in angiosarcomas suggests that the antibody to VEGF, bevacizumab, or inhibitors of VEGFR tyrosine kinases such as sunitinib, sorafenib, and pazopanib might help to control the disease in selected patients.[464] The c-kit protein has been detected in four of five postirradiation angiosarcomas in two series,[460,465] but the angiosarcoma reported by Wang et al.[290] did not stain for the protein. The presence of c-kit in a few cases raises the possibility that administration of imatinib might play a role of the treatment of certain patients with postirradiation angiosarcoma.

Postirradiation Cutaneous Vascular Lesions Other than Angiosarcoma

Benign vascular lesions arising in the skin of the chest wall following postmastectomy radiotherapy were reported in 1968 by Kurwa and Waddington[466] as "post mastectomy lymphangiomatosis" and in 1978 by Prioleau and Santa Cruz[467] as "lymphangioma circumscriptum." Other terms such as "benign lymphangiomatous papules"[468] and "cutaneous lymphangiectases"[469] have also been suggested. With the widespread use of irradiation as a component of breast conservation therapy, similar tumors have been observed in the radiation field overlying the breast. These nodules have been referred to as "atypical vascular lesions," a term first proposed by Fineberg and Rosen[408] because they were sometimes mistaken for angiosarcoma and their relationship to mammary angiosarcoma arising in irradiated mammary skin has not been fully characterized. Similar benign lesions arise in the skin at other sites of therapeutic irradiation.[358,468–471]

Clinical Presentation

AVLs following irradiation for breast carcinoma have developed in women aged 29[450] to 91 years.[472] The average age ranges from 52[473] to 68 years.[408] The radiation had been administered as a component of breast conservation therapy, following mastectomy, or as the sole treatment. To the extent that it can be determined, radiation doses have fallen within the customary range. AVLs typically develop 2 to 5 years after radiotherapy, but intervals as long as 27 years have been reported.[474]

The lesions present as single or multiple pink or brown papules in the skin of the breast, axilla, or chest wall and usually span 5 mm or less. Plaques, vesicles, and cystic examples have been observed much less commonly.[468,471,473,475] In one patient, approximately 30 papules became evident 6 years after irradiation.[476] Another patient, who underwent bilateral mastectomies for metachronous breast carcinomas, developed bilateral AVLs on the chest wall 12 and 78 months following irradiation.[473] Bilateral involvement occurred in one patient in the series of Santi et al.[475] Rare cases have spanned as much as 2.0 cm,[358] and one AVL[472] was described as 60 mm in size, although the authors questioned the accuracy of that clinical measurement. Clinical diagnoses included recurrent carcinoma, angiosarcoma, dermatofibroma, lymphangioma, and epidermal cyst. Rarely, AVL develops in the breast parenchyma (Fig. 39.51).

Microscopic Pathology

Histologic examination reveals a focal proliferation of dilated, anastomosing vascular channels typically centered in the papillary and reticular dermis and lined by a single layer of endothelial cells. The overlying epidermis appears normal or displays mild acanthosis. The superficial vascular channels often appear dilated, whereas those in the deeper reaches look smaller and compressed. On the basis of the characteristics of the small vessels, Patton et al.[472] identified two types of AVLs: lymphatic AVL and vascular AVL. In this series, lymphatic AVLs constituted 70% of the 32 cases. Lymphatic-type AVLs (Figs. 39.52 and 39.53) usually form a circumscribed collection of ectatic, clustered, thin-walled vessels lined by flat or slightly protuberant (hobnail) endothelial cells within the superficial dermis. In a minority of cases, the vessels grow in a serpiginous or somewhat infiltrative manner and extend into the deep dermis or subcutis. The neoplastic vessels can surround preexisting vessels or skin adnexa and infiltrate the arrector pili. The vascular spaces usually are empty, but occasionally there are lymphocytes in the stroma or in the vascular lumens (Fig. 39.54). Tufts of stroma typically project into the vascular lumens. Gengler et al.[473] subdivided the lymphatic type of AVLs into three subtypes: a lymphangioma circumscriptum-like pattern in which dilated vessels in the superficial dermis create an exophytic bulging papule, a lymphangioendothelioma-like pattern in which narrow slit-like vessels occupy the dermis, and a pattern in which the vessels resemble those of a hobnail hemangioma. Certain AVLs display a combination of these patterns. Vascular-type AVLs (Fig. 39.55) consist of irregular collections of round to linear capillaries growing within the superficial or deep dermis and surrounded by pericytes. In certain respects, vascular AVLs resemble capillary hemangiomas, although the former lack the lobular pattern characteristic of the latter. The "capillary lobule" described by Di Tommaso and Rosai[477] is a type of AVL.

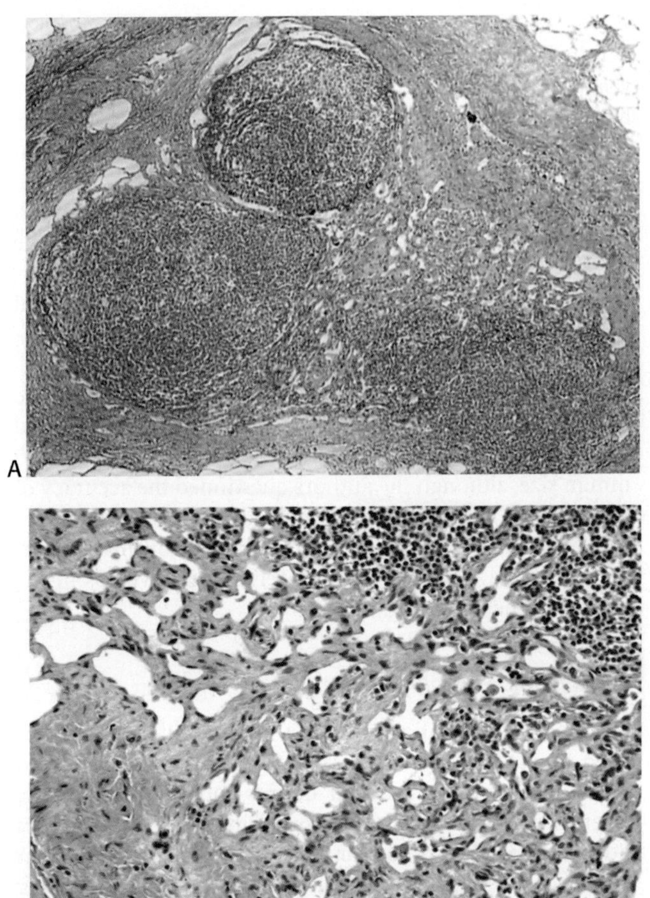

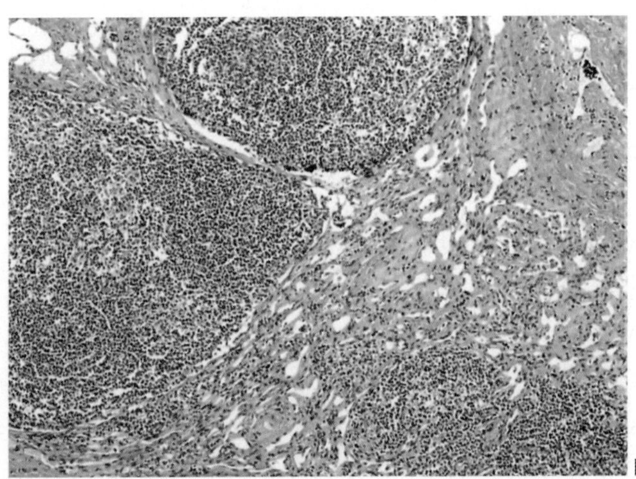

FIG. 39.51. ***Atypical vascular lesion, breast.*** **A:** This tumor was well circumscribed and it contained lymphoid follicles with germinal centers. **B,C:** Open, vascular spaces are present between the lymphoid follicles.

The vessels in the vascular type of AVL do not usually appear to communicate with each other in the manner of an angiosarcoma. The stroma often contains chronic inflammatory cells, including mast cells and occasionally plasma cells. Hemorrhage or stromal hemosiderin deposition occurs frequently. The background stromal cells in all types of AVL often display cellular atypia characteristic of radiation damage.

The endothelial cells lining the vessels appear bland. The nuclei can appear slightly hyperchromatic, but they do not demonstrate enlargement, angulation of their contours, or prominence of the nucleoli. Stratification of the endothelial cells is not usually present but may occur.[473] Mitotic figures are rarely seen, and if they are present the possibility that low-grade angiosarcoma is present increases.

Immunohistochemistry

The endothelial cells of the lymphatic type of AVL stain for CD31 and D2-40 and they stain variably for CD34; those of the vascular type of AVL stain for CD31 and CD34, but they do not stain for D2-40.[449,472,478] Reactivity for factor VIII–related antigen has been described.[358,468] The endothelial cells do not stain for Ki67.[471,478] One tumor did not stain for HHV-8 LNA-1.[474] Santi et al.[475] demonstrated immunohistochemical staining for p53 in 9 of 10 AVLs and alterations in the *p53* gene in 10 of 12 AVLs.

Electron Microscopy

An ultrastructural study[468] revealed vascular spaces lined by slender endothelial cells containing pinocytotic vesicles, thin filaments, rare mitochondria, and scant endoplasmic reticulum. The contacts between endothelial cells appeared poorly developed, and in many regions, the cells simply overlapped and did not form junctions at all. Collagen rather than laminin surrounded the endothelial cells, and thin anchoring fibrils terminated directly on the abluminal surface of the cell membrane. Pericytes were observed only rarely. The vascular lumen contained granular amorphous material and a few lymphocytes.

The differential diagnosis of AVL includes acquired progressive lymphangioma,[479] which rarely involves the skin of the breast in the absence of antecedent radiotherapy, reactive angioendotheliomatosis,[480] which usually occurs on the limbs in association with a systemic disease, and patch-stage Kaposi sarcoma, which typically exhibits the presence of erythrocytes, hemosiderin, and plasma cells. AVLs must also be distinguished from postirradiation angiosarcomas. AVLs tend to occur earlier and to form smaller masses

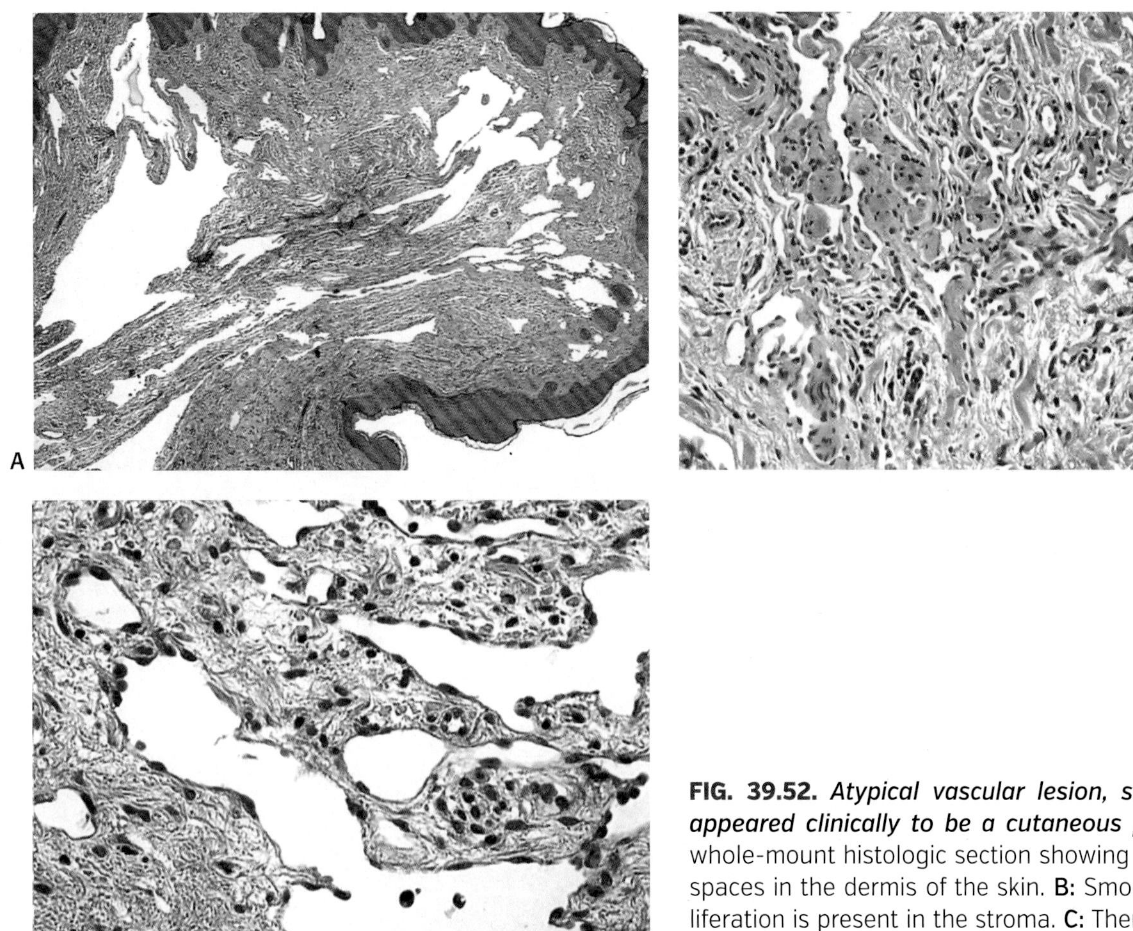

FIG. 39.52. ***Atypical vascular lesion, skin. This lesion appeared clinically to be a cutaneous papilloma.*** **A:** A whole-mount histologic section showing dilated vascular spaces in the dermis of the skin. **B:** Smooth muscle proliferation is present in the stroma. **C:** There is a mild lymphocytic infiltrate between serpiginous vascular spaces.

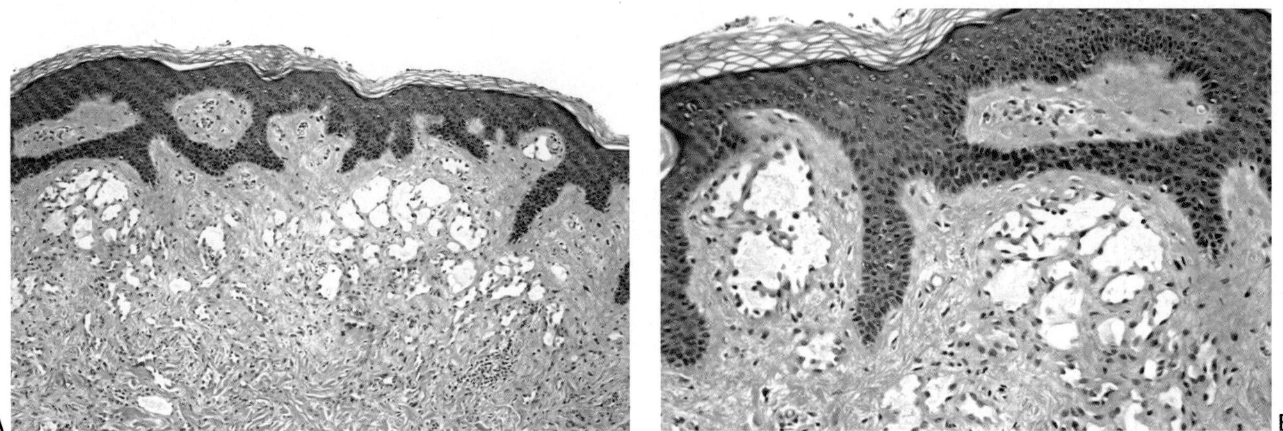

FIG. 39.53. ***Atypical vascular lesion, skin.*** **A,B:** Empty, dilated anastomosing vascular spaces are shown in the superficial dermis. This lesion appeared in a 54-year-old woman 3 years after excision and radiation therapy for invasive duct carcinoma. **C:** A small papule in the mammary skin of another patient found 6 years after breast-conserving surgery and radiotherapy. **D:** Serpiginous vascular channels in the dermis. **E,F:** Nodular lesions in the deep dermis of the patient with the superficial dermal lesion shown in **(C)**.

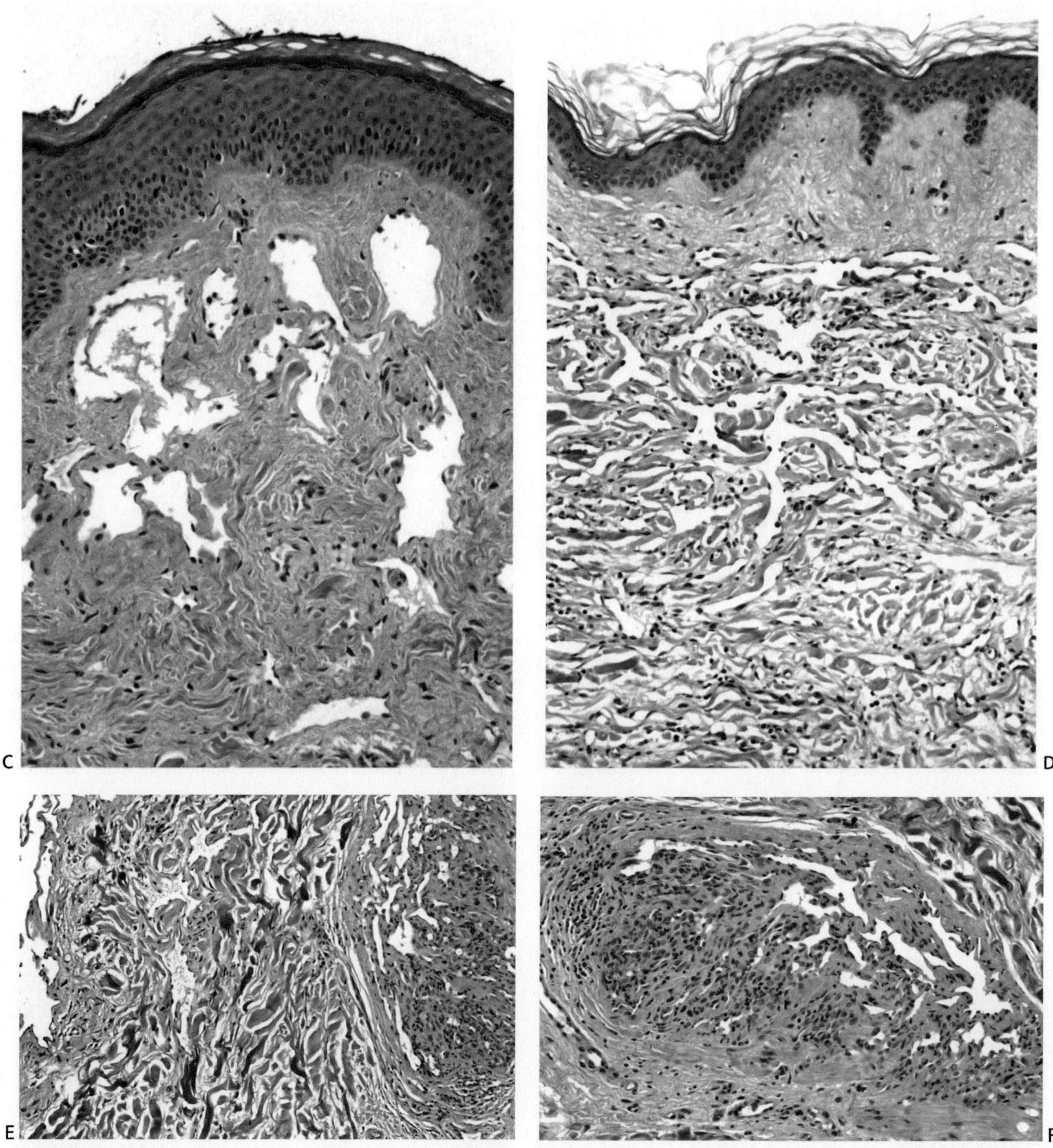

FIG. 39.53. *[Continued]*

compared to angiosarcomas; however, both parameters show considerable overlap between the two entities, and the differentiation ultimately rests on histologic characteristics. None of the AVLs from 32 patients showed the amplification of *MYC* characteristic of postirradiation angiosarcomas,[449–451] and only one case displayed immunoreactivity for MYC, which was seen in just a few cells.[450] Table 39.2 lists histologic features that aid in distinguishing these two lesions.

Treatment and Prognosis

In their study of AVL, Fineberg and Rosen[408] did not find evidence that these benign lesions evolved into angiosarcoma in patients who had been followed for as long as 10 years; however, local recurrences of AVLs were reported in this publication and others. One patient developed another AVL 17 months after excision of the first lesion.[408] A second patient had a 1-cm lesion in her mastectomy scar 35

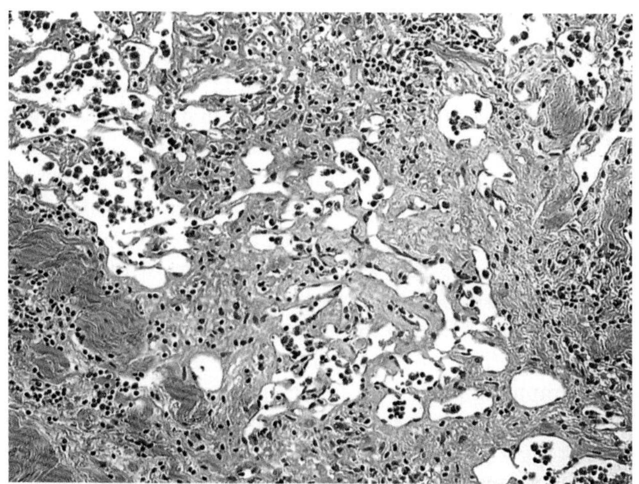

FIG. 39.54. ***Atypical vascular lesion, skin.*** Lymphocytes are present in the stroma and in the vascular spaces.

months after radiotherapy accompanied by smaller satellite nodules.[478] Fourteen months later, a second crop of lesions appeared nearby. Although both areas were diagnosed as acquired progressive lymphangioma, they most likely represent AVLs.[479] In a third case, multiple lesions arose in the parasternal area and axilla 10 years after mastectomy and ALN dissection followed by radiotherapy.[481] Additional lesions appeared in the same area and on the arm outside the radiation field 4 years later. Biopsies on both occasions were interpreted as lymphangiosarcoma. The lesions continued "waxing and waning" thereafter, and on subsequent review the diagnosis was revised to a "lymphedema-related dilatation or proliferation of lymph vessels, resembling lymphangioma circumscripta" (H. Peterse, personal communication [letter], May 20, 1996). In the study of Brenn and Fletcher,[358] 2 of 11 patients with AVLs involving the skin of the breast had recurrences of benign AVLs at the site of the initial lesion or in the radiation field. Both women remained disease-free after excision of the recurrent AVLs. Gengler et al.[473] noted recurrences of AVLs in 5 of 31 patients. One woman in this series developed more than 40 papules, which appeared in "3 efflorescences" 6, 12, and 24 months following irradiation. Four months after seemingly complete excision, another nodule appeared in the same region. Mentzel et al.[450] recorded the recurrence of an AVL in one patient. In contrast, spontaneous regression of an AVL occurred in one woman.[473]

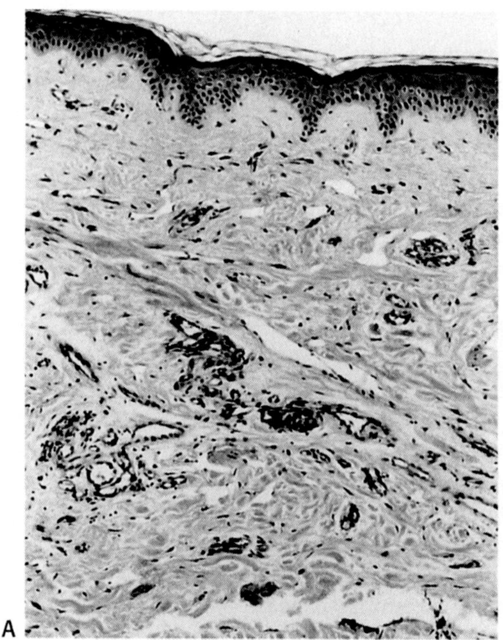

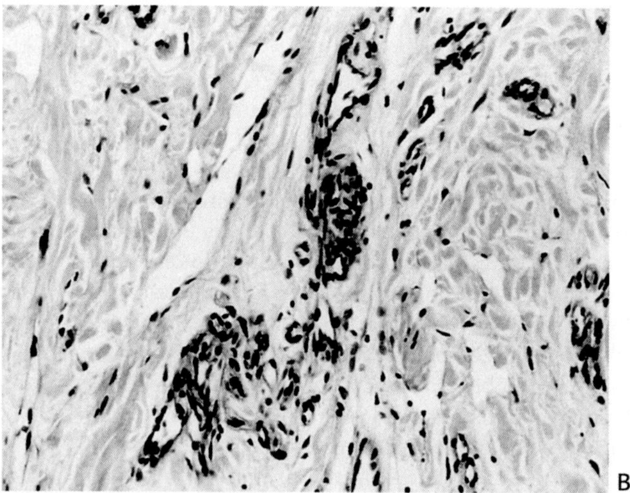

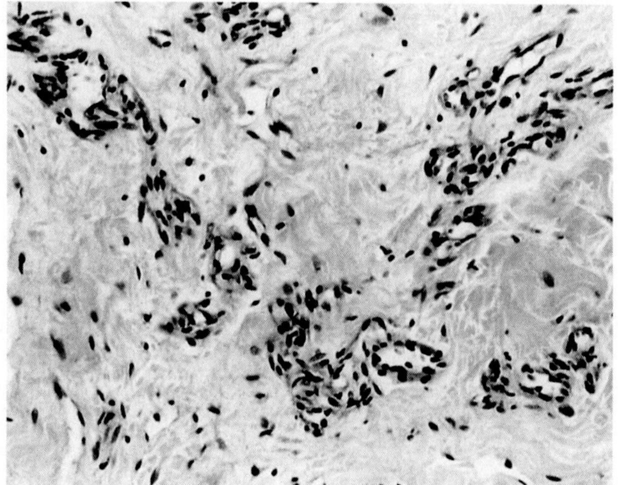

FIG. 39.55. ***Atypical vascular lesion of skin, capillary type.*** **A,B:** The atypical capillary proliferation stands out from the surrounding tissue. **C:** Loosely connected capillaries in which endothelial cells have hyperchromatic nuclei are shown.

TABLE 39.2 Histopathologic Characteristics of AVL and Cutaneous Angiosarcoma (AS)

	AVL	AS
Infiltration of subcutis	−	+++
"Blood lakes"	−	+++
Papillary endothelial hyperplasia	−	+++
Prominent nucleoli	−	+++
Mitotic figures	−	+++
Marked cytologic atypia	−	+++
Anastomotic vessels	++	+++
Chronic inflammation	+++	+
Hyperchromatic endothelial cells	+++	++
Dissection of dermal collagen	+/−	+++
Relative circumscription	+++	−
Projection of stroma into lumen	+++	−

−, absent; +/−, rare focal finding; +, occasionally present; ++, present in most cases; +++, present in all cases.

Relationship with Angiosarcoma

The Senior Editor has encountered additional examples of AVLs that had focal areas of cytologic atypia and even rare mitotic figures associated with entirely bland, typical AVLs. In one case, the patient had multiple recurrent atypical lesions that were focally indistinguishable from low-grade angiosarcoma. The vascular proliferation was found to be entirely limited to the skin when a mastectomy was performed. The study of Gengler at al.[473] includes 10 patients who had AVLs with atypical features: focal nuclear hyperchromasia of endothelial cells, prominence of nucleoli, or an infiltrative pattern of growth. None of the patients developed angiosarcomas despite incomplete excision in two of the cases. Patton et al.[472] noted "significant cytologic atypia" in 4 of the 10 vascular-type AVLs in their study. One patient developed angiosarcoma, and one developed additional AVLs with atypical features.

The published evidence suggests that AVLs have a benign nature, but a few observations raise the possibility that they might progress to angiosarcomas in rare circumstances. The presence of AVL-like formations in angiosarcomas,[451] the mingling of possible AVLs with angiosarcomas,[450] and the presence of mutations in the *p53* gene in both AVLs and angiosarcomas[449–451] suggest a pathogenetic link between the two lesions. The clinical course in rare cases raises the possibility that rare AVLs could progress to angiosarcomas. Six years after radiotherapy for breast carcinoma, a 56-year-old woman included in the report of Brenn and Fletcher[358] developed lymphatic-type AVLs, which were histologically atypical but "did not fulfill criteria for malignancy." The patient subsequently underwent a mastectomy in which low-grade angiosarcoma was found. At the time of the report, she had not had a recurrence with 42 months of follow-up. Two patients with AVLs in the study of Patton et al.[472] developed angiosarcomas. One AVL, which displayed atypical features, belonged to the vascular category. The lesion progressed to conventional epithelioid high-grade angiosarcoma in 14 months. The second angiosarcoma originated in a lymphatic-type AVL. In a series of four biopsy specimens collected over a 5-year period, the authors witnessed the evolution of the angiosarcoma from its origin in a solid focus of hobnail endothelium in "an otherwise classic [lymphatic type] AVL." These observations led the authors to suggest that lymphatic-type AVLs "presenting as localized lymphangiectasis do not seem to present any short-term risk of developing of angiosarcoma. The fact that one of our cases displays a clonal outgrowth of hobnail endothelium over a period of 5 years leading to a diagnosis of angiosarcoma, however, indicates that the lesions are not totally innocuous. . . . Lesions with 'hemangiomatous features' are more problematic. . . . those lesions that display atypia appear at increased risk to develop angiosarcoma and require a more aggressive approach to therapy and clinical surveillance."[472]

POSTMASTECTOMY ANGIOSARCOMA (STS)

Angiosarcoma arising in the lymphedematous upper extremity is not a primary breast neoplasm, but the majority of cases have developed as a complication of the treatment of mammary carcinoma. Since the report by Stewart and Treves in 1948,[482] the relationship of postmastectomy angiosarcoma with lymphedema of the upper arm has been referred to as the "Stewart–Treves syndrome." Although this clinical setting represents the most common one, angiosarcomas can arise in extremities rendered lymphedematous by other conditions and in other anatomic sites. The first description of the association between angiosarcoma and an edematous extremity[483] involved a 58-year-old woman with posttraumatic edema of the upper extremity following a blow by a heavy bundle of grapevines (*Rebenbündels*), and a publication 12 years later[484] detailed the case of a 44-year-old woman with edema of the right lower extremity since childhood who developed an angiosarcoma in the affected limb. Other examples affecting both men and women and involving congenital factors,[485–488] parasitic infestation of the regional lymph nodes,[489] regional surgery,[490–494] vascular surgery,[495] regional irradiation,[496–498] and immobility[485] have been reported. In one instance,[499] angiosarcoma arose in the edematous abdominal wall of a morbidly obese woman. The origin of these vascular sarcomas in lymphedematous limbs led to the use of the term "lymphangiosarcoma"; however, the lesions are similar to high-grade angiosarcomas that arise at other sites, and their microscopic characteristics most closely resemble those of angiosarcomas that occur in the mammary skin and breast after excision and radiotherapy.

The pathogenesis of angiosarcoma in areas of chronic lymphedema is unknown. It is unlikely that irradiation contributes directly to this process, because the lesion develops in the absence of radiotherapy, and in irradiated patients, it originates outside the treated field. Impaired immune responsiveness has been demonstrated in anatomic areas affected by lymphatic obstruction.[489,500] Hence, the lymphedematous limb may be a relatively privileged site immunologically, subject to neoplastic transformation,[501–504] a situation that may also contribute to the development of malignant lymphoma in this setting.[505,506]

The estimated frequency of STS ranges from 0.07%[507] to 0.45%.[508] A population-based study of sarcomas in Swedish women with breast carcinoma found that 30 angiosarcomas arose in edematous arms and 2 were present in conserved breasts.[509] Most of the patients were treated in the era prior to widespread breast conservation. The development of angiosarcoma in the ipsilateral arm was not significantly associated with the amount of radiation. When compared with control women who did not have lymphedema, the odds ratio for developing Stewart–Treves angiosarcoma was 12.0 (95% confidence interval [CI], 3.5 to 41.0). The incidence of STS has declined with the growing use of breast-conserving surgery and SLN sampling.

A distinction should be made between angiosarcoma in the STS and postirradiation angiosarcoma of the skin and soft tissue of the chest wall.[510–512] The latter arises after mastectomy on the chest wall in the irradiation field and is one of several types of radiation-induced sarcomas.[513] Most patients with radiation-induced angiosarcoma of the chest wall have not had lymphedema of the ipsilateral arm,[510,511] but this complication was present in one case.[512] The interval to the onset of postirradiation angiosarcoma of the chest wall has been less than 10 years, with most tumors having arisen in 3 to 6 years. Also excluded from STS are patients who develop angiosarcoma of the mammary skin or mammary parenchyma following breast-conserving surgery and irradiation. These forms of angiosarcoma, discussed earlier in this chapter, are not specifically related to postirradiation edema of the breast.

Clinical Presentation

The average age at diagnosis of STS is approximately 65 years (range, 44 to 84 years). Nearly 65% of patients who developed STS had irradiation of the chest wall and axilla after a radical mastectomy. The average interval between the treatment of mammary carcinoma and the clinical appearance of Stewart–Treves angiosarcoma in the arm is approximately 10 years,[492,500,514] although periods as short as 1 year[515,516] and as long as 49 years[517] have been reported.

STS occurs most commonly in women, but two reports[518,519] document cases in men. The initial lesions appear on the upper inner or medial arm in at least 75% of cases,[500] but they also have been found on the forearm and elbow. They often consist of purplish discoloration of the skin, which may be mistaken for an ecchymosis. These subtle changes evolve into plaques that enlarge into blue or blue-red nodules (Fig. 39.56). Superficial vesicles or bullae containing hemorrhagic fluid tend to develop before the surface ulcerates and often ooze serosanguineous fluid or blood. Usually there is rapid progression from the initial lesion with spread in the skin to involve the chest wall and forearm, but rarely the evolution of the disease can have a chronic course.

Imaging Studies

CT scans display increased density of the subcutaneous tissue and may reveal a mass.[487,497] Contrast administration may define the mass and may reveal thickening of fibrous septa, nodular thickening of the skin, or a honeycomb pattern resulting from encapsulated lakes of fluid associated with soft tissues. On MRI studies,[497,520,521] the edema appears as a diffuse increase in signal on T2-weighted images. The tumor exhibits an inhomogeneous low T2-weighted signal and an intermediate signal on T1-weighted studies. Contrast administration leads to enhancement of the tumor. Dynamic

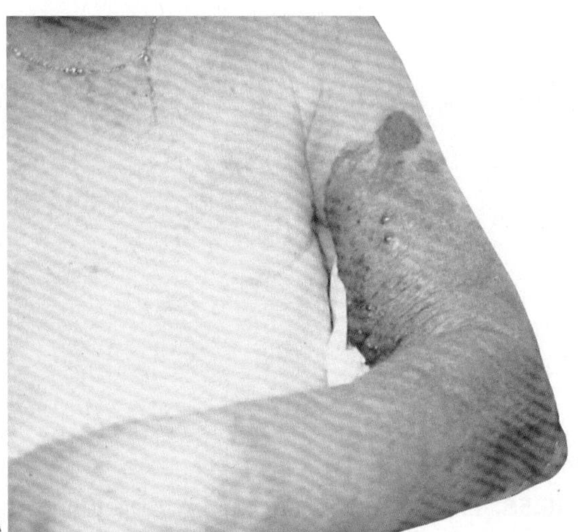

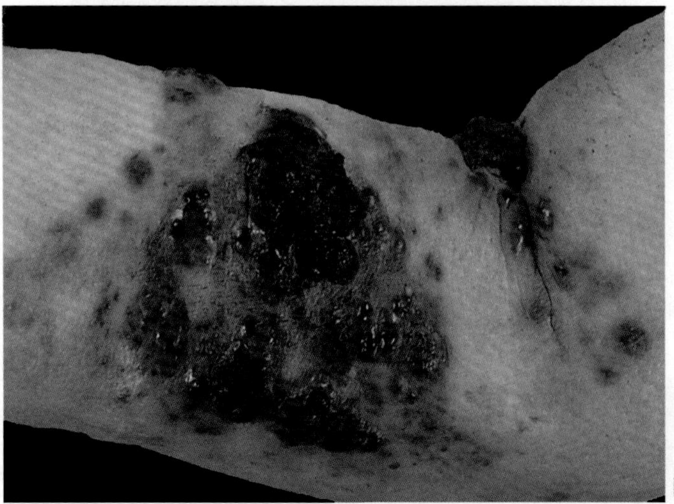

FIG. 39.56. ***Postmastectomy angiosarcoma.*** **A:** Clinical picture showing a sharply demarcated lesion in an edematous upper extremity. **B:** Hemorrhagic masses involving the distal upper arm and proximal forearm are shown in an amputation specimen.

studies show enhancement in the early phase, which persists in the delayed phase. PET scans may prove especially useful in defining the extent of the disease and revealing other sites of involvement.[485,496,522]

Gross Pathology

Biopsies obtained at an early stage before the development of nodules and plaques reveal lesions limited to the dermis of the skin and the superficial subcutaneous tissues. The lesions usually consist of punctate hemorrhagic foci with little or no induration. When surgery is performed in a more advanced case, there are usually hemorrhagic tumor nodules, involving muscles, subcutaneous fat, and skin (Fig. 39.57). The gross distribution of satellite cutaneous and deep soft-tissue lesions suggests that either they develop from in-transit metastases or there may be multiple sites of origin. Stewart and Treves[482] noted that deep tumors were associated with blood vessels and that in some instances tumor was present in large veins.

Microscopic Pathology

This form of angiosarcoma presents heterogeneous histologic appearances. Flat discolored or faintly infiltrated skin lesions may reveal inconspicuous findings. Diffuse alterations related to the underlying chronic lymphedema consist of dilatation of lymphatic vessels, edema and collagenization of the dermis, proliferation of capillaries in the dermis, and focal lymphocytic infiltrates in the superficial dermis, which tend to have a perivascular distribution (Fig. 39.58). A subtle proliferation of small vessels in the superficial dermis commonly occurs in chronic lymphedema (Fig. 39.59). The earliest evidence of angiosarcoma usually consists of the focal proliferation of irregular vascular channels lined by somewhat prominent endothelial cells, which have hyperchromatic nuclei and demonstrate mitotic figures (Fig. 39.60). Erythrocytes can be seen in these vessels and also in the surrounding dermal stroma. These early lesions may be indistinguishable from Kaposi sarcoma, a diagnostic problem emphasized by Stewart and Treves.[482]

FIG. 39.57. *Postmastectomy angiosarcoma.* In this hemisected amputation specimen, angiosarcoma involves the subcutaneous tissue and underlying muscle.

The formation of interconnecting vascular channels, papillary endothelial proliferation, and hemorrhage are indicative of more fully developed lesions (Figs. 39.61 and 39.62). In advanced cases, endothelial growth may be so exuberant that the accumulated cells form nodules (Fig. 39.63). When such foci have an epithelial appearance, the lesions can be difficult to distinguish from carcinoma by light microscopy (Fig. 39.64). A diagnosis of retrograde metastasis of mammary carcinoma may be suggested by such lesions, but it is usually possible to identify areas with a distinct vascular component, often with a prominent papillary configuration. Spindle cell

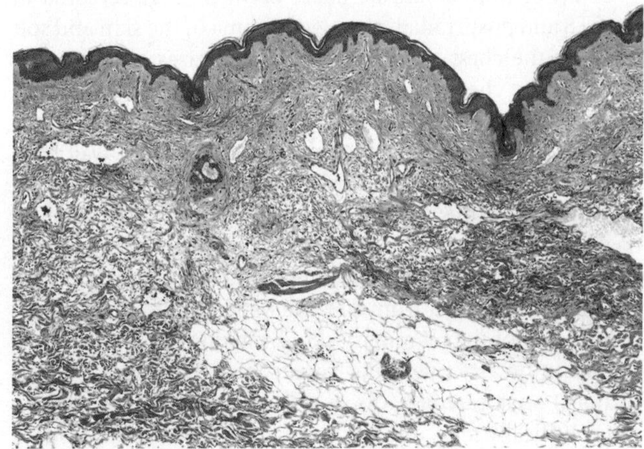

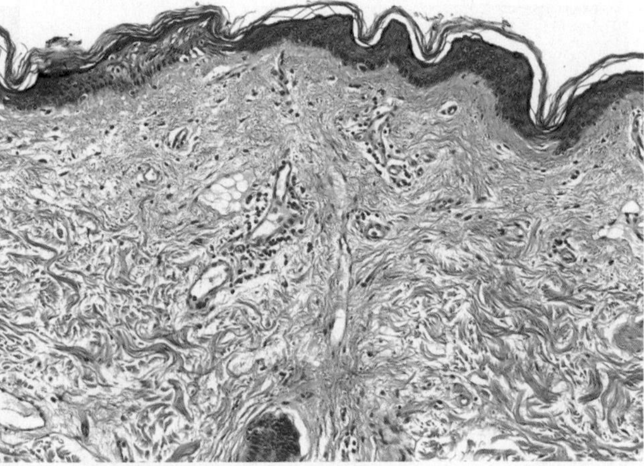

FIG. 39.58. *Chronic lymphedema.* **A:** Dilatation of lymphatic vessels, vascular proliferation, and collagenization of the superficial dermis are evident. **B:** The superficial dermis displays an increased number of small blood vessels and a slight perivascular lymphocytic infiltrate.

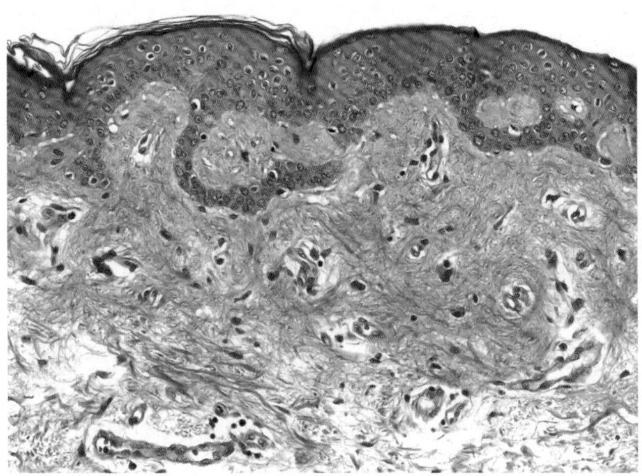

FIG. 39.59. ***Chronic lymphedema.*** Proliferation of small blood vessels and collagen deposition can be seen in the papillary dermis.

sarcomatous elements may be found in association with lesions that have an epithelial growth pattern and as independent lesions. Larger veins appear to become involved most often as a result of intramural neoplastic proliferation rather than as a consequence of transmural invasion by extrinsic tumor cells. Embolic spread of angiosarcoma has been found at distant sites such as the lung and kidney.

Cytology

Cytologic specimens demonstrate dyshesive cells in a clean background. The neoplastic cells have long, spindly, crescentic shapes, and they contain oval nuclei and prominent nucleoli.[523]

Immunohistochemistry

Factor VIII–related antigen has been detected in cells lining well-formed neoplastic vascular channels,[493,495,499,521,524–530] but it has been absent[524,526] or minimally expressed[510] in poorly differentiated foci. It is often difficult to distinguish well-differentiated neoplastic vascular channels from reactive vessels associated with chronic lymphedema. Both may be factor VIII–related antigen immunoreactive. Anti-CD34 and CD31 are also reactive with the majority of angiosarcomas, but they are less specific because they also stain other types of sarcoma (Fig. 39.65). D2-40 is immunoreactive with lymphatic channels and with angiosarcoma, but not with mammary carcinoma.[531] Three angiosarcomas stained for

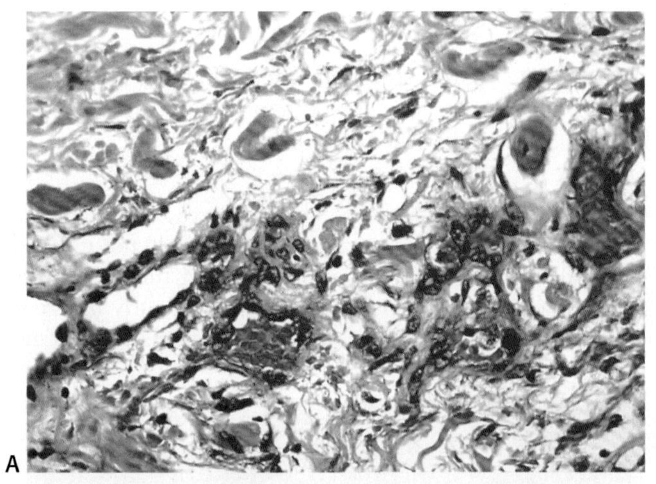

A

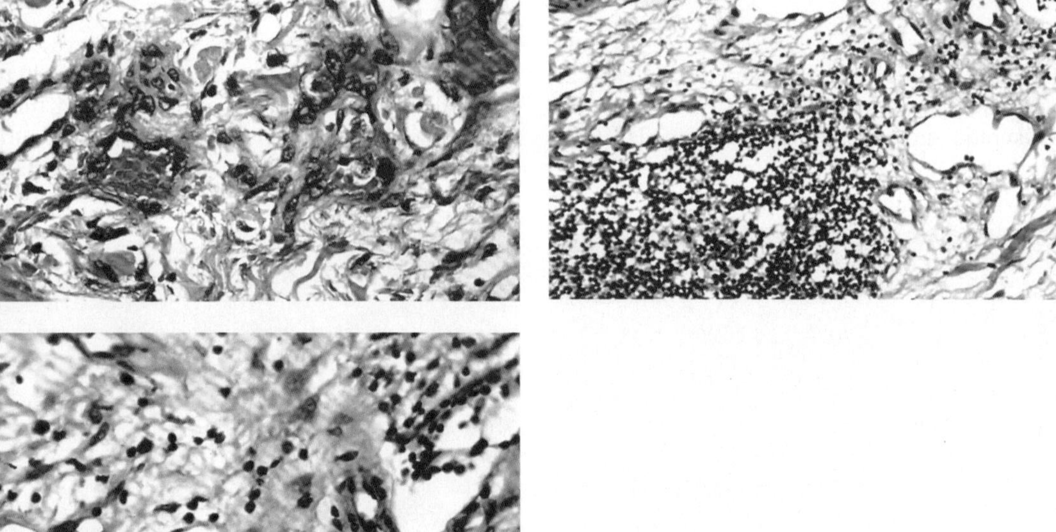

B

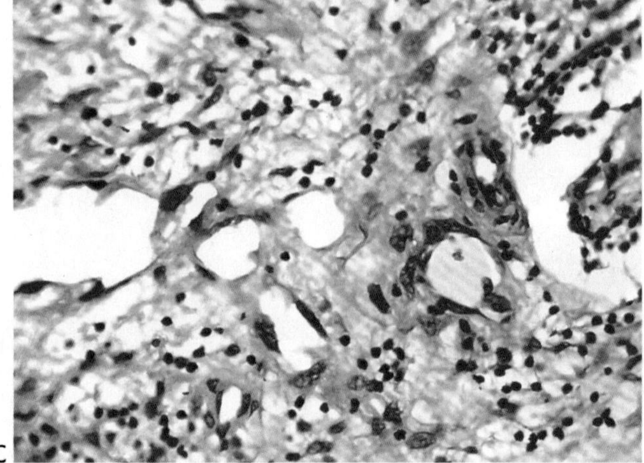

C

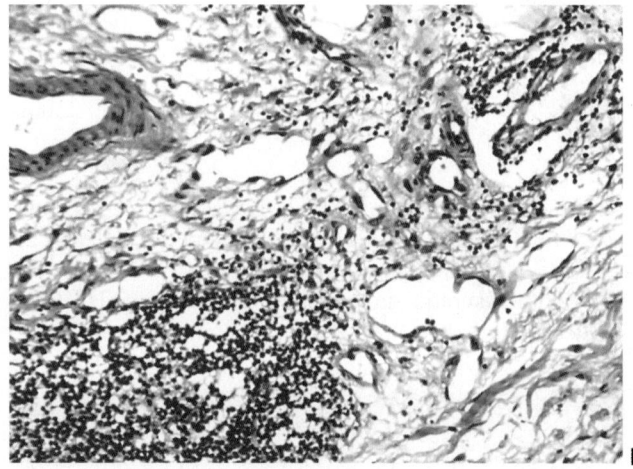

FIG. 39.60. ***Postmastectomy angiosarcoma, early lesions.*** **A:** Congested capillaries with atypical endothelial cells. **B,C:** The small, dilated, empty vascular channels have atypical endothelial cells, and there is focal lymphocytic infiltration.

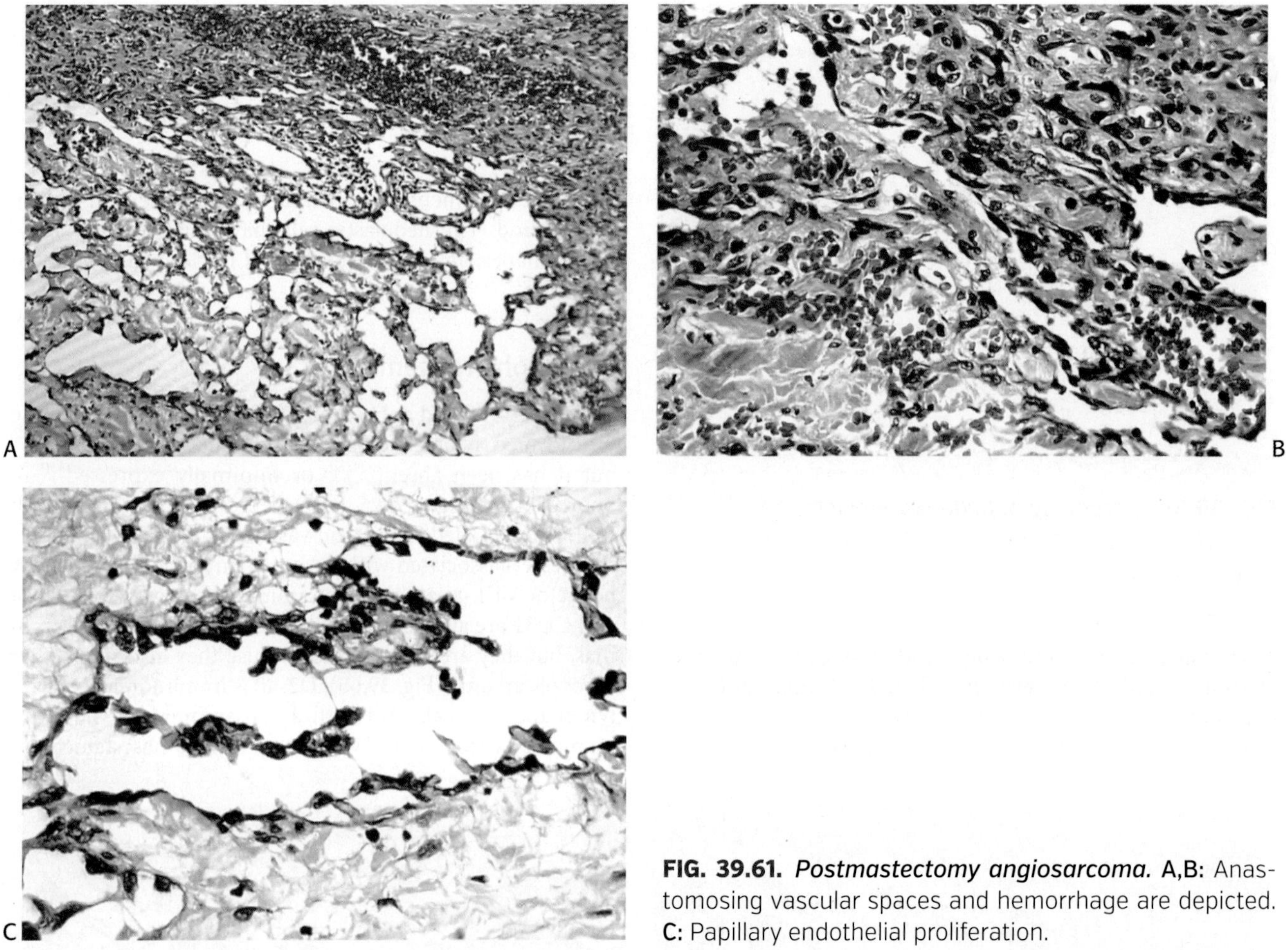

FIG. 39.61. ***Postmastectomy angiosarcoma.*** **A,B:** Anastomosing vascular spaces and hemorrhage are depicted. **C:** Papillary endothelial proliferation.

laminin.[495,529] Staining for HLA-DR was observed in one case[528] for FLI-1 in another,[496] and for type IV collagen in a third.[529] Isolated cases did not stain for CAM5.2, keratin AE1/3, other keratin molecules, EMA, melanin, HMB45, S-100, and HHV-8.[493,496,528–530]

The distinction between Stewart–Treves angiosarcoma and recurrent mammary carcinoma is usually not difficult clinically, but biopsies of undifferentiated tumor nodules can present problems for the pathologist. Poorly differentiated recurrent carcinoma generally contains little or no

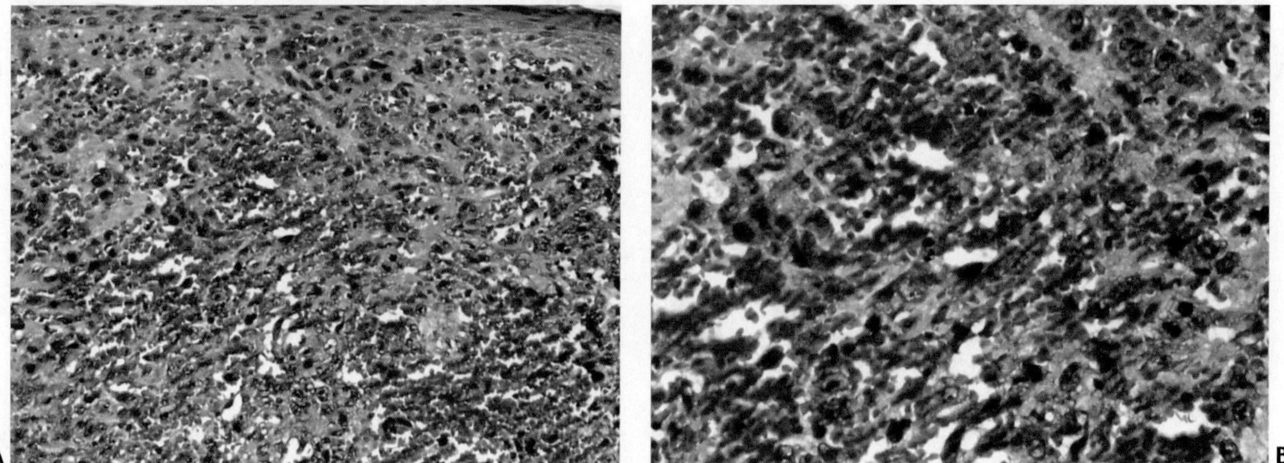

FIG. 39.62. ***Postmastectomy angiosarcoma.*** **A:** A hemorrhagic tumor nodule that developed in the soft tissue of the arm. **B:** The tumor cells have poorly differentiated nuclei with vesicular chromatin and prominent nucleoli.

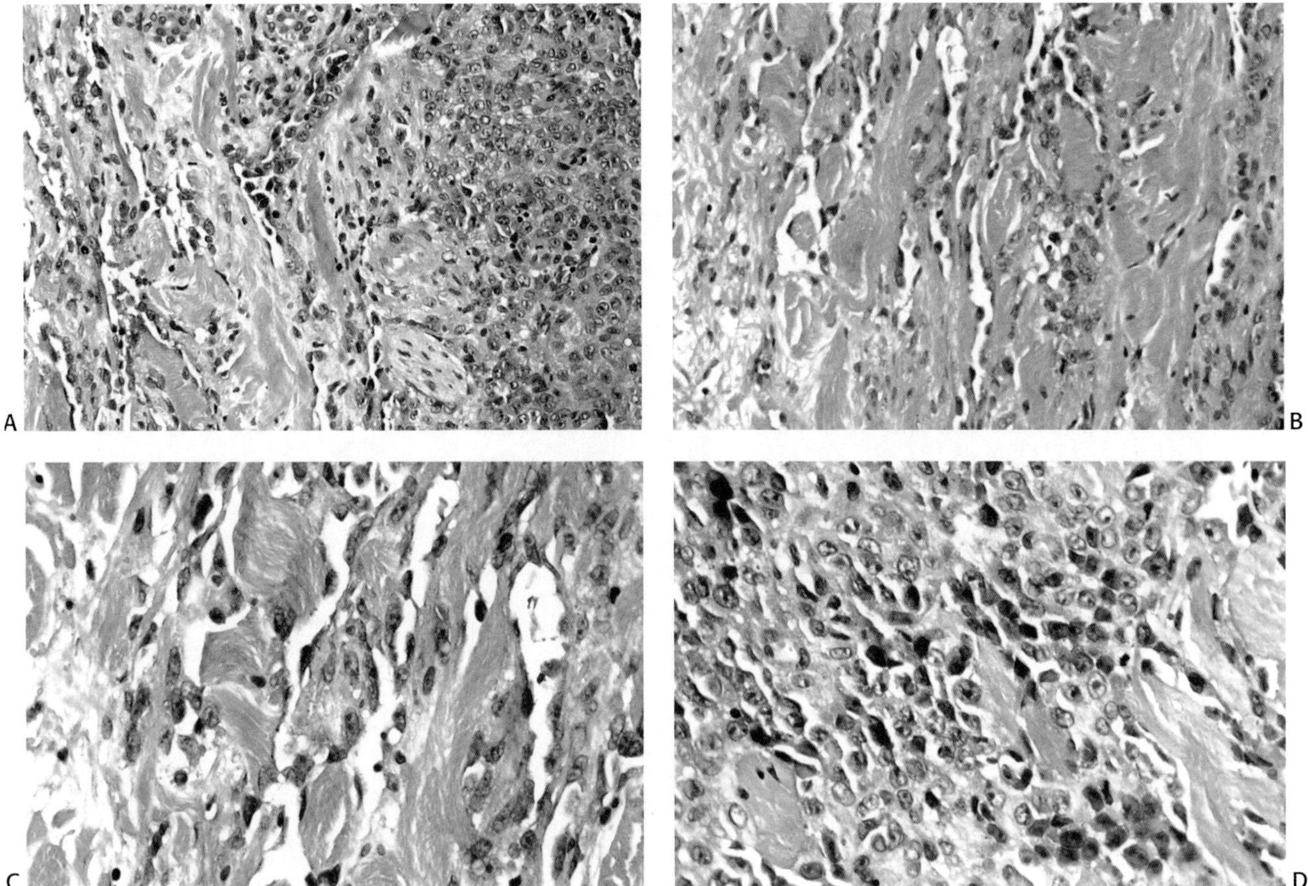

FIG. 39.63. *Postmastectomy angiosarcoma.* **A:** This tumor nodule has slit-shaped vascular spaces and a solid epithelioid component. **B,C:** A vascular area. **D:** An epithelioid area. Nucleoli are more prominent in this part of the lesion.

mucin, but the tumor cells are almost always immunoreactive to cytokeratin.[532] Vimentin reactivity is absent from many carcinomas and present in angiosarcomas.[524,528,529] Staining for the blood group antigen UEA-1 has resulted in strong immunoreactivity in vascular components and variable immunoreactivity in solid undifferentiated areas of Stewart–Treves angiosarcoma[495,524,525,527,529]; however, immunoreactivity for UEA-1 has also been found in mammary carcinomas.[533]

Immunohistochemical studies are also helpful in the diagnosis of other malignant neoplasms, which may arise in the lymphedematous limb. Two reported instances of malignant lymphoma were immunoreactive for markers of lymphoid cells such as L26, a protein associated with B cells.[505,506] An example of malignant melanoma that arose in the skin of an arm with postmastectomy lymphedema predated modern IHC, but one would expect melanoma to be reactive for S-100 protein, HMB45 antigen, and possibly vimentin.[534] Several cases of Kaposi sarcoma have presented in women with lymphedematous upper extremities following treatment for breast carcinoma.[535–538] Testing for HHV-8 reveals the presence of viral proteins or DNA and permits the proper diagnosis in such cases. After careful evaluation of the clinical presentation and a thorough assessment of histologic sections, it is usually possible to distinguish Stewart–Treves angiosarcoma from the exceedingly rare retrograde metastatic carcinoma and other malignant neoplasms.

Electron Microscopy

Several studies established the heterogeneous ultrastructural features of Stewart–Treves angiosarcoma.[495,499,524–526,528,529,539–541] The electron microscopic findings were typical for a malignant vascular tumor. In angiomatous areas, endothelial cells resting on a basement membrane were joined by well-formed junctional complexes. The nuclei appeared large and they possessed peripherally located chromatin and one to three nucleoli. The cytoplasm contained pinocytotic vesicles, clusters of intermediate filaments, and Weibel–Palade bodies. With loss of differentiation, Weibel–Palade bodies and pinocytotic vesicles became less numerous. Solid portions of the tumors were composed of round and spindle cells arranged in a loosely cohesive fashion and joined by desmosomes. Erythrocytes were seen in neoplastic vascular lumens and between neoplastic cells in poorly differentiated areas. Pericytic cells were reportedly not evident,[525] or present only in well-differentiated areas.[539,540,542]

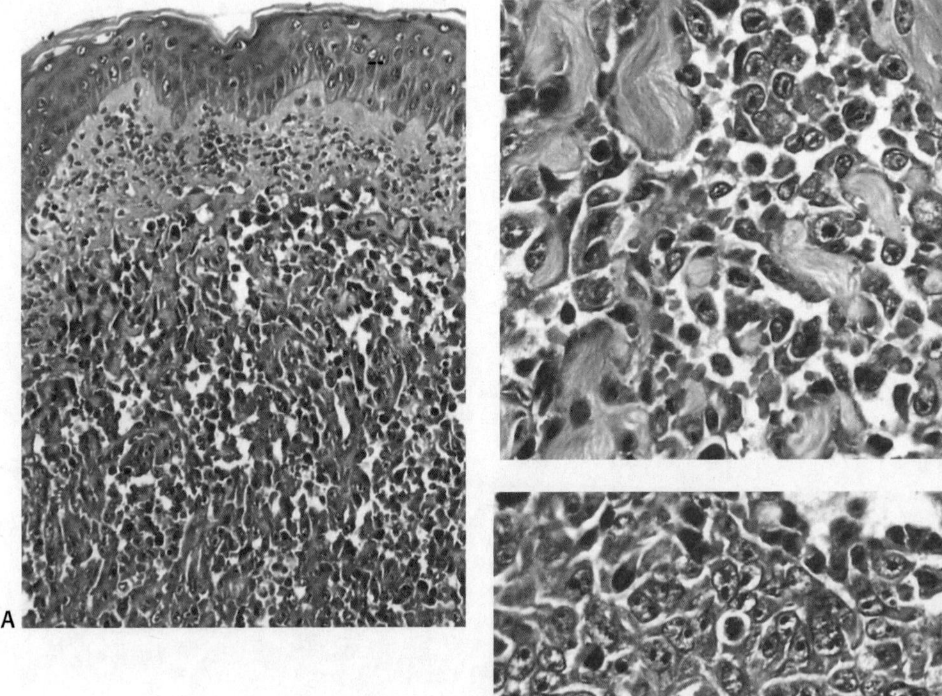

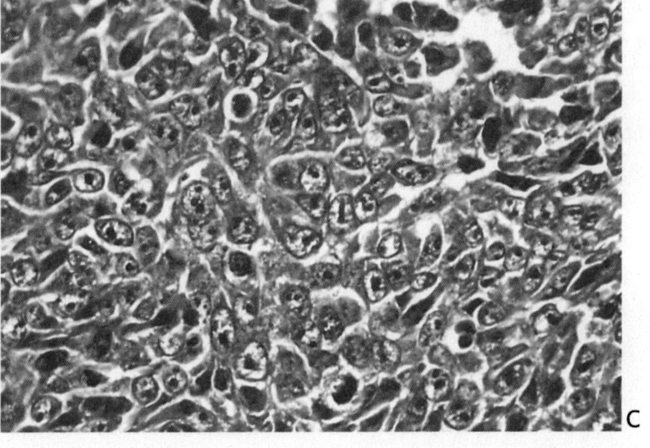

FIG. 39.64. *Postmastectomy angiosarcoma, epithelioid type.* **A,B:** The tumor composed of epithelioid cells had a vascular pattern in this region. **C:** Part of the sarcoma had epithelioid cells arranged in sheets.

Immunohistochemical and ultrastructural observations have led to the widely held conclusion that the neoplastic cells in Stewart–Treves angiosarcoma have properties more typically associated with blood vascular than with lymphatic endothelium. The features that characterize blood vascular endothelium include fenestrated cells, Weibel–Palade bodies, pinocytotic activity, and pericytic cells.

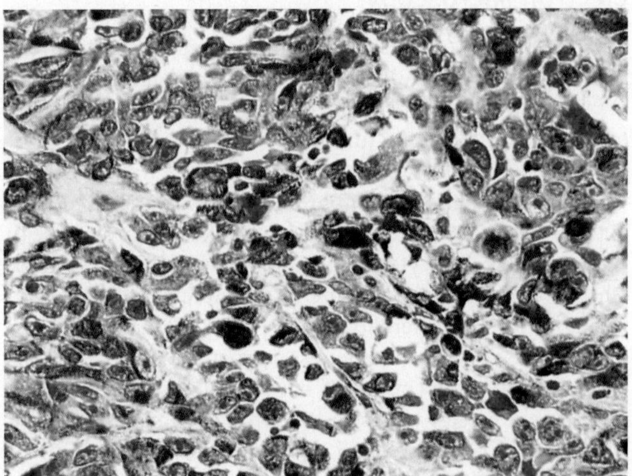

FIG. 39.65. *Postmastectomy angiosarcoma, CD31.* Intense immunostaining for CD31 is shown.

Genetic Studies

Chromosome analysis of 32 cells in one cases of STS[529] showed a large number of chromosomal alterations. Thirteen cells had a normal karyotype, 6 cells showed random losses of a single chromosome, and 13 cells showed many nonclonal alterations, which included 17 unique markers types resulting from different translocations and deletions.

Treatment and Prognosis

Patients with STS have a poor prognosis. Most have died of metastatic sarcoma within 2 years from the time of diagnosis, and only 10% to 15% of reported patients have survived for 5 years. Woodward et al.[500] assembled survival data on 129 patients from the literature prior to 1972, including their series of women treated at the Mayo Clinic. The median survival was 19 months. Eleven patients (9%) survived for 5 years.

Several authors have recommended amputation as the primary surgical treatment of patients with STS.[492,498,500,526,543] In a recent study, Roy et al.[498] reported that "early radical surgery," which consisted of amputation, led to disease-free intervals between 3 and 135 months in three women. One woman developed recurrences on the chest wall 6 months after amputation; she remained free of disease 23 months after resection of the recurrent disease. Grobmyer et al.[544] analyzed the relationship between the initial treatment and survival in 92 cases published since 1966. The workers did not detect a significant difference in survival between patients initially treated with wide excision and those treated with amputation, but both surgical procedures resulted in better survival than either radiation or chemotherapy as the primary treatment.

Irradiation and chemotherapy have been used as primary treatments in patients for whom surgery is not acceptable and as components of salvage therapy in patients with relapses. The chemotherapeutic agents used include 5-fluorouracil, methotrexate, vincristine, actinomycin D, cyclophosphamide, doxorubicin, dacarbazine, bleomycin, paclitaxel, sorafenib, ifosfamide, and etoposide. Occasional patients have shown responses to certain of these drugs.[544] Kaufmann et al.[545,546] reported long-term survival in two women treated with combined radiation therapy and actinomycin D. One woman initially underwent an amputation, but rapid recurrence on the chest wall led to treatment with radiation and chemotherapy. She remained free of disease for 19 years. The second woman did not undergo amputation; instead she received irradiation of the arm and chemotherapy. The angiosarcoma did not reappear during the ensuing 13 years. The few cases such as these notwithstanding, the role of irradiation and conventional cytotoxic chemotherapy remains undefined.

In one series of eight women with STS treated with hyperthermic isolated limb perfusion using tumor necrosis factor and melphalan instead of surgery, five remained free of disease 6 to 115 months after infusion, two died of metastatic angiosarcoma, and one died of an unrelated stroke.[547] Intra-arterial infusion of mitoxantrone and paclitaxel led to a complete response at the primary site in a 72-year-old woman. Six months later, a recurrence was treated similarly, and she subsequently remained free of disease.[548] In one patient,[549] primary treatment with pegylated liposomal doxorubicin led to "almost complete" clinical and radiologic response, but progression of the disease occurred 7 months later and death ensued soon thereafter. A second patient also treated with pegylated liposomal doxorubicin in combination with paclitaxel experienced "an excellent clinical and subjective response."[522] Immunotherapy was used to treat the pleural effusion caused by pulmonary metastases in a 56-year-old woman with STS.[527] The treatment led to transient symptomatic improvement.

Systemic metastases invariably involve the lungs and often occur in bones, the liver, and other sites. The brain is rarely involved by metastases. Other malignant neoplasms, particularly contralateral mammary carcinoma, may occur in patients with STS.[492,546]

REFERENCES

Sarcoma

1. Zelek L, Llombart-Cussac A, Terrier P, et al. Prognostic factors in primary breast sarcomas: a series of patients with long-term follow-up. *J Clin Oncol* 2003;21:2583–2588.
2. Huang J, Mackillop WJ. Increased risk of soft tissue sarcoma after radiotherapy in women with breast carcinoma. *Cancer* 2001;92:172–180.
3. Yap J, Chuba PJ, Thomas R, et al. Sarcoma as a second malignancy after treatment for breast cancer. *Int J Radiat Oncol Biol Phys* 2002;52:1231–1237.
4. Mery CM, George S, Bertagnolli MM, et al. Secondary sarcomas after radiotherapy for breast cancer: sustained risk and poor survival. *Cancer* 2009;115:4055–4063.
5. Balzer BL, Weiss SW. Do biomaterials cause implant-associated mesenchymal tumors of the breast? Analysis of 8 new cases and review of the literature. *Hum Pathol* 2009;40:1564–1570.
6. Al-Benna S, Poggemann K, Steinau HU, et al. Diagnosis and management of primary breast sarcoma. *Breast Cancer Res Treat* 2010;122:619–626.
7. Bousquet G, Confavreux C, Magné N, et al. Outcome and prognostic factors in breast sarcoma: a multicenter study from the rare cancer network. *Radiother Oncol* 2007;85:355–361.
8. Adem C, Reynolds C, Ingle JN, et al. Primary breast sarcoma: clinicopathologic series from the Mayo Clinic and review of the literature. *Br J Cancer* 2004;91:237–241.
9. Barrow BJ, Janjan NA, Gutman H, et al. Role of radiotherapy in sarcoma of the breast—a retrospective review of the M.D. Anderson experience. *Radiother Oncol* 1999;52:173–178.
10. Blanchard DK, Reynolds CA, Grant CS, et al. Primary nonphylloides breast sarcomas. *Am J Surg* 2003;186:359–361.
11. Pandey M, Mathew A, Abraham EK, et al. Primary sarcoma of the breast. *J Surg Oncol* 2004;87:121–125.
12. Berg JW, Decrosse JJ, Fracchia AA, et al. Stromal sarcomas of the breast. A unified approach to connective tissue sarcomas other than cystosarcoma phyllodes. *Cancer* 1962;15:418–424.
13. Gutman H, Pollock RE, Ross MI, et al. Sarcoma of the breast: implications for extent of therapy. The M. D. Anderson experience. *Surgery* 1994;116:505–509.
14. Glenn J, Kinsella T, Glatstein E, et al. A randomized, prospective trial of adjuvant chemotherapy in adults with soft tissue sarcomas of the head and neck, breast, and trunk. *Cancer* 1985;55:1206–1214.
15. Mazanet R, Antman KH. Sarcomas of soft tissue and bone. *Cancer* 1991;68:463–473.
16. McGregor GI, Knowling MA, Este FA. Sarcoma and cystosarcoma phyllodes tumors of the breast—a retrospective review of 58 cases. *Am J Surg* 1994;167:477–480.
17. Sheth GR, Cranmer LD, Smith BD, et al. Radiation-induced sarcoma of the breast: a systematic review. *Oncologist* 2012;17:405–418.

Stromal Sarcoma

18. Berg JW, Decrosse JJ, Fracchia AA, et al. Stromal sarcomas of the breast. A unified approach to connective tissue sarcomas other than cystosarcoma phyllodes. *Cancer* 1962;15:418–424.
19. Christensen L, Schiodt T, Blichert-Toft M, et al. Sarcomas of the breast: a clinico-pathological study of 67 patients with long term follow-up. *Eur J Surg Oncol* 1988;14:241–247.
20. Terrier P, Terrier-Lacombe MJ, Mouriesse H, et al. Primary breast sarcoma: a review of 33 cases with immunohistochemistry and prognostic factors. *Breast Cancer Res Treat* 1989;13:39–48.
21. Rao AC, Geetha V, Khurana A. Periductal stromal sarcoma of breast with lipoblast-like cells: a case report with review of literature. *Indian J Pathol Microbiol* 2008;51:252–254.
22. Burga AM, Tavassoli FA. Periductal stromal tumor: a rare lesion with low-grade sarcomatous behavior. *Am J Surg Pathol* 2003;27:343–348.
23. Tomas D, Jankovic D, Marusic Z, et al. Low-grade periductal stromal sarcoma of the breast with myxoid features: immunohistochemistry. *Pathol Int* 2009;59:588–591.
24. Callery CD, Rosen PP, Kinne DW. Sarcoma of the breast. A study of 32 patients with reappraisal of classification and therapy. *Ann Surg* 1985;201:527–532.
25. Fujita N, Kimura R, Yamamura J, et al. Leiomyosarcoma of the breast: a case report and review of the literature about therapeutic management. *Breast* 2011;20:389–393.

26. Adem C, Reynolds C, Ingle JN, et al. Primary breast sarcoma: clinicopathologic series from the Mayo Clinic and review of the literature. *Br J Cancer* 2004;91:237–241.
27. Bouropoulou V, Markaki S, Prevedorou D, et al. Sarcomas of the breast. A clinicopathologic, histochemical and immunohistochemical study of ten cases. *Breast Disease* 1989;2:1989.

Leiomyosarcoma

28. Confavreux C, Lurkin A, Mitton N, et al. Sarcomas and malignant phyllodes tumours of the breast—a retrospective study. *Eur J Cancer* 2006;42:2715–2721.
29. Christensen L, Schiodt T, Blichert-Toft M, et al. Sarcomas of the breast: a clinico-pathological study of 67 patients with long term follow-up *Eur J Surg Oncol* 1988;14:241–247.
30. Blanchard DK, Reynolds CA, Grant CS, et al. Primary nonphylloides breast sarcomas. *Am J Surg* 2003;186:359–361.
31. Bousquet G, Confavreux C, Magné N, et al. Outcome and prognostic factors in breast sarcoma: a multicenter study from the rare cancer network. *Radiother Oncol* 2007;85:355–361.
32. Zelek L, Llombart-Cussac A, Terrier P, et al. Prognostic factors in primary breast sarcomas: a series of patients with long-term follow-up. *J Clin Oncol* 2003;21:2583–2588.
33. Allison JG, Dodds HM. Leiomyoma of the male nipple. A case report and literature review. *Am Surg* 1989;55:501–502.
34. Nascimento AG, Karas M, Rosen PP, et al. Leiomyoma of the nipple. *Am J Surg Pathol* 1979;3:151–154.
35. Tsujioka K, Kashihara M, Imamura S. Cutaneous leiomyoma of the male nipple. *Dermatologica* 1985;170:98–100.
36. Hernandez FJ. Leiomyosarcoma of male breast originating in the nipple. *Am J Surg Pathol* 1978;2:299–304.
37. Parham DM, Robertson AJ, Hussein KA, et al. Leiomyosarcoma of the breast; cytological and histological features, with a review of the literature. *Cytopathology* 1992;3:245–252.
38. Cameron HM, Hamperl H, Warambo W. Leiomyosarcoma of the breast originating from myothelium (myoepithelium). *J Pathol* 1974;114:89–92.
39. Pardo-Mindan J, Garcia-Julian G, Eizaguirre Altuna M. Leiomyosarcoma of the breast. Report of a case. *Am J Clin Pathol* 1974;62: 477–480.
40. Alessi E, Sala F. Leiomyosarcoma in ectopic areola. *Am J Dermatopathol* 1992;14:165–169.
41. Visfeldt J, Scheike O. Male breast cancer. Histologic typing and grading of 187 Danish cases. *Cancer* 1973;32:985–990.
42. Falconieri G, Della Libera D, Zanconati F, et al. Leiomyosarcoma of the female breast: report of two new cases and a review of the literature. *Am J Clin Pathol* 1997;108:19–25.
43. Kusama R, Fujimori M, Hama Y, et al. Stromal sarcoma of the breast with leiomyosarcomatous pattern. *Pathol Int* 2002;52:534–539.
44. Stafyla VK, Gauvin JM, Farley DR. A 53-year-old woman with a leiomyosarcoma of the breast. *Curr Surg* 2004;61:572–575.
45. Vu LT, Luce J, Knudson MM. Image of the month—leiomyosarcoma of the breast. *Arch Surg* 2006;141:1263–1264.
46. Jayaram G, Jayalakshmi P, Yip CH. Leiomyosarcoma of the breast: report of a case with fine needle aspiration cytologic, histologic and immunohistochemical features. *Acta Cytol* 2005;49:656–660.
47. De la Pena J, Wapnir I. Leiomyosarcoma of the breast in a patient with a 10-year-history of cyclophosphamide exposure: a case report. *Cases J* 2008;1:301.
48. Shinto O, Yashiro M, Yamada N, et al. Primary leiomyosarcoma of the breast: report of a case. *Surg Today* 2002;32:716–719.
49. Liang WC, Sickle-Santanello BJ, Nims TA, et al. Primary leiomyosarcoma of the breast: a case report with review of the literature. *Breast J* 2003;9:494–496.
50. Hussien M, Sivananthan S, Anderson N, et al. Primary leiomyosarcoma of the breast: diagnosis, management and outcome. A report of a new case and review of literature. *Breast* 2001;10:530–534.
51. Nielsen BB. Leiomyosarcoma of the breast with late dissemination. *Virchows Arch A Pathol Anat Histopathol* 1984;403:241–245.
52. Markaki S, Sotiropoulou M, Hanioti C, et al. Leiomyosarcoma of the breast. A clinicopathologic and immunohistochemical study. *Eur J Obstet Gynecol Reprod Biol* 2003;106:233–236.
53. Barnes L, Pietruszka M. Sarcomas of the breast: a clinicopathologic analysis of ten cases. *Cancer* 1977;40:1577–1585.
54. Jun Wei X, Hiotis K, Garcia R, et al. Leiomyosarcoma of the breast: a difficult diagnosis on fine-needle aspiration biopsy. *Diagn Cytopathol* 2003;29:172–178.
55. Bhagat P, Kline TS. The male breast and malignant neoplasms. Diagnosis by aspiration biopsy cytology. *Cancer* 1990;65:2338–2341.
56. Wei CH, Wan CY, Chen A, Tseng HH. Epithelioid leiomyosarcoma of the breast: report of a case. *J Formos Med Assoc* 1993;92:379–381.
57. González-Palacios F. Leiomyosarcoma of the female breast. *Am J Clin Pathol* 1998;109:650–651.
58. Gupta RK, Kenwright D, Naran S, et al. Fine needle aspiration cytodiagnosis of leiomyosarcoma of the breast. A case report. *Acta Cytol* 2000;44:1101–1105.
59. Székely E, Madaras L, Kulka J, et al. Leiomyosarcoma of the female breast. *Pathol Oncol Res* 2001;7:151–153.
60. Arista-Nasr J, Gonzalez-Gomez I, Angeles-Angeles A, et al. Primary recurrent leiomyosarcoma of the breast. Case report with ultrastructural and immunohistochemical study and review of the literature. *Am J Clin Pathol* 1989;92:500–505.
61. Terrier P, Terrier-Lacombe MJ, Mouriesse H, et al. Primary breast sarcoma: a review of 33 cases with immunohistochemistry and prognostic factors. *Breast Cancer Res Treat* 1989;13:39–48.
62. Waterworth PD, Gompertz RH, Hennessy C, et al. Primary leiomyosarcoma of the breast. *Br J Surg* 1992;79:169–170.
63. Lee J, Li S, Torbenson M, et al. Leiomyosarcoma of the breast: a pathologic and comparative genomic hybridization study of two cases. *Cancer Genet Cytogenet* 2004;149:53–57.
64. Boscaino A, Ferrara G, Orabona P, et al. Smooth muscle tumors of the breast: clinicopathologic features of two cases. *Tumori* 1994;80:241–245.
65. Chen KT, Kuo TT, Hoffmann KD. Leiomyosarcoma of the breast: a case of long survival and late hepatic metastasis. *Cancer* 1981;47:1883–1886.
66. Yatsuka K, Mihara S, Isobe M, et al. Leiomyosarcoma of the breast—a case report and an electron microscopic study. *Jpn J Surg* 1984;14:494–498.
67. Rane SU, Batra C, Saikia UN. Primary leiomyosarcoma of breast in an adolescent girl: a case report and review of the literature. *Case Rep Pathol* 2012;2012:491984.
68. Lonsdale RN, Widdison A. Leiomyosarcoma of the nipple. *Histopathology* 1992;20:537–539.
69. Falconieri G. Leiomyosarcoma of the female breast (letter). *Am J Clin Pathol* 1999;109:651.

Liposarcoma

70. Austin RM, Dupree WB. Liposarcoma of the breast: a clinicopathologic study of 20 cases. *Hum Pathol* 1986;17:906–913.
71. Powell CM, Rosen PP. Adipose differentiation in cystosarcoma phyllodes. A study of 14 cases. *Am J Surg Pathol* 1994;18:720–727.
72. Carpanelli JB, Lempel G, Gatta C. Sobre un caso de liposarcoma de glandula mamaria. *Sem Med* 1963;123:321–322.
73. Parikh BC, Ohri A, Desai MY, et al. Liposarcoma of the breast—a case report. *Eur J Gynaecol Oncol* 2007;28:425–427.
74. Vivian JB, Tan EG, Frayne JR, et al. Bilateral liposarcoma of the breast. *Aust N Z J Surg* 1993;63:658–659.
75. Hummer CD Jr, Burkart TJ. Liposarcoma of the breast. A case of bilateral involvement. *Am J Surg* 1967;113:558–561.
76. Lifvendahl RA. Liposarcoma of the mammary gland. *Surg Gynecol Obstet* 1930;50:81–84.
77. Nandipati KC, Nerkar H, Satterfield J, et al. Pleomorphic liposarcoma of the breast mimicking breast abscess in a 19-year-old postpartum female: a case report and review of the literature. *Breast J* 2010;16:537–540.
78. Pant I, Kaur G, Joshi SC, Khalid IA. Myxoid liposarcoma of the breast in a 25-year-old female as a diagnostic pitfall in fine needle aspiration cytology: report of a rare case. *Diagn Cytopathol* 2008;36:674–677.
79. Foust RL, Berry AD III, Moinuddin SM. Fine needle aspiration cytology of liposarcoma of the breast. A case report. *Acta Cytol* 1994;38:957–960.
80. Arbabi L, Warhol MJ. Pleomorphic liposarcoma following radiotherapy for breast carcinoma. *Cancer* 1982;49:878–880.
81. Demaria S, Yee HT, Cangiarella J, et al. Fine needle aspiration of primary pleomorphic liposarcoma of the breast. A case report. *Acta Cytol* 1999;43:1131–1136.

82. Charfi L, Driss M, Mrad K, et al. Primary well differentiated liposarcoma: an unusual tumor in the breast. *Breast J* 2009;15:206–207.
83. Mazaki T, Tanak T, Suenaga Y, et al. Liposarcoma of the breast: a case report and review of the literature. *Int Surg* 2002;87:164–170.
84. Sanfeliu Torres E, Sáez Artacho A, Villajos Fernández MA, et al. Liposarcoma mixoide de mama. A propósito de un caso y revisión de la literatura. *Rev Esp Patol* 2011;44:55–59.
85. McGregor JK. Liposarcoma of the breast: case report and review of literature. *Can Med Assoc J* 1960;82:781–783.
86. Mardi K, Gupta N. Primary pleomorphic liposarcoma of breast: a rare case report. *Indian J Pathol Microbiol* 2011;54:124–126.
87. Kanemoto K, Nakamura T, Matsuyama S, et al. Liposarcoma of the breast, review of the literature and a report of a case. *Jpn J Surg* 1981;11:381–384.
88. Odom JW, Mikhailova B, Pryce E, et al. Liposarcoma of the breast. Report of a case and review of the literature. *Breast Dis* 1991;4:293–298.
89. Rasmussen J, Jensen H. Liposarcoma of the breast. Case report and review of the literature. *Virchows Arch A Pathol Anat Histol* 1979;385:117–124.
90. Kristensen PB, Kryger H. Liposarcoma of the breast. A case report. *Acta Chir Scand* 1978;144:193–196.
91. Padilla-Rodriguez AL, Padilla-Villalta A, Arandia Y. Synchronous benign and malignant mesenchymal breast tumor. *Breast J* 2007;13:314–315.
92. Pollard SG, Marks PV, Temple LN, et al. Breast sarcoma. A clinicopathologic review of 25 cases. *Cancer* 1990;66:941–944.
93. Bouropoulou V, Markaki S, Prevedorou D, et al. Sarcomas of the breast. A clinicopathologic, histochemical and immunohistochemical study of ten cases. *Breast Disease* 1989;2:59–70.
94. Barnes L, Pietruszka M. Sarcomas of the breast: a clinicopathologic analysis of ten cases. *Cancer* 1977;40:1577–1585.
95. Callery CD, Rosen PP, Kinne DW. Sarcoma of the breast. A study of 32 patients with reappraisal of classification and therapy. *Ann Surg* 1985;201:527–532.
96. Terrier P, Terrier-Lacombe MJ, Mouriesse H, et al. Primary breast sarcoma: a review of 33 cases with immunohistochemistry and prognostic factors. *Breast Cancer Res Treat* 1989;13:39–48.
97. Adair FE, Herrmann JB. Sarcoma of the breast. *Surgery* 1946;19:55–73.
98. Christensen L, Schiodt T, Blichert-Toft M, et al. Sarcomas of the breast: a clinico-pathological study of 67 patients with long term follow-up *Eur J Surg Oncol* 1988;14:241–247.

Osteosarcoma and Chondrosarcoma

99. Silver SA, Tavassoli FA. Primary osteogenic sarcoma of the breast: a clinicopathologic analysis of 50 cases. *Am J Surg Pathol* 1998;22:925–933.
100. Trihia H, Valavanis C, Markidou S, et al. Primary osteogenic sarcoma of the breast: cytomorphologic study of 3 cases with histologic correlation. *Acta Cytol* 2007;51:443–450.
101. Argus A, Halton L. Case of the season: osteosarcoma of the breast. *Semin Roentgenol* 2011;46:4–6.
102. Bahrami A, Resetkova E, Ro JY, et al. Primary osteosarcoma of the breast: report of 2 cases. *Arch Pathol Lab Med* 2007;131:792–795.
103. Coussy F, Le Scodan R, Guinebretiere JM, et al. Breast mass with intense 99mTc-diphosphonate uptake revealing primary breast osteosarcoma. *J Clin Oncol* 2011;29:e428–e430.
104. Fiori E, Burza A, Izzo L, et al. Primary osteosarcoma of the breast. *Breast J* 2010;16:656–658.
105. Irshad K, Mann BS, Campbell H. Primary osteosarcoma of the breast. *Breast* 2003;12:72–74.
106. Middela S, Jones M, Maxwell W. Primary osteosarcoma of the breast—a case report and review of literature. *Indian J Surg* 2011;73:363–365.
107. Murakami S, Isozaki H, Shou T, et al. Primary osteosarcoma of the breast. *Pathol Int* 2009;59:111–115.
108. Nugent E, Wang LM, McCormack O, et al. Pure primary osteosarcoma of the breast. *Breast J* 2011;17:425–426.
109. Sabaté JM, Gómez A, Torrubia S, et al. Osteosarcoma of the breast. *AJR Am J Roentgenol* 2002;179:277–278.
110. Vanhoeij M, Bourgain C, Lamote J. Primary osteogenic sarcoma of the breast: a rare and fatal case. *Breast J* 2011;17:97–99.
111. Yang JG, Li CL, Hao RR, et al. Primary osteogenic sarcoma of breast detected on Tc-99m MIBI scintigraphy and Tc-99m MDP skeletal scintigraphy. *Ann Nucl Med* 2008;22:79–82.
112. Zils K, Ebner F, Ott M, et al. Extraskeletal osteosarcoma of the breast in an adolescent girl. *J Pediatr Hematol Oncol* 2012;34:e261–e263.
113. Dragoumis D, Bimpa K, Assimaki A, et al. Primary osteogenic sarcoma of the breast. *Singapore Med J* 2008;49:e315–e317.
114. Ogundiran TO, Ademola SA, Oluwatosin OM, et al. Primary osteogenic sarcoma of the breast. *World J Surg Oncol* 2006;4:90.
115. Khan S, Griffiths EA, Shah N, et al. Primary osteogenic sarcoma of the breast: a case report. *Cases J* 2008;1:148.
116. Jacob S, Japa D. Primary osteogenic sarcoma of the breast. *Indian J Pathol Microbiol* 2010;53:785–786.
117. Rakha EA, Tan PH, Shaaban A, et al. Do primary mammary osteosarcoma and chondrosarcoma exist? A review of a large multi-institutional series of malignant matrix-producing breast tumours. *Breast* 2013;22:13–18.
118. Thilagavathi G, Subramanian S, Samuel AV, et al. Primary chondrosarcoma of the breast. *J Indian Med Assoc* 1992;90:16–17.
119. Gupta S, Gupta V, Aggarwal PN, et al. Primary chondrosarcoma of the breast: a case report. *Indian J Cancer* 2003;40:77–79.
120. Meunier B, Leveque J, Le Prise E, et al. Three cases of sarcoma occurring after radiation therapy of breast cancers. *Eur J Obstet Gynecol Reprod Biol* 1994;57:33–36.
121. Rudman F Jr, Stanec S, Stanec M, et al. Rare complication of breast cancer irradiation: postirradiation osteosarcoma. *Ann Plast Surg* 2002;48:318–322.
122. Gurleyik E, Yildirim U, Gunal O, et al. Malignant mesenchymal tumor of the breast: primary chondrosarcoma. *Breast Care (Basel)* 2009;4:101–103.
123. Mertens HH, Langnickel D, Staedtler F. Primary osteogenic sarcoma of the breast. *Acta Cytol* 1982;26:512–516.
124. Brown AL, Holwill SD, Thomas VA, et al. Case report: primary osteosarcoma of the breast: imaging and histological features. *Clin Radiol* 1998;53:920–922.
125. Verfaillie G, Breucq C, Perdaens C, et al. Chondrosarcoma of the breast. *Breast J* 2005;11:147–148.
126. Savage AP, Sagor GR, Dovey P. Osteosarcoma of the breast: a case report with an unusual diagnostic feature. *Clin Oncol* 1984;10:295–298.
127. Lee JK, Sun SS. *Primary osteogenic sarcoma of the breast demonstrated by Tc-99m MDP scintigraphy. Clin Nucl Med* 1998;23:619.
128. Lumsden AB, Harrison D, Chetty U, et al. Osteogenic sarcoma—a rare primary tumour of the breast. *Eur J Surg Oncol* 1985;11:183–186.
129. Going JJ, Lumsden AB, Anderson TJ. A classical osteogenic sarcoma of the breast: histology, immunohistochemistry and ultrastructure. *Histopathology* 1986;10:631–641.
130. Ladefaged C, Nielsen BB. Primary chondrosarcoma of the breast: a case report and review of the literature. *Breast* 1984;10:26–28.
131. Guymar S, Ferlicot S, Genestie C, et al. Chondrosarcome du sein: a propos d'un cas. *Ann Pathol* 2001;21:168–171.
132. De Padua M, Bhandari TP. Primary mesenchymal chondrosarcoma of the breast. *Indian J Pathol Microbiol* 2009;52:129–130.
133. Lakshmikantha A, Kawatra V, Varma D, et al. Primary breast chondrosarcoma. *Breast J* 2010;16:553–554.
134. Patterson JD, Wilson JE, Dim D, et al. Primary chondrosarcoma of the breast: report of a case and review of the literature. *Breast Dis* 2011;33:189–191.
135. Beltaos E, Banerjee TK. Chondrosarcoma of the breast. Report of two cases. *Am J Clin Pathol* 1979;71:345–349.
136. Kennedy T, Biggart JD. Sarcoma of the breast. *Br J Cancer* 1967;21:635–644.
137. Mufarrij AA, Feiner HD. Breast sarcoma with giant cells and osteoid. A case report and review of the literature. *Am J Surg Pathol* 1987;11:225–230.
138. Benediktsdottir K, Lagerberg F, Lundell L, et al. Osteogenic sarcoma of the breast. Report of a case. *Acta Pathol Microbiol Scand A* 1980;88:161–165.
139. Pettinato G, Manivel JC, Petrella G, et al. Primary osteogenic sarcoma and osteogenic metaplastic carcinoma of the breast. Immunocytochemical identification in fine needle aspirates. *Acta Cytol* 1989;33:620–626.
140. Muller AG, Van Zyl JA. Primary osteosarcoma of the breast. *J Surg Oncol* 1993;52:135–136.
141. Remadi S, Doussis-Anagnostopoulu I, Mac Gee W. Primary osteosarcoma of the breast. *Pathol Res Pract* 1995;191:471–474; discussion 475–477.

142. Gonzalez-Licea A, Yardley JH, Hartmann WH. Malignant tumor of the breast with bone formation. Studies by light and electron microscopy. *Cancer* 1967;20:1234–1247.
143. Aubrey DA, Andrews GS. Mammary osteogenic sarcoma. *Br J Surg* 1971;58:472–474.
144. Teich S, Brecher IN. Osteogenic sarcoma of the breast: a case report. *Breast* 1985;11:11–15.

Malignant Fibrous Histiocytoma and Fibrosarcoma

145. Jones MW, Norris HJ, Wargotz ES, et al. Fibrosarcoma-malignant fibrous histiocytoma of the breast. A clinicopathological study of 32 cases. *Am J Surg Pathol* 1992;16:667–674.
146. Bahrami A, Folpe AL. Adult-type fibrosarcoma: a reevaluation of 163 putative cases diagnosed at a single institution over a 48-year period. *Am J Surg Pathol* 2010;34:1504–1513.
147. Adem C, Reynolds C, Ingle JN, et al. Primary breast sarcoma: clinicopathologic series from the Mayo Clinic and review of the literature. *Br J Cancer* 2004;91:237–241.
148. Kijima Y, Umekita Y, Yoshinaka H, et al. Stromal sarcoma with features of giant cell malignant fibrous histiocytoma. *Breast Cancer* 2007;14:239–244.
149. Christensen L, Schiodt T, Blichert-Toft M, et al. Sarcomas of the breast: a clinico-pathological study of 67 patients with long term follow-up. *Eur J Surg Oncol* 1988;14:241–247.
150. Bouropoulou V, Markaki S, Prevedorou D, et al. Sarcomas of the breast. A clinicopathologic, histochemical and immunohistochemical study of ten cases. *Breast Dis* 1989;2:59–70.
151. Terrier P, Terrier-Lacombe MJ, Mouriesse H, et al. Primary breast sarcoma: a review of 33 cases with immunohistochemistry and prognostic factors. *Breast Cancer Res Treat* 1989;13:39–48.
152. Pollard SG, Marks PV, Temple LN, et al. Breast sarcoma. A clinicopathologic review of 25 cases. *Cancer* 1990;66:941–944.
153. Blanchard DK, Reynolds CA, Grant CS, et al. Primary nonphylloides breast sarcomas. *Am J Surg* 2003;186:359–361.
154. Bousquet G, Confavreux C, Magné N, et al. Outcome and prognostic factors in breast sarcoma: a multicenter study from the rare cancer network. *Radiother Oncol* 2007;85:355–361.
155. Zelek L, Llombart-Cussac A, Terrier P, et al. Prognostic factors in primary breast sarcomas: a series of patients with long-term follow-up. *J Clin Oncol* 2003;21:2583–2588.
156. Rossen K, Stamp I, Sorensen IM. Primary malignant fibrous histiocytoma of the breast. A report of four cases and review of the literature. *APMIS* 1991;99:696–702.
157. Gutman H, Pollock RE, Ross MI, et al. Sarcoma of the breast: implications for extent of therapy. The M.D. Anderson experience. *Surgery* 1994;116:505–509.
158. Kraft R, Altermatt HJ, Nguyen-Tran Q, et al. Primäres malignes fibröses Histiozytom einer Mamma virilis. *Pathologe* 1988;9:334–339.
159. Jeong YJ, Oh HK, Bong JG. Undifferentiated pleomorphic sarcoma of the male breast causing diagnostic challenges. *J Breast Cancer* 2011;14:241–246.
160. van Niekerk JL, Wobbes T, Holland R, et al. Malignant fibrous histiocytoma of the breast with axillary lymph node involvement. *J Surg Oncol* 1987;34:32–35.
161. Ostyn C, Spector I, Bremner CG. Malignant fibrous histiocytoma of the breast. A case report. *S Afr Med J* 1987;71:665–666.
162. Remer S, Tartter PI, Schawrtz IS. Malignant fibrous histiocytoma of the breast. A case report and review of the literature. *Breast Dis* 1987;1:37–45.
163. Dirix LY, Fierens H, Langerock G, et al. Radiation related malignant fibrous histiocytoma. *Acta Clin Belg* 1988;43:204–208.
164. Meunier B, Leveque J, Le Prise E, et al. Three cases of sarcoma occuring after radiation therapy of breast cancers *Eur J Obstet Gynecol Reprod Biol* 1994;57:33–36.
165. Brady MS, Garfein CF, Petrek JA, et al. Post-treatment sarcoma in breast cancer patients. *Ann Surg Oncol* 1994;1:66–72.
166. Laskin WB, Silverman TA, Enzinger FM. Postradiation soft tissue sarcomas. An analysis of 53 cases. *Cancer* 1988;62:2330–2340.
167. Tsuneyoshi M, Enjoji M. Postirradiation sarcoma (malignant fibrous histiocytoma) following breast carcinoma: an ultrastructural study of a case. *Cancer* 1980;45:1419–1423.
168. Vera-Sempere F, Llombart-Bosch A. Malignant fibrohistiocytoma (MFH) of the breast. Primary and postirradiation variants —an ultrastructural study. *Pathol Res Pract* 1984;178:289–296.
169. Hardy TJ, An T, Brown PW, et al. Postirradiation sarcoma (malignant fibrous histiocytoma) of axilla. *Cancer* 1978;42:118–124.
170. Kuten A, Sapir D, Cohen Y, et al. Postirradiation soft tissue sarcoma occurring in breast cancer patients: report of seven cases and results of combination chemotherapy. *J Surg Oncol* 1985;28:168–171.
171. Luzzatto R, Grossmann S, Scholl JG, et al. Postradiation pleomorphic malignant fibrous histiocytoma of the breast. *Acta Cytol* 1986;30:48–50.
172. Horii R, Fukuuchi A, Nishi T, et al. A case of malignant fibrous histiocytoma after breast conserving therapy for breast cancer. *Breast Cancer* 2000;7:75–77.
173. Callery CD, Rosen PP, Kinne DW. Sarcoma of the breast. A study of 32 patients with reappraisal of classification and therapy. *Ann Surg* 1985;201:527–532.
174. Stanley MW, Tani EM, Horwitz CA, et al. Primary spindle-cell sarcomas of the breast: diagnosis by fine-needle aspiration. *Diagn Cytopathol* 1988;4:244–249.
175. MR Jr, Mills AS, DeMay RM, et al. Malignant fibrous histiocytoma of the breast. A case report and review of the literature. *Cancer* 1984;54:558–563.
176. Prasad PR, Kumar B, Kumar S, et al. Primary stromal sarcoma of breast with malignant fibrous histiocytoma-like features causing diagnostic dilemma on fine-needle aspiration cytology in a patient with squamous cell carcinoma of cervix: a case report. *Diagn Cytopathol* 2011;39:223–228.
177. Leader M, Patel J, Collins M, et al. Anti-alpha 1-antichymotrypsin staining of 194 sarcomas, 38 carcinomas, and 17 malignant melanomas. Its lack of specificity as a tumour marker. *Am J Surg Pathol* 1987;11:133–139.
178. Lentini M, Grosso M, Carrozza G, et al. Fibrohistiocytic tumors of soft tissues. An immunohistochemical study of 183 cases. *Pathol Res Pract* 1986;181:713–717.
179. Elson BC, Ikeda DM, Andersson I, et al. Fibrosarcoma of the breast: mammographic findings in five cases. *AJR Am J Roentgenol* 1992;158:993–995.
180. Kim MS, Kim KS, Han HY, et al. Fibrosarcomatous transformation in dermatofibrosarcoma protuberans of the breast—a case report. *J Clin Ultrasound* 2009;37:420–423.
181. Crocker DJ, Murad TM. Ultrastructure of fibrosarcoma in a male breast. *Cancer* 1969;23:891–899.
182. Lee JY, Kim DB, Kwak BS, et al. Primary fibrosarcoma of the breast: a case report. *J Breast Cancer* 2011;14:156–159.
183. Borman H, Safak T, Ertoy D. Fibrosarcoma following radiotherapy for breast carcinoma: a case report and review of the literature. *Ann Plast Surg* 1998;41:201–204.

Rhabdomyosarcoma

184. Barnes L, Pietruszka M. Sarcomas of the breast: a clinicopathologic study of ten cases. *Cancer* 1977;40:1577–1785.
185. Hajdu SI, Urban JA. Cancers metastatic to the breast. *Cancer* 1972;29:1691–1696.
186. Howarth CB, Caces JN, Pratt CB. Breast metastases in children with rhabdomyosarcoma. *Cancer* 1980;46:2520–2524.
187. Wakely PE Jr, Powers CN, Frable WJ. Metachronous soft-tissue masses in children and young adults with cancer: correlation of histology and aspiration cytology. *Hum Pathol* 1990;21:669–677.
188. Hays DM, Donaldson SS, Shimada H, et al. Primary and metastatic rhabdomyosarcoma in the breast: neoplasms of adolescent females, a report from the Intergroup Rhabdomyosarcoma Study. *Med Pediatr Oncol* 1997;29:181–189.
189. Oberman HA. Sarcomas of the breast. *Cancer* 1965;18:1233–1243.
190. Evans RW. Rhabdomyosarcoma of breast. *J Clin Pathol* 1953;6:140–144.
191. Woodard BH, Farnham R, Mossler JA, et al. Rhabdomyosarcoma of the breast. *Arch Pathol Lab Med* 1980;104:445–446.
192. Herrera LJ, Lugo-Vicente H. Primary embryonal rhabdomyosarcoma of the breast in an adolescent female: a case report. *J Pediatr Surg* 1998;33:1582–1584.
193. Li DL, Zhou RJ, Yang WT, et al. Rhabdomyosarcoma of the breast: a clinicopathologic study and review of the literature. *Chin Med J (Engl)* 2012;125:2618–2622.
194. Nogi H, Kobayashi T, Kawase K, et al. Primary rhabdomyosarcoma of the breast in a 13-year-old girl: report of a case. *Surg Today* 2007;37:38–42.

195. Kyriazis AP, Kyriazis AA. Primary rhabdomyosarcoma of the female breast: report of a case and review of the literature. *Arch Pathol Lab Med* 1998;122:747–749.
196. d'Angelo P, Carli M, Ferrari A, et al. Breast metastases in children and adolescents with rhabdomyosarcoma: experience of the Italian soft tissue sarcoma committee. *Pediatr Blood Cancer* 2010;55:1306–1309.
197. Dausse F, Balu-Maestro C, Chapellier C, et al. Rhabdomyosarcoma of the breast. *Clin Imaging* 2005;29:337–341.
198. Reale D, Guarino M, Sgroi F, et al. Rabdomiosarcoma embrionale primitivo della mammella. Descrizione di un caso. *Pathologica* 1994;86:98–101.
199. da Silva BB, Lopes-Costa PV, dos Santos LG, et al. Primary embryonal rhabdomyosarcoma of the breast. *South Med J* 2007;100:226–227.
200. Italiano A, Largillier R, Peyrottes I, et al. Primary embryonal rhabdomyosarcoma of the breast in an adult female. *Breast J* 2005;11:214.
201. Copeland LJ, Sneige N, Stringer CA, et al. Alveolar rhabdomyosarcoma of the female genitalia. *Cancer* 1985;56:849–855.
202. Deeley TJ. Secondary deposits in the breast. *Br J Cancer* 1965;19:738–743.
203. Pappo I, Zamir O, Ron N, et al. Alveolar rhabdomyosarcoma in young females presenting as breast tumor: two case reports and review of the literature. *Breast Dis* 1994;7:69–77.
204. Torres V, Ferrer R. Cytology of fine needle aspiration biopsy of primary breast rhabdomyosarcoma in an adolescent girl. *Acta Cytol* 1985;29:430–434.

Hemangiopericytoma

205. Stout AP, Murray MR. Hemangiopericytoma: a vascular tumor featuring Zimmermann's pericytes. *Ann Surg* 1942;116:26–33.
206. Arias-Stella J Jr, Rosen PP. Hemangiopericytoma of the breast. *Mod Pathol* 1988;1:98–103.
207. Jiménez-Ayala M, Diez-Nau MD, Larrad A, et al. Hemangiopericytoma in a male breast. Report of a case with cytologic, histologic and immunochemical studies. *Acta Cytol* 1991;35:234–238.
208. Mittal KR, Gerald W, True LD. Hemangiopericytoma of breast: report of a case with ultrastructural and immunohistochemical findings. *Hum Pathol* 1986;17:1181–1183.
209. Tavassoli FA, Weiss S. Hemangiopericytoma of the breast. *Am J Surg Pathol* 1981;5:745–752.
210. Volmer J, Pickartz H, Jautzke G. Vascular tumors in the region of the breast. *Virchows Arch A Pathol Anat Histol* 1980;385:201–214.
211. Callery CD, Rosen PP, Kinne DW. Sarcoma of the breast. A study of 32 patients with reappraisal of classification and therapy. *Ann Surg* 1985;201:527–532.
212. Kanazawa N, Ono A, Nitou G, et al. Primary malignant hemangiopericytoma of the breast: report of a case. *Surg Today* 1999;29:939–944.
213. Gengler C, Guillou L. Solitary fibrous tumour and haemangiopericytoma: evolution of a concept. *Histopathology* 2006;48:63–74.
214. Kauffman SL, Stout AP. Hemangiopericytoma in children. *Cancer* 1960;13:695–710.
215. Wang CS, Li H, Gao CF, et al. Hemangiopericytoma of the adult male breast. *Saudi Med J* 2011;32:1193–1195.
216. Talwar S, Prasad N, Gandhi S, et al. Haemangiopericytoma of the adult male breast. *Int J Clin Pract* 1999;53:485–486.
217. Kudawara I, Ueda T, Araki N, et al. Malignant hemangiopericytoma of the breast. *J Comput Assist Tomogr* 2001;25:319–321.
218. Meoli FG, Kopitnik NL. Hemangiopericytoma of the breast. *J Am Osteopath Assoc* 1991;91:606–613.
219. van Kints MJ, Tham RT, Klinkhamer PJ, et al. Hemangiopericytoma of the breast: mammographic and sonographic findings. *AJR Am J Roentgenol* 1994;163:61–63.
220. Coarasa-Cerdán A, Palomo-Jimenez M, Montero-Montero A, et al. Hemangiopericytoma of the breast: mammographic and sonographic findings. *J Clin Ultrasound* 1998;26:155–158.
221. Buecker B, Kapsimalakou S, Stoeckelhuber BM, et al. Malignant hemangiopericytoma of the breast: a case report with a review of the literature. *Arch Gynecol Obstet* 2008;277:357–361.
222. Breitbart AS, Harris MN, Vazquez M, et al. Metastatic hemangiopericytoma of the breast. *N Y State J Med* 1992;92:158–160.
223. Spatola C, Privitera G. Recurrent intracranial hemangiopericytoma with extracranial and unusual multiple metastases: case report and review of the literature. *Tumori* 2004;90:265–268.
224. Panda A, Dayal Y, Singhal V, et al. Haemangiopericytoma. *Br J Ophthalmol* 1984;68:124–127.
225. Kindblom LG, Ullman A. Malignant hemangiopericytoma with admixed glandular structures in breast and lung metastases. A light and electron microscopic and histochemical study of a case. *Appl Pathol* 1983;1:50–59.
226. Battifora H. Hemangiopericytoma: ultrastructural study of five cases. *Cancer* 1973;31:1418–1432.
227. Ruhland B, Dittmer C, Thill M, et al. Metastasized hemangiopericytoma of the breast: a rare case. *Arch Gynecol Obstet* 2009;280:491–494.

Dermatofibrosarcoma Protruberans

228. Ahmed AA, Ostlie D, Fraser JD, et al. Dermatofibrosarcoma protuberans in the breast of a 2-year-old girl. *Ann Diagn Pathol* 2010;14:279–283.
229. Cottier O, Fiche M, Meuwly JY, et al. Dermatofibrosarcoma presenting as a nodule in the breast of a 75-year-old woman: a case report. *J Med Case Rep* 2011;5:503.
230. Chen X, Chen YH, Zhang YL, et al. Magnetic resonance imaging and mammographic appearance of dermatofibrosarcoma protuberans in a male breast: a case report and literature review. *J Med Case Rep* 2009;3:8246.
231. Lee SJ, Mahoney MC, Shaughnessy E. Dermatofibrosarcoma protuberans of the breast: imaging features and review of the literature. *AJR Am J Roentgenol* 2009;193:W64–W69.
232. Kim MS, Kim KS, Han HY, et al. Fibrosarcomatous transformation in dermatofibrosarcoma protuberans of the breast—a case report. *J Clin Ultrasound* 2009;37:420–423.
233. Fukushima H, Suda K, Matsuda M, et al. A Case of dermatofibrosarcoma protuberans in the skin over the breast of a young woman. *Breast Cancer* 1998;5:407–409.
234. Kim T, Choi YL, Park HY, et al. Dermatofibrosarcoma protuberans of the breast skin. *Pathol Int* 2010;60:784–786.
235. Lin JY, Sheen-Chen SM, Hsu W, et al. Dermatofibrosarcoma protuberans of the breast. *Tumori* 2008;94:861–863.
236. Sandberg AA, Anderson WD, Fredenberg C, et al. Dermatofibrosarcoma protuberans of breast. *Cancer Genet Cytogenet* 2003;142:56–59.
237. Swan MC, Banwell PE, Hollowood K, et al. Late recurrence of dermatofibrosarcoma protuberans in the female breast: a case report. *Br J Plast Surg* 2005;58:84–87.
238. Sin FN, Wong KW. Dermatofibrosarcoma protuberans of the breast: a case report. *Clin Imaging* 2011;35:398–400.
239. Kamiya T, Saga K, Kaneko R, et al. Postradiation dermatofibrosarcoma protuberans. *Acta Derm Venereol* 2006;86:152–153.
240. Park TH, Seo SW, Kim JK, et al. Reconstructive challenge of dermatofibrosarcoma protuberans in the female breast. *World J Surg Oncol* 2011;9:1.
241. Lee HJ, Kim MJ, Choi J, et al. Dermatofibrosarcoma protuberans arising on the skin of the breast. *Breast J* 2011;17:93–95.
242. Oberman HA. Sarcomas of the breast. *Cancer* 1965;18:1233–1243.
243. Djilas-Ivanovic D, Prvulovic N, Bogdanovic-Stojanovic D, et al. Dermatofibrosarcoma protuberans of the breast: mammographic, ultrasound, MRI and MRS features. *Arch Gynecol Obstet* 2009;280:827–830.
244. Sakuragi T, Fujiwara K, Akashi-Tanaka S, et al. A case of dermatofibrosarcoma protuberans in the skin over the breast. *Breast Cancer* 1997;4:53–56.
245. Liu SZ, Ho TL, Hsu SM, et al. Imaging of dermatofibrosarcoma protuberans of breast. *Breast J* 2010;16:541–543.
246. Ramakrishnan V, Shoher A, Ehrlich M, et al. Atypical dermatofibrosarcoma protuberans in the breast. *Breast J* 2005;11:217–218.
247. Dragoumis DM, Katsohi LA, Amplianitis IK, et al. Late local recurrence of dermatofibrosarcoma protuberans in the skin of female breast. *World J Surg Oncol* 2010;8:48.
248. Karcnik TJ, Miller JA, Fromowitz F, et al. Dermatofibrosarcoma protuberans of the breast: a rare malignant tumor simulating benign disease. *Breast J* 1999;5:262–263.
249. Zee SY, Wang Q, Jones CM, et al. Fine needle aspiration cytology of dermatofibrosarcoma protuberans presenting as a breast mass. A case report. *Acta Cytol* 2002;46:741–743.
250. Tsang AK, Wong FC, Ng PW, et al. Fine needle aspiration cytology of dermatofibrosarcoma protuberans in the breast: a case report. *Pathology* 2005;37:84–86.
251. Bulliard C, Murali R, Chang LY, et al. Subcutaneous dermatofibrosarcoma protuberans in skin of the breast: may mimic a primary breast lesion. *Pathology* 2007;39:446–448.

252. Çavuşoğlu T, Yavuzer R, Tuncer S. Dermatofibrosarcoma protuberans of the breast. *Aesthetic Plast Surg* 2003;27:104–106.
253. Callery CD, Rosen PP, Kinne DW. Sarcoma of the breast. A study of 32 patients with reappraisal of classification and therapy *Ann Surg* 1985;201:527–532.

Sarcomas of Peripheral Nerve Sheath

254. Malas S, Krawitz HE, Sur RK, et al. Von Recklinghausen's disease associated with a primary malignant schwannoma of the breast. *J Surg Oncol* 1995;59:273–275.
255. Medina-Franco H, Gamboa-Dominguez A, de La Medina AR. Malignant peripheral nerve sheath tumor of the breast. *Breast J* 2003;9:332.
256. Dhingra KK, Mandal S, Roy S, et al. Malignant peripheral nerve sheath tumor of the breast: case report. *World J Surg Oncol* 2007;5:142.
257. Wang H, Ge J, Chen L, et al. Melanocytic malignant peripheral nerve sheath tumor of the male breast. *Breast Care (Basel)* 2009;4:260–262.
258. Berrada R, Chahtane A, Lakhdar Z, et al. Schwannome malin du sein. *J Gyneol Obstet Biol Reprod* 1998;27:441–444.
259. Catania S, Pacifico E, Zurrida S, et al. Malignant schwannoma of the breast. *Eur J Surg Oncol* 1992;18:80–81.
260. Hauser H, Beham A, Steindorfer P, et al. Malignant schwannoma of the breast. *Langenbecks Arch Chir* 1995;380:350–353.
261. Thanapaisal C, Koonmee S, Siritunyaporn S. Malignant peripheral nerve sheath tumor of breast in patient without Von Recklinghausen's neurofibromatosis: a case report. *J Med Assoc Thai* 2006;89:377–379.
262. Pollard SG, Marks PV, Temple LN, et al. Breast sarcoma. A clinicopathologic review of 25 cases *Cancer* 1990;66:941–944.
263. Salvadori B, Greco M, Galluzzo D, et al. Surgery for malignant mesenchymal tumors of the breast: a series of 31 cases. *Tumori* 1982;68:325–329.
264. Visfeldt J, Scheike O. Male breast cancer. Histologic typing and grading of 187 Danish cases. *Cancer* 1973;32:985–990.
265. Zelek L, Llombart-Cussac A, Terrier P, et al. Prognostic factors in primary breast sarcomas: a series of patients with long-term follow-up. *J Clin Oncol* 2003;21:2583–2588.

Miscellaneous Sarcomas

266. Chuthapisith S, Prasert W, Warnnissorn M, et al. Ewing's sarcoma and primitive neuroectodermal tumour (ES/PNET) presenting as a breast mass. *Oncol Lett* 2012;4:67–70.
267. da Silva BB, Lopes-Costa PV, Pires CG, et al. Primitive neuroectodermal tumor of the breast. *Eur J Obstet Gynecol Reprod Biol* 2008;137:248–249.
268. Sezer O, Jugovic D, Blohmer JU, et al. CD99 positivity and EWS-FLI1 gene rearrangement identify a breast tumor in a 60-year-old patient with attributes of the Ewing family of neoplasms. *Diagn Mol Pathol* 1999;8:120–124.
269. Tamura G, Sasou S, Kudoh S, et al. Primitive neuroectodermal tumor of the breast: immunohistochemistry and fluorescence in situ hybridization. *Pathol Int* 2007;57:509–512.
269a. Ko K, Kim EA, Lee ES, et al. Primary primitive neuroectodermal tumor of the breast: a case report. *Korean J Radiol* 2009;10:407–410.
269b. Vindal A, Kakar AK. Primary primitive neuroectodermal tumor of the breast. *J Clin Oncol* 2010;28:e453–455.
270. Kwak JY, Kim EK, You JK, et al. Metastasis of primitive neuroectodermal tumor to the breast. *J Clin Ultrasound* 2002;30:374–377.
270a. Majid N, Amrani M, Ghissassi I, et al. Bilateral ewing sarcoma/primitive neuroectodermal tumor of the breast: a very rare entity and review of the literature. *Case Rep Oncol* Med 2013.doi:10.1155/2013/964568.
271. Vega AR, Vetto JT, Kinne DW. Primary sarcomas of the breast in women under 20 years of age. *NY State J Med* 1992;92:497–498.
272. Wu J, Brinker DA, Haas M, et al. Primary alveolar soft part sarcoma (ASPS) of the breast: report of a deceptive case with xanthomatous features confirmed by TFE3 immunohistochemistry and electron microscopy. *Int J Surg Pathol* 2005;13:81–85.
273. Pollard SG, Marks PV, Temple LN, et al. Breast sarcoma. A clinicopathologic review of 25 cases. *Cancer* 1990;66:941–944.
274. Hanna NN, O'Donnell K, Wolfe GR. Alveolar soft part sarcoma metastatic to the breast. *J Surg Oncol* 1996;61:159–162.
275. Lim HS, Heo SH, Park JG, et al. Metastatic alveolar soft part sarcoma of the breast. *J Ultrasound Med* 2006;25:929–932.
276. Muzumdar GA, Murthy AK. Bilateral mammary metastasis of alveolar soft part sarcoma—a case report. *Indian J Pathol Microbiol* 1996;39:325–327.
277. Madrigrano A, Beach B, Wheeler A, et al. Metastases to the breast: alveolar soft part sarcoma in adolescents. *Clin Breast Cancer* 2008;8:92–93.
278. Oberman HA. Sarcomas of the breast. *Cancer* 1965;18:1233–1243.
279. Tormo V, Andreu FJ. Primary breast synovial sarcoma: a rare primary breast neoplasm. *Clin Transl Oncol* 2009;11:854–855.
280. Yoshitani K, Kido A, Honoki K, et al. Pelvic metastasis of breast synovial sarcoma. *J Orthop Sci* 2009;14:219–223.
281. González-Palacios F, Enriquez JL, San Miguel P, et al. Myofibroblastic tumors of the breast: a histologic spectrum with a case of recurrent male breast myofibrosarcoma. *Int J Surg Pathol* 1999;7:11–17.
282. Lučin K, Mustać E, Jonjić N. Breast sarcoma showing myofibroblastic differentiation. *Virchows Arch* 2003;443:222–224.
283. Morgan PB, Chundru S, Hatch SS, et al. Uncommon malignancies: case 1. Low-grade myofibroblastic sarcoma of the breast. *J Clin Oncol* 2005;23:6249–6251.
284. Taccagni G, Rovere E, Masullo M, et al. Myofibrosarcoma of the breast: review of the literature on myofibroblastic tumors and criteria for defining myofibroblastic differentiation. *Am J Surg Pathol* 1997;21:489–496.
285. Ng CS, Taylor CB, O'Donnell PJ, et al. Case report: mammographic and ultrasound appearances of Kaposi's sarcoma of the breast. *Clin Radiol* 1996;51:735–736.
286. Fisher C, Magnusson B, Hardarson S, et al. Myxoid variant of follicular dendritic cell sarcoma arising in the breast. *Ann Diagn Pathol* 1999;3:92–98.

Angiosarcoma

287. Rosen PP, Kimmel M, Ernsberger D. Mammary angiosarcoma. The prognostic significance of tumor differentiation. *Cancer* 1988;62:2145–2151.
288. Rainwater LM, Martin JK Jr, Gaffey TA, et al. Angiosarcoma of the breast. *Arch Surg* 1986;121:669–672.
289. Shackelford RT. Surgical disorders of the breast. In: Shackelford RT, ed. *Diagnosis of surgical disease*, vol. 1. Philadelphia: WB Saunders, 1968:439–551.
290. Wang ZS, Zhan N, Xiong CL, et al. Primary epithelioid angiosarcoma of the male breast: report of a case. *Surg Today* 2007;37:782–786.
291. Yadav RV, Sahariah S, Mittal VK, et al. Angiosarcoma of the male breast. *Int Surg* 1976;61:463–464.
292. Mansouri H, Jalil A, Chouhou L, et al. A rare case of angiosarcoma of the breast in a man: case report. *Eur J Gynaecol Oncol* 2000;21:603–604.
293. Fraga-Guedes C, Gobbi H, Mastropasqua MG, et al. Primary and secondary angiosarcomas of the breast: a single institution experience. *Breast Cancer Res Treat* 2012;132:1081–1088.
294. Luini A, Gatti G, Diaz J, et al. Angiosarcoma of the breast: the experience of the European Institute of Oncology and a review of the literature. *Breast Cancer Res Treat* 2007;105:81–85.
295. Chen KT, Kirkegaard DD, Bocian JJ. Angiosarcoma of the breast. *Cancer* 1980;46:368–371.
296. Donnell RM, Rosen PP, Lieberman PH, et al. Angiosarcoma and other vascular tumors of the breast. *Am J Surg Pathol* 1981;5:629–642.
297. Vorburger SA, Xing Y, Hunt KK, et al. Angiosarcoma of the breast. *Cancer* 2005;104:2682–2688.
298. Gatcombe HG, Olson TA, Esiashvili N. Metastatic primary angiosarcoma of the breast in a pediatric patient with a complete response to systemic chemotherapy and definitive radiation therapy: case report and review of the literature. *J Pediatr Hematol Oncol* 2010;32:192–194.
299. van Geel AN, den Bakker MA. Bilateral angiosarcoma of the breast in a fourteen-year-old child. *Rare Tumors* 2009;1:e38.
300. Benda JA, Al-Jurf AS, Benson AB III. Angiosarcoma of the breast following segmental mastectomy complicated by lymphedema. *Am J Clin Pathol* 1987;87:651–655.
301. Batchelor GB. Haemangioblastoma of the breast associated with pregnancy. *Br J Surg* 1959;46:647–649.
302. Horne WI, Percival WL. Hemangiosarcoma of the breast. *Can J Surg* 1975;18:81–84.
303. Khanna SD, Manchanda RL, Saigal RK, et al. Hemangioendothelioma (angiosarcoma) of the breast. *Arch Surg* 1964;88:807–809.
304. Masin M, Masin F. Cytology of angiosarcoma of the breast. A case report. *Acta Cytol* 1978;22:162–164.

305. Cao Y, Panos L, Graham RL, et al. Primary cutaneous angiosarcoma of the breast after breast trauma. *Proc (Bayl Univ Med Cent)* 2012;25:70–72.
306. Jennings TA, Peterson L, Axiotis CA, et al. Angiosarcoma associated with foreign body material. A report of three cases. *Cancer* 1988;62:2436–2444.
307. Kotton DN, Muse VV, Nishino M. Case records of the Massachusetts General Hospital. Case 2-2012. A 63-year-old woman with dyspnea and rapidly progressive respiratory failure. *N Engl J Med* 2012;366: 259–269.
308. Cuesta-Mejías T, de León-Bojorge B, Abel de la Peña J, et al. Angiosarcoma de la mama en paciente con cirugias multiples e implante mamario. Informe de un caso. *Ginecol Obstet Mex* 2002;70:76–81.
309. Takenaka M, Tanaka M, Isobe M, et al. Angiosarcoma of the breast with silicone granuloma: a case report. *Kurume Med J* 2009;56:33–37.
310. Bundred NJ, O'Reilly K, Smart JG. Long term survival following bilateral breast angiosarcoma. *Eur J Surg Oncol* 1989;15:263–264.
311. Nascimento AF, Raut CP, Fletcher CD. Primary angiosarcoma of the breast: clinicopathologic analysis of 49 cases, suggesting that grade is not prognostic. *Am J Surg Pathol* 2008;32:1896–1904.
312. Fujita T, Taira N, Ogasawara Y, et al. Bilateral angiosarcoma of the breast detected by magnetic resonance imaging during pregnancy. *Int J Clin Oncol* 2009;14:560–563.
313. Pai MR, Upadhyaya K, Naik R, et al. Bilateral angiosarcoma breast diagnosed by fine needle aspiration cytology. *Indian J Pathol Microbiol* 2008;51:421–423.
314. Kumar A, Gupta S, Chopra P, et al. Bilateral angiosarcoma of the breast: an overview. *Aust N Z J Surg* 1990;60:341–345.
315. Al-Salam S, Balalaa N, Faour I, et al. HIF-1alpha, VEGF and WT-1 are protagonists in bilateral primary angiosarcoma of breast: a case report and review of literature. *Int J Clin Exp Pathol* 2012;5:247–253.
316. Marchant LK, Orel SG, Perez-Jaffe LA, et al. Bilateral angiosarcoma of the breast on MR imaging. *AJR Am J Roentgenol* 1997;169:1009–1010.
317. Kar A, Mukhopadhyay D, Das SS, et al. Cytodiagnosis of angiosarcoma of breast. *Indian J Pathol Microbiol* 2008;51:427–429.
318. Gupta RK, Naran S, Dowle C. Needle aspiration cytology and immunocytochemical study in a case of angiosarcoma of the breast. *Diagn Cytopathol* 1991;7:363–365.
319. Mazzocchi A, Foschini MP, Marconi F, et al. Kasabach-Merritt syndrome associated to angiosarcoma of the breast. A case report and review of the literature. *Tumori* 1993;79:137–140.
320. Bernathova M, Jaschke W, Pechlahner C, et al. Primary angiosarcoma of the breast associated Kasabach-Merritt syndrome during pregnancy. *Breast* 2006;15:255–258.
321. Kim YS, Kim YJ, Yim KI, et al. A case report of primary breast angiosarcoma with fatal pulmonary hemorrhage due to thrombocytopenia. *J Korean Surg Soc* 2012;82:251–255.
322. Moussa SH, Oliveira AL, de Amorim AP, et al. Angiosarcoma of the breast associated with Kasabach-Merritt syndrome. *Arch Gynecol Obstet* 2002;267:43–45.
323. Rozen WM, Mann GB. Angiosarcoma arising in an unirradiated breast with subsequent pituitary metastasis. *Clin Breast Cancer* 2007;7:811–813.
324. Britt LD, Lambert P, Sharma R, et al. Angiosarcoma of the breast. Initial misdiagnosis is still common. *Arch Surg* 1995;130:221–223.
325. Ni Y, Xie X, Bu H, et al. Concurrent primary angiosarcoma and invasive ductal carcinoma in the same breast. *J Clin Pathol* 2013;66:263–264.
326. Ryan JF, Kealy WF. Concomitant angiosarcoma and carcinoma of the breast: a case report. *Histopathology* 1985;9:893–899.
327. Markidou S, Karydas I, Papadopoulos S, et al. Fine needle aspiration cytology in primary breast angiosarcoma: a case report. *Acta Cytol* 2010;54:764–770.
328. Gentile-Fradet A, Pallud C, Le Doussal V, et al. Hemangioendotheliosarcome mammaire. A propos de deux observations, dont une avec etude ultrastructurale. *Arch Anat Cytol Pathol* 1981;29:149–153.
329. West JG, Weitzel JN, Tao ML, et al. BRCA mutations and the risk of angiosarcoma after breast cancer treatment. *Clin Breast Cancer* 2008;8:533–537.
330. Liberman L, Dershaw DD, Kaufman RJ, et al. Angiosarcoma of the breast. *Radiology* 1992;183:649–654.
331. Yang WT, Hennessy BT, Dryden MJ, et al. Mammary angiosarcomas: imaging findings in 24 patients. *Radiology* 2007;242:725–734.
332. Lvoff NM, Leung JW. Case of the season: primary angiosarcoma of the breast: correlative imaging and pathology. *Semin Roentgenol* 2007;42:208–210.
333. Schnarkowski P, Kessler M, Arnholdt H, et al. Angiosarcoma of the breast: mammographic, sonographic, and pathological findings. *Eur J Radiol* 1997;24:54–56.
334. Glazebrook KN, Morton MJ, Reynolds C. Vascular tumors of the breast: mammographic, sonographic, and MRI appearances. *AJR Am J Roentgenol* 2005;184:331–338.
335. Kikawa Y, Konishi Y, Nakamoto Y, et al. Angiosarcoma of the breast—specific findings of MRI. *Breast Cancer* 2006;13:369–373.
336. Jozefczyk MA, Rosen PP. Vascular tumors of the breast. II. Perilobular hemangiomas and hemangiomas. *Am J Surg Pathol* 1985;9:491–503.
337. Grant EG, Holt RW, Chun B, et al. Angiosarcoma of the breast: sonographic, xeromammographic, and pathologic appearance. *AJR Am J Roentgenol* 1983;141:691–692.
338. Cucci E, Ciuffreda M, Tambaro R, et al. MRI findings of large low-grade angiosarcoma of the breast with subsequent bone metastases: a case report. *J Breast Cancer* 2012;15:255–257.
339. Murakami S, Nagano H, Okubo K, et al. Angiosarcoma of the breast. Report of a case and its findings of MRI *Breast Cancer* 2001;8:254–258.
340. Glazebrook KN, Magut MJ, Reynolds C. Angiosarcoma of the breast. *AJR Am J Roentgenol* 2008;190:533–538.
341. Sanders LM, Groves AC, Schaefer S. Cutaneous angiosarcoma of the breast on MRI. *AJR Am J Roentgenol* 2006;187:W143–W146.
342. Zeng W, Styblo TM, Li S, et al. Breast angiosarcoma: FDG PET findings. *Clin Nucl Med* 2009;34:443–445.
343. Sher T, Hennessy BT, Valero V, et al. Primary angiosarcomas of the breast. *Cancer* 2007;110:173–178.
344. Scow JS, Reynolds CA, Degnim AC, et al. Primary and secondary angiosarcoma of the breast: the Mayo Clinic experience. *J Surg Oncol* 2010;101:401–407.
345. Hill RP, Stout AP. Sarcoma of the breast. *Arch Surg* 1942;44:723–759.
346. Merino MJ, Carter D, Berman M. Angiosarcoma of the breast. *Am J Surg Pathol* 1983;7:53–60.
347. Shin SJ, Lesser M, Rosen PP. Hemangiomas and angiosarcomas of the breast: diagnostic utility of cell cycle markers with emphasis on Ki-67. *Arch Pathol Lab Med* 2007;131:538–544.
348. Macias-Martinez V, Murrieta-Tiburcio L, Molina-Cardenas H, et al. Epithelioid angiosarcoma of the breast. Clinicopathological, immunohistochemical, and ultrastructural study of a case. *Am J Surg Pathol* 1997;21:599–604.
349. Carter E, Ulusaraç O, Dyess DL. Axillary lymph node involvement in primary epithelioid angiosarcoma of the breast. *Breast J* 2005;11:219–220.
350. Fariña MC, Casado V, Renedo G, et al. Epithelioid angiosarcoma of the breast involving the skin: a highly aggressive neoplasm readily mistaken for mammary carcinoma. *J Cutan Pathol* 2003;30:152–156.
351. Muzumder S, Das P, Kumar M, et al. Primary epithelioid angiosarcoma of the breast masquerading as carcinoma. *Curr Oncol* 2010;17:64–69.
352. Ewing J. *Neoplastic diseases: A textbook on tumors.* Philadelphia: WB Saunders, 1919:223–224.
353. Borrmann R. Metastasenbildung bei histologisch gutartigen Geschwülsten: fall von metastasierendem Angiom. *Ziegler's Bertäg z Allg Path u Path Anat* 1906;40:372–392.
354. Rosen PP. Vascular tumors of the breast. III. Angiomatosis. *Am J Surg Pathol* 1985;9:652–658.
355. Rosen PP, Ridolfi RL. The perilobular hemangioma. A benign microscopic vascular lesion of the breast. *Am J Clin Pathol* 1977;68:21–23.
356. Carson KF, Hirschowitz SL, Nieberg RK, et al. Pitfalls in the cytologic diagnosis of angiosarcoma of the breast by fine-needle aspiration: a case report. *Diagn Cytopathol* 1994;11:297–299; discussion 299–300.
357. Kiyozuka Y, Koyama H, Nakata M, et al. Diagnostic cytopathology in type II angiosarcoma of the breast: a case report. *Acta Cytol* 2005;49:560–566.
358. Brenn T, Fletcher CD. Radiation-associated cutaneous atypical vascular lesions and angiosarcoma: clinicopathologic analysis of 42 cases. *Am J Surg Pathol* 2005;29:983–996.
359. Burgdorf WH, Mukai K, Rosai J. Immunohistochemical identification of factor VIII-related antigen in endothelial cells of cutaneous lesions of alleged vascular nature. *Am J Clin Pathol* 1981;75:167–171.
360. Guarda LA, Ordonez NG, Smith JL Jr, et al. Immunoperoxidase localization of factor VIII in angiosarcomas. *Arch Pathol Lab Med* 1982;106:515–516.
361. Yonezawa S, Maruyama I, Sakae K, et al. Thrombomodulin as a marker for vascular tumors. Comparative study with factor VIII and Ulex europaeus I lectin. *Am J Clin Pathol* 1987;88:405–411.

362. De Young BR, Wick MR, Fitzgibbon JF, et al. CD31: an immunospecific marker for endothelial differentiation in human neoplasms. *Appl Immunohistochem Mol Morphol* 1993;1:97–100.
363. El-Gohary YM, Silverman JF, Poppiti RJ, et al. D2-40 expression in cutanous angiosarcoma arising after radiotherapy treatment of breast carcinoma. *Modern Pathol* 2006;19(Suppl. 1):26A.
364. Gennaro M, Valeri B, Casalini P, et al. Angiosarcoma of the breast and vascular endothelial growth factor receptor. *Tumori* 2010;96:930–935.
365. Shet T, Malaviya A, Nadkarni M, et al. Primary angiosarcoma of the breast: observations in Asian Indian women. *J Surg Oncol* 2006;94:368–374.
366. Kallen ME, Nunes Rosado FG, Gonzalez AL, et al. Occasional staining for p63 in malignant vascular tumors: a potential diagnostic pitfall. *Pathol Oncol Res* 2012;18:97–100.
367. Brentani MM, Pacheco MM, Oshima CT, et al. Steroid receptors in breast angiosarcoma. *Cancer* 1983;51:2105–2111.
368. Antman KH, Corson J, Greenberger J, et al. Multimodality therapy in the management of angiosarcoma of the breast. *Cancer* 1982;50:2000–2003.
369. Hunter TB, Martin PC, Dietzen CD, et al. Angiosarcoma of the breast. Two case reports and a review of the literature. *Cancer* 1985;56:2099–2106.
370. Alvarez-Fernandez E, Salinero-Paniagua E. Vascular tumors of the mammary gland. A histochemical and ultrastructural study. *Virchows Arch A Pathol Anat Histol* 1981;394:31–47.
371. Hamazaki M, Tanaka T. Hemangiosarcoma of the breast—case report with scanning electron microscopic study. *Acta Pathol Jpn* 1978;28:605–613.
372. Toth B, Malick L. Scanning electron-microscopic study of the surface characteristics of neoplastic endothelial cells of blood vessels. *J Pathol* 1976;118:59–63.
373. Baumhoer D, Gunawan B, Becker H, et al. Comparative genomic hybridization in four angiosarcomas of the female breast. *Gynecol Oncol* 2005;97:348–352.
374. Barber KW Jr, Harrison EG, Clagett OT, et al. Angiosarcoma of the breast. *Surgery* 1960;48:869–878.
375. Steingaszner LC, Enzinger FM, Taylor HB. Hemangiosarcoma of the breast. *Cancer* 1965;18:352–361.
376. Rosner D. Angiosarcoma of the breast: long-term survival following adjuvant chemotherapy. *J Surg Oncol* 1988;39:90–95.
377. Savage R. The treatment of angiosarcoma of the breast. *J Surg Oncol* 1981;18:129–134.
378. Myerowitz RL, Pietruszka M, Barnes EL. Primary angiosarcoma of the breast. *JAMA* 1978;239:403.
379. Massé SR, Mongeau CJ, Rioux A. Angiosarcoma of the breast. *Can J Surg* 1977;20:341–343.
380. Bae SY, Choi MY, Cho DH, et al. Large clinical experience of primary angiosarcoma of the breast in a single Korean medical institute. *World J Surg* 2011;35:2417–2421.
381. Epstein JB, Knowling MA, Le Riche JC. Multiple gingival metastases from angiosarcoma of the breast. *Oral Surg Oral Med Oral Pathol* 1987;64:554–557.
382. Win KK, Yasuoka T, Kamiya H, et al. Breast angiosarcoma metastatic to the maxillary gingiva. Case report. *Int J Oral Maxillofac Surg* 1992;21:282–283.
383. Poulopoulos AK, Antoniades K, Kiziridou A. Bilateral metastatic breast angiosarcoma to the mandibular gingiva: case report. *Oral Oncol* 2001;37:199–201.
384. Souza FF, Katkar A, den Abbeele AD, et al. Breast angiosarcoma metastatic to the ovary. *Case Rep Med* 2009;2009:381015.
385. Sedgely MG, Ostor AG, Fortune DW. Angiosarcoma of breast metastatic to the ovary and placenta. *Aust N Z J Obstet Gynaecol* 1985;25:299–302.
386. Baum JK, Levine AJ, Ingold JA. Angiosarcoma of the breast with report of unusual site of first metastasis. *J Surg Oncol* 1990;43:125–130.
387. Kessler E, Kozenitzky IL. Haemangiosarcoma of breast. *J Clin Pathol* 1971;24:530–532.
388. Kaklamanos IG, Birbas K, Syrigos KN, et al. Breast angiosarcoma that is not related to radiation exposure: a comprehensive review of the literature. *Surg Today* 2011;41:163–168.
389. Nanus D, Kaufman R. Angiosarcoma of the breast: adjuvant chemotherapy with actinomycin D. *Proc Am Soc Clin Oncol* 1986;5:73.
390. Kopp HG, Kanz L, Hartmann JT. Complete remission of relapsing high-grade angiosarcoma with single-agent metronomic trofosfamide. *Anticancer Drugs* 2006;17:997–998.
391. Biswas T, Tang P, Muhs A, et al. Angiosarcoma of the breast: a rare clinicopathological entity. *Am J Clin Oncol* 2009;32:582–586.
392. Huang J, Mackillop WJ. Increased risk of soft tissue sarcoma after radiotherapy in women with breast carcinoma. *Cancer* 2001;92:172–180.
393. Davies JD, Rees GJ, Mera SL. Angiosarcoma in irradiated post-mastectomy chest wall. *Histopathology* 1983;7:947–956.
394. Hamels J, Blondiau P, Mirgaux M. Cutaneous angiosarcoma arising in a mastectomy scar after therapeutic irradiation. *Bull Cancer* 1981;68:353–356.
395. Maddox JC, Evans HL. Angiosarcoma of skin and soft tissue: a study of forty-four cases. *Cancer* 1981;48:1907–1921.
396. Otis CN, Peschel R, McKhann C, et al. The rapid onset of cutaneous angiosarcoma after radiotherapy for breast carcinoma. *Cancer* 1986;57:2130–2134.
397. Abbott R, Palmieri C. Angiosarcoma of the breast following surgery and radiotherapy for breast cancer. *Nat Clin Pract Oncol* 2008;5:727–736.
398. Marchal C, Weber B, de Lafontan B, et al. Nine breast angiosarcomas after conservative treatment for breast carcinoma: a survey from French comprehensive Cancer Centers. *Int J Radiat Oncol Biol Phys* 1999;44:113–119.
399. West JG, Qureshi A, West JE, et al. Risk of angiosarcoma following breast conservation: a clinical alert. *Breast J* 2005;11:115–123.
400. Andrews S, Wilcoxon R, Benda J, et al. Angiosarcoma following MammoSite partial breast irradiation. *Breast Cancer Res Treat* 2010;124:279–282.
401. Mery CM, George S, Bertagnolli MM, et al. Secondary sarcomas after radiotherapy for breast cancer: sustained risk and poor survival. *Cancer* 2009;115:4055–4063.
402. Georgiannos SN, Sheaff M. Angiosarcoma of the breast: a 30 year perspective with an optimistic outlook. *Br J Plast Surg* 2003;56:129–134.
403. Billings SD, McKenney JK, Folpe AL, et al. Cutaneous angiosarcoma following breast-conserving surgery and radiation: an analysis of 27 cases. *Am J Surg Pathol* 2004;28:781–788.
404. Strobbe LJ, Peterse HL, van Tinteren H, et al. Angiosarcoma of the breast after conservation therapy for invasive cancer, the incidence and outcome. An unforseen sequela. *Breast Cancer Res Treat* 1998;47:101–109.
405. Torres KE, Ravi V, Kin K, et al. Long-term outcomes in patients with radiation-associated angiosarcomas of the breast following surgery and radiotherapy for breast cancer. *Ann Surg Oncol* 2013;20:1267–1274.
406. Cafiero F, Gipponi M, Peressini A, et al. Radiation-associated angiosarcoma: diagnostic and therapeutic implications—two case reports and a review of the literature. *Cancer* 1996;77:2496–2502.
407. Blanchard DK, Reynolds C, Grant CS, et al. Radiation-induced breast sarcoma. *Am J Surg* 2002;184:356–358.
408. Fineberg S, Rosen PP. Cutaneous angiosarcoma and atypical vascular lesions of the skin and breast after radiation therapy for breast carcinoma. *Am J Clin Pathol* 1994;102:757–763.
409. Timmer SJ, Osuch JR, Colony LH, et al. Angiosarcoma of the breast following lumpectomy and radiation therapy for breast carcinoma: Case report and review of the literature. *Breast J* 1997;3:40–47.
410. Monroe AT, Feigenberg SJ, Mendenhall NP. Angiosarcoma after breast-conserving therapy. *Cancer* 2003;97:1832–1840.
411. Perin T, Massarut S, Roncadin M, et al. Radiation-associated angiosarcoma: diagnostic and therapeutic implications—two case reports and a review of the literature. *Cancer* 1997;80:519–521.
412. Molitor JL, Spielmann M, Contesso G. Angiosarcoma of the breast after conservative surgery and radiation therapy for breast carcinoma: three new cases. *Eur J Cancer* 1996;32A:1820.
413. Mobini N. Cutaneous epithelioid angiosarcoma: a neoplasm with potential pitfalls in diagnosis. *J Cutan Pathol* 2009;36:362–369.
414. Hodgson NC, Bowen-Wells C, Moffat F, et al. Angiosarcomas of the breast: a review of 70 cases. *Am J Clin Oncol* 2007;30:570–573.
415. Hui A, Henderson M, Speakman D, et al. Angiosarcoma of the breast: a difficult surgical challenge. *Breast* 2012;21:584–589.
416. Wijnmaalen A, van Ooijen B, van Geel BN, et al. Angiosarcoma of the breast following lumpectomy, axillary lymph node dissection, and radiotherapy for primary breast cancer: three case reports and a review of the literature. *Int J Radiat Oncol Biol Phys* 1993;26:135–139.
417. Badwe RA, Hanby AM, Fentiman IS, et al. Angiosarcoma of the skin overlying an irradiated breast. *Breast Cancer Res Treat* 1991;19:69–72.
418. Moskaluk CA, Merino MJ, Danforth DN, et al. Low-grade angiosarcoma of the skin of the breast: a complication of lumpectomy and radiation therapy for breast carcinoma. *Hum Pathol* 1992;23:710–714.

419. Rubin E, Maddox WA, Mazur MT. Cutaneous angiosarcoma of the breast 7 years after lumpectomy and radiation therapy. *Radiology* 1990;174:258–260.
420. Taat CW, van Toor BS, Slors JF, et al. Dermal angiosarcoma of the breast: a complication of primary radiotherapy? *Eur J Surg Oncol* 1992;18:391–395.
421. Bolin DJ, Lukas GM. Low-grade dermal angiosarcoma of the breast following radiotherapy. *Am Surg* 1996;62:668–672.
422. de Giorgi V, Santi R, Grazzini M, et al. Synchronous angiosarcoma, melanoma and morphea of the breast skin 14 years after radiotherapy for mammary carcinoma. *Acta Derm Venereol* 2010;90:283–286.
423. Hanna G, Lin SJ, Wertheimer MD, et al. Unresolved, atraumatic breast hematoma: post-irradiation or secondary breast angiosarcoma. *Breast Dis* 2011;33:139–142.
424. Lim RF, Goei R. Best cases from the AFIP: angiosarcoma of the breast. *Radiographics* 2007;27(suppl. 1):S125–S130.
425. Rao J, Dekoven JG, Beatty JD, et al. Cutaneous angiosarcoma as a delayed complication of radiation therapy for carcinoma of the breast. *J Am Acad Dermatol* 2003;49:532–538.
426. Feigenberg SJ, Mendenhall NP, Reith JD, et al. Angiosarcoma after breast-conserving therapy: experience with hyperfractionated radiotherapy. *Int J Radiat Oncol Biol Phys* 2002;52:620–626.
427. Perez-Ruiz E, Ribelles N, Sanchez-Muñoz A, et al. Response to paclitaxel in a radiotherapy-induced breast angiosarcoma. *Acta Oncol* 2009;48:1078–1079.
428. Deutsch M, Rosenstein MM. Angiosarcoma of the breast mimicking radiation dermatitis arising after lumpectomy and breast irradiation: a case report. *Am J Clin Oncol* 1998;21:608–609.
429. Poellinger A, Landt S, Diekmann F, et al. Rapid growth of an exophytic angiosarcoma of the breast. *Breast J* 2006;12:80–82.
430. Zucali R, Merson M, Placucci M, et al. Soft tissue sarcoma of the breast after conservative surgery and irradiation for early mammary cancer. *Radiother Oncol* 1994;30:271–273.
431. Roncadin M, Massarut S, Perin T, et al. Breast angiosarcoma after conservative surgery, radiotherapy and prosthesis implant. *Acta Oncol* 1998;37:209–211.
432. Hanasono MM, Osborne MP, Dielubanza EJ, et al. Radiation-induced angiosarcoma after mastectomy and TRAM flap breast reconstruction. *Ann Plast Surg* 2005;54:211–214.
433. Williams SB, Reed M. Cutaneous angiosarcoma after breast conserving treatment for bilateral breast cancers in a BRCA-1 gene mutation carrier—a case report and review of the literature. *Surgeon* 2009;7:250.
434. de Bree E, van Coevorden F, Peterse JL, et al. Bilateral angiosarcoma of the breast after conservative treatment of bilateral invasive carcinoma: genetic predisposition? *Eur J Surg Oncol* 2002;28:392–395.
435. Lindford A, Böhling T, Vaalavirta L, et al. Surgical management of radiation-associated cutaneous breast angiosarcoma. *J Plast Reconstr Aesthet Surg* 2011;64:1036–1042.
436. Moore A, Hendon A, Hester M, et al. Secondary angiosarcoma of the breast: can imaging findings aid in the diagnosis? *Breast J* 2008;14:293–298.
437. Vesoulis Z, Cunliffe C. Fine-needle aspiration biopsy of post-radiation epithelioid angiosarcoma of breast. *Diagn Cytopathol* 2000;22:172–175.
438. Seo IS, Min KW. Postirradiation epithelioid angiosarcoma of the breast: a case report with immunohistochemical and electron microscopic study. *Ultrastruct Pathol* 2003;27:197–203.
439. Cunha AL, Amendoeira I. High-grade breast epithelioid angiosarcoma secondary to radiotherapy metastasizing to the contralateral lymph node: unusual presentation and potential pitfall. *Breast Care (Basel)* 2011;6:227–229.
440. Liu YC, Fung MA. Angiosarcoma with pseudoepidermotropism in a patient with breast cancer: a mimic of epidermotropic metastatic adenocarcinoma. *Am J Dermatopathol* 2011;33:400–402.
441. Layfield LJ, Dodd LG. Cytologic findings in a case of postirradiation angiosarcoma of the breast. *Acta Cytol* 1997;41:612–614.
442. Gherardi G, Rossi S, Perrone S, et al. Angiosarcoma after breast-conserving therapy: fine-needle aspiration biopsy, immunocytochemistry, and clinicopathologic correlates. *Cancer* 2005;105:145–151.
443. Pfeiffer DF, Bode-Lesniewska B. Fine needle aspiration biopsy diagnosis of angiosarcoma after breast-conserving therapy for carcinoma supported by use of a cell block and immunohistochemistry. *Acta Cytol* 2006;50:553–556.
444. Weed BR, Folpe AL. Cutaneous CD30-positive epithelioid angiosarcoma following breast-conserving therapy and irradiation: a potential diagnostic pitfall. *Am J Dermatopathol* 2008;30:370–372.
445. Sener SF, Milos S, Feldman JL, et al. The spectrum of vascular lesions in the mammary skin, including angiosarcoma, after breast conservation treatment for breast cancer. *J Am Coll Surg* 2001;193:22–28.
446. Nakamura R, Nagashima T, Sakakibara M, et al. Angiosarcoma arising in the breast following breast-conserving surgery with radiation for breast carcinoma. *Breast Cancer* 2007;14:245–249.
447. Gil-Benso R, Lopez-Gines C, Soriano P, et al. Cytogenetic study of angiosarcoma of the breast. *Genes Chromosomes Cancer* 1994;10: 210–212.
448. Manner J, Radlwimmer B, Hohenberger P, et al. MYC high level gene amplification is a distinctive feature of angiosarcomas after irradiation or chronic lymphedema. *Am J Pathol* 2010;176:34–39.
449. Guo T, Zhang L, Chang NE, et al. Consistent MYC and FLT4 gene amplification in radiation-induced angiosarcoma but not in other radiation-associated atypical vascular lesions. *Genes Chromosomes Cancer* 2011;50:25–33.
450. Mentzel T, Schildhaus HU, Palmedo G, et al. Postradiation cutaneous angiosarcoma after treatment of breast carcinoma is characterized by MYC amplification in contrast to atypical vascular lesions after radiotherapy and control cases: clinicopathological, immunohistochemical and molecular analysis of 66 cases. *Mod Pathol* 2012;25:75–85.
451. Fernandez AP, Sun Y, Tubbs RR, et al. FISH for MYC amplification and anti-MYC immunohistochemistry: useful diagnostic tools in the assessment of secondary angiosarcoma and atypical vascular proliferations. *J Cutan Pathol* 2012;39:234–242.
452. Morgan EA, Kozono DE, Wang Q, et al. Cutaneous radiation-associated angiosarcoma of the breast: poor prognosis in a rare secondary malignancy. *Ann Surg Oncol* 2012;19:3801–3808.
453. Jallali N, James S, Searle A, et al. Surgical management of radiation-induced angiosarcoma after breast conservation therapy. *Am J Surg* 2012;203:156–161.
454. Seinen JM, Styring E, Verstappen V, et al. Radiation-associated angiosarcoma after breast cancer: high recurrence rate and poor survival despite surgical treatment with R0 resection. *Ann Surg Oncol* 2012;19:2700–2706.
455. Palta M, Morris CG, Grobmyer SR, et al. Angiosarcoma after breast-conserving therapy: long-term outcomes with hyperfractionated radiotherapy. *Cancer* 2010;116:1872–1878.
456. Slotman BJ, van Hattum AH, Meyer S, et al. Angiosarcoma of the breast following conserving treatment for breast cancer. *Eur J Cancer* 1994;30A:416–417.
457. Edeiken S, Russo DP, Knecht J, et al. Angiosarcoma after tylectomy and radiation therapy for carcinoma of the breast. *Cancer* 1992;70:644–647.
458. Buatti JM, Harari PM, Leigh BR, et al. Radiation-induced angiosarcoma of the breast. Case report and review of the literature. *Am J Clin Oncol* 1994;17:444–447.
459. Raina V, Sengar M, Shukla NK, et al. Complete response from thalidomide in angiosarcoma after treatment of breast cancer. *J Clin Oncol* 2007;25:900–901.
460. Komdeur R, Hoekstra HJ, Molenaar WM, et al. Clinicopathologic assessment of postradiation sarcomas: KIT as a potential treatment target. *Clin Cancer Res* 2003;9:2926–2932.
461. Chiarelli A, Boccone P, Goia F, et al. Gingival metastasis of a radiotherapy-induced breast angiosarcoma: diagnosis and multidisciplinary treatment achieving a prolonged complete remission. *Anticancer Drugs* 2012;23:1112–1117.
462. Gambini D, Visintin R, Locatelli E, et al. Paclitaxel-dependent prolonged and persistent complete remission four years from first recurrence of secondary breast angiosarcoma. *Tumori* 2009;95:828–831.
463. Mano MS, Fraser G, Kerr J, et al. Radiation-induced angiosarcoma of the breast shows major response to docetaxel after failure of anthracycline-based chemotherapy. *Breast* 2006;15:117–118.
464. Park MS, Ravi V, Araujo DM. Inhibiting the VEGF-VEGFR pathway in angiosarcoma, epithelioid hemangioendothelioma, and hemangiopericytoma/solitary fibrous tumor. *Curr Opin Oncol* 2010;22:351–355.
465. Miettinen M, Sarlomo-Rikala M, Lasota J. KIT expression in angiosarcomas and fetal endothelial cells: lack of mutations of exon 11 and exon 17 of C-kit. *Mod Pathol* 2000;13:536–541.
466. Kurwa A, Waddington E. Post mastectomy lymphangiomatosis. *Br J Dermatol* 1968;80:840.

467. Prioleau PG, Santa Cruz DJ. Lymphangioma circumscriptum following radical mastectomy and radiation therapy. *Cancer* 1978;42:1989–1991.
468. Diaz-Cascajo C, Borghi S, Weyers W, et al. Benign lymphangiomatous papules of the skin following radiotherapy: a report of five new cases and review of the literature. *Histopathology* 1999;35:319–327.
469. Ambrojo P, Cogolludo EF, Aguilar A, et al. Cutaneous lymphangiectases after therapy for carcinoma of the cervix—a case with unusual clinical and histological features. *Clin Exp Dermatol* 1990;15:57–59.
470. Jappe U, Zimmermann T, Kahle B, et al. Lymphangioma circumscriptum of the vulva following surgical and radiological therapy of cervical cancer. *Sex Transm Dis* 2002;29:533–535.
471. Requena L, Kutzner H, Mentzel T, et al. Benign vascular proliferations in irradiated skin. *Am J Surg Pathol* 2002;26:328–337.
472. Patton KT, Deyrup AT, Weiss SW. Atypical vascular lesions after surgery and radiation of the breast: a clinicopathologic study of 32 cases analyzing histologic heterogeneity and association with angiosarcoma. *Am J Surg Pathol* 2008;32:943–950.
473. Gengler C, Coindre JM, Leroux A, et al. Vascular proliferations of the skin after radiation therapy for breast cancer: clinicopathologic analysis of a series in favor of a benign process: a study from the French Sarcoma Group. *Cancer* 2007;109:1584–1598.
474. Mattoch IW, Robbins JB, Kempson RL, et al. Post-radiotherapy vascular proliferations in mammary skin: a clinicopathologic study of 11 cases. *J Am Acad Dermatol* 2007;57:126–133.
475. Santi R, Cetica V, Franchi A, et al. Tumour suppressor gene TP53 mutations in atypical vascular lesions of breast skin following radiotherapy. *Histopathology* 2011;58:455–466.
476. Kim PS, Neff AG, Mutasim DF, et al. Multiple lymphatic-type, atypical vascular lesions of the breast following radiation therapy. *Int J Dermatol* 2013;52:195–197.
477. Di Tommaso L, Rosai J. The capillary lobule: a deceptively benign feature of post-radiation angiosarcoma of the skin: report of three cases. *Am J Dermatopathol* 2005;27:301–305.
478. Rosso R, Gianelli U, Carnevali L. Acquired progressive lymphangioma of the skin following radiotherapy for breast carcinoma. *J Cutan Pathol* 1995;22:164–167.
479. Guillou L, Fletcher CD. Benign lymphangioendothelioma (acquired progressive lymphangioma): a lesion not to be confused with well-differentiated angiosarcoma and patch stage Kaposi's sarcoma: clinicopathologic analysis of a series. *Am J Surg Pathol* 2000;24:1047–1057.
480. McMenamin ME, Fletcher CD. Reactive angioendotheliomatosis: a study of 15 cases demonstrating a wide clinicopathologic spectrum. *Am J Surg Pathol* 2002;26:685–697.
481. Janse AJ, van Coevorden F, Peterse H, et al. Lymphedema-induced lymphangiosarcoma. *Eur J Surg Oncol* 1995;21:155–158.

Postmastectomy Angiosarcoma (StewartTreves Syndrome)

482. Stewart FW, Treves N. Lymphangiosarcoma in postmastectomy lymphedema; a report of six cases in elephantiasis chirurgica. *Cancer* 1948;1:64–81.
483. Löwenstein S. Der äetiologische Zusammengang zwischen akutem einmalignem Trauma und malignem Sarkom. *Beiträge zur klinischen Chirurgie; Mitteilungen aus der chirurgischen Klinik zu Tübingen* 1906;780–824.
484. Kettle EH. Tumours arising from endothelium. *Proc R Soc Med* 1918;11:19–34.
485. Dawlatly SL, Dramis A, Sumathi VP, et al. Stewart-Treves syndrome and the use of positron emission tomographic scanning. *Ann Vasc Surg* 2011;25:699 e691–e693.
486. Hulme SA, Bialostocki A, Hardy SL, et al. Stewart-Treves syndrome in a congenitally lymphedematous upper limb. *Plast Reconstr Surg* 2007;119:1140–1141.
487. Kazerooni E, Hessler C. CT appearance of angiosarcoma associated with chronic lymphedema. *AJR Am J Roentgenol* 1991;156:543–544.
488. Merrick TA, Erlandson RA, Hajdu SI. Lymphangiosarcoma of a congenitally lymphedematous arm. *Arch Pathol* 1971;91:365–371.
489. Muller R, Hajdu SI, Brennan MF. Lymphangiosarcoma associated with chronic filarial lymphedema. *Cancer* 1987;59:179–183.
490. Case records of the Massachusetts General Hospital. Weekly clinicopathological exercises. Case 18-1993. A 57-year-old man with chronic lymphedema and enlarging purple cutaneous nodules of the leg. *N Engl J Med* 1993;328:1337–1343.
491. Komorowski AL, Wysocki WM, Mitus J. Angiosarcoma in a chronically lymphedematous leg: an unusual presentation of Stewart-Treves syndrome. *South Med J* 2003;96:807–808.
492. Sordillo PP, Chapman R, Hajdu SI, et al. Lymphangiosarcoma. *Cancer* 1981;48:1674–1679.
493. Chen KT, Bauer V, Flam MS. Angiosarcoma in postsurgical lymphedema. An unusual occurrence in a man. *Am J Dermatopathol* 1991;13:488–492.
494. di Meo N, Drabeni M, Gatti A, et al. A Stewart-Treves syndrome of the lower limb. *Dermatol Online J* 2012;18:14.
495. Hultberg BM. Angiosarcomas in chronically lymphedematous extremities. Two cases of Stewart-Treves syndrome. *Am J Dermatopathol* 1987;9:406–412.
496. McHaffie DR, Kozak KR, Warner TF, et al. Stewart-Treves syndrome of the lower extremity. *J Clin Oncol* 2010;28:e351–e352.
497. Nakazono T, Kudo S, Matsuo Y, et al. Angiosarcoma associated with chronic lymphedema (Stewart-Treves syndrome) of the leg: MR imaging. *Skeletal Radiol* 2000;29:413–416.
498. Roy P, Clark MA, Thomas JM. Stewart-Treves syndrome—treatment and outcome in six patients from a single centre. *Eur J Surg Oncol* 2004;30:982–986.
499. Krause KI, Hebert AA, Sanchez RL, et al. Anterior abdominal wall angiosarcoma in a morbidly obese woman. *J Am Acad Dermatol* 1986;15:327–330.
500. Woodward AH, Ivins JC, Soule EH. Lymphangiosarcoma arising in chronic lymphedematous extremities. *Cancer* 1972;30:562–572.
501. Futrell JW, Albright NL, Myers GH Jr. Prevention of tumor growth in an "immunologically privileged site" by adoptive transfer of tumor-specific transplantation immunity. *J Surg Res* 1972;12:62–69.
502. Lambert PB, Frank HA. Bellman S,et al. The role of the lymph trunks in the response to allogeneic skin transplants. *Transplantation* 1965;3:62–73.
503. Schreiber H, Barry FM, Russell WC, et al. Stewart-Treves syndrome. A lethal complication of postmastectomy lymphedema and regional immune deficiency. *Arch Surg* 1979;114:82–85.
504. Stark RB, Dwyer EM, de Forest M. Effect of surgical ablation of regional lymph nodes on survival of skin homografts. *Ann NY Acad Sci* 1960;87:140–148.
505. d'Amore ES, Wick MR, Geisinger KR, et al. Primary malignant lymphoma arising in postmastectomy lymphedema. Another facet of the Stewart-Treves syndrome. *Am J Surg Pathol* 1990;14:456–463.
506. Waxman M, Fatteh S, Elias JM, et al. Malignant lymphoma of skin associated with postmastectomy lymphedema. *Arch Pathol Lab Med* 1984;108:206–208.
507. Fitzpatrick PJ. Lymphangiosarcoma and breast cancer. *Can J Surg* 1969;12:172–177.
508. Schirger A. Postoperative lymphedema: etiologic and diagnostic factors. *Med Clin North Am* 1962;46:1045–1050.
509. Karlsson P, Holmberg E, Samuelsson A, et al. Soft tissue sarcoma after treatment for breast cancer—a Swedish population-based study. *Eur J Cancer* 1998;34:2068–2075.
510. Davies JD, Rees GJ, Mera SL. Angiosarcoma in irradiated post-mastectomy chest wall. *Histopathology* 1983;7:947–956.
511. Hamels J, Blondiau P, Mirgaux M. Cutaneous angiosarcoma arising in a mastectomy scar after therapeutic irradiotation. *Bull Cancer* 1981;68:353–356.
512. Lo TC, Silverman ML, Edelstein A. Postirradiation hemangiosarcoma of the chest wall. Report of a case. *Acta Radiol Oncol* 1985;24:237–240.
513. Chen KT, Hoffman KD, Hendricks EJ. Angiosarcoma following therapeutic irradiation. *Cancer* 1979;44:2044–2048.
514. Styring E, Fernebro J, Jonsson PE, et al. Changing clinical presentation of angiosarcomas after breast cancer: from late tumors in edematous arms to earlier tumors on the thoracic wall. *Breast Cancer Res Treat* 2010;122:883–887.
515. Birge RF, Peisen CJ, Thornton FE, et al. Angiosarcoma in postmastectomy lymphedema. *J Iowa State Med Soc* 1957;47:491–495.
516. Sternby NH, Gynning I, Hogeman KE. Postmastectomy angiosarcoma. *Acta Chir Scand* 1961;121:420–432.
517. Scott RB, Nydick I, Conway H. Lymphangiosarcoma arising in lymphedema. *Am J Med* 1960;28:1008–1012.
518. Oettlé AG, van Blerkp PJP. Postmastectomy lymphostatic endothelioma of Stewart and Treves in a male. *Br J Surg* 1963;50:736–743.

519. Ramsey HE, Lucas JC Jr, Gray G Jr. Post-mastectomy angiosarcoma in the male. *J Natl Med Assoc* 1968;60:468–470.
520. Chopra S, Ors F, Bergin D. MRI of angiosarcoma associated with chronic lymphoedema: Stewart Treves syndrome. *Br J Radiol* 2007;80: e310–e313.
521. Schindera ST, Streit M, Kaelin U, et al. Stewart-Treves syndrome: MR imaging of a postmastectomy upper-limb chronic lymphedema with angiosarcoma. *Skeletal Radiol* 2005;34:156–160.
522. Almond MH, Jones RL, Thway K, et al. Atypical metastatic profile in Stewart-Treves syndrome. *Acta Oncol* 2010;49:1388–1390.
523. Shimizu M, Hirokawa M, Fukuya T, et al. Postmastectomy angiosarcoma (Stewart-Treves syndrome). *Acta Cytol* 1997;41:1865–1866.
524. Miettinen M, Lehto VP, Virtanen I. Postmastectomy angiosarcoma (Stewart-Treves syndrome). Light-microscopic, immunohistological, and ultrastructural characteristics of two cases. *Am J Surg Pathol* 1983;7:329–339.
525. Capo V, Ozzello L, Fenoglio CM, et al. Angiosarcomas arising in edematous extremities: immunostaining for factor VIII-related antigen and ultrastructural features. *Hum Pathol* 1985;16:144–150.
526. Tomita K, Yokogawa A, Oda Y, et al. Lymphangiosarcoma in postmastectomy lymphedema (Stewart-Treves syndrome): ultrastructural and immunohistologic characteristics. *J Surg Oncol* 1988;38:275–282.
527. Furue M, Yamada N, Takahashi T, et al. Immunotherapy for Stewart-Treves syndrome. Usefulness of intrapleural administration of tumor-infiltrating lymphocytes against massive pleural effusion caused by metastatic angiosarcoma. *J Am Acad Dermatol* 1994;30:899–903.
528. Kanitakis J, Bendelac A, Marchand C, et al. Stewart-Treves syndrome: an histogenetic (ultrastructural and immunohistological) study. *J Cutan Pathol* 1986;13:30–39.
529. Kindblom LG, Stenman G, Angervall L. Morphological and cytogenetic studies of angiosarcoma in Stewart-Treves syndrome. *Virchows Arch A Pathol Anat Histopathol* 1991;419:439–445.
530. Malhaire JP, Labat JP, Simon H, et al. One case of Stewart-Treves syndrome successfully treated at two years by chemotherapy and radiation therapy in a 73-year-old woman. *Acta Oncol* 1997;36:442–443.
531. El-Gohary YM, Silverman JF, Poppiti RJ, et al. D2-40 expression in cutanous angiosarcoma arising after radiotherapy treatment of breast carcinoma. *Modern Pathol* 2006;19(Suppl. 1):26A.
532. Hashimoto K, Matsumoto M, Eto H, et al. Differentiation of metastatic breast carcinoma from Stewart-Treves angiosarcoma. Use of anti-keratin and anti-desmosome monoclonal antibodies and factor VIII-related antibodies. *Arch Dermatol* 1985;121:742–746.
533. Lee AK, DeLellis RA, Rosen PP, et al. ABH blood group isoantigen expression in breast carcinomas--an immunohistochemical evaluation using monoclonal antibodies. *Am J Clin Pathol* 1985;83:308–319.
534. Sarkany I. Malignant melanomas in lymphoedematous arm following radical mastectomy for breast carcinoma (an extension of the syndrome of Stewart and Treves). *Proc R Soc Med* 1972;65:253–254.
535. Allan AE, Shoji T, Li N, et al. Two cases of Kaposi's sarcoma mimicking Stewart-Treves syndrome found to be human herpesvirus-8 positive. *Am J Dermatopathol* 2001;23:431–436.
536. Salameire D, Templier I, Charles J, et al. An "anaplastic" Kaposi's sarcoma mimicking a Stewart-Treves syndrome. A case report and a review of literature. *Am J Dermatopathol* 2008;30:265–268.
537. Merimsky O, Chaitchik S. Kaposi's sarcoma on a lymphedematous arm following radical mastectomy. *Tumori* 1992;78:407–408.
538. Ron IG, Amir G, Marmur S, et al. Kaposi's sarcoma on a lymphedematous arm after mastectomy. *Am J Clin Oncol* 1996;19:87–90.
539. McWilliam LJ, Harris M. Histogenesis of post-mastectomy angiosarcoma--an ultrastructural study. *Histopathology* 1985;9:331–343.
540. Lagacé R, Leroy JP. Comparative electron microscopic study of cutaneous and soft tissue angiosarcomas, post-mastectomy angiosarcoma (Stewart-Treves syndrome) and Kaposi's sarcoma. *Ultrastruct Pathol* 1987;11:161–173.
541. Marsch WC. Das Stewart-Treves-Syndrom: ein Hämangiosarkom bei chronischem Lymphödem. Ultrastrukturelle Analyse differenter klinischer Entwicklungsstadien. *Hautarzt* 1987;38:82–87.
542. Silverberg SG, Kay S, Koss LG. Postmastectomy lymphangiosarcoma: ultrastructural observations. *Cancer* 1971;27:100–108.
543. Chung KC, Kim HJ, Jeffers LL. Lymphangiosarcoma (Stewart-Treves syndrome) in postmastectomy patients. *J Hand Surg Am* 2000;25:1163–1168.
544. Grobmyer SR, Daly JM, Glotzbach RE, et al. Role of surgery in the management of postmastectomy extremity angiosarcoma (Stewart-Treves syndrome). *J Surg Oncol* 2000;73:182–188.
545. Yap BS, Yap HY, McBride CM, et al. Chemotherapy for postmastectomy lymphangiosarcoma. *Cancer* 1981;47:853–856.
546. Kaufmann T, Chu F, Kaufman R. Post-mastectomy lymphangiosarcoma (Stewart-Treves syndrome): report of two long-term survivals. *Br J Radiol* 1991;64:857–860.
547. Lans TE, de Wilt JH, van Geel AN, et al. Isolated limb perfusion with tumor necrosis factor and melphalan for nonresectable Sewart-Treves lymphangiosarcoma. *Ann Surg Oncol* 2002;9:1004–1009.
548. Breidenbach M, Rein D, Schmidt T, et al. Intra-arterial mitoxantrone and paclitaxel in a patient with Stewart-Treves syndrome: selection of chemotherapy by an ex vivo ATP-based chemosensitivity assay. *Anticancer Drugs* 2000;11:269–273.
549. Tassone P, Tagliaferri P, Cucinotto I, et al. Pegylated liposomal doxorubicin is active in Stewart-Treves syndrome. *Ann Oncol* 2007;18: 959–960.

CHAPTER 40

Lymphoid and Hematopoietic Neoplasms of the Breast

JUDITH A. FERRY

LYMPHOMAS OF THE BREAST

Primary lymphoma of the breast is generally defined as lymphoma involving one or both breasts with or without ipsilateral axillary lymph node (ALN) involvement, without evidence of disease elsewhere at presentation, in a patient without a history of lymphoma. Tissue should be adequate for pathologic examination, and the lymphoma should be seen in close proximity to mammary tissue,[1] although some authorities have not required this last criterion if the diagnostic specimen is a needle biopsy.[2] Others have accepted cases as primary if clinically the lesion was a breast mass, even if the biopsy contained fat but no mammary epithelial elements.[3] Some investigators also accept cases in which staging reveals more distant lymph node or bone marrow involvement, so long as clinically the primary or major manifestation of the lymphoma is the breast.[4]

The breast is a very uncommon primary site for lymphoma, possibly correlating with the very sparse endogenous lymphoid tissue in this site. Primary lymphoma of the breast accounts for 0.1% to 0.15%[4–7] of all malignant neoplasms of the breast, for 0.34% to 0.85% of all non-Hodgkin lymphomas (NHLs),[4,6,8–10] and for less than 2% of all extranodal NHLs.[4] Certain types of lymphoma are more likely to involve the breast as primary breast lymphomas, while others are more likely to involve the breast secondarily, that is, secondary to spread from another primary site, in the setting of widespread disease, and/or in the form of a relapse. Different types of lymphoma are discussed separately in the following sections.

Primary Lymphoma of the Breast

Clinical Presentation

Most patients with primary lymphoma of the breast are middle-aged to elderly women, although occasionally young women and, rarely, adolescents are affected,[1,5,11–14] with a median age in the sixth or seventh decade in most series.[2–3,6–10,15–23] Approximately 2% of primary breast lymphoma patients are males.[2,6–10,16–23] Occasionally the disease affects pregnant or lactating women. Rarely patients have had prior breast carcinoma.[1]

Most patients present with a palpable breast mass with or without ipsilateral axillary lymphadenopathy.[2–3,6,8,17,19,22] The lesions are typically painless, but occasionally they are painful.[22,24] A few patients have been asymptomatic, and have had the lymphoma detected by mammography. Lymphomas detected initially by routine mammography are typically low-grade lymphomas.[6,12–13,15] Constitutional symptoms are uncommon, being found in zero[8,15,17,19,25] to 4%[21] of patients in different series. In some reports, right-sided lymphoma was more common than left-sided lymphoma.[3,26] In 0% to 25% of cases in different series, patients present with bilateral disease. Overall, slightly less than 10% of primary breast lymphomas are bilateral.[1,3,5,7,9–10,18–19,21,23,25,27] A few patients have a history of autoimmune disease, diabetes mellitus, or mastitis.[4,6–7,17] Several human immunodeficiency virus (HIV)-positive patients have developed lymphoma presenting with involvement of the breast.[28] However, most patients have no underlying illness, and specific factors predisposing to lymphoma of the breast have not been identified.[2,10,27]

On physical examination, the patient usually has a discrete, mobile mass. The overlying skin is involved infrequently, but occasionally it is thickened,[22] erythematous, or inflamed,[5,29] potentially mimicking inflammatory carcinoma. Skin retraction and nipple discharge are virtually never found. The proportion of cases with ipsilateral axillary lymphadenopathy varies widely among series from 11%[12] to about 50%.

Pathology and Clinico-Pathologic Correlates

In most series, diffuse large B-cell lymphoma is the most common type, comprising 43% to 94% of cases in different series, and approximately 60% of cases overall.[2,5–9,14–15,19–20,30,31] The remainder are mainly low-grade lymphomas (extranodal mucosal-associated lymphoid tissue [MALT] lymphoma or follicular lymphoma [FL]). However, recent studies suggest that low-grade B-cell lymphomas may be more prevalent, with MALT lymphoma being more common, followed by FL, at least in some series.[7,13] In different series, extranodal marginal zone lymphoma (MALT lymphoma) accounts for 0% to 50% of cases,[2,4–9,12,15,19,20,30] and for approximately 9% of cases in one large series.[32] FLs make up approximately 14% of primary breast lymphomas.[32] It is possible that a larger number of low-grade lymphomas are being detected because of identification of asymptomatic lesions by mammography,[13] and because with the wider recognition of marginal zone lymphomas and larger number of immunostains and molecular assays for paraffin-embedded tissue, pathologists are now better able to recognize and diagnose these lymphomas. Burkitt lymphoma is uncommon. T-cell lymphoma is very rare.[2,13]

Although breast lymphomas often appear grossly circumscribed, on microscopic examination they often show invasion into surrounding tissues at the periphery of the lesion.[3,12] The neoplastic cells tend to infiltrate around and within mammary ducts and lobules, sometimes with obliteration of these structures. In a few cases, histologic changes of lymphocytic mastitis were described in association with primary breast lymphoma.[27,33]

B-Cell Lymphomas

Diffuse Large B-Cell Lymphoma

Clinical Presentation

Diffuse large B-cell lymphoma primary in the breast affects women (and a few men) over a wide age range, including some young patients,[6,14,17,21,23] with a median age in the sixth decade.[31] Lesions range from 1 to 20 cm in greatest dimension, with a median size of 4 to 5 cm. A few patients have diffuse breast enlargement.[9,10,17,19,21,23,31] These lymphomas are thus larger on average than mammary carcinomas. They have been described as discrete, hard, rubbery,[18] soft or fleshy masses[5] that may be rapidly enlarging.[1,18,29]

Pathology

The lymphomas are composed of a diffuse infiltrate of large lymphoid cells (Fig. 40.1). When these diffuse large B-cell lymphomas have been subclassified, the majority are centroblastic, a minority are immunoblastic,[2,5,20,34] and rare cases are diffuse large B-cell lymphoma, anaplastic variant,

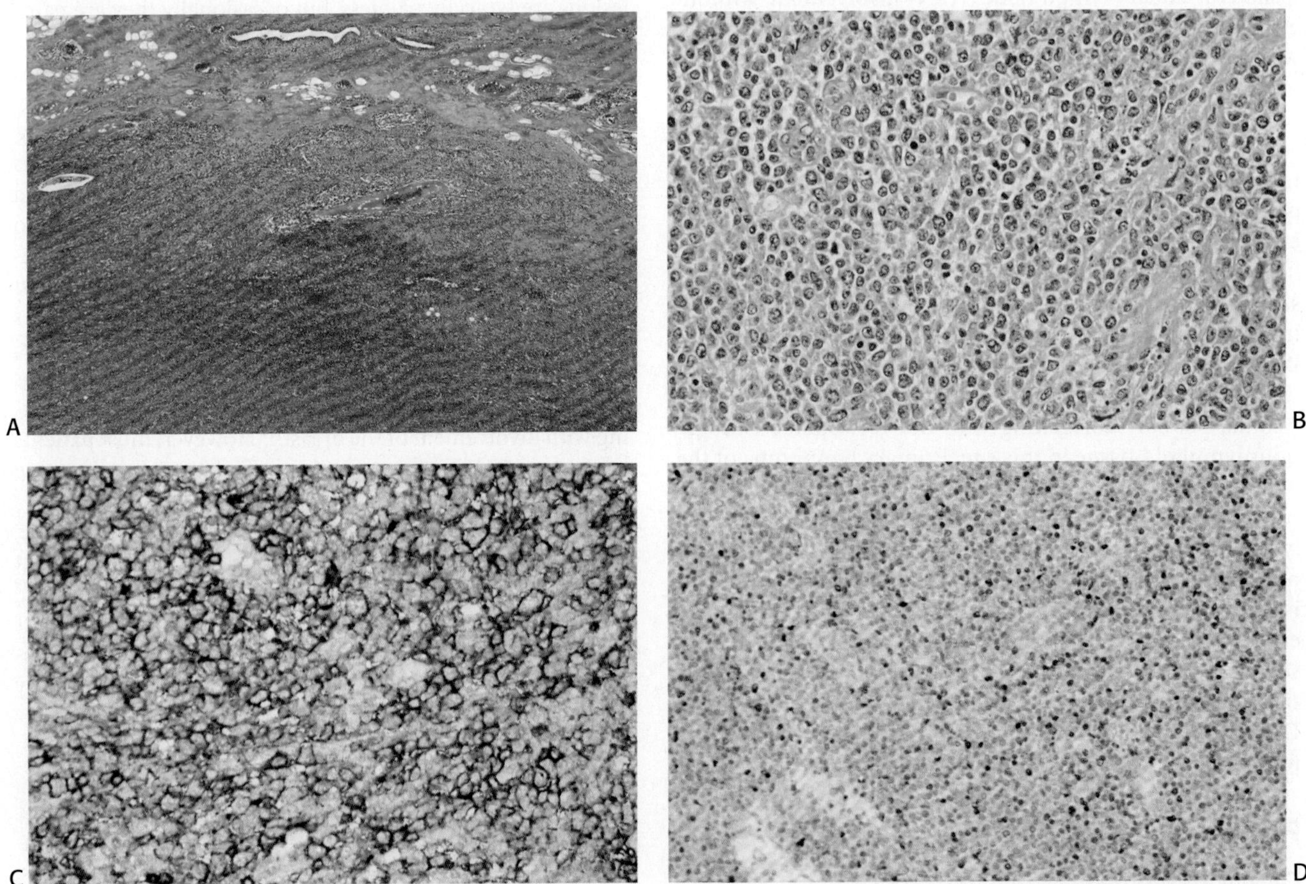

FIG. 40.1. ***Diffuse large B-cell lymphoma.*** **A:** Low power shows a dense, diffuse infiltrate of lymphoid cells involving breast parenchyma; ductules are present adjacent to the lymphoma (*top* of image). **B:** High power shows closely packed large lymphoid cells with oval vesicular nuclei. Condensation of chromatin along the nuclear membrane, occasional distinct nucleoli, and scant cytoplasm, an appearance consistent with centroblasts. Mitoses are frequent. **C:** Large lymphoid cells are CD20+. **D:** Most large lymphoid cells show positive nuclear staining for MUM1/IRF4. This lymphoma had a nongerminal center immunophenotype (**C** and **D**, immunoperoxidase technique on paraffin sections).

co-expressing CD30.[10] A few cases of diffuse large B-cell lymphoma have had a component of MALT lymphoma, consistent with large cell transformation of the low-grade lymphoma.[21,23,35] A case of intravascular large B-cell lymphoma presenting with breast involvement has been reported (Fig. 40.2).[36] The lymphomas are CD45+, CD20+, with rare CD5+ cases.[23] CD10 is expressed in a small minority, bcl-6 is expressed in approximately half of the cases, bcl-2 is expressed in the majority of cases, and MUM1/IRF4 is expressed in nearly all cases (Fig. 40.1).[2,7,17,23,25] The majority of cases thus have a nongerminal center B-cell (non-GCB) immunophenotype (CD10−, bcl-6+, MUM1/IRF4+, or CD10−, bcl-6−), while a minority have a germinal center B-cell (GCB) phenotype (CD10+, bcl-6+ or CD10−, bcl-6+, MUM1/IRF4−) (Table 40.1).[2] In one recent large series, 77% of cases had a non-GCB immunophenotype and 23% had a GCB immunophenotype[31]; in another, 95% of cases were non-GCB-like.[37] The proliferation index is fairly high (60% to 95% in one

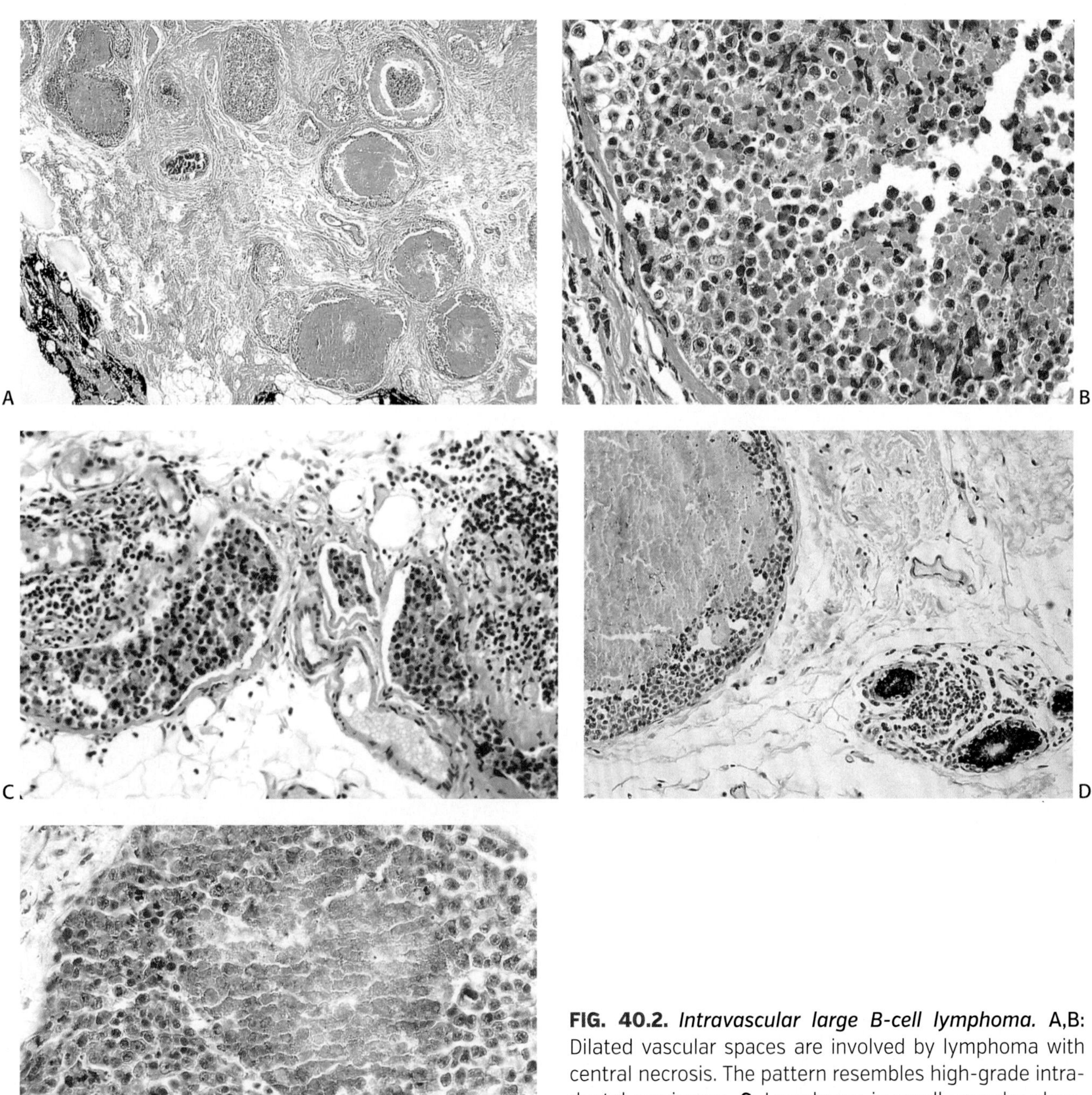

FIG. 40.2. ***Intravascular large B-cell lymphoma.*** **A,B:** Dilated vascular spaces are involved by lymphoma with central necrosis. The pattern resembles high-grade intraductal carcinoma. **C:** Lymphoma in small vascular channels easily mistaken for carcinomatous lymphatic tumor emboli. **D:** The immunostain for cytokeratin shows reactivity limited to the epithelium of a small lobule (CAM5.2). **E:** The tumor cells are immunoreactive for CD45 (LCA).

TABLE 40.1 Lymphomas of the Breast: Principal Features

Type of Lymphoma	Patients Affected	Histology	Neoplastic Cells, Usual Immunophenotype	Genetic, Cytogenetic Features	Clinical Behavior
Diffuse large B-cell lymphoma	Adults, females >> males, broad age range; few pregnant	Diffuse proliferation of large lymphoid cells; CB more common than IB	CD45+, CD20+, CD10 usually −, bcl-6+/−, bcl-2 and MUM1/IRF4 usually +, Ki67 high; non-GC > GC	Rare *MALT1* rearrangements; trisomy 18 in some; possible NFκB activation in a minority	Aggressive; CNS, opposite breast: most common sites of relapse; best outcomes with CHOP or CHOP-like chemo +/− RT
Extranodal marginal zone lymphoma (MALT lymphoma)	Middle-aged and older adults; females >> males	Marginal zone B cells, variable plasma cells, and reactive follicles may be present. LELs are often not prominent	CD45+, CD20+, CD5−, CD10−, CD23−, CD43+/−, bcl-2+/−, cyclin D1−, cIg+/−	Rare *MALT1* rearrangements; Minority of cases: trisomy 3, 12, and/or 18	Good prognosis. Localized extranodal relapses may occur. Few have large cell transformation. Few die of lymphoma
Follicular lymphoma (FL)	Middle-aged and older women	Similar to lymph nodal FL	CD45+, CD20+, CD10+, CD5−, CD23−, CD43−, bcl-2+, cyclin D1−, sIg+, occasionally bcl-2−	n/a	Prognosis less good than MALT lymphoma. Behavior similar to nodal FL
Burkitt lymphoma	Young to middle-aged, few older women, some pregnant or lactating	Diffuse infiltrate of medium-sized round cells, many mitoses, and starry sky	CD45+, CD20+, CD10+, bcl-6+, bcl-2−, Ki67 ~100%[a]	Translocation of *MYC* with *IGH* [t(8;14)], less often with *IGK* or *IGL*[a]	Very aggressive; disease is often widespread
B- and T-lymphoblastic lymphoma/leukemia	Mostly adolescents and young adults, often with concurrent acute lymphoblastic leukemia	Diffuse infiltrate of small- to medium-sized cells with oval or irregular nuclei, fine chromatin, small nucleoli, and scant cytoplasm	B lineage: CD19+, CD20−, CD10+, TdT+[a] T lineage: Variable expression of T-cell markers, but often CD3+, CD7+, CD4+/CD8+ (double+), CD1a+, TdT+[a]	Variable	Aggressive disease with relatively good prognosis depending on underlying genetic abnormalities, if optimally treated
ALCL, ALK−, associated with implant	Women with saline or silicone implants, for cosmetic purposes or following mastectomy; lymphoma occurs years after implant; seroma rather than discrete mass	Large atypical, pleomorphic cells in a background of fibrosis, debris, and, sometimes, chronic inflammation	CD30+, ALK1−, CD45−/+, CD4+/−, CD43+/−, CD3−/+, CD5−/+, CD8−, EMA+/−, TIA1+/−, granzyme B +/−, EBV−, HHV8−	*TCR*: clonal *IGH*: polyclonal	Very good prognosis in absence of a discrete mass or spread beyond breast

TABLE 40.1 Lymphomas of the Breast: Principal Features *(continued)*

Type of Lymphoma	Patients Affected	Histology	Neoplastic Cells, Usual Immunophenotype	Genetic, Cytogenetic Features	Clinical Behavior
Classical Hodgkin lymphoma (CHL)	Rare; breast involvement virtually always secondary to lymph nodal disease	Reed–Sternberg cells and variants in a reactive background	CD15+, CD30+, CD45–, PAX5 dim+, CD20–, CD3–, ALK1–	*TCR*: polyclonal *IGH*: polyclonal	Outcome likely similar to other CHL of same stage

CB, centroblastic; IB, immunoblastic; non-GC, nongerminal center immunophenotype; GC, germinal center immunophenotype; CHOP, cytoxan, adriamycin, vincristine, prednisone; RT, radiation therapy; cIg, monotypic cytoplasmic immunoglobulin; sIg, monotypic surface immunoglobulin; *IGH*, immunoglobulin heavy-chain gene; *IGK*, immunoglobulin kappa light-chain gene; *IGL*, immunoglobulin lambda light-chain gene.

[a]Based in part on data on same types of lymphoma in other sites.

series).[23] Immunostaining for p50 and p65 has shown nuclear localization of p50 in a minority, suggesting NFκB activation in a subset of cases.[34] *In situ* hybridization for Epstein–Barr virus (EBV) using a probe for EBER is typically negative.[23]

Genetic and cytogenetic features have not been extensively studied. The available data show rare cases with evidence of *MALT1* rearrangement, similar to most mammary marginal zone lymphomas.[34,35] Chromosomal trisomies have been described in a subset of cases, with trisomy 18 representing the most common trisomy in one series.[35] *IGH* variable region gene mutational analysis has shown a mutation frequency of 1% to 10%, generally without ongoing somatic mutation. In conjunction with results of immunophenotyping, these findings suggest that neoplastic cells typically correspond to a postgerminal center stage of B-cell differentiation.

Staging, Treatment, and Outcome

Most large studies of diffuse large B-cell lymphoma primary in the breast include only those cases with lymphoma confined to the breast or with spread to ipsilateral ALNs.[10,21,31,37] The relative proportion of cases with stage I (confined to breast) and II (with ALN involvement) disease varies among series, but overall more than 60% of patients have stage I disease. Most of the remainder have stage II disease and a few have stage IV (bilateral breast) disease.[8,16–18,20,21,23,30,31] Diffuse large B-cell lymphoma patients are currently typically treated with combination chemotherapy, accompanied in some cases by radiation therapy. By far the most common chemotherapeutic regimen used is CHOP (cyclophosphamide, doxorubicin, vincristine, and prednisone). Among patients treated in recent years, Rituxan has often been used in addition to CHOP chemotherapy. The impact of Rituxan on outcome is not clear; improved outcome with Rituxan has been reported by some authors,[25] but not by others.[31]

Relapses may involve lymph nodes and a wide variety of extranodal sites. Among the latter, the central nervous system (CNS) and the ipsilateral and contralateral breast are most common (Table 40.1).[5,8,9,14,16,17,20,21,23,34] However, the proportion of cases with CNS involvement varies significantly among different series, with some reporting no CNS involvement.[31] CNS involvement is associated with a very poor prognosis[16,20,37]; for this reason some authorities advocate the addition of CNS prophylaxis to the treatment regimen.[17,20]

A variety of clinical and pathologic features impact prognosis. Patients treated with only local therapy have a worse outcome than those receiving combination chemotherapy.[7,9,16,17,21] In some studies the addition of radiation is associated with decreased risk of local relapse and an improved outcome.[9,16,21] Mastectomy does not improve survival. Obtaining a large enough biopsy for optimal pathologic evaluation is the only surgery needed.[17,19,21] Men and women have a similar prognosis.[21] Diffuse large B-cell lymphoma arising from marginal zone lymphoma and *de novo* diffuse large B-cell lymphoma do not appear to have a different prognosis.[21] In a number of studies tumor size and stage (I vs. II) did not affect prognosis,[16,17,21] although other investigators have described an inferior outcome for those with stage II disease compared to stage I disease.[14] A trend toward a worse outcome for patients with bilateral disease has been observed.[21] A worse outcome has been described with younger age (less than 45 years) by some,[14] although others have not made this observation. Some reports suggest a better outcome for patients with CD10+, bcl-6+ lymphomas than with CD10–, bcl-6– lymphomas[17] and a worse outcome for those with a non-GCB immunophenotype.[2] Others found no survival benefit for patients with GCB-like diffuse large B-cell lymphoma compared to those with a non-GCB immunophenotype.[31]

In one study only the stage-adjusted International Prognostic Index impacted overall survival (OS).[37] A 10-year OS of up to approximately 80% for optimally treated patients has been reported,[16] although most other series report less favorable outcomes.[2,21] Other recent reports, for example, described an 82% 3-year OS[37] and 66% 5-year disease-free survival (DFS)[31] for stage I and II diffuse large B-cell lymphoma of the breast. Traditionally, diffuse large B-cell lymphoma arising in the breast has been considered to have a worse prognosis than primary lymph nodal diffuse large B-cell lymphoma, but a recent comparison suggests that their outcomes are not significantly different in patients treated with CHOP plus Rituxan.[37]

Extranodal Marginal Zone Lymphoma of Mucosa-Associated Lymphoid Tissue (MALT Lymphoma)

Clinical Presentation

Extranodal marginal zone lymphoma (MALT lymphoma) arising in the breast was first reported by Lamovec in 1987.[5] MALT lymphoma mainly affects middle-aged and older women and rarely men,[4–6,8,12,26,30,35,38,39] with a median age of 68 years in one large series (Table 40.1).[32] Occurrence in a premenopausal patient is somewhat unusual, and association with pregnancy or lactation is exceptional.[32] In contrast to MALT lymphomas arising in other sites, where specific infectious agents or underlying autoimmune diseases have been identified as risk factors, patients with MALT lymphoma of the breast typically have no recognized factors predisposing to lymphoma. One exception to this general rule is a case report of MALT lymphoma presenting in the breast of a patient with Sjögren syndrome, an autoimmune disease known to be associated with MALT lymphomas in the parotid gland and other sites.[40] MALT lymphoma patients present with a lesion that is typically unilateral, and may be detected by physical examination or by mammography. Constitutional symptoms are almost never present.[32]

Pathology

A description of features on gross examination is only available in a few cases, but the lymphomas range from less than 1 to 20 cm, with a median size of approximately 3 cm.[5,8,12,30,32,38,39] Their histologic features are similar to those of MALT lymphomas in other sites. The lymphomas have a vaguely nodular to diffuse appearance on low power examination. They are composed of small to medium-sized cells with slightly irregular nuclei and scant to abundant quantity of pale cytoplasm. Reactive follicles, sometimes with follicular colonization (infiltration and partial to complete replacement by neoplastic marginal zone cells), and plasmacytic differentiation, sometimes accompanied by Dutcher bodies (intranuclear protrusions of cytoplasm containing immunoglobulin), are found in some cases. Mitotic activity is low, except in residual reactive follicles (Fig. 40.3). Necrosis and sclerosis are typically absent. Infiltration of epithelial structures by lymphocytes may be seen, but well-formed lymphoepithelial lesions (LELs) are less conspicuous than in marginal zone lymphomas involving some other sites.[2,6,12,34] Infrequently MALT lymphomas with plasmacytic differentiation are associated with localized deposition of amyloid[41]; this phenomenon has been documented rarely in the breast.[5,40]

The neoplastic cells are typically CD45+, CD20+, CD5−, CD10−, CD23−, CD43+/−, bcl-2+/−, and cyclin D1−, with monotypic cytoplasmic immunoglobulin in those cases with plasmacytic differentiation (Fig. 40.3).[7,26,38] The proliferation index is low. If there are remnants of reactive follicles, the germinal center cells are CD10+, bcl-6+, and bcl-2−, with a high proliferation index. Markers of follicular dendritic cells (CD21, CD23) typically show underlying follicular dendritic meshworks, which are often expanded and disrupted. The presence of follicular dendritic cell meshworks tends to correlate with a vaguely nodular growth pattern in MALT lymphomas.

There are several specific or nearly specific, mutually exclusive chromosomal translocations that may be found in MALT lymphomas, with a frequency that varies depending on the anatomic site. Two of these translocations involve the *MALT1* gene: t(11;18), involving *API2* and *MALT1*; and t(14;18), involving *IGH* and *MALT1*. They are believed to contribute to the pathogenesis of MALT lymphoma through activation of the NFκB pathway. In MALT lymphomas arising in the breast, in nearly all studies, fluorescence *in situ* hybridization (FISH) studies have been negative for rearrangements of *MALT1*.[34,42,43] In one recent Italian study three of nine MALT lymphomas of the breast showed the presence of the t(11;18) and one showed the t(14;18).[26] Trisomies of chromosomes 3, 12, and 18 are relatively common in MALT lymphomas arising in a variety of sites, and each of these trisomies has been documented in a minority of cases of MALT lymphoma of the breast (Table 40.1).[35,42] The absence of nuclear p50 and p65 expression has been reported. This suggests a lack of NFκB activation, but this study was among those showing no translocation involving

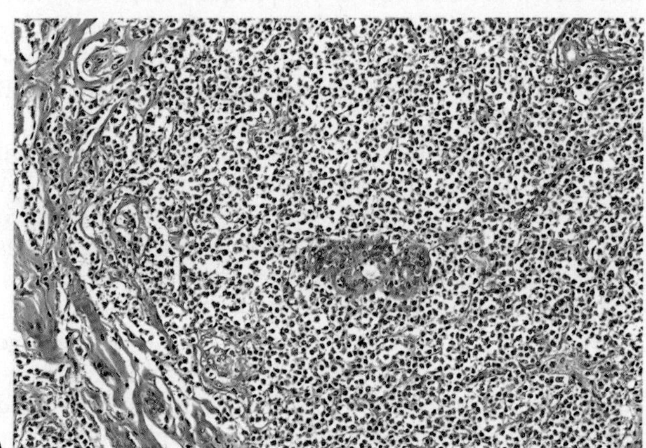
A

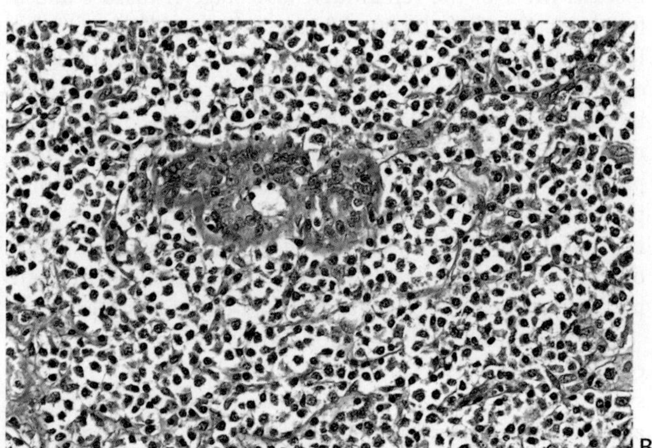
B

FIG. 40.3. *MALT lymphoma.* **A,B:** The lymphomatous infiltrate around a mammary duct consists of small cells with plasmacytic features. **C:** The tumor cells are reactive for CD43. **D:** Immunoreactivity for CD79 is shown. **E:** Immunoreactivity for kappa is shown. **F:** There was no reactivity for lambda.

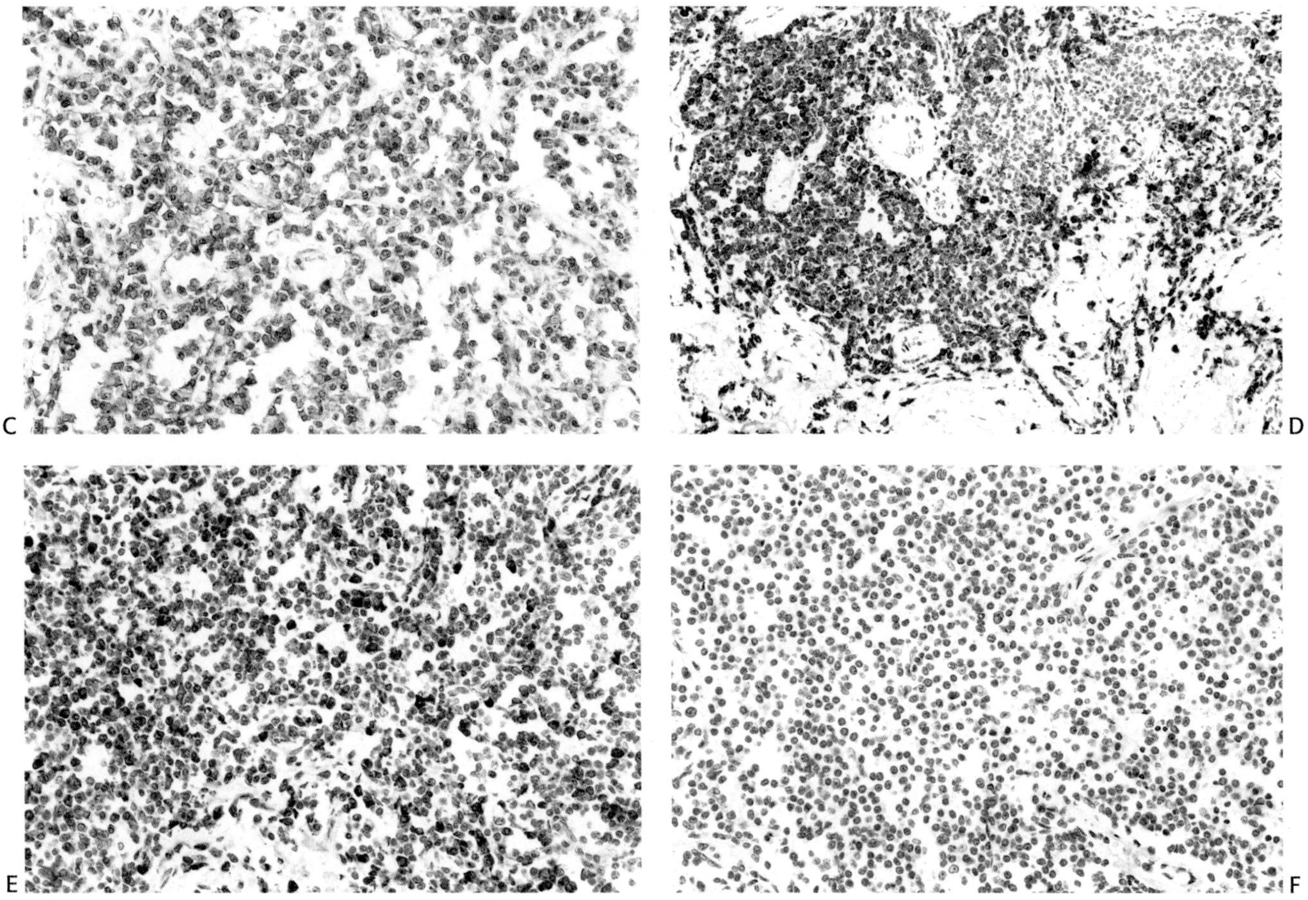

FIG. 40.3. *(Continued)*

MALT1.[34] The genetic defects leading to the development of MALT lymphoma of the breast are uncertain, and its etiology is not understood. The possibility of lymphoma arising from MALT acquired during lactation has been proposed.[7]

Staging, Treatment, and Outcome

Most patients present with Ann Arbor stage I disease, with lymphoma confined to the breast. A minority have involvement of ipsilateral ALNs (stage II), and patients rarely have more distant spread.[2,4,6–8,20,38,39] Some patients have been treated with surgery only (excisional biopsy or mastectomy), some with radiation, and others with chemotherapy. MALT lymphoma patients typically remain well after treatment or develop relapses that are usually extranodal (same or opposite breast, subcutis, larynx, chest wall, lacrimal gland), but occasionally involving lymph nodes as well, although usually without generalized disease.[4,5,30,39] Progression to diffuse large B-cell lymphoma has been reported.[5,12] A small proportion of patients die of lymphoma, sometimes following large cell transformation.[12] In one study, the median DFS was 31 months and median OS was 118 months.[2] In another study of nine patients with a mean follow-up time of 51 months at last follow-up, only two patients were alive and well. Six patients were alive with lymphoma and one had died of lymphoma.[26] In a series of 24 patients with primary MALT lymphoma of the breast, progression-free survival was 56% at 5 years and 34% at 10 years, while cause-specific survival was 100% at 5 years and 80% at 10 years.[32] Thus, as for MALT lymphomas arising in other sites, relapses are fairly common, but death due to lymphoma is infrequent.[4,5,12,20,32]

Follicular Lymphoma

Clinical Presentation

FL mainly affects middle-aged and older women,[8,12,30] and rarely men,[32] with a median of 62 years (range, 32 to 88 years) in one large series.[32] Patients present with lesions that are unilateral in roughly 95% of cases, typically unaccompanied by constitutional symptoms.[32]

Pathology

The tumor size ranges from less than 1 to 9 cm, with a median of about 2 to 3 cm.[8,12,30,32] Histologic and immunophenotypic features are similar to those of nodal FLs. The lymphomas take the form of poorly delineated lymphoid follicles, usually occupied by a relatively monotonous population of centrocytes (small cleaved cells) with a variable admixture of centroblasts (large noncleaved cells). FLs of all grades (1 to 3) have been reported.[12,13,17,19] Atypical lymphoid cells may also be found infiltrating tissue unassociated with follicles, in a diffuse pattern. Associated sclerosis is common (Figs. 40.4 and 40.5). Single cell epithelial

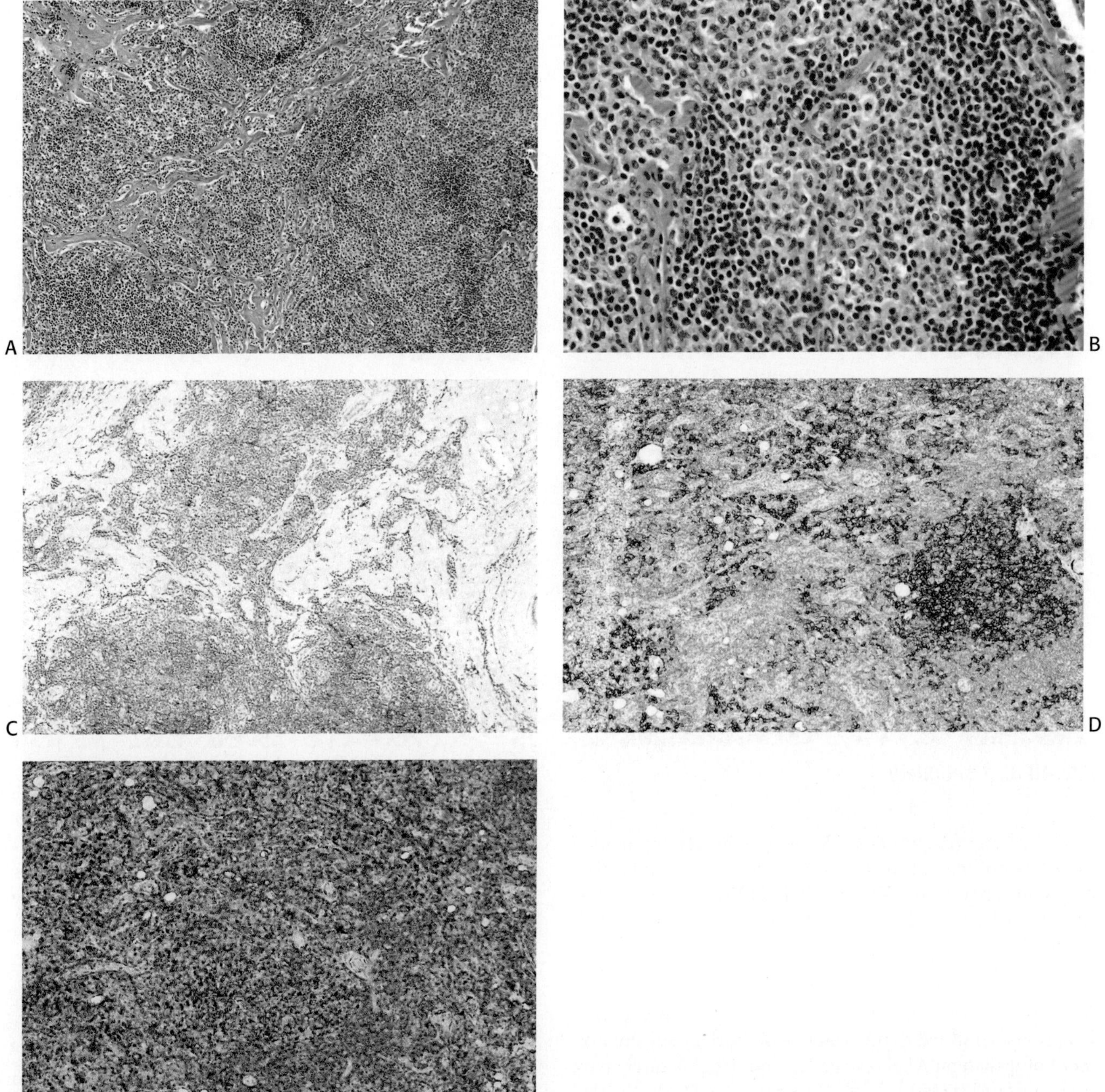

FIG. 40.4. ***Follicular lymphoma, grade 1 to 2 of 3, follicular and diffuse pattern.*** **A:** Low power shows poorly delineated follicular aggregates of atypical lymphoid cells that are slightly larger, with slightly more pale cytoplasm, than admixed non-neoplastic small lymphocytes. The lymphoid infiltrate is associated with prominent sclerosis. Strands and small clusters of atypical lymphoid cell appear to be present outside follicles. **B:** Higher magnification shows one atypical follicle composed mainly of small to medium-sized centrocytes with irregular nuclei and only rare large centroblasts with oval, vesicular nuclei. Most of the atypical follicle is surrounded by small lymphocytes. **C:** Distorted, fragmented CD21+ follicular dendritic cell meshworks highlight the neoplastic follicles. **D:** Atypical lymphoid cells in a follicle (*right midportion* of image) are CD10+. Multiple cords and clusters of CD10+ B cells are present outside the follicle. **E:** The atypical B cells coexpress bcl-2 (**C–E**, immunoperoxidase technique on paraffin sections).

infiltration has been described that could potentially be mistaken for LELs.[7] Neoplastic follicles are typically CD45+, CD20+, CD10+, bcl-6+, CD5−, CD23−, CD43−, bcl-2+, cyclin D1− (Fig. 40.4, Table 40.1).[7] Demonstration of monotypic immunoglobulin light-chain expression typically requires evaluation by flow cytometry. The breast lymphomas are occasionally bcl-2–negative (Fig. 40.5). Follicular architecture can be highlighted with antibodies to follicular dendritic cells (CD21, CD23). B cells (CD20+) expressing germinal center markers (CD10, bcl-6) can often be found outside follicles (Figs. 40.4 and 40.5), a feature helpful in distinguishing FL from follicular hyperplasia.

Staging, Treatment, and Outcome

Patients present with disease involving the breast, sometimes accompanied by axillary lymph nodal involvement. Occasional patients have more widespread disease.[6–8,12,20,30] Treatment has not been uniform, and patients have been treated with surgery, radiation, and/or chemotherapy. The prognosis appears to be less favorable than that of MALT lymphoma,[12,20] and possibly also worse than for limited-stage FL arising in lymph nodes.[32] In one series of 36 patients with FL primary in the breast, progression-free survival was 49% at 5 years and 28% at 10 years, while cause-specific survival was 79% at 5 years and 66% at 10 years.[32]

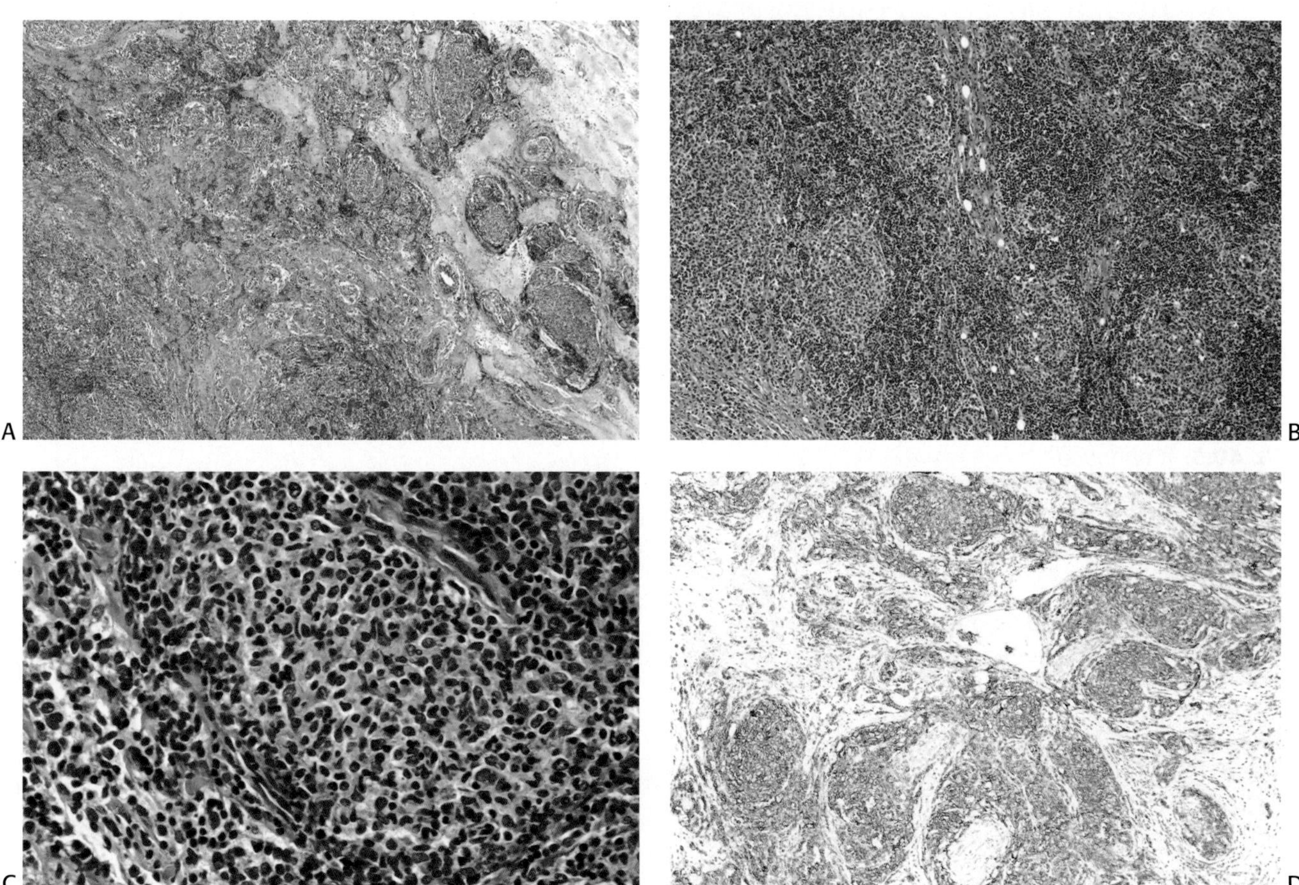

FIG. 40.5. ***Follicular lymphoma, follicular and diffuse pattern, grade 1 to 2 of 3.*** **A:** The lymphoma is composed of multiple poorly delineated follicles, as well as clusters of atypical cells outside atypical follicles. The infiltrate is associated with sclerosis. Atypical lymphoid cells surround small lobules (*top, center* of image). **B:** Scattered small, ill-defined follicles in a background of nonneoplastic small lymphocytes. **C:** High magnification shows one small, poorly delineated follicle composed almost entirely of centrocytes. Centrocytes are scattered outside the follicle as well. **D:** The atypical cells are CD20+ and present primarily in a follicular pattern. **E:** CD21 highlights small, tightly organized follicular dendritic cell meshworks. **F:** Atypical B cells are positive for bcl-6. In addition to numerous bcl-6+ B cells in follicles, there are many bcl-6+ cells outside follicles (*left* of image). **G:** Atypical B cells are negative for bcl-2. **H:** The proliferation index is low in this small atypical follicle. Although bcl-2 co-expression is not a feature of this case, a diagnosis of lymphoma can be made because of the atypical appearance of the follicles with a monotonous cellular composition, low proliferation index, and the presence of many bcl-6+ B cells outside follicles.

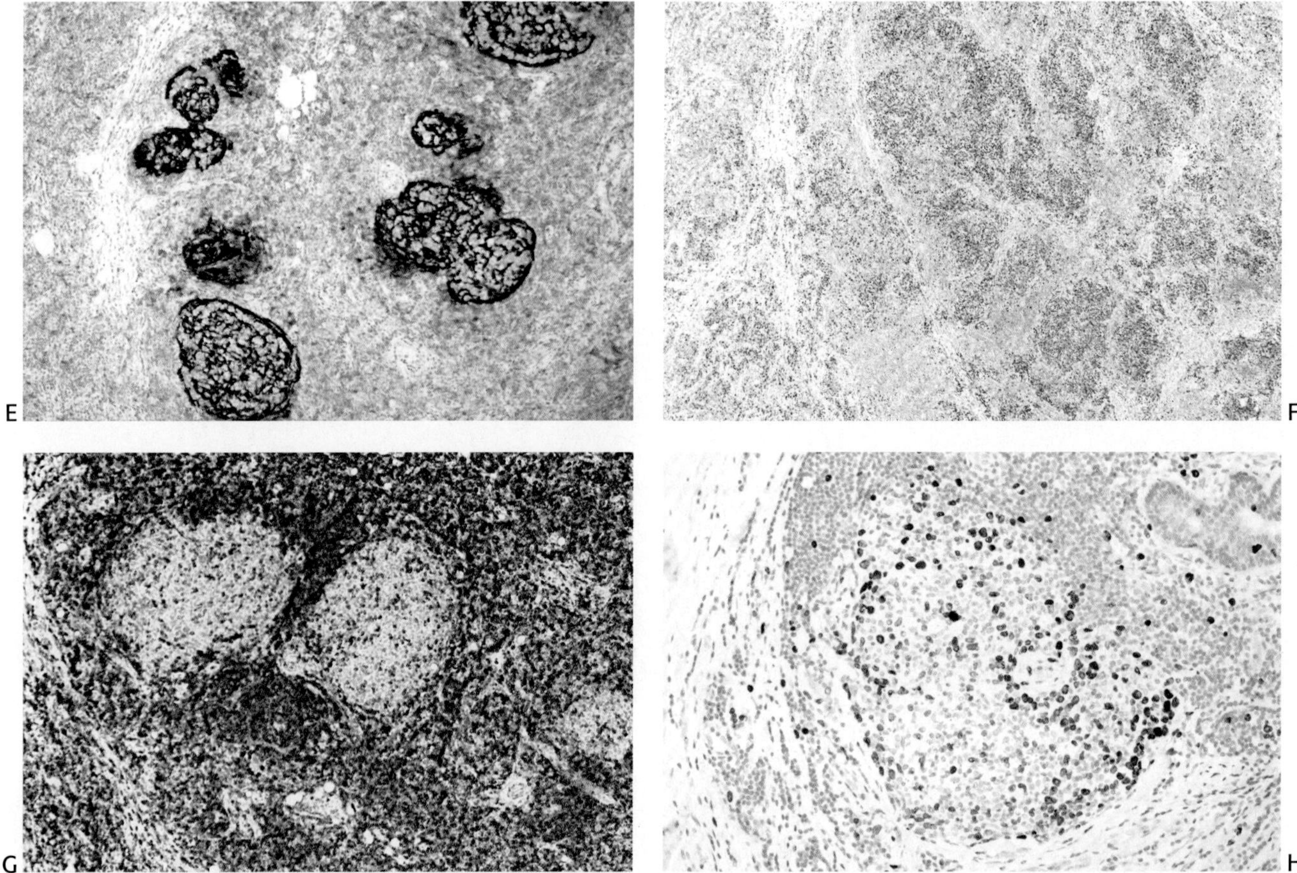

FIG. 40.5. *(Continued)*

Burkitt Lymphoma

Clinical Presentation

Burkitt lymphoma occurs in one of three clinical settings: endemic Burkitt lymphoma, occurring mainly in equatorial Africa, where malaria is endemic; sporadic Burkitt lymphoma, occurring worldwide in individuals without immunodeficiency; and immunodeficiency-associated Burkitt lymphoma, occurring in immunodeficient individuals. The most common cause of immunodeficiency in the third scenario is HIV infection.[44] The breast can be affected in any of these clinical settings.

Burkitt lymphoma mainly affects young to middle-aged females[6,19,20,45]; some have been pregnant or are postpartum at the time of diagnosis.[6,19,20] Cases of endemic Burkitt lymphoma resulting in marked, bilateral mammary enlargement in African women who were sometimes pregnant or lactating were recognized by Burkitt.[46] Premenarchal girls are uncommonly affected.[47] Burkitt lymphoma is a highly proliferative, aggressive neoplasm, but with optimal treatment that consists of aggressive combination chemotherapy, the prognosis is now more favorable.

Pathology

Burkitt lymphoma is typically composed of a dense, diffuse proliferation of uniform, medium-sized cells with round nuclei, clumped chromatin, several nucleoli, and a scant to moderate amount of cytoplasm that is deeply basophilic on Giemsa staining. The lymphoma is highly cellular with minimal intervening stroma. The mitotic rate is very high, and there is abundant apoptotic debris related to rapid turnover of neoplastic cells. Burkitt lymphoma has many interspersed pale tingible body macrophages containing apoptotic debris in a background of deep blue neoplastic cells, creating the characteristic starry sky pattern (Table 40.1, Fig. 40.6).[44]

Burkitt lymphoma also has a characteristic immunophenotype. The neoplastic cells are almost always CD20+, CD10+, bcl-6+, bcl-2−, monotypic surface immunoglobulin (IgM)+, with virtually all cells positive for Ki67 (proliferation). As for other types of lymphoma, successful demonstration of surface immunoglobulin usually requires fresh tissue for flow cytometry. The underlying genetic event is a translocation involving *MYC* on chromosome 8 and *IGH* on chromosome 14. In a minority of cases the rearrangement involves *MYC* and the gene for κ or λ immunoglobulin light chain rather than the immunoglobulin heavy-chain (*IGH*) gene. The neoplastic cells almost always harbor EBV in endemic Burkitt lymphoma; sporadic and immunodeficiency-associated Burkitt lymphoma are each EBV-associated, with EBV present in about one-third of the cases.[44]

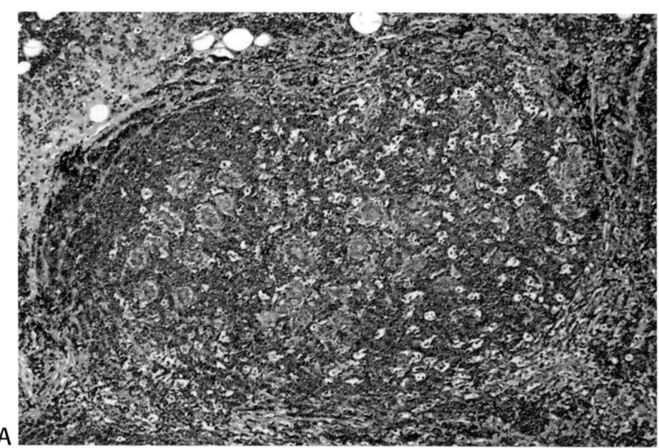

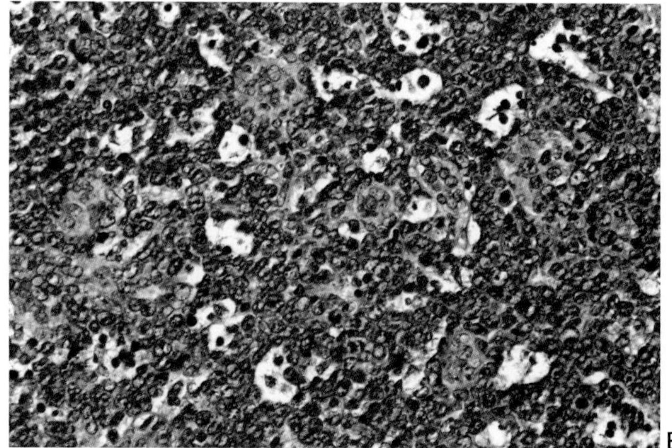

FIG. 40.6. ***Burkitt lymphoma, with bilateral breast involvement in a young woman.*** **A:** A lobule is surrounded and infiltrated by deeply basophilic, atypical lymphoid cells, with scattered tingible body macrophages creating a "starry sky" pattern. **B:** High magnification shows numerous medium-sized lymphoid cells with occasional distinct nucleoli, as well as scattered tingible body macrophages.

T-Cell Lymphomas

Primary breast lymphoma of T lineage is very uncommon, accounting for only about 2% to 3% of cases.[2,6,18] As for most other breast lymphomas, patients typically present with a unilateral mass. Bilateral disease is uncommon initially. Some are ALK-negative anaplastic large cell lymphomas (ALK– ALCLs) arising in association with breast implants (see section Lymphoma of the Breast in Association with Implants). Others include ALK+ ALCL, peripheral T-cell lymphoma, not otherwise specified, including CD4+ and CD8+ cases, and T-lymphoblastic lymphoma.[2,6,24,48–51] Despite aggressive therapy in at least some cases, the lymphomas often disseminate and result in death. Based on the small number of cases, the prognosis appears poor, with behavior that is overall more aggressive than B-cell lymphomas in this site. An exception to this are the ALCLs that arise in association with implants, which have a relatively good prognosis (see below). T-cell lymphomas involving the breast in the setting of widespread disease are more common than primary T-cell breast lymphomas.[52]

Anaplastic Large Cell Lymphoma

Clinical Presentation

Most ALCLs arising in the breast are associated with implants and they are almost always ALK– (discussed in more detail in a later section, Lymphoma of the Breast in Association with Implants). Rare cases of ALK+ ALCL involving the breast in teenage girls and young adult women, and in one case in an adult male, unassociated with implants have been reported.[49,51–54] In these cases, when staging information was available, one patient had disease confined to the breast,[52] while other patients had concurrent ALN involvement,[53] or widespread disease, at presentation and in one case at the time of relapse.[54] In cases with follow-up, patients have died of lymphoma or were alive with lymphoma.[49,53–54] One case of ALK+ ALCL that was initially misinterpreted as adenocarcinoma on the basis of a fine-needle aspiration (FNA) cytology specimen has been described, with no follow-up reported.[55]

ALCL, ALK–, has also presented with breast involvement in rare instances unassociated with implants.[53] Breast involvement by ALCL representing spread from primary cutaneous ALCL has also been reported.[54]

Pathology

The term "anaplastic large cell lymphoma" encompasses three distinct forms of T-cell lymphoma: ALCL, ALK+; ALCL, ALK–; and primary cutaneous ALCL, each with distinct clinical features.[56–58] ALCL, ALK–, arising in association with implants has features distinct from the usual systemic ALCL, ALK–. The microscopic features of the types of ALCL overlap, and it may be difficult to distinguish them without judicious immunophenotyping and careful clinical correlation. ALCL is typically composed of a diffuse proliferation of large atypical lymphoid cells with oval, irregular, bean-shaped, or donut-shaped nuclei, smooth to vesicular chromatin, small nucleoli, and moderately abundant pink cytoplasm. Because of the abundant cytoplasm, neoplastic cells sometimes appear cohesive. "Hallmark cells" with indented nuclei and a small rounded paranuclear eosinophilic zone can usually be identified. The neoplastic cells are CD30+ often with loss of multiple pan–T-cell antigens. By definition, ALCL, ALK+, is associated with the expression of ALK protein, with staining most often in a nuclear and cytoplasmic pattern. ALCL, ALK+, and ALCL, ALK–, are often epithelial membrane antigen + (EMA+), while primary cutaneous ALCL is typically EMA–.

ALCLs are more likely than other types of lymphoma to be mistaken for nonlymphoid neoplasms because of their relatively abundant cytoplasm and apparent cohesive growth. Carcinoma, melanoma, and histiocytic neoplasms can be considered in the differential diagnosis. Immunophenotyping establishes a diagnosis.

Subcutaneous Panniculitis-Like T-Cell Lymphoma

Rare cases of subcutaneous panniculitis-like T-cell lymphoma involving the breast and forming a breast mass have been reported.[30,52] Patients may have involvement of subcutaneous tissue in other sites in addition to breast involvement.[59] This type of lymphoma is characterized by an interstitial and diffuse proliferation of atypical lymphoid cells, usually with dark, irregular nuclei and a scant to moderate quantity of pale cytoplasm in fat, with sparing of the epidermis and dermis. The neoplastic cells often show "rimming" of individual fat cells. Interspersed apoptotic debris may be abundant (Fig. 40.7). Immunostains typically reveal the following results: TCRαβ+, CD3+, CD4–, CD8+, CD56–, cytotoxic granule protein (granzyme B and/or perforin)+, TdT–. There is clonal rearrangement of T-cell receptor (TCR) genes. The prognosis is fairly good, with an estimated 5-year survival of 80%,[60] although in one reported case the patient died of lymphoma.[52]

The differential diagnosis includes other T-cell lymphomas, especially primary cutaneous γδ T-cell lymphoma, and panniculitis, especially lupus profundus. Primary cutaneous γδ T-cell lymphoma is a more aggressive lymphoma with a poor prognosis, with some histologic and immunophenotypic overlap with subcutaneous panniculitis-like T-cell lymphoma. In contrast to subcutaneous panniculitis-like T-cell lymphoma, primary cutaneous γδ T-cell lymphoma may involve the epidermis and/or dermis as well as the subcutaneous fat. The neoplastic cells are γδ T cells that are characteristically TCRγδ+, and typically CD3+, CD5–, CD4–, CD8–, CD56+, and cytotoxic granule protein+.

Panniculitides show prominent subcutaneous tissue involvement, but lack significant cytologic atypia, an atypical immunophenotype, and clonal *TCR* gene rearrangement. Lupus profundus often has a lobular pattern of involvement with preservation of septae, areas of hyalinization or fibrinoid change of stroma, inconspicuous rimming of fat cells by lymphoid cells, and an admixture of B cells, sometimes with lymphoid follicles, plasma cells, and CD4+ and CD8+ T cells. On the other hand, there is a marked CD8+ T-cell preponderance in subcutaneous panniculitis-like T-cell lymphoma.

Lymphoblastic Leukemia/Lymphoma

Lymphoblastic leukemia/lymphoma rarely involves the breast. Patients are mostly adolescents and young adults. Breast involvement by a lymphoblastic neoplasm may occur at the time of initial diagnosis or in the form of a relapse after therapy. Frequently, other sites are involved by acute

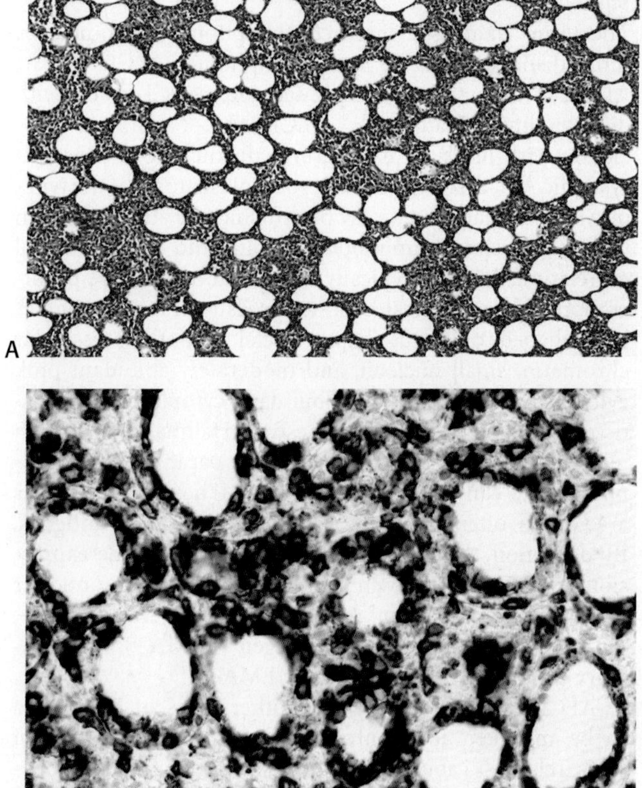

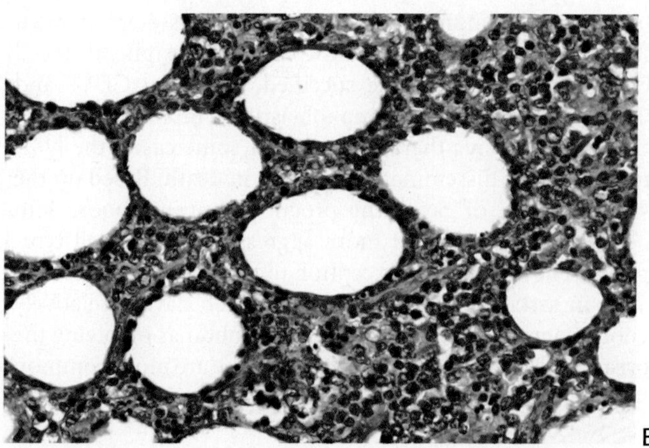

FIG. 40.7. ***Subcutaneous panniculitis-like T-cell lymphoma, presenting as a breast mass.*** **A:** Low magnification shows a prominent interstitial infiltrate of dark lymphoid cells. **B:** Higher magnification shows atypical, medium-sized, dark lymphoid cells with rimming of fat cells, with interspersed apoptotic debris. **C:** Antibody to CD8 highlights the atypical cells, with prominent rimming of fat cells (immunoperoxidase technique on paraffin sections).

lymphoblastic leukemia concurrent with breast involvement. The sites most commonly involved include the bone marrow, CNS, lymph nodes, female genital tract, and skin and subcutaneous tissue[61]; disease may be widespread at the time of breast involvement (see also the section Secondary Lymphomas of the Breast)[52] Examples of both B- and T-lineage lymphoblastic leukemia involving the breast have been documented (Table 40.1).[52,61] Many cases in the older literature predate the era of immunophenotyping.[61] Rare cases of B-lymphoblastic leukemia associated with t(9;22) (BCR/ABL) and t(4;11) involving the *MLL* gene have been reported.[61] Rarely, B-lymphoblastic lymphoma[2] presents with localized involvement of the breast.[2]

Hodgkin Lymphoma

Rare cases of classical Hodgkin lymphoma (CHL), most often nodular sclerosis CHL, have involved the breast at the time of presentation.[2] In one such case the lymphoma likely arose in an intramammary lymph node rather than as an extranodal primary.[62] Breast involvement at the time of relapse has also been reported.[2,62–64] Typically, Hodgkin lymphoma involves the breast in the setting of concurrent lymph node involvement, and sometimes widespread disease (Table 40.1). Relapse in the form of isolated breast involvement is very rare, but has been described.[64]

Breast involvement is usually unilateral, but occasionally bilateral.[63] As in other sites, Hodgkin lymphoma in the breast takes the form of a mixed infiltrate of reactive cells in varying proportions (lymphocytes, histiocytes, eosinophils, plasma cells, and/or neutrophils) with scattered large atypical uninucleated, binucleated, or multinucleated Reed–Sternberg cells and variants with large oval or irregular nuclei, inclusion-like reddish nucleoli, paranucleolar haloes, and scant to moderate quantity of pale cytoplasm (Fig. 40.8). The neoplastic cells typically are CD15+, CD30+, PAX5 dim+, CD20−, CD3−, and ALK1−. Because of the rarity of Hodgkin lymphoma involving the breast, the diagnosis should be made with extreme caution, particularly in the absence of concurrent lymph nodal involvement by Hodgkin lymphoma, or in the absence of a history of Hodgkin lymphoma.

Lymphoma of the Breast in Association with Implants

Clinical Presentation

Lymphoma has rarely arisen adjacent to breast implants used for both cosmetic purposes and reconstruction after mastectomy for carcinoma (Table 40.1).[30,52,54,65–67] Such lymphomas account for only a small proportion of all lymphomas of the breast. Only 2% of cases in each of two large series of lymphoma involving the breast arose in association with an implant.[2,30]

Determining the relative risk of lymphoma in association with breast implants is difficult. The number of cases may be underestimated if protocols for examining capsulectomy specimens require few sections be taken for microscopic examination so that abnormal areas are not sampled, or if the pathologist overlooks the abnormal lymphoid infiltrate that may be focal, subtle, or masked by nonspecific inflammation. Despite the distinctive clinical and pathologic features of lymphoma in this setting, there is no convincing evidence of an increased risk of NHL overall in association with breast implants in large epidemiologic studies.[68] In one study the risk of developing an implant-associated ALCL was estimated to be 0.1 to 0.3 per 100,000 individuals per year, with an odds ratio of 18.2 for developing implant-associated ALCL.[45] Thus there may be a slightly increased risk of developing ALCL, ALK−, in the breast in women with implants, but the risk is very low.

Affected patients are adults, with a broad age range. The implants have been of saline and silicone types. However, saline-containing implants typically have a silicone capsule, leading some to speculate about a role for silicone in the pathogenesis of lymphoma through an immunologic mechanism.[65–66,69–72] The interval from insertion of the implant to diagnosis of lymphoma has ranged from 3 to 32 years, with a median ranging from 7 to 11 years in larger series.[30,45,51,65,73–80]

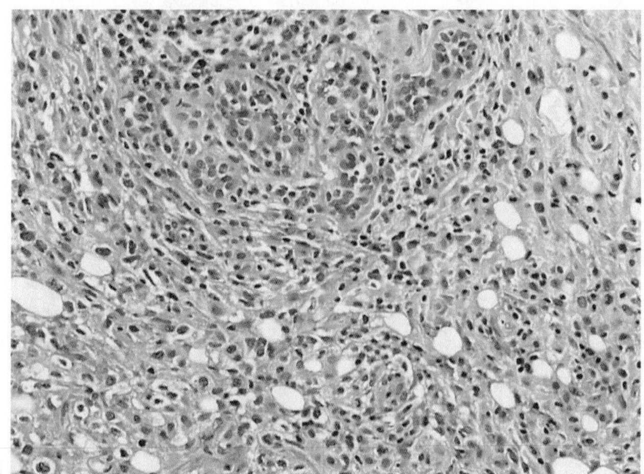
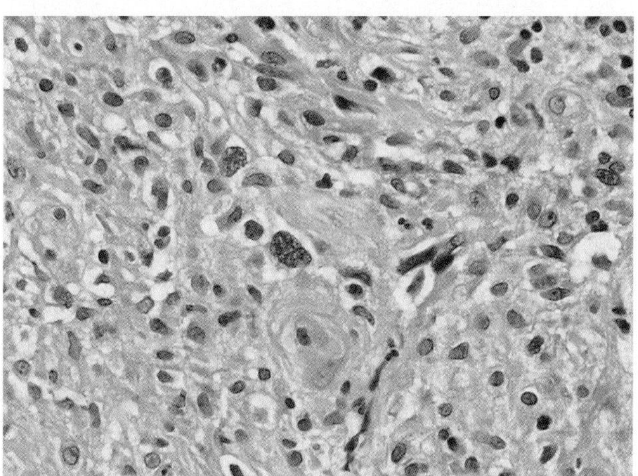

FIG. 40.8. ***Hodgkin lymphoma.*** **A,B:** Breast involvement in a patient with a diagnosis previously established in a cervical lymph node.

Surprisingly, in contrast to the marked preponderance of B-cell lymphomas among breast lymphomas, the vast majority of lymphomas arising in patients with implants have been ALK− ALCLs. In general, these patients have no history of lymphoma, although rare instances of implant-associated ALCL arising in the setting of prior CD30+ cutaneous lymphoproliferative disorders have been reported.[73] Patients with ALCL typically present with swelling related to a fluid collection between the implant and the fibrous capsule surrounding the implant. This is sometimes accompanied by tenderness or pain, and by erythema, warmth, or ulceration of the overlying skin, but a discrete mass is typically abs ent.[30,54,65–67,73–78,80] The presentation can mimic mastitis.[52] In some instances patients present with capsular contracture, which may or may not be accompanied by a fluid collection.[81] Capsular contracture occurring years after the original surgery, or requiring multiple revisions, should be viewed with suspicion and investigated to exclude neoplasia.[81] Patients usually present with localized disease,[65,66,76] although in occasional cases there has been spread to ALNs[45,73] or more widespread disease[45] by the time of presentation.

Pathology

Microscopic examination reveals large, atypical, pleomorphic, mitotically active cells with oval or irregular nuclei, prominent nucleoli, and moderately abundant cytoplasm, often accompanied by a mixed inflammatory infiltrate composed of lymphocytes, plasma cells, histiocytes, and sometimes eosinophils, neutrophils, and giant cells. The neoplastic cells typically form a thin, discontinuous layer along the inner aspect of the fibrous capsule, sometimes with foci of more abundant tumor cells, in a background of necrotic debris or fibrinoid material.[66] The neoplastic cells may become entrapped within the fibrous capsule,[67,74,78] but typically they do not invade through the fibrous capsule, and do not actually come into direct contact with breast parenchyma.[73] A cell block prepared from the fluid is very useful for visualizing the abnormal cellular population. Cytologic examination of fluid from the seroma may reveal large numbers of neoplastic cells. Refractile silicone may be identified adjacent to the infiltrate,[52,78] although some cases have no evidence of damage to the prosthesis in the form of leakage of silicone (Fig. 40.9).

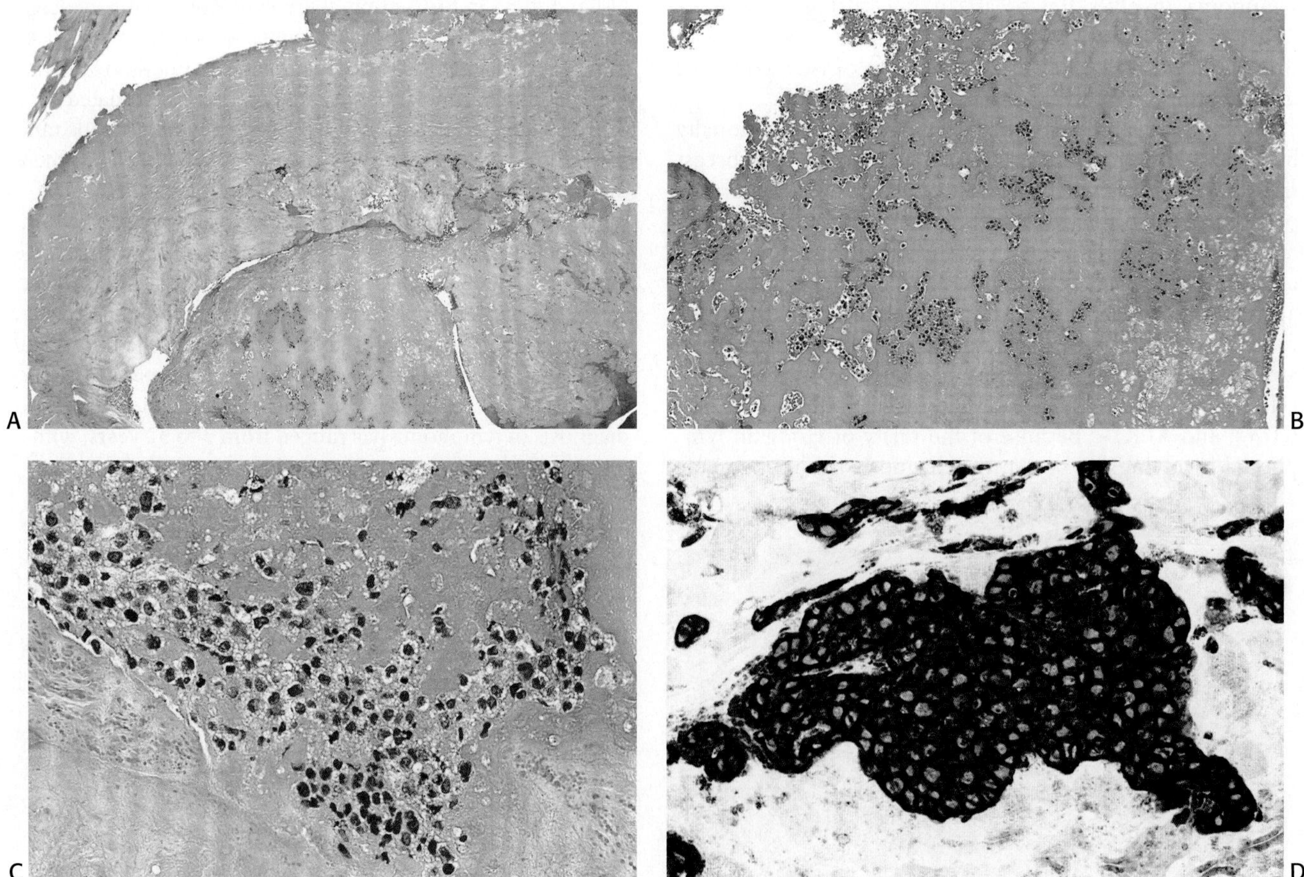

FIG. 40.9. ***Anaplastic large cell lymphoma, ALK−, arising in association with a breast implant.*** **A:** Low power shows a hypocellular fibrous pseudocapsule (*top* of image) overlying an area with hyaline material in which there are a few clusters of cells. **B:** Clusters of atypical cells are scattered in a background of hyalinized collagen and amorphous debris. **C:** High magnification shows large atypical cells with oval and irregular nuclei in a background of debris. **D:** The large atypical cells are intensely positive for CD30 (immunoperoxidase technique on a paraffin section).

In a minority of cases there is deviation from this classic scenario. In these cases patients have a discrete mass in addition to an effusion, and the mass may penetrate the capsule and involve breast tissue.[51,73] In one case the patient had a mass adjacent to her implant unassociated with an effusion. The mass was excised, which recurred later with an associated effusion. In one case the patient presented with a painful mass and constitutional symptoms.[79] Involvement has generally been unilateral, but a case with bilateral, metachronous involvement of breasts with implants by lymphoma has been reported.[79] The size of the masses has only occasionally been given, but it has been described as relatively small (1 to 2.5 cm).[73]

The ALCLs have been CD30+, ALK−, CD45+/−, except for a single case of ALK+ ALCL that arose adjacent to an implant.[51] T-cell antigens are variably expressed, almost always with loss of one or more pan-T-cell antigens. CD4 and CD43 are usually positive, while CD3, CD5, CD7, and CD8 are often negative. Expression of EMA is common. Rare CD15+ cases are reported. Cytotoxic granule proteins such as TIA1 and granzyme B are often expressed. EBV and human herpes virus 8 (HHV8) are absent.[54,65–67,73–75,77–80] Keratin and melanoma-associated markers are not expressed. The proliferation index is high (90% in one case).[79] Clonal rearrangement of the TCR γ chain gene can usually be demonstrated, while clonal B cells are not found.[65,66,73,75,78]

Treatment has varied, but has usually included removal of the implant with or without additional therapy that may include combination chemotherapy, radiation, or both, or, in a few instances of aggressive disease, stem cell or bone marrow transplantation.[51,65,73,75,76,78–80] Follow-up is uneventful in most cases.[65,76–78] Patients presenting with the classical picture—ALCL, ALK− associated with an effusion without a discrete mass, and with localized disease, without a history of lymphoma—appear to have an excellent prognosis. It is possible that excision of the implant and capsulectomy, with close follow-up to monitor for recurrence, would constitute sufficient therapy for these patients. In a few cases, however, there have been local recurrences[51,73] or progression to systemic involvement,[51,75,80] sometimes resulting in the death of the patient.[73,79] Patients with more aggressive disease appear to correspond to those who present with a discrete mass, or who present with spread beyond the breast, and these patients likely require aggressive therapy. One patient presenting with constitutional symptoms died of lymphoma,[79] and hence systemic symptoms may represent an additional predictor of poor outcome. A single case of ALK+ ALCL arising adjacent to an implant relapsed with widespread disease after being treated with combination chemotherapy. The patient eventually achieved a sustained complete remission after additional chemotherapy and stem cell transplant.[51] It is difficult to draw definite conclusions because the number of cases is small and patients have not been treated uniformly.

Some investigators have suggested that ALCL in this setting is reminiscent of primary cutaneous ALCL rather than ALK− ALCL of systemic type, which is an aggressive lymphoma with a poor prognosis.[65] In contrast to most primary cutaneous ALCLs, however, these lymphomas have often been EMA+. Primary cutaneous ALCL secondarily involving the breast in association with an implant has also been described.[54]

Establishing a diagnosis may be problematic. The manner of presentation can lead to a clinical impression of inflammation, infection, or leaking implant. The associated inflammation may obscure the neoplastic population. The neoplastic lymphoid cells may be mistaken for carcinoma, particularly in women previously treated for breast carcinoma. Familiarity with the rare occurrence of ALCL arising in association with a breast implant will assist the pathologist in establishing a diagnosis.

Other types of lymphoma rarely involve the breast in association with an implant. In one remarkable case, a 46-year-old woman developed a HHV8+ primary effusion lymphoma in an artificial cavity adjacent to the capsule of a silicone breast implant. The lymphoma had anaplastic cytologic features, expressed CD30, CD45, and CD43, lacked other B- and T-cell-associated markers, and showed clonal rearrangement of the *IGH* gene.[82] Four cases of mycosis fungoides/Sézary syndrome (beginning in three cases in the skin overlying the implant)[70,72] and one case each of FL,[69] lymphoplasmacytic lymphoma,[71] and extranodal natural killer (NK)/T-cell lymphoma, nasal type (EBV+),[83] have affected patients with breast implants. The two B-cell lymphomas were widespread at presentation and likely did not represent primary breast lymphomas.[69,71]

Differential Diagnosis of Mammary Lymphoma

The diagnosis of lymphoma of the breast is almost never suspected preoperatively. The clinical impression is typically carcinoma, but may also be fibroadenoma (FA) or phyllodes tumor.[29] Selected problems in differential diagnosis are discussed above in regard to certain lymphoma subtypes. More general issues are discussed in this section.

On average, lymphoma forms a larger mass than carcinoma, with a mean or median diameter of about 4 cm.[3,31] Occasionally, lymphomas can present with a clinical picture that mimics inflammatory carcinoma[84] or mastitis.[85,86]

A number of problems in the differential diagnosis of lymphoma of the breast may arise, particularly when the specimen submitted is small or a diagnosis is requested on a frozen section (FS).

Extranodal Versus Lymph Nodal Lymphoma

Differentiating lymphoma in a low axillary or intramammary lymph node from lymphoma involving the breast parenchyma itself is important, as the frequencies of the various types of lymphoma involving the breast parenchyma and lymph nodes differ. The distinction may be difficult, particularly if the biopsy specimen is small. Identifying a discrete capsule, patent sinuses, or areas of residual uninvolved lymph node confirms lymph nodal involvement, while finding the lymphoid infiltrate in continuity with ducts or lobules indicates breast parenchymal involvement.

High-Grade Lymphomas Versus Carcinoma

Differentiating lymphoma from carcinoma may be difficult, especially in cases of invasive lobular carcinoma (ILC) with dyscohesive cells with a linear growth pattern,[17] since lymphoma can occasionally mimic this arrangement. In some instances, mastectomy and ALN dissection have been performed because of a mistaken diagnosis of carcinoma.[25] Careful study of the histologic features should raise the consideration of lymphoma. The presence of cohesive growth or lumen formation by the tumor, and the presence of ductal carcinoma *in situ* (DCIS) or lobular carcinoma *in situ* (LCIS) favor a diagnosis of carcinoma. A basic panel of immunostains, with antibodies to cytokeratin (CK) and B- and T-cell–associated markers, should establish the diagnosis.

Lymphoepithelioma-Like Carcinoma and Medullary Carcinoma Versus Lymphoma

Lymphoepithelioma-like carcinoma and medullary carcinoma of the breast are associated with a dense lymphoid infiltrate. In this setting neoplastic cells may be obscured by the lymphoid infiltrate or mistaken for large lymphoid cells. Lymphoepithelioma-like carcinoma produces an ill-defined mass with infiltrative borders. Neoplastic cells may be present singly, or in cords, nests, or sheets associated with a dense lymphoid infiltrate that can contain reactive follicles.[87] Medullary carcinoma takes the form of a well-circumscribed mass containing neoplastic epithelial cells with high nuclear grade and numerous mitoses, growing in a syncytial pattern in a background of numerous lymphoid cells.[29] Atypical lobular hyperplasia and LCIS have been reported in association with lymphoepithelioma-like carcinoma, and the presence of atypical epithelium in lobules may provide a clue to the diagnosis of carcinoma rather than lymphoma.[87] Immunostains for CK and lymphoid-associated antigens will delineate reactive and neoplastic components in cases of carcinoma.[87]

Low-Grade Lymphomas Versus Chronic Inflammatory, Reactive Lymphoid Infiltrates

Dense reactive lymphoid infiltrates potentially mimicking lymphoma are unusual in the breast. One condition that may cause difficulty in differential diagnosis is diabetic mastopathy. This is an uncommon, reactive, fibroinflammatory process mainly encountered in women, but also occasionally in men, who typically have long-standing type 1 diabetes mellitus. A few patients have had type 2 diabetes mellitus.

Similar lesions occur in patients with various immunologic disorders or in those who are otherwise well. In these instances, the condition may be referred to as autoimmune mastopathy or lymphocytic mastitis. Diabetic mastopathy, or lymphocytic mastitis, usually presents as unilateral or less often as bilateral palpable breast mass(es) in young or middle-aged women, although older women may be affected.[88–90] Recurrences occur in some patients and may be unilateral or bilateral.[88] Microscopic examination reveals a perilobular and/or periductal infiltrate of small lymphocytes and a variable number of plasma cells. The infiltrate may also be perivascular and may invade small blood vessels. Reactive lymphoid follicles may be present. Some cases also show lobular atrophy and dense, keloidal fibrosis, in some cases with reactive epithelioid fibroblasts. Immunophenotyping reveals that lymphocytes are predominantly B cells with varying numbers of T cells. LELs composed of B cells are found in some cases. No clonal B-cell population is identified using immunophenotyping or polymerase chain reaction.[89,90] The tight perilobular or periductal distribution, lack of cytologic atypia, lack of clonal B cells, and the characteristic sclerosis help to distinguish this disorder from lymphoma (Fig. 40.10).

In the differential diagnosis between MALT lymphoma and chronic inflammation, findings favoring lymphoma are the presence of large numbers of B cells outside follicles with the morphology of marginal zone cells, and monotypic immunoglobulin expression by the lymphoid cells or by

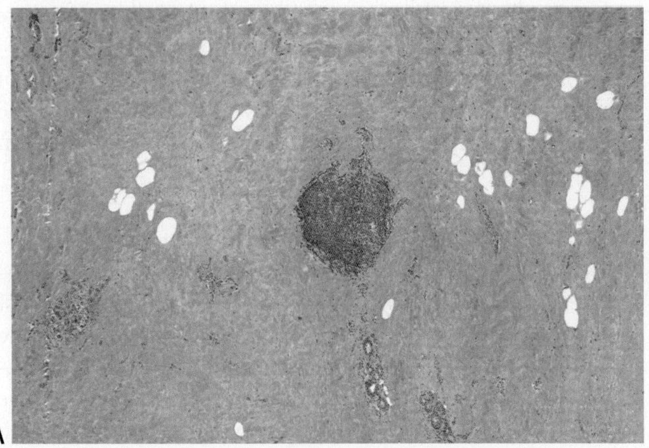

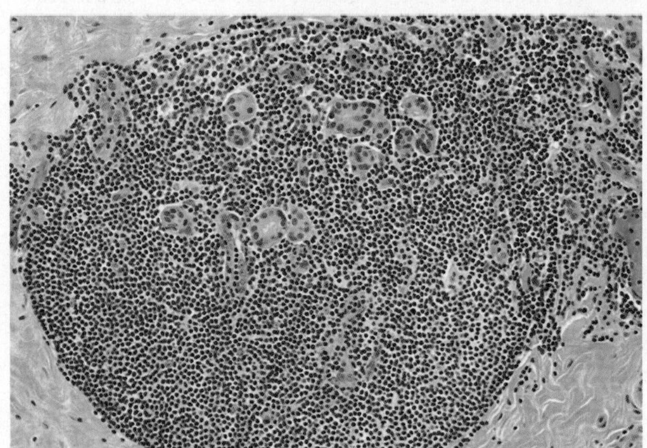

FIG. 40.10. ***Diabetic mastopathy*** **A:** A tight perilobular aggregate of lymphoid cells is present in a background of collagenized fibrous tissue. **B:** Higher magnification shows a well-delineated aggregate of small, mature lymphocytes surrounding and infiltrating a lobule.

admixed plasma cells. In distinguishing follicular hyperplasia from FL, criteria similar to those used in lymph nodes can be utilized.

Secondary Lymphomas of the Breast

Clinical Presentation

Secondary lymphoma of the breast includes lymphoma relapsing in the breast or cases presenting with widespread disease including the breast, so that the breast is unlikely to be the primary site. Lymphoma is reported to be the most common type of neoplasm to involve the breast secondarily.[91] In a number of studies that have included any lymphoma involving the breast, there have been more secondary lymphomas than primary lymphomas,[2,6,12,92] suggesting that secondary involvement of the breast by lymphoma is more common than primary breast lymphoma. In common with primary lymphoma, most patients are women, but a few men are affected.[2,6,12,30,92] Patients often present with a mass,[30] although radiologic evaluation more often reveals multicentric disease in the breast,[2,22] with lesions that tend to be smaller than in cases of primary breast lymphoma.[22]

Pathology

The vast majority of cases are B-cell lymphomas of a variety of types. The most common are diffuse large B-cell lymphoma, FL, and MALT lymphoma.[2,6,12,14,30,92] Primary mediastinal large B-cell lymphoma presenting during pregnancy with a breast mass has been described (Fig. 40.11).[93] Less commonly, small lymphocytic lymphoma/chronic lymphocytic leukemia (SLL/CLL), mantle cell lymphoma, and B-lymphoblastic lymphoma involve the breast secondarily.[2,12,13,94] We have seen a case in which the breast was the site of Richter transformation in a patient with a history of chronic lymphocytic leukemia. The breast was involved by SLL/CLL in addition to diffuse large B-cell lymphoma. In another patient hairy cell leukemia spread to involve the

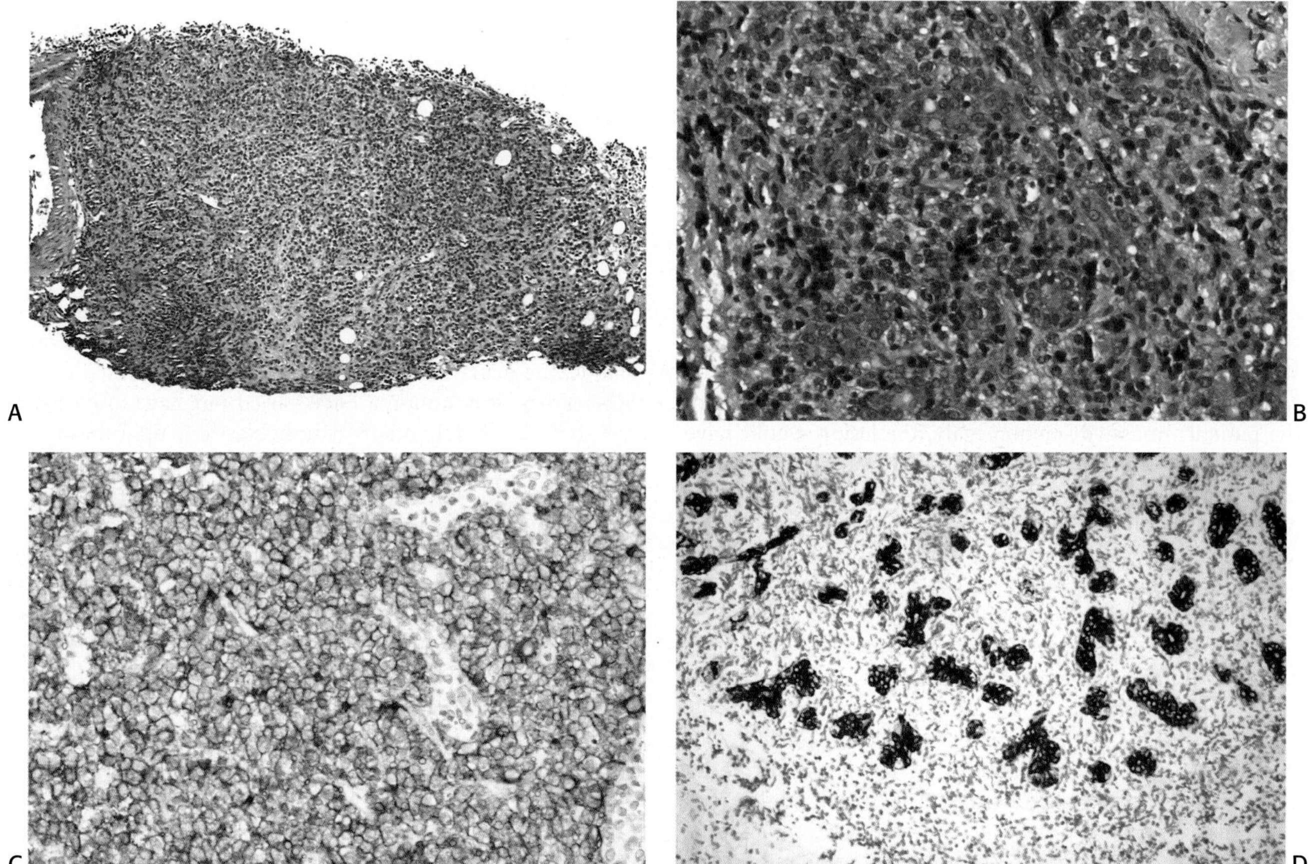

FIG. 40.11. ***Mediastinal large B-cell lymphoma presenting as a breast mass.*** **A:** Dense infiltrate of large atypical lymphoid cells invades a lobule in this core biopsy sample. **B:** The neoplastic lymphoid cells are only slightly larger than the epithelial cells of the lobule. **C:** Large lymphoid cells are diffusely positive for CD20. **D:** Residual lobular elements are positive for cytokeratin (**C** and **D**, immunoperoxidase technique on paraffin sections).

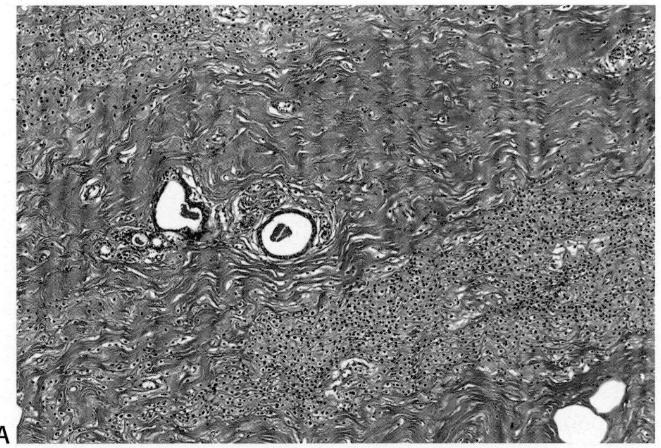

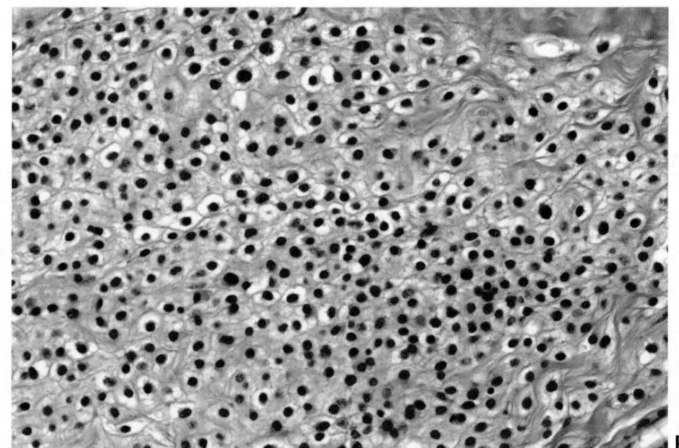

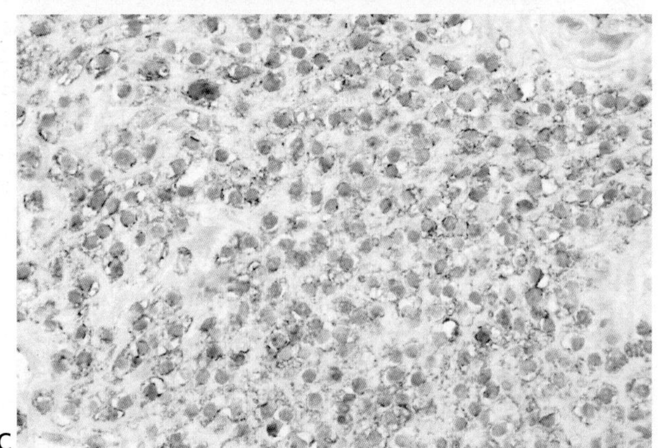

FIG. 40.12. *Hairy cell leukemia involving the breast.* **A:** Low magnification shows a monotonous population of mononuclear cells infiltrating breast parenchyma. **B:** Higher magnification shows medium-sized cells with oval nuclei, smooth dark chromatin, and abundant pale cytoplasm. The atypical cells have the "fried egg" appearance that is typical for hairy cell leukemia and may also be found in some mammary carcinomas. **C:** Neoplastic cells are CD20+ (immunoperoxidase technique on paraffin sections).

breast (Fig. 40.12). Without knowledge of the patient's history, the distinction from marginal zone lymphoma or even ILC would have been difficult.[67] When splenic marginal zone lymphoma involved the breast, without knowledge of the patient's massive splenomegaly, the lesion would have been virtually indistinguishable from extranodal marginal zone lymphoma (Fig. 40.13). A case of mantle cell lymphoma that was initially interpreted as probable diffuse large B-cell lymphoma on breast biopsy has been reported.[94] Staging revealed widespread disease, and additional evaluation confirmed a diagnosis of mantle cell lymphoma.

T-cell lymphomas secondarily involving the breast are rare, and are also of a variety of types. They include peripheral T-cell lymphomas[12,14,52,92] and T-lymphoblastic lymphoma.[2,95] ALK+, ALK− and primary cutaneous ALCLs involving the breast at relapse or in the setting of widespread disease have been described.[2,54] Cases of adult T-cell leukemia/lymphoma occurring in patients from an area endemic for HTLV1, and involving the breasts unilaterally and bilaterally, are reported.[30,52] We have encountered angioimmunoblastic T-cell lymphoma with breast involvement late in the course of the disease, occurring shortly before the patient died of lymphoma. A case of EBV+ NK cell lymphoma presenting with widespread disease, including breast involvement, has been reported[96] and CHL secondarily involving the breast[2] has been described.

The primary sites for the extranodal marginal zone lymphomas that spread to the breast tend to be the salivary glands, the ocular adnexa, or soft tissue.[12] Primary sites for other types of lymphoma have varied but have often been lymph nodal. Rarely, the B-lymphoblastic lymphomas have occurred in patients with chronic myelogenous leukemia who developed lymphoblastic blast crisis.[2]

The outcome for patients with secondary lymphoma of the breast tends to be worse overall than that for patients with primary breast lymphoma.[14] Extranodal marginal zone lymphoma patients, however, may have isolated relapses in the breast and in other extranodal sites, and still have a long survival.[12] Patients with marginal zone lymphoma with large cell transformation may succumb to the disease.[2]

Lymphoma in ALNs in Patients with Breast Cancer

Lymphomas of a wide variety of types can involve ALNs. Infrequently, lymphoma is discovered as an incidental finding in patients who have ALNs excised during evaluation and treatment of carcinoma of the breast. In general, the possibility of lymphoma in this setting may be considered if the lymph nodes are enlarged unrelated to the presence of metastatic carcinoma and if nodal architecture is distorted or obliterated by an atypical lymphoid proliferation. The most common lymphoid neoplasm to encounter as an incidental

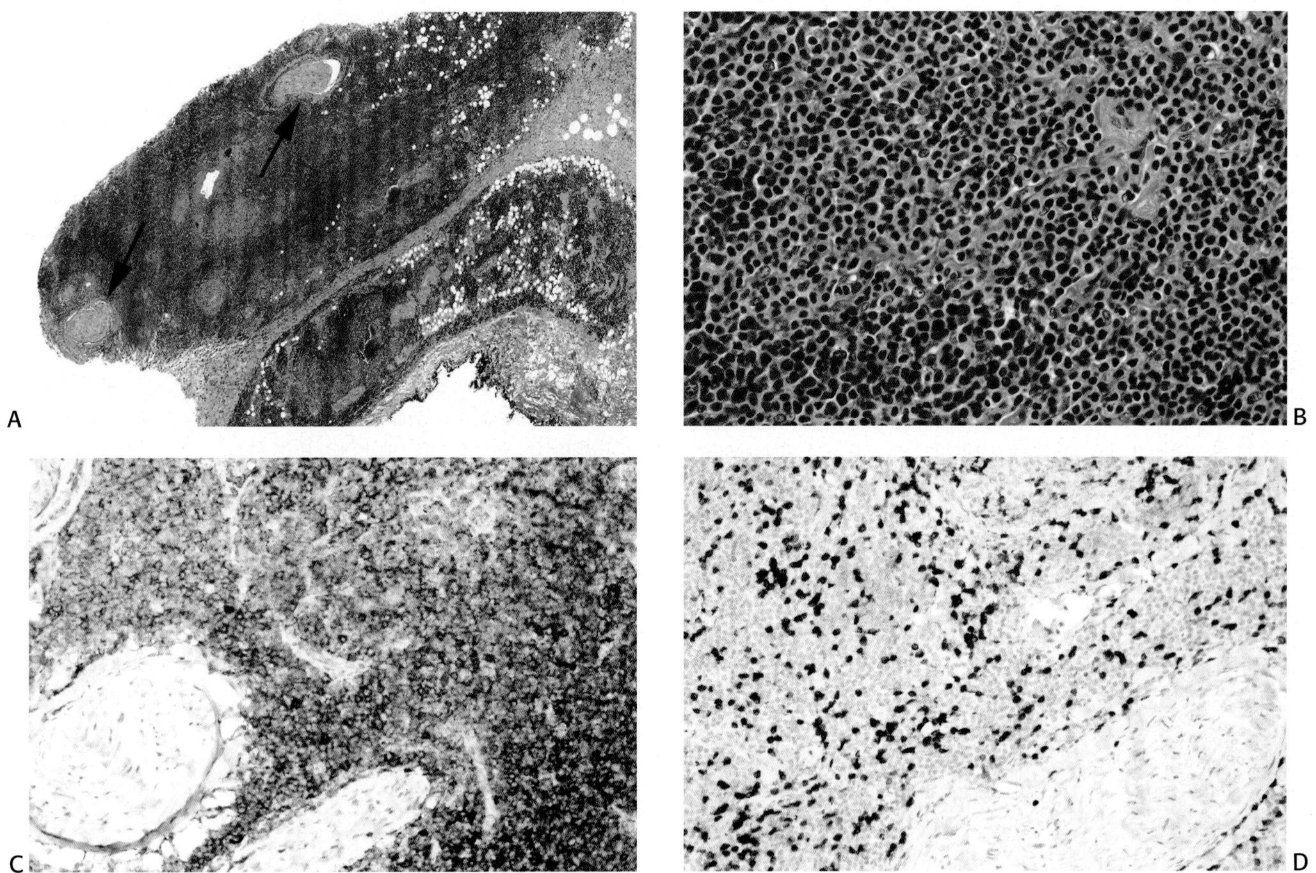

FIG. 40.13. ***Splenic marginal zone lymphoma involving the breast.*** **A:** The lymphoma takes the form of large nodules of lymphoid cells surrounding epithelial elements and nerves (*arrows*). **B:** The neoplastic cells are small and monotonous, with oval nuclei, dark chromatin, and scant pale cytoplasm. A few interspersed plasma cells are present. The slightly larger more irregular cells in the *left lower* corner of the image represent the remnants of a reactive germinal center. **C:** The lymphoma is composed of CD20+ B cells. **D:** A few nonneoplastic CD3+ T cells are admixed (**C** and **D**, immunoperoxidase technique on paraffin sections).

finding is most likely SLL/CLL. Involved lymph nodes typically show an expanded interfollicular area or diffuse obliteration of nodal architecture with a proliferation of small lymphocytes, sometimes with scattered, ill-defined proliferation centers (pseudofollicles) composed of medium-sized and occasional large cells. The neoplastic cells are CD20+ (sometimes dim), CD5+ (usually dimmer than admixed nonneoplastic T cells), CD10−, CD43+, and cyclin D1−. Patients often have lymphocytosis in the peripheral blood, so that correlation with laboratory studies may be helpful.

PLASMA CELL NEOPLASMS

Clinical Presentation

Breast involvement by plasma cell neoplasia is much less common than involvement by lymphoma. Plasmacytoma of the breast can develop very uncommonly in patients with plasma cell myeloma, and exceptionally as an isolated extramedullary plasmacytoma. Extramedullary neoplastic plasmacytic infiltrates can occur at many sites as part of disseminated multiple myeloma; the mammary gland infrequently appears among these sites. No breast infiltrates were found in two large autopsy studies of myeloma patients,[97,98] and only one patient had a breast lesion in a third series.[99]

Most reports of plasmacytoma of the breast described the occurrence in patients with an established diagnosis of plasma cell myeloma. These patients were mostly middle-aged and older adults who were almost all over 40 years. Most patients were women,[100–105] but myeloma with involvement of the male breast has been documented.[104] Patients present with painless or painful nodules within the breast. Usually the nodules are multiple and bilateral, but may be unilateral.[103]

Plasmacytoma of the breast rarely presents as an isolated initial manifestation of systemic disease. There are several reports of patients who each presented with a single unilateral breast tumor as the first manifestation of plasma cell myeloma.[106] One was a 50-year-old woman with a 2-cm right breast lesion who proved on clinical evaluation to have osseous and other soft tissue plasma infiltrates, amyloidosis, and plasma cell leukemia with IgGλ paraproteinemia. A second woman was 49 years old when she presented with a 2-cm plasmacytoma of the right breast. Work-up revealed IgGκ paraproteinemia and osseous lesions. A third patient was a 59-year-old woman who presented with a single 2-cm breast plasmacytoma; a staging marrow revealed plasma cell myeloma.[102]

Approximately 3% to 5% of plasma cell neoplasms are extraosseous (extramedullary) tumors unassociated with plasma cell myeloma, with the majority occurring in the upper respiratory tract.[107] Extraosseous plasmacytoma limited to the breast has been described in a very small number of cases. Innes and Newall[99] referred to a 43-year-old woman with bilateral breast lesions and no evidence of systemic involvement. Serum electrophoresis was not performed. Proctor et al.[108] described a 63-year-old woman with normal serum protein and immunoglobulin levels who remained disease-free 46 months after excision and local radiotherapy of a solitary right breast tumor. A 37-year-old woman with an isolated IgAκ+ plasmacytoma in the right breast, with no paraprotein, was well 15 months after surgical excision alone.[109] In one unique case a 27-year-old woman was found to have a 5-cm mass that was an infiltrating ductal carcinoma (IFDC) with an extramedullary plasmacytoma forming a portion of the lesion. This patient had no abnormal serum protein and no evidence of extramammary plasma cell neoplasia.[110]

Several women with apparently isolated mammary plasmacytomas have had abnormal serum proteins. In one case, a 70-year-old woman with a solitary tumor had mildly increased serum IgG and IgM levels but no monoclonal spike or urinary Bence Jones protein.[111] Nine years following a radical mastectomy, she remained well except for an excision of a nasal plasmacytic polyp 6 years after treatment of the breast tumor. Another patient was an 85-year-old woman with monoclonal kappa gammopathy, a 5-cm breast tumor, and no clinical evidence of lesions outside the breast.[112] A third patient was a 73-year-old woman with a single tumor and elevated serum IgG with a monoclonal lambda peak.[113] IgM and IgA levels were normal. Bone marrow aspiration revealed that "plasma cells were present but not conspicuously increased." Forty months after excision and local mammary radiation the patient remained well. In a fourth case, a 49-year-old woman presented with two tumors in the left breast measuring 3 and 4 cm, respectively.[114] IgD and λ were demonstrated in the tumor cells by immunohistochemistry (IHC), and the serum contained IgDλ monoclonal protein. The bone marrow contained only normal plasma cells. Two weeks after a mastectomy, a plasmacytoma of the nasal cavity was identified, and this regressed after combination chemotherapy. The patient reportedly had no evidence of myeloma 12 months later.

Mammography reveals a circumscribed mass that is hypoechoic and solid on sonography.[100,102,104,109] In some cases, mammography of patients with myeloma has disclosed a larger number of lesions than were appreciable on physical examination.

Gross Pathology

Solitary plasmacytomas of the breast have generally measured between 2 and 4 cm in diameter. Tumors less than 1 cm have been described in patients who have multiple lesions. The masses are typically well-circumscribed and tan or brown. Plasmacytomas that developed in patients with multiple myeloma were usually described as firm and rubbery, whereas solitary extramedullary tumors were typically soft or fleshy.[109]

Microscopic Pathology

The diagnosis has often been made on an incisional or excisional biopsy of the lesion, but some authors have reported making the diagnosis on FNA biopsy.[100,102,104] FNA is especially useful in patients already carrying an established diagnosis of plasma cell myeloma (Fig. 40.14). The histologic features of the breast lesions in systemic and solitary plasmacytomas are similar. They are composed of a variable admixture of mature plasma cells with clock-face chromatin and absent nucleoli, as well as enlarged, immature plasma cells, sometimes with distinct central nucleoli (Figs. 40.14 and 40.15). Mitoses, Russell bodies, nuclear pleomorphism, and bi- and multinucleated plasma cells may be seen. Mammary epithelial structures are largely effaced in the region where the plasma cell infiltrate is most concentrated. The neoplastic cells spread microscopically into the mammary parenchyma and fat beyond the grossly evident mass. Immunohistochemical analysis reveals plasma cells staining for CD138 and expressing monotypic immunoglobulin light chain that may be either κ or λ. Neoplastic plasma cells are negative for CK, but they may express EMA.

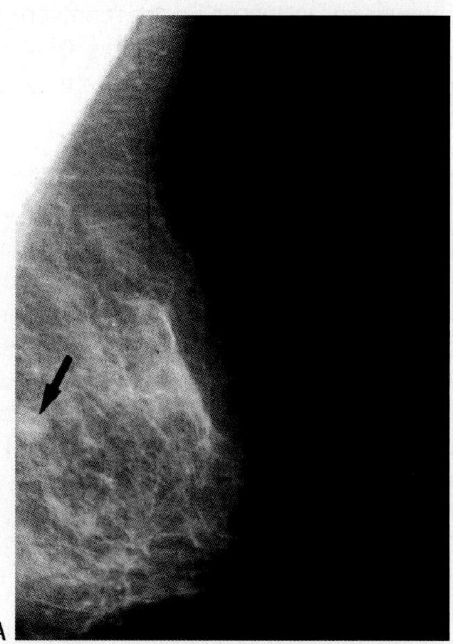

FIG. 40.14. ***Plasmacytoma of the breast in a patient with plasma cell myeloma.*** **A:** The mammogram of a breast of this 64-year-old woman with multiple myeloma revealed a discrete parenchymal nodule (*arrow*). **B,C:** The FNA smear revealed mature and immature plasma cells.

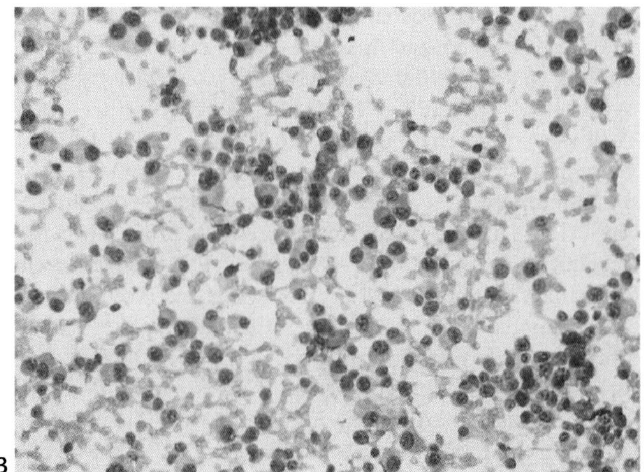

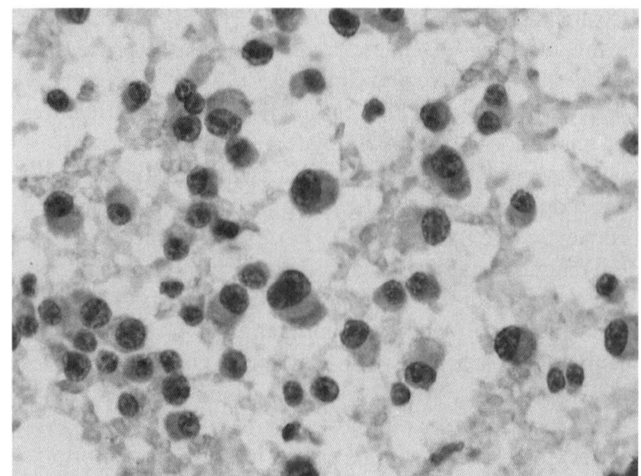

FIG. 40.14. *(Continued)*

Differential Diagnosis

Histologically, mammary plasmacytoma should be distinguished from plasma cell mastitis, amyloid tumor, MALT lymphoma with plasmacytic differentiation, and poorly differentiated carcinoma. Mass-forming lesions with a reactive lymphoplasmacytic infiltrate, previously classified as plasma cell granuloma or as pseudolymphoma, may also enter the differential diagnosis of plasmacytoma (see Chapter 3). If appropriate samples are available, immunohistochemical studies for immunoglobulin heavy and light chains may be

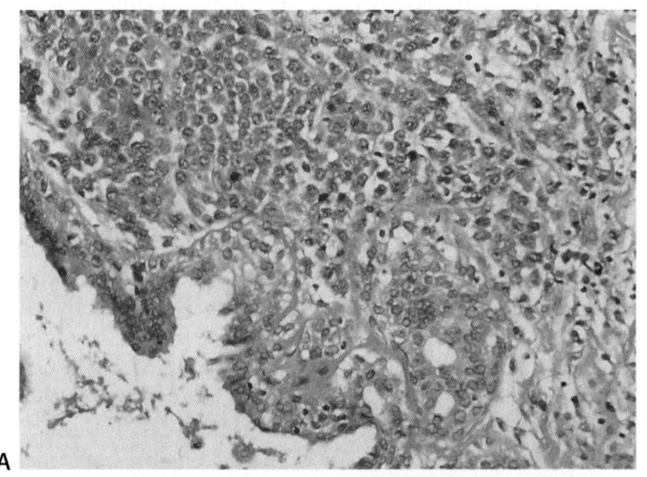

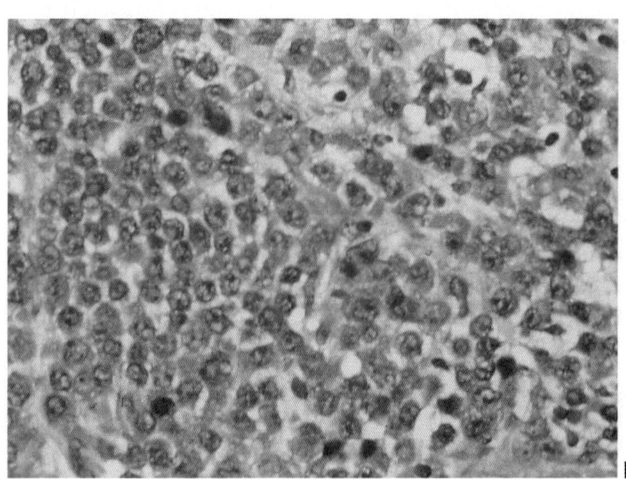

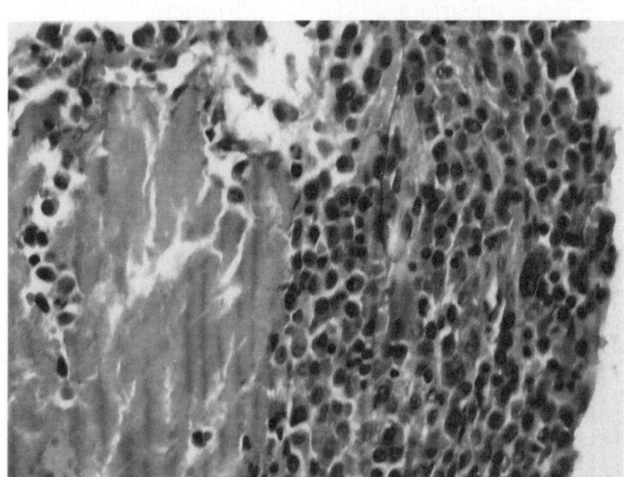

FIG. 40.15. ***Plasmacytoma of the breast in a patient with plasma cell myeloma.*** **A,B:** Immature plasma cells that formed a tumor in the breast of a 66-year-old woman. The tumor cells stained for lambda chains but not for kappa, and they were positive with methyl green pyronine. **C:** This biopsy of the bone marrow revealed mature and immature plasma cells.

performed on the tissue to determine whether the infiltrate has the monoclonal character of a neoplastic process or whether it is a reactive polyclonal lesion.

Plasma cell mastitis is a periductal process that features duct dilation, a mixed inflammatory infiltrate, and abscess formation (see Chapter 3). Mammary amyloid tumor is also discussed in Chapter 3. MALT lymphomas with prominent plasmacytic differentiation may be considered in the differential diagnosis of plasmacytoma. In favor of plasmacytoma is the presence of a pure population of monotypic plasma cells, while the presence of a population of B cells with the morphology of marginal zone cells and of lymphoid follicles favors lymphoma. MALT lymphoma is most often IgM+, whereas plasmacytoma is most often IgG+ or IgA+; IgM+ plasmacytoma is exceedingly rare. The somewhat monotonous, dyscohesive infiltrate of plasma cells can be mistaken for carcinoma, especially ILC, particularly on FS.[102,109]

Treatment and Prognosis

Following the histologic diagnosis of a plasmacytic tumor of the breast, the patient should be evaluated for evidence of systemic involvement. The prognosis and treatment will depend on the type and extent of the underlying disorder. Treatment may consist of excision and local radiation in patients who prove to have a lesion limited to the breast. The prognosis for patients with solitary mammary plasmacytoma appears to be excellent, but extended follow-up and study of more cases will be necessary to determine whether these patients are at risk to ultimately develop systemic disease. Among patients who develop plasmacytoma of the breast in the setting of an established diagnosis of myeloma, the prognosis is guarded. As these patients have often had plasma cell myeloma for a number of years and have often already been treated, the breast involvement typically represents relapsed or progressive disease, and the patients have often succumbed to complications of myeloma less than 1 year after the diagnosis of plasmacytoma of the breast.[100,102,104,105]

MYELOID SARCOMA OF THE BREAST

Myeloid sarcoma, previously called chloroma, granulocytic sarcoma, or extramedullary myeloid tumor, is a mass-forming neoplasm composed of myeloid blasts with or without maturation occurring at a site other than the bone marrow.[115,116] Myeloid sarcoma can occur in any of a wide variety of anatomic sites; myeloid sarcoma involving the breast is rare.

Clinical Presentation

Myeloid sarcoma of the breast can occur in one of several clinical scenarios. It can occur as an isolated finding in a patient with no history of a myeloid neoplasm; this accounts for a minority of cases.[117,118] It can occur in a patient with concurrent acute myeloid leukemia (AML) or concurrent myeloid sarcoma in other sites, or as a relapse of AML in a patient previously treated for AML.[61,118–121] Myeloid sarcoma may also arise in patients with other myeloid neoplasms such as myeloproliferative neoplasms or myelodysplastic syndrome.[118] When myeloid sarcomas occur in this setting, they may represent the first sign of progression to AML/blast crisis.

Whatever the clinical scenario, myeloid sarcoma of the breast has a marked female preponderance, with men accounting for only about 5% of cases.[61] Patients have a wide age range, although most are adolescents or young adults. An estimated 90% are younger than 50 years.[61] Patients present with a mass lesion or swelling of the breast unassociated with nipple discharge or retraction of the overlying skin. The lesions are usually unilateral, but bilateral mammary myeloid sarcoma has been described.[61,121] Most are in the range of 1 to 6 cm.[116–121] Concurrent ipsilateral ALN involvement is common.[61,118,121] Among patients with sites of extramedullary disease other than the breast, including disease occurring before, concurrent with, or after the diagnosis of myeloid sarcoma of the breast, the most common sites are skin and subcutaneous tissue, the female genital tract, CNS, and lymph nodes (axillary and nonaxillary).[61]

Clinical outcome has been variable. Patients who present with isolated breast myeloid sarcoma appear to have a favorable outcome, particularly if they receive systemic chemotherapy.[117,118] Those patients with widespread disease have a guarded prognosis,[116–118] although the clinical course is strongly dependent on the underlying molecular genetic and cytogenetic abnormalities of the AML.

Pathology

Myeloid sarcomas in the breast and in other sites are composed of primitive myeloid and/or monocytic cells. In a subset of cases there is some maturation of the neoplastic clone to more mature myeloid forms. On microscopic examination the tumors typically have a diffuse pattern, usually with sparing of mammary epithelial structures. In some instances, neoplastic cells infiltrate stroma as a string of single cells. They can also surround nonneoplastic ducts and lobules in a "targetoid" pattern. Mitoses are usually easily found. In a minority of cases there are scattered tingible body macrophages, imparting a "starry sky" pattern.[117,118,120] Some authorities have subclassified myeloid sarcomas as well differentiated, poorly differentiated, and blastic, depending on the presence and extent of maturation within the tumor.[118] The neoplastic cells are dyscohesive, with round, oval, irregular, or reniform, medium-sized nuclei that have finely dispersed chromatin and variably prominent nucleoli (Fig. 40.16). The cytoplasm ranges from scant in primitive cells to moderately abundant, sometimes with a distinct eosinophilic color due to the presence of granules if there is some maturation of the blasts. There may be admixed eosinophils and precursors.

At least a subset of neoplastic cells is usually positive for chloroacetate esterase. On IHC analysis, the neoplastic cells are usually positive for myeloperoxidase, lysozyme, CD117, and CD43, and often for CD34. CD45 (leukocyte common

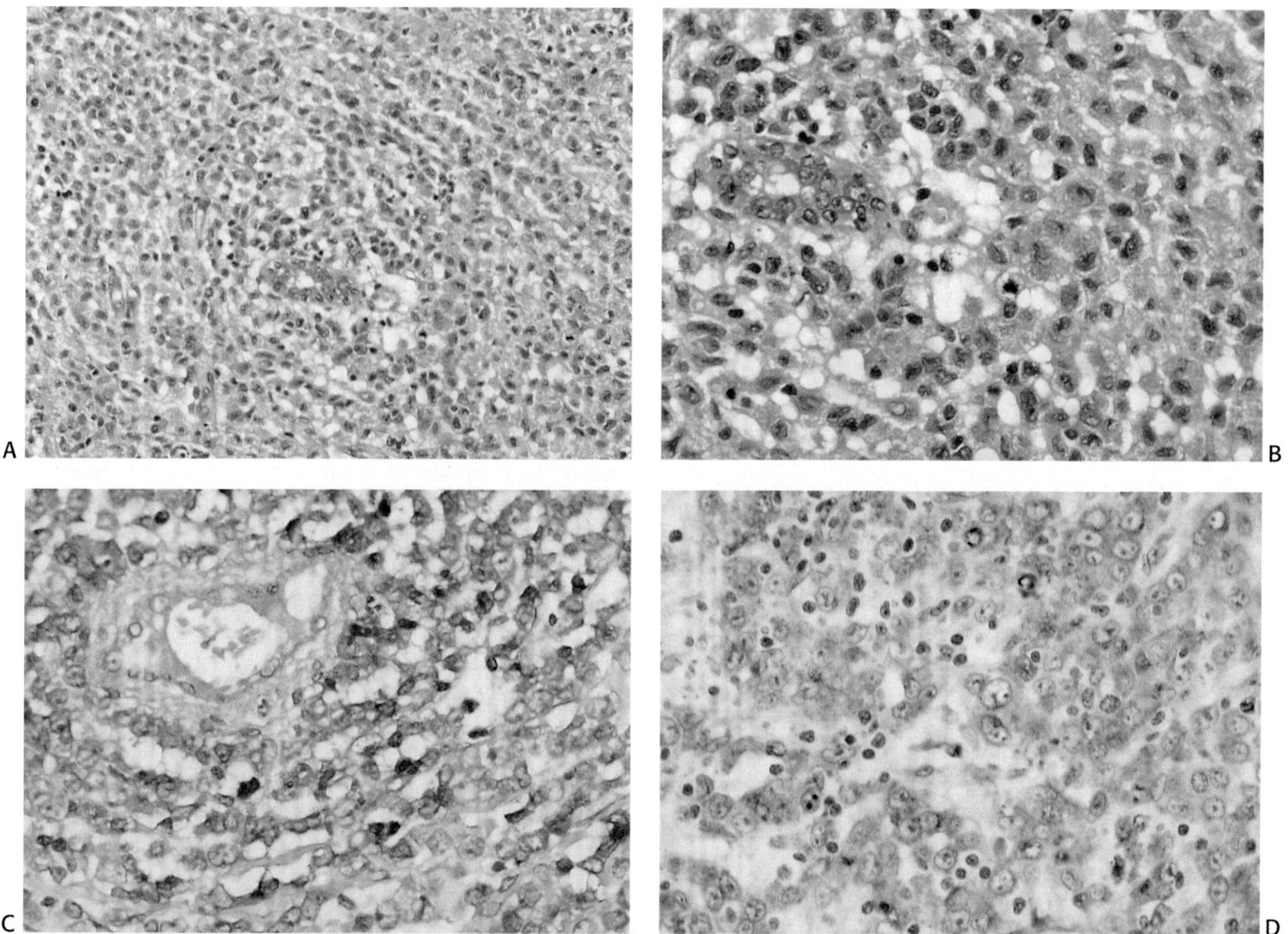

FIG. 40.16. *Myeloid sarcoma.* **A,B:** This periductal infiltrate of undifferentiated granulocytic cells could be mistaken for carcinoma. **C:** A few tumor cells are reactive (*red*) with naphthol-ASD-chloroacetate esterase stain. Undifferentiated cells are not stained. **D:** The differentiated cells are positive with the immunostain for muramidase (lysozyme).

antigen) is often expressed, but may be dim. Myeloid sarcomas composed exclusively of monocytes and their precursors (monocytic sarcoma) are CD68+, lysozyme+, but are negative for myeloperoxidase and often for CD34 and CD117. Tumor cells are negative for CD20, CD3, and keratins. In a few cases, there may be an expression of one or more lymphoid-associated antigens, such as TdT, CD79a, or PAX5; a broad panel of immunostains, including myeloid markers, will help avoid misinterpretation of such cases as lymphoblastic lymphoma.[117,118,120]

When there has been an associated AML, it usually has been classified according to the FAB Classification. AML of M0, M1, M2, M3, M4 (including M4Eo), and M5 types has been reported. AML, M1 (myeloblastic without maturation), and AML, M2 (myeloblastic with maturation), appear to be most common.[61,118] A few AMLs associated with t(15;17), t(8;21), inv(16), and del(5) have been described.[61] A case of AML with mutated NPM1 and a FLT3 internal tandem duplication, in which the patient developed a relapse in the form of a breast myeloid sarcoma, has been described.[119]

Differential Diagnosis

The main entity in the differential diagnosis of myeloid sarcoma is lymphoma, especially diffuse large B-cell lymphoma. On routinely stained sections, large lymphoid cells typically have slightly larger nuclei, with either more vesicular or more coarsely clumped chromatin, and less delicate nuclear membranes than the neoplastic cells of myeloid sarcoma. Differentiation into recognizable maturing myeloid elements, when present, helps to identify a neoplasm as myeloid sarcoma. Immunophenotyping with an appropriate panel of lymphoid and myeloid antigens will confirm the diagnosis.

Occasionally, myeloid sarcoma, particularly when composed predominantly of primitive monocytes, is characterized by large, pleomorphic cells, raising the question of a histiocytic neoplasm, such as histiocytic sarcoma, or one of the histiocytic proliferations discussed in the following section. There may be a good deal of overlap in the pathologic features of entities in these categories. The presence of circulating blasts in the peripheral blood and diffuse marrow involvement supports a diagnosis of myeloid sarcoma/AML.

When myeloid sarcoma grows in a linear or targetoid pattern, it can mimic carcinoma, particularly ILC. The presence of *in situ* carcinoma makes myeloid sarcoma less likely.[118] Areas with cohesive neoplastic cells or formation of tubules or lumens supports carcinoma. A history of myeloid neoplasm should prompt consideration of myeloid sarcoma. Of note, a small subset of patients treated for breast carcinoma with chemotherapy develops therapy-related AML; hence a history of carcinoma does not exclude the possibility of AML/myeloid sarcoma.

EXTRAMEDULLARY HEMATOPOIESIS

Extramedullary hematopoiesis, or myeloid metaplasia, can occur in a wide variety of sites, usually in association with an underlying hematologic disorder. Breast masses formed by extramedullary hematopoiesis are rare, but have been reported in middle-aged and elderly female patients, most of whom carry a diagnosis of a chronic myeloproliferative neoplasm that is often primary myelofibrosis (formerly known as chronic idiopathic myelofibrosis and as myelofibrosis with myeloid metaplasia).

Extramedullary hematopoiesis also occurs rarely in the breast in women with no prior hematologic disorder. It has been described in the breast and in ALNs of previously healthy women following neoadjuvant chemotherapy for breast carcinoma (Fig. 40.17)[122,123] and in a FA.[124] Among those with primary myelofibrosis, breast involvement has occurred 5 to 16 years after the diagnosis of myelofibrosis.[125–129] The lesions measured 1.8 to 8 cm. One patient reportedly had no other tumorous manifestations of myeloid metaplasia except hepatic enlargement.[127] Most other patients had splenomegaly. Mammography revealed bilateral confluent densities in two cases.[128,129] The lesions were smooth, homogeneous, and hypoechoic on sonography.

Microscopic examination reveals a diffuse infiltrate of mature and maturing hematopoietic cells. There is a variable admixture of cells of myeloid, erythroid, and megakaryocytic lines, with a predominance of myeloid elements described in some cases. In patients with primary myelofibrosis, the megakaryocytes are often large, hyperchromatic, and atypical or even bizarre. The extramedullary hematopoiesis may be associated with sclerosis of the mammary stroma.[129,130] Mammary extramedullary hematopoiesis has been described in postmortem examinations of patients with myelofibrosis.[126]

Differential Diagnosis

Establishing a diagnosis of extramedullary hematopoiesis can be challenging in the absence of clinical information concerning an underlying hematologic disorder, particularly

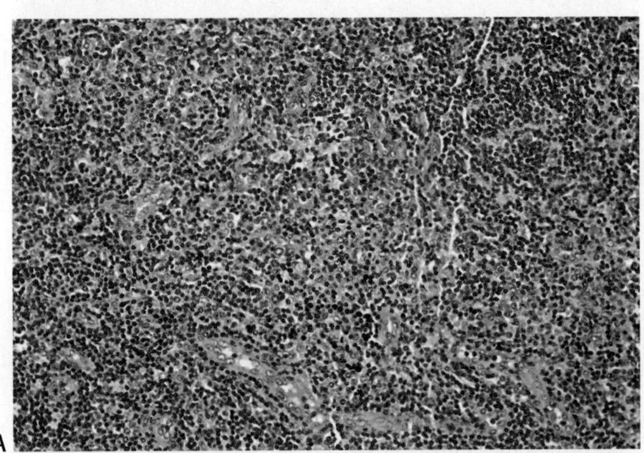

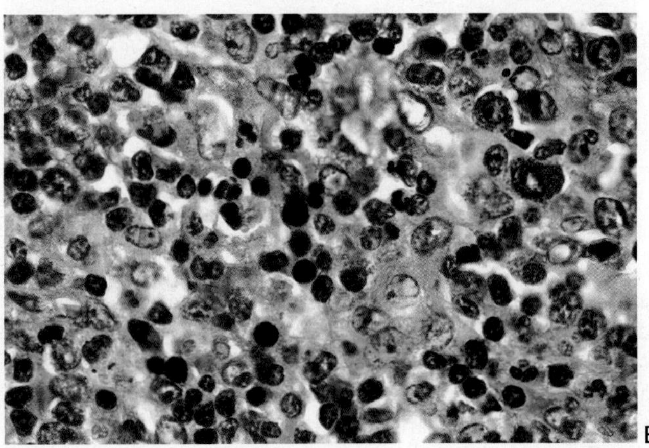

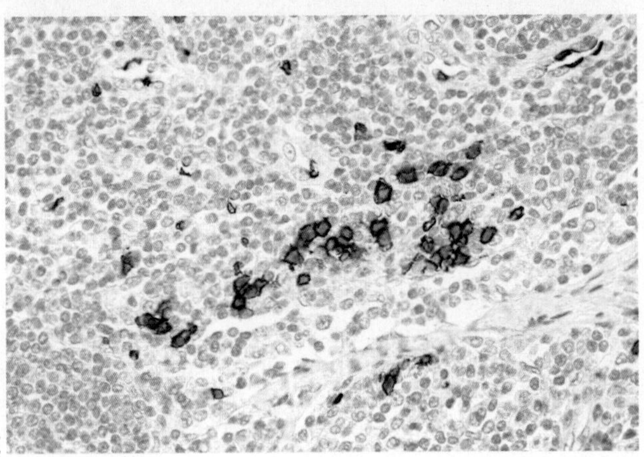

FIG. 40.17. ***Extramedullary hematopoiesis in an axillary sentinel lymph node.*** **A:** The interfollicular area is expanded by maturing myeloid and erythroid elements. **B:** High magnification shows scattered eosinophil precursors with coarse red granules, and nucleated red blood cells with homogeneous dark, nearly black, nuclei scattered singly and forming small strands. **C:** Glycophorin highlights the erythroid elements (immunoperoxidase technique on a paraffin section).

on FS or on FNA biopsy.[129,130] The hematopoietic elements can be mistaken for carcinoma, especially lobular carcinoma or lymphoma, and other neoplasms. The megakaryocytes set in a mixed background of smaller cells can be mistaken for Reed–Sternberg cells. The diagnosis is facilitated by knowledge of the clinical history, careful examination of routine sections, and awareness of the possibility of extramedullary hematopoiesis affecting the breast.

HISTIOCYTIC PROLIFERATIONS OF THE BREAST

Rosai–Dorfman Disease of the Breast

Rosai–Dorfman disease (sinus histiocytosis with massive lymphadenopathy) is an uncommon disorder of unknown etiology that typically presents with lymphadenopathy. Some patients have extranodal involvement in addition to lymphadenopathy, and in a minority it involves extranodal sites alone. The more commonly involved extranodal sites include skin, bone, soft tissue, and ocular adnexa.

Breast involvement by Rosai–Dorfman disease is very unusual. Rosai–Dorfman disease can affect children and adults; most patients with Rosai–Dorfman disease involving the breast are adults, with rare occurrence during adolescence. Patients with breast involvement ranged from 15 to 84 years of age, with a median age in the early 50s at presentation.[131–134] There is a marked female preponderance. Rosai–Dorfman disease of the breast in men has been reported, but these cases account for no more than 10% of all cases.[132,133,135] Patients often present with a firm, painless, ill-defined or irregular breast mass.[131,133] The lesions have been detected on screening mammography.[132] In rare instances retraction of skin and inflammation overlying the lesion have been described.[131] The tumors range in size from 1 to 6.5 cm (median, 3 cm).[132] The lesions are usually single and unilateral, but a few cases with multifocal or bilateral breast involvement have been described.[131–133,135] Most patients have Rosai–Dorfman disease confined to the breast, but a minority have more widespread disease that may involve ALNs,[131,136] multiple different lymph node groups, and/or extranodal sites.[131] Patients with bilateral breast involvement appear more likely to have Rosai–Dorfman disease beyond the breast than those with unilateral involvement.[131,133] A woman with a history of Rosai–Dorfman disease involving a lymph node and the thigh who developed breast involvement in the form of multiple bilateral subcentimeter nodules has been reported.[137]

Microscopic examination of the lesions reveals a dense infiltrate of lymphocytes, plasma cells, histiocytes, and sometimes lymphoid follicles. The histiocytes are large with large oval nuclei, open chromatin, distinct nucleoli, and abundant cytoplasm. Some of the large histiocytes show emperipolesis, which may be translated as "inside round about wandering," in which intact cells, usually lymphocytes, but sometimes plasma cells, red blood cells, and neutrophils, are present within the cytoplasm. A clear halo may surround the engulfed cells (Fig. 40.18). This is in contrast to phagocytosis, in which ingested cells are digested. Although the large nuclei of the histiocytes give them an atypical appearance, mitoses and necrosis are absent. Eosinophils are very infrequent. Abscess formation and granulomas are absent. In lymph nodes, the large histiocytes are mainly confined to

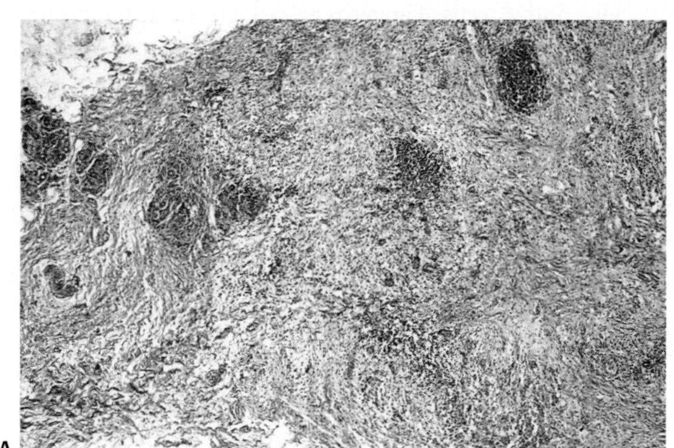

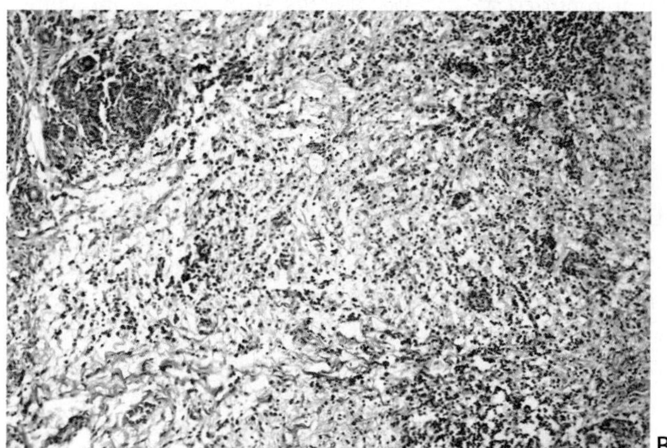

FIG. 40.18. ***Rosai–Dorfman disease.*** **A:** The lesion forms an unencapsulated nodule within breast tissue. A few lobules are present in the *upper* portion of the image. **B:** Medium magnification shows a proliferation of histiocytes with abundant pale cytoplasm and a patchy infiltrate of lymphocytes and plasma cells. A lobule is present in the *upper right* corner of the image. **C:** High magnification shows scattered large histiocytes with large, somewhat atypical nuclei, vesicular chromatin, small nucleoli, and abundant pale finely fibrillar cytoplasm. Occasional histiocytes appear to have intracytoplasmic lymphocytes (*arrows*). **D:** S-100 highlights the characteristic histiocytes and facilitates identification of intracytoplasmic lymphocytes, many of which are surrounded by a clear halo (immunoperoxidase technique on a paraffin section).

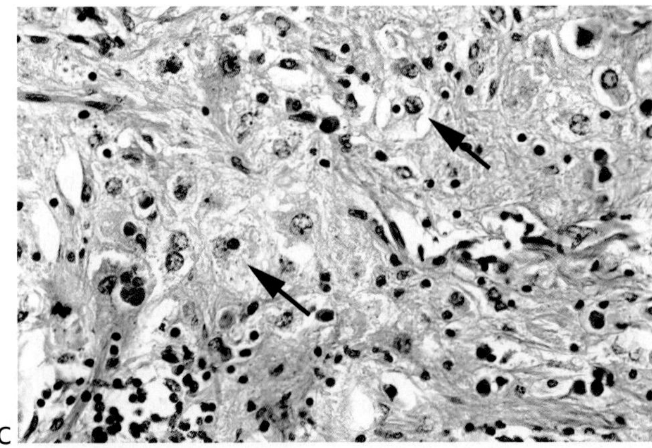

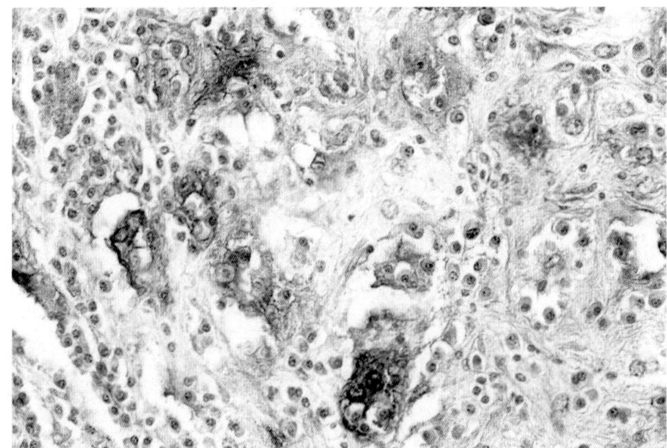

C D

FIG. 40.18. *(Continued)*

expanded sinuses (sinus histiocytosis with massive lymphadenopathy). Emperipolesis may be more difficult to identify in extranodal sites than in lymph nodes. Examination of touch preps may help with identification of emperipolesis. The lesions may be associated with fibrosis, which may become prominent and may be band-like. Fibrosis is overall more prominent in extranodal sites than in Rosai–Dorfman disease in lymph nodes. The distinctive histiocytes are positive for S-100 and for histiocytic markers such as CD68, and are negative for CD1a. The S-100 stain can be helpful in highlighting cells with emperipolesis (Fig. 40.18).[131–133,135,136]

Long follow-up is not often available in cases of Rosai–Dorfman disease involving the breast. When follow-up is available, patients have typically been alive and well.[132,133] The breast lesions may persist for months to years if not excised, however.[134,136] Recurrence after excision has also been reported.[134,136] Rare patients with disease involving the breast and other sites at presentation have had persistent or progressive disease. One death due to widespread Rosai–Dorfman disease that involved the breast has been reported.[131]

Erdheim–Chester Disease

Erdheim–Chester disease is a rare non-Langerhans cell histiocytosis characterized by xanthomatous features. Nearly all cases show involvement of long bones of the lower extremities that is associated with characteristic radiographic features. About half of the patients have extraskeletal involvement in sites that may include the skin, orbit, lung, and other tissues. Breast involvement is very rare, but when it occurs, it can take the form of mass lesions clinically mimicking carcinoma. Histologic examination shows CD68+ xanthomatous histiocytes, scattered Touton-type giant cells, admixed lymphocytes, and fibrosis.[138]

Langerhans Cell Histiocytosis

Langerhans cell histiocytosis, formerly called histiocytosis X, is a clonal proliferation of Langerhans cells that in general affects children more than adults and can present as unifocal or multifocal disease in one of three clinical patterns: unifocal disease (previously referred to as eosinophilic granuloma), multifocal disease (formerly referred to as Hand–Schüller–Christian disease), or multifocal disease with disseminated or visceral involvement (formerly called Letterer–Siwe disease).[139] Breast involvement by Langerhans cell histiocytosis is rare. The case of an adult woman with widespread involvement by Langerhans cell histiocytosis has been reported.[140] The patient presented with a 5-cm lesion of the nipple and areola with an appearance on physical examination that was suspicious for Paget disease. Biopsy showed an infiltrate of large pale cells with large pale nuclei with longitudinal or complex folds and moderately abundant pale cytoplasm filling the dermis. The large cells were CD1a+, S-100+. There was a background inflammatory cell infiltrate of eosinophils, B cells, and T cells. Langerhans cell histiocytosis is rarely found in association with Hodgkin or NHL. A case of FL involving the breast with nodules of Langerhans cells present within the lymphoma has been reported.[141]

Differential Diagnosis of Histiocytic Proliferations in the Breast

Clinically and radiographically Rosai–Dorfman disease can mimic carcinoma, fibrocystic changes, and even FA.[131,132,136] On pathologic evaluation it is first important to determine whether the specimen represents a lymph node or breast parenchyma, as Rosai–Dorfman disease much more commonly involves lymph nodes than breast tissue. The differential diagnosis includes low-grade B-cell lymphoma with plasmacytic differentiation, particularly extranodal marginal zone lymphoma (MALT lymphoma). Misdiagnosis as lymphoma may occur if one focuses on the lymphoplasmacytic component of the infiltrate and overlooks the distinctive histiocytic component. A case of Rosai–Dorfman disease initially misinterpreted as MALT lymphoma has been reported.[134] In another instance, a core biopsy was suspicious for lymphoma, but the excision specimen proved to represent Rosai–Dorfman disease.[136]

In Rosai–Dorfman disease, there is no significant cytologic atypia or immunophenotypic abnormality or evidence of clonality of the lymphoplasmacytic component of the infiltrate. Other differential diagnostic considerations include inflammatory lesions such as acute or chronic mastitis and granulomatous mastitis. Rosai–Dorfman disease has been described in a patient with type 2 diabetes mellitus[132]; the lymphoid infiltrate in conjunction with a history of diabetes could raise the question of diabetic mastopathy. However, none of these inflammatory processes contains the histiocytes characteristic of Rosai–Dorfman disease. A case of diabetic mastopathy associated with an unusually exuberant lymphohistiocytic infiltrate with granuloma formation that was initially misdiagnosed as Rosai–Dorfman disease has been reported.[142] Characteristic periductal, perilobular, and perivascular lymphoid infiltrates supported diabetic mastopathy despite the presence of unusual features; this cellular distribution is not seen in Rosai–Dorfman disease.

Rosai–Dorfman histiocytes have large nuclei and distinct nucleoli, and can mimic malignant cells. Some malignant neoplasms have abundant pale cytoplasm and may mimic histiocytic proliferations. Renal cell carcinoma and melanoma metastatic to the breast could result in such a problem in differential diagnosis if a history of these neoplasms is not available. The fact that melanoma is typically S-100+ may increase the chance of it being mistaken for Rosai–Dorfman disease. Carcinomas and melanoma typically have more pronounced cytologic atypia and lack the distinctive cytoplasmic features of Rosai–Dorfman histiocytes. The low N:C ratio, and the presence of emperipolesis in some of the distinctive histiocytes, will allow the correct diagnosis to be made.[131]

An unusual type of breast carcinoma, histiocytoid carcinoma, is characterized by a proliferation of atypical epithelial cells with abundant finely vacuolated, granular, or ground glass cytoplasm that may be scattered singly, loosely clustered, or present in sheets. These cells can be mistaken for histiocytes, but they are CK+ on immunostaining and the cytoplasm may stain with mucicarmine.[143]

Rosai–Dorfman disease can also be considered in the differential diagnosis of other histiocytic proliferations, including Langerhans cell histiocytosis and Erdheim–Chester disease. In Langerhans cell histiocytosis, cytologic features are different: the histiocytes have more elongate nuclei with prominent grooves and less abundant cytoplasm without emperipolesis. Langerhans cells express CD1a and langerin in addition to S-100. In contrast to Rosai–Dorfman disease, eosinophils are often admixed in Langerhans cell histiocytosis. Both clinical and histologic features of Erdheim–Chester disease (see above) are different from those of Rosai–Dorfman disease, and the distinction is usually not difficult.

Fat necrosis is a common finding compared to the histiocytic proliferations noted above, but careful examination of well-prepared slides should allow distinction between fat necrosis, Langerhans cell histiocytosis, and Rosai–Dorfman disease.

REFERENCES

1. Wiseman C, Liao K. Primary lymphoma of the breast. *Cancer* 1972;29:1705–1712.
2. Talwalkar SS, Miranda RN, Valbuena JR, et al. Lymphomas involving the breast: a study of 106 cases comparing localized and disseminated neoplasms. *Am J Surg Pathol* 2008;32:1299–1309.
3. Brustein S, Filippa DA, Kimmel M, et al. Malignant lymphoma of the breast. A study of 53 patients. *Ann Surg* 1987;205:144–150.
4. Hugh J, Jackson F, Hanson J, et al. Primary breast lymphoma—an immunohistologic study of 20 new cases. *Cancer* 1990;66:2602–2611.
5. Lamovec J, Jancar J. Primary malignant lymphoma of the breast—lymphoma of the mucosa-associated lymphoid tissue. *Cancer* 1987;60:3033–3041.
6. Domchek SM, Hecht JL, Fleming MD, et al. Lymphomas of the breast: primary and secondary involvement. *Cancer* 2002;94:6–13.
7. Farinha P, Andre S, Cabecadas J, et al. High frequency of MALT lymphoma in a series of 14 cases of primary breast lymphoma. *Appl Immunohistochem Mol Morphol* 2002;10:115–120.
8. Cabras MG, Amichetti M, Nagliati M, et al. Primary non-Hodgkin's lymphoma of the breast: a report of 11 cases. *Haematologica* 2004;89:1527–1528.
9. Lin Y, Guo XM, Shen KW, et al. Primary breast lymphoma: long-term treatment outcome and prognosis. *Leuk Lymphoma* 2006;47:2102–2109.
10. Vigliotti ML, Dell'olio M, La Sala A, et al. Primary breast lymphoma: outcome of 7 patients and a review of the literature. *Leuk Lymphoma* 2005;46:1321–1327.
11. Liu M, Hsieh C, Wang A, et al. Primary breast lymphoma: a pooled analysis of prognostic factors and survival in 93 cases. *Ann Saudi Med* 2005;25:288–293.
12. Mattia A, Ferry J, Harris N. Breast lymphoma: a B-cell spectrum including the low grade B-cell lymphoma of mucosa associated lymphoid tissue. *Am J Surg Pathol* 1993;17:574–587.
13. Wang LA, Harris NL, Ferry JA. Lymphoma of the breast and the role of mammography in the detection of low-grade lymphomas. *Mod Pathol* 2004;17:276A.
14. Lin YC, Tsai CH, Wu JS, et al. Clinicopathologic features and treatment outcome of non-Hodgkin lymphoma of the breast—a review of 42 primary and secondary cases in Taiwanese patients. *Leuk Lymphoma* 2009;50:918–924.
15. Lyons J, Myles J, Pohlman B, et al. Treatment and prognosis of primary breast lymphoma—a review of 13 cases. *Am J Clinical Oncol* 2000;23:334–336.
16. Aviles A, Delgado S, Nambo MJ, et al. Primary breast lymphoma: results of a controlled clinical trial. *Oncology* 2005;69:256–260.
17. Fruchart C, Denoux Y, Chasle J, et al. High grade primary breast lymphoma: is it a different clinical entity? *Breast Cancer Res Treat* 2005;93:191–198.
18. Uesato M, Miyazawa Y, Gunji Y, et al. Primary non-Hodgkin's lymphoma of the breast: report of a case with special reference to 380 cases in the Japanese literature. *Breast Cancer* (Tokyo, Japan) 2005;12:154–158.
19. Vignot S, Ledoussal V, Nodiot P, et al. Non-Hodgkin's lymphoma of the breast: a report of 19 cases and a review of the literature. *Clin Lymphoma* 2005;6:37–42.
20. Ribrag V, Bibeau F, El Weshi A, et al. Primary breast lymphoma: a report of 20 cases. *Br J Haematol* 2001;115:253–256.
21. Ryan G, Martinelli G, Kuper-Hommel M, et al. Primary diffuse large B-cell lymphoma of the breast: prognostic factors and outcomes of a study by the International Extranodal Lymphoma Study Group. *Ann Oncol* 2008;19:233–241.
22. Sabate JM, Gomez A, Torrubia S, et al. Lymphoma of the breast: clinical and radiologic features with pathologic correlation in 28 patients. *Breast J* 2002;8:294–304.
23. Yoshida S, Nakamura N, Sasaki Y, et al. Primary breast diffuse large B-cell lymphoma shows a non-germinal center B-cell phenotype. *Mod Pathol* 2005;18:398–405.
24. Kebudi A, Coban A, Yetkin G, et al. Primary T-lymphoma of the breast with bilateral involvement, unusual presentation. *Int J Clin Prac* 2005;95–98.
25. Pisani F, Romano A, Anticoli Borza P, et al. Diffuse large B-cell lymphoma involving the breast. A report of four cases. *J Exp Clin Cancer Res* 2006;25:277–281.

26. Liguori G, Cantile M, Cerrone M, et al. Breast MALT lymphomas: a clinicopathological and cytogenetic study of 9 cases. *Oncol Rep* 2012;28:1211–1216.
27. Aozasa K, Ohsawa M, Saeki K, et al. Malignant lymphoma of the breast. Immunologic type and association with lymphocytic mastopathy. *Am J Clin Pathol* 1992;97:699–704.
28. Chanan-Khan A, Holkova B, Goldenberg AS, et al. Non-Hodgkin's lymphoma presenting as a breast mass in patients with HIV infection: a report of three cases. *Leuk Lymphoma* 2005;46:1189–1193.
29. Jeon H, Akagi T, Hoshida Y, et al. Primary non-Hodgkin's malignant lymphoma of the breast. *Cancer* 1992;70:2451–2459.
30. Gualco G, Bacchi CE. B-cell and T-cell lymphomas of the breast: clinical–pathological features of 53 cases. *Int J Surg Pathol* 2008;16:407–413.
31. Aviles A, Neri N, Nambo MJ. The role of genotype in 104 cases of diffuse large B-cell lymphoma primary of breast. *Am J Clin Oncol* 2012;35:126–129.
32. Martinelli G, Ryan G, Seymour JF, et al. Primary follicular and marginal-zone lymphoma of the breast: clinical features, prognostic factors and outcome: a study by the International Extranodal Lymphoma Study Group. *Ann Oncol* 2009;20:1993–1999.
33. Rooney N, Snead D, Goodman S, Webb A. Primary breast lymphoma with skin involvement arising in lymphocytic lobulitis. *Histopathology* 1994;24:81–84.
34. Talwalkar SS, Valbuena JR, Abruzzo LV, et al. MALT1 gene rearrangements and NF-kB activation involving p65 and p50 are absent or rare in primary MALT lymphomas of the breast. *Mod Pathol* 2006;19:1402–1408.
35. Kuper-Hommel MJ, Schreuder MI, Gemmink AH, et al. T(14;18)(q32;q21) involving MALT1 and IGH genes occurs in extranodal diffuse large B-cell lymphomas of the breast and testis. *Mod Pathol* 2013;26:421–427.
36. Monteiro M, Duarte I, Cabecadas J, et al. Intravascular large B-cell lymphoma of the breast. *Breast* (Edinburgh, Scotland) 2005;14:75–78.
37. Yhim HY, Kim JS, Kang HJ, et al. Matched-pair analysis comparing the outcomes of primary breast and nodal diffuse large B-cell lymphoma in patients treated with rituximab plus chemotherapy. *Int J Cancer* 2012;131:235–243.
38. Duman BB, Sahin B, Guvenc B, et al. Lymphoma of the breast in a male patient. *Med Oncol* 2011;28(suppl. 1):S490–S493.
39. Ghetu D, Membrez V, Bregy A, et al. Expect the unexpected: primary breast MALT lymphoma. *Arch Gynecol Obstet* 2011;284:1323–1324.
40. Kambouchner M, Godmer P, Guillevin L, et al. Low grade marginal zone B cell lymphoma of the breast associated with localised amyloidosis and corpora amylacea in a woman with long standing primary Sjogren's syndrome. *J Clin Pathol* 2003;56:74–77.
41. Ryan RJ, Sloan JM, Collins AB, et al. Extranodal marginal zone lymphoma of mucosa-associated lymphoid tissue with amyloid deposition: a clinicopathologic case series. *Am J Clin Pathol* 2012;137:51–64.
42. Joao C, Farinha P, da Silva MG, et al. Cytogenetic abnormalities in MALT lymphomas and their precursor lesions from different organs. A fluorescence in situ hybridization (FISH) study. *Histopathology* 2007;50:217–224.
43. Mulligan S, Hu P, Murphy A, et al. Variations in MALT1 Gene Disruptions Detected by FISH in 109 MALT Lymphomas Occurring in Different Primary Sites. *J Assoc Genet Technol* 2011;37:76–79.
44. Leoncini L, Raphael M, Stein H, et al. Burkitt lymphoma In: Swerdlow S, Campo E, Harris N, et al., eds. *WHO classification tumours of haematopoietic and lymphoid tissues.* 4th ed. Lyon: World Health Organization-IARC; 2008:262–264.
45. de Jong D, Vasmel WL, de Boer JP, et al. Anaplastic large-cell lymphoma in women with breast implants. *JAMA* 2008;300:2030–2035.
46. Burkitt D, Wright D. *Burkitt's lymphoma.* 1st ed. Edinburgh and London: E and S Livingstone; 1970.
47. Lingohr P, Eidt S, Rheinwalt KP. A 12-year-old girl presenting with bilateral gigantic Burkitt's lymphoma of the breast. *Arch Gynecol Obstet* 2009;279:743–746.
48. Vakiani E, Savage DG, Pile-Spellman E, et al. T-Cell lymphoblastic lymphoma presenting as bilateral multinodular breast masses: a case report and review of the literature. *Am J Hematol* 2005;80:216–222.
49. Aguilera NS, Tavassoli FA, Chu WS, et al. T-cell lymphoma presenting in the breast: a histologic, immunophenotypic and molecular genetic study of four cases. *Mod Pathol* 2000;13:599–605.
50. Briggs JH, Algan O, Stea B. Primary T-cell lymphoma of the breast: a case report. *Cancer Investigation* 2003;21:68–72.
51. Popplewell L, Thomas SH, Huang Q, et al. Primary anaplastic large-cell lymphoma associated with breast implants. *Leuk Lymphoma* 2011;52:1481–1487.
52. Gualco G, Chioato L, Harrington WJ Jr, et al. Primary and secondary T-cell lymphomas of the breast: clinico-pathologic features of 11 cases. *Appl Immunohistochem Mol Morphol* 2009;17:301–306.
53. Daneshbod Y, Oryan A, Khojasteh HN, et al. Primary ALK-positive anaplastic large cell lymphoma of the breast: a case report and review of the literature. *J Pediatr Hematol Oncol* 2010;32:e75–e78.
54. Miranda RN, Lin L, Talwalkar SS, et al. Anaplastic large cell lymphoma involving the breast: a clinicopathologic study of 6 cases and review of the literature. *Arch Pathol Lab Med* 2009;133:1383–1390.
55. Iyengar P, Reid-Nicholson M, Moreira AL. Pregnancy-associated anaplastic large-cell lymphoma of the breast: a rare mimic of ductal carcinoma. *Diagn Cytopathol* 2006;34:298–302.
56. Delsol G, Falini B, Muller-Hermelink H, et al. Anaplastic large cell lymphoma (ALCL), ALK-positive. In: Swerdlow S, Campo E, Harris N, et al., eds. *WHO classification tumours of haematopoietic and lymphoid tissues.* 4th ed. Lyon: World Health Organization-IARC; 2008:312–316.
57. Mason D, Harris N, Delsol G, et al. Anaplastic large cell lymphoma (ALCL), ALK-negative. In: Swerdlow S, Campo E, Harris N, et al., eds. *WHO classification tumours of haematopoietic and lymphoid tissues.* 4th ed. Lyon: World Health Organization-IARC; 2008:317–319.
58. Ralfkiaer E, Willemze R, Paulli M, et al. Primary cutaneous CD30-positive T-cell lymphoproliferative disorders. In: Swerdlow S, Campo E, Harris N, et al., eds. *WHO classification tumours of haematopoietic and lymphoid tissues.* 4th ed. Lyon: World Health Organization-IARC; 2008:300–301.
59. Schramm N, Pfluger T, Reiser MF, Berger F. Subcutaneous panniculitis-like T-cell lymphoma with breast involvement: functional and morphological imaging findings. *Br J Radiol* 2010;83:e90–e94.
60. Jaffe E, Gaulard P, Ralfkiaer E, et al. Subcutaneous panniculitis-like T-cell lymphoma In: Swerdlow S, Campo E, Harris N, et al., eds. *WHO classification tumours of haematopoietic and lymphoid tissues.* 4th ed. Lyon: World Health Organization-IARC; 2008:294–295.
61. Cunningham I. A clinical review of breast involvement in acute leukemia. *Leuk Lymphoma* 2006;47:2517–2526.
62. Hoimes CJ, Selbst MK, Shafi NQ, et al. Hodgkin's lymphoma of the breast. *J Clin Oncol* 2010;28:e11–e13.
63. Ergul N, Guner SI, Sager S, et al. Bilateral breast involvement of Hodgkin lymphoma revealed by FDG PET/CT. *Med Oncol* 2012;29:1105–1108.
64. Park J, Rizzo M, Jackson S, et al. Reed–Sternberg cells in breast FNA of a patient with left breast mass. *Diagn Cytopathol* 2010;38:663–668.
65. Roden AC, Macon WR, Keeney GL, et al. Seroma-associated primary anaplastic large-cell lymphoma adjacent to breast implants: an indolent T-cell lymphoproliferative disorder. *Mod Pathol* 2008;21:455–463.
66. Wong AK, Lopategui J, Clancy S, et al. Anaplastic large cell lymphoma associated with a breast implant capsule: a case report and review of the literature. *Am J Surg Pathol* 2008;32:1265–1268.
67. Farkash EA, Ferry JA, Harris NL, et al. Rare lymphoid malignancies of the breast: a report of two cases illustrating potential diagnostic pitfalls. *J Hematop* 2009;2:237–244.
68. Lipworth L, Tarone RE, McLaughlin JK. Breast implants and lymphoma risk: a review of the epidemiologic evidence through 2008. *Plast Reconstr Surg* 2009;123:790–793.
69. Cook PD, Osborne BM, Connor RL, et al. Follicular lymphoma adjacent to foreign body granulomatous inflammation and fibrosis surrounding silicone breast prosthesis. *Am J Surg Pathol* 1995;19:712–717.
70. Duvic M, Moore D, Menter A, et al. Cutaneous T-cell lymphoma in association with silicone breast implants. *J Am Acad Dermatol* 1995;32:939–942.
71. Kraemer DM, Tony HP, Gattenlohner S, et al. Lymphoplasmacytic lymphoma in a patient with leaking silicone implant. *Haematologica* 2004;89:ELT01.
72. Sendagorta E, Ledo A. Sezary syndrome in association with silicone breast implant. *J Am Acad Dermatol* 1995;33:1060–1061.
73. Aladily TN, Medeiros LJ, Amin MB, et al. Anaplastic large cell lymphoma associated with breast implants: a report of 13 cases. *Am J Surg Pathol* 2012;36:1000–1008.
74. Fritzsche FR, Pahl S, Petersen I, et al. Anaplastic large-cell non-Hodgkin's lymphoma of the breast in periprosthetic localisation 32 years after treatment for primary breast cancer—a case report. *Virchows Arch* 2006;449:561–564.

75. Gaudet G, Friedberg JW, Weng A, et al. Breast lymphoma associated with breast implants: two case-reports and a review of the literature. *Leuk Lymphoma* 2002;43:115–119.
76. Newman MK, Zemmel NJ, Bandak AZ, et al. Primary breast lymphoma in a patient with silicone breast implants: a case report and review of the literature. *J Plast Reconstr Aesthet Surg* 2008;61:822–825.
77. Olack B, Gupta R, Brooks GS. Anaplastic large cell lymphoma arising in a saline breast implant capsule after tissue expander breast reconstruction. *Ann Plast Sur* 2007;59:56–57.
78. Sahoo S, Rosen PP, Feddersen RM, et al. Anaplastic large cell lymphoma arising in a silicone breast implant capsule: a case report and review of the literature. *Arch Pathol Lab Med* 2003;127:e115–e118.
79. Carty MJ, Pribaz JJ, Antin JH, et al. A patient death attributable to implant-related primary anaplastic large cell lymphoma of the breast. *Plast Reconstr Surg* 2011;128:112e–118e.
80. Taylor KO, Webster HR, Prince HM. Anaplastic large cell lymphoma and breast implants: five Australian cases. *Plast Reconstr Surg* 2012;129:610e–617e.
81. Lazzeri D, Zhang YX, Huemer GM, et al. Capsular contracture as a further presenting symptom of implant-related anaplastic large cell lymphoma. *Am J Surg Pathol* 2012;36:1735–1736; author reply 6–8.
82. Said JW, Tasaka T, Takeuchi S, et al. Primary effusion lymphoma in women: report of two cases of Kaposi's sarcoma herpes virus-associated effusion-based lymphoma in human immunodeficiency virus-negative women. *Blood* 1996;88:3124–3128.
83. Aladily TN, Nathwani BN, Miranda RN, et al. Extranodal NK/T-cell lymphoma, nasal type, arising in association with saline breast implant: expanding the spectrum of breast implant-associated lymphomas. *Am J Surg Pathol* 2012;36:1729–1734.
84. Anne N, Pallapothu R. Lymphoma of the breast: a mimic of inflammatory breast cancer. *World J Surg Oncol* 2011;9:125.
85. Antoniou SA, Antoniou GA, Makridis C, et al. Bilateral primary breast lymphoma masquerading as lactating mastitis. *Eur J Obstet Gynecol Reprod Biol* 2010;152:111–112.
86. Sun LM, Huang EY, Meng FY, et al. Primary breast lymphoma clinically mimicking acute mastitis: a case report. *Tumori* 2011;97:233–235.
87. Sanati S, Ayala AG, Middleton LP. Lymphoepithelioma-like carcinoma of the breast: report of a case mimicking lymphoma. *Ann Diagn Pathol* 2004;8:309–315.
88. Ely KA, Tse G, Simpson JF, et al. Diabetic mastopathy. A clinicopathologic review. *Am J Clin Pathol* 2000;113:541–545.
89. Valdez R, Thorson J, Finn WG, et al. Lymphocytic mastitis and diabetic mastopathy: a molecular, immunophenotypic, and clinicopathologic evaluation of 11 cases. *Mod Pathol* 2003;16:223–228.
90. Brogi E, Harris N. Lymphomas of the breast: pathology and clinical behavior. *Semin Oncol* 1999;26:357–364.
91. Vizcaino I, Torregrosa A, Higueras V, et al. Metastasis to the breast from extramammary malignancies: a report of four cases and a review of literature. *Eur Radiol* 2001;11:1659–1665.
92. Duncan VE, Reddy VV, Jhala NC, et al. Non-Hodgkin's lymphoma of the breast: a review of 18 primary and secondary cases. *Ann Diagn Pathol* 2006;10:144–148.
93. Shulman LN, Hitt RA, Ferry JA. Case records of the Massachusetts General Hospital. Case 4-2008. A 33-year-old pregnant woman with swelling of the left breast and shortness of breath. *N Engl J Med* 2008;358:513–523.
94. Windrum P, Morris TC, Catherwood MA, et al. Mantle cell lymphoma presenting as a breast mass. *J Clin Pathol* 2001;54:883–886.
95. Vandenberghe G, Claerhout F, Amant F. Lymphoblastic lymphoma presenting as bilateral gigantomastia in pregnancy. *Int J Gynaecol Obstet* 2005;91:252–253.
96. Lima M, Goncalves C, Teixeira MA, et al. Aggressive natural-killer cell lymphoma presenting with skin lesions, breast nodule, suprarenal masses and life-threatening pericardial and pleural effusions. *Leuk Lymphoma* 2001;42:1385–1391.
97. Hayes DW, Bennett WA, Heck FJ. Extramedullary lesions in multiple myeloma; review of literature and pathologic studies. *AMA Arch Pathol* 1952;53:262–272.
98. Pasmantier MW, Azar HA. Extraskeletal spread in multiple plasma cell myeloma. A review of 57 autopsied cases. *Cancer* 1969;23:167–174.
99. Innes J, Newall J. Myelomatosis. *Lancet* 1961;1:239–245.
100. Pasquini E, Rinaldi P, Nicolini M, et al. Breast involvement in immunolymphoproliferative disorders: report of two cases of multiple myeloma of the breast. *Ann Oncol* 2000;11:1353–1359.
101. Ross JS, King TM, Spector JI, et al. Plasmacytoma of the breast. An unusual case of recurrent myeloma. *Arch Intern Med* 1987;147:1838–1840.
102. Kumar PV, Vasei M, Daneshbod Y, et al. Breast myeloma: a report of 3 cases with fine needle aspiration cytologic findings. *Acta Cytol* 2005;49:445–448.
103. Escobar PF, Patrick RJ, Hicks D, et al. Myeloma of the breast. *Breast J* 2006;12:387–388.
104. Daneshbod Y, Bagheri MH, Zakernia M, et al. Multiple myeloma recurrence presenting as bilateral breast masses. *Breast J* 2007;13:310–311.
105. Fayyaz A, Ghani UF. Multiple breast masses in a case of multiple myeloma. *J Coll Physicians Surg Pak* 2009;19:529–530.
106. Ben-Yehuda A, Steiner-Saltz D, Libson E, et al. Plasmacytoma of the breast. Unusual initial presentation of myeloma: report of two cases and review of the literature. *Blut* 1989;58:169–170.
107. McKenna R, Kyle R, Kuehl W, et al. Plasma cell neoplasms. In: Swerdlow S, Campo E, Harris N, et al., eds. *WHO classification tumours of haematopoietic and lymphoid tissues*. 4th ed. Lyon: World Health Organization-IARC; 2008:200–213.
108. Proctor NS, Rippey JJ, Shulman G, et al. Extramedullary plasmacytoma of the breast. *J Pathol* 1975;116:97–100.
109. De Chiara A, Losito S, Terracciano L, et al. Primary plasmacytoma of the breast. *Arch Pathol Lab Med* 2001;125:1078–1080.
110. Cao S, Kang HG, Liu YX, et al. Synchronous infiltrating ductal carcinoma and primary extramedullary plasmacytoma of the breast. *World J Surg Oncol* 2009;7:43.
111. Merino MJ. Plasmacytoma of the breast. *Arch Pathol Lab Med* 1984;108:676–678.
112. Alhan E, Calik A, Kucuktulu U, et al. Solitary extramedullary plasmocytoma of the breast with kappa monoclonal gammopathy. *Pathologica* 1995;87:71–73.
113. Kirshenbaum G, Rhone DP. Solitary extramedullary plasmacytoma of the breast with serum monoclonal protein: a case report and review of the literature. *Am J Clin Pathol* 1985;83:230–232.
114. Momiyama N, Ishikawa T, Doi T, et al. Extramedullary plasmacytoma of the breast with serum IgD monoclonal protein: a case report and review of the literature. *Breast Cancer* (Tokyo, Japan) 1999;6:217–221.
115. Pileri S, Orazi A, Falini B. Myeloid sarcoma In: Swerdlow S, Campo E, Harris N, et al., eds. *WHO classification tumours of haematopoietic and lymphoid tissues*. Lyon: World Health Organization-IARC; 2008:140–141.
116. Jelic-Puskaric B, Ostojic-Kolonic S, Planinc-Peraica A, et al. Myeloid sarcoma involving the breast. *Coll Antropol* 2010;34:641–644.
117. Azim HA Jr, Gigli F, Pruneri G, et al. Extramedullary myeloid sarcoma of the breast. *J Clin Oncol* 2008;26:4041–4043.
118. Valbuena JR, Admirand JH, Gualco G, et al. Myeloid sarcoma involving the breast. *Arch Pathol Lab Med* 2005;129:32–38.
119. Choschzick M, Bacher U, Ayuk F, et al. Immunohistochemistry and molecular analyses in myeloid sarcoma of the breast in a patient with relapse of NPM1-mutated and FLT3-mutated AML after allogeneic stem cell transplantation. *J Clin Pathol* 2010;63:558–561.
120. Lim HS, Park MH, Heo SH, et al. Myeloid sarcoma of the breast mimicking hamartoma on sonography. *J Ultrasound Med* 2008;27:1777–1780.
121. Toumeh A, Phinney R, Kobalka P, et al. Bilateral myeloid sarcoma of the breast and cerebrospinal fluid as a relapse of acute myeloid leukemia after stem-cell transplantation: a case report. *J Clin Oncol* 2012;30:e199–e201.
122. Wang J, Darvishian F. Extramedullary hematopoiesis in breast after neoadjuvant chemotherapy for breast carcinoma. *Ann Clin Lab Sci* 2006;36:475–478.
123. Millar EK, Inder S, Lynch J. Extramedullary haematopoiesis in axillary lymph nodes following neoadjuvant chemotherapy for locally advanced breast cancer—a potential diagnostic pitfall. *Histopathology* 2009;54:622–623.
124. Harbin LJ, Burnett S, Ghilchik M, et al. Extramedullary haematopoiesis in a hyalinized mammary fibroadenoma. *Histopathology* 2002;41:475–477.
125. Brooks JJ, Krugman DT, Damjanov I. Myeloid metaplasia presenting as a breast mass. *Am J Surg Pathol* 1980;4:281–285.
126. Glew RH, Haese WH, McIntyre PA. Myeloid metaplasia with myelofibrosis. The clinical spectrum of extramedullary hematopoiesis and tumor formation. *Johns Hopkins Med J* 1973;132:253–270.
127. Martinelli G, Santini D, Bazzocchi F, et al. Myeloid metaplasia of the breast. A lesion which clinically mimics carcinoma. *Virchows Arch A Pathol Anat Histopathol* 1983;401:203–207.

128. Zonderland HM, Michiels JJ, ten Kate FJ. Case report: mammographic and sonographic demonstration of extramedullary haematopoiesis of the breast. *Clin Radiol* 1991;44:64–65.
129. Cufer T, Bracko M. Myeloid metaplasia of the breast. *Ann Oncol* 2001;12:267–270.
130. Al-Nafussi A, Al-Okati D, Alsewan M. Extramedullary haematopoietic tumour of the breast: a case report in a woman with secondary myelofibrosis following essential thrombocythaemia. *Histopathology* 2004;44:625–626.
131. Green I, Dorfman RF, Rosai J. Breast involvement by extranodal Rosai-Dorfman disease: report of seven cases. *Am J Surg Pathol* 1997;21:664–668.
132. Morkowski JJ, Nguyen CV, Lin P, et al. Rosai-Dorfman disease confined to the breast. *Ann Diagn Pathol* 2010;14:81–87.
133. Bansal P, Chakraborti S, Krishnanand G, et al. Rosai-Dorfman disease of the breast in a male: a case report. *Acta Cytol* 2010;54:349–352.
134. Wu YC, Hsieh TC, Kao CH, et al. A mimic of breast lymphoma: extranodal Rosai-Dorfman disease. *Am J Med Sci* 2010;339:282–284.
135. Baladandapani P, Hu Y, Kapoor K, et al. Rosai-Dorfman disease presenting as multiple breast masses in an otherwise asymptomatic male patient. *Clin Radiol* 2012;67:393–395.
136. Tenny SO, McGinness M, Zhang D, et al. Rosai-Dorfman disease presenting as a breast mass and enlarged axillary lymph node mimicking malignancy: a case report and review of the literature. *Breast J* 2011;17:516–520.
137. Gwin K, Cipriani N, Zhang X, et al. Bilateral breast involvement by disseminated extranodal Rosai-Dorfman disease. *Breast J* 2011;17:309–311.
138. Provenzano E, Barter SJ, Wright PA, et al. Erdheim-chester disease presenting as bilateral clinically malignant breast masses. *Am J Surg Pathol* 2010;34:584–588.
139. Jaffe E, Weiss L, Facchetti F. Tumours derived from Langerhans cells. In: Swerdlow S, Campo E, Harris N, et al., eds. *WHO classification of tumours of haematopoietic and lymphoid tissues*. 4th ed. Lyon: World Health Organization-IARC; 2008:358–360.
140. Ansari B, Purdie CA, Brown DC. Adult Langerhans cell histiocytosis mimicking Paget's disease of the nipple. *Breast J* 2005;11:281–282.
141. Adu-Poku K, Thomas DW, Khan MK, et al. Langerhans cell histiocytosis in sequential discordant lymphoma. *J Clin Pathol* 2005; 58:104–106.
142. Fong D, Lann MA, Finlayson C, et al. Diabetic (lymphocytic) mastopathy with exuberant lymphohistiocytic and granulomatous response: a case report with review of the literature. *Am J Surg Pathol* 2006;30:1330–1336.
143. Tan PH, Harada O, Thike AA, et al. Histiocytoid breast carcinoma: an enigmatic lobular entity. *J Clin Pathol* 2011;64:654–659.

CHAPTER 41

Pathologic Effects of Therapy

ELENA BRACHTEL • FREDERICK C. KOERNER

RADIATION

Radiation and Hodgkin Lymphoma

The breasts may be exposed secondarily to radiation during multiple diagnostic procedures such as mammography and fluoroscopy,[1] or in the course of radiotherapy administered to another organ, such as mediastinal radiotherapy for Hodgkin lymphoma.[2–5] The radiation exposure in these situations has been associated with an increased risk of the subsequent development of breast carcinoma.[2,6–9] Wendland et al.[10] reported that the standard incidence ratio (SIR) of breast carcinoma among Hodgkin lymphoma patients who received radiotherapy was 3.17, with a 95% confidence interval (CI) of 2.66 to 3.79 when compared to the general population. The SIR of breast carcinoma in irradiated female Hodgkin lymphoma patients compared to nonirradiated patients was 1.90. In the same study, the SIR of breast carcinoma in nonradiated Hodgkin lymphoma patients when compared to the general population was also elevated (1.67; 95% CI, 1.24 to 2.20). Each of these differences was statistically significant, indicating that women treated for Hodgkin lymphoma have an elevated risk of breast carcinoma that is enhanced in irradiated women.

In one study, the relative risk (RR) of developing breast carcinoma in women irradiated for Hodgkin lymphoma before the age of 15 years was 136 (95% CI, 34 to 371) compared to the general population, whereas among those treated at ages 15 to 19, 20 to 24, and 25 to 29 years, the RRs were 19, 19, and 7.3, respectively.[11] Swerdlow et al.[9] reported a very high SIR of breast carcinoma in patients treated at the age of 14 years (47.2), with 95% CI of 28.0 to 79.8. These results suggest greater susceptibility to breast carcinoma when radiation exposure is near puberty. Others reported the cumulative probability of developing breast carcinoma to be 35% by age 40 (95% CI, 17.4 to 52.6).[3] Another study of women with Hodgkin lymphoma treated before age 21 found an RR of 26.2 (95% CI, 15.0 to 42.6) with a 20-year actuarial risk of 9.2%.[12]

Estimates of radiation dosage to the breasts during the treatment of Hodgkin lymphoma indicate that the exposure is at a potentially carcinogenic level.[13,14] Kowalski and Smith[15] studied the distribution of radiation with an anthropomorphic phantom. Some regions of the breast in the treatment fields had more than 70% of the prescribed dose, whereas blocked regions received 2% to 29% of the prescribed dose. Newer approaches to irradiation for Hodgkin lymphoma with mediastinal involvement utilize lower doses than the traditional mantle field irradiation (35 to 45 Gy) and more targeted irradiation. These techniques result in reduced exposure of other organs.[16,17]

Most studies report breast carcinoma after irradiation for Hodgkin lymphoma in women, but in rare instances breast carcinoma may also occur in men. The first author has studied one case in which breast carcinoma developed in a 55-year-old man who had undergone irradiation for Hodgkin lymphoma at the age of 12 years. His mother also developed carcinoma of the breast at the age of 50 years, and other members of the family suffered from carcinomas of other organs.

Data from the studies by Cutuli et al.[18–20] included 189 patients who developed a total of 214 breast carcinomas after radiotherapy for Hodgkin lymphoma. The median age at diagnosis of Hodgkin lymphoma was 25 years. The median age at diagnosis of breast carcinoma was 42 years, with a median interval of 18.6 years. The frequency of bilaterality was 13.2%; most contralateral tumors were metachronous. Axillary lymph node (ALN) metastases occurred in 32% of the invasive carcinomas for which axillary dissection was performed.

Patients who received supradiaphragmatic radiotherapy for the treatment of Hodgkin lymphoma are candidates for surveillance for the early detection of breast carcinoma. Mammography is reported to have high sensitivity for detecting carcinomas in the breast of women irradiated for Hodgkin lymphoma, especially when calcifications are present.[21–24] Ultrasonography may be employed as an adjunct to mammography, but one cannot rely on this technique as a primary screening modality because of a relatively high frequency of false-positive findings.[25] Magnetic resonance imaging (MRI) is effective for detecting tumor-forming, largely invasive carcinomas in women with genetic and other high-risk predispositions to breast carcinoma, but it has less sensitivity than mammography for detecting ductal carcinoma *in situ* (DCIS).[26,27] On this basis, MRI has been shown to be useful for screening irradiated Hodgkin lymphoma patients.[28]

No structural changes attributable to the level of radiation exposure after treatment for Hodgkin lymphoma are evident when the mammary glandular tissue is examined histopathologically. Except for a trend to less desmoplastic reaction in carcinomas that arose in irradiated women, Dvoretsky et al.[29] found no histologic difference between tumors in women previously irradiated for postpartum mastitis and a control group. Carcinomas in patients treated for Hodgkin lymphoma tend to be poorly differentiated, but in other respects they are not significantly different pathologically from tumors in women without prior irradiation.[5,30] Nearly all carcinomas have been ductal, with very rare examples of infiltrating lobular and special types such as mucinous carcinoma.[19,20] Approximately 15% of the carcinomas are DCIS. The carcinomas are more likely to be bilateral, and both synchronous and metachronous bilateral carcinomas have been reported.[20,23,31]

Mastectomy is still performed more often than lumpectomy for the primary surgical treatment of breast carcinoma that develops after Hodgkin lymphoma treated with radiotherapy, although these breast carcinomas are now more likely to be detected at a lower stage.[30,32] Deutsch et al.[33] described 12 patients successfully treated with lumpectomy and radiation with "good to excellent cosmetic results" and "no significant acute adverse reactions and no late sequelae" after a median follow-up of 46 months.

Radiation and Breast Conservation Therapy

Radiation of the breast as a component of breast conservation treatment for mammary carcinoma is usually performed after surgery to decrease the risk of ipsilateral recurrence.[34] Conventional irradiation protocols involve levels of exposure of 45 to 50 Gy often with a boost of 10 to 16 Gy to the site of the excision.[35] In selected cases of early-stage breast carcinoma, partial breast irradiation (PBI) is currently performed in some centers for selected patients who meet the eligibility recommendations set out by the American Society for Radiation Oncology.[36,37]

Long-term clinical effects of therapeutic mammary radiation on the normal breast evolve over a period of months to years,[38] and the extent to which these occur varies among individuals. Some women ultimately exhibit diffuse increased firmness or sclerosis of the breast, but in the majority this is mild and the tissue remains elastic. Ptosis, a natural change of aging, is less pronounced in the irradiated breast. Cutaneous atrophy and telangiectasia are likely to be more conspicuous in areas that received a radiation boost.[38,39] The irradiated breast is usually unable to lactate but the untreated breast is unaffected.[40,41] Radiation can be delivered effectively to the breast containing an implant, although there may be a tendency for more frequent fibrous encapsulation of the prosthesis or for infection to occur.[42,43] The adverse clinical effects of radiation may be more severe in patients who have a collagen vascular disease such as scleroderma, systemic lupus erythematosus, or other related conditions.[44,45]

After breast-conserving treatment for breast carcinoma, patients are screened following national guidelines for ipsi- or contralateral recurrence. Imaging of the operated and irradiated breast poses challenges and is considered less sensitive for the detection of abnormalities than imaging of the the untreated breast. However, common benign post-treatment changes such as fat necrosis, parenchymal distortion, and scarring often can be distinguished from recurrence radiographically.[46,47] MRI studies, in which focal enhancement of the treated breast is expected, are of limited use in the immediate post-treatment period. This modality shows high sensitivity and specificity when used to distinguish scar tissue from tumor recurrence at least 12 months after the last intervention in the breast.[47–49]

Coarse, scattered benign-appearing calcifications may be found in 25% of irradiated breasts, and these are generally of little concern.[50] On the other hand, new, clustered pleomorphic calcifications present a significant problem.[51] Calcified sutures in the biopsy site may mimic the pattern of calcifications associated with carcinoma, although rarely suture calcifications have a distinctive knotted configuration.[52] Fat necrosis, which often has a stellate configuration and may contain calcifications, is often recognized as such radiologically.[53,54] Localized, encapsulated fat necrosis with a cystic appearance has been described at the site of iridium implantation[50] (Fig. 41.1). Other forms of brachytherapy or intraoperative radiation are also associated with increased fat necrosis.[55,56] Occasionally, fat necrosis causes an enhancing lesion on MRI in the area of the scar that is not easily distinguishable from recurrent tumor.

Cases exhibiting a new mass, a suspicious area of enhancement on MRI, a change in an existing postoperative scar, or the appearance of new, pleomorphic calcifications warrant a biopsy to exclude recurrence of the carcinoma. Early detection of a local recurrence has been shown to be associated with improved long-term outcome.[57] Recurrences that may present as invasive or *in situ* carcinoma most often occur

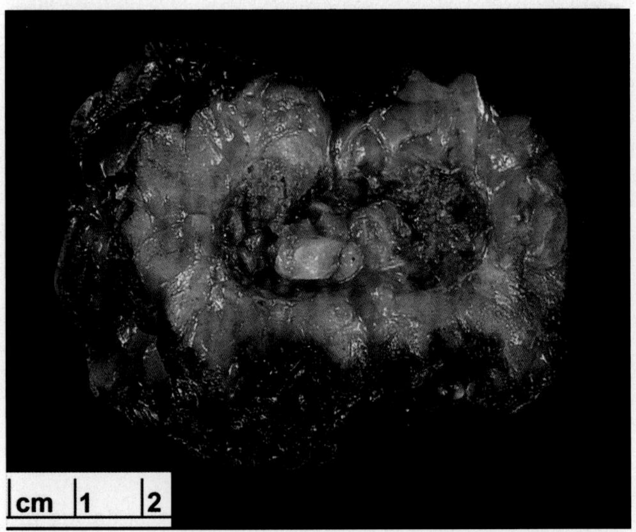

FIG. 41.1. ***Radiation-induced fat necrosis.*** Cystic fat necrosis at the site of prior interstitial and external beam radiation therapy after lumpectomy for invasive ductal carcinoma.

2 to 6 years after completion of breast-conserving treatment and are typically located close to the site of prior operation. Carcinomas that develop more than 10 years following treatment and those that arise distant from the scar more likely represent new primary carcinomas.[46]

The risk of second malignant neoplasms that develop after radiotherapy as part of breast conservation therapy was studied by Obedian et al.[58] The authors compared the outcomes of 1,029 patients treated by lumpectomy with radiation (LRT) and 1,387 patients treated by mastectomy (MAST). The median follow-up was 14.6 and 16 years, respectively. The risk of contralateral carcinoma was 10% in both cohorts. For women 45 years or younger at the time of treatment, the risks of contralateral carcinoma were not significantly different (LRT, 10%; MAST, 7%) after 15 years of follow-up. The frequency of contralateral carcinoma was lower in women who received adjuvant hormonal therapy, but the difference was not statistically significant. During an interval of 15 years, nonmammary malignant neoplasms were diagnosed in 11% of LRT patients and 10% of MAST patients. The risk of lung carcinoma was higher among smokers than among nonsmokers who received radiotherapy ($p = 0.06$). Radiotherapy for breast carcinoma has also been associated with a significantly increased RR of carcinoma of the esophagus and lung.[59,60] A small increased risk of acute myeloid leukemia after locoregional radiation for breast carcinoma was enhanced by chemotherapy.[61] However, the overall incidence of such neoplasms appears to be low, with about 160 cases observed in a cohort of 33,763 women with breast carcinoma who had radiotherapy.[59] The relationship of breast irradiation to the development of angiosarcoma is discussed in Chapter 39.

Microscopic Pathology

Radiation-induced histologic changes in benign breast tissue must be distinguished from recurrent carcinoma in the interpretation of a post-treatment biopsy specimen. When compared to a pre-radiation specimen, the major changes in normal breast are apparent in terminal duct–lobular units[50,62,63] (Figs. 41.2 and 41.3). These include collagenization of intralobular stroma; thickening of periacinar and periductular basement membranes; severe atrophy of acinar and ductular epithelium; cytologic atypia of residual epithelial cells; and relatively prominent acinar myoepithelial cells, which seem to be preserved to a greater extent than the epithelial cells. In a minority of specimens, one may also find atypical fibroblasts in the interlobular stroma (Fig. 41.4). Apocrine epithelium is susceptible to developing severe cytologic atypia after therapeutic radiotherapy, especially in

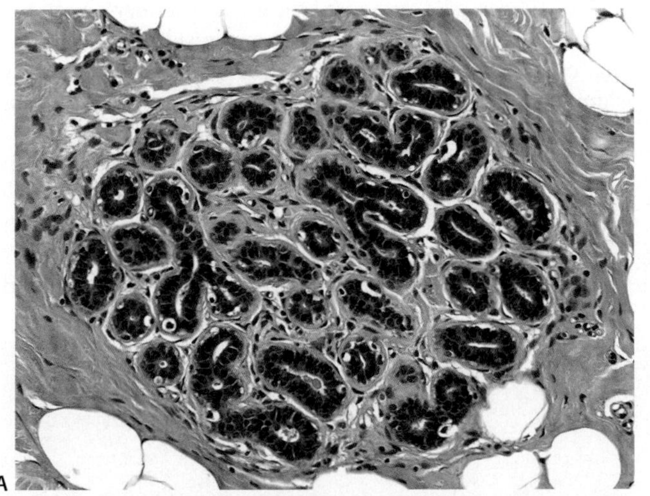

A

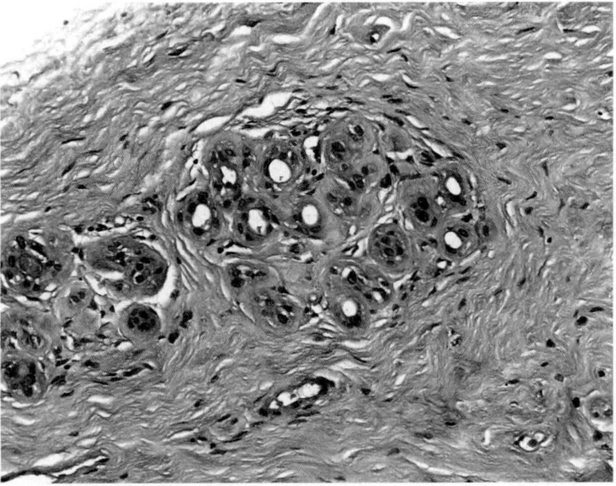

B

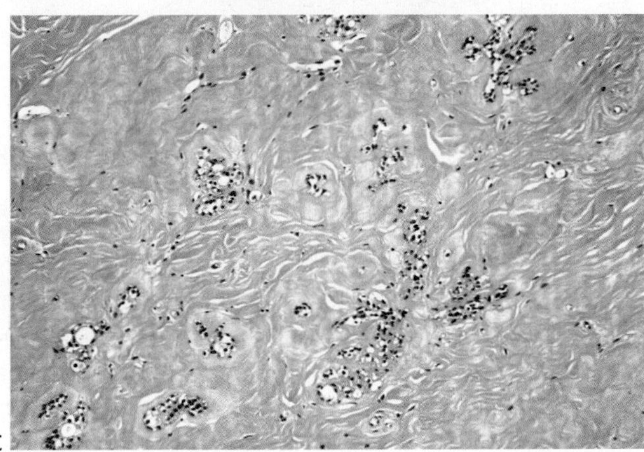

C

FIG. 41.2. ***Radiation effect in normal breast.*** **A:** A normal lobule from a 47-year-old woman prior to irradiation. **B:** A lobule from the same patient 18 months after treatment exhibits epithelial atrophy, thickening of basement membranes, and intralobular sclerosis. **C:** Marked lobular atrophy in a 40-year-old woman after irradiation.

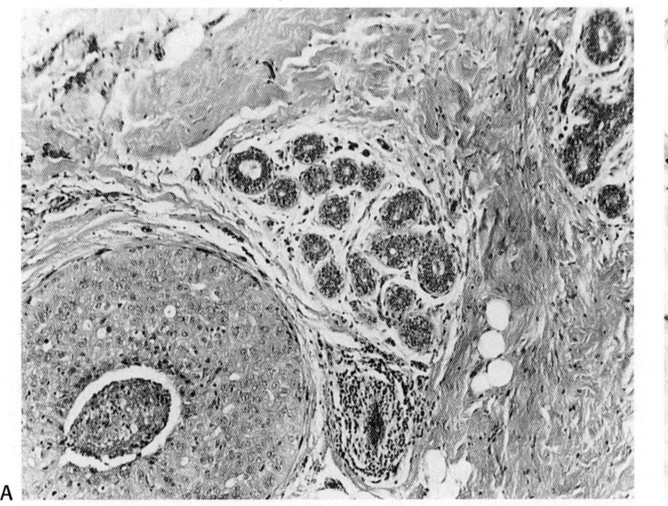

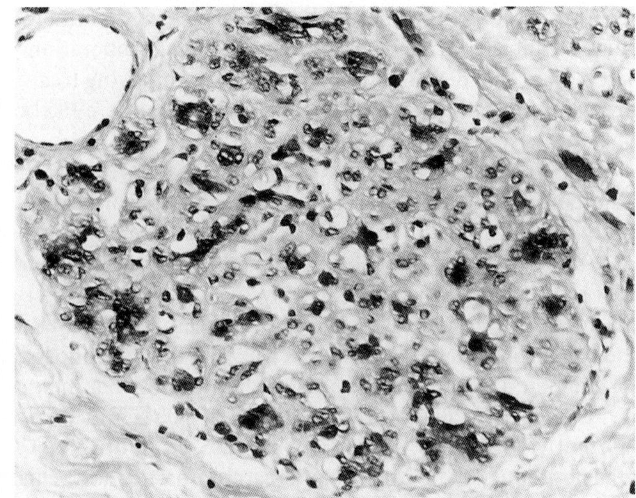

FIG. 41.3. ***Radiation effect in normal breast.*** **A:** DCIS and adjacent normal lobules in a 37-year-old woman. **B:** A lobule from the same patient after external beam radiotherapy exhibits epithelial atrophy and intralobular sclerosis. Persisting epithelial nuclei are hyperchromatic and pleomorphic.

hyperplastic foci. When evaluating a post-treatment biopsy sample, it is useful to examine the pre-treatment specimen for evidence of apocrine metaplasia. Knowledge that apocrine metaplasia was present in the pre-treatment specimen can be helpful in correctly interpreting the post-treatment biopsy with radiation atypia in apocrine metaplasia.

Generally, the effects on the larger ducts appear less pronounced than those in lobules (Fig. 41.5). Substantial variation in the severity of changes in the lobules can be observed from one patient to another, and on occasion the changes may be so slight as to be virtually indistinguishable from physiologic atrophy. In any one patient, most of the glandular tissue responds in a uniform fashion if the entire breast has been irradiated. Extreme variation in different parts of the breast is not commonplace. In one study, differences in radiation effects between individual patients were not correlated with radiation dose, patient age, post-treatment interval, or the use of adjuvant chemotherapy.[62]

Moore et al.[63] studied 120 breast specimens obtained at various intervals (less than 1 year to more than 6 years) after radiotherapy. They observed statistically significant differences between pre- and post-treatment specimens, with the latter showing pathologic alterations resulting from irradiation. However, radiation-induced changes did not vary significantly in the time intervals, indicating absence of regression.

When studied *in vitro*, atypical fibroblasts isolated from irradiated human mammary stroma expressed oncofetal fibronectin and an α-actin isoform specific for smooth muscle cells indicative of myofibroblastic differentiation.[64] A study of benign breast tissue samples obtained before and

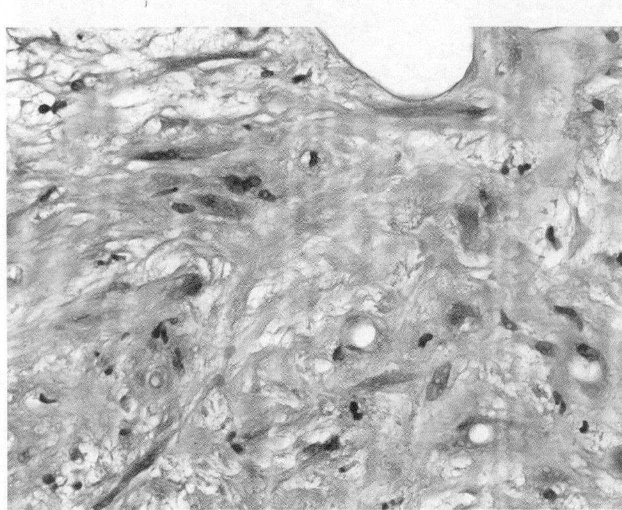

FIG. 41.4. ***Radiation atypia in stromal fibroblasts.***

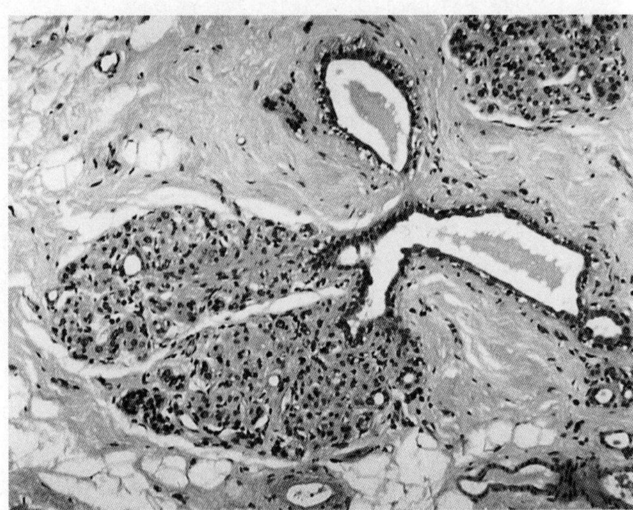

FIG. 41.5. ***Duct and lobule in irradiated breast.*** In contrast to lobular sclerosis, the duct in this post-irradiation breast appears unaffected

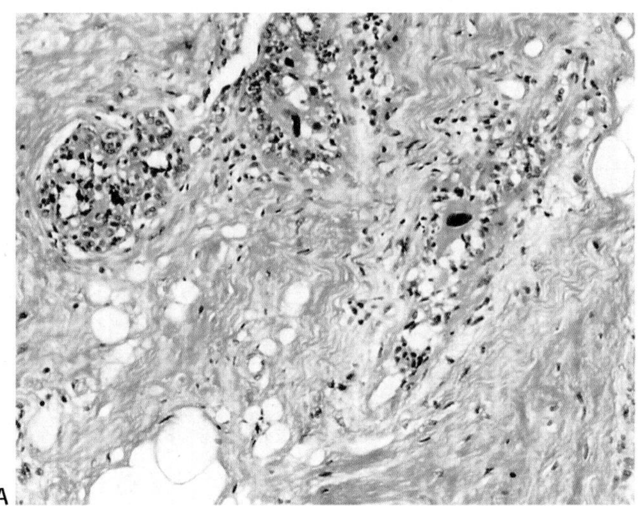

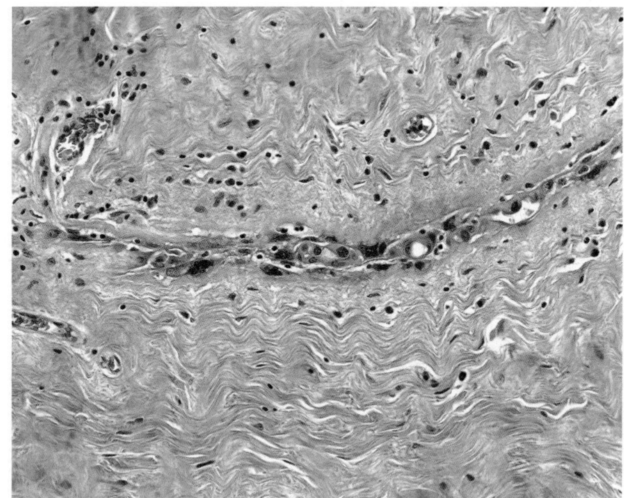

FIG. 41.6. ***Radiation atypia in ducts.*** **A:** Epithelial atrophy is evident. Note large atypical cells. **B:** Luminal cells lining the ducts have pleomorphic, large, irregular nuclei.

after adjuvant radiotherapy for breast carcinoma revealed increased immunohistochemical expression of p53 and increased proliferative activity assessed by Ki67 expression as long as 10 years after radiotherapy.[65]

When a radioactive implant or external boost has been used to give more intense treatment to the biopsy site, histologic changes in this area may be more severe than those in the surrounding breast. Fat necrosis and atypia of stromal fibroblasts are more common in proximity to such "boosted" or implanted areas.[50,55,56] Radiation-induced vascular changes are not ordinarily seen after external beam radiotherapy, but they may occur when a boost dose has been delivered. Cytologic and architectural indications of radiation effect in larger blood vessels include fragmentation of elastica, endothelial atypia, and myointimal proliferation that leads to vascular sclerosis. Prominent, cytologically atypical endothelial cells are also apparent in capillaries. In boosted areas, epithelial atypia may occur in the larger ducts of the breast and it may even be superimposed on existing hyperplasia (Fig. 41.6) or apocrine metaplasia (Fig. 41.7).

Cytologic atypia can create diagnostic problems, even if one is aware of the typical appearance of radiation-induced atrophy of the breast.[66–68] False-positive fine-needle aspiration (FNA) cytology diagnoses have been attributed to radiation atypia.[69] In one series, the diagnostic yield with incisional or needle core biopsy was considerably higher than with aspiration cytology.[70] The aspirate from a breast with radiation changes alone tends to be sparsely cellular because of treatment-induced atrophy. Filomena et al.[71] reported that all carcinomas recurrent in irradiated breasts that were diagnosed by FNA had at least 5 epithelial cell clusters and more than 15 single epithelial cells

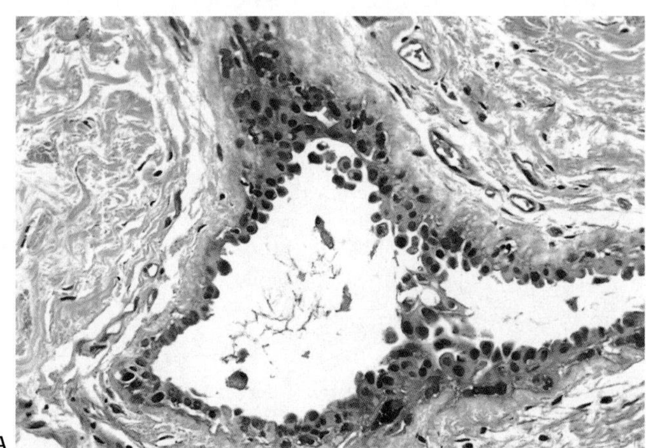

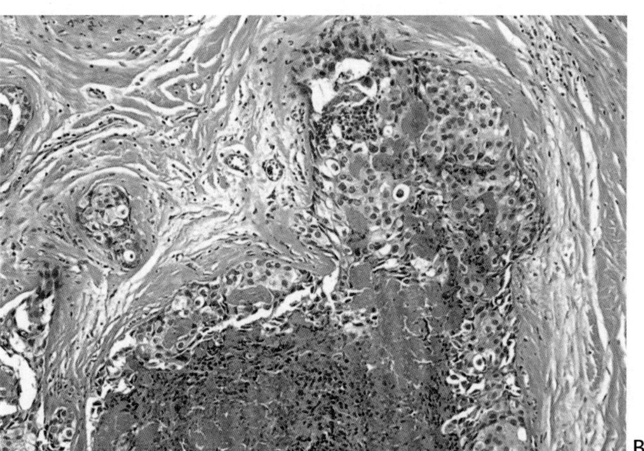

FIG. 41.7. ***Radiation atypia in duct with apocrine metaplasia.*** **A:** Epithelial nuclei are enlarged and hyperchromatic. Images **(B–D)** are from the same patient. **B:** In 1994, the patient underwent breast-conserving surgery and radiotherapy for DCIS shown here. **C:** Coincidental with DCIS in 1994, the breast also had foci of apocrine metaplasia shown here in a lobule. **D:** Biopsy performed in 1998 showed apocrine metaplasia with cytologic atypia. There was no recurrent carcinoma.

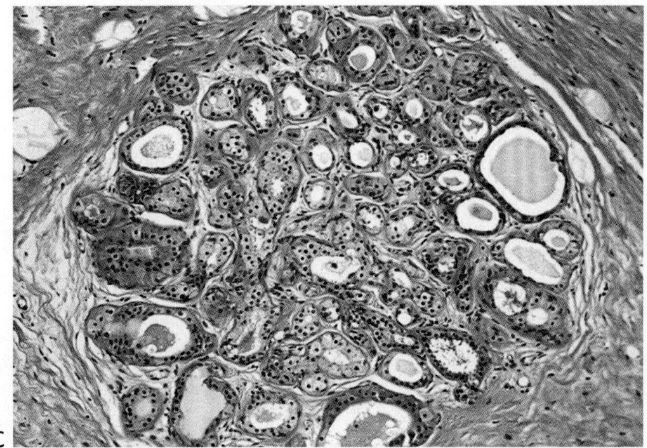

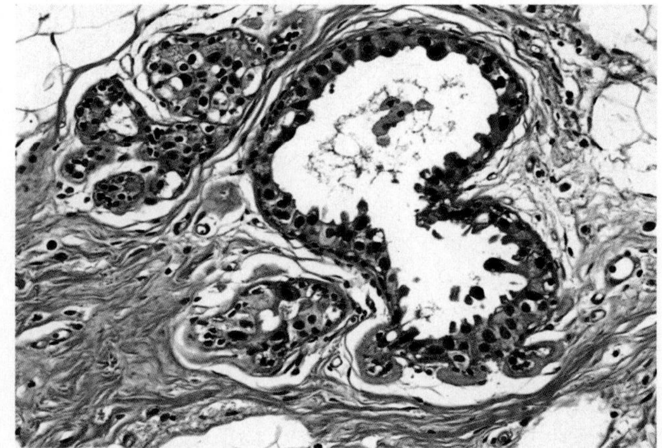

FIG. 41.7. *(Continued)*

on the slides. Usually, there were two diagnostic slides per case. Cytologic features of benign irradiated epithelial cells were frequently very atypical and usually displayed nuclear enlargement, increase in the nuclear-to-cytoplasmic ratio, and prominence of the nucleoli. Loss of cohesion, irregularity of the nuclear borders, and necrosis are features associated with carcinoma.[72] Although core biopsy has replaced FNA biopsy in many settings,[73] the difficulties distinguishing the cytologic alterations produced by irradiation from the cellular atypia of irradiated carcinoma and tumor recurrence are also encountered in these samples.

In situ lobular and ductal carcinomas persisting after radiation therapy are largely intact; consequently, the affected lobules and ducts appear filled and, often, expanded with the neoplastic population. In one study,[74] the grade of recurrent DCIS was the same as the pre-treatment lesion in 95 (84%) of 113 cases. Frequently, little or no microscopic change attributable to treatment is evident when pre- and postradiation samples of *in situ* carcinoma are compared (Figs. 41.8 and 41.9). Greater cytologic atypia after treatment is encountered in a minority of cases. Comparison with the histologic appearance of the tumor and noncancerous tissue prior to treatment is necessary in difficult cases.

In a study of invasive breast recurrences after conservation therapy with radiotherapy in women 40 years or younger at diagnosis, Sigal-Zafrani et al.[75] found no significant differences in histologic type, grade, and hormone receptor expression between primary and recurrent tumors. New carcinomas that arose outside the index quadrant were more likely to differ from the initial primary tumor than

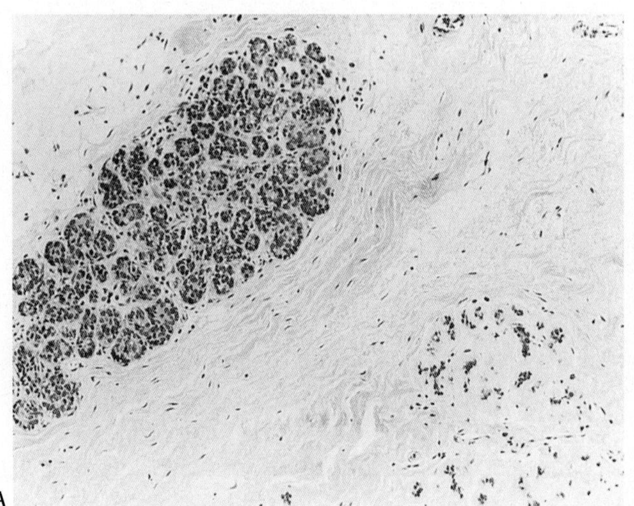

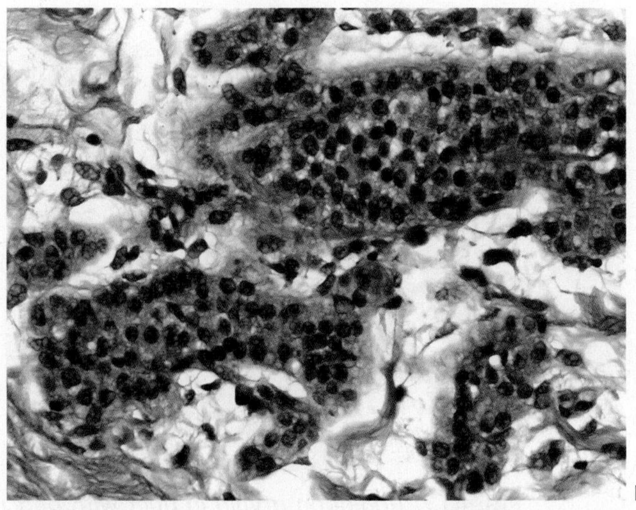

FIG. 41.8. ***Lobular carcinoma in situ after radiation therapy.*** **A:** The *in situ* carcinoma appears unaffected by the treatment. A lobule not involved by carcinoma showing radiation atrophy is present in the *lower right* corner. **B:** Irradiation has not affected the lobular carcinoma *in situ* in another case.

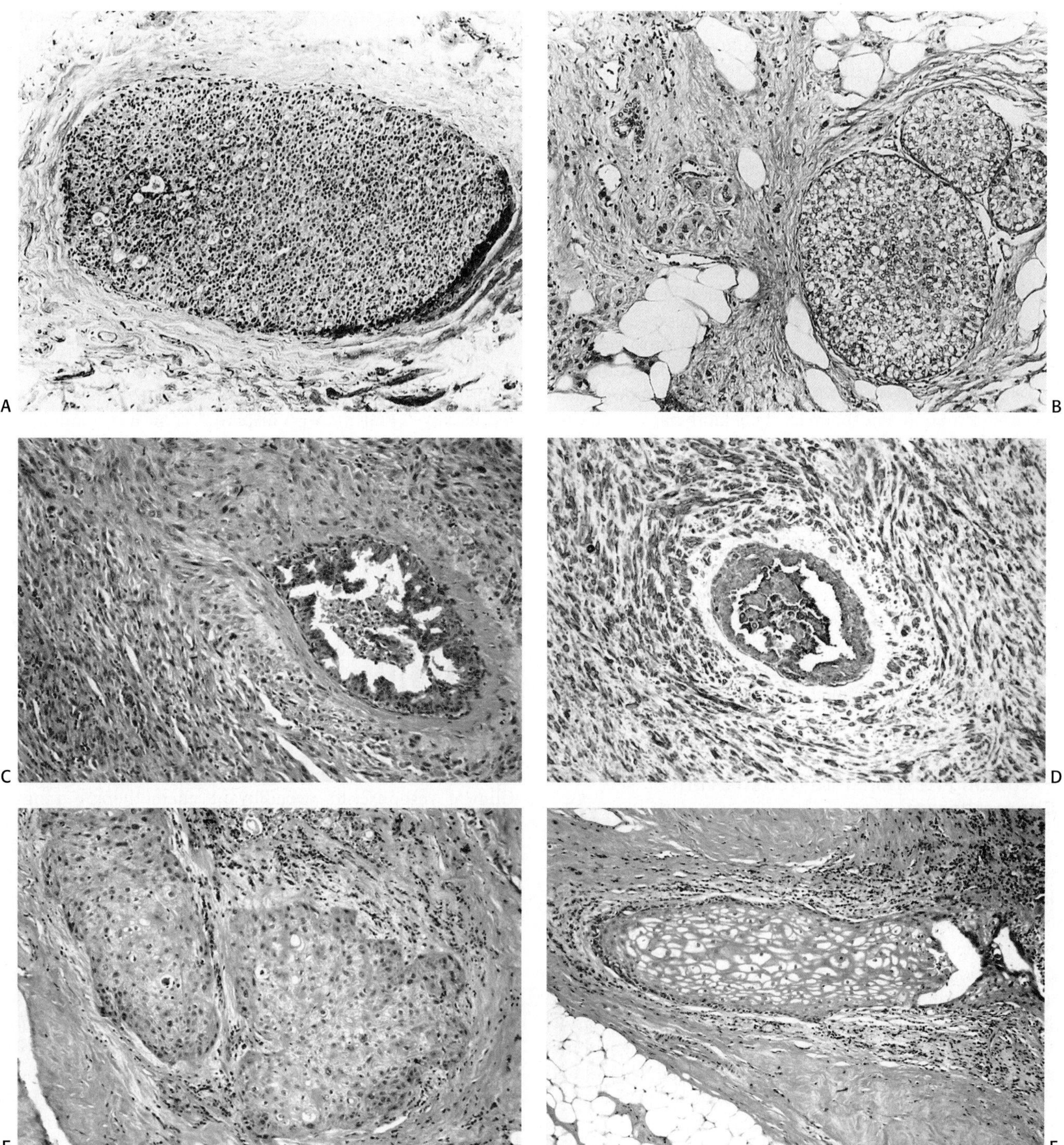

FIG. 41.9. ***Radiation effect in DCIS.*** **A:** DCIS prior to radiotherapy. **B:** Recurrent carcinoma in the same patient 2 years after treatment. The DCIS closely resembles the pre-treatment lesion. Invasive carcinoma is present on the *left*. **C–F:** After a lumpectomy with negative margins for DCIS, this patient was treated with radiotherapy. Three years later she developed recurrent DCIS similar to the original lesion, which was accompanied by invasive spindle cell metaplastic carcinoma **(C)**. CK7 immunoreactivity is demonstrated in the spindle cell carcinoma **(D)**. Intraductal squamous carcinoma was also present **(E,F)**.

were recurrences in the same quadrant. From time to time, irradiated invasive carcinoma cells contain multiple hyperchromatic nuclei, or there is focal necrosis that was not seen in the pre-treatment biopsy. These findings suggest that the cells represent residual carcinoma showing radiation effects. The relationship of breast irradiation to the development of angiosarcoma is discussed in Chapter 39.

NEOADJUVANT CHEMOTHERAPY

Neoadjuvant chemotherapy refers to chemotherapy administered before surgery; adjuvant chemotherapy, in contrast, refers to chemotherapy administered after surgery. Longitudinal studies such as the National Surgical Adjuvant Breast and Bowel Project (NSABP) B18 and B27 showed that the long-term outcome is similar if chemotherapy is administered before or after surgery and established the equal value of systemic treatment irrespective of its pre- or postsurgical application.[76] In earlier times, neoadjuvant chemotherapy was given predominantly for locally advanced breast carcinomas in an effort to reduce the size of the tumor and thereby to allow complete excision.[77] The indication for neoadjuvant chemotherapy has broadened in the recent decade to include its use in the treatment of earlier stages of breast carcinoma.[78] The excision or mastectomy specimen after neoadjuvant chemotherapy displays a range of histologic changes in both the residual carcinoma and benign mammary tissue.[79]

Predicting Response to Neoadjuvant Chemotherapy

Most of the current chemotherapy regimens use a combination of cytotoxic agents, which include anthracyclines and taxanes, often in combination with fluoropyrimidines and cyclophosphamide.[78,80] One cannot attribute specific histologic responses to the use of any of these cytotoxic drug combinations except that successful treatment means disappearance of tumor cells by histopathologic evaluation (pathologic complete response, pCR). With the arrival of targeted treatments, nomograms or prediction algorithms are used to match a breast carcinoma subtype determined from the pre-treatment core biopsy specimen with the most promising combination of cytotoxic agents.

In specific treatment protocols, it is possible to develop nomograms based on factors such as histologic grade, hormone receptor status, clinical stage, and treatment cycles for predicting the likelihood of achieving a complete pathologic response.[81] Neoadjuvant chemotherapy for a human epidermal growth factor 2 (HER2)-amplified carcinoma, for example, may include targeted anti-HER2 treatment, for which a high rate of complete response has been reported.[82] A high response rate to neoadjuvant chemotherapy also characterizes a proportion of triple negative breast carcinomas, those that do not express estrogen receptor (ER), progesterone receptor (PR), or HER2.[83] A subset of triple negative breast carcinomas also responded well to chemotherapeutic agents containing cisplatinum that are not routinely utilized in breast carcinoma treatment.[84] On the other hand, there is evidence that invasive lobular carcinomas, which are mostly ER positive, rarely have a complete pathologic response to neoadjuvant chemotherapy.[85] High-grade tumors were shown to respond better to neoadjuvant chemotherapy in the NSABP B18 cohort.[86] Pu et al.[87] investigated the use of pathologic features for predicting a complete pathologic response to neoadjuvant chemotherapy in a pre-treatment needle core biopsy specimen. Among complete responders, 80% had tumor necrosis in the core biopsy sample, whereas necrosis was found in only 17% of nonresponders.

A study of patients with primary operable breast carcinoma staged as T2 to T4, N0 or N1, and M0 employed needle core biopsy sampling to investigate the relationship of proliferative markers to response to neoadjuvant chemotherapy.[88] Patients who displayed clinical or pathologic response to treatment or who were nonresponders did not have significant differences in median Ki67 and apoptotic indices determined on samples taken before, during, and at the end of treatment. In this study, Ki67 and apoptotic indices were not predictive of response to the neoadjuvant chemotherapy. When stratified according to molecular breast carcinoma subtypes, a greater reduction of Ki67 rate after neoadjuvant chemotherapy was observed in HER2-positive and triple-negative breast carcinomas when compared to hormone receptor–positive breast carcinomas.[89]

Clinical Assessment of Chemotherapy Response

Clinical response to neoadjuvant chemotherapy ranges from complete disappearance of a previously palpable mass to unchanged size or even continued growth of a mass.[86] The greatest histopathologic alterations are usually found in patients who appear to have complete resolution of their neoplasm by clinical examination.[90,91] However, it is not unusual to observe dissociation between the clinical picture after therapy and the histologic findings, for example, when the patient seems to have had a complete clinical response but histologic examination of the breast reveals residual carcinoma, or the patient presents with a residual palpable mass in which there is no histologic evidence of residual carcinoma.[92] In the study of 43 patients from the NSABP B18 cohort reported by Sharkey et al.,[93] only about 50% of the tumors had histopathologic changes of treatment effect.

Mammography may suggest a response in patients treated with neoadjuvant chemotherapy, but this procedure is not reliable for predicting the pathologic status of the breast. Vinnicombe et al.[94] reported that five of eight patients judged by mammography to have a complete response had residual carcinoma pathologically. Mammographically detected calcifications associated with the carcinoma may increase or decrease in number or remain unchanged after neoadjuvant chemotherapy.[95] MRI is reported to be a more effective method than mammography for detecting residual carcinoma in the breast after neoadjuvant chemotherapy.[96] Yeh et al.[97] reported that agreement as to the quality of postchemotherapy response when compared to pathology findings was 19%, 26%, 35%, and 71% for clinical examination, mammography, sonography, and MRI, respectively. Positron emission tomography (PET) appears to be a specific but less sensitive method for identifying patients with complete pathologic responses early in the course of chemotherapy treatment.[98] Placement of a clip at the tumor site is necessary as a guide for following tumor regression radiographically and for locating the position of a tumor after complete regression.[79,99]

Histopathologic Assessment of Chemotherapy Response

The histologic effects of chemotherapy are most easily appreciated by comparing samples taken before and after treatment. The fundamental manifestation of treatment effect is a decrease in tumor cellularity accompanied by chronic inflammation, histiocyte accumulation, and stromal fibrosis and elastosis (Fig. 41.10). Rajan et al.[100] observed a decrease in median tumor cellularity from 40% in pre-treatment core biopsies to 10% in tumors resected after neoadjuvant chemotherapy. There was considerable variation in changes in cellularity among clinical response categories. Many tumors appeared to have a pronounced decrease in cellularity but only minimal reduction in size. Ogston et al.[101] compared breast tumor cellularity pre- and post-neoadjuvant chemotherapy and correlated the post-treatment tumor cellularity with long-term survival.

In the most favorable situation, no residual carcinoma may be detectable, an occurrence reported in 6.7%[91] and 13%[102] of cases in cohorts with mixed subtypes of carcinoma. Breast carcinoma cohorts that are enriched for certain subtypes and treatments can show much higher rates of pathologic complete response. For example, the pCR rate of HER2-positive breast carcinomas treated with trastuzumab and chemotherapy was 65% in the study by Buzdar et al.[82] Definitions of pathologic complete response vary between studies.[80] The NSABP trials distinguished between the absence (pCR) and the presence of residual invasive carcinoma (pINV) in the breast and noted that long-term outcome also depends on the extent of lymph node involvement.[92] Residual DCIS in the absence of invasive carcinoma is typically included in the prognostically favorable group of pCR. Several pathologic response algorithms require the absence of not only invasive tumor in the breast but also carcinoma in the lymph nodes to classify a response as pCR.[103,104]

If the breast of a patient who has a complete histologic and clinical response is examined histologically soon after treatment, residual degenerated and infarcted necrotic invasive carcinoma may be recognized by the loss of normal staining properties and decreased architectural detail. With the passage of time, the degenerated invasive carcinoma is absorbed. Healed sites of previous infiltrating carcinoma

A

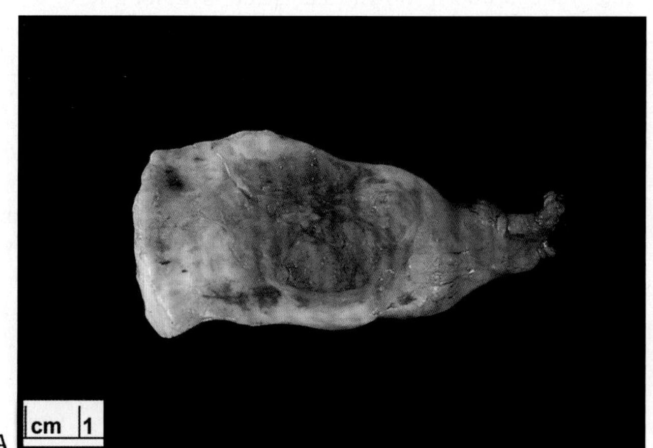

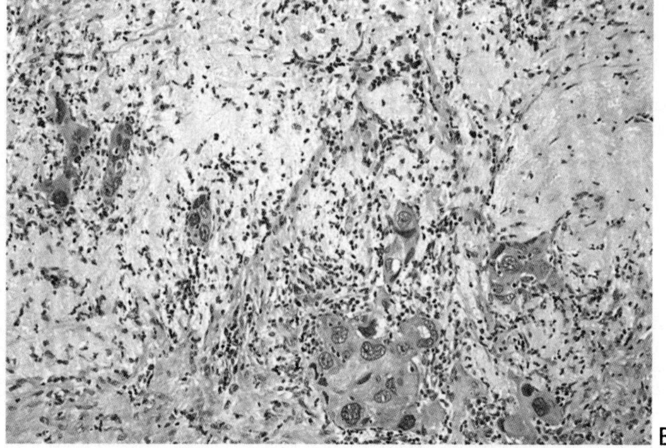

B

C

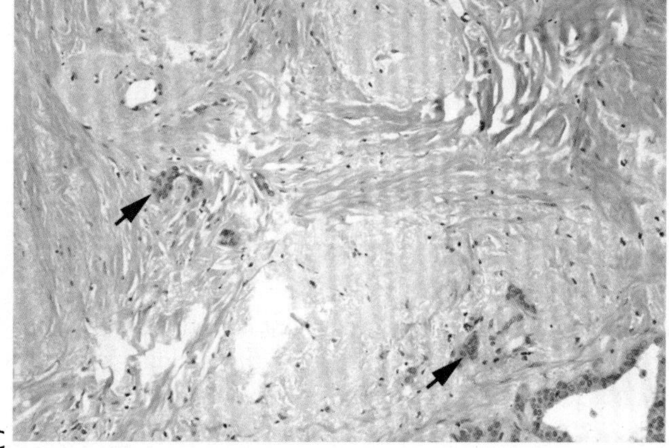

FIG. 41.10. ***Chemotherapy effect in invasive ductal carcinoma.*** **A:** This excisional biopsy performed after neoadjuvant therapy reveals a persistent 2-cm mass. Prior to treatment, the carcinoma measured nearly 5 cm. **B:** Stromal elastosis has replaced tumor destroyed by the treatment. The remaining carcinoma cells have large vesicular and pleomorphic nuclei. **C:** Marked stromal elastosis in which there are small nests of carcinoma cells (*arrows*) after chemotherapy.

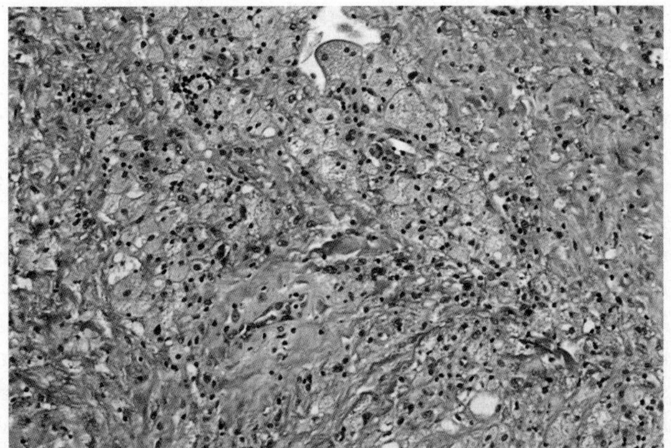

FIG. 41.11. ***Complete disappearance of carcinoma following chemotherapy.*** Histiocytes, lymphocytes, and fibrous tissue have taken the place of carcinoma cells.

may be appreciated because of architectural distortion characterized by fibrosis, stromal edema, increased vascularity composed largely of thin-walled vessels, and a chronic inflammatory cell infiltrate (Fig. 41.11).[105] Histologic identification of the tumor bed is necessary, especially in the absence of residual carcinoma, and finding a radiologic marker placed at the time of the core biopsy often helps to localize the site of the former tumor.[79] Reparative changes from the prior core biopsy can be difficult to identify on gross and histologic examination when the core biopsy preceded the excision by several months. At this time, the biopsy site typically becomes largely resorbed or merged with the scar tissue of the tumor bed. Sometimes a small area of scarring accompanied by scattered hemosiderin granules remains as the only trace of the core biopsy.

Residual invasive carcinoma cells can appear morphologically unaltered after neoadjuvant therapy, but in most cases they exhibit cytologic changes that reflect treatment effect.[90,106] The alterations may be more pronounced after combined chemoradiotherapy than following either form of treatment alone.[107] The invasive carcinoma cells usually appear enlarged as a result of increased cytoplasmic volume (Fig. 41.12). The cytoplasm often contains vacuoles or eosinophilic granules.[108] Cell borders are typically well defined, and the cells tend to shrink from the stroma. The cells contain large, hyperchromatic, pleomorphic nuclei, and multinucleated cells and abnormal mitotic figures may be encountered (Fig. 41.13).[109] The altered carcinoma cells can mimic histiocytes, especially when present individually, but they retain immunohistochemical reactivity for cytokeratin (CK) and epithelial membrane antigen (EMA). In certain cases, the residual invasive carcinoma cells appear smaller than those in the pre-treatment specimen (Fig. 41.14). Such cells contain scant eosinophilic cytoplasm and small collapsed nuclei. CK immunostaining is essential for the detection of minimal invasive residual carcinoma (Fig. 41.15).

An analysis comparing the components of histologic grading in a small series of pre- and post-chemotherapy specimens did not reveal significant differences in nuclear pleomorphism, tubule formation, or mitotic count.[102] Others[93] reported that nuclear grade was increased in 32% of cases. An increased score for nuclear pleomorphism after neoadjuvant chemotherapy might be combined with a lower mitotic or proliferation score. In some cases, the overall tumor grade is lower after neoadjuvant chemotherapy than before. In the majority of cases, it is feasible to determine histologic grade in residual carcinoma after neoadjuvant chemotherapy, and grade has been shown to correlate with long-term outcome.[110] Morphologic comparison of the tumor cells in the residual carcinoma with those in the prechemotherapy core biopsy specimen may help determine a possible difference or discrepancy.

Aneuploid carcinomas are more likely than diploid tumors to exhibit histologic and cytologic changes from chemotherapy.[90] The effect of chemotherapy on tumor cell proliferation as measured with the Ki67 antibody and mitotic counts is variable and was not shown to be

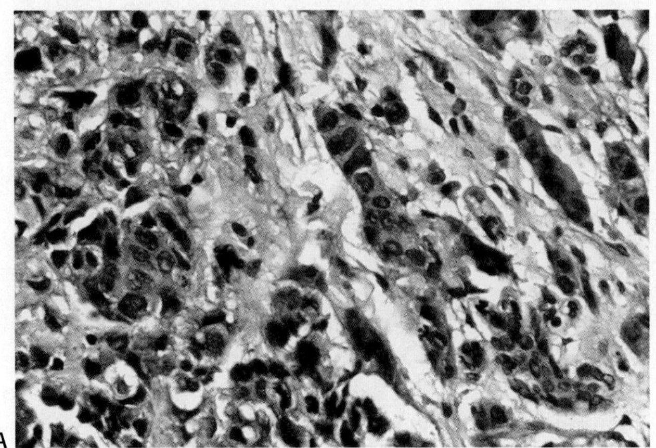

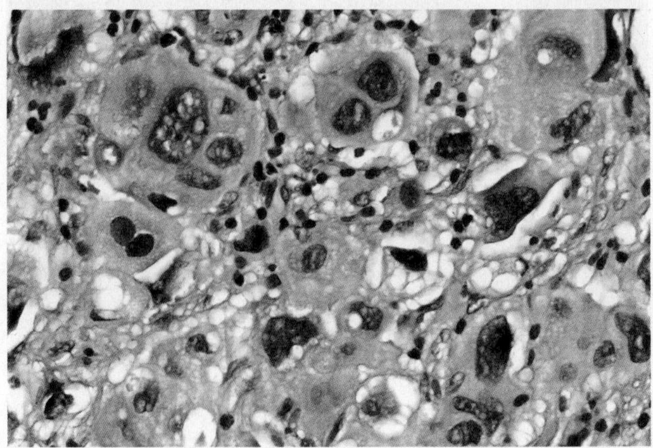

FIG. 41.12. ***Chemotherapy effect in invasive ductal carcinoma.*** **A:** The pre-treatment core biopsy specimen contains high-grade invasive ductal carcinoma. **B:** After chemotherapy, the residual invasive carcinoma cells appear enlarged and they possess bizarre and markedly pleomorphic nuclei.

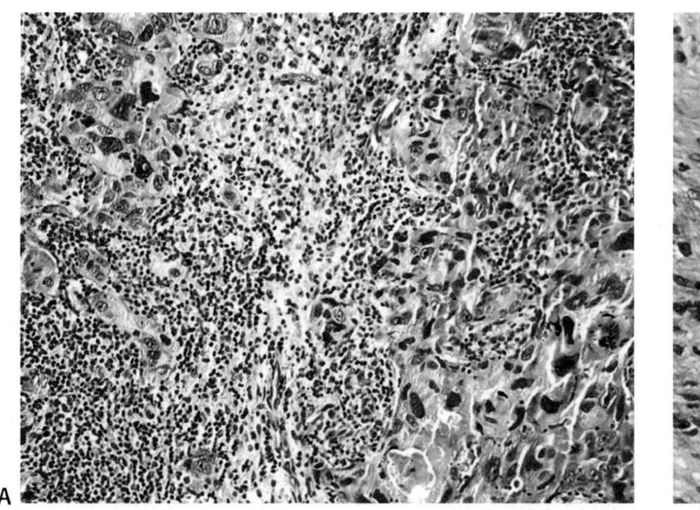
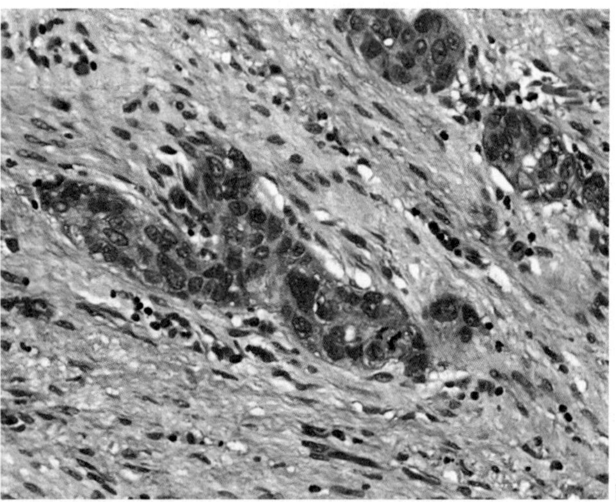

FIG. 41.13. ***Chemotherapy effect in invasive ductal carcinoma.*** **A:** The tumor cells have very pleomorphic nuclei. Some nuclei are hyperchromatic or have nucleoli. Note focal necrosis in the tumor (*lower right*). **B:** Residual carcinoma after chemotherapy showing mitotic activity and marked cytologic atypia.

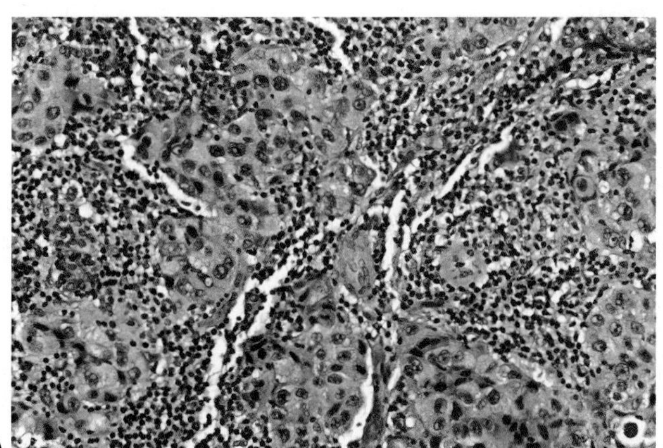
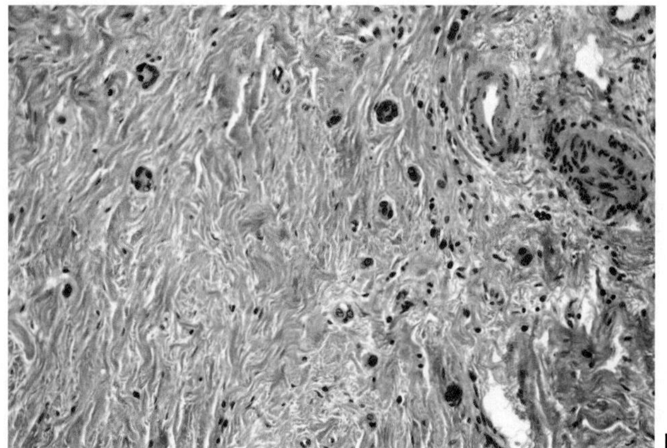

FIG. 41.14. ***Chemotherapy effect in invasive ductal carcinoma.*** **A:** The pre-treatment core biopsy specimen discloses high-grade invasive ductal carcinoma accompanied by a lymphocytic response. **B:** The postchemotherapy specimen contains only scattered groups of small carcinoma cells in sclerotic stroma, which is virtually devoid of lymphocytes.

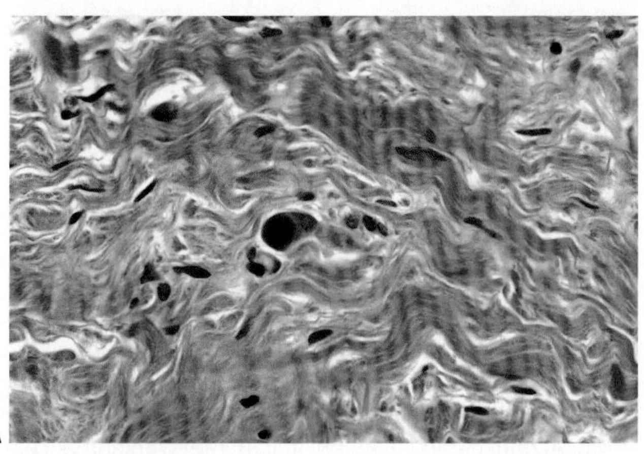
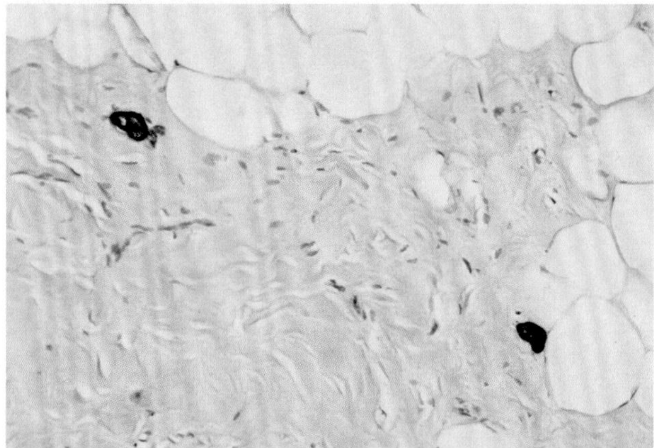

FIG. 41.15. ***Detection of residual invasive carcinoma using immunohistochemical staining for cytokeratin.*** **A:** Occasionally, the rare dispersed residual tumor cells seen after chemotherapy can be difficult to detect in hematoxylin and eosin–stained sections. **B:** The CK stain highlights residual tumor cells in the background of scar tissue.

associated with pathologic response.[109] Proliferative rates may be increased, decreased, or remain unchanged in the course of neoadjuvant chemotherapy. Although some studies indicate changes in receptor and HER2 status before and after neoadjuvant chemotherapy, larger series indicate that most breast carcinomas maintain the pre-treatment profile. Burcombe et al.[111] examined breast carcinomas from 118 patients and observed a shift in ER or PR classification in 8%. Immunohistochemical overexpression of HER2 was maintained in all cases, whereas changes between 2+ and 3+ HER2 scores occurred in a few cases. The Ki67 score was lower after neoadjuvant chemotherapy. Proliferation scores with Ki67 are also utilized to predict response and outcome after endocrine therapy has been administered in a neoadjuvant setting.[112]

In a minority of instances, the only residual carcinoma found after neoadjuvant chemotherapy consists of DICS, lymphatic tumor emboli, or both. Sharkey et al.[93] reported finding "unusually prominent intraductal and/or intralymphatic tumor" in 40% of specimens obtained after preoperative doxorubicin/cyclophosphamide consistent with relative resistance of carcinoma in these tissue compartments. Residual DCIS sometimes demonstrates marked cellular enlargement and extreme nuclear pleomorphism (Fig. 41.16). These bizarre cells can form confluent collections overlying a layer of easily recognized myoepithelial cells, or they can persist as individual cells and small clusters scattered among benign cells in the epithelium of ducts and lobules. Rabban et al.[113] reported a series of cases in which intralymphatic carcinoma was the only form of residual carcinoma (Fig. 41.17). This scenario can provide problems in classification of the neoadjuvant response because residual carcinoma is still present, albeit in the absence of stromal invasion. Carcinoma in lymphatic vessels is associated with lymph node metastases, which independently have a negative effect on long-term prognosis.

Nonneoplastic breast parenchyma is also altered following cytotoxic chemotherapy, but the changes are more subtle than those induced in the tumor. The glandular elements undergo diffuse atrophy causing a reduction in the size of existing lobules, loss of acinar luminal cells, shrinkage of the acini, and condensation of the basement membrane (Fig. 41.18).[93,108,114]

Lymph Nodes and Neoadjuvant Chemotherapy

Cytologic assessment of ALNs before neoadjuvant chemotherapy has been shown to be a minimally invasive and reliable technique for initial breast carcinoma staging.[115,116] The subsequent assessment of the ALNs after neoadjuvant chemotherapy is of great importance for long-term outcome but can be challenging for various reasons. Patients whose mammary tumors respond usually exhibit decreased clinical evidence of axillary disease that may be manifested

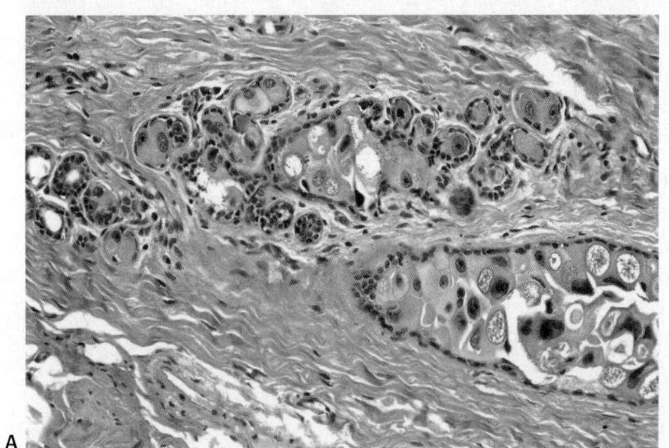

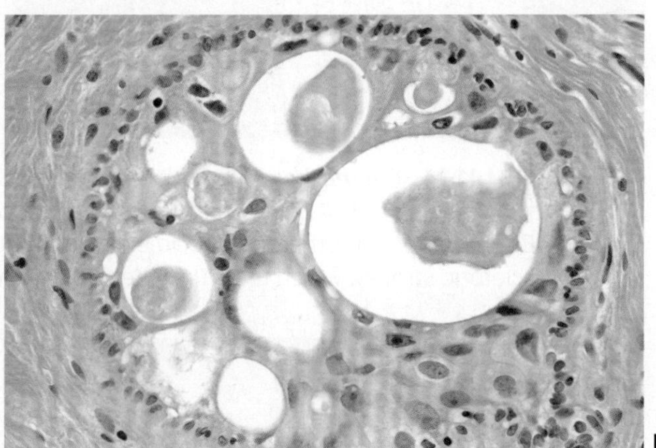

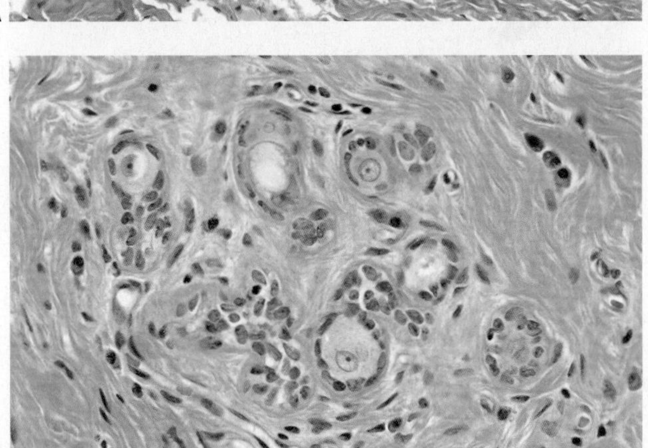

FIG. 41.16. ***Chemotherapy effect in DCIS.*** **A:** Persistent DCIS with lobular extension after chemotherapy displays marked epithelial atypia. Numerous myoepithelial cells form a noticeable layer encircling the carcinoma cells. **B:** The carcinoma cells fill and distend a small duct. Note the prominent myoepithelial cells. **C:** Scattered carcinoma cells with abundant cytoplasm and prominent nucleoli are present in the epithelium of acini within a lobule.

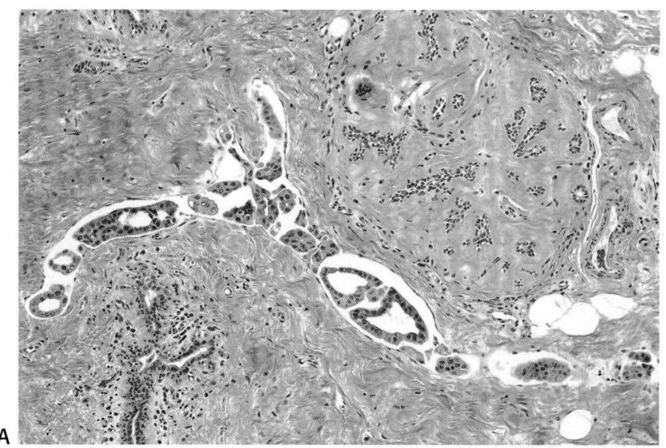

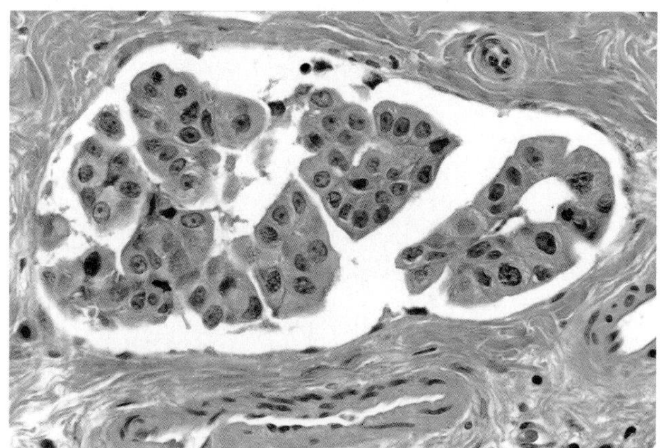

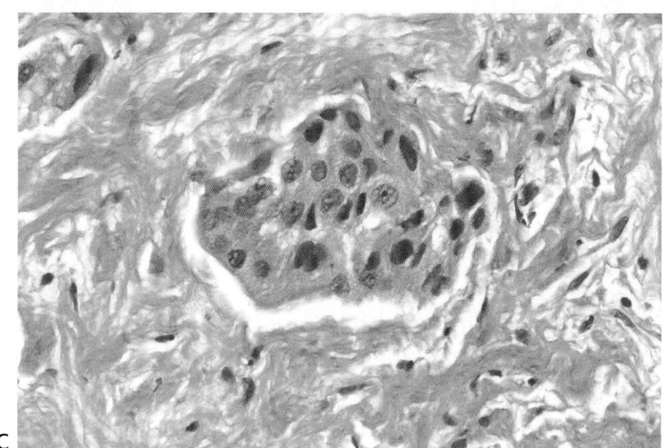

FIG. 41.17. ***Post-chemotherapy carcinoma confined to lymphatic vessels.*** **A:** The residual carcinoma cells are present only in lymphatic vessels. **B:** The intralymphatic carcinoma cells appear unaltered when compared to those in the pre-treatment specimen (**C**). **C:** The pre-treatment core biopsy specimen contains intermediate-grade invasive ductal carcinoma.

by smaller metastases in fewer lymph nodes than were present prior to treatment.[117,118] Neuman et al.[119] found that women who received neoadjuvant chemotherapy were more likely to have fewer than 10 lymph nodes harvested in an axillary dissection than were women who did not have chemotherapy before surgery. Clinical downstaging after neoadjuvant chemotherapy may actually suggest absence of nodal metastases leading to a decision to restrict the axillary staging to sentinel node biopsy.[120,121] Kuerer et al.[117] found that ultrasonography was significantly more sensitive (62%) than physical examination (45%) for detecting persistent axillary metastases after neoadjuvant therapy. On the other hand, physical examination, correct in 84% of cases, had higher specificity than ultrasonography (70%), but the difference was not statistically significant. In this study, 55 patients with locally advanced carcinoma were considered to have negative lymph nodes when evaluated clinically and by ultrasonography. Histologic examination revealed nodal metastases in 29 of the 55 patients after axillary dissection. Metastases were found either in one to three lymph nodes or limited to foci 2 to 5 mm in diameter in 28 of these 29 cases.

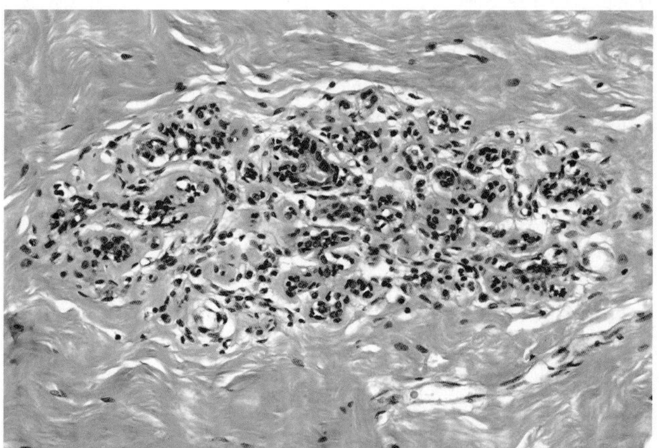

FIG. 41.18. ***Chemotherapy effect in a normal lobule.*** The acini have small diameters and only barely detectable lumens. The luminal cells possess scant cytoplasm, and the myoepithelial cell cytoplasm appears pale. The basement membranes are thickened.

Chemotherapy effects in axillary nodal metastases are similar to those affecting the primary tumor. Metastatic carcinoma can disappear completely leaving behind only areas of scarring and lymphohistiocytic infiltration[79,93] (Fig. 41.19A). Small clusters of carcinoma cells may remain embedded in regions of fibrosis and chronic inflammation (Figs. 41.19B, C). Immunohistochemical staining for CK will facilitate the detection of minimal residual metastatic carcinoma. Regressive changes may also be found in the uninvolved lymph nodes.[93]

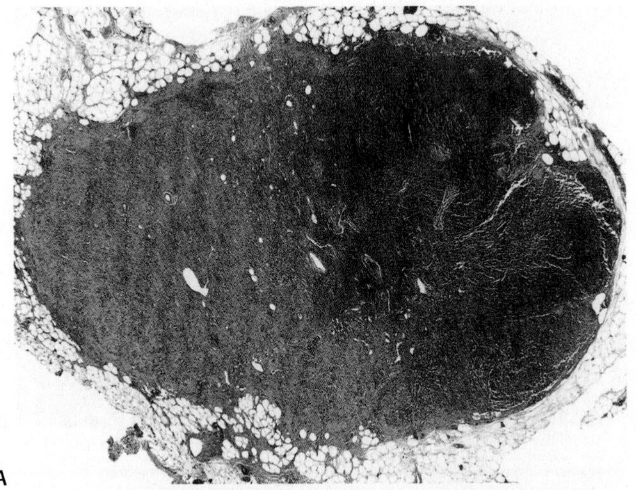

A

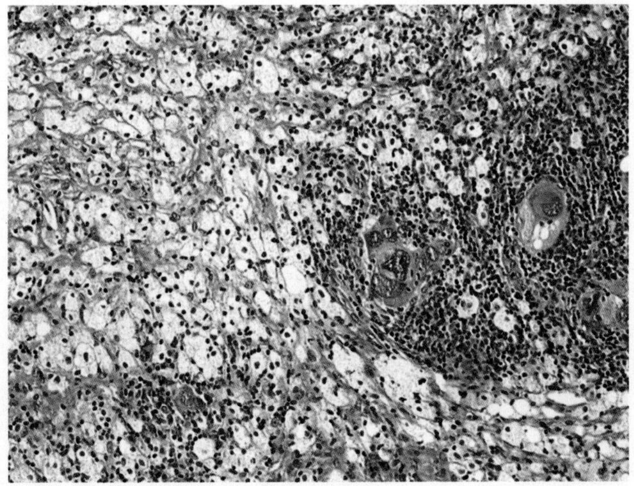

B

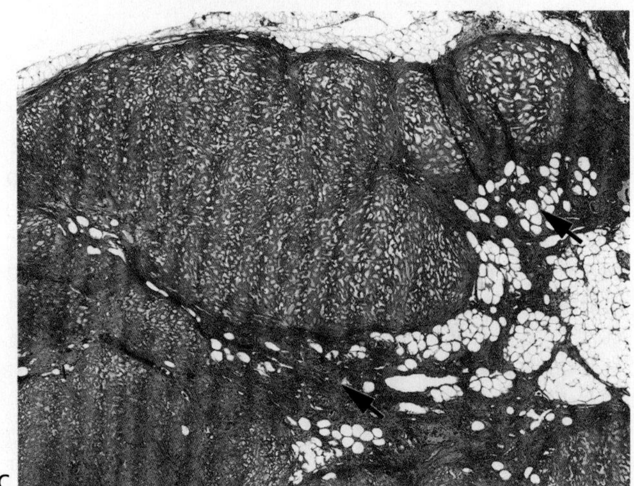

C

FIG. 41.19. ***Chemotherapy effect, lymph node.*** **A:** Scarring and lymphohistiocytic infiltration mark the site of a metastasis destroyed by chemotherapy. **B:** Small groups of carcinoma cells with pleomorphic nuclei persist in this lymph node where most of the tumor, destroyed by treatment, has been replaced by histiocytes. This is from the case shown in Figures 41.10A, B. **C:** Hyalin material has replaced most of the metastatic carcinoma; however, one can still detect the nested pattern of the carcinoma, and a few intact glands (*arrows*) remain at the periphery of the lymph node.

Prognosis

Prognosis is related to the completeness of pathologic response and appears to be especially favorable at 5 years in patients with the least evidence of tumor in the breast or lymph nodes after therapy.[92,122] Feldman et al.[91] reported a 93% 5-year survival in patients with no gross tumor in the breast or ALNs compared to a 30%, 5-year survival in those with grossly evident residual tumor. Others[92,106] found a 5-year disease-free survival (DFS) of 87% after complete clinical regression and 65% when regression was incomplete.[92,106] Not only the number of involved lymph nodes but also the size of the metastases after treatment correlated with long-term outcome.[123]

The study of 372 patients with locally advanced breast carcinoma by Kuerer et al.[122] found that 60 patients (16%) had a complete pathologic tumor response after neoadjuvant chemotherapy and that 43 (12%) had no histologic evidence of carcinoma in the breast or axillary nodes. There was a significant correlation between complete pathologic response in the breast tumor and in the ALNs. Pre-treatment factors predictive of complete pathologic response were poorly differentiated nuclear grade, anaplastic or poorly differentiated histologic grade, and absence of ER. Patients with a complete pathologic response had significantly better 5-year OS and DFS rates (89% and 87%, respectively) than those with a partial pathologic response (64% and 58%, respectively).

Residual carcinoma may be detected by CK staining in lymph nodes that appear to show a complete histologic response in routine histologic sections.[79,120] Since extent and size of metastatic disease influence long-term prognosis,[92,123] it is important to find even small foci of metastatic disease. Kuerer et al.[120] studied 191 patients with locally advanced carcinoma treated with neoadjuvant chemotherapy after axillary metastases were documented by FNA. Routine histologic sections of lymph nodes obtained after treatment did not reveal metastases in 43 (23%). CK immunostaining of histologically negative lymph nodes in 39 cases revealed occult micrometastases in 4 (10%). Patients without occult micrometastases had a better 5-year DFS (87%) than those with occult metastases (75%) and those with residual nodal disease (51%). Factors associated with conversion to negative nodal status were absence of ER in the tumor and complete pathologic response of the primary tumor.

HORMONAL THERAPY

Estrogens and androgens have been used to treat mammary carcinoma for several decades. In 1949, Adair et al.[124] described the pathologic effects of sex steroid hormones noting that changes in the tumor tissue attributed to treatment consisted of "degenerative changes in the nucleus and cytoplasm of the carcinoma cells and fibroblastic proliferation and sclerosis of the connective tissue." It was also observed that the vaginal mucosa exhibited cytologic changes of maturation in response to estrogen, whereas androgens caused atrophy. Similar effects of hormones on breast carcinoma were illustrated by Taylor et al.[125]

The results of a detailed examination of the effects of therapeutic doses of estrogen on noncancerous mammary glandular tissue were reported by Huseby and Thomas in 1954.[126] In postmenopausal women, normal breast epithelium was stimulated to proliferate with the elongation of small terminal ducts and the formation of lobules. Epithelial changes were accompanied by the accumulation of interlobular connective tissue. The authors also commented that "the reaction to estrogen administration of certain abnormal, but nonmalignant, epithelial structures was one of proliferation and thus more like that of the normal breast epithelium than like that of the cancerous epithelium." The clinical and pathologic response of the carcinomas to treatment did not correlate with the extent or degree of change that occurred in normal breast tissue. It was observed that two patients with "excellent regressions of breast carcinoma" showed "no evidence of stimulation of the normal breast epithelium."

Further studies of the morphologic changes associated with tumor regression in hormone-treated patients were reported by Emerson et al.[127] They confirmed the observation that low-grade tumors were more likely to respond to treatment and also noted that the duration of regression was longer. Apparently viable tumor cells were found in mammary lymphatics of patients whose primary tumors were undergoing regression. Persistent DCIS was also noted in some cases. These findings suggested that tumor cells at these sites might be less responsive or that they may be exposed to less effective levels of hormone.

Since the antiestrogen tamoxifen was shown to be effective in reducing tumor size and inducing remissions in women with advanced breast carcinoma,[128] hormonal therapy with tamoxifen has become a mainstay of breast carcinoma treatment. Tamoxifen was specifically shown to improve long-term outcome for patients whose breast carcinomas express ER, the majority of breast carcinomas.[129] Hormone receptor–negative carcinomas do not benefit from antiestrogen treatment.

Although the selective ER modulator tamoxifen exerts its antagonistic function by competitive action at the ER, more recently developed agents show antiestrogen effects by inhibiting synthesis of the protein. A class of substances referred to as aromatase inhibitors block the aromatization step in the synthesis of estrogen.[130]

Most hormonal treatment is administered after local treatment is completed to prevent relapse. Antiestrogen treatment with aromatase inhibitors has also been given in a neoadjuvant setting and has been shown to allow breast-conserving surgery in patients who present with large tumors.[112,131] In the observational study by Dixon et al.,[131] the aromatase inhibitor letrozole was given to 61 patients with ER-positive invasive lobular carcinomas for a median duration of 9 months. The investigators observed a reduction in tumor volume in two-thirds of cases after 3 months.

Hormonal therapy is also used to prevent breast carcinoma from occurring in women at high risk. Clinical trials and epidemiologic studies have shown that an antiestrogen such as tamoxifen can be effective in reducing the frequency of breast carcinoma in high-risk women.[132] Women who had been treated for ER-positive DCIS were shown to have a lower risk of subsequent breast carcinomas over 10 years of follow-up when treated with tamoxifen.[133]

The effects of tamoxifen on normal breast tissue have received little attention. Walker et al.[134] examined tissues from breast carcinoma patients treated with tamoxifen for 4 days to 3 weeks prior to surgery and observed increased immunoreactivity for ER in ductal and lobular epithelium when compared with untreated patients.

With the advent of classification schemes based on molecular subtypes, breast carcinomas are increasingly categorized in the framework of hormone receptor and HER2 expression.[135] Testing for these proteins in clinical practice is done primarily by immunohistochemical methods on tumor samples, but the use of a variety of molecular assays is increasing.

ABLATION METHODS

Several techniques for ablating carcinomas in the breast have been investigated. The two most studied are radiofrequency ablation (RFA) and cryoablation, but additional methods include interstitial laser therapy, microwave ablation, and high-intensity–focused ultrasound.[136] All of these procedures use an image-guided technique to insert a probe into the lesion. Cryoablation destroys the tumor by freezing. The other methods destroy the tumor with heat generated by various energy sources to temperatures of at least 50°C. Histologic changes induced by these procedures are limited to the lesion and the immediate surrounding tissue. At present, these techniques are considered investigational. As practice with ablation methods extends beyond the exploratory stage, not all ablated lesions will be removed surgically so that histopathologic correlation may remain incomplete. An important limitation to the use of ablation is that tissue for receptor analysis and other studies must be obtained before the tumor is ablated.

Radiofrequency Ablation

In situ thermal destruction of breast carcinoma has been achieved by applying radiofrequency energy with probes inserted into the breast tumor. Histologic examination immediately after RFA of carcinomas in five patients revealed heat-induced necrosis of much of the tumor, but tumor cells that seemed viable when stained with NADH-diaphorase immunohistochemistry remained.[137] Cell death after RFA can be delayed by as much as 48 hours. In the study by Noguchi et al.,[138] recurrences were not detected during a mean follow-up of 60 months in 19 patients who underwent RFA. Cosmesis was considered good or excellent, but a hard lump persisted in about half of the patients.[138]

Other applications include RFA of breast carcinomas without subsequent removal of the masses but surveillance for recurrence based on MRI and sonography.[139] In an exploratory study[140] with the goal to reduce local recurrence after breast-conserving surgery, RFA has been applied not to the tumor itself but to the excision cavity with subsequent histopathologic correlation and staining for proliferating cell nuclear antigen.[140] Klimberg et al.[140] concluded that RFA is "best suited for small, deep, localized, discretely visualized invasive ductal carcinomas" but not for invasive lobular carcinomas because of their more diffuse growth pattern.

Cryoablation

The histologic effects of cryoablation are well established by 7 days after treatment at which time the affected tissue displays coagulative necrosis surrounded by a zone of fat necrosis and scar formation.[141] Residual *in situ* or invasive carcinoma may be found beyond the perimeter of the necrotic tissue. Cryoprobe-assisted lumpectomy is a procedure in which freezing is used to convert a nonpalpable ultrasound-detected lesion into a palpable target ("ice ball") that can be excised without the need for wire localization.[142] The tissue is affected in much the same manner as occurs when cryoablation is performed, but excisional surgery is done promptly after procedure while the tissue is still frozen. In a study of six specimens obtained by this method, Sahoo et al.[143] found that alterations in the tissue caused by freezing compromised grading of carcinomas and interfered with distinguishing between *in situ* and invasive components, assessing mitoses, detecting vascular invasion, and testing for hormone receptors. Cryoablation instead of surgical removal has been reported for fibroadenomas (FAs) and for breast carcinoma in patients who were not good candidates for surgery.[144,145]

Other Ablation Methods

Laser-induced thermal therapy has been investigated as a method for causing the thermal destruction of small primary breast carcinomas.[146–148] Thermal energy is generated with a laser probe inserted into the tumor. Bloom et al.[149] studied the pathologic changes associated with laser tumor ablation after delayed excision and observed a series of concentric rings around the laser probe tract: a cavity corresponding to the laser tip (zone 1), a coagulated area showing changes similar to cautery artifact with "wind-swept nuclei" (zone 2), a region of CK-negative tumor cells (zone 3), an area of necrotic tumor (zone 4), and an outermost layer of vascular proliferation around the necrotic mass (zone 5).

High-intensity–focused ultrasound therapy applies thermal energy via a transducer through the skin. The application of this technique is exploratory and was successfully demonstrated on 12 FAs under MRI guidance.[150]

Vogl et al.[151] reported results comparing microwave, radiofrequency, and laser ablation techniques for breast carcinoma metastatic to the liver.

REFERENCES

1. Yaffe MJ, Mainprize JG. Risk of radiation-induced breast cancer from mammographic screening. *Radiology* 2011;258:98–105.
2. Anderson N, Lokich J. Bilateral breast cancer after cured Hodgkin's disease. *Cancer* 1990;65:221–223.
3. Bhatia S, Robison LL, Oberlin O, et al. Breast cancer and other second neoplasms after childhood Hodgkin's disease. *N Engl J Med* 1996;334:745–751.
4. O'Brien PC, Barton MB, Fisher R. Breast cancer following treatment for Hodgkin's disease: the need for screening in a young population. Australasian Radiation Oncology Lymphoma Group (AROLG). *Australas Radiol* 1995;39:271–276.
5. Yahalom J, Petrek JA, Biddinger PW, et al. Breast cancer in patients irradiated for Hodgkin's disease: a clinical and pathologic analysis of 45 events in 37 patients. *J Clin Oncol* 1992;10:1674–1681.
6. Boice JD Jr, Monson RR. Breast cancer in women after repeated fluoroscopic examinations of the chest. *J Natl Cancer Inst* 1977;59:823–832.
7. Hildreth NG, Shore RE, Dvoretsky PM. The risk of breast cancer after irradiation of the thymus in infancy. *N Engl J Med* 1989;321:1281–1284.
8. Little MP, Boice JD Jr. Comparison of breast cancer incidence in the Massachusetts tuberculosis fluoroscopy cohort and in the Japanese atomic bomb survivors. *Radiat Res* 1999;151:218–224.
9. Swerdlow AJ, Cooke R, Bates A, et al. Breast cancer risk after supradiaphragmatic radiotherapy for Hodgkin's lymphoma in England and Wales: a National Cohort Study. *J Clin Oncol* 2012;30:2745–2752.
10. Wendland MM, Tsodikov A, Glenn MJ, et al. Time interval to the development of breast carcinoma after treatment for Hodgkin disease. *Cancer* 2004;101:1275–1282.
11. Hancock SL, Tucker MA, Hoppe RT. Breast cancer after treatment of Hodgkin's disease. *J Natl Cancer Inst* 1993;85:25–31.
12. Wolden SL, Lamborn KR, Cleary SF, et al. Second cancers following pediatric Hodgkin's disease. *J Clin Oncol* 1998;16:536–544.
13. Janjan NA, Zellmer DL. Calculated risk of breast cancer following mantle irradiation determined by measured dose. *Cancer Detect Prev* 1992;16:273–282.
14. Janjan NA, Wilson JF, Gillin M, et al. Mammary carcinoma developing after radiotherapy and chemotherapy for Hodgkin's disease. *Cancer* 1988;61:252–254.
15. Kowalski A, Smith S. Measurement of radiation dose delivered to breast tissue during mantle field irradiation for Hodgkin's disease. *Med Dosim* 1998;23:31–36.
16. Hodgson DC, Koh ES, Tran TH, et al. Individualized estimates of second cancer risks after contemporary radiation therapy for Hodgkin lymphoma. *Cancer* 2007;110:2576–2586.
17. De Bruin ML, Sparidans J, van't Veer MB, et al. Breast cancer risk in female survivors of Hodgkin's lymphoma: lower risk after smaller radiation volumes. *J Clin Oncol* 2009;27:4239–4246.
18. Cutuli B. Radiation-induced breast cancer after treatment for Hodgkin's disease. *J Clin Oncol* 1998;16:2285–2287.
19. Cutuli B, Dhermain F, Borel C, et al. Breast cancer in patients treated for Hodgkin's disease: clinical and pathological analysis of 76 cases in 63 patients. *Eur J Cancer* 1997;33:2315–2320.
20. Cutuli B, Kanoun S, Tunon De Lara C, et al. Breast cancer occurred after Hodgkin's disease: clinico-pathological features, treatments and outcome: analysis of 214 cases. *Crit Rev Oncol Hematol* 2012;81:29–37.
21. Dershaw DD, Yahalom J, Petrek JA. Breast carcinoma in women previously treated for Hodgkin disease: mammographic evaluation. *Radiology* 1992;184:421–423.
22. Diller L, Medeiros Nancarrow C, Shaffer K, et al. Breast cancer screening in women previously treated for Hodgkin's disease: a prospective cohort study. *J Clin Oncol* 2002;20:2085–2091.
23. Tardivon AA, Garnier ML, Beaudre A, et al. Breast carcinoma in women previously treated for Hodgkin's disease: clinical and mammographic findings. *Eur Radiol* 1999;9:1666–1671.
24. Howell SJ, Searle C, Goode V, et al. The UK national breast cancer screening programme for survivors of Hodgkin lymphoma detects breast cancer at an early stage. *Br J Cancer* 2009;101:582–588.
25. Teh W, Wilson AR. The role of ultrasound in breast cancer screening. A consensus statement by the European Group for Breast Cancer Screening. *Eur J Cancer* 1998;34:449–450.
26. Orel SG, Mendonca MH, Reynolds C, et al. MR imaging of ductal carcinoma *in situ*. *Radiology* 1997;202:413–420.

27. Neubauer H, Li M, Kuehne-Heid R, et al. High grade and non-high grade ductal carcinoma *in situ* on dynamic MR mammography: characteristic findings for signal increase and morphological pattern of enhancement. *Br J Radiol* 2003;76:3–12.
28. Saslow D, Boetes C, Burke W, et al. American Cancer Society guidelines for breast screening with MRI as an adjunct to mammography. *CA Cancer J Clin* 2007;57:75–89.
29. Dvoretsky PM, Woodard E, Bonfiglio TA, et al. The pathology of breast cancer in women irradiated for acute postpartum mastitis. *Cancer* 1980;46:2257–2262.
30. Elkin EB, Klem ML, Gonzales AM, et al. Characteristics and outcomes of breast cancer in women with and without a history of radiation for Hodgkin's lymphoma: a multi-institutional, matched cohort study. *J Clin Oncol* 2011;29:2466–2473.
31. Cutuli B, Borel C, Dhermain F, et al. Breast cancer occurred after treatment for Hodgkin's disease: analysis of 133 cases. *Radiother Oncol* 2001;59:247–255.
32. Wolden SL, Hancock SL, Carlson RW, et al. Management of breast cancer after Hodgkin's disease. *J Clin Oncol* 2000;18:765–772.
33. Deutsch M, Gerszten K, Bloomer WD, et al. Lumpectomy and breast irradiation for breast cancer arising after previous radiotherapy for Hodgkin's disease or lymphoma. *Am J Clin Oncol* 2001;24:33–34.
34. Darby S, McGale P, Correa C, et al. Effect of radiotherapy after breast-conserving surgery on 10-year recurrence and 15-year breast cancer death: meta-analysis of individual patient data for 10,801 women in 17 randomised trials. *Lancet* 2011;378:1707–1716.
35. Bartelink H, Horiot JC, Poortmans PM, et al. Impact of a higher radiation dose on local control and survival in breast-conserving therapy of early breast cancer: 10-year results of the randomized boost versus no boost EORTC 22881-10882 trial. *J Clin Oncol* 2007;25:3259–3265.
36. Wilkinson JB, Beitsch PD, Shah C, et al. Evaluation of current consensus statement recommendations for accelerated partial breast irradiation: a pooled analysis of William Beaumont Hospital and American Society of Breast Surgeon MammoSite((R)) Registry trial data. *Int J Radiat Oncol Biol Phys* 2012;85:1179–1185.
37. McCormick B. Partial breast radiation for early-stage breast cancer. *Curr Opin Obstet Gynecol* 2012;24:31–37.
38. Pierquin B, Grimard L, Marinello G. Normal-tissue tolerance in the irradiation of female breast. *Front Radiat Ther Oncol* 1989;23:341–348.
39. Barnett GC, Wilkinson JS, Moody AM, et al. The Cambridge breast intensity-modulated radiotherapy trial: patient- and treatment-related factors that influence late toxicity. *Clin Oncol (R Coll Radiol)* 2011;23:662–673.
40. Higgins S, Haffty BG. Pregnancy and lactation after breast-conserving therapy for early stage breast cancer. *Cancer* 1994;73:2175–2180.
41. Varsos G, Yahalom J. Lactation following conservation surgery and radiotherapy for breast cancer. *J Surg Oncol* 1991;46:141–144.
42. Ryu J, Yahalom J, Shank B, et al. Radiation therapy after breast augmentation or reconstruction in early or recurrent breast cancer. *Cancer* 1990;66:844–847.
43. Ho A, Cordeiro P, Disa J, et al. Long-term outcomes in breast cancer patients undergoing immediate 2-stage expander/implant reconstruction and postmastectomy radiation. *Cancer* 2012;118:2552–2559.
44. Robertson JM, Clarke DH, Pevzner MM, et al. Breast conservation therapy. Severe breast fibrosis after radiation therapy in patients with collagen vascular disease. *Cancer* 1991;68:502–508.
45. Lin A, Abu-Isa E, Griffith KA, et al. Toxicity of radiotherapy in patients with collagen vascular disease. *Cancer* 2008;113:648–653.
46. Chansakul T, Lai KC, Slanetz PJ. The postconservation breast: part 2, Imaging findings of tumor recurrence and other long-term sequelae. *AJR Am J Roentgenol* 2012;198:331–343.
47. Chansakul T, Lai KC, Slanetz PJ. The postconservation breast: Part 1, Expected imaging findings. *AJR Am J Roentgenol* 2012;198:321–330.
48. Morakkabati N, Leutner CC, Schmiedel A, et al. Breast MR imaging during or soon after radiation therapy. *Radiology* 2003;229:893–901.
49. Li J, Dershaw DD, Lee CH, et al. Breast MRI after conservation therapy: usual findings in routine follow-up examinations. *AJR Am J Roentgenol* 2010;195:799–807.
50. Girling AC, Hanby AM, Millis RR. Radiation and other pathological changes in breast tissue after conservation treatment for carcinoma. *J Clin Pathol* 1990;43:152–156.
51. Rebner M, Pennes DR, Adler DD, et al. Breast microcalcifications after lumpectomy and radiation therapy. *Radiology* 1989;170:691–693.
52. Davis SP, Stomper PC, Weidner N, et al. Suture calcification mimicking recurrence in the irradiated breast: a potential pitfall in mammographic evaluation. *Radiology* 1989;172:247–248.
53. Clarke D, Curtis JL, Martinez A, et al. Fat necrosis of the breast simulating recurrent carcinoma after primary radiotherapy in the management of early stage breast carcinoma. *Cancer* 1983;52:442–445.
54. Rostom AY, el-Sayed ME. Fat necrosis of the breast: an unusual complication of lumpectomy and radiotherapy in breast cancer. *Clin Radiol* 1987;38:31.
55. Piroth MD, Fischedick K, Wein B, et al. Fat necrosis and parenchymal scarring after breast-conserving surgery and radiotherapy with an intraoperative electron or fractionated, percutaneous boost: a retrospective comparison. *Breast Cancer* 2012. doi:10.1007/s12282-012-0418-2
56. Rivera R, Smith-Bronstein V, Villegas-Mendez S, et al. Mammographic findings after intraoperative radiotherapy of the breast. *Radiol Res Pract* 2012;2012:758371.
57. Lu WL, Jansen L, Post WJ, et al. Impact on survival of early detection of isolated breast recurrences after the primary treatment for breast cancer: a meta-analysis. *Breast Cancer Res Treat* 2009;114:403–412.
58. Obedian E, Fischer DB, Haffty BG. Second malignancies after treatment of early-stage breast cancer: lumpectomy and radiation therapy versus mastectomy. *J Clin Oncol* 2000;18:2406–2412.
59. Roychoudhuri R, Evans H, Robinson D, et al. Radiation-induced malignancies following radiotherapy for breast cancer. *Br J Cancer* 2004;91:868–872.
60. Zablotska LB, Neugut AI. Lung carcinoma after radiation therapy in women treated with lumpectomy or mastectomy for primary breast carcinoma. *Cancer* 2003;97:1404–1411.
61. Curtis RE, Boice Jr JD, Stovall M, et al. Risk of leukemia after chemotherapy and radiation treatment for breast cancer. *N Engl J Med* 1992;326:1745–1751.
62. Schnitt SJ, Connolly JL, Harris JR, et al. Radiation-induced changes in the breast. *Hum Pathol* 1984;15:545–550.
63. Moore GH, Schiller JE, Moore GK. Radiation-induced histopathologic changes of the breast: the effects of time. *Am J Surg Pathol* 2004;28:47–53.
64. Brouty-Boye D, Raux H, Azzarone B, et al. Fetal myofibroblast-like cells isolated from post-radiation fibrosis in human breast cancer. *Int J Cancer* 1991;47:697–702.
65. Poeze M, von Meyenfeldt MF, Peterse JL, et al. Increased proliferative activity and p53 expression in normal glandular breast tissue after radiation therapy. *J Pathol* 1998;185:32–37.
66. Pedio G, Landolt U, Zobeli L. Irradiated benign cells of the breast: a potential diagnostic pitfall in fine needle aspiration cytology. *Acta Cytol* 1988;32:127–128.
67. Bondeson L. Aspiration cytology of radiation-induced changes of normal breast epithelium. *Acta Cytol* 1987;31:309–310.
68. Peterse JL, Thunnissen FB, van Heerde P. Fine needle aspiration cytology of radiation-induced changes in nonneoplastic breast lesions. Possible pitfalls in cytodiagnosis. *Acta Cytol* 1989;33:176–180.
69. Dornfeld JM, Thompson SK, Shurbaji MS. Radiation-induced changes in the breast: a potential diagnostic pitfall on fine-needle aspiration. *Diagn Cytopathol* 1992;8:79–80; discussion 80–81.
70. Solin LJ, Fowble BL, Schultz DJ, et al. The detection of local recurrence after definitive irradiation for early stage carcinoma of the breast. An analysis of the results of breast biopsies performed in previously irradiated breasts. *Cancer* 1990;65:2497–2502.
71. Filomena CA, Jordan AG, Ehya H. Needle aspiration cytology of the irradiated breast. *Diagn Cytopathol* 1992;8:327–332.
72. Peterse JL, Koolman-Schellekens MA, van de Peppel-van de Ham T, et al. Atypia in fine-needle aspiration cytology of the breast: a histologic follow-up study of 301 cases. *Semin Diagn Pathol* 1989;6:126–134.
73. Nassar A. Core needle biopsy versus fine needle aspiration biopsy in breast—a historical perspective and opportunities in the modern era. *Diagn Cytopathol* 2011;39:380–388.
74. Millis RR, Pinder SE, Ryder K, et al. Grade of recurrent *in situ* and invasive carcinoma following treatment of pure ductal carcinoma *in situ* of the breast. *Br J Cancer* 2004;90:1538–1542.
75. Sigal-Zafrani B, Bollet MA, Antoni G, et al. Are ipsilateral breast tumour invasive recurrences in young (< or =40 years) women more aggressive than their primary tumours? *Br J Cancer* 2007;97:1046–1052.
76. Rastogi P, Anderson SJ, Bear HD, et al. Preoperative chemotherapy: updates of National Surgical Adjuvant Breast and Bowel Project Protocols B-18 and B-27. *J Clin Oncol* 2008;26:778–785.

77. Morrow M, Braverman A, Thelmo W, et al. Multimodal therapy for locally advanced breast cancer. *Arch Surg* 1986;121:1291–1296.
78. Thompson AM, Moulder-Thompson SL. Neoadjuvant treatment of breast cancer. *Ann Oncol* 2012;23(suppl. 10):x231–x236.
79. Pinder SE, Provenzano E, Earl H, et al. Laboratory handling and histology reporting of breast specimens from patients who have received neoadjuvant chemotherapy. *Histopathology* 2007;50:409–417.
80. Huober J, von Minckwitz G. Neoadjuvant therapy—what have we achieved in the last 20 years? *Breast Care (Basel)* 2011;6:419–426.
81. Rouzier R, Pusztai L, Delaloge S, et al. Nomograms to predict pathologic complete response and metastasis-free survival after preoperative chemotherapy for breast cancer. *J Clin Oncol* 2005;23:8331–8339.
82. Buzdar AU, Ibrahim NK, Francis D, et al. Significantly higher pathologic complete remission rate after neoadjuvant therapy with trastuzumab, paclitaxel, and epirubicin chemotherapy: results of a randomized trial in human epidermal growth factor receptor 2-positive operable breast cancer. *J Clin Oncol* 2005;23:3676–3685.
83. Liedtke C, Mazouni C, Hess KR, et al. Response to neoadjuvant therapy and long-term survival in patients with triple-negative breast cancer. *J Clin Oncol* 2008;26:1275–1281.
84. Silver DP, Richardson AL, Eklund AC, et al. Efficacy of neoadjuvant Cisplatin in triple-negative breast cancer. *J Clin Oncol* 2010;28:1145–1153.
85. Cristofanilli M, Gonzalez-Angulo A, Sneige N, et al. Invasive lobular carcinoma classic type: response to primary chemotherapy and survival outcomes. *J Clin Oncol* 2005;23:41–48.
86. Fisher B, Bryant J, Wolmark N, et al. Effect of preoperative chemotherapy on the outcome of women with operable breast cancer. *J Clin Oncol* 1998;16:2672–2685.
87. Pu RT, Schott AF, Sturtz DE, et al. Pathologic features of breast cancer associated with complete response to neoadjuvant chemotherapy: importance of tumor necrosis. *Am J Surg Pathol* 2005;29:354–358.
88. Burcombe R, Wilson GD, Dowsett M, et al. Evaluation of Ki-67 proliferation and apoptotic index before, during and after neoadjuvant chemotherapy for primary breast cancer. *Breast Cancer Res* 2006;8:R31.
89. Matsubara N, Mukai H, Fujii S, et al. Different prognostic significance of Ki-67 change between pre- and post-neoadjuvant chemotherapy in various subtypes of breast cancer. *Breast Cancer Res Treat* 2013;137:203–212.
90. Briffod M, Spyratos F, Tubiana-Hulin M, et al. Sequential cytopunctures during preoperative chemotherapy for primary breast carcinoma. Cytomorphologic changes, initial tumor ploidy, and tumor regression. *Cancer* 1989;63:631–637.
91. Feldman LD, Hortobagyi GN, Buzdar AU, et al. Pathological assessment of response to induction chemotherapy in breast cancer. *Cancer Res* 1986;46:2578–2581.
92. Fisher ER, Wang J, Bryant J, et al. Pathobiology of preoperative chemotherapy: findings from the National Surgical Adjuvant Breast and Bowel (NSABP) protocol B-18. *Cancer* 2002;95:681–695.
93. Sharkey FE, Addington SL, Fowler LJ, et al. Effects of preoperative chemotherapy on the morphology of resectable breast carcinoma. *Mod Pathol* 1996;9:893–900.
94. Vinnicombe SJ, MacVicar AD, Guy RL, et al. Primary breast cancer: mammographic changes after neoadjuvant chemotherapy, with pathologic correlation. *Radiology* 1996;198:333–340.
95. Esserman LE, d'Almeida M, Da Costa D, et al. Mammographic appearance of microcalcifications: can they change after neoadjuvant chemotherapy? *Breast J* 2006;12:86–87.
96. Abraham DC, Jones RC, Jones SE, et al. Evaluation of neoadjuvant chemotherapeutic response of locally advanced breast cancer by magnetic resonance imaging. *Cancer* 1996;78:91–100.
97. Yeh E, Slanetz P, Kopans DB, et al. Prospective comparison of mammography, sonography, and MRI in patients undergoing neoadjuvant chemotherapy for palpable breast cancer. *AJR Am J Roentgenol* 2005;184:868–877.
98. Tateishi U, Miyake M, Nagaoka T, et al. Neoadjuvant chemotherapy in breast cancer: prediction of pathologic response with PET/CT and dynamic contrast-enhanced MR imaging—prospective assessment. *Radiology* 2012;263:53–63.
99. Baron LF, Baron PL, Ackerman SJ, et al. Sonographically guided clip placement facilitates localization of breast cancer after neoadjuvant chemotherapy. *AJR Am J Roentgenol* 2000;174:539–540.
100. Rajan R, Poniecka A, Smith TL, et al. Change in tumor cellularity of breast carcinoma after neoadjuvant chemotherapy as a variable in the pathologic assessment of response. *Cancer* 2004;100:1365–1373.
101. Ogston KN, Miller ID, Payne S, et al. A new histological grading system to assess response of breast cancers to primary chemotherapy: prognostic significance and survival. *Breast* 2003;12:320–327.
102. Frierson HF Jr, Fechner RE. Histologic grade of locally advanced infiltrating ductal carcinoma after treatment with induction chemotherapy. *Am J Clin Pathol* 1994;102:154–157.
103. Symmans WF, Peintinger F, Hatzis C, et al. Measurement of residual breast cancer burden to predict survival after neoadjuvant chemotherapy. *J Clin Oncol* 2007;25:4414–4422.
104. Chollet P, Abrial C, Durando X, et al. A new prognostic classification after primary chemotherapy for breast cancer: residual disease in breast and nodes (RDBN). *Cancer J* 2008;14:128–132.
105. Addington S, Sharkey F, Fowler L, et al. Effects of preoperative chemotherapy on the morphology of resectable breast carcinoma. *Lab Invest* 1994;70:12A.
106. McCready DR, Hortobagyi GN, Kau SW, et al. The prognostic significance of lymph node metastases after preoperative chemotherapy for locally advanced breast cancer. *Arch Surg* 1989;124:21–25.
107. Rilke F, Veronesi U, Luini A, et al. Preoperative chemotherapy alone and combined with preoperative radiotherapy in small-size breast cancer. *Breast J* 1996;2:176–180.
108. Aktepe F, Kapucuoglu N, Pak I. The effects of chemotherapy on breast cancer tissue in locally advanced breast cancer. *Histopathology* 1996;29:63–67.
109. Rasbridge SA, Gillett CE, Seymour AM, et al. The effects of chemotherapy on morphology, cellular proliferation, apoptosis and oncoprotein expression in primary breast carcinoma. *Br J Cancer* 1994;70:335–341.
110. Amat S, Abrial SC, Penault-Llorca F, et al. High prognostic significance of residual disease after neoadjuvant chemotherapy: a retrospective study in 710 patients with operable breast cancer. *Breast Cancer Res Treat* 2005;94:255–263.
111. Burcombe RJ, Makris A, Richman PI, et al. Evaluation of ER, PgR, HER-2 and Ki-67 as predictors of response to neoadjuvant anthracycline chemotherapy for operable breast cancer. *Br J Cancer* 2005;92:147–155.
112. Ellis MJ, Suman VJ, Hoog J, et al. Randomized phase II neoadjuvant comparison between letrozole, anastrozole, and exemestane for postmenopausal women with estrogen receptor-rich stage 2 to 3 breast cancer: clinical and biomarker outcomes and predictive value of the baseline PAM50-based intrinsic subtype—ACOSOG Z1031. *J Clin Oncol* 2011;29:2342–2349.
113. Rabban JT, Glidden D, Kwan ML, et al. Pure and predominantly pure intralymphatic breast carcinoma after neoadjuvant chemotherapy: an unusual and adverse pattern of residual disease. *Am J Surg Pathol* 2009;33:256–263.
114. Kennedy S, Merino MJ, Swain SM, et al. The effects of hormonal and chemotherapy on tumoral and nonneoplastic breast tissue. *Hum Pathol* 1990;21:192–198.
115. Krishnamurthy S, Sneige N, Bedi DG, et al. Role of ultrasound-guided fine-needle aspiration of indeterminate and suspicious axillary lymph nodes in the initial staging of breast carcinoma. *Cancer* 2002;95:982–988.
116. Chang MC, Crystal P, Colgan TJ. The evolving role of axillary lymph node fine-needle aspiration in the management of carcinoma of the breast. *Cancer Cytopathol* 2011;119:328–334.
117. Kuerer HM, Newman LA, Fornage BD, et al. Role of axillary lymph node dissection after tumor downstaging with induction chemotherapy for locally advanced breast cancer. *Ann Surg Oncol* 1998;5:673–680.
118. Lenert JT, Vlastos G, Mirza NQ, et al. Primary tumor response to induction chemotherapy as a predictor of histological status of axillary nodes in operable breast cancer patients. *Ann Surg Oncol* 1999;6:762–767.
119. Neuman H, Carey LA, Ollila DW, et al. Axillary lymph node count is lower after neoadjuvant chemotherapy. *Am J Surg* 2006;191:827–829.
120. Kuerer HM, Sahin AA, Hunt KK, et al. Incidence and impact of documented eradication of breast cancer axillary lymph node metastases before surgery in patients treated with neoadjuvant chemotherapy. *Ann Surg* 1999;230:72–78.
121. Schwartz GF, Tannebaum JE, Jernigan AM, et al. Axillary sentinel lymph node biopsy after neoadjuvant chemotherapy for carcinoma of the breast. *Cancer* 2010;116:1243–1251.
122. Kuerer HM, Newman LA, Smith TL, et al. Clinical course of breast cancer patients with complete pathologic primary tumor and axillary lymph node response to doxorubicin-based neoadjuvant chemotherapy. *J Clin Oncol* 1999;17:460–469.
123. Klauber-DeMore N, Ollila DW, Moore DT, et al. Size of residual lymph node metastasis after neoadjuvant chemotherapy in locally advanced breast cancer patients is prognostic. *Ann Surg Oncol* 2006;13:685–691.

124. Adair FE, Mellors RC, et al. The use of estrogens and androgens in advanced mammary cancer; clinical and laboratory study of 105 female patients. *J Am Med Assoc* 1949;140:1193–1200.
125. Taylor SG III, Slaughter DP, Smejkal W, et al. The effect of sex hormones on advanced carcinoma of the breast. *Cancer* 1948;1:604–617.
126. Huseby RA, Thomas LB. Histological and histochemical alterations in the normal breast tissues of patients with advanced breast cancer being treated with estrogenic hormones. *Cancer* 1954;7:54–74.
127. Emerson WJ, Kennedy BJ, Taft EB. Correlation of histological alterations in breast cancer with response to hormone therapy. *Cancer* 1960;13:1047–1052.
128. Ward HW. Anti-oestrogen therapy for breast cancer: a trial of tamoxifen at two dose levels. *Br Med J* 1973;1:13–14.
129. Davies C, Godwin J, Gray R, et al. Relevance of breast cancer hormone receptors and other factors to the efficacy of adjuvant tamoxifen: patient-level meta-analysis of randomised trials. *Lancet* 2011;378:771–784.
130. Goss PE, Strasser K. Aromatase inhibitors in the treatment and prevention of breast cancer. *J Clin Oncol* 2001;19:881–894.
131. Dixon JM, Renshaw L, Dixon J, et al. Invasive lobular carcinoma: response to neoadjuvant letrozole therapy. *Breast Cancer Res Treat* 2011;130:871–877.
132. Fisher B, Costantino JP, Wickerham DL, et al. Tamoxifen for prevention of breast cancer: report of the National Surgical Adjuvant Breast and Bowel Project P-1 Study. *J Natl Cancer Inst* 1998;90:1371–1388.
133. Allred DC, Anderson SJ, Paik S, et al. Adjuvant tamoxifen reduces subsequent breast cancer in women with estrogen receptor-positive ductal carcinoma *in situ*: a study based on NSABP protocol B-24. *J Clin Oncol* 2012;30:1268–1273.
134. Walker KJ, Price-Thomas JM, Candlish W, et al. Influence of the antioestrogen tamoxifen on normal breast tissue. *Br J Cancer* 1991;64:764–768.
135. Sorlie T, Perou CM, Tibshirani R, et al. Gene expression patterns of breast carcinomas distinguish tumor subclasses with clinical implications. *Proc Natl Acad Sci U S A* 2001;98:10869–10874.
136. Sharma R, Wagner JL, Hwang RF. Ablative therapies of the breast. *Surg Oncol Clin N Am* 2011;20:317–339.
137. Jeffrey SS, Birdwell RL, Ikeda DM, et al. Radiofrequency ablation of breast cancer: first report of an emerging technology. *Arch Surg* 1999;134:1064–1068.
138. Noguchi M, Motoyoshi A, Earashi M, et al. Long-term outcome of breast cancer patients treated with radiofrequency ablation. *Eur J Surg Oncol* 2012;38:1036–1042.
139. Oura S, Tamaki T, Hirai I, et al. Radiofrequency ablation therapy in patients with breast cancers two centimeters or less in size. *Breast Cancer* 2007;14:48–54.
140. Klimberg VS, Boneti C, Adkins LL, et al. Feasibility of percutaneous excision followed by ablation for local control in breast cancer. *Ann Surg Oncol* 2011;18:3079–3087.
141. Roubidoux MA, Sabel MS, Bailey JE, et al. Small (<2.0-cm) breast cancers: mammographic and US findings at US-guided cryoablation—initial experience. *Radiology* 2004;233:857–867.
142. Tafra L, Smith SJ, Woodward JE, et al. Pilot trial of cryoprobe-assisted breast-conserving surgery for small ultrasound-visible cancers. *Ann Surg Oncol* 2003;10:1018–1024.
143. Sahoo S, Talwalkar SS, Martin AW, et al. Pathologic evaluation of cryoprobe-assisted lumpectomy for breast cancer. *Am J Clin Pathol* 2007;128:239–244.
144. Nurko J, Mabry CD, Whitworth P, et al. Interim results from the FibroAdenoma Cryoablation Treatment Registry. *Am J Surg* 2005;190:647–651; discussion 651–652.
145. Littrup PJ, Jallad B, Chandiwala-Mody P, et al. Cryotherapy for breast cancer: a feasibility study without excision. *J Vasc Interv Radiol* 2009;20:1329–1341.
146. Dowlatshahi K, Fan M, Gould VE, et al. Stereotactically guided laser therapy of occult breast tumors: work-in-progress report. *Arch Surg* 2000;135:1345–1352.
147. Dowlatshahi K, Francescatti DS, Bloom KJ. Laser therapy for small breast cancers. *Am J Surg* 2002;184:359–363.
148. van Esser S, Stapper G, van Diest PJ, et al. Ultrasound-guided laser-induced thermal therapy for small palpable invasive breast carcinomas: a feasibility study. *Ann Surg Oncol* 2009;16:2259–2263.
149. Bloom KJ, Dowlat K, Assad L. Pathologic changes after interstitial laser therapy of infiltrating breast carcinoma. *Am J Surg* 2001;182:384–388.
150. Hynynen K, Pomeroy O, Smith DN, et al. MR imaging-guided focused ultrasound surgery of fibroadenomas in the breast: a feasibility study. *Radiology* 2001;219:176–185.
151. Vogl TJ, Farshid P, Naguib NN, et al. Thermal ablation therapies in patients with breast cancer liver metastases: a review. *Eur Radiol* 2013;23:797–804.

CHAPTER 42

Cutaneous Neoplasms

FREDERICK C. KOERNER

MELANOCYTIC LESIONS OF MAMMARY SKIN AND BREAST

Melanocytic lesions of the mammary gland occur in several forms: cutaneous nevus, cutaneous melanoma, primary melanoma of the mammary parenchyma, and benign melanocytic lesions of the mammary parenchyma.

Cutaneous Nevus

Like the skin covering the rest of the body, the skin of the breast gives rise to commonplace nevi. Those arising in the mammary skin do not differ from nevi of other locations in their general histologic classification (junctional, compound, and intradermal types) or their division into well-recognized variants. Rongioletti et al.[1] compared 101 nevi from mammary skin with 97 nevi from other sites, mainly the back and extremities, excluding those of the palms of the hands and soles of the feet. There was no significant difference in the frequencies of different types. The four most common types of mammary cutaneous nevi (Clark nevi, compound nevi, lentiginous compound nevi, and congenital nevi) accounted for two-thirds of the lesions. Eighty percent of mammary cutaneous nevi were from women. The age distribution of patients with mammary cutaneous nevi (range, 8 to 81 years; mean, 31.5 ± 12.7 years) was not significantly different from patients with nevi at other sites. In this study, nevi of the skin of the breast had atypical features significantly more often than nevi from other sites. For this reason, dermatopathologists regard such nevi as members of a group termed "nevi of special sites," a category that also includes nevi of the genital, acral, and flexural locations.[2,3] Special site nevi may show architectural features overlapping with melanoma; consequently, pathologists can misinterpret these nevi as dysplastic nevi or even melanomas. Special site nevi of the breast more frequently display intraepidermal melanocytes above the basal layer, melanocytic atypia, and dermal fibrosis than do nevi in other locations.[1] The presence of these features does not seem to foretell any unusual biologic behavior. Pathologists should take note of these peculiarities so as to avoid raising undue alarm.

Cutaneous Melanoma

Cutaneous melanoma represents the most common malignant melanocytic lesion involving the breast. It occurs more often in men than in women.[4–7] The ages of the patients range from 16 to 86 years. The average age of women is the mid-30s and of men the 40s.[6] Any region may be affected, but the upper quadrants and especially the upper inner quadrant represent favored locations in women.[8] Approximately two-thirds of melanomas arise medial to the midclavicular line or in the central region, where exposure to the sun is greatest.[6,8] The left and right breasts of women are involved with equal frequency.[8] Origin in the nipple–areola complex (Figs. 42.1A, B) is relatively uncommon.[9–12] When the patient reports a recent change in a long-standing pigmented lesion, the presence of an antecedent nevus is suspected and is often confirmed histologically. Some patients with malignant melanoma of the nipple or areola reported a change in an existing "mole," but in most cases a new pigmented lesion was described.[4,9,11] Origin of a malignant melanoma of the mammary skin at the site of a tattoo in the skin of the breast has been reported.[13]

There is no predilection for any subtype of malignant melanoma to arise in the skin of the breast. Superficial spreading melanomas occur most frequently, but nodular and ulcerated types have been described, also.[8,14] Melanomas of the skin of the breast demonstrate the macroscopic features seen in melanomas arising in other cutaneous sites, and the histologic characteristics of mammary cutaneous melanomas do not differ from those of other cutaneous melanomas. The diagnosis of melanoma of the skin of the breast is based on the same criteria generally employed to assess cutaneous melanocytic lesions at other sites.

Melanomas involving the mammary skin do not always represent primary tumors, for melanomas arising in extramammary sites can spread to the skin of the breast.[14] Attention to the clinical history will keep one from mistaking the cutaneous metastasis of a melanoma for a primary tumor.

Treatment and Prognosis of Mammary Cutaneous Melanoma

Metastases from mammary cutaneous melanomas occur in axillary lymph nodes in about 50% of patients, and they are more frequently associated with lateral tumors than with medial ones. Supraclavicular lymph node metastases derive from tumors of the infraclavicular region or upper half of the breast. Internal mammary lymph node metastases were not found in 19 patients subjected to dissection of these

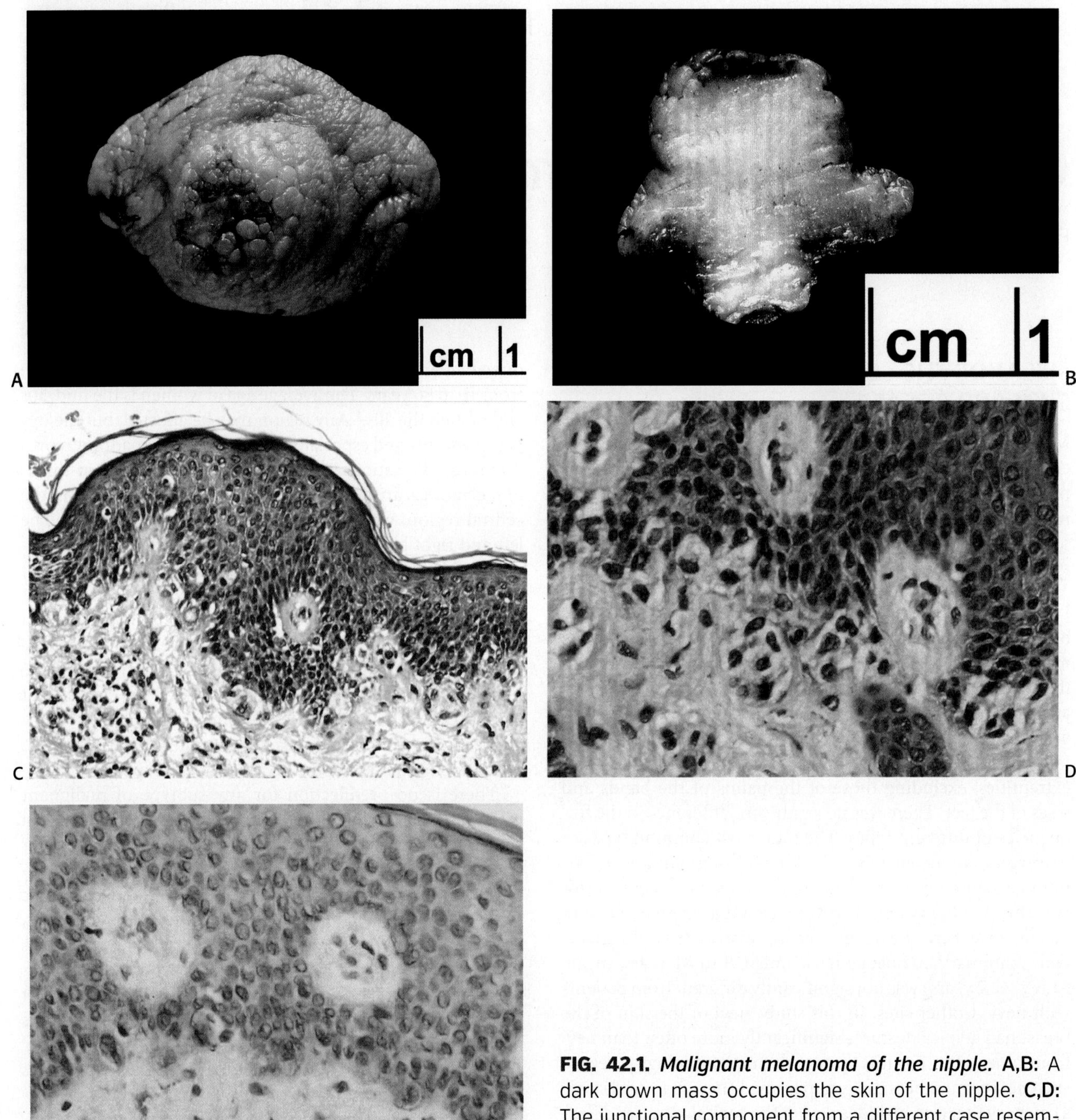

FIG. 42.1. ***Malignant melanoma of the nipple.*** **A,B:** A dark brown mass occupies the skin of the nipple. **C,D:** The junctional component from a different case resembles Paget disease. **E:** The tumor cells are immunoreactive for S-100 protein.

nodes.[5,6] Only 6 of 16 patients with widely disseminated malignant melanoma at autopsy had metastases in internal mammary lymph nodes.[6] The frequencies of regional lymph node involvement and 5-year disease-free survival (DFS) are inversely related to the thickness of the primary lesion as determined by Clark level of invasion[6] and to the stage at diagnosis. In the largest series, about 60% of all patients remained disease free 5 years after treatment. When axillary lymph nodes were not involved, the 5-year DFS was nearly 90%, and it dropped to about 25% when there were axillary nodal metastases.[6] When stratified by stage, there were no significant differences in outcomes between men and women or between patients with medial and lateral lesions.

Most patients in retrospective series were treated by mastectomy and axillary dissection regardless of the location of the primary lesion. Although mastectomy might be necessary in some cases, many patients can be treated with wide excision that may include some underlying breast parenchyma.[6,7] Origin in the nipple–areola complex is not considered a contraindication to wide excision if a cosmetically acceptable result can be obtained.[9] Axillary dissection, when performed, should include the tail of Spence, to ensure excision of all lymph nodes. Sentinel lymph node mapping is a reliable method to assess the axilla and other lymph node sites in patients with malignant melanoma of the mammary skin.

Melanin Pigmentation of Mammary Carcinoma in the Skin (Melanocytic Colonization of Mammary Carcinoma)

Conventional breast carcinomas involving the skin of Caucasian, Oriental, and African American individuals can become so heavily pigmented that they mimic melanomas.[15] On occasion, the melanin resides only in melanocytes and melanophages that have heavily colonized the region of the carcinoma. Saitoh et al.[16] described such a pigmented tumor excised from the right nipple of a 63-year-old man. The tumor was located in the breast and dermis without Paget disease of the epidermis. Histologically, the tumor was described as a ductal carcinoma infiltrated by pigment-containing dendritic melanocytes. Immunoreactivity for S-100 and HMB45 was limited to the melanocytes, which were not stained by markers of epithelial differentiation. Mele et al.[17] described a striking example of this phenomenon in a 74-year-old woman with a massive carcinoma of the breast with extensive involvement of lymphatic vessels and cutaneous metastases. Melanocytic colonization is not limited to breast carcinomas involving the skin. It has been described in other epithelial tissues such as the oral mucosa and minor salivary glands[18] and the epithelium overlying an anorectal carcinoma.[19]

Besides accumulating melanin within their cytoplasm, the colonizing melanocytes can transfer it to the carcinoma cells. In their description of a mammary carcinoma involving the nipple and areola of a 50-year-old woman, Sau et al.[20] noted that "a few granules of melanin pigment were present in some of the tumor cells." This phenomenon occurs commonly when mammary carcinoma cells infiltrate the papillary dermis, breach the epidermal–dermal junction, and make contact with the basal melanocytes. The melanocytes migrate into the dermis, where they surround the carcinoma cells. Release of melanin from the melanocytes with uptake of the pigment by the neoplastic cells leads to pigmentation of the carcinoma. Ultrastructural studies demonstrated intimate juxtaposition of the melanocytes and the carcinoma cells.[21,22] Researchers suggested that the close apposition of the plasma membranes of the two types of cells allows the melanocytes to transfer melanosomes to the carcinoma cells in a process analogous to the transfer of melanosomes from epidermal melanocytes to normal epidermal basal and squamous cells. Ordinarily, the carcinoma cells contain only traces of melanin, but occasional carcinomas become so heavily pigmented that they mimic melanomas. This phenomenon has occurred in the setting of primary breast carcinomas,[20,21] local cutaneous recurrences,[23–25] and cutaneous metastases at various sites.[26–29] Azzopardi and Eusebi[26] noted that melanocytes can mingle with clumps of carcinoma cells within lymphatic vessels. This phenomenon might explain the origin of the melanin pigment in the pulmonary metastasis reported by Blaustein.[30] Release of melanin from intraepidermal melanocytes (melanin "incontinence") without melanocytic proliferation and uptake by macrophages and carcinoma cells can also create a pigmented carcinoma.[31]

Pigmented Paget Disease of the Nipple

The diagnosis of melanoma of the nipple–areola complex presents a more challenging problem. Both the clinical findings and the histologic features of melanomas (Figs. 42.1C, D) can mimic those seen in Paget disease of the nipple (see Chapter 30). One cannot rely on the mere presence of melanin to differentiate these lesions from each other because Paget cells can acquire melanin.[32–34] Culbertson and Horn[32] detected the pigment in the cytoplasm of Paget cells in 10 of 25 cases (40%) of Paget disease of the nipple, and Neubecker and Bradshaw[34] observed pigment granules in 8 of 13 similar cases (62%). The latter authors noted, "these granules were present only in isolated cells and were generally few in number."[34] However, the pigmentation can become intense and give rise to the condition known as *pigmented Paget disease.* The literature contains only a small number of reports of this uncommon condition, and a publication by Soler et al.[35] lists selected clinical and pathologic findings of 17 cases published before 2011. The brown macules or nodules seen in pigmented Paget disease can mimic either a cutaneous nevus[36] or a melanoma[37–41] on both physical and dermoscopic examinations[39,42–44] in Caucasian and African American men and women. The presence of ductal carcinoma in the breast and lactiferous ducts of the nipple[21] as well as reactivity for one or more epithelial markers such as cytokeratin (CK), epithelial membrane antigen, or mucin provides convincing evidence to support the diagnosis of pigmented Paget disease rather than melanoma. A strongly positive S-100 stain is suggestive of malignant melanoma, but confirmatory evidence is necessary to establish the diagnosis confidently in the skin of the nipple. Malignant melanoma is S-100 positive in virtually all instances (Fig. 42.1E), and it is usually reactive for HMB45. Melanoma is not reactive for human epidermal growth factor 2 (HER2), which stains the carcinoma cells in more than 90% of cases of Paget disease of the nipple. Although these generalizations usually hold, Park et al.[45] reported a case of pigmented Paget disease in which the carcinoma cells stained for HMB45 and S-100.

Malignant Melanoma in the Mammary Parenchyma

Before a diagnosis of primary malignant melanoma of the breast parenchyma can be established with confidence, one must exclude the presence of both an extramammary malignant melanoma that could be the source of a metastasis in the breast and a pigmented adenocarcinoma of the breast.

Metastatic Melanoma

Among metastatic tumors in the breast, melanoma stands out as the most frequent46,47 (see Chapter 34). Nonmammary cutaneous melanomas accounted for nearly 40% of the primary malignancies in a series of 169 patients with mammary metastases from the MD Anderson Cancer Center47 and 33% of the cases in the study from the Washington University School of Medicine.46 Most patients had primary lesions on the skin of the upper body, usually the upper arm. In one report,48 the primary site of an apparently metastatic amelanotic melanoma (CK negative, S-100/HMB45 positive) remained undetected despite careful clinical assessment. The median interval between the diagnosis of the primary melanoma and the diagnosis of a mammary metastasis was 52.5 months, but intervals as long as 18 years were observed.49 Almost all patients had other foci of metastatic melanoma.

Although these findings demonstrate that most melanomas involving the mammary parenchyma represent metastatic nodules presenting in the setting of disseminated disease, solitary metastases limited to the breast sometimes occur. Bacchi et al.[50] described the findings of 20 cases of metastatic melanoma clinically presenting as breast carcinoma. Thirteen of the 20 tumors featured predominantly epithelioid or mixed epithelioid/spindle cell morphology, and most cases demonstrated necrosis. Poorly differentiated carcinoma was the most common provisional diagnoses, but lymphoma, sarcoma, and medullary carcinoma were all given initial consideration. Knowledge of the patient's history and the results of immunohistochemical staining for CK, Melan-A, and HMB45 pointed to the correct diagnosis.

Melanin-Producing Carcinoma of the Mammary Parenchyma

A melanin-containing malignant tumor in the breast parenchyma could also represent a primary metaplastic pigmented breast carcinoma. The literature contains several examples of mammary carcinomas in which the carcinoma cells expressed metaplastic melanocytic properties, including the ability to form melanin pigment. Romanelli and Toncini[51] reported a "pigmented papillary carcinoma of the male breast" that arose in the subareolar region and "did not affect the overlaying skin." A woman of 72 years underwent mastectomy for a T2N1 tumor with lymph node metastases documented by axillary dissection.[52] The neoplasm was composed of nonpigmented, invasive ductal carcinoma with ductal carcinoma *in situ* (DCIS) and an invasive heavily pigmented melanocytic component. Epithelial markers (CAM5.2 and CA19-9) were expressed only in the adenocarcinoma, whereas staining for HMB45 and vimentin was limited to the melanocytic regions. S-100 was detected in both portions of the tumor. The pigment was stained black with the Fontana–Masson method and bleached with potassium permanganate. Melanosomes and premelanosomes were demonstrated by electron microscopy. The patient died of metastatic tumor about 18 months after diagnosis, and at autopsy some metastases were "brown-black" grossly. No evidence of an extramammary primary melanoma was detected. Microdissected samples of DCIS and invasive ductal carcinoma from areas with melanocytic differentiation and from metastases were obtained for polymerase chain reaction-based microsatellite analysis with 37 markers. Loss of heterogeneity was detected on multiple chromosome arms, with similar patterns in all components. This result suggests that the adenocarcinomatous and melanocytic aspects of the tumor derived from a single neoplastic clone and that the genetic alterations leading to melanocytic metaplasia occurred in the *in situ* phase of the neoplasm. Padmore et al.[53] studied melanocytic tumors from two women 41 and 44 years old at the time of diagnosis. One patient had a 3-cm tumor and no axillary metastases. She remained disease free 1 year after mastectomy. The second patient had a 3-cm cystic tumor and two lymph nodes with metastases that exhibited carcinomatous and melanomatous features. Cells with an epithelial phenotype were immunoreactive for CK (CAM5.2) and S-100 protein, whereas reactivity for HMB45 was limited to melanin-containing spindle cells in both tumors. Ruffolo et al.[54] described a 4-cm tumor from a 34-year-old woman treated by breast-conserving surgery. Metastatic carcinoma without melanomatous features involved two axillary lymph nodes. The patient died of metastases after chemotherapy. Nonpigmented cells with an epithelial phenotype in this tumor were reactive for CK but not for S-100 or HMB45, whereas the pigmented cells stained with S-100 and HMB45. Yen et al.[55] described a metaplastic breast carcinoma with melanocytic, squamous, and osseous differentiation, and Noske et al.[56] a metaplastic carcinoma containing regions of adenoid cystic carcinoma, spindle cell carcinoma, and melanoma. The Senior Editor has studied other examples of melanin-containing mammary carcinomas (Fig. 42.2). Electron microscopy demonstrated melanosomes in one of these tumors. (For additional information about melanin-producing metaplastic mammary carcinoma, see Chapter 16.)

Accumulation of melanin does not account for the brown color of every pigmented carcinoma. A potential source of melanin-like pigmentation is the accumulation of abundant lipofuscin in carcinoma cells (Fig. 42.3). Grossly, the tumor may appear tan or light brown, but it will not have the dark brown or black color of a melanocytic lesion.[57]

Primary Melanoma Arising in the Mammary Parenchyma

If one excludes the possibilities of metastatic melanoma and a primary pigmented metaplastic adenocarcinoma, then one can entertain the diagnosis of primary melanoma of the mammary parenchyma if pathologic findings fit with that diagnosis. Histologic evidence of a precursor lesion would strengthen that suggestion considerably.

Primary malignant melanoma of the breast parenchyma has been reported, but the precise nature of these lesions has not been well documented.[58–61] Two of these patients died within a year of detection of the breast lesion with widespread metastatic melanoma, leaving considerable doubt as to the primary site.[58,60] The third patient had a solitary metastasis in the ileum resected 3 years after mastectomy for the melanocytic breast lesion, and she remained well 14 years after the time of the mastectomy.[59] An intriguing aspect of the latter case is the notation that the

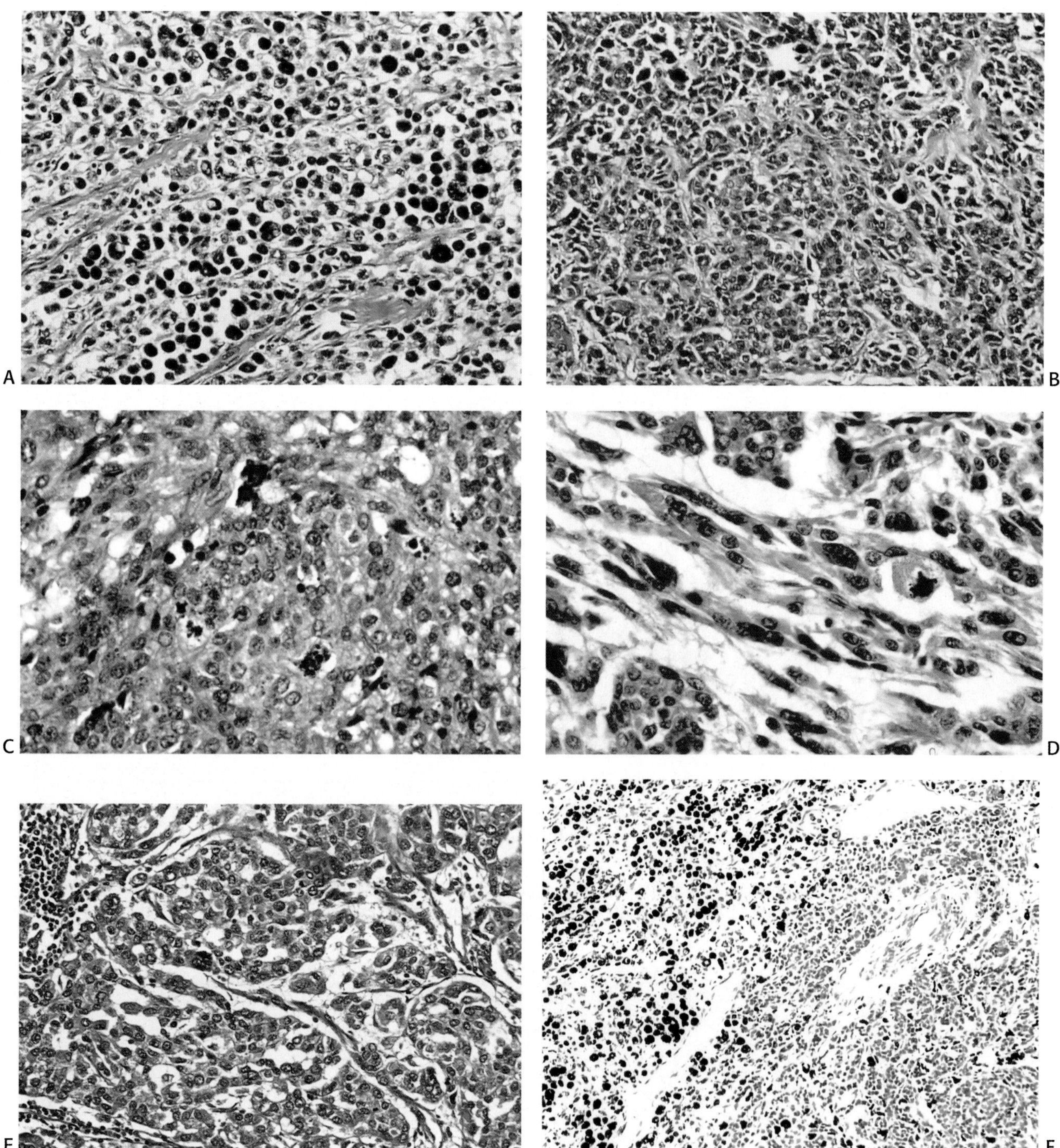

FIG. 42.2. ***Malignant neoplasm with melanocytic and epithelial features.*** The tumor was a 5-cm, partly necrotic and cystic parenchymal breast mass that did not involve the skin in a 47-year-old woman. The patient developed systemic metastases and died within 2 years of diagnosis. No primary cutaneous, ocular, or mucosal lesion was identified. An autopsy was not performed. **A:** Part of the tumor consisted of round, poorly cohesive cells that contained abundant black pigment. **B,C:** An area with an alveolar arrangement composed of tumor cells with little pigment. **D:** Part of the tumor with spindle cells. **E:** Invasive poorly differentiated carcinoma without melanin in the tumor. **F:** Cells in the pigmented portion of the tumor are stained black with the Fontana–Masson stain. **G:** The tumor cells shown in (**E**) were immunoreactive for AE1/3. **H:** Immunoreactivity for HMB45. **I:** Immunoreactivity for S-100. (Courtesy of Dr. B. Shmookler.)

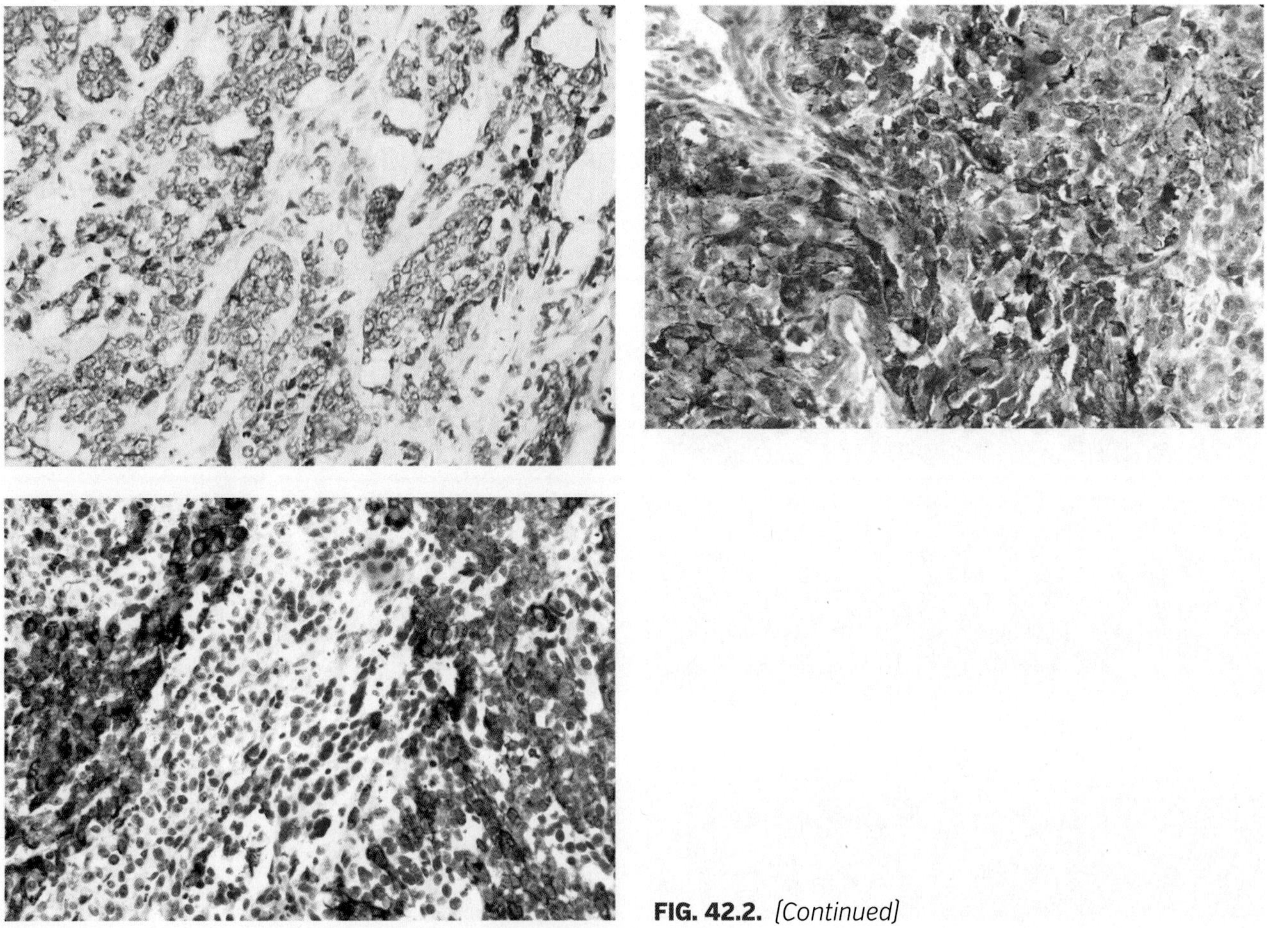

FIG. 42.2. *(Continued)*

patient was aware of the breast tumor for 2 years and that "it has grown steadily" before she presented for treatment. The microscopic description does not mention any nevus-like features in the primary lesion. A fourth patient presented with a 4-cm mass in the lower inner quadrant of the left breast at the site of an excision carried out 18 months earlier.[61] The excision specimen contained a 4 × 3 cm necrotic mass. The tumor cells did not contain melanin, but they stained for S-100 and HMB45 and did not stain for markers of epithelial or mesenchymal cells. Sections

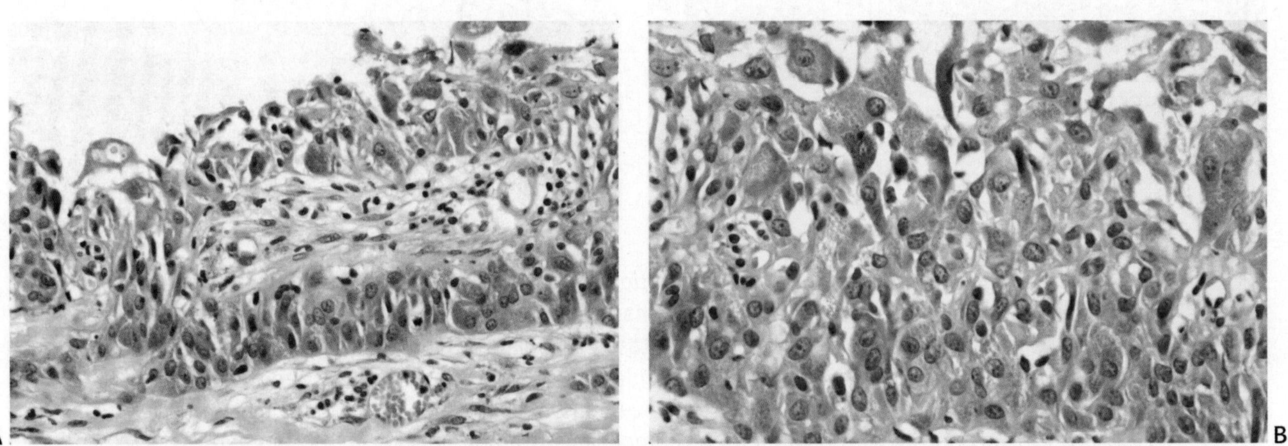

FIG. 42.3. ***Carcinoma with lipofuscin pigment.*** **A,B:** The cavity of the cystic tumor is lined by a thick layer of *in situ* carcinoma with apocrine and clear cell differentiation. Brown, granular pigment is present in some tumor cells. **C:** The brown granular pigment is stained magenta with the periodic acid–Schiff reaction. **D:** The tumor cells are reactive for CK. Melanocytic markers were negative. **E:** Part of the carcinoma showing cribriform growth. **F:** Immunoreactivity for S-100 in a gland-forming area.

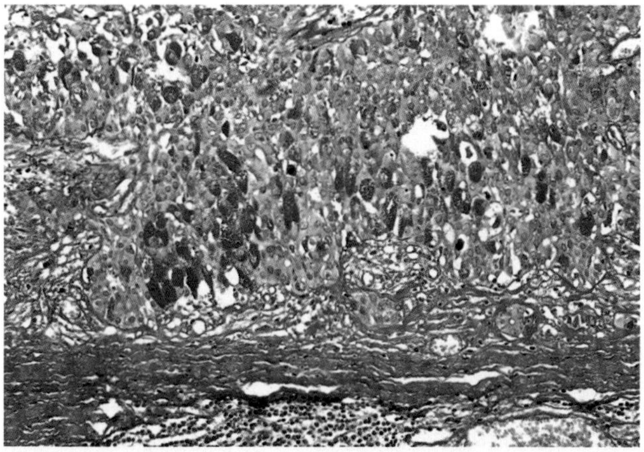

FIG. 42.3. *(Continued)*

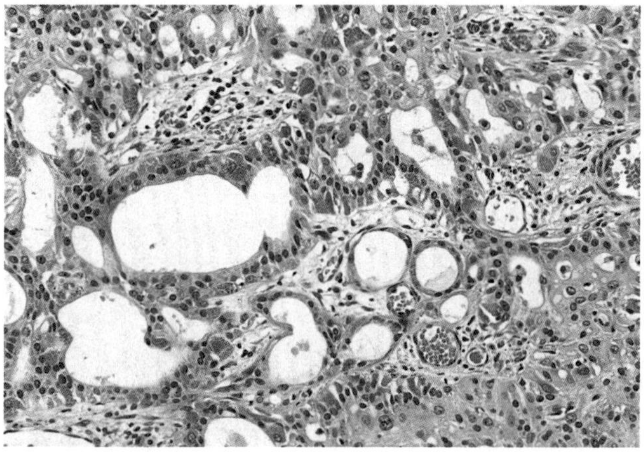

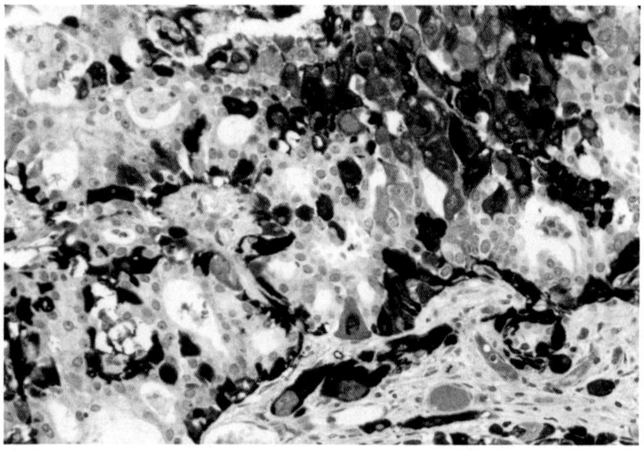

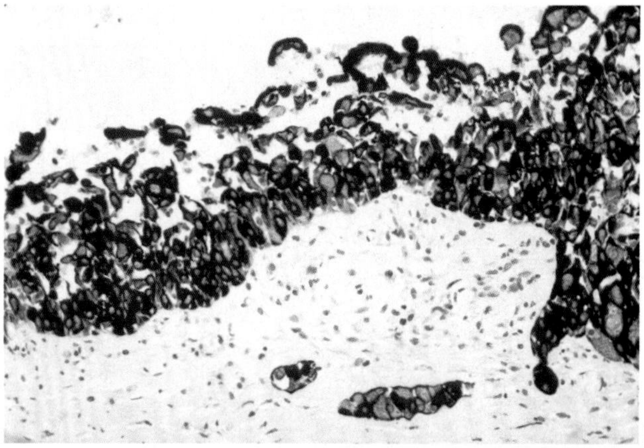

of the original mass were not available for study, so the presence of a precursor lesion could not be established. Metastatic melanoma involved 1 of 13 resected lymph nodes. Clinical evaluation described as "careful examination of the skin and mucosa" did not disclose a primary lesion, and abnormalities were not found in a "metastatic workup." The patient was treated with irradiation and immunotherapy, and remained free of disease during a short period of follow-up.

Benign Melanocytic Lesions of the Mammary Parenchyma

Benign melanocytic lesions of the mammary parenchyma are very uncommon. Blue nevi have been found in the breast (Fig. 42.4), and they may be associated with axillary lymph nodes (see Chapter 43). An exceedingly unusual example of a cellular blue nevus of the breast was studied by the Senior Editor (Fig. 42.5). The lesion was identical to the cellular

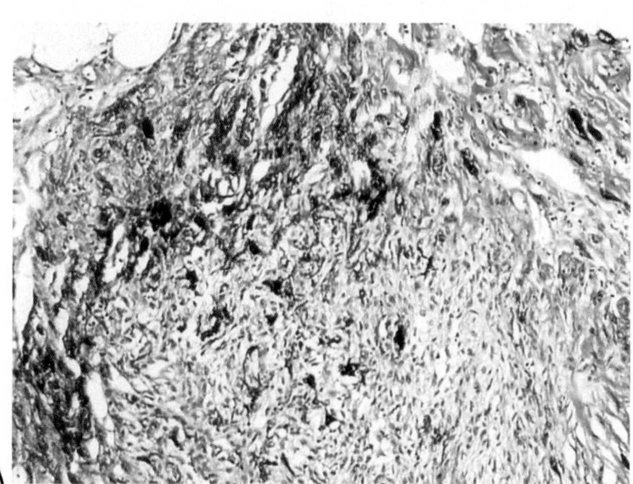
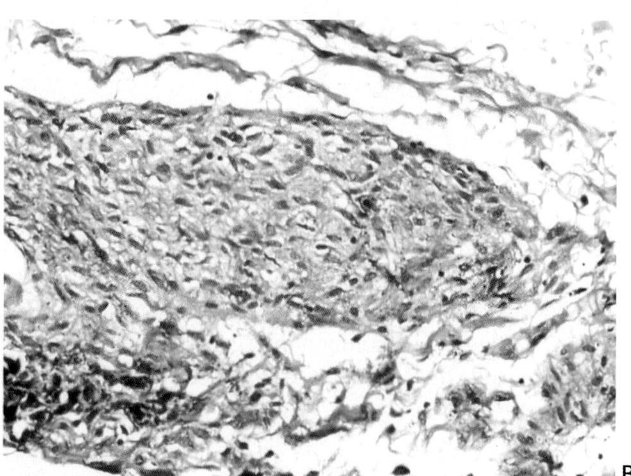

FIG. 42.4. ***Blue nevus of the breast.*** **A:** A heavily pigmented blue nevus found in the breast. **B:** The lesion was associated with a nerve.

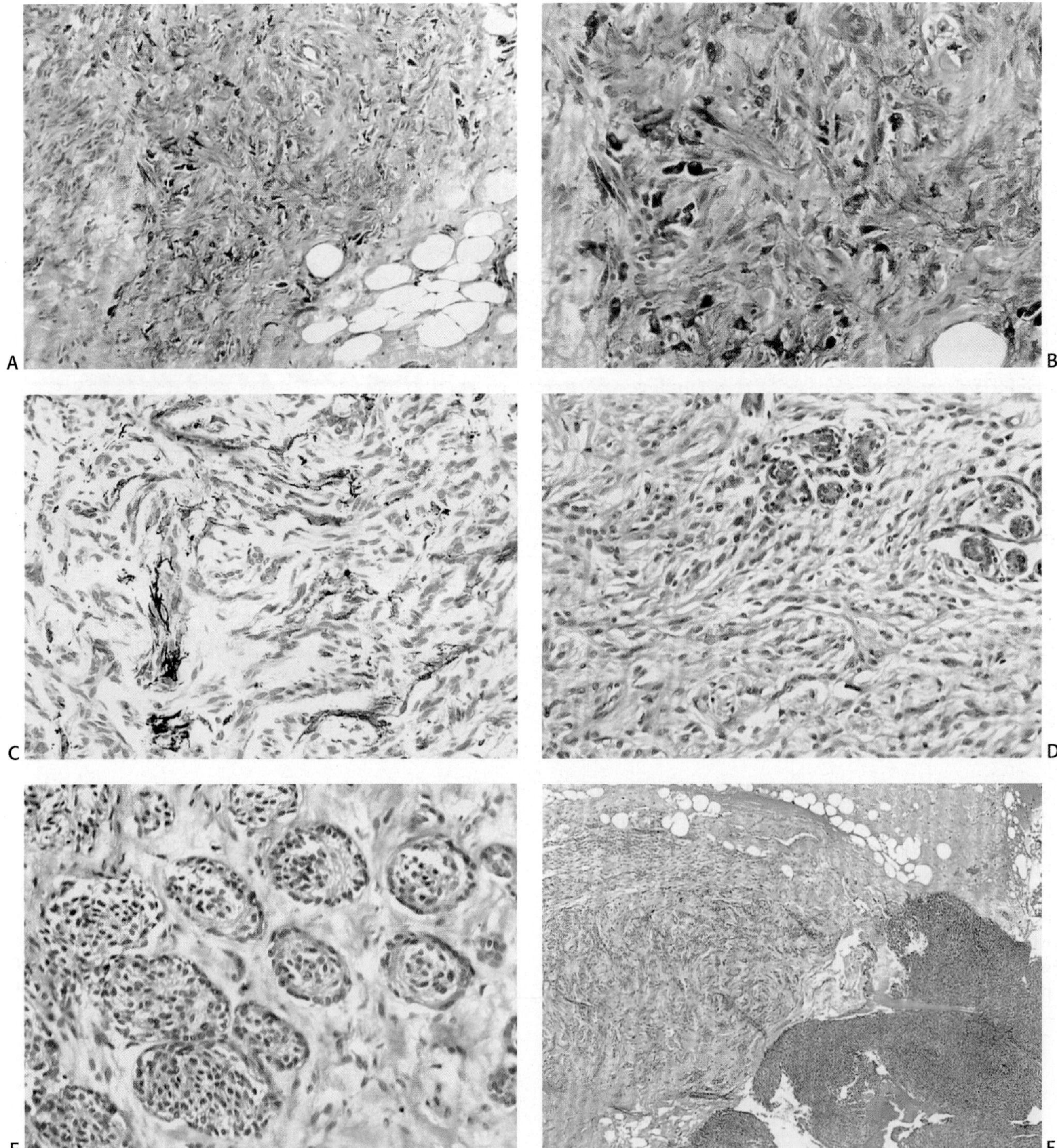

FIG. 42.5. ***Cellular blue nevus of the breast.*** **A,B:** A portion of the lesion was composed of heavily pigmented spindle cells. **C:** The pigment was black with the Fontana-Masson stain. **D:** The spindle cell portion of the tumor invaded mammary glandular parenchyma. **E:** Alveolar nests were formed among the spindle cells. **F:** The cellular portion of the tumor on the *right* contrasts sharply with the blue nevus component. **G:** In the cellular region, the cells have oval nuclei, inconspicuous nucleoli, and very few mitoses. **H:** Electron microscopy revealed aberrant melanosomes. (**H:** Courtesy of Dr. R. A. Erlandson.)

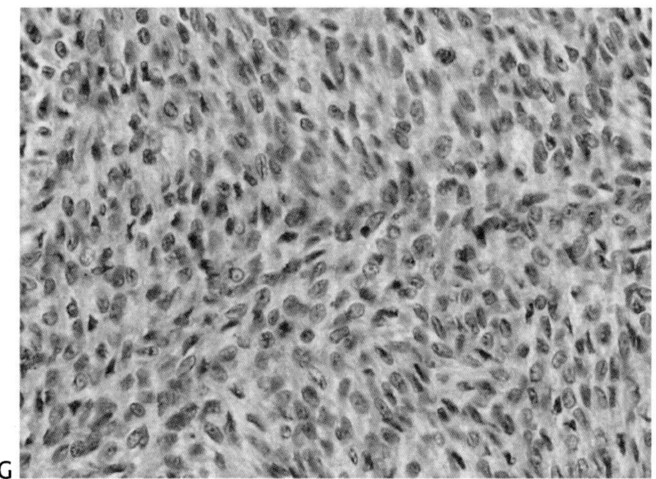

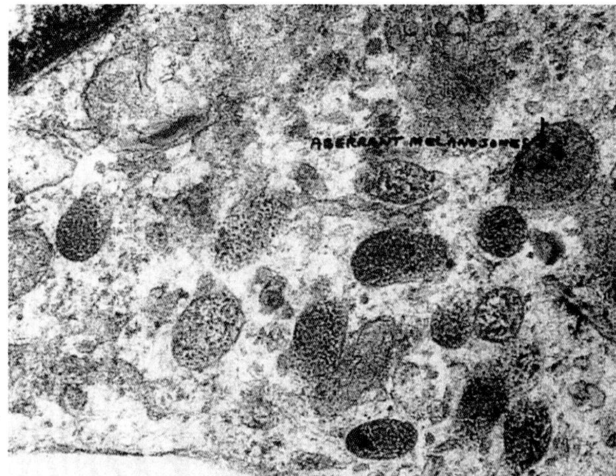

FIG. 42.5. *(Continued)*

blue nevi described by Rodriguez and Ackerman[62] in a series that included two tumors of the "chest and breast" and to a case reported by Busam et al.[63] Malignant melanoma has arisen from cellular blue nevi in other organs, and this lesion could conceivably be the substrate for primary malignant melanoma of the breast.[64,65] Geschickter[66] referred to a malignant mammary tumor with melanin pigment as a melanosarcoma.

NONMELANOCYTIC CUTANEOUS MAMMARY LESIONS

Benign and malignant neoplasms that arise at various cutaneous sites may also be found in the skin and subcutaneous tissue of the mammary region.[67] Seborrheic keratoses and cutaneous hemangiomas represent the most common benign tumors of the mammary skin. Shamsadini et al.[68] described an extraordinary example of the sign of Leser-Trelat (eruptive seborrheic keratoses associated with visceral malignancy) in which the sudden appearance of many seborrheic keratoses in the skin of the right breast of a 48-year-old woman preceded the diagnosis of ipsilateral Paget disease and associated DCIS.

Basal Cell Carcinoma

The upper medial skin of the female breasts, the "cleavage" area, receives more sun exposure than other parts of the breast and may be predisposed to develop nonmelanocytic neoplasms such as basal cell carcinoma (BCC).[69] The majority of patients with BCC of the mammary skin reported in the literature were men. Wong and Smith[70] described a woman with bilateral BCCs. Gombos et al.[71] reported an example of clinically cryptic BCC of the mammary skin that was detected only after calcifications were noted in the skin on the patient's mammogram.

Therapeutic irradiation can also predispose individuals to the development of BCC. One patient, who received superficial irradiation to her thighs, face, and trunk for generalized hirsutism, developed approximately 150 cutaneous BCCs on her face and chest, including several involving the skin overlying both breasts.[72] She also developed a cutaneous squamous cell carcinoma (SQC) and an adenocarcinoma of the breast. A squamous carcinoma of the mammary skin reported by Watanabe et al.[73] was the highly aggressive adenoid variety, which emerged from a well-differentiated SQC that probably had been present for more than 20 years. The carcinoma spawned widespread metastases and killed the patient in 8 months. Alzaraa et al.[74] described a Merkel cell carcinoma involving the deep dermis of the breast of a 74-year-old man. Yavuzer et al.[75] reported a microcystic adnexal carcinoma of the lower inner quadrant of the left breast of an 83-year-old woman.

Pilosebaceous Neoplasms

Several types of tumors arising from the hair apparatus have presented in the skin of men and women overlying the breast. *Pilomatrixoma*, a tumor derived from cells of the outer sheath of the hair follicle root, typically affects the face, head, neck, and upper extremities of young adults. The literature contains about a dozen reports of cases involving the skin of the breast.[76–86] The patients' ages have ranged from 12[83] to 83 years,[78] and the tumor has affected women and men equally. The patients usually seek attention because of a mass of a few months' duration, although a symptomatic interval of 4 years was described in one case.[76] The presence of pain is not usually mentioned. The nodules typically span 1 to 2 cm. The largest, a tumor present for 3 years, measured 12 cm.[82] The masses may become attached to the skin, but they do not become fixed to the chest wall. Except for its attachment to the nodule, the skin often looks normal. In one case, the skin displayed the phenomenon of anetoderma,[83] and in another it appeared "discoloured, unhealthy, and about to ulcerate."[82] The nodules are usually described as hard. The findings of the physical examination can suggest the diagnosis of carcinoma.[77,79,82] On mammography, the mass usually has well-defined margins, but a partially ill-defined margin was reported once.[84] Calcifications can appear pleomorphic[81,86] large and irregular,[78] or small and punctate.[80] On sonographic studies, the masses have shown variable echo patterns.[76,80–82] Posterior shadowing was recorded in two cases.[76,81] The imaging findings also can suggest the diagnosis of malignancy.[76,78,81,85] Most reports do not describe the macroscopic characteristics of the masses (Fig. 42.6A). Ismail et al.[82] wrote: "Macroscopically the tumour weighed 551 g and measured 12 × 10 × 7 cm . . . The tumour was too hard [to] cut, so was sawn instead." Another report[77] described a "grayish-white" mass. Two nodules, 0.4 and 0.5 cm in greatest dimension, were noted by Rousselot et al.[86] Microscopic examination reveals the features of pilomatrixomas seen in tumors from the common locations: peripherally placed basaloid cells, central cells with abundant eosinophilic cytoplasm and small or absent nuclei (ghost cells), keratinous debris, multinucleate giant cells, and calcifications (Fig. 42.6B). Smears prepared from a needle aspiration specimen appear cellular and display the cellular constituents seen in tissue sections.[77,84] Although benign, pilomatrixomas in this location can recur.[86]

Trichoblastomas present as superficial, well-defined masses, which can contain calcifications evident on mammography.[87–89] The tumors consist of nests or cords of cells resembling follicular germinative cells set in a collagenous or myxoid stroma. The cells have indistinct cell borders and dark nuclei, and those in the larger nests may display a palisade arrangement. The stroma forms abortive hair papillae (papillary mesenchymal bodies), which consist of indentations of the stroma into nests of epithelial cells. Pathologists can confuse trichoblastomas with both BCCs and primary breast carcinomas when studying either needle aspiration specimens[89] or core biopsy specimens.[88] Examination of an excision specimen containing the entire mass will usually reveal the diagnostic features.[88] Uchida et al.[90] described a 10-cm *malignant proliferating trichilemmal tumor*, which was first thought to represent a primary SQC of the breast. Attention to the presence of trichilemmal keratinization, the lobulated and well-circumscribed contour of the mass, and the presence of cysts led to the proper diagnosis.

Cutaneous *sebaceous carcinomas* of the breast can mimic an infected sebaceous cyst[91] or a BCC.[92] Sebaceous carcinomas of the skin can arise spontaneously or as part of a hereditary cancer syndrome known as Muir-Torre syndrome, a subtype of Lynch Type II hereditary nonpolyposis colon cancer.

Eccrine Proliferations

The sweat glands of the mammary skin give rise to the types of reactive and neoplastic proliferations that develop in extramammary sites. Yoshii et al.[93] reported a case of *syringoma-like eccrine sweat duct proliferation* occurring in the field of irradiation following a mastectomy for mammary carcinoma. The lesion consisted of papules composed of eccrine ducts, cystic structures, epithelial clusters, and sclerotic collagen. The papules appeared during the period of radiation therapy and spread to involve the entire chest, but they resolved without treatment upon completion of irradiation. Syringoma-like eccrine sweat duct proliferation is considered a reactive process that develops in the setting of inflammatory, neoplastic, and scarring disorders of the skin.

Sweat gland carcinoma is one of the most common types of the adnexal tumor and the one that creates the most diagnostic difficulties[94] (Figs. 42.7 to 42.10). Eccrine carcinomas of the mammary skin are occasionally large enough to impinge upon the breast tissue, thereby obscuring their origin from the skin. When the differential diagnosis includes carcinoma of skin adnexal gland or mammary origin, the biopsy sample should be thoroughly examined for evidence of mammary glandular tissue and for the presence of an *in situ*

A 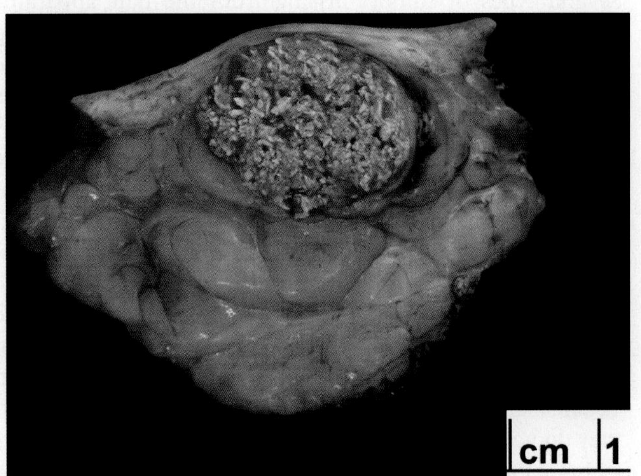

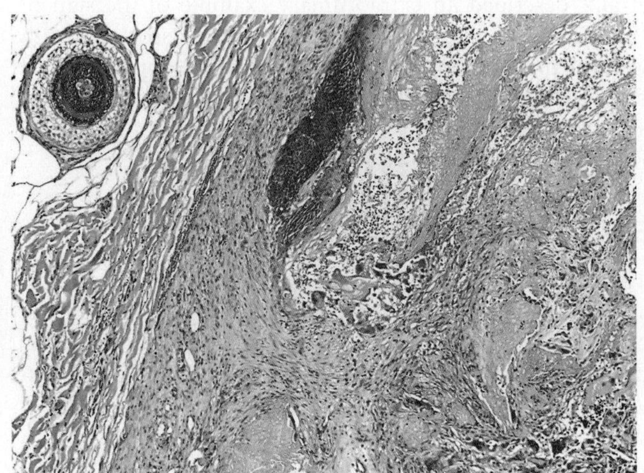 B

FIG. 42.6. ***Pilomatrixoma overlying the breast.*** **A:** The gross appearance of a bisected, circumscribed tumor that impinged on the underlying breast tissue. **B:** This smoothly outlined mass contains a cluster of basaloid cells [*upper center*] and many anucleate cells with eosinophilic cytoplasm ("ghost cells") [*right*] associated with a reactive fibroblastic stroma containing multinucleate giant cells.

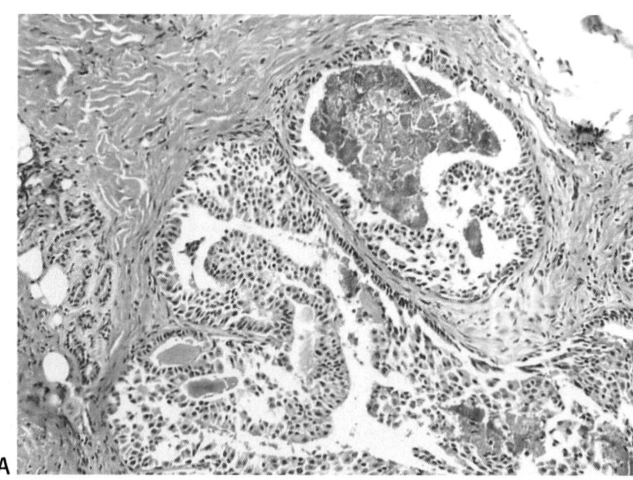

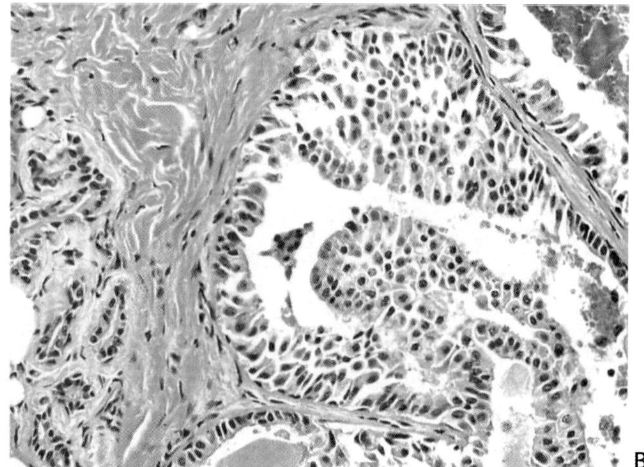

FIG. 42.7. ***Adnexal gland carcinoma, papillary type.*** **A,B:** Orderly papillary carcinoma. An uninvolved sweat gland is shown on the *left*.

component in skin appendages or breast parenchyma. If it is present, the distribution of an *in situ* component can be helpful in determining the primary tissue of origin (Figs. 42.11 and 42.12). When ectopic mammary glandular tissue mingles with skin appendage glands in the dermis of the skin, particularly in the axilla, it is especially difficult to pinpoint the origin of a carcinoma found in these structures even if an *in situ* element is identified. In some of these

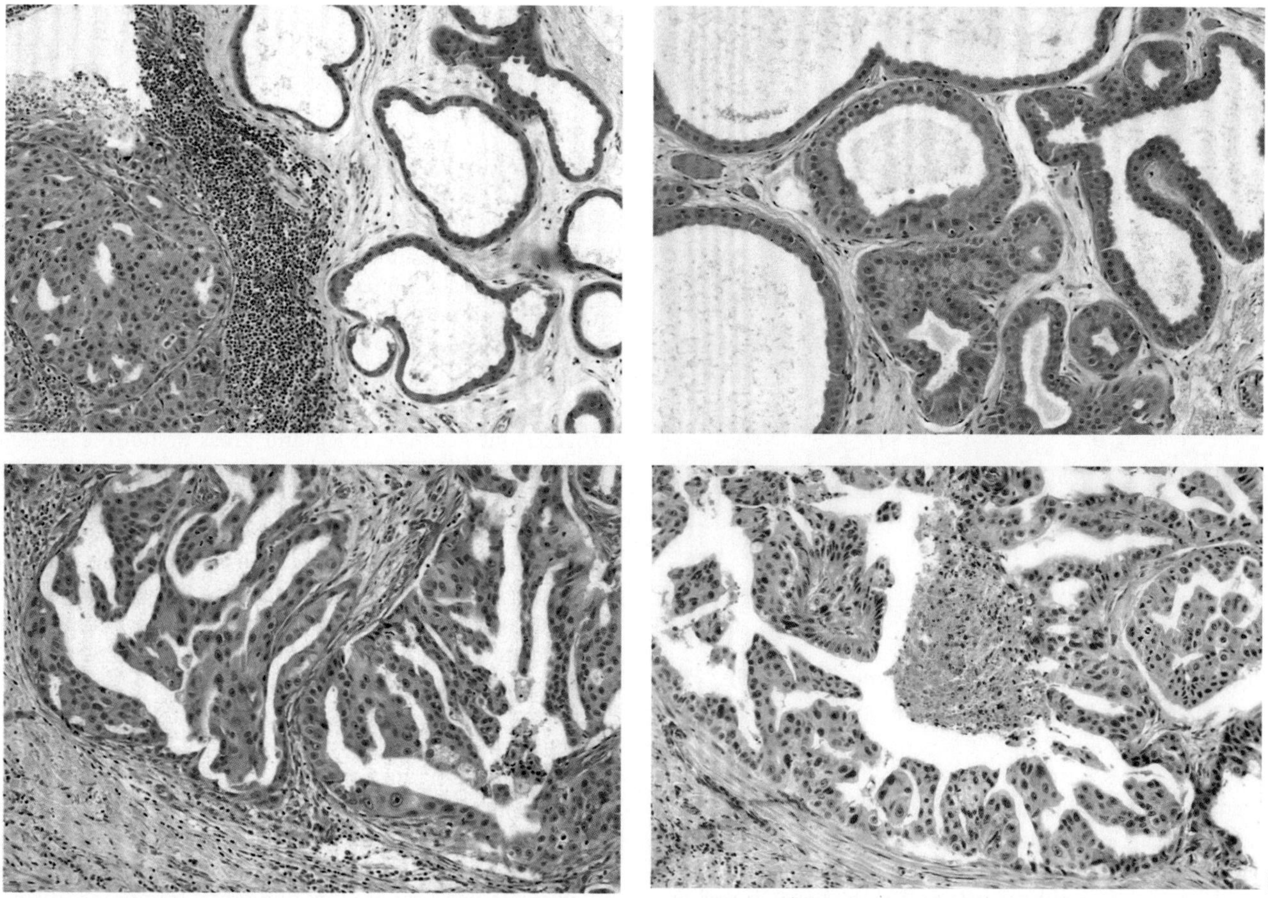

FIG. 42.8. ***Adnexal gland carcinoma, apocrine type.*** All images are from a single subcutaneous axillary tumor. **A:** Apocrine carcinoma is shown adjacent to axillary apocrine glands. **B:** Mild epithelial hyperplasia in apocrine glands. **C:** Papillary apocrine carcinoma. **D:** Micropapillary DCIS with necrosis.

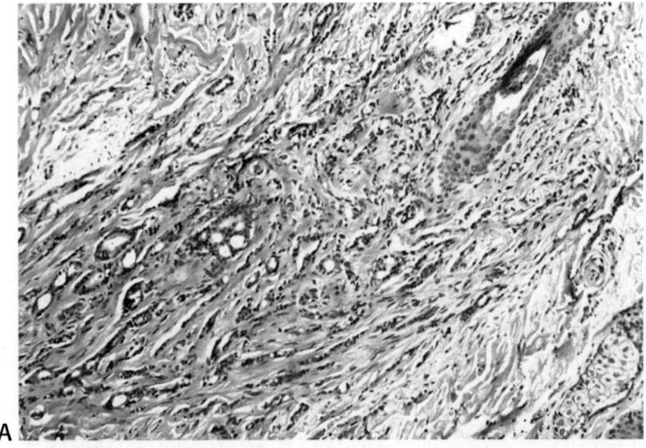

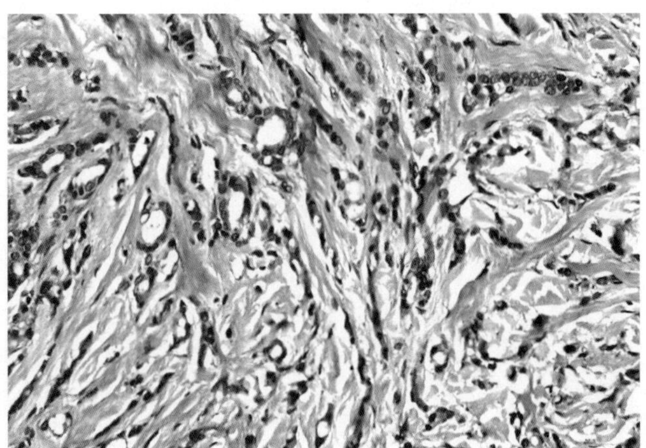

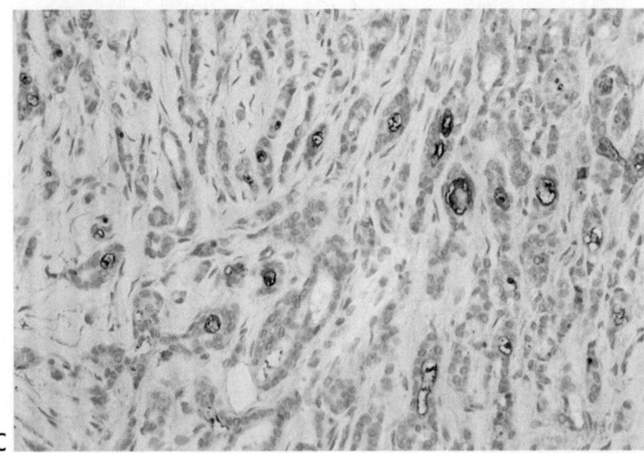

FIG. 42.9. ***Adnexal gland carcinoma, tubulolobular type.*** **A,B:** Invasive carcinoma with tubulolobular growth in the dermis of the scalp. Hair and sebaceous structures are present. **C:** Immunoreactivity for GCDFP-15 is shown in tumor glands. This patient had been treated previously for mucinous mammary carcinoma. The scalp lesion was interpreted as a primary adnexal tumor.

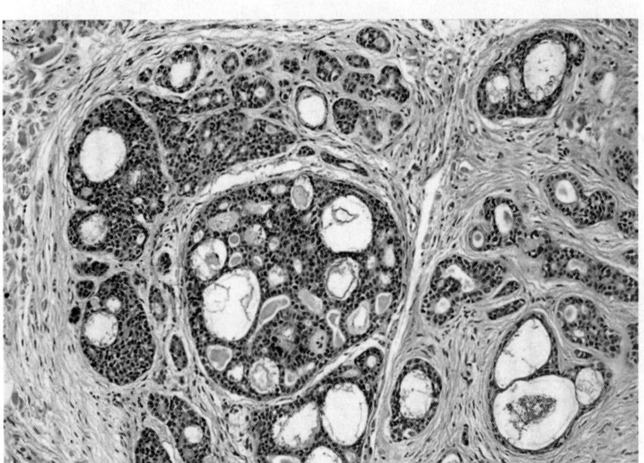

FIG. 42.10. ***Adnexal gland carcinoma, cribriform.*** This image is from a 1-cm discrete tumor in the dermis of the axillary skin.

situations, the distinction between primary or metastatic mammary carcinoma and sweat gland carcinoma cannot be made with absolute certainty, and a judgment that takes into consideration clinical factors as well as the location and the histopathology of the lesion must be made.

For the most part, immunohistochemical markers give similar results in mammary and sweat gland carcinomas (Figs. 42.13 and 42.14).[95] A particularly vexing problem arises if a patient had a prior or has a concurrent carcinoma of the mammary glandular parenchyma and is later found to have an adenocarcinoma in the skin of the axilla or breast or in the skin at a distant site. Wallace et al.[96] studied a series of skin lesions, which included metastatic mammary carcinoma and carcinomas of skin adnexal gland origin. The patterns of immunoreactivity for estrogen receptor (ER), progesterone receptor (PR), and gross cystic disease fluid protein 15 (GCDFP-15) did not differ sufficiently to distinguish the two groups of lesions. Wick et al.[95] not only detected GCDFP-15 significantly more often in breast carcinomas than in eccrine sweat gland carcinomas but also reported finding GCDFP-15 reactivity in sweat gland carcinomas of apocrine type. In the same study, carcinoembryonic antigen was expressed more often by sweat gland carcinomas than by breast carcinomas.

Busam et al.[97] analyzed immunoreactivity for ER, PR, and epidermal growth factor receptor (EGFR) in 42 primary sweat gland carcinomas and breast carcinoma. EGFR reactivity was present in 81% of sweat gland carcinomas and in only 17% and 22%, respectively, of the primary and metastatic breast carcinoma samples. The expressions of ER and PR in sweat gland carcinomas and breast carcinomas did not differ. Hanby et al.[98] studied 12 examples of primary mucinous carcinoma of the skin and found all of the tumors to be strongly immunoreactive for ER. PR was also detected in the 12 tumors, but staining was heterogeneous and weak in some

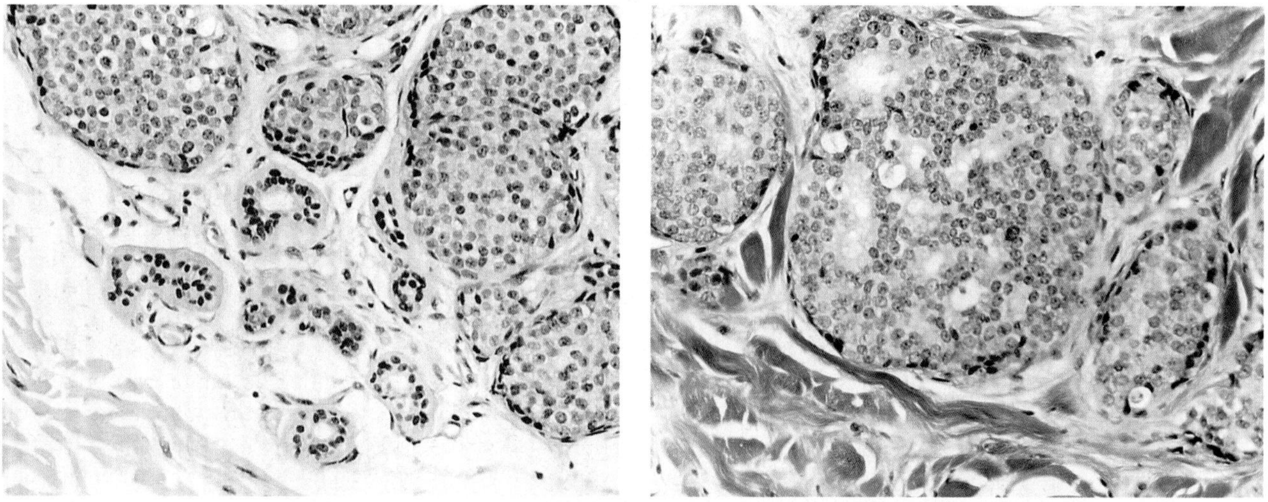

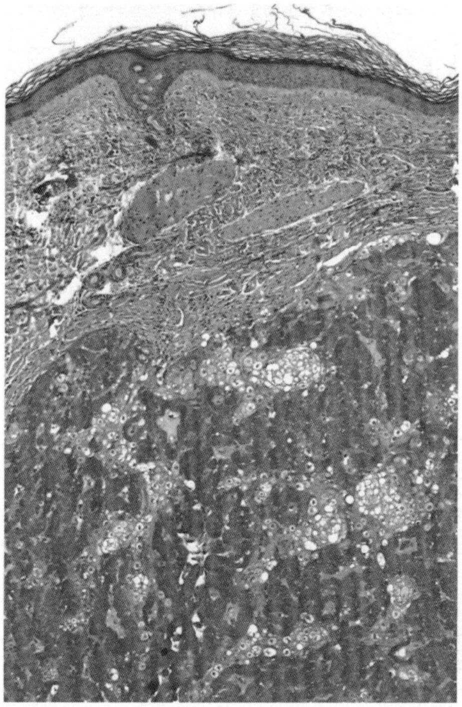

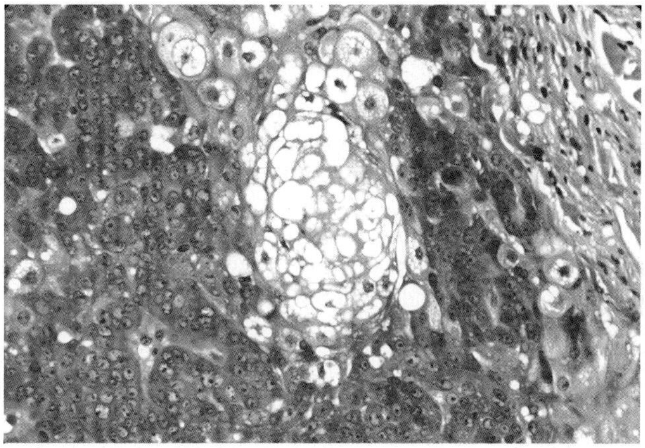

FIG. 42.11. ***Adnexal gland carcinoma.*** **A:** The *in situ* portion of this neoplasm resembles mammary lobular carcinoma *in situ*. Uninvolved sweat gland structures are shown in the *center*. **B:** The invasive component among dermal collagen fibers has a cribriform structure. **C,D:** Another adnexal carcinoma with sebaceous differentiation.

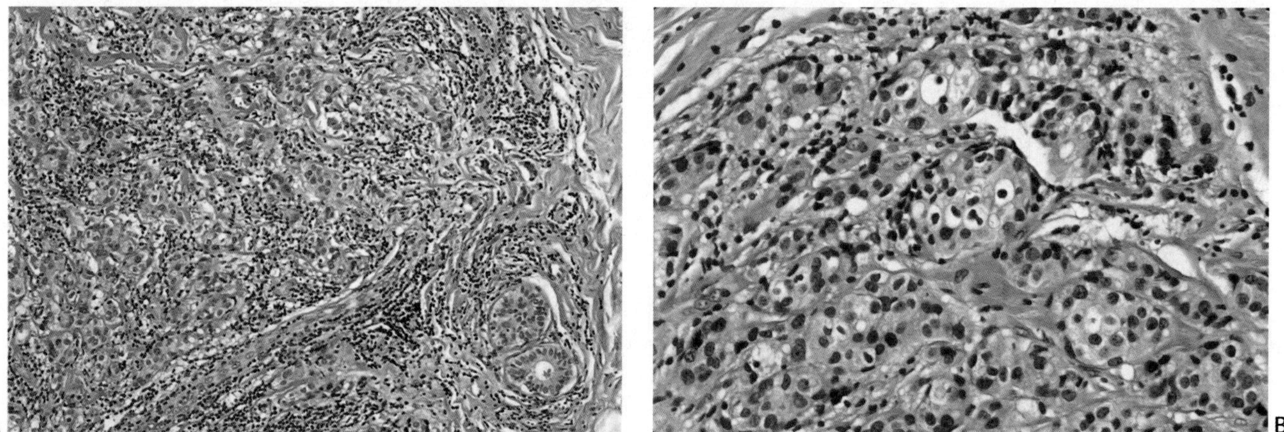

FIG. 42.12. ***Adnexal gland carcinoma with DCIS.*** **A,B:** Invasive carcinoma is shown next to two skin adnexal gland structures. One of these glands has hyperplastic epithelium. **C:** DCIS in an adnexal gland duct.

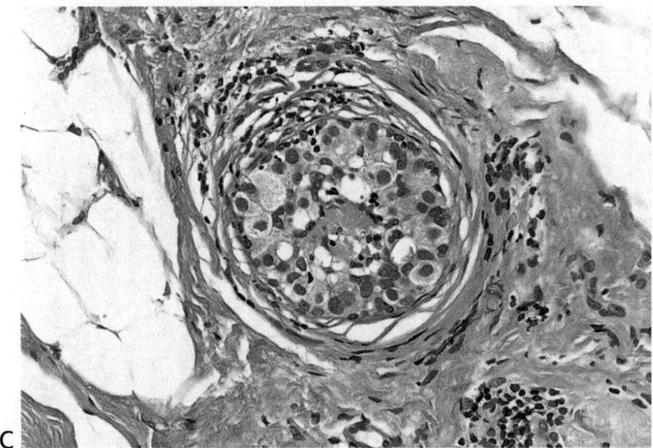

FIG. 42.12. *(Continued)*

instances. Two of the tumors resembled type B mucinous mammary carcinoma, which tends to manifest neuroendocrine differentiation. Both of the type B cutaneous mucinous carcinomas were argyrophilic with the Grimelius stain. The 12 primary cutaneous mucinous carcinomas were also immunoreactive for the mucus-associated peptide TFF1 but not for TFF2, and they expressed TFF1 and TFF3 mRNA. TFF1 and TFF3, members of the trefoil factor family, are peptides upregulated by ER. The presence of mRNA for these proteins indicates the functionality of the ER in these tumors.

Another type of mammary-like carcinoma reported to have arisen in the axillary skin, presumably from sweat glands, is histiocytoid signet ring cell carcinoma. One example found in a 55-year-old man was CK7 positive and not reactive for E-cadherin or hormone receptors.[99] No ectopic breast tissue was present. The neoplasm involved the full thickness of the dermis, giving rise to secondary Paget disease in the overlying epidermis.

Brandt et al.[100] described secretory carcinoma that arose in the axillary skin of a girl. The tumor was present for 2 years before it was excised, when the child was 11 years old. It was located in the dermis of the skin where the intraductal component involved sweat gland ducts. No mammary glandular parenchyma was detected.

The *endocrine mucin-producing sweat gland carcinoma* of the skin,[101] which occurs on the eyelids and face, duplicates the histologic appearance of solid papillary carcinoma of the mammary parenchyma (see Chapter 14). Occurrence of this type of carcinoma in the skin of the breast has not been reported.

Eccrine spiradenomas arise in the skin of the breast only very rarely, and when they do so, they may be mistaken on ultrasound examination for an epidermal cyst[102] or a breast carcinoma.[67] The tumor grows as a well-defined cellular mass surrounded by basement membrane material and composed of closely packed nests of cells in a jigsaw puzzle pattern. The nests consist of peripherally situated small cells with dark

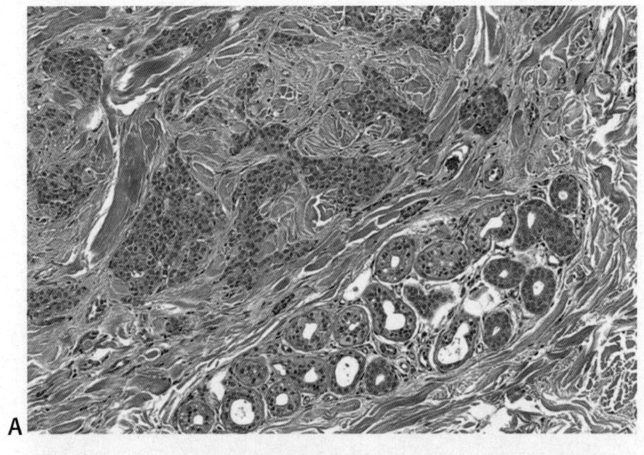

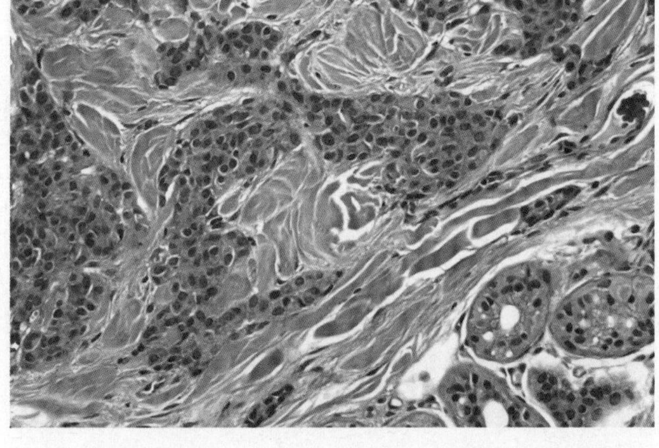

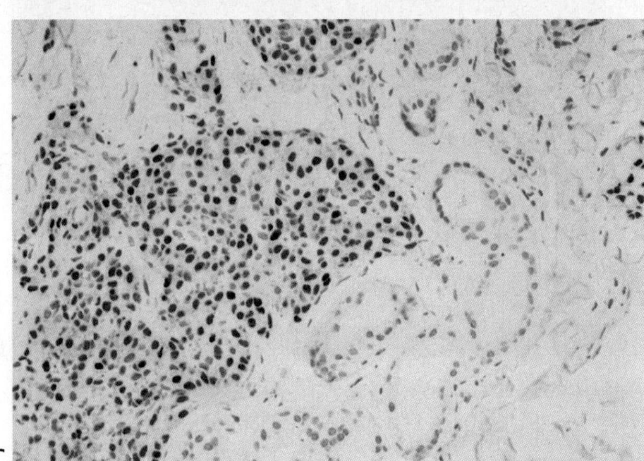

FIG. 42.13. ***Adnexal gland carcinoma in the axillary skin.*** **A,B:** The histologic appearance of this carcinoma shown next to a sweat gland is indistinguishable histologically from mammary carcinoma. **C:** Nuclear reactivity for ER is present only in the carcinoma, which was also immunoreactive for PR and CK7.

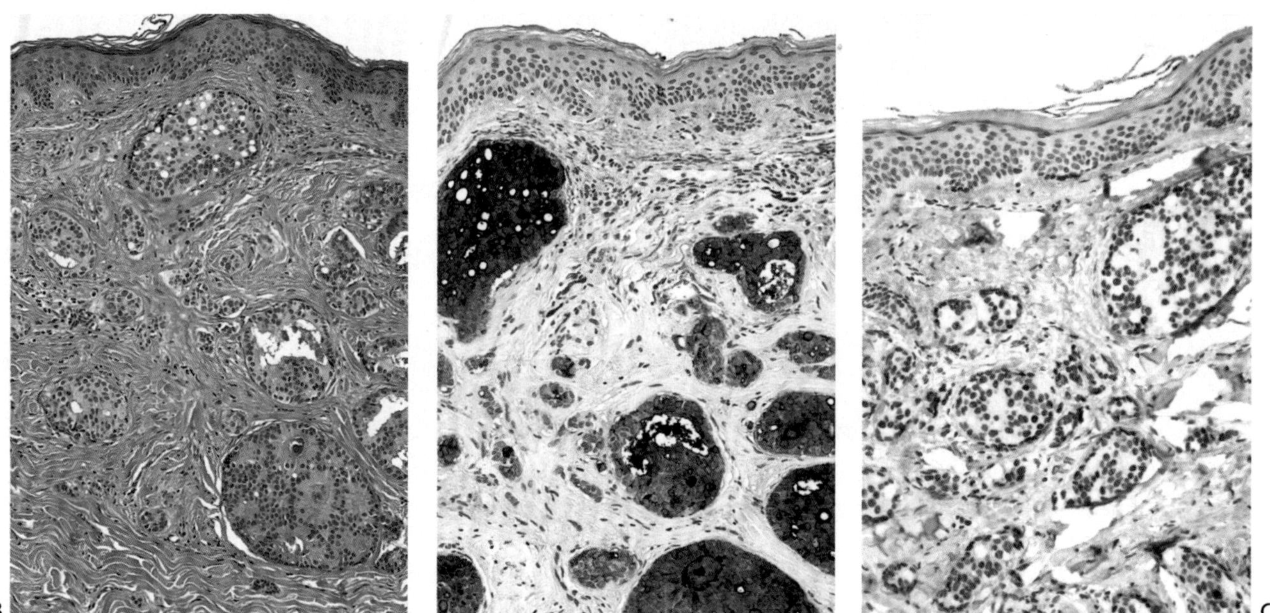

FIG. 42.14. ***Adnexal gland carcinoma of chest wall skin.*** The lesion was an 8-mm cutaneous nodule in the upper mid-chest. No breast tissue was present. **A:** Carcinoma, partly cribriform. Calcifications are present in the gland *at the bottom*. A trace of sebaceous differentiation is evident in the gland just beneath the epidermis. **B:** The tumor was strongly reactive for GCDFP-15. **C:** Nuclear reactivity for ER is shown.

nuclei and central larger cells with pale cytoplasm.[103] Lesions described as primary benign or malignant spiradenomas of the breast parenchyma[104,105] appear to be forms of solid papillary carcinoma or other malignant neoplasms of the breast. The development of spiradenocarcinoma in a long-standing spiradenoma leading to invasion of the underlying breast parenchyma has been reported. Transition to a malignant neoplasm is usually heralded by rapid growth.[106–108] Thomas et al.[108] detailed the case of a 42-year-old woman with a recurrent eccrine spiradenoma that eventually became malignant and spread to three axillary lymph nodes. Saboorian et al.[107] described a 68-year-old woman with a 50-year history of a mass in the upper outer quadrant of the right breast. Recent sudden increase in size, erythema of the overlying skin, and the presence of a nipple discharge led to an excision. The specimen contained an eccrine spiradenoma associated with malignant tumor containing both carcinomatous and sarcomatous elements. In a case published by Tanaka et al.,[109] metastatic malignant eccrine spiradenoma derived from a primary tumor in the abdominal skin and involving an intramammary lymph node simulated a primary breast tumor. Eccrine spiradenomas also arise in the skin of the axilla (Fig. 42.15).

Hidradenomas arise in mammary skin,[110] often near the nipple[111] (Fig. 42.16). These tumors form well-defined partly cystic and partly solid gray-white masses composed of two types of cells in varying proportion: polyhedral cells with round nuclei and slightly basophilic cytoplasm, and round cells with clear cytoplasm, which frequently contains glycogen. Duct-like structures resembling eccrine ducts or displaying squamous metaplasia are often present. Hidradenomas can simulate carcinomas on clinical examination[110,112] and cytologic study.[110,112,113] Hidradenomas seem to arise within the mammary parenchyma, also. Ohi et al.[114] reported one such case in a 55-year-old woman. Domoto et al.[113] detailed a hidradenoma deeply located in the breast of a 44-year-old man. The presence of intraductal components in this case and in the one recounted by Ohi et al.[114] makes it likely that these tumors arose from mammary glandular tissue.

Whether cutaneous or mammary glandular in origin, hidradenomas occur more frequently in women and usually present between the fourth and eighth decades of life.

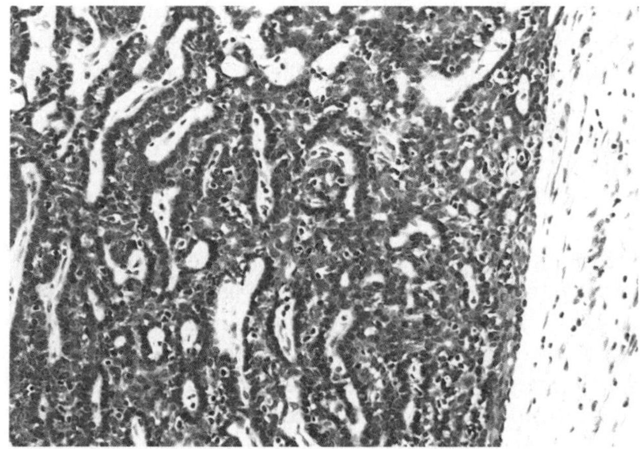

FIG. 42.15. ***Eccrine spiradenoma of axillary skin.***

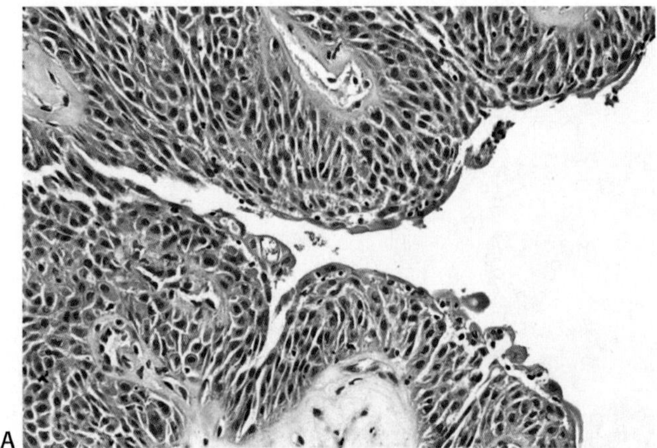
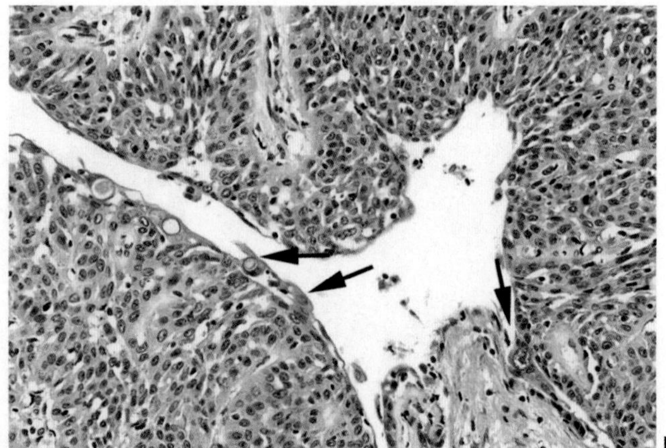

FIG. 42.16. *Hidradenoma, subareolar.* A,B: The tumor was solid and cystic. Note vacuolated superficial cells that contain mucin demonstrated with the mucicarmine stain in (B) (*arrows*).

Grampurohit et al.[115] reported an exceptional case involving the skin of the breast of a man of 18 years. Most examples are benign, but even these tumors can recur if incompletely excised.[116] In the single reported case tested,[117] a hidradenoma arising within the breast demonstrated the t(11;19) translocation seen in approximately 50% of cutaneous hidradenomas.[118] One might note in passing that Japanese patients account for a large proportion of the cases of hidradenoma of the mammary skin or parenchyma reported in the literature.[114]

The literature contains only rare reports of *syringocystadenoma papilliferum* arising from the skin of the breast such as the one by Yamane et al.,[119] who described a 77-year-old woman with three skin lesions of the right breast: a syringocystadenoma papilliferum, a nevus sebaceous, and a tubular apocrine adenoma.

In 2001, Gokaslan et al.[120] described a solitary, primary, parenchymal breast neoplasm showing the typical histologic features of a type of skin adnexal tumor referred to as *cylindroma* (*dermal analog tumor*). (Although the term *cylindroma* has been used to refer to adenoid cystic carcinomas in earlier times, it has since come to designate a skin appendage tumor unrelated to adenoid cystic carcinoma.) During the decade following the first description of this type of mammary tumor, observers added reports of 10 more cases to the literature.[121–124] All patients have been women. With two exceptions, their ages ranged from 62 to 85 years. In the remaining two patients, the tumors appeared at the ages of 37[123] and 59 years[124] as a manifestation of the autosomal dominant, multiple cylindromatosis (Brooke-Spiegler) syndrome. Several of the tumors have arisen close to the nipple. They form well-defined pink-tan to white, rubbery to firm nodules that range from 0.5 to 1.6 cm in greatest dimension. Histologic study reveals epithelial cells in nests of variable size and shape disposed in a "jigsaw puzzle" pattern (Fig. 42.17). Eosinophilic basement membrane–like material (type IV collagen) surrounds each nest and accumulates in small aggregates within the epithelial clusters. The clusters contain two types of epithelial cells: peripheral small basaloid cells with scant cytoplasm and dark nuclei and larger cells with pale cytoplasm and granular nuclei. One could confuse a cutaneous cylindroma with an adenoid cystic carcinoma of the solid type. The presence of nuclear atypia and mitotic figures and the absence of peripheral bands of basement membrane material characterize adenoid cystic carcinoma and differentiate it from cylindroma.[121] Although rare cylindromas have become malignant, but those that arose in the breast have not done so.

LESIONS OF THE NIPPLE

Cutaneous lesions of the nipple have attracted specific attention, and much of the literature devoted to cutaneous lesions of the breast centers on those in this location.

Hyperkeratosis

Benign conditions include several varieties of hyperkeratosis of the nipple and areola. This rare skin condition occurs in three clinical settings[125,126]: as an extension of an epidermal nevus; in association with other skin disorders such as ichthyosis, acanthosis nigricans, lymphoma, chronic eczema, seborrheic keratoses, or Darier disease; and as a process unrelated to other skin disorders. This third variety, known as *nevoid hyperkeratosis*, occurs only very rarely. The literature contains reports of approximately 50 cases, and a review by Pérez-Izquierdo et al.[127] collates details from many of the reports. The lesion typically affects women in their second or third decades of life, usually after menarche[128,129] or during pregnancy.[126,130,131] A few cases have developed in men whose ages range from 24[132] to 75 years.[133] Two men developed nevoid hyperkeratosis during treatment with diethylstilbestrol for prostatic carcinoma,[134,135] and one during treatment of prostatic hyperplasia with finasteride,[136] but others did not receive estrogenic medications or display evidence of endocrine abnormalities.[132,133,137] Two men developed nevoid hyperkeratosis in the setting of generalized cutaneous T-cell lymphoma.[138,139] Treatment of the lymphoma led to resolution of the nevoid hyperkeratosis in both men.[138,139] In two women,[140,141] the presence of intraepidermal collections of lymphocytes suggested the possibility of

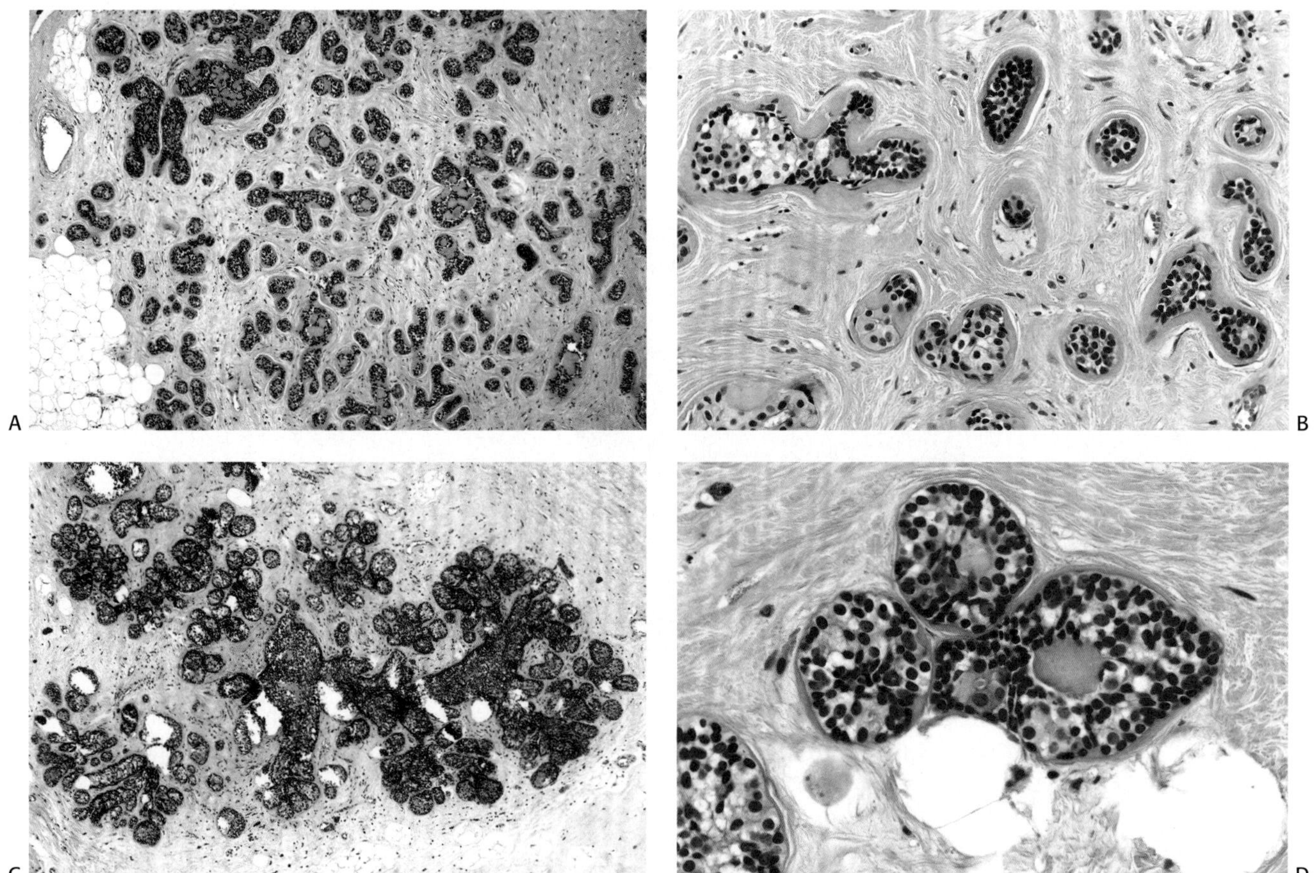

FIG. 42.17. ***Primary mammary neoplasm resembling cutaneous cylindroma.*** **A:** The mass consists of aggregates of cells surrounded by dense eosinophilic, basement membrane–like material. **B:** Two types of cells compose the nests: small basaloid cells with small nuclei and scant cytoplasm and larger glandular cells with more abundant pale cytoplasm. **C:** The neoplastic cells grew within ducts and lobules. **D:** The *in situ* nests do not demonstrate peripheral bands of collagen.

cutaneous T-cell lymphoma, but the clinical courses do not support that suggestion.

Although nevoid hyperkeratosis typically involves both breasts, cases of unilateral involvement have been reported.[127,131,132,142] Unilateral involvement can progress to bilateral involvement after pregnancy.[127] The lesion presents as hyperpigmented hyperkeratotic thickening of the skin of the nipple or areola.[130,134] Yellowish discoloration,[143] desquamation,[127] and crusting[144] have been noted. The lesions are often described as verrucous and they can resemble acanthosis nigricans (Fig. 42.18A), but other lesions such as Paget disease, superficial BCC, dermatophytosis, and Bowen disease can produce similar clinical findings.[145] The changes involve the nipple and areola in 58% of cases, the nipple alone in 17% of cases, and the areola alone in 25% of cases.[137] Histologic examination reveals orthokeratotic hyperkeratosis and keratotic plugging. The epidermis shows marked elongation of the rete ridges with consequent filiform acanthosis and papillomatosis, and horn cysts can form within the elongated rete ridges. The basal layer demonstrates hyperpigmentation without melanocyte proliferation. A mild lymphocytic infiltrate surrounds small blood vessels of the dermis in certain cases (Fig. 42.18B).

Once formed, the signs and symptoms do not usually change, although pregnancy may exaggerate them.[128] In one unusual case,[146] unilateral involvement of the areola appeared during pregnancy, spontaneously disappeared following delivery, reappeared during a subsequent pregnancy, and again resolved spontaneously. In another,[129] the lesion appeared after puberty, improved during the patient's one and only pregnancy, and worsened with the start of oral contraceptive therapy. Nevoid hyperkeratosis does not usually bother the patient except for dissatisfaction with the appearance of the affected regions. One man complained of itching,[137] and two women could not breast feed.[127,128] Treatment with topical keratolytic agents or cryotherapy has been recommended, but the results have varied.[130,133,136,144,147] Single reports of the use of topical retinoic acid,[127,143,144] oral vitamin A,[143] steroid gel,[144] and oral etretinate[148] document variable results.

Adenoma

Benign cutaneous neoplasms involving the nipple include *apocrine poroma*,[149] *sebaceous adenoma* (Fig. 42.19), and *syringomatous adenoma* (see Chapter 15).

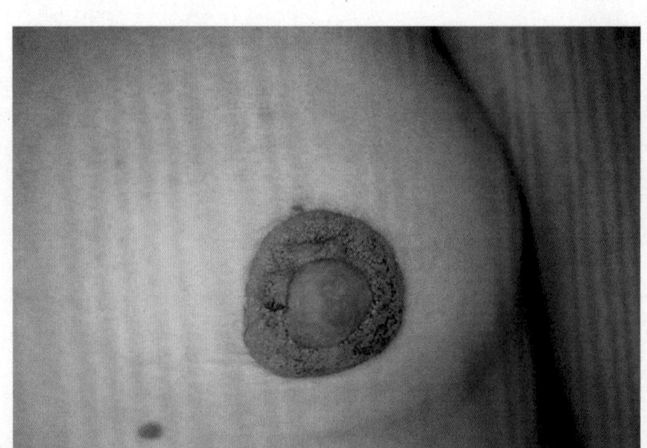

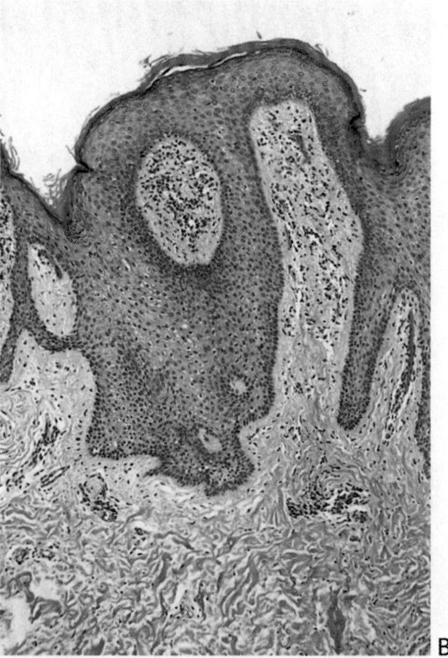

FIG. 42.18. ***Nevoid hyperkeratosis of the areola.*** **A:** The skin of the areola is thickened and focally pigmented. **B:** This biopsy from a nonpigmented area shows papillary hyperplasia of the epidermis, with hyperkeratosis and a mild dermal lymphocytic reaction. The patient was 29 years old. The skin changes were present for "several years."

Basal Cell Carcinoma

On rare occasions, the skin of the nipple gives rise to nonpigmented neoplasms that commonly develop in sun-exposed skin. Approximately 34 examples of *BCC* of the nipple have been reported since the first description in 1893 by Robinson[150] (Fig. 42.20). Selected details of these cases have been tabulated by Takeno et al.[151] Like BCCs developing in common sites, those in the nipple arise more commonly

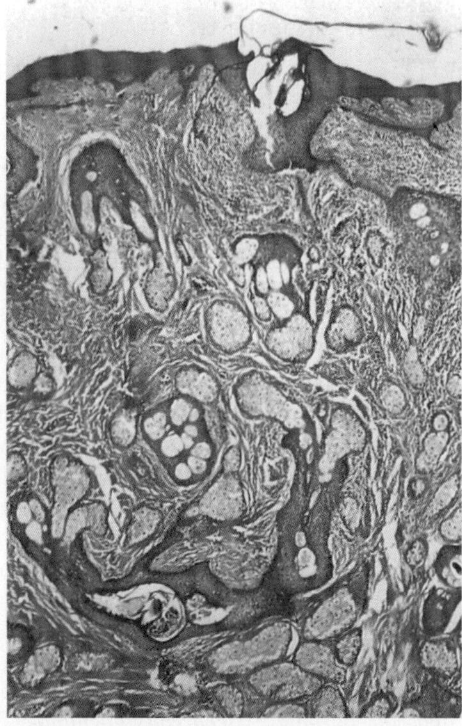

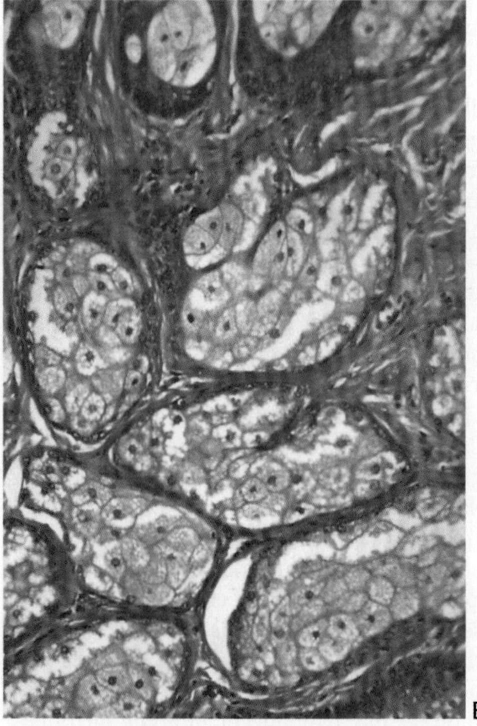

FIG. 42.19. ***Sebaceous adenoma of the nipple.*** **A,B:** A nodular tumor formed by adenomatous proliferation of sebaceous glands.

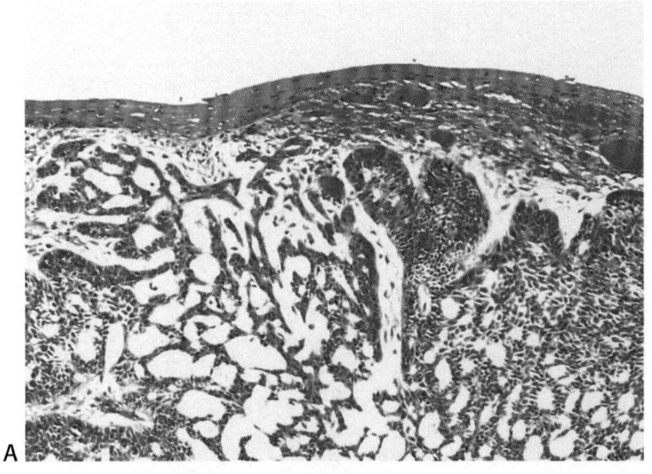

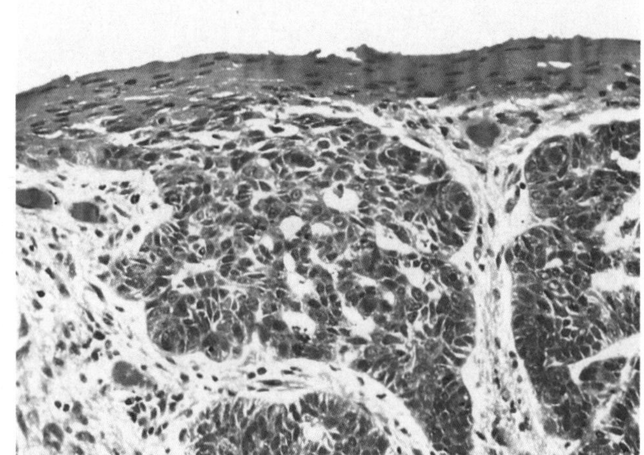

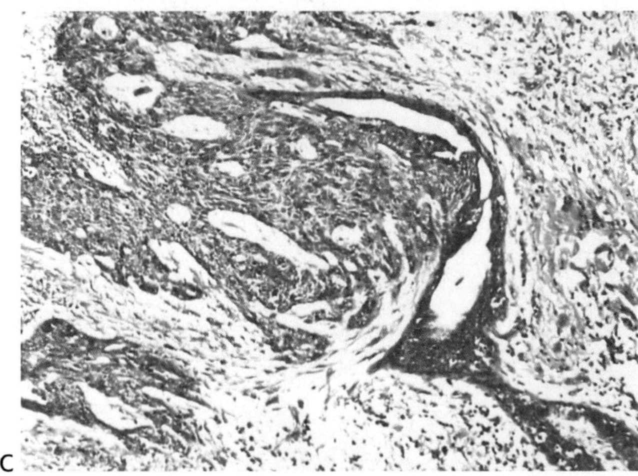

FIG. 42.20. ***Basal cell carcinoma of the nipple.*** **A:** BCC growing beneath the attenuated nipple epidermis. **B:** Carcinoma with an adenoid pattern attached to the epidermis. **C:** BCC invading a major lactiferous duct.

in men (63%) than in women (37%). This sex distribution probably reflects the greater exposure to the sun of the male breast. The ages of the patients have ranged from 35[69] to 86 years[152] with a median age of 59.5 years. One-half of the patients have been younger than 50 years at the time of diagnosis. Three patients had BCCs at another site.[153–155] In one patient,[156] the carcinoma grew in skin damaged by a "soap burn." Two men recounted unusual amounts of sun exposure to the breasts,[153,157] one woman reported brief periods of topless sunbathing,[158] and a man worked in the desert for 30 years, usually wearing a shirt.[155] The carcinomas affected the right and left breasts with equal frequency. Mammograms disclosed calcifications in the nipple in two cases[159,160] and in the periareolar area of a third case.[161]

Reported BCCs of the nipple spanned from 0.4 cm[162] to "9–10" cm[163] and include an 8-cm BCC involving the nipple of a 71-year-old man.[164] They presented as scaling red, eczematous areas, which the patients had noted for as long as 20 years before seeking medical attention.[165] In one case,[163] the signs mimicked those of Paget disease, and a pigmented BCC suggested the diagnosis of pigmented Paget disease.[161] Ulceration, plaque-like thickening of the skin, and nodular lesions have been reported. Robinson described the seminal tumor as "an ulcerated patch, the size of a half crown, with everted edges."[150] The clinical differential diagnosis includes inflammatory conditions, florid papillomatosis of the nipple, Bowen disease, and Paget disease.[166] A biopsy is necessary to establish the diagnosis.

There does not appear to be a predilection for a particular type of BCC to arise in the nipple, since various patterns have been described. Basaloid proliferation originating in the epidermis is a diagnostic feature, and this form of growth is accompanied by lateral spread within the dermis and the nipple stroma. Intraepithelial extension into or invasion of lactiferous ducts is sometimes observed (Fig. 42.20C).[153,160,167] Keratinization occurs in solid as well as cystic foci. Rarely, the entire tumor may exhibit basal and squamous differentiation (Fig. 42.21).

Most patients with BCC of the nipple have been treated successfully by wide excision, occasionally supplemented by irradiation. Three patients underwent Mohs micrographic surgery,[154,158,168] and one patient, who initially refused surgery and irradiation, received retinoids.[169] A mastectomy carried out 4 months later did not disclose residual carcinoma. Mastectomy may be performed when patients develop axillary nodal metastases, an event reported on two occasions.[170,171] In one instance, a 46-year-old man had a single lymph node metastasis detected after a mastectomy for a 1.5-cm tumor.[171] In the second case, axillary nodal enlargement became apparent 4 years after a BCC of the nipple

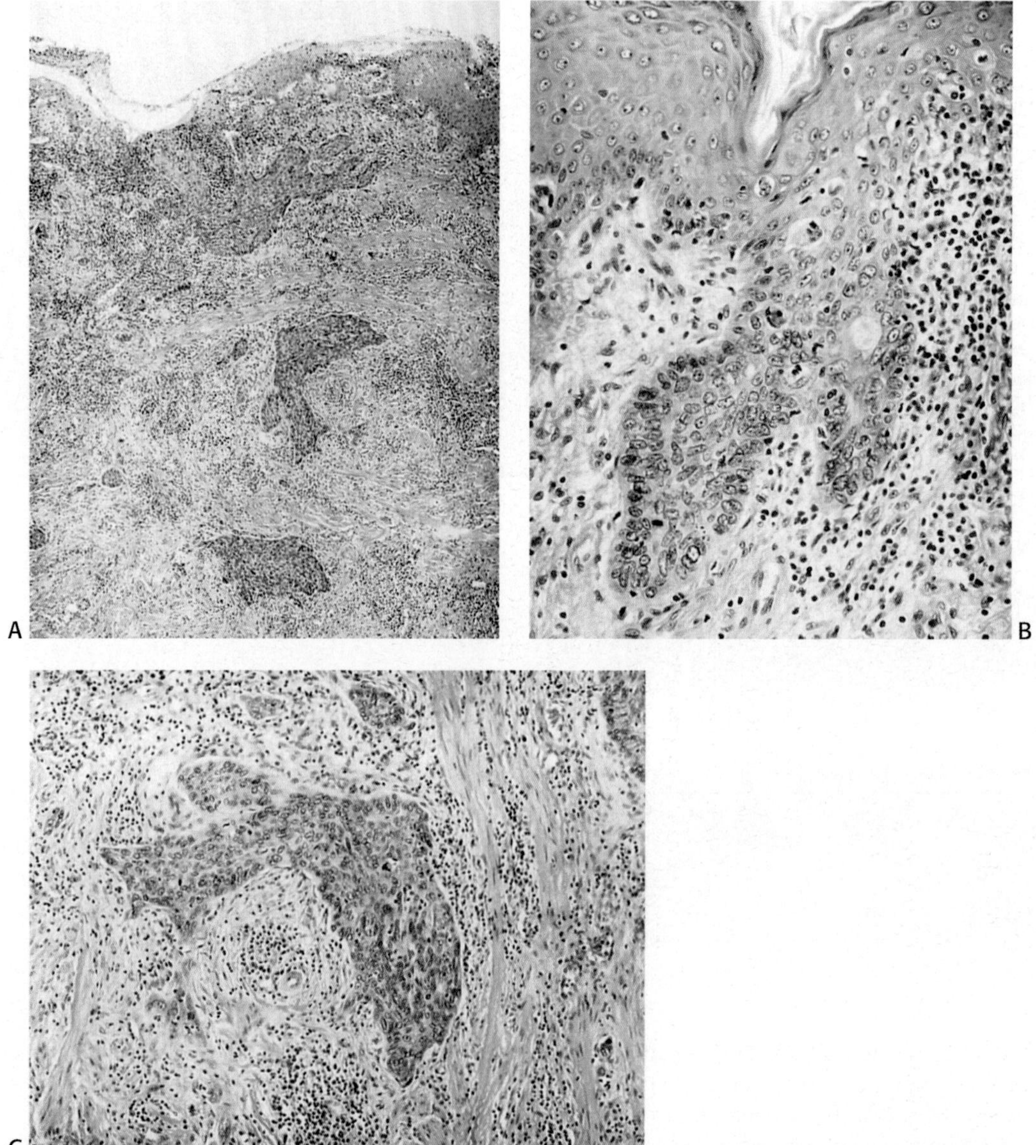

FIG. 42.21. ***Basal squamous carcinoma of the nipple.*** This ulcerated lesion in the nipple of a woman was thought to be Paget disease clinically. **A:** In the *center* of the lesion, carcinoma involves the full thickness of the epidermis and invades the stroma of the nipple. **B:** *In situ* carcinoma arising from the basal layer of the epidermis. **C:** Invasive carcinoma with squamous differentiation.

was treated by excision and radiation. Axillary dissection revealed metastatic tumor in three lymph nodes.[170]

Squamous Carcinoma (Bowen Disease)

Squamous carcinomas arise in the nipple even more rarely than BCCs. To date, the literature contains six cases of intraepidermal squamous carcinoma (Bowen disease) of the nipple.[172–176] The patients, five women and one man, ranged from 41 to 84 years in age. One woman gave a 3-year history of itching and crusting of the right nipple,[172] and the others described a rash of several months' duration, which had not responded to topical treatments. The man had a 20-year history of acquired immunodeficiency syndrome.[176] Clinical diagnoses included the usual dermatoses, Paget disease of the nipple, and melanoma. Histologic examination disclosed atypical squamous epithelium occupying the full thickness of the epidermis, hyperkeratosis, parakeratosis, acanthosis with elongation of the rete ridges, and a dermal chronic inflammatory cell infiltrate. In two cases,[175,176] the malignant squamous cells extended into lactiferous sinuses. Wide excision cured three of these patients, and a mastectomy[176] cured the fourth. Photodynamic treatments and cryotherapy[172] seemingly cured the fifth patient. One poorly differentiated squamous carcinoma grew rapidly as an exophytic mass in the nipple of a 73-year-old woman.[174] The carcinoma showed only minimal invasion of the dermis and it did not involve the lactiferous sinuses. The tumor cells expressed chromogranin A and synaptophysin, and electron microscopy demonstrated tonofilaments and neurosecretory granules. The patient remained well five years after a mastectomy.

Other Carcinomas of the Skin of the Nipple

Other rare carcinomas of the nipple include a *Merkel cell carcinoma*[177] and a *sebaceous carcinoma.*[178] Metastatic neoplasms, especially metastatic carcinomas, involving mammary skin, can mimic primary cutaneous carcinomas of the breast.[179]

REFERENCES

1. Rongioletti F, Urso C, Batolo D, et al. Melanocytic nevi of the breast: a histologic case-control study. *J Cutan Pathol* 2004;31:137–140.
2. Elder DE. Precursors to melanoma and their mimics: nevi of special sites. *Mod Pathol* 2006;19(Suppl. 2):S4–S20.
3. Mason AR, Mohr MR, Koch LH, et al. Nevi of special sites. *Clin Lab Med* 2011;31:229–242.
4. Jochimsen PR, Pearlman NW, Lawton RL, et al. Melanoma of skin of the breast: therapeutic considerations based on six cases. *Surgery* 1977;81:583–587.
5. Lee YT, Sparks FC, Morton DL. Primary melanoma of skin of the breast region. *Ann Surg* 1977;185:17–22.
6. Papachristou DN, Kinne DW, Rosen PP, et al. Cutaneous melanoma of the breast. *Surgery* 1979;85:322–328.
7. Roses DF, Harris MN, Stern JS, et al. Cutaneous melanoma of the breast. *Ann Surg* 1979;189:112–115.
8. Bono A, Baldi M, Maurichi A, et al. Distribution of melanoma on breast surface suggests its etiology. *Int J Cancer* 2003;105:434.
9. Papachristou DN, Kinne D, Ashikari R, et al. Melanoma of the nipple and areola. *Br J Surg* 1979;66:287–288.
10. D'Aiuto G, Del Vecchio S, Mansi L, et al. Malignant melanoma of the nipple: a case studied with radiolabeled monoclonal antibody. *Tumori* 1991;77:449–451.
11. Kinoshita S, Yoshimoto K, Kyoda S, et al. Malignant melanoma originating on the female nipple: a case report. *Breast Cancer* 2007;14:105–108.
12. Lin CH, Lee HS, Yu JC. Melanoma of the nipple mimicking Paget's disease. *Dermatol Online J* 2007;13:18.
13. Lee YT, Craig JR. Melanoma in a tattoo of the breast. *J Surg Oncol* 1984;25:100–101.
14. Kurul S, Tas F, Buyukbabani N, et al. Different manifestations of malignant melanoma in the breast: a report of 12 cases and a review of the literature. *Jpn J Clin Oncol* 2005;35:202–206.
15. Wyatt AJ, Agero AL, Delgado R, et al. Cutaneous metastatic breast carcinoma with melanocyte colonization: a clinical and dermoscopic mimic of malignant melanoma. *Dermatol Surg* 2006;32:949–954.
16. Saitoh K, Saga K, Okazaki M, et al. Pigmented primary carcinoma of the breast: a clinical mimic of malignant melanoma. *Br J Dermatol* 1998;139:287–290.
17. Mele M, Laurberg T, Engberg Damsgaard T, et al. Melanocyte colonization and pigmentation of breast carcinoma: pathological and clinical aspects. *Case Report Pathol* 2012;2012:427628.
18. Dunlap CL, Tomich CE. Melanocyte colonization of oral squamous cell carcinoma. *Oral Surg Oral Med Oral Pathol* 1981;52:524–530.
19. Chumas JC, Lorelle CA. Melanotic adenocarcinoma of the anorectum. *Am J Surg Pathol* 1981;5:711–717.
20. Sau P, Solis J, Lupton GP, et al. Pigmented breast carcinoma. A clinical and histopathologic simulator of malignant melanoma. *Arch Dermatol* 1989;125:536–539.
21. Fernandez-Figueras MT, Puig L, et al. Pigmented epidermotropic ductal carcinoma of the breast in a male. Untrastructural evidence of melanocytic colonization and melanin transfer to the tumor. *J Cutan Pathol* 1995;22:276–280.
22. Lloreta-Trull J, Ordonez NG, Mackay B. Pigmented carcinoma of the breast: an ultrastructural study. *Ultrastruct Pathol* 2000;24:109–113.
23. Gadkari R, Pangarkar MA, Lele VR, et al. Florid melanocytic colonization in a metastasis of breast carcinoma. A case report. *Acta Cytol* 1997;41:1353–1355.
24. Bourlond A. Pigmented epidermotropic metastasis of a breast carcinoma. *Dermatology* 1994;189(Suppl. 2):46–49.
25. Konomi K, Imayama S, Nagae S, et al. Melanocyte chemotactic factor produced by skin metastases of a breast carcinoma. *J Surg Oncol* 1992;50:62–66.
26. Azzopardi JG, Eusebi V. Melanocyte colonization and pigmentation of breast carcinoma. *Histopathology* 1977;1:21–30.
27. Poiares-Baptista A, De Vasconcelos AA. Cutaneous pigmented metastasis from breast carcinoma simulating malignant melanoma. *Int J Dermatol* 1988;27:124–125.
28. Brasanac D, Boricic I, Todorovic V. Epidermotropic metastases from breast carcinoma showing different clinical and histopathological features on the trunk and on the scalp in a single patient. *J Cutan Pathol* 2003;30:641–646.
29. Hamada M, Toyoshima S, Duan H, et al. Pigmented cutaneous metastasis of mucinous carcinoma of the breast to the scalp mimicking malignant melanoma. *Eur J Dermatol* 2006;16:592–593.
30. Blaustein RL. Fine-needle aspiration of a metastatic breast carcinoma in the lung with melanin pigmentation: a case report. *Diagn Cytopathol* 1990;6:364–365.
31. Shamai-Lubovitz O, Rothem A, Ben-David E, et al. Cutaneous metastatic carcinoma of the breast mimicking malignant melanoma, clinically and histologically. *J Am Acad Dermatol* 1994;31:1058–1060.
32. Culberson JD, Horn RC Jr. Paget's disease of the nipple; review of twenty-five cases with special reference to melanin pigmentation of Paget cells. *AMA Arch Surg* 1956;72:224–231.
33. Ho TC, St Jacques M, Schopflocher P. Pigmented Paget's disease of the male breast. *J Am Acad Dermatol* 1990;23:338–341.
34. Neubecker RD, Bradshaw RP. Mucin, melanin, and glycogen in Paget's disease of the breast. *Am J Clin Pathol* 1961;36:49–53.
35. Soler T, Lerin A, Serrano T, et al. Pigmented paget disease of the breast nipple with underlying infiltrating carcinoma: a case report and review of the literature. *Am J Dermatopathol* 2011;33:e54–e57.
36. Tang X, Umemura S, Kumaki N, et al. A case report of pigmented mammary Paget's disease mimicking nevus of the nipple. *Breast Cancer* 2011;Jan 7 [Epub ahead of print]. doi:10.1007/s12282-010-0249-y.
37. Mitchell S, Lachica R, Randall MB, et al. Paget's disease of the breast areola mimicking cutaneous melanoma. *Breast J* 2006;12:233–236.
38. Peison B, Benisch B. Paget's disease of the nipple simulating malignant melanoma in a black woman. *Am J Dermatopathol* 1985;7(Suppl.):165–169.
39. Pizzichetta MA, Canzonieri V, Massarut S, et al. Pigmented mammary Paget's disease mimicking melanoma. *Melanoma Res* 2004;14:S13–S15.
40. Stretch JR, Denton KJ, Millard PR, et al. Paget's disease of the male breast clinically and histopathologically mimicking melanoma. *Histopathology* 1991;19:470–472.
41. Oiso N, Kawara S, Inui H, et al. Pigmented spots as a sign of mammary Paget's disease. *Clin Exp Dermatol* 2009;34:36–38.
42. Longo C, Fantini F, Cesinaro AM, et al. Pigmented mammary Paget disease: dermoscopic, in vivo reflectance-mode confocal microscopic, and immunohistochemical study of a case. *Arch Dermatol* 2007;143:752–754.
43. Meyer-Gonzalez T, Alcaide-Martin A, Contreras-Steyls M, et al. Pigmented mammary Paget disease mimicking cutaneous melanoma. *Int J Dermatol* 2010;49:59–61.
44. Yanagishita T, Tamada Y, Tanaka M, et al. Pigmented mammary Paget disease mimicking melanoma on dermatoscopy. *J Am Acad Dermatol* 2011;64:e114–e116.
45. Park JS, Lee MJ, Chung H, et al. Pigmented mammary Paget disease positive for melanocytic markers. *J Am Acad Dermatol* 2011;65:247–249.
46. Vaughan A, Dietz JR, Moley JF, et al. Metastatic disease to the breast: the Washington University experience. *World J Surg Oncol* 2007;5:74.
47. Williams SA, Ehlers RA II, Hunt KK, et al. Metastases to the breast from nonbreast solid neoplasms: presentation and determinants of survival. *Cancer* 2007;110:731–737.
48. Roy S, Dhingra K, Mandal S, et al. Unusual presentation of metastatic amelanotic melanoma of unknown primary origin as a solitary breast lump. *Melanoma Res* 2008;18:447–450.

49. Ravdel L, Robinson WA, Lewis K, et al. Metastatic melanoma in the breast: a report of 27 cases. *J Surg Oncol* 2006;94:101–104.
50. Bacchi CE, Wludarski SC, Ambaye AB, et al. Metastatic melanoma presenting as an isolated breast tumor: a study of 20 cases with emphasis on several primary mimickers. *Arch Pathol Lab Med* 2013;137:41–49.
51. Romanelli R, Toncini C. Pigmented papillary carcinoma of the male breast. *Tumori* 1986;72:105–108.
52. Nobukawa B, Fujii H, Hirai S, et al. Breast carcinoma diverging to aberrant melanocytic differentiation: a case report with histopathologic and loss of heterozygosity analyses. *Am J Surg Pathol* 1999;23:1280–1287.
53. Padmore RF, Lara JF, Ackerman DJ, et al. Primary combined malignant melanoma and ductal carcinoma of the breast. A report of two cases. *Cancer* 1996;78:2515–2525.
54. Ruffolo EF, Koerner FC, Maluf HM. Metaplastic carcinoma of the breast with melanocytic differentiation. *Mod Pathol* 1997;10:592–596.
55. Yen H, Florentine B, Kelly LK, et al. Fine-needle aspiration of a metaplastic breast carcinoma with extensive melanocytic differentiation: a case report. *Diagn Cytopathol* 2000;23:46–50.
56. Noske A, Schwabe M, Pahl S, et al. Report of a metaplastic carcinoma of the breast with multi-directional differentiation: an adenoid cystic carcinoma, a spindle cell carcinoma and melanoma. *Virchows Arch* 2008;452:575–579.
57. Shin SJ, Kanomata N, Rosen PP. Mammary carcinoma with prominent cytoplasmic lipofuscin granules mimicking melanocytic differentiation. *Histopathology* 2000;37:456–459.
58. Bernardo MM, Mascarenhas MJ, Lopes DP. Primary malignant melanoma of the breast. *Acta Med Port* 1980;2:39–43.
59. Gatch WD. A melanoma, apparently primary in a breast; its single known metastasis in the small bowel. *AMA Arch Surg* 1956;73:266–268.
60. Stephenson SE Jr, Byrd BF Jr. Malignant melanoma of the breast. *Am J Surg* 1959;97:232–235.
61. Biswas A, Goyal S, Jain A, et al. Primary amelanotic melanoma of the breast: combating a rare cancer. *Breast Cancer* 2010;Oct 27 [Epub ahead of print]. doi:10.1007/s12282-010-0231-8.
62. Rodriguez HA, Ackerman LV. Cellular blue nevus. Clinicopathologic study of forty-five cases. *Cancer* 1968;21:393–405.
63. Busam KJ, Woodruff JM, Erlandson RA, et al. Large plaque-type blue nevus with subcutaneous cellular nodules. *Am J Surg Pathol* 2000;24: 92–99.
64. Connelly J, Smith JL Jr. Malignant blue nevus. *Cancer* 1991;67: 2653–2657.
65. Loffler KU, Witschel H. Primary malignant melanoma of the orbit arising in a cellular blue naevus. *Br J Ophthalmol* 1989;73:388–393.
66. Geschickter CF. Mammary sarcoma. In: *Diseases of the breast: diagnosis, pathology, treatment.* 2nd ed. Philadelphia: J.B. Lippincott, 1943:390.
67. Ilie B. Neoplasms in skin and subcutis over the breast, simulating breast neoplasms: case reports and literature review. *J Surg Oncol* 1986;31:191–198.
68. Shamsadini S, Wadji MB, Shamsadini A. Surrounding ipsilateral eruptive seborrheic keratosis as a warning sign of intraductal breast carcinoma and Paget's disease (Leser Trelat sign). *Dermatol Online J* 2006;12:27.
69. Nunez M, Marques A, de las Heras ME, et al. Bilateral basal cell carcinoma of the breasts in a woman. *J Dermatol* 1995;22:226–228.
70. Wong SW, Smith JG Jr, Thomas WO. Bilateral basal cell carcinoma of the breasts. *J Am Acad Dermatol* 1993;28:777.
71. Gombos EC, Esserman LE, Poppiti RJ Jr. Basal cell carcinoma of the skin presenting as microcalcifications on screening mammography. *Breast J* 2005;11:149.
72. Schwartz RA, Burgess GH, Milgrom H. Breast carcinoma and basal cell epithelioma after x-ray therapy for hirsutism. *Cancer* 1979;44:1601–1605.
73. Watanabe K, Mukawa A, Saito K, et al. Adenoid squamous cell carcinoma of the skin overlying the right breast. An autopsy case clinically manifested with rapid growth and widely spreading metastases. *Acta Pathol Jpn* 1986;36:1921–1929.
74. Alzaraa A, Thomas GD, Vodovnik A, et al. Merkel cell carcinoma in a male breast: a case report. *Breast J* 2007;13:517–519.
75. Yavuzer R, Boyaci M, Sari A, et al. Microcystic adnexal carcinoma of the breast: a very rare breast skin tumor. *Dermatol Surg* 2002;28: 1092–1094.
76. Becker TS, Moreira MA, Lima LA, et al. Pilomatrixoma mimicking breast cancer in man. *Breast J* 2010;16:89–91.
77. Bhalotra R, Jayaram G. Fine-needle aspiration cytology of pilomatrixoma: a case report. *Diagn Cytopathol* 1990;6:280–283.
78. Gilles R, Guinebretiere JM, Gallay X, et al. Pilomatrixoma mimicking male breast carcinoma on mammography. *AJR Am J Roentgenol* 1993;160:895.
79. Hamilton A, Young GI, Davis RI. Pilomatrixoma mimicking breast carcinoma. *Br J Dermatol* 1987;116:585–586.
80. Hubeny CM, Sykes JB, O'Connell A, et al. Pilomatrixoma of the adult male breast: a rare tumor with typical ultrasound features. *J Clin Imaging Sci* 2011;1:12.
81. Imperiale A, Calabrese M, Monetti F, et al. Calcified pilomatrixoma of the breast: mammographic and sonographic findings. *Eur Radiol* 2001;11:2465–2467.
82. Ismail W, Pain S, al-Okati D, et al. Giant pilomatricoma simulating carcinoma of the male breast. *Int J Clin Pract* 2000;54:55–56.
83. Lloyd-Lavery A, Espinosa O, Asher R, et al. 'Once seen, never forgotten'. *Clin and Experimental Dermatol* 2011;37:692–694.
84. Pascual A, Casado I, Colmenero I, et al. Fine needle aspiration cytology of pilomatrixoma of the breast. *Acta Cytol* 2000;44:274–276.
85. Reynaud P, Orliaguet T, Robin YM, et al. Un pilomatricome mammaire simulant cliniquement un carcinome. *Ann Pathol* 1997;17:213–214.
86. Rousselot C, Tourasse C, Samimi M, et al. Pilomatricomes mammaires reveles par des microcalcifications a la mammographie: a propos de deux cas. *J Radiol* 2007;88:978–980.
87. Craig S, Bui-Mansfield LT, Lusk JD. Radiology pathology conference of Brooke Army Medical Center: trichoblastoma of breast. *Clin Imaging* 2009;33:311–313.
88. Sherley-Dale AC, Chachlani N, Sanders DS, et al. Trichoblastoma of the breast detected by screening mammography: a diagnostic pitfall. *Am J Surg Pathol* 2010;34:748–754.
89. Shimazaki H, Anzai M, Aida S, et al. Trichoblastoma of the skin occurring in the breast. A case report. *Acta Cytol* 2001;45:435–440.
90. Uchida N, Tsuzuki Y, Ando T, et al. Malignant proliferating trichilemmal tumor in the skin over the breast: a case report. *Breast Cancer* 2000;7:79–82.
91. Alzaraa A, Ghafoor I, Yates A, et al. Sebaceous carcinoma of the skin of the breast: a case report. *J Med Case Rep* 2008;2:276.
92. Ascari-Raccagni A, Dondas A, Padovani F, et al. A case of giant sebaceous carcinoma localized in the breast area of a male patient. *Indian J Dermatol Venereol Leprol* 2011;77:403.
93. Yoshii N, Kanekura T, Churei H, et al. Syringoma-like eccrine sweat duct proliferation induced by radiation. *J Dermatol* 2006;33:36–39.
94. Urso C, Bondi R, Paglierani M, et al. Carcinomas of sweat glands: report of 60 cases. *Arch Pathol Lab Med* 2001;125:498–505.
95. Wick MR, Ockner DM, Mills SE, et al. Homologous carcinomas of the breasts, skin, and salivary glands. A histologic and immunohistochemical comparison of ductal mammary carcinoma, ductal sweat gland carcinoma, and salivary duct carcinoma. *Am J Clin Pathol* 1998;109: 75–84.
96. Wallace ML, Longacre TA, Smoller BR. Estrogen and progesterone receptors and anti-gross cystic disease fluid protein 15 (BRST-2) fail to distinguish metastatic breast carcinoma from eccrine neoplasms. *Mod Pathol* 1995;8:897–901.
97. Busam KJ, Tan LK, Granter SR, et al. Epidermal growth factor, estrogen, and progesterone receptor expression in primary sweat gland carcinomas and primary and metastatic mammary carcinomas. *Mod Pathol* 1999;12:786–793.
98. Hanby AM, McKee P, Jeffery M, et al. Primary mucinous carcinomas of the skin express TFF1, TFF3, estrogen receptor, and progesterone receptors. *Am J Surg Pathol* 1998;22:1125–1131.
99. Misago N, Shinoda Y, Okawa T, et al. Histiocytoid and signet-ring cell carcinoma of the axilla: a type of cutaneous apocrine carcinoma equivalent to histiocytoid lobular carcinoma of the breast? *Clin Exp Dermatol* 2011;36:874–877.
100. Brandt SM, Swistel AJ, Rosen PP. Secretory carcinoma in the axilla: probable origin from axillary skin appendage glands in a young girl. *Am J Surg Pathol* 2009;33:950–953.
101. Zembowicz A, Garcia CF, Tannous ZS, et al. Endocrine mucin-producing sweat gland carcinoma: twelve new cases suggest that it is a precursor of some invasive mucinous carcinomas. *Am J Surg Pathol* 2005;29:1330–1339.
102. Lee HH, Park SH, Choi HY, et al. Eccrine spiradenoma arising in the breast misdiagnosed as an epidermal inclusion cyst. *Korean J Radiol* 2011;12:256–260.
103. Bosch MM, Boon ME. Fine-needle cytology of an eccrine spiradenoma of the breast: diagnosis made by a holistic approach. *Diagn Cytopathol* 1992;8:366–368.

104. Draheim JH, Neubecker RD, Sprinz H. An unusual tumor of the breast resembling eccrine spiradenoma. *Am J Clin Pathol* 1959;31:511–516.
105. Panico L, D'Antonio A, Chiacchio R, et al. An unusual, recurring breast tumor with features of eccrine spiradenoma: a case report. *Am J Clin Pathol* 1996;106:665–669.
106. Ribeiro-Silva A, Shaletich C, Careta RS, et al. Spiradenocarcinoma of the breast arising in a long-standing spiradenoma. *Ann Diagn Pathol* 2004;8:162–166.
107. Saboorian MH, Kenny M, Ashfaq R, et al. Carcinosarcoma arising in eccrine spiradenoma of the breast. Report of a case and review of the literature. *Arch Pathol Lab Med* 1996;120:501–504.
108. Thomas B, Duwel V, Proot L, et al. An uncommon breast tumour: the malignant eccrine spiradenoma. A case report. *Acta Chir Belg* 1993;93:295–298.
109. Tanaka Y, Bhunchet E, Shibata T. A case of malignant eccrine spiradenoma metastatic to intramammary lymph node. *Breast Cancer* 2008;15:175–180.
110. Kumar N, Verma K. Clear cell hidradenoma simulating breast carcinoma: a diagnostic pitfall in fine-needle aspiration of breast. *Diagn Cytopathol* 1996;15:70–72.
111. Finck FM, Schwinn CP, Keasbey LE. Clear cell hidradenoma of the breast. *Cancer* 1968;22:125–135.
112. Mote DG, Ramamurti T, Naveen Babu B. Nodular hidradenoma of the breast: a case report with literature review. *Indian J Surg* 2009;71:43–45.
113. Domoto H, Terahata S, Sato K, et al. Nodular hidradenoma of the breast: report of two cases with literature review. *Pathol Int* 1998;48:907–911.
114. Ohi Y, Umekita Y, Rai Y, et al. Clear cell hidradenoma of the breast: a case report with review of the literature. *Breast Cancer* 2007;14:307–311.
115. Grampurohit VU, Dinesh U, Rao R. Nodular hidradenoma of male breast: cytohistological correlation. *J Cytol* 2011;28:235–237.
116. Girish G, Gopasetty M, Stewart R. Recurrent clear cell hidradenoma of the breast: a case report. *Internet J Surg* 2007;10:1–5.
117. Kazakov DV, Vanecek T, Belousova IE, et al. Skin-type hidradenoma of the breast parenchyma with t(11;19) translocation: hidradenoma of the breast. *Am J Dermatopathol* 2007;29:457–461.
118. Winnes M, Molne L, Suurkula M, et al. Frequent fusion of the CRTC1 and MAML2 genes in clear cell variants of cutaneous hidradenomas. *Genes Chromosomes Cancer* 2007;46:559–563.
119. Yamane N, Kato N, Yanagi T, et al. Naevus sebaceus on the female breast accompanied with a tubular apocrine adenoma and a syringocystadenoma papilliferum. *Br J Dermatol* 2007;156:1397–1399.
120. Gokaslan ST, Carlile B, Dudak M, et al. Solitary cylindroma (dermal analog tumor) of the breast: a previously undescribed neoplasm at this site. *Am J Surg Pathol* 2001;25:823–826.
121. Albores-Saavedra J, Heard SC, McLaren B, et al. Cylindroma (dermal analog tumor) of the breast: a comparison with cylindroma of the skin and adenoid cystic carcinoma of the breast. *Am J Clin Pathol* 2005;123:866–873.
122. Mahmoud A, Hill DH, O'Sullivan MJ, et al. Cylindroma of the breast: a case report and review of the literature. *Diagn Pathol* 2009;4:30.
123. Nonaka D, Rosai J, Spagnolo D, et al. Cylindroma of the breast of skin adnexal type: a study of 4 cases. *Am J Surg Pathol* 2004;28:1070–1075.
124. Wang N, Leeming R, Abdul-Karim FW. Fine needle aspiration cytology of breast cylindroma in a woman with familial cylindromatosis: a case report. *Acta Cytol* 2004;48:853–858.
125. Lévy-Franckle A. Les hyperkératoses de l'aréole et du mamelon. *Paris Med* 1938;28:63–66.
126. Mehregan AH, Rahbari H. Hyperkeratosis of nipple and areola. *Arch Dermatol* 1977;113:1691–1692.
127. Pérez-Izquierdo JM, Vilata JJ, Sánchez JL, et al. Retinoic acid treatment of nipple hyperkeratosis. *Arch Dermatol* 1990;126:687–688.
128. Alpsoy E, Yilmaz E, Aykol A. Hyperkeratosis of the nipple: report of two cases. *J Dermatol* 1997;24:43–45.
129. Marín-Bertolín S, González-Martínez R, Marquina Vila P. Nevoid hyperkeratosis of the areola. *Plast Reconstr Surg* 1998;102:275–276.
130. Revert A, Bañuls J, Montesinos E, et al. Nevoid hyperkeratosis of the areola. *Int J Dermatol* 1993;32:745–746.
131. Vestey JP, Bunney MH. Unilateral hyperkeratosis of the nipple: the response to cryotherapy. *Arch Dermatol* 1986;122:1360–1361.
132. Mitxelena J, Raton JA, Bilbao I, et al. Nevoid hyperkeratosis of the areola in men: response to cryotherapy. *Dermatology* 1999;199:73–74.
133. Kuhlman DS, Hodge SJ, Owen LG. Hyperkeratosis of the nipple and areola. *J Am Acad Dermatol* 1985;13:596–598.
134. Mold DE, Jegasothy BV. Estrogen-induced hyperkeratosis of the nipple. *Cutis* 1980;26:95–96.
135. Schwartz RA. Hyperkeratosis of nipple and areola. *Arch Dermatol* 1978;114:1844–1845.
136. English JC III, Coots NV. A man with nevoid hyperkeratosis of the areola. *Cutis* 1996;57:354–356.
137. Kubota Y, Koga T, Nakayama J, et al. Naevoid hyperkeratosis of the nipple and areola in a man. *Br J Dermatol* 2000;142:382–384.
138. Ahn SK, Chung J, Soo Lee W, et al. Hyperkeratosis of the nipple and areola simultaneously developing with cutaneous T-cell lymphoma. *J Am Acad Dermatol* 1995;32:124–125.
139. Allegue F, Soria C, Rocamora A, et al. Hyperkeratosis of the nipple and areola in a patient with cutaneous T-cell lymphoma. *Int J Dermatol* 1990;29:519–520.
140. Roustan G, Yus ES, Simon A. Nevoid hyperkeratosis of the areola with histopathological features mimicking mycosis fungoides. *Eur J Dermatol* 2002;12:79–81.
141. Soden CE. Hyperkeratosis of the nipple and areola. *Cutis* 1983;32:69–71, 74.
142. D'Souza M, Gharami R, Ratnakar C, et al. Unilateral nevoid hyperkeratosis of the nipple and areola. *Int J Dermatol* 1996;35:602–603.
143. Ollague W. Hyperkeratosis of the nipple. *Arch Dermatol* 1979;115:111.
144. Mayock P. Hyperkeratosis of the nipples. Arch Dermatol 1978;114:1245.
145. Xifra M, Lagodin C, Wright D, et al. Nevoid keratosis of the nipple *J Am Acad Dermatol* 1999;41:325–326.
146. Rodallec J, Morel P, Guilaine J, et al. Hyperkératose de l'aréole mammaire unilatérale recidivante chez une femme enceinte. *Ann Dermatol Venereol* 1978;105:527–528.
147. Krishnan RS, Angel TA, Roark TR, et al. Nevoid hyperkeratosis of the nipple and/or areola: a report of two cases and a review of the literature. *Int J Dermatol* 2002;41:775–777.
148. Ortonne JP, el Baze P, Juhlin L. Nevoid hyperkeratosis of the nipple and areola mammae: ineffectiveness of etretinate therapy. *Acta Derm Venerol* 1986;66:175–177.
149. Azma A, Tawfik O, Casparian JM. Apocrine poroma of the breast. *Breast J* 2001;7:195–198.
150. Robinson H. Rodent ulcer of the male breast. *Trans Pathol Soc Lond* 1893;44:147–148.
151. Takeno S, Kikuchi N, Miura T, et al. Basal cell carcinoma of the nipple in male patients with gastric cancer recurrence: report of a case. *Breast Cancer* 2010;Aug 11 [Epub ahead of print]. doi:10.1007/s12282-010-0217-6.
152. Nirodi NS, Mudd DG. Basal cell carcinoma of the male nipple. *J R Coll Surg Edinb* 1986;31:121–123.
153. Gupta C, Sheth D, Snower DP. Primary basal cell carcinoma of the nipple. *Arch Pathol Lab Med* 2004;128:792–793.
154. Nouri K, Ballard CJ, Bouzari N, et al. Basal cell carcinoma of the areola in a man. *J Drugs Dermatol* 2005;4:352–354.
155. Benharroch D, Geffen DB, Peiser J, et al. Basal cell carcinoma of the male nipple. Case report and review of the literature. *J Dermatol Surg Oncol* 1993;19:137–139.
156. Farrow JH. Benign and malignant lesions of the nipple. *CA Cancer J Clin* 1958;8:16–19.
157. Bruce S, Tschen JA, Goldberg LH. Basal-cell carcinoma of the nipple. *J Dermatol Surg Oncol* 1985;11:424–425.
158. Rosen N, Muhn CY, Bernstein SC. A common tumor, an uncommon location: basal cell carcinoma of the nipple and areola in a 49-year-old woman. *Dermatol Surg* 2005;31:480–483.
159. Cooper RA, Eilers DB. Mammographic findings in basal cell carcinoma of the male nipple. *AJR Am J Roentgenol* 2000;175:1065–1066.
160. Yamamoto H, Ito Y, Hayashi T, et al. A case of basal cell carcinoma of the nipple and areola with intraductal spread. *Breast Cancer* 2001;8:229–233.
161. Jung HJ, Jun JH, Kim HY, et al. Pigmented basal cell carcinoma of the nipple-areola complex in an elderly woman. *Ann Dermatol* 2011;23:S201–S204.
162. Lupton GP, Goette K. Basal cell carcinoma of the nipple. *Arch Dermatol* 1978;114:1845.
163. Mikhaimer NC, Kahler KC, Schwarz T, et al. Giant basal cell carcinoma of the breast mimicking paget's disease: complete remission after photodynamic therapy. *Onkologie* 2010;33:613–615.
164. Wyatt AP. Basal cell carcinoma of the male breast. *Proc R Soc Med* 1965;58:509–510.

165. Sanchez-Carpintero I, Redondo P, Solano T. Basal cell carcinoma affecting the areola-nipple complex. *Plast Reconstr Surg* 2000;105:1573.
166. Davis AB, Patchefsky AS. Basal cell carcinoma of the nipple: case report and review of the literature *Cancer* 1977;40:1780–1781.
167. Cain RJ, Sau P, Benson PM. Basal cell carcinoma of the nipple. Report of two cases. *J Am Acad Dermatol* 1990;22:207–210.
168. Weber PJ, Moody BR, Foster JA. Series spiral advancement flap: an alternative to the ellipse. *Dermatol Surg* 2001;27:64–66.
169. Jones R, Wayte DM, Mitchell E, et al. Basal-cell carcinoma of the breast—treatment with retinoids. *Clin Exp Dermatol* 1991;16: 448–450.
170. Shertz WT, Balogh K. Metastasizing basal cell carcinoma of the nipple. *Arch Pathol Lab Med* 1986;110:761–762.
171. Baker M, Kim H-K, Todd M. Basal cell carcinoma masquerading as breast cancer in a male breast. *Breast* 1985;11:25–27.
172. Brookes PT, Jhawar S, Hinton CP, et al. Bowen's disease of the nipple—a new method of treatment. *Breast* 2005;14:65–67.
173. Cremer H, Paulussen F. Die Bowensche erkrankung der mamille. *Geburtsh Frauenheilk* 1982;42:590–592.
174. Hosaka N, Uesaka K, Takaki T, et al. Poorly differentiated squamous cell carcinoma of the nipple: a unique case for marked exophytic growth, but little invasion with neuroendocrine differentiation. *Med Mol Morphol* 2011;44:174–178.
175. Venkataseshan VS, Budd DC, Un Kim D, et al. Intraepidermal squamous carcinoma (Bowen's disease) of the nipple. *Hum Pathol* 1994;25:1371–1374.
176. Sharma R, Iyer M. Bowen's disease of the nipple in a young man with AIDS: a case report. *Clin Breast Cancer* 2009;9:53–55.
177. Asioli S, Dorji T, Lorenzini P, et al. Primary neuroendocrine (Merkel cell) carcinoma of the nipple. *Virchows Arch* 2002;440:443–444.
178. Cibull TL, Thomas AB, Badve S, et al. Sebaceous carcinoma of the nipple. *J Cutan Pathol* 2008;35:608–610.
179. Hajdu SI, Urban JA. Cancers metastatic to the breast. *Cancer* 1972;29: 1691–1696.

CHAPTER 43

The Pathology of Axillary and Intramammary Lymph Nodes

SYED A. HODA

This chapter is devoted to diverse pathologic changes other than metastatic carcinoma that affect the axillary and intramammary lymph nodes. It is, of course, also possible for these lymph nodes to harbor another synchronous disease process in addition to metastatic carcinoma. Additional information about axillary lymph nodes (ALNs) can be found in Chapters 12 and 44 as well as various chapters that discuss the pathology of lymph nodes in relation to specific disease entities.

HETEROTOPIC EPITHELIAL INCLUSIONS

Types of Inclusions

Benign heterotopic epithelial tissue has been found in or associated with lymph nodes at various sites other than the axilla. A frequent example of this phenomenon is inclusion of salivary gland tissue in cervical lymph nodes.[1] Heterotopic glandular inclusions (endosalpingiosis) in pelvic and periaortic lymph nodes are derived from pelvic müllerian epithelium and the peritoneum.[2–4] In the axilla, heterotopic mammary-type glands can appear to be histologically normal except for their aberrant location, or they may develop fibrocystic changes (FCCs), including epithelial hyperplasia, apocrine metaplasia, cysts, and sclerosing adenosis (SA). A minority of glandular inclusions in ALNs have müllerian-like features, including microvilli.[5] Other inclusions consist of squamous epithelium that is usually cystic, or a mixture of glandular and squamous elements. Heterotopic epithelial inclusions in ALNs are found in the capsule or parenchyma of a lymph node.[6–16] Epithelial inclusions have also been found in intramammary lymph nodes,[11,17] including those with müllerian-like epithelium.[18] Since this patient was found to have a borderline serous carcinoma of the peritoneum 3 years after the intramammary lymph node was excised, the müllerian-like epithelial gland in the lymph node was probably metastatic rather than a benign inclusion.

With the exception of heterotopic intranodal inclusions, the finding of orderly glands distributed singly or in small groups within a subcapsular sinus or in the substance of an ALN should be regarded as evidence of metastatic carcinoma. Well-differentiated metastatic carcinoma in ALNs that has been mistakenly diagnosed as glandular heterotopia usually occurs in patients with invasive well-differentiated ductal carcinoma or in patients with intraductal carcinoma who have undergone a needling procedure that results in epithelial displacement.[13] Rarely, well-differentiated nodal metastases represent a minor, inconspicuous component of a primary tumor, most of which is histologically different and less well-differentiated (Figs. 43.1 and 43.2). Ohsie et al.[19] described an unusual nodal inclusion in a patient with classical invasive lobular carcinoma of one breast. The ipsilateral sentinel lymph node (SLN) contained scattered orderly glands that lacked myoepithelium. Complete sampling of the mastectomy with 366 paraffin blocks failed to uncover an invasive duct carcinoma comparable to the glands in the lymph node. A contralateral mastectomy revealed only FCCs. On the basis of the images provided in this case report, it was not possible to determine whether the glands in the lymph node had müllerian-type epithelium, as might be suspected from the findings as reported.

Histogenesis of Epithelial Inclusions

There is no association between glandular heterotopia and the presence of accessory breast tissue in the axilla.

The histogenesis of glandular heterotopia associated with ALNs is unknown. One hypothesis suggests that heterotopic intranodal epithelium results from isolated cells or fragments of tissue that were displaced by a prior procedure and were transported by lymphatic flow to the lymph node. Since it has been well-documented that epithelial displacement occurs as a result of needle core biopsy procedures (see Chapter 44), this process could explain some cases of nodal heterotopic epithelium. However, the absence of prior procedures in many patients, and the fact that early reports of nodal heterotopia predated the use of needle core biopsies, means that this explanation does not apply in many cases.

Displaced epithelium would not explain the orderly structure of mammary-type glands in which the epithelium is encircled by myoepithelial cells. The latter finding supports the alternative hypothesis that the inclusions derive from epithelial rests that are the result of embryologic maldevelopment.

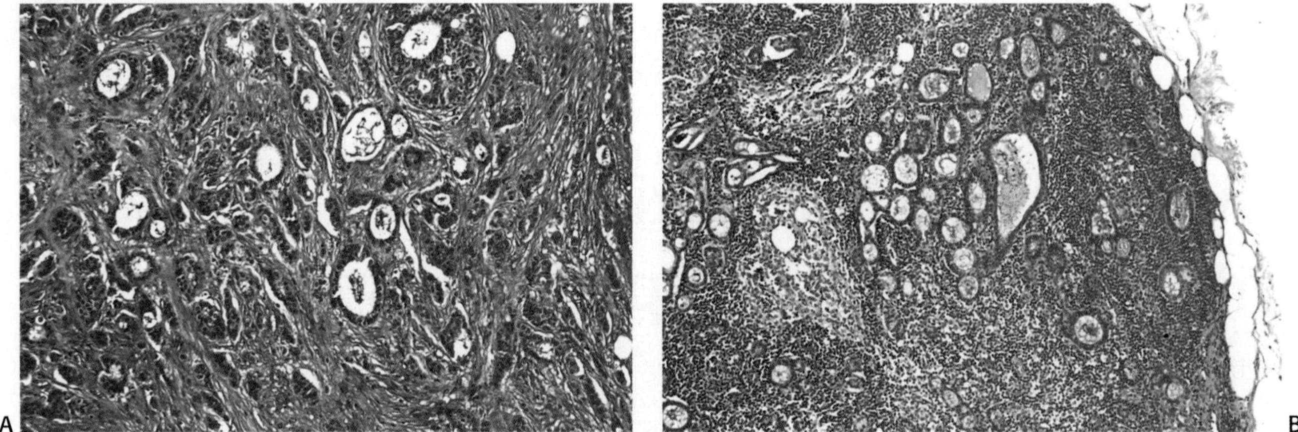

FIG. 43.1. ***Metastatic carcinoma mistaken for heterotopic glands in axillary lymph node.*** **A:** Well-differentiated glandular elements with open lumens are distributed in the midst of moderately differentiated infiltrating duct carcinoma in the primary tumor. **B:** The nodal metastasis consisting only of the well-differentiated glands was initially mistakenly diagnosed as glandular heterotopia.

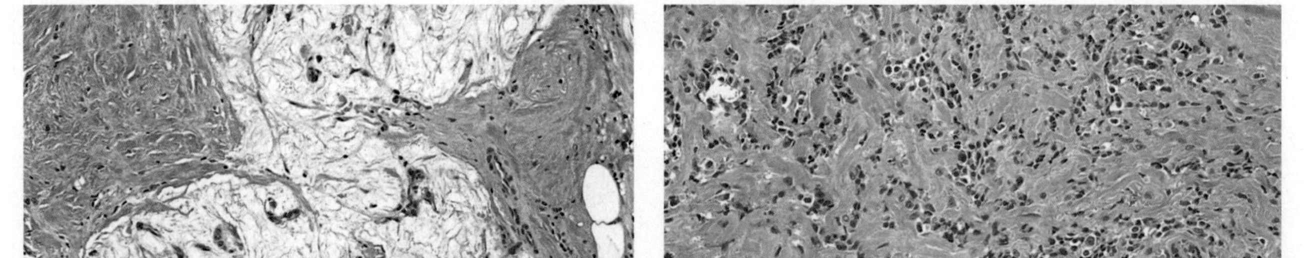

FIG. 43.2. ***Metastatic carcinoma in the capsule of a sentinel lymph node mistaken for a heterotopic gland inclusion.*** **A,B:** The primary tumor had a mixed growth pattern consisting almost entirely of (**A**) mucinous and (**B**) classical infiltrating lobular carcinoma. **C:** Less than 5% of the tumor had this well-differentiated structure. **D:** Metastatic carcinoma, found only in the capsule and adjacent tissue of this SLN, had well-differentiated glands that were misdiagnosed as heterotopic inclusions.

However, neither hypothesis provides an explanation for the presence of glands composed of müllerian-like cells in the absence of a demonstrated neoplasm of the female genital tract.

Clinical Presentation

The occurrence of benign heterotopic epithelium in ALNs is rare.[20] In a study of autopsy material, no epithelial inclusions were identified in 8,825 slides prepared from 3,904 lymph nodes obtained from 160 postmortem axillary dissections. Each lymph node was grossly cut at 0.2-cm interval, and histologic sections were prepared at 100-μm interval.[21]

Almost all reported examples of heterotopic epithelial tissue associated with ALNs have occurred in women. Before the era of SLN biopsy, patients with no prior surgery sometimes presented with an axillary mass, but in many instances the affected lymph nodes were clinically inapparent. They were detected in grossly normal lymph nodes removed as part of a surgical procedure. One patient underwent a mastectomy for carcinoma of the left breast 10 years before an enlarged right ALN that contained heterotopic glandular tissue was excised.[8] Kadowaki et al.[16] described a patient who presented with a 1.8-cm axillary tumor 8 years after she underwent excision of a "nipple adenoma" from the ipsilateral breast. Mammography revealed calcifications in the axillary lesion. When excised after a 2-year delay, the lymph node was found to be extensively involved by a complex, multicystic inclusion with glandular and squamous components.

Since the advent of SLN biopsy of the axilla in women with breast carcinoma, heterotopic epithelial inclusions have received closer scrutiny. Maiorano et al.[20] described seven examples of heterotopic epithelial inclusions in axillary SLNs in a total of 3,500 specimens analyzed in a 6-year period. Six of the patients had invasive carcinoma and one had ductal carcinoma *in situ* (DCIS), but none had had prior surgery of a needling procedure. Three of the lymph nodes had coincidental metastatic or micrometastatic carcinoma and four had no metastases. In some instances, the heterotopic tissue exhibited proliferative FCCs, including adenosis, duct hyperplasia, apocrine metaplasia, and cystic squamous metaplasia. Immunoreactive myoepithelial cells were detected in foci regarded as heterotopic glandular epithelium. As expected, no myoepithelium was found around the cystic squamous inclusions, and the squamous epithelium was immunoreactive for p63.

Gross Pathology

Lymph nodes found to harbor epithelial inclusions are usually grossly unremarkable, but enlarged lymph nodes that measured up to 3 cm have been described in a few instances. Some have contained grossly apparent cysts that were filled with "colorless or brownish fluid,"[7] "greenish yellow necrotic-like,"[9] or "cottage-cheese-like material."[11] Calcified keratotic debris may be present in cysts lined by squamous epithelium.[16]

Microscopic Pathology

Cystic epithelial inclusions in lymph nodes have been lined by glandular, squamous, or apocrine epithelium[6,7,11] (Fig. 43.3). Discharge of keratin from cystic squamous inclusions can elicit a granulomatous reaction.[11] Inclusions that appear to be derived from skin appendage glands may exhibit sebaceous differentiation. Proliferative changes in the glandular inclusions have included apocrine metaplasia and duct hyperplasia.[20] Heterotopic lobular glands altered by SA involving the capsules and superficial nodal tissue have been reported in two SLNs from a single patient. Myoepithelium was demonstrated in both foci by p63 and CD10 immunostains. Benign mammary ductal structures are a rare form of heterotopia (Fig. 43.4).

One case report described papillary carcinoma that seemed to arise from a benign intranodal mammary glandular inclusion. This conclusion was based on the observation that some glands associated with the papillary carcinoma in the lymph node appeared to be benign. However, the authors reported that the patient also had in one breast "a small intraductal papillary carcinoma . . . differing cytologically and architecturally from the nodal carcinoma." Because of the apparently noninvasive character of the mammary lesions, and differences in the histologic appearance of the two processes, they were regarded as independent lesions, but metastatic involvement of the ALN from the existing mammary papillary carcinoma cannot be ruled out. The possibility that mammary carcinoma could arise from heterotopic glandular inclusions in ALNs is considered more fully in the discussion of occult carcinoma presenting as an axillary nodal metastasis (see Chapter 33).

The distinction between heterotopic mammary glandular epithelium and metastatic carcinoma is usually not difficult (Fig. 43.5). The glandular structures typically occur outside or within the lymph node capsule or in the lymphoid tissue rather than in nodal sinusoids. Myoepithelial cells and specialized intralobular stroma are evident in most heterotopic glands and ducts of the mammary type. On the other hand, they are absent from müllerian-type heterotopic glands and from squamous inclusions. In the absence of myoepithelial cells, glands in ALNs usually represent metastatic carcinoma, even if the growth pattern is extremely well-differentiated. These metastatic foci are typically distributed as isolated glands or small groups of glands in the lymphoid tissue of the lymph node, or in the capsule and subcapsular lymphatic spaces (Figs. 43.1 and 43.2). A collagenous band that resembles a basement membrane may be found around part or all of such metastatic glands. Metastatic tubular carcinoma mistakenly diagnosed as "benign epithelial lined tubules" within a lymph node was illustrated in a published report.[22] Histologic identification of ciliated cells and "peg" cells is helpful to recognize the müllerian type of inclusion. Immunoreactivity for Wilms tumor 1 (WT-1) and PAX8 can be used to support the diagnosis.[5]

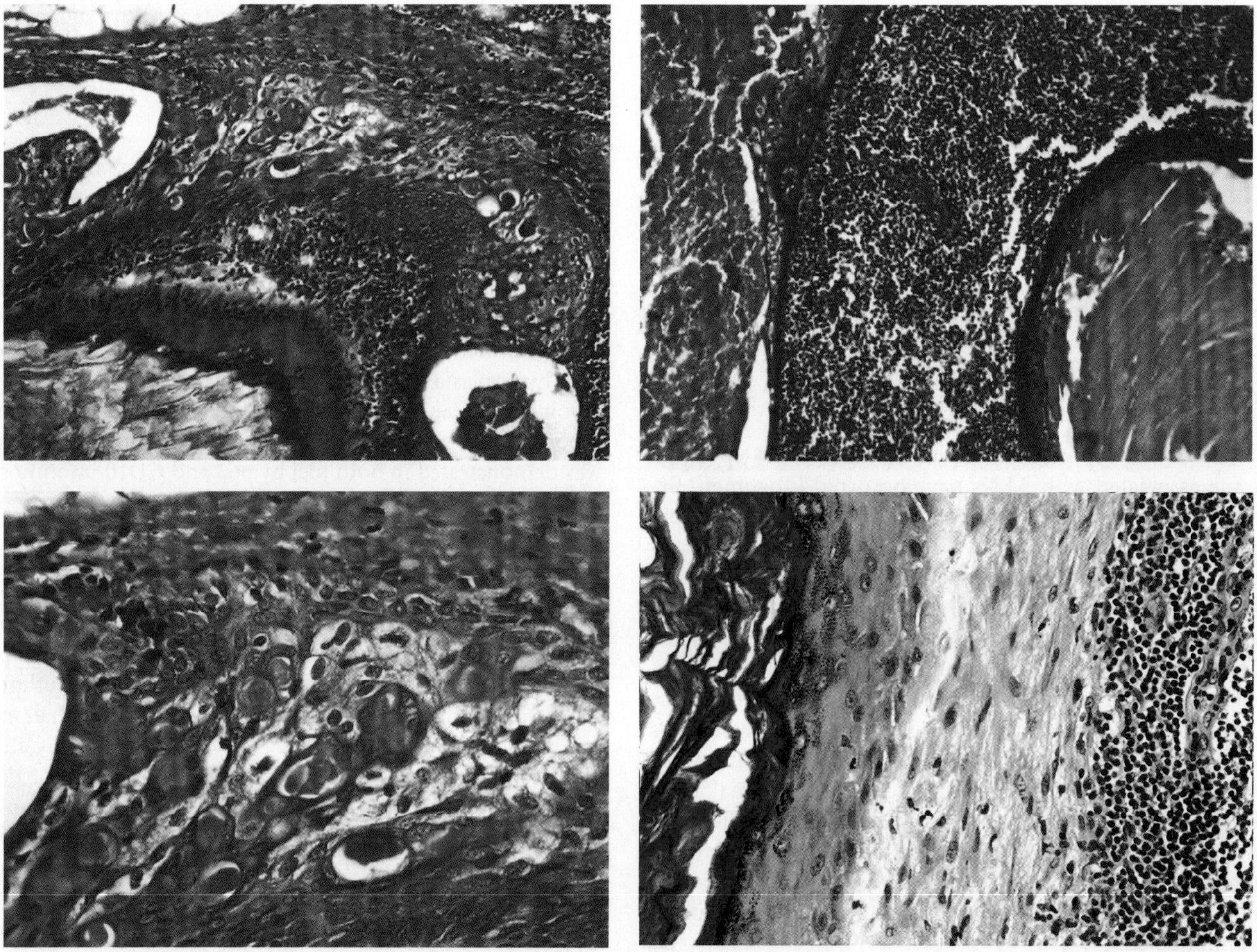

FIG. 43.3. ***Heterotopic glands in axillary lymph node. This glandular complex may be of sweat gland origin.*** **A:** Cystic glands with squamous metaplasia in a lymph node. The lymph node capsule is at the *upper* border of the picture. **B:** Cysts within the lymph node. **C:** Sebaceous metaplasia in the nodal inclusion. **D:** Squamous epithelium in a cyst with hyperkeratosis and pigmentation.

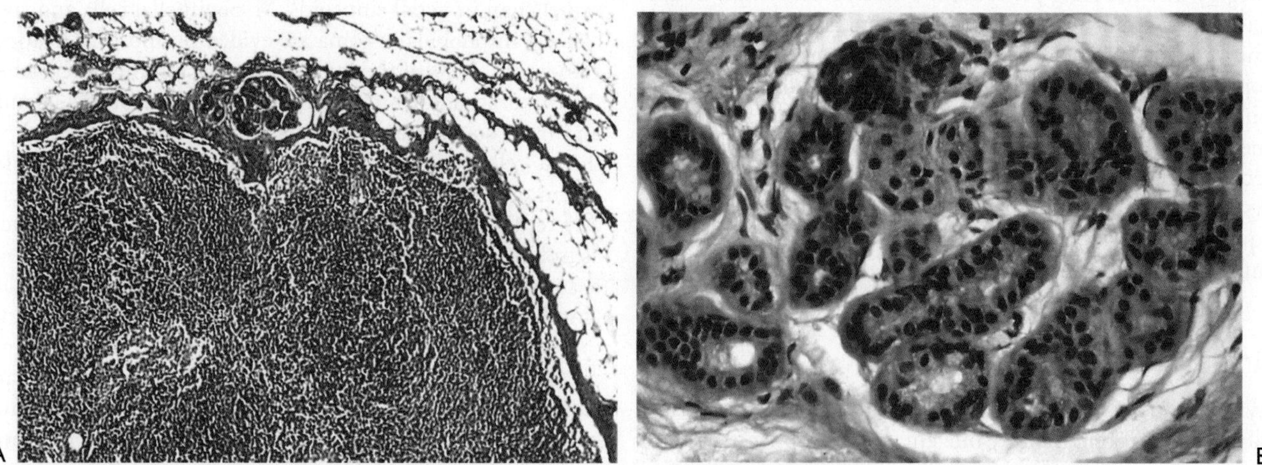

FIG. 43.4. ***Heterotopic lobule associated with lymph nodes.*** **A ,B:** Myoepithelial cells outline this benign lobule in the capsule of an ALN. The 39-year-old patient had fibromatosis. **C:** A skin adnexal gland adjacent to an ALN.

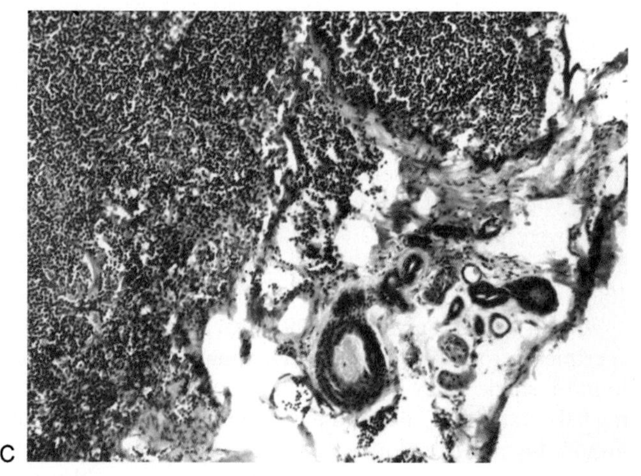

FIG. 43.4. *(Continued)*

NEVUS CELL AGGREGATES

Collections of cells that resemble cutaneous nevi can be found in the capsules of lymph nodes in various areas of the body, including the axilla. Because of their usual association with the lymph node capsule rather than the lymphoid parenchyma in most cases, these groups of cells have been termed "nevus cell aggregates" (NCA), rather than the frequently used term "nevus cell inclusions."[23] A minority of NCA are found within the cortical and medullary lymphoid tissue where they appear to be associated with stromal septa that originate in the capsule.

Etiology

The etiology of NCA is unknown, but it has been suggested that they originate in the lymph node capsule. One investigator has presented evidence of origin from cells in the

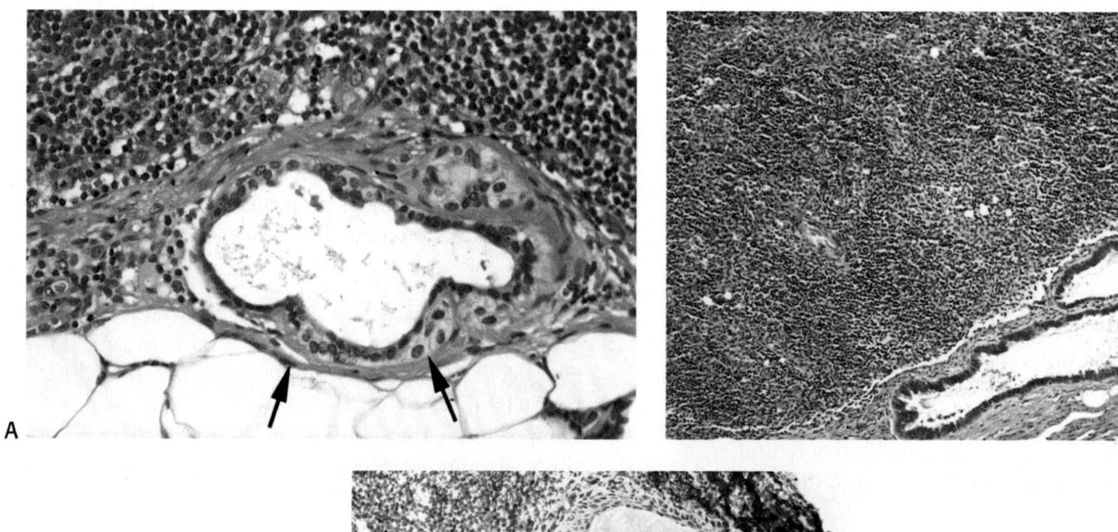

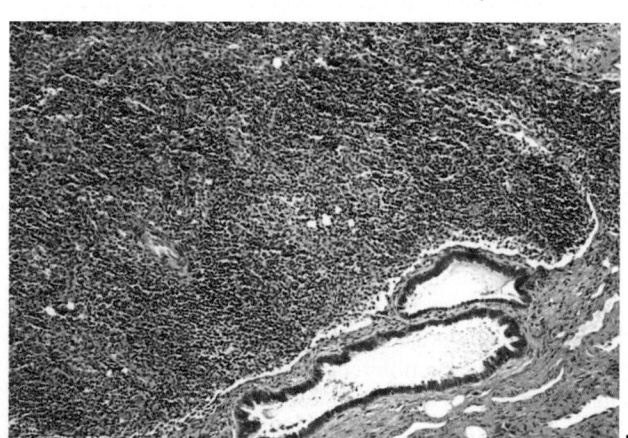

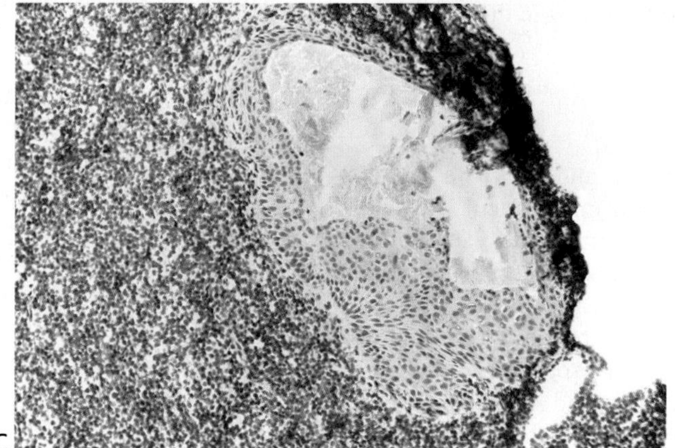

FIG. 43.5. ***Heterotopic ductal and squamous epithelial tissue associated with axillary lymph nodes.*** **A,B:** Two examples of mammary-type ducts in the capsules of lymph nodes. Myoepithelial cells (*arrows*) are evident around the duct in **(A)**. Micropapillary hyperplasia is evident in **(B)**. **C:** Squamous epithelium-lined cystic inclusion in an SLN. Note the granular cell layer in the epithelium and intracystic keratinous debris. This inclusion was detected on frozen section examination. This photograph is from the frozen section slide that was subsequently destained, and restained for estrogen receptor (ER). The inclusion is ER-negative. The ipsilateral moderately differentiated invasive carcinoma was ER-positive.

walls of vessels in the lymph node capsule.[24] This observation is consistent with the view that NCA are angioglomic structures derived from perithelial cells with glomus properties around vessels in the lymph node capsule.[25] It has also been hypothesized that NCA arise by a process of "benign metastasis" in which cells are transported (presumably via lymphatic channels) from benign cutaneous nevi to the lymph node. Rarely, these patients have a notable contiguous cutaneous nevus.[26] The fact that a few individuals have had prominent nevi or melanomas in the nearby skin suggests that some factor or factors may predispose particular individuals to develop NCA and melanocytic skin lesions. It is not known whether such patients have NCA in nodal areas anatomically unrelated to the known cutaneous lesion because it is not possible to sample lymph nodes at other sites. If NCA were "benign metastases" from clinically inapparent or inconspicuous cutaneous nevi, it is difficult to envision the mechanism by which such "metastases" would almost always be localized to the nodal capsule, since one expects that cellular elements transported via the lymphatics should be deposited in nodal sinuses. The most likely explanation for the histogenesis of NCA is that they are the result of embryologic maldevelopment or that they arise from angioglomic structures that are normally present.

Although NCA have some glomoid structural features, the presence of melanin pigment (verified by electron microscopy) and the existence of heavily pigmented NCA with a blue nevus configuration are indicative of nevocellular differentiation. As discussed in subsequent text, electron microscopy has documented many similarities between the cells of NCA and cutaneous nevi, but it has failed to detect smooth muscle differentiation commonly seen in glomus cells.[27] Consequently, it seems more likely that NCA develop from melanocytic cells arrested in migration from the neural crest to the skin, or from primitive neural crest-derived cells that may be normally present in the capsules of superficial lymph nodes.[28]

Frequency

NCA were first described by Stewart and Copeland[29] in the hilar region of an ALN obtained from a patient with von Recklinghausen disease, a bathing trunk nevus, and malignant melanoma. Stewart[30] commented on three additional axillary NCA in 1960. The first series of six cases was reported by Johnson and Helwig,[31] who noted that NCA often contained pigments with the staining properties of melanin. Two of the patients were women who had ALNs removed in the treatment of breast carcinoma, and a third woman had fibrocystic mastopathy. NCA were also found in ALNs obtained from men with basal cell carcinoma and malignant melanoma, and in a cervical lymph node from a man with an epidermal inclusion cyst. Pigmented NCA were subsequently described in an inguinal lymph node from an 8-year-old child with juvenile melanoma,[32] and in a cervical lymph node from a man with squamous carcinoma of the larynx.[33]

In 1974, McCarthy et al.[34] described 24 patients who had NCA, including 15 who were treated for malignant melanoma. The majority of NCA were associated with ALNs, but inguinal nodes were affected in seven cases and cervical nodes in two cases. The ages of the patients ranged from 17 to 70 years. The series included four women with axillary NCA who had been treated for breast carcinoma. Pigmented nevi were present in the skin drained by the lymph nodes with NCA in 21 cases. McCarthy et al.[34] reported that NCA were present in 6.2% of 129 axillary and in 4.0% of 50 inguinal lymph node dissections. No NCA were found in 130 dissections of thoracic, abdominal, or iliac lymph nodes.

Ridolfi et al.[23] reviewed 909 consecutive mastectomy specimens from patients with mammary carcinoma and found a single NCA in each of three cases (0.33%) affecting 0.017% (3 of 17,504) of the lymph nodes examined. One hundred lymph node dissections from patients with malignant melanoma obtained from various sites were also reviewed, yielding NCA in 3 of 2,607 lymph nodes (0.12%). Another study in which lymph nodes were examined by immunohistochemistry as well as routine histology reported that NCA were present in 49 (22%) of 226 lymph node dissections.[35] Seventy-eight percent of NCA were detected by routine histology and 22% by staining for S-100 protein. ALNs were the most frequent sites of NCA (22%), followed by cervical (18%) and inguinal (11%) nodes. Bautista et al.[36] also used the S-100 stain to study 300 axillary dissections. They reported finding NCA in 7.3% of the specimens and in 0.54% of 5,186 lymph nodes examined.

Several conclusions can be drawn from the foregoing data:

1. NCA occur in association with superficial lymph node groups that drain the skin as well as other organs. If they ever occur in visceral lymph nodes, it is extraordinarily unusual.
2. Lymph nodes that contain NCA are most frequent in the axilla and less often found in the groin and cervical regions.
3. NCA have been detected in lymph nodes from men, women, and children. Most of the patients have had malignant neoplasms, but NCA have been found in lymph nodes from individuals with benign neoplasms and nonneoplastic conditions. They may be more frequent in ALNs from patients with malignant melanoma than in the ALNs of women with mammary carcinoma.
4. Although some patients with NCA have a contiguous skin lesion such as malignant melanoma or a conspicuous nevus, the majority of these patients have no notable skin lesions.

Clinical Presentation

The majority of NCA are small, often microscopic, structures that do not cause palpable enlargement of lymph nodes or any other clinical symptoms. Consequently, their presence is unsuspected until resected lymph nodes have been examined microscopically after excision. Rare examples of diffuse intranodal NCA have caused grossly evident lymph node enlargement.

Gross Pathology

NCA are rarely visible grossly. Heavily pigmented NCA have been described grossly on rare occasions. In one instance, the gross findings suggested anthracotic pigment.[37] Another example occurred in an inguinal lymph node removed incidentally during treatment of varicose veins that contained "three darkly pigmented nodules, the largest being 0.3 cm in diameter."[38] A third 0.8-cm lymph node from the axilla of a woman with breast carcinoma contained "a golden-brown crescentic lesion . . . that occupied approximately one-third of the perimeter"[28] (Fig. 43.6). In each of these instances, the microscopic configuration of the NCA was that of a blue nevus.

Microscopic Pathology

Two distinct microscopic patterns of NCA have been described: NCA that resemble intradermal nevi and NCA with the appearance of blue nevi. The former are much more common, with fewer than 10% of NCA having the blue nevus structure. Patients with the two types of NCA do not differ appreciably with respect to age distribution, associated diseases, or the frequency of multinodal involvement.

Intradermal Nevus Type of NCA

NCA of the intradermal nevus type have a flat or nodular configuration in the lymph node capsule (Fig. 43.7). In most cases, a single lymph node is affected, but in rare instances NCA are found in two or more lymph nodes from a nodal group.[25,31,39–41] In a single plane of section, nevus-type NCA occupy a fraction of the perimeter of a lymph node. They often appear to have a discontinuous distribution and may extend into the node itself usually along fibrous trabeculae. Any portion of the capsule may be affected, and there does not seem to be a predilection to involve the hilar region. Rarely, these NCA lie entirely within the lymphoid parenchyma of the lymph node.[23,36,42] Nevus-type NCA have not been encountered as isolated structures in the peripheral sinus of a lymph node.

The architecture of nevus-type NCA is demonstrated in sections prepared with the reticulin stain. The cells that form an NCA are cytologically very similar to cells of an ordinary intradermal nevus. They tend to be tightly clustered into defined masses separated by, or sometimes seemingly centered about, thin-walled capillaries. When they have a particularly angular configuration, these capillaries may be mistaken for artifactual spaces. The outer, peripheral portion of nevus-type NCA is usually sharply defined, whereas at the inner margin NCA cells may merge with capsular tissue.

Cytologically, nevus-type NCA cells are typically oval or spindle-shaped with indistinct cytoplasmic borders (Fig. 43.8). Polygonal or epithelioid cells are found in some cases. The central nuclei have fine, diffuse chromatin and are surrounded by pale or clear cytoplasm. Nucleoli are small and indistinct or absent. Intranuclear inclusions may be evident. Mitoses are not seen, and less than 1% of the cells express Ki67.[42] Multinucleated cells of the type sometimes found in intradermal nevi are not a feature of nevus-type NCA.

Fine brown pigment granules can be detected in the cytoplasm of a few scattered cells in a minority of NCA. This pigment gives a negative Perls Prussian blue reaction for iron, and it is blackened with the Fontana Masson and Grimelius stains, indicating the presence of melanin (Fig. 43.9). NCA contain no mucin when studied with mucicarmine, periodic acid–Schiff (PAS), or Alcian blue stains. Immunohistochemical studies have revealed strong reactivity for S-100 protein and MART1/MelanA, but not for HMB45.[42] There is also absence of staining for cytokeratin (CK), hormone receptors, or epithelial membrane antigen (Fig. 43.10).

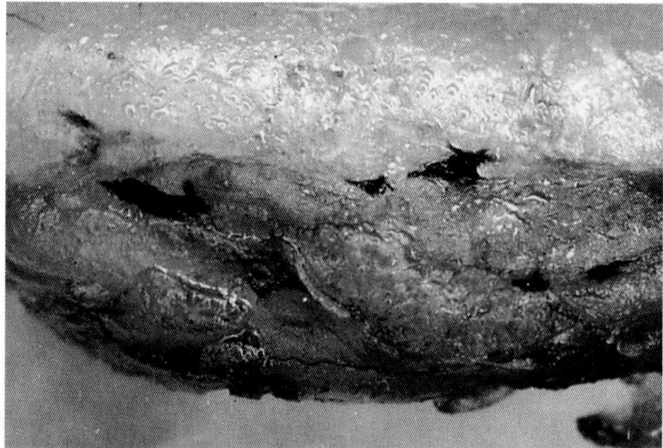

FIG. 43.6. ***Nevus cell aggregate, gross appearance.*** This blue nevus-type lesion had abundant black melanin pigment. [Reproduced from Epstein JI, Erlandson RA, Rosen PP. Nodal blue nevi. A study of three cases. *Am J Surg Pathol* 1984;8:907–915.]

Blue Nevus Type of NCA

NCA of the blue nevus variety have poorly defined borders. These heavily pigmented lesions, which occupy the lymph node capsule and radiate into surrounding fat, may also extend into the nodal lymphoid tissue[28,37,38,43] (Fig. 43.11). The finely granular pigment is golden or dark brown. It fills and often obscures the cytoplasm of many cells in the lesion, especially the closely packed elongated cells with dendritic processes. At the outer, peripheral edges of blue nevus type of NCA, these slender cells extend into the perinodal fat. It is unusual for blue nevus type of NCA to extend along trabeculae into the substance of a lymph node. Scattered singly and in small groups among the spindle cells are polygonal cells with pale cytoplasm that contains coarsely clumped pigment. These epithelioid cells resemble pigmented histiocytes. Blue nevus-type NCA differ from nevus-type NCA in being immunoreactive for HMB45.[44] They are also immunoreactive for S-100 protein and MART1/MelanA. Mitotic figures and multinucleated giant cells are absent from the blue nevus type of NCA.

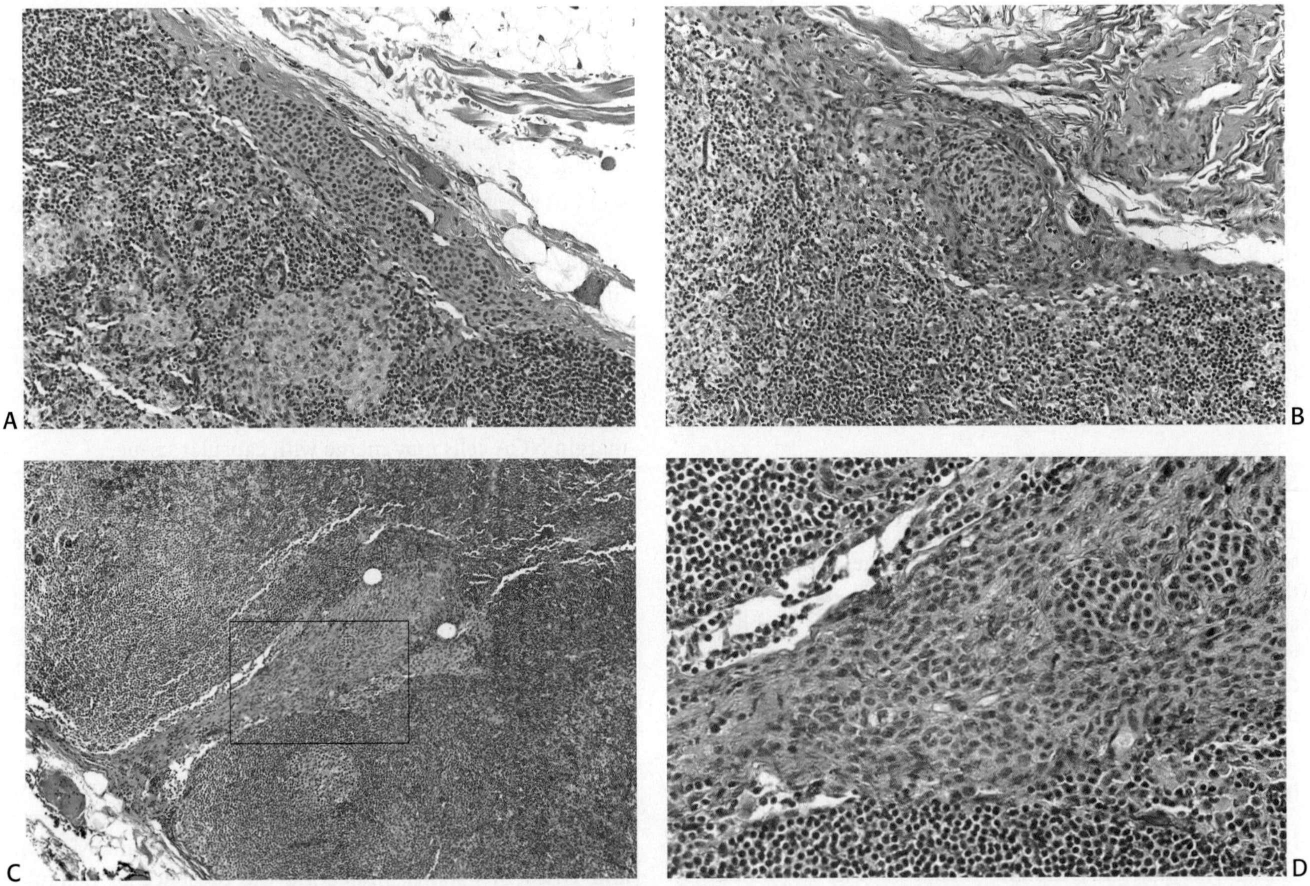

FIG. 43.7. ***Nevus cell aggregate, flat and nodular types.*** **A:** This relatively flat lesion forms a band along the outer border of the lymph node capsule. **B:** A minute NCA that forms a nodule in the capsule of the lymph node. The apparent structural difference between the NCA in **(A)** and **(B)** may simply result from the plane of section since **(B)** may be a transverse section through an NCA such as **(A)** that is seen in the longitudinal plane. **C,D:** This NCA extends into the lymph node along fibrous trabeculum. **(D)** depicts area within the *box* in **(C)**.

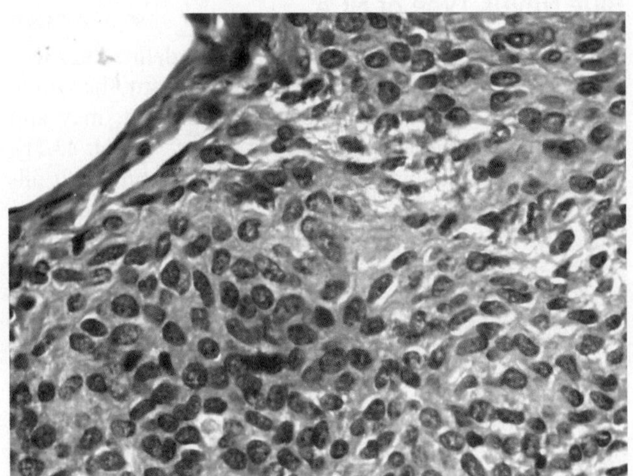

FIG. 43.8. ***Nevus cell aggregate, cytology.*** The cells have oval nuclei with finely granular chromatin. They are identical to cells typically found in a cutaneous dermal nevus.

Differential Diagnosis

Because the indication for a lymph node dissection is almost always a regional malignant neoplasm, it is important that NCA not be mistakenly interpreted as metastatic tumor.[45] The deceptively bland histologic appearance of some melanoma metastases can simulate an NCA. Since NCA as well as most melanomas express S-100 and MART1/MelanA, these stains are not helpful in the differential diagnosis. However, melanoma has a high percentage of Ki67-positive cells, whereas less than 1% of cells in NCA are Ki67-positive. When uncertainty persists, fluorescence *in situ* hybridization (FISH) testing for chromosomal alterations that are commonly found in melanoma may be helpful.[46]

In patients with mammary carcinoma, NCA most closely resemble metastatic lobular carcinoma. Features that help to distinguish NCA from mammary carcinoma include the capsular location, the presence of fine brown pigment with the staining properties of melanin, the absence of mucin,

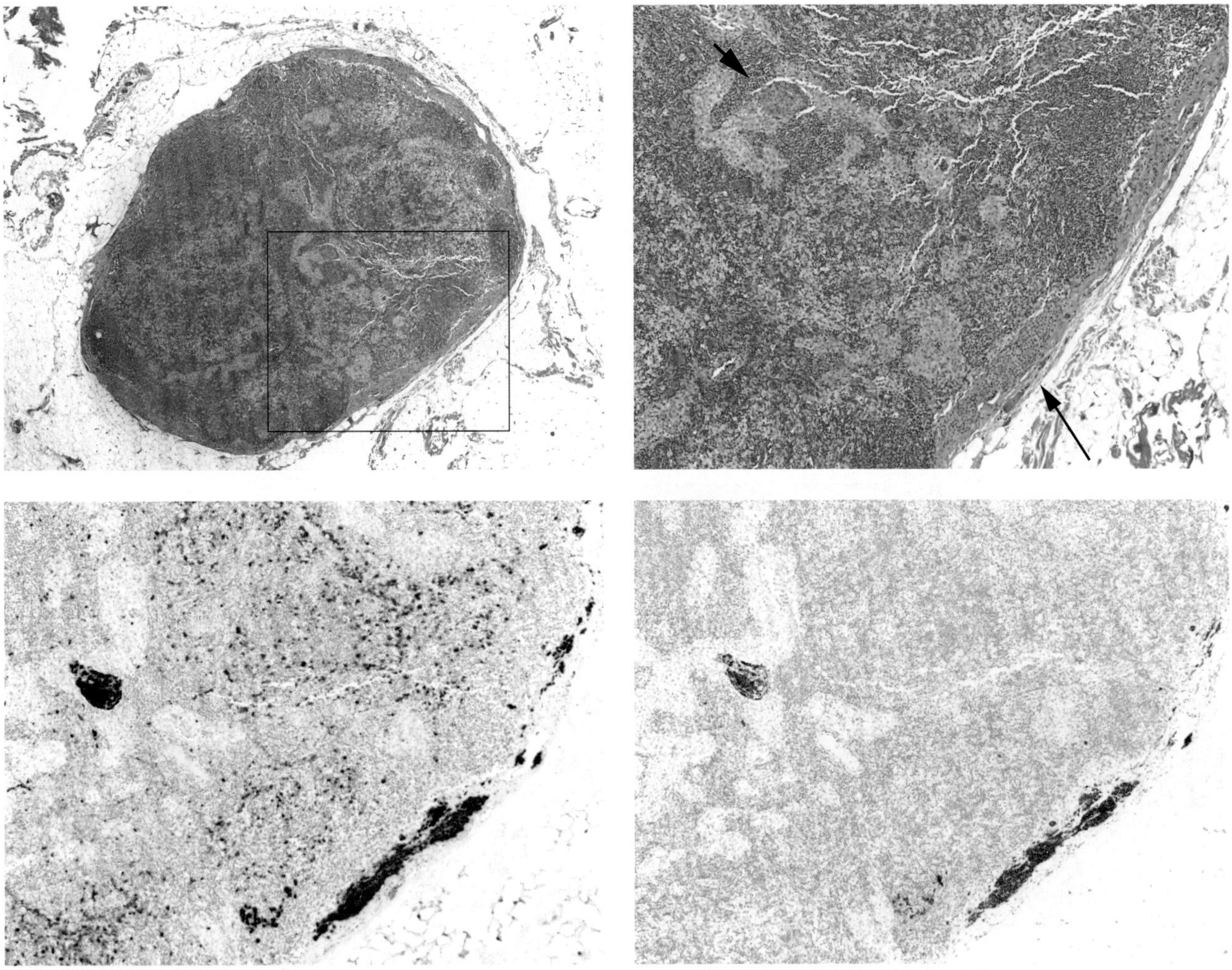

FIG. 43.9. ***Nevus cell aggregate, S-100 protein and A103 immunostains.*** **A,B:** The NCA in this lymph node lies along the capsule (long arrow) as well as centrally (*short arrow*) in the intranodal trabecular extension of the capsule. Box outlines area shown in **(B)**. **C,D:** Immunoreactivity for S-100 protein **(C)** and A103 **(D)**. Note the decoration of dendritic reticular cells and perinodal adipocytes with S-100 protein **(C)**.

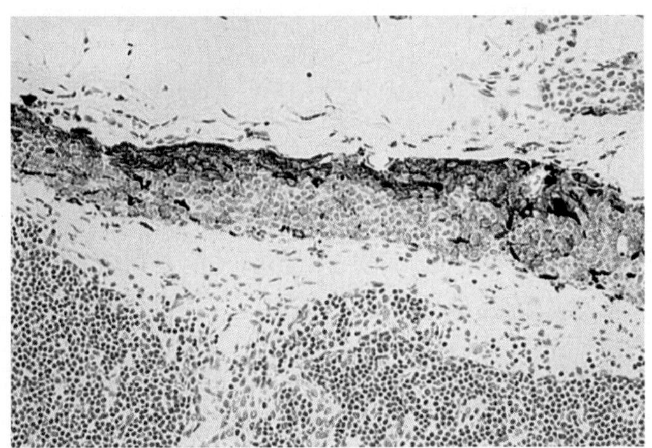

FIG. 43.10. ***Nevus cell aggregate, Fontana Masson stain.*** The pigment stains black.

and immunohistochemical reactivity consistent with neuroepithelial rather than glandular histogenesis. Rarely, a lymph node may contain an NCA and metastatic tumor.

Electron Microscopy

Ultrastructural studies of two NCA have been published. The first report described a dermal nevus type of NCA in the ALN of an 82-year-old woman with mammary carcinoma.[27] The NCA consisted of nests of round cells that contained round nuclei with fine, dispersed marginated chromatin. Widely scattered electron-dense mature melanosomes were found in the cytoplasm of occasional cells. Ultrastructural study of compound, intradermal, and junctional cutaneous nevi revealed cells resembling those in the NCA. A blue nevus type of NCA studied by electron microscopy contained

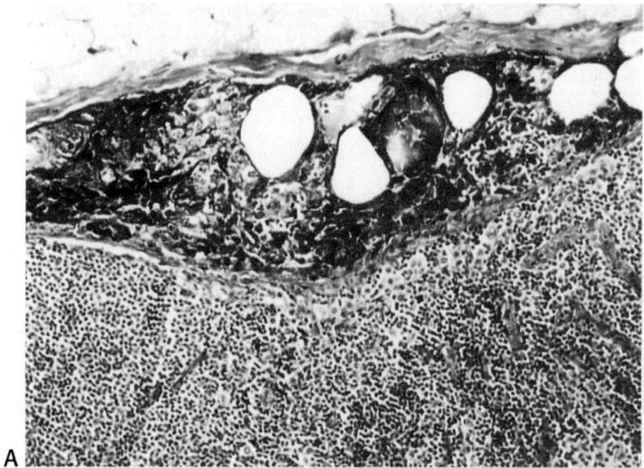

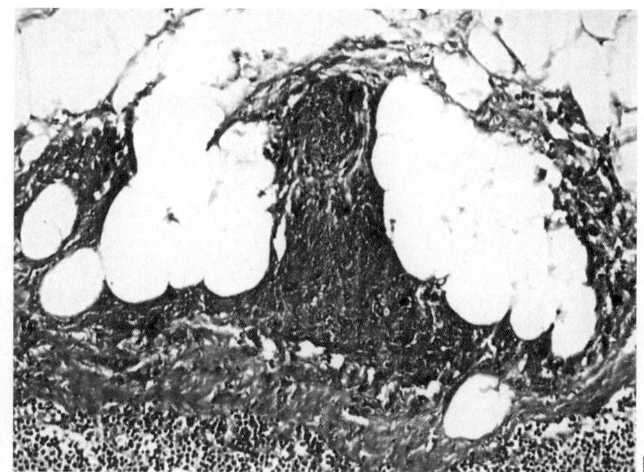

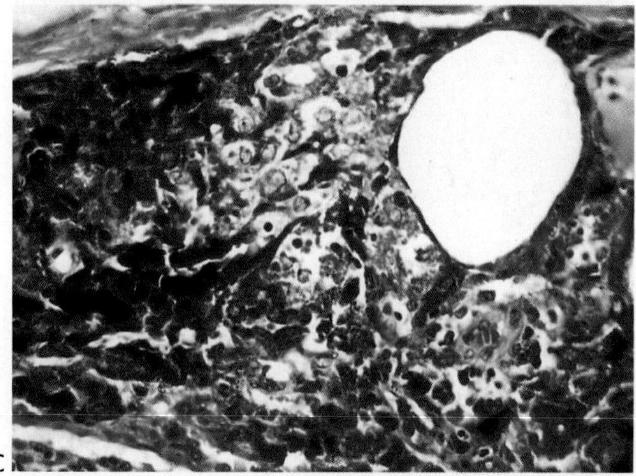

FIG. 43.11. ***Nevus cell aggregate, blue nevus type.*** **A,B:** Two heavily pigmented NCA that radiate into the perinodal fat. **C:** Many of the cells are obscured by *brown* pigment.

round and elongated cells with abundant cytoplasmic, spherical, electron-dense, mature stage IV melanosomes as well as smaller, membrane-limited melanosomes in clusters.[28]

Prognosis

NCA could theoretically be the source of some malignant melanomas detected in lymph nodes in the absence of a demonstrable cutaneous primary. There is no evidence that the presence of NCA in the lymph nodes of patients with an associated malignant neoplasm affects the prognosis of the neoplasm, or that such individuals are predisposed to develop any particular type of neoplasm subsequently.

SINUS HISTIOCYTOSIS

Sinus histiocytosis has been defined as the "distention of the sinusoids of the lymph nodes by elongated histiocytes that have finely granular, eosinophilic-staining cytoplasm in a syncytial arrangement"[47] (Fig. 43.12). Various schemes have been devised to grade or subclassify the intensity of sinus histiocytosis, including 3-point,[47] 5-point,[48] and 2-point scales.[49] In a 3-point grading system, sinus histiocytosis is described as minimal or absent, intermediate when sinusoids are widened by three to four elongated histiocytes, and marked when the breadth of sinusoids is greater than four cells.[47] Grading has been determined from the most severe change seen among the lymph nodes on a single slide[47] by

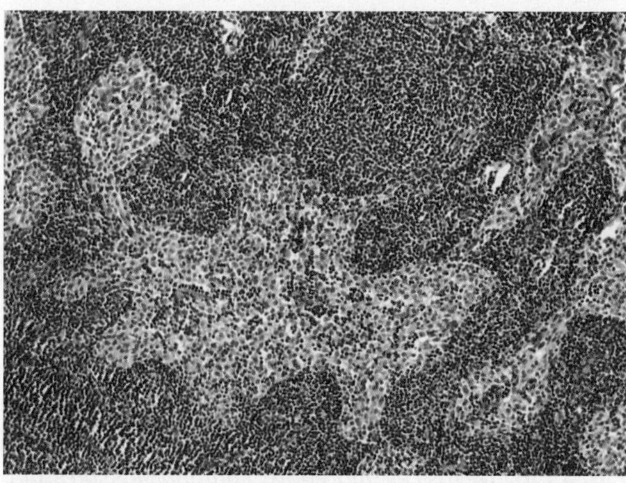

FIG. 43.12. ***Sinus histiocytosis.*** The lymph sinuses are distended by broad syncytial sheets of histiocytes.

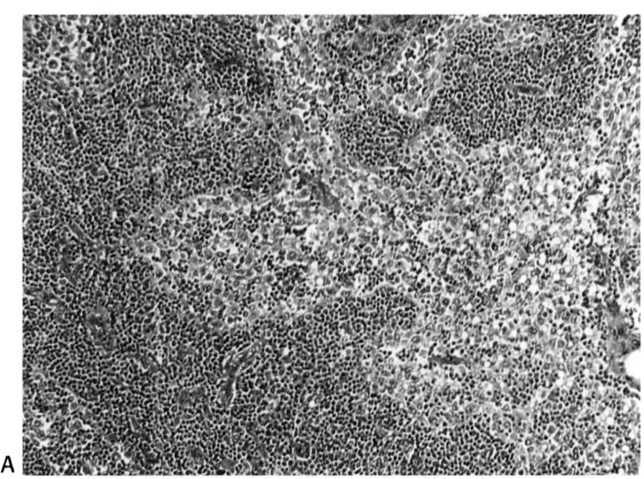
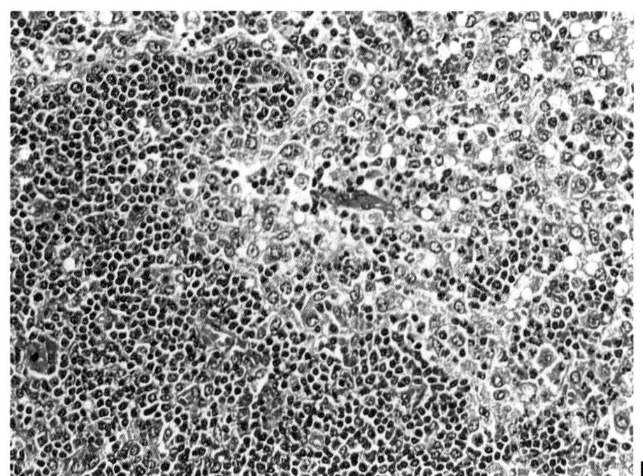

FIG. 43.13. *Sinus histiocytosis, inflammatory.* **A:** Red blood cells are dispersed in the sinusoids. **B:** Red blood cells, leukocytes, and lymphocytes mingle with the histiocytes.

assessing each lymph node separately and then calculating the mean intensity of reaction,[48] or on the basis of the lymph node that showed the most extreme sinus histiocytosis.[49] Lymph nodes exhibiting inflammatory sinus histiocytosis, characterized by sinusoidal edema or erythrophagocytosis and polymorphonuclear leukocytes, should be excluded from evaluation (Fig. 43.13). Lipid transported from the lactating breast to ALNs accumulates in histiocytes, causing a variant of inflammatory sinus histiocytosis referred to as lactational histiocytosis (Fig. 43.14).

A nodal infiltrate of histiocytosis with signet ring cell features can mimic metastatic lobular carcinoma.[50] In this rare condition, the histiocytes have crescentic nuclei as a result of being displaced by an intracytoplasmic vacuole. The contents of the vacuole may be weakly mucin-positive. These cells are not immunoreactive for epithelial markers such as CK and hormone receptors. Their histiocytic nature can be confirmed by demonstrating immunoreactivity to CD68.

It has been suggested that sinus histiocytosis is a manifestation of a cell-mediated immune reaction. Marked sinus histiocytosis in the ipsilateral ALNs of patients with breast carcinoma has been associated with an enhanced cellular response to autologous breast carcinoma tissue[51] and to clinically evident enlargement of contralateral ALNs.[48] Several studies, largely carried out by Black et al.[48,51–53] and Cutler et al.,[54,55] reported a correlation between the grade of sinus histiocytosis and survival. Patients with the most intense, high-grade reaction had the most favorable prognosis. Marked sinus histiocytosis was associated with a better prognosis in node-negative and node-positive patients,[53,54] with the effect more pronounced when nodal metastases were present.[55] Silverberg et al.[49] found that marked sinus histiocytosis indicated a favorable prognosis in women with moderately or poorly differentiated tumors and in those with fewer than nine positive lymph nodes. There was no correlation with outcome in women who had well-differentiated tumors, negative lymph nodes, or more than eight positive nodes. Friedell et al.[56] found that the ALNs of Japanese women with breast carcinoma had marked sinus

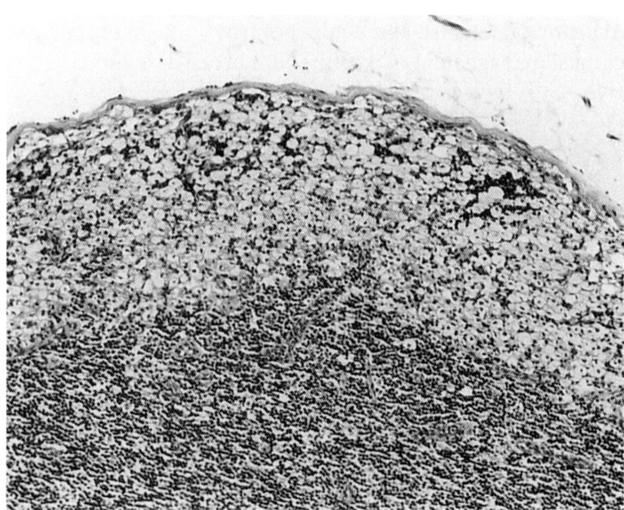

FIG. 43.14. *Sinus histiocytosis, lactational.* Histiocytes filled with lipid have accumulated in the sinusoids.

histiocytosis more often than the lymph nodes from British women, regardless of the presence or absence of nodal metastases, and suggested that this phenomenon contributed to racial differences in survival. However, survival analysis was not reported for the patients studied.

Others have not been able to confirm the association between sinus histiocytosis and prognosis. Berg[57] concluded that nodal status and factors associated with lymph node metastases were more significant for prognosis. Moore et al.[58] were unable to find a difference in the pattern of sinus histiocytosis between patients who survived and those who died of metastatic breast carcinoma. DiRe and Lane,[59] Schiodt,[60] and Kister et al.[61] also concluded that sinus histiocytosis was not a significant indicator of prognosis.

Failure of investigators to find a consistent relationship between sinus histiocytosis and prognosis in breast cancer may reflect significant technical problems in the histologic evaluation of this phenomenon. A major difficulty is the growing trend to biopsy the breast tumor days or weeks prior to the axillary dissection. As a consequence, the lymph nodes exhibit reactive inflammatory alterations resulting from the earlier procedure. Furthermore, in the current era of SLN biopsy the small number of lymph nodes removed by this procedure does not provide an adequate sample for assessing the character of sinus histiocytosis.

It is also necessary to have good quality sections of well-fixed tissue, and such preparations are not always available. Investigators have not used consistent grading schemes, and there is no consensus on the measurement, grading, or reporting of sinus histiocytosis. Finally, the evaluation of sinus histiocytosis has proven to be a highly subjective endeavor with considerable interobserver and intraobserver variability. In one study, an "experienced observer" achieved 70% self-reproducibility in two separate reviews of the same lymph nodes.[47] Two less-experienced pathologists agreed with the average grade of the two reviews of the "experienced observer" in 55% and 61% of cases, respectively. Presently, the evaluation of sinus histiocytosis as a prognostic indicator is largely of historical interest, and it does not play a role in the current clinical management of patients with breast carcinoma.

ROSAI–DORFMAN DISEASE

Rosai–Dorfman disease, also referred to as sinus histiocytosis with massive lymphadenopathy, is an idiopathic benign histiocytic proliferative disorder that most commonly affects the cervical lymph nodes. The disease can rarely affect the breast as an isolated process,[62] or as part of a disseminated extranodal process,[63] with or without the involvement of ALNs.[64,65] Nodal disease is microscopically characterized by sheets of histiocytes alternating with mature lymphocytes. The histiocytes bear inconspicuous nuclei and abundant pale and foamy cytoplasm, and are immunoreactive for S-100 protein. Emperipolesis is characteristic of this disease. This peculiar finding is manifested by the presence of lymphocytes demarcated by a clear halo in the cytoplasm of histiocytes. Additional information about Rosai–Dorfman disease can be found in Chapter 40.

SILICONE LYMPHADENITIS

Clinical Presentation

Silicone, a polymer of dimethylsiloxane, is used in the manufacture of breast prostheses. This material is nonbiodegradable and stable, although it elicits a variable foreign body inflammatory reaction. Reaction to silicone transported to lymph nodes has been described in association with orthopedic prostheses,[66,67] cosmetic injection of silicone in the breast and other sites, and from silicone breast implants.[68,69] Silicone lymphadenitis can be the result of leakage from an intact implant, rupture of an implant, or shedding of silicone particles from the exterior surface of an implant. Even "third-generation" silicone implants can leak or rupture, albeit rarely.

In the mammary region, clinically symptomatic silicone lymphadenopathy is manifested by nontender or painful axillary nodal enlargement. Asymptomatic silicone lymphadenitis may be encountered when a patient with a silicone-containing prosthesis undergoes an axillary dissection or lymph node biopsy for another condition such as mammary carcinoma.[68] Involvement of an intramammary lymph node by silicone can produce mammographic changes that mimic carcinoma.[70] Enlargement of ipsilateral and contralateral internal mammary, mediastinal, para-aortic, and pelvic lymph nodes due to silicone lymphadenitis related to silicone mammary implants has been reported.[71–74] The abnormal lymph nodes may suggest metastatic carcinoma in imaging studies.

Gross Pathology

Affected lymph nodes generally do not manifest specific or distinctive gross features. In some cases, the lymph nodes are enlarged and firmer than normal. In extreme examples of silicone lymphadenitis, the cut surface reveals a distorted nodal architecture and fibrosis.[66] The gross appearance of lymph nodes with silicone lymphadenitis is also affected by concurrent diseases such as metastatic carcinoma or malignant lymphoma.

Microscopic Pathology

There is considerable variation in the extent of lymph node involvement in a given case.[75] Some may be diffusely affected and others spared entirely. In most instances, silicone lymphadenitis has a patchy distribution in involved lymph nodes. In a study of ALNs from 96 women who had silicone implants, Katzin et al.[75] found histologic evidence of silicone in 86 (90%) of cases and refractile material consistent with polyurethane in 16 (17%). By means of spectroscopy, the presence of silicone was confirmed in 71 (74%) and polyurethane in 2 (2%).

Histologic examination reveals diffuse follicular hyperplasia. Histiocytes with clear, vacuolated cytoplasm are scattered throughout the lymphoid tissue but tend to be concentrated in sinusoidal regions. Coalescent groups of clear cells are associated with the formation of empty vacuoles and the accumulation of foreign body giant cells[68,69] (Fig. 43.15). Refractile and nonbirefringent particles may be present in the giant cells. Silicone lymphadenitis caused by material from orthopedic devices is typically characterized by a prominent granulomatous reaction with clumps of granular yellowish refractile material, whereas silicone gel from mammary prostheses ordinarily produces finer vacuolated deposits that resemble soap suds. Asteroid bodies, star-shaped structures within the cytoplasm of multinucleated histiocytes, have been observed in lymphadenitis associated with silicone-containing mammary implants and orthopedic prostheses implants.[66,76]

The differential diagnosis of silicone lymphadenitis includes various causes of granulomatous lymphadenitis, adenitis associated with lymphangiography, and congenital storage diseases. The presence of silicone compounds in

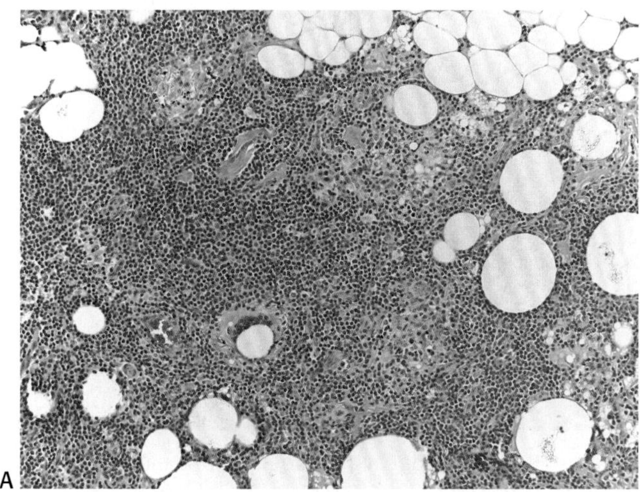
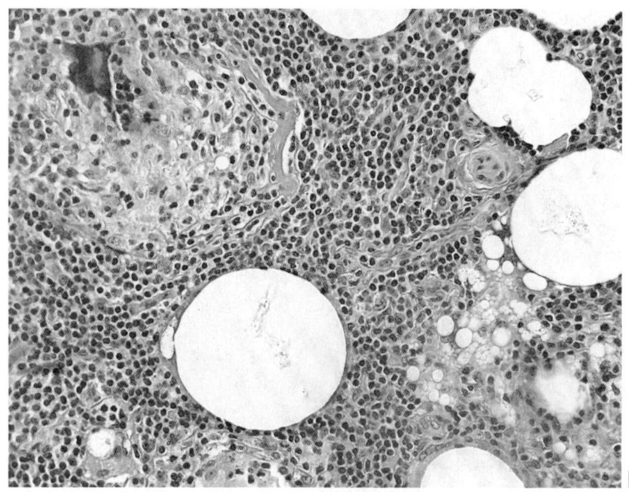

FIG. 43.15. ***Silicone lymphadenitis.*** **A,B:** The lymph node architecture is distorted by material from an implant that has accumulated in histiocytes with vacuolated cytoplasm and large clear spaces. Minute particles of refractile material are evident in some spaces.

lymph nodes and other tissues can be confirmed by electron microprobe analysis using transmission or scanning electron microscopy[66,69,77] and other techniques for microanalysis.[78] A method for detecting silica in lymph nodes and other tissue samples by incineration has been described.[79]

Routine histochemical and immunohistochemical procedures do not stain silicone in tissue sections. Most specific granulomatous reactions and sarcoidosis lack the vacuolated histiocytic reaction seen in silicone lymphadenitis. The distinction from lymphangiogram effect and storage diseases can usually be made on the basis of clinical information. One lymph node from a patient with silicone lymphadenitis reportedly exhibited histologic features of Kikuchi necrotizing lymphadenitis.[80]

PIGMENT DEPOSITS IN ALNS AND THE BREAST

Several types of pigmented material have been detected in ALNs. Histiocytes may contain black anthracotic pigment that apparently accumulates as a result of retrograde flow from thoracic to axillary lymphatics (Fig. 43.16). The pigment is usually not abundant and tends to be more prominent in apical rather than in low ALNs. Cserni[81] described a patient in whom anthracotic pigment in a lymph node was grossly mistaken for staining with dye injected for SLN mapping. Anthracotic and melanin pigment may not be grossly distinguishable in an ALN.

Prior surgical trauma, or an underlying systemic condition such as hemosiderosis, can cause accumulation of brown iron pigment. Dermatopathic lymphadenitis features melanin pigment transported from inflammatory skin lesions. Pigment from cutaneous tattoos can also be transported to ALNs (Fig. 43.17). Tattoo pigment in an ALN may resemble calcification on mammography.[82] Patients who received systemic gold therapy for rheumatoid arthritis have reportedly developed gold deposits in lymph nodes that were visualized by mammography.[83,84] In one case, the particles appeared to be within the breast radiologically and were thought to be microcalcifications that suggested carcinoma.[84] At operation, gold deposits were found within an intraparenchymal lymph node.

Ochronotic pigment is deposited in connective tissues of patients with ochronosis. The condition is caused by an autosomal recessive genetic defect that results in the accumulation of homogentisic acid detectable in the urine as alcaptonuria. Ochronotic pigment in synovium is associated with the development of arthritis. Tumorous lesions resulting from ochronotic pigment deposition in the mammary stroma are brown to black, grossly resembling malignant melanoma.[85] Histologic examination reveals dense fibrous tissue containing yellow-brown pigment that stains black with the Fontana Masson and methenamine silver stains.[85] The lesions are hypocellular and lack the cytologic features of malignant melanoma.

Material derived from cutaneous solar elastosis that can mimic mucin has been described in ALNs.[86]

VASCULAR LESIONS

Hemangiomas

Hemangiomas are the most frequent benign vascular neoplasms encountered in ALNs. Most are found in lymph nodes removed in the course of axillary dissections or SLN biopsy and are chance findings, although they can measure up to 0.5 cm.[87] They may occupy the nodal hilum or parenchyma and sometimes extend to perinodal tissues. Nodal hemangiomas are typically of the capillary variety, but cavernous and cellular or epithelioid features[88] may also be present (Fig. 43.18). Although usually solitary, multiple microscopic nodal hemangiomas are occasionally encountered.

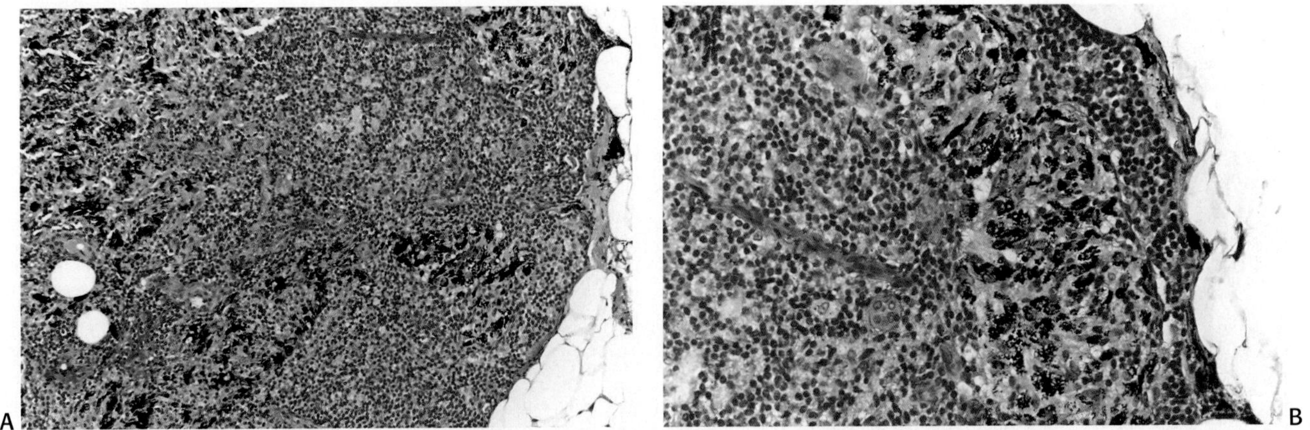

FIG. 43.16. ***Anthracotic pigment.*** **A,B:** Coarse black pigment in sinusoidal histiocytes that has elicited a granulomatous reaction. The histologic appearance of this ALN resembles a typical pulmonary lymph node.

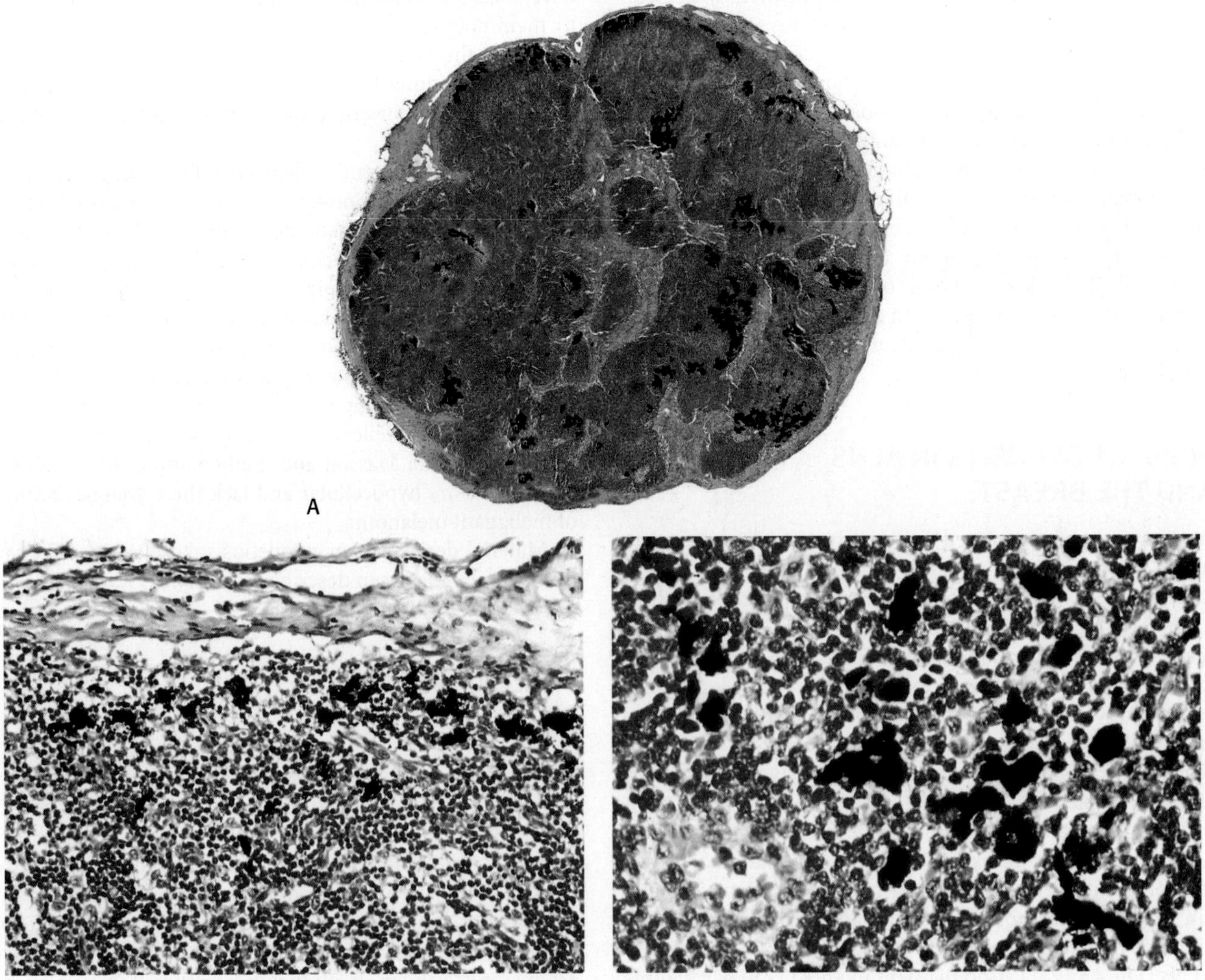

FIG. 43.17. ***Tattoo pigment.*** **A,B:** Pigment-laden histiocytes are evident in widely scattered groups in the parenchyma of lymph nodes. Note the *bright green* pigment particle in **(C)**.

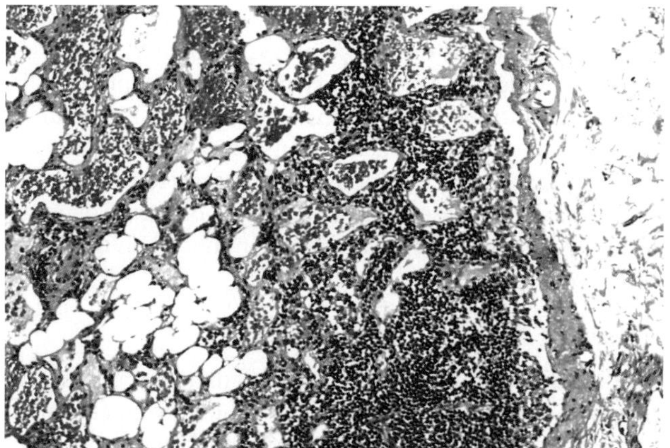

FIG. 43.18. ***Nodal hemangioma.*** A capillary hemangioma fills the center of this lymph node.

Breast tissue removed at the same time or previously may contain one or more perilobular hemangiomas, and in this setting, care should be exercised to avoid misinterpreting the findings as evidence of angiosarcoma. Clinically evident nodal enlargement caused by a hemangioma has been reported.[89] Lymphangiomas of lymph nodes are almost always associated with involvement of other organs.

Kaposi Sarcoma

This vascular neoplasm that involves skin and many parenchymal organs can arise primarily in lymph nodes, including those in the axilla.[90,91] Primary Kaposi sarcoma of lymph nodes was described prior to the recognition of the association between this neoplasm and AIDS. Patients who present with Kaposi sarcoma in lymph nodes usually have involvement of several nodal sites, although rarely the condition is clinically limited to one lymph node.

Vascular Transformation or Nodal Angiomatosis

A Kaposi-like proliferative lesion termed "vascular transformation" or "nodal angiomatosis" is sometimes found incidentally in one or more lymph nodes removed from the axilla and other sites.[92,93] This condition features the formation of complex capillary and cavernous vascular channels in the lymph sinuses. In most instances, vascular transformation is an incidental microscopic finding in lymph nodes removed for another disease. However, the condition can cause nodal enlargement that is clinically apparent.[94] Common sites include the cervical, axillary, and supraclavicular lymph nodes. Involvement of mediastinal, inguinal, and various abdominal lymph node groups has also been reported.[95] Vascular transformation has been found in ALNs from patients with breast carcinoma.[94,96] Rarely, there have been hemangiomas in the skin and other tissues drained by the lymph nodes affected by vascular transformation. An unusual instance has been seen in which there was a vasoproliferative condition in the dermis of the skin overlying an infiltrating breast carcinoma in a patient with vascular transformation of the ipsilateral ALNs. The cutaneous lesion was histologically similar to the nodal vascular abnormality.

The histologic features of nodal vascular transformation are variable. The condition occurs mainly in lymphoid sinuses, largely sparing the lymph node capsule. Blood vessels in perinodal tissues may have a thickened muscular layer. Several vasoformative patterns found in differing proportions in individual cases include the formation of narrow vascular slits, open round spaces, solid foci composed of spindle and polygonal cells, and a plexiform pattern of interconnecting vascular spaces (Fig. 43.19). Red blood cells are found in many but not all vascular channels. Extravasation of red blood cells, fibrin deposits, and thrombosis are variably present. Endothelial cells display little or no cytologic atypia, papillary endothelial hyperplasia is absent, and there is minimal mitotic activity.

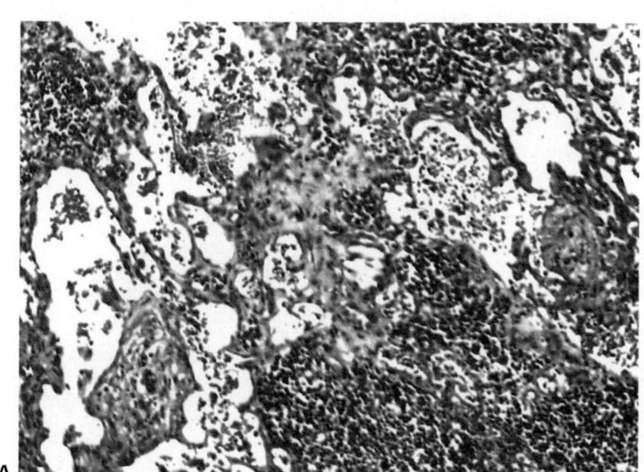

A

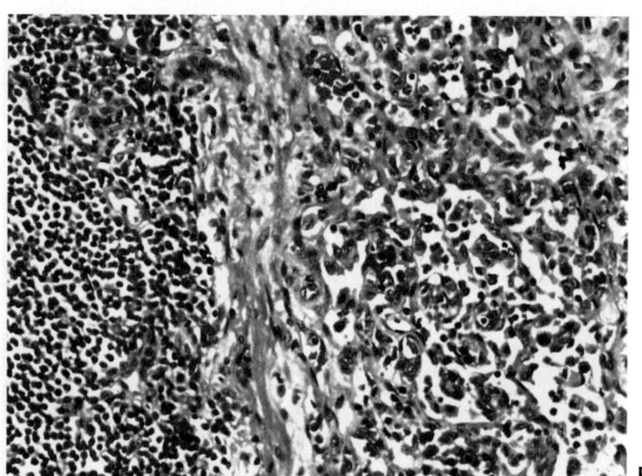

B

FIG. 43.19. ***Vascular transformation of axillary lymph nodes.*** **A:** The lymph sinuses have been transformed into dilated vascular channels separated by fibrous stroma. Red blood cells are present in the vascular spaces. **B:** An area in which angioendothelial proliferation fills a lymph sinus (right).

The etiology of nodal vascular transformation is not known, but the appearance of the lesions suggests a proliferative response to an angiogenic stimulus that may be derived from an associated neoplasm in some cases.

INTRAMAMMARY LYMPH NODES

Intramammary lymph nodes are completely surrounded by breast tissue, and are located outside the axilla. The typical intramammary lymph node is impalpable, and usually comes to clinical attention radiographically. The mammogram shows an ovoid structure with a lucid center and a hilar notch, and sonogram demonstrates an iso- to hypoechoic cortex and an echogenic linear hilum.

Intramammary lymph nodes are most often located deep in the outer quadrants of the breast.[97] They are typically 1 cm or smaller,[98] but have been reported to measure up to 3 cm when involved by metastatic carcinoma. In the latter circumstance, it may become difficult to distinguish between a primary carcinoma with lymphocytic reaction and a lymph node enlarged by metastatic carcinoma. Jadusingh[98] reported finding intramammary lymph nodes in 5 (0.7%) of 681 breast specimens personally examined grossly.

Imaging Studies

Mammographic examination usually reveals a well-circumscribed mass that may have a lucent center and a peripheral "hilar" notch[99] (Figs. 43.20 and 43.21). Lymphoid hyperplasia in intramammary lymph nodes has been associated with rapid contrast uptake in contrast-enhanced magnetic resonance imaging (MRI) studies, a result that may suggest carcinoma.[100,101] Intramammary lymph nodes are sometimes identified in the course of SLN biopsy of the axilla.[102–104] Jansen et al.[103] reported finding intramammary SLNs in 3 of 113 patients. Metastatic carcinoma has been found in intramammary SLNs.[102,104] Metastases in an intramammary lymph node can distort its radiologic characteristics so that it may masquerade as a primary mammary neoplasm.[105,106] Changes in intramammary lymph nodes documented in serial mammograms may also be an indication of otherwise clinically inapparent carcinoma.[107] These alterations include enlargement, increased density, and loss of the hilar notch, resulting from metastatic carcinoma in the lymph node.

Cytology and Needle Core Biopsy

Fine-needle aspiration (FNA) of a benign intramammary lymph node yields a heterogeneous cellular specimen similar to material from a lymph node at any other site.[108] Lymphocytes are the dominant cellular elements. The diagnosis of an intramammary lymph node in a needle core biopsy sample is facilitated by finding portions of the lymph node capsule, subcapsular sinusoids, and germinal centers.

Clinical Studies and Pathology

Enlargement of intramammary lymph nodes may be caused by inflammatory conditions such as sinus histiocytosis,[109] reaction to dermatitis,[110] tuberculosis,[111] foreign material such as gold,[112] or by neoplasms, including lymphoma[113,114] (Fig. 43.22), metastatic melanoma,[109] and metastatic carcinoma.[109,115,116] The distinction between medullary carcinoma and metastatic carcinoma in an intramammary lymph node is sometimes difficult. This issue can arise in the breast proper and in the axillary region. The presence of a capsule, subcapsular sinus, and sinusoidal structure is the best indication of a lymph node involved by carcinoma. Germinal centers suggest a lymph node, but are rarely present at sites of primary carcinoma. The underlying architecture of a lymph node is usually revealed by a reticulin stain, whereas the presence of intraductal carcinoma, a prominent plasmacytic reaction, syncytial growth, and necrosis characterizes

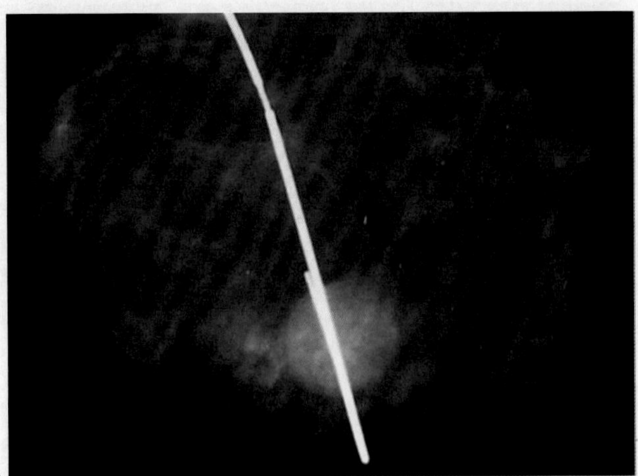

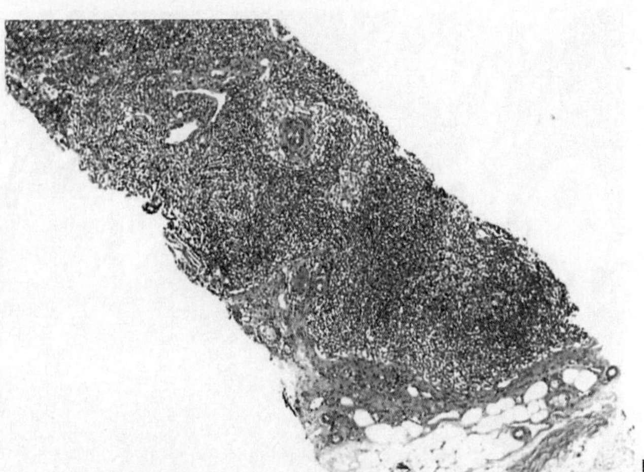

FIG. 43.20. ***Intramammary lymph node detected by mammography.*** **A:** A radiograph of a breast biopsy specimen that contains a lymph node with a localization wire in place. **B:** The tissue sample obtained by needle core biopsy of a radiologically detected intramammary lymph node.

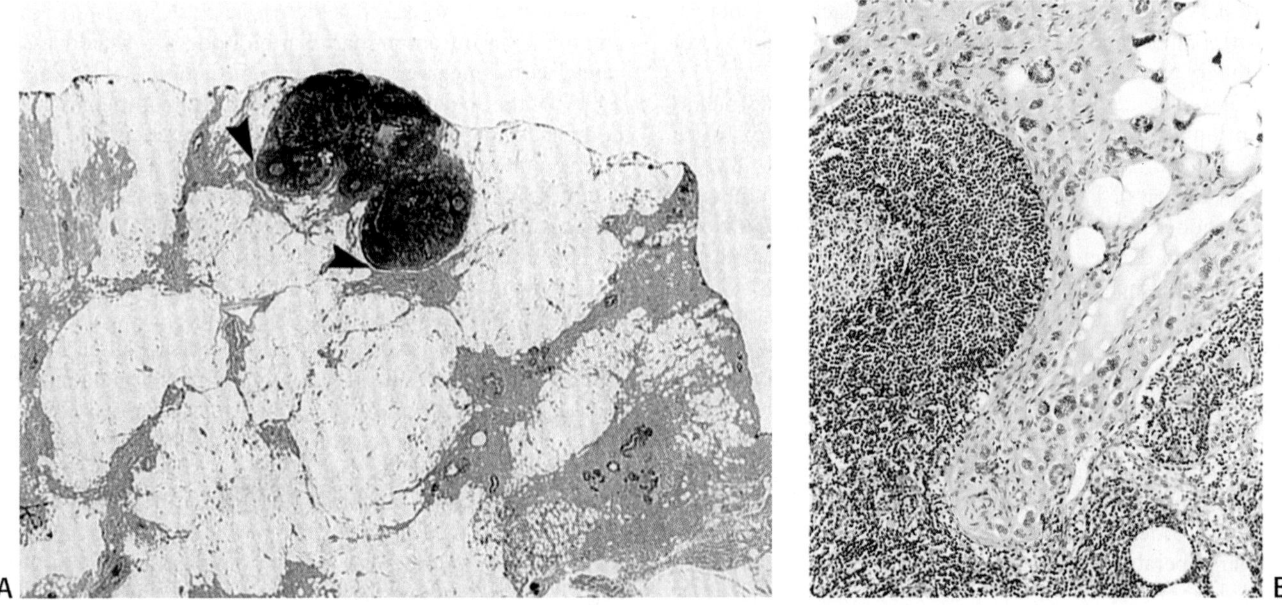

FIG. 43.21. ***Intramammary lymph node.*** **A:** Whole-mount histologic section of breast tissue from a mastectomy specimen. A bean-shaped lymph node with a hilar "notch" is located next to invasive carcinoma [*arrows*]. **B:** Carcinoma invading the lymph node capsule. [**A:** Reproduced from Rosen PP, Oberman HA. Tumors of the mammary gland. [*AFIP Atlas of Tumor Pathology*, 3rd series, vol. 7.] Baltimore: American Registry of Pathology, 1993.]

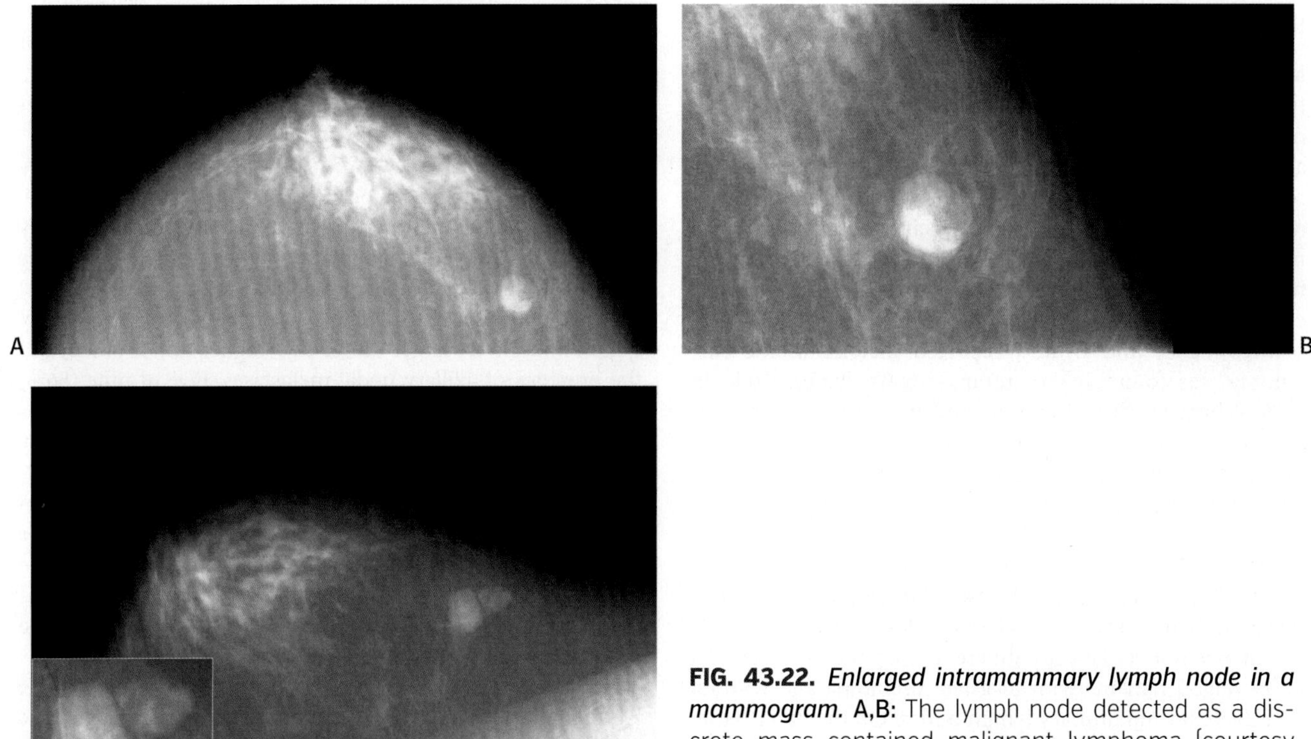

FIG. 43.22. ***Enlarged intramammary lymph node in a mammogram.*** **A,B:** The lymph node detected as a discrete mass contained malignant lymphoma [courtesy of Bela Ben-Dor, MD]. **C:** Two lymph nodes involved by chronic lymphocytic leukemia [*inset* shows detail].

medullary carcinoma. If the carcinoma lacks a syncytial growth pattern and is not cytologically high grade, it is not medullary carcinoma.

Dawson et al.[117] reviewed 18 patients with clinically palpable intramammary lymph nodes seen at one institution over a 6-year period. The patients ranged in age from 22 to 58 years (mean, 32 years). Three lumps were painful. The number of lymph nodes in the palpable lesions varied from one to six, with a mean diameter of 0.8 cm. Pathologic findings in the lymph nodes included fibrosis, lymphoid hyperplasia, sinus histiocytosis, melanin pigmentation (seven cases), fatty infiltration, and a capsular NCA (one case).

McSweeney and Egan[116] found intramammary lymph nodes in 52 (30%) of 173 breasts evaluated by whole-organ serial sectioning, specimen radiography, and pathologic examination. A lymph node was classified as intramammary only if "completely surrounded by breast tissue." Lymph nodes were identified in 45 (29%) of 158 breasts removed for primary operable breast carcinoma. The size of lymph nodes ranged from 3 to 15 mm. A total of 72 lymph nodes were found, with nine being the largest number in a single case. This patient had at least one lymph node in each of three quadrants. The distribution of lymph nodes in the breast quadrants was as follows: upper outer, 26 (36%); lower outer, 21 (29%); upper inner, 11 (15%); central, 8 (11%); and lower inner, 6 (8%). Seven breasts with carcinoma had one or more intramammary lymph nodes in the same quadrant as the primary tumor, and eight had lymph nodes in other quadrants.

METASTATIC CARCINOMA IN INTRAMAMMARY LYMPH NODES

Metastatic carcinoma in intramammary lymph node typically originates in the ipsilateral breast, but extramammary origin, from an abdominal eccrine spiradenoma, has also been reported.[118] In a study of 1,655 retrospectively reviewed mammograms from patients with breast carcinoma, 16 (0.9%) had metastatic carcinoma in an intramammary lymph node detected radiologically.[119] All lymph nodes with carcinoma were larger than 1.0 cm, and one had calcifications.

McSweeney and Egan[116] reported that metastatic carcinoma was found in an intramammary lymph node in 10% of breasts with carcinoma and in 33% of breasts that had an intramammary lymph node and carcinoma. Lymph nodes that contained metastatic carcinoma were not especially enlarged, measuring 3 to 10 mm. Positive intramammary lymph nodes occurred in six patients who were otherwise clinically stage I, and in nine who were stage II. Twelve stage I patients with invasive carcinoma and negative intramammary lymph nodes had a 66% survival at 10 years, which was not statistically different from the 74% survival of 49 stage I patients with invasive carcinoma and without detectable intramammary lymph nodes. On the other hand, only 33% of six stage I patients with a positive intramammary lymph node survived 10 years.

Shen et al.[120] found that the presence of metastatic carcinoma in an intramammary lymph node was usually associated with concurrent axillary nodal metastases. However, 2 (5%) of the 36 patients with positive intramammary lymph nodes had negative ALNs. In this study, metastatic carcinoma in an intramammary lymph node was associated with a significantly less-favorable prognosis when compared to patients with a negative intramammary lymph node.

The unfavorable prognostic significance of metastatic carcinoma in an intramammary lymph node was confirmed in a study of 57 patients by Nassar et al.,[121] who attributed the less favorable prognosis to the fact that patients with metastatic carcinoma in an intramammary lymph node were more likely than those with a negative intramammary lymph node to have metastatic carcinoma in ALNs. These observations indicate that the finding of metastatic carcinoma in an intramammary lymph node is a strong predictor of the presence of ALN metastases. The prognostic significance of metastases in an intramammary lymph node in patients with negative ALNs is uncertain.

Metastases in intramammary lymph nodes are regarded as equivalent to axillary nodal involvement representing stage II disease in the seventh edition of the AJCC-UICC *TNM Staging System*. The issue of clinical management when SLN mapping localizes a lymph node to an intramammary location has been addressed in multiple publications.[122–127]

Cox et al.[122] reported an analysis of 91 patients who had intramammary SLN. Eight (9%) of these patients who had isolated foci of metastatic carcinoma in the intramammary lymph node had negative ALNs. These results led the authors to conclude that complete axillary dissection was not necessary in patients with a positive intramammary SLN and a negative axillary SLN. Pugliese et al.[125] also reported that patients with a positive intramammary lymph node and a negative axillary SLN had no additional axillary nodal metastases when an axillary dissection was performed.

Nassar et al.[123] reviewed 57 examples of intramammary lymph nodes that were associated with mammary carcinoma. Metastatic carcinoma was found in 32% of the intramammary lymph nodes from patients with invasive carcinoma. A positive intramammary lymph node was found in one of eight (13%) patients with DCIS. Predictors of positive intramammary lymph nodes were larger tumor size, higher tumor grade, and the presence of axillary nodal metastases. Five of nine (56%) patients with a positive axillary SLN had a positive intramammary lymph node. Among 21 patients with a negative axillary SLN, 3 (14%) had a positive intramammary lymph node. Analysis of follow-up revealed that patients with a positive intramammary lymph node had a significantly poorer disease-free and overall survival, regardless of axillary nodal status. On the other hand, the presence of metastatic carcinoma in an intramammary lymph node did not have a significant effect on the outcome of women with a positive axillary SLN.

In a meta-analysis of reports published prior to 2012, Abdullgaffar et al.[128] concluded that patients with metastatic carcinoma in intramammary lymph nodes had a significantly less favorable prognosis regardless of the status of their

ALNs. However, the authors cautioned that this conclusion was based on relatively few reports consisting of heterogeneous patient groups subject to various treatment programs.

Subject to revision resulting from additional data, some tentative conclusions can be drawn about the management of patients with a positive intramammary lymph node:

1. Patients with a positive intramammary lymph node have a nearly 65% chance of having one or more positive ALNs.
2. When carcinoma is found in an intramammary lymph node, a full axillary dissection is not necessary if no metastatic carcinoma is found in the concurrent axillary SLN.
3. Although the data are not conclusive, evidence has been presented to indicate that the presence of a positive intramammary lymph node has an unfavorable influence on prognosis in patients with negative ALNs. This is consistent with the current classification of such patients as having stage II disease.
4. The impact of a positive intramammary lymph node on the prognosis of a patient with one or more positive ALNs has not been determined.

Additional information about intramammary SLN can be found in Chapter 44.

EXTRAMEDULLARY HEMATOPOIESIS

Extramedullary hematopoiesis (EMH) is the occurrence of one or more of the trilineage of precursor cells outside the bone marrow. When present in a lymph node, erythroid and myeloid precursors singly or in small groups can blend inconspicuously with the lymphocytic and histiocytic cells in lymph node. Scattered, isolated megakaryocytes are more easily detected because of their large, typically multilobulated hyperchromatic nuclei, with inconspicuous nucleoli and abundant eosinophilic cytoplasm. In this setting, megakaryocytes can be mistaken for metastatic carcinoma cells in an excisional or needle core biopsy specimen, or in FNA cytology material, especially after neoadjuvant chemotherapy.[129–132] Additional information about EMH in axillary lymph nodes can be found in Chapter 40.

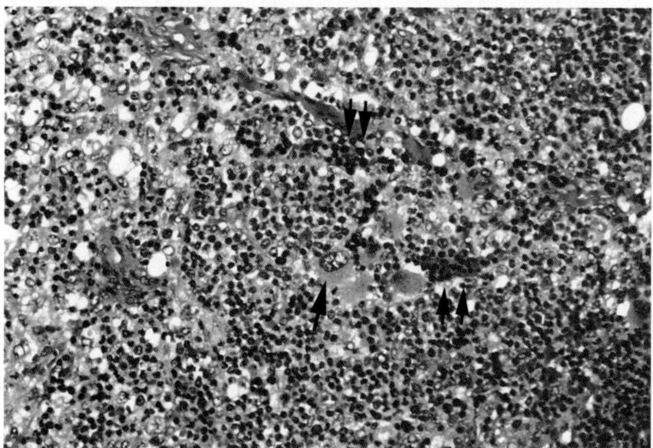

FIG. 43.23. ***Extramedullary hematopoiesis.*** A megakaryocyte (*arrow*) surrounded by erythrocyte precursors with small dark nuclei (*double arrows*) in an ALN.

The ALNs can be the site of EMH in a patient with myelofibrosis or other hematopoietic disorder (Fig. 43.23). Rarely, EMH is found in the ALNs of a patient with no known cause. Bhusnurmath et al.[133] described three patients who had megakaryocytes in sentinel ALNs that were obtained from patients after neoadjuvant chemotherapy. Each of the patients also had metastatic carcinoma in the SLN. Megakaryocytes are immunoreactive for CD31, CD41, CD42b, CD51, and CD61 and negative for CK.

REFERENCES

Heterotopic Glands

1. Brown RB, Gaillard RA, Turner JA. The significance of aberrant or heterotopic parotid gland tissue in lymph nodes. *Ann Surg* 1953;138:850–856.
2. Karp LA, Czernobilsky B. Glandular inclusions in pelvic and abdominal para-aortic lymph nodes. *Am J Clin Pathol* 1969;52:212–218.
3. Kempson RL. Consultant case: benign glandular inclusions in iliac lymph nodes. *Am J Surg Pathol* 1978;2:321–325.
4. Schnurr RC, Delgado G, Chun B. Benign glandular inclusions in para-aortic lymph nodes in women undergoing lymphadenectomies. *Am J Obstet Gynecol* 1978;130:813–816.
5. Corben AD, Nehhozina T, Garg K, et al. Endosalpingiosis in axillary lymph nodes: a possible pitfall in the staging of patients with breast carcinoma. *Am J Surg Pathol* 2010;34:1211–1216.
6. Edlow DW, Carter D. Heterotopic epithelium in axillary lymph nodes: report of a case and review of the literature. *Am J Clin Pathol* 1973;59:666–673.
7. Garret R, Ada AEW. Epithelial inclusion cysts in an axillary lymph node. Report of case simulating metastatic adenocarcinoma. *Cancer* 1957;10:173–178.
8. Holdsworth PJ, Hopkinson JM, Leveson SH. Benign axillary epithelial lymph node inclusions—a histological pitfall. *Histopathology* 1988;13:226–228.
9. Zhang C, Xiong J, Quddus MR, et al. A rapidly enlarging squamous inclusion cyst in an axillary lymph node following core needle biopsy. *Case Rep Pathol* 2012;2012:418070.
10. Walker AN, Fechner RE. Papillary carcinoma arising from ectopic breast tissue in an axillary lymph node. *Diagn Gynecol Obstet* 1982;4:141–145.
11. Layfield LJ, Mooney E. Heterotopic epithelium in an intramammary lymph node. *Breast J* 2000;6:63–67.
12. Resetkova E, Hoda SA, Clarke JL, et al. Benign heterotopic epithelial inclusions in axillary lymph nodes: histological and immunohistochemical patterns. *Arch Pathol Lab Med* 2003;127:e25–e27.
13. Silton RM. More glandular inclusions. *Am J Surg Pathol* 1979;3:285–286.
14. Fellegara G, Carcangiu ML, Rosai J. Benign epithelial inclusions in axillary lymph nodes: report of 18 cases and review of the literature. *Am J Surg Pathol* 2011;35:1123–1133.
15. Zynger DL, McCallum JC, Everton MJ, et al. Paracortical axillary sentinel lymph node ectopic breast tissue. *Pathol Res Pract* 2009;205:427–432.
16. Kadowaki M, Nagashima T, Sakata H, et al. Ectopic breast tissue in axillary lymph node. *Breast Cancer* 2007;14:425–428.
17. Nakaguro M, Suzuki Y, Ichihara S, et al. Epithelial inclusion cyst arising in an intramammary lymph node: case report with cytologic findings. *Diagn Cytopathol* 2009;37:199–202.

18. Rousselot C, Chapiron C, Blechet C, et al. Mullerian "inclusions" within an intramammary lymph node. *Ann Pathol* 2006;26: 204–206.
19. Ohsie SJ, Moatamed NA, Chang HR, et al. Heterotopic breast tissue versus occult metastatic carcinoma in lymph node, a diagnostic dilemma. *Ann Diagn Pathol* 2010;14:260–263.
20. Maiorano E, Mazzarol GM, Pruneri G, et al. Ectopic breast tissue as a possible cause of false-positive axillary sentinel lymph node biopsies. *Am J Surg Pathol* 2003;27:513–518.
21. Iken S, Schmidt M, Braun C, et al. Absence of ectopic epithelial inclusions in 3,904 axillary lymph nodes examined in sentinel technique. *Breast Cancer Res Treat* 2012;132:621–624.
22. Fisher CJ, Hill S, Millis RR. Benign lymph node inclusions mimicking metastatic carcinoma. *J Clin Pathol* 1994;47:245–247.

Nevus Cell Aggregates

23. Ridolfi RL, Rosen PP, Thaler H. Nevus cell aggregates associated with lymph nodes: estimated frequency and clinical significance. *Cancer* 1977;39:164–171.
24. Nodl F. Uber anastomosen und epitheloide Gefaswandzellen hautnaher Lymphknoten. *Arch Derm Res* 1977;257:319–326.
25. Micheau C, Contesso G. Formations d'aspect angioglomique dans les ganglions lymphatiques axillaires. *Arch Anat Pathol* 1971;19: 167–175.
26. Lambert WC, Brodkin RH. Nodal and subcutaneous cellular blue nevi. *Arch Dermatol* 1984;120:367–370.
27. Erlandson RA, Rosen PP. Electron microscopy of a nevus cell aggregate associated with an axillary lymph node. *Cancer* 1982;49: 269–272.
28. Epstein JI, Erlandson RA, Rosen PP. Nodal blue nevi. A study of three cases. *Am J Surg Pathol* 1984;8:907–915.
29. Stewart FW, Copeland MM. Neurogenic sarcoma. *Am J Cancer* 1931; 15:1235–1320.
30. Stewart FW. Early cancer (Thayer lecture, The Johns Hopkins University, 1960) as cited by Wood S Jr, Holyoke ED, Yardley JH, *Can Cancer Conf* 1960;4:167–223, New York, Academic Press.
31. Johnson WT, Helwig EB. Benign nevus cells in the capsule of lymph nodes. *Cancer* 1969;23:747–753.
32. Lerman RI, Murray D, O'Hara JM, et al. Malignant melanoma of childhood. *Cancer* 1970;25:436–449.
33. Hart WR. Primary nevus of a lymph node. *Am J Clin Pathol* 1971; 55:88-92.
34. McCarthy SW, Palmer AA, Bale PM, et al. Nevus cells in lymph nodes. *Pathology* 1974;6:351–358.
35. Carson K, Wen DR, Cochran AJ. Nodal nevi are frequent and selectively located in melanoma-draining nodes: implications for their etiology. *Lab Invest* 1994;70:44A.
36. Bautista NC, Cohen S, Anders KH. Benign melanocytic nevus cells in axillary lymph nodes. A prospective incidence and immunohistochemical study with literature review. *An J Clin Pathol* 1994;102:102–108.
37. Azzopardi JG, Ross CM, Frizzera G. Blue nevi of lymph node capsule. *Histopathology* 1977;1:451–461.
38. Gray GF Jr, Dineen P. Benign nevus in lymph node. *NY State J Med* 1976;76:754–755.
39. Bertrand G, Rabreau M, George P. Presence de cellules naeviques dans les ganglions lymphatiques. *Arch Anat Cytol Pathol* 1980;28:58–62.
40. Goldman RL. Blue nevus of lymph node capsule. Report of a unique case. *Histopathology* 1981;5:445–450.
41. Nodl F. Spindelzelliger blauer Naevus mit Lymphknoten-"Metastasen." *Arch Dermatol* 1979;264:179–184.
42. Biddle DA, Evans HL, Kemp BL, et al. Intraparenchymal nevus cell aggregates in lymph nodes. A possible diagnostic pitfall with malignant melanoma and carcinoma. *Am J Surg Pathol* 2003;27:673–681.
43. Lamovec J. Blue nevus of the lymph node capsule. Report of a new case with review of the literature. *Am J Clin Pathol* 1984;81:367–372.
44. Dohse L, Ferringer T. Nodal blue nevus: a pitfall in lymph node biopsies. *J Cutan Pathol* 2010;37:102–104.
45. Douglas-Jones AG. Benign lymph node inclusions mimicking metastatic carcinoma. *J Clin Pathol* 1994;47:868–869.
46. Dalton SR, Gerami P, Kolaitis NA, et al. Use of fluorescence *in situ* hybridization (FISH) to distinguish intranodal nevus from metastatic melanoma. *Am J Surg Pathol* 2010;34:231–237.

Sinus Histiocytosis

47. Cutler SJ, Black MM, Friedell GH, et al. Prognostic factors in cancer of the female breast. II. Reproducibility of histopathologic classification. *Cancer* 1966;19:75–82.
48. Black MM, Asire AJ. Palpable axillary lymph nodes in cancer of the breast. Structural and biologic considerations. *Cancer* 1969;23:251–259.
49. Silverberg SG, Chitale AR, Hind AD, et al. Sinus histiocytosis and mammary carcinoma. Study of 366 radical mastectomies and an historical review. *Cancer* 1970;26:1177–1185.
50. Pathi R, Lawrence WD, Barroeta JE. Signet ring cell histiocytosis in axillary lymph nodes: a sheep in wolves' clothing? A potentially underrecognized pitfall in the diagnosis of metastatic breast cancer. *Breast J* 2009;15:302–303.
51. Black MM, Leis HP Jr. Cellular responses to autologous breast cancer tissue. Correlation with stage and lymphoreticular reaction. *Cancer* 1971;28:263–273.
52. Black MM, Opler SR, Speer FD. Survival in breast cancer cases in relation to structure of primary tumor and regional lymph nodes. *Surg Gynecol Obstet* 1955;100:543–551.
53. Black MM, Speer FD. Sinus histiocytosis of lymph nodes in cancer. *Surg Gynecol Obstet* 1958;106:163–175.
54. Cutler SJ, Black MM, Goldenberg IS. Prognostic factors in cancer of the female breast. I. An investigation of some interrelations. *Cancer* 1963;16:1589–1597.
55. Cutler SJ, Black MM, Mork T, et al. Further observations on prognostic factors in cancer of the female breast. *Cancer* 1969;24:653–667.
56. Friedell GH, Soto EA, Kumaoka S, et al. Sinus histiocytosis in British and Japanese patients with breast cancer. *Lancet* 1974;304:1228–1229.
57. Berg JW. Sinus histiocytosis: a fallacious measure of host resistance to cancer. *Cancer* 1956;9:935–939.
58. Moore RD, Chapnick R, Schoenberg MD. Lymph nodes associated with carcinoma of the breast. *Cancer* 1960;13:545–549.
59. DiRe JJ, Lane M. The relation of sinus histiocytosis in axillary lymph nodes to surgical curability of carcinoma of the breast. *Am J Clin Pathol* 1963;40:508–515.
60. Schiodt T. *Breast carcinoma. A histologic and prognostic study of 650 followed-up cases.* Copenhagen: Munksgaard, 1966.
61. Kister SJ, Sommers SC, Haagensen CD, et al. Nuclear grade and sinus histiocytosis in cancer of the breast. *Cancer* 1969;23:570–575.

Rosai-Dorfman Disease

62. Morkowski JJ, Nguyen CV, Lin P, et al. Rosai-Dorfman disease confined to the breast. *Ann Diagn Pathol* 2010;14:81–87.
63. Gwin K, Cipriani N, Zhang X, et al. Bilateral breast involvement by disseminated extranodal Rosai-Dorfman disease. *Breast J* 2011;17: 309–311.
64. da Silva BB, Lopes-Costa PV, Pires CG, et al. Rosai-Dorfman disease of the breast mimicking cancer. *Pathol Res Pract* 2007;203:741–744.
65. Tenny SO, McGinness M, Zhang D, et al. Rosai-Dorfman disease presenting as a breast mass and enlarged axillary lymph node mimicking malignancy: a case report and review of the literature. *Breast J* 2011;17: 516–520.

Silicone Lymphadenitis

66. Benjamin E, Ahmed A, Rashid ATMF, et al. Silicone lymphadenopathy: a report of two cases one with concomitant malignant lymphoma. *Diagn Histopathol* 1982;5:133–141.
67. Harvey T, Leahy M. Silicone lymphadenopathy: a complication of silicone elastomer finger joint prostheses. *J Rheumatol* 1984;11:104–105.
68. Hausner RJ, Schoen FJ, Mendez-Fernandez MA, et al. Migration of silicone gel to axillary lymph nodes after prosthetic mammoplasty. *Arch Pathol Lab Med* 1981;105:371–372.
69. Wintsch W, Smahel J, Clodius L. Local and regional lymph node responses to ruptured gel-filled mammary prostheses. *Br J Plastic Surg* 1978;31:349–352.
70. Rivero MA, Schwartz DS, Mies C. Silicon lymphadenopathy involving intramammary lymph nodes: a new complication of silicone mammaplasty. *AJR Am J Roentgenol* 1994;162:1089–1090.
71. Gil T, Mettanes I, Aman B, et al. Contralateral internal mammary silicone lymphadenopathy imitates breast cancer metastasis. *Ann Plast Surg* 2009;63:39–41.

72. Kao CC, Rand RP, Holt CA, et al. Internal mammary silicone lymphadenopathy mimicking recurrent breast cancer. *Plast Reconstr Surg* 1997;99:225–229.
73. Maricevich M, Grams J, Aleff PA, et al. Mediastinal silicone lymphadenopathy secondary to a ruptured breast implant. *Breast J* 2011;17:674–675.
74. Patel CN, Macpherson RE, Bradley KM. False-positive axillary lymphadenopathy due to silicone granuloma on FDG PET/CT. *Eur J Nucl Med Mol Imaging* 2010;37:2405.
75. Katzin WE, Centeno JA, Feng LJ, et al. Pathology of lymph nodes from patients with breast implants. A histologic and spectroscopic evaluation. *Am J Surg Pathol* 2005;29:506–511.
76. Balco MT, Ali SZ. Asteroid bodies in silicone lymphadenitis on fine-needle aspiration. *Diagn Cytopathol.* 2007;35:715–716.
77. Truong LD, Cartwright J Jr, Goodman MD, et al. Silicone lymphadenopathy associated with augmentation mammaplasty. Morphologic features in nine cases. *Am J Surg Pathol* 1988;12:484–491.
78. Greene WB, Raso DS, Walsh LG, et al. Electron probe microanalysis of silicon and the role of the macrophage in proximal (capsule) and distant sites in augmentation mammaplasty patients. *Plast Reconstr Surg* 1995;95:513–519.
79. Vaamonde R, Cabrera JM, Vaamonde-Martin RJ, et al. Silicone granulomatous lymphadenopathy and siliconomas of the breast. *Histol Histopathol* 1997;12:1003–1011.
80. Sever CE, Leith CP, Appenzeller J, et al. Kikuchi's histiocytic necrotizing lymphadenitis associated with ruptured silicone breast implant. *Arch Pathol Lab Med* 1996;120:380–385.

Pigment Deposits in Axillary Lymph Nodes and the Breast

81. Cserni G. Misidentification of an axillary sentinel lymph node due to anthracosis. *Eur J Surg Oncol* 1998;24:168.
82. Honegger MM, Hesseltine SM, Gross JD, et al. Tattoo pigment mimicking axillary lymph node calcifications on mammography. *AJR Am J Roentgenol* 2004;183:831–832.
83. Bruwer A, Nelson GW, Spark RP. Punctate intranodal gold deposits simulating microcalcifications on mammograms. *Radiology* 1987;163:87–88.
84. Carter TR. Intramammary lymph node gold deposits simulating microcalcifications on mammogram. *Hum Pathol* 1988;19:992–994.
85. Lefer LG, Rosier PP. Ochronosis in the breast. *Am J Clin Pathol* 1979;71:349–352.
86. Pulitzer MP, Gerami P, Busam K. Solar elastotic material in dermal lymphatics and lymph nodes. *Am J Surg Pathol* 2010;34:1492–1497.

Benign Vascular Lesions

87. Chan JKC, Frizzera G, Fletcher CD, et al. Primary vascular tumors of lymph nodes other than Kaposi's sarcoma. Analysis of 39 cases and delineation of two new entities. *Am J Surg Pathol* 1992;16:335–350.
88. Elgoweini M, Chetty R. Primary nodal hemangioma. *Arch Pathol Lab Med* 2012;136:110–112.
89. Kasznica J, Sideli RV, Collins MH. Lymph node hemangioma. *Arch Pathol Lab Med* 1989;113:804–807.

Kaposi Sarcoma

90. Lubin J, Rywlin AM. Lymphoma-like lymph node changes in Kaposi's sarcoma. *Arch Pathol* 1971;92:338–341.
91. Ramos CV, Taylor HB, Hernandez BA, et al. Primary Kaposi's sarcoma of lymph nodes. *Am J Clin Pathol* 1976;66:998–1003.

Vascular Transformation or Nodal Angiomatosis

92. Haferkamp O, Rosenau W, Lennert K. Vascular transformation of lymph node sinuses due to venous obstruction. *Arch Pathol* 1971;92:81–83.
93. Ostrowski ML, Siddiqui T, Barners RE, et al. Vascular transformation of lymph node sinuses, a process displaying a spectrum of histological features. *Arch Pathol Lab Med* 1990;114:656–660.
94. Chan JKC, Warnke RA, Dorfman R. Vascular transformation of sinuses in lymph nodes. A study of its morphological spectrum and distinction for Kaposi's sarcoma. *Am J Surg Pathol* 1991;15:732–743.
95. Pirola S, Shenjere P, Nonaka D, et al. Combined usual and nodular types of vascular transformation of sinuses in the same lymph node. *Int J Surg Pathol* 2012;20:175–177.
96. Fayemi AO. Nodal angiomatosis. *Arch Pathol* 1975;99:170–172.

Intramammary Lymph Nodes

97. Kalisher L. Xeroradiography of axillary lymph node disease. *Radiology* 1975;114:67–71.
98. Jadusingh IH. Intramammary lymph nodes. *J Clin Pathol* 1992;45:1023–1026.
99. Meyer JE, Kopans DB, Lawrence WD. Normal intramammary lymph nodes presenting as occult breast masses. *Breast* 1982;40:30–32.
100. Gallardo X, Sentis M, Castaner E, et al. Enhancement of intramammary lymph nodes with lymphoid hyperplasia: a potential pitfall in breast MRI. *Eur Radiol* 1998;8:1662–1665.
101. Kinoshita T, Yashiro N, Yoshigi J, et al. Inflammatory intramammary lymph node mimicking the malignant lesion in dynamic MRI. A case report. *J Clin Imaging* 2002;26:258–262.
102. Upponi S, Kalra S, Poultsidis A, et al. The significance of intramammary nodes in primary breast cancer. *Eur J Surg Oncol* 2001;27:707–708.
103. Jansen L, Doting MHE, Rutgers EJ, et al. Clinical relevance of sentinel lymph nodes outside the axilla in patients with breast cancer. *Br J Surg* 2000;87:920–925.
104. Tytler I, Hayes A, Kissin M. Intramammary sentinel nodes in early breast cancer: can we find them and do they matter? *Eur J Surg Oncol* 2003;29:6–8.
105. Solorzano S, Seidler M, Mesurolle B. Metastatic intramammary lymph node as a synchronous benign-appearing breast nodule detected in a patient with breast cancer. *AJR Am J Roentgenol* 2009;192:W349.
106. Hale MP, Peponis NT, Anker RL, et al. AIRP best cases in radiologic–pathologic correlation: primary invasive lobular carcinoma of the breast manifesting with an associated intramammary lymph node metastasis. *Radiographics* 2011;31:1101–1106.
107. Cawson J, Rose AK. Intramammary lymph node metastases—a rare presenting sign of breast cancer. *Breast* 1995;4:122–126.
108. Layfield LJ, Glasgow BJ, Hirschcowitz S, et al. Intramammary lymph nodes: cytologic findings and implications for fine-needle aspiration cytology diagnosis of breast nodules. *Diagn Cytopathol* 1997;17:223–229.
109. Hyman LJ, Abellera M. Carcinomatous lymph nodes within breast parenchyma. *Arch Surg* 1974;109:759–761.
110. Kopans DB, Meyer JE, Murphy GF. Benign lymph nodes associated with dermatitis presenting as breast masses. *Radiology* 1980;137:15–19.
111. Arnaout AH, Shousha S, Metaxas N, et al. Intramammary tuberculous lymphadenitis. *Histopathology* 1990;17:91–93.
112. Carter JR. Intramammary lymph node gold deposits simulating microcalcifications on mammogram. *Hum Pathol* 1988;19:992–994.
113. Meyer JE, Kopans DB, Long JC. Mammographic appearance of malignant lymphoma of the breast. *Radiology* 1980;135:623–626.
114. Laforga JB, Chorda D, Sevilla F. Intramammary lymph node involvement by mycosis fungoides diagnosed by fine-needle aspiration biopsy. *Diagn Cytopathol* 1998;19:124–126.
115. Lindfors KK, Kopans DB, McCarthy KA, et al. Breast cancer metastasis to intramammary lymph nodes. *AJR Am J Roentgenol* 1986;146:133–136.
116. McSweeney MB, Egan RL. Prognosis of breast cancer related to intramammary lymph nodes. *Recent Results Cancer Res* 1984;90:166–172.
117. Dawson PM, Shousha S, Burn JI. Lymph nodes presenting as breast lumps. *Br J Surg* 1987;74:1167–1168.
118. Tanaka Y, Bhunchet E, Shibata T. A case of malignant eccrine spiradenoma metastatic to intramammary lymph node. *Breast Cancer* 2008;15:175–180.
119. Gunhan-Bilgen I, Memis A, Ustun EE. Metastatic intramammary lymph nodes: mammographic and ultrasonographic features. *Eur J Radiol* 2001;40:24–29.
120. Shen J, Hunt KK, Mirza NQ, et al. Intramammary lymph node metastases are an independent predictor of poor outcome in patients with breast carcinoma. *Cancer* 2004;101:1330–1337.
121. Nassar A, Cohen C, Cotsonis G, et al. Significance of intramammary lymph nodes in staging of breast cancer; correlation with tumor characteristics and outcome. *Mod Pathol* 2006;19(Suppl. 1):36A.

122. Cox CE, Cox JM, Ramos D, et al. Intramammary sentinel lymph nodes: what is the clinical significance? *Ann Surg Oncol* 2008;15:1273–1274.
123. Nassar A, Cohen C, Cotsonis G, et al. Significance of intramammary lymph nodes in the staging of breast cancer: correlation with tumor characteristics and outcome. *Breast J* 2008;14:147–152.
124. Fujii T, Yajima R, Matsumoto A, et al. Implication of an intramammary sentinel lymph node in breast cancer: Is this a true sentinel node? A case report. *Breast Care (Basel)* 2010;5:102–104.
125. Pugliese MS, Stempel MM, Cody HS III, et al. Surgical management of the axilla: do intramammary nodes matter? *Am J Surg* 2009;198:532–527.
126. Toesca A, Luini A, Veronesi P, et al. Sentinel lymph node biopsy in early breast cancer: the experience of the European Institute of Oncology in Special Clinical Scenarios. *Breast Care (Basel)* 2011;6: 208–214.
127. Diaz R, Degnim AC, Boughey JC, et al. A positive intramammary lymph node does not mandate a complete axillary node dissection. *Am J Surg* 2012;203:151–155.
128. Abdullgaffar B, Gopal P, Abdulrahim M, et al. The significance of intramammary lymph nodes in breast cancer: a systematic review and meta-analysis. *Int J Surg Pathol* 2012;20:555–563.

Extramedullary Hematopoiesis

129. Longano A. Nodal extramedullary haemopoiesis: a diagnostic conundrum in core biopsies. *Pathology* 2009;41:605–607.
130. Meara RS, Jhala N, Eltoum I, et al. Fine needle aspiration of an axillary lymph node in a patient suspected of having metastatic cancer of unknown primary. *Cytopathology* 2008;19:192–196.
131. Millar EK, Inder S, Lynch J. Extramedullary haematopoiesis in axillary lymph nodes following neoadjuvant chemotherapy for locally advanced breast cancer—a potential diagnostic pitfall. *Histopathology* 2009;54:622–623.
132. Hoda SA, Resetkova E, Yusuf Y, et al. Megakaryocytes mimicking metastatic breast carcinoma. A potential trap in the interpretation of sentinel lymph nodes. *Arch Pathol Lab Med* 2002;126:618–620.
133. Bhusnurmath S, Balazs L, Pritchard E, et al. Megakaryocytes in sentinel lymph node may detract from identification of metastatic breast cancer or may be misdiagnosed as metastatic carcinoma. *Mod Pathol* 2007;20(Suppl. 2):25A.

CHAPTER 44

Pathologic Examination of Breast and Lymph Node Specimens, Including Sentinel Lymph Nodes

SYED A. HODA • ERIKA RESETKOVA

The purpose of this chapter is to highlight clinically important aspects of the pathologic examination of breast specimens. It is not intended to be a presentation of all differing points of view, nor should this material be regarded as a laboratory "workbook." The handling and examination of breast specimens should continually evolve to reflect changes in the understanding of breast diseases and alterations in clinical practice. As an example, neoadjuvant chemotherapy is an increasingly exercised option for the management of not only locally advanced but also primary breast carcinoma. Neoadjuvant chemotherapy may "down stage" larger carcinomas. It allows for breast conservation in cases where it might otherwise not be possible, and the assessment of tumor response to neoadjuvant chemotherapy also offers prognostic information. The examination of specimens obtained after neoadjuvant chemotherapy presents a particular set of challenges.

The complexity of pathology reports has increased substantially in the last three decades to accommodate the need for detailed individualized information about breast and related specimens. This has been necessitated by the availability of, and the need for, increasingly personalized medicine, that is, a course of tailored treatment most likely to be beneficial for a given patient with a particular tumor. Consequently, a greater number of findings are now recorded for each specimen. With the routine establishment of sentinel lymph node (SLN) biopsy, greater attention is also given to the handling and evaluation of lymph nodes. Immunohistochemical and other emerging procedures have extended the pathologist's role to assessing biologic as well as morphologic prognostic markers, and most of these results also appear in the routine pathology report.

Various structured forms of pathology reports have been devised to present the data that a pathologist documents by gross and microscopic examination. These reports have the advantage of ensuring that key observations are reported. They assist the clinical staff by providing comprehensive documentation, and can be the source of a database for studies. A disadvantage of most structured reports is that they are inflexible with the order in which information is presented, in that regardless of its importance for an individual patient a particular finding always appears in the same part of the report. This requires that the entire report be read to ensure that a critical finding that might appear near the end of the report is not overlooked. Some reporting formats have addressed this issue by offering a free-text summary of the diagnosis that highlights the most significant findings as well as a formatted full listing of observations. Additional information about pathology reporting—including information on the reporting of newer clinically relevant data, various staging dilemmas, and significant unexpected findings—may be found in several reviews and position papers.[1–11]

NEEDLE CORE AND INCISIONAL BIOPSY

Needle core biopsy (NCB) or incisional biopsy specimens should be processed for histopathologic examination in their entirety. Those who perform the biopsy procedure must exercise care not to crush the specimen. An electrocautery-type scalpel should not be used to perform an incisional biopsy (see subsequent text). These samples can be examined by frozen section, but it must be understood that limited information about the lesion is typically obtained from such small specimens. The histologic details can be altered by the frozen section process, and this may impede interpretation of subsequent permanent sections. Consequently, frozen section examination (FSE) is not recommended for incisional biopsy or NCB samples unless there are exceptional clinical circumstances. The samples are suitable for immunohistochemical analysis if not damaged by cautery and if appropriately fixed. Unless frozen section or some other study that requires fresh tissue is intended, small (needle core and incisional) biopsy specimens should be placed immediately in fixative after acquisition.

Newer vacuum-assisted needle biopsy devices (Mammotome, Suros, Breast Lesion Excision System, etc.) are more effective than older NCB instruments for the sampling calcifications,[12] and are also being used to "excise" lesions proven in an earlier biopsy to be benign, for example, fibroadenoma, radial sclerosing lesion, papilloma.[13] The advantages of such radiologically conducted excisions include shorter procedure, minimal anesthesia, low complication rate, gratifying patient tolerance, and negligible cutaneous scarring. On the other hand, a major disadvantage is the removal of lesion in a "piecemeal" manner, which precludes assessment of totality of excision and adequacy of margins in the event that carcinoma is detected, and may also preclude the precise assessment of the extent of invasive carcinoma.[14]

EXCISIONAL BIOPSY

Many factors influence the manner in which excisional biopsy specimens are handled. Paramount among these are logistical considerations relating to when and where the procedure was performed and the particular clinical circumstances. Hence, the material presented in this section should be regarded as guidelines that may need to be modified in some situations. Additional perspectives on handling excisional biopsy specimens can be found elsewhere.[15]

Gross Examination of Excisional Biopsy

The pathologist is responsible for the detailed description of tissue removed from a patient. This can most accurately be accomplished if the excised specimen is delivered to the pathology laboratory intact, promptly, and unfixed. The pathologist should ensure that all initial handling, including specimen accessioning and preliminary gross examination of breast excisional specimens, be expedited so as to minimize "cold ischemia time." The latter term refers to the time interval between specimen removal and formalin fixation, which should be kept under 1 hour as recommended by American Society of Clinical Oncology and the College of American Pathologists (ASCO–CAP).[16] Minimizing cold ischemia time optimizes not only histologic preparations but also key immunohistochemical and *in situ* hybridization studies.[17–19]

The size of an excisional biopsy specimen should be recorded in three dimensions, and the general shape (e.g., ovoid, spherical) should be described. Since the overall dimensions of an excisional biopsy specimen cannot be reliably determined after the tissue has been sliced open or dissected by the surgeon, the specimen should be intact when delivered to the laboratory. Contrary to traditional thinking, formalin fixation does not "shrink" excisional biopsies of breast,[20] although specimen distortion can occur. In the latter event, specimen dimensions can be misleading *vis-à-vis* orientation. Recording of the "actual specimen volume" using water displacement technique has been proposed as the "gold standard" for certain oncoplastic surgeries wherein volume considerations are important.[21] For all other specimens, documentation of dimensions and weight of breast specimens should suffice.

Ideally, the intact excisional biopsy specimen should be promptly delivered to the pathology laboratory. It is preferable that the tissue be unfixed in order to not preclude the possibility of performing a frozen section or to obtain material for other studies. If a delay is anticipated, the tissue may be chilled (in a refrigerator or placed on ice), but freezing of the entire specimen compromises histologic examination. Even if a frozen section is not requested, the tissue should be examined promptly by a pathologist to determine whether a tumor, that is, a grossly identifiable lesion, is present. If a tumor is found, the size should be recorded in three dimensions. Because of the critical prognostic significance of tumor size, this measurement should be made prior to removing for frozen section or other studies. It may be difficult to accurately measure the tumor if the specimen is received previously sliced or otherwise disrupted. The gross character of the tumor (shape, consistency, appearance of cut surface) should be described. Whether or not a distinct lesion is found, the appearance of the native breast parenchyma should be noted (consistency, relative proportions of fat and fibrous tissue, cysts or other lesions).

Intraoperative Evaluation, Including FSE

Presently, the majority of breast carcinomas are diagnosed prior to surgery by an NCB procedure. As a consequence, FSE of a primary tumor is a relatively less commonly requested procedure than in previous decades, and is likely to be done only if samples obtained by the needling procedure are not diagnostic or if the presence of invasive carcinoma could not be determined in the prior sampling. In the absence of a grossly apparent mass, routine FSE of a seemingly benign breast biopsy specimen is not recommended. Although a small proportion of such specimens harbor grossly inapparent *in situ* or invasive carcinoma, these foci will usually not be detected in the random frozen section.[22,23]

The appropriateness of FSE for the diagnosis of nonpalpable, mammographically detected lesions has been a subject of controversy. Some reports encompassing large groups of cases have described little difficulty in performing FSE in this setting.[24–26] Others have recommended that FSE not be routinely performed on such specimens because the lesions are likely to present problems in diagnosis, the tissue may be distorted by freezing and could be rendered more difficult to interpret in permanent sections, and some portion of the tissue may be irretrievably lost in the process of preparing frozen sections.[1]

Those who recommend using FSE to evaluate nonpalpable lesions caution that a frozen section diagnosis of *in situ* carcinoma or of a benign lesion should be regarded as "preliminary" because of the potential for sampling. This issue was studied by Niemann et al.,[27] who compared the results from 440 consecutive biopsies, of which 98% were examined by frozen section, with those from 604 biopsies, among which only 310 with gross lesions larger than 1.0 cm were submitted for frozen section. In the first group, the false-negative rate was 3.3%, with a sensitivity of 84%, whereas in the second more-selected series the false-negative rate was 1%, with a sensitivity of 96%. The authors concluded that "frozen section examination should be limited to cases with distinct gross lesions >1.0 cm."

FSE is recommended only if the resultant diagnosis will have an immediate effect on the surgical management, and it is not recommended for the diagnosis of nonpalpable mammographically detected lesions or for biopsy specimens in which a distinct lesion cannot be identified. It is preferable to limit FSE to tumors 1 cm in size or larger, and in all instances a portion of the grossly evident lesion should not be frozen.

The use of touch imprint cytology (TIC) can be a valuable adjunct to FSE, and it has been advocated not only in grossly evident lesions but also for the routine assessment of lumpectomy margins.[28] It should be noted, however, that TIC alone can lead to false-negative results in lower-grade carcinomas and invasive carcinoma. The decreased sensitivity of TIC for lobular carcinoma has been reported with regard to the assessment of margins[29] as well as SLNs.[30]

Sampling of the Excisional Biopsy (Lumpectomy) Specimen

The number of samples that should be taken for histologic examination from an excisional biopsy specimen varies greatly with the clinical circumstances, gross appearance of the tissue, and the results of a frozen section, if performed. No fixed rule (e.g., "x" number of samples should be examined per 5 g or cm^3 of tissue) can be reasonably applied to all specimens. The tissue used for frozen section must be saved, processed into a paraffin-embedded permanent section, and identified by a term such as the "frozen section control" (FSC). Distinct tumors that appear grossly to be carcinomas 2 cm in size or smaller in greatest extent should be entirely submitted for histology, with samples taken to demonstrate peripheral features of the tumor. In general, tumor tissue should be "banked" only if the distinct lesion exceeds 2 cm in greatest extent. Adjacent breast tissue must also be sampled adequately to enable histologic evaluation for evidence of tumor emboli in lymphovascular channels, *in situ* carcinoma outside the lesion, and the status of surgical margins.

When no distinct tumor is present, some advocate processing the entire specimen. This may be appropriate in selected situations, owing to clinical, radiologic, or pathologic findings. However, the cost of this approach can become prohibitive, and judgment must be exercised. Specimen radiography can be helpful in this regard, particularly if the targeted lesion had been radiologically detected. This technique has been shown to reliably confirm the excision of the target in 99% of cases[31] and contribute to the assessment of resection margins without increased sampling.[32] To establish criteria for sampling grossly negative breast biopsies, Schnitt and Wang[33] carried out a retrospective study of 384 specimens entirely submitted for histologic examination from biopsies performed for clinically palpable lesions in which no tumor was evident on gross pathologic examination. One to 80 blocks were required to submit entire specimens, resulting in 3,342 blocks (average, 8.7 per case; median, 6 per case). Carcinoma was found in 23 specimens (6%) and atypical hyperplasia in 3 others (0.8%). Eighty percent of the blocks consisting of fibrous parenchyma contained all carcinomas, and two of the three atypical ductal hyperplasias (ADHs). One focus of atypical lobular hyperplasia (ALH) was present among the 20% of the specimens, which consisted entirely of fat. If sampling had been limited to five blocks per case, 41% fewer blocks would have been prepared, but 6 of the 26 (23%) significant lesions would have been missed. By submitting up to 10 blocks of fibrous parenchyma per case, it would have been possible to detect 25 of the 26 significant lesions, with an 18% reduction in blocks. Only a single microscopic focus of lobular carcinoma *in situ* (LCIS) was overlooked by this selection. Mathematical analysis indicated that "it is not necessary to increase proportionately the actual number of blocks submitted to achieve the same probability of detecting carcinoma or ADH in larger specimens as for smaller specimens."[33] The authors recommended submitting up to 10 samples of fibrous parenchyma or, if the specimen is entirely fat, a similar number of samples. If carcinoma or ADH is found in the first set of slides, the remaining tissue may be processed.

Owings et al.[34] investigated the problem of tissue sampling from needle localization excisional breast biopsies. They examined 157 consecutive specimens, among which 32% contained carcinoma. All specimens were entirely submitted for histologic examination. Forty-nine of 50 (98%) carcinomas and 14 of 19 (74%) ADHs were directly related to mammographically detected foci of calcification. All carcinomas and 17 of 19 (89%) ADHs were detected in samples selected from regions of calcification and all fibrous parenchyma.

Although the data from the foregoing studies provide useful guidelines for initial tissue examination, it may be necessary to obtain additional samples to determine the extent of the lesion if initial sections show carcinoma or atypia. The margins of excision should be examined at the time of initial tissue evaluation. These samples may, of necessity, consist of fatty, nonfibrous breast tissue. It should also be remembered that excisional biopsies obtained from elderly women are generally fatty, and those from younger women are mostly fibrous.

Reexcision specimens obtained because a prior biopsy procedure had microscopically positive or close margins may not have grossly apparent tumor. Abraham et al.[35] reviewed 97 grossly negative reexcision specimens from which all tissue was submitted for histologic examination to develop guidelines for processing such specimens. Overall, 1,867 tissue blocks were processed (range, 3 to 74; mean, 19.2). Ten or more blocks were prepared in 67% of the cases. Residual *in situ* or invasive carcinoma was present in 47 reexcisions (48%). The number of blocks with residual carcinoma ranged from 1 to 41, representing 2.4% to 100% of blocks of reexcision tissue. The authors calculated that submitting two sections per centimeter of maximal tissue dimension from grossly benign reexcision specimens detected 97% of lesions having a major clinical impact on treatment with 315 (17%) fewer paraffin blocks.

Issues relating to the processing and reporting of specimens after neoadjuvant therapy have been addressed in published recommendations.[36] The fundamental principles that ought to guide the evaluation of such specimens can be summarized as follows: (1) the clinical history of neoadjuvant chemotherapy, including the specific agents used, must be provided by the surgeon; (2) the site of primary tumor (tumor bed) must be identified grossly; (3) the tumor bed must be adequately sampled; and (4) the pathology report must include assessment of residual invasive and *in situ* carcinoma, tumor size, cellularity, lymphovascular channel involvement, and margins of excision. The effects of therapy in the breast and lymph nodes should be recorded. The assessment of hormone receptors, proliferation rate *via* Ki67, and human epidermal growth factor 2 (HER2) status is indicated but may not be possible when scanty tumor remains.

Gross Description of Excisional Biopsy

The gross description of an excisional biopsy specimen is part of the pathology report. Included in this section must be an index of the tissue samples taken for microscopic examination, indicating the number of tissue blocks and providing a key to explain abbreviations used, if any, to designate individual samples. Each sample taken from a specimen should be identified with a unique letter and number, which ought to appear on the paraffin block and corresponding histologic slide. All samples taken from a specimen should be identified with a common letter, and each should be further labeled with a subnumber. For example, in this system a left breast biopsy specimen would be recorded as specimen "A" and the samples in paraffin blocks and corresponding histologic slides designated as "A1," "A2," etc. A second biopsy specimen of the right breast would be listed as "B," with samples in paraffin blocks and histologic slides designated as "B1," "B2," etc. Alternatively, specific designations such as "A-MM," instead of consecutive letters, which might indicate "Medial Margin," should be recorded in the aforementioned index. This information is essential to understand the significance of individual slides and the relationship of the findings in these slides to the overall diagnosis.

Some pathology reports do not provide an adequate index of samples (tissue blocks and slides) from a specimen, or do so in a confusing manner. Because of the growing mobility of patients and their slides, it is no longer acceptable to adhere to idiosyncratic labeling practices unique to a given facility. One unsatisfactory method is to label specimen samples taken for histology with consecutive letters without further differentiation. If presented with the slides labeled "A–P," a pathologist may not have any indication that they represent multiple specimens, conceivably from both breasts. Even with a copy of the pathology report in hand, it requires close attention to segregate the slides corresponding to each specimen. This task would be facilitated by numbering specimens separately as described previously.

Assessing Lumpectomy Margins

The definition of an adequate surgical margin remains elusive, and the extent of acceptable clearance varies considerably. The presence of invasive carcinoma at ink is regarded as a positive margin. Invasive carcinoma at the inked margin is associated with increased ipsilateral tumor recurrence.[37] Ductal carcinoma *in situ* (DCIS), particularly of the micropapillary type, can exhibit "discontinuous spread," and a more generous extent of margin clearance may be required.[38]

Technical factors complicate the microscopic evaluation of margins. The surface is often irregular, and it has a large area relative to the sampling that can be represented even in multiple histologic sections. The uneven surface sometimes contains defects or crevices that obviously do not represent the true margin. Definitions of positive and "close" margins have not been standardized. Techniques based on optical scatter spectroscopy that are independent of pathologic examination show potential for intraoperative surgical guidance of margin assessment,[39] but it is unlikely that this methodology will be adopted in the near future.

Because the contours and orientation of tissue slices may be altered in the course of preparing histologic sections, it is necessary to mark surfaces corresponding to the margin so that they can be identified microscopically. This is most easily accomplished with finely particulate reagents such as India ink or similar dyes that remain adherent to the tissue throughout processing and are visible through the microscope. Various colors can be used to designate specified margins. If applied carefully, the ink or dye is unlikely to seep into crevices in the tissue surface. The tissue should not be dipped into ink or dye, since this practice leads to seepage into crevices in the surface that can be mistaken for margins microscopically. The pigments adhere better to fresh tissue that has been blotted free of blood than to formalin-fixed tissue. If properly applied to the intact specimen, the surface pigment should not contaminate the interior of the specimen (Fig. 44.1). An excisional biopsy specimen that has been previously sliced by the surgeon cannot be reliably reassembled in order to "ink" the margins. This is an important reason for submitting intact biopsy specimens to the pathologist.

Once "inked" and the blotted dry, the specimen should be serially incised in a plane that will transect the longest palpable dimension. The gross impression of the relationship of an evident tumor to the margins should be reported, although this may underestimate the frequency of involved margins because microscopic foci of invasive and *in situ* carcinoma at the margins are usually not grossly apparent.[40,41] Specimen radiography is not a reliable method for assessing the margins of excision at the time of operation.[42] Frozen sections of margins are not indicated unless the tumor appears grossly close to a margin and confirming this intraoperatively will have an immediate impact on treatment. Random frozen sections of margins that appear grossly unremarkable are not recommended. In one study, the sensitivity of this procedure was only 77%.[43] Notwithstanding the reportedly successful experience of routine frozen sections for margin evaluation in selected settings,[44,45] this labor intensive and time-consuming practice is impractical for most laboratories.

Weber et al.[46] described the results of a study in which frozen sections were performed on samples obtained from the surface of the cavity left after an excisional biopsy. Five samples were taken from each biopsy cavity in 140 cases. Carcinoma was found in one or more biopsy cavity samples from 21 of the patients (15%). In 14 of the 21 cases, negative

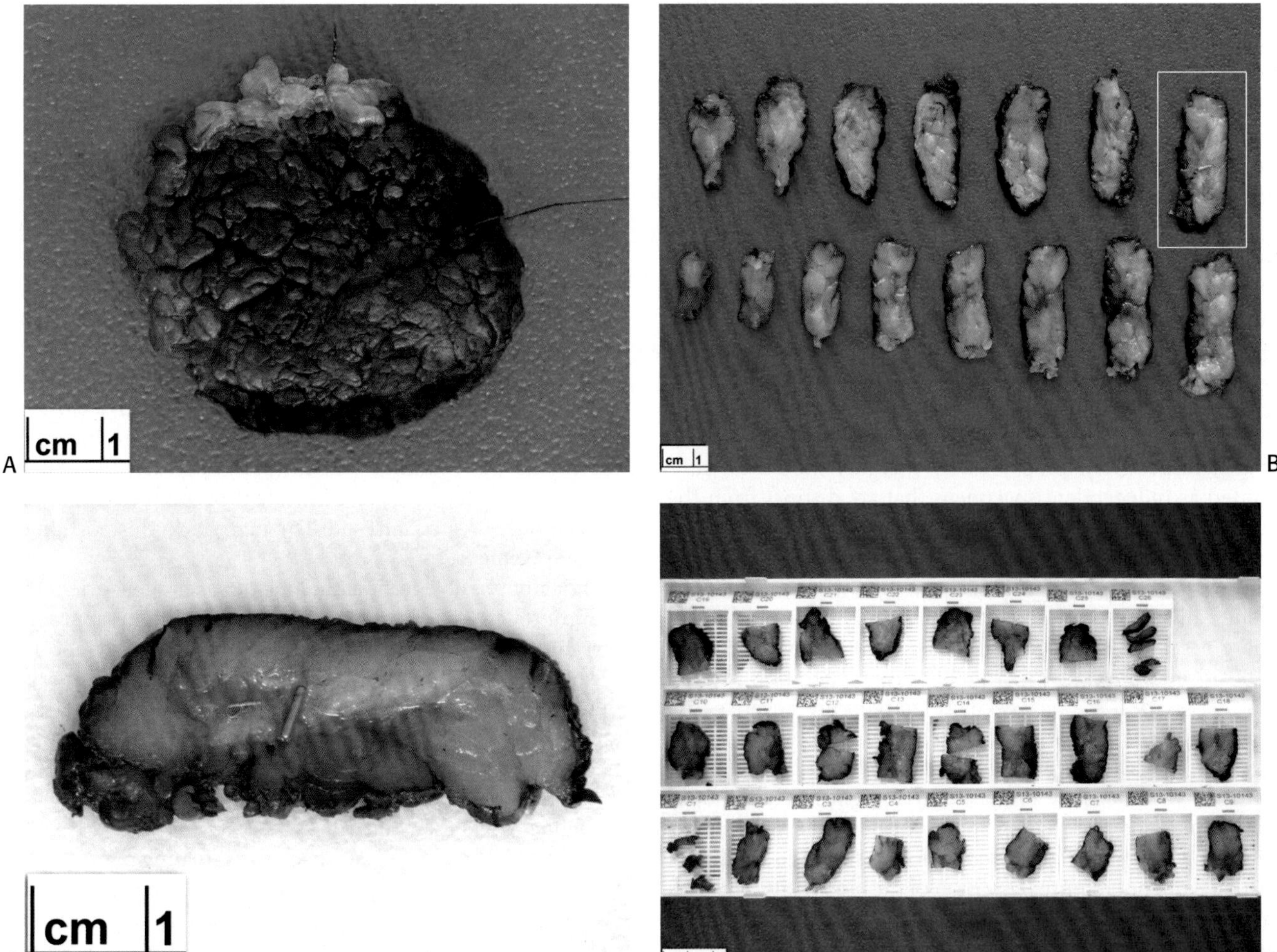

FIG. 44.1. ***Inking an excisional biopsy specimen.*** **A:** Variously colored permanent inks applied to an excisional biopsy (lumpectomy) specimen. The long suture on the surface (*right*) designates the lateral margin, and the short suture on the surface (*top*) indicates the superior surface. Six colors are typically used. Five (*yellow*, superior; *green*, anterior; *black*, inferior; *orange*, medial; *blue*, lateral) are shown here. **B:** The specimen has been sequentially sectioned from the medial to the lateral aspect, at approximately 2-mm interval. The slices show ink to be limited to the outer surface of the tissue. The slices are shown laid out in a counterclockwise sequence, starting at bottom-left. The "slice" showing the radiographic clip (indicating site of prior NCB) and the radioactive seed (placed immediately before surgery to assist in the surgical localization of the target lesion) is boxed. **C:** Magnified view of the specimen "slice" showing the radiographic clip and the radioactive seed. **D:** The specimen slices have been placed in cassettes for histologic processing. Some of the larger central slices have been bisected and placed in two cassettes. Note that the most lateral and medial slices, shown at top-right and bottom-left, respectively, have been serially sectioned in a manner perpendicular to the inked edge. (Courtesy of Dr. Paul DiMaggio.)

margins were achieved by reexcision. Three patients found to have persistent involvement of margins underwent immediate mastectomy. This procedure was questioned by Esserman and Weidner[47] on its cost-effectiveness, difficulty of distinguishing atypical hyperplasia from DCIS, and conversion of planned excisional surgery to an immediate mastectomy.

It is important to distinguish between *pathologic* "shaved" and "perpendicular" margins when reporting the margin status of a biopsy. A shaved margin is a thin slice of tissue taken parallel to the inked surface of the specimen as a separate sample. Shave samples are sectioned *en face*, and the margin is considered positive if carcinoma cells are detected anywhere in the corresponding histologic section. It is important that the inked aspect of such shaved margins be sectioned for microscopic evaluation to be representative of the true margin. Samples designated as "inked" margins are taken perpendicular to the surface and considered to be positive when carcinoma cells are seen microscopically at the inked edge.

A *surgical* "shaved" margin (also known as biopsy cavity margins) is a sample obtained by a surgeon intraoperatively from the exposed surface of the biopsy cavity. In recent years, the practice of taking multiple "cavity margins" has gained wide acceptance.[48] Cavity margins help in determining the true status of margins by averting the histopathologic pitfalls associated with interpretation of margins in the main lumpectomy specimen—such as ink trickling into crevices and cautery artifact. As many as six cavity margins can be taken, although some surgeons[49] may not take an additional anterior margin and posterior margin if these surfaces abut the overlying subcutaneous tissue or underlying fascial plane, respectively. Biopsy cavity margins should be submitted as independent specimens that are distinct from the lumpectomy specimen.

Biopsy cavity margins can be oriented with a suture, clip, or ink to indicate the final margin and processed histologically with this orientation in mind. These additional margin samples have proved to be useful for patients with a positive lumpectomy margin because reoperation is often not necessary if the biopsy cavity margins are negative.[50–52] Cao et al.[52] found that 52 of 103 patients (50.5%) had carcinoma at or within 2 mm of a lumpectomy margin, leaving 51 (49.5%) with negative lumpectomy margins. When biopsy cavity margins were taken into consideration, 61 patients (59%) had negative final margins. As a result nine additional patients did not require reexcision of the biopsy site. Features associated with finding residual carcinoma in biopsy cavity margins were high-grade carcinoma, extensive DCIS in the lumpectomy specimen, and multiple involved lumpectomy margins. Women with positive biopsy cavity margins had a lower mean age at diagnosis (55.2; range, 31 to 88 years) than did those with negative margins (60.6; range, 42 to 85 years).

The presence of negative lumpectomy margins does not provide complete assurance that all carcinoma in the region of the primary site was removed. Evidence for this comes from the analysis of biopsy cavity shave margins obtained from patients with negative lumpectomy margins. Guidi et al.[53] found that 39% of patients with a positive shave margin had negative lumpectomy margins, and that the likelihood of having a positive lumpectomy margin increased with more frequent positive shave margins in a given case. Rubin et al.[54] reported finding carcinoma in 9% of tumor bed biopsies from 135 consecutive patients with histologically negative margins in the lumpectomy specimens. Cao et al.,[52] who considered a lumpectomy margin to be negative if carcinoma was more than 2 mm from the margins, reported that 9.7% of patients with negative lumpectomy margins had carcinoma in biopsy cavity shave margins.

Various technical circumstances may create false-positive lumpectomy margins. Ink that seeps into defects in the tissue may come in proximity with carcinoma that is not at the true margin on the tissue surface.[7,52] Detached fragments of carcinoma displaced into ink can be misinterpreted as a positive margin. There is also evidence that compression of excised breast tissue during specimen radiography may create false-positive lumpectomy margins by compressing normal tissue at the surface of the specimen.[52,55] Tissue compression during specimen radiography invariably leads to some degree of "pancaking" of lumpectomy tissue.[56] The latter phenomenon generally leads to artifactual reduction of margin clearance of two (compressed) margins and artifactual increment in margin clearance of the other four (expanded) margins. Dooley and Parker[55] studied this phenomenon in a series of 220 lumpectomy specimens that were consistently oriented during specimen radiography so that compression was applied only to the skin surface and deep margin. Reexcisions were performed in cases with close or positive margins. No residual carcinoma was found in 12 cases with a close or positive deep margin. When other margins were involved, carcinoma was found in 5 of 14 (35.7%) reexcisions. These results were interpreted as evidence that compression of the deep surface created false-positive margins in this portion of some specimens.

It is not possible for a pathologist to accurately orient the margins of an excisional biopsy specimen without appropriate guidance from the surgeon. This can be easily accomplished if the surgeon places a short suture at the superior margin and a long stitch laterally (Fig. 44.1). The use of orienting sutures has been widely adopted; however, this practice has been shown to have an overall "disorientation" rate of 31%, and a remarkably higher rate (78%) on specimens with a volume of less than 20 cm^3.[57]

One widely practiced approach to evaluating margins histologically employs samples taken perpendicular to each of six inked surfaces (superior, inferior, medial, lateral, superficial, and deep), with additional samples of margins determined by the gross findings. Different colors of ink can be used to distinguish individual margins, but a single color will suffice if margin samples are clearly labeled. Typically, at least two perpendicular sections are taken from each margin surface. The recognition of "true" colors can occasionally be a problem under the microscope, for example, interpretation as green at the interface of blue and yellow or mistaking orange or yellow as red. In such situations, review of the colors as they appear in the corresponding tissue block can be helpful.[58] As an aside, inking of NCBs before histologic processing has gained acceptance as a method to reduce specimen "mix-up."[59]

Carter[60] recommended "peeling" the entire external surface from the specimen, a procedure that is technically challenging. Taking "shaved" samples from the specimen surface has been adopted in some laboratories as an alternative to the peel method. Usually, these shaved samples are sectioned parallel to the surface, and the finding of carcinoma is considered a positive margin, although it may not be in contact with ink. Typically, carcinoma will be within 2 mm of the inked surface when present in a shaved specimen margin.

Cytologic methods for examining the margins of resection have been investigated, but none have proven to be more reliable than histologic sections. In particular, the use of TIC alone can lead to false-negative results in lower grade carcinomas, particularly invasive lobular carcinoma of the classical type. Cox et al.[43] employed touch preparations from the surfaces of lumpectomy specimens to assess the margins. There were three false-positive interpretations. FSE yielded five false-negative and no false-positive results in the same series of specimens. Veronesi et al.[61] explored the use of the B72.3 as a means of detecting carcinoma cells at the margins of excisional biopsies. Cytospin preparations were made from specimens obtained by scraping the biopsy surface. One significant limitation of this procedure was the fact that only 57% of the primary carcinomas were B72.3-positive. Immunoreactive cells were detected in 33% of the cytospin specimens containing a B72.3-positive tumor, whereas only 12% had histologically positive margins. The clinical significance of finding B72.3-positive cells cytologically on the surface of a specimen with histologically negative margins remains undetermined. England et al.[62] also described a method for evaluating the margins of a lumpectomy specimen by cytologic examination of cells obtained by scraping the surface of the tissue.

The interpretation of margins is directed at the distribution of intraductal or invasive carcinoma in relation to the various margins. The proximity of LCIS of the classical type or proliferative lesions to the margin of resection has not been proven to be a risk factor for local recurrence after breast conservation therapy.[63] Nonetheless, the presence of classical LCIS should be noted in the report. It has been recommended that margin status should be reported for the pleomorphic variant of LCIS[64] and for its florid variant because there is some evidence that it may be a marker for local recurrence (see Chapter 31). A 2-mm clearance can be regarded as "negative" margin in these, as in most other, settings.

There is no standardized system for reporting the microscopic appearance of margins obtained perpendicular to the tissue surface. Tumor transected at an "inked" surface clearly represents a "positive" margin (Fig. 44.2). This criterion applies equally to *in situ* and to invasive carcinoma. Borderline situations occur in which tumor closely approaches the margin, but is not transected (Fig. 44.3). One useful convention in these situations is to regard foci less than 1 high-power field as "close to the margin." Others have defined tumor as close to the margin when it is within 3 mm of the inked surface.[65] The actual microscopic distance in millimeters between carcinoma and a margin can be reported. The nature of the carcinoma at or close to the margin (*in situ* or invasive) should be stated, and some estimate of the extent should be given. It is possible to describe the quantity of carcinoma at or near the margins by specifying the histologic findings in the relevant

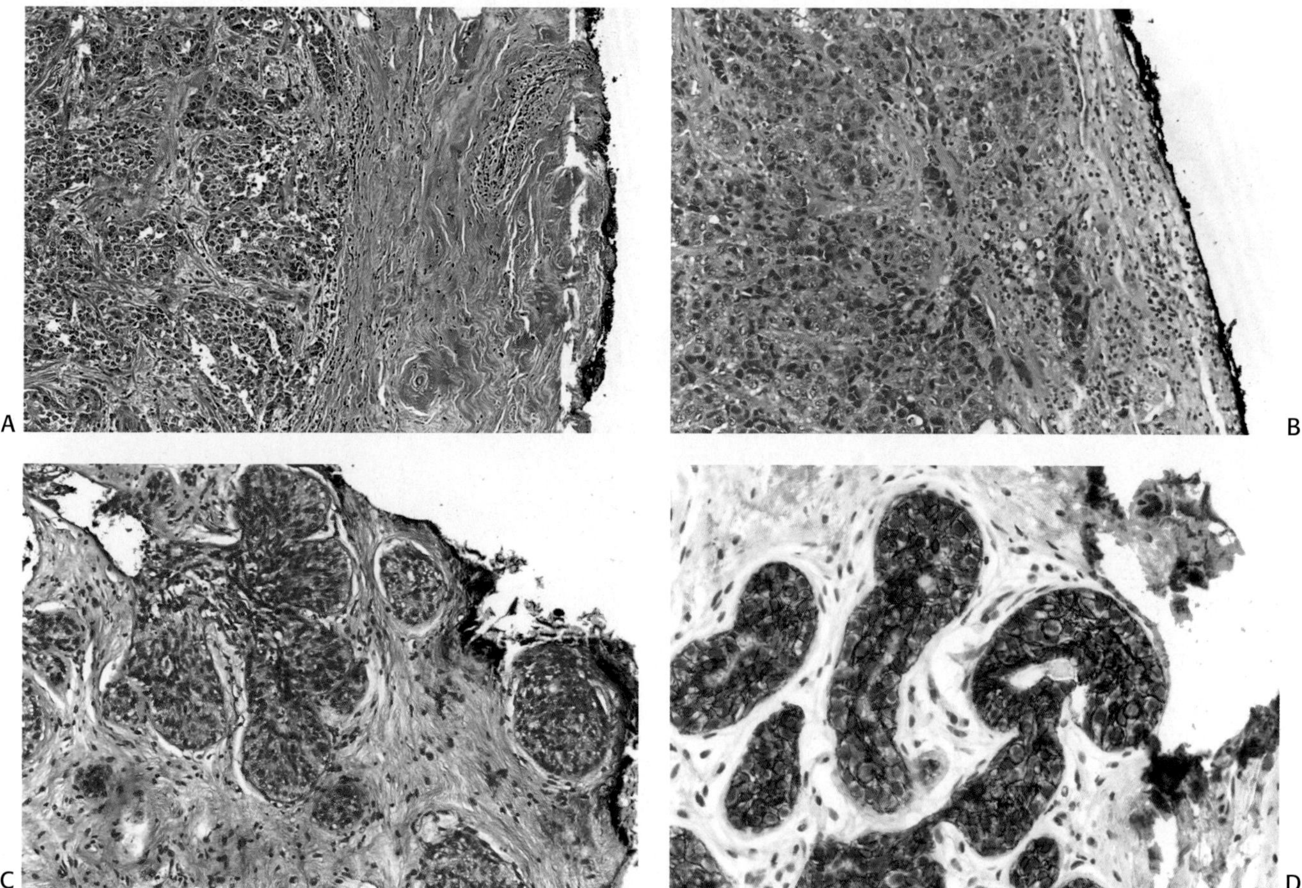

FIG. 44.2. ***Microscopic appearance of inked margins.*** **A:** Invasive ductal carcinoma 1 mm from the inked margin. **B:** Invasive ductal carcinoma less than 1 mm from the inked margin. **C:** DCIS of the solid type at the inked margin. The lesion was misinterpreted as LCIS. **D:** E-cadherin reactivity indicates ductal differentiation in the lesion shown in **(C)**.

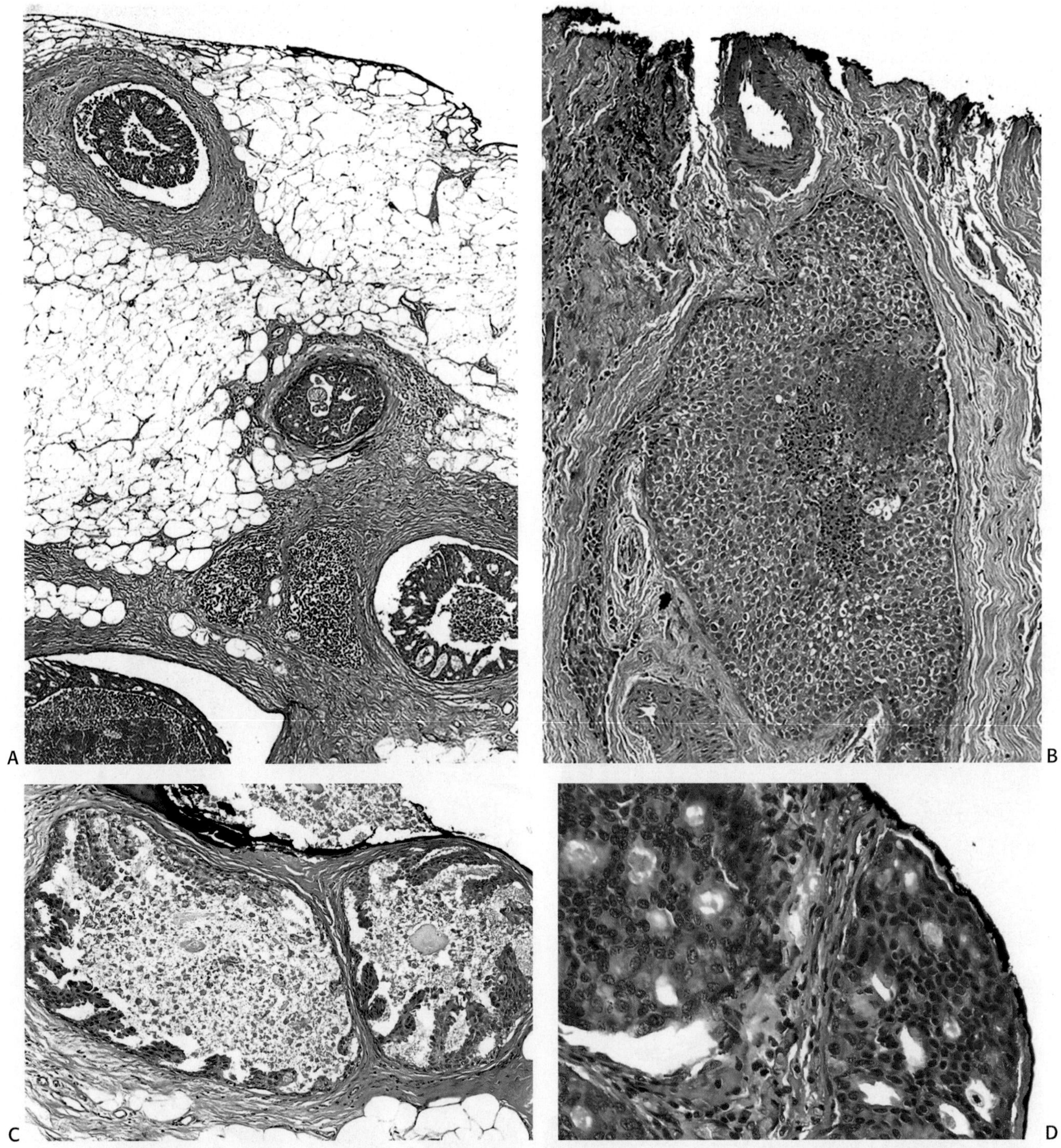

FIG. 44.3. ***Carcinoma "close" to inked margins.*** **A,B:** DCIS less than 1 mm from the inked margin. **C:** About 0.1 mm of collagen and the basement membrane separate this DCIS from the inked margin. **D:** Only basement membrane lies between the inked margin and DCIS. Typically, such "close" margins require reexcision to obtain wider "clearance" (usually regarded as 2 mm).

slides. For example, the report can be worded as follows: "Invasive ductal carcinoma involves the medial margin along a 1-mm plane and DCIS of the cribriform type is present in rare isolated ducts at the superior and lateral margins. Invasive carcinoma extends to within 1 mm of the lateral margin."

Clinical Significance of Margin Assessment

The clinical importance of making a distinction between tumor transected at the margin or "close" to the margin is uncertain. Schnitt et al.,[66] who defined a close margin as carcinoma within 1 mm of the inked margin, reported local recurrence rates at 5 years after lumpectomy and radiation for patients with negative and close margins to be 0% and 4%, respectively. In this series, the margin was considered to be "focally" positive when carcinoma was "present at the margins in three or fewer low-power microscopic fields using a 4× objective" and "more than focally" positive if greater than three low-power fields were involved. The local recurrence rates for "focal" and "more than focal" involvement were 6% and 21%, respectively. The presence of an extensive component of DCIS did not significantly increase the risk of local recurrence in patients with negative, close, or focally involved margins. However, the combination of extensive DCIS and more than focal margin involvement was associated with a 50% local failure rate. These observations were confirmed in a subsequent analysis of a larger series by these investigators.[67]

The number of margins with carcinoma is significantly related to the likelihood of finding residual tumor at the time of reexcision. DiBiase et al.[68] reported that the number of positive margins diagnosed in biopsy cavity samples was a significant factor for local tumor control and overall survival (OS). Local control was inferior for women with two or more positive margins when compared to those with negative margins or only one positive margin. An assessment of the margins of excisional biopsy specimens yielded similar data in a study by Papa et al.[69] Residual carcinoma was found in 70% of reexcisions after excision with positive margins (tumor at inked surface), and in 25% after excisions with close margins (tumor smaller than 2 mm from inked surface). Residual tumor was found in 12.5%, 37.5%, and 47.9% of reexcision specimens after initial biopsies with 1, 2, or 3 positive margins, respectively. In other reports, residual carcinoma was found in 32% to 62% of reexcision specimens obtained after positive lumpectomy margins.[70–74] The likelihood of finding residual carcinoma and the amount of carcinoma in the reexcision specimen were usually a function of the size of the initial tumor and the status of the original resection margins.

A related study of margin status and outcome was reported by Pittinger et al.[65] In this analysis, a "close" margin was defined as tumor detected microscopically within 3 mm of the inked margin of the initial excisional biopsy. When a reexcision was performed, residual carcinoma was found in 0%, 24%, 44%, and 48% of patients whose margin status for the initial biopsy was negative, close, positive, and unknown, respectively. A margin of 3 mm or wider has been shown to have a 6.1% (95% CI, 41% to 8.2%) rate of ipsilateral breast events after a median follow-up of 6.2 years in 565 patients with low- to intermediate-grade DCIS not treated with radiation.[75] In the same study, the recurrence rate was 15.3% (95% CI, 8.2% to 22.5%) with a median follow-up of 6.7 years for high-grade carcinomas. The authors concluded that 3 mm may be considered as a reassuring extent of clearance in rigorously evaluated and appropriately selected cases but offered the caveat that "further follow-up is necessary to document long-term results." It is our opinion that it would be premature to draw any conclusions about the long-term outcome of patients in this study because of the relatively indolent clinical course of low-grade DCIS and invasive carcinomas.

The status of lumpectomy margins is an important prognostic indicator for breast recurrence after breast conservation therapy. Multivariate analysis of 869 patients with stage I and stage II breast carcinoma treated by breast conservation with radiotherapy revealed that margin status was the only significant predictor for local control.[76] Among women with positive margins, local control was improved when the dose of radiation to the tumor bed was increased ("boosted"). Mansfield et al.[77] also found positive margin status to be a significant predictor of local failure in a multivariate analysis of patients with stage I and stage II disease after a median follow-up of 40 months.

The local recurrence rate is lower if margins are negative than if they are positive or unknown,[65,78,79] but it is well documented that margins reported to be negative do not provide complete assurance that local recurrence will not occur in patients given equivalent treatment.[80] The initial breast recurrence rates for patients treated for "small" invasive carcinomas in a trial comparing lumpectomy to quadrantectomy, in which all patients received radiotherapy, were 8.6% and 4.5%, respectively.[61] In a subsequent report, the 10-year estimated breast recurrence rate after lumpectomy was 18.6%, and 7.4% after quadrantectomy.[81] Margin status, reported to be positive in 16.3% of patients who underwent lumpectomy and in 4.5% who underwent quadrantectomy, was not significantly related to recurrence in the breast, despite the fact that reexcision was not performed when margins were involved.

A study by the National Surgical Adjuvant Breast and Bowel Project (NSABP)[82] revealed a breast recurrence rate of nearly 40% in women with negative margins treated by lumpectomy without radiotherapy. In the NSABP, a margin was negative if tumor was not present at the inked surface. Patients with negative margins who received radiotherapy had a 10% local recurrence rate at 8 years. Others have reported local recurrence rates (after radiation therapy) of 28%,[83] 13%,[84] 9%,[85] 3.7%,[79] 3%,[65] 2%,[43] and 0%[66] when margins were negative. Final margin status that takes into account reexcision or shaved biopsy cavity samples is a more reliable predictor of local control than original excision margins alone.[78]

Pittinger et al.[65] found that after a follow-up of 3 years or more, the frequency of breast recurrence following excision and radiotherapy was the same in those with negative and close margins. The authors concluded that "reexcision of close margins is not necessary in patients" treated by breast conservation therapy. Kunos et al.[86] reported that a negative margin with a clearance of 2 mm or more resulted in a significantly lower frequency of breast recurrence (2.1%) than a margin of less than 2 mm in women who also received chemotherapy and hormonal therapy.

Prognostic Significance of Local Breast Recurrence

The relationship of local recurrence in the breast to the occurrence of distant metastases and death due to breast carcinoma is controversial. Several studies have shown no significant difference in distant disease-free survival (DFS) between women who did and did not have a breast recurrence after conservation therapy. Others have reported a less favorable outcome after local recurrence itself that has been attributed to an initially more aggressive primary tumor causing local as well as distant metastases rather than the local recurrence itself giving rise to systemic disease.[87–92]

Fortin et al.[93] evaluated survival in patients treated by breast conservation with radiotherapy and concluded that local failure could be a source of distant metastases. The study included 2,030 patients with a median follow-up of 6 years. The local control rate at 10 years was 87%. Patients with local failure had a significantly less favorable 10-year survival rate (55%) than those who did not experience a breast recurrence. Local failure was a significant predictor of poor survival in multivariate analysis. The relative risk (RR) of death due to breast carcinoma was 3.6 for women with local recurrence, and their RR of systemic metastases was 5.6, when compared to the RRs for those who did not experience local failure. Additional evidence for local recurrence as a possible source of distant metastases came from analysis of the timing of systemic recurrences. The rate of systemic recurrences was higher among women with local breast recurrences than among those without local failure. The rates of systemic recurrence were parallel for 2 years after treatment, but they rose thereafter among those with local recurrence, reaching a peak around 6 years. By comparison, the group with local control had a declining rate of systemic spread more than 2 years after treatment (Fig. 44.4). Consequently, the mean time until systemic recurrence was significantly shorter among women with local failure (1,050 days) than in the group with local control (1,650 days). In this series, patients with close or positive margins had a higher local failure rate (15.7%) than those with negative margins. The presence of tumor at, or close to, the margin was associated with more frequent systemic recurrence (28%) than negative margins (17%).

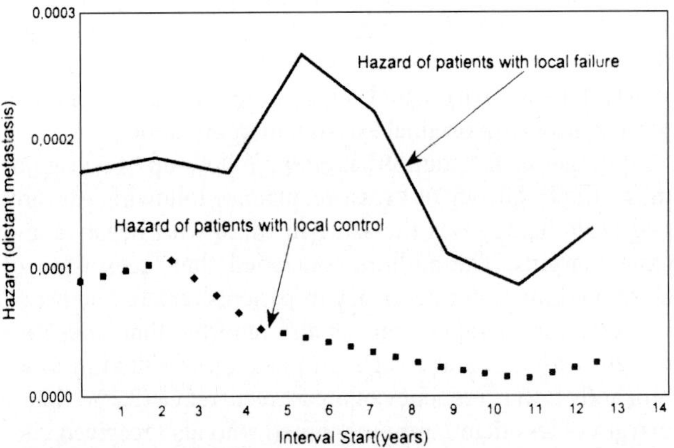

FIG. 44.4. ***Local breast recurrence after conservation therapy and the hazard rate of distant metastases.*** Patients with local control after primary therapy had a lower risk of systemic metastases than those with local failure. (From Fortin A, Larochelle M, Laverdiere J, et al. Local failure is responsible for the decrease in survival for patients with breast cancer treated with conservative surgery and postoperative radiotherapy. *J Clin Oncol* 1999;17:101–109, with permission.)

Studies of margin status as a predictor of local control vary greatly in terms of the uniformity of surgical procedures performed, the completeness of pathologic evaluation, the forms of adjunctive therapy such as irradiation, and the length of follow-up. Differences can be found in these variables between studies and also in the selection of treatment for patients within a given study. For example, Solin et al.[94] treated patients with grossly positive or diffusely positive microscopic margins by mastectomy. Among patients selected for breast conservation, there were significant differences in the total radiation dosages administered to women with negative, positive, close, or unknown margins.

Clinical Follow-up after Breast-Conserving Surgery

Mammography is an important element in the clinical follow-up of patients after breast conservation therapy.[95] In one study, 47 of 189 (25%) breast recurrences in patients without systemic metastases were detected by mammography alone. As might be expected, mammographically detected lesions were smaller than those detected by palpation or other signs. Patient outcome was significantly correlated with the size of recurrent tumors. The 5-year frequencies of death and of systemic metastases were 38% and 30.7%, respectively, for patients with tumors 10 mm or less in diameter, whereas for patients with recurrent tumors larger than 10 mm, the frequencies were 46% and 54.4%, respectively. These results suggest that the detection of breast recurrence as soon as possible after conservation therapy might be beneficial to the overall prognosis in this group.

Reexcision of Biopsy Site

Reexcision of the biopsy site is indicated when the margins of the initial excision are involved grossly by carcinoma, if breast conservation is desired, and if an acceptable cosmetic result can be achieved. Other relative indications for reexcision are the finding of residual microcalcifications at the biopsy site in the postbiopsy mammogram, carcinoma microscopically at or close to the margins, the presence of "extensive" intraductal component associated with in an invasive carcinoma (defined later in text) in the initial excision specimen, and inability to assess the margin status of the first excision. The likely cosmetic effect of reexcision and whether radiation will be employed can further influence the decision to recommend reexcision.

The reexcision specimen should be handled by the surgeon and pathologist in the same fashion as a primary lumpectomy. The specimen should be submitted intact with orientation markers such as sutures, and the external surfaces should be inked in the same manner as in a primary lumpectomy. FSE of the margins of reexcision specimens is rarely indicated except to confirm a gross impression of carcinoma extending to a margin. The gross assessment of the amount of carcinoma, if any, remaining at the biopsy site can be unreliable because regional fat necrosis, fibrous scarring, and organizing hemorrhage in this region can produce a palpable alteration that may be mistaken for carcinoma. Most reexcision specimens, especially those 3 cm or less in greatest extent, can be entirely submitted for histologic examination. The extent of sampling of larger reexcision specimens depends on the gross findings and the particular indications for reexcision in each case, but should generally follow the guidelines for primary lumpectomy as enunciated above.

Extensive DCIS Component of an Invasive Carcinoma

Extensive intraductal component (EIC) of an invasive carcinoma has been defined as the presence of DCIS making up more than 25% of the entire area of the invasive carcinoma and the presence of DCIS in the surrounding breast tissue.[2] Residual carcinoma, especially DCIS, is more likely to be found in a reexcision if the primary invasive carcinoma was accompanied by EIC.[72] Among patients with a microscopically positive margin in the primary excision, there is a substantially greater likelihood of finding residual carcinoma in the reexcision if the initial specimen has EIC.[2] The presence of EIC has been shown to be a predictor of increased risk of local recurrence in the breast by some investigators.[2,65,83,96–98] Sinn et al.[96] defined EIC as being present if the extent of the intraductal component was at least twice the size of the invasive carcinoma or the tumor was predominantly intraductal. The presence of EIC in this study was associated with low tumor grade, positive resection margins, and multifocal invasive carcinoma. In multivariate analysis, the factors associated with local recurrence were EIC (RR, 1.9), high-grade tumor (RR, 1.76), invasive lobular carcinoma (RR, 1.65), age at diagnosis less than or equal to 40 years (RR, 1.39), and "angioinvasion" (RR, 1.34). Others have not reported a higher local recurrence rate in women with EIC, or they have found that it was a significant predictor in univariate but not in multivariate analysis.[66,67,78,84]

Ohtake et al.[99] developed a computerized method for mapping the distribution of DCIS in patients with invasive carcinoma. The procedure used graphics to create a three-dimensional reconstruction of the ductal system from information obtained with subgross serial sections of the specimen. In most cases, intraductal extension tended to be distributed from the invasive lesion toward the nipple. Anastomosing ductal branches connecting otherwise independent ductal systems were found in breast tissue not involved by DCIS, and in one case such a connecting branch provided the bridge for extension of DCIS beyond a single ductal system. Further development of such systems could provide a method for mapping DCIS in clinical practice.

Many breast tumors are presently diagnosed initially by NCB, especially when the lesion is not palpable. The samples obtained by this procedure typically include portions of the main lesion as well as peripheral tissue. Jimenez et al.[100] reported that the relative proportions of DCIS and invasive carcinoma in needle biopsy samples were significantly correlated with the distribution of these components in corresponding surgical excisions. An NCB was deemed to have EIC if the ratio of ducts with DCIS to the number of cores was greater than 0.5. A specimen with a ratio of 0.5 or less was considered to be EIC-negative. EIC was present in 70% of excisions after core biopsies, with a ratio greater than 0.5, and in 36% when the ratio was less than or equal to 0.5. EIC was present in only 2 of 29 (7%) excisional biopsies obtained after the core biopsy specimen with invasive carcinoma had no DCIS. These findings suggest that describing the proportion of NCB samples involved by DCIS may predict the presence of EIC and be useful for planning the extent of surgical excision.

TNM Staging

Tumor (size), regional node (involvement), (distant) metastases (TNM) staging according to erstwhile criteria of the American Joint Committee on Cancer–Union for International Cancer Control (AJCC–UICC) may be inaccurate when based only on the initial excision if the patient has positive margins and residual tumor is detected in a reexcision specimen. Evidence to support this supposition was presented by Brenin and Morrow,[101] who found a significantly greater frequency of nodal metastases in patients who had residual invasive tumor in a reexcision than when no tumor remained. The analysis was controlled for major predictors of lymph node metastases and compared patients on the basis of tumor size measured only in the initial excision. The authors concluded that understaging may occur, especially among patients with T1a–b (i.e., invasive carcinoma measuring 1.0 cm or smaller) tumors, if invasive carcinoma remains in a reexcision, and they suggested this be considered in planning treatment. No method was offered for arriving at a tumor size based on measurements from both the excision and reexcision specimens.

This issue is difficult to resolve, since breast carcinomas are usually not spherical and it is uncertain whether the diameter of residual tumor should be added to the largest diameter of the primary lesion. Any size increment, howsoever minimal, could have a major impact on treatment for example by changing staging from T1a to T1b, or from T1b to T1c. In the latest TNM Staging System, the grossly positive margin of a carcinoma cannot be "T" staged. On the other hand, "T" staging can be based on a measurement of the gross carcinoma when the margins are positive only miscroscopically.[101]

Refinements in radiographic techniques offer promise for preoperative staging, and have the potential to improve the accuracy of surgical excision. Magnetic resonance imaging (MRI) has proven more useful than mammography for evaluating possible invasion of the pectoral muscle in patients with a deep or posterior tumor. A study of 19 patients with this clinical presentation revealed that 12 had mammographic findings suggestive of muscle involvement.[102] MRI showed extension to the prepectoral fat plane and muscle enhancement in five of these cases that proved to be the only ones with muscle invasion demonstrated surgically.

MRI also has the potential for detecting the presence and distribution of EIC or multifocal and multicentric carcinoma. Esserman et al.[103] analyzed 44 cases in which MRI and mammography had been performed. The MRI interpretation was in concordance with the pathologic findings in each of 19 patients with a unicentric tumor, all 10 patients with multifocal or multicentric carcinoma, and in 7 of 8 patients (88%) with EIC. The false-positive rate, representing an MRI determination of more extensive tumor than was detected pathologically, and the false-negative rate were each about 3%. Ultrasonography has also proven to be effective for detecting multifocal or multicentric carcinoma that was not apparent in conventional mammograms.[104]

Lymphovascular Tumor Emboli and Breast Recurrence after Conservation Therapy

The presence of lymphovascular tumor emboli associated with a primary carcinoma or in a reexcision specimen was associated with a significantly increased risk of local recurrence in patients treated by lumpectomy and radiotherapy[60,61] in some reports,[69,82,83,85] but others reported no association.[67,95] The influence of radiotherapy and systemic adjuvant therapy on the risk of breast recurrence associated with lymphovascular tumor emboli has not been determined. However, various forms of treatment may be a factor in the different results reported in previously cited studies.

Specimen Radiography

The radiologic examination of excised breast tissue has been employed for nearly 75 years.[105] As early as 1913, Salomon,[106] a surgeon at the University of Berlin, reported on the use of x-rays to study mastectomy specimens. He employed serial sections of specimens in order to correlate histologic and radiologic features of breast carcinoma. He described radiologically detected calcifications in breast carcinomas, but the clinical significance of this finding was not appreciated until several decades later.[107] In 1951, Leborgne[108] commented on a case in which "roentgenographic study of the operative specimen also permitted the localization of the tiny calcifications for histopathological study, and thus aided in finding a small cancer."

The increasing use of mammography is a major factor in the progressively earlier stage of breast carcinomas detected in the last three decades.[109] Carcinomas are detected mammographically because of an abnormal soft tissue structure, the presence of calcifications, or both. Soft-tissue alterations in the breast may be distorted in the excised specimen, rendering them less suitable to specimen x-ray study. Changes in the relationships of structures in the compressed breast at the time of mammography and the altered orientation in an excised specimen make it difficult to accurately compare these features in clinical and specimen x-rays. Clinical mammographic findings that do not lend themselves to specimen radiography are alterations in parenchymal pattern, skin changes, vascular abnormalities, and ill-defined lesions.[110,111] Specimen compression devices are useful for localizing noncalcified lesions in specimen radiographs,[112] and image quality may be improved further if the specimen is immersed in water[112–114] (Fig. 44.5). Sonography has also been employed to assess biopsy specimens obtained after preoperative sonographic localization of nonpalpable lesions.[115]

The availability of corresponding mammogram and specimen radiograph is helpful in ensuring radiologic–pathologic correlation (Figs. 44.6 to 44.8). The presence of calcifications associated with a lesion provides an intrinsic marker that can be visualized in clinical and specimen radiographs. Specimen radiography provides a method for proving that a nonpalpable lesion has been removed, and it is an efficient technique for pinpointing the area for histologic examination.[116]

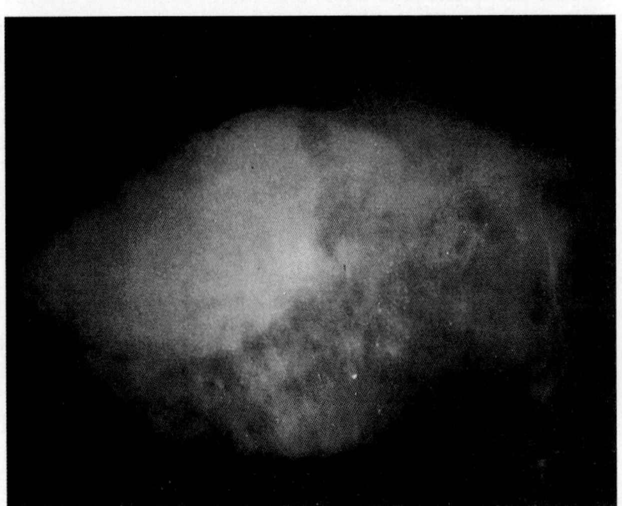

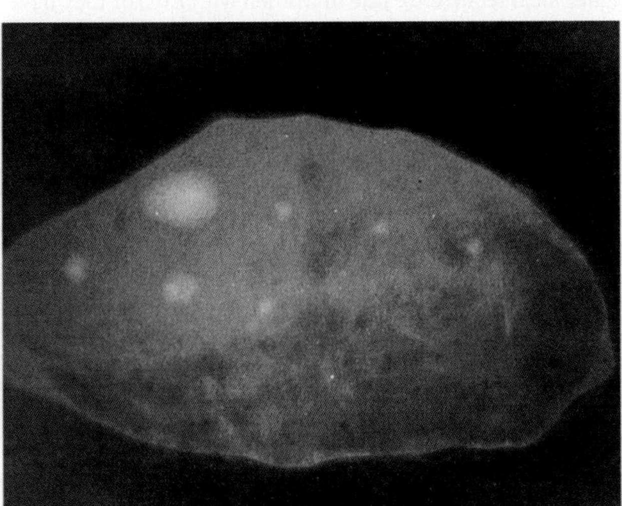

FIG. 44.5. ***Specimen radiography with compression.*** **A:** A specimen radiograph taken without compression. No discrete lesions are apparent. **B:** A radiograph of the specimen shown in (A) taken with compression. Seven discrete nodules can be seen. The largest nodule was a fibroadenoma; the others were cysts. Specimen compression can compromise the precise evaluation of margins.

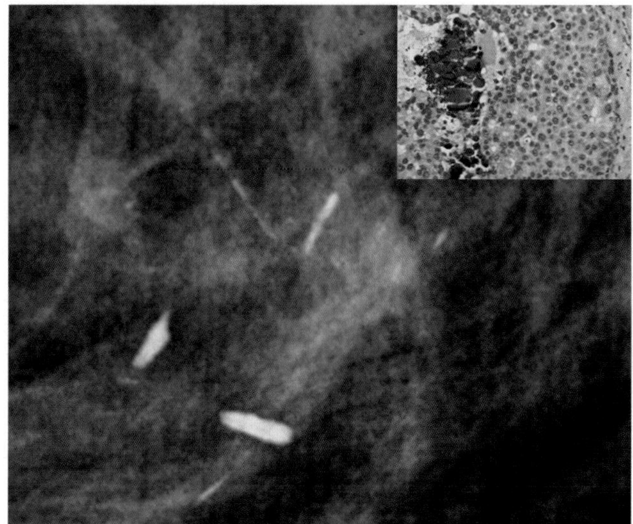

FIG. 44.6. ***Radiologic–pathologic correlation.*** Magnified view of a mammogram of the left breast from a 54-year-old woman reveals linear-branching cast-like calcifications that upon excision corresponded to calcifications in DCIS of the solid type with high-grade nuclei and central necrosis [*inset*]. (Courtesy of Dr. Shabnam Momtahen.)

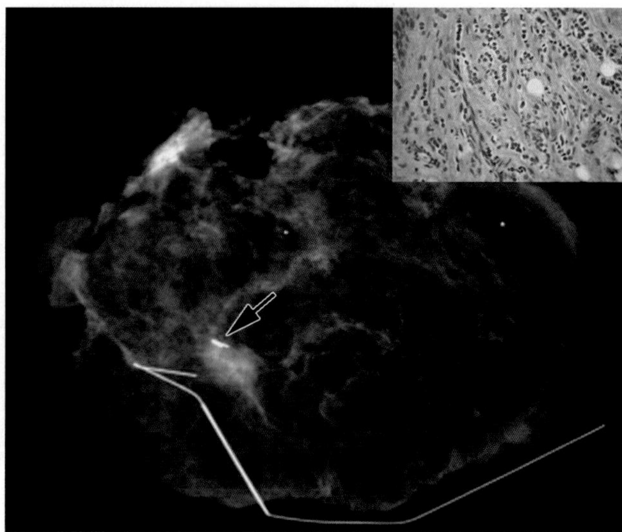

FIG. 44.8. ***Radiologic–pathologic correlation.*** The specimen radiograph of a needle-localized lumpectomy specimen from a 57-year-old woman shows a clip [*arrow*] marking the site of prior NCB in the targeted asymmetric and irregular soft tissue density that was invasive lobular carcinoma of the classical type [*inset*].

Carcinoma is found in approximately 25% of nonpalpable lesions biopsied because the mammogram reveals a pattern of calcification that suggests carcinoma.[110,111,117]

In order to effectively evaluate a breast specimen radiograph, it is helpful to have the clinical mammogram simultaneously available. A variety of procedures have been described for specimen radiography, and this chapter will not address their advantages or disadvantages, which primarily depend on the availability of personnel, equipment, and other resources in a given institution. Thus, the processing and interpretation of specimen radiographs may be the responsibility of a pathologist, a surgeon, or a radiologist. However, certain principles enunciated below apply in most situations.

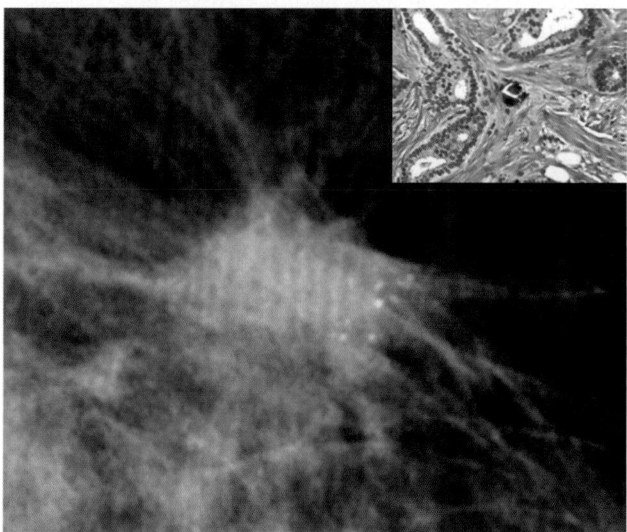

FIG. 44.7. ***Radiologic–pathologic correlation.*** Magnified view of mammogram of the right breast from a 63-year-old woman reveals a stellate soft tissue density that upon excision corresponded to an invasive well-differentiated ductal carcinoma [*inset*]. Calcifications within the lesion seen in the mammogram corresponded to stromal calcifications.

An x-ray of the intact excisional biopsy specimen should be obtained, and if possible, it should be compared with the mammogram. If the tissue is dissected prior to obtaining a specimen x-ray, disruption of the pattern of calcifications may occur. Changes in the position, that is, orientation, of the specimen may make it difficult to locate calcifications. Radiographs of NCB specimens should also be obtained (Fig. 44.9).

It is recommended that nonpalpable mammographically detected lesions be processed solely for permanent sections, and that frozen sections be performed only in exceptional situations.[1] In one study of 359 mammographically detected lesions, frozen section yielded a correct diagnosis in 68% of cases, 17.3% did not have a frozen section, 1.9% of frozen sections yielded false-negative results, and 0.6% were false-positive diagnoses.[118]

The immediate goal of specimen radiography is to confirm that a nonpalpable lesion has been excised. Ideally, this should be determined intraoperatively. If the lesion is not present in the specimen, the surgeon may elect to obtain more tissue at that time or a postoperative mammogram at a later date. Postoperative clinical mammography is reportedly useful to evaluate patients with a negative or inconclusive specimen radiograph following biopsy of a lesion with or without calcifications.[119] Others recommend delaying postoperative mammography for 6 to 12 weeks after biopsy to minimize

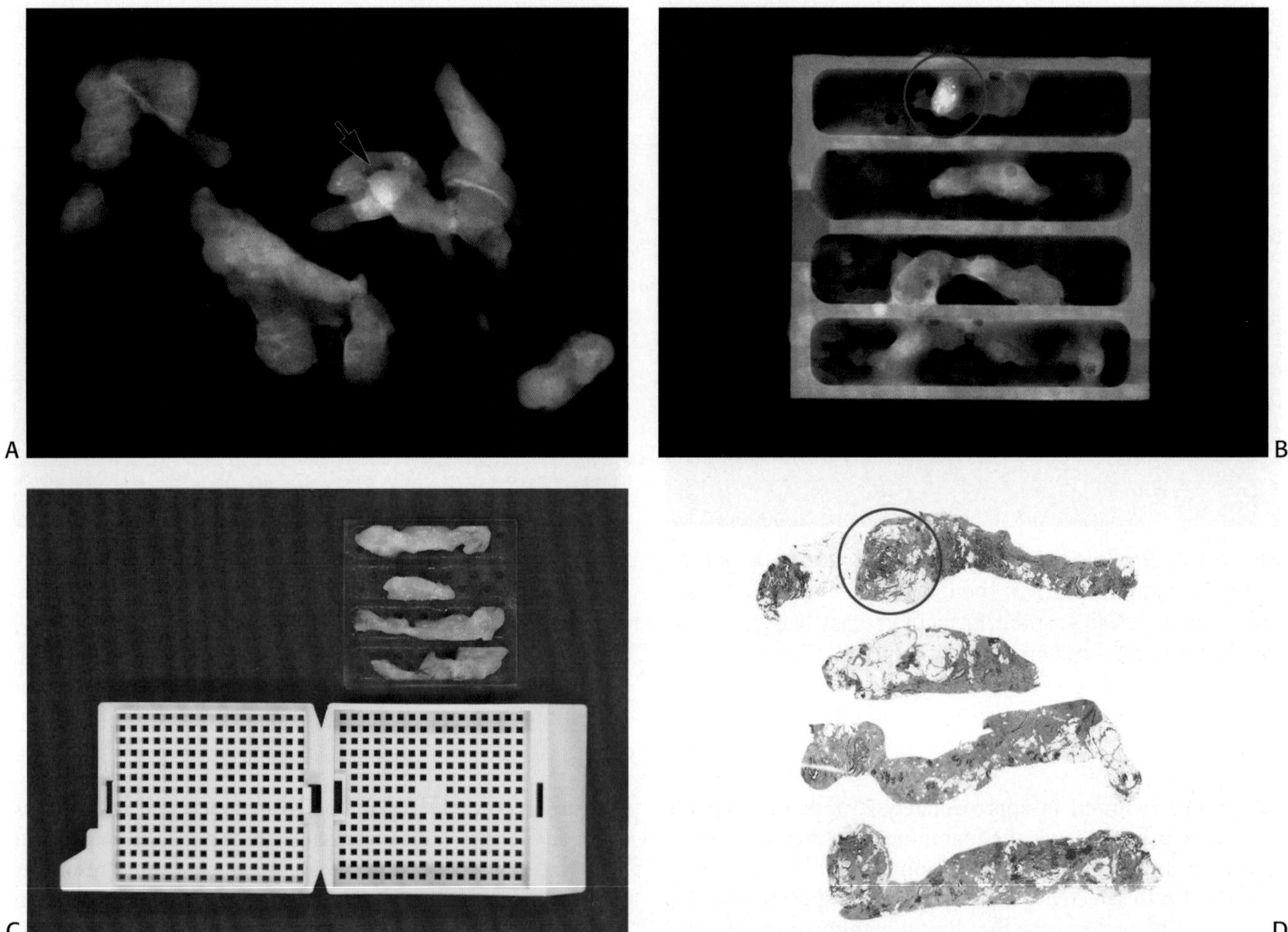

FIG. 44.9. ***Radiologic–pathologic correlation in a needle core biopsy specimen.*** A commercially available tissue "tray" can facilitate radiology–pathology correlation mainly by allowing the usually fragile biopsied tissue to maintain its orientation and integrity.[160] **A:** A set of NCB samples in a specimen radiograph. The *arrow* indicates the suspicious lesion. **B:** The individual NCB specimens have been placed into one of the four separate slots in the "tray." This radiograph of the tray indicates the location of the lesional tissue (*circle*). **C:** The tray fits into a standard tissue cassette for histologic processing. The biopsies are embedded into the tissue block with the same orientation as in the "tray." **D:** The corresponding histologic slides have the tissue samples with similar orientation, allowing ready radiologic–pathologic comparison of the circled calcifications and density. (Courtesy of Dr. O. Tawfik.)

discomfort associated with the procedure and to allow subsidence of postsurgical inflammation that may obscure the mammogram.[120] Missed lesions have been reported in up to 13.6% of needle localization biopsies,[121] but in most series this occurred in 5% or less of cases.[122–124]

False-negative specimen radiographs may occur because the lesion has been distorted by the operation, by dissection after excision, or as a result of positioning of the specimen that obscured the lesion when the image was obtained. The specimen radiograph may also be negative because of inaccurate preoperative localization or loss of localization resulting from displacement of a needle or wire used in this procedure. Finally, the position of calcifications may be misjudged in conventional mammographic views if localization has not been performed. Cutaneous calcifications can be misinterpreted as an intraparenchymal lesion.[125] Tangential views and stereotactic imaging are useful for confirming the cutaneous position of such calcifications.[126] One unusual cutaneous abnormality that may mimic calcifications in the breast is a skin tattoo.[127] Tattoo powder applied to specimens to mark margins is an iatrogenic source of microcalcification-like particles that may interfere with the interpretation of a specimen radiograph.[128]

A variety of procedures are available to mark areas in the breast preoperatively in order to guide the surgeon in excision of the lesion and to minimize the size of the specimen required. These include the placement of one or more needles or hooked wires in proximity to the lesion[129,130] and, some years earlier, the injection of dyes.[131,132] Presently, almost all localization procedures employ either a wire or a needle placement technique with ultrasound or stereotactic guidance or radioactive seed localization. The latter procedure is an effective approach, and it may be used in the surgical excision of previously biopsied radiographically identified lesions, and serve an alternative to the placement of marker "clips," which can "migrate." Radioactive seed localization is an increasingly utilized approach that is as acceptable to patients, radiologists, and surgeons as the wire or needle localization approach, and it may offer the considerable added benefit of a lower positive margin rate.[133] This method of localization has been successfully used to guide surgery following neoadjuvant chemotherapy—in unifocal as well as multifocal tumors.[134] The principles for the safe handling of radioactive seeds in breast specimens have been outlined.[135]

The various aforementioned techniques for localization assist the surgeon and the pathologist in finding the targeted lesion. Before the position of the specimen is changed after imaging, the site of the radiographically detected calcifications or a density should be identified grossly. This targeted portion of the tissue should be excised *en bloc* from the specimen and labeled. The remainder of the tissue must also be dissected, since occasionally calcifications lie in a benign process near an unanticipated carcinoma fortuitously included in an excisional biopsy.

It is essential that the localization wire or wires remain within the excisional biopsy specimen when it is delivered to the pathology laboratory. The pathologist must describe the wire or wires in the gross specimen report. It is advisable that the length of wire or wires be measured. Localization wires have occasionally been inadvertently transected intraoperatively, or they may retract into the breast preoperatively and migrate from the lesion in question.[136,137] In one remarkable case, a retracted wire reportedly migrated to the subcutaneous tissue of the ipsilateral buttock.[137]

Most of the lesions that are the target of a wire localization biopsy procedure are microscopic. Unless there is a compelling clinical need, FSE is not recommended in these cases.[1] If a decision is made to attempt a frozen section and the diagnosis is not readily apparent immediately, further sectioning should not be carried out and the remaining tissue must be fixed for permanent sections. The surgeon must defer to the pathologist's judgment as to the feasibility of obtaining a diagnosis by frozen section in this, as in any other, situation.

The identification of calcifications in NCB specimens can be facilitated by the provision of the corresponding specimen radiograph (Fig. 44.9). The latter also provides evidence for the removal of the target calcification, and guides the pathologist in correlating the microscopic finding with the radiologic appearance of the lesion.

PATHOLOGY OF MAMMARY CALCIFICATIONS

Calcium Phosphate Calcifications

Microcalcifications found in breast tissue were thoroughly described and classified by Frappart et al.,[138,139] and the basic characteristics of calcifications in breast lesions were outlined by Tse et al.[140] The majority of calcifications detected in mammograms are basophilic concretions of varying size composed of calcium phosphates largely in the form of hydroxyapatite[141] (Fig. 44.10). These type II calcifications of Frapport are not birefringent. They react with the von Kossa stain and with alizarin red at pH 4.2 and 7.0.[142] A black precipitate is formed with silver nitrate/rubeanic acid, but not after pretreatment with 5% acetic acid.[142,143]

Foschini et al.[144] described the patterns of calcium phosphate calcifications in DCIS. Granular calcifications were formed by deposition of calcium on nuclear debris or on secreted

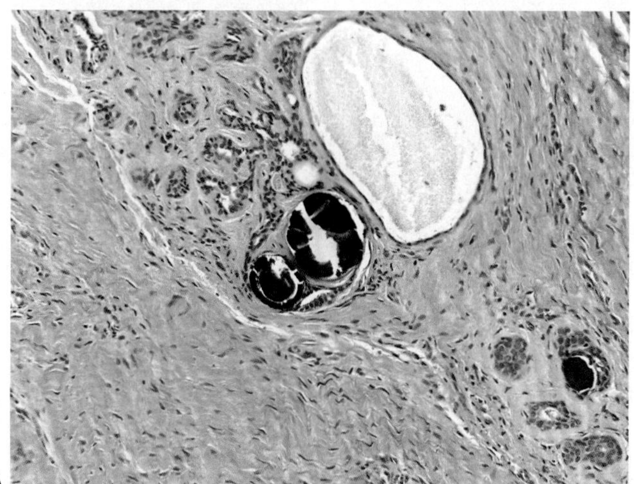
A

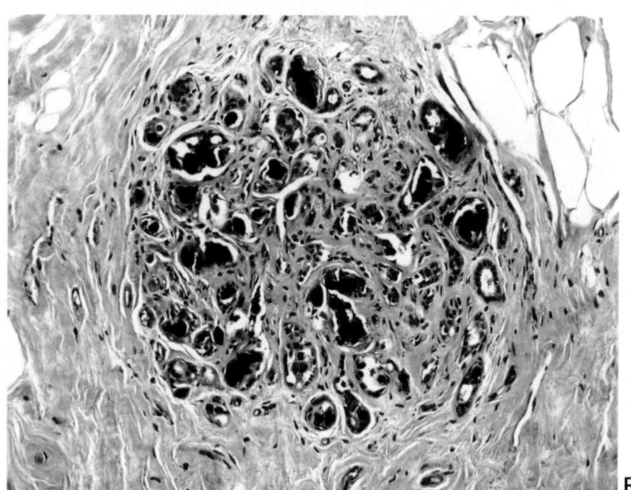
B

FIG. 44.10. ***Calcification in breast tissue.*** Various configurations of phosphate calcifications are depicted. **A:** Microcalcifications of the psammomatous type in lobules. **B:** Calcifications in sclerosing adenosis (SA). **C:** An "ossifying" type of calcification in DCIS. **D:** Calcifications in extreme glandular atrophy. The patient was a nanogenerian. **E:** Calcifications of the fine powdery and coarsely granular types are seen in a mucin-filled cyst. A mucocele-like lesion (*not shown*) was present in the vicinity. **F:** Arterial intramural calcification. **G:** Dense stromal calcifications. **H:** Coarse calcifications in a lobule in a case with complete pathologic response following neoadjuvant chemotherapy.

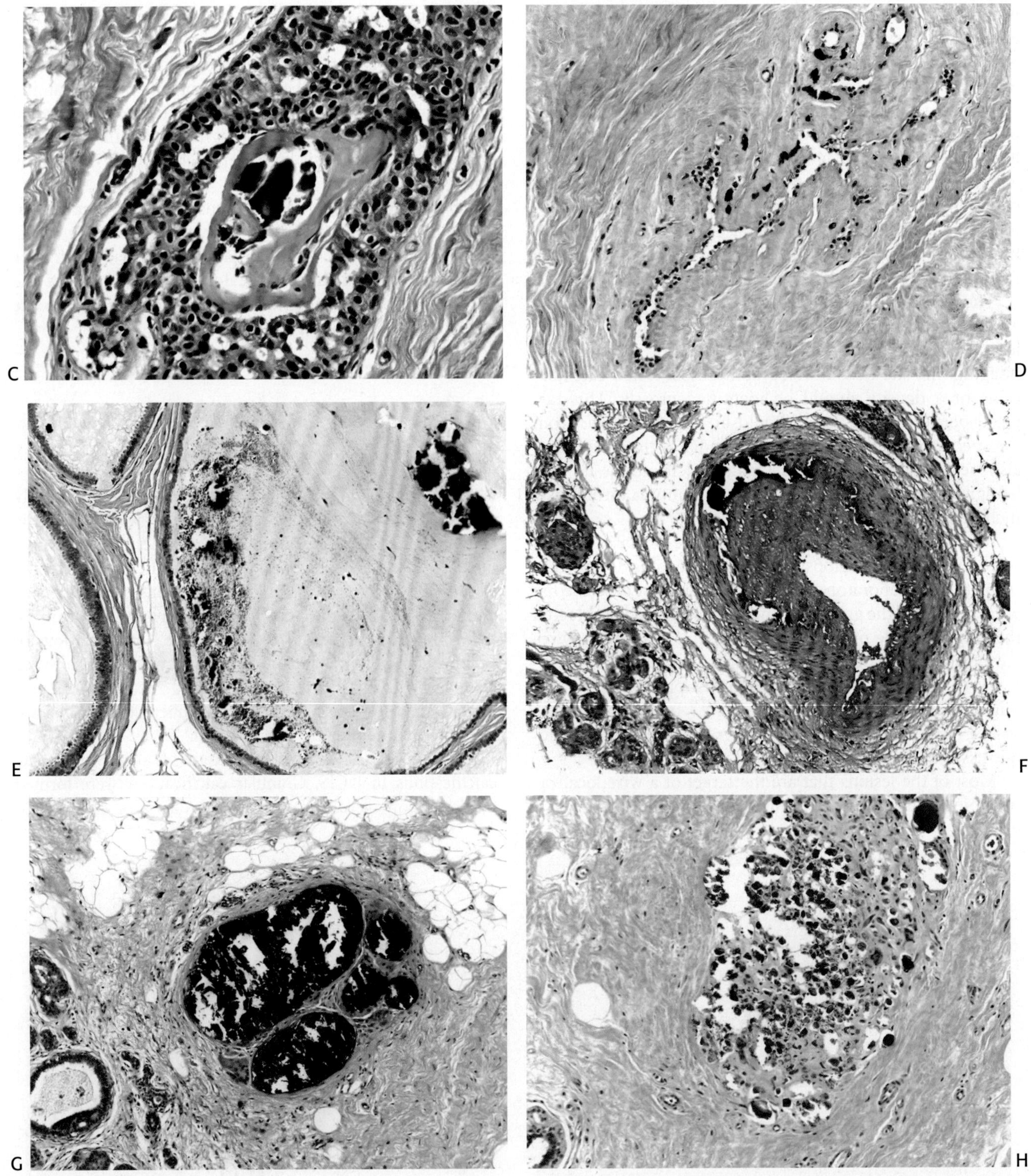

FIG. 44.10. *(Continued)*

mucosubstances. Lamellar calcifications resulted from deposits of calcium on proteinaceous or mucoid material arranged in concentric layers. Calcification on nuclear debris was found only in DCIS with necrosis of intermediate or poorly differentiated grade, whereas the other types of calcification were present mainly in well to moderately differentiated lesions.

Calcium Oxalate Calcifications

Type I microcalcifications of Frappart composed of calcium oxalate dihydrate crystals (Weddelite) are birefringent, nonbasophilic, von Kossa–negative crystals[141,143,145] (Fig. 44.11). The term "Weddelite" derives from the fact that calcium

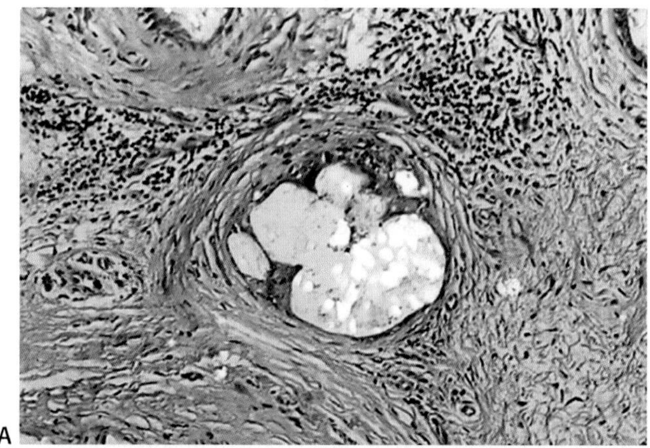
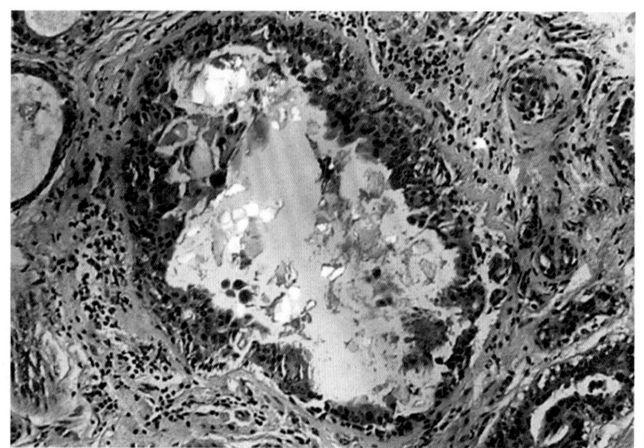

FIG. 44.11. ***Calcium oxalate calcifications.*** **A:** The calcifications appear as bright birefringent crystals in a duct in this section of mastitis. **B:** Calcium oxalate crystals are birefringent in this duct with apocrine epithelium (polarized illumination).

oxalate used commercially was originally extracted from the Weddell Sea, located south of the Falkland Islands, named after the British explorer James Weddell (1787 to 1834).[146] Calcium oxalate calcifications are not stained by alizarin red at pH 4.2, and at pH 7.0 alizarin red staining is weak or absent. Black staining is observed with silver nitrate/rubeanic acid, with or without pretreatment with 5% acetic acid.[143] Because they are colorless, calcium oxalate crystals are difficult to identify in hematoxylin and eosin (H&E)–stained sections with standard light microscopy. They tend to fragment and are sometimes accompanied by multinucleated giant cells. Intact crystals assume various configurations including overlapping plates, rosettes, sheaves, rods, and geometric shapes such as pyramids or diamonds (Fig. 44.12).

In one series, 9 of 66 (13.6%) mammographically detected calcifications identified histologically consisted of calcium oxalate crystals, 72.7% were calcium phosphate, and 13.6% were a mixture of calcium oxalate and calcium phosphate.[141] Similar frequencies of calcium phosphate and oxalate calcifications have been found by other investigators.[147] Tornos et al.[143] reported finding calcium oxalate calcifications alone in 2% and in combination with calcium phosphate calcifications in 10.4% of 153 specimens. Calcium oxalate crystals have been responsible for 7.3%[145] and 12%[148] of mammographically localized calcifications that led to biopsy. Calcium oxalate crystals can rarely appear in fine-needle aspiration (FNA) biopsy specimens of breast, wherein they usually appear in clusters and are strongly birefringent under polarizing microscopy.[149]

Calcium phosphate calcifications and calcium oxalate crystals appear as conventional calcifications in specimen radiographs and in clinical mammograms. Calcium phosphate calcifications typically have high to medium density, and they may have irregular or distinct shapes suggestive of carcinoma in a mammogram, whereas calcium oxalate crystals are likely to appear as polyhedral deposits of low- to medium density.[150] An analysis of 2,000 screening mammograms revealed that 3% of women examined had two or more polyhedral microcalcifications.[151]

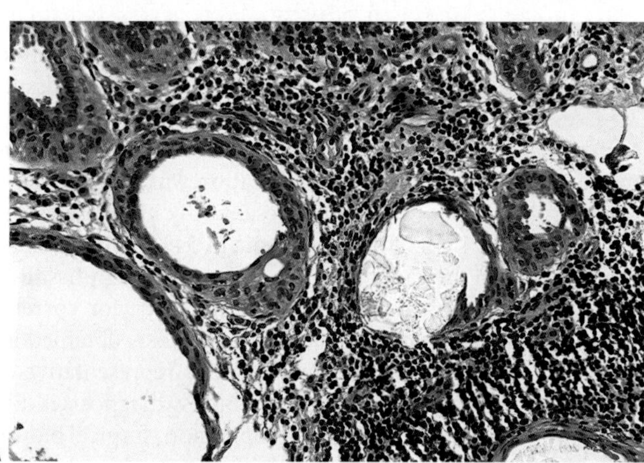
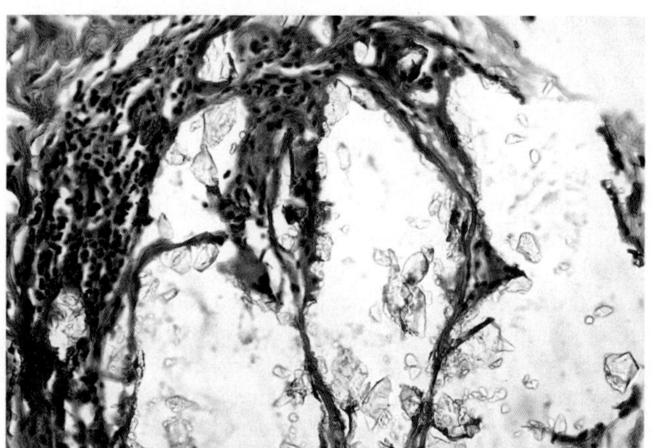

FIG. 44.12. ***Calcium oxalate calcification.*** **A:** The visibility of these crystals was enhanced when the tissue was examined with the microscope condenser lowered to heighten refractivity. **B:** Fragmented crystals in a duct with surrounding inflammation.

Calcium oxalate crystals are most frequently seen in benign cysts, especially those lined by apocrine epithelium, and in dilated ducts (Figs. 44.11 and 44.12).[141,143,145,147,152,153] This association suggests that apocrine epithelium is able to synthesize or concentrate and secrete oxalic acid or calcium oxalate. In some cases, calcium phosphate calcifications have been present coincidentally with calcium oxalate deposits in proliferative lesions. It is unusual for calcium oxalate crystals to develop in carcinoma.[139,152] Calcium oxalate crystals have been described in papillary DCIS.[154]

Calcium oxalate crystals probably account for the majority of instances in which "calcifications" are reportedly not present in histologic sections of breast biopsies obtained for calcifications found in a mammogram.[155,156] In this situation, sections should be examined with polarized light. Fragments of birefringent material may be the only residual evidence of larger crystalline deposits that are sometimes shattered or partially dissolved during processing of the tissue.

Localizing Calcifications in Tissue Blocks

Radiographic examination of paraffin-embedded tissue blocks is an essential procedure if a biopsy has been performed for calcifications and they are not evident in the histologic sections.[157] Calcifications are easily identified in the resultant x-ray images of the blocks. This allows the pathologist to select blocks for deeper sections. Radiographs should be obtained to document the presence of calcifications in NCB samples.[158,159] A novel, recently described device ensures maintenance of orientation of NCB samples from procurement through microscopic evaluation (Fig. 44.9). After mammographic identification of calcifications, the NCBs are harvested, placed in tissue trays, and then x-rayed to confirm calcifications. The tray with the corresponding radiograph is submitted to the laboratory, where the core biopsies are placed into cassettes without "disturbing" the orientation of the cores. This procedure facilitates the ready identification of calcifications in NCB specimens.[160]

Calcifications may be lost in the course of trimming paraffin blocks that is part of the process of preparing routine histologic sections. Winston et al.[161] documented the presence of calcifications in microtome shavings, including some particles larger than the thickness of paraffin sections that were apparently fractured and then knocked out of the tissue by the microtome blade.

The number of sections taken from tissue blocks for the evaluation of calcifications in NCBs remains a matter of some debate. The need to conserve tissue for any immediate or future ancillary studies is a major consideration, as are factors relating to resources and finances. Be that as it may, it is recommended that at least two H&E-stained levels, cut approximately 50 μm apart, be evaluated initially. Additional levels could be obtained if needed. Lee et al.[162] have proposed that while the histologic examination of multiple levels is useful in the evaluation of calcifications, the examination of one level alone may suffice for cases in which the biopsies were taken for reasons other than calcifications.

BI-RADS Classification of Calcifications

Image analysis has been used to study calcifications as they appear in mammograms in order to refine the characterization of calcification associated with benign and malignant lesions.[163–166] Features examined included the number of particles in a cluster, the number of clusters, distances between calcifications in a cluster, and the area of clusters. Data from these analyses may lead to the development of automated image screening systems for calcifications, but such procedures cannot replace the interpretation of noncalcific parenchymal alterations.

Calcifications in clinical mammography are currently reported according to the American College of Radiology Breast Imaging Reporting and Data System (BI-RADS) classification.[167] The BI-RADS lexicon definitions range from category 1 (*normal*) to categories 5 (*highly suspicious*) and 6 (*histologically proven malignancy*). Variability in the application of BI-RADS can lead to classification errors, especially in category 3 lesions, that is, those interpreted to be probably benign, needing short-term follow-up.[168]

Calcifications classified as ductal are typically linear if associated with carcinoma, and often branching, whereas benign ductal calcifications are described as "rod-like." Nonductal calcifications are typically punctate, pleomorphic, or coarse irregular deposits. The distribution is usually reported as clustered, linear, segmental, or regional.

Relationships of Calcifications to Primary and Recurrent Carcinoma

The precise microanatomic distribution of calcifications is an important consideration when correlating imaging findings with the pathologic diagnosis. Although the presence of calcifications may contribute to the radiologic impression that leads to a biopsy procedure and the finding of carcinoma, some of the calcifications may not be located in the carcinoma. This becomes a concern especially when an NCB procedure is performed to sample a lesion with intermediate (BI-RADS 3) or suspicious (BI-RADS 4) calcifications. In some instances the needle biopsy sample shown to contain calcifications by specimen x-ray and histologic examination can be an unrepresentative specimen of peritumoral tissue. To assess this issue, Selim and Tahan[169] studied the distribution of calcifications in benign tissue surrounding carcinomas and in the carcinomas. Calcification was limited to the carcinoma in 31% of cases and present only in benign components within 1 cm of the carcinoma in 34%. Calcifications were present in the carcinoma and adjacent benign tissue in 35%. These observations underscore the need for correlation between mammography and the diagnosis obtained by NCB to determine whether the sample is representative of the radiographic image. If the benign biopsy diagnosis is discordant with the mammographic impression, surgical biopsy should be considered, even if calcifications were obtained and documented in the NCB.

Calcifications are often an important clue to the presence of recurrent carcinoma in the breast after conservation therapy. Dershaw et al.[170] found that at least 10 calcifications were present in 17 of 22 (77%) breast recurrences. The patterns of calcification were classified as highly suspicious for carcinoma (BI-RADS 5) in 77% of cases and as suggestive of carcinoma requiring biopsy (BI-RADS 4) in the remaining cases. Less worrisome punctate and coarse calcifications were also present in 36% and 14% of cases, respectively, but these were always coincidental with malignant patterns of calcification. Other investigators have not observed the same degree of calcification specificity in the breast after conservation therapy.[171] When an NCB sample from the site of a possible breast recurrence shows calcifications and benign histologic changes, the results must be integrated with the radiologic and mammographic findings in order to determine if surgical excision should be performed.

In recent years, the technique of procuring NCBs of the breast has evolved toward the use of vacuum-assisted devices with larger (8- to 11-G) needles rather than that of semiautomatic guns with smaller (14- to 18-G) needles. Also, markers made of titanium, stainless steel, or carbon-coated ceramic are increasingly being deployed during the procedure to indicate the biopsy site. These markers serve to guide subsequent radiologic studies (mainly for follow-up purposes), surgical procedures (especially to guide subsequent wire localization and excisional biopsy), and pathologic examination (particularly to indicate the tumor bed in the event neoadjuvant chemotherapy leads to apparent dissolution of the tumor mass). However, the use of larger needles and vacuum-assisted techniques removes relatively larger volume of tissue, leaving a large biopsy cavity. Marker clips placed in this setting have been reported to become displaced or "migrate" a distance of more than 1 cm from the biopsy site in 28% of cases.[172] In an attempt to prevent migration, clips "with grips" and those surrounded by bioresorbable collagen "plug" material have been devised. The plug has a distinctive "collagen-like" histologic appearance, and it elicits only minimal reactive changes. However, microcalcifications formed in these plugs within 7 to 14 months can hinder subsequent radiologic follow-up (see later).

Changes in Number of Calcifications in Clinical Mammograms

Spontaneous "disappearance" of calcifications has been documented *in vivo* with serial mammograms.[173,174] The composition of calcifications prone to this process is not known, but follow-up studies suggest that the associated lesions are usually benign.[173] A study of NCB specimens revealed that radiographically detectable calcifications could no longer be seen in x-rays of the specimens after several days of storage in aqueous solutions, including 10% formalin, whereas the calcifications were preserved in samples stored in ethanol.[175]

An increase in the number and extent of calcifications raises concern for the presence of carcinoma. Rapid expansion of the area of calcifications has been associated with high-grade DCIS with necrosis (i.e., comedo DCIS), whereas slower growth of calcifications characterizes noncomedo DCIS.[176] The mean doubling time for all DCIS based on the extent of calcifications was 118.0 ± 111.2 days (range, 18 to 539 days). The mean diameters of noncomedo and comedo DCIS based on the distribution of calcifications were 255.8 ± 71.1 μm and 302.7 ± 232.0 μm, respectively, using a computerized image analysis system.

Calcifications and Systemic Diseases

Mammographically detected calcifications can be a manifestation of systemic conditions.[177] Awareness of various patterns of calcifications as well as other forms of radiologic abnormalities in various systemic diseases can aid in differentiating primary mammary lesions from systemic diseases. In one case, a diagnosis of Klippel–Trénaunay syndrome (characterized by nevus flammeus, vascular malformations, and hypertrophy of soft and bony tissue) was made after calcifications found in a routine mammogram were shown to be localized to subcutaneous vascular structures.[178] Chronic renal failure can be associated with "metastatic" calcifications in soft tissues and blood vessels at various sites including the breast.[179,180]

The relationship of arterial calcifications to cardiovascular disease and diabetes mellitus has been the subject of a number of studies. Arterial calcifications were found in 9% of mammograms from women aged 50 to 68 years at entry into a screening program, and in 15.4% of the women studied who had diabetes mellitus.[181] Overall excess cardiovascular mortality of 40% was found after 16 to 19 years of follow-up among women with arterial calcifications (hazard ratio [HR], 1.4; 95% CI, 1.1 to 1.8), and in the group with diabetes excess mortality due to cardiovascular disease was 90% (HR, 1.9; 95% CI, 1.1 to 3.2).

Maas et al.[182] studied risk factors associated with mammographically detected arterial calcifications in a cohort derived from a breast cancer–screening program. Arterial calcifications were found in 194 of 1,699 women (11%). The frequency increased with age. After adjusting for age, the presence of arterial calcifications was associated with parity, being present in 2.5% of nulliparous women, 9% with one or two children, and in 17% of women with three or more children. Arterial calcifications were significantly related to breast-feeding. Maas et al.[183] have also reported that the prevalence of arterial calcifications in mammograms from a cohort of women with increased risk of cardiovascular disease was 23%. The risk of arterial calcifications was 58% greater in diabetics than in nondiabetics. Kataoka et al.[184] found that arterial calcifications detected in screening mammograms were associated with prevalent coronary artery disease, with an odds ratio of 2.54 (95% CI, 1.03 to 6.30). There was an inverse relation to smoking, an observation also reported by Maas et al.[182] These and other studies[185,186] suggest that mammographically detected vascular calcifications may be an indicator of coronary heart disease, especially in women with diabetes mellitus.

Noncalcified Crystalloids

Noncalcified crystalloids found in the salivary gland ducts also occur very rarely in mammary ducts or lobules, and

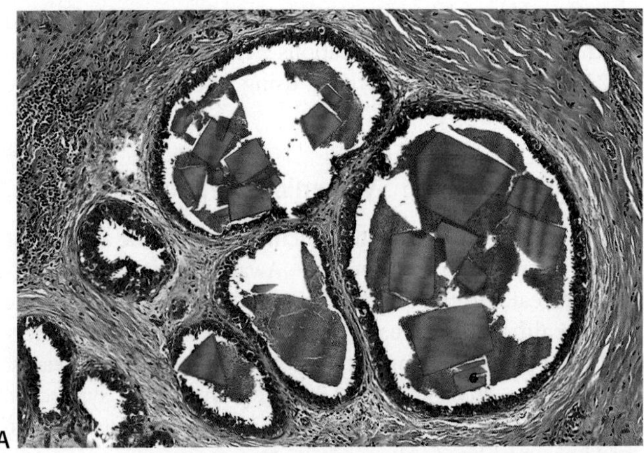

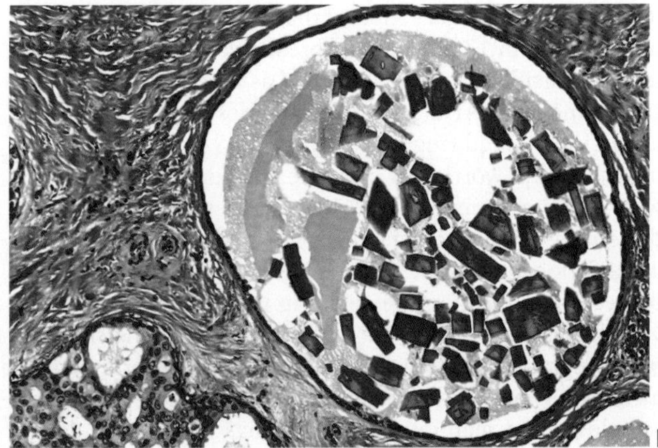

FIG. 44.13. ***Noncalcified crystalloids.*** **A,B:** Characteristic rectangular and triangular shapes are shown associated with proteinaceous secretion in small cysts. **B:** A gland contiguous to one with crystalloids shows ADH.

they may be associated with DCIS.[187] These deposits are not visualized in mammograms and are not birefringent. Histologic examination reveals eosinophilic, variously shaped crystal-like deposits (needles, rhomboid, hexagonal, plate, and tetrahedral) measuring up to 500 μm with an average size of 20 μm (Fig. 44.13). Secretion on the surfaces of crystalloids is stained with Alcian blue, mucicarmine, periodic acid–Schiff (PAS), and the antibody for epithelial membrane antigen (EMA). Crystalloids are electron-dense when examined by electron microscopy, and they do not contain calcium phosphate hydroxyapatite or calcium oxalate. The source of crystalloids in the breast is not known, but it has been speculated that they are formed by crystallization of protein–carbohydrate complexes in abnormal secretions produced by the epithelium.

Liesegang-like rings, concentric structures formed by a complex chemical reaction, can occasionally be encountered in benign mammary glands with pregnancy-like changes.[188] These rings may not be mammographically evident, unless there is a calcified center therein.

NCB AS AN INITIAL DIAGNOSTIC PROCEDURE

The increasing use of ultrasound-directed or stereotactic-guided core biopsies has made it possible to reliably sample a growing number of nonpalpable radiographically detected lesions. In one series of 100 such lesions at least 5 mm in diameter, NCB procedures correctly identified 35 of 36 carcinomas that were confirmed by surgical biopsy.[189] Five to six core biopsy specimens obtained with a 14-G needle provide adequate samples for the diagnosis of most lesions. Liberman et al.[190] found that six cores proved to be diagnostic in 92% of mammographic lesions with calcifications, whereas five cores were sufficient for 99% of mass lesions.

There is generally a high level of concordance between the diagnosis obtained with stereotactic NCB and the subsequent surgical excision. Gisvold et al.[191] reported a slightly higher concordance rate for benign (90%) than for malignant lesions (85%) if at least five cores were obtained. When there were fewer than five cores, the concordance rates decreased to 66% and 34% for benign and carcinomatous lesions, respectively. The positive predictive value (PPV) of stereotactic NCB for the presence of invasion in patients with carcinoma was 98% in 48 cases.[192] In the one discordant instance, a fragment of DCIS displaced into fat in a core biopsy sample was mistakenly interpreted as invasive carcinoma (Fig. 44.14). Intrinsic invasive carcinoma was found in 3 of 15 excisional biopsy specimens from other patients who had only DCIS in needle biopsy samples. Liberman[193] has reviewed the diagnostic reliability of NCB procedures. A high level of concordance

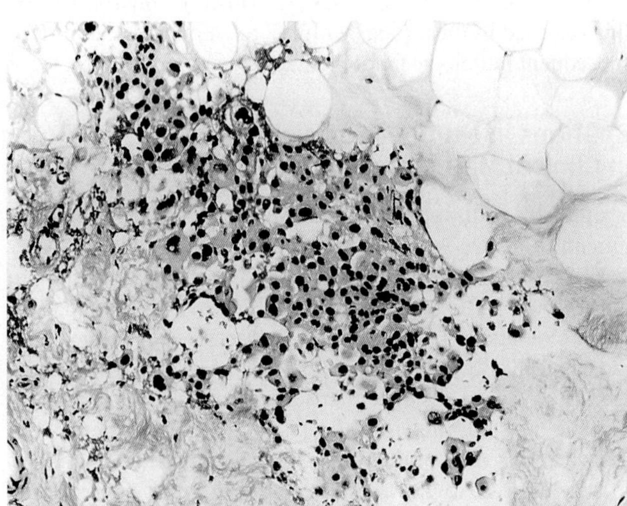

FIG. 44.14. ***Displaced carcinoma in a stereotactic needle core biopsy sample.*** This specimen was mistakenly interpreted as invasive carcinoma. It shows carcinoma displaced in fat. The subsequent excisional biopsy showed only DCIS with additional displaced epithelium.

between tumor type and grade, as well as hormone receptors and HER2 status between NCB and the subsequent surgical excision, is generally obtained.

Pathologic Changes Attributable to Needling Procedures

The placement of localizing wires has become precise with the widespread use of stereotactic procedures. Direct penetration of the lesion is sought when biopsy is combined with localization. Follow-up mammography performed 6 months after stereotactic 14-G biopsy revealed no mammographically detectable architectural distortion attributable to the procedure in 24 patients studied by Kaye et al.[194] In two instances, there were fewer calcifications in postbiopsy mammograms, and a 6-mm fibroadenoma contained a 3 × 2 mm^2 defect. These and other observations suggest that the procedure, at least when performed conservatively, usually does not cause longstanding structural changes in the breast that might interfere with later radiographic studies.

Nonetheless, some traumatic changes invariably occur in the breast tissue as a result of needle localization and biopsy procedures (Figs. 44.14 to 44.26). Displacement of benign or malignant epithelium into the breast stroma can be found in subsequent excisional biopsies. Fragments of cutaneous squamous epithelium displaced by needles into the breast can form epidermal inclusion cysts.[195] Conversely, rare instances of carcinoma displaced to the skin as a result of NCB procedures have been reported. In one instance, carcinoma cells accompanied by hemosiderin-laden macrophages were found in dermal lymphatic channels after an NCB, and mastectomy revealed DCIS with carcinomatous epithelial displacement in the needle track and in lymphatics of the breast.[196] Carcinomatous deposits in the dermis of the skin after "multiple-puncture biopsy" were reported in two patients by Stolier et al.[197] One of these patients developed a clinical skin recurrence 34 months after the procedure. Chao et al.[198] described two patients with subcutaneous recurrence of carcinoma in the site of a prior NCB procedure. The recurrences were detected 12 and 17 months postbiopsy. A third patient was found to have microscopic deposit of carcinoma in the skin in a mastectomy specimen.

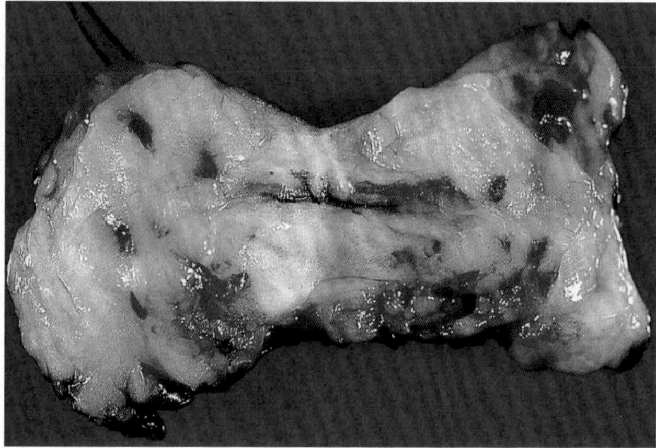

FIG. 44.15. ***Traumatic effects of needle core biopsy.*** This excisional biopsy specimen was obtained after stereotactic biopsies were performed. The specimen has been incised to expose the interior. The punctate *red* foci are needle tracks.

Displaced DCIS cells have been observed in breast stroma and within vascular channels in breast specimens obtained subsequent to needling procedures. In patients with DCIS, these displaced carcinoma fragments can mimic stromal invasion, and, in some circumstances, they represent a potential source of misdiagnosis of intrinsic invasive carcinoma. Histologic findings suggesting displacement of DCIS include the presence of scattered, isolated fragments of carcinomatous epithelium in artifactual spaces within breast stroma, accompanied by hemorrhage, fat necrosis, inflammation, hemosiderin-laden macrophages, or granulation tissue. Calcifications and "foamy" histiocytes of the type commonly seen in intraductal lesions may be associated with displaced carcinomatous epithelium in the stroma or in vascular channels. The extent to which breast needling procedures might contribute lymphovascular dispersal of tumor cells has not been determined.

Papillary lesions are especially vulnerable to epithelial displacement after needling procedures because of their intrinsic fragile structure.[199,200] Reactive changes at needling sites in papillary lesions may evolve into nodular foci of spindle cell proliferation that are composed of proliferating myofibroblasts and blood vessels, as well as inflammatory cells.[201] Benign and carcinomatous papillary epithelium may be found embedded in such nodules.

Boppana et al.[202] reviewed 100 consecutive breast carcinomas that had been subjected to prior FNA, and noted displaced epithelial fragments in 36% of cases. Youngson et al.[203,204] reviewed slides from 43 consecutive cases in which surgical biopsy and/or mastectomy had been performed following an initial 14-G core biopsy diagnosis of breast carcinoma, and identified displaced epithelial fragments outside of the primary lesion in 12 of the cases (28%). However, multiple needling procedures (e.g., local anesthetic injection in all 43 cases, needle localization in 22 of 43 cases, suture placement in 18 of 43 cases, and FNA in 1 of 43 cases) had been performed in each of the cases reviewed. Hoorntje et al.[205] reported finding displaced carcinoma cells in 11 of 22 (50%) needle tracks after 14-G needle biopsy procedures. Prospectively, these authors found displaced carcinoma in 7 (64%) or 11 needle tracks examined 7 to 35 days (median interval, 25 days) after 14-G needle biopsy. The frequency of epithelial displacement in the needle track has been reduced substantially but not eliminated since the introduction of vacuum-assisted stereotactic biopsy with an 11-G needle.[193]

The clinical significance of epithelial displacement remains largely uncertain. Chen et al.[206] investigated the potential role of NCB as a factor predisposing to breast recurrence after conserving surgery with radiotherapy. The breast recurrence rate was lower (2.3%) in women who underwent excision after a diagnostic NCB procedure than in those who had a needle-localized excisional biopsy without prior core

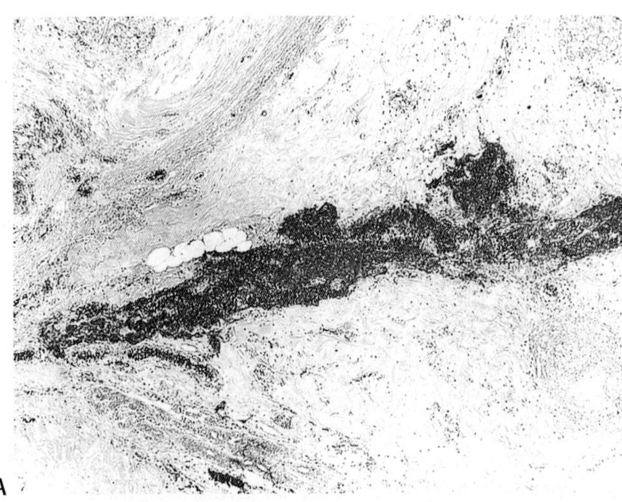

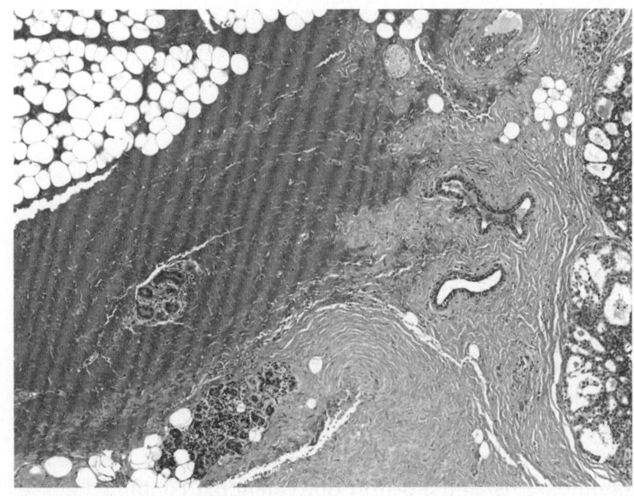

FIG. 44.16. ***Traumatic effects of needle core biopsy.*** **A:** Hemorrhage along a needle track is shown. **B:** This excisional biopsy specimen was obtained 2h after a radiographic needle localization procedure. Note fresh hemorrhage in a linear track and blood in a duct.

biopsy (5.4%) and patients with palpable tumors who had a nonimaged guided excision (10.3%). Although other factors such as margin status and tumor size probably influenced these results, they suggest that epithelial displacement that occurs in a substantial number of NCB sites is not a major factor contributing to breast recurrence. In many instances, the potential risk of local recurrence posed by displaced carcinoma is ameliorated because the biopsy site and needle track are removed in the subsequent excision.

Epithelial displacement presents a challenging diagnostic histopathologic problem. Eliciting a history of a previous needling procedure may help prevent an erroneous diagnosis of invasive carcinoma. A diagnosis of carcinoma should not be based solely on the presence of epithelium within stroma, since epithelial displacement has been observed following needling procedures in benign breast lesions, notably papillary ductal hyperplasia and intraductal papilloma.

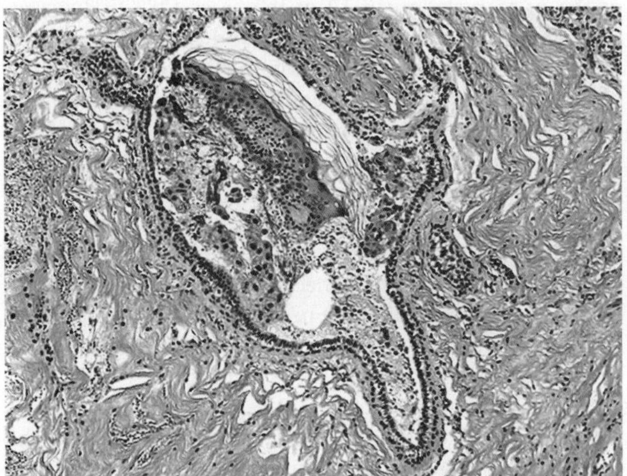

FIG. 44.17. ***Displaced apocrine epithelium and skin.*** Fragments of apocrine epithelium and epidermis from the skin have been displaced into the lumen of a duct.

The significance of carcinomatous lymphovascular emboli in the setting of epithelial displacement remains uncertain. Until further clinical information becomes available, the finding of lymphatic tumor emboli is considered to be a risk factor for transport of carcinoma cells to axillary lymph nodes (ALNs), even when conventional stromal invasion cannot be identified. As a general principle, the presence of carcinoma cells in a lymph node capsule or subcapsular sinus should be considered to represent metastatic carcinoma, even when no intrinsic stromal invasion is found in the breast. These cases often have carcinoma cells in lymphovascular spaces in the breast parenchyma in the vicinity of the needling procedure. One unusual patient presented with a clinically enlarged ALN diffusely involved by metastatic carcinoma 7 years after a mastectomy for DCIS that had been diagnosed by needle biopsy. Lymph nodes removed from the axilla at the time of mastectomy had no carcinoma identified in routine sections. Upon review, the site of the NCB in the breast exhibited carcinoma cells in lymphatic channels. The viability of DCIS or invasive carcinoma cells that may have been traumatically displaced into lymphovascular channels and possibly deposited in sites outside the breast is unknown, but the case just described raises the possibility that such cells could persist for a substantial period.

THERMAL (ELECTROCAUTERY) DAMAGE IN BIOPSY SPECIMENS

Electrocautery instruments used for the excision of tissue from the breast and other sites decrease blood loss from dissected tissues because the surfaces are coagulated as they are separated by the cutting edge. When used to perform an excisional breast biopsy, these instruments reduce the risk of

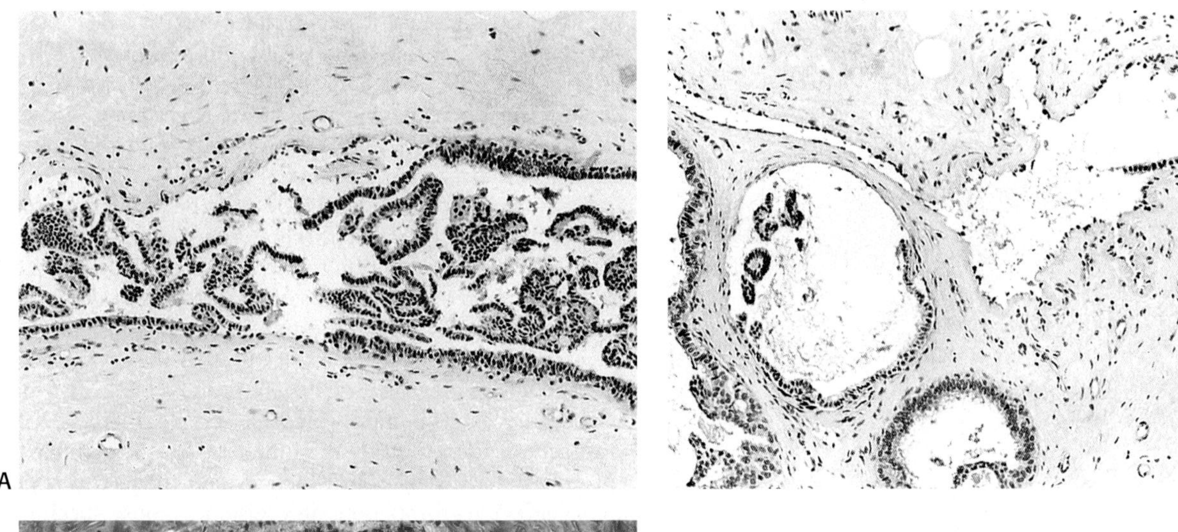

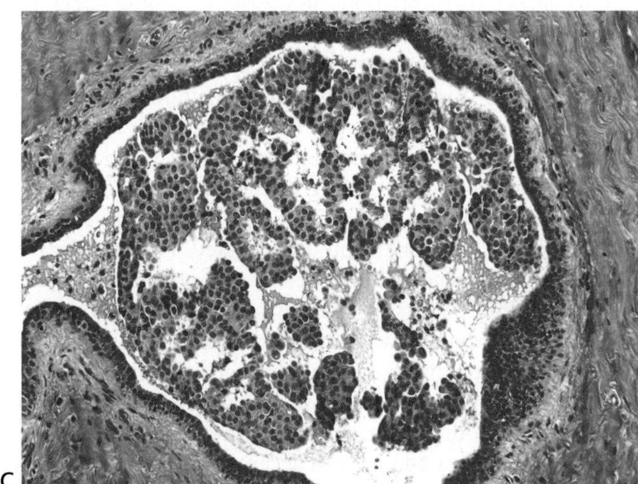

FIG. 44.18. ***Displaced epithelium within ducts.*** These photographs illustrate ductal epithelium displaced by FNA procedures. **A:** Fragments of ductal epithelium that were stripped off the basement membrane have been displaced into the ductal lumen. The detached epithelium resembles a papillary proliferation. **B:** Part of the duct shown in (A) is present in the *upper right* corner. There is detached epithelium in the cyst on the *left*. **C:** Papillary fragments of apocrine carcinoma are shown displaced into the lumen of an inactive duct after an FNA procedure.

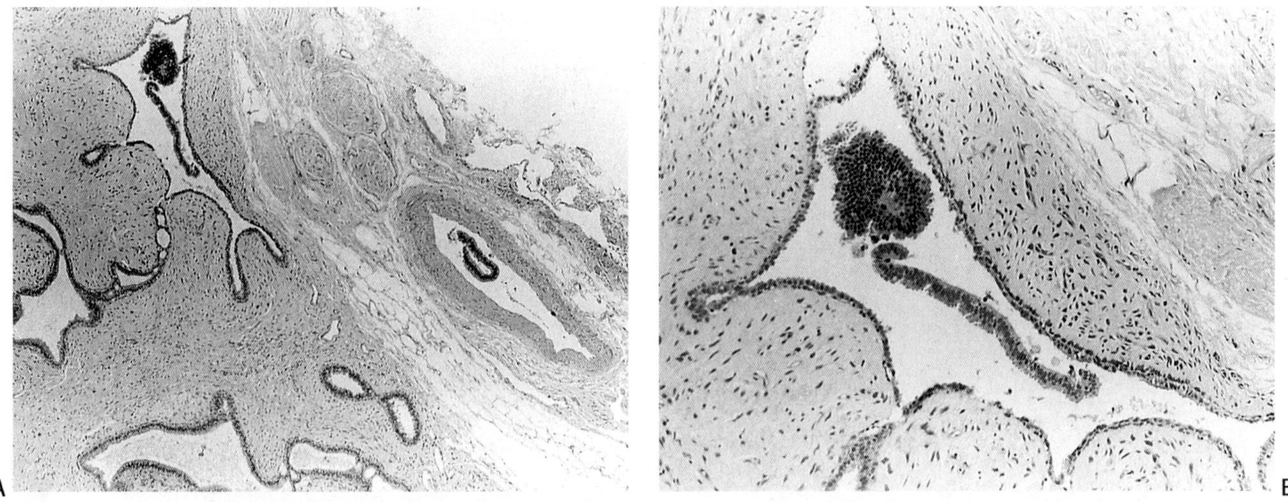

FIG. 44.19. ***Displaced benign epithelium in a fibroadenoma.*** **A:** Detached epithelium in an epithelial cleft in the tumor and in an artery on the *right* after an FNA biopsy. **B:** Epithelium in the cleft. **C:** Benign epithelium in the artery.

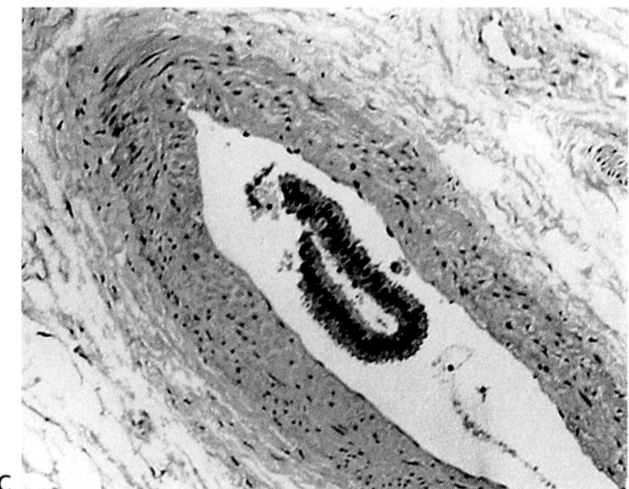

FIG. 44.19. *(Continued)*

hematoma formation in the biopsy cavity, and the operation can be completed in a shorter period of time.[207]

The thermal effect may produce significant changes in the tissues. Reduced biochemically measured estrogen receptor (ER) activity had been described some years ago when such testing was the norm,[208–210] with the decrease in receptor activity sufficient to result in a false-negative report.[211] Immunohistochemical study of breast (and prostate) specimens after electrocautery treatment also reveals a decrease in steroid binding[208,209](Fig. 44.27).

The histologic changes in the breast caused by thermal injury are similar to those seen at other sites. Thermal damage is most severe at the surface of the specimen, generally penetrating not more than 1 mm. The manner in which the instrument is used, the character of the tissue, and the size of the specimen removed influence the intensity and depth of the effect. The most significant effects are alterations in cytologic detail. Microscopic architecture may be so distorted that the distinction between normal, hyperplastic, and neoplastic tissues is impossible (Figs. 44.28 and 44.29). Because the damage is maximal at the edges or surfaces of the tissues, thermal artifacts can severely limit the assessment of the margins of excision (Figs. 44.28 and 44.30). If an excision is carried out with little or no breast parenchyma surrounding a carcinoma, thermal damage may occur in the tumor itself. In addition to the risk of altering results of receptor activity testing, the histologic artifacts can interfere with the diagnosis or classification of the tumor, and with the assessment of microscopic features of the tumor such as histologic grade (Figs. 44.29, 44.31, and 44.32). Thermal artifacts may make it impossible to determine whether DCIS is present in tissue outside the tumor mass. It is possible to encounter rare instances in which cautery-induced changes are so egregious throughout an excisional biopsy specimen that no diagnosis could be rendered and the presence of carcinoma could not be affirmed or refuted (Figs. 44.28 and 44.29). In this situation, the patient may undergo reexcision to determine whether carcinoma remains at the biopsy site. Since the features of the primary tumor are critical for assessing prognosis and determining therapy, such a patient is left not knowing whether she had carcinoma, what her prognosis might be, and how she should be treated. Fortunately, this scenario is infrequent, but it serves as a reminder that the primary purpose of a surgical biopsy is to obtain a specimen for histologic diagnosis, and that the procedure should be performed in a manner most likely to achieve this goal.

The use of ultrasonic dissecting instruments that enable safe (if slower) dissection and better hemostasis, as well as less artifact, has gained limited acceptance in breast surgery. Ultrasonic dissection utilizes high-frequency vibrations within the "harmonic" frequency range to cut and coagulate tissues. It induces lesser thermal artifact because of lower operating temperature than electrocautery.[212,213]

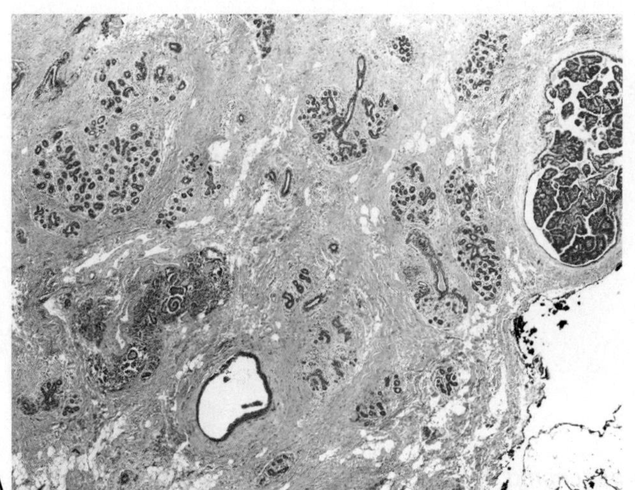

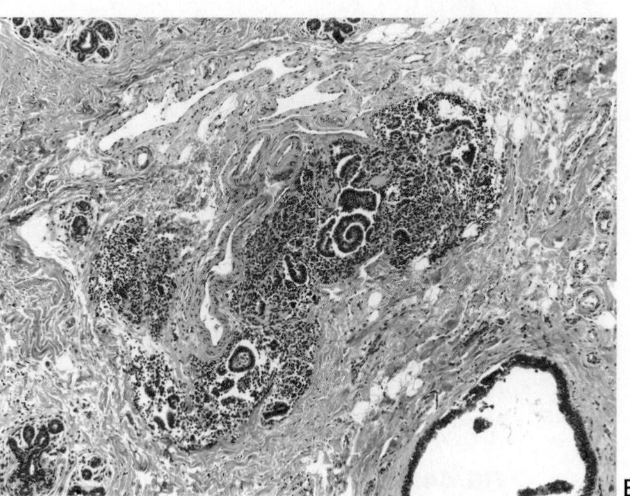

FIG. 44.20. ***Displaced fragments of papilloma.*** **A:** Detached fragments of papillary epithelium appear in the stroma (*left*) in this excisional biopsy obtained 1 week after an NCB had been performed for a lesion that proved to be an intraductal papilloma (*right*). **B:** Magnified view of displaced benign papillary epithelium.

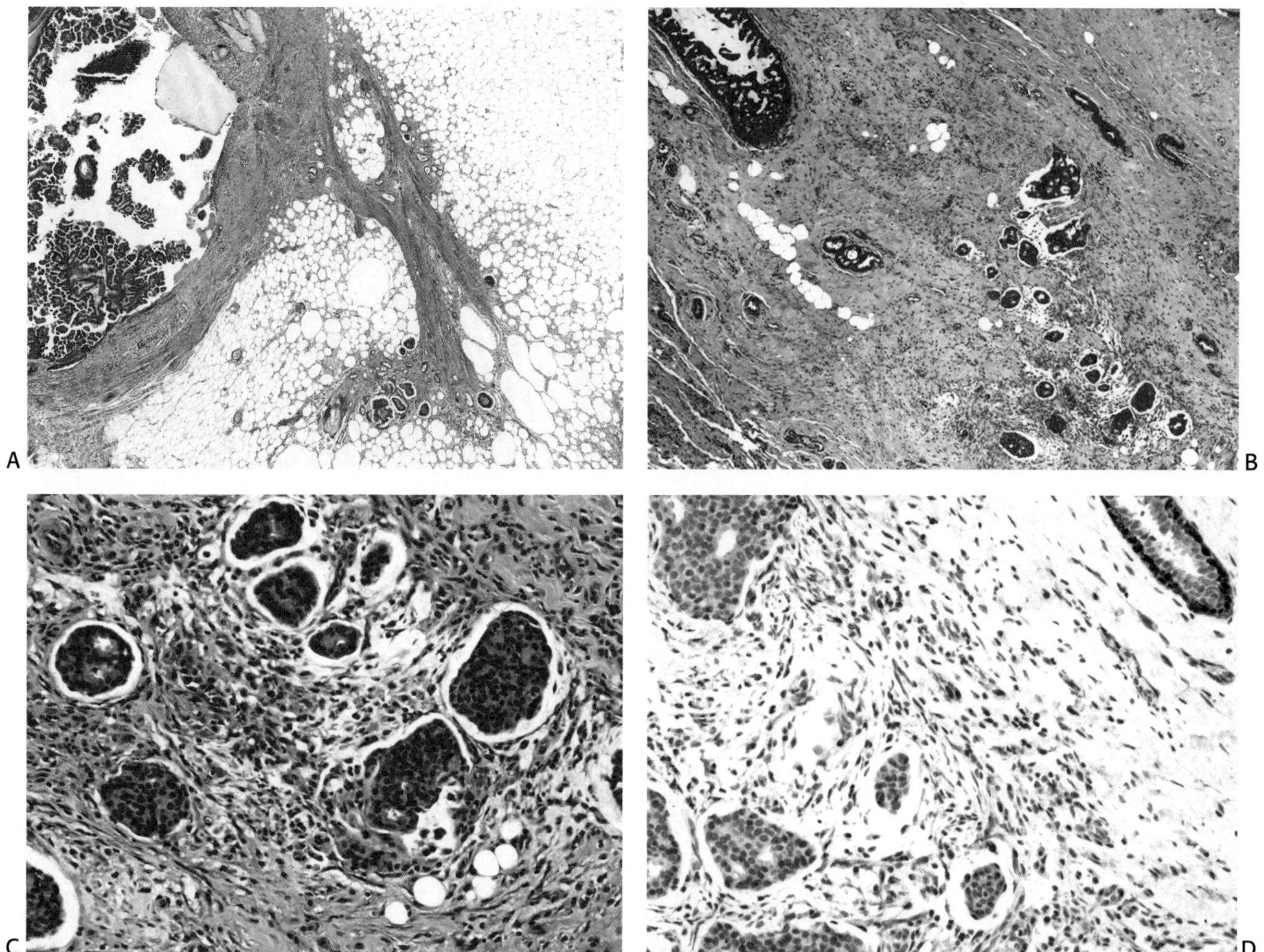

FIG. 44.21. ***Displaced papillary carcinoma.*** **A:** Intracystic papillary carcinoma (*left*), status-post NCB, with seeding of the needle track (*right*) in a healing biopsy site with fat necrosis. Images **(B–D)** are from a case of a noninvasive micropapillary carcinoma, status-post NCB. **B:** DCIS (*upper left*) and displaced DCIS in the needle biopsy track (*right*). **C:** Magnified view of the displaced DCIS. **D:** The smooth muscle actin immunostain shows no evidence of myoepithelial cells around the displaced clusters of carcinoma cells. Myoepithelial reactivity is evident in a benign duct (*upper right*). Myofibroblasts in the stroma around the displaced carcinoma are also immunoreactive. In some cases, myoepithelial cells may be detected by appropriate immunostains in clusters of displaced DCIS cells.

THE MASTECTOMY SPECIMEN

Multiple variations of the mastectomy procedure can be performed—including those of the radical, modified radical, simple, nipple-sparing, skin-sparing, and partial types. In general, mastectomy has evolved from the taking of larger specimens to smaller specimens, that is, from one considered as a "mutilation" to an "aid to breast reconstruction."[214] The surgeon should specify the type of mastectomy performed in each instance, since this information cannot always be ascertained from gross examination of the specimen.

The purpose of the gross description of a mastectomy specimen is to document the extent of the operation and the characteristics of the tissue removed. A standard radical mastectomy can usually be oriented on the basis of landmarks in the specimen, especially the position of the muscle segments. This may not be so easily accomplished with various types of modified radical mastectomies that have almost replaced the radical mastectomy. It is important that the surgeon indicate if there is anything unusual about the specimen and that important landmarks such as levels of ALNs be identified.

The external description of the specimen should include the following: overall size, dimensions and appearance of the skin with measurement of scars or incisions, appearance of the nipple and areola (if present), presence of muscle and

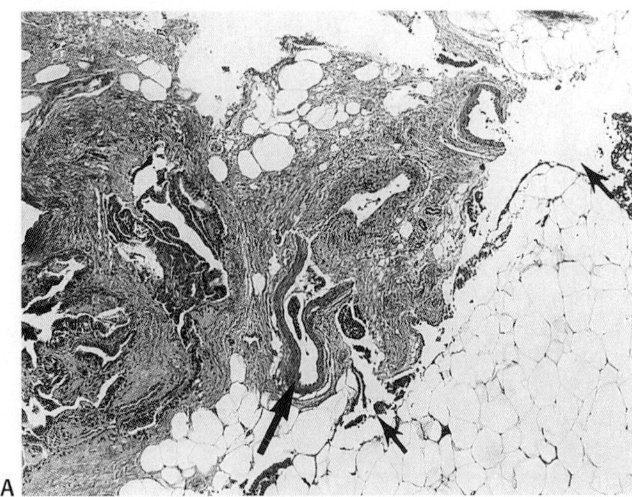

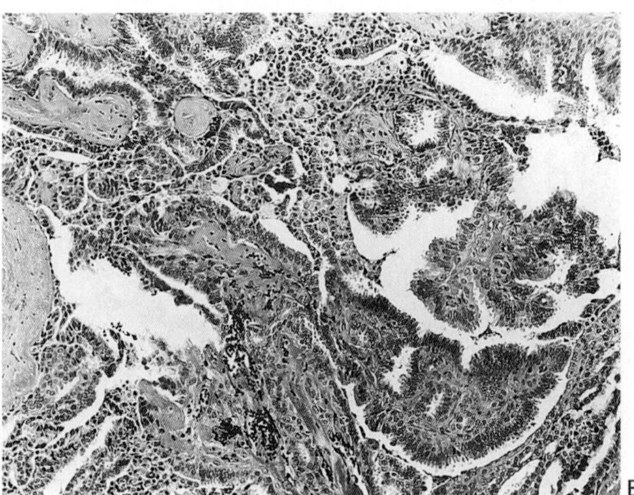

FIG. 44.22. ***Displaced papillary carcinoma in an artery.*** **A:** Part of the needle track resulting from an NCB procedure is shown on the *right and lower center* (*small arrows*). Displaced carcinoma is present in an artery (*large arrow*) and in the stroma in the *center*. The papillary tumor is shown on the *left*. **B:** A portion of the papillary carcinoma that was disrupted by the needling procedure.

axillary tissue, and location of any distinct palpable lesion. There is an increasing trend to take a minimal central portion of the skin of the breast or to remove no skin with the mastectomy specimens.

Dissection of the specimen is easily accomplished by placing it skin-side down anatomically oriented in order to identify the quadrants. One visualizes the findings as if one were looking through the patient from back to front. The external noncutaneous surfaces should be inspected and palpated for evidence of tumor involvement and inked. For a standard radical mastectomy, the cut edge of the sternal attachment of the pectoralis major muscle marks the medial side. In such a specimen, the fascia between the major and minor pectoralis muscles should be dissected to identify interpectoral (Rotter) lymph nodes.

The breast is sectioned by a series of parallel incisions at least 5 mm apart through the posterior surface up to the skin. A tumor, if present, should be described in the same fashion as for a biopsy specimen. The size and character of a biopsy site should be noted, including areas of induration. It is preferable that these fibrotic areas not be identified as tumor, since the reaction in a healing biopsy cavity may be grossly indistinguishable from carcinoma. The appearance of the remaining breast parenchyma is also recorded, including relative proportions of fat and fibrous parenchyma, the size, location and character of any discrete lesions, and the presence or absence

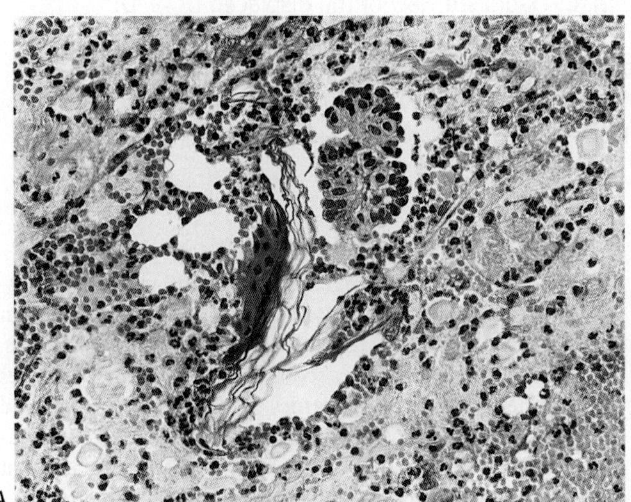

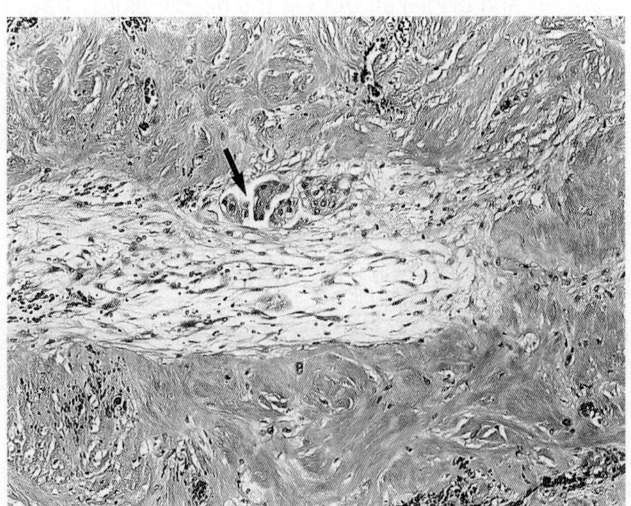

FIG. 44.23. ***Displaced intraductal carcinoma in a needle track.*** **A:** Detached fragments of papillary carcinoma and squamous epithelium (presumably from the skin) are shown surrounded by inflammatory cells in a needle track. **B:** Detached fragments of DCIS (*arrow*) are shown in granulation tissue at the site of a healing needle track.

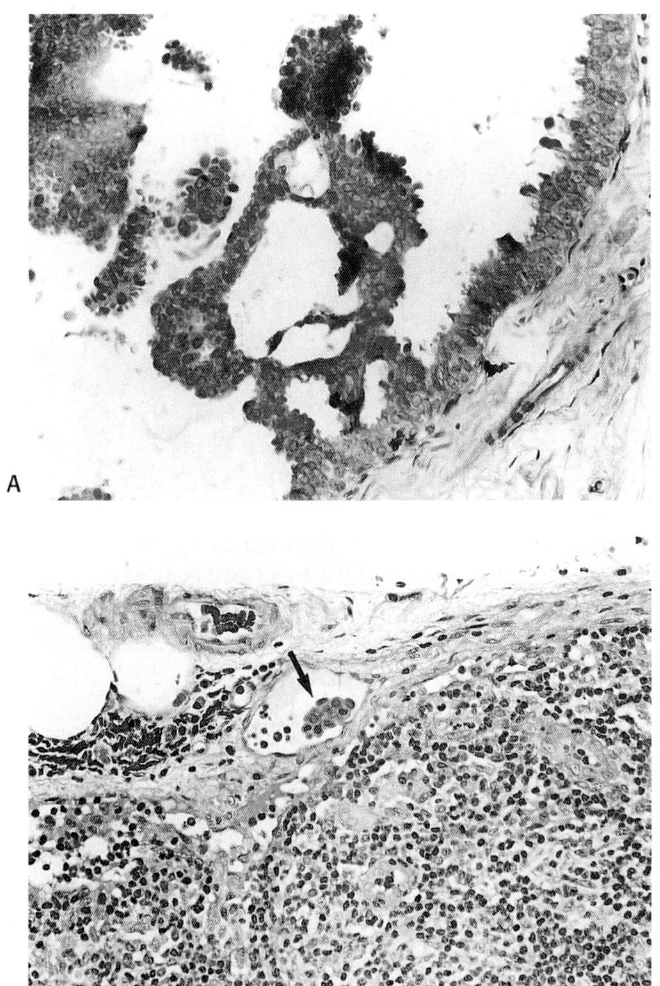
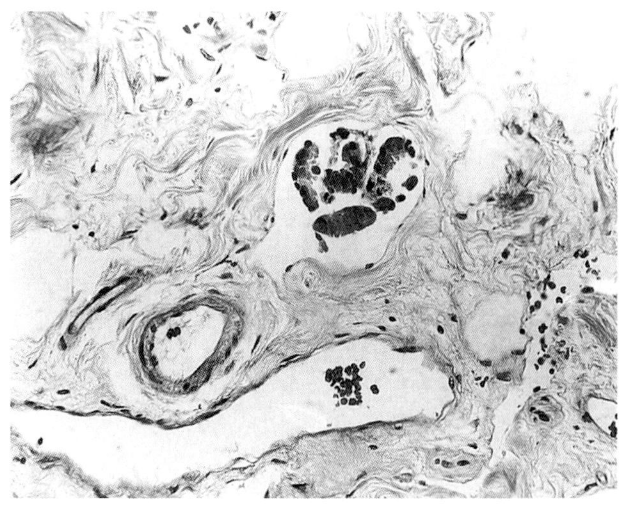

FIG. 44.24. ***Displaced intraductal carcinoma in lymphatic spaces of the breast and carcinoma in axillary lymph nodes.*** The patient had an FNA biopsy and stereotactic localization before this excisional biopsy was performed. **A:** Micropapillary DCIS. **B:** Clusters of DCIS cells in a lymphatic channel. **C:** An axillary dissection performed after intralymphatic carcinoma was found in the breast biopsy revealed small clusters of carcinoma cells in the capsular lymphatics of lymph nodes such as the one shown here (*arrow*) and in peripheral sinusoids.

of cysts. It is generally recommended that samples for histologic examination be taken from the tumor and/or biopsy site, nipple, skin, quadrants, and the margins, including the deep surface under the tumor as well as the superficial surface not covered by skin. However, the value of random sampling was questioned by Sikand et al.,[215] who studied more than 200 consecutive mastectomy specimens. Multifocality was found in 21% of breasts with invasive carcinoma but in none of 34 breasts with DCIS. Overall, when Paget disease of the nipple and carcinoma in the quadrants were considered, multifocality was found in 7% of mastectomies. The authors concluded that careful gross examination would detect about 50% of multifocal carcinoma and that the information was rarely clinically important. United Kingdom's National Health Service Breast Screening Programme guidelines indicate that routine sampling of the nipple and quadrants is not mandatory and should be done if "resources permit."[216] However, sampling of the grossly unremarkable nipple and quadrants is recommended in the United States since samples from these sections may reveal unsuspected invasive carcinoma.

A vertical section of the nipple will usually suffice to detect Paget disease or direct involvement of the nipple by carcinoma, even when it is not clinically suspected. With more elaborate sectioning of the nipple, unsuspected foci of carcinoma may be detected, but these are generally Paget disease or DCIS in lactiferous ducts that are of negligible clinical significance for a patient treated by mastectomy. Hence, preparing multiple sections of the nipple is not cost-effective for routine use. Nipple-sparing mastectomies are generally not indicated in tumors that are centrally located.[217] FSE of the nipple margin is a useful procedure, and can help ensure a low recurrence rate following a nipple-sparing mastectomy.[218,219]

Generally, two sections are taken randomly from the breast per quadrant, but more extensive sectioning may be indicated by the gross findings, or if the mastectomy were performed for DCIS, LCIS, or as a "prophylactic" procedure.

CLINICAL STAGING OF THE ALNS

Optimal staging of the axilla requires histopathologic examination of at least 10 lymph nodes.[220] Typically, a dissection of axillary level I and II lymph nodes should yield about 15 lymph nodes, and one including level III should approach

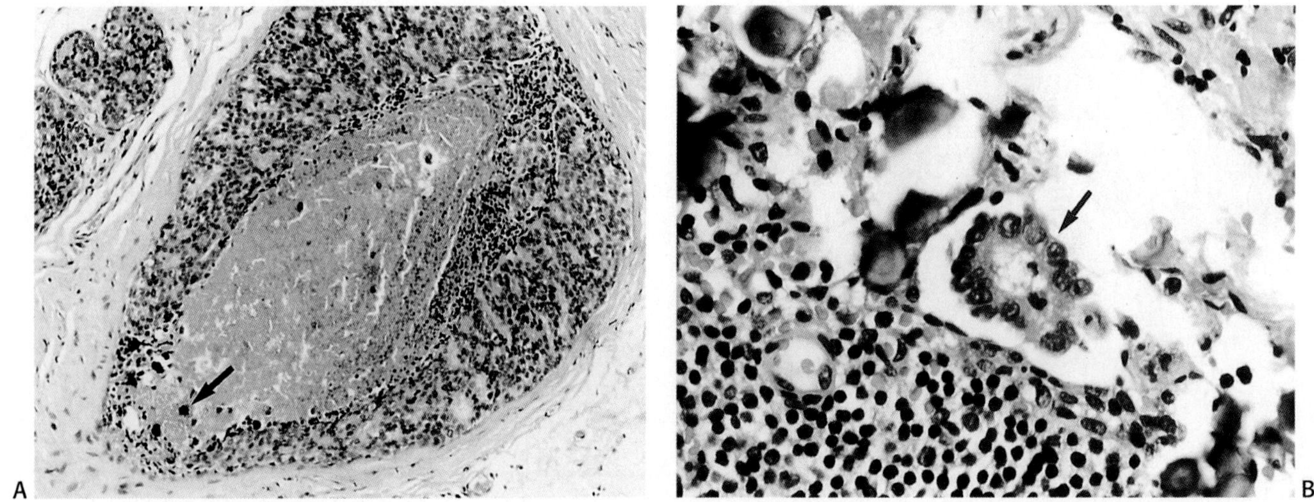

FIG. 44.25. ***Displaced intraductal carcinoma in the breast and carcinoma in axillary lymph nodes.*** **A:** Comedo DCIS in an excisional biopsy specimen after a stereotactic NCB and needle localization for nonpalpable mammographically detected calcifications. Small granular calcifications are present in the DCIS (*arrow*). **B:** A cluster of carcinoma cells (*arrow*) and several calcifications in the peripheral sinus of an ALN obtained after the procedure that yielded the DCIS shown in **(A)**.

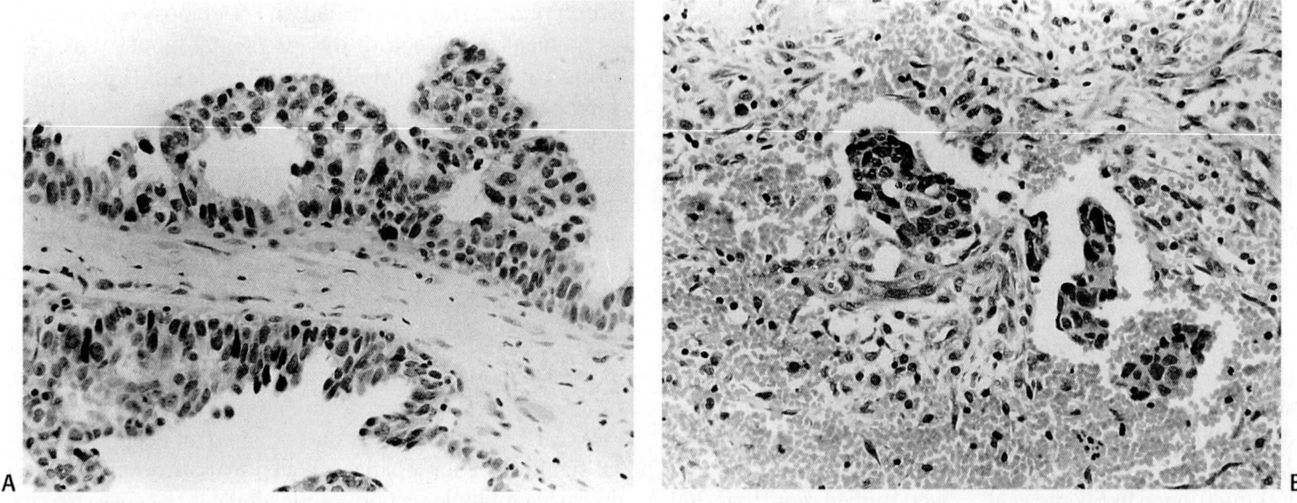

FIG. 44.26. ***Displaced intraductal carcinoma in the breast and a subsequent axillary lymph node metastasis.*** **A:** In 1987, this patient had an FNA biopsy obtained for mammographically detected calcifications. An excisional biopsy performed shortly thereafter revealed DCIS of the papillary and cribriform types shown here. **B,C:** Fragments of displaced DCIS were present in the biopsy specimen. **D:** These clusters of displaced carcinoma cells were present in granulation tissue at the excisional biopsy site in the subsequent mastectomy specimen. No intrinsic invasive carcinoma was found in the breast, and no metastatic carcinoma was identified in eight ALNs included with the 1987 mastectomy specimen. **E:** In 1994, the patient presented with an ipsilateral axillary tumor that proved to be metastatic mammary carcinoma in a lymph node. The growth pattern duplicated that of the previous DCIS. A likely explanation for this set of circumstances is that DCIS displaced to the lymph node in 1987 survived and, in the intervening 7 years, progressed to invasive carcinoma. No carcinoma was detected in the contralateral breast.

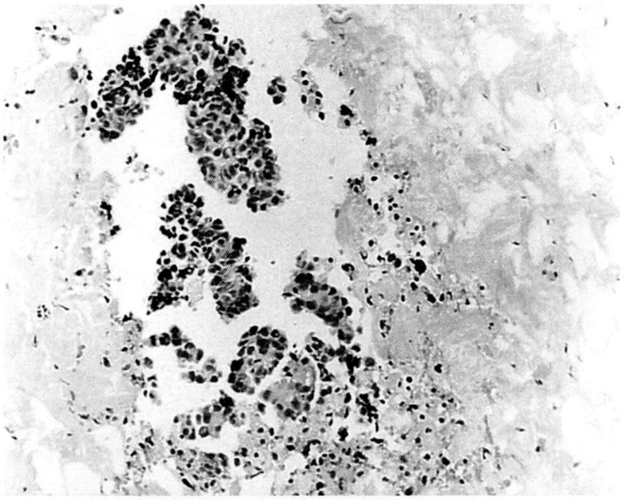

FIG. 44.26. *(Continued)*

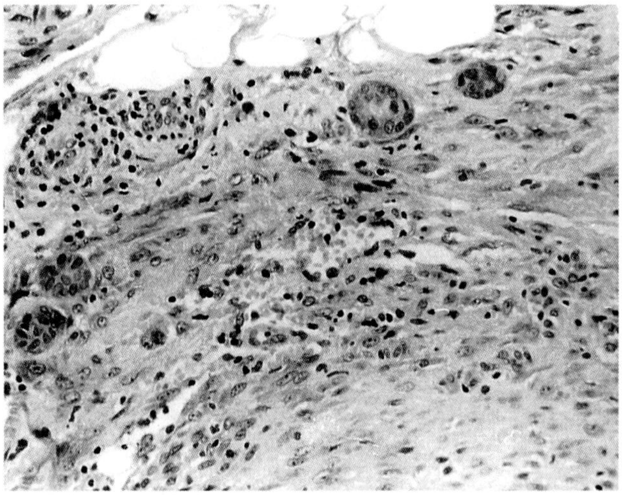

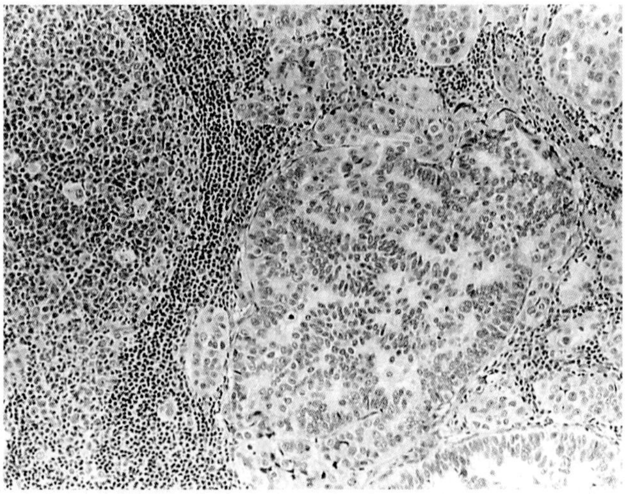

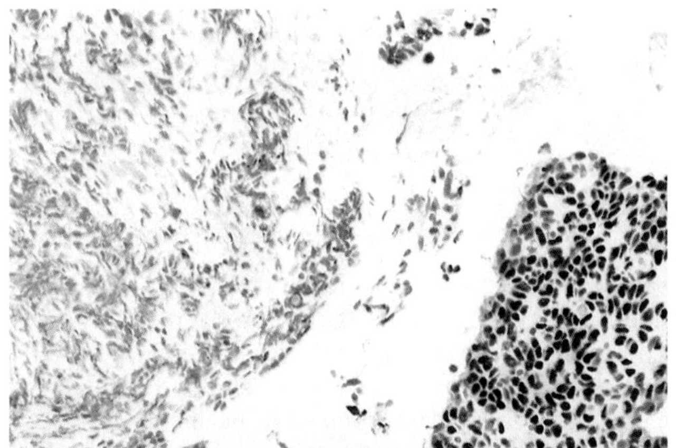

FIG. 44.27. ***Cautery effect and estrogen receptors.*** This biopsy sample shows nuclear reactivity in intact carcinoma on the *right*. No staining is present in cauterized carcinoma on the *left*.

20 lymph nodes. Some aspects of the pathology of ALNs are discussed in Chapter 43. SLN biopsy is discussed in a separate section later in this chapter.

Nonsurgical Imaging Methods for Staging of the ALNs

Clinical methods for detecting metastatic carcinoma in ALNs preoperatively have been in development for several years, but have thus far not been sufficiently effective to be used routinely.[221] These procedures have involved injection of radioactive tracers such as technetium Tc 99m,[222–225] computed tomography (CT),[226,227] MRI,[228–230] positron emission tomography (PET) with radiolabeled glucose analogs,[231,232] and sonography.[233,234]

Yoshimura et al.[229] used MRI to evaluate ALNs preoperatively in 202 patients. They were able to detect lymph nodes in 200 of the patients (99%). When compared with clinical assessment, MRI was more accurate (88% vs. 79%) in predicting axillary nodal status. Computer programs have been

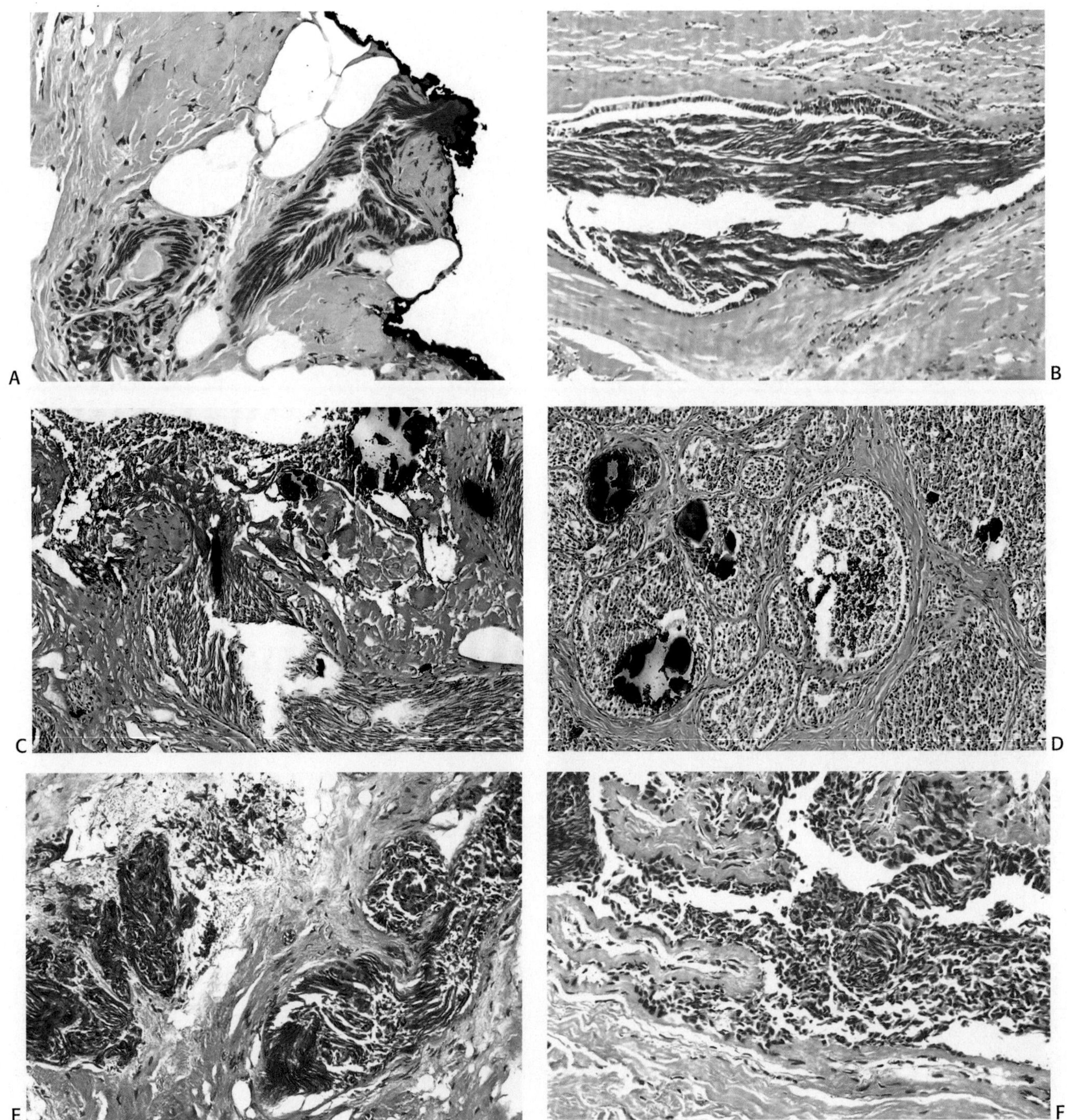

FIG. 44.28. ***Cautery effect.*** **A,B:** The smudged appearances of ductal epithelium and stromal hyalinization are typical changes resulting from severe cautery damage. No diagnosis can be given for this tissue. **C:** Calcifications and a duct with severe cautery effect are present at the inked margin. This part of the margin was not interpretable. **D:** Tissue deeper in the specimen depicted in (**C**) shows cautery-induced disruption of an intraductal proliferation with calcifications. A specific diagnosis was not possible. **E:** The most severe cautery-associated changes in this biopsy specimen are on the *left*, near the surface of the tissue. **F:** A duct deeper in the specimen shown in (**E**) with slightly less severe cautery effect. No diagnosis can be made on the tissues shown in (**E**) and (**F**).

developed to select lymph node regions of interest (ROI) for automated screening of MR images, and in one study the maximum enhancement ratio of automated ROI was a strong predictor of axillary nodal status.[230]

CT scanning has been compared with SLN biopsy as a method for staging the axilla. Miyauchi et al.[226] studied 51 women who had a full axillary dissection after CT scanning and SLN biopsy. False-negative SLN biopsy occurred in 3 of

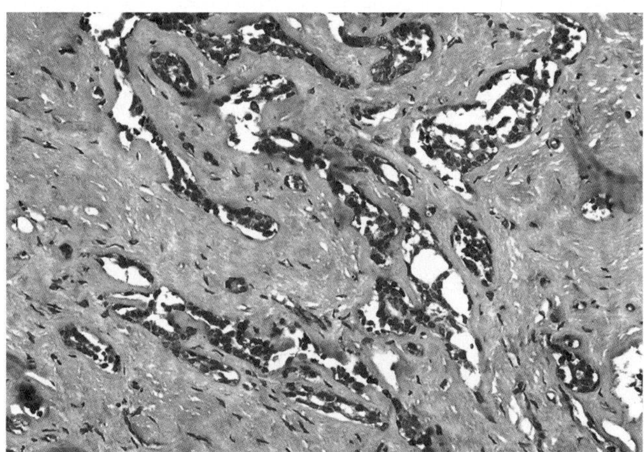

FIG. 44.29. ***Cautery effect.*** Loss of cellular cohesion, shrinkage of cells, and detachment of the epithelium characterize cautery effect in this glandular proliferation. Carcinoma could not be ruled out, but no specific diagnosis was made. Immunostaining was unreliable because of severe background reactivity and loss of specific cellular localization.

51 cases (6%) when non-SLNs (NSLNs) contained metastatic carcinoma after the SLN biopsy was negative. False-negative CT interpretations were recorded in 10 cases (19.7%). CT scans were able to identify the SLN in 42 of 51 cases (82.4%). Hata et al.[227] investigated thin-section CT as a method for improving the detection of ALN metastases and reported 93.8% sensitivity for detecting positive lymph nodes. However, specificity (detection of node-negative cases) remained relatively low (82.1%) because the procedure was unable to detect micrometastases.

PET scanning detected 19 of 24 patients (79%) with histologically documented lymph node metastases in a series of 51 women studied after injection of 2-deoxy-2-fluoro[^{18}F]-d-glucose (FDG).[231] In this series, PET imaging was 96% correct in identifying women without axillary nodal metastases. Among women with tumors larger than 2 cm, PET accurately identified 94% of women with nodal metastases (sensitivity) and 100% with negative lymph nodes (specificity). In the pathologic T1 (pT1) group with tumors smaller than 2 cm, PET had a sensitivity of only 33%. The authors concluded that PET imaging was not a "substitute for histopathologic analysis in detecting ALN metastases."

A prospective multicenter study of axillary staging by PET imaging obtained satisfactory data from 308 of 360 enrolled women (86%).[232] The positive and negative predictive values were 62% (60% to 64%) and 79% (76% to 81%), respectively.

Sonography has also been investigated as a method for staging ALNs. Alvarez et al.[233] reviewed 16 published reports and concluded that "axillary sonography is moderately sensitive and fairly specific." When lymph node size was used as the diagnostic criterion in women with clinically negative axillae, sensitivity in various reports ranged from 48.8% to 87.1% and specificity from 55.6% to 97.3%. Using lymph node morphology, sensitivity ranged from 26.4% to 75.9% and specificity from 88.4% to 98.1%. Ultrasound-guided core biopsy and FNA cytology are useful procedures for confirming the presence of metastatic carcinoma in lymph nodes.[233,234] FNA cytology of ALNs conducted under ultrasound guidance has been shown to have a PPV of 98.7% and a negative predictive value (NPV) of 81.8% in untreated cases.[235] The cytologic aspirates can be processed as air-dried Diff-Quik- or as alcohol-fixed Papanicolaou- or H&E-stained smear preparations or as ThinPrep slides.[236] TIC can be a valuable adjunct to the evaluation of ALNs after neoadjuvant chemotherapy.[237]

Surgical Staging of Axilla by Endoscopic Axillary Dissection

Endoscopic ALN dissection is an interesting, potentially useful, minimally invasive technique for surgical staging of the axilla. In an investigational setting, endoscopic axillary

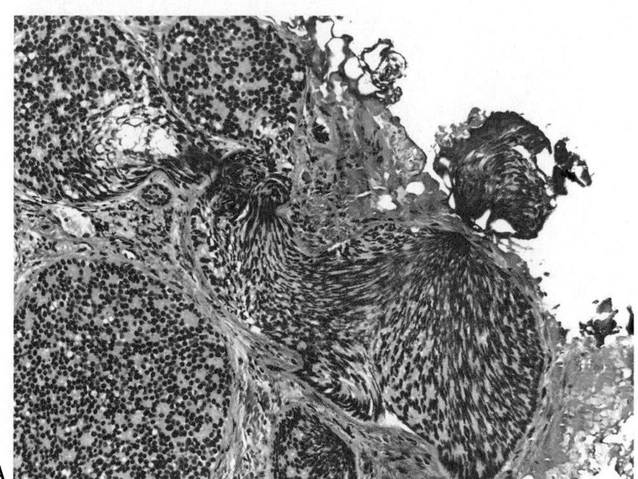

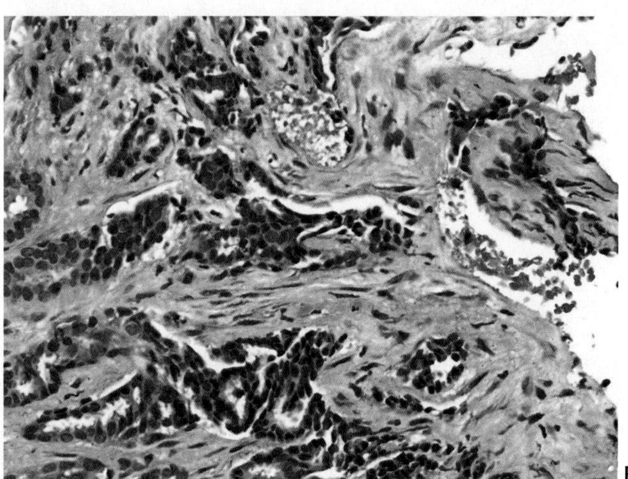

FIG. 44.30. ***Cautery effect.*** **A:** The tissue is distorted by cautery effect at the margin. This area can be reasonably interpreted as showing DCIS at the margin because it is continuous with underlying carcinoma. **B:** This isolated distorted area at the edge of another specimen can, in the appropriate context, be reasonably interpreted as invasive ductal carcinoma.

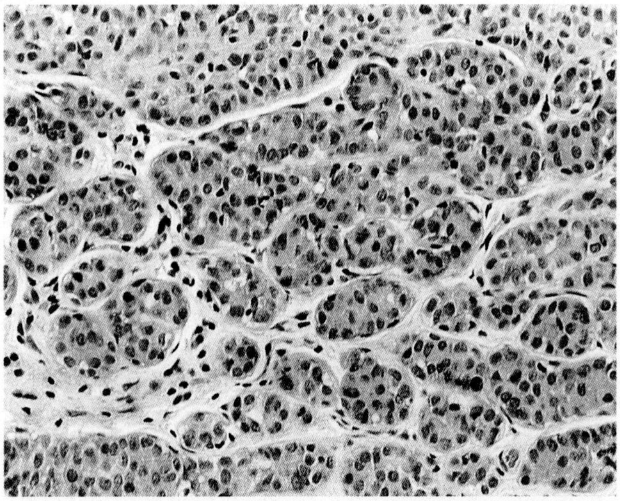

FIG. 44.31. ***Cautery effect, lobular carcinoma in situ.*** **A:** The patient had LCIS in SA shown here. **B:** The area in the *upper part* of the photograph near the margin is uninterpretable because of cautery effect. *In situ* carcinoma in SA is present *below*. **C:** A nondiagnostic lobule in which the epithelial cells were destroyed by thermal damage. All images are from a single specimen.

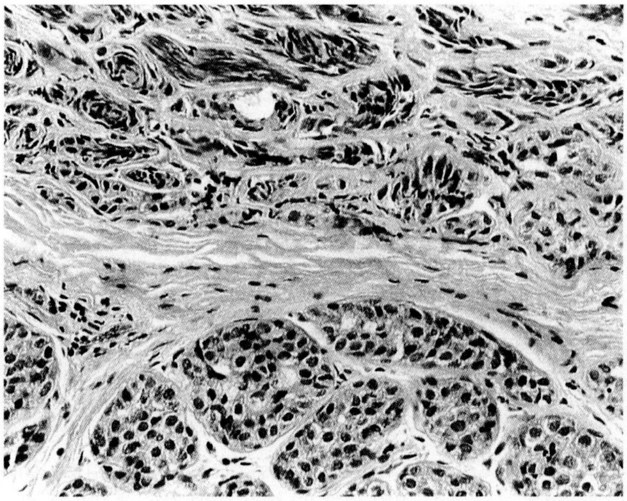

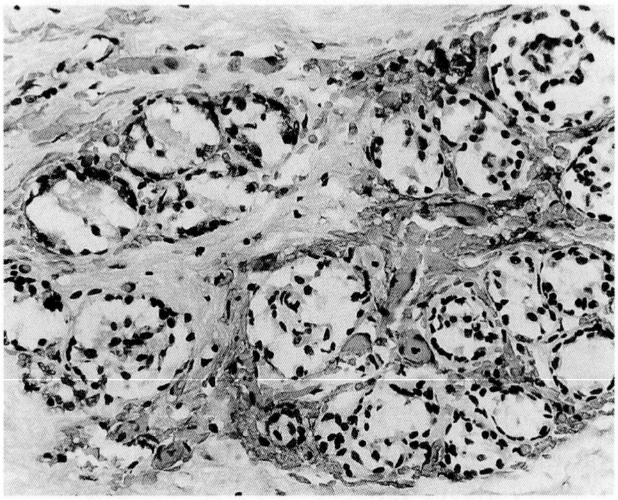

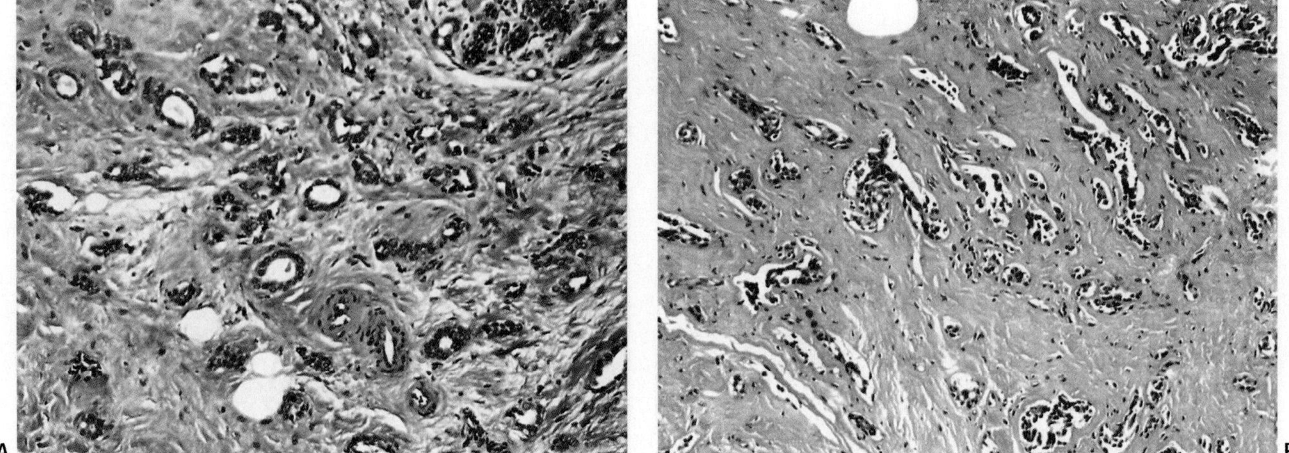

FIG. 44.32. ***Cautery effect, tubular carcinoma.*** **A:** Tubular carcinoma in the center of a biopsy specimen. **B,C:** Adjacent portions of the specimen shown in (**A**) exhibiting cautery effect. The glandular configuration is evident in (**C**) and this is probably part of the carcinoma. The interpretation of (**B**) is uncertain. **D:** Severe cautery effect at the surface of the specimen. No diagnosis can be made in the region of the inked margin at the *top*.

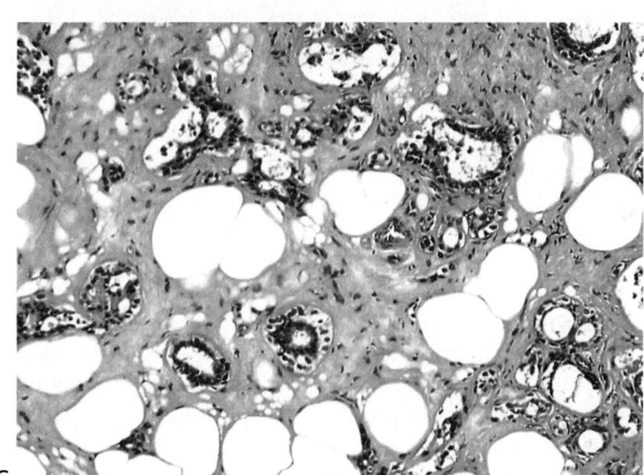

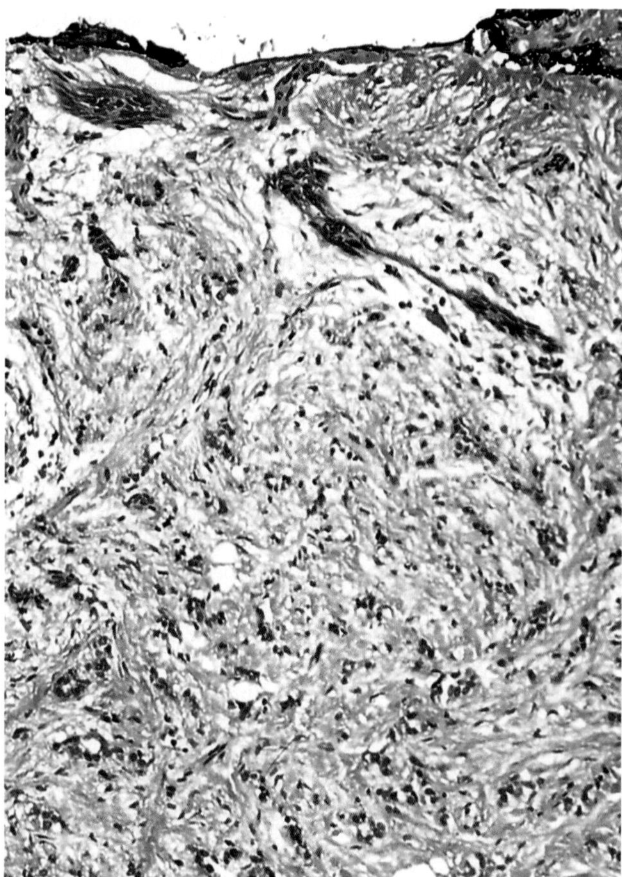

FIG. 44.32. *(Continued)*

dissections were performed in 12 cadavers yielding an average of 9.9 ± 7.2 lymph nodes (range, 2 to 22).[238]

Lim and Lam[239] performed endoscopic axillary dissection in 30 patients and obtained an average of 15 lymph nodes (range, 7 to 25). Follow-up of patients after endoscopic axillary dissection was reported by Langer et al.[240] Endoscopic dissection yielded positive lymph nodes in 30 of 52 women (57.6%). After follow-up of 11 to 96 months (median, 71.9 months), 2 of 52 patients (4%) developed recurrent carcinoma at the endoscopic port site, and 1 of these women also had an axillary recurrence. The patient with axillary and port-site recurrences had negative lymph nodes in the endoscopic dissection specimens. These authors expressed concern that port-site recurrences might be related to failure to perform an *en bloc* dissection. Kuehn et al.[241] considered the long operating time, which exceeded 1 hour, to be a serious drawback of endoscopic axillary dissection.

Axillary Staging Based on Clinicopathologic Factors

Clinical and pathologic factors have been studied extensively in an effort to define parameters that could identify patients with the lowest risk of axillary metastases. The goal of this effort has been to establish criteria that would serve as a basis for not performing axillary dissection if the probability of there being nodal metastases was sufficiently low. Silverstein[242] emphasized the importance of distinguishing between palpable and nonpalpable tumors in these analyses. Overall, nodal metastases were found in 45 of 364 patients (12.3%) with nonpalpable and in 450 of 1,217 (37%) with palpable T1 and T2 tumors, respectively.

By combining palpability with other tumor characteristics, Barth et al.[243] identified a subset that represented 13% of more than 900 patients with T1 tumors, among whom 3% had axillary nodal metastases. The authors concluded that axillary dissection should be omitted for patients with this clinicopathologic presentation, "especially if the decision for adjuvant treatment was not altered by the results of ALND" (axillary lymph node dissection). Other studies reported that lymphovascular channel involvement was an important factor associated with nodal metastases in patients with small T1 tumors. In three separate studies, when lymphovascular tumor emboli were absent, the reported frequency of positive ALNs was 9% for tumors smaller than 10 mm,[244] 7% for tumors 5 mm or less with low nuclear grade,[245] and 4.8% for tumors smaller than 5 mm.[246] Port et al.[247] reported that 30 of 247 T1a and T1b patients (12.1%) had ALN metastases (T1a, 7.4%; T1b, 14.5%). The presence of lymphovascular involvement was a significant predictor of nodal involvement

(27.8% vs. 10.9%) for the entire group. The authors did not feel that these data defined "a subgroup at acceptably low risk of nodal positivity" that would not require ALN staging. Shoup et al.[248] found ALN metastases in 4.3%, 16.4%, and 31.7% of patients with T1a, T1b, and T1c tumors, respectively. Other factors that contributed significantly to increased risk of nodal involvement were high-grade nuclei and lymphovascular involvement. Morrow's[249] review of the problem of identifying patients at low risk for axillary metastases led her to conclude that "tumor size, whether alone or in combination with other prognostic factors, cannot reliably identify a group of breast cancers with a less than 5% risk of axillary nodal metastases."

The idea that tumor size can be used as the sole determinant of the risk of ALN metastases remains controversial. One group of investigators found axillary metastases in 3 of 66 women (4.5%) who had T1a tumors, and in a literature review of combined data for single-institution trials reported axillary involvement in 3.9% of 256 patients.[250] The authors concluded that "our data support abandoning routine axillary dissection in T1a breast cancer." Similar results were reported by Pandelidis et al.,[251] who detected ALN metastases in 2 of 54 T1a cases (3.7%). On the other hand, McGee et al.[252] reviewed data from three large urban hospitals with a total series of 3,077 breast carcinoma cases and reported finding ALN metastases in 8 of 74 patients (12.2%) with T1a tumors. The authors felt that "these results justify axillary node dissections even for very small invasive cancers."

GROSS PATHOLOGIC EXAMINATION OF ALNS

With the exception of the now virtually extinct procedure of radical mastectomy, it is not possible to determine, by anatomic orientation alone, the position or level of lymph nodes in axillary contents received with a mastectomy specimen. If this information is desired clinically, the lymph node groups should be tagged or submitted as separate specimens. In properly oriented, complete axillary dissection specimens, the distribution of lymph node metastases generally follows a consistent pattern. Typically, metastases are found in a stepwise fashion in the low, mid-, and upper axillary zones. Several authors reported that discontinuous or "skip" metastases that do not follow this distribution were found in 2% or less of all patients or in less than 5% of patients with axillary nodal metastases.[253–255] In a study of more than 1,000 patients with a mean follow-up of 97 months, who underwent complete axillary dissection (levels I, II, and III), tumor size, the number of involved lymph nodes, and the level of involvement were independent predictive factors for survival.[256]

Careful manual blunt dissection of the unfixed axillary fat is the most cost-effective method for isolating lymph nodes for microscopic study. In this process, firm portions of fat and fibrous tissue may be mistaken for lymph nodes. Although the gross description should include an approximate count of samples thought to be lymph nodes that were submitted for histology, the final number of nodes is determined microscopically. The gross character and dimensions of lymph nodes should be described. It is generally advisable to avoid stating that metastases are grossly present or absent, since uncertainty arises when the microscopic results differ from the gross impression. Lymph nodes with reactive hyperplasia, or those with fatty infiltration, are a common cause for a false-positive interpretation on gross pathologic and clinical examination (Fig. 44.33).

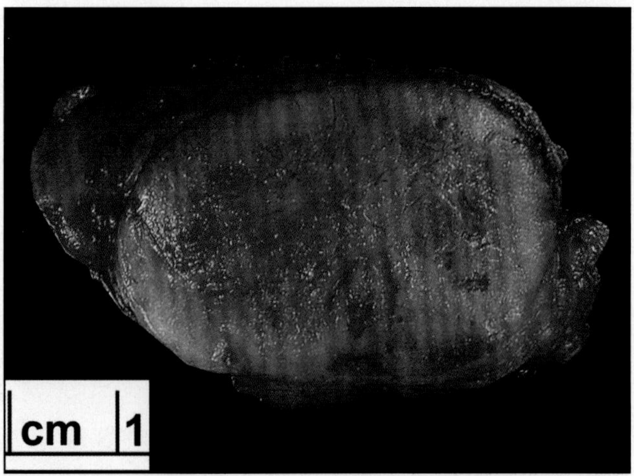

FIG. 44.33. ***Fatty infiltration of a lymph node.*** The lymph node is grossly enlarged by a lipomatous mass of fat that fills the hilum. Lymphoid tissue forms a thin brown band at the periphery.

Procedures available to facilitate the isolation of lymph nodes from the axillary fat include obtaining x-rays of the fat,[257,258] fixing the fat in Bouin solution, which stains fat intensely yellow but leaves the lymph nodes white, and clearing the fat by a process that renders it relatively translucent so that solid structures such as lymph nodes stand out.[259–261] These techniques increase the yield of lymph nodes obtained by locating smaller lymph nodes that may be missed on palpation. Although it is possible that an occasional patient may be incorrectly staged because a positive lymph node was missed in manual dissection,[260,261] the considerable time and expense required for clearing of axillary fat cannot be justified as a routine practice.

Lymph nodes larger than 0.5 cm should be bisected in the long axis. Lymph nodes larger than 1.0 cm should be serially sectioned into multiple portions. There is no consensus on whether it is necessary to histologically examine all lymph node tissue. The gross description should state how this issue has been handled. All tissue from a lymph node divided into two or more parts should be processed together in one or more separately designated tissue blocks. Consequently, each lymph node will require at least one cassette in order that multiple portions of metastatic carcinoma from a single subdivided lymph node not be mistakenly interpreted as two or more involved lymph nodes. Alternatively, the capsular surfaces of smaller (those smaller than 0.5 cm) lymph nodes could be painted with different colored inks and processed in one cassette. Such inking does not hinder microscopic evaluation. If a lymph node contains grossly unequivocal metastatic carcinoma, it is not necessary to process the entire lymph node for histologic study, but the samples should be taken in a manner (i.e., with liberal sampling of nodal capsule) that would be most likely to demonstrate extranodal spread, if present.

There is no consensus as to the optimum procedure to use when submitting tissue from grossly benign lymph nodes that are too large to process entirely for histologic examination. This will generally apply to lymph nodes 1.0 cm or larger. Recommendations include submitting one-half of a bisected lymph node, submitting a representative sample, or processing up to one cassette of tissue per large lymph node.[262–264]

An important concern in considering the need to process all tissue from large, grossly negative lymph nodes is the cost of this effort relative to the amount of useful additional information. This issue was investigated by Niemann et al.[265] in a study of consecutive lymph node dissections from various anatomical regions that yielded 2,915 lymph nodes from 149 patients. Lymph nodes too large to be processed intact were divided into two or more samples. The series included 50 patients who underwent axillary dissection for mammary carcinoma. Additional lymph node tissue representing material that would not be included if only one sample per lymph node had been examined histologically uncovered metastatic carcinoma in nine lymph nodes deemed to be negative in the initial sample from seven patients. Each of these patients already had metastases detected in routine sections of other lymph nodes, and the additional information raised the stage in only two cases, both with cervical metastases from oropharyngeal carcinoma. No changes in staging occurred among the 50 women with mammary carcinoma. The estimated cost for preparing and examining the 808 additional tissue blocks needed for all lymph node tissue was estimated, in 1998 terms, to be $5935.62, or $847.94 per case with an additional positive lymph node. The authors concluded that "whether these results justify the expense incurred remains an open question."

Portions of grossly negative lymph nodes may be reserved for ancillary studies. Presently, these are investigational procedures to detect submicroscopic metastases in SLNs by molecular techniques such as the reverse transcriptase–polymerase chain reaction (RT–PCR). Smith et al.[266] investigated the potential impact on axillary staging that might result from examining one-half of each SLN histologically if the other half were reserved for molecular analysis. The study was based on 227 patients included in a SLN biopsy protocol in which all patients also underwent a complete axillary dissection. As part of the study design, all lymph nodes larger than 8 mm were bisected and the two halves were submitted for histologic examination separately. Sixty patients had axillary nodal metastases totaling 230 lymph nodes. On review, 107 of the positive lymph nodes (46.5%) were found to have been bisected. Carcinoma was present in both halves of 64 lymph nodes (59.8%) and in only one-half of 43 lymph nodes (40.2%). Both halves were more likely to be involved if a patient had metastases in multiple lymph nodes. In 12 patients (20% of those with nodal metastases), the only evidence of metastatic carcinoma was contained in one-half of one lymph node. These data suggest that failing to process both halves of a bisected lymph node for histologic study could affect the accuracy of lymph node staging. Heterogeneous distribution of metastatic carcinoma explains some of the discrepant results between molecular and histologic examination of a lymph node.

ALN Ratios

Among patients staged by axillary dissection prior to the era of SLN biopsy, the total number of lymph nodes obtained was found to be prognostically significant. Weir et al.[267] reported that there was a significant inverse relationship between the number of lymph nodes removed and the regional relapse rate in women staged as node negative who did not receive systemic adjuvant therapy. Bélanger et al.[268] reported retrieval of a median number of 10.0 lymph nodes (range, 0 to 38) in 107 patients who had received neoadjuvant chemotherapy compared to 12.5 (range, 0 to 30) lymph nodes in the control group of 176 patients who had not received chemotherapy.[268] Salama et al.[269] reported that recovery of fewer than 10 negative lymph nodes in the axillary dissection of women who underwent mastectomy with little or no adjuvant therapy was associated with a 10% to 15% lower DFS when compared to women from whom 10 or more lymph nodes were obtained.

The ALN ratio is the percentage of lymph nodes involved by metastatic carcinoma. Woodward et al.[270] reviewed published reports on the prognostic significance of nodal ratios. The studies varied considerably in terms of the numbers of patients studied and tumor stage, and generally demonstrated that the nodal ratio was equivalent to or better than the absolute number of positive lymph nodes for predicting recurrence and survival.

SLN BIOPSY

Intraoperative mapping of the lymphatic drainage from the breast has proved to be an effective method for locating one or more lymph nodes most likely to harbor metastatic carcinoma, the so-called sentinel lymph nodes. An important advantage of SLN biopsy when compared with conventional axillary dissection is reduced postoperative morbidity.[271] Patients experience significantly less lymphedema and other symptoms after SLN biopsy than after axillary dissection.

The procedures widely employed involve injection of a vital blue dye, a radioactive tracer such as technetium Tc 99m sulfur colloid, or a combination of these reagents. Blue dye transported to the SLN can be identified visually. Allergic reactions to the blue dye are infrequent and generally mild. Retrograde migration of the dye may cause it to remain in dermal lymphatics, resulting in a bluish hue in the skin. Radiocolloid localization can be identified preoperatively by lymphoscintigraphy and intraoperatively by using a probe to detect irradiation. Lymphoscintigraphy can alert the surgeon to the location of SLN in the axilla and in extra-axillary sites.

Extra-Axillary SLNs

Extra-axillary "hot spots" on lymphoscintigraphy usually represent SLNs outside the axillary lymphatic drainage. Involvement of internal mammary lymph node metastases most often occurs in patients with medial tumors or in those who have axillary metastases. In a review of 7,070 patients reported in published studies, Morrow and Foster[272] found that 347 (4.9%) had metastatic carcinoma limited to internal mammary lymph nodes. Harlow et al.[273] detected extra-axillary hot spots by lymphoscintigraphy in 44 of 680 patients (6.5%) who had SLN biopsy, including 9 (1.3%) whose only hot spot was extra-axillary. The most common site of extra-axillary localization was in the internal mammary lymph nodes. Other locations of extra-axillary hot spots were supraclavicular, interpectoral, infraclavicular, intramuscular (pectoralis major), thyroid gland, and chest wall. Surgical biopsy revealed lymph nodes in 35 (79.5%) hot spot sites; no lymph nodes were found in nine sites. Three of the 35 (8.6%) extra-ALNs contained metastatic carcinoma, including two patients with negative axillary SLN. van Rijk et al.[274] reported the presence of lymphoscintigraphy-detected SLN sites other than the axilla and internal mammary region in 91 of 785 patients (12%). Unusual hot sites included breast (n:58), infraclavicular fossa (n:38), interpectoral or Rotter lymph nodes (n:22), and supraclavicular lymph nodes (n:6). Metastatic carcinoma was found in 18 (17%) of these lymph nodes.

Hill et al.[275] reported extra-axillary hot spots in 35 of 195 patients (17%) examined by lymphoscintigraphy. All of the extra-axillary sites had an internal mammary distribution. Five of these patients (2%) also had supraclavicular localization and in 8 (4%), the only activity was in the internal mammary lymph node region. Internal mammary lymph nodes were mapped in 36 of 1,470 patients (2.4%) studied by Dupont et al.[276] The primary tumor was in an inner quadrant in 24 cases (67%). Five (14%) patients had at least one positive internal mammary lymph node.

There is no consensus on the clinical management of extra-axillary nodal hot spots, especially those with an internal mammary distribution. Harlow et al.[273] recommended "removal of these nodes . . . to improve staging." Cody[277] suggested that internal mammary SLN biopsy be considered for "medially placed tumors . . ., if either lymphoscintigraphy or the interoperative gamma probe suggests internal mammary drainage of isotope." Veronesi[278] reported that 6 of 380 patients (1.6%) had internal mammary hot spots and that these patients all had negative ALNs. He noted that "their prognostic significance is as great as that of the axillary nodes."

From the foregoing data, it is apparent that at least 75% of extra-axillary "hot spots" prove to be lymph nodes. However, the routine use of preoperative lymphoscintigraphy remains controversial. Teal et al.[279] found that lymphoscintigraphy underestimated the number of SLNs in a study of 12 patients who had 129 SLNs identified by preoperative imaging, whereas 209 radioactive SLNs were found at surgery. There is also no consensus as to the clinical benefit derived from extirpating internal mammary lymph nodes, the most common site of extra-axillary SLNs, except in selected situations.[280,281]

Success Rate for Detecting SLNs

Numerous papers have been published describing technical aspects of SLN biopsy in breast carcinoma.[277,282–286] With experience, most reports describe successful identification of one or more SLN in 90% or more patients. Radioisotope localization appears to find SLN more frequently than the blue dye technique alone, and the combination of both procedures has proven to be superior to either alone. Guenther et al.[287] observed a substantial risk of nodal metastasis in women with no detectable SLN. Positive lymph nodes were found in 33.3% of these patients, including some women with five or more affected nodes.

In a review of 1,564 patients who underwent SLN biopsy described in 16 reports, Cody[277] found that SLNs were detected in 76% of cases by the blue dye method, 90% by an isotope procedure, and 93% with a combined technique. A meta-analysis of reports through 2003 prepared by Kim et al.[288] summarized the results of SLN biopsy in 8,059 patients documented in published reports. The success rate was 96%, yielding a positive SLN in 17% to 74% (average, 42%) of cases. The false-negative rate averaged 7.3% (range, 0% to 29%) and was inversely related to operator experience as reflected in the number of procedures performed.

Injections of blue dye and radiocolloid may be performed separately in the breast parenchyma around the tumor site. Successful SLN biopsy is also achieved by subdermal injection of radiocolloid[289,290] or intradermal injection of blue dye[291] over the tumor site. Rodier et al.[292] reported a higher rate of SLN detection by lymphoscintigraphy after periareolar injection of a radiolabeled tracer than after peritumoral injection. Prior excisional biopsy is not a contraindication to SLN biopsy as long as the injection is placed in breast parenchyma around the biopsy cavity.[277,286] However, a large biopsy cavity, especially in the upper outer quadrant, may compromise lymphatic drainage in the region and has been associated with unsuccessful or false-negative SLN biopsy.[277]

The frequency of detecting a positive SLN increases with tumor size. In one study, the frequency of positive SLN was 4.3%, 19.5%, and 23.8% for T1a, T1b, and T1c tumors, respectively, and 48.9% and 66.7% for T2 and T3 tumors, respectively.[293] Bass et al.[294] reported the following frequencies of positive SLN biopsy in relation to tumor size: T1a, 13 of 69 (18.8%); T2, 108 of 202 (53.5%); and T3, 22 of 25 (88%).

Patients with nonpalpable invasive breast carcinoma diagnosed by percutaneous NCB are excellent candidates for SLN biopsy. When compared with women who had carcinoma diagnosed by surgical excision or FNA, patients diagnosed by NCB have a similar success rate with SLN biopsy.[295] Liberman et al.[296] reported that SLNs were identified in 30 of 33 women (91%) with nonpalpable infiltrating carcinomas (0.5 to 2.2 cm; median, 1 cm) who underwent

SLN biopsy with combined blue dye and radiocolloid injection. One measure of the utility of SLN biopsy for axillary staging is the clinical follow-up of patients who had negative SLNs. Langer et al.[297] described the prospective analysis of patients after 236 SLN procedures. Macrometastases were found in 74 of mapped cases (33%) and 27 (12%) had micrometastases. Adjuvant chemotherapy was administered about equally to SLN-negative patients and those with micrometastases. None of the patients with micrometastases or negative SLNs had an axillary dissection. After follow-up of 12 to 64 months (median, 42 months), no axillary recurrences were diagnosed clinically in the micrometastasis group. One patient (0.7%) with a negative SLN experienced an axillary recurrence. Chung et al.[298] reported on 208 procedures with negative SLNs and a median follow-up of 26 months. Axillary recurrences were documented in three of the procedures (1.4%). When these results were added to those of four other reports cited by Chung et al.,[298] axillary recurrences were recorded in 4 of 743 (0.5%) SLN biopsy procedures with median follow-up of 22 to 39 months. In a retrospective review of 647 patients with a median follow-up of 33 months (range, 2 to 73 months), 4 patients (0.62%) developed an ALN recurrence after staging by SLN biopsy alone. Three of these patients had had negative SLNs, and in one there had been a 0.25-mm focus of carcinoma in a SLN. The only patient who received adjuvant chemotherapy had a negative SLN.

Within the range of follow-up currently available, these data indicate that clinical axillary recurrence is a rare event when axillary dissection is not performed after SLNs are found to be negative or involved by micrometastases.[299]

SLNs and the Type of Preoperative Biopsy Procedure

The possibility that dispersal of carcinoma cells caused by a preoperative biopsy procedure could result in the detection of micrometastases in SLN has been the subject of concern. As noted earlier in this chapter, displacement of DCIS cells resulting from needling procedures was occasionally associated with the presence of carcinoma cells in peritumoral lymphatic spaces and in ALNs in the pre-SLN era.

Clinical studies of this issue have provided conflicting results. Hansen et al.[300] investigated 663 patients who had a preoperative diagnosis by FNA, NCB, or excisional biopsy prior to SLN biopsy. Using multivariate analysis, the authors found SLN metastases significantly more often after FNA (odds ratio [OR], 1.531) and NCB (OR, 1.018) than after excisional biopsy. Peters-Engl et al.[301] investigated 1,890 patients and concluded that the presence or absence of a preoperative biopsy and the method of biopsy were not associated with SLN status. Chagpar et al.[302] reached the same conclusion on the basis of a study of 3,853 patients, but did not analyze cases with only immunohistochemically positive SLN separately.

Prior excisional biopsy has been associated with an increased frequency of immunohistochemically positive SLN when compared to patients with an antecedent needle biopsy.[303,304] Newman et al.[303] found that this association was limited to SLNs that were positive by immunohistochemistry (IHC) alone. A study by Moore et al.[304] included a control group of patients who had no biopsy procedure prior to SLN biopsy. The frequency of an immunohistochemical-only positive lymph node was highest after excisional biopsy (4.6%), intermediate after NCB (3.8%), and lowest when there had been no antecedent biopsy (1.2%).

Massage of the breast after injection of dye or a radiolabeled tracer can be used to enhance flow of the marker to the lymph node basin. Diaz et al.[305] found isolated tumor cells (ITCs) or tumor cell clusters significantly more often in the SLNs of patients who had breast massage than in nodes of patients who did not have breast massage. The authors concluded that their observations support the hypothesis that mammary carcinoma cells can, under some circumstances, be transported mechanically to ALNs.

As discussed earlier in this chapter, displacement of carcinomatous epithelium by biopsy procedures was first documented by Youngson et al.[203,204] Subsequently, Carter et al.[306] introduced the term "benign transport" to describe instances that they concluded were iatrogenic displacement of carcinoma cells to ALNs. It was suggested that benign transport could be recognized by the absence of reactive changes at the site of carcinomatous nodal involvement and the presence of foamy histiocytes.

Disruption of breast tissue by biopsy procedures causes displacement of benign as well as carcinomatous epithelial cells. This is most noticeable when the biopsied tissue contains a papilloma or papillary ductal hyperplasia. Clusters of papillary epithelial cells may be found at these sites not only in the needle track but also in the adjacent lymphovascular channels. Because SLN biopsy is not performed after a benign breast biopsy, the frequency of this event, if it occurs at all, cannot be ascertained. Data collected by Bleiweiss et al.[307] in patients with coexisting benign papillary lesions and carcinoma provide circumstantial evidence to support the hypothesis that cells displaced from a benign papillary lesion could be transported to an ALN. The study described a series of cases in which epithelial cells in the SLN appeared to be cytologically benign and differed in marker expression from the primary carcinoma. In 13 cases the primary carcinomas were ER positive and the nodal epithelial cells were ER negative. The authors concluded that epithelial cells in the SLN derived from the benign papillary lesions rather than from the carcinomas.

At present there is no objective method for determining with certainty whether a microdeposit of epithelial cells arrived in a SLN as a result of intrinsic invasion at the primary site or because of iatrogenic mechanical displacement. Even if the phenomenon of mechanical transport were proven to occur, the clinical significance of displaced carcinoma cells in SLNs or other ALNs remains uncertain. The indeterminate nature of these findings was highlighted by Carter and Page[308] who stated that "they look forward to the future development of laboratory assays that will correctly differentiate small lymph node deposits that are truly metastatic from those minimal deposits that are unlikely to have any significant impact on the patient and those deposits that have been benignly transported to the lymph node . . . ." Each case requires careful scrutiny of the histologic and immunohistochemical appearances of the primary tumor and epithelial deposits in the lymph node and of epithelial displacement at the primary site. In most cases, the evidence supports interpreting the lymph nodes as containing metastatic carcinoma, but rarely the findings may suggest displacement of benign epithelium.

SLNs and DCIS

This subject is also discussed in Chapter 11.

Several reports have presented data on the frequency of positive SLNs in patients with DCIS. In 1998, Cox et al.[285] reported finding positive SLNs in 11 of 150 patients (7.3%) with DCIS. The DCIS with positive lymph nodes were mainly of the high-grade type with necrosis. A subsequent analysis by these investigators described finding positive SLNs in 18 of 200 patients (9%) with DCIS.[294] Pendas et al.[309] reported that 5 of 87 patients (6%) with DCIS in their series had immunohistochemically positive SLN, and they recommended SLN biopsy for patients with relatively large, high-grade DCIS.

In a meta-analysis of 22 published series, the incidence of SLN positivity in 366 patients was 7.4% in those with a preoperative diagnosis of DCIS, and 3.7% in patients with a postoperative, that is, definitive, diagnosis of DCIS.[310] The data reflect the fact that 10% to 30% of patients with a preoperative NCB diagnosis of DCIS will be diagnosed with invasive carcinoma upon excision.

SLNs and Microinvasive Carcinoma

Results of SLN biopsy have also been reported for a number of patients with microinvasive carcinoma. Dauway et al.[286] described nine women with T*mic* tumors (invasion less than or equal to 1 mm) who underwent SLN biopsy, with detection of micrometastases by IHC in three (33%). Complete axillary dissection in these three patients did not uncover additional positive lymph nodes. Zavotsky et al.[311] performed SLN biopsy in 14 women with microinvasive carcinoma. Invasive foci were less than or equal to 1 mm in 11 cases. Positive SLNs were identified in two cases (14%), both associated with 4.5-cm high-grade DCIS, which had invasion less than or equal to 1 and 2 mm, respectively. Neither had additional positive ALNs, but one later developed a malignant pleural effusion. Two of the 15 patients (13.3%) had one positive ALN each. In a series of 13 patients with microinvasive lobular carcinoma, ALN biopsies (including 9 SLN samplings) were all negative.[311,312]

The largest series to date of SLN biopsies in patients with microinvasive carcinoma was reported by Lyons et al.[313] Positive SLNs were found in 14 of 112 cases (12.5%), including 3 (2.7%) with macrometastases. The other patients had micrometastases (five cases) or ITCs (six cases). Completion axillary dissection revealed additional positive lymph nodes in two of the three patients with a macrometastasis in a SLN.

The authors concluded that "as we are not able to reliably predict which patients with microinvasive carcinoma are most likely to have a positive SLN, it appears reasonable to perform a SLNB [SLN biopsy] only on those in whom the presence of positive SLN will influence management." Unfortunately, this conclusion provides no guidance since clinical management will be determined by the results of the SLN procedure in most cases, with completion axillary dissection and adjuvant chemotherapy most likely to be recommended for patients found to have a macrometastasis or possibly those found to have SLN with micrometastases.

SLNs and Multifocal and Multicentric Invasive Carcinoma

The presence of multiple foci of invasive carcinoma may be a risk factor of SLN metastases. In one study, 15 of 25 patients (60%) with multifocal invasion (5 lobular, 10 ductal) had a positive SLN.[314] However, the risk of having positive SLN appears to depend on the size of the largest invasive focus, and when stratified on this basis, it may not differ appreciably from patients with a unifocal tumor of equivalent size. The likelihood of there being positive NSLNs was greater when the SLN was positive (53%) than when the SLN was negative (10%). Veronesi et al.[315] reported finding positive ALNs in 31 of 46 patients (67%) who had multicentric or extensively multifocal carcinomas. Three of these patients had a negative SLN. False-negative rates for SLN biopsy of multifocal carcinoma reported in other studies were 8%,[316] 4%,[317] and 0%.[318] Knauer et al.[317] observed that when compared to patients with unicentric carcinoma, those with multicentric carcinoma had a higher frequency of positive SLN, but there was not a statistically significant difference in false-negative rates. A similar conclusion was reached by Tousimis et al.,[316] who noted that false-negative SLNs were more likely to be found in patients with a dominant tumor larger than 5 cm or a palpable ALN. They recommended that despite a negative SLN, patients with the latter clinical findings should undergo axillary dissection for accurate staging. Multifocal or multicentric invasive carcinoma is not a technical contraindication to SLN biopsy[281,319]; indeed, a systematic review of the topic found that this procedure is as successful in multifocal and multicentric carcinomas as in unifocal tumors.[320]

SLNs and Neoadjuvant Therapy

SLN biopsy is being increasingly performed in patients who have received neoadjuvant chemotherapy. Cumulative data suggest that SLN biopsy in this setting is a safe and feasible procedure, and is accurately predictive of the axillary nodal status.[321–323]

Schrenk et al.[324] described 21 patients who had SLN biopsy prior to neoadjuvant therapy and full axillary dissection following the completion of systemic therapy. The mean number of SLNs per case was 1.9. Twelve SLNs were negative and nine had metastatic carcinoma. Examination of the axillary dissections revealed additional involved lymph nodes in six of the nine patients with positive SLN. None of the patients with a negative SLN had metastases in the remaining lymph nodes. In a retrospective analysis, Jones et al.[325] reported a higher rate of unsuccessful SLN mapping if the procedure was performed after neoadjuvant treatment (19.4%) than if it was done before therapy (0%). A clinically positive axilla confirmed by axillary dissection was documented in six of the seven women who failed to map. Among those with a negative SLN, two (11%) were found to have metastases at axillary dissection (false-negative SLN biopsy).

Concern about the reliability of SLN biopsy in this setting is based on several factors:

1. destruction of metastatic tumor by the chemotherapy;
2. altered pathways of lymphatic drainage caused by fibrosis in the breast, in lymphatic channels and in lymph nodes; and
3. blockage of lymphatics by nonviable tumor tissue.

Despite these potential drawbacks, several reports (in addition to those cited above) have described successful SLN biopsy for the majority of candidates in this clinical setting. Haid et al.[326] described SLN biopsy in 29 of 33 cases (88%), resulting in positive SLN in 18 and negative SLN in 11. No SLNs were detected by preoperative lymphoscintigraphy in nine of the patients, five of whom had positive SLNs identified surgically. The results of SLN examination were confirmed in all cases by axillary dissection (100% sensitivity, 100% NPV). Julian et al.[327] were able to identify a SLN in 29 of 31 patients (93.5%) after neoadjuvant chemotherapy. A positive SLN was found in 11 (38%) and in 5 the SLN was the only positive lymph node.

Tafra et al.[328] studied 968 patients entered into a SLN biopsy protocol, including 29 who had had prior chemotherapy. Biopsy was successful in 27 of the 29 (93%) patients who had had prior chemotherapy and in 822 of 939 women (88%) who had not had prior chemotherapy. Positive SLNs were found more often in patients who had neoadjuvant chemotherapy (15 of 29, 52%) than in the untreated group (200 of 939, 21%). After the results of axillary dissection were taken into consideration, the false-negative rate was 13% in the untreated group, and there were no false negatives in the adjuvant chemotherapy cohort. Schwartz and Meltzer[329] reported 100% success in the SLN biopsy of 21 patients after neoadjuvant chemotherapy. When the results of SLN biopsy and axillary dissection were compared, one patient with a negative SLN was found to have a nodal metastasis in the axillary dissection (9% false-negative rate). Kang et al.[330] had a lower success rate with SLN biopsy after neoadjuvant chemotherapy (61 of 80, 76.3%) with three false-negative procedures (7.3% false-negative rate). Kinoshita et al.[331] reported successful SLN biopsy in 72 of 77 patients (93.5%) post-chemotherapy, with a false-negative rate of 11.1%.

The largest series of patients was reported from the NSABP B27 protocol for neoadjuvant therapy.[332] Data were available for 343 patients who underwent SLN biopsy followed by axillary dissection. SLNs were positive in 125 patients, including 70 (56%) whose only metastasis was a SLN. Fifteen of 218 patients with a negative SLN had lymph node metastases in the axillary dissection (NPV, 93.1%). Overall, the SLN procedure accurately predicted axillary nodal status in 328 of 343 patients (95.6% accuracy). In this study the false-negative rate was not significantly related to patient characteristics, clinical tumor stage, type of SLN biopsy procedure, or chemotherapy response.

In an effort to detect factors associated with additional axillary nodal involvement after postneoadjuvant therapy–positive SLN biopsy, Jeruss et al.[333] analyzed 104 patients. In multivariate analysis, the following features were associated with additional axillary metastases: clinically positive lymph nodes, the presence of lymphovascular invasion, multicentric carcinoma, and tumor size.

The foregoing data indicate that SLN biopsy can be successfully performed after neoadjuvant chemotherapy, with a success rate that is not significantly different from when the procedure is employed in untreated patients. The false-negative rate is comparable in both situations. These studies do not adequately address the question of the frequency with which neoadjuvant treatment completely destroys nodal metastases and thereby converts an N1 patient to the N0 category (understaging). If the pretreatment nodal status is necessary to plan management, the SLN procedure should be performed prior to the initiation of chemotherapy.

SLN Biopsy and Other Special Circumstances

Drainage to contralateral ALNs has been documented in isolated cases. Two patients described by Agarwal et al.[334] had previously undergone ipsilateral breast-conserving surgery with radiotherapy and negative axillary dissections. Repeat SLN biopsy, when recurrent carcinoma was detected, revealed drainage to the contralateral axilla. One lymph node contained micrometastatic carcinoma and the other was uninvolved. Another instance of contralateral axillary metastasis after prior breast surgery was described by Lim et al.[335] SLN biopsy in both axillae with the detection of metastases bilaterally was reported by Allweis et al.[336] Jansen et al.[337] identified SLN in the ipsilateral axilla and contralateral internal mammary lymph nodes, yielding metastatic carcinoma only at the latter site.

Prior surgery on the breast and axilla affects the pattern of lymphatic drainage.[338] As noted previously, this can result in drainage to aberrant sites, such as the contralateral axilla, but aberrant drainage has been demonstrated in the absence of prior surgery. In practice, SLN biopsy has been accomplished successfully in the management of recurrent breast carcinoma after prior surgery on the ipsilateral breast.[295,339] Dinan et al.[340] were able to evaluate 16 women who had SLN biopsy with lymphoscintigraphy for new primary or recurrent carcinoma after breast-conserving surgery with radiotherapy. Axillary surgery initially consisted of partial or complete dissection in 14 and SLN biopsy in 2. At the time of the second carcinoma, SLN biopsy was successful in 11 of 16 cases (69%). Drainage was identified at the following sites: ipsilateral axilla, 4 (25%); contralateral axilla, 3 (19%); ipsilateral supraclavicular, 2 (13%); contralateral posterior cervical/supraclavicular, 1 (6%); and internal mammary, 1 (6%). One intramammary lymph node was also located. All SLNs proved to be negative.

Cox et al.[319] reported SLN biopsy in more than 50 patients with "breast implants." The same authors described successful SLN biopsy in four patients with tumors outside the pedicle flap after breast reduction procedures by the inferior pedicle technique. Biopsy was not successful in one patient whose tumor was inside the pedicle flap. Failure of SLN biopsy was reported in 25% of patients who had prior axillary surgery.[339]

SLN biopsy has been done at the time of prophylactic mastectomy because of the risk of occult carcinoma.[341] Cox et al.[319] detected occult carcinoma in 14 of 245 (5.7%) unilateral prophylactic mastectomies. Two patients (0.8%) had metastatic carcinomas in a SLN. No positive SLNs were found in 15 patients who underwent bilateral prophylactic mastectomy. Boughey et al.[342] reviewed 436 prophylactic mastectomies performed at the M. D. Anderson Cancer Center between 2000 and 2005. SLN biopsy was successful in 106 of 108 patients (98%) in which it was undertaken. The SLN was negative in one patient with a 2-mm occult invasive carcinoma. Another patient had a 9-mm metastatic SLN focus on the side of a carcinoma-free prophylactic mastectomy, derived from a contralateral inflammatory carcinoma. In the entire series, including patients who did not undergo SLN biopsy, carcinoma was identified in 19 of 382 (5%) contralateral prophylactic mastectomies (12 intraductal, 7 invasive) and in 3 of 54 (5.6%) bilateral prophylactic mastectomies (2 intraductal, 1 invasive). Hence, 8 of the 436 (1.8%) prophylactic mastectomies harbored an occult invasive carcinoma. King et al.[343] found occult carcinoma in 13 of 163 (8%) prophylactic mastectomy specimens (9 intraductal, 4 invasive). Two patients with occult invasive carcinoma each had a positive SLN. Among 130 women who did not have occult carcinomas in the prophylactic mastectomy specimens, one (0.8%) had a positive SLN on the prophylactic side, which probably derived from stage IIIC carcinoma in the other breast. In a cohort of 99 patients, Nasser et al.[344] reported the presence of occult contralateral carcinoma in eight patients (8.1%), of whom six (75%) had DCIS alone. A positive SLN was found on the prophylactic side in two patients (2%). Both had inflammatory carcinoma in the opposite breast.

Data from the foregoing studies suggest that the likelihood of finding a positive SLN on the side of a prophylactic mastectomy is 2% or less, and that SLN biopsy can be generally omitted in prophylactic mastectomies, although it may be undertaken in the setting of contralateral inflammatory carcinoma.

For a discussion of SLN biopsy in male carcinoma, see Chapter 36.

Radiation Exposure during SLN Biopsy

Radiation exposure of the patient and medical personnel is not considered to be an issue of concern when a radioactive tracer is employed in SLN biopsies.[315,345,346] It has been estimated that the radiation dose to the tissue at the injection site is about 45 rad/mCi.[345] Excision of the SLN, frequently concurrent with the tumor site, greatly reduces local radiation in the patient. Dosimetry studies obtained intraoperatively have measured exposure to the surgeon's hands to be 9.4 ± 3.6 mrem per operation.[346] Low exposure levels can be expected for pathology personnel, since the radiation dose is minimal and contact with specimens is brief. Veronesi et al.[315] found that absorbed radiation dose for the surgeon, calculated in terms of exposure during 100 operations per year, was within the dose limits for the general population when compared with recommendation of the International Commission on Radiological Protection. Veronesi and colleagues[347] have also reported on the "safety of sentinel lymph node biopsy in pregnant patients with breast cancer, when performed with a low-dose lymphoscintigraphic technique." Nonetheless, it would be prudent to follow institutional, local, and national regulatory guidelines with respect to radiation safety.

PATHOLOGY OF SLNS

Intraoperative Diagnosis of SLNs

Intraoperative histologic diagnosis of SLNs is appropriate only if management of the patient will be immediately influenced by the results. For example, permission to perform an axillary dissection may be dependent on detecting carcinoma in the SLN, or the operation may be terminated if the frozen section of the SLN is reported to be negative. Intraoperative diagnosis of SLN can be accomplished by FSE, TIC, or a combination of the two techniques.

Touch Imprint Cytology (TIC) of SLN

Advocates of TIC feel that preparing a frozen section is wasteful of tissue because portions of the frozen samples are customarily trimmed in the microtome to obtain a surface suitable for sectioning. Some lymph nodes are difficult to cut for frozen section, especially when there is fatty infiltration. TIC not only spares tissue but also makes it possible to obtain specimens from multiple cut surfaces of a lymph node, thereby allowing a wider sampling of the tissue than would be achieved by frozen section. TIC is also potentially less time-consuming than frozen section, although optimal cytologic screening can be a painstakingly slow process. A significant drawback is that many pathologists are not skilled in cytology, and it may be difficult to recognize sparse carcinoma cells in the highly cellular background of lymph node imprints. Imprint preparations can be stained rapidly with H&E, Diff-Quik, Wright–Giemsa, or other methods. The choice of staining procedure depends on individual preference.

Several studies have documented the use of TIC for the diagnosis of SLN with varying success.[348–353] Two separate reports from different institutions each described results obtained in 55 patients who had SLN specimens diagnosed intraoperatively with H&E-stained slides.[349,350] The results for both studies were similar, with one false-negative interpretation (0.8%) in each report. The NPV was 99.2%, sensitivity was 95.7%, specificity was 100%, and PPV was 100%. Moes et al.[352] reported on 66 patients who had 175 SLNs examined intraoperatively with H&E-stained cytologic preparations made by scraping the cut surfaces of bisected lymph nodes. The cytologic diagnosis corresponded to the histologic diagnosis in 167 of 175 (95.4%) SLNs. There were six false-negative and one false-positive cytologic interpretations, but the latter patient had another lymph node which was cytologically and histologically positive. Ku et al.[348] reported an intraoperative false-negative TIC diagnosis on 10 of 103 (10%) SLNs and one false-positive diagnosis for an accuracy of 91%. Jeruss et al.[353] evaluated diagnosis in 342 consecutive patients who had SLN biopsy in which the SLNs were examined by imprint cytology and routine postoperative histology. The SLNs were positive by both methods in 32 patients (9.3%), and 2 patients (0.5%) had positive TIC with negative histology. SLNs were diagnosed as negative by both methods in 265 (77.5%). Metastatic carcinoma was detected histologically in 43 SLNs reported to be negative by imprint cytology, representing 14% of TIC negative cases. The sensitivity and specificity of TIC proved to be 42.7% and 99.3%, respectively.

These results suggest that TIC is a useful adjunct intraoperative technique for the diagnosis of SLN, with low sensitivity and high specificity. Because of the low sensitivity, negative TIC cannot be relied upon as the only intraoperative method for evaluating SLNs in breast cancer patients and should be combined with FSE if further surgical treatment is dependent on the results.

Frozen Section of SLN

FSE of the SLN has been evaluated in several studies, and the results have proven to be generally satisfactory. Hill et al.[275] reported on a study of 405 patients who had a SLN examined by FSE. Metastatic carcinoma was detected in 68 patients (17%), but final sections were positive in 78, yielding 10 false-negative FSE reports (13%). False-negative rates for FSE of SLN reported in other studies were 18 of 75 (17%),[289] 19 of 225 (8%),[354] and 3 of 50 (6%).[355]

Comparison of Frozen Section and Touch Imprint Cytology of SLN

A direct comparison of the results of FSE and TIC was reported by van Diest et al.[356] False-negative diagnoses were obtained in 4 of 31 (13%) SLNs examined by FSE and in 10 of 26 (38%) examined by TIC. In 11 cases, the imprint preparations were deemed unsatisfactory for diagnosis. There was 88% concordance between FSE and TIC, but 7 of 23 (30%) SLNs diagnosed as positive on FSE had a negative imprint. The sensitivity and overall accuracy of FSE (87%; 95%) were substantially greater than those of TIC (62%; 83%). Turner et al.[357] evaluated the results of combined FSE and TIC. The overall accuracy was 93.2%. The combined diagnostic approach detected 87% of SLNs with macrometastases (smaller than 2 mm), but only 28% of micrometastases were found by H&E on paraffin sections.

Data from the various studies described in this section demonstrate that metastatic carcinoma can be detected in SLNs from many patients intraoperatively by either FSE or TIC. These procedures are approximately equivalent for detecting macrometastases (larger than 2 mm) in more than 90% of cases, and neither is especially reliable for identifying micrometastases that are the major source of false-negative intraoperative diagnoses. In cases where the diagnosis may be difficult, having TIC as well as FSE available can be useful. Despite these limitations, intraoperative diagnosis of SLNs makes an important contribution because patients with a positive SLN can undergo a complete axillary dissection, if it is clinically indicated, without a second trip to the operating room.

Recent studies have questioned the clinical and pathologic significance of finding micrometastases in SLN, particularly in intraoperative consultations. As a result, the practice of using TIC or FSE on SLN has waned. Nevertheless, the pathologist is obligated to accede to clinically appropriate requests for intraoperative evaluation (i.e., FSE) of SLN. In this context, the reporting of such evaluations can be limited to assessment of metastatic deposits that are larger than 0.2 cm (more than micrometastasis). Thus, the FSE diagnosis in this setting can take either of two forms: *negative*, negative for metastases that are larger than 0.2 cm; and *positive*, positive for metastases larger than 0.2 cm. In the later event, completion axillary dissection can be performed in the same operative procedure in the appropriate clinical setting. Adoption of this reporting practice obviates the problem of false-negative results that are inherent to the practice of FSE of SLN on account of the occasional inevitable missed diagnosis of ITCs and micrometastasis.

Methods for Histologic Examination of SLNs

As noted in the preceding discussion, metastatic carcinoma can be readily detected in routine H&E slides of an appropriately sectioned lymph node if it is a macrometastasis (larger than 2 mm). Additional ("enhanced") procedures such as obtaining multiple "levels" or cytokeratin (CK) IHC contribute largely to the finding of micrometastases in SLN that appear to be histologically negative in a routine H&E section, and less frequently to the finding of a macrometastasis that is eccentrically positioned. These procedures have assumed greater importance with SLN biopsy that identifies the lymph node or nodes most likely to harbor metastatic carcinoma.

Various protocols combining multiple sections and CK IHC have been employed to examine SLN, but there is no consensus as to which is most labor- and cost-effective. Some of the procedures used include two H&E levels separated by 40 μm and one CK IHC section[357]; serial sectioning with every sixth level taken for H&E, and the succeeding two levels for CK and EMA IHC[358]; H&E and CK IHC on paired sections separated by 40 μm[359]; CK IHC on serial sections taken at 0.25-mm intervals through the block[360]; one H&E section and CK IHC at four additional levels not otherwise specified[361]; three H&E levels "100–500 μm apart"[289]; multiple H&E sections (from 4 to 20) without IHC[290]; at least four H&E levels and CK IHC[293]; and serial sections of the entire lymph node at 0.5-mm intervals stained with H&E and CK IHC.[358] Another study suggests that three H&E sections taken at levels 25%, 50%, and 75% into the tissue block would detect virtually all metastatic foci in a lymph node.[362] A survey of European pathology laboratories found that 71% used IHC to evaluate SLNs found to be negative in H&E sections.[363] Overall, an astonishing 123 different protocols were described by 240 respondents.

The routine use of IHC for the diagnosis of SLN is somewhat controversial, at least in part because of the uncertain clinical significance of micrometastases and ITCs that are the major contribution of this procedure. An earlier retrospective study by Chagpar et al.[364] described the follow-up of 84 patients with H&E-negative SLN, including 15 who had metastatic carcinoma detected in the SLN by IHC only. Adjuvant chemotherapy was given on the basis of primary tumor characteristics, including only 5 of the 15 with an IHC-positive SLN. After a median follow-up of 40.2 months, there was no significant difference in OS or metastasis-free survival between chemotherapy-treated patients with negative and IHC-positive SLN. Guidelines published by the College of American Pathologists,[365] the American Society of Clinical Oncology,[366] and others[367–369] state that IHC examination is not required. A differing viewpoint has been expressed by some investigators.[370–373]

Regardless of the foregoing controversy, there is some practical value to IHC because it more sharply defines the extent of metastatic foci, and this allows for the more accurate measurement of metastases. Furthermore, most pathologists with experience in the diagnosis of SLNs can recount surprising instances where IHC highlighted metastatic foci, sometimes measuring more than 2 mm, that were overlooked because of being intimately mingled with native nodal lymphoid tissue or being mistaken for postcapillary venules or histiocytes. In some instances, IHC detects more than one adjacent metastatic focus in a SLN that had only one metastasis identified in an H&E section, resulting in an aggregate size exceeding 0.2 or 2 mm. Finally, IHC is essential if one is to estimate the number of ITCs, because the cells may be widely distributed in a SLN. This dispersed pattern of metastases is characteristically encountered with infiltrating lobular carcinoma.[374] Therefore, despite the present uncertainty as to the therapeutic and prognostic significance of micrometastases and ITCs, IHC is recommended here as part of the standard work-up of SLN in order to maximize information from these limited specimens and to more precisely define the extent of nodal involvement when it is present. A broad-spectrum CK (AE1/3) is well-suited for this purpose. Low-molecular-weight CK (such as CAM5.2) may immunoreact for dendritic reticular cells and can, on this account, cause diagnostic difficulty.

An interesting study of an enhanced pathology protocol for SLN was reported by Fortunato et al.[375] The authors retrospectively reviewed slides from 416 consecutive breast cancer patients who had SLNs examined according to the following protocol: The first section was stained with H&E and if it was negative, three pairs of sections were prepared at 100-μm intervals for H&E and CK stains at each level. The SLN was found to be positive in the initial H&E section in 106 of 416 cases (25%). As a result of the enhanced protocol in the remaining 310 cases, 61 additional nodal metastases were detected, representing 15% of the initial 416 cases and 20% of the 310 cases with negative lymph nodes in the initial H&E section. Thirty-seven of the 61 additional metastases (60.6%) were found in the first 100-μm level, 17 (28%) at the second 100-μm level, and 7 (11.4%) at the third level. Classification of the 61 additional metastatic foci was as follows: 22 (36%) micrometastases, 38 (62%) ITCs, and 1 (2%) macrometastasis. The authors reported that all micrometastases were found in H&E sections, whereas most ITCs were detected by CK IHC. Because of the low yield at the third 100-μm level, the authors concluded that very little additional information would be gained from sections beyond the three 100-μm levels specified in their protocol.

Optimal Pathologic Processing of SLNs

The mean number of SLNs biopsied in each procedure is generally estimated to be about 2, and it is unusual to receive more than four SLNs. Most surgeons consider those lymph nodes with radioactive counts more than 10% of the hottest node as SLN, although some contend that all "hot and blue" lymph nodes should be designated as such. The removal of more than four lymph nodes as SLN carries the risk of complications that are typically associated with ALND.

All SLNs should be serially sliced along their long axis at 2-mm intervals. All slices should be submitted for histologic evaluation. If three or more slices result from such sectioning, then alternate sections should be placed face-down in the tissue cassette.[376] This process ensures the detection of the great majority of macrometastases, that is, those that span more than 2 mm. *In toto* submission of SLNs that span 3 mm or more or mere bisection of SLNs that span more than 5 mm may not detect significant nodal metastases. Unfortunately, more attention is usually paid to following histologic protocols (step sections and immunostains) in the processing of SLNs than to protocols for their gross handling.

As noted previously, there is also no consensus on the histologic sectioning protocol to be used in examining SLNs.[377] Step-sectioning is recommended in some, but not all, guidelines published by national and international organizations. When step-sectioning is recommended, there are often differences as to the spacing of sections. Sectioning at 200-μm intervals or less is considered to be necessary to detect metastases measuring at least 2 mm.

If the aforementioned gross protocol for SLN handling is followed, then the use of multiple H&E-stained sections can be omitted. The use of CK immunostain, preferably CK AE1/3, is helpful for the detection of smaller subtle metastases. Metastases from carcinomas of the classical lobular type, and particularly after neoadjuvant chemotherapy, can be readily identified with the CK immunostain, which can be of utmost value in the assessment of the size of metastases, and micrometastases can also be optimally assessed.

Relationship between SLNs and NSLNs

Positivity of SLN and the extent of SLN involvement are strong predictors of the presence of metastases in NSLNs, a fact that validates the SLN concept. This was convincingly demonstrated by Turner et al.,[357] who studied 103 patients who underwent SLN biopsy, followed by dissection of level I to II lymph nodes. Routine H&E study of the SLN revealed metastatic carcinoma in 33 patients (32%). CK IHC detected micrometastases in a SLN from 10 of the remaining 70 patients (14.3%) whose SLN appeared negative with the H&E staining, leaving 60 women with negative SLN after H&E and immunohistochemical staining. None of the 1,087 NSLNs from these 60 patients was found to have metastatic carcinoma in H&E sections, and only 0.09% had micrometastasis demonstrated by IHC. Consequently, only 1 of 60 patients (1.7%) with a SLN negative in H&E- and immunohistochemical sections had a positive NSLN. On the other hand, 18 of 43 patients (41.9%) with a positive SLN had NSLN metastases.

The distinction between a true-positive SLN on frozen section and a false-negative SLN is also a significant predictor of the presence of metastases in NSLNs, since the true-positive group usually has macrometastases (>2 mm) and the false-negative group mainly has micrometastases (≤2 mm). Turner et al.[378] reported that the frequency of positive NSLN was 64% when the SLN was positive intraoperatively and 18% when the SLN diagnosis during surgery was falsely negative.

The size of SLN metastases is a significant predictor for the likelihood of metastases in NSLN.[379–382] Viale et al.[383] found NSLN metastases in 18.8% of patients with micrometastatic SLN and in 54.8% of women with SLN macrometastases (larger than 2 mm). van Rijk et al.[379] reported that NSLN metastases were found in 20 of 106 patients (19%) who had micrometastases (less than or equal to ≤2 mm) detected in a SLN. In 16 of these cases, the NSLN harbored macrometastases (larger than 2 mm). Axillary dissection was also performed in 54 patients with a SLN "submicrometastasis," usually referring to ITCs detected by IHC. Metastatic carcinoma was found in NSLNs in four cases (8%) (two macrometastases, two micrometastases). Jakub et al.[380] detected metastases in the NSLN of 9 of 62 patients (14.5%) who underwent axillary dissection after finding of micrometastases only by IHC in a SLN. In a study of patients with ITCs in a SLN, Calhoun et al.[381] reported finding metastatic carcinoma in 3 of 58 (4.9%) axillary dissections (1 macrometastasis, 2 micrometastases). No axillary recurrences were detected in 17 women who did not have an axillary dissection after a mean follow-up of 80.5 months. Fifteen of the 17 patients received systemic adjuvant therapy.

Rutledge et al.[382] investigated the size of SLN metastases identified intraoperatively as a predictive factor for metastases in NSLN. Among 19 women with micrometastatic lymph nodes diagnosed by frozen section, 1 (5%) had a positive NSLN, whereas 21 of 34 patients (62%) with a macrometastatic SLN had positive NSLN.

The risk of NSLN metastases appears to be influenced not only by the size of SLN metastasis but also by the number of positive SLNs. Chu et al.[384] detected micrometastases by IHC in H&E-negative NSLNs in 11.8% of cases where there was one positive SLN and in 29.4% when more than one SLN contained metastatic carcinoma. Other pathologic factors associated with NSLN metastases in univariate analysis were tumor size and lymphovascular tumor involvement, but only tumor size and number of positive SLNs were significant risk factors in multivariate analysis. Viale et al.[385] also found that the number of positive SLNs as well as the size of the SLN metastasis was predictive of the likelihood of positive NSLNs.

Other factors reported to be associated with a significantly increased risk of NSLN metastases in patients with a positive SLN included the presence of lymphovascular involvement at the primary tumor site,[385,386] extranodal extension by metastatic tumor in the SLN that is almost always associated with macrometastases,[386,387] and a poorly differentiated or HER2-positive carcinoma.[387]

Nomograms have been developed for predicting the probability of NSLN metastases based on various factors, including the degree of SLN positivity as well as the characteristics of the primary tumor.[388,389] Degnim et al.[389] applied a nomogram developed at Memorial Sloan-Kettering Cancer Center (MSKCC)[388] to sets of patients from two institutions and were able to predict NSLN metastases in 72% and 86%, respectively. Chagpar et al.[390] described a less-complex model that was developed to predict which patients had metastases limited to SLN. Multivariate analysis of 1,253 cases revealed that tumor size, the number of positive SLNs, and the proportion of the SLNs that were involved were significant predictors. In the resultant model, each of these factors was assigned a point score. A 95% probability of having negative NSLN was obtained in 19 of 1,253 cases (1.4%), consisting of patients with T1a tumors, one positive SLN, and at least three SLNs removed. Overall, the model was predictive in only 68.1% of cases. Validation of the MSKCC nomogram was reported in a subsequent analysis.[390,391]

At least four breast cancer nomograms that are currently being used to calculate the predictive probability of non-sentinel ALN metastasis in cases with positive SLN. These nomograms include those developed by MSKCC, Paris's Tenon Hospital, Cambridge University, and Stanford University. All are easily accessible through Google with links to their respective Web sites. Multiple studies have compared the predictive value of these nomograms. Sanjuan et al.[392] found the MSKCC and Paris nomograms to be similar according the area under receiver operating characteristics (ROC) curve, and Moghaddam et al. found no significant differences between the MSKCC, Cambridge, and Stanford models.[393] Gur et al. found the MSKCC to be more predictive than the Paris, Cambridge, and Stanford models[394]; however, it should be noted that the latter three models are simpler to use, using three rather than eight pathology parameters.

Limited information is presently available about patients with a positive SLN who do not have an axillary dissection performed. Hwang et al.[395] reviewed 3,366 patients with invasive breast carcinoma who underwent SLN biopsy at the M. D. Anderson Cancer Center. A positive SLN was found in 750 patients (22%) among whom 196 (26% of positive SLN cases) did not undergo a completion axillary dissection because of "clinician and patient preference." Positive SLNs were identified in H&E sections in 126 (64.3%) and by IHC in 70 of the 196 patients (35.7%). The sizes of SLN metastases were as follows: ITCs with no foci larger than 0.2 mm in 67 (34%), micrometastases between 0.2 and 2 mm in 90 (46%), and macrometastases larger than 2 mm in 39 (20%) patients. In conjunction with breast-conserving surgery or mastectomy, 70% of the patients received chemotherapy and 58% had radiotherapy. Axillary radiation therapy was administered to 56 of the 196 patients (29%). When analyzed with two nomogram models for predicting the likelihood of finding NSLN metastases, the study group was found to have a low risk (9.8% in one model) for having additional nodal metastases. After a median follow-up of 29.5 months (range, 1.3 to 62.3 months), none of the patients had developed an axillary recurrence and one patient had a supraclavicular recurrence. Two other studies of patients with a positive SLN, typically smaller than a macrometastasis, reported no axillary recurrences after median follow-ups of 30 months[396] and 27.4 months.[397]

The foregoing data support the use of completion axillary dissection in most patients with macrometastatic carcinoma in one or more SLNs. The evidence also favors axillary dissection if more than one SLN is involved by micrometastatic carcinoma. If a single SLN harbors a micrometastasis or ITCs, axillary dissection has become distinctly uncommon as a result of studies that are discussed subsequently. Axillary dissection may be recommended in selected patients with a micrometastatic SLN if the primary tumor is poorly differentiated or has lymphovascular tumor emboli, but many of these patients will not need further axillary surgery, especially if they receive systemic adjuvant chemotherapy and/or regional radiotherapy. Follow-up of 5 to 10 years is needed to more accurately assess the actual risk of axillary recurrence in women with any category of positive SLN who do not undergo axillary dissection. Currently available nomograms are adjunctive, albeit imperfect, tools that are useful for decision-making in ambiguous cases.

Measuring Metastatic Carcinoma in SLNs

A deposit of metastatic carcinoma in a lymph node is described as a micrometastasis if it measures more than 0.2 mm and less than 2 mm, and as a macrometastasis if 2 mm or larger. The term "isolated tumor cells" was originally suggested by Hermanek et al.[398] to describe "single tumor cells or small cluster" that might be found in blood, lymph fluid, bone marrow, or lymph nodes. According to these authors, ITCs are not in contact with vessel or lymph sinus walls, they do not penetrate a vessel or lymph sinus wall, and they are not associated with stromal reaction. In the current staging of ALNs, ITC refers to 200 or fewer number of tumor cells distributed individually or in small clusters measuring 0.2 mm (i.e., 200 μm) or less.[399,400]

As discussed by Rivera et al.,[400] there are metastatic patterns encountered in SLNs and NSLNs that do not readily fit into the categories of ITC or micrometastases. Multiple metastases in a single lymph node are usually characterized on the basis of the largest focus, and a lymph node may, therefore, be classified as having an ITC or a micrometastasis, although the aggregate diameter of the tumor deposits may appear to exceed 2 mm. Other issues cited by Rivera et al.[400] include the staging of lymph nodes when carcinoma is found only in capsular lymphatic channels and when there are mitoses and/or stromal reactive changes in metastatic foci that qualify as ITC on the basis of size. In the TNM Staging System, the distinction between ITC and micrometastasis can serve to distinguish node-negative and node-positive status; however, this distinction can be subject to interobserver variation in interpretation of guidelines.[401] The interpretation of metastases from invasive lobular carcinoma can be particularly problematic.[402] Turner et al.[403] have reported improvement in reproducibility of results of nodal staging by use of "standardized histologic criteria and image-based training."

Distribution of Metastatic Carcinoma in SLN

The flow of lymph into lymph nodes occurs through channels that drain predominantly into subcapsular sinusoids and then to parenchymal sinusoids. This pattern of physiologic and anatomical function is responsible for the frequent observation that small metastatic deposits identified in H&E sections are located in the subcapsular sinusoids (Fig. 44.34). Consequently, pathologists devote particular attention to this region during histologic examination of SLNs. ITCs, particularly those lacking pleomorphic cytologic features, can be difficult to separate from histiocytes that normally populate the sinusoids (Fig. 44.35). Some metastatic carcinoma cells appear to undergo changes that suggest degenerative alterations represented by nuclear pyknosis and increased eosinophilia of the cytoplasm. These cells are often indistinguishable from histiocytes in H&E-stained sections, and it is usually necessary to rely on CK IHC to determine whether epithelial cells are present (Fig. 44.36).

Clusters of carcinoma cells are more readily recognized in sinusoids than are isolated cells, in part because of a tendency for the cohesive carcinoma cells to separate from the surrounding histiocytes, causing them to appear to be located in a lacunar space (Figs. 44.34, 44.36, and 44.37). By itself, this is not a completely reliable diagnostic criterion because carcinoma cells vary in their cohesiveness and histiocytes are sometimes aggregated in clumps. Metastatic lobular carcinoma is notorious in this regard because it is characterized by loss of cell surface adhesion proteins such as E-cadherin and it tends to involve lymph nodes in a dispersed fashion without particular regard to sinusoidal distribution, although occasionally the metastases in such cases may be predominantly subcapsular (Fig. 44.38).

One of the interesting observations to result from intense histologic examination of SLNs with multiple sections and IHCs is that isolated micrometastases can be found in the lymphoid stroma without detectable subcapsular deposits (Figs. 44.35 and 44.39). These parenchymal micrometastases are particularly difficult to appreciate in H&E sections, and they are usually detected only after CK IHC sections have been prepared. This distribution of metastatic carcinoma

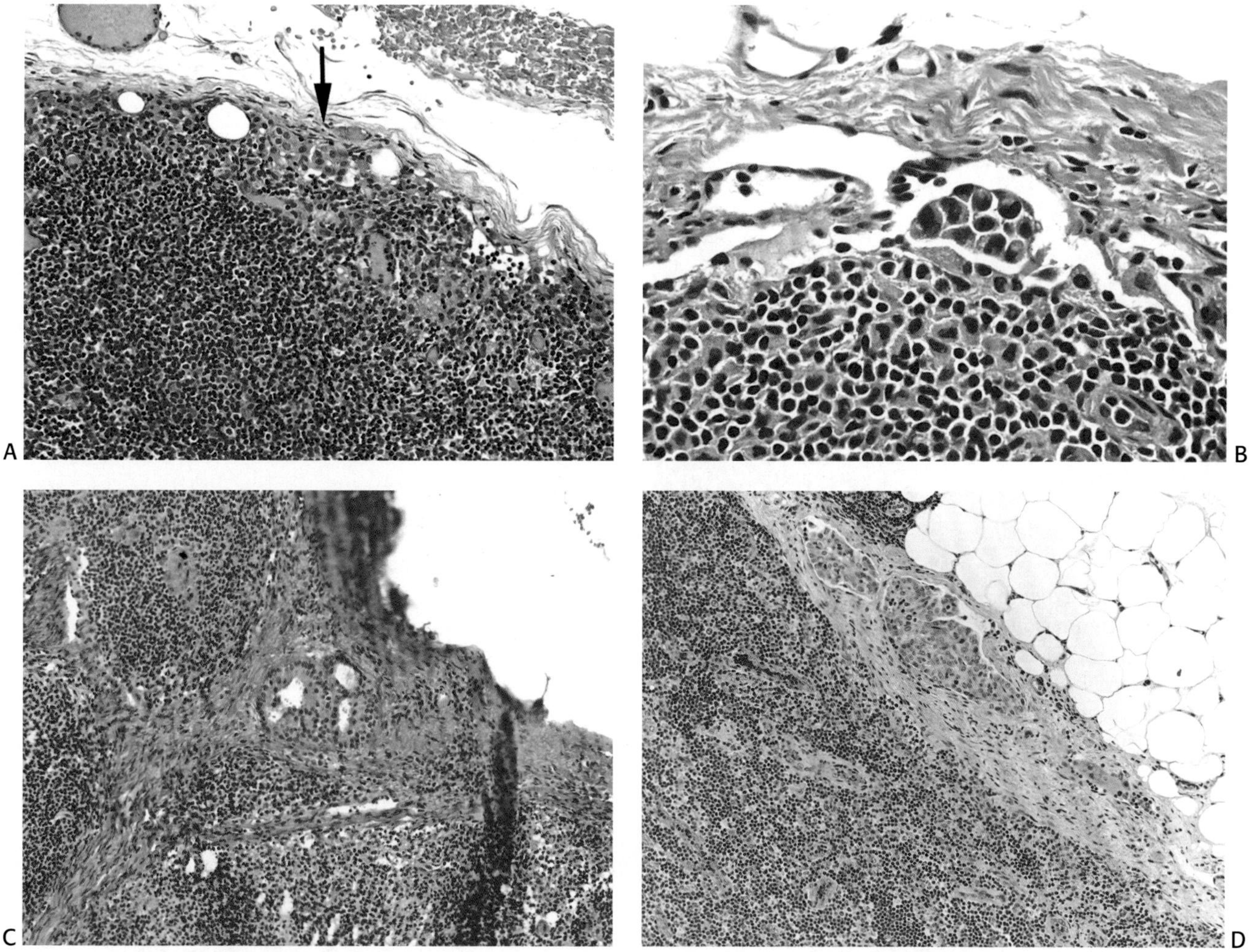

FIG. 44.34. ***Sentinel lymph nodes, isolated tumor cells (A,B) and micrometastasis (C,D) in peripheral sinusoids.*** **A,B:** Deposits of metastatic carcinoma (<0.2 mm) are present in peripheral sinusoids of two lymph nodes. The less-distinct metastasis in **(A)** is indicated by an *arrow*. CK immunostaining is usually not needed to detect such metastases. **C,D:** Deposits of micrometastatic carcinoma (>0.2 mm) are present in peripheral sinusoids of two SLNs. Image **(C)** is from a frozen section preparation. **(D)** is a permanent section preparation from another case.

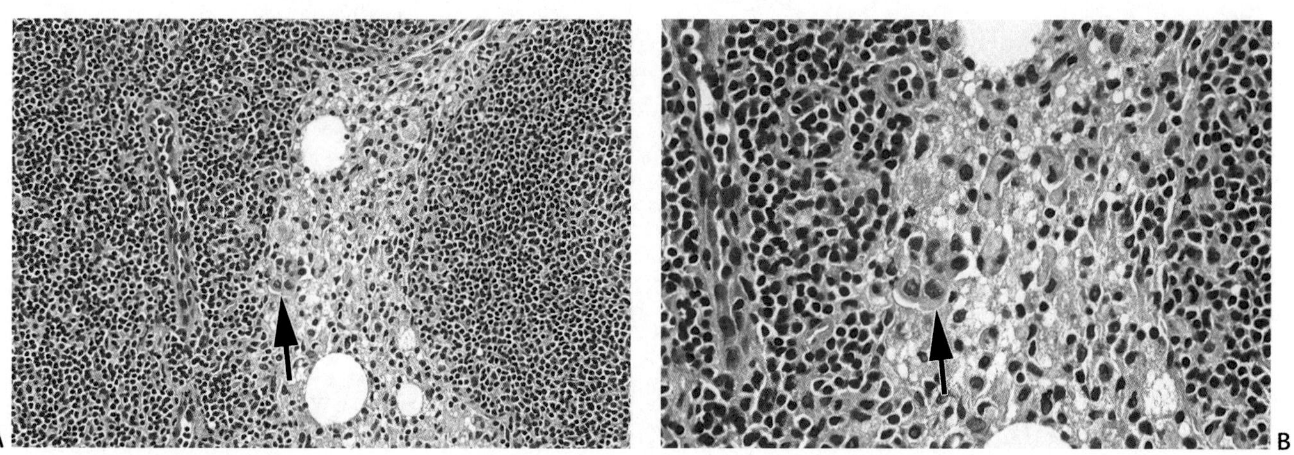

FIG. 44.35. ***Sentinel lymph nodes, isolated tumor cells in central sinusoids.*** **A,B:** Two large lipid vacuoles are present among histiocytes that fill a central sinusoid. A cluster of "suspicious" cells located between the lipid vacuoles is indicated by the *arrows.* **C:** The immunostain for CK7 on a replicate section discloses two clusters of immunoreactive cells near the upper lipid vacuole. The lower CK7-positive cell group is in the location of the "suspicious" cells in **(B)**.

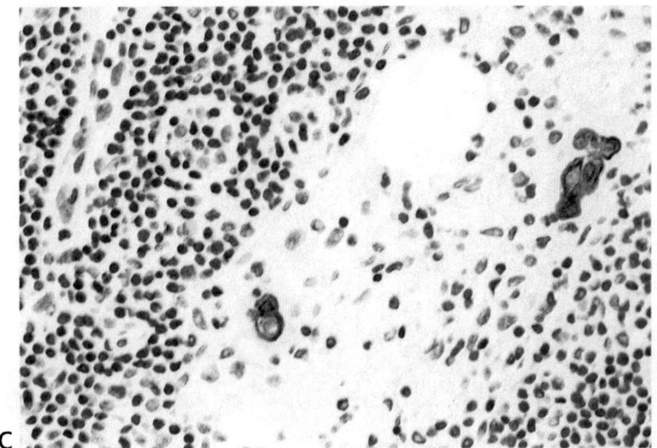

FIG. 44.35. *(Continued)*

has been associated with, but is not specific for, lobular carcinoma. Di Tommaso et al.[404] found that the site of micrometastases in SLNs as well as their size was a predictor of metastases in NSLNs. The frequency of positive NSLN was 3% (1 of 31) when micrometastases were sinusoidal and 29% (9 of 31) when they were intranodal.

Metastatic Carcinoma and Structural Changes in SLN

SLNs that harbor micrometastases may undergo subtle structural changes. Ribatti et al.[405] evaluated angiogenesis and mast cell concentration in SLN with and without micrometastases. Using the CD34 and antitryptase antibodies to detect angiogenesis and mast cells, respectively, they found that both were significantly increased in the presence of micrometastases. It is possible that mast cells, attracted to lymph nodes containing micrometastases, contribute to angiogenesis since these cells contain angiogenic factors and cytokines.

Histology of Metastatic Carcinoma in SLN

Metastatic carcinoma in SLNs and NSLNs usually duplicates the cytologic and histologic features of the primary tumor. Knowledge of the appearance of the primary tumor is, therefore, useful in screening lymph nodes in general, and especially SLNs, for metastatic carcinoma. Comparison of cytologic features can be done with small micrometastases and even single cells, whereas architectural comparison

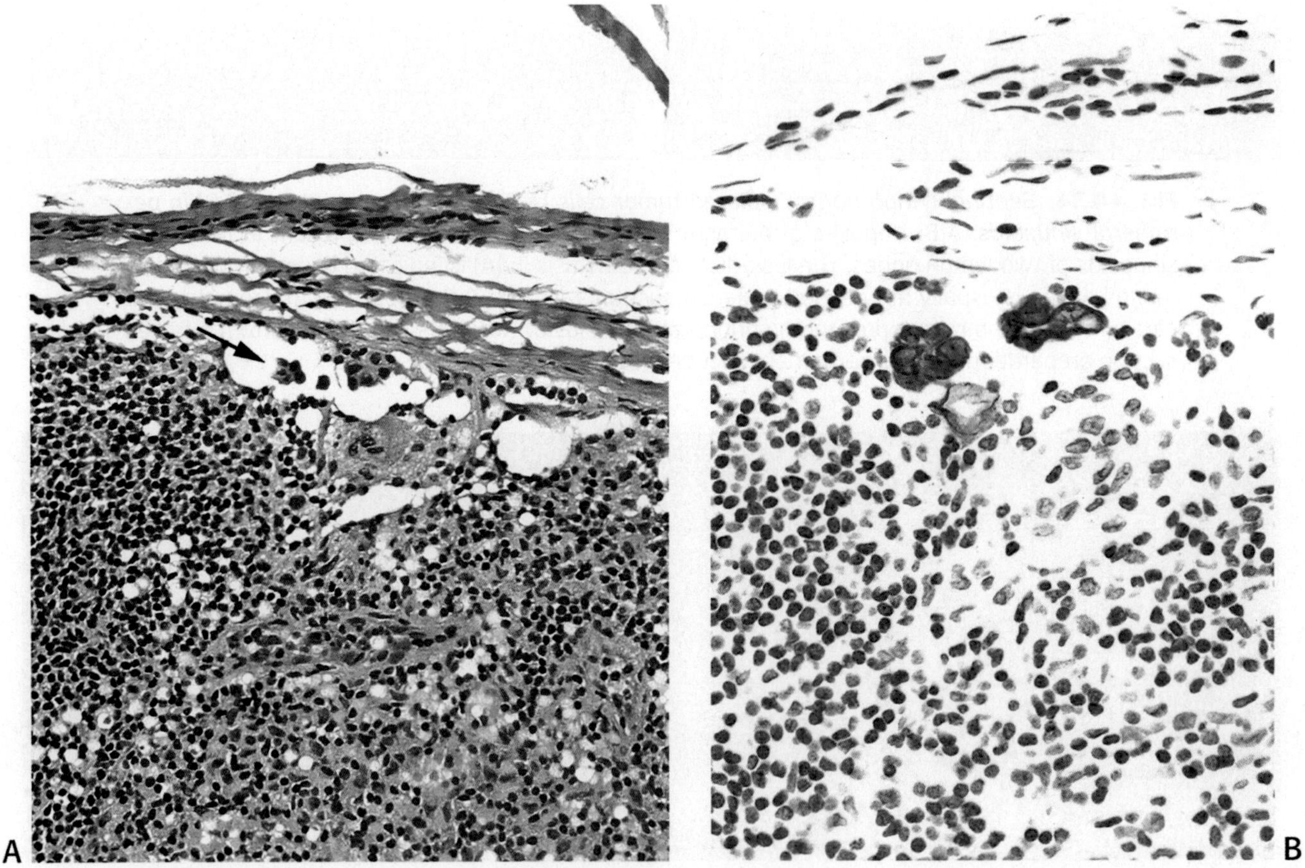

FIG. 44.36. ***Sentinel lymph node, isolated tumor cells.*** **A:** The minute clusters of cells *(arrow)* in the peripheral sinusoid of this lymph are not clearly diagnostic of metastatic carcinoma in this H&E section. **B:** Reactivity for CK7 is shown, establishing the epithelial character of the cells depicted in **(A)**. **C:** A cluster of about three carcinoma cells is located just beneath the lymph node capsule *(arrow)*. Two small clusters of carcinoma cells are located just beneath the lymph node capsule *(arrows)*.

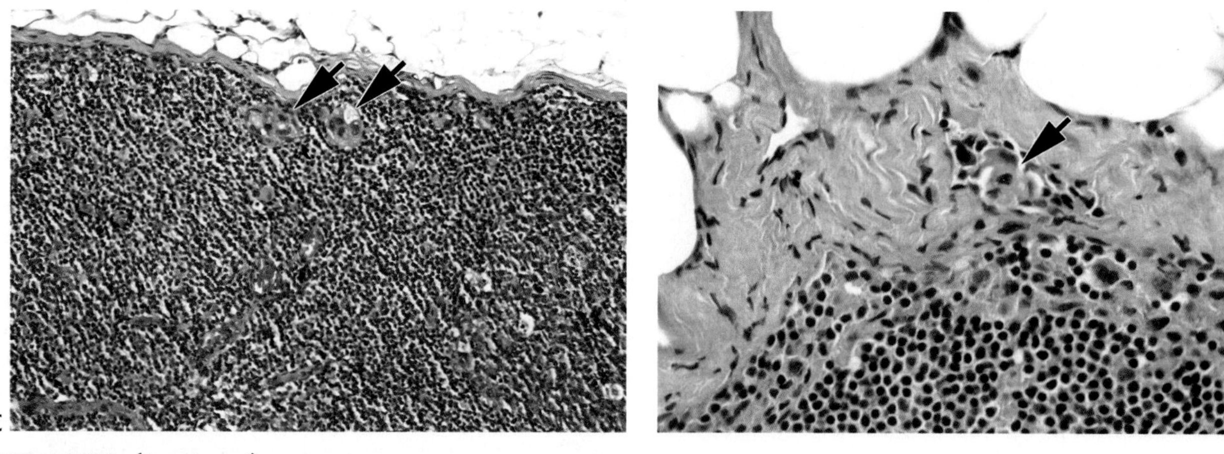

FIG. 44.36. *(Continued)*

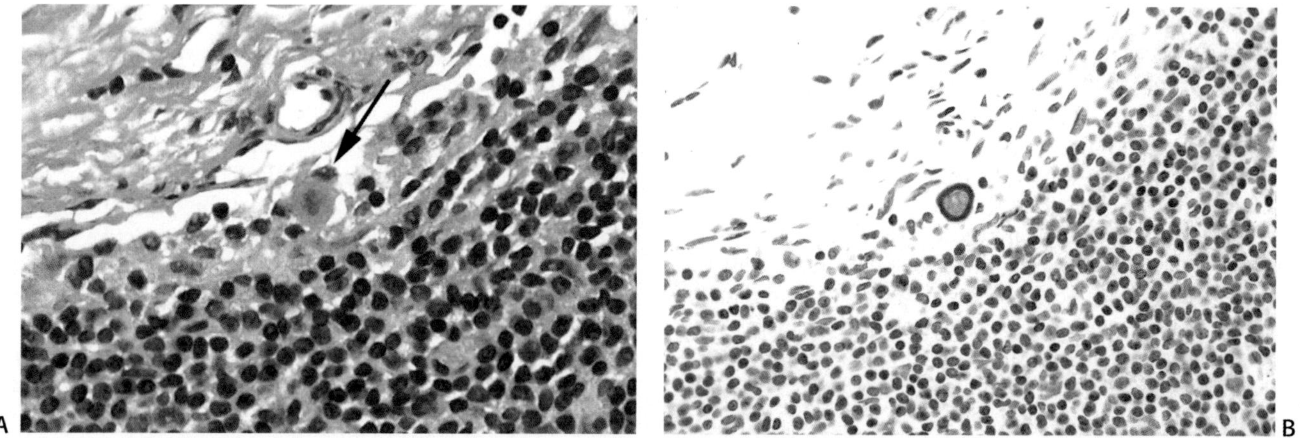

FIG. 44.37. ***Sentinel lymph nodes with isolated cell metastasis.*** The patient had comedo DCIS with microinvasion. **A:** The nature of the solitary cell (*arrow*) identified in the peripheral sinus was uncertain. **B:** The cell was immunoreactive with the CK immunostain AE1/3.

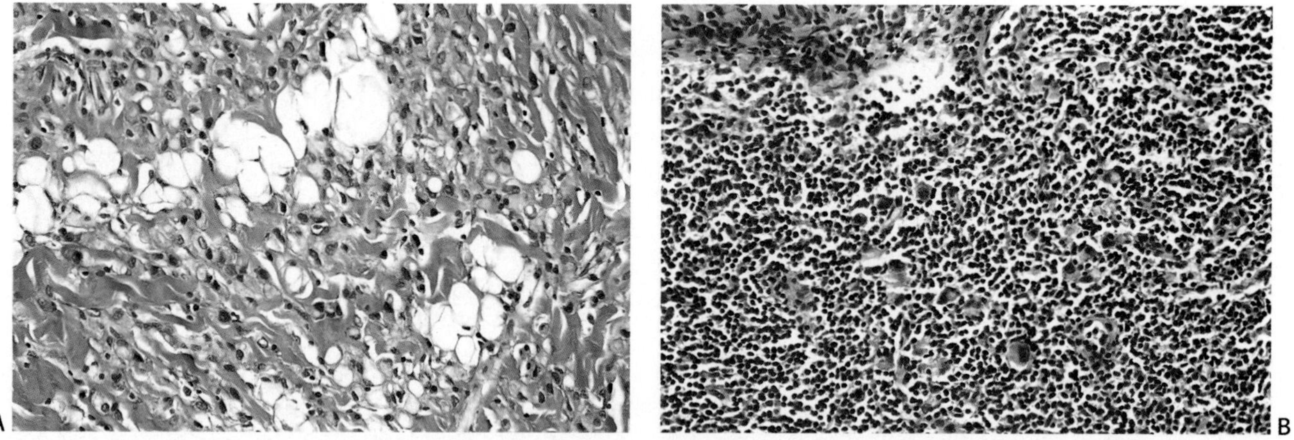

FIG. 44.38. ***Sentinel lymph node in invasive lobular carcinoma.*** **A:** A 7-mm invasive lobular carcinoma in the breast. **B:** Cells with hyperchromatic nuclei in the lymphoid tissue of the SLN. **C:** Numerous isolated cells in the lymphoid tissue are reactive for CK7 and the peripheral sinusoids are devoid of CK-positive cells. More than 200 such cells, counted in a single section, would constitute a micrometastasis per current staging AJCC–UICC guidelines.

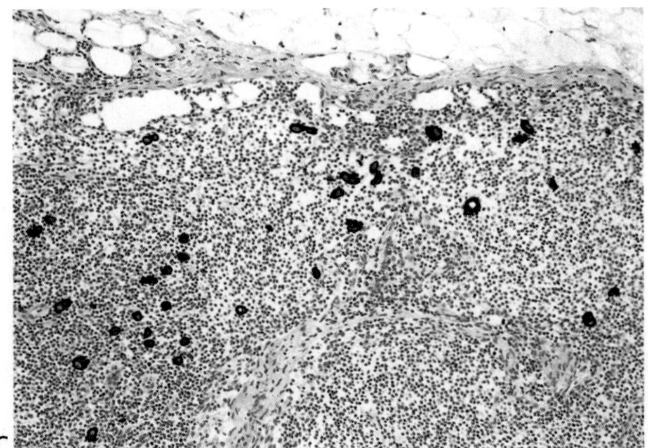

FIG. 44.38. *[Continued]*

frequently requires metastatic foci of 1 to 2 mm or larger. Because of the possibility of heterogeneity in the primary tumor, having a substantial sample of tissue from the excised primary tumor specimen is preferable to reliance on the limited material in an NCB specimen (Fig. 44.40). Marked histologic disparity between the breast tumor and a lymph node metastasis can be indicative of a second, inapparent focus of carcinoma in the breast (Fig. 44.41). Despite the expectation that higher-grade tumors are more likely than lower-grade tumors to be the source of axillary nodal metastases, the reverse situation can occur. As discussed previously, data on the expected frequency of SLN metastases in patients with microinvasive carcinoma are limited. Involvement of the SLN is typically micrometastatic and often inapparent without CK IHC.

Confounding Lesions in the Diagnosis of SLN

The vast majority of metastatic foci in lymph nodes are readily identified as carcinoma and distinguishable from rarely occurring "noncarcinomatous glandular inclusion." Difficulty arises when glands in the lymph node or in perinodal tissue have a close resemblance to nonneoplastic mammary lobules or ducts. In the majority of instances, these nodal foci are very well-differentiated metastatic carcinoma, usually originating in a tubular or tubulolobular carcinoma (Fig. 44.42). These metastatic foci may be in the lymphoid stroma or in the lymph node sinuses. For a discussion of heterotopic glands in ALNs and their distinction from metastatic carcinoma, see Chapter 43.

Another benign lesion encountered in SLNs, as well as in lymph nodes generally, is the "nevus cell aggregate." These neuroepithelial structures localized to the lymph node capsule, rarely extending into perinodal tissue or along fibrovascular tissue into the lymph node, are not immunoreactive for CK. Because of their cytologic features, the pathologist inexperienced in the appearance of nevus cell aggregates may interpret this finding as metastatic lobular carcinoma. A complete discussion of nevus cell aggregates can be found in Chapter 43.

"Dendritic cells," interstitial reticulum cells, are elements in the reticulohistiocytic system involved in presenting antigens to CD34(+) T cells. Dendritic cells are present throughout the lymphoid tissue, especially in subcapsular, paracortical, and medullary regions. These cells are immunoreactive for CK8 and CK18 but not for CK19. Increased numbers of dendritic cells can be found in reactive lymph nodes. In contrast to most carcinoma cells, they are not located in the sinusoids and they have irregular shapes with branching dendritic processes (Fig. 44.43).

The "pseudosentinel" lymph node is a source of concern. It is a lymph node with the clinical characteristics of a SLN (distinct labeling with blue dye, radiocolloid, or both agents) that does not contain metastatic carcinoma or harbors micrometastases in a patient who proves to have macrometastases in NSLN. The lymph node found to act as a SLN has most likely assumed this function secondarily because lymphatic drainage in the original true SLN has been obstructed by metastatic carcinoma. Unfortunately, a "pseudosentinel" lymph

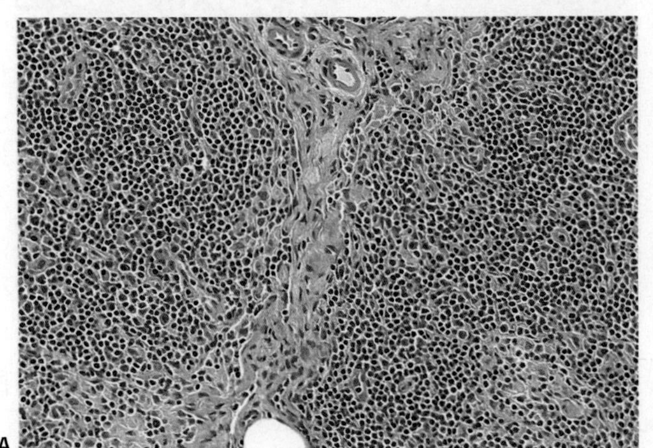

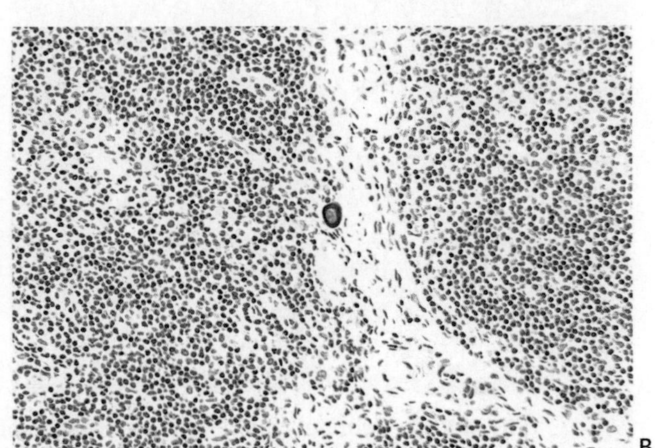

FIG. 44.39. ***Sentinel lymph node, isolated tumor cell.*** **A,B:** Replicate sections of fibrous stroma within a lymph node. The immunostain for AE1/3 revealed a single CK AE1/3-positive cell **(B)** that was not evident in the H&E section **(A)**.

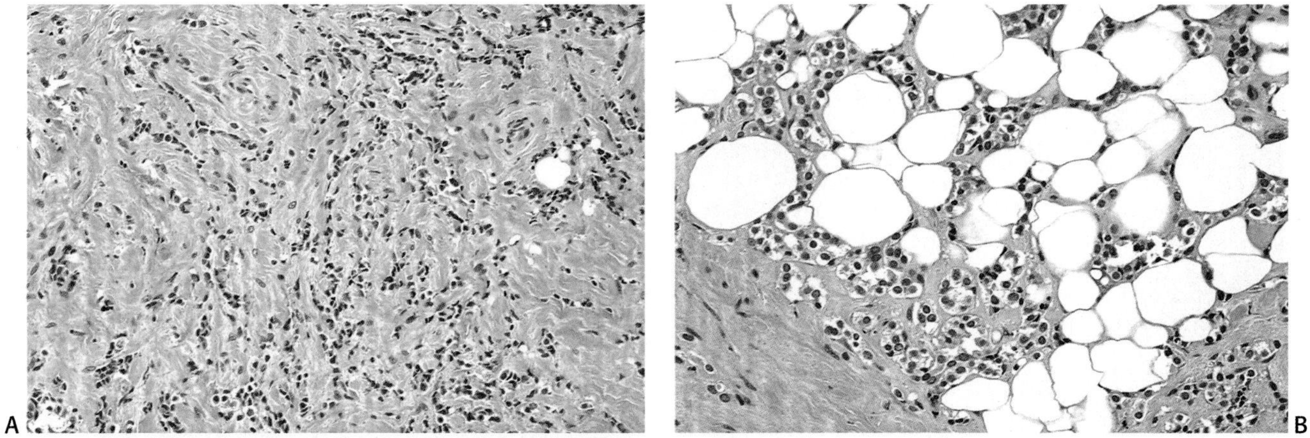

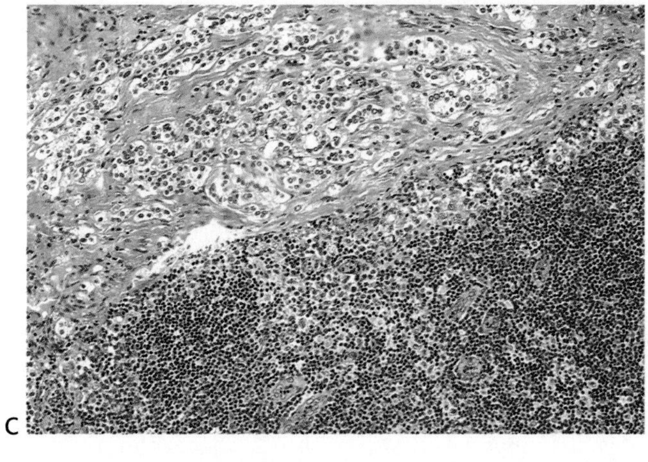

FIG. 44.40. ***Sentinel lymph node and heterogeneous carcinoma.*** The primary carcinoma had two growth patterns. **A:** Infiltrating lobular carcinoma. **B:** Infiltrating gland-forming ductal carcinoma composed of clear cells. **C:** The SLN displayed only the gland-forming pattern, largely in the lymph node capsule.

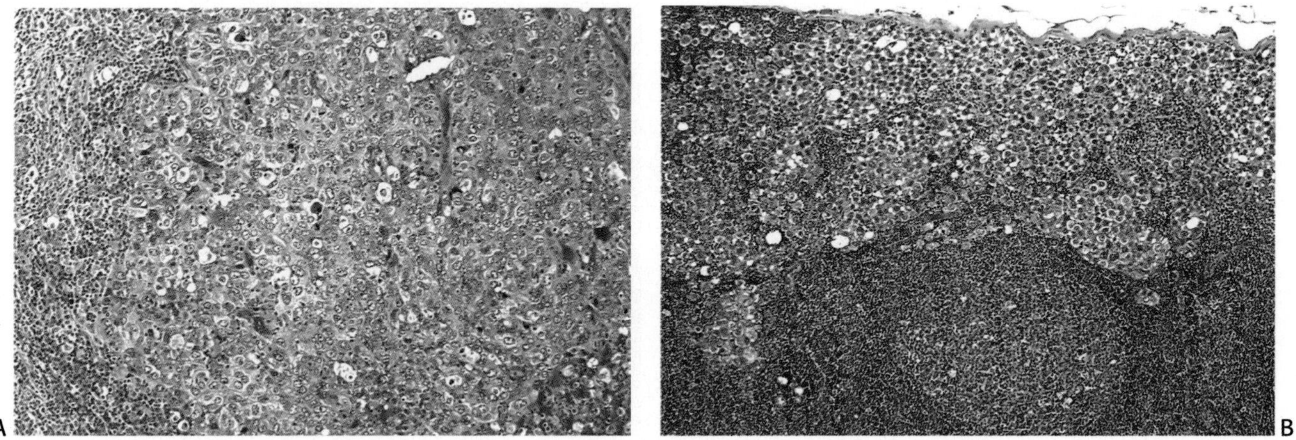

FIG. 44.41. ***Sentinel lymph nodes with heterogeneous metastases.*** Images (**A–C**) are from a single case. **A:** The primary tumor was poorly differentiated invasive ductal carcinoma. **B:** Part of the SLN contained metastatic carcinoma similar to the primary tumor. **C:** The lymph node also contained metastatic papillary apocrine carcinoma. This pattern was not found in the primary breast tumor and presumably derived from a second undetected breast carcinoma. Images (**D–G**) are from a patient who had two histologically different breast carcinomas in one breast. **D:** One tumor was well-differentiated invasive ductal carcinoma. **E:** Metastatic ductal carcinoma was found in one SLN (*arrow*). **F:** The second tumor was invasive lobular carcinoma, classical type. **G:** Metastatic lobular carcinoma in another SLN. **H:** This image shows a SLN from another case. The metastatic deposit in this lymph node is reminiscent of intraductal carcinoma. No myoepithelial cell layer could be demonstrated around this solitary metastatic deposit by either p63 or myosin immunostains. No intraductal carcinoma component was identified in the ipsilateral primary invasive poorly differentiated ductal carcinoma.

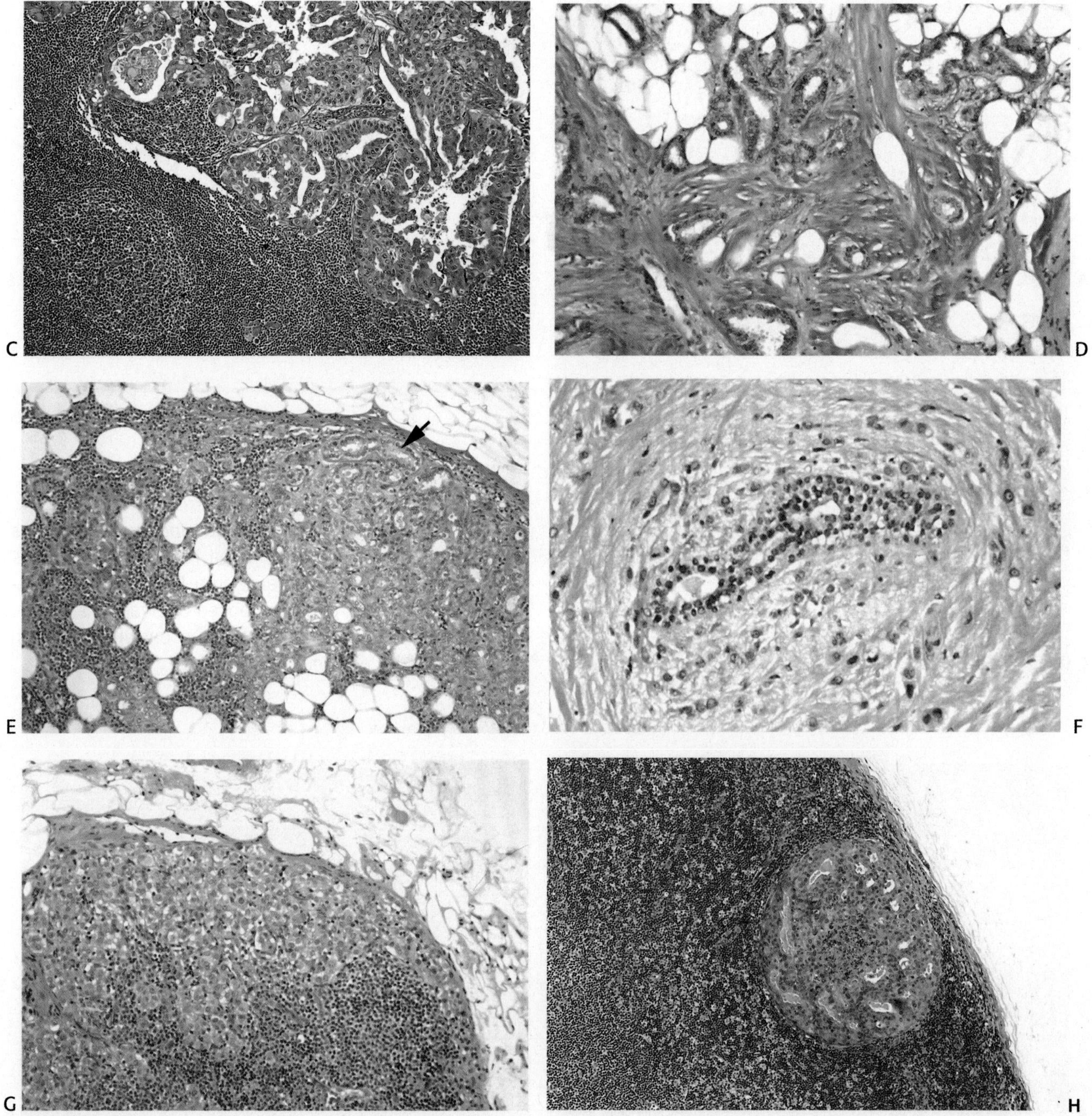

FIG. 44.41. *(Continued)*

node cannot be distinguished from a true SLN unless the status of the other lymph nodes is known.

Molecular Studies of SLNs to Detect Micrometastases

RT-PCR is an ultrasensitive method for detecting mRNA associated with specific markers at extremely low levels of expression. The technique is capable of detecting one carcinoembryonic antigen (CEA)–positive cell among 1×10^6 mononuclear cells[406] or one carcinoma cell among 1×10^6 lymphocytes.[407,408]

RT-PCR has been studied for several years as a method for detecting micrometastases in ALNs. Some of this work antedated the introduction of SLN biopsy and, therefore, the early results are not specific for the SLN. Noguchi et al.[409,410] reported two studies of CK 19 (CK19) expression determined by RT-PCR in ALNs from women with breast carcinoma. In one study, CK19 expression was seen in all lymph nodes with histologically documented metastatic carcinoma but in only 5 of 53 (9%) lymph nodes lacking metastatic carcinoma.[409] The authors also reported that mucin-1.[1,409] RNA was detectable in all lymph nodes that had metastatic carcinoma and

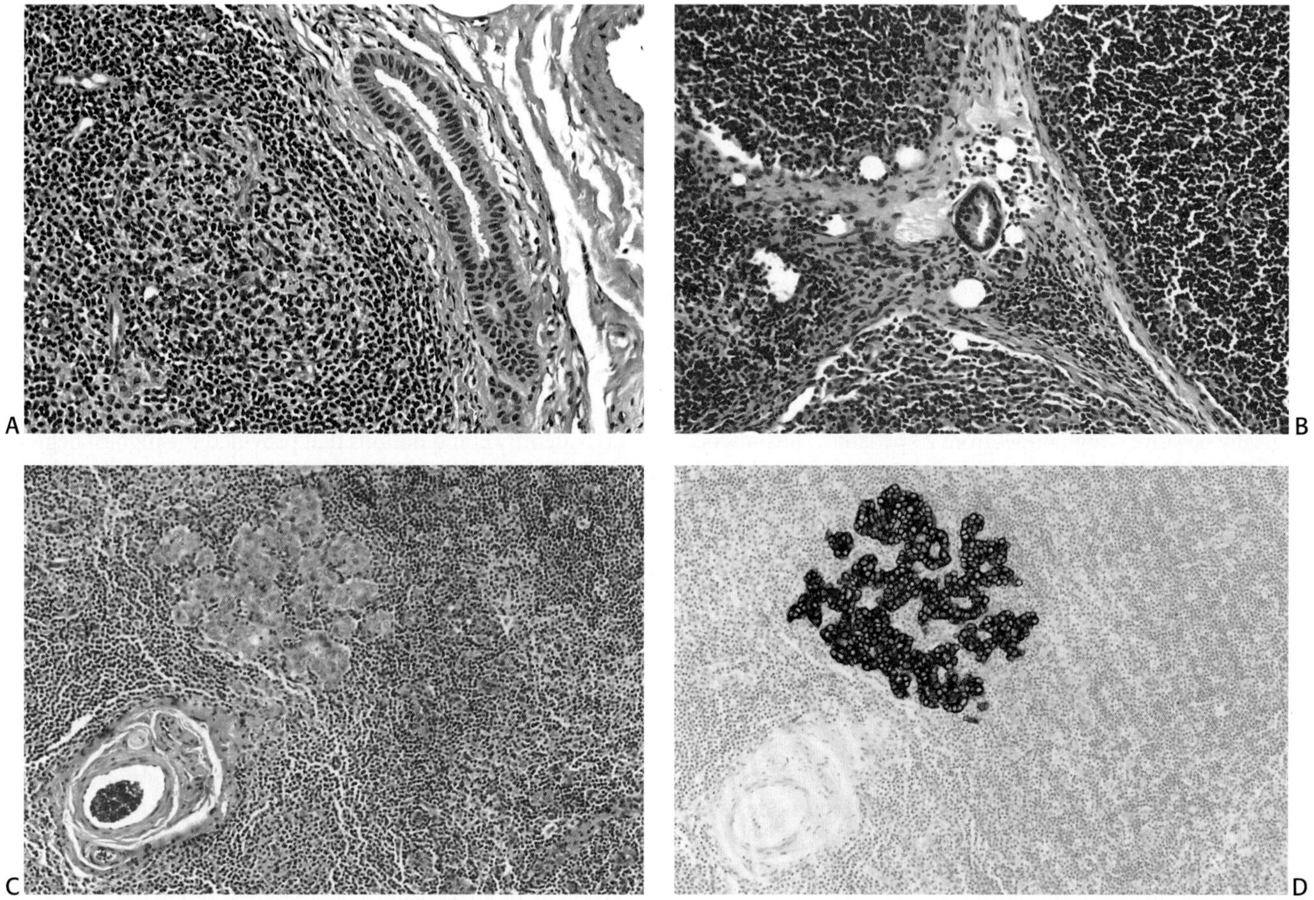

FIG. 44.42. ***Sentinel lymph node, well-differentiated carcinoma.*** **A:** Metastatic well-differentiated ductal carcinoma in the capsule of a SLN. Foci such as this are sometimes misinterpreted as benign ductal inclusions. Myoepithelial cells were not present in this metastatic gland. **B:** Metastatic well-differentiated ductal carcinoma deep in the fibrous trabeculum of a SLN. **C,D:** Metastatic well-differentiated ductal carcinoma deep in the paracortical region of a SLN. The subtle metastatic deposit was readily highlighted by a CK AE1/3 immunostain **(D)**.

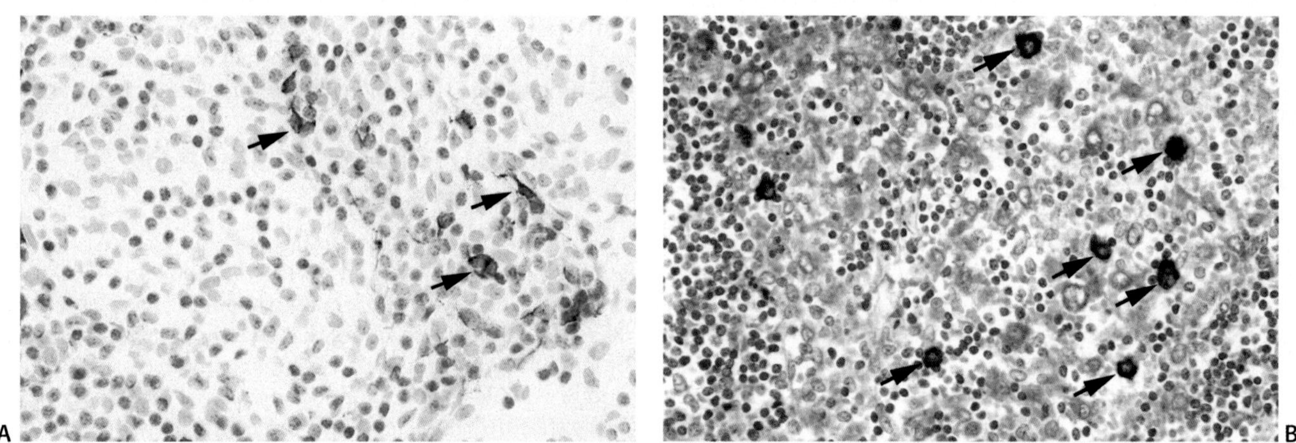

FIG. 44.43. ***Sentinel lymph node, dendritic cells and plasma cells.*** **A:** Dendritic cells in the lymphoid tissue are immunoreactive for CAM5.2 CK (*arrows*). By comparison with metastatic carcinoma, these cells have sparse cytoplasm and ill-defined cytoplasmic borders. **B:** Plasma cells scattered in this lymph node are reactive for EMA (*arrows*). This could lead to a false-positive diagnosis of metastatic carcinoma. For this reason, the EMA stain should not be used to detect carcinoma cells in lymph nodes. The plasma cells were also immunoreactive for lambda immunoglobulin.

in 6% of histologically negative lymph nodes. A second report documented similar results, with CK19 detected in 90% of positive lymph nodes and in 14% of negative lymph nodes.[410] Lymphatic invasion was present in primary tumors associated with histologically positive (70%) and CK19 RT-PCR–positive/histologically negative (53%) lymph nodes significantly more often than when the lymph nodes were histologically and CK19 RT-PCR negative (18%).

Schoenfeld et al.[411] studied 530 histologically negative lymph nodes from 75 consecutive patients for CK19 mRNA by RT-PCR. CK19 was detected in 106 (20%) of the 530 histologically negative lymph nodes from 23 patients. The presence of CK19 mRNA in histologically negative lymph nodes was significantly correlated with tumor size and histologic grade.

The value of a multimarker panel for the RT-PCR study of lymph nodes was explored by Lockett et al.[412] These investigators studied ALNs from 621 consecutive patients for three markers CK19, C-Myc, and prolactin-inducible protein (PIP). Lymph nodes larger than 1 cm were bisected, with the halves used for histopathologic and molecular analysis, respectively. Metastatic carcinoma was detected in lymph nodes from 24 patients by routine histologic examination. RT-PCR detected at least one of the three tumor markers in 22 (92%) of the histologically positive lymph nodes; two histologically positive lymph nodes were RT-PCR negative. RT-PCR demonstrated one or more epithelial markers in 15 (40%) of histologically negative cases. The distribution of RT-PCR positivity varied among the three molecular markers. In the 22 histologically positive, RT-PCR–positive cases, the frequencies of expression for C-Myc, CK19, and PIP were 41%, 73%, and 32%, whereas in 15 histologically negative, RT-PCR–positive cases, the frequencies of expression were 93%, 13%, and 20%, respectively. The fact that no marker was positive in every histologically positive lymph node underscores the value of using a multigene panel for RT-PCR detection of micrometastases.

RT-PCR has been used in the study of SLNs. Bostick et al.[413] evaluated the expression of CEA, CK19, CK20, gastrointestinal tumor-associated antigen 733.2 (GA733.2), and MUC-1 using RT-PCR to analyze frozen section samples of SLNs. They reported that CK20 was the only marker not detected in control lymph nodes from patients who did not have carcinoma. In 12 SLNs classified as negative in H&E sections and by immunostaining for CK, marker expression by RT-PCR was detected for GA733.2, MUC-1, CK19, CEA, and CK20 in 92%, 83%, 67%, 42%, and 8%, respectively, of the samples analyzed. The frequencies of detecting these markers in histologically or immunohistochemically positive SLNs were 70%, 70%, 80%, 70%, and 20%, respectively, for GA733.2, MUC-1, CK19, CEA, and CK20. Another study by Bostick et al.[414] explored the detection of three other mRNA tumor markers c-met, P97, and 4GalNac-T (4-*N*-acetyl galactosaminyl transferase). One of 17 SLNs with histologically documented metastases did not express any of these three mRNA markers. The markers were expressed individually in 53% to 83% of histologically negative SLNs, and all three markers were expressed in 43% of negative SLNs.

A multimarker study reported by Nissan et al.[415] employed RT-PCR to assay SLNs and other tissues for CK19, NY-BR-1, and mammaglobin B. The specimens examined were 30 SLNs, 3 breast carcinomas, 31 lymph nodes from women with benign breast disease, and peripheral blood lymphocytes from 10 normal volunteers. Amplification of all markers was detected in the three carcinomas and in 15 of 30 SLNs (50%). Routine histologic examination found metastatic carcinoma in 6 (20%) of SLNs, and 8 (27%) were positive by IHC.

Automated RT-PCR analysis of SLN was reported by Hughes et al.,[416] who screened a panel of 43 potential markers to identify combinations that provided the highest degree of sensitivity and specificity. After a series of tests, the authors determined that the combination of the genes for PIP and TACSTDI provided 96.3% sensitivity and 100% specificity with 97.9% accuracy for detecting positive SLNs.

Failure to detect mRNA markers in histologically positive lymph nodes is probably due to sampling error. The significance of markers detected in SLNs with no histologically identified carcinoma is unknown. The ideal mRNA marker that is expressed only by tumor cells and not in normal lymph nodes has not been identified. Therefore, detection of mRNA markers in histologically negative lymph nodes cannot be interpreted as indicative of metastatic carcinoma.

Two molecular-based intraoperative diagnostic techniques for lymph node metastases were developed in recent years. The first test using a combination of CK19 and mammaglobin as markers is no longer available.[417] The second test is a one-step nucleic acid amplification (OSNA) test that amplifies CK19 mRNA (OSNA, Sysmex, Kobe, Japan). The latter test is designed to detect a metastasis that spans more than 0.2 mm, and has been shown to have sensitivity per patient of 91.4% and specificity of 93.3% in a prospective multicenter study.[418] The OSNA assay has also been shown to detect more sentinel nodal micrometastases than FSE.[419] At the present time when minimal metastases in SLNs may or may not lead to axillary nodal dissection, the semiquantitative results of OSNA provide a "unique opportunity to tailor intraoperative surgical decision-making to the individual patient based on the relative lymph node tumor burden."[420]

Studies of ALN Micrometastases Prior to the Era of SLN Biopsy

In addition to detecting metastatic carcinoma in ALNs and establishing the level of involvement, histologic examination can provide other information about the metastatic foci. The number of lymph nodes that contain metastases should be documented. Prognosis is significantly decreased as the number of affected lymph nodes increases. Patients are generally stratified in the following three categories: one to three (pN1a), four to nine (pN2 or pN2a), and 10 or more (pN3 or pN3a) affected lymph nodes.[399,421]

Historically, several investigators assessed the prognostic significance of the size of metastatic foci in ALNs. In these studies, micrometastases were 2 mm or smaller in diameter; larger metastases were macrometastases.[422–425] Micrometastases may be detected in routine sections of lymph nodes, in serial sections of initially negative lymph nodes, or by CK IHC. Metastases found by the latter two methods have been referred to as "occult micrometastases." The frequency with which occult micrometastases have been detected varies from 9%[426,427] to 33%,[428] with a median of 17% in eight reports reviewed.[427] Studies that did not take the number of involved lymph nodes and/or the size of the primary tumor into consideration led to the conclusion that patients with macrometastases had a less favorable prognosis than those with micrometastases.[422–424] It has also been further suggested that the prognosis of women with micrometastases did not differ significantly from that of women with negative lymph nodes.[422,429–431]

Analyses that evaluate the size of metastases and number of affected lymph nodes are difficult to perform and most meaningful when limited to patients with single nodal metastases classified as either a macro- or micrometastasis. If two lymph nodes are involved, three categories are possible (2 micro, 2 macro, or 1 micro and 1 macro), and with more extensive metastases the stratification becomes impractical. One study analyzed the prognostic significance of solitary nodal metastases in T1N1 and T2N1 patients with an average follow-up of 10 years.[425] When the T1N1 and T2N1 patients with a single nodal metastasis were analyzed together, there was a significantly poorer prognosis among patients with a single macrometastasis in comparison with those having a micrometastasis. A major prognostic difference was apparent after stratification by tumor size. During the first 6 years of follow-up, T1 patients with negative nodes and those with a single micrometastasis had similar survival curves, significantly better than those with a macrometastasis. With additional follow-up, the DFS of patients with a micrometastasis became nearly identical to that of patients with a macrometastasis, and significantly worse than that of patients with negative lymph nodes. Conversely, T2 patients with negative lymph nodes or a single micrometastasis had survival rates that did not differ significantly throughout the 10-year follow-up. Both groups had an outcome significantly better than T2 patients with a single macrometastasis. These observations demonstrate that tumor size, length of follow-up, and the number of involved lymph nodes together influence the prognostic significance of axillary micrometastases.

de Mascarel et al.[432] used a serial-sectioning technique to restudy lymph nodes initially reported as negative. DFS and OS were similar for patients with a single micrometastasis and a single macrometastasis detected in this fashion, and significantly less favorable than among the patients with negative lymph nodes.

The significance of occult micrometastases in ALNs was reported in 1990 in a Ludwig Breast Cancer Study Group prospective cooperative adjuvant chemotherapy trial that included 921 patients judged to have negative ALNs in routine sections.[427] Additional sections of the lymph nodes were prepared at six levels. Occult micrometastases in a single lymph node were found in 83 (9%) of the cases. Factors significantly associated with the detection of occult micrometastases were tumor size larger than 2 cm, peritumoral vascular invasion, and diagnosis before age 50. Occult micrometastases were detected with nearly equal frequency in patients with invasive ductal and lobular carcinoma. Five-year DFS and OS were significantly lower in patients with a single micrometastasis, whether or not the metastasis was found in routine or serial sections, than in patients whose lymph nodes were negative after more sections were made. Multivariate analysis revealed that the unfavorable prognostic effect of solitary occult micrometastases was significantly correlated with the following: invasive ductal carcinoma, high-grade tumors, tumors larger than 2 cm, and peritumoral vascular invasion.

A second study published in 1999 by the Ludwig Breast Cancer Study Group employed CK immunostaining (AE1 and CAM5.2) as well as serial sectioning of histologically negative lymph nodes.[433] Lymph node samples were available for 736 patients. Occult nodal metastases were found in 52 patients (7%) by serial sectioning and in 149 (20%) by IHC. Both methods were positive in 45 cases (6%) and both were negative in 581 (79%). Among the 110 discrepant cases (15%), 103 were positive only by IHC and 7 only in serial sections. Immunostaining was more sensitive for detecting occult metastases than serial sections among all histologic types. This was especially true for infiltrating lobular carcinoma in which 39% (20 of 51) patients with histologically negative lymph nodes were found to have occult metastases. The yield of IHC-detected occult metastases in patients with infiltrating ductal, special types, and mixed ductal–lobular carcinomas was 13%, 16%, and 38%, respectively. Occult metastases detected by serial sectioning or by IHC were associated with a significantly less favorable DFS and OS in postmenopausal but not in premenopausal women. Occult micrometastases detected by IHC were also a significant risk factor for recurrence in multivariate analysis.

The identification in routine sections of isolated metastatic cells or small groups of cells originating from infiltrating lobular carcinoma presents a particularly vexing problem. These small cells may be difficult to distinguish from histiocytes in a lymph node stained with H&E. To investigate this issue, Bussolati et al.[434] prepared new sections of lymph nodes reported to be negative from 50 patients with infiltrating lobular carcinoma. By using antibodies to three epithelial-associated immunohistochemical markers (EMA, human milk-fat globule membrane 2 [HMFG-2], and CK), the authors were able to detect metastatic carcinoma in 26 lymph nodes (3.3%) from 12 (24%) of the 50 patients. Because carcinoma cells were evident in H&E-stained duplicate sections of seven lymph nodes from five patients, the net contribution of the immunohistochemical studies was to detect tumor cells in 2.4% of the lymph nodes from 14% of the patients. The positive cells were, for the most part, present individually in sinuses or in the lymphoid tissue. Recurrences occurred in 2 of 12 (17%) immunocytochemically positive cases and in 7 of 38 (18%) negative cases.

Trojani et al.[435] applied a mixture of five monoclonal antibodies to existing histologic sections of lymph nodes reported to be negative from 150 consecutive patients with average follow-up of 10 years. Overall, 21 patients (14%) were found to have occult micrometastases. The yield of positive lymph nodes was greater in patients with invasive lobular carcinoma (38%) than in those with invasive ductal carcinoma (11%). The finding of occult micrometastases was not related to tumor grade or lymphatic tumor emboli. It is notable that instances of plasma cells with positive staining with anti-EMA were present, a phenomenon previously reported by Delsol et al.[436] Among patients with invasive ductal carcinoma, death due to disease was significantly more frequent in the group with micrometastases (23%) than in those with immunohistochemically negative lymph nodes (6.3%).

Another retrospective study of ALNs previously reported to be negative in 208 patients yielded occult metastases in 51 cases (24.5%) studied with a combination of resectioning and IHC.[437] Occult metastases were detected more often in lymph nodes from patients with lobular (38%) than with ductal (25%) carcinoma and in women younger than 50 years (41%) than in women 50 years and older (19%). Although the presence and increasing size of occult metastases were significantly associated with decreased DFS in multivariate analysis, these factors were not significant predictors of OS.

The weight of evidence from the foregoing retrospective studies indicates that the presence of micrometastases detected in routine H&E sections of ALNs predicts an adverse prognosis when compared with patients who have histologically negative lymph nodes.[438–440] The same observation applies to occult micrometastases uncovered by serial sections and/or IHC in histologically negative lymph nodes. The frequency of detecting occult micrometastases is higher for infiltrating lobular and ductal–lobular carcinoma than for infiltrating ductal carcinoma. However, occult micrometastases have been detected in histologically negative lymph nodes from patients with prognostically favorable special types of carcinoma. The presence of lymphovascular tumor emboli in the breast is a factor associated with occult micrometastases. The size of the primary tumor is directly correlated with detection of occult micrometastases.

Longer follow-up data on SLN patients will be needed to fully assess the prognostic significance of micrometastases in SLN. Prospective studies have been initiated to assess the prognostic significance of micrometastases in SLNs.[277] Because of the overall favorable prognosis of many patients who undergo SLN biopsy with the finding of histologically negative SLN, it will require large numbers of patients with long-term follow-up to determine the extent to which occult micrometastases in the SLN alter prognosis. If the aforementioned retrospective studies are a reliable guide, it is likely that SLN micrometastases will be prognostically meaningful. It is unfortunate that SLNs cannot be identified retrospectively because they were inevitably included in the total ALN specimens submitted by prior investigators for serial sections and IHC. Based on information obtained from thousands of SLN biopsy procedures, it is highly likely that lymph nodes found to harbor micrometastases in retrospective serial sectioning and immunohistochemical studies were SLNs. For this reason, the many retrospective studies of the prognostic significance of micrometastases are relevant in the current era of SLN biopsy and options for treatment.[441]

The survival of metastatic carcinoma in lymph nodes depends on many factors such as the angiogenic capacity of the cells and the microenvironment of the lymph node.[442] The survivability of micrometastatic carcinoma cells has been questioned, a concern supported in some instances by the degenerated appearance of the cells in histologic sections. A method developed for isolating micrometastatic carcinoma cells for *in vitro* culture may prove useful for investigating this question.[443] At present the issue remains unsettled and this dilemma is unlikely to be resolved soon. Speculative opinions unsupported by follow-up information, such as the statement that "we believe that this phenomenon in itself does not carry risk of future metastatic behavior," referring to epithelial cells in some lymph nodes as resulting from "benign transport," are premature.[444]

The TNM Staging System distinguishes the presence of "ITCs" from micrometastases.[398,399] The term "isolated tumor cells" refers to individual tumor cells not numbering more than 200, or small cell clusters not greater than 0.2 mm, that are usually detected by IHC, which may be verified by the H&E stain. It has been suggested that ITCs do not usually show evidence of malignant activity, for example, proliferation or stromal reaction, and that ITCs differ from micrometastases in having no contact with a vascular or lymph sinus wall and showing no invasion of a vascular lymph sinus wall.[404] These putative distinguishing criteria are meaningless since both ITCs and micrometastases often lack mitoses and stromal reaction. Invasion of the walls of lymph sinuses is rarely evident in micrometastases or where ITCs are located.

SLN BIOPSY: CHANGES IN CLINICAL PRACTICE ON THE BASIS OF RESULTS FROM CLINICAL TRIALS

Clinical Significance and TNM Staging of Micrometastases Today

SLN biopsy is currently the accepted method of axillary nodal staging in clinically node-negative disease. Cumulative data indicate that a SLN is the only positive lymph node in about 75% of cases of invasive breast carcinoma. About 25% of SLNs are positive on standard single-section (one-level) H&E evaluation. This rate increases to 40% or so if either additional H&E-stained level or CK immunohistochemical evaluation is added, with upstaging occurring in up to 20% of cases. Thus, enhanced assessment of SLN can result in "stage migration," primarily because of detection of low-volume nodal disease, that is, ITCs and micrometastases.

The significance of occult metastases, that is, metastases detected by enhanced assessment techniques, remains controversial. The American College of Surgeons Oncology Group (ACOSOG) Z0010 trial found occult metastases in 10.5% of patients with no difference in DFS or OS.[445] The NSABP B32 trial identified occult metastases in 16% of patients with a significant difference in OS of 1.2%.[446] In the MIRROR ("Micrometastases and Isolated tumor cells: Relevant and Robust or Rubbish") study from the Netherlands, reduced DFS was found with both ITCs and micrometastases in patients who did not receive adjuvant therapy, and follow-up showed a higher axillary recurrence rate for micrometastases but not ITCs (5.6% vs. 2.0%), but again significant only in patients who did not receive adjuvant therapy.[447] In De Boer's[448] meta-analysis, there was an increased RR of 1.55 for recurrence and 1.45 for decreased OS associated with the occult metastases.

The tumor burden in a SLN is a continuous variable extending from the presence of a single CK-positive cell to a macrometastasis. In the latest seventh edition of the AJCC–UICC Staging Manual, the categorization of ITCs and micrometastasis is determined by size alone, and not by location as was done in the immediately preceding edition.[449] In this staging system, ITC has been renamed "isolated tumor cell clusters" and includes two categories: confluent cell clusters smaller than or equal to 0.2 mm and single cells that number less than or equal to 200. Micrometastasis includes confluent cell clusters measuring 0.2 to 2.0 mm, and now also allows single dispersed cells or minute noncohesive clustered cells if the number of cells is more than 200 per single nodal cross section. The former scenario is typically encountered with metastatic lobular carcinoma, and the latter with metastases from invasive micropapillary carcinoma.

It is notable that ITCs are regarded in the current staging system as node-negative disease (N0(i+)), whereas micrometastasis is considered to be node-positive (N1*mic*). Thus, it is important that the two disease categories be reliably distinguished. The European Working Group for Breast Cancer Screening recommends that an even distribution of cells and clusters be regarded as a single collective deposit.[450] The current AJCC–UICC guidelines would regard such cells and clusters to be separate individual deposits unless the cells are embedded in a desmoplastic stromal reaction. However, these efforts to substratify minimal nodal involvement appear to be moot in view of the results of some studies that show no difference in survival between patients with ITCs or micrometastases.[451,452] Furthermore, in various published series, as summarized by Galimberti et al.,[453] the frequency of NSLN involvement when the SLN contains macrometastatic carcinoma ranges from 46% to 80%, and when it is micrometastatic, it ranges from 0% to 80%. The frequency of NSLN involvement ranges from 15% to 19% when the SLN contains ITC.[453]

Thus, the cumulative data suggest that the clinical significance of low-volume nodal disease remains uncertain despite the fact that it is increasingly being regarded clinically as negligible. There is an increasing trend toward omission of ALND in selected SLN-positive cases. This was first evident from Surveillance Epidemiology and End Results (SEER) data (1998 to 2005) that showed a 20% drop in ALND in the group of patients with micrometastases in SLN.[454] Nevertheless, ALND in this setting does optimize staging and offers additional prognostic information. It may also dictate the use of subsequent adjuvant chemotherapy and radiotherapy, and may also offer some degree of therapeutic benefit.

The declining rate of ALND is reflective of several factors. These factors include (1) increasing use of nomograms to predict the risk of NSLN involvement in the event of a positive SLN; (2) increasing use of primary tumor characteristics (such as tumor size, grade, ER, and HER2 status) rather than results of axillary staging in making decisions regarding adjuvant therapy; (3) increasing reliance on chemotherapy and radiation therapy, rather than surgery, to treat axillary nodal disease in cases wherein such treatment modalities are already indicated; and (4) the increasing realization that nodal staging can be accomplished by SLN biopsy alone. The rate of ALND is likely to drop precipitously following the wide acceptance of ACOSOG Z0011 trial results that have seriously challenged the need for ALND in patients with positive SLNB.

Reduced Frequency of ALND

The ACOSOG Z0011 trial, which was closed early due to poor recruitment and a low event rate, examined ALND versus no ALND in T1–T2 patients with two or fewer positive nodes treated conservatively with whole-breast radiation.[455,456] The 6-year follow-up results showed no difference in DFS, OS, or axillary recurrences with or without ALND.[457] Ninety-six percent of patients had received adjuvant therapy—including adjuvant chemotherapy and radiotherapy. The latter would have included level I and II nodes in most patients. The role of axillary radiation as a substitute for ALND is being examined in the AMAROS ("After Mapping of Axilla: Radiotherapy Or Surgery") study.[458]

With the drop in the rate of ALND, there has been a concomitant reduction in the need for intraoperative assessment of SLN. In a study analyzing the trend of FSE of SLN and completion ALND over 10 years (1997 to 2006) at MSKCC in New York City, a diminished rate of frozen sections for SLN was reported, and for patients with low-volume SLN involvement there were fewer ALNDs.[459] This trend suggests a "more nuanced" approach to management of the axilla. The authors calculated that if the selection criteria for ACOSOG Z0011 trial had been applied to the cohort, then 66% of SLN frozen sections and 48% of ALNDs would have been avoided. Between 2008 and 2013, ALND has been reduced to approximately one-half, and requests for intraoperative consultation for SLN have been reduced by two-third at Weill Cornell Medical Center in New York City (unpublished data). This trend was summed up by Benson and Wishart,[460] who stated that "intraoperative node examination may be more difficult to justify for all patients in the context of contemporary practice which either deselects patients for SLN biopsy or dictates that completion ALND is performed alongside definitive or additional breast surgery."

With this decreasing rate of ALND, largely regardless of the results of SLN evaluation, the need for the application of special techniques such as rapid intraoperatively performed immunohistochemical staining for CK and the use of RT-PCR in the same setting has also become questionable, and may even become obsolete at least in the clinical setting.

As outlined above, clinical and pathologic concepts regarding SLN and minimal metastases have evolved considerably over the last 15 years or so. The management of the axilla continues to change based on the results of various clinical trials including those conducted in Europe.[461]

The considerable practical impact of these trials has been outlined in several publications.[462–467] These publications can influence the broader approach to axillary management, but it is only with an individually tailored approach that the optimal management plan can be devised for each patient.

EXTRANODAL EXTENSION OF METASTASES

The prognostic significance of the spread of metastatic carcinoma from a lymph node to the surrounding axillary tissues, so-called extranodal extension, has been investigated extensively (Fig. 44.44). It has been difficult to analyze this feature independently of other factors such as the number of involved lymph nodes or the size of the primary tumor. Extranodal extension is associated with tumors larger than 2 cm, the presence of carcinoma in four or more lymph nodes, and peritumoral lymphovascular channel involvement.[468] Several studies reviewed here demonstrated that extranodal extension indicates a higher risk of systemic or local recurrence in patients already predisposed to these events because of other unfavorable prognostic factors. The reports do not provide compelling evidence that extranodal extension is a high-risk factor for axillary recurrence in women who have a complete axillary dissection. Extranodal extension appears to have a negative effect on relapse-free survival and OS. In some studies, this effect is influenced by the number of lymph nodes involved by metastases (fewer than 4 or greater than or equal to ≥4). There does not appear to be a consensus favoring axillary radiation in these patients. It is likely that virtually all patients with extranodal extension will be offered systemic chemotherapy because of their TMN stage.

Several retrospective studies found extranodal extension to be prognostically unfavorable in women treated by mastectomy and axillary dissection. Hultborn and Tornberg[469] described a series of patients treated by mastectomy and postoperative radiotherapy. The 10-year survival of women with extranodal extension (19%) was substantially lower than that of patients with metastases limited to their axillary nodes (52%). Pierce et al.[470] reported that microscopic

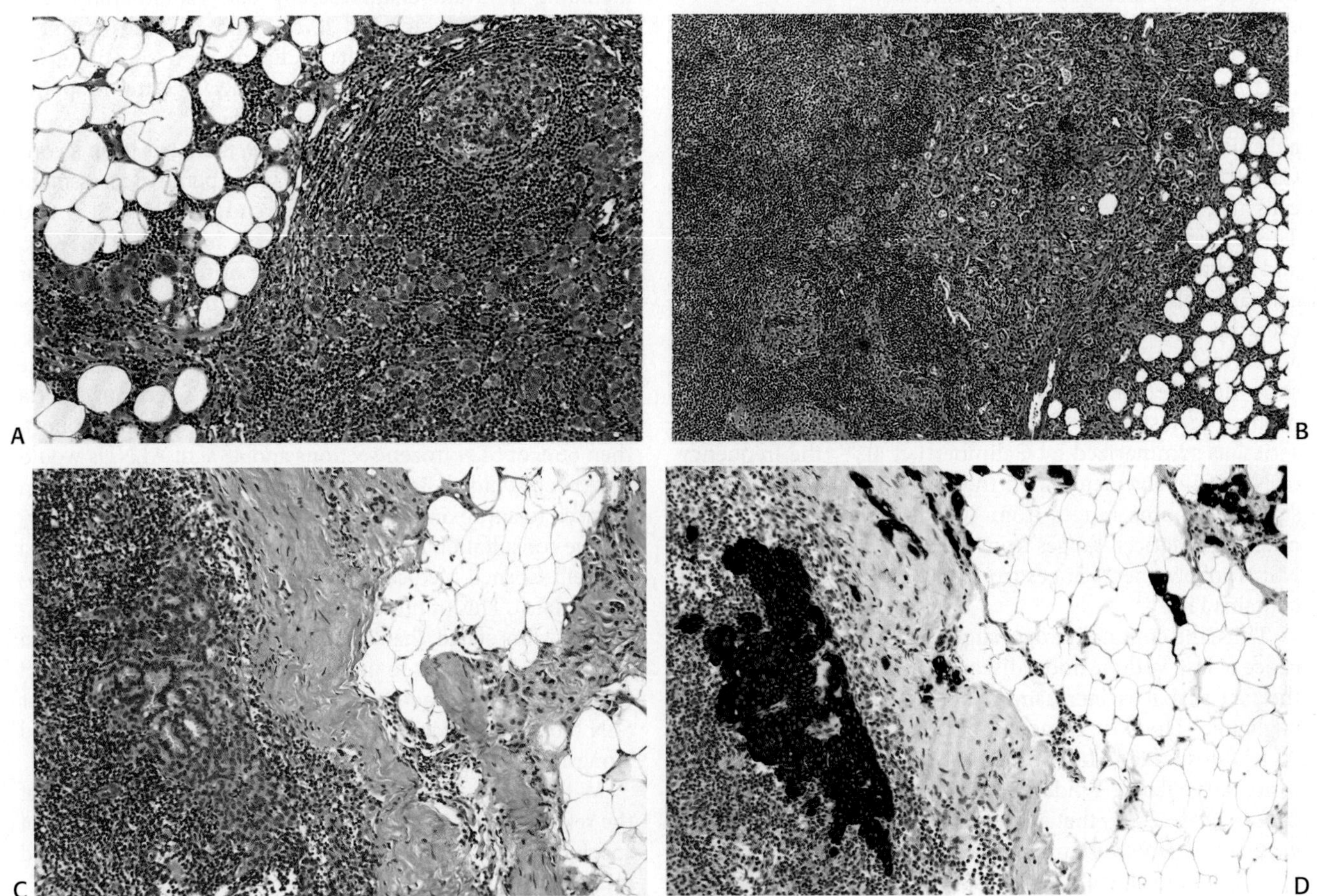

FIG. 44.44. ***Extranodal extension.*** **A:** Invasive lobular carcinoma surrounds a germinal center and invades perinodal fat. **B:** Invasive ductal carcinoma has destroyed the lymph node capsule and extended into perinodal fat (*right*). **C:** Metastatic ductal carcinoma in a lymph node with no apparent extranodal extension in perinodal adipose tissue on H&E-stained section. **D:** The CK AE1/3 immunostain highlights extranodal extension of the metastatic carcinoma in perinodal adipose tissue (same lymph node shown in **C**).

extranodal extension was significantly more frequent in women with four or more nodal metastases and that it was a significant predictor of systemic rather than local axillary recurrence. Fisher et al.[471] also found that extranodal extension was significantly more frequent in patients who had four or more lymph nodes with metastases. In this prospective study by Fisher et al.,[471] patients with extranodal extension had a significantly higher frequency of short-term relapse, but the analysis did not demonstrate that the tendency to treatment failure associated with extranodal extension was independent of the extent of nodal involvement.

A series of 308 positive-node patients treated by mastectomy without adjuvant radiation or chemotherapy with 10 years of follow-up were evaluated at the Milan National Cancer Institute.[472] The frequency of extranodal (extracapsular) extension was significantly related to the number of involved lymph nodes (one to three nodes positive, 27% extracapsular; four or more nodes positive, 51% extracapsular). Further analysis revealed that extracapsular extension of nodal metastases did not have an impact on prognosis when only one lymph node was involved, but if two or more lymph nodes were affected, extracapsular extension was associated with a significantly higher systemic recurrence rate.

Leonard et al.[473] reported that extranodal tumor extension was significantly more frequent in patients with tumors larger than 2 cm, high-grade carcinomas, when there were more than three lymph node metastases, and when there was lymphatic or vascular invasion at the primary tumor site. This study did not detect an increased risk of axillary recurrence associated with extranodal extension, regardless of treatment with axillary radiation or systemic chemotherapy. Multivariate analysis revealed that the presence of extranodal extension and more than three nodal metastases were significant independent prognostic factors, with the number of involved lymph nodes having a stronger effect. Mignano et al.[474] found no axillary recurrences among 43 patients with extracapsular extension treated by mastectomy, axillary dissection, and chemotherapy without radiation.

"Minimal" extranodal extension has been defined as perinodal extension of tumor 1 mm beyond the lymph node capsule, and "extensive" extranodal extension as penetration of metastatic tumor more than 1 mm into perinodal soft tissues. However, the clinical value of the use of these terms largely undetermined, other than implying that extensive extranodal extension is more likely to be associated with metastases in multiple additional lymph nodes.[475]

The diagnosis of extranodal extension of metastatic carcinoma can be difficult to render in the hilar region of the lymph node, a region that commonly shows fatty infiltration, and is devoid of a continuous and well-defined capsule.

PATHOLOGIC CHANGES IN ALNS THAT MIMIC METASTATIC CARCINOMA

Signet Ring Histiocytes

Vacuolated histiocytes that resemble signet ring adenocarcinoma cells present a troublesome diagnostic problem.[476–478] The histiocytes stain positively with antichymotrypsin, anti-α_1-trypsin, lysozyme,[478] and for CD68. They are weakly positive or negative with stains for mucin (mucicarmine, PAS) and negative for CKs (AE1/3) and (gross cystic disease fluid protein 15 [GCDFP-15])[477,478] (Fig. 44.45). Electron microscopy in one case revealed a single cytoplasmic vacuole in each cell that in some cells, contained amorphous electron-dense material interpreted to be lipid.[477] The nature of the vacuolar material is unknown, but does not appear to be related to breast carcinoma. One patient was found to have signet ring sinus histiocytosis after coronary bypass surgery with no documented evidence of mammary carcinoma.[476]

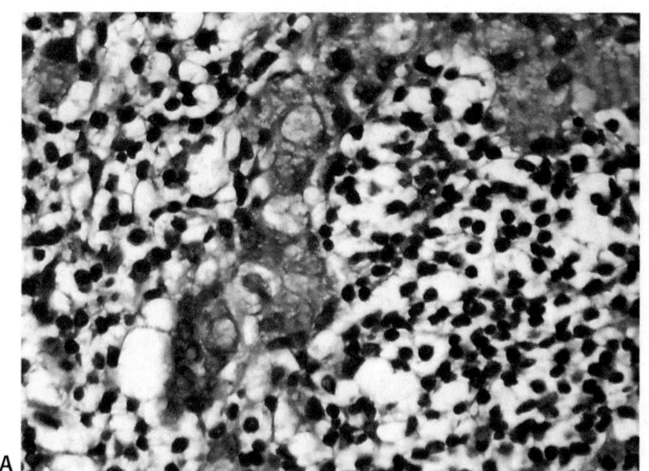

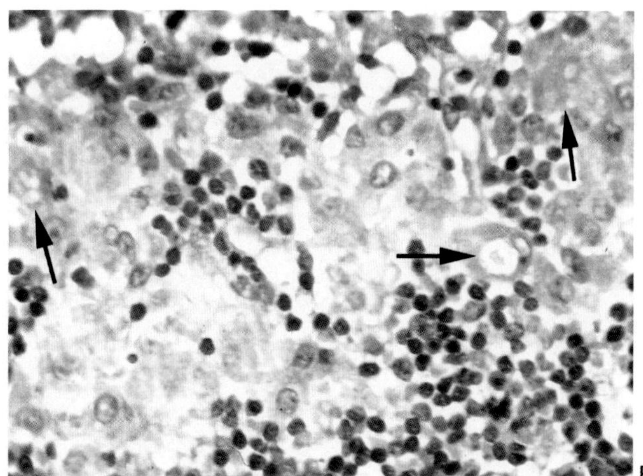

FIG. 44.45. ***Vacuolated histiocytes.*** **A:** The intracytoplasmic lumens suggest signet ring cells. **B:** The cytoplasm is very weakly stained with the mucicarmine stain (*arrows*). **C:** Metastatic lobular carcinoma with signet ring cells in the subcapsular sinusoids of a lymph node. This type of metastasis can mimic vacuolated histiocytes. A CK immunostain may be required for definitive diagnosis in such cases.

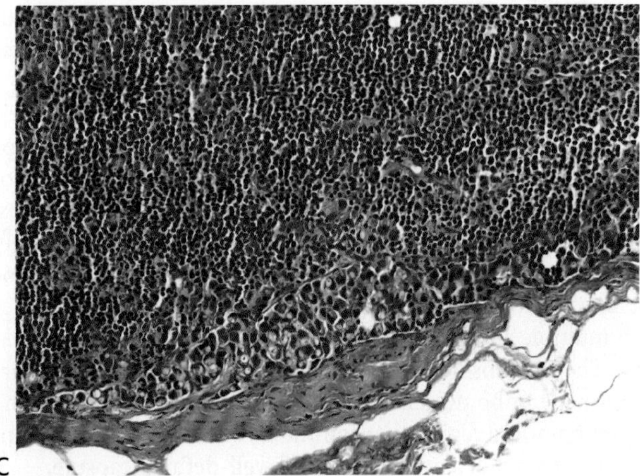

FIG. 44.45. *(Continued)*

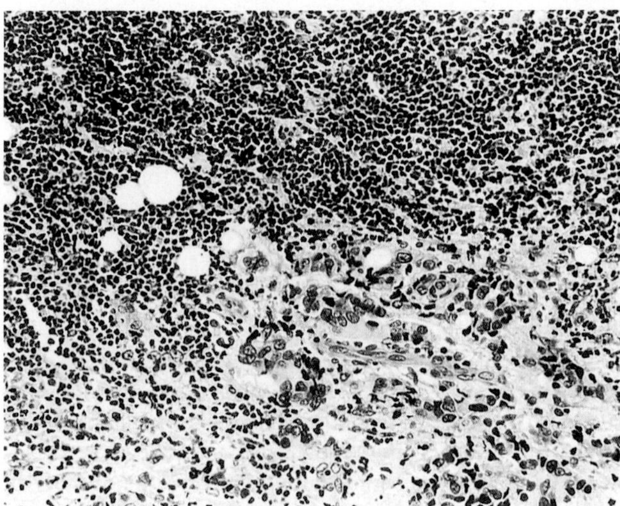

FIG. 44.47. ***Metastatic carcinoma and chronic lymphocytic leukemia in an axillary lymph node.*** The leukemic infiltrate is shown *above*, merging with metastatic lobular carcinoma *below*.

Hematologic Disorders

The differential diagnosis of signet ring histiocytes in ALNs also includes lymphangiogram effect,[479] silicone lymphadenitis,[480] Whipple disease,[481] signet ring cell melanoma,[482] and lymphoma.[483]

Hematologic disorders involving ALNs may be confused with or they can obscure metastatic carcinoma. These conditions include extramedullary hematopoiesis (Fig. 44.46) and coexisting lymphoma or leukemia (Fig. 44.47). Nevus cell aggregates usually occur in the lymph node capsule but may also extend into the lymph node parenchyma (see Chapter 43).

DETECTION OF MICROMETASTASES IN BONE MARROW

Another clinically important application of the immunohistochemical detection of micrometastases is in the study of bone marrow. This procedure is more likely to detect occult metastases in patients with lobular than with ductal carcinoma.[484] IHC with EMA has been used to identify micrometastases in tissue sections of bone marrow.[485] The authors found alkaline phosphatase conjugates preferable to horseradish peroxidase and were able to effectively block endogenous alkaline phosphatase with 20% acetic acid. EMA-positive cells were detected in 15 aspirates, but malignant cells were recognized in only eight Giemsa-stained samples from the same aspirates. EMA-positive cells were found in marrow aspirates from 9 of 24 patients (38%) with known bone marrow metastases, 4 of 20 (20%) with nonosseous systemic metastases, and 2 of 30 (7%) not known to have metastatic disease.

Repeat follow-up marrow aspirations have been described in two series of patients. Positive aspirations were obtained

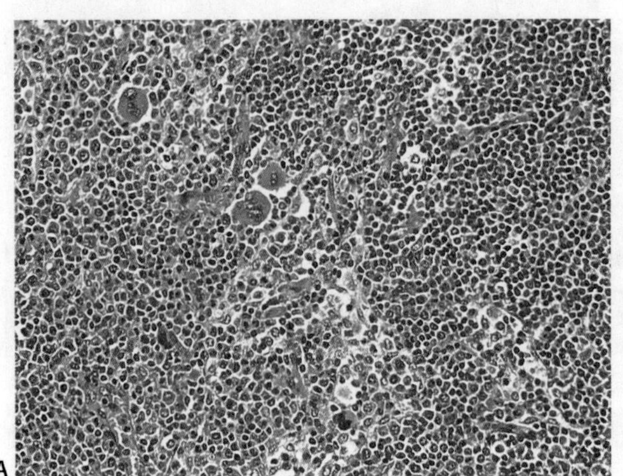

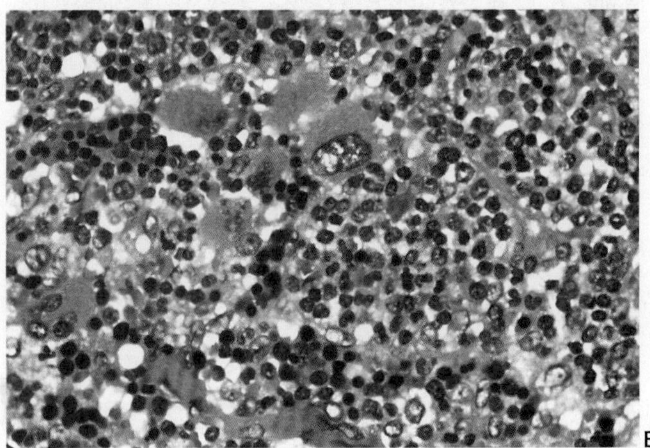

FIG. 44.46. ***Extramedullary hematopoiesis in an axillary lymph node.*** The patient had invasive ductal carcinoma, and no hematologic disorder was detected. **A:** Immature hematopoietic cells and megakaryocytes are present among the lymphocytes. **B:** Megakaryocytes and erythroid precursors in the lymph node.

initially in 21 (26%) of the cases studied by Mansi et al.[486] After a median follow-up of 18 months, only 2 of the 82 patients (2.4%) who remained clinically disease free had tumor cells detected in a second marrow aspirate, both having had carcinoma cells in their initial marrow samples. One of these women had received adjuvant chemotherapy and the other had not been so treated. During the course of follow-up, 6 of the 82 patients developed a recurrence, 4 having had bone micrometastases initially, including 1 of the 2 women with a subsequent positive marrow. Among 16 additional patients with local recurrence, 3, or 19%, had a positive marrow aspirate at the time of recurrence, whereas the aspirate was positive in 30% at the time of nonosseous systemic recurrence and in all patients with radiologically evident bone metastases.

A second study of patients with initial and follow-up bone marrow aspirations examined by IHC involved 59 women with inflammatory or locally advanced carcinoma.[487] Immunostains detected CK-positive cells in marrow samples from 29 (49.2%) of the patients before systemic chemotherapy. Overall 26 patients (41%) had a CK-positive marrow after chemotherapy, with no significant difference in the number of CK-positive cells before (17 per 2×10^6 leukocytes) and after (12 per 2×10^6 leukocytes) treatment. The presence of CK-positive cells in the marrow was significantly correlated with higher frequency of systemic metastases and shorter survival.

A larger study by Braun et al.[488] presented data on bone marrow samples obtained from patients with stage I to III breast carcinoma. CK-positive cells were detected in specimens from 199 of the 552 patients (36%) and also in 2 of 191 control samples (1%) from patients not known to have carcinoma. The presence or absence of axillary nodal metastases was not predictive of marrow status. After follow-up of 4 years, systemic recurrence and death due to breast carcinoma were significantly more frequent in women with a CK-positive marrow, regardless of axillary nodal status. After adjustment for systemic adjuvant chemotherapy, the RR of death due to breast carcinoma was 4.17 (95% CI, 2.51 to 6.94) for women with a CK-positive marrow when compared to those with a CK-negative specimen.

Wiedswang et al.[489] prospectively analyzed bone marrow aspirates taken from 817 patients at the time of primary surgery using the anti-CK AE1/3 antibody. The median follow-up was 49 months. CK-positive cells were found overall in 13.2% of patients. The likelihood of having a positive marrow was significantly related to tumor size and nodal status. The presence of carcinoma cells in the marrow aspirate was significantly related to an increased risk of clinical bone and liver metastases during follow-up. Bone marrow micrometastases increased the risk of systemic metastases but not of local or regional recurrences in node-positive patients. Systemic recurrence was not significantly increased among node-negative patients with bone marrow micrometastases who received adjuvant chemotherapy.

An analysis of the clinical significance of persistent bone marrow micrometastases was reported by Janni et al.[490] using an antibody cocktail to CK8/18 and CK8/19. The patients had various surgical and adjuvant treatment programs, including a substantial proportion who did not receive adjuvant chemotherapy. Ten of 102 patients (10%) with an initially negative marrow aspirate were found to have marrow micrometastases in a follow-up specimen. Nine of 31 (29%) with an initially positive marrow had persistent micrometastases in a subsequent specimen, and the remaining 22 patients (71%) had negative second aspirates. DFS was significantly related to the status of the follow-up bone marrow aspirate, with a mean recurrence-free survival of 149.7 months when the follow-up sample was negative and 86.5 months when there were micrometastases.

Evidence for the clinical significance of bone marrow micrometastases comes from the analysis of pooled data from published studies that included 4,703 patients with median follow-up of 5.2 years.[491] Micrometastases were found in 30.6% of the patients. The presence of bone marrow micrometastases was significantly associated with larger tumors, the presence of axillary nodal metastases, high-grade tumors, and negative hormone receptor status. Micrometastases were significantly related to increased deaths due to breast cancer, with a mortality ratio of 2.44. DFS was significantly reduced by the presence of marrow micrometastases among patients who had endocrine adjuvant therapy (mortality ratio, 3.22), chemotherapy (mortality ratio, 2.32), and among T1N0 patients who did not receive adjuvant therapy (mortality ratio, 3.65).

A consensus statement regarding bone marrow micrometastases prepared by the German, Australian, and Swiss Societies of Senology was published in 2006.[492] Major conclusions presented in this report include the following:

1. IHC with an alkaline phosphatase–based CK antibody and levamisole to block endogenous peroxidase was recommended to detect micrometastases.
2. The test material should consist of two to four slides containing 2×10^6 cells and a negative control preparation also with 2×10^6 cells.
3. A specimen is considered to be positive if one or more cells "with disseminated tumor cell morphology" are found in the test preparation, with no such cells in the control sample.
4. Prognosis is "impaired" in clinically disease-free stage I to III patients who have microscopically demonstrated bone marrow micrometastases.
5. Examination of marrow aspirates for micrometastases by IHC is not "a routine procedure" for the management of breast cancer patients.
6. The presence of micrometastases in the marrow is not currently a basis for treatment of disease-free patients outside of a clinical trial.

On the basis of their analysis of data from more than 400 patients, Braun et al.[491] stated that clinical trials would be useful to determine "whether the presence or absence of micrometastases suffices for a decision on the need for therapy and to predict the outcome of treatment in certain subgroups." Janni et al.[490] concluded that "prospective trials should investigate the benefit of secondary adjuvant treatment on the basis of bone marrow status." In this context, the detection of disseminated tumor cells in the marrow has been shown to predict survival after neoadjuvant therapy in primary breast cancer.[493]

Small breast epithelial mucin (SBEM), a recently described gene product, shows promise as a biomarker.[494] As outlined above, PCR amplification of tissue or tumor selective mRNA is the most powerful analytical tool for detection of bone marrow micrometastasis. Valladares-Ayerbes et al.[495] found SBEM-specific transcript in bone marrow in 26% of breast cancer patients—a number that is largely similar to that of patients with tumor cells detected using IHC. Furthermore, SBEM mRNA in marrow aspirates in the study was significantly associated with presence of clinically active disease, including locally advanced and metastatic patients.

Finally, the results of the ACOSOG Z0010 trial, designed to determine the association between survival and metastases detected by immunohistochemical staining of sentinel node and marrow specimens from patients with early-stage breast cancer, are notable. One-hundred and four of 3,413 (3.0%) marrow specimens were positive in this study.[496] At a median follow-up of approximately 6 years, 435 patients had died, and 376 had recurred. Marrow metastasis, although a rare finding in this trial, was associated with decreased OS, but was not found to be statistically significant on multivariate analysis. The remarkably low incidence of marrow involvement found in this trial was the main factor that led the authors not to recommend incorporation of marrow evaluation into routine practice.

EXAMINATION OF PROSTHETIC BREAST IMPLANTS

A standard policy for the handling of breast prosthetic devices should be established in each surgical pathology laboratory. The prosthetic device should be accessioned as a specimen. The patient should be informed by the surgeon that this will occur and that the prosthesis will be retained only for a limited period of time, typically 4 weeks or as otherwise stated in the aforementioned policy. The patient may request return of the device during this time. However, the device may not be handed to the patient until it has been examined by the pathology department.

Prostheses with adherent or detached soft or calcified tissue visible on gross inspection require placement in a standard laboratory fixative such as 10% buffered formalin. Implants returned to the patient should be sealed in a labeled biohazard container. A release form signed by the patient should be used to document receipt of the specimen. The patient should be informed about the possible biohazard risks associated with the specimen.

The pathology report for an explanted prosthetic device should include all clinical history and information supplied in the accompanying requisition. It is preferable that photographic documentation be obtained for all explanted devices. When any photograph is taken, it is essential to include the identity of the patient as well as the serial number, brand name, or other visible identifying markings pertaining to the specimen. These markings should also be stated in the pathology report.

The gross description should include salient features of the device. The dimensions in centimeters and the weight in grams of the prosthesis should be recorded, and the shape should be reported. The appearance of the external surface (smooth, textured, etc.) should be recorded, and a statement should be made about the apparent integrity of the surface. The prosthesis may be intact. If disrupted, the extent of the defect if grossly evident should be described. The contents should be described if visible.

Any tissue received with the prosthesis, either attached or detached, must be described grossly and sampled for microscopic study. In most instances, the tissue largely constitutes the fibrous capsule formed around the device (Fig. 44.48). To the extent possible, the weight in grams and dimensions

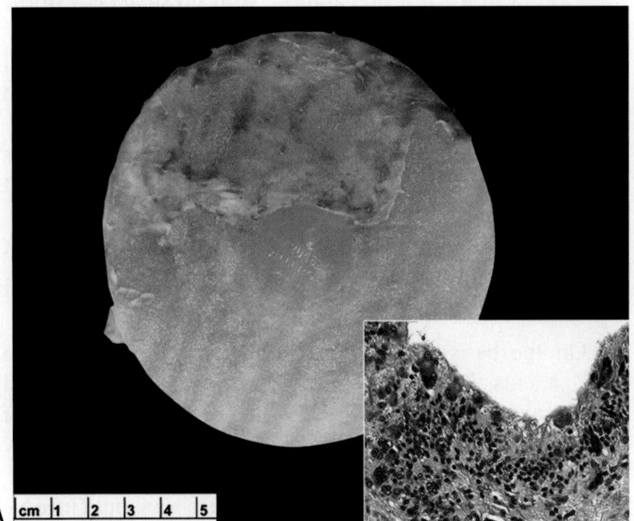

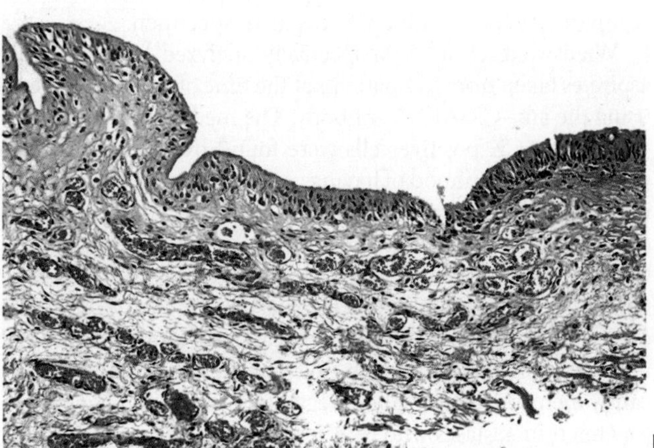

FIG. 44.48. ***Implant capsule with synovial-like metaplasia.*** **A:** The gross specimen of an implant with 'capsule' formation. Inset shows the histopathological appearance of the 'capsule' with formation of synovial-like metaplasia and multinucleated giant cells. **B–E:** Implant capsule with fibromatosis in a 19-year-old girl. **B,C:** Part of the implant capsule with typical reactive changes and synovial metaplasia on the surface. **D,E:** Fibromatosis involving the wall of the implant capsule *below* synovial metaplasia and invasion of adjacent pectoral muscle.

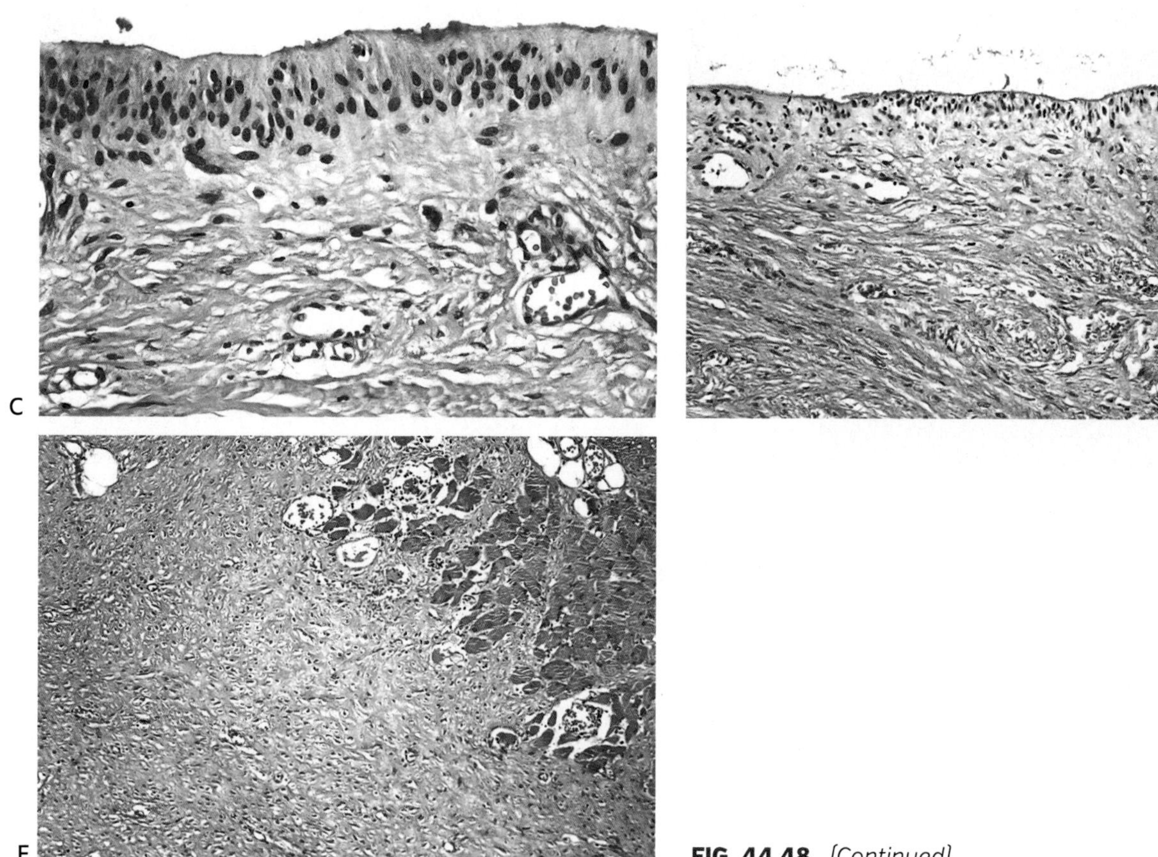

FIG. 44.48. *(Continued)*

in centimeters of the tissue should be recorded. The character of the inner surface of capsular tissue, if identifiable, should be described. Significant gross features such as hemorrhage, calcification, or foreign nontissue material attached to the specimen should be reported. Capsular contracture, the most common complication of mammary implant placement, tends to be less common with textured shells of either saline or silicone prostheses, and with the placement in the subcapsular versus the subglandular plane.[497]

The microscopic report should describe the general histologic features of the specimen such as fibrosis, type of inflammatory reaction, foreign material, and calcification. Microscopic changes on the capsular surface including the presence or absence of synovial metaplasia should be reported. The specific identification of foreign material is best reserved for spectroscopic analysis and other such procedures,[498,499] although it is possible to identify most commonly encountered material. Peri-implant and chest wall fibromatosis,[500,501] angiosarcoma,[502] and malignant lymphoma of various types[503,504] (see Chapter 40) can arise around a prosthetic breast implant (Fig. 44.48). Carcinoma[505] has been unexpectedly detected in an implant capsule specimen.

OTHER FOREIGN BODIES

A number of foreign bodies may be found in the breast. Some of these are the consequence of medical procedures. Spongioma (also referred to as gauzoma or gossypiboma) that occurs due to inadvertent retention of surgical sponges after surgery occurs relatively rarely in the breast.[506,507] Smaller foreign bodies in the iatrogenic category are localizing wires or needles that can break during a procedure or be transected intraoperatively.[508,509] Cardiac tamponade occurring as a delayed complication of cardiac injury resulting from migration of a retained hook wire 2 years after needle-localized breast biopsy has been reported.[510] Portions of catheters used for drainage of abscesses or after surgery may also be inadvertently detached, unknowingly retained, and detected mammographically as asymptomatic abnormalities.[511–513] In one case, a retained folded Penrose drain caused localized inflammation without a palpable mass 7 years following a biopsy for "benign disease" (Fig. 44.49).[514] Linear calcifications were seen mammographically. Calcifications in retained sponges or in sutures may mimic the mammographic appearance of calcifications in carcinoma (Fig. 44.50). Remnants of sutures with calcifications may suggest recurrent carcinoma mammographically.[515] The nature of such calcifications is readily appreciated when these have a knotted configuration or a smooth linear distribution on mammogram. Dense fibrous scarring and suture material detected histologically with or without calcifications should alert the pathologist to the site of a prior surgical procedure. The surgeon may fail to inform the pathologist that a biopsy was previously performed in a given case, and may be unaware of such a procedure. Tattoo pigments in the skin of the breast[516] and soap crystals containing calcium on the skin[517] can also mimic intramammary calcifications.

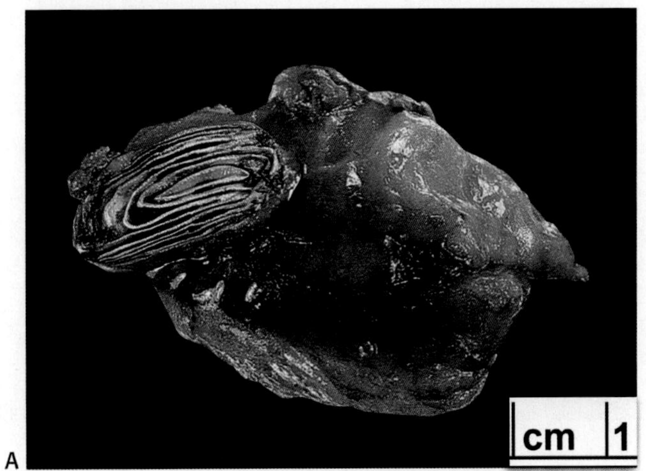

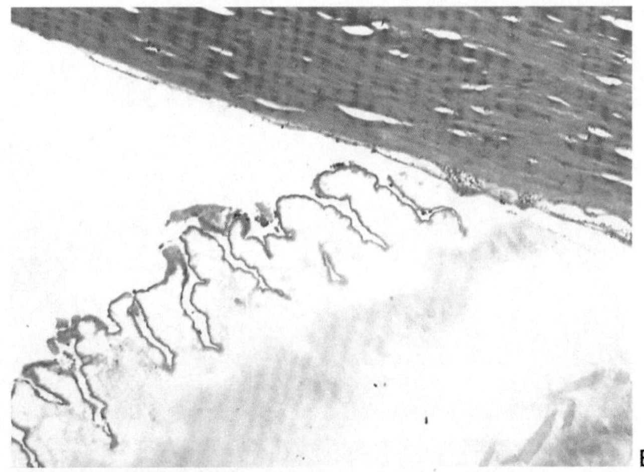

FIG. 44.49. ***Unusual foreign body.*** **A:** This mammographically detected foreign body is a retained, sequestered drain inserted 35 years earlier to evacuate an abscess. **B:** The histologic appearance of the degenerated drain and surrounding fibrous capsule.

An unusual case report described the finding of metallic fragments and a suspicious 2-cm mass with calcifications in the baseline mammogram of a 38-year-old woman.[518] An NCB revealed metallic particles and fibrous material composed of cotton fibers with a giant cell foreign body reaction. By history the patient had sustained a gunshot wound in the breast causing a portion of her clothing as well as bullet fragments to be embedded in the wound.

Various nonmedical foreign bodies of factitious or accidental origin have been described in the breast. These include glass,[519] needles,[520] hairpins,[520] stones,[521] and sewing machine needle.[522] Chinese herbal treatment of a breast abscess has been associated with intramammary punctate lead-containing deposits on mammography.[523] Foreign material injected directly into the breast for cosmetic enhancement can still occasionally be encountered. Such material includes silicone oil which has been banned by Food and Drug Administration (FDA) for this purpose since 1976.[524]

EXAMINATION OF REDUCTION MAMMAPLASTY SPECIMENS

Reduction mammaplasties are relatively commonly encountered in most surgical pathology laboratories. Most such procedures are performed for abnormal enlargement of both breasts without history of significant breast disease. Reduction procedures can also be performed in women with

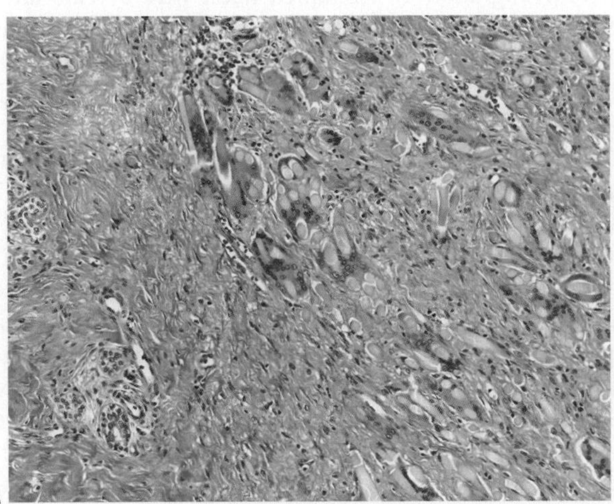

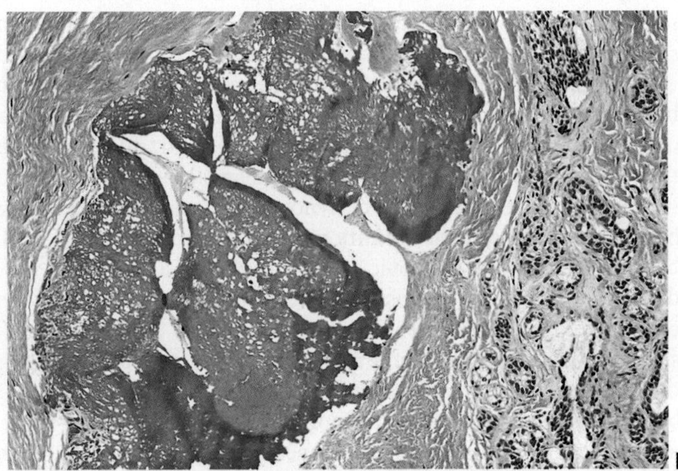

FIG. 44.50. ***Suture granuloma.*** **A:** Suture material surrounded by a mild fibrous and foreign body–type giant cell granulomatous reaction. The suture remained from an operation performed 3 weeks earlier. **B:** Calcified suture material in a healed biopsy site. Surgery had been performed at the site years earlier.

unilateral (or bilateral) carcinoma as part of "balancing" and reconstruction surgeries. In a study by Clark et al.,[525] 11.2% of 562 patients who underwent reduction mammaplasties had a history of breast carcinoma.

The incidence of occult significant pathology encountered in reduction mammaplasties reportedly ranges from 4% to 12.4%.[526–528] Based on the results of these studies, it can be concluded that in this setting DCIS and invasive carcinomas are identified with nearly equal frequency. Furthermore, carcinoma is more likely to be detected in patients older than 40, and those with a history of ipsilateral or contralateral carcinoma. The likelihood of uncovering significant disease obviously also depends on the degree of radiologic, gross and microscopic scrutiny of the specimens. The foregoing information should be duly considered in the establishing guidelines for the evaluation of reduction mammaplasty specimens.

PATHOLOGY OF BIOPSY SITE MARKERS

As discussed earlier in this chapter, a wide spectrum of reactive histopathologic alterations can be encountered following needle core, incisional, and excisional biopsies of the breast. The pathology of breast biopsy site–marking devices was reviewed by Guarda and Tran.[529] The radiographic clip placed after core biopsy to facilitate subsequent surgical excision is typically embedded in one of two types of substances: pellets of resorbable copolymer of polylactic acid/polyglycolic acid or plugs of bovine collagen (Fig. 44.51). Grossly, the pellets resemble rice grains, whereas collagen plugs appear sponge-like. Microscopically, the pellets elicit an initial cell-poor fibrotic reaction around empty spaces followed by a granulomatous reaction. The collagen plugs consist of eosinophilic, hyalinized, acellular material and are usually accompanied by a mixed inflammatory cell infiltrate. The collagen plug is usually devoid of a pronounced multinucleate giant cell reaction. Microcalcifications can form in collagen-based breast markers.[530] The biopsy site markers do not usually interfere with either tissue processing or histopathologic interpretation. It is likely that biopsy site–marking devices will be increasingly deployed[531] and newer types thereof will be introduced, with possibly distinctive reactive patterns.

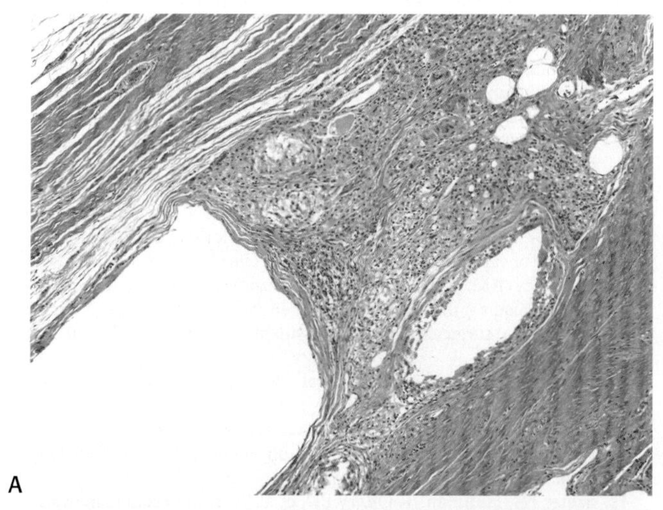
A

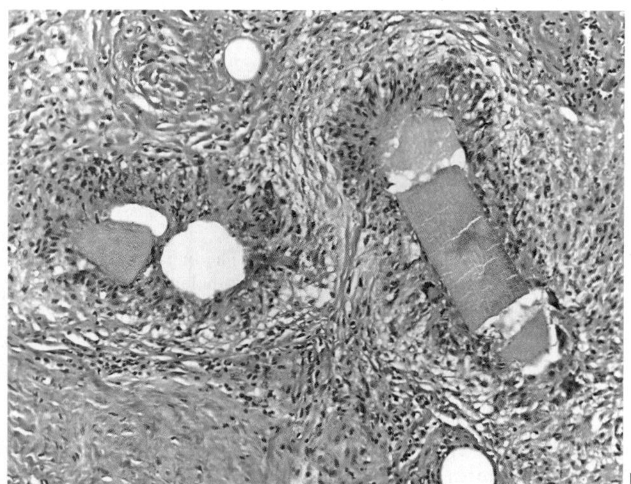
B

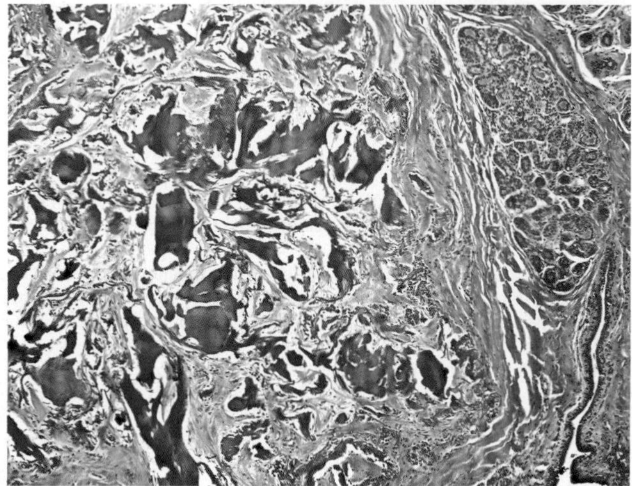
C

FIG. 44.51. ***Changes in excisional biopsy specimen following the placement of biopsy site markers.*** **A:** This site where a marker pellet was placed is characterized by a space surrounded by fibrosis and granulomatous reaction. **B:** Granulomatous reaction at the site of a polymer pellet. **C:** Fibrosis in and around the collagen plug at the site where a radiographic marker was placed.

REFERENCES

1. Association of Directors of Anatomic and Surgical Pathology. Immediate management of mammographically detected breast lesions. *Am J Surg Pathol* 1993;12:850–851.
2. Connolly JL, Schnitt SJ. Evaluation of breast biopsy specimens in patients considered for treatment by conservative surgery and radiation therapy for early breast cancer. *Pathol Annu* 1988;23(Pt. 1):1–23.
3. National Cancer Institute. Standardized management of breast specimens. Recommended by Pathology Working Group. Breast Cancer Task Force. *Am J Clin Pathol* 1973;60:789–798.
4. Schmidt WA. The breast. In: *Principles and techniques of surgical pathology*. Boston, MA: Butterworth, 1983:362–388.
5. Schnitt SJ, Connolly JL. Processing and evaluation of breast excision specimens. A clinically oriented approach. *Am J Clin Pathol* 1992;98:125–137.
6. Association of Directors of Anatomic and Surgical Pathology. Recommendations for the reporting of breast carcinoma. *Am J Clin Pathol* 1995;104:614–619.
7. Fitzgibbons PL, Connolly JL, Page DL, et al. Updated protocol for the examination of specimens from patients with carcinomas of the breast. A basis for checklists. *Arch Pathol Lab Med* 2000;124:1026–1033.
8. Lucirica R. Intraoperative assessment of the breast. Guidelines and potential pitfalls. *Arch Pathol Lab Med* 2005;129:1565–1574.
9. Fitzgibbons PL, Page DL, Weaver D. Prognostic factors in breast cancer. College of American Pathologists Consensus Statement 1999. *Arch Pathol Lab Med* 2000;124:966–978.
10. Nakhleh RE, Myers JL, Allen TC, et al. Consensus statement on effective communication of urgent diagnoses and significant, unexpected diagnoses in surgical pathology and cytopathology from the College of American Pathologists and Association of Directors of Anatomic and Surgical Pathology. *Arch Pathol Lab Med* 2012;136:148–154.
11. Adams AL, Dabbs DJ. Commonly encountered dilemmas in breast cancer reporting and staging. *Semin Diagn Pathol* 2012;29:109–115.
12. Lacambra MD, Lam CC, Mendoza P, et al. Biopsy sampling of breast lesions: comparison of core needle- and vacuum-assisted breast biopsies. *Breast Cancer Res Treat* 2012;132:917–923.
13. Allen SD, Nerurkar A, Della Rovere GU. The breast lesion excision system (BLES): a novel technique in the diagnostic and therapeutic management of small indeterminate breast lesions? *Eur Radiol* 2011;21:919–924.
14. Edwards HD, Oakley F, Koyama T, et al. The impact of tumor size in breast needle biopsy material on final pathologic size and tumor stage: a detailed analysis of 222 consecutive cases. *Am J Surg Pathol* 2013;37:739–744.
15. Huo L. A practical approach to grossing breast specimens. *Ann Diagn Pathol* 2011;15:291–301.
16. Hammond ME. ASCO-CAP guidelines for breast predictive factor testing: an update . *Appl Immunohistochem Mol Morphol* 2011;19:499–500.
17. Li X, Deavers MT, Guo M, et al. The effect of prolonged cold ischemia time on estrogen receptor immunohistochemistry in breast cancer. *Mod Pathol* 2013;26:71–78.
18. Portier BP, Wang Z, Downs-Kelly E, et al. Delay to formalin fixation 'cold ischemia time': effect on ERBB2 detection by *in-situ* hybridization and immunohistochemistry. *Mod Pathol* 2013;26:1–9.
19. Khoury T. Delay to formalin fixation alters morphology and immunohistochemistry for breast carcinoma. *Appl Immunohistochem Mol Morphol* 2012;20:531–542.
20. Krekel NM, van Slooten HJ, Barbé E,et al. Is breast specimen shrinkage really a problem in breast-conserving surgery? *J Clin Pathol* 2012;65:224–227.
21. Yip JM, Mouratova N, Jeffery RM, et al. Accurate assessment of breast volume: a study comparing the volumetric gold standard (direct water displacement measurement of mastectomy specimen) with a 3D laser scanning technique. *Ann Plast Surg* 2012;68:135–141.
22. Rosen PP, Senie R, Schottenfeld D, et al. Noninvasive breast carcinoma: frequency of unsuspected invasion and implication for treatment. *Ann Surg* 1979;89:98–103.
23. Speights VO Jr. Evaluation of frozen sections in grossly benign breast biopsies. *Mod Pathol* 1994;7:762–765.
24. Bianchi S, Palli D, Ciatto S, et al. Accuracy and reliability of frozen section diagnosis in a series of 672 nonpalpable breast lesions. *Am J Clin Pathol* 1995;103:199–205.
25. Ferreiro JA, Gisvold JJ, Bostwick DG. Accuracy of frozen-section diagnosis of mammographically directed breast biopsies. Results of 1,490 consecutive cases. *Am J Surg Pathol* 1995;19:1267–1271.
26. Tinnenmans JGM, Wobbes T, Holland HJH, et al. Mammographic and histopathologic correlation of nonpalpable lesions of the breast and the reliability of frozen section diagnosis. *Surg Gynecol Obstet* 1987;165:523–529.
27. Niemann TH, Lucas JG, Marsh WL Jr. To freeze or not to freeze. A comparison of methods for the handling of breast biopsies with no palpable abnormality. *Am J Clin Pathol* 1996;106:225–228.
28. Esbona K, Li Z, Wilke LG. Intraoperative imprint cytology and frozen section pathology for margin assessment in breast conservation surgery: a systematic review. *Ann Surg Oncol* 2012;19:3236–3245.
29. Valdes EK, Boolbol SK, Ali I, et al. Intraoperative touch preparation cytology for margin assessment in breast-conservation surgery: does it work for lobular carcinoma? *Ann Surg Oncol* 2007;14:2940–2945.
30. Lorand S, Lavoué V, Tas P, et al. Intraoperative touch imprint cytology of axillary sentinel nodes for breast cancer: a series of 355 procedures. *Breast* 2011;20:119–123.
31. Britton PD, Sonoda LI, Yamamoto AK, et al. Breast surgical specimen radiographs: how reliable are they? *Eur J Radiol* 2011;79:245–249.
32. Young ES, Hogg DE, Krontiras H, et al. Specimen radiographs assist in identifying and assessing resection margins of occult breast carcinomas. *Breast J* 2009;15:521–523.
33. Schnitt S, Wang HH. Histologic sampling of grossly benign breast biopsies. How much is enough? *Am J Surg Pathol* 1989;13:505–512.
34. Owings DV, Hann L, Schnitt SJ. How thoroughly should needle localization breast biopsies be sampled for microscopic examination? A prospective mammographic/pathologic correlative study. *Am J Surg Pathol* 1990;14:578–583.
35. Abraham SC, Fox K, Fraker D, et al. Sampling of grossly benign breast reexcisions: a multidisciplinary approach to assessing adequacy. *Am J Surg Pathol* 1999;23:316–322.
36. Sahoo S, Lester SC. Pathology of breast carcinomas after neoadjuvant chemotherapy: an overview with recommendations on specimen processing and reporting. *Arch Pathol Lab Med* 2009;133:633–642.
37. Kreike B, Hart AA, van de Velde T, et al. Continuing risk of ipsilateral breast relapse after breast-conserving therapy at long-term follow-up. *Int J Radiat Oncol Biol Phys* 2008;71:1014–1021.
38. Goldhirsch A, Ingle JN, Gelber RD, et al. Thresholds for therapies: highlights of the St Gallen International Expert Consensus on the primary therapy of early breast cancer 2009. *Ann Oncol* 2009;20:1319–1329.
39. Laughney AM, Krishnaswamy V, Rizzo EJ, et al. Scatter spectroscopic imaging distinguishes between breast pathologies in tissues relevant to surgical margin assessment. *Clin Cancer Res* 2012;18: 6315–6325.
40. Pezner RD, Terz J, Ben-Ezra J, et al. Now there are two effective conservation approaches for patients with stage I and II breast cancer: how pathological assessment of inked resection margins can provide valuable information for the radiation oncologist. *Am J Clin Oncol* 1990;13:175–179.
41. Sauter ER, Hoffman JP, Ottery FD, et al. Is frozen section analysis of reexcision lumpectomy margins worthwhile? Margin analysis in breast reexcisions. *Cancer* 1994;73:2607–2612.
42. Aitken RJ, Going JJ, Chetty U. Assessment of surgical excision during breast conservation surgery by intraoperative two-dimensional specimen radiology. *Br J Surg* 1990;77:322–323.
43. Cox CE, Ku NN, Reintgen D, et al. Touch preparation cytology of breast lumpectomy margins with histologic correlation. *Arch Surg* 1991;126:490–493.
44. Novita G, Filassi JR, Ruiz CA, et al. Evaluation of frozen-section analysis of surgical margins in the treatment of breast cancer. *Eur J Gynaecol Oncol* 2012;33:498–501.
45. Jorns JM, Visscher D, Sabel M, et al. Intraoperative frozen section analysis of margins in breast conserving surgery significantly decreases reoperative rates: one-year experience at an ambulatory surgical center. *Am J Clin Pathol* 2012;138:657–669.
46. Weber S, Storm FK, Stitt J, et al. The role of frozen section analysis of margins during breast conservation surgery. *Cancer J Sci Am* 1997;3:273–277.
47. Esserman L, Weidner N. Is routine frozen section assessment feasible in the practice environment of the 1990s? *Cancer J Sci Am* 1997;3:266–267.

48. Hewes JC, Imkampe A, Haji A, et al. Importance of routine cavity sampling in breast conservation surgery. *Br J Surg* 2009;96:47–53.
49. Mullen R, Macaskill EJ, Khalil A, et al. Involved anterior margins after breast conserving surgery: is re-excision required? *Eur J Surg Oncol* 2012;38:302–306.
50. Barthelmes L, Al Awa A, Crawford DJ. Effects of cavity margin shavings to ensure completeness of excision on local recurrence rates following breast conservation surgery. *Eur J Surg Oncol* 2003;29:644–648.
51. Malik HZ, George WD, Mallon EA, et al. Margin assessment by cavity shaving breast-conserving surgery: analysis and follow-up of 543 patients. *Eur J Surg Oncol* 1999;25:464–469.
52. Cao D, Lin C, Woo SH, et al. Separate cavity margin sampling at the time of initial breast lumpectomy significantly reduces the need for reexcisions. *Am J Surg Pathol* 2005;29:1625–1632.
53. Guidi AJ, Connolly JL, Harris JR, et al. The relationship between shaved margin and inked margin status in breast excision specimens. *Cancer* 1997;79:1568–1573.
54. Rubin P, O'Hanlon D, Browell D, et al. Tumour bed biopsy detects the presence of multifocal disease in patients undergoing breast conservation therapy for primary breast carcinoma. *Eur J Surg Oncol* 1996;22:23–26.
55. Dooley WC, Parker J. Understanding the mechanisms creating false positive lumpectomy margins. *Am J Surg* 2005;190:606–608.
56. Graham RA, Homer MJ, Katz J, et al. The pancake phenomenon contributes to the inaccuracy of margin assessment in patients with breast cancer. *Am J Surg* 2002;184:89–93.
57. Molina MA, Snell S, Franceschi D, et al. Breast specimen orientation. *Ann Surg Oncol* 2009;16:285–288.
58. Ginter P, Jones JG, Hoda SA. True colors. *Int J Surg Pathol* 2011;19:494–496.
59. Renshaw AA, Kish R, Gould EW. The value of inking breast cores to reduce specimen mix-up. *Am J Clin Pathol* 2007;127:271–272.
60. Carter D. Margins of "lumpectomy" for breast cancer. *Hum Pathol* 1986;17:330–332.
61. Veronesi U, Farante G, Galimberti V, et al. Evaluation of resection margins after breast conservative surgery with monoclonal antibodies. *Eur J Surg Oncol* 1991;17:338–341.
62. England DW, Chan SY, Stonelake PS, et al. Assessment of excision margins following wide local excision for breast carcinoma using specimen scrape cytology and tumour bed biopsy. *Eur J Surg Oncol* 1994;20:425–429.
63. Ciocca RM, Li T, Freedman GM, et al. Presence of lobular carcinoma *in situ* does not increase local recurrence in patients treated with breast-conserving therapy. *Ann Surg Oncol* 2008;15:2263–2271.
64. Downs-Kelly E, Bell D, Perkins GH, et al. Clinical implications of margin involvement by pleomorphic lobular carcinoma *in situ*. *Arch Pathol Lab Med* 2011;135:737–743.
65. Pittinger TP, Maronian NC, Poulter CA, et al. Importance of margin status in outcome of breast-conserving surgery for carcinoma. *Surgery* 1994;116:605–609.
66. Schnitt SJ, Abner A, Gelman R, et al. The relationship between microscopic margins of resection and the risk of local recurrence in patients with breast cancer treated with breast-conserving surgery and radiation therapy. *Cancer* 1994;74:1746–1751.
67. Gage I, Schnitt SJ, Nixon AJ, et al. Pathologic margin involvement and the risk of recurrence in patients treated with breast-conserving therapy. *Cancer* 1996;78:1921–1928.
68. DiBiase SJ, Komarnicky LT, Schwartz GF, et al. The number of positive margins influences the outcome of women treated with breast preservation for early stage breast carcinoma. *Cancer* 1998;82:2212–2220.
69. Papa MZ, Zippel D, Koller M, et al. Positive margins of breast biopsy: is reexcision always necessary? *J Surg Oncol* 1999;70:167–171.
70. Gwin JL, Eisenberg BL, Hoffman JP, et al. Incidence of gross and microscopic carcinoma in specimens from patients with breast cancer after re-excision lumpectomy. *Ann Surg* 1993;218:729–734.
71. McCormick B, Kinne D, Petrek J, et al. Limited resection for breast cancer: a study of inked specimen margins before radiotherapy. *Int J Radiat Oncol Biol Phys* 1987;13:1667–1671.
72. Schnitt SJ, Connolly JL, Khettry U, et al. Pathologic findings on re-excision of the primary site in breast cancer patients considered for treatment by primary radiation therapy. *Cancer* 1987;59:675–681.
73. Solin LJ, Fowble B, Martz K, et al. Results of re-excisional biopsy of the primary tumor in preparation for definitive irradiation of patients with early stage breast cancer. *Int J Radiat Oncol Biol Phys* 1986;12:721–725.
74. Stotter AT, McNeese MD, Ames FC, et al. Predicting the rate and extent of locoregional failure after breast conservative therapy for early breast cancer. *Cancer* 1989;64:2217–2225.
75. Hughes LL, Wang M, Page DL, et al. Local excision alone without irradiation for ductal carcinoma *in situ* of the breast: a trial of the Eastern Cooperative Oncology Group. *J Clin Oncol* 2009;27:5319–5324.
76. Heimann R, Powers C, Halpern HJ, et al. Breast preservation in stage I and II carcinoma of the breast. The University of Chicago experience. *Cancer* 1996;78:1722–1730.
77. Mansfield CM, Komarnicky LT, Schwartz GF, et al. Ten-year results in 1070 patients with stages I and II breast cancer treated by conservative surgery and radiation therapy. *Cancer* 1995;75:2328–2336.
78. Smitt MC, Nowels KW, Zdeblick MJ, et al. The importance of the lumpectomy surgical margin status in long term results of breast conservation. *Cancer* 1995;76:259–267.
79. Spivack B, Khanna MM, Tafra L, et al. Margin status and local recurrence after breast-conserving surgery. *Arch Surg* 1994;129:952–957.
80. Veronesi U. How important is the assessment of resection margins in conservative surgery for breast cancer? *Cancer* 1994;74:1660–1661.
81. Mariani L, Salvadori B, Marubini E, et al. Ten year results of a randomised trial comparing two conservative treatment strategies for small size breast cancer. *Eur J Cancer* 1998;34:1156–1162.
82. Fisher ER, Sass R, Fisher B, et al. Pathologic findings from the National Surgical Adjuvant Breast Project (Protocol 6). II. Relation of local breast recurrence to multicentricity. *Cancer* 1986;57:1717–1724.
83. Fourquet A, Campana F, Zafrani B, et al. Prognostic factors of breast recurrence in the conservative management of early breast cancer: a 25-year follow-up. *Int J Radiat Oncol Biol Phys* 1989;17:719–725.
84. Ryoo MC, Kagan AR, Wollin M, et al. Prognostic factors for recurrence and cosmesis in 393 patients after radiation therapy for early mammary carcinoma. *Radiology* 1989;172:555–559.
85. Anscher MS, Jones P, Prosnitz LR, et al. Local failure and margin status in early-stage breast carcinoma treated with conservation surgery and radiation therapy. *Ann Surg* 1993;218:22–28.
86. Kunos C, Latson L, Overmoyer B, et al. Breast conservation surgery achieving ≥≥2 mm tumor-free margins results in decreased local-regional recurrence rates. *Breast J* 2006;12:28–36.
87. Veronesi U, Marubini E, Del Vecchio M, et al. Local recurrences and distant metastases after conservative breast cancer treatments: partly independent events. *J Natl Cancer Inst* 1995;87:19–27.
88. Haffty BG, Reiss M, Beinfield M, et al. Ipsilateral breast tumor recurrence as a predictor of distant disease: implications for systemic therapy at the time of local relapse. *J Clin Oncol* 1996;14:52–57.
89. Noguchi S, Koyama H, Kasugai T, et al. A case-control study on risk factors for local recurrences or distant metastases in breast cancer patients treated with breast-conserving surgery. *Oncology* 1997;54:468–474.
90. Fisher B, Anderson S, Fisher ER, et al. Significance of ipsilateral breast tumour recurrence after lumpectomy. *Lancet* 1991;338:327–331.
91. Silvestrini R, Daidone MG, Luisi A, et al. Biologic and clinicopathologic factors as indicators of specific relapse types in node-negative breast cancer. *J Clin Oncol* 1995;13:697–704.
92. Francis M, Cakir B, Ung O, et al. Prognosis after breast recurrence following conservative surgery and radiotherapy in patients with node-negative breast cancer. *Br J Surg* 1999;86:1556–1562.
93. Fortin A, Larochelle M, Laverdiere J, et al. Local failure is responsible for the decrease in survival for patients with breast cancer treated with conservative surgery and postoperative radiotherapy. *J Clin Oncol* 1999;17:101–109.
94. Solin LJ, Fowble BL, Schultz DJ, et al. The significance of the pathology margins of the tumor excision on the outcome of patients treated with definitive irradiation for early stage breast cancer. *Int J Radiat Oncol Biol Phys* 1991;21:279–287.
95. Voogd AC, van Tienhoven G, Peterse HL, et al. Local recurrence after breast conservation therapy for early stage breast carcinoma: detection, treatment, and outcome in 266 patients. Dutch Study Group on Local Recurrence after Breast Conservation (BORST). *Cancer* 1999;85:437–446.
96. Sinn HP, Anton HW, Magener A, et al. Extensive and predominant *in situ* component in breast carcinoma: their influence on treatment results after breast-conserving therapy. *Eur J Cancer* 1998;34:646–653.
97. Peterse JL, van Dongen JA, Bartelink H. Recurrence of breast carcinoma after breast conserving treatment. *Eur J Surg Oncol* 1988;14:123–126.
98. Zafrani B, Vielh P, Fourquet A, et al. Conservative treatment of early breast cancer: prognostic value of the ductal *in situ* component and

other pathological variables on local control and survival. Long-term results. *Eur J Cancer Clin Oncol* 1989;25:1645–1650.
99. Ohtake T, Abe R, Kimijima I, et al. Intraductal extension of primary invasive breast carcinoma treated by breast-conservation surgery. Computer graphic three-dimensional reconstruction of the mammary duct-lobular systems. *Cancer* 1995;76:32–45.
100. Jimenez RE, Bongers S, Bouwman D, et al. Clinicopathologic significance of ductal carcinoma *in situ* in breast core needle biopsies with invasive cancer. *Am J Surg Pathol* 2000;24:123–128.
101. Brenin DR, Morrow M. Accuracy of AJCC staging for breast cancer patients undergoing re-excision for positive margins. American Joint Committee on Cancer. *Ann Surg Oncol* 1998;5:719–723.
102. Morris EA, Schwartz LH, Drotman MB, et al. Evaluation of pectoralis major muscle in patients with posterior breast tumors on breast MR images: early experience. *Radiology* 2000;214:67–72.
103. Esserman L, Hylton N, Yassa L, et al. Utility of magnetic resonance imaging in the management of breast cancer: evidence for improved preoperative staging. *J Clin Oncol* 1999;17:110–119.
104. Berg WA, Gilbreath PL. Multicentric and multifocal cancer: whole-breast US in preoperative evaluation. *Radiology* 2000;214:59–66.
105. Rosen PP. Specimen radiography and the diagnosis of clinically occult mammary carcinoma. *Pathol Annu* 1980;15(Pt. 1):225–237.
106. Salomon A. Beitrag zur Pathologie und Klinik der mammacarcinome. *Arch Klin Chir* 1918;101:573–668.
107. Gershon-Cohen J, Colcher AE. An evaluation of the roentgen diagnosis of early carcinoma of the breast. *JAMA* 1937;108:867–871.
108. Leborgne R. Diagnosis of tumors of the breast by simple roentgenography: calcifications in carcinoma. *AJR Am J Roentgenol* 1951;65:1–11.
109. Cody III HS. The impact of mammography in 1096 consecutive patients with breast cancer, 1979–1993. *Cancer* 1995;76:1579–1584.
110. Rosen PP, Snyder RE, Urban JA, et al. Correlation of suspicious mammograms and x-rays of breast biopsies during surgery. Results in 60 cases. *Cancer* 1973;31:656–659.
111. Snyder RE, Rosen PP. Radiography of breast specimens. *Cancer* 1971;28:1608–1611.
112. Chilcote WA, Davis GA, Suchy P, et al. Breast specimen radiography: evaluation of a compression device. *Radiology* 1988;168:425–427.
113. Eastgate RJ, Gilchrist KW, Matallana RH. Enhancement of tissue structure visualization in breast specimen radiography. *Radiology* 1979;132:744–746.
114. Philip J, Harris WG, Rustage JH. Radiography of breast biopsy specimens. *Br J Surg* 1982;69:126–127.
115. Birdwell RL, Ikeda DM, Jeffrey SS. Value of sonographic identification of breast masses in excised specimens in the breast imaging department: report of 7 cases. *Breast Dis* 1996;9:93–99.
116. Bauermeister DE, Hall MH. Specimen radiography—a mandatory adjunct to mammography. *Am J Clin Pathol* 1973;59:782–788.
117. Meyer JE, Eberlein TJ, Stomper PC, et al. Biopsy of occult breast lesions. Analysis of 1261 abnormalities. *JAMA* 1990;263:2341–2343.
118. Tinnemans JGM, Wobbes T, Holland R, et al. Mammographic and histopathologic correlation of nonpalpable lesions of the breast and the reliability of frozen section diagnosis. *Surg Gynecol Obstet* 1987;165:523–529.
119. Pastakia B, Chang V, McDonald H, et al. Immediate post-excision mammography for occult noncalcified breast lesions. *South Med J* 1990;83:30–33.
120. Reid SE Jr, Scanlon EF, Bernstein JR, et al. An alternative approach to nonpalpable breast biopsies. *J Surg Oncol* 1990;44:93–96.
121. Norton LW, Zeligman BF, Pearlman NW. Accuracy and cost of needle localization breast biopsy. *Arch Surg* 1988;123:945–950.
122. Leis HP, Cammarata A, LaRaja RD, et al. Breast biopsy and guidance for occult lesions. *Int Surg* 1985;70:115–118.
123. Meyer JE, Sonnenfeld MR, Greene RA, et al. Preoperative localization of clinically occult breast lesions. Experience at a referral hospital. *Radiology* 1988;169:627–628.
124. Symmonds RF Jr, Roberts JW. Management of nonpalpable breast abnormalities. *Ann Surg* 1987;205:520–528.
125. Kopans DB, Meyer JE, Homer MJ, et al. Dermal deposits mistaken for breast calcifications. *Radiology* 1983;149:592–594.
126. Linden SS, Sullivan DC. Breast skin calcifications: localization with a stereotactic device. *Radiology* 1989;171:570–571.
127. Brown RC, Zuehlke RL, Ehrhardt JC, et al. Tattoos simulating calcifications on xeroradiography of the breast. *Radiology* 1981;138:583–584.
128. Lager DJ, O'Connor JC, Robinson RA, et al. Factitious microcalcifications in breast biopsy material: laboratory-induced error by use of tattoo powder for specimen mammography. *J Surg Oncol* 1989;40:281–282.
129. Frank HA, Hall FM, Steer ME. Preoperative localization of nonpalpable breast lesions demonstrated by mammography. *N Engl J Med* 1976;295:259–260.
130. Silverstein MJ, Gamagami P, Rosser RJ, et al. Hooked-wire-directed breast biopsy and overpenetrated mammography. *Cancer* 1987;59:715–722.
131. Czarmecki DJ, Feider HK, Splittgerber GF. Toluidine blue dye as a breast localization marker. *Am J Radiol* 1989;153:261–263.
132. Hirsch JI, Banks WL Jr, Sullivan JS, et al. Noninterference of isosulfan blue on estrogen-receptor activity. *Radiology* 1989;171:109–110.
133. Alderliesten T, Loo CE, Pengel KE, et al. Radioactive seed localization of breast lesions: an adequate localization method without seed migration. *Breast J* 2011;17:594–601.
134. Gobardhan PD, de Wall LL, van der Laan L, et al. The role of radioactive iodine-125 seed localization in breast-conserving therapy following neoadjuvant chemotherapy. *Ann Oncol* 2013;24:668–673.
135. Graham RP, Jakub JW, Brunette JJ, et al. Handling of radioactive seed localization breast specimens in the pathology laboratory. *Am J Surg Pathol* 2012;36:1718–1723.
136. Davis PS, Wechler RJ, Feig SA, et al. Migration of breast biopsy localization wire. *AJR Am J Roentgenol* 1988;150:787–788.
137. Owen AWMC, Kumer EN. Migration of localizing wires used in guided biopsy of the breast. *Clin Radiol* 1991;43:251.
138. Frappart L, Boudeulle M, Boumendil J, et al. Structure and composition of microcalcifications in benign and malignant lesions of the breast: study by light microscopy, transmission and scanning electron microscopy, microprobe analysis, and X-ray diffraction. *Hum Pathol* 1984;15:880–889.
139. Frappart L, Remy I, Hu CL, et al. Different types of microcalcifications observed in breast pathology. Correlations with histopathologic diagnosis and radiologic examination of operative specimens. *Virchows Arch [A]* 1986;410:179–187.
140. Tse GM, Tan PH, Pang AL, et al. Calcification in breast lesions: pathologists' perspective. *J Clin Pathol* 2008;61:145–151.
141. Radi MJ. Calcium oxalate crystals in breast biopsies. An overlooked form of microcalcification associated with benign breast disease. *Arch Pathol Lab Med* 1989;113:1367–1369.
142. Symonds DA. Use of the von Kossa stain in identifying occult calcifications in breast biopsies. *Am J Clin Pathol* 1990;94:44–48.
143. Tornos C, Silva E, El-Naggar A, et al. Calcium oxalate crystals in breast biopsies. The missing microcalcifications. *Am J Surg Pathol* 1990;14:961–968.
144. Foschini MP, Fornelli A, Peterse JL, et al. Microcalcifications in ductal carcinoma *in situ* of the breast: histochemical and immunohistochemical study. *Hum Pathol* 1996;27:178–183.
145. Going JJ, Anderson TJ, Crocker PR, et al. Weddellite calcification in the breast: eighteen cases with implications for breast cancer screening. *Histopathology* 1990;16:119–124.
146. Ortiz-Hidalgo C. Dihydrate birefringent calcium oxalate or Weddellite calcification (Letter). *J Clin Pathol* 2000;53:84–85.
147. Winston JS, Yeh I-T, Evers K, et al. Calcium oxalate is associated with benign breast tissue. *Am J Clin Pathol* 1993;100:488–492.
148. Truong LD, Cartwright J Jr, Alpert L. Calcium oxalate in breast lesions biopsied for calcification detected in screening mammography: incidence and clinical significance. *Mod Pathol* 1992;5:146–152.
149. Panjwani P, Tirumalae R, Emmanuel A. Calcium oxalate crystals—an unexpected finding in a breast aspirate. *Diagn Cytopathol* 2011; 39:349–351.
150. Frouge C, Meunier M, Guinebretière J-M,et al. Polyhedral-shaped microcalcification on mammography: histologic correlation with calcium oxalate. *Radiology* 1993;186:681–684.
151. Frouge C, Guinebretière J-M, Juras J, et al. Polyhedral microcalcifications on mammograms: prevalence and morphometric analysis. *AJR Am J Roentgenol* 1996;167:621–624.
152. Gonzalez JEG, Caldwell RG, Valaitis JO. Calcium oxalate crystals in the breast. Pathology and significance. *Am J Surg Pathol* 1991;15: 586–591.
153. Feirt N, Vazquez MF. Indeterminate microcalcifications (BIRAD 3): what do they represent pathologically? *Mod Pathol* 2000;13:21A.
154. Singh N, Theaker JM. Calcium oxalate crystals (Weddellite) within the secretions of ductal carcinoma *in situ*—a rare phenomenon. *J Clin Pathol* 1999;52:145–146.

155. Stein MA, Karlan MS. Calcification in breast biopsy specimens: discrepancies in radiologic-pathologic identification. *Radiology* 1991;179:111–114.
156. Surratt JR, Monsees BS, Mazoujian G. Calcium oxalate microcalcifications in the breast. *Radiology* 1991;181:141–142.
157. Rebner M, Helvie MA, Pennes DR, et al. Paraffin tissue block radiography: adjunct to breast specimen radiography. *Radiology* 1989;173:695–696.
158. Brem RF, Askin FB, Gatewood OM. Selection of core biopsy specimens for pathologic evaluation of targeted microcalcifications. *AJR Am J Roentgenol* 1999;173:901–902.
159. Liberman L, Evans WP III, Dershaw DD, et al. Specimen radiography of microcalcifications in stereotactic mammary core biopsies. *Radiology* 1994;190:223–225.
160. Gallagher R, Schafer G, Redick M, et al. Microcalcifications of the breast: a mammographic-histologic correlation study using a newly designed Path/Rad Tissue Tray. *Ann Diagn Pathol* 2012;16:196–201.
161. Winston JS, Geradts J, Liu DF, et al. Microtome shaving radiography: demonstration of loss of mammographic microcalcifications during histologic sectioning. *Breast J* 2004;10:200–203.
162. Lee AH, Villena Salinas NM, Hodi Z, et al. The value of examination of multiple levels of mammary needle core biopsy specimens taken for investigation of lesions other than calcification. *J Clin Pathol* 2012;65:1097–1099.
163. Wu YC, Freedman MT, Hasegawa A, et al. Classification of microcalcifications in radiographs of pathologic specimens for the diagnosis of breast cancer. *Acad Radiol* 1995;2:199–204.
164. Wu Y, Doi K, Giger ML, et al. Computerized detection of clustered microcalcifications in digital mammograms: applications of artificial neural networks. *Med Phys* 1992;19:555–560.
165. Ng KH, Looi LM, Bradley DA. Microcalcification clustering parameters in breast disease: a morphometric analysis of radiographs of excision specimens. *Br J Radiol* 1996;69:326–334.
166. Zhang W, Doi K, Giger ML, et al. Computerized detection of clustered microcalcifications in digital mammograms using a shift-invariant artificial neural network. *Med Phys* 1994;21:517–524.
167. American College of Radiology (ACR). *Breast imaging reporting and data system (BI-RADS)*. 4th ed. Reston, VA: American College of Radiology, 2003.
168. Boyer B, Canale S, Arfi-Rouche J, et al. Variability and errors when applying the BIRADS mammography classification. *Eur J Radiol* 2013;82:388–397.
169. Selim A, Tahan SR. Microscopic localization of calcifications in and around breast carcinoma: a cautionary note for needle core biopsies. *Ann Surg* 1998;228:95–98.
170. Dershaw DD, Giess CS, McCormick B, et al. Patterns of mammographically detected calcifications after breast-conserving therapy associated with tumor recurrence. *Cancer* 1997;79:1355–1361.
171. Mitnick JS, Vazquez MF, Roses DF, et al. Recurrent breast cancer: stereotaxic localization for fine-needle aspiration biopsy. Work in progress. *Radiology* 1992;182:103–106.
172. Trop I, David J, El Khoury M, et al. Microcalcifications around a collagen-based breast biopsy marker: complication of biopsy with a percutaneous marking system. *AJR Am J Roentgenol* 2011;197:W353–W357.
173. Homer MJ, Slowinski J. Spontaneously disappearing calcifications in the breast: incidence appearance and implications. *Breast Dis* 1992;5:251–258.
174. Parker MD, Clark RL, McLelland R, et al. Disappearing breast calcifications. *Radiology* 1989;172:677–680.
175. Moritz JD, Luftner-Nagel S, Westerhof JP, et al. Microcalcifications in breast core biopsy specimens: disappearance at radiography after storage in formaldehyde. *Radiology* 1996;200:361–363.
176. Matsunaga T, Nakamura Y, Mimuro M, et al. Chronological changes of microcalcifications of breast carcinoma. *Breast Cancer* 1998;5:269–277.
177. Cao MM, Hoyt AC, Bassett LW. Mammographic signs of systemic disease. *Radiographics* 2011;31:1085–1100.
178. Apestegía L, Pina L, Inchusta M, et al. Klippel-Trenaunay syndrome: a very infrequent cause of microcalcifications in mammography. *Eur Radiol* 1997;7:123–125.
179. Evans SE, Whitehouse GH. Extensive calcification in the breast in chronic renal failure. *Br J Radiol* 1991;64:757–759.
180. Resnikoff LB, Mendelson EB, Tobin CE, et al. Breast imaging case of the day. Metastatic calcification in the breast from secondary hyperparathyroidism induced by chronic renal failure. *Radiographics* 1996;16:1512–1513.
181. Kemmeren JM, Beijerinck D, van Noord PA, et al. Breast arterial calcifications: association with diabetes mellitus and cardiovascular mortality. Work in progress. *Radiology* 1996;201:75–78.
182. Maas AHEM, van der Schouw YT, Beijernick D, et al. Arterial calcifications seen on mammograms: cardiovascular risk factors, pregnancy, and lactation. *Radiology* 2006;240:33–38.
183. Maas AHEM, van der Schouw YT, Mali WPThM, et al. Prevalence and determinants of breast arterial calcium in women at high risk of cardiovascular disease. *Am J Cardiol* 2004;94:655–659.
184. Kataoka M, Warren R, Luben R. How predictive is breast arterial calcification of cardiovascular disease and risk factors when found at screening mammography? *AJR Am J Roentgenol* 2006;187:73–80.
185. van Noord PA, Beijerinck D, Kemmeren JM, et al. Mammograms may convey more than breast cancer risk: breast arterial calcification and arteriosclerotic related diseases in women of the DOM cohort. *Eur J Cancer Prev* 1996;5:483–487.
186. Crystal P, Crystal E, Leon J, et al. Breast artery calcium on routine mammography as a potential marker for increased risk of CVD. *Am J Cardiol* 2000;86:216–217.
187. Ro JY, Ngadiman S, Sahin A, et al. Intraluminal crystalloids in breast carcinoma. Immunohistochemical, ultrastructural, and energy-dispersive x-ray element analysis in four cases. *Arch Pathol Lab Med* 1997;121:593–598.
188. Islam MT, Ou JJ, Hansen K, et al. Liesegang-like rings in lactational changes in the breast. *Case Report Pathol* 2012;2012:268903.
189. Elvecrog EL, Lechner MC, Nelson MT. Nonpalpable breast lesions: correlation of stereotaxic large-core needle biopsy and surgical biopsy results. *Radiology* 1993;188:453–455.
190. Liberman L, Dershaw DD, Rosen PP, et al. Stereotaxic 14-gauge breast biopsy: how many core biopsy specimens are needed? *Radiology* 1994;192:793–795.
191. Gisvold JJ, Goellner JR, Grant CS, et al. Breast biopsy: a comparative study of stereotaxically guided core and excisional techniques. *AJR Am J Roentgenol* 1994;162:815–820.
192. Liberman L, Dershaw DD, Rosen PP, et al. Stereotaxic core biopsy of breast carcinoma: accuracy at predicting invasion. *Radiology* 1995;194:379–381.
193. Liberman L. Impact of image-guided core biopsy on the clinical management of breast disease. In: Rosen PP, Hoda SA, eds. *Breast pathology: diagnosis by needle core biopsy*. 2nd ed. New York: Lippincott Williams & Wilkins, 2006:314–324.
194. Kaye MD, Vicinanza-Adami CA, Sullivan ML. Mammographic findings after stereotaxic biopsy of the breast performed with large-core needles. *Radiology* 1994;192:149–151.
195. Davies JD, Nonni A, Costa HFD. Mammary epidermoid inclusion cysts after wide-core needle biopsies. *Histopathology* 1997;31:549–551.
196. Diaz NM, Mayes JR, Vrcel V. Breast epithelial cells in dermal angiolymphatic spaces: a manifestation of benign mechanical transport. *Hum Pathol* 2005;36:310–313.
197. Stolier A, Skinner J, Levine EA. A prospective study of seeding of the skin after core biopsy of the breast. *Am J Surg* 2000;180:104–107.
198. Chao C, Torosian MH, Boraas MC, et al. Local recurrence of breast cancer in the stereotactic core needle biopsy site: case reports and review of the literature. *Breast J* 2001;7:124–127.
199. Nagi C, Bleiweiss I, Jaffer S. Epithelial displacement in breast lesions. A papillary phenomenon. *Arch Pathol Lab Med* 2005;129:1465–1469.
200. Douglas-Jones AG, Verghese A. Diagnostic difficulty arising from displaced epithelium after core biopsy in intracystic papillary lesions of the breast. *J Clin Pathol* 2002;55:780–783.
201. Gobbi H, Tse G, Page DL, et al. Reactive spindle cell nodules of the breast after core biopsy or fine-needle aspiration. *Am J Clin Pathol* 2000;113:288–294.
202. Boppana S, May M, Hoda, S. Does prior fine-needle-aspiration cause diagnostic difficulties in histologic evaluation of breast carcinomas? *Lab Invest* 1994;70:13A.
203. Youngson BJ, Cranor M, Rosen PP. Epithelial displacement in surgical breast specimens following needling procedures. *Am J Surg Path* 1994;18:896–903.
204. Youngson BJ, Liberman L, Rosen PP. Displacement of carcinomatous epithelium in surgical breast specimens following stereotaxic core biopsy. *Am J Clin Pathol* 1995;103:598–602.
205. Hoorntje LE, Schipper MEI, Kaya A, et al. Tumor cell displacement after 14G breast biopsy. *Eur J Surg Oncol* 2004;30:520–525.

206. Chen AM, Haffty BG, Lee CH. Local recurrence of breast cancer after breast conservation therapy in patients examined by means of stereotactic core needle biopsy. *Radiology* 2002;225:707–712.
207. Pilnik S, Steichen F. The use of the hemostatic scalpel in operations upon the breast. *Surg Gynecol Obstet* 1986;162:589–591.
208. Bloom ND, Johnson F, Pertshuck L, et al. Electrocautery: effects on steroid receptors in human breast cancer. *J Surg Oncol* 1984;25:21–24.
209. Pertshuck LP, Tobin EH, Tanapat P, et al. Histochemical analyses of steroid hormone receptors in breast and prostate carcinoma. *J Histochem Cytochem* 1980;28:799–810.
210. Rosenthal LJ. Discrepant estrogen receptor protein levels according to surgical technique. *Am J Surg* 1979;138:680–681.
211. Rosen PP. Electrocautery induced artifacts in breast biopsy specimens: an iatrogenic source of diagnostic difficulty (Letter to the editor). *Ann Surg* 1986;204:612–613.
212. Hung SH, Chu D, Chen FM, et al. Evaluation of the harmonic scalpel in breast conserving and axillary staging surgery. *J Chin Med Assoc* 2012;75:519–523.
213. Currie A, Chong K, Davies GL, et al. Ultrasonic dissection versus electrocautery in mastectomy for breast cancer—a meta-analysis. *Eur J Surg Oncol* 2012;38:897–901.
214. Zurrida S, Bassi F, Arnone P, et al. The changing face of mastectomy (from mutilation to aid to breast reconstruction). *Int J Surg Oncol* 2011;2011:980158.
215. Sikand K, Lee AHS, Pinder SE, et al. Sections of the nipple and quadrants in mastectomy specimens for carcinoma are of limited value. *J Clin Pathol* 2005;58:543–545.
216. The UK national coordinating committee for breast screening pathology. Pathology reporting of breast disease. Sheffield: National Health Service Breast Screening Programme and the Royal College of Pathologists, 2005.
217. D'Alonzo M, Martincich L, Biglia N, et al. Clinical and radiological predictors of nipple-areola complex involvement in breast cancer patients. *Eur J Cancer* 2012;48:2311–2318.
218. Kaplan RE, Swistel A, Hoda S. Occult involvement of nipple by malignancy occurs in 14% of therapeutic nipple-sparing mastectomies. *Breast J*. In press.
219. Jensen JA, Orringer JS, Giuliano AE. Nipple-sparing mastectomy in 99 patients with a mean follow-up of 5 years. *Ann Surg Oncol* 2011;18:1665–1670.
220. Edge SB, Byrd DR, Compton CC, et al. (eds). AJCC Cancer Staging Manual. 7th ed. New York: Springer, 2010.
221. Bombardieri E, Crippa F, Maffioli L, et al. Nuclear medicine approaches for detection of axillary lymph node metastases. *Q J Nucl Med* 1998;42:54–65.
222. Lam WWM, Yang WT, Chan YL, et al. Detection of axillary lymph node metastases in breast carcinoma by technetium-99m sestamibi breast scintigraphy, ultrasound and conventional mammography. *Eur J Nucl Med* 1996;23:498–503.
223. Tolmos J, Khalkhali I, Vargas H, et al. Detection of axillary lymph node metastasis of breast carcinoma with technetium-99m sestamibi scintimammography. *Am Surg* 1997;63:850–853.
224. Taillefer R, Robidoux A, Turpin S, et al. Metastatic axillary lymph node technetium-99m-MIBI imaging in primary breast cancer. *J Nucl Med* 1998;39:459–464.
225. Danielsson R, Bone B, Perbeck L, et al. Evaluation of planar scintimammography with 99mTc-MIBI in the detection of axillary lymph node metastases of breast carcinoma. *Acta Radiol* 1999;40:491–495.
226. Miyauchi M, Yamamoto N, Imanaka N, et al. Computed tomography for preoperative evaluation of axillary nodal status in breast cancer. *Breast Cancer* 1999;6:243–248.
227. Hata Y, Ogawa Y, Nishioka A, et al. Thin section computed tomography in the prone position for detection of axillary lymph node metastases in breast cancer. *Oncol Rep* 1998;5:1403–1406.
228. Harika L, Wessleder R, Poss K, et al. Macromolecular intravenous contrast agent for MR lymphography: characterization and efficacy studies. *Radiology* 1996;198:365–370.
229. Yoshimura G, Sakurai T, Oura S, et al. Evaluation of axillary lymph node status in breast cancer with MRI. *Breast Cancer* 1999;6:249–258.
230. Mussurakis S, Buckley DL, Horsman A. Prediction of axillary lymph node status in invasive breast cancer with dynamic contrast-enhanced MR imaging. *Radiology* 1997;203:317–321.
231. Avril N, Dose J, Jänicke F, et al. Assessment of axillary lymph node involvement in breast cancer patients with positron emission tomography using radiolabeled 2-(Fluorine-18)-fluoro-2-deoxy-D-glucose. *J Natl Cancer Inst* 1996;88:1204–1209.
232. Wahl RL, Siegel BA, Coleman E, et al. Prospective multicenter study of axillary nodal staging by positron emission tomography in breast cancer: a report of the Staging Breast Cancer with PET Study Group. *J Clin Oncol* 2004;22:277–285.
233. Alvarez S, Añorbe E, Alcorta P, et al. Role of sonography in the diagnosis of axillary lymph node metastases in breast cancer: a systemic review. *AJR Am J Roentgenol* 2006;196:1342–1348.
234. Britton PD, Goud A, Godward S, et al. Use of ultrasound-guided axillary node core biopsy in staging of early breast cancer. *Eur Radiol* 2009;19:561–569.
235. Chang MC, Crystal P, Colgan TJ. The evolving role of axillary lymph node fine-needle aspiration in the management of carcinoma of the breast. *Cancer Cytopathol* 2011;119:328–334.
236. Jing X, Wey E, Michael CW. Diagnostic value of fine needle aspirates processed by ThinPrep® for the assessment of axillary lymph node status in patients with invasive carcinoma of the breast. *Cytopathology*. 2012. doi:10.1111/cyt.12022.
237. Jegaraj A, Kadambari D, Srinivasan K, et al. Imprint cytology of axillary lymph nodes in breast carcinoma following neoadjuvant chemotherapy. *Acta Cytol* 2010;54:685–691.
238. Brunt LM, Jones DB, Wu JS, et al. Endoscopic axillary lymph node dissection: an experimental study in human cadavers. *J Am Coll Surg* 1998;187:158–163.
239. Lim SML, Lam FL. Laparoscopic-assisted axillary dissection in breast cancer surgery. *Am J Surg* 2005;190:641–643.
240. Langer I, Kocher T, Guller U, et al. Long-term outcomes of breast cancer after endoscopic axillary lymph node dissection: a prospective analysis of 52 patients. *Breast Cancer Res Treat* 2005;90:85–91.
241. Kuehn T, Santjohanser C, Grab D, et al. Endoscopic axillary surgery in breast cancer. *Br J Surg* 2001;88:698–703.
242. Silverstein MJ. Predicting axillary nodal positivity in 1787 patients with invasive breast carcinoma. *Breast J* 1998;4:324–329.
243. Barth A, Craig PH, Silverstein MJ. Predictors of axillary lymph node metastases in patients with T1 breast carcinoma. *Cancer* 1997;79:1918–1922.
244. Chadha M, Chabon AB, Friedmann P, et al. Predictors of axillary lymph node metastases in patients with T1 breast cancer. A multivariate analysis. *Cancer* 1994;73:350–353.
245. Mustafa IA, Cole B, Wanebo HJ, et al. The impact of histopathology on nodal metastases in minimal breast cancer. *Arch Surg* 1997;132:384–390.
246. Olivotto IA, Jackson JS, Mates D, et al. Prediction of axillary lymph node involvement of women with invasive breast carcinoma: a multivariate analysis. *Cancer* 1998;83:948–955.
247. Port ER, Tan LK, Borgen PI, et al. Incidence of axillary lymph node metastases in T1a and T1b breast carcinoma. *Ann Surg Oncol* 1998;5:23–27.
248. Shoup M, Malinzak L, Weisenberger J, et al. Predictors of axillary lymph node metastasis in T1 breast carcinoma. *Am Surg* 1999;65:748–752.
249. Morrow M. Management of the axillary nodes. *Breast Cancer* 1999;6:1–12.
250. Chontos AJ, Maher DP, Ratzer ER, et al. Axillary lymph node dissection: is it required in T1a breast cancer? *J Am Coll Surg* 1997;184:493–498.
251. Pandelidis SM, Peters KL, Walusimbi MS, et al. The role of axillary dissection in mammographically detected carcinoma. *J Am Coll Surg* 1997;184:341–345.
252. McGee JM, Youmans R, Clingan F, et al. The value of axillary dissection in T1a breast cancer. *Am J Surg* 1996;172:501–504.
253. Lloyd LR, Waits RK, Schroder D, et al. Axillary dissection for breast carcinoma. The myth of skip metastases. *Ann Surg* 1989;55:381–384.
254. Rosen PP, Lesser ML, Kinne DW, et al. Discontinuous or "skip" metastases in breast carcinoma: analysis of 1228 axillary dissections. *Ann Surg* 1983;197:276–283.
255. Veronesi U, Rilke F, Luini A, et al. Distribution of axillary node metastases by level of invasion. An analysis of 539 cases. *Cancer* 1987;59:682–687.
256. Zurrida S, Morabito A, Galimberti V, et al. Importance of the level of axillary involvement in relation to traditional variables in the prognosis of breast cancer. *Int J Oncol* 1999;15:475–480.
257. Anderson J, Jensen J. Lymph node identification: specimen radiography of tissue predominated by fat. *Am J Clin Pathol* 1977;68:511–572.
258. Groote AD, Oosterhuis JW, Molenaar WM, et al. Radiographic imaging of lymph nodes in lymph node dissection specimens. *Lab Invest* 1985;52:326–329.

259. Durkin K, Haagensen CD. An improved technique for the study of lymph nodes in surgical specimens. *Ann Surg* 1980;191:419–429.
260. Morrow M, Evans J, Rosen PP, et al. Does clearing of axillary lymph nodes contribute to accurate staging of breast carcinoma? *Cancer* 1984;53:1329–1332.
261. Hartveit F, Samonsen G, Tanqen M, et al. Routine histological investigation of the axillary lymph nodes in breast cancer. *Clin Oncol* 1982;8:121–126.
262. Schmidt WA. *Principles and techniques of surgical pathology*. Menlo Park: Addison-Wesley, 1983:362–388.
263. Silverberg SG, Masood S. The breast. In: *Principles and practice of surgical pathology and cytopathology*. New York: Churchill Livingston, 1997:579.
264. Rosai J. *Ackerman's Surgical Pathology*. St. Louis: Mosby, 1996:2682.
265. Niemann TH, Yilmaz AG, Marsh WLJ, et al. A half a node or a whole node: a comparison of methods for submitting lymph nodes. *Am J Clin Pathol* 1998;109:571–576.
266. Smith PA, Harlow SP, Krag DN, et al. Submission of lymph node tissue for ancillary studies decreases the accuracy of conventional breast cancer axillary node staging. *Mod Pathol* 1999;12:781–785.
267. Weir L, Speers C, D'yachkova Y, et al. Prognostic significance of the number of axillary lymph nodes removed in patients with node-negative breast cancer. *J Clin Oncol* 2002;20:1793–1799.
268. Bélanger J, Soucy G, Sidéris L, et al. Neoadjuvant chemotherapy in invasive breast cancer results in a lower axillary lymph node count. *J Am Coll Surg* 2008;206:704–708.
269. Salama JK, Heimann R, Lin F, et al. Does the number of lymph nodes examined in patients with lymph node-negative breast carcinoma have prognostic significance? *Cancer* 2005;103:664–671.
270. Woodward WA, Vinh-Hung V, Ueno NT, et al. Prognostic value of nodal ratio in node-positive breast cancer. *J Clin Oncol* 2006;24:2910–2916.
271. Schrenk P, Rieger R, Shamiyeh A, et al. Morbidity following sentinel lymph node biopsy versus axillary lymph node dissection for patients with breast carcinoma. *Cancer* 2000;88:608–614.
272. Morrow M, Foster RS Jr. Staging of breast cancer: a new rationale for internal mammary node biopsy. *Arch Surg* 1981;116:748–751.
273. Harlow S, Krag D, Weaver D, et al. Extra-axillary sentinel lymph nodes in breast cancer. *Breast Cancer* 1999;6:159–165.
274. van Rijk MC, Tanis PJ, Nieweg OE, et al. Clinical implications of sentinel nodes outside the axilla and internal mammary chain in patients with breast cancer. *J Surg Oncol* 2006;94:281–286.
275. Hill AD, Tran KN, Akhurst T, et al. Lessons learned from 500 cases of lymphatic mapping for breast cancer. *Ann Surg* 1999;229:528–535.
276. Dupont EL, Salud CJ, Peltz ES, et al. Clinical relevance of internal mammary node mapping as a guide to radiation therapy. *Am J Surg* 2001;182:321–324.
277. Cody HL. Sentinel lymph node mapping in breast cancer. *Breast Cancer* 1999;6:13–22.
278. Veronesi U. The sentinel node and breast cancer. *Br J Surg* 1999;86:1–2.
279. Teal CB, Slocum JP, Akin EA, et al. Correlation of lymphoscintigraphy with the number of sentinel lymph nodes identified interoperatively in patients with breast cancer. *Am J Surg* 2005;190:567–569.
280. Cody HS III. Clinical aspects of sentinel node biopsy. *Breast Cancer Res* 2001;3:104–106.
281. Ozmen V, Cabioglu N. Sentinel lymph node biopsy for breast cancer: current controversies. *Breast J* 2006;12(Suppl. 2):S134–S142.
282. Miltenburg DM, Miller C, Karamlou TB, et al. Meta-analysis of sentinel lymph node biopsy in breast cancer. *J Surg Res* 1999;84:138–142.
283. Haigh PL, Hsueh EC, Giuliano AE. Sentinel lymphadenectomy in breast cancer. *Breast Cancer* 1999;6:139–144.
284. McMasters KM, Giuliano AE, Ross MI, et al. Sentinel-lymph-node biopsy for breast cancer—not yet the standard of care. *N Engl J Med* 1998;339:990–995.
285. Cox CE, Haddad F, Bass S, et al. Lymphatic mapping in the treatment of breast cancer. *Oncology* 1998;12:1283–1292.
286. Dauway EL, Giuliano R, Pendas S, et al. Lymphatic mapping: a technique providing accurate staging for breast cancer. *Breast Cancer* 1999;6:145–154.
287. Guenther JM, Krishnamoorthy M, Tan LR. Sentinel lymphadenectomy for breast cancer in a community managed care setting. *Cancer J Sci Am* 1997;3:336–340.
288. Kim T, Giulliano AE, Lyman GH. Lymphatic mapping and sentinel lymph node biopsy in early-stage breast carcinoma. *Cancer* 2006;106:4–16.
289. Veronesi U, Paganelli G, Galimberti V, et al. Sentinel-node biopsy to avoid axillary dissection in breast cancer with clinically negative lymph-nodes. *Lancet* 1997;349:1864–1867.
290. Sandrucci S, Mussa A. Sentinel lymph node biopsy and axillary staging of T1-T2 N0 breast cancer: a multicenter study. *Semin Surg Oncol* 1998;15:278–283.
291. Borgstein PJ, Meijer S, Pijpers R. Intradermal blue dye to identify sentinel lymph-node in breast cancer. *Lancet* 1997;349:1668–1669.
292. Rodier J-F, Velten M, Wilt M, et al. Prospective multicentric randomized study comparing periareolar and peritumoral injection of radiotracer and blue dye for the detection of sentinel lymph node in breast sparing procedures: FRANSENODE trial. *J Clin Oncol* 2007;25:3664–3669.
293. Reynolds C, Mick R, Donohue JH, et al. Sentinel lymph node biopsy with metastasis: can axillary dissection be avoided in some patients with breast cancer? *J Clin Oncol* 1999;17:1720–1726.
294. Bass SS, Lyman GH, McCann CR, et al. Lymphatic mapping and sentinel lymph node biopsy. *Breast J* 1999;5:288–295.
295. Haigh PI, Hansen NM, Qi K, et al. Biopsy method and excision volume do not affect success rate of subsequent sentinel lymph node dissection in breast cancer. *Ann Surg Oncol* 2000;7:21–27.
296. Liberman L, Cody HS, Hill AD, et al. Sentinel lymph node biopsy after percutaneous diagnosis of nonpalpable breast cancer. *Radiology* 1999;211:835–844.
297. Langer I, Marti WR, Guller U, et al. Axillary recurrence rate in breast cancer patients with negative sentinel lymph node (SLN) or SLN micrometastases. Prospective analysis of 150 patients after SLN biopsy. *Ann Surg* 2005;241:152–158.
298. Chung MA, Steinhoff MM, Cady B. Clinical axillary recurrence in breast cancer patients after a negative sentinel node biopsy. *Am J Surg* 2002;184:310–314.
299. Swenson KK, Mahipal A, Nissen MJ, et al. Axillary disease recurrence after sentinel lymph node dissection for breast carcinoma. *Cancer* 2005;104:1834–1839.
300. Hansen NM, Ye X, Grube BJ, et al. Manipulation of the primary breast tumor and the incidence of sentinel node metastases from invasive breast cancer. *Arch Surg* 2004;139:634–640.
301. Peters-Engl C, Konstantiniuk P, Tausch C, et al. The impact of preoperative breast biopsy on the risk of sentinel lymph node metastases: analysis of 2502 cases from the Austrian sentinel node biopsy study group. *Br J Cancer* 2004;91:1782–1786.
302. Chagpar AB, Scoggins CR, Sahoo S, et al. Biopsy type does not influence sentinel lymph node status. *Am J Surg* 2005;190:551–556.
303. Newman EL, Kahn A, Diehl KM, et al. Does the method of biopsy affect the incidence of sentinel lymph node metastases? *Breast J* 2006;12:53–57.
304. Moore KH, Thaler HT, Tan LK, et al. Immunohistochemically detected tumor cells in the sentinel lymph nodes of patients with breast carcinoma: biologic metastasis or procedural artifact? *Cancer* 2004;100:929–934.
305. Diaz NM, Cox CE, Ebert M, et al. Benign mechanical transport of breast epithelial cells to sentinel lymph nodes. *Am J Surg Pathol* 2004;28:1641–1645.
306. Carter BA, Jensen RA, Simpson JF, et al. Benign transport of breast epithelium into axillary lymph nodes after biopsy. *Am J Clin Pathol* 2000;113:259–265.
307. Bleiweiss IJ, Nagi CS, Jaffer S. Axillary sentinel lymph nodes can be falsely positive due to iatrogenic displacement and transport of benign epithelial cells in patients with breast carcinoma. *J Clin Oncol* 2006;24:213–218.
308. Carter BA, Page DL. Sentinel lymph node histopathology in breast cancer: minimal disease versus artifact. *J Clin Oncol* 2006;24:1978–1979.
309. Pendas S, Dauway E, Giuliano R, et al. Sentinel node biopsy in ductal carcinoma in situ patients. *Ann Surg Oncol* 2000;7:15–20.
310. Ansari B, Ogston SA, Purdie CA, et al. Meta-analysis of sentinel node biopsy in ductal carcinoma *in situ* of the breast. *Br J Surg* 2008;95:547–554.
311. Zavotsky J, Hansen N, Brennan MB, et al. Lymph node metastasis from ductal carcinoma *in situ* with microinvasion. *Cancer* 1999;85:2439–2443.
312. Ross DS, Hoda SA. Microinvasive (T1mic) lobular carcinoma of the breast: clinicopathologic profile of 16 cases. *Am J Surg Pathol* 2011;35:750–756.

313. Lyons JM III, Stempel M, Van Zee KJ, et al. Axillary node staging for microinvasive breast cancer: is it justified? *Ann Surg Oncol* 2012;19:3416–3421.
314. Kaptain S, Montgomery LL, Son T, et al. Sentinel lymph node (SLN) metastases in multifocal invasive breast carcinoma (MIBC). *Mod Pathol* 2000;13:24A.
315. Veronesi U, Paganelli G, Viale G, et al. Sentinel lymph node biopsy and axillary dissection in breast cancer: results in a large series. *J Natl Cancer Inst* 1999;91:368–373.
316. Tousimis E, Van Zee KJ, Fey JV, et al. The accuracy of sentinel lymph node biopsy in multicentric and multifocal invasive breast cancers. *J Am Coll Surg* 2003;197:529–535.
317. Knauer M, Konstantiniuk P, Haid A, et al. Multicentric breast cancer: a new indication for sentinel node biopsy—a multi-institutional validation study. *J Clin Oncol* 2006;24:3374–3380.
318. Schrenk P, Wayand W. Sentinel-node biopsy in axillary lymph node staging for patients with multicentric breast cancer. *Lancet* 2001;357:122.
319. Cox CE, White L, Stowell N, et al. Clinical considerations in breast cancer sentinel lymph node mapping: a Moffitt review. *Breast Cancer* 2004;11:225–232.
320. Spillane AJ, Brennan ME. Accuracy of sentinel lymph node biopsy in large and multifocal/multicentric breast carcinoma—a systematic review. *Eur J Surg Oncol* 2011;37:371–385.
321. Gimbergues P, Abrial C, Durando X, et al. Sentinel lymph node biopsy after neoadjuvant chemotherapy is accurate in breast cancer patients with a clinically negative axillary nodal status at presentation. *Ann Surg Oncol* 2008;15:1316–1321.
322. Schwartz GF, Tannebaum JE, Jernigan AM, et al. Axillary sentinel lymph node biopsy after neoadjuvant chemotherapy for carcinoma of the breast. *Cancer* 2010;116:1243–1251.
323. Canavese G, Dozin B, Vecchio C, et al. Accuracy of sentinel lymph node biopsy after neo-adjuvant chemotherapy in patients with locally advanced breast cancer and clinically positive axillary nodes. *Eur J Surg Oncol* 2011;37:688–694.
324. Schrenk P, Hochreiner G, Fridrik M, et al. Sentinel node biopsy performed before preoperative chemotherapy for axillary lymph node staging in breast cancer. *Breast J* 2003;9:282–287.
325. Jones JL, Zabicki K, Christian RL, et al. A comparison of sentinel node biopsy before and after neoadjuvant chemotherapy: timing is important. *Am J Surg* 2005;190:517–520.
326. Haid A, Tausch C, Lang A, et al. Is sentinel lymph node biopsy reliable and indicated after preoperative chemotherapy in patients with breast carcinoma? *Cancer* 2001;92:1060–1064.
327. Julian TB, Patel N, Dusi D, et al. Sentinel lymph node biopsy after neoadjuvant chemotherapy for breast cancer. *Am J Surg* 2001;182:407–410.
328. Tafra L, Verbanac KM, Lannin DR. Preoperative chemotherapy and sentinel lymphadenectomy for breast cancer. *Am J Surg* 2001;182:312–315.
329. Schwartz GF, Meltzer AJ. Accuracy of axillary sentinel lymph node biopsy following neoadjuvant (induction) chemotherapy for carcinoma of the breast. *Breast J* 2003;9:374–379.
330. Kang SH, Kang JH, Choi EA, et al. Sentinel lymph node biopsy after neoadjuvant chemotherapy. *Breast Cancer* 2004;11:233–241.
331. Kinoshita T, Takasugi M, Iwamoto E, et al. Sentinel lymph node biopsy examination for breast cancer patients with clinically negative axillary lymph nodes after neoadjuvant chemotherapy. *Am J Surg* 2006;191:225–229.
332. Mamounas EP, Brown A, Anderson S, et al. Sentinel node biopsy after neoadjuvant chemotherapy in breast cancer: results from National Surgical Adjuvant Breast and Bowel Project Protocol B-27. *J Clin Oncol* 2005;23:2694–2702.
333. Jeruss JS, Ayers GD, Cristofanilli AM, et al. Positive sentinel nodes after neoadjuvant chemotherapy: what factors predict additional disease in the axilla? *J Clin Oncol* 2006;24:28S.
334. Agarwal A, Heron DE, Sumkin J, et al. Contralateral uptake and metastases in sentinel lymph node mapping for recurrent breast cancer. *J Surg Oncol* 2005;92:4–8.
335. Lim I, Shim J, Goyenechea M, et al. Drainage across midline to sentinel nodes in the contralateral axilla in breast cancer. *Clin Nucl Med* 2004;329:346–347.
336. Allweis TM, Parson B, Klein M, et al. Breast cancer draining to bilateral axillary sentinel lymph nodes. *Surgery* 2003;134:506–508.
337. Jansen L, Neiweg OR, Valdes-Olmos RA, et al. Improved staging of breast cancer through lymphatic mapping and sentinel node biopsy. *Eur J Surg Oncol* 1998:28;445–446.
338. Perre CI, Hoefnagel CA, Kroon BBR, et al. Altered lymphatic drainage after lymphadenectomy or radiotherapy of the axilla in patients with breast cancer. *Br J Surg* 1996;83:1258.
339. Port ER, Fey J, Gemignani ML, et al. Reoperative sentinel lymph node biopsy: a new option for patients with primary or locally recurrent breast carcinoma. *J Am Coll Surg* 2002;195:167–172.
340. Dinan D, Nagle CE, Pettinga J. Lymphatic mapping and sentinel node biopsy in women with an ipsilateral second breast carcinoma and a history of breast and axillary surgery. *Am J Surg* 2005;190:614–617.
341. Dupont EL Kuhnam, McCann C, et al. The role of sentinel lymph node biopsy in women undergoing prophylactic mastectomy. *Am J Surg* 2000;180:274–277.
342. Boughey JC, Khakpour N, Meric-Bernstam F, et al. Selective use of sentinel lymph node surgery during prophylactic mastectomy. *Cancer* 2006;107:1440–1447.
343. King TA, Ganaraj A, Fey JV, et al. Cytokeratin-positive cells in sentinel lymph nodes in breast cancer are not random events. Experience in patients undergoing prophylactic mastectomy. *Cancer* 2004;101:926–933.
344. Nasser SM, Smith SG, Chagpar AB. The role of sentinel node biopsy in women undergoing prophylactic mastectomy. *J Surg Res* 2010;164:188–192.
345. Glass EC, Essner R, Giuliano AE. Sentinel node localization in breast cancer. *Semin Nucl Med* 1999;29:57–68.
346. Miner T, Shriver C, Flicek P, et al. Guidelines for the safe use of radioactive materials during localization and resection of the sentinel lymph node. *Ann of Surg Oncol* 1999;6:75–82.
347. Gentilini O, Cremonesi M, Toesca A, et al. Sentinel lymph node biopsy in pregnant patients with breast cancer. *Eur J Nucl Med Mol Imaging* 2010;37:78–83.
348. Ku NK, Ahmad N, Smith PV, et al. Intraoperative imprint cytology of sentinel lymph nodes in breast cancer. *Acta Cytol* 1997;41:1606–1607.
349. Rubio IT, Korourian S, Cowan C, et al. Use of touch preps for intraoperative diagnosis of sentinel lymph node metastases in breast cancer. *Ann Surg Oncol* 1998;5:689–694.
350. Ratanawichitrasin A, Biscotti CV, Levy L, et al. Touch imprint cytological analysis of sentinel lymph nodes for detecting axillary metastases in patients with breast cancer. *Br J Surg* 1999;86:1346–1348.
351. Litz C, Miller R, Ewing G, et al. Intraoperative sentinel lymph node touch imprints are not sensitive in detecting metastatic carcinoma. *Mod Pathol* 2000;13:26A.
352. Moes GS, Guibord RS, Weaver DL, et al. Intraoperative cytologic evaluation of sentinel lymph nodes in breast cancer patients. *Mod Pathol* 2000;13:28A.
353. Jeruss JS, Hunt KK, Xing Y, et al. Is intraoperative touch imprint cytology of sentinel lymph nodes in patients with breast cancer cost effective? *Cancer* 2006;107:2328 2336.
354. Turner RR, Giuliano AE. Intraoperative pathologic examination of the sentinel lymph node. *Ann Surg Oncol* 1998;5:670–672.
355. Flett MM, Going JJ, Stanton PD, et al. Sentinel node localization in patients with breast cancer. *Br J Surg* 1998;85:991–993.
356. van Diest PJ, Torrenga H, Borgstein PJ, et al. Reliability of intraoperative frozen section and imprint cytological investigation of sentinel lymph nodes in breast cancer. *Histopathology* 1999;35:14–18.
357. Turner RR, Ollila DW, Krasne DL, et al. Histopathologic validation of the sentinel lymph node hypothesis for breast carcinoma. *Ann Surg* 1997;226:271–276.
358. Cserni G. Metastases in axillary sentinel lymph nodes in breast cancer as detected by intensive histopathological work up. *J Clin Pathol* 1999;52:922–924.
359. Turner RR, Ollila DW, Stern S, et al. Optimal histopathologic examination of the sentinel lymph node for breast carcinoma staging. *Am J Surg Pathol* 1999;23:263–267.
360. Dowlatshahi K, Fan M, Bloom KJ, et al. Occult metastases in the sentinel lymph nodes of patients with early stage breast carcinoma: a preliminary study. *Cancer* 1999;86:990–996.
361. Czerniecki BJ, Scheff AM, Callans LS, et al. Immunohistochemistry with pancytokeratins improves the sensitivity of sentinel lymph node biopsy in patients with breast carcinoma. *Cancer* 1999;85:1098–1103.
362. Zhang PJ, Reisner RM, Nangia R, et al. Effectiveness of multiple-level sectioning in detecting axillary nodal micrometastasis in breast cancer:

a retrospective study with immunohistochemical analysis. *Arch Pathol Lab Med* 1998;122:687–690.
363. CserniG, Amendoeira I, Apostolikas N, et al. Discrepancies in current practice of pathological evaluation of sentinel lymph nodes in breast cancer. results of a questionnaire-based survey by the European Working Group for Breast Screening Pathology. *J Clin Pathol* 2004;57:695–701.
364. Chagpar A, Middleton LP, Sahin AA, et al. Clinical outcome of patients with lymph node-negative breast carcinoma who have sentinel lymph node micrometastases detected by immunohistochemistry. *Cancer* 2005;103:1581–156.
365. Fitzgibbons PL, Page DL, Weaver D, et al. Prognostic factors in breast cancer. College of American Pathologists consensus statement 1999. *Arch Pathol Lab Med* 2000;124:966–978.
366. Lyman GH, Giuliano AE, Somerfield MR, et al. American Society of Clinical Oncology guideline recommendations for sentinel lymph node biopsy in early-stage breast cancer. *J Clin Oncol* 2006;22:7703–7720.
367. Schwartz GF, Giulliano AE, Veronesi U; the Consensus Conference Committee. Proceedings of the Consensus Conference on the Role of Sentinel Lymph Node Biopsy in Carcinoma of the Breast, April 19 to 22, 2001, Philadelphia, Pennsylvania. *Hum Pathol* 2002;33:579–585.
368. Silverberg SG. Sentinel node processing. Recommendations for pathologists. *Am J Surg Pathol* 2002;26:383–385.
369. Klevesath MB, Bobrow LG, Pinder SE, et al. The value of immunohistochemistry in sentinel lymph node histopathology in breast cancer. *Br J Cancer* 2005;92:2201–2205.
370. Kollias J, Gil PG, Chatterton B, et al. Sentinel node biopsy in breast cancer: recommendations for surgeons, pathologists, nuclear physicians and radiologists in Australia and New Zealand. *Aust N Z J Surg* 2000;70:132–136.
371. Cserni G. Surgical pathological staging of breast cancer by sentinel lymph node biopsy with special emphasis on the histological work-up of axillary sentinel lymph nodes. *Breast Cancer* 2004;11:242–249.
372. Treseler P. Pathologic examination of the sentinel lymph node: what is the best method? *Breast J* 2006;12(Suppl.):S143–S151.
373. Cserni G. Histopathologic examination of the sentinel lymph nodes. *Breast J* 2006;12(Suppl.):S152–S156.
374. de Mascarel I, Soubeyran I, Macgrogan G. Immunohistochemically detected lymph node metastases from breast carcinoma. Practical considerations about the New American Joint Committee on Cancer Classification. *Cancer* 2005;103:1319–1322.
375. Fortunato L, Amini M, Costarelli L, et al. A standardized lymph node enhanced pathology protocol (SEPP) in patients with breast cancer. *J Surg Oncol* 2007;96:470–473.
376. Weaver DL. Pathology evaluation of sentinel lymph nodes in breast cancer: protocol recommendations and rationale. *Mod Pathol* 2010;23(Suppl. 2):S26–S32.
377. Weaver DL. Pathological evaluation of sentinel lymph nodes in breast cancer: a practical academic perspective from America. *Histopathology* 2005;46:697–706.
378. Turner RR, Hansen NM, Stern SL, et al. Intraoperative examination of the sentinel lymph node for breast carcinoma staging. *Am J Clin Pathol* 1999;112:627–634.
379. van Rijk MC, Peterse JL, Nieweg OE, et al. Additional axillary metastases and stage migration in breast cancer patients with micrometastases or submicrometastases in sentinel lymph nodes. *Cancer* 2006;107:467–471.
380. Jakub JW, Diaz NM, Ebert MD, et al. Completion axillary lymph node dissection minimizes the likelihood of false negatives for patients with invasive breast carcinoma and cytokeratin positive only sentinel lymph nodes. *Am J Surg* 2002;184:302–306.
381. Calhoun KE, Hansen NM, Turner RR, et al. Nonsentinel node metastases in breast cancer patients with isolated tumor cells in the sentinel node: implications for completion axillary node dissection. *Am J Surg* 2005;190:588–591.
382. Rutledge H, Davis J, Chiu R, et al. Sentinel node micrometastasis in breast carcinoma may not be an indication for complete axillary dissection. *Mod Pathol* 2005;18:762–768.
383. Viale G, Renne G, Pruneri G, et al. The axillary lymph node status in breast carcinoma patients with micrometastatic sentinel nodes. *Mod Pathol* 2000;13:49A.
384. Chu KU, Turner RR, Hansen NM, et al. Sentinel node metastasis in patients with breast carcinoma accurately predicts immunohistochemically detectable nonsentinel node metastasis. *Ann Surg Oncol* 1999;6:756–761.
385. Viale G, Maiorano E, Pruneri G, et al. Predicting the risk of additional axillary metastases in patients with breast carcinoma and positive sentinel lymph node biopsy. *Ann Surg* 2005;241:319–325.
386. Abdessalam SF, Zervos EE, Prasad M, et al. Predictors of positive axillary lymph nodes after sentinel lymph node biopsy in breast cancer. *Am J Surg* 2001;182:316–320.
387. Changsri C, Prakash S, Sadweiss L, et al. Prediction of additional axillary metastasis of breast cancer following sentinel lymph node surgery. *Breast J* 2004;10:392–397.
388. van Zee JK, Mannasseh DM, Bevilacqua JL, et al. A nomogram for predicting the likelihood of additional nodal metastases in breast cancer patients with a positive sentinel node biopsy. *Ann Surg Oncol* 2003;10:1140–1151.
389. Degnim AC, Reynolds C, Pantvaidya G, et al. Nonsentinel node metastasis in breast cancer patients: assessment of an existing and a new predictive nomogram. *Am J Surg* 2005;190:543–550.
390. Chagpar AB, Scoggins CR, Martin RCG II, et al. Prediction of sentinel lymph node-only disease in women with invasive breast cancer. *Am J Surg* 2006;192:882–887.
391. Bevilaqua JLH, Kattan MW, Fey JV, et al. Doctor, what are my chances of having a positive sentinel node? A validated nomogram for risk estimation. *J Clin Oncol* 2007;25:3670–3679.
392. Sanjuán A, Escaramís G, Vidal-Sicart S, et al. Predicting non-sentinel lymph node status in breast cancer patients with sentinel lymph node involvement: evaluation of two scoring systems. *Breast J* 2010;16:134–140.
393. Fant JS, Grant MD, Knox SM, et al. Preliminary outcome analysis in patients with breast cancer and a positive lymph node who declined axillary dissection. *Ann Surg Oncol* 2003;10:126–130.
394. Jeruss JS, Sener SE, Brinkmann EM, et al. Axillary recurrence after sentinel node biopsy. *Ann Surg Oncol* 2005;12:34–40.
395. Hwang RF, Gonzalez-Angulo AM, Yi M, et al. Low locoregional failure rates in selected breast cancer patients with tumor-positive sentinel lymph nodes who do not undergo completion axillary dissection. *Cancer* 2007;110:723–730.
396. Moghaddam Y, Falzon M, Fulford L, et al. Comparison of three mathematical models for predicting the risk of additional axillary nodal metastases after positive sentinel lymph node biopsy in early breast cancer. *Br J Surg* 2010;97:1646–1652.
397. Gur AS, Unal B, Johnson R, et al. Predictive probability of four different breast cancer nomograms for nonsentinel axillary lymph node metastasis in positive sentinel node biopsy. *J Am Coll Surg* 2009;208: 229–235.
398. Hermanek P, Hutter RVP, Sobin LH, et al. Classification of isolated tumor cells and micrometastasis. *Cancer* 1999;86:2668–2673.
399. Greene FL, Page DL, Fleming ID, et al. , eds. *AJCC Cancer staging handbook—TNM Classification of malignant tumors*. 6th ed. New York: Springer Verlag, 2002:221–240.
400. Rivera M, Merlin S, Hoda RS, et al. Minimal involvement of sentinel lymph node in breast carcinoma: prevailing concepts and challenging problems. *Int J Surg Pathol* 2004;12:301–306.
401. Cserni G, Amendoeira I, Bianchi S, et al. Distinction of isolated tumour cells and micrometastasis in lymph nodes of breast cancer patients according to the new Tumour Node Metastasis (TNM) definitions. *Eur J Cancer* 2011;47:887–894.
402. van Deurzen CH, Cserni G, Bianchi S, et al. Nodal-stage classification in invasive lobular breast carcinoma: influence of different interpretations of the pTNM classification. *J Clin Oncol* 2010;28:999–1004.
403. Turner RR, Weaver DL, Cserni G, et al. Nodal stage classification for breast carcinoma: improving interobserver reproducibility through standardized histologic criteria and image-based training. *J Clin Oncol* 2008;26:258–263.
404. Di Tommaso L, Arizzi C, Rahal D, et al. Anatomic location of breast cancer micrometastasis in sentinel lymph node predicts axillary status. *Ann Surg* 2006;243:706–707.
405. Ribatti D, Finato N, Crivellato E, et al. Angiogenesis and mast cells in human breast cancer sentinel lymph nodes with and without micrometastases. *Histopathology* 2007;51:837–842.
406. Burchill SA, Bradbury MF, Pittman K, et al. Detection of epithelial cancer cells in peripheral blood by reverse transcriptase-polymerase chain reaction. *Br J Cancer* 1995;71:278–281.
407. Mori M, Mimori K, Inoue H, et al. Detection of cancer micrometastases in lymph nodes by reverse transcriptase-polymerase chain reaction. *Cancer* Res 1995;55:3417–3420.

408. Noguchi S, Aihara T, Nakamori S, et al. The detection of breast carcinoma micrometastases in axillary lymph nodes by means of reverse transcriptase-polymerase chain reaction. *Cancer* 1994;74:1595–1600.
409. Noguchi S, Aihara T, Motomura K, et al. Detection of breast cancer micrometastases in axillary lymph nodes by means of reverse transcriptase-polymerase chain reaction. Comparison between MUC1 mRNA and keratin 19 mRNA amplification. *Am J Pathol* 1996;148:649–656.
410. Noguchi S, Aihara T, Motomura K, et al. Histologic characteristics of breast cancers with occult lymph node metastases detected by keratin 19 mRNA reverse transcriptase-polymerase chain reaction. *Cancer* 1996;78:1235–1240.
411. Schoenfeld A, Luqmani Y, Sinnett HD, et al. Keratin 19 mRNA measurement to detect micrometastases in lymph nodes in breast cancer patients. *Br J Cancer* 1996;74:1639–1642.
412. Lockett MA, Baron PL, O'Brien PH, et al. Detection of occult breast cancer micrometastases in axillary lymph nodes using a multimarker reverse transcriptase-polymerase chain reaction panel. *J Am Coll Surg* 1998;187:9–16.
413. Bostick PJ, Chatterjee S, Chi DD, et al. Limitations of specific reverse-transcriptase polymerase chain reaction markers in the detection of metastases in the lymph nodes and blood of breast cancer patients. *J Clin Oncol* 1998;16:2632–2640.
414. Bostick PJ, Huynh KT, Sarantou T, et al. Detection of metastases in sentinel lymph nodes of breast cancer patients by multiple-marker RT-PCR. *Int J Cancer* 1998;79:645–651.
415. Nissan A, Jager D, Roystacher M, et al. Multimarker RT-PCR assay for the detection of minimal residual disease in sentinel lymph nodes of breast cancer patients. *Br J Cancer* 2006;94:681–685.
416. Hughes SJ, Xi L, Raja S, et al. A rapid, fully automated, molecular-based assay accurately analyzes sentinel lymph nodes for the presence of metastatic breast cancer. *Ann Surg* 2006;243:389–398.
417. Mansel RE, Goyal A, Douglas-Jones A, et al. Detection of breast cancer metastasis in sentinel lymph nodes using intra-operative real time GeneSearch BLN Assay in the operating room: results of the Cardiff study. *Breast Cancer Res Treat* 2009;115:595–600.
418. Le Frère-Belda MA, Bats AS, Gillaizeau F, et al. Diagnostic performance of one-step nucleic acid amplification for intraoperative sentinel node metastasis detection in breast cancer patients. *Int J Cancer* 2012;130:2377–2386.
419. Osako T, Iwase T, Kimura K, et al. Intraoperative molecular assay for sentinel lymph node metastases in early stage breast cancer: a comparative analysis between one-step nucleic acid amplification whole node assay and routine frozen section histology. *Cancer* 2011;117:4365–4374.
420. Feldman S, Krishnamurthy S, Gillanders W, et al. A novel automated assay for the rapid identification of metastatic breast carcinoma in sentinel lymph nodes. *Cancer* 2011;117:2599–2607.
421. Jatoi I, Hilsenbeck SG, Clark GM, et al. Significance of axillary lymph node metastasis in primary breast cancer. *J Clin Oncol* 1999;17:2334–2340.
422. Attiyeh FF, Jensen M, Huvos AG, et al. Axillary micrometastases and macrometastases in carcinoma of the breast. *Surg Gynecol Obstet* 1977;144:839–842.
423. Fisher ER, Palekar A, Rockette H, et al. Pathologic findings from the National Surgical Adjuvant Breast Project (Protocol No.4). V. Significance of axillary nodal micro- and macrometastases. *Cancer* 1978;42:2032–2038.
424. Huvos AG, Hutter RVP, et al. Significance of axillary macrometastases and micrometastases in mammary cancer. *Ann Surg* 1971;173:44–46.
425. Rosen PP, Saigo PE, Braun DW, et al. Axillary micro- and macrometastases in breast cancer. Prognostic significance of tumor size. *Ann Surg* 1981;194:585–591.
426. Friedman S, Bertin F, Mouriesse H, et al. Importance of tumor cells in axillary node sinus margins (‘clandestine’ metastases) discovered by serial sectioning in operable breast carcinoma. *Acta Oncol* 1988;27:483–487.
427. International (Ludwig) Breast Cancer Study Group. Prognostic importance of occult axillary lymph node micrometastases from breast cancers. *Lancet* 1990;1:1565–1568.
428. Saphir O, Amromin GD. Obscure axillary lymph-node metastasis in carcinoma of the breast. *Cancer* 1948;1:238–241.
429. Fisher ER, Swamidos S, Lee CH, et al. Detection and significance of occult axillary node metastases in patients with invasive breast cancer. *Cancer* 1978;45:2025–2031.
430. Pickren JW. Significance of occult metastases. A study of breast cancer. *Cancer* 1961;14:1266–1271.
431. Wilkinson EJ, Hause LL, Hoffman RG, et al. Occult axillary lymph node metastases in invasive breast carcinoma: characteristics of the primary tumor and significance of the metastases. *Pathol Annu* 1982;17(Pt. 2):67–91.
432. de Mascarel I, Bonichon F, Coindre JM, et al. Prognostic significance of breast cancer axillary lymph node micrometastases assessed by two special techniques: reevaluation with longer follow-up. *Br J Cancer* 1992;66:523–527.
433. Cote RJ, Peterson HF, Chaiwun B, et al. Role of immunohistochemical detection of lymph-node metastases in management of breast cancer. International Breast Cancer Study Group. *Lancet* 1999;354:896–900.
434. Bussolati G, Gugliotta P, Morra I, et al. The immunohistochemical detection of lymph node metastases from infiltrating lobular carcinoma of the breast. *Br J Cancer* 1986;54:631–636.
435. Trojani M, de Mascarel I, Bonichon F, et al. Micrometastases to axillary lymph nodes from carcinoma of breast: detection by immunohistochemistry and prognostic significance. *Br J Cancer* 1987;55:303–306.
436. Delsol G, Gatter KC, Stein H, et al. Human lymphoid cells express epithelial membrane antigen. Implications for diagnosis of human neoplasms. *Lancet* 1984;2:1124–1128.
437. McGuckin MA, Cummings MC, Walsh MD, et al. Occult axillary node metastases in breast cancer: their detection and prognostic significance. *Br J Cancer* 1996;73:88–95.
438. Dowlatshahi K, Fan M, Snider HC, et al. Lymph node micrometastases from breast carcinoma: reviewing the dilemma. *Cancer* 1997;80:1188–1197.
439. Siziopikou KP, Schnitt SJ, Connolly JL, et al. Detection and significance of occult axillary metastatic disease in breast cancer patients. *Breast J* 1999;5:221–229.
440. Steinhoff MM. Axillary node micrometastases detection and biologic significance. *Breast J* 1999;5:325–329.
441. Recht A. Should irradiation replace dissection for patients with breast cancer with clinically negative axillary lymph nodes? *J Surg Oncol* 1999;72:184–192.
442. Santin AD. Lymph node metastases: the importance of the microenvironment. *Cancer* 2000;88:175–179.
443. Scheunemann P, Izbicki JR, Pantel K. Tumorigenic potential of apparently tumor-free lymph nodes. *N Engl J Med* 1999;340:1687.
444. Carter BA, Jensen RA, Simpson JF, et al. Benign transport of breast epithelium into axillary lymph nodes post biopsy. *Am J Clin Pathol* 2000;113:259–265.
445. Giuliano AE, Hawes D, Ballman KV, et al. Association of occult metastases in sentinel lymph nodes and bone marrow with survival among women with early-stage invasive breast cancer. *JAMA* 2011;306:385–393.
446. Weaver DL, Ashikaga T, Krag DN, et al. Effect of occult metastases on survival in node-negative breast cancer. *N Engl J Med* 2011;364:412–421.
447. Pepels MJ, de Boer M, Bult P, et al. Regional recurrence in breast cancer patients with sentinel node micrometastases and isolated tumor cells. *Ann Surg* 2012;255:116–121.
448. de Boer M, van Dijck JA, Bult P, et al. Breast cancer prognosis and occult lymph node metastases, isolated tumor cells, and micrometastases. *J Natl Cancer Inst* 2010;102:410–425.
449. Singletary SE, Greene FL, Sobin LH. Classification of isolated tumor cells: clarification of the 6th edition of the American Joint Committee on Cancer Staging Manual. *Cancer* 2003;98:2740–2741.
450. Cserni G, Bianchi S, Boecker W, et al. Improving the reproducibility of diagnosing micrometastases and isolated tumor cells. *Cancer* 2005;103:358–367.
451. Cserni G, Bianchi S, Vezzosi V, et al. Variations in sentinel node isolated tumour cells/micrometastasis and non-sentinel node involvement rates according to different interpretations of the TNM definitions. *Eur J Cancer* 2008;44:2185–2191.
452. de Mascarel I, MacGrogan G, Debled M, et al. Distinction between isolated tumor cells and micrometastases in breast cancer: is it reliable and useful? *Cancer* 2008;112:1672–1678.
453. Galimberti V, Chifu C, Rodriguez Perez S, et al. Positive axillary sentinel lymph node: is axillary dissection always necessary? *Breast* 2011;20(Suppl. 3):S96–S98.
454. Bilimoria KY, Bentrem DJ, Hansen NM, et al. Comparison of sentinel lymph node biopsy alone and completion axillary lymph

node dissection for node-positive breast cancer. *J Clin Oncol* 2009;27:2946–2953.

455. Giuliano AE, Hunt KK, Ballman KV, et al. Axillary dissection vs no axillary dissection in women with invasive breast cancer and sentinel node metastasis: a randomized clinical trial. *JAMA* 2011;305:569–575.
456. Grube BJ, Giuliano AE. Observation of the breast cancer patient with a tumor-positive sentinel node: implications of the ACOSOG Z0011 trial. *Semin Surg Oncol* 2001;20:230–237.
457. Giuliano AE, McCall L, Beitsch P, et al. Locoregional recurrence after sentinel lymph node dissection with or without axillary dissection in patients with sentinel lymph node metastases: the American College of Surgeons Oncology Group Z0011 randomized trial. *Ann Surg* 2010;252:426–432.
458. Straver ME, Meijnen P, van Tienhoven G, et al. Sentinel node identification rate and nodal involvement in the EORTC 10981-22023 AMAROS trial. *Ann Surg Oncol* 2010;17:1854–1861.
459. Weber WP, Barry M, Stempel MM, et al. A 10-year trend analysis of sentinel lymph node frozen section and completion axillary dissection for breast cancer: are these procedures becoming obsolete? *Ann Surg Oncol* 2012;19:225–232.
460. Benson JR, Wishart GC. Is intra-operative nodal assessment essential in a modern breast practice? *Eur J Surg Oncol* 2010;36:1162–1164.
461. Veronesi U, Viale G, Paganelli G, et al. Sentinel lymph node biopsy in breast cancer: ten-year results of a randomized controlled study. *Ann Surg* 2010;251:595–600.
462. Olson JA Jr, McCall LM, Beitsch P, et al. Impact of immediate versus delayed axillary node dissection on surgical outcomes in breast cancer patients with positive sentinel nodes: results from American College of Surgeons Oncology Group Trials Z0010 and Z0011. *J Clin Oncol* 2008;26:3530–3535.
463. Caudle AS, Hunt KK, Tucker SL, et al. American College of Surgeons Oncology Group (ACOSOG) Z0011: impact on surgeon practice patterns. *Ann Surg Oncol* 2012;19:3144–3151.
464. Patani N, Mokbel K. The clinical significance of sentinel lymph node micrometastasis in breast cancer. *Breast Cancer Res Treat* 2009;114:393–402.
465. Patani N, Mokbel K. Clinical significance of sentinel lymph node isolated tumour cells in breast cancer. *Breast Cancer Res Treat* 2011;127:325–334.
466. Pazaiti A, Fentiman IS. Which patients need an axillary clearance after sentinel node biopsy? *Int J Breast Cancer* 2011;2011:195892.
467. Cody HS III, Houssami N. Axillary management in breast cancer: what's new for 2012? *Breast* 2012;21:411–415.
468. Altinyollar H, Berberoglu U, Gülben K, et al. The correlation of extranodal invasion with other prognostic parameters in lymph node positive breast cancer. *J Surg Oncol* 2007;95:567–571.
469. Hultborn KA, Tornberg B. Mammary cancer: the biologic character of mammary carcinoma studied in 517 cases by a new form of malignancy grading. *Acta Radiol* 1960;(Suppl. 196):1–146.
470. Pierce LJ, Oberman HA, Strawderman MH, et al. Microscopic extracapsular extension in the axilla: is this an indication for axillary radiotherapy? *Int J Radiat Oncol Biol Phys* 1995;33:253–259.
471. Fisher ER, Gregorio RM, Redmond C, et al. Pathologic findings from the National Surgical Adjuvant Breast Project (Protocol No. 4). III. The significance of extranodal extension of axillary metastases. *Am J Clin Pathol* 1976;65:439–449.
472. Cascinelli N, Greco M, Bufalino R, et al. Prognosis of breast cancer with axillary node metastases after surgical treatment only. *Eur J Cancer Clin Oncol* 1987;23:795–799.
473. Leonard C, Corkill M, Tompkin J, et al. Are axillary recurrence and overall survival affected by axillary extranodal tumor extension in breast cancer? Implications for radiation therapy. *J Clin Oncol* 1995;13:47–53.
474. Mignano JE, Zahurak ML, Chakravarthy A, et al. Significance of axillary lymph node extranodal soft tissue extension and indications for postmastectomy irradiation. *Cancer* 1999;86:1258–1262.
475. Palamba HW, Rombouts MC, Ruers TJ, et al. Extranodal extension of axillary metastasis of invasive breast carcinoma as a possible predictor for the total number of positive lymph nodes. *Eur J Surg Oncol* 2001;27:719–722.
476. Cappellari J, Islandar S, Woodruff R. Signet ring cells sinus histiocytosis. *Am J Clin Pathol* 1990;94:800–801.
477. Frost AR, Shek YH, Lack EE. "Signet ring" sinus histiocytosis mimicking metastatic adenocarcinoma: a report of two cases with immunohistochemical and ultrastructural study. *Mod Pathol* 1992;5:497–500.
478. Gould E, Perez J, Albores-Saavedra J, et al. Signet ring cell sinus histiocytosis. A previously unrecognized histologic condition mimicking metastatic adenocarcinoma in lymph nodes. *Am J Clin Pathol* 1989;92:509–512.
479. Ravel R. Histopathology of lymph nodes after lymphangiography. *Am J Clin Pathol* 1966;46:335–340.
480. Truong L, Cartwright J, Goodman D, et al. Silicone lymphadenopathy associated with augmentation mammoplasty. Morphologic features in nine cases. *Am J Surg Pathol* 1988;12:484–491.
481. Chears W, Smith A, Ruffin J. Diagnosis of Whipple's disease by peripheral lymph node biopsy: report of a case. *Am J Med* 1959;27: 351–353.
482. Livolsi VA, Brooks JJ, Soslow R, et al. Signet cell melanocytic lesions. *Mod Pathol* 1992;5:515–520.
483. Kim K, Dorfman RF, Rappaport H. Signet ring cell lymphoma: a rare morphologic and functional expression of nodular (follicular) lymphoma. *Am J Surg Pathol* 1978;2:119–132.
484. Dunphy CH. The role of wide-spectrum cytokeratin staining of bone marrow cores in patients with ductal carcinoma of the breast. *Mod Pathol* 1996;10:955–958.
485. Dearnaley DP, Sloane JP, Ormerod MG, et al. Increased detection of mammary carcinoma cells in marrow smears using antisera to epithelial membrane antigen. *Br J Cancer* 1981;44:85–90.
486. Mansi JL, Berger U, McDonnell T, et al. The fate of bone marrow micrometastases in patients with primary breast cancer. *J Clin Oncol* 1989;7:445–449.
487. Braun S, Kentenich C, Janni W, et al. Lack of effect of adjuvant chemotherapy on the elimination of single dormant tumor cells in bone marrow of high-risk breast cancer patients. *J Clin Oncol* 2000;18:80–86.
488. Braun S, Pantel K, Muller P, et al. Cytokeratin-positive cells in the bone marrow and survival of patients with stage I, II, or III breast cancer. *N Engl J Med* 2000;342:525–533.
489. Wiedswang G, Borgen E, Karesen R, et al. Detection of isolated tumor cells in bone marrow is an independent prognostic factor in breast cancer. *J Clin Oncol* 2003;21:3469–3478.
490. Janni W, Rack B, Schindlbeck C, et al. The persistence of isolated tumor cells in bone marrow from patients with breast carcinoma predicts an increased risk of recurrence. *Cancer* 2005;103:884–891.
491. Braun S, Vogl FD, Naume B, et al. A pooled analysis of bone marrow micrometastasis in breast cancer. *N Engl J Med* 2005;353:793–802.
492. Fehm T, Braun S, Muller V, et al. A concept for the standardized detection of disseminated tumor cells in bone marrow from patients with primary breast cancer and its clinical implementation. *Cancer* 2006;107;885–902.
493. Hall C, Krishnamurthy S, Lodhi A, et al. Disseminated tumor cells predict survival after neoadjuvant therapy in primary breast cancer. *Cancer* 2012;118:342–348.
494. Skliris GP, Hubé F, Gheorghiu I, et al. Expression of small breast epithelial mucin (SBEM) protein in tissue microarrays (TMAs) of primary invasive breast cancers. *Histopathology* 2008;52:355–369.
495. Valladares-Ayerbes M, Iglesias-Díaz P, Díaz-Prado S, et al. Diagnostic accuracy of small breast epithelial mucin mRNA as a marker for bone marrow micrometastasis in breast cancer: a pilot study. *J Cancer Res Clin Oncol* 2009;135:1185–1195.
496. Giuliano AE, Hawes D, Ballman KV, et al. Association of occult metastases in sentinel lymph nodes and bone marrow with survival among women with early-stage invasive breast cancer. *JAMA* 2011;306:385–393.
497. Schaub TA, Ahmad J, Rohrich RJ. Capsular contracture with breast implants in the cosmetic patient: saline versus silicone—a systematic review of the literature. *Plast Reconstr Surg* 2010;126:2140–2149.
498. Raso DS, Greene WB, Metcalf JS. Synovial metaplasia of a periprosthetic breast capsule. *Arch Pathol Lab Med* 1994;118:249–251.
499. Raso DS, Crymes LW, Metcalf JS. Histological assessment of fifty breast capsules from smooth and textured augmentation and reconstruction mammoplasty prostheses with emphasis on the role of synovial metaplasia. *Mod Pathol* 1994;7:310–316.
500. Mátrai Z, Tóth L, Gulyás G, et al. A desmoid tumor associated with a ruptured silicone breast implant. *Plast Reconstr Surg* 2011;127:1e–4e.
501. Henderson PW, Singh SP, Spector JA. Chest wall spindle cell fibromatosis after breast augmentation. *Plast Reconstr Surg* 2010;126: 94e–95e.

502. Kotton DN, Muse VV, Nishino M. Case records of the Massachusetts General Hospital. Case 2-2012. A 63-year-old woman with dyspnea and rapidly progressive respiratory failure. *N Engl J Med* 2012;366:259–269.
503. Eaves F III, Nahai F. Anaplastic large cell lymphoma and breast implants: FDA report. *Aesthet Surg J* 2011;31:467–468.
504. Nichter LS, Mueller MA, Burns RG, et al. First report of nodal marginal zone B-cell lymphoma associated with breast implants. *Plast Reconstr Surg* 2012;129:576e–578e.
505. Sahoo S, Rosen PP, Feddersen RM, et al. Anaplastic large cell lymphoma arising in a breast implant capsule. A case report and review of the literature. *Arch Pathol Lab Med* 2003;127:e115–e118.
506. Wu CL, Tiu CM, Chen JD, et al. Gauzoma of the breast. *Breast J* 2011;17:678–679.
507. Salemis NS, Gemenetzis G, Lagoudianakis E. Gossypiboma of the breast. *Am Surg* 2012;78:E125–E126.
508. O'Doherty AJ. Spontaneous fracture of the wire tip during breast localization. *Br J Radiol* 1991;64:1154–1156.
509. Homer MJ. Transection of localization hooked wire during breast biopsy. *AJR Am J Roentgenol* 1983;141:929–930.
510. Seifi A, Axelrod H, Nascimento T, et al. Migration of guidewire after surgical breast biopsy: an unusual case report. *Cardiovasc Intervent Radiol* 2009;32:1087–1090.
511. Barzilai M, Roisman I. Foreign bodies in the breast. *Breast Dis* 1995;8:179–183.
512. Hoda SA, Borgen P, Rosen PP. Unanticipated clinical presentation of unusual foreign body in the breast. *Breast Dis* 1994;7:227–230.
513. Holt RW, Potter JF. Retained Groshong catheter cuff presenting as a breast mass. *Breast Dis* 1993;6:153–155.
514. de Souza GA. Penrose drain as a foreign body in the breast. *Breast J* 1999;5:208–210.
515. Davis SP, Stomper PC, Weidner N, et al. Suture calcification mimicking recurrence in the irradiated breast: a potential pitfall in mammographic evaluation. *Radiology* 1989;172:247–248.
516. Brown RC, Zuehlke RL, Ehrhardt JC, et al. Tattoos simulating calcifications on xeroradiographs of the breast. *Radiology* 1981;138:583–584.
517. Thomas DR, Fisher MS, Caroline DF. Case report: soap—another artefact that can mimic intramammary calcifications. *Clin Radiol* 1995;50:64–66.
518. Wakabayashi M, Reid JD, Bhattacharjee M. Foreign body granuloma caused by prior gunshot wound mimicking malignant breast mass. *AJR Am J Roentgenol* 1999;173:321–322.
519. Kupic EA. Glass foreign body in the breast simulating a hyperdense nodule on mammography. *AJR Am J Roentgenol* 1992;159:1125.
520. Schwartz DL, So HB, Schneider KM, et al. Chronic insertion of foreign bodies into the mature breast. *J Pediatr Surg* 1977;12:743–744.
521. Sampson D. Unusual self-inflicted injury of the breast. *Postgrad Med* 1975;51:116–118.
522. Sunamak O, As A, Cetin A, et al. Long standing accidental foreign body (sewing-machine needle) in breast tissue. *Breast J* 2009;15:662–663.
523. Moon WK, Park JM, Im J-G, et al. Metallic punctate densities in the breast after Chinese herbal treatment: mammographic findings. *Radiology* 2000;21:890–894.
524. Sánchez-Ponte A, Martí E, Rubio J, et al. Illegal injection of industrial silicone oil for breast augmentation: risks, solutions and results. *Breast J* 2012;18:174–176.
525. Clark CJ, Whang S, Paige KT. Incidence of precancerous lesions in breast reduction tissue: a pathologic review of 562 consecutive patients. *Plast Reconstr Surg* 2009;124:1033–1039.
526. Freedman BC, Smith SM, Estabrook A, et al. Incidence of occult carcinoma and high-risk lesions in mammaplasty specimens. *Int J Breast Cancer* 2012;2012:145630.
527. Ambaye AB, MacLennan SE, Goodwin AJ, et al. Carcinoma and atypical hyperplasia in reduction mammaplasty: increased sampling leads to increased detection. A prospective study. *Plast Reconstr Surg* 2009;124:1386–1392.
528. Dotto J, Kluk M, Geramizadeh B, et al. Frequency of clinically occult intraepithelial and invasive neoplasia in reduction mammoplasty specimens: a study of 516 cases. *Int J Surg Pathol* 2008;16:25–30.
529. Guarda LA, Tran TA. The pathology of breast biopsy-site marking devices. *Am J Surg Pathol* 2005;29:814–819.
530. Trop I, David J, El Khoury M, et al. Microcalcifications around a collagen-based breast biopsy marker: complication of biopsy with a percutaneous marking system. *AJR Am J Roentgenol* 2011;197:W353–W357.
531. Thomassin-Naggara I, Lalonde L, et al. A plea for the biopsy marker: how, why and why not clipping after breast biopsy? *Breast Cancer Res Treat* 2012;132:881–893.

CHAPTER 45

Molecular Classification and Testing of Breast Carcinoma

YUN WU • AYSEGUL A. SAHIN

Carcinomas of the breast constitute a heterogeneous group of tumors with marked variation in regard to clinical presentation, biologic behavior, and response to therapy. For the past several decades, the classification and management of breast carcinoma were primarily based on clinicopathologic (morphology, size, grade, nodal status, etc.) characteristics. Even among phenotypically similar tumors, these characteristics could not always offer accurate prognostic and predictive information. Over the last few decades, the immunophenotypical (principally estrogen receptor [ER] and human epidermal growth factor 2 [HER2]) profile of a breast carcinoma assumed greater prognostic and predictive importance. Cumulative data indicated that ER(+) and ER(−) breast carcinomas were fundamentally different not only in clinically behavior but also in molecular profiles.[1,2] Likewise, HER2(+) and HER2(−) tumors exhibited mostly dissimilar clinical and molecular characteristics. However, over the years, it became increasingly evident that there was some degree of clinical, pathologic, and molecular heterogeneity within each of these groups of tumors; that is, breast carcinomas with similar ER and HER2 profiles could have differing clinical outcomes and exhibit dissimilar pathologic features as well as divergent molecular profiles. Thus, there was a need for more efficient and effective prognostic and predictive tools. In recent years, advances have been made to craft such tools using molecular pathology techniques. This chapter is intended to provide an overview of these advances—especially as applied to the classification and testing of breast carcinomas.

MOLECULAR CLASSIFICATIONS OF BREAST CARCINOMA

Intrinsic Molecular Classification

The pioneering molecular classification system for breast carcinoma was developed by Perou et al.[1] in 2000. This group performed cDNA microarray analysis on 65 samples from 42 patients. Therein, hierarchical data revealed distinctly variable gene expression patterns in different tumors, but similar patterns among paired samples of the same tumor. The "intrinsic" gene expression pattern was characteristic of an individual tumor—as opposed to those that varied as a function of tissue sampling. In this study, four molecular subtypes of breast carcinomas were identified: "luminal," "HER2-enriched", "basal-like", and "normal breast-like". The "*luminal* group" of carcinomas were largely hormone receptor (1) and express luminal epithelial genes—traits similar to those of normal luminal epithelial cells. The "HER2-enriched group" was mainly composed of breast carcinomas with amplification of the HER2 gene. The "basal-like group" was ER(−), and frequently corresponded to the triple negative breast carcinomas (TNBCs, i.e., ER(−), PR(−), and HER2(−)). This group of tumors was immunoreactive for cytokeratin (CK) 5/6 and CK17, similar to the reactivity pattern observed in myoepithelial cells of the normal breast epithelium (i.e., "basal" cells, hence the term applied to this group). The category of tumors called "normal breast-like" had a gene expression pattern similar to that observed in normal breast tissue. It subsequently became evident that the latter group most likely resulted from contamination of tissue samples with high levels of normal breast tissue, and may not exist at all.

A year later, Sorlie et al.[2] performed 85 cDNA microarray analyses on 78 breast carcinoma samples. The results thereof further refined the intrinsic molecular classifier and proposed the division of ER(+) luminal group of breast carcinomas into "luminal A" and "luminal B" subgroups. Although both groups expressed hormone receptors, the luminal B subgroup had a higher proliferation rate and lesser expression of ER-related genes relative to those observed in luminal A group of tumors. Some luminal B tumors overexpressed the HER2/*neu* gene. Luminal B tumors responded less to hormonal therapy, and more to chemotherapy, relative to luminal A tumors. In general, luminal B tumors had a poorer prognosis than did luminal A tumors. The "HER2-enriched" subtype was characterized by high expression of ERBB2 and genes in the ERBB2 amplicon at 17q22.24, including GRB7. Among HER2-overexpressed/amplified tumors, a significant proportion (50% or so) were ER(+), and ER(+)/HER2(+) tumors were classified as luminal B subgroup by both intrinsic classification systems. Additional studies also suggested that ER(+) and HER2(+) (luminal B) breast carcinomas had high levels of genes often expressed by normal luminal epithelial cells, whereas ER(−)/HER2(+) (HER2-enriched) carcinomas had high levels of genes expressed by progenitor and stem cell–like cells.[3,4] These studies suggested that ER(+)/HER2(+) (luminal B) and ER(−)/HER2(+) (HER2-enriched) breast carcinomas were biologically distinct. These two groups of tumors not only showed distinct patterns of responses to chemotherapy and HER2-targeted therapy but also displayed relatively distinctive time to and sites of relapse. ER(−)/HER2(+) tumors tended to recur in the first 5 years, and recurrence after 5 years was low. In contrast, ER(+)/HER2(+) tumors had lower recurrence rate during the first 5 years, but their tendency for recurrence persisted for 15 or more years. ER(−)/HER2(+) tumors recurred more often in visceral organs, whereas ER(+)/HER2(+) tumors recurred more often in bone. The latter pattern was also observed in ER(+) luminal-type tumors. In addition, ER(+)/HER2(+) tumors had a lower rate of pathologic complete response (pCR) after neoadjuvant chemotherapy with or without trastuzumab than did ER(−)/HER2(+) tumors, but ER(+)/HER2(+) tumors did not seem to have poorer prognosis, compared with ER(−) / HER2(+) tumors.[5,6] The clinical, pathologic, and molecular features of the basic molecular subtypes of breast carcinomas are summarized in Table 45.1.

Intrinsic Molecular Subtype 50-Gene Classifier (Prediction Analysis of Microarray)

Parker et al.[7] narrowed down the classifier gene list to 50 genes on the basis of gene expression microarray data for the intrinsic molecular classification for breast carcinomas. A quantitative reverse transcription–polymerase chain reaction (qRT-PCR) assay for these 50 genes was developed to assign intrinsic subtypes (luminal A, luminal B, HER2-enriched, basal-like, and normal breast-like) for formalin-fixed paraffin-embedded (FFPE) samples. The prognostic value of prediction analysis of microarray (i.e., PAM50, termed as such due to its reproducibility in subtype classification) was later validated on an additional 786 breast carcinomas and shown to be superior to that of routine clinicopathologic factors.[8] In the National Cancer Institute of Canada Clinical Trials Group MA.12 study, the PAM50 assay also showed predictive value for adjuvant tamoxifen treatment in addition to offering prognostic value.[9] The MA.12 study was a prospective, randomized trial of premenopausal women with stage I to III breast carcinomas post–adjuvant chemotherapy to evaluate the effect of tamoxifen versus placebo. Intrinsic subtypes assigned by PAM50 showed independent prognostic value in addition to standard clinicopathologic variables. In addition, patients with the luminal A subtype defined by PAM50 showed greater benefit from adjuvant tamoxifen.

Molecular Classification of TNBCs

In 2011, Lehmann et al.[10] reported their analyses of 587 TNBCs from 14 human breast carcinoma gene expression datasets (*n*: 2,353, TNBC: 386) as the discovery set, and seven different gene expression datasets (*n*: 894, TNBC: 201) as the validation set. The group identified six TNBC subtypes: basal-like 1 (BL1), basal-like 2 (BL2), immunomodulatory (IM), mesenchymal (M), mesenchymal stem-like (MSL), and luminal androgen receptor (LAR) subtypes (Fig. 45.1).

TABLE 45.1 Clinical, Pathologic, and Molecular Differences between Molecular Subtypes of Breast Carcinomas

	Luminal A	Luminal B	HER2-Enriched	Basal-like
Prognosis	Good	Intermediate	Poor	Poor
Distant relapse	Peak at 4 y, and risk of relapse prolongs over 10–15 y		Peak at 4–6 y, but risk persistent over 10–15 y	Peak at 2 y, then reduced to minimal in 10 y
Most common site of relapse	Bone	Bone	Visceral organ	Visceral organ
Response to hormonal therapy	Good	Poor with hormonal therapy only	No response	No response
Response to chemotherapy	Poor (pCR = 8%–10%)	Intermediate (pCR = 20%)	Good and better with trastuzumab (pCR = 30%–60%)	Good (pCR = 25%–30%)
Histologic grade	Low to intermediate	Intermediate	High	High
Ki67 proliferation rate	Low	Intermediate to high	High	High
Common genetic abnormality	PI3K mutation common, p53 mutation rare	p53 mutation more common	PI3K mutation (20%)	p53 mutation frequent PI3K mutation less common
Oncotype DX/ MammaPrint	Low risk	High risk	High risk	High risk

pCR=pathological Complete Response

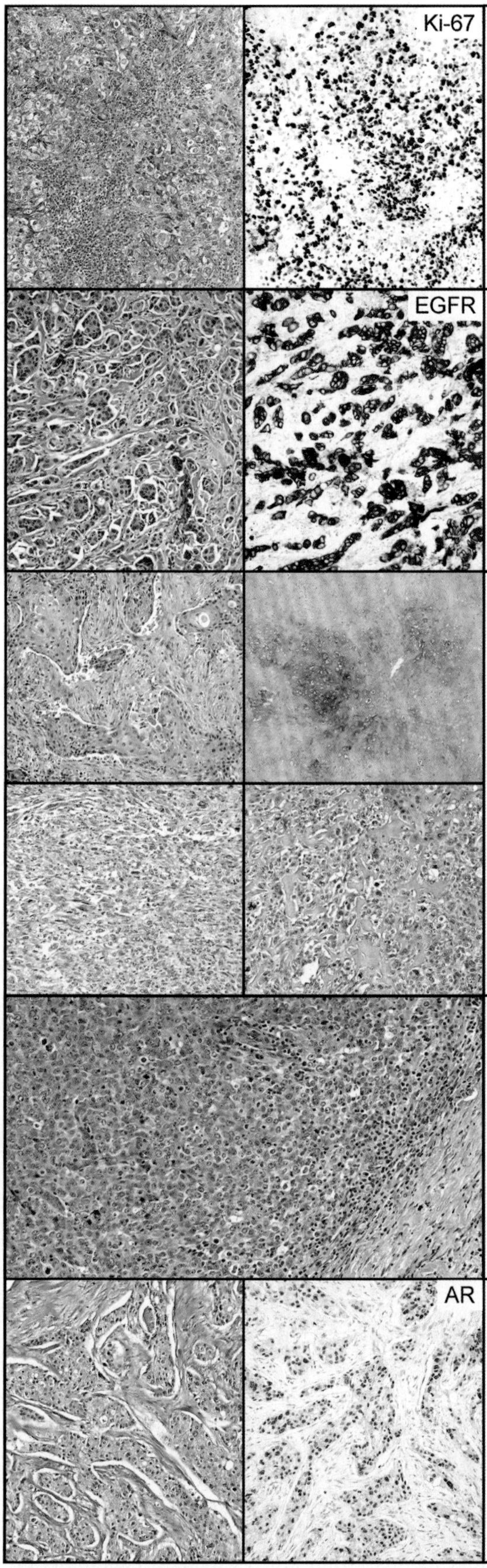

		Key Features	Aberrant Pathways	Potential Targeted Therapy
BL1	Ki-67	• High Ki-67 (average 70%) • High pCR rate	• Cell cycle • DNA replication	• Antimitotic agent: taxanes • DNA-PK inhibitors • TORC inhibitors
BL2	EGFR	• High Ki-67 (average 70%) • High pCR rate	• EGF/NGF/MET/ WNT/IGF1R	• Antimitotic agent: taxanes • Growth factor receptor inhibitors
M/MSL		• Metaplastic carcinoma • MSL, low level of proliferation, low expression of claudins and enrichment of stem cells	• ECM/EMT • Pathway involved in cell motility	• PI3K/mTOR inhibitors
IM		• Medullary carcinoma	• Immune signaling	• PAPP inhibitors
LAR	AR	• High AR and luminal cytokeratin expression	• AR pathway	• Androgen antigonists

FIG. 45.1. ***Molecular subtypes of triple negative breast carcinomas.*** Molecular abnormalities in each subtype can be potential targets for therapy. pCR=pathological Complete Response.

These subtypes were reported to display distinct gene expressions and had different clinical outcomes.

The "BL1" subtype showed enrichment of cell cycle–related gene expression, and the "BL2" subtype showed elevated expression of genes involved in growth factor signaling (including EGF, NGF, MET, and IGF1R). The BL2 subtype was suggestive of basal/myoepithelial differentiation, with high levels of p63 and CD10 expression. Both BL1 and BL2 had a high Ki67 proliferation rate and a higher pCR rate (63%) after neoadjuvant taxane treatment. "M" and "MSL" subtypes had enrichment expression of genes involved in cell motility and cell differentiation pathways. Metaplastic carcinomas (which included matrix-producing, sarcomatoid, and squamous cell carcinomas) shared molecular features with M and MSL subtypes. Compared with the M subtype, the MSL subtype showed lower levels of proliferation genes and shared molecular features of claudin-low subtype (see later).[10] The "IM" subtype had enrichment of genes involved in immune cell responses and showed substantial overlap with the gene signature for medullary breast carcinoma—a TNBC with a good prognosis.[11] The "LAR" subtype expressed luminal CK18 and had elevated expression of genes involved in hormonal pathways, including androgen receptor. The LAR subtype corresponded to the molecular apocrine subtype described previously by Farmer et al.[12] Lehmann et al.'s study indicated that each of the molecular subtypes in TNBC has distinct "druggable" targets for potential targeted therapy. This finding could change the current "one size fits all" chemotherapy regimen usually employed for TNBC to individually targeted therapy based on specific molecular subtypes. Their study also showed that TNBC does not consist only of basal-type breast carcinoma and that TNBC was a heterogeneous group, which included basal-like (47%), luminal A (17%), luminal B (6%), normal breast-like (12%), HER2 (6%), and unclassified (12%) carcinomas as categorized by the intrinsic classification.

Most of the initial molecular classifications were based on analyses of relatively small cohorts of retrospectively collected breast carcinomas, and did not include low-incidence subtypes. Claudin-low tumor, a recently identified molecular subtype, is characterized by low gene expression of tight-junction proteins claudins 3, 4, and 7 and E-cadherin. Claudin-low tumors have been shown to express low to absent luminal epithelial markers and high epithelial–mesenchymal transition (EMT) markers.[3] Tumor-initiating cells/stem-like cells (CD44(+)/CD24(-/low)) sorted from primary breast carcinomas show exclusive features of claudin-low molecular subtype and are resistant to chemotherapy.[13] The MSL subtype identified from TNBC by Lehmann et al.[10] shared features similar to those of the claudin-low molecular subtype.

Other Molecular Classifiers

Curtis et al.,[14] using integrated copy number alteration (CNA) and gene expression, analyzed over 2,000 breast carcinoma samples and found 10 integrative subgroups with distinct clinical outcomes. The group also identified additional heterogeneity within the intrinsic subtypes defined by gene expression alone. The integrative classification also identified the putative molecular drivers in each subgroup, for example, loss of expression of the *PPP2R2A* gene, a B-regulatory subunit of the PP2A mitotic exit holoenzyme complex located on chromosomal 8p21 that is highly associated with luminal B breast carcinomas.

With technologic advancement and bioinformatic integration, one can expect the development of additional molecular classifiers. However, owing to technologic complexity and cost considerations, immunohistochemical (IHC) surrogates for molecular classification have been devised (Fig. 45.2). These surrogate markers have been endorsed by the St. Galen Consensus Conference.[15] Notably, these IHC surrogates are not always accurate, particularly when applied to the TNBC group. Not all TNBCs are of the basal-type and not all basal-type tumors are triple negative. Due caution should be exercised when employing IHC-based surrogates for molecular classification.

Clinical Significance of Molecular Classifications

The various molecular classifications of breast carcinomas attempt to capture the intrinsic biologic variances among these tumors and stratify them into clinically relevant groups beyond those possible by ER/PR/HER2 testing. Most significantly, molecular classifications seek to stratify breast carcinomas into molecularly distinct subtypes with an aim to employ "druggable" targeted therapy.

As stated earlier, until recently, the classification and management of breast carcinomas were primarily based on clinicopathologic features. These features included tumor size, histologic grade, and lymph node status, as well as ER/PR/HER2 status. Typically, systemic chemotherapy was applied to high–clinical stage breast carcinomas regardless of histologic grade or immunophenotypical profile. Even among patients with early-stage breast carcinomas, about 60% received systemic chemotherapy—usually of the generic type.[16]

The management of breast carcinoma is increasingly been driven by molecular pathobiologic characteristics, and in this respect clinicopathologic features are of increasingly lesser consideration. Patients with a better prognostic molecular subtype of tumor, for example, luminal A, may be spared chemotherapy. Patients who have tumors with worse prognostic subtypes, for example, basal-type, could potentially benefit from systemic chemotherapy, even if these are "small."

Furthermore, the identification of distinct molecular aberrations in each subtype of breast carcinoma may serve as potential therapeutic targets. It has been shown that some TNBCs respond well to neoadjuvant chemotherapy, with 5-year survival exceeding 90%, whereas other TNBCs that did not respond to chemotherapy had a worse outcome, with a 5-year survival of 30%.[17] Basal-like subtypes (BL1 and BL2) have higher expressions of cell cycle and DNA response genes, and preferentially respond to antimitotic agents.[10] The MSL subtype expresses low levels of proliferation genes, and tumors in this group are resistant to chemotherapy. Chemoresistant breast carcinomas possess a high proportion of stem-like cells.[13] Nevertheless, the MSL subtype of carcinoma

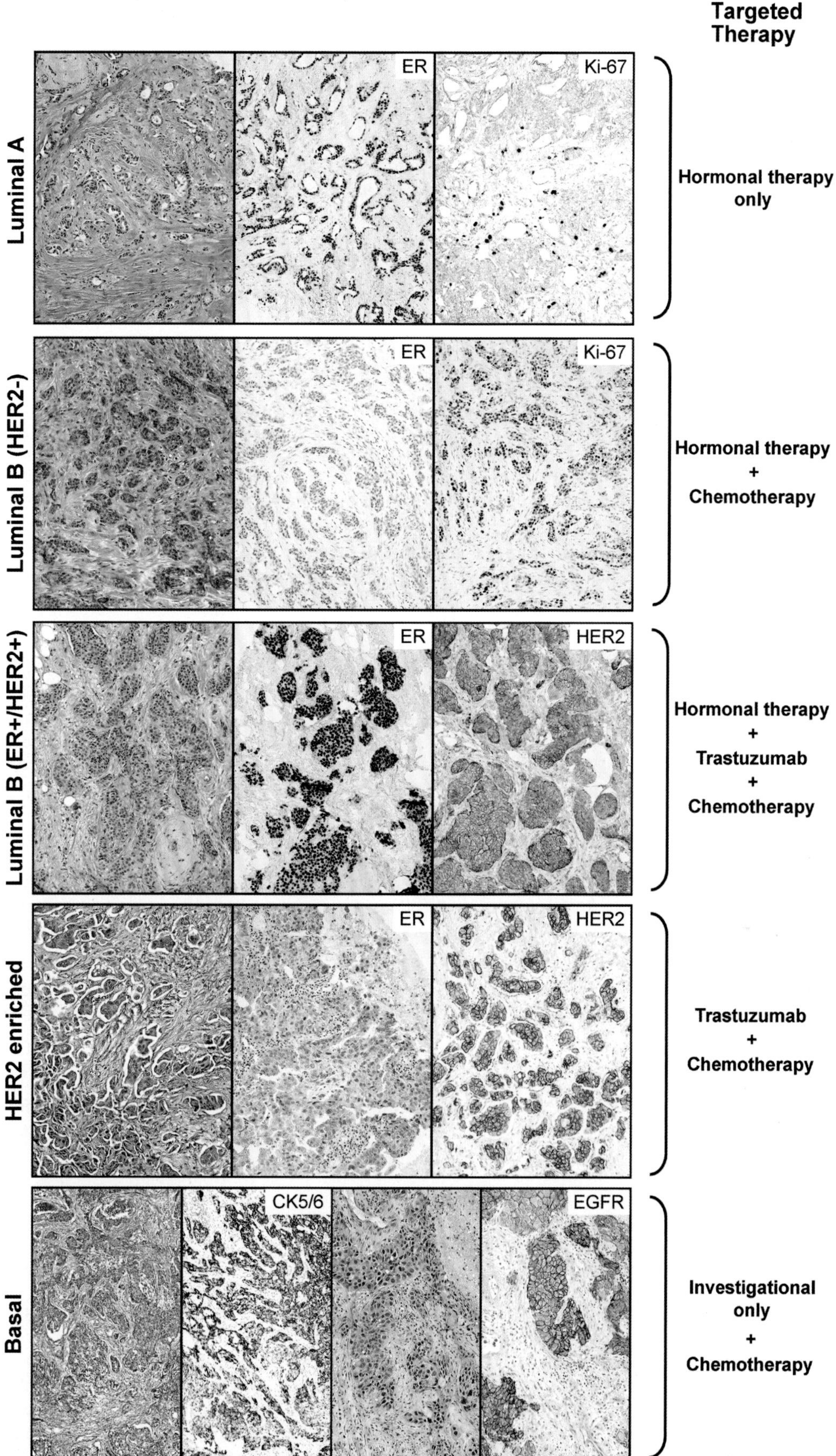

FIG. 45.2. *Immunohistochemical surrogates for intrinsic subtypes of breast carcinomas.* Luminal A: low histologic grade, ER(+), PR(+), HER2(−), low Ki67 (<15%). Luminal B HER2(−): grade 2, ER(+), PR(+), high Ki67 (≥15%). Luminal B HER2(+): ER(+), grade 2/3, high Ki67 (>15%). HER2-enriched: ER(−), PR(−), HER2(+), grade 3, high Ki67 (>15%). Basal: ER(−), PR(−), HER2(−), "basal" markers (CK5/6) (+), epidermal growth factor receptor (EGFR)(+).

has increased expression of genes involved in growth factor pathways, and could respond to PI3K/mTOR inhibitors and abl/src kinase inhibitors.

PROGNOSTIC AND PREDICTIVE MOLECULAR TESTS IN BREAST CARCINOMA

The key features of current commercially available prognostic and predictive multigene tests for invasive breast carcinomas are listed in Table 45.2.

70-Gene Prognostic Signature (MammaPrint)

This prognostic signature was developed by The Netherlands Cancer Institute, from the gene expression array analyses of 78 untreated and node-negative breast carcinomas that were 5 cm or smaller in size, from women younger than 55 years.[18] By comparing the gene expressions of 44 tumors from patients who were disease-free after 5 years with those from patients who developed distant recurrence within 5 years, the investigators identified 70 genes that could identify patients with poor prognosis. This prognostic signature was further validated in three large-scale studies with cohorts of several hundred patients with node-positive and node-negative diseases.[19–21] The 70-gene prognostic signature has been shown to be a better prognostic predictor than routine clinicopathologic risk assessments.[19,21] This 70-gene signature has been developed as a commercially available test ("MammaPrint" by Agendia, Amsterdam, the Netherlands) and has been approved by Food and Drug Administration (FDA).

76-Gene Prognostic Signature

This prognostic signature was developed by Wang et al. at Veridex, LLC (Raritan, NJ) and Erasmus University (Rotterdam, the Netherlands). In contrast to the development of the 70-gene signature, the investigators separated the microarray analyses between the ER(+) and ER(−) breast carcinomas and identified 60 prognostic genes in the

TABLE 45.2 Commercially Available Prognostic/Predictive Multigene Tests for Invasive Breast Carcinomas

	MammaPrint	PAM50 (Breast Bioclassifiers)	MapQuant Dx/Simplified	Oncotype DX	Breast Cancer Index (HOXB13:IL17BR/MGI)
Analysis	Microarray	qRT-PCR	Microarray/qRT-PCR	qRT-PCR	qRT-PCR
Provider	Agendia (Amsterdam, the Netherlands)	NanoString Technologies (Seattle, WA)	Ipsogen (Marseille, France)	Genomic Health (Redwood City, CA)	bioTheranostics (San Diego, CA)
Assay	70-Gene signature	50-Gene signature	97-Gene signature or 8-gene PCR	21-Gene RS	Two-gene HOXB13:IL17R/five-gene MGI
Tissue type	Fresh or frozen	FFPE	Fresh or frozen or FFPE	FFPE	FFPE
Clinical indications	• 0–3 node positive • <5 cm • All ages • ER(+) or ER(−)	• Stage I–III • All ages • ER(+) or ER(−)	• ER(+) • Histologic grade 2	• ER(+) • 0–3 node positive • Treated with tamoxifen • Postmenopausal, treated with AIs	• ER(+) • Node negative • All ages
Prognostic/predictive value	• Prognostic for early distant recurrence within first 5 y after diagnosis • Predictive for chemoresponse in poor prognostic group	• Prognostic based on assigned intrinsic molecular subtypes • Predictive for tamoxifen benefit in luminal cancers	• Prognostic in ER(+) tumors • Predictive for chemoresponse in high GGI tumors	• Prognostic for distant recurrence in 10 y • Predictive for chemoresponse in high RS group	• Prognostic in ER(+) tumors • Predictive for tamoxifen response in low-risk group

FFPE=Formalin-Fixed Paraffin-Embedded

ER(+) group and 16 genes in the ER(−) group that could predict the likelihood of distant metastasis within 5 years. The signature was initially developed from 115 breast carcinomas, and validated using a different set of 171 node-negative patients.[22] It was revalidated in a multi-institutional study of 180 node-negative, chemotherapy-naive patients[23] and further validated independently in a cohort of 198 patients.[24] This prognostic 76-gene signature can apply to all node-negative breast carcinomas in all age groups, and in tumors of different sizes, and has been shown to outperform National Institutes of Health (NIH) or St. Gallen clinicopathologic criteria in identifying patients at low risk for disease recurrence who can be spared chemotherapy.[23] This prognostic signature system can also identify higher-risk patients who may benefit from adjuvant tamoxifen therapy.[25]

Genomic Grade Index

The genomic grade index (GGI) was developed by Sotiriou et al.[26] Using publicly available microarray data from 64 ER(+) breast carcinomas of known histologic grade (grade 1:33 and grade 3:31), this group identified a 97-gene signature that can classify breast carcinomas into low- and high-grade groups. This signature can segregate histologic grade 2 tumors into either low or high grade and eliminate the histologically intermediate group. This prognostic signature was later validated in over 1,100 ER(+) patients.[27] Breast carcinomas with high GGI respond to chemotherapy and have a higher complete pathologic response rate, but still show poorer prognosis than tumors with low GGI in ER(+) carcinomas.[28] GGI has prognostic value only in ER(+) tumors that have received neither neoadjuvant hormonal therapy nor chemotherapy. This signature has been made available as a commercially available test (MapQuant Dx Genomic Grade, Ipsogen SA, Marseille, France).

Oncotype DX Test

Oncotype DX (Genomic Health, Redwood, CA) is the most commercially successful qRT-PCR test developed to date. This test measures gene expression in FFPE samples for the purpose of predicting clinical outcome and response to therapy. The developers of the test chose a panel of 21 genes (16 cancer-related genes and 5 housekeeping control genes) from their initial study of a 92-gene panel[29] and generated a recurrence score (RS) algorithm from the qRT-PCR assay of these 21 genes.[30] The RS was based on well-characterized FFPE samples from the National Surgical Adjuvant Breast and Bowel Project (NSABP) B20 trial and validated using the NSABP B14 trial to estimate the distant recurrence rate at 10 years in ER(+) and node-negative patients who received tamoxifen treatment.[30] RS is a continuous variable that estimates the likelihood of distant recurrence within 10 years in patients who are ER(+) and node negative and who received tamoxifen treatment. RS stratifies patients into three risk groups: low risk (RS less than 18), intermediate risk (RS 18 to 30), and high risk (RS, 31 or greater), with 10-year distant recurrence rates of 6.8%, 14.3%, and 30.5%, respectively. RS also correlates with chemotherapy benefit: the high RS group benefited from the adjuvant chemotherapy, whereas the low-risk group did not.[31] Oncotype DX was revalidated in an independent Eastern Corporative Oncology Group (ECOG) E2197 trial with a cohort of ER(+) and chemotherapy-treated early breast carcinomas with 0-3+ nodes.[32] Subsequently the Southwest Oncology Group (SWOG) 8814 trial, a randomized study of tamoxifen with or without anthracyclin-based chemotherapy for postmenopausal women with node-positive breast carcinomas, further validated the predictive value for chemoresponse in the high RS group in both node-negative and node-positive patients.[33] The study also indicated that not all patients with node-positive and ER-positive breast carcinomas benefited from chemotherapy, thereby challenging the current treatment dogma in node-positive breast carcinomas. RS was also later shown to be of prognostic value in ER(+) patients treated with aromatase inhibitors (AIs) in the Arimidex, Tamoxifen, alone or in Combination (ATAC) trial.[34] The indication for the Oncotype DX test has recently been expanded to include ER(+) patients with up to three positive lymph nodes and treated with either tamoxifen or AIs. There are significant numbers of ER(+) tumors (up to 50%) that lie in the intermediate RS category, which *per se* obfuscates management decisions. Although a clinical trial (TAILORx; NCT00310180) is under way to evaluate whether the intermediate category patients will benefit from hormonal therapy only or need additional chemotherapy (see later), a two-gene expression ratio (HOXB13:IL17BR) by RT-PCR may provide further biologic insight into tamoxifen resistance. HOXB13 and IL17BR are reversely regulated by estradiol; therefore, the ratio of these two genes serves as a surrogate marker for dysfunctional ER pathways.[35]

Breast Carcinoma Index (HOXB13:IL17R/ Five-Gene Molecular Grade Index)

The HOXB13:IL17R two-gene ratio assay was first developed by Ma et al.[35] to predict hormonal therapy response in ER(+) patients. This group performed gene expression microarray analyses on 60 fresh tissues from ER(+) carcinomas (matched by size, grade, and nodal status). The group compared tumors from patients who received tamoxifen treatment and experienced early recurrence within 5 years with tumors from patients without recurrence. Thus, the two-gene ratio, HOXB13:IL17BR (H/I), which was predictive and prognostic for hormonal resistance and early recurrence, was identified. This two-gene ratio was validated by qRT-PCR in 20 FFPE breast carcinoma samples. The prognostic value and prediction of tamoxifen resistance using a high HOXB13:IL17BR ratio were further validated in two large independent cohorts from the North Central Cancer Treatment Group Adjuvant Tamoxifen trial (NCCTG 89-30-52, $n = 206$)[36] and Baylor College of Medicine ($n = 852$).[37] The latter study also demonstrated that the HOXB13:IL17BR ratio was an independent prognostic marker for ER(+) and node-negative breast carcinomas irrespective of tamoxifen therapy.

Ma et al. subsequently developed a five-gene (RRM2, BUB1B, RACGAP1, CENPA, and NEK2, all involved in the cell cycle) molecular grade index (MGI), by qRT-PCR, to add to the two-gene ratio H/I test. The MGI and the H/I two-gene ratio were found to be complementary prognostic factors in early-stage ER(+) breast carcinomas. The two aforementioned qRT-PCR tests were combined to create the Breast Cancer Index test.[38]

Sensitivity to Endocrine Therapy Index

There are fewer predictive molecular models compared to prognostic signatures. The sensitivity to endocrine therapy (SET) index was developed as a predictive test for hormonal therapy responses in ER(+) breast carcinomas. It was developed by investigators at M.D. Anderson Cancer Center from microarrays of 400 ER(+) breast carcinomas from patients who had received 5 years of hormonal therapy. The index is calculated from the gene expression of 165 ER-related genes, and is prognostic in patients with ER(+) carcinomas receiving hormonal therapy—but not in those not receiving hormonal therapy.[39] This recently developed predictive model is awaiting independent validation.

Clinical Trials and Personalized Therapy for Breast Carcinomas

In the recent past, a node-negative, 10-cm "classical" type of invasive lobular carcinoma (low grade, strongly ER(+)) would have been treated with chemotherapy in addition to hormonal therapy—primarily because of its large size. At this time, this type of tumor would be considered highly sensitive to endocrine therapy. Despite the large size of the tumor, only minimal benefit from chemotherapy could be expected.

A node-negative, 0.5-cm, HER2(+) breast carcinoma could now receive trastuzumab plus chemotherapy per the St. Galen Consensus[15] despite its relatively small size.

A node-positive, 2.5-cm, grade 2, ER(+) invasive ductal carcinoma would likely have received chemotherapy plus hormonal therapy in the past; however, now the decision on whether systemic chemotherapy is needed may depend on the Oncotype DX RS. The National Comprehensive Cancer Network (NCCN) guidelines and the 2011 St. Galen Consensus Conference both recommend that Oncotype DX test be incorporated into treatment decision making.[40,41] In the aforementioned case, if RS is high, chemotherapy would reduce distant recurrence risk by 50%. If RS is low, hormonal therapy alone could be the best option. If RS is intermediate, no statistically significant chemotherapy benefit could be expected, and the decision on its use could be left to the patient and the treating physician. The question of whether this intermediate group of ER(+) early-stage breast carcinoma patients can be spared from systemic chemotherapy is being addressed by the ongoing prospective Trial Assigning Individualized Options for Treatment (Rx) (TAILORx, NCT00310180) (Fig. 45.3A). The intermediate-risk group with an RS of 11 to 25 will be randomized to receive hormonal therapy alone or in combination of chemotherapy. In this trial, 10,500 patients are expected to be screened using the Oncotype DX test, with about 5,000 randomized for the study, and results are expected to be available in 2013. Until then, intermediate-risk tumors by Oncotype DX test may require a second biomarker test (e.g., MapQuant Dx, GGI, and Breast Carcinoma Index) to differentiate high risk and low risk. GGI can further stratify intermediate tumors into a "low-risk" or "high-risk" group in about 80% of cases (approximately 70% to low-risk group and approximately 10% to high-risk group), and the H/I–MGI may further categorize the intermediate tumors to low or high risk in about 60% of cases (approximately 45% to the low-risk group and approximately 15% to the high-risk group) (personal communication with D. Sgroi, MD, Massachusetts General Hospital, Boston, MA, May 2009).

The "microarray in node-negative and 1 to 3 positive lymph node disease may avoid chemotherapy" (MINDACT) trial is another ongoing trial (Fig. 45.3B). This prospective trial, which plans to enroll 10,000 patients, will compare the predictive value for chemotherapy benefit of the 70-gene signature from MammaPrint with clinicopathologic factors from Adjuvant! Online.[42] Patients with low risk by both Adjuvant! Online and genetic text will receive hormonal therapy alone; patients with high risk by both criteria will receive chemotherapy with or without hormonal therapy depending on the expression of hormone receptor. The patients with discordant results from the two predictive tools will be randomized to be treated based on either Adjuvant! Online risk assessment or 70-gene signature risk assignment. The final study result is pending, but a preliminary result from 800 enrolled patients was released, which showed that, in the discordant group, there were significantly more numbers of patients with clinically high risk/genetically low risk than those with clinically low risk/genetically high risk.[43] Therefore, if the study hypothesis is validated in this study, more patients can be spared chemotherapy.

CHALLENGES AND FUTURE DIRECTIONS

Molecular tests and traditional clinicopathologic factors that can be currently utilized for the purpose of optimizing patient management are outlined in Figure 45.4.

A revolution in the management of breast carcinomas, brought by molecular biologic testing, is upon us. The incorporation of molecular pathology tests into daily decision making for breast carcinoma treatment is becoming increasingly evident. However, molecular testing is fraught with problems. Discordance between clinicopathologic assessment and molecular testing presents one such challenge (Case in Point 1, Fig. 45.5A). The yield of equivocal or indeterminate results with both clinicopathologic as well as molecular assessments offers another (see Case in Point 2, Fig. 45.5B). At this time, management decisions in such scenarios are generally rendered on either the bases of available evidence or personal experiences of physicians. The results of the MINDACT and TAILORx trials could help in objectively meeting these challenges.

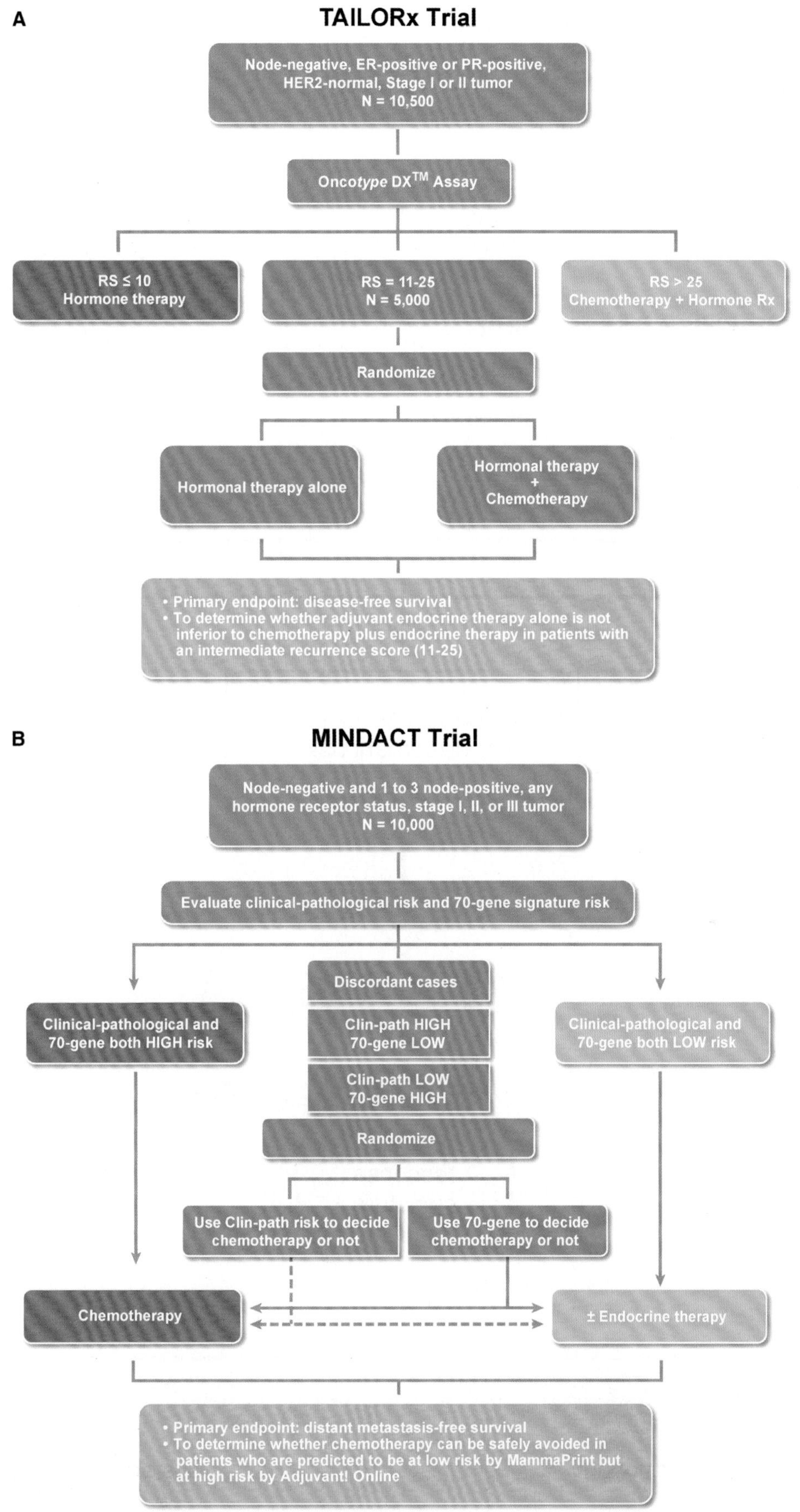

FIG. 45.3. *A,B: Ongoing prospective clinical trials using multigene molecular tests.* **A:** TAILORx trial. **B:** MINDACT trial.

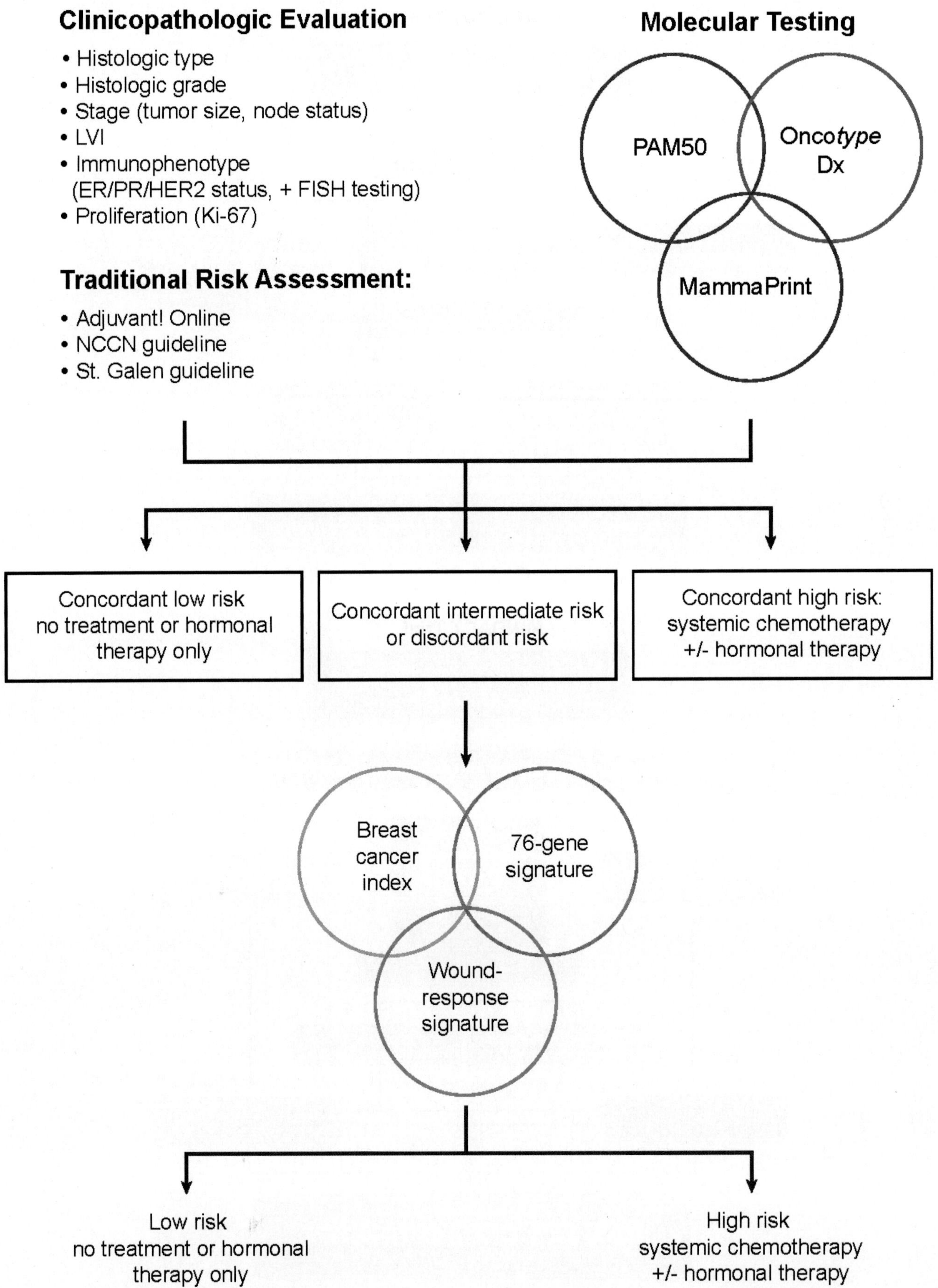

FIG. 45.4. ***Outline of comprehensive molecular and clinicopathologic evaluation that could be used for guiding individualized therapy.*** Wound-response signature is another genetic model for prognostic prediction.[44]

Case in point #1

- 50 year-old female
- Invasive lobular carcinoma
- Nottingham histologic grade 2
- 5 cm
- ER/PR+, HER2-, Ki-67 15%
- S/P total mastectomy
- Sentinel lymph node biopsy showed 1 negative node

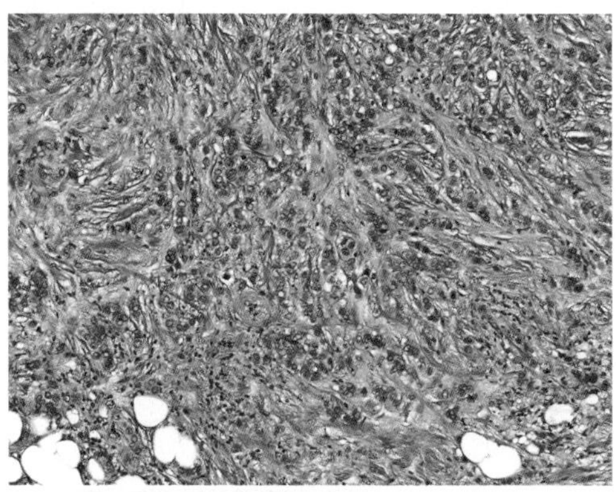

Adjuvant! Online

- Without systemic therapy: 45% chance of recurrence within 10 years
- With 5 year hormonal therapy: 30% chance of recurrence within 10 years
- With systemic chemotherapy plus 5 year hormonal therapy: 16% chance of of recurrence within 10 years

MammaPrint

MammaPrint

GENE PROFILE RESULTS:
Breast Cancer Recurrence Assay
70-gene signature
Prognostic and predictive tumor analysis

LOW RISK

Low risk: 10 year Distant Metastasis-Free Survival (DMFS) prior to treatment ~90%; these patients can expect their risk to be reduced up to 50% with adjuvant hormomal therapy.

BluePrint

MOLECULAR SUBTYPING RESULTS::
Molecular Subtyping Assay
80-gene signature
Profiles Basal, Luminal and HER2 subtypes

Luminal-type

Luminal-type cancers are typically hormone receptor positive tumors predictive for hormonal therapy sensitivity:
MammaPrint 'Low Risk' and Luminal-type: predicted to have a clinical course similar to luminal A, usually treated with hormonal therapy.
MammaPrint 'High Risk' and Luminal-type: predicted to have a clinical course similar to luminal B patients who usually benefit from more aggressive treatment which may include chemotherapy.

Challenge

There is discordance between traditional clinicopathologic risk assessment and molecular risk assessment. How should this patient be treated based on these conflicting assessments?

Pending MINDACT trial results

FIG. 45.5. *A,B: Challenges in incorporating molecular testing in breast carcinoma management.*

Case in point #2

- 60 year-old female
- Invasive ductal carcinoma
- Nottingham histologic grade 2
- 2 cm
- ER/PR+, HER2-, Ki-67 15%
- S/P segmental mastectomy with clear margins
- Sentinel lymph node biopsy showed 3 negative nodes

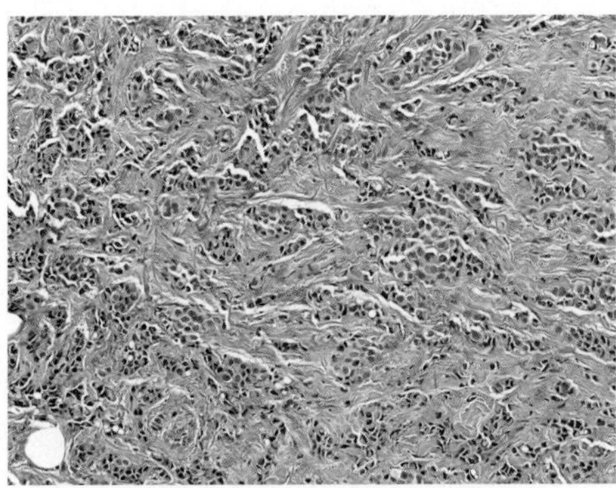

Adjuvant! Online

- Without systemic therapy: 25% chance of recurrence within 10 years
- With 5 year hormonal therapy: 16% chance of recurrence within 10 years
- With systemic chemotherapy plus 5 year hormonal therapy: 10% chance of recurrence within 10 years

Onco*type* Dx

Recurrence Score = 22

Test Results should be interpreted using the Clinical Experience information contained in this report which is derived from clinical studies involving patient populations with specific clinical features as noted in each section of the Clinical Experience. It is unknown whether the findings summarized in the Clinical Experience are applicable to patients with features different from those described.

CLINICAL EXPERIENCE: PROGNOSIS FOR NODE NEGATIVE, ER-POSITIVE PATIENTS

The Clinical Validation study included female patients with Stage I or II, Node Negative, ER-Positive breast cancer treated with 5 years of tamoxifen. Those patients who had a Recurrence Score of 16 had an Average Rate of Distant Recurrence of 14% (95%CI: 11%-18%)

The following results are from a clinical validation study of 668 patients from the NSABP B-14 study. *N Engl J Med* 2004; 351: 2817-26.

Recurrence Score vs Distant Recurrence in NODE NEGATIVE, ER-Positive Breast Cancer Prognosis

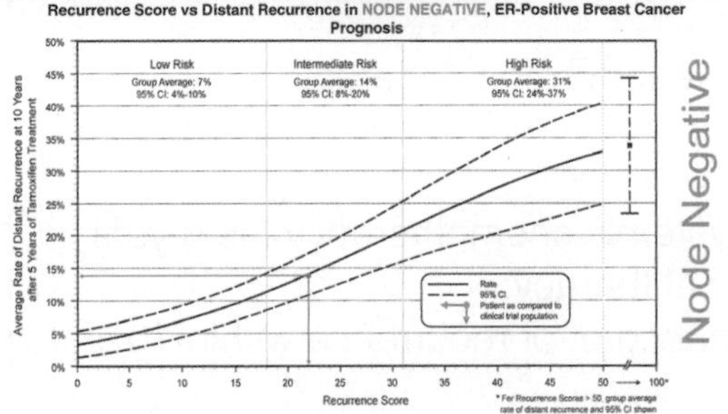

NODE NEGATIVE, ER-Positive Breast Cancer Chemotherapy Benefit

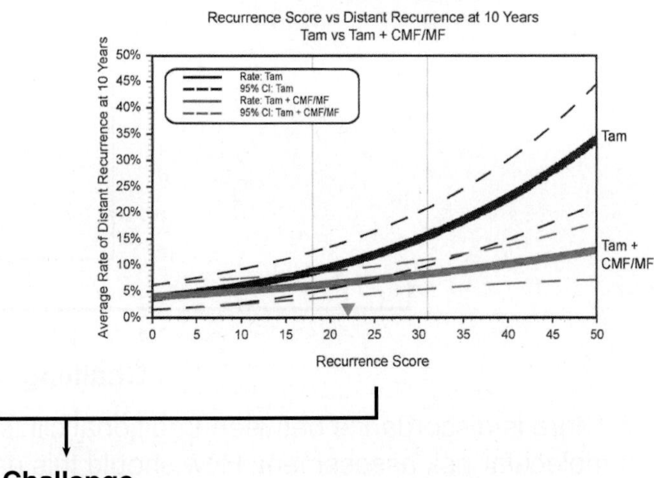

Challenge

Patient will benefit from hormornal therapy, and there will be small increment of benefit from aditional systemic chemotherapy. Question is whether this small amount of benefit from systemic chemotherapy outweights the cytotoxicity of the chemotherapy?

Pending TAILORx trial results

FIG. 45.5. *(Continued)*

The management of breast carcinoma will likely become increasingly personalized and targeted. This approach will ensure that patients are neither overtreated nor undertreated. With maturity of next-generation sequencing technology and decreasing costs, it is foreseeable that such testing will become commonplace.

REFERENCES

1. Perou CM, Sorlie T, Eisen MB, et al. Molecular portraits of human breast tumours. *Nature* 2000;406(6797):747–752.
2. Sorlie T, Perou CM, Tibshirani R, et al. Gene expression patterns of breast carcinomas distinguish tumor subclasses with clinical implications. *Proc Natl Acad Sci U S A* 2001;98:10869–10874.
3. Prat A, Parker JS, Karginova O, et al. Phenotypic and molecular characterization of the claudin-low intrinsic subtype of breast cancer. *Breast Cancer Res* 2010;12:R68.
4. Korkaya H, Paulson A, Iovino F, et al. HER2 regulates the mammary stem/progenitor cell population driving tumorigenesis and invasion. *Oncogene* 2008;27:6120–6130.
5. Romond EH, Perez EA, Bryant J, et al. Trastuzumab plus adjuvant chemotherapy for operable HER2-positive breast cancer. *N Engl J Med* 2005;353:1673–1684.
6. Untch M, Gelber RD, Jackisch C, et al. Estimating the magnitude of trastuzumab effects within patient subgroups in the HERA trial. *Ann Oncol* 2008;19:1090–1096.
7. Parker JS, Mullins M, Cheang MC, et al. Supervised risk predictor of breast cancer based on intrinsic subtypes. *J Clin Oncol* 2009;27:1160–1167.
8. Nielsen TO, Parker JS, Leung S, et al. A comparison of PAM50 intrinsic subtyping with immunohistochemistry and clinical prognostic factors in tamoxifen-treated estrogen receptor-positive breast cancer. *Clin Cancer Res* 2010;16:5222–5232.
9. Chia SK, Bramwell VH, Tu D, et al. A 50-gene intrinsic subtype classifier for prognosis and prediction of benefit from adjuvant tamoxifen. *Clin Cancer Res* 2012;18:4465–4472.
10. Lehmann BD, Bauer JA, Chen X, et al. Identification of human triple-negative breast cancer subtypes and preclinical models for selection of targeted therapies. *J Clin Invest* 2011;121:2750–2767.
11. Bertucci F, Finetti P, Cervera N, et al. Gene expression profiling shows medullary breast cancer is a subgroup of basal breast cancers. *Cancer Res* 2006;66:4636–4644.
12. Farmer P, Bonnefoi H, Becette V, et al. Identification of molecular apocrine breast tumours by microarray analysis. *Oncogene* 2005;24:4660–4671.
13. Creighton CJ, Li X, Landis M, et al. Residual breast cancers after conventional therapy display mesenchymal as well as tumor-initiating features. *Proc Natl Acad Sci U S A* 2009;106:13820–13825.
14. Curtis C, Shah SP, Chin SF, et al. The genomic and transcriptomic architecture of 2,000 breast tumours reveals novel subgroups. *Nature* 2012;486:346–352.
15. Goldhirsch A, Wood WC, Coates AS, et al. Strategies for subtypes—dealing with the diversity of breast cancer: highlights of the St. Gallen International Expert Consensus on the Primary Therapy of Early Breast Cancer 2011. *Ann Oncol* 2011;22:1736–1747.
16. Early Breast Cancer Trialists' Collaborative Group (EBCTCG). Effects of chemotherapy and hormonal therapy for early breast cancer on recurrence and 15-year survival: an overview of the randomised trials. *Lancet* 2005;365:1687–1717.
17. Liedtke C, Mazouni C, Hess KR, et al. Response to neoadjuvant therapy and long-term survival in patients with triple-negative breast cancer. *J Clin Oncol* 2008;26:1275–1281.
18. van 't Veer LJ, Dai H, van de Vijver MJ, et al. Gene expression profiling predicts clinical outcome of breast cancer. *Nature* 2002;415:530–536.
19. van de Vijver MJ, He YD, van 't Veer LJ, et al. A gene-expression signature as a predictor of survival in breast cancer. *N Engl J Med* 2002;347:1999–2009.
20. Mook S, Schmidt MK, Viale G, et al. The 70-gene prognosis-signature predicts disease outcome in breast cancer patients with 1-3 positive lymph nodes in an independent validation study. *Breast Cancer Res Treat* 2009;116:295–302.
21. Buyse M, Loi S, van 't Veer L, et al. Validation and clinical utility of a 70-gene prognostic signature for women with node-negative breast cancer. *J Natl Cancer Inst* 2006;98:1183–1192.
22. Wang Y, Klijn JG, Zhang Y, et al. Gene-expression profiles to predict distant metastasis of lymph-node-negative primary breast cancer. *Lancet* 2005;365:671–679.
23. Foekens JA, Atkins D, Zhang Y, et al. Multicenter validation of a gene expression-based prognostic signature in lymph node-negative primary breast cancer. *J Clin Oncol* 2006;24:1665–1671.
24. Desmedt C, Piette F, Loi S, et al. Strong time dependence of the 76-gene prognostic signature for node-negative breast cancer patients in the TRANSBIG multicenter independent validation series. *Clin Cancer Res* 2007;13:3207–3214.
25. Zhang Y, Sieuwerts AM, McGreevy M, et al. The 76-gene signature defines high-risk patients that benefit from adjuvant tamoxifen therapy. *Breast Cancer Res Treat* 2009;116:303–309.
26. Sotiriou C, Wirapati P, Loi S, et al. Gene expression profiling in breast cancer: understanding the molecular basis of histologic grade to improve prognosis. *J Natl Cancer Inst* 2006;98(4):262–272.
27. Loi S, Haibe-Kains B, Desmedt C, et al. Definition of clinically distinct molecular subtypes in estrogen receptor-positive breast carcinomas through genomic grade. *J Clin Oncol* 2007;25:1239–1246.
28. Liedtke C, Hatzis C, Symmans WF, et al. Genomic grade index is associated with response to chemotherapy in patients with breast cancer. *J Clin Oncol* 2009;27:3185–3191.
29. Cronin M, Pho M, Dutta D, et al. Measurement of gene expression in archival paraffin-embedded tissues: development and performance of a 92-gene reverse transcriptase-polymerase chain reaction assay. *Am J Pathol* 2004;164:35–42.
30. Paik S, Shak S, Tang G, et al. A multigene assay to predict recurrence of tamoxifen-treated, node-negative breast cancer. *N Engl J Med* 2004;351:2817–2826.
31. Paik S, Tang G, Shak S, et al. Gene expression and benefit of chemotherapy in women with node-negative, estrogen receptor-positive breast cancer. *J Clin Oncol* 2006;24:3726–3734.
32. Goldstein LJ, Gray R, Badve S, et al. Prognostic utility of the 21-gene assay in hormone receptor-positive operable breast cancer compared with classical clinicopathological features. *J Clin Oncol* 2008;26:4063–4071.
33. Albain KS, Barlow WE, Shak S, et al. Prognostic and predictive value of the 21-gene recurrence score assay in postmenopausal women with node-positive, oestrogen-receptor-positive breast cancer on chemotherapy: a retrospective analysis of a randomised trial. *Lancet Oncol* 2010;11:55–65.
34. Dowsett M, Cuzick J, Wale C, et al. Prediction of risk of distant recurrence using the 21-gene recurrence score in node-negative and node-positive postmenopausal patients with breast cancer treated with anastrozole or tamoxifen: a TransATAC study. *J Clin Oncol* 2010;28:1829–1834.
35. Ma XJ, Wang Z, Ryan PD, et al. A two-gene expression ratio predicts clinical outcome in breast cancer patients treated with tamoxifen. *Cancer Cell* 2004;5:607–616.
36. Goetz MP, Suman VJ, Ingle JN, et al. A two-gene expression ratio of homeobox 13 and interleukin-17B receptor for prediction of recurrence and survival in women receiving adjuvant tamoxifen. *Clin Cancer Res* 2006;12:2080–2087.
37. Ma XJ, Hilsenbeck SG, Wang W, et al. The HOXB13:IL17BR expression index is a prognostic factor in early-stage breast cancer. *J Clin Oncol* 2006;24:4611–4619.
38. Ma XJ, Salunga R, Dahiya S, et al. A five-gene molecular grade index and HOXB13:IL17BR are complementary prognostic factors in early stage breast cancer. *Clin Cancer Res* 2008;14:2601–2608.
39. Symmans WF, Hatzis C, Sotiriou C, et al. Genomic index of sensitivity to endocrine therapy for breast cancer. *J Clin Oncol* 2010;28:4111–4119.
40. http://www.nccn.org/professionals/physician_gls/pdf/breast.pdf. Accessed April 21, 2013.
41. Gnant M, Harbeck N, Thomssen C. St. Gallen 2011: summary of the consensus discussion. *Breast Care (Basel)* 2011;6:136–141.
42. Adjuvant! Online. www.adjuvantonline.com. Accessed March 13, 2013.
43. Rutgers E, Piccart-Gebhart MJ, Bogaerts J, et al. The EORTC 10041/BIG 03-04 MINDACT trial is feasible: results of the pilot phase. *Eur J Cancer* 2011;47:2742–2749.
44. Chang HY, Nuyten DSA, Sneddon JB, et al. Robustness, scalability, and integration of a wound-response gene expression signature in predicting breast cancer survival. *Proc Natl Acad Sci* 2005;102:3738-3743.

LIST OF ABBREVIATIONS

Note: Abbreviations apply to singular and plural context.

ADASP	Association of Directors of Anatomic and Surgical Pathology
AdCC	adenoid cystic carcinoma
ADH	atypical ductal hyperplasia
AFB	acid-fast bacilli
AFIP	Armed Forces Institute of Pathology
AIDS	acquired immunodeficiency syndrome
AJCC	American Joint Committee on Cancer
ALH	atypical lobular hyperplasia
ALN	axillary lymph node
AME	adenomyoepithelioma
AR	androgen receptor
AS	angiosarcoma
ASCO	American Society of Clinical Oncology
ASCP	American Society of Clinical Pathology
AVL	atypical vascular lesion
BCC	basal cell carcinoma
BDA	blunt duct adenosis
BI-RADS	Breast Imaging-Reporting and Data System
BPT	benign phyllodes tumor
BRCA	breast cancer (gene)
BSE	breast self-examination
CALGB	Cancer and Leukemia Group B
CAP	College of American Pathology
CBE	clinical breast examination
CCH	columnar cell hyperplasia
CEA	carcinoembryonic antigen
CGH	comparative genomic hybridization
CHH	cystic hypersecretory hyperplasia
CIS	carcinoma *in situ*
CK	cytokeratin
CSL	complex sclerosing lesion
DCIS	ductal carcinoma *in situ*
DFS	disease-free survival
DFSP	dermatofibrosarcoma protuberans
EGFR	epidermal growth factor receptor
EMA	epithelial membrane antigen
ER	estrogen receptor
FA	fibroadenoma
FCC	fibrocystic change
FEA	flat epithelial atypia
FISH	fluorescence *in situ* hybridization
FNA	fine-needle aspiration
FS	frozen section
GCDFP	gross cystic disease fluid protein
GMS	Gomori-Grocott methenamine silver
HCG	human chorionic gonadotrophin
HER2/*neu*	human epidermal growth factor/*neu* receptor
HIV	human immunodeficiency virus
HPF	high-power field
IBC	inflammatory breast carcinoma
IDC/IFDC	infiltrating ductal carcinoma
IHC	immunohistochemistry
ILC	invasive lobular carcinoma
ITC	isolated tumor cell
JP	juvenile papillomatosis
LCIS	lobular carcinoma *in situ*
LGASC	low-grade adenosquamous carcinoma
LOH	loss of heterozygosity
LVI	lymphovascular involvement
MAC	*Mycobacterium avium* complex
MALT	mucosal-associated lymphoid tissue
MBRG	modified Bloom–Richardson (Nottingham) grading system
MFH	malignant fibrous histiocytoma (pleomorphic sarcoma)
MGA	microglandular adenosis
MLL	mucocele-like lesion
MPT	malignant phyllodes tumor
MRI	magnetic resonance imaging
MSA	muscle-specific actin
NHL	non-Hodgkin lymphoma
OS	overall survival
p53	protein 53 (tumor protein 53)
PAS	periodic acid–Schiff
PASH	pseudoangiomatous stromal hyperplasia

PCNA proliferating cell nuclear antigen
pCR pathological complete remission
PCR polymerase chain reaction
PET–CT positron emission tomogram–computerized tomogram
PLCIS pleomorphic lobular carcinoma *in situ*
PLH pregnancy-like hyperplasia
PPV positive predictive value
PR progesterone receptor
PSA prostate-specific antigen
PSAP prostate-specific acid phosphatase
RFS relapse-free survival
RR relative risk
RSL radial sclerosing lesion (radial scar)
s/p status-post
SA sclerosing adenosis
SCC small cell carcinoma
SEER Surveillance Epidemiology and End Results
SLN sentinel lymph node
SMA smooth muscle actin
SMM-HC smooth muscle myosin-heavy chain
SPF S-phase fraction
SQC squamous cell carcinoma
SSDH subareolar sclerosing duct hyperplasia
TDLU terminal duct lobular unit
TMA tissue microarray
TNM tumor (size), regional node (involvement), (distant) metastases
TRAM transverse rectus abdominus muscle (flap)
TTF-1 thyroid transcription factor 1
UICC *Union Internationale Contre le Cancer* (International Union Against Cancer)
VEGF vascular epidermal growth factor
VNPI Van Nuys prognostic index
WHO World Health Organization
WT-1 Wilms tumor 1

INDEX

Note: Page numbers followed by "f" indicate figures; page numbers followed by "t" indicate tabular material.

B

C

E

F

G

H

M

O